Cardiological Society of India

CARDIOLOGY

UPDATE 2023

Cardiological Society of India

CARDIOLOGY

UPDATE 2023

Volume 1

Editor-in-Chief

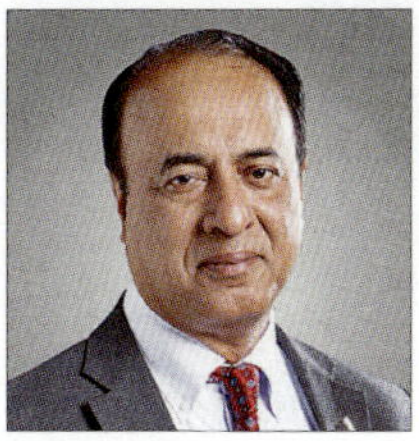

Pratap Chandra Rath
MD DM FICC FESC FACC FRCP (London) FRCP (Edinburgh)
Senior Consultant Cardiologist and HOD
Department of Cardiology
Apollo Hospital, Jubilee Hills
Hyderabad, Telangana
Apollo Hospital
Bhubaneshwar, Odisha, India

Co-Editors

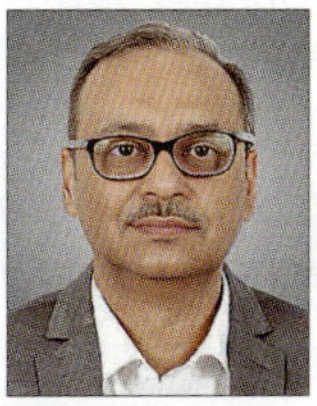

Manoj Kumar Agarwala
MD (PGI) DM (PGI) FACC
Consultant Cardiologist
Department of Cardiology
Apollo Hospital, Jubilee Hills
Hyderabad, Telangana, India

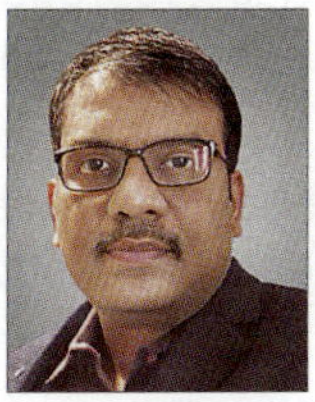

Sundar Chidambaram
MD DNB DM FNB
Senior Consultant Interventional Cardiologist
Kauvery Hospital
Chennai, Tamil Nadu, India

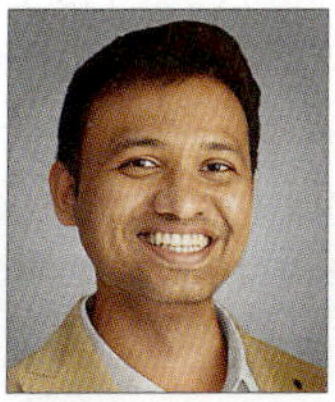

Shabbir Ali Shaik
MD DM FNB
Fellow Interventional Cardiologist
Department of Cardiology
Apollo Hospital, Jubilee Hills
Hyderabad, Telangana, India

Foreword

Alain Cribier

JAYPEE

JAYPEE BROTHERS MEDICAL PUBLISHERS
The Health Sciences Publisher
New Delhi | London

JAYPEE Jaypee Brothers Medical Publishers (P) Ltd

Headquarters
EMCA House
23/23-B, Ansari Road, Daryaganj
New Delhi 110 002, India
Landline: +91-11-23272143, +91-11-23272703
+91-11-23282021, +91-11-23245672
E-mail: jaypee@jaypeebrothers.com

Corporate Office
Jaypee Brothers Medical Publishers (P) Ltd.
4838/24, Ansari Road, Daryaganj
New Delhi 110 002, India
Phone: +91-11-43574357
Fax: +91-11-43574314
E-mail: jaypee@jaypeebrothers.com

Overseas Office
JP Medical Ltd.
83, Victoria Street, London
SW1H 0HW (UK)
Phone: +44-20 3170 8910
Fax: +44(0)20 3008 6180
E-mail: info@jpmedpub.com

Website: www.jaypeebrothers.com
Website: www.jaypeedigital.com

Inquiries for bulk sales may be solicited at: jaypee@jaypeebrothers.com

CSI Cardiology Update 2023 (Volume 1) / Pratap Chandra Rath

First Edition: **2024**

ISBN: 978-93-5696-437-2

Printed at: Samrat Offset Pvt. Ltd.

DEDICATION

The CSI Update Book 2023 is dedicated to all cardiologists and students in particular

Pratap Chandra Rath

CONTRIBUTORS

Editor-in-Chief

Pratap Chandra Rath MD DM FICC FESC FACC FRCP (London) FRCP (Edinburgh)
Senior Consultant Cardiologist and HOD
Department of Cardiology
Apollo Hospital, Jubilee Hills
Hyderabad, Telangana
Apollo Hospital
Bhubaneshwar, Odisha, India

Co-Editors

Manoj Kumar Agarwala MD (PGI) DM (PGI) FACC
Consultant Cardiologist
Department of Cardiology
Apollo Hospital, Jubilee Hills
Hyderabad, Telangana, India

Sundar Chidambaram MD DNB DM FNB
Senior Consultant Interventional Cardiologist
Kauvery Hospital
Chennai, Tamil Nadu, India

Shabbir Ali Shaik MD DM FNB
Fellow Interventional Cardiologist
Department of Cardiology
Apollo Hospital, Jubilee Hills
Hyderabad, Telangana, India

Contributing Authors

Aarya Naik MBBS
Research Assistant
Marengo CIMS Hospital
Ahmedabad, Gujarat, India

Abdul S Talpur MD
Research Student
Department of Cardiology
West Virginia University School of Medicine
Morgantown, WV, USA

Abha Bajaj Nee Sheth MS
Associate Professor
Department of Anatomy
Dr Harvansh Singh Judge Institute of Dental Sciences and Hospital
Panjab University
Chandigarh, India

Abhinav Shrivastava MD DM
Consultant
Maharaja Agrasen Hospital
Punjabi Bagh, New Delhi, India

Abhishek MD DM
Resident, Department of Cardiology
Dayanand Medical College and Hospital
Unit Hero DMC Heart Institute
Ludhiana, Punjab, India

Abraham Oomman MD DM (Cardiology)
Senior Consultant Interventional Cardiologist
Department of Cardiology
Apollo Main Hospital
Chennai, Tamil Nadu, India

Aditi Parimoo MD
Senior Resident
Department of Cardiology
KEM Hospital, Parel
Mumbai, Maharashtra, India

Aditi Rastogi DNB (Medicine) DM-PDT
Postdoctoral Trainee
Department of Cardiology
Medical College
Kolkata, West Bengal, India

Aditi Singhvi MBBS Fellowship in Cardiovascular Medicine (USA)
Consultant – Heart Failure and Transplant Cardiology
Narayana Institute of Cardiac Sciences
Narayana Health City
Bengaluru, Karnataka, India

Aditya Goyal MD (Medicine)
DM Cardiology Resident 2nd Year
Mahatma Gandhi Medical College and Hospital
Jaipur, Rajasthan, India

Aftab Khan MD (Medicine) DM (Cardiology) DNB (Cardiology)
Consultant Interventional Cardiologist
Director Electrophysiology Services
Apollo Multispeciality Hospitals
Kolkata, West Bengal, India

Ajay Bahl DM FRCP
Professor
Department of Cardiology
Postgraduate Institute of Medical Education and Research
Chandigarh, India

Ajay Naik MD DM DNB FACC FHRS
Cardiac Electrophysiologist
Room 1, CIMS East
Marengo CIMS Hospital
Ahmedabad, Gujarat, India

Ajit Desai MD (Medicine) DM DNB (Cardiology)
Additional Director
Jaslok Hospital
Consultant Cardiologist
HN Reliance, Breach Candy, Nanavati, Asian Heart Hospitals
Mumbai, Maharashtra, India

Ajit S Mullasari MD DM
Director
Department of Cardiology
Institute of Cardio Vascular Diseases
The Madras Medical Mission Hospital
Professor of Practice
Indian Institute of Technology – Madras
Chennai, Tamil Nadu, India

Ajoe John Kattoor MD
Staff Cardiologist
Division of Cardiovascular Medicine
Northwest Health
La Porte and Porter, IN, USA

Akash MD (Radiodiagnosis)
Senior Resident
Department of Imaging
Fortis Escort Heart Institute
New Delhi, India

AK Pancholia MD FACC FESC FCSI FISH FIMSA MAMS
Head
Department of Medicine, Clinical and Preventive Cardiology
Arihant Hospital
Indore, Madhya Pradesh, India
BC Roy and Charak Awardee of MPIMA

Alain Cribier MD FACC FESC
Emeritus Professor of Medicine
Former Head
Department of Cardiology
University Hospital Charles Nicolle
Rouen, France
Adviser for Cardiology Programs
Rouen Normandy Medical Training Center

Alla Gopala Krishna Gokhale MS MCh DNB SMP (IIM-C) DSc (Hon)
Cardiothoracic and Transplant Surgeon, Apollo Hospitals, Jubilee Hills
Hyderabad, Telangana, India

Amal Kumar Khan MD MNAMS DM
Former Professor of Cardiology
WBMES
Visiting Consultant
AMRI Hospital, Salt Lake
Kolkata, West Bengal, India

Aman Makhija MD DM
Senior Consultant Cardiologist
Sir Ganga Ram Hospital
New Delhi, India

Aman T Patel MD DM
Consultant Interventional Cardiologist, Apex Heart Institute
Ahmedabad, Gujarat, India

Amartya Khan MD
RMO Clinical Tutor
JNM Medical College, Kalyani
Kolkata, West Bengal, India

Amitabha Chattopadhyay DCH DNB Fellowship in Pediatric Cardiology (Australia)
Chief Pediatric Cardiologist and Clinical Lead Eastern India
Department of Pediatric Cardiology
Narayana Superspeciality Hospital
Howrah, West Bengal, India

Amit Garg MD (Radiodiagnosis)
Senior Consultant
Department of Imaging
Fortis Escort Heart Institute
New Delhi, India

Amit Kumar Chaurasia MD DM FESC FAPSIC
Unit Chief (1), Chief Cath Lab, Chief TAVR and Structural Heart Disease
Artemis Hospital
Gurugram, Haryana, India

Amit Patel MD
Cardiologist
Magnum Heart Institute
Nashik, Maharashtra, India

Amritesh Biswas MD
Postdoctoral Trainee
Institute of Postgraduate Medical Education and Research
Kolkata, West Bengal, India

Anand M MD DM (Cardiology) Fellowship in EP
Associate Professor
Christian Medical College Hospital
Vellore, Tamil Nadu, India

Anantharaman Rajaram MRCP FRCP CCT (Cardiology)
Senior Consultant Interventional Cardiologist
Clinical Lead
Advanced Heart Failure, Cardiomyopathy and Transplantation, Transcatheter Valve Therapy
Kauvery Hospital
Chennai, Tamil Nadu, India

(Col) Anil Dhall Sena Medal MD (Medicine) DM (Cradiology) FACC FESC FAHA FRCP (Edinburgh) FSCAI FHRS FCSI
Professor and Head
Department of Cardiology
Janakpuri Super Speciality Hospital
New Delhi, India

Anil J MD DNB (Cardiology)
Former Professor and Head
Deaprtment of Cardiology
Dutta Meghe Institute of Medical Sciences
Wardha, Maharashtra, India

Anil Sharma MD (Medicine) DM (Cardiology) FAPSC (Taiwan), DSc FWSIM FSCAI (USA) FACC (USA) Advanced Fellowship in Complex Angioplasty (Italy)
Professor, Head and Senior Consultant and Interventional Cardiologist
Department of Cardiology
Bombay Hospital and Medical Research Centre
Mumbai, Maharashtra, India

Anil Sivadasan Radha MD DCH DNB (Pediatrics) DNB (Cardiology)
Senior Consultant and Head
Department of Pediatric Cardiology
Lisie Hospital
Kochi, Kerala, India

Anirban Das MD DM
Senior Resident
Burdwan Medical College
Burdwan, West Bengal, India

Anirudda Deshpande MD (Internal Medicine) DM (Neurology) FRCP (London) FRCP (Edinburgh) DNB Neurology Fellowship in Stroke (Canada)
Consultant Neurologist
Vinayaka Neuro Multispecialty Centre
Warangal, Telangana, India

Anita Saxena MD DM FACC
Vice Chancellor
Pt BD Sharma University of Health Sciences
Rohtak, Haryana, India

Anju Nohria MD
Director
Cardio-Oncology and Cancer Survivorship Program
Dana Farber Cancer Institute
Cardiovascular Division
Brigham and Women's Hospital
Harvard Medical School
Boston, MA, USA

Ankit Gulia DNB
Senior Resident
Department of Cardiology
Dayanand Medical College and Hospital
Ludhiana, Punjab, India

Ankur Gautam MD DM (Cardiology)
Assistant Professor
Department of Cardiology
GB Pant Institute of Postgraduate Medical Education and Research
New Delhi, India

Ankush Gupta MD DM FACC
Professor of Medicine and Interventional Cardiologist
Department of Cardiology
Army Institute of Cardio Thoracic Sciences (AICTS)
Pune, Maharashtra, India

Anoop Agrawal MBBS MD FACC
American Board Certified in Internal Medicine, Cardiovascular Diseases, and Interventional Cardiology
Consultant Cardiologist
Krishna Institute of Medical Sciences
Secunderabad, Telangana, India

Anuj Gupta MBBS
All India Institute of Medical Sciences
Bhopal, Madhya Pradesh, India

Anuradha D MD DNB (Cardiology)
Junior Consultant
Apollo Hospital
Visakhapatnam, Andhra Pradesh, India

Anushree D Kumbhalkar MD (Medicine)
Senior Resident
Department of Cardiology
Bombay Hospital and Medical Research Centre
Mumbai, Maharashtra, India

Aqdas Mumtaz MD
Senior Resident
Department of Cardiology
Institute of Medical Sciences
Banaras Hindu University
Varanasi, Uttar Pradesh, India

Aravind Duruvasal MD DM
Consultant Interventional Cardiologist
SNN Specialities Clinic and SNN Diagnostic Centre
Chennai, Tamil Nadu, India

Aravind MS MPH
Research Associate
Department of Public Health
Amrita Institute of Medical Science
Kochi, Kerala, India

Arijit Ghosh MD DM
Consultant Interventional Cardiologist
Department of Cardiology
AMRI Hospital, Salt Lake
Kolkata, West Bengal, India

Arijit Kumar Ghosh MD DM FACC FESC FSCAI FAPSIC FAPVS FICC
Professor and Head
Department of Cardiology
All India Institute of Medical Sciences
Nagpur, Maharashtra, India

Arijt Ghosh MD DM (Cardiology)
In-charge, Cath Lab
AMRI Hospital
Kolkata, West Bengal, India

Arshdeep Singh Sandhu MD (Medicine) DM-PDT
Postdoctoral Trainee
Department of Cardiology
Medical College
Kolkata, West Bengal, India

Arun Kumar MD DM (Cardiology)
Fellow Peripheral Vascular and Aortic Intervention
Christian Medical College
Vellore, Tamil Nadu, India

Arun Mohanty MD DM
Professor, Sir Ganga Ram Hospital
New Delhi, India

Arup Dasbiswas MD DM (Cardiology) FACC FESC FSCAI
Director, Cath Lab
BMRC Hospital
Ex-Director, ICVS, IPGME&R
Ex-Professor and Head
Department of Cardiology
IPGME&R and SSKM Hospital
Kolkata, West Bengal, India

Asesh Haldar MD DM
Consultant, Medica Institute of Cardiology Sciences
Kolkata, West Bengal, India

Asha Mahilmaran MD DNB DM FCSI FACC FESC FSCAI
Senior Interventional Consultant Cardiologist, Apollo Hospitals
Chennai, Tamil Nadu, India

Asha Moorthy MD DM FCCP FIACM FICP FIMSA FICC
Professor and Head
Sri Ramachandra Medical College and Saveetha Medical College (Former)
Chennai, Tamil Nadu, India

Ashesh Halder MD (Medicine, Gold Medalist) DM (Cardiology) Fellowship in Electrophysiology
Consultant – Medica Institute of Cardiology Services
Medica Institute of Cardiac Science
Kolkata, West Bengal, India

Ashish Deshpande MD DM (Cardiology) FACC
Consultant Interventional Cardiologist
Oriion Citicare Superspeciality Hospital
Ex-Professor and Head
MGM Medical College and Hospital
Aurangabad, Maharashtra, India

Ashish Jai Kishan MD DNB
Senior Consultant Interventional Cardiology
Fortis Escorts Heart Institute
New Delhi, India

Ashish Kumar MD DM
Associate Consultant
Division of Interventional Cardiology
Medanta Heart Institute
Medanta – The Medicity
Gurugram, Haryana, India

Ashish Kumar Jain MD DNB (Cardiology)
Associate Consultant Cardiologist
Sir Ganga Ram Hospital
New Delhi, India

Ashok Seth FRCP FACC MSCAI FAPSIC DSc
Chairman
Fortis Escorts Heart Institute
New Delhi, India

Ashraf SM MD DM FACC
Professor and Head
Department of Cardiology
GMC Kannur, Hrudayalaya
Kannur, Kerala, India

Ashwin B Mehta MD FACC FCCP FISE FICP
Interventional Cardiologist
Director of Cardiology
Jaslok Hospital and Research Centre
Mumbai, Maharashtra, India

Ashwin Mahesh MD
Cardiovascular Disease Fellow
UPMC Harrisburg
Harrisburg, PA, USA

Asit Das MD DM (Cardiology)
Associate Professor
IPGME&R and SSKM Hospital
Kolkata, West Bengal, India

Asmita Samal MD DNB (Medicine)
Senior Resident
DY Patil Medical College
Pune, Maharashtra, India

Asok Kumar Kar MD DM FACC
Senior Interventional Cardiologist
Peerless Hospitals
Kolkata, West Bengal, India

Atul Mathur MD DM
Executive Director Interventional Cardiology and Chief of Cardiac Cath Labs
Fortis Escorts Heart Institute
New Delhi, India

Auriom Kar MD DM
Consultant
Department of Cardiology
Narayana Multispeciality Hospital
Kolkata, West Bengal, India

Avani Jain MD
Medical Officer
DNS Hospital
Indore, Madhya Pradesh, India

Ayan Kar DNB (General Medicine) DNB (Cardiology)
Interventional Cardiologist and Clinical Lead in Heart Failure Services
Narayana Health-Rabindranath Tagore
International Institute of Cardiac Sciences
Kolkata, West Bengal, India

Babu Reddy MD DM (Cardiology)
Associate Professor
Department of Cardiology
Sri Jayadeva Institute of Cardiovascular Sciences and Research
Bengaluru, Karnataka, India

Badrinarayana Tumula MD DM FICC FESC FIAMS LICC
Senior Consultant Cardiologist
Apollo Hospital, Jubilee Hills
Hyderabad, Telangana, India

Bagirath Raghuraman MD DNB DM (Cardiology) FESC FSCAI FHFA
Senior Consultant Cardiologist and Program Director
Heart Transplant
Narayana Institute of Cardiac Sciences
Narayana Health City
Bengaluru, Karnataka, India

Bahuleyan CG MD DM FRCP FSCAI
Chairman
Cardiovascular Centre
Ananthapuri Hospitals and Research Institute
Thiruvananthapuram, Kerala, India

Baruah DK DM FACC FSCAI FICC FCSI
Senior Consultant and Director
Catheterization Laboratory
Apollo Hospital, Health City
Visakhapatnam, Andhra Pradesh, India

BC Srinivas MD DM (Cardiology)
Professor
Department of Cardiology
Sri Jayadeva Institute of Cardiovascular Sciences and Research
Bengaluru, Karnataka, India

Bharat Vijay Purohit MD DM
Senior Consultant and Director of Cathlab
Department of Cardiology
Yashoda Hospital Hitech City
Hyderabad, Telangana, India

B Hygriv Rao MD DM FACC FESC
Senior Consultant Cardiologist and Director
Division of Pacing and Electrophysiology
KIMS Group of Hospitals,
Hyderabad, Telangana, India

Biswajit Majumder MD DM FACC
Professor and Head
Department of Cardiology
RG Kar Medical College and Hospital
Kolkata, West Bengal, India

Biswaranjan Mishra MD DM FCSI FIAE FICC
Senior Consultant Cardiologist
Max Diagnostic
Cuttack, Odisha, India

BKS Sastry MD DM FACC
Head
Department of Cardiology
CARE Hospital
Hyderabad, Telangana, India

Blessvin Jino MD DM
Consultant Cardiologist
Meditrina Hospital
Kollam, Kerala, India

Brian Pinto MD DM FACC FSCAI
Director and Consultant Interventional Cardiologist
Holy Family Hospital, Breach Candy, Khar Hinduja, Saifee, Nanavati
Mumbai, Maharashtra, India

B Srinivas MD DM
Professor and Head
Department of Cardiology
NIMS
Hyderabad, Telangana, India

BVA Ranga Reddy MD DM
Consultant Cardiologist
Apollo Hospital, Jubilee Hills
Hyderabad, Telangana, India

Byomakesh Dikshit MD DM (Cardiology)
Senior Consultant
Apollo Hospitals
Bhubaneswar, Odisha, India

Chhabi Satpathy MD DM
Professor and Head
Division of Cardiology
MKCG Medical College
Berhampur, Odisha, India

Chaitanya Gupta MBBS
Final Year Student
Santosh University
Ghaziabad, Uttar Pradesh, India

Chakradhar P MD DM
Consultant, Apollo Hospital
Visakhapatnam, Andhra Pradesh, India

Chandan Kumar Das MD (Medicine) DNB (Cardiology)
Assistant Professor
Advance Cardiology Institute
Pt JNM Medical College
Raipur, Chhattisgarh, India

Chandrakanta Mishra MD (Medicine) DM (Cardiology) FACC FCSI FICC FESC
Associate Professor
Department of Cardiology
SCB Medical College and Hospital
Cuttack, Odisha, India

Chandrashekhar K Ponde MD DM (Medicine) DNB (Cardiology)
Consultant Cardiologist
Head
Department of Cardiology
PD Hinduja National Hospital and MRC
Mumbai, Maharashtra, India

Chan KS Mike BSc (Science) Researcher Stem Cell
Professor, Researcher and Author
Founder
European Wellness Biomedical Group
Germany

Chinmay Gupta MBBS FICC MBA (Hospital Administration)
Clinical Associate (Cardiology)
Indraprastha Apollo Hospitals
New Delhi, India

CM Nagesh MD DM (Cardiology)
Professor
Department of Cardiology
Sri Jayadeva Institute of Cardiovascular Sciences and Research
Bengaluru, Karnataka, India

C Narasimhan MD DM
Head
Department of Cardiac Electrophysiology
AIG Hospital
Hyderabad, Telangana, India

C Venkata S Ram MD MACP FACC FASH
Director
Apollo Institute for Blood Pressure Management
Apollo Group of Hospitals
Hyderabad, Telangana, India
Professor of Internal Medicine
University of Texas Southwestern Medical Center
Dallas, TX, USA

Darshan Krishnappa MD DM FACC
Assistant Professor
Sri Jayadeva Institute of Cardiac Sciences and Research
Bengaluru, Karnataka, India

Dayasagar Rao V DM FRCP (Canada) FRCP (Edinburgh)
Consultant Cardiologist
KIMS Hospital
Secunderabad, Telangana, India

Debabrata Dash MD DM FICC FAPSC FCCP FSCAI FACC FESC
Director and Consultant Interventional Cardiologist
Department of Cardiology
Aster Hospital Mankhool
Dubai, Al Quasis, UAE

Debabrata Roy MD DM (Cardiology) FACC FESC FSCAI FAHA
Senior Consultant Interventional Cardiologist and Academic Co-ordinator
NH-RTIICS
Kolkata, West Bengal, India

Debasish Roychoudhury MD FACC FASE
Clinical Associate Professor
Department of Medicine
Weill Cornell University
New York, NY, USA

Debdatta Bhattacharyya MD MRCP CCST (Cardiology)
Senior Interventional Cardiologist
Clinical Director and Chief of Cathlab Services
Narayana Health RN Tagore Hospital
Kolkata, West Bengal, India

Debika Chatterjee MD
Senior Consultant and Head
Department of Noninvasive Cardiology
NH RTIICS
Kolkata, West Bengal, India

Debopriyo Mondal MD (Internal Medicine, Gold Medalist) DM (Cardiology)
Consultant Interventional Cardiologist
Medica Institute of Cardiac Science
Kolkata, West Bengal, India

Deepak Padmanabhan DM (Cardiology) Fellowship in Electrophysiology and Advanced Adult Cardiology (USA)
Assistant Professor
Department of Electrophysiology
Sri Jayadeva Institute of Cardiac Sciences and Research
Bengaluru, Karnataka, India

Deepak Ranjan Das MD DM (Cardiology)
Associate Professor
SCB Medical College and Hospital
Cuttack, Odisha, India

Deepanjan Bhattacharya MD DM
Senior Consultant
Advanced Cardiac Centre
BR Singh Hospital and Centre for Medical Education and Research
Eastern Railways
Kolkata, West Bengal, India

Deepesh Agarwal MD (Medicine) DM (Cardiology)
Professor, Department of Cardiology
Mahatma Gandhi Medical College and Hospital
Jaipur, Rajasthan, India

Devanu Ghosh Roy MD DM MRCP (UK) FRCP (London)
Senior Consultant
Advanced Cardiac Centre
BR Singh Hospital and Centre for Medical Education and Research
Eastern Railways
Kolkata, West Bengal, India

Devesh Kumar MD DM
Senior Resident
Department of Cardiology
All India Institute of Medical Sciences
New Delhi, India

Dev Pahlajani MD FACC FSCAI
Head
Department of Cardiology
Breach Candy Hospital
Mumbai, Maharashtra, India

Devyani Dogra MBBS
Student
American International College of Arts and Science
Antigua

Dheeraj Kela MD
Senior Resident
Department of Cardiology
Institute of Medical Sciences
Banaras Hindu University
Varanasi, Uttar Pradesh, India

Dhiman Kahali MD Dip (Cardiology) DM (Cardiology)
Senior Consultant and Director
BM Birla Heart Research Centre
Kolkata, West Bengal, India

Dibya Kumar Baruah MD DM (CMC, Vellore) FACC FSCAI FAPSC FCSI
Senior Consultant Cardiologist and Director
Interventional Cardiology and Cardiac Catheterization Laboratory
Apollo Hospitals, Health City
Visakhapatnam, Andhra Pradesh, India

Dilip Kumar MD DM FACC FRCP (Glasgow) FSCAI FESC FICC FHRS FHFA Certified Cardiac Device Specialist (CCDS, HRS, USA)
Director – Cardiac Cath Lab Services
Senior Consultant Interventional Cardiologist and Electrophylogist
Chief Academic Co-ordinator
Medica Institute of Cardiac Science
Kolkata, West Bengal, India

Dipanjan Chatterjee MD FNB (Cardiac Anaesthesia)
Head, Department of Cardiopulmonary Critical Care
Director
ECMO and Transplant Programme (Heart and Lungs)
Medica Institute of Cardiac Science
Kolkata, West Bengal, India

Dipankar Ghosh Dastidar DCH MD (Medicine) DM (Cardiology) FESC FACC FICP FCSI FSCAI
Associate Professor and Head
Department of Cardiology
Burdwan Medical College
Burdwan, West Bengal, India

Dixit Goyal MD
Senior Resident
Department of Cardiology
GB Pant Hospital
New Delhi, India

Donovon Allen MD
Internal Medicine Resident
Department of Medicine
University of Alabama
Birmingham, AL, USA

Dorairaj Prabhakaran MD DM (Cardiology) MSc FRCP FNASc FNA DSc (Honoris Causa)
Executive Director, Centre for Chronic Disease Control (CCDC)
Distinguished Professor – Public Health Foundation of India (PHFI)
New Delhi, India
Professor, Department of Epidemiology
London School of Hygiene and Tropical Medicine, UK
Adjunct Professor, Rollins School of Public Health, Emory University, USA

DP Sinha MD DM
Head, Department of Cardiology
ILS Hospital
Dumdum, West Bengal, India

DS Gambhir MD DM FAMS FCSI FICC FCAPSC FSCAI FACC (USA)
Padma Shri Awardee
Group Director, Cardiology
Kailash Health Care Ltd
Director
Kailash Hospital and Heart Institute
Noida, Uttar Pradesh, India

Evgeniya V Shalaeva MD MPH CHES
Dean, School of Medicine, Central Asian University
Tashkent, Uzbekistan

Filippo Crea MD
Department of Cardiovascular Medicine
Fondazione Policlinico Universitario Agostino Gemelli IRCCS
Department of Cardiovascular and Pulmonary Sciences, Catholic University of the Sacred Heart
Rome, Italy

Florian A Wenzl MD
Research Assistant
Center for Molecular Cardiology
University of Zurich
Switzerland and Zurich Heart House
Zürich, Switzerland

Franz H Messerli MD HonD FACC FESC
Department of BioMedical Research
University of Bern, Switzerland
Jagiellonian University Krakow, Poland

G Ashok MD DM
Associate Professor and Senior Interventional Cardiologist
Chettinad Academy of Research and Education
Chettinad Super Speciality Hospital
Chennai, Tamil Nadu, India

Ganesh Jagdale MD
Cardiologist
Magnum Heart Institute
Nashik, Maharashtra, India

Gaurav Agarwal MD DM
Consultant
Department of Cardiology
Narayana Multispeciality Hospital
Kolkata, West Bengal, India

Gaurav Kumar Arora MD DM
Assistant Professor
Department of Cardiology
Vardhman Mahavir Medical College and Safdarjung Hospital
New Delhi, India

George Wuni MD
Postgraduate Year 3 Resident
Department of Internal Medicine
Harlem Hospital Center in affiliation with Columbia University
New York, NY, USA

Girish B Navasundi MD DNB
Senior Consultant Cardiologist
Director, Cath Lab
Apollo Hospital
Bengaluru, Karnataka, India

Girish MP MD DM
Professor
Department of Cardiology
GB Pant Hospital
New Delhi, India

Giuseppe Mancia MD PhD
Emeritus Professor of Medicine
University of Milano-Bicocca
Milan, Italy

G Justin Paul MD DNB (Medicine) DM DNB (Cardiology) FACC FESC
Director and Head (i/c)
Department of Cardiology
Madras Medical College
Chennai, Tamil Nadu, India

GN Mahapatra FRCP (Glasgow) DRM (Delhi University) FCSI (India) FCCP (USA) FRSH (UK) Spl Train Nucl Med (University of Texas, MD Anderson, Houston)
Consultant and Head
Department of Nuclear Medicine and PET-CT
SPECT–CT Seven Hills Hospital (JCI, USA Accredited)
Mumbai, Maharashtra
Director
Department of Nuclear Medicine and PET-CT
Sri Aurobindo Institute of Medical Sciences (SAIMS)
Indore, Madhya Pradesh, India
President – World Federation of Cardiac Imaging and Clinical Cardiology

Gopala Krishna Koduru MD DM
Consultant Cardiologist
Aayush Hospitals
Vijayawada and Eluru, Andhra Pradesh, India

Gopal Chandra Ghosh DM (Cardiology) FACC FESC FSCAI
Consultant Interventional Cardiologist
Director, Cath Lab
Rabindranath Thakur Diagnostic and Medical Care Center
Berhampore, West Bengal, India

Gourav Bhattacharya MD DM (Cardiology)
Senior Resident
Department of Cardiology
Burdwan Medical College and Hospital
Burdwan, West Bengal, India

Goutam Datta MD DNB DM MRCP (UK) FESC FSCAI
Professor
Institute of Postgraduate Medical Education and Research
Kolkata, West Bengal, India

Guido Grassi MD
Clinica Medica
University of Milano-Bicocca
Milan, Italy

Gunjan Ghodeshwar DM (Cardiology)
Assistant Professor
Department of Cardiology
All India Institute of Medical Sciences
Nagpur, Maharashtra, India

Gurpreet Singh Wander MD DM FACC FAMS
Professor
Department of Cardiology
Dayanand Medical College and Hospital
Unit Hero DMC Heart Institute
Ludhiana, Punjab, India

G Venkateshwara Reddy MD DM
Head
Department of Cardiology
Star Pinnacle Heart Centre
Visakhapatnam, Andhra Pradesh, India

Harendra Kumar MD (Medicine) PhD (Medicine) FICP FIAE FCSI FICC
National Professor of Medicine, Senior Consultant Cardiologist, Ex-Director
Indira Gandhi Institute of Cardiology
Patna Medical College Campus
Visiting Senior Consultant Cardiologist
Jeevak Heart Hospital
Patna, Bihar, India

Haresh G Mehta MD (Medicine) DNB (Cardiology) FACC FESC FSCAI
Director of Cardiology
Healing Hearts
Mumbai, Maharashtra, India

Harikrishnan S DM FACC FRCP FAMS
Head and Professor
Department of Cardiology
SCTIMST
Thiruvananthapuram, Kerala, India

Harshit Khare MD DM (Cardiology)
Assistant Professor
Department of Cardiology
Sanjay Gandhi Postgraduate Institute of Medical Sciences
Lucknow, Uttar Pradesh, India

Hemant K Satpathy MD
Maternal-Foetal- Medicine (MFN) Specialist
Methodist Women's Hospital
Omaha, NE, USA

Himanshu Dabral MD DM
Director
Division of Interventional Cardiology
Medanta Heart Institute
Medanta – The Medicity
Gurugram, Haryana, India

Himanshu Jain MD
Senior Resident
Department of Gastroenterology
Superspeciality Hospital
MGM Medical College
Indore, Madhya Pradesh, India

HK Chopra MD DM FRCP FACC FISC FISCU FASE FCSI FIAE FIMSA
Senior Consultant Cardiologist
Medanta Moolchand Heart Institute
New Delhi, India
Past President – National CSI
Past Editor – IHJ, JIAE
Past President – National IAE
Country Head, AHA
President, WHA, WWF

Ilayaraja U MD DM
Cardiologist
Billroth Hospital
Chennai, Tamil Nadu, India

Indrani Mandal MD
Consultant Pediatrician
WBHS
Midnapore, West Bengal, India

I Sathyamurthy MD DM FACC FRCP DSc (Honoris Causa)
Senior Interventional Cardiologist
Department of Cardiology
Apollo Main Hospitals
Chennai, Tamil Nadu, India

IB Vijayalakshmi MD DM DSc FICC FIAE FICP FCSI FIAMS FAMS FISH FRCP (London)
Professor Emeritus
Former Professor and Head
Department of Pediatric Cardiology
Sri Jayadeva Institute of Cardiovascular Sciences and Research
Bengaluru, Karnataka, India

Jagdish C Mohan MD DM
Interventional Cardiologist
Department of Cardiology
Institute of Heart and Vascular Diseases
Jaipur Golden Hospital
Rohini, Delhi, India

Jaideep C Menon DM (Cardiology)
Professor
Department of Adult Cardiology
Amrita Institute of Medical Science
Kochi, Kerala, India

Jain T Kallarakkal MD DM FRCP
Senior Interventional Cardiologist
Sree Narayana Institute of Medical Sciences
Eranakulam, Kerala, India

Jasneet Singh MBBS
Senior Resident
Department of Cardiology
Janakpuri Super Speciality Hospital
New Delhi, India

Jasur B Babadjanov C MD MScPHS
Division of Public Health Science
Westminster International University
Tashkent, Uzbekistan

Jayagopal PB MD DM DNB FACC FICC FCSI FESC FSCAI FRCP(E)
Director, Head and Senior Interventional Cardiologist
Lakshmi Hospital,
Palakkad, Kerala, India

Jayanta Sharma MD FCSI
Consultant Cardiologist
Apollo Gleneagles Hospital
Kolkata, West Bengal, India

Jenu Rose Jose E MD (Pediatrics) DNB (Pediatrics) DM (Cardiology) PDF (Pediatric Cardiology)
Junior Consultant
Department of Pediatric Cardiology
Lisie Hospital
Kochi, Kerala, India

Jesu Krupa MD DM (Cardiology)
Faculty
Department of Cardiology
Christian Medical College
Vellore, Tamil Nadu, India

Johann Christopher MD DNB FACC
Director of Cardiac Imaging
Care Hospital
Hyderabad, Telangana, India

John Jose MD DM Fellowship in Interventional Cardiology (Germany)
Professor and Head
TAVI and Structural Heart Interventions
Department of Cardiology Unit-2
Christian Medical College Hospital
Vellore, Tamil Nadu, India

John Roshan Jacob MD DM (Cardiology) CEPS CCDS Fellowships in Adult and Pediatric EP
Professor
Christian Medical College Hospital
Vellore, Tamil Nadu, India

Jo Joseph MD DM
Senior Consultant Cardiologist
Department of Cardiology and Vascular Medicine
Lisie Heart Institute, Lisie Hospital
Kochi, Kerala, India

JPS Sawhney DM FESC FACC FRCP
Chairperson
Department of Cardiology
Dharma Vira Heart Center
Sir Ganga Ram Hospital
New Delhi, India

Juhi Singh MD DNB (Medicine)
Senior Resident
Department of Cardiology
Dharma Vira Heart Center
Sir Ganga Ram Hospital
New Delhi, India

Kabir Sethi MD DM
Consultant, Department of Cardiology
Delhi Heart and Lung Institute
New Delhi, India

Kajal Ganguly MD DM FACC
Consultant Interventional Cardiologist
Department of Cardiology
AMRI Hospital, Salt Lake
Kolkata, West Bengal, India

Kamal K Sethi MD DM FACC FHRS FCSI FISE
Director of Cardiology
Chairman and Managing Director
Delhi Heart and Lung Institute
New Delhi, India

Karthikeyan Balakrishnan MD DM
Consultant Cardiologist
Hindu Mission Hospital
Chennai, Tamil Nadu, India

Karunakar Rapolu MD DM
Consultant Cardiologist
Apollo Hospital, Jubillee Hills
Hyderabad, Telangana, India

Kashinath Ghosh Hazra MD DM DNB (Cardiology) MNAMS FNB (Interventional Cardiology)
Senior Consultant Interventional Cardiologist
NH-Rabindranath Tagore International Institute of Cardiac Sciences
Kolkata, West Bengal, India

Kavish Chopda MD
Physician
Magnum Heart Institute
Nashik, Maharashtra, India

Kayan Siodia DNB (Medicine) DNB (Cardiology)
Consultant Cardiologist
Healing Hearts
Mumbai, Maharashtra, India

K Durga Devi MD DM
Assistant Professor and Senior Interventional Cardiologist
Chettinad Academy of Research and Education
Chettinad Super Speciality Hospital
Chennai, Tamil Nadu, India

Kesavamoorthy MD DM
Consultant
Department of Interventional Cardiology
Meenakshi Hospital
Thanjavur, Tamil Nadu, India

Kiran Gaur MSc PhD
Associate Professor and Head
Department of Statistics, Mathematics and Computer Science
Government SKN Agriculture University
Jaipur, Rajasthan, India

Kiran Gopinath MD DM
Senior Consultant Cardiologist
NIMS Heart Foundation
Thiruvananthapuram, Kerala, India

Kiran Kumar G MD DM
Interventional Cardiologist
Care Hospitals
Hyderabad, Telangana, India

K Meenakshi MD (General Medicine) DM (Cardiology)
Professor and Head
Department of Cardiology
Saveetha Medical College
Chennai, Tamil Nadu, India

KN Srinivasan MD DNB (Cardiology) FCSI FESC FSCAI
Senior Interventional Cardiologist
Department of Cardiology
Apollo Main Hospitals
Chennai, Tamil Nadu, India

Kousalya Gopalsamy MBBS
DMO, Department of Cardiology
Meenakshi Hospital
Thanjavur, Tamil Nadu, India

Krishnaswamy Chandrasekaran MD FACC FASE
Senior Consultant
Department of Cardiovascular Diseases, Apollo Hospitals
Chennai, Tamil Nadu, India
Professor of Medicine, Mayo Clinic
Rochester, MN, USA

K Sivakumar MD DCH DNB (Pediatrics) DM DNB (Cardiology)
Head
Department of Pediatric Cardiology
Institute of Cardio Vascular Diseases
The Madras Medical Mission Hospital
Chennai, Tamil Nadu, India

Kunal Patankar MD (Medicine)
Senior Resident
Department of Cardiology
PD Hinduja National Hospital and MRC
Mumbai, Maharashtra, India

K Venugopal MD DM FCSI FICC FACC FESC
Senior Consultant Cardiologist
SP Fort Hospital, Thiruvananthapuram
Former Professor and Head
Department of Cardiology
Government Medical College
Kozhikode, Kerala, India

Lekha Adik Pathak MD (Medicine) DM (Cardiology) FRCP (Edinburgh)
Director and Head
Department of Cardiology
Nanavati Max Super Speciality Hospital
Mumbai, Maharashtra, India

Madhumanti Panja MD DNB (Cardiology)
Consultant Interventional Cardiologist
Belle Vue Clinic, AMRI Hospital
Kolkata, West Bengal, India

Madhu Shukla MBBS PhD
Head of Noninvasive Cardiology
Department of Cardiology
Institute of Heart and Vascular Diseases
Jaipur Golden Hospital
Rohini, New Delhi, India

Madhu Sreedharan MD DM MRCP (UK) FRCP FACC
Director
NIMS Heart Foundation
Thiruvananthapuram, Kerala, India

Madhuvanthi Rajendran DNB
Registrar in Cardiology
Kovai Medical Center and Hospital
Coimbatore, Tamil Nadu, India

Mahendra Chouhan DNB (Medicine) DrNB
Senior Resident
Department of Cardiology
Janakpuri Super Speciality Hospital
New Delhi, India

Mahesh Nalin Kumar MD DrNB FACC FESC
Head and Senior Consultant Cardiology
St Gregorios Medical Mission Hospital
Parumala, Kerala, India

Mainak Mukhopadhyay MD MRCP DM FESC CCDS
Consultant Interventional Cardiologist
Department of Cardiology
AMRI Hospital, Salt Lake
Kolkata, West Bengal, India

Maitreyee Bhattacharyya MD DM
Assistant Professor
LPS Institute of Cardiology
Kanpur, Uttar Pradesh, India

Mandava Satya Sahitya MD
Fellow
Department of Cardiology
Advanced Cardiac Centre
Postgraduate Institute of Medical Education and Research
Chandigarh, India

Manik Chopra MD DM
Clinical Lead – Structural Heart Disease Interventions
Department of Cardiology
Narayana Multispeciality Hospital
Ahmedabad, Gujarat, India

Manish Bansal MD DNB (Cardiology) FACC FASE
Senior Director
Department of Clinical and Preventive Cardiology
Medanta Heart Institute
Medanta – The Medicity
Gurugram, Haryana, India

Manish Chokhandre MD
Consultant Pediatric Cardiologist
Swasthyam Superspeciality Hospital
Nagpur, Maharashtra, India

Manoj Chopda MD DM (Cardiology)
Consultant Interventional Cardiologist
Director
Magnum Heart Institute
Nashik, Maharashtra, India

Manoj Kumar Agarwala MD (PGI) DM (PGI) FACC
Consultant Cardiologist
Department of Cardiology
Apollo Hospital, Jubilee Hills
Hyderabad, Telangana, India

Manoranjan Mandal MD Dip Card DM (Cardiology)
Professor and Head
Department of Cardiology
Medical College
Kolkata, West Bengal, India

Mansi Kaushik MBBS PGDCC FNIC
Consultant
Department of Clinical and Preventive Cardiology
Medanta Heart Institute
Medanta – The Medicity
Gurugram, Haryana, India

Manu Gupta MBBS
JR (Academic)
Department of Medicine
Peoples College of Medical Sciences
Bhopal, Madhya Pradesh, India

Manu Rajendran MD DM
Consultant Cardiologist
Meditrina Hospital
Kollam, Kerala, India

Marsha Barreto MD DM
Cardiology Resident
Department of Cardiology
Amrita Institute of Medical Sciences
Kochi, Kerala, India

Mayuri Mhatre MD DNB (Emergency Medicine)
Senior Clinical Associate
Department of Cardiology
PD Hinduja National Hospital and MRC
Mumbai, Maharashtra, India

M Chokkalingam MD DNB FACC FESC
Professor and Senior Interventional Cardiologist
Chettinad Academy of Research and Education
Chettinad Super Speciality Hospital
Chennai, Tamil Nadu, India

Meeraji Rao MD DM (Cardiology)
Senior Conultant and Head
Cardiology
Continental Hospital
Hyderabad, Telangana, India

Meetu Arora MBBS PGDCC (Cardiology) CCEBDM (Diabetes)
Consultant
Department of Cardiac Sciences
Max Super Speciality Hospital
Patparganj, New Delhi, India

Meghna Gupta MD (Psychiatry)
Senior Resident
Department of Psychiatry
All India Institute of Medical Sciences (AIIMS)
Bathinda, Punjab, India

Mohammed Abdul Azeez Asad MD DNB FNB
Consultant Cardiologist
Bahrain Specialist Hospital – Apollo Heart Centre
Juffair, Manama, Bahrain

Mohit D Gupta MD DM
Professor, Department of Cardiology
GB Pant Hospital
New Delhi, India

Mohsin Wali MD FACC
Professor and Senior Consultant
Department of Internal Medicine
Sir Ganga Ram Hospital
New Delhi, India

Mona Bhatia MD FRCR (UK) FSCCT (USA) FSCMR (USA)
Principal Director and Head
Department of Radiodiagnosis and Imaging
Fortis Escorts Heart Institute
New Delhi, India
Convener, Multimodality Imaging, Cardiological Society of India
Chair, International Regional Committee, India Chapter
Society of Cardiovascular CT, USA

Monotosh Panja MD FACC (USA) FCSI FICP DM (Cardiology)
Senior Consultant Interventional Cardiologist
Belle Vue Clinic
BM Birla Heart Institute
Ex-Director, ICVS, IPGME&R and SSKM Hospital
Kolkata, West Bengal, India

Moukthika KVN MD DM PDF (Electrophysiology)
Consultant Cardiologist and Electrophysiologist
Apollo Hospital
Bengaluru, Karnataka, India

Mrinalini Alla MD
Resident
Department of General Surgery
Flushing Hospital Medical Center
Queens, NY, USA

Mrinal Kanti Das MD DM FICP FICC FCSI FACC FESC
Consultant Cardiologist
CK Birla Hospitals (BMB/CMRI)
Kolkata, West Bengal, India

MS Ravi MD DM (Cardiology)
Former Director of Cardiology
Madras Medical College and Rajiv Ghandhi Government General Hospital
Chennai, Tamil Nadu, India

Mufaddal Lunawadawala DNB (Medicine) DrNB Cardiology
Senior Clinical Associate
Department of Cardiology
PD Hinduja National Hospital and MRC
Mumbai, Maharashtra, India

Musna PJ MD DM
Consultant Cardiologist
Department of Cardiology
St Mary's Hospital
Thodupuzha, Kerala, India

Mustafa Sajjad Cheema MBBS
Research Fellow
Department of Cardiology
West Virginia University School of Medicine
Morgantown, WV, USA

Nagamani AC MD DM
Professor
Department of Cardiology
Sri Jayadeva Institute of Cardiovascular Sciences and Research
Bengaluru, Karnataka, India

Nagaraj Desai MD (Medicine) DM (Cardiology)
Adjunct Professor
Department of Cardiology
JSSAHER, Mysuru
Director
Namana Medical Centre
Bengaluru, Karnataka, India

Nagendra Boopathy Senguttuvan MD DM FACC FSCAI
Professor of Cardiology and Senior Consultant Interventional Cardiologist
Sri Ramachandra Institute of Higher Education and Research
Chennai, Tamil Nadu, India

Nagendra Singh Chouhan MD DNB FNB
Senior Director
Division of Interventional Cardiology
Medanta – The Medicity
Gurugram, Haryana, India

Naima Parveen PhD
Research Coordinator
Harmony – Dr Sachin's 360 Degree Diabetes Care
Bhopal, Madhya Pradesh, India

Nandhakumar Vasu MD DNB (Cardiology) FNB (Interventional Cardiology)
Consultant, Department of Cardiology
Institute of Cardio Vascular Diseases
The Madras Medical Mission Hospital
Chennai, Tamil Nadu, India

Narra Lavanya MD (General Medicine) DrNB (Cardiology)
Cardiologist
Department of Cardiology
Apollo Main Hospital
Chennai, Tamil Nadu, India

Natisha Arora MD DNB
Senior Resident
Department of Imaging
Fortis Escort Heart Institute
New Delhi, India

Navanil Biswas MD (General Medicine) DrNB (Cardiology)
Consultant Interventional Cardiologist
Apollo Multispeciality Hospital
Kolkata, West Bengal, India

Navanil Biswas MD DNB (Cardiology)
Senior Resident
Department of Cardiology, NH-RTIICS
Kolkata, West Bengal, India

Naveen Garg MD DM DNB MNAMS FACC FSCAI FCSI
Professor, Department of Cardiology
Sanjay Gandhi Postgraduate Institute of Medical Sciences
Lucknow, Uttar Pradesh, India

Navin C Nanda MD DSc (Hon) DSc (Medicine) (Hon) FACC FAHA FASE FISCU (D)
Distinguished Professor of Medicine and Cardiovascular Disease
University of Alabama
Birmingham, AL, USA

Neusha Gopal MD DNB (Cardiology)
Associate Consultant Cardiologist
Remedy Hospital
Hyderabad, Telangana, India

Nihar Mehta MD DNB (Medicine) DNB (Cardiology)
Consultant Cardiologist
Jaslok, HN Reliance, Breach Candy Hospitals
Mumbai, Maharashtra, India

Nihar P Mehta MD (Medicine) DNB (Medicine) DNB (Cardiology) FICP FRCP (London)
Consultant Cardiologist, TAVI Specialist
Jaslok Hospital and Research Centre
Mumbai, Maharashtra, India

Nishad Chitnis MD MRCP DNB
Interventional Cardiologist
Heart Care Clinic
Kolhapur, Maharashtra, India

Nishank P Nooli MBBS
Assistant Professor
Department of Anesthesia
University of Alabama
Birmingham, Alabama, USA

Nishit Chandra MD DM
Director Cardiology
Fortis Escorts Heart Institute
New Delhi, India

Nitin Bajaj DM (Cardiology)
Associate Professor
Department of Cardiology
AICTS/AFMC
Pune, Maharashtra, India

Nitin J Burkule MD DM DNB FACC FASE FSCMR
Director, Department of Cardiology
Jupiter Hospital
Thane, Maharashtra, India

Nitin K Kabra MD DM FACC
Professor and Head
Department of Cardiology
Gandhi Medical College Hospital
Secunderabad, Telangana, India

Nitin Kumar Parashar MD DM
Consultant Cardiology
Artemis Hospital
Gurugram, Haryana, India

Nitish Naik MD DM
Professor
Department of Cardiology
All India Institute of Medical Sciences
New Delhi, India

NN Khanna MD DM FRCP (London, Glasgow, Edinburgh) FACC FSCAI FESC FAPSIC FCCP FEISI FICC FCSI
Senior Consultant Cardiologist
Indraprastha Apollo Hospital
New Delhi, India
Chairman – Asia Pacific Vascular Society
Advisor – Apollo Group of Hospitals in India

Panagiotis I Georgianos MD PhD
Assistant Professor
Department of Nephrology
School of Medicine
Aristotle University of Thessaloniki
Thessaloniki, Greece

Panchanan Sahoo MD (Medicine) DM (Cardiology) FACC FESC FICC FISE
Professor, Senior Consultant and Electrophysiologist
Department of Cardiology
Kalinga Institute of Medical Sciences
Bhubaneshwar, Odisha, India

Panigrahi NK MD DM FACC FSCAI FICC FCSI
Senior Consultant and Director Interventional Cardiology
Head, Division of Cardiology
Apollo Hospital, Health City
Visakhapatnam, Andhra Pradesh, India

Pankaj Harkut MD DM (Cardiology) FACC FESC
Consultant Interventional Cardiologist
Swasthyam Superspeciality Hospital
Nagpur, Maharashtra, India

Pankaj Lakhwan MSc CEPS
Lead Clinical Scientist
Nference Labs Pvt Ltd
Bengaluru, Karnataka, India

Pankaj Manoria MD DM FACC FESC
Director
Manoria Heart and Critical Care Hospital
Bhopal, Madhya Pradesh, India

Parayaru Kottayil Asokan MD DM FRCP FACC FESC FSCAI FICC
Chief Consultant Interventional Cardiologist
Fathima Hospital
Kozhikode, Kerala, India

Parth Mashru MD (Medicine)
DM Cardiology Resident 2nd Year
Mahatma Gandhi Medical College and Hospital
Jaipur, Rajasthan, India

Parveen Kumar MD EDiR DICRI FRCR
Ex-Attending Consultant
Department of Radiodiagnosis and Imaging
Fortis Escort Heart Institute
New Delhi, India

Paul V George MD DM
Senior Professor
Department of Cardiology Unit-2
Christian Medical College Hospital
Vellore, Tamil Nadu, India

PC Manoria MD DM FACC FESC FCAPSC
Director
Manoria Heart and Critical Care Hospital
Bhopal, Madhya Pradesh, India

PLN Kapardhi MD DM
Senior Interventional Cardiologist
Care Hospitals
Hyderabad, Telangana, India

Prabhakar Koregol MD DM (Cardiology)
Senior Consultant Cardiologist
Fortis Hospitals
Bengaluru, Karnataka, India

Pradeep Kumar MD DNB
Associate Consultant Cardiologist
Apollo hospital, Jubilee Hills
Hyderabad, Telangana, India

Prafulla G Kerkar MD DM FCSI FACC FESC
Professor Emeritus
Department of Cardiology
KEM Hospital, Parel
Mumbai, Maharashtra, India

Prakas Chandra Mondal MD MRCP (UK, Ireland) MRRCPS (Glasgow) DM (Cardilogy) DNB (Cardiology) FACC (USA)
Consultant Interventional Cardiologist and Head
Department of Cardiology
Apolo Multispeciality Hospital
Kolkata, West Bengal, India

Praneeth S MD DM
Consultant Cardiologist
Apollo Hospital
Bengaluru, Karnataka, India

Prasant Kumar Sahoo MD DM FRCP (London and Glasgow) FACC FESC FSCAI FAPSIC FCSI FICC
Senior Consultant and Director
Interventional Cardiology
Apollo Hospitals
Bhubaneswar, Odisha, India

Prasit Maity DNB
Attending Consultant
Department of Imaging
Fortis Escort Heart Institute
New Delhi, India

Pratap Chandra Rath MD DM FICC FESC FACC FRCP (London) FRCP (Edinburgh)
Senior Consultant Cardiologist and HOD
Department of Cardiology
Apollo Hospital, Jubilee Hills
Hyderabad, Telangana
Apollo Hospital
Bhubaneshwar, Odisha, India

Prathap Kumar MD DM
Chief Interventional Cardiologist
Meditrina Hospital
Kollam, Kerala, India

Pratibha Misra MD (Biochemistry)
Molecular Biologist and Head
Department of Laboratory Sciences
Base Hospital
Guwahati, Assam, India

Praveen Chandra MD DM FACC FESC FSCAI FAPSIC
Chairman
Department of Cardiology
Medanta – The Medicity
Gurugram, Haryana, India

Prayaag Kini MD (Medicine) DNB (Cardiology) Fellow (Interventional Cardiology) FSCAI
Additional Senior Consultant
Department of Cardiology
Sri Sathya Sai Institute of Higher Medical Sciences
Bengaluru, Karnataka, India

Preetish Rath PhD
Candidate (Computer Science)
Tufts University, Medford
Massachusetts, USA

PS Banerjee MD DM (Cardiology) FACC
Chief Interventional Cardiologist
Manipal Hospital
Former Head
Department of Cardiology
Medical College
Kolkata, West Bengal, India
Immediate Past President
Cardiological Society of India

Purneshwar Kumar Pandey MD DM
Associate Consultant
Max Super Specialty Hospital
Saket, New Delhi, India

P Vijay Shekar MD DM
Consultant Cardiologist and Electrophysiologist
Division of Cardiac Pacing and Electrophysiology
Department of Cardiology
Apollo Speciality Hospitals
Tiruchirappalli, Tamil Nadu, India

Raghuram Palaparti MD DM
Consultant Cardiologist
Aayush Hospitals
Vijayawada and Eluru
Andhra Pradesh, India

Rahul Shewale MD
Cardiologist
Magnum Heart Institute
Nashik, Maharashtra, India

Rajan Joseph Manjuran MD DM PGDHRM FICC FIAE FISE FCSI FACC
Emeritus Professor of Cardiology
Pushpagiri Medical College
Thiruvalla, Kerala, India

Rajeev Garg MD (Medicine) Dip Card (NIMS) DNB (Cardiology) MNAMS FSCAI FESC FACC Diplomate National Board
Senior Consultant Interventional Cardiologist
Aware Gleneagles Global Hospital
Hyderabad, Telangana, India

Rajeev Gupta MD DM (Cardiology)
Professor and Head
Department of Cardiology
Gandhi Medical College
Bhopal, Madhya Pradesh, India

Rajeev Gupta MD PhD
Chairman
Department of Preventive Cardiology and Medicine
Eternal Heart Care Centre and Research Institute
Jaipur, Rajasthan, India

Rajendra Kumar Jain MD DM DIU (Paris)
Founder Director
KIMS Group of Hospitals
Hyderabad, Telangana, India

Rajesh Natuva MD DrNB (Cardiology)
Consultant Interventional Cardiologist
Star Hospital, Jubilee Hills
Hyderabad, Telangana, India

Rajesh Thachathodiyl MD DM FACC
Senior Interventional Cardiologist
Professor and Head
Department of Cardiology
Amrita Institute of Medical Sciences
Kochi, Kerala, India

Rajesh Vijayvergiya MD DM FSCAI FACC FESC FISES
Professor
Department of Cardiology
Advanced Cardiac Centre
Postgraduate Institute of Medical Education and Research
Chandigarh, India

Rajeswari K Dip Echo MBA
Echo Technologist
Billroth Hospital
Chennai, Tamil Nadu, India

Rajiv Agarwal MD MS
Professor
Department of Medicine
Division of Nephrology
Indiana University School of Medicine and Richard L Roudebush Veterans Administration Medical Center
Indianapolis, IN, USA

Rajneesh Kapoor MD DNB FACC
Chairman
Division of Interventional Cardiology
Medanta Heart Institute
Medanta – The Medicity
Gurugram, Haryana, India

Rakesh Yadav MD DM
Professor
Department of Cardiology
All India Institute of Medical Sciences
New Delhi, India

Ramakrishna Janapati MD DM
Consultant Cardiologist
Apollo Hospital, Jubilee Hills
Hyderabad, Telangana, India

Ramesh Daggubati MD
Vice Chair and Chief of Interventional Cardiology
Department of Cardiology,
West Virginia University School of Medicine
Morgantown, WV, USA

Rana Rathor Roy MD (General Medicine) DM (Cardiology)
Senior Consultant Interventional Cardiologist
Medica Institute of Cardiac Science
Kolkata, West Bengal, India

Ranjan Modi MD DM (Cardiology)
Senior Consultant and Unit Head
Department of Cardiology
Sarvodaya Healthcare
Faridabad, Haryana, India

Rathindra Nath Karmakar MD DM
Consultant
Department of Cardiology
Narayana Multispeciality Hospital
Kolkata, West Bengal, India

Ratul Ghosh MD
Postdoctoral Trainee
Department of Cardiology
RG Kar Medical College and Hospital
Kolkata, West Bengal, India

Ravi Kant T MD DM
Consultant, Apollo Hospital
Visakhapatnam, Andhra Pradesh, India

Ravinder Singh Rao MD DM FACC FSCAI
Chairman and Managing Director
Department of Cardiology
Rajasthan Hospital Limited
Jaipur, Rajasthan, India

Ravi R Kasliwal MD DM FASE FIMSA MNAMS
Chairman
Department of Clinical and Preventive Cardiology
Medanta Heart Institute
Medanta – The Medicity
Gurugram, Haryana, India

Raymond R Townsend MD FAHA
Professor of Medicine
University of Pennsylvania
Philadelphia, PA, USA

Reeta Varyani MD (Medicine) DNB (Cardiology) Fellow (Interventional Cardiology) FSCAI
Senior Consultant and In-Charge
Department of Cardiology
Sri Sathya Sai Institute of Higher Medical Sciences
Bengaluru, Karnataka, India

Reinhold Kreutz MD PhD
Charité - Universitaetsmedizin Berlin
Corporate Member of Freie Universitaet Berlin and Humboldt-Universitaet zu Berlin
Institute of Clinical Pharmacology and Toxicology
Berlin, Germany

Riccardo Rinaldi MD
Department of Cardiovascular and Pulmonary Sciences
Catholic University of the Sacred Heart
Rome, Italy

Rishika Mehta MD (Pediatrics) DrNB (Pediatric Cardiology)
Pediatric Cardiologist
Department of Pediatric Cardiology
Narayana Superspeciality Hospital
Howrah, West Bengal, India

Ritesh Acharya MD (Medicine) DM (Cardiology)
Assistant Professor
Department of Cardiology
Pursuing Fellowship in Electrophysiology
Kalinga Institute of Medical Sciences
Bhubaneshwar, Odisha, India

Ritwik Ghosal MBBS
Resident
Department of Cardiology
IPGME&R and SSKM Hospital
Kolkata, West Bengal, India

Rocco A Montone MD PhD
Department of Cardiovascular Medicine
Fondazione Policlinico Universitario Agostino Gemelli IRCCS
Rome, Italy

Rohit Mody MD DM
Director of Cardiology
Department of Cardiology
Max Super Specialty Hospital
Bathinda, Punjab, India

Ronak V Ruparelia DNB (Medicine) DNB (Cardiology)
Interventional Cardiologist
Bankers Super Speciality Hospital
Vadodara, Gujarat, India

Rony Mathew MD DM DNB (Medicine) DrNB (Cardiology) FACC FESC FCSI FRCP (London)
Head, Department of Cardiology and Vascular Medicine
Lisie Heart Institute, Lisie Hospital
Kochi, Kerala, India

Roopali Khanna MD DM
Professor, Sanjay Gandhi Postgraduate Institute of Medical Sciences
Lucknow, Uttar Pradesh, India

R Rameshwar MD (General Medicine)
PG in DM Cardiology
Saveetha Medical College
Chennai, Tamil Nadu, India

R Ravi Kumar MD DM
Senior Consultant and Clinical Lead – Heart Failure and Heart Transplantation
MGM Healthcare
Chennai, Tamil Nadu, India

Rufus Demel X MD DNB (Cardiology) FNB (Interventional Cardiology)
Chief Consultant Cardiologist
Devaki Heart Center
Madurai, Tamil Nadu, India

RVA Ananth MD (General Medicine) PGDCC
Department of Cardiology
Government Medical College, Virudhunagar
Consultant Cardiologist
Jeyalakshmi Heart Center
Madurai, Tamil Nadu, India

Sabari Krishnan MD DM
Consultant, Department of Interventional Cardiology
Meenakshi Hospital
Thanjavur, Tamil Nadu, India

Sabyasachi Rout MD DM (Cardiology)
Consultant Cardiologist
Apollo Hospitals
Bhubaneswar, Odisha, India

Sachin Chittawar MD DM (Endocrinology)
Former Associate Professor
Gandhi Medical College
Director, Harmony – Dr Sachin's 360 Degree Diabetes Care
Bhopal, Madhya Pradesh, India

Sachin Raiya MD
Senior Resident
Department of Imaging
Fortis Escort Heart Institute
New Delhi, India

Sagar R Makode DM (Cardiology)
Assistant Professor
Department of Cardiology
All India Institute of Medical Sciences
Nagpur, Maharashtra, India

Saibal Kar MD DM FACC FSCAI
Program Director, Cardiology
Los Robles Regional Medical Center
National Physician Director
Interventional Cardiology
HCA Healthcare
Thousand Oaks, CA, USA

Sai Satish MD DM
Senior Interventional Cardiologist
Clinical Lead – Transcatheter Heart Valve Therapeutics
Apollo Hospitals
Chennai, Tamil Nadu, India

Sajan Narayanan MD DM FESC
Consultant and Interventional Cardiologist
Little Flower Heart Institute, Angamaly
Kochi, Kerala, India

Sameer S Ambar MD DM
Associate Professor
Department of Cardiology
JN Medical College, KAHER
Belgavi, Karnataka, India

Samir B Pancholy MD FAHA FACC MSCAI
Professor of Medicine
Geisinger Commonwealth School of Medicine
Program Director, Fellowship in Cardiovascular Diseases
The Wright Center for Graduate Medical Education
Scranton, PA, USA

Sandeep Bansal MD DM DNB MNAMS FESC FSCAI
Professor and Head
Department of Cardiology
Vardhman Mahavir Medical College and Safdarjung Hospital
New Delhi, India

Sanjay C Shah MD DM
Director
Department of Cardiology
Apex Heart Institute
Ahmedabad, Gujarat, India

Sanjay Kumar Chugh MD DM (Cardiology) FACC FSCAI FIMSA FCSI
Associate Director and Senior Consultant
Cardiology and Interventional Cardiology
Narayana Healthcare Superspeciality Hospital
Gurugram, Haryana, India

Sanjay Mehrotra MD DM
Consultant and Interventional Cardiologist
NH Institute of Cardiac Sciences
Bengaluru, Karnataka, India

Sanjay Tyagi MD DM (Cardiology) FAMS FESC FSCAI FRCP FACC (USA)
Clinical Director
Department of Cardiology
Apollo Hospital Groups - North
Ex-Director Professor and Head
Department of Cardiology
GB Pant PGI and Dean MAMC
New Delhi, India

Sanjeeb Roy MD DM
Director Cardiology
CK Birla Hospital
Jaipur, Rajasthan, India

S Anne Princy MD DM
Assistant Professor,
Department of Cardiology
Tamil Nadu Government Multi Super Speciality Hospital
Chennai, Tamil Nadu, India

Santosh Kumar Singh MD DNB
Associate Consultant
Max Super Specialty Hospital
Saket, New Delhi, India

Santosh Palled MD DM
Interventional Cardiologist
Care Hospitals
Hyderabad, Telangana, India

Sarju Ganatra MD
Director
Cardio-Oncology Program
Division of Cardiovascular Medicine
Vice Chair, Department of Medicine
Lahey Hospital and Medical Center
Beth Israel Lahey Health
Burlington, MA, USA

Saro Avedikian MD MPH
Resident Physician, Internal Medicine
Los Robles Regional Medical Center
HCA Healthcare
Thousand Oaks, CA, USA

Sarumathi Thangavel MD FACC
Consultant
Advanced Heart Failure and Transplant Cardiology
MGM Healthcare
Chennai, Tamil Nadu, India

Satyanarayan Routray MD DM FICC FCSI FACC FSCAI
Professor
SCB Medical College and Hospital
Cuttack, Odisha, India

Satyendra Tewari MD DM (Cardiology) FACC FSCAI FCAPSC FESC FCSI FICC
Professor
Department of Cardiology
Sanjay Gandhi Postgraduate Institute of Medical Sciences
Lucknow, Uttar Pradesh, India

Saumitra Ray MD FRCP FCSI FICP FESC FACC FSCAI
Ex-Professor, Vivekananda Institute of Medical Sciences
Director – Invasive Cardiology
Advanced Medical Research Institute(S)
Kolkata, West Bengal, India

Saurabh Dhumale MD DrNB (Cardiology)
Consultant Interventional Cardiologist
Narayana Health RN Tagore Hospital
Kolkata, West Bengal, India

SB Gupta MD FCSI FICP FISE FACC
Ex-Consultant Physician Cardiologist
Asian Heart Institute Mumbai
Former Head
Department of Medicine and Cardiology
Central Railway Headquarters Hospital
Mumbai, Maharashtra, India

Selvamani S DNB (Cardiology)
Senior Consultant and Interventional Cardiologist
Meenakshi Mission Hospital and Research Centre
Madurai, Tamil Nadu, India

Sengottuvelu G MD (General Medicine) DM (Cardiology) DNB (Cardiology) FRCP (Glasgow, London) Fellowship in Interventional Cardiology (France) FMMC FSCAI FCSI
Clinical Lead
Structural Heart Disease Program
Apollo Hospitals Group
Chennai, Tamil Nadu, India

Senthilraj Thangasami MD (General Medicine), DM (Cardiology)
Interventional Cardiologist
Apollo Hospitals
Chennai, Tamil Nadu, India

S Gnansambandam MD (Pediatrics) DCH DM (Cardiology)
Professor of Cardiology
Head
Department of Pediatric Cardiology
Institute of Child Health and Hospital for Children, Egmore
Chennai, Tamil Nadu, India

Shabbir Ali Shaik MD DM FNB
Fellow Interventional Cardiologist
Department of Cardiology
Apollo Hospital, Jubilee Hills
Hyderabad, Telangana, India

Shanmugam K MD DM (Cardiology)
Assistant Professor
Department of Cardiology
Sri Jayadeva Institute of Cardiovascular Sciences and Research
Bengaluru, Karnataka, India

Shanmugasundaram S MD DM
Cardiologist
Billroth Hospital
Chennai, Tamil Nadu, India

Shantanu P Sengupta MD DNB PhD FACC FASE
Heart Failure Specialist
Director, Sengupta Hospital and Research Institute
Nagpur, Maharashtra, India

Shashank C MD DM
Consultant
Apollo Hospital
Visakhapatnam, Andhra Pradesh, India

Shibba Takkar Chhabra MD DM
Professor
Department of Cardiology
Hero DMC Heart Institute
Dayanand Medical College and Hospital
Ludhiana, Punjab, India

Shibsankar Sarkar MD
Postdoctoral Trainee
Department of Cardiology
RG Kar Medical College and Hospital
Kolkata, West Bengal, India

Shifas Babu M MD DM DNB MNAMS
Senior Consultant Cardiologist
Cardiovascular Centre
Ananthapuri Hospitals and Research Institute
Thiruvananthapuram, Kerala, India

Shirisha Reddy Kommareddy MD DrNB (Cardiology)
Junior Consultant Cardiologist
KIMS
Hyderabad, Telangana, India

Shirley Adivi MD
Research Student, Department of Cardiology, West Virginia University School of Medicine
Morgantown, WV, USA

Shishu Shankar Mishra MD FAIMS MCAM DoCM FCCP FIAE FICC FCSI
Professor and Director
SOA University, Bhubaneswar
Professor and Director
Dreams Health Sciences and Padmini Care Hospital
Director Med-n-Heart Clinic
Cuttack, Odisha, India

Shivangi Tiwari MBBS
Resident Doctor Final Year (Medicine)
Department of Medicine
RD Gardi Medical College
Ujjain, Madhya Pradesh, India

Shunmuga Sundaram Ponnusamy MD DM CEPS
Associate Professor
Department of Cardiology
Velammal Medical College Hospital and Research Institute
Madurai, Tamil Nadu, India

Shyam Prasad Sahoo MBBS
Medical Officer, SRM Medical College Hospital and Research Centre
Chennai, Tamil Nadu, India

Sibaram Panda MD (Medicine) DM (Cardiology)
Assistant Professor
Department of Cardiology
Veer Surendra Sai Institute of Medical Science and Research
Burla Sambalpur, Odisha, India

Siddhartha Mani MD DM FSCAI
Consultant
Department of Adult Cardiology
RN Tagore Hospital
Kolkata, West Bengal, India

Siddharth Bajaj MD DM
Consultant Cardiologist
Apollo Hospital, Jubillee Hills
Hyderabad, Telangana, India

Siddharth Chinta MD
Research Fellow
Division of Cardiac Imaging/Cardiology
Tufts Medical Center
Boston, USA

Siddhant Gupta MBBS
Resident Doctor Final Year (Medicine)
Department of Medicine
RD Gardi Medical College
Ujjain, Madhya Pradesh, India

Siddarth Varshney MD DM
Associate Consultant
Division of Interventional Cardiology
Medanta – The Medicity
Gurugram, Haryana, India

S Kumaran MD (General Medicine) DCH DM (Cardiology)
Associate Professor
Department of Cardiology
Institute of Child Health and Hospital for Children, Egmore,
Chennai, Tamil Nadu, India

Smit Shrivastava MD PGDHHM DM (Cardiology) FACC FSCAI FESC FICP FIMSA FICN FISE
Professor and Head
Advance Cardiac Institute
Pt JNM Medical College and Dr BRAM Hospital
Raipur, Chhattisgarh, India

Sneha Karekar MD (Medicine) DrNB
Cardiology Resident, Manipal Hospital
Bengaluru, Karnataka, India

SN Narasingan MD FRCP (Edinburgh and Glasgow) FACP FICP FCCP (USA)
Managing Director
SNN Specialities Clinic and SNN Diagnostic Centre
Chennai, Tamil Nadu, India
Vice Chairman, Lipid Association of India
Vice President, World Hypertension League

Soma Sen MD FACC
Consultant Cardiologist and Director of Nuclear Imaging
Park Nicollet Health Partners Care Group and Methodist Hospital
Bloomington, MN, USA

Sonu Abraham MD
Clinical and Research Fellow
Cardio-Oncology Program
Division of Cardiovascular Medicine
Department of Medicine
Lahey Hospital and Medical Center
Beth Israel Lahey Health
Burlington, MA, USA

Soumen Devidutta MD DM PDF
Consultant Cardiologist and Electrophysiologist
Apollo Hospitals
Hyderabad, Telangana, India

Soumen Prasad Behera MD DM (Cardiology)
Consultant Cardiologist
Hitech Medical College and Hospital
Rourkela, Odisha, India

Sourabh Agstam MD DM
Assistant Professor
Department of Cardiology
All India Institute of Medical Sciences
New Delhi, India

Sourav Das MD
PDT Cardiology
Medica Superspecialty Hospital
Kolkata, West Bengal, India

Sradhananda Rout MD DM (Cardiology)
Senior Resident
SCB Medical College and Hospital
Cuttack, Odisha, India

Sreenivas Kumar A MD DM FACC
Senior Consultant Cardiologist and Director
Department of Cardiology and Clinical Research
Apollo Hospital, Jubilee Hills
Hyderabad, Telangana, India

Sridhar Kasturi MD DM FACC FESC FSCAI FICC
Head
Department of Cardiology and Cardiothoracic Surgery
KIMS – Sunshine Hospitals
Secunderabad, Telangana, India

Srijani Thannir MBBS
Research Fellow
Division of Cardiology
University of Alabama
Birmingham, AL, USA

Srina Ray MBBS (Cal)
Clinical Assistant
Heart Clinic
Kolkata, West Bengal, India

Srinivasa Rao Malladi MD (General Medicine) DM (Cardiology) DNB (Cardiology)
Professor
Department of Cardiology
Andhra Medical College/King George Hospital
Visakhapatnam, Andhra Pradesh, India

Srinivas Kudva MD (Medicine) DNB (Cardiology)
Consultant Cardiologist
Healing Hearts
Mumbai, Maharashtra, India

Srinivas Ramaka MD DM FIAE FACC FAHA FCSI
Honorary Professor IMA
Consultant Cardiologist
Srinivasa Heart Centre
Chairman and Managing Trustee
Srinivasa Heart Foundation
Warangal, Telangana, India

SR Sharath Shanmugam MD (General Medicine)
PG in DM Cardiology
Sri Ramachandra Medical College
Chennai, Tamil Nadu, India

SS Binu MD (Medicine) DNB (Medicine) DM (Cardiology) FSCAI FESC
Senior Consultant Cardiologist
Sree Gokulam Medical College and Research Foundation
Thiruvananthapuram, Kerala, India

SS Iyengar DM (Cardiology)
Consultant Cardiologist
Manipal Hospital
Bengaluru, Karnataka, India

S Sunilkumar MD DM (Cardiology)
Professor and Head
Department of Cardiology
JSSMC, JSSAHER
Mysuru, Karnataka, India

Subasis Dash DNB (Medicine) DNB (Cardiology) MNAMS
Consultant Cardiologist
Apollo Hospitals
Bhubaneswar, Odisha, India

Subhasish Singh MD DM
Associate Professor
Division of Cardiology
MKCG Medical College
Berhampur, Odisha, India

Subhasis Roy Chowdhury MD DM
Consultant Interventional Cardiologist
Department of Cardiology
AMRI Hospital, Salt Lake
Kolkata, West Bengal, India

Subroto Mandal MD DM DC FACC FICC FCPCI FSCAI
Professor and Head
Department of Cardiology
Director, Cath Lab
Ubuntu Heart and Super Specialty Hospital
Bhopal, Madhya Pradesh, India

Sudhir Chandra Sinha MD DM FACC
Senior Consultant Cardiologist
Star Pinnacle Heart Centre
Visakhapatnam, Andhra Pradesh, India

Sudhir Lakamsani MD (General Medicine) DrNB (Cardiology)
Cardiology Registrar
Department of Cardiology
Apollo Main Hospital
Chennai, Tamil Nadu, India

Suganthi Jaganathan BDS MPH PhD (Pursuing)
Senior Research Associate
Centre for Health Analytics Research and Trends (CHART)
Trivedi School of Biosciences, Ashoka University
Institute of Environmental Medicine, Karolinska Institute
Stockholm, Sweden
Centre for Chronic Disease Control
New Delhi, India

Suman Bhandari MD DM FACC FESC FSCAI FIMSA
Director
Department of Cardiology
Fortis Escorts Heart Institute
New Delhi, India

Sumanth Khadke MD
Research Fellow
Cardio-Oncology Program
Division of Cardiovascular Medicine
Department of Medicine
Lahey Hospital and Medical Center
Beth Israel Lahey Health
Burlington, MA, USA

Sunandan Sikdar MD DM FACC
Consultant
Department of Cardiology
Narayana Multispeciality Hospital
Kolkata, West Bengal, India

Sundar Chidambaram MD DNB DM FNB
Senior Consultant Interventional Cardiologist
Kauvery Hospital
Chennai, Tamil Nadu, India

Sunil Kumar Sharma MD (Medicine) DM (Cardiology) FACC
Professor and Head
Department of Cardiology
Veer Surendra Sai Institute of Medical Science and Research
Burla Sambalpur, Odisha, India

Sunil Modi MD DM FACC FICC FCSI
Senior Consultant
Department of Cardiology
Indraprastha Apollo Hospital
New Delhi, India

Surendra Poonia DM (Cardiology)
Senior Consultant Interventional Cardiology
Apex Hospital
Bikaner, Rajasthan
Consultant Interventional Cardiologist
Holy Family Hospital
Mumbai, Maharashtra, India

Suresh V Patted MD DM FACC FCSI FAPSIC
Professor and Head
Department of Cardiology
JN Medical College, KAHER
Belgavi, Karnataka, India

Sushant Mishra MD DM (Cardiology)
Consultant Cardiology
Meditrina Hospitals
Gurugram, Haryana, India

Suvro Banerjee MD MRCP (UK) FRCP (London) FRCP (Edinburgh) FCSI FICC FSCAI FESC FACC
Senior Consultant Cardiologist
Apollo Multispeciality Hospitals
Kolkata, West Bengal, India

Swasthi S Kumar MD
Senior Resident, Department of Cardiology, SCTIMST
Thiruvananthapuram, Kerala, India

Swati Singh MD DM (Cardiology)
Consultant Cardiology
Meditrina Hospitals
Gurugram, Haryana, India

Syed Imamuddin MD DM FACC FESC FSCAI FCSI
Professor and Head
Department of Cardiology
Osmania Medical College/Osmania General Hospital
Director
Heart Beat
Hyderabad, Telangana, India

Tanmay Mukhopadhyay MD DM (Cardiology) FESC FSCAI
Associate Professor
Department of Cardiology
Burdwan Medical College and Hospital
Burdwan, West Bengal, India

Tejas M Patel MD DM FCSI FACC FESC FSCAI
Chairman and Chief Interventional Cardiologist
Apex Heart Institute
Ahmedabad, Gujarat, India

T Govindan Unni MD DM
Professor
Department of Cardiology
Jubilee Mission Medical College and Research Institute
Thrissur, Kerala, India

Thajfeer UM MD
Senior Resident
Department of Cardiology
GMC Kannur, Hrudayalaya
Kannur, Kerala, India

Thomas Alexander MD DM
Head of Cardiology
Kovai Medical Center and Hospital
Coimbatore, Tamil Nadu, India

Thomas F Lüscher MD FRCP FESC
Director of Research, Education and Development
Royal Brompton and Harefield Clinical Group,
Guy's and St Thomas' NHS Foundation Trust
Professor of Cardiology
Imperial College and King's College London
London, United Kingdom

Thomas Xavier Paulsingh JS DM FNB (Interventional Cardiology)
Associate Consultant and Interventional Cardiologist
Meenakshi Mission Hospital and Research Centre
Madurai, Tamil Nadu, India

Tiny Nair MD DM FACC FRCP
Head, Department of Cardiology
PRS Hospital
Thiruvananthapuram, Kerala, India

Trinath K Mishra MD DM
Professor, Division of Cardiology
MKCG Medical College
Berhampur, Odisha, India

Tripti Deb MD DNB
Senior Consultant Cardiologist
Apollo Health City, Jubilee Hills
Hyderabad, Telangana, India

U Ankur B Pharma M Pharma Toxicology
Senior Safety Scientist, Project Coordinator, Safety Science Specialist
Department of Pharmacology and Toxicology
Durham College
Oshawa, Canada

Umesh C Samal MD FACC FIACM FICC FIAE FISE FISC FAPVS FEAC
Former Professor of Cardiology and Head
Department of Medicine
Patna Medical College
Patna, Bihar, India

V Amuthan MD DM FACC FASE FEACVI FCSI FIAE
Emeritus Professor of Cardiology
The Tamil Nadu Dr MGR Medical University
Formerly Professor and Head
Department of Cardiology
Madurai Medical College
Director
4D Echo Lab, Jeyalakshmi Heart Center
Senior Interventional Cardiologist
Vadamalayan Hospital
Madurai, Tamil Nadu, India

Vaibhav Bandil MD (Medicine) DrNB (Cardiology)
Associate Consultant
Department of Cardiology
Fortis Escorts Heart Institute
New Delhi, India

Vardhini Vijaykumar BDS MDS
Hyderabad, Telangana, India

Varsha Kiron MD DM (Cardiology) DNB (Cardiology) FSCAI FESCC
Consultant Cardiologist
Apollo Health City
Hyderabad, Telangana, India

Varun Bhatia MD DM
Consultant – Structural Heart Interventions
Department of Cardiology
Aster Medicity Hospital
Kochi, Kerala, India

Varun Gupta MD (Thoracic Surgery)
Resident – Thoracic Surgery
Lungenklinik Hemer
Hemer, Germany

Varun Marimuthu MD DM
Assistant Professor
Department of Cardiology
Sri Jayadeva Institute of Cardiovascular Sciences and Research
Bengaluru, Karnataka, India

Vasudeva Murthy Sindgi M Pharm PhD
Principal and Professor
Department of Phamacology
Jayamukhi College of Pharmacy
Narsampet, Telangana, India

Vemuri S Murthy MD MS FAHA FICS
Associate Professor (Adjunct)
Department of Emergency Medicine
University of Illinois College of Medicine
Chicago, IL, USA

Venkata RS Subrahmanya Sarma MD DM
Consultant Cardiologist
Aayush Hospitals
Vijayawada and Eluru
Andhra Pradesh, India

Venkatesh CR MD (Medicine)
Assistant Professor
Department of Medicine
JSSMC, JSSAHER,
Mysuru, Karnataka, India

Vidyut Jain MD FSCAI FACC FESC
Consultant Cardiologist
Choithram Hospital
Indore, Madhya Pradesh, India

Vigyan Vijay Bang MD FACC
Interventional and Structural Cardiologist
Freeman Heart and Vascular Institute
Joplin, MO, USA

Vijay Garg MD FIAE FICP FCSI FICA (USA) FISE FACC (USA) FACP (USA) FIMSA FISC FESC (EUROPE)
Professor, Department of Medicine
RD Gardi Medical College
Ujjain, Madhya Pradesh, India

Vijayadithyan Jaganathan MD
Research Fellow, Division of Cardiology
University of Alabama
Birmingham, AL, USA

Vijayakumar Subban MD DM FNB
Senior Consultant
Interventional Cardiologist
Clinical Lead – Cardiac Imaging Services
Apollo Hospitals
Chennai, Tamil Nadu, India

Vijayanand B Metgudmath MD DNB (Cardiology)
Associate Professor
Department of Cardiology
JN Medical College, KAHER
Belgavi, Karnataka, India

Vijay Bang MD DM FCSI FESC FSCAI FACC
Senior Interventional Cardiologist
Lilavati Hospital and Research Center
Honorable Professor and Head
Grant Medical College and
Sir JJ Group of Hospitals (Former)
Mumbai, Maharashtra, India

Vijay Iyer MD PhD FACC FSCAI
Chief
Division of Cardiovascular Medicine
Department of Medicine
Jacobs School of Medicine and Biomedical Sciences
University at Buffalo
Buffalo, NY, USA

Vijay Kumar MD DNB (Cardiology)
Director, Interventional Cardiology
Fortis Escorts Heart Institute
New Delhi, India

Vijaykumar JR MD DM DNB (Cardiology)
Associate Professor
Department of Cardiology
Sri Jayadeva Institute of Cardiovascular Sciences and Research
Bengaluru, Karnataka, India

Vikas Agrawal MD DNB (Cardiology)
Professor
Department of Cardiology
Institute of Medical Sciences
Banaras Hindu University
Varanasi, Uttar Pradesh, India

Vinay Wasan
Business Major
James Madison University
Harrisonburg, VA, USA

Vineet Bhatia MD DM DNB (Cardiology) MNAMS
Director
Department of Cardiac Sciences
Max Super Specialty Hospital
Patparganj, New Delhi, India

Vishal Batra MD DM (Cardiology)
Associate Professor
Department of Cardiology
GB Pant Institute of Postgraduate Medical Education and Research
New Delhi, India

Vishal Rastogi MD DM (Cardiology)
Director Interventional Cardiology
Fortis Escorts Heart Institute
New Delhi, India

Vitull K Gupta MD (Medicine) FICP FCSI FACP FIACM
Health and Human Rights Activist
Consultant, Kishori Ram Hospital and Diabetes Care Centre
Honorary Teaching Faculty
All India Institute of Medical Sciences (AIIMS)
Bathinda, Punjab, India

Viveka Kumar MD DM FSCAI FACC FECS FAPSIC FRCP (Edinburgh)
Principal Director and Chief of Cath Labs
Max Super Specialty Hospital
Saket, New Delhi, India

Vivekanand S Gajapati MD DM
Consultant Cardiologist
SDM Naryana Heart Centre
Dharwad, Karnataka, India

Vivek Gupta MD DM FACC FESC FSCAI FAPSIC FEAPCI FIEIC FCSI FICC FIC (France)
Senior Interventional Cardiologist
Indraprastha Apollo Hospitals
New Delhi, India
Scientific Course Chairman, Indo European Course on Revascularization (IECR)

V Jacob Jose MD DM (Cardiology) FACC FASE FCCP MS
Consultant Cardiologist
Naruvi Hospitals
Vellore, Tamil Nadu, India

VK Bahl MD DM (Cardiology)
Director, Cardiac Sciences
MS Ramaiah Medical College
Bengaluru, Karnataka, India

VS Ramchandra MD DM FACC
Electrophysiologist
Sri Sri Holistic Hospitals
Hyderabad, Telangana, India

V Suryaprakasa Rao MD DM FACC FSCAI
Senior Interventional Cardiologist
Care Hospitals
Hyderabad, Telangana, India

W Sunil MD DNB (Cardiology)
Associate Professor
Department of Cardiology
Super Speciality Hospital, GMC
Nagpur, Maharashtra, India

Yasar Satar MD
Fellow in Cardiovascular Disease
Department of Cardiology
West Virginia University School of Medicine
Morgantown, WV, USA

Yashaswi Koguru MBBS
Observer, Clinical Electrophysiology
University of Alabama
Birmingham, Alabama, USA

Y Chandrashekhar MD FACC
Professor, Department of Medicine
University of Minnesota/VAMC
Minneapolis, MN, USA

Yogesh Kolamkar MD DrNB (Cardiology)
Consultant Interventional Cardiologist
Swasthyam Superspeciality Hospital
Nagpur, Maharashtra, India

Yogesh Om Sharma MD DM
Consultant Cardiologist
Artemis Hospital
Gurugram, Haryana, India

Yogesh Varma MD DM (CMCH Vellore)
Former Professor and Head
Director Cardiac Science Centre
Department of Cardiology
Dean, Gandhi Medical College
Bhopal, Madhya Pradesh, India

Zoofi Shan MBBS
Resident, Department of Cardiology
Dayanand Medical College and Hospital
Unit Hero DMC Heart Institute
Ludhiana, Punjab, India

FOREWORD

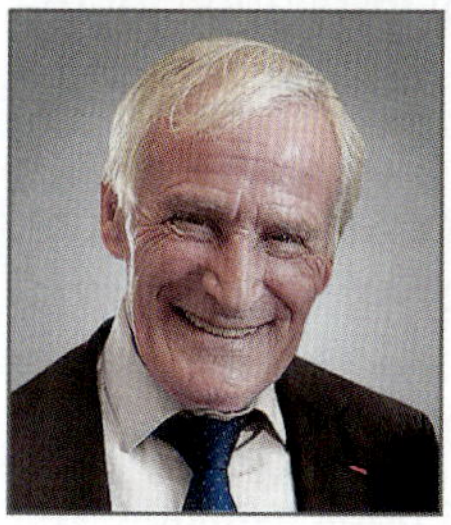

Alain Cribier MD
Emeritus Professor of Medicine
Past-Chief of the Department of Cardiology
Consultant for the Rouen Normandy Medical Training Center
Charles Nicolle Hospital, University of Rouen, France

It is an honor and a pleasure for me to preface this 2023 edition of the CSI Update Book. This is an outstanding edition, covering in no less than 2 volumes and 217 chapters the current state and most advanced aspects of general cardiology and interventional cardiology worldwide and particularly in India.

In over 20 years, accelerating technological, therapeutic, and organizational advances have changed the face of cardiology. Thanks to scientific discoveries in recent years, new gains in life expectancy can be achieved. Decisive victories have been won in cases of myocardial infarction, stroke, rhythm disorders, valvular diseases, and heart failure. Nevertheless, it should be remembered that cardiovascular disease (CVD) remains the world's leading cause of mortality and is set to grow exponentially as the population ages. Over the past 10 years, cardiovascular deaths have soared worldwide, rising from 12.1 million in 1990 to 29.5 million in 2021, according to the report of the World Heart Association, with 4 out of 5 deaths occurring in low- or mid-income countries. These are also the countries where the coronavirus disease 2019 (COVID-19) has had the most devastating impact.

The challenges of the future must include progresses in primary and secondary prevention methods and the fight against risk factors, such as smoking, alcohol, sedentary lifestyle, hyperlipidemia, diabetes, and high blood pressure, and adapt them to the considerable disparity of medical and social situations around the world. In countries with limited economic resources the challenge is particularly high due to the often-insurmountable difficulties of acceding to preventive and therapeutic measures.

These subjects are superbly covered in the first volume of the book in which the current state of prevention and treatment of CVD in India is fully documented.

The second volume of the book is dedicated to "Interventional Cardiology" which includes a special overview of the situation in India. The history of interventional medicine is short with an explosion of innovative treatments emerging at the end of the 20th century and dramatically expanding in the 21st century. For the newer generation of interventional specialists, with the armamentarium of these strategies at their fingertips, it is intellectually impossible to imagine what it was like treating CVD less than 50 years ago. Conceptually described by Dotter and Judkins in 1964, the crucial milestone has been the first coronary angioplasty performed by Andreas Gruentzig in September 1977 (who initiated at the same time the specialty of "interventional cardiology"), a great source of inspiration for many others. Coronary stent implantation was launched 10 years later by Jacques Puel in France who performed the first case. This technique has been dramatically expanding to become a routine daily procedure in the whole world and particularly in India.

"Structural Heart diseases" covers all noncoronary heart diseases and their dedicated interventional techniques and valve replacement and repair that have been the fastest developing areas. Following the footsteps of trans-catheter treatment of congenital pulmonic (1979) and aortic valvular stenosis (1983), mitral valvuloplasty (1984) and aortic valvuloplasty in adults by our group (1985), and then pulmonic valve replacement in degenerated conduits (2000), the technique of transcatheter aortic valve implantation (TAVI) for the transcatheter treatment of degenerative aortic stenosis, initiated by us after 15 years of research, emerged in 2002 to profoundly alter the landscape of cardiovascular medicine. Helene Eltchaninoff and I have the pleasure of describing the amazing odyssey of TAVI development in one of the chapters of this volume. Over the last 20 years, this breakthrough lifesaving procedure has been constantly improved and used in about 3 million of patients worldwide, with expanding indications. Since 2011, the year of the first case performed in India, the number of cases has been steadily but rather slowly increasing due to several obstacles including high cost and lack of coverage by insurance companies. However, thousands of patients have benefited from TAVI in the country to date. TAVI, in turn, became a strong source of inspiration for the development of new interventional techniques aimed at treating other valvular diseases, such as mitral and tricuspid insufficiency by repairing or replacing the diseased valve.

The most recent technical and procedural advances, the issues of patient's selection, procedural techniques, prevention and treatment of complications, and the latest scientific results obtained in all aspects of interventional cardiology are fully overviewed in the book.

The sum of information provided in this edition of the CSI Update Book 2023 is a real achievement, thanks to the Editor and the outstanding contribution of all expert authors. There is no doubt that having this book available will immensely benefit anyone working in the field of healthcare in India and far beyond.

PREFACE

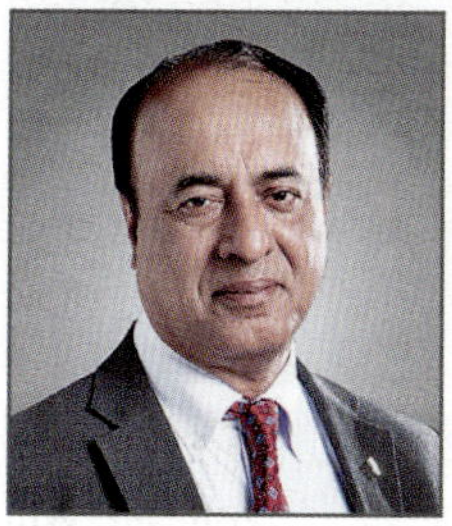

Pratap Chandra Rath MD DM FICC FESC FACC FRCP (London) FRCP (Edinburgh)
Senior Consultant Cardiologist and HOD
Department of Cardiology
Apollo Hospital, Jubilee Hills
Hyderabad, Telangana
Apollo Hospital
Bhubaneshwar, Odisha, India

As a President Elect of the Cardiology Society of India (CSI), it is my immense pleasure and privilege to introduce the book *Cardiology Update 2023* which aims to provide a comprehensive and up-to-date overview of the entire cardiology field. Our goal is to produce a clinically oriented book including all the major cardiovascular advances.

Over the years, interventional and preventive cardiology has revolutionized the management of cardiovascular diseases, offering different prevention strategies, new medical management guidelines, and minimally invasive procedures that have transformed the lives of countless patients. The development of wearable devices, smartphone applications, and telemedicine platforms has made remote monitoring and management of cardiovascular conditions a reality. Patients can now actively participate in their own care. From the early days of balloon angioplasty to the more recent advancements in percutaneous coronary interventions, the field has witnessed remarkable progress. There has been an explosion of structural interventions such as transcatheter aortic valve replacement (TAVR), transcatheter mitral valve replacement (TMVR), MitraClip, and left atrial appendage (LAA) occluder in the last decade. These recent trends are reflected in the book and are covered in great detail.

This book serves as a valuable resource for both aspiring and experienced interventional cardiologists, clinical cardiologists, and other healthcare professionals. The book is divided into sections that deal with specific themes involving various topics.

The chapters in this book are written by pioneers in the field who have dedicated their careers to advancing the practice of cardiology. We have recruited young cardiologists as authors of many key topics with an eye on the future. Each chapter provides a concise yet comprehensive overview of a specific aspect of interventional cardiology, supported by evidence-based research and clinical experience. We hope that this edition of *Cardiology Update 2023* will provide guidance and education to cardiologists of various disciplines and primarily students. Please enjoy reading the update and adopt this as a resource in your daily practice.

CONTENTS

VOLUME 1

SECTION 1: ARTIFICIAL INTELLIGENCE IN CARDIOLOGY

SECTION 2: GENERAL CARDIOLOGY

SECTION 4: HYPERTENSION

SECTION 6: LIPIDS

SECTION 8: CHRONIC CORONARY SYNDROMES

SECTION 9: CARDIOMYOPATHY

SECTION 10: CARDIO DIABETES

SECTION 11: CARDIO-OBSTETRICS

SECTION 12: CARDIO-ONCOLOGY

SECTION 13: ECHOCARDIOGRAPHY

SECTION 18: MISCELLANEOUS

VOLUME 2

SECTION 19: CORONARY INTERVENTION

SECTION 20: STRUCTURAL INTERVENTION

Scan the QR code to access references of all the chapters.

SECTION

1

Artificial Intelligence in Cardiology

CHAPTER

1

Artificial Intelligence and Machine Learning in Cardiovascular Disease

Thomas F Lüscher, Florian A Wenzl

ABSTRACT

Intelligence, a key characteristic of humans, has enabled them to survive and develop tools, weapons, agriculture, and modern technology. However, today's world is flooded with data, making computers increasingly useful. Artificial intelligence (AI) and machine learning (ML) have become useful tools in everyday life, technology, and medicine. This chapter reviews AI/ML applications in diagnostics, prognostication, and treatment in cardiovascular medicine.

Keywords: Artificial intelligence, machine learning, deep learning, precision medicine, personalized care.

INTRODUCTION

Intelligence is a characteristic of humans *(homo sapiens sapiens)*, which distinguishes our species from others in nature. Human intelligence, together with the socialization in groups, allowed this species to survive in spite of an overall fragile physical constitution. Indeed, intelligent thinking allowed humankind to use tools and weapons, develop agriculture, and eventually, modern technology, and medicine.

However, today's world is flooded by a huge amount of data that are difficult for the human brain to comprehend or analyze effectively. Therefore, computers are now increasingly used to handle more and more data points, seemingly without an upper limit. As conventional basic analyses alone proved inefficient, within the last decades, specific algorithms were developed that went beyond traditional statistics. Importantly, these models are able to learn while analyzing increasing numbers of parameters. As such, artificial intelligence (AI) and machine learning (ML) have developed into useful tools in many aspects of everyday life, technology, and medicine. This chapter reviews current AI/ML applications and their utility as well as reliability in diagnostics, prognostication, and treatment in cardiovascular medicine.

DATA REVOLUTION

Over the last decades, an ever-increasing amount of patient data has been collected in medicine, and cardiology in particular. It started in the 1950s with only 14,000 individuals living in Framingham, a suburb of Boston, where data on cardiovascular risk factors, such as age, blood pressure, cholesterol, diabetes, and the like were systematically recorded to investigate their role in disease development. Over time, the number and size of such cohorts have increased dramatically, reaching half a million subjects in the United Kingdom (UK) biobank and even higher numbers in several other cohorts. As a consequence, epidemiology and data science have gained increasing importance in medicine and developed into independent disciplines dedicated to the investigation of demographics, health status, and outcomes of huge populations. While initially, mainly demographics and basic clinical parameters, as well as the electrocardiogram (ECG) and some blood values have been collected in cardiovascular registries, later, imaging findings of different modalities have been included, particularly echocardiography and vascular ultrasound, followed by nuclear scans, computer tomography (CT), and magnetic resonance imaging (MRI). These enormous datasets required new analytical tools data and helped the implementation of computer algorithms for diagnostication, outcome prediction, and patient management in clinical practice.[1]

More recently, the analysis of genes and epigenetic modifications yielded huge datasets containing the information of the whole genome and epigenome, respectively. These developments in molecular biology have shed more light on the complex relationship between genotype and phenotype and have shown that phenotypes are not only dependent on the deoxyribonucleic acid (DNA) sequence but also on environmental factors. Thus, the complexity of genes and genetics, environmental factors, and demographics make personalized medicine a real challenge and require novel data analysis tools, as have been provided by AI/ML.

MAJOR APPLICATIONS OF ARTIFICIAL INTELLIGENCE/MACHINE LEARNING

Based on the above, AI/ML has proved helpful in analyzing biomedical, imaging, and clinical data, as well as in the prediction of outcomes in certain patient populations. Indeed, thanks to the sheer unlimited number of parameters that can be simultaneously analyzed, AI/ML is able to provide efficient means to much more specific or much more personalized diagnostics, predictions, and/or treatment recommendations.

Echocardiography

Echocardiography is the working horse of cardiology diagnostics as it can be applied in almost every patient, is available in any hospital, and it provides important information on cardiac structure and function. Over the years, automatic echocardiographic assessment of left ventricular ejection fraction (LVEF) using AI/ML has been developed[2] and, in several studies, has shown to be noninferior to experienced sonographers.[3] The advantages of this automated image analysis are its speed, unbiased approach, and impressive precision **(Figs. 1A and B)**. Obviously, the algorithm relies heavily on the image quality of the echo exam being insufficient but it can be improved using contrast medium. Furthermore, robotic arms are in development that automatically search for the optimal probe position to enhance image quality, thereby further improving AI/ML-guided echocardiography. As such, the number of patients who can be examined in a given time can be substantially increased and eventually the reproducibility of the exams improved.

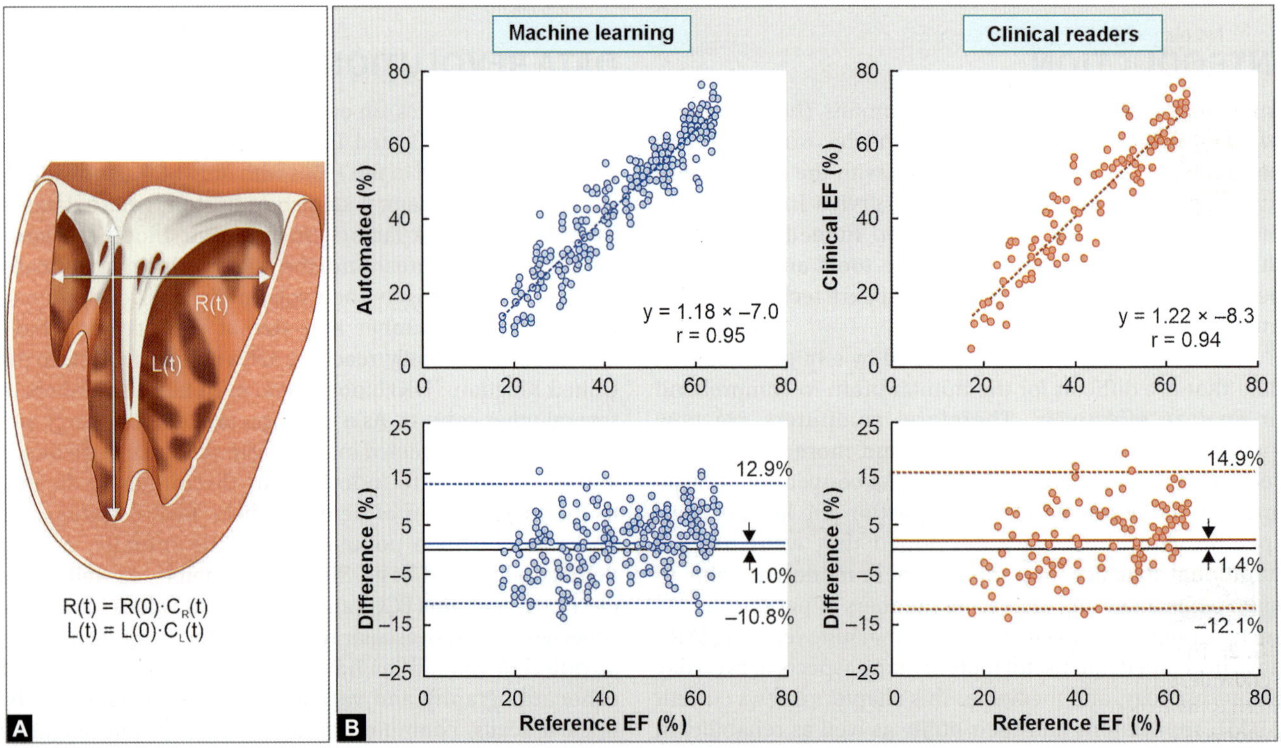

FIGS. 1A AND B: Schematic representation of the left ventricle with its longitudinal and radial dimensions L and R, which change over time from its initial values at time 0, namely L(0) and R(0) according to dimensionless, time-dependent contraction coefficients $C_L(t)$ and $C_R(t)$, which can be used to calculate ejection fraction (EF) (A). Agreement between the machine learning-based automated EF (B) measurements (B left), side-by-side with the clinical measurements (B right) against reference values obtained by averaging measurements by a panel of three experts: linear regression (B top) and Bland–Altman analysis (B bottom).

Computer Tomography

Computer tomography is a cross-sectional imaging modality with high resolution and excellent contour detection, allowing for three-dimensional (3D) reconstruction of the acquired images. As the images are standing frames, CT lends itself particularly well to automated analysis with or without the help of AI/ML.

In particular, in CT coronary angiography, AI/ML algorithms have made a huge impact. Specifically, the analysis of fat attenuation in the perivascular area has provided new insights into the inflammatory status of plaques within the coronary circulation. Indeed, inflamed atherosclerotic plaques, by releasing cytokines and chemokines, initiate the digestion of fat cells surrounding the adventitia of the coronary vascular wall. This can be detected with CT, as the so-called fat attenuation index (FAI; **Fig. 2**).[3,4] Of note, this analysis goes far beyond what any radiologist can see with naked eye (*"see what you can't see"*) and provides, thanks to AI models developed at the University of Oxford by Charalambos Antoniades and his team, impressive outcome predictions that sets the basis for much more granular assessments and personalized management in primary and secondary prevention.

Cardiac Magnetic Resonance Imaging

Cardiac MRI is a highly complex imaging procedure requiring data based on magnet-induced changes in the atomic structure of various tissues. In cardiology, obviously, function and structure as well as perfusion of the heart muscle, cardiac chambers, and valves can be obtained. Cardiac contrast perfusion MRI is able to assess not only cardiac volumes and wall thicknesses with high precision, but also myocardial texture, coronary perfusion, and the presence or absence of myocardial ischemia. Late gadolinium enhancement (LGE) allows for precise detection and quantification of myocardial scars and coupled with T2 sequences and novel analysis software for high-resolution imaging of myocardial pathologies.

In the past, the quantitative analysis of MRI scans was rather tedious and time consuming; however, with AI/ML algorithms, volumes, and volume changes, as well as ejection fraction are calculated within seconds, allowing for more rapid and highly standardized image analysis.

Facial Recognition

For any physician, facial recognition of a patient entering surgery, assessment of his body shape and language, position,

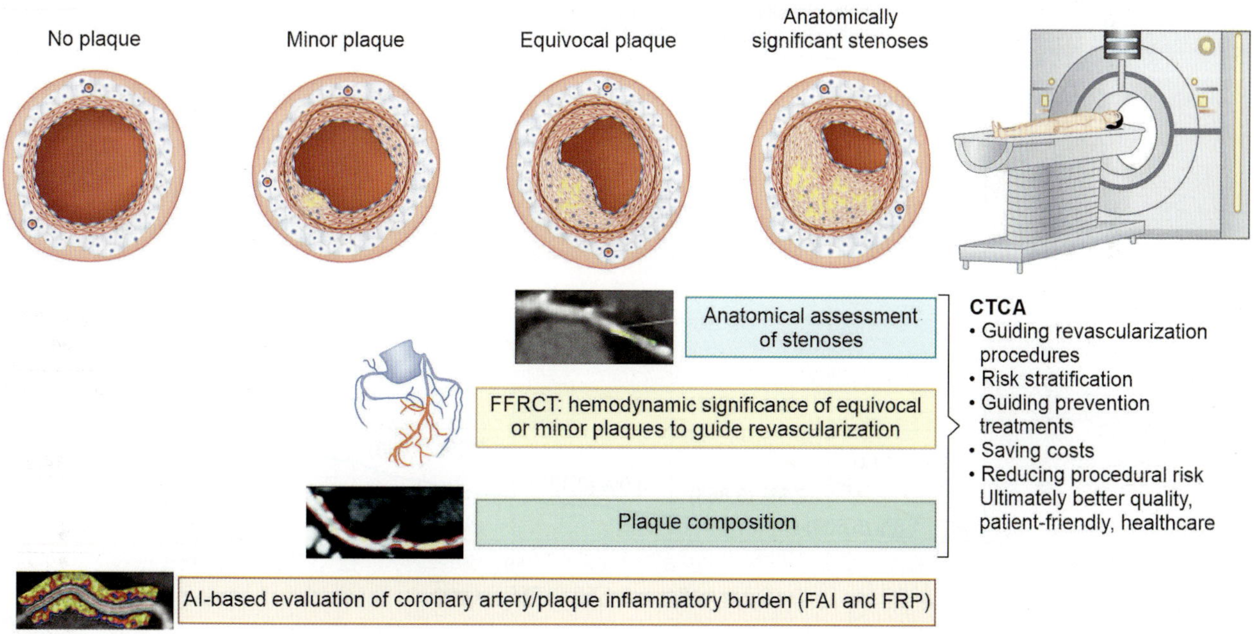

FIG. 2: The CTCA is rapidly becoming a "one-stop shop" for the investigation of patients with stable chest pain. With the rise of CTCA worldwide, distinct groups of patients will be frequently encountered; those with no detectable atherosclerosis, those with atherosclerosis which is minor, those with atherosclerosis of questionable hemodynamic importance, and those with obstructive disease clearly visible on anatomical assessment. FFRCT is likely to be most useful for patient care and resource minimization in the minor and equivocal stenosis groups where FFRCT can be a gatekeeper for invasive procedures. Within the group with no atherosclerosis, only new AI-based technologies, such as FAI, will be useful for adding yield to the CTCA through enhanced risk stratification, and such technologies can also be applied across all stages of disease.[5]

(AI: artificial intelligence; CTCA: computed tomography coronary angiography; FAI: fat attenuation index; FFRCT: fractional flow reserve computed tomography; FRP: fat radiomic profile)

and gait speed within a blink of an eye allows for a first basic, but often highly useful assessment of the overall health status of a given patient. Based on this impression, experienced physicians assess a patient's health status at a glance.

With the development of facial recognition for many other purposes in everyday life, be it at the airport or at other sites, the technology has now also been applied to patient face recognition analysis. Indeed, several studies have shown the feasibility of detecting coronary disease and predicting outcomes based on a single facial photo with reasonable precision **(Fig. 3)**.[6] The algorithm analyses hair structure and density, wrinkles on the forehead, around the eyes, and the chin and derives a comprehensive analysis of the obtained information and relates it to clinical outcomes [e.g., major adverse cardiovascular events (MACE)] derived from large patient populations.[8] Thus, this technology takes advantage of previous studies, showing that visible age-related signs, such as baldness, ear lobe crease, xanthelasma, as well as their combination allows for rather accurate prediction of cardiovascular outcomes beyond traditional risk factors, such as blood pressure, dyslipidemia, or diabetes.

Electrocardiogram

After the stethoscope, the ECG is the oldest cardiac examination tool that is used by physicians worldwide, billions of times every year, in patients with various health conditions. The interpretation of the ECG belongs to the basic skills of most physicians and of cardiologists, in particular. However, the paper version of the ECG hides a large amount of information contained in the electronic vector ECG that can be analyzed further by AI/ML in large cohorts. The Mayo Clinic has pioneered this field and has analyzed more than 650,000 ECGs of patients with various cardiac conditions, allowing for the developed AI/ML algorithms to learn and derive important clinically useful information.[9] For instance, only based on a few heartbeats, the AI/ML algorithm is able to determine whether a patient is male or female, what his or her biological age is, and whether there is evidence of left ventricular dysfunction **(Fig. 4)**,[7] prior episodes of atrial fibrillation (AF), significant aortic stenosis, or amyloid heart disease. Finally, it has been shown that a completely normal ECG practically excludes the presence of a coronavirus disease 2019 (COVID-19) infection and possibly of other acute infectious diseases.

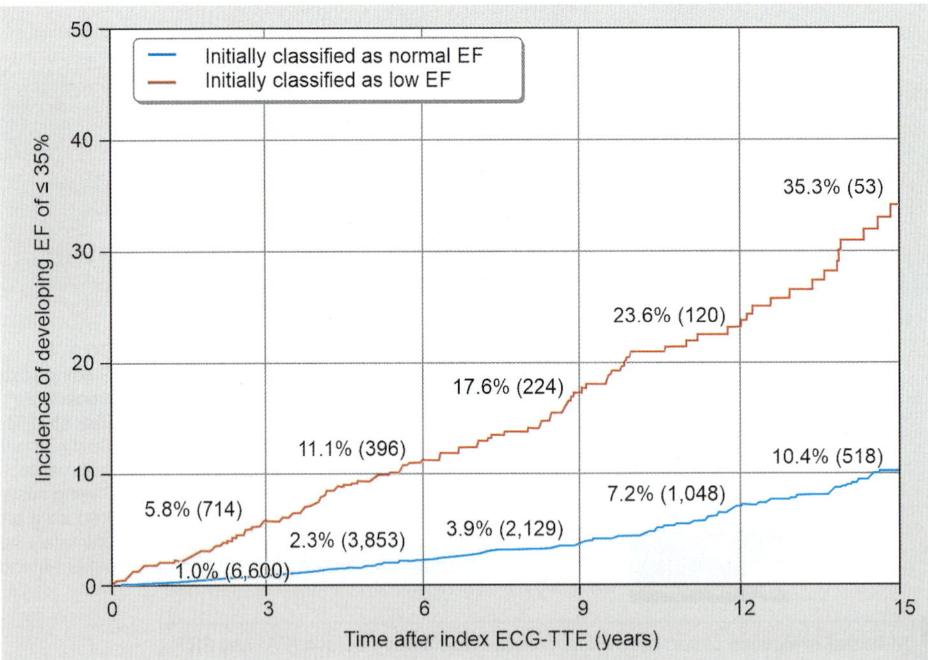

FIG. 3: Long-term incidence of developing an ejection fraction (EF) of ≤35% in patients with an initially normal EF stratified by AI classification. Long-term outcome of patients with an echocardiographic EF of ≥50% at the time of initial classification, stratified by the initial network classification. The ordinate shows the cumulative incidence of developing a low EF (35%) and the abscissa indicates years from the time of index electrocardiogram (ECG)–transthoracic echocardiogram (TTE) evaluation. A fourfold risk of future-low EF was present when the AI algorithm defined the ECG as abnormal [age- and sex-adjusted hazard ratio (HR) 4.1, $p < 0.001$), compared with patients with an echocardiographic normal EF who were classified as having a normal EF by the ECG network. The numbers reported along the cumulative incidence curves reflect the estimated cumulative incidence (and number at risk, in parentheses) for each group at the times indicated along the axis.[7]

Diagnosis of Arrhythmias

The diagnosis of arrhythmias is largely based on the analysis of an ECG at rest, during exercise, or in the electrophysiology lab. AI/ML is also here of utmost importance.[11] Most impressively, an ECG algorithm developed by Paul Friedman and his team is able to detect previous episodes of AF in patients who are in sinus rhythm at the time of the examination.[12] This obviously has important clinical implications in patients presenting with stroke or transient ischemic attacks (TIAs) and may guide physician to consider a nonvitamin K antagonist oral anticoagulant (NOAC).

Speech Analysis

We all intuitively hear differences in the voice pattern of individuals and suspect a cold, mood changes, and alike based on changes in sound of speech. It, therefore, comes as no surprise that AI/ML is able provide information about the health status of a patient based on speech analysis.

Indeed, automated speech analysis technology can identify voice alterations, reflecting heart failure decompensation, thus providing clinical value for outpatient follow-up. Indeed, acute decompensation of heart failure affects both larynx function and respiratory rate, and thereby the quality of speech.[13] Often, so-called mel-frequency cepstral coefficient (MFCC) features, used to model the human voice, as well as glottal features and their combination are used to distinguish acute heart failure speech from healthy speech. In this context, MFCC features yielded even higher classification accuracies than glottal features.

In another study in patients hospitalized for acutely decompensated heart failure, 1,484 discharge recordings were tagged as distinctly different from baseline (i.e., compensated state) in 94% of cases, with distinct differences shown for all five speech measures in 87.5% of cases, thereby providing promising information for early detection of evolving decompensation.[14]

In another prospective study enrolling patients with persistent AF admitted for cardioversion were enrolled and asked to pronounce the vowels "Ahh" and "Ohh" which were then recorded synchronously with an ECG tracing. An algorithm was developed to provide an "AF indicator" for detection of AF from the speech signal **(Fig. 3)**.[10] And indeed, the investigators were able to demonstrate the feasibility and reliability of voice-based identification of AF with acceptable accuracy. The values at sinus rhythm were significantly more homogenous compared to AF. The area under the receiver operating characteristic curve was >0.98 and >0.89 for "Ahh" and "Ohh", respectively.

OUTCOMES PREDICTION

The prediction of outcomes of patients with various cardiac conditions is of utmost importance in guiding management strategies, particularly in secondary prevention, but more and more also in primary prevention. Indeed, many

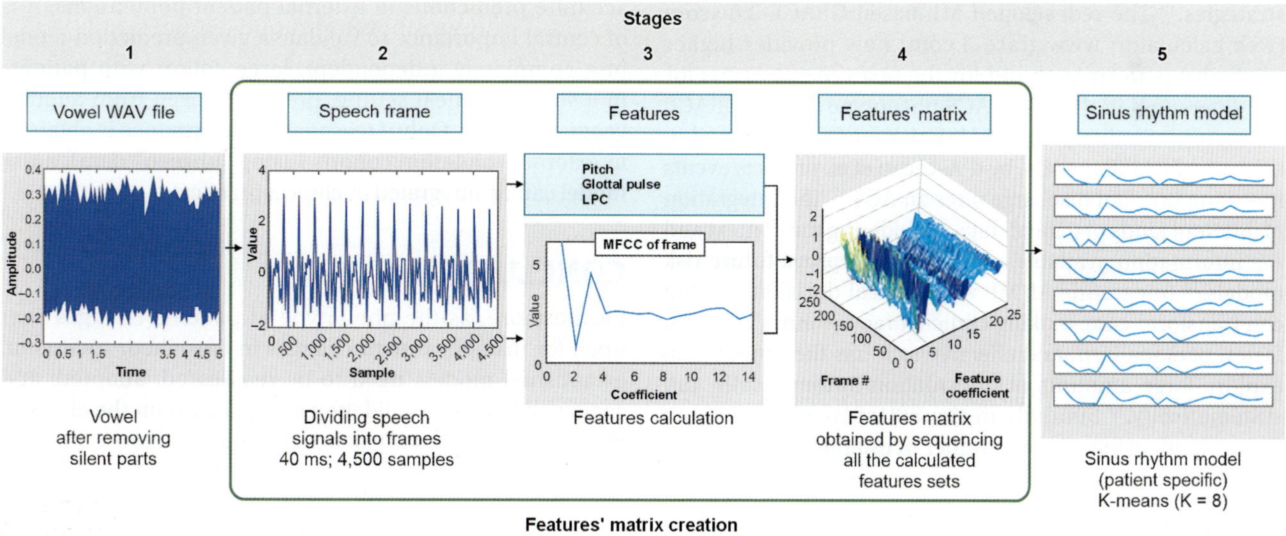

FIG. 4: Creation of the "sinus rhythm model." The patient sinus rhythm-specific model was created in five stages using sinus rhythm recordings.[10]

(LPC: linear prediction coefficient; MFCC: mel-frequency cepstral coefficient)

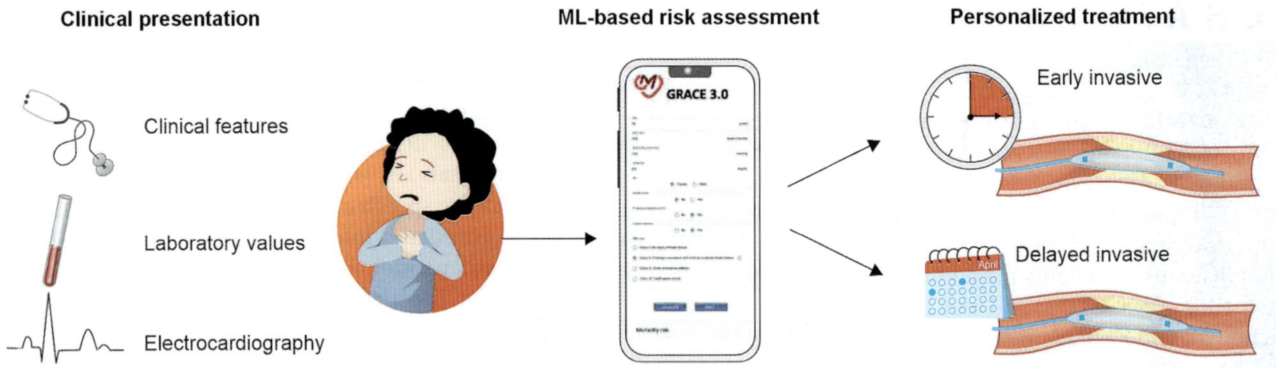

FIG. 5: Machine learning (ML)-based risk assessment for personalized care of patients with non-ST-segment elevation acute coronary syndromes.[16]

established risk models, which are based on conventional statistics fail to account for nonlinear and potential high-dimensional relationships of patient features and provide limited predictive performance. Thus, there is a real unmet medical need to improve risk prediction. Using not just basic demographics and a few CV risk factors, but also a comprehensive set of parameters derived from clinical examination, facial presentation, ECG recordings, biomarker analyses, laboratory results, and imaging studies hold promise to improve future risk models. Such huge amounts of patient data require modern AI/ML algorithms for efficient analysis. In a nationwide investigation in the UK involving over 400,000 patients with non-ST-elevation acute coronary syndrome (NSTE-ACS), the predictive performance of the GRACE 2.0 score could be significantly improved using ML strategies.[15] The redeveloped ML-based GRACE 3.0 score (web calculator: www.grace-3.com) now provides higher predictive performance and for the first time accounts for sex differences in the NSTE-ACS phenotype (**Fig. 5**; GRACE 3.0 score).[15] Similarly, the PRAISE risk models developed in the in the PRAISE registry, by d'Ascenzo et al. predicts events following hospital discharge after an ACS.[17] The integration of different kinds of patient data, considering the context and the information available, may help to improve future risk models.[18] Integrating AI/ML with clinical decision-making can transform care, making clinical practice more efficient, faster, personalized, and effective as it has the potential to explore large amounts of information automatically and systematically.[19] Similarly in the SPUM-ACS cohort from Switzerland, using a large number of established and novel biomarkers [including trimethylamine N-oxide (TMAO) among others], AI/ML was superior to conventional risk assessment after ACS.[20]

VALIDATION OF ARTIFICIAL INTELLIGENCE/MACHINE LEARNING ALGORITHMS

As ML is able to learn independently, considering increasing amounts of data provided to the algorithm, vigorous independent validation of the results obtained is of utmost importance. Indeed, for a nonexpert investigator, the AI/ML algorithm is like a black box where he feeds data in and obtains a result. To assure the reproducibility of accurate predictions in external patient populations, it is of central importance to validate a given prediction model in a completely independent, large cohort with patients in a similar clinical setting, preferably even from another geographic area. Only if reasonable performance is obtained in external validation cohorts (using "unseen" data), a risk model can be integrated in clinical practice.

CONCLUSION

Furthermore, as the phenotype of patients changes over time, for instance due to changes in lifestyle or treatment, established models need to be reassessed, adapted, and again validated in a validation cohort based on the changed phenotype of presenting patients, as outlined earlier.

ONLINE REFERENCES

Please scan the QR code provided at the end of the table of contents for References of this chapter.

CHAPTER 2

Artificial Intelligence in Echocardiography: Usefulness and Limitations

George Wuni, Vinay Wasan, Navin C Nanda

ABSTRACT

Artificial intelligence (AI) has the potential to improve the efficacy and efficiency of echocardiography studies by replicating human logic and making precise decisions. In this chapter, we will discuss the usefulness and limitations of AI in the field of echocardiography.

Keywords: Echocardiography, artificial intelligence, left ventricular function, stress echocardiography, valvular heart disease.

INTRODUCTION

Since its discovery in the 1950s, echocardiography has been pivotal in the evaluation and management of heart diseases.[1] Its noninvasive nature, coupled with its wide availability and cost effectiveness, has made echocardiography the most-performed cardiac imaging modality worldwide.[2] However, it has not been without setbacks. When compared to other forms of cardiac imaging, it is most often influenced by interobserver and intraobserver variation, with excessive reliance on the skill and experience of both the sonographer and the reading clinician.[3] Sometimes, even with the same sonographer and patient, there is variation in the reproducibility of two-dimensional transthoracic echocardiography (2DTTE) images.[2] Standard guidelines recommend capturing over 100 images for an extensive and complete study.[1] This is unfortunately not the case in most echocardiography laboratories for some of these reasons: (1) Lack of ample time allotted for each study. The American Society of Echocardiography (ASE) recommends 45–60 minutes for a standard echocardiogram in normal patients. Complicated cases or patients with pathologies might even require up to 90 minutes.[4] (2) High-patient load, coupled with sonographer fatigue and burnout. (3) Inadequate experience of some sonographers. All these increase discrepancies among studies. It is, therefore, crucial to employ ways to mitigate these challenges and hence improve the efficacy and efficiency of echocardiography studies. The relatively recent introduction of artificial intelligence (AI) in cardiology and echocardiography may provide a much-needed solution to some of these problems. In this chapter, we discuss the usefulness as well as limitations of AI in the context of echocardiography.[5]

DEFINITION OF AI TERMS (TABLES 1 AND 2; FIGS. 1 TO 3)

Artificial intelligence is transforming cardiology by replicating human logic and making precise decisions. It utilizes computer algorithms and machine learning (ML) to process data and improve over time. ML allows echocardiographic equipment to enhance its performance by learning from patterns in the data. By comparing images during examinations, the machine updates its "templates," leading to faster and more accurate results. ML algorithms use supervised, unsupervised, semisupervised, and reinforcement learning models.[3,6,7]

Supervised learning, which is used for diseases with well-established diagnostic criteria, involves using categorized data to train the machine to recognize and analyze patterns and produce desired outcomes. On the other hand, unsupervised learning, which is used for understanding rare diseases with unclear diagnostic criteria, involves providing

TABLE 1: Basic AI definitions with some advantages and limitations.

Artificial intelligence (AI)	• *Definition*: The science of making intelligent machines and computer programs that execute tasks comparable to, or beyond the capabilities of a human brain • *Advantages*: Possibility of accurate, faster, less cumbersome, and easily reproducible results • *Limitations*: We must standardize AI. Because of its limited generalizability, AI cannot be applied to many situations right away. Definitions of privacy and legal obligations are necessary. Results' plausibility is also difficult to determine
Artificial neural networks (ANNs)	• *Definition*: Complex networks of nodes, similar to the communication of neurons in the human brain. It has the capacity to modify its own algorithms, gaining new knowledge by handling fresh data. Convolutional neural network (CNN) is a specific type of ANN used mostly in AI applications • *Advantages*: Can examine big, varied, and dynamic datasets • *Limitations*: It is necessary to use algorithms that are acceptable and have large, high-quality input data
Machine learning (ML)	• *Definition*: A division of AI that uses a multilayer convolutional neural network algorithm, typically containing three layers or less • *Advantages*: Aiming to enhance AI, ML can analyze more data and increase the accuracy of the generated model • *Limitations*: The data must be of high quality and quantity, and the methods must be suitable
Deep learning (DL)	• *Definition*: A subdivision of ML. It uses convolutional neural networks that have more than three layers and typically several hundred hidden nodes to process input • *Advantages*: Aiming to enhance ML, DL can handle more data than ML and enhance the accuracy of the generated models even more • *Limitations*: A huge training dataset is required. Time-consuming (using particular techniques to set up the neural network, requiring longer training times to increase algorithm precision). Data overfitting
Supervised learning (SL)	• *Definition*: Implies that human beings label data because predictions are made using the selected algorithm • *Advantages*: Excellent for classifying problems and addressing regression problems • *Limitations*: Time consuming since it calls for manual labeling
Unsupervised learning (UL)	• *Definition*: Aims to combine unlabeled data such that pattern recognition might occur freely • *Advantages*: Can distinguish novel features from attributes in a concealed sample without human labeling. Suitable for understanding rare diseases with unclear diagnostic criteria • *Limitations*: Since it may be challenging to identify the first cluster model, it must be validated across different cohorts to guard against biases. For example, some entangled data may need to be "disentangled" by human coding for final validation, which may necessitate supervised training in order to ultimately find the best method
Convolutional neural network (CNN)	• *Definition*: A highly efficient deep learning approach for evaluating visual input. The way neurons are arranged in the human brain, especially in the visual cortex, is similar to how connections are made in a CNN • *Advantages*: Allows for analysis of complex data • *Limitations*: Black box phenomenon applied in its use is poorly understood
Black box	• *Definition*: A complicated system whose inputs and outputs but not interior workings may be observed. Its internal workings are either concealed or difficult for the user to comprehend • *Advantages*: Allows for analysis of complex data • *Limitations*: Concealed nature. Its full "mechanism of action" raises questions about the validity of its results

raw, unlabeled data for the machine to process and develop its own set of templates.[6] Semisupervised learning combines aspects of both supervised and unsupervised learning, leveraging labeled and unlabeled data.[5] Reinforcement learning is a trial-and-error process where a machine interacts with its environment, rewarding desired outputs, and penalizing undesired ones. It is useful in robotics and has limited use in clinical practice but has not been applied to echocardiography.

Deep learning (DL), a subdivision of ML, handles large datasets by using complex networks of nodes like the human brain's neurons. Artificial neural networks (ANNs) in DL (space) learn from extensive datasets and generate precise predictions about new or unknown data. The initial dataset must be comprehensive, encompassing various demographics and disease conditions, to ensure higher accuracy while minimizing confounders and bias.[3] Convolutional neural networks (CNNs) are a specific type of

ANN used in AI applications, including echocardiography. CNNs excel in image analysis and pattern recognition. They consist of convolutional layers that analyze smaller sectional images derived from the input image, passing the details to deeper layers for further analysis. Multiple CNN layers collaborate to produce the final outcome, incorporating studies at each level.[3,8]

Table 2: Machine learning versus deep learning.

Machine learning	Deep learning
Able to complete tasks with lesser amounts of data	Usually benefits from large volumes of data
To draw a conclusion, it is reliant on a certain function	Can learn extremely complicated functions in order to reach a decision
An expert is usually needed to identify important features	The most significant attributes are determined by the neural network and do not need to be selected by an expert
Shorter time required for training	Longer time required for training
Improves with experience by employing statistical approaches	Imitates the behavior of neural networks in the human brain

ARTIFICIAL INTELLIGENCE IN ECHOCARDIOGRAPHY (TABLE 3)

Left Ventricular Ejection Fraction, Dimensions, and Mass

The assessment of left ventricular (LV) function is one of the most common parameters obtained from an echocardiogram. It carries important prognostic value.[9-18] LV ejection fraction (LVEF) is the measure that is most frequently used to assess LV function. LVEF may be evaluated using a variety of echocardiographic techniques. The most common technique in use is the modified Simpson's biplane method, which often serves as the "gold standard" for LVEF assessment by echocardiography. Its usage entails manually tracing the end-systolic and end-diastolic borders of the LV in the apical two- and four-chamber views. This approach can be cumbersome for the untrained or inexperienced sonographer since it relies heavily on excellent apical view images and the time taken to properly trace the endocardial borders of the LV, which in itself is not without error.[16] Also, the modified Simpson biplane method is predicated on the notion that the LV is made up of cylindrical disks and ignores structural and morphological diversity, which might be seen in patients with significant/extensive wall motion abnormalities and

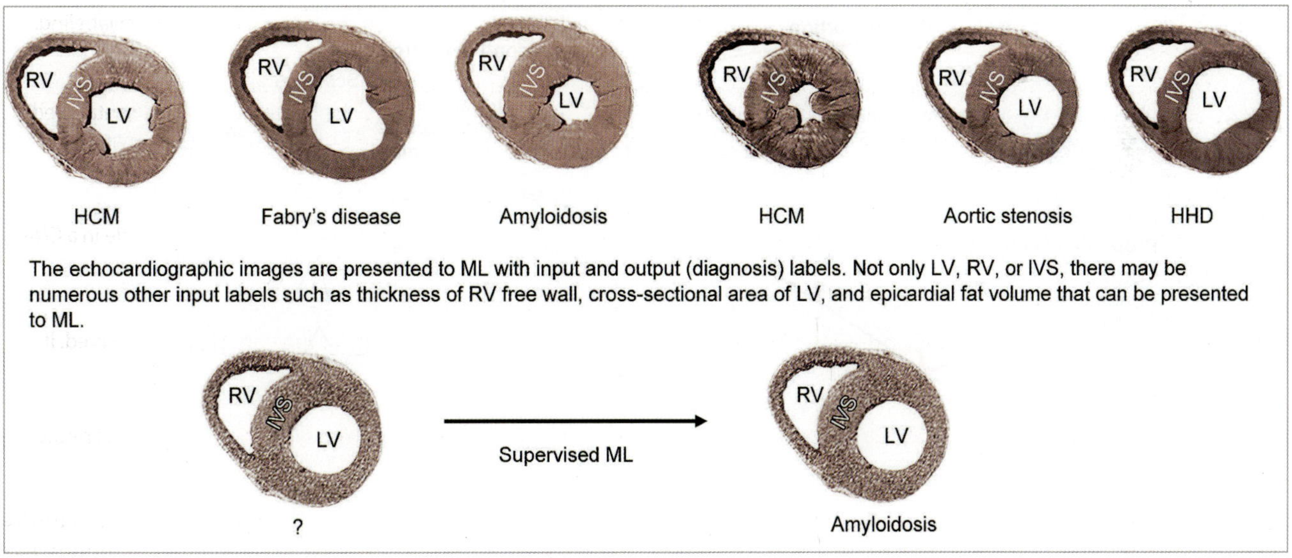

FIG. 1: Supervised machine learning (ML). The echocardiographic images are presented to ML with input and output (diagnosis) labels. Not only left ventricle (LV), right ventricle (RV), or interventricular septum (IVS), there may be numerous other input labels such as thickness of RV free wall, cross-sectional area of LV, and epicardial fat volume that can be presented to ML.

(HCM: hypertrophic cardiomyopathy; HHD: hypertensive heart disease)

Source: Reproduced with permission from Karakuş G, Degirmencioglu A, Nanda NC. Artificial intelligence in echocardiography: Review and limitations including epistemological concerns. Echocardiography. 2022;39(8):1044-53.

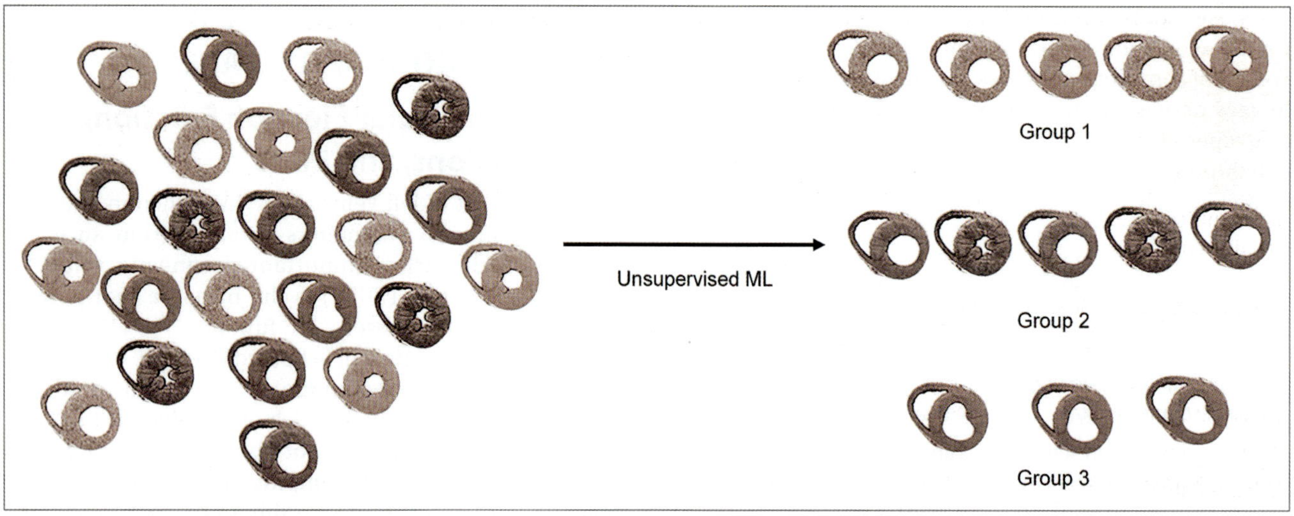

FIG. 2: Unsupervised machine learning (ML). This analyzes and clusters unlabeled datasets. These algorithms find hidden patterns in data without the need for human intervention. The data is presented to ML without any explanation of "what is what" (e.g., "the etiology of this hypertrophied LV is amyloidosis"-output label-) or "these findings are important" (e.g., "if the septum thickness is >20 mm, the etiology is unlikely to be athlete's heart" or "asymmetric LV hypertrophy is unlikely to be amyloidosis"-input label-). Unsupervised ML is especially helpful in clustering; it groups similarities and differences in the echo images presented. As seen in the figure, ML determines that the hypertrophied ventricles in group 1 share features and may have the same etiology (without specifying its name). Unsupervised ML generates its own findings, whereas supervised ML provides predictions based on labels provided by the researcher.

Source: Reproduced with permission from Karakuş G, Degirmencioglu A, Nanda NC. Artificial intelligence in echocardiography: Review and limitations including epistemological concerns. Echocardiography. 2022;39(8):1044-53.

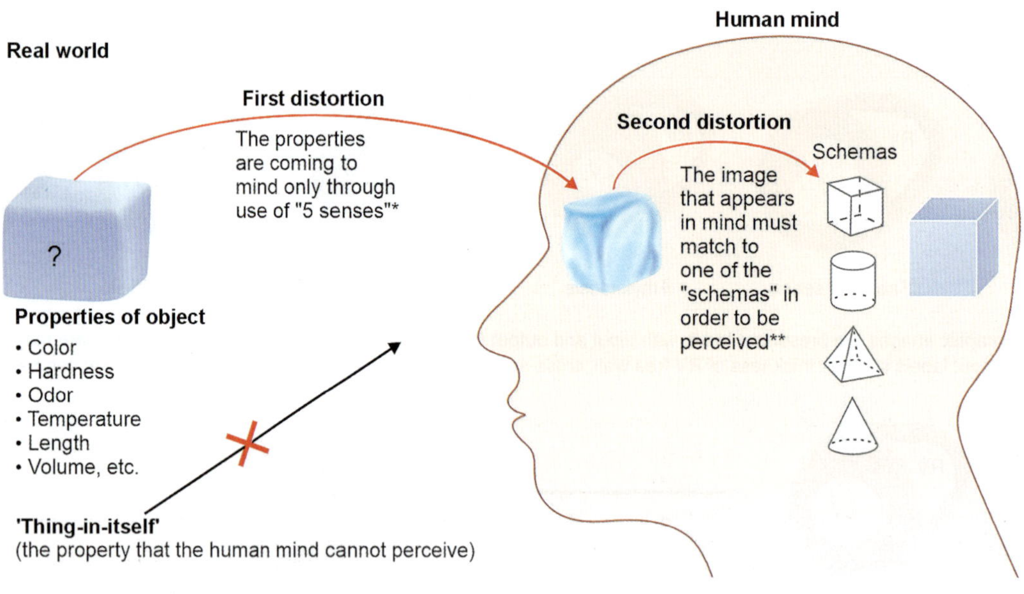

*Those properties must be within certain limits in order to enter the mind. Otherwise, like a "thing-in-itself," they cannot reach the mind. The human eye, for example, cannot detect wavelengths beyond 400–700 nanometers (visible light).

**The features of the perceived image have lower power than the real properties of the actual world, e.g., spatial resolution.

FIG. 3: Simplified illustration of Kant's epistemology. A "thing it itself," according to Kant, is a property of an object that the human mind cannot perceive. When the image of the object reaches the human mind, it only enters with its perceptible features; this causes the first distortion in the object's knowledge. Then, the mind arranges this first raw image according to its own schemes, resulting in a second distortion. In short, there are important differences between the object in real word and what we perceive.

Source: Reproduced with permission from Karakuş G, Degirmencioglu A, Nanda NC. Artificial intelligence in echocardiography: Review and limitations including epistemological concerns. Echocardiography. 2022;39(8):1044-53.

TABLE 3: Application of artificial intelligence (AI) in various echocardiographic parameters.

		Mode of echo-cardiography	Method of AI used in studies	Accuracy (agreement with experienced examiner)	Time saver/ rapidity	Repro-ducibility	Aid in diagnosis	Prognosis/ prediction of mortality
Left ventricular ejection fraction and volumes		2D, 3D, and speckle tracking	DL, unsupervised ML, and CNN	++	++ (<2 seconds)	++	++	N/A
Left ventricular mass		2D and 3D	DL and CNN	++ (comparable with CMR)	++	++	++	N/A
LV global longitudinal strain		2D	DL and CNN	++	++ (~15 seconds)	++	++	N/A
Left atrial strain		2D	DL, unsuper-vised ML and CNN	++	++	++	++	++
Diastology		2D	DL and CNN	++	++	++	++	++
Stress echocardiography and coronary artery disease		2D and 3D	DL and CNN	++ (comparable with CMR)	++	++	++	+
Right ventricular function		2D and 3D	DL and CNN	++	++	++	++	++
Valvular heart disease	Aortic stenosis severity	2D and 3D	DL and CNN	++ (comparable with CT)	++	++	++	++
	Mitral regurgitation severity	2D and 3D	DL and CNN	++	++	++	++	++
	Rheumatic heart disease screening	2D	DL and CNN	++	++	++	++	+
	TAVR planning	2D, 3D, and TEE	DL and CNN	++ (comparable with CT)	++	++	++	N/A
Amyloidosis and sarcoidosis		2D, 3D, and speckle tracking	DL and CNN	++	++	++	++	N/A
Intracardiac masses		2D and TEE	DL, ANN, and supervised CNN	++	++	++	++	N/A

(2D: 2-dimensional; 3D: 3-dimensional; ANN: artificial neural network; CMR: cardiac magnetic resonance; CNN: convolutional neural network; CT: computed tomography; DL: deep learning; ML: machine learning; N/A: not applicable at this time; TAVR: transcatheter aortic valve replacement; TEE: transesophageal echocardiography; ++: very good; +: fair)

LV aneurysms, and this results in poor LVEF correlation with the so-called gold-standard cardiac magnetic resonance (CMR) imaging.[16] In addition, only two apical views are used to calculate LVEF, omitting all other views. Aside from these, it is also prone to interobserver variability. Newer AI algorithms can accurately determine LVEF in one cardiac cycle in <2 seconds, even with poor-quality images. When results were compared to those of expert sonographers, they were found to be more reproducible than results from human experts.[9-18] In the first ever blinded randomized noninferiority clinical trial, investigators sought to test the influence of AI's DL model in the interpretation workflow by comparing AI with the sonographer's initial evaluation of LVEF. The major outcome metric was the difference in LVEF between the final cardiologist assessment and the AI or sonographer evaluation. AI was found to be noninferior and even superior to sonographer assessment of LVEF when compared to the gold standard used in this trial (final cardiologist assessment). The AI method used was the DL model (Siemens Syngo VA40D). The study's key strength is the possibility of using a well-trained and proven AI system in the context of limited cardiological expertise.[10,11]

It remains uncertain whether AI can help in accurately assessing LVEF and LV volumes in patients with poor acoustic windows and poorly defined or incomplete endocardial borders.[10] Unlike 2D TTE, LV mass measurements and analysis by AI-derived models have been found to be accurate and similar to CMR imaging.[14] Also, LV chamber dimensions and wall thickness measurements are automated by AI algorithms, resulting in time saving and greater accuracy.[11,12,16,18] To the best of our knowledge, there are no studies showing the superiority of AI in assessing LV volumes, or specific superiority studies that compare the use of AI in 2D TTE versus three-dimensional (3D) TTE. There is, however, exciting progress on AI-generated automated echo reporting. AI-based reporting solutions have the potential to revolutionize echocardiography by lowering physician effort while increasing report turnaround time and accuracy. However, issues such as data protection, cost, and the risk of over-reliance on AI must be thoroughly evaluated and handled.[9]

Left Ventricular Global Longitudinal Strain

Systolic strain refers to the deformation of the myocardium that occurs as a result of cardiac contraction. It is useful for the identification of subclinical ventricular dysfunction that conventional 2D TTE may miss.[19] It is widely used to identify chemotherapy-related cardiotoxicity early.[16,20] DL models have been applied in the assessment of left ventricular global longitudinal strain (LVGLS). When they were compared to the traditional time-consuming speckle tracking software, LV strain was assessed faster with DL models in as little as 15 seconds, as opposed to 5-10 minutes with conventional methods. Results obtained from both were comparable.[16,21] In another study, the within-patient test-retest repeatability of the LVGLS evaluated by cutting-edge AI in repeated echocardiograms captured by various echocardiographers was compared to the outcomes by manual assessments. AI techniques decreased test-retest variability and eliminated reader bias in both test-retest datasets.[21] In another study, AI-derived classification confidence (CC) was used to objectively assess echocardiographic image quality for monitoring cancer therapeutics-related cardiac dysfunction (CTRCD). The CC of the apical 4-chamber view was linked to the consistency and dependability of automated LVGLS. It also showed great promise for being used as a filter to select consecutive echocardiographic studies in individual patients and decreased the CTRCD false positive detection rate.[22]

Left Atrial Strain

In time-series data of the left atrial (LA) strain, investigators sought to know if unsupervised ML algorithms might be able to discern if clinically significant phenogroups were linked with the likelihood of developing adverse outcomes. The ML models correctly identified clinically relevant predictive information over conventional risk factors.[23]

Diastology

Diastolic dysfunction is common, and its assessment is laboriously challenging. Guidelines recommend the measurement of six distinct echocardiographic metrics, a review of numerous complicated flowcharts, and correlation with an appropriate clinical picture. The diagnosis can still be challenging, and there is still a considerable element of uncertainty, despite all these guidelines.[16,24] AI has offered creative methods for the evaluation of diastology. AI-derived algorithms have successfully been used to assess diastology using three out of the six conventional parameters. The results obtained were comparable to those of a human heart failure expert.[25] AI innovation has also contributed to the improvement of diastolic function phenotyping, which has led to better prediction of outcomes. The development of quick and precise screening tools for diastolic dysfunction has also shown promise. In one study, a prescreening test for diastolic heart failure was effectively developed using intrabeat dynamic variations in the LA and LV.[26] All these have contributed to the early detection, monitoring, and prediction of mortality associated with heart failure.[27] AI algorithms have also been successfully used to automatically annotate and accurately assess mitral valve inflow velocity measured by pulsed Doppler (E') to mitral valve annulus velocity measured by tissue Doppler (e'). These findings, when compared to similar tasks executed by top human experts, were found to be similar.[15] AI has also been used to track the deformation of left-sided cardiac chambers, providing precise data for the noninvasive measurement of LV-filling pressures and Doppler-independent phenotypic characterization of LV diastolic performance.[28]

Stress Echocardiography and Coronary Artery Disease

Stress echocardiography is a helpful method for determining whether or not coronary artery disease (CAD) is present; however, there is a great deal of interobserver diversity, it requires extensive knowledge, and incorporates a sizeable amount of qualitative information into its evaluation.[29] CNN has been used to create models on both dobutamine and post-exercise stress echocardiograms that can distinguish patients with CAD, which can be seen angiographically.[13,30] Findings were comparable to those of human experts.[29] 3D TTE DL modules have been successfully used to accurately ascertain the existence of coronary artery calcification (CAC)

as well as identify high amounts of coronary calcium with great precision. These discoveries were similar to the CAC assessed by CT. These findings highlight the potential future use of AI for CAD risk categorization, which might help direct preventive treatments.[31] Beyond the limitations of the traditional visual wall motion scoring index, AI-derived assessment of LVEF and LVGLS by contouring contrast-enhanced and unenhanced dobutamine and post-exercise stress echocardiograms independently has been shown to improve the detection of obstructive CAD.[32]

Right Ventricular Function

Assessment of the right ventricle (RV) carries great clinical relevance but can be challenging due to its asymmetric crescent form, poor 2D TTE visualization, and the discrepancies that exist in the assessment of RV parameters.[33] AI-based models have provided quick, accurate, and consistent volumetric and nonvolumetric assessments of RV systolic function.[34,35] Postimplantation of a left ventricular assist device (LVAD) is complicated by the development of RV failure in up to a third of all patients. This is partly explained by the LVAD's increased RV preload and the interventricular septum's drastic leftward shift, which decreases the interventricular septum's contribution to RV contraction. AI models have proven highly beneficial in the advancement of predictive tools for the identification and assessment of RV failure post-LVAD implantation.[35] These aid clinicians to take precautionary measures in their decision making.[16,36]

Valvular Heart Disease

Current standard techniques employed in valvular function assessment are complicated and time intensive, making them ideal for AI development and growth. The emphasis of AI in the sphere of valvular heart diseases (VHDs) focuses on the echocardiographic assessment of the degree of valve disorders as well as the recognition of high-risk patients.[37] Four primary categories define the suitable e-application of AI to echocardiographic images in patients with VHD: image acquisition, view recognition, image segmentation, and disease state identification.[38] Through the creation of software applications that direct acquisition of images, AI has the ability to enhance valvular assessments. The focus of such AI-assisted image acquisition is now on fundamental noncolor images such as the parasternal and apical views.[39] Automated image analysis powered by AI largely increases reproducibility and accuracy through image segmentation, which refers to identifying a specific structure in an image, determining its boundaries, and taking measurements.[38] Precise and dependable quantitative analysis of stenosis and regurgitation is critical for determining severity, prognosis, and for evaluation for possible surgical intervention. The proximal isovelocity surface area (PISA) technique is commonly used to calculate regurgitant volume and measure the area of the mitral valve orifice. The traditional PISA technique of 2D echocardiography is based on the incorrect assumption that the geometry of the proximal flow region is hemispheric. AI-assisted techniques allow for direct PISA measurements, thereby decreasing errors.[40]

ML has also been employed to create highly sensitive and precise innovative techniques for assessing mitral valvular dysfunction based on 2D echocardiographic fine patterns and image-processing methods.[8,41,42] AI has allowed for automated identification and quantification of mitral regurgitation severity, as well as rheumatic heart disease involving the aortic and mitral valves.[41] These algorithms are also capable of effective and quick identification of prosthetic mitral valves from native valves in conventional 2D echocardiographic images with nearly 100% accuracy. This, therefore, goes a long way toward improving the assessment of prosthetic mitral valve dysfunction.[43] AI-guided color Doppler has been used to facilitate the assessment of rheumatic heart disease by nonexperts, performing much better for mitral valve evaluation than aortic valve assessment.[44]

Highly precise algorithms are also being employed to aid in the detection of aortic stenosis (AS), characterization of its severity, and identification of higher-risk patients, like those with increased aortic valve calcium scores and prominent late gadolinium enhancement. This was useful in decreasing the time from diagnosis to intervention.[37] AI can closely imitate human measurement of all essential parameters in the assessment of AS severity. This reduces interscan discrepancies, enhances diagnosis and interpretation of AS, and enables precise and repeatable recognition and care of AS patients.[45] AI 3D echocardiography models have made it possible to measure the aortic annulus and root with extreme accuracy in patients receiving transcatheter aortic valve replacement. This is essential for the accurate implantation of the prosthesis. Results obtained were similar to those obtained with CT, making way for decreased radiation exposure from CT imaging.[46] AI has been employed in VHD phenotyping which is a growing field showing much promise. AI phenotyping applications are being utilized in certain special situations where valvular evaluation and assessment might be difficult, such as in the recognition of low-flow, low-gradient AS, or in e-quantification of disease in mixed valve diseases.[38]

Amyloidosis and Sarcoidosis

Artificial intelligence techniques have been employed to identify uncommon cardiac diseases such as sarcoidosis and amyloidosis (CA), which may be missed by routine echocardiography.[47] CNN algorithms using echocardiography have accurately identified cardiac sarcoidosis patients from healthy individuals with excellent sensitivity. It is anticipated to be a viable technique for its diagnosis.[5,48] The evaluation of LVGLS and LVEF is crucial for the diagnosis of CA. Fully automated AI calculations of these parameters in patients before and at the time of diagnosis of CA were similar to human assessments. However, AI offered a more rapid assessment.[49]

Intracardiac Masses

It might be challenging but crucial to accurately identify the cause of intracardiac masses using echocardiography.[20] Intracardiac mass evaluation by echocardiography is subjective and requires substantial training.[16] AI-derived models in echocardiography have been used to automatically identify, characterize, and differentiate various intracardiac tumors and thrombi and were able to show higher accuracy, sensitivity, and specificity than pre-existing software.[50,51] Further AI algorithms applied in transesophageal echocardiography (TEE) have been proven to be more effective than existing conventional methods for detecting LA thrombi in patients with atrial fibrillation.[51]

LIMITATIONS

Although using AI in cardiology and medicine has many benefits, it is important to delve into the concerns surrounding the "black box" nature of AI models and the epistemological implications of their outputs. AI algorithms construct complex models directly from raw data, leading to a lack of transparency and understanding regarding how factors are combined to produce predictions, even for the designers themselves. This inherent opacity makes it challenging for users to comprehend and validate the outputs of AI models from a clinical standpoint, contributing to the "black box" nature of AI.[20,52] The "black box" concern extends beyond interpretability to epistemological concerns. AI models generate predictions and decisions based on patterns learned from training data, but the reasoning behind these predictions remains elusive. This lack of explicit reasoning poses challenges in terms of justifying and trusting the outcomes produced by AI algorithms. It raises questions about how much confidence we can place in the decisions made by AI models, especially in critical medical contexts where explanations and justifications are essential.

Epistemology is a philosophical field that investigates the nature of knowledge and its relationship to the human mind. What can and cannot the human mind, which is the foundation of knowledge, know?. According to Immanuel Kant, an influential philosopher, the structures and causations we perceive originate in our minds and not in the physical or real world.[5,53,54] The human mind generates knowledge by mixing a priori of associative patterns (categories) and experimental evidence to produce what we finally "see". If this is true, then some epistemological concerns raised with regards to AI are valid. The DL design is comparable to that of a human neural system, and it too uses sensory information and its own distinctive internal schemas to filter relevant data, detect objects in noisy and chaotic settings, and establish causation. They build knowledge by integrating inductive and deductive reasoning. As a result, it is critical to exercise caution when AI makes judgments regarding reality.[5,53,54]

Furthermore, the reliance on labeled data in some ML models introduces potential bias in the labeling process. Scientists or real-world data are considered the source of indisputable truth for labeling, although biases may exist. This reliance on labeled data raises concerns about the objectivity and accuracy of the AI models' predictions, as they may inherit or perpetuate biases present in the training data.[20,55] The requirement for high-quality data for training AI algorithms is another challenge. AI requires large databases of excellent images to refine its algorithms, but when applied to real-world imaging, which may be imperfect or variable, the analysis can be compromised. Imperfections or variations in image quality can affect the performance and accuracy of AI models, highlighting the importance of rigorous data curation and preprocessing.[2,56,57]

A significant limitation in AI's application in medicine is the scarcity of prospective studies with reliable clinical outcomes. While retrospective studies comparing AI-derived measurements and findings to traditional techniques are available, comprehensive clinical trials assessing the effect of AI on direct patient care are lacking. To date, only one blinded, randomized clinical trial has been conducted.[10,11] The absence of prospective studies limits our understanding of the true effectiveness and safety of AI applications in clinical practice.[16,58] Ethical and legal challenges also arise from the use of large databases and registries containing sensitive patient data for AI applications. These databases are necessary for training AI models using ML methods, but they raise concerns about data security and the potential for unauthorized disclosure of confidential patient information. Increasing security breaches can erode patient trust and hinder participation in prospective studies, thus impeding further advancements in AI research.[20,59-61]

While AI has greatly impacted echocardiography, there is a concern that it may erode the skills and artistry of experienced echocardiographers and reading clinicians. The visual and dexterity aspects of echocardiography, honed through years of practice, may be gradually diminished as AI assumes a greater role in the field. Finally yet importantly, AI's automated generation of clinical and/or management decisions fails to take into account each patient's unique clinical, physical, environmental, and social situations. Although scientifically relevant, the results may not always directly correspond to patient care. This goes to stress the point that this form of intelligence, though helpful, still remains "artificial".

CONCLUSION

In conclusion, the use of AI in medicine, particularly in cardiology and echocardiography, is rapidly developing and has the potential to completely transform patient treatment. The identification, classification, and diagnosis of cardiac diseases may be aided by AI algorithms. It is quite promising

in the world of echocardiography, as it increases workflow efficiency, repeatability, and diagnostic accuracy. By early identification of subtle changes in cardiac hemodynamics, AI promises to aid clinicians in the near future to better predict, anticipate, and probably curtail mortality from cardiac diseases.

However, AI also raises critical concerns related to the "black box" nature of AI models with the opacity of their outputs, the potential biases inherited from training data, the possibility of providing inaccurate information with potentially serious patient care consequences, and epistemological limitations. These concerns highlight the need for ongoing research, transparency, ethical considerations, and the integration of human expertise to ensure the responsible application of AI. For now, AI is unlikely to fully replace clinicians.

ONLINE REFERENCES

Please scan the QR code provided at the end of the table of contents for References of this chapter.

CHAPTER

3 Wearable Devices and Artificial Intelligence in the Diagnosis and Management of Arrhythmias

Pankaj Lakhwan, Darshan Krishnappa, Deepak Padmanabhan

ABSTRACT

In the current age of technology, wearable devices with advanced machine learning (ML) algorithms have paved the way for medicine and healthcare. The combination of artificial intelligence (AI) and wearable devices is transforming healthcare by enabling continuous monitoring, personalized interventions, and data driven decision making. These complex ML algorithms have continuously been validated with multiple clinical trials and all these trials over the period of the time have proven the accuracy and efficiency of these models over human experts and other linear regression ML models. There are ML models for risk stratification and prediction in cardiac electrophysiology and arrhythmia management which are continuously being developed and validated. ML models have been used in computational research on cardiac electrophysiology, assessing cardiac activation from electroanatomical and body surface potential mapping, ventricular arrhythmia research and clinical decision support, atrial fibrillation research and clinical decision support, electrocardiogram (ECG) interpretation, and ECG based diagnosis. With all the advantages that AI has to offer, there are some challenges and considerations as well which are discussed. Data quality and reliability, explainability, and clinical validation reliability remain a challenge. Ethical considerations, algorithm bias, and regulatory and legal considerations cannot be overlooked as well. We have discussed the future directions of AI in cardiac electrophysiology and arrhythmia management. It is essential to focus our future research efforts in data privacy and security, interoperability, data harmonization, and validation of these ML models for improving healthcare management and assisting in clinical decision making and managing patients.

Keywords: Artificial intelligence, machine learning, wearable devices, arrhythmia management, prediction, cardiac electrophysiology, electrocardiogram, echocardiogram.

INTRODUCTION

Arrhythmias are abnormal heart rhythms that can range from harmless to life-threatening conditions. Early diagnosis and effective management are crucial to prevent adverse outcomes and improve a patient's quality of life. A retrospective study[1] found that early identification of high-risk patients with atrial fibrillation (AF) and initiation of appropriate anticoagulant therapy significantly reduced the risk of stroke and mortality. Early diagnosis and management of arrhythmias can prevent disease progression in AF.[2,3] Research has shown that personalized treatment approaches, including genetic testing influenced treatment decisions in patients with long QT syndrome, leading to more effective management.[4] Early diagnosis facilitates the identification and management of risk factors associated with arrhythmias like AF.[5] Timely diagnosis and effective management can lead to cost savings for healthcare systems by preventing hospitalizations and emergency department visits related to arrhythmia-related complications.[6]

OVERVIEW OF WEARABLE DEVICES AND ARTIFICIAL INTELLIGENCE IN HEALTHCARE

Wearable devices are transforming healthcare by enabling continuous monitoring, real-time data analysis, and personalized interventions. This integration of wearable devices and artificial intelligence (AI) is revolutionizing patient care, disease management, and medical research. They come in a variety of form factors and measure physiological parameters outside traditional clinical settings which has implications for chronic disease management and post-surgery recovery. Consumers use wearable devices for tracking fitness goals, sleep patterns, and overall wellness, promoting a proactive approach to health.

Artificial intelligence using machine learning (ML) algorithms has the potential to analyze vast amounts of patient data derived from traditional sources such as electronic medical records (EMRs) and nontraditional sources such as wearables. This aids in the detection of patterns hitherto unseen and not understood. This can predict disease progression, identify high-risk patients, and recommend personalized treatment plans. It is also postulated to aid in new drug discovery by analyzing vast datasets and identifying potential therapeutic compounds.

The integration of wearables and the recorded data analyzed by AI algorithms enable real-time data analysis providing edge level information aiding clinicians and patients in a variety of decision-making scenarios. For instance, AI-powered wearable electrocardiogram (ECG) devices can detect arrhythmias and alert patients or healthcare providers to potential cardiac events. AI powered stethoscopes can provide clinicians with information about murmurs, asymptomatic left ventricular dysfunction, and AF thereby aiding triage of patient and selection of appropriate investigation to proceed with.[7-9]

The combination of wearable devices and AI has the potential to transform healthcare by enabling continuous monitoring, personalized interventions, and data-driven decision-making. As research and development continue, the potential impact of wearable devices and AI in healthcare is likely to expand even further, improving patient outcomes and healthcare delivery.

WEARABLE DEVICES FOR ARRHYTHMIA DIAGNOSIS AND MONITORING

Electrocardiogram Wearables

Electrocardiogram wearables are portable devices designed to continuously monitor the heart's electrical activity, providing real-time data on cardiac rhythms and patterns **(Figs. 1A to D)**. ECG wearables offer continuous monitoring of the heart's electrical signals over an extended period, ranging from several hours to several days. Modern ECG wearables are equipped with wireless communication

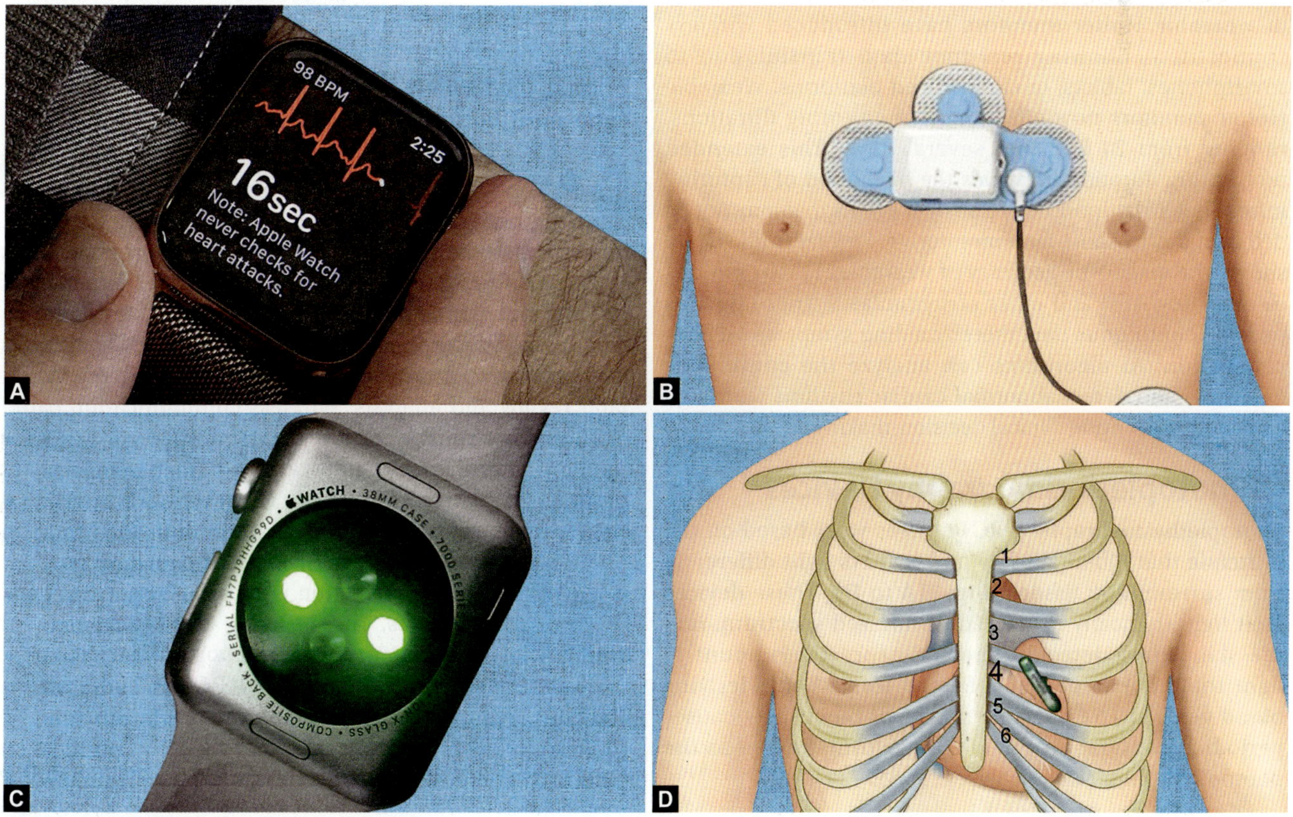

FIGS. 1A TO D: Examples of common wearables in clockwise order from top left; electrogram wearable, wearable Holter monitor, implantable cardiac monitor, and photoplethysmography device.

capabilities, allowing real-time transmission of data to a smartphone or cloud-based platform. This feature enables remote monitoring by healthcare professionals, facilitating prompt intervention in case of abnormal cardiac events. ECG wearables are highly valuable in the diagnosis and management of arrhythmias. They are instrumental in remote patient monitoring, allowing healthcare providers to track the cardiac status of patients outside traditional healthcare settings and particularly beneficial for patients with chronic cardiovascular conditions in remote settings or where hospital visits are challenging.[10]

Numerous studies have demonstrated the accuracy of ECG wearables in detecting AF. For instance, the mHealth Screening to Prevent Strokes (mSToPS)[11,12] trial found that a wrist-worn ECG wearable exhibited high sensitivity and specificity in identifying AF compared to traditional methods. A study[13] compared wearable ECG monitoring to traditional Holter monitors and found comparable diagnostic yield, suggesting that wearable devices could replace or complement conventional monitoring methods.

Wearable Holter Monitors

Holter monitors have been widely used for continuous ambulatory electrocardiogram monitoring to detect arrhythmias and assess cardiac health **(Figs. 1A to D)**. Traditional Holter monitors involve cumbersome devices with multiple leads and limited wearability. Advancements in wearable Holter monitors have introduced wireless connectivity, allowing real-time data transmission to smartphones, tablets, or cloud-based platforms. Wearable Holter monitors now offer longer monitoring durations, ranging from 24 hours to several days. This extended monitoring duration improves the likelihood of capturing infrequent arrhythmias and transient events that may not be detected during short-term monitoring. Several studies have shown the diagnostic accuracy of wearable Holter monitors in detecting AF[14] and other arrhythmias.[15] These devices provide continuous data thereby aiding symptom-rhythm correlation. AI algorithms can analyze the continuous ECG data and detect abnormal cardiac rhythms with high accuracy, supporting clinical decision-making.

Photoplethysmography Devices

Photoplethysmography (PPG) devices work based on the principle that blood absorbs and scatters light differently from surrounding tissues **(Figs. 1A to D)**. These devices emit light, typically in the red or infrared spectrum, into the skin. Photodetectors then measure the amount of light that is absorbed or reflected from the underlying blood vessels. The pulsatile nature of blood flow causes periodic variations in the PPG waveform, known as the photoplethysmogram.

Recent advancements have led to the development of wearable PPG devices, such as smartwatches and fitness trackers. These wearables integrate PPG sensors, enabling continuous monitoring of physiological parameters, such as heart rate and blood oxygen saturation (SpO_2), throughout daily activities. Traditional PPG devices measure blood flow at a single wavelength, multiwavelength PPG devices use multiple light sources to capture data at different wavelengths, providing more accurate measurements of SpO_2 and enhancing diagnostic capabilities.

Photoplethysmography devices are widely used for heart rate monitoring. A study[16] compared the accuracy of heart rate measurements using PPG and ECG in healthy subjects and found high correlation between PPG and ECG heart rate measurements, demonstrating the reliability of PPG devices in heart rate monitoring. PPG devices integrated into wearable sleep trackers can provide insights into sleep patterns, including sleep duration, quality, and disturbances. These devices aid in diagnosing sleep disorders and promoting healthy sleep habits.[17,18] Advancements in PPG technology have enabled the estimation of blood pressure through cuffless measurements.[19,20]

There are efforts to detect P-waves, which represent atrial depolarization, using PPG-derived pulse transit time which aided in the detection of AF by analyzing P-wave characteristics. The ubiquitous PPG-based detection of AF has since been confirmed by several studies.[21,22]

Implantable Cardiac Monitors

Implantable cardiac monitors (ICMs) are implanted subcutaneously or submuscularly in the chest area and can provide long-term arrhythmia monitoring **(Figs. 1A to D)**. They are equipped with highly sensitive sensors that continuously record the heart's electrical signals. This prolonged monitoring duration allows for the detection of intermittent and asymptomatic arrhythmias that may be missed during short-term monitoring. Advanced algorithms can automatically detect and record arrhythmic events for later review and analysis. Wireless communication capabilities allowing the transmission of enables real-time monitoring and prompt intervention in case of significant arrhythmic events. CRYSTAL AF trial[23] demonstrated the effectiveness of ICMs in detecting AF in patients with cryptogenic stroke. The trial showed that ICMs provided a higher yield in AF detection compared to conventional monitoring methods, highlighting the importance of continuous monitoring in this patient population.

Comparative studies between ICMs and other monitoring methods have been conducted to evaluate the diagnostic yield, accuracy, and clinical utility of ICMs in detecting arrhythmias and managing cardiac conditions.[24-28]

ARTIFICIAL INTELLIGENCE IN ARRHYTHMIA DIAGNOSIS AND RISK PREDICTION

Arrhythmia Detection Algorithms

Artificial intelligence algorithms powered by ML leverage advanced computational techniques to analyze electrocardiogram signals and identify abnormal heart rhythms with high accuracy.[29-31]

A few advanced analysis tools are as follows:

- *Convolutional neural networks (CNNs)* are deep learning algorithms widely used in image and signal processing tasks, including ECG analysis. CNNs use convolutional layers to automatically learn spatial features from ECG signals and identify specific patterns associated with different arrhythmias. They excel in feature extraction and have demonstrated high accuracy in arrhythmia detection.
- *Recurrent neural networks (RNNs)* are another class of deep learning algorithms commonly used in sequence data analysis, such as time-series ECG signals. RNNs can capture temporal dependencies in ECG data, making them suitable for detecting arrhythmias based on the dynamic patterns of heart rhythms.
- *Long short-term memory (LSTM) networks* are a type of RNN that address the vanishing gradient problem, allowing them to capture long-term dependencies in time-series data such as ECG signals. LSTM networks are effective in modeling irregular and long-duration arrhythmias, providing high accuracy in arrhythmia detection.
- *Support vector machines (SVMs)* is a classical ML algorithm that has been applied to ECG data for arrhythmia classification. SVM aims to find the optimal hyperplane that best separates different arrhythmia classes based on extracted features from ECG signals.
- *Random forest (RF)* is an ensemble learning algorithm that builds multiple decision trees and combines their outputs to make predictions. RF has been applied to ECG data to identify arrhythmias by utilizing a diverse set of features.

Several studies have investigated the accuracy of AI algorithms compared to human experts in various medical domains, including arrhythmia detection **(Table 1)**.

TABLE 1: Examples of several studies validating the machine learning (ML) algorithms predicting different outcomes.

Study	Type of study	Outcome	ML model	ML performance
Chang et al.[32]	Development of an ML model from surface ECG using 3,628 waves of premature ventricular complex (VPCs) from 731 patients	Idiopathic VAs	CNN	• AUC 0.963 • Sensitivity 90.7% • Specificity 92.3%
Yong et al.[33]	Development of an ML model using raw digital data of 2,412 12-lead ECGs	AF during sinus rhythm	RNN	• AUC 0.79 • Accuracy 72.8 • Specificity 78%
Katshushika et al.[34]	Development of an ML model using 151 echocardiographic movies from 50 cardiac sarcoidosis patients and 151 from 149 healthy subjects	Cardiac sarcoidosis	CNN	AUC 0.842
Samad et al.[35]	Retrospective study including 1.7 million unselected patients with 3.3 million echocardiograms in large regional health system	Predicting survival from large echo and electronic health records (EHRs)	Nonlinear RF	• AUC > 0.82 • Accuracy 96%
König et al.[36]	Retrospective analysis of inpatient heart failure (HF) cases which were nonelectively admitted	In hospital mortality in HF patients	Random forest (RF), gradient boosting machine (GBM), single layer neural network (NNET), extreme gradient boosting (XBoost)	• AUC (RF) 0.875 • AUC (GBM) 0.882 • AUC (NNET) 0.866 • AUC (XBoost) 0.882
Zhu et al.[37]	Randomized retrospective cohort study of 0.18 million 10 seconds, 12 channel ECGs from adult patients which were classified into 21 rhythms	Heart rhythm or conduction abnormalities	CNN	• AUC 0.983 • Accuracy 80% • Sensitivity 68.7% • Specificity 99.5%

Continued

Continued

Study	Type of Study	Outcome	Machine learning model	Machine learning performance
Rodriguez et al.[38]	Prospective cohort of 140 participants with nonischemic cardiomyopathy as part of the German autonomic regulation trial (ART) study	Sudden cardiac death or survived arrest	Laplacian support vector machines (LSVM)	• AUC 0.965 • Accuracy 99%
Okada et al.[39]	Prospective observational US registry from three sites with 122 participants with ischemic cardiomyopathy and left ventricular ejection fraction <35%	Ventricular arrhythmias	Laplacian support vector machines	• AUC 0.72 • Accuracy 81%
Vergara et al.[40]	Retrospective analysis of 1,753 participants undergoing catheter ablation for previous sustained VT (disease agnostic) from 12 international sites making up the International VT Ablation Center Collaborative Group (1,251 development cohort, 502 validation cohort)	VT recurrence	Random forest	AUC 0.84
Doldi et al.[41]	Retrospective artificial intelligence (AI)-based analysis	Long QT syndrome	Xception time model	• AUC 0.97 • Accuracy 91.8% • Sensitivity 92.9% • Specificity 90.8%

(AF: atrial fibrillation; AUC: area under the curve; CNN: convolutional neural network; ECG: electrocardiogram; RNN: recurrent neural network; VA: ventricular arrhythmia)

Risk Stratification and Prediction

The AI techniques can analyze large and complex datasets, including patient demographics, medical history, genetic information, imaging data, and sensor-based measurements, to provide more accurate and personalized risk assessments.

Using a combination of traditional risk factors, along with novel biomarkers and genetic data, to predict an individual's risk of developing cardiovascular diseases (CVDs) is possible. These predictive models enable healthcare providers to identify high-risk patients who may benefit from targeted interventions and lifestyle modifications.

AI-driven Risk Stratification and Prediction Models in Arrhythmia and Cardiac Electrophysiology (Fig. 2)

There are multiple applications of AI driven models in cardiac electrophysiology and arrhythmia for risk stratification and prediction. Some of the models under consideration are discussed here.

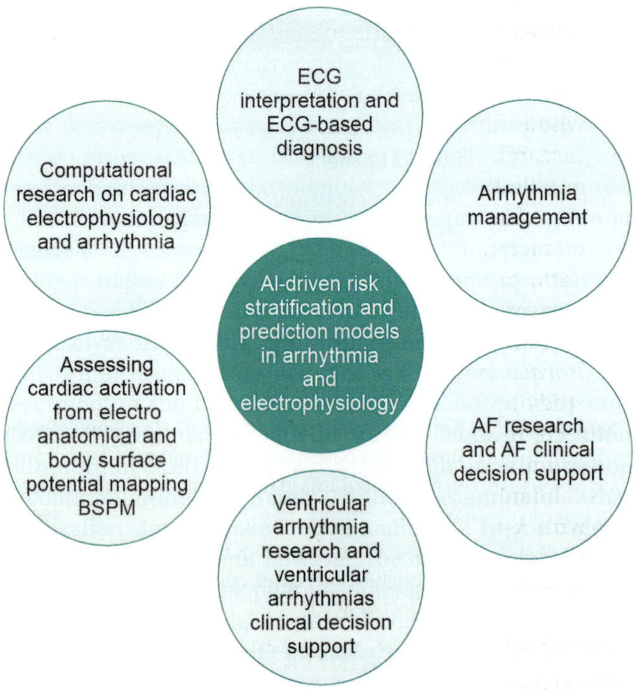

FIG. 2: Possible use cases of artificial intelligence (AI) driven risk stratification and prediction models in arrhythmia and cardiac electrophysiology.

Use of AI in Computational Research on Cardiac Electrophysiology and Arrhythmia

- *Investigate the factors that underlie emergent electrophysiological behaviors and reentrant dynamics in cardiac tissue:*[42-45] ML is used to analyze variability in *in silico cell electrophysiology*, particularly in the kinetic properties of ion channel recovery, which modulates the dynamics of arrhythmias. ML has also been used to detect reentrant activity and its termination in tissue models and to locate reentrant drivers from electrograms in a model of AF. In these studies, an interesting use of ML is the classification of simulated electrophysiological data, such as classifying clinical phenotypes in simulated ECGs for patients with hypertrophic cardiomyopathy (HCM).

- *Classify phenotypes from in silico electrophysiological activity in cardiac disease*:[46,47] Two ECG-based HCM phenotypes are explained by distinct mechanisms—ionic remodeling and action potential prolongation in hypertrophied apical and septal areas lead to T wave inversion with normal QRS complexes, whereas abnormal Purkinje-myocardial coupling causes abnormal QRS morphology in V4–V6. These findings have potential implications for patients' management as they point toward different arrhythmia mechanisms in different phenotypes.
- *Create activation maps from sparse data*:[48] Physics-informed artificial neural networks (ANNs) accounting for the underlying wave propagation dynamics have also been used to generate full electrical activation maps from sparse synthetic activation data.
- *Link AF spatial pattern to re-entrant driver (RD) localization*:[49] The mechanisms underlying persistent AF in patients with atrial fibrosis are poorly understood. Zahid et al. used patient-derived atrial models to test the hypothesis that AF RDs persist only in regions with specific fibrosis patterns. Patient-derived models demonstrate that AF in fibrotic substrates is perpetuated by RDs persisting in fibrosis boundary zones characterized by specific regional fibrosis metrics [high fibrosis entropy (FE) and fibrosis density (FD)].
- *Personalize cardiac models*:[50-54] Personalization of whole-heart models has been an active avenue of research that utilizes ML approaches. Personalization entails the incorporation, within a model of cardiac electrical activity, features and characteristics that are extracted from the patient's clinical records, imaging data, or invasive or noninvasive electrophysiological measurements.
- *Localize atrial ectopic beats from simulated body surface P-wave maps*[55] *and predict AF ablation outcome*:[56] In a study by Albero et al., using clustering and classifying techniques to localize atrial triggering sites provided promising and useful results for physicians. Their validated atrial-torso multiscale model used together with k-means clustering algorithms and classifying models based on multiclass SVM providing an accuracy of up to 97%.

Use of ML in Assessing Cardiac Activation from Electroanatomical and Body Surface Potential Mapping

- *Reconstruct epicardial maps from endocardial catheter recordings*:[57-59] In one of the early ML applications, where electroanatomical maps were used to estimate cardiac activation, ML reconstructed epicardial maps from endocardial catheter recordings in the ventricles using experimental data from a dog animal model, to localize the onset of focal ventricular activations.
- *Estimate activation patterns from three-dimensional (3D) echocardiographic images*:[60] Prakosa et al. estimated contraction forces and activation times from 3D echocardiographic images. This model is then applied to two 3D echocardiographic sequences (one in sinus rhythm and other in LV pacing) for which strains and displacement were estimated using incompressible diffeomorphic demons for nonrigid registration.
- *Reconstruct heart surface potentials from body surface potential mapping (BSPM)*:[61-64] Inverse electrographic imaging, which involves calculating potentials or activation maps on the heart surfaces from BSPMs, is a promising noninvasive tool to detect abnormal electrical activity on the surfaces of the heart. It has also seen its share of ML applications providing data-driven approaches in lieu of inverse problem calculations in determining ventricular surface activations from BSPMs.

Use of ML in Ventricular Arrhythmia Research and Ventricular Arrhythmias Clinical Decision Support

- *Predict risk of ventricular arrhythmias using texture analysis of late gadolinium enhancement magnetic resonance imaging (LGE-MRI),*[39,65] *analysis of electronic health records (EHRs),*[66] *device-measured physical activity,*[67] *and ventricular monophasic action potential recordings.*[68] As structural remodeling (scar, fibrosis) characterizes several heart diseases that result in VA, texture feature analysis of LGE-MRI scans has been used to assess VA risk in HCM; VA risk has been assessed from EHRs of HCM patients, where ML identified 10 new variables, in addition to 12 known, as VA risk predictors, and from physical activity time-series data of patients with implantable cardioverter-defibrillator (ICDs). Rogers et al. used an SVM to predict risk of ventricular tachycardia (VT)/ventricular fibrillation in patients from recordings of ventricular monophasic action potentials acquired during an electrophysiological study; the independent test C statistic was 0.90.
- *Short-term prediction of hypotension and ventricular fibrillation*:[69] Tsuji et al. proposed a method for predicting acute clinical deterioration triggered by hypotension, ventricular fibrillation, and an undiagnosed multiple disease condition using biological signals, such as heart rate, respiratory rate (RR) interval, and blood pressure. The results showed that the proposed method has a prediction accuracy of 92.5% for patients with acute hypotension and can predict the occurrence of ventricular fibrillation 5 minutes before it occurs with an accuracy of 82.5%. In addition, a multiple disease condition can be predicted 7 minutes before they occur, with an accuracy of over 90%.

- *Locate VT exit site or the origin of ventricular activation*:[70-74] Yokokawa et al. were the first to demonstrate the feasibility of using ML in localizing the exit site of a scar-related VT from paced 12-lead ECGs during the ablation procedure's pace-mapping. Sapp et al. presented two independent methods based on multiple linear regression model to progressively approach the site of origin of early LV activation. Extending the latter ML approach to localization of idiopathic VA origin on the patient-specific geometry of LV, RV, and neighboring vessels, Zhou et al. achieved, in a recent study, a mean localization accuracy of 3.6 mm.
- *Learning from images to predict VT ablation targets*:[75] Lozoya et al. presented a model-based feature augmentation scheme to improve the performance of a learning algorithm for the detection of cardiac radiofrequency ablation (RFA) targets with respect to learning from images alone.
- *Identifying patients with left ventricular systolic dysfunction (LVSD)*[76] *and predicting left ventricular ejection fraction (LVEF)*: AI-enabled ECG can identify patients with LVSD and predict LVEF. Addedinsewo et al. retrospectively applied and validated ML model to a cohort of 1,606 patients aged ≥18 years who presented in emergency department with dyspnea for the identification of LVSD (LVEF ≤ 35%). AI-enabled ECG algorithm identified LVSD with are under the receiver operating characteristics curve of 0.89 and accuracy of 85.9%.
- *Diagnostics of cardiac sarcoidosis using multichamber wall motion analyses*:[77] Eckstein et al. utilized a cardiac MRI for a support vector ML-based diagnostic approach to cardiac sarcoidosis.

Use of ML in AF Research and AF Clinical Decision Support

- *Predict which patients will experience AF from EHRs*[78,79] *and by using a smartphone camera*:[80] Tiwari et al. developed and tested an ML model to predict 6-month incidence of AF using EHR data. The study used EHR data sampled from over 2.2 million individuals and found using the 200 most common EHR features provided the optimal classification of AF risk (area under the curve of 0.8). Hill et al. sought to evaluate novel and conventional statistical and ML models for risk predication of AF in a cohort study of nearly 3 million adults without a history of AF. These two studies offer hope that ML can be used directly to guide targeted screening of patients at risk of AF. In that vein, an interesting approach for AF screening used an iPhone camera to detect and analyze photoplethysmographic signals from the face and index finger of 217 in-hospital patients by extracting subtle beat-to-beat variations of skin color that reflect the cardiac pulsatile signal. The patterns in the photoplethysmographic waveform were classified using a previously trained algorithm.
- *Predict stroke risk from a daily AF burden signature*:[81] Using continuous remote monitoring data from cardiac implantable electronic devices (CIEDs), Han et al. evaluated that ML and ensemble methods that incorporate daily AF burden signature provides incremental prognostic value for risk stratification beyond CHA_2DS_2-VASc for near-term risk of stroke.
- *Define AF clinical phenotypes with various treatment patterns and outcomes*:[82] AF is typically classified based on disease subtype; however, such characterization does not fully capture AF heterogeneity. An ML cluster analysis on 9,749 patients with AF revealed different classifications of patients—(1) a cluster with low comorbid burden; (2) a younger/behavioral disorder cluster; (3) a cluster who resembled patients with tachycardia-bradycardia and had ICDs; and (4) a cluster defined by atherosclerotic comorbidities. The authors underscored that the groupings were not driven by conventional classifications and had different risks for adverse clinical outcomes.
- *Predict AF recurrence after catheter ablation from clinical records*,[83,84] *from atrial shape changes*,[85,86] *and from the combination of AF simulation results and imaging features*:[87] A series of research articles focused on using ML to predict risk of AF recurrence after the first catheter ablation procedure. Identifying patients who are unlikely to remain in sinus rhythm after the ablation is an important pathway toward improving ablation success rates and avoiding ineffective procedures. These are based on preprocedural shape of the patient's atria, patients' laboratory, and clinical parameters and by conducting simulations of AF induction in atrial models.
- *Identifying patients who may benefit from AF cardioversion response*:[88] Vinter et al. showed modest predictive performance for successful electrical cardioversion using sex-specific ML and logistic regression models.

Use of ML in Arrhythmia Management

- *Reduce false arrhythmia alarms in the intensive care unit*[89] *and in ICD therapy*:[90,91] According to Zhang et al., use of robust heart rate estimation and automatic templates of electrogram morphology can lessen the rate of false critical arrhythmia alarms. There are different studies to reduce ICD inappropriate therapies using patients' intrinsic rhythm and a fuzzy logic-based detection algorithm to decrease false ICD therapies.
- *Identify the implantable anti-arrhythmia device implanted in the patient*:[92] Howard et al. developed an ML system which identifies the manufacturer and even the model group of a pacemaker or defibrillator from a chest radiograph. Using radiographic images of 1,676

devices, a CNN classified the images with 99.6% and 96.4% accuracy (manufacturer and model, respectively).

Use of ML in ECG Interpretation and ECG-based Diagnosis

- *Classify heart rhythms*[93-98] *and detect subtle changes in ECG morphology*:[99,100] There are multiple studies and proposals for using ECG dataset in diagnosing arrhythmia disease and classifying arrhythmia in ambulatory electrograms, improving recognition of sustained VTs, recognition of late potentials, improving conventional arrhythmia detection algorithms, differentiation of wide QR provide better performances than traditional algorithms but demand more resources such as higher computational power and more memory.
- *Detect AF*:[101-104] Most of the times, AF goes undetected because it is frequently asymptomatic but is associated with stroke, heart failure, and death. There are methods to detect AF, but efficacy and yield of those methods limit their usage. Attia et al. were able to predict AF within a period of 30 days utilizing a single 10s 12-lead sinus rhythm ECG using a CNN.
- *Predict VT 1 hour before occurrence*:[105] Lee et al. developed an early prediction model that can predict VTs 1 hour before its onset using 14 parameters obtained from heart rate variability (HRV) and respiratory rate variability (RRV) analysis.
- *Predict cardiac resynchronization therapy (CRT) outcomes*:[106-109] Different ML models have been developed to predict the response of CRT therapies using echocardiography and other clinical parameters. There are ML models to predict 1- to 5- year all-cause mortality post-CRT implantation.
- *Identify (hidden) disease state signatures*[105,110-115] *mortality*[116,117] *and clinical deterioration*:[118] AI application has enabled us to identify many diseased states such as contractile and relaxation dysfunction, premature ventricular contractions (PVCs), hyperkalemia, likelihood of future Parkinson's disease, and nocturnal hypoglycemic events from the 12-lead ECG signatures which are often hidden from human naked eye.
- *Estimate blood pressure*[119] *and age (physical age vs. chronological) and sex*:[120] Monika et al. developed a method to estimate systolic blood pressure, diastolic blood pressure, and mean arterial pressure using ML models trained on ECG sensor data. Attia et al. trained a neural network using 10 seconds sample from 12-lead ECG from 0.5 million patients to predict age and sex.
- *Classification of hypertrophic heart diseases*:[121] Julian et al. assessed deep learning model performance of single-lead, 2-lead, and 12-lead ECG data to classify cardiac amyloidosis (AUH 0.95), HCM (AUH 0.92), aortic stenosis (AUH 0.90), hypertensive left ventricular hypertrophy (AUH 0.76), and another left ventricular hypertrophy (AUH 0.69).
- *Detection of patients with long QT syndrome*:[41] Doldi et al. performed a retrospective AI-based analysis using a 12-lead ECG of 124 genetically confirmed LQTS patients, including 41 patients with a concealed LQTS (33%), and validated against a control cohort (n = 161 of patients) without known LQTS or without QT-prolonging drug treatment but any other CVDs.
- *Early detection of patients with cardiac amyloidosis*:[122-124] Grogan et al. used single-lead and 6-lead ECG data sets to train a deep neural network to predict the presence of cardiac amyloidosis. Goto et al. also presented a pipeline using AI models with ECG or echocardiogram as inputs for cardiac amyloidosis detection. Agibetov et al. used cardiac magnetic resonance images to detect the potential patterns of cardiac amyloidosis.

AI-POWERED DECISION SUPPORT SYSTEMS

Applications of AI-based Decision Support Systems in Arrhythmia Management (Box 1)

The AI-based decision support systems leverage AI algorithms to analyze patient data and provide valuable insights to healthcare providers. They have been the subject of numerous studies evaluating their effectiveness in improving patient outcomes, particularly in the field of arrhythmia management which have demonstrated promising results, showcasing the potential of AI to enhance diagnostic accuracy, risk prediction, and treatment planning.

Challenges and Considerations in Implementing AI in Clinical Decision-making (Box 2)

Implementing AI in clinical decision-making poses several challenges and considerations that need to be addressed to ensure its successful integration and safe usage in healthcare settings.

Despite the challenges, implementing AI in clinical decision-making holds immense potential to transform healthcare by improving diagnostic accuracy, personalized treatment planning, and patient outcomes. Addressing the considerations mentioned above is crucial to maximize the benefits of AI while safeguarding patient safety, privacy, and equitable access to quality healthcare. Collaboration between clinicians, data scientists, ethicists, and policymakers is essential to develop robust AI solutions that align with clinical needs and ethical standards.

BOX 1 Applications of AI-based decision support system in arrhythmia management.

Applications of ML models in arrhythmia management

- Arrhythmia detection and diagnosis
- Risk stratification and prediction
- Personalized treatment planning
- Implantable device programming
- Remote monitoring and telemedicine
- Identification of underlying conditions
- Predicting response to medications
- Clinical research and data analysis

(AI: artificial intelligence; ML: machine learning)

BOX 2 Challenges and considerations in implementing AI in clinical decision-making.

- Data quality and availability
- Interoperability and integration
- Interpretability and explainability
- Ethical considerations and bias
- Regulatory and legal frameworks
- Limited clinical validation
- Workflow integration and user acceptance
- Continuous learning and maintenance
- Liability and accountability

(AI: artificial intelligence)

AI AND WEARABLES IN ARRHYTHMIA THERAPY

Personalized Therapy Delivery

- *Personalized antiarrhythmic drug therapy*: AI-driven algorithms can analyze patient-specific data, including ECG signals, genetic information, and medical history, to predict individual responses to antiarrhythmic medications. By tailoring drug selection and dosage based on patient characteristics, AI-guided personalized therapy delivery aims to improve treatment efficacy while minimizing adverse effects.
- *Optimization of ablation procedures*: For patients undergoing catheter ablation procedures to treat arrhythmias, AI algorithms can analyze imaging data and electrophysiological signals to assist in identifying the optimal ablation targets. This personalized approach may lead to more successful outcomes and reduce the need for repeat procedures.
- *Closed-loop cardiac implantable devices*: Closed-loop systems, where AI algorithms continuously monitor patient data and adjust therapy delivery in real-time, are being investigated for CIEDs. These AI-guided devices could dynamically respond to changes in heart rhythm patterns, automatically adjusting pacing or defibrillation parameters as needed.
- *Predictive risk stratification*: AI-guided risk stratification models can analyze wearable device data, genetic markers, and other clinical information to predict an individual's risk of experiencing adverse arrhythmic events. This approach may enable targeted interventions for high-risk patients to prevent potential complications.
- *Personalized remote monitoring*: AI algorithms can analyze data from wearable devices and other remote monitoring systems to create personalized patient profiles. These profiles can be used to tailor the frequency and intensity of remote monitoring based on the patient's risk level, optimizing the use of healthcare resources.
- *Mobile health (mHealth) applications for therapy delivery*: mHealth applications incorporating AI-driven decision support systems could help patients manage their arrhythmia treatments more effectively. These applications may remind patients to take medications, monitor symptoms, and provide personalized self-care recommendations.
- *Clinical trials and treatment response prediction*: AI-guided models can assist in predicting patient responses to specific arrhythmia treatments, which may aid in patient selection for clinical trials. This personalized approach could lead to more efficient and successful trial outcomes.

It is important to note that while AI-guided personalized therapy delivery holds promise, its implementation in clinical practice requires extensive validation and careful consideration of ethical, regulatory, and practical implications. Researchers continue to explore the potential benefits and challenges of AI-guided personalized therapy delivery in arrhythmia management through clinical trials and real-world studies.

Benefits and Potential Drawbacks of AI-driven Therapy Adjustments

The AI-driven therapy adjustments offer several benefits in healthcare, including in the management of arrhythmias. However, there are also potential drawbacks and challenges **(Table 2)** that need to be considered. Some benefits and potential drawbacks of AI-driven therapy adjustments are discussed in the **Table 2**.

Closed-loop Systems

Prospects and potential developments in closed-loop systems for arrhythmia management:

- *Improved arrhythmia detection and classification:* AI-based closed-loop systems can continuously learn from patient data and adapt their algorithms to better identify various arrhythmias, including rare or challenging cases.
- *Personalized therapy* to patients' conditions may optimize therapy delivery and improve patient outcomes.

TABLE 2: Benefits and potential drawbacks of AI-driven therapy adjustments.

Benefits	Potential drawbacks
Personalized treatment	Data quality and reliability
Real-time decision making	Limited explainability
Optimization of drug dosages	Ethical considerations
Reduced healthcare costs	Algorithm bias
Enhanced patient engagement	Lack of clinical validation
	Reliability of data sources
	Regulatory and legal considerations

(AI: artificial intelligence)

- *Integration of multiple physiological signals*: Beyond ECG, providing a more comprehensive assessment of the patient's cardiac health.
- *Remote monitoring and telemedicine*: Real-time adjustments to therapy
- *Closed-loop drug delivery*: AI algorithms could control drug dosing based on real-time physiological feedback, optimizing medication administration, and minimizing side effects.
- *Multimodal sensing and actuation*: Future closed-loop systems may integrate various sensors and actuators to enable more versatile and sophisticated control of arrhythmia.

CHALLENGES AND FUTURE DIRECTIONS

Data Privacy and Security

- *Data minimization*: Collect only the minimum necessary data.
- *Informed consent*: Obtain explicit and informed consent.
- *Anonymization and pseudonymization*: Anonymize or pseudonymize personal data to remove or replace identifying information.
- *Data encryption*: Use strong encryption methods to safeguard data.
- *Secure data storage*: Implement robust access controls, authentication mechanisms, and encryption to protect data from unauthorized access.
- *Transparency and explainability*: Ensure that users understand how their data is used.
- *User control and access rights*: Allow users to have control over their data. Provide options for data deletion, access, and the ability to modify their preferences for data sharing.
- *Regular security audits and assessments*: Conduct regular security audits and privacy impact assessments to identify vulnerabilities and address potential risks proactively.
- *Adherence to regulations*: Comply with relevant data protection and privacy regulations applicable locally.
- *Ethical considerations*: Uphold ethical principles in the design to ensure that user interests are prioritized minimizing bias.
- *Data sharing agreements*: To outline how the data will be used and protected.
- *Regular updates and patching*: Better iteration based on previous learning and solving exposed vulnerabilities.
- *User education*: Educate users about data privacy risks and best practices for protecting their personal information.

Interoperability and Integration

Enhancing interoperability among different wearable devices and AI platforms by standardization is a critical aspect of advancing healthcare technology and improving patient care. Standardization provides a common language that enhances collaboration and allows developers to build applications that can interact with various devices and platforms effortlessly.

Open APIs and SDKs also play a pivotal role to empower third-party developers to access and integrate their functionalities into a broader healthcare ecosystem encouraging innovation and allowing for the creation of custom solutions that cater to specific healthcare needs.

Data harmonization by that consistent data formats and terminologies are used. This facilitates a more comprehensive view of patient health, enabling healthcare providers to make well-informed decisions and deliver more personalized care.

To validate and encourage interoperability, it is essential to establish testing and certification programs fostering trust among stakeholders and provide an added layer of assurance about reliability.

Validation and Clinical Trials

Rigorous validation and clinical trials **(Box 3)** are of utmost importance when evaluating wearable devices and AI

BOX 3 Key reasons why rigorous validation and clinical trials are essential when evaluating wearable devices and machine learning algorithms in healthcare.

- Safety assurance
- Efficacy evaluation
- Regulatory compliance
- Generalizability of results
- Identifying limitations and improvements
- Evidence-based medicine
- Building trust
- Cost-effectiveness assessment
- Ethical considerations

algorithms in healthcare. These processes play a critical role in ensuring the safety, efficacy, and reliability of these technologies before they are used in real-world patient care.

ETHICAL CONSIDERATIONS AND PATIENT SAFETY IN CLINICAL RESEARCH INVOLVING AI

Clinical research involving AI holds immense potential to advance healthcare, but it also comes with ethical responsibilities. Some of them are listed in **Box 4**.

BOX 4 Ethical considerations.

- Informed consent
- Data privacy and confidentiality
- Bias mitigation
- Safety monitoring and oversight
- Transparency and open communication
- Beneficence and nonmaleficence
- Respect for autonomy
- Compliance with ethical guidelines
- Public trust and collaboration
- Social responsibility

CONCLUSION

Wearable devices provide a stream of continuous unique data that needs data processing capability to aid clinical usage. AI driven by a variety of advanced data management techniques as well as learning algorithms provides an opportunity to place this data in context. Together this symbiosis allows for an opportunity to enhance patient care and management.

ONLINE REFERENCES

Please scan the QR code provided at the end of the table of contents for References of this chapter.

CHAPTER 4

ChatGPT and Large Language Models: The Potential to Improve the Practice of Cardiology

Varsha Kiron, Preetish Rath

ABSTRACT

Large language models (LLMs) like ChatGPT (Chat Generative Pre-trained Transformer) are artificial intelligence (AI) systems which have an ability to interact with human intuition and computer-like intelligence. There is a huge potential of the role of LLMs in the practice of medicine ranging from medical education, diagnosis, and decision support to in manuscript preparation and editing. In the administrative standpoint, it helps in automation of various tasks, thereby streamlining the patient care and overall improvement in hospital experience. There has been immense interest in the field of cardiology to explore the role of LLMs in various aspects. Very often, the patient education domain is where the clinicians fail to meet the patients' expectation and such gaps can be filled by optimal utilization of newer technologies. There is published literature validating the efficiency of ChatGPT in educating patients undergoing procedures like coronary angiogram. Harnessing the power of AI will not only make the clinician efficient but also more accessible and cordial toward patients.

Keywords: LLMs (large language models), ChatGPT, artificial intelligence in cardiology.

"Technology is unlikely to replace the humans in the practice of clinical medicine, but humans who are unable to use technology may easily be replaced!"

—Anonymous

INTRODUCTION

Artificial intelligence (AI) is the area of computer science where machines are trained to perform tasks that require human-like intelligence, such as recognizing speech, writing documents, or real world decision-making. Language models are AI systems with the capacity to analyze and generate text in a manner akin to human thought processes. They achieve this by undergoing training on extensive text datasets using machine learning models.[1] OpenAI's Chat Generative Pre-trained Transformer (ChatGPT) has taken the global stage by storm, demonstrating remarkably intuitive text analysis and report generation capabilities. These capabilities are so refined that the outputs often seamlessly resemble human interactions.[2] The scope of large language models (LLMs) like ChatGPT is very wide, starting from entertainment industry in creating stories/lyrics for songs to education industry in creating and correcting test papers and also in medical industry which will be discussed in detail in this chapter.

Large language models are created by training large models (with millions of parameters) on a diverse range of sources like books, articles, websites, and more. It does this by analyzing the patterns, structures, and relationships within the text. Speech recognition, speech-to-text conversion, language conversion, and summarization are few of the basic tasks performed by the LLMs.[3]

Upon asking ChatGPT to write a 200-word introduction to this chapter, we received a certain output as shown in **Box 1**.[4]

Language models are increasingly used in medical field and have a huge potential in various aspects of medical care such as analysis of symptoms and laboratory data to aid in diagnosis and treatment, summarizing physician interaction

BOX 1 A ChatGPT output.

In the ever-evolving landscape of modern medicine, technology continues to play an increasingly vital role in enhancing diagnostic accuracy, treatment efficacy, and patient care across diverse medical specialties. In the realm of cardiology, a discipline critically concerned with heart health, a transformative force has emerged in the form of ChatGPT—an advanced artificial intelligence language model.

The "Role of ChatGPT in Cardiology" article delves into the dynamic synergy between cutting-edge artificial intelligence (AI) technology and the intricate domain of heart-related health. As the medical community seeks innovative tools to augment its capabilities, ChatGPT has emerged as a potent asset, offering insights, guidance, and collaboration that can potentially redefine the standard of care.

This article embarks on an exploratory journey into the multifaceted roles ChatGPT assumes within cardiology, ranging from aiding clinicians in rapid and precise diagnostics to facilitating patient education and engagement. By contextualizing the nuances of ChatGPT's applications within cardiology, this piece illuminates the symbiotic relationship between human expertise and AI proficiency, ultimately amplifying the potential for early detection, personalized treatment strategies, and improved patient outcomes.

Through a comprehensive analysis of real-world use cases, ethical considerations, and future prospects, this article endeavors to cast a spotlight on the transformative influence of ChatGPT in shaping the landscape of cardiology, ushering in a new era of synergy between technology and healthcare that promises to revolutionize the way heart health is understood and managed.

to facilitate electronic medical records (EMRs), personalized patient education, and automation of various administrative tasks.[5] We aim to review some of the uses of LLMs specific to the field of cardiology in the current chapter.

USES OF LARGE LANGUAGE MODELS IN CARDIOLOGY

Medical Diagnosis and Decision Support

In a busy clinical practice, a lot of obvious symptoms and signs are overlooked and there is an increasing dependence on laboratory tests and investigations. LLMs help in integrating the symptomatology and help identify a potential red flag in a given patient. It also helps the clinician in asking the right questions to make the appropriate diagnosis keeping the prognosis in mind which eventually influences the treatment options.[6] Additionally, images of electrocardiogram (ECG), echocardiogram (ECHO), angiograms, etc., could be analyzed by AI-powered applications to identify abnormalities and facilitate early diagnosis even prior to the engagement of a cardiologist.[7] Language models have the power to identify patterns in data which are not perceived by human thinking and thereby help identifying new associations and risk factors not previously acknowledged. ChatGPT helps the clinician ask the appropriate questions.

Large language models leverage their natural language understanding capabilities to assist in the following ways:

- *Symptom analysis*: A healthcare practitioner can input a patient's symptoms in natural language into ChatGPT. The model can process the input, recognize key medical terms, and identify potential patterns or associations with specific medical conditions.[2,8]
- *Medical history review*: By providing the patient's relevant medical history, such as past illnesses, surgeries, allergies, and medications, ChatGPT can take into account the patient's preexisting conditions, which can be crucial in determining the most accurate diagnosis and treatment options.[9]
- *Risk assessment*: Based on the symptoms and medical history, ChatGPT can evaluate the potential risks associated with different conditions and treatments, helping the healthcare provider make informed decisions.[8]
- *Treatment recommendations*: ChatGPT can propose treatment options based on the patient's condition, including medication choices, lifestyle modifications, and potential referrals to specialists for further evaluation and treatment.[10]
- *Continual learning*: As ChatGPT interacts with healthcare professionals, it can continually update its knowledge base, learning from each interaction and staying up to date with the latest advancements in medical research.[11]

For example, upon asking about a patient presenting with dyspnea and chest pain, ChatGPT prompted with certain responses as given in **Figures 1 and 2**.[4]

Upon asking to list the potential red flag clinical features, ChatGPT immediately prompts with a response as given in **Figure 2**.[4]

This highly intuitive analysis and communication not only helps the primary physician, but also the patients themselves in seeking appropriate timely care. A major concern of use of AI in medicine is the potential for self-treatment at the hands of patients. It is noteworthy how ChatGPT prompts the patients to seek medical attention rather than start medication although it is guideline recommendation. We hereby, show an example of "what medication should I take for heart failure?"[4] The disclaimer upfront is very evident; however, the answer does provide a basic insight into the pharmacotherapy in heart failure. It remains a clinical judgement in choosing the right therapy which is pertinent to the given patient, e.g., avoidance of ARNI/ACE/ARB (angiotensin receptor neprilysin inhibitor/angiotensin-converting enzyme/angiotensin receptor blocker) in renal failure and preference to Ismo/Hydralazine, dosages of individual drugs and so on. One must also notice the incompleteness in the response as newer agents like vericiguat and omecamtiv mecarbil are not mentioned as they are not routinely used in clinical practice yet **(Fig. 3)**.

When a patient presents with dyspnea (shortness of breath) and chest pain, it's important to gather as much information as possible to help determine the underlying cause and severity of their symptoms. Here are some key questions to ask:

1. **Onset and Duration:**
   - When did the symptoms start?
   - How long have you been experiencing these symptoms?
2. **Quality of Pain:**
   - Can you describe the chest pain? (e.g., sharp, stabbing, dull, crushing)
   - Does the pain radiate to any other parts of your body, like your arm, jaw, or back?
3. **Severity:**
   - On a scale of 0 to 10, how would you rate the severity of your chest pain and dyspnea?
   - Has the intensity of the symptoms changed since they started?
4. **Triggers and Aggravating Factors:**
   - Did anything specific trigger these symptoms? (e.g., physical activity, stress, eating)
   - Does anything make the symptoms worse or better?
5. **Associated Symptoms:**
   - Do you feel lightheaded, dizzy, or faint?
   - Have you experienced nausea, vomiting, or sweating?
6. **Medical History:**
   - Do you have a history of heart problems, such as angina, heart attack, or heart failure?
   - Have you been diagnosed with any lung conditions, like asthma or chronic obstructive pulmonary disease (COPD)?
   - Are you taking any medications or have any allergies?
7. **Risk Factors:**
   - Do you smoke?
   - Do you have a family history of heart disease or other related conditions?
   - Are you currently under a lot of stress?
8. **Recent Activities:**
   - Have you engaged in any strenuous physical activities or exercises recently?
   - Have you traveled recently, especially to areas with high altitudes?
9. **Current Health Status:**
   - Have you been feeling unwell or had any other symptoms recently?
10. **Changes Over Time:**
    - Have the symptoms improved, worsened, or remained the same since they started?

Remember, these questions serve as a starting point for gathering information, but it's essential to adapt and ask follow-up questions based on the patient's responses. This information will help guide your assessment and help determine whether the symptoms are related to a cardiac, pulmonary, or other medical condition, and whether immediate medical attention is required. Always seek medical help if the symptoms are severe or if there's any doubt about the patient's condition.

FIG. 1: ChatGPT response to "management of patient presenting with dyspnea and chest pain".

In patients presenting with dyspnea (shortness of breath) and chest pain, certain "red flags" or warning signs can indicate a potentially serious or life-threatening condition. These signs suggest that urgent medical attention is needed. If you encounter any of these red flags, it's crucial to seek immediate medical assistance. Some of the red flags include:

1. **Severe Chest Pain:** Intense, crushing, or squeezing chest pain that persists or worsens, especially if it radiates to the arm, jaw, neck, or back, could indicate a heart attack (myocardial infarction).
2. **Difficulty Breathing at Rest:** Severe shortness of breath even when the person is not exerting themselves could be a sign of heart failure, pulmonary embolism, or a severe lung condition.
3. **Cyanosis:** Bluish or grayish discoloration of the lips, face, or extremities indicates inadequate oxygenation and could be a sign of severe respiratory or cardiovascular issues.
4. **Sudden Onset:** Rapid onset of chest pain and dyspnea can be a sign of aortic dissection, pulmonary embolism, or tension pneumothorax.
5. **Associated Symptoms:** Presence of symptoms such as dizziness, lightheadedness, fainting, profuse sweating, or nausea/vomiting suggests a potentially serious cardiac event.
6. **Hemoptysis:** Coughing up blood could indicate conditions such as pulmonary embolism, severe pneumonia, or lung cancer.
7. **Recent Trauma:** If the patient has recently experienced trauma, especially to the chest, it raises concerns for possible rib fractures, pneumothorax, or cardiac injury.
8. **History of Heart Disease:** A known history of heart disease, including angina, heart attack, or heart failure, increases the risk of serious cardiac events.
9. **History of Blood Clots:** A history of deep vein thrombosis (DVT) or pulmonary embolism increases the suspicion of pulmonary embolism.
10. **High-Risk Factors:** High-risk factors such as older age, smoking, obesity, diabetes, and hypertension raise the likelihood of cardiovascular or respiratory issues.
11. **Physical Examination Findings:** Abnormal vital signs, such as low blood pressure or rapid heart rate, along with clinical signs like decreased breath sounds or asymmetrical chest expansion, could indicate serious underlying conditions.
12. **Previous Thromboembolic Events:** A history of blood clots, especially if not adequately treated, increases the risk of recurrent events.
13. **History of Cancer:** Patients with a history of cancer are at higher risk of certain conditions, including pulmonary embolism.
14. **History of Recent Surgery or Immobilization:** Recent surgery or prolonged immobility increases the risk of deep vein thrombosis and subsequent pulmonary embolism.
15. **History of Travel:** Recent travel, especially long flights or car rides, increases the risk of blood clots and pulmonary embolism.

These red flags are not exhaustive, and clinical judgment is crucial when evaluating patients with dyspnea and chest pain. If you encounter any of these warning signs, it's essential to prioritize immediate medical evaluation and intervention to ensure the patient's safety and well-being.

FIG. 2: ChatGPT response to "red flags in a patient with dyspnea".

I am not a doctor, but I can provide you with some general information about medications commonly used in the treatment of heart failure. It's important to consult a healthcare professional before starting or changing any medication regimen, as the appropriate treatment will depend on your specific condition, medical history, and other factors. Here are some common classes of medications used to manage heart failure:

1. **Angiotensin-Converting Enzyme (ACE) Inhibitors:** These medications help relax blood vessels, reduce blood pressure, and improve the heart's pumping ability. Examples include lisinopril, enalapril, and ramipril.
2. **Angiotensin II Receptor Blockers (ARBs):** Similar to ACE inhibitors, ARBs also relax blood vessels and lower blood pressure. They are often used as an alternative if ACE inhibitors cause side effects. Examples include losartan, valsartan, and candesartan.
3. **Beta-Blockers:** These medications slow down the heart rate, reduce blood pressure, and improve the heart's pumping function. They can also help relieve symptoms and improve exercise tolerance. Examples include carvedilol, metoprolol, and bisoprolol.
4. **Diuretics:** Diuretics help reduce fluid buildup in the body, which can alleviate symptoms of fluid retention such as swelling and shortness of breath. Common diuretics used include furosemide, bumetanide, and spironolactone.
5. **Aldosterone Antagonists:** These medications, such as spironolactone and eplerenone, help block the effects of aldosterone, a hormone that can contribute to fluid retention and heart damage in heart failure.
6. **Hydralazine and Isosorbide Dinitrate:** This combination can be used in certain cases, particularly for patients who cannot tolerate ACE inhibitors or ARBs. It helps relax blood vessels and improve blood flow.
7. **Digoxin:** Digoxin helps strengthen the heart's contractions and can improve symptoms of heart failure, particularly in cases where the heart's pumping function is weakened.
8. **Sacubitril/Valsartan (Entresto):** This is a newer medication that combines an angiotensin receptor-neprilysin inhibitor (ARNI). It helps relax blood vessels and increase levels of beneficial hormones.
9. **Ivabradine:** This medication helps lower heart rate and may be used in certain cases to improve symptoms and exercise tolerance.
10. **Anticoagulants and Antiplatelet Medications:** These may be prescribed to reduce the risk of blood clots, which can be a concern in some heart failure cases.

It's important to note that treatment for heart failure may involve a combination of these medications, along with lifestyle changes and other interventions. Your doctor will determine the most appropriate treatment plan based on your individual needs and medical history. Regular follow-up appointments and close communication with your healthcare provider are crucial for managing heart failure effectively.

FIG. 3: ChatGPT response to "what are the medication for heart failure?"

Despite the seemingly simple interface and utility, it has some important limitations. Symptomatology is not often clear as a lot of patients often underrepresent their symptoms and the LLMs analyze only the data that is provided to them. LLMs are incapable of accounting for specific rare pathologies which may not be statistically likely for the given patient, however, there could be glaring clinical likelihood of the same. This may lead to a lot of redundant diagnostic recommendations with little relevance to the patient.

Summarizing Physician Interaction: Facilitation of Electronic Health Record

Application of natural language processing (NLP) to electronic health record (EHR) is a game changer and has varied clinical utilities such as: medical documentation, patient education, improved data extraction and analysis, clinical entity recognition, and medical translation. There are numerous companies which enable the auto text-to-speech to facilitate digital documentation of clinical encounter with patients thereby saving time and eliminating writing/typing errors.

Helping Physicians Stay Up to Date with the Latest Advancements in Cardiology

Large language models are proficient in natural language understanding and generation. They can process vast amounts of text, including research articles, medical journals, and conference proceedings related to cardiology. A recent study evaluated ChatGPT's performance in a core curriculum exam consisting of 120 multiple choice questions developed by the European Society of Cardiology.[12] ChatGPT achieved nearly 58.8% accuracy in questions testing knowledge of pathophysiology, clinical reasoning, and guideline-recommended medical management. While ChatGPT has only been trained on data until 2021, newer versions of the model such as GPT-4 would incorporate more recent studies and inevitably increase accuracy on such standardized exams. Furthermore, cardiologists may have varying levels of expertise and interest in specific subfields within cardiology. LLMs can adapt to the individual's preferences and offer customized learning paths, focusing on areas that are most relevant and interesting to the practitioner. Apart from ChatGPT, LLMs trained specifically on biomedical text such as BioBERT have shown promise due to the ability to fine-tune them for more specialized clinical tasks such as causal relation detection.[13] BioBERT could similarly be fine-tuned on specifically the latest studies in cardiology to further their usage as an up-to-date educational resource for clinicians.

Patient Education

Since LLMs like ChatGPT are known to encode medical knowledge, they could prove to be a valuable resource for patients in understanding their medical diagnosis. The diagnosis by a cardiologist often contains medical jargon summarizing the cardiovascular functioning and treatment recommendations. In a recent study, the utility of ChatGPT in patient education regarding coronary angiogram was evaluated and was found to be very efficient.[14] **Box 2** shows

BOX 2 Case study.

Question: Could you help me understand the result of my 2D echo:

Dilated cardiomyopathy, all four chambers are dilated, global LV dysfunction (EF-25%), severe MR and severe TR with RV dysfunction.

Answer: Of course, I can help you understand the results of your 2D echo. Based on the information you provided, here's what each finding means:

1. Dilated cardiomyopathy: This is a condition where the heart's muscle becomes weakened and enlarged. As a result, the heart chambers become dilated, which means they are larger than normal.
2. Global LV dysfunction: LV stands for the left ventricle, which is the main pumping chamber of the heart. Global LV dysfunction means that the left ventricle is not pumping effectively, resulting in reduced cardiac output.
3. EF-25%: EF stands for Ejection Fraction, which is a measure of how much blood the left ventricle pumps out with each contraction. A normal EF is typically around 55–70%. An EF of 25% indicates that only 25% of the blood in the left ventricle is being pumped out with each heartbeat. This indicates severe impairment of the heart's pumping function.
4. Severe MR (Mitral Regurgitation): The mitral valve is a valve that separates the left atrium from the left ventricle. In mitral regurgitation, the valve does not close properly, causing blood to leak back from the left ventricle into the left atrium during each heartbeat. Severe MR means a significant amount of blood is flowing back, which can further decrease the heart's efficiency.
5. Severe TR (Tricuspid Regurgitation): The tricuspid valve separates the right atrium from the right ventricle. Similar to MR, TR involves the improper closure of the valve, leading to the backflow of blood from the right ventricle into the right atrium during each heartbeat. Severe TR can cause additional strain on the right side of the heart.
6. RV Dysfunction: RV refers to the right ventricle, which is also affected in your condition. RV dysfunction means that the right ventricle is not pumping blood effectively, likely due to the effects of severe TR.

Continued

Continued

In summary, the 2D echo results indicate that you have Dilated Cardiomyopathy with significant dilation of all four heart chambers, impaired pumping function of the left ventricle (global LV dysfunction) with an ejection fraction of only 25%, and severe regurgitation of blood in both the mitral and tricuspid valves, leading to further heart dysfunction. The right ventricle is also affected, likely due to the severe tricuspid regurgitation. These findings collectively suggest that your heart is not functioning optimally and requires appropriate medical management and further evaluation by a cardiologist to determine the most suitable treatment plan.

Question: What does this conclusion of my examination:

BP-90/60 mm Hg, CVS-PSM+ at apex

Answer:

The conclusion of your examination includes two main findings: blood pressure (BP) and CVS-PSM.

1. Blood Pressure (BP): The recorded blood pressure is 90/60 mm Hg. Blood pressure is measured in two values: the systolic pressure (the higher number) and the diastolic pressure (the lower number). In your case, the systolic pressure is 90 mm Hg, and the diastolic pressure is 60 mm Hg.

   A blood pressure of 90/60 mm Hg falls within the range of low blood pressure or hypotension.
2. CVS-PSM+ at Apex: CVS stands for Cardiovascular System, and PSM stands for Precordial Systolic Murmur. "PSM+" indicates the presence of a precordial systolic murmur.

A precordial systolic murmur is an abnormal sound heard during a stethoscope examination of the heart. It occurs during the systolic phase of the cardiac cycle when the heart is contracting. A murmur can be indicative of abnormal blood flow across the heart valves or within the chambers of the heart. There are various grades and types of murmurs, and additional testing and evaluation by a cardiologist are usually required to determine the cause and significance of the murmur.

Question: What are some treatment recommendations for my diagnosis?

Answer:

Treatment recommendations will depend on the severity of your condition, your overall health status, and other factors. Here are some potential treatment options for the conditions mentioned:

Dilated Cardiomyopathy:

Medications: Your doctor may prescribe medications such as ACE inhibitors, beta-blockers, diuretics, and aldosterone antagonists to improve heart function and manage symptoms.

Lifestyle Changes: Adopting a heart-healthy lifestyle is essential. This includes a balanced diet, regular exercise, smoking cessation, and limiting alcohol consumption.

Implantable Devices: In severe cases, your doctor may recommend devices like implantable cardioverter-defibrillators (ICDs) or cardiac resynchronization therapy (CRT) devices to help regulate heart rhythms.

Cardiac Rehabilitation: A supervised exercise program and education about heart health can be beneficial in managing dilated cardiomyopathy.

Mitral Regurgitation (MR) and Tricuspid Regurgitation (TR):

Medications: Medications can be used to manage symptoms and prevent further deterioration. Diuretics may help reduce fluid retention, and vasodilators can ease the workload on the heart.

Valve Repair or Replacement: In severe cases, surgical repair or replacement of the affected heart valves may be necessary to reduce regurgitation and improve heart function.

Percutaneous Valve Repair: For some patients, minimally invasive procedures, such as transcatheter mitral valve repair, may be an option.

RV Dysfunction:

Treating the Underlying Cause: Addressing the cause of RV dysfunction is essential. In your case, it may involve managing severe TR and optimizing overall heart function.

Medications: Medications like diuretics and medications to improve heart function may be prescribed to manage RV dysfunction.

Supportive Measures: Oxygen therapy, if necessary, and lifestyle modifications may also be recommended.

It's crucial to work closely with your cardiologist or a heart failure specialist to develop a comprehensive treatment plan tailored to your specific needs. They will consider your medical history, test results, and other relevant factors to provide the best possible care for your condition. Regular follow-ups and adherence to the prescribed treatment plan are essential to monitor progress and manage your heart health effectively.

Continued

Continued

Question: What are your thoughts on these treatment recommendations?

- Carnitor 500 mg twice daily
- Carvedilol 3.125 mg half tablet
- Dytor plus 20 mg thrice daily
- Restrict fluid intake to 1 liter per day
- Restrict salt intake

Answer:

Here's an overview of the medications and recommendations you mentioned:

Carnitine (Carnitor) 500 mg twice daily:

Carnitine is a naturally occurring substance in the body that helps in the utilization of fatty acids for energy. It is sometimes used as a supplement in certain heart conditions, including cardiomyopathies. However, the use of carnitine for dilated cardiomyopathy can vary depending on the individual's specific condition and response to other treatments. Its efficacy may not be universally established, so it's essential to discuss its use with your doctor.

Carvedilol 3.125 mg half tablet:

Carvedilol is a beta-blocker that is commonly prescribed for heart failure. It helps in reducing the workload on the heart and improving cardiac function. The starting dose is often low to minimize side effects, and it is gradually increased as tolerated. Carvedilol has been shown to be effective in managing heart failure symptoms and improving outcomes in certain patients.

Dytor Plus 20 mg thrice daily:

Dytor Plus is a combination medication that contains torsemide (a diuretic) and spironolactone (an aldosterone antagonist). Diuretics help in removing excess fluid from the body and can be beneficial in managing fluid retention and symptoms associated with heart failure. Spironolactone, in particular, can also help in reducing the progression of heart failure and improving survival in certain cases.

Restrict fluid intake to 1 liter per day:

Limiting fluid intake is often recommended for patients with heart failure to prevent excessive fluid accumulation in the body. This can help reduce symptoms like shortness of breath and swelling. The recommended fluid restriction may vary depending on individual factors, so it's crucial to follow your doctor's guidance on this.

Restrict salt intake:

Reducing salt (sodium) intake is important for heart failure patients to minimize fluid retention and manage blood pressure. Excessive salt consumption can lead to fluid buildup and worsen heart failure symptoms. Following a low-sodium diet can be beneficial in managing the condition.

Again, I must emphasize that these treatment recommendations are general in nature and may not be suitable for everyone. Your healthcare provider will tailor the treatment plan based on your specific condition, medical history, and other relevant factors. It's essential to communicate openly with your doctor about any concerns or questions you may have regarding your treatment regimen. They can provide the most appropriate guidance and monitor your progress to ensure the best possible outcomes for your heart health.

an example of a case study, where a patient could use ChatGPT to understand their diagnosis.

Automation of Administrative Tasks

Large language models help in automation of various administrative tasks like discharge summaries, International Classification of Diseases (ICD) coding of diagnoses, and patient communication.

We hereby present a sample discharge summary written by ChatGPT for a 60-year-old gentleman who presented with acute anterior wall ST-elevation myocardial infarction (STEMI) and underwent a primary percutaneous coronary intervention (PTCA) to left anterior descending artery (LAD) and discharged in moderate left ventricular (LV) systolic dysfunction **(Box 3)**.[4]

LIMITATIONS OF LARGE LANGUAGE MODELS

While LLMs like ChatGPT have enormous potential in assisting with the practice of cardiology, their limitations must be accounted for before any widespread adoption. Here are some possible pitfalls:

- Insufficient fine-tuning on the latest advancements in the field leading to inaccuracies in responses and irrelevant recommendations for medical practice. Moreover, the fine-tuning task itself would require careful aggregation of the relevant literature and technical expertise.
- LLMs cannot replace the judgment of clinicians: While LLMs can be useful in understanding patient summaries,

BOX 3 A sample discharge summary by ChatGPT.

Patient Name: [Patient's Full Name] Date of Admission: [Date of Admission] Date of Discharge: [Date of Discharge] Age: 60 years Medical Record Number: [MRN] Diagnosis: Anterior Wall ST-Elevation Myocardial Infarction (STEMI) with Moderate Left Ventricular Dysfunction

Clinical Course: Mr. [Patients Last Name] was admitted to [Hospital Name] on [Date of Admission] with complaints of severe chest pain and difficulty breathing. He was diagnosed with an anterior wall ST-elevation myocardial infarction (STEMI) based on clinical presentation and electrocardiogram (ECG) findings. Urgent revascularization was initiated, and the patient underwent a primary percutaneous coronary intervention (PTCA) to the left anterior descending artery (LAD). The procedure was successful in restoring coronary blood flow, and subsequent angiography revealed a patent LAD with no significant residual stenosis.

Treatment and Management: Upon admission, the patient was immediately started on dual antiplatelet therapy (aspirin and clopidogrel) and intravenous heparin. Echocardiography confirmed moderate left ventricular (LV) dysfunction with an ejection fraction (EF) of [EF%], consistent with the location and extent of the myocardial infarction. The patient was closely monitored in the coronary care unit (CCU), and appropriate heart failure medications, including beta-blockers, ACE inhibitors (or ARBs), and diuretics, were initiated and titrated to optimize LV function and manage symptoms.

Discharge Plan: Following a [length of stay] in the hospital, Mr. [Patient's Last Name] has made significant clinical improvement. His symptoms of chest pain and shortness of breath have alleviated. Repeat echocardiography prior to discharge confirms moderate LV dysfunction with an improved ejection fraction of [EF%]. The patient has been educated about heart-healthy lifestyle modifications, including a low-sodium diet, regular exercise, smoking cessation, and medication adherence.

Medications at Discharge:

- Aspirin [Dose]
- Clopidogrel [Dose]
- [Beta-Blocker Name] [Dose]
- [ACE Inhibitor or ARB Name] [Dose]
- [Diuretic Name] [Dose]
- [Other Medications, if applicable]

Follow-Up: Mr. [Patient's Last Name] is scheduled for regular follow-up appointments with Dr. [Cardiologist's Name] at [Hospital/Clinic Name] on [Date]. He will undergo further assessment of his LV function and optimization of his medical regimen as needed. The patient has been advised to monitor his blood pressure, weight, and any signs of worsening heart failure symptoms. In case of any concerning symptoms or emergent issues, he is instructed to seek immediate medical attention.

Instructions: The patient and his family have been educated about the importance of adhering to medications, lifestyle modifications, and regular follow-up appointments. They have received comprehensive instructions on recognizing warning signs of heart-related complications and have been provided with emergency contact information.

Conclusion: Mr. [Patient's Last Name] has been successfully treated for an anterior wall STEMI with primary PTCA to the LAD. His LV dysfunction has improved with medical management, and he is being discharged with a comprehensive plan for ongoing care and rehabilitation.

Discharging Physician: [Your Name] [Your Title] [Date of Discharge]

This discharge summary is meant to provide a general template. Please consult with the patient's healthcare team to ensure accurate and personalized information is included in the summary.

they cannot directly replace the expertise of healthcare professionals. For example, one study showed that ChatGPT gave inappropriate responses pertaining to inclisiran and low-density lipoprotein (LDL) levels, which could potentially result in misunderstanding of patient diagnosis and suggest incorrect treatment recommendations.[10]

- The use of LLMs in research, particularly for writing scientific papers or grant proposals, raises ethical concerns. Validation of information generated by LLMs through human domain experts becomes crucial.

CONCLUSION

ChatGPT is one of the many language models which continues to evolve and has a huge potential in medical field including cardiology. These models help in addressing the shortcomings of present practice and streamline the patient care in future. Although there are a lot of obstacles in the form of accessibility, validation, medicolegal implications, etc., there seems to be never-ending enthusiasm among physicians and patients in this area which is going to be the future of healthcare and not just another recreational application.

ONLINE REFERENCES

Please scan the QR code provided at the end of the table of contents for References of this chapter.

CHAPTER 5

Digital Technology in Heart Failure Management: Hope, Hype, or just Hep?

Prayaag Kini, Reeta Varyani

ABSTRACT

Heart failure (HF) patient cohort is an ever-growing population owing to higher longevity in current times. HF management has grown by leaps and bounds with the advent of the "Fantastic Four" concept of pharmacological management; yet there is a growing need of managing HF remotely after patient discharge to facilitate "continuity of care". The use of drugs such as angiotensin receptor-neprilysin inhibitor (ARNI) and sodium-glucose cotransporter-2 inhibitors (SGLT-2Is) combined with electronic devices for HF management has thrown up new vistas; however, there is need of continuous innovation to facilitate patient-end management and remotely monitor data from physician perspective. Also COVID epidemic brought in an urgent need to remotely manage disease in various dimensions and in a unique way facilitated the advent and use of more Artificial Intelligence (AI)-based healthcare management in general. AI has in last few years to a decade demonstrated significant capability to radically change nearly all areas of HF including diagnosis, device-guided accurate "measurement" and monitoring, eventually leading to better management. AI possesses the capability to perform tasks using similar-to-human capability by receiving input data, learning semantics from observing patterns in it, predicting results based on variates appearing repeatedly and thus formulating an analysis using various algorithms and cognitive computing eventually culminating in creation of an algorithm. In the cardiac sphere, AI can analyse raw image data from cardiac imaging techniques like electrocardiography, echocardiography, computed tomography, cardiac MRI amongst others to generate input data. AI and machine learning (ML)-based HF diagnosis using AI-Clinical Decision Support System (AI-CDSS), and deep learning with convolutional neural networks for image analysis are other exciting topics of ongoing research. The use of decision trees by rough Sets (RS), and logistic regression (LR) methods utilized to construct decision-making model to diagnose congestive HF, and role of AI in early detection of future mortality and destabilization episodes has played a vital role in optimizing cardiovascular disease outcomes. Wearables for HF and rhythm monitoring such as Apple Watch, the wearable Zio patch and the wear-on μCor patch should be accurate for clinical use, and considered more than just fancy gadgetry. Remote monitoring with devices such as remote dielectric sensing (ReDS) and intrathoracic impedance monitoring devices for HF are already on the horizon for clinical use. Eventual patient management should remain in clinical domain with digital technology playing a supportive role for the same.

Keywords: Digital health, heart failure, remote monitoring, wearables, sustainability.

INTRODUCTION

Clinical medicine, especially cardiovascular medicine, has made tremendous strides in both diagnostic and therapeutic armamentaria, leading to higher longevity and more patients surviving to older ages in the last two decades. The fallout is a unique challenge of managing a new and ever-increasing cohort of heart failure (HF) patients that has worldwide led to higher morbidity and financial implications. It is estimated that by 2030, 9.8 million people ≥18 years of age will be living with HF, representing ~50% increase in prevalence compared to 2012,[1,2] with almost half of the patients dying within 5 years of initial diagnosis.[2,3] Despite the availability of newer, effective, evidence-based treatment options such as angiotensin receptor-neprilysin inhibitor (ARNI) and the gliflozins, the prognosis remains uncertain for this subset of patients. This has ushered in the need of digital health and remote monitoring (RM) at home post-discharge, including but not limited to implantation of electronic devices which primarily use artificial intelligence (AI) for their functioning.

Where is the trade-off between expensive "fancy" digital healthcare (DH) gadgetry and effective management of HF, as of circa 2023?

RISE OF DIGITAL HEALTHCARE DESPITE THE OBITUARY OF IBM WATSON

Just over a decade ago, AI made one of its showier forays into the public's consciousness when IBM's Watson computer appeared on the American quiz show Jeopardy! that subsequently led its foray into making a bigger splash in oncological disease and management.[4] Although the machine triumphed comfortably, the next decade exemplified the numerous shortcomings of applying AI to healthcare. The brouhaha finally ended in 2022 when it was realized that data entry could be time-consuming and labor-intensive for a relatively small payoff, leading to MD Anderson finally backing out of its partnership with Watson. The two key failures of the Watson cited were interoperability and data collection and management. Watson XAI (using eXplainable AI) has resurfaced in the last 2 years—this "simpler" version of Watson based on machine learning (ML), holding more real-life applicability as per IBM.[5]

ADVENT OF DIGITAL TECHNOLOGY AND ARTIFICIAL INTELLIGENCE FOR HEART FAILURE MANAGEMENT

Digital health entails the use of various forms of information and communications technology to monitor patient health with the aim of improving outcomes of care for HF at the patient end, even after he or she is physically distanced from the treating primary physician. Mobile healthcare or "mHealth," a subset of digital health, involves the use of mobile wireless technologies to the same end[6,7] and has been applied to even diagnosis of HF using ML techniques.[7] There is ample evidence today that supports the potential role of digital health across the entire spectrum of HF, including primary prevention, early detection, and treatment options for HF, eventually reducing associated morbidity and mortality.

The diagnosis of HF can be difficult, even for HF specialists. Artificial Intelligence-Clinical Decision Support System (AI-CDSS) was designed with the potential to assist physicians in HF diagnosis using a hybrid (expert-driven and ML-driven) approach of knowledge acquisition to evolve the knowledge base with HF diagnosis. A retrospective cohort of 1,198 patients with and without HF was used for the development of AI-CDSS (training dataset, $n = 600$) and to test the performance (test dataset, $n = 598$). A prospective clinical pilot study of 97 patients with dyspnea was used to assess the diagnostic accuracy of AI-CDSS compared with that of non-HF specialists. In retrospective cohort, the concordance rate was 98.3% in the test dataset. The concordance rate for patients with HF with reduced ejection fraction (EF), HF with mid-range EF, HF with preserved EF, and no HF was 100%, 100%, 99.6%, and 91.7%, respectively. In a prospective pilot study of 97 patients presenting with dyspnea to the outpatient clinic, the concordance rate between AI-CDSS and HF specialists was a whopping 98%, whereas that between non-HF specialists and HF specialists was 76%. Thus, AI-CDSS showed a high diagnostic accuracy for HF and may be useful especially when HF specialists are not immediately available.

DID CORONAVIRUS DISEASE 2019 OPEN UP THE CASCADE OF DIGITAL HEALTHCARE AVENUES?

As more of the medical world becomes digitally empowered and "cloud connected," technology can reach the patient's bedside remotely for better HF management. OptiVol[8] and CardioMEMS[9] were two evidence-based devices already in use for RM for fluid management in HF patients. The coronavirus disease 2019 (COVID-19) pandemic forced healthcare systems to reevaluate the widespread adoption of DH approaches to HF diagnosis and care.[10] Self-monitoring of blood glucose (SMBG) or management of sugars in diabetic patients using sensors had already opened new avenues to active patient participation with limited physician contact.[11] This was closely followed by self-management of blood pressure to reduce the risk of HF rehospitalization and mortality due to HF. Reimbursement mechanisms were also forced to keep pace parallelly to enhance the usage of these DH technologies.[12]

APPLICATION OF ARTIFICIAL INTELLIGENCE-BASED DIGITAL TOOLS FOR MANAGEMENT OF HEART FAILURE

Digital technology that incorporates clinical data recording, combined with clinician feedback and structured follow-up, appears to be more efficacious and has been proven to reduce hospital readmissions.[12] Multiple forms of noninvasive mobile digital technology are now available to assist in the optimal management of HF patients, such as teleconsultations, SMS systems, smartphone applications, wearables, and RM systems **(Figs. 1 and 2)**.

Teleconsultation

Teleconsultation employs the facilities of enhanced communications technology to enable the physician to consult with patients at a distance and has been a possible solution to overburdened outpatient HF clinics. The ESC has even set guidelines on the management of HF via RM much before its enhanced popularity with the advent of the COVID-19 pandemic.[13,14]

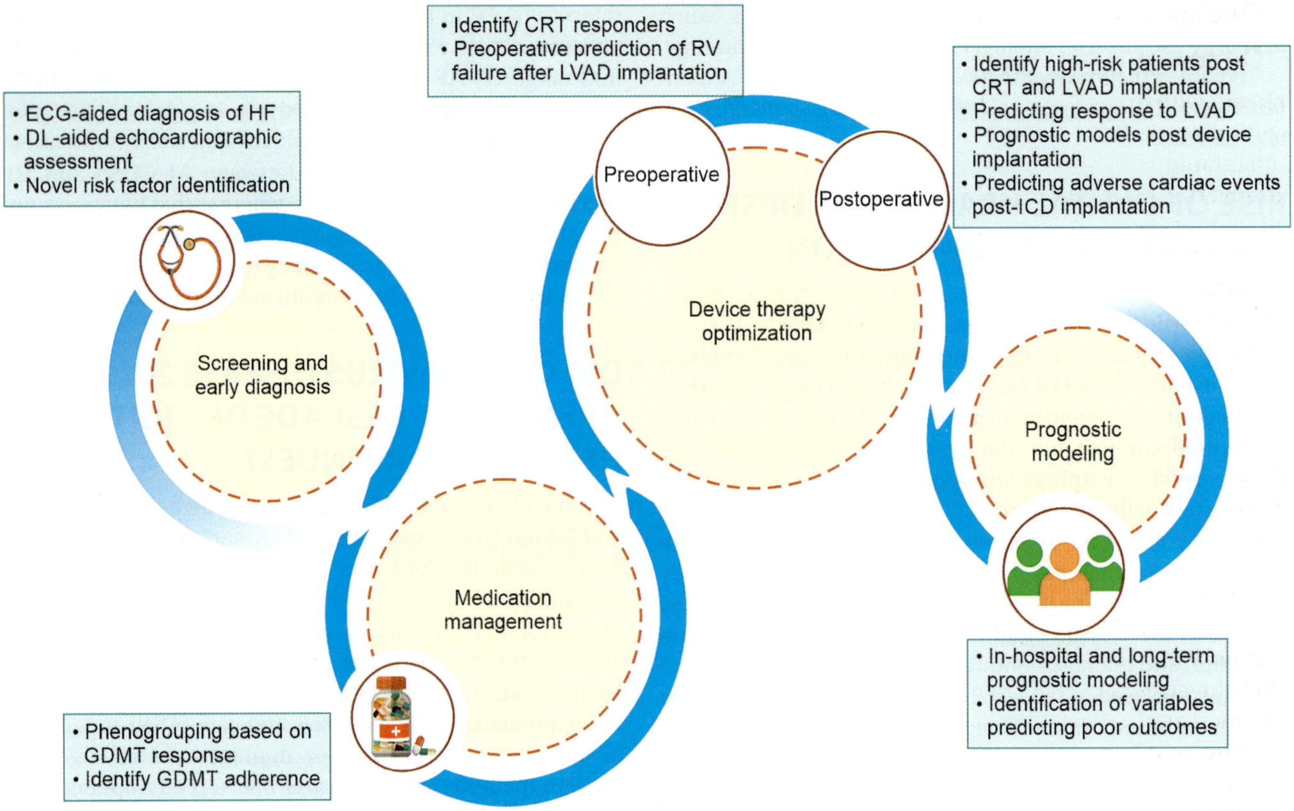

FIG. 1: Spectrum of applications of AI in HF management.

(AI: artificial intelligence; CRT: cardiac resynchronization therapy; DL: deep learning; ECG: electrocardiogram; GDMT: guideline-directed medical therapy; HF: heart failure; ICD: implantable cardioverter defibrillator; LVAD: left ventricular assist device; RV: right ventricular)

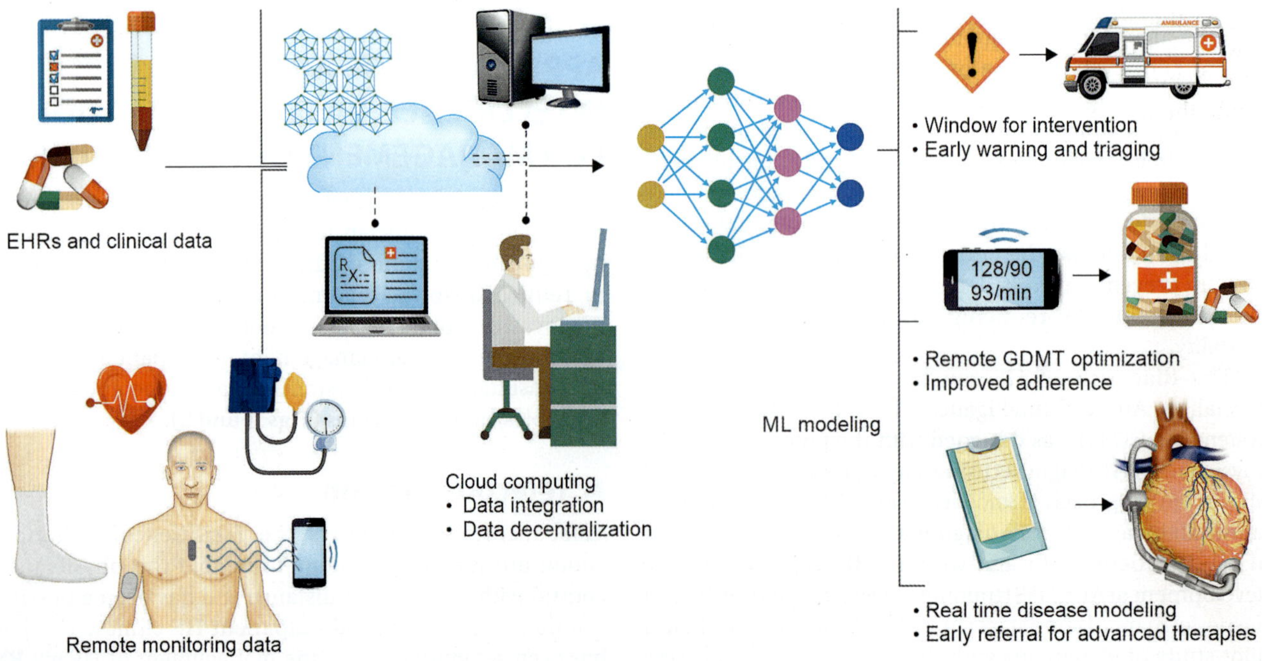

FIG. 2: Managing data accrued from remote monitoring facilities.

(EHRs: electronic health records; GDMT: guideline-directed medical therapy; ML: machine learning)

Device-based Monitoring for Decompensation of Heart Failure

Patients with symptomatic HF with severely reduced left ventricular ejection fraction (LVEF) are advised cardiac implantable electronic devices such as an implantable cardioverter defibrillator (ICD) or cardiac resynchronization therapy (CRT). These devices are periodically "interrogated" to monitor device alerts for arrhythmias, therapies provided by the machine, and device longevity and elective replacement indicators such as battery voltage. Most modern devices can wirelessly be monitored from a central healthcare specialist facility or heart station by enabling Bluetooth facilities using smartphone applications.

Intrathoracic impedance monitoring (IIM) correlates well with pulmonary fluid content, multiparametric monitoring incorporating detection of heart sounds and concomitantly studying intrathoracic impedance, patient heart rate, and heart rate variability with physical activity carries more promise scientifically **(Fig. 3)**.

The LIMIT-CHF (Lung Impedance Monitoring in Treatment of Chronic Heart Failure) trial[15] randomized to either the active group (IIM alarm turned on and diuretic dose increased by 50% for 1 week in the event of alarm sounding) or the control group (IIM alarm turned off) found no unplanned HF visits in the active group versus 0.1 ± 0.3 per patient in the control group. In another study, patients were studied with an implantable device at nine English hospitals over an average of 2.8 years to adjust therapies based on temporal results. Though it failed to show a clear mortality benefit, refined iterations of this model in time to come may prove beneficial with larger data volume. Ongoing studies may expand the choice of location of IIM, allowing a more personalized approach. Implant sites currently under investigation in first-in-human safety trials include the inferior vena cava (FUTURE-HF trial) and the left atrium [VECTOR-HF (V-LAP™ Left Atrium Monitoring systEm for Patients With Chronic sysTOlic and Diastolic Congestive heaRt Failure) trial]. Placed in the interatrial septum, preliminary results from the left atrial pressure sensor show it is likely to be safe—the readings showing a strong correlation with invasive pulmonary artery pressure (PAP) measurements and improvement in New York Heart Association (NYHA) class based on device-guided therapy.[16]

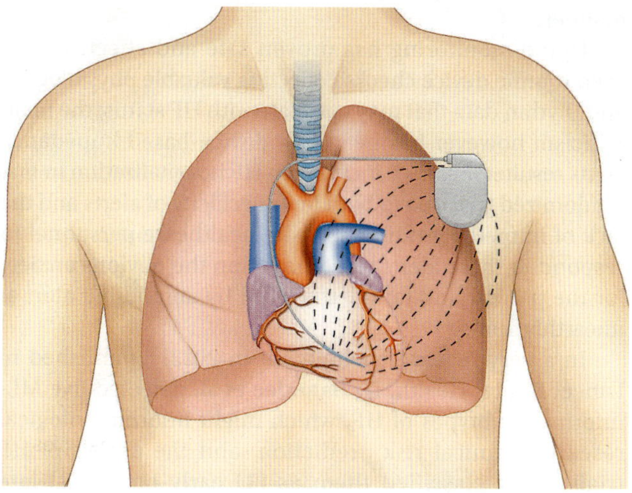

FIG. 3: Intrathoracic impedance monitoring (IIM).

The HeartLogic algorithm (Boston Scientific) was able to identify HF decompensation with a sensitivity of 70% and an unexplained alert rate of only 1.47 per patient-year, with a median lead time of 34 days before the HF event.[17] Implantable hemodynamic monitors have shown promise at preventing HF hospitalization with early detection of rise in PAP in response to increasing intracardiac left ventricular (LV) end-diastolic pressures typically preceding symptoms by up to 2–3 weeks.

Remote Dielectric Sensing (ReDS™) (Sensible Medical, USA) is an easy-to-use, noninvasive system for the monitoring and management of lung fluid in patients with HF and other chronic diseases requiring lung fluid level monitoring. ReDS technology originated in the defense technology that allows the military to see through walls and find survivors in the rubble of collapsed buildings. This was adapted for medical use by creating a system to see through the "walls" of the chest and inside the lungs of HF patients. It takes less than a minute to get a ReDS measurement at the hospital, clinic, or even in the comfort of a patient's home **(Fig. 4)**.

The use of the ReDS noninvasive lung fluid monitoring system to assess readiness for discharge in patients hospitalized with acute HF was evaluated in a pilot study by Bensimhon et al. who performed[18] ReDS measurement for all patients once they were deemed ready for discharge. Patients in the treatment arm with residual lung congestion defined by ReDS ≥ 39% had HF consultation and further diuresis. Of 108 HF patients [50% male, age 73.6 ± 12.6 years, body mass index (BMI) 29.3 ± 4.3 kg/m^2, EF 38.5 ± 15.1%, B-type natriuretic peptide (BNP) 1138 ± 987 pg/mL], 32% demonstrated residual lung congestion at the time of proposed hospital discharge. ReDS guided therapy triggered additional diuresis in 30% of the patients in the treatment arm (average weight loss 5.6 pounds, $p = 0.02$). Patients discharged as planned with residual lung congestion with ReDS ≥ 39% had higher 30-day readmission rate compared to patients who were adequately decongested at discharge with ReDS < 39% (11.8% vs. 1.4%, $p = 0.03$). They concluded that ReDS testing demonstrated that 32% of HF patients deemed ready for discharge have clinically significant residual lung congestion which was associated with a higher risk of readmission. ReDS-guided management was associated with significant decongestion but not a reduction in HF readmissions in this sample.

A further meta-analysis on the efficacy of ReDS in the prevention of HF rehospitalizations was presented by Sattar et al. among 985 patients across seven studies.[19] Patients with HF monitored with ReDS had significantly lower odds

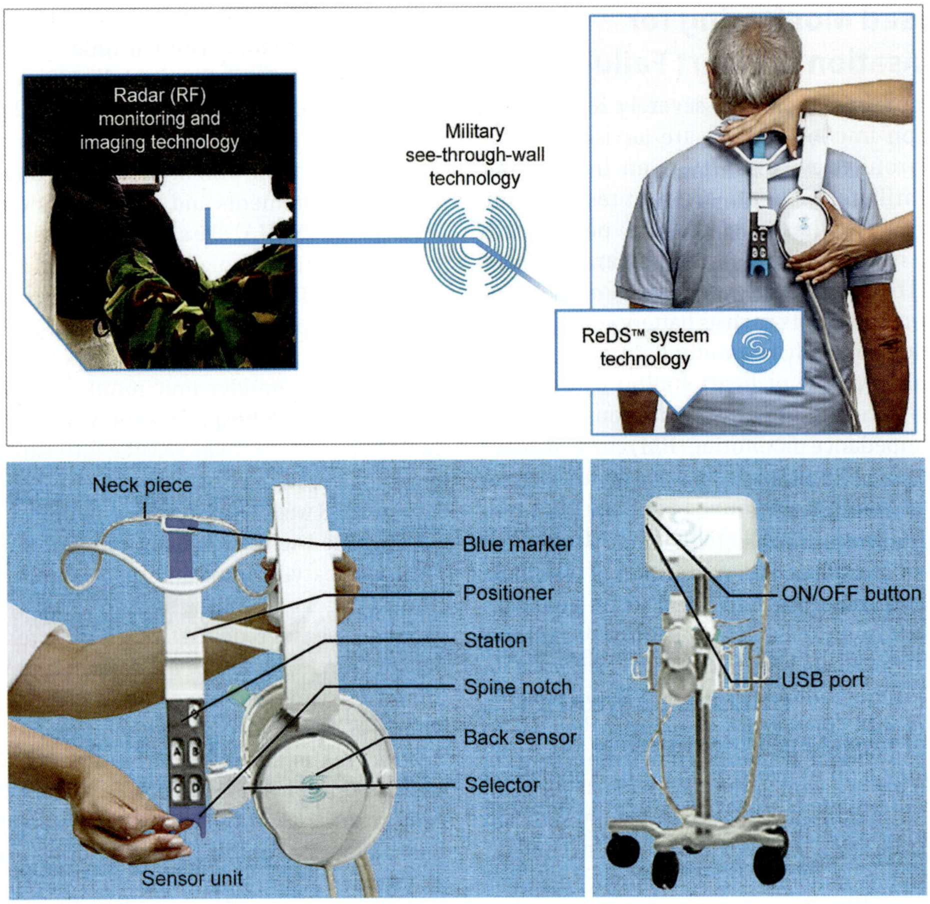

FIG. 4: Remote Dielectric Sensing (ReDS) for heart failure (HF).

of hospital readmission compared with non-ReDS patients. Subgroup analysis based on the duration of follow-up showed lower odds of readmission within 30 days as well as between 1 and 3 months. ReDS effect of lower readmissions of HF was observed irrespective of the duration of follow-up (<1 month vs. 1–3 months). ReDS monitoring significantly lowered the odds of HF readmission within 3 months compared to participants not using ReDS.

As mentioned earlier, remote daily PAP monitoring in CardioMEMS device-implanted patients had already been facilitating titration of medications, mitigating the need to be subsequently hospitalized by up to 30% and ushering in the era of AI-based fluid management.[9] The MultiSense study, MANAGE-HF (Multiple Cardiac Sensors for Management of Heart Failure) trial, and GUIDE-HF (Hemodynamic-GUIDEd Management of Heart Failure) randomized trial are more such instances in the pipeline and will impact clinical practice in the coming years.[17,20]

The European registry database shows a recent decompensation of HF portended to a 24% increased risk of death within 1 year—identification of the event before patients deteriorate therefore carries obvious implications. Simple avenues of self-monitoring by patients for their symptoms, pedal edema, weight, and blood pressure do not require complex training and can be managed even by an educated family member, and hence have been a mainstay of HF management for over two decades now and can subvert a "too little, too late" situation with patients having lost crucial time in instituting therapies in a timely manner.[21,22]

Home monitoring has proven safe and effective with even routine device checks collecting valuable physiological and rhythm data that may correlate with HF status; the main criticism however has been that device-based impedance alerts resulted in a 79% increase in HF hospitalization in one randomized trial due to both low specificity of alerts and the lack of immediate trained on-site healthcare personnel to respond to these alerts not to mention the obvious anxiety for the patient and family triggered by an audible alert at unearthly hours.[21]

In a very recent development in 2023,[22] published in Lancet Digital Health, Dr Banerjee et al. detected five ML-informed subtypes of HF, which might inform etiological research, clinical risk prediction, and the design of HF trials. They classified them as (1) early onset, (2) late onset, (3) atrial fibrillation (AF) related, (4) metabolic, and

(5) cardiometabolic. In the external validity analysis, *late onset* and *cardiometabolic subtypes* of HF were the most similar and strongly associated for hypertension, myocardial infarction, and obesity. They have developed a prototype app for routine clinical use and enable its effectiveness—large-scale use of this is eagerly awaited.

Remote Monitoring

Remote Monitoring is the use of telecommunication technologies to monitor patient status at a distance **(Fig. 5)**. In structured telephone support (STS), patients are called by a member of the HF team to discuss symptoms, drug therapy, and compliance with lifestyle measures.[23,24] STS is relatively labor intensive and costly due to gadgetry and logistic requirements, and a 2015 meta-analysis reported only a marginal mortality benefit [risk ratio (RR) 0.87 for all-cause mortality; 95% confidence interval (CI) 0.77–0.98] and reduction in HF hospitalizations (RR 0.85; 95% CI 0.77–0.93) with no effect on all-cause hospitalizations.

One randomized trial of telemonitoring in 1,571 HF patients with NYHA Class II–III symptoms and HF hospitalization in the preceding 12 months compared a wireless system, transmitting daily readings of weight, blood pressure, oxygen saturations, heart rate, and a health status questionnaire, with usual care. The composite outcome of all-cause mortality and percentage days hospitalized was reduced (RR 0.8; 95% CI 0.65–1.00). A meta-analysis of smaller randomized telemonitoring trials showed a small mortality benefit also. (RR 0.80 for all-cause mortality; 95% CI 0.68–0.94).[25]

Apps and Wearables

The last decade has seen a rapid proliferation of health apps. In 2017, it was estimated that 325,000 health apps were available on smartphones.[26] Despite this, very few of them have been designed specifically for HF patients; a 2019 review identified 10 apps focused on HF self-care available on the Apple App Store and Google Play Store. Four of these were developed by scientific societies [including the American Heart Association (AHA)] and predominantly aimed at patient education, symptom tracking, and prompting users to seek early self-care in HF.[27] While RM systems are generally "prescribed" by clinicians and often reimbursed by healthcare systems or insurance companies, apps and wearables are largely marketed directly to consumers as tools for health and lifestyle maintenance. Consumer wearables are devices that record and transmit physiological signals that can be worn, such as activity trackers and smartwatches, and these are becoming increasingly popular. Some products such as the Fitbit[28] are user-friendly and also offer irregular pulse detection, single-lead ECG, blood pressure, and oxygen saturation monitoring, and carry potential in HF self-care. The fact though remains that these wearables and HF apps have not been actually evaluated in randomized clinical trials (RCTs), and without quality evidence and clear app standards, there is need for regulation in this field.

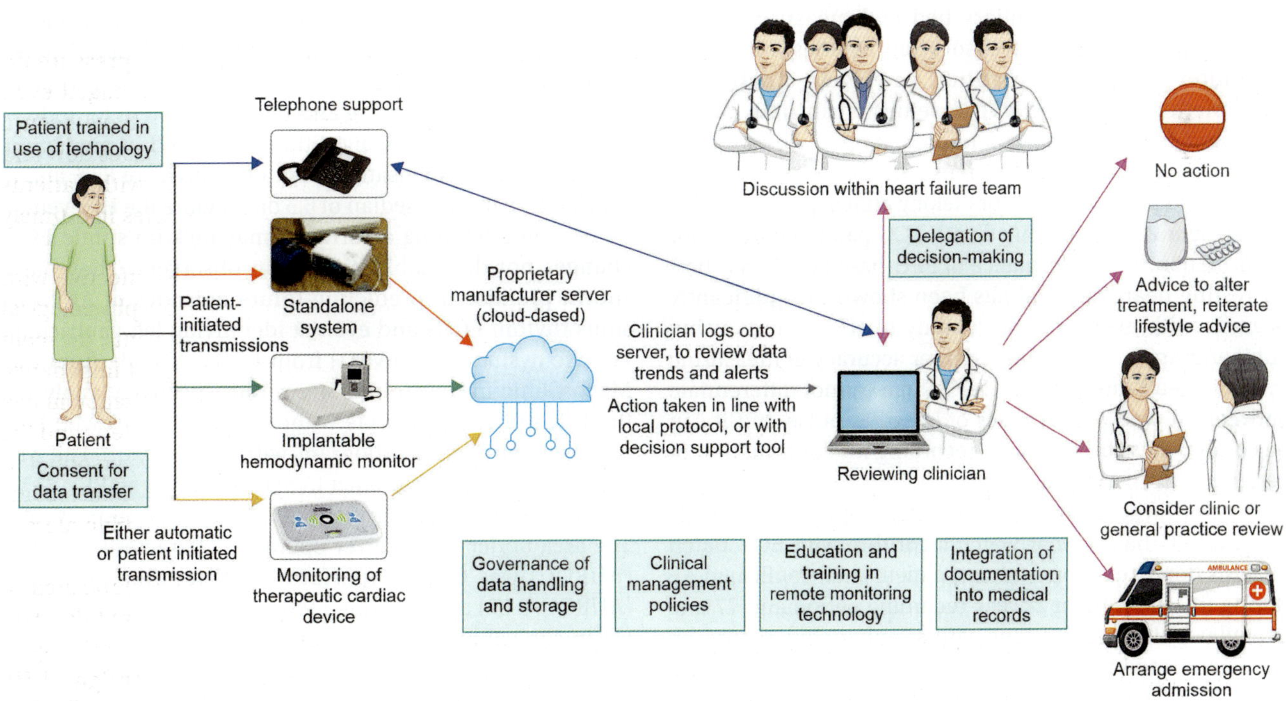

FIG. 5: Remote monitoring system's workflow for heart failure (HF) monitoring.

USING DATA FROM WEARABLES IN HEART FAILURE PATIENTS

Physical activity is an important prognostic parameter in HF and a measure of functional limitation. 6-minute walk test performance is a strong predictor of subsequent cardiac death in HF patients but is rarely used outside of research as it is cumbersome to measure. A retrospective study of 189 patients with self-reported HF showed a significant negative association between physical activity and mortality, and a prospective Japanese study of 170 HF patients showed a step count of <4,889 steps/day was a stronger predictor of mortality than VO_2 max (peak oxygen consumption, an important marker of cardiopulmonary fitness) on exercise testing.[29] However, prospective evidence of using activity monitors to guide therapy and adherence to exercise therapy in HF is lacking and not endorsed widely by authoritative bodies.[29,30] Patient acceptability of wearables, including a watch or other wrist-worn devices, is also likely to be variable.[28-30]

INCORPORATING DIGITAL TECHNOLOGY INTO ELECTRONIC HEALTH RECORDS: THE WAY AHEAD

Activity monitors in the form of a wristband/watch that use accelerometry are the most common form of wearable devices and have found easy acceptance with lay population, despite the fact that these devices have less accurate performance at low ambulation speeds.[30] Wearable heart rate monitors use photoplethysmography that relies on illumination of a capillary bed and measurement of pulsatile changes in light absorption as does an oxygen saturation probe in most critical care units. Analysis of photoplethysmogram (PPG) waveforms can help detect irregularities in pulse and therefore potentially be used for AF screening and critical decisions regarding rate or rhythm control, and potential need for lifelong anticoagulation—this especially if PPG is combined with ECG patch recording for confirmation.[31-33] Performance of PPG-based devices is best for resting heart rate and has been shown to significantly degrade with exertion, and a study of HF patients using Fitbit and Apple Watch showed poor accuracy in measuring dynamic heart rate changes. PPG alone cannot differentiate between AF and other causes of irregular pulse, but it can be combined with ECG patch recording for confirmation in patients with an irregular pulse.[32-34]

In the large-scale AF screening, Apple Heart Study using a PPG-based smartwatch algorithm with ECG patch analysis done, up to one-third of patients had confirmed AF during the subsequent 2-week recording period and 77% of irregular pulse notifications with simultaneous recording were confirmed to be AF, with atrial ectopy making up the majority of the remainder. The HEARTLINE study, recruiting 150,000 patients aged over 65 years, is investigating whether the irregular pulse detection algorithm and ECG feature lead to a reduction in stroke and death in a real-world setting.[35]

In addition to PPG and ECG features, miniature wrist oscillometric sphygmomanometers can now be incorporated into a smartwatch for blood pressure monitoring; the first such device to be licensed showed high accuracy when compared with manual blood pressure measurement at rest.[36]

MACHINE LEARNING AND DIGITAL HEALTH FOR PATIENT CARE IN HEART FAILURE

Most implanted devices can only provide short daily samples of data, but noninvasive monitors linked with smartphones can transmit continuously and allow for larger, richer datasets for analysis. ML is the proverbial "new kid on the block" in medicine, though it has been existing for decades in other fields of digital technology. ML bases itself on computers training themselves on large sample datasets to build predictive mathematical models. As the systems are able to incorporate these data with electronic health records, the resulting datasets offer the potential of studying unknown disease patterns and predictors and potentially leading to "customized" solutions (precision medicine). Algorithms using convoluted neural networks and deep learning are gaining big time on ECG and ECHO image analysis for creating stencils for more accurate, faster, and earlier diagnosis based on big data input and are exciting tools to look forward to in the future.

The LINK-HF study, for instance, investigated the use of a multisensor patch continuously measuring ECG signals, thoracic impedance, body temperature, and accelerometry in 100 HF patients with real-time continuous data uploaded to the cloud via a smartphone to create a personalized ("customized") monitoring and response system for individual patients.[37] The ML algorithm succeeded in predicting impending decompensation with a sensitivity of 88% and a specificity of 86%, a median of 6.5 days before the HF event.

Machine learning algorithms may pick up subtle ECG changes not detectable by human observers. They have shown promise in predicting future episodes of AF from sinus rhythm ECGs and even at identifying left ventricular systolic dysfunction (LVSD) from ECGs. A study from the Mayo Clinic in the United States retrospectively analyzed the ECGs of 1,606 patients without known LVSD who had a subsequent echocardiogram within 30 days.[38] The ML algorithm was able to predict LVSD (defined as an EF < 35%) with a sensitivity and specificity of 74% and 87%, respectively. The area under the receiver operating characteristic curve (AUROC) was 0.89, outperforming N-terminal pro-BNP (AUROC: 0.80) at predicting LVSD. Such algorithms are not yet in clinical practice and would need to be certified as a medical device before they would be able to be used, but they may form part of decision and diagnostic aids in the near future.

The μCor patch (Zoll) **(Fig. 6)** and Zio patch **(Fig. 7)**, equipped with an ECG monitor and radiofrequency

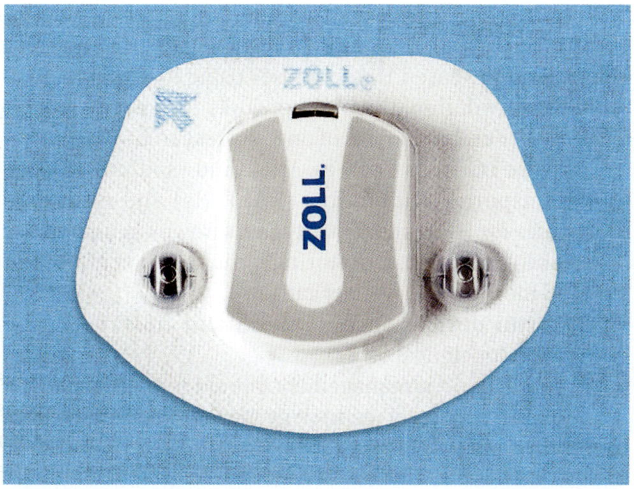

FIG. 6: μCor wear-on patch (Zoll) patch for detection of abnormal heart rhythms.

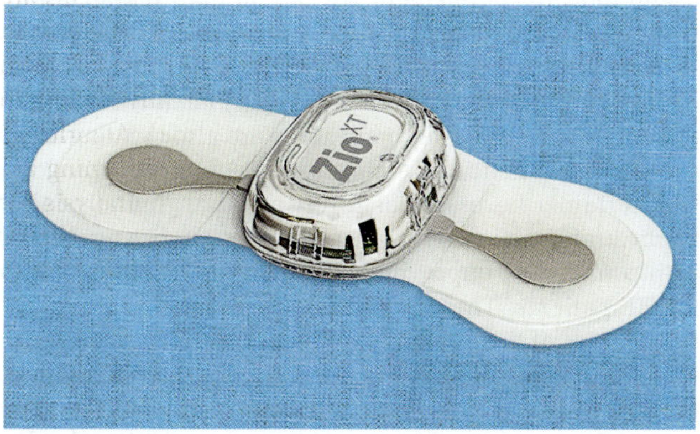

FIG. 7: Wearable Zio patch for atrial fibrillation (AF) detection.

transmitter measuring pulmonary fluid content, are under investigation for its ability to predict HF event, and a smart-textile vest with multiple electrodes measuring similar parameters to HeartLogic (heart rate, heart rate variability, respiratory rate, and thoracic impedance) is also under study.[39,40] Big data analysis will be required to determine whether such algorithms can be used to trigger an appropriate intervention to prevent the need for HF hospitalizations.

PSYCHOSOCIAL SUPPORT USING TELEMEDICINE-BASED COUNSELING IN HEART FAILURE

Artificial intelligence-enabled psychological support plays a large role in RM of HF patient cohort. Interactive voice response (IVR) allows patients to communicate with clinicians asynchronously using a mobile or landline telephone. Based on their responses, the patients can receive tailored feedback during the same call from the physician and also facilitate peer-to-peer support among older adults with HF by contacting them once a week using a toll-free IVR phone system.[41] Studies have noted positive effects and an improvement in depressive symptoms. In a study of HF patients using IVR by Zan et al., it was found that HF-related quality of life (QOL) scores improved from baseline in almost all participants, with the latter feeling more connected to their healthcare provider team. Studies by Clark et al. demonstrated a high acceptability rate of 78% for IVR system-(IVRS)-based technologies, especially in elderly patients due to increased engagement and support that may alleviate loneliness and social isolation.

There is ample evidence today for the benefit in HF patients accruing from tele-based psychological support and counseling. The BEAT-HF (Better Effectiveness After Transition–Heart Failure) study by Ong et al. in 2016 offered detailed HF patient education and counseling on medicines prior to hospital discharge to the patient and family, regularly scheduled telephone coaching, and home telemonitoring of symptoms and concluded that telephone support improved the QOL for patients 180 days after hospital discharge.[42] Kolasa et al. in 2020 have shown that telephone contact to a trained nurse with access to a family physician can prevent hospitalization in a quarter of HF patients. In a multisite RCT of the CASA (Collaborative Care to Alleviate Symptoms and Adjust to Illness) intervention by Bekelman et al. in 2018, it was found that secondary outcomes of depression and fatigue, both difficult symptoms to treat in HF, did improve by telecounseling.[43] In yet another RCT by Pekmezaris in 2018 that compared telemedicine versus a comprehensive outpatient management program, there was a demonstrated reduction in both anxiety and depression over the study period of 90 days.[44] Koehler et al., in the TIM-HF2 (Telemedical Interventional Management in Patients with Heart Failure) study in 2018, studied the efficacy of a structured remote patient management intervention in HF patients—there was significant improvement in the QOL and reduction in the rate of lost days due to unplanned hospital admissions for cardiovascular causes and mortality from any cause.[45] Studies by Mao-Huan et al. and Kuan et al. found that HF patients who received diet, medication, and lifestyle teaching via real-time IVRS with nurses improved their mental health status, QOL scores, and decreased rehospitalization over a 1-year period.[46,47]

BARRIERS TO "BLANKET APPLICATION" OF DIGITAL TECHNOLOGY FOR HEART FAILURE PATIENTS

Healthcare is human science and technology ought to reflect the clinical nature of it. Technology firms marketing health apps and wearable devices "sell" their products online as "health and wellness" products rather than tools for disease management. Currently, there is no clinical regulatory authority checking their claims and accuracy and few RCTs have validated their use in large-scale populations—for the common man, they are more appealing and fancier than the need to be truly reflective of devices used for improving healthcare status.[48] "Black-box decisions" made by programs such as IBM Watson could not explain clinical real-life events, leading to their questionability. Artifacts during recording or transmission add to fear and confusion, impeding their wider applicability, especially for AF detection. Privacy policies and legalities involved due to data protection regulations of many medical apps and wearables may not meet standards set for data storage, control, and processing by the Food and Drug Administration (FDA).[13,49] Incorporating wearable data into electronic health records needs a dedicated and savvy workforce since it requires manual input.

Second Big Barrier in the Sustainability of this Healthcare System[49,13]

Digitalization and use of technology comes with a cost—the "COST"!! Teleconsultation following the detection of an abnormal rhythm or alert is associated with a significant start-up cost for equipment and requires personnel training and software licenses. Following the COVID-19 pandemic, there has been a big push on this front, but still RM systems need to prove themselves on both counts, clinical and cost-effectiveness, in different healthcare settings, both in nations where third-party payment for healthcare facilities is the norm and in countries such as India where it is not and patients pay out of their pocket for the same.

KEY POINTS

- HF cohort is an ever-increasing population with continuing research happening into its myriad etiologies, early diagnosis, treatment, and avenues for home monitoring after discharge.
- AI- and ML-based HF diagnoses using AI-CDSS and DL with convolutional neural networks for image analysis are other exciting topics of ongoing research.
- The use of drugs such as ARNI and sodium-glucose cotransporter-2 inhibitors (SGLT-2Is) and electronic devices for HF management have thrown up new vistas; wearables for HF monitoring should be accurate and used more than just fancy gadgetry.
- RM with devices such as ReDS and IIM are on the horizon for clinical use.
- Eventual patient management should remain in clinical domain with digital technology playing a supportive role for the same.

CONCLUSION

Digital health technologies have emerged as potentially useful tools to complement HF care in both research and clinical realms. As they continue to play an increasing role in transforming healthcare delivery at the patient bedside by allowing RM facilities and bringing healthcare at the patient bedside after discharge, they are also creating their own framework for effective use. Regulatory practices will certainly be essential to ensure that digital health applications maintain accuracy and patient privacy along with consistently improving outcomes and enhancing care for HF patients. They should not encroach upon clinical sensibilities of the treating physicians by always keeping in mind that medicine is eventually a science on humans and not tech gadgetry.

ONLINE REFERENCES

Please scan the QR code provided at the end of the table of contents for References of this chapter.

CHAPTER 6

Prediction of Sudden Cardiac Death and Application of Machine Learning

Aftab Khan, Navanil Biswas

ABSTRACT

Sudden cardiac death (SCD) is one of the major and unexpected ailments in the cardiovascular disease spectrum affecting the community, causing a lot of suffering and devastation to the affected families. Predicting SCD is one of the more important research targets undertaken, which has unfortunately yielded very poor results till now. With the advent of artificial intelligence (AI) and machine learning (ML), however, this scenario is about to undergo a momentous change, more so because of the ability of these deep learning programs to assess and interpret huge volumes of data, well outside the scope of human interpretation. This chapter deals with the basic understanding of SCD and the progress made by ML in predicting SCD, so that proper preventive steps can be taken to recognize as well as alleviate this "Bolt from the Blue".

Keywords: Sudden cardiac death, risk prediction, primary prevention, artificial intelligence.

INTRODUCTION

Sudden cardiac death (SCD) remains the most common cause of death worldwide, and accounts for >50% of all cardiovascular deaths. It manifests as unexpected cardiovascular collapse from an underlying cardiac cause. Prediction of this entity is all the more important because most episodes occur in persons without any history of cardiac ailments. SCD may occur in both in the community and in the healthcare setting, but in either case, the outcomes are very dismal. On an average, only around 8% of those who receive community-based resuscitation measures survive, and in the hospitals, the outcomes are only slightly better. These outcomes can be improved by better training of the general population in basic resuscitation measures, increasing availability of defibrillators in public places, wider use of preventive measures by the physicians, and improving postresuscitation care protocols in the hospitals. However, the main interest in recent times is on the prediction of these SCD events, and with the rise of artificial intelligence (AI)and advent of machine learning (ML) in healthcare, this field is gaining prominence.

SUDDEN CARDIAC DEATH: A BRIEF DISCUSSION

In common parlance, SCD may be described as a sudden and unexpected pulseless event, which occurs in the absence of any noncardiac cause. However, a proper and standardized definition was required which was provided by Fisher et al. They divided SCD into two nomenclatures—"Established SCD" is defined as an unexpected death without obvious extracardiac cause, occurring with a rapid witnessed collapse, or if unwitnessed, occurring within 1 hour after the onset of symptoms. A "Probable SCD" is an unexpected death without an obvious extracardiac cause that occurred within the previous 24 hours.[1] In either of these cases, it should not occur in the setting of any end-stage chronic disease. SCD should be differentiated from the term "Sudden Cardiac Arrest" which is used to describe SCD cases, in which there is availability of specific resuscitation records, or if the individual has survived the cardiac arrest.

Sudden cardiac death usually occurs in the background of a high-risk anatomical or electrophysiological substrate, aggravated by an identifiable or unidentifiable trigger.

However, in most cases, this trigger remains unknown. The most common substrates and triggers are enumerated in **Table 1** and **Box 1**. It has been seen that in 40–50% cases, SCD is unheralded by any symptoms, and in around 30–40% cases, they are unwitnessed.

Sudden cardiac death usually occurs due to some electrical disturbance, which might be ventricular tachycardia (VT), ventricular fibrillation (VF), pulseless electrical activity (PEA), or complete asystole. Among them, VF is the underlying mechanism behind most episodes of cardiac arrest. Studies have shown that survival declines by around 10% per minute for patients in VF. Recent evidences have revealed that the prevalence of SCD cases presenting with VF is decreasing, while those with PEA are increasing. Based on the underlying arrhythmia, the survival rates also varies, with around >25% survival for VF and <2% for PEA.

Coming to the incidence of SCD, in the western world, the annual incidence of SCD varies between 50 and 100 per 100,000 population. The mean age of the affected individuals is in the mid-sixth decade, with around 40% of them having an SCD episode before 65 years. However, these are all estimates, as the recording and documentation of SCD are imprecise at best, even in the developed countries. Measures to obtain data include "verbal autopsy" which is defined as "a systematic retrospective inquiry of family members about the symptoms and signs of illness prior to death". Using this and other methods, Rao et al.[2] conducted a comprehensive study including 22,724 subjects in south India, and obtained some interesting results. They saw that 10.3% of total mortality was contributed by SCD. The mean age of SCD subjects was 60.8 ± 14 years (35–85 years), which was around 5–8 years younger than the western population. Coronary artery disease (CAD) was found to be present in 38% cases, with MI documented in at least 17% of SCD deaths. A huge majority (80.6%) had at least one major CAD risk factor among hypertension, diabetes, and smoking.

TABLE 1: Most common substrates identified in SCD subgroup.

Primary anatomical substrates	Primary electrophysiological substrates
Ischemic heart disease	Long QT syndromes
Nonischemic cardiomyopathy	Short QT syndromes
Hypertrophic cardiomyopathy	Ventricular pre-excitation (WPW syndrome)
Arrhythmogenic right ventricular dysplasia	Idiopathic VF
Valvular heart disease	Brugada syndrome
Congenital heart disease	CPVT
Anomalous coronary artery origin	

(CPVT: catecholaminergic polymorphic ventricular tachycardia; SCD: sudden cardiac death; VF: ventricular fibrillation; WPW: Wolff–Parkinson–White)

BOX 1 Common conditions identified as triggers in the occurrence of SCD.

Common triggers:
- Ischemia
- Changes in autonomic tone
- Hypoxia
- Physical exertion
- Drugs
- Dyselectrolytemia
- Myocardial toxins

(SCD: sudden cardiac death)

PREDICTING DEATH: PREDICTION AND PREVENTION OF SCD

From the above discussion, it is evident that SCD represents a sudden, unexpected, and dynamic event, which in most cases turns out to be fatal. Even in the western world, with better developed emergency medical response system, 90–95% patients do not survive this event. So, besides focusing on resuscitation, the interest has turned toward predicting this fatal event, taking recourse to the age old adage "Prevention is better than cure". A stumbling block to this approach is the paucity of information on the epidemiology, risk factors, prognosis, and the temporal trends of this condition. Both population-based and healthcare-based approaches have been studied, with emphasis on ascertaining the phenotype of the individual at risk of SCD.

In the pursuit of this objective, numerous invasive and noninvasive techniques have been developed over time to identify patients at risk of SCD. Previously, left ventricular ejection fraction (LVEF) was the common parameter used in this regard. Those who had significant LV systolic dysfunction (EF < 35%) were categorized as high risk, and advised implantable cardioverter-defibrillator (ICD), which demonstrated reduction in total, cardiac, and arrhythmic mortality, as proven by numerous clinical trials. However, recent studies confirm that LVEF is insufficient as an effective SCD risk predictor, because it lacks both sensitivity and specificity. Also, it has been seen only a very small minority (2–5% annually) of ICD qualifiable candidates actually suffer an SCD event. Furthermore, taking into account that at least 55% of men and 68% of women suffering an SCD have no clinically recognizable heart disease, identification of other risk predictors has become of paramount importance.

Since SCD results mainly from some form of electrical disturbance, there has been growing interest in using markers for prediction that reflect the arrhythmic substrate more directly, and hence enrich the prediction of SCD events. Numerous markers have been derived mainly from surface ECG that have been correlated with SCD, cardiac, as well as total mortality over the last three decades.[3] These can be classified as:

- *Indices of abnormal autonomic modulation of cardiovascular function*: Heart rate variability (HRV), heart rate turbulence, heart rate recovery from exercise, and baroreflex sensitivity
- *Indices of abnormal impulse conduction*: Signal-averaged ECG and QRS fractionation
- *Indices of abnormal repolarization*: Microvolt T-wave alternans, QT interval dynamicity, and various measures of T-wave morphology and dispersion

Among them, T-wave alternans appear to be the most accurate, as it appears to predict SCD-related events with the greatest negative predictive value. However, all the available experience derived from numerous studied suggests that multiple risk markers used in combination provides a more robust prediction of events, which is expected when one considers the complexity and diversity of electroanatomic substrates underlying SCD. Other clinical risk markers, that have been identified, but have failed clinical trials and hence not currently used for risk stratification, include LV hypertrophy, QTc prolongation, diabetes mellitus, and elevated resting heart rate. Significant ongoing efforts to identify biomarkers as well as imaging techniques that can identify key events related to inflammation and vulnerable plaque pathways, for predicting SCD due to CAD, are also underway.

Recently, a number of studies have been published which provide strong evidence for independent genetic contributions to risk of SCD, thus lending momentum to efforts aimed at the identification of variants that confer genetic susceptibility.[1] The first SCD risk predictor is genome-wide association study (GWAS) that has identified determinants of intermediate-risk traits for SCD such as the QT interval. Variants in *NOS1AP* gene have been identified as modest predictors of risk (odds ratios ≈ 1.3). Another initial GWAS from the Oregon Sudden Unexpected Death Study has identified a novel genetic locus (glypican 5) that is actually protective against SCD. A risk locus at chromosome 21q21 has been identified in patients of myocardial infarction as a significant predictor. The role of genes encoding ion channel pore-forming (e.g., *SCN5A,119 KCNQ1120*) and accessory subunits (e.g., *CACNB2121* and *SCN4B122*), as well as cytoskeletal (*SNTA1123 ANK2,124 ANK3125*) and trafficking (*CAV3126*) proteins has also been looked at as predictors of SCD. Common variants of these genes are being studied as modulators of SCD-related phenotypes: *KCNE1 D85N* as a risk factor for drug-induced torsades or the congenital long QT syndrome and *SCN5A S1103Y* as a modulator of SCD and of sudden infant death syndrome risk in African Americans are some examples of this effort.

New imaging techniques have also come into use for assessing a range of myocardial pathophysiological processes that might be implicated in the pathways leading up to SCD. Magnetic resonance-based imaging (cardiac MRI) has the ability to quantify cardiac structure and function and the presence and extent of myocardial fibrosis and ischemia. New imaging tracers using positron emission tomography can also provide measures for assessing cardiac sympathetic function. Though these sophisticated imaging techniques are promising but they still have not been tested to date in large studies, and their effectiveness as predictors of SCD remain unknown.

Thus, we see that the current methods of clinical risk prediction are inadequate and there is increasing recognition of a conspicuous lack of studies that combine panels of SCD risk markers to assess additive or synergistic effects on risk. There is an urgent need for discovery of novel risk predictors early in the natural history of conditions that predispose to SCD from large population-based studies. Facilitation of studies that combine novel risk markers and testing to create risk scores for prediction of SCD is the need of the hour. Also, it has been increasingly recognized that a viable strategy for prediction and prevention of SCD will require tools for serial assessment of risk markers over a prolonged period of time. That is where the role of AI and ML comes into being.

TERMINATOR TO THE RESCUE: THE ROLE OF ARTIFICIAL INTELLIGENCE AND MACHINE LEARNING

Currently, we are living in the era of smartphones and smart devices. Their influence has percolated into the world of cardiac devices as well. This has led to the increasing availability of electrophysiological signals collected through conventional methods (e.g., ECG) and digital health technologies (e.g. wearable devices). There already exists staggering volume of *healthcare* data—clinical notes, wearable and sensor data, medication lists, imaging, and much more—and it continues to increase astronomically, with 2 zettabytes (1 zettabyte = 1 trillion gigabytes) being produced in 2020 alone. To put it simply "the complexity of medicine now exceeds the capacity of the human mind", ML is the use of computer algorithms that can learn complex patterns from these vast amount of data.[4] There are several types of ML algorithms, from decision trees and support vector machines to highly complex, data-hungry algorithms called neural networks. Neural networks are used in deep ML [deep learning (DL)] and their ability to analyze large amounts of highly complex data. DL, therefore, refers to the part of a broader family of ML methods, which is based on artificial neural networks with representation learning. The adjective "deep" in DL refers to the use of multiple layers in the network. Methods used can be either supervised, semi-supervised, or unsupervised. The EAGLE (ECG AI-Guided Screening for Low Ejection Fraction) trial[5] was among the first to specifically evaluate the use of an AI-tool for screening of heart failure patients in an integrated, real-world workflow using ECG. The EAGLE trial successfully demonstrated that use of the AI-ECG model significantly increased the number of low LVEF diagnoses. Similarly, the use of all the available healthcare data in combination with novel predictive analytics using ML and DL holds incredible potential for personalized predictions of arrhythmic events, and by extension in the prediction and prevention of SCD **(Fig. 1)**.

Two important concepts in DL are: (1) *convolutional neural networks* (CNNs) and (2) *recurrent neural networks (RNNs)*. In brief, the neural network is a mathematical model that is constructed with units that simulate the function of neuron cells. The unit takes multiple inputs and multiplies the input with internal weights. After summing the results, the number is inputted into a function called the activation function. The training process adjusts the internal weights such that the output approaches the given target. CNNs are designed to recognize images. It has convolutions inside, which see the edges of an object recognized on the image. RNNs are designed to recognize sequences, for example, a speech signal or a text. CNN is applied to extract features and reduce computation time in classification of patients having heart conditions using their ECG signals. CNNs are well-known in pattern recognition technique that combines feature extraction, feature reduction, and classification techniques with the use of multiple convolution layers, pooling layers, and a fully connected layer. Using these concepts, attempts have been made for risk stratification and prediction of SCD with varying levels of success, some of which have been discussed in the following text.

Zhi Yu et al.[6] developed an ML approach that uses time-dependent variables and incorporates complex interactions between risk factors, the Random Forest for Survival, Longitudinal, and Multivariate Data (RF-SLAM), to predict SCD. Time-varying variables collected at four visits were used, and 17 predictors were taken into account for prediction models. These included clinical characteristics (diabetes, prior myocardial infarction, prior stroke, and prior heart failure), electrophysiologic variables (T-wave abnormality in any of leads I, aVL, and V_6, and ST junction and segment depression in any of leads I, aVL, or V_6), medication (antihypertensive medications and antidiabetic medications), biomarkers (N-terminal pro-B-type natriuretic peptide, troponin T, troponin I, and creatinine), subclinical atherosclerotic indices (carotid intima media thickness), as well as race, sex, and visit. Predictive accuracy of this model was assessed by area under the receiver operating characteristic curve [area under the curve (AUC)]. RF-SLAM model improved prediction (mean AUC 0.83) compared to poisson regression (cross-validated mean AUC 0.75).

Yasuyuki Shiraishi et al.[7] conducted a prospective observational study in four tertiary care hospitals in Tokyo enrolling 2,559 patients hospitalized for HF, using ML to predict risk of SCD in HF patients. They used the WET-HF Registry (West Tokyo Heart Failure Registry) **(Fig. 2)** and proposed whether the combination of the ECG-AI index and conventional predictors of SCD would improve the SCD stratification among HF patients. The AI model to predict 3-year SCD was constructed using a combination of CNN and long short-term memory (LSTM), a variant of RNN. The ECG-AI index plus classical predictive guidelines (i.e., LVEF ≤35%, NYHA Class II and III) significantly improved the discriminative value of SCD [receiver operating characteristic area under the curve (ROC-AUC), 0.66 *vs.* 0.59; $p = 0.017$; Delong's test] with good calibration ($p = 0.11$; Hosmer–Lemeshow test) and improved net reclassification [36%; 95% confidence interval (CI) 9–64%; $p = 0.009$].

A lot of work in predicting SCD in the in-hospital setting has been done by Fujita, UR Acharya et al.[8] They used nonlinear features [Fractal dimension (FD), Hurst's exponent (H), detrended fluctuation analysis (DFA), approximate entropy (ApproxEnt), sample entropy (SampEnt), and correlation dimension (CD)], which were first extracted from the second-level discrete wavelet transform (DWT) decomposed ECG signal. The extracted nonlinear features were ranked using *t*-value and then, a combination of highly ranked features are used in the formulation and employment of an integrated sudden cardiac death index (SCDI). This calculated novel SCDI can be used to accurately predict SCD (4 minutes before the occurrence) by using just one numerical value 4 minutes before the SCD episode. The study results show accuracy of 94.7%, sensitivity of 95%, and specificity of 94.4% using three HRV signal features. They have also been able to predict SCD by analyzing 4 minutes of ECG signals (separately for each 1 minute interval) prior to SCD using the same methods, and have been able to achieve an accuracy of 97.3%, 89.4%, 89.4%, and 94.7% for prediction of SCD 1, 2, 3, and 4 minutes prior to the SCD onset respectively using SVM classifier. Thus, using all these proposed techniques, they were able to identify the

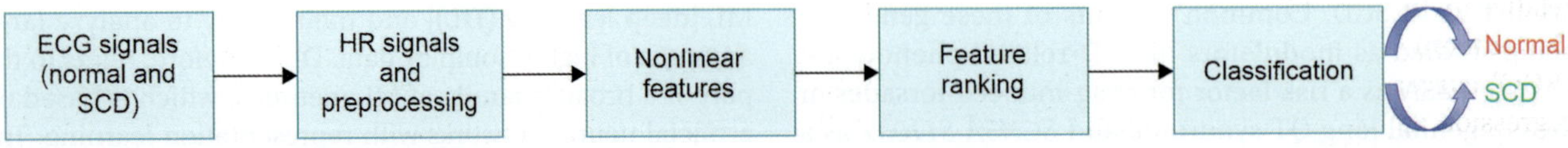

FIG. 1: Algorithm for predicting SCD using AI.

(AI: artificial intelligence; ECG: electrocardiography; HR: heart rate; SCD: sudden cardiac death)

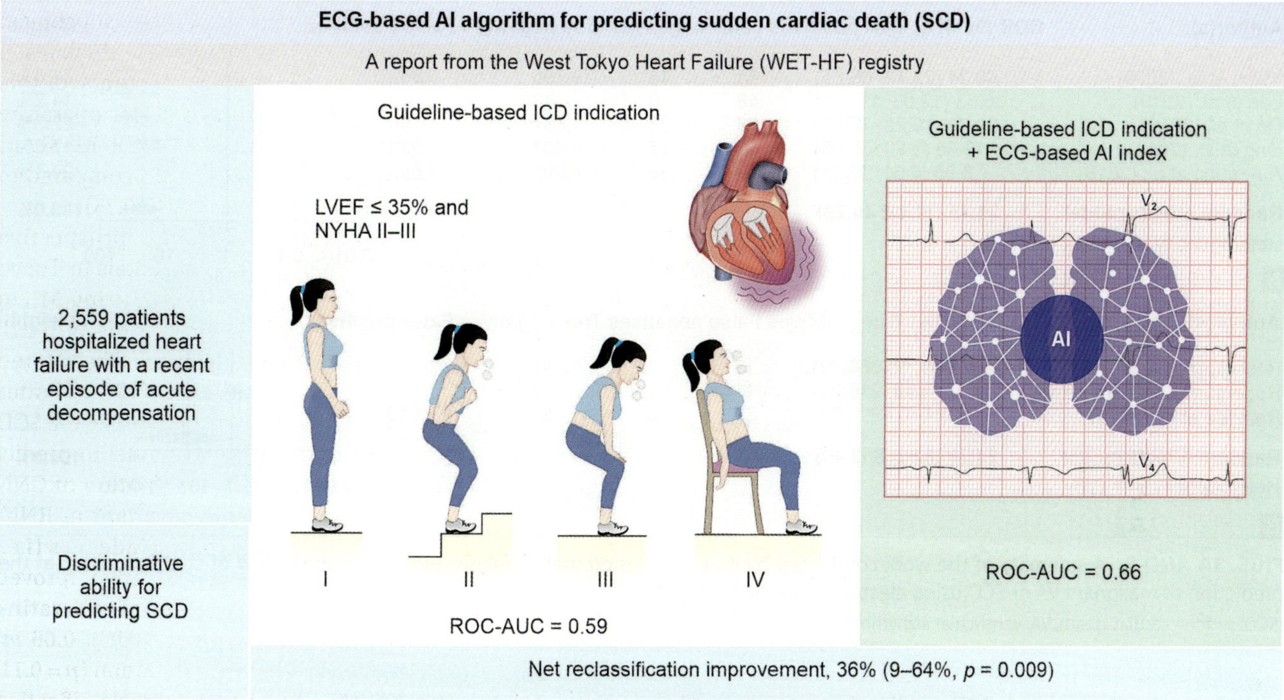

FIG. 2: Study conducted determining efficacy of AI when ECG-AI index was combined with HF parameters.

(AI: artificial intelligence; ECG: electrocardiography; HF: heart failure; ICD: implantable cardioverter-defibrillator; ROC-AUC: receiver operating characteristic area under the curve)

person at risk of developing SCD even 4 minutes earlier, thereby providing sufficient time for the emergency doctors to respond with preventive treatment in intensive care units (ICUs) and other wards. This proposed technique in the near future can thus serve as a valuable tool for increasing the survival rate of many cardiac patients.

Finally, it is important to mention the work done by Kolk et al.[9] who searched the MEDLINE (Ovid), EMBASE (Ovid), Scopus, Web of Science, and Cochrane Library Databases electronic databases to identify studies published before August 2021 that developed an ML or DL model for prediction of malignant ventricular arrhythmia (VA) or SCD using electrophysiological signals. The search identified 2,194 studies of which 46 were included in the systematic review and 32 in the meta-analysis. Pooled estimates of the diagnostic odds ratio (DOR) and summary area under the curve (AUROC) were calculated and taken into consideration. Meta-analyses were performed separately for studies using publicly available, ad-hoc datasets, and versus targeted clinical data acquisition. The DOR describes the odds of a positive prediction in those with the outcome, relative to, the odds of a positive prediction in those without the outcome. Summary receiver operator characteristic (ROC) curves were also constructed based on a bivariate regression approach. Using parametric bootstrapping, the 95% CIs around the AUROC were calculated. It was seen that most commonly, studies used HRV as model input. Other ECG features were related to the ECG morphology, such as intervals and amplitude of the QRS complex and ventricular repolarization features (e.g., T-wave alternans). Predictions horizons ranged from a time-to-event of 20 seconds until 3 hours. The pooled DOR of the seven best performing models for each of the (combination of) datasets was 282.04 (95% CI 62.96–1263.40) and the summary AUROC was 0.919 (95% CI 0.867–0.952). Pooling of individual models demonstrated a summary AUROC of 0.856 (95% CI 0.755–0.909) for short-term (time-to-event up to 72 hours) prediction and AUROC of 0.876 (95% CI 0.642–0.980) for long-term prediction (time-to-event up to years) **(Fig. 3)**.

Their work proved that ML and DL models appear to accurately predict malignant VA and SCD. They also found that the predictive performance of individual ML and DL models were generally high, and, in particular, ML and DL models derived from publicly available datasets had superior accuracy. However, these studies were characterized by a high risk of bias and methodological limitations that hinder their potential translation to clinical practice.[10]

CONCLUSION

The prediction and prevention of SCD still remain an enormous challenge. Though groundbreaking work on the remarkable insight into the genetic basis and regulation of cardiac excitability has been done, translation of this knowledge into novel strategies to identify the majority of individuals at risk of SCD is lacking. AI has the potential

Author(s)	DOR (95 CI%)	True positives	False negatives	True negatives	False positives	Weight
Kwon et al. (2020)	40.24 (23.72; 68.26)	63	18	9,795	852	21.6%
Lee et al. (2016)	36.63 (12.03; 111.54)	46	6	43	9	14.2%
Do et al. (2019)	30.89 (19.22; 49.63)	58	33	1,687	96	22.3%
Ong et al. (2012)	13.46 (5.90; 30.66)	36	7	607	232	17.8%
Au-Yeung et al. (2018)	8.95 (6.61; 12.11)	173	58	4,995	1,665	24.1%
Random effects model	**21.45 (11.42; 40.29)**					**100.0%**
Heterogeneity: I^2 = 89%						

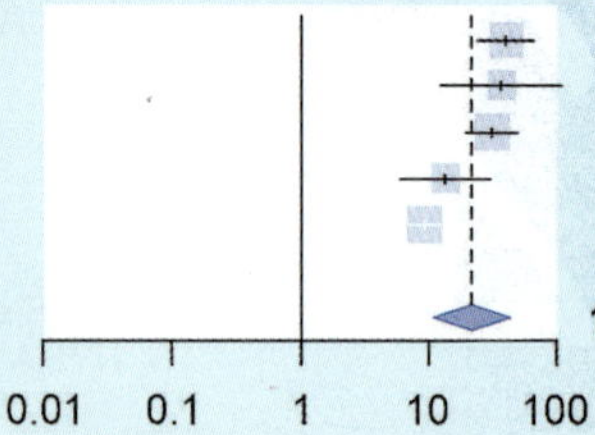

A

Author(s)	DOR (95 CI%)	True positives	False negatives	True negatives	False positives	Weight
Rodriguez et al. (2019)	624.00 (36.50; 10,666.79)	13	1	48	1	30.2%
Rogers et al. (2020)	34.38 (5.46; 216.35)	11	2	25	4	33.6%
Ramirez et al. (2015)	0.86 (0.42; 1.78)	39	10	99	449	36.1%
Random effects model	**21.79 (0.52; 913.46)**					**100.0%**
Heterogeneity: I^2 = 93%						

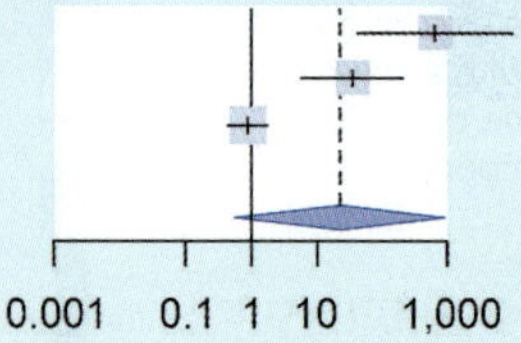

B

FIGS. 3A AND B: A summary of the work conducted by Kolk et al. using meta-analysis and systematic review of studies looking at the prediction of malignant VA or SCD using electrophysiological signals.

(SCD: sudden cardiac death; VA: ventricular arrhythmia)

to help us in this regard. ML applications can now, by using simple measures of heart and breathing rates, detect imminent collapse or hypotension within minutes. Though ML will never replace the clinician, it has the ability to provide better tools for personalized medicine—an evolving trend for over a decade, and predict the risk of SCD in high-risk individuals. Predictive models, such as the SCDI and others developed using AI, achieve high performance and enable automated and personalized predictions. However, methodological limitations have consequences for the generalizability, clinical utility, and reproducibility of these models. In order for research on the intersection of medicine and AI to be relevant and useful in clinical practice, further work has to be done.

ONLINE REFERENCES

Please scan the QR code provided at the end of the table of contents for References of this chapter.

SECTION

2 General Cardiology

CHAPTER

7

Obstructive Sleep Apnea, Blood Pressure, and Cardiovascular Outcomes: An Overview

Nagaraj Desai, Venkatesh CR, S Sunilkumar, Prabhakar Koregol

ABSTRACT

Sleep-disordered breathing as a spectrum has a significant impact on health, with obstructive sleep apnea (OSA) being its most severe form. It is imperative that a caregiver should recognize it and institute appropriate measures to mitigate its contribution to the overall clinical outcomes. Untreated OSA can potentially result in cardiovascular disease, atrial fibrillation, and hypertension. Though the exact mechanisms of development of these conditions are not fully deciphered, putative mechanisms that largely explain these changes have been proposed. Screening with questionnaires such as STOP-BANG and home sleep apnea testing (HSAT), though imperfect, are reasonable alternatives to more elaborate gold-standard polysomnography. Evidence on the treatment of OSA to prevent cardiovascular disease, atrial fibrillation, and hypertension with positive airway pressure (PAP) therapy is presented. The clinically intuitive approach to intervene early and prevent poor outcomes is still to be established more firmly with large-scale randomized controlled trials.

Keywords: Obstructive sleep apnea (OSA), OSA screening, cardiovascular disease, hypertension, atrial fibrillation, positive airway pressure (PAP) therapy.

INTRODUCTION

Sleep-disordered breathing encompasses a broad spectrum of sleep-related breathing disorders, which include obstructive sleep apnea (OSA), central sleep apnea, sleep-related hypoventilation, and hypoxemia. OSA is the most common form of sleep-disordered breathing and is highly prevalent and grossly underdiagnosed. It is characterized by episodic collapse of the upper airway during sleep, resulting in periodic reductions or cessations in ventilation, consequent hypoxia, hypercapnia, or arousals from sleep. OSA has emerged as a major cardiovascular (CV) risk in recent times. Sleep-disordered breathing and cardiovascular disease (CVD) commonly co-occur, reflecting both causal relationships and shared risk factors, such as male sex, older age, and obesity. Sleep-disordered breathing is common in people with, or at risk of, CVD, including those who are obese or have hypertension (HTN), coronary disease, heart failure, or atrial fibrillation (AF). With poorer interest among clinicians, fueled by poorer unawareness of sleep-disordered breathing among the care seekers, possibly, it is the tip of iceberg that typically gets the attention in clinical practice.

EPIDEMIOLOGY

Culturally, patients do not consider sleepiness a relevant topic to be discussed with healthcare providers.[1] The prevalence statistics are mind boggling, given the rarity of patients receiving a diagnosis of OSA. It is estimated that 10% men and 3% women aged 30–49 years have OSA, whereas the prevalence steadily increases to 17% men and 9% women in the population aged 50–70 years. The disease is grossly underdiagnosed. There are an estimated 24 million persons in the United States alone who have not received a diagnosis.[2]

Apart from resulting in symptoms such as excessive fatigue, nonrefreshing sleep, daytime sleepiness, nocturia, morning headache, irritability, and memory loss, in the long term, OSA has been found to result in CVD, metabolic disorders, cognitive impairment, and depression.[3]

PROPOSED PATHOPHYSIOLOGICAL MECHANISMS EXPLAINING THE LINK BETWEEN OBSTRUCTIVE SLEEP APNEA, CARDIOVASCULAR DISEASE, AND HYPERTENSION

The exact mechanisms of the associations between OSA and CVD are yet to be fully deciphered. Nevertheless, several important intermediate mechanisms are proposed. The role of sustained sympathetic activation, changes in the intrathoracic pressure, and nocturnal hypoxia and reoxygenation cycles due to upper airway obstruction resulting in vascular inflammation are postulated.[3]

Development of Hypertension

It is postulated that repetitive apnea or hypopnea events cause ensuing arterial desaturation and hypercapnia, which activates the sympathetic nervous system. This leads to increased systolic blood pressure (SBP) that might progress to HTN or exacerbate this condition.[4] Vasoconstriction and impaired blood pressure (BP) regulation secondary to higher levels of endothelin and lower levels of nitric oxide have been found in OSA, which may contribute to development of HTN.[5]

Another putative contribution is that of aldosterone excess in OSA. Aldosterone promotes sodium-water reabsorption. There is an overnight fluid shift to the neck in the supine position, potentially resulting in pharyngeal edema and upper airway obstruction. Clinical studies have shown a significant reduction of neck girth along with the reduction in plasma aldosterone concentration (PAC) and BP with aldosterone blockade.[6-9] Additionally, taste sensitivity for sodium chloride (NaCl) could be abnormal in aldosterone excess, thus favoring more salt intake, causing water-sodium retention.[10] Besides, significantly increased secretion of cortisol in patients with primary aldosteronism (PA) and excess aldosterone impeding myogenesis are other potential mechanisms.[11-13]

Development of Coronary Artery Disease and Atrial Fibrillation

Due to upper airway obstruction, there would be periods of hypoxia and reoxygenation. Reactive oxygen species (ROS) are induced by hypoxia, which produces hypoxia-inducible factor 1, a transcriptional activator. This activator of transcription could result in increased gene expression to transcribe proteins promoting adaptation to hypoxia. Inflammatory and immune responses are also induced by activation of endothelial cells, leukocytes, and platelets. These elaborate adhesion molecules and proinflammatory cytokines, which result in endothelial injury and dysfunction. No doubt, over a period of time, these mechanisms may eventually result in CV morbidity.[5] This has been evidenced by premature atherosclerosis, increased arterial stiffness, increased coronary calcium scores, and coronary plaque instability observed in patients with OSA.[5]

DIAGNOSIS OF OBSTRUCTIVE SLEEP APNEA

Attended in-hospital polysomnography (PSG) is currently the gold standard test for the diagnosis of sleep apnea. Apart from detecting apneas and hypopneas, it has the advantage of staging sleep, quantifying sleep fragmentation, and identifying other sleep-related phenomena.[1]

Episodes of apnea and hypopnea define sleep-disordered breathing. A complete or almost complete (>90%) cessation of airflow (measured by nasal pressure) lasting 10 seconds or longer is defined as an apnea.[3] However, the definition of hypopnea is much more complex.

Hypopnea is defined if all of the following criteria are met:

- Peak signal excursions drop by at least 30% of pre-event baseline using nasal pressure (diagnostic study), positive airway pressure (PAP) device flow (titration study), or an alternative hypopnea sensor (diagnostic study)
- Duration of at least 30% drop in the signal excursion is 10 or more seconds.
- There is 3% or greater oxygen desaturation from pre-event baseline and/or the event is associated with an arousal.

Obstructive sleep apnea is defined by ≥5 apnea and hypopnea events per hour of sleep associated with excessive sleepiness.

The apnea-hypopnea index (AHI) is widely used to diagnose and assess the severity of OSA. The AHI refers to the mean number of apneas or hypopneas per hour of sleep. An AHI of >5 on overnight PSG study is required for the diagnosis of OSA.[1,2]

The American Academy of Sleep Medicine classifies OSA as mild (AHI = 5–14.9/h), moderate (AHI = 15–29.9/h), and severe (AHI ≥ 30/h).[14] Though the classification is somewhat arbitrary, it is still very valuable in categorizing patients who potentially would benefit from PAP therapy.

SCREENING FOR OBSTRUCTIVE SLEEP APNEA

Obstructive sleep apnea is a widely underdiagnosed disease, and this cannot be overemphasized. There are logistical and financial barriers and other confounding variables that significantly hinder screening. Screening for OSA should be routine in patients with CVD given its high prevalence and as a comorbidity among such patients.[3]

To overcome the painstaking screening of patients with PSG and to triage at-risk individuals, reasonably easy-to-administer screening questionnaires have been developed. These include the Berlin questionnaire, STOP (snoring, tiredness during daytime, observed apnea and high blood pressure), STOP-BANG [STOP + BMI >35 kg/m^2 (or 30 kg/

m^2), age > 50 years, neck circumference > 40 cm and male gender], Epworth Sleepiness Scale (ESS), and 4-Variable screening tool (4-V) to name a few. These questionnaires include the assessment of OSA symptoms and risk factors. Among these, the STOP-BANG has emerged as the most sensitive screening tool and one of the easiest to administer quickly in the clinical setting.[15] However, these OSA screening questionnaires have limited specificity and poorer diagnostic accuracy in certain groups such as in women and in patients with underlying CVD. These inaccuracies have made these questionnaires less trustworthy for screening.[14] Therefore, OSA screening questionnaires, though useful, are not recommended as a replacement for formal sleep testing to diagnose or exclude OSA.[16]

A reasonable alternative to PSG is home sleep apnea testing (HSAT). This modality has the advantage of lower cost and is technically lesser complex.[17-19] It has certain limitations. Though HSAT cannot calculate an AHI, it rather provides a respiratory event index (REI). REI is calculated by the sum of apneas and hypopneas divided by the estimated sleep time. HSAT lacks the sensitivity of in-laboratory PSG. Additionally, HSAT REI-based OSA diagnosis and categorization use the same scale as the AHI cutoffs, though in reality it does not calculate AHI. REI may potentially underestimate apnea or hypopnea events per hour of sleep, thereby misclassifying OSA and denial of beneficial therapy. In patients with significant cardiopulmonary disease, HSAT methods are generally not recommended.[16] Also, a negative, inconclusive, or technically inadequate result may require a confirmatory in-laboratory PSG.

PREVALENCE OF OBSTRUCTIVE SLEEP APNEA IN CORONARY ARTERY DISEASE

The evidence on the complex relationship of OSA with coronary artery disease (CAD) is still evolving. Many studies have been added to the literature recently. It would be reasonable to expect OSA as a modifiable risk factor, with the opportunity to reduce the early signs of endothelial dysfunction and atherosclerosis and improve CV outcomes with continuous positive airway pressure (CPAP) administration, currently the gold-standard treatment of OSA.[2]

DEVELOPMENT OF CARDIOVASCULAR DISEASE IN OBSTRUCTIVE SLEEP APNEA

Obstructive sleep apnea is not an uncommon occurrence. It is found to be prevalent in approximately 3–7% in men and 2–5% in women and in ≥50% of patients with cardiac or metabolic disorders in the same study.[20] Patients with OSA may not present with the cardinal signs of the disease, such as excessive sleepiness and obesity, posing diagnostic challenges, even in patient populations where OSA is highly prevalent, such as those with CV disorders.

Sixty-three percent of the patients admitted to the cardiac intensive care unit (CICU) for acute coronary syndrome (ACS) were diagnosed with OSA.[21] In a study by Martinez et al.[22] in a small cohort of 55 patients to verify the association between OSA and angiographically proven CAD, after excluding patients older than 65 years with a body mass index (BMI) higher than 40 kg/m^2, diabetes mellitus, and history of smoking in the last year, AHI was determined for patients with and without CAD. 29 patients without CAD had an AHI of 11 ± 11/h, whereas of the 26 patients with CAD, the AHI was 23 ± 14/h ($p = 0.001$). In this study, they used a binary logistic regression to predict CAD, after controlling for all the above risk factors. They concluded that without smoking, morbid obesity, or diabetes, AHI was the main predictor of CAD. This strongly suggests that sleep apnea should be integrated into the set of risk factors routinely assessed in the clinical investigation for CAD risk stratification.

Forty consecutive patients with acute myocardial infarction (MI) who underwent PSG and CV magnetic resonance imaging within 5 days and 12 weeks after the event to assess sleep apnea and cardiac function were studied by Buchner et al.[23] The prevalence of OSA (AHI ≥ 15) within 5 days after MI was about 55%. Also, AHI was significantly more reduced in patients in whom ejection fraction (EF) improved in comparison to those in whom it remained unchanged ($p = 0.036$). This reduction was based on a significant alleviation of obstructive events ($p = 0.009$), while the reduction of central events was similar between groups ($p = 0.906$). They concluded that improvement in cardiac function early after MI was associated with an alleviation of sleep apnea.[23]

Schäfer et al.[24] performed overnight nonlaboratory-monitoring-system recordings to detect OSA in 223 male patients with angiographically proven CAD. They found that >30% of patients with CAD had OSA, whereas OSA was observed in almost up to 20% of patients in the control group and found that OSA of moderate severity (AHI ≥ 20) was independently associated with MI.

Fan et al.[25] in a prospective landmark cohort study of 804 patients studied the association of OSA with subsequent CV events after ACS onset, major adverse cardiovascular and cerebrovascular events (MACCE), including CV death, MI, stroke, ischemia-driven revascularization, or hospitalization for unstable angina or heart failure as primary outcomes. OSA was present in 50.1% patients. During a median follow-up of 1 year, the cumulative incidence of MACCE was significantly higher in the OSA group than in the non-OSA group (log-rank $p = 0.041$). OSA was nominally associated with the incidence of MACCE [adjusted hazard ratio (HR) 1.55; 95% confidence interval (CI) 0.94–2.57; $p = 0.085$]. Patients with OSA had 3.9 times the risk of incurring a MACCE after 1 year (adjusted HR 3.87; 95% CI 1.20–12.46;

$p = 0.023$), but no increased risk was found within 1 year of follow-up (adjusted HR 1.18; 95% CI 0.67–2.09; $p = 0.575$). Also, the hospitalization rate for unstable angina was higher in the OSA group than in the non-OSA group. However, no significant differences were found in the incidence of CV death, MI, and ischemia-driven revascularization.

Indian data regarding OSA and CAD is sparse. In a study by Mahajan et al.[26] on OSA prevalence among patients admitted with ACS, 66 patients were subjected to overnight PSG within 8 weeks of the index ACS event. The prevalence of OSA (AHI ≥ 5/h) was 78.8% (95% CI 67.0–87.9), while 31 (46.9%) patients with ACS had moderate-to-severe OSA, emphasizing a significantly higher prevalence of moderate-to-severe OSA among ACS patients.

DEVELOPMENT OF HYPERTENSION IN OBSTRUCTIVE SLEEP APNEA

Untreated OSA carries a risk of developing HTN, which is at least two to three times greater as compared to general population.[27] About 50% of OSA patients are hypertensive and 30% of hypertensive patients also have OSA.[28-30] HTN and OSA often coexist. OSA can often precede the development of HTN.[31] The normal nocturnal fall in BP is blunted by OSA.[32] Nondipping of nocturnal BP has been linked with an increase in all-cause mortality.[33] 80% of patients with resistant hypertension (RHTN) have OSA.[34] OSA has thus emerged as an independent risk factor for RHTN.[35] An increase in AHI was found to be linearly matched by an increase in 24-hour BP.[36]

Primary aldosteronism is found to coexist with OSA. In earlier retrospective studies, although an increased prevalence of PA was found in OSA, PSG was only conducted in those with snoring and was possibly an underestimated prevalence.[37] OSA occurred more frequently in patients with RHTN with PA than those without PA (59.4% vs. 42.4%) in the RESIST-POL study.[38] In another study of 3,003 patients with HTN, 321 patients had PA, among whom 45.8% were found to have OSA.[39] PA in OSA has been found in several studies with no ethnic differences.[37-42] In a study of 207 patients with PA, the prevalence of OSA was 67.6%, and there was no obvious difference in the prevalence between different ethnic groups (White and Chinese) (64.4% vs. 70%).[41] Similar results were reported from a Japanese study with a OSA prevalence of 55% among 71 patients with PA. Additionally, BMI and higher triglyceride levels increased the risk of OSA in PA patients [odds ratio (OR) 1.27 and 1.01, respectively].[40]

Management of PA improved OSA symptoms. Wolley et al.[43] in their study demonstrated improvement in the mean AHI from 22.5 to 12.3 events/h ($p = 0.02$) after an 8-month follow-up surgical treatment with adrenalectomy or medical treatment with spironolactone, amiloride, or both. Another retrospective study on 83 PA patients (48 surgically managed and 35 medically managed) also showed a significant reduced OSA probability assessed by the Berlin questionnaire after PA treatment (from 64 to 35%, mean Berlin score 1.64–1.35, $p < 0.001$) with the follow-up duration up to 2.6 years. Both obese and nonobese patients showed significant decreases in OSA probability.[44]

TREATMENT OF OBSTRUCTIVE SLEEP APNEA TO PREVENT ADVERSE OUTCOMES

Obstructive sleep apnea is known to be associated with a variety of poor health outcomes, including increased mortality.[45] PAP therapy is an effective form of treatment for OSA and is considered to be standard first-line therapy. In the following section, we discuss the evidence pertaining to use of PAP therapy on different CV benefits and the recommendations for its use as per the international consensus statement on OSA.[46]

POSITIVE AIRWAY PRESSURE THERAPY AND CARDIOVASCULAR AND ALL-CAUSE MORTALITY RISK REDUCTION

ISAACC study: Impact of sleep apnea syndrome in the evolution of ACS—effect of intervention with CPAP by Sánchez-de-la-Torre et al.[47] Their study included 1,264 Spanish patients hospitalized for ACS and AHI > 15. They were randomized to CPAP treatment plus usual care versus usual care alone. No significant benefit with CPAP therapy for CV mortality (HR 0.83) or all-cause mortality (HR 0.82) was observed; however, the mean adherence to CPAP therapy was only 2.78 h/night.

Huang et al.[48] studied 83 patients in a randomized controlled trial (RCT). They were randomized to CPAP versus no therapy. There was a nonsignificant trend toward lower severe CV and cerebrovascular events with one death in the control group.

A systematic review by Patil et al.,[49] which included four RCTs comparing CPAP to no CPAP and nine nonrandomized trials comparing PAP versus control group, was done recently. A meta-analysis of RCTs showed that CPAP therapy did not reduce all-cause mortality (risk ratio: 0.96); however, there was variability in CPAP adherence. A meta-analysis of nonrandomized trials demonstrated a clinically significant reduction in all-cause mortality (risk ratio: 0.4).

Sleep Apnea Cardiovascular Endpoints (SAVE) study,[50] an international, multicenter, randomized, parallel-group, open-label trial, with blinded endpoint assessment, recruited 2,717 patients at 89 clinical centers in 7 countries of 45–75 years of age with a diagnosis of CAD or cerebrovascular disease and a diagnosis of moderate-to-severe OSA. A home sleep-study screening device was employed. Therapy with CPAP plus usual care, as compared with usual care alone, did not prevent CV events in patients with moderate-to-severe OSA and established CVD.

These studies underline the fact that treatment with CPAP is not consistently associated with reduction in CV and all-cause mortality in available studies, although CPAP adherence was variable in the studies and severe OSA and excessively sleepy patients were excluded in the RCTs. Modest reductions in mortality have been demonstrated in nonrandomized studies. Based on the best available evidence, benefits are unclear and harms are minimal for PAP therapy in reducing CV and all-cause mortality. Hence, PAP therapy for mortality benefit is currently only optional. There is potential for the reduction in CV and all-cause mortality with PAP therapy in patients with severe OSA, excessive daytime sleepiness, and adherent PAP use as per the OSA consensus statement.[46]

POSITIVE AIRWAY PRESSURE THERAPY AND CONTROL OF HYPERTENSION

In a meta-analysis of 16 RCTs by Bazzano et al.[51] ($n = 818$) with low heterogeneity, OSA treated with CPAP for at least 2 weeks (and up to 24 weeks, with good adherence in most studies) was selected. OSA controls (who were on sham-CPAP, pill, or usual care) served as controls in these studies. OSA was mostly of moderate-severe intensity. 11 studies had data of ambulatory BP, while five studies did not have data of ambulatory BP measurement. It was observed that mean SBP decreased by 2.46 mm Hg (95% CI –4.31 to –0.62), mean diastolic blood pressure (DBP) by 1.83 mm Hg (95% CI –3.05 to –0.61), and mean arterial pressure (MAP) by 2.22 mm Hg (95% CI –4.38 to –0.05) with CPAP. Decreases in nocturnal and daytime BP were not statistically different. A dose-response relationship between mean hourly usage of CPAP and reduction in SBP was noted.

Fava et al.,[52] in their meta-analysis of 29 RCTS ($n = 1,820$) included patients with moderate heterogeneity, who were treated for OSA with CPAP (good adherence in most studies) for 2–52 weeks. With similar subjects to the previous meta-analysis, mean SBP decreased by 2.6 ± 0.6 mm Hg and DBP by 2.0 ± 0.4 mm Hg ($p < 0.001$) with CPAP. Daytime SBP and DBP fell by 2.2 ± 0.7 and 1.9 ± 0.6 mm Hg, respectively, and nighttime SBP and DBP by 3.8 ± 0.8 and 1.8 ± 0.6 mm Hg, respectively. It was observed that higher severity of OSA was associated with a greater decline in mean SBP.

Patil et al.,[49] in their meta-analysis of 26 RCTs ($n = 2,444$) comprising OSA patients treated with CPAP (many with suboptimal adherence) compared them with control group of OSA patients treated with sham-CPAP, pill, or usual care. OSA was mostly of moderate-severe intensity. Five studies included subjects with HTN and five included patients with RHTN. Mean nighttime SBP and DBP fell by 4.2 mm Hg (95% CI –6.0 to –2.5) and 2.3 mm Hg (95% CI –3.7 to –0.9), respectively, with CPAP. Mean daytime SBP and DBP fell by –2.8 mm Hg (95% CI –4.3 to –1.2) and –2.0 mm Hg (95% CI –3.0 to –0.9), respectively; 24-hour SBP, DBP, and mean BP all decreased significantly. In those with HTN, nighttime SBP and DBP, daytime SBP and DBP, and 24-hour SBP and mean BP all decreased. In those with RHTN, significant reductions in nighttime SBP and DBP, daytime BP, 24-hour SBP and DBP, but no clinically significant reduction in daytime SBP was noted.[49]

In another meta-analysis (two observational studies, $n = 44$; four RCTs, $n = 320$) with moderate heterogeneity by Iftikhar et al.,[53] OSA and RHTN treated with CPAP for 2–6 months was compared with OSA and RHTN not treated. OSA was mostly severe. CPAP adherence was good. All but one study used ambulatory BP monitoring. 24-hour SBP decreased by 7.21 mm Hg (95% CI –9.04 to –5.38; $p < 0.001$) and DBP by 4.99 mm Hg (95% CI –6.01 to –3.96; $p < 0.001$) with CPAP. Ambulatory SBP and DBP from four RCTs showed a decrease of 6.74 mm Hg (95% CI –9.98 to –3.49; $p < 0.001$) and 5.94 mm Hg (95% CI –9.40 to –2.47; $p = 0.001$), respectively.

Bratton et al.[54] in their meta-analysis of 51 studies ($n = 4,888$) with moderate heterogeneity included OSA, on CPAP, OSA, on oral appliance (OA) as compared to OSA with inactive control. Follow-up of the subjects ranged between 4 and 157 weeks, with variable adherence to CPAP. Many studies had subjects with HTN, including RHTN. Forty-four studies compared CPAP to inactive control, three compared OA to inactive control, one compared CPAP to OA, and three compared those on CPAP, OA, and inactive control. CPAP reduced SBP by 2.5 mm Hg (95% CI –1.5 to –3.5; $p < 0.001$) and DBP by 2.0 mm Hg (95% CI –1.3 to –2.7; $p < 0.001$) versus inactive control; a dose-response relationship between hours of usage of CPAP and reduction in SBP/DBP was noted. OA reduced SBP by 2.1 mm Hg (95% CI –0.8 to –3.4; $p = 0.002$) and DBP by 1.9 mm Hg (95% CI –0.5 to –3.2; $p = 0.008$). There were no significant differences in reduction in SBP/DBP between CPAP and OA in the network meta-analysis.

It is strongly recommended that successful treatment of OSA with CPAP leads to reduction in BP. Antihypertensive medications will likely still be required. Patients with OSA, particularly those with moderate-to-severe OSA and/or RHTN, should be offered CPAP to help decrease BP as per the OSA consensus statement.[46]

POSITIVE AIRWAY PRESSURE THERAPY AND CONTROL OF ATRIAL FIBRILLATION

Several observational studies have evaluated the association of CPAP treatment for OSA with the risk of recurrent AF following electrical cardioversion or ablation procedures.

A recent randomized clinical trial by Traaen et al.[55] shed light on the use of PAP therapy in patients with OSA with AF. Patients with paroxysmal AF, screened for sleep apnea with two nights of home respiratory polygraphy with a mean AHI ≥ 15, and use of CPAP ≥ 4 hours on each night of a 7-night run-in period were recruited to the study. There were two groups: Usual care alone (n = 54, no dropouts), baseline AF burden 5.0% and the other being usual care plus CPAP (n = 55, one dropout), baseline AF burden 5.6%; mean CPAP use 4.4 (SD 1.9) h/night. The primary outcome was to evaluate difference in change in AF burden (percent of time in AF) between the groups from the 1-month period prior to treatment to the final 3 months of the 5-month treatment period. Also, the secondary outcome was to assess the percentage of patients with a ≥25% reduction in AF burden. In post-hoc analyses, the frequency of AF episodes and duration of AF episodes were also assessed. AF burden decreased from 5.0 to 4.3% in the control group and from 5.6 to 4.1% in the CPAP group (adjusted mean difference –0.6%; 95% CI –2.6 to +1.3%; p = 0.52). There was no significant difference in "per protocol" analysis including only those using CPAP ≥ 4 h/night. 41% of patients in the CPAP group and 31% in the usual care group had a ≥25% reduction in AF burden (adjusted mean difference –9.3%; 95% CI –26.4 to +8.7%; p = 0.33). No significant difference in frequency or duration of AF events was observed. Serious adverse events occurred in 13% of CPAP and 4% of control subjects.

Hojo et al.[56] in their cohort study recruited 100 patients undergoing pulmonary vein isolation (PVI) for AF. PSG was done in all at baseline. All patients had a second PVI procedure at 6 months, after which CPAP was recommended based on local guidelines. 11 patients with treated OSA, 23 patients with untreated OSA, and 66 patients without OSA were followed up. No significant difference among groups was noted in the rate of AF recurrence (12.1% in no OSA group, 9.1% untreated OSA group, 8.7% in untreated OSA group).

The overall quality of evidence favoring diagnosis and treatment of OSA solely for the prevention of recurrent AF without cardioversion or ablation is generally weak, with no adequately powered randomized clinical trials. Patients with paroxysmal AF did not demonstrate AF burden reduction with CPAP therapy. Patients who are undergoing cardioversion or catheter ablation for AF may benefit from adjunctive treatment of OSA with CPAP to prevent AF recurrence. Shared decision-making regarding CPAP treatment is suggested to weigh individual patient symptoms, preferences, and comorbidities. PAP therapy is optional as per the OSA consensus statement.[46]

CONCLUSION

Obstructive sleep apnea is a widely underdiagnosed disease. Efforts to screen for the disease would bear the fruits of alleviating risks of development of CVD, AF, and HTN. With proper management of these diseases, it would potentially translate to improved all-cause mortality and cerebrovascular disease. To date, PAP is the undisputed and only therapy that would potentially yield the above said benefits, if properly used with proper care and for the proper duration of sleep. Future studies should aim at establishing the exact mechanisms of development of complications in OSA, which would result in the development of alternate therapies that afford better patient compliance and comfort.

ONLINE REFERENCES

Please scan the QR code provided at the end of the table of contents for References of this chapter.

CHAPTER 8

Point-of-care Cardiac Ultrasound: Current Capabilities and the Cardiologist's Perspective

Chandrashekhar K Ponde, Mufaddal Lunawadawala, Mayuri Mhatre, Kunal Patankar

ABSTRACT

Point-of-care cardiac ultrasound (POCUS) has emerged as a pivotal diagnostic tool in contemporary clinical practice, revolutionizing the approach to cardiovascular assessment and patient management. This chapter presents a comprehensive overview of the significant strides made in the field of POCUS cardiac echocardiography, highlighting its role in expediting accurate diagnoses, improving treatment decisions, and optimizing patient outcomes. A central focus of the chapter is the expanding array of clinical applications that POCUS cardiac echocardiography enables. From rapid assessment of cardiac function in emergency settings to guiding interventional procedures with real-time visualization, POCUS has proven invaluable in scenarios ranging from critical care units to remote and resource-limited environments. Moreover, the chapter underscores POCUS's role in enhancing bedside monitoring of hemodynamic changes, evaluating valvular pathologies, and providing crucial insights into cardiac performance during and after surgical interventions. In conclusion, this chapter highlights the transformative impact of POCUS cardiac echocardiography on contemporary medical practice. By enabling rapid and precise cardiac assessments at the point of care, this technology has redefined diagnostic and therapeutic paradigms, empowering healthcare professionals to make informed decisions and significantly improve patient outcomes. The ongoing integration of advanced technologies and expanding clinical applications further solidify POCUS cardiac echocardiography as an indispensable tool in the modern medical arsenal.

Keywords: Cardiac ultrasound, point of care.

"The successful warrior is the average man, with a laser-like FOCUS."

—Bruce Lee

INTRODUCTION

With the ever-changing landscape of healthcare delivery, a greater proportion of patients are receiving their initial care and diagnostic testing in emergency departments (EDs). With this change, significant efforts have been made to improve the speed and accuracy of diagnostic testing, particularly by using point-of-care testing, to minimize the delay between onset of symptoms and initiation of definitive therapy. Expediting triage and time to diagnosis are crucial to decreasing morbidity and mortality in critically ill patients. Point-of-care testing has been shown to achieve these goals, leading to improved diagnostic efficiency and, ultimately, better patient outcomes.[1]

Point-of-care cardiac ultrasound (POCUS) is structured to answer a focused clinical question (or a set of questions), and therefore it transcends specialty boundaries and can be adopted by a physician, anesthesiologist, casualty medical officer, and intensivist. POCUS has revolutionized the field of cardiovascular medicine by providing rapid and accessible bedside imaging capabilities. POCCUS, also known as focused cardiac ultrasound or bedside echocardiography, allows healthcare providers to directly visualize and assess the structure and function of the heart in real time. It serves as a valuable tool in critical care settings, EDs, and perioperative care settings, enabling prompt diagnosis and facilitating timely interventions for improved patient outcomes.

Point-of-care cardiac ultrasound offers several advantages over traditional comprehensive echocardiography:

- It enables healthcare providers to quickly assess patients in critical situations by bedside.
- Additionally, POCUS is relatively easy to learn and can be performed by a range of healthcare professionals, including emergency room physicians, intensivists, anesthesiologists, and critical care nurses, among others. This widespread accessibility empowers frontline clinicians to make rapid decisions based on real-time imaging information, potentially saving lives and improving patient outcomes.

The clinical applications of POCUS are vast and encompass various aspects of cardiac assessment. It aids in the evaluation of cardiac function, detection of structural abnormalities, assessment of volume status and hemodynamics, identification of pericardial effusions and cardiac tamponade, diagnosis and monitoring of myocardial infarction (MI) and heart failure, and evaluation of pulmonary embolism (PE). By providing immediate and actionable information at the bedside, POCUS complements the clinical examination and other diagnostic tools, enabling a comprehensive assessment of cardiac status.[2]

PRINCIPLES OF POINT-OF-CARE CARDIAC ULTRASOUND

Point-of-care cardiac ultrasound relies on the fundamental principles of ultrasound imaging to visualize and assess the structure and function of the heart. Ultrasound uses high-frequency sound waves that are transmitted into the body and reflected back to create real-time images. In the case of cardiac ultrasound, a handheld ultrasound device is used along with a transducer or probe that emits and receives the sound waves.

The components of a POCUS system include the handheld or truly portable ultrasound device, which is compact and designed for easy use at the bedside. The device typically features a screen for displaying the ultrasound images and user-friendly controls for adjusting settings and optimizing image quality. The transducer, attached to the device, contains piezoelectric crystals that generate sound waves and receive the echoes produced by the tissues. These echoes are then converted into electrical signals that are processed by the device's software to generate the ultrasound images.

Point-of-care cardiac ultrasound devices often offer different imaging modalities to assess cardiac structures and function. Two-dimensional (2D) imaging provides real-time, cross-sectional images of the heart and its chambers, allowing clinicians to assess chamber size and wall thickness and identify structural abnormalities such as intracardiac thrombus and vegetations. Motion mode (M-mode) provides a single-line display of motion over time, enabling the assessment of ventricular wall motion and valve function. Color Doppler imaging is used to visualize blood flow, with colors representing the direction and velocity of blood flow within the heart and blood vessels.

Caution: While POCUS provides valuable real-time imaging, it is important to note that it may not offer the same level of detail as comprehensive echocardiography performed by specialized sonographers or cardiologists. The images obtained through POCUS may be limited in their field of view and resolution. Additionally, the operator's experience and expertise play a significant role in obtaining high-quality images and interpreting them accurately.

Overall, POCUS serves as a rapid and accessible tool for bedside cardiac assessment, providing valuable information about the heart's structure and function. Its portable nature and user-friendly design make it a valuable asset in critical care settings, enabling prompt diagnostic decisions and facilitating timely interventions for improved patient outcomes.[2]

CLINICAL APPLICATIONS OF POINT-OF-CARE CARDIAC ULTRASOUND

Cardiac Ultrasound Indications

Point-of-care cardiac ultrasound can be used in the following indications:

- Medically ill patient with significant electrocardiogram (EKG) changes
- ST-segment elevation myocardial infarction/non-ST-segment elevation myocardial infarction (STEMI/NSTEMI)
- Acute breathlessness
- Hypotension and shock
- Medically ill patient with a new heart murmur
- Cardiac arrest (assess for cardiac standstill)

Point-of-care cardiac ultrasound has a wide range of clinical applications, particularly in critical care settings, EDs, and perioperative care. Its real-time imaging capability allows for immediate assessment and diagnosis, enabling healthcare providers to make timely decisions and interventions. The key clinical applications of POCUS in cardiac assessment are as follows:

- *Evaluation of cardiac function*: POCUS plays a crucial role in evaluating cardiac function at the bedside. It allows for the assessment of left ventricular (LV) systolic and diastolic function, enabling clinicians to evaluate ejection fraction (EF) (visual EF), wall motion abnormalities, and ventricular filling patterns. POCUS can also assess right ventricular function [visual EF and tricuspid annular plane systolic excursion (TAPSE)-derived EF] and insights into the presence and severity of pulmonary hypertension.
- *Detection of structural abnormalities*: POCUS aids in the detection of various structural abnormalities of the heart. It allows clinicians to assess valve function and detect abnormalities such as stenosis, regurgitation, and

valve vegetations. POCUS is also valuable in identifying congenital heart defects, such as septal defects, patent ductus arteriosus, and abnormalities of the great vessels. Furthermore, POCUS can detect cardiac masses, including tumors and thrombi.

- *Assessment of volume status and hemodynamics*: POCUS is useful in assessing volume status and hemodynamics, particularly in critically ill patients. It can assist in determining the adequacy of fluid resuscitation by evaluating parameters such as inferior vena cava (IVC) diameter and collapsibility (surrogate of central venous pressure), LV filling patterns, and E/e′ [surrogate of pulmonary capillary wedge pressure (PCWP)].
- *Evaluation of pericardial effusions and cardiac tamponade*: POCUS is highly effective in the evaluation of pericardial effusions and the detection of cardiac tamponade. It allows clinicians to visualize the size and characteristics of pericardial effusions, assess their hemodynamic significance, and guide pericardiocentesis procedures by identifying the optimal site for needle entry and confirming needle tip position during pericardiocentesis.
- *Diagnosis and monitoring of MI and heart failure*: POCUS can aid in the diagnosis and monitoring of MI and heart failure. It allows for the assessment of regional wall motion abnormalities (RWMA), identifying areas of ischemia or infarction. Additionally, POCUS enables the evaluation of LV function and chamber dimensions, providing crucial information for diagnosing and managing heart failure.
- *Assessment of PE*: POCUS is increasingly used in the evaluation of suspected PE. It identifies right heart dysfunction and evaluates for signs of elevated pulmonary artery pressures. POCUS is particularly useful in risk stratification and guiding decisions regarding further imaging or therapy.

In each of these applications, POCUS provides immediate and actionable information at the bedside, facilitating prompt diagnosis and treatment decisions. It complements the clinical examination and other diagnostic tools, allowing for a comprehensive assessment of cardiac status in critically ill.[3]

CLINICAL SCENARIOS AND THE RESPECTIVE RELEVANT INFORMATION THAT POCUS CAN OFFER

Acute Chest Pain

- Distinct RWMA
- Mechanical complications of acute myocardial infarction (AMI) (ventricular septal rupture) **(Fig. 1)**
- Minimal pericardial effusion in pericarditis **(Fig. 2)**
- Aortic dissection **(Fig. 3)**

Acute Breathlessness

- Pericardial tamponade **(Figs. 4A and B)**
- Acute PE **(Figs. 5 to 7)**
- Severe LV dysfunction
- Severe valvular regurgitation

Shock

- Collapsed IVC with hyperdynamic LV (hypovolemic shock) **(Fig. 8)**
- Severe LV systolic dysfunction with plethoric IVC (cardiogenic shock) **(Fig. 9)**
- Severe valvular regurgitation (tricuspid regurgitation) **(Fig. 10)**
- Dilated right atrium/right ventricle (RA/RV) with pulmonary arterial hypertension (PAH) with hyper-contractile RV apex (McConnell's sign in acute PE) **(Fig. 11)**

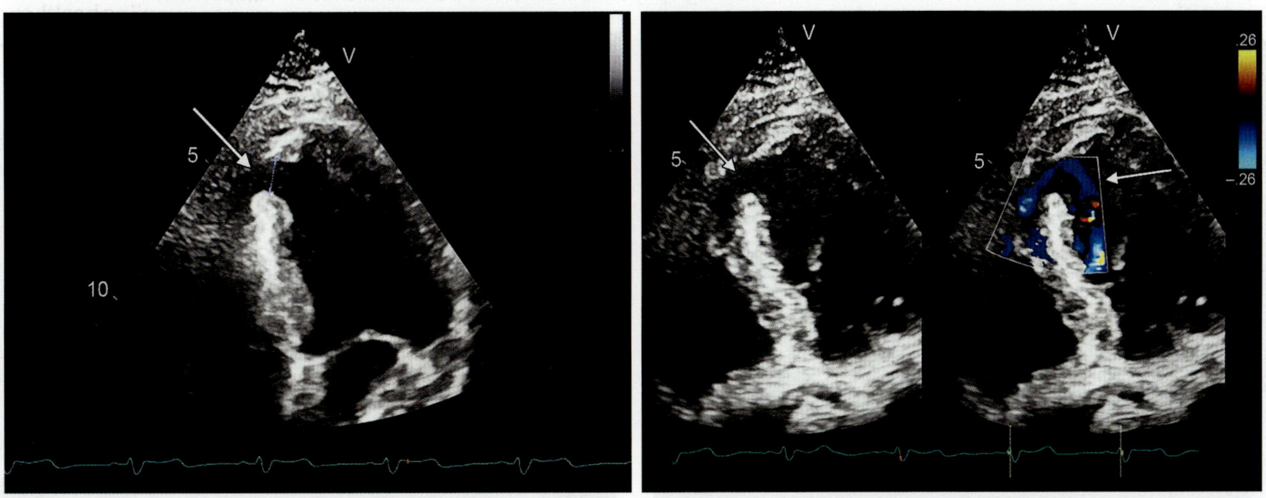

FIG. 1: A four-chamber two-dimensional (2D) echocardiography view of the heart showing ventricular septal defect as shown by the white arrows.

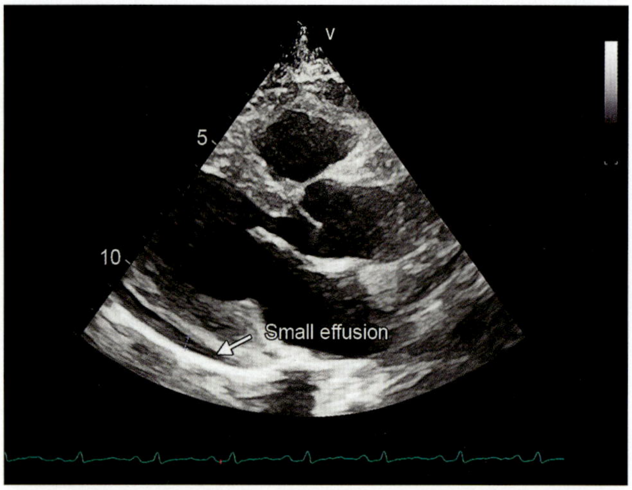

FIG. 2: Parasternal long-axis on two-dimensional (2D) echocardiography showing small pericardial effusion (white arrow).

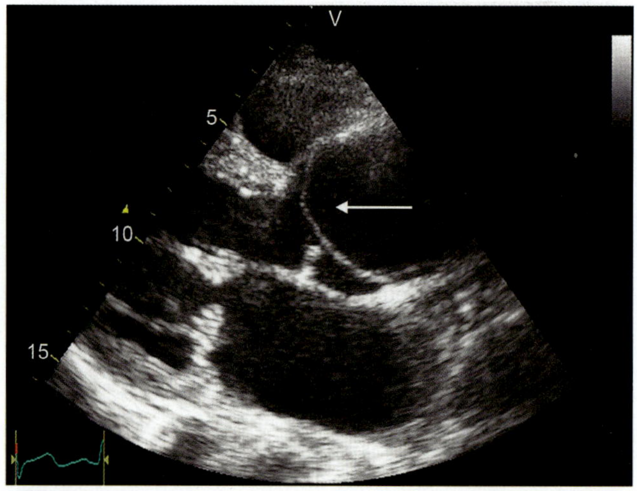

FIG. 3: Parasternal long-axis of the heart showing type A aortic dissection diagnosed by TTE (white arrow).

(TTE: transthoracic echocardiography)

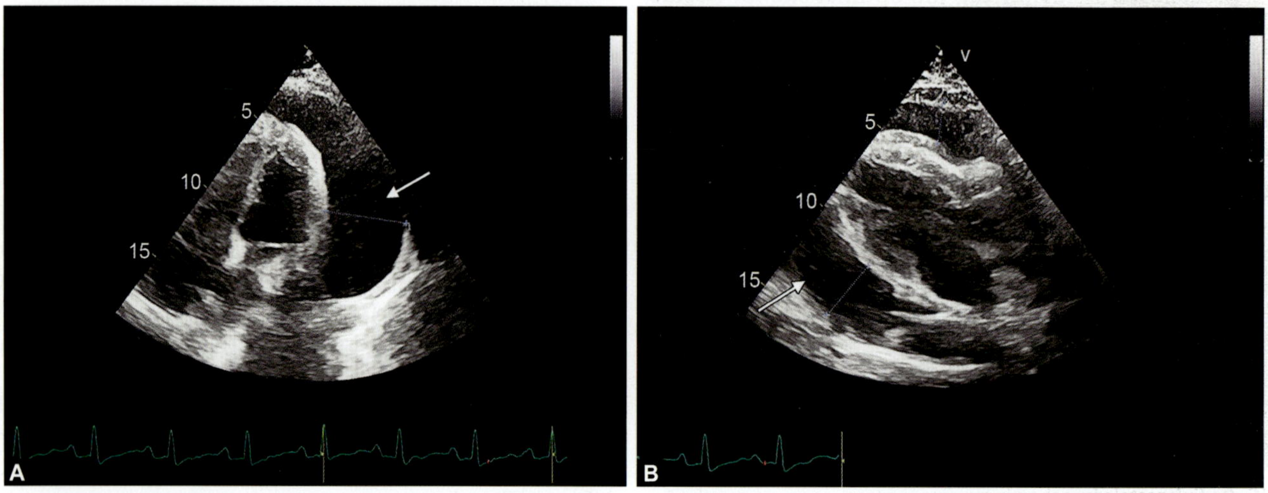

FIGS. 4A AND B: (A) Four-chamber view of the heart on two-dimensional (2D) echocardiography showing massive pericardial effusion (tamponade); (B) Long-axis parasternal view on 2D echocardiography showing massive pericardial effusion (tamponade).

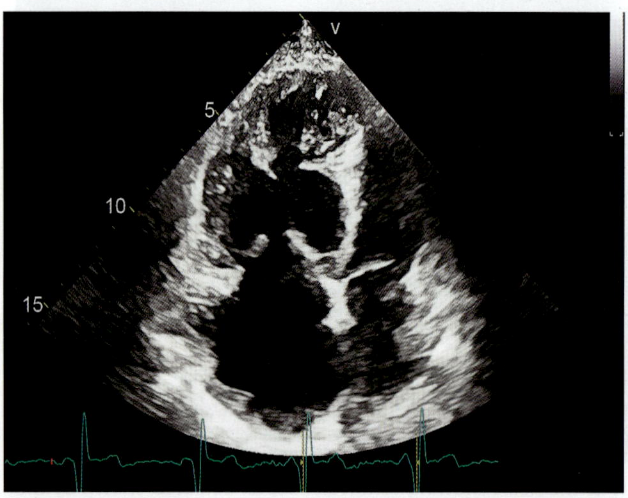

FIG. 5: Four-chamber view of the heart showing dilated right atrium (RA) and right ventricle (RV) in acute pulmonary embolism.

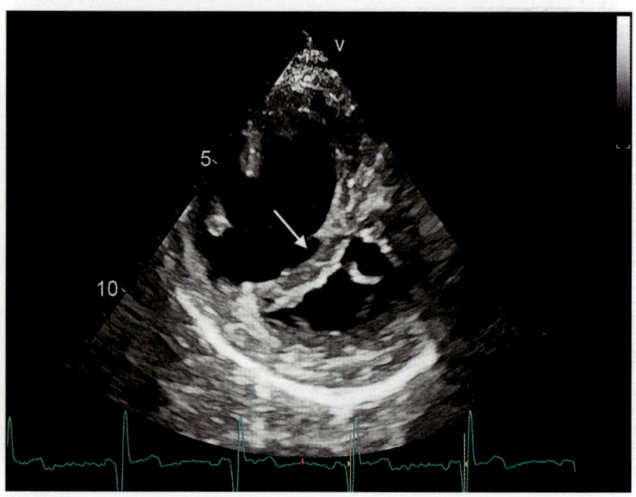

FIG. 6: Short-axis of the heart showing "D"-shaped septum.

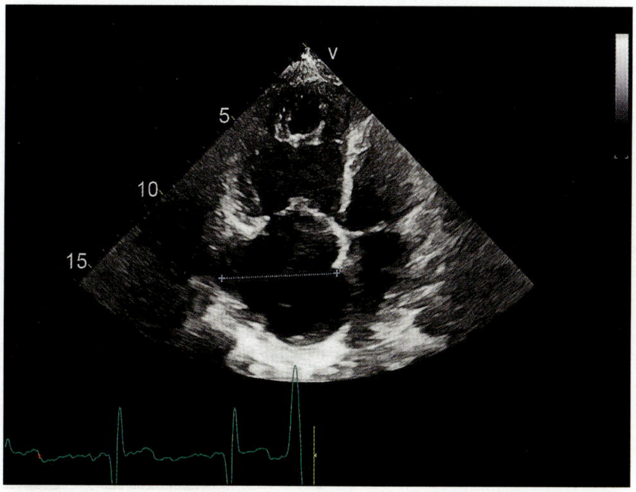

FIG. 7: Four-chamber view of the heart showing dilated right atrium (RA).

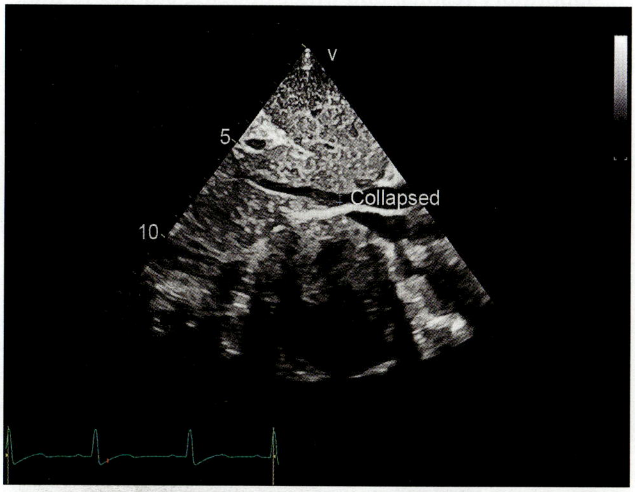

FIG. 8: Subcostal view showing collapsed inferior vena cava (IVC).

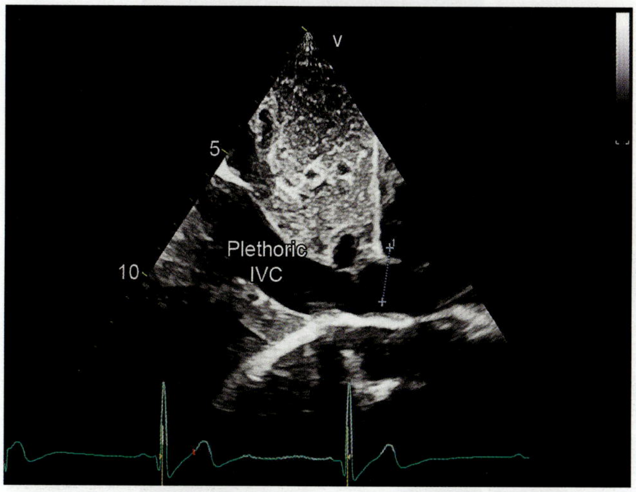

FIG. 9: Subcostal view showing plethoric (dilated) inferior vena cava (IVC).

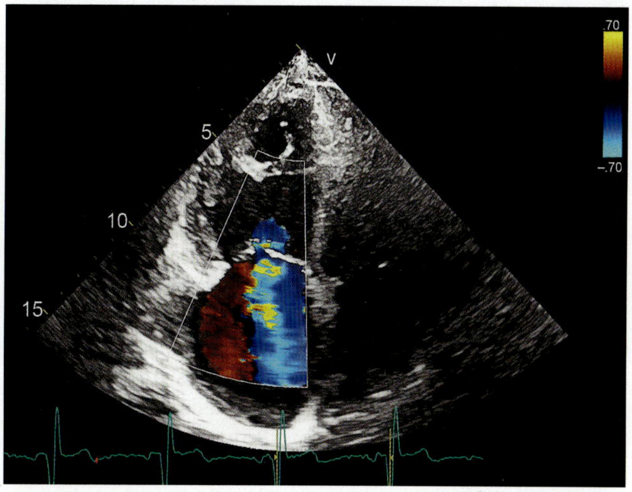

FIG. 10: Four-chamber view of the heart showing severe valvular (tricuspid) regurgitation.

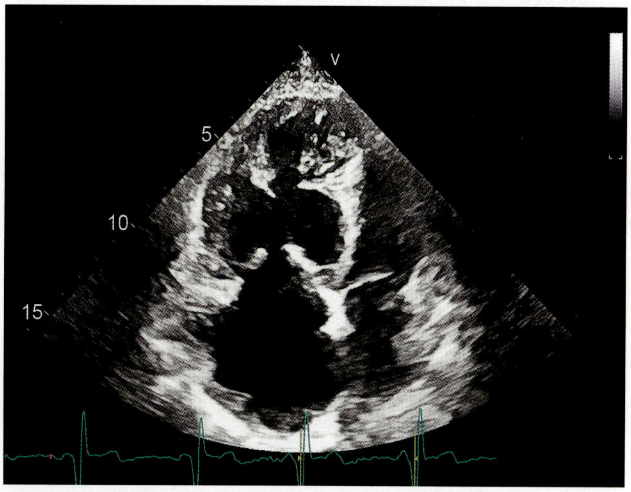

FIG. 11: Four-chamber view showing hypercontractile right ventricle (RV) apex (McConnell's sign).

Pulseless Patient with Nonshockable Rhythm

- Tamponade
- Acute pulmonary thromboembolism (PTE)
- Pulseless electrical activity (PEA)
- Fine ventricular fibrillation (VF) versus asystole

PERFORMING POINT-OF-CARE CARDIAC ULTRASOUND

Key aspects to consider when performing POCUS are as follows:

- *Training and competency*: Healthcare providers performing POCUS should receive appropriate training and demonstrate competency in cardiac ultrasound. This training can be obtained through courses, workshops, and hands-on practical sessions. Organizations such as the American Society of Echocardiography (ASE) and the American College of Emergency Physicians (ACEP) offer educational resources and certification programs to help clinicians develop proficiency in POCUS.

- *Standardized protocols and guidelines*: To ensure standardized image acquisition and interpretation, several professional societies have developed protocols and guidelines for performing POCUS examinations. These guidelines provide step-by-step instructions on probe placement, imaging views, and relevant measurements. Adhering to these guidelines helps ensure consistency in POCUS examinations and facilitates accurate interpretation of the obtained images.
- *Image acquisition techniques*: Proper image acquisition techniques are essential for obtaining high-quality cardiac ultrasound images. The choice of probe and imaging windows depends on the specific cardiac structures being assessed. Different views, such as parasternal long-axis, parasternal short-axis, apical four-chamber, and subcostal views, provide comprehensive visualization of cardiac anatomy and function. Healthcare providers should have a good understanding of probe manipulation and patient positioning to optimize image acquisition.
- *Image optimization*: Optimizing the ultrasound image is crucial to enhancing diagnostic quality. Adjustments in gain, depth, focus, and image settings may be required to obtain the best possible image quality. Healthcare providers should be familiar with the functions of the ultrasound device and its software to optimize the images appropriately. Proper image optimization aids in visualizing cardiac structures, identifying abnormalities, and accurately assessing cardiac function.
- *Image interpretation*: Interpreting POCUS images requires knowledge of normal and abnormal cardiac anatomy and function. Providers should be able to identify key structures, assess chamber sizes, evaluate valve function, and detect any structural abnormalities or wall motion abnormalities. It is important to correlate the findings with the patient's clinical presentation and integrate the POCUS findings with other clinical information.
- *Clinical integration*: POCUS findings should be interpreted and integrated into the overall clinical context. POCUS is a valuable adjunct to the clinical examination and other diagnostic tools. Providers should consider the patient's history, physical examination findings, laboratory results, and other imaging studies to make comprehensive diagnostic and treatment decisions.

By following standardized protocols, mastering image acquisition techniques, optimizing image quality, and integrating findings into the clinical context, healthcare providers can effectively perform POCUS. Continuous practice, ongoing education, and adherence to quality assurance programs further enhance proficiency in POCUS, ensuring accurate and meaningful cardiac assessment at the bedside **(Fig. 12)**.[4]

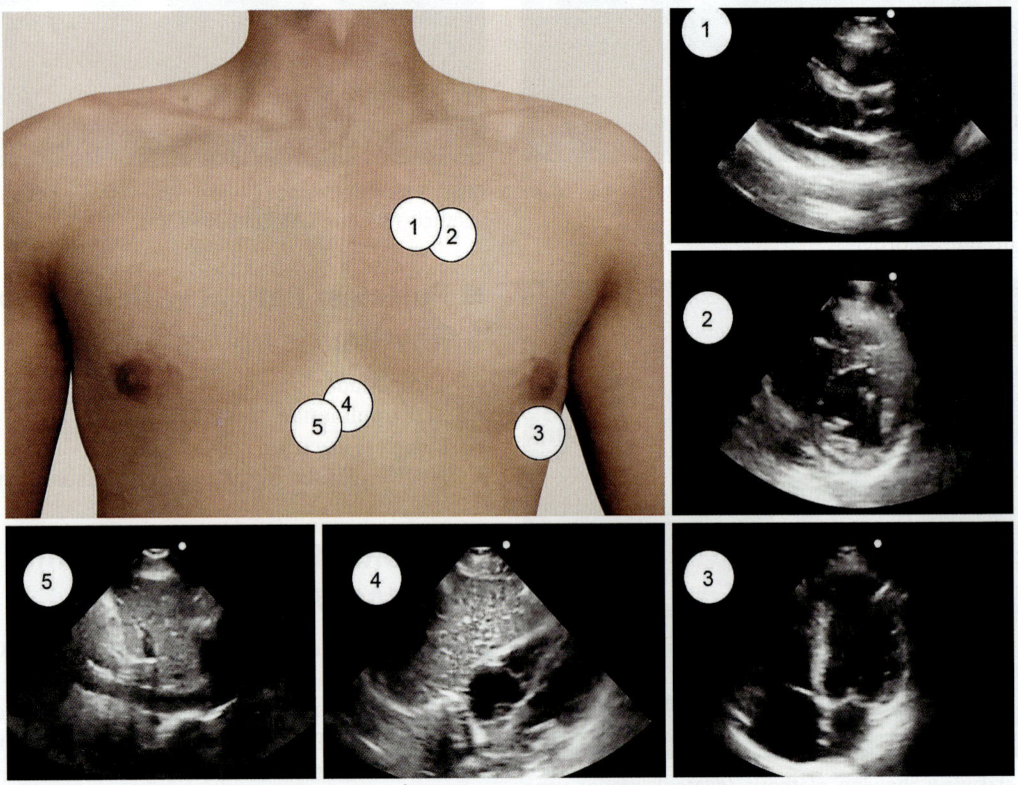

FIG. 12: Transducer probe locations and respective echocardiographic views.

Courtesy: The human body with landmarks is attritubed to google images, Rest echo pics are own images.

WHAT DO THE GUIDELINES SAY?

The ASE has developed guidelines for the use of POCUS in various clinical scenarios. The ASE guidelines provide recommendations for the appropriate use of POCUS in the evaluation and management of cardiac conditions. Some key points from the ASE POCUS guidelines are as follows:

- *Training and education*:
  - Providers performing POCUS should have appropriate training, including didactic and practical experience, to ensure competency in image acquisition and interpretation.
  - Training programs should follow standardized curricula, and providers should participate in ongoing educational activities to maintain proficiency.
- *Equipment and transducers*:
  - POCUS examinations should be performed using high-quality ultrasound machines capable of producing adequate image resolution for accurate interpretation.
  - Different transducers may be needed for various cardiac views and specific clinical scenarios.
- *Image acquisition and interpretation*:
  - Providers should follow standardized imaging protocols to acquire appropriate cardiac views and optimize image quality.
  - Image interpretation should include a comprehensive assessment of cardiac structures, function, and pathology, according to established guidelines and criteria.
- *Clinical applications*:
  - ASE guidelines cover a wide range of clinical applications of POCUS, including evaluation of LV function, detection of pericardial effusion and cardiac tamponade, assessment of valvular heart disease, identification of right ventricular dysfunction, and detection of structural abnormalities.
  - The guidelines provide specific recommendations for image acquisition techniques, interpretation criteria, and clinical decision-making based on the specific cardiac condition being evaluated.
- *Reporting and documentation*:
  - POCUS findings should be documented thoroughly in the patient's medical record, including images, measurements, and interpretations.
  - Clear and concise reporting of POCUS findings is important for communication with other healthcare providers and continuity of care.
- *Quality assurance*:
  - Quality assurance programs should be in place to ensure consistent and accurate performance of POCUS examinations.
  - Regular case review, feedback, and continuous quality improvement initiatives are recommended.[2]

LIMITATIONS AND FUTURE PERSPECTIVES

While POCUS has significant advantages, it also has limitations. Additionally, ongoing advancements in technology and evolving perspectives provide exciting opportunities for the future of POCUS. Here are the key aspects to explore in this section:

- *Limitations of POCUS*:
  - *Operator dependence*: The quality of POCUS images and interpretation can vary depending on the operator's experience and skill level. Inadequate image acquisition or suboptimal interpretation may lead to diagnostic errors or missed findings.
  - *Limited field of view*: POCUS provides a limited field of view compared to comprehensive echocardiography. Moreover, some structures or regions may be challenging to visualize, especially in patients with obesity, lung disease, or poor acoustic windows.
  - *Image quality*: POCUS devices may have limitations in image resolution and depth penetration, potentially affecting the visualization of subtle cardiac abnormalities or small structures.
  - *Lack of quantitative analysis*: POCUS may not offer advanced quantitative measurements like comprehensive echocardiography, limiting its ability to provide detailed assessments of cardiac function and hemodynamics.
  - *Operator fatigue and ergonomics*: Performing POCUS examinations can be physically demanding, particularly during busy, hectic emergency rooms (ERs) potentially leading to operator fatigue and decreased image quality.
- *Advancements in POCUS technology*:
  - Improved image quality
  - Integration of artificial intelligence (AI)
  - Miniaturization and portability
  - Wireless and cloud connectivity
- *Expansion of POCUS applications*:
  - *Remote monitoring*: POCUS has the potential to enable remote monitoring of cardiac patients, allowing for real-time assessment and guidance by experts located remotely.
  - *Telemedicine and teleconsultation*: POCUS can be integrated into telemedicine platforms, enabling remote consultation between healthcare providers and patients, especially in underserved areas.
  - *Point-of-care decision support*: AI-powered POCUS platforms can assist healthcare providers in real time by providing automated analysis, clinical decision support, and guidance during examinations.
  - *Training and education*: Continued development of POCUS training programs and educational resources will ensure widespread competency among

healthcare providers, leading to more consistent and accurate use of POCUS in clinical practice.

- *Cost-effectiveness and workflow integration*: Future perspectives for POCUS involve optimizing cost-effectiveness and workflow integration. Streamlining POCUS procedures, integrating POCUS data into electronic health records, and demonstrating its value in improving patient outcomes and reducing healthcare costs will further enhance its adoption and integration into routine clinical practice.

In conclusion, while POCUS has its limitations, ongoing technological advancements, expanding applications, and evolving perspectives offer exciting opportunities for the future. By addressing these limitations and embracing the possibilities of AI, telemedicine, remote monitoring, and continued training, POCUS can continue to advance bedside cardiac assessment and improve patient care.[3]

CONCLUSION

Point-of-care cardiac ultrasound has emerged as a game-changing technology in cardiovascular medicine, bringing the power of cardiac imaging directly to the patient's bedside. Its portability, ease of use, and real-time imaging capabilities have transformed the way healthcare providers assess and manage cardiac conditions in critical care settings, EDs, and perioperative care. By providing immediate visual information about cardiac structure and function, POCUS facilitates prompt diagnostic decisions and timely interventions, potentially leading to improved patient outcomes.

The clinical applications of POCUS are extensive, encompassing the evaluation of cardiac function, detection of structural abnormalities, assessment of volume status and hemodynamics, identification of pericardial effusions and cardiac tamponade, diagnosis and monitoring of MI and heart failure, and evaluation of PE. POCUS serves as a valuable adjunct to the clinical examination, enabling healthcare providers to make comprehensive and well-informed decisions at the bedside.

While POCUS offers numerous advantages, it is important to acknowledge its limitations. Operator dependence, limited field of view, and potential variability in image quality and interpretation must be taken into account. However, ongoing advancements in POCUS technology, including improved image resolution, integration of AI, and wireless connectivity, hold great promise for overcoming these limitations and enhancing the utility of POCUS in clinical practice.

The future of POCUS is exciting, with opportunities for expanding its applications in remote monitoring, telemedicine, and point-of-care decision support. Integration of POCUS into electronic health records, optimization of workflow integration, and demonstrating its cost-effectiveness will further drive its adoption and integration into routine clinical practice.

To maximize the benefits of POCUS, continued training and education are crucial. Healthcare providers should strive for proficiency in image acquisition, interpretation, and integration of POCUS findings into the overall clinical context. Ongoing quality assurance programs and adherence to standardized protocols and guidelines will ensure the consistent and accurate use of POCUS.

In conclusion, POCUS has revolutionized cardiac assessment by providing rapid and accessible imaging capabilities at the bedside. Its ability to deliver immediate visual information about the heart empowers healthcare providers to make timely decisions and interventions. With ongoing technological advancements and expanding applications, POCUS is poised to play an increasingly prominent role in cardiovascular care, improving patient outcomes and enhancing the delivery of bedside cardiac assessment.

ONLINE REFERENCES

Please scan the QR code provided at the end of the table of contents for References of this chapter.

CHAPTER

9

Mitral Annular Calcification: Significance in Clinical Practice

Rajan Joseph Manjuran

ABSTRACT

Mitral annular calcification (MAC) is considered to be an active atherosclerotic process. Females are more affected than males. Chronic kidney disease patients are at high risk of developing MAC. Patients with MAC can progress to mitral valve dysfunction, needing mitral valve surgery. Transcatheter mitral valve replacement is being tried in these patients. Atrioventricular conduction abnormalities and atrial fibrillation are more frequent in MAC patients. Caseous mitral annulus calcification (CMAC) is a variant of MAC. CMAC must be differentiated from cardiac tumor or cyst.

Keywords: Mitral annular calcification (MAC), caseous mitral annulus calcification (CMAC).

INTRODUCTION

Mitral annular calcification (MAC) **(Figs. 1 and 2)** is a degenerative process affecting the fibrous tissue of the mitral annulus.[1] Initially MAC was thought to be an age-related change. Subsequent studies have indicated that MAC is an active process and could be compared to atherosclerotic calcification.[2] MAC prevalence increases with age. It affects females more frequently than males. Posterior part of mitral annulus is more often affected than the anterior annulus.[3] Echocardiography is the cheapest and most frequently used investigation to detect MAC. The two-dimensional echocardiography can localize and assess the extent of MAC.[4] Cardiac computed tomography (CT) is superior to two-dimensional echocardiography for localization of MAC.[5] Simple fluoroscopy can also detect MAC.

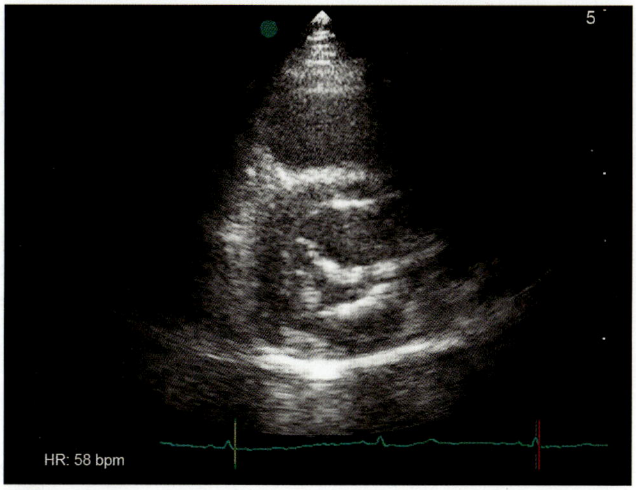

FIG. 1: Mitral annular calcification (MAC) involving posterior and anterior mitral annulus.

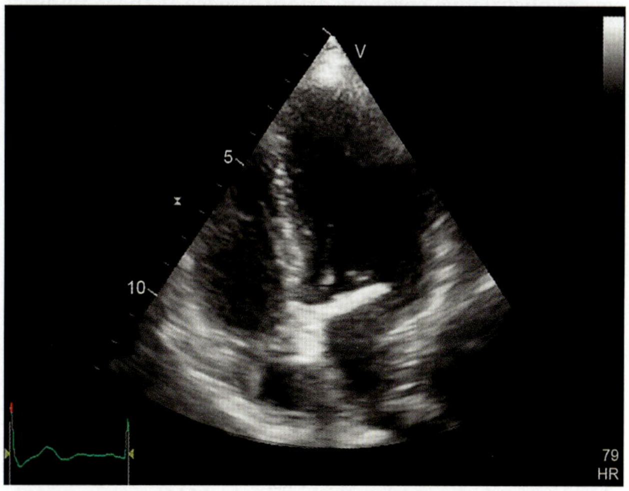

FIG. 2: Mitral annular calcification (MAC) involving anterior mitral leaflet and spreading to interventricular and interatrial septa.

ASSOCIATION

Initially, MAC was thought to be a degenerative process. Now, it is considered an active process with similarity to atherosclerotic process.[2] A number of risk factors of atherosclerosis play a vital role in the MAC process. MAC has a strong association with atherosclerosis.[6] Conditions which increase the stress on the mitral valve such as systemic hypertension, aortic stenosis, and hypertrophic obstructive cardiomyopathy predispose for MAC.[1] Left ventricular hypertrophy is frequently seen in MAC patients.[7] Mitral valve prolapse and mitral valve replacement patients have higher frequency of MAC.[1,8] Chronic renal failure is an important risk factor for MAC. Abnormal calcium and phosphorus metabolism may be the underlying pathogenesis of MAC in these patients.[9] Marfan and Hurler syndromes are hereditary disorders with higher prevalence of MAC.[1,10] Even though atherosclerosis and aortic stenosis are more frequent in males, MAC is more frequent in females.[11]

CLINICAL SIGNIFICANCE OF MITRAL ANNULUS CALCIFICATION

Most of the patients of MAC are asymptomatic. MAC in majority of the cases is an accidental finding in patients undergoing two-dimensional echocardiographic examination.

Cardiovascular Disease and Mitral Annulus Calcification

There is a correlation between MAC and cardiovascular disease (CVD). In patients without CVD, the prevalence of MAC was 8–15%, while in CVD patients, it was as high as 42%.[12] MAC is associated with increased risk of CVD. In the Framingham Heart Study, MAC was found to be associated with CVD risk, cardiovascular death, and all-cause mortality.[13] In the study by Atar et al., MAC was correlated with more severe obstructive coronary artery disease.[14] These findings indicate that MAC may be a marker of atherosclerosis.[15] There is higher incidence of stroke in MAC patients. This correlated with carotid atherosclerosis and atheroma and atrial fibrillation (AF) in MAC patients.[15]

Mitral Valve Disease and Mitral Annulus Calcification

In advanced MAC, where the calcific process extends into valve leaflets and subvalvular apparatus, mitral valve dysfunction in the form of mitral regurgitation or mitral stenosis or combination of both can happen. MAC is a progressive disease and over 10 years, one-third of MAC patients progressed to severe calcification and associated mitral valve dysfunction.[16] In the Euro Heart Study, in the elderly population with mitral stenosis, MAC was present in 60%.[17]

Mitral annulus calcification was found to coexist with calcific aortic stenosis (CAS). In patients undergoing transcatheter aortic valve implantation, severe MAC was observed in 9.5% of patients.[18]

An association between progression of CAS and MAC was observed by Willner et al.[16] This observation indicates that MAC and CAS may have common risk factors leading to simultaneous progression of the disease.

Infective endocarditis (IE) is uncommon in MAC patients. Fulkerson et al.[19] have reported three cases of IE out of 80 MAC patients during follow-up.

Mitral Valve Surgery and Mitral Annulus Calcification

Mitral annulus calcification patients undergoing mitral valve surgery have higher risk of atrioventricular rupture and paravalvular regurgitation.[20] Debridement of calcium in patients of MAC during surgery can result in injury to circumflex coronary artery.[3] MAC patients are more likely to undergo mitral valve replacement than repair.[8] In order to reduce the surgical complication of MAC, it is recommended to avoid annular calcium debridement. However, this can lead to smaller-sized prosthetic valve replacement and higher incidence of perivalvular leak. For good surgical benefit, MAC patients may be subjected for complete annular dissection, followed by reconstruction of the annulus with atrial flap or pericardial patch.[3]

Interventional approach in the form of MitraClip and transcatheter mitral valve replacement (TMVR) can become alternative treatment options for MAC patients with severe mitral regurgitation and high surgical risk.[21] However, lack of complete annular calcification and risk of annular rupture are the problems faced during TMVR.

Cardiac Arrhythmias and Mitral Annulus Calcification

Atrioventricular conduction abnormalities have been reported in patients of MAC.[1] This may be as a sequela to the extension of calcific process to the conduction system.[22] It is also suggested that in MAC patients, there may be primary conduction system disease.[23]

Mitral annulus calcification patients have higher incidence of AF. In the analysis of 1,126 patients of MAC from Framingham Heart Study, there was higher risk of AF in these patients.[24] The mechanisms leading to AF in these patients could be atrial enlargement due to mitral valve disease and/or atrial conduction abnormalities.[23]

Caseous Mitral Annulus Calcification

Caseous MAC (CMAC) is an uncommon variant of MAC. In 1970, 7 out of 256 MAC patients were reported to have CMAC by Pomerance in an autopsy series.[25] In 1983, Kronzon et al. reported five cases of CMAC out of 9,000 echocardiograms.[26] CMAC presents as a round, echo-dense mass with central echolucency. It simulates a periannular mass. It is mostly located in the posterior annulus of the mitral valve. CMAC was seen in 0.63–0.64% of MAC patients.[27] In autopsy studies, CMAC was detected in 2.7% of the MAC patients.[25] The exact mechanism of caseation in CMAC is ill understood.[28] CMAC may be associated with systemic embolization thought to be due to embolization of small calcium particles or ulceration of the surface of the mass, leading to thrombus formation and consequent embolization.[29] In CMAC, the mass is seen to bulge from the posterior region of the mitral annulus into the left atrial or left ventricle. The CMAC can be diagnosed by echocardiography, cardiac magnetic resonance imaging, and CT.[27] CMAC is to be differentiated from other intracardiac masses such as tumor or abscess or IE vegetations.[27]

TREATMENT

Caseous MAC can sometimes resolve spontaneously.[28] Medical management can be followed for CMAC as long as there is no obstruction to left atrial emptying.[29] Anticoagulation is indicated in patients of CMAC with embolic episodes.[29,30]

CONCLUSION

Mitral annulus calcification was initially thought to be a degenerative, age-related disease. Now, it is considered to be an active atherosclerotic process. Increased mitral valve stress as in systemic hypertension or aortic stenosis or hypertrophic obstructive cardiomyopathy can predispose for MAC. Chronic kidney disease patients are at high risk of MAC. MAC patients are at high risk of CVD. MAC patients can develop mitral valve dysfunction, mitral regurgitation, or mitral stenosis or both. Symptomatic patients with MAC need surgical treatment. Patients of MAC undergoing surgical treatment require modification of the surgical technique. Percutaneous techniques like Mitraclip or TMVR are other alternative treatment options. Conduction abnormalities and AF are more frequent in MAC patients. CMAC is an uncommon variant of MAC. Not recognizing this condition can lead to misdiagnosis and sometimes unnecessary surgical treatment.

ONLINE REFERENCES

Please scan the QR code provided at the end of the table of contents for References of this chapter.

CHAPTER 10

Electrocardiogram Yesterday, Today, and Tomorrow

SB Gupta

ABSTRACT

Electrocardiogram (ECG) invention by Einthoven, then its clinical application, and newer and newer developments is history by itself. Refining the techniques of taking ECG, proper classification, and identifying various waveforms and putting them into clinical practice have been the boon to mankind. ECG has not lost its sheen even after a century of its birth and its role in acute coronary syndrome (ACS) and in identifying various arrhythmias is unparallel. Stress ECG and ambulatory ECG recording are the developments of today. Future lies in improved ECG instrumentation and use of artificial intelligence (AI) in ECG interpretation **(Fig. 1)**.

Keywords: ECG, history, artificial intelligence.

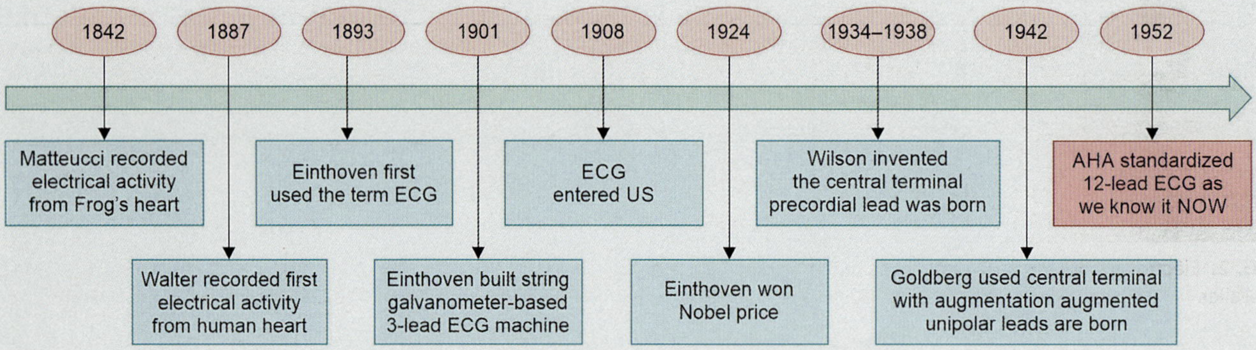

FIG. 1: Timeline of clinically pertinent landmarks in the development of electrocardiogram (ECG).

INTRODUCTION

History of electrocardiogram (ECG) goes back to 1856 and Einthoven coined the term ECG in 1893 and got the Nobel prize for the same in 1924. Since then, various ECG forms have been recognized and the clinical applications of ECG has kept on increasing. Though various imaging modalities have come for better diagnostics for cardiovascular diseases, ECG, though more than 100 years old, still remains the first line investigation for the diagnosis of acute coronary syndrome (ACS) and in the management of arrhythmias. Stress ECG and ambulatory recording of ECG has improved the diagnostic yield in ACS and arrhythmias. With the advent of artificial intelligence, there will be revolutionary changes in the usefulness of ECG.

ELECTROCARDIOGRAM YESTERDAY

In 1856, the history of ECG started when Köllicker and Müller discovered the electrical activity of the heart muscle. Muirhead, in London, recorded the first human ECG with a siphon instrument in 1869 or 1870.[1]

Luigi Luciani in 1873 noted cardiac group beating and recorded second-degree atrioventricular (AV) blocks in frog hearts. Same year, Alfred Lewis Galabin demonstrated AV block in humans using apexcardiogram.

Augustus Waller invented an ECG machine in 1887, consisting of a capillary electrometer and recorded the first human ECG and the tracing revealed only two deflections which were labeled by him V_1 and V_2 indicating ventricular events **(Fig. 2)**.[2]

In 1893, Willem Einthoven **(Fig. 3)**, a Dutch physician and physiologist introduced the term "electrocardiogram" at a meeting of Dutch Medical Association.[3]

Einthoven, in 1895, using an improved electrometer and a correction formula developed independently of Burch, distinguished five deflections which he named P, Q, R, S, and T.[3]

Why PQRST and not ABCDE?

The four deflections prior to the correction formula were labeled ABCD and the five derived deflections were labeled PQRST. The choice of P is a mathematical convention dating from Descartes (as used also by Du Bois-Reymond in his galvanometer's "disturbance curve" 50 years previously) by using letters from the second half of the alphabet. N has other meanings in mathematics and O is used for the origin of the Cartesian coordinates. In fact, Einthoven used O.....X to mark the timeline on his diagrams. P is simply the next letter. A lot of work had been undertaken to reveal the true electrical waveform of the ECG by eliminating the damping effect of the moving parts in the amplifiers and using correction formulae. If you look at the diagram in Einthoven's 1895 paper, you will see how close it is to the string galvanometer recordings and the ECGs we see today **(Fig. 4)**. The image of the PQRST diagram may have been striking enough to have been adopted by the researchers as a true representation of the underlying form. It would have then been logical to continue the same naming convention when the more advanced string galvanometer started creating ECGs a few years later.[4]

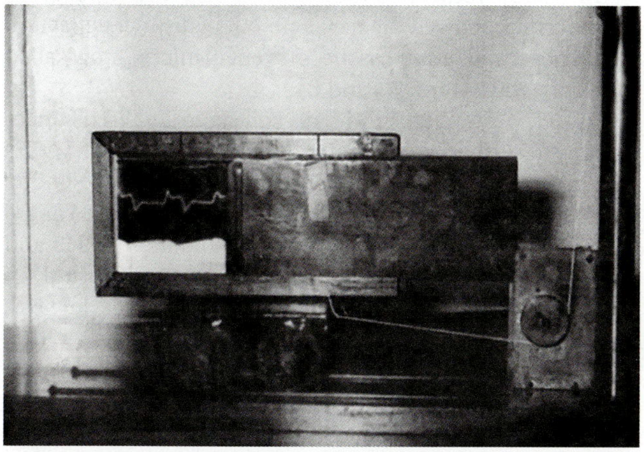

FIG. 2: Electrocardiogram (ECG) tracing as recorded by Augustus D Waller.

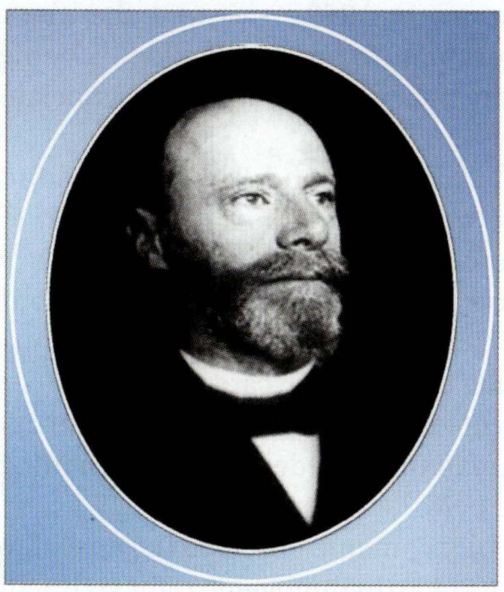

FIG. 3: Willem Einthoven—the inventor of electrocardiogram (ECG).

Einthoven, in 1901, with his invention of the string galvanometer weighing 600 pounds, a device that could accurately measure ECG signals **(Figs. 5 and 6)** and published the first ECG in 1902.[5]

In 1905, he introduced U wave. Clinical use of the ECG and a lot of information depicting various ECG patterns and arrhythmias were described by him in 1906.[6] Three leads were invented by him and gave the uniformity of the recording process and he won the Nobel Prize for the same in 1924.[7]

In 1912, Einthoven outlined the equilateral triangle formed by standard leads I, II, and III (Einthoven triangle).[8]

In 1920, Louis Sigurd Fridericia brought the concept of QT interval correction and used the cube root of RR interval (Fridericia formula),[9] while in the same year Henry Cuthbert Bazett related the corrected QT interval to the square root of the RR interval (Bazett formula).[10]

In 1930, Wolff L, Parkinson J, and White PD published 11 cases of the description "Bundle Branch Block with Short

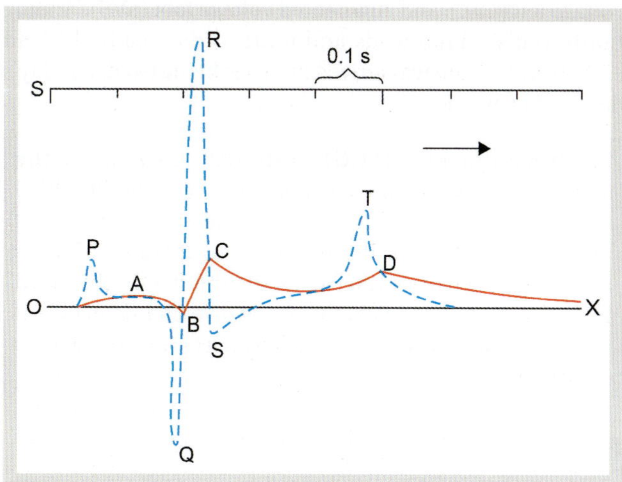

FIG. 4: Uncorrected and corrected electrocardiogram (ECG) tracing as labeled by Willem Einthoven.

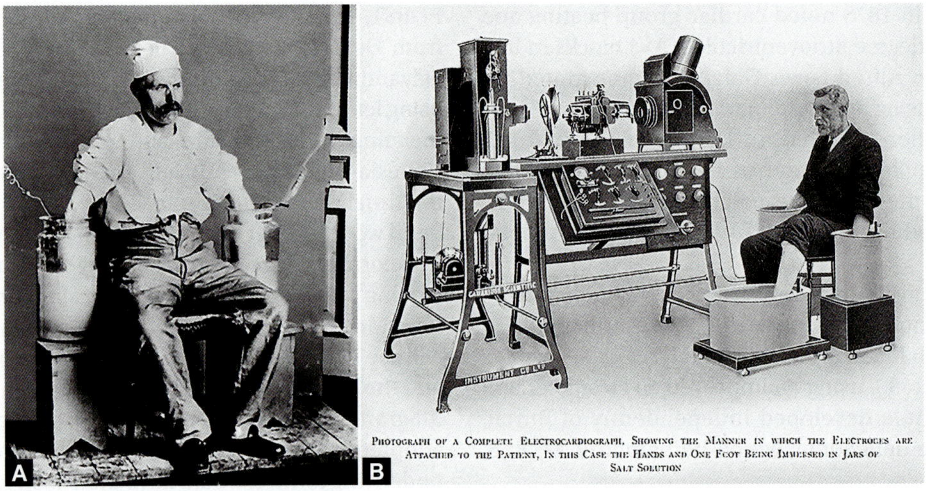

FIGS. 5A AND B: Electrocardiography being taken by Einthoven and the first string galvanometer.

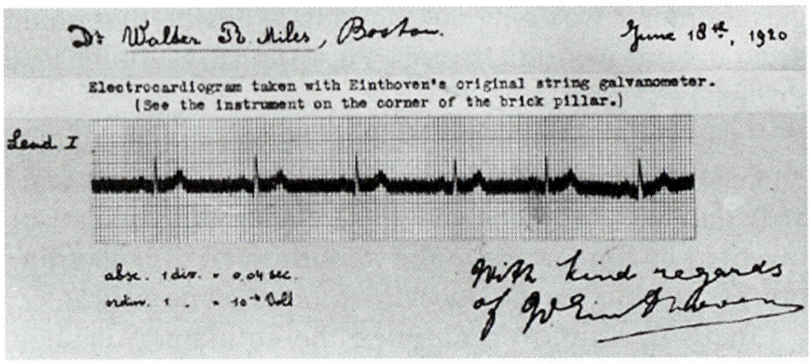

FIG. 6: First electrocardiography (ECG) by Einthoven by his original string galvanometer in 1920.

P-R interval in Healthy Young People Prone to Paroxysmal Tachycardia"—known as WPW syndrome.[11]

Precordial leads were introduced in 1931.[12]

In 1942, Emanuel Goldberger incremented the voltage of Wilson's unipolar leads by 50% and created the augmented limb leads augmented voltage right (aVR), augmented voltage left (aVL), and augmented voltage foot (aVF). Adding Einthoven's 3 limb leads and 6 precordial leads, 12-lead electrocardiogram was arrived at that is being used in today's day-to-day practice.[13]

Electrocardiogram (ECG) yesterday showed us the evolution of ECG to the current status and the first ECG reported by Einthoven in 1920 looks exactly the same as of ECG today. From 3 leads, it saw the augmented unipolar limb leads, then precordial leads and the standard 12-lead ECG. Concept of 15-lead ECG was evolved for detection of ischemic changes in certain hidden areas in acute coronary insufficiency.

ELECTROCARDIOGRAM TODAY

In 1949, Norman Jeff Holter invented ambulatory electrocardiography, popularly known as Holter monitoring currently. The first ECG radio transmitter with batteries weighed >38 kg.[14]

In 1953, John J Osborn, studying the effects of hypothermia, showed the development of distinct deflection at the j point and termed as the "current of injury", now called as Osborn wave **(Figs. 7A and B)**.[15]

In 1957, Anton Jervell with his colleague and Fred Lange-Nielsen described a congenital long QT syndrome (LQTS) with severe bilateral sensorineural hearing loss and sudden death, an autosomal recessive syndrome—Jervell and Lange-Nielsen syndrome (JLNS).[16] Cesarino Romano in 1963 and in 1964 Owen Conor Ward independently reported an autosomal dominant congenital LQTS without hearing loss, now known as Romano-Ward syndrome[17,18].

In 1966, first case of "torsade de pointes" was published by François Dessertenne.[19]

In 1968, Henry JL "Barney" Marriott introduces the modified CL or MCL system (M for modified, C for chest, and L for left arm) for constant monitoring of patients in coronary intensive care units.[20]

Rosenbaum, in 1969, reviewed the classification of ventricular premature beats and added a benign form that arises from the right ventricle and is not associated with heart disease.[21]

In 1974, Gozensky and Thorne introduce the term "rabbit ears" to electrocardiography. Rabbit ears describe the appearance of the QRS complex in lead V_1 with an Rsr' pattern (good rabbit) being typical of right bundle branch block and an RSr' (bad rabbit) suggesting a ventricular origin, i.e., ventricular ectopy/tachycardia.[22]

Use of right-sided precordial leads in the diagnosis of right ventricular infarction was described by Erhardt, Sjögren, and Wahlberg in 1976.[23]

In 1977, Guy Fontaine observed the epsilon waves in 30% of the patients of arrhythmogenic right ventricular dysplasia (ARVD)[24].

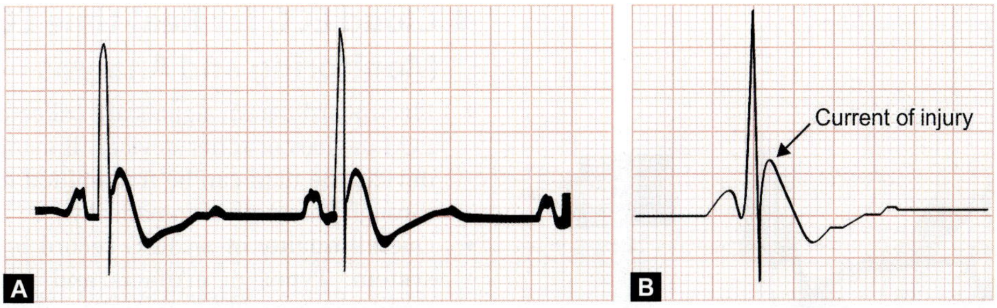

FIGS. 7A AND B: Osborn waves—"current of injury".

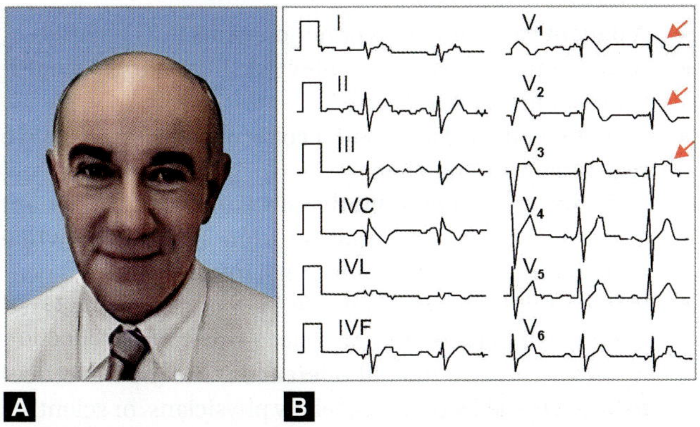

FIGS. 8A AND B: Pedro Brugada and his description of Brugada syndrome.

In 1992, Pedro Brugada **(Figs. 8A and B)** and Joseph Brugada of Barcelona publish a series of eight cases of sudden death, right bundle branch block pattern and ST elevation in V_1-V_3 in apparently healthy individuals—Brugada syndrome.[25]

The concept of 15-lead ECG containing V_4R, V_8, and V_9 for better ECG prediction in ACS was brought by Zalenski RJ in 1993.[26]

In 1996, Elena B Sgarbossa proposed a set of ECG criteria for the diagnosis of acute myocardial infarction (MI) in patients with chest pain with left bundle branch block (LBBB).[27] The criteria was modified by SW Smith in 2012.[28]

Physicians from the Mayo Clinic describe a new hereditary form of short QT syndrome associated with syncope and sudden death that they discovered in 1999.[29]

In 2018, using Apple Smart Watch >400,000 persons were enrolled to identify irregular heart rhythm suggestive of atrial fibrillation (AF).[30]

STRESS ELECTROCARDIOGRAM TESTING

In 1918, Bousfield observed ST depression during angina.[31]

1928, Feil and Siegel reported ST changes during exercise (sit-ups), associated with chest pain.

In 1929, Master introduced first standard exercise protocol—Master's step test[32] **(Figs. 9A and B)**.

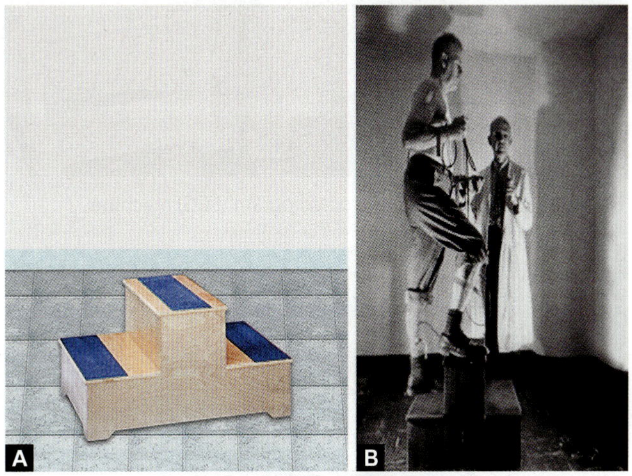

FIG. 9A AND B: Master's step test.

Missal (1938) studied normal persons by having them run up from three to six flight of stairs.[33]

In 1942, The "Harvard Step Test" was introduced to assess the fitness.

Yu and Soffer (1952) described criteria for changes in ECG on exercise indicating ischemia.[34]

In 1956, modern exercise ECG test using a motor-driven treadmill was introduced **(Fig. 10)**.

In 1963, Robert Bruce **(Fig. 11)** and colleagues described their multistage treadmill exercise test, later known as the Bruce Protocol.[35]

> Electrocardiogram (ECG) today focuses more in the area of acute coronary syndrome and detection of various arrhythmias. Continuous ambulatory ECG recording (Holter monitoring) and development of stress ECG testing took place in the current era. Various characteristic ECG patterns such as Osborn waves, Epsilon waves, and Brugada syndrome were described. Congenital long QT syndrome and its relation with sudden cardiac death were observed. Rosenbaum presented the classification of ventricular extrasystoles. Finally, the Apple Watch was introduced for detection of arrhythmias, especially atrial fibrillation.

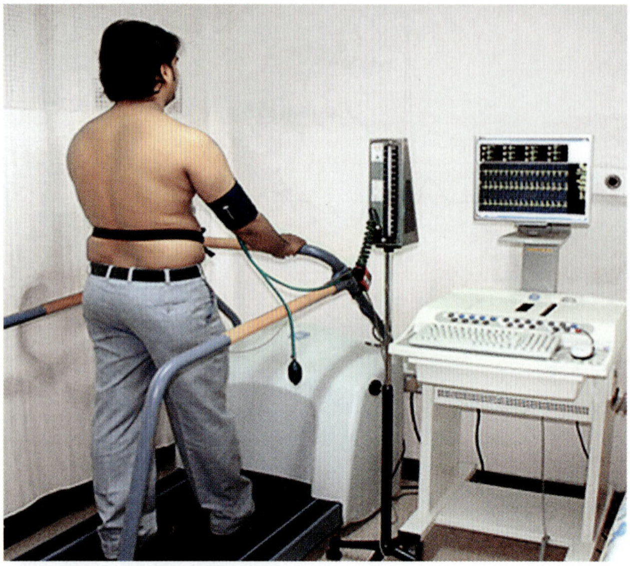

FIG. 10: Modern stress electrocardiogram (ECG) machine.

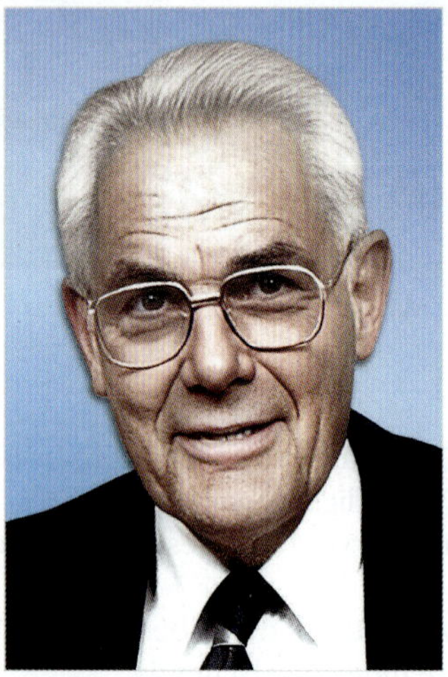

FIG. 11: Robert Bruce—"Father of Stress Electrocardiography".

ELECTROCARDIOGRAM TOMORROW

Computer-aided ECG diagnostic tool:[36]

- To reduce the analysis time needed for the busy physician especially when there are multiple diagnoses, and in cases of large numbers of ECGs to be analyzed
- To assist the physician in ECG analysis and improve his/her diagnostic accuracy
- To facilitate handling of large numbers of ECGs
- To simplify ECG storage and retrieval in a database
- More sophisticated, less expensive with an increasing number of available programs

Cloud ECG software: ECG data was uploaded to the web server from a mobile phone at a certain frequency and analysis was performed in real time using the server **(Fig. 12)**.

Cloud ECG for Real-time ECG Monitoring and Analysis—Advantages

- Electrocardiogram signals are collected using wearable ECG devices or other devices. If using a wearable ECG device, the data can be transmitted to a mobile phone through Bluetooth automatically.
- Overall quality of an ECG record is evaluated by the system. Types of artifacts and potential electrode misplacement will be identified and reported.
- ECG records can be viewed online.
- Critical parameters such as the heart beat rate and RR interval are estimated.
- A patient can browse his or her previous ECG records.
- A patient can submit selected ECGs to a health professional for diagnosis.
- A doctor can have access to records of the users that have registered with him/her.
- A doctor can make tentative decision about a patient and ask for a second opinion from a colleague while withholding the patient's personal information.
- Once a final decision is made by a doctor, the related patient will immediately have access to the results.
- A doctor can also upload reference ECGs (open-source) to be accessed by patients, fellow physicians, or scientists for purpose of education and research.

FUTURE OF ECG LIES WITH THE USE OF ARTIFICIAL INTELLIGENCE IN ECG INTERPRETATION

Artificial intelligence (AI) has revolutionized the science by predictions using computer-based algorithms, no one expected. Machine learning is the basis of AI where computers are allowed to learn, directly from the vast data. In medicine, the principle is utilized to differentiate between healthy and diseased. In healthcare system, AI is being used for screening, disease detection and classification, risk-stratification and proper therapy selection.

Computers are made to work like human brain with interconnected nodes called as neurons, arranged in a network layout. This process is called *deep learning* and the network is called *convolutional neural network* (CNN). Basically, there are three steps of deep learning:

1. Training
2. Internal validation
3. Testing

For example, lacs of ECGs of males are being fed so that machine learns to identify the ECG of males. Similarly, lacs of ECGs of females are fed for the machine to learn the ECG of females. Then, a set of ECGs, again in lacs, are being fed and machine identifies whether the ECG is of male or female and the accuracy is estimated. This process is known as internal validation. If accuracy is acceptable, then the machine is subjected to the test the data given.

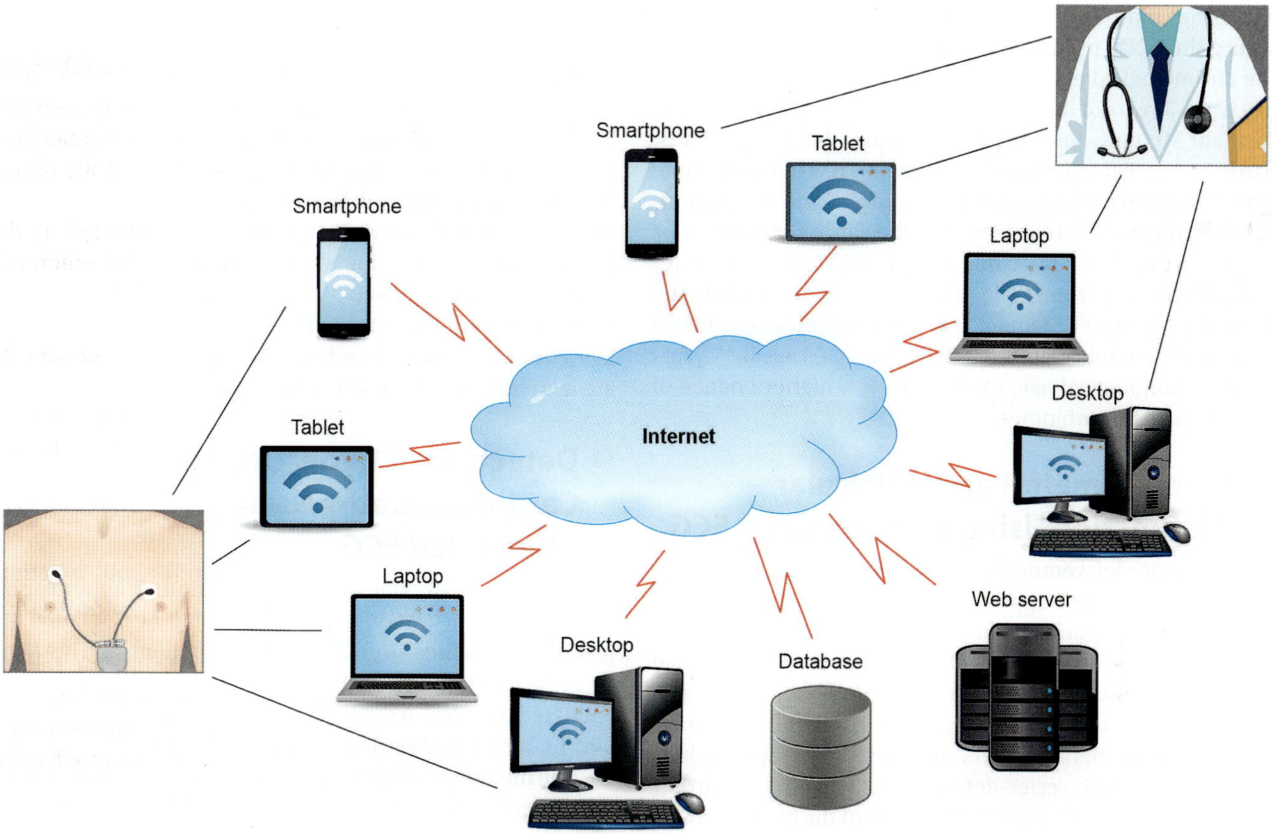

FIG. 12: Electrocardiogram (ECG) transmission from patient to physician using newer technologies.

Age and Sex Estimation Using AI from Standard 12-lead ECGs

Convolutional neural networks were trained to predict age and sex using 10-second 12-lead ECG from 499,727 patients by Attia et al.[37] 399,750 patients were in the training set and 99,977 patients were in the internal validation set. Mean age of the patients was 58.6 ± 16.2 years and 52% were males. Then, 275,056 ECGs were the testing set. Apart from the above data set, 100 patients were selected randomly and their multiple ECGs over two decades were also tested for their chronological age against CNN-predicted age at that year of life.

For all patients, clinical history was extracted for previous history of diabetes, hypertension, coronary artery disease (CAD), MI, low ejection fraction (EF), arrhythmias, and any cardiac surgery. For the set of 100 patients, in the follow-up period, history for any incident events were recorded like history of hospitalizations for any hemodynamic shock, new diagnosis of CAD, heart failure (HF), any thromboembolic events, and cardiac transplantation.

For each ECG, the algorithm output gave a probability number for sex determination. Number closer to 0 had high probability of being female, and number closer to 1 means high probability of being male. The overall accuracy was 90.4%, 90.6% for females, and 90.3% for males. When 10% of the ECGs with intermediate probability ($0.31 < p < 0.69$) were rejected, the accuracy improved to 94.3% and if the 20% ECGs with p values between 0.17 and 0.83 were excluded, the accuracy for sex determination further improved to 96.8%. Sex differentiation was more accurate in younger patients (<45 years of age) as compared to patients older than 55 years, 93% versus 89% respectively. Lower accuracy of sex determination in older individuals can be due to changes in the hormonal status and its effect on the ECGs. Another limitation was the comparison of the data with the self-reported sex.

The output of the age estimation network was a continuous variable. The mean absolute error was 6.9 ± 5.6 years ($p < 0.0001$). The area under the curve (AUC) was 0.94 for detection of age ≥40 years, with 87.8% sensitivity, 86.8% specificity, and accuracy of 87%. It was noted that where CNN-predicted age was >7 years from the chronological age, the patients had a higher incidence of preexisting comorbidities like previous MI, low EF, CAD, hypertension, and AF. It appears that CNN-predicted age is more of physiological age of a person than just the chronological age and is a better marker. In the cohort of 100 patients where multiple ECGs were taken over decades, a sicker cohort of patients with a need of serial ECGs. There were no significant morbidities and patients were otherwise healthy where the CNN-predicted age was <7 years or ±7 years of the chronological age. However, where the CNN-predicted age was >7 years of the chronological age, new-onset low EF, incident MI, new-onset hypertension and diabetes mellitus, cardiac transplantation, and major events like hemodynamic shock occurred during follow-up period. In one patient, CNN-predicted age decreased after the cardiac transplant.

Attia et al.[37] concluded that using CNN, trained computer can identify the from 12-lead standard ECG whether the individual is male or female and can determine age within 7 years of the actual age. And if CNN-predicted age is >7 years of the chronological age, there is likely a higher chance of cardiovascular morbidities.

Asymptomatic Left Ventricular Dysfunction Using an AI-enabled ECG

Asymptomatic left ventricular dysfunction (ALVD) is common in elderly population, approximately 9% and 3–6% in general population and leads to increased morbidity and mortality and reduced life expectancy. Identification of ALVD can lead to proper medical treatment with angiotensin-converting enzyme inhibitors (ACEI), angiotensin receptor blockers (ARBs) and/or beta blockers and device therapy such as implantable cardioverter-defibrillators (ICDs) and cardiac resynchronization therapy (CRT) to retard the progression of the disease to symptomatic HF, thereby reducing mortality. Currently, we do not have a noninvasive, inexpensive tool to determine ALVD and either echocardiography or estimation of B-type natriuretic peptide (BNP) levels are the basic investigations to identify it. Using AI-enabled ECG with paired 12-lead ECG and echocardiogram data, Attia et al.[38] hypothesized to identify ALVD.

A cohort of 625,326 patients with paired ECG and transthoracic echocardiogram (TTE) were screened for analysis and finally, 97,829 patients where ECG and echocardiography were performed within 2 weeks constituted the analysis data set, with 89% within 1 day: 35,970 patients in training set, 8,989 patients in internal validation set, and 52,870 patients in testing set. The mean age of the patient population was 61.8 ± 16.5 years. In the testing data set, EF ≤ 35% was present in 4,131 patients (7.8%), 6,740 (12.7%) patients had EF between 35 to <50%, and 41,999 (79.5%) patients had EF ≥ 50%.

Higher degree of discrimination between EF ≤ 35% and EF, 35% was seen in the test data with the overall accuracy of 85.7%, sensitivity of 86.3%, and specificity of 85.7%. When patients with no known comorbidities were analyzed separately, the accuracy improved to 92.5%, with 95.6% sensitivity and 92.4% specificity. Across all age and sex groups, the network performance was strong.

Total 1,335 patients, having normal EF on echocardiogram, were labeled as having low EF on CNN-ECG (false positive), when followed up, 147 patients developed left ventricular (LV) dysfunction over a median follow-up of 3.4 years, suggesting that the network identified the ECG abnormalities of LV dysfunction earlier before the overt LV dysfunction. Such "false positive" patients who had normal EF, but network reported low EF, had a four-fold increased risk of developing ventricular dysfunction over next 5 years. AUC of CNN-predicted low EF was 0.93 as compared to AUC for BNP and N-terminal pro-B-type natriuretic peptide (NTproBNP) to screen for systolic and diastolic function was 0.60 and 0.70, respectively.

To conclude, AI-enabled ECG screening for ALVD is a low-cost, powerful tool and can identify the individuals who are at increased risk for developing LV dysfunction in future.

Detection of Hypertrophic Cardiomyopathy Using AI-enabled ECG

Ko et al.[39] published a study for detection of hypertrophic cardiomyopathy (HCM) using AI-enabled ECG. Digital 12-lead ECG, obtained from 2,448 verified patients of HCM and 51,153 non-HCM age- and sex- matched controls trained and validated the CNN. A separate dataset from 612 HCM patients and 12,788 control subjects were used as the testing set.

The mean age for HCM group was 54.8 ± 15.9 years and for the control group 57.5 ± 15.5 years. The AUC of CNN was 0.96 with 87% sensitivity and 90% specificity. In younger patients, the performance of CNN was better with 95% sensitivity and 92% specificity.

To conclude, AI-based algorithm can detect HCM on ECG by trained and validated CNN with high diagnostic accuracy.

Noninvasive Detection of Hyperkalemia from AI-enabled ECG

Hyperkalemia is a medical emergency, if not detected early and treated appropriately. Seen commonly in patients with HF, chronic kidney disease, and with the medications to treat these conditions. Hyperkalemia carries high arrhythmia risk and mortality. ECG changes have been described in hyperkalemia, but not consistent and appear late. As patients are mostly asymptomatic, diagnosis of hyperkalemia is challenging.

Electrocardiogram and serum potassium levels within 12 hours of ECG were extracted from Mayo Clinic Data between 1994 and 2017. 709,000 patients, 2.1 million ECGs, and 4.0 million serum potassium values made the data for the study. 5.0 mmol/L was taken as the threshold and repeated positive results were taken to avoid false positive tests. Finally, 20,196 positive and 2.0 million negative tests were the dataset. Using ECG leads I and II, deep neural network was trained with AI algorithm to detect hyperkalemia. Tests were performed on 698,939 ECGs from 224,690 patients and the AUC was 0.87, with 85% sensitivity and 72% specificity.[40]

The study concluded that AI algorithm is a viable tool for detecting even mild hyperkalemia from a two-lead ECG.

Detection of Aortic Stenosis Using an AI-enabled ECG

Almost 263,570 patients with ECG and echocardiogram performed within 180 days were the study dataset. CNN was trained to detect at least moderate AS (aortic valve velocity ≥3 m/s and/or area ≤1.5 cm^2) using 12-lead ECG. 50% of the patients were used for the training, 10% for internal validation, and 40% for the testing. Out of 105,461 testing patients, 5,088 (4.8%) patients were of at least moderate AS category and were labeled as "positive". CNN could identify at least moderate AS with 75% accuracy, 78% sensitivity and 75% specificity.[41]

To conclude, AI-enabled ECG can be used to detect AS early and can become a powerful tool for screening of asymptomatic AS in community using 12-lead ECG.

Artificial Intelligence-enabled ECG Algorithm for Atrial Fibrillation

Atrial fibrillation is the most common type of cardiac arrhythmia and affects 1–4% of the general population and is important risk factor for stroke,[42] HF, and mortality. Prevalence of AF is predicted to double over the next 30 years and is associated with a five-fold increased risk of ischemic stroke.[43] Screening for AF remains a challenge, as the present common screening methods like single ECG or 24 hours ambulatory ECG recording (Holter) have very low yield.

Identifying AF from a sinus rhythm ECG using AI seems to be a good proposition. From the Mayo Clinic dataset between December 31st 1993 and July 21st 2017, digital standard 12-lead ECG having sinus rhythm of patients, 18 years or older was the study material. If they had at least one ECG of AF or atrial flutter, they were taken as positive for AF. 180,922 patients were included with 649,931 sinus rhythm ECGs, 454,789 ECGS from 126,526 patients were used for the training set; 6,430 ECGS from 18,116 patients used for internal validation and 130,802 ECGs from 36,280 patients comprised the testing dataset. 3,051 (8.4%) patients of testing dataset had verified AF or atrial flutter. Patients were categorized into two categories: first, having AF within 31 days of the index ECG (window of interest) and second, AF later than 31 days.

Overall AUC was 0.87, accuracy of 79.4% with 79.0% sensitivity and 79.5% specificity. If taken for ECGs within window of interest, AUC improved to 0.90 with overall accuracy of 83.3%, sensitivity of 82.3%, and 83.4% specificity. For the second group of patients where the AF occurred beyond 31 days of index ECG, the AUC remained at 0.90.[44]

Study concluded that AI-enabled ECG in sinus rhythm can identify patients with history of AF or impending AF, quiet accurately.[44]

Super-human diagnostic abilities have been provided to the clinicians by the application of AI to the ECG interpretation.[45]

> Future of electrocardiogram (ECG) lies in the development of better and better instrumentation and quick transmission of ECG from patient to physician so that the patient can get the correct advice faster. Application of artificial intelligence will bring the revolution in the ECG interpretation.

CONCLUSION

Electrocardiogram has not lost its sheen in spite of >100 years old and it is the first investigation of choice in any suspected case of chest pain to rule in or rule out ACS and in the evaluation of various arrhythmias. The 12-lead surface ECG can indicate pathological changes even before structural changes in the heart can be diagnosed by other methods. There have been many historical events that have happened in the long journey of ECG. Many advancements have come especially in the recording of ECG and its transmission between the patients and the physicians. AI is going to change the total outlook of ECG interpretation.

ONLINE REFERENCES

Please scan the QR code provided at the end of the table of contents for References of this chapter.

CHAPTER

11

Learnings from the M-PAC Registry

S Anne Princy, G Justin Paul

ABSTRACT

Cardiac disease remains a major cause of morbidity and mortality during pregnancy and postpartum. Even in low- and middle-income countries (LMICs), the prevalence of heart disease during pregnancy is increasing and is slowly dominating as an important contributor to maternal mortality.

Proper evaluation of the clinical characteristics of the patient, early triaging, and periodic close follow with an appropriate plan of care play a key role in the management of these pregnant women with heart disease (PWWHD). The above components can be achieved only through appropriate preconception counseling and multidisciplinary teamwork, which is not often a priority, especially in the resource-limited setting of LMICs.

This chapter enlightens the inception of the Madras Medical College Pregnancy and Cardiac (M-PAC) registry, the largest single-center prospective study of PWWHD in an LMIC setting. The results of the registry, risk predictors, and maternal and fetal outcomes are briefly delineated. We display the learnings from the registry so as to highlight the gaps in the knowledge of managing PWWHD and the future outlooks.

Keywords: Pregnancy, heart disease, cardio-obstetrics, MMR, maternal mortality.

INTRODUCTION

Pregnancy complicated by heart disease accounts for 1–4% of pregnancies[1] and has now become a leading cause of maternal mortality and morbidity in both high-income country (HIC) and low- and middle-income countries (LMICs). During pregnancy, the intricate interplay between the maternal cardiovascular system and heart disease can lead to complex challenges. Pregnancy not only alters the hemodynamics of preexisting heart conditions but can also predispose women to new-onset heart disease. Pregnancy is not only known to alter the hemodynamics of an underlying heart disease but also can predispose to new-onset heart disease. This is because the increased cardiac demands during pregnancy and the associated altered physiological milieu increase morbidity and mortality in women with underlying heart disease and can also predispose to new-onset heart disease. Pregnant women with heart disease (PWWHD) faces a higher incidence of adverse outcomes, including abortions, stillbirths, preterm births, and low birth weight infants. In this chapter, we discuss the rationale of conducting the Madras Medical College Pregnancy and Cardiac (M-PAC) study and the key learning points from the study.

NEED FOR FOCUSING ON PREGNANT WOMEN WITH HEART DISEASE

There are many reasons why a developing nation like India needs to focus on care of PWWHD. Firstly, the number of women presenting with heart disease and cardiovascular risk factors during pregnancy has been increasing over the past few decades. This is related to the increased prevalence of unhealthy lifestyle habits, advancing maternal age, and improved survival of women with complex congenital and rheumatic heart disease (RHD) to childbearing age secondary to advances in diagnosis and management of these cardiac conditions.

Secondly, India presently falls in the stage III and IV of obstetric transition,[2] which is a transition from a predominance of direct obstetric causes of maternal mortality to an increasing proportion of indirect causes and noncommunicable causes. With improved management of bleeding, infective and hypertensive causes of maternal death, cardiovascular disease is becoming an increasingly important nonobstetric cause of maternal death in LMICs.

Thirdly, a large proportion of maternal deaths[3] (30–68%) attributable to cardiac disease in pregnancy can be prevented by improved care during pregnancy. The review of maternal death reviews and audits indicates that delayed and wrong diagnosis, inadequate and inappropriate treatment, delayed recognition of high-risk markers, and failure to offer timely referral to appropriate specialists as some of the areas of concern that need improvement.

NEED FOR REGISTRIES OF PREGNANT WOMEN WITH HEART DISEASE

Registries involving PWWHD help in assessing the current clinical practices and the outcomes in actual scenarios at the field level. They are an essential tool to improve and reinforce the delivery of quality healthcare. They also provide an opportunity to ensure quality assurance and help indicate the healthcare system, the areas that need intervention to optimize standard of care delivery. There are large-scale registries that provide information on risk predictors and outcomes in PWWHD from HIC,[4] whereas in LMICs only scare reports are available.

In addition, patient's characteristics and the profile of cardiovascular conditions are different in LMICs compared to that of HICs. Congenital heart disease (CHD) is the most common heart disease in pregnant women in HIC, while it is RHD in LMICs.[5] Because PWWHD in LMICs has a diverse profile of heart illnesses and lives in a different sociocultural milieu with a restricted healthcare system, observations from affluent countries may not adequately address their needs.

Thus, the M-PAC registry was initiated to address the issue of lack of contemporary data from the LMICs, gaps in knowledge pertaining to PWWHD, and to provide contemporary information on the profile of cardiovascular diseases during pregnancy, their impact on maternal and fetal outcomes and to identify the risk predictors relevant to a LMIC population.

A BRIEF OVERVIEW OF THE METHODOLOGY OF THE MADRAS MEDICAL COLLEGE PREGNANCY AND CARDIAC REGISTRY[6]

The M-PAC registry is a single-center prospective observational registry conducted at a tertiary care public hospital in Tamil Nadu, India between the period of July 2016 and December 2019. All pregnant women with known or newly diagnosed structural heart disease, aortic disease, pulmonary vascular disease, and cardiac rhythm disturbances, seeking care in our institution, during the antenatal period or 1-week postpartum and willing to partake were included in the registry. Enrolment for patients with peripartum cardiomyopathy was allowed up to 6-month postpartum. To be eligible for inclusion with cardiac arrhythmia as the primary diagnosis, patient must have had symptomatic sustained tachyarrhythmia or bradyarrhythmia with a structurally normal heart, requiring treatment before pregnancy. All patients underwent a detailed baseline questionnaire-based assessment, clinical evaluation, electrocardiography, and echocardiography at enrolment. Patients were grouped according to the modified World Health Organization (mWHO) classification to classify the maternal risk of pregnancy associated with specific cardiovascular conditions. Routine obstetric and cardiac care were followed as per existing hospital protocol. Patients were followed up through pregnancy and 1-week postpartum. Those belonging to mWHO class III and IV had a closer follow-up antenatally and for at least 6-month postpartum. All newborns were examined by pediatrician and neonatal echocardiographic evaluation was done for those with suspected cardiac abnormalities.

Left ventricular ejection fraction, valvular area, transvalvular gradients, and severity of valvular regurgitation were measured using validated methods and standardized criteria. Tricuspid regurgitation jet velocity-driven estimate of the right ventricular systolic pressure (RVSP) in the absence of pulmonary stenosis was used to classify pulmonary hypertension (PH) as per existing institutional protocol.

Outcomes

All-cause maternal mortality and a composite of maternal cardiac events (MCEs) during pregnancy and first week postpartum constituted the primary outcomes. Fetal loss (defined as abortions or stillbirths) and a composite of adverse fetal events (AFEs) were the secondary outcomes. Fetal loss, preterm birth, small-for-gestational-age, and congenital anomalies in the newborn were included in AFEs.

Analysis

Baseline characteristics were analyzed for all the pregnancies included in the study. Differences in the baseline characteristics between the pregnancies with and without cardiac event/death were analyzed. An additional analysis of outcome predictors was done after excluding the pregnancies that did not continue beyond 24 weeks of gestation. The high-risk factors specifically evaluated in the M-PAC registry are given in **Box 1**.

Categorical data were presented as frequencies and percentages and compared using chi-square tests. Continuous data were presented as mean and standard deviation and were compared using independent samples t-tests. Parameters with $p < 0.1$ in univariable analysis and parameters considered to influence various outcomes were analyzed with multivariable logistic regression model. We

BOX 1 High-risk factors in the M-PAC registry.

- Left ventricular systolic dysfunction (LVSD) (ejection fraction ≤45%)
- *High-risk valve lesions*: Left ventricular outflow tract (LVOT) obstruction with mean gradient ≥20 mm Hg, severe mitral stenosis with mitral valve area ≤1.5 cm^2, or moderate-to-severe regurgitation of aortic or mitral valves
- Moderate or severe PH (RVSP >45 mm Hg in the absence of right ventricular outflow obstruction)
- Mechanical heart valves
- Maternal cyanosis
- Diagnosis during current pregnancy
- Prior cardiac procedures
- NYHA class at presentation

(M-PAC: Madras Medical College Pregnancy and Cardiac; NYHA: New York Heart Association; PH: pulmonary hypertension; RVSP: right ventricular systolic pressure)

generated adjusted odds ratio (OR) and their 95% confidence interval (CI) and *p*-value. Hosmer–Lemeshow test was used to confirm the goodness-of-fit. Significance was assumed at a two-sided value of $p < 0.05$. We assessed the ability of the mWHO classification to predict the maternal outcome and fetal outcome in our cohort, using the receiver operating characteristic (ROC) curves and c-statistic values.

RESULTS

Out of the 152,415 pregnancies registered in our institution, 1,154 pregnancies (0.8%) involved women with heart disease. Our study population was predominantly young with 41% of them <25 years of age. Only 2.3% were above 35 years of age. Heart disease was diagnosed for the first-time during pregnancy in 60.5% of women. Most of the pregnancies involved asymptomatic or minimally symptomatic women, with only 8.7% having NYHA class III or IV symptoms. All mWHO categories were represented in our population, with 63.8% of the pregnancies in high-risk mWHO II–III, III, and IV categories. Almost a third of the pregnancies (34.2%) had PH. Almost one-fifth (20.5%) of pregnancies were in mothers who had undergone a surgical or interventional procedure prior to conception.

Profile of Heart Disease

Valvular heart disease was the most common cardiac illness present in 54.1% of our study population, of which RHD (77.7%) was the predominant cause. Mitral valve involvement was most common, with combined mitral stenosis and mitral regurgitation accounting for 30%. CHD was the next largest group (33.6%) of which shunt lesions (76.3%) predominated, the most common being atrial septal defect followed by ventricular septal defect. Complex CHDs were relatively low in our population. Only 3.1% of our patients had cyanotic CHDs.

Maternal Outcome

About 38.8% were delivered by cesarean section. MCEs were observed in 156 pregnancies and maternal deaths in 20. New or worsening heart failure was the most common MCE, followed by thromboembolic events. Peripartum cardiomyopathy was the most common cause of heart failure followed by valvular heart disease. The multivariable analysis showed that the presence of prosthetic heart valve (PHV), left ventricular systolic dysfunction (LVSD), and PH was predictors of MCEs and maternal death. Severe mitral stenosis was a predictor of MCEs but not maternal death. The 72 pregnancies that did not progress beyond 24 weeks also had a high MCE rate (13.9%) and mortality (1.4%).

Fetal Outcome

Around 91.2% of pregnancies resulted in live births. AFEs occurred in 33.7% of pregnancies and fetal loss occurred in 8.8% pregnancies. AFEs were more common in pregnancies involving higher NYHA class, higher mWHO category > II, cyanotic heart disease, PHV, severe mitral stenosis, moderate or severe PH, and in those on prior cardiac medications. Maternal cyanosis, presence of PHV, and severe mitral stenosis were the multivariable predictors of AFEs and fetal loss. PH was a predictor of AFEs but not fetal loss.

COMPARATIVE EVALUATION WITH OTHER PROSPECTIVE REGISTRIES

Comparing the data[7] for M-PAC, ROPAC, and CARPREG II, the following key findings were noted. Patients in M-PAC were older with half of them being diagnosed to have heart disease during current pregnancy. The proportion of CHD was lower, with a greater representation of patients belonging to higher risk mWHO categories III and IV **(Table 1)**.

LESSONS FROM M-PAC REGISTRY

The M-PAC registry identified that presence of severe mitral stenosis, LV systolic dysfunction, mechanical prosthetic valve, PH, NYHA class > II, mWHO grade > II, and diagnosis during current pregnancy was associated with adverse maternal cardiac outcome. In addition, it was shown that 60% of women come to know about their heart disease for the first time during their pregnancy. Apart from the disease-specific risk and the above-mentioned risk predictors, there are many other inferences that were drawn from the M-PAC study which are discussed below. Some of the contributors to higher mortality in PWWHD include lack of coordination among the various disciplines involved in the management of PWWHD, lack of uniform guidelines in managing PWWHD, nonuniform distribution of healthcare facilities, and lack of awareness among the public and healthcare providers.

TABLE 1: Pregnancy outcomes in WWHD—data from prospective registries.

Parameters		M-PAC	ROPAC	CARPREG II
Baseline characteristic	Age, mean	26.0	29.5	30.6
	Nulliparity	53.5%	39.7%	51%
	Diagnosis during current pregnancy	50.1%	8.2%	NA
Main diagnosis	CHD	33.6%	57.4%	63.7%
	VHD	54.1%	28.7%	NA
	Others	12.3%	13.9%	36.3%
Modified World Health Organization (mWHO) classification	mWHO I	21.4%	20.6%	13%
	mWHO II	14.8%	14.4%	26%
	mWHO II–III	26.9%	47.0%	38%
	mWHO IV	17.8%	10.3%	10%
	mWHO V	19.1%	7.1%	5%
Maternal death		1.9%	0.6%	0.6%
Maternal cardiac event (MCE)		15.2%	16.5%	15.8%
Type of MCE	HF	10.0%	10.6%	6.2%
	Arrhythmia	0.9%	3.3%	9.3%
	Thrombotic	2.0%	1.5%	1.4%
Cesarean delivery		39.0%	46.7%	NA
Fetal outcome	Fetal mortality	1.9%	1.3%	NA
	Preterm	4.8%	15.8%	NA
	LBW	20.2%	11.7%	NA

(CHD: congenital heart disease; RHD: rheumatic heart disease; HF: heart failure; LBW: low birth weight; NA: not available)

OTHER INFERENCES

In addition to unveiling new insights into the profiles and outcomes of PWWHD in LMICs, the experience gained from conducting the M-PAC registry shed light on the sociocultural aspects of the lives of PWWHD, exposed limitations in the available healthcare systems, and identified areas for improvement.

Need for Improved Coordination among the Various Disciplines

One significant challenge in providing quality care for PWWHD is the lack of coordination and effective communication among the involved healthcare disciplines.

Additionally, in many institutions, including ours, cardiac care and obstetric facilities are geographically separate, requiring patients and medical personnel to travel between these locations. Establishing a coordinated cardio-obstetric team following a predefined working model can effectively address these limitations.

The cardio-obstetric team (also called the Maternal Cardiology Team or Pregnancy Heart Team) comprises a multidisciplinary team of dedicated professionals involved in providing care and expertise in the management of PWWHD from preconception to postpartum. The team includes at a minimum, subspecialists from the following disciplines—cardiologist, obstetrician, anesthetist, and pediatrician/neonatologist. Additional members such as cardiothoracic surgeons, cardiac intensivists, blood bank, and perfusion specialists may be added to the CO team while dealing with pregnant women with complex and high-risk conditions. The PH team should take up a wide range of responsibilities including preconception counseling and risk stratification of PWWHD, antenatal, intranatal, and postpartum care of women with known and newly detected heart disease during pregnancy, management of cardiac emergencies during pregnancy and postpartum, contraception, and long-term follow-up in women with adverse pregnancy outcomes.

We established a social media group comprising cardiologists, obstetricians, and anesthetists within our institution to facilitate seamless and rapid coordination in managing PWWHD. This platform enables us to formulate the patient's care plan, discuss the frequency of follow-up evaluations, admission timing, mode of delivery, and anticipated complications.

In addition to regular cardiac consultations, we conducted need-based additional consultations, as determined by our group discussions. This approach significantly improved communication and collaboration between obstetrics and cardiology, even though they are located in different premises.

Need for Uniform Management Guidelines

We identified a lack of uniformity in the treatment protocols in managing PWWHD, particularly in areas such as anticoagulant management for women with PHVs and heart failure management. We also perceived that some maternal adverse events could be attributed to the lack of standardized protocols. To address this issue, we organized multiple awareness and education sessions for both obstetricians and cardiologists involved in PWWHD care. We also established consistent treatment guidelines throughout our institution. As a result, we observed a reduction in adverse MCEs among subsequent PWWHD patients treated in our institution.

Need for Cardio-obstetric Training and Awareness

Many PWWHDs lack access to healthcare facilities equipped with the necessary infrastructure for their specialized management. To address this gap, it is essential to identify high-risk cardiac cases early and refer them to tertiary or quaternary centers staffed with multidisciplinary cardio-obstetric teams for optimized care. Achieving this goal necessitates providing ongoing training in cardio-obstetrics to all healthcare professionals, starting from the foundational level. This training not only equips them with the knowledge needed to identify high-risk cases requiring advanced care but also helps in preventing unnecessary referrals for mWHO I and II cases that can be appropriately managed in secondary care centers

Thus, the M-PAC registry made it evident that to provide comprehensive care for PWWHD, the cardiologists and obstetricians require ongoing Continuous Medical Education (CME) programs beyond their initial graduation.

However, we also noted a deficiency in existing CME programs of both specialties, as they often lacked sufficient emphasis on cardio-obstetrics training.

As a recommendation, we suggest that cardiology and obstetrics conferences, as well as CME programs, incorporate dedicated sessions to address the management challenges encountered in caring for PWWHD.

Preconception Counseling

Preconception counseling is crucial for planning a healthy pregnancy in women with heart disease. Every woman with a known heart condition should receive timely counseling. Informed decision-making by the mother is key, considering not only her heart health but also psychological, ethical, and social factors. Contraception advice is vital and should be discussed before conception. Counseling should involve both the patient and her family, providing guidance on treatment, medical options, drug therapy, interventions, and potential outcomes. Unfortunately, this step is often overlooked. Institutions caring for these women should not only offer preconception counseling but also ensure that those providing it are well-trained in cardio-obstetrics.

Patients with heart disease may receive counseling on contraception and pregnancy at various points in their healthcare journey: after early cardiac surgery or interventional procedures, before marriage, before planning pregnancy, after conception, or after termination of pregnancy. Ideally, preconception counseling should be offered before planning for pregnancy. However, it is concerning that only half of women with CHD receive this crucial guidance.[8]

Regrettably, we also observed that counseling advice was not always appropriate. This was particularly evident in cases where termination of pregnancy advice was given after conception or contraception advice was provided postdelivery. Surprisingly, high-risk women with CHD were more likely to miss out on contraceptive advice.[8]

PSYCHOSOCIAL INFERENCES

In many developing countries, including our own, there is a strong cultural emphasis on marrying off daughters, while having a heart disease is often stigmatized. Unfortunately, in some healthcare settings in these countries, counseling about heart disease is directed toward parents rather than the affected child. In their eagerness to marry off their daughters, parents of girls with heart disease may choose not to disclose the condition to their daughters or to prospective grooms and their families. This situation leads to women becoming pregnant before their heart condition can be properly addressed, putting their health at risk. It can also create mistrust among all parties involved, potentially leading to marital problems and domestic conflicts. Additionally, societal pressures to become a mother drive many women with high-risk heart diseases to pursue pregnancies against medical advice, further increasing the health risks for PWWHD.

NEED FOR REGIONAL CLASSIFICATIONS AND RISK SCORES APPLICABLE TO INDIAN POPULATION

The widely used mWHO classification has been developed predominantly based on the profile and outcome of cardiac disease in the Western population. The limitation of its applicability to Indian population has been brought about the M-PAC study, where it overpredicted maternal risk in mWHO categories I, II–III, and IV and underpredicted in category III. The discriminative power mWHO classification to predict maternal risk was moderate (c-statistic of 0.794; 95% CI 0.763–0.826) and fetal risk was low-to-moderate (c-statistic of 0.646; 95% CI 0.610–0.682). It calls for a more simple and regionally applicable classification suitable for our population.

Pulmonary Hypertension

We also observed that categorization of all forms and degrees of PH into class IV mWHO may be a significant limitation. We have earlier shown that pregnancies in women with left-to-right shunt lesions had a better outcome despite associated PH. We also noticed that though women with PH due to left heart disease had a higher proportion of adverse events, they fared better than those with primary PH and Eisenmenger syndrome. This indicates a need for a modification in the recommendation that all patients with PH have a prohibitive risk of pregnancy and should be counseled against pregnancy.

HIGH-RISK CONDITIONS CAN BE MADE NOTIFIABLE

The most high-risk and vulnerable pregnant women, requiring continuous monitoring, include those with PHVs, depressed left ventricular function (particularly peripartum cardiomyopathy), and those with cyanotic heart disease. These patient groups accounted for the majority of cardiac events documented in the M-PAC registry. We recommend designating these cardiac conditions as notifiable, which would encourage treating physicians to prioritize a comprehensive team-based approach to their management.

PUBLIC HEALTH IMPACT OF THE M-PAC REGISTRY

Based on preliminary data shared from this study, the Government of Tamil Nadu State has organized the formation of pregnancy and heart disease teams in all government medical colleges, provided echocardiographic machines for all their antenatal care units and initiated sensitization programs to improve coordinated care of these women. The Tamil Nadu Pregnancy and Heart Disease Registry, a multicenter study involving 29 public and private hospitals funded by the Indian council of Medical Research with administrative support from the Government has been initiated in the State of Tamil Nadu to further understand the needs and improve the care of PWWHD.

CONCLUSION

We envision a comprehensive continuum of care for women with heart disease, spanning from infancy to pregnancy. This highlights the necessity for a robust tracking system to facilitate early diagnosis and effective management of cardiac conditions before a woman embarks on motherhood. Identifying underlying heart conditions prior to pregnancy is crucial for optimizing clinical outcomes and providing relevant preconception counseling. In cases, where antenatal diagnosis is absent, and hence preconception counseling is not possible, it is imperative to ensure that systems are in place to grant PWWHD access to advanced medical care for safe pregnancy management.

In conclusion, we emphasize the need for LMICs to prioritize several key areas such as establishing a continuum of care system to detect heart disease in women early, providing disease-specific preconception counseling, offering psychological support and marital counseling for women in the reproductive age group and their families, empowering healthcare systems to deliver multidisciplinary care during pregnancy, providing postdelivery counseling, and addressing contraception needs. Additionally, we stress the importance of developing nation-specific classification schemes and risk stratification tools for PWWHD, with input from diverse regions within the country.

ONLINE REFERENCES

Please scan the QR code provided at the end of the table of contents for References of this chapter.

CHAPTER 12

Relevance of Chest X-ray in Current Cardiology Practice

Sunil Kumar Sharma, Sibaram Panda

ABSTRACT

Early recognition and confirmation of acute heart failure or acute decompensation of chronic heart failure is highly essential to prevent adverse cardiovascular mortality and morbidity. Pulmonary congestion is the leading cause of mortality and hospitalization in heart failure. Accurate assessment and objective demonstration of the presence of congestion is the basic step for effective management and are challenging even for the most experienced and highly skilled physician. Signs and symptoms may be a poor indicator of underlying congestion and sometimes misleading. Chest X-ray (CXR) is often the first-line investigation in patients because of its relative low cost and wide availability. As the pulmonary vasculature is in direct continuity with the left atrium (LA), the rise in LA and pulmonary venous pressure results in various radiographic changes, and the radiologic findings on chest radiography reflect the anatomopathologic alterations. As the severity of congestion increases, the sequence of signs visible on chest radiographs are: (1) vascular opacity "redistribution" toward the upper lobes and distention of the upper pulmonary veins; (2) enlargement and loss of definition of hilar structures; (3) septal lines in the lower lung, indicated as Kerley B lines and around the hilum as Kerley A lines; (4) peribronchial and perivascular cuffing with widening and blurring of the margins; (5) thickening of interlobar fissures with subpleural fluid accumulation; and ultimately (6) alveolar edema. The pulmonary venous pressure can be roughly evaluated from different radiographic changes. Hence, CXR is a very simple, noninvasive, and bedside tool for the evaluation of pulmonary congestion, and correlation with clinical findings can help emergency physicians detect acute heart failure early and prevent the adverse mortality and morbidity associated with acute heart failure.

Keywords: Chest X-ray, pulmonary venous congestion, acute chest pain.

INTRODUCTION

Early evaluation and diagnosis of different conditions presenting with acute pain in the chest and shortness of breath (SOB) in emergency and outpatient settings is crucial for proper management and prevention of morbidity and mortality associated with such medical emergencies. Acute left ventricular failure (LVF), acute decompensation of chronic heart failure, exacerbation of bronchial asthma, chronic obstructive pulmonary disease (COPD), acute pulmonary embolism, spontaneous pneumothorax pleural effusion, and chest infection (both bacterial and viral) are some of the common conditions associated with acute SOB. Acute decompensated heart failure (ADHF) is a frequent emergency condition that often represents a diagnostic challenge for emergency physicians. Unless recognized and treated early, it is associated with fatal adverse events and mortality. The evaluation of decompensation in chronic heart failure is challenging, even for highly skilled clinicians.[1,2] Decompensation is clinically silent in most patients with chronic heart failure and is often not recognized until conditions develop that require hospital admission; this critical delay in diagnosis justifies the need for more sensitive diagnostic tools.[3] Pulmonary congestion, rather than low cardiac output, is considered the leading cause of hospital admissions and death among patients with heart failure.[3,4] Signs and symptoms provide only poor sensitivity for the detection of elevated left heart pressures.[5,6] Accurate assessment and objectively demonstrating the presence of congestion is the basic step for the effectiveness of medical treatment in reducing pulmonary congestion in patients with ADHF and in the subset of heart failure with preserved ejection fraction (diastolic heart failure). The inferior vena cava (IVC) diameter > 21 mm and its collapsibility < 50% are used as indicators of systemic congestion as the IVC is in indirect continuity with the right atrium (RA) and reflects the RA pressure and hence the central venous pressure.[7] The pulmonary vasculature is also in direct continuity with the left atrium (LA), and a rise in LA pressure results in dilatation and engorgement of the pulmonary veins. Echocardiographic measurement of pulmonary veins can be used as an indicator of pulmonary venous congestion, but there is no guideline or method for measuring pulmonary veins to assess pulmonary congestion. Elevated N-terminal pro-B-type natriuretic peptide (NT-proBNP) is a powerful neurohormonal predictor and prognostic marker of heart failure. Echocardiography helps in the noninvasive evaluation of left ventricular filling pressure by measuring the E/e′ ratio. But it is not widely available in our country and may not be affordable for the vast majority of our population. Both investigations evaluate hemodynamic congestion but do not provide direct evidence of pulmonary congestion. Lung ultrasound (LUS) through B-line evaluation (formerly ultrasound lung comets) has recently been proposed as a simple, noninvasive, and semiquantitative tool to assess lung congestion by evaluating extravascular lung water.[5,6,8] But many of our hospitals are not equipped with manpower to perform these tests in the emergency department, so they may not be useful for routine use. Hence, there is a need to objectively evaluate pulmonary congestion as soon as possible to prevent further clinical deterioration and reduce mortality and morbidity. The pulmonary vasculature is also in direct continuity with the LA, and a rise in LA pressure results in dilatation and engorgement of the pulmonary vein, which is reflected roentgenographically by the generalized dilatation of the pulmonary arteries and veins. The introduction of digital chest X-ray (CXR) has improved the quality of CXR, and we can now directly visualize the pulmonary veins converging at the hilum, and interstitial edema can be evaluated by Kerley lines. The CXR remains by far the most widely used test for detecting pulmonary edema.[9]

COMPARISON OF THE DIFFERENT DIAGNOSTIC TOOLS FOR EVALUATION OF PULMONARY CONGESTION

Elevated NT-proBNP has emerged as one of the most powerful neurohormonal diagnostic and prognostic markers in heart failure[10] and is very helpful for titration of further medical treatment and guiding the intensity of medical treatment. It is a marker for elevated filling pressure, raised LA pressure, and hemodynamic congestion. But it is not widely available in our country and may not be affordable for the vast majority of our population. Echocardiography helps in the noninvasive evaluation of left ventricular filling pressure, which is a precursor for the development of pulmonary congestion.[11,12] The ratio of early diastolic mitral inflow velocity to early diastolic velocity of the mitral annulus (E/e') is one of the most frequently used parameters to assess LV pressures and estimate hemodynamic congestion.[13] Hemodynamic congestion is related to high left ventricular filling pressure, a condition that precedes pulmonary congestion. Pulmonary congestion is the result of high hydrostatic pressure in the pulmonary vasculature and is usually, but not always, related to high LV filling pressure and hemodynamic congestion. Hence, diastolic dysfunction or the detection of high filing pressure is not equivalent to pulmonary congestion. Thus, these two commonly used diagnostic tools identify hemodynamic congestion but not true pulmonary congestion.

With the onset of the accumulation of fluid in the interstitium, there is a change in the normal balance between the air and fluid pulmonary content when air is lost and fluid is increased. The multiple and small air–fluid interfaces, due to small water-rich structures surrounded by air, present in the lung periphery, create a reverberation phenomenon represented on the screen by multiple B-lines in the LUS.[6] B-line evaluation by LUS provides direct insight into the pulmonary interstitium and allows one to differentiate a condition of pure hemodynamic congestion from pulmonary interstitial edema. LUS through B-line evaluation (formerly ultrasound lung comets) has recently been proposed as a simple, noninvasive, and semiquantitative tool to assess lung congestion by evaluating extravascular lung water.[8] LUS appears to be particularly useful in differentiating between exacerbations of COPD, a condition that does not show B-lines, and decompensated heart failure.[5,6]

In the acute phase of decompensated heart failure, the early pulmonary alteration is congestion of the vascular bed (pulmonary congestion) due to a progressive increase in capillary hydrostatic pressure. When pressure increases further and the lymphatic vessels become congested, fluids begin to accumulate in the interstitium around arteries, veins, and airways, particularly in the interlobular septa. The CXR detects the change in pulmonary interstitial fluid by detecting Kerley lines and dilatation of the pulmonary vasculature. The CXR remains by far the most widely used test for detecting pulmonary edema.[9] CXR is the traditional first-line procedure to assess because of its ability to recognize pulmonary vascular congestion and other subsets of chest opacity. It is widely and easily available as a diagnostic tool in all emergency and outpatient departments. Chest radiography has the great advantage of combining relative low cost with a panoramic view that allows the exclusion of many pulmonary conditions that come into the differential diagnosis. Another advantage of CXR is its portability, so that investigations can be done at the bedside. All the medical professionals are familiar with the investigation tool. The recent addition of digital CXR has increased the resolution and sharpness of images and can detect subtle findings without adding artifacts. The main reason for this limitation is that CXR is not very sensitive (50-68%), and heart failure cannot be ruled out with certainty in the presence of a normal radiologic pattern. The absence of radiological evidence for decompensated heart failure in the chronic outpatient evaluation does not exclude elevated filling pressures.[2] There is a lot of interobserver variability in the interpretation of radiologic signs, such as vascular opacity, redistribution, and interstitial edema. Hence, according to the American Heart Association/American College of Cardiology guidelines, serial CXRs are not recommended in the assessment of pulmonary congestion in chronic heart failure.[14,15]

Before interpreting CXR, ensure that the exposure and rotation are proper and that it is a full inspiratory film. Failure to expose the film at full inspiration can also result in an apparent redistribution of pulmonary blood flow. The caliber of arteries and veins running through the lung parenchyma is greatly affected by lung volume, and the expansion of the lung determines the extent to which the lung parenchyma pulls on the walls of the arteries and veins.[16,17] Therefore, the radiograph should be exposed at full inspiration (total lung capacity) with the patient standing erect; otherwise, there will be features of apparent redistribution of pulmonary blood flow. In a CXR taken in a supine or semi-erect position, the gravitational difference between the apex and the lung bases will be less, and in the supine position, there will be equalization of blood flow, which may give the false impression of redistribution. Hence, for proper evaluation, it is essential to compare the present CXR with old films and good-quality normal CXR to detect any minor changes. Always interpret the CXR in conjunction with the clinical findings. Whenever CXRs are reviewed and interpreted, a systematic approach should always be used. It is preferable to use an inside-out approach from central to peripheral. First, the heart figure is evaluated, followed by the mediastinum and hila. Subsequently, the lungs, lung borders, and, finally, the chest wall and abdomen are examined.

RADIOGRAPHIC FEATURES OF NORMAL VASCULATURE

Normally, blood flow in the pulmonary vasculature is caudal because of gravity, and in an upright posture, the pressure differential between the base and apex is around 22 mm Hg. Hence, normally very little vascularity is seen above the hilum, and vessels seen in the upper lung fields are smaller and fewer in number than those supplying the lung bases **(Figs. 1A and B)**. The upper lobe vessels have a diameter of around 1-2 mm, and vessel sizes > 3 mm are suggestive of dilated vasculature. Thus, a significant component of the available pulmonary vascular reserve exists in the upper lung zones. This reserve can be recruited to handle increased volume loads in the pulmonary vascular bed. An increase in flow is recognized in chest radiographs by an increase in the size and number of vessels supplying a given area of the lung.[18,19] Normally, the vessels in the upper lobes are smaller than the accompanying bronchus, with a ratio of 0.85. At the level of the hilum, they are equal, and in the lower lobes, the arteries are larger, with a ratio of 1.35. When there is a redistribution of pulmonary blood flow, there will be an increased pulmonary artery bronchus ratio in the upper and middle lobes. This is best visible in the perihilar region.

The normal hilar shadow is for 99% composed of vessels—pulmonary arteries and, to a lesser extent, veins. The vessel margins are smooth, and the vessels have branches. The normal right hilum can be divided into upper and lower halves. The upper half is composed mainly of the descending right upper lobe vein and the lower half is primarily formed

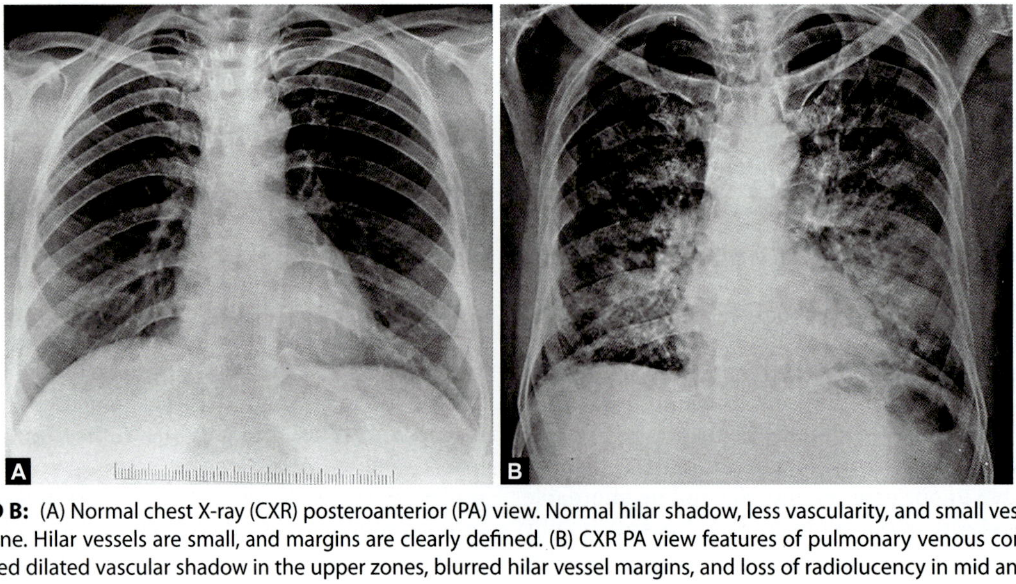

FIGS. 1A AND B: (A) Normal chest X-ray (CXR) posteroanterior (PA) view. Normal hilar shadow, less vascularity, and small vessel seen in the upper lung zone. Hilar vessels are small, and margins are clearly defined. (B) CXR PA view features of pulmonary venous congestion: Hazy hilum, increased dilated vascular shadow in the upper zones, blurred hilar vessel margins, and loss of radiolucency in mid and lower zones.

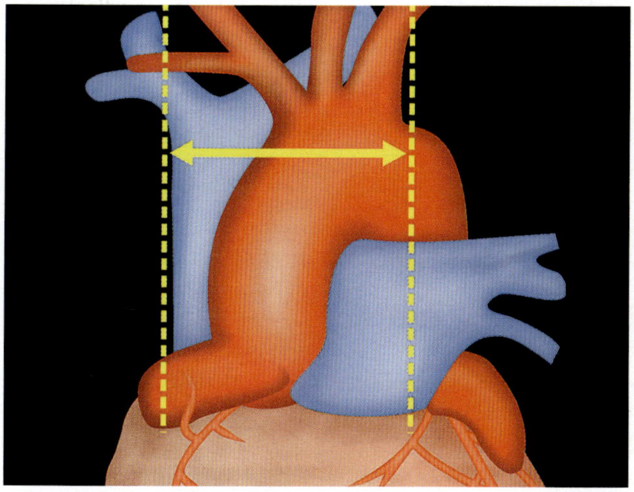

FIG. 2: Vascular pedicle. The vascular pedicle is bordered on the right by the superior vena cava and on the left by the left subclavian artery origin.

by the main trunk of the descending pulmonary artery. An angle is formed where these vessels overlap, which divides the hilum into its two components. Enlargement of the pulmonary veins, as seen in pulmonary venous hypertension, will theoretically obliterate the normal hilar angle and provide a useful sign of pulmonary venous hypertension.[20]

The vascular pedicle is bordered on the right by the superior vena cava and on the left by the left subclavian artery origin **(Fig. 2)**.[21] In 90% of normal CXRs, the vascular pedicle width (VPW) is <60 mm on a posteroanterior (PA) chest radiograph. The vascular pedicle is an indicator of the intravascular volume. A VPW of >85 mm is pathologic in 80% of cases. A 5-mm increase in diameter corresponds to a 1-L increase in intravascular fluid. An increase in the width of the vascular pedicle is accompanied by an increase in the width of the azygos vein. The diameter of the azygos vein varies according to positioning. In the standing position, a diameter > 7 mm is most likely abnormal, and a diameter > 10 mm is definitely abnormal. In a supine patient, a diameter > 15 mm is abnormal. An increase of 3 mm in comparison to previous films is suggestive of fluid overload. The VPW can help in differentiating the different forms of pulmonary edema.[21] Pulmonary edema with a normal pedicle is suggestive of increased capillary permeability or acute heart failure, whereas a wide pedicle is observed in chronic heart failure or fluid overload (e.g., renal failure).

RADIOLOGICAL FEATURES OF PULMONARY VENOUS HYPERTENSION (PULMONARY CONGESTION)

Acute heart failure with alveolar edema interferes with gas exchange, resulting in a state of hypoxemia. Alveolar hypoxia causes pulmonary vessels to constrict. Since there is greater hypoxemia at lung bases than apices, the basilar vessels constrict significantly, forcing blood to flow upward through the veins (redistribution, cephalization). With progressive pulmonary venous hypertension, the relationship between the upper and lower lungs equalizes or then reverses, such that the upper lung ABR exceeds the lower lung ABR in heart failure. As venous pressure rises, the redistribution of flow increases, and vessels in the upper lung fields become equal in size to those in the lower lung fields, which manifests radiographically as the enlargement of upper lobe vessels (cephalization) **(Figs. 3 and 4)**.[22,23] The chest roentgenographic changes that reflect this altered physiology are said to be generalized pulmonary venous engorgement and a disparity between the dilated upper zone vessels and constricted lower zone vessels. While the most striking changes in redistribution are noted in chronic settings, less severe changes may be noted with milder elevations in pulmonary venous pressure. When pulmonary vascular pressure exceeds plasma oncotic pressure (normally approximately 25 mm Hg), fluid begins to leak from the vessels into the vascular bed at the lung bases, resulting in the development of congestion of the vascular bed. When pressure increases further and the lymphatic vessels become congested, fluids begin to accumulate in the interstitial tissue around arteries, veins, and airways, particularly in the interlobular septa and peribronchial interstitium. When fluid leaks into the peripheral interlobular septa, it is seen as Kerley B or septal lines (as shown in **Fig. 5**), which are seen as peripheral, short, 1–2 cm horizontal lines near the costophrenic angle running perpendicular to the pleura.[24-28] Leaking and accumulation of fluids into the peribronchovascular interstitium are seen as thickening of the bronchial walls (peribronchial cuffing) and as a loss of definition of these vessels (perihilar haze) **(Figs. 6A and B)**. The radiologic findings at chest radiography reflect the anatomopathologic alterations. As the severity of congestion increases, the sequence of signs visible on chest radiographs is as follows: (1) Vascular opacity "redistribution" toward the upper lobes and distention of the upper pulmonary veins; (2) enlargement and loss of definition of hilar structures; (3) septal lines in the lower lung, indicated as Kerley B lines and around the hilum as Kerley A lines **(Table 1)**; (4) peribronchial and perivascular cuffing with widening and blurring of the margins; and (5) thickening of interlobar fissures with subpleural fluid accumulation **(Figs. 7A and B)**.

The final stage of congestion is characterized by continued fluid leakage into the interstitium, which cannot be compensated by lymphatic drainage. This eventually leads to fluid leakage in the alveoli (alveolar edema) **(Figs. 8A and B)** and leakage into the pleural space (pleural effusion). When congestion increases and becomes alveolar edema, chest radiography shows bilateral and usually symmetric parenchymal opacities with a central or basilar distribution without an air bronchogram **(Fig. 9)**. One of

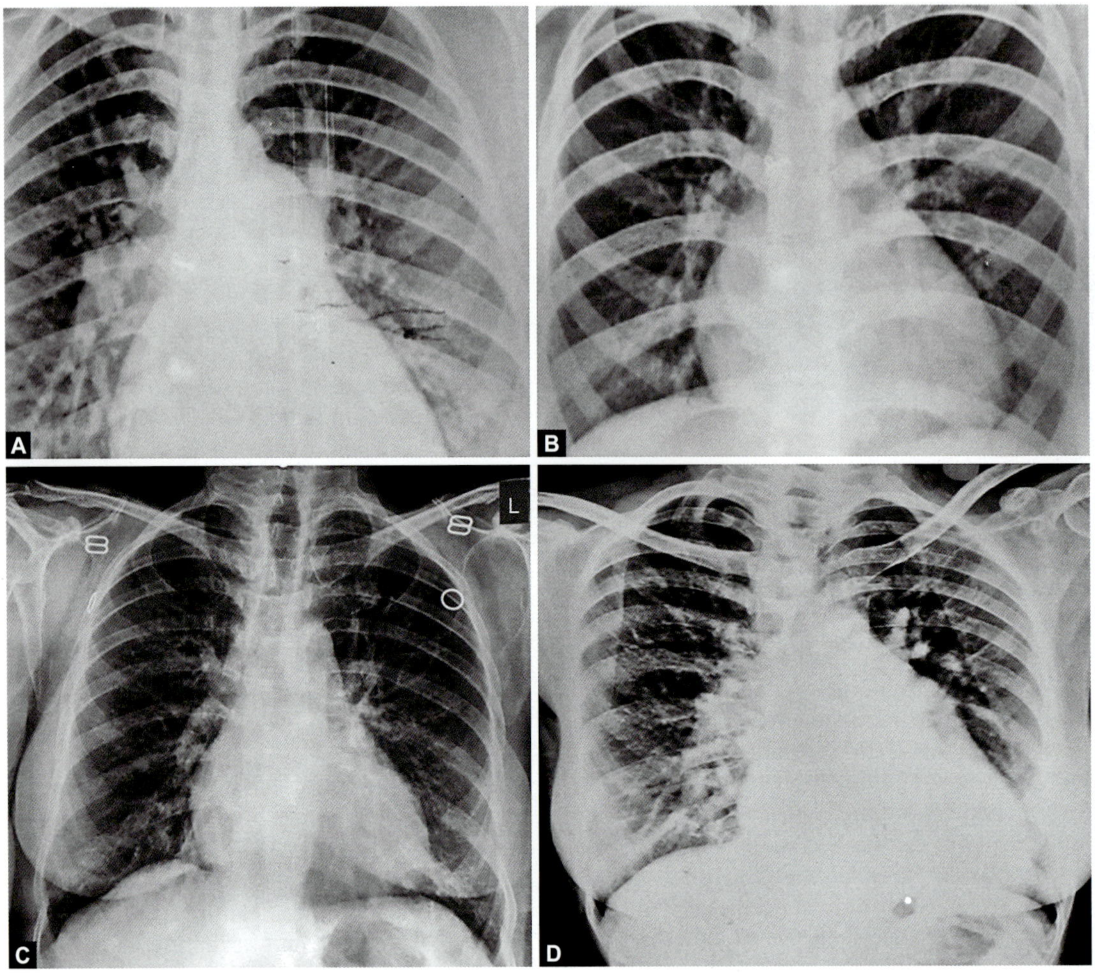

FIGS. 3A TO D: (A and B) Chest X-ray (CXR) showing evidence of prominent vasculature in the upper lung zones, where there is normally less vascularity. Vessels are dilated in both upper, mid, and lower zones, which occurs early in the stage of pulmonary congestion (cephalization, redistribution). (C and D) CXR of patients presenting with shortness of breath shows evidence of left atrial enlargement with features of dilated veins in the upper zones converging at the hilum.

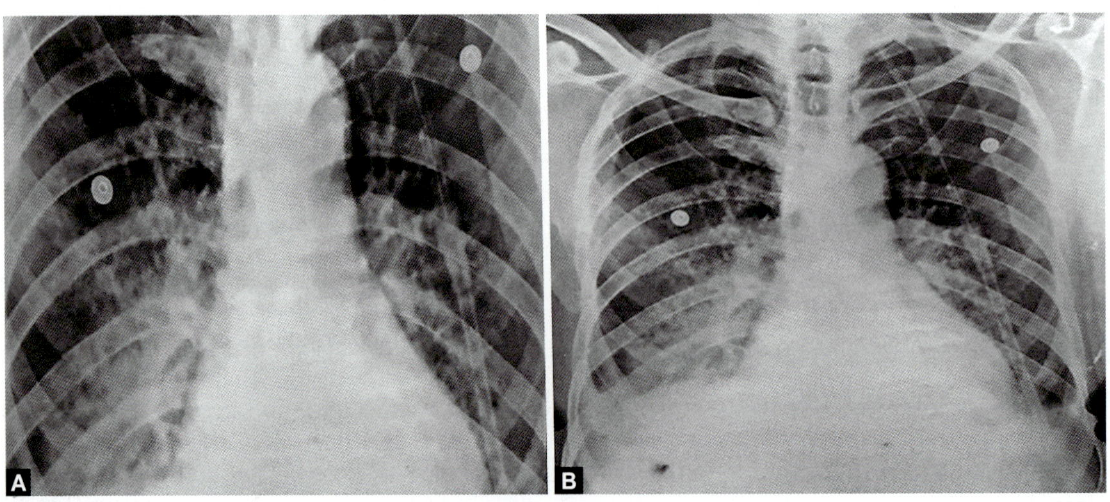

FIGS. 4A AND B: Chest X-ray (CXR) showing increased vascularity of the upper lung zones with the presence of dilated pulmonary veins and of perihilar haze.

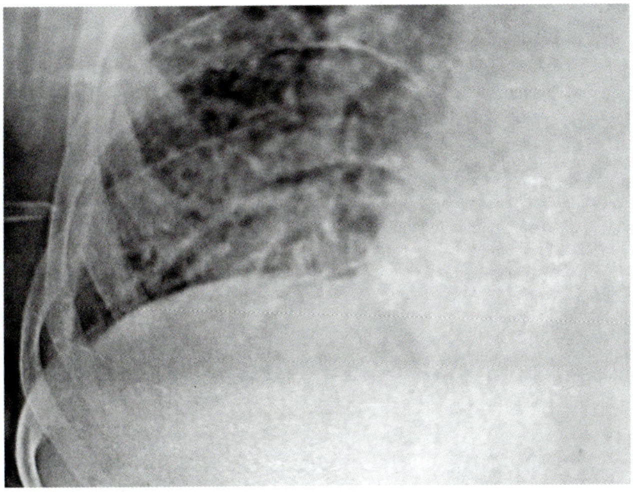

FIG. 5: Horizontal septal lines are seen in lower and midzones (Kerley B lines). Reticular shadows in the mid and lower zone and perihilar haziness are features of early changes of raised pulmonary wedge pressure.

the most frequent radiological signs of early pulmonary edema is the blurring of vascular margins, pulmonary clouding, loss of definition of vascular marking extending from the right hilum to the right hemidiaphragm, and loss of radiolucency of lung bases **(Figs. 4A and B)**.[24] In the case of acute myocardial infarction (MI) that impairs the function of the papillary muscle and hence the mitral valve, a regionally asymmetric distribution of pulmonary edema may produce atypical radiologic patterns that mimic noncardiogenic edema or, in some cases, even pneumonia **(Box 1 and Figs. 10 and 11)**.

Signs of pulmonary congestion on chest radiography may even precede clinical symptoms. Conversely, pulmonary edema may be visible radiographically for hours or even days after hemodynamic recovery. After the elevation of the wedge pressure secondary to LVF, a finite time period is required for pulmonary edema to accumulate, either in the interstices or the alveoli. Usually, a lag of around 12 hours is required for the radiographic manifestations of moderate LVF to occur. The major cause of the lack of correlation between the chest

TABLE 1: Kerley lines.

Kerley lines	Definition
Kerley B lines	They are defined as fine parallel linear densities, 2 cm or more in length, in the peripheral lung fields perpendicular to the pleural surface and are usually seen in the lower part around the costophrenic angle. They are divided into distinct when B lines are 2 cm or more and indistinct when they are short and ill-defined. Distinct Kerley B lines may be mild if they are few in number and severe if there are many B lines. Engorgement of the pulmonary veins and lymphatics leads to the development of Kerley lines, which are thought to be due to thickened interlobular septa from interstitial edema
Kerley A lines	They are defined as lines radiating toward the hilar regions for a distance of 2 inches or more without branching. They are caused by the distension of anastomotic channels between peripheral and central lymphatics. These lines are seen only in acute episodes of interstitial edema and, hence, are transient, whereas Kerley B lines are present for long time and clinically more useful than Kerley A lines
Kerley C lines	These are reticular opacities at the lung base, representing Kerley B lines en face

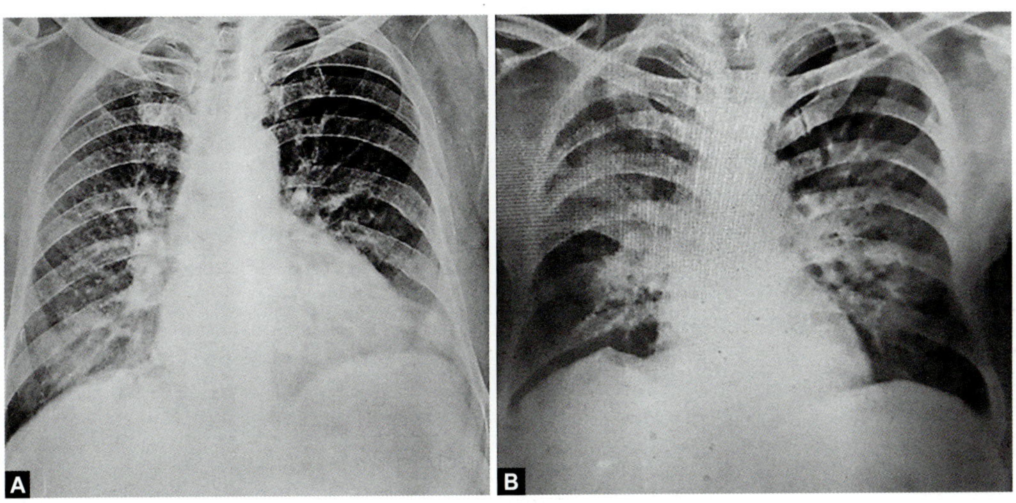

FIGS. 6A AND B: Chest X-ray (CXR) showing the presence of perihilar haziness with a loss of definition of vessel margins and reticular shadows in the lower and midzones on the right side, suggestive of venous hypertension.

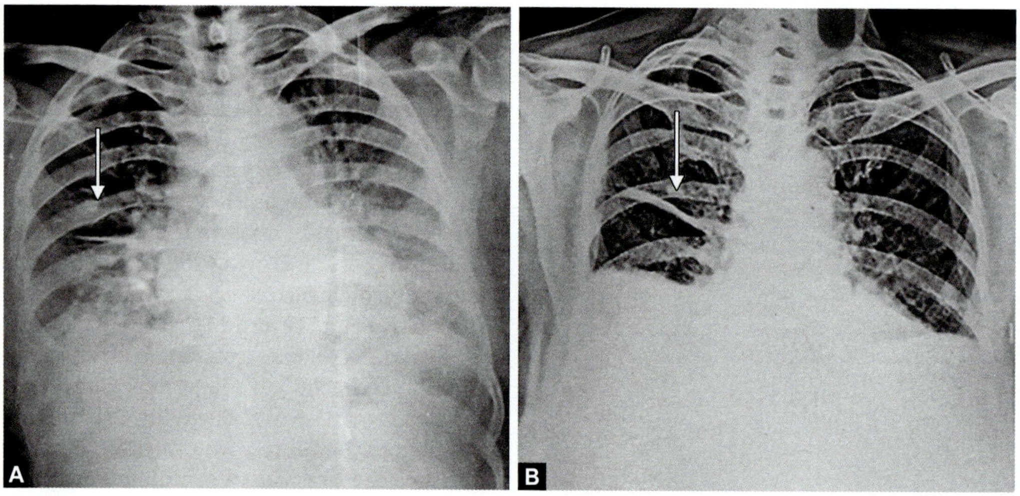

FIGS. 7A AND B: Chest X-ray (CXR) showing hilar haziness extending to both lower zones, thickening of interlobar fissure (fissure edema) (white arrowhead), prominent vasculature in the upper zones, and pleural effusion.

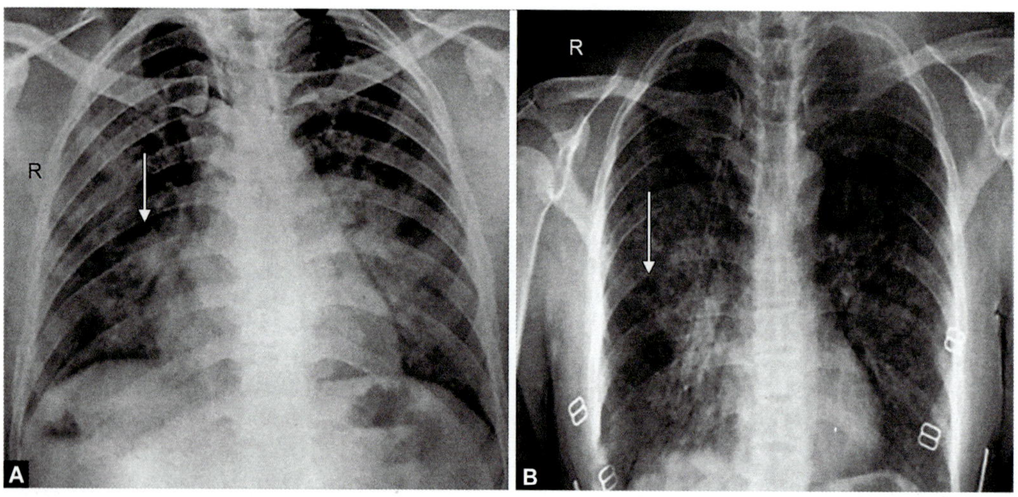

FIGS. 8A AND B: Early radiological features of alveolar edema with the presence of bilateral symmetrical opacities extending from the hilum to the midzone.

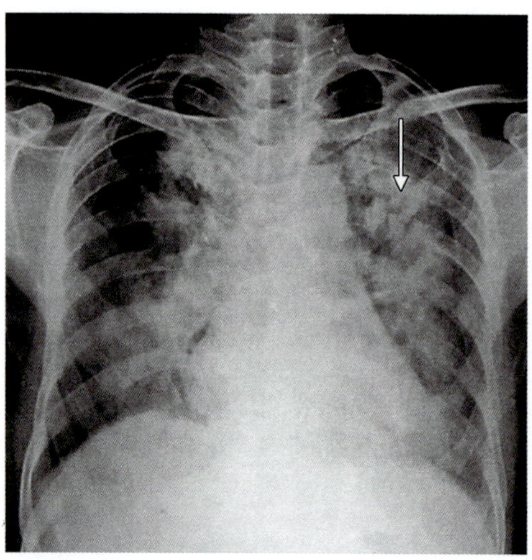

FIG. 9: Chest X-ray (CXR) showing opacities that typically involve the central hilar portion of the lungs, suggestive of alveolar edema, producing batwing appearance.

BOX 1 Radiographic features of raised pulmonary venous pressure.

- Vascular opacity "redistribution" toward the upper lobes and distention of the upper pulmonary veins
- Enlargement and loss of definition of hilar structures
- Septal lines in the lower lung, indicated as Kerley B lines and around the hilum as Kerley A lines
- Peribronchial and perivascular cuffing with widening and blurring of the margins
- Thickening of interlobar fissures with subpleural fluid accumulation
- Fluid leakage in the alveoli (alveolar edema) and leakage into the pleural space (pleural effusion)

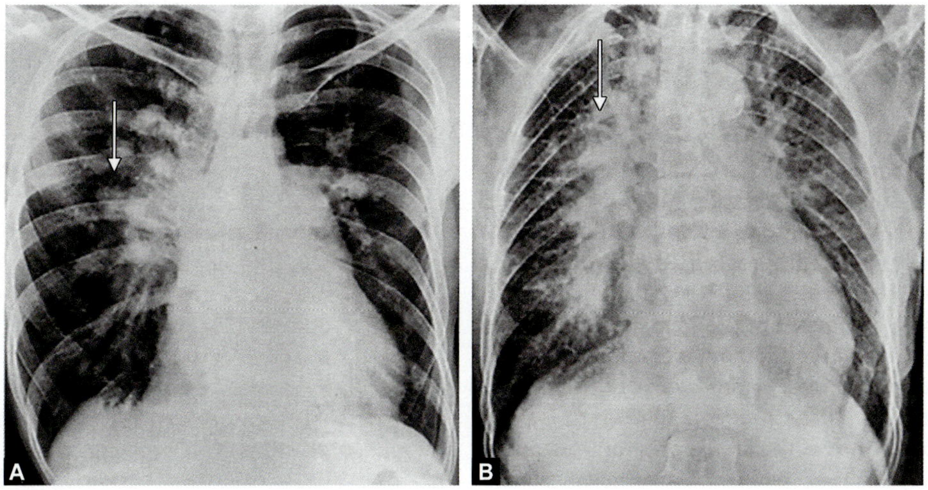

FIGS. 10A AND B: Chest X-ray (CXR) showing prominent shadows on the right side than the left side, suggesting early radiographic features of alveolar edema rather than infective pathology (white arrowheads).

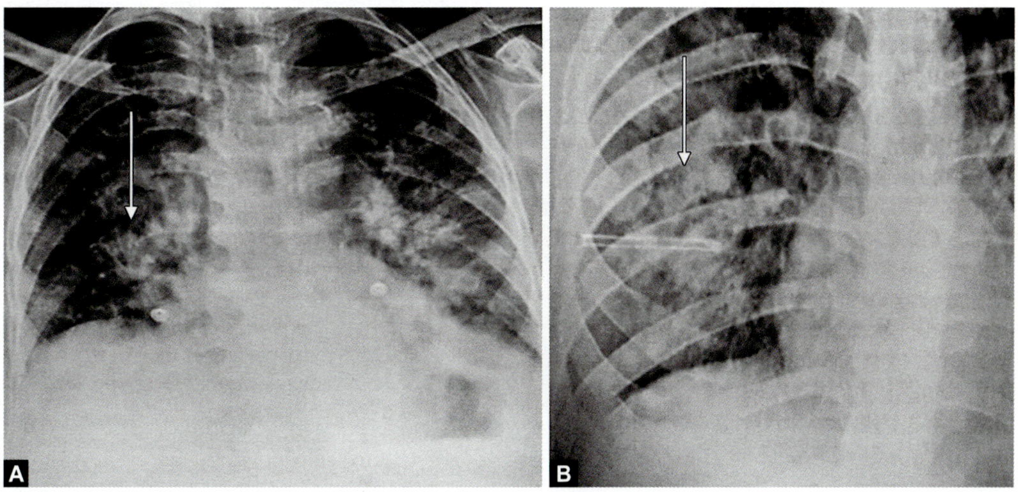

FIGS. 11A AND B: Chest X-ray (CXR) showing soft shadows involving the perihilar region [A (white arrowhead)], and shadows are mostly in the mid-lateral and upper zone, but there is also associated loss of definition in the margin of perihilar vessel [B (white arrowhead)] in two patients having acute shortness of breath (SOB) in the setting of myocardial infarction.

roentgenogram and hemodynamic state in acute LVF in acute MI probably lies in the rapidity with which the hemodynamic changes take place and the inability of chest radiographic changes to reflect this faithfully. Specifically, the left ventricular decompensation that occurs with acute MI may require up to 12 hours to manifest itself radiographically. Similarly, a "post-therapeutic phase lag" has been demonstrated by McHugh et al., and a lag of up to 4 days for these signs to clear. This post-therapeutic phase lag undoubtedly occurs because of the time required for the edema fluid to be resorbed after returning to normal wedge pressure.[29,30]

HEMODYNAMIC CORRELATION OF WEDGE PRESSURE WITH RADIOGRAPHIC FEATURES

The chest roentgenogram has been helpful in evaluating the degree of pulmonary venous hypertension in patients with mitral valve disease.[31,32] The appearance of the pulmonary vasculature has been thought to reflect the severity of the elevated pulmonary capillary wedge pressure **(Table 2)**. A redistribution of blood flow occurs in the early phase, with increased blood flow through the upper lobe vessels and a diminution in the blood flow through the lower lobes.[33,34] The level of wedge pressure at which lower zone venous constriction occurs has been placed somewhere between 12 and 18 mm Hg.[22] Transudation of plasma from the capillaries into the interstitial space occurs when capillary pressure exceeds the colloid osmotic pressure of blood (25 mm Hg). One manifestation of this is Kerley B lines, which are usually said to appear with a minimal mean left atrial pressure of 18 mm Hg.[28,26,27] Other signs of interstitial edema, including the loss of definition of the hilar and peripheral pulmonary vessels, perivascular and peribronchial cuffing, and peripheral clouding, have not been correlated with hemodynamic data.[23,35,36] The range of 18–25 mm Hg has been suggested by Simon for the appearance of these early signs of interstitial pulmonary edema.[23] Alveolar pulmonary edema occurs when pulmonary wedge pressure greatly exceeds the colloid osmotic pressure of plasma. Although interstitial fluid is present at this time, the great majority of edema is in the alveoli.[29,36,37] The critical wedge pressure necessary for the appearance of alveolar pulmonary edema has been postulated as 22–25 mm Hg by McHugh et al.[29] and as 25–35 mm Hg by Simon et al.[23]

TABLE 2: Correlation of chest X-ray (CXR) with pulmonary capillary wedge pressure.

Pulmonary cap wedge pressure (mm Hg)	CXR findings
5–12	Normal
12–17	Cephalization of pulmonary vessels
17–20	Kerley lines
>25	Pulmonary edema

ROLE OF CHEST X-RAY IN EVALUATION OF CHEST PAIN AND BREATHLESSNESS

The main objective of chest evaluation in the emergency department or outpatient care is to confirm or rule out coronary artery disease, acute LVF as the cause of pain in the chest and SOB. The other objective is to evaluate the immediate prognosis and rule out noncardiac causes of acute pain and SOB. CXR is a very important tool for alternative diagnoses such as pleurisy, pleural effusion **(Figs. 12A and B)**, pneumothorax **(Fig. 13)**, and pneumonic consolidation

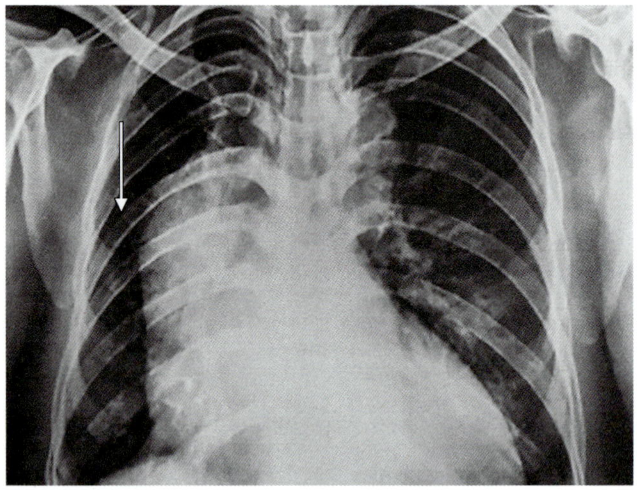

FIG. 13: Chest X-ray (CXR) showing underlying pneumothorax (white arrowhead) in right-sided thorax in a patient having recent onset of acute chest pain and shortness of breath, with a past history of percutaneous coronary intervention (PCI) to left anterior descending (LAD) 5 years back.

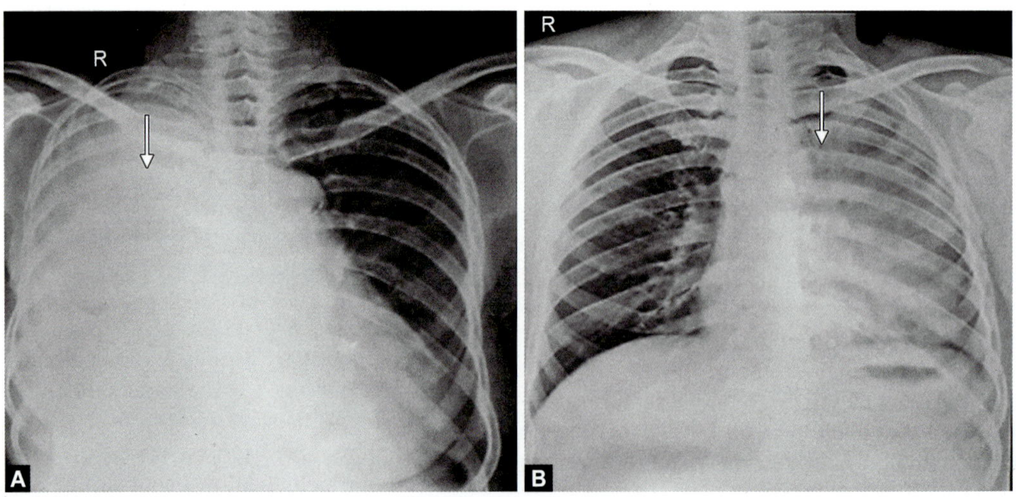

FIGS. 12A AND B: Chest X-ray (CXR) showing a large right-sided pleural effusion [A (white arrowhead)] and a veil-like shadow of pleurisy in the left hemithorax [B (white arrowhead)] in a patient complaining of acute chest pain and shortness of breath.

(Figs. 14 and 15). It is commonly insensitive, nonspecific, and normal in acute pulmonary embolism. Occasionally, dilatation of pulmonary vessels proximal to the embolism, along with a paucity of pulmonary vasculature in the diseased lung, sometimes with a sharp cutoff, i.e., the Westermark sign, can be observed in pulmonary embolism. A triangular or rounded pleural-based infiltrate with the apex toward the hilum, usually located adjacent to the hilum, is known as Hampton's hump and can rarely be observed. CXR can sometimes prove useful in detecting life-threatening causes such as dissection of the aorta. CXR features suggestive of dissection of the aorta include widening of the mediastinum, widening of the aortic contour, kinking of the aorta, and the presence of the calcium sign, which is defined as the separation of intimal calcification from the outer aortic soft-tissue border by 10 mm. Although it is observed in 14% of patients with dissection of the aorta, it is very specific for dissection.[38] CXR has limited sensitivity (64%) and specificity (86%) in the diagnosis of aortic diseases.[39]

ROLE OF CHEST X-RAY IN PERIOPERATIVE EVALUATION

Perioperative cardiovascular evaluation is now a routine practice in the perioperative evaluation of patients undergoing nonvascular surgery. The number of patients referred for perioperative evaluation is increasing in many tertiary care hospitals. Routine CXRs will help the cardiologist avoid time-consuming tests such as echocardiography and evaluate patients quickly. A proper history, routine electrocardiogram (ECG), and CXR can screen out the vast majority of normal patients. A normal 12-lead ECG and CXR, with no cardiomegaly, normal vascularity, normal main pulmonary artery, and a normal left border of the heart, will exclude many underlying structural heart diseases and avoid echocardiographic evaluation. Comparison with previous CXR (when available) can detect new-onset subtle disease. Asymptomatic primary myocardial disease, mitral stenosis, and pulmonary hypertension may escape clinical detection unless searched carefully. Routine CXR can give clue to the presence of such subsets **(Figs. 16 to 18)**. Hence, routine CXR can be a part of all perioperative evaluations.

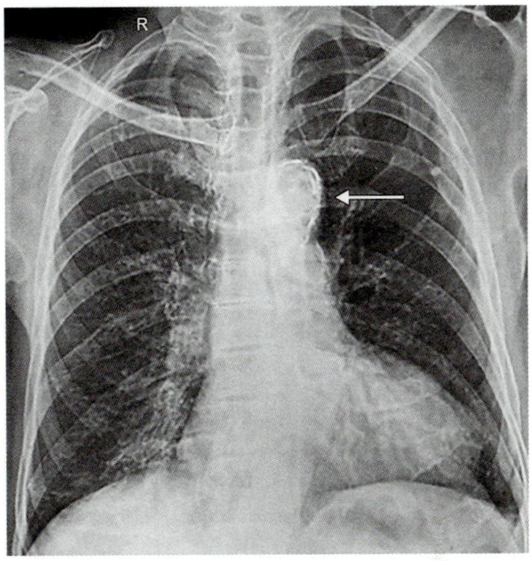

FIG. 15: Chest X-ray (CXR) posteroanterior (PA) view showing calcification (white arrowhead) at aortic knuckle (separation of the calcification >10 mm can give clue to the presence of aortic dissection).

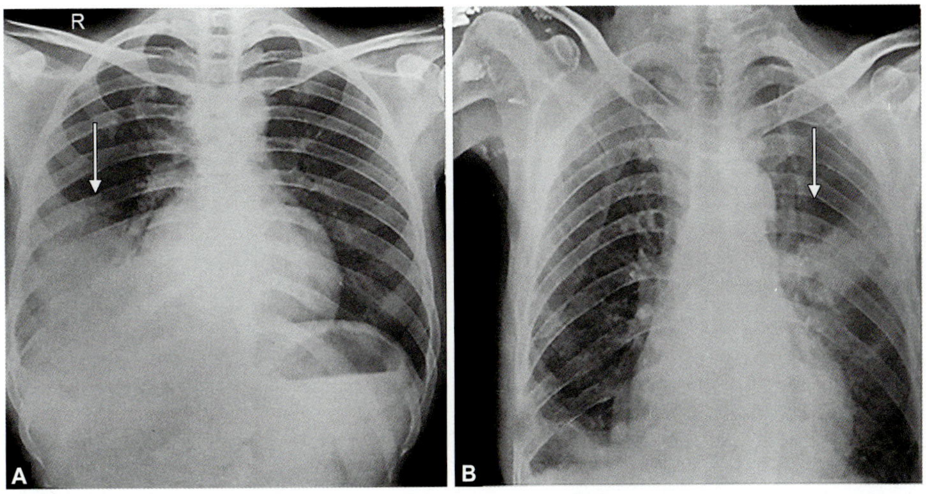

FIGS. 14A AND B: Chest X-ray (CXR) showing pneumonic consolidation in the (A) right middle lobe (RML) (white arrowhead) and (B) left upper lobe (LUL) (white arrowhead) in patients with chest pain and shortness of breath (SOB).

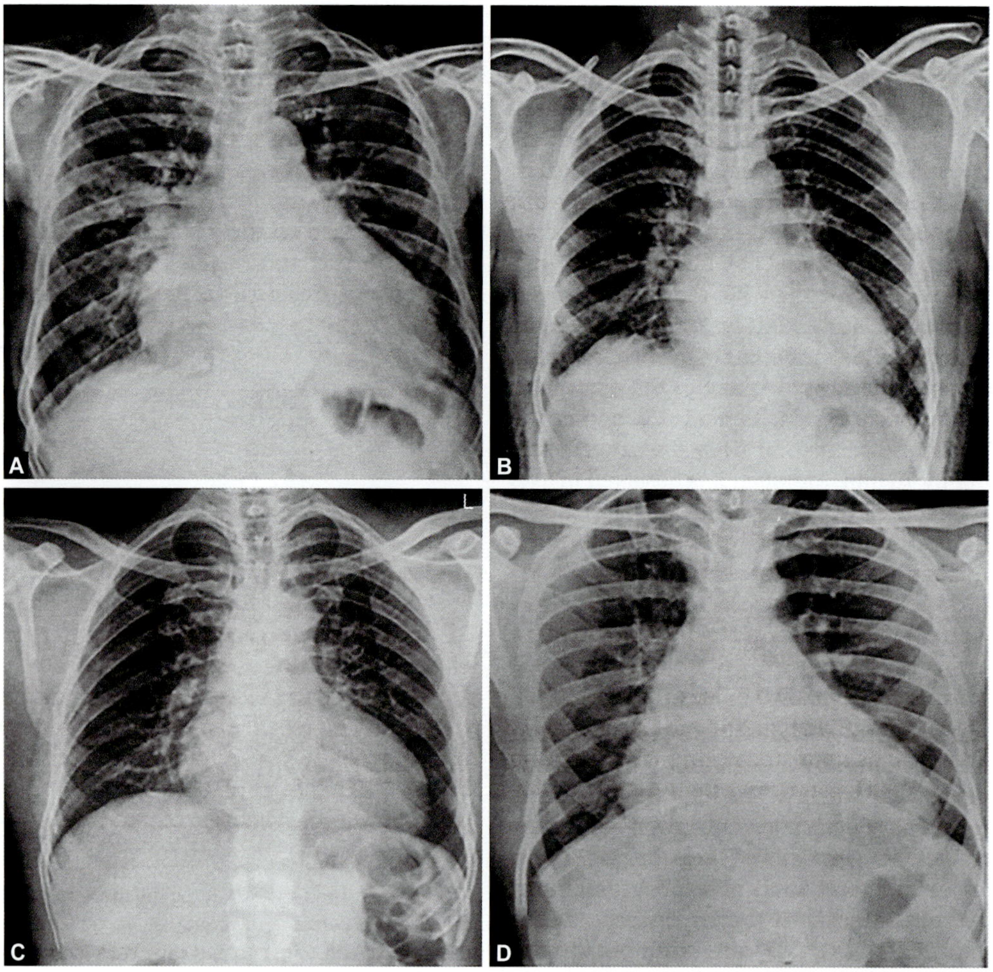

FIGS. 16A TO D: Routine chest X-ray (CXR) of four patients presenting for preoperative evaluation for noncardiac surgery. Presence of cardiomegaly (A, B, and D), straightening of the left border of the heart (B), and prominent vascular shadows (A, B, and C) in the upper zones can identify the presence of underlying diseases such as cardiomyopathy, mitral stenosis, and pericardial effusion.

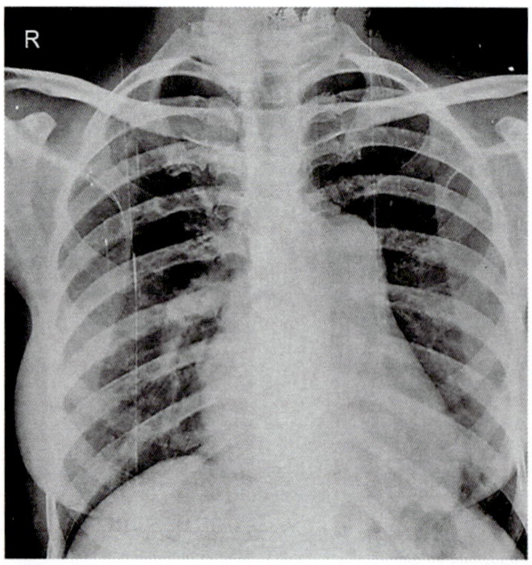

FIG. 17: Chest X-ray (CXR) showing dilated main pulmonary artery (MPA), normal vascularity of the upper zones, and tapering of the right pulmonary artery, suggestive of underlying pulmonary arterial hypertension (PAH) in a 32-year-old female presented for routine preoperative evaluation for intra-abdominal surgery.

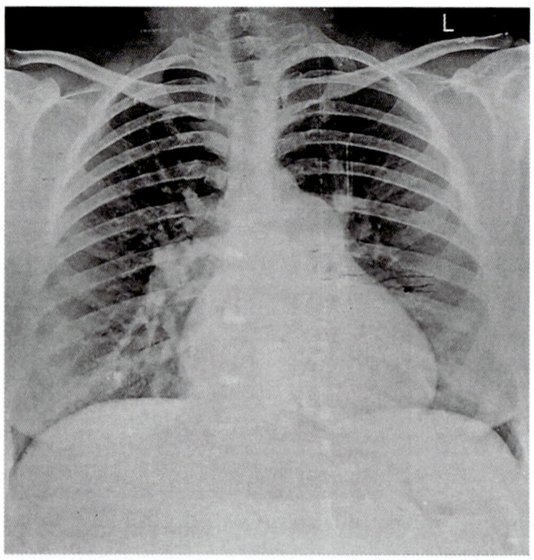

FIG. 18: A 34-year-old female presented for evaluation of palpitations and shortness of breath (SOB). Chest X-ray posteroanterior (PA) view showing dilated main pulmonary artery (MPA) increased vascularity suggestive of an underlying atrial septal defect (ASD).

CONCLUSION

Thus, CXR is the traditional first-line procedure to assess, as it is widely and easily available as a diagnostic tool in all emergency and outpatient departments. Till date, CXR represents the first-line imaging examination in patients presenting to the emergency department complaining of acute dyspnea because of its ability to recognize pulmonary vascular congestion and other subsets of chest opacity. Chest radiography has the great advantage of combining relative low cost, easy availability, portability, and the familiarity of medical professionals with the investigation tool. CXR has the ability to take a panoramic view of the chest, which allows for the exclusion of many pulmonary conditions that come into the differential diagnosis. In doubtful cases, LUS has been shown to be of value in assessing pulmonary congestion by the evaluation of vertical comet tail artifacts, named B-lines. A computed tomography (CT) thorax is required only for confirmation or exclusion of pulmonary embolism. Digital X-ray has improved the imaging quality and removed many artifacts. For proper evaluation and to exclude artifacts, CXR should be properly exposed, rotation should be normal, and the film should be taken in full inspiration. CXR should always be interpreted along with a clinical examination of the patient.

ONLINE REFERENCES

Please scan the QR code provided at the end of the table of contents for References of this chapter.

CHAPTER 13

Chronic Aortic Regurgitation: Timing of Intervention and Effect of AVR on Outcomes

Dayasagar Rao V, Rajesh Natuva

ABSTRACT

Aortic regurgitation (AR) is due to failure of normal coaptation of aortic leaflets and is caused by two major pathologies primary aortic valve diseases and disease of aortic root, the former being more common than later. Infrequently AR may also be seen after surgical or catheter-based interventions on aortic valve. AR leads to increase in left ventricle (LV) preload and afterload (LV wall stress) proportional to severity.

The LV responds to this hemodynamic abnormality by increase in LV end-diastolic dimension (LVEDD) and improved compliance in an attempt to maintain forward cardiac output and normal LV end-diastolic pressure. With progression of valve regurgitation, reactive interstitial fibrosis develops in LV myocardium which leads to systolic myocardial dysfunction and elevated end-diastolic pressure leading to onset of symptoms. The combination of increased myocardial oxygen demand (consequence of increased LVEDD) and reduced coronary blood supply (consequence of low aortic diastolic pressure) may cause angina [even in absence of coronary artery disease (CAD)] and contribute to myocardial dysfunction. Optimal timing of valve surgery in patients with chronic severe AR is recognition of LV dysfunction before it becomes irreversible with advanced cardiac imaging like cardiac magnetic resonance (CMR) in addition to 2D echo and 3D echo.

The results of aortic valve replacement (AVR) in present era even in patients with severe LV dysfunction [ejection fraction (EF) < 35%] are very good—mortality <1% and recovery of LV function in majority of patients, a consequence of significant advances in every branch of cardiac sciences—surgical techniques, myocardial protection, anesthetic techniques, postoperative care, and drug therapy and thus should not be denied of benefits of surgery. Role of transcatheter aortic valve replacement (TAVR) is evolving and not yet established as alternative therapy to AVR.

Keywords: Chronic severe aortic regurgitation, advanced cardiac imaging, symptoms, LV dysfunction, aortic valve replacement.

INTRODUCTION

Aortic regurgitation (AR) is characterized by reflux of blood flow from aorta to left ventricle (LV) in diastole and is a consequence of incomplete/inappropriate coaptation of aortic leaflets. Etiology of chronic AR falls in to two broad categories, i.e., aortic leaflet pathology (thickening, eversion, and perforation) and abnormal dilatation of aortic root—former more common than later. Assessing severity of AR is generally done by echo Doppler using following parameters: vena contracta (VC) (>6 mm width), effective regurgitant orifice area (EROA) (>30 mm^2), regurgitant volume (>60 mL), and regurgitant fraction (>50%). In multivalvular heart disease, flow independent parameters (VC and EROA) are used for quantification of severity of AR. Cardiac magnetic resonance (CMR) is very useful in patients with poor acoustic window and is more accurate in measuring LV volumes, strain, and are more reproducible. Thus, CMR is more useful in the follow-up of patients with chronic AR. Further it is very reliable in assessing aortic pathology and its progression.

Chronic severe AR induces LV remodeling with chamber dilatation, improved compliance, and eccentric hypertrophy, with ultimate goal of maintaining forward output and normal end-diastolic pressure of LV. Earlier observational studies assumed that remodeling of LV and rate of progression was uniform and independent of age and sex.[1] Recent studies have shown that older patients and women have smaller LV volumes for same degree of regurgitation compared to young male patients. Women have less body surface area (BSA) and less likely to reach non-indexed LV dimensions large enough to meet surgical indications. Thus they are more likely to be referred late with more advanced New York Heart Association (NYHA) class and hence poor surgical outcomes. Further studies using CMR have shown that remodeling of LV involves complex geometric changes which are not captured by linear dimensions measured by echocardiography. These initial compensatory adaptive remodeling of LV maintain the hemodynamic parameters and functional capacity to near normal levels.

Over a period of time the adaptive remodeling leads to maladaptive remodeling characterized by increased reactive interstitial fibrosis with increased fibronectin[2] and noncollagen components, which if uncorrected is followed by myocyte apoptosis and replacement fibrosis. This loss of myocytes coupled with increased replacement fibrosis leads to impaired LV function and worsening of physical work capacity of patients (functional class). There is not only systolic dysfunction but also diastolic dysfunction[3] in patients with chronic severe AR, which contributes to the functional disability. This diastolic dysfunction was evaluated by analyzing the left atrial strain (LAS) function by speckle tracking. This LASct (conduit function) along with LASr (reservoir function) correlated with LV end-diastolic pressure (LVEDP), left atrial (LA) pressure, and N-terminal pro b-type natriuretic peptide (NT-proBNP) levels. This decreased LASct may be related to increase in stiffness of LV, a consequence of myocardial fibrosis. Several studies correlated CMR parameters[3] [native T1, T1 after gadolinium, extracellular volume (ECV) indexed to BSA (iECV) measures on 3T, and replacement fibrosis by late gadolinium enhancement (LGE)] with morphological alterations in myocardium (surgically removed during valve surgery). This study showed inverse correlation between interstitial fibrosis with functional improvement and long-term prognosis. These findings suggest that presence of replacement fibrosis is marker of adverse ventricular remodeling that lead to further functional deterioration even after successful AVR.

NATURAL HISTORY—AORTIC REGURGITATION

Understanding the natural history of disease like chronic AR helps in the appropriate management of disease including timing of intervention.[4]

Progression of AR (from stage-B to C/D) is slow, that seldom results in catastrophic clinical event. The rate of progression in isolated AR is influenced by etiology of disease (slow in degenerative and rheumatic) (2–5% year) and faster in bicuspid aortic valve disease. The progression of AR can be faster in patients with moderate AR at initial presentation. The overall 10 years progression of mild AR to stage C/D stage was 12% in patients with trivial/moderate AR, 30% in patients with moderate AR at baseline. The total percentage of progression over 4.5 years was 2% and rate of progression was 4.2 mm/year for ERO and 9.9 mL/year for regurgitant volume. These faster progressions experienced rapid chamber remodeling and decline in functional class. The anatomical determinants of faster progression included aortic annular size and size of sinotubular junction.[5]

Moderate-to-severe AR has favorable progression in the absence of symptoms and LV dysfunction. Asymptomatic patients with normal LV function need AVR at rate of 4% per year with 90% patients remain asymptomatic at 3 years, 81% at 5 years, and 75% at 7 years. In asymptomatic patients, the rate of progression to symptomatic LV dysfunction is <3.5% year and risk of sudden death is 0.2%. The duration of symptoms and/or LV dysfunction before AVR are important, as longer duration results in poorer surgical results with residual postoperative LV dysfunction. After development of symptoms progression to LV dysfunction occurs rapidly approaching nearly 25% per year. Once symptoms develop, the survival rates without surgical intervention—AVR is 28% at 4 years in patients with class III and IV.[6]

Some patients decrease their physical activity as means to overcome the worsening of valvular heart disease like severe AR while in others symptoms are equivocal (class II or III). Under those circumstances it is useful to assess functional capacity and unmasking of symptoms by stress testing which additionally may reveal presence of contractile reserve which if absent is predictive of LV systolic dysfunction both at follow-up and post AVR. Exercise testing is also useful (in patients with more than moderate AR) in advising participation of sports and athletic activities. Exercise testing with cardiac imaging also helpful in identifying patients with early systolic dysfunction.

It is desirable to perform exercise testing with electrocardiography and cardiac imaging to evaluate earlier mentioned parameters. One study has shown that ST depression of >1 mm during stress testing is associated with lower resting ejection fraction (EF) and greater end-systolic dimension (ESD) compared to those not having ST changes.[7]

Exercise echocardiography can be used to measure incremental change in EF and LV dimensions in severe AR. Change of >5 units (5%) correlates with preserved LV systolic function, while failure to increase EF indicates LV systolic dysfunction. Other studies revealed decrease in resting right ventricle (RV) strain and exercise tricuspid annular plane systolic excursion (TAPSE) of tricuspid valve was independently associated with need for earlier AVR. LV strain [global longitudinal strain (GLS)] is used to determine LV systolic dysfunction as it precedes onset of decrease in LVEF and thus need for timing of AVR. Not all adult patients have good acoustic window for complete echo study in which case cardiac MRI can be used. Cardiac magnetic resonance imaging (CMRI) can evaluate aortic valve anatomy, severity of AR, and remodeling of LV chamber in response to severe AR, in addition to evaluation of aortic pathology. Further more evaluation of LGE, reveals degree of fibrosis and thus reversibility of LV size and function. CMR can also evaluate LV volumes (rather than longitudinal measurement) which is better parameter of LV dilatation and LV remodeling.

TIMING OF AORTIC VALVE REPLACEMENT

Optimal timing of surgery should be determined from the perspective of short- and long-term outcome postsurgery. Management of severe AR usually requires AVR (aortic valve replacement). However in selected patients and surgical centers of excellence, aortic valve repair and Ross procedure (pulmonic autograft in aortic position, with prosthetic pulmonic valve) are other options. In some selected patients, TAVR has also been used in therapy of severe AR.

The following data is required in the evaluation of AR before considering aortic valve intervention:

- AR-severity (by echo and/or CMR)
- Mechanism of AR (consideration of aortic valve repair)
- Associated aortic pathology

When all parameters of severe AR are met by transthoracic echocardiogram (TTE) no further investigation is required in patients with symptoms and/or LV dysfunction. When TTE parameters are discordant no official recommendations exist to resolve the issue.[8] The cardiovascular medicine unit at Cleveland Clinic developed and proposed hierarchical model for grading severity of AR using end-diastolic volume (EDV) index as primary parameters, with VC, relative regurgitant width, and holodiastolic flow reversal as secondary parameters. Severe AR is deemed to be present if LVEDD (indexed) is increased and if one of the three secondary parameters is in severe range. Moderate AR is present if LVEDV is in normal range and none of secondary parameters are in severe range. This hierarchical scheme when tested against gold standard CMR has good correlation ($r = 0.90$) and less interobserver variability (kappa +0.70). Age is an important modulating factor in LV response to overload. In an experimental model of AR, younger animals rapidly normalized LV diastolic pressure by LV dilatation whereas this response was absent in older animals.

Adjustment of LV size to body size is important, as AR can occur in individuals at extreme body size distribution (like in Marfan syndrome and women). In practice, we adjust parameters to BSA for variations in body size. Even indexed values can be affected at extremes of height, as volumes [LV end-systolic volume (ESV) and EDV] are proportional to cube of body height and BSA is proportional to square of height. Recent studies of chronic severe AR have paid considerable attention for adjusting the LV functional parameters body size (indexed to BSA–iEDD). In USA and Europe where BSA is 1.9–2.0 m^2 an LVESD index >25 mm/m^2 may be an appropriate cut-off values whereas in Asian countries where BSA is 1.6–1.7 m^2 indexed values may be over corrected and thus may not be appropriate. Thus cut-off indexed LVESD values may be different in people at extremes of body size. This is reflected in the European Society of Cardiology (ESC) guidelines 2017 where annotation was added that cut-off LVESD index value of 20 mm/m^2 may be more appropriate in patients with small BSA. More data is needed to determine threshold value of LV systolic diameter for predicting the postoperative outcome in patients with smaller BSA.[9]

Novel biomarkers are advocated to help refining indications for intervention and risk stratification. In patients with severe AR, advanced echocardiographic modalities (like GLS) and CMR imaging have shown promise in providing new tools to depict the switch from adaptive to maladaptive myocardial changes in response to severe AR. Present understanding in therapy of valvular heart disease is shifting of focus from indirect parameters of LV functions to structural alterations of myocardium by advanced imaging. Long-term follow-up results are required to show incremental prognostic utility of morphological changes (by advanced imaging) in prediction of postoperative survival and morbidity. Observational study in 865 patients with chronic severe AR and preserved LVEF (EF > 50%) who underwent aortic valve surgery (aortic valve replacement and aortic valve repair) and follow-up for a median period of 6.9 years showed that LV-GLS value less than –19% was associated with reduced survival postoperatively. LVEF normalized in 91% patients but only 31% had GLS better than –19%. An absolute worsening of 5% LV-GLS from baseline was associated with increased mortality in long-term follow-up. This study indicates that LV-GLS is better predictor of immediate and long-term outcomes in patients with severe AR undergoing aortic valve surgery.

The goals of intervention are to (see **Table 1**):

- Improve outcome (morbidity and mortality)
- Improve symptoms
- Prevent development heart failure and dysrhythmias

Several investigations have identified preoperative predictors of outcome and LV function after AVR. The most consistent measures are functional class, and LV function [LVEF, end-systolic dimension (LV), and GLS].[5]

In one study from Mayo clinic published in 2019, an analysis of 748 patients with severe AR done. The average age of this cohort was 58 years (58 + 17 years) with 18% women and 382 patients (52%) of this cohort did not under go AVR. The referral for surgery was driven by class I indication (symptoms and LV dysfunction) in 86% and 14% [by class II indication (echo criteria without symptoms)]. This study showed LV end-systolic dimension index (ESDi) was the only criteria linked to mortality and risk of death increased when ESDi > 20 mm/m^2. This ESDi was important

TABLE 1: STS database (2011–2018) of AVR in chronic severe AR.[11,12]

STS database 2011–2018		
Analysis 12,564 patients: • 50% symptomatic • 27% reduced EF Outcomes: • Operative mortality 1% • Major morbidity 8.2%	Operative mortality—disease stage: • Stage C1: 0.4% • Stage C2: 0.7% • Stage D: 1.6%	
Risk increased		
Symptomatic	↓ EF	Prior MI
× 2.3	× 1.2	× 1.6

(AR: aortic regurgitation; AVR: aortic valve replacement; EF: ejection fraction; MI: myocardial infarction; STS: Society of Thoracic Surgeons)

variable in identifying asymptomatic high-risk surgical candidates, especially women and elderly. Large LV (EDD > 75 mm) was associated with poor outcomes with increased perioperative mortality and unsatisfactory LV function recovery.

Symptom onset is a clear indication for AVR, irrespective of LV function, but should establish that they are related to severe AR (and not due to other associated comorbidities). However, if serial studies reveal progressive LV dilatation and decrease in EF, nearing lower limit of normal, surgery should be considered. Onset of symptoms and/or signs of LV dysfunction are definitive indications for AVR, with good recovery of function and size of LV and long-term survival. Long-term results in patients with poor functional class (NYHA class IV), with extremely enlarged ventricles and poor LV function (EF 35% or less) will have poor recovery of LV function and long-term survival. Even in these sick patients AVR and subsequent medical therapy is better alternative than long-term medical therapy alone or cardiac transplantation.

Asymptomatic patients with LV dysfunction (EF < 50%, ESD > 50 mm) are at high risk for symptomatic heart failure within 2–3 years and likelihood of LV dysfunction normalizing decreases with increased duration of LV dysfunction, thus need for prompt surgical intervention (AVR). Asymptomatic patients with normal LV systolic function at rest and LV dilatation (EDD > 65 mm) have increased risk of sudden cardiac death. Their prognosis after AVR is excellent and should be referred for AVR if surgical risk is low (<1%).

Moderate-to-severe AR should have AVR, having heart surgery for another indication [coronary artery bypass graft (CABG)/aortic aneurysm/other valve surgeries].

Use of GLS of LV (in patients with normal EF) exercise testing and biomarkers (NT-proBNP) may be used as an additional tool in determining optimal time of surgery in patients where conventional indications for surgery are equivocal but should not be used as primary determinants of indications of AVR surgery. AVR confers survival benefit with recovery of LV function and favorable ventricular remodeling.

AMERICAN COLLEGE OF CARDIOLOGY–AMERICAN HEART ASSOCIATION GUIDELINES—(2020) OF AORTIC VALVE REPLACEMENT AVR (FLOWCHART 1 AND BOX 1)

- *Class I indication*:
  - Symptomatic patients with severe AR
  - Asymptomatic patients with severe AR and LVEF < 55%
  - Severe AR having heart surgery for another indication
- *Class II indication [asymptomatic patients with preserved LVEF (>55%) AVR is recommended]*:
  - LVESD > 50 mm, LV ESDi 25 mm/m^2
  - Moderate AR who are undergoing other cardiac surgery
  - Progressive LV dilatation LVEDD > 65 mm if surgical risk is low [class II(b)]

EFFECT OF AVR ON LV REMODELING AND SURVIVAL[10]

Aortic regurgitation—chronic and severe results in increase preload (in LVEDD) and afterload (LV wall stress) which leads series of compensatory changes including LV dilatation and hypertrophy. AVR for AR corrects the hemodynamic abnormality resulting in reverse remodeling (decrease in LV size) and recovery of LV function in majority of patients with improvement in functional class but is some patients the LV dilatation and dysfunction persists in spite of AVR. The freedom from major adverse cardiac events (MACEs) including cardiac death, hospitalization heart failure, and lethal arrhythmias were 94.4% at 5 years and 92.5% at 10 years in remodeling group and 60% at 5 years and 46.7% at 10 year in nonremodeling group perhaps consequence of myocardial fibrosis and irreversible LV dysfunction. This recovery of size and function may take as long as 5 years. Thus favorable LV remodeling after AVR had good clinical long-term results, than those with no remodeling. The predictors of adverse remodeling were cases with LVESD > 55 mm, EF < 50%, and extremely dilated LV (EDD > 75–80 mm) are indicators of irreversible myocardial damage.

TRANSCATHETER AORTIC VALVE REPLACEMENT IN AORTIC REGURGITATION[13]

Transcatheter aortic valve replacement in pure and isolated severe valvular AR has not been tested in any randomized clinical trials and has been one of exclusion criteria in many randomized controlled trials (RCTs) of TAVR. One study

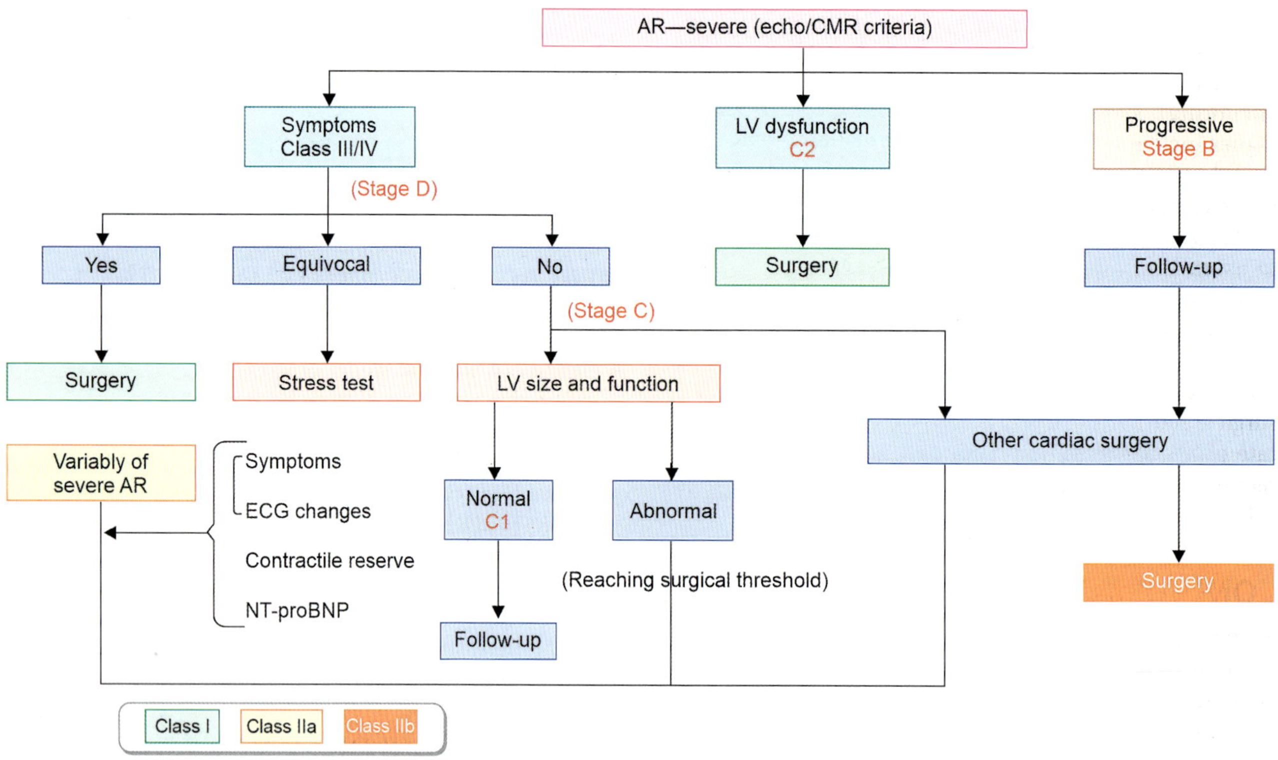

FLOWCHART 1: Decision algorithm for aortic valve replacement in severe AR.
(AR: aortic regurgitation; CMR: cardiac magnetic resonance; ECG: electrocardiogram; LV: left ventricle; NT-proBNP: N-terminal pro b-type natriuretic peptide)

BOX 1 Parameters of severe AR for AVR.

- LV dysfunction: EF < 55%
- LV dilatation:
  - LVESD > 50 mm
  - LV ESDi > 25 mm/m^2
  - LVEDD > 65 mm
- Other cardiac surgery:
  - Other valve surgery
  - CABG
  - Aortic root surgery

ESC-EACTS-2021—Asymptomatic patients with LVESD > 20 mm/m^2, especially in patients with small BSA if surgical risk is low (class IIb, LOE–c)

Other indications for AVR are similar to ACC–AHA guidelines

(ACC: American College of Cardiology; AHA: American Heart Association; AR: aortic regurgitation; AVR: aortic valve replacement; BSA: body surface area; CABG: coronary artery bypass graft; EACTS: European Association for Cardio-Thoracic Surgery; EF: ejection fraction; ESC: European Society of Cardiology; LOE: level of evidence; LV: left ventricle; LVEDD: LV end-diastolic dimension; LVESD: LV end-systolic dimension; LV ESDi: LV end-systolic dimension index)

from Heart, Vascular, and Thoracic Institute at Cleveland Clinic tracked data from 11,000 patients with pure AR and underwent TAVR or surgical aortic valve replacement (SAVR) from 2016 to 2019. In this study, 10.5% patients with isolated severe noncalcific severe valvular AR underwent TAVR and the remaining 89.5% underwent surgical AVR. Inhospital mortality and 30 days mortality and stroke were comparable between TAVR and SAVR. However, after follow-up of 31 months TAVR patients were associated with higher mortality and higher risk of redo AVR. In another international registry study involving 18 centers across Europe, UK, USA, and Canada using transcatheter heart valve (THV) for treatment noncalcific pure native aortic valve regurgitation (NAVR) and failing bioprosthetic surgical heart valves (SHVs). This study revealed THV in pure severe AR was associated with less device implantation success (85% with complication of device embolization and migration) and more frequent paravalvular regurgitation (moderate-to-severe paravalvular regurgitation of 10%).[14]

These differences could be related to anatomical abnormalities of native valve. Higher incidence of bicuspid aortic valve and annular and root dilatation, with relatively less/no calcification, which will interfere with optimal anchoring, and apposition of THR and lead to device migration, embolization, and paravalvular leak. Recommendation to oversize THV in AR is associated with increased risk of rupture and conversion to SAVR which occurred in 1% of TAVR patients.

Dedicated transcatheter aortic valve for therapy of AR has been created like JenaValve trilogy. JenaValve trilogy comprises self-expanding nitinol stent with porcine pericardial valve. This valve has "locators" attached to valve frame that clip on to leaflets up on deployment facilitating anchoring, without relying on annular calcification (for anchoring). Hemodynamic results are excellent but with higher incidence of conduction disturbances. One clinical trial ALIGN, AR study, is ongoing with recruitment of patients from 30 sites. This study is prospective single-arm Investigation Device Exemption (IDE) study, designed to assess the safety and efficacy of JenaValve trilogy for treatment of severe and symptomatic AR. 180 patients have been recruited and the results are awaited.

Correction of AR is most often by surgical valve replacement with either mechanical or biological valve with low surgical mortality of 1% in centers of excellence and stroke rate of 2%. TAVR in isolated severe native valve AR is not recommended but may be considered for failed biologic valves, with high surgical risk.

CONCLUSION

Aortic regurgitation is characterized by reflux of blood flow from aorta to LV in diastole due to failure of appropriate coaptation of aortic valve leaflets. Etiology of AR falls into two broad categories, i.e., primary aortic valvular pathology and abnormalities aortic root preventing coaptation of normal aortic leaflets, the former being more common than later.

Aortic regurgitation results in increase in preload (volume overload) and afterload (wall stress) of LV proportional to severity of AR with little change in ESV and end-diastolic pressure until they develop LV dysfunction.

There is paradigm shift in therapy of valvular heart disease in general including severe AR—shift from functional parameters to myocardial structural alterations in LV to identify patients before development of irreversible LV dysfunction. The role of advanced echocardiography (GLS) and CMR (T1 mapping, LGE postcontrast, and strain) is evolving in identifying early reversible LV dysfunction. Presently there are no randomized clinical trials testing this hypothesis in chronic severe AR.

Appropriate timing of AVR surgery in chronic severe AR traditionally dictated by presence of symptoms and LV dysfunction (class I indications) and in presence of need for another cardiac surgery (CABG/aortic dilatation). These were dictated by long-term postoperative follow-up studies.

Early surgical intervention during phase of reversible LV dysfunction results in better long-term results. Majority of patients undergo AVR, while selected subgroup undergo aortic valve repair in surgical centers of excellence.

Role of TAVR in therapy of chronic severe AR is evolving, with availability of dedicated valves for AR like JenaValve trilogy. TAVR for severe AR may be considered in high-risk patients with failed biologic aortic valves.

ONLINE REFERENCES

Please scan the QR code provided at the end of the table of contents for References of this chapter.

CHAPTER 14

Coronary Artery Disease in Women: How is it Different?

Shibba Takkar Chhabra, Ankit Gulia

ABSTRACT

CAD in women differs from men given its unique risk factor profile and varied clinical presentation. Moreover, a diffuse atherosclerotic pattern with minimal calcification, nonobstructive plaques with different morphology and outward remodeling characterize CAD in women. As CAD rates rise and assume alarming proportion of mortality in women; it's imperative for the treating physicians to acclimatize themselves to the women specific diagnostic and management algorithms. A women targeted approach to CAD in this subset would not just aid in prompt diagnosis but also yield favorable short- and long-term morbidity and mortality outcomes.

Keywords: Women, coronary artery disease, nonobstructive coronary artery disease (NOCAD), variant, atherosclerosis.

INTRODUCTION

Cardiovascular ailments continue to be the leading cause of mortality among women.[1] Acute myocardial infarction (AMI) mortality has decreased in both sexes, although younger women, under the age of 55 years, still have the greatest mortality rate with no discernible improvement over the past two decades.[1,2]

Despite immense progress in treating focal and obstructive atherosclerotic lesions, gender-specific differences in coronary artery disease (CAD) continues to be under-recognized and overlooked. Sex disparities in women presenting with acute coronary syndrome (ACS) are widely documented. Women with CAD have different clinical manifestations, are older, and have more comorbidities than men. Most of the women are still treated on the same lines as men in ischemic heart disease (IHD) with rare emphasis on prevalent nonobstructive coronary artery disease (NOCAD) and coronary microvascular dysfunction in the fair sex. Women have variant plaque structure, lesser obstruction, and minimal calcification and a diffuse atherosclerotic pattern with outward remodeling in comparison to men.[3]

EPIDEMIOLOGY

Coronary artery disease is very common in both developed and developing world. Despite being responsible for causing 35% of deaths in women each year, cardiovascular disease (CVD) in women remains understudied, under-recognized, underdiagnosed, and undertreated, with women under-represented in clinical trials. Globally, it was estimated that in 2020, 244.1 million people were living with IHD, and it was more prevalent in males than in females (141.0 and 103.1 million people, respectively).[1] The Global Burden of Disease (GBD) study reported that in the year 2017 in India, CVD caused 2.64 million deaths (women 1.18; men 1.45 million) and IHD 1.54 million (women 0.62; men 0.92 million). The burden of IHD-related disability-adjusted life years (DALYs) was 36.99 million (women 13.80; men 23.19 million). From 2000 to 2017, the annual IHD mortality increased from 0.85 to 1.54 million (+81.1%) with a greater increase in women (0.32–0.62 million, +93.7%) compared to men (0.53–0.92 million, +73.6%). An increase in age-adjusted IHD mortality rate/100,000 was also more in women (62.9–92.7, +47.4%) than in men (97.5–129.5, +32.8%).[4]

RISK FACTORS (FIG. 1 AND TABLE 1)

Women have both traditional and women-specific CAD risk factors. Traditional cardiac risk factors of diabetes, smoking, obesity, and hypertension affect the cardiovascular system differently in men and women **(Box 1)**.

Hypertension prevalence is the same in women and men. Women are less likely to receive medical treatment for hypertension and have poorer blood pressure control.[5]

Women using oral contraceptives had a two to three times rise in the incidence of hypertension. Moreover, compared to men, hypertension in women beyond 60 years has a more severe influence on CVD.[6]

Compared to men, women are more at risk for CAD from diabetes mellitus.[5] Additionally, diabetes mellitus increases the adjusted hazard ratio (HR) of fatal CAD in diabetic women more than it does in diabetic men [HR 3.77; 95% confidence interval (CI) 2.52–5.65] (HR 14.74; 95% CI 6.16–35.27). Also, there is a gender difference in the extent of cardiovascular risk reduction in women with diabetes, inclusive of lesser medication use and poorer glycated hemoglobin (HbA1c) levels.[7]

Women are more likely than men to suffer from dyslipidemia. Menopausal transition is linked to negative changes in the lipid profile. Women's levels of total cholesterol, low-density lipoprotein, and apolipoprotein B significantly rise following menopause, according to the SWAN (Study of Women's Health Across the Nation) study. Additionally, an increase in high-density lipoprotein (HDL),

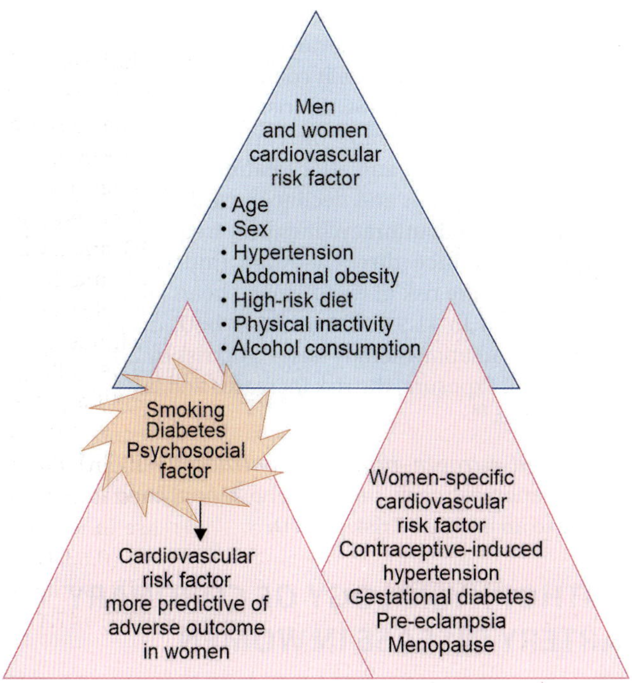

FIG. 1: Coronary artery disease (CAD) risk factors in men and women.

TABLE 1: Cardiovascular disease (CVD) risk factors and conditions in female sex.

Female-specific CVD risk factors	Female-predominant CVD risk factors

• Adverse pregnancy outcomes
• Pregnancy-related gestational hypertension:
  ○ Preeclampsia
  ○ Eclampsia
  ○ Gestational diabetes mellitus
  ○ Preterm delivery
• Polycystic ovarian syndrome
• Functional hypothalamic amenorrhea
• Reproductive hormones
	• Autoimmune inflammatory diseases:
	  ○ Rheumatoid arthritis
	  ○ Systemic lupus erythematosus
	  ○ Scleroderma
	• Breast cancer

Female-specific CVD conditions	**Female-predominant CVD conditions**

Peripartum cardiomyopathy	• Myocardial infarction with nonobstructive coronary arteries
	  ○ Takotsubo cardiomyopathy/ nonobstructive coronary artery disease (NOCAD)
	  ○ Microvascular dysfunction
	  ○ Endothelial dysfunction
	• Heart failure with preserved ejection fraction
	• Spontaneous coronary artery dissection
	• Postural orthostatic tachycardia syndrome
	• Coronary vasospasm
	• Pulmonary hypertension

BOX 1 Variant ischemic heart disease (IHD) pattern in women.

- Nonobstructive coronary artery disease (NOCAD), a predominant presentation
- Functional disorders of the coronary (micro-) circulation
- Clinically relevant sex differences in plaque morphology at all ages:
    - Fewer calcifications
    - Less focal obstruction
    - More diffuse pattern of atherosclerosis
    - Outward remodeling and "soft" plaques
- Distinct presentation of angina symptoms warranting a more gender-sensitive diagnostic and therapeutic approach

which has athero-protective qualities in the premenopausal period, has been discovered to be paradoxically related to an increase in atherosclerosis progression in the postmenopausal phase.[8]

Since >10 years ago, sex-related dimorphisms in CVDs and atherosclerosis have been noted. Vascular remodeling is caused by inflammatory mediators such as cytokines, endothelial dysfunction, vascular smooth muscle cell migration, and proliferation, although sex has varying effects on each of these processes. Men are more likely than women to die from CVDs each year, and they also tend to be impacted sooner in life (40–70 years old), whereas women mostly have difficulties from atherosclerosis after menopause (60+ years).[9] Smoking is the leading preventable cause of cardiovascular death in the general population. As compared to men, smoking has a higher detrimental effect on the onset of IHD in women. Moreover, a younger age of current smoking predisposes women to develop premature CAD.

Age strongly predicts CAD. Although the prevalence of CAD rises with age in both men and women, women typically present with CVD 10 years later than men.[7]

There are more clusters of traditional vascular disease risk factors in postmenopausal women than in nonpostmenopausal women. This suggests that sex differences in CAD are caused by variations in endogenous sex hormones. Obesity and a sedentary lifestyle are two additional risk factors that might be modified. These new risk factors are more prevalent in women and increase the likelihood of developing CAD and having unfavorable cardiovascular outcomes.

Pregnancy-associated Risk Factors

Various medical conditions of pregnancy may predict an increase in the risk of future cardiovascular events in women.

An increased risk of future cardiovascular events, cardiovascular mortality, coronary heart disease (CHD), CHD death, and stroke is linked to preterm delivery (before 37 weeks of gestation). Comparing those with a history of preterm delivery to those without one, the adjusted risk was between 1.4 and 2 times higher. Preterm births that take place before 32 weeks of gestation are most at risk.[9] It has been discovered that gestational hypertension in any form raises the risk of CVD, be in heart failure, myocardial damage, stroke, and mortality or death.[10]

A comprehensive review of the literature on the relationship between severe maternal morbidity (severe preeclampsia, eclampsia, amniotic fluid embolism, and postpartum hemorrhage) and CVD demonstrated a higher future risk of any CVD in women who suffer severe maternal morbidity during pregnancy.[11]

Gestational diabetes increases the risk of both future diabetes and CVD.[12]

Spontaneous pregnancy loss (miscarriage) or stillbirth has an increased risk of atherosclerotic cardiovascular disease (ASCVD) in the future, particularly CHD. It may be related to procoagulant and proinflammatory conditions associated with recurrent miscarriages. Pregnancy loss is also linked to an increased risk of hypertension and type 2 diabetes mellitus (T2DM).[13]

Other pregnancy complications associated with an increased risk of subsequent CVD include low birth weight, placental abruption, and maternoplacental syndrome.

Other Conditions Associated with Cardiovascular Disease Risk in Women

Timing of menarche: Either early or late menarche appears to be associated with future ASCVD risk. A history of menarche before the age of 10 years and delayed menarche after the age of 25 years are associated with an increased risk of CVD.[14]

Early menopause: Early menopause (occurring at <40 years of age), either naturally, surgically, or chemically, is associated with an increased risk of ASCVD. Alterations in estrogen during menopause may lead to alterations in a woman's CVD risk. Estrogen reduction during menopause has been linked to changes in body fat distribution, endothelial dysfunction, vascular inflammation, sympathetic tone, and insulin resistance.

Polycystic ovary syndrome is strongly associated with metabolic syndrome and diabetes mellitus, increasing the risk of CVD in an indirect way.

Autoimmune diseases: Rheumatoid arthritis, systemic lupus erythematosus (SLE), and antiphospholipid antibody syndrome are more common in females and are associated with an increased risk of ASCVD.[15]

Breast cancer: There is an elevated risk of ASCVD mortality in females with breast cancer. It could be due to the combined effects of underlying ASCVD risk factors, direct adverse effects of cancer therapy on cardiac function, lifestyle perturbations during and after treatment, and concomitant metabolic alterations and decline in cardiovascular reserve. Trastuzumab and anthracyclines, two frequently prescribed drugs, can induce direct cardiac injury. When taking trastuzumab, the risk of experiencing heart failure increases to 32.1% and to 41.9% when taking both drugs together. Moreover, radiation therapy raises CVD risk by 7.4%. Within a few years of exposure, the risk increases and lasts for roughly two decades.[16]

Combined estrogen-progestin contraceptives: The use of combination estrogen-progestin hormonal contraception is linked to an increased risk of CVD.

PATHOPHYSIOLOGY OF CORONARY ARTERY DISEASE IN WOMEN

There is evidence that vasculopathy in women with CAD is different and more severe compared to that in men. Atherosclerosis is usually found to be less extensive in women. Plaque erosion is the most frequent cause of ACS in women, while in men, it is plaque rupture. Women's coronary arteries are structurally smaller than men's, with a smaller caliber size. However, plaques burden eccentricity, and calcification in atherosclerotic plaques is identical in both men and women.

Women have a distinct coronary vasculature in terms of its functional characteristics. The pathogenesis of CAD in women is significantly influenced by sex hormones. Sex hormones can affect the smooth muscle and endothelium's vascular responsiveness. The coronary vasculature is subject to dramatic changes as a result of the powerful hormonal impacts that women experience throughout their lifetime. Studies on vascular imaging have revealed detrimental changes that occur during the menopausal transition and go beyond the effects of aging.

One hundred sixty-three women who were referred for coronary angiography to look into a possible myocardial ischemia were evaluated for coronary reactivity as part of the WISE (Women's Ischemia Syndrome Evaluation) project. According to the study, 50% of women who reported having chest discomfort but who did not have an obstructive CAD had coronary artery dysfunction. The findings demonstrated reduced coronary vasomotor response to acetylcholine, which indicated coronary endothelial dysfunction. Regardless of the severity of CAD, coronary endothelial dysfunction independently predicted worse cardiovascular outcomes.[17]

CLINICAL PRESENTATION OF CORONARY ARTERY DISEASE IN WOMEN

There have been numerous reports of sex variations in the clinical presentation of CAD. Women are less likely than men to arrive with an AMI (6% vs. 10%) and are more likely to experience angina pectoris as their initial sign of CAD (47% vs. 32%).[5]

It is well recognized that myocardial ischemia causes some "typical" symptoms. These are radiation to the left arm precordial chest discomfort and sensation of heaviness or fullness. For many years, it was believed that women with ACS frequently have "atypical" symptoms. An ACS presentation without chest pain was more common in women, according to prior research. More recent data indicate that there are no gender differences in the symptoms of ACS. The VIRGO (Variation in Recovery: Role of Gender on Outcomes of Young AMI Patients) study examined sex disparities in the manifestation of symptoms in young myocardial infarction (MI) patients (55 years old). The findings showed that chest pain was the most common complaint among both men and women (87.0% vs. 89.5%; $p = 0.19$). Additionally, women were more likely to have more than three ACS-related symptoms, such as shortness of breath, pain in a different body area, pain that radiates to the jaw, vomiting, exhaustion, and general weakness. According to the study, women were also much less likely than males to have their symptoms classified as having a cardiac origin (53% vs. 37%, $p = 0.001$) and significantly more likely to attribute their discomfort to stress or anxiety (20.9% vs. 11.8%, $p = 0.001$).[18]

A significant disparity among treating healthcare professionals was noticed who rarely attributed women's symptoms as health worsened. MI trends were stable in men and increased in women.

Women typically present with an AMI at an older age than men do and frequently have more cardiovascular risk factors (CVRFs) than men. But in recent years, a considerably younger age range has become a population at a higher risk. The YOUNG-MI registry looked at this cohort and discovered that younger women (50 years old) with MI had a considerably higher percentage of rheumatological, diabetes, and depressive problems than their male counterparts. During the average follow-up of 11.2 years, these women had a considerably higher all-cause mortality rate than men.[19]

OBSTRUCTIVE VERSUS NONOBSTRUCTIVE CORONARY ARTERY DISEASE

Women might exhibit both chronic coronary syndrome (CCS) and ACS, much like males. CAD might be nonobstructive or obstructive in each of these clinical settings. NOCAD is more common in women with CCS. The majority of ACS patients, regardless of gender, have obstructive CAD.

Nonobstructive Coronary Artery Disease

The paradox of IHD in women has been attributed to the fact that, although having higher rates of myocardial ischemia and mortality than males, anatomically they have less obstructive CAD. This is particularly obvious in younger women. Microvascular disease causes greater vascular dysfunction and ischemia with no obstructive coronary artery disease (INOCA) in women. Plaque erosion and microvascular dysfunction are the proposed pathophysiology.

In the WISE trial, NOCAD was found in 57% of the women with stable symptomatic CAD who also had symptoms and evidence of ischemia.[19] Women are at least twice as likely as males to have NOCAD (defined as 50% diameter stenosis of all main epicardial arteries).[5]

The mechanism of myocardial infarction with nonobstructive coronary artery disease (MINOCA) is atherothrombosis with the possible contribution of coronary artery spasm and/or endothelial dysfunction, and thus secondary prevention of atherosclerosis is vital in these patients. Lack of awareness of gender differences in pathophysiology may adversely impact CAD diagnosis in women. Women with NOCAD with MI are less likely to be administered drugs for the secondary prevention of MI despite the poor prognosis of MINOCA.

The MINOCA/INOCA syndromes are becoming more widely known. In over 6% of individuals with AMI, MINOCA is the initial symptom.[20,21] According to data from the ACTION Registry-GWTG, women are more likely to experience this entity (10.5% vs. 3.4%; $p = 0.0001$) than males. Women are reported to have a greater mortality rate than males among patients with obstructive CAD (3.9% vs. 2.4%; $p = 0.0001$), while there is no sex difference in mortality observed among patients with MINOCA (1.1% vs. 1.0%; $p = 0.84$).[22]

Takotsubo cardiomyopathy needs to be considered in the differential diagnosis of MINOCA. Over 90% of the cases of this transient ventricular apical ballooning syndrome are in females. Catecholamine surge rather than atherosclerotic disease is the pathogenesis. The catecholamine surge causes a predominantly microvascular dysfunction—due to multiple factors including microvascular spasm and ensuring myocardial stunning, direct catecholamine cardiotoxicity, and an increase in the myocardial energy demand.

Obstructive Coronary Artery Disease

The majority of women presenting with ACS have evidence of obstructive CAD. Atherosclerotic disease is the primary cause of ACS in women. Compared to ST-elevation myocardial infarction (STEMI), non-ST-elevation myocardial infarction (NSTEMI) is more common in women with ACS.[18] In comparison to men, women with STEMI experience longer delays in presentation, diagnosis, and treatment administration.[23]

When treating women with ACS, one should consider spontaneous coronary artery dissection (SCAD). Up to 4% of female MIs are caused by it, and it mostly affects women. The coronary artery wall spontaneously separates in SCAD, occluding the coronary lumen with an intramural hematoma. It predominates in young women and accounts for 43% of all MIs related to pregnancy.[24] During coronary angiography, intravascular imaging can be done by visualizing the artery wall. As opposed to atherosclerotic coronary disease, it has different treatment and prognosis implications.[24]

Noninvasive Testing

Several noninvasive tests can be used to evaluate female individuals suspected of having CAD. For intermediate-risk patients with normal baseline cardiograms, an exercise stress test is routinely employed. The negative predictive value of an exercise stress test by electrocardiography (ECG) remains high in women; however, women have reduced sensitivity and specificity for identifying obstructive CAD. Endogenous estrogen in women contributes to ST segment depression, particularly in premenopausal women, which can increase the likelihood of a false-positive exercise stress test. Regardless of the patient's gender, the diagnostic and prognostic yield of a stress echocardiography is comparable.

Myocardial perfusion imaging (MPI) with single-photon emission computed tomography (SPECT) also has good diagnostic accuracy in both men and women; however, artifacts due to breast attenuation and decreased left ventricular (LV) size can complicate data interpretation. Women who have a positive stress imaging test and later find out that they have NOCAD should be closely monitored due to their increased risk of future cardiovascular events. Given the higher mortality and cardiovascular event rates recorded in women with NOCAD and normal epicardial coronary arteries, they should not be dismissed as false positives. The stress MPI test may increase diagnostic accuracy for obstructive CAD even further **(Flowchart 1)**.

Stress cardiac magnetic resonance (CMR) imaging has a similar higher diagnostic sensitivity in women for assessing CAD. In a study of women with angina who did not have epicardial CAD, stress CMR revealed indications of subendocardial hypoperfusion. Computed tomography coronary angiography (CTCA) has the same diagnostic accuracy in both sexes for diagnosing anatomical obstructive as well as nonobstructive coronary atherosclerotic plaques **(Flowchart 2)**.

Fractional flow reserve (FFR) measurements can determine the hemodynamic relevance of coronary artery stenoses. Compared to men, coronary arteries of women are smaller and supply a smaller amount of myocardium even after adjusting for vessel size, which may explain the overall higher FFR value of women. In an analysis of revascularization deferral after FFR assessments, long-term outcomes during 5-year follow-up differed significantly between women and men in favor of women **(Fig. 2)**.[25]

TREATMENT GAPS

Data demonstrates that women with ACS are more likely to experience a delay in reperfusion and are less likely to receive medical therapy based on guidelines.[26] The ACS international guidelines state that men and women should receive the same care.[27] However, compared to men, women frequently receive less intensive therapy and subsequent preventative care, which has a negative impact on prognosis and outcomes. The majority of individuals should receive percutaneous coronary intervention (PCI) for the treatment of AMI. Similar to men, early invasive therapy in women improves outcomes with lower mortality and recurrent MI and/or ischemic episodes. After accounting for advanced age and an increased burden of comorbidities, there are no sex differences in clinical outcomes among ACS patients who are not receiving PCI.[28]

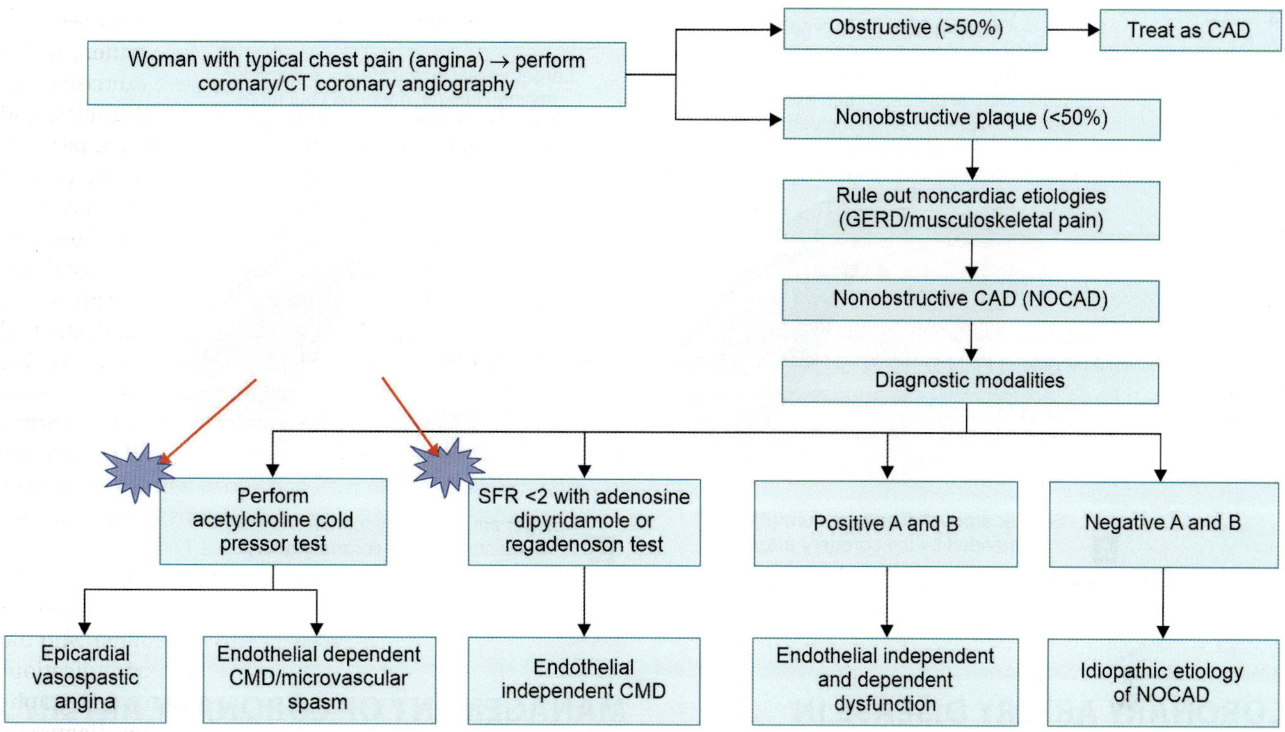

FLOWCHART 1: Evaluation of coronaries in a woman presenting with typical chest pain (obstructive/nonobstructive).

(CAD: coronary artery disease; CFR: coronary flow reserve; CMD: coronary microvascular dysfunction; CT: computed tomography; GERD: gastroesophageal reflux disease)

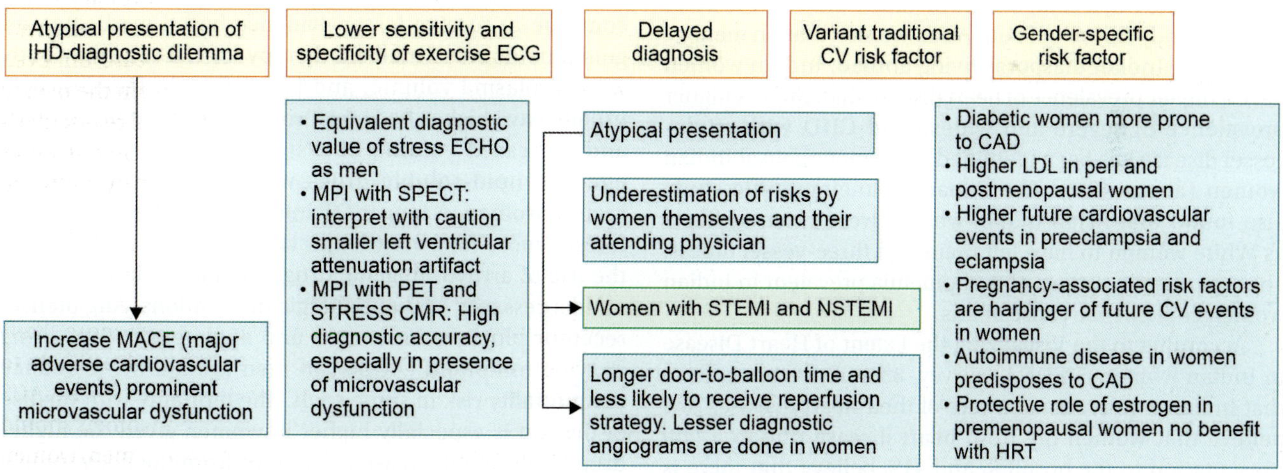

FLOWCHART 2: Pertinent issues in a coronary artery disease (CAD) assessment in women.

(CMR: cardiac magnetic resonance; CV: cardiovascular; ECG: electrocardiography; ECHO: echocardiography; HRT: hormone replacement therapy; IHD: ischemic heart disease; LDL: low-density lipoprotein; MPI: myocardial perfusion imaging; NSTEMI: non-ST-segment elevation myocardial infarction; PET: positron emission tomography; SPECT: single-photon emission computed tomography; STEMI: ST-segment elevation myocardial infarction)

Women with MINOCA are particularly affected by the treatment differences between men and women because they are less likely to be given drugs for the secondary prevention of MI. Women under the age of 55 years are particularly affected by this gender disparity because they are less likely to obtain the proper medical care after an ACS occurrence. Instead of reduced treatment adherence, lower treatment initiation is the culprit.

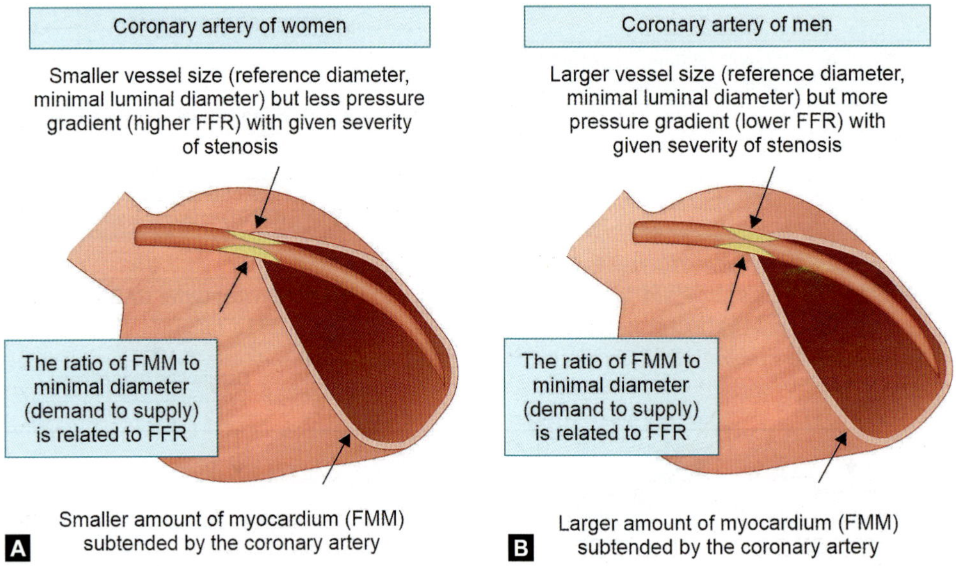

FIGS. 2A AND B: Higher FFR in women with given severity of stenosis compared to men.
(FFR: fractional flow reserve; FMM: fractional myocardial mass)

CORONARY ARTERY DISEASE IN WOMEN: INDIAN SCENARIO

Asian Indian women had an eightfold greater mortality rate from CAD than Chinese and White women in the 30–39 years age group. Similarly, South Asian women have a higher CAD mortality rate when compared to men. The drop in CAD rates is significantly slower in South Asian women than in men.

Among Indian diasporas living abroad, Indian women have a higher prevalence of heart disease than men. A higher prevalence of severe and widespread CHD with triple-vessel disease has been identified in premenopausal Indian women (about 40%). The Canadian angiographic study also found that Asian Indian women were twice as likely as White women to have left main and three-vessel illness. The atherogenic pattern of dyslipidemia prevalent in Indian women could be the cause of this.

According to the Visualizing the Extent of Heart Disease in Indian women (VEDNA) survey, 83% of doctors believe that Indian women are unaware of their heart disease, 76% believe that women die from heart disease due to a late presentation to the hospital, and 41% believe that there is an alarming 10–15% increase in CVD among Indian women, particularly in the premenopausal age group of 20–40 years.

The Queen of Heart campaign in 2013 targeted 450 million Indian women to raise CVD awareness. From 2001 to 2003, the Million Death Study (MDS) identified CVD as a primary cause of mortality among women. Higher mortality was associated with risk assessment issues, delayed diagnosis and management, a variety of clinical presentations, poor-quality ACS therapies, long-term management, and secondary prevention programs.

MANAGEMENT OF CORONARY ARTERY DISEASE IN WOMEN

Conservative Management

Despite equivalent benefits with the use of aspirin, statins, and beta-blockers in the established guidelines, women continue to receive lesser evidence-based medicine and guideline-directed medical therapy for IHD. A lower body weight, plasma volume, and blood flow in females, who usually have higher body fats, contribute to a quicker onset and increased volume of distribution and a persistent effect of lipid-soluble drugs with more adverse effects seen in women. A longer QT interval in women might also foresee more fatal ventricular tachycardia, especially with the use of arrhythmogenic drugs such as antiarrhythmics, antidepressants, and antiallergic medications. Angiotensin receptor blockers in women and angiotensin-converting enzyme inhibitors (ACEIs) in men are known to reduce the mortality risk in some trials. The mortality with the use of digoxin is especially higher in women given the higher drug levels and decreased clearance from the body. At any given dose, the women tend to respond more with the use of beta-blockers, ACEIs, or diuretics. Also, they experience more adverse effects, hereby leading to less adherence to the medication schedule. Women also tend to have greater benefit and atheroma regression with the use of statins. However, the adverse effects with statins are also more reported by women, again leading to less adherence and disruption of the usual dosage pattern. Conservative management of SCAD is usually preferred, despite the high risk of per-procedural complications with underlying weak coronary artery structure prone to iatrogenic dissection. The attempts of performing percutaneous intervention might be associated with the propagation of SCAD.

Percutaneous Transluminal Coronary Angioplasty

Though men and women may derive equivalent benefits with an invasive interventional therapy, women are less likely to receive the revascularization strategy for the management of coronary events. Female sex has been considered as an independent predictor of poorer outcomes, especially with higher periprocedural MI and a higher risk of in-hospital events. This could be due to more elderly women undergoing revascularization, higher comorbidities and coexistent CVRFs, smaller coronary arteries, and delayed revascularization. Delays in symptoms-to-door and door-to-balloon time have been noted by several registries across different countries for STEMI presentation in women. The women also have a tendency of having residual persistent symptoms with a poor quality of life (QOL) post PCI given there are more microvascular and functional coronary artery dysfunction and diffuse pattern of atherosclerosis. Women are also reported to have higher restenosis rates after the intervention and higher access site complications as compared to men.

Coronary Artery Bypass Grafting

Female sex is again an independent risk factor for a patient undergoing coronary artery bypass grafting (CABG). Women continue to be under-represented in randomized as well as observational trials for CABG. Women needing surgical revascularization are generally older than their male counterparts and have more comorbidities. Also, postsurgical QOL continues to be poorer as compared to men with pre- and postoperative complications, increased mortality, and longer durations to recovery. Just like post-PCI, the post-CABG women also experience more residual symptoms and poor QOL given a diffused pattern of atherosclerosis and less likely complete revascularization. Women experience higher in-hospital mortality compared to men and greater postoperative problems, such as renal failure and neurological issues, even after controlling for confounding variables. These sex disparities are especially obvious in younger women (<50 years old) having coronary bypass surgery.[29]

Cardiac Rehabilitation

Participating in cardiac rehabilitation (CR) programs has been shown to significantly lower cardiovascular mortality and repeat hospitalizations. According to suggestions in worldwide practice guidelines, patients after a MI should be referred to CR.[30] Women receive less referral for primary and secondary preventive treatment programs and rehabilitation programs. Even after having received a referral, they continue to have low attendance rates and lesser access and completion of CR programs as compared to men. Though women may benefit more as regards to mortality reduction with CR as compared to men, women still continue to be less enrolled in CR programs. Socioeconomic factors, the time constraints placed on women as the primary caregiver for the home, and the low rates of proper physician referral are a few of the explanations put out for this. It is essential and necessary to put into practice strategies to boost women's referral and adherence to CR.

PROGNOSIS

In comparison to men, women with CCS have less atherosclerotic diseases, and their prognosis is better. Women with ACS and those who have undergone coronary revascularization experience longer hospital stays, higher in-hospital mortality, and higher readmission rates during the first 30 days following hospitalization than males.[25] In the clinical setting of STEMI, female sex stands alone as a poor predictive factor.[23] Women are more prone to experiencing mechanical issues and subsequent heart failure following an AMI.

Over the last 20 years, the rate of 30-day major adverse cardiac events and in-hospital complications among women with ACS is decreasing.[31] The prevalence of CVRFs and the outcomes of CVD are inversely linked with socioeconomic status (SES). Women may be more susceptible to income and education when it comes to CVD incidence. Men may be more susceptible to income and education than those from low- and middle-income nations when it comes to CVD mortality.[32]

CONCLUSION

Coronary artery disease in women has a variant risk factor profile and clinical presentation. Moreover, women differ in their plaque structure and have lesser obstruction and minimal calcification with a diffuse atherosclerotic pattern and outward remodeling in comparison to men. As CAD contributes to a rising and alarming proportion of mortality in women, these differences in clinical presentation and diagnostic and management strategies need a readdresal. Women-targeted guidelines for CAD management shall sensitize the physicians for a focused approach culminating into favorable outcomes in women with CAD.

ONLINE REFERENCES

Please scan the QR code provided at the end of the table of contents for References of this chapter.

CHAPTER 15

Diet as a Driver for Coronary Artery Disease

Jaideep C Menon, Aravind MS

ABSTRACT

Diet and nutrition play a crucial role in determining our health and can impact the development of chronic diseases like coronary artery disease. Macronutrients (proteins, carbohydrates, and fats) and micronutrients (vitamins and minerals) are essential for the body's growth, metabolism, and repair. Global food shifts toward sugary, fatty, and animal-based diets, seen more in low-middle income countries, drive unhealthy eating habits due to modern food environments. Starting with breastfeeding, healthy diets from early life curb obesity and noncommunicable diseases (NCDs). Balanced diets rich in veggies, legumes, fish, and whole grains, lower the risk of cardiovascular disease (CVD) by 31%. Conversely, Western diets, high in processed meat, sugary treats, and red meat, elevate the risk by 14%. A balanced diet can help prevent NCDs such as diabetes, heart disease, stroke, and cancer as well as all types of malnutrition. The two biggest hazards to health worldwide are an improper diet and insufficient exercise.

Keywords: Cardiovascular disease (CVD), coronary artery disease (CAD), macronutrient, micronutrient, trans-fatty acids, polyunsaturated fatty acids, monounsaturated fatty acids.

INTRODUCTION

In 1826, the renowned French gastronome and lawyer Jean Anthelme Brillat-Savarin is attributed to have coined the phrase "Dis-moi ce que tu manges, je te dire ce que tu es," which can be roughly translated to "tell me what you eat, and I will tell you who you are." Over the time, this sentiment has evolved into the commonly heard phrase "You are what you eat." This proverb is especially true for noncommunicable, chronic, and to a lesser extent, some communicable disorders; however, its relevance is arguably most pronounced in the context of coronary artery disease.

Diet and nutrition are foundational elements for the well-being of populations. The concept of "diet" refers to the habitual food choices an individual makes, while "nutrition" pertains to the essential nutrients that our bodies require daily to function optimally. Diet encompasses the overall quantity of food consumed, whereas nutrition involves the process of utilizing food to facilitate growth, metabolism, and tissue repair. The relationship between diet, nutrition, and health is bidirectional, wherein health status can be influenced by nutrient deficiencies and vice versa. To promote a diet that meets nutritional needs and prevents diet-related illnesses, evidence-based dietary guidelines have been established to offer recommendations for food and beverage consumption at a population level.

Nutrients are categorized into two main types based on the human body's requirements for normal metabolic functioning, growth, and overall physical well-being. Macronutrients comprise proteins, carbohydrates, and fats, with fats being the most energy-dense. Carbohydrates, quantitatively speaking, serve as the primary dietary energy source for the majority of populations. Proteins, essential for the growth, cellular repair, and overall health, are vital components of every cell. Micronutrients encompass vitamins and minerals, are present in trace amounts in most foods, and play a critical role in maintaining normal metabolic functions.[1]

WORLD HEALTH ORGANIZATION RECOMMENDATIONS ON DIET

The key points are summarized as follows:

- Maintaining a balanced diet is a key to preventing malnutrition and reducing the risk of noncommunicable diseases (NCDs).[2]

- Global health concerns include eating a poor diet and not exercising enough.
- The good eating habits begin in childhood.
- The consumption of calories should be balanced with the expenditure of energy to prevent undesirable weight gain. The recommendation is that the overall intake of fats should be <30%,[3-5] saturated fats <10%, and trans fats <1% of the total energy intake. There should be a transition in fat consumption patterns, moving away from saturated and trans fats toward unsaturated fats,[5] with the ultimate objective of eliminating industrially-generated trans fats[6-8]
- Restricting the consumption of free sugars to below 10% of the total energy intake.[2,9]
- Maintaining a daily salt intake of <5 g (equivalent to an intake of <2 g of sodium) is effective in averting hypertension and reducing the risk of heart disease and stroke among adults.[10]
- World Health Organization (WHO) member states have reached a consensus to decrease global salt consumption by 30% before 2025 in addition to preventing the prevalence of diabetes, hypertension, and obesity.[11,12]

Adopting a nutritious diet throughout the life course plays a crucial role in preventing various forms of malnutrition and a spectrum of NCDs and ailments; however, the increased production of processed foods, rapid urbanization, and evolving lifestyles have prompted a shift in dietary habits. Presently, individuals are consuming a greater quantity of energy-dense foods, fats, free sugars, and salt/sodium, while insufficiently incorporating fruits, vegetables, and dietary fiber sources like whole grains into their diets.

The precise composition of a diversified, well-balanced, and healthful diet will differ based on the individual attributes (e.g., age, gender, lifestyle, and levels of physical activity), cultural environment, locally accessible food options, and dietary traditions. But the essential ideas of what makes up a healthy diet stay the same.

For adults, the recommendations for a healthy and nutritious diet from the WHO are as follows:

- Whole grains such as unprocessed maize, millet, oats, wheat, and brown rice as well as fruits, vegetables, legumes (such as lentils and beans), nuts, and legumes.
- About 400 g or five servings (minimum) of fruit and vegetables each day, omitting potatoes, sweet potatoes, cassava, and other starchy roots.
- An intake of free sugars should be limited to 50 g (~12 levels of teaspoons) for an individual with a healthy body weight who consumes approximately 2,000 calories each day.[4,9]
- Fats in a diet to below 30% of the total energy intake[3-5] with unsaturated fats, found in foods such as fish, avocados, nuts, and oils such as sunflower, soybean, canola, and olive oils are being recommended. It is advised to limit the consumption of saturated fats, which are present in fatty meats, butter, palm and coconut oil, cream, cheese, *ghee*, and lard as well as all forms of trans fats.[7] In particular, industrially-produced trans fats should be entirely avoided as they have no place in a healthful diet.[6,8]
- About <5 g (or around one teaspoon) of salt per day. Salt should be iodized.

AVAILABLE EVIDENCE ON THE ASSOCIATION OF HEART DISEASE WITH DIET

There is a lot of controversy with regard to what constitutes a cardiac-friendly diet. Data relating diet to cardiovascular diseases (CVDs) has predominantly been generated from high-income countries (HIC), whilst > 80% of CVD deaths occur in low- and middle-income countries (LMIC) from where data is sparse.[13,14]

The rising burden of NCDs in LMICs is attributed to the lifestyle shifts linked with heightened urbanization, economic progress, and global integration. The Global Burden of Disease study identifies diet as a primary driver of conditions such as hypertension, diabetes, obesity, and other components of CVD.[15] Presently, there are over 500 million people classified as obese,[16,17] and nearly 2 billion individuals globally are either overweight or obese.[18]

There is a consensus on the fact that poor quality diets are high in refined grains, added sugars, excessive salt, unhealthy fats, and animal-derived foods. Conversely, they lack adequate quantities of whole grains, fruits, vegetables, legumes, fish, and nuts. These diets often feature heavily processed food items, usually packaged and designed for a quick consumption, while minimizing the inclusion of whole foods and freshly prepared meals. The proliferation of these unhealthy dietary patterns is facilitated by contemporary food environments, which are becoming more prevalent even in LMICs.[17,19,20]

ROLE OF GLOBAL FOOD SYSTEMS AND THE INDUSTRY

The transition to a global food system was initially propelled by the governmental investments and interventions in markets, infrastructure, and research aimed at boosting productivity within the agricultural sector.[21-25] In most LMICs, this took a different form, involving measures, such as food subsidies, agricultural product taxes, and systems to manage the supply and marketing of key commodities.[26-29] The 1960s marked a significant agricultural transformation in LMICs with initiatives like the "Green Revolution" and the "White Revolution," which aimed to enhance the productivity of essential crops, such as corn, rice, wheat, and milk.[30] Alongside, substantially increasing the calorie supply, the resulting surge in productivity also laid the foundation for inexpensive livestock feed and economical inputs for processed foods, thus fostering incentives for the growth of processed food manufacturers,[31-35] the rise of supermarket retailing, and the proliferation of fast-food establishments.[36-38] Conversely, the production of less processed foods such as coarse grains (e.g., millet and sorghum), roots, tubers, and legumes witnessed a decline,[39,40] while the production of animal-source foods experienced a significant upsurge.[41]

DIETARY IMPACTS

Noticeable disparities have emerged in people's eating habits. The prevalence of snacking and the consumption of snack foods have escalated in both frequency and variety.[42-47] Meal frequency has risen, and there is a substantial surge in eating occasions taking place outside the home, in restaurants, fast-food establishments, and through take-out options, particularly in LMICs.[46,48] The overall proportion of highly processed foods in diets has expanded.[49,50] This trend is significantly boosted by the rapid proliferation of online food delivery systems.

This in turn has led to a shift to refined carbohydrates and added sugars. In Asia, there has been a transition toward white rice as a staple, displacing legumes, and coarse grains.[51-54] Low- or middle-income countries have witnessed a significant rise in the added sugar consumption, particularly increased consumption of sugar-sweetened beverages (SSBs) and processed foods.[55-58]

Also, there has been an increasing intake of vegetable oils, including processed vegetable oils, and a decline in the consumption of animal fats.[14,59] Oilseeds have now become some of the most extensively traded crops, also undergoing processing to generate margarine, and vegetable shortenings as well as partially hydrogenated fats and refined, deodorized oils employed in processed foods. Between 1958 and 1996, there was a substantial change in the types and amounts of fats accessible around the world, with conventional sources such as butter, tallow, and lard being replaced by soybean, palm, and rapeseed/canola oils. Initially, from 1958 to 1962, soybean, palm, and rapeseed/canola oils accounted for 20% of the total 29 million metric tons of fat produced globally each year, while butter, lard, and tallow represented 37%. However, from 1996 to 2001, these oils escalated to 52% of the global fat production of 103 million metric tons annually, while butter, lard, and tallow comprised only 20%.[60] Palm oil (deodorized) serves as a source of saturated fatty acids, while partially hydrogenated fats are the primary contributors to trans-fatty acids. Between 1990 and 2010, dietary cholesterol, trans fats, and saturated fat intakes worldwide were largely consistent (trans fat consumption increased in LMIC and decreased in HIC).[14] Vegetable oil consumption remains twice as high in HIC as in LMIC. However, the consumption of trans fats remains remarkably high in many LMICs, even as it has been significantly declining in HIC. In India, for example, *vanaspati* (a type of vegetable *ghee*) used in baked goods, fried snacks, and street-vendor foods as well as bakery shortening, constitute significant sources of trans fats.

There is an increasing global consumption of meat, which has been made economically feasible by the subsidized production of crops for animal feed—most importantly corn and soybeans (soybean oil is a byproduct of soymeal production for animals).[61-64] At minimal levels of consumption, animal-derived foods can offer benefits by providing high-quality protein and iron. However, in HIC, excessive intake of animal-derived foods might lead to detrimental health effects, particularly when it involves processed meats.[65,66]

The dietary consumption patterns of various protein sources have shown a diverse trend. From 1973 to 1997, per capita dairy consumption in LMIC rose by 48%, and it is anticipated to nearly double (a projected increase of 93%) by 2020. On an average, the consumption of fish is two to three times greater in HIC as compared to LMIC.

A fourth is the noticeable increase in sales of all packaged goods and drinks. All LMIC markets are seeing an acceleration of this phenomenon.[67-69] There is also a marked growth in purchases of all the packaged foods and beverages. This process is accelerating across all LMIC markets.[67-69] The frequency and variety of snacking and snack foods have experienced a notable expansion.[42-47] Overall, diets now contain a greater proportion of highly processed foods.[49,50,58,70]

The shift in how LMICs are seeing a significant increase in added sugar in beverages is another trend related to the added sugar change that has been previously noticed. Between the years 1985 and 2005, HIC witnessed a significant rise in added sugar intake.[54] However, in more recent times, considerable increases have been observed in LMICs, particularly in the consumption of SSBs and ultra-processed foods.

Intake of fruits and vegetables has also continued to be insufficient. Consumption of fruits and vegetables is significantly greater in HIC than LMIC.[71]

MACRONUTRIENTS, FOODS, AND CVD RISK FACTORS (FLOWCHART 1)

Association of Cardiovascular Disease with Classes of Food

- *Carbohydrates*: Research demonstrates an association between refined carbohydrates, such as corn syrup; and the development of type 2 diabetes mellitus (T2DM) and obesity.[72] Evidence from systematic reviews and randomized controlled trials (RCTs) supports the adverse impact of highly-refined, high-glycemic load (GL) carbohydrates. High-glycemic index (GI) meals may raise chance of developing T2DM, according to a meta-analysis of the observational studies.[73,74]

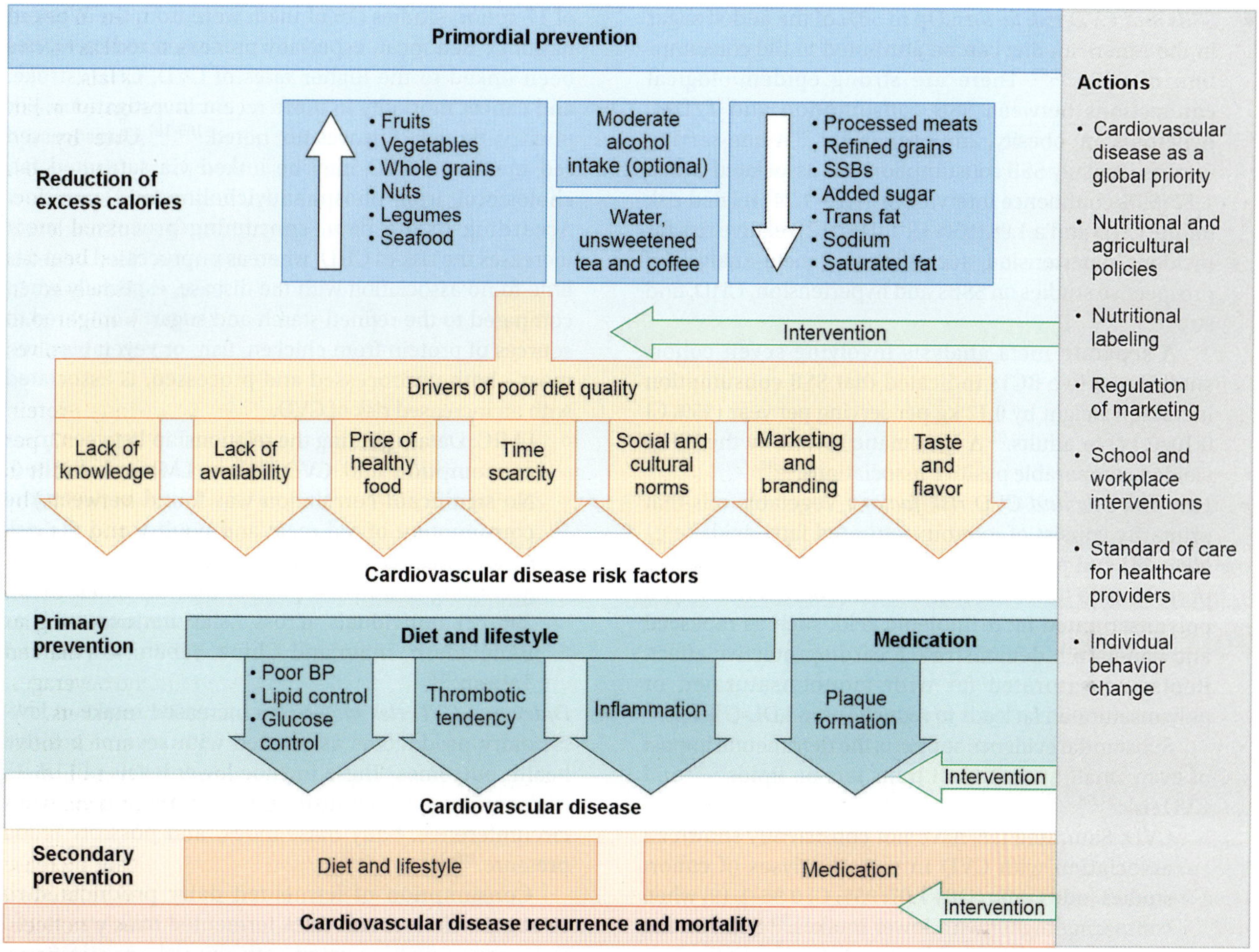

FLOWCHART 1: Role of dietary factors and its association with CVD.

Note: Avoiding excess calories is an integral part of halting the development of cardiovascular disease risk factors (i.e., primordial prevention). Unfavorable eating patterns are driven by a variety of biological, social, economic, and psychological factors, and a robust intervention from all the levels of society may steer populations toward a healthier diet and prevent disease progression. Diet and other lifestyle changes remain crucial steps in primary and secondary prevention of cardiovascular disease, although the relative importance of medication and clinical procedures increases over time with disease progression.

(CVD: cardiovascular disease; SSB: sugar-sweetened beverage)

Source: Yu E, Malik VS, Hu FB. Cardiovascular Disease Prevention by Diet Modification: JACC Health Promotion Series. J Am Coll Cardiol. 2018;72(8):914-26.

Individuals with the highest GL and lowest cereal fiber diet face a 2.5-fold higher risk of T2DM compared to those with the lowest GL and highest cereal fiber intake.[75] According to a large Danish prospective cohort research, switching from saturated fats to high-GI carbohydrates increases the risk of myocardial infarction (MI) by 33%.[76] Another meta-analysis encompassing 10 prospective cohort studies found that increased GL is associated with a 27% elevated risk of coronary heart disease (CHD) and MI.[77]

Traditional foods in LMIC are now highly refined such as polished white rice and refined flours, in contrast to their former abundance in whole grains and dietary fiber.[78,79] Higher intake of refined grains was connected to the higher waist circumference, systolic and diastolic blood pressure, fasting glucose, triglycerides, insulin resistance, and lower high-density lipoprotein cholesterol (HDL-C) values in the CURES 57 (Chennai Urban Rural Epidemiology trial 57).[80] Substituting brown rice for white rice (50 g/day) resulted in a 16% decrease in T2DM risk,[81] and replacing beans with white rice had reduced the odds of metabolic syndrome by 35%.[77]

Promoting an increase in the whole grain and cereal fiber consumption while decreasing total and high-GI carbohydrate intake, emerges as a beneficial strategy for preventing T2DM and CVD in the general population.[82,83] Furthermore, low-GI diets show improvements in the glycemic control and serum lipids in RCTs involving participants with T2DM, indicating significant implications for reducing the CHD risk in this rapidly growing vulnerable population segment.[84-87]

- *SSBs and CVD risk factors*: Up to 50% of the added sugar in the American diet can be attributed to the consumption of SSBs.[88,89] There are strong epidemiological connections between SSB consumption and T2DM, hypertension, obesity, and overweight.[90] A one-serving increase in daily SSB consumption was associated with a 1.17 [95% confidence interval (CI) 1.10–1.24] related risk for the CHD and a 1.08 (95% CI 1.04–1.12) relative risk for incident hypertension, according to a meta-analysis of prospective studies on SSBs and hypertension, CHD, and stroke.[91]

  A separate meta-analysis involving seven cohort studies and five RCTs indicated that SSB consumption increased weight by 0.12 kg per serving per year (95% CI 0.10–0.14) in adults.[92] A systematic review by the WHO yielded comparable positive associations.[93,94]
- *Fats and oils and CVD risk factors*: Vegetable oils that primarily consist of monounsaturated fatty acids (e.g., olive oil) and polyunsaturated fatty acids have shown a propensity to lower the risk of CHD. Sources rich in N-3 polyunsaturated fat α-linolenic acid, such as rapeseed and canola oil, demonstrate a cardioprotective effect. Replacing saturated fat with monounsaturated or polyunsaturated fat leads to reductions in LDL-C levels.[95]

  Substantial evidence supports the detrimental impact of even small quantities of trans fats on lipids[95,96] and CVD risk.[97,98]
  - CVD: Saturated fats have not consistently shown an association with CVD in meta-analyses of cohort studies [odds ratio (OR) 1.07; 95% CI 0.96–1.19] when comparing higher with lower intakes.[99] Substituting saturated fat with highly-refined carbohydrates does not lead to a lower CHD risk, whereas replacing saturated fat with polyunsaturated fat does reduce CHD risk.[100,101]

  Incorporating plant oils into a Mediterranean diet has been shown to reduce CVD risk in two RCTs. The Lyon Diet Heart Study demonstrated that regular consumption of α-linolenic acid (found in canola oil), has significantly reduced cardiac deaths and nonfatal CHD.[102] Similarly, the PREDIMED (Prevención con Dieta Mediterránea) RCT indicated that a Mediterranean diet supplemented with 50 g/day of extra-virgin olive oil reduced CVD events by 30% over 5 years.[103] Palm oil, being a dominant fat globally, has relatively high-saturated fat content. Unsaturated fatty acids could replace palm oil to reduce the incidence of CHD, according to the controlled feeding studies that looked at changes in the blood lipids,[96] but that palm oil would be preferable to partially hydrogenated oils high in trans-fatty acids. A case-control research conducted in Costa Rica indicated that intake of soybean oil was associated with a decreased risk of acute MI compared to the consumption of the palm oil.[104]

  Red and processed meat consumption increased the incidence of T2DM and CHD, according to a meta-analysis of 17 cohort studies (16 of them were from the Western nations). Red meat, especially processed red meat, has been linked to the higher rates of CVD, CHD, stroke, and cancer mortality in more recent investigations. For poultry, though, this was not noted.[105-107] Unprocessed red meat and CVD may be linked via saturated fat, cholesterol, iron, phosphatidylcholine, and carnitine. According to the data, consuming processed meat increases the risk of CHD, whereas unprocessed beef has little to no association with the disease, especially when compared to the refined starch and sugar. Compared to sources of protein from chicken, fish, or vegetables, red meat—both unprocessed and processed, is associated with an increased risk of CVD.
  - LMIC: Data regarding the relationship between meat consumption and CVD risk in LMICs is limited. No significant correlation was found between the consumption of red meat and poultry and the risk of CVD, cancer mortality, or all-cause mortality, according to a recent pooled analysis of data from 296,721 individuals across Asian nations, such as Bangladesh, mainland China, Japan, Korea, and Taiwan.[108]
- *Dairy and CVD risk factors*: An increased intake of low-fat dairy products is associated with several positive health outcomes. These include lower levels of LDL-C, triglycerides, plasma insulin, insulin resistance, waist circumference, body mass index, and possibly blood pressure.[109-117]

  Consumption of fermented dairy products such as yogurt, cheese, and thick fermented milk was found to be inversely associated with the risk of T2DM in a meta-analysis that included cohort studies with over 13,000 incident cases and the EPIC InterAct (European Prospective Investigation into Cancer and Nutrition) case-cohort study with about 12,000 incident cases. On analysis of a large dataset, milk consumption was not associated with CHD or stroke.[108] A prospective cohort study of 53,387 Japanese men and women indicated that higher dietary calcium from dairy (173 mg/day vs. none) reduced the risk of hemorrhagic stroke, ischemic stroke, and stroke mortality by approximately 50% over a 10-year follow-up.[118] In summary, the available studies do not strongly or consistently suggest a clear relationship between the consumption of dairy products and the risk of T2DM and CVD risk.
- *Eggs*: Eggs serve as a relatively inexpensive and low-calorie source of protein, folate, and B vitamins.[119] However, eggs also contain dietary cholesterol, with a medium-sized egg containing about 225 mg of cholesterol.[120] A meta-analysis indicated that egg consumption can lead to increased total cholesterol (TC), HDL-C, and the TC:HDL-C ratio.[121] However, The intake of eggs did not have a significant effect on these parameters[122-124] or endothelial function, according to subsequent RCTs

involving five investigations.[125,126] The effects of egg consumption on CVD events have not been studied in RCTs. Egg consumption was not linked to the total CVD, CHD, stroke, or CHD or stroke death in a meta-analysis of 16 prospective cohort studies with 90,735 participants. Generally, consuming eggs in moderation (about 1 egg/day) appears to have a neutral effect on CVD.

- LMIC: Unpublished findings from three major international studies—PURE (Prospective Urban and Rural Epidemiological Study), ONTARGET (Ongoing Telmisartan Alone and in Combination with Ramipril Global Endpoint Trial), and INTERHEART (a global study of risk factors for acute myocardial infarction)—collectively involving around 200,000 individuals and encompassing 22,000 CVD events, reveal that consuming eggs in moderation seems to have a neutral or potentially protective effect against CVD. These studies encompass diverse regions including China, India, and Africa.

The evidence suggesting that fish consumption is protective against CVD primarily comes from studies conducted in HIC.[127-131] Unpublished data from three major international studies—PURE, ONTARGET, and INTERHEART, which reveals significant variations in the relationship between fish intake and CVD outcomes. In the PURE trial, fish consumption had a negative correlation (RR 0.76–0.84) with CVD outcomes in places, such as South America, China, North America, and Europe. However, in South Asia, a positive association was observed (RR 1.97). Interestingly, no significant associations between fish consumption and CVD outcomes were observed in a high-risk secondary population in the ONTARGET study. In the INTERHEART study, fish intake was found to be beneficial in North America and Europe (RR 0.73; 95% CI 0.62–0.87) but potentially harmful in the Middle East (RR 1.59; 95% CI 1.32–1.93). More research is needed, especially in countries such as China and India, to comprehensively understand the effects of various regional types and preparation methods of fish on CVD outcomes.

The existing evidence indicates potential cardiovascular advantages linked to the consuming fish in the secondary prevention cases, yet there is inconclusiveness in terms of primary prevention.

The DART-1 (Diet and Reinfarction trials 1), conducted for secondary prevention, and DART-2, involving men with stable angina, are the sole randomized trials investigating the connection between fish consumption and CVD outcomes, yielding conflicting results. DART-1 demonstrated that fish reduced overall mortality and exhibited a tendency to lower CVD events within 2 years.[132] Conversely, in the DART-2 trial, oily fish did not impact all-cause mortality or CVD events over 3–9 years, while it led to increased sudden cardiac death, primarily within the subgroup receiving fish oil capsules.[133] No primary prevention trial on fish intake and CVD outcomes exists, but a meta-analysis of RCTs focusing on fish oil supplements presents a neutral outcome.[134]

- *Nuts*: Clinical trials demonstrate that nuts have a positive impact on the serum lipids.[135-137] Observational studies indicate that nuts lower the risk of CHD[138-140] and hypertension,[140] but not stroke.[130,140] In one meta-analysis of prospective cohorts, no association between nuts and T2DM was found,[141] while another showed a protective effect.[130] Despite having a high energy density, nuts do not increase weight, alter waist circumference, or cause obesity. This may be because they have a satiating effect and cause more fecal energy excretion.[142,143]

  Observational studies[144-148] and RCTs[103,149-151] demonstrate that a Mediterranean diet containing nuts reduces the risk of CVD. However, there have been no RCTs evaluating the specific impact of nut consumption alone on CVD events. In LMIC, unpublished data from the PURE cohort indicate that nut consumption remains scarce (60% of the individuals consuming one or fewer servings per week).
- *Legumes*: Consuming legumes has shown improvement in the CVD risk markers such as waist circumference, cholesterol levels, blood pressure, C-reactive protein, and glucose in both the observational studies and RCTs. Additionally, legume consumption offers protection against T2DM.[152-159] A meta-analysis of 26 RCTs involving 1,037 participants revealed that consuming 130 g of legumes per day (approximately one serving) resulted in a reduction of 0.17 mmol/L in LDL cholesterol (95% CI –0.25 to –0.09).[156] Furthermore, an analysis of 8 RCTs indicated that legumes lowered systolic blood pressure by 2 mm Hg and mean arterial pressure.[159] An RCT involving participants with diabetes showed that a legume-rich diet led to a decrease in glycated hemoglobin (HbA1c) by –0.3% (95% CI –1.4 to –0.1%).[154]
  - CVD: An observational meta-analysis of five studies suggests that consuming 100 g of legumes four times/week is inversely linked to CHD risk (RR 0.86; 95% CI 0.78–0.94).[160] In LMIC, soy consumption in China was negatively correlated with TC and LDL-C.[161] An Indian cross-sectional study found legume consumption linked to a reduced T2DM risk for women (OR 0.55; 95% CI 0.34–0.88).[162] Similar trends were observed for men (OR 0.70; 95% CI 0.39–1.26).[162] In a Shanghai study, increased legume intake by around 50 g/day over 4.6 years reduced T2DM risk by 38% (RR 0.62; 95% CI 0.51–0.74).[163] Another study showed that Chinese women consuming 11.2 g/day of soy protein had lower CHD risk (RR 0.25; 95% CI 0.10–0.63) compared to those consuming 4.5 g/day.[164]
  - Summary of major protein sources: Reducing red meats, especially processed ones, and increasing fish, nuts, legumes, and possibly fermented dairy can have potential benefits.

- *Fruits and vegetables and CVD risk factors*: In the DASH (Defeat Alcoholic Steatohepatitis) RCT, increased fruit and vegetable intake, in a typical Western diet or the DASH plan, lowered blood pressure, TC, LDL-C, and HDL-C without affecting triglycerides.[165] A meta-analysis of three cohorts (3,415 cases) showed strong adherence to the DASH diet reduced T2DM risk by 27%.[166] Robust observational evidence supports that high consumption of fruits and vegetables lowers risks of CHD and stroke.[138]
    - LMIC: Global studies and systematic reviews affirm the protective role of fruits and vegetables against CVD.[167-169] Unpublished INTERHEART data showed a 12% decreased MI risk per fruit serving (RR 0.88) and 5% per vegetable serving (RR 0.95). Meta-analyses support 5–10% CVD mortality reduction per serving/day,[169] and green leafy vegetable's protective effect on T2DM (RR 0.87).[170]

    To sum up, rising refined carbs and added sugar correlate with obesity and T2DM. Focus on low-GI whole grains, legumes, nuts, fruits, and vegetables, and limit high-GI refined grains and added sugars, including SSBs.
- *Dietary sodium*: Sodium is essential for normal physiological function.[171-173] Excessive intake elevates blood pressure[166,174,175] and CVD mortality.[176-178] In LMIC, sodium sources include table salt, additives, and spices, while processed foods dominate in HIC. Short-term RCTs show blood pressure reduction with lower sodium intake.[179-181] No RCTs have established if low sodium intake reduces CVD events compared to the moderate intake.[171] Meta-analyses of CVD event trials did not significantly reduce CVD with lower sodium intake, likely due to underpowered trials.[182] Cohort studies show a J-shaped sodium-CVD association, consistent across estimation methods.[183-189]
- *Beverages*: The relationship between alcohol and CVD risk follows a U-shaped pattern, where both abstainers and heavy drinkers exhibit an increased risk compared to moderate drinkers.[190] The specific point of the lowest risk (nadir) varies based on the factors such as age, gender, ethnicity, and existing health conditions,[191] but the consistent finding is that individuals consuming 1–2 drinks/day have the lowest risk.[192] Moderate alcohol consumption has been found to raise levels of HDL-C, apolipoprotein A1, and adiponectin, while reducing fibrinogen levels.[193,194]

CONCLUSION

Principal component and factor analyses have consistently identified two primary dietary patterns that account for the majority of variations in population-level eating habits—prudent and Western. Prudent diets are characterized by substantial consumption of fruits, vegetables, legumes, whole grains, fish, and poultry. On the other hand, Western diets are characterized by a high intake of processed meat, French fries, sugary desserts, SSBs, red meat, and high-fat dairy products.[195] A comprehensive meta-analysis involving 22 cohort studies revealed that individuals adhering to a prudent diet at the highest level experienced a 31% lower risk of CVD in comparison to those with the lowest adherence. Conversely, a Western dietary pattern was associated with a 14% increase in the CVD risk.[196] The remarkable consistency of these findings across diverse countries and various dietary factors and indices as well as the concurrence of results from intervention trials provides substantial evidence supporting the causal relationship between a high-quality diet and the prevention of CVD.[197,198]

- *Carbohydrates*: Both the quality and quantity of carbohydrates play crucial roles in maintaining a healthy dietary pattern. Diets characterized by high glycemic index and glycemic load—measures reflecting the postprandial glucose level response—have been linked to an elevated risk of CHD, while diets with low glycemic index or load have shown an inverse relationship with CHD risk.[199] Elevated consumption of added sugars appears to elevate CVD risk independently of body weight or other dietary components.[200]
- *Dietary fiber* consistently demonstrates its capacity to lower CVD risk and enhance cardiovascular risk factors, as evidenced by both observational studies[201] and dietary intervention trials.[202,203]
- *Dietary fat*: Among the three main types of dietary fats—trans-fatty acids, saturated fatty acids, and unsaturated fatty acids (which include mono- and polyunsaturated fats)—trans-fatty acids have demonstrated the most pronounced connection with unfavorable cardiovascular outcomes.[204,205]

In studies employing substitution models, it has been observed that replacing either carbohydrates or saturated fats with unsaturated fats leads to a reduced risk of CVD, with polyunsaturated fats consistently yielding a greater magnitude of benefit **(Fig. 1)**.[206] Supplementation with long-chain omega-3 fatty acids, a specific type of polyunsaturated fat primarily sourced from fish oil, has yielded mixed outcomes in research,[207,208] and further confirmation is required regarding the potential benefits of omega-3 fatty acids in reducing the risk of sudden cardiac death. Long-chain omega-3 fatty acids have demonstrated effects in maintaining cell membrane fluidity, decreasing blood viscosity and clotting propensity, and promoting the generation of anti-inflammatory mediators.[209,210]

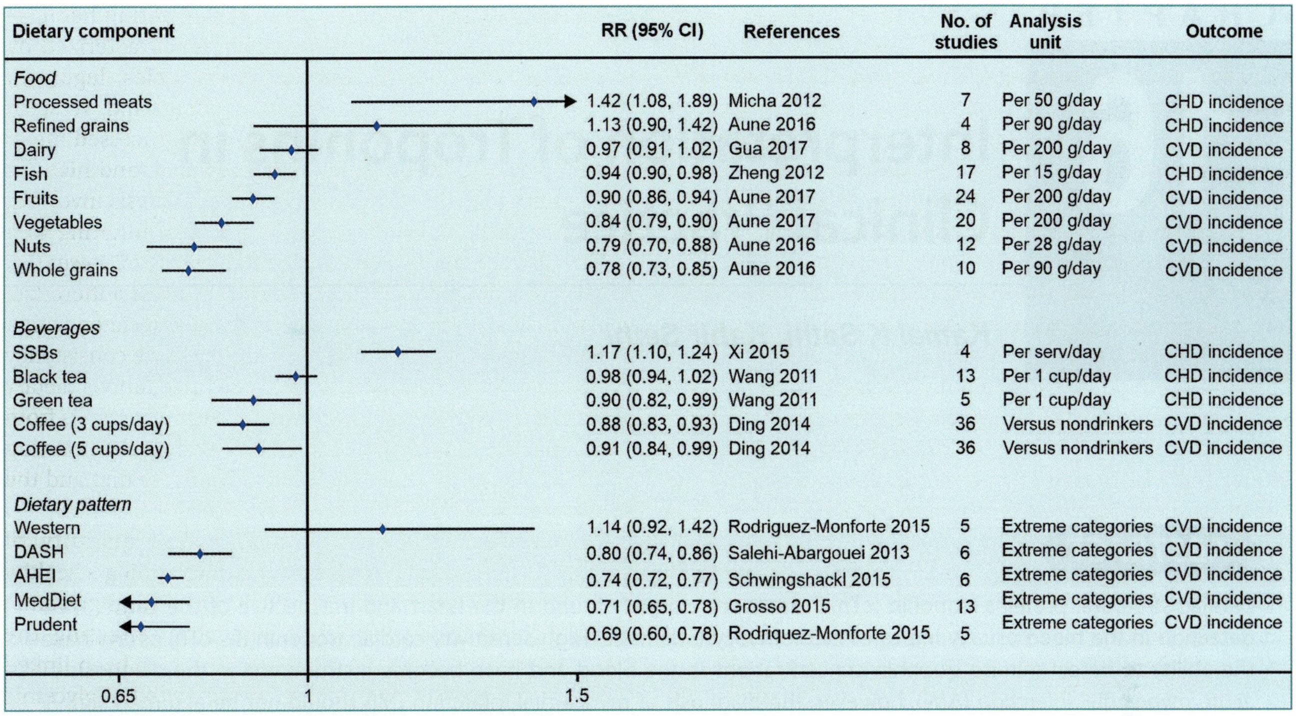

FIG. 1: Summary of various meta-analyses showing the association of dietary factors with CVD.

Note: High amounts of processed meat, SSBs, and refined grain consumption are associated with greater CVD incidence; moderate coffee and alcohol intake, and high fruit/vegetable, dairy (low-fat), whole grain, fish, and nut intake are associated with lower incidence. High adherence to Mediterranean, DASH, AHEI, and prudent dietary patterns are significantly predictive of lower CVD incidence.

(AHEI: Alternative Healthy Eating Index; CHD: coronary heart disease; CI: confidence interval; CVD: cardiovascular disease; DASH: Dietary Approaches to Stop Hypertension; Med diet: Mediterranean diet; RR: risk ratio; SSB: sugar-sweetened beverage)

Source: Yu E, Malik VS, Hu FB. Cardiovascular Disease Prevention by Diet Modification: JACC Health Promotion Series. J Am Coll Cardiol. 2018;72(8):914-26.

ONLINE REFERENCES

Please scan the QR code provided at the end of the table of contents for References of this chapter.

CHAPTER

16

Interpretation of Troponins in Clinical Practice

Kamal K Sethi, Kabir Sethi

ABSTRACT

Cardiac structural proteins troponin (cTn) T and I are uniquely found in the heart and irrespective of the cause, their detection in the blood usually indicates cardiomyocyte damage. High-sensitivity cardiac troponin (hs-cTn) assays have the ability to detect minute troponin concentrations in the blood and have become instrumental in the diagnosis of acute myocardial infarction (AMI), however, the diagnosis of myocardial infarction (MI) should not be assumed simply based on laboratory values. Minor troponin release secondary to cardiomyocyte damage can be seen in a number of acute and chronic conditions. However, substantial elevation in hs-cTn levels is largely restricted to AMI, myocarditis, stress cardiomyopathy, and critical illness. Regardless of the cause, an elevated cTn almost always indicates a poor prognosis. This chapter attempts to highlight the differential diagnosis of elevated cTn and their interpretation and clinical implications.

Keywords: High-sensitivity cardiac troponin, cardiomyocyte damage, myocarditis, acute myocardial infarction, stress cardiomyopathy.

INTRODUCTION

Ever since the European Society of Cardiology and the American College of Cardiology Committee jointly redefined myocardial infarction (MI) as clinical evidence of myocardial ischemia in conjunction with elevation of cardiac troponin T (cTnT) or I (cTnI), the two have emerged as preferred biochemical markers for the diagnosis of myocardial infarction,[1] because high-sensitivity cardiac troponin (hs-cTn) assays have the ability to detect minute troponin concentrations, its elevation can be noted in a number of potential diseases including pulmonary embolism (PE), heart failure, myocarditis, end stage renal disease, and so forth. Regardless of the release mechanics, elevated cTnT and cTnI almost always imply a poor prognosis. This review will provide context for how hs-cTn assays might be applied beyond "acute myocardial infarction (AMI) diagnostic evaluation."

WHAT ARE CARDIAC TROPONINS?

The troponin complex, located on the myofibrillar thin (actin) filament of striated (skeletal and cardiac) muscle consists of three subunits—troponin C, troponin I, and troponin T. Of these, the isoforms T and I are found in the cardiac muscle and form the cardiac troponin (cTn) complex which regulates the excitation–contraction coupling in the heart. Near about 4–5% of cTn is found in the cytosol, while the rest is found in the sarcomere.[2] Following myocyte injury, the initial release of troponin occurs from cytoplasm followed by a slower and more continuous release from the rest of the contractile apparatus.[2]

Even though cardiomyocyte injury and irreversible cell death have been deemed necessary for the release of cTn into the circulation, other mechanisms not requiring cell death and necrosis have been suggested, in particular those leading to chronic myocardial injury **(Fig. 1)**.

CHARACTERISTICS OF HIGH-SENSITIVITY CARDIAC TROPONIN ASSAYS

Enhancements in assay technology and widespread availability has made cTn the biomarker of choice for evaluating patients with suspected acute myocardial injury.

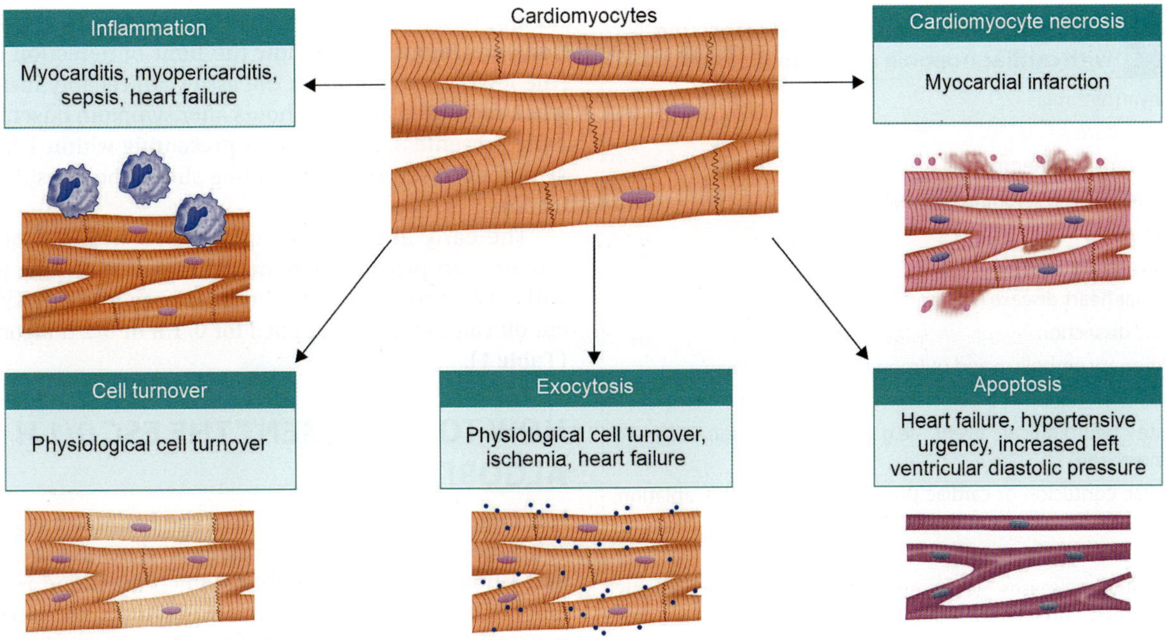

FIG. 1: Mechanism of cardiomyocyte injury and associated disease states.

Note: The mechanism of troponin release may differ across conditions and disease states and includes ischemia, inflammation, cell turnover, exocytosis, and apoptosis.

Source: Raber I, McCarthy CP, Januzzi JL Jr. A Test in Context: Interpretation of High-Sensitivity Cardiac Troponin Assays in Different Clinical Settings. J Am Coll Cardiol. 2021;77(10):1357-67.

Instrumental in the diagnosis of AMI is a rise and/or fall of cTn with at least one value above the 99th percentile from a normal population.[3,4] Clinically, the most relevant point to understand is that a value above the 99th percentile of a hs-cTn assay is indicative of myocardial injury.[3] Myocardial injury is considered acute if there is a rise and/or fall of cTn concentration over serial measurements and chronic if the cTn level remains elevated without significant rise or fall **(Box 1)**.[3]

Patient characteristics are likely to have an influence on hs-cTn values. Men, due to increased left ventricle size and more prevalent subclinical cardiovascular disease have higher hs-cTn concentrations than women.[5] Thus, the 99th percentile cut-off is higher for men than women. Other conditions known to be associated with increased levels of hs-cTn include older age, left ventricular hypertrophy (LVH), hypertension, chronic kidney disease (CKD), critical illness, sepsis, acute respiratory distress syndrome, and stroke **(Box 2)**.[6-11] High-sensitivity assays are recommended, as their diagnostic accuracy is higher. Assays run on automated platforms in the laboratory are much more sensitive than point-of-care tests, and are preferable.

BOX 1 Clinical implications of hs-cTn assays.

Compared with standard cardiac troponin assays, hs-cTn assays:

- Have higher NPV for AMI
- Reduce the "troponin-blind" interval, leading to earlier detection of AMI
- Result in ~4% absolute and ~20% relative increases in the detection of type 1 MI and a corresponding decrease in the diagnosis of unstable angina
- Are associated with a twofold increase in the detection of type 2 MI

Levels of hs-cTn should be interpreted as quantitative markers of cardiomyocyte damage (i.e., the higher the level, the greater the likelihood of MI):

- Elevations beyond fivefold—the upper reference limit have high (>90%) PPV for acute type 1 MI
- Elevations up to threefold—the upper reference limit have only limited (50–60%) PPV for AMI and may be associated with a broad spectrum of conditions
- It is common to detect circulating levels of cardiac troponin in healthy individuals

Rising and/or falling cardiac troponin levels differentiate acute (as in MI) from chronic cardiomyocyte damage (the more pronounced the change, the higher the likelihood of AMI)

(AMI: acute myocardial infarction; hs-cTn: high-sensitivity cardiac troponin; MI: myocardial infarction; NPV: negative predictive value; PPV: positive predictive value)

Source: With permission from Collet et al. (2021).[15]

HIGH-SENSITIVITY CARDIAC TROPONIN IN THE DIAGNOSIS OF MYOCARDIAL INFARCTION

According to the Fourth Universal Definition,[3] to diagnose MI in the presence of acute myocardial injury (elevated

BOX 2 Conditions other than type 1 MI associated with cardiac troponin elevation.

- Tachyarrhythmias
- Heart failure
- Hypertensive emergencies
- Critical illness (e.g., shock/sepsis/burns)
- Myocarditis*
- Takotsubo syndrome
- Valvular heart disease (e.g., aortic stenosis)
- Aortic dissection
- Pulmonary embolism and pulmonary hypertension
- Renal dysfunction and associated cardiac disease
- Acute neurological event (e.g., stroke or subarachnoid hemorrhage)
- Cardiac contusion or cardiac procedures (CABG, PCI, ablation, pacing, cardioversion, or endomyocardial biopsy)
- Hypo- and hyperthyroidism
- Infiltrative diseases (e.g., amyloidosis, hemochromatosis, sarcoidosis, and scleroderma)
- Myocardial drug toxicity or poisoning (e.g., doxorubicin, 5-fluorouracil, herceptin, snake venoms)
- Extreme endurance efforts
- Rhabdomyolysis

*Includes myocardial extension of endocarditis or pericarditis.

Note: Bold is used for most frequent conditions.

[CABG: coronary artery bypass graft(ing); MI: myocardial infarction; PCI: percutaneous coronary intervention]

Source: With permission from Collet et al. (2021).[15]

cTn), there must also be evidence of myocardial ischemia with at least one of the following present: (1) Symptoms of myocardial ischemia, (2) new ischemic changes on the electrocardiogram (ECG), (3) new pathological Q waves, (4) new ischemic regional wall motion abnormalities on cardiac imaging, or (5) acute coronary thrombus on coronary angiography. Not only do the cardiac troponins allow for more sensitive diagnosis of AMI but also indicate the adverse prognostic risk associated with its elevation. Multiple randomized studies and several meta-analyses have substantiated the adverse outcome associated with elevated cTn with higher odds (3.44-fold) of death and MI at 30 days in patients with elevated cTn in comparison to those presenting with unstable angina.[12] In order to understand the characteristics of an abnormal hs-cTn better, clinicians should look at cTn as a continuous value with higher concentrations more likely linked to acute MI. All efforts must be made to measure the biomarker serially, seeking a rise and/or fall in concentration **(Fig. 1)**. The European Society of Cardiology (ESC) 2020 non-ST-segment elevation acute coronary syndrome (ACS) guideline favours hs-cTn testing at 0 hour and 1 hour using the the ESC 0/1-h algorithm with later sampling (e.g., at 2 or 3 hours) as reasonable alternatives.[12] Using the ESC 0/1-h algorithm, MI may be excluded when single sample hs-cTn concentrations are found to be below the limit of detection (LoD) (the lowest concentration the assay can reliably measure) when measured at least 3 hours after symptom onset.[13,14] In early presenters, i.e., the ones presenting within 1 hour of symptom onset, repeat sampling should be considered at 3 hours.[15]

The early absolute changes of cTn within 1 hour or 2 hours can provide incremental diagnostic value jointly with ECG and clinical findings. However, assay specific cut off values must be applied for 0/1 h or 0/2 h algorithms **(Table 1)**.

HOW TO IMPLEMENT THE ESC 0/1 H ALGORITHM?

It is important to understand that the ESC 0/1 h algorithm is irrespective of the local turnaround time and the 0 hour and 1 hour refer to the point at which the blood is drawn and not to the time from the onset of symptoms. In order to maximize the safety and feasibility of the process, the nursing team should obtain samples for cTn following the 0/1 h algorithm irrespective of other clinical details and pending results. Documentation of the 0 hour blood draw allows exact determination of the time window of the 1 hour blood draw (±10 min). If the 1 hour blood draw is not feasible then blood should be drawn at 2 hours and ESC 0/2 hour algorithm must be applied **(Fig. 2)**.[15]

HIGH-SENSITIVITY CARDIAC TROPONIN TESTING IN AMBULATORY INDIVIDUALS

In seemingly healthy, ambulatory individuals, hs-cTn concentrations above the 99th percentile are usually suggestive of nonischemic cardiovascular injury and studies examining the mechanism of cTn elevation in this population have demonstrated a stronger association with LVH in comparison to coronary artery disease (CAD).[16-18] When measured in the outpatient setting, studies **(Table 2)** have demonstrated a strong association between hs-cTn levels and risk of future cardiovascular events (incident heart failure and CAD), cardiovascular death and all-cause mortality.[19-24]

In the ARIC (Atherosclerosis Risk In Communities) study which enrolled 8,838 participants, those who exhibited > 50% increment in hs-cTnT level (spaced 6 years apart) had higher rates of incident heart failure (HF) [hazard ratio (HR) 1.60; 95% confidence interval (CI) 1.35–1.91], coronary heart disease (HR 1.28; 95% CI 1.09–1.52), and death (HR 1.39; 95% CI 1.22–1.59).[19] Likewise, lowering hs-cTnT by >50% from the baseline, lowers risk for HF (HR 0.73; 95% CI 0.54–0.97) and cardiovascular death (HR 0.71; 95% CI 0.52–0.97).[20] When combined with LVH, hs-cTn may

TABLE 1: Assay specific cut-off levels in ng/L within the 0/1 h and 0/2 h algorithms.

0/1 h algorithm	Very low	Low	No 1 h Δ	High	1 h Δ
hs-cTnT (Elecsys; Roche)	<5	<12	<3	≥52	≥5
hs-cTnI (Architect; Abbott)	<4	<5	<2	≥64	≥6
hs-cTnI (Centaur; Siemens)	<3	<6	<3	≥120	≥12
hs-cTnI (Access; Beckman Coulter)	<4	<5	<4	≥50	≥15
hs-cTnI (Clarity; Singulex)	<1	<2	<1	≥30	≥6
hs-cTnI (Vitros; Clinical Diagnostics)	<1	<2	<1	≥40	≥4
hs-cTnI (Pathfast; LSI Medience)	<3	<4	<3	≥90	≥20
hs-cTnI (Triage True; Quidel)	<4	<5	<3	≥60	≥8
0/2 h algorithm	**Very low**	**Low**	**No 2 h Δ**	**High**	**2 h Δ**
hs-cTnT (Elecsys; Roche)	<5	<14	<4	≥52	≥10
hs-cTnI (Architect; Abbott)	<4	<6	<2	≥64	≥15
hs-cTnI (Centaur; Siemens)	<3	<8	<7	≥120	≥20
hs-cTnI (Access; Beckman Coulter)	<4	<5	<5	≥50	≥20
hs-cTnI (Clarity; Singulex)	<1	TBD	TBD	≥30	TBD
hs-cTnI (Vitros; Clinical Diagnostics)	<1	TBD	TBD	≥40	TBD
hs-cTnI (Pathfast; LSI Medience)	<3	TBD	TBD	≥90	TBD
hs-cTnI (Triage True; Quidel)	<4	TBD	TBD	≥60	TBD

(hs-cTn: high-sensitivity cardiac troponin; TBD: to be determined)

Source: With permission from Collet et al. (2021).[15]

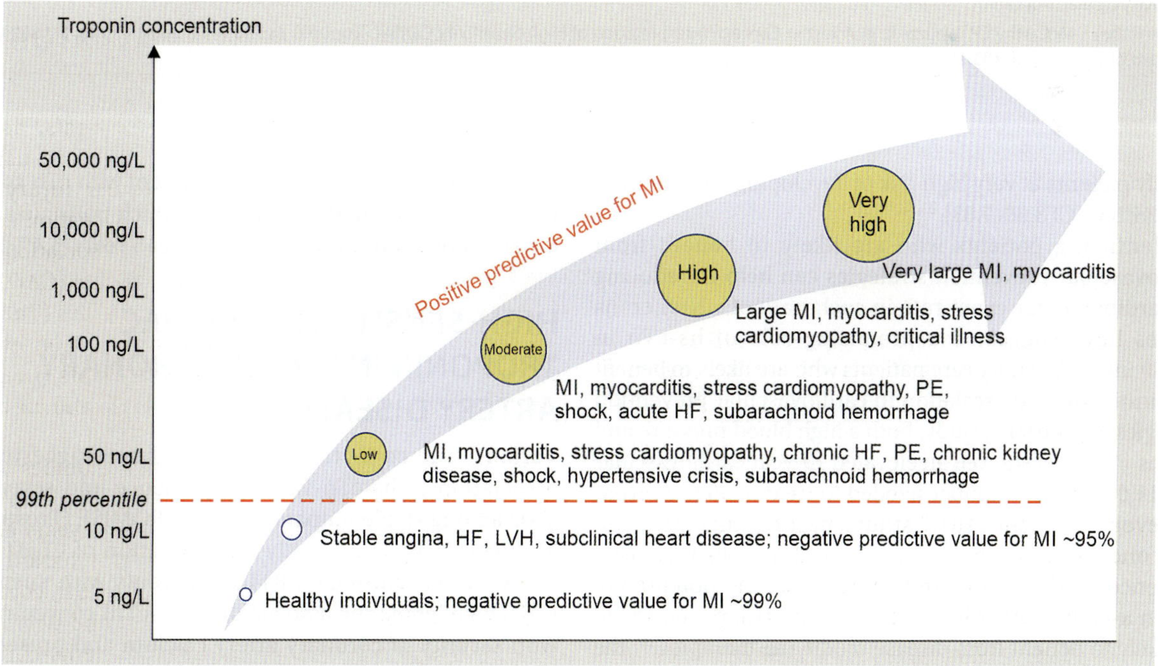

FIG. 2: Range of diagnoses across hS-cTn concentrations.

(HF: heart failure; hS-cTn: high-sensitivity cardiac troponin; LVH: left ventricular hypertrophy; MI: myocardial infarction; PE: pulmonary embolism)

Source: Raber I, McCarthy CP, Januzzi JL Jr. A Test in Context: Interpretation of High-Sensitivity Cardiac Troponin Assays in Different Clinical Settings. J Am Coll Cardiol. 2021;77(10):1357-67.

TABLE 2: hs-cTn levels in ambulatory patients.

First author (reference #), year	*n*	Cardiac troponin cutoff, ng/L	Troponin assay	% individuals above troponin cutoff	Outcome	Adjusted HR (95% CI)
deFilippi et al. (2010) [36]	4,221	hs-cTnT ≥ 13	Roche Elecsys	17	11.8-year incident HF	2.5 (2.0–3.0)
deFilippi et al. (2010) [36]	4,221	hs-cTnT ≥ 13	Roche Elecsys	17	11.8-year CV mortality	2.9 (2.4–3.6)
de Lemos et al. (2010) [8]	3,546	hs-cTnT ≥ 14	Roche Elecsys	2	6.4-year all-cause mortality	2.8 (1.4–5.2)
Saunders et al. (2011) [37]	9,698	hs-cTnT ≥ 14	Roche Elecsys	7	10-year all-cause mortality	4.0 (3.2–4.9)
Saunders et al. (2011) [37]	9,698	hs-cTnT ≥ 14	Roche Elecsys	7	10-year CV mortality	7.6 (3.8–15.3)
Saunders et al. (2011) [37]	9,698	hs-cTnT ≥ 14	Roche Elecsys	7	10-year incident HF	6.0 (4.5–7.9)
McEvoy et al. (2016) [7]	8,838	hs-cTnT ≥ 5	Roche Elecsys	56	14-year incident CHD	1.4 (1.2–1.6)
McEvoy et al. (2016) [7]	8,838	hs-cTnT ≥ 5	Roche Flecsys	56	14-year incident HF	2.0 (1.6–2.4)
McEvoy et al. (2016) [7]	8,838	hs-cTnT ≥ 5	Roche Elecsys	56	14-year mortality	1.5 (1.3–1.7)
Welsh et al. (2019) [38]	19,501	hs-cTnT ≥ 5	Rache Elecsys	Not reported	7.8-year CVD composite	1.0 (0.8–1.2)
Welsh et al. (2019) [38]	19,501	hs-cTnI ≥ 5	Abbott Architect	Not reported	7.8-year CVD composite	1.5 (1.2–1.9)
Yan et al. (2020) [40]	48,455	hs-cTnI ≥ 3.2	Abbott Architect	3l	6.6-year incident HF	1.6 (1.3–2.0)
Blankenberg et al. (2016) [39]	74,738	hs-cTnI ≥ 6.0	Abbott Architect	Highest quintile	12.1-year all-cause mortality	1.6 (1.5–1.8)
Blankenberg et al. (2016) [39]	74,738	hs-cTnI ≥ 6.0	Abbott Architect	Highest quintile	13.8-year CV mortality	2.6 (2.3–2.9)

Note: The reference numbers cited in square brackets are from the original article and do not correspond with the current bibliography.

(CHD: coronary heart disease; CI: confidence interval; CV: cardiovascular; CVD: cardiovascular disease; HF: heart failure; HR: hazard ratio; hs-cTn: high-sensitivity cardiac troponin)

Source: Raber I, McCarthy CP, Januzzi JL Jr. A Test in Context: Interpretation of High-Sensitivity Cardiac Troponin Assays in Different Clinical Settings. J Am Coll Cardiol. 2021;77(10):1357-67.

identify patients at very high risk of developing HF (adjusted HR 5.35; 95% CI 3.66–7.83).[25,26]

Identifying patients who are likely to benefit from cardiovascular prevention strategies can help in reducing the cardiovascular event rate in such patients. Numerous studies have suggested a promising role of hs-cTn in identifying ambulatory care patients who are likely to benefit from initiation and escalation in cardiovascular prevention strategies. In one such study, both a high blood pressure and high hs-cTn level showed an elevated 10-year cardiovascular risk (11.0%) with a number needed to treat of 36 to prevent one event.[27] In the ARIC study, participants with hs-cTn concentration above 8 ng/L exhibited an increased incidence of diabetes there by reiterating the potential of hs-cTn as a biomarker in identifying high-risk patients who are likely to benefit from disease modifying therapies.[28] The WOSCOPS (West of Scotland Coronary Prevention Study) randomized men with no history of MI and raised low-density lipoprotein (LDL) cholesterol to pravastatin 40 mg once daily or placebo for 5 years[29] and demonstrated a greater benefit with pravastatin treatment with cTn concentration reduction by 13% ($p < 0.001$) which translated into a lower risk of future coronary events over 5 years (1.4%).

HIGH-SENSITIVITY CARDIAC TROPONIN IN STABLE CORONARY ARTERY DISEASE

Various studies in the recent past have suggested the association of hs-cTn with the presence and severity of CAD among stable outpatients. The PROMISE (Prospective Multicenter Imaging Study for Evaluation of Chest Pain) study, which enrolled 1,844 outpatients with suspected CAD, highlighted the association of hs-cTnI concentrations with severity of coronary artery calcium and presence of obstructive CAD (odds ratio 1.25 per interquartile range increase; *p* ¼ 0.001).[30] In a subsequent analysis performed in a larger cohort of 4,021 patients in the PROMISE study, hs-cTnI concentrations independently predicted death,

TABLE 3: hs-cTn in "stable" coronary artery disease.

First author (reference #), year	*n*	Cardiac troponin cutoff, ng/L	Troponin assay	% individuals above troponin cutoff	Outcome	Adjusted HR (95% CI)
deFilippi et al. (2010) [36]	4,221	hs-cTnT ≥ 13	Roche Elecsys	17	11.8-year incident HF	2.5 (2.0–3.0)
deFilippi et al. (2010) [36]	4.221	hs-cTnT ≥ 13	Roche Elecsys	17	11.8-year CV mortality	2.9 (2.4–3.6)
de Lemos et al. (2010) [8]	3,546	hs-cTnT ≥ 14	Roche Elecsys	2	6.4-year all-cause mortality	2.8 (1.4–5.2)
Saunders et al. (2011) [37]	9,698	hs-cTnT ≥ 14	Roche Elecsys	7	10-year all-cause mortality	4.0 (3.2–4.9)
Saunders et al. (2011) [37]	9,698	hs-cTnT ≥ 14	Roche Elecsys	7	10-year CV mortality	7.6 (3.8–15.3)
Saunders et al. (2011) [37]	9,698	hs-cTnT ≥ 14	Roche Elecsys	7	10-year incident HF	6.0 (4.5–7.9)
McEvoy et al. (2016) [7]	8,838	hs-cTnT ≥ 5	Roche Elecsys	56	14-year incident CHD	1.4 (1.2–1.6)
McEvoy et al. (2016) [7]	8,838	hs-cTnT ≥ 5	Roche Elecsys	56	14-year incident HF	2.0 (0.6–2.4)
McEvoy et al. (2016) [7]	8,838	hs-cTnT ≥ 5	Roche Elecsys	56	14-year mortality	1.5 (1.3–1.7)
Welsh et al. (2019) [38]	19,501	hs-cTnT ≥ 5	Roche Elecsys	Not reported	7.8-year CVD composite	1.0 (0.8–1.2)
Welsh et al. (2019) [38]	19,501	hs-cTnI ≥ 5	Abbott Architect	Not reported	7.8-year CVD composite	1.5 (1.2–1.9)
Yan et al. (2020) [40]	48,455	hs-cTnI ≥ 3.2	Abbott Architect	31	6.6-year incident HF	1.6 (1.3–2.0)
Blankenberg et al. (2016) [39]	74,738	hs-cTnI ≥ 6.0	Abbott Architect	Highest quintile	12.1-year all-cause mortality	1.6 (1.5–1.8)
Blankenberg et al. (2016) [39]	74,738	hs-cTnI ≥ 6.0	Abbott Architect	Highest quintile	13.8-year CV mortality	2.6 (2.3–2.9)

Note: The reference numbers cited in square brackets are from the original article and do not correspond with the current bibliography.

(CHD: coronary heart disease; CI: confidence interval; CV: cardiovascular; CVD: cardiovascular disease; HF: heart failure; HR: hazard ratio; hs-cTn: high-sensitivity cardiac troponin)

Source: Raber I, McCarthy CP, Januzzi JL Jr. A Test in Context: Interpretation of High-Sensitivity Cardiac Troponin Assays in Different Clinical Settings. J Am Coll Cardiol. 2021;77(10):1357-67.

acute MI, or hospitalization for unstable angina (HR 1.54 per increase in log-hs-cTnI inter quartile range; $p < 0.001$) and cardiovascular death or acute MI (HR 1.52 per increase in log-hs-cTnI interquartile range; $p < 0.001$).[31] Longer-term results among patients with stable CAD have **(Table 3)** shown an independent link between the higher concentrations of hs-cTn and the risk of MI, stroke, progression of CAD, and death.[31-37] Increased hs-cTI concentrations at baseline and at 6 months in diabetic patients with history of ACS in the past have been found to be associated with increased risk of cardiovascular death, MI, or stroke.[38] In the same cohort, hs-cTnI $16 ng/L for women and hscTnI $33 ng/L for men were associated with an increased risk of a composite outcome of cardiovascular death, HF hospitalization, initiation of loop diuretic agents, or elevated N-terminal prohormone B-type natriuretic peptide.[39] With the expanding role of antidiabetic drugs with proven cardiovascular benefits, identification of diabetic patient sat high risk and initiation of cardiovascular preventive and/or protective strategies in these patients can translate into huge clinical benefit in the long run.

HIGH-SENSITIVITY CARDIAC TROPONIN IN HEART FAILURE

High-sensitivity cardiac troponin concentrations are often elevated in patients with acute and chronic HF, and apart from predicting a worse outcome in these patients, it may offer additional prognostic information in both settings **(Tables 4 and 5)**.[40-50]

Even though cTn measurement is recommended in patients presenting with acute heart failure (to rule out type 1 MI as a precipitant), interpretation of an elevated hs-cTn in the clinical setting of heart failure poses a huge challenge. The rise and/or fall of cTn can occur even in the absence of type 1 MI owing to mechanisms leading to demand/supply mismatch and noncoronary myocardial injury. Troponin release can also be seen in conditions enhancing the cardiac

TABLE 4: Effect of hs-cTn on prognosis in heart failure.

First author (reference #), year	*n*	Cardiac troponin cutoff, ng/L	Troponin assay	% individuals above troponin cutoff	Outcome	Adjusted HR (95% CI)
Nakamura et al. (2014) [68]	444	hs-cTnT ≥ 28	Roche Elecsys	50	15-month CV mortality	4.0 (1.9–8.3)
Nakamura et al. (2014) [68]	444	hs-cTnT ≥ 28	Roche Elecsys	50	15-month all-cause mortality	2.9 (1.6–5.0)
Felker et al. (2015) [69]	1,074	Doubling in peak change in hs-cTnT	Roche Elecsys	–	180-day CV mortality	1.4 (1.2–1.6)
Diez et al. (2016) [76]	187	hs-cTnT > 42	Roche Elecsys	50	30-day mortality or readmission	1.7 (0.9–3.0)
Fudim et al. (2018) [70]	139	Per doubling of baseline hs-cTnI	Beckman Coulter Access	–	Emergency room visits, readmissions, and death at day 60	1.2 (1.0–1.4)
Aimo et al. (2019) [80]	1,499	hs-cTnT ≥ 43	Roche Elecsys	50	All-cause mortality at 2 years	1.9 (1.3–2.8)

Note: The reference numbers cited in square brackets are from the original article and do not correspond with the current bibliography.

(CI: confidence interval; CV: cardiovascular; HR: hazard ratio; hs-cTn: high-sensitive cardiac troponin T)

Source: Raber I, McCarthy CP, Januzzi JL Jr. A Test in Context: Interpretation of High-Sensitivity Cardiac Troponin Assays in Different Clinical Settings. J Am Coll Cardiol. 2021;77(10):1357-67.

TABLE 5: hs-cTn and long-term risk in heart failure.

First author (reference #), year	*n*	Cardiac troponin cutoff, ng/L	Troponin assay	% individuals above troponin cutoff	Outcome	Adjusted HR (95% CI)
Latini et al. (2007) [71]	4,053	Per increments of hs-cTnT 10	Roche Elecsys	–	2-year all-cause mortality	1.05 (1.0–1.1)
Alehagen et al. (2010) [72]	470	hs-cTnT > 18 (men) hs-cTnT > 8 (women)	Roche Elecsys	37	10-year CV mortality	2.2 (1.5–3.4)
Tentzeris et al. (2011) [73]	172	hs-cTnT > 14	Roche Elecsys	58	3.5-year all-cause mortality or HF hospitalization	1.9 (1.1–3.3)
Eggers et al. (2011) [74]	103	hs-cTnT > 13.5	Roche Elecsys	36	2-year all-cause mortality	2.0 (1.3–3.1)
Eggers et al. (2011) [74]	103	hs-cTnI > 14.4	Beckman Coulter	48	2-year all-cause mortality	1.9 (1.2–2.8)
Masson et al. (2012) [78]	554	Per 1-U increment in hs-cTnT on log scale	Roche Elecsys	–	2-year all-cause mortality	1.6 (1.4–1.8)
Egstrup et al. (2012) [75]	416	hs-cTnT > 18 (men) hs-cTnT > 8 (women)	Roche Elecsys	57	4.4-year all-cause mortality	1.7 (1.2–2.5)
Aimo et al. (2018) [60]	7,382	hs-cTnT > 18	Roche Elecsys	–	2.4-year CV hospitalization	1.4 (1.4–1.5)
Aimo et al. (2018) [60]	7,553	hs-cTnT > 18	Roche Elecsys	–	2.4-year CV death	1.4 (1.3–1.5)
Aimo et al. (2018) [60]	9,283	hs-cTnT > 18	Roche Elecsys	–	2.4-year all-cause mortality	1.5 (1.4–1.6)
Welsh et al. (2018) [77]	1,853	Per 1-SD hs-cTnT	Roche Elecsys	–	28-month all-cause mortality	1.6 (1.5–1.8)
Welsh et al. (2018) [77]	1,853	Per 1-SD hs-cTnT	Roche Elecsys	–	28-month HF hospitalization or CV death	1.6 (1.5–1.7)

Note: The reference numbers cited in square brackets are from the original article and do not correspond with the current bibliography.

(CI: confidence interval; CV: cardiovascular; HF: heart failure; hs-cTn: high-sensitive cardiac troponin; HR: hazard ratio; SD: standard deviation)

Source: Raber I, McCarthy CP, Januzzi JL Jr. A Test in Context: Interpretation of High-Sensitivity Cardiac Troponin Assays in Different Clinical Settings. J Am Coll Cardiol. 2021;77(10):1357-67.

preload without accompanying ischemia.[51] Irrespective of the cause, an increased hs-cTn concentration in the setting of acute heart failure predicts risk. For instance, in a study of 1,499 patients with acute HF, patients with hs-cTnT > 43 ng/L had higher rates of all-cause death at 6, 12, and 24 months.[52] Similar cardiovascular outcomes with hs-cTn concentrations can also be seen in patients with chronic HF. A meta-analysis of 10 studies showed a strong association between hs-cTn values and risk of cardiovascular hospitalizations (HR 1.42; 95% CI 1.36–1.49), cardiovascular mortality (HR 1.40; 95% CI 1.33–1.48), and all-cause mortality (HR 1.48; 95% CI 1.41–1.55)[53] even in the absence of CAD. Patients with heart failure with reduced ejection fraction and chronically elevated hs-cTn are likely to have a further decline in the left ventricular (LV) function during a year of follow-up, as reported by Motiwala et al.[54] Although most studies have examined the prognostic utility of hs-cTn in patients with heart failure with reduced ejection fraction (HFrEF), a small number of studies have demonstrated its utility in predicting adverse clinical outcomes in patients with heart failure with preserved ejection fraction (HFpEF) as well.[42,55]

HIGH-SENSITIVITY CARDIAC TROPONIN IN PULMONARY EMBOLISM

Cardiac troponin elevation can be seen in 50% of the individuals with acute PE. Even though it has emerged as an important prognostic tool for risk stratification of patients with PE the real reason for its elevation after PE remains unclear. It is believed that an abrupt increase in the pulmonary artery pressure owing to the mechanical obstruction causes abrupt dilatation of the right ventricle (RV) which in turn leads to injury to RV myocardial cells resulting in the troponin release. Other plausible mechanisms include reduced coronary perfusion, hypoxemia from perfusion-ventilation mismatch, systemic hypoperfusion, or a combination of these factors. What is noteworthy is that in patients with PE peak cTn is lower and persists for a shorter duration in comparison to cTn elevations in AMI patients.[56] This is primarily because the cTn appearance in the blood in PE is due to efflux of the free cytosolic pool of cTn owing to transient membrane leakage in contrast to irreversible myocardial damage in patients with ACS.[56,57] Giannitsis et al. showed that troponin elevation in the setting of PE was associated with a more complicated course in the hospital with higher odds of prolonged hypotension, cardiogenic shock, need for resuscitation and death.[58] Conversely, normal troponin values are associated with a good outcome. PE patients with hemodynamic instability and RV dysfunction, in the background of elevated cTn are at an increased risk of adverse outcome and should be considered for a more aggressive treatment approach with either thrombolysis or embolectomy.

CARDIAC TROPONIN RELEASE IN SEPSIS/SEPTIC SHOCK AND SYSTEMIC INFLAMMATORY RESPONSE SYNDROME

Cardiac troponin values in patients with sepsis and/or systemic inflammatory response syndrome (SIRS) provide prognostic information and tend to correlate with the severity of disease process [more so with the degree of hypotension and acute physiology and chronic health evaluation (APACHE) II score] and have been linked with an adverse outcome. hS-cTn concentrations in the blood are quite prevalent in patients being treated in the intensive care unit (ICU) for sepsis, septic shock, or SIRS and can be detected in 36% (cTnT > 0.1 ng/mL) to 85% (cTnI > 0.1 ng/mL) of the cases.[59] This wide range of prevalence can be attributed to the different underlying causes of sepsis, the use of different troponin assays, and the different cut-off values that are applied. The absence of significant CAD in vast majority of these cases indicates other mechanisms responsible for troponin elevations such as oxygen supply-demand mismatch which usually occurs as a result of increased oxygen-demand of the myocardium owing to the fever and tachycardia which is widely prevalent in patients with sepsis and/or SIRS. The simultaneous reduction in the oxygen supply of the myocardium due to systemic hypoxemia, respiratory failure, microcirculatory dysfunction, hypotension and at times anemia further contributes to the troponin release. In addition, the direct myocardial injury owing to the cytotoxic effects of the bacterial toxins, proinflammatory cytokines, local, and circulating inflammatory markers including tumor necrosis factor, interleukin 6 and reactive oxygen species, further results in troponin release.[59]

HIGH-SENSITIVITY CARDIAC TROPONIN IN RENAL DISEASE

Patients living with renal dysfunction have chronically elevated troponin level[8] as a result interpreting hs-cTn levels in this population becomes very challenging. Since these individuals exhibit a higher incidence and prevalence of myocardial infarction and carry a worse prognosis in comparison to their counterparts,[60] it becomes extremely important and relevant to recognize MI in this subset of patients and ensure appropriate treatment in order to improve the outcome. The pathophysiology of chronic troponin elevation in patients with CKD is not fully understood, however, is likely to be multifactorial, as patients with CKD often have coexistent coronary atherosclerosis,[61] LV hypertrophy,[62] HF,[53] and hypertension,[7] all of which can contribute to elevation of hs-cTn. Notably, among patients with impaired renal function, cTnT concentrations are more commonly elevated when compared with cTnI using both conventional and high sensitivity assays.[63,64] Abnormal hs-cTn levels in patients with CKD reduces the specificity of the assay for MI using both hscTnT and hs-cTnI assays thereby making it difficult to diagnose MI in this subset of patients.[65] However, despite difficulties in interpreting troponins in CKD, the 0/1 h and 0/2 h algorithms can be applied for diagnosis of acute MI with appropriate clinical symptoms and ECG changes suggestive of ischemia. Elevated troponins should not be dismissed as irrelevant in patients with CKD as incidence of ACS is quite high, requiring a thorough judgment for early treatment. The 0/1 h and 0/2 h protocols have been tested in CKD and found to be equally effective compared to patients without renal disease **(Flowcharts 1 and 2)**.[65]

CONCLUSION

Measurement of hs-cTn has improved our understanding of cardiac as well as noncardiac conditions causing myocyte necrosis both in acute and chronic settings. It is particularly relevant to mention that use of hscTn should be preferred, but diagnosis of MI should not be assumed just on the basis of a laboratory value. A good patient history, ECG findings and an astute clinical judgment is required to differentiate a type 1 infarction from myriad conditions causing elevated troponins. The value of troponins is strongly associated with prognosis, irrespective of pathology, and calls for appropriate investigations and implementation of modern therapies.

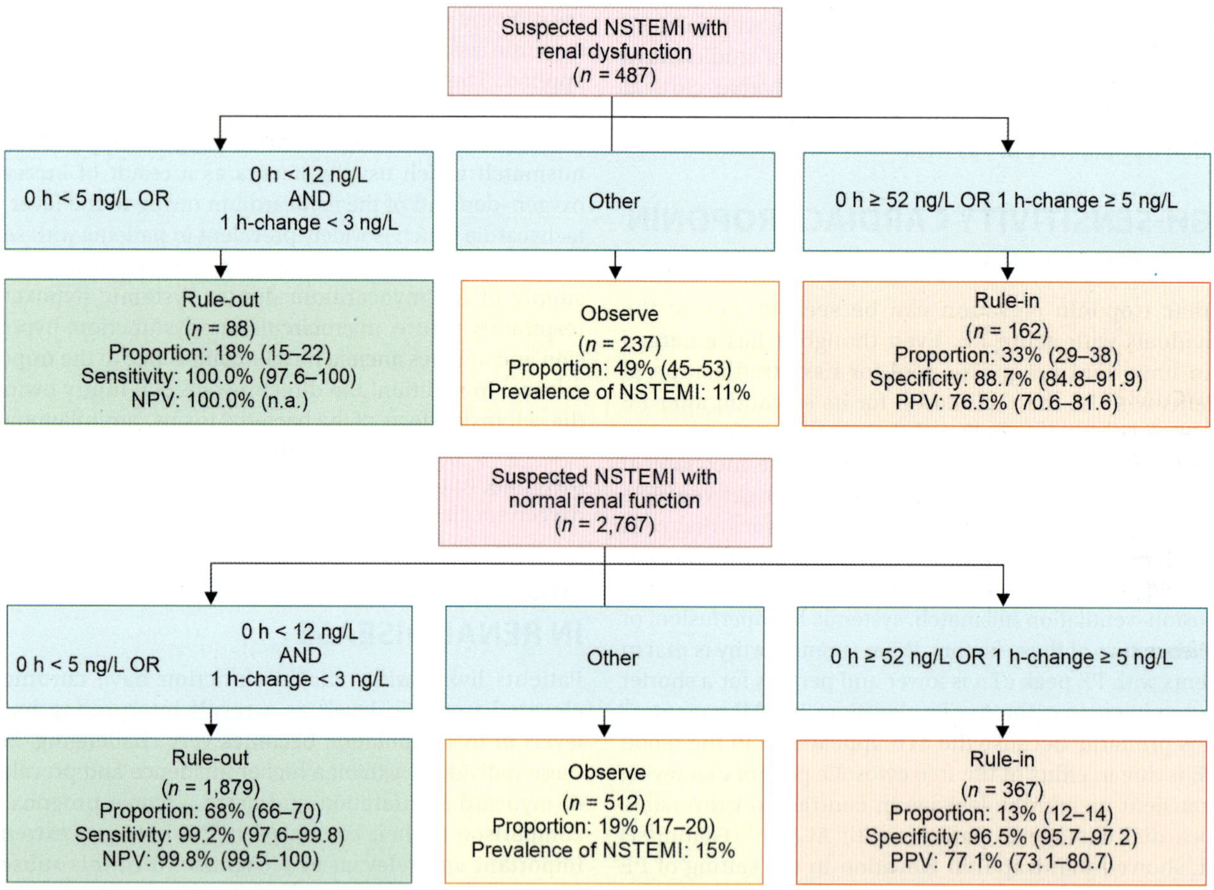

FLOWCHART 1: ESC 0/1 h algorithm using high-sensitivity cardiac troponin T in patients with and without renal dysfunction.
(ESC: European Society of Cardiology; NPV: negative predictive value; NSTEMI: non-ST-elevation myocardial infarction; PPV: positive predictive value)
Source: With permission from Twerenbold et al. (2018).[65]

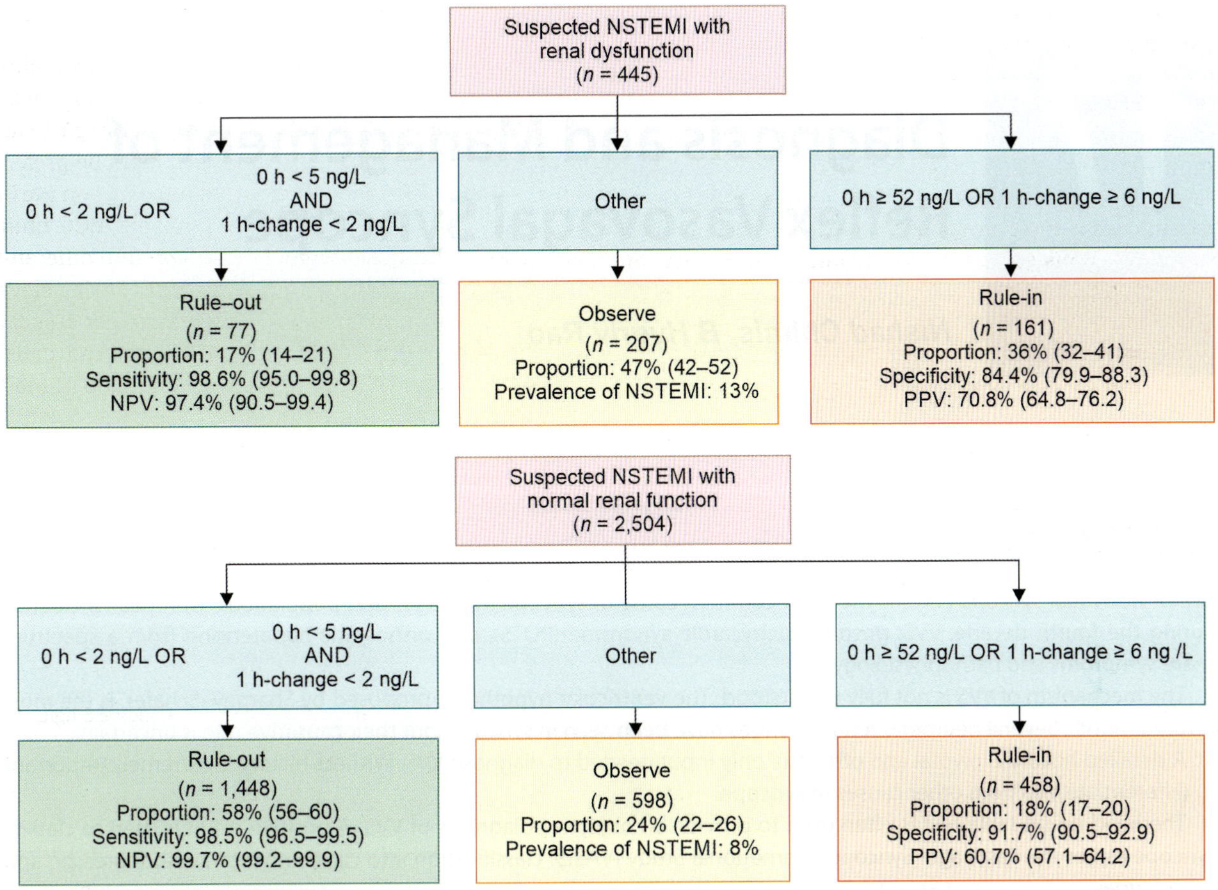

FLOWCHART 2: ESC 0/1 h algorithm using high sensitivity cardiac troponin I in patients with and without renal dysfunction.
(ESC: European Society of Cardiology; NPV: negative predictive value; NSTEMI: non-ST-elevation myocardial infarction; PPV: positive predictive value)
Source: With permission from Twerenbold et al. (2018).[65]

ONLINE REFERENCES

Please scan the QR code provided at the end of the table of contents for References of this chapter.

CHAPTER

17

Diagnosis and Management of Reflex Vasovagal Syncope

Nishad Chitnis, B Hygriv Rao

ABSTRACT

Reflex vasovagal syncope (VVS) is the most common cause of syncope in all ages and populations, with peak incidence during the fourth decade. VVS, postural tachycardia syndrome (POTS), and orthostatic hypotension from a spectrum share symptoms and pathophysiology.

The mechanism of VVS is not fully understood. The ventricular hypothesis, proposed by Sharpey–Schafer, is the most favored model. Several neuroendocrine changes have been seen in syncope, but their causative role is uncertain.

A detailed history is pivotal and often the only input needed to diagnose VVS. Witness history is extremely important to differentiate VVS from other causes of syncope.

The head-up tilt table test is often used to provide an objective diagnosis of VVS. A positive result is used to classify syncope as per the Vasovagal Syncope International Study (VASIS) classification into cardioinhibitor, vasodepressor, and mixed types.

Nonpharmacological interventions form the mainstay of management. Maintaining adequate hydration, withdrawing some medications, compression garments, and physical counter pressure maneuvers and reassurance are most important measures.

Pharmacological therapy has a limited role. The role of yoga in the management is being increasingly recognized; particularly a yoga maneuver—*tadasana*, which is easy to learn and practice has been shown to be effective in reducing syncopal and presyncopal events. Pacemakers are useful in patients who have severe cardio inhibitory response or asystole. Cardioneuroablation has evolved as a new tool in select patients.

Keywords: Vasovagal syncope, neurocardiogenic syncope tilt table test, *tadasana*, yoga.

INTRODUCTION

Syncope is a commonly encountered clinical situation and it is estimated that about 30–40% of people at some point in their lifetime have reported having experienced an episode of syncope.[1] Reflex vasovagal syncope (VVS) is by far the commonest cause of syncope even in patients with structural heart disease.[2] Though no age is exempt, this is seen more often in the younger population and the incidence increases with age, peaking in the fourth decade.

Vasovagal syncope, orthostatic hypotension (OH), and postural tachycardia syndrome (POTS) share a similar pathophysiology and their management too rests on common principles. They probably should be considered as a spectrum of the same clinical syndrome rather than distinct entities. Syncope in OH occurs in the first 3 minutes of assuming upright posture in contrast to VVS which occurs late. Hence, a bedside measurement of blood pressure in supine and upright postures suffices for the diagnosis of OH. The standard definitions of these conditions are summarized in **Table 1**.

Patients with syncope were found to have a 1.3 increased risk of all-cause mortality in the Framingham Heart Study.[3] Patients with cardiac syncope have a consistently higher 1-year mortality than patients with noncardiac or unexplained syncope.[4] Therefore, differentiation between reflex syncope and other varieties of syncope, especially cardiac syncope (Stokes–Adams syndrome) is vital.

TABLE 1: Definitions: 2017 ACC/AHA guidelines.[5]

Syncope	A symptom that presents with an abrupt, transient, complete loss of consciousness, associated with inability to maintain postural tone, with rapid and spontaneous recovery. The presumed mechanism is cerebral hypoperfusion. There should not be clinical features of other non-syncope causes of loss of consciousness, such as seizure, antecedent head trauma, or apparent loss of consciousness (i.e., pseudosyncope)[3]
Reflex syncope	Syncope due to a reflex that causes vasodilation, bradycardia, or both[3]
Vasovagal syncope	The most common form of reflex syncope mediated by the vasovagal reflex. VVS: (1) may occur with upright posture (standing or seated or with exposure to emotional stress, pain, or medical settings); (2) typically is characterized by diaphoresis, warmth, nausea, and pallor; (3) is associated with vasodepressor hypotension and/or inappropriate bradycardia; and (4) is often followed by fatigue. Typical features may be absent in older patients. VVS is often preceded by identifiable triggers and/or by a characteristic prodrome. The diagnosis is made primarily on the basis of a thorough history, physical examination, and eyewitness observation, if available[3]
Orthostatic hypotension	A drop in systolic BP of ≥20 mm Hg or diastolic BP of ≥10 mm Hg with assumption of an upright posture[3]
Postural (orthostatic) tachycardia syndrome (POTS)	A clinical syndrome usually characterized by all of the following: (1) Frequent symptoms that occur with standing (e.g., light-headedness, palpitations, tremulousness, generalized weakness, blurred vision, exercise intolerance, and fatigue); and (2) an increase in heart rate of ≥30 bpm during a positional change from supine to standing (or ≥40 bpm in those 12–19 years of age); and (3) the absence of OH (>20 mm Hg reduction in systolic BP). Symptoms associated with POTS include those that occur with standing (e.g., light-headedness, palpitations); those not associated with particular postures (e.g., bloating, nausea, diarrhea, abdominal pain); and those that are systemic (e.g., fatigue, sleep disturbance, and migraine headaches). The standing heart rate is often >120 bpm[3]

(ACC: American College of Cardiology; AHA: American Heart Association; VVS: vasovagal syncope)

PATHOPHYSIOLOGY OF VASOVAGAL SYNCOPE

The mechanism of VVS remains incompletely understood. Of all the animals, VVS is seen only in humans and this possibly is the price for the upright posture during evolution. Though some people appear to be susceptible, there is a wide variation and inconsistency in this susceptibility to different triggers. An individual, who develops syncope with a trigger at one time, may not experience an episode with the same trigger at another time. Genetic predisposition appears to have a role but does not explain temporal variation in the same person. Neurohormonal changes are seen in most cases of syncope, but there is doubt as to which are contributory and which are compensatory.[6]

Ventricular Hypothesis

The ventricular hypothesis (or Sharpey-Schafer model) is the most accepted hypothesis for the mechanism of cerebral hypoperfusion.[7] This is shown in **Flowchart 1**.

This model gives a good explanation for the four phases of syncope seen clinically.[8]

- *Phase 1*: Early phase of stabilization during standing
- *Phase 2*: Circulatory instability
- *Phase 3*: Terminal hypotension and syncope
- *Phase 4*: Recovery

The model also explains the observation that conditions that reduce cardiac output (CO), such as dehydration, blood loss, hypotension producing drugs, etc., increase the susceptibility to syncopal episodes.

Neurohormonal Changes

Several neurohormonal changes are seen during syncope:[6]

- Epinephrine and norepinephrine levels are increased; however, it is uncertain whether this is causative. High epinephrine to norepinephrine ratio seems related to episodes. But adrenergic blockers are inconsistent in preventing episodes.
- Arginine vasopressin levels increase but do not appear protective for unknown reasons.
- Endothelin-1 levels are raised in VVS, but not other types of syncope.
- Adrenomedullin (a peptide vasodilator) paradoxically appears to be protective.
- B-type natriuretic peptide and A-type natriuretic peptide levels show inconsistent relationship with syncopal events.
- Pancreatic polypeptide levels are raised but appear to denote increase vagal activity rather than a causative relationship.
- Cyclic adenosine monophosphate (AMP) levels are raised, probably due to rise in catecholamine levels.
- Endogenous opioids have been proposed as triggers of VVS, data is inconsistent.
- Renin-angiotensin-aldosterone axis insufficiency has been suggested but remains uncertain.

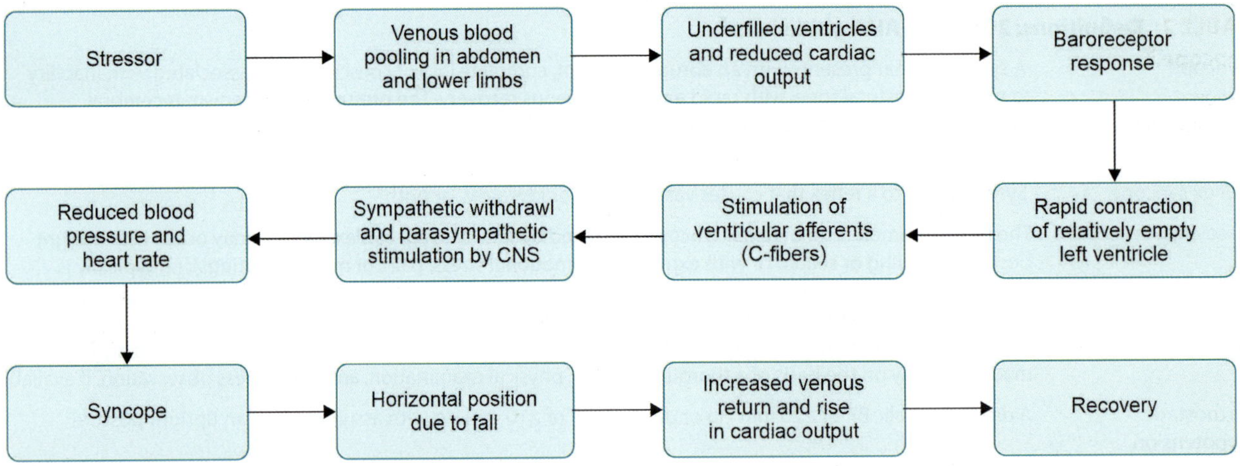

FLOWCHART 1: Sharpey–Schafer model of syncope.
(CNS: central nervous system)

- Increased serotonin response in the CNS has been proposed to be one of the causative mechanisms for syncope, but the effect of serotonin receptor antagonists is inconsistent.

To conclude, the pathophysiology of reflex syncope remains incompletely understood.

DIAGNOSIS

In general, the main objective of evaluation of a patient with syncope is to identify and rule out those conditions which can contribute to mortality. This is important as VVS is more common but relatively benign. Patients with cardiac causes of syncope have more mortality than those without and hence, cardiac evaluation should be the first step in syncope evaluation.

DIAGNOSTIC WORKUP

History

A detailed history is pivotal and most often the only input needed to diagnose VVS. It is necessary to make all efforts to obtain detailed history of the syncopal event from a witness. The patient is unlikely to give the most reliable sequence of events which are important for diagnosis. Longer duration of loss of consciousness (LOC) is unlikely in VVS, and a history of tongue bite may denote a seizure but does not exclude VVS. A detailed physical examination is needed to pick up evidence of trauma resulting from the episode of syncope.

None of the tests which follow can give an unequivocal diagnosis of VVS. Ruling out each alternative diagnosis is difficult, expensive, and may even be impossible. The following features support the diagnosis of VVS:[5]

- Young age of onset
- Long duration of history
- No known cardiac illness
- Syncope in standing/sitting position
- Syncope during assuming upright posture after prolonged recumbency
- Prodromal symptoms such as nausea, vomiting, feeling of warmth
- Triggers such as dehydration, pain, emotional distress, witnessing blood
- Situational triggers (seen in situational syncope) such as laugh, micturition
- Frequent recurrence with similar history for most episodes.

Vasovagal syncope in the catheterization laboratory deserves a special mention. It can occur during a procedure, or later during removal of cannulation sheaths (especially femoral arterial sheaths). The syncope occurs in supine position, is frequently triggered by pain or anxiety, and usually includes bradycardia and hypotension.

The 2018 ESC guidelines for syncope give the following recommendations for initial evaluation based on history **(Table 2)**.

Initial Evaluation

After a physical examination, including a detailed cardiovascular examination, basic biochemistry should be obtained in all patients, including estimation of B12 levels. A 12-lead ECG and 2D echocardiogram are most important investigations to be done as these help to exclude many causes of syncope associated with sudden death and overall mortality. Neurological imaging is rarely indicated after history suggests diagnosis of VVS and certainly does not need to be ordered routinely.

Head-up Tilt Table Test

The head-up tilt table (HUTT) test is an important objective tool to diagnose VVS. The test entails strapping down the patient on the tilt-table and incrementally increasing the angle of tilt of the table. Heart rate and blood pressure are

TABLE 2: Recommendations for initial evaluation of syncope.[9]

Reflex syncope and OH	VVS is highly probable if syncope is precipitated by pain, fear, or standing, and is associated with typical progressive prodrome (pallor, sweating, and/or nausea)
	Situational reflex syncope is highly probable if syncope occurs during or immediately after specific triggers
	Syncope due to OH is confirmed when syncope occurs while standing and there is concomitant significant OH
	In the absence of the above criteria, reflex syncope and OH should be considered likely when the features that suggest reflex syncope or OH are present and the features that suggest cardiac syncope are absent
Cardiac syncope	Arrhythmic syncope is highly probable when the ECG shows: • Persistent sinus bradycardia <40 bpm or sinus pauses >3 s in awake state and in absence of physical training • Mobitz II second- and third-degree AV block • Alternating left and right BBB • VT or rapid paroxysmal SVT • Non-sustained episodes of polymorphic VT and long or short QT interval; or • Pacemaker or ICD malfunction with cardiac pauses
	Cardiac ischemia-related syncope is confirmed when syncope presents with evidence of acute myocardial ischemia with or without myocardial infarction
	Syncope due to structural cardiopulmonary disorders is highly probable when syncope presents in patients with prolapsing atrial myxoma, left atrial ball thrombus, severe aortic stenosis, pulmonary embolus, or acute aortic dissection

(ECG: electrocardiogram; ICD: implantable cardioverter-defibrillator; OH: orthostatic hypotension; SVT: supraventricular tachycardia; VVS: vasovagal syncope)

monitored throughout. The aim is to document changes in heart rate and blood pressure during upright tilt and to confirm whether the said changes correlate with reproduction of the patient's symptoms during the test **(Fig. 1)**.

Certain precautions should be taken while performing HUTT. Conditions such as dehydration, anemia, and renal failure should be ruled out by routine examination and investigations in order to avoid false-positives and eliminate confounding factors. Usually, a couple of hours nil-by-mouth is preferred to reduce the risk of vomiting and consequent aspiration. Various protocols exist. Choice of protocol depends on the investigator's choice and the patient's clinical condition. Emergency equipment including external defibrillator must be present in the proximity as a prolonged cardio inhibitory response may lead to ventricular fibrillation.

Head-up Tilt Table Test Protocols

- *Classic HUTT:* A supine phase of 5 minutes with baseline BP and HR measurements is done. Head-up tilt between 60° and 80° is given for duration of 45 minutes without provocation or 40 minutes with nitroglycerin provocation given at 20-minute mark. Test is terminated early if symptoms occur, and HR and BP response is documented.[10]
- *Nitroglycerin protocol:* Proposed by Raviele et al., this protocol of the nitroglycerin consists of a maximum of five successive stages of 5 minutes in the supine position plus 10 minutes 80° upright tilt at progressively increasing infusion rates (increments of 0.86 μg/kg/h every stage).[11] A year later, the team modified the protocol to use 0.3 mg of sublingual nitroglycerin 45 minutes after baseline tilt.[12] A "short protocol" variation of the test has also been proposed in which non-medicated step is skipped and nitroglycerin is given before starting tilt in supine position.[13]
- *Italian protocol:* In this protocol, 400 μg sublingual nitroglycerin spray is administered after a 20-minute baseline phase.[14]
- *Westminster protocol:* This protocol entails prolonged (45 min) tilt of 60°.[15]
- *Newcastle protocol:* There are three Newcastle protocols. All start with supine position for 20 minutes.[16]
  - Drug-free passive tilt test: Supine position is followed by 70° tilt for 40 minutes.
  - Isoproterenol HUTT: After supine, 5 minutes 70° tilt followed by 5 minutes supine. Isoproterenol is infused for 5 minutes at rate of 1 μg/min in supine, followed by 5 minutes 1 μg/min infusion at 70° tilt. The infusion is discontinued in supine for 2 minutes. Infusion is restarted at 3 μg/min for 5 minutes in supine followed by 5 minutes with 3 μg/min infusion at 70° tilt.
  - Glyceryl trinitrate HUTT: After supine rest, two metered doses of sublingual glyceryl trinitrate (GTN) spray of 400 μg and 800 μg are administered. After another 5 minutes of supine, the patient is tilted to 70° for 20 minutes.
- Edrophonium, adenosine, and clomipramine have been used as provocative agents recently.[4]

Vasovagal Syncope International Study Classification (Table 3)

A positive HUTT result is used to classify syncope as per the Vasovagal Syncope International Study (VASIS) classification based on predominance of hypotensive or bradycardic response and sequence of events.

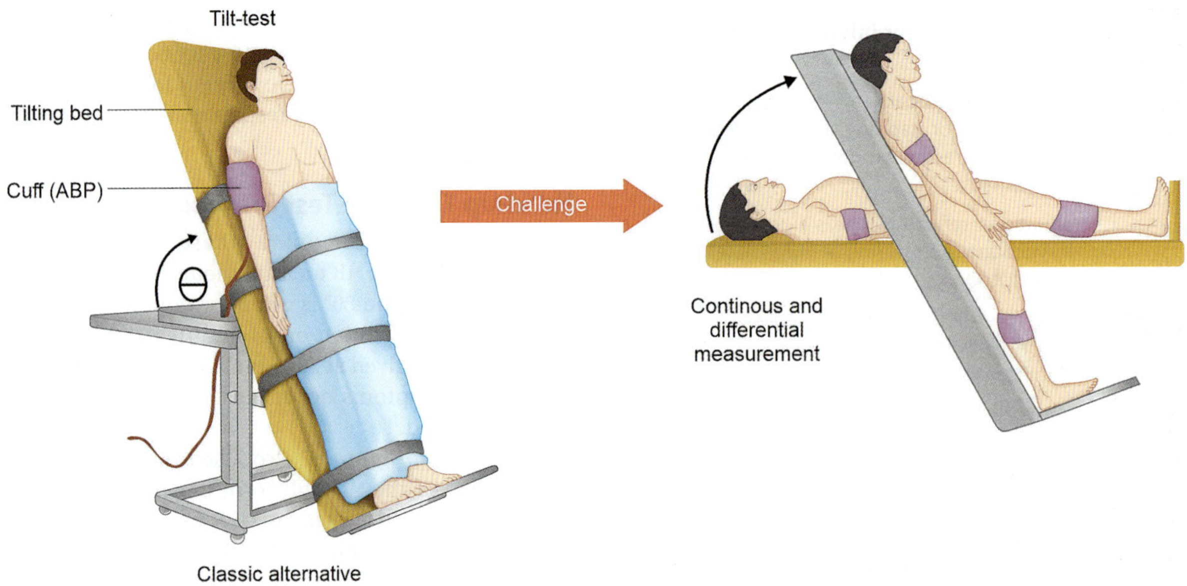

FIG. 1: The head-up tilt table test.

Source: Regueiro-Busoch C, Busoch Morlán CB, Castro FH, Diaz Martínez RJ, Regueiro-Gómez A. A novel method for non-invasive measurement of blood pressure in differential and continuous mode during tilt table test. Biomed Eng Int. 2020;2(1):0049-57.

TABLE 3: VASIS classification.[17]

Type 1	*Mixed*: Heart rate falls during syncope but does not fall to <40 bpm or falls to <40 bpm for <10 s. Blood pressure falls before the heart rate falls
Type 2A	*Cardioinhibition without asystole*: Heart rate falls to <40 bpm for >10 s but asystole of >3 s does not occur. Blood pressure falls before the heart rate falls
Type 2B	*Cardioinhibition with asystole*: Asystole occurs for >3 s. Blood pressure fall coincides with or occurs before the heart rate fall
Type 3	*Vasodepressor*: Heart rate does not fall >10% from its peak at the time of syncope
Exception 1	*Chronotropic incompetence*: No heart rate rise during tilt testing (i.e., <10% from the pre-tilt rate)
Exception 2	*Excessive heart rate rise*: An excessive rise in heart rate both at the onset of the upright position and throughout its duration before syncope (i.e., >130 bpm)

(VASIS: Vasovagal Syncope International Study)

Importance of Head-up Tilt Table Test

Head-up tilt table test is an important part of the work-up of syncope. There are many merits of HUTT in patients suspected to have VVS. Firstly, it is an objective tool to arrive at a diagnosis replicating the VVS episode in controlled surroundings. This contributes to increasing the confidence of the patient and his family, who are often psychologically distressed by the episodes. Further, it ensures compliance with treatment. Secondly, although rare, cardio inhibitory type of VVS can be diagnosed to select patients who may need a permanent pacemaker. Thirdly, conditions like POTS can be diagnosed which are otherwise difficult to identify. Lastly, a positive result saves time and expense by negating the need for extensive and expensive investigations.

Limitations of Head-up Tilt Table Test

Head-up tilt table test has several limitations which reduce its utility. As per the authors' experience, the reproducibility of the test is low, sometimes resulting in diagnostic confusion. Specificity and sensitivity are limited and VVS cannot be fully confirmed or ruled out. In patients with confounding conditions such as anemia or dehydration, false positive results are common. Availability of HUTT and clinicians familiar with conducting HUTT are limited, while VVS is extremely common. Finally, the protocols are not yet fully standardized, and head-to-head comparisons between most protocols are lacking.

Despite the limitations, the role of HUTT in evaluation of syncope is very important.

MANAGEMENT OF VASOVAGAL SYNCOPE

General Measures

The most important component of the management of VVS is patient reassurance and education. The patient and his family should be counselled that this is benign and a common condition. It is not a life-threatening condition and does not affect the longevity of life. Though not a serious condition, the injuries associated with syncopal episodes can be life threatening. Hence, syncope avoidance maneuvers should be taught to the patient. This includes switch to a supine position when they feel a prodrome of syncope. Simple measures can improve the quality of life in most patients. They should avoid triggers like prolonged standing or suddenly standing up from a sitting or lying down position.[7]

Counter-maneuvers can be attempted during the prodrome to abort the syncope.[7]

Nonpharmacological Therapy

- *Fluid and salt intake:* Fluid and salt intake should be liberalized to increase blood volume and consequently venous return (ESC 2018 Class 1, AHA 2017 Class 2b). Around 3 L of fluid should be consumed per day, mainly in the form of water. Salt intake should be around 8–10 g/day, preferably through food, alternatively via salt tablets. In patients with heart failure, these goals may not be achievable[7].
- *Medication review and withdrawal:* Patients' medication should be reviewed, and possible offending medications should be withdrawn or reduced (ESC 2018 Class 2a, AHA 2017 Class 2b). Diuretics and vasodilators such as nitrates and alpha-adrenergic blockers are especially prone to precipitate reflex syncope. Regardless, all antihypertensives and several neurological and neuropsychiatric drugs can precipitate VVS and OH. Dosage reduction or switching over to alternative agents may be required.[7]
- *Compression garments:* Compression garments reduce venous pooling and increase venous return. A pressure of 20–30 mm Hg can be beneficial in reducing frequency of syncope (ESC 2018, AHA 2017 Class 1). Since abdominal venous pooling plays a major role in the pathophysiology of VVS, waist-high, pantyhose style garments are recommended. These are uncomfortable and often not tolerated. In such cases, athletic compression wear can be advised.[7]
- *Physical Counterpressure maneuvers:* Physical counter pressure maneuvers are useful in patients with prodrome to abort a syncopal episode (ESC 2018, AHA 2017 Class 2a). Two maneuvers are commonly used. In case syncope still comes on, the patient should take a supine position (get down and stay down).[7]
    - *Leg crossing and lower body muscle testing* is done in standing position. The legs are crossed, and the muscles of the legs, buttocks, and abdomen are tensed.
    - *Arm tensing* is done by linking one's hands in front of the body and pulling them apart.
- *Tilt training:* Tilt training (ESC 2018, AHA 2017 Class 2b) is used in highly motivated patients. Patients are subjected to progressively longer duration of upright posture in order to develop advantageous physiologic regulatory mechanisms. An example is 30 minutes vertical wall stand for 6 days a week for at least 4 weeks. A simple home tilt training method is head-up sleeping.[7]

Pharmacological Therapy

The role of drug therapy in the treatment of VVS is limited. None of the drugs proposed have been consistent with preventing syncope. Consequently, there is no drug which has a Class 1 recommendation. Drugs are only recommended in patients who are symptomatic despite nonpharmacological measures, with the caveat that they may not benefit from drugs either. The drugs used in the treatment of reflex syncope are given in **Table 4**.

Yoga in the Management of Vasovagal Syncope

Recent studies have demonstrated the benefits of yoga for the therapy of syncope. Several studies have demonstrated the benefits of yoga on autonomic modulation by achieving a balance between the sympathetic and parasympathetic tone.[18]

Gunda et al. were the first to demonstrate the benefits of yoga in reducing the incidence and severity of syncope and improving quality of life in 2015.[19] In 2021, Jayprakash Shenthar et al. demonstrated a similar benefit in a randomized trial.[20] The LIVE-Yoga study conducted by AIIMS, New Delhi similarly demonstrated an impressive reduction in VVS frequency and improvement in quality of life.[18]

TABLE 4: Drugs used for treatment of syncope.[5]

Drug	Class of recommendation	Indications
Midodrine	IIA	This alpha agonist is recommended in recurrent VVS with no hypertension, HF or urinary retention
Fludrocortisone	IIB	This mineralocorticoid is used in recurrent VVS with inadequate response to salt and water. Hypokalemia can occur
Beta blockers	IIB	Patients of 42 years or older with recurrent VVS
Selective serotonin reuptake inhibitors (SSRI)	IIB	Fluoxetine and paroxetine have shown some benefit in small RCTs. They may be considered in recurrent VVS

(RCTs: randomized controlled trials; VVS: vasovagal syncope)

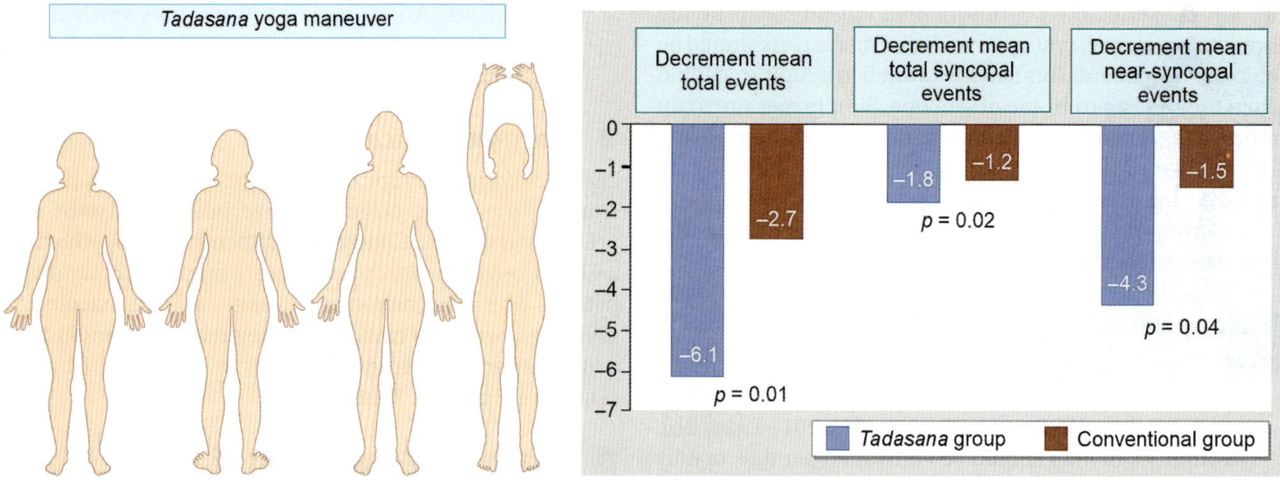

FIG. 2: (Left) *Tadasana* steps. (1) Stand straight with feet together and arms by the side against wall with support; (2) and (3) Alternate dorsiflexion and plantar flexion of the ankle and foot; (4) Isometric contraction of quadriceps—stand on toes keeping shoulders relaxed and straight; extend arms upward to keep them facing and parallel to each other. Breathe normally for 10 seconds. (Right) Comparison of decrement of total events, syncopal events, and near-syncopal events in the *tadasana* and conventional groups in relation to pretreatment event burden. The *tadasana* group demonstrated greater reduction in all three event categories.

Source: With permission from Rao BH et al. 2022.[21]

However, a commonality in all these studies is the use of guided yoga sessions consisting of several *yogasanas* done daily with a daily session of 30–60 minutes. Real world compliance with such sessions is likely to be quite low. A pilot study by our group has demonstrated the benefit of a single *asana*, viz., *tadasana* in reducing VVS frequency. Eight to twelve cycles of *tadasana* were advised twice a day. Compliance with this simple regimen is far more likely in the real world.[21] The method of *tadasana* is shown in **Figure 2**.

Pacemaker Implantation

Implantation of dual-chamber pacemaker has been used for treatment of syncope. Pacemakers have shown benefit only in patients with predominantly cardioinhibitory syncope with asystole (VASIS classification type 2B) on HUTT. Patients with predominantly vasodepressor or a mixed response do not benefit from pacemaker implantation.[5]

Cardioneuroablation Therapy

Cardioneuroablation (CNA) is being evaluated as therapy for refractory syncope. CNA entails radiofrequency cardiac ablation of postganglionic parasympathetic neurons located in the epicardial fat pads and atrial walls.[22] While early results are promising, this is an evolving technique and its eventual place in the therapy of VVS is yet to be defined.

CONCLUSION

Vasovagal syncope is a very common clinical problem. History obtained from a witness is the main stay of diagnosis. The HUTT is a very useful investigation for diagnosis and obviates the need for multiple expensive investigations. Treatment of VVS consists mainly of nonpharmacological measures. Yoga, especially *tadasana*, shows promise in the treatment of VVS.

ONLINE REFERENCES

Please scan the QR code provided at the end of the table of contents for References of this chapter.

CHAPTER

18

Newer Antiarrhythmic Drugs

Soumen Devidutta

ABSTRACT

Antiarrhythmic drugs in contemporary use although effective are limited by their adverse effects which are broadly proarrhythmia and chronic toxicity. Nonselective action of antiarrhythmic drugs results in occasional serious ventricular arrhythmias. Progressive organ dysfunction is specifically a limitation associated with long-term amiodarone use caused by its large iodine moiety. Newer antiarrhythmics are being explored to circumvent these limitations. Atrial specific drugs are being developed which target channels expressed predominantly in the atria. Such drugs are devoid of ventricular proarrhythmia. Some amiodarone congeners have been developed with similar antiarrhythmic potential but avoid its tissue toxicity as they do not have the iodine portion.

Keywords: Newer antiarrhythmics, atrial specific antiarrhythmics, novel antiarrhythmics.

INTRODUCTION

Antiarrhythmic drugs are broadly classified into four categories on the basis of their mode of action (1) blockade of sodium (class I), (2) potassium (class III), or (3) calcium (class IV) channels, or (4) inhibition of sympathetic stimulation (class II). Class III drugs are broad-spectrum antiarrhythmic and are used widely for ventricular and supraventricular arrhythmias. Class Ia and Ib are used mainly for ventricular tachycardia (VT) while class Ic agents are used mainly for atrial fibrillation (AF) and tachycardia. Class II and IV agents are more commonly used for AF rate control, because of their atrioventricular node-blocking properties. Their antiarrhythmic effects are mild.

Contemporary antiarrhythmics especially for AF rhythm control have some particular safety concerns. The major concern is that of antiarrhythmic drug-related proarrhythmia. Class Ic agents (propafenone and flecainide) can cause serious proarrhythmias in patients with ischemic heart disease, with myocardial infarction, or in those with severe left ventricular (LV) systolic dysfunction. On the other hand class Ia and class III agents need to be monitored for their QT prolonging effects and consequent risk of torsade de pointes (TdP). Class Ia agents (e.g., quinidine and disopyramide) primarily inhibit of sodium channels (I_{Na}). They also block delayed potassium rectifier (I_{Kr}) channels, prolonging repolarization and increasing risk of TdP. Although potent antiarrhythmics, they have a narrow therapeutic window and can be proarrhythmic without monitoring. The major class III agents, sotalol, dofetilide, and ibutilide, increase the risk of TdP although being effective drugs for the control of AF. Amiodarone is a class III agent and is a highly effective agent for the control of AF[1] and ventricular arrhythmias.[2] Despite markedly blocking the I_{Kr} and prolonging the QT interval,[3] it rarely causes proarrhythmia. Clearly, the prolongation is negated by reducing the dispersion of repolarization which protects against torsades.[4]

A critical limitation with amiodarone is that of its potentially serious adverse effects such as thyroid dysfunction, pulmonary fibrosis, hepatic fibrosis, and peripheral neuropathy. Hence, it is important to focus on the development of newer antiarrhythmic drugs with equal potency but devoid of the limiting side effects.

An ideal antiarrhythmic should exhibit the following:

- Restores sinus rhythm
- Effective for atrial and ventricular arrhythmias

- Effective for arrhythmia of any mechanism
- Reduces ventricular rate during AF episodes
- Prolongs effective refractory period myocytes without risk of proarrhythmia (TdP)
- Reduces drug-induced dispersion of myocardial refractoriness
- Reduces induction of early after depolarization
- Has no negative inotropic effect or has positive inotropic effect.
- Has a favorable or neutral impact on survival
- Exhibits long-term efficacy without major adverse effects or organ toxicity
- Minimal interaction with other cardioactive drugs.

ATRIAL SELECTIVE ANTIARRHYTHMICS

There is a significant interest in this group of antiarrhythmic recently to minimize the ventricular proarrhythmic effects [TdP or ventricular fibrillation (VF)]. Thus, atrial selective agents should ideally be devoid of significant Na^+-channel-blocking or QT prolonging properties in the ventricular myocardium.

Better understanding of the pathophysiology of AF[5] has paved the way for these atrial selective drugs.[6] The ultrarapid delayed rectifier (I_{Kur}) current is expressed exclusively in the atria. This has allowed the prospect of developing atrial-selective drugs devoid of ventricular proarrhythmia in treatment of patients with AF. These atrial-selective agents include I_{Kur} blockers, atrial-selective sodium channel blockers, muscarinic receptor (M2) blockers, and serotonin type 4 (5-HT4) receptor antagonists.

- *Vernakalant* is an activation-dependent sodium and early-activating potassium channel blocker.[7] It was developed as an atrial-selective antiarrhythmic for both acute restoration of sinus rhythm in patients with AF and maintenance of sinus rhythm. The acute version is done with intravenous form. It has been shown to be safe and effective for chemical cardioversion of AF.[8,9] But it is less effective for more organized atrial flutter. An oral form of vernakalant is under development for the maintenance of sinus rhythm following cardioversion.

  AVE0118 is an atrial-selective potassium channel blocker under development, inhibiting I_{Kur} and the transient outward current (I_{to}), which is expressed predominantly in atria. In animals studies have shown AVE0118 to prolong atrial refractoriness, notably in electrically remodeled atria, inhibit AF inducibility, and acutely convert persistent AF to sinus rhythm without altering the QT interval.[10]

  AZD7009 is a mixed ion-channel blocker blocking the delayed rectifier potassium channel (I_{Kr}), the sodium current (I_{Na}), and the I_{Kur}. These effects are predominantly on atrial tissue.[11] Both an intravenous and oral forms for acute conversion and long-term treatment of AF are being developed and are now in phase II trials.

  Venakalant is the first of such atrial selective molecules and is effective in the conversion of AF to sinus rhythm when administered intravenously.[7,8] The other molecules in pipeline will make the options of atrial selective antiarrhythmics more robust. They could bring in a paradigm change in AF management if they can consistently maintain sinus rhythm as they would eliminate the constant threat of proarrhythmia and organ toxicity of the contemporary agents.

AMIODARONE CONGENERS

Amiodarone and sotalol have remained the two leading antiarrhythmic agents for decades, especially for AF. Amiodarone's broad-spectrum antiarrhythmic efficacy in maintaining sinus notwithstanding, its adverse effects have been a serious limitation and the reason to look for newer agents and congeners. The large iodine moiety of amiodarone is responsible for the chronic organ effects.

Dronedarone is a noniodinated amiodarone benzofuran[12,13] with similar antiarrhythmic properties. It inhibits sodium, potassium, and calcium currents, including the I_{Kr} and acetylcholine-activated potassium currents (I_{KAch}) and the L-type calcium current. Dronedarine is also an antagonist of α- and β-adrenoreceptors. It has a shorter half-life than amiodarone, can be loaded more rapidly, and is distributed less in tissues. 800 mg of, in a study, dronedarone has a 55% relative risk reduction of AF relapse compared to placebo.[14] Higher doses (1,200 and 1,600 mg daily) were poorly tolerated, with gastrointestinal side effects. However, thyroid, ocular or pulmonary toxicity was not seen and no proarrhythmia was reported.[14] In the pooled analysis of two large multinational trials, EURIDIS and ADONIS, evaluating dronedarone in maintenance of sinus rhythm in 1,250 patients with either paroxysmal (70%) or persistent AF (compared with placebo), the time to AF recurrence was 2.3–2.7 times longer after treatment with dronedarone 400 mg twice daily.[15] Dronedarone also significantly slowed the ventricular rates during AF recurrences adding to its merits. Though safety outcomes were promising, but notably patients with advanced heart failure were excluded from these two trials. ATHENA trial established the safety and efficacy of dronedarone in treatment of AF in high risk patients.[16] There is a particular interest around dronedarone as it potentially maintains the potent antiarrhythmic efficacy of amiodarone eliminating the unwanted thyroid and pulmonary effects. The nonspecific antiadrenergic and calcium-channel-blocking actions of dronedarone confer a bonus ventricular rate control in AF recurrences.

- *SSR149744C* is another noniodinated amiodarone derivative under study that exhibits similar electrophysiological and hemodynamic properties to dronedarone.[17]
- *ATI-2042* is another under trial amiodarone congener with retained iodine moiety.

OTHER ANTIARRHYTHMICS

- *Azimilide* is a selective class III antiarrhythmic drug that blocks both the rapid (I_{Kr}) and the slow (I_{Ks}) delayed rectifier potassium channel.[17] Azimilide prolongs cardiac action potential duration (APD) and refractory periods in both the atria and the ventricles.

  It has a long half-life allowing for once daily dosing. Studies have proven its efficacy in prolonging the symptomatic[18] arrhythmia-free interval in patients with AF or atrial flutter with 100 and 125 mg doses being equally effective.[19,20] Azimilide also significantly reduces the recurrence of VT or ventricular fibrillation (VF) and implantable cardioverter-defibrillator (ICD) therapies.[21]
- *Ibutilide* is a pure class III agent only available in the intravenous form and is used for cardioversion of AF and flutter. It is structurally similar to sotalol and derives its action by inhibiting rapid component of delayed rectifier potassium current (I_{Kr}).[22] It prolongs the APD and the QT interval as well in a dose-dependent manner. It increases the refractoriness of both atria and ventricles.[23-25] It is given as a 0.01 mg/kg bolus, usually 1 mg bolus over 10 minutes is recommended for patients over 60 kg and 0.01 mg/kg for patients below 60 kg. Most of the patients converting within 30 minutes of the start of drug infusion. A second bolus can be repeated in 10 minutes if sinus is not restored necessary, monitoring QT interval and proarrhythmia. It is more successful for atrial flutter than AF. Predictors of successful arrhythmia conversion include the duration of arrhythmia before treatment as well as left atrial size. It is an effective agent for postcardiac surgery AF and atrial flutter.[26] Baseline QT prolongation, hypokalemia, severe LV dysfunction, combining with other QT prolonging agents increases the risk of TdP or VF and caution should be exercised in such patients.
- *Ranolazine* inhibits late phase of the I_{Na} and delayed I_{Kr} during cardiac repolarization.[27] Its clinical effects and those on QT prolongation as a standalone drug are modest but can be significant with other repolarization active drugs. It has been studied and used as an adjunct antiarrhythmic in combination with more potent drugs such as amiodarone and dronedarone[28] for paroxysmal or new onset AF to good effect, the combination being better than the main drug alone. As a standalone drug for persistent AF it does not seem to prolong AF-free duration.
- *Tedisamil*, an antianginal agent, possesses multiple ion-channel effects, including blockade of I_{to}, I_{Kr}, I_{Ks}, I_{Kur}, $I_{K\text{-}ATP}$, and even I_{Na}.[29,30] The drug also causes reverse, rate-dependent QT interval prolongation. Intravenous form is about 50% effective in chemical cardioversion.[31] Some safety concerns due to proarrhythmia led to the interruption of the trials.

  Rotigaptide is a specific gap-junction-modifying drug. It is a novel therapeutic target and has been tried in canine hearts. It is being currently evaluated in a phase II trial.

  As per recent data serotonin 5-HT4 receptor antagonists could be promising drugs in patients with AF. Further atrial-specific 5-HT4 receptor subtype is present in the atria but not in the ventricles, allowing the possibility to pharmacologically exclude ventricular adverse effects.

CONCLUSION

Poor efficacy in restoring or maintaining sinus rhythm, nonselective antiarrhythmic action leading to serious proarrhythmia (ventricular arrhythmias) or long-term organ toxicities are limitations of the currently used antiarrhythmics paving way for the newer agents. Newer antiarrhythmic drugs including atrial-selective agents like vernakalant and agents with multiple channel-blocking properties like dronedarone hold promise for improving upon these shortcomings and afford better control with lesser safety concerns.

ONLINE REFERENCES

Please scan the QR code provided at the end of the table of contents for References of this chapter.

CHAPTER

19

Degenerative Mitral Valve

Madhu Shukla, Jagdish C Mohan

ABSTRACT

Degenerative mitral valve disease (DMVD) is a spectrum of valvulopathy in which morphologic changes in the connective tissue of the mitral valve cause structural alterations that prevent normal functioning of the mitral valve apparatus. Three distinct types of mitral valve degeneration have been described—myxomatous degeneration, fibroelastic deficiency, and mitral annular calcification. All these have unique clinical and echocardiographic characteristics although a little bit of overlap is possible. DMVD is acquiring epidemic proportions because of increased longevity and pervading risk factors. This review describes salient aspects of DMVD, its epidemiology, and pathogenesis with therapeutic implications.

Keywords: Pathobiology of mitral valve, fibroelastic degeneration, myxomatous valve, calcific mitral valve, degeneration, mitral annulus calcification.

INTRODUCTION

Valvular heart disease (VHD) of any severity is an important cause of physical disability and reduced life span. Prevalence of VHD is on the rise largely due to increased longevity, greater recognition, and pervading dysmetabolism. The burden of nonrheumatic VHD is disproportionately increasing in the world; degenerative valvulopathy accounts for majority of the hemodynamically significant VHD in the developed countries.[1] Moderate or severe VHD affects ~2.5% of the US population, with a prevalence that increases steeply with age, affecting up to 12% of persons ≥75 years old.[2] There is a significant geographic variation in prevalence and the exact estimates are not available from India. The lack of comprehensive estimates of nonrheumatic VHD burden is attributable in part to a limited number of population-based studies of prevalence as well as underdiagnosis of asymptomatic VHD. Significant VHD portends bad prognosis, and is associated with a 35–75% higher risk of death compared with those without significant VHD.[2] Degenerative VHD, unlike conventional assumption, is not topped by aortic stenosis but by mitral valve disease. It has been estimated that about 24 million people worldwide suffer from degenerative mitral valve disease (DMVD).[3] Structural valve degeneration is a permanent valve dysfunction resulting from factors both intrinsic and extrinsic leading to degeneration and/or hemodynamic dysfunction. While aging is an important risk factor for progression in some subtypes, calcific mitral valve degeneration may be an active biological process similar to atherosclerosis with common risk factors such as hypertension, diabetes, dyslipidemia, smoking, obesity, and chronic kidney disease, etc.[4-7] Noncalcific DMVD which affects connective tissue of the leaflets and chordae tendineae usually and paradoxically spares other fibrous skeleton of the heart and is not associated with atherosclerotic risk factors.

ANATOMY OF MITRAL VALVE

Mitral valve directs blood flow from the left atrium to the left ventricle during diastole and closes during systole in coordination with aortic valve opening. It has two asymmetrical leaflets attached to the fibrous ring (annulus) sandwiched between aortic annulus anteriorly and the tricuspid annulus to the right and anterior **(Figs. 1 to 4)**. The fibrous skeleton of the heart is in continuity with the annulus fibrosa that constitutes the common fibrous support system of the tricuspid, mitral, and aortic valves.[8] The leaflets have specialized subvalvar supporting structures which synchronize and coordinate their movements. The supporting tendinous cords or chordae tendineae (three different types with different functions) on the ventricular aspect of the valve leaflets usually insert into two

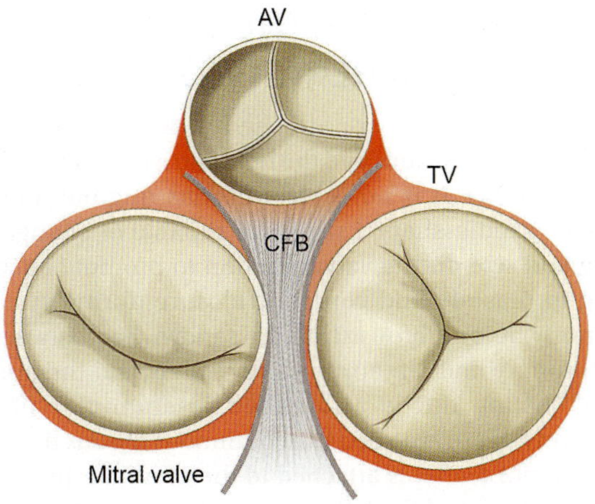

FIG. 1: Schematic cross-sectional diagram showing the relationship between annuli of mitral, aortic, and tricuspid valves.
(AV: aortic valve; CFB: central fibrous body; TV: tricuspid valve)

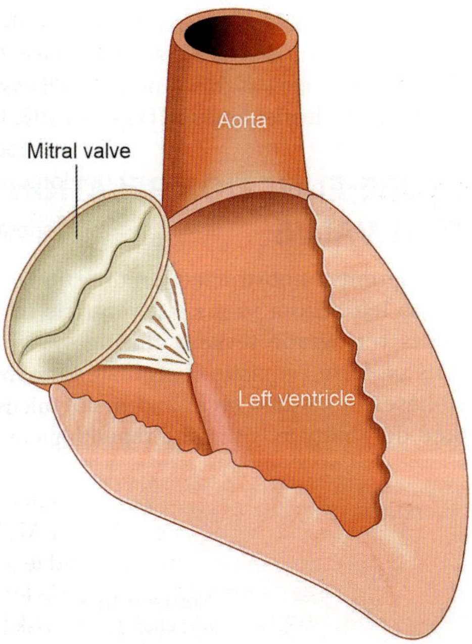

FIG. 2: Schematic diagram showing the entire mitral apparatus.

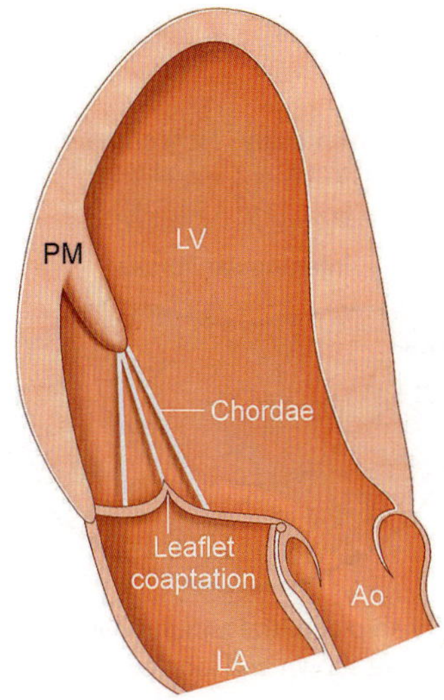

FIG. 3: Schema as in Figure 2.
Note the plane of coaptation and coaptation height of leaflets.
(Ao: aorta; LA: left atrium; LV: left ventricle; PM: papillary muscle)

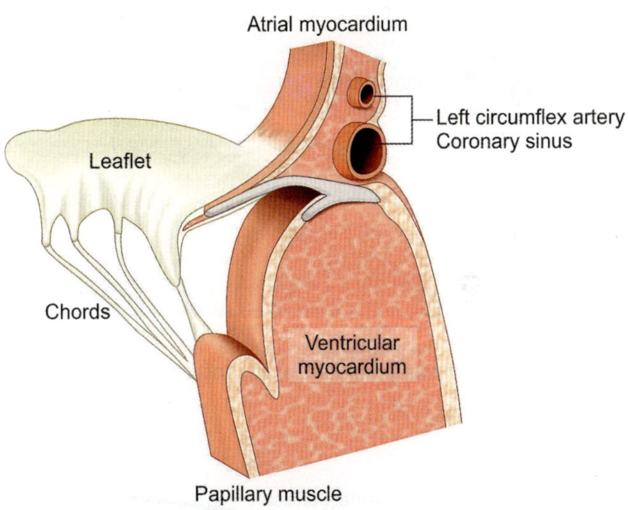

FIG. 4: Attachment of posterior mitral valve leaflet directly to the muscular atrioventricular junction without any well-defined continuous fibrous ring.

well-defined muscle pillars called papillary muscles which are continuous with the left ventricular myocardium **(Fig. 3)**. The leaflets are made of highly organized extracellular matrix, interstitial cells, and with surface-overlying endothelial cell layer.[8] The extracellular matrix consists of elastin, collagen, and proteoglycans/aminoglycans which provide unique biomechanical character to the entire valve apparatus **(Figs. 5 and 6)**. The valve interstitial cells in adults have very low activity in health but participate in additional matrix laying only during physicochemical insult.[9] Expansion of the spongiosa containing glycosaminoglycans right in the middle of the leaflet is the harbinger of myxomatous change which is a unique type of degeneration.[9] The anterior leaflet has much larger area while the posterior leaflet covers much more circumference. The posterior or mural leaflet has three indentations along the free edge which variably divide it into three segments or scallops (P1, P2, and P3). The anterior leaflet is also divided arbitrarily into three regions labelled A1, A2, and A3 corresponding to the adjacent regions of the posterior leaflet. Three zones of the leaflet surface from the annulus toward free margin are called basal, clear, and rough zones. The rough zone participates in coaptation.[10] The average thickness of the leaflets does not exceed 2 mm normally and it is more at base and near the free margin which is called the rough zone.

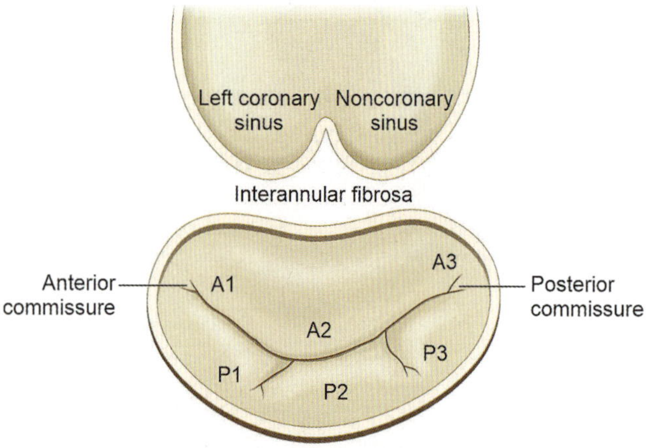

FIG. 5: The relationship of mitral annulus with interannular fibrosa. The leaflet scallops are shown and labeled.

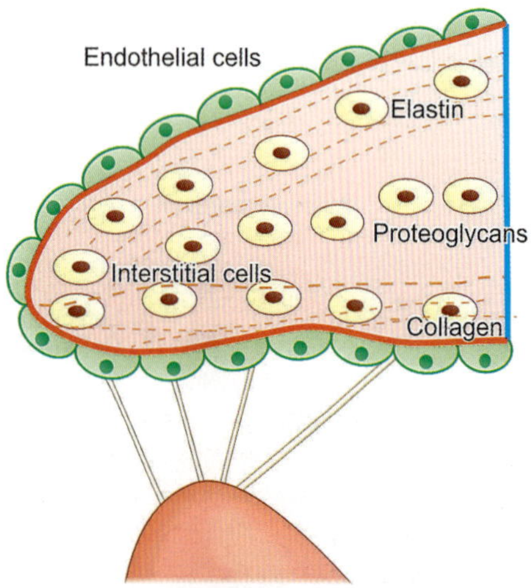

FIG. 6: Schema showing different layer constituents of the leaflet structure.

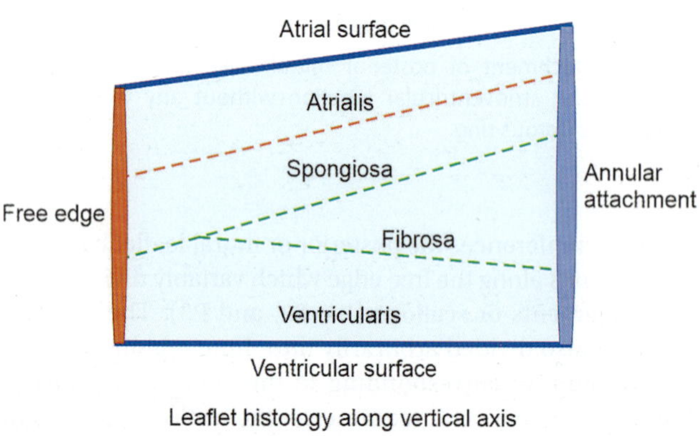

FIG. 7: The layer concept of the leaflet structure.

MITRAL ANNULUS: THE CORE OF CALCIFIC DEGENERATIVE PROCESS

Bases of the leaflets are attached to a junctional tissue between the left atrium and the left ventricle which has been called annulus. It is not a rigid fibrous ring but a pliable elliptical saddle-shaped structure capable of changing its shape and size during valvar motion to promote adequate filling in diastole and complete closure during systole.[10] Anteriorly, it is a fibrous structure sandwiched between the noncoronary and left aortic valve leaflets and the anterior mitral leaflet and is also called interannular fibrosa. Posteriorly, there is no definite continuous fibrous tissue and the posterior leaflet is attached to the muscular junction of the left atrium and the left ventricle. This posterior junction has fibrofatty tissue and is adjacent to the left circumflex artery and the coronary sinus. Hence, this circumferential basal attachment of the leaflets called the annulus, which is oval in shape, is only partly fibrous and two-thirds almost muscular allowing it to dilate, contract (20–30% reduction in area during systole), and displace downward. Degeneration and calcification initiates at this junction and progresses inward impairing the leaflet function **(Figs. 7 to 9)**.

STRUCTURE-FUNCTION RELATIONSHIP IN MITRAL VALVE

Mitral valve permits unobstructed, unidirectional forward flow from the left atrium to the left ventricle in diastole and prevents retrograde leakage during systole. Valve components perform exquisite coordinated movement in different phases of cardiac cycle and maintain adequate tensility and durability to withstand repetitive mechanical

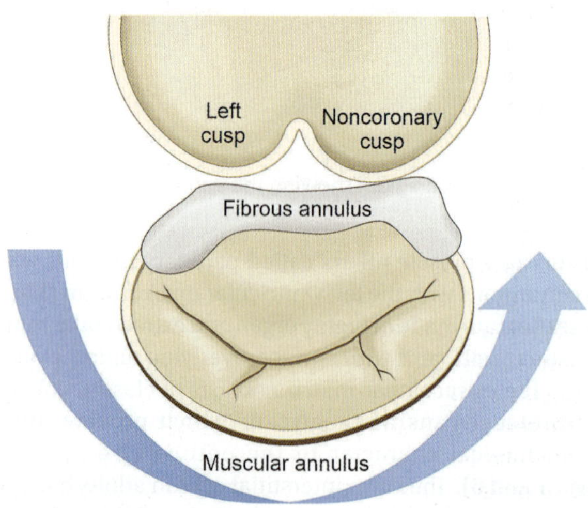

FIG. 8: Schematic depiction of mitral annulus. The concept of virtual ring.

stress and strain over life time. The functional requirements of the heart valves are accomplished by a specialized set of cells and heterogeneous extracellular matrix, arrayed in a spatially distinct and differentiated tissue structure, that are temporally dynamic and highly responsive to the external biomechanical environment.[11] Mitral valve opens and closes ≈40 million times a year and 3 billion times over an average lifetime.[12] The leaflets undergo flexion, shear stress, and tension in every beat. Mitral valve is slightly thicker than the tricuspid valve because of the sequelae of shear, compressive, and longitudinal stress.[13]

PATHOBIOLOGICAL TYPES OF DEGENERATIVE MITRAL VALVE

Resident cells of the mitral valve leaflets have a mixed population (surface endothelium and interstitial cells) and play a role in maintaining structure and function of the valves. The interstitial cells are bioactive heterogenous population of cells that can transform into fibroblasts and myofibroblasts, may express cytoskeletal and muscle proteins and participate in processes that may ultimately initiate degeneration and calcification when faced with obnoxious stimuli.[14] Normally, these cells participate in synthesis of elastin, collagen, proteoglycans, glycosaminoglycans, cytokines, and matrix-regulating enzymes. The intracellular calcium responses to vasoactive agents indicate that a number of receptor signaling pathways exist. These pathways underscore the role of myofibroblasts and other fibroblast phenotypes in valve function/dysfunction.[15] Inflammation, extracellular matrix remodeling, turbulent flow, and mechanical stress and strain contribute to the myofibroblastic, osteogenic and hypersecretory phenotypic differentiation of valve endothelial and interstitial cells. Increased valvular interstitial cell mass and uncontrolled synthesis of catalytic enzymes such as matrix metalloproteinases alter the homeostasis between collagen, elastin and proteoglycan components and provide a biomechanical basis for myxomatous degeneration.

Degeneration of the mitral valve has distinct phenotypes and is characterized by extracellular matrix dysregulation, cellular disarray, and sometimes calcification. Inherent embryogenic issues may account for some degeneration in later life as in Barlow's disease. In mitral annular calcification (MAC), the interstitial cells of the annulus undergo myofibroblastic differentiation, apoptosis and necrosis in response to injurious stimuli and the cellular degradation products attract calcium deposition.[16]

There is emerging evidence that disruption of the valvular extracellular matrix initiates diverse signaling pathways that lead to maladaptive matrix remodeling and consequently valve disease of at least three types:

1. Myxomatous degeneration of the mitral valve (MDMV)
2. Fibroelastic deficiency (FED)
3. Calcific degeneration of the mitral annulus (MAC)

Valve histopathology in degenerated leaflets may have two main patterns—*myxomatous* change or *fibrotic*

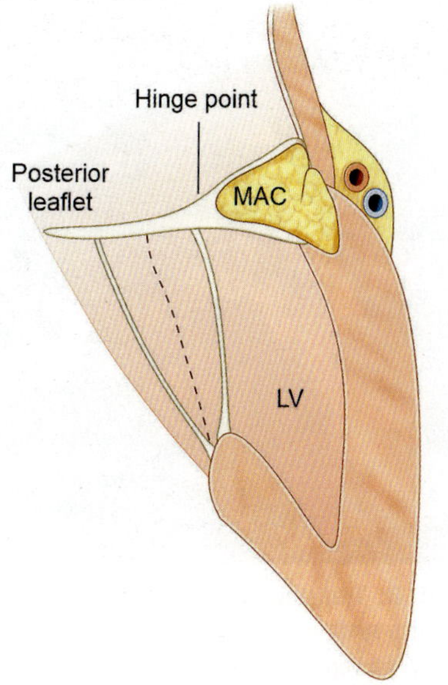

FIG. 9: Schema of the mitral annular calcification (MAC). Deposition of calcium in cellular degradation products of dying interstitial cells of the annulus.

change. Myxomatous degeneration is characterized by proteoglycan accumulation, collagen degradation, and elastic fiber fragmentation.[17] These changes result in a voluminous valve that is prone to prolapse and regurgitation **(Figs. 10 and 11)**. Conversely, fibrosis as seen in FED is characterized by collagen accumulation, proteoglycan degradation, and elastic fiber fragmentation with thinning of the valve leaflets.[17] Histologically, MDMV is characterized by thickening and proliferation of the spongiosa with pooling of glycosaminoglycans that expand to eliminate the fibrosa, giving the appearance of cystic spaces and less dense collagen **(Flowchart 1)**.[17]

Degeneration can be arbitrarily classified as follows:

- *Stage 0*: No change in valve
- *Stage 1*: Morphological change without hemodynamic change. Focal leaflet thickening or calcification
- *Stage 2*: Moderate stenosis and/or regurgitation along with morphometric changes
- *Stage 3*: Severe stenosis and/or regurgitation with gross leaflet changes

MYXOMATOUS DEGENERATION OF THE MITRAL VALVE

Myxomatous degeneration is a noninflammatory progressive disease of the valve structure caused by a defect in the biomechanical integrity of the leaflet due to the altered synthesis and/or remodeling by collagen and excess of proteoglycans in the spongiosa layer. It is characterized by:

- Voluminous and thickened leaflets **(Figs. 10 to 12)**
- Elongated, thickened, and fleshy chordae tendineae with or without rupture

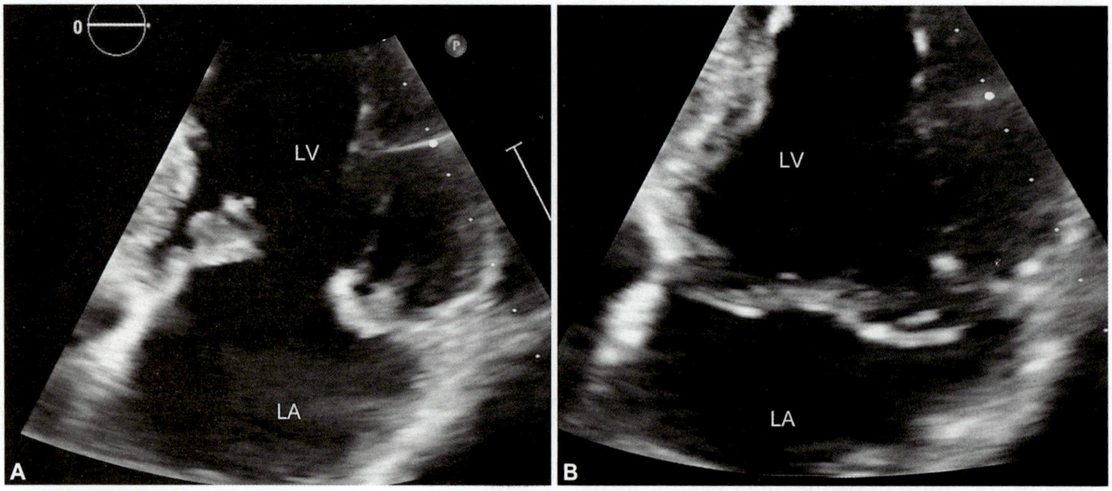

FIGS. 10A AND B: Transthoracic apical four-chamber view in diastole (panel A) and systole (panel B) showing thick and voluminous mitral valve leaflets with systolic superior displacement. Classic myxomatous degeneration with enlarged left atrium due to mitral regurgitation.
(LA: left atrium; LV: left ventricle)

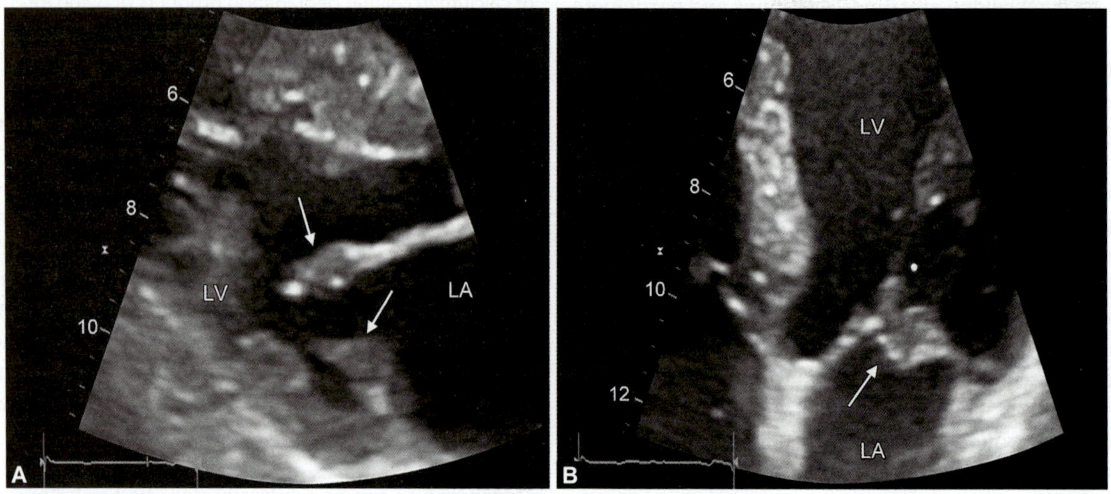

FIGS. 11A AND B: Transthoracic parasternal long-axis view (panel A) in diastole and four-chamber view in systole (panel B) showing thickening of the leaflets confined to rough zones. Another variant of myxomatous degeneration.
(LA: left atrium; LV: left ventricle)

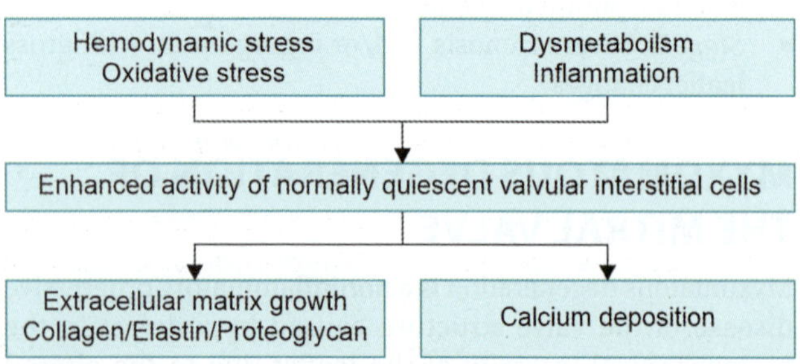

FLOWCHART 1: Mechanism of degeneration.

- Normal or mildly enlarged annulus
- No commissural fusion
- More often involvement of the posterior leaflet
- Hypermobility of the tensor apparatus
- Occasional tumor-like focal leaflet proliferative thickening

Myxomatous degeneration accounts for about 10% cases undergoing surgery for valvular regurgitation,[18] mostly involving mitral valve followed by aortic valve and then combined mitral and aortic regurgitation. Isolated tricuspid

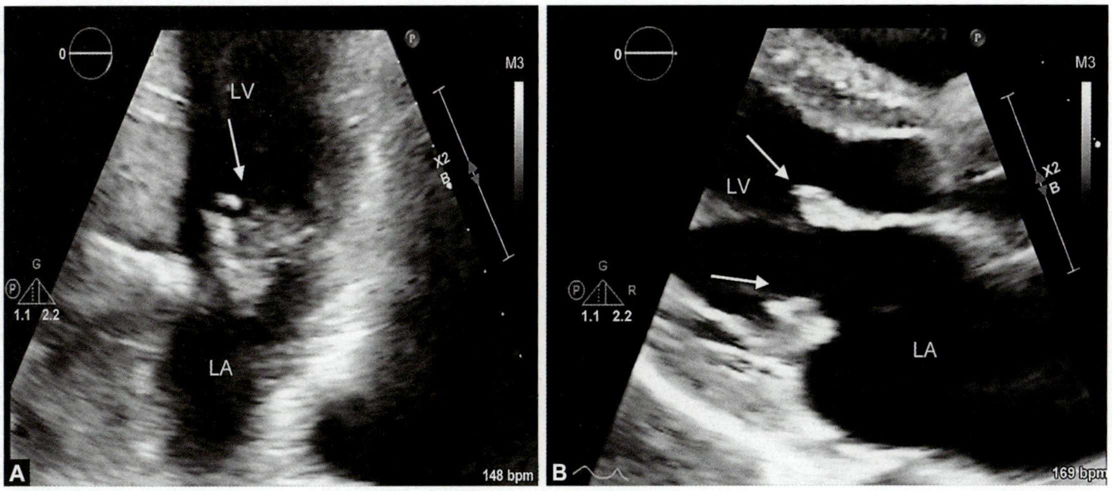

FIGS. 12A AND B: Transthoracic apical two-chamber view (panel A) and parasternal long-axis view (panel B) showing markedly tumor-like thickened mitral valve leaflets.

(LA: left atrium; LV: left ventricle)

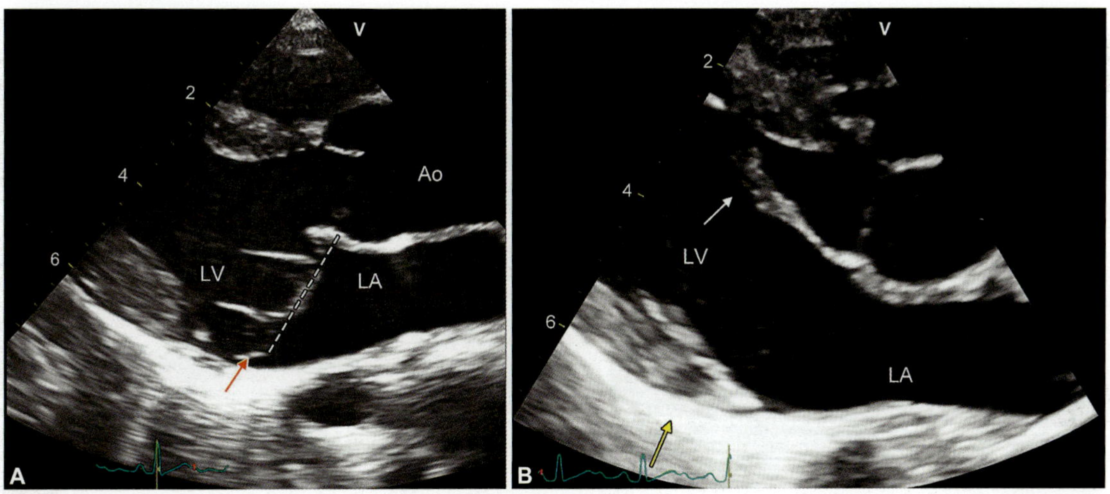

FIGS. 13A AND B: Transthoracic parasternal long-axis view showing bileaflet systolic prolapse beyond the marked annular plane (interrupted line) in panel A. Panel B shows leaflet thickening of the rough zones in diastole. Red arrow points toward atrioventricular discontinuity of the myocardium.

(Ao: aorta; LA: left atrium; LV: left ventricle)

valve involvement is uncommon but combined mitral and tricuspid involvement is frequently seen. The three prominent features of myxomatous valve are leaflet thickening, prolapse, and chordal rupture. Precise diagnostic criterion of prolapse is systolic atrial displacement of the valve leaflets by ≥2 mm beyond the annular plane in the echocardiographic long-axis view[19] as shown in **Figure 13**. Thickening of leaflets is defined as focal or diffuse leaflet thickness exceeding 3 mm.

Myxomatous degeneration can be confined to a single segment of the leaflet **(Figs. 14 and 15)** or may involve all segments of the mitral valve. The leaflets in advanced myxomatous degeneration are voluminous and aneurysmal, and the number of prolapsing segments is proportional to the degree of displacement of the mitral annulus. Hypermobility of the tension apparatus leads to increased mechanical stress on the leaflet tissue, with subsequent secondary thickening and elongation of both leaflets and chordae tendineae.

Myxomatous degeneration is not synonymous with mitral valve prolapse although the two coexist frequently. Myxomatous degeneration with or without leaflet prolapse is the commonest Mendelian cardiovascular abnormality in humans with varying spectrum. Mitral valve prolapse occurs in 2–3% of the general population and can be inherited or acquired.[19] Myxomatous degeneration represents the result of multiple genetic and/or acquired pathways alterations and may be syndromic and nonsyndromic.[20] Familial, inherited forms of mitral valve prolapse (MVP) present more frequently as a Barlow disease, with abundant, myxomatous

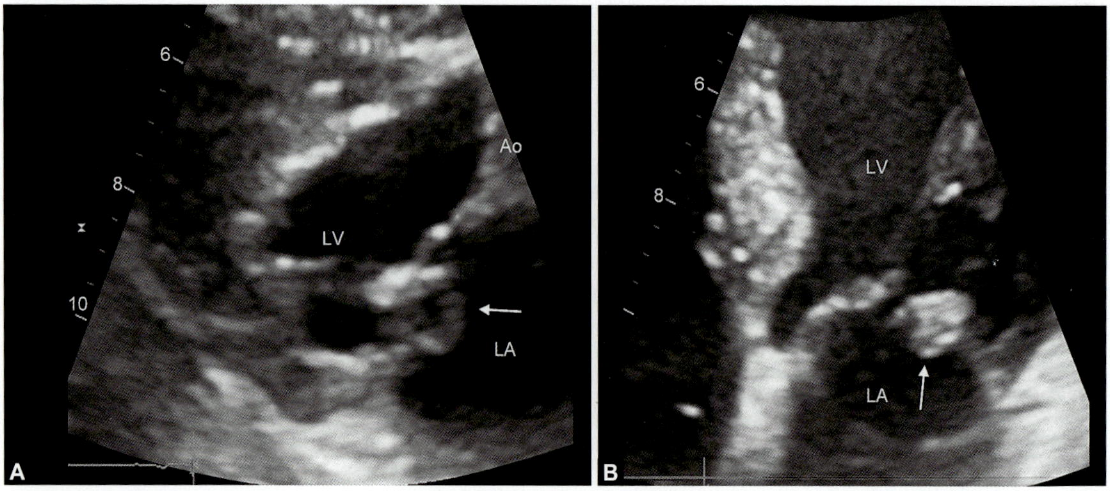

FIGS. 14A AND B: Parasternal long-axis view in systole (panel A) and apical four-chamber view in diastole (panel B) showing isolated involvement of P2 segment.
(LA: left atrium; LV: left ventricle)

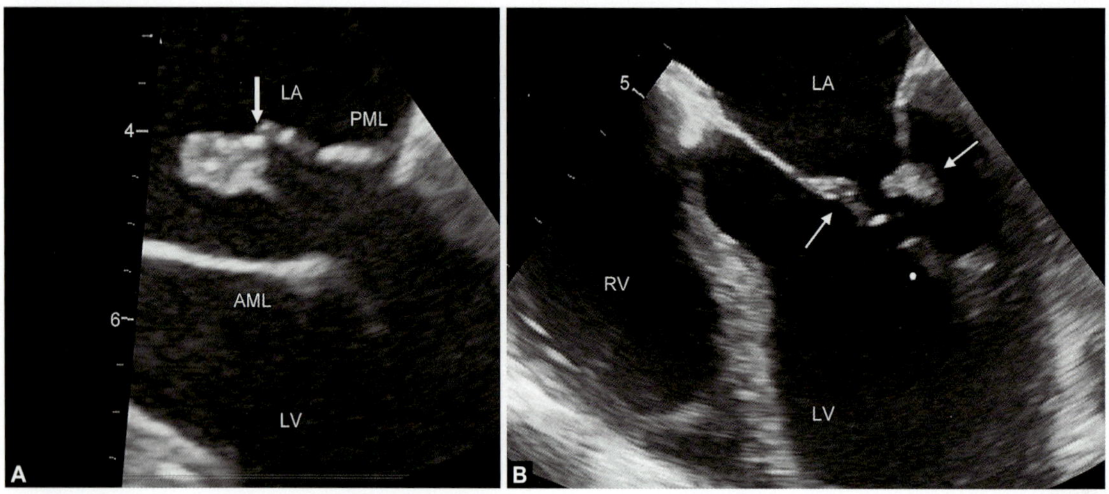

FIGS. 15A AND B: Transesophageal four-chamber view showing P2 thickening confined to a small portion of the leaflet giving tumor-like appearance with flail leaflet (thick arrow) in panel A and B.
(AML: anterior mitral leaflet; LA: left atrium; LV: left ventricle; PML: posterior mitral leaflet)

leaflets, the sporadic, degenerative forms generally show the features common to FED.[20] Finally, myxomatous mitral valve disease (MMVD) may present as a unique component of the cardiovascular disease involving a significant proportion of patients affected by connective tissue diseases such as Marfan syndrome, Loeys-Dietz syndrome, Ehlers-Danlos syndrome, osteogenesis imperfecta, pseudoxanthoma elasticum and also with trisomy and Down syndrome.[21] Thus, apart from sporadic form, myxomatous mitral valve is a dominantly inherited condition with incomplete and age-dependent penetrance, that can also be an X chromosome inherited disease **(Figs. 16 and 17)**.

The patients with syndromic MMVD are usually much younger, have a specific genetic transmission and associated cardiac and extracardiac abnormalities. Sporadic MMVD is much more common than syndromic one. A malignant variety of MMVD has been described which is characterized by young age, bileaflet prolapse, mitral annulus dysjunction **(Figs. 16 and 17)**, systolic inward curling of the basal inferolateral wall, fibrosis of the papillary muscle, electrocardiographic repolarization abnormalities in inferolateral leads, ventricular arrhythmias, and occasional sudden cardiac death.[22]

FIBROELASTIC DEFICIENCY

Clinicians distinguish classically two main types of DMVD—fibroelastic degeneration which occurs in the elderly, and myxomatous degeneration also called Barlow disease which develops earlier in the lifespan.[23,24] In contrast to Barlow

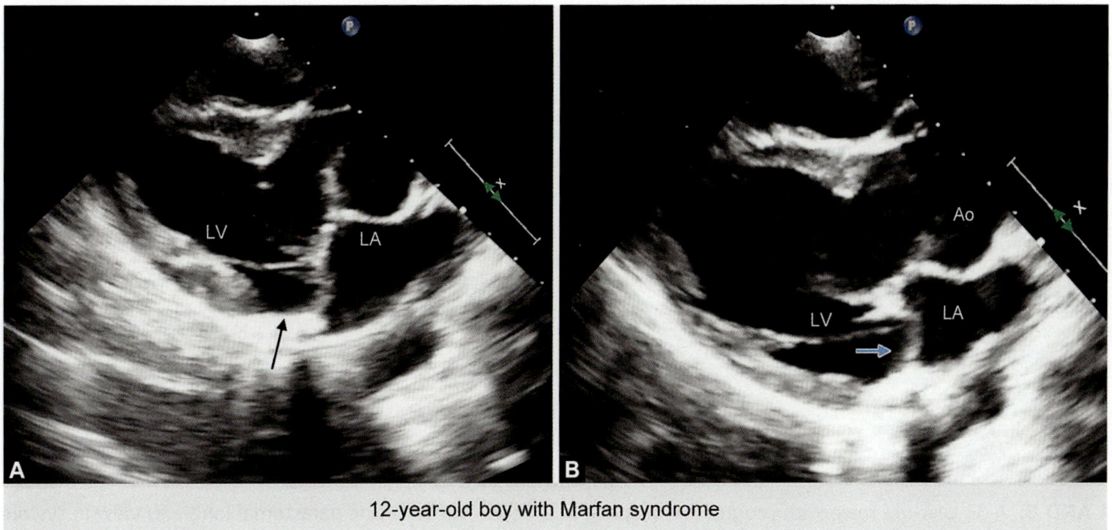

FIGS. 16A AND B: Transthoracic parasternal long-axis view showing mitral annulus dysjunction in systole (black arrow) and prolapse of the posterior leaflet (blue arrow).
(LA: left atrium; LV: left ventricle)

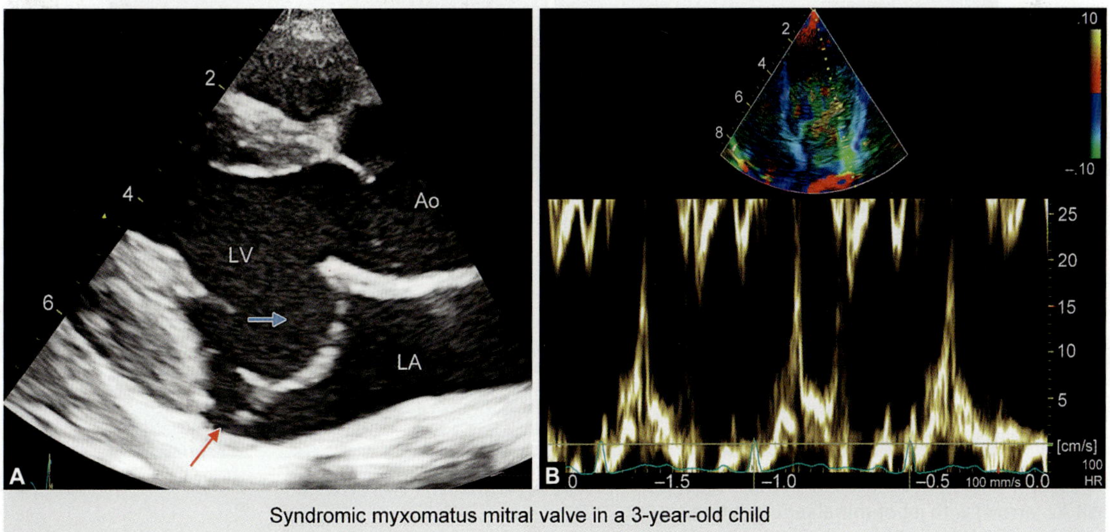

FIGS. 17A AND B: Transthoracic parasternal long-axis view in systole in a 3-year-old child with annuloaortic ectasia (panel A) showing bileaflet prolapse (blue arrow), mitral annulus dysjunction (red arrow), and tissue Doppler Pickelhaube sign with sample volume placed at lateral edge of the mitral annulus (panel B).
(LA: left atrium; LV: left ventricle)

disease, patients with mitral regurgitation due to FED have a lack of connective tissue as the pathological mechanism that triggers leaflet and chordal thinning and eventual chordal rupture. Typical findings in FED are:

- Thin leaflets and chordae
- Normal or near-normal valve size
- Typically single segment prolapse, most commonly of the middle scallop of the posterior leaflet (P2) **(Figs. 18 and 19)**.
- The prolapsing segment may appear to be distended, thickened, and elongated, while the adjacent segments appear normal in height and consistency.
- Billowing of nonprolapsing segments is not observed.
- Bi-leaflet dysfunction is not seen.
- There is no mitral annulus dysjunction.

Fibroelastic degeneration is characterized by thinning of the leaflets due to reduced production of elastin, proteoglycans, and collagen. The three-layer architecture of the leaflet is preserved. Primarily, there is elastin deficiency. Secondary myxomatous changes may occur in the prolapsed segment but is not mandatory. Rupture of thin, deficient chords is the usual mechanism of regurgitation in affected patients. The affected segment is unsupported and flailed and there is no billowing.

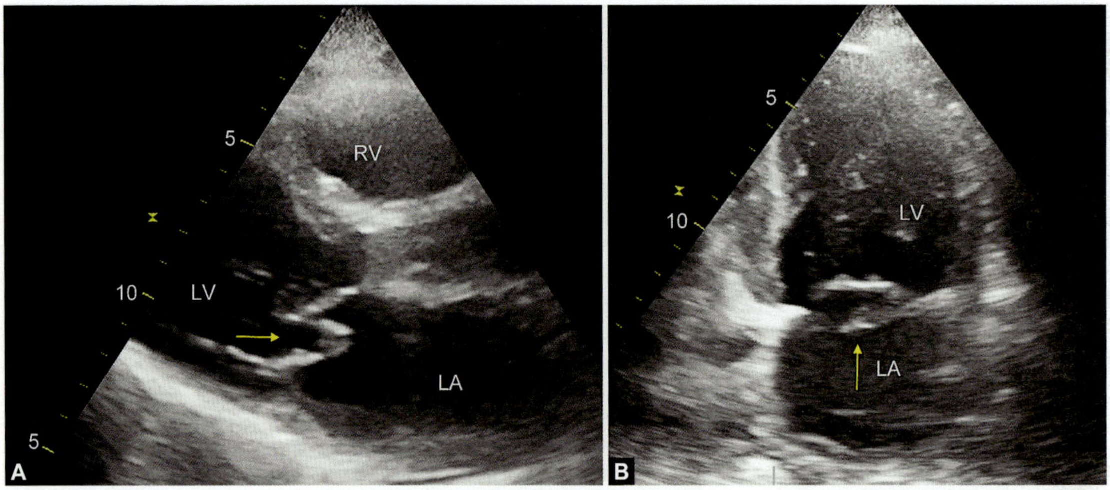

FIGS. 18A AND B: A 58-year-old male with progressive dyspnea of 3 years. Transthoracic parasternal long-axis view in systole (panel A) and apical four-chamber view (panel B) showing isolated prolapse of flail P2 segment of the posterior leaflet (yellow arrows). The anterior leaflet shows no thickening or prolapse.

(LA: left atrium; LV: left ventricle; RV: right ventricle)

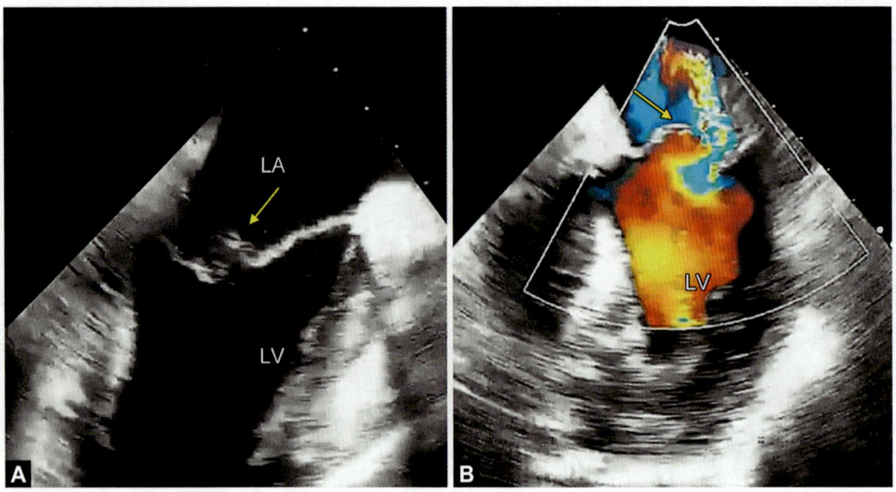

FIGS. 19A AND B: A 63-year-old male with heart failure. Transesophageal two-chamber view (panel A) and four-chamber view (panel B) showing flail A2 (arrow) with jet of mitral regurgitation.

(LA: left atrium; LV: left ventricle)

MITRAL ANNULAR CALCIFICATION AND DEGENERATIVE MITRAL VALVE

Mitral annular calcification represents an increasingly complex degenerative process which starts in the annulus and in later stages, extends into the leaflets. Its prevalence is estimated between 8 and 15%,[25] mostly in patients with advancing age, atherosclerotic disease, diabetes, chronic kidney disease, etc. It is independently associated with increased prevalence of cardiovascular disease and poor prognosis.[26] It may result in mitral stenosis (MS) or regurgitation **(Figs. 20 and 21)**. Uncommonly, it provides nidus for intracardiac thrombus formation.[27] In 25% cases, there is extra-annular calcification involving the ventricular walls, papillary muscles, and posterior leaflet.[28]

Mitral annular calcification usually starts in the posterior part of the annulus **(Fig. 22)**. Posteriorly, the fibrous layer of the mitral annulus is discontinuous and periodically interrupted by fat tissue. Interstitial cells present at the junction or annulus posteriorly undergo apoptosis and necrosis with age or as a consequence of calcium dysmetabolism. Cellular degradation products invite calcium deposition. Some interstitial cells undergo myofibroblastic differentiation and penetrate the basal portions of the atrioventricular junction.

Although 2D echocardiography is the initial imaging modality for MAC, computed tomography (CT) represents the gold standard with regard to presence of MAC, its extent and classification **(Fig. 23)**. Initially, a qualitative echocardiographic classification was proposed wherein MAC

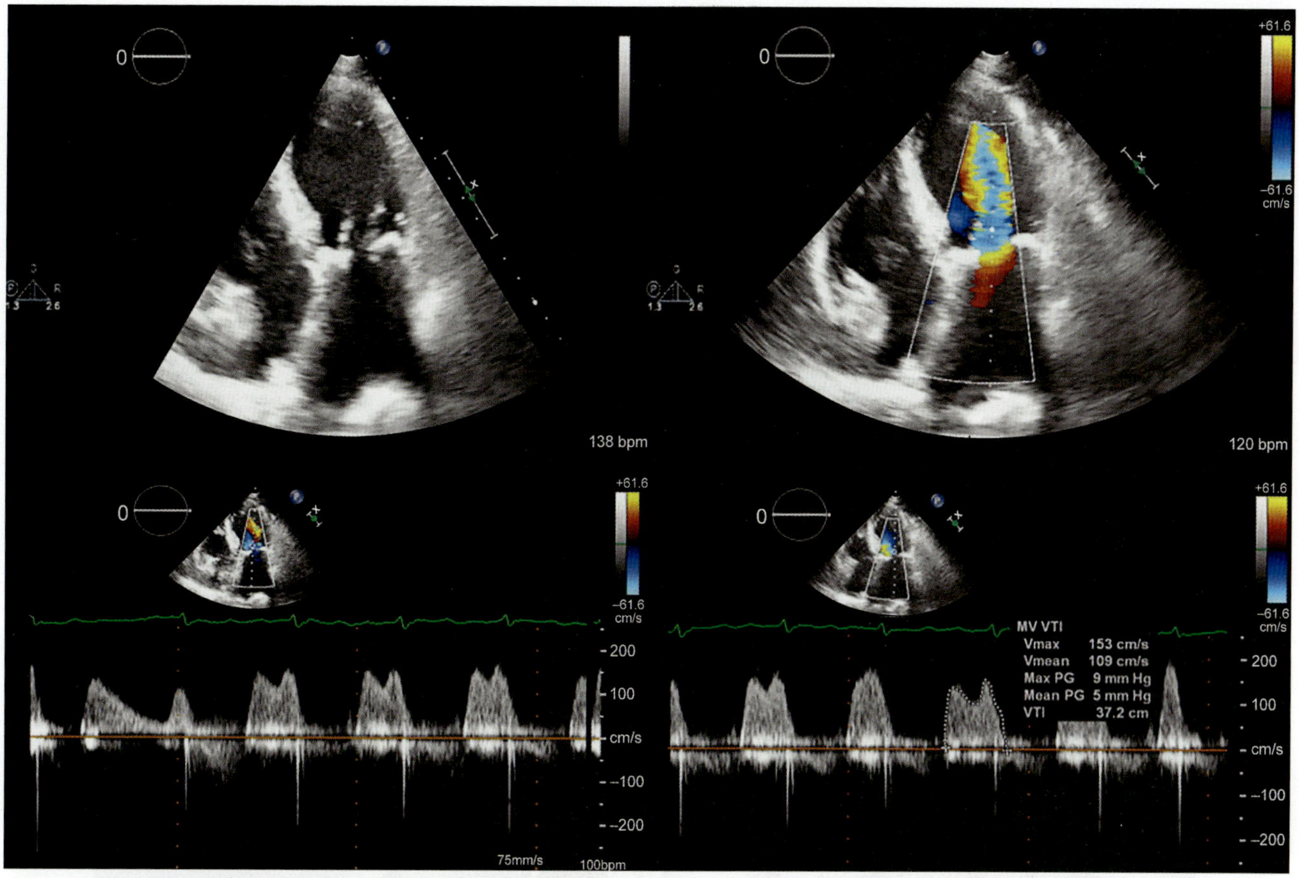

FIG. 20: Mitral annular calcification (MAC) in an 84-year-old female. Upper panels represent transthoracic apical four-chamber view and show narrowed left ventricular inflow. The lower panels show a mean transmitral diastolic gradient of 5 mm Hg on continuous-wave Doppler examination.

was defined as "mild" in presence of only focal calcifications, confined to mitral annulus, "moderate" when >1/3 but <1/2 of mitral annulus is involved and "severe" when more than half of ring circumference is affected, with calcifications intrusion into left ventricular wall.[29] A comprehensive score system based upon computerized tomography is the standard method to evaluate MAC and its suitability for surgical versus transcatheter intervention **(Fig. 24)**. Four characteristics are taken into account—calcium thickness, calcium distribution in the annulus circumference, calcification of one or both fibrous trigones, and leaflet involvement. The sum of points acquired in each of these categories makes the final score, with a score of 3 or less representing mild MAC, 4–6 moderate MAC, and 7 or more severe MAC.[30]

Mitral stenosis is more frequent in MAC than regurgitation. MS occurs due to decreased diastolic motion of the annulus, restricted leaflet motion, and calcium extending into the leaflets. Unlike rheumatic MS, there is no commissural fusion, leaflet thickening or subvalvular fusion. Despite apparently severe MS, valvular impedance may not be severe and high transmitral pressure gradients may denote higher net left atrioventricular stiffness. MAC is associated with at least 50% higher cardiovascular mortality and morbidity compared to matched controls.[31] When MAC is associated with significant MS or regurgitation and needs operative intervention, there are risks of rupture of atrioventricular junction, perivalvular leaks, atrioventricular blocks, injury to the left circumflex artery, and embolism.[25] Nonsurgical methods including transcatheter mitral valve repair or replacement are promising techniques albeit with higher mortality.

HEMODYNAMIC QUANTIFICATION

Transthoracic echocardiography (TTE) is the initial imaging modality for assessing the mechanism, etiology, severity, and repair probability of DMVD. CT imaging is an integral part of evaluating MAC, its severity and operability. When TTE leaves doubts about quantification, cardiac magnetic resonance (CMR) imaging and/or transesophageal echocardiography (TEE) provide complementary and incremental information. TEE helps in grading MR severity, although its incremental value over TTE or CMR is to provide a comprehensive assessment of the anatomical lesions and mechanism of MR.

Assessment of degenerative mitral regurgitation is no different from regular cases of valvular regurgitation. The

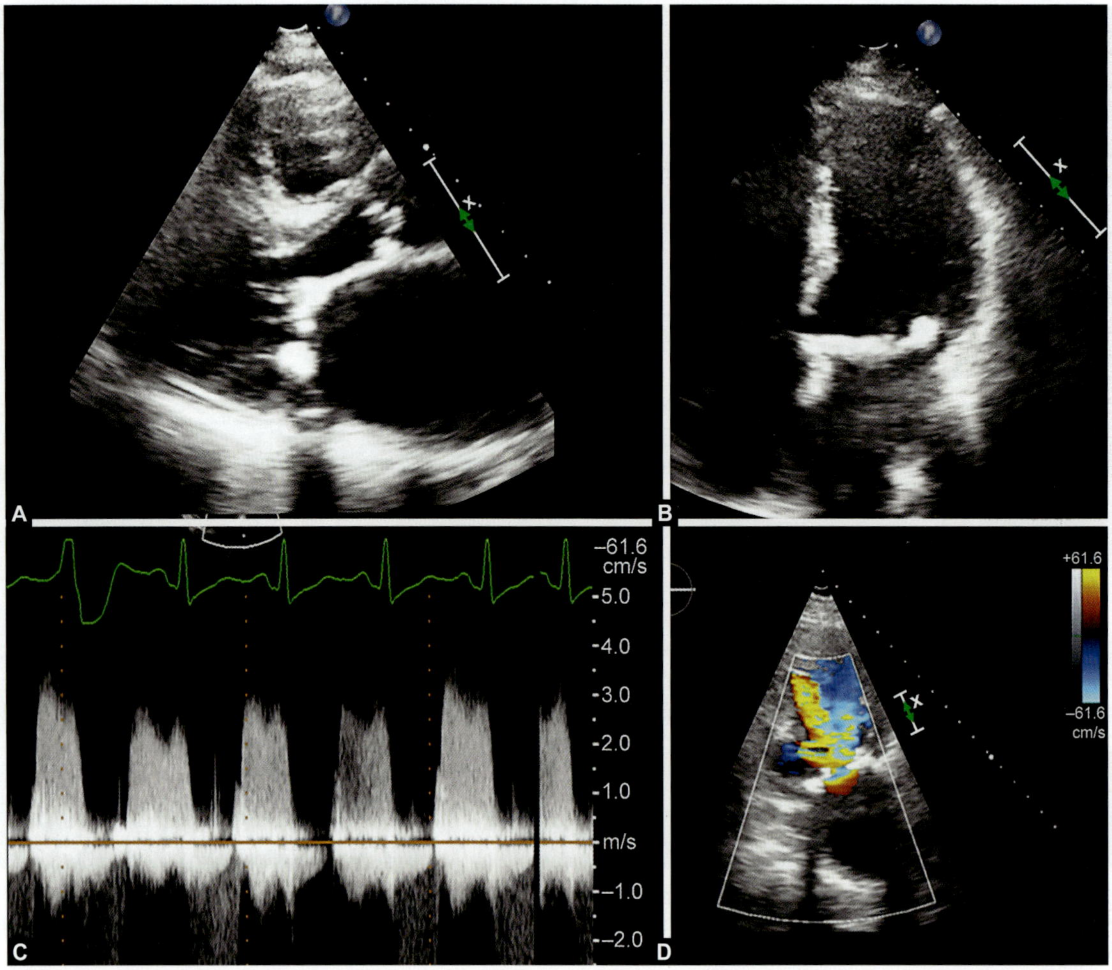

FIGS. 21A TO D: Mitral annular calcification (MAC) in a 67-year-old male. Panel A shows calcification of mitral and aortic annulus in parasternal long-axis view. Panel B shows a horizontal bar of hyperechoic tissue in place of annulus in apical four-chamber view. Panel C shows a peak transmitral velocity of 3.2 m/s while panel D shows turbulent color Doppler flow across the mitral orifice.

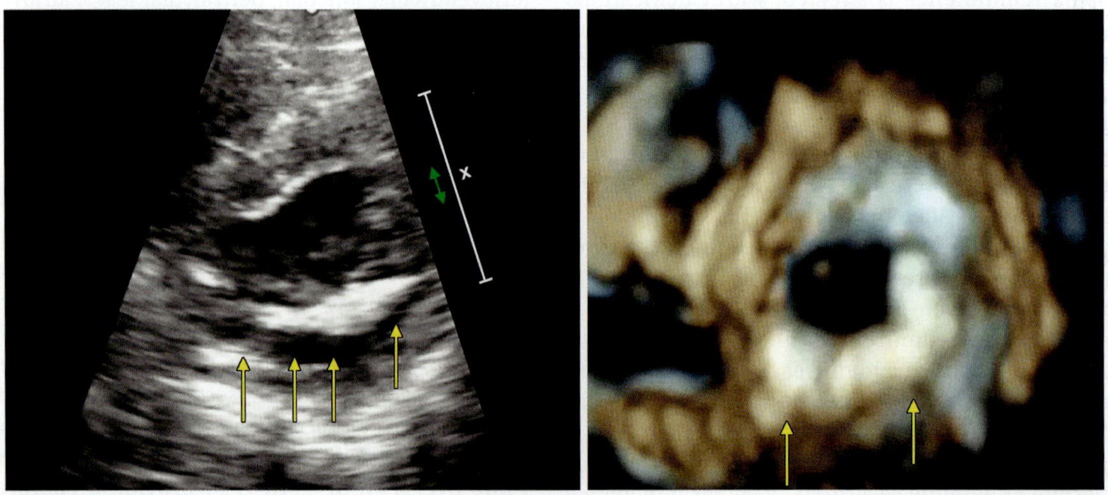

FIG. 22: 2D (left) and 3D (right) parasternal short-axis views showing MAC involving the posterior annulus with an arch of about 180°. The anterior annulus is spared.

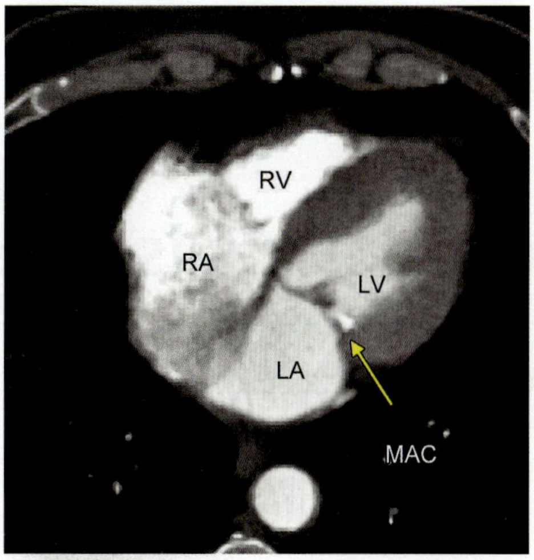

FIG. 23: A speck of calcium in posterior mitral annulus in computerized tomographic (CT) axial view (yellow arrow).
(LA: left atrium; LV: left ventricle; RA: right atrium; RV: right ventricle)

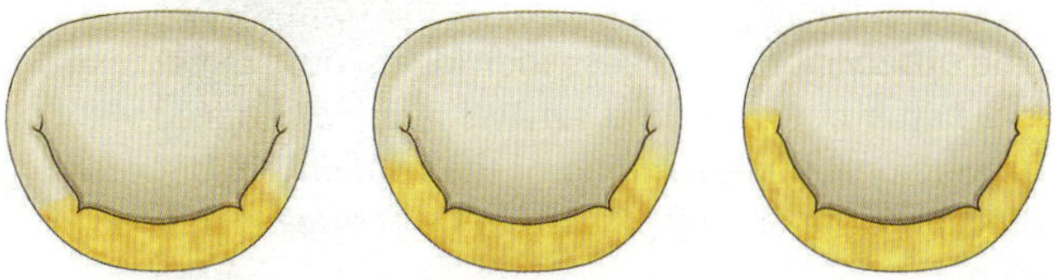

FIG. 24: Schema showing CT-based grading of the mitral annular calcification (MAC). The yellow portion represents calcium in the annulus.

estimation of mitral regurgitation by semi-quantitative and quantitative methods is imperative in every case. Grading severity of regurgitation may be challenging as in late-systolic MR, bi-leaflet prolapse with multiple jets or extensive leak, wall-hugging eccentric jet or in multi-mechanism mitral insufficiency.

Calcific MS secondary to MAC is hard to quantify by usual echocardiographic methods. Valvular impedance may be surpassed by left ventricular diastolic dysfunction. Higher transmitral gradients need not necessarily represent severe MS because stiffer left atrium, associated morbidities and local accelerative forces can increase initial driving pressure resulting in high mean pressure gradients.[32] Low stroke volume due to associated heart failure with preserved ejection fraction which is common in these patients, can result in overestimation of severity of valve area by continuity equation.

SURGICAL OR TRANSCATHETER APPROACH

Indication for surgery or transcatheter intervention is based on the severity of MS and/or regurgitation and the presence of symptoms, LV dilatation and dysfunction, atrial fibrillation or pulmonary hypertension. Mitral valve repair is preferred over mitral valve replacement and successful possibility of repair decides the indication and timing of surgery. The feasibility of mitral valve repair largely depends on the complexity of mitral valve pathology, and the surgical approach is often different between FED and MMVD according to the mitral valve lesions. Usually an annuloplasty is performed using a ring to stabilize the annulus in both types of patients. Additional surgical repair techniques, such as annular plication, leaflet resection, leaflet sliding, and neochord implantation have been developed with the aim of correcting any leaflet prolapse, as well as taking care of excessive leaflet tissue and preventing systolic anterior motion of the mitral valve. Inspection of the valve during surgery reveals differences between FED and Barlow disease, and while in most FED cases neochordae implantation is sufficient, Barlow's valves often require different resecting techniques. Repair in some cases may be complex and less than satisfactory.

Patients with MAC and significant mitral valve disease represent a high-risk surgical population with an increased risk of atrioventricular junction rupture, circumflex artery injury, atrioventricular blocks, and embolism.[25] As a consequence, transcatheter mitral valve replacement has been proposed as a safer alternative. Newer devices, specifically designed to fit the complex shape of mitral annulus, are being developed in order to treat mitral valve disease in patients deemed too high risk to undergo conventional surgery. In the complex anatomical and clinical context of patients with MACs and significant mitral valve disease, conventional surgery still represents, in eligible subjects, the gold standard of treatment, capable of ensuring durable results.

CONCLUSION

Degenerative mitral valve disease accounts for significant valvular interventions in the current scenario. MAC, a unique type of valve apparatus degeneration, is on the rise due to increasing longevity, chronic kidney disease, and other conventional risk factors of atherosclerosis. This variety poses unique challenges in management of the patients and is associated with high morbidity and mortality.

ONLINE REFERENCES

Please scan the QR code provided at the end of the table of contents for References of this chapter.

CHAPTER 20

Obesity Paradox in Heart Disease

Vikas Agrawal, Dheeraj Kela, Aqdas Mumtaz

ABSTRACT

Obesity has long been recognized as a significant risk factor for various health conditions, including cardiovascular disease. However, recent studies have shed light on a counterintuitive phenomenon known as the "obesity paradox" in the context of heart disease. The obesity paradox refers to the observation that obese individuals, despite being at a higher risk for developing cardiovascular disease, tend to have better outcomes and survival rates when faced with certain cardiac conditions. This paradox has challenged our conventional understanding of the relationship between obesity and heart disease. In this chapter, we will explore the concept of the obesity paradox in heart disease and delve into the possible explanations behind this intriguing phenomenon.

Keywords: Obesity, cardiorespiratory fitness, obesity paradox, body composition, cardiovascular disease.

INTRODUCTION

Obesity is a global public health problem. The most severe effects of obesity are currently being felt by the healthcare systems of poor countries as a result of the adoption of western dietary practices with a sedentary lifestyle. Nearly 13.5 crore Indians are currently obese. In India, the obesity epidemic has grown to affect 11.8–31.3% of the population; abdominal obesity is also common among this group, with prevalence rates ranging from 16.9 to 36.3%.[1] It has reached epidemic proportions and is an independent risk factor for several noncommunicable diseases, including heart diseases.[2]

However, in patients with established cardiovascular disease (CVD), the link between obesity and clinical outcomes has not always been clear, leading to reports of an obesity paradox. The obesity paradox is particularly important for heart failure (HF) and coronary heart disease (CHD)[3] but is also reported in other CVDs, such as hypertension (HTN), pulmonary arterial hypertension (PAH), and atrial fibrillation (AF).

The body mass index (BMI) is a commonly used index for diagnosing obesity, and increased BMI is the surrogate marker of increased adiposity. However, BMI-based measurement represents both fat mass (FM) and non-FM; therefore, it does not differentiate between increased FM and increased lean mass (LM) or a combination of both. Moreover, the distribution of body fat cannot be assessed with BMI, which is crucial, since it is the visceral adiposity that is associated with poor cardiovascular (CV) health.[3,4] Furthermore, the understanding of body composition (BC) (LM or FM) as a predictor of patient outcomes with established CVD has an important implication in guiding weight management. We will review about obesity paradox in CVDs, the role of cardiorespiratory fitness (CRF), and weight loss in determining the prognosis in patients with obesity and established CVD.

COMPARTMENTALIZING OBESITY

Obesity is defined as *excess body fat that impairs health*.[5] The BMI is a commonly used index for diagnosing obesity, and increased BMI $\geq$ 30 kg/m^2 is the surrogate marker of increased adiposity.[3,5]

The simplest BC model divides body weight into two compartments, FM and fat-free mass (FFM), which assumes that both remain constant during the course of our lives and/or in the setting of pathophysiologic conditions and that the composition of FFM does not change over time. FFM is the largest BC compartment, and it includes total body water, bones, and skeletal muscle mass (SMM); the latter and total body water compose LM **(Fig. 1)**.[6-8]

The assessment of FM is crucial to determine excess adiposity and, therefore, to characterize obesity. However, LM is regarded as the ideal surrogate for SMM. The assessment of SMM or its surrogates has recently been acknowledged as a significant part of the nutritional status assessment. Lower SMM, especially in the extremities (i.e., appendicular SMM), is linked to decreased functioning and exercise intolerance[9,10] and is referred to as sarcopenia,[11] a condition that is linked to a poor prognosis in a number of chronic diseases. It is also important to note that obesity and sarcopenia can coexist when there is excessive adiposity and a decline in SMM and its functionality (i.e., sarcopenic obesity),[12] which is linked to even worse results **(Fig. 2)**.

In addition to not assessing BC, BMI also does not evaluate FM distribution. Indirect measurements of excess visceral adiposity, such as waist circumference (WC) or waist-to-hip ratio, have been found to be more strongly associated with cardiometabolic risk than BMI alone.[13]

WHAT IS OBESITY PARADOX?

The obesity paradox was first described by Gruberg et al.[14] nearly two decades ago where they observed better outcomes in overweight and obese patients with CHD undergoing

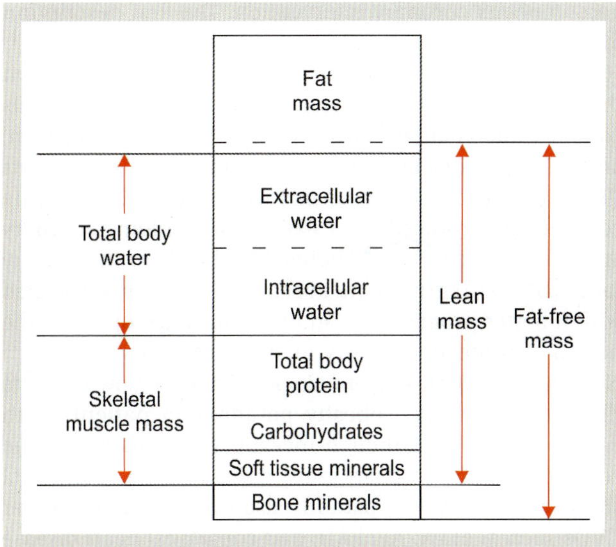

FIG. 1: Body composition models. Total body mass can be divided into different body composition compartments. The most commonly used model is the two-compartment model, which divides total body mass into fat mass and fat-free mass. Fat-free mass can be divided into lean mass and bones. Lean mass, the best surrogate for skeletal muscle mass, can be further divided into body water (extracellular and intracellular), total body protein, carbohydrates, and soft tissue minerals.

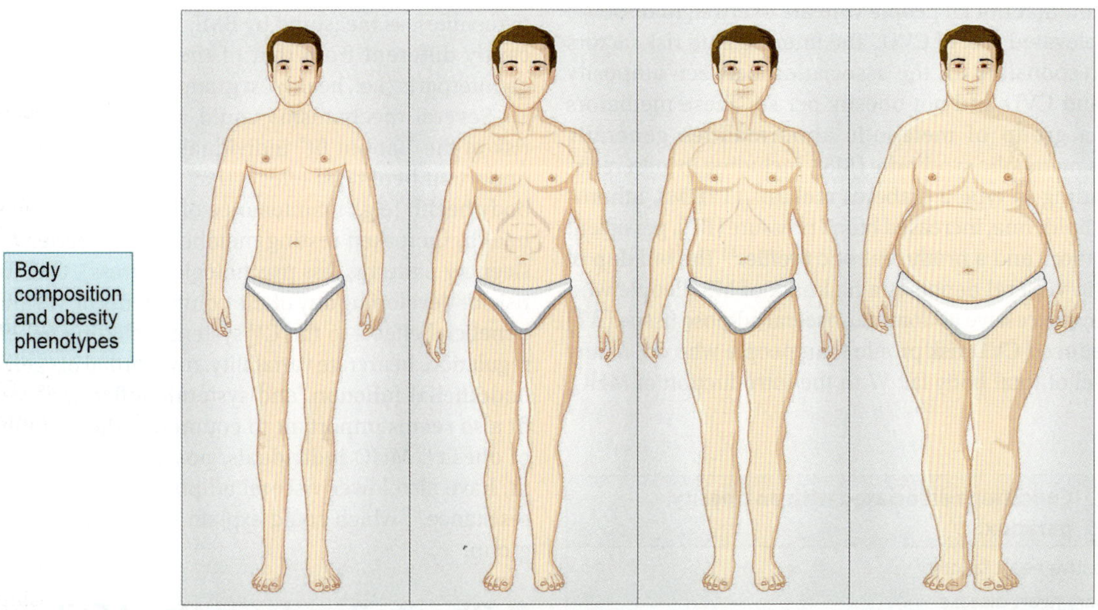

	Normal weight	Athlete	Nonsarcopenic obese	Sarcopenic obese
BMI (kg/m^2)	18.5–25	>30	>30	>30
Fat mass	Normal	Decreased	Decreased	Increased
Lean mass	Normal	Increased	Increased	Decreased
CRF	Normal	Increased	Mild impairment	Severe impairment

FIG. 2: Various phenotypes of increased BMI according to the proportion of fat and lean mass.
(BMI: body mass index; CRF: cardiorespiratory fitness)

percutaneous coronary intervention. The first description of obesity paradox in HF was given by Horwich et al.[15] "Obesity paradox" was coined to describe this association that obese patients with systolic HF[15] or postpercutaneous coronary intervention[14] have a better prognosis. Since then, an obesity paradox has been reported in overweight patients (BMI range of 25.0–30.0 kg/m^2) with stable CHD,[16] acute coronary syndromes,[17,18] or patients undergoing coronary artery bypass grafting.[19] Higher BMI levels in the obesity range (BMI >30 kg/m^2) have not consistently been associated with a better prognosis.[20] Other groups have opposed the notion of protective obesity in stable coronary patients.[21] Nonetheless, ample epidemiological evidence now supports the presence of an "obesity paradox" in patients with established CVD. Although investigated primarily in the context of HF and coronary artery disease (CAD), recent data shows that the obesity paradox also exists in various other CVDs such as HTN, AF, PAH, and congenital heart disease (**Box 1**).[22]

Metabolically Healthy Obesity

While the "obesity paradox" seems to be an epidemiological finding associated with the limitations of BMI, clinical evidence suggests that a subgroup of obese individuals [defined either by BMI or by body fat percentage (BF%) criteria] is indeed characterized by low CVD risk. The idea of metabolically healthy obesity (MHO) evolved from the observation that not all people who are overweight or obese have an elevated risk of CVD. The intermediate risk factors may be responsible for the association between adiposity indices and CVD and not obesity per se. These mediators include a group of metabolic abnormalities generally known as metabolic syndrome (MS), including insulin resistance leading to type 2 diabetes mellitus (T2DM), atherogenic dyslipidemia, increased blood pressure (BP), persistent inflammation, and a prothrombotic profile.[23] The buildup of extra fat in visceral depots is a hallmark of MS. People who do not have excessive abdominal visceral adipose tissue (AT) have a reduced CVD risk profile than people who do, at any given level of total body fat. With the introduction of MHO, an individualistic approach to treating obesity has replaced the "one-size-fits-all" approach in which not only the total quantity of body fat but also its geographical distribution has become of utmost importance.

It is currently estimated that the prevalence of the MHO is close to 12% of obese individuals (or 7 million of European adults).[24] Obese individuals (by BMI or BF%) with one of the following criteria: (1) No metabolic abnormalities (based on MS criteria), (2) no insulin resistance (based on homeostatic model assessment, quantitative insulin sensitivity check index, or hyperinsulinemic–euglycemic clamp measurements), (3) high CRF levels (based on maximal oxygen consumption during exercise treadmill test or muscle strength which is also a good surrogate), (4) low visceral AT volume (by imaging), and possibly also (5) low levels of systemic inflammatory mediators could be classified as MHO.[25]

BOX 1 **Conditions associated with an obesity paradox.**

- Congestive heart failure
- Coronary heart disease
- Following percutaneous coronary intervention
- Following coronary artery bypass grafting
- Hypertension
- Hypertensive emergency
- Pulmonary arterial hypertension
- Atrial fibrillation
- End-stage renal disease

Cardiorespiratory Fitness and the "Fat but Fit" Phenomenon

It has been suggested that being fit might attenuate some of the adverse consequences of obesity, independent of some key potential confounders. Studies conducted in the late 1990s offered the first proof of the phenomenon known as "fat but fit."[2] These studies showed that the all-cause and CVD mortality risk in obese people who are fit (i.e., have CRF levels above the age-specific and sex-specific 20th percentile), as measured by BMI, BF%, or WC, is not significantly different from that of their normal-weight and fit counterparts (i.e., healthiest group possible).

Several mechanisms could account for the low CVD risk of the "fat but fit" individuals. Exercise has numerous important beneficial effects that are associated with whole body health (e.g., maintenance of muscle mass and skeletal health, increased resting metabolic rate, better mood and sleeping patterns, less psychological stress). CRF lowers the risk for developing any of the components of MS and confers beneficial effects to the CV system including benefits in BP regulation, heart rate variability, myocardial oxygen demand, endothelial function, and systemic inflammation.[26] Being fit also seems important to counteract the metabolic perils of obesity. MHO individuals, possibly as a result of being fit, have also lower visceral adiposity and systemic insulin resistance,[27] which could explain the lower CVD risk in this group.

Obesity Paradox in Heart Failure

The obesity paradox in HF was initially observed in patients with advanced disease where the coexistence of overweight or obesity was associated with improved prognosis compared to normal weight or underweight patients.[15] In a meta-analysis involving 22,807 patients with chronic HF followed up for a mean duration of 2.85 years, the risk for total mortality, CV mortality, and hospitalization was highest in underweight patients with chronic HF and lowest in overweight subjects.[28] The association of BMI with risk of mortality was found to be graded in a cohort of acute decompensated HF patients. It was observed that for every 5 kg/m^2 increase in BMI, 30-day mortality was reduced by 11%, and 1-year mortality was reduced by 9%.[29] Subsequent studies have confirmed the obesity paradox in both HF with reduced left ventricular ejection fraction (LVEF) [heart failure with reduced ejection fraction (HFrEF)] and heart failure with preserved ejection fraction (HFpEF).[30]

Several workers indicate that the relationship between adiposity and survival in patients with HF maybe modified by the degree of CRF.[31-35] In an analysis of 4,623 patients from the Italian MECKI Score Research Group, the protective impact of BMI disappeared after adjustment for peak oxygen consumption (peak VO_2).[35] In another study, in patients with HFrEF who underwent cardiopulmonary exercise testing, BMI was a significant predictor of improved survival in the low-fitness group defined as peak VO_2 <14 mL/kg/min but not in the high-fitness group.[32] Thus in the unfit population, obese HF patients have better outcomes, whereas this benefit is lost when compared to groups with preserved fitness.

The obesity paradox has also been studied in light of new HF therapies. The effect of sodium-glucose cotransporter-2 inhibitor (SGLT-2I), dapagliflozin, according to baseline BMI in the DAPA-HF trial showed a U-shaped relationship seen with higher risk with both low and very high BMI. The lowest rate of primary outcome was found in patients of BMI around 30 kg/m^2.[36] A similar pattern was seen for the other outcomes of interest including CV death, worsening HF, and all-cause death. Thus, the obesity paradox persisted in HFrEF patients treated with dapagliflozin. However, no significant association between BMI and all-cause death or hospitalizations for HF was apparent after adjustment for different variables was seen in patients with HFrEF who were receiving sacubitril/valsartan.[37]

The mechanisms through which obesity improves prognosis in patients with HF are incompletely understood; however, several hypotheses have been proposed. Particularly, the increased LM in obese individuals may play a crucial role as it has been associated with improved long-term outcomes.[9] LM as a surrogate for SMM is a major predictor of CRF in HF,[10] and because greater BMI is typically associated with an increase in FM paralleled by increased LM and SMM, the increased BMI may be protective because of greater LM (**Flowchart 1**). The inaccuracy of BMI in obese patients differentiating BC compartments is a major limitation. Patients with excess adiposity and reduced LM do not do as well as those with an increase in both compartments.[38] The obesity paradox in HF disappears in those with relatively good CRF,[31,32] suggesting that independent of their BMI and BC, improving CRF should be prioritized when treating patients with HF.

Obesity Paradox in Hypertension

The AT has components of the renin-angiotensin-aldosterone system (RAAS), which explains why its activation is greater in obese people. This increased activation ultimately leads to glomerular damage, decreased natriuresis, increased fluid retention, and HTN.[39] Increased sympathetic nervous system (SNS) activity is also associated with obesity, especially visceral adiposity, which is linked to HTN. A physical renal compression caused by a rise in intra-abdominal pressure and accumulation of fat around and inside the kidney can also raise BP.[40]

Once HTN is detected, being overweight or obese has been proven to give some degree of protection, particularly when CHD is also present. Initial explanations for this obesity paradox included other confounding elements such as smoking and increased alcohol consumption.[41] Outcomes in 22,576 patients with HTN and CHD showed that despite worse control of BP, all-cause mortality was 30% lower in overweight and obese HTN patients compared with their leaner counterparts.[42] According to a recent meta-analysis involving 489,222 HTN participants, there is an 8% relative risk reduction for all-cause mortality for every 5-unit increase in BMI, and there is a substantial dose-dependent relationship between BMI and lower risk for CVD mortality.[43] The mechanisms by which obesity exerts beneficial effects in HTN are unknown. However, given that higher levels of renin are frequently linked to worse outcomes, the relatively lower levels of renin reported in obese patients may be accountable, at least in part, for this protection.

Obesity Paradox in Coronary Heart Disease

Increased atherosclerotic plaque load, characterized by macrophage infiltration and plaque erosion, has been linked to excess visceral adiposity.[44,45] The persistent systemic low-grade inflammation associated with obesity appears to be a key factor, despite the fact that the underlying mechanisms are not fully known. Patients who are obese exhibit an excessive activation of the inflammasome, which produces interleukin (IL)-1 and IL-18. In addition to cardiac cells and FM, these proinflammatory cytokines can also be produced by cells of the innate immune system in response to stimuli like free fatty acids, particularly saturated ones, and cholesterol crystals, both of which are elevated in the presence of obesity.[46] Additionally, obesity is linked to significant CHD risk factors, such as T2DM and dyslipidemia.

Although obesity is a major risk factor for CHD, patients with established CHD and a higher BMI have a more favorable prognosis, forming an obesity paradox similar to that seen in HF.[16,47,48] A metanalysis of 89 studies including >1.3 million CHD patients confirmed an obesity paradox. Such protective effects were seen mainly in overweight/

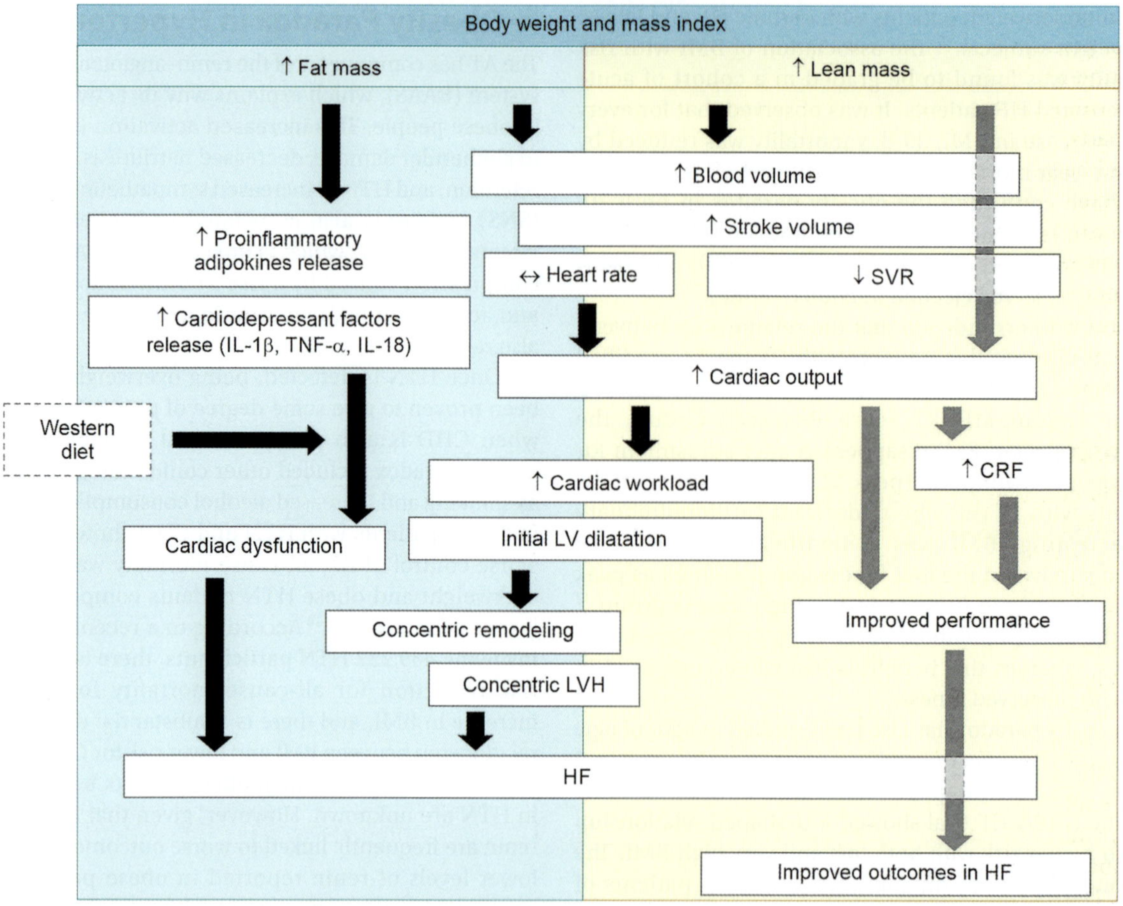

FLOWCHART 1: Potential mechanisms driving obesity to HF and the "obesity paradox" in patients with diagnosed HF. The detrimental effects of body composition compartments (i.e., fat mass and lean mass) on cardiac function are indicated by the black arrows. The gray arrows indicate the potential mechanisms by which body composition compartments (i.e., lean mass) improve CRF.

(CRF: cardiorespiratory fitness; HF: heart failure; IL: interleukin; LV: left ventricular, LVH: left ventricular hypertrophy; SVR: systemic vascular resistance; TNF: tumor necrosis factor).

mildly obese (BMI = 25–35 kg/m^2) patients, and interestingly, they started to disappear after approximately 5 years. However, in a study, patients with CAD and moderate/severe obesity (BMI > 35 kg/m^2) had higher mortality during long-term follow-up.[49]

The effect of BC has been rarely studied; however, more LM and FM have been linked to a better prognosis,[50] debunking the concept that LM would be the only protective BC compartment. Conversely, a worse prognosis was linked to lower levels of LM and FM. After myocardial infarction, obese elderly patients have reported lower in-hospital death rates in an interesting study.[48]

As was mentioned for HF, further explanation is needed for the obesity paradox in CHD. In CHD, CRF is a more significant independent predictor than BMI and WC, especially in patients with higher CRF.[51,52] In comparison to calorie restriction-induced weight reduction techniques not linked to exercise training, therapeutics meant to improve CRF, such as cardiac rehabilitation and increased physical activity, should be used more frequently and possibly given priority.[53] Compared to dieting alone, which typically results in FM as well as LM losses,[54] cardiac rehabilitation improves BC by increasing LM or preventing its loss, increasing physical activity, and building muscle strength.[55] Reducing the amount and functionality of LM in patients with sarcopenia, sarcopenic obesity, or those at high risk for such conditions can worsen outcomes.

Obesity Paradox in Pulmonary Arterial Hypertension

Obesity and a chronic insulin-resistant state typically resulting from excess adiposity have been recently associated with an increased risk of PAH.[56,57] PAH has also been associated with chronic systemic low-grade inflammation,[58,59] which is also characteristic of obesity. Recent studies suggest that the prevalence of obesity in PAH can reach up to 30%.[60]

The effects of obesity on prognosis in studies suggest a neutral or perhaps a protective role of obesity. A nationwide 9-year survey revealed lower in-hospital mortality among patients with PAH and obesity (3.5%) than nonobese (8.1%) counterparts.[61] In a recent study, patients with PAH who were obese had better prognosis with the exception of those who were severely obese and under 65 years old.[60] Obesity was linked to the lowest risk of in-hospital death in a registry of >18,000 patients with PAH, confirming an obesity paradox in this cohort. Another study of 267 PAH patients indicated that being overweight was linked to the lowest mortality rate, followed by obesity and morbid obesity, with normal-weight and underweight patients having the worst survival rates.[62]

Obesity Paradox in Atrial Fibrillation

Obesity is considered to be an independent risk factor for AF and obese patients have been shown to have a 50% increased risk of developing AF.[63] Obesity and especially severe obesity are associated with left atrial enlargement, conduction abnormalities, interstitial atrial fibrosis, and reduced posterior left atrial endocardial voltage, which are associated with a greater risk for AF.[64] The risk of AF is further increased by the high prevalence of HTN and HF in this population. A chronic low-grade systemic inflammation linked to the activation of the NLRP3 (NOD-,LRR- and pyrin domain-containing protein 3) inflammasome pathway has also been linked to the pathogenesis of AF.[65]

An obesity paradox has been demonstrated in patients with AF. Despite clear evidence supporting the increased risk for AF in obese patients, once AF is diagnosed, multiple studies have demonstrated that obese patients present an improved long-term prognosis. A registry-based study involving 9,606 patients with AF demonstrated lower all-cause mortality with higher BMI in patients with AF.[66] In about 2,500 patients with AF, overweight and obesity were associated with the lowest risk for all-cause mortality as well as CVD mortality during a mean follow-up of 3 years.[67] In a study of almost 18,000 patients with AF, visceral adiposity was also assessed using WC and the ones who were defined obese using BMI and WC presented an improved prognosis.[68]

The relationship between CRF and concurrent obesity and AF has also been reported. Greater CRF enhances the positive effects of deliberate weight loss in a cohort by being associated with reduced AF-related complications (i.e., recurrent arrhythmia).[69] These findings support the idea that in patients with obesity and AF, the main objective of lifestyle and pharmacological therapy should be to increase CRF.

BIOLOGICAL HYPOTHESIS AND MECHANISMS FOR OBESITY PARADOX

Numerous mechanisms have been proposed to explain why the obesity paradox exists.

Body structure and BC: Higher body weight by supplying enough muscular and adipose reserves may be able to thwart the metabolic effects of diseases and their treatments.[70]

Lipid metabolism: While individuals with CHF and low total serum cholesterol levels are more susceptible to endotoxemia and its inflammatory effects because of bacterial/endotoxin translocation from gut wall edema, high levels of total cholesterol and lipoproteins may ameliorate the endotoxin-scavenging impact.[71]

N-terminal pro-B-type natriuretic peptide (NT-proBNP): Due to increased wall strain, cardiomyocytes release NT-proBNP, which may be viewed as a key prognostic marker for mortality in acute coronary syndrome. After myocardial infarction, NT-proBNP levels are significantly lower in patients who are overweight or obese compared to subjects with a lower BMI.[18]

Prothrombotic factors: Since endothelial function, which affects the generation of prothrombotic factors like thromboxane B2, is paradoxically better in subjects with obesity than in nonobese people, there is a negative correlation between BMI and leptin.[18]

Ghrelin production/sensitivity: Increased ghrelin production/sensitivity has been demonstrated to be a compensatory mechanism that prevents HF from progressing.[72]

Cytokines production: An increase in the production of cytokines, such as tumor necrosis factor (TNF), is linked to cardiometabolic risk. Obese individuals produce less-soluble TNF receptors I and II from subcutaneous AT, which is associated with BMI and BF% in patients with HF.[73]

Endothelial/Vascular aspects: Increased endothelial progenitor cell mobilization may prevent atherogenesis in very obese patients by enhancing the repair of damaged myocardium and the growth of new blood vessels.[74]

The Obesity Paradox may not be a Paradox at all

There is a presence in the literature of potential methodological explanations for the obesity paradox, such as misclassification bias caused by confounders, using BMI as a measure of obesity, reverse causation, or a form of selection bias[75] called collider stratification bias. This has led to observations which question the presence of obesity paradox.[76-78]

Role of Confounders

The obesity paradox may be a spuriously observed finding based on retrospective analysis of observational studies.[79] A variety of confounding factors have been suggested, including the earlier onset of HF in obese patients due to more severe symptoms, better tolerability of cardioprotective medications due to HTN or the higher volume of distribution, the attenuated response of the RAAS, less sarcopenia and cachexia, and implications for CRF.

Body Mass Index as a Measure of Obesity

It is important to acknowledge that the vast majority of studies that examined the obesity paradox in HF patients have used BMI values to assess its magnitude. This may be partly due to the ease of calculating the BMI but also because BMI $\geq$ 25 kg/m^2 is recognized as overweight worldwide. On the other hand, the limitations of the anthropometric measure BMI have to be kept in mind because BMI is an index that fails to account for BC consisting of muscle, fat, and bone. Also, it does not reflect the distribution of fat in the body, such as visceral, subcutaneous, or ectopic fat.[79] Consequently, some authors have recently questioned the existence of an obesity paradox,[80] while others have suggested to speak of an "obesity paradigm" because its existence appears so very clear.[81] In light of this, alternative anthropometric indices to BMI, such as WC and waist-to-hip ratio, require closer scrutiny as these may more accurately reflect central obesity and may be less influenced by skeletal muscle.[82] A recent study debunked the idea that there is an "obesity paradox" in patients of HF and that adiposity assessed by the waist-to-height ratio (WHtR) more definitely eliminates the paradox.[83]

Reverse Causation and Collider Stratification Bias

Another possible explanation includes the bias due to the so-called reverse causation where antecedent weight loss due to chronic illness like cancer may elevate mortality risk.[84,85] It has been proposed that excess AT may act as a metabolic reservoir, in a way protecting exposure of additional tissues to lipotoxicity and ectopic fat deposition along with acting as a buffer for dietary fat influx.

It is well documented that collider stratification bias can potentially reverse the direction of an effect, making a harmful exposure appear protective.[86-88] The selection bias results from conditioning on a variable affected by exposure and sharing common causes with the outcome (known as collider). Thus, apparently, the obesity paradox is simply the result of collider stratification, a source of selection bias. Thus, patients with CVD stratified into different categories based on BMI introduce selection bias and differ on account of unmeasured/unknown risk factors. This distorts the true association of BMI with deaths leading to a spurious conclusion of the protective effect of obesity.

CONCLUSION

The obesity paradox in heart disease presents a fascinating and complex puzzle that challenges our preconceived notions about the relationship between obesity and CV outcomes. Despite the well-established link between obesity and increased CV risk, the paradoxical finding of improved outcomes in certain cardiac conditions among obese individuals demands further investigation. Understanding the underlying mechanisms and factors contributing to this paradox can potentially lead to the development of personalized treatment strategies and targeted interventions that consider the complex interplay between obesity, CV health, and patient outcomes. As research in this field continues to evolve, it is crucial to remain open to new perspectives and embrace the complexity of the obesity paradox in order to enhance our understanding of CVD and improve patient care.

ONLINE REFERENCES

Please scan the QR code provided at the end of the table of contents for References of this chapter.

SECTION 3

Antiplateletes and Anticoagulants

CHAPTER

21

Newer Antiplatelet Agents

Suresh V Patted, Sameer S Ambar, Vijayanand B Metgudmath

ABSTRACT

As the chase for ideal antiplatelet drugs continues for the cardiologist, we appraise the antiplatelet drugs and also upcoming newer antiplatelet drugs along with current approvals in the treatment of ischemic heart disease.

Keywords: P2Y12 receptor antagonists, platelet glycoprotein GP IIb/IIIa, thrombosis, receptor, PAR-1, platelet aggregation.

INTRODUCTION

Antiplatelet medications play a crucial role in treating cardiovascular diseases. Although the currently approved drugs have significantly reduced the morbidity and mortality, still there are signs of undesirable bleeding, recurrent ischemia, and heart attacks. Many of the drugs are manufactured with the aim to target surface receptors or enzymes in the platelet to prevent undesirable clot formation after initial platelet activation. In antiplatelet therapy, the role of aspirin was to target the cyclooxygenase-1 (COX-1).[1] In spite of evolution in alternative drugs to inhibit platelet activity, the pharmacokinetics and pharmacodynamics of those suggest that aspirin will remain a key component of antiplatelet therapy in the future. Currently, a combined regimen of aspirin and clopidogrel is the standard treatment for prevention of thrombosis, platelet activation, and stroke.[2] However, many of the present available antiplatelet drugs have restrictions in their use because of genetic differences in metabolizing prodrugs (such as Clopidogrel) resistance and allergic response as conceded with aspirin. Currently approved antiplatelet agents have a narrow therapeutic window and the efficacy is limited.[3]

CLASSIFICATION OF ANTIPLATELETS[4] (FLOWCHART 1, FIG. 1, AND TABLE 1)[5-8]

Cyclooxygenase Inhibitors

Aspirin is the most widely used drug in medicine. It is also one of the many ancient drugs known to mankind, with the history dating back to the period of Hippocrates and Galen.[9]

In 1971, aspirin's mode of action was discovered. Aspirin irreversibly inhibits cyclooxygenase (COX) and leads to suppression of thromboxane A2.

International Study of Infarct Survival (ISIS-2) trial[10] first demonstrated the role of aspirin in reducing recurrent myocardial infarction (MI) and its mortality. In this study, there was significant reduction in stroke, reinfarction, and 5-week mortality. In ISIS-2 trial, 1,000 patients of acute MI were treated with 1 month of low-dose aspirin. This trail came to conclusion that aspirin therapy prevented 25 deaths and 10–15 nonfatal infarcts and strokes per thousand treated patients.

In 2002, the Antithrombotic Trialists' Collaboration[11] analyzed 16 trials. They analyzed 17,000 patients treated with long-term aspirin with doses ranging from 50 to

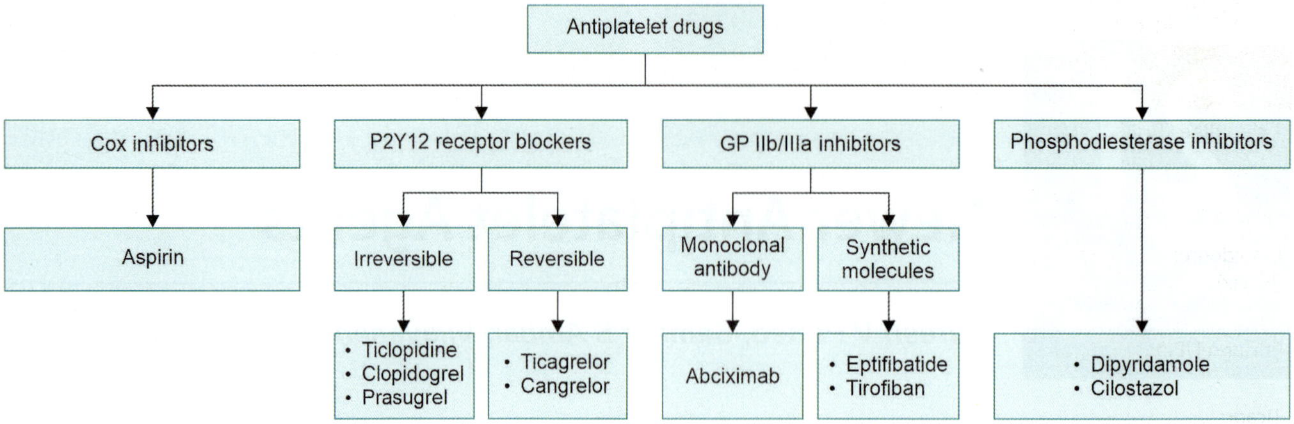

FLOWCHART 1: Classification of antiplatelets.
(Cox: cyclooxygenase; GP: glycoprotein)

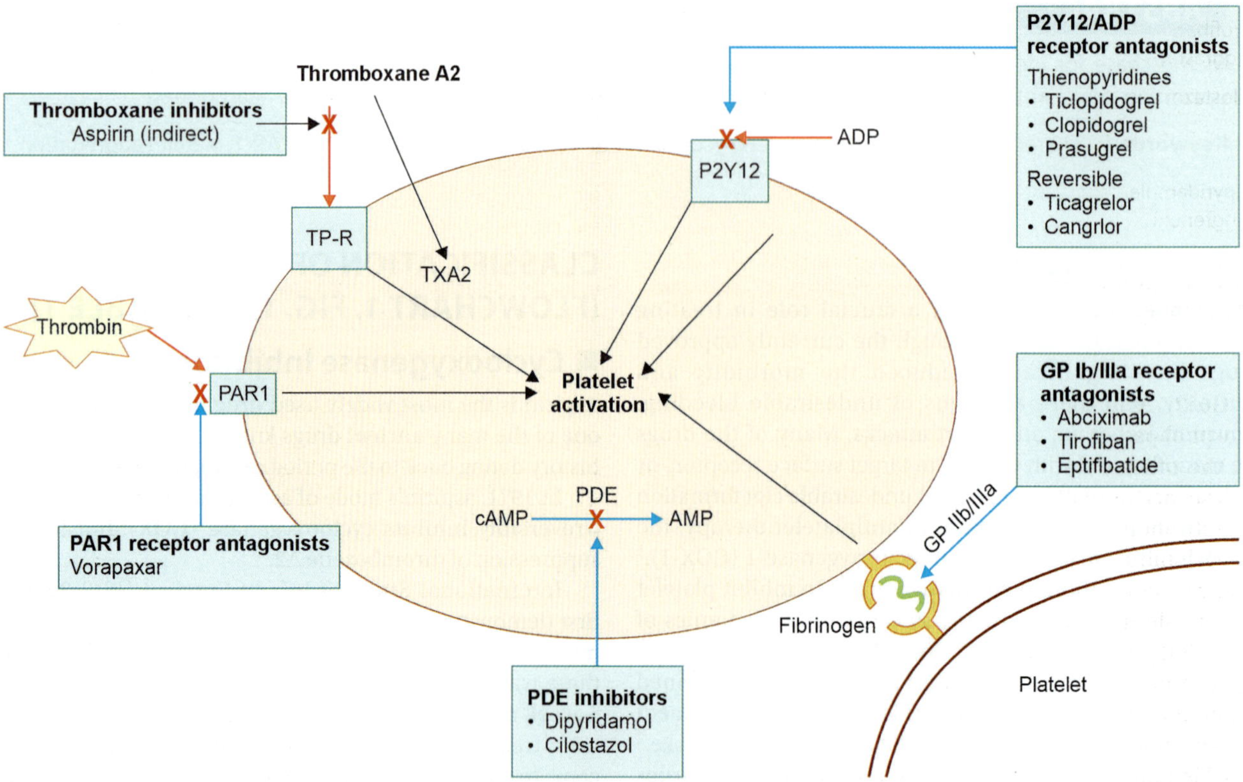

FIG. 1: Sites of action of different antiplatelet drugs.[5-7]
(AMP: adenosine monophosphate; cAMP: cyclic adenosine monophosphate; PAR1: protease-activated receptor 1; PDE: phosphodiesterase; TP-R: thromboxane receptor)

1,500 mg/day for secondary prevention of cardiovascular events. This analysis showed there was reduction in stroke and coronary events in both men and women. Major associations well accepted aspirin used in secondary prevention of cardiovascular events.

P2Y12 Inhibitors

The P2Y12 receptors, which belong to the P2 family, are purinergic receptors that are G-protein-coupled receptors (GPCR). Within platelets, there are two receptors, namely P2Y1 and P2Y12. P2Y1 is a GPCR, while P2Y12 is coupled

TABLE 1: Approved antiplatelet drugs.[8]

Drug	Target	Half-life	Side effects	Bioavailability	Use
Ticlopidine (Ticlid)	P2Y12 receptor	12 hours	Bleeding, rash, neutropenia, thrombotic thrombocytopenic purpura (rare), nausea, vomiting, heartburn, and indigestion	Oral	Transient ischemic attacks, patients undergoing PCI
Clopidogrel (Plavix)	P2Y12 receptor	6–8 hours	Bleeding, rash, neutropenia, thrombotic thrombocytopenic purpura (rare)	Oral	NSTEMI, STEMI, PCI, recent stroke, or established PAD
Prasugrel (Effient)	P2Y12 receptor	8 hours	Bleeding	Oral	Patients with ACS undergoing PCI
Ticagrelor (Brilinta)	P2Y12 receptor	6–12 hours	Dyspnea	Oral	STEMI and ACS
Abciximab (ReoPro)	GP IIb/IIIa receptor	<10–30 minutes	Bleeding, thrombocytopenia, EDTA-induced pseudothrombocytopenia	IV	PCI
Eptifibatide (Integrilin)	GP IIb/IIIa receptor	~2.5 hours	Bleeding, thrombocytopenia, EDTA-induced pseudothrombocytopenia	IV	NSTEMI, PCI, and unstable angina
Tirofiban (Aggrastat)	GP IIb/IIIa receptor	2 hours	Bleeding, thrombocytopenia, EDTA-induced pseudothrombocytopenia	IV	NSTEMI, PCI, and unstable angina
Cilostazol (Pletal)	PDE3	11–13 hours	Headache, dizziness, hypotension, flushing, nausea, vomiting, diarrhea, and abdominal pain	Oral	Intermittent claudication, PAD, and PCI
Dipyridamole (Aggrenox)	PDE3 and inhibition of adenosine uptake	10 hours	Bleeding, headache, diarrhea, palpitations, dizziness, rash, and pancytopenia	Oral	Transient ischemic attacks

(ACS: acute coronary syndromes; EDTA: ethylenediaminetetraacetic acid; GP: glycoprotein; IV: intravenous; NSTEMI: non-ST-elevation myocardial infarction; PAD: peripheral arterial disease; PCI: percutaneous coronary intervention; PDE: phosphodiesterase; STEMI: ST-elevation myocardial infarction)

to Gαi2. Activation of P2Y1 triggers the signaling of phospholipase β pathway leading to calcium mobilization.[12] On the other hand, activation of P2Y12 inhibits adenylyl cyclase, activates phosphoinositide 3-kinase,[13] and leads to the activation of αIIbβ3 receptor.[14]

Ticlopidine is a first-generation thienopyridine drug that requires metabolism by cytochrome P450 (CYP1A). It has irreversible antagonistic effects on platelet reactivity through the P2Y12 receptor. The maximum inhibition of platelet aggregation is seen after 3–5 days after administration of ticlopidine because of metabolism of the prodrug. Clinical trials such as Canadian-American Ticlopidine Study (CATS) and Ticlopidine Aspirin Stroke Study (TASS) have shown that ticlopidine is more effective than aspirin alone, but it is associated with significant minor bleeding (<1%).[15] Moreover, patients treated with ticlopidine often discontinue the treatment due to various secondary adverse events such as diarrhea, skin rash, and neutropenia.

Clopidogrel is oral thienopyridine of second generation that also requires metabolism of a pro-drug by CYP2C19. The active metabolite irreversibly binds to and inhibits the P2Y12 receptor through a disulfide bridge. The CURE trial[16] has showed as compared to aspirin alone the clinical benefit of dual therapy with clopidogrel and aspirin, significantly reduced nonfatal MI, mortality, or stroke in patients with unstable angina. But dual therapy was associated with an increased risk of bleeding when compared to placebo. The CAPRIE trial,[17] which evaluated the efficacy of clopidogrel monotherapy versus dual therapy with clopidogrel and aspirin, demonstrated that clopidogrel treatment reduces primary endpoints. The presence of poor metabolizers for clopidogrel has helped to explain the reduced effectiveness in patients with an altered CYP2C19 allele. Diminished platelet inhibition (clopidogrel resistance) is seen in poor metabolizers of clopidogrel, resulting in more incidence of adverse cardiovascular events. Invention of clopidogrel marked the death of ticlopidine in clinical practice.

Prasugrel is an oral drug, third-generation thienopyridine. It is pro-drug and requires activation through the action of enzymes CYP450, esterase, CYP2, and CYP3A4. Prasugrel is more potent than clopidogrel. The adenosine diphosphate (ADP)-induced platelet aggregation is selectively and irreversibly inhibited by adenosine triphosphate (ATP) analog. The irreversible binding occurs through the disulfide bond between the active metabolite's reactive thiol group and the cysteine residue of the P2Y12 receptor.

In TRITON TIMI 38 trial,[18] prasugrel demonstrated favorable secondary endpoints, with lower incidences of rehospitalization due to recurrent ischemia, nonfatal MI, and cardiovascular death. Ticagrelor is an oral cyclopentyl-triazolo-pyrimidine analog that directly and reversibly inhibits the P2Y12 receptor. It is a pro-drug form activated by CYP3A. Ticagrelor works by binding to a site on the P2Y12 receptor separate from the ADP-binding site, making it an allosteric inhibitor. PLATO trial[18] compared ticagrelor to clopidogrel and demonstrated a reduction in the primary composite endpoints (MI, stent thrombosis, and cardiovascular death) in patients with acute coronary syndromes (ACS), regardless of ST-elevation. Major bleeding rates did not significantly differ between the two agents, but ticagrelor was related with an increase in spontaneous or nonprocedural-related bleeding. Additionally, ticagrelor use has been linked to effects such as dyspnea and asymptomatic ventricular pauses. Overall, ticagrelor has demonstrated supremacy over other antiplatelets, in terms of rapid onset of action, safety profile, and effectiveness in reducing primary endpoints in ACS patients. With the rise of ticagrelor, the complication of stent thrombosis post percutaneous coronary intervention (PCI) has drastically come down.

Cangrelor is an intravenous nonthienopyridine and reversible P2Y12 inhibitor. As compared to clopidogrel, it has more rapid onset of action and greater platelet inhibition, thus being preferred in primary PCI with cardiogenic shock or patients with nausea and vomiting where Cangrelor bypasses first-pass metabolism. Platelet inhibition is reversible within 2 hours of stopping the drug infusion and, therefore, the risk of bleeding and need for antidote are minimized and if the patient requires emergency CABG, patient can be taken up for the surgery without any additional risk of bleeding. Other advantages of Cangrelor include that no dosage adjustment is required in patients with deranged renal or hepatic parameters which is very common scenario in the elderly population who presents with ACS with multiple comorbidities and are undergoing PCI. It can also be used as a bridge therapy in patients undergoing noncardiac surgery to minimize the risk of stent thrombosis. Evaluation of Cangrelor in the CHAMPION-PCI, CHAMPION-PLATFORM, and CHAMPION-PHOENIX trials showed reduction in the primary endpoint of death, MI, or ischemia-driven revascularization within 48 hours after PCI.[19] The morbidity rate of major bleeding was higher with Cangrelor as compared to clopidogrel in both studies. The recommended dosage of Cangrelor is 30 μg/kg IV bolus followed immediately by a 4 μg/kg/min IV infusion. Initiate the bolus infusion prior to PCI. The maintenance infusion should normally be continued for at least 2 hours or for the duration of PCI, whichever is longer.[20]

Elinogrel is a direct-acting reversible P2Y12 receptor inhibitor. It is currently under clinical investigation (INNOVATE-PCI)[21] to evaluate its efficacy and safety in patients undergoing PCI. As per preclinical data, it has been suggested that intravenous or oral administration of Elinogrel has higher efficacy than clopidogrel and has minimal impact on bleeding times. Additionally, a single dose of Elinogrel has been shown to overcome high platelet reactivity in PCI patients who do not respond to clopidogrel. Elinogrel shows promise as a next-generation P2Y12 antagonist.

BX 667 is a reversible P2Y12 receptor antagonist that can be taken orally. It undergoes metabolism by esterases to produce the active form, BX 048. In laboratory studies, BX 667 has demonstrated potent inhibition of ADP-induced platelet aggregation. However, the effects and safety of this antagonist have not yet been assessed in healthy people.[22]

Glycoprotein Antagonists

GP IIb/IIIa Antagonists

Glycoprotein GP IIb/IIIa (αIIbβ3) is the most abundant protein found on the surface of platelets. It plays a role in platelet signaling. When fibrinogen or von Willebrand factor (VWF) binds to αIIbβ3, it leads to platelet adhesion, aggregation, and activation of integrin signaling, resulting in granule secretion, stabilized platelet adhesion, aggregation, and clot retraction.

Abciximab is an antibody derived from a murine-human chimera c7E3 Fab. It specifically targets the αIIbβ3 integrin, preventing its binding to fibrinogen and VWF. Abciximab has a high affinity for its target and a slow dissociation rate. The intravenous administration of abciximab rapidly inhibits platelet function, but its effects diminish within 12–24 hours after discontinuation. Clinical trials such as EPIC, CAPTURE, and EPILOG have shown mixed results, with some demonstrating no additional benefit over placebo and others showing reduced ischemic complications and mortality, particularly in patients who had raised troponin levels. Monitoring for bleeding and thrombocytopenia is required when using abciximab.[23]

Eptifibatide is derived from snake venom which is cyclic heptapeptide and it selectively recognizes αIIbβ3. The IMPACT-II study revealed limited efficacy with eptifibatide when a single bolus dose followed by continuous infusion was used. However, the ESPRIT trial, which employed a double bolus followed by a maintenance infusion, demonstrated significant reductions in MI, target vessel revascularization, and death. Parallel findings were seen in the PURSUIT trial. However, there was an increased incidence of major bleeding in patients with acute coronary syndrome (ACS) undergoing PCI in the ACUITY trial.[24]

Tirofiban is a tyrosine-derivative nonpeptide mimetic. It is reversible inhibitor of αIIbβ3 that competitively binds to the platelet receptor. When given in combination with heparin and aspirin in patients with ACS, it significantly reduced the incidence of death, MI, or recurrent ischemia. Tirofiban was also superior in ACS patients undergoing invasive coronary angiography.[25] However, in the context of PCI, tirofiban was shown to be inferior to abciximab in terms of the composite endpoint of death, nonfatal MI, and urgent target vessel revascularization.[26]

Z4 A5 is a novel αIIbβ3 peptide antagonist presently in developmental process. It has exhibited the ability to inhibit platelet-induced aggregation and thrombus formation. With advent of newer potent antiplatelets drugs such as Prasugrel and Ticagrelor, the use of GP IIb/IIIa inhibitor has come down.

Additional Glycoprotein Inhibitors

Additional target is VWF, a multimeric glycoprotein, that acts as a bridge between damaged endothelial sites and platelet glycoprotein receptors. VWF binds to active αIIbβ3 on the platelet surface. Interactions between VWF and αIIbβ3 are important in final step, irreversible binding of platelets to the damaged subendothelium, and play a pivotal role in platelet aggregation. Another target that has gained notice for potential antiplatelet therapy is glycoprotein VI (GPVI), the receptor for collagen. When collagen binds to GPVI, it initiates subsequent tyrosine phosphorylation of the Fc receptor γ chain's immunoreceptor tyrosine-based activation motif. This triggers platelet activation or aggregation.

GPVI Receptor Antagonists

PR-15 is a soluble, dimeric glycoprotein (GPVI-Fc) that adheres to exposed collagen in endothelial lesions, precluding binding to platelet GPVI receptors. It has shown extensive reduction in collagen-induced platelet adhesion and plaque formation. In mice, infusion of GPVI-Fc in vascular injury prevents stable arrest and aggregation of platelets.[27] A Phase I of clinical trial has shown the safety and permissibility of IV administration of PR-15 in healthy volunteers.

DZ-697b is an orally active inhibitor of collagen and ristocetin, currently under clinical investigation. In a Phase I clinical trial, it showed potential benefits by decreasing bleeding time as compared to the usage of clopidogrel.[28]

GPIb Receptor Antagonists

Novel targets under investigation include h6B4-Fab, GPGP-290, and SZ2. h6B4-Fab is a murine monoclonal antibody.[3]

Phosphodiesterase Antagonists

Platelet inhibitors known as phosphodiesterase (PDE) antagonists act in regulating platelet activation and thrombosis. There are three PDE isoenzymes expressed in platelets, namely PDE2, PDE3, and PDE5. Platelet activation depends on the degradation of cyclic adenosine monophosphate (cAMP) and cyclic guanosine monophosphate (cGMP), making the regulation of these secondary messengers essential.[29]

Cilostazol is an oral inhibitor that selectively targets PDE3 (type III PDE). By inhibiting adenosine uptake, cilostazol increases the concentration of adenosine, which then stimulates A2 receptors and raises cAMP levels. Cilostazol effectively inhibits platelet aggregation. However, despite its benefits in reducing repeated revascularization and restenosis after PCI, cilostazol has not shown superiority in reducing adverse cardiovascular events post DES implantation. Moreover, the drug's side effects, including headaches, gastrointestinal symptoms, and skin rash, often lead to discontinuation.

Dipyridamole is PDE antagonist and acts both as antiplatelet and vasodilator. Like cilostazol, it inhibits cyclic nucleotide phosphodiesterase and blocks adenosine uptake, leading to increased cAMP levels. Clinical trials such as ESPS-2 and ESPRIT have demonstrated that combining dipyridamole with aspirin significantly reduces the risk of death or stroke as compared to aspirin alone. Consequently, dipyridamole has got FDA approval for stroke prevention.[30]

Thromboxane A2 Receptor Antagonists

Platelets express the thromboxane receptor α (TPα), a G protein-coupled receptor (GPCR), that activates platelet signaling pathways upon interaction with thrombin or collagen. Various intracellular pathways are involved, reinforcing primary platelet activation. S18886 (terutroban) and Z-335 are oral inhibitors of TPα.[31,32] Z-335 demonstrated the inhibition of platelet aggregation induced by U46619 in healthy volunteers.

BM-573 is TPα inhibitor under investigation that has been effective in halting the progression of atherosclerosis in animal models. Preclinical studies have shown complete inhibition of arachidonic acid-induced platelet aggregation with BM-573. Clinical investigations of this compound are presently ongoing.[33]

Thrombin Receptor Antagonists

Platelet activation through protease activated receptors (PARs) plays a significant role in thrombin-mediated platelet activation. PAR1 and PAR4 are the two main receptors activated by thrombin. These receptors recruit prothrombotic signaling events, and their inhibition is being explored as a therapeutic target to control platelet activation.[34]

SCH 530348 (Vorapaxar) is a synthetic analog of himbacine.[35] It competitively binds with high affinity to PAR1. Preclinical studies have shown inhibition of thrombin-induced platelet aggregation. Animal study treatment with SCH 530348 alone or in combination with aspirin and clopidogrel did not experience increased bleeding times. The TRA-PCI study confirmed that adding SCH 530348 to standard antiplatelet therapy did not increase thrombolysis or bleeding. However, Phase III trials (TRA-CER and TRA 2°P-TIMI) assessing the impact of vorapaxar on stroke, MI, cardiovascular death, and recurrent vascular events failed due to unforeseen intracranial bleeding.[36,37]

E5555 (Atopaxar) is a PAR1 antagonist that has shown significant extension of bleeding times in guinea pigs.[36] It reduced the expression of various platelet surface markers involved in platelet aggregation. Clinical studies have shown that E5555 diminishes thrombin-induced platelet aggregation but not ADP-induced aggregation.[38]

Other PAR1 antagonists, such as SCH 205831 and SCH 602539, are still being investigated in preclinical models. Early data suggests that these compounds inhibit platelet deposition and thrombosis in animal models.[39,40]

CURRENT RECOMMENDATIONS OF ANTIPLATELET AGENTS IN REPERFUSION ERA

In patients who have undergone recent PCI, DAPT therapy with combination of aspirin with P2Y12 inhibitors forms the foundation of medical therapy post PCI and forms class 1 indication.

1. *Primary PCI*: Loading dose of aspirin 162–325 mg plus clopidogrel 300–600 mg OR Prasugrel 60 mg OR ticagrelor 180 mg should be given.
2. Primary PCI with vomiting/unconscious patient—loading with intravenous Cangrelor
3. Patients receiving fibrinolytic therapy—loading dose of aspirin 162–325 mg plus clopidogrel 300 (age <75 years) or 75 mg (age >75 years)

   The dosages of aspirin and P2Y12 inhibitors in patients undergoing primary PCI or PCI as adjunctive to PCI are given in **Table 2**.
4. Acute coronary syndrome PCI with DES/BMS—dual antiplatelet therapy with aspirin plus prasugrel or ticagrelor for 12 months.
5. Stable coronary artery disease with drug-eluting stent (DES)/bare metal stent (BMS)—dual antiplatelet therapy with aspirin plus clopidogrel for 6 months.

   Duration of the therapy depends on the various factors such as indication for PCI, ischemic burden, and the bleeding risk. Observations from the landmark trials such as CURE and DAPT have shown the benefit of reduced stent thrombosis and major adverse cardiac occurrences with the use of dual antiplatelet therapy for a minimum duration of 12 months. However, the recent trials, STOP DAPT2, TWILIGHT, and GLOBAL LEADERS trials, have emphasized on the shorter duration of dual antiplatelet therapy for duration of 1-3 months followed by monotherapy with P2Y12 inhibitors in patents with increased bleeding risk with related effects. The duration

TABLE 2: Duration of antiplatelet therapy for 1 year post PCI.

Antiplatelet drug	Initial therapy (class of recommendation, level of evidence)	Continued therapy (class of recommendation, level of evidence)
Antiplatelet therapy adjunctive to primary percutaneous intervention (PCI)		
Aspirin	162–325 mg should be given to all patients before primary PCI (I,B)	• 81–1,325 mg maintenance dose indefinitely (I,A) • 81 mg as preferred maintenance dose with ticagrelor (I,B)
P2Y12 inhibitors	Loading dose should be given as early as possible or at the time of primary PCI in patients with STEMI *Options*: • Clopidogrel 300–600 mg (I,B) • Prasugrel 60 mg (I,B) • Ticagrelor 180 mg (I,B) • Prasugrel should not be given to patients with a history of stroke or transient ischemic attack (III,B)	Maintenance dose should be continued for 1 year following a drug-eluting or bare metal stent placement *Options*: • Clopidogrel 75 mg daily (I,B) • Prasugrel 10 mg daily (I,B) • Ticagrelor 90 mg twice daily (I,B) • Continue P2Y12 inhibitor beyond 1 year may be considered in patients with drug-eluting stent placement (IIa,C)
Antiplatelet therapy adjunctive to PCI after fibrinolytic therapy		
Aspirin	162–325 mg should be given to all patients who receive fibrinolytic therapy (I,A)	• 81–1,325 mg maintenance dose indefinitely (I,A) • 81 mg is preferred maintenance dose (IIa,B)

P2Y12 inhibitors	Clopidogrel loading dose based an age in all patients who receive fibrinolytic therapy (I,A)
	• Age ≤75:300 mg
	• Age >75:75 mg
		If drug-eluting stent is placed:
		• Continue P2Y12 inhibitor for at least 1 year with either
		  ○ Clopidogrel 75 mg daily (I,C)
		  ○ Prasugrel 10 mg daily (IIa,B)

(PCI: percutaneous coronary intervention; STEMI: ST-elevation myocardial infarction)

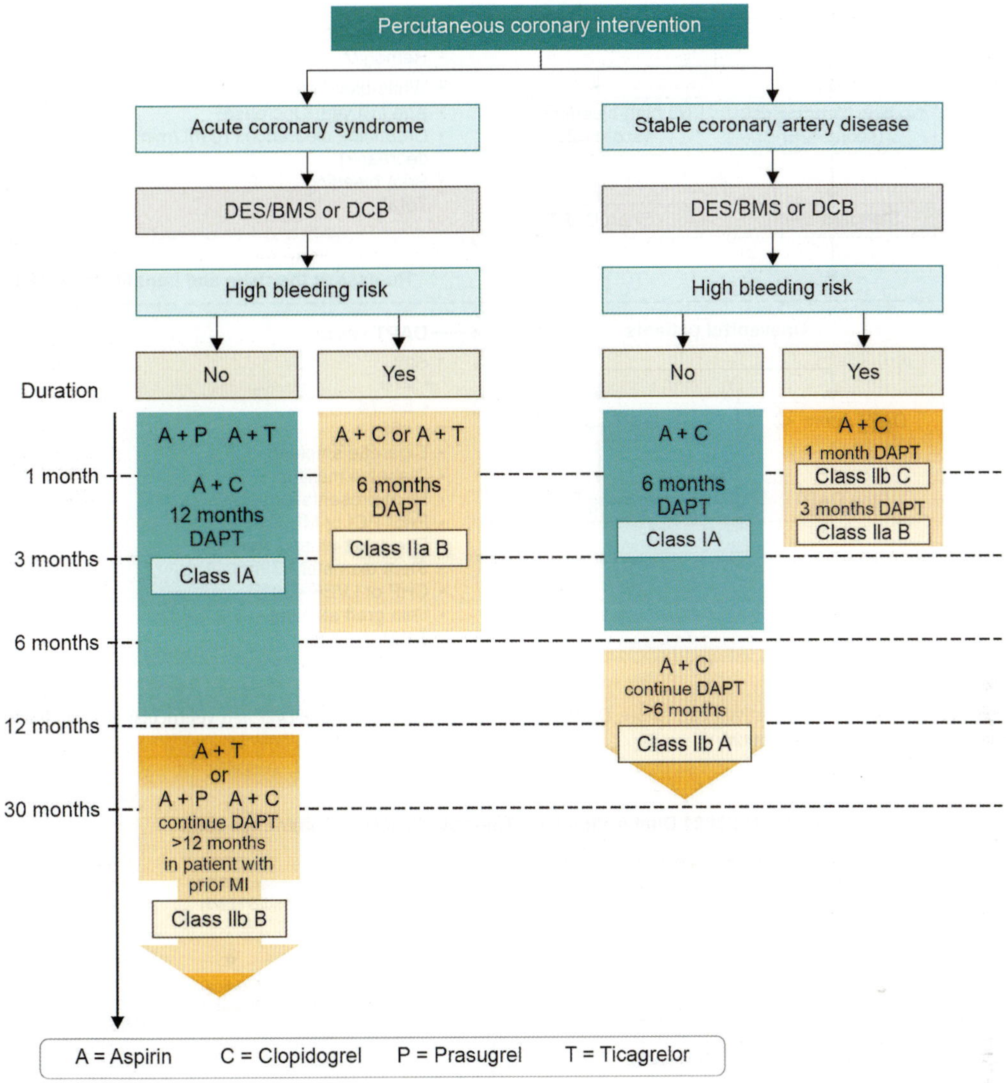

FLOWCHART 2: Duration of antiplatelet agents post PCI.
(BMS: bare metal stent; DAPT: dual antiplatelet therapy; DCB: drug-coated balloon; DES: drug-eluting stent)

and the antiplatelet agents recommended post PCI as per American College of Cardiology (ACC)/American Heart Association (AHA) are given in following **Flowchart 2**.

The recommendations by ACC/AHA slightly differ among patients with stable ischemic heart disease post PCI patients. Among patients with stable ischemic heart disease with previous history of PCI, it is reasonable to start with DAPT with aspirin and clopidogrel combination for 6 months if DES was used or 1 month if BMS was used. In post CABG patients, it is prudent to give DAPT for minimum duration of 12 months as shown in **Figure 2**. However, if patient is at increased risk of bleeding with increased DAPT score, it may be reasonable to stop aspirin after 1–3 months of therapy and continuing with clopidogrel.

6. Post PCI with DAPT score >2—continue dual antiplatelet therapy. Aspirin plus clopidogrel 75 mg OD or prasugrel 10 mg OD or ticagrelor 60 mg BD **(Flowchart 3)**
7. Post PCI with DAPT score <2—monotherapy with aspirin or clopidogrel

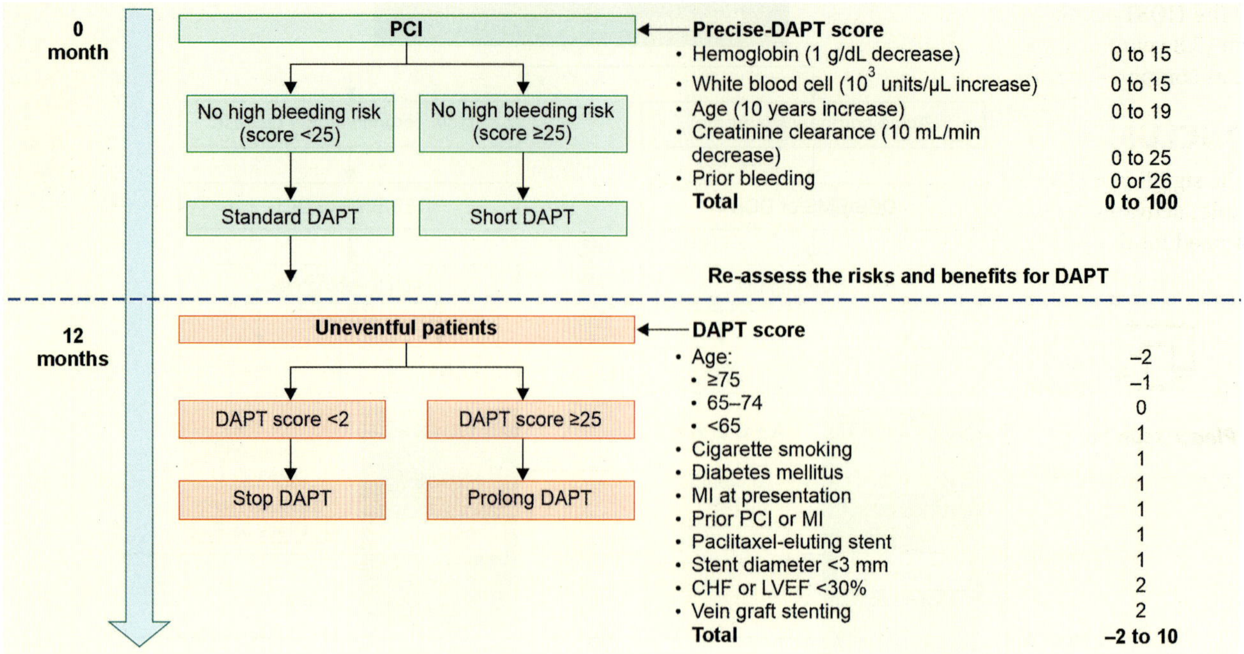

FIG. 2: AHA, 2021 DAPT score.

(AHA: American Heart Association; CHF: congestive heart failure; DAPT: dual antiplatelet therapy score; LVEF: left ventricular ejection fraction; MI: myocardial infarction; PCI: percutaneous coronary intervention)

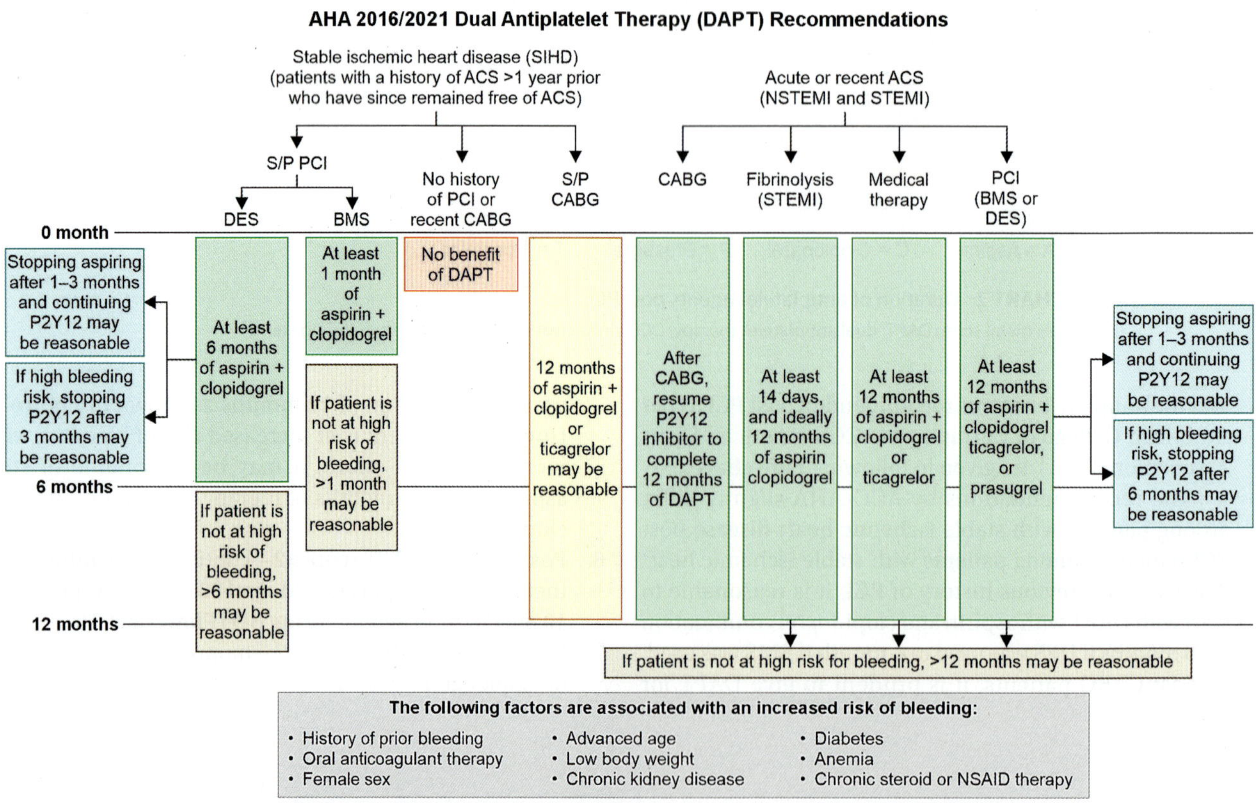

FLOWCHART 3: Duration of antiplatelet therapy for 1 year post PCI.

Note: Medical therapy—treatment with aspirin, statins, and aggressive risk factor management (e.g., hypertension and diabetes).

[ACS: acute coronary syndrome defined as myocardial infarction or unstable angina; BMS: bare metal stent; CABG: coronary artery bypass grafting; DAPT: dual antiplatelet therapy (aspirin + P2Y12 inhibitor); DES: drug-eluting stent; NSAID: nonsteroidal anti-inflammatory drug; PCI: percutaneous coronary intervention; STEMI: ST-elevation myocardial infarction]

The HOST-EXAM-extended trial has shown good long-term (5.8 years) results with clopidogrel monotherapy post PCI as compared to aspirin monotherapy.

CONCLUSION

While significant progress has been made in understanding platelet activation and its role in thrombus formation, there is a need for the development of new antiplatelet therapies. The current standard, aspirin has limitations due to its irreversible action and the increased risk of bleeding when combined with dual therapy. Novel compounds targeting alternative platelet sites are being developed to reduce bleeding events and MIs. However, the complexity of platelet signaling necessitates exploration of new therapeutic targets with fewer off-target effects to effectively manage cardiovascular disease.

ONLINE REFERENCES

Please scan the QR code provided at the end of the table of contents for References of this chapter.

CHAPTER

22 Antiplatelet Use in Chronic Kidney Disease Patients

Gopal Chandra Ghosh, Suvro Banerjee

ABSTRACT

Antiplatelets are an essential therapeutic option both for treatment and prevention of cardiovascular diseases. Presence of chronic kidney disease (CKD) alters hemostatic parameters and affects the effectiveness and safety of antiplatelet therapy. Randomized trials data are lacking regarding the safety and effectivity of antiplatelets in patients of CKD. Majority of evidence is extrapolated from non-CKD studies. In future, dedicated randomized controlled trials of antiplatelets in CKD patients are necessary. Till then, selection of an antiplatelet agent in patients with CKD should be individualized on the basis of patient risk factor profiles, tolerance, and other clinical characteristics.

Keywords: Chronic kidney disease, coronary artery disease, antiplatelets, DAPT, high bleeding risk.

INTRODUCTION

Chronic kidney disease (CKD) affects 10–16% of adult population worldwide. CKD is a progressive condition characterized by the gradual loss of kidney function.[1] Cardiovascular disease is an important cause of morbidity and mortality in CKD patients. Antiplatelet therapy plays a crucial role in the prevention and management of cardiovascular events. However, the use of antiplatelet agents in CKD patients requires careful consideration due to altered platelet function and the risk of bleeding complications.

BENEFICIAL EFFECTS OF ANTIPLATELET AGENTS IN CKD PATIENTS

- *Cardiovascular events*: Antiplatelet agents have been shown to reduce the risk of cardiovascular events, including myocardial infarction and stroke, in the general population.
- *Atherothrombotic events*: CKD patients are at an increased risk of atherothrombotic events, and antiplatelet therapy can help to decrease this risk.
- *Maintain patency of arteriovenous fistulas*: Antiplatelet agents have been shown to improve the patency of arteriovenous fistulas in CKD patients undergoing hemodialysis.

CONSIDERATIONS FOR ANTIPLATELET THERAPY IN CKD PATIENTS

- *Altered platelet function*: CKD can cause platelet dysfunction. CKD state leads to impaired platelet aggregation and increased platelet activation. This altered platelet function may impact the efficacy of antiplatelet therapy.
- *Bleeding risk*: CKD patients may have an increased risk of bleeding complications, primarily due to uremic platelet dysfunction, vascular calcification, and the use of anticoagulants.
- *Individualized approach*: The decision to initiate antiplatelet therapy in CKD patients should be based on a careful assessment of the balance between the potential benefits and bleeding risks.

CLINICAL EVIDENCE AND RECOMMENDATIONS

- *Aspirin*: The Antithrombotic Trialists' Collaboration meta-analysis demonstrated that aspirin reduces the risk of serious vascular events in patients with established cardiovascular disease, even those with existing CKD.[2]

  A post hoc analysis of the Folic Acid for Vascular Outcome Reduction in Transplantation (FAVORIT) trial found that aspirin reduced the risk of cardiovascular events in kidney transplant recipients with CKD.[3] A systematic review and meta-analysis of observational studies indicated that aspirin use was associated with a reduced risk of all-cause mortality in CKD patients.[2]

The use of low-dose aspirin (75–100 mg/day) may be considered in CKD patients with a high risk of cardiovascular events. However, the benefits should be weighed against the bleeding risks, especially in patients with advanced CKD or on hemodialysis.

- *Clopidogrel*: Clopidogrel is an alternative to aspirin in CKD patients who cannot tolerate or have contraindications to aspirin. It may be preferred over aspirin in patients with a high risk of bleeding. The Prevention of Serious Adverse Events Following Angiography (PRESERVE) trial demonstrated that clopidogrel, in combination with aspirin, did not reduce the incidence of major adverse cardiovascular events in patients with moderate-to-severe CKD undergoing angiography. However, a meta-analysis of randomized controlled trials indicated that dual antiplatelet therapy (DAPT) with clopidogrel and aspirin reduced the risk of major adverse cardiovascular events in CKD patients with acute coronary syndrome.
- *Dual antiplatelet therapy*: The use of DAPT (aspirin plus clopidogrel) in CKD patients should be individualized, considering the specific clinical scenario and bleeding risk. The DAPT trial, which included patients with and without CKD, found that DAPT with clopidogrel and aspirin reduced the risk of major adverse cardiovascular and cerebrovascular events but increased the risk of major bleeding compared to aspirin alone. A meta-analysis of randomized controlled trials demonstrated that DAPT reduced the risk of major adverse cardiovascular events but increased bleeding complications, in CKD patients undergoing percutaneous coronary intervention (PCI).[4]

The 2019 Kidney Disease: Improving Global Outcomes (KDIGO) Clinical Practice Guideline for Diabetes Management in CKD recommends considering low-dose aspirin for primary prevention of cardiovascular events in CKD patients with a high risk of cardiovascular disease. The decision to initiate antiplatelet therapy in CKD patients should be individualized. The potential benefits need to be assessed against the bleeding risks based on the patient's clinical characteristics and preferences.[5]

POTENTIAL MECHANISMS FOR REDUCED EFFICACY OF ANTIPLATELET AGENTS IN CKD PATIENTS

The reason why some CKD patients respond less favorably to antiplatelet agents is not known. Impaired platelet aggregability, polymorphism of cytochrome P450 monooxygenase system (CYP) enzymes, alteration in other system of drug metabolism (like liver metabolism) due to presence of uremia, and increased von Willebrand factor (VWF) antigen and impaired VWF activity are some of the potential mechanistic pathways that require further discussion.[6]

CURRENT RECOMMENDATIONS

The National Kidney Foundation (NKF) task force has evaluated strategies for preventing and treating cardiovascular diseases in patients with CKD. Unfortunately, these recommendations have not been updated recently. Evidence to support the efficacy of aspirin in patients with CKD is limited, and the NKF recommendation for the usual aspirin dose in patients with CKD and coronary artery disease (CAD) was based on extrapolation of the benefits of aspirin in the general population in patients with pre-existing cardiovascular disease. Furthermore, the 2009 KDIGO practice guidelines for secondary prevention of cardiovascular events in kidney transplant recipients with diabetes or cardiovascular disease suggest use of low-dose aspirin based on very poor quality of evidence. The American Heart Association (AHA) Task Force and American College of Cardiology (ACC) and US Preventive Task Force make no specific recommendations for the use of antiplatelet agents in CKD patients, as because there is lack of sufficient data to support. A recent study reported that >75% of published CAD trials have excluded CKD patients. Evidence is "level C" at best. This is especially concerning given that antiplatelet agents are the third most commonly prescribed medications that lead to adverse drug events and hospitalizations.[7]

The American Heart Association (AHA)/American College of Cardiology (ACC) guidelines encourage the performance of appropriately designed clinical trials to identify the optimal clopidogrel loading dose, realizing that there is considerable interpatient variability in clopidogrel response, and in the presence of CKD, a wide range of inhibition of platelet aggregation after a given dose may happen. But till now, the ideal techniques for monitoring for poor clopidogrel response and the appropriate dosing strategy are yet to be established. The AHA does not suggest routine platelet function testing to guide antiplatelet therapy, as it is expensive and not routinely covered by health insurance. However, platelet function testing can be of help for those undergoing coronary interventions and are at high risk, such as those with underlying CKD. However, no specific recommendations are currently available as there is a lack of controlled studies to prove that routine platelet function testing will improve hard clinical outcomes.[7]

Overall, selection of an antiplatelet agent should be individualized on the basis of patient risk factor profiles, tolerance, and other clinical characteristics. Because CKD patients are at higher risk for not only thrombotic but also bleeding events, there is an urgent need for future trials to guide antiplatelet therapy in CKD patients.

CURRENT LIMITATIONS

A major limitation of our current understanding and interpretation of the available evidence result from the heterogeneity of the published studies. The existing studies are not powered to address the safety and efficacy of antiplatelet agents in CKD patients. The majority of evidence is from subgroup or post hoc analyses. Furthermore, we are still clueless to know if antiplatelet therapy is efficacious in some CKD patients but not others, then how to identify such subgroups. Clinicians also face the dilemma of choosing the correct type, correct dose, duration, and combination of antiplatelet agents in order to lower the side effects while maximizing cardiovascular and survival benefits. Gaps still exist in our knowledge and understanding of the pharmacodynamics of platelet aggregation and inhibition by antiplatelet agents in the CKD population. Published studies lacked data on proven adherence to antiplatelet medications, were underpowered, and used nonstandardized cut-offs to measure residual platelet aggregability thus limiting the interpretation of these results. Many studies actually did not have control for body mass index, sex, other factors that are known to affect platelet aggregability.[7]

There is a large methodological heterogeneity in assessing platelet function. Numerous in vitro or ex vivo laboratory assays are available for platelet functional assessment, but whole blood platelet aggregation (WBPA) measured by ex vivo impedance aggregometry via chrono-log or multiplate aggregometers appear to be one of the better tests for assessing platelet function compared with the traditional light transmittance method using platelet-rich plasma. WBPA is more sensitive and faster, and does not require centrifugation that can result in platelet injury.[8,9]

Clinicians face uncertainty at how to best choose antiplatelet agents for both prevention of cardiovascular disease and treatment of atherothrombotic events in CKD population. High residual platelet reactivity on antiplatelets is a novel modifiable risk factor which predicts future cardiovascular events, and this is also true in patients with CKD. This area needs further research to prevent events which occur in patients already on antiplatelet agents.[9]

Currently, we have limited data regarding platelet aggregability in pre-dialysis CKD patients to guide current clinical practice. The ACC/AHA recommends conducting randomized clinical trials to determine whether routine platelet function testing would be helpful to guide antiplatelet therapy, with special focus on high-risk patients such as those with CKD.

Whatever current evidence is available to guide antiplatelet management in CKD patients, we could follow the below mentioned principles. First, low-dose aspirin monotherapy should be used for secondary prevention and for primary prevention in appropriately selected patients. Be cautious to use higher aspirin doses, as we have limited data on added benefits and there is concern for increased adverse events. Second, DAPT with aspirin and clopidogrel should be considered for secondary prevention in patients undergoing PCIs and patients with ischemic strokes and other high-risk events. The optimal duration of dual therapy is still unclear in patients with CKD. To date, there is no adequate data on added benefit of administering higher loading or maintenance doses of clopidogrel. Third, platelet function testing could be considered in those patients who experience thrombotic events despite dual therapy to guide treatment. Newer agents could be tried in patients who demonstrate higher residual platelet aggregability on standard antiplatelet treatment. There remains an urgent need for more studies to assess the pharmacodynamics and pharmacokinetics of antiplatelet agents, and their long-term safety and efficacy profile in CKD patients.

FUTURE DIRECTIONS

The management of antiplatelet therapy in CKD patients is an evolving field. Future research should focus on refining risk stratification models, optimizing dosing regimens, and assessing the long-term benefits and risks associated with antiplatelet agents in this population.

CONCLUSION

Antiplatelet therapy plays a significant role in the prevention and management of cardiovascular events in CKD patients. Aspirin has demonstrated benefits in reducing cardiovascular risks in CKD patients, while the evidence for clopidogrel and DAPT is more complex and requires careful consideration. It is crucial to balance the potential benefits with the bleeding risks associated with antiplatelet therapy in CKD patients. Individualized approaches, considering patient-specific factors, are necessary for decision-making. Future research should focus on how to predict the efficacy and safety of antiplatelets in CKD patients.

ONLINE REFERENCES

Please scan the QR code provided at the end of the table of contents for References of this chapter.

CHAPTER 23

De-escalation of Antiplatelet Therapy in Post-PCI Patients: Time to Change Our Strategy?

Arijit Kumar Ghosh, Nitin Bajaj, Sagar R Makode, Gunjan Ghodeshwar, Pratibha Misra

ABSTRACT

Dual antiplatelet therapy (DAPT) with aspirin and a P2Y12 inhibitor is a cornerstone in the treatment of patients of coronary artery disease (CAD) undergoing percutaneous coronary intervention (PCI). Post-PCI DAPT leads to a decrease in rates of ischemic events at the expense of increased bleeding risk. Over the years, DAPT has seen significant changes in the agents utilized and duration of therapy as trials have raced to keep up with advancements made in stent technology and our understanding of bleeding and ischemic risk. Novel therapeutic strategies have been proposed to mitigate the bleeding risk associated with DAPT. Antiplatelet de-escalation (guided or unguided) to less potent P2Y12 inhibitors or monotherapy after a short-term DAPT post-PCI has been shown to be a feasible and safe alternative. Recent studies showing antiplatelets' de-escalation to less potent P2Y12 inhibitors after a short period of more potent ones and P2Y12 inhibitor monotherapy are associated with improved outcomes compared to DAPT or aspirin. Recent data from large clinical trials have shifted the traditional paradigm of 6- or 12-month antiplatelet therapy after PCI. Antiplatelet regimens of shorter duration and variable intensity, based on individual risk factors, comorbidities, and bleeding/ischemic risks, appear to be the next antiplatelet frontier post-PCI. There has been a shift toward more individualized antiplatelet regimens to meet patient-specific risk profiles.

Keywords: Dual antiplatelet therapy, percutaneous coronary intervention, P2Y12 inhibitors, antiplatelet de-escalation, guided and unguided de-escalation, short-term antiplatelet therapy.

INTRODUCTION

In patients with coronary artery disease (CAD), percutaneous coronary interventions (PCI) are the cornerstone of treatment for those presenting with an acute coronary syndrome (ACS) and PCI has also been largely adopted in patients with chronic coronary syndromes (CCSs) on failure of guideline-directed medical therapy (GDMT). Dual antiplatelet therapy (DAPT) for a period of 6–12 months constitutes the standard of care after PCI. Post-PCI DAPT leads to a decrease in rates of ischemic events at the expense of increased bleeding risk. DAPT consisting of the combination of aspirin and a P2Y12 inhibitor is currently the cornerstone in the prevention of ischemic events following PCI for ACS and CCS.[1]

The synergistic effect of cyclooxygenase-1 receptor blocking and P2Y12 signaling inhibition has demonstrated a strong antithrombotic efficacy coupled with a relatively favorable safety profile.[2,3] Ticlopidine and clopidogrel were the first P2Y12 inhibitors to demonstrate reduced ischemic events in patients with unstable angina, non-ST-segment elevation myocardial infarction (NSTEMI), or ST-segment elevation myocardial infarction (STEMI), as well as those undergoing angioplasty and stenting for symptomatic stable ischemic heart disease (SIHD).[3-6] Novel P2Y12 inhibitors, ticagrelor and prasugrel, have shown to further reduce ischemic events in patients with ACS, compared to clopidogrel, at the cost of increased bleeding risk.[7-9]

The benefits of DAPT from randomized clinical trials (RCTs) have translated into a strong recommendation from the 2018 European Society of Cardiology (ESC) as well the 2022 American College of Cardiology/American Heart Association guidelines for DAPT for a period of at least

12 months for ACS and at least 6 months for stable CAD, followed by a lifelong aspirin monotherapy in patients at low bleeding risk.[10,11]

However, bleeding complications have always been the Achilles' heel of antiplatelet drugs. Bleeding events remain one of the most frequent complications post-PCI and are associated with increased risk of subsequent myocardial infarction (MI) and death. Approximately 5% of post-PCI patients are readmitted for bleeding, with the highest incidence occurring within a month of discharge. Patients having postdischarge bleeding are at increased risk for subsequent death or MI, with the highest risk occurring within the first 2 months after a bleeding-related hospitalization.[12] These findings emphasize the importance of bleeding risk identification and the need for individualized antiplatelet therapy (APT) strategies. At least 6 scores have been developed that predict long-term bleeding risk in patients taking APT.[13] The duration of DAPT has always been an area of ongoing research with the aim of minimizing both the ischemic complications as well as the bleeding risk with DAPT. In recent years, new anti-ischemic strategies for high bleeding risk (HBR) patients have been evolved and investigated in clinical trials. Such approaches, known as dual antiplatelet (DAP) shortening and de-escalation, represent a strategy to maintain anti-ischemic benefits of DAPT while mitigating bleeding risks.

ISCHEMIC RISK VERSUS BLEEDING RISK

The duration of DAPT is based on an assessment of the ischemic risk [risk of stent thrombosis (ST), repeat ACS] balanced with a risk of bleeding complications, especially major life-threatening bleeds associated with DAPT. This risk assessment can be done based on clinical and procedural features which can be defined qualitatively as well as quantified by means of various scoring systems.[14-16] The bleeding and the ischemic risk can be assessed by several clinical, procedural, and laboratory factors, which have been proven in various retrospective studies and included in the scores and definitions for risk assessment **(Fig. 1)**. It is important to note that many patients are at risk of both increased bleeding and ischemic events; when these are concordant, observational data suggest that bleeding, more than ischemic risk, should inform the decision-making on the duration of DAPT [17] Guidelines also recommend that the bleeding risk of an individual patient be the key determinant in defining DAPT duration.

ANTIPLATELET THERAPY DE-ESCALATION

The ischemic risk is believed to be greatest during the acute and subacute phase after the index procedure, while bleeding

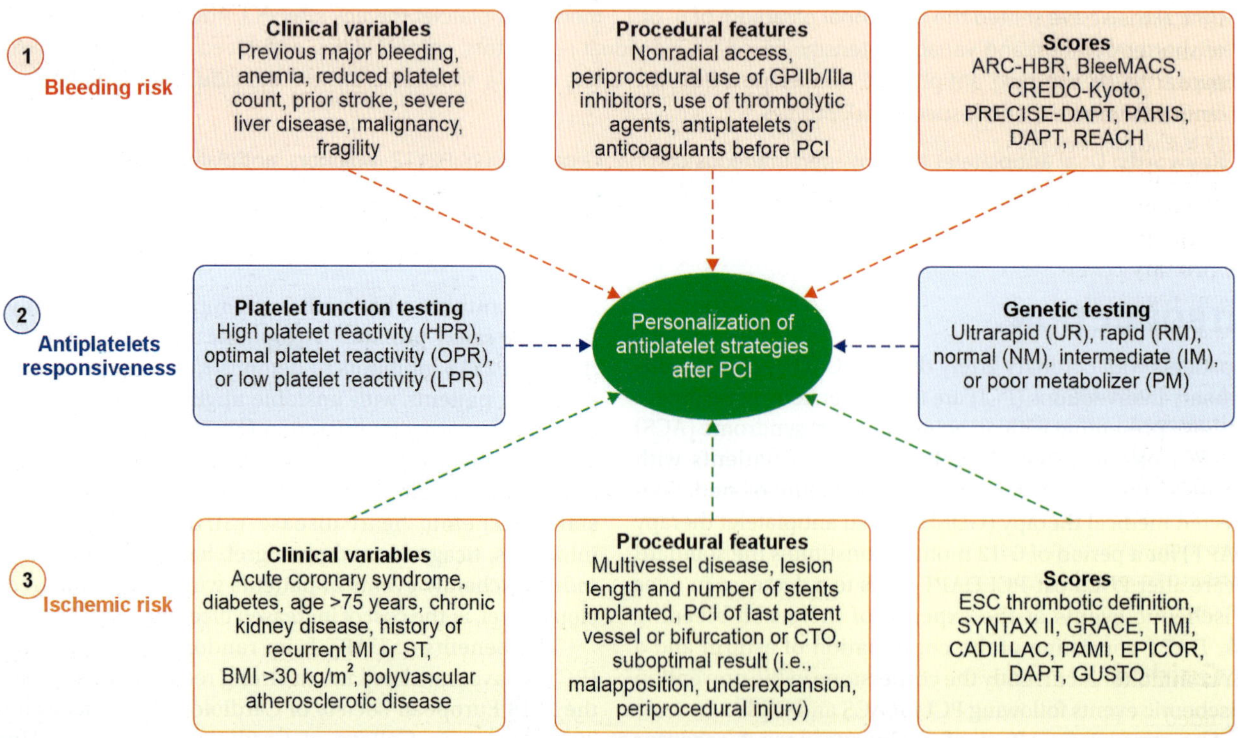

FIG. 1: Risk assessment to guide antiplatelet therapy among percutaneous coronary disease patients. Bleeding and ischemic risk assessments are based on clinical variables, procedural features, and the use of scores/definitions. Antiplatelet responsiveness can be assessed by either platelet function or genetic testing.[1]

(BMI: body mass index; CTO: chronic total occlusion; DAPT: dual antiplatelet therapy; ESC: European Society of Cardiology; GP: glycoprotein; MI: myocardial infarction; PCI: percutaneous coronary intervention; ST: stent thrombosis; TIMI: thrombolysis in myocardial infarction)

risk remains stable throughout the therapy period. More potent P2Y12 inhibitors (i.e., ticagrelor and prasugrel) have previously been shown to reduce ischemic events in patients with ACS compared to clopidogrel, particularly early after PCI, at the cost of increased bleeding risk.[7-9] De-escalation of P2Y12 inhibitor therapy consists of de-escalation from more potent P2Y12 inhibitor such as prasugrel or ticagrelor to a less potent drug such as clopidogrel or the dose of the potent P2Y12 inhibitor is reduced after a short course of DAPT, with an aim to reduce the risk of bleeding events albeit with a trade-off in an increased risk of ischemic events. This is in reference to ACS patients where more potent P2Y12 inhibitors are recommended as a standard of care.

Two different therapeutic strategies for antiplatelet de-escalation have been described in the literature—guided or unguided. In the guided strategy, de-escalation is assisted by platelet function tests (PFTs) and genetic testing for *CYP2C19* gene variants. On the other hand, in the unguided strategy, changes are made without any platelet function or genetic testing.

Unguided De-escalation

Current guidelines recommend at least 12 months of potent P2Y12 inhibitor (i.e., ticagrelor or prasugrel) for ACS patients managed with PCI.[10] Unguided de-escalation has been studied in a few RCTs in patients of ACS who have been given ticagrelor or prasugrel after PCI. The open-label, monocentric, the TOPIC (Timing of Platelet Inhibition after Acute Coronary Syndrome) trial evaluated the benefit of switching DAPT from aspirin plus a more potent P2Y12 inhibitor (ticagrelor or prasugrel) to aspirin plus clopidogrel 1 month after ACS.[18] There were 646 patients with STEMI and NSTEMI ACS at low-to-moderate bleeding risk randomly assigned to the switched DAPT group or to the unchanged DAPT group. At 1-year follow-up, the de-escalation strategy was superior to the standard DAPT strategy with regard to the primary composite endpoint of cardiovascular death, urgent revascularization, stroke, and Bleeding Academic Research Consortium (BARC) ≥ 2 bleeding. No significant differences were reported in ischemic endpoints, while BARC ≥ 2 bleeding occurred in significantly less patients in the switched DAPT group.

The TALOS-AMI (TicAgrelor Versus CLOpidogrel in Stabilized Patients with Acute Myocardial Infarction) trial from 32 institutes in South Korea, comparing de-escalation from ticagrelor to clopidogrel 1 month after PCI versus standard ticagrelor-based DAPT among 2,697 East Asian ACS patients, showed similar results.[19]

Guided De-escalation

A guided de-escalation strategy has been tested in RCTs in patients of ACS. In TROPICAL-ACS (Testing Responsiveness to Platelet Inhibition on Chronic Antiplatelet Treatment for Acute Coronary Syndrome) trial, which was the largest of the studies using platelet function testing, in 2,610 ACS patients undergoing PCI, guided de-escalation was noninferior for the primary composite endpoint of net adverse clinical event (NACE) as compared to standard of care, with a trend toward reduced bleeding at 12 months compared to the standard group.[20] On the basis of the TROPICAL-ACS trial, the latest ESC guidelines on myocardial revascularization upgraded their recommendation to Class IIb for the use of PFT for guided de-escalation, especially in patients who deemed to not be good candidates for 12 months of potent APT.[11] In the POPULAR GENETICS (Genotype-Guided Strategy for Oral P2Y12 Inhibitors in Primary PCI) trial, the benefit of *CYP2C19* genetic testing-guided DAPT de-escalation was evaluated.[21] There were 2,488 patients undergoing primary PCI with stent implantation for STEMI; they were randomly assigned to receive either a P2Y12 inhibitor on the basis of early *CYP2C19* genetic testing (genotype-guided group) or standard treatment with either ticagrelor or prasugrel (standard-treatment group) for 12 months. At 12 months, guided de-escalation was noninferior to standard DAPT in terms of clinical events. However, unlike the TROPICAL-ACS trial, bleeding rates were significantly reduced in the de-escalation group compared to the standard group.

Individual RCTs have limited power to assess the ischemic and bleeding endpoints. A recent meta-analysis overcoming such limitations found that a strategy of guided de-escalation of APT is associated with a 19% reduction of any bleeding, driven by a reduction of minor bleeding, without any trade-off in efficacy, as compared to standard selection of APT among patients undergoing PCI.[20] A recent meta-analysis has shown that both guided and unguided de-escalation reduce bleeding without any trade-off in ischemic events.[19]

SHORT-TERM DUAL ANTIPLATELET THERAPY: WHAT IS THE EVIDENCE?

The risk of bleeding in post-PCI patients, especially in HBR cases, has led to various trials where a strategy of shorter DAPT has been studied in comparison to the standard DAPT. The shortening of DAPT traditionally consists of the withdrawal of the P2Y12 inhibitor before the recommended standard period of DAPT, usually 3 or 6 months after PCI. Alternatively, shortened DAPT can also occur due to the discontinuation of aspirin while maintaining P2Y12 inhibitor monotherapy.

Until a few years ago, bare-metal stents (BMSs) were used for PCI in patients at HBR or those unable to tolerate long-term DAPT. That strategy allowed for a shorter duration of DAPT, 1 month for stable CAD, and 6 months for ACS, at the cost of higher rates of ST and repeat revascularization when compared to drug-eluting stent (DES).[22] As recently as 2014, BMS were used in ~20% of coronary-stenting procedures in patients over the age of 65 years in the USA, with 18.2% of BMS recipients having a predicted bleeding risk of >5% per year.[23]

Three recent RCTs comparing DES and BMS with 1 month of DAPT in patients perceived to be at increased bleeding risk provided the evidence to swift this paradigm. In the LEADERS FREE (Polymer-Free Drug-Coated Coronary Stents in Patients at High Bleeding Risk) trial, 2,466 HBR patients undergoing PCI were randomized to receive either a polymer-free and carrier-free drug-coated stent or a BMS.[24] Both groups were treated with DAPT for 1 month followed by a single antiplatelet agent thereafter. The primary safety endpoint, tested for both noninferiority and superiority, was a composite of cardiac death, MI, or ST. The primary efficacy endpoint was clinically driven target lesion revascularization. At 390 days, the primary safety endpoint had occurred in 9.4% of patients in the drug-coated-stent group and in 12.9% of patients in the BMS group. During the same period, clinically driven target-lesion revascularization was needed in 5.1% of the drug-coated-stent group versus 9.8% of the BMS group.

Similar results were observed in a prespecified analysis from the ZEUS (Zotarolimus-Eluting Endeavor Sprint Stent in Uncertain DES Candidates) trial,[25] as well as in the DES in elderly patients with CAD (the SENIOR trial).[26] In the multinational, randomized single-blinded ZEUS trial, 828 HBR patients were randomized to receive a Zotarolimus DES or BMS. Both groups were treated with 1 month of DAPT followed by a single-agent APT. At 12 months, DES implantation provided superior efficacy and safety as compared with conventional BMS. In the SENIOR trial, 1,200 HBR patients over the age of 75 years were randomized to receive either DES or BMS. DAPT was administered in both groups for 1 month followed by single APT. The primary endpoint consisting of all-cause mortality, MI, stroke, and ischemia-driven target lesion revascularization occurred less frequently in the DES group versus the BMS group. No significant difference was observed in bleeding complications or ST rates. Following these three trials, there have been multiple subsequent studies evaluating a shorter course of DAPT in patients treated with DES such as the XIENCE Short DAPT, ONYX ONE, and EVOLVE Short DAPT.[27-29]

Various RCTs have studied shorter DAPT to the conventional DAPT in the last few years. In the GLOBAL LEADERS trial, patients undergoing PCI with a Biolimus A9-eluting stent for stable CAD or ACS were randomly assigned (1:1) to 75–100 mg aspirin daily plus 90 mg ticagrelor twice daily for 1 month, followed by 23 months of ticagrelor monotherapy, or standard DAPT with 75–100 mg aspirin daily plus either 75 mg clopidogrel daily (for patients with stable CAD) or 90 mg ticagrelor twice daily (for patients with ACS) for 12 months. The primary endpoint at 2 years was a composite of all-cause mortality or nonfatal centrally adjudicated new Q-wave MI as assessed by a core lab in a blinded manner. The secondary endpoint was BARC grade 3 or 5 bleeding as reported by the sites. This study concluded that 1-month DAPT with aspirin and ticagrelor followed by ticagrelor monotherapy was not superior to standard 12-month DAPT and there was no significant difference in the bleeding events. Although the trial failed to reach superiority for the primary endpoint events at 2 years, it did demonstrate noninferiority. Bleeding rates were similar between the two groups in the trial.[30]

The TWILIGHT (Ticagrelor with Aspirin or Alone in High-Risk Patients after Coronary Intervention) trial enrolled patients who were high risk for either a thrombotic or a bleeding risk after a PCI were enrolled. A total of 7,119 patients were enrolled in the study. They all were given 3 months of DAPT with aspirin and ticagrelor 90 mg BID. After 3 months, all patients who did not have any major bleeding or ischemic events were randomized to either receive an addition 12 months of ticagrelor with either aspirin or a placebo. This trial concluded that after an initial 3 months of DAPT with aspirin and ticagrelor, ticagrelor monotherapy was associated with a lower incidence of clinically relevant bleeding without an increased risk of death, stroke, or MI.[31]

The STOPDAPT-2 trial tested for clopidogrel monotherapy after 1 month of DAPT versus standard DAPT. This trial showed that 1 month of DAPT was associated with significantly lesser number of composite endpoint of cardiovascular death, MI, definite ST, ischemic and hemorrhagic stroke, or thrombolysis in myocardial infarction (TIMI) major or minor bleeding. The difference was driven due to increased number bleeding episodes with the standard 12-month DAPT.[32] The STOPDAPT-2-ACS trial tested the same hypothesis of clopidogrel monotherapy after 1 month of DAPT versus standard 12-month DAPT in patients of ACS. This study showed no significant difference in composite endpoint of cardiovascular death, MI, definite ST, ischemic and hemorrhagic stroke, or TIMI major or minor bleeding.[33]

The TICO trial tested ticagrelor monotherapy after 3 months of DAPT versus standard DAPT in patients of ACS who were treated with ultrathin bioresorbable polymer sirolimus-eluting stent (Orsiro). This trial showed that 3 months DAPT followed by ticagrelor monotherapy was superior to standard DAPT in this population in reducing composite ischemic and bleeding endpoints.[34] The MASTER-DAPT (Management of High Bleeding Risk Patients Post Bioresorbable Polymer Coated Stent Implantation with an Abbreviated versus Standard DAPT Regimen) was the first RCT to selectively enroll HBR patients. In the MASTER-DAPT trial, 4,579 patients at HBR were randomized after 1 month of DAPT to abbreviated (DAPT stopped and 11 months single APT or 5 months in patients with oral anticoagulants) or nonabbreviated APT (DAPT for minimum 3 months) strategies. There were two subgroups with presence or absence of recent ACS (in the past 12 months). The study showed that abbreviated DAPT had significantly fewer bleeding events with no significant increase in the ischemic event rates in this population.

Overall, the results of the individual studies, as well as pooled analyses of RCTs, showed the early withdrawal of P2Y12 inhibitor-reduced bleeding, including major bleeding without any significant increase of thrombotic events.[35]

However, it has been argued that many of the studies enrolled patients at low ischemic risk or that the studies were not powered for hard ischemic endpoints; whether a trade-off in thrombotic complication can be ruled out in high-risk settings remains to be fully defined. The recent ARC-HBR trade-off model may represent a useful tool to balance bleeding and ischemic risks.[36] In fact, patients with ACS had an increase in MI with 6 months compared with 12 months of DAPT.[37] Overall, these considerations are the reason for which shortened DAPT durations should be reserved for HBR patients for whom the benefits are more likely to outweigh the risks. Further studies are warranted to support shortened DAPT among high-risk populations for both bleeding and thrombotic events.

Short-DAPT versus Antiplatelet De-escalation

A recent network meta-analysis aimed at comparing short DAPT and de-escalation strategies being performed.[38] 29 randomized trials of DAPT modulation strategies encompassing 50,602 patients with ACS undergoing PCI were included. No significant difference was observed in all-cause mortality between short DAPT and de-escalation. De-escalation strategy reduced the risk for net adverse cardiovascular events, whereas short DAP decreased major bleeding events. The comparisons of short DAPT versus de-escalation relied on indirect evidence and, therefore, the consistency in treatment estimates for direct versus indirect evidence cannot be checked. Further randomized studies comparing the two strategies are still required.

P2Y12 Monotherapy with Clopidogrel after Short DAPT

Three large RCTs have explored the benefit of clopidogrel monotherapy after short DAPT in patients undergoing PCI. In the SMART-CHOICE (Effect of P2Y12 Inhibitor Monotherapy vs. Dual Antiplatelet Therapy on Cardiovascular Events in Patients Undergoing PCI) trial, 2,993 patients undergoing PCI were randomly assigned to 3 months of DAPT, followed by monotherapy with a P2Y12 inhibitor or DAPT for 12 months.[39] There were 58.2% of the study participants who presented with ACS and 49.5% had multivessel disease. Clopidogrel was used as the P2Y12 inhibitor in 76.9% of the patients in the P2Y12 inhibitor monotherapy group and 77.6% in the DAPT group. At 12 months, short DAPT with P2Y12 monotherapy was shown to be noninferior to standard DAPT with respect to the primary ischemic endpoint (composite of all-cause death, MI, or stroke). Additionally, no statistically significant difference in the rates of the individual endpoints was observed between the two groups. Of note, the rate of bleeding was significantly lower in the P2Y12 inhibitor monotherapy group compared to the DAPT group. The STOPDAPT-2 (Effect of 1-Month Dual Antiplatelet Therapy Followed by Clopidogrel vs. 12-Month Dual Antiplatelet Therapy on Cardiovascular and Bleeding Events in Patients Receiving PCI) Japanese study randomized 3,045 low-to-moderate bleeding risk patients undergoing PCI.[32] ACS composed 38% of the study population. The experimental group received 1 month of DAPT followed by clopidogrel monotherapy, while the control group received 12 months of DAPT with aspirin and clopidogrel. Despite the even shorter duration of DAPT, 1-month DAPT was both noninferior and superior to 12-month DAPT for the primary composite endpoint of cardiovascular death, MI, ischemic or hemorrhagic stroke, definite ST, or major or minor bleeding at 12 months. Short DAPT was also superior to 12-month DAPT with regard to major secondary bleeding with the endpoint occurring in 0.41% of the patients in the 1-month DAPT group and 1.54% of patients in the 12-month DAPT group. Despite the promising safety data for short clopidogrel monotherapy, the STOPDAPT-2 ACS (Comparison of Clopidogrel Monotherapy after 1 to 2 Months of Dual Antiplatelet Therapy with 1 Month of Dual Antiplatelet Therapy in Patients with ACS) study suggested that the benefit does not apply to unstable patients.[33] Randomizing 4,169 patients with ACS undergoing PCI to either 1–2 months of DAPT followed by clopidogrel monotherapy (n = 2,078) or to 12 months of DAPT with aspirin and clopidogrel, this trial failed to meet the primary noninferiority endpoint (combined endpoint of cardiovascular death, MI, any stroke, or definite ST) at 12 months. Additionally, patients in the short DAPT group exhibited numerical increase in cardiovascular event rates; although this difference did not meet statistical significance, despite reduction in bleeding events. The abovementioned trials demonstrated the benefit of clopidogrel monotherapy after short DAPT in reducing bleeding risk while maintaining a safe ischemic profile in stable patients with mixed bleeding risks. The MASTER DAPT (Management of High Bleeding Risk Patients Post Bioresorbable Polymer-Coated Stent Implantation with an Abbreviated versus Standard DAPT Regimen) trial was the first one to investigate the benefit of clopidogrel monotherapy after short DAPT in patients only at HBR.[40] 1 month after undergoing implantation of a biodegradable-polymer sirolimus-eluting coronary stent, 4,434 patients were randomly instructed to discontinue DAPT immediately (abbreviated therapy) or to continue it for at least 2 additional months (standard therapy). The three ranked primary outcomes were NACEs (a composite of death from any cause, MI, stroke, or major bleeding), major adverse cardiac or cerebral events (a composite of death from any cause, MI, or stroke), and major or clinically relevant nonmajor bleeding. At 11 months of follow-up, clopidogrel monotherapy, after 1 month of DAPT, was noninferior to the continuation of DAPT for at least 2 additional months with regard to the occurrence of NACEs and major adverse cardiac or cerebral events. Furthermore, abbreviated therapy resulted in a lower incidence of major or clinically relevant nonmajor bleeding.

P2Y12 Monotherapy with Ticagrelor after Short Dual Antiplatelet Therapy

Following the promising results for clopidogrel monotherapy, multiple clinical trials have explored a potential role for ticagrelor monotherapy after short DAPT following stent placement. The GLOBAL LEADERS (ticagrelor plus aspirin for 1 month, followed by ticagrelor monotherapy for 23 months versus aspirin plus clopidogrel or ticagrelor for 12 months, followed by aspirin monotherapy for 12 months after implantation of a drug-eluting stent) study was the first to randomize patients undergoing PCI for SIHD or ACS with a Biolimus A9-eluting stent, to aspirin plus ticagrelor for 1 month, followed by 23 months of ticagrelor monotherapy, or standard DAPT with aspirin plus either clopidogrel (for patients with stable CAD) or ticagrelor twice daily (for patients with ACS) for 12 months, followed by aspirin monotherapy for 12 months.[30] The primary endpoint at 2 years was a composite of all-cause mortality or nonfatal centrally adjudicated new Q-wave MI as assessed by a core lab in a blinded manner. The key secondary safety endpoint was site-reported bleeding assessed according to the BARC criteria (grade 3 or 5). Patients at low bleeding risk and mixed ischemic risk were included. Although the trial failed to reach superiority for the primary endpoint events at 2 years, it did demonstrate noninferiority. Bleeding rates were similar between the two groups in the trial. Comparable findings were demonstrated in the GLASSY (GLOBAL LEADERS Adjudication Sub-study), including all consecutive patients from the 20 highest recruiting sites.[41] The co-primary efficacy endpoint was broadened to include a composite of death, MI, stroke, or urgent target vessel revascularization (TVR). The co-primary safety endpoint was a composite of BARC 3 or 5 bleeding events. At 2 years, ticagrelor monotherapy after 1-month DAPT was noninferior, but not superior to conventional treatment in the prevention of ischemic events. Rates of BARC 3 or 5 bleeding did not differ between the groups. Interestingly, a time-dependent treatment effect was observed with the experimental strategy being associated with a lower risk of MI and definite ST after 1-year post-PCI. The TWILIGHT (Ticagrelor with or without Aspirin in High-Risk Patients after PCI) trial provided further large body of evidence for monotherapy with ticagrelor.[31] There were 7,119 patients at high risk for bleeding or an ischemic event randomized 3 months after receiving DAPT with ticagrelor plus aspirin to receive aspirin or placebo for 1 year in addition to ticagrelor. The primary endpoint was BARC type 2, 3, or 5 bleeding. The composite endpoint of death from any cause, nonfatal MI, or nonfatal stroke was also evaluated. Ticagrelor monotherapy, after 3 months of DAPT, was associated with a 44% lower risk of BARC type 2, 3, or 5 bleeding over 1 year compared to ticagrelor plus aspirin. Additionally, there was no increase in the risk of death, MI, or stroke among patients who received ticagrelor monotherapy compared to those who received ticagrelor plus aspirin. The treatment effect with respect to both bleeding and ischemic endpoints was consistent across subgroups.

Data from TWILIGHT and GLASSY studies were analyzed together in the collaborative individual patient data meta-analysis (SIDNEY), including a total of 14,628 patients undergoing DES implantation.[42] BARC type 3 or 5 bleeding occurred in fewer patients receiving ticagrelor monotherapy compared to DAPT. The composite of all-cause death, MI, or stroke was similar between groups. However, ticagrelor monotherapy was associated with lower risk for all-cause and cardiovascular mortality. Rates of MI, ST, and stroke did not differ.

Focusing exclusively on patients with ACS, the TICO (Effect of Ticagrelor Monotherapy vs. Ticagrelor with Aspirin on Major Bleeding and Cardiovascular Events in Patients with ACS) RCT was designed to prospectively compare ticagrelor monotherapy to DAPT specifically in ACS population[34] There were 3,056 patients with ACS treated with DES randomized to ticagrelor monotherapy after 3 months of DAPT or ticagrelor-based 12 months of DAPT. Importantly, only patients at low bleeding risk were included in the study. At 1 year, ticagrelor monotherapy after 3 months of DAPT resulted in a modest but statistically significant reduction in a composite outcome of major bleeding and cardiovascular events. Nevertheless, the lower than anticipated event rate of the primary outcome led to a lower-than-expected power, limiting the generalizability of the study findings.

P2Y12 Monotherapy with Prasugrel after Short DAPT

There are currently limited clinical data on the use of prasugrel as monotherapy after short DAPT. In the ASET Pilot study (Aspirin-Free Prasugrel Monotherapy Following Coronary Artery Stenting in Patients with Stable CAD), 201 patients undergoing PCI for SIHD with SYNTAX score < 23 were included.[43] All participants were on standard DAPT at the time of index PCI. Aspirin was discontinued on the day of the index procedure but given prior to the procedure. Prasugrel was administered in the catheterization laboratory immediately after the successful procedure, and aspirin-free prasugrel became the therapy regimen after that. Patients were treated solely with prasugrel for 3 months. The primary ischemic endpoint was the composite of cardiac death, spontaneous target vessel MI, or definite ST, and the primary bleeding endpoint was BARC types 3 and 5 bleeding. At 3 months, the primary ischemic and bleeding endpoints occurred in one patient (0.5%). No ST events occurred. However, this was a pilot study with no direct comparison group and a small sample size.

P2Y12 Monotherapy in Complex Percutaneous Coronary Intervention

Several studies have already demonstrated the benefits of P2Y12 monotherapy after short DAPT in overall PCI population receiving newer generation DES. However, the application of these findings to patients undergoing complex PCI has been limited. Recently, a meta-analysis of 22,941 patients undergoing complex PCI from five trials provided further data in this area.[44] After an initial period of DAPT (which ranged from 1 to 3 months across trials), patients either discontinued aspirin and continued with P2Y12 monotherapy or continued with standard DAPT for 12 months. Complex PCI was defined as any of the six criteria: 3 vessels treated, ≥3 stents implanted, ≥3 lesions treated, bifurcation with 2 stents implanted, total stent length > 60 mm, or chronic total occlusion. The primary efficacy endpoint was all-cause mortality, MI, and stroke. The key safety endpoint was BARC 3 or 5 bleeding. Overall, the primary efficacy endpoint occurred more often in the complex PCI group compared with the noncomplex PCI group. Additionally, the risk of the key safety endpoint of BARC 3 or 5 bleeding was numerically, but not statistically significantly higher in complex PCI patients. Nevertheless, there was no significant difference observed in the primary efficacy endpoint between P2Y12 inhibitor monotherapy and DAPT among patients with complex PCI and noncomplex PCI. Compared with DAPT, P2Y12 inhibitor monotherapy consistently reduced BARC 3 or 5 bleeding in complex PCI and noncomplex PCI patients.

CURRENT GUIDELINES

The findings presented in the abovementioned trials have significantly affected the recommendations for antiplatelet regimens post-PCI and DAPT duration in both the American College of Cardiology/American Heart Association as well as the ESC guidelines. In the 2021 American College of Cardiology/American Heart Association revascularization guideline, discontinuation of aspirin after 1–3 months of DAPT with continuation of P2Y12 monotherapy for at least 12 months is now a Class IIa indication for patient with SIHD or ACS.[10] Additionally, in patient at high risk for bleeding or with overt bleeding, P2Y12 discontinuation is reasonable at 3 months for SIHD (Class IIb) or at 6 months after ACS PCI (Class IIb). Finally, routine platelet function testing and genetic testing in patients treated with DAPT are still not recommended (Class III: no benefit) **(Flowchart 1)**. Similarly, aspirin discontinuation at 3–6 months after balancing the risks of bleeding and ischemic events is now a Class IIa recommendation in the 2020 ESC Society of Cardiology non-STE ACS guidelines.[45] In patients at high risk for bleeding, discontinuation of the P2Y12 receptor inhibitor after 3 months can be considered (Class IIa). Finally, de-escalation of the P2Y12 receptor inhibitor treatment either unguided and based on clinical judgement or guided by platelet function testing or *CYP2C19* genotyping testing may be considered (Class IIb).

CONCLUSION

Antiplatelet therapy represents the cornerstone of treatment for the prevention of local and systemic ischemic complications in patients with CAD undergoing PCI. Prolonged DAPT has been the mainstay therapy after PCI for more than two decades. The development of newer generation DES, as well as more potent P2Y12 antiplatelet agents, has led to a decrease in ischemic events and a safer therapeutic profile post-PCI. Over the past many years, different antiplatelet regimens using aspirin and P2Y12 inhibitors have been developed and implemented. A better understanding of the ischemic and bleeding risk profile, as well as individual responsiveness to antiplatelet agents, has been instrumental in defining the optimal regimen for the individual patient. In particular, the intensity and the duration of aspirin and P2Y12 inhibiting therapy should be adjusted to reduce the risk of ischemic complications while minimizing the risk of bleeding. Nevertheless, an increase in bleeding events remains the Achilles' heel of long DAPT or more potent P2Y12 inhibitors. Novel antiplatelet strategies aimed at decreasing bleeding rates through shortening duration of DAPT and antiplatelet de-escalation have been extensively studied and described in the past decade. A strong body of evidence from multiple clinical trials supports these two strategies, shifting the therapeutic paradigm post-PCI. Recent data from large clinical trials have shifted the traditional paradigm of 6- or 12-month APT after PCI. Antiplatelet regimens of shorter duration and variable intensity, based on individual risk factors, comorbidities, and bleeding/ischemic risks, appear to be the next antiplatelet frontier post-PCI. Strategies developed to mitigate the risk of bleeding include shortening DAPT duration, P2Y12 inhibitor monotherapy, and de-escalation.

In the absence of HBR, patients at increased ischemic risk may consider prolonging intensified antithrombotic therapy. The use of platelet function and genetic testing can indeed be of aid in the selection of P2Y12 inhibitor therapy. An integrated approach, including scores/definitions to define ischemic and bleeding risk, procedural characteristics, characteristics of stents used, and tools to help assess drug response, represents the most promising approach for a personalized selection of antiplatelet agents among patients undergoing PCI. Personalized antiplatelet strategies and DAPT durations, based on ischemic and bleeding profiles, appear to be the next frontier of pharmacotherapy in PCI.

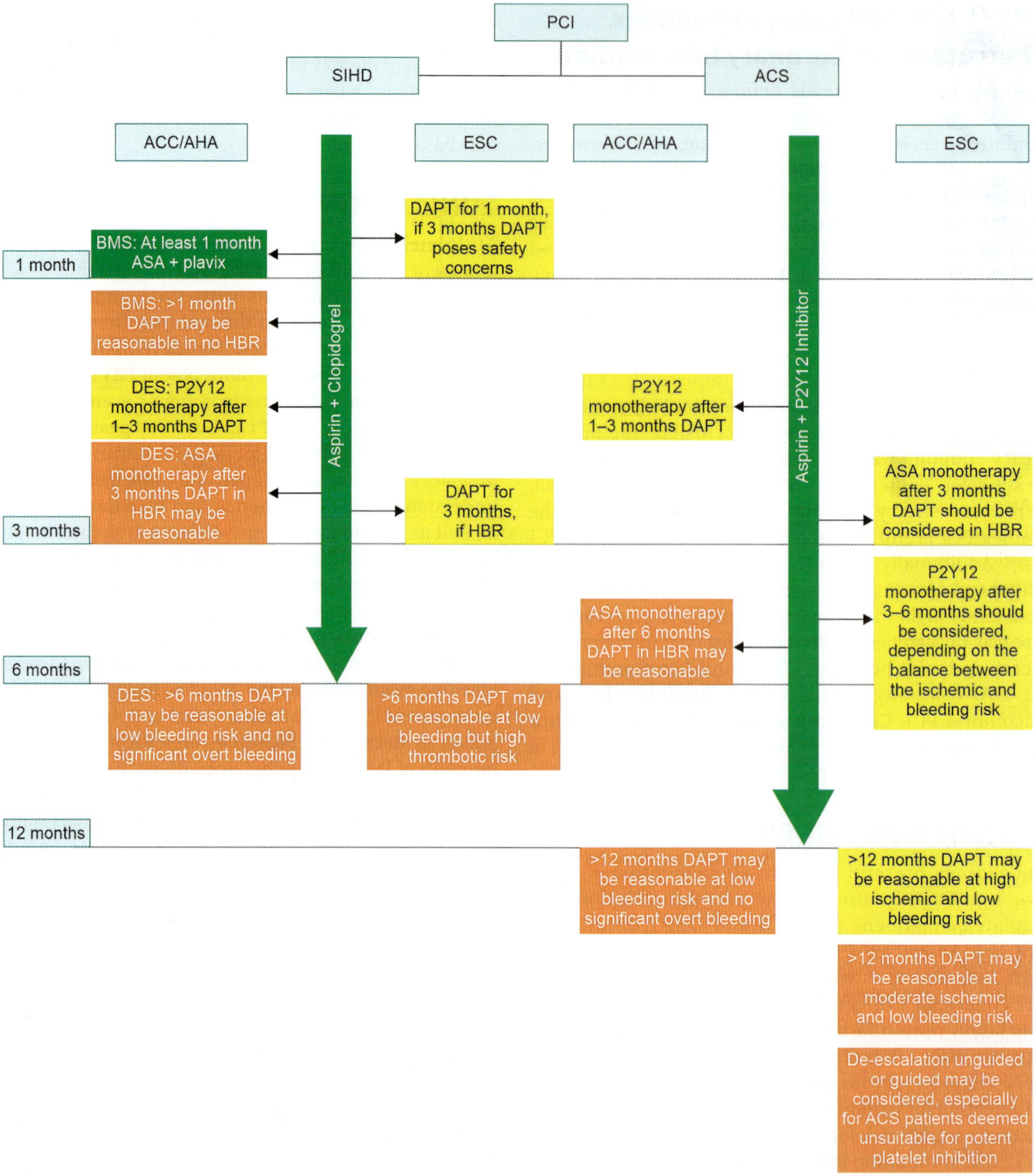

FLOWCHART 1: Antithrombotic strategies according to the American College of Cardiology/American Heart Association as well as the ESC guidelines.

Note: *Green*: Class I; *Yellow*: Class IIa; *Orange*: Class IIb

(ACC/AHA: American College of Cardiology/American Heart Association; ACS: acute coronary syndrome; ASA: acetylsalicylic acid; BMS: bare-metal stent; DAPT: dual antiplatelet therapy; DES: drug-eluting stent; ESC: European Society of Cardiology; HBR: high bleeding risk; PCI: percutaneous coronary intervention; SIHD: stable ischemic heart disease)

ONLINE REFERENCES

Please scan the QR code provided at the end of the table of contents for References of this chapter.

CHAPTER 24

Landscape of Oral Anticoagulation in Valvar and Nonvalvar Atrial Fibrillation

Gaurav Kumar Arora, Sandeep Bansal

ABSTRACT

Atrial fibrillation (AF) is the most common arrhythmia worldwide that can cause stroke leading to morbidity and mortality. The pathologic basis of stroke in atrial fibrillation is the manifestation of left atrial appendage thrombus. Hence oral anticoagulation is the cornerstone therapy for the prevention of stroke in patients with atrial fibrillation. Assessment of stroke risk and bleeding risk helps in individualizing the need for oral anticoagulation. Valvar atrial fibrillation includes atrial fibrillation in patients with moderate-to-severe mitral stenosis or mechanical heart valve and they require long-term anticoagulation with vitamin K antagonists. Non-vitamin K antagonist oral anticoagulants are preferred agents in the rest of the patients owing to their fixed dose and safety profile.

Keywords: Atrial fibrillation, NOAC, valvar AF.

INTRODUCTION

Atrial fibrillation (AF) is the most common incessant arrhythmia that accounts for an increased risk of stroke. There is no effective contraction of atria in AF, leading to stasis in these low-pressure cardiac chambers. This results in a fertile ground for thrombus formation, usually in the left atrial appendage (LAA). Such a thrombus upon dislodgement can cause thromboembolism to intracranial circulation leading to a cardioembolic stroke. Hence oral anticoagulation (OAC) is advised for preventing stroke in patients with AF after assessment of stroke risk and bleeding risk.

STROKE RISK ASSESSMENT IN ATRIAL FIBRILLATION

Atrial fibrillation carries a greater risk of stroke than sinus rhythm, and the quantum of risk depends on coexisting risk factors for stroke. Prior stroke/transient ischemic attack (TIA)/systemic embolism, hypertension, aging (per decade), structural heart disease, diabetes mellitus, vascular disease, LV dysfunction/congestive heart failure, and female sex are the most commonly studied risk factors of stroke in AF.[1]

Moreover, impaired renal function, obstructive sleep apnea, smoking, malignancy, hypertrophic cardiomyopathy, thyroid disease, aortic atherosclerosis, metabolic syndrome, or degenerative disease of the heart and brain, like amyloidosis carry a greater risk of stroke in AF.[2] AF in hypertrophic cardiomyopathy or hyperthyroidism should be offered anticoagulation for stroke prevention.[3]

The CHA_2DS_2-VASc score **(Table 1)** is a practical bedside tool for stroke risk assessment in nonvalvar AF. Those identified as low-risk [CHA_2DS_2-VASc 0 (males), or score of 1 (females)] consistently have a low ischemic stroke or mortality rate (<1%/year) and do not need any stroke prevention treatment. **Table 2** illustrates the stroke risk with the corresponding CHA_2DS_2-VASc risk score. Stroke risk must be re-evaluated at each follow-up visit. About 15% of low-risk patients would have ≥1 nonsex CHA_2DS_2-VASc risk factor at 6 months–1 year follow-up.[4,5] OAC is recommended in when CHA_2DS_2-VASc score is ≥2 in men and ≥3 in women.

Ineffective atrial mechanical contraction in AF predisposes thrombus formation in the LAA. Thromboembolism from the heart can present as a stroke. LAA characteristics such as peak LAA anterograde flow velocity <20 cm/s (normal >50 cm/s), nonchicken wing morphology, and the presence of LAA thrombus are risk factors for stroke. Compared with chicken wing, cactus was 4.08 times (p = 0.046), windsock was 4.5 times (p = 0.038), and

TABLE 1: CHA_2DS_2-VASc score.

Risk factors and definitions		Points awarded	Comment
C	Congestive heart failure: Clinical HF, or objective evidence of moderate-to-severe LV dysfunction, or HCM	1	Recently decompensated HF irrespective of LVEF, or the presence (even if asymptomatic) of moderate-severe LV systolic dysfunction; HCM confers a high stroke risk and OAC is beneficial for stroke reduction[6]
H	*H*ypertension or on antihypertensive therapy	1	A history of hypertension may result in vascular changes predisposing to stroke, and a well-controlled BP today may not be well-controlled over time. Uncontrolled BP—the optimal BP target associated with the lowest risk of ischemic stroke, death, and other cardiovascular outcomes is 120–129/<80 mm Hg[6]
A	*A*ge 75 years or older	2	The risk rises from age 65 years upward. The risk of stroke may rise from age 50–55 years upward and that a modified CHA_2DS_2-VASc score may be used in Asian patients.[7] Age-related risk is a continuum, but for reasons of simplicity and practicality, 1 point is given for age 65–74 years and 2 points for age ≥75 years
D	*D*iabetes mellitus: Treatment with oral hypoglycemic drugs and/or insulin or fasting blood glucose >125 mg/dL (7 mmol/L)	1	Diabetes mellitus is a well-established risk factor for stroke, and more recently stroke risk has been related to duration of diabetes mellitus and presence of diabetic target organ damage, e.g., retinopathy
S	*S*troke: Previous stroke, TIA, or thromboembolism	2	Previous stroke, systemic embolism, or TIA confers a particularly high risk of ischemic stroke, hence weighted 2 points. Although excluded from RCTs, AF patients with ICH (including hemorrhagic stroke) are at very high risk of subsequent ischemic stroke
V	*V*ascular disease: Angiographically significant CAD, previous myocardial infarction, PAD, or aortic plaque	1	Vascular disease (PAD or myocardial infarction) confers a 17–22% excess risk, particularly in Asian patients. Angiographically significant CAD is also an independent risk factor for ischemic stroke among AF patients. Complex aortic plaque on the descending aorta, as an indicator of significant vascular disease, is also a strong predictor of ischemic stroke
A	*A*ge 65–74 years	1	See above
S	*S*ex category (female)	1	A stroke risk modifier rather than a risk factor

(CAD: coronary artery disease; HCM: hypertrophic cardiomyopathy; ICH: intracranial hemorrhage; LVEF: left ventricular ejection fraction; OAC: oral anticoagulant; PAD: peripheral artery disease; RCTs: randomized controlled trials; TIA: transient ischemic attack)

TABLE 2: Stroke risk based on CHA_2DS_2-VASc score.

CHA_2DS_2-VASc score	Annual adjusted stroke risk (%)
0	0
1	1.3
2	2.2
3	3.2
4	4.0
5	6.7
6	9.8
7	9.6
8	6.7
9	15.2

cauliflower was 8.0 times ($p = 0.056$) more likely to have had a stroke/TIA.[8,9]

More complex clinical scores such as Global Anticoagulant Registry in the FIELD—atrial fibrillation (GARFIELD-AF)[10] and those including biomarkers such as anticoagulation and risk factors in AF (ATRIA),[11] Intermountain Risk Score[12] or ABC-stroke (age, biomarkers, clinical history)[13] improves stroke risk prediction statistically significantly but not substantially, at an additional burden of healthcare costs.

BLEEDING RISK ASSESSMENT

All OAC agents carry a finite bleeding risk. The risk factors for bleeding should be assessed as per **Table 3** for every individual considered for OAC. The modifiable risk factors may be worked upon to reduce bleeding risk. HAS-BLED

TABLE 3: Risk factors for bleeding in patients with atrial fibrillation.

Nonmodifiable	Potentially modifiable	Modifiable	Biomarkers
Age >65 years	Extreme frailty ± excessive risk of falls	Hypertension/elevated SBP	GDF-15
Previous major bleeding	Anemia	Concomitant antiplatelet/NSAID	Cystatin
Severe renal impairment (on dialysis or renal transplant)	Reduced platelet count or function	Excessive alcohol intake	C/CKD-EPI
Severe hepatic dysfunction (cirrhosis)	Renal impairment with CrCl <60 mL/min	Nonadherence to OAC	cTnT-hs
Malignancy	VKA management strategy	Hazardous hobbies/occupations	von Willebrand factor (+ other coagulation markers)
Genetic factors (e.g., CYP2C9 polymorphisms)		Bridging therapy with heparin	
Previous stroke, small-vessel disease, etc.		INR control (target 2.0–3.0), target TTR >70%	
Diabetes mellitus		Appropriate choice of OAC and correct dosing	
Cognitive impairment/ dementia			

(CKD-EPI: chronic kidney disease epidemiology collaboration; CrCl: creatinine clearance; cTnT-hs: high-sensitivity troponin T; CYP: cytochrome P; GDF-15: growth differentiation factor-15; INR: international normalized ratio; NSAID: nonsteroidal anti-inflammatory drug; OAC: oral anticoagulant; SBP: systolic blood pressure; TTR: time in therapeutic range; VKA: vitamin K antagonist)

TABLE 4: HASBLED score.

Risk factors and definitions		Points
H	Uncontrolled *h*ypertension: SBP >160 mm Hg	1
A	*A*bnormal renal and/or hepatic function dialysis, transplant, serum creatinine >200 μmol/L, cirrhosis, bilirubin >2 × upper limit of normal, AST/ALT/ALP >3 × upper limit of normal	1 point for each
S	*S*troke: Previous ischemic or hemorrhagica stroke	1
B	*B*leeding history or predisposition: Previous major hemorrhage or anemia or severe thrombocytopenia	1
L	*L*abile INR: TTR <60% in patient receiving VKA	1
E	*E*lderly: Aged >65 years or extreme frailty	1
D	*D*rugs or excessive alcohol drinking: Concomitant use of antiplatelet or NSAID; and/or excessive alcohol per week	1 point for each

(ALP: alkaline phosphatase; ALT: alanine transaminase; AST: aspartate transaminase; INR: international normalized ratio; NSAID: nonsteroidal anti-inflammatory drug; TTR: time in therapeutic range; VKA: vitamin K antagonist)

score **(Table 4)** has the best evidence for predicting bleeding risk in this situation.[14] HAS-BLED is better in identifying patients at low risk of bleeding (HAS-BLED 0–2). The bleeding risk can vary and must be reassessed at each follow-up visit. Prospective monitoring and reassessment using the HAS-BLED score reduces major bleeding events and increase OAC uptake.[15]

ABSOLUTE CONTRAINDICATION TO ORAL ANTICOAGULANTS

The absolute contraindications to OAC include severe active bleeding, associated comorbidities such as severe thrombocytopenia <50 platelets/μL, severe anemia under investigation, or a recent high-risk bleeding event such as intracranial hemorrhage (ICH). Nondrug options like LAA closure devices may be considered in such cases.

Oral Anticoagulants

Vitamin K antagonist (VKA) therapy (primarily warfarin) reduces stroke risk by 64% and mortality by 26% in selected AF patients.[16] VKA requires frequent prothrombin time international normalized ratio (INR) monitoring and corresponding dose adjustments owing to their narrow therapeutic range. Quality of VKA management, quantified using the time in therapeutic range based on the Rosendaal method, or the percentage of INRs in therapeutic range, correlates with the outcome of hemorrhagic and thromboembolic rates.[17] Numerous factors (including genetics, concomitant drugs, etc.), influence the anticoagulant effect of VKA. SAMe-TT_2R_2 score [sex (female), age (<60 years), medical history of ≥2 comorbidities (hypertension, diabetes mellitus, coronary artery disease (CAD)/myocardial infarction, peripheral artery disease (PAD), HF, previous stroke, pulmonary disease, and hepatic or renal disease), treatment (interacting drugs, e.g., amiodarone), tobacco use, race (non-Caucasian)] helps to identify patients who are less likely to achieve a good time in therapeutic range (TTR) on VKA therapy (score >2).[18]

Non-vitamin K antagonist oral anticoagulants (NOACs) are associated with a similar ischemic stroke risk reduction compared with VKAs, 51% reduction in hemorrhagic stroke, and 10% reduction in all-cause mortality in cases of nonvalvar AF.[19] Persistence with NOAC therapy is generally higher than that with VKAs, owing to no regular monitoring required for NOAC. Hence NOACs have become the OAC of choice for most patients **(Table 5)**.

ATRIAL FIBRILLATION AND VALVAR AND NONVALVAR ATRIAL FIBRILLATION

Valvar AF is defined as AF present in case of "moderate-to-severe mitral stenosis or mechanical heart valve" in the guidelines.[20,21] The term "nonvalvar AF" does not imply the absence of valvular heart disease but AF in the absence of moderate-to-severe mitral stenosis or a mechanical heart valve. Nonvalvar AF includes all the patients with AF who have evidence for the use NOAC for stroke prevention. In the clinical trials, up to 20% of patients had various valvular defects, including mild mitral stenosis, mitral regurgitation, aortic regurgitation, aortic stenosis, or tricuspid regurgitation; some had undergone valve repair, valvuloplasty, or bioprosthetic valves. NOACs reduced stroke and systemic embolism compared with warfarin, but with favorable bleeding risk.[22]

Patients with valvar AF require anticoagulation with VKA. NOAC is ineffective in stroke prevention in these patients and may lead to higher ischemic events than warfarin.[23,24] The mechanism due to which NOACs are ineffective in this sub-group is unclear as the patients with mitral stenosis and mechanical heart valves were excluded from large randomized trials.[25]

PATIENTS WITH ATRIAL FIBRILLATION AND CONGENITAL HEART DISEASE

Oral anticoagulant treatment is recommended for all patients with cyanotic congenital heart disease, intracardiac repair, systemic right ventricle, or Fontan palliation. Patients with AF and other congenital heart diseases should follow the general risk stratification for OAC use in AF.[26]

Periprocedural Stroke Risk Management in Patients Undergoing Rhythm Control Interventions

Patients undergoing cardioversion of AF (>12–48-hour duration) are at increased risk of stroke. Mechanisms of the increased propensity to pericardioversion thromboembolism include the presence of preexisting thrombus (especially if not anticoagulated), change in the atrial mechanical function with the restoration of sinus rhythm, atrial stunning post-cardioversion, and a transient prothrombotic state.[27]

Cardioversion can be scheduled after 3 weeks of therapy of VKA (INR 2-3)/NOAC. If there is no atrial thrombus on transesophageal echocardiography (TEE), cardioversion can be done upon administration of heparin. OAC is continued postcardioversion for 4 weeks. After that, anticoagulation is advised based on the CHA_2DS_2-VASc score, as rhythm

TABLE 5: Dosage of nonvitamin K antagonists oral anticoagulants.

	Dabigatran	Rivaroxaban	Apixaban	Edoxaban
Standard dose	150 mg BID	20 mg OD	5 mg BID	60 mg OD
Lower dose	110 mg BID			
Reduced dose		15 mg OD	2.5 mg BID	30 mg OD
Dose-reduction criteria	Dabigatran 110 mg BID in patients with: • Age ≥80 years • Concomitant use of verapamil, or • Increased bleeding risk	CrCl 15–49 mL/min	At least two of three criteria: • Age ≥80 years, • Body weight ≤60 kg, or • Serum creatinine ≥1.5 mg/dL (133 μmol/L)	If any of the following: • CrCl 15–50 mL/min, • Body weight ≤60 kg, • Concomitant use of dronedarone, cyclosporine, erythromycin, or ketoconazole

(CrCl: creatinine clearance; BID: twice daily; OD: once daily)

control strategies have not been shown to reduce stroke risk. AF ablation, when planned is done while the patient is on therapeutic anticoagulation with heparin.[28]

CORONARY ARTERY DISEASE AND ATRIAL FIBRILLATION

After stopping aspirin within a week, dual therapy with OAC and an antiplatelet drug (preferably clopidogrel) is recommended for the first 12 months after percutaneous coronary intervention (PCI) for acute coronary syndrome or 6 months after PCI in patients with chronic coronary syndrome.[29] After that, OAC monotherapy can be continued. In 1-year event-free AF patients with CAD and no PCI, OAC monotherapy is recommended.[30]

ACUTE ISCHEMIC STROKE WHILE ON ORAL ANTICOAGULATION IN ATRIAL FIBRILLATION

Thrombolytic therapy with recombinant tissue plasminogen activator (rt-PA) is approved within 4.5 hours of onset of stroke symptoms but should not be administered in patients on full anticoagulation (INR ≥1.7 in VKA).[31] Thrombolytic therapy cannot be given within 24 hours after the last intake of an NOAC due to their plasma half-lives, which may even be prolonged in renal dysfunction. After reversal and assessment of coagulation status, intravenous thrombolysis within 4.5 hours of onset of moderate-to-severe stroke can be done.[32] Endovascular thrombectomy may be considered in selected patients, but there is a risk of hemorrhagic transformation of ischemic stroke.[33]

TIMING TO REINITIATE ANTICOAGULATION AFTER ISCHEMIC STROKE

There is no evidence from RCTs to prefer one NOAC over the other or to switch from one NOAC to another in patients with a history of ischemic stroke under NOAC therapy. By consensus, infarct size/stroke severity is used clinically to guide the timing of OAC initiation.[21] OAC using an NOAC may be continued (according to prescription and label) or started 1 day after a TIA, ≥3 days after an ischemic stroke. In patients with moderate stroke, anticoagulation may be started ≥6–8 days, and in patients with severe stroke at ≥12–14 days, after excluding secondary hemorrhagic transformation.[31] Earlier OAC administration within 48 hours after a minor or moderate stroke or on day 6 or 7 after a major stroke led to better primary composite outcomes of a composite of recurrent ischemic stroke, systemic embolism, major extracranial bleeding, symptomatic ICH, or vascular death at 30 days.[34]

ACTIVE BLEEDING ON ANTICOAGULATION

General assessment should include detection of the bleeding site, assessment of bleeding severity, and evaluation of the time-point of last OAC intake, antithrombotic drugs, alcohol abuse, and renal function. Specific coagulation tests for NOACs include diluted thrombin time, ecarin clotting time, or ecarin chromogenic assay for dabigatran, and chromogenic anti-factor Xa assay for rivaroxaban, apixaban, and edoxaban and the serum drug levels are usually not readily available.

For minor bleeding, delay VKA till INR <2, and delay NOAC dose for one dose or day. In case of severe bleeding fluids and blood replacement is needed. For VKA, vitamin K administration followed by prothrombin complex concentrate/fresh frozen plasma may be considered. For severe bleeding with NOAC, specific antidotes such as idarucizumab, a monoclonal antibody fragment that binds dabigatran,[35] can be administered as 5 g intravenous (IV), divided in two doses, given up to 15 minutes apart.[36,37] Andexanet alfa is administered as an antidote for factor Xa inhibitors. Low dose andexanet alfa [400 mg IV bolus over 15 minutes, followed by 480 mg IV infusion (4 mg/min) over 2 hours] is administered if not >5 mg apixaban or 10 mg rivaroxaban is administered 8 hours prior to bleeding. If a higher dose of apixaban/rivaroxaban is received within 8 hours, then a high dose of andexanet alfa [800 mg IV bolus over 30 minutes, followed by 960 mg IV infusion (8 mg/min) over 2 hours] is administered.[38,39] Ciraparantag is a synthetic drug that binds and inhibits the direct factor Xa inhibitors, dabigatran, and heparin. Ciraparantag (100–300 mg single dose) may potentially provide a broader reversal of anticoagulation.[40]

MANAGEMENT OF PATIENTS WITH ATRIAL FIBRILLATION POST-INTRACRANIAL HEMORRHAGE

Intracranial hemorrhage survivors with AF are at high risk of ischemic stroke and recurrent ICH.[31] Whereas the risk of ischemic stroke depends on the presence of associated clinical stroke risk factors and can be assessed using the CHA_2DS_2-VASc score, the risk of recurrent ICH is highly variable (1.3–7.4%) and multifactorial.[41] Traumatic intracranial bleeding has a lower risk of recurrent intracranial bleeding.[42] Patients with a history of recent ICH were excluded from RCTs of stroke prevention in AF. However, observational data suggest AF patients would benefit from reinstitution of OAC about 2–4 weeks after intracranial hemorrhagic stroke [class II LOE (level of evidence) C].[3] Treatment decision to restart OAC in AF patients after an ICH requires multidisciplinary-team input from cardiologists, stroke specialists, neurosurgeons, patients, and their family.

CONCLUSION

Anticoagulation in AF is vital for stroke prevention in high stroke risk patients. CHA_2DS_2-VASc score and HAS-BLED score should be used to assess the stroke risk and bleeding risk at the first visit and on follow-up to account for development of new risk factors. NOACs are safe and effective OACs for all patients except valvar AF. VKAs are recommended in patients with valvar AF which include moderate-to-severe mitral stenosis or mechanical heart valve.

ONLINE REFERENCES

Please scan the QR code provided at the end of the table of contents for References of this chapter.

CHAPTER

25

Factor XI Inhibitors

Dipankar Ghosh Dastidar

ABSTRACT

Vitamin K antagonists (VKAs) are commonly associated with bleeding complications. The equally efficacious direct oral anticoagulants (DOACs) also cause gastrointestinal bleeds. A search for a novel anticoagulant is on, which will be efficacious against pathological thrombosis without affecting hemostasis. Factor XI (FXI) inhibition has been found to have a more important role in thrombosis than hemostasis. This uncoupling of thrombosis from hemostasis has led to the use of several FXI inhibitors in several phase 2 and 3 studies in a variety of clinical thrombotic scenarios. The results show great potential for the revolutionary development of FXI inhibitors as a novel anticoagulant.

Keywords: Factor XI inhibitors, DOACS, antisense oligonucleotides, osocimab, milvexian.

INTRODUCTION

Traditional anticoagulants such as heparin and vitamin K antagonists (VKAs) are potent but cause major bleeding. Recently, direct oral anticoagulants (DOACs) targeting specific factors in the coagulation cascade became available. They were found to be equally efficacious but caused much less bleeding than the traditional anticoagulants. Still, DOACs were found ineffective in certain situations such as prosthetic mechanical heart valves, antiphospholipid syndrome (APS), or rheumatic mitral stenosis with atrial fibrillation. They were ineffective in situations where atherothrombosis mainly involved contact pathway activation such as exposure of blood to artificial surfaces like catheters, cardiopulmonary bypass, and mechanical valves. Factor XI (FXI) is a protein in the intrinsic or contact pathway whose levels are found to be increased in cases of pathological atherothrombosis but whose deficiency seems to cause only minor bleeds. FXI reduces the formation of pathologic thrombi while preserving the ability to form clots in response to bleeding. This ability of FXI to uncouple thrombosis from hemostasis provided an opportunity to target them as potential anticoagulants.[1]

LIMITATIONS OF DIRECT ORAL ANTICOAGULANTS

Direct oral anticoagulants, such as apixaban, dabigatran, edoxaban, and rivaroxaban, were shown in randomized trials to be at least as effective as heparins and VKAs for the prevention of stroke in patients with atrial fibrillation and the prevention and treatment of venous thromboembolism (VTE).[2-5] Moreover, they cause less major bleeds than VKAs and also have more predictable pharmacokinetics. All of these translate into reduced mortality with the use of DOACs over VKAs. Additionally, low-dose rivaroxaban in combination with antiplatelet therapy is also used in chronic coronary or peripheral artery disease.[6,7] They can be given orally in fixed doses without the need for routine coagulation monitoring, and they have a low propensity for food and drug interactions. Hence, DOACs are the preferred anticoagulants. However, they are still not used as anticoagulants in prosthetic mechanical heart valves,[8] in the APS,[9] and in rheumatic mitral stenosis with atrial fibrillation.[10] They are not used in extremes of renal function, impaired liver function, and extremes of body weight. They still cause bleeding, particularly gastrointestinal bleeds.

TARGETING THE CONTACT PATHWAY

Our knowledge of targeting the contact pathway for more effective thrombosis prevention without increasing the risk of bleeding stems from the fact that FXI-deficient patients present with reduced risk of thrombosis with only minor bleeding tendency. FXI deficiency, also known as hemophilia C (or Rosenthal disorder), was first described in the 1950s in four generations of patients experiencing bleeding during surgery or dental extractions.[11] Its prevalence is 1 in 100,000 people, although a higher frequency of 8–9% has been reported in Ashkenazi and Iraqi Jews.[12] FXI deficiency increases the activated partial thromboplastin time (aPTT) but not the prothrombin time.[13] Though FXI deficiency causes minimal bleeding, it has been observed that FXI levels are elevated in atherothrombotic events such as myocardial infarction.[14] In pathological thrombus, naturally occurring polyanions, such as deoxyribonucleic acid (DNA) extruded from activated neutrophils [neutrophil extracellular traps (NETs)] or inorganic phosphates (polyphosphates) from activated platelets, further amplify thrombin formation via the FXI-mediated contact pathway. Hence, it is prudent to target FXI-mediated contact pathway. FXI is more activated when thrombosis is triggered by exposure of blood to artificial surfaces such as catheters, cardiopulmonary bypass, and mechanical valves **(Figs. 1A and B)**.

PHARMACOLOGICAL PROPERTIES OF FACTOR XI INHIBITORS (FIG. 2)

There are five types of FXI inhibitors in development:

1. Antisense oligonucleotides (ASOs)
2. Monoclonal antibodies (mAb)
3. Small molecules
4. DNA aptamers
5. Natural inhibitors

Antisense Oligonucleotides

Antisense oligonucleotides are small pieces of ribonucleic acid (RNA) or DNA that can bind to specific portion of RNA, thereby blocking specific protein synthesis. Two anti-FXI ASOs, IONIS-FXIRX and fesomersen, have been tested in clinical trials. IONIS-FXIRX blocks hepatic FXI messenger ribonucleic acid (mRNA). Maximum reduction in FXI levels occurs 3–4 weeks after the start of therapy, and the effect lasts for months after treatment discontinuation.[16] Fesomersen is a more potent blocker of hepatic FXI mRNA. These ASOs are administered by the subcutaneous route on a monthly basis. They do not have any drug interactions. However, ASOs can have proinflammatory effects and can cause nephrotoxicity, hepatotoxicity, and thrombocytopenia.[17]

Monoclonal Antibodies

Monoclonal antibodies are artificially created proteins that behave like in vivo antibodies and bind to target proteins to neutralize them.

Osocimab is a human immunoglobulin G1 mAb that binds near the active site of FXI.[18] Abelacimab binds to the catalytic site of FXI.[19] Xisomab 3G3 binds to the apple 2 (A2) domain of FXI blocking FXI activation.[20] However, thrombin-mediated activation of FXI remains unchallenged. Hence, it prevents pathological thrombosis without disturbing natural hemostasis. Xisomab 3G3 has been tested in end-stage renal disease (ESRD) patients with anticoagulant effect lasting over

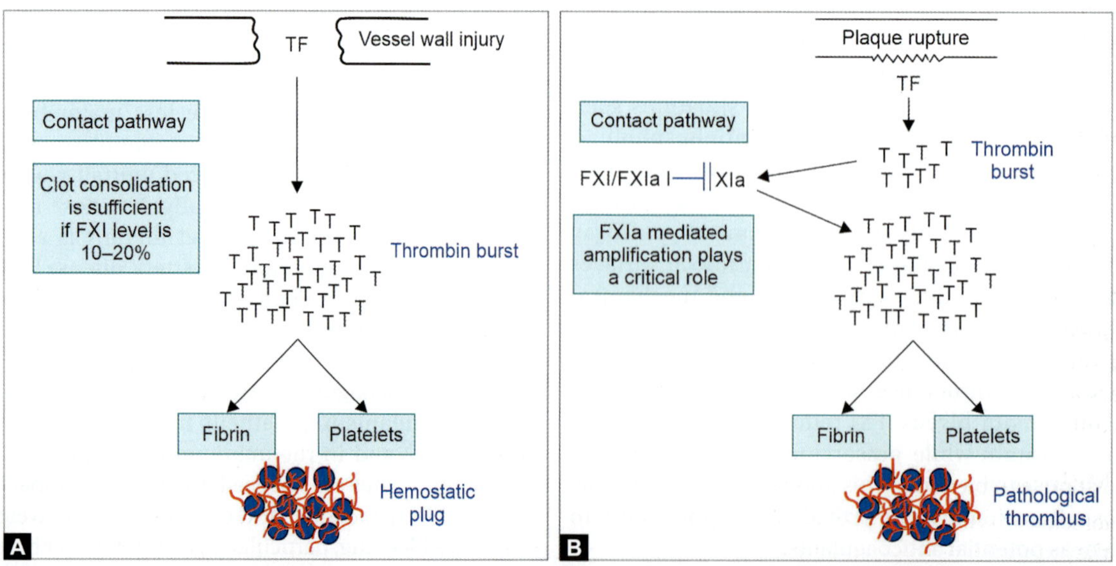

FIGS. 1A AND B: Uncoupling of hemostasis from thrombosis in the presence of factor XI (FXI) inhibition. (A) Traumatic vessel wall injury is sufficient to induce hemostatic plug formation without requiring amplification of thrombin generation via the contact pathway. (B) Conversely, disruption of atherosclerotic plaque requires amplification via the contact pathway to induce pathological thrombus formation. Factor XI inhibitors may thus achieve thrombosis inhibition without impairing hemostasis.[1,15]

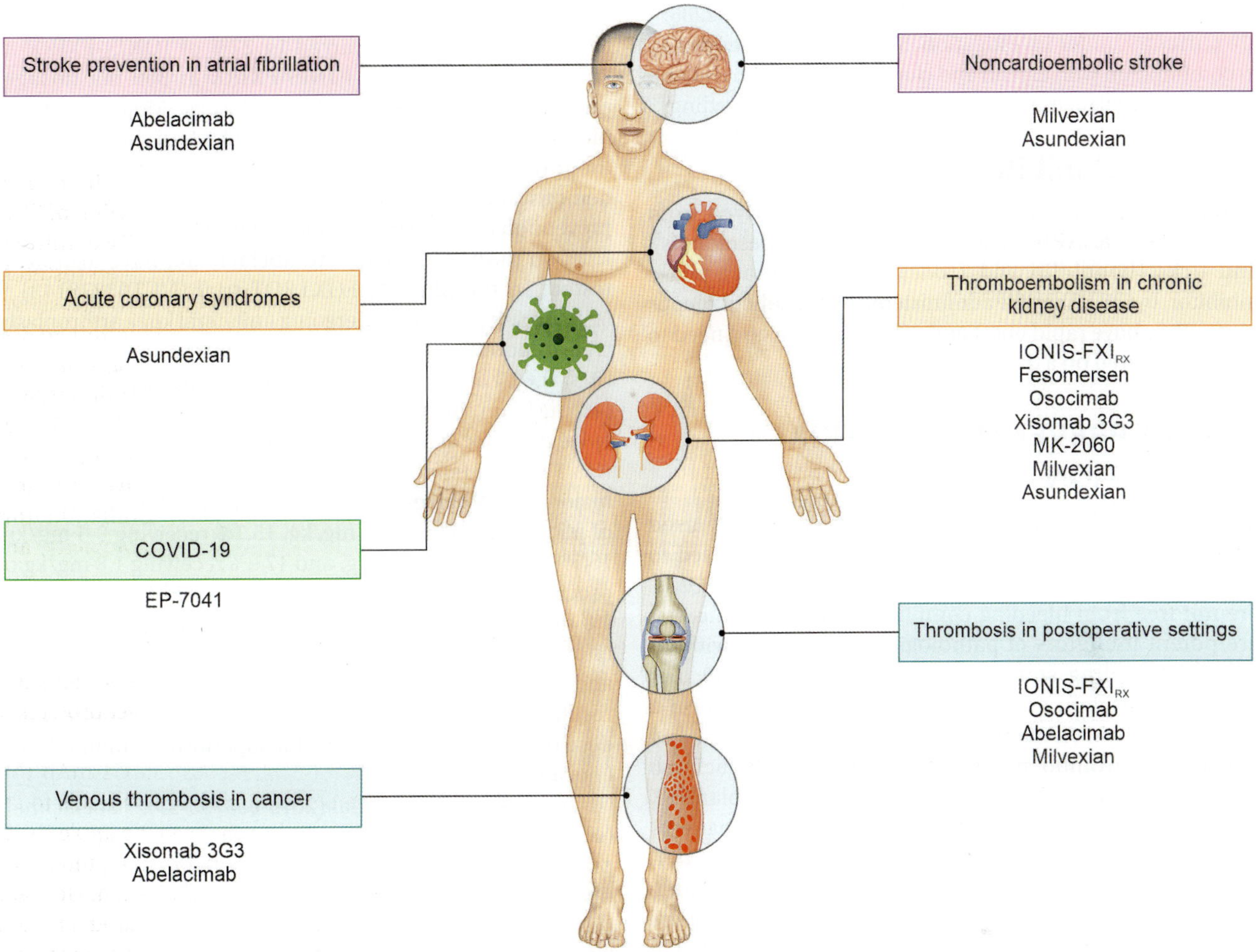

FIG. 2: Factor XI inhibitors in clinical development for a variety of thrombotic scenarios.[15]

a month after the last dosage. mAb can be immunogenic and can cause acute injection site and autoimmune reactions **(Fig. 3)**.[21]

Deoxyribonucleic Acid Aptamers

Aptamers are short, single-stranded DNA or RNA (ssDNA or ssRNA) molecules that can selectively bind to specific targets. The Factor ELeven Inhibitory APtamer (FELIAP) is a DNA aptamer that binds near the active site of FXI.[22] Two RNA aptamers (11.16 and 12.7) were developed as noncompetitive inhibitors of FXIa, binding the FXIa anion-binding site (ABS2) of the catalytic domain.[23] However, the aptamers are renally excreted making them unsuitable for use in ESRD patients.[24]

Small Molecules

Small molecules have a low molecular weight (<900 daltons). Hence, they can diffuse across membranes and have a rapid onset and offset of action. Another advantage is that they can be administered orally. Small molecules target activated FXI sparing the catalytic site, which has structural similarities to prekallikrein.[25] Milvexian is an oral, highly selective, reversible inhibitor of human FXI.[26] It reached peak plasma concentrations in 3–4 hours with a half-life of 8–13 hours. Asundexian is another orally administered small molecule.[27]

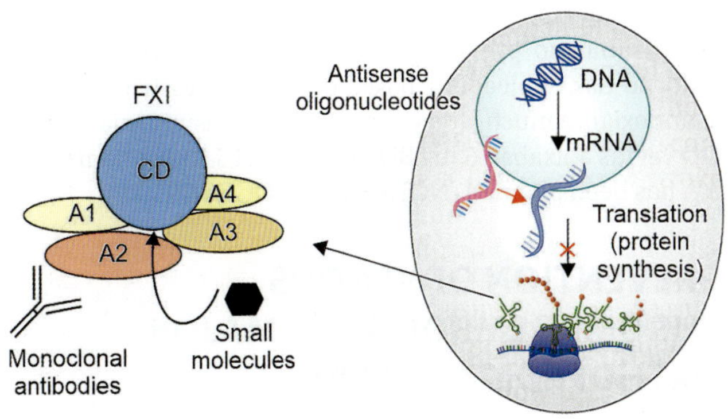

FIG. 3: Mechanism of action of factor XI (FXI)a inhibitors currently in development.[15]

(A: apple domain; CD: catalytic domain; DNA: deoxyribonucleic acid; mRNA: messenger ribonucleic acid)

Two other oral small molecules, ONO-7684[28] and SHR2285,[29] are currently under investigation. SHR2285 has been tested in combination with aspirin and clopidogrel or ticagrelor and seems to be well tolerated with no increased risk of bleeding.[30]

Natural Inhibitors

Natural FXIa inhibitors include molecules derived from nematodes (acaNAP10), snakes (fasxiator), bats (desmolaris), and ticks (boophilin and *Ixodes ricinus* contact phase inhibitor, Ir-CPI). They are administered by the subcutaneous route. They have rapid onset and offset of action and need to be administered on a daily basis.[31]

STROKE PREVENTION IN ATRIAL FIBRILLATION

Direct oral anticoagulants are the most commonly used agents apart from VKAs, whose use is mainly restricted to valvular AF and mechanical heart valves. However, DOACs are not free from bleeding complications. FXIa inhibitors are potent inhibitors of pathological thrombosis without altering bleeding status. Abelacimab (120 or 180 mg) subcutaneously on a monthly basis has been tested in a phase 2 study in AF patients with low risk of cerebral and peripheral thromboembolism.[19] A study of abelacimab against rivaroxaban in AF patients has also been planned. Another study of milvexian versus apixaban in AF patients (LIBREXIA AF) has also been planned.[32] A multicenter, randomized, active comparator-controlled, double-blind, parallel-group, dose-finding phase 2 study comparing the safety of asundexian (20–50 mg/day, administered orally) to apixaban in patients with atrial fibrillation (NCT04218266, PACIFIC-AF) was conducted.[33] The study demonstrated that asundexian 20- and 50-mg OD dosage was as potent as apixaban to prevent cerebral embolism with a much reduced risk of bleeding. Based on the impressive results of asundexian, a much larger phase 3 study of asundexian 50 mg OD versus apixaban 5 mg BD, in around 15,000 patients with AF, has been planned (NCT05643573, OCEANIC AF).

PREVENTION OF VENOUS THROMBOEMBOLISM IN MAJOR ORTHOPEDIC SURGERY

The ASO IONIS-FXIRX has been tested in phase 2 trials in patients undergoing elective primary unilateral total knee arthroplasty (NCT01713361).[34] 300 patients undergoing elective primary unilateral total knee arthroplasty were randomly allocated to treatment with IONIS-FXIRX (at the dosage of 200 or 300 mg, administered three times per week during the first week of treatment, followed by weekly administrations) or enoxaparin (40 mg/day). The primary outcome was a decrease in VTE incidence, while the principal safety outcome was to look for major or clinically relevant nonmajor (CRNM) bleeding events. VTE events occurred in 27% of IONIS-FXIRX at 200-mg dosage, 4% in IONIS-FXIRX at 300-mg dosage, and 30% in enoxaparin at 40-mg dosage. Major or CRNM bleeding events occurred in 3, 3, and 8% of the patients in the three study groups, respectively. This study effectively demonstrated the superior efficacy of FXI inhibitors in VTE prevention as compared to traditional anticoagulants.[34]

Two mAb, osocimab and abelacimab, have also been tested. In the phase 2 FOXTROT trial (NCT03276143),[35] 52,813 adult patients undergoing unilateral knee arthroplasty were randomized to receive single intravenous osocimab (0.3, 0.6, 1.2, or 1.8 mg/kg), subcutaneous enoxaparin (40 mg/day), or two daily doses of oral apixaban (2.5 mg twice daily) for at least 10 days. The primary efficacy outcome was VTE incidence, while the primary safety outcome was major or CRNM bleed. The VTE incidence occurred in 23.7% of patients receiving 0.3 mg/kg, 15.7% receiving 0.6 mg/kg, 16.5% receiving 1.2 mg/kg, and 17.9% receiving 1.8 mg/kg of osocimab; in 29.9% receiving 0.3 mg/kg and 11.3% receiving 1.8 mg/kg of osocimab preoperatively; in 26.3% receiving enoxaparin and 14.5% receiving apixaban. The 0.6, 1.2, and 1.8 mg/kg osocimab dosages given post-operatively resulted noninferior to enoxaparin, while the preoperative dose of 1.8 mg/kg met criteria for superiority compared with enoxaparin.

In another phase 2 trial (2019-003756-37),[36] abelacimab (single intravenous postoperative dose of 30, 75, or 150 mg) or enoxaparin (40 mg/day SC) was tested in 51,412 patients undergoing total knee arthroplasty. The primary efficacy and safety outcomes were VTE and major or CRNM bleeding up to 30 days after surgery, respectively. VTE occurred in 13, 5, and 4% of patients in the 30-, 75-, and 150-mg abelacimab groups, respectively, as compared with 22% in the enoxaparin group. The single intravenous 30-mg abelacimab regimen proved noninferior to enoxaparin, and the 75- and 150-mg regimens were superior to enoxaparin.

In another phase 2 trial (AXIOMATIC-TKR trial),[37] the small molecule milvexian (25, 50, 100, or 200 mg BD or 25, 50, or 200 mg OD, administered orally) or enoxaparin (40 mg/day, SC) was tested in 1,242 patients undergoing knee arthroplasty. VTE occurred in 21, 11, 9, and 8% of patients receiving milvexian 25, 50, 100, and 200 mg twice daily, respectively, and in 25, 24, and 7% of those on 25, 50, and 200 mg once daily, as compared with 21% in patients taking enoxaparin. Bleeding events were negligible in both arms.

PREVENTION AND TREATMENT OF CANCER-ASSOCIATED VENOUS THROMBOEMBOLISM

A phase 2 trial is ongoing to assess the efficacy and safety of the recombinant humanized mAb xisomab 3G3 for the prevention of catheter-associated thrombosis in patients with cancer receiving chemotherapy (NCT04465760).

Two other phase 2 trials comparing the mAb abelacimab with dalteparin for VTE prevention in gastrointestinal/genitourinary cancer (MAGNOLIA trial, NCT05171075) and with apixaban in the treatment of cancer-associated VTE (ASTER trial, NCT05171049) are ongoing.

PREVENTION OF CARDIOVASCULAR EVENTS IN PATIENTS WITH END-STAGE RENAL DISEASE OR UNDERGOING HEMODIALYSIS

Chronic kidney disease increases the risk of atherothrombosis with increased bleeding risk. DOACs are relatively contraindicated in ESRD patients. ASOs and mAbs are not excreted by the kidney and are not removed by dialysis, making them attractive candidates for use in patients with advanced kidney disease. Small molecule inhibitors are protein-bound and minimally cleared by the kidneys.

The ASO IONIS-FXIRX has been tested in phase 2 trials in patients with ESRD on hemodialysis (NCT02553889—EMERALD trial).[38] Hemodialysis has no effect on IONIS-FXIRX pharmacokinetics and tolerability, and that the treatment effectively reduces dialysis circuit clotting events. Fesomersen is undergoing phase 2 trial on ESRD patients requiring hemodialysis (NCT04534114—RE-THINc ESRD trial). Three different regimens of fesomersen (40, 80, or 120 mg administered subcutaneously every 4 weeks for up to 48 weeks) or placebo were given in 307 patients with ESRD on hemodialysis. Fesomersen achieved the primary safety outcome of no increase in the risk of major bleeding and CRNM bleeds.

The mAb osocimab is under investigation in a phase 2 trial in patients with kidney failure requiring hemodialysis (CONVERT trial—NCT04523220). Another phase 2 study with a single dose of xisomab 3G3 (0.25 or 0.5 mg/kg), administered at the beginning of a regular hemodialysis procedure, in ESRD patients on chronic hemodialysis (NCT03612856) is ongoing. It showed less catheter thrombosis.[39]

In a phase 1 study, the safety and tolerability of asundexian (25 mg) have been investigated in patients with renal impairment, including those on hemodialysis (NCT04510987). Another phase 1/phase 2 study assessed the safety and tolerability of single oral doses of the small molecule milvexian as compared with enoxaparin or unfractionated heparin in patients with ESRD on chronic hemodialysis (NCT03000673).

SECONDARY PROPHYLAXIS OF ISCHEMIC STROKE

The AXIOMATIC-SSP study (NCT03766581) is a phase 2, randomized, double-blind, placebo-controlled, dose-finding study of milvexian for the secondary prevention of new ischemic stroke in patients following acute nonhemorrhagic infarcts or a transient ischemic attack who are already on 1 month of dual antiplatelet therapy (DAPT) followed by long-term aspirin. PACIFIC-STROKE (NCT04304508) is a global phase 2 randomized double-blind, placebo-controlled, dose-ranging study of asundexian for secondary prevention of new ischemic stroke in about 1,800 patients following acute nonhemorrhagic stroke or a transient ischemic attack who are treated with standard antiplatelet therapy. The higher doses of milvexian were associated with more major bleeds than placebo, but the differences for both symptomatic stroke and major bleeding were not statistically significant.[33] As was the case in AF subjects, a phase 3 study comparing asundexian with apixaban in noncardioembolic ischemic stroke or high-risk ischemic attack (OCEANIC-STROKE) has been planned.

SECONDARY PROPHYLAXIS AFTER A MYOCARDIAL INFARCTION

Dual antiplatelet therapy, particularly aspirin with P2Y12 inhibitors, is the pillar of long-term therapy in acute coronary syndrome patients. However, there is much evidence of persistent thrombin generation in post-ACS subjects. Different DOACs have been tried to this end. Only rivaroxaban in ATLAS ACS 2-TIMI 51 trial has been shown to be beneficial.[40] Still, the combination is associated with a higher risk of major bleeding and intracranial hemorrhage. Asundexian has been used in combination with DAPT in acute myocardial infarction (AMI) subjects in a phase 2 dose-finding study (PACIFIC-AMI, NCT04304534). Asundexian was associated with no increased bleeding risk compared to placebo.[41] A phase 3 study of asundexian 50 mg daily on top of DAPT in AMI subjects has been planned (OCEANIC-AMI). The target is aimed for >20% reduction of cardiovascular death, myocardial infarction, and stroke with no relevant impact on bleeding.

THROMBOPROPHYLAXIS IN COVID-19 PATIENTS

The small molecule EP-7041 has been used as thromboprophylaxis in COVID-19 patients in an intensive care unit setup (NCT05040776).[30]

PREVENTION OF CENTRAL VENOUS CATHETER THROMBOSIS

Preclinical animal studies have revealed that FXII and FXI blockade prevents catheter thrombosis, while blocking FVII has no effect. In rabbit models, catheters coated with corn trypsin inhibitor, a specific inhibitor of FXIIa, remained patent longer than uncoated catheters.[42] A phase 2 study of xisomab 3G3 is underway for the prevention of catheter-associated thrombosis in patients with cancer receiving chemotherapy (NCT04465760).

PROPHYLAXIS IN DEVICE-RELATED CLOTTING EVENTS

Chronic heart failure patients often require left ventricular assist device (LVAD) support. The use of extracorporeal membrane oxygenation (ECMO) particularly in COVID-19 patients has also increased. A major limitation to the prolonged use of such devices has been the development of thrombotic complications. DOACs have been quite ineffective in these situations primarily because of the activation of contact pathway in the coagulation cascade in these situations. FXI inhibitors are particularly promising alternative anticoagulants in these situations. Similarly, FXI inhibitors can also be tried in patients with mechanical heart valves, for whom the standard of care is represented by VKAs, given the negative results of the Re-ALIGN study with dabigatran.[8]

PREVENTION OF THROMBOSIS IN ANTIPHOSPHOLIPID SYNDROME PATIENTS

A "two-hit" thrombosis model is proposed to explain thrombus formation in APS. A "first hit" injury to the endothelium needs to happen to have a "second hit" that potentiates the thrombus formation. APS patients who carry a triple positivity for lupus anticoagulant, anticardiolipin, and anti-β2-glycoprotein I antibodies are at an increased thrombotic risk. The phase III rivaroxaban in TRAPS (Thrombotic Antiphospholipid Syndrome) trial,[43] which was conducted in high-risk APS patients triple-positive for lupus anticoagulant, anticardiolipin, and anti-β2-glycoprotein I antibodies of the same isotype, was terminated prematurely after the enrollment of 120 patients because of an excess rate of arterial thromboembolic events in patients on rivaroxaban: 12% (four ischemic strokes and three myocardial infarctions) versus 0% in patients on warfarin, after 569 days of follow-up. In May 2019, the European Medicines Agency (EMA) issued a guidance statement recommending against the use of direct-acting oral anticoagulants (including rivaroxaban, apixaban, edoxaban, and dabigatran etexilate) for patients with a history of thrombosis who are diagnosed with APS, in particular those who are triple positive.[44] Till date, VKAs are the only anticoagulant approved for use in APS patients. FXI inhibitors act by the intrinsic pathway only. Hence, it is assumed that they will be of limited benefit in APS subjects.

CONCLUSION

The search for a novel anticoagulant that will be more efficacious against pathological thrombosis without affecting hemostasis was always on. Several phase 1 and phase 2 studies have conclusively proven FXI inhibition to have a more important role in thrombosis than in hemostasis in a variety of thrombotic scenarios. VKAs are associated with bleeding risks. DOACs, which are equipotent, are still not without bleeding risks, particularly gastrointestinal bleeds. Moreover, they are ineffective in certain situations such as prosthetic mechanical heart valves, APS, or rheumatic mitral stenosis with atrial fibrillation. FXI inhibitors have a unique mechanism of action of blocking the intrinsic or contact pathway without affecting the tissue pathway. They uncouple thrombosis from hemostasis. Advanced phase 3 studies are underway in a variety of thrombotic scenarios to look into efficacy and safety issues. One particular concern is the potential difficulty in antagonizing FXI inhibitors with FXI concentrates, which can be thrombogenic, or with prothrombin complex concentrates, which may be ineffective.[45] Further results of the ongoing clinical trials are awaited before this molecule could be launched as a wonder drug in the field of anticoagulation.

ONLINE REFERENCES

Please scan the QR code provided at the end of the table of contents for References of this chapter.

CHAPTER 26

Single Antiplatelet Therapy in Percutaneous Intervention: Current Evidence

Sajan Narayanan

ABSTRACT

Early studies which assessed outcomes of patients who underwent percutaneous intervention (PCI) considered a dual antiplatelet therapy (DAPT) duration of 12 months as safe time period which balanced risks of recurrent ischemia and bleeding. These trials were conducted in bare metal stent (BMS) and first generation drug-eluting stent (DES) era. In fact certain reports raised serious concerns about safety of this duration with reports of increased very late stent thrombosis (occurring >1 year) with first generation DES. Subsequently, there has been continuous evolution of platforms, polymers, and drugs which made stents much safer. Development of prasugrel and ticagrelor made incidence of stent thrombosis (ST) even lower. Scientific community became more and more aware about bleeding hazard of DAPT. Reports suggested worse outcomes in patients who develop a bleeding complication following PCI. There has been a deluge of drugs which were shown to reduce ischemic events in last decade (e.g., PCSK9i, SGLT-2i, GLP-1A, ARNI, etc.) which are not associated with risk of bleeding. With advances in development of safe stent platforms and other secondary prevention drugs, interest has now shifted to shorten standard 12-month DAPT duration. This review will discuss latest evidence on single antiplatelet strategies after PCI.

Keywords: De-escalation, acute coronary syndrome, high bleeding risk, DAPT.

INTRODUCTION

The synergistic blockade of platelet cyclooxygenase-1 (COX-1) and P2Y12 signaling pathways with use of aspirin, also known as acetylsalicylic acid (ASA) and P2Y12 inhibitors (clopidogrel, prasugrel, and ticagrelor) is called dual antiplatelet therapy (DAPT).[1] DAPT is the cornerstone in the management of patients who present with acute coronary syndrome (ACS), especially after percutaneous intervention (PCI). The combination is useful to prevent early ischemic complications after PCI in chronic coronary syndromes (CCS) as well. DAPT has played an important role in optimizing outcomes after PCI.[2] Patients who undergo PCI are exposed to high risk for ischemic complications due to activation of platelets and coagulation system. Since platelets play a key role in thrombus formation, administration of powerful combination of antiplatelets is associated with bleeding. There has been considerable evolution of antiplatelet strategies over last three decades, coupled with improvements in stent designs, greater use of imaging guidance, and other preventive treatments (e.g., stains, PCSK9i, and antidiabetic drugs) which has reduced the ischemic complications in patients undergoing coronary interventions. Numerous investigations have helped to identify profile of patients who are at high risk for ischemic and bleeding complications. This review will discuss on contemporary abbreviated DAPT strategy (shorter than recommended duration by major guidelines) with focus on single antiplatelet therapy (SAPT).

ASSESSMENT OF ISCHEMIC AND BLEEDING RISK AFTER PERCUTANEOUS INTERVENTION

- European Society of Cardiology/European Association for Cardio-Thoracic Surgery (ESC/EACTS) guidelines have defined high ischemic risk considering clinical and procedural characteristics.[3] Broadly it includes clinical variables [diabetes, chronic kidney disease (CKD), history of ST-elevation myocardial infarction (STEMI), prior stent thrombosis] and procedural characteristics [>3 stents implanted, >3 lesions treated, bifurcation treated with 2-stent strategy, total stent length >60 mm, treatment of chronic total occlusion (CTO), and stenting of last remaining coronary artery].

- Academic research consortium (ARC) has defined high bleeding risk (HBR) characteristics in patients receiving antiplatelet agents[4] which is defined according to at least one major or two minor criteria.
- Specific clinical, procedural, and laboratory factors have been identified, which would help to define optimal DAPT duration after PCI considering both ischemic and bleeding risks.[5,6]
- PRECISE DAPT score is calculated at time of index PCI, a score of >25 defines patients at high risk for bleeding and identifies patients who would benefit from shortening of DAPT.[7]
- DAPT score is calculated at 12 months in patients who have successfully completed 1 year of DAPT without adverse events. A score of >2 identifies category of patients who are at high ischemic risk and benefit from extending DAPT up to 30 months.[8]

RATIONALE FOR SINGLE ANTIPLATELET THERAPY AFTER PERCUTANEOUS INTERVENTION IN CONTEMPORARY PRACTICE

European Society of Cardiology guidelines for choice and duration of DAPT after PCI are shown in **Figure 1**.[9,10]

- Introduction of clopidogrel along with aspirin following PCI dramatically reduced early ischemic events; especially stent thrombosis rates. Individual clopidogrel response is affected by several pharmacokinetic and pharmacodynamic interactions, with some patients especially in certain ethnic groups having variable response to the drug.[11,12]
- Prasugrel and ticagrelor significantly reduced ischemic endpoints (especially stent thrombosis rates) when compared to clopidogrel in pivotal studies which tested efficacy of new P2Y12i.[13,14]
- The impressive reduction in ischemic events with new P2Y12i were obtained at a price of increased bleeding events.[13,14]
- A bleeding event has significant impact on immediate and overall outcomes in patients receiving DAPT. In a pooled

Presentation	Before PCI	In Cath lab	Duration
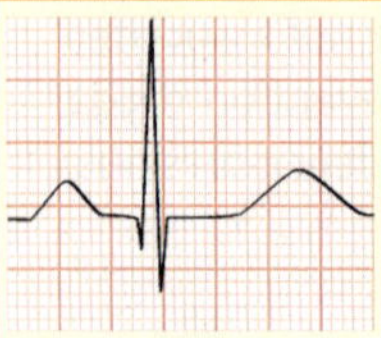 CCS	ASA I A Clopidogrel IIb C	Clopidogrel I A Prasugrel/Ticagrelor High ischemic risk IIb C	DAPT 6 months I A >6 months—high ischemic risk IIa A 3 months DAPT ASA (HBR) IIa A 1 month DAPT ASA (HBR) IIb C
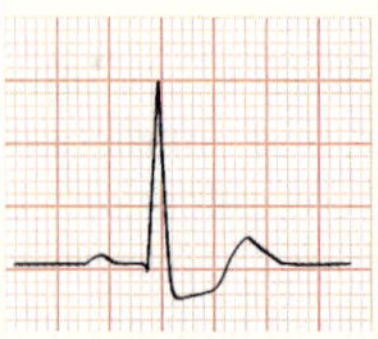 NSTE ACS	ASA I A Routine P2Y12i III A	Prasugrel I B Ticagrelor I B Clopidogrel I C Prasugrel over Ticagrelor IIa B	DAPT–12 months I A 3–6 months DAPT→ P2Y12i IIa A Prasu/Tica → Clopidogrel IIb A 1 month DAPT (HBR) → ASA/clopi IIb B
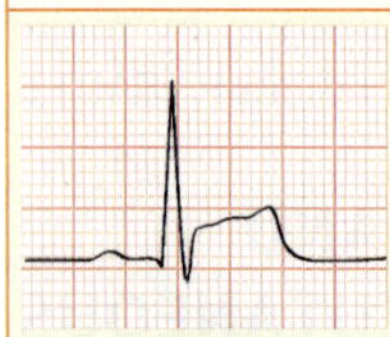 STEMI	ASA I B Prasugrel/Ticagrelor I A Clopidogrel if pras/Tica not tolerated I C		DAPT for 12 months I A 3–6 months DAPT→ P2Y12i IIa A Prasu/Tica → Clopidogrel IIb A 1 month DAPT (HBR) → ASA/clopi IIb B

FIG. 1: European Society of Cardiology recommendations for oral antiplatelet agents in patients undergoing PCI.

(ACS: acute coronary syndromes; ASA: aspirin; CCS: chronic coronary syndrome; DAPT: dual antiplatelet therapy; PCI: percutaneous intervention) analysis of patients undergoing stent implantation and subsequent DAPT, long duration of DAPT was beneficial only in subgroup that did not have HBR features. In this study, a short duration of DAPT was better in patients with HBR regardless of the complexity of the PCI and ischemic risk.[15]

- Pharmacodynamic substudy of patients enrolled in TWILIGHT trial showed that ticagrelor monotherapy yielded similar antithrombotic effect, assessed as ex vivo platelet rich thrombus formation as compared to a combination of ticagrelor with aspirin;[16] raising questionsover added benefit of adding aspirin to a newer P2Y12i.
- The incidence of ischemic complications following PCI is highest in initial postprocedural period. Risk for thrombotic complications wanes off after about 3 months while bleeding risk persists. Hence, in addition to platelet agent administered, the duration of DAPT is an important determinant of bleeding risk after PCI **(Fig. 2)**.
- Different strategies have been studied to balance early ischemic risk and late bleeding events by modulation of DAPT regimen **(Flowchart 1)**. Most important among the strategies tested is discontinuation of one of the agents from DAPT after a variable period ranging from 1-6 months after PCI. These are aimed at mitigating early ischemic events with use of DAPT and de-escalating later to reduce bleeding events.

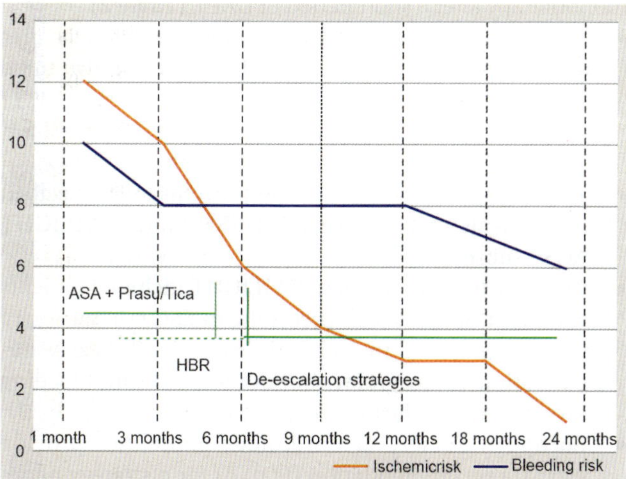

FIG. 2: Ischemic risk is maximum in the initial 1–3 months following PCI, after which the risk comes down. Bleeding risk is also high in initial postprocedural period but risk remains largely static over time. Aspirin + powerful P2Y12i help to reduce high initial ischemic risk. De-escalation strategies would help to balance ischemic and bleeding risks beyond 3–6 months. De-escalation strategies may be considered earlier (may be 1–3 months after PCI) in HBR patients.

(HBR: high bleeding risk; PCI: percutaneous intervention; Prasu: prasugrel; Tica: ticagrelor)

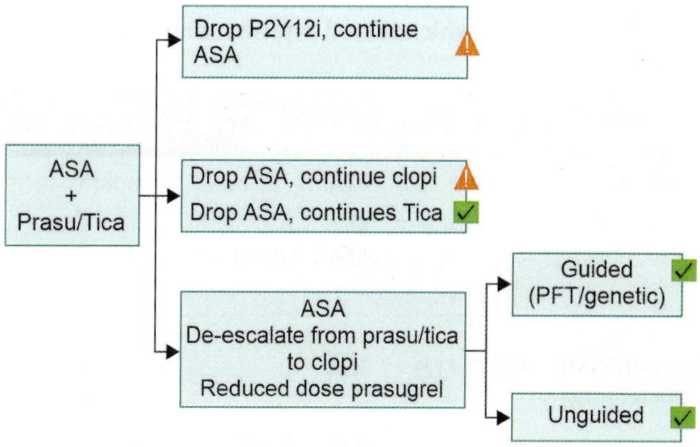

FLOWCHART 1: De-escalation strategies tested in clinical trials. Strategies which showed positive outcomes for experimental arm are indicated in green.

(ASA: aspirin; Clopi: clopidogrel; Prasu: prasugrel; Tica: ticagrelor)

SINGLE ANTIPLATELET THERAPY IN ACUTE CORONARY SYNDROMES AFTER PERCUTANEOUS INTERVENTION

- In ACS patients undergoing PCI, standard duration of DAPT is 12 months. Prasugrel and ticagrelor are preferred over clopidogrel.[9]
- Shortening of DAPT before recommended duration is referred to as de-escalation.
- De-escalation can be dropping either aspirin or P2Y12i, usually 3-6 months after PCI or substituting prasugrel/ticagrelor with clopidogrel (guided by platelet function tests or genetic analysis for cytochrome P450 polymorphisms).[17] Latter strategy is beyond scope of this review.

SHORT DUAL ANTIPLATELET THERAPY FOLLOWED BY ASPIRIN MONOTHERAPY

There are three studies which tested the strategy of stopping P2Y12i between 3-6 months after PCI and continuing on aspirin monotherapy compared to standard DAPT of 12 months in exclusive ACS population **(Table 1)**.

Major drawbacks of these studies are:

- Noninferiority design
- Not powered to verify safety of de-escalation with regard to ischemic endpoints
- Enrolled patients with predominantly non-complex lesions (ACC/AHA B2 lesions in 37% and C-25% in DAPT STEMI, multi-lesion-25%, and multivessel-19.4% in SMART DATE) undergoing PCI. Safety of early discontinuation of P2Y12i in patients who have complex lesions cannot be inferred.

TABLE 1: Studies which tested aspirin monotherapy after short dual antiplatelet therapy (DAPT) in acute coronary syndrome (ACS).

Study (duration)	Patients (*n*)	Comparison	Timing of de-escalation	1° endpoint	Result	Drawbacks
DAPT STEMI (18 months)	STEMI (1,100)	ASA vs. ASA + P2Y12i	6 months	Composite: • All-cause mortality • MI, stroke • Any revasc, bleeding	• SAPT: 4.8% • DAPT: 6.6% • $p = 0.004$ • Noninferior	• Noninferiority design • Composite of ischemic and bleeding • Included noncomplex lesion subsets
SMART DATE (18 months)	ACS (2,712)	ASA vs. ASA + clopidogrel	6 months	• 1° composite: Mortality, MI, stroke • 2° composite: • ST, bleeding	• SAPT: 4.7% • DAPT: 4.2% • $p = 0.03$ • Noninferior	• TV and non-TV MI more in SAPT • Increase in stent thrombosis
REDUCE (12 months)	ACS (1,496)	ASA vs. ASA + P2Y12i	3 months	• 1° composite: • All cause death • MI, ST, stroke • TVR, bleeding	• SAPT: 8.2% • DAPT: 8.4% • Noninferior	• Higher ST in SAPT arm (p = NS) • Higher cardiac mortality in SAPT (p = NS)

(ASA: aspirin; DAPT: dual antiplatelet therapy; SAPT: single antiplatelet therapy)

- DAPT STEMI[18] showed no difference in ischemic endpoints between two arms, while in both SMART DATE[19] and REDUCE,[20] there was an increase in stent thrombosis (ST) rates in SAPT arm. SMART DATE study reported higher incidence of both target and non-target vessel myocardial infarction (MI) rates in SAPT arm. REDUCE trial had higher incidence of cardiovascular (CV) death in SAPT arm.
- Individual patient data meta-analysis comparing short (3- or 6-month DAPT) versus standard DAPT (12 months) in 11,473 patients from six trials, there was an interaction between presenting diagnosis of ACS and incidence of MI and ST, (3-month DAPT was associated with higher rates of MI or ST and <6-month DAPT was associated with a trend toward increased rates of MI or ST at 1 year) while there was no such interaction seen with CCS.[21]
- Hence, a strategy of early de-escalation (3–6 months) from DAPT to aspirin monotherapy in ACS patients undergoing PCI may be associated with higher rates of MI and ST.

Clopidogrel Monotherapy

The STOP DAPT-2 ACS[22] noninferiority study focused on ACS patients in whom 12-month DAPT was compared with DAPT for 1–2 months followed by clopidogrel monotherapy (n = 2,078). Clopidogrel monotherapy was *not* noninferior to control arm for primary endpoint [3.2% vs. 2.8%; absolute difference, 0.37%, (95% CI -0.68% to 1.42%) HR 1.14; 95% CI 0.8–1.62]. Major secondary ischemic endpoints of CV death, MI, any stroke or definite ST was increased in clopidogrel monotherapy arm [2.8% vs. 1.9%, absolute difference, 0.9%, (95% CI -0.02% to 1.82%) HR 1.5, 95% CI 0.99–2.26]. Early de-escalation of DAPT to clopidogrel monotherapy in ACS patients undergoing PCI may be associated with higher ischemic events.

Ticagrelor Monotherapy

There are three studies that analyzed benefit of ticagrelor monotherapy after a short period of DAPT **(Table 2)**.

- A strategy of stopping ASA and continuing ticagrelor after a period of 1–3 months after PCI has been shown to be safe and effective in randomized controlled trials (RCT) which included both ACS and CCS (GLOBAL LEADERS,[23] TWILIGHT[24]) as well as those focused on ACS (TICO[25]).
- There was no trade off in ischemic events in prespecified subanalysis of GLOBAL LEADERS[26] and TWILIGHT ACS[27] subsets.
- Contrary to other studies, TWILIGHT included patients with high ischemic risk according to ESC criteria. There was no increase in ischemic events with early de-escalation to ticagrelor monotherapy, while bleeding events were significantly reduced.
- European Society of Cardiology guidelines provide class IIa recommendation (LOE B) for a strategy of de-escalation to ticagrelor monotherapy after 3-month DAPT in NSTE ACS **(Fig. 1)**.[9]

SINGLE ANTIPLATELET THERAPY IN CCS AFTER PCI

European Society of Cardiology guidelines[28] for DAPT strategy after PCI in patients with CCS are illustrated in **Table 3**.

TABLE 2: Trials which tested a strategy of ticagrelor monotherapy after short dual antiplatelet therapy (DAPT).

Study (duration)	Patients	Comparison	Timing of de-escalation	1° endpoint	Result	Drawbacks
GLOBAL LEADERS ACS substudy (2 years)	ACS	Ticagrelor vs. ASA + Tica	1 month	Composite: • All cause death • New Q wave MI Safety endpoint: • BARC 3/5 bleeding	3.92% vs. 4.52% ($p = 0.189$) 1.95% vs. 2.68% ($p = 0.037$)	Substudy of an RCT
TWILIGHT ACS substudy	ACS	Ticagrelor vs. ASA + Tica	3 months	BARC 2, 3, 5 bleeding All cause death, nonfatal MI/stroke	3.6% vs. 7.6% ($p < 0.001$) 4.3% vs. 4.4% ($p = 0.84$)	• Substudy of RCT • Ischemic + bleeding EP
TICO (12 months)	ACS	Ticagrelor vs. ASA + Tica	3 months.	Composite : TIMI major bleed + MACE	3.9% vs. 5.9% ($p = 0.01$) Major bleed: 1.7% vs. 3% ($p = 0.001$)	• Primary EP–composite • Low ischemic risk • Multivessel PCI subset – no benefit

(ASA: aspirin; BARC: Bleeding Academic Research Consortium; Tica: ticagrelor)

TABLE 3: Studies which tested short versus standard dual antiplatelet therapy (DAPT) in all comer population.

			Clinical presentation %					
Study	**Year**	**Patients (*n*)**	**ACS**	**CCS**	**DAPT duration**	**1° endpoint (EP)**	**1° EP met?**	**Duration**
EXCELLENT	2012	1,443	51	49	6 vs. 12 months	CV death, MI, ischemia-driven, TOR	Yes	12 months
RESET	2012	2,148	54	46	3 vs. 12 months	CV death, MI, ST, TLR, bleeding	Yes	12 months
OPTIMIZE	2013	3,211	32	68	3 vs. 12 months	All death, MI, stroke, bleeding	Yes	12 months
SECURITY	2014	1,404	39	61	6 vs. 12 months	• CV death, MI, stroke, ST • BARC 3–5 bleed	Yes	12 months
ISAR SAFE	2015	4,005	39	61	6 vs. 12 months	• All death, MI, ST, stroke • TIME major bleed	Yes	9 months
I-LOVE-IT	2016	1,829	85	15	3 vs. 12 months	CV death, TVMI, TLR	Yes	18 months
NIPPON	2017	3,773	32	68	6 vs. 12 months	All death, MI, stroke, major bleed	Yes	36 months
OPTIMA-C	2018	1,368	51	49	6 vs. 12 months	All death, MI, TLR	Yes	12 months
1-month DAPT	2021	3,020	39	61	1 vs. 6–12 months	CV death, MI, TVR, stroke, bleeding	Yes	12 months
HOST IDEA	2023	2,013	56.6	43.4	3 vs. 6 months	Cardiac death, TVMI, TLR	Yes	12 months

Short Dual Antiplatelet Therapy Followed by Aspirin Monotherapy

Ten studies tested a strategy of dropping clopidogrel and continuing aspirin at a variable time from 3–6 months. These studies enrolled a mixed population of ACS and CCS and none focused entirely on CCS population. The studies have consistently shown reduction in bleeding endpoints with short DAPT without a trade off in ischemic events.

Short Dual Antiplatelet Therapy Followed by Clopidogrel Monotherapy

- Studies which tested short DAPT followed by clopidogrel monotherapy are illustrated in **Table 4**.
- Subanalysis of STOP DAPT2[29] study suggested clopidogrel monotherapy after 1-month DAPT was superior in major bleeding and noninferior in primary end point

TABLE 4: Studies which tested short dual antiplatelet therapy (DAPT) followed by clopidogrel monotherapy.

Study		Endpoints	Results
STOP DAPT – 2 CCS (62.3%) ACS (37.7%)	Multicenter, open label, RCT Noninferiority design 1-month DAPT → clopidogrel vs. 12-month DAPT	1° EP: Composite (1 year) • CV death, MI, definite ST • Ischemic/hemorrhagic stroke • TIMI major/minor bleed	2.36% vs. 3.7% Absolute difference: 1.34% (95% CI 2.57–0.11%) HR 0.64 ($p < 0.001$ – noninferiority) $p = 0.04$ - superiority
SMART CHOICE CCS (41.8%) ACS (58.2%)	Open label noninferiority design 3-month DAPT followed by P2Y12i (clopidogrel–76.9%) vs. 12-month DAPT (clopidogrel–77.6%)	• 1° EP: Composite (1 year) • All cause death, MI or stroke • 2° EP: BARC 2–5 bleed	2.9% vs. 2.5% $p = 0.007$ (noninferiority) Bleed: 2% vs. 3.4% (HR 0.58) 95% CI 0.36–0.92 ($p = 0.02$)

(ACS: acute coronary syndrome; CCS: chronic coronary syndrome; DAPT: dual antiplatelet therapy)

of CV death, MI, definite ST, any stroke or bleeding compared to 12-month DAPT regardless of ACS or CCS presentation.

Short Dual Antiplatelet Therapy Followed by Ticagrelor Monotherapy

- No RCTs tested ticagrelor monotherapy after a short course of DAPT in exclusive CCS subset.
- GLOBAL LEADERS enrolled a mixed population of ACS and CCS patients. Tested a strategy of 1-month DAPT followed by ticagrelor monotherapy for 23 months (experimental arm) and compared to standard DAPT (ASA + ticagrelor for 12 months followed by ASA alone).
- Broadly, there was no difference in primary endpoint (all death, MI) between experimental arm and control arm. No differences in bleeding endpoints [BARC (Bleeding Academic Research Consortium) 3 or 5] were noted.
- When stratified by presentation, only ACS subset showed a reduction in bleeding endpoints in favor of experimental arm while there were no differences in bleeding between comparator arms (ticagrelor monotherapy vs. standard DAPT) in patients who presented with CCS.[26]
- TWILIGHT study: Risk of BARC 2, 3, or 5 bleed were significantly reduced in favor of experimental arm at 1 year. There was no heterogenicity with regard to benefit according to mode of presentation in this study.[27]
- SHARE study: 3 months DAPT was noninferior to 12 months DAPT[30]

Short Dual Antiplatelet Therapy Followed by Prasugrel Monotherapy

- The strategy of prasugrel monotherapy has not been adequately tested in large RCTs.
- ASET pilot study[31] included 201 patients (low SYNTAX score) with low ischemic and bleeding risk, who underwent PCI with platinum chromium DES to discontinue aspirin immediately after PCI and to continue only on prasugrel. At 3 months, the rate of ischemic and bleeding events was extremely low in both treatment arms.

SINGLE ANTIPLATELET THERAPY STRATEGIES IN SPECIAL SUBSETS

High Bleeding Risk

- MASTER DAPT[32] study enrolled patients with >1 HBR criteria undergoing PCI with thin strut biodegradable polymer DES to standard DAPT versus abbreviated DAPT **(Flowchart 2)**.
- Choice of SAPT after recommended duration of DAPT in either arm was left to treating physician. Clopidogrel was the P2Y12i administered in 53.8% of abbreviated arm and 78.7% of standard DAPT arm—reflecting physician's choice of P2Y12i in HBR patients.
- Net adverse clinical events (composite of death from any cause, MI, stroke or major bleed): 7.5% (abbreviated group) versus 7.7% (standard group) - $p < 0.001$ for non-inferiority.
- Major adverse cardiac or cerebral events (death, MI, stroke): 6.1% versus 5.9% - $p < 0.001$ for noninferiority.
- Major (BARC 3 or 5) or clinically relevant non-major bleed (BARC 2, 3, 5 bleed): 6.5% versus 9.4% - $p < 0.001$ for superiority.
- A subgroup analysis showed there was no increase in ischemic events with abbreviated DAPT. There was significant reduction in bleeding endpoints regardless of procedure complexity or presentation as ACS.[33]
- In patients who had an indication for oral anticoagulation (OAC), net adverse clinical outcomes or major adverse cardiac and cerebral events did not differ between abbreviated versus standard DAPT regimens. BARC 2, 3, 5 bleed did not differ between arms in patients with an indication for OAC; while bleeding was lower in sub group without an OAC indication.[34]

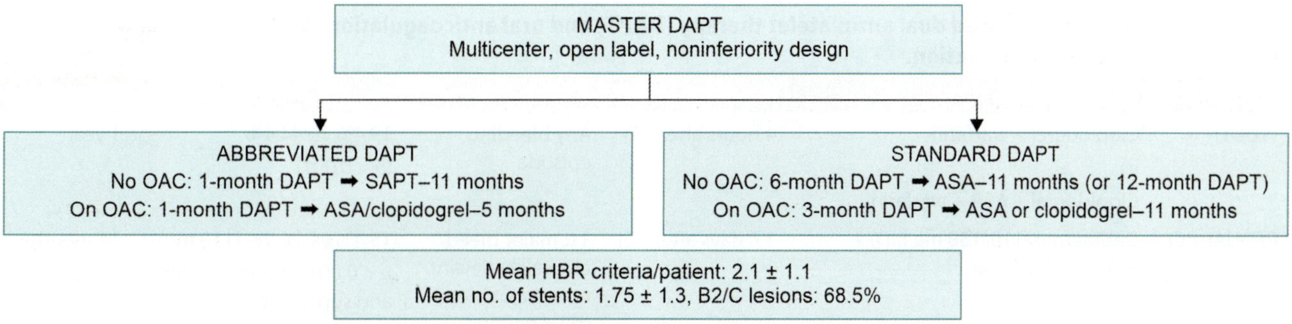

FLOWCHART 2: MASTER DAPT study.

(ASA: aspirin; DAPT: dual antiplatelet therapy; OAC: oral anticoagulation; SAPT: single antiplatelet therapy)

- A systematic meta-analysis of 11 studies which comparing abbreviated (very short) 1 month or short (3 months) with standard DAPT (>6 months) in HBR patients without an indication for OAC showed that abbreviated strategy significantly reduced the bleeding events compared with standard DAPT with no differences in ischemic events. The beneficial effect of SAPT was consistent regardless of clinical presentation (ACS vs. CCS) and the type of SAPT continued (ASA vs. P2Y12i).[35]
- ESC guidelines **(Fig. 1)**:
  - NSTE ACS + HBR – ASA monotherapy after *1-month* DAPT – Class IIa LOE B
  - STEMI + HBR – ASA monotherapy after *6-month* DAPT – Class IIa LOE B
  - CCS – ASA monotherapy after *3-month* DAPT – Class IIa LOE A
  - CCS – ASA monotherapy after *1-month* DAPT – Class IIb LOE C

PATIENTS WITH CONCOMITANT ATRIAL FIBRILLATION/INDICATION FOR ORAL ANTICOAGULATION

- Atrial fibrillation (AF) is seen in about 5–8% of patients undergoing PCI.[36]
- Concomitant DAPT with OAC [called triple therapy (TT)] leads to high bleeding risk compared to single antiplatelet with OAC (dual therapy - DAT).
- There are five studies which tested combination and duration of DAPT (majority of patients received clopidogrel as P2Y12i) in patients with an indication for OAC **(Table 5)**.
- WOEST[37] tested warfarin (plus clopidogrel alone vs. clopidogrel + ASA) while other four studies tested efficacy and safety of NOACS versus warfarin with different durations of DAPT.
- All studies were powered only for bleeding endpoints.
- Studies broadly agree that a combination of (N)OAC and clopidogrel (DAT) provides maximum reduction in bleeding endpoints.
- Optimal timing of discontinuation of aspirin is unclear from the trials so far with regard to ischemic efficacy endpoint.
- AUGUSTUS by its 2 × 2 factorial design provides certain insights into optimal timing of discontinuation of aspirin and the duration of triple therapy. ASA was discontinued in patients randomized to dual therapy group by 14 days and mean duration of triple therapy was 6.6 days.[38] About 80% of definite/probable ST events occurred within 30 days of PCI; coinciding with discontinuation of aspirin. Kaplan–Meier curves of severe ischemic events started to diverge immediately after PCI. On the other hand, Kaplan–Meier curves of severe bleeding events were similar with DAT or TT during first weeks after PCI, starting to diverge only thereafter in favor of DAT.[39,40]
- A landmark analysis of ENTRUST-AF PCI, comparing very early dual therapy (DAT) to a TT strategy from 0–14 days and from 15 days to 1 year after randomization found composite endpoint of NACE (CV death, stroke, systemic embolic events, MI, ST, and major bleeding) to be reduced with TT in 1st 14 days, but to be similar between treatment arms from 15 days to 1 year.[41]
- Numerically higher rates of MI and ST were observed in ACS subgroup with dabigatran 110 mg dual therapy versus warfarin triple therapy in a subanalysis of REDUAL PCI study although this was not statistically significant,[42] raising concerns about early discontinuation of aspirin. However there was a consistent reduction in bleeding endpoints with both doses of dabigatran (110 mg BID and 150 mg BID) versus warfarin.
- Systematic review and meta-analysis showed that all NOAC-based short DAT was associated with higher risk of stent thrombosis.[43]
- Hence, an optimal duration of triple therapy (NOAC + ASA + clopidogrel) in patients undergoing PCI and who have an indication for oral anticoagulation may be 1 month. A combination of NOAC and clopidogrel (stopping aspirin) after 1 month provides best tradeoff between bleeding and ischemia, especially in patients who undergo complex PCI **(Table 5)**.

TABLE 5: Studies which tested dual antiplatelet therapy (DAPT) and oral anticoagulation (OAC) in patients with an indication for oral anticoagulation.

Study	Comparators	Randomization	1° endpoint	Results	Time
WOEST	Clopidogrel + warfarin vs. Clopidogrel + ASA + warfarin	4 hours after PCI	Any bleeding episode	19.4% vs. 44.4% ($p < 0.001$)	1 year
REDUAL PCI	Dabigatran (110/150 mg BID) + P2Y12i (Clop/Tica) vs. Warfarin + ASA + P2Y12i (Clop/Tica)	1.6 days after PCI	1st major bleed/ clinically relevant non-major bleed (ISTH defined)	15.4% vs. 26.9% (110 mg) $p < 0.001$ – noninferiority and superiority 20.2% vs. 25.7% (150 mg) $p < 0.001$ for noninferiority	14 months
PIONEER AF	• Group 1: P2Y12i (1, 6 or 12 months) + Riva 15 mg OD • Group 2: P2Y12i (1, 6 or 12 months) + Riva 2.5 mg BID + ASA 75–100 mg • Group 3: P2Y12i (1, 6 or 12 months) + Warfarin + ASA 75–100 mg	1.6 days after PCI	TIMI major/minor bleed	Group 1: 16.8% vs. Group 3: 26.7% $p < 0.001$ Group 2: 18.0% vs. Group 3: 26.7%. $p \leq 0.001$	12 months
AUGUSTUS	2×2 factorial design P2Y12i (6 months) + ASA vs. placebo *(arm 1)* P2Y12i (6 months) + Apixaban vs. warfarin *(arm 2)*	6.6 days	Major/minor bleed (ISTH defined)	10.5% (apixaban arm) vs. 14.7% (warfarin arm) $p < 0.001$ 16.1% (aspirin arm) vs. 9% (placebo arm) $p < 0.001$	6 months
ENTRUST AF	Edoxaban + P2Y12i (12 months) Warfarin + P2Y12i + ASA (12 months) (ASA – minimum 1 month)	2.2 days	Major/minor bleed (ISTH defined)	17% (edoxaban) vs. 20% (Warfarin) $p = 0.001$ (noninferiority)	12 months

(ASA: aspirin; Clop: clopidogrel; PCI: percutaneous intervention; Prasu: prasugrel; Tica: ticagrelor)

- European Society of Cardiology guidelines for diagnosis and management of AF provides recommendation for early discontinuation of aspirin (<1 week) and continuation of dual therapy with OAC and a P2Y12i (preferably clopidogrel) up to 12 months if risk of stent thrombosis is low and concerns about bleeding risk is high and prevails over concerns of stent thrombosis (Class I LOE A) in both ACS and CCS patients with AF undergoing PCI.[44]
- Triple therapy (OAC + ASA + clopidogrel) for at least 1 month in patients who are considered to have higher risk of ST, outweighing risk for bleeding (Class IIa LOE C), in both ACS and CCS patients undergoing PCI.[44]

SAPT STRATEGIES IN LONG-TERM PREVENTION OF CARDIOVASCULAR EVENTS

- Antiplatelet therapy is the cornerstone in the long-term prevention of recurrent atherosclerotic events.
- Evidence for use of aspirin in secondary prevention of atherothrombotic events in patients with established atherosclerosis is compelling.[45,46]
- CAPRIE was first large randomized controlled trial which compared aspirin with clopidogrel in secondary prevention. Trial included broad group of patients with established coronary, cerebrovascular, and peripheral atherosclerosis. Subgroup analysis showed significant 23.8% reduction in events for patients with peripheral vascular disease (PVD).[47] More importantly, incidences of gastrointestinal complications were lower with clopidogrel monotherapy as compared to aspirin.
- HOST EXAM study (prospective, randomized, open label, and multicenter trial) randomized patients who underwent PCI with new generation DES having completed 6–18 months of DAPT to maintenance therapy with aspirin (100 mg daily) versus clopidogrel (75 mg daily). Primary endpoint (composite of all cause death, nonfatal MI, stroke, recurrent ACS, and major bleeding) at 24 months was 5.7% (clopidogrel) versus 7.7% (aspirin)

(HR 0.73; 95% CI 0.59–0.9) *p* -0.0035. There was an absolute risk reduction of 2% in favor of clopidogrel with number needed to treat (NNT) = 51 patients. Any bleeding (>BARC type 2) occurred in 2.3% (clopidogrel) versus 3.3% (aspirin).[48]

- Long-term follow-up of patients enrolled in HOST EXAM (HOST EXAM extended) study (median 5.8 years) showed maintenance of superiority of clopidogrel over asprin in secondary prevention of events in patients who underwent PCI. The results were same in diabetic subsets as well.[49] OPT BRISK[30] presented at ESC 2023 showed similar results.
- P2Y12i monotherapy was superior to aspirin monotherapy in secondary prevention of atherothrombotic events in a large meta-analysis of seven trials which compared aspirin versus P2Y12i in long-term prevention of cardiovascular events in patients with CAD.[50] Treatment effect for primary efficacy outcomes (CV death, MI, and stroke) favored P2Y12i monotherapy while risk of major bleed was similar between the groups.[50]
- 2019 ESC guidelines[51] **(Table 6)** and 2023 ACC AHA guidelines agree on use of aspirin as drug of choice for prevention of atherosclerotic events in patients with CCS. ACC AHA guidelines provide class 2a LOE A for a strategy of short DAPT of 3 months followed by P2Y12i monotherapy in CCS patients undergoing PCI.[52]

TABLE 6: ESC guidelines for event prevention in CCS.

Recommendation	Class	Level
Aspirin 75–100 mg daily is recommended in patients with a previous MI/revascularization	I	A
Clopidogrel 75 mg daily is recommended as an alternative to aspirin in patients with aspirin intolerance	I	B
Clopidogrel 75 mg daily may be considered in preference to aspirin in symptomatic/asymptomatic patients, with either PAD or history of ischemic stroke or TIA	IIb	B
Aspirin 75–100 mg daily may be considered in patients without a history of MI/revascularization, but with definitive evidence of CAD on imaging	IIb	C

CAD: coronary artery disease; CCS: chronic coronary syndrome; ESC: European Society of Cardiology; MI: myocardial infarction; PAD: peripheral artery disease; TIA: transient ischemic attack)

CONCLUSION

- In ACS patients undergoing PCI, standard DAPT duration is 12 months. A strategy of Ticagrelor based monotherapy after 3-month DAPT is safe with reduction in bleeding events.
- In CCS patients undergoing PCI, standard DAPT duration is 6 months. A P2Y12i based monotherapy (clopidogrel/ticagrelor) after 1–3 months of DAPT is proven to be safe and effective.
- In special subset of patients with increased bleeding risk who undergo PCI, P2Y12i of choice is clopidogrel and studies report safety of 1-month DAPT.
- In long-term secondary prevention of patients who have underwent PCI, aspirin monotherapy is recommended. Evidence is emerging in favor of P2Y12i monotherapy which is reported to be better tolerated.
- Furthur reading on the topic - References.[52,53]

ONLINE REFERENCES

Please scan the QR code provided at the end of the table of contents for References of this chapter.

SECTION

4

Hypertension

CHAPTER 27

Blood Pressure Measurement Methods: Which One is the Best for a Clinician?

Abhishek, Gurpreet Singh Wander, Zoofi Shan

ABSTRACT

There are three common sources of error in the measurement of blood pressure (BP), i.e., faulty equipment, observer bias, and failure to standardize the technique of measurement. Despite the proper guidelines on BP measurement technique, there are large interobserver variations, both among physicians and nursing group as well as between the two groups. Moreover, technical errors might occur related to the equipment used in practice, and this can influence BP reading. International studies confirm that training, teaching, and knowledge toward BP measurement and apparatus for healthcare professional are suboptimal. These gaps in training are continuing in medical education and among interns and practitioners. In this chapter, we provide a concise summary of the BP measurement along with different types of devices, location of BP measurement, techniques, and recent advances.

Keywords: Blood pressure measurement, errors, recent advances.

INTRODUCTION

India, with a population of >1.40 billion, is experiencing increasing cardiovascular disease (CVD) along with increased mortalities, which is driven mainly by uncontrolled hypertension. Hypertension is directly responsible for 24% of all coronary artery disease deaths and 57% of all stroke deaths in India.[1] Hypertension is a common condition that does not have specific clinical symptoms until target organ damage develops.[2-4] It confers a substantial risk of CVD much of which is at least partially reversible with treatment. Screening of adults to be done to detect hypertension in early stage and initiate treatment before onset of target organ damage occurs.[4,5] The teaching, training, and knowledge of BP measurement and apparatus for healthcare professional are suboptimal.[6-8] These gaps in training exist for medical students, nursing, and other paramedical staff who need to know the correct technique.[1]

BLOOD PRESSURE MEASUREMENT DEVICES

The accurate measurement of BP is correlated to better hypertension management and a decrease in cardiovascular morbidity and mortality.[9] Overestimates of BP are associated with issues such as psychological effects of misdiagnosis, side effects of antihypertensive medications, higher treatment costs, and increased insurance. Having said that, the aftermath of underestimates of BP could not only deprive patients of therapy but could also potentially increase the current levels of fatal strokes and myocardial infarctions.[10] One of the major reasons for inaccurate measurement of BP has to do with the equipment itself.[11,12] Three most widely accepted devices for the measurement of BP are the mercury sphygmomanometer (MS), the aneroid sphygmomanometer (AS), and the automatic digital monitor (DM).

Mercury sphygmomanometer **(Fig. 1)** has been considered as the gold standard of BP measurement for >100 years. Its advantage is its accuracy, minimal calibration requirement, and infrequent breakdown.

Aneroid sphygmomanometer **(Fig. 2)** uses mechanical springs and dashpot systems. These use the same auscultatory method of measurement as that of MS but are prone to run out of calibration within 6 months to a year due to loosening of springs, especially in heavy use environments of hospitals.[13-15] Once spring becomes loose, these are nearly impossible to recalibrate. In a study conducted by McKay et al.,[16] among 114 physicians, it was found that nearly 40% of AS were out of calibration by at least 4 mm Hg while just 8% of MS were off calibration by the same degree.

Automatic digital sphygmomanometers (oscillometric) **(Fig. 3)** are most popular as home-use self-monitoring devices. They use the oscillometric method of BP measurement, which measures the mean pressure accurately, but systolic and diastolic pressures are derived based on different empirical and signal processing methods, which vary from company to company and are mostly maintained as trade secrets.[17] When the aneroid and the digital BP monitor were pitted against each other, it was seen that the sensitivity and specificity of the aneroid device are higher than the digital device by 6.7% and 31%, respectively.[18] The aneroid and oscillometric types are still inadequate compared to the accuracy or reliability of the MS.[19] Mercury device is being banned not because of the invention of any new technology of BP measurement but because of the harmful effects of mercury. Advisory has been issued as far back as 2010 to avoid usage and procurement of the MS,[10] and India is required to ban MS by end of year 2020.[10] However, MSs are still widely used in India as there is an unmet need for a more reliable replacement of MS which is not being fulfilled by aneroid and oscillometric types and is the cause behind resilience of clinicians to still stick to the MS.

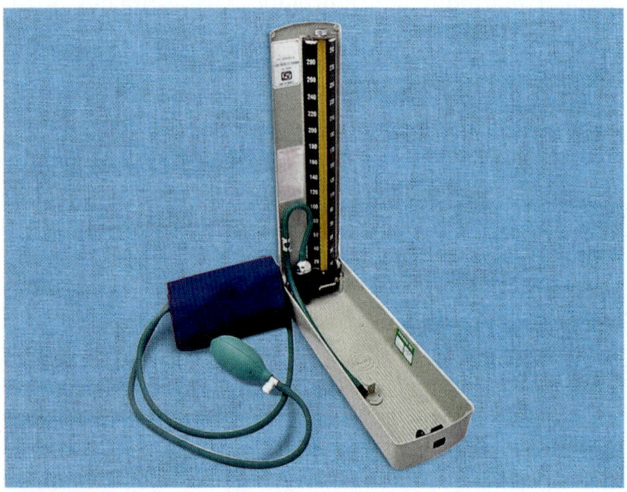

FIG. 1: Mercury sphygmomanometer (MS).

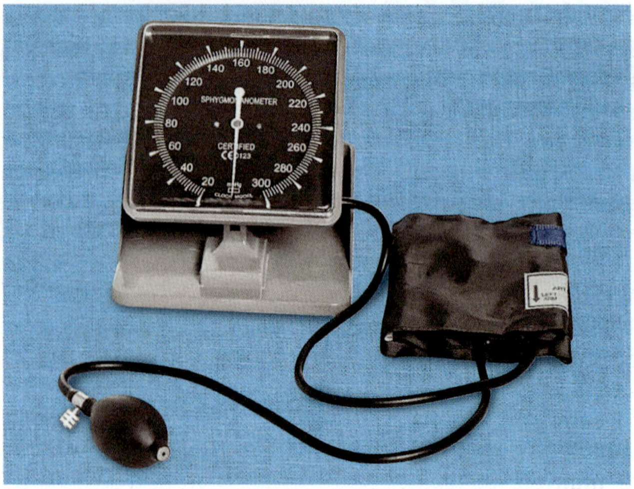

FIG. 2: Aneroid sphygmomanometer.

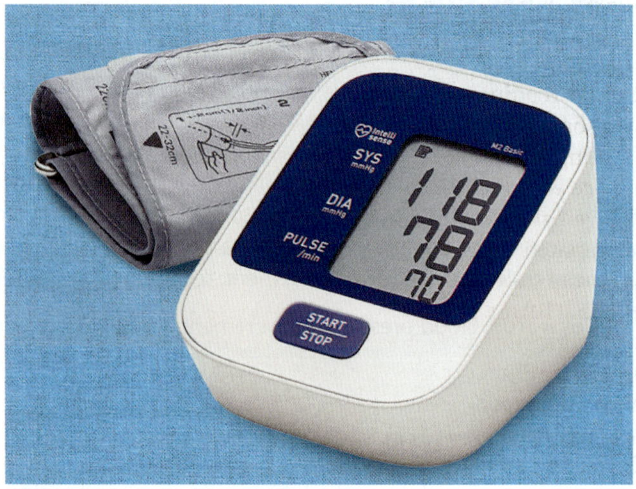

FIG. 3: Automatic digital sphygmomanometers.

According to recent guidelines, i.e., European Society of Hypertension (ESH), 2023,[20] automatic electronic, upper-arm cuff devices are recommended for office and out-of-office BP measurement (home and ambulatory) as a class-1 recommendations.

BLOOD PRESSURE MEASUREMENT LOCATION

Office Blood Pressure Measurement

It is measured using a brachial pressure cuff and auscultation of the brachial artery to identify the appearance and disappearance of Korotkoff sounds. Office blood pressure measurement (OBPM) is recommended for diagnosis of hypertension as per guidelines, because it is the one method by which hypertension-related risk, benefits of antihypertensive treatment, and treatment-related BP thresholds and goals are based.[20] Triplicate measurements should be taken and the average of the last two should be referred to as the representative value.[20] It is recommended to diagnose hypertension during at least two separate office visits (within 4 weeks) unless office BP indicates grade-3 hypertension (≥180/110 mm Hg) or patient presents with hypertension-related symptoms or there is evidence of hypertension-mediated organ damage (HMOD) or CVD.[20] At the first office visit, BP should be measured in both arms. A consistent between-arm systolic blood pressure (SBP) difference of >15–20 mm Hg suggests atheromatous disease and is associated with increased cardiovascular (CV) risk. All subsequent measurements should be made on the arm with the higher BP readings.[20] Out-of-office BP is a source of multiple BP-related information before and during treatment. It is, therefore, recommended to obtain additional information on BP values by ambulatory blood pressure measurement (ABPM) or home blood pressure measurement (HBPM) or both if available.[20]

Automated office blood pressure (AOBP) means that the BP readings recorded with a fully automated device.[19] The basic principles of AOBP include mean of multiple readings to be taken with a fully automated BP recording device with the patient resting alone in a quiet room. When above principles are followed, white coat hypertension is eliminated and AOBP exhibits a much stronger correlation with the awake ambulatory BP as compared with routine manual BP measurements. Unlike routine manual BP, AOBP also correlates as well with left ventricular mass as does the awake ambulatory BP.[21] Over the last years, automated BP measurement devices have reached the market and are now widely accepted. Presently, these are expensive and cannot be recommended for wide usage.

Devices

These are MSs, ASs, and automated blood pressure measurement devices.

Advantages

Office blood pressure measurement has been the cornerstone of hypertension diagnosis and management for over 100 years and it is also method of choice in most of research work even important trials such as SPRINT and HOPE-3 trials were based on OBPM.[16,17] Office BP is recommended for diagnosis of hypertension, because it is the one method by which hypertension-related risk, benefits of antihypertensive treatment, and treatment-related BP thresholds and goals are based.[20]

Disadvantages

A single office BP reading does not represent a patient's correct BP. Errors may be due to clinic ambience that can lead to white coat hypertension. OBPM is an act like a snapshot that gives information of BP of single visit but it lacks information on BP during usual daytime activities and during sleep. Moreover, it is more prone to a variety of procedural error that can lead to false measurement that can be due to faulty position such as legs crossed, back or arm unsupported, talking during the measurement or insufficient number of readings. False measurement can be due to use of nonvalidated devices.

Home Blood Pressure Measurement

Proper and accurate BP measurement is necessary for screening, diagnosis, and management of hypertension.[22] HBPM provides an easy, reliable, convenient, and cost-effective methods for measurement of BP.[22] In fact, in previous studies, it was found that patients were more comfortable with self-reading at home ranked higher than repeated measurements by staff or a doctor.[22] Despite the wider community increasingly recognizing the importance of HBPM, explicit recommendations and proper guidance for accurate HBPM are lacking in many countries/regions in Asia.[22]

Device and Measurement Technique

The standard type of monitor for home use is an oscillometric device that records BP from the brachial artery. Use of the arm cuff is preferred over wrist and finger monitors.[23] HBPM should be measured twice daily for a 3- to 7-day period for diagnosis of hypertension; first day values are typically not used, to allow patients to acclimatize to the process.[23] A good regimen is to measure HBPM twice in the morning after 5 minutes of rest before breakfast (preferably between 6:00 and 10:00 AM) and twice in the evening (also preferably between 6:00 and 10:00 PM), while the patient is sitting at rest for 5 minutes, and with an empty bladder.[23] However, the Japanese Society of Hypertension guidelines for self-monitoring of BP at home propose that the measurements be made after 1–2 minutes of rest as seen in **Box 1**. Equipment must be calibrated against a mercury manometer, with the difference in measurement compared with the auscultatory method being 5 mm Hg or less. It is also recommended that the device be calibrated annually.[23] Every measurement should be documented, along with the pulse rate, time, and date; devices with an attached printer or an integrated memory are helpful to avoid selection bias.[23]

Advantages

Home blood pressure measurement eliminates white coat hypertension, and it can help in diagnosing the masked hypertension. It can provide information that cannot be provided with OBPM, that it provides BP changes during activity. As HBPM is not influenced by observer bias and its reproducibility has been found better than office measurements.[23] Integration of HBPM in practice can provide a promising tool that can aid in diagnosis and treatment of hypertension. It also helps in to find out risk of CVD and

BOX 1 Japanese Society of Hypertension guidelines for home blood pressure monitoring.[24]

- Arm-cuffs based on the oscillometric method devices are recommended. They should be validated and confirmed for accuracy in each individual
- Blood pressure should be measured in the upper arm. Finger cuff devices and wrist-cuff devices should not be used for home blood pressure measurements
- Devices for home BP measurement should be validated by the American Association Medical Instrumentation standards and the British Hypertension Society guidelines. In addition, the difference between the blood pressure measured by the auscultatory method and that measured using the device should be 5 mm Hg or less
- The morning BP measurement should be made within 1 hour after waking, after micturition, sitting after 1–2 minutes of rest, before drug ingestion, and before breakfast. The evening measurement should be made just before going to bed, sitting after 1–2 minutes of rest
- All home BP measurements should be documented without selection or omission and include the date, time, and pulse rate. Use of a device with a printer or an integrated circuit memory is useful to avoid selection bias

complications of hypertension than hospital measure BP.[23] It can help in patients with chronic kidney disease, diabetics to diagnose the resistant or refractory hypertension.[23] HBPM can also help in research work like onset and duration of antihypertensive drugs and their side effects. And, it is more useful to detect or to prevent hypertension mediated organ damage.[23] More than diagnostic and prognostic values, it also offers awareness of treatment and to remain active in management of BP.[23]

Disadvantage

Home blood pressure measurement has many advantages, but still has some disadvantages. HBPM needs awareness about device and measurement techniques. Poverty and illiteracy were one of the common reasons for not using HBPM which is higher side in our country. The main disadvantage is that this HBPM cannot measure night BP, so it lacks prognostic value about dipping patterns.

Ambulatory Blood Pressure Measurement

In this method, BP will be measured automatically at regular intervals (mostly every 20 minutes at day time and every 30 minutes at night time) over 24 hours.

Device and Techniques

Patients are provided with an ABPM device, which measures BP during 24–72 hours at predefined time intervals. If one arm gives a higher reading at baseline, then this arm should be used subsequently;[25] however, in general, the nondominant arm will lead to as little interference with daily activities as possible. ABPM monitors include a cuff and bladder connected to electronic sensors which detect changes in cuff pressure and allow BP to be measured oscillometrically.[25] Systolic and diastolic pressure readings are deduced from the shape of these oscillometric pressure changes using a specific algorithm. The cuff is inflated by a battery-powered compressor.[25] Devices differing in size, weight, noise level, data manipulation, and costs are available.[25] They should be validated and internationally recommended.[25] The recommended frequency of measurements is 20 minutes during day and night to minimize the risk of missing day or night periods.[20]

Advantage

This method can overcome disadvantages of both OBPM and HBPM methods. With this, we can monitor the profile of BP behavior with respect to daily activities. As mentioned earlier, in this method, BP will not be influenced by clinic ambience and we can monitor BP during night also. It is also superior to clinic BP measurement. ABPM is recommended to identify white coat hypertension, masked hypertension, and nocturnal BP phenotypes.[20] Repeated ABPM may be necessary because these phenotypes have a limited reproducibility.[20] ABPM should be used to diagnose true resistant hypertension.[20] It should be done before starting antihypertension drugs. Moreover, it is now recognized as the best method for predicting the risk of cardiovascular events in relations to patient's BP.[26] The relation between ABPM and risk of cardiovascular events is continuous, consistent, and independent of other risk factors.[26]

Disadvantage

The main disadvantage is cost and limited availability. Moreover, it can cause discomfort to patient especially during sleep or sexual activity and patients may be reluctant to use it.

Figure 4 summarizes the uses of OBPM, HBPM, and ABPM in clinical practice according to the guidelines.

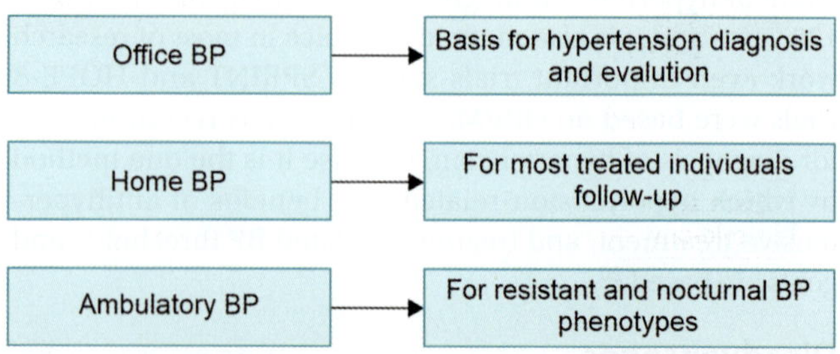

FIG. 4: Uses of OBPM, HBPM, and ABPM in clinical practice according to the guidelines.

(ABPM: ambulatory blood pressure measurement; HBPM: home blood pressure measurement; OBPM: office blood pressure measurement)

BLOOD PRESSURE MEASUREMENT TECHNIQUE

Failure to standardize the technique of measurement is one of the most common error in BP measurement. As previous Indian studies showed, training, teaching, and knowledge toward BP apparatus and measurement for healthcare professional are suboptimal.[1] A study conducted by Mohan B et al.[1] showed that out of 400 individuals, only 5.8% of the medical staff had excellent knowledge, 74.5% had good knowledge, and 19.6% had poor knowledge of correct measurement technique. However, only 1.47% had accurate practices and among paramedical staff, only 0.5% had accurate practice. This shows that although the knowledge of a correct method of BP measurement is reasonable, the practice is in adequate and often the due precautions are not taken.

Figure 5 shows the various precautions one needs to take for correct BP readings. The various aspects are discussed below.

Posture

- Blood pressure should be measured in sitting position. If measured in supine position, SBP will increase by 3 mm Hg and diastolic blood pressure (DBP) will be recorded lower by 3 mm Hg.[1]
- Patient should be comfortably sitting with bare arm at the heart level. The legs should be uncrossed and the feet flat on floor with back supported. The arm should be resting on a desk.[1]

Conditions

- Patient should be resting comfortably for at least 5 minutes in a quiet room.
- Pain, strenuous exercise, cold temperature, food consumption, smoking, caffeine ingestion, and emotional stress are to be avoided 30 minutes before taking measurements.
- Urinary bladder should be empty.

Measurements

- Blood pressure cuff length should be two-thirds of the arm circumference. If size of cuff is small as in the case of obese person, the SBP will be recorded falsely high (up to 8 mm Hg).[1]
- Systolic pressure is first estimated through palpation so that the systolic gap which may be present in some individuals does not get missed. Also, we can diagnose pseudohypertension due to significant artery calcifications as in elderly.
- Blood pressure should be measured in both arms at initial visit. The arm with higher BP should be used subsequently.[20]
- Cuff should be inflated up to 30 mm Hg more than the estimated SBP.
- Rate of deflation should be 2 mm/s.
- First appearance of sound (phase I) is used to define SBP.
- The disappearance of sound (phase V) is used to define DBP.

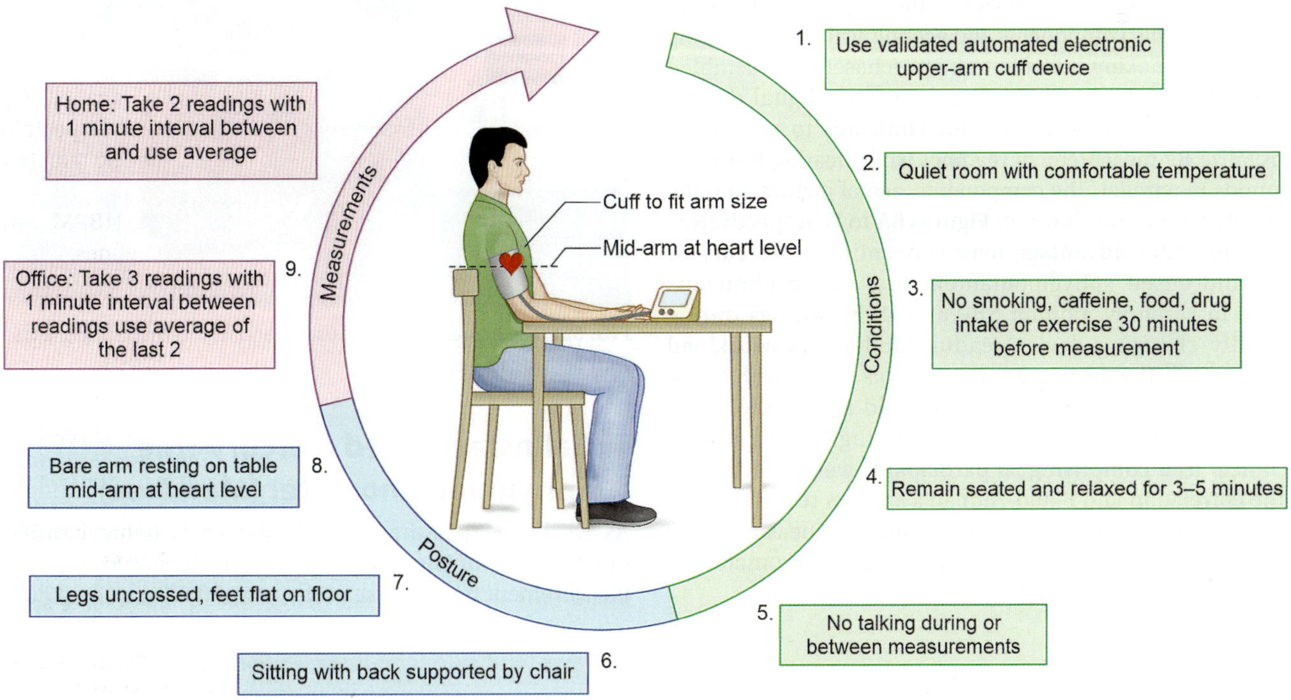

FIG. 5: Technique of blood pressure measurement.

RECENT ADVANCES

Cuffless Blood Pressure Devices

Conventional BP cuffs and methods have some limitations, as they provide only snapshot of BP value and ignore the variability with daily life activities. Inappropriate cuff size is one of the common causes of error. To overcome these errors, there is recent advance of cuffless measuring devices. These work with a sensor, signal processing, and machine learning along with other technologies. All of these are embedded in a wearable device, pocket devices, and smartphones and these have potential to improve awareness of hypertension. However, there are lot of issues that need to be addressed before using these devices in clinical practice. Major issue is validation of cuffless BP devices, as these require periodic calibrations. The standard validation protocols are for cuff BP devices and are not valid for cuffless device. Due to above-mentioned reasons, at present, cuffless devices should not be used for diagnosis and treatment of hypertension as per ESH, 2023 guidelines.[20] However, cuffless devices definitely will have a bright future after standard validation protocols are developed.

Digital Auscultatory BP Measurement Device (Auscl-D)

Recently, digital devices have been developed for BP measurement. Once such device is Auscl-D, which displays BP reading digitally, like oscillometric devices, but measurements are performed using auscultation method employing traditional stethoscope and manual pumping system as in an aneroid device.[27] The device is made from easily available components and economical manufacturing processes, making it viable to be purchased or assembled even in areas with limited resources.[27] Its digital display provides direct line of sight for clinicians to accurately visualize BP measurement readings while hearing Korotkoff sounds in parallel. The components, actual picture, and the use of Auscl-D are shown in **Figures 6A to C**, respectively.[27] This provides advantage over conventional mercury or aneroid-based sphygmomanometers, where clinicians have to carefully monitor SBP and DBP readings during rapidly changing device reading under high-workload condition.[27] The device performance was on par with MS in laboratory conditions and with aneroid and oscillometric sphygmomanometer in clinical setting.[27] Preliminary clinical trial comprising 30 participants was conducted.[27] The correlation and Bland–Altman's analysis reveal that the performance of Auscl-D for both SBP and DBP measurements is comparable to commonly used sphygmomanometers in hospitals.[27]

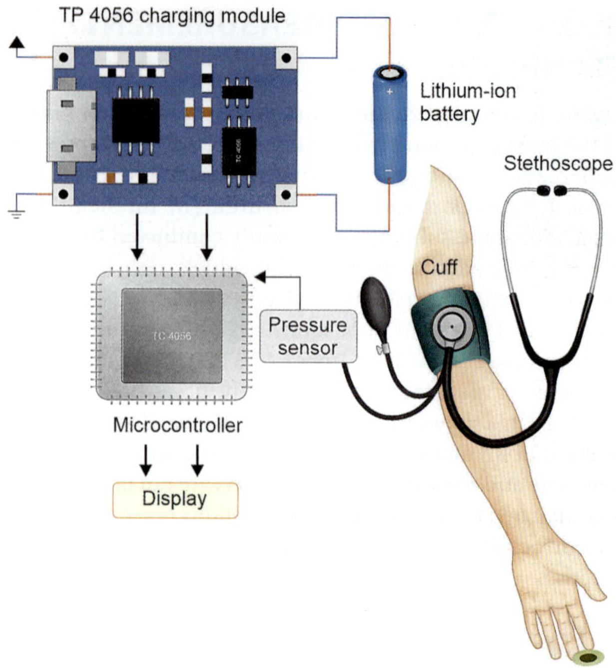

FIG. 6A: The components of the digital BP device Auscl-D and their functioning.
(BP: blood pressure)

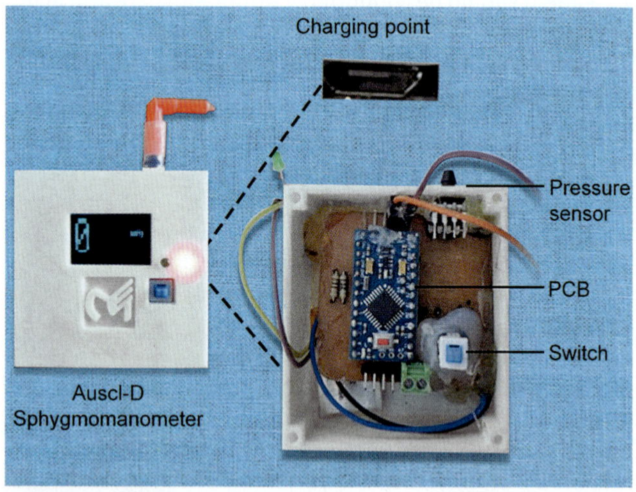

FIG. 6B: The actual image of Auscl-D and its internal components.
(PCB: printed circuit board)

Galinstan-based Mercury-free Sphygmomanometer (Merkfree)

As we know that the mercury device is being banned not because of the invention of any technology of BP measurement but because of the harmful effects of mercury

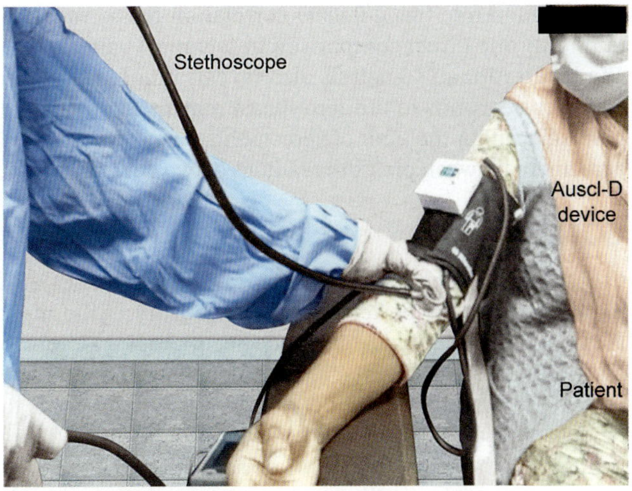

FIG. 6C: Auscl-D being used clinically for measurement of BP. The small and convenient size of the device is visible.

and there is an unmet need in the market for a mercury-free sphygmomanometer with the same structure and principle of operation as of MS after the mercury ban due to Minamata convention comes into effect. India is a signatory to this convention undertaking and is obliged to eliminate mercury-based products in medical equipment.[28]

Galinstan is a promising substitute for mercury. It is a nontoxic alloy of gallium, indium, and tin and its density is about half that of the mercury, and a melting point of approximately –19°C.[29] Galinstan is being used in various areas of applications such as in microdevices,[30] actuators, electrochemistry, 3D patterning, microfluidics, elastomeric composites, soft electronics,[29] integrated liquid cooling system,[31] and generation of electrically conductive composites for electronic applications.

The components of the Merkfree device are shown in **Figure 7A** and the actual size of the BP apparatus is shown in **Figure 7B**. This device is double the size of MS as shown

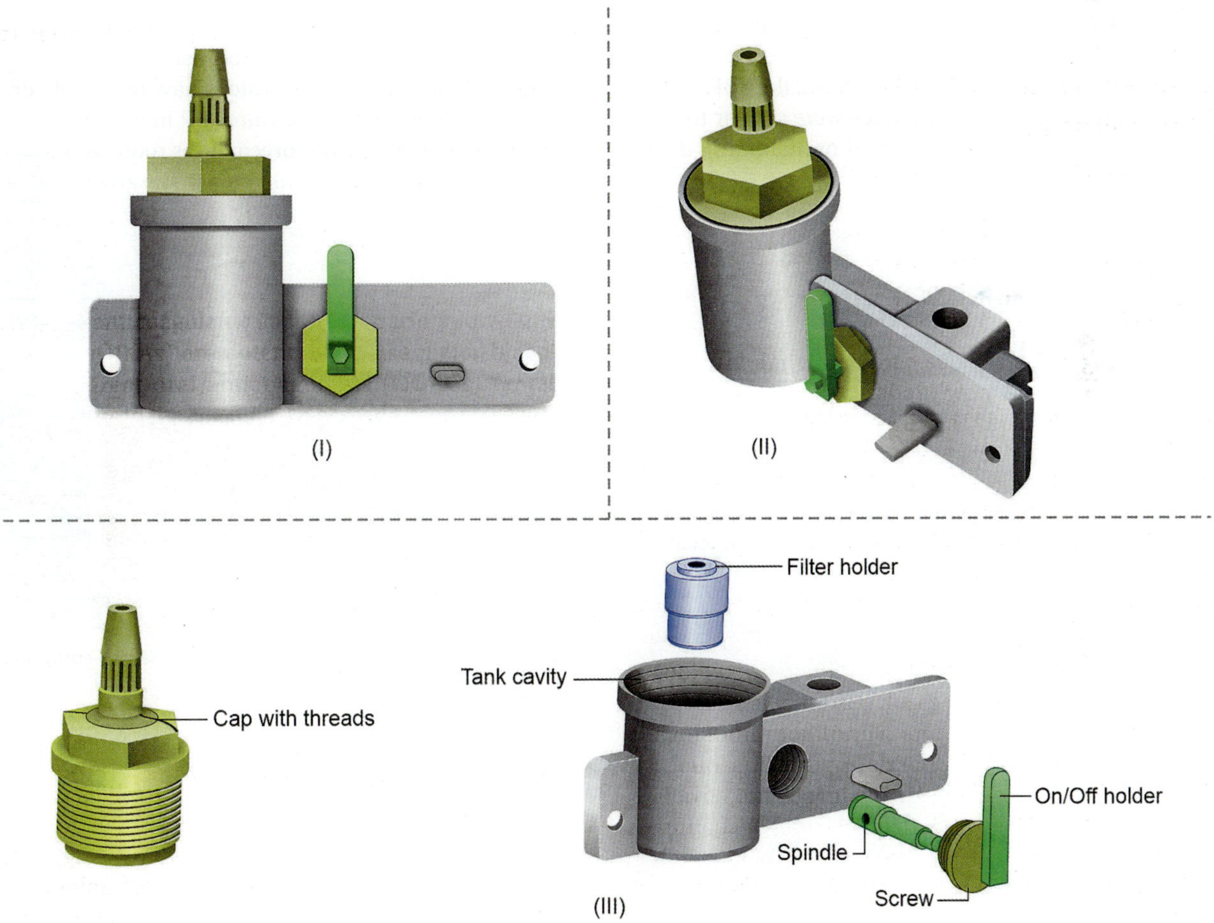

FIG. 7A: The Merkfree device components. Container tank for Galinstan and the on–off knobs.

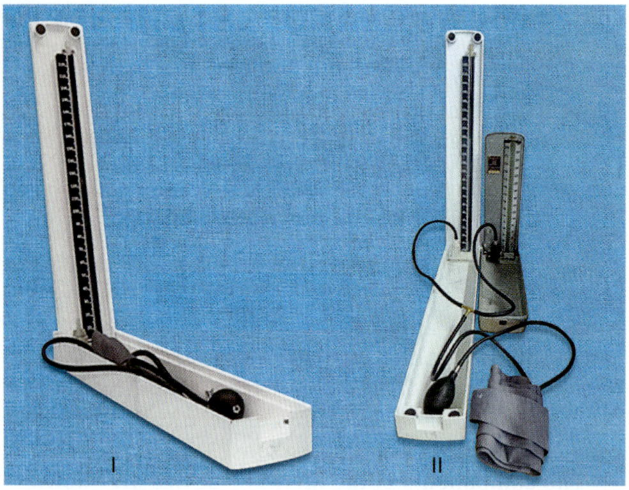

FIG. 7B: The size of the Merkfree device is double of the mercury sphygmomanometer which is seen in the picture.

in the figure.[28] All methods were performed in accordance with the relevant guidelines and regulations.[28] In clinical trials in a total of 252 participants, across various age groups (12–80 years, mean ± standard deviation = 41.23 ± 15.56 years) and sex (143 males and 109 females), the SBP and the DBP measurements with the Merkfree were similar to those taken with MS and a validated digital oscillometric device (WatchBP Office, Microlife).[28]

The Merkfree has a 0.9999 correlation factor with MS in one-to-one direct comparison in technical validation.[28] The bland Altman's analysis also reveals that bias is zero, which corresponds to the zero-measurement error, all data points lie within the limit of agreements and show the good agreement between pressure readings of two devices.[28]

CONCLUSION

Correct BP measurement is important for diagnosis and management of hypertension. Hypertension is the most common noncommunicable public health disease. Errors in diagnosis can result in either lack of treatment or unnecessary usage of drugs. The technique, though it is simple, needs to be respected and all due precautions are to be taken. There is shift from the conventional MS device which we have used for a century to the oscillometric automatic device which is now most commonly used for OBPM. The aneroid BP device can also be used in the office. Reliable and validated devices should be used for measurement. Various international bodies like the British Hypertension Society have given a list of devices that are validated. The Indian government is also making validation of BP measurement devices mandatory. Clinicians should stop using the MS and shift to the oscillometric devices. Besides having reliable device, it is equally important to measures BP in a quiet room and take multiple readings. The precautions required for correct measurement have been highlighted in the article above.

ONLINE REFERENCES

Please scan the QR code provided at the end of the table of contents for References of this chapter.

CHAPTER 28

Current Trends in Hypertension Epidemiology and Blood Pressure Control in India

Rajeev Gupta, Kiran Gaur

ABSTRACT

Hypertension has emerged as one of India's most important chronic disease risk factors. It is endemic in the country. Unique epidemiological features of hypertension in India are (1) increasing trends in mean systolic blood pressure (BP) and prevalence of hypertension with a more rapid increase in rural and young populations; (2) substantial geographic variations with greater prevalence in more developed states and districts of the country; (3) emergence of young-age or premature hypertension, especially in less developed states of the country; (4) significantly greater mortality from hypertension-related cardiovascular disease as compared to the more developed countries; (5) low levels of hypertension awareness, treatment, and control and inequitable distribution; and (6) low focus on strategies to reduce target-organ damage in hypertension. In this narrative review, we highlight recent nationwide studies and discuss evidence highlighting the unique features of hypertension in India and suggest strategies for better hypertension management and control.

Keywords: Hypertension, India, epidemiology, hypertension management.

INTRODUCTION

High blood pressure (BP) of hypertension has traditionally been considered a disease of developed countries and a problem among the upper socioeconomic classes in developing countries. In the last 50 years, however, it has emerged as a more important problem in less developed countries.[1] World Health Organization (WHO) reported that presently the highest prevalence of hypertension is in low and lower-middle-income countries of Africa and Asia and the lowest in high-income countries of Europe and North America.[2] In the Prospective Urban Rural Epidemiology (PURE) study, at 11-year follow-up, it was reported that both in women and men, the rates of cardiovascular events as well as mortality were higher in low and lower-middle-income countries compared to the higher-income countries.[3] Data also show that hypertension-related mortality in low-income countries (South Asia and Africa) is >3–4 times than in high-income countries.[1,2] In the PURE study it was also reported that rates of hypertension awareness, treatment, and control were significantly lower in low and lower-middle-income countries.[4] India was part of the low-income countries at the initiation of the PURE study (2002–2003) and greater event rates and cardiovascular deaths due to hypertension have attracted worldwide attention. Hypertension has now emerged as the most important cause of death and disability in India according to the Global Burden of Diseases (GBDs) study.[5,6] In the current narrative review, we focus on salient aspects of hypertension epidemiology in India and suggest remedial measures to reverse the increasing trends in adverse cardiovascular events and deaths due to hypertension in our country.

INCREASING HYPERTENSION PREVALENCE IN INDIA

Hypertension epidemiology in India has more than a 100-year history of investigation.[7] Almost 30 years ago, we performed a meta-analysis of data on hypertension epidemiology in India using available population-based studies in urban and rural populations.[7] Hypertension was diagnosed using the then prevalent WHO criteria of systolic BP ≥160 and/or diastolic BP ≥95 mm Hg. These levels correspond to stage II hypertension in the current guidelines. A significant increase in the prevalence of hypertension in both urban ($R^2 = 0.47$) and rural populations ($R^2 = 0.21$) was observed

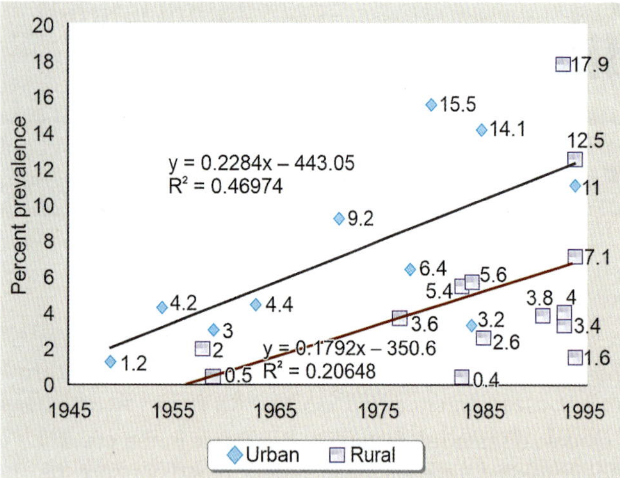

FIG. 1: Fifty-year trends in hypertension prevalence in urban and rural Indian populations. Hypertension was diagnosed using older WHO criteria (BP ≥160 and/or ≥95 mm Hg), presently equivalent to stage-II hypertension.

(BP: blood pressure; WHO: World Health Organization)

Source: With permission from Gupta et al. (1996).[7]

(Fig. 1). In a second meta-analysis using hypertension prevalence studies following revised BP cut-offs for the diagnosis of hypertension—systolic BP ≥140 and/or diastolic BP ≥90 mm Hg), we reported that the increasing trend of hypertension continued.[8] These findings were confirmed in another, more recent meta-analysis.[9] We performed a third meta-analysis which showed an urban-rural convergence of hypertension in India with a more rapid increase in rural as compared to urban populations.[10] Limitations of these meta-analyses were multiple and were regarding the inclusion of studies that were performed in disparate study locations with variable methodology and nonstandardized reporting.

There have been a number of multisite studies regarding hypertension prevalence in India in recent years **(Table 1)**.[11-21] Most of these studies used identical methodology and reporting standards and diagnosed hypertension according to the recent definition (systolic BP ≥140 and/or diastolic BP ≥90 mm Hg). The prevalence of hypertension in these studies ranges from 25 to 35% in urban populations and 15–20% in rural populations.

Much larger studies with a standardized methodology and nationwide scope have been performed by Indian governmental agencies in recent years.[22-26] Five such studies are: (1) Annual Health Survey-3/District Level Health Survey-4 (AHS-3/DLHS-4, 2009–2011);[22] (2) National Family Health Survey-4 (NFHS-4, 2012-2013);[23] (3) National NCD Monitoring Survey (NNMS, 2017–2018);[24] (4) Longitudinal

TABLE 1: Hypertension prevalence in multisite studies from India.

Study acronym	Location	Year reported	Sample size	Hypertension prevalence		
				Men	Women	Total
India Industrial Population Study[11]	Mixed	2006	10,442	29.3	25.2	27.7
India Migration Study[12]	Rural	2010	1,983	20.0	22.0	21.0
ICMR Integrated Disease Surveillance[13]	Urban	2010	15,223	30.2	25.7	28.0
ICMR Integrated Disease Surveillance[13]	Rural	2010	13,517	22.3	20.6	21.4
ICMR Integrated Disease Surveillance[13]	Periurban	2010	15,751	27.3	22.3	24.8
India Women's Health Study[14]	Urban	2013	2,008	–	56.8	56.8
India Women Health Study[14]	Rural	2013	2,616	–	24.6	24.6
India Heart Watch[15]	Urban	2014	6,106	32.5	30.4	31.1
ICMR study[16]	Tribal	2015	47,401	27.1	26.4	26.9
ICMR-INDIAB (Phase 1)[17]	Mixed	2015	14,059	NA	NA	26.3
NNMB study[18]	Rural	2016	7,531	18.0	16.0	17.0
PURE South Asia Study[19]	Mixed	2017	33,423	31.5	32.6	32.1
Great India BP Survey[20]	Urban	2019	180,335	34.2	23.7	30.7
ICMR-INDIAB Study[21]	Mixed	2023	111,439	NA	NA	35.5

(BP: blood pressure; ICMR: Indian Council of Medical Research; INDIAB: Indian Diabetes; NNMB: National Nutrition Monitoring Bureau; PURE: Prospective Urban Rural Epidemiology)

TABLE 2: Hypertension prevalence in India in the recent nationwide studies.

	Years performed	Age-group screened	Sample size	Age-adjusted prevalence (%)		
				Men	Women	Total
AHS-3/DLHS-4[22]	2009–2011	>15 years	1,320,555	27.4	20.0	25.3
NFHS-4[23]	2012–2013	15–49 (W); 15–54 (M)	799,228	13.8	8.8	10.8
NNMS[24]	2017–2018	18–69	10,593	27.0	29.4	28.5
LASI[25]	2017–2019	>45 years	64,427	39.6	43.7	41.9
NFHS-5[26]	2019–2021	>15 years	825,954	24.0	21.3	22.4

(AHS-3/DLHS-4: Annual Health Survey-3/District Level Health Survey-4; LASI: Longitudinal Aging Study in India; M: men; NFHS: National Family Health Survey; NNMS: National NCD Monitoring Survey; W: women)

Aging Study in India (LASI, 2017-2019);[25] and (5) National Family Health Survey-5 (NFHS-5, 2019-2021).[26] All the studies used standardized methodology but included adults of different age groups. The AHS/DLHS and NFHS-5 screened for hypertension in all adults >15 years while NFHS-4 was confined to women 15-49 years and men 15-54 years, LASI was performed in adults >45 years while NNMS included all adults >20 years. The prevalence of hypertension in these studies is shown in **Table 2**. It is observed that the prevalence of hypertension in both rural and urban populations is high and successive studies have shown an increasing trend in age-group-specific rates of hypertension. The prevalence of hypertension in the more ambitious ICMR-INDIAB national study,[21] has been reported to be even higher than many of the other national studies.

The Non-Communicable Disease Risk Factor Studies Collaboration (NCD-RiSC) calculated hypertension burden across the globe using meta-regression of various regional and local epidemiological studies. It was reported that from the 1990s to 2015 the mean systolic BP declined in almost all regions of the world (high-income western, central and eastern Europe, Latin America and the Caribbean, high-income Asia Pacific, and Southeast Asia) except South Asia in both women and men.[27] Increasing hypertension is an important concern in India and a challenge for healthcare professionals, bureaucrats and policy makers.[1,28] It has been well said that hypertension is a social disease and needs social solutions.[29] Population-level intervention and focus on social determinants of health (hypertension) are needed to curb the increasing mean systolic BP and hypertension levels in the country **(Table 3)**.

TABLE 3: Population-level interventions for hypertension control in India.

Policy domain	Examples
Public health policies	• Universal and free primary and secondary healthcare • Socialized and state-funded health services • Health literacy • BP screening programs and medicine availability
Food policies	• Policies to curb the intake of salt, sugars, transfats, etc. • Promotion of BP healthy foods —fruits and vegetables • Tobacco and alcohol control policies
Maternal and child health policies	• Maternal and fetal nutrition • Evidence-based food supplementation policies • Promotion of breastfeeding • Curbing salt and sugar intake in early childhood
Poverty eradication, income support policies	• Universal social support systems • Universal basic income guarantee schemes
Education and employment guarantee schemes	• Right to high-quality education • Employment guarantee schemes

GEOGRAPHIC VARIATION IN HYPERTENSION PREVALENCE AND NFHS-5

In almost all the large countries of the world, geographic variations in hypertension prevalence have been reported. In the early 2000s WHO reported that hypertension prevalence was more in Sub-Saharan African and South-East Asian countries,[2] while the NCD-RiSC reported that in 2018 the highest prevalence of hypertension was in Eastern European, Central Asian, and Eastern Asian countries.[27,30] GBD estimated that hypertension-related deaths were significantly less in more developed countries.[31] Within-country variation has also been reported from large countries such as China, USA, Brazil, Indonesia, Pakistan, UK, and in the European region.[30,32-37] Epidemiological studies have also reported a district (county) level variation from the USA and UK.[38,39] It is important to note that the studies from USA, UK, and China have reported greater hypertension prevalence in less developed regions and districts.

Variations in the prevalence of hypertension have been reported in earlier meta-analyses as well as in recent national studies from India.[7,9,23,40] All the national studies **(Table 2)** have reported significant state-level variation and urban-rural differences in hypertension prevalence. The AHS-3/DLHS-4 study highlighted important geographic differences and reported more hypertension in south India, north-eastern Indian states and a few states in north India.[22] Similar geographic distribution has been reported in other national studies (NFHS-4, NNMS, and LASI) with greater hypertension prevalence in southern, northeastern, and some north Indian states, in the young as well as the elderly.

The more recent NFHS-5 study reported hypertension prevalence among men and women >15 years in all the states of the country.[41] Age-adjusted prevalence (%) of hypertension among women and men in different states of India is depicted in **Figure 2**. There is significant state-level variation in hypertension prevalence. In women the highest prevalence is in Sikkim (34.5%), Punjab (31.2%), and Goa (27.5%) and the lowest in Rajasthan (15.4%), Ladakh (15.7%), and Bihar (15.9%). In men the highest prevalence is in Sikkim (41.6%), Punjab (37.7%), and Manipur (33.2%) while the lowest is in Ladakh (17.4%), Rajasthan (17.9%), and Bihar (18.4%) **(Fig. 3)**. These variations are only slightly different from the previous studies (AHS-3/DLHS-4) but show an increasing trend in hypertension in most of the states of the country. Empirical calculations show that the number of patients with hypertension in India is currently about 20–25 crores, this is more than any other country (except China). For the first time, the NFHS-5 reported hypertension prevalence in almost all the districts of India.[41] There is a significant district-level variation with greater prevalence in most western and southern districts in women and western, southern, and eastern districts in men. A significant concern is the very high prevalence in some districts of Punjab, eastern and northeastern states, and central India.

Understanding geographic variations in hypertension prevalence at the state and district level in India is important as healthcare is a state subject. The knowledge regarding geographic variation informs the policymakers regarding the targeted deployment of health systems geared to take care of these patients. We believe that not only manpower deployment and pharmaceutical supply chain are important, but equally important is focusing on

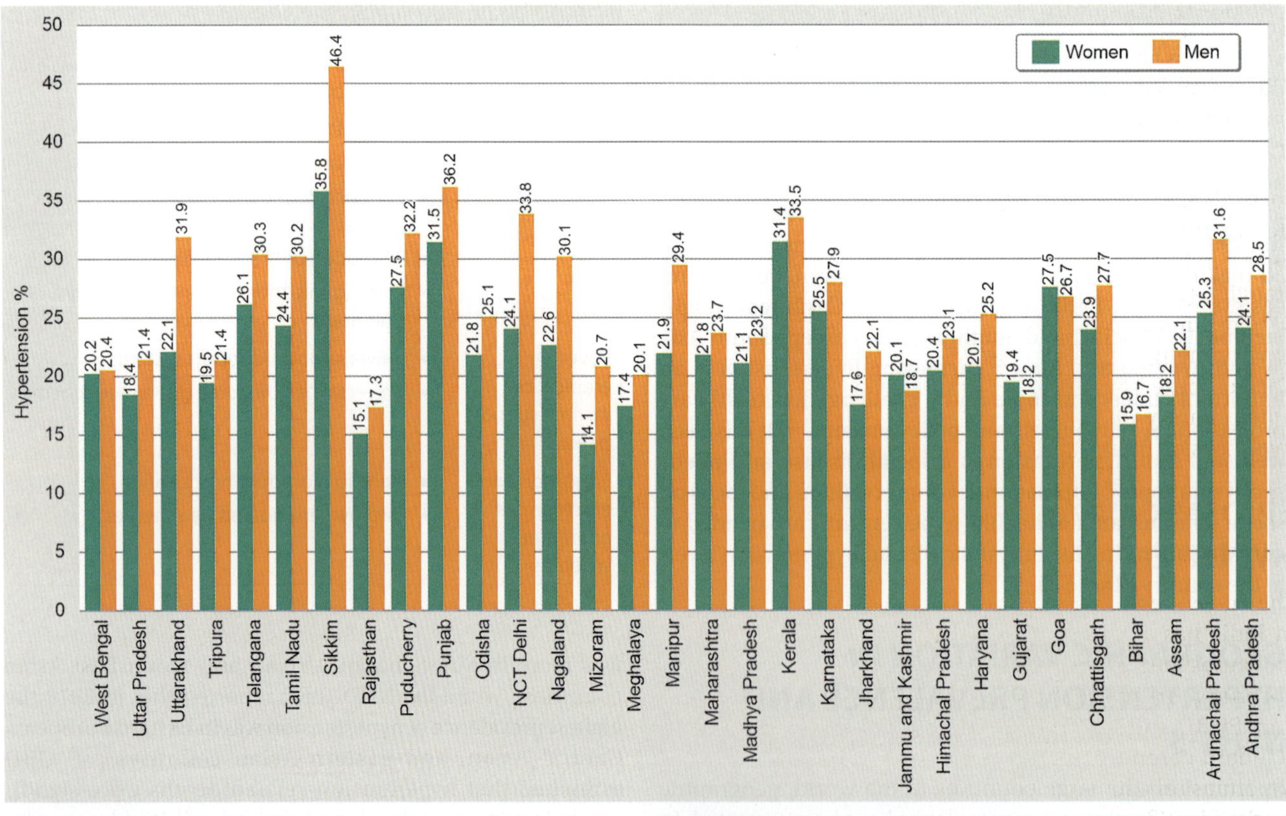

FIG. 2: Hypertension prevalence among women and men in various districts of India.

Source: With permission from National Family Health Survey-5.[26]

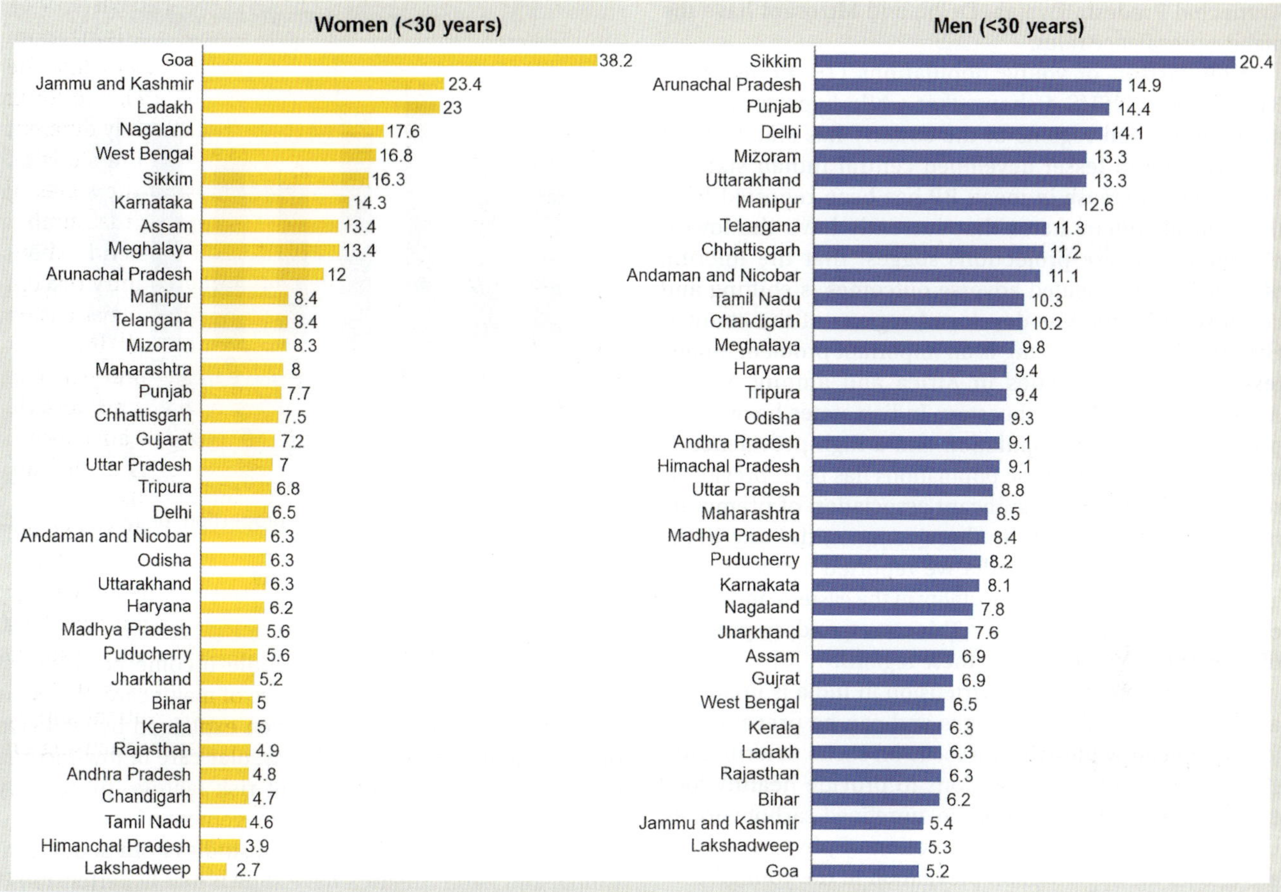

FIG. 3: Prevalence of premature hypertension (age <30 years) in various states of India.
Source: With permission from National Family Health Survey-5.[26]

social determinants to reduce hypertension-related disparities in the country. Social interventions have recently been highlighted and include (1) focus on economic stability, (2) education, (3) social and community context of noncommunicable diseases, (4) neighborhood and built environment, and (5) healthcare access and quality.[42,43] Each of these interventions is important in India, as in any other country, to mitigate geography-related variation in hypertension morbidity and mortality.

EPIDEMIC OF PREMATURE HYPERTENSION

The current epidemic of premature cardiovascular deaths in India has attracted widespread attention and a search for causes thereof.[44] There are multiple causes of premature coronary artery disease in India and INTERHEART and PURE studies have highlighted the importance of standard coronary risk factors—the most important being hypertension and lipid abnormalities.[44] Prospective studies for the identification of cardiovascular diseases in India are limited. PURE study investigators reported long-term follow-up data on 33,583 individuals (85% from India) without CAD at baseline and identified 12 common risk factors that predicted cardiovascular diseases.[45] Population-attributable fractions were calculated and important risk factors identified were hypertension, raised non-high-density lipoprotein (non-HDL) cholesterol, diabetes, low education, abdominal obesity, indoor air pollution, tobacco use, etc. This study also reported that raised non-HDL cholesterol, diabetes, low education, indoor air pollution, and unhealthy diet were more important in South Asians as compared to participants from high and upper-middle-income countries. The AHS-3/DLHS-4 study reported that mean levels of systolic BP were more in young participants (<40 years) of this survey as compared to countries in central and eastern Europe, high-income western world, and other South Asian countries.[22]

We obtained data on the state-level distribution of premature hypertension (<30 years age) in India from NFHS-5 **(Fig. 3)**.[41] It is observed that young-age hypertension is much more prevalent in the northern and northeastern states of the country. Among women, the highest prevalence is in Goa, Jammu and Kashmir, Ladakh, Nagaland, and West Bengal while in men states of Sikkim,

Arunachal Pradesh, Punjab, Delhi, and Mizoram have the highest prevalence rates.

Comparison of young populations (15–49 years) in NFHS-5 with NFHS-4 shows that while hypertension in many developed regions of the country has stabilized, it is increasing in lesser developed central Indian states.[46] The largest increase in mean BP has been reported from the central Indian states that currently have the lowest prevalence. These projections suggest that the fulcrum of hypertension-related adverse outcomes is shifting and could soon be the less developed regions of the country. Hypertension in the young is an important problem among less developed societies in Africa and among African Americans in USA. Northeastern Indian states have a very proportion of tribal population and a high prevalence of hypertension among these populations has been previously reported.[16] There is a significant association of premature hypertension with stroke in these communities and in the Million Death Study in India we reported a significantly greater stroke burden and mortality in the eastern and north-eastern states of the country.[47] This corresponds to presence of premature hypertension in these regions.

Focus on premature hypertension in India is important as it is a silent killer at all ages and can be prevented by focus on healthy lifestyles via focus on social determinants **(Table 3)**.[44] Policy interventions to provide healthy food choices and reduce salt, tobacco, unrefined carbohydrates, transfats, and alcohol and promotion of physical activity are crucial for hypertension prevention in the young.[1,6,29,43] Opportunistic measurement of BP at every clinical encounter is an important policy and clinical intervention for the early detection of young hypertension.

HYPERTENSION AND CARDIOVASCULAR MORTALITY

There are multiple causes of hypertension-related deaths and disability. These include cardiac (coronary artery disease, heart failure, and arrhythmias), cerebral (hemorrhagic stroke, subarachnoid hemorrhage and ischemic strokes), renal (chronic renal failure), and others. In >90% of cases, the deaths are due to cardiovascular causes. GBD study has reported that cardiovascular deaths as a proportion of all-cause deaths (%) are >90% in almost all regions of the world except the Americas **(Fig. 4)**.[48] This variation could be due to more deaths due to noncardiovascular causes in North American and Latin American countries compared to other regions.

The PURE study reported that deaths from hypertension-related complications were significantly greater in lower-middle-income and low-income countries **(Fig. 4)**.[3] Significantly more cardiovascular deaths have also been reported among the four low-income countries in the PURE study (India, Pakistan, Bangladesh, and Zimbabwe) compared to 13 upper and middle-income countries.[49] This was despite a lower prevalence of major cardiovascular risk factors. This paradox has been explained by evidence of lower quality general cardiovascular care in low-income countries with lower control of risk factors, principally hypertension, and gaps in the management of acute cardiovascular events.[50] Recent PURE substudies from South Asia, China, and Latin America have shown that hypertension is the most important contributor to cardiovascular deaths in all the regions,[45,51,52] and low levels of treatment and control are responsible for higher cardiovascular events and deaths.

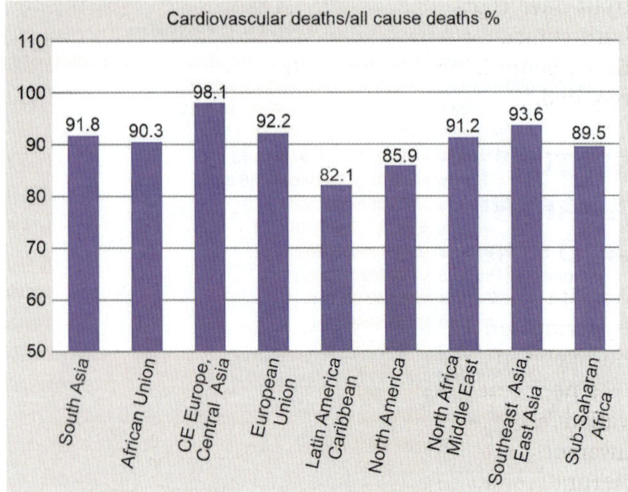

FIG. 4: Cardiovascular causes as proportion of deaths due to hypertension in various global regions.
Source: Global Burden of Diseases study 2019.

Prospective studies that report the association of hypertension with cardiovascular events, cardiovascular mortality and all-cause deaths in India are very few. Four large population-based studies (Mumbai,[53] Kerala,[54,55] and Andhra Pradesh[56]) reported cardiovascular deaths and events at follow-up of 5–7 years. Million death study reported that presence of hypertension was associated with 6–8-fold increase in ischemic heart disease mortrality.[57] Mumbai Cohort Study reported 5 year prospective outcomes of various levels of BP in an urban cohort.[53] It was reported that increasing BP levels (prehypertension, stage I hypertension, and stage II hypertension) were associated with successively greater cardiovascular deaths in both men and women.[53] These are important observations and suggest lower targets for BP control in India, however, no randomized trials exist in India that have reported the association of BP lowering with adverse cardiovascular outcomes in prehypertension and stage I hypertension.

It is well known that hypertension control by drugs and other measures can significantly reduce related mortality and events by 20–30%.[58] Multiple meta-analyses of clinical trials have reported a significant reduction in deaths and hard clinical events at 2–5 years of follow-up. To achieve these, better hypertension treatment and control rates are required.

STATUS OF HYPERTENSION AWARENESS, TREATMENT, AND CONTROL

A meta-analysis of multiple regional population-based hypertension epidemiological studies in India focusing on hypertension awareness, treatment, and control rates was performed some years ago.[40] A significant regional variation was observed and it was reported that hypertension awareness rates varied from 30 to 50% in urban and 20–40% in rural populations. Hypertension treatment rates varied from 20 to 40% on a population level and from 50 to 70% in those aware of hypertension. The BP control rates were also low and varied from 8 to 15% in rural and 10–30% in urban locations on a population scale and about 20–30% among those on treatment.[40]

More recently, the PURE-South Asia study, one of the larger multisite studies, reported that hypertension awareness, treatment, and control rates were low.[19] The study was conducted among >33,000 middle aged individuals (35–70 years of age) and reported that in urban vs. rural populations rates of hypertension awareness (45.9% vs. 32.5%), treatment (37.5% vs. 23.6%) and control (15.4% vs. 9.3%) were low, although the status of treatment and control was better among those with known hypertension. Similar awareness levels has been reported from other studies.[40]

In India, more recent NFHS-4 and LASI studies **(Table 2)** provide national data on hypertension awareness, treatment, and control. While the NFHS-4 was focused on young individuals (men and women 15–49 years),[59] LASI determined risk factors among older individuals ≥44 years.[60] Both the studies reported low rates of hypertension awareness, treatment, and control with significantly lower rates in the younger compared to the older individuals **(Fig. 5)**. An interesting observation in NFHS-4 is that despite the recall of screening for hypertension in 76.1% of participants, the recall rate of hypertension awareness was only half (44.7%). An almost identical hypertension treatment cascade has been reported in the NNMS.[61]

In a series of cross-sectional Jaipur Heart Watch studies, we reported 25-year trends in hypertension awareness, treatment, and control in urban cohorts in Jaipur **(Fig. 6)**.[62] It was observed that the awareness of hypertension increased from <10% in 1980s to 55–60% in mid-2010s. The treatment status also improved from 9–15% to 35–40%, and among participants who were aware of hypertension from 45–50% to 65–70%. Hypertension control rates increased from 5–10% to 15–20%, among participants who were aware of hypertension from 12–15% to 35–40% and among the treated hypertensives from 10–15% to 45–50%. We projected that at the current rates, hypertension treatment and control rates would be 65% and 40% in the year 2030, these rates are much lower than suggested by WHO. These control rates are also much lower than control rates of >50–70% reported in many high-income and middle-income countries.[62]

The NCD-RiSC investigators collated 1,173 population-representative studies with 104 million participants

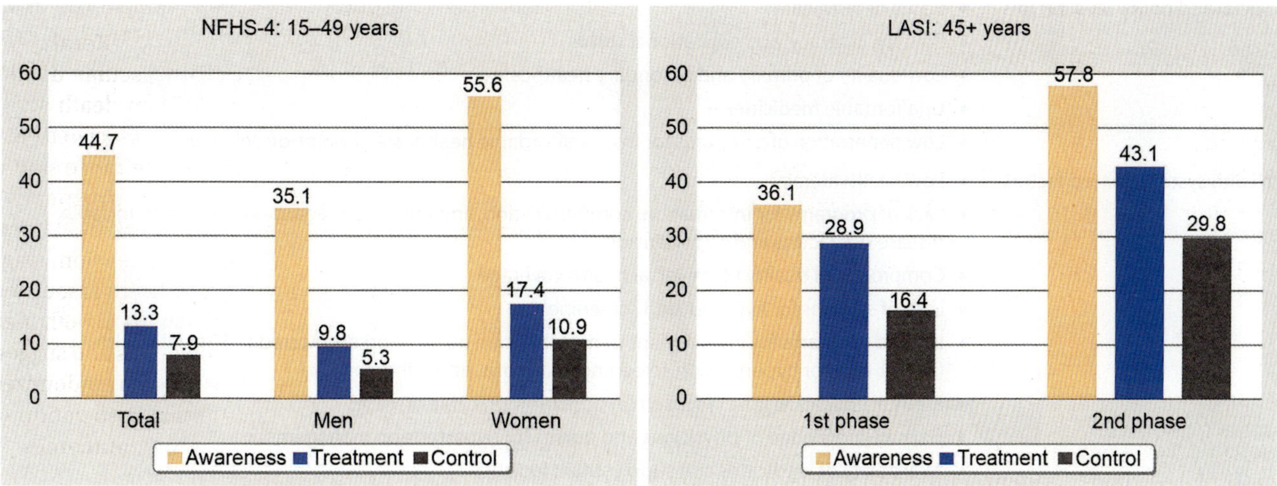

FIG. 5: Country-wide hypertension awareness, treatment, and control status in epidemiological studies in India. NFHS-4 was focused on young individuals (15–49 years) and LASI evaluated older individuals (45+ years).

(LASI: Longitudinal Ageing Study in India; NFHS-4: fourth National Family Health Survey)

Source: With permission from Prenissl et al. (2019)[59] and Lee et al. (2022).[60]

and reported secular trends in hypertension awareness, treatment and control globally, and in various regions of the world from 1990 to 2018.[63] It was reported that globally while the prevalence of undiagnosed hypertension remained static from 1990 to 2018, the prevalence of treated and controlled hypertension have increased. Substantial regional variations were observed. Undiagnosed hypertension has declined in most high-income and upper middle-income countries but increased in South Asia, Sub-Saharan Africa and Oceania. Hypertension treatment and control rates have increased rapidly in most high and middle-income countries but have increased only slowly in South Asian countries including India.

Multiple factors are responsible for low rates of hypertension awareness and treatment and control in India and include multiple social determinants and health system-related and individual-level factors.[64,65] Some of these factors are listed in **Table 4**.

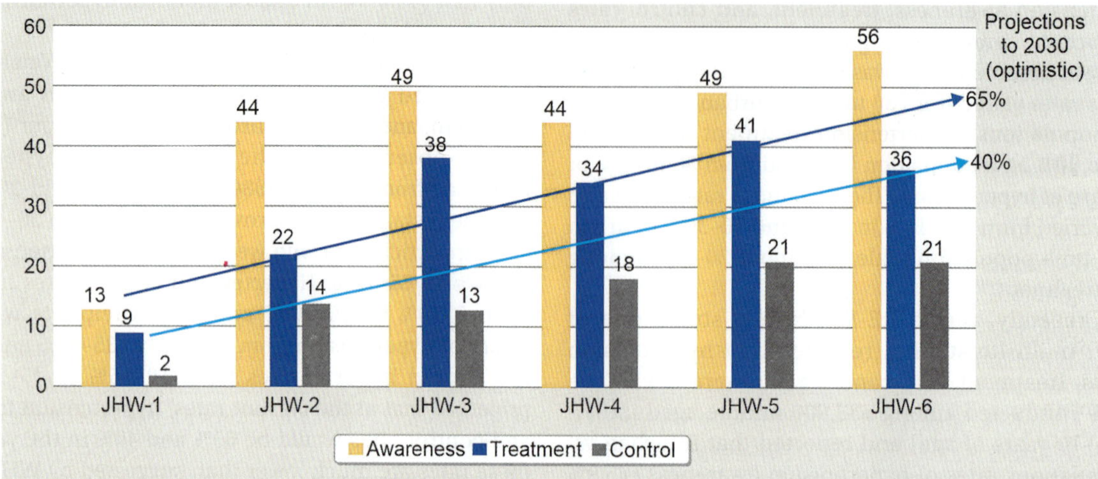

FIG. 6: 25-year trends in hypertension awareness, treatment, and control in Jaipur Heart Watch studies from 1991 to 2016 and projections for awareness (65%) and treatment (40%) to the year 2030.

TABLE 4: Factors responsible for low status of hypertension awareness, treatment, and control in India.

	Variables
Social and policy level factors	• Social determinants • Poverty, illiteracy, and educational status • Low quality of primary and secondary healthcare • Unaffordable medicines • Low penetration of programs for free or affordable healthcare at point-of-delivery
Health system-related factors	• Low health literacy • Lack of programs for information, communication, and education regarding noncommunicable disease risk factors and hypertension • Compromised quality of universal health coverage • Lack of systems for hypertension screening • Limited programs for involvement of nonphysician health workers, Accredited Social Health Activist (ASHA), etc., for hypertension screening, diagnosis, and adherence • Medical education is not focused on noncommunicable diseases • Gaps in knowledge of physicians and nurses for hypertension management • Availability of medicines and supply-chain logistics • Free or subsidized medicines at point of care

Continued

Continued

	Variables
Physician level factors	• Lack of opportunistic screening protocols • Low guidelines awareness, lack of officially sponsored continuing medical education • Gaps in physician knowledge and application; inertia • Inappropriate choice of drugs, failure to promote single-pill multidrug combinations • Poor time management
Patient level factors	• Low health literacy • Age and aging and physical inactivity • Low affordability of high-quality foods (vegetables, fruits, nuts, etc.) • *Addictions*: Salt, tobacco, alcohol, etc. • Poor access to care and low adherence

REDUCING CARDIOVASCULAR RISK IN HYPERTENSION

Blood pressure management is the cornerstone of cardiovascular risk reduction. Multiple randomized clinical studies and meta-analyses over the past seven decades have consistently reported benefits of BP control in high-risk as well as low-risk patients with hypertension. Interventions to promote hypertension control are in **Table 3** and barriers that have to be overcome are listed in **Table 4**. International guidelines using available studies have been promulgated and are widely available.[66] Western guidelines (American, European, and UK)[67-69] are directed to the respective countries. Guidelines from the International Society of Hypertension[70] and WHO[71] provide evidence-based recommendations for hypertension diagnosis and management in high-income as well as lower-income countries. Indian Hypertension guidelines are consensus statements adopted from the available international guidelines.[72] A life-course approach for better management of hypertension has also been recommended.[73] Major barrier in India and elsewhere is the implementation of guidelines into practice. Context- and culture-specific strategies to overcome the barriers are urgently needed.[74]

Strategies to reduce overall cardiovascular risk are also important for the prevention of cardiovascular deaths, coronary events, and strokes in patients with hypertension. Patients with hypertension can be classified into low-medium-, and high-risk based on BP levels as well as associated cardiovascular risk factors **(Fig. 7)**. Interventions include the adoption of healthy lifestyles (physical activity and exercise, healthy diet, smoking cessation, salt and alcohol moderation), guideline-supported target-oriented BP control, lipid management with a focus on use of statins, diabetes management, antithrombotic strategies, and anti-inflammatory therapies (e.g., aspirin and colchicine) in a select few, and multifactorial interventions in high and moderate risk individuals.

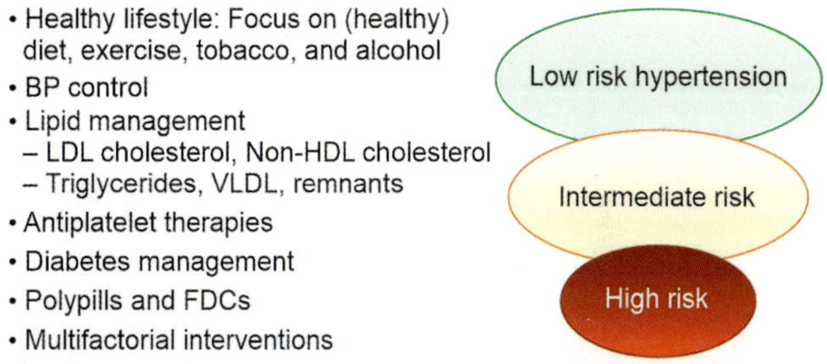

FIG. 7: Strategies for reducing cardiovascular risk in hypertension.
(BP: blood pressure; FDCs: fixed-dose combinations; HDL: high-density lipoprotein; LDL: low-density lipoprotein; VLDL: very low-density lipoprotein)

Addressing social determinants is important for prevention and control of hypertension and prevents cardiovascular complications.[42] Social and financial policies are important and can lead to significant changes in cardiovascular health. Specific policy interventions relevant to India are shown in **Table 3**. We believe that healthcare policies that include promulgation of state-funded health services, high-quality universal healthcare, health insurance for select groups (poor, marginalized, elderly, etc.), drug price control and production of high-quality generics and free medicine supply in public health systems are important. Technological interventions are important for the empowerment of basic healthcare workers and the patients,[64,65] but need more studies before implementation. Blood pressure control is a challenge to healthcare systems worldwide, more so in low and lower-middle-income countries, including India. A multipronged approach involving population-wide and clinic-based approaches is required to reduce the mortality and morbidity burden of hypertension.

CONCLUSION

Hypertension is the most important chronic disease risk factor in India. This review shows some unique features of hypertension in India. There is increasing hypertension prevalence (both in absolute and proportionate terms) with a more rapid increase in rural and young populations. There are substantial geographic variations with greater prevalence in more developed states and districts of the country. A concerning feature is the emergence of young-age or premature hypertension, especially in less developed states of the country and significantly greater mortality from hypertension-related cardiovascular disease as compared to the more developed countries. Levels of hypertension awareness, treatment, and control are low with an inequitable distribution among rural and young individuals. Hypertension is a social as well as a biological disease and strategies for better hypertension management and control should include a focus on social determinants as well as individual-level precision medicine approaches.

ONLINE REFERENCES

Please scan the QR code provided at the end of the table of contents for References of this chapter.

CHAPTER 29

2023 Hypertension Guidelines of the European Society of Hypertension: An Abridged Narrative

Giuseppe Mancia, Guido Grassi, Reinhold Kreutz

ABSTRACT

This chapter focuses on some of the novelties of the 2023 hypertension guidelines of the European Society of Hypertension. Mention is made that these guidelines are more ponderous than previous guidelines because they address issues never or only marginally addressed before, including hypertension diagnosis and treatment in a large number of conditions frequently associated with blood pressure (BP) elevation. Concerning the specific novelties, they provide a critical review of the advantages and limitations of the multiple approaches to BP measurement currently available, although still recommending office BP as the gold standard because of its use in proving the benefits of antihypertensive treatment and the related threshold and target for BP-lowering interventions. However, out-of-office BP measurements are upgraded, i.e., recommended whenever they are feasible because of the amount and importance of the clinical information provided. Other important aspects are the addition of new cardiovascular risk factors, the expansion of the use of organ damage measures, the upgrading of beta-blockers to the level of major antihypertensive drugs, and the wider choice of drug combinations (including single-pill combinations) between the major drugs, with confirmation of their strategic role as first-line and subsequent treatments in most patients. Polypills are also considered an option, and this is also the case for renal denervation in resistant hypertension. Sequential BP thresholds and targets are indicated for treatment strategies based on treatment tolerability, and their differences across clinical subgroups are reported. Diagnostic and treatment approaches are described for many specific conditions, with mention of treatment specificity and the use of a number of new drugs, particularly but not exclusively in resistant hypertension, heart failure, and kidney disease. Special attention is reserved for follow-up modalities, including the assessment of nonadherence as a fundamental barrier to long-term BP control.

Keywords: Antihypertensive agents, blood pressure, cardiovascular diseases, evidence-based guidelines, hypertension management, prevention and control, treatment guidelines.

INTRODUCTION

The first hypertension guidelines of the European Society of Hypertension (ESH) were published in the *Journal of Hypertension* in 2003.[1] The publication was very well received by the medical community, making it the most widely cited paper in the medical field over the following years. Further ESH guidelines were published in 2007, 2009, 2013, and 2018,[2] always raising great interest not only in Europe but also internationally, with an extremely high citation rate. The latest guidelines were presented at the 2023 meeting of the ESH and have been published in the September issue of the *Journal of Hypertension*.[3] The scientific and ethical principles on which these guidelines are based are similar to those of the previous guidelines. This is also the case for the format which, as in the past, aims at combining education with a practical purpose, the former being achieved by discussing the sometimes complex and nonunivocal scientific evidence from which recommendations are derived and the latter being the translation of the evidence into concise diagnostic and treatment advice. However, these guidelines extend to issues and areas unaddressed or only marginally touched by previous guidelines. In particular, they also extend recommendations to more or less common comorbidities associated with hypertension that can make the antihypertensive treatment approach different from that recommended for hypertension alone. This makes the 2023 guidelines more ponderous than the previous guidelines, with a total of 22 sections (subdivided into multiple subsections), about 200 pages, more than 1,700 references, 27 tables, 21 figures, and 47 recommendation tables, almost one per section or subsection addressed. In this chapter, we will review some novelties of the new guidelines but also mention a few important areas where previous recommendations have been confirmed. For guidelines, confirmation of previous recommendations is not less important than the presentation of novelties, because it shows that previous evidence is not contradicted by new scientific evidence and approaches and thus stands the test of time.

BLOOD PRESSURE MEASUREMENTS

The 2023 guidelines devote space to the description and recommendations on how to measure blood pressure (BP). Current technological progress is addressed, along with the mention of future developments, such as nighttime BP measurements by home devices[4] as well as cuffless BP measurements, which may avoid the BP alterations and discomfort associated with cuff pressurization.[5] Various BP measurement approaches are described, addressing their technical, clinical, or logistic limitations. In the end, however, the ESH guidelines strongly emphasize the superior value of office BP measurement on which virtually all available data on the risk of hypertension and the benefits of treatment depend. The suggested definition of hypertension, the BP classification, the BP threshold for the use of antihypertensive drugs, and the BP target for treatment are all based on office BP. Meanwhile, according to the 2023 guidelines, other BP measurements in the office (e.g., unattended BP, central BP, exercise BP) have a less important and a substantially complementary role.

An important aspect of the 2023 European guidelines is that they take a clear position on the role of out-of-office BP in the management of hypertension. In the previous guidelines,[2] home and/or ambulatory BP were recommended for the confirmation of a hypertension state after an initial office BP elevation, as an alternative to further office measurements through repeated medical visits. In the 2023 guidelines, emphasis is given to the absence of outcome-based randomized trials using out-of-office BP, which prevents their use for evidence-based hypertension diagnosis and treatment guidance. Nevertheless, it is recognized that both home and ambulatory BP are a source of important clinical information, e.g., improved reproducibility of BP values, identification of white coat hypertension, masked hypertension, nocturnal BP patterns [with their specific levels of cardiovascular (CV) risk], BP control throughout between-visit intervals, treatment-related hypotensive episodes, and more accurate risk stratification when used on top of office BP values. Therefore, the 2023 ESH guidelines recommend the use of out-of-office BP at any time this is feasible or allowed by the healthcare facilities of the medical practice environment where the physician operates. It is advised to collect data, if possible, on both home and ambulatory BP because evidence shows that in a number of patients, these values may be discrepant (home but not 24-hour BP elevation or vice versa) and that combined or discrepant home and ambulatory BP elevations may have prognostic relevance.[6]

QUANTIFICATION OF CARDIOVASCULAR RISK

The 2023 guidelines confirm that quantification of total CV risk is important because of its impact on several aspects of hypertension management, such as the frequency of medical visits, the frequency of laboratory or instrumental examinations, BP threshold and target for treatment, cotreatments, and choice of antihypertensive drugs as well as the choice of antihypertensive treatment strategies. They advise calculating the total CV risk using the SCORE2 and SCORE2-OP algorithms based on European data.[7] However, mindful of the fact that this algorithm is largely based on a limited number of CV risk factors [sex, age, smoking, level of systolic blood pressure (SBP), and non-high-density lipoprotein (HDL) cholesterol], they suggest a wider search for factors that may contribute to the risk of a CV event in patients with a BP elevation even if these factors have not been included in the algorithm used for total risk quantification. Some of these risk factors can be identified by laboratory examinations in addition to the basic examinations traditionally recommended for hypertension. Others rely on an accurate collection of patient history. Both are listed in a table format in the sections that address CV risk stratification. This comprehensive information is necessary to have full knowledge of the patient's medical status, calibrate the intensiveness (and type) of treatment, and properly organize the patient's follow-up.

Like in the past, the 2023 guidelines give great importance to the search for subclinical organ damage, based on the evidence that subclinical organ damage affects a large fraction of the hypertensive population[8] and that its presence is usually associated with a high CV risk.[9] Old and new measures of organ damage are described, and a list of those to search for is provided, with a subdivision based on their complexity, cost, and availability. The recommendation is issued to search for damage in different organs because multiple-organ damage associates with a greater increase of CV risk compared to single-organ damage.[9] It is also mentioned that in some instances, different measures of damage in a single organ (e.g., increased urinary protein excretion and decline of glomerular filtration rate) have an additive prognostic effect.[10] A table is also provided with the available evidence of the relationship between treatment-induced reduction of organ damage and subsequent reduction of CV outcomes. Compared to a few years ago, this evidence has increased and now extends to the protective effect of regression of left ventricular hypertrophy, reduction albuminuria, decline of glomerular filtration rate, and, although somewhat more controversial, also regression of arterial stiffening or carotid artery thickening.[11,12] The 2023 guidelines strongly support research in this area and call for stronger evidence on the prognostic relevance of all recommended measures of subclinical organ damage, including the regression of an abnormal ankle-brachial index and retinal microvascular alterations. It is emphasized that this information may fill, at least in part, the gaps in knowledge associated with the use of outcome-based trials as the only evidence of treatment benefits. This has substantially limited the evidence on the benefits of antihypertensive treatment in patients aged <40 years, where outcomes are rare and trials are affected by insufficient statistical power. At that age, the protection offered by BP-lowering interventions can be more appropriately documented by reduced progression of functional or structural organ alterations that will progressively increase CV risk beyond age and, in some patients, emerge as an overt event years later.

BLOOD PRESSURE THRESHOLD AND TARGET FOR TREATMENT

The office BP threshold for treatment in the general hypertensive population is not different in the 2023 guidelines compared to previous guidelines, i.e., it remains ≥140 mm Hg SBP or ≥90 mm Hg diastolic blood pressure (DBP). This does not hold, however, for all subgroups of patients, the exceptions being patients aged 80+ years, patients with isolated systolic hypertension, patients defined as frail, and patients with coronary heart disease. In the former two groups, drug treatment is recommended as mandatory when office SBP is ≥160 mm Hg, based on the results of dedicated outcome trials.[13,14] Because of meta-analyses based on both trials and trial subgroups, however, an additional, although less strong, recommendation is issued to consider treatment initiation also in the 140–159 mm Hg SBP range, if regarded as appropriate and feasible by the patient's physician.[15] In frail people, guidelines openly admit the absence of relevant evidence because frail and other vulnerable patients are usually excluded from trials. The guidelines rely on the clinical judgment of the physician in individual cases. Meanwhile, in patients with a very high CV risk, it is recommended to implement antihypertensive treatment also when BP is in the high normal range (130–139/85–89 mm Hg). Support for this recommendation still comes from a meta-analysis of trials (or trial subgroups) published years ago,[16] which showed that in patients with a high normal BP and a previous CV event (mainly a myocardial infarction), antihypertensive treatment lowers the risk of stroke or stroke plus coronary events although it does not exert any beneficial effect in lower CV risk patients.[16] In this context, an appropriate note of the guidelines is that coronary heart disease patients with a high normal BP should almost invariably be treated with antihypertensive drugs, which are given for protective effects that are independent of their BP-lowering ability. The practical problem faced by the physician under these circumstances is thus not to use or not use antihypertensive drugs but rather to ensure that their use brings BP to the target value of <130/80 mm Hg.

The 2023 guidelines consider two different levels of target office BP in the general hypertension population. The first and "must" target is to lower office BP to <140/80 mm Hg, based on the evidence that this BP target accounts for a large fraction of the treatment-dependent CV benefit.[17] However, evidence demonstrates that further SBP reduction is associated with an incremental, albeit quantitatively smaller, benefit, which justifies the second recommendation to lower SBP to <130 mm Hg if treatment is well tolerated. However, this does not hold for patients aged 80+ years and patients with isolated systolic hypertension in whom the target BP values recommended by the guidelines are more conservative, i.e., the "must" SBP target is between 149 and 140 mm Hg while the second target (to be pursued if treatment is well tolerated) is between 139 and 130 mm Hg. A more conservative target (SBP <140 but not <130 mm Hg) is also recommended for patients with left ventricular hypertrophy, based on the evidence that, probably because of the anatomical and functional disadvantages of an increased left ventricular mass, a SBP reduction to <130 mm Hg may not be accompanied by greater patient protection.[18] Finally, no predefined target is recommended for frail patients due to the absence of any evidence from controlled trials as well as for the suggestion offered by observational studies that in older frail patients, low BP values have detrimental effects.[19] Under all circumstances, the guidelines recommend not to actively pursue a BP reduction to <120/70 mm Hg because these lower BP values are usually associated with a marked increase of serious side effects, leading to treatment discontinuation and thus to the loss of patients' protection. Furthermore, in several post hoc analyses of outcome trials, a SBP <120 mm Hg or a DBP <70 mm Hg has been associated with an increased risk of events, particularly coronary events.[20] Although the post hoc approach does not allow to discriminate whether this J-curve phenomenon is due to reduced vital organ perfusion or a greater baseline risk that favors excessive BP reduction and events during treatment,[20] the existence of this patient subgroup is real and cannot be ignored. It should be mentioned that the position of the 2023 guidelines to avoid an active pursue of on-treatment BP values <120/70 is in contrast with the report of an individual patient-based meta-analysis of randomized trials, which has concluded that antihypertensive drug treatment is beneficial independent of the baseline BP values, including a systolic BP <120 mm Hg.[21] The limitations of this meta-analysis have been discussed in a recent paper.[22]

It is important to mention that, in a separate section, the 2023 guidelines acknowledge that issuing recommendations on the target BP values to be reached with treatment is a challenging task because the results of dedicated trials (those comparing higher with lower BP targets) are not univocal, their nature is often heterogeneous because of different methodological and BP-measuring approaches, and the heterogeneity extends to patients' demographic and clinical characteristics. In addition, a conceptual difficulty is that the optimal office BP target for treatment (i.e., the BP level at which outcomes are maximally reduced) is likely to vary between patients and probably even within patients with age and progression of anatomical and functional organ damage. This is why the guidelines prefer to indicate, as BP targets, ranges of values; in a figure that addresses target BP in the general hypertensive population, the 2023 guidelines mention that these values are 139–120 mm Hg for SBP and 79–70 mm Hg for DBP.

The 2023 ESH guidelines recognize as an additional problem the definition of optimal home or ambulatory BP targets because of the absence of outcome-based trials using these BP measurement approaches. The home, 24-hour, daytime, and nighttime mean BP values corresponding to office BP values to be reached with treatment (120/80–140/90 mm Hg) are reported via a table provided by the last hypertension guidelines of the American College of Cardiology and the American Heart Association.[23] However, a warning is issued that this indirect approach has obvious limitations and should be interpreted with caution, also because office and out-of-office BP can have a limited correlation. Hence, in individual patients, there can be marked deviations in office and out-of-office BP differences from the corresponding mean values.

ANTIHYPERTENSIVE TREATMENT

Drugs

Like the previous European guidelines, the 2023 ESH guidelines favor a liberal approach to the choice of antihypertensive drugs to be used in hypertension. They consider antihypertensive drugs suitable for the initiation and maintenance of antihypertensive treatment if evidence from randomized outcome-based trials indicates that they (1) effectively lower BP, (2) reduce outcomes in placebo-controlled trials, and (3) exhibit a reduction of treatment-related risk of events that, for a similar BP reduction, is similar to that of other major antihypertensive agents. Based on these principles, they recommend five drug classes for the general hypertensive population, i.e., angiotensin-converting enzyme inhibitors (ACEIs), angiotensin receptor antagonists, calcium channel blockers, diuretics, and beta-blockers. At variance from some other guidelines, no preference is given to thiazides versus thiazide-like diuretics. Furthermore, and also at variance from other guidelines, beta-blockers are placed at the level of the other major antihypertensive agents. Mention is further made that beta-blockers have a large number of specific indications and that these indications include CV diseases or conditions (some of which are very common in patients with a BP elevation, e.g., increased heart rate) but also extend to a large number of noncardiovascular abnormalities or diseases in which the use of beta-blockers is preferred or is mandatory in clinical practice. Mention is also made of the potential advantages of cardioselective beta-blockers and beta-blockers with a direct vasodilating mode of action for their ability to minimize some well-known drawbacks of classical beta-blockers, such as dysmetabolic effects. Nevertheless, it is acknowledged that beta-blockers can be validated as an important drug class and no more be regarded as drugs typically associated with adverse effects such as depression or contraindications such as peripheral artery or obstructive lung disease. Other antihypertensive drugs [mineralocorticoid receptor antagonists (MRAs), central agents, alpha-blockers, loop diuretics, and vasodilators] are also mentioned, but their use is advised in combination with the previous drugs (when they are not fully effective) and/or in specific conditions, similar to what has been done in previous guidelines. As a general principle, the 2023 guidelines support the view that, except for a few specific conditions (e.g., the greater renal protective effect in diabetic or nondiabetic nephropathy by blockers of the renin–angiotensin system), the protective effect of antihypertensive treatment is largely accounted for by BP lowering "per se," no matter how it is obtained. According to the 2023 guidelines, this implies that the greater the number of valid BP-lowering drug options, the greater is the chance of achieving an effective BP reduction and a treatment tailored to the patient's needs.

Treatment Strategies

The 2023 ESH guidelines describe the major treatment strategies that can be adopted in hypertension to reduce the elevated BP, i.e., switching from one monotherapy to another monotherapy, combination of antihypertensive drugs administered following initial monotherapy, treatment initiation with two drugs, and use of four antihypertensive agents at very low doses (quadpill) to improve treatment tolerability. It is acknowledged that all treatment strategies can lead to a reduction of the elevated BP. However, the 2023 ESH guidelines offer their strongest support to the combination of two or three antihypertensive drugs with different mechanisms of action, which can markedly enhance antihypertensive effects[24] because of the multimechanistic nature of hypertension. In some groups of patients [frail patients, very old patients, very high-risk patients with a high normal BP, or patients with a low risk and modest BP elevation (i.e., in the low range of grade 1 hypertension)], combination treatment is recommended as an uptitration of initial monotherapy, because in these conditions, monotherapy can alone provide the relatively limited BP reduction necessary to achieve BP control and make treatment safe. However, in a far greater portion of the hypertensive population, initial combination treatment with two drugs is strongly recommended as the first treatment step, followed by an increase in the dosing of the combination components and a shift to a three-drug combination, the uptitration being guided by the need to achieve BP control and the preservation of treatment tolerability. This confirms the treatment strategy recommended by the 2018 guidelines with a larger body of favorable evidence derived from real-life studies. These studies indicate that compared to initial monotherapy, the initial two-drug combination therapy is accompanied by a striking reduction of therapeutic inertia (a factor that prevents treatment uptitration despite the absence of BP control), an improvement of long-term adherence to treatment, an improvement of long-term BP control, and a reduction in the risk of CV hospitalization and death in the treated population. The guidelines also strengthen the recommendation to use single-pill combinations of two or three drugs whenever they are available because of the increased evidence that this treatment simplification markedly increases adherence to treatment and the resulting patients' protection.[25,26] At variance from previous guidelines,[2] however, the new guidelines not only acknowledge the importance of the use of single-pill combination of a blocker of the renin–angiotensin system along with a diuretic or a calcium channel blocker but also mention other newly developed single-pill combinations such as a calcium channel blocker with a diuretic or a blocker of the renin–angiotensin system with a beta-blocker, i.e., combinations that also have evidence of a protective effect from trials and can be preferred in a number of specific conditions. Further expansion in the availability of single-pill two- and three-drug combinations containing different types and doses of the combination components is strongly supported to offer treatments with a maximum level of flexibility and use in different clinical conditions.

Unlike previous guidelines, the present treatment recommendations express a favorable opinion on the possible use of polypills based on two antihypertensive agents and a statin with or without a low dose of acetylic acid, depending on their use in the secondary or primary prevention setting, respectively. It has always been acknowledged that combining antihypertensive and lipid-lowering treatments has a valid rationale because of (1) the frequent concomitance of high BP and dyslipidemia and (2) the evidence that in hypertension, lipid-lowering drugs exert an additional CV protective effect.[27] However, the new favorable attitude of the guidelines regarding the polypill is based on new trials that have shown improved adherence and reduction of outcomes following the use of a variety of polypills in primary and secondary CV prevention.[28]

Device-based Treatment

In the 2018 European guidelines, a number of devices that had shown BP-lowering effects were not recommended for the treatment of hypertension. This was the case also for renal denervation because after a series of observational studies with favorable results, a randomized trial showed no difference in BP reduction between resistant hypertensive patients with renal denervation and patients who had been subjected to sham denervation.[29] This has been modified in the 2023 guidelines, which now recognize renal denervation as a possible treatment option in resistant hypertension based on (1) a substantial amount of favorable BP data (ambulatory and office BP reductions) from trials comparing renal denervation with the sham procedure and (2) evidence from a dedicated registry and few post-trial long-term observations that the BP reduction persists after 3 years, with no emergence of safety problems.[30] The 2023 ESH guidelines mention that renal denervation can be considered a treatment option in patients with true resistant hypertension. The role of sodium-glucose cotransporter-2 inhibitors (SGLT-2Is) and the nonsteroidal MRA finerenone in patients with chronic kidney disease, i.e., a condition that accounts for a large proportion of patients with resistant hypertension and in which these new drugs appear to have a clear BP-independent renal protective effect, is also acknowledged and implemented in the treatment algorithm. Concerning renal denervation, mention is made that the inability to predict responders to renal denervation treatment is a disadvantage, and that this is the case also for the limited BP-lowering effect of the procedure and the absence of data documenting to what extent the BP reduction translates into a reduction of the high CV risk typical of resistant hypertension. Guidelines also briefly describe other old and new BP-lowering devices without recommending their use in resistant or difficult-to-treat hypertension.

BLOOD PRESSURE PHENOTYPES

A novelty of the 2023 guidelines is a section on the BP phenotypes, i.e., the conditions characterized by selective increases of SBP or DBP in the younger fraction of the population as well as by only office, out-of-office, or nighttime BP elevation. Description is made of their prevalence (often high), CV risk (usually increased), and diagnostic and treatment approaches. Treatment recommendations, however, are usually limited to accurate search for risk factors, close follow-up, and correction of inappropriate lifestyles due to the absence of outcome-based trials on the protective effect of drug-related BP reductions. Use of drugs is suggested, with a lower level of evidence, only if CV risk is high, possibly because of organ damage. An interesting recommendation is to make use of central BP in young people with isolated systolic hypertension because normality of this BP value may favor the clinical innocence of this condition. Importantly, in conditions characterized by selective increases of office or out-of-office BP, the recommendation is to always achieve their identification by repeated BP measurements because of the recent evidence of their poor reproducibility.[31,32]

HYPERTENSION IN OTHER CONDITIONS

The epidemiology of hypertension and its diagnostic and treatment approaches are extended to a large number of additional conditions. One set of conditions refers to different demographic situations, i.e., the specific problems of hypertensive children and adolescents, the difficulty for a patient with BP abnormalities to cope with the transition period from pediatric to medical adult-governed care, the sex differences for the consequences and treatment of hypertension, and the problems posed by old and very old age and those associated with ethnicity differences. Another set of conditions refers to (1) the complex diagnostic and treatment problems posed by BP disorders in pregnancy as well as by their possible long-term consequences for the affected women, (2) hypertension urgencies and emergencies, and (3) proper medical conduct in hypertensive patients who plan or have to undergo surgery. The problems related to the frequent coexistence of hypertension with cardiac or vascular disorders, including BP-lowering interventions in acute hemorrhagic or ischemic stroke and the chronic maintenance of BP after a cerebrovascular accident, are addressed in a third separate section. Moreover, additional sections are devoted to the coexistence of hypertension with diabetes, kidney disease, and obesity as well as with conditions unfrequently or never addressed by general hypertension guidelines such as respiratory, rheumatic, and autoimmune diseases), or the new important problem of the pressogenic effect of some cancer therapies. Although it is impossible for this chapter to go into details, it is important to mention that in a large number of specific conditions, the treatment algorithm importantly differs from the treatment algorithm recommended for the more general hypertensive population. The difference not only involves the preferred drugs but also extends to the strategy used, the dosing and timing of the intervention, the speed of BP control, the target BP value, and the need to consider interactions with other treatments. A pertinent example is the coexistence of hypertension with atrial fibrillation, which requires a treatment algorithm that makes use of drugs that reduce the risk of atrial fibrillation episodes, guarantees an adequate control of heart rate, and accounts for the need to implement effective antihypertensive treatment in a timely manner to avoid the administration of anticoagulants at BP levels that increase the risk of hemorrhage.[33] Another example is the coexistence of hypertension with heart failure, which in patients with reduced ejection fraction is now treated with a combination of old and new drugs, i.e., an ACEI or angiotensin receptor neprilysin inhibitor, a beta-blocker, MRA, a diuretic, and an SGLT-2 agent, not only to reduce the risk of mortality or hospitalization but also to contain symptoms. A simultaneous increase in BP is unusual under these circumstances also because the reduction of cardiac performance and cardiac output decapitates previously elevated BP levels. If hypertension persists, however, treatment must be based on algorithms strikingly different from the more general one.

FOLLOW-UP

A last element of the novelties of the 2023 ESH guidelines that we would like to mention is the attention devoted to the follow-up of hypertensive patients, a topic which is usually not given adequate space and attention by hypertension guidelines, despite its fundamental importance for the persistent success of antihypertensive treatment. Recommendations on follow-up strategies suffer from the paucity of adequate and controlled studies, but some good evidence is available and can lead, with the contribution of an expert consensus, to helpful realistic recommendations. The ESH guidelines for the follow-up recommend (1) very frequent visits during the initial 3-month period, where the effectiveness and tolerability of treatment are tested and BP control is pursued; (2) visits spaced by 3–6 months in the following year; and (3) more rarefied visits after 1 year, with a frequency that depends on the severity of hypertension, the consistency of BP control, and the trust of the physician on adherence to the prescribed treatment regimen. Excessive visit rarefaction is discouraged (unlike the recommendations issued by some guidelines for low-risk patients with mild hypertension) to avoid the deterioration or loss of a good patient–doctor relationship. Recommendations are also issued with regard to the time intervals of out-of-office BP measurements and laboratory or instrumental medical examinations (again dependent on the patient's status), with the consideration that the instrumental examinations that measure organ damage may provide the physician with valuable information on the long-term clinical effectiveness of the prescribed treatment and the possible need of changes in the adopted follow-up. Finally, the follow-up section of the ESH guidelines includes subsections on adherence to treatment and measures of nonadherence at the patient's bedside, an area that is now considered a fundamental aspect of chronic antihypertensive treatment. Attention is also given to follow-up strategies that may in the future replace or complement the follow-up model now largely prevalent in Europe, i.e., a follow-up partly based on the contribution of the pharmacists, the accountability of nurses or other health professionals, and the use of medical teams with different areas of expertise. Mention is made that this may relieve the problem of the excessive workload to which physicians are exposed, a large part of which depends on the time required for chronic treatments.

CONCLUSION

The 2023 ESH guidelines have been formulated based on evidence not only from outcome-based randomized trials but also from other sources, including real-life research and data, when needed. The guidelines retain their emphasis on several previous recommendations while also providing novel insights based on evidence that has emerged post-2018. Deriving practical application value from trial findings, the ESH guidelines can serve as a reference not only for practicing physicians but also for hypertension experts and investigators.

ONLINE REFERENCES

Please scan the QR code provided at the end of the table of contents for References of this chapter.

CHAPTER 30

Is Hypertension an Inflammatory Disorder?

Tiny Nair

ABSTRACT

Abnormal salt handling by the kidneys are at the core of development of hypertension, which in turn amplifies renin–angiotensin axis, increases blood volume, and stiffens arteries leading to progression of hypertension and target-organ damage. Recent data indicate that development and progression of such pathology could be closely linked with an abnormal immune system, leading to low-grade inflammation. This chapter reviews the data of hypertension and its connection with immune dysregulation.

Keywords: Hypertension, immunity, inflammation.

INTRODUCTION

A seminal paper by Dr Lewis K Dahl in 1968 in the circulation research highlighted the connection between salt in diet and blood pressure levels in an animal model for the first time. Subsequent experiments pointed to kidney as the focal point of etiopathogenesis of hypertension. Clinical data showed that altered renal blood flow, or a parenchymal damage to the kidney, resulted in elevation of blood pressure. It was subsequently hypothesized that mishandling of renal sodium was the key to the development and progression of hypertension.[1]

Alteration of the immune status is well known to cause renal damage. Subsequent work with both animal and human models identified subtle kidney damage in many inflammatory diseases, resulting from altered T and B cells immunity, as well as altered cytokine levels. Over time, it was realized that most cases of hypertension, be it sympathetic or renin–angiotensin system (RAS) driven, volume overloaded or vasoconstricted, progression of hypertension and target-organ damage is mediated by immune-mediated mechanism to a large extent.[1,2]

LINKING HYPERTENSION TO INFLAMMATION

Experiments with rat model treated with deoxycorticosterone acetate (DOCA) and fed with high salt diet are standard model for hypertension studies. Experiments in athymic rat models in the past have shown resistance to development of hypertension despite treatment with salt loading and DOCA. These data connected the dots pointing to an unusual nexus between the neurohormones produced by the kidneys and its complex connection with the immune system. Today we know about the precise neurohormonal pathways that are responsible for hypertension. Immunostimulation, in a complex way, initiates and drives hypertension and results in progressive target-organ damages and atherosclerosis.[3]

CONCEPT OF IMMUNE STIMULATION

The human immune system could be divided as general and specific. General (innate) immunity is always 'on', considered first line, but is less targeted and less specific. The more specific adaptive immunity is mounted on demand, normally triggered by a stimulated response from innate immunity. While innate immunity is myeloid, like neutrophils, macrophage, monocyte, and dendritic cells (DCs), adaptive immunity involves lymphoid tissues—thymus, spleen, tonsils and lymph nodes, circulating lymphocytes, and T and B cells.[3,4]

Innate Immunity

Innate immunity involves activation of myeloid cells—a slow, less specific, and first-line defense. It needs very little training and is "first line." Neutrophils, monocytes, and macrophage constitute the mainstay of innate immunity. Detection of DC and their relationship with major histocompatibility complex (MHC) has advanced knowledge in this field.

Pattern Recognition Receptor Systems

Pattern recognition receptors (PRRs) are designed to fight infection. Small peptides and particles of "pathogens" sensed by these receptors called "toll-like receptors" (TLRs) activate innate immune system. They are found on the surface of DC. The system of recognizing pathogen signature is called pathogen-associated molecular pattern (PAMP). A similar system recognizes abnormal peptides and particles that are not from infective source is the damage-associated molecular pattern (DAMP). DAMP are produced by reactive oxygen species, a change of redox potential, altered nucleic acid proteins, as well as damaged endothelial cells. These stimulate the innate immunity in the short run but through expression of MHC, they end up in the activation of adaptive immunity as well.[3,4]

Dendritic Cells

Dendritic cells have multiple receptors that get activated during an infection. They have on their surface TLRs that sense PAMP and DAMP and activated MHC to deliver parts of antigen "peptide" to the naïve T cells. This in turn cascades to activation of the adaptive immunity.[3-5]

Adaptive Immunity

Upon activation by MHC, the activated T cells produced differentiate into subclasses such as the cluster of differentiation 4 (CD4) positive "helper" T lymphocytes (TL) and the CD8 "cytotoxic" TL **(Box 1)**. Different cytokines are involved in maturation process of the subclass of T helper cell clones which in turn secrete more cytokines. These cytokines can damage renal vasculature, activating abnormal salt handling by the kidneys, and activation of RAS **(Fig. 1)**. The altered immune system also damages the arterial wall which stiffens the arterial wall to further percolate hypertension.[5]

BOX 1 **Cytokine release and T lymphocyte activation by CD4 T cells.**

- IL-12—TH1
- IL-4 and IL-6—TH2
- TGF-β—TH17
- TGF-β—Tregs

List of cytokines released (partial list):

- CD8: Cluster of differentiation 8
- Th1: T helper cell 1
- Th17: T helper cell 17
- Tregs: T regulatory cells
- IL: Interleukin
- TNF: Tumor necrosis factor
- TGF: Transforming growth factor

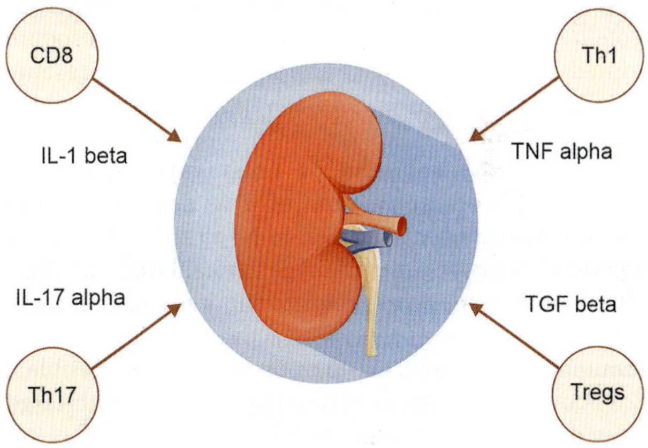

FIG. 1: Effect of different T cells on kidney.

(CD8: cluster of differentiation 8; Th1: T helper cell 1; Th17: T helper cell 17; Tregs: T regulatory cells; IL: interleukin; TNF: tumor necrosis factor; TGF: transformin growth factor)

TARGET-ORGAN DAMAGE

The hemodynamic precursor of hypertension is well known. Vasoconstriction, volume overload, exaggerated, sympathetic renin–angiotensin, and neprilysin axis are the key drivers of hypertension. But a defective salt handling in the kidneys is at the core that results in salt retention, volume expansion, and stimulation of RAS. An activated RAS and resultant elevation of angiotensin II create salt retention and vasoconstriction in general, as well as glomerular efferent artery constriction in the kidneys. This results in increased glomerular pressure which causes progressive deterioration of renal function and further worsening of hypertension. Meanwhile salt retention in medium and large-sized arteries results in stiffening of arteries. This too adds up to an increase in systolic blood pressure. All this hemodynamic stress on the endothelium in general and kidneys in particular ends up in release of various DAMP. The DAMP are sensed by the TLR on the surface of the DC. Complex changes happen, including epitope stimulation, attachment to MHC, and finally stimulation of T cells.

The MHC-bound peptide and the CD28 express on its surface to bind naïve T cells, activating them. The naïve T cells are then transformed to "pathogenic effector T cells" which are now programmed against the vessel wall proteins. They localize in vessel wall, secrete cytokines, and amplify the target-organ damage.[3-5]

Dahl developed mouse with salt-sensitive hypertension models. Salt-sensitive mouse models had shown a stronger immune response and a more profound immunogenic organ damage compared to salt resistant animals. This indirectly shows the link between kidney, sodium handling, and the activated immune stimulation. This results in progression of hypertension with more profound target-organ damage. In 2010, Vihn et al. used cytotoxic T cell antigen immunoglobulin G (IgG) in a mouse model to show its effects on both angiotensin II as well as DOCA-induced hypertension. The results showed not just reduction of blood pressure but a better redox state and suppression of the immune excitement loop that results in progression of hypertension. In the mouse model, dissociation between activated RAS axis and immune stimulation resulted in target-organ protection in hypertension.[5]

NOVEL THERAPIES AND TREATMENT TARGETS

The DC carry and present altered body proteins as antigens that are sensed as DAMP and recognized by the PRR system. Heat shock protein 70 as well as isolevuglandin (isoLG) protein adducts are being considered as putative. A sodium-primed DC tends to react abnormally to the presented proteins, setting up an abnormal inflammatory cascade is a prevailing theory.

2-hydroxybenzylamine, a chemical that involves IsoLG-mediated activation of DC and subsequent immune activation, has shown to be effective in reducing hypertensive target-organ damage in initial trials. Similarly, A20—a ubiquitin editor—tends to suppress nuclear factor-kappa B (NF-κB) and subsequent activation of DC-mediated immunity is of benefit. Deletion of the gene responsible for A20 activation results in severe hypertension with target-organ damage in an animal model.[6]

The CANTOS (Canakinumab Anti-Inflammatory Thrombosis Outcome Study) trial looked at the effect of canakinumab, an interleukin 1β inhibitor in patients with a history of myocardial infarction and residual inflammation as evidenced by increased C-reactive protein (CRP). After a follow-up of 4 years, there was a substantial reduction of cardiovascular events by 15%. This was accompanied by a parallel reduction of CRP also. A subsequent analysis of data looked into incident hypertension. Surprisingly, there was no reduction of hypertension on treatment with canakinumab.[5]

Renin–angiotensin system has long been considered a target of therapy with monoclonal antibodies. Recent advances in therapeutics in this field show promise in use of anti-inflammatory therapy in the long term. The ribonucleic acid (RNA) therapeutic agents tend to target RNA of a specific gene to produce specific and more targeted results. Advantage of such therapy includes longer duration and lack of side effects in the treatment of hypertension.

These agents under focus are short-interfering RNA (siRNA) and antisense oligonucleotide (ASO).[6,7]

Short-interfering Ribonucleic Acid

Short-interfering ribonucleic acids are short segments of double-stranded RNA which interfere with the expression of a specific gene (angiotensinogen) by binding to a specific complimentary segment of a messenger RNA of that gene.

Zilebesiran, a small molecule siRNA, targets and destroys messenger RNA (mRNA) responsible for synthesis of angiotensinogen, the precursor of angiotensin II. It is conjugated to N-acetylgalactosamine (GalNAc) which avidly binds to asialoglycoprotein receptor found abundantly in the liver. Because of this, it is specific to liver with minimal extrahepatic suppression of renin–angiotensin axis. Preliminary studies have shown encouraging results.[7]

Antisense Oligonucleotide

Antisense oligonucleotide is a single-stranded DNA that binds to a specific mRNA. Enzyme such as ribonuclease H1 (RNase H1) is activated and it destroys the mRNA. The IONIS-AGT-L is such an agent being tried in clinical trials.[6]

Being new agents that act on mRNA, concerns about their long-term safety are yet to be proven. In case of emergency such as shock or hypotension or pregnancy where activation of RAS is actively called for, the effects of siRNA can be nullified by a new reversal agent.[5,7]

CONCLUSION

There is a complex connection and interplay between neurohormonal stimulation, kidneys, and the immune system. There is clear evidence of immune dysregulation with development and progression of hypertension as well as hypertensive target-organ damage. Suppression of immune dysregulation remains an interesting solution for treatment of hypertension. Recent trial data shows a promising new therapeutic future in the management of hypertension.

ONLINE REFERENCES

Please scan the QR code provided at the end of the table of contents for References of this chapter.

CHAPTER 31

From Hypertension to Left Ventricular Hypertrophy to Heart Failure Continuum

Debabrata Roy, Navanil Biswas

ABSTRACT

Hypertension is a major determinant of heart failure. Though left ventricular hypertrophy is a cardinal manifestation of hypertensive heart failure, it is neither an obligatory feature nor the only pathophysiological mechanism for this disease. Remodeling of both atria, right ventricle, and large and small arteries can contribute to hypertensive heart failure also. Proper medication is necessary for management of hypertensive heart failure and the target blood pressure should be maintained within a narrow range to avoid reverse J-curve effect.

Keywords: Hypertension, left ventricular hypertrophy, heart failure.

INTRODUCTION

Hypertension (HTN) is the leading cause of cardiovascular morbidity and mortality worldwide. More than 7.5 million deaths per year are attributable to HTN. Untreated and uncontrolled HTN may lead to a wide cohort of cardiovascular diseases including heart failure (HF), myocardial ischemia, stroke, and atrial fibrillation. In fact, HTN antedated the development of HF in 91% of all newly diagnosed HF patients. Data from the landmark Framingham Heart Study revealed that hypertensive subjects had a two- to threefold risk of HF when compared with normotensive subjects. Multivariate analyses from this study using time-dependent modeling for HTN and other risk factors showed that among all the risk factors, HTN carried the greatest population attributable risk for the development of HF (39% of cases of HF in men and 59% in women). A meta-analysis conducted among 23 blood pressure (BP)-lowering trials revealed that 28.9% of the patients developed HF, which amounted to approximately 8.5 events per 1,000 patients.[1,2]

What is hypertensive heart failure (HHF)?

No universal practical definition of HHF is available till date. The definition of HHF proposed in 1979 by the New York Heart Association (NYHA) as "an anatomofunctional alteration characterized by left ventricular hypertrophy (LVH) and cardiac failure in patients with systemic HTN" fails to differentiate HHF from HF.[2] More recently, HHF is defined as "a form of decompensated HF characterized by complex myocardial alterations, including disruptions in cardiac function and electrical activity, and/or coronary flow abnormalities resulting from response to biochemical stress imposed on the LV by chronic and progressive increase in BP".[3] The Working Group of the Spanish Society of Cardiology (SSC) proposed that a clinically meaningful definition of HHF should include myocardial alterations induced by—(1) a chronic BP elevation; (2) alterations to the left ventricle (LV); (3) myocardial ischemia; and (4) atrial fibrillation.[2] It is pertinent to note that LVH, though a cardinal manifestation of HHF, is neither an obligatory characteristic nor the only pathophysiological mechanism for HHF.[1]

PATHOPHYSIOLOGY: FROM HYPERTENSIVE HEART DISEASE TO HYPERTENSIVE HEART FAILURE

Left ventricular hypertrophy is a cardinal intermediate phenotype in the transition of hypertensive heart disease (HHD) to HHF. As proposed by Messerli et al., classically, a patient of HTN gradually progresses through escalating degrees of severity, initiating from normal LV structure with diastolic dysfunction (Degree I) to LVH with diastolic dysfunction (Degree II), and then clinical HF with heart

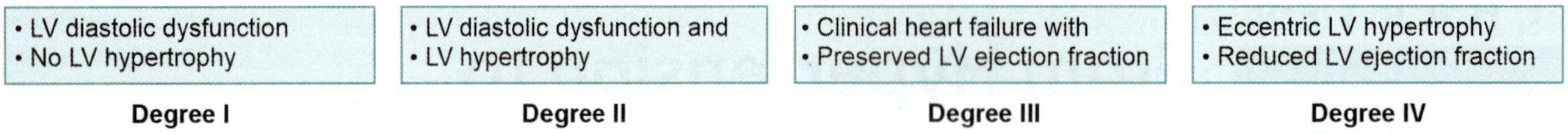

FIG. 1: Degrees of severity of hypertensive heart disease.
(LV: left ventricle)
Source: With permission from Messerli et al. (2017).[4]

failure with preserved ejection fraction (HFpEF) (Degree III), ultimately culminating into eccentric LVH and heart failure with reduced ejection fraction (HFrEF) (Degree IV) **(Fig. 1)**.[4]

HYPERTENSION TO LEFT VENTRICULAR HYPERTROPHY

The main contributors to development of LVH in a hypertensive patient are: (1) increase in the size of the cardiomyocyte; (2) alterations in extracellular matrix (ECM) with interstitial fibrosis; and (3) medial hypertrophy and perivascular fibrosis along with other abnormalities of intramyocardial coronary vasculature.[2] BP accounts for <20% of this increase in LV mass.[1] Other important mechanisms contributing to LVH are: (1) neurohormones—angiotensin II, norepinephrine, epinephrine, increased peripheral and cardiac sympathetic drive; (2) cytokines; (3) growth factors; and (4) profibrotic and prohypertrophic genetic pathways.[5] Every increase of LV mass by 39 g/m^2 is associated with an independent 40% increase in major cardiovascular event risk in HHF patients.[2] Pathological hypertrophy is differentiated from physiological hypertrophy by presence of inflammation and fibrosis.[6]

LEFT VENTRICULAR HYPERTROPHY TO HYPERTENSIVE HEART FAILURE (FIG. 2)

Classically HTN progresses into concentric LVH [increased LV mass and relative wall thickness (RWT), without LV dilatation] which culminates into HFpEF (pathway 1 and 6).[7] This is mainly contributed by: (1) increased LV mass, especially the interstitial fibrosis that limits the end-diastolic muscle fiber length and thus reduces myocardial force of contraction; and (2) myocardial ischemia due to acceleration of systemic and coronary arteriosclerosis as well as increase in cardiomyocyte size without proportional proliferation of the capillaries. The resultant demand supply mismatch leads to cardiac myocyte dysfunction or death.[2]

Ahmed et al. demonstrated that such progression to HFpEF may depend on matrix metalloproteinase (MMP) and tissue inhibitor of matrix metalloproteinase (TIMP) levels in the plasma. In hypertensives without LVH or HF, plasma levels of MMP and TIMP are normal, whereas HTN with LVH is associated with decreased levels of MMP-2 and -13 and increased level of MMP-9 (that activates profibrotic pathways) leading to more fibrosis. In hypertensives with LVH and HF, there is increase in plasma level of TIMP-1 which

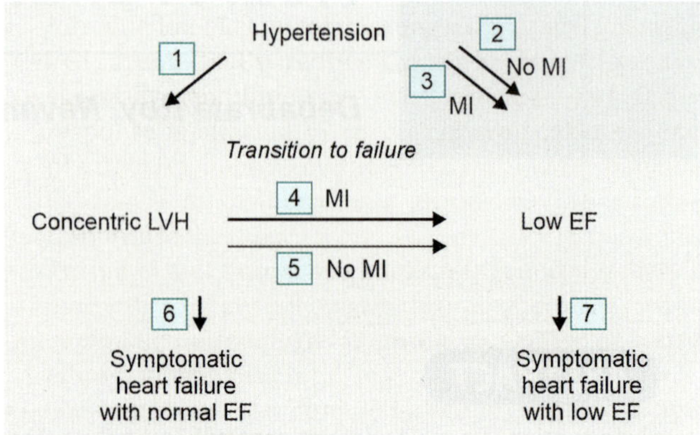

FIG. 2: Pathways of progression of hypertension to heart failure.
(EF: ejection fraction; LVH: left ventricular hypertrophy; MI: myocardial infarction)
Source: With permission from Drazner (2011).[7]

reduces proteolysis of ECM resulting in its accumulation. In fact, TIMP-1 level above 1,200 ng/mL is predictive of CHF.[8] A novel index obtained by cardiac MRI-remodeling index $\left(RI = \frac{\sqrt[3]{\text{end-diastolic volume}}}{\text{maximum wall thickness}}\right)$ may serve as another predictor of HFpEF in hypertensives. Goh et al. showed that hypertensives with LVH and low RI are associated with higher indexed LV mass, more fibrosis, and elevated biomarkers of myocardial injury and HF as compared to hypertensives with/without LVH and high RI.[9]

Progression of concentric LVH to eccentric LVH (increased LV mass normal RWT with LV cavity dilatation) and consequent HFrEF with or without intervening myocardial infarction (MI) is uncommon (pathways 4, 5, and 7).[7] Milani et al. showed that over a period of 3 years, only 13% of concentric LVH will progress to HFrEF and 42.5% of this transition is accounted by MI.[10] In fact, recent studies revealed concentric LVH and eccentric LVH are results of two different pathophysiological mechanisms and consequently are two distinctly different entities. Khouri et al., based on cardiac MRI assessment of LV geometry, proposed a novel 4-tiered classification of LVH: (1) thick hypertrophy; (2) thick and dilated hypertrophy; (3) dilated hypertrophy; and (4) indeterminate (not thick/dilated) hypertrophy (first two falling under concentric LVH and last two falling under eccentric LVH by standard classification) **(Fig. 3)**.[11]

The thick, dilated variety is associated with lower LV ejection fraction and higher N-terminal prohormone of

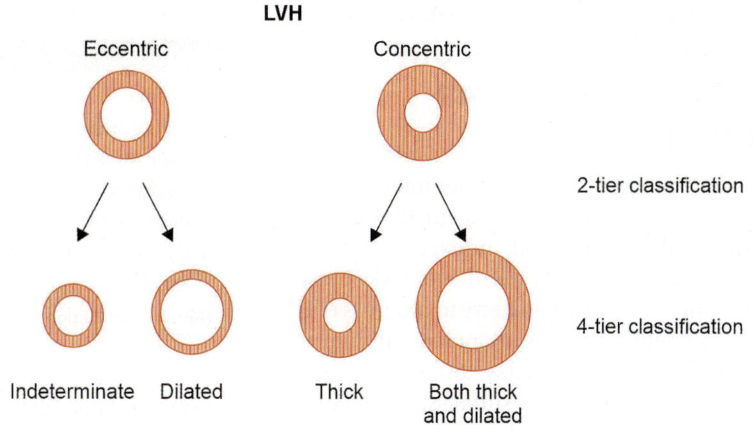

	Indeterminate	Dilated	Thick	Both thick and dilated
• Increased LV mass/height	+	+	+	+
• Increased LV mass/volume (concentricity)	–	–	+	+
• Increased LVEDV/BSA	–	+	–	+

FIG. 3: 4-tier classification of LVH.

(LVH: left ventricular hypertrophy; LVEDV: left ventricular end-diastolic volume; BSA: body surface area)

Source: With permission from Khouri et al. (2010).[11]

brain natriuretic peptide (NT-proBNP) and BNP levels as compared to thick variety but forms only 5% of the total concentric LVH.

Among eccentric remodeling, dilated variety makes up the minority fraction and is associated with lower LV ejection fraction and higher troponin T, NT-proBNP, and BNP levels as compared to indeterminate variety. Therefore in both concentric and eccentric LVH, dilated phenotype determines HHF.[11]

Eccentric LVH is likely the result of increased wall stress and endothelial dysfunction and is associated with biomarkers such as NT-proBNP, MMP-2, tumor necrosis factor receptor 2 (TNFR2), and junctional adhesion molecule A (JAM-A). On the other hand, concentric LVH owes its origin most probably to oxidative stress and inflammation and is associated with expression of biomarkers such as tumor necrosis factor receptor 1 (TNFR1), urokinase plasminogen activator surface receptor (U-PAR), paraoxonase 3 (PON), and P-Selectin (SELP). The TNFR1:TNFR2 ratio may determine concentric or eccentric remodeling with increased TNFR1 favoring concentric LVH and vice versa.[12] Eccentric LVH may also be associated with lesser number of cardiomyocytes.[13]

Several demographic and genetic factors, comorbidities, and pattern of neurohormonal activation also determine progression of hypertensives into concentric or eccentric hypertrophy **(Table 1)**.

TABLE 1: Factors influencing concentric or eccentric LVH.

Concentric versus eccentric LVH	
• *Pressure load*: Severity, duration, and rapidity of onset • Volume load • *Demographic factors*: Age, race/ethnicity, and gender • *Concomitant medical conditions*: Coronary artery disease, diabetes mellitus, obesity, valvular heart disease • Neurohormonal milieu • Alterations of the extracellular matrix • Genetic factors	• Concentric: ○ Black population ○ Female ○ Elderly ○ Isolated systolic hypertension ○ Higher SBP ○ Higher ambulatory BP ○ Higher total peripheral resistance ○ Higher plasma renin activity ○ Diabetes • Eccentric: ○ Male ○ CAD ○ Obesity ○ Low plasma renin activity

(CAD: coronary artery disease; LVH: left ventricular hypertrophy; SBP: systolic blood pressure)

Sources: With permission from Oh and Cho (2020)[1]; Milani et al. (2011).[10]

HYPERTENSIVE HEART DISEASE TO HYPERTENSIVE HEART FAILURE: BEYOND LEFT VENTRICULAR HYPERTROPHY

Hypertensives may progress to HF without intervening LVH or MI (Pathway 2).[7] Patients with concentric remodeling, which is associated with normal indexed LV mass but increased RWT, have an intermediate risk between concentric LVH and normal LV geometry to progress to HHF. In concentric remodeling, there is no increase in interstitial fibrosis or impairment in myocardial systolic strain. However, it is associated with increased aortic stiffness.[9] Aortic stiffness impairs Windkessel function with resultant increase in systolic BP and decrease in diastolic BP thereby producing diastolic dysfunction by the following mechanisms: (1) impairment of myocardial microcirculation due to reduced coronary flow in diastole; (2) myocyte hypertrophy and collagen deposition as a result of increased LV wall stress because of increased afterload; and (3) prolonged LV relaxation due to changed LV ejection phase.[14] Aortic stiffness by increasing pulse wave velocity induces adverse eutrophic remodeling (increased media-to-lumen ratio with unchanged total wall tissue) of small arteries thereby causing rarefaction of microvasculature—a phenomenon termed large artery and small artery crosstalk. This microcirculation damage further begets more aortic stiffness thus initiating a vicious cycle.[15]

Recently, it is revealed that HHD involves a range of target organ damage beyond LVH that includes remodeling of atria, right ventricle, and, as described above, of the arterial system. The changes are as follows:

- *Right atrium (RA)*: RA enlargement and dysfunction
- *Left atrium (LA)*: LA myopathy and dysfunction
- *Right ventricle (RV)*: RV hypertrophy and systolic and diastolic dysfunction
- *Arteries*: Aortic stiffness; smaller arterial increased wall thickness and stiffness

All these can lead to HHF. The pathophysiological mechanisms responsible are: (1) neurohormonal activation; (2) growth factors; (3) cytokines; (4) mitochondrial dysfunction/reactive oxygen species; (5) endothelial dysfunction; and (6) abnormal calcium handling.[15]

RISK STRATIFICATION OF HYPERTENSIVE HEART FAILURE

Hemodynamic and nonhemodynamic factors that contribute to increase in LV mass may also lead to progression and destabilization of atherosclerotic plaques. This can predispose HHF patients to myocardial ischemia and arrhythmias. Thus, HF in hypertensives seldom occurs in isolation and is often seen in combination with ischemia and/or atrial fibrillation. To stratify hypertensive patients according to this cumulative risk, the working group of Spanish Society of Cardiology proposed the VIA classification for HHD, similar to the widely used TNM staging for cancer **(Table 2)**. This classification is based on the main complications occurring in the heart induced by chronic blood pressure elevation, and encompasses—(1) alterations to the left ventricle (V), (2) myocardial ischemia (I), and (3) atrial fibrillation (A). A score of 1 to 3 is assigned to each of these three main headings to grade the cumulative cardiac risk in increasing order, from mild or early to more severe or later ones.[16]

TABLE 2: VIA classification.

Ventricle	Ischemia	Arrhythmia
0: Normal	0: Not clinically apparent	0: No or banal extrasystole
1: Left ventricular hypertrophy	1: Angina/Microvascular ischemia	1: Paroxystic AF
2: Dysfunction or diastolic HF	2: Angina/Macrovascular ischemia	2: Permanent AF
3: Dysfunction or systolic HF	3: Acute coronary syndrome	3. AF and embolism

(AF: atrial fibrillation; HF: heart failure)

CLINICAL IMPLICATIONS OF LEFT VENTRICULAR HYPERTROPHY REGRESSION IN THE MANAGEMENT OF HYPERTENSIVE HEART FAILURE

Regression of LVH can reduce the risk of cardiovascular events by as much as 59%.[1] Fortunately, progression of HTN from one stage to other happens over a prolonged period thereby offering enough "window period" for instituting appropriate lifestyle modifications and medicines to effect favorable prognosis. It takes an average of 7 years 10 months for transition from normal/elevated BP to stage 1 HTN, and 1 year 8 months for transition from stage 1 HTN to stage 2 HTN. In the WHO-SAGE longitudinal study, the probability of stage 1 HTN of recovering to normal/elevated BP (47.3%) was greater than progressing to stage 2 HTN (31.6%).[17]

Though a recent meta-analysis of 3,632 patients showed that any class of antihypertensive medication in HHF patients provides a protective effect against future cardiovascular events and the onset of HF compared to placebo, not all antihypertensives are equal in its efficacy to prevent progression of HHD to HHF.[2,4] Renin-angiotensin-aldosterone system (RAAS) inhibitors and diuretics are the preferred agents for preventing HHF. Among the diuretics, chlorthalidone, thiazide, and indapamide are most effective. Beta-blockers have no effect and can increase the risk of stroke by 19% in the elderly; calcium channel blockers increases the risk for HF as compared to diuretics though decreases the risk for stroke as compared to angiotensin-converting enzyme inhibitor (ACEI)/angiotensin receptor blocker (ARB); and alpha-blockers, particularly doxazosin, increase both the risks of HF and stroke. Hence, these agents should not be used as first-line agents for preventing progression of HHD to HHF.[4]

Established HHF should receive the mainstays of HF therapy—angiotensin receptor-neprilysin inhibitor (ARNI) or ACEI/ARB, vasodilating beta-blocker, and sodium-glucose cotransporter-2 inhibitor (SGLT-2I), along with loop diuretic. As adjunct therapy, spironolactone and thiazide diuretic can be added for both HFrEF and HFpEF while calcium channel blockers can be added for HFpEF and doxazosin for HFrEF.[4] The LV geometry influences the effect of uptitration of some of these drugs on mortality, e.g., eccentric LVH is associated with favorable response on uptitration of beta-blockers and ACEI/ARBs[12] **(Flowchart 1)**.

The target BP should be kept within a narrow range as risks of mortality and readmission can increase both for too low and too high BP. This phenomenon is termed as reverse J-curve hypothesis and exists for both HFrEF and HFpEF. Korean Society of Hypertension guideline suggested 130/80 mm Hg as an optimal BP in HHF.[1] Too low BP can be a result of increased aortic stiffness or can lead to decreased diastolic coronary perfusion, both of which can contribute to adverse events.[18]

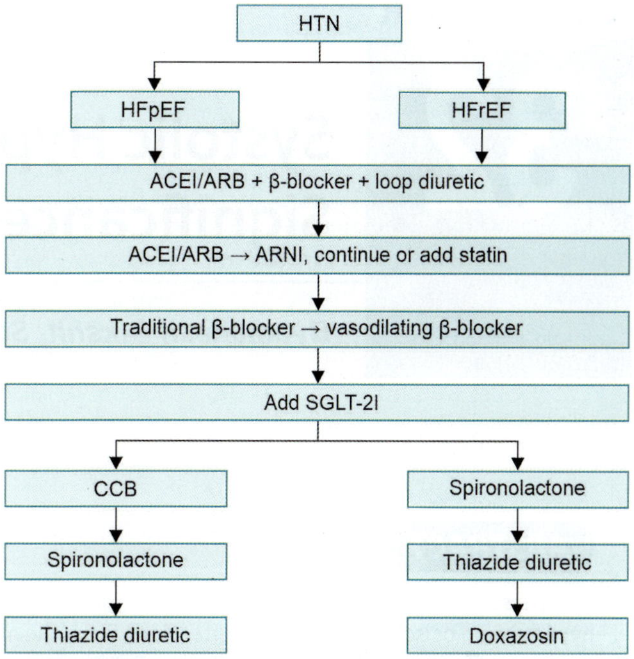

FLOWCHART 1: Treatment algorithm for HHF.

(ACEI: angiotensin-converting enzyme inhibitor; ARB: angiotensin receptor blocker; ARNI: angiotensin receptor-neprilysin inhibitor; CCB: calcium channel blocker; HTN: hypertension; HFrEF: heart failure with reduced ejection fraction; HFpEF: heart failure with preserved ejection fraction; SGLT-2I: sodium-glucose cotransporter-2 inhibitor)

Source: With permission from Messerli et al. (2017).[4]

CONCLUSION

Hypertension is a leading cause of cardiovascular disease, stroke, and death. It affects a substantial proportion of the population worldwide, and remains underdiagnosed and undertreated. HTN causes both structural and functional changes in the heart that affect both the atrial and the ventricular myocardium, as well as the epicardial and intramural coronary arteries. Adequate blood pressure control must be achieved in patients with HTN to prevent progression to overt HF. The presence of LVH and concentric LV geometry are strong predictors of poor prognosis because of increased risk of major cardiovascular events. LV geometry is a significant factor determining the progression to HHF. However, HHD can progress to HHF even in absence of LVH. Not all antihypertensives are equally effective for preventing progression to HF. Established HHF should receive the mainstays of HF therapy and the treatment goal should be achieving a BP of 130/80 mm Hg.

ONLINE REFERENCES

Please scan the QR code provided at the end of the table of contents for References of this chapter.

CHAPTER

32

Systolic Hypertension: Clinical Significance and Management

Byomakesh Dikshit, Soumen Prasad Behera, Sabyasachi Rout

ABSTRACT

Any person >65 years old, with normal blood pressure, has a 90% lifetime risk of developing hypertension. Systolic hypertension or isolated systolic hypertension (ISH) is the most common form of hypertension in the elderly. ISH develops as a result of decreased arterial compliance. This is seen commonly among the elderly. However, ISH is also observed in the young. Most cases of systolic hypertension are primary. In this review of literature, we will be discussing the definition, clinical significance, and management of ISH in young as well as in the elderly.

Keywords: Isolated systolic hypertension, definition of ISH, grading of ISH, systolic diastolic hypertension, ISH in the elderly, ISH in the young.

INTRODUCTION

Systolic hypertension or isolated systolic hypertension (ISH) is the most common form of hypertension in the elderly. It is also observed in young males. ISH develops as a result of decreased arterial compliance, which means the volume of arteries remains the same because of the loss of elasticity and it causes a big gap between the systolic and the diastolic blood pressure (DBP). This is seen commonly among the elderly as there is increased deposition of calcium and collagen in the arterial wall and arteries lose elasticity. Most cases of systolic hypertension are primary. ISH remains an important public health concern as untreated cases, carries significant mortality and morbidity.

DEFINITION

As per the European Society of Hypertension guidelines 2023, ISH is defined as systolic blood pressure (SBP) of >140 mm Hg and DPB of <90 mm Hg.[1]

Isolated systolic hypertension in the youth[2] (0–15 years) is defined as SBP ≥95th and DBP <90th percentile for age, height, and sex. In those aged 16 years and over, ISH is said to be present if the SBP ≥140 mm Hg and DBP <90 mm Hg.[3]

The grading of ISH is given in **Table 1**.

TABLE 1: Grading of isolated systolic hypertension.

Grading of ISH based on office BP measurement	
Category	**SBP (mm Hg)**
Grade I	140–159
Grade II	160–179
Grade III	>180
Diastolic BP is <90 mm Hg in all grades	
(BP: blood pressure; SBP: systolic blood pressure)	

EPIDEMIOLOGY

The prevalence of ISH increases with age, such that two-thirds of the population >60 years and three-fourths of people above 75 years of age have ISH. As per the Framingham Heart Study data, people having normal BP who reach >65 years have a 90% lifetime risk of developing hypertension if they live for another 20–25 years and that too mostly of predominant systolic type.[4] It is more common in the urban population than rural population. However, because of rapid industrialization, the difference is becoming insignificant.[5]

In a study by Staessen et al.,[6] the prevalence of ISH was 2–8% in those aged around 30 years, it was 0.1–0.8% in the age group between 40 and 50 years and the prevalence was 12.6% in those over 70 years of age. In another study by Sorof et al.,[7] among 2,460 school children between the age group of 12 and 16 years,17% were found to be hypertensive out of which 88% had ISH.

Young males are more likely to develop hypertension. However, after the age of 50 years, the prevalence of ISH is more in females. This may be because of the loss of the protective effects of progesterone and estrogen.[8-10]

In a study carried out in France in 2003 by Mallion et al.,[11] it was found that the prevalence of ISH is more in young males as compared to females. Similar findings were also reported in three different studies, viz., the ENIGMA[12] study done in 2005 among young adults in the UK, the Atherosclerosis Risk in Young Adults (ARYA) study[13] done in Europe and the HARVEST[14] study done in Italy.

RISK FACTORS FOR ISOLATED SYSTOLIC HYPERTENSION

In the elderly, ISH can be due to modifiable and hereditary risk factors. It can also occur as a result of pathophysiological changes in aging.[15] Burned-out diastolic hypertension in long-term essential hypertension can also result in ISH in the elderly. Other determinants of ISH in the elderly are advancing age, overweight and female sex, and aging of the proximal aorta.

In the young, ISH is more likely to occur in persons with a history of smoking, lower education status, and obese people, those who are more engaged in sports and those who have a high resting heart rate and African-American race.

However, the risk factors of ISH in the Asian population are quite varied. In a national survey carried out in Korea, ISH was more frequently found in people with high body mass index (BMI), high triglyceride levels, and alcohol intake.[16] In yet another study done in China, ISH was more frequently found in females, people with history of smoking and alcohol intake, high salt intake, and high BMI.[15]

Other causes of ISH in both the elderly and young people are accelerated atherosclerosis from chronic kidney disease, hyperthyroidism, peripheral vascular disease, osteoporosis with vascular calcification, and repaired coarctation of the aorta.

PATHOPHYSIOLOGY

Pathophysiology of Isolated Systolic Hypertension in the Elderly

As age increases, there is progression of atherosclerosis which results in calcium and collagen deposition in the arterial wall. There is also fraying of the arterial elastin. This causes a loss of elasticity and compliance of the arterial wall which subsequently leads to a decrease in the lumen-to-wall ratio and there is an increase in arterial stiffness. The renin-angiotensin-aldosterone system (RAAS) affects the arterial elastin-collagen content and leads to vascular stiffening and loss of arterial wall contractility, the proliferation of arterial smooth muscle cells and fibrotic remodeling of vascular intima increases vascular thickening. These changes are predominantly seen in large arteries and the aorta. There is a fast rise in peak SBP in the noncompliant stiffened arterial tree and there is greater decline of DBP due to limited recoil of the arterial wall.

Pathophysiology of Isolated Systolic Hypertension in the Young

Various mechanisms have been proposed which contribute to ISH in youth.

The earlier studies on ISH in the young were described by O'Rourke et al.[17] and Mahmud and Feely.[18] In their studies, they found that individuals with elevated brachial BP have normal central aortic pressures. The SphygmoCor system was used in both studies to estimate central BP. As per their studies, systolic hypertension in the young is spurious systolic hypertension and is a result of highly elastic arteries with low peripheral vascular resistance and low wave reflection. Later on, it was by McEniery et al.[12] who described that the individuals with ISH actually amplify an already elevated central SBP rather than amplifying a normal central SBP. Waveform analysis of the distal arterial sites was used by McEniery et al.[12] for estimating the central aortic pressures.

Another mechanism for ISH in the young is the overactivation of the sympathetic nervous system. One of the first investigators who proposed this mechanism was Stevo Julius in the Tecumseh study.[19] Hyperactivated sympathetic nervous system in the youth leads to increased cardiac output and tachycardia and thus the development of hypertension. Data from the Framingham Heart Study[20] also supports the same mechanism for ISH in the young. Similar findings were also found in the HARVEST study[21] during a 6-year follow-up period.

The "white coat effect" also causes ISH in the young. Stress leads to a hyperkinetic state and subsequently leads to ISH. Pulse pressure amplification leads to higher systolic BP in these situations.[22] Another proposed mechanism for ISH in the young was described by the ENIGMA study.[12] It is one of the largest studies to date on ISH in young. As per the study, elevated cardiac output was the hemodynamic parameter more strongly associated with systolic hypertension in lean individuals. The study did not include African-Americans descent blacks who tend to have high peripheral vascular resistance from a younger age. Thus, the data from ENIGMA study cannot be generalized to all ethnic groups. About 20% of ISH young individuals do not have increased cardiac output or stroke volume and as such in these patients, premature aortic stiffening is the cause of systolic hypertension. Premature aortic stiffening leads to an increase in pulse wave velocity thereby raising the SBP.

IMPACT OF ISOLATED SYSTOLIC HYPERTENSION

Isolated systolic hypertension in the elderly is an independent and strong risk factor for cardiovascular disease which includes myocardial infarction and various cardiomyopathies. It is also an important risk factor for cerebrovascular accidents (both ischemic and hemorrhagic stroke), dementia, cognitive impairment, end-stage renal disease, retinopathy, and erectile dysfunction.

However, only a few studies have been carried out to know the impact of ISH in the young. The best strong current evidence for the long-term impact of ISH in the young comes from the Chicago Heart Association Detection in Industry Programme[23] in which 15,868 males and 11,213 females in the age group between 18 and 49 years were studied for a period of 31 years and in that study, it was found ISH is associated with increased risk for cardiovascular disease and coronary artery disease mortality.

MANAGEMENT OF ISOLATED SYSTOLIC HYPERTENSION IN THE ELDERLY

Various trials have shown that the treatment of ISH in the elderly reduces the risk of cardiovascular events and stroke. The Hypertension in the Very Elderly Trial (HYVET)[24] showed a marked reduction of deaths from any cause and cardiovascular death in the treatment group. Studies on ISH were also conducted in the Asian population. One of the studies was the VALISH study[25] which was conducted in Japan. Another study was the FEVER study[26] which was conducted in the Chinese population. Both studies showed that treatment of ISH in the elderly reduces the risk of cardiovascular death and stroke.

Management of ISH includes:
- Nonpharmacological therapy
- Pharmacotherapy
- Nonpharmacological treatment

It includes various lifestyle modifications which include:
- *Weight loss*: BP increases with an increase in weight. Obesity also results in sleep apnea in a majority of individuals which in turn causes hypertension. Hence weight loss is one of the most effective nonpharmacological therapies for BP control.
- *Regular physical activity*: In the absence of any contraindication, regular physical activity should be encouraged in all hypertensive individuals. It should be 30 minutes a day for 5 days a week. This may include walking, cycling, jogging, dancing, or swimming. Regular physical exercises decrease BP by 5–8 mm Hg.
- *Healthy diet*: A diet rich in whole grains, vegetables, and fruits should be encouraged in hypertensive individuals. Diet may also include a small amount of poultry, fish, legumes, seeds, and nuts a few times a week. The diet should be low in salt, saturated fats, transfats, and whole fats.
- *Decrease in alcohol intake*: Alcohol intake should be less than one drink per day for females and less than two drinks per day for males. This can potentially lower the BP by around 4 mm Hg. Alcohol intake also reduces the effectiveness of the drugs.
- *Stop smoking and tobacco intake*: Cigarette smoking and tobacco intake cause a rise in BP and so it should be stopped.

Pharmacotherapy

The primary aim of pharmacotherapy is to achieve optimal BP control and that too with a minimal drug regimen that has fewer side effects.

The common antihypertensive medications for the treatment of ISH are:
- *Calcium channel blockers (CCBs)*: These are highly efficacious, safest, and first-line drugs for the treatment of hypertension in the elderly as proved in various clinical trials.
- *Diuretics*: Thiazide and thiazide like diuretic groups of drugs are highly efficacious for the initial management of ISH.
- *Angiotensin-converting enzyme inhibitor/angiotensin receptor blockers (ACEI/ARBs)*: These are the group of antihypertensive drugs used in the presence of comorbidities (as given in **Table 2**).
- *Beta-blockers*: In the elderly, these drugs should not be used for initial treatment and are to be used when associated with a comorbidity as given in **Table 2**.

General Guidelines of Treatment[27]

- Antihypertensives drugs need to be started with lower initial doses (approximately one-half that in younger patients) to minimize the risk of side effects.
- If hypertensive emergency is unlikely, BP need to be lowered gradually over a period of 3–6 months rather than hours to days to minimize the risk of ischemic

TABLE 2: Preference of drugs in specific comorbidities.

Indication	Specific drugs
Postmyocardial infarction	• ACEI • Beta-blockers
Heart failure	ACEI/ARBs, diuretics
Risk of CAD	ACEI/ARBs, beta blockers, calcium channel blockers, diuretics
Chronic kidney disease	Calcium channel blockers
Diabetes mellitus	• ACEI/ARBs • Beta-blockers • Calcium channel blockers • Diuretics

(ACEI: angiotensin-converting enzyme inhibitor; ARB: angiotensin receptor blocker; CAD: coronary artery disease) symptoms, particularly in patients with orthostatic hypotension as older adults have sluggish baroreceptor and sympathetic neural responses along with impaired cerebral autoregulation.

- Extra caution needs to be taken when treating frail elderly hypertensive patients to avoid overtreating them as orthostatic hypotension is common in elderly patients with ISH posing an increased risk of hip fracture during the initial months of therapy.
- Cardiovascular risk reduction is affected by BP reduction, not by the choice of antihypertensive drugs. This principle of equivalent efficacy in cardiovascular outcomes applies to monotherapy, not to combined antihypertensive therapy. The combination of ACEI/ARB and a long-acting dihydropyridine CCB appears to significantly reduce cardiovascular events at the same attained BP as an ACEI/ARB and a thiazide diuretic as observed in (ACCOMPLISH) trial of combination therapy.[28]

The stepwise approach of ISH treatment is like any other case of hypertension is given in **Box 1**.

Management of ISH in the Young

Data on the management of ISH in the young are lacking. Lifestyle modifications in the form of dietary salt restriction, increasing physical activity, quitting smoking, and weight reduction are the first-line options advised in young ISH patients, even if pharmacotherapy is necessary. **Flowchart 1** shows the management approach for ISH in the young.

CONCLUSION

Isolated systolic hypertension is a common problem in the elderly population and needs to be addressed properly to reduce cardiovascular risk and also all-cause mortality. ISH is also a growing issue among the young nowadays due to changes in lifestyle and diet. So nonpharmacological management as described and close follow-up and initiation of drugs, when required, needs to be followed for their management as ISH in the young with raised central BP is more likely to develop systolic/diastolic hypertension in future.

BOX 1 Stepwise approach to ISH treatment.

Stepwise approach to ISH:

Grade I ISH

- Lifestyle modification
- Monitor blood pressure (BP) at home
- If target BP not achieved, start with single drug therapy
- CCB/thiazide/thiazide like diuretic/ACEI/ARB

Grade II or III ISH

- Lifestyle modification and two-drug therapy
- CCB + thiazides/thiazide like diuretics
- CCB+ACEI/ARB
- ACEI/ARB + thiazides/thiazide like diuretics
- If target BP not achieved, then three-drug therapy
- CCB + ACEI/ARB + thiazides/thiazide like diuretics
- If still target BP not achieved then add spironolactone/eplerenone or nebivolol

(ACEI: angiotensin-converting enzyme inhibitor; ARB: angiotensin receptor blocker; CCB: calcium channel blocker; ISH: isolated systolic hypertension)

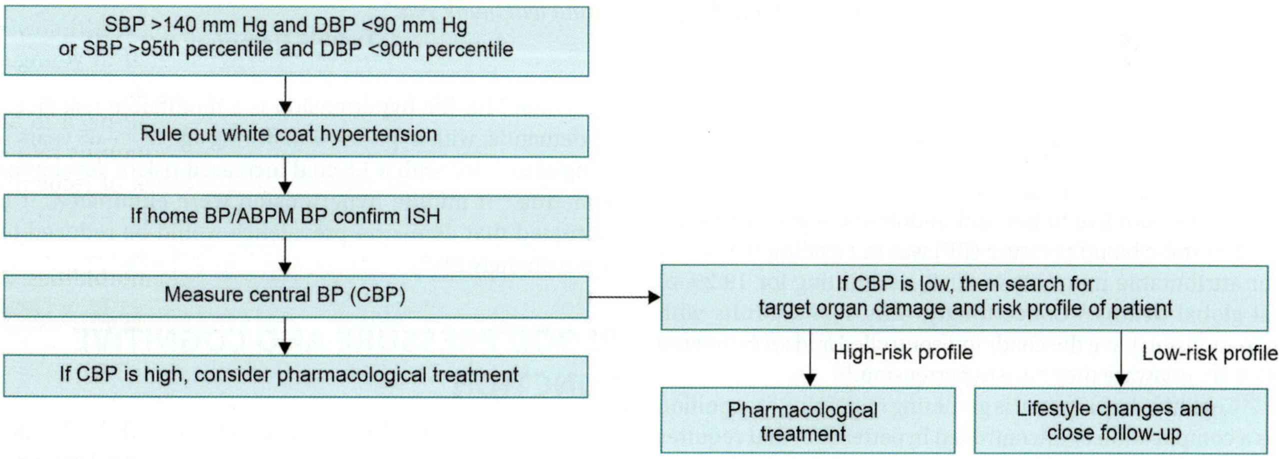

FLOWCHART 1: Approach to ISH in the young.

(ABPM: ambulatory blood pressure monitoring; DBP: diastolic blood pressure; ISH: isolated systolic hypertension; SBP: systolic blood pressure)

ONLINE REFERENCES

Please scan the QR code provided at the end of the table of contents for References of this chapter.

CHAPTER

33

Hypertension and Cognitive Impairment

C Venkata S Ram, Mohsin Wali

ABSTRACT

Worldwide, the number of people living with dementia is projected to climb rapidly in the coming decades. As dementia cannot be cured, preventive strategies are required to stem the rise in cases. Midlife hypertension is a modifiable risk factor for the development of dementia later in life and early control of blood pressure (BP) is currently the only pharmacological strategy known to reduce the risk of late-life cognitive decline. Prompt diagnosis and aggressive management of hypertension is needed to reduce the burden of dementia and cognitive decline, particularly in aging populations and those with limited healthcare access.

Keywords: Hypertension, complications, neurological damage, brain function, dementia, cognitive impairment.

"Take care of your mind, your body will thank you,
take care of your body, your mind will thank you."

—Debbie Hampton

INTRODUCTION

The global burden of hypertension continues to escalate with 1.56 billion people projected to be affected by 2025, two-thirds of whom live in low and middle-income countries.[1,2] High systolic blood pressure (BP) was the leading risk factor for attributable mortality in 2019, accounting for 19.2% of all global deaths.[1] Concerningly, only 1 in 5 adults with hypertension have the condition controlled and an estimated 46% are unaware they have hypertension.[1,3]

Cognitive impairment is garnering increasing recognition as a complication of uncontrolled hypertension that requires urgent attention. Worldwide, it is estimated that the number of people with dementia will increase from 57.4 million in 2019 to 152.8 million in 2050.[4] This rapid rise in cases has substantial geographic disparities, for example, it is estimated that dementia will increase in India and China by 197% from 2019 to 2050.[4]

Dementia cannot currently be cured; and diagnosing and treating hypertension early is one of the few therapeutic avenues available to slow the increasing prevalence of dementia. Mid-life hypertension is a modifiable risk factor for dementia, with hypertension during age of 45–65 years is being associated with a 1.6-fold increased risk of developing dementia.[5] If midlife hypertension were eliminated, it is estimated that dementia prevalence would be reduced by approximately 2%.[5]

BLOOD PRESSURE AND COGNITIVE FUNCTION

One of the first studies linking elevated BP with poor cognitive outcomes occurred in the 1970s.[6] During a 10-year period, diastolic hypertension was correlated with a significant intellectual decline in people in their 60s, but not in age-matched peers with a normal or mildly elevated BP. Cognitive impairment is also a frequent finding in patients with hypertension, with one meta-analysis estimating the overall prevalence of mild cognitive impairment (MCI) in people with hypertension to be 30%.[7] Numerous epidemiological studies have shown strong associations between hypertension and decreased cognitive function, thereby suggesting a causal link between elevated BP and impaired cognitive ability in susceptible individuals later in life.

Epidemiological Evidence

The Framingham study provided robust epidemiological evidence of an association between hypertension and cognitive decline.[8] Five BP measurements taken between 1956 and 1964 from 1,702 participants aged 55–88 years were examined and their relationship with neuropsychological tests administered between 1976 and 1978 was assessed. Both BP levels and duration of hypertension were inversely related to the cognitive composite score and for measures of attention and memory. This early study is interesting because the data was collected during a period when hypertension was largely untreated in the general population.

More recent data from a longitudinal study of a 70-year-old in Sweden assessed the relationship between BP and dementia onset over 15 years.[9] It was found that the participants aged 79–85 years old who developed dementia had both increased systolic BP (178 vs. 164 mm Hg, $p = 0.034$) and increased diastolic BP (101 vs. 92 mm Hg, $p = 0.004$) at the age of 70 years, compared to the participants who did not develop dementia. Increased diastolic BP was also recorded at the age of 70 years for the participants who had developed Alzheimer's disease (AD), and at the age of 75 years for those who had developed vascular dementia. Furthermore, the presence of white matter lesions (WMLs) at the age of 85 years was associated with an increased BP at the age of 70 years, compared to those that did not have WML.

Midlife Hypertension is a Risk Factor

The association between hypertension and BP control on dementia onset in different age groups was examined in a Korean cohort study.[10] This study enrolled 428,976 participants aged 40–79 years without a prior history of a dementia or a stroke. During the mean follow-up of 7.3 years, 2.2% of the cohort was diagnosed with a dementia. For every 10 mm Hg increase in systolic BP, the dementia risk increased by 22% for participants aged 40–59 years and by 8% for those aged 60–69 years. An increased duration of exposure to hypertension was also associated with an elevated dementia risk with a hazard ratio (HR) of 1.09/10% increase.

Another study that performed dose-response meta-analyses found stronger associations between midlife hypertension and cognitive decline than with late-life hypertension.[11] A midlife systolic BP >130 mm Hg was associated with a 34% increased risk of cognitive impairment and dementia. Specifically, significant associations were found between midlife hypertension and deficits in global cognition and executive function, but not with a memory.

The potential cognitive benefit of controlling hypertension in midlife was demonstrated by a 20-year follow-up of the Atherosclerosis Risk in Communities cohort who were aged 48–67 at a study entry.[12] It was concluded that hypertension in midlife and elevated midlife systolic BP was associated with a greater cognitive decline over the 20-year study, however, an elevated systolic BP during late-life was not.

> **BOX 1 Dementia prevention possible.**
> The clinical significance of midlife hypertension being a risk factor for late-life dementia is that it provides a potential 15–20-year therapeutic window in which to prevent dementia onset.

Treated Hypertension

People with controlled hypertension also have a decreased risk of developing dementia, compared to those with untreated hypertension. A French study of 1,373 participants aged 59–71 years assessed the association between elevated baseline BP (systolic BP ≥160 mm Hg or diastolic BP ≥95 mm Hg) and cognitive decline over a 4-year period.[13] Among participants with elevated baseline BP, the odds ratio (OR) of cognitive decline was 4.3 for those who were not receiving antihypertensive treatment and 1.9 in those who were receiving BP treatment. In those with elevated BP at the baseline and at the 2-year assessment, the OR of cognitive decline for untreated participants was 6, compared to 1.3 for those receiving the treatment.

A study of 3,703 Japanese–American men in the Honolulu Heart Program in 1965–1971 examined participants for dementia in 1991.[14] After adjusting for age, education, apolipoprotein epsilon allele, smoking and alcohol intake, in patients who were never treated for hypertension, the OR for dementia was 4.3 for a diastolic BP ≥95 mm Hg, compared to those with a diastolic BP of 80–89 mm Hg. In participants with a systolic BP ≥160 mm Hg, the risk of dementia was 4.8 compared to those with a systolic BP ≤139 mm Hg. However, in participants with treated BP, there was no association between BP and dementia risk.

A large meta-analysis that included more recent data also reported that the use of antihypertensive medicines was associated with a 21% reduction in dementia risk.[11]

Hypertension in Early Life

Evidence is accumulating that early-life exposure to cardiovascular (CV) risk factors is also associated with deficits in cognition later in life.[15-19] For example, a cohort study of 3,596 children followed at 3–9-year intervals since 1980 found that elevations in systolic BP and total serum cholesterol as well as smoking from childhood were independent risk factors for a decreased cognitive performance in midlife, particularly relating to memory and learning.[19]

A prospective study of 3,381 adults aged 18–30 years at a study entry, found that the primary predictors of cognitive deficits at year 25 were cumulative exposure to elevations in systolic and diastolic BP, and elevations in blood glucose and total cholesterol.[15] It is possible that a detrimental effect of elevated BP at a young age may be detected early as young adults with hypertension tend to have lower cognitive test performances than normotensive controls, although they are not considered to be cognitively impaired.[16]

Hypertension and Stroke Risk

Hypertension is the most significant and prevalent risk factor for stroke and multiple studies have demonstrated that stroke is strongly associated with cognitive impairment and dementia.[20-23] In a case-control study involving 22 countries with patients with an acute first stroke (78% ischemic stroke and 22% intracerebral hemorrhage) hypertension was a significant risk factor for all the stroke with an OR of 2.64.[20]

Following a stroke and to a lesser extent transient ischemic attack (TIA), the risk of cognitive impairment is dramatically increased. A prospective incidence study of 92,728 people living in the United Kingdom found that among 2,305 stroke patients, the dementia incidence was 34.4% in 1 year after a severe stroke.[21] Compared to a matched population, the risk of dementia was increased by nearly 50-fold following a major stroke. Poststroke cognitive impairment may not; however, be immediately recognizable as dementia. A meta-analysis of 21 studies found that in the first year following a stroke, 4 out of 10 patients exhibited cognitive impairment that was not sufficient to meet the diagnostic criteria of dementia.[22]

Hypertension and Alzheimer's Disease

The evidence that hypertension is a risk factor for AD is less clear, partially because of the difficulty in distinguishing AD from other forms of dementia. Most cases of cognitive impairment or dementia are found to have multiple pathologies and cerebrovascular disease is a frequent finding.[24,25] In a study of 50 people with dementia, 38% had AD and infracts, 30% were assessed as having pure AD and 12% had vascular dementia.[25] Furthermore, cerebral amyloid angiopathy appears to increase the risk of microhemorrhage and microinfarction, as well being a marker for the onset of AD.[26] It is likely that multiple pathologies overlap to increase the risk of cognitive impairment and dementia.

Longitudinal data from population studies indicate that a systolic BP ≥ 160 mm Hg in midlife is associated with an increased risk of AD later in life, compared to normotensive individuals.[27] In particular, the combination of an elevated systolic BP and high serum cholesterol significantly increased the odds of people developing AD, compared to those with only one of these risk factors. The association between midlife hypertension and AD has also been confirmed by a meta-analysis that found moderate-to-high evidence that midlife hypertension was a risk factor for AD, as was elevated midlife diastolic BP.[11] When a stratified analysis was performed, a diastolic BP > 90 mm Hg was associated with a 51% increase in the risk of developing AD.

THE CEREBROVASCULAR PATHOPHYSIOLOGY OF HYPERTENSION

The long-term effects of persistent hypertension on the cerebrovascular system are wide-reaching and profound. Importantly, this includes structural adaptations to the cerebral arteries and arterioles to protect the distal micro-circulation from the increase in transmural pressure.[2,28] Endothelial dysfunction, neurovascular uncoupling and damage to the blood–brain barrier are also likely to contribute to impairments in cerebral blood supply, neuroinflammation and the promotion of amyloid pathologies.[28,29]

Cerebral small vessel disease (cSVD) is the most notable consequence of a long-term exposure of the cerebrovasculature to persistent elevations in BP.[2] The most common manifestations of cSVD are deep perforator arteriopathy and cerebral amyloid angiopathy, both of which are thought to cause ischemic stroke, intracerebral hemorrhage, and vascular cognitive impairment.[30,31] cSVD is associated with WML on magnetic resonance imaging (MRI), lacunar infarcts, cerebral microhemorrhage and enlarged perivascular spaces as well as cognitive impairment and dementia.[28,32]

Endothelial Dysfunction

Long-term hypertension provokes changes in the vascular endothelium that stimulate vasospasm, promote thrombosis, macrophage infiltration, cellular growth, and inflammation, all of which contribute to atherosclerosis.[33] Impaired endothelium-dependent vasodilation has also been associated with WML in a small group of older people with cardiovascular disease (CVD).[34] Furthermore, endothelial dysfunction may be predictive of the severity of cSVD, as assessed by the presence of WML and microhemorrhages.[35] It has also been suggested that long-term exposure to hypertension may cause dysfunctional endothelium-mediated neurovascular coupling responses, potentially impairing the regulation of the cerebral blood flow (CBF).[28]

White Matter Lesions

The presence of WML indicates alterations in the water content of the white matter's tracts and fibres.[36] Pronounced WML are thought to represent demyelination and degradation of axons.[28] Clinically, the presence of WML on MRI **(Figs. 1A and B)** is considered to be a marker of cSVD, although because multiple pathologies can result in an increased white matter signal intensity, the presence of WML may not confirm a diagnosis of cSVD.[31]

The causes of WML include disrupted cerebrovascular autoregulation, ischemia, inflammation, endothelial activation and gliosis, all of which may be driven by underlying hypertension.[28,32]

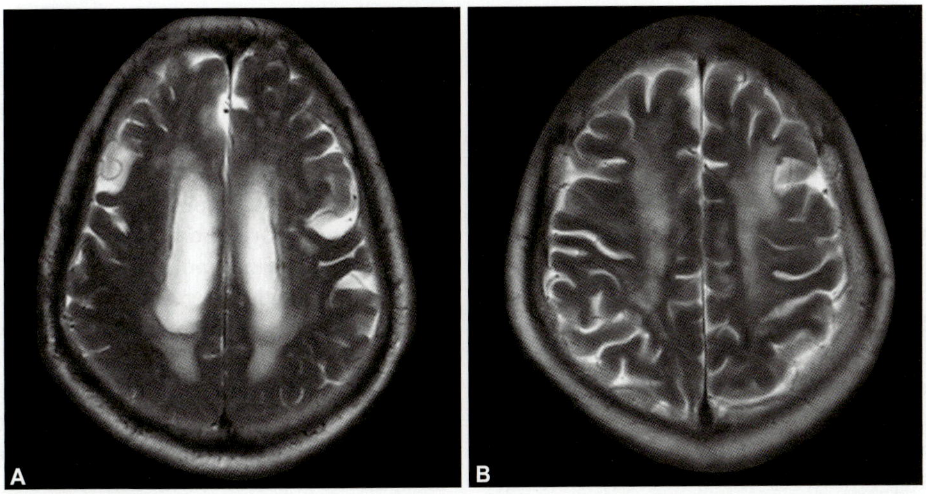

FIGS. 1A AND B: White matter lesions (WMLs). (A) Periventricular WMLs on a T2-weighted magnetic resonance imaging (MRI) and (B) Subcortical WMLs on a T2-weighted MRI.[32]

People aged >60 years with hypertension have increased rates of subcortical and periventricular WML on MRI, compared to normotensive people of the same age.[37] In people with >20 years of exposure to hypertension, the relative risk of subcortical and periventricular WML was 24.3 and 15.8 times higher, respectively, compared to normotensive individuals. Additional studies, have shown that not only that is hypertension associated with an increased risk of WML, individuals with treated or controlled hypertension have a decreased risk of WML, compared to those with uncontrolled hypertension.[38,39] Furthermore, a 3-year study of 639 older patients without disability found that severe age-related white matter changes independently and strongly predicted a rapid decline in global cognitive function.[40] Data from 1,077 people aged 60–90 years in the Rotterdam Scan study also indicate that WML, especially periventricular WML, are associated with an increased risk of dementia.[41]

Lacunar Infarcts

It is estimated that cSVD is the underlying factor in one-quarter of all acute ischemic strokes, most of which are lacunar infarcts.[31] Approximately 90% of subclinical brain infarcts are also thought to be lacunar infarcts.[28]

Hypertension-related cSVD is thought to be the primary cause of lacunar infarcts, following progressive stenosis and/or spontaneous thrombosis of the distal vasculature supplying blood to the deep white matter, basal ganglia, thalamus, and pons.[28,31] These subcortical infarctions are generally small and although they are thought to occur due to disease within the small deep perforating arteries, they may occasionally be caused by brain ischemia following cardiac embolism or carotid artery stenosis.[31] Lacunar infarcts are considered to be a feature of cSVD, along with WML.[28]

Despite their relatively small size (<1.5–2 cm in axial diameter), lacunar strokes are associated with similar rates of MCI or dementia following the event as nonlacunar strokes.[42] A meta-analysis found that up to 4 years after a lacunar stroke, the prevalence of dementia was 20% and the incidence of MCI or dementia was 37%. MCI or dementia was present in similar proportions with lacunar and nonlacunar stroke. Given that lacunar strokes are small, it is likely that the concurrent presence of cSVD contributes to their association with a declining cognitive function.[31,42]

Cerebral Microhemorrhage

Cerebral microhemorrhage is the most common hemorrhagic radiological feature of cSVD.[2] These are focal hemorrhages <5 mm in diameter caused by fissures in small intracerebral blood vessels, visible due to deposition of paramagnetic material.[2,28] The pathology underlying cerebral microhemorrhages is suggested by their pattern of distribution. Microhemorrhages deep within the basal ganglia and brainstem are associated with hypertension and its sequelae such as left ventricular hypertrophy and arterial stiffening, while a purely lobar distribution is associated with cerebral amyloid angiopathy, thought to be caused by β-amyloid accumulation in small cortical and leptomeningeal vessels. Systolic BP, diastolic BP and age are independent risk factors for cerebral microhemorrhages and a correlation has also been reported between hypertension severity and the number of microhemorrhages.[43,44] Data from the Framingham study also indicates that the prevalence of microhemorrhages increases with an increased duration of exposure to hypertension.[45] A weaker association has been reported in hypertension and lobar hemorrhage in patients with cerebral amyloid angiopathy, which is consistent with hypertension aggravating but not causing this condition.[2]

Alzheimer Pathology

Determining how vascular and AD pathologies might interact is challenging. As previously noted, >50% of the patients with

AD have vascular lesions, and mixed dementia comprising AD and vascular pathology is the most frequent form of late-life dementia.[46] There is evidence that vascular disease may precede the onset of AD, as midlife but not late-life hypertension is associated with cerebral amyloid deposition in older individuals.[47]

The potential mechanisms by which hypertension may influence the amyloid deposition and neurodegeneration seen in AD patients remain controversial. Rodent models suggest that hypertension is associated with increased cerebral accumulation of β-amyloid, hyperphosphorylated tau and cognitive impairment.[48-50] Additional studies suggest that antihypertensives may slow the onset of AD pathology in murine models and improve spatial learning.[51,52]

Blood–brain barrier dysfunction has also been suggested as an important step toward AD onset, whereby molecules toxic to both the neuronal and cerebrovascular architecture accumulate within the brain, resulting in reduced CBF, hypoxia, and potential neurodegeneration.[53] This hypothesis is supported by evidence that reduced glucose transport into the brain of mice overexpressing the β-amyloid precursor protein leads to AD pathology, reduced β-amyloid clearance, behavioral deficits, and neuronal degeneration.[54]

It is also possible that the vascular and neurodegenerative pathologies seen in many older patients with dementia is bidirectional.[55] Deposition of β-amyloid may therefore be a consequence and a cause of cSVD and the two processes may be intwined in a destructive cycle, driving the onset and progression of a mixed dementia.

PREVENTING OR MODIFYING COGNITIVE DECLINE

Longitudinal epidemiological studies have clearly established hypertension as a risk factor for cognitive decline and dementia during later life. However, little is known as to the extent to which treating hypertension can prevent, modify, or even potentially reverse the pathology underlying late-life cognitive deterioration. This is partially due to the design of the relevant randomized controlled trials (RCTs), where the primary outcomes of interest were major cardiovascular events (MACE), stroke, and mortality, rather than cognitive function.[56]

Prospective Trials with Cognitive Decline as Primary Outcome

Results from early RCTs involving antihypertensive treatment with cognitive decline as a primary outcome have provided mixed results. In some cases, study design or early study termination may have contributed to these equivocal findings.

The Syst-Eur (Systolic Hypertension in Europe) trial was a double-blind, placebo-controlled study designed to determine whether antihypertensive medicines could reduce the incidence of dementia.[57] The study enrolled participants aged >60 years with isolated systolic hypertension and compared placebo (n = 1,180) to active treatment (n = 1,238) with nitrendipine and potentially enalapril and/or hydrochlorothiazide to reduce systolic BP < 150 mm Hg. After a median follow-up of 2 years, a 50% reduction in dementia incidence was reported in the active treatment arm, from 7.7 to 3.8 cases per 1,000 patient-years (p = 0.05). Extrapolated, this result suggested that if 1,000 patients with hypertension received antihypertensives for 5 years, 19 cases of dementia might be prevented.

Conversely, the PROGRESS (Perindopril Protection Against Recurrent Stroke Study) did not detect a statistically significant decrease in dementia.[58] This study randomized 6,105 patients with prior stroke or TIA to perindopril and indapamide or placebo, with dementia and cognitive decline being the primary outcomes. Over a mean of 3.9 years of follow-up, dementia was documented in 6.3% of those actively treated and 7.1% of placebo-treated participants (p = 0.2). A statistically significant difference in cognitive decline was detected, however, with a rate of 9.1% in the active treatment group and 11% in the placebo group (p = 0.01)

The HYVET (Hypertension in the Very Elderly Trial) assessed the risks and benefits of antihypertensive treatment in older patients, including an assessment of cognitive function.[59] HYVET did not detect a statistically significant reduction in dementia associated with antihypertensive treatment, although the study was stopped prematurely due to a 21% reduction in all-cause mortality in the treatment arm. At 2 years, there was a mean decrease of –15 mm Hg systolic BP and –5.9 mm Hg diastolic BP between the active treatment and placebo arms with respective rates of incident dementia of 33 and 38 per 1,000 patient-years.

Evidence from Meta-analyses

While HYVET did not detect a statistically significant effect of antihypertensive treatment on dementia incidence, when the results were combined with three other RCTs [Syst-Eur, PROGRESS, and the SHEP (Systolic Hypertension in Elderly Patients) trial] a significant effect was detected in favor of antihypertensive treatment.[59]

A more recent Cochrane review with 30,412 participants included eight studies comparing active treatment with placebo and four nonplacebo trials comparing intensive versus standard BP treatment.[60] The meta-analysis found low certainty evidence that pharmacological treatment of hypertension in patients without prior cerebrovascular disease results in reduced cognitive decline and very low evidence that the treatment in the same patient group prevents dementia.

In contrast, the first individual patient data meta-analysis from placebo-controlled RCTS to assess the effects of antihypertensive treatment on dementia prevention did find class I evidence supporting the use of BP-lowering treatments in mid and later life to reduce the risk of dementia.[61]

The synthesized data included 28,008 participants from 20 countries with 861 cases of incident dementia recorded over a median follow-up of 4.3 years. The adjusted OR in favor of antihypertensive treatment was 0.87 [95% confidence interval (CI) 0.75–0.99] with a mean BP reduction of 10/4 mm Hg.

Sprint Mind Trial

Perhaps the most significant RCT assessing the effect of antihypertensives on the risk of dementia is SRINT MIND (Systolic Blood Pressure Intervention Trial–Memory and Cognition in Decreased Hypertension). An important feature of this trial is that it is the only relevant prospective trial to date that has employed expert adjudicated assessment of dementia or cognitive decline.[24]

The SPRINT MIND randomized 9,361 participants aged ≥50 years with hypertension but without diabetes or stroke history to a systolic BP target of <120 or <140 mm Hg.[62] The primary outcome was adjudicated probable dementia. The trial was stopped early due to reductions in CV events and all-cause mortality associated with intensive treatment, therefore, the median intervention duration was 3.3 years. Over a median follow-up of 5.1 years, dementia was detected in 149 patients receiving intensive treatment and 176 in those receiving standard care (HR 0.83; 95% CI 0.67–1.04; $p = 0.1$) **(Fig. 2)**. Intensive BP control did significantly reduce the risk of MCI (14.6 vs. 18.3 cases per 1,000 person-years; HR 0.81; 95% CI 0.69–0.95) and the composite rate of MCI or probable dementia (20.2 vs. 24.1 cases per 1,000 person-years; HR 0.85; 95% CI 0.74–0.97). It is possible that the early termination of the study and the fewer than expected cases of incident dementia meant that the study was under-powered with respect to its primary outcome.

A subset analysis was performed on 673 volunteers from SPRINT MIND to determine the effect of intensive versus standard BP control on AD-related brain biomarkers.[63] Patients receiving intensive treatment underwent a small but statistically significant reduction in hippocampal volume, compared to those receiving standard treatment. Significant differences between the groups were not detected for AD regional atrophy, CBF, or mean fractional anisotropy. Interestingly, the reduction in mean hippocampal volume was consistent with a reduction in total brain volume associated with intensive BP-lowering treatment that was reported by another study.[64]

Another subset analysis of SPRINT MIND assessed the influence of intensive systolic BP control versus standard control on whole brain CBF.[65] This study found that intensive treatment was associated with an increased CBF from the baseline, compared to the standard BP management. Additionally, the increase in CBF associated with intensive management was largest in those with a history of CVD.

Blood Pressure Variability

It has been proposed that blood pressure variability (BPV) may be a more important risk factor for cognitive decline and dementia than elevated BP.[24] To investigate this hypothesis, a post hoc analysis of SPRINT MIND was undertaken in which BPV was calculated as tertiles of systolic BP standard deviation.[66] In patients with excellent BP control, the respective dementia rates were 2.4, 3.6, and 5.4% ($p < 0.001$)

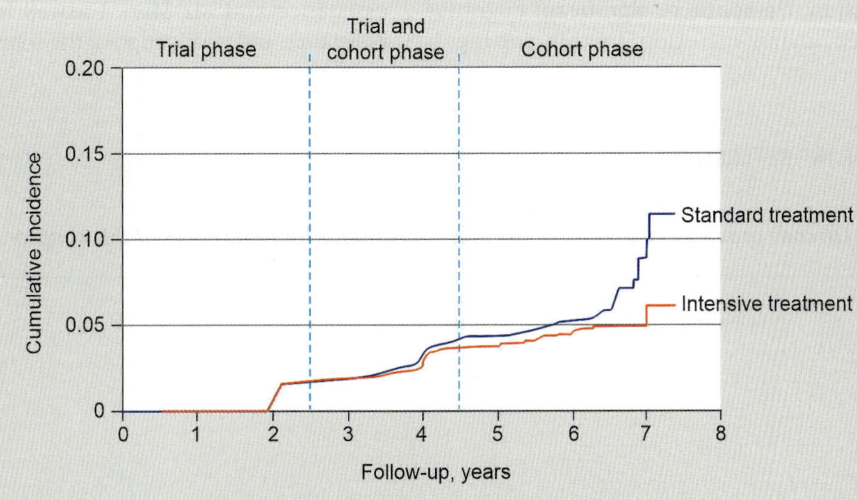

No. at risk									
Standard treatment	4,285	4,282	4,168	3,886	2,829	2,107	989	87	0
Intensive treatment	4,278	4,277	4,171	3,917	2,893	2,189	1,027	93	0

FIG. 2: Probable dementia in patients undergoing intensive or standard blood pressure control.[62]

for ascending tertiles of BPV and compared to the lowest tertile, the adjusted HR for dementia in the highest tertile was 1.69 (95% CI 1.25–2.28).

The results of the post hoc analysis of SPRINT MIND were corroborated by a meta-analysis that found the mean BPV effect size with regards to dementia and cognitive impairment was stronger than the mean effect size of BP.[67]

FUTURE UNANSWERED QUESTIONS

Currently, our understanding of the effect of hypertension on cognitive decline and dementia onset is limited by a lack of robust prospective trials with vascular dementia as the primary outcome. Methodological criticisms have also arisen as to whether the cognitive tests used in many of the trials are the most appropriate way to detect dementia with a vascular component,[24] for example, the domains of cognitive function thought to be most severely impaired by hypertension are abstract reasoning and/or executive function, memory, and mental processing speed.[28] WMLs associated with cSVD have also been specifically linked to a reduced information processing speed and executive function.[36] The mini-mental state examination (MMSE) used to assess cognitive function in many studies evaluates attention and orientation, memory, registration, recall, calculation, language, and drawing ability, and is thought to be relatively insensitive to executive function and declining processing speed.[24,68] Furthermore, a lack of specialist adjudication in the diagnosis of cognitive impairment and dementia, as was used in SPRINT MIND, also calls into question the accuracy of many of the diagnoses in the trials data.

Patients with dementia are routinely excluded from clinical trials assessing the effect of antihypertensives on cognitive function. Dementia or significant cognitive impairment as exclusion criterion in this setting is understandable, not least because the safety of aggressive BP control in this population that is likely to have cerebrovascularpathology is unknown. The consequence of these exclusion criteria, however, is that it is not possible to determine to what extent cognitive impairment with a vascular cause is reversible.

Additional questions that need to be addressed in the future studies include:

- What is the optimal stage of life to initiate antihypertensive interventions to prevent the onset of cognitive decline?
- Which antihypertensive medicines are the most effective at improving cognitive outcomes?
- Can biomarkers and/or genetic testing identify individuals at high-risk of developing dementia who may benefit from early and aggressive BP control?

CONCLUSION

Hypertension has long been recognized as a major risk factor for stroke and midlife hypertension is now established as a modifiable risk factor for late-life dementia.[5] As dementia cannot be cured and there are currently no pharmacological interventions known to prevent or reverse dementia, the potential benefits of early BP control in aging populations cannot be overstated. Increasingly this point is being recognized with improving CV health in the general population recommended as a strategy to lower the prevalence and incidence of cognitive decline.[69]

ACKNOWLEDGMENT

The authors thank Ms Madhavi Lata for her secretarial assistance and Mr Mark Caswell for his expert editorial assistance and verification of the source references.

ONLINE REFERENCES

Please scan the QR code provided at the end of the table of contents for References of this chapter.

CHAPTER

34

Pulse Wave Velocity as an Indicator of Cardiovascular Disease in Hypertension

Mansi Kaushik, Ravi R Kasliwal, Manish Bansal

ABSTRACT

Hypertension is one of the most significant risk factors for cardiovascular diseases (CVDs). In hypertensive individuals, arterial stiffness is high and requires high pressure to stretch to a similar degree as in normotensive individuals. Arterial stiffness implies loss of arterial compliance and alterations in vessel wall properties affecting the flow and pressure at the peripheral sites. Consequently, there is a short capillary transit time and reduced metabolic exchange, causing tissue damage to the target organs.

Arterial stiffness can be determined by measuring pulse wave velocity (PWV), a noninvasive and reproducible method accepted widely. Since pathophysiological effects of arterial stiffness is mainly observed in aorta, carotid-femoral PWV (cfPWV), along the aortic and aortoiliac pathway, is considered to be the most clinically important measure of arterial stiffness.

The measurement of arterial stiffness has been recommended by the European Society of Hypertension-European Society of Cardiology Guidelines and American Heart Association for the management of hypertension. The interplay between aging, blood pressure, and arterial stiffness is a complex process. Role of angiotensin II and other growth factors on arterial stiffness provides a direction for future research areas for prevention of hypertension and cardiovascular (CV) events.

Keywords: Pulse wave velocity, hypertension, arterial stiffness.

INTRODUCTION

Hypertension is one of the most significant risk factors for cardiovascular diseases (CVDs), which include coronary artery disease, left ventricular hypertrophy, valvular heart diseases, and cardiac arrhythmias. Studies have demonstrated an independent association between increase in blood pressure and the incidence of several cardiovascular (CV) events such as stroke, myocardial infarction (MI), sudden death, heart failure, and peripheral arterial disease[1-3] in patients of all ages and ethnic groups.[3,4] Further, the association between blood pressure and consequent CV morbidity and mortality is modified by presence of metabolic risk factors such as lipid abnormalities and glucose intolerance or type 2 diabetes mellitus.[5,6]

EFFECT OF AGING ON BLOOD PRESSURE

Longitudinal and cross-sectional studies have observed that prevalence of hypertension increases with increasing age. Framingham heart study has underlined the association between advancing age and increase in prevalence of hypertension.[6,7] The systolic blood pressure (SBP) rises relatively more than the diastolic blood pressure (DBP) with advancing age.

While SBP keeps on rising until 80–90 years of age, the DBP, on the contrast, reaches a plateau around 50 years of age and then tends to decrease with advancing age. As an aftereffect to decrease in DBP after 60 years of age, there is a gradual increase in pulse pressure (PP) with advancing age. Whereas, the increase in SBP and DBP before 50 years of age is considered due to increase in peripheral vascular resistance, increase in large artery stiffness is the most likely cause of fall in DBP after the age of 60 years.[8-13] For reasons explained above, isolated systolic hypertension (SBP > 140 mm Hg and DBP < 90 mm Hg) is a commonly observed form of hypertension in elderly subjects > 60 years of age. The blood pressure pattern between men and women also varies with age. It is observed that the women have a lower prevalence of hypertension then men during young age. Blood pressure is lower in young women (age < 40 years) than men, and reaches similar values around 40 years of age and keeps rising as the age progresses. It is further noticed that BP, in women around 70 years of age, is higher than in men.[14]

ARTERIAL STIFFNESS, STIFFNESS GRADIENT, WAVE REFLECTION, AND CENTRAL BLOOD PRESSURE

Arterial stiffness implies loss of arterial compliance and alterations in vessel wall properties. Compliance of large arteries in normal physiological state is characterized by their ability to dampen the pulsatility of ventricular ejection and to convert a pulsatile pressure/pulsatile flow in ascending aorta into a continuous pressure/flow in arterioles, maintaining the organ perfusion, and reducing the energy expenditure. The ventricular systole pushes forward part of stroke volume to peripheral tissues, while part of stroke volume transitorily remains in the aorta and central arteries, stretching or distending their walls and raising the local blood pressure. During ventricular diastole, the stretched aorta recoils back, squeezing the blood forward into peripheral tissues thereby maintain a continuous flow.

The stiffness and geometry of the arteries determine the effectiveness of above function.[15,16] In normotensive individual, arterial stiffness is low and adequate elasticity and distensibility of arterial wall facilitate continuous perfusion of peripheral tissues at a lower pressure as explained above. However, in hypertensive individuals, arterial stiffness is high and requires high pressure to stretch to a similar degree as in normotensive individuals.

A higher arterial stiffness means an intermittent flow and pressure at the peripheral sites. It is because a greater fraction of stroke volume will flow down the arterial system and peripheral tissues during systole, giving rise to excessive flow and pressure pulsatility at the distal small resistance arteries and capillaries. Consequently, there is a short capillary transit time and reduced metabolic exchange, causing tissue damage to the target organs. The pressure pulsatility further amplify the wave reflection as described in below section.[15,16]

Stiffness Gradient, Wave Reflection, and Central BP

The difference in elastic properties of proximal large arteries and distal medium sized arteries creates a stiffness gradient along the arterial tree. In normotensive subjects, the distensibility of arteries decreases as blood flows down from proximal large arteries to distal medium-sized arteries. This is because the proximal arteries have relatively higher amount of vascular smooth muscle cells (VSMCs) and extracellular matrix (ECM) (specifically elastic lamellae) in its media, than the distal muscular arteries.[15,17]

The difference between the elasticity, distensibility and therefore the stiffness gradient between elastic proximal arteries and stiffer medium size muscular arteries creates a mismatch in impedance, thereby generating a partial wave reflections, i.e., partial reflection of forward pressure waves travelling back to the central aorta (also called as reflected wave). Additionally, geometric tapering, branching of arteries, and microvascular network contribute to the phenomenon of wave reflection.[8,16,18] Partial wave reflection is a protective phenomenon as it limits the transmission of pulsatile energy to the periphery and protects the peripheral microcirculation. In hypertensive patients, the stiffness gradient diminishes due to increase in stiffness and the reflected wave travels more swiftly. Less wave reflections are generated. The early reflected waves superimpose on the forward wave and boost the systolic pressure further. This is how increase in central PP and SBP is observed due to early return of reflected waves in late systole in cases of hypertension-induced arterial stiffening. Moreover, pulsatile pressure is not sufficiently dampened and is transmitted toward periphery, damaging the microcirculation.

Cellular and Molecular Determinants of Arterial Stiffness

Intrinsic structural abnormalities are considered to be the likely cause of increase in arterial stiffness, which leads to rise in PP and decrease in DBP with aging. These structural abnormalities include breaking or fragmentation of elastin fibers, crosslinking of elastin network, increase in collagen, necrosis of medial smooth muscle, and calcification in vascular wall of large arteries.[10,19-21]

Measurement of Arterial Stiffness

Arterial stiffness can be determined by measuring the pulse wave velocity (PWV), a noninvasive, and reproducible method accepted widely. Arterial stiffness can be measured at both regional and local arterial level. Since pathophysiological effects of arterial stiffness are mainly observed in aorta, carotid-femoral PWV (cfPWV), along the aortic and aortoiliac pathway, is considered to be the most clinically important measure of arterial stiffness. cfPWV is calculated by foot-to-foot velocity method as cfPWV = D [meters/Δt (seconds)], where D is the distance covered by the waves, i.e., surface distance between the two recording sites from various wave forms, and Δt is the transit time or time delay.

The PWV in the arterial system in normotensive human subjects reveals an increasing trend from ascending aorta (4–5 m/s) to abdominal aorta (5–6 m/s) and even higher in iliac and femoral arteries (8–9 m/s).[15,22] Further, a decreasing order is observed in cross-sectional distensibility when measured in thoracic aorta (40 $kPa^{-1} \times 10^{-3}$), to carotid and brachial arteries (25 $kPa^{-1} \times 10^{-3}$), common femoral artery (10–15 $kPa^{-1} \times 10^{-3}$), and radial artery (5 $kPa^{-1} \times 10^{-3}$).[17,23-29]

Age and blood pressure are the key determinants of cfPWV. Several studies[26,30-34] have observed a higher cfPWV in hypertensive patients as compared to normotensive subjects for a given age.

Methods/Equipment to Measure Pulse Wave Velocity

Pulse wave velocity can be measured with several methods. These can be classified into four categories: (1) devices that use a probe or tonometer to record the pulse wave with a transducer, e.g., tonometry-based techniques (e.g., the SphygmoCor device, AtCor Medical, West Ryde, NSW, Australia) using a piezoelectric Millar tonometer that is placed at any two sites where a pulse is detectable. Mechano-transducer-based techniques (e.g., Complior, ALAM Medical, Vincennes, France) use similar principles and allow simultaneous measurement between sites with distention sensors. The Complior software provides an online pulse wave recording and automatic calculation of the PWV.[18] Other devices (e.g., PulsePen, DiaTecne, Milan, Italy) use an ECG signal and a handheld tonometer (similar to the SphygmoCor). (2) Devices which use cuffs placed around the limbs or the neck that record arrival of the pulse wave oscillometrically (e.g., VP1000, Omron Healthcare, Kyoto, Japan). These devices calculate brachial-ankle PWV (baPWV; measured in meters per second). (3) Ultrasonography methods; ultrasonography can estimate vessel distention and stiffness indexes or flow waveforms to calculate PWV. Distention waveforms can be assessed on the carotid and femoral sites (e.g., ARTLAB, ESAOTE, Genoa, Italy). (4) Magnetic resonance imaging (MRI)-based method; MRI can be used similar to ultrasonography to determine distention-based indexes or PWV. It has the advantage of being able to assess almost any vessel and providing more accurate distance and area estimates (vessels can always be "cut" in a perpendicular manner). However, these advantages are offset by poorer time and spatial resolution and cost. **Table 1 and Figures 1A and B** provide recordings of PWV in a patient.

Arterial Stiffness/PWV and Cardiovascular Mortality: Mechanism

Several mechanisms, as given in **Flowchart 1**, may help us understand how increased PWV leads to CV complications.

PROGNOSTIC VALUE AND CLINICAL USEFULNESS OF PULSE WAVE VELOCITY

The measurement of arterial stiffness has a clinical importance and has been recommended by the European Society of Hypertension-European Society of Cardiology Guidelines for the Management of Hypertension.[35-37] The cfPWV is considered a gold standard for determining arterial stiffness, and it has been shown to have an independent predictive value for all-cause CV mortality, fatal and nonfatal coronary events and fatal strokes in general population, and patients with type 2 diabetes mellitus, hypertension, end-stage renal disease (ESRD).[26,30-32,38] Aortic stiffness, according to American Heart Association, is considered a true surrogate endpoint for CV events.[39]

An analysis of Framingham Heart Study by Kaess et al. (2012) revealed that in a 7-year follow-up, cfPWV was a predictor of incident hypertension, and high blood pressure at baseline was not linked to progressive arterial stiffening.[40] The analysis suggests that arterial stiffness is not a consequence of hypertension, but a cause.[40,41] Antihypertensive drugs such as angiotensin-converting enzyme inhibitors (ACEIs) have been shown to reduce arterial stiffness and thus can attenuate the process of vascular ageing.[42] However, there is no clear evidence if lowering blood pressure reduces the stiffness or it is due to direct effect of drugs on the arterial wall.

EVIDENCE: PWV AS PROGNOSTIC INDICATOR FOR CARDIOVASCULAR RISK IN HYPERTENSION

Blacher et al. (1999) conducted a cross-sectional study on a cohort of 710 patients with essential hypertension.[43] The objective of the study was to assess the potential of aortic PWV as a marker of individual CV risk, and to ascertain high-risk patients from a hypertensive population who may or may not have been treated with an antihypertensive agents. *Study Cohort*: It comprised of 710 hypertensive patients (412 men and 298 women) with mean age (±SD) of 60 ± 13 years, with or without previously identified atherosclerotic alterations (AA). Out of the 710 patients, 605 (85%) patients at inclusion were treated with antihypertensive therapy, which included calcium antagonists, β-blockers, diuretics, ACEI, central-acting agents, angiotensin II antagonists, and α-blockers, either alone or in combination. A total of 108 (15%) patients were treated for dyslipidemia with statins or

TABLE 1: Values of pulse wave velocity recorded at different sites against the reference values in a patient.

Cardiovascular risk analysis

Interpretation summary*

- Estimated functional vascular age: 41–43 years
- Framingham risk analysis: Risk of coronary event in 10 years is 1%

Cardiovascular interpretation*

Total cardiovascular risk grade: Borderline with no arterial stiffness

Clinical recommendations

- Modify lifestyle: Weight reduction required
- Check for Heart rate

Therapeutic suggestions**

Lifestyle modification recommended: Modify lifestyle and control lipid levels

*To be clinically correlated.

**Suggestive therapy only. Actual therapy must be decided by the Physician. Please ensure compatibility and avoid contra-indications.

Test report and observations

Parameter	Unit	Normal value	Observed value	Significance*
Heart rate	BPM	60–100	52.0	HR is low. Bradycardia suspected
Blood pressure	mm Hg	120/80	129/75	Normal blood pressure
Pulse pressure	mm Hg	<50	54	PP high by 4 mm Hg: borderline risk
Right baPWV	cm/s	<1369.52	1,205.2	Normal right baPWV
Left baPWV	cm/s	<1369.52	1,252.3	Normal left baPWV
C-F PWV	cm/s	<947.68	790.6	Normal PWVcf
R Bra ASI	mm Hg	20–70	38.0	Normal rbASI
L Bra ASI	mm Hg	20–70	32.3	Normal lbASI
R Ank ASI	mm Hg	20–70	51.0	Normal raASI
L Ank ASI	mm Hg	20 –70	53.3	Normal laASI
R-ABI	–	0.9–1.35	1.17	ABI normal: Peripheral ASO may be absent
L-ABI	–	0.9–1.35	1.10	ABI normal: Peripheral ASO may be absent
Ao Sys	mm Hg	<119	109	Normal aortic systolic pressure
Ao PP	mm Hg	<37	34	Normal aortic pulse pressure
Ao Dia	mm Hg	>72	74	Normal aortic diastolic pressure
Ao AugP	mm Hg	<8	5	Normal aortic augmentation pressure
Alx (Alx@HR75)	%	<18(27)	15(24)	Normal aortic Alx pressure

*This may be clinically correlated.

Also refer to Waveforms and Osc. Envelopes to depict CV risk.

Pressure waveforms with sharp peak (Fast Rise and fall) are normal. Blunted peaks and flat waveforms are abnormal.

Oscillometric envelopes with a temple shape are normal. Other shapes depict abnormal conditions of various types.

(Alx: augmentation index; ASI: arterial stiffness index; ASO: atherosclerosis obliterans; Ao: Aortic; baPWV: brachial ankle PWV; CA: central arterial; C-F PWV: carotid femoral PWV; PA: peripheral arterial; PWV: pulse wave velocity)

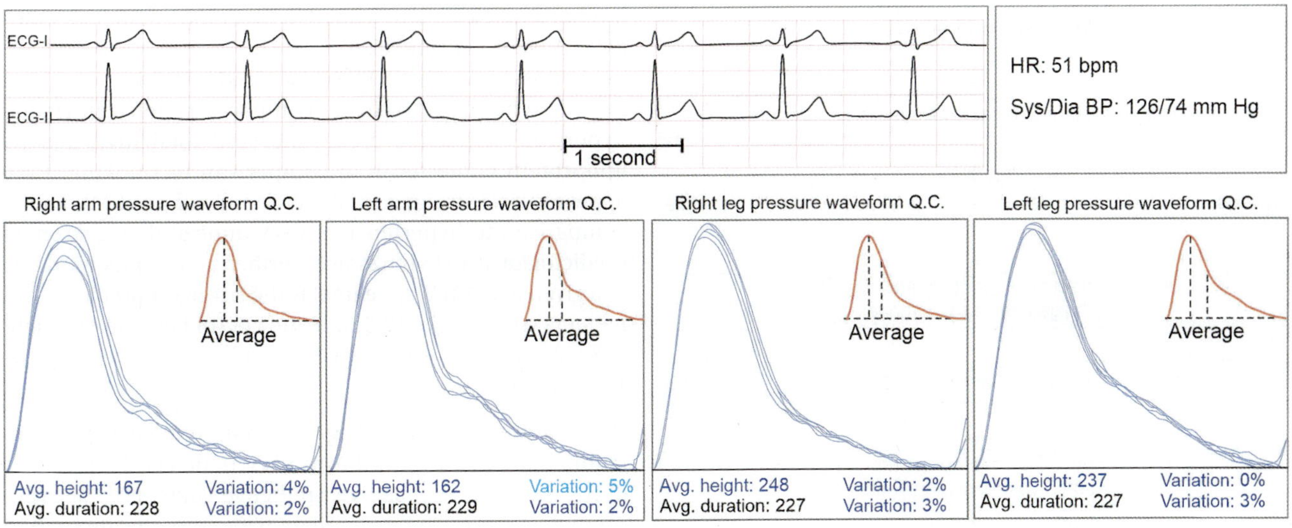

Est. central aortic parameter values

Central aortic parameter	Observed value	Normal value for patient
Aortic systolic pressure	109 mm Hg	Less than 119
Aortic systolic pressure	74 mm Hg	Greater than 72
Aortic pulse pressure	34 mm Hg	Less than 37
Aortic pressure augmentation	5 mm Hg	Less than 8
Aortic augmentation index	15%	Less than 18%
Aortic augmentation index @HR75	24%	Less than 27%
Carotid femoral pulse wave velocity	790.6 cm/s	Less than 947.68 cm/s

Acceptable quality control (Q.C) values:
Avg. waveform height > 40
Height and duration variation < 10%

Observations

Physician

A

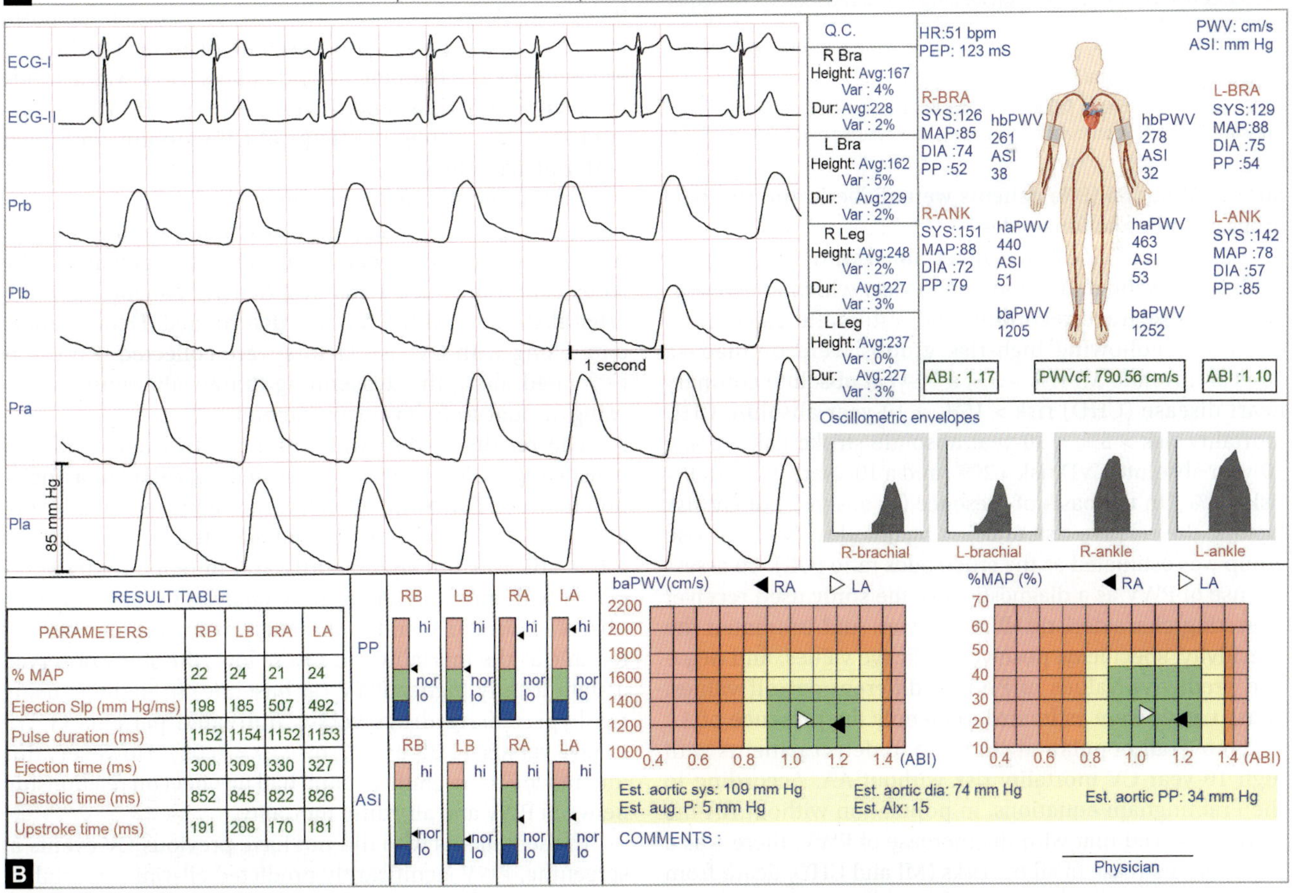

PARAMETERS	RB	LB	RA	LA
% MAP	22	24	21	24
Ejection Slp (mm Hg/ms)	198	185	507	492
Pulse duration (ms)	1152	1154	1152	1153
Ejection time (ms)	300	309	330	327
Diastolic time (ms)	852	845	822	826
Upstroke time (ms)	191	208	170	181

B

FIGS. 1A AND B: Shows pressure wave forms in all four limbs. Pressure wave forms with sharp peak (fast rise and fall) are normal. Blunted peaks and flat waveforms are abnormal.

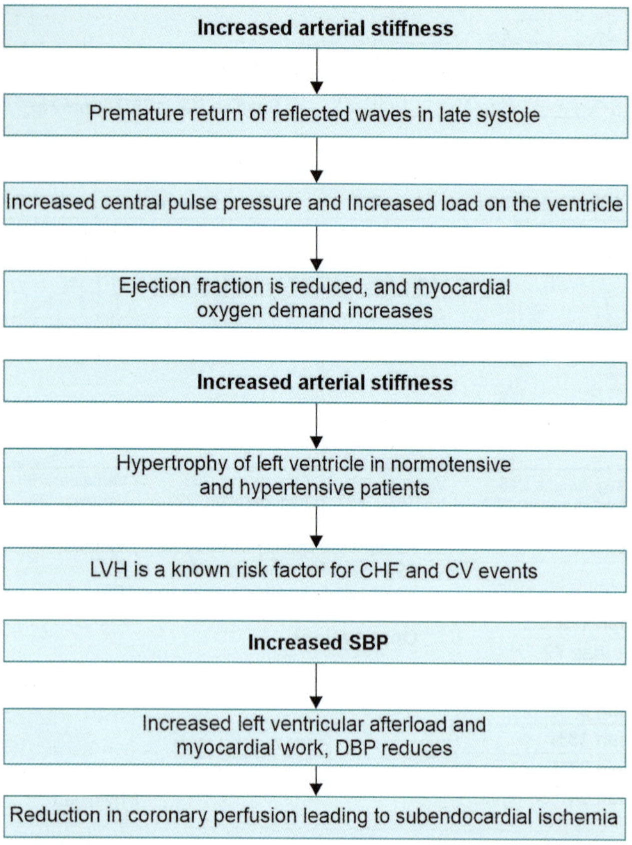

FLOWCHART 1: Several mechanisms of arterial stiffness/PWV and cardiovascular mortality.

(CHF: congestive heart failure; CV: cardiovascular; DBP; diastolic blood pressure; LVH: left ventricular hypertrophy; SBP: systolic blood pressure)

fibrate. About 66 (9%) patients were diabetic and received drugs including sulfonamides and/or biguanides).

Pulse wave velocity was determined with the Complior (Colson), a validated automatic device, which allowed an online pulse wave recording and automatic calculation of PWV.[35] Following high-risk groups were defined—a 10-year absolute MI risk > 5%, a 10-year absolute coronary heart disease (CHD) risk > 15%, a 10-year absolute CHD mortality risk > 5%, a 10-year absolute stroke risk > 5%, a 10-year absolute CVD risk > 20%, and a 10-year CV mortality risk > 5%. On the basis of presence (or absence) of CV risk factors, the relative risk of being included in the high-risk group was estimated as the crude odds ratio (OR). To assess the use of PWV as a diagnostic test, the study used receiver operating characteristic (ROC) curves, and estimated the sensitivity, specificity, positive predictive values, and negative predictive values of PWV at different cut-off values. These values were estimated to identify the presence of AA in the overall population, and also to detect patients with high 10-year CV mortality risk without AA. According to the Framingham equations, in population without AA the study observed that with the increase of PWV, there was a persistent increase of all the risks (MI and CHD, death from CHD, stroke, CVD, and death from CVD), with the same level of statistical significance (correlation coefficients ranging between 0.44 and 0.50).

In this study, aortic PWV appeared a stronger predictor for any type of CV risks, as compared to left ventricular hypertrophy, plasma creatinine, and total/high-density lipoprotein cholesterol; in comparison to smoking, PWV appeared as a stronger predictor for all risks but MI; and in comparison to hypertension, PWV appeared as a stronger predictor for all risks but stroke. Furthermore, for CV mortality at a given age, PWV appeared as the strongest predictor. For patients with PWV > 13.5 m/s, the OR (of being in the high-risk CV mortality) was 7.1 [95% confidence interval (CI) 4.5–11.3].

Pulse wave velocity as a diagnostic test: In the overall population, optimal cut-off value of PWV to detect the presence of AA was 13 m/s [positive predictive value 39%; negative predictive value 84% sensitivity 62%; and specificity 67% (area under ROC curve = 0.69 ± 0.07)].

In the patients' subgroup without AA (age 74 years), PWV cutoff value, to identify patients with high 10-year CV mortality risk, was 13 m/s [(60% sensitivity, 84% specificity, positive predictive value 67%, and negative predictive value 80% (area under ROC curve = 0.78 ± 0.07)].

Overall, the findings of this study suggest that (in treated or untreated subjects with essential hypertension) aortic PWV was strongly related to the presence and extent of AA, including CHD, cerebrovascular disease, abdominal aorta aneurysm, and peripheral vascular disease. Further, as estimated by the Framingham equations, PWV was a strong predictor of CV risks, and the presence of a PWV >13 m/s, appeared as a strong predictor of CV mortality with high performance values.

Laurent et al. (2001) investigated whether aortic stiffness could predict CV and all-cause mortality after CV risk factors have been controlled in hypertensive patients.[30] The study cohort included 1,980 hypertensive patients in whom arterial stiffness with PWV was determined. Demographic data along-with CV risk factors were collected. PWV was estimated along the descending thoracoabdominal aorta using the foot-to-foot velocity method.[35,44]

The results of the study, in a multivariate model of logistic regression analysis, suggested a significant association between PWV with all-cause mortality, independent of age, heart rate, previous CVD, and diabetes. On the contrary, PP or SBP was not significantly and independently associated with mortality. A separate analysis in men only also observed similar results. The analysis in women was not feasible as the mortality rates were low. The study observed a significantly higher PWV (at baseline) in patients using antihypertensive drugs versus untreated patients (11.79 ± 3.64 versus 11.39 ± 3.27 m/s, p = 0.02). However, this difference was insignificant and had no effect on relationship between PWV and all-cause mortality.

In the patients who did not have previous CV events at screening, PWV significantly predicted all-cause mortality. The OR for an increase in PWV of 5 m/s was 1.79 (95% CI

1.45–2.14; $p < 0.001$) in these patients. The study reported a significant association between PWV and CV mortality in a univariate model of logistic regression analysis. PWV, independent of previous CVD, age, and diabetes, was significantly associated with CV mortality in a multivariate model of logistic regression analysis.

When antihypertensive treatment at the original screening was included in a multivariate model of logistic regression analysis, in addition to previous CVD and age, the OR for an increase in PWV of 5 m/s was 1.40 (95% CI 1.08–1.80; $p = 0.01$) for CV mortality. In the multivariate model of logistic regression analysis, the OR for an increase in PWV of 5 m/s was 1.40 (95% CI 1.08–1.80; $p = 0.01$) for CV mortality, when antihypertensive treatment, in addition to previous CVD and age, was included in the analysis. In the patients who did not have previous CV events at entry, PWV significantly predicted CV mortality. The OR, in univariate analysis for an increase in PWV of 5 m/s was 1.60 (95% CI 1.12–2.13; $p = 0.011$).

The study demonstrated that a direct measurement of stiffness may be more helpful than an indirect index, i.e., PP, in the evaluation of the individual risk in hypertensive patients; estimation of aortic stiffness retains predictive power with respect to all-cause and CV deaths, even after other risk factors have been taken into account.

Kawai et al (2012) conducted a prospective cohort study in hypertensive individuals with the objective to determine the cut-off values of baPWV to predict CV prognosis in hypertensive patients.[45] The study was part of NOn-invasive Atherosclerotic Evaluation of Hypertension (NOAH) study,[46] which enrolled patients with essential hypertension. A total of 440 patients with essential hypertension were analyzed with a mean follow-up period of 6.3 ± 0.1 years (study part 1). A second part of the study analyzed 400 patients with essential hypertension, who did not have a past history of CVD/stroke (40 patients with a past history of CVD/stroke were excluded). The mean follow-up in the second part of study was 6.4 ± 0.1 years (study part 2). baPWV was determined using model FCP-4731(Fukuda Denshi Co., Tokyo Japan). The results from the study revealed that in study 1, 30 cases of CVD, 62 stroke + CVD, 35 strokes were reported during the mean follow-up period of 6.3 ± 0.1 years. In study 2, 25 cases of CVD, 48 cases of CVD + stroke, 26 strokes, and 17 deaths were reported during a mean follow-up period of 6.4 ± 0.1 years. ROC analysis was done to obtain cut-off value of baPWV to predict stroke, CVD, and death. ROC curves suggested that a baPWV cut-off value of 1736.0 cm/s predicted CVD (AUC: 0.59,215, sensitivity: 0.6,000, and specificity: 0.6,195). baPWV cut-off value of 1794.0 cm/s predicted stroke + CVD (AUC: 0.59,215, sensitivity: 0.5,323, and specificity: 0.7,037). ROC analysis in second part of the study revealed that baPWV cut-off value of 1,735.0 cm/s predicted CVD (AUC: 0.57,568, sensitivity: 0.5,600, and specificity: 0.6,240). baPWV cut-off value of 1,794.0 cm/s predicted stroke + CVD (AUC: 0.59,129, sensitivity: 0.7,059, and specificity: 0.7,045). From the above results authors concludes that 1,750.0 cm/s is an appropriate cut-off baPWV value for predicting prognosis or onset of stroke, CVD, and stroke + CVD. baPWV higher than 1,750 cm/s is a significant and independent risk factor for the onset of stroke + CVD.

Shlomo et al (2014) conducted a meta-analysis of prospective observational data of 17,635 subjects with 1,785 CVD events from 16 studies.[47] The systematic review determined study-specific association of aPWV with CVD outcomes using Cox proportional hazard models and random effect models to estimate pooled effects. All the studies included in the analysis had a cohort design with at least 1 year of follow-up. Aortic stiffness was assessed by measuring cfPWV. The study observes that aPWV can be useful in predicting future CV events and mortality. aPWV has a stronger predictive value in young subjects versus older subjects, and is not modifiable by hypertension sex, diabetes, smoking, or renal disease. The study further observes that aPWV improved the risk classification particularly in younger subjects at intermediate risk as it improved the 10-year classification by 13%. The observations in this meta-analysis also confirm results of another meta-analysis [Vlachopolous et al, (2010)] in role of aPWV in predicting fatal and nonfatal CV events. The findings from the study suggest that there is a 7% increase in risk of CV events with a 1 m/s increase in aPWV in a nonsmoker, nondiabetic patient aged about 60 years and who is not on any blood pressure medication, etc.

The study observed that among younger individuals that aPWV was a stronger risk factor, although it has a predictive value in older individuals, and that aPWV has less predictive value in models already having systolic pressure included.

Further, the authors suggests that in younger subjects aPWV is a stronger risk factor than SBP, which is a better surrogate of aortic stiffness in older subjects, and therefore aPWV may not provide any additional predictive value to SBP in elderly patients. In other words, systolic pressure or PP is considered to be a poor surrogate for stiffness in younger individuals.[48]

Vlachopolous et al. (2010), in a meta-analysis of 17 longitudinal studies,[31] which followed-up 15,877 subjects for a mean of 7.7 years, calculated the quantitative estimates of the predictive value of aPWV for future CV events (CV deaths and nonfatal CV events, e.g., MI, stroke, revascularization, aortic syndromes, and all-cause mortality) and all-cause mortality. A separate meta-analyses was performed for total CV events, CV mortality, and all-cause mortality. Pooled RRs were calculated for high versus low aortic PWV. The study also estimated pooled RRs for increases in aortic PWV per 1 m/s and 1 SD, as the data showed a linear-graded association between aortic PWV and clinical events.

Total CV events: The extent of risk was significantly higher in individuals with high aPWV versus individuals with low aPWV. For high aPWV, pooled RRs were 2.26 (95% CI 1.89–2.70) for total CV events. The RR of total CV events was 1.14 (95% CI 1.09–1.20) for an increase in aortic PWV by 1 m/s. Additionally, in a population-specific analysis, the results revealed a significant increase in the RR for high aortic PWV in ESRD groups and in hypertensive individuals versus general population (RR 2.81; 95% CI 1.97–4.02 in ESRD groups vs. RR 2.46; 95% CI 1.93–3.13 in hypertensive individuals vs. RR 1.68; 95% CI 1.45–1.96 in general population subject; $p = 0.01$ for ESRD vs. general population subjects and $p = 0.009$ for hypertensive individuals vs. general population subjects). Further, the study found a significant increase in the RR for high aortic PWV in patients with hypertension and ESRD versus general population subjects (RR 2.46; 95% CI 1.93–3.13 in hypertensive individuals vs. RR 2.81; 95% CI 1.97–4.02 in ESRD groups vs. RR 1.68; 95% CI 1.45–1.96 in general population subjects; $p = 0.01$ for ESRD vs. general population subjects and $p = 0.009$ for hypertensive individuals vs. general population subjects).

Cardiovascular mortality: The pooled risk ratios of CV mortality for high aortic PWV were higher versus low aortic PWV subjects (RR 2.02; 95% CI 1.68–2.42). The risk ratios of CV mortality were 1.15 (95% CI 1.09–1.21) and 1.47 (95% CI 1.29–1.66) for an increase in aortic PWV by 1 m/s and 1 SD, corresponding to a risk increase of 15 and 47%, respectively. The RR for high aortic PWV in high-risk populations was higher versus low-risk populations (RR 2.48; 95% CI 1.94–3.18 vs. RR 1.68; 95% CI 1.41–2.01, respectively; $p = 0.013$).

The study noted a higher pooled RRs of CV mortality for high aPWV versus low aPWV (RR 2.02; 95% CI 1.68–2.42). The RRs of CV mortality were 1.15 (95% CI 1.09–1.21) and 1.47 (95% CI 1.29–1.66) for an increase in aortic PWV by 1 m/s and 1 SD, which corresponds to an increase in risk by 15 and 47%, respectively. Higher pooled values of RRs of CV mortality were observed for high aPWV versus low aPWV (RR 2.02; 95% CI 1.68–2.42). The RRs of CV mortality were 1.15 (95% CI 1.09–1.21) and 1.47 (95% CI 1.29–1.66) for an increase in aortic PWV by 1 m/s and 1 SD, which corresponds to an increase in risk by 15 and 47%, respectively. For an increase in aPWV by 1 m/s and 1 SD, the RRs of CV mortality were 1.15 (95% CI 1.09–1.21) and 1.47 (95% CI 1.29–1.66), which corresponds to an increase in risk by 15 and 47%, respectively. The study observed that aortic PWV has predictive value, which is independent of classic CV risk factors.

The study demonstrated that predictive value of aPWV is independent of other typical CV risk factors, and arterial stiffness may potentially integrate effect of genetic background[49] as well as other risk factors on the arterial wall to translate into real risks over a long period of time. The authors observe that their study results highlight that arterial stiffness could be a potential treatment target in patient groups. Overall, the study demonstrates the ability of aPWV in predicting adverse outcomes in subjects with higher baseline CV risks, such as hypertension, CAD, and renal disease as compared to subjects with lower risks.

ANTIHYPERTENSIVE THERAPY AND EFFECT ON ARTERIAL STIFFNESS

Ming Liu et al. (2013) reviewed the findings of 27 clinical trials, which investigated the efficacy of antihypertensive drugs in reducing arterial stiffness (assessed by PWV) and wave reflections [assessed by augmentation index (Aix)].[42] The results of these trials revealed a significant effect of ACEI and angiotensin receptor blockers (ARBs) as compared to other antihypertensive drugs on arterial stiffness. β-blockers were found to have the least effect on reducing AIx, in comparison to all the other classes of antihypertensive drugs. The authors were of the view that these studies were of short duration and in small sample size, and therefore effect of these drugs on CV protection should be investigated further.

Chen et al. (2015) conducted a systematic review and meta-analysis of 10 randomized controlled trials to analyze the clinical benefits of various antihypertensive drugs on reducing the arterial stiffness in hypertensive patients.[50] The review observed no difference in efficacy of antihypertensive drugs in reducing arterial stiffness. Further, efficacy of ARBs was found to be better than other drugs in reducing AIx.

Gismondi et al. (2015), in a clinical trial, compared efficacy of ACEI (benazepril) and ARBs (losartan).[51] The results showed a similar efficacy of both the drugs on PWV and AIx. A slightly higher (45% increase, $p = 0.057$) flow-mediated vasodilation (FMD) response in the ACEI group as compared to the ARB group losartan group (19% increase, $p = 0.132$) was noted in the study.

CONCLUSION

The interplay between aging, blood pressure, and arterial stiffness is complex process, which occurs at a cellular and molecular level. Role of angiotensin II and other growth factors on the cellular and molecular proinflammatory pathophysiology underlying the arterial stiffness has given a direction for future research areas for prevention of hypertension, atherosclerosis, and other CV events.

Though, limited evidence suggests that ACEI may produce blood pressure independent reduction in PWV, much larger studies and meta-analysis will be required in future to establish the same.

ONLINE REFERENCES

Please scan the QR code provided at the end of the table of contents for References of this chapter.

CHAPTER

35 Orthostatic Hypotension: Evaluation and Management

SS Binu

ABSTRACT

Orthostatic hypotension (OH) is a very common and disabling cardiovascular disorder. It can be with or without association with an underlying neurodegenerative disease. OH is diagnosed based on the extent of systolic/diastolic blood pressure decrease during an orthostatic challenge. The prevalence increases with age, ranging from <5% in under 50s to >30% in over 70s. OH can cause disabling symptoms and lead to traumatic injuries as a result of falls. It affects the overall quality of life. The extent of symptoms can range from the asymptomatic and mildly distressing to the severely incapacitating. Nonpharmacological measures alone or a combination of nonpharmacological plus pharmacological treatments may be needed to ameliorate the symptoms and to prevent complications. This chapter attempts to discuss the prevalence, classification, evaluation, and management of OH.

Keywords: Orthostatic hypotension, syncope, autonomic dysfunction, midodrine, fludrocortisone.

INTRODUCTION

Orthostatic intolerance defines the inability to tolerate the upright posture as a consequence of autonomic dysfunction. It can be classified into three categories as follows:

1. Orthostatic hypotension (OH)
2. Reflex syncope
3. Postural tachycardia syndrome (POTS)

This chapter deals with OH only.

PREVALENCE

The prevalence increases with advancing age. This is due to normal physiological decline in baroreceptor sensitivity as well as due to age-associated increased prevalence of autonomic neurodegenerative disease. The prevalence ranges from 5% in patients <50 years of age to 30% in those above 70 years.[1-4]

Orthostatic hypotension is the second most common etiology of syncope, occurring in about 15% of syncope presentations. It frequently affects older people and patients who have neurodegenerative disease, diabetes, or hypertension.

CLASSIFICATION

Orthostatic hypotension can be classified as either primary or secondary **(Box 1)**.[5,6]

Orthostatic hypotension can also be classified on the basis of pathophysiology into two categories: structural (neurogenic) and functional (non-neurogenic). Neurogenic OH is a result of autonomic failure due to primary

BOX 1 Etiological classification of OH.

Primary:
- Parkinsonism, multiple system atrophy, pure autonomic failure, autoimmune autonomic ganglionopathy, etc.

Secondary:
- Iatrogenic (drug induced), DM, cardiovascular diseases such as sinus node dysfunction, AV blocks, heart failure, aortic stenosis, PAH, etc.
- Renal failure, volume depletion, venous pooling, endocrine disorders, etc.

(AV: atrioventricular; DM: diabetes mellitus; OH: orthostatic hypotension; PAH: pulmonary arterial hypertension)

neurodegenerative disorders such as pure autonomic failure, Parkinsonism, and multiple system atrophy. It can also be associated with neurological dysfunction secondary to systemic disorders such as diabetes, amyloidosis, and severe kidney disease.[7]

In case of functional or non-neurogenic OH, the causes include treatment with vasodilators, tricyclic antidepressants, diuretics, or chemotherapeutic agents; absolute or relative reduction in circulating blood volume; venous pooling; rhythm disorders, heart failure, and valvular heart diseases, etc.[8,9]

On the basis of temporal changes, three different clinical variants of OH are as follows:

1. *Classic OH*: It is defined as a sustained reduction in systolic blood pressure (SBP) of at least 20 mm Hg and/or diastolic blood pressure (DBP) of at least 10 mm Hg, within 30–180 seconds of active standing or during a head-up tilt test of at least 60°.[10] However, in patients with supine hypertension, a reduction in supine BP of at least 30 mm Hg may be a more appropriate criterion. Classic OH only rarely has symptoms of autonomic failure.
2. *Delayed OH*: There is a slow and progressive drop in BP ≥ 20/10 or ≥ 30/15 mm Hg in hypertensive patients, between 3 and 45 minutes. This disorder may be a less severe or an early form of autonomic failure.[11,12] Absence of bradycardia or pauses differentiates delayed OH from reflex syncope.
3. *Initial OH*: It is defined as a transient BP decrease ≥ 40/20 mm Hg within 15 seconds of standing.[13] It is more common in younger patients,[14] exclusively associated with active standing. The BP fall is not significant during passive tilting. The mechanism may be a short-duration mismatch between a sudden decrease in venous return and neurally mediated compensatory vasoconstriction.[15]

PROGNOSTIC SIGNIFICANCE

Disorders of postural hemodynamic control can predict all-cause mortality and cardiovascular disease incidence.[7,16-18] It could be prognostically more relevant than the ambulatory blood pressure monitoring (ABPM)-derived nocturnal reverse dipping.[19] Higher diurnal BP variability and supine hypertension, which are associated with OH, may lead to intermittently raised afterload, leading to end-organ damage such as left ventricular hypertrophy, left ventricular dysfunction, and renal dysfunction. An association between the higher incidence of atrial fibrillation and presence of hypertension and OH has been noted. However so far, no firm data is there to conclude whether OH is a causative factor or simply a marker or measure of disease severity.

CLINICAL PRESENTATION

The symptoms typically occur when there is sudden orthostatic change but can also occur after meals, exertion, and prolonged standing. These are due to cerebral hypoperfusion and include generalized weakness, light headedness, dizziness, blurred vision, and syncope. "Coat-hanger headache"—neck pain and headache localized in the suboccipital, posterior cervical, and shoulder region—is reportedly seen in about 50–90% patients. Symptoms are often precipitated by warm environments due to peripheral vasodilation. Standing quickly after prolonged sitting results in a sudden redistribution of 500–1,000 mL of blood to the lower extremities and can precipitate severe orthostatic intolerance or even syncope.

Some patients have severe incapacitating symptoms and are unable to leave the supine position without experiencing presyncope or syncope.

In patients with autonomic failure, symptoms are worse in early mornings. Nocturnal diuresis can lead to early morning hypotension, a reversal of the normal circadian variation in BP.[20]

EVALUATION

The diagnosis of OH is based on a single principle—demonstration of significant persistent BP decrease during orthostatic position. This can be done either by a simple bedside active-standing test or by using a head-up tilting test. The testing is done when the clinical picture is suggestive of OH, such as the presence of characteristic postural symptoms, unexplained syncope, or falls. But a significant percentage of people with OH are asymptomatic and may be picked up during routine screening.

The threshold of BP reduction for diagnosis of OH is 20 mm Hg or more in SBP and 10 mm Hg or more in DBP. The BP is taken initially in supine posture after 5 minutes of rest in supine position and then again after the patient is made to stand for 2–5 minutes. Continuous BP monitoring may be needed for some symptomatic patients not identifiable by the initial supine-stand BP measurements. This is performed by using plethysmography that avoids multiple inflations of a sphygmomanometer cuff.

Blood pressure measurement with tilt-table testing may be done to identify patients with delayed OH. In such patients, about half of them have hypotension coming on after 5 minutes of tilt and in 40%, it occurs after 10 minutes.

Heart rate (HR) typically increases as a compensatory mechanism. In non-neurogenic OH, due to volume depletion, it normally rises immediately on standing. If this is absent, it is a useful clinical clue to the presence of neurogenic OH in the setting of autonomic failure.

The ratio of HR increase to BP decrease is a sensitive and specific bedside differentiator between neurogenic and non-neurogenic OH **(Table 1)**.

Increase in HR of >30 beats/min in the absence of OH suggests POTS, which usually does not include OH.

Additional tests may be performed to identify other treatable conditions that could be contributing to OH and to distinguish between neurogenic and non-neurogenic OH.

TABLE 1: Differences between non-neurogenic and neurogenic OH.

	Non-neurogenic OH	Neurogenic OH
Age	65 years or older	40–60 years
Causes	Physical deconditioning, antihypertensives, intravascular volume depletion, and heart failure	Reduced norepinephrine release from sympathetic postganglionic nerves
Prognosis	Resolves with correction of underlying cause	Chronic
Increase in HR on standing	Pronounced	Mild or absent
Change in HR/SBP	>0.5 beats/min/mm Hg	<0.5 beats/min/mm Hg
BP overshoot in phase IV Valsalva	Present	Reduced or absent
Other symptoms of autonomic failure	None	Present

(BP: blood pressure; HR: heart rate; OH: orthostatic hypotension; SBP: systolic blood pressure)

HISTORY AND PHYSICAL EXAMINATION

A detailed history should be taken regarding medications, especially diuretics, adrenergic antagonists such as alpha- and beta-blockers, nitric oxide-mediated vasodilators (nitroglycerine and sildenafil), renin–angiotensin–aldosterone system (RAAS) inhibitors, calcium channel blockers, sodium-glucose cotransporter-2 inhibitors (SGLT-2Is), and psychiatric medications such as antipsychotics and antidepressants (including amitriptyline and serotonin inhibitors).

- Recent medical history of potential volume loss (e.g., vomiting, diarrhea, febrile illness, and fluid restriction)
- History of congestive heart failure (CHF), malignancy, diabetes mellitus (DM), and alcoholism
- Evidence on neurologic history and examination or family history of disorders, such as Parkinsonism, ataxia, and peripheral neuropathies
- Almost one-third of patients will have no identifiable causes after extensive evaluation.

LABORATORY TESTS

Basic tests such as hematocrit, electrolytes, blood urea nitrogen (BUN) and creatinine, glucose, and electrocardiogram (ECG) should be obtained in most patients. This helps to evaluate for underlying problems such as anemia, dehydration, and cardiac or renal disease.

Plasma norepinephrine concentration should be estimated. This helps in guiding medication selection for patients being planned for pharmacotherapy.

In suspected neuropathy, electromyography and nerve conduction studies may be conducted.

To identify patients with baroreflex dysfunction, noninvasive autonomic testing including beat-to-beat BP and HR changes induced by Valsalva maneuver or other standardized stimuli can be obtained to ascertain abnormal baroreflex function. This helps to distinguish them from those with volume depletion or severe physical deconditioning.

COMPLICATIONS

Falls: Increased risk of recurrent falls is there especially when OH is symptomatic in the elderly. This can result in considerable morbidity and mortality in the frail, elderly population.

Cardiovascular disease: Some population-based studies have shown that OH is a risk factor for cardiovascular and all-cause mortality.[7,21,22] This could be due to a combination of the underlying causes and associated diseases. A prospective study using ABPM in 374 elderly people found that systolic OH was a strong predictor of future cardiovascular events.[19] OH has also been linked to increased risk of CHF[23,24], and to incident atrial fibrillation.[25]

Cognitive impairment: OH has been associated with the development of cognitive impairment and dementia. A Swedish longitudinal population-based cohort analysis of 2,532 older adults[26] and Atherosclerosis Risk in Communities (ARIC) study of 11,709 participants[27] showed that OH patients tend to have higher prevalence of cognitive impairment and dementia.

MANAGEMENT

The first step in the management of OH is the evaluation of the severity and frequency of symptoms. Asymptomatic OH is the most prevalent form.

The steps in the management of OH can be classified as:

- Patient education
- Correction of aggravating factors
- Nonpharmacological management
- Pharmacological management

Patient Education

Patients should be educated on the basis of postural physiology and mechanisms of orthostatic intolerance. They should be made aware of the aggravating factors (e.g., warm ambient temperatures, hot baths or showers, straining, especially with breath holding, sudden moves from the supine or seated position to the upright posture, and ingestion of large meals) and learn how to avoid conditions that can trigger symptoms and syncope. They should be trained on physical countermeasures to prevent fall in BP (e.g., leg-crossing, stooping, squatting, and tensing of the muscles of the legs, arms, abdomen, buttocks, or whole body). Patient education regarding prompt recognition of warning signs and symptoms is also very important. Physical activity and exercise should be encouraged to avoid deconditioning.

Correction of Aggravating Factors

Correction of aggravating factors is important in the management of OH patients and should be done as the first step.

Drugs: Medications that reduce intravascular volume or cause vasodilation can lead to OH. These include nitrates, tricyclic antidepressants, diuretics, calcium channel blockers, beta-blockers, alpha-blockers (often prescribed as associated prostatic hypertrophy is common in this age), sildenafil/tadalafil for erectile dysfunction, and centrally acting alpha-2 agonists such as clonidine. Drugs used for Parkinsonism such as levodopa and other dopamine agonists can also cause OH.

Anemia: Anemia of chronic disease is common in these age groups. It reduces blood viscosity and oxygen-carrying capacity and therefore worsens OH. Hemoglobin is a scavenger of nitric oxide, a potent vasodilator.[28] Thus, nitric oxide-mediated mechanisms may enhance vasodilation in patients with OH and concomitant anemia.[29]

Nonpharmacologic Management

Volume expansion: Adequate plasma volume is essential for orthostatic tolerance. It can be increased by increasing sodium intake with high-sodium foods or salt tablets and by increasing fluid intake. Patients should have a dietary intake of at least 2–3 g of sodium per day. Fluid intake should be 2–2.5 L/day.[30-32] A 24-hour urinary sodium excretion of >170 mEq/24 h and a urinary volume of >1,500 mL is considered to indicate adequate salt and fluid intake.

Bolus water drinking: Rapid ingestion of approximately 500 mL water (over 3–4 min) has a fast pressor effect, with the BP increasing within 5–10 minutes. This is useful as a rescue effort, but the effect is relatively short (30–45 min) and usually not very marked in young people.[33] The mechanisms underlying this effect have not been well established. However, it has been observed that venous plasma norepinephrine and muscle sympathetic nerve activity increase after water ingestion and also there is pressor response attenuation after ganglionic blockade with trimethaphan.[34] These suggest a role for sympathetic nervous system activation.

Sleeping with the head of the bed elevated: This is based on observations in studies from the 1940s.[35,36] This intervention was noted to decrease nocturnal water and sodium excretion and reduces the overnight fluid loss. The intervention is particularly effective in whom supine hypertension is associated. Typically, the head end of the bed is raised by 10–20°. The use of pressor agents should be avoided within at least 4 hours before bedtime.

Compression garments: Elastic compression stockings apply counterpressure to the lower limbs and abdomen, reducing venous pooling.[37] Limb and abdomen compression improves orthostatic tolerance in up to 40% of symptomatic patients. The recommended compression pressure is 30–50 mm Hg for legs and 20–30 mm Hg for the abdomen. Leg compression alone is not as effective as abdomen compression since the venous compartment of the legs is smaller than that of the splanchnic region.[38,39] Therefore, "the higher, the better" principle should be applied. But the disadvantage is that the elderly patients, those with movement disorders, etc., will find it difficult to put on these garments.

Pharmacologic Management

The goal of pharmacotherapy is to relieve symptoms. It is not necessary to restore normotension.

The agents used can be classified into three:

1. Drugs that increase blood volume
2. First-line sympathomimetic agents
3. Second-line sympathomimetic agents

Blood Volume-increasing Agents

Fludrocortisone

9-alpha-fludrocortisone is a synthetic steroid with mineralocorticoid activity that enhances sodium reabsorption from renal tubules and urinary excretion of potassium with hydrogen exchange. However, the effects of fludrocortisone on volume expansion through renal sodium reabsorption last for only a few weeks. The main mechanism of action is believed to be sensitization of smooth muscles in the blood vessels to circulating catecholamines.[40,41]

Fludrocortisone usually requires at least 7 days of treatment to exert significant clinical effects. The dosage is usually 0.05–0.2 mg once a day. Higher dosages do not improve therapeutic effects but may lead to significantly increased side effects. The short-term side effects are frequent and include supine hypertension, hypokalemia, and ankle edema.[40] Long-term use exacerbates hypertension and leads to target-organ damage, such as left ventricular hypertrophy and renal failure.[42,43] Long-term use of fludrocortisone and consequent activation of renal mineralocorticoid receptors can result in inflammation and fibrosis and may have a direct nephrotoxic effect, leading to renal failure and worsening of hypertension.[43] Steroid-induced diabetes and secondary adrenal insufficiency are uncommon at usual doses for OH.

The use of this drug is contraindicated in patients with heart failure, kidney failure, or severe hypertension.

Desmopressin

It is a synthetic analog of an endogenous pituitary hormone, 8-arginine vasopressin [antidiuretic hormone (ADH)]. It increases water reabsorption in the renal-collecting ducts by acting on vasopressin receptor type 2. Patients with OH who also have nocturnal polyuria are candidates for desmopressin therapy.

It is usually administered as a nasal spray (5–40 µg) at nighttime.[44] The oral dosage is 100–800 µg. Adverse events include water intoxication and hyponatremia.[45]

Erythropoietin

Orthostatic hypotension patients with autonomic failure sometimes have associated normocytic normochromic anemia, possible due to sympathetic denervation to the kidney.[46-48] Recombinant human erythropoietin administered subcutaneously or intravenously corrects the normochromic anemia, increases standing BP, and improves orthostatic tolerance in patients with OH.[49,50] The dosage used is between 25 and 75 U/kg three times a week until the patient's hematocrit returns to normal. Lower maintenance doses (25 U/kg three times a week) may be continued thereafter. Supine hypertension may accompany the use of erythropoietin.

Sympathomimetic Agents: First-line Drugs

Orthostatic hypotension is largely due to a failure to release norepinephrine appropriately. Therefore, administration of sympathomimetic agents is a central part of the management of patients with OH. If symptoms of orthostatic intolerance persist once the intravascular volume has been replenished, then sympathomimetic drugs should be considered.

The first-line drugs include midodrine and droxidopa.

Midodrine

It is an oral prodrug that is converted peripherally into the active metabolite desglymidodrine, a selective alpha-1 adrenoceptor agonist, which constricts arteriolar and venous vasculature, thus increasing the BP. It was approved by the Food and Drug Administration (FDA) in 1996 for the treatment of symptomatic OH after clinical trials proved its effect on improving orthostatic tolerance.[51] Unlike fludrocortisone, midodrine is a short-acting agent. Standing BP increases by 10–30 mm Hg approximately 1 hour after a 10-mg dose. The effects may persist up to 3 hours. Dosages start with 2.5–5 mg three times a day. They can be increased up to 10 mg thrice a day. Supine hypertension can occur; therefore, the last dose should be taken 3–4 hours before bedtime.

A multicenter, double-blind registration study for midodrine demonstrated that 10 mg three times a day increased standing BP by 21.8 mm Hg and resulted in improvement of symptoms such as light-headedness and fatigue.[52] Another double-blind, placebo-controlled study also showed that this same dosage increased standing BP by 22 mm Hg and improved symptoms including dizziness, fatigue, syncope, inability to stand, and depression in patients with neurogenic OH due to various causes.[53]

Common adverse reactions include supine hypertension, itching (especially scalp itching), pilomotor activation (goose bumps), urinary retention, and headaches.

Droxidopa

It is a synthetic amino acid that is metabolized by DOPA decarboxylase to yield norepinephrine. Therefore, its pharmacological effects are likely to be through an increased level of norepinephrine, resulting in peripheral vasoconstriction. The short-term efficacy of droxidopa has been proven in several multicenter, placebo-controlled studies showing that patients on droxidopa had higher standing BP and symptomatic improvement compared with placebo.[54-56]

Droxidopa was approved in Japan in 1989 for the treatment of neurogenic OH in hereditary amyloidosis, Parkinson disease, and multiple system atrophy.[57] The FDA approved this drug in 2014.

The recommended starting dose is 100 mg t.i.d., which can be titrated to a maximum dose of 600 mg t.i.d. The dosing can be individualized based on the needs of each patient. For example, a patient with movement disorder and OH, who is active only in the morning hours, can do with a single morning dose and skip the afternoon and evening doses. It is well tolerated in most patients with common adverse effects being supine hypertension, headaches, dizziness, and nausea. DOPA decarboxylase inhibitors such as carbidopa can theoretically reduce the effects of droxidopa by decreasing its metabolic conversion to norepinephrine. But this has not been shown to be significant clinically.

Sympathomimetic Agents: Second-line Drugs

This category includes drugs such as pyridostigmine and atomoxetine.

Pyridostigmine

It is a reversible cholinesterase inhibitor that enhances cholinergic neurotransmission in sympathetic and parasympathetic ganglia. The signal transmission normally has low activity in supine position, but its activity increases with postural changes. Pyridostigmine increases BP as well as peripheral vascular resistance in a standing position.[58] A double-blind, placebo-controlled, single-dose study showed 60 mg of pyridostigmine reduced fall in standing DBP.[59]

The efficacy of pyridostigmine is limited in clinical practice and it is commonly chosen as an adjunctive drug. A combination of 5 mg midodrine along with 60 mg of pyridostigmine was more effective than pyridostigmine alone. A combination of pyridostigmine and atomoxetine also appears to have synergistic effect.

Atomoxetine

It is a selective norepinephrine transporter blocker. This increases the synaptic norepinephrine concentrations in postganglionic sympathetic neurons.

Short-term, controlled clinical trials have shown that atomoxetine (10–18 mg b.d.) increases standing BP and improves symptoms compared to placebo in neurogenic OH.[60-62] The efficacy of this drug is more when the norepinephrine levels are higher. This makes it useful for neurogenic OH caused by autonomic decentralization (like multiple system atrophy). On the other hand, lower supine plasma norepinephrine levels predict a greater response to droxidopa.

In patients with refractory neurogenic OH, atomoxetine can be combined with droxidopa or midodrine, with or without fludrocortisone or pyridostigmine. However, extreme caution is advised and no safety data are available.

Supplementary Agents

Other agents from diverse classes that can be used along with first- and second-line sympathomimetic agents include nonselective beta-blockers with intrinsic sympathomimetic activity (e.g., pindolol and xamoterol) and alpha-2 receptor antagonists (e.g., yohimbine). However, none of these has been studied well in trials.

Supine Hypertension

Supine hypertension is present in up to 50% of patients with neurogenic OH. The underlying mechanisms include residual sympathetic activity, angiotensin II elevation, inappropriate mineralocorticoid receptor activation, etc.[63-65] The treatment of supine hypertension includes nonpharmacological and pharmacological interventions. Nonpharmacological interventions include raising the head end of bed at night, small snacks to induce postprandial hypotension, etc. Pharmacotherapy involves usage of low doses of short-acting angiotensin-converting enzyme inhibitors, short-acting calcium-channel blockers, etc.

CONCLUSION

Orthostatic hypotension is a common disorder seen in general population with a prevalence ranging from 5% in those under 50 years of age and going up to 30% in those over 70 years old. In the elderly, this is often the result of drug effects, volume depletion, or cardiovascular deconditioning. Patients with minor symptoms can be managed nonpharmacologically, but moderate-to-severe symptoms need a combination of pharmacological and nonpharmacological therapies. Often, the results of treatment are less than fully satisfactory and further research is needed to develop newer and more effective therapies.

ONLINE REFERENCES

Please scan the QR code provided at the end of the table of contents for References of this chapter.

CHAPTER 36

Hypertension in Old Age and Very Old Age Patients

Aditya Goyal, Parth Mashru, Deepesh Agarwal

ABSTRACT

Along with major cardiovascular events such as myocardial infarction, stroke, and heart failure, hypertension (HTN) is frequently a comorbid precursor factor. Due to aging and/or obesity, it is predicted that a third of the world's population will have HTN, indicating a large worldwide burden of this ailment.[1] Age-related poor outcomes in older persons are exacerbated by neurohormonal and autonomic dysregulation, deteriorating renal function, arterial stiffness, and mechanical hemodynamic change. This chapter focuses on the most recent research findings and recommendations on HTN in older adults. It is essential to customize HTN care plans for each patient, taking into account their level of frailty, psychosocial issues, and other comorbidities. Diuretics, angiotensin-converting enzyme inhibitors (ACEI), and calcium channel blockers (CCBs) have been shown to improve cardiovascular outcomes in elderly individuals. It is crucial to address the prevention of HTN with aging by lifestyle change in younger generations.

Keywords: Hypertension, octogenarians, elderly, frail.

INTRODUCTION AND EPIDEMIOLOGY

More subjects have been classified as hypertensive as a result of discrepancies in the guidelines for defining pressure targets (particularly for older persons); nonetheless, for the senior population, European Society of Cardiology (ESC)/European Society of Hypertension (ESH)[2] recommends a range of 130/70–139/79 mm Hg [compared to American College of Cardiology (ACC)/American Heart Association (AHA's) 130/80 mm Hg].[3] Cardiovascular event outcomes such as myocardial infarction, heart failure, and stroke are affected by hypertension (HTN).[4] Systemic HTN's asymptomatic nature can delay diagnosis and initiation of the best treatments.

According to the present data, the prevalence in urban areas is 33.8% and in rural areas, it is 27.6% with an overall prevalence of 29.8%.[5]

Prevalence of HTN has been increasing in the last 20 years **(Fig. 1)**.[5]

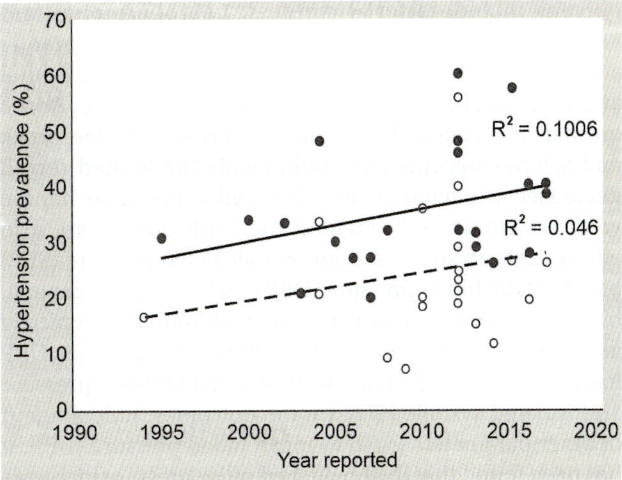

FIG. 1: Prevalence of hypertension in India over last four decades—increasing trend in hypertension in India is urban (top panel) and rural (bottom panel) populations according to cross-sectional regional studies from 1990s to the date.[5]

Hypertension is more common in people over the age of 80 years than it is in persons under the age of 60 years (74% vs. 27%, respectively), suggesting that HTN prevalence rises with aging. The Framingham Heart Study[6] revealed that 90% of the study's subject pool of participants who were under the age of 55 years at the time of enrollment eventually developed HTN, with the prevalence of the condition rising with advancing age and females being more susceptible than males in the population over the age of 70 (65% males vs. 75% females).

Numerous studies have continued to emphasize HTN guidelines and screening for people under the age of 80 years, which has led to a lack of more precise guidelines for the management of HTN in patients over the age of 80 years.

The results of treating HTN in older persons may improve the outcomes of treating cardiovascular disease (CVD), according to certain recent research completed around the world. [Among the studies are the Systolic HTN in the Elderly Program (SHEP),[7] Systolic HTN in Europe trial (Syst-Eur),[8] SPRINT, Medical Research Counsel Working Party,[9] HTN in the Very Elderly Trial (HYVET),[10] and the UK Prospective Diabetes Study (UKPDS).[11]] Therefore, doctors should give priority to identifying and treating HTN in elderly patients. The difficulties in assessing and managing HTN in elderly people are discussed in this chapter. In addition, we draw attention to the different guidelines and how, in our experience, they affect the management of HTN.

PATHOPHYSIOLOGY OF HYPERTENSION AND COMPLICATIONS IN OLDER ADULTS

The main underlying mechanics that cause HTN in elderly persons include arterial stiffness, neurohormonal and autonomic dysregulation, mechanical hemodynamic alterations, and the aging kidney.[12] Aging leads to structural and functional changes in the arterial vasculature. Aortic intimal hyperplasia is seen when elastic lamellae break and arteries become stiff, additionally the limited recoil, decreased capacitance, and reduced capacity to handle volume variations throughout the cardiac cycle are also effects of artery stiffness. Both, systolic blood pressure (SBP) and diastolic blood pressure (DBP) rise with age in general, but at the point of central arterial predominance (typically around the age of 60 years), SBP continues to rise while DBP has been found to decrease with age.[13] Wider pulse pressure and isolated systolic HTN are the outcomes. Independent of other parameters [such as mean blood pressure (BP)], it has been found that the broadened pulse pressure increases with age. In the elderly population without CVD, Sasaki et al.[14] have demonstrated that N-terminal pro-B-type natriuretic peptide (NT-proBNP) concentrations may serve as a measure for arterial stiffness. In their presentation, they demonstrated that NT-proBNP was positively associated with SBP whereas DBP and NT-proBNP were found to have a U-shaped association.

An increase in pulse wave velocity and pressure as well as a decrease in aortic flexibility are all the effects of hemodynamic mechanical changes that alter wave reflection. The alteration in arterial shape results in an increase in the forward and reflected pressure waves in the ascending aorta, which raises the central SBP even more.

Endothelial dysfunction, which develops with age, affects arterial dilation by increasing endothelin-1 and decreasing nitric oxide availability.[15] Another neurohormonal mechanism that contributes to worse CVD outcomes is the decline of renin–angiotensin aldosterone system at the age of 60 years (40–60% drop compared to earlier age grops).[16] This mechanism causes individuals to experience drug-related hyperkalemia by lowering plasma aldosterone levels.[17]

Age has been associated with an increase in peripheral plasma norepinephrine,[18,19] which is thought to be a compensatory mechanism for the decline in β-adrenergic responsiveness that comes with aging.[20] Kidney aging is accompanied by an increase in salt sensitivity. This is due to the reported drop in sodium, potassium, and calcium adenosine triphosphate pump's function, which finally leads to vasoconstriction and vascular resistance.[21] Along with the aforementioned conditions, HTN in older persons is linked to the atrial fibrillation, chronic renal and retinal illness, ischemic and hemorrhagic strokes,[22,23] vascular dementia, coronary artery disease (CAD),[24] and Alzheimer's disease.[25]

HYPERTENSION DIAGNOSIS

Hypertension is diagnosed by taking a blood pressure reading while the patient is relaxed (sitting in a chair with their arms at their sides for at least 5 minutes prior to the readings). A positive diagnosis requires two high blood pressure readings on two different occasions.[3] According to AHA guidelines precautions and things are to be kept in mind while blood pressure measurement has been depicted in **Figure 2**.[26]

One of the most frequent causes of white coat HTN in elderly adults is thought to be arterial stiffness. If the in-office blood pressure readings are only modestly elevated,[2,27] it is crucial to confirm the readings in this subgroup of patients in an ambulatory/out-of-office situation. The ACC's 2017 criterion for a positive HTN diagnosis is a blood pressure reading of >130/80 mm Hg, but the European Society of HTN's norm is >140/90 mm Hg.[1,2] According to 2018 ESC/ESH blood pressure guidelines older adults were divided in two subgroups; elderly is >65–79 years and very elder >80 years **(Table 1)**. The guidelines recommends that pharmacologic treatment should be offered to all older patients having SBP >160 mm Hg. Lower therapeutic target of SBP 130–139 and DBP 70–79 mm Hg can also be considered in elderly (>65 and <80 years) patients, however in very old (>80 years) patients pharmacologic treatment can be considered in fit individuals with SBP >160 mm Hg and/or DBP >90 mm Hg with a

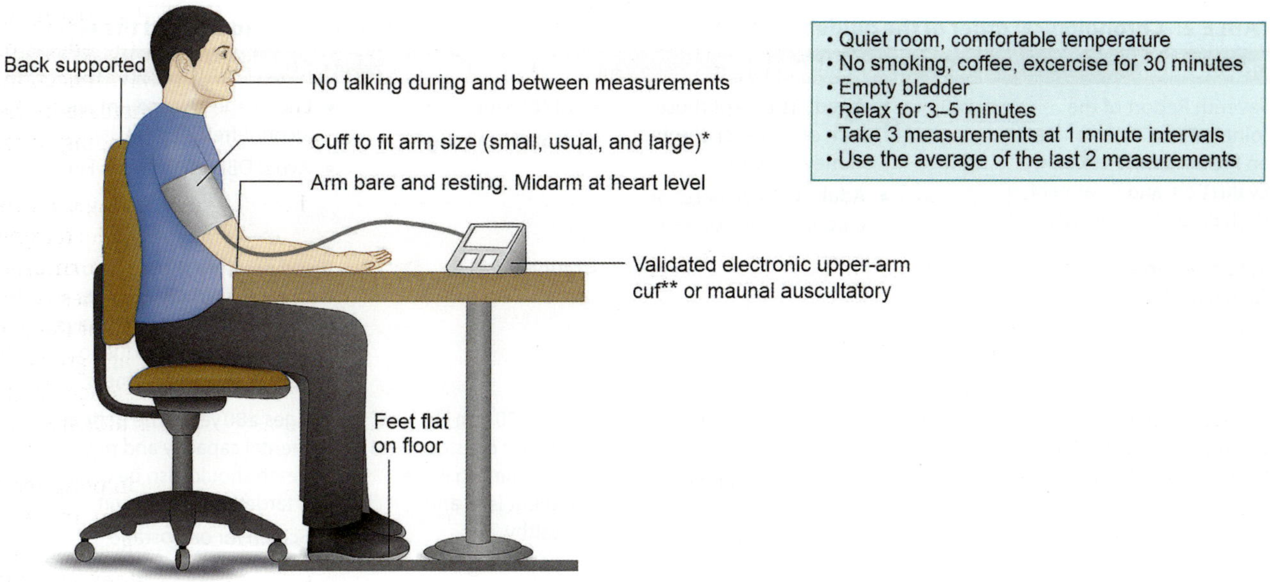

*For manual auscultatory devices the inflatable bladder of the cuff must cover 75–100% of the individual's arm circumference. For electronic devices use cuffs according to device instructions.

**See validated electronic devices.

FIG. 2: According to American Heart Association (AHA) guidelines precautions and things to be kept in mind while blood pressure measurement.[26]

TABLE 1: Definition of old age according to different guidelines, blood pressure (BP) for initiation of therapy, BP targets.

	ACC/AHA 2017	ACP/AAFP 2017	ESC/ESH 2018	ESH 2023[30]
Definition of older patients	≥65 years	≥60 years	• Elderly 65–79 years • Very old ≥80 years	• Elderly ≥65 years • Very old ≥80 years
BP threshold for initiation of pharmacotherapy	≥130/80 mm Hg	SBP ≥150 mm Hg	• Elderly ≥140/90 mm Hg • Very old ≥160/90 mm Hg	• ≥60 years SBP >140 mm Hg • ≥80 years SBP ≥160 mm Hg
BP target	<130/80 mm Hg	SBP <150 mm Hg	• SBP 130–139 mm Hg • DBP 70–79 mm Hg	• For 65–75 years <140/80 mm Hg • For ≥80 years SBP 140–150 mm Hg • DBP <80 mm Hg

(AAFP: American Academy of Family Physicians; ACC: American College of Cardiology; ACP: American College of Physicians; AHA: American Heart Association; DBP: diastolic blood pressure; ESC: European Society of Cardiology; ESH: European Society of Hypertension; SBP: systolic blood pressure)

target blood pressure of 130–139 mm Hg/70–79 mm Hg.[2] Decision regarding treatment should be made after keeping comorbidities in mind and thorough clinical assessment. Since HTN is typically asymptomatic, systematic community programs frequently diagnose a large number of unknowing HTN patients.[28,29]

European Society of Cardiology hypertension guideline 2023 stats that patients >60–79 years with SBP >140 mm Hg should be started on antihypertensive treatment regardless of DBP and, in >80 years threshold for treatment should be >160 mm Hg and starting treatment at SBP >150 mm Hg may be considered. Very old age patients who are currently on anti-hypertensive treatment should continue the medications as tapering of antihypertensive treatment may lead to rebound HTN and increase CVD risk.[30]

DIRECTIVES FOR MANAGING HIGH BLOOD PRESSURE IN ADULTS AND THE ELDERLY

There are numerous publications that offer guidelines for the management of HTN in adults of all ages, including the elderly, and the majority of them take the age and comorbidities of the patients into account when setting blood pressure reduction targets. In **Table 2** summary, some of these are listed in chronological order.

TABLE 2: Chronological order of the guidelines for the management of high blood pressure in adults and the elderly.

Organization	Year	Population	Target blood pressure	Considerations for the elderly
Seventh Report of the Joint National Committee on Prevention, Detection, Evaluation, and Treatment of High Blood Pressure (JNC 7)[31]	2003	• All adults except those with diabetes or chronic kidney disease • Adults with diabetes or chronic kidney disease	• <140/90 mm Hg • <130/80 mm Hg	• Encourage low sodium and alcohol-free lifestyle • Avoid DBP <50–60 mm Hg
Indian Hypertension Guideline II	2007		<140/90 mm Hg	Blood pressure should be measured with care in elderly subjects as some older patients may have falsely high readings due to excessive vascular stiffness
European Society of Hypertension/European Society of Cardiology (ESH/ECS)[32]	2013	• All adults except those with diabetes • Adults with diabetes	• 140–150 mm Hg systolic; consider <140 mm Hg if the patient is fit and healthy • <85 mm Hg DBP	• Ages ≥80 years, the patient's mental capacity and physical heath should also be considered if targeting to <140 mm Hg • Screen for orthostatic hypotension before initiating therapy • Avoid DBP < 55 mm Hg
Prevention, Detection, Evaluation, and Treatment of High Blood Pressure[33]	2014	Adults age <60 years and those >18 with diabetes or chronic kidney disease	<140/90 mm Hg	• Adults age ≥ 60 years • Goal: <150/90 mm Hg • If CKD or DM <140/90 mm Hg
American Heart Association/American College of Cardiology/Centers for Disease Control and Prevention (AHA/ACC/CDC)[34]	2014	All adults	<140/90 mm Hg	No age-specific guidelines
American Society of Hypertension/International Society of Hypertension (ASH/ISH)[34]	2014	Adults ages 18–79 years	• BP target for treatment of hypertension in adults of age 18-79 years is <140/90 mm Hg • BP target of <130/80 mm Hg may be considered in younger adults	• Adults ages ≥80 years • Diagnose of HTN only if SBP >150 mm Hg • Goal: <150/90 mm Hg
Department of Veterans Affairs/Department of Defense (VA/DoD)[35]	2014	• All adults • Adults with diabetes	• <150/90 mm Hg • <150/85 mm Hg	No age-specific guidelines
American Heart Association/American College of Cardiology/American Society of Hypertension (AHA/ACC/ASH)[36]	2015	• Adults with CAD, except as noted below • Adults with MI, stroke, TIA, carotid artery disease, peripheral artery disease or abdominal aortic aneurysm	• <140/90 mm Hg • <130/80 mm Hg	• Adults ages >80 years • Goal: <150/90 mm Hg
American College of Cardiology/American Heart Association (ACC/AHA)[3]	2017	All adults	<130/80 mm Hg	• ≥65 + ambulatory: Goal <130 mm Hg • ≥65 + high burden of comorbidity, limited life expectancy, clinical judgment, patient preference—assess risk/benefit
Hypertension Canada[37]	2017	All adults	<140/90 mm Hg	• Age 60–79: Goal <140/90 mm Hg • Age > 79: Goal <150/90

Continued

Continued

Organization	Year	Population	Target blood pressure	Considerations for the elderly
American College of Physicians—elderly[38]	2017			≥60 years: Goal <150 mm Hg, if TIA <140 mm Hg
European Society of Hyper-tension/European Society of Cardiology (ESH/ECS)[2]	2018	All adults	<140/90 mm Hg	≥60 years: Goal <150/90 mm Hg, if tolerate <140 mm Hg do not change therapy
Indian guideline of hypertension—IV[5]	2019	All adults	• <130/80 mm Hg in <60 years • 130–140/80–90 and it needs to be individualized in ≥60 years	• Treatment in >80 years has been shown to be beneficial • Patients of CAD and heart failure, therapy may be started beyond 130/80
ESC Guidelines For Management of Hypertension[30]	2023	All adults	• For 65–75 years <140/80 mm Hg • For ≥80 years SBP 140–150 mm Hg, DBP <80 mm Hg	• >60 years SBP >140 mm Hg • >80 years SBP >160 mm Hg

(CAD: coronary artery disease; CKDL: chronic kidney disease; DBP: diastolic blood pressure; DM: diabetes mellitus; MI: myocardial infarction; TIA: transient ischemic attack)

GERIATRIC CARDIOLOGY DIFFICULTIES

Personalized medicine has a clear place in geriatric cardiology. Clinical decision-making in this field is difficult since several cofounding factors, including the patient's age, general health, physical condition, social situation, and mental health, must be taken into account to increase the odds of a favorable clinical response to a treatment. Frailty, concurrent medical conditions, cognitive impairment,[39] polypharmacy,[40] age-related changes in pharmacokinetics and pharmacodynamics, orthostatic hypotension, any visual or auditory limitations, cost of treatment, side effects, and/or the availability of social support or caregivers are some of the factors the doctor will need to take into account.[41-43] Furthermore, in the case of resistant HTN, it is crucial to get the right diagnosis and rule out additional reasons, such as pseudo/masked/situational HTN.

WHEN TO START TREATMENT?

All recommendations concur that patients with grade 2 or 3 HTN should receive lifestyle modifications in addition to antihypertensive medication therapy.[2,26,44-46] Consistent with guidelines, individuals with grade 1 HTN and a high cardiovascular (CV) risk should be treated with BP-lowering medications as well as lifestyle changes. It has been rejected in the past and is still debatable whether or not to prescribe BP-lowering medications to patients with grade 1 HTN and low-to-moderate CV risk [no CVD, diabetes, chronic kidney disease (CKD), or hypertension-mediated organ damage (HMOD)]. Furthermore, in patients with grade 1 HTN and low CV risk, certain randomized controlled trial (RCT)-based meta-analyses failed to detect a significant treatment-related CV benefit.[46] However, three more recent meta-analyses[47] found that patients with grade 1 HTN experienced significantly fewer CV events and deaths as a result of treatment. The second meta-analysis[48] (five RCTs with 8,974 patients) demonstrated that untreated patients with grade 1 HTN and a real low risk condition showed a combined 34% reduction in stroke and CAD with an approximate 7 mm Hg SBP drop **(Flowchart 1)**.

It was likewise not the case for the third meta-analysis,[49] which showed that lowering blood pressure in patients with baseline blood pressure in the range of grade 1 HTN decreased death and CVD. The HOPE-3 trial data,[50] which showed a 27% reduction in major CV events when SBP was lowered by 6 mm Hg in a sample of patients primarily (80%) untreated, at intermediate CV risk, and with baseline SBP values >143.5 mm Hg (average 154 mm Hg), provide additional support for these findings. Based on the aforementioned information, we advise that, regardless of the CV risk, grade 1 hypertensive patients should receive both lifestyle counseling and BP-lowering medication treatment.

However, it may be possible to start the treatment with merely lifestyle changes in patients with grade 1 HTN in their lower blood pressure range, no HMOD, and a low CV risk. A lifestyle-based intervention alone may last for several months (e.g., 6 months). Drug therapy will be required if blood pressure control is not obtained after a few months of a lifestyle-based strategy **(Table 3)**.

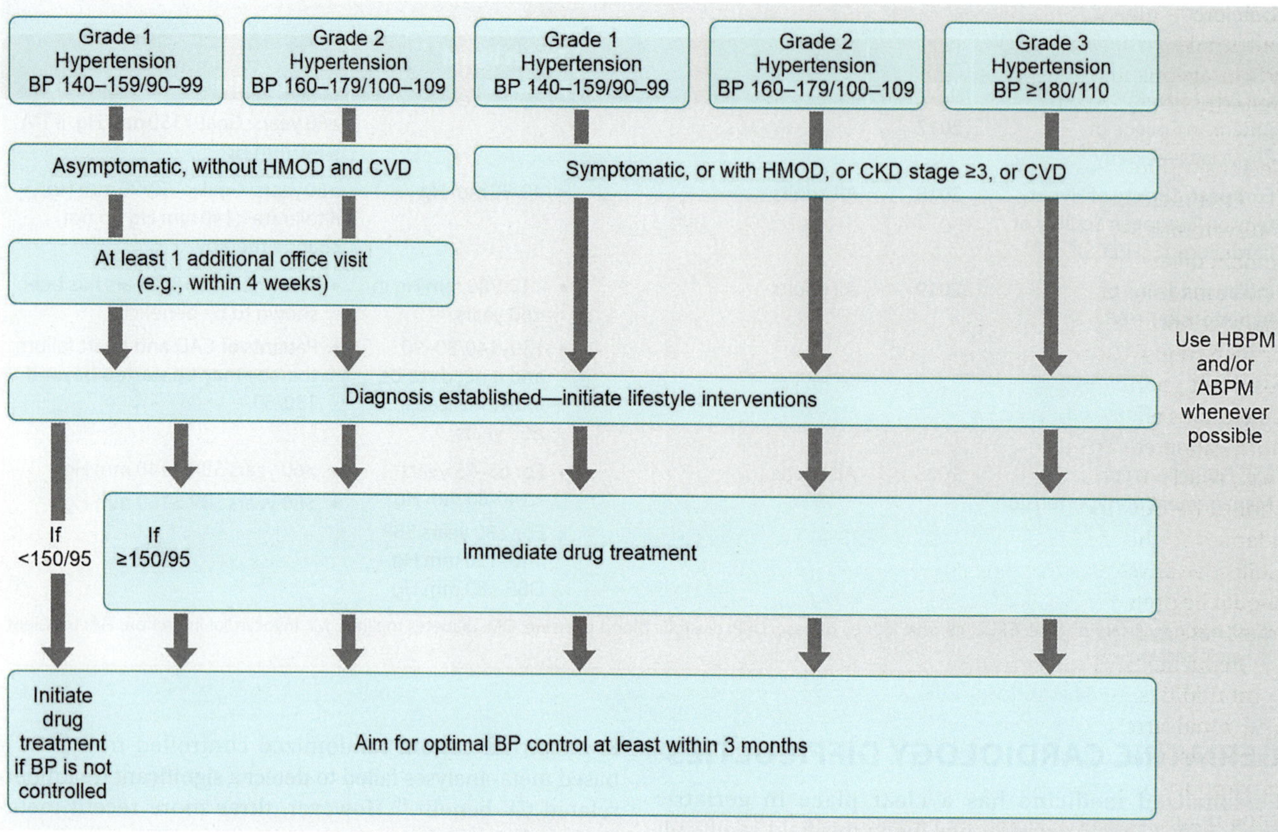

FLOWCHART 1: Initial management of hypertension.[30]

(ABPM: ambulatory blood pressure monitoring; BP: blood pressure; CKD: chronic kidney disease; CVD: cardiovascular disease; HBPM: home blood pressure monitoring; HMOD: hypertension-mediated organ damage)

TABLE 3: Office BP thresholds for drug treatment initiation.[30]

Recommendations and statements	CoR	LoE
In patients 18–79 years, the recommended office threshold for initiation of drug treatment is 140 mm Hg for SBP and/or 90 mm Hg for DBP	I	A
In patients ≥80 years, the recommended office SBP threshold for initiation of drug treatment is 160 mm Hg	I	B
However, in patients ≥80 years a lower SBP threshold in the range 140–160 mm Hg may be considered	II	C
The office SBP and DBP thresholds for initiation of drug treatment in frail patients should be individualized	I	C
In adult patients with a history of CVD, predominantly CAD, drug treatment should be initiated in the high-normal BP range (SBP ≥130 or DBP ≥80 mm Hg)	I	A

(CAD: coronary artery disease; CoR: class of recommendation; CVD: cardiovascular disease; DBP: diastolic blood pressure; LoE: level of evidence; SBP: systolic blood pressure)

HYPERTENSION MANAGEMENT IN THE ELDERLY

Nonpharmacological Interventions

According to the evidence that is currently available, stress reduction, regular physical exercise, alcohol consumption decrease, smoking cessation, and weight control are recommended nonpharmacological interventions that assist reduce blood pressure.[51]

Diet: A Mediterranean diet that is vegetarian, low in carbohydrates, and heart healthy is also a suggested intervention. It is also advised to consume less salt and to take calcium, magnesium, and potassium supplements. Garlic, tea, coffee, fish oil, probiotics, fiber, flaxseeds, and dark chocolate are some foods that are advised.[51]

Weight loss and sodium intake restriction to 1,000 mg/day are efficient and secure ways to lower blood pressure in HTN patients. A counterargument, however, has been made in certain papers on the effectiveness, albeit negative, impacts of the low sodium intake strategy on cardiovascular outcomes that may be related to the activation of the renin–angiotensin–aldosterone system (RAAS).[52,53] The above counterargument was disproved by Burto et al., in their meta-analysis, which also demonstrated that cutting salt intake to fewer than 1,200 mg/day is thought to be advantageous and safe for lowering blood pressure.[54] The majority of the data has been used to support the Dietary Approaches to Stop Hypertension (DASH) diet regimen for decreasing blood pressure.[51]

Treatment of older patients should make use of lifestyle interventions as in younger patients. Overweight and obesity remain deleterious for CV and metabolic health, weight loss programs may lead to muscle mass loss, sarcopenia, and malnutrition. Therefore, except for the case of severe obesity or with robust old people, weight loss is not recommended. Also, salt restriction may contribute to loss of appetite with deleterious effects on nutritional status and therefore should not be adopted, except in cases of very high salt consumption (e.g., NaCl >10 g day). In these patients, a particular effort should be devoted to the promotion of physical activity, adapted to the individual's capacity and cultural context. Collective physical activities (e.g., dance, Tai-chi, or walking) should be preferred to also promote social contacts and fight loneliness and social isolation in older people.

Reducing HTN also requires appropriate management of comorbidities, such as primary aldosteronism, sleep apnea, and renal artery stenosis. The clinician should perform a cross-examination of any medications that are known to support or cause comorbidities, notably those listed underneath [e.g., steroids, tyrosine kinase (TKN) inhibitors, nonsteroidal anti-inflammatory drugs (NSAIDs), anti-depressants, hormone replacement therapy, angiogenesis inhibitors, etc.].[55] Before deciding on a course of action for HTN therapy, it is important to comprehend the patient's usage of recreational drugs and caffeine consumption patterns.

Pharmacological Intervention

Before administering the drug to treat uncontrolled HTN in older individuals, it is important to carefully evaluate factors such the complexity of the patient's existing treatment plan, concomitant conditions, patient fragility, and electrolyte and renal function.[3] Angiotensin II receptor blockers (ARB), thiazide diuretics, calcium channel blockers (CCBs), and angiotensin-converting enzyme inhibitor (ACEI) have all been proven to improve CVD outcomes in older patients. Older patients are more susceptible to side effects associated with β-blockers (BBs), most importantly fatigue, sleep-related disorders (unusual dreams or insomnia) and depression[56] that can negatively impact on the quality of life therefore, BBs should not be thought of as first-line alternatives until clinically required to treat comorbidities such as atrial fibrillation, ischemic heart disease, and heart failure.[9] It is also advised to steer clear of α-blockers and loop diuretics given their connection to patients fall incidents.[57] It has been observed that many of the elderly patients are suffering from benign prostatic hyperplasia (BPH) and are on α-blocker treatment; these patients should be monitored and should not to be given aggressive antihypertensive treatment so as to prevent orthostatic hypotension. Because of stiff vessels and atherosclerosis some patients are labeled falsely as hypertensive, these patients should be started on antihypertensive cautiously.

According to the ESH/ESC recommendations, treating solitary HTN in older individuals with a calcium antagonist or diuretic is advised.[58] Evidence from the ALLHAT[59] trial, which found that low-dose daily chlorthalidone was most effective for the older population, and the combination of CCB + ACEI in the ASCOT-BPLA[60] have both demonstrated a significant reduction in overall mortality in those over the age of 60 years.

Because older patients (even those in healthy conditions) experience more drug-related side effects compared with younger patients,[61] medical efforts should aim at achieving the blood pressure goal and at the same time avoid side effects, the risk of which increases with the number of prescribed drugs. Therefore, in old patients and particularly frail patients, initial monotherapy should be considered the first treatment step more frequently than in younger patients, especially with grade 1 HTN. However, because controlling the SBP elevation of older patients is particularly difficult, even in grade 1 HTN, physicians should consider an initial two-drug combination treatment or be prepared to up titrate treatment with the addition of a second and, if needed, a third drug. Combination treatment is necessary in the vast majority of the patients with grade 2 or 3 HTN, and in these patients, it can usually be considered as first step treatment because initial combination treatment favors better adherence to treatment and reduced treatment inertia,[62] also in old patients. This is particularly important because due to their multimorbidity, more than half of older patients are exposed to polypharmacy, i.e., are treated with at least five agents.[63,64] As a general rule, and although delayed achievement of blood pressure control should be avoided, it may be wise to start antihypertensive drugs with lower doses and up titrate treatment somewhat more slowly in older than in younger patients.

According to the most recent clinical research, the best combination is RAAS blockers and CCB/thiazide, while other combinations may also work.[65]

It is strongly advised to gradually increase the dose while taking the patient's tolerance into account and monitoring for orthostatic hypotension. Up until the dosage is changed, renal function should be monitored to look for any substantial changes in glomerular filtration rate (GFR) or serum creatinine levels. The medical team should keep an eye on any known adverse effects of prescription medications or drug combinations that have a higher potential for incidence or flare-up than what has been documented in the literature such as hypokalemia with the use of diuretics.

Management Strategies

In light of the increased SBP variability in older age group, home blood pressure monitoring (HBPM) should be used to help identify the variation in blood pressure values.

These assessments can be suggested for patients with Alzheimer's disease and other neurocognitive disorders as well as patients with mild-to-moderate dementia. The ambulatory blood pressure monitoring (ABPM) can be helpful in identifying hypotensive episodes and determining the presence and severity of the nighttime blood pressure decline, especially in patients who take many medications.

In patients who are 80 years or older there is only one outcome-based RCT, the HYVET trial,[66] which demonstrated that antihypertensive treatment was associated with a decreased risk of CV events and all-cause mortality in hypertensive patients aged 80 years old or more. Overall, BP-lowering medication appears to have similar benefits in moderately weak octogenarians as it does in fit older persons. Additionally, the SPRINT research noted that the effect of intensive blood pressure control was seen in a subgroup of patients older than 75 years regardless of their level of frailty.[67] Last but not least, according to a recent analysis of a sizable real-life population from northern Italy, elderly patients who are considered frail due to a high risk of mortality within a short period of time showed a lower risk of passing away if their compliance with antihypertensive drug prescriptions was high.[68] Antihypertensive medication should be used alongside lifestyle changes such as the promotion of light physical activity, in very elderly HTN patients who can be considered fit for their age or just mildly frail, preferably in a group setting. Even if blood pressure readings are lower than those advised by guidelines, a well-tolerated treatment regimen should not be lowered or discontinued in extremely old patients. According to a number of observational studies, the degree of frailty affects the link between blood pressure and mortality,[69,70] and among the most frail elderly patients, rates of morbidity and death are higher at low blood pressure (mostly SBP <130). Frailty and functionality at age of 80 years old should be included as part of the diagnostic process **(Table 4)**.

TABLE 4: Additional safety recommendations for drug treatment.[30]

Recommendations and statements	CoR	LoE
Additional safety recommendations		
In frail patients, the treatment target for office SBP and DBP should be individualized	I	C
Do not aim to target office SBP below 120 mm Hg or DBP below 70 mm Hg during drug treatment	III	C
However, in patients with low office DBP, i.e., below 70 mm Hg, SBP should be still lowered, albeit cautiously, if on-treatment SBP is still well above the target values	II	C
Reduction of treatment of can be consider in patient aged 80 years old or older with a low SBP (<120 mm Hg) or in the presence of severe orthostatic hypotension or a high frailty level	III	C

(CoR: class of recommendation; DBP: diastolic blood pressure; LoE: level of evidence; SBP: systolic blood pressure)

FUTURE DIRECTION

The key to preventing HTN in older people is lifestyle adjustment in the younger population. The physiological and physical factors that increase the prevalence of HTN with age cannot be controlled, but it is evident that behavioral factors (such as quitting smoking, maintaining a healthy weight, managing diabetes mellitus, no tobacco use, and avoid drinking alcohol) can lessen the likelihood of developing HTN as we age. In order to enhance lifestyle adjustment, it is essential to educate the younger population about the CVD events (such as heart failure, renal failure, cognitive impairment, stroke, and others) that follow HTN.

Recent clinical trials focusing on polypill may offer a way to improve adherence because it would reduce the number of pills needed. Answers regarding the use of technology to manage patients from home, the use of telemedicine, and text messages to trend blood pressure medications will be addressed via the HoME trial.[71] Other researchers are examining the relationship between the gut bacteria and HTN and weight management. The enrollment phase of a new clinical trial assessing medications (such as MK-8266 and fimasartan) for the treatment of HTN in older persons is about to be completed.[71] Studies are also being done on invasive techniques like renal denervation.[71]

CONCLUSION

The prevalence of HTN is rising in the senior population. In order to give effective therapy based on guidelines, minimize the use of unnecessary antihypertensives, and improve people's quality of life, it is vital for both the general public and practicing physicians to raise knowledge of this. Programs for education and awareness at community centers, houses of worship (temples, churches, synagogues, and mosques), and companies will continue to have an impact. The burden of HTN on our senior patients can be diminished by the use of guideline-driven management, improved access to care, and blood pressure elevation screening. Since just a small percentage of people over 85 years old are included in the majority of clinical trials, more research on this area is required.

ONLINE REFERENCES

Please scan the QR code provided at the end of the table of contents for References of this chapter.

CHAPTER

37 Clinical Evaluation and Management of True Resistant Hypertension

SS Iyengar, Sneha Karekar

ABSTRACT

Hypertension continues to be one of the leading causes of mortality and morbidity globally. It is a major modifiable risk factor for coronary artery disease, heart failure, cerebrovascular disease (including dementia), peripheral vascular disease, and chronic kidney disease. Despite availability of safe and effective drugs and devices, uncontrolled hypertension continues to be a clinical problem. Amongst uncontrolled hypertensive patients on treatment, "apparent treatment resistant hypertension" and "pseudo-resistant hypertension" have to be carefully excluded before labelling it as "true resistant hypertension". Resistant hypertension enhances the risk of target organ damage. Early identification and effective strategies to treat resistant hypertension will improve outcome. There is another phenotype "refractory hypertension" to describe a subgroup of patients of resistant hypertension whose BP remains poorly controlled and are at an extremely high risk of complications; these patients are reported to typically exhibit increased sympathetic nervous system activity.

Keywords: Resistant hypertension, pseudoresistance, mineralocorticoid receptor antagonists (MRA), renal sympathetic denervation (RDN), carotid baroreflex activation.

"Continued persistence overcomes almost all resistance."

— Mark Victor Hansen

INTRODUCTION

Hypertension is a global problem of great magnitude. The World Health Organization (WHO) report states that 1.28 billion people between the age of 30 and 79 years are affected by hypertension worldwide and two-thirds of them are from low to middle income countries. The global prevalence is 34% in men and 32% in women, the prevalence being higher in women following menopause.[1]

At least one in four persons in India are known to have hypertension,[2] although only around 12% of them have their blood pressure under control, 20% in urban and 11% in rural population[3,4] By 2025, India's target is to achieve 25% relative reduction in the prevalence of hypertension.[5]

Amongst hypertensives, it is important to identify and treat patients of "true resistant hypertension (RH)" as they are at a much greater risk of premature cardiovascular events, chronic kidney disease (CKD), and other hypertension-mediated organ damage.

DEFINITION OF TRUE RESISTANT HYPERTENSION

Resistant hypertension is defined as BP that remains above goal (target BP <130/80 mm Hg as per ACC/AHA guidelines[6,7] and <140/90 as per ESC/ESH[8] guidelines) despite three antihypertensive drugs of different classes, with one of them being a diuretic appropriate for renal function and all the drugs are used at maximally tolerable doses.

Limitation of the definition: Surprisingly no definition mentions the duration of therapy to be given before labelling it as RH. It is reasonable to state a period of 3–6 months on maximal optimal treatment in a compliant patient (Personal Communication – Dr C Venkat Ram).

Resistant hypertension has to be differentiated from pseudoresistance by confirming with appropriate BP measuring technique in office or by using ambulatory BP monitoring or home BP monitoring.[9] The recent European

Society of Hypertension (ESH) guidelines[10] add that the inadequate BP control should be confirmed by out-of-office BP measurement showing an uncontrolled 24-hour BP of 130/80 mm Hg or more. Adherence to therapy has to be ensured and secondary causes of hypertension have to be excluded before diagnosing RH. By this process, apparent RH and pseudo-resistant hypertension get eliminated. Some cases with RH may have reversible causes and may benefit from specific diagnostic and therapeutic approaches.[11]

PREVALENCE OF RESISTANT HYPERTENSION

With the new target BP given by ACC/AHA guidelines which is defined as systolic blood pressure (SBP) <130 mm Hg and diastolic blood pressure (DBP) <80 mm Hg for all adults <65 years of age,[6,7] RH was seen in 19.7% (in USA) with almost 3% of adults taking thiazide like diuretic and 9% taking mineralocorticoid receptor antagonist.[11] In India, according to a study done in JIPMER institute between December 2018 and February 2020, RH was seen in 11% of individuals according to the new target BP definition. There was a fourfold increase in prevalence of RH after considering the new definition of target BP.[12] However, it is difficult establish true prevalence of RH since white coat hypertension (WCH) and pseudohypertension may not have been factored in many prevalence studies.

PATHOGENESIS OF RESISTANT HYPERTENSION

The pathophysiology of RH is not fully understood. RH has been associated with three major underlying mechanisms which include—fluid retention, sympathetic system activation, and arterial stiffness.[13] Increased aldosterone production, impaired renal natriuresis and excessive salt consumption all contribute to excessive fluid retention.[13] Aldosterone is of special importance in RH due to its ability to enhance fluid and salt retention as well as other non-genomic proinflammatory actions that contribute to pharmacological resistance.[14,15] As a result, mineralocorticoid receptor antagonist (MRA) becomes significantly more crucial in the treatment of RH.[6,7]

The next mechanism which plays an important role in the pathogenesis of RH is sympathetic system activation.[16] Several studies have demonstrated that norepinephrine regional spillover technique resulted in significant activation of renal sympathetic system in RH patients as compared to both healthy individuals and those with non-RH.[17]

Finally, arterial stiffness is also considered to be a significant mechanism in the pathophysiology of RH. Factors that contribute to arterial stiffness include endothelial dysfunction, excessive salt consumption, and sympathetic signalling.[18] RH patients had increased arterial stiffness when compared to those with controlled hypertension.[19-21] It is a vicious cycle which consists of increased arterial stiffness leading to increased BP which further enhances the arterial stiffness.[20,21]

There are certain peculiar features associated with RH, notably obesity, diabetes, CKD, obstructive sleep apnea (OSA), non-dippers on ambulatory blood pressure monitoring (ABPM) and hyperuricemia **(Table 1)**.[22-27]

TABLE 1: The list of peculiar features associated with RH and its prevalence according to various studies.[22-27]

Peculiar features	Prevalence of RH
Demographic correlates	
Black race	27.3%
Older age	≥ 69 years, (72.9 ± 11.0 years)
Male sex	49.6%
Comorbidities	
Obesity: BMI >35–<40 kg/m² ≥ 40 kg/m²	 16.2% 26.5%
Left ventricular hypertrophy	40%
Albuminuria	27%
Diabetes mellitus	49%
CKD	20% (serum creatinine >1.5 mg/dL)
Higher Framingham 10 year risk score	21.7 ± 3%
OSA	60–84%
Physiological aberration	
Peripheral and carotid atherosclerosis	65%
Impaired endothelial dysfunction	40%
Reduced arterial compliance and raised systemic vascular resistance	42.3%
Attenuated normal nocturnal decline BP, non-dipping ambulatory BP, reverse dipping in BP	43–65%
Metabolic derangements	
Hyperuricemia	63.6% (serum uric acid >6.8 mg/dL)
Hyperaldosteronism	20%
Suppressed circulating renin levels	67%

(BMI: body mass index; CKD: chronic kidney disease; OSA: obstructive sleep apnea; RH: resistant hypertension)

GENETICS IN RESISTANT HYPERTENSION

Mutations in two beta and gamma epithelial sodium channel (*ENaC*) gene variants were significantly more prevalent in RH individuals.[28] Mutations in 11 beta hydroxysteroid dehydrogenase type 2 which plays an important role in cortisol and corticosterone metabolism has been associated with RH in African Americans.[29]

DIAGNOSIS OF RESISTANT HYPERTENSION

The definition of RH which is previously stated should be fulfilled.

First Step: Rule Out Pseudoresistance[6-8]

Pseudoresistance:[11,30-32] The common causes include–

- *Inappropriate BP measurement technique*: In a study conducted by Bhatt et al.[33] found that 33% of the 130 patients enrolled in the study were mislabeled to have uncontrolled BP. The apt technique to measure BP is to make the patient sit with back supported and feet on the floor for minimum of 5 minutes and then check the BP with appropriate size cuff using either a sphygmomanometer or automated BP machine.[7,8,34-38]
- Suboptimal antihypertensive prescription (clinical inertia) is defined as failure of physician to escalate the level of care as needed.[37] In spite of the fact that 40% of the patients had raised blood pressure readings during their clinic appointments, only 6.7% of the sessions saw the BP regimes escalated as advised, according to a study of 800 male patients getting care at five outpatient department of veterans affairs centers. A second study of a significant ambulatory care survey with over 19,000 patients revealed that clinicians were not administering antihypertensives in accordance with the guidelines. Some of the causes of clinician inertia include an overestimation of the care, unsubstantiated decisions as well as a lack of understanding of how to reach BP objectives.[39-42]
- White coat hypertension is described as a rise in BP noticed when an individual comes to the clinic. The prevalence of WCH ranges between 15 and 40% in outpatients. According to European guidelines, WCH is defined as office systolic/diastolic BP of 140/90 mm Hg or more and a 24-hour BP <130/80 mm Hg. To distinguish between true hypertension and WCH, the individual should be advised ABPM or home BP monitoring.[41]
- Poor adherence to therapy is one of the causes of poorly controlled BP. A total of 40% of naïve hypertension patients discontinue the therapy within 1 year.[42,43] Adherence can be measured via indirect and direct means. The techniques used are (i) medication event monitoring system (MEMS)—a sensor is placed in the vial cap which records every time the cap is opened, (ii) self-reported questionnaire, (iii) liquid chromatography, (iv) mass spectroscopy, and (v) pill count.[44]

Employing correct technique of measuring BP with validated instruments, use of ABPM or home monitoring to exclude WCH, appropriate escalation of therapy during visits and emphasizing adherence to therapy are various measures to deal with the issue of pseudohypertension.

Second Step: Assessment for Secondary Causes of Hypertension

Almost 5–10% of RH patients are associated with secondary hypertension. It is not feasible to screen all patients for secondary hypertension. The common causes are primary aldosteronism, renal parenchymal disease and renovascular disease, and less frequently encountered ones are Cushing syndrome, pheochromocytoma or coarctation of the aorta.[10] A comprehensive clinical examination followed by relevant laboratory and radiological tests would identify a cause for secondary hypertension.[45] The causes of secondary hypertension along with the relevant screening tests used for diagnosis of each of them are shown in **Table 2**.[6,46,47]

Third Step: Exclude Interfering Substances

There are certain drugs and substances which interfere with the regulation of BP and can result in increased BP. These substances/factors need to be excluded **(Table 3)**.[48-66]

TABLE 2: The list of causes of secondary hypertension and the relevant screening tests used for diagnosis of each of them.[6,46,47]

Causes of secondary hypertension	Relevant screening tests
Acromegaly	Serum growth hormone
Thyroid disease	TSH and free T4
Cushing's disease	24 hours free urinary cortisol and late night salivary cortisol
Coarctation of aorta	CT angiogram
Renal artery stenosis	Renal artery Doppler
Pheochromocytoma	Serum metanephrine and 24-hour urine catecholamines
Obstructive sleep apnea	Polysomnography
Renal parenchymal disease	Serum creatinine
Hyperaldosteronism	Serum renin–aldosterone ratio

(TSH: thyroid-stimulating hormone)

TABLE 3: The list of interfering substances and its effect on BP studies.[48,66]

	Interfering substances/drugs	Effect on BP
Drugs	NSAID	Causes 5 mm Hg increase in MAP. They blunt the action of all antihypertensives except that of CCBs
	Selective COX-2 inhibitors	Rise in BP occurs secondary to inhibition of renal prostaglandin production, particularly PGE_2 and PC_{I2} which results in sodium and water retention
	Sympathomimetics such as nasal decongestants, OCPs, glucocorticoids, erythropoietin	• Sympathetic amines increase BP by activation of the sympathetic nervous system • Recombinant human erythropoietin can increase BP by complex mechanisms in a dose-dependent fashion, resulting in hypertension in 20–33% of recipients
	Cyclosporine	• Cyclosporine increase BP by inducing systemic and renal vasoconstriction and sodium retention
Substance abuse	• Black licorice present in oral tobacco products • Herbal supplements such as *ma huang*	Causes rise in BP by stimulation of mineralocorticoid receptors via suppressing the metabolism of cortisol.
	Cocaine and amphetamine	BP elevation is caused by intense sympathetic activation.
	Alcohol (>3–4 drinks/day)	• Has a dose-related effect on BP, in both normal and hypertensive individuals • Cessation of alcohol resulted in 7.2/6.6 mm Hg decrease in SBP/DBP readings in 24 hour ABPM
Diet	Salt intake	>10 g/day was associated with RH

(ABPM: ambulatory blood pressure monitoring; CCBs: calcium channel blockers; DBP: diastolic blood pressure; MAP: mean arterial pressure; NSAID: non-steroidal anti-inflammatory drug; OCPs: oral contraceptive pills; PCI_2: prostacyclin 2; PGE_2: prostaglandin E2; SBP: systolic blood pressure)

TREATMENT OF RESISTANT HYPERTENSION (FLOWCHART 1)

The treatment goal is to maintain BP at <130/80 mm Hg according to 2018 AHA guidelines.[7] In patients with RH, BP should be reduced <140/90 mm Hg and <130/80 mm Hg, if tolerated.[10] In patients with CKD according to Kidney Disease: Improving Global Outcomes (KDIGO) recommendation the target BP should be 120 mm Hg systolic or less.[67] However, for patients after proteinuria sets in, European guidelines[10] suggest that the BP targets be the same for proteinuric diabetics and nondiabetics. The target BP recommended for both the groups is a SBP of <130 mm Hg and DBP <80 mm Hg, if well tolerated. This offers protection against CKD progression and mortality in most. Caution needs to be exercised in patients with advanced CKD in stage 4 and 5 with careful monitoring of estimated glomerular filtration rate (eGFR), as lower BP may cause decline in GFR.

The treatment options in patients with RH include:

- Optimization of nonpharmacologic intervention and pharmacological intervention
- Additional drugs
- Device-based therapies
- Management of comorbidities
- Newer strategies

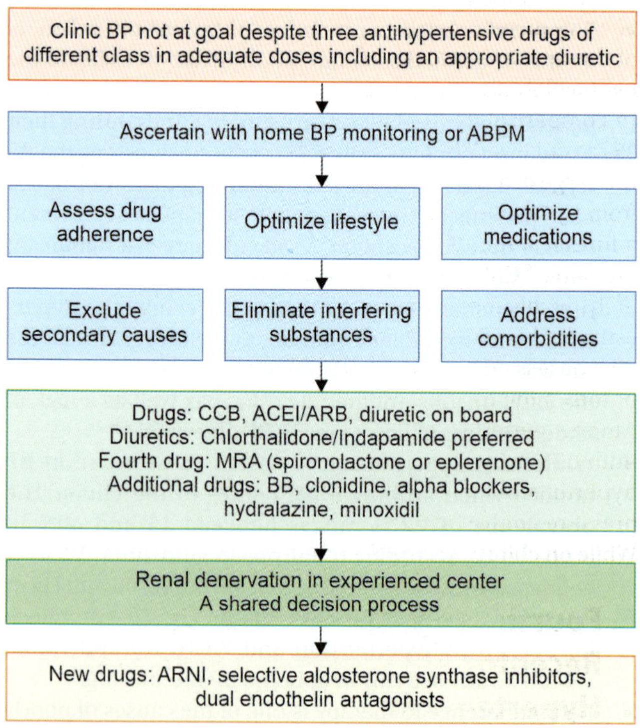

FLOWCHART 1: Management of resistant hypertension: Stepwise approach.

Optimization of Nonpharmacological Intervention

This includes lifestyle modification in the form of weight reduction, daily exercise, and dietary changes in the form of consumption of food rich in fiber, low salt, less fat, increased potassium intake, smoking cessation, and reduction in alcohol intake. These measures need to be emphasized, enhanced, and reinforced, and this in turn may reduce the number of drugs required to achieve BP control.[68]

Optimization of Pharmacotherapy

General Principles

Prior medication effects, adverse event histories, intolerances, allergies, budgetary constraints, and the presence of diabetes, chronic renal disease, and other comorbidities are all the factors that should be taken into account.

Commonly used antihypertensive drugs in these patients are calcium channel blockers (CCB), angiotensin-converting enzyme inhibitors (ACEI)/angiotensin receptor blockers (ARBs), and diuretics. The drugs should be used in maximally tolerated doses along with an appropriate diuretic less.[69-71]

Diuretics in the Treatment of Resistant Hypertension

As prolonged volume expansion contributes to RH, an effective diuretic continues to be the fundamental component of therapy. Chlorthalidone appears to be more potent than hydrochlorothiazide (HCTZ) and is preferred over the latter. In comparison to HCTZ 50 mg once daily, chlorthalidone 25 mg once daily showed a higher ambulatory BP drop, with the largest difference occurring overnight.[72-74] Changing from hydrochlorothiazide (HCTZ) to chlorthalidone caused a further 8 mm Hg decline and achieved the target blood pressure.[74] Chlorthalidone should be started at 12.5 mg once daily, with subsequent titration up to 25 mg daily. With an estimated GFR of <30 mL/min/1.72 m^2, thiazide diuretics may be less effective, and loop diuretics such as furosemide or torsemide may be necessary for effective volume control. Among patients with CKD and GFR of 15 to <30 mL/min/1.73 m^2 of body-surface area and poorly controlled hypertension, chlorthalidone therapy improved blood-pressure control at 12 weeks as compared with placebo.[75] While on chlorthalidone, hypokalemia has to be monitored.[9]

Fourth Drug: Mineralocorticoid Receptor Antagonists in Resistant Hypertension

Once a diagnosis of RH is made, a fourth drug is needed after use of a calcium antagonist, diuretic, and renin-angiotensin-aldosterone system (RAAS) blocker. A mineralocorticoid inhibitor such as spironolactone has shown significantly favorable effect in controlling BP in these patients.[9] In ASPIRANT trial, 111 patients who were all on diuretics and mostly using beta-blockers, calcium channel blockers, and either an ACEI or ARB were included in the study. SBP significantly decreased in subjects who were randomly assigned to receive 25 mg of spironolactone in both the office (8.6 mm Hg) and ambulatory readings (6.5 mm Hg).[76]

The PATHWAY-2 trial, double-blind, placebo-controlled, crossover trial, patients of RH received spironolactone, doxazosin, bisoprolol, and a placebo for 12 weeks cycle. Spironolactone was found to be the most effective add-on drug and there was no significant difference in adverse events between the agents.[77]

In a meta-analysis of 12 randomized controlled clinical trials (RCTs) (1,655 patients of RH)[78] spironolactone significantly lowered BP compared with other agents.

Irrespective of age, sex, smoking, diabetes status, in the BP-lowering arm of the ASCOT study, patients who received spironolactone as the fourth-line antihypertensive medicine for uncontrolled BP experienced a 21.9/9.5 mm Hg decline in BP. Spironolactone has the benefit of lowering blood pressure even when aldosterone levels are normal or low.[9,79,80]

Other Mineralocorticoid Receptor Antagonists

Spironolactone has side effects like painful gynecomastia and sexual impotence in men, and menstrual irregularities in women. Eplerenone, another steroidal MRA interferes less with progesterone or androgen receptors and can be used as an alternative though less potent than spironolactone.[81]

Some nonsteroidal MRAs are under study in patients with hypertension, diabetes or CKD,

finerenone being one of them. It is effective in reducing BP with favorable cardiac and kidney outcomes.[82]

Other Potassium Sparing Diuretics

Amiloride is a potassium-sparing diuretic and was used for uncontrolled or RH in the PATHWAY-2[77] and PATHWAY-3[83] studies. In PATHWAY-3 study, amiloride and HCTZ did not differ much in reducing BP. But the combination of low doses of amiloride (5–10 mg) and HCTZ (12.5–25 mg) showed greater reductions of BP than with the higher dose of HCTZ alone. A higher dose of amiloride (10–20 mg once daily) was as effective as spironolactone in reducing BP with no serious adverse events.

Triamterene is another potassium-sparing diuretic, but has not been adequately studied independently in hypertension[84]

Other Drugs

In situations where MRAs are not tolerated or contraindicated (i.e., in CKD stage 4, eGFR <30 mL/min) or additional drugs are required for BP control, the following drugs may be considered.

- Bisoprolol (5–10 mg/day) is less effective than spironolactone in reducing BP as was seen in the PATHWAY-2 trial.[77] In a real-world retrospective cohort study where 6,626 received MRA and 73,972 were on beta blockers as the fourth antihypertensive drug, there was no difference in cardiovascular risk between the two (23% nonsignificant effect in favor of spironolactone) and the MRA had more adverse events.[85] The study was probably underpowered.
- Doxazosin, an alpha blocker, reduces BP though less effectively than spironolactone events.[77] An observational small study applied electronic health record data of 8,639 patients with RH who received MRAs or BBs or alpha-1 blockers.[86] In the risk of the primary outcome there was a nonsignificant difference in favor of BBs compared with spironolactone and a significant difference in favor of alpha-1 blockers. Unmeasured confounding, small cohort size, and a low number of observed outcomes were the limitations of the study.
- Clonidine, a centrally acting alpha adrenergic receptor agonist (0.1–0.3 mg twice a day) has shown BP-lowering effect similar to spironolactone as the fourth agent in patients of RH in a randomized study.[87]
- Hydralazine or minoxidil which are direct vasodilators should be used in these patients with caution as they may lead to fluid retention and tachycardia.[10]

It may be surmised from these various studies that MRAs are underused and there is a need for more data to clearly define the role of MRAs in long term CV outcomes and safety. There is need to identify more effective strategies for managing RH.

Newer Drugs

Sacubitril-valsartan: It is the combined angiotensin receptor–neprilysin inhibitor. In a post-hoc analysis of "PARAGON-HF" trial,[88] 15% were found to have apparent RH. Sacubitril–valsartan was effective in reducing blood pressure in patients with apparent RH and also in those with an elevated SBP despite treatment with at least four drugs including an MRA.

Selective aldosterone synthase inhibitors: Aldosterone synthase controls the synthesis of aldosterone. Baxdrostat is a selective aldosterone synthase inhibitor. In a phase 2 trial,[89] Baxdrostat resulted in significant reductions in SBP and DBP in patients with treatment-RH. It also avoids the adverse effects of aldosterone by reducing its synthesis rather than blocking its effects on mineralocorticoid receptors.

Dual endothelin antagonist aprocitentan: In patients with RH, aprocitentan was well tolerated and superior to placebo in lowering blood pressure at week 4 and the effect was sustained at 40 weeks. Adverse effects were mild-to-moderate edema and fluid retention.[90]

Management of Comorbidities

Comorbidities are frequent in patients with RH. The common ones are obesity, OSA, and heart failure with preserved ejection fraction (HFpEF). These should be managed appropriately.

OSA: Continuous positive airway pressure (CPAP) treatment is beneficial in patients with RH and OSA. Those showing good adherence, increased nighttime spent with oxygen <90% (CT 90% value), the presence of severe OSA, i.e., apnea-hypopnea index (AHI) >30 events/h, and higher baseline BP were the features associated with a more favorable BP reduction and CPAP may confer cardiovascular protection.[91]

Obese patients: Sodium-glucose cotransporter-2 inhibitors (SGLT-2I) and glucagon-like peptide-1 (GLP-1) receptor agonists reduce body weight and BP modestly and have established their efficacy in improving cardiovascular (CV) and renal outcomes in patients with diabetes or with CV disease. Bariatric surgery has shown a favorable effect on BP, CV risk factors, and risk of CV events in severely obese patients and consequently may reduce the pill-burden in RH.[92-98]

DEVICE-BASED THERAPIES FOR RESISTANT HYPERTENSION

The device techniques that have been developed for the treatment of RH are:
- Catheter-based ablation of renal sympathetic nerves
- Electrical stimulation of carotid baroreflex system
- Central iliac arteriovenous anastomosis (CAV anastomosis)

These device-based therapies have undergone trials in patients with uncontrolled hypertension. Of all these, renal sympathetic denervation (RDN) has been found to be safe and effective.

Catheter-based Radiofrequency Ablation of Renal Sympathetic Nerves

The discovery of RDN therapy, which targets the ablation of renal (efferent and afferent) nerves penetrating the renal artery, has revitalized the pathophysiological theory behind surgical sympathectomy which was practiced earlier. Vasoconstrictor and volume/sodium retention mechanisms as well as renal afferent and efferent nerve stimulation cause blood pressure to increase.[99] RDN counters these mechanisms.

Recent RCTs have shown that endovascular RDN can be associated with a significant, though not of great magnitude reduction in office and ambulatory BP readings in patients with uncontrolled hypertension.

The RADIANCE-HTN SOLO study[100] showed that endovascular ultrasound renal denervation reduced ambulatory blood pressure at 2 months in patients with hypertension in the absence of medications compared with a sham procedure.

In SPYRAL HTN-OFF MED (SPYRAL Pivotal study),[101] a sham controlled trial examined the efficacy of catheter-based renal denervation in the absence of antihypertensive medications in 331 patients. At 3 months of follow-up, it was found to be safe and effective.

Endovascular ultrasound renal denervation was studied in 136 patients with RH. They were randomly assigned to either renal denervation (n = 69) or a sham procedure (n = 67). At 2 months, RDN reduced day time ambulatory SBP significantly as compared to the sham procedure, with no difference in the safety outcome between the two arms.[102]

In patients with hypertension, who were not on antihypertensive medication, ultrasound renal denervation reduced daytime ambulatory SBP at 2 months versus a sham procedure without safety issues.[103]

The registry data of hypertensive patients receiving renal denervation have clearly shown that the BP reduction is long lasting without safety concerns.[104,105]

European Society of Cardiology (ESC) Council on Hypertension and the European Association of Cardiovascular Interventions (EAPCI)[106,107] have proposed the following in their consensus statement:

- RDN may be used in adult patients with uncontrolled RH (office BP ≥140/≥90 mm Hg, confirmed by 24-hour ambulatory systolic BP ≥130 mm Hg or daytime systolic BP ≥135 mm Hg) treated with ≥3 antihypertensive drugs and an eGFR ≥40 mL/min/1.73 m^2.
- RDN may be a possible treatment option for patients unable to tolerate antihypertensive drugs in the long term or patients who express a preference to undergo RDN in a tailored, shared decision-making process.
- It is not advisable to employ RDN in the following:
    - The renal transplant patients
    - Patients with severely impaired kidney function (KDIGO stage G4 and G5)
    - Patients with fibromuscular dysplasia
    - Untreated secondary hypertension
    - A single functioning kidney
    - Patients requiring hemodialysis

The ESC/ESH guidelines[10] have given RDN a Class II B recommendation as an additional treatment option in patients with RH if eGFR is >40 mL/min/1.73 m^2.

Renal sympathetic denervation had its ups and downs and has finally has its footprints. Unfortunately, there is no easily measurable and validated method to indicate the success or otherwise of the renal nerve ablation periprocedurally. The procedure should be performed in experienced centers and it should be a shared decision.

Other devices: Carotid baroreceptor stimulation, arteriovenous anastomoses, and cardiac neuromodulation therapy (via a dedicated pacemaker) are the other modes of device therapy for RH, but are not recommended at present.[10]

CONCLUSION

Resistant hypertension carries a higher cardiovascular and renal risk. While pathophysiology of RH needs to be understood better and, more effective therapeutic strategies have to be developed, it is important in the meantime for the clinician to avoid "clinical inertia", ensure medication adherence, exclude pseudoresistant hypertension, and detect secondary hypertension. Therapeutic lifestyle measures and drug therapy have to be optimized using appropriate diuretics, MRAs, and other drugs. Renal denervation therapy looks promising, has a role and its use should be a shared decision process.

ONLINE REFERENCES

Please scan the QR code provided at the end of the table of contents for References of this chapter.

CHAPTER 38

The Choice of a Diuretic in the Treatment of Hypertension: An Updated Narrative

Evgeniya V Shalaeva, Jasur B Babadjanov, Franz H Messerli, C Venkata S Ram

ABSTRACT

Diuretics, which promote the excretion of sodium and water from the body, have served as an essential component of blood pressure management regimens for decades. They are effective, affordable, and provide favorable cardiovascular outcomes. This chapter provides an overview of currently used diuretics, which can be divided into five classes—thiazides, loop diuretics, potassium-sparing diuretics, carbonic anhydrase inhibitors, and osmotic diuretics. It highlights the pharmaceutical profiles of key antihypertensive medications from these classes. Further, it provides supporting evidence and the rationale behind their use in monotherapy or combination therapy for different groups of patients with hypertension, attempting to resolve the debate regarding diuretic selection for hypertension control. Accordingly, the chapter provides key insights into the value of diuretics in hypertension management.

Keywords: Diuretics, hypertension, blood pressure, excretion, kidney function, antihypertensive agents, cardiovascular outcomes.

INTRODUCTION

According to the World Health Organization (WHO), an estimated 1.28 billion adults aged 30–79 years worldwide have hypertension, accounting for 16% of the global population. An estimated 46% of adults with hypertension are unaware that they have this condition and only 21% of patients have their hypertension under control.[1]

Salt retention is the primary mechanism underlying elevated blood pressure (BP) in all monogenic forms of hypertension. Increasing urine sodium excretion is a reasonable and important aspect of hypertension treatment. In fact, modifying the Na^+ balance through dietary salt reduction is among the earliest approaches for hypertension control.

In this context, diuretics are one of the most frequently prescribed medications for the treatment of arterial hypertension.[2] They can be divided into five classes (thiazides, loop diuretics, potassium-sparing diuretics, carbonic anhydrase inhibitors, and osmotic diuretics) based on the specific nephron segment they target and their effects on ion reabsorption and excretion **(Table 1)**.[3] According to international guidelines, diuretics can be used in first-line therapies for individuals with essential hypertension **(Table 2)**.[4-11]

The American College of Cardiology/American Heart Association (ACC/AHA) hypertension guidelines focus on the reduction in clinical events as the primary outcome of antihypertensive drug treatment.[8] According to several studies, the hypotensive effect of diuretics is not inferior to that of angiotensin-converting enzyme inhibitors (ACEIs), calcium channel blockers (CCBs), and angiotensin receptor blockers (ARBs).[12-17]

Thiazide diuretics are one of the three equally weighted first-line antihypertensive treatments, alongside CCBs and ARBs. They can be further subdivided into compounds containing the benzothiadiazine ring structure (thiazide-type diuretics, such as hydrochlorothiazide) and those lacking the benzothiadiazine ring (thiazide-like diuretics, such as chlorthalidone and indapamide).[18] Regardless of class heterogeneity, they are equally effective as monotherapy in a majority of hypertensive patients and augment the efficacy of other classes of antihypertensives when used in combination therapy. Thiazides remain underutilized, and currently, they

TABLE 1: Five classes of diuretics and their mechanisms of action.

Classes	Key drugs	Main mechanism	Nephron target sites	Molecular sites of action	Potassium excretion
• Thiazides • Thiazide-like diuretics	• Hydrochlorothiazide • Indapamide and chlorthalidone	Sodium excretion	Distal convoluted tubule	Na^+–Cl^- symporters	K^+ ↑
Loop diuretics	Furosemide and torasemide	Sodium excretion	Loop of Henle	Na^+–K^+–$2Cl^-$ symporter	K^+ ↑
Potassium-sparing diuretics	• Triamterene • Spironolactone	Sodium excretion	Late distal tubule and collecting duct	• Epithelial Na^+ channels • Mineralocorticoid receptors	K^+ ↓
Carbonic anhydrase inhibitors	Acetazolamide	Sodium excretion	Proximal tubule	Carbonic anhydrase	K^+ ↑
Osmotic diuretics	Mannitol	Osmosis	Unspecific	Unspecific	K^+ ↑

(↑ increased; ↓ decreased)

TABLE 2: Summary of the guideline recommendations for the use of diuretics in primary hypertension.

Guidelines	Years	Recommendations
Adults		
ACC/AHA[8]	2018	Selection among three medication classes: 1. Thiazide-type diuretics 2. ACEI/angiotensin receptor antagonists 3. CCBs (long-acting)
JNC 8[92]	2014	Selection among four medication classes: 1. Thiazide-type diuretics 2. ACEI 3. Angiotensin receptor antagonists 4. CCBs (long-acting)
ESH/ESC[93]	2013	Selection among five medication classes: 1. Thiazide-type diuretics 2. ACEI 3. Angiotensin receptor antagonists 4. CCBs (long-acting) 5. Beta-blockers
NICE[2]	2011	• Individuals aged >55 years or of African–American/Caribbean descent • Thiazide-type diuretics, if CCBs are not suitable, owing to a high risk of heart failure • Combination of an ACEI or ARB and a CCB • Thiazide-type diuretics
Canadian guidelines[94]	2014	Selection among four medication classes: 1. Thiazide-type diuretics 2. Beta-blockers (<60 years) 3. ACEI 4. CCBs (long-acting)
WHO[95]	2003	Thiazide-type diuretics
Management of hypertension in black individuals[96]	2010	• Thiazide-type diuretics • CCBs

Continued

Continued

Guidelines	Years	Recommendations
Pediatric guidelines		
Task force 4th report[97]	2004	No preferred agents, diuretics can be considered
ESH[98]	2009	No preferred agents, diuretics can be considered

(ACC/AHA: American College of Cardiology/American Heart Association; ACEI: angiotensin-converting enzyme inhibitor; ARB: angiotensin receptor blocker; CCBs: calcium channel blockers; ESH/ESC: European Society of Hypertension/European Society of Cardiology, JNC: Joint National Committee; NICE: National Institute for Health and Clinical Excellence; WHO: World Health Organization)

are used to treat only one-third of all hypertensive patients. Nevertheless, for many patients, a thiazide is indispensable for achieving adequate BP control.

THIAZIDES

Thiazide diuretics initially act by decreasing extracellular volume after interacting with a thiazide-sensitive sodium-chloride cotransporter (NCC; *SLC12A3*) expressed in the distal convoluted tubule (DCT) of nephrons, enhancing Na^+ excretion in the urine and decreasing cardiac output. However, their hypotensive effects are maintained during long-term therapy due to decreased vascular resistance. The cardiac output returns to pretreatment values and the extracellular volume returns to almost normal due to compensatory responses, such as the activation of the renin-angiotensin system (RAS). The reason behind the long-term vasodilation induced by thiazide diuretics is unknown.[19]

Hydrochlorothiazide

Hydrochlorothiazide is a thiazide-type diuretic that has been used clinically for more than half a century. It acts on DCTs and inhibits the NCC system.[20] It can open Ca^{2+}-activated K^+ channels, leading to the hyperpolarization of vascular smooth muscle cells, which, in turn, leads to the closing of L-type Ca^{2+} channels and inhibits their opening. Together, these effects result in decreased Ca^{2+} entry and reduced vasoconstriction. Hydrochlorothiazide also inhibits vascular carbonic anhydrase, potentially altering the systolic pH of smooth muscle cells and thereby, opening Ca^{2+}-activated K^+ channels.

Hydrochlorothiazide enhances chloride instead of bicarbonate excretion.[21] Recent studies have shown that therapeutic intervention with this drug exerts effects on the kidney beyond the proximal tubule, indicating that its activity affects chloride excretion in the distal tubule.[22]

When administered acutely, hydrochlorothiazide lowers BP by promoting diuresis and decreasing plasma volume. However, following chronic use, it appears to reduce BP by decreasing peripheral resistance. How the drug induces vasodilation is not known, but laboratory evidence suggests that it could inhibit the enzyme carbonic anhydrase, desensitizing smooth muscle receptors to calcium elevations, or preventing autoregulation in the kidneys.[20] These actions lead to diuretic effects and the loss of potassium in the urine. The half-life of the drug varies from 6 to 12 hours.

Numerous studies have shown that at doses of 12.5–25 mg/day, hydrochlorothiazide lowers systolic BP by 5–7 mm Hg and diastolic BP by 4–5 mm Hg over a 24-hour period. While this magnitude of BP lowering is smaller than that achieved by ACEIs, CCBs, and beta-blockers, the effects of hydrochlorothiazide are more consistent and reliable in almost all populations. At doses of 50 mg, hydrochlorothiazide provides effects that are similar to those seen with CCBs (verapamil), beta-blockers (metoprolol), and ACEIs (enalapril).[23-26]

Regarding the potential minimization of cardiovascular risk, hydrochlorothiazide is not as effective as CCBs and ARBs/ACEIs in reducing harm from cardiovascular disease (CVD). Some studies show that while hydrochlorothiazide can lower BP, it does not always reduce left ventricular hypertrophy in patients with hypertension. Further, evidence suggests that when compared to CCBs, hydrochlorothiazide is associated with a higher risk of adverse cardiovascular events for any given lowering of systolic BP.[25,27,28]

Notably, in patients with renal dysfunction, hydrochlorothiazide can cause azotemia.[29] It can also cause electrolyte and/or fluid imbalances, including hypokalemia, hyponatremia, hypercalcemia, and/or hypomagnesemia.[29] The exacerbation of systemic lupus erythematosus with the use of hydrochlorothiazide has been reported in the literature.[30] This drug can also cause acute transient myopia and acute angle-closure glaucoma, which may occur hours to weeks after drug initiation. Risk factors for these adverse events include a history of sulfonamide or penicillin allergy.[31,32]

Hyperuricemia leading to acute gout may also occur due to hydrochlorothiazide. Another potential adverse effect is hyperglycemia, and this drug has been known to unmask latent diabetes and increase cholesterol and triglyceride levels in patients.[33,34] Overall, thiazides have been linked, in a dose-dependent manner, to deleterious metabolic consequences such as hypokalemia, hyperglycemia, hyponatremia, hyperuricemia, hyperlipidemia, and hypomagnesemia.[35-37]

Low blood potassium was found to be a risk factor for sudden cardiac death after thiazide therapy in a case-control study[37] and could impair the effects of the drug in preventing major cardiovascular events.[38] Additionally, potassium reductions were linked to higher blood sugar levels.[39]

Chlorthalidone

Chlorthalidone is a thiazide-like sulfonamide-derived diuretic that was first approved by the Food and Drug Administration (FDA) for hypertension management in 1960.[40] It is a first-line agent for the treatment of hypertension.[41] Due to its prolonged elimination half-life, which averages at 50–60 hours with chronic dosage, chlorthalidone appears superior to other thiazides and can be used in once-daily dosage forms.[42] Virtually, all of the drug irreversibly binds to carbonic anhydrase in erythrocytes, resulting in a huge volume of distribution and the creation of a storage reservoir for chlorthalidone. Hence, just 1.4% of the total drug administered is detected in the plasma.[43]

Chlorthalidone enables BP management by decreasing intravascular volume through increased diuresis. The 2017 guidelines for the prevention, detection, evaluation, and management of high BP state that chlorthalidone can be used as a first-line agent in the setting of hypertension if no contraindications or contributory comorbidities are present.[44]

Several well-controlled outcome trials, including the Treatment of Mild Hypertension Study (TOMHS)[44] and Systolic Blood Pressure Intervention Trial (SPRINT),[45] have clearly demonstrated the protective effects of chlorthalidone against hypertension. In addition to its long duration of action, chlorthalidone provides target-organ protection (e.g., left ventricular hypertrophy regression) and improved cardiovascular/clinical outcomes. Specifically, it reduces the risk of heart failure and cerebrovascular damage[45] and can control nocturnal hypertension, further demonstrating its chronobiological value.[46]

It is important to note that unlike in other countries, chlorthalidone is available in low-dosage forms (6.25 and 12.5 mg) in India. Hypokalemia is believed to be the most common adverse effect associated with chlorthalidone use.[47] Other reported adverse effects of this drug include hyponatremia, hypersensitivity, and precipitation of acute gout attacks. These known derangements make the periodic monitoring of serum electrolytes essential for patients receiving chlorthalidone throughout hypertensive management. However, it must be noted that studies examining the adverse effects and renal risks of chlorthalidone are typically based on chlorthalidone doses of 12.5 mg and higher. Hence, the risk of hypokalemia and other adverse events can be mitigated using 6.25 mg chlorthalidone or adding a potassium-sparing agent to the treatment regimen.[46,48] It may thus be appropriate to say, based on the overall published evidence from numerous clinical trials, that chlorthalidone is the superior choice among all diuretics for hypertension control, especially in India, given its widespread availability and cost-effective nature.

Indapamide

Indapamide has a dual mechanism of action; it exerts a diuretic effect at the level of the distal tubule in the kidney and also produces direct vascular effects. The sustained-release (SR) formulation of indapamide contains a hydrophilic matrix, which provides a smoother pharmacokinetic profile. This prevents unnecessary peak plasma concentrations, which are often associated with side effects. Indapamide SR is now extensively used in hypertensive patients, including those at increased risk of cardiovascular events, such as older patients and patients with diabetes. It has been shown to decrease BP, particularly systolic BP, with 24-hour efficacy, allowing a once-daily dosage. Studies have demonstrated that indapamide SR is as effective at lowering BP as all major therapeutic drug classes, including more recently developed antihypertensive drugs. Beyond BP reductions, indapamide SR can also provide protection against hypertension-induced target-organ damage in the heart and kidneys and has a favorable metabolic profile. A broad evidence base supports the benefits of indapamide 1.5 mg SR in hypertensive patients, alone or as part of combination therapy, as recommended by the majority of guidelines.[49]

The pharmacokinetic profile of indapamide falls between that of chlorthalidone and hydrochlorothiazide. It has a substantial (25 L) volume of distribution throughout the body and is strongly bound (76%) to plasma proteins, including erythrocyte carbonic anhydrase (98%).[46] With a biphasic terminal half-life of around 16 hours, it has a substantially longer half-life than hydrochlorothiazide, and it is extensively metabolized in the liver (7% eliminated as unaltered drug in urine).[46,47]

OTHER DIURETICS

Mineralocorticoid receptors, also known as aldosterone receptors, are expressed in the DCT cells of the kidney. Spironolactone and aldosterone compete with one another to bind to this receptor. When spironolactone binds to the receptor, it prevents aldosterone-dependent sodium–potassium exchange, causing sodium and water to be excreted and potassium to be retained. Since spironolactone is a mild diuretic, it is frequently administered in combination with another drug that acts on the proximal tubules to promote diuresis. Spironolactone intake can result in hyperkalemia in some patients and has nontarget effects such as gynecomastia because it binds to both androgen and progesterone receptors.[48] Spironolactone and eplerenone are both effective antihypertensive medications;[50-52] however, they are not frequently used in combination with thiazides.

A recent study aimed to compare the use of thiazide diuretics alone and in combination with potassium-sparing diuretics in the treatment of arterial hypertension. It showed that thiazides plus potassium-sparing diuretics are more effective at lowering BP while minimizing hypokalemia and hyperglycemia. Hence, combining thiazides with potassium-sparing diuretics, such as spironolactone, eplerenone, amiloride, or triamterene, may reduce the risk of treatment-induced hypokalemia, decreased glucose tolerance, and abrupt death.[53]

According to a systematic review of six double-blind randomized controlled trials (RCTs) encompassing a total of 496 individuals, amiloride and triamterene provide comparable reductions in BP.[54] However, in two separate studies, amiloride was found to enhance hydrochlorothiazide's ability to reduce BP.[53,55] Hence, amiloride may be helpful in managing resistant hypertension,[56] especially at larger dosages.[57]

Loop diuretics are not recommended as part of hypertension guidelines largely due to the limited availability of outcome data. Nevertheless, they have been shown to lower BP and offer potential advantages over thiazide-type diuretics. Torsemide has a longer duration of action with once-daily dosing (vs. furosemide and bumetanide) and has more reliable bioavailability (vs. furosemide). Research is needed to fill current gaps in knowledge and address misconceptions about loop diuretic use in hypertension and to determine their place in the antihypertensive arsenal.[58]

RANDOMIZED CONTROLLED TRIALS FOR DIURETICS

The Antihypertensive and Lipid-Lowering Treatment to Prevent Heart Attack Trial [(ALLHAT); *n* = 33,357] compared the long-term effects of treatment with chlorthalidone, amlodipine, and lisinopril in patients with hypertension.[54] In the cohort of hypertensive patients with at least one other coronary heart disease risk factor, the trial found no significant between-group differences in the primary outcome (combined fatal coronary heart disease or nonfatal myocardial infarction) or all-cause mortality. However, no J-curve association was detected between stroke risk and systolic or diastolic BP, and the association remained linear down to a BP level of 110/55 mm Hg. Hence, for stroke prevention, the old BP adage "the lower the better" holds true. This is a pivotal take-home message for practicing cardiologists—were it not risky for the heart, the brain would prefer an optimally cerebroprotective systolic BP of 110–120 mm Hg.[59] The value of treatment with chlorthalidone is further supported by the subanalysis of ALLHAT data in patients at least 65 years of age (*n* = 19,173).[54] Moreover, while higher fasting glucose levels have been observed after treatment with chlorthalidone, there is no conclusive evidence that this modestly increased risk of diabetes mellitus increases the risk of other clinical events.[60]

In contrast, ALLHAT revealed differences in secondary outcomes among the different therapeutic classes. The 6-year relative risk (RR) of heart failure was higher with amlodipine than with chlorthalidone [RR 1.38 (95% CI 1.25–1.52)]. Further, the RR of CVD, stroke, and heart failure was significantly higher with lisinopril than with chlorthalidone [RR 1.10 (95% CI 1.05–1.16); RR 1.15 (95% CI 1.02–1.30); RR 1.20 (95% CI 1.09–1.34)], respectively.[54] Indeed, diuretics are specifically recommended in patient groups that are especially responsive to these agents, such as patients with diabetes, older patients, patients of African origin, and patients with a history of stroke or low renin levels, as well as patients with heart failure, isolated systolic hypertension, or resistant hypertension.

Two major trials support the preferred use of chlorthalidone and indapamide in the elderly. The placebo-controlled Systolic Hypertension in the Elderly Program [(SHEP); *n* = 4,736], which enrolled hypertensive patients aged at least 60 years, showed that patients treated with chlorthalidone 12.5–25 mg (with atenolol as needed) for 4.5 years had significantly lower rates of stroke [RR 0.63 (95% CI 0.49–0.82)], myocardial infarction [RR 0.67 (95% CI 0.47–0.96)], coronary heart disease [RR 0.75 (95% CI 0.60–0.94)], heart failure [RR 0.51 (95% CI 0.37–0.71)], and all-cause mortality [RR 0.87 (95% CI 0.73–1.05)] than patients treated with placebo.[61] Safety evaluations after 3 years showed that although treatment led to statistically significant effects on laboratory parameters, these changes were not clinically significant in most patients, as the incidence of diabetes development after chlorthalidone treatment was not greatly affected.[62] The rate of hypokalemia (3.9% vs. 0.8% with placebo) was, however, higher in the chlorthalidone group.[61] Nevertheless, chlorthalidone performed significantly better than amlodipine for heart failure. Moreover, in the comparison with lisinopril, chlorthalidone still performed significantly better for preventing heart failure, the combined endpoint for coronary heart disease, and the combined endpoint for CVD.

The results of the Hypertension in the Very Elderly Trial [(HYVET); *n* = 3,845][63] and the HYVET extension study dispelled any uncertainty about the benefits of treating hypertension in much older patients. In patients at least 80 years of age, 2 years of treatment with indapamide SR 1.5 mg (and perindopril as needed to reach a BP target of 150/80 mm Hg) reduced the risk of stroke [unadjusted heart rate (HR) 0.70 (95% CI 0.49–1.01); $p = 0.06$], cardiovascular events [unadjusted HR 0.66 (95% CI 0.53–0.82); $p < 0.001$], heart failure [unadjusted HR 0.36 (95% CI 0.22–0.58); $p < 0.001$], cardiovascular mortality [unadjusted HR 0.77 (95% CI 0.60–1.01); $p = 0.06$], mortality from stroke [unadjusted HR 0.61 (95% CI 0.38–0.99); $p < 0.05$], and all-cause mortality [unadjusted HR 0.79 (95% CI 0.65–0.95); $p = 0.02$] compared with placebo. Additionally, no significant differences in the levels of serum potassium, uric acid, glucose, and creatinine were noted after indapamide treatment.[63]

Chlorthalidone is similar to thiazide diuretics with respect to its mechanism of action, although it has a mildly altered chemical structure. It inhibits sodium reabsorption at the level of the DCT via NCC inhibition and thus affects chloride levels. By attenuating sodium reabsorption at this site, it allows the retention of sodium. This lack of reabsorption alters the osmotic gradient and shifts fluid distribution from the outside of the tubule to the inside of the tubule. The increased osmotic load from the increased sodium concentration leads to elevated intratubular volume, thus inducing diuretic effects. The increased excretion of sodium and extracellular fluid decreases intravascular water and solute concentrations. By lowering the intravascular volume and osmotic gradient, the drug reduces hydrostatic pressure, leading to a clinical reduction in BP.

According to recent studies, chlorthalidone shows beneficial effects in managing arterial hypertension in patients with comorbidities. Among patients with advanced chronic kidney disease (CKD) and poorly controlled hypertension, chlorthalidone therapy improved BP control at 12 weeks of study when compared with placebo.[64] Moreover, the use of chlorthalidone to reduce BP in patients with stage 4 CKD and hypertension, especially those with significant proteinuria, was shown to provide high treatment with high efficacy.[65]

Hydrochlorothiazide appears to be less potent per milligram for BP reduction than chlorthalidone (hydrochlorothiazide 50 mg is equipotent to chlorthalidone 12.5–25 mg).[26,66,67] A 2014 meta-analysis of 26 trials (n = 4,683), for example, showed that to decrease office systolic BP by 10 mm Hg, 8.6 mg of chlorthalidone or 26.4 mg of hydrochlorothiazide was needed.[67] In addition, a 2014 Cochrane database analysis showed that a reduction of 8.7–11.9 mm Hg in systolic BP could be reached after treatment with a 1.5–5 mg dose of indapamide, and that for systolic BP, indapamide SR 1.5 mg was roughly equipotent to hydrochlorothiazide 25–50 mg.[26] This analysis also suggested that the effects of indapamide and chlorthalidone on BP are not dose dependent over the 1–5 and 12.5–75 mg ranges, respectively, whereas reductions in systolic BP with hydrochlorothiazide treatment increase with the dose from <5 mm Hg at the 6.25 mg dose to 10.5 mm Hg at the 50 mg dose.[66]

A 2015 systematic review demonstrated that chlorthalidone alleviates hypertensive burden by about 5.1 mm Hg of systolic BP more than hydrochlorothiazide, suggesting that chlorthalidone is more potent than hydrochlorothiazide.[68] Conversely, in a recent study, chlorthalidone use was not associated with significant cardiovascular benefits when compared with hydrochlorothiazide, while its use was associated with greater risk of renal and electrolyte abnormalities.[69] However, the study used 12.5 mg of chlorthalidone, and the results may not be applicable to lower-dose formulations of chlorthalidone, such as those available in India.

A 2022 study also showed that patients receiving chlorthalidone do not have a lower occurrence of major cardiovascular outcome events or non-cancer-related deaths than those receiving hydrochlorothiazide.[70] The participants were selected among patients in the Department of Veterans Affairs health system (aged 65 years or older) who had been receiving hydrochlorothiazide at a daily dose of 25 or 50 mg. They were randomized to continue therapy with hydrochlorothiazide or switch to chlorthalidone at a daily dose of 12.5 or 25 mg. The primary outcome was a composite of nonfatal myocardial infarction, stroke, and heart failure, resulting in hospitalization, urgent coronary revascularization for unstable angina, and non-cancer-related death.

A total of 13,523 patients underwent randomization. At baseline, hydrochlorothiazide at a dose of 25 mg/day had been prescribed to 12,781 patients (94.5%). The mean baseline systolic BP in each group was 139 mm Hg. At a median follow-up of 2.4 years, there was little difference in the occurrence of primary-outcome events between the chlorthalidone [702 patients (10.4%)] and hydrochlorothiazide groups [675 patients (10.0%)]. There were no between-group differences in the occurrence of any primary outcome, and the results showed that patients who received chlorthalidone did not have a lower occurrence of major cardiovascular outcome events or non-cancer-related deaths than patients who received hydrochlorothiazide. However, a careful analysis of the data shows that although the protective effects of chlorthalidone and hydrochlorothiazide were comparable **(Fig. 1)**, the dosage of the latter was higher. Furthermore, in patients with preexisting CVD, the benefits provided by chlorthalidone were significantly greater than those of hydrochlorothiazide **(Fig. 2)**, although the duration of treatment with chlorthalidone was shorter **(Fig. 3)**.[47] Hence, these data suggest that even a shorter duration of chlorthalidone treatment can prevent hypertension complications in a manner comparable to long-term,

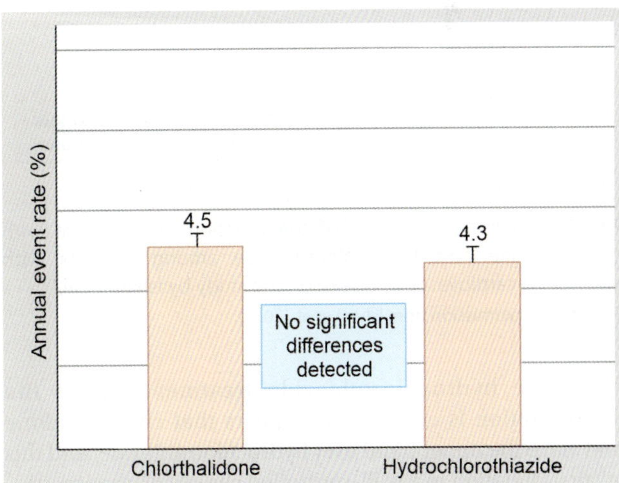

FIG. 1: Comparison of annual event rate between the chlorthalidone and hydrochlorothiazide groups in the study by Ishani et al.,[70] showing that the protective effects of chlorthalidone and hydrochlorothiazide were similar when the dosage of hydrochlorothiazide was higher.

Source: With permission from Ishani et al. (2022).

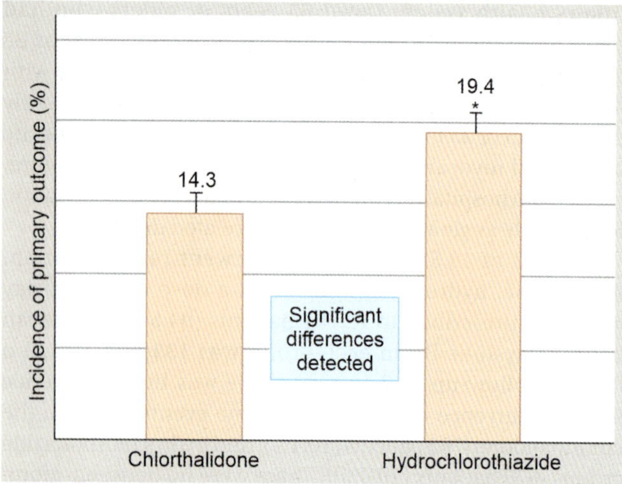

*<0.05

FIG. 2: Comparison of the benefits of chlorthalidone and hydrochlorothiazide among patients with preexisting cardiovascular disease in the study by Ishani et al.,[70] showing that chlorthalidone provided greater protection in this group.
Source: With permission from Ishani et al. (2022).

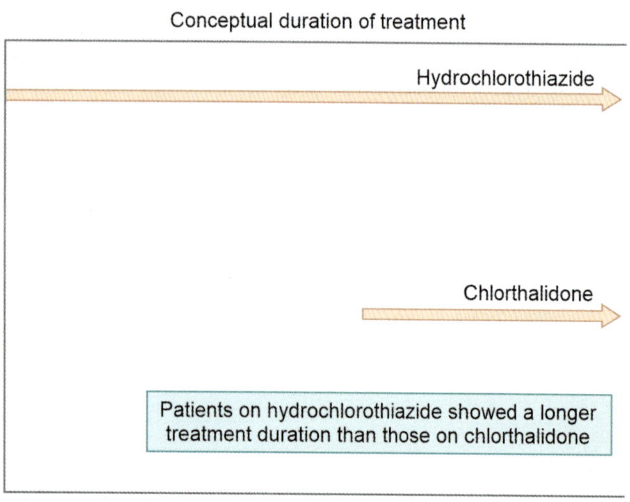

FIG. 3: Schematic depicting of the duration of treatment with chlorthalidone and hydrochlorothiazide among patients with preexisting cardiovascular disease in the study by Ishani et al.[70]
Source: With permission from Ishani et al. (2022).

high-dose hydrochlorothiazide treatment. While the interpretation is complex, it appears that chlorthalidone may have the upper hand over hydrochlorothiazide, and this awaits validation in a well-controlled clinical environment.

In addition to potency, studies have demonstrated that chlorthalidone holds a longer duration of action than hydrochlorothiazide (24 h vs. 6–12 h). This increased duration of action allows for an increased flexibility of dosing.[68] As a result of this longer duration of action, chlorthalidone is 1.5–2.0 times more effective at lowering systolic BP than hydrochlorothiazide (comparative antihypertensive effects between hydrochlorothiazide and chlorthalidone on ambulatory and office BP).[71]

When examining an antihypertensive medication, the effect on cardiovascular outcomes is of the highest priority. The ALLHAT trial showed a decreased risk of heart failure exacerbation and cerebrovascular incidents with chlorthalidone when compared to amlodipine and lisinopril, respectively.[27,45,72]

Additionally, a meta-analysis including over 100,000 patients concluded that chlorthalidone and thiazide-like diuretics lower the risk of heart failure and cardiovascular events by 21% and 12%, respectively. In comparison, the thiazide-type hydrochlorothiazide did not provide improved outcomes compared to placebo. Together, these data demonstrate the superiority of chlorthalidone as a diuretic for hypertension management.

Indapamide is frequently referred to as a thiazide-like diuretic, since it is more comparable to chlorthalidone than to hydrochlorothiazide.[73] Hence, it is unlikely to be used in a direct comparison trial with either of these drugs. Thus, data on these comparisons are limited.

DIURETICS FOR RESISTANT ARTERIAL HYPERTENSION

Resistant arterial hypertension (RAH) is a serious condition that leads to severe cardiovascular complications, such as myocardial infarction, stroke, and death. It is defined as the persistence of above-goal elevated BP despite the concurrent use of three or more classes of antihypertensive medications administered at maximum or maximally tolerated doses and at appropriate dosing frequency.[11]

Calcium channel blockers, RAS blockers (ARBs or ACEIs), and diuretics [thiazide diuretic, if renal function is normal or loop diuretic, in case of CKD with estimated glomerular filtration rate (eGFR) 30 mL/min] are considered first-choice agents for RAH treatment. Spironolactone (25–50 mg daily), a mineralocorticoid receptor antagonist, should be administered if resistant hypertension is verified. Spironolactone, eplerenone, and canrenone (not available in the United States) are three mineralocorticoid receptor antagonists that can be used to treat hypertension. For instance, the addition of spironolactone as the fourth medicine to treat RAH can provide a significant antihypertensive effect, with mean BP reductions frequently reaching 20/10 mm Hg.[74,75]

In the PATHWAY-2 (Prevention and Treatment of Hypertension with Algorithm-based Therapy-2) study, the standardized triple-drug combination of a RAS inhibitor, amlodipine, and a thiazide-like diuretic was used as baseline therapy. This study also showed the superiority of spironolactone when added as a fourth drug.[50] It has not been scientifically proven that combining spironolactone with medications other than an ACEI or ARB, amlodipine, chlorthalidone, or indapamide is advantageous. In participants with normal renal function (eGFR >45 mL/min and mean eGFR 91.1 mL/min), spironolactone was well tolerated. Although study participants were only exposed to spironolactone for 3 months, no side effects were documented during the investigation.[50]

Similar to this, patients with good renal function have a low risk of spironolactone-induced hyperkalemia, particularly if they concurrently take the potassium excretion-promoting drug chlorthalidone. However, the risk of hyperkalemia increases as renal function deteriorates.[76] Hence, a beta-blocker, an alpha-blocker, or a medication with central antihypertensive action should be provided if spironolactone is contraindicated or side effects appear.[77]

Clinical inertia, often referred to as the undertreatment of hypertension, is a typical problem that worsens as the number of drugs recommended rises.[76] Undertreatment of hypertension includes inadequate treatment intensification in uncontrolled individuals.[78] Using electronic medical data, Egan et al.[79] found that >44,000 individuals enrolled in community-based clinics in the Southeast of the United States had evident uncontrolled resistant hypertension. Only 15% of them had been given diuretics and two additional antihypertensive medications at <50% of the maximum dosage advised for managing hypertension.[79]

Khosla and colleagues showed that switching from hydrochlorothiazide to chlorthalidone in patients whose BP is uncontrolled by multiple drug combinations results in further BP reduction and increases overall BP control rates.[80] Approximately 20% of patients with RAH have increased aldosterone levels,[81-84] and the excess of aldosterone may underlie resistance to antihypertensive therapy.[74,85-87]

DIURETIC USE IN PATIENTS WITH CHRONIC KIDNEY DISEASE

The AHA's recommendation for daily dietary sodium intake of <1,500 mg/day is strongly supported by a thorough meta-analysis of clinical trials based on a novel statistical method. However, it also suggests that any decrease in sodium intake is likely to be advantageous. According to this meta-analysis, the thiazide-like diuretic chlorthalidone (as add-on medication) significantly reduces BP in individuals with stage 4 renal disease compared to placebo. It has been demonstrated that nonsteroidal mineralocorticoid receptor antagonists decrease BP and significantly reduce the risk of CVD.[88]

However, spironolactone usage may be restricted in patients with CKD due to hyperkalemia. Modern potassium-binding medicines address the risk of hyperkalemia, allowing patients with severe CKD and resistant hypertension to continue taking spironolactone, a powerful BP-lowering supplement. Thanks to patiromer, patients with CKD and resistant hypertension are more likely to continue spironolactone therapy with mitigated hyperkalemia. The treatment of resistant hypertension in this population of patients with prolonged spironolactone has clinical relevance.[89,90]

A recent investigation showed that in patients with heart failure with preserved ejection fraction (HFpEF) and resistant hypertension, but not in those without resistant hypertension, spironolactone use was associated with a decreased risk of composite cardiovascular events. Spironolactone usage decreased hospitalization for heart failure and death from all causes in patients with HFpEF and resistant hypertension. Patients with resistant hypertension and nonresistant hypertension both saw drops in BP, following spironolactone administration, but those with HFpEF with resistant hypertension did not. In summary, patients with HFpEF and resistant hypertension had a lower risk of composite cardiovascular events, all-cause mortality, and heart failure hospitalization when they used spironolactone. However, this trend was not noted in patients without resistant hypertension. Therefore, patients with HFpEF and resistant hypertension who are currently on ACEIs/ARBs, CCBs, and diuretics may benefit from the supplementary administration of spironolactone.[91]

CONCLUSION

Diuretics are critical agents for the management of hypertension and their efficacy, even in hypertensive patients with other comorbidities, is well established. Studies have confirmed that the use of diuretics, both as monotherapy and combination therapy, lowers BP and reduces hypertension-related complications and target-organ damage, thus improving cardiovascular outcomes. Chlorthalidone has emerged as a superior diuretic given its versatile nature, long-duration of action, and clinical protection, especially when used in combination with potassium-sparing diuretics. Owing to these advantages and its unique benefits in the Indian context, chlorthalidone now seems to be the answer to the long-standing debate on diuretic choice in hypertension management.

ACKNOWLEDGMENT

The authors thank Ms Zeba Khatri for her editorial assistance and reference verification.

ONLINE REFERENCES

Please scan the QR code provided at the end of the table of contents for References of this chapter.

CHAPTER 39

Basic Therapeutic Principles in the Management of Hypertension in Patients with Chronic Kidney Disease

Panagiotis I Georgianos, Rajiv Agarwal

ABSTRACT

In patients with chronic kidney disease (CKD), hypertension is very common and remains often poorly controlled. Nonpharmacological interventions, such as dietary sodium restriction, should be the initial step to the management of hypertension. When blood pressure (BP) remains unresponsive to nonpharmacological therapy, initiation of antihypertensive medications is the next step to achieve an adequate BP control. In CKD patients with severely-increased albuminuria, guidelines consistently and strongly recommend the preferential use of an agent blocking the renin–angiotensin system (RAS) as first-line treatment. Patients who fail to achieve BP control despite adherence to triple therapy with a RAS blocker, a long-acting dihydropyridine calcium channel blocker and a diuretic fulfill the diagnostic criteria of resistant hypertension. In such patients, the steroidal mineralocorticoid receptor antagonist (MRA) spironolactone is recommended by guidelines as the standard of care treatment, when the levels of estimated glomerular filtration rate are >45 mL/min/1.73 m^2 and the levels of serum potassium <4.5 mmol/L. For patients with poorly controlled hypertension and CKD not on dialysis, including patients with treatment-resistant hypertension, chlorthalidone is effective in lowering ambulatory BP and in improving albuminuria. Novel therapies, such as sodium-glucose cotransporter-2 inhibitors and the nonsteroidal MRA finerenone, have been added to our therapeutic armamentarium. These agents are not indicated for their BP-lowering effects, but guidelines strongly recommend their broad utilization for the improvement of cardiorenal outcomes. In this chapter, we will discuss the basic principles in the diagnosis, classification, and management of hypertension in patients with CKD who are not on dialysis.

Keywords: Blood pressure, CKD, hypertension, RAS blockade, spironolactone, chlorthalidone.

INTRODUCTION

Hypertension is very common in patients with chronic kidney disease (CKD) and remains often inadequately controlled despite the intensive treatment with multiple blood pressure (BP)-lowering medications.[1] Several epidemiological studies have shown that the prevalence of high BP increases with worsening stage of CKD,[2] generating the impression that the severity of hypertension goes hand-in-hand with the progressive decline in the levels of estimated glomerular filtration rate (eGFR). However, a growing body of evidence suggests that independently from eGFR, albuminuria is more closely associated with the severity of hypertension.[3,4] Uncontrolled BP is an established risk factor for faster progression of kidney injury to end-stage kidney disease (ESKD).[5,6] Lack of an adequate BP control also magnifies the risk of cardiovascular disease,[5,6] which is the leading cause of mortality in the CKD population.[7]

In this chapter, we will review the basic principles in the diagnosis, classification, and management of hypertension in patients with CKD who are not yet on dialysis.

DIAGNOSIS

Office Blood Pressure Measurements

The first principle for the adequate diagnosis and management of hypertension is to get the BP measurement in the right way **(Table 1)**. Accordingly, guidelines recommend the use of standardized instead of routine BP measurements in the office environment.[8-10] The rationale for this guidance is that all major trials that guide our therapeutic decisions were

TABLE 1: Methods for the measurement of BP in the office and outside of the office.

Parameter	Routine office BP	Unattended automated office BP	Home BP	Ambulatory BP
Description	Manual or automated oscillometric measurements without specification of seated rest and with an observer in the room	Multiple automated oscillometric measurements after a 5-minute seated and without observer in the room	BP recordings obtained twice daily by the patients themselves at home typically with a validated oscillometric device	Automated BP measurements every 20 minutes during the daytime and nighttime periods
Monitoring schedule	Office visit	Office visit	At least 3 and preferably 7 days	24-hour recording on a usual day
White-coat effect	Yes	Reduced versus routine recordings	No	No
Assessment of nocturnal hypertension	No	No	No	Yes
Association with target organ damage	Poor	Moderate	Moderate	Strong
Association with cardiorenal outcomes	Poor	Few outcome data	Superior to routine office BP	Strong
Need for patient training	No	No	Yes	Yes
Availability in daily clinical practice	Yes	Limited	Yes	Limited
Diagnostic threshold according to the 2017 AHA/ACC guidelines[10]	≤130/80 mm Hg	≤130/80 mm Hg	≤130/80 mm Hg	• 24-hour: ≤125/75 mm Hg • Awake: ≤130/80 mm Hg • Asleep: ≤110/65 mm Hg
Diagnostic threshold according to the 2023 ESH/ESC guidelines[9]	≤140/90 mm Hg	≤135/85 mm Hg	≤135/85 mm Hg	• 24-hour: ≤130/80 mm Hg • Awake: ≤135/85 mm Hg • Asleep: ≤120/70 mm Hg

(ACC: American College of Cardiology; AHA: American Heart Association; BP: blood pressure; ESC: European Society of Cardiology; ESH: European Society of Hypertension)

based on office BP recordings obtained with standardized protocols. For example, SPRINT was a landmark trial demonstrating that among nondiabetic adults with a high risk for cardiovascular disease, as compared with a conservative systolic BP (SBP) target of <140 mm Hg, targeting a SBP <120 mm Hg provoked a 25% reduction in the risk of cardiovascular morbidity and mortality.[11] However, BP in SPRINT was measured with a research-grade technique that specified 5 minutes of seated rest in a quiet room followed by multiple oscillometric BP measurements taken without the presence of an observer in the room.[11] A diagnostic test study investigated the relationship of this research-grade BP measurement methodology with routine office BP in a cohort of 275 patients CKD.[12] On average, research-grade office SBP was 12.7 mm Hg lower than routine office SBP. The 95% limits of agreement between these two techniques were wide, indicating that differences from routine office SBP can range from 46.1 mm Hg lower up to 20.7 mm Hg higher at a population level.[12] Research-grade office SBP underestimated daytime ambulatory SBP by 7.9 mm Hg, once again with wide 95% limits of agreement (–33.2 to 17.4 mm Hg). As compared with routine office SBP, research-grade office SBP and ambulatory daytime SBP were more strongly associated with echocardiographically documented left ventricular hypertrophy.[12] Taken together, these data indicate that if the intensive SBP target of SPRINT is to be implemented in daily clinical practice, then a minimum requirement would be the adoption of this research-grade technique in our daily practices. Without attention to details on how BP is measured, implementation of BP guidelines can be dangerous.

Out-of-office Blood Pressure Measurements

International guidelines recommend the use of out-of-office BP measurements as a complement to standardized office BP recordings for the confirmation of the diagnosis and classification of the severity of hypertension.[8-10]

As shown in **Table 1**, ambulatory BP monitoring (ABPM) is considered as the "gold standard" technique, because the average of these BP measurements is valid, reproducible, and provides strong prognostic associations with the risk for adverse cardiovascular and kidney outcomes.[13,14] During ABPM, a cuff of appropriate size is fitted to the nondominant arm for 24 hours and BP is typically recorded every 20 minutes during daytime and every 20–30 minutes during nighttime. In contrast to the other techniques that obtain BP measurements only during periods of rest, ABPM enables the measurement of BP during periods of activity.[13] Another unique advantage is the availability of BP measurements during sleep that enables the diagnosis of nocturnal hypertension and identification of patients with abnormal diurnal variation of BP (i.e., nondippers or reverse dippers).[13] These BP phenotypes are commonly diagnosed in patients with CKD and are associated with accelerated target organ damage and potentially increased cardiorenal risk.[15-17] There are some drawbacks of ABPM that need to be mentioned. For example, the equipment is expensive and the technique is not broadly available in daily clinical practice. The acceptability rate for repeated measurements is low; therefore, compared to home or clinic BP measurements, ABPM is less feasible for the long-term assessment and management of hypertension.[13]

Home BP monitoring (HBPM) is a more practical approach to obtain BP recordings outside of the office. This technique requires that patients will be trained to measure their BP at home under standardized conditions with the use of validated automated devices.[18] The optimal HBPM schedule includes a set of two BP measurements in the morning and a set of two BP measurements in the evening for at least 3, and preferably 7 consecutive days. Prospective observational studies have shown that as compared with office BP, 1-week averaged home BP is superior in prognosticating the long-term risk for adverse cardiorenal outcomes.[19,20] A drawback is that HBPM is less reproducible than ABPM in diagnosing masked uncontrolled hypertension (MUCH) in patients with CKD.[21] An important advantage of HBPM over ABPM is that this technique can be repeatedly performed over a long-term period to guide the intensification of antihypertensive therapy, offering the potential for less therapeutic inertia that leads to a small, but clinically meaningful improvement in BP control.[22]

CLASSIFICATION

White-coat/Masked Hypertension

The concomitant use of office and out-of-office BP measurements enables the identification of white-coat and masked hypertension **(Table 2)**.[23] A meta-analysis of six studies incorporating data from 980 patients with CKD showed that the use of office BP measurements alone results in a substantial misclassification of hypertension.[24] Overall, 40.4% of patients who had CKD and were thought to have normotension (or adequately controlled hypertension), in fact had abnormal BP outside of the office. Conversely, 30% of patients who had CKD and were thought to have hypertension, in fact had normotension when out-of-office BP monitoring was used concomitantly with office BP recordings for the classification of hypertension.[24]

The prevalence of MUCH in patients with CKD varies considerably, if different methods are used to diagnose hypertension. In a prospective observational study including 333 US veterans with CKD and normal BP when they came to the clinic, the prevalence of MUCH was 26.7% when the threshold of 135/85 mm Hg for daytime ambulatory BP was used to define hypertension.[21] It was 32.8% when hypertension was defined as 24-hour ambulatory BP ≥ 130/80 mm Hg, 56.1% when hypertension was defined as either daytime ambulatory BP ≥ 135/85 mm Hg or nighttime ambulatory BP ≥ 120/70 mm Hg, whereas the prevalence of MUCH was 50.8% when the threshold of 135/85 mm Hg for 1-week averaged home BP was used.[21] The prevalence of MUCH increased progressively with increasing levels of office SBP: 2% in the 90–110 mm Hg subgroup, 17% in the 110–119 mm Hg subgroup, 37% in the 120–129 mm Hg, and 66% in the 130–139 mm Hg subgroup. Therefore, MUCH is uncommon in CKD patients who have repeatedly low BP (90–110 mm Hg range) in the office. In contrast, the suspicion of MUCH should be raised when office BP is within the prehypertensive range. Standardized office SBP provided a high accuracy in diagnosing MUCH. Paradoxically, 1-week averaged home SBP was not superior to standardized office SBP in diagnosing MUCH.[21] One plausible explanation might be that HBPM is often performed without the required attention to details, such as 5 minutes of seated rest before the BP measurement. Accordingly, ABPM is necessary for the confirmation of the diagnosis of MUCH. HBPM cannot be used as a substitute. Most importantly, the phenotype of MUCH is not innocent. Prospective observational studies conducted specifically in patients with CKD demonstrated that the risk of adverse cardiorenal outcomes attributable to MUCH is at least similar or even higher than the cardiorenal risk of patients with sustained uncontrolled hypertension.[14,25]

Resistant Hypertension

As shown in **Table 2**, apparent treatment-resistant hypertension (aTRH) is diagnosed in patients with above-goal BP despite the concurrent use of ≥3 antihypertensive medications from different classes, one of which should be a diuretic. Patients receiving treatment with ≥4 antihypertensive medications also fulfill the diagnostic criteria of aTRH irrespective of BP levels.[26] International guidelines require the exclusion of common causes of pseudoresistance to aid the identification of true-resistant hypertension. Accordingly, the diagnostic work-up of patients with aTRH includes the use of HBPM or ABPM for the exclusion of the white-coat effect. In addition, suboptimal adherence to the prescribed antihypertensive regimen is another common cause of pseudoresistance that should be properly excluded.[26,27]

TABLE 2: Classification of hypertension into phenotypes.

Blood pressure (BP) classification*	Office BP**	Daytime ambulatory or home BP
Normotension	<140/90 mm Hg	<135/85 mm Hg
White-coat hypertension	≥140/90 mm Hg	<135/85 mm Hg
Masked hypertension	<140/90 mm Hg	≥135/85 mm Hg
Sustained hypertension	≥140/90 mm Hg	≥135/85 mm Hg
Difficult-to-control BP	**Definition**	
Apparent treatment-resistant hypertension	Uncontrolled BP despite the concurrent use of ≥3 BP-lowering medications from different categories, inclusive of a diuretic or use of ≥4 antihypertensive medications regardless of BP levels	
True-resistant hypertension	Exclusion of the white-coat effect and confirmation of medication adherence in a patient with apparent treatment-resistant hypertension	
Refractory hypertension	Uncontrolled BP despite the concurrent use of at least 5 antihypertensive medication classes, one of which should be a diuretic	

*For patients with drug-treated hypertension, the BP classification is controlled hypertension, white-coat uncontrolled hypertension, masked uncontrolled hypertension, and sustained uncontrolled hypertension.

**According to the BP thresholds recommended by the 2023 guidelines of the European Society of Hypertension (ESH).

In a meta-analysis of 91 studies involving a total of 3.2 million patients with drug-treated hypertension, the prevalence of aTRH was 14.7%, the prevalence of pseudoresistant hypertension was 10.3%, whereas the prevalence of true-resistant hypertension was 10.3%.[28] True-resistant hypertension is more commonly diagnosed in patients with CKD than in the general hypertensive population.[29] For example, a prospective observational study from Italy included 436 hypertensive CKD patients who underwent ABPM. Using the threshold of 125/75 mm Hg for 24-hour ambulatory BP in conjunction with the diagnosis of aTRH (defined as office BP ≥130/80 mm Hg despite adherence to treatment with ≥3 antihypertensives, inclusive of a diuretic, or adherence to therapy with ≥4 antihypertensives), patients were classified in four different BP phenotypes.[30] Controlled hypertension was diagnosed in 27.1% of patients, pseudoresistant hypertension in 7.1% of patients, sustained uncontrolled hypertension in 42.9% of patients, whereas the prevalence of true-resistant hypertension was 22.9%.[30] In a longitudinal part of this study, adverse cardiorenal outcomes were monitored over a median follow-up of 57 months. Using those with controlled hypertension as a reference category, the hazard ratio (HR) for the composite outcome of fatal or nonfatal cardiovascular events was 1.24, 1.11, and 1.98 in patients with pseudoresistant, sustained uncontrolled, and true-resistant hypertension, respectively.[30] As compared with the referent category of controlled hypertension, the HR for the composite outcome of ESKD or death was 1.18 in patients with pseudoresistance, 2.14 in patients with sustained uncontrolled hypertension and 2.66 in those with true-resistance to antihypertensive therapy.[30] Accordingly, in CKD, patients with true-resistant hypertension carry the highest risk for adverse cardiorenal outcomes.

Refractory Hypertension

Refractory hypertension is a rare, but severe phenotype of complete antihypertensive treatment failure that has been defined in population-based studies as uncontrolled BP in patients who are being treated with ≥5 antihypertensive medication classes, one of which should be a diuretic.[31] The prevalence and prognostic significance of refractory hypertension were investigated in 3,147 hypertensive patients enrolled in the Chronic Renal Insufficiency Cohort (CRIC) study.[32] Of the overall population, 136 patients (4.3%) fulfilled the diagnostic criteria of refractory hypertension at baseline. As compared to patients with aTRH, those with refractory hypertension were more likely to be Black, have established cardiovascular disease, have lower serum potassium levels, and receive more aggressive treatment with second-line antihypertensive medications.[32] In fully adjusted analysis, relative to aTRH, refractory hypertension was associated with 1.73-fold higher risk for the composite kidney outcome of sustained ≥50% decline in eGFR from baseline or ESKD across the whole spectrum of follow-up.[32] As compared with aTRH, refractory hypertension was also associated with 2.72-fold higher risk for the composite cardiovascular outcome of nonfatal stroke, nonfatal myocardial infarction (MI), or hospitalization for heart failure (HF) over the later years of follow-up.[32] Prior studies revealed that the cardiorenal risk is higher in patients with than in those without aTRH. These data from the CRIC study indicate that cardiorenal risk is further magnified in patients with the more severe phenotype of refractory hypertension.

MANAGEMENT

Blood Pressure Targets

In the CKD population, the optimal target BP levels remain an area of controversy **(Table 3)**.[23] The guideline recommendations released over the last years were based mainly on the results of three landmark trials, i.e., MDRD, AASK, and SPRINT.[33-35] In the MDRD trial,[34] 840 nondiabetic patients with moderate-to-advanced CKD [glomerular filtration rate (GFR): 13–55 mL/min/1.73 m^2] were randomized to a usual protein or a low-protein diet and to achieve a standard or an intensive BP goal (mean arterial pressure: ≤107 vs. ≤92 mm Hg) in a 2 × 2 factorial design. In the overall analysis, over a mean follow-up of 2.2 years, the risk of CKD progression did not differ between the standard BP and intensive BP arm.[34] Exploratory subgroup analyses showed a slower rate of GFR decline in patients who had proteinuria >1 g/day at trial initiation.[34] In the AASK trial,[35] 1,094 African-Americans with hypertensive nephrosclerosis were randomized to two different levels of BP control (mean arterial pressure: 102–107 vs. ≤92 mm Hg) and to initial anti-hypertensive treatment with a regimen containing either metoprolol (50–200 mg/day), or ramipril (2.5–10 mg/day), or amlodipine (5–10 mg/day) in a 2 × 3 factorial design. As compared with the standard BP arm, intensive BP-lowering did not improve the composite outcome of sustained ≥50% decline in GFR from baseline, ESKD, or death until the completion of the randomized phase of the trial.[35] However, a post hoc analysis incorporating long-term follow-up data from AASK participants showed that the treatment effect of intensive BP-lowering differed according to the levels of proteinuria at baseline.[36] In the subgroup of patients with a urinary protein-to-creatinine ratio ≥0.22, initial randomization to the intensive BP arm was associated with 27% reduction in the risk of progression of CKD.[36] Despite the fact that these potential benefits were derived from post hoc and/or subgroup analyses, the Kidney Disease: Improving Global Outcomes (KDIGO) 2012 guidelines differentiated the therapeutic targets in patients CKD, according the presence or absence of proteinuria. In proteinuric CKD, the KDIGO 2012 guidelines provided a Level 2D recommendation for a tighter BP target of <130/80 mm Hg.[37] In nonproteinuric CKD, there was a recommendation for a conservative BP target of <140/90 mm Hg.[37]

Published in 2017, a prespecified subgroup analysis of the SPRINT trial reported the treatment effects of intensive BP-lowering in 2,646 patients with nondiabetic CKD and a high cardiovascular risk profile.[33] Over a median follow-up of 3.3 years as compared with a SBP target of <140 mm Hg, targeting a SBP of <120 mm Hg was associated with a 19% relative risk reduction in the primary composite cardiovascular outcome of nonfatal MI, nonfatal stroke, acute decompensated HF, and death from cardiovascular causes. In addition, the risk of all-cause mortality was lower

TABLE 3: Treatment algorithms for the management of hypertension in patients with CKD according to recently released international guidelines.

Guideline/ Year	BP target	Office BP measurement	First-line therapy	Second-line therapy	Third-line therapy	Fourth-line therapy
AHA/ACC 2017	<130/80 mm Hg	Standardized	ACEI or ARB in those with very high albuminuria	CCB or diuretic	Diuretic or CCB	Spironolactone*
ISH 2020	<130/80 mm Hg (<140/90 mm Hg in elderly patients)	Standardized	ACEI or ARB	CCB or diuretic	Diuretic or CCB	Spironolactone*
ESC 2021	Systolic <140 down to 130 mm Hg, if tolerated	Standardized	Initial combination of an ACEI or an ARB + CCB or diuretic		Combination therapy with ACEI or ARB + CCB + diuretic	Spironolactone*
KDIGO 2021	Systolic <120 mm Hg, when tolerated	Standardized	ACEI or ARB in those with very high albuminuria			
ESH 2023	<130/80 mm Hg in most CKD patients, if tolerated	Standardized	Initial combination of an ACEI or an ARB + CCB or diuretic		Combination therapy with ACEI or ARB + CCB + diuretic	*CKD stage 1–3*: spironolactone (CKD stage 4–5ND: chlorthalidone)

*The use of spironolactone as fourth-line therapy is discouraged in patients with eGFR <45 mL/min/1.73 m^2 or with a serum potassium concentration of >4.5 mmol/L.

(ACEI: angiotensin-converting enzyme inhibitor; ACC: American College of Cardiology; AHA: American Heart Association; ARB: angiotensin receptor blocker; BP: blood pressure; CCB: calcium channel blocker; CKD: chronic kidney disease; ESC: European Society of Cardiology; eGFR: estimated glomerular filtration rate; ESH: European Society of Hypertension; ISH: International Society of Hypertension; KDIGO: Kidney Disease: Improving Global Outcomes; ND: non-dialysis) by 27% in the intensive BP arm than in the standard BP arm.[33] The benefits of intensive BP-lowering on cardiovascular outcomes and all-cause mortality were not modified by the presence or absence of CKD at baseline. SPRINT trial was not adequately powered to investigate the effect of intensive BP lowering on kidney outcomes. Therefore, it is not surprising that the secondary kidney failure outcome occurred in few patients; sustained ≥50% decline in eGFR from baseline or ESKD occurred in only 15 patients in the intensive BP arm and 16 patients in the standard BP arm.[33]

This impressive cardioprotective benefit of intensive BP-lowering in SPRINT has substantially influenced the guideline recommendations released over the subsequent years. The 2017 American College of Cardiology/American Heart Association (ACC/AHA) guidelines reappraised the definition/classification of hypertension and recommended a tight SBP target of <130 mm Hg for all hypertensive patients at high risk of cardiovascular disease, including patients with CKD.[10] However, the results of SPRINT may not be generalizable to the whole spectrum of the CKD population. For example, patients with diabetes, autosomal dominant polycystic kidney disease, severely increased proteinuria >1 g/day, or advanced CKD (those with eGFR <30 mL/min/1.73 m^2) were not included in this landmark trial.[11] In these large subgroups of the CKD population, the optimal BP target for the management of hypertension still remains unknown.

Another important issue is the algebraic manipulation of the SBP target in the intensive arm of SPRINT. The 2017 ACC/AHA guidelines used a correction factor of 10 mm Hg to adjust the mean difference between the research-grade BP measurement methodology that guided the intensification of antihypertensive therapy in SPRINT and routine BP recordings that continue to form the basis for the management of hypertension in daily clinical practice.[10] However, as mentioned earlier, diagnostic test studies have shown that the 95% limits of agreement between research-grade and routine office SBP are wide (ranging from –46.1 mm Hg lower up to 20.7 mm Hg higher).[12] Therefore, algebraic adjustment for the mean difference cannot capture the much larger range of differences between these two techniques at an individual level. In this particular aspect, we believe that the 2021 KDIGO guidelines take, perhaps, a more straightforward position.[8] According to the KDIGO 2021 recommendation, SBP in patients with CKD should be targeted to levels <120 mm Hg, if this is tolerated and with the use of standardized office BP measurements.[8] The key is how we measure BP in the office.

Nonpharmacological Therapy

The 2021 KDIGO guidelines recommend that in patients with high BP and CKD, dietary sodium intake should be restricted to levels lower than 2 g of sodium per day (or <90 mmol of sodium per day).[8] The effects of this intervention were investigated in a 2021 Cochrane meta-analysis of 21 studies incorporating data from 1,197 patients with CKD.[38] With high-certainty evidence this meta-analysis showed that reducing dietary sodium intake by 73.51 mmol/day provokes an average reduction of 6.91/3.91 mm Hg in office BP and a 36% improvement in albuminuria.[38] Secondary analysis of randomized controlled trials also showed that dietary sodium restriction magnifies the albuminuria-lowering effect of the renin–angiotensin system (RAS) inhibitors.[39] Since the currently available studies had short-term follow-up periods, the effect of dietary sodium restriction on "hard" cardiovascular and kidney outcomes remains uncertain. In a recent open-label, cluster-randomized trial including 20,995 patients who had a history of stroke or were 60 years of age or older and had high BP, as compared with regular salt use (100% NaCl), the consumption of a potassium-containing salt substitute (75% NaCl and 25% KCl) provoked a 14% reduction in the risk of stroke, a 13% reduction in the risk of major adverse cardiovascular events and a 12% reduction in the risk of all-cause death.[40] However, these data from trials conducted in the general hypertensive population may not be applicable to patients with CKD.[41] In the CKD setting, salt substitutes that are rich in potassium may aggravate the risk for hyperkalemia-related adverse events.[42] Other nonpharmacological interventions with favorable effects on BP control are weight loss and moderate-intensity physical exercise for a cumulative duration of at least 150 minutes per week.[8-10] Lastly, patients with CKD should be advised to avoid the use of over-the-counter medications, such as nonsteroidal anti-inflammatory drugs, because these agents may lead to worsening of BP control and deterioration of kidney function.[8-10]

Pharmacotherapy

The KDIGO 2021 guidelines provided a strong (Level 1B) recommendation that in diabetic or nondiabetic patients with hypertension, CKD and severely increased albuminuria, angiotensin-converting enzyme inhibitors (ACEIs) or angiotensin receptor blockers (ARBs) should be preferably used as first-line antihypertensive therapy.[8] As shown in **Table 3** and **Box 1**, the use of ACEIs/ARBs as antihypertensive agents of first choice in patients with albuminuric CKD is also recommended by all major hypertension guidelines on the basis of solid evidence from large outcome trials.[9,10] Among 1,513 patients with CKD associated with type 2 diabetes mellitus (T2DM), the RENAAL trial showed that as compared with placebo, losartan reduced by 16% the risk of doubling of serum creatinine, ESKD, or death.[43] The Irbesartan Diabetic Nephropathy Trial (IDNT) showed that among 1,715 hypertensive patients with T2DM and albuminuric CKD, irbesartan was more effective than placebo and active treatment with amlodipine in slowing the progression diabetic kidney disease.[44] Among 1,094 Black patients with hypertensive CKD, the AASK trial showed that ramipril provoked reductions of 22% and 38%

BOX 1 Pharmacological management of hypertension in patients with CKD.

- A single antihypertensive agent to control BP in patients with CKD is rare
- ACEI/ARB plus dihydropyridine CCB/diuretic in most patients
- Use single-pill combinations to increase adherence to therapy
- The thiazide-like diuretic chlorthalidone is effective in CKD, if the patient is not on dialysis. If the patient is on a loop diuretic, start chlorthalidone at a dose of 6.25 mg once daily. If the patient is not on a loop diuretic, start chlorthalidone at a dose of 12.5 mg once daily
- Monitor the patient for adverse events, such as hyponatremia, hypokalemia, orthostatic hypotension, and reversible deterioration in kidney function
- Spironolactone raises the risk of hyperkalemia. Chlorthalidone can mitigate this risk to enable the combined use of spironolactone in patients with difficult-to-control BP
- β-blockers and doxazosin are also effective and can be used as add-on therapy in patients with CKD and resistant hypertension

(ACEI: angiotensin-converting enzyme inhibitor; ARB: angiotensin receptor blocker; BP: blood pressure; CCB: calcium channel blocker; CKD: chronic kidney disease)

in the composite outcome of sustained ≥50 decrease in GFR from baseline, ESKD, or death relative to metoprolol and amlodipine, respectively.[35] In the absence of persuasive evidence to demonstrate the renoprotective effect of RAS-blockade in nondiabetic patients with moderately-increased albuminuria, the preferential use of ACEIs or ARBs as first-line antihypertensive therapy is not strongly recommended by guidelines in this setting.[8] In addition, combination therapy with an ACEI and an ARB is contraindicated.[8] The VA-NEPHRON-D trial was stopped early due to safety reasons. As compared to monotherapy with losartan, the combination of losartan and lisinopril increased the risk of hyperkalemia and acute kidney injury.[45] The ALTITUDE trial was also prematurely terminated, because the addition of the direct renin inhibitor aliskiren to standard therapy with an ACEI or an ARB magnified the risk of hyperkalemia and hypotension.[46]

The 2021 KDIGO guidelines provided a clinical practice recommendation that in patients with advanced CKD who are nearing the initiation of kidney replacement therapy, reducing the dose or discontinuation of ACEIs/ARBs can be considered as an intervention aiming to mitigate the uremic symptoms and provide the appropriate time for the preparation of dialysis.[8] This guidance was based on low-quality evidence from observational studies showing the discontinuation of RAS inhibitor therapy to be associated with better preservation of kidney function in patients with advanced CKD.[47-49] In the STOP-ACEi trial, 411 patients with advanced and progressive CKD were randomized either to stop or to continue RAS inhibitor therapy.[50] At 3 years of follow-up, the least squares mean eGFR was 12.6 ± 0.7 mL/min/1.73 m^2 in the discontinuation group versus 13.3 ± 0.6 mL/min/1.73 m^2 in the continuation group. There was a between-group difference of –0.7 mL/min/1.73 m^2 that was in favor of continuation of RAS inhibitor therapy.[50] As compared with continuation, stopping ACEIs/ARBs was associated with a nonsignificant increase of 28% in the risk of ESKD or initiating dialysis.[50] Therefore, among patients with advanced CKD, discontinuation of RAS inhibitor therapy does not result in stabilization of the long-term decline in kidney function and does not delay the initiation of kidney replacement therapy. In contrast, a trend toward earlier dialysis was observed.

The majority of patients with CKD need therapy with multiple antihypertensive medications to achieve adequate BP control. On this basis, the second-line agent can be either a long-acting dihydropyridine calcium channel blocker (CCB) or a diuretic, with the latter being a more suitable choice for patients with clinically overt hypervolemia.[5,9,10] As the next step in the treatment algorithm, guidelines recommend the combination of a RAS blocker, a dihydropyridine CCB and a diuretic.[5,9,10] With respect to diuretic therapy, there is an established belief that loop diuretics should be administered when the levels of eGFR fall below the threshold of 30 mL/min/1.73 m^2, because thiazide or thiazide-like diuretics are generally considered as less effective or ineffective in advanced CKD.[9,10] This therapeutic approach has been reappraised after the publication of the CLICK trial.[51] In this trial, 160 patients with stage 4 CKD and poorly controlled hypertension were randomly assigned in a 1:1 ratio to double-blind treatment with the thiazide-like diuretic chlorthalidone (at an initial dose of 12.5 mg/day) or with placebo.[51] Between the baseline and week 12 of follow-up, chlorthalidone provoked a placebo-subtracted reduction of 10.5 mm Hg in 24-hour ambulatory SBP. In parallel, relative to placebo, chlorthalidone lowered by 50% the urinary albumin excretion, a favorable effect that is suggestive of a potential cardiorenal protective benefit of this agent.[51] With respect to safety, hypokalemia, reversible increases in the levels of serum creatinine, hyperglycemia, hyperuricemia, dizziness, and orthostatic hypotension were adverse events that occurred more commonly in the chlorthalidone group than in the placebo group. The incidence of these adverse events was higher in the subgroup of patients who were concomitantly treated with a loop diuretic.[51] In such patients, we recommend the use of chlorthalidone at an even lower starting dose (i.e., 6.25 mg daily) as an approach to mitigate the risk of adverse events.[52]

The steroidal mineralocorticoid receptor antagonist (MRA) spironolactone is recommended by guidelines for use as fourth-line agent in patients with resistant hypertension.[9,10] Evidence to support this guidance was provided by the PATHWAY-2,[53] a double-blind, randomized, and crossover trial that demonstrated the superiority of add-on therapy with spironolactone versus placebo or active treatment with bisoprolol and doxazosin in reducing home BP in patients with resistant hypertension.[53] Notably, this additive BP-lowering effect was observed in patients receiving optimal background therapy with maximally tolerated doses of a RAS blocker, a CCB, and a diuretic. However, PATHWAY-2 trial excluded patients with moderate-to-advanced CKD.[53] Accordingly, international guidelines discourage the administration of spironolactone when eGFR is <45 mL/min/1.73 m^2 or when serum potassium is >4.5 mmol/L.[9,10] In this subgroup of high-risk patients the prevalence of resistant hypertension is high,[54,55] but the use of spironolactone is often restricted, mainly due to the associated risk of hyperkalemia.[56,57]

The AMBER trial randomized 295 patients with uncontrolled resistant hypertension and moderate-to-advanced CKD to receive either placebo or the potassium-binding polymer, patiromer, in addition to open-label therapy with spironolactone (25–50 mg/day) and their background BP-lowering medications for 12 weeks.[58] As compared with placebo, patiromer effectively mitigated the risk of hyperkalemia and enabled more patients to continue treatment with spironolactone. Over the course of the AMBER trial, add-on therapy with spironolactone was associated with a clinically meaningful reduction of 11–12 mm Hg in unattended automated office SBP.[58] However, even with the concomitant administration of a potassium-lowering therapy, one in three patients who received spironolactone developed hyperkalemia over 12 weeks of follow-up.[58]

Taking into consideration that newer potassium-binding polymers cannot fully eliminate the risk of hyperkalemia arising from the use of spironolactone, the 2023 guidelines of the European Society of Hypertension (ESH) recommend the administration of chlorthalidone as the preferred fourth-line agent for the management of resistant hypertension in patients with eGFR <30 mL/min/1.73 m^2.[9] A secondary analysis of CLICK involving 113 patients with resistant hypertension at the initiation of the trial showed that chlorthalidone provoked a placebo-subtracted reduction of 13.9 mm Hg in 24-hour ambulatory SBP over 12 weeks of follow-up.[59] An important advantage of chlorthalidone relative to spironolactone is that the risk of hyperkalemia is practically nonexistent.[52] However, in patients who have low baseline levels of serum potassium, the risk of hypokalemia may become a concern. Careful monitoring of BP, serum electrolytes, and kidney function is essential for the prevention of adverse events associated with the use of chlorthalidone.[52]

According to guidelines,[9,10] β-blockers are not recommended for use as monotherapy or first-line therapy in patients with uncomplicated hypertension. However, these agents are effective in improving cardiovascular outcomes and should be considered for the treatment of hypertension in patients with specific cardiovascular indications for β-blocker use, such as in patients with atrial fibrillation, HF with reduced ejection fraction, angina, or after an acute MI.[60] β-blockers are also useful as add-on therapy in the management of resistant hypertension. In the PATHWAY-2 trial,[53] the β-blocker bisoprolol was more effective than placebo in improving home BP when added to the baseline antihypertensive regimen.

Novel Therapies for Cardiorenal Protection in Patients with Chronic Kidney Disease

Sodium-glucose cotransporter-2 inhibitors (SGLT-2Is) originally received approval by regulatory agencies for use as glucose-lowering medications, but it was later discovered that cardiorenal protection is the main therapeutic effect of this novel drug class.[61] A triad of landmark phase 3 trials (CREDENCE, DAPA-CKD, and EMPA-KIDNEY) demonstrated that in patients with albuminuric CKD who are already treated with a RAS blocker, SGLT-2I therapy resulted in an impressive improvement in cardiovascular and kidney outcomes as compared with placebo.[62-64] The magnitude of benefit was similar in patients with or without T2DM.[62,63] In addition, in a large phase 3 clinical trial program involving 13,026 patients with T2DM and a broad spectrum of CKD, as compared with placebo, the nonsteroidal MRA finerenone provoked a 23% relative risk reduction in the composite kidney outcome of sustained ≥57% eGFR decline from baseline or renal death.[65-67] Finerenone also improved by 14% the composite cardiovascular outcome of cardiovascular death, nonfatal MI, nonfatal stroke, or hospitalization for HF.[65-67] Preliminary evidence suggests a synergistic effect of SGLT-2Is and finerenone and less hyperkalemia when finerenone is administered in combination with an SGLT-2I.[68,69]

Although neither of these two novel drug categories is indicated for the treatment of hypertension, the BP-lowering properties of these agents require a closer examination. In a meta-analysis of seven trials including a total of 2,381 patients with T2DM, SGLT-2Is lowered 24-hour ambulatory SBP by 3.62 mm Hg relative to placebo.[70] The reduction in 24-hour ambulatory SBP in response to SGLT-2I therapy was comparable to that seen with low-dose hydrochlothiazide.[70] In sharp contrast, the nonsteroidal MRA finerenone exerts a much more potent BP-lowering effect. This was illustrated in a recent post hoc analysis of the ARTS-DN trial.[71] In this phase 2b trial, 823 patients with albuminuric CKD and T2DM were randomly assigned to receive placebo or finerenone (1.25–20 mg once daily in the morning). A subgroup of 240 patients underwent ABPM at screening, day 60, and day 90.[72] The placebo-subtracted reduction in 24-hour ambulatory SBP at day 90 was 8.3 mm Hg for finerenone 10 mg/day, 11.2 mm Hg for finerenone 15 mg/day, and 9.9 mm Hg for finerenone 20 mg/day.[72] Despite its short plasma half-life, the BP-lowering effect of finerenone persisted during both awake and asleep periods.[72] This indirect comparison suggests that hemodynamic effects of SGLT-2Is and finerenone may substantially differ. Accordingly, BP-lowering may be a more important mediator of cardiorenal protection afforded by finerenone, whereas the benefits of SGLT-2Is on cardiorenal outcomes may be independent from their BP-lowering action.

CONCLUSION

In conclusion, the diagnosis and management of hypertension in patients with CKD should rely on standardized BP measurements in the office environment. The concomitant use of office and out-of-office BP measurements enables the classification of the severity of hypertension and facilitates the better stratification of cardiorenal risk. ACEIs or ARBs remain the backbone of pharmacotherapy of hypertension, particularly in patients with severely increased albuminuria. Patients with uncontrolled BP despite adherence to triple therapy with a RAS blocker, a long-acting dihydropyridine CCB and a diuretic fulfill the diagnostic criteria of resistant hypertension. In this setting, spironolactone is the standard-of-care treatment, if the eGFR is >45 mL/min/1.73 m^2 and the serum potassium is <4.5 mmol/L. Since the associated risk of hyperkalemia restricts the broad utilization of spironolactone in moderate-to-advanced CKD, the 2023 ESH guidelines recommend the use of the thiazide-like diuretic chlorthalidone as the preferred fourth-line therapy for patients with resistant hypertension and eGFR <30 mL/min/1.73 m^2. However, once again, this agent should be used sensibly and with careful monitoring of the patients for the prevention of adverse events. Novel agents, such as SGLT-2Is and the nonsteroidal MRA finerenone, have been added to our therapeutic armamentarium. These therapies are not indicated for their BP-lowering effects, but their broad utilization in daily clinical practice is essential for the mitigation of cardiorenal risk in CKD patients with or without T2DM.

CONFLICTS OF INTEREST

Rajiv Agarwal reports personal fees and nonfinancial support from Bayer Healthcare Pharmaceuticals, Akebia Therapeutics, Boehringer Ingelheim, Eli Lilly, Relypsa, Vifor Pharma, and Diamedica; is a member of data safety monitoring committees for Vertex and Chinook; has served as an associate editor of the American Journal of Nephrology and Nephrology Dialysis and Transplantation and has been an author for UpToDate; and has received research grants from the National Institutes of Health and the US Veterans Administration.

Panagiotis I Georgianos has nothing to disclose.

FINANCIAL SUPPORT

Rajiv Agarwal is supported by the National Heart Lung and Blood Institute (grant R01 HL126903).

ONLINE REFERENCES

Please scan the QR code provided at the end of the table of contents for References of this chapter.

CHAPTER

40 Renal Denervation for Hypertension Therapy: Lessons Learnt and Future Prospects

Raymond R Townsend

ABSTRACT

The sympathetic nervous system is one of the several regulators of the blood pressure (BP) in a man. Although, several classes of antihypertensive medications address sympathetic mechanisms, their actual impact is limited, in part by tolerability, and in part by counterregulatory mechanisms such as sodium retention. Consequently, alternative means of interrupting sympathetic nerve activity such as renal denervation (RDN) have been undertaken over the last two decades. RDN as a therapy for hypertension is based on the current understanding of the neural connections between the kidney and the vasomotor centers in the brainstem. This is supported by several animal models that show improvement or amelioration of hypertension following RDN. Moreover RDN studies have a combined experience of more than 20,000 human subjects treated with this procedure over the last 15 years. In this chapter we will begin with the historical basis for sympathetic interruption as an antihypertensive treatment. We will include supporting data from animal models, and review the clinical efficacy of RDN in humans in both clinical trials and registry experience. A brief segment will walk the reader through an RDN procedure using current radiofrequency, or ultrasound, or neurolytic ablation techniques. We will consider the safety of the RDN procedure, and potential patient preferences for the procedure. Finally, we will conclude with some thoughts about what the future may hold for this device-based approach to high BP management.

Keywords: Renal denervation, review, clinical trials, hypertension, human.

INTRODUCTION

Historical Aspects

The role of the sympathetic nervous system in circulatory hemodynamics has a long history. Sympathetic excitation increases heart rate and blood pressure (BP), and was an early target of both surgical and medication approaches to reducing extreme elevations in BP that were associated with rapid target organ compromise, particularly heart failure and death.

The early antisympathetic medication approaches typically blunted sympathetic ganglion function and were associated with many side effects, including orthostasis, depression, bowel and bladder issues and sexual function impairment.[1] Although they paved the way for the development of α- and β-blocking drugs, and the central α-agonists currently used in hypertension treatment, the degree of sympathetic blockade with all these drugs is frequently limited by similar side effects to the earlier blockers.

An alternative attempt at the interrupting sympathetic flow was to surgically sever the connections between the sympathetic ganglia and other organs, such as the blood vessels and kidney. These involved thoracic and lumbar incisions to undertake this "sympathectomy" as pioneered by surgeons like Smithwick for which such approaches were named.[2] It is worth a moment to detail one large surgical series of such cases, as it was one of the earliest attempts at denervation, short of actual nephrectomy.

This study involved patients who underwent thoracolumbar splanchnicectomy, a two stage procedure in which the thoracic and lumbar sympathetic chains are interrupted.[3] In a series of 1,266 such patients, who underwent this procedure for hypertension, the authors used a scoring system based on hypertensive-mediated organ damage where patients were assigned values ranging from 1 to 4 that reflected the underlying severity of their hypertension.[4] The actual BP level was not part of the scoring process. The patients who underwent the procedure were compared with patients who were offered the procedure, but who declined to undergo surgery, as a sort of convenience control group. The point made by the authors was that the mortality rate was substantially better, particularly in groups with values of 2 and 3, compared with the "control" group.

Several lessons were learned from these surgical endeavors. The procedures did prolong survival, even among those whose BPs were minimally affected, when compared with the "control" group. The adverse effects were substantial. Though perhaps not appreciated as such at the time, the organ denervation in these surgical series included the kidney, though it is not known the degree to which this aspect contributed to any reduction in BP, or the mortality outcomes, that were observed in this study.

A second set of observations are important to note. Nephrologists are well aware of the occasional hemodialysis patient who, despite volume reduction via ultrafiltration during dialysis sessions and the use of copious amounts of antihypertensive medications, nonetheless remains hypertensive and prone to hospitalizations and hypertension-mediated organ damage,[5,6] such patients show elevated levels of sympathetic neural activity as registered by muscle sympathetic nerve activity.[7] Bilateral native nephrectomy, though infrequently done, can be curative of the hypertension excess in this situation.[8] This was particularly evident in young Black American patients with malignant hypertension on dialysis who were transplanted in the precyclosporine era, where the removal of the native kidneys and the insertion of a kidney transplant not only relieved the patient of needing dialysis, it also cured their hypertension.[9]

The current approach to renal denervation (RDN) owes its physiologic underpinnings to the proof-of-principle observations noted in the pharmacologic and surgical approaches outlined above. The challenge was to overcome the drastic surgical procedure morbidity and mortality while at the same time disabling the sympathetic traffic in the nerves located in the renal artery periadventitial compartments. The outcome of this planning was the construction of the first radiofrequency emitting catheter, which served as the tool for research in porcine models of hypertension.[10] The adult pig kidney is roughly similar in size and anatomy to the human kidney. Having shown the ability to safely denervate the pig kidney without visible damage to the renal artery, this set the stage for the first uncontrolled human trial of catheter-based RDN followed in 2009.[11]

In this beginning phase of deploying a catheter approach for denervation, it involved placing a radiofrequency emitting electrode in the vicinity of the renal nerves, using a femoral approach. In the first human trials, only one kidney artery was treated, and this treatment involved placing the unipolar electrode distally in the main renal artery, performing an ablation, withdrawing the catheter about 5 mm, turning it 90° and performing a second ablation and repeating that over about 2 cm of renal artery.[11] The goal was to deliver the energy in a quadrant-shaped fashion, and by withdrawing, rotating, and repeating, there would be a net circumferential ablation undertaken, hopefully encompassing two full quadrants, and undertaken in the main renal artery segment only. The branches and accessory arteries were not ablated in the early series of patients. After a month, in the first 10 patients of the original series in the Lancet, and following an arteriogram showing the circulation in the denervated side to be in reasonably good shape, the other kidney would be treated.[11] To this author's knowledge [renal replacement therapy (RRT)], there has not been a series of unilateral only approaches to RDN. The presence of a single kidney excludes a patient from receiving the procedure, as does the presence of significant (>50% narrowing) atherosclerotic plaque. The original catheter was designed to allow blood flow in the artery while in use, since the native blood flow served to cool the artery, and reduce the effects of the temperature increase mediated by emitting the radiofrequency energy.

A bit more on the first trial of denervation is warranted here. This was an uncontrolled investigation of drug-resistant patients with hypertension.[11] In this undertaking, 50 patients with office systolic BP higher than 160 mm Hg on at least three antihypertensive medications at maximally tolerated dosages were treated with bilateral RDN using radiofrequency energy. The magnitude of the BP reduction was impressive. Although the original outcome endpoint of systolic BP reduction was determined at 6 months, a surprising and welcome finding, repeated consistently since this early observation, is the continued, though modest, reduction of systolic BP over time. As of this writing, the durable effect of denervation in this original cohort is 9 years.[12]

When Murray Esler gave the 2009 Ludwig Lecture, he did an excellent job of outlining the key steps in the elucidation of the role of the sympathetic nervous system in the control of circulatory physiology.[13] Summarizing this data, and the contributions of researchers like Gerald DiBona and Ulla Kopp in Iowa,[14,15] and Karen Griffin and Anil Bhidani at Loyola[16,17] a number of key observations were elucidated that support the physiologic basis for RDN. Sympathetic nerves travel with arteries and arterioles and contribute a tonic constrictor influence on these vessels. Stimulation of the renal sympathetic nerves, in a progressively more intense fashion yields three observations:[18]

1. A release of renin from the juxtaglomerular apparatus at low levels of stimulation
2. An increase in renal sodium reabsorption at moderate levels of stimulation
3. Constriction of the afferent arterioles at the upper levels of stimulation

These findings provided the impetus for a number of animal-based experiments, using various models of hypertension, providing additional evidence of the importance of the renal nerves. Selected examples of this research are summarized next.

BASIS FOR RENAL DENERVATION AS THERAPY FOR ELEVATED BLOOD PRESSURE

- *Animal studies showing amelioration of established high BP by RDN*: Minipigs made hypertensive by a deoxycorticosterone acetate (DOCA) implant and a high salt diet have shown reductions in established BP increases following RDN using either RDN by a radiofrequency catheter method,[19] or surgical sectioning of renal nerves.[20] The use of topical phenol, which is neurotoxic, to the nerves on the surface of the renal artery, in rats born under conditions of reduced uterine perfusion during their gestation, also ameliorates elevated BP.[21] In a renovascular hypertension dog model, using either the one kidney one clip, or the two-kidney one-clip models, the BP was reduced by the use of adventitial stripping and application of phenol to the renal nerves.[22]
- *Reduction of expected BP increase by RDN*: In a dog model of elevated BP following unilateral nephrectomy and infusion of adenosine, the magnitude of BP increase from adenosine is blunted following RDN.[23]
- *Nerves that travel on the renal artery*: In the early phases of the current denervation trials, it was thought that circumferential ablation of the renal nerves through a catheter placed in the main renal artery, before its bifurcation, was adequate to provide sufficient damage to the afferent and efferent nerve traffic from the kidney to the central nervous system vasomotor centers leading to BP reduction. After the failure of HTN-3 to achieve its primary endpoint (discussed later), more attention was paid to the distribution and functional aspects of the renal nerves.[24,25] Importantly, it was subsequently observed that some nerves from the sympathetic ganglia near the kidney arteries, touch down on the main kidney artery and then leave before entering the renal parenchyma, and some nerves touch further down the renal artery circulation at the distal main renal artery and in the first order branches bypassing the early-middle main renal artery, and go on to innervate the renal parenchyma.[26] The biologic significance of these findings is still unclear. Work in normotensive porcine models, whose kidney size and innervation patterns are similar to humans,[25] suggest that ablating these more distal nerves in conjunction with main renal artery ablations, results in a greater reduction of parenchymal norepinephrine content than ablation focused on the main renal alone.[27]

What can be said at this point in the discussion of renal nerve anatomy?

- The porcine and human renal innervation patterns are similar, validating the use of a porcine model
- There are fewer nerves in the periadventitial space as one move distally down the renal artery into the bifurcations, but ablation of these more distal nerves seems to produce greater depletion of parenchymal catecholamine content that restricting ablations to the main renal artery segment.
- To date, the magnitude of BP reduction following denervation (by whatever approach, discussed underneath) has been similar across technologies even though some technologies only treat the main renal artery segment. Thus, the role of nuances in renal nerve distribution, and the role of branch artery denervation in the efficacy of RDN remains an open question. Findings from the DYSTAL study, which focuses on denervating only the distal segments of the kidney circulation, may shed more light on this (https://classic.clinicaltrials.gov/ct2/show/NCT04311086).

MORE ON THE EARLY HUMAN EXPERIENCE WITH SYMPATHETIC DENERVATION

Before the era of effective and safe long-term medication therapy for hypertension, many patients had little or no intervention to manage their BP until it entered an accelerated or malignant phase. One approach to managing this phase of hypertension, in which mortality approached 100% at 1 year,[28] was to perform thoracolumbar sympathetic denervation as noted earlier. It is a curious thing that *prior* to the era of effective and long-term pharmacologic therapy for hypertension, the two nondrug approaches found most effective for BP treatment were (1) rigorous low salt/low fat diets[29] and (2) surgical procedures that either sought to nullify the sympathetic nervous system effect on vessels through lumbodorsal sympathectomy, or sought to remove hormones such as catecholamines and mineralocorticoid/glucocorticoids through bilateral adrenalectomy.[30] It seems curious to me because establishing and maintaining low salt/low fat diets in hypertensive is a substantial challenge today, and drugs which work through antiadrenergic mechanisms or mineralocorticoid blockade are often fourth-line treatments in the pharmacologic toolbox.

RENAL DENERVATION ERA

The ability to denervate the kidney through the use of an endovascular approach eliminated the need for extensive surgery, with its attendant morbidity and mortality, to accomplish denervation. The field has been, basically, through three "phases" (by the author's classification) of efficacy testing. These are shown in **Table 1**. The first phase used the first generation radiofrequency Ardian® unipolar catheter. The second phase used the more flexible Symplicity® unipolar catheter. The third phase expanded to include studies using the third-generation Spyral® catheter, designed to overcome the failure to achieve four quadrant ablations in the HTN-3 study,[31] along with publications of the ultrasound and ablative approaches to RDN.

Phase 1

In the first phase was a demonstration of proof-of-principle in patients with the most difficult to manage hypertension. The original series of 45 patients treated with RDN for severe, drug-resistant hypertension on five antihypertensive drugs whose office systolic BP remained above 160 mm Hg.[11] There was no control group in this study, and the reduction in office

TABLE 1: Listing of RDN clinical trials.

Study	Year	N (D)	RDN system	HTN	MED[#]	Time to primary	SHAM	Δ 24 SBP RDN (mm Hg)	Δ 24 SBP CTL (mm Hg)
Phase 1									
HTN-1[11]	2009	45	RFA 1st	Res	5	6 months	No	22[$]	+14[$]
HTN-2[32]	2010	100 (49)	RFA 1st	Res	5	6 months	No	32[$]	1[$]
Phase 2									
HTN-3[35]	2014	535 (364)	RFA 2nd	Res	5	6 months	Yes	7	5
DENERHTN[37]	2015	106 (53)	RFA 2nd	Res	3	6 months	No	16	10
Prague[53]	2015	106 (52)	RFA 2nd	Res	5	6 months	No	9	8
Desch[54]	2015	71 (35)	RFA 2nd	Res	4	6 months	Yes	7	4
DENERVHTA[55]	2016	27 (13)	RFA 2nd	Res	4	6 months	No	5	23
ReSET[56]	2016	69 (36)	RFA 2nd	Res	4	6 months	Yes	6	4
Phase 3									
SPYRAL OFF MED pilot[57]	2017	80 (38)	RFA Spyral	Unc	None	3 months	Yes	6	1
SPYRAL OFF MED pivotal[38]	2017	331 (166)	RFA Spyral	Unc	None	3 months	Yes	5	1
RADIANCE HTN SOLO[39]	2018	146 (74)	US Paradise	Unc	None	2 months	Yes	9[%]	2[%]
SPYRAL ON MED pilot[58]	2018	80 (38)	RFA Spyral	Unc	1–3	6 months	Yes	9	2
RADIOSOUND[59]	2018	120 (120)	US Paradise vs RFA Spyral	Res	5	3 months	No	10[%]	N/A
REDUCE HTN REINFORCE[60]	2020	51 (34)	RFA Vessix	Unc	None	2 months	Yes	5	9
RADIANCE-TRIO[45]	2021	136 (69)	US Paradise	Res	3	2 months	Yes	8[%]	3[%]
REQUIRE[61]	2021	143 (72)	US Paradise	Res	4	3 months	Yes*	7	7
RADIANCE II[62]	2023	224 (150)	US Paradise	Unc	1–2	2 months	Yes	8[%]	2[%]
TARGET BP OFF MED[40]	2023	106 (50)	ABL Peregrine	Unc	None	2 months	Yes	3	2
SPYRAL ON MED expansion	2023	337 (206)	RFA Spyral	Unc	1–3	6 months	Yes	7	5

[#] Number.
[Δ] Change.
[$] Office only (ABPM not done in study).
[%] Daytime ABPM (not 24 hours).
*REQUIRE was single blinded; investigators were aware of group assignment.

[ABL: ablative catheter (injects neurolytics); CTL: control group; HTN: hypertension; MED: blood pressure medications; N (D): number in study (number in denervation group); RDN: renal denervation; Res: resistant hypertension; SBP: systolic blood pressure; Unc: uncontrolled hypertension; US: ultrasound catheter; 1st: first-generation RFA catheter ("Ardian®"; unipolar); 2nd: second generation RFA catheter ("Symplicity®"; unipolar)] systolic BP at 6 months from an average of 177 mm Hg to an average of 155 mm Hg. This initial publication was followed by a great deal of enthusiasm and technology development. A second study of denervation, HTN-2, this time randomized (but not sham-controlled, discussed underneath) observed a 32 mm Hg office systolic BP reduction at 6 months in the 49 subjects undergoing denervation, compared with a 1 mm Hg office systolic BP reduction in the 51 subjects in the nondenervated group, confirming the findings of the earlier HTN-1 trial.[32] Following HTN-2, the expectations were that office systolic BP levels in patients on multiple (usually 5) drugs for hypertension would experience ~25 mm Hg systolic BP fall 6 months after a denervation procedure. Although not all were convinced by such large BP reductions,[33] the findings in this first phase of denervation were the preliminary data supporting a sham-controlled trial in which drug-resistant hypertensive patients would be randomized to receive either RDN, or undergo all the same procedures (hospitalization, angiography, and conscious sedation) but stopping short of an actual denervation procedure.[34]

Phase 2

Following on the dramatic reductions in systolic BP noted in HTN-1 and HTN-2, a large randomized sham-controlled study was undertaken in the USA to determine the comparative reductions of office systolic BP after RDN in drug-resistant hypertensive patients.[34] In 90 centers in the USA, 535 hypertensive subjects with an office systolic BP of at least 160 mm Hg, on an average of five antihypertensive medications were randomized 2:1 (RDN:sham-control) and were followed for 3 years.[35] The primary endpoint was office systolic BP change at 6 months. In those undergoing RDN, the office systolic BP reduction was 14 mm Hg. In the sham-control group the systolic BP reduction was 12 mm Hg. The difference was not statistically significant (p = 0.26). After HTN-3 results were disclosed, investigators, clinical trialists, biostatisticians, and basic scientists met in a series of conferences reviewing the design and conduct of HTN-3. Prior to the publication of HTN-3 many countries had approved RDN as a clinical procedure. After publication of HTN-3, RDN usage declined dramatically and entered a hiatus. During this time, several problems were identified in HTN-3, particularly variations in the procedure using the original unipolar catheter, variations in antihypertensive drug usage within the protocol, and nuances of the study population leading to the use of ambulatory blood pressure monitoring (ABPM) to minimize the placebo effects.[31,36] About a year after HTN-3 was published, the DENERHTN (Renal Denervation for Hypertension) trial, undertaken in French hypertension centers and conducted in a similar timeframe to HTN-3, was published.[37] This trial was open-label, with blinded outcome assessment. Although, the control group did not undergo angiography or denervation, the investigators showed that in a study where medication was administered, stepwise to triple therapy (indapamide, ramipril or irbesartan, and amlodipine), and office BP remained eligible for inclusion in the trial, the RDN group had about a 6 mm Hg larger reduction in 24 hours ABPM compared with medication alone. Other phase two studies are shown in the **Table 1**. Taking the lessons learned from HTN-3 and the encouragement from DENERHTN, RDN entered the next phase.

Phase 3

It is characterized by three different endovascular approaches to RDN. The largest experience is with (1) radiofrequency ablation, followed by (2) ultrasound ablation, and more recently (3) neurolytic ablation. The procedures are further described in the section following this one.

There have been >20,000 patients treated with RDN during and since the phase 1 experience. **Table 1** summarizing much of the current literature provided for the reference. Phase 3 studies have concentrated on providing full circumferential ablations so that all surfaces of the kidney artery (dorsal, ventral, anterior, and posterior) are denervated. Accessory arteries with ≥3 mm lumens are now denervated. Diastolic BP is typically 90 mm Hg or higher in the office, and white coat effects are minimized by ABPM requirements (typically a 24-hour ABPM systolic of 135–140 to 170 mm Hg). All current approaches do multiple ablations at each activation, or injection. Medication usage, when medications are permitted, is surveilled by drug testing in the blood and urine. Denervation centers typically restrict the procedure to one or two proceduralists to reduce operator heterogeneity. Finally, current trials focus on uncontrolled hypertension, defined as an office systolic BP > 150–180 mm Hg, whether on, or off, medication. When medications are permitted, no more than three separate classes are allowed. The performance of denervation trials on no medications (OFF MED, SOLO, and TARGET BP OFF) are meant to confirm the efficacy of the denervation procedure. The performance of denervation trials on medications (ON MED, TRIO, RADIANCE II, etc.), are meant to evaluate the efficacy of the denervation procedure when medications are present.

Rather than reviewing each study in the **Table 1** not covered so far, the readers are advised to focus on the last two columns on the right side in phase 3, as this represents the current state of the art in the field. As you can see, the typical daytime or a 24-hour ABPM systolic BP reduction within the denervation groups is, on average, about 7 mm Hg. The typical daytime or a 24-hour ABPM systolic BP reduction within the sham-control groups is quite variable, ranging from 1 to 9 mm Hg. Loss of BP data due to escape mandated changes in BP medication and changes in BP medication within and outside the protocol (detected by urine and drug screening) account for a significant portion of the sham-control group responses.

In general, the magnitude of systolic BP reduction is proportional to the starting office systolic BP, which (to date) has been the only consistent predictor of BP change. Early RDN studies showed 20–30 mm Hg of office systolic BP reduction. Subsequent studies generally show an office systolic BP reduction of about 10 mm Hg, whether ascertained at 2 or 3 months in off-medication trials,[38-40] or at a 6-month time point. ABPM studies show that about two out of three patients assigned to denervation therapy have a 5 mm Hg, or more, systolic BP reduction and this has been found across all three different approaches to denervation.

Another point to make about the systolic BP efficacy of RDN is the role of time passage. The largest experience is with the Global Symplicity Registry (GSR).[41] This Registry will have over 3,000 patients undergoing clinical-indicated RDN and followed for 3 years. There is no "control" group. The decline in office systolic BP over time (baseline office systolic BP average was 166 mm Hg) on more than 2,000 patients enrolled in the GSR, as presented by Professor Mahfoud at the May 2022 EuroPCR meeting in Paris, was:

- At 6 months = 13 mm Hg (n = 2,208)
- At 1 year = 14 mm Hg (n = 2,092)
- At 2 years = 15 mm Hg (n = 1,607)
- At 3 years = 17 mm Hg (n = 1,270)

These changes in systolic BP were not due to intensification of the antihypertensive medication regimen. The average number of antihypertensive medication over the time period had shown actually fell slightly from 4.9 to 4.8 agents taken daily.

It takes about a month to see a decline in BP values after denervation, and most longer term studies of at least 3 years duration show a continued decline in office and ABPM systolic BP, counter to what would be expected from aging alone, which tends to increase systolic BP.[42,43] This is not due to additional medication usage; if anything medications tend to be slightly reduced over time. Additionally, concern is often expressed about durability, from concerns that the nerves may regrow. Two studies that have followed patients for 9 years after RDN provide support for the notion that if nerves regrow, this is not attended by a return of BP to predenervation levels.[12,44]

HOW DENERVATION IS DONE?

Here, briefly, is what happens during a denervation procedure (see for more details).[38,40,45]

For *radiofrequency ablation*, a patient is brought to a catheterization suite (cardiologic or radiologic) a peripheral IV is inserted and the femoral site is prepped for catheter insertion. Conscious sedation and anticoagulation are used throughout the procedure. Usually a six French sheath is inserted in the femoral artery, a soft-tipped wire is advanced to the kidney artery, and angiography confirms suitable anatomy and is used to plan sequential denervations in the main artery, and branches, with vessel diameters of 3–8 mm. Next, the denervation catheter inserted over the wire and location confirmed radiologically. The denervation catheter has four electrodes **(Fig. 1)** and when the wire is retracted the catheter assumes a spiral shape so that each electrode comes into contact with the endothelial lining, confirmed by the generator. The catheter allows blood to flow through the center of the spiral, which cools the arterial wall. Then the electrodes are activated by the generator, confirmed by continuous impedance, emitting 45–60 seconds of radiofrequency energy. This is repeated at each of the planned denervation sites, and the same process used in the other kidney's arterial circulation. At this time, with branch denervations, about 24–28 ablations are done in each kidney artery. Care is taken that the electrodes do not overly kidney parenchyma. A final angiogram is done and the catheter system removed and attention is paid to hemostasis at the femoral puncture site. The denervation process takes up to 90 minutes and uses about 150 cc of the contrast media.

For *ultrasound ablation*, the preparation process is similar, using a peripheral IV and femoral access. The main differences are that the catheter used for ultrasound ablation is a balloon that expands blocking blood flow while emitting four concentric rings of ultrasound energy, and circulates a coolant within the balloon portion to protect the arterial wall **(Fig. 2)**. The duration of emission is 7 seconds. Lastly, the ultrasound approach usually performs two sets of four ablations in the main kidney artery of both sides. The denervation process takes up to 80 minutes and uses about 135 cc of contrast media.

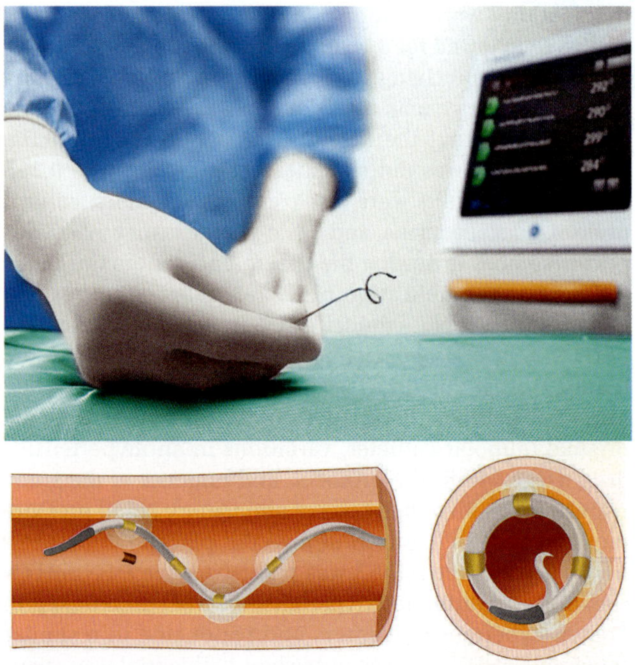

FIG. 1: Radiofrequency quadripolar ablation catheter (upper half) shown in hand of operator. Radiofrequency generator seen on the right side. Below, left, is catheter deployed in artery. Below, right, is en face view showing catheter conformed to inner arterial wall with channel in center for blood flow.

For *neurolytic ablation*, again the preparation process is similar. The difference with this procedure is that once the catheter is position, three "subcatheters" emerge from the central catheter and land on the inner arterial wall **(Fig. 3)**. Through these portals microneedles are advanced that pierce the artery wall and extend into the periadventitial space. Through these microneedles 0.6 mL (0.2 mL at each microneedle) of absolute ethanol is injected. The microneedles and the subcatheters are retracted. A surveillance angiogram is performed and, as mentioned earlier, the catheter system is removed and attention is paid to femoral hemostasis. The denervation process takes about 60 minutes, and uses about 100 cc of the contrast media.

Safety

Unlike medications or lifestyle measures used in the treatment of hypertension, denervation procedures are invasive, and safety concerns have been an important focus throughout the development of this area of BP therapy. Three aspects of safety have been a part of the clinical programs in developing these technologies, and include:

1. Periprocedural safety
2. Device safety
3. Long-term safety

Periprocedural Safety

This involves all the aspects of an invasive procedure using femoral access sites, introducing catheters, anticoagulation and conscious sedation and includes arterial puncture, kidney vessel access, intraprocedural pain, catheter deployment and hemostasis during the denervation procedure, and the first month of the clinical follow-up. The potential complications include pseudoaneurysm formation of the femoral artery, potential vascular puncture

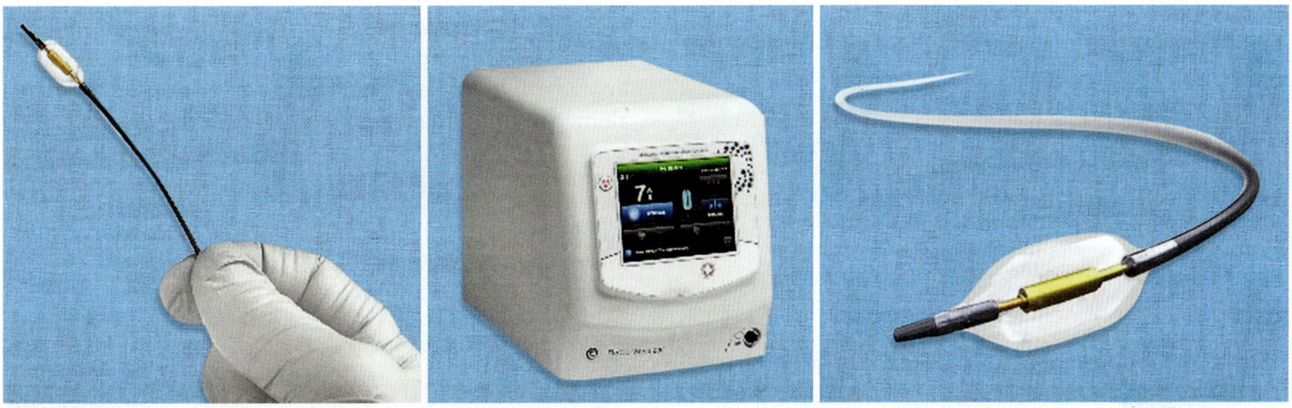

FIG. 2: Ultrasound ablation catheter (left) shown in hand of operator. Ultrasound generator is seen in the center. Larger view of ultrasound catheter is shown (right) for detail.

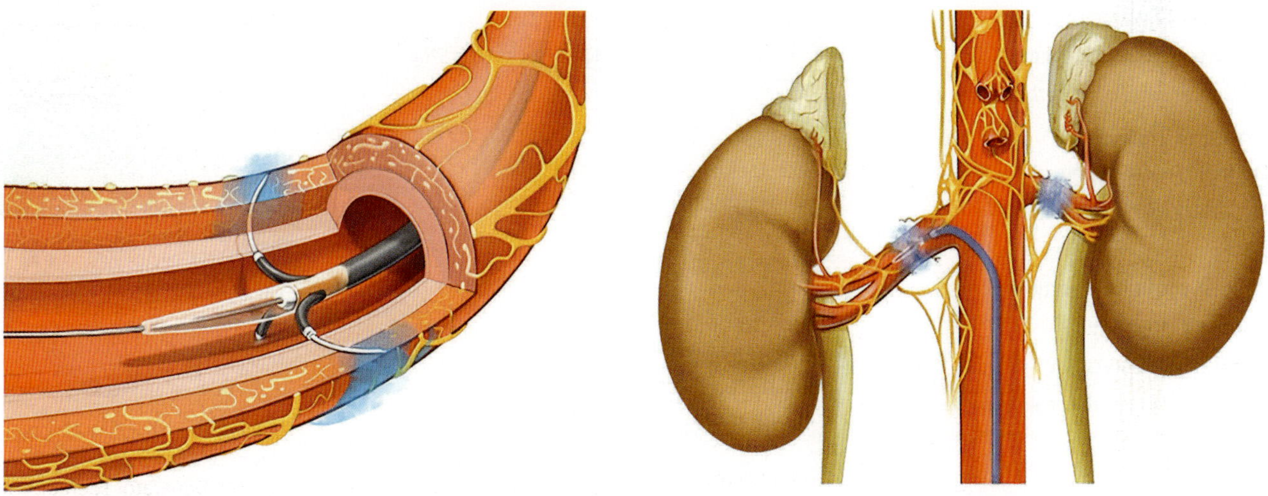

FIG. 3: Neurolytic-delivering ablation catheter (left) seen in situ in artery with microneedles deployed. Blue shading shows area of 95% ethanol spread in periadventitial space. On right side are a typical central artery locations for microneedle deployment.

or dissection of the renal artery by the guide wire, persistent pain associated with the ablation itself, bleeding, and clinical outcomes related to BP. **Table 2** shows the general safety profile of RDN, including the periprocedural and longer-term considerations. The most common safety events relate to the complications of accessing the femoral artery (pseudoaneurysms and bleeding), and pain (in the back, or in the groin) that persists for >2 days. In general RDN appears to have an acceptable periprocedural safety profile.

Device Safety

Events in this category would include items, such as catheter breakage, generator faults, and excessive heating of the artery. To date, to my knowledge, there are no reported device safety issues with any of the three technologies.

Long-term Safety

Occurrence of these events typically encompass the time period from 1 to 6 months after the baseline visit. Most of the short-term and long-term clinical safety reports have focused on the interval medical history, laboratory (creatinine) surveillance, and imaging modalities to monitor the kidney artery, which include Doppler ultrasound, magnetic resonance angiography, and computed tomographic angiography. These typically include surveillance for death, renal artery stenosis, and/or changes in the kidney function, heart attack, stroke, and admissions for the heart failure.

One of the primary concerns for long-term safety has the potential to promote atherosclerosis in the kidney arteries. We specifically evaluated this in a meta-analysis that included >5,000 patients who had undergone RDN using radiofrequency ablation. Our observations were that the incidence of renal artery stenosis requiring an intervention occurred at a rate of 0.2%/year during the 2 years after denervation follow-up period.[46] This is at, or below, the occurrence of symptomatic renovascular disease (0.5–1%/year) in similar hypertension populations. We also observed that most events (23 of 34 published instances) occurred within 6 months of denervation.[46]

Data from the GSR have been used to assess longer-term safety in patients who received RDN, largely outside of randomized clinical trials. Several GSR reports have focused on safety issues,[47] and these consistently show no significant impact on long-term renal function changes out to 3 years postprocedure, supporting further the reasonable safety profile of radiofrequency ablation denervation.[43] In particular, kidney function changes over time in those with, compared to those without, preexisting chronic kidney disease, show that the radiofrequency denervation does not impair kidney function irrespective of the starting estimated glomerular filtration rate.[48]

PATIENT PREFERENCE

Studies assessing whether patients would opt for denervation therapy to manage high BP have been conducted in Europe,

TABLE 2: Representative safety events associated with renal denervation.

Trial name	SOLO[39]		OFF MED[58]		TRIO[45]		ON MED		TARGET BP OFF[40]	
Periprocedural (includes denervation day and up to 30 days after)										
Enrolled	D = 74	S = 72	D = 166	S = 165	D = 69	S = 67	D = 206	S = 131	D = 50	S = 56
Femoral vascular injury					1 (1%)		2 (1%)	1 (1%)		1 (2%)
Pain > second postprocedure	8 (11%)	8 (11%)			12 (17%)	10 (15%)				
Postprocedural (1–6 months after denervation)										
Death					1 (1%)***					
Doubling of creatinine					1 (1%)**					
Hypertensive emergency			1 (1%)						1 (2%)	
Stroke				1 (<1%)				1 (1%)		
Acute myocardial infarction					1 (1%)					
Coronary intervention						1 (1%)				
Renal angioplasty/stent	1 (1%)*									

*Subject had preexisting renal artery stenosis.
**Doubling of creatinine was unrelated to study (was due to spironolactone usage).
***Death was unrelated to study.

Asia, and the USA. Three examples should give the reader a sense of the aggregate findings.

The first patient preference study evaluated the attitudes of physicians and patients about denervation. Investigators used market surveys conducted in Western Europe and the USA which gathered data from >1,900 physicians and >2,700 patients. They observed that physicians believe that a therapy like denervation should be desirable to patients when their BP is substantially elevated and their medication burden is large. Patients felt that uncontrolled BP, irrespective of medication usage, including not being on medication at all, and drug side effects were factors that they considered important to opt for denervation.[49]

Almost 2,400 Japanese hypertensive patients, on medications, participated in a web-based survey that included a question about whether they would undergo denervation. A little of >30% patients said they would consider it, especially when their BP was elevated, if there were problems with drug adherence, or if they experienced side effects from antihypertensive medications.[50]

Finally, a discrete choice patient preference study was conducted in the US using the internet on 400 patients with uncontrolled hypertension, with no prior participation in a denervation trial. The survey presented options that asked the patient to choose additional medication, denervation, or no further treatment, and evaluated the importance of a number of factors including how much BP reduction could be expected, device risks, drug risks, and other factors. The clearest factor influencing the choice of patients, who chose denervation 15–30% of the time, was the magnitude of BP reduction.[51]

CONCLUSION

Several lessons would seem apparent from the last decade and a half of clinical investigation in the field of RDN. These are:

- The optimal candidate for RDN still remains to be defined
- There is still no accepted marker that indicates the denervation was "complete"
- The employment of a sham-control arm has led to a number of improvements both in the understanding or renal neuroanatomy, and the role of human behavior (adherence) in BP outcomes
- The value of blood and urine antihypertensive drug testing is helpful to understand unexpectedly large reductions in BP in sham-control arms
- Registry follow-up, now reaching to 9 years in some centers, supports a durable duration of BP reduction and, to date, likely indicates a lack of functional reinnervation of the human kidney following denervation

A recent editorial in circulation nicely encapsulated the challenges that yet remain in the denervation space. Optimum selection of patients, preferential ablation of vasopressor nerve fibers, and improvement in understanding the mechanisms by which denervation works, and understanding why it takes so long for efficacy to emerge remain in "holy grail" status in the clinical arena of RDN.[52]

ACKNOWLEDGMENT

I am grateful to Wanpen Vongpatanasin, MD, at UT Southwestern in Dallas, TX for help organizing the **Table 1** of RDN studies.

ONLINE REFERENCES

Please scan the QR code provided at the end of the table of contents for References of this chapter.

SECTION

5

Heart Failure

CHAPTER

41

Heart Failure in India

T Govindan Unni

ABSTRACT

Heart failure (HF) is a growing problem in India and is likely to worsen in the future. We have the dual burden of rheumatic heart disease (RHD) and coronary artery disease (CAD) contributing to HF. The mean age of our patients is almost 10 years lower than in the developed countries. In spite of the younger population, mortality is high. Adherence to guideline-directed medical treatment (GDMT) is poor. CAD is the most common etiology. Hence, adherence to GDMT for acute coronary syndrome (ACS) management also needs improvement. The major HF registries are all conducted in tertiary care centers in urban/semiurban areas. So, data from the rural areas where most of our HF patients live are nonexistent. Prevention essentially involves managing CAD risk factors such as hypertension (HTN), diabetes mellitus (DM), obesity, dyslipidemia, and smoking. Appropriate, guideline-directed treatment of ACS is also important. Even though at present, HF with reduced ejection fraction (HFrEF) is the predominant type of HF, we can expect increasing numbers of HF with preserved ejection fraction (HFpEF) as the longevity of the population increases.

Keywords: Heart failure, India.

INTRODUCTION

Age is the most important predisposing factor for heart failure (HF). With the rising elderly population, HF is likely to be one of the most important health burdens in India. Coronary artery disease (CAD) is the most common predisposing factor for HF. The rising incidence of hypertension (HTN), diabetes mellitus (DM), dyslipidemia, and obesity is likely to increase the incidence of CAD and thus of HF. Specialized HF clinics and HF specialists are confined to urban areas. The poor insurance cover denies the rural population of the benefits of costly drugs and devices. General practitioners across the thousands of villages in India have no access to knowledge about the benefits of guideline-directed medical treatment (GDMT). All these factors contribute to the rising number of HF patients in India and their increasing mortality.

HEART FAILURE ENTITIES PECULIAR TO A REGION

Heart failure entities peculiar to a region will be determined by the local factors producing an endemic disease (such as endomyocardial fibrosis in Uganda and Chagas disease in Brazil) and the stage of epidemiological transition that the region is in. There are four stages of epidemiological transition.[1,2] Stage 1 is the age of pestilence and famines. Malnutrition and infectious diseases predominate. The mortality from cardiovascular disease (CVD) will be low (<10%). The dominant diseases are infectious and nutritional. The main CVD will be rheumatic and nutritional. The etiology of HF will be rheumatic heart disease (RHD), nutritional like Beriberi, and infectious like diphtheria. The primary victims of CVD will be from the higher class. Stage 2 is the age of receding pandemics. There are better public health systems, improved sanitation, increased availability of vaccines and antibiotics. Mortality from communicable diseases decreases. Longevity increases and CVD mortality will gradually increase to about 10–35%. While communicable diseases will start receding, noncommunicable diseases start rising. Thus, there will be the dual burden of both these groups of diseases. Contribution of CVD to overall mortality will rise to around 15–35%. The pattern of CVD will include stroke (especially hemorrhagic stroke), in addition to rheumatic and nutritional diseases. Thus, in this stage, we will have HF from nutritional and infectious causes, RHD and HF due to uncontrolled HTN, poorly treated ischemic heart disease (IHD), and other noncommunicable diseases. Both higher and lower classes of people start getting affected by CVD. Stage 3 is the age of degenerative and human made mortality. CVD mortality increases to 35–65% and becomes more than mortality from communicable diseases. The dominant diseases will be chronic midlife diseases. The contribution of CVD to overall mortality will cross 50%. CAD and stroke become the pattern of CVD. Victims will primarily belong to lower class. The causes of HF will be mainly IHD with a significant contribution from RHD also. Infectious and nutritional causes slowly decline. In Stage 4, the age of delayed degenerative diseases, cancer, and CVDs is the predominant cause of death. CVD contributes about 40% of all deaths. In general, there is a declining trend in death rates. The dominant disease will be chronic elderly diseases. The contribution of CVD to overall mortality falls below 50% and malignancies and other degenerative diseases start dominating. Coronaries and stroke continue to be the predominant CVD. There is better survival of patients with CAD and, hence, HF incidence increases. The primary victims of CVD will be the lower class. Heart failure with preserved ejection fraction (HFpEF) becomes the dominant form of HF in this stage. With better treatment of IHD, heart failure with reduced ejection fraction (HFrEF) starts decreasing.

While in stage 1, the average life span is around 35 years, in stage 2, it will increase to about 50 years. By stage 3, life expectancy increases to around 60 years and will cross 70 years in stage 4.

India is a large and socioeconomically diverse country. Hence, the HF burden in India is likely to be diverse across various regions. The country has areas in all stages of epidemiological transition. There will be areas in India which are still in stage 1 of the epidemiological transition and there will be areas which are already in stage 4. However, the striking features of HF epidemiology in India across all areas are the high mortality rates, the younger age at which they present (whatever the etiology is), the major contribution from IHD, and the increasing burden.

Etiology of HF in India has changed tremendously during the last several years. When Vakil and colleagues[3] presented their first data in 1949, the primary causes of HF in 1,281 hospitalized patients were HTN and IHD which contributed 31%, RHD contributed 29%, syphilis 12%, and pulmonary disease 9%. Presently, nearly 70% of HF is due to IHD, and RHD contributes only <10%. It must be remembered, however, that several infectious diseases epidemics continue to ravage the country. Dengue fever and leptospirosis epidemics during monsoon result in good number of myocarditis and acute HF. Coronavirus disease 2019 (COVID-19) pandemic was also responsible for myocarditis cases.

Current estimates of HF in India vary widely from 1.3 to 23 million.[4] It is likely to increase in the near future because all the major risk factors for HF are increasing. This includes the aging population, rising number of CAD, rising number of people with other risk factors such as HTN, DM, persistence of diseases such as RHD, and increasing number of untreated patients with congenital heart disease who survive to adulthood. We also have a younger population with HF. Mean age of patients in Trivandrum Heart Failure Registry (THFR),[4] Medanta Registry,[5] and INTER-CHF (Indian subset)[6] were 61.2, 58.9, and 56 years, respectively. This is in contrast to the ADHERE data from USA,[7] where the mean age was 72.4 years. Male-to-female ratio was 70:30 in THFR[4] and 83:17 in Medanta Registry[5] while in USA[7] it was almost 50:50. In THFR,[4] HFpEF constituted 25% of all HF patients. HFrEF was the predominant form of HF reflecting the epidemiological stage. IHD is the most common etiology of HF, in both USA and India. RHD continues to be a major contributor of HF in India, but not in USA (8% of cases in THFR[4] and 5% in the Medanta Registry[5]). As expected, DM was much more prevalent among Indians than in the West.[4] Majority of the Indian patients are from low socioeconomic states, less educated, and are younger. They spend out-of-pocket for their treatment, unlike in the West, where insurance coverage is more universal.

The prognosis in Indian patients was worse than in the West, probably, reflecting the less-than-optimal utilization of GDMT. In Trivandrum Registry,[4] only 25% received GDMT at the time of discharge. The in-hospital mortality observed in the THFR[4] was 8.4% compared to 4% in the ADHERE[7] registry of the USA. 30-day mortality is similar at 30% in both US and India.

The challenges we face in India are, hence, multifaceted. On top of the list will be making quality healthcare services accessible and affordable to a socioeconomically and linguistically diverse population of >1.3 billion spread over 3.287 million km^2. Unfortunately, in most parts of the country, we have inadequate infrastructure to deliver the services. Strict quality control measures are lacking. Villages, where 72% of the population lives, have poor access by roads or rail. Only basic healthcare facilities are available at most of the primary health centers. These centers are often understaffed and their services overstretched. Tertiary healthcare resources are mostly concentrated in the large cities. Thus, there is gross inequality in healthcare distribution across the country.

There are mainly five major published registries on HF from India.[8] They are (1) THFR,[4] (2) CSI Kerala Heart Failure Registry (CSI-KHFR),[9] (3) National Heart Failure Registry (NHFR),[10] (4) Indian College of Cardiology National Heart Failure Registry (ICCNHFR),[11] (5) and the Medanta Registry.[5] The last one is a single-center study while the first four are multicenter. But all these studies are conducted at tertiary care centers, manned by cardiologists, in urban/semiurban areas, while the large number of HF patients in India resides in the villages looked after by primary care physicians in primary care centers. Hence, it is questionable as to how much these data actually represent what happens at the ground level.

Trivandrum Heart Failure Registry[4]

Trivandrum Heart Failure Registry is the first organized HF registry in India, with follow-up data up to 5 years available. Mean age of patients was 61.2 years. The etiology was IHD (72%), dilated cardiomyopathy (DCM) (13%), and RHD (8%). Among the CV risk factors, current tobacco use was 16%, alcohol use was 19%, HTN 58%, DM 55%, chronic obstructive pulmonary disease (COPD) 15%, and chronic kidney disease (CKD) 18%. It is important to note the high prevalence of HTN and DM. The rhythm was sinus in 85%. Atrial flutter or fibrillation (AF) was present in 15%. Nearly, a quarter (26%) had HFpEF, defined as left ventricular ejection fraction (LVEF) >45%. The majority were HFrEF. During hospitalization, 54% received beta-blockers, 46% received angiotensin-converting enzyme inhibitors (ACEI) or angiotensin receptor blockers (ARB), and 44% received mineralocorticoid receptor antagonists (MRAs). Only 19% with left ventricular systolic dysfunction received GDMT during hospitalization. The number of patients receiving GDMT at the time of hospital discharge was only 25%. In-hospital mortality was 8.5%. The 30 and 90-day mortality rates were 12.5% and 18.1%, respectively. As expected, those who did not receive GDMT at the time of discharge experienced higher mortality than those who did. This was evident even at the end of 5 years.

It is interesting to note that in THFR, there were only 4% of patients above the age of 85 years. It was 25% in the US-based ADHERE data.[7] More than half (57%) of patients were below the age of 65 years in THFR. In the ADHERE data only, 29% were below 65 years. These data show the large number of young people affected by HF in India.

The main etiological factor in THFR was IHD, as already mentioned. The Kerala ACS registry[12] data showed that less than half of acute coronary syndrome (ACS) patients in Kerala received optimal discharge medications at the time of discharge. So, one of the important aspects of preventing HF will be identifying ACS patients who are at risk of developing HF and targeting them for better management.

Literacy rate in Kerala is one of the highest in India. But among HF patients, majority have a low educational level. Obviously, chronic conditions such as HF are no longer limited to the higher socioeconomic group.

One of the most important determinants of prognosis was GDMT during hospitalization and at the time of discharge.

At the end of 1 year, cumulative all-cause mortality was 30.8%.[13] Greatest risk of mortality was in the first 3 months (18.1%). Nearly two-thirds (61%) of those who died were <70 years. One out of every three (30.2%) were readmitted at least once over 1 year. Lack of GDMT after index hospitalization and New York Heart Association (NYHA) functional class IV were associated with increased likelihood of readmissions. Propensity for hospital readmission was 30% higher in those who did not receive GDMT at the time of discharge. Hospital readmissions and lack of GDMT were independently associated with increased mortality. Prescription of GDMT at the time of discharge from the index hospitalization is, thus, of paramount importance and significantly affects patient outcomes even long term.

At the end of 3 years,[14] mortality was 44.8%. Those who survived index hospitalization and had no hospital readmissions were less likely to die. Patients with HFrEF and discharged on GDMT were less likely to die.

At the end of 5 years,[15] the unadjusted mortality rate was 59%. It was 61.3%, 60.5%, and 46.8% in HFrEF, HF with mildly reduced EF (HFmrEF), and HFpEF, respectively. Median survival time was only 3.1 years. Among death in HFrEF, 48% died from sudden cardiac death (SCD) and 48% from worsening HF. Higher survival rate was noticed in those discharged from index hospitalization on GDMT even at the end of 5 years. The hospital readmission rate was 49% over the 5-year period. In those who had no hospital readmissions, the 5-year cumulative mortality rate was only 50% compared to 69% in individuals with more than one readmission. Most deaths were due to worsening HF or SCD. In contrast, CV deaths were less common in HF in high-income countries. CV deaths are being increasingly replaced by causes related to infections or neoplasms in these countries. Adequate GDMT and appropriate device therapy may be the key reasons for lower CV deaths in high-income countries.

CSI Kerala HF Registry[9]

This was a registry of 7,507 patients with acute HF from 50 hospitals in Kerala. At the time of discharge, 28% of patients with HFrEF were on GDMT. In-hospital mortality was 7%. The patients who were on GDMT had survival advantage. Majority were HFrEF (67.5%). There were nearly equal number of HFmrEF (17.6%), and HFpEF (14.9%). The mean age was 64 ± 12.9 years with male predominance (63%) in HFrEF and HFmrEF. No significant sex difference was noted in HFpEF. CAD was the most common etiology (65.5%) and RHD contributed to 3.1% of patients. Majority had DM (61.5%) and HTN (53%). The salient epidemiological features in the registry were the relatively younger age of patients, higher rates of HFrEF, high prevalence of DM and CAD, surprisingly low rehospitalization rates and low rates of AF and stroke.

National Heart Failure Registry[10]

The mean age was 59.9 years with women constituting less than one-third (31%). More than three-fourths (74.4%) were *de novo* HF. Nearly two-thirds (65.2%) had HFrEF with HFmrEF in 22% and HFpEF in 12.7%. Etiological factor in 72% was IHD, DCM in 18%, and RHD in 5.9%. It was a pleasant surprise that 47.5% of HFrEF patients received GDMT, a very significant improvement from previous HF registries in India. The setting up of registries and dissemination of its results itself probably improved adherence to GDMT. In-hospital

TABLE 1: Comparison of the four multicenter registries.

	THFR[4]	CSI-KHFR[9]	NHFR[10]	ICCNHFR[11]
Age in years (mean)	61.2	64	59.9	61.9
IHD	72%	65.5%	72%	75.44%
RHD	8%	3.1%	5.9%	4.88%
HFrEF	74%	67.5%	65.7%	68.3%

(HFrEF: heart failure with reduced ejection fraction; IHD: ischemic heart disease; RHD: rheumatic heart disease)

TABLE 2: Comparison of the four multicenter registries.

	THFR[4]	CSI-KHFR[9]	NHFR[10]	ICCNHFR[11]
GDMT at discharge	25%	28%	47.5%	24.93%
In-hospital mortality	8.5%	7%	6.7%	6.98%
Atrial flutter/fibrillation	15%	14%	9.5%	8.78%

(GDMT: guideline-directed medical treatment)

mortality was 6.7% (7.6% and 6.7% in women and men respectively). Patients with HFrEF and HFmrEF who did not receive GDMT experienced higher mortality. Low educational level was also found to be a determinant of mortality.

Indian College of Cardiology National Heart Failure Registry[11]

Mean age of the patient population was 61.90 ± 13.85 years. Males predominated (67.09%). Mean duration of hospitalization was 5.74 ± 4.74 days. The most common underlying disease was IHD (75.44%). In 12.83% and 4.88%, DCM and RHD were the underlying diseases, respectively. In 68.29% of patients LVEF was <40%. In-hospital mortality rate was 6.98%. At discharge, 24.99% of patients received GDMT. There was high incidence of DM (51.53%) and HTN (52.27%). **Tables 1 and 2** are a comparison of the four multicenter registries.

However, these data may not be applicable to several areas of India. These are applicable only to urban/semiurban areas and tertiary hospitals. Data from eastern India[16] shows the mean age of HF patients was only 50.70 years. While IHD continued to be the most important cause of HF, it contributed only 58.6%. Significantly, 14.7% were valvular heart disease, mostly RHD. Surprisingly, 46.3% had HF with preserved EF. This data from eastern India suggests that in the rural areas of India, we have even younger patients than shown by these registries. The mortality rate is likely to be worse and contribution from RHD may be more than that projected in the registries.

PREVENTION

Prevention of HF in India should concentrate on prevention and adequate treatment of CAD. Thus primordial, primary, and secondary prevention of risk factors for CAD is of utmost importance. The major risk factors include HTN, DM, dyslipidemia, smoking, and obesity. Treating ACS properly also will reduce the incidence of HF. Adequate control of blood pressure is of utmost importance in preventing HFpEF. Importantly, RHD, though the incidence is decreasing, continues to be a significant contributor of HF, at least in some pockets in India. Primary and secondary prophylactic measures to prevent RHD should also be instituted.

CONCLUSION

India is on the verge of an HF epidemic. We have the dual burden of RHD and IHD contributing to HF. The mean age of HF patients in India is a decade less than the western population. The burden is mostly in those <65 years. Nearly 70% of the population affected are males. The main contributor is CAD, followed by DCM. Contribution from RHD varies widely across the country ranging from 4 to 10%. In-hospital mortality is higher, reflecting the suboptimal utilization of GDMT. Approximately, a quarter are HFpEF. Treating CAD appropriately and aggressive control of HTN, DM, obesity, dyslipidemia, and smoking will go a long way in reducing the incidence of HF. With the increase in the aging population, we should be ready to meet an epidemic of HFpEF.

ONLINE REFERENCES

Please scan the QR code provided at the end of the table of contents for References of this chapter.

CHAPTER

42

Heart Failure in Women: How Different than Men

Harendra Kumar

ABSTRACT

Heart failure (HF) may occur in both sexes—young or old, but women are at high risk of HF. Concomitant diabetes also increases risk of death. Hypertension is the most common cause of HF in women. Owing to silent nature of hypertension, diabetes, etc., people do not go for medical advice.

- Rheumatic heart disease (RHD) is the commonest cause of HF in India.
- Severe anemia also contributes in causing HF in women.
- Obesity, sedentary life, and smoking also increase the chances of HF.

Keywords: Heart failure, rheumatic heart disease (RHD), hypertension.

INTRODUCTION

Marked differences have been observed in the males and females.[1,2] Women generally have preserved left ventricular (LV) functions, men have underlying coronary artery disease (CAD)[3] with reduced left ventricular ejection fraction (LVEF) life time risk of developing heart failure (HF) at 40 years of age both in men and women is one in five, i.e., 20%.

Incidence

Johansson et al. (2015)[4] in their large study ($n \geq 36{,}000$), had follow-up of 1.9 years, and mostly were hypertensive. In this study, impact of diabetes mellitus (DM) on mortality was also observed. A total of 24% were diabetic and 39% women. Hypertension was more common in females (63%) versus 58 in males in this study.

Coronary artery disease was more prevalent in males (62%) versus 54% in women.

This study also showed that diabetic women had higher risk of HF, but importantly[4] diabetic women had higher mortality.[4] Prevalence of HF in older women (>75 years) was 10.9% and in men of the same age group was 9.8%.[5]

Occurrence of acute myocardial infarction (AMI) in a diabetic person is harmful in both sexes, but within 6 years of AMI in women, 46% ladies are disabled while only 22% of males had this adversity.[5] Women have less sudden cardiac death.[3] Once a woman with HF with diabetes[3] develops CAD mortality risk becomes higher, but HT as cause of heart failure kills large number of patients.

In a large study in Mumbai, India on stage-II hypertensive men (n = 87,459) and women (n = 59,368) 14% of cardiovascular deaths in men and 25% in women were attributed to hypertension. So, women suffered more than men.[6]

SOME COMMON CAUSES OF HEART FAILURE IN GENERAL

- Increasing age
- Rheumatic heart disease (RHD) (especially in India)
- Non-RHD valvular heart disease
- Hypertension
- CAD
- DM
- HF with preserved ejection fraction
- Cardiomyopathies (includes stress CMPs, i.e., apical ballooning syndrome)
- Severe anemia

- Atrial fibrillation
- Obesity
- Smoking
- Sedentary life
- Hypothyroidism
- Chronic kidney disease (CKD)
- Peripartum CMP
- Apical ballooning syndrome

IMPACT OF DIFFERENT ETIOLOGICAL FACTORS: DIFFERENCE IN MALE/ FEMALE IN SYMPTOMS

- Women are more dyspneic on exertion.
- Quicker relief in dyspnea on treatment in women
- Higher chance of edema in females[7]

The Framingham study[8] has shown reduction in the incidence of HF in women, but not in men over the last 50 years.

Usually women survive longer than men.[9,10]

Best survival is with non-ischemic HF.

IMPACT OF AGING ON HEART FAILURE

Incidence of HF increases with increasing age. Prevalence of HF at any age is higher in males than females, but overall risk of HF is 20% for both sexes. By age of 80 years, the risk of HF equalizes.

Etiology of HF also influences the future course. Females who had myocardial infarction (MI), 46% of them are disabled due to HF whereas disability occurs in 22% males only.[5]

INDIAN STUDIES ON HEART FAILURE

Unlike Western World, RHD is the commonest cause of HF in India (52% of hospitalized patients followed by CAD 17%) (Chaturvedi et al.).[11] Women contributed 43% of HF, CAD as cause of HF was more common in men (67.4%) versus 46% in women. Since RHD affects young population, 22.5% patients were <30 years of age and 14.9% >50 years. Valvular heart disease and dilated CMP as causes of HF are more common in women (18.8% and 22% than men 10.6% and 15%).

Another important thing for India is that anemia also causes HF or acts as contributor of HF in women especially in rural areas.[12]

IMPACT OF OBESITY (AS CAUSE OF HEART FAILURE)

Heart failure due to obesity [body mass index (BMI)] >30 kg/M^2 has been estimated to increase by 0.3% in women and 0.5% in men. Reddy et al. estimated prevalence of obesity in Delhi, Haryana to be 6.8%.[13]

But, this is old data, whenever one goes to Delhi, obese women and men (less) are visible in contrast, people of rural India are generally not obese.

IMPACT OF ETHNICITY AND RACE

In white women of USA, the prevalence rate of HF was 1.8%; in contrast, African-American women had 3%.[3]

In multiethnic Asian population, women were more hypertensive, CAD was less and had HF with preserved ejection fraction.[14]

HAVE ANATOMICAL DIFFERENCES IN CARDIOVASCULAR SYSTEM AN IMPACT ON HEART FAILURE

Magnetic resonance imaging (MRI) studies of nonhypertensive males have been done.

Left ventricular end-diastolic and end-systolic volumes LV, mass, LVEF, LV wall, and length were studied.[15]

Result: All dimensions from the—

- Framingham cohort were greater in men even when normalized for height.
- Volumes were greater in men than women after adjustment for body surface area.

DIFFERENCES IN BIOMARKERS OF HEART FAIL: MEN VERSUS WOMEN

Women have comparatively higher levels of natriuretic peptides and galectin-3 and lower levels of cardiac stress marker ST2. N-terminal pro–B-type natriuretic peptide (NT-proBNP) levels have shown clinical importance because their high levels indicate high risk of HF.[16]

IMPACT OF DIABETES: MALE VERSUS FEMALE

Diabetes is a risk factor in both sexes but a study (Johansson)[4] has found slightly higher risk in women. But, it is understandable that any additional risk factor is bound to increase the risk.

LOWER AFFORDABILITY OF TREATMENT IN WOMEN

- In women, less angiotensin-converting enzyme inhibitors (ACEI), angiotensin receptor blocker (ARB), and statin were prescribed.[4]
- Referral to higher center was less.
- Revascularization was less in CAD cases.

- Implantation of implantable cardioverter-defibrillator (ICD) was also less in women.[17]
- Lastly, representation of women is only 20% in studies. So here also they lag behind.

ACUTE BALLOONING SYNDROME (ALSO CALLED STRESS, CMP, AND BROKEN HEART SYNDROME)

- In 90% cases it occurs in females, especially post-menopausal women average at 61–76 years of age.
- Ballooning of LV occurs.
- LVEF is usually 35–50% which returns to normal in 95 cases in a few weeks.

CONCLUSION

Heart failure can be prevented/controlled with lifestyle management which includes exercise which may be as simple as walking. Secondly, in this era we have sodium-glucose cotransporter-2 (SGTL-2) inhibitors and other drug for DM. But we should not forget old landmark trials—4S, CARE, etc., which reduced incidence of HF, presumably by decreasing vulnerability of atherosclerotic plaque. We know the benefit of treating diabetic patients with ACEI or now ARBI is available, which is decreasing the incidences of HF. Mineralocorticoid receptor antagonist (MRA) and angiotensin receptor neprilysin inhibitor (ARNI) are also available in this era.

ONLINE REFERENCES

Please scan the QR code provided at the end of the table of contents for References of this chapter.

CHAPTER

43 Etiology and Management of Heart Failure in Pediatric Population

Anita Saxena

ABSTRACT

Heart failure is defined as an abnormality of cardiac structure or function leading to failure of the heart to deliver oxygen at a rate commensurate with the requirements of the metabolizing tissues, despite normal filling pressures (or only at the expense of increased filling pressures). In children, heart failure is often a transient state that is secondary to an underlying condition. Pediatric heart failure has different etiologies as compared to causes in adults and hence the management strategies may be different. Congenital heart diseases (CHDs) are the cause of heart failure in majority, followed by cardiomyopathies. The signs and symptoms of heart failure may be mistaken for common diseases in children such as pneumonia and sepsis and a high index of suspicion must be kept to diagnosed heart failure in children, especially in infants. A combination of tachycardia, tachypnea, and hepatomegaly may indicate heart failure in a young child. Diagnostic work-up should include echocardiography in addition to X-ray chest and electrocardiogram (ECG). Elevated biomarkers not only help in diagnosing cardiac cause of symptoms but also help in guiding therapy and prognostication. Most data on pharmacologic treatment is derived from experience in adults but more and more trials are being conducted in children. Conventional therapy consists of angiotensin-converting enzyme inhibitors/angiotensin receptor blockers, aldosterone antagonists, and beta-blockers. Diuretic therapy is used to alleviate symptoms of congestion. Digoxin is often not used in current day practice. Newer drugs include ivabradine, sacubitril-valsartan, sodium-glucose cotransporter-2 (SGLT-2) inhibitors, vericiguat, etc. Adequate attention must be paid to fluid balance and nutritional supplementation for optimal growth of children. Anemia should be treated and infection, if present, controlled. Nonpharmacologic methods such as ventricular assist devices (VADs), pulmonary artery banding, and cardiac transplantation are reserved for children with end-stage heart failure.

Keywords: Pediatric, heart failure, pharmacological treatment.

INTRODUCTION

Heart failure is defined as an abnormality of cardiac structure or function leading to failure of the heart to deliver oxygen at a rate commensurate with the requirements of the metabolizing tissues, despite normal filling pressures (or only at the expense of increased filling pressures). In case of children, this requirement includes "growth and development". It is a clinical syndrome resulting from ventricular dysfunction, and volume or pressure overload, alone or in combination and encompasses a diverse population of patients. In children, heart failure is often a transient state that is secondary to an underlying condition. Some pediatric heart failure specialists believe that pulmonary overcirculation secondary to a large left to right shunt should not be labeled as heart failure.

Pediatric heart failure has different etiologies as compared to causes in adults and hence the management strategies may be different. In fact, due to the diverse nature of underlying etiology in children, therapeutic approaches need to be tailored. Right heart failure is also more common in children, could be associated with tetralogy of Fallot, atrial septal defect, Ebstein anomaly, and single ventricle physiology. Since underlying congenital heart disease (CHD) is the cause in majority, surgical or transcatheter treatment can resolve symptoms with normalization of structure and function of the heart. Myocardial causes such as myocarditis, genetic cardiomyopathies, and metabolic diseases have different clinical course and require long-term therapies.

INCIDENCE AND PREVALENCE

True global incidence and prevalence are difficult to estimate due to lack of standard definition of heart failure. CHD may account for 25–75% of pediatric heart failure cases.[1] Dilated cardiomyopathy is an important cause of heart failure at any age, its incidence has been reported between 0.87 and 7.4/100,000 children in a systematic literature review.[2] The prevalence in the Pediatric Cardiomyopathy Registry in the USA and Australia has been 1.2/100,000 children at a peak incidence at a median age of 1.8 years.[3,4] Dilated cardiomyopathy is a leading cause of pediatric heart transplantation.

STAGING OF HEART FAILURE

The American College of Cardiology and the American Heart association staging of heart failure is often used in adult patients for categorizing. Unlike New York Heart Association (NYHA) classification, staging represents the onset and progression of the disease. Similar staging has been recommended for pediatric patients with heart failure by the International Society for Heart and Lung Transplantation guidelines, published in 2004[5] and is given in the **Table 1**. Those with prior symptoms would fall in heart failure stage C. This staging may not be always applicable to children as a number of children with heart failure will recover from stage C or even D. For example, children with large left to right shunts will completely recover after closure of the shunt. Similarly, heart failure may completely resolve in children with acute myocarditis.

TABLE 1: Proposed heart failure staging for infants and children.

Stage	Interpretation
A	Patients with increased risk of developing HF, but who have normal cardiac function and no evidence of cardiac chamber volume overload. For examples, previous exposure to cardiotoxic agents, family history of heritable cardiomyopathy, univentricular heart, and congenitally corrected transposition of the great arteries
B	Patients with abnormal cardiac morphology or cardiac function, with no symptoms of HF, past or present. For examples, aortic insufficiency with LV enlargement, history of anthracycline with decreased LV systolic function
C	Patients with underlying structural or functional heart disease, and past or current symptoms of HF
D	Patients with end-stage HF requiring continuous infusion of inotropic agents, mechanical circulatory support, cardiac transplantation, or hospice care

(HF: heart failure; LV: left ventricular)

ETIOLOGY

The various etiologies can be grouped under three main categories. The most common cause is CHD, which be a simple large left to right shunt or a complex single ventricle. The second common category is primary muscle disease, cardiomyopathy. The third category is of acquired heart disease such as rheumatic heart disease. Rare causes include arrhythmias, metabolic causes, etc. The underlying etiology varies with the region. In India and other low- and middle-income countries (LMIC), unoperated CHDs and rheumatic heart disease are common causes. In high-income countries (HIC), cardiomyopathies and postoperated CHD are common causes of pediatric heart failure. Brazil and Africa have high prevalence of HIV-related cardiac disease as the cause of heart failure. The various causes of heart failure in children are shown in **Box 1**. The underlying etiology tends to vary at different ages. The various causes which are more likely at different ages are shown in **Table 2**. As one can see from the **Table 2**, heart failure in fetal life or on day one of life are mostly not due to CHD. Critical obstructive lesions tend to present in first week of life and large shunt lesions, in second week or later. Acquired heart disease is more common in toddlers or in older children. Arrhythmias are also important cause of heart failure and may be missed as neonates and infants tend to have high heart rates even normally.

BOX 1 Etiology of pediatric heart failure.

Volume overload with preserved systolic ventricular function (over circulation HF):
- *Large left to right shunt*: VSD, AVSD, and PDA
- *Admixture lesions with high PBF*: TGA, TAPVC, and truncus
- *Regurgitant lesions*: MR and AR (rheumatic/congenital/IE)
- Anemia, AV fistula, beriberi, etc.

Myocyte dysfunction with abnormal ventricular contractile function (pump failure):
- *Pressure overload*: Severe LVOT, RVOT obstruction, and CoA
- *DCM*: Idiopathic, neuromuscular, familial, and metabolic
- *Inflammatory*: Myocarditis, Chaga's, and HIV related
- *Rhythm disturbances*: Tachycardiomyopathy and CHB
- *Ischemic*: ALCAPA
- *Postoperated*: Fontan, ToF with severe PR
- *Others*: LV noncompaction, hypocalcemia, anthracycline toxicity, and sepsis

(ALCAPA: anomalous origin of left coronary artery from pulmonary artery; AR: aortic regurgitation; AV: arteriovenous; AVSD: atrioventricular septal defect; CHB: complete heart block; IE: infective endocarditis; LV: left ventricle, LVOT: left ventricular outflow tract; MR: mitral regurgitation; PDA: patent ductus arteriosus; PR: pulmonary regurgitation; RVOT: right ventricular outflow tract; TGA: transposition of great arteries; ToF: tetralogy of Fallot; TAPVC: total anomalous pulmonary venous connection; VSD: ventricular septal defect)

TABLE 2: Causes of heart failure at different ages.

Day 1 of life/fetal		1–2 months	
• Asphyxia • Systemic AV fistula • Myocarditis	• Metabolic arrhythmias • Ebstein anomaly	• VSD and AVSD • Transposition and malposition complexes • ALCAPA	• PDA • Aorto-pulmonary window • Unobstructed TAPVC
First week of life (after day 1)		**2–6 months**	
• Critical AS/PS HLHS • Adrenal insufficiency	• Obstructed TAPVC • Coarctation • Hypertension • TGA IVS	• Causes at 1–2 months, coarctation, critical and AS/PS • *Metabolic*: Hypocalcemia/beriberi	
Second week of life		**Older children**	
• Large VSD • AV septal defect • Unobstructed TAPVC	• Large PDA • Persistent truncus arteriosus	• Rheumatic heart disease • Cardiomyopathies • Palliated CHD/postoperative • Corrected transposition great arteries • Severe PS/AS with ventricular dysfunction • Severe hypertension • Aortoarteritis	
Tachycardiomyopathy can present at any age			

(ALCAPA: anomalous origin of left coronary artery from pulmonary artery; AS: aortic stenosis; AV: arteriovenous; AVSD: atrioventricular septal defect; CHD: congenital heart disease; HLHS: hypoplastic left heart syndrome; IVS: Intact ventricular septum; PDA: patent ductus arteriosus; PS: pulmonary stenosis; TGA: transposition of great arteries; TAPVC: total anomalous pulmonary venous connection; VSD: ventricular septal defect)

CLINICAL FEATURES

The signs and symptoms of heart failure may be mistaken for common diseases in children such as pneumonia and sepsis. A gastroenteritis may be suspected in a child having nausea and vomiting due to an enlarged congested liver. Common cardiac symptoms include breathlessness on exertion, fatigue, palpitations, and abdominal pain. Parents may notice tachypnea and respiratory distress in infants. Failure to gain weight, feeding difficulties, suck-rest-suck cycle, and sweating overhead especially during feeds is other symptoms noted in infants. Examination may not reveal classical signs of heart failure such as raised jugular venous pressure (JVP) and pedal edema in small children. A triad of tachypnea, tachycardia, and hepatomegaly may be indicative of heart failure in infants. A gallop rhythm may also be present. All patients must also be evaluated for arterial oxygen saturation by using a pulse oximeter. In severe cases, signs of poor perfusion, such as delayed capillary refill and cool distal extremities, may be seen. A careful precordial examination helps in making a diagnosis of underlying CHD such as a large ventricular septal defect. A murmur of mitral regurgitation may be audible in some cases of dilated cardiomyopathy. Common signs and symptoms of heart failure in children are given in **Table 3**.

TABLE 3: Common signs and symptoms of heart failure in children.

Age	Common signs and symptoms	Less common signs and symptoms
Infant	Growth failure, persistent tachypnea, tachycardia, feeding difficulties, diaphoresis, subcostal recession, and hepatomegaly	Cyanosis, palpitation, syncope, seizures, and wheeze
Toddlers	Respiratory distress, tachypnoea, tachycardia, fatigue, and hepatomegaly	Poor appetite, palpitations, and edema
School age	Fatigues, effort intolerance, poor appetite, orthopnea, abdominal pain, nausea, vomiting, hepatomegaly, and raised JVP	Palpitations, chest pain, leg edema, ascites, and basal crepts
Adolescents	Effort intolerance, poor appetite, abdominal pain, orthopnea, and hepatomegaly	Nausea, vomiting, leg edema, and ascites

The conventional NYHA functional classification is not applicable to children under 6 years of age. For this reason, modified Ross classification is used for assessment of younger children.[6] A comparison of two classifications is given in **Table 4**.

DIAGNOSTIC WORKUP

A chest X-ray and an electrocardiogram (ECG) must be done for all patients with heart failure. These investigations help to pinpoint cardiac cause for nonspecific symptoms such as tachypnea, effort intolerance, and feeding difficulties. X-ray chest will show cardiomegaly, increased vascularity (in CHDs with increased pulmonary blood flow), and pulmonary venous hypertension of varying severity **(Fig. 1)**. Pleural effusion may be present, especially on the right side. In addition, lung parenchyma can be evaluated for evidence of any evidence of an infective etiology, such as bronchiolitis and consolidation. ECG often shows sinus tachycardia and ventricular hypertrophy, volume overload in some cases depending on the underlying heart disease. Nonspecific ST T wave changes may be present in those with cardiomyopathy. ECG is almost diagnostic in children with anomalous origin of left coronary artery from pulmonary artery as it shows a myocardial infarct pattern in anterior and lateral leads, otherwise a very uncommon finding in children. Rhythm alterations, such as supraventricular tachycardia **(Fig. 2)**, atrial flutter, and atrial fibrillation could be the cause of heart failure in some children and ECG gives away the diagnosis.

TABLE 4: New York Heart Association (NYHA) and modified Ross heart failure classification for children.

	NYHA	Modified Ross
Class I	No limitations of physical activity	No limitations or symptoms
Class II	May experience fatigue, palpitations, dyspnea, or angina during moderate exercise but not during rest	• *Infants*: Mild tachypnea or diaphoresis with feeding • *Older children*: Mild-to-moderate dyspnea on exertion
Class III	Symptoms with minimal exertion that interfere with normal daily activity	• *Infants*: Growth failure and marked tachypnea or diaphoresis with feeding • *Older children*: Marked dyspnea on exertion
Class IV	Unable to carry out any physical activity because they typically have symptoms at rest that worsen with any exertion	Symptoms at rest such as tachypnea, retractions, grunting, or diaphoresis

Echocardiography is the most useful investigation as it provides the precise diagnosis in most cases and is widely available. It provides information on function of right and left ventricle, size cardiac chambers, and wall thickness, severity of valvular stenosis, or incompetence, if present and associated structural abnormality of heart and great vessels. Infants presenting with dilated cardiomyopathy like picture **(Fig. 3)** must be evaluated for any coronary anomaly. Pericardial effusion and intracardiac thrombi are also easily seen on echocardiography. Information obtained on echocardiography is crucial to make correct diagnosis and also to guide appropriate management.

Laboratory tests include serum electrolytes, renal function tests, etc., may be impaired, either due to heart failure or due to diuretic therapy and need to be monitored. Complete blood counts and hemoglobin (Hb) should be determined and anemia treated if present. Serum calcium, liver function tests, thyroid profile, antistreptolysin titer, erythrocyte sedimentation rate (ESR), and C-reactive protein (CRP) may be required to be tested in specific cases. Newborns presenting with heart failure may require screening for sepsis.

Biomarkers

Brain natriuretic peptide (BNP) and or its cleavage product amino-terminal pro-BNP (NT-proBNP) are often elevated in children with heart failure. BNP or amino terminal,

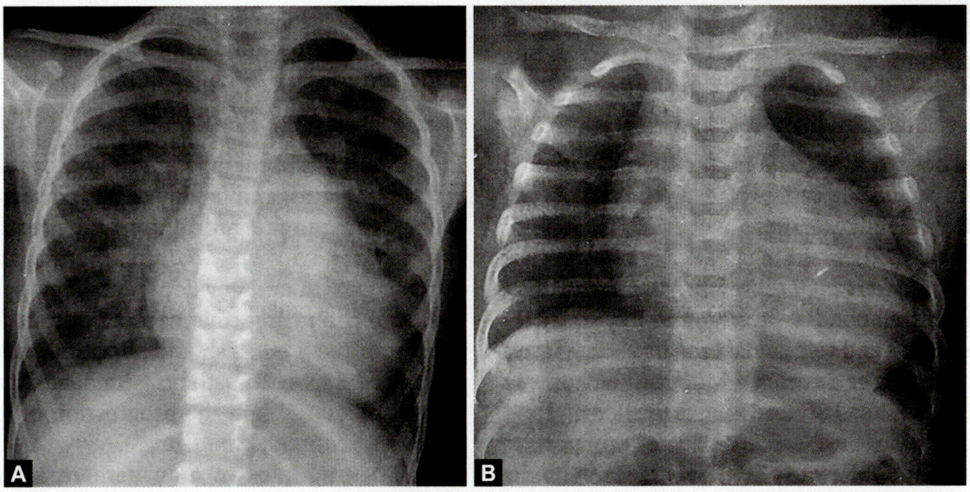

FIGS. 1A AND B: X-ray chest from two infants with heart failure. (A) Secondary to a large ventricular septal defect; and (B) Secondary to dilated cardiomyopathy.

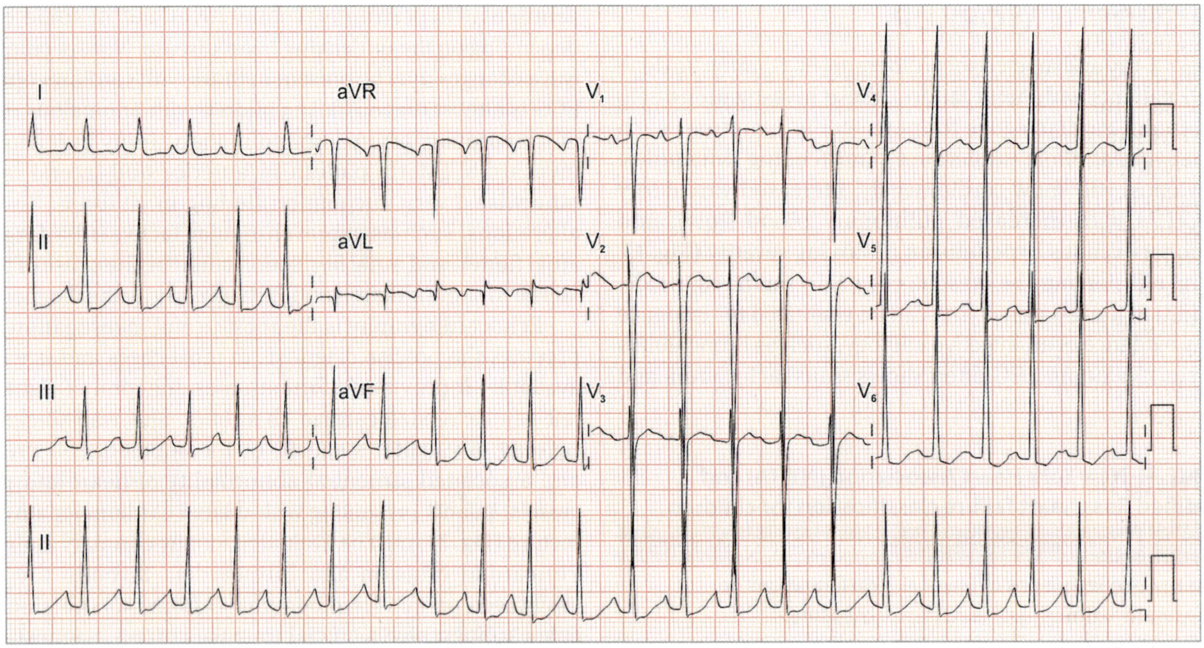

FIG. 2: ECG from a 10-year-old boy showing supraventricular tachycardia at a rate of 150 beats/min.

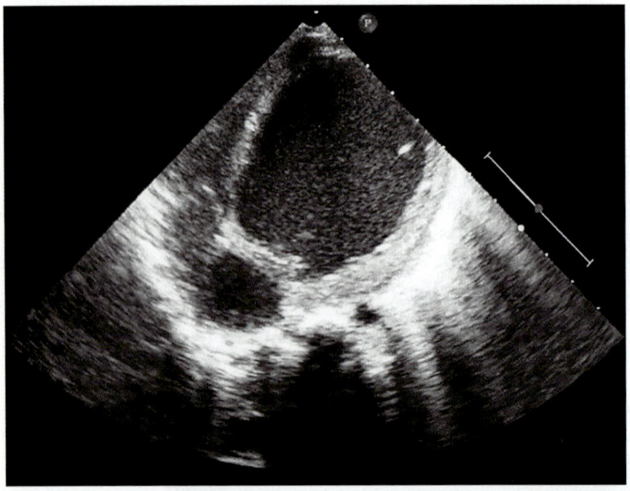

FIG. 3: 2D echocardiogram from an infant with dilated cardiomyopathy showing a dilated left ventricle (LV).

NT-proBNP has been shown to be of use in differentiating heart failure from pulmonary causes of respiratory distress in acute settings. Data on utility of these biomarkers in children on prognosis is emerging. According to some studies, higher levels of these biomarkers may represent poor prognosis.[7] Similarly strong correlation has been found between NT-proBNP and symptoms and ventricular function.[8] High levels of these biomarkers may be associated with worst outcome in heart failure, high likelihood of admission to the hospital and high chances of need for mechanical circulatory support, or heart transplant. Serial BNP or NT-proBNP measurements may be useful for monitoring the progress of the patient.

Other Investigations

Second line tests may be required in some specific cases for making a diagnosis. These include cardiac magnetic resonance imaging (MRI), computed tomography (CT) angiography, endomyocardial biopsy, Holter monitoring, metabolic and genetic testing, viral pathogenic screening, etc. Cardiac catheterization for assessing hemodynamics is hardly ever required but it is particularly useful for quantifying pulmonary artery pressure and identifying the cause of pulmonary hypertension. A number of therapeutic interventions to manage heart failure are performed in the catheterization laboratory. Examples include balloon dilation of critically narrow valves (aortic/pulmonary stenosis), closure of shunts and fistulae, balloon dilation and/or stenting of vessels (coarctation of aorta, peripheral pulmonary artery stenosis, etc.).

MANAGEMENT OF HEART FAILURE

The main goals of therapy are to improve hemodynamics, functional status, and quality of life, correct the underlying cause, and reduce morbidity and mortality. In infant and children with heart failure, therapy should allow for somatic growth and development. Therapy should reduce congestion and improve cardiac output and end-organ perfusion. The preload should be optimized without causing volume depletion. In patients with dilated cardiomyopathy, treatment should halt the progression of disease through improved ventricular modeling.

Main principles of management include treatment of underlying cause, e.g., shunts, valvar stenosis/

regurgitation, coronary anomaly, etc. A number of comorbidities can precipitate heart failure and these include anemia, intercurrent infections, electrolyte imbalance (hypocalcemia, hypoglycemia, and acidosis), arrhythmias, active rheumatic carditis, infective endocarditis, and drug toxicity or interaction. Active search should be made for these precipitating factors and, if present, appropriately treated.

Management includes supplemental oxygen therapy, nutrition supplements, and fluid management. Pharmacologic agents form the backbone of treatment. Extracorporeal membrane oxygenation (ECMO), left ventricular assist devices (LVADs), and other advanced therapies may be required in cases not responding to conventional management.

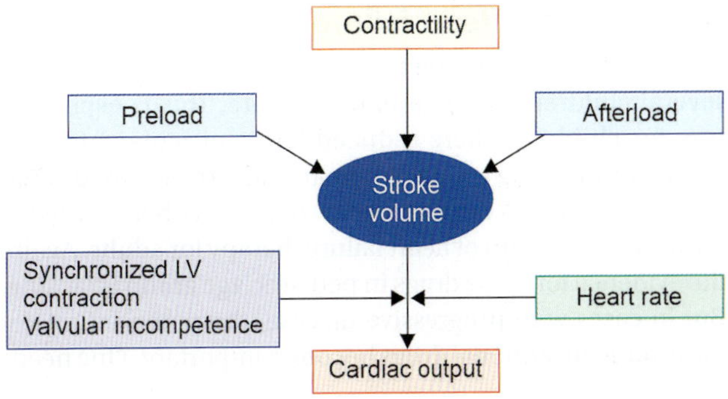

FIG. 4: Pharmacologic targets for treatment of heart failure. (LV: left ventricular)

Nutrition

In infants' calorie intake of 120–150 kcal/kg/day is recommended with a fluid intake of 100 mL/kg/day. Many patients are unable to tolerate this amount of fluid. Calorie dense food, adding fat to feeds (coconut oil or medium chain triglyceride), frequent small feeding, and at times feeding through the nasogastric tube may achieve adequate calories. Nutrition supplementation is easier in older children where protein content of the diet is increased along with optimal fats and carbohydrates. Calcium and vitamin D3 supplements should be prescribed. Unlike in adults, dietary restriction of sodium is generally not recommended in children unless there is severe edema which is not responding to diuretic therapy. Frequent weight measurement is encouraged, especially in infants, to assess their nutritional status.

Fluid Management

Fluid intake is generally not restricted unless child has acute heart failure with significant lung congestion and edema despite diuretics. Fluid restriction may also be required in cases with hyponatremia.

Bed Rest

This is generally not required. In fact, some amount of physical activity should be encouraged in children with controlled heart failure.

Correction of Anemia

A large proportion of these children are anemic due to various reasons and these should receive iron and vitamin supplements. If Hb is <7 or 8 g/dL, blood transfusion is recommended.

Pharmacological Therapy

Most of the recommendations for chronic pediatric heart failure therapy are extrapolated from adult heart failure trials. A number of obstacles exist for conducting trials for heart failure drugs in children. These include widely varied etiologies of heart failure, complexities of CHDs, changes in child's weight due to growth, nonavailability of pediatric drug formulations, dose selection, comorbid conditions, and the large number of patients required to be recruited. Medical therapy for heart failure has been based on the neurohormonal paradigm. Impairment of heart function activates the compensatory mechanisms. The adrenergic nervous system, the renin-angiotensin system, and the cytokine system are activated leading to secondary end-organ damages which worsen symptoms and a vicious cycle is set up leading to decompensation and heart failure. Drugs which can block this pathway can break this cycle and prevent the further deterioration and may improve symptoms of heart failure, hospitalization, and even death. **Figure 4** depicts the pharmacologic targets for treatment of heart failure.

Several studies in adults have shown role of diuretics, angiotensin-converting enzyme inhibitors (ACEIs), mineralocorticoid antagonists, angiotensin receptor blockers (ARBs), and beta-blockers in heart failure management to relieve symptoms and improve survival. Despite the lack of such robust data in pediatrics, drugs commonly used in adults, i.e., diuretics, ACEIs, ARBs, and aldosterone antagonists (spironolactone or eplerenone) are the current standard of care therapy for chronic heart failure. The addition of a β-adrenergic receptor antagonist (β-blocker) for both asymptomatic and symptomatic patients with chronic heart failure is less well supported in the pediatric literature, but is being increasingly used in practice. Digoxin is not routinely recommended, but can be reserved for patients who remain symptomatic despite maximum doses of above stated drugs and in those with tachyarrhythmia such as atrial fibrillation.

Table 5 provides the most common pediatric heart failure drugs and doses.

Table 6 provides information on four randomized clinical trials on drugs, with key findings, which have been performed in children with heart failure till date.[9-12]

New Drugs for Heart failure

With conventional therapy as per recommendations, several children continue to deteriorate. This is especially true for children where reduced left ventricular function is the underlying cause of heart failure, as in dilated cardiomyopathy. A number of new drugs have been added to the armamentarium of heart failure therapy for adults. Again, the evidence for these drugs in pediatric age group is lacking. But in cases with progressive disease, the potential role of these nonconventional drugs becomes important. One needs to be familiar with the doses and possible side effects of the new pharmacologic agents in pediatric age group. Some of the newer drugs are discussed below.

TABLE 5: Conventional pharmacotherapy of chronic heart failure in children.

Drug	Standard dose
Captopril	0.5–2 mg/kg/dose, 2–5 times/day (max 25 mg/dose)
Enalapril	0.1–0.5 mg/kg/day (max 20 mg/dose)
Lisinopril	0.05–2 mg/kg/day once or twice/day
Losartan	0.5–2 mg/kg/day
Metoprolol	0.1 mg/kg 2 times/day (max 1 mg/kg dose)
Bisoprolol	0.05–0.2 mg/kg/day 1–2 times/day
Propranolol	0.2–0.5 mg/kg/dose 3 times/day
Carvedilol	0.025 mg/kg/dose twice a day, max 0.5 mg/kg/dose BD
Furosemide	0.5–2 mg/kg/day
Spironolactone	0.5–2 mg/kg/day twice a day, max 200 mg/day
Hydrochlorothiazide	0.5–1 mg/kg/day
Digoxin	3–5 µg/kg dose twice a day

Ivabradine

Ivabradine is an inhibitor of the funny channels located in the sinoatrial node that slows the rate of phase-4 depolarization, thereby reducing the heart rate. Though tachycardia is a common compensatory mechanism in heart failure, high heart rates have been known to be associated with higher mortality in heart failure and are directly related to the risk of cardiovascular death or admission to the hospital in these patients.[13] Ivabradine has been well studied in adult population with heart failure, in the SHIFT and BEAUTIFUL trials.[14] Ivabradine improved clinical outcomes in patients with left ventricular dysfunction, despite the primary clinical presentation. As in adults with heart failure, elevated heart rates has been shown to increase risk of death and cardiac transplant in registry data of children with dilated cardiomyopathy.[15] A randomized, double-blind, placebo-controlled, phase II/III clinical trial of children with stable heart failure reported safety of ivabradine in children.[12] The trial showed reduction of the resting heart rate and an increase in the left ventricular ejection fraction (LVEF). Following this trial, ivabradine has been approved by the Food and Drug Administration (FDA) in the year 2019 for treatment in children with symptomatic heart failure >6 months of age. The recommended dose is 0.02–0.05 mg/kg twice a day for children under 40 kg and 2.5 mg twice a day for children >40 kg.

Sacubitril–valsartan

This drug is a combination of a neprilysin inhibitor with an angiotensin II receptor antagonist. The enzyme neprilysin degrades natriuretic peptides, which decrease

TABLE 6: Randomized controlled trials for pediatric heart failure.

Author/Year	Title	Key findings
Lewis AB, et al. 1993[9]	The effect of treatment with angiotensin-converting enzyme inhibitors (ACEIs) on survival of pediatric patients with dilated cardiomyopathy	*n* = 80; (26 = ACEI, 54 = digoxin plus diuretics). 1-and 2-year survival with ACEI was better than digoxin group
Shaddy RE, et al. 2007[10]	Carvedilol for children and adolescent with heart failure: A randomized controlled trial	*n* = 161; no significant difference between treatment versus placebo group in primary endpoint (clinical improvement) or secondary endpoint (ventricular function or serum BNP)
Hsu DT, et al. 2010[11]	Enalapril in infants with single ventricle	*n* = 230; no improvement in somatic growth, ventricular function, and heart failure severity. Routine use of enalapril in SV CHD patients with RV is not recommended as systemic ventricle
Bonnet D, et al. 2017[12]	Ivabradine in children with dilated cardiomyopathy and symptomatic chronic heart failure	*n* = 116; primary endpoint reached by 51 of 73 children taking ivabradine (70%); ivabradine safely reduced the resting heart rate of children with chronic HF and dilated cardiomyopathy; improvement in ejection fraction, functional class, and NT-pro-BNP was noted

(BNP: brain natriuretic peptide; CHD: congenital heart disease; HF: heart failure; SV: single ventricle)

the sympathetic tone and aldosterone levels. Inhibition of neprilysin prevents degradation of natriuretic peptides, thereby promoting sodium excretion and lowering blood pressure. The combination of a neprilysin inhibitor with an angiotensin II receptor antagonist provides inhibition of neprilysin as well as blockade of the renin–angiotensin–aldosterone system. This combination is available as sacubitril/valsartan. A large trail conducted in adults, PARDIGM-HF (2009-2014), recruited >8,000 patients. They alternatively received sacubitril/valsartan or enalapril. The results were very encouraging. The sacubitril/valsartan group showed a reduction of 3.7% in the primary endpoint of death from cardiovascular causes or hospitalization for heart failure and a 3.2% reduction in overall mortality.[16] These encouraging results led to initiation of an international multicenter study in the pediatric population, the PANORAMA-HF study. It was designed to assess the pharmacokinetics and pharmacodynamics of sacubitril/valsartan and to evaluate the superiority of sacubitril/valsartan over enalapril for the treatment of heart failure in children.[17] Based on the analysis of interim data in 110 subjects, FDA approved the use of this drug in October 2019 for children, 1 year of age or older, with symptomatic heart failure with left ventricular systolic dysfunction. This was based on comparable reduction in NT-proBNP between enalapril and sacubitril/valsartan. Dosing recommendations for younger children are yet to be defined. The trial has enrolled 393 children and it is waiting for all enrolled patients to complete 52 weeks of therapy before the data is analyzed. Till the final results become available, sacubitril/valsartan can be used safely in pediatric patients in place of ACEIs, if required. The starting dose for children <40 kg is 1.6 mg/kg of the combined amount of both valsartan and sacubitril. The dose is titrated upward every 2 weeks from 2.3 mg/kg up to a maximum dose of 3.1 mg/kg based on tolerance.

Sodium-glucose Cotransporter-2 Inhibitors

Drugs included under this group are canagliflozin, dapagliflozin, and empagliflozin. These were initially developed for patients with diabetes mellitus. The mechanism of action is to inhibit the sodium-glucose cotransporter (SGLT) situated in the kidney, and to promote glucose excretion and improve sugar control in a diabetic patient. However, the trial also showed a reduction in heart failure-related events in these patients and this led to further trials, specifically addressing the issue of improvement in heart failure and reducing other cardiovascular events. A multicenter randomized trial on 4,744 patients further showed that dapagliflozin reduces the risk of worsening heart failure or death from cardiovascular problems compared to a placebo, independent of the presence of diabetes. A more recent, larger trial, named EMPEROR-Reduced confirmed the finding of improved outcome in heart failure patients, seen as early as within 12 weeks of therapy.[18] Similar results have been seen with canagliflozin in the CHIEF-HF trial where 476 adults with heart failure were randomized.[19] The first description of use of SGLT-2 inhibitor use in pediatric age group was reported in the year 2021.[20] 38 patents were included and dapagliflozin was added to the heart failure therapy regimen. The drug was well tolerated and there were no report of experiencing hypovolemia or hypoglycemia. However, six patients reported a symptomatic urinary tract infection requiring antibiotic treatment. The left ventricular function improved in 26 patients who had dysfunction initially. The ejection fraction of left ventricle significantly improved from 32 to 37.2%. More data in pediatric heart failure is required before recommending this drug for heart failure. The dose in pediatric age group is 0.1–0.2 mg/kg once daily with a maximum of 10 mg.

Vericiguat

Vericiguat is a novel oral soluble guanylate cyclase stimulator, an enzyme responsible for the production of nitrogen monoxide (NO). This enzyme plays a role in arteriolar vasodilation and inhibits fibrosis. It is also known to reduce mechanical and oxidative vascular stress. In a recent trial in adult patients with chronic symptomatic heart failure, this drug reduced the risk of cardiovascular death, all-cause death, and hospitalization due to heart failure. The study, called VICTORIA, enrolled 5050 patients who had an ejection fraction of <45%.[21] A recent meta-analysis study compared sacubitril/valsartan, vericiguat, and SGLT-2 inhibitors in adult patients with heart failure and reduced ejection fraction. The risk of heart failure hospitalization was not significantly different between patients on SGLT-2 inhibitors or sacubitril/valsartan. However, dapagliflozin was superior to vericiguat in this meta-analysis.[22] No data are currently available for children. A clinical trial about the safety, efficacy, and pharmacokinetics of vericiguat in pediatric heart failure is being initiated. No information on pediatric dosing is available.

Omecamtiv Mecarbil

This drug is the first small molecule which is an activator of cardiac myosin. Omecamtiv mecarbil is the first-in-class drug, with demonstrated selective ability to increase cardiac myosin ATPase activity. It improves myocardial function by directly augmenting cardiac sarcomere function and increases the systolic function of ventricle in patients with reduced ejection fraction. One trial in adult patients, called GALACTIC-HF trial, recruited 8,256 adult patients with symptomatic chronic heart failure, ejection fraction of 35% or less. Omecamtiv mecarbil was compared to a placebo, in addition to standard heart failure therapy. Omecamtiv mecarbil significantly decreased the primary endpoint (time-to-first heart failure event or death due to cardiovascular causes), more so in the group of patients with ejection fraction of <22%. Overall, there was a 16% reduction in the time-to-first heart failure event or cardiovascular death [hazard ratio (HR) 0.84; 95% confidence intervals (CI) 0.77–0.92; p = 0.0003].[23] These findings are very encouraging for patients with more severe heart failure as the benefits are likely to be more in this group. However, no data is currently available for children and there is no ongoing trial. No information on pediatric dosing is available.

Investigational Supplement Drugs

Recently published data suggest that coenzyme Q10 (a potent antioxidant) improves cardiac function. Its mechanism of action is to stabilize myocardial calcium-dependent ion channels and to prevent the consumption of some of the essential metabolites.[24] Another study has shown the role of ubiquinol supplementation in the dose of 10 mg/kg/day for 24 weeks in improving ejection fraction and NYHA class of 10 pediatric patients with dilated cardiomyopathy.[25]

Which Drug for Which Patient: The Logical Approach

It seems reasonable to start with a drug in ACEI or ARB group, except in patients having heart failure secondary to obstructive lesions. For patients with dilated cardiomyopathy, an aldosterone antagonist drug may also be added. There is evidence that sacubitril/valsartan is tolerated well in this setting, and so this may become the preferred option in place of ACEI in future. It is also important to use the maximal tolerated doses of vasodilators to reap maximum benefit of these drugs. Generally, the doses can be escalated rapidly in stable patients with chronic heart failure. This can be followed by a β-blocker. β-blockers can be started prior to discharge in hospitalized patients. Those treated in the outpatient can be given a lower dose to ensure tolerability and the dose is gradually increased. Target dosing of ACEIs can be achieved within 6–7 days in most patients, but optimizing dose of β-blockers generally takes longer. For those having high heart rate despite β-blockers or intolerant to β-blockers, additional treatments with ivabradine may be prescribed. Diuretics may be prescribed for reducing pulmonary or systemic congestion in symptomatic patients, the dosage may be given daily or as and when required. Indications for SGLT-2 inhibitors are not very clear at this stage for children. Based on excellent results in adults, these drugs may be used in adolescent patients with reduced function of the left ventricle due to dilated cardiomyopathy who have persistent symptoms.

Monitoring Pharmacologic Therapy

Monitoring the response to therapy has been conventionally done by relief of symptoms, resolution of clinical features of heart failure such as tachypnea, tachycardia, and hepatomegaly. Assessment of laboratory parameters such as kidney function tests and electrolytes also needs monitoring when on diuretic therapy. Patients and their caregivers should be told about the side effects of various drugs which have been prescribed and careful watch kept for side effects during follow-up visits. There is some evidence in children that BNP or NT-proBNP can act as surrogate markers of the likelihood of admission to hospital, the need of mechanical circulatory support, or heart transplant after admission due to heart failure.[7] Recently, data published by Pediatric Cardiomyopathy Registry has suggested added value of incorporating a panel of multiple serum biomarkers in the risk assessment of children presenting with heart failure.[26]

Advanced Nonpharmacologic Therapy

Device Therapy

Device therapy in heart failure includes pacemaker therapy, cardiac resynchronization therapy (CRT), and mechanical circulatory support.

- *Cardiac resynchronization therapy:* This device therapy is indicated in adults who have LVEF of <35%, dilated left ventricle, and NHYA classes II, III, and IV despite maximization of drug therapy and QRS duration of >120 ms. A clear benefit has been shown with CRT in terms of slower progression of heart failure due to the improvement of cardiac motion and a reduced risk of sudden death. There is also general improvement in quality of life. CRT may be useful in adolescents and young adults as per 2013 European Heart Rhythm Association (EHRA) and Association for European Paediatric and Congenital Cardiology (AEPC) guidelines. The QRS duration should be >98th percentile for age and patient should have a systemic left ventricle, complete left bundle branch block pattern. A specific evaluation for mechanical dyssynchrony should be made before CRT is offered.[27]
- *Implantable cardioverter-defibrillator (ICD):* This device is implanted for patients with a history of cardiac arrest or symptomatic sustained ventricular tachycardia in association with CHD. Some pediatric patients with a history of severe left ventricular dysfunction (LVEF <30%) with or without documented ventricular arrhythmias may benefit from a combination of CRT and ICD, so called defibrillator-associated CRT (CRT-D).
- *Permanent pacemaker implantation* is recommended for advanced second- or third-degree atrioventricular block associated with ventricular dysfunction.

Extracorporeal Membrane Oxygenation and Ventricular Assist Device

This approach has been widely used in acute settings of cardiopulmonary arrest, especially when the cause of heart failure is likely to be reversible, such as fulminant myocarditis. ECMO or a VAD is used as a temporizing measure allowing ventricular function to recover. ECMO is also often used in emergency during perioperative period if there is ventricular pump failure. Patients who require a long-term support as a bridge to cardiac transplantation, VAD is increasingly being used. VAD can offer isolated left or right ventricular support or biventricular circuit support. However, VADs have high complication rates including thrombosis, bleeding, infections, and more so in infants with a body weight of <10 kg. Patients can stay on VAD till a heart becomes available for transplantation but have high morbidity and mortality.

Cardiac Transplantation

Heart transplantation is to be considered only for end-stage heart failure which is refractory to surgical and medical therapy. The most common indication is cardiomyopathy, other indication is uncorrectable CHD, such as hypoplastic left heart syndrome or failed Fontan due to ventricular dysfunction. Approximately 600–700 pediatric heart transplantation procedures are performed worldwide each year. Complications include systemic viral infections (cytomegalovirus, Epstein–Barr virus, and adenovirus), acute rejection, vasculopathy with graft failure, and hypertension. Malignancy-like lymphoproliferative disorders are other major complications of cardiac transplantation in children. Advances in immunosuppression have reduced episodes of rejection and have resulted in improved survival and quality of life. Survival is >70% at 5 years, a large number of children survive for over 20 years. Major limitation to cardiac transplantation is the inadequate donor supply.

Pulmonary Artery Banding

Pulmonary artery banding is a palliative procedure reserved for patients with large left to right shunts when it is not possible to repair the shunt lesion. Recently, it has been used in selected infants or toddlers with dilated cardiomyopathy, as a bridge-to-recovery or to more definitive therapy such as cardiac transplantation. The mechanism of action of pulmonary artery band in improving left ventricular function has been described by Schranz et al.[28] Band results in right ventricular pressure overload, which straightens the interventricular septum, thereby improving the filling of left ventricle, its end-diastolic volume, and pressure. This improves LVEF. A multicenter survey reported 70 patients from 15 centers in 11 countries.[29] 60% of the patients showed a clinical improvement after pulmonary artery banding, and 48% showed a functional recovery in 1 year. Right ventricular function must be normal for this modality of pulmonary artery banding to be of use. The best response is obtained in children <1 year, normal pulmonary artery pressure, and normal or mild left atrial dilatation.

A patient-tailored approach to end-stage heart failure in infants and children has been proposed.[30] For patients <1 year with left ventricular dysfunction but preserved right ventricular function, and normal pulmonary artery pressures, pulmonary artery banding should be considered. The band should be tightened to obtain right ventricular pressure 70% of left ventricular pressure. Patients <10 years and <20 kg can be managed with left or biventricular Berlin Heart. Those above 10 years or >20 kg should undergo placement of intracorporeal HeartWare VAD (HVAD). In future, miniaturization of VADs will make implantation possible even in smaller patients, reducing complications and recovery times.

CONCLUSION

Heart failure in children is a complex syndrome resulting from diverse etiologies and varied clinical presentation. Correction of underlying heart disease can reverse heart failure in a large number of cases. A systematic clinical approach is necessary to the exact clinical diagnosis. Treatment has evolved in last three decades or so. However, most of the pharmacotherapy for heart failure in children is extrapolated from data in adults. In future, pediatric specific data should be developed with the goal of identifying individualized management regimen.

ONLINE REFERENCES

Please scan the QR code provided at the end of the table of contents for References of this chapter.

CHAPTER 44

Heart Failure and Left Ventricular Remodeling: Current Understanding

Abraham Oomman, Narra Lavanya, Sudhir Lakamsani

ABSTRACT

Heart failure (HF) is a clinical condition resulting from structural and functional impairment of ventricular filling or ejection of blood resulting in reduced ability of the heart to provide adequate tissue perfusion.[1] The burden of HF driven by traditional risk factors is increasing. HF is a leading cause of cardiovascular (CV) mortality and morbidity. Left ventricular (LV) remodeling is one of the pathological situations encountered in the progression of HF. The process of LV remodeling includes structural, functional, cellular, and molecular changes involving cardiac myocytes and the interstitial collagen matrix. This article highlights the mechanism of LV remodeling, reverse remodeling, latest diagnostic tools, and effective treatment options for patients with HF and LV remodeling.

Keywords: Heart failure, cardiovascular diseases, left ventricular remodeling, LV reverse remodeling.

INTRODUCTION

Heart failure (HF) is a clinical state characterized by anatomical and functional abnormalities in ventricular filling or ejection of blood. The most common causes of HF include hypertension, diabetes mellitus, valvular heart disease, myocardial ischemia, cardiomyopathy, pulmonary hypertension, sleep apnea, excessive drug or alcohol use, obesity, and congenital heart disease.[2] The prevalence of HF increases with advancing age. It affects a substantial proportion of the global population thus negatively impacting the society.

Heart failure is categorized based on left ventricular ejection fraction (LVEF). Nearly one-half of patients with HF have HF with preserved ejection fraction (HFpEF) with an LVEF ≥50%, while the remaining account for HF with reduced ejection fraction (HFrEF) with an LVEF ≤40%.[3] HF with mid-range ejection fraction (HFmrEF) with an ejection fraction (EF) ranging from 41 to 49% accounts for 10–25% of the population.[4] HF with recovered EF (HFrecEF) is increasingly recognized and refers to patients with improvement in LVEF spontaneously or that which occurs after the use of guideline-directed medical therapy (GDMT) and device therapy.[5]

Left ventricular remodeling is a progressive condition in the journey of HF. It involves alteration in architecture of the ventricle. In 1806, Corvisart described two types of ventricular dilatation—active and passive; active dilatation with thick walls and increased force and passive with thinned ventricles and reduced force.[6] LV remodeling is determined by three important parameters: (1) alteration in myocyte biology, (2) myocardial changes, and (3) alteration in LV chamber geometry. It was originally described after myocardial infarction (MI), but it can develop in response to various forms of myocardial insult.[7,8]

MECHANISM OF HF AND LV REMODELING

The LV acts as a pump which generates pressures for circulation. The major determinants of LV performance are the preload, afterload, and myocardial contractility.[9] The ventricular dysfunction in HF is systolic (impaired cardiac contractility) or diastolic (impaired cardiac relaxation/filling). Systolic dysfunction triggers hemodynamic changes which lead to neurohormonal activation and cardiac remodeling. The progressive decline in compliance eventually produces diastolic dysfunction in patients with advanced HF.[10] The major neurohumoral systems involved in the response to HF are the sympathetic nervous system, the renin–angiotensin-aldosterone system (RAAS), and antidiuretic hormone (ADH).[11]

Remodeling can be physiologic or pathological and involves increase in myocardial mass. Physiological remodeling refers to changes in the heart dimensions in response to physiologic stimuli such as exercise (athletes heart) and pregnancy. Pathological remodeling, on the other hand, occurs secondary to underlying cardiac stressor. It can be a volume overload condition like valvular regurgitation or a pressure overload situation like hypertension or aortic stenosis. Pathologic remodeling can also occur post-myocardial injury as seen in MI. Initially compensatory, in the long run, patients with myocardial injury transition to irreversible changes with worsening LV stress and LV dysfunction.[12]

Remodeling is associated with various changes at the cellular level which in turn are the reflection of underlying molecular events. Cellular changes include myocyte hypertrophy, necrosis, or apoptosis of myocytes and fibrocyte proliferation eventually leading to fibrosis. Changes at the molecular level include increase in inflammatory cytokines, oxidative stress, and increased activity of matrix metalloproteinases (MMPs). The levels of inflammatory cytokines such as tumor necrosis factor-alpha (TNF-α), interleukin (IL)-6, 2, and 1β increase as the myocardial function worsens with degradation of extracellular matrix (ECM).[13,14]

Remodeling mainly involves alterations in the LV geometry. LV dilatation and wall thinning, change in LV shape from ellipsoidal to more spherical, and mitral valve incompetence are the effects of both cellular and molecular events **(Fig. 1)**.[15]

ASSESSMENT OF LV REMODELING

Cardiac biomarkers, echocardiography, radionucleotide imaging, and cardiac magnetic resonance (CMR) imaging are the various modalities used in clinical practice in assessing ventricular remodeling.

Cardiac Biomarkers (Fig. 2)

N-terminal Pro-brain Natriuretic Peptide

Increasing ventricular wall stress, worsening LV function, and increasing LV volumes increase the circulating N-terminal pro-brain natriuretic peptide (NT-proBNP) levels. PROTECT (ProBNP Outpatient Tailored Chronic HF Therapy) trial showed that greater improvement in the LVEF and reduced LV volumes was seen in patients with greater reduction in NT-proBNP levels ≤1,000 pg/mL.[16]

High-sensitivity Troponin

Elevated high-sensitivity troponin (hsTn) levels indicate myocardial injury and ongoing cardiomyocyte loss. hsTn T values < 11 pg/mL and hsTn I < 11 pg/mL were associated with lower CV event rate and higher frequency reverse remodeling.[17,18]

Echocardiography

The most commonly used metric to assess cardiac function in clinical practice is LVEF assessed by echocardiography (Echo). Two-dimensional (2D) Echo is widely available and easy-to-use tool at the bedside. 2D Echo measurements have been proven to be superior over M-mode in normal subjects and in those with abnormal LV geometry.[19] 2D Echo is subject to geometric assumptions and is operator dependent. These limitations are overcome by 3D Echo. 3D Echo measurements of LV mass, volume, and LVEF correlate well with CMR.[20] Contrast-enhanced and speckle tracking Echo allow rapid quantification of global LV dyssynchrony.[21]

Left ventricular global longitudinal strain (LVGLS) is a sensitive marker of LV systolic function and left atrial reservoir strain (LARS) of LV diastolic function. Improvement of these parameters indicates response to treatment and reverse remodeling.[22,23] GLS is useful in reclassifying the

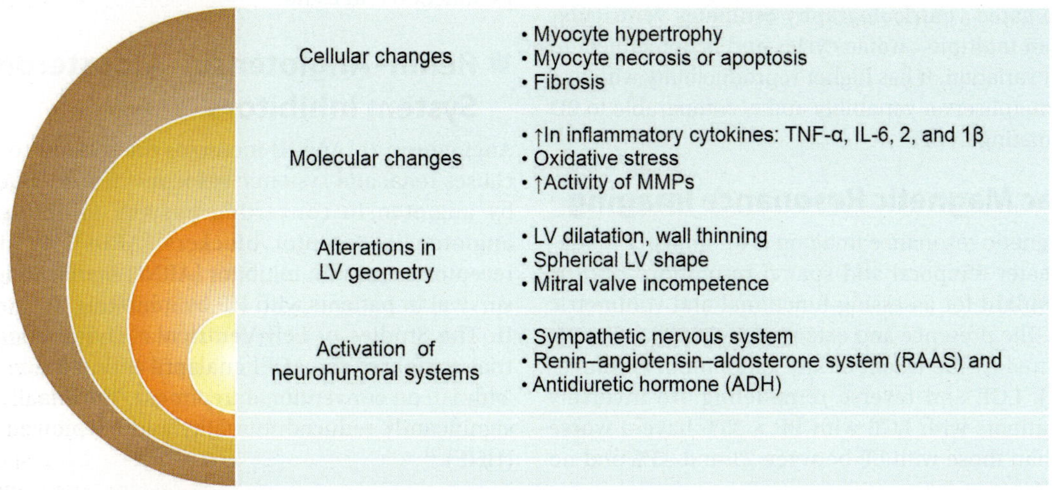

FIG. 1: Mechanism of LV remodeling.
(IL: interleukin; LV: left ventricular; MMPs: matrix metalloproteinases; TNF: tumor necrosis factor)

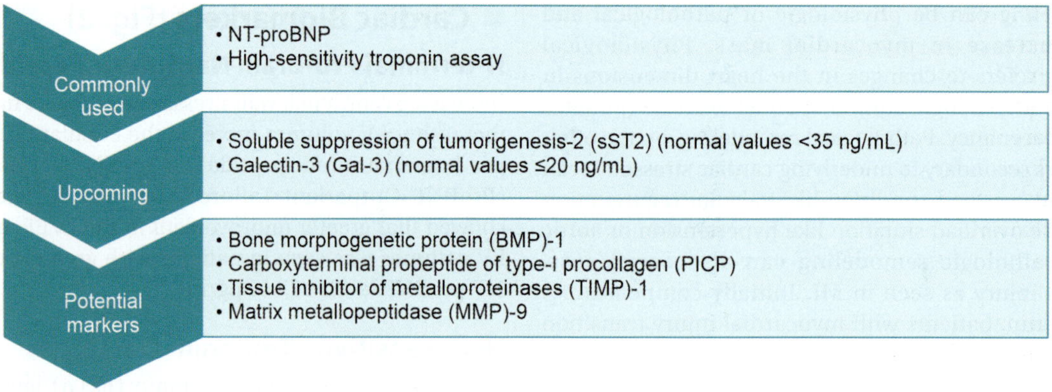

FIG. 2: Cardiac biomarkers for evaluating LV remodeling.
(NT-proBNP: N-terminal pro-brain natriuretic peptide; LV: left ventricular)

baseline function at every EF and may predict mortality better especially when EF > 35%.[24]

The Echo substudy of the VALIANT trial defined four patterns of LV remodeling in patients with HF and LVEF ≤ 35%, based on LV mass index (LVMI) and relative wall thickness (RWT): (1) Normal geometry where LVMI and RWT are normal, (2) concentric remodeling with normal LVMI and increased RWT, (3) concentric hypertrophy with increased LVMI and RWT, and (4) eccentric hypertrophy with increased LVMI and normal RWT. These patterns have prognostic implications with concentric hypertrophy having the worst composite CV outcome.[25]

In the Val-HeFT trial, outcomes and response to therapy were associated with the severity of LV remodeling. Worse LV internal diastolic diameter (LVIDd) and EF are associated with highest risk. LVEF, end-diastolic volume (EDV), and end-systolic volume (ESV) were each independent predictors of events.[26]

Radionuclide Ventriculography

Equilibrium gated ventriculography estimates ventricular volumes from multiple cardiac cycles and is not subject to beat-to-beat variation. It has higher reproducibility with less intra- and interobserver variability and is comparable to 2D Echo in estimating LVEF.[27]

Cardiac Magnetic Resonance Imaging

Cardiac magnetic resonance imaging is an imaging modality with greater temporal and spatial resolution. CMR is the gold standard for assessing functional and volumetric parameters. The presence and extent of myocardial fibrosis are determined by the extent of late gadolinium enhancement (LGE). LGE and reverse remodeling are inversely related.[28] Patients with LGE with EF > 35% have a worse prognosis than those with EF between 21 and 35% and no LGE. This gives us a new approach in considering implantable cardioverter-defibrillator (ICD), especially in nonischemic dilated cardiomyopathy (DCM).

Although guidelines suggest that LGE-negative patients with LVEF between 21 and 35% should receive a primary prevention ICD, these patients had a lower risk for arrhythmic events and sudden cardiac death. Conversely, among patients with LVEF > 35%, the presence of LGE with high-risk distribution was associated with intermediate to high risk, suggesting that these patients might benefit from ICD.[29] Contrast-enhanced CMR can predict the risk of adverse remodeling post-MI.[30]

EFFECT OF DRUGS ON LVRR

Left ventricular reverse remodeling (LVRR) can occur either by withdrawing the noxious stimulus causing cardiac injury or by introducing therapies that can halt or slow LV remodeling. Neurohormonal activation is the main culprit in LV remodeling and its inhibition is associated with improved LV function and LVRR.

Renin–Angiotensin–Aldosterone System Inhibitors

Angiotensin II (Ang II) increases the sodium retention and causes renal and systemic vasoconstriction. RAAS blockade by angiotensin-converting enzyme inhibitors (ACEIs), angiotensin receptor blockers (ARBs), or angiotensin receptor–neprilysin inhibitor (ARNI) significantly improved survival in patients with HF by inhibiting the action of Ang II. The Studies of Left Ventricular Dysfunction (SOLVD) trial compared the ACEI enalapril with placebo in patients with HF on conventional treatment. The enalapril arm had significantly reduced mortality and hospitalization for HF (HHF).[31]

The HOPE (Heart Outcomes Prevention Evaluation) trial assessed the role of the ACEI, ramipril, in patients who were at high risk of CV events but with no LV dysfunction or HF. Patients on ramipril had reduced rate of death from CV causes when compared with placebo (6.1% vs. 8.1%, respectively). There was a lower rate of MI, stroke, cardiac arrest, and HF in those patients who received ramipril.[32]

In the CHARM-Alternative trial (Candesartan in Heart failure: Assessment of Reduction in Mortality and morbidity), candesartan was generally well tolerated and reduced CV mortality and morbidity in patients with symptomatic HF and intolerance to ACEIs.[33]

Angiotensin Receptor–Neprilysin Inhibitor

In a study by Moon et al.,[34] addition of ARNI to GDMT in patients with HFrEF was associated with low rate of CV death and HHF. There was also improvement in the LVGLS and LARS within a period of 6 months.

In the PARADIGM-HF trial, ARNI was found to be superior to enalapril in reducing HHF, CV mortality, and all-cause mortality in patients with HFrEF.[35] Sacubitril/valsartan arm was associated with a reduction in NT-proBNP concentrations but its association with LV remodeling was not established.

The PROVE-HF (Prospective study of Biomarkers, Symptom Improvement and Ventricular Remodeling during Sacubitril/Valsartan therapy for heart failure) study showed that there was reduction in NT-proBNP levels following treatment with even lowest doses of sacubitril–valsartan. There was increase in LVEF and reduction in LA volume index (LAVI) and E/e' (filling pressures). Most patients in this study were on contemporary GDMT, yet initiation of ARNI was associated with reverse remodeling suggesting that patients with NT-proBNP reduction following ARNI initiation are likely to experience reverse cardiac remodeling.[36] ARNI may be associated with more LVEF improvement with reverse remodeling compared to other GDMT.

Beta-blockers

Beta-blockers (β-blockers) reduce the systemic catecholamine stimulation and reduce the heart rate, myocardial energy demand, and also reduce LV remodeling by reducing LV mass. The LVRR by β-blockers improves the LV shape, function, and reduces functional mitral regurgitation (MR).[37] The addition of cardioselective β-blockers carvedilol (US Carvedilol Heart Failure Study Group), metoprolol (MERIT-HF Study Group), or bisoprolol (The Cardiac Insufficiency Bisoprolol Study II) to standard GDMT reduced mortality in large-scale trials in patients with both ischemic and nonischemic HF.[38-40]

Mineralocorticoid Receptor Antagonists

Mineralocorticoid receptor antagonists (MRAs) reduce the endothelial dysfunction, salt and water retention, and electrolyte imbalance. Addition of selective or nonselective MRAs to GDMT reduces the rate of HHF, mortality, and sudden cardiac death.[41] The RALES (Randomized Aldactone Evaluation Study) trial studied the effect of adding 25 mg of spironolactone to GDMT in patients with HFrEF. Patients in the spironolactone arm had lower CV mortality, lower HHF, and improved HF symptoms.[42]

Sodium-glucose Cotransporter-2 Inhibitors

Sodium-glucose cotransporter-2 inhibitors (SGLT-2Is) reduce LV remodeling in HF by decreasing ECM synthesis and myocardial fibrosis. Both dapagliflozin and empagliflozin have been shown to reduce ECM remodeling and promote antifibrotic markers thus reducing LV remodeling and progression of HF.[43]

The EMPA-TROPISM study demonstrated that empagliflozin significantly reverses LV remodeling by reducing LV volumes and LV hypertrophy, increasing LVEF and causing lesser structural remodeling as compared to placebo in nondiabetic HFrEF patients.[44] The EMPA-HEART trial on the other hand reported LV mass regression in diabetic population without HF.[45] The REFORM trial in contrast showed no improvement in LV remodeling with dapagliflozin in diabetic HF patients owing to the fact that it included patients with greater LVEF (46%) and lesser dilated LV (LVEDV 180 mL).[46] However, the DAPA-MODA trial showed beneficial effects on remodeling with dapagliflozin.

Vericiguat

The HF is associated with low-soluble guanylate cyclase (sGC) activity leading to reduced intracellular cyclic guanosine monophosphate (cGMP) generation and disturbed cGMP-dependent signaling with unfavorable effects on the cardiac system. Vericiguat is a novel molecule that stimulates the activity of sGC restoring the reduced cGMP levels. The VICTORIA echocardiographic substudy showed significant improvements in LV structure and function over 8 months in both vericiguat and placebo in a high-risk HFrEF population with recent worsening HF.[47] Further studies are needed to establish the benefits of vericiguat on LVRR.

DEVICE THERAPY IN LVRR

Cardiac Resynchronization Therapy

Left bundle branch block (LBBB) causes intraventricular dyssynchrony of the septum and paradoxical septal motion.

This dyssynchrony promotes pathologic LV remodeling by increasing LV volumes, reducing diastolic filling, and prolonging the duration of MR. Cardiac resynchronization therapy (CRT) has become an established treatment for selected patients with refractory symptomatic HF.[48]

In patients with symptomatic HFrEF with LVEF < 35% and LBBB with QRS duration >150 ms despite optimal GDMT, CRT improves symptoms and reduces morbidity and mortality (Class I level A recommendation). Similarly in patients with LBBB and QRS duration of >139–149 ms despite GDMT, CRT improves symptoms and reduces morbidity and mortality (Class IIa, level B recommendation). The extent of LVRR is one of the most important mechanisms of action of CRT.[49]

Percutaneous Repair of the Mitral Valve

Significant MR is an independent adverse predictor of progressive LV remodeling. Moderate-to-severe MR persisting despite GDMT or CRT is associated with poor prognosis. These patients should be evaluated for therapeutic strategies such as percutaneous repair of the mitral valve (i.e., MitraClip).[50] The COAPT trial revealed that LVRR at 6 months was associated with better clinical outcomes in patients with HF and severe MR but was not altered by transcatheter edge-to-edge repair or the extent of residual MR at the end of 2 years.[51]

Left Ventricular Assist Device

Left ventricular assist device (LVAD) is a mechanical circulatory support (MCS) system which can cause significant LVRR especially in younger HF patients, women, and in those with nonischemic HF with short duration of symptoms. The degree of LVRR has been seen to the extent of withdrawal of LVAD therapy but relapses have been noted. The lower rates of remission and the occurrence of relapses are due to the persistent changes at molecular and cellular levels. Even so, improvement in biventricular function reduces the rate of HHF and improves exercise tolerance in patients on LVAD.[52]

POST-MYOCARDIAL INFARCTION LVRR

Post-MI timely revascularization by thrombolysis, percutaneous coronary intervention (PCI), or coronary artery bypass grafting (CABG) is of paramount importance to attenuate adverse remodeling. Various surgical approaches and devices were studied for ventricular restoration and reconstruction post-MI. Various techniques were used such as resection (Batista procedure), plication (Revivient), approximation (Coapsys), cinching (AccuCinch), and ventricular exclusion. The ventricular exclusion procedure involved percutaneous placement of a covered frame to partition the ventricular cavity. The parachute and Heartech devices have been studied in this regard.[53]

The Parachute first-in-man (FIM) study demonstrated a sustained improvement in LV function with significant reduction in the LV end-systolic volume index (LVESVi) and LV end-diastolic volume (LVEDV) after implantation of the Heartech device for up to 12 months.[54] These therapies accelerate LVRR. However, in spite of clinical improvement, changes in LV geometry, matrix, and myocytes may persist and withdrawal of GDMT may result in worsening HF **(Fig. 3)**.

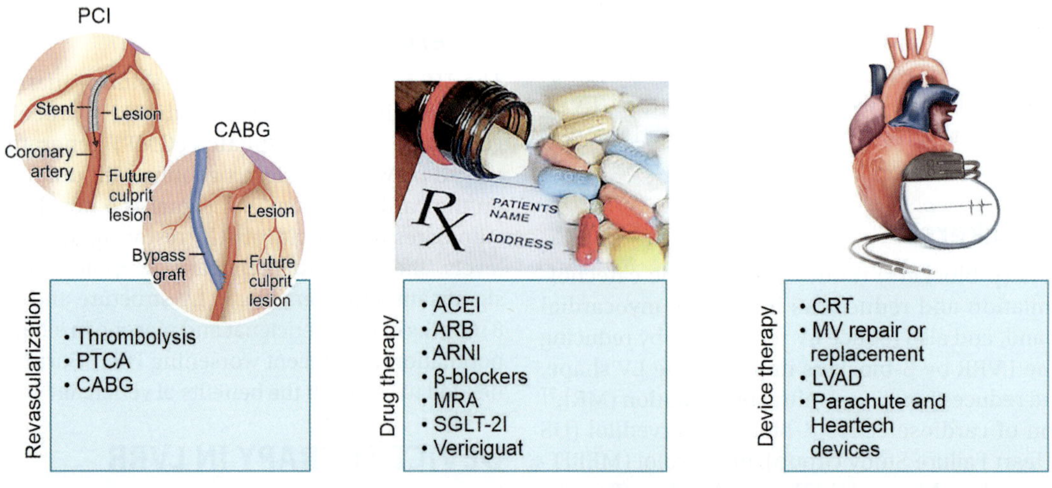

FIG. 3: Therapies for LVRR.

(ACEI: angiotensin-converting enzyme inhibitor; ARB: angiotensin receptor blocker; ARNI: angiotensin receptor–neprilysin inhibitor; CABG: coronary artery bypass grafting; CRT: cardiac resynchronization therapy; LVAD: left ventricular assist device; LVRR: left ventricular reverse remodeling; MRA: mineralocorticoid receptor antagonist; PTCA: percutaneous transluminal coronary angioplasty; SGLT-2I: sodium-glucose cotransporter-2 inhibitor)

CONCLUSION

Left ventricular remodeling and its role in the progression of HF are well established. Biomarkers and imaging with Echo and CMR are widely incorporated tools in assessment of this process. Predictors of adverse remodeling include male sex, ischemic etiology, longer HF duration, higher LVEF, presence of LGE, and high or rising biomarker levels. Whereas predictors of reverse remodeling include female sex, nonischemic etiology, shorter HF duration, lower LVEF, no LGE, and lower or falling biomarker levels.[55] Predictors of LV remodeling and LVRR should be assessed using a multimodality approach.

Attenuation of LV remodeling and progression to LVRR can be achieved by drugs and device therapy. Timely drug and device therapy is shown to slow or even reverse the process of ventricular remodeling. The need of the hour is better standardization of protocols and incorporation of LGE/fibrosis in diagnostic algorithms. Future studies are needed to develop more effective therapies to reverse LVRR.

A key driver of HF progression is LVRR. Reverse remodeling is protective and can be augmented by GDMT. Reverse remodeling may be further enhanced by device-based therapy. HF events and mortality correlate with the pace and extent of reverse remodeling. One has to keep in mind that reverse remodeling and improvement in LVEF are not equivalent to recovery and not be hasty in withdrawing therapy.

ONLINE REFERENCES

Please scan the QR code provided at the end of the table of contents for References of this chapter.

CHAPTER

45

Cardiac Biomarkers-based Reclassification of Preheart Failure Staging

Jayagopal PB, Jain T Kallarakkal

ABSTRACT

Heart failure (HF) is the leading problem in current-day cardiology practice. It is only the right approach to identify pre-HF so as to prevent or delay the onset of HF. Various investigations and novel diagnostic tools are being studied. The most studied and effective strategies are the evaluation of cardiac biomarkers. This manuscript discusses the currently available biomarkers, namely N-terminal pro-B-type natriuretic peptide (NT-proBNP) and high-sensitivity troponins in identifying this high group category. This when performed on these vulnerable groups of individuals with diabetes mellitus and high blood pressure may be a very effective preventive tool in the future.

Keywords: Preheart failure, cardiac bio-markers in HF, HF classification.

INTRODUCTION

Preheart failure is an area that has not been really analyzed well. It is a known fact that various comorbid conditions such as diabetes mellitus, hypertension, and chronic kidney disease ultimately lead to heart failure (HF) and various complications. Once set in HF is a relentlessly progressive disease with poor outcomes. The concept of identifying pre-HF and adequately using the appropriate drugs would go a long way in preventing this condition from progressing to overt HF. Thus there is a need to identify and risk stratify these groups of patients. This article discusses the currently available and validated markers that could be utilized in a broader group of individuals.

CLASSIFICATION OF HEART FAILURE STAGES

The 2022 American Heart Association/American College of Cardiology/Heart Failure Society of America Guideline for the Management of Heart Failure proposed a more standardized classification of HF.[1] HF progression is classified into different stages. This looks into the development and progression of HF, and the idea is to identify those at greatest risk of HF. This is useful in guiding preventive and therapeutic strategies. The stages of HF from the 2013 American College of Cardiology/American Heart Association guidelines define the spectrum of the disease as in **Table 1**.

TABLE 1: Stages of heart failure (HF).

Stages	Descriptions
A	At high risk for HF but without structural heart disease or symptoms of HF
B	Structural heart disease but without signs or symptoms of HF
C	Structural heart disease with prior or current symptoms of HF
D	Refractory HF requiring specialized interventions

Source: Yancy CW, Jessup M, Bozkurt B, Buttler J, Casey Jr DE, Drazner MH, et al. 2013 ACCF/AHA guideline for the management of Heart Failure. Circulation. 2013;128(16):e240-327.

Cardiac markers such as natriuretic peptides and highly sensitive troponins have been noticed to be elevated in pre-HF stage itself. Thus this could be a useful tool in classifying and defining stages of HF. Stage B HF is categorized by B-type natriuretic peptide (BNP) ≥35 pg/mL or N-terminal pro-B-type natriuretic peptide (NT-proBNP) of ≥125 pg/mL in an ambulatory setting. There may have persistently elevated levels of high-sensitivity cardiac troponins.

The impact of incorporating cardiac biomarkers to reclassify HF in 5,324 participants without prevalent HF enrolled in the ARIC (Atherosclerosis Risk In Communities)[2] study was assessed along with the prognosis of Stage B using cardiac biomarkers by Xiaoming Jia et al., recently published in JACC. This study has shown its utility in reclassifying a good percentage of patients into more advanced stages when cardiac markers like NT-proBNP was analyzed in them. About >20% thus needed a change in the classification. When additional echocardiographic parameters, if performed in this category of individuals, then the chance of further risk assessment becomes even more stronger. When cardiac biomarkers and abnormal echo parameters are present, these groups have high risk for the future events and death. Isolated elevation of biomarkers or abnormal echocardiographic abnormalities only translates into higher HF events, but not death. Thus, it provides significant improvement in the risk stratification.

Despite advances in the management of HF carries very high morbidity and mortality. The utility of cardiac biomarkers are indeed a newer tool to identify high-risk population, these groups otherwise could never have been identified. Cardiac biomarkers are further helpful in risk stratification across various blood pressure ranges.[3] It is clear that the best benefit for preventing HF is for individuals with elevated biomarker levels. SPRINT (Systolic Blood Pressure Intervention Trial) study showed that intensive blood pressure control in people with elevated NT-proBNP and/or troponin T highly sensitive (hs-TnT) led to a larger absolute risk reduction in HF and mortality.[4] Similarly, CANVAS (Canagliflozin Cardiovascular Assessment Study) showed that treatment with the sodium-glucose cotransporter-2 inhibitor (SGLT-2I) canagliflozin reduced further increase of natriuretic peptides and cardiac troponins in diabetic patients among older adults with type 2 diabetes mellitus.[5]

Cardiac biomarkers, along with echocardiography, help further in the risk stratification of individuals with Stage B HF. Various structural and functional abnormalities obtained on echocardiography are useful. Although HF and death were associated with biomarker and echo abnormalities, isolated structural or functional derangements may not be associated with an increased risk. The biomarkers have been associated with structural cardiovascular phenotypes in earlier studies. Elevated cardiac troponin and NT-proBNP are associated with fibrosis and changes in the left ventricular structure and pose a risk for subsequent HF.[6]

Echocardiography has revolutionized the diagnosis and risk assessment in cardiology practice and its role in HF diagnosis and treatment is really unmatched by any other investigation. However, the role of high-sensitivity troponins in acute coronary syndrome has improved the diagnostic yield. With the major contributor being ischemic heart disease in HF, it is only rational to think of this as another valuable diagnostic test. NT-proBNP in HF today is like what troponins are in coronary syndromes. It is at present expensive and the cost is likely to come down in coming years. This test could then be routinely used for early diagnosis. This has the potential of diagnosing overt HF, but also identifying pre-HF. Use of both biomarkers are useful as shown by Xiaoping Jia et al. They showed how the positivity of diagnosis in asymptomatic young individuals increased from 19 to 33% from visit two to four when these biomarkers were used. Thus these are valuable tools to identify this high-risk group. This will perhaps be utilized like prostatic surface antigen in prostate malignancy screening. One must also remember that HF once established has a poorer prognosis than carcinoma prostate and breast cancer.

CONCLUSION

Cardiac biomarkers have an established role in HF diagnosis and management. It is now well recognized that various comorbidities such as diabetes mellitus, hypertension, and chronic kidney disease all ultimately develop HF. The usefulness of cardiac biomarkers in pre-HF is a giant leap forward. The future HF guidelines would need to incorporate this based on current evidence.

ONLINE REFERENCES

Please scan the QR code provided at the end of the table of contents for References of this chapter.

CHAPTER 46

Role of Four Pillars of Pharmacotherapy in HFrEF: When and How to Initiate?

Satyendra Tewari, Harshit Khare

ABSTRACT

The current therapy of heart failure with reduced ejection fraction (HFrEF) has evolved from the time when once beta blockers (BBs) were considered redundant to the present where BB along with angiotensin receptor-neprilysin inhibitors (ARNIs), mineralocorticoid receptor antagonists (MRAs) and sodium-glucose cotransporter-2 inhibitors (SGLT-2Is) reduce mortality in this cohort significantly. This all hails to the continued progress in understanding of pathophysiology behind the HFrEF. The recent European Society of Cardiology (ESC) 2021 heart failure (HF) and American Heart Association (AHA) 2022 HF guidelines recommend all four drugs to be initiated in HFrEF cohort as early as possible and to be uptitrated to their maximum doses within 3–6 months. However, the uptitration of these drugs is more of an art than science. It needs patient understanding and monitoring while ensuring compliance as well. Various sequencing methods have been suggested for these classes of drugs and most suitable way seems to be rapid sequencing starting with low-dose BB and SGLT-2I simultaneously and then adding MRA and ARNI in graded way within a month, providing the patients the benefit of these drugs as early and rapidly as possible, while avoiding adverse effects.

Keywords: HFrEF, pharmacotherapy, sequencing.

INTRODUCTION

The therapy for heart failure with reduced ejection fraction (HFrEF) in the present time has seen complete turnaround from the times when digoxin formed the basis of heart failure (HF) pharmacotherapy to the present era of disease-modifying drugs like sodium-glucose cotransporter-2 inhibitors (SGLT-2Is) and angiotensin receptor-neprilysin inhibitors (ARNIs). From "nonpharmacologic era" before 1980s, the timeline of HFrEF treatment changed to "pharmacologic era" in 1980s, with the advent of radical thinking, when drugs to alter the natural history of HFrEF and improve the quality of life evolved.[1]

The present therapy of HFrEF is based on understanding that following a myocardial insult, when HFrEF develops, there are continuous adverse hemodynamic and pathophysiologic changes due to secondary response in the form of neurohormonal activation of renin–angiotensin system (RAS), leading to direct cellular injury and ventricular remodeling. This in turn leads to further deterioration of ventricular pump function, and it is a vicious cycle. This formed the basis of development of neurohormonal antagonism therapy in HFrEF patients. Subsequently angiotensin-converting enzyme inhibitors (ACEis), angiotensin receptor blockers (ARBs), ARNI, and mineralocorticoid receptor antagonist (MRA) were developed to alter the ventricular remodeling and disease progression. Beta blockers (BBs) also proved beneficial through attenuation of adverse left ventricular (LV) remodeling mediated by chronic sympathetic activity. Recent addition to this armamentarium of drugs, were SGLT-2I, which have pleotropic effects, preventing deteriorating clinical course across all strata of HF. Together these four now form the pillars of HF therapy among HFrEF patients.

EVIDENCES FROM CLINICAL TRIALS

Renin–Angiotensin Inhibitors with or without Neprilysin Inhibitor

Evidence for RAS inhibition comes from various clinical trials from the past. The earliest trial Cooperative North

Scandinavian Enalapril Survival Study (CONSENSUS) enrolling New York Heart Association (NYHA) IV patients compared enalapril (target does of 20 mg twice daily) with placebo, and at 6 months showed absolute mortality risk reduction by 18%.[2] Further in the SOLVD (Studies of Left Ventricular Dysfunction) treatment trial, enalapril in doses of 2.5–20 mg twice daily showed reduction in mortality and the risk of hospitalization for worsening HF, even in patients of NYHA class II or III with an left ventricular ejection fraction (LVEF) ≤ 35%.[3] Similarly, captopril in the doses of 12.5 mg to a maximum of 50 mg thrice daily showed mortality reduction of 19% in SAVE (Survival and Ventricular Enlargement) trial.[4] In the V-HeFT and V-HeFT II trials, there was a trend toward increased survival with isosorbide dinitrate and hydralazine, but treatment with enalapril reduced mortality by 7% compared to isosorbide dinitrate and hydralazine.[5,6]

The traditional strategy for ACEI dosing was to initiate at a low dose and increase the dose over 1–2 weeks, up to the maximum target dose used in trials. Patients are to be monitored for hypotension, hyperkalemia, and decrease in renal function during the titration. Patients who are at high risk for side effects like creatinine clearance (CrCl) <30 mL/min, or with requirement for an increase in diuretic dose in the past, or had treatment with a potassium-sparing diuretic, were to be initiated at a lower dose. However, there is now criticism for this approach as it takes time to build up the required dosing.

The evidence for ARBs came from Val-HeFT trial and CHARM (Candesartan in Heart Failure Assessment of Reduction in Mortality and morbidity) trial, both of which showed reduction in composite end point of cardiovascular death and HF hospitalization with valsartan and candesartan, respectively, although the results were driven mainly by reduction in hospitalization.[7,8] Like ACEI, ARB therapy is started with a low dose and titrated up as tolerated by doubling the dose to the target.

The more recent, concluded trial named PARADIGM-HF (Prospective Comparison of ARNI with ACE Inhibitor to Determine Impact on Global Mortality and Morbidity in Heart Failure) compared sacubitril/valsartan (ARNI) in target dose of 97/103 mg twice daily to enalapril and showed risk reduction of cardiovascular death or HF hospitalization by 20%.[9] Further, even among patients with acutely decompensated HF, the addition of sacubitril–valsartan therapy led to a greater reduction in the N-terminal pro-B-type natriuretic peptide (NT-proBNP) concentration compared to enalapril therapy, while the rate of adverse events were similar between the two groups.[10] However, the initiation of ARNI therapy and uptitration to target dose is often limited due to intolerance caused by symptoms of hypotension and can lead to discontinuation. This is overcome by initiating at a lower dose as low as 50 mg twice daily and then uptitrating as tolerated.

Beta Blockers

There is huge body of evidence now backing up the beneficial role of BBs in HFrEF that is in addition to ACEI/ARBs/ARNI. The earliest trial was United States (US) Carvedilol Heart Failure Study that showed significant mortality relative risk reduction of 65% attributable to carvedilol (target dose 25 mg twice daily) in patients of LVEF ≤ 35% who were already on diuretics, digoxin, and ACEI.[11] Later even in patients of LVEF ≤ 25%, carvedilol reduced the combined risk of death or hospitalization for HF by 31% and days of hospital stay for HF by 40% over a period of 6 months of therapy. Carvedilol-treated group was also less likely to have sudden death or ventricular tachycardia.[12] The evidence for other two BBs (bisoprolol and metoprolol) came from CIBIS II (Cardiac Insufficiency Bisoprolol Study II) and MERIT-HF studies, respectively. The CIBIS II demonstrated 34% relative risk reduction in mortality with bisoprolol (target dose 10 mg once daily) in patients with an LVEF ≤ 35% and there was 36% risk reduction for hospitalization due to worsening HF.[13] The MERIT-HF study showed 34% relative risk reduction in all-cause mortality, 22% relative risk reduction in sudden death, and 49% relative risk reduction in death from worsening HF, with metoprolol (target dose of 200 mg once daily).[14] As mentioned in the above studies, the mortality benefit with BBs is not a class effect, but rather seen only with carvedilol, bisoprolol, and metoprolol. BBs can be started at low doses and uptitrated gradually to target doses if tolerable adverse effects include acute worsening of HFrEF, fatigue, bradycardia, or heart block, and hypotension. However, it should be noted that the initial fluid retention or worsening HFrEF seen with BBs does not require withdrawal of treatment as it may negate the potential long-term benefit of these drugs. This can be managed with diuretic dose adjustment.

Mineralocorticoid Receptor Antagonists

The RALES (Randomized Aldactone Evaluation Study) provided the earliest evidence for MRA showing 30% risk reduction in both mortality and hospitalization with spironolactone in the daily doses of 25–50 mg, in patients with an LVEF of ≤35% and in NYHA functional Class III or IV.[15] Later the results of EMPHASIS-HF (Eplerenone in Mild Patients Hospitalization and Survival Study in Heart Failure) trial extended these benefits to even patients with milder symptoms and an LVEF of ≤35%, showing 37% significant risk reduction in the primary composite endpoint of time to first HF hospitalization or cardiovascular death.[16] The impressive results of RALES and EMPHASIS-HF, and later EPHESUS (Eplerenone Post-Acute Myocardial Infarction Heart Failure Efficacy and Survival Study) trial provided benefit of MRA in LV dysfunction in post-myocardial infarction also; all these results have established MRA as the third pillar of current pharmacotherapy for HFrEF.

Sodium-glucose Cotransporter-2 Inhibitors

Sodium-glucose cotransporter-2 inhibitor discovery is an interesting story in itself. While evaluating cardiovascular safety of newer drug empagliflozin for diabetes mellitus, in EMPA-REG trial there is significant reduction in primary outcome of HF hospitalization and major adverse cardiovascular events (MACEs), but mortality reduction was not separately significant.[17] Similar results were seen in CANVAS trial for canagliflozin[18] and DECLARE-TIMI 58 (Dapagliflozin Effect on Cardiovascular Events-Thrombolysis in Myocardial Infarction 58) trial for dapagliflozin.[19]

These results paved way for evaluation of efficacy of SGLT-2I in HFrEF patients regardless of their diabetes status, as in the DAPA-HF (Dapagliflozin and Prevention of Adverse Outcomes in Heart Failure) and EMPEROR-reduced trials. The DAPA-HF trial showed 18% cardiovascular mortality reduction and 30% reduction in HF hospitalization with dapagliflozin, and also showed significant reduction in all-cause mortality.[20] Similarly, in EMPEROR-reduced trial, with empagliflozin, there were similar results.[21]

With these beneficiary results of SGLT-2I in HFrEF patients, both American College of Cardiology (ACC)/ AHA and ESC guidelines support the use of an SGLT-2I (dapagliflozin or empagliflozin at a dose of 10 mg once daily) as the fourth foundational therapy for patients with symptomatic HFrEF.

TIMING AND UPTITRATION

The traditional way of including all four drug classes in HF therapy is to escalate them individually to the doses that were tested in previous clinical trials and then add other classes of drug one by one. It is recommended to start with ACEI or ARB first, followed by a BB, and then MRA and finally, a SGLT-2I. It is advocated to titrate the dose of each drug class to the target dose used in large-scale trials before initiating the other class of drug. This sequencing method emphasizes on fixed way of escalating the recommended HF therapy.

The current approach suffers from many other drawbacks as well. Firstly, it is assumed that the most efficient way of providing the recommended therapy is to start all classes of drugs all at once. Secondly, we assume that the HF therapy is effective only when maximized to trial-defined target doses. Thirdly, the clinical trial cohorts of HF patients studied were not themselves on guideline-directed medical therapy.

Thus, traditional approach of sequencing these drugs has caused giving up on the beneficial effects of disease-modifying therapies for HFrEF. This is because if we take time to add and escalate each drug class before initiating treatment with the other, it can take >6 months to prescribe all guideline-recommended therapies. This means that physicians will have to compromise in their practice while adopting such recommendations because of patient intolerance. More importantly, even if the current guideline-recommended approach was fully adopted, one has to have a delay of >6 months to achieve that target and we also know by trial results that these four classes of drugs have shown promise of reducing morbidity and mortality within 30 days of initiating therapy. So, by adopting such an approach we may have absence of one or more therapy, resulting in poor clinical outcomes in the future.

CURRENT GUIDELINE RECOMMENDATIONS

European Society of Cardiology 2021 HF Congress recommended ARNI (or ACEI/ARB), BB, SGLT-2I, and MRA as class I indication for HFrEF to reduce risk of mortality. ARNI was to be preferred over ACEI as class I recommendation.

2021 ACC Expert gave class I recommendation for BB and ACEI/ARB/ARNI in patients newly diagnosed with stage C HFrEF. They suggested that BB and ARNI can be started in any order of preference with BB to be more suitable to start in "dry" state, and after that MRA and SGLT-2I can be added. Each class has to be uptitrated to maximum tolerated dose.

SEQUENCING OF FOUNDATIONAL TREATMENTS

The current European Society of Cardiology (ESC) and AHA HF management guidelines give class I recommendation for each of these four classes of drugs, i.e., ARNI, BBs, MRA, and SGLT-2I in HFrEF therapy. These drugs are recommended to be escalated to their maximum tolerable doses first before adding remaining classes of drugs. However, this leads to loss of crucial time period before the benefits of each of these four classes of drugs can be achieved. This is important especially when we also know that the benefit of each of these classes of drug starts within 30 days of administration and is independent of each other. Further even the low doses of these drugs can offer nearly same benefit of reducing morbidity and mortality as noted in their large-scale trials before protocol-mandated increase in dose was achieved. Therefore, a proper sequencing of these drug classes while offering to the patient can greatly improve their safety, efficacy, and tolerability. Packer and Murray suggested a novel algorithm to achieve therapy with all four classes of these drugs within 4 weeks. They suggested to start with simultaneous administration of BB and an SGLT-2I. While BBs are known to be effective for prevention of sudden cardiac death, SGLT-2I class has benefit of reducing HF hospitalization risk. In the second step, we can add ARNI in low dose within 1 or 2 weeks of first step and monitor patient for hypotension and angioedema. If patient tolerates, then in the third step, before we escalate doses of added drugs, we add MRA in next 1 or 2 weeks and look for potassium levels and renal function. If this is tolerated then, we can consider uptitration of doses of individual classes of drugs. If we relook at this proposition, it is so beautiful that how within a span of 4 weeks, we will achieve the goal of administer all four classes of drugs to the HFrEF patients. This algorithm also highlights the freedom we can have in administering low doses of one/two classes of drugs initially and then adding on as early as tolerated by the patient on an individual basis.[22] This sequencing also increases the chance of implementing HF therapy in a manner that rapidly prevents deaths and hospitalizations and promotes the tolerability of drugs administered.

CONCLUSION

The present HFrEF therapy has been built upon evidence from a large series of clinical trials, and it appears that with the recent addition of SGLT-2I and ARNI, in future, we may see increasing population of surviving HF patients. The key lies in proper sequencing of these drugs while administering and ensuring patient compliance. However, despite all the treatment modalities at hand, the burden of HF may remain quite significant and that will call for search other disease-modifying drugs in the field.

ONLINE REFERENCES

Please scan the QR code provided at the end of the table of contents for References of this chapter.

CHAPTER

47 Implication of the Rapid Initiation of Quadruple Therapy in Heart Failure

PS Banerjee, Tanmay Mukhopadhyay, Gourav Bhattacharya

ABSTRACT

Heart failure (HF) is a complex clinical syndrome occurring from structural and functional derangement of ventricular filling or ejection of blood. HF is categorized into HF with preserved ejection fraction (HFpEF), HF with mid-range ejection fraction (HFmrEF), and HF with reduced ejection fraction (HFrEF) according to ejection fraction. Quadruple therapy for HF is the mainstay of therapy in the HFrEF phenotype. Conventional approach of achieving treatment with all four drug classes is to start with angiotensin-converting enzyme inhibitor (ACEI) or angiotensin receptor blockers (ARBs), to be followed by a beta-blocker, then a mineralocorticoid receptor antagonist (MRA), then an angiotensin receptor–neprilysin inhibitor (ARNI), and, finally, a sodium-glucose cotransporter-2 inhibitor (SGLT-2I). There are several limitations of this conventional sequencing. So, the concept of simultaneous or rapid initiation and titration of guideline-directed medical therapy (GDMT) for HFrEF has been proposed which involves three steps, viz., simultaneous initiation of beta-blocker and SLLT-2I, followed by ARNI within 1–2 weeks and MRA thereafter within 2 weeks of step 2. This proposed new sequencing can result in improved tolerance, better safety profile and reduced major adverse cardiovascular event (MACE).

Keywords: Heart failure, quadruple therapy, HFrEF, HFpEF, HFmrEF, rapid sequencing, pillars of HF therapy.

INTRODUCTION

Heart failure (HF) is a pathophysiological condition in which an abnormal of cardiac function results in failure of the heart to pump blood at a rate commensurate with the need of the metabolizing cells of the body or does so only at higher filling pressures.[1]

American College of Cardiology/American Heart Association (ACC/AHA) defines HF as a complex clinical syndrome resulting from structural and functional impairment of ventricular filling or ejection of blood.[2]

The European Society of Cardiology (ESC) guidelines define HF as "a clinical syndrome characterized by typical symptoms (e.g., breathlessness, ankle swelling, and fatigue) that may be accompanied by signs (e.g., elevated jugular venous pressure, pulmonary crackles, and peripheral edema) caused by a structural and/or functional cardiac abnormality, resulting in a reduced cardiac output and/or elevated intracardiac pressures at rest or during stress.[3]

Traditionally, HF has been divided into distinct phenotypes based on the measurement of left ventricular ejection fraction (LVEF). Reduced LVEF defined as ≤40%, i.e., those with a significant reduction in LV systolic function are designated as HF with reduced ejection fraction (HFrEF). Patients with a LVEF between 41% and 49% have mildly reduced LV systolic function, i.e., HF with mid-range ejection fraction (HFmrEF). Those with symptoms and signs of HF, with evidence of structural and/or functional cardiac abnormalities consistent with the presence of LV diastolic dysfunction/raised LV filling pressure and/or raised natriuretic peptides, and with an LVEF ≥50%, have HF with preserved ejection fraction (HFpEF).

Quadruple therapy for HF is the cornerstone of therapy in the HFrEF phenotype.

EPIDEMIOLOGY

In developed countries, the age-adjusted incidence of HF may have decreasing trend, mainly due to better management of cardiovascular (CV) disease, but because of aging, the overall incidence is rising.[4] The prevalence of HF appears to be 1–2% overall.[4] It increases with age from around 1% for those aged <55 years to 10% in those aged 70 years or over.[5,6] Of those with HF, about 50% have HFrEF and 50% have HFpEF/HFmrEF, mainly based on studies in hospitalized patients.[6] In USA, there has been a 26% increase in HF hospitalizations and number of patients hospitalized with HF.[7]

Based on disease-specific estimates, Huffman and Prabhakar in their projections showed that the prevalence of HF in India due to coronary heart disease, hypertension, obesity, diabetes mellitus, and rheumatic heart disease (RHD) is in the range from 1.3 to 4.6 million, with an annual incidence of 0.4–1.8 million.[8]

Patients with HF are younger than in the high-income countries, with a mean average age of around 60 years at presentation. They also have a higher in-hospital mortality and 1-year mortality, which are significantly more than that in the high-income countries. HFpEF is seen in 25% of the population. Most common etiology is coronary artery disease followed by idiopathic dilated cardiomyopathy (DCM). RHD accounts for 10% of the cases which is more than any developed country.[9,10]

PATHOPHYSIOLOGY

Heart failure results due to loss of functional myocardial cells (ischemia, myocarditis, and cardiomyopathies) and also due to extramyocardial diseases (valvular heart diseases, pericardial diseases, and systemic hypertension). Chronically, the extramyocardial diseases also affect the myocardial function by creating pressure and volume overload.

Heart failure due to any etiology is characterized by activation of compensatory mechanisms that causes a change in vascular function, fluid volume, and neurohormonal status, which initially restores the balance, but ultimately becomes detrimental over a long term.

DIAGNOSTIC EVALUATION

The patients of HF must undergo robust evaluation for etiology, prognostication, and assessment of treatable comorbidities. After a detailed clinical evaluation, all patients suspected of having HF should have an electrocardiogram (ECG), chest X-ray, echocardiogram done and N-terminal pro-B-type natriuretic peptide (NT-proBNP) assayed. Most of the HF patients can be diagnosed and prognosticated on the basis of these investigations. Other high-end investigations such as cardiac magnetic resonance imaging (MRI), cardiac computed tomography (CT), coronary angiogram, and genetic studies are needed for specific occasions.

MANAGEMENT OF HEART FAILURE WITH REDUCED EJECTION FRACTION

Management of HFrEF patients mainly consists of pharmacological and nonpharmacological intervention and device

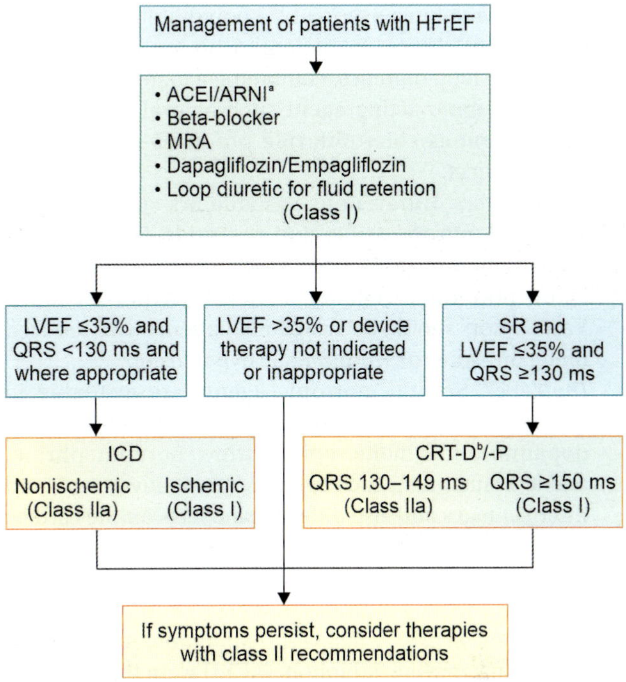

[a] As a replacement of ACEI.
[b] Where appropiate.

FLOWCHART 1: Treatment of HFrEF.

(ACEI: angiotensin-converting enzyme inhibitor; ARNI: angiotensin receptor–neprilysin inhibitor; CRT: cardiac resynchronization therapy; HFrEF: heart failure with reduced ejection fraction; ICD: implantable cardioverter-defibrillator; LVEF: left ventricular ejection fraction; MRA: mineralocorticoid receptor antagonist)

therapies. **Flowchart 1** depicts the algorithm for the treatment strategy, including drugs and devices in patients with HFrEF.

- *Nonpharmacological intervention*: Lifestyle modification occupies an important place in HF therapy. However, most of the recommendations are based on consensus expert opinion or are derived from limited trial data. Different lifestyle interventions include sodium and fluid restriction, weight reduction, multivitamin and mineral supplementation, relaxation techniques such as meditation and yoga, physical conditioning by exercise training, etc.
- *Pharmacological treatment*: Pharmacotherapy is the mainstay of treatment for HFrEF and should be started before considering device therapy, and simultaneous initiation of nonpharmacological interventions.

There are three main aims of treatment for HFrEF patients—(1) survival benefit, (2) prevention of hospitalizations for worsening HF, and (3) betterment in clinical status, functional capacity, and quality of life (QOL).[11]

Conventional Therapy

- *Optimizing volume status*: Current guidelines recommend intravenously administered diuretics as first-line therapy for volume overload.[12] Loop diuretics are initial diuretics of choice. In patients who are refractory to high-dose loop diuretics, combining a loop diuretic with a distal tubule acting agent such as oral metolazone or intravenous chlorothiazide produces a synergistic diuretic effect.

- *Vasodilators*: Intravenous vasodilators such as nitroglycerine, nitroprusside, and nesiritide often provide rapid symptom resolution, especially in patients with acute pulmonary edema or severe hypertension.[13] Vasodilators should be avoided in patients with reduced filling pressures or symptomatic hypotension.
- *Inotropes*: Several inotropic agents are available in the armamentarium of HF therapy viz., dobutamine, dopamine, milrinone, epinephrine, norepinephrine, and levosimendan. Each agent has their advantages and disadvantages and also differential effects on the cardiac output, mean arterial pressure, pulmonary capillary wedge pressure, systemic vascular resistance, and heart rate.
- *Renin–angiotensin system (RAS) inhibition*: Angiotensin-converting enzyme inhibitors (ACEI) were the first class of drugs which reduced both mortality and morbidity in patients with HFrEF alongside improvement of symptoms.[14]

Angiotensin receptor blockers (ARBs) in the management of HFrEF are now recommended for patients who cannot tolerate ACEI or angiotensin receptor–neprilysin inhibitor (ARNI) because of serious side effects. They have demonstrated reduction in CV death and HF hospitalization. However, no ARB has reduced all-cause mortality in any trial.[15,16]

- *Beta-blockers*: Evidence-based beta-blockers (bisoprolol, carvedilol, and metoprolol succinate) have been shown to decrease mortality and morbidity and improve symptoms in patients with HFrEF, in addition to other guideline-directed medical therapy (GDMT).[17-20] There is unifying agreement that ACEI and beta-blockers can be started together as soon as the diagnosis of symptomatic HFrEF is established. There is no data suggesting the initiation of a beta-blocker before an ACEI and vice versa.
- *Mineralocorticoid receptor antagonists*: MRAs (spironolactone or eplerenone) are recommended, in addition to an ACEI and a beta-blocker, in all patients with HFrEF to reduce mortality and the risk of HF hospitalization. They also improve symptoms.[21,22]
- *Hydralazine and isosorbide dinitrate*: There is no proper data to suggest the use of this fixed-dose combination therapy in all patients with HFrEF. Two randomized controlled trials (RCTs), V-HeFT I (Vasodilator-Heart Failure Trial) and A-HeFT (African-American Heart Failure Trial), established benefit of the combination of hydralazine-isosorbide dinitrate in self-identified African Americans. Also, this combination may be considered in symptomatic patients with HFrEF who cannot tolerate or there is contraindication to any of an ACEI, ARNI, or an ARB in order to reduce mortality (Veterans Administration Cooperative Study).
- *Digoxin*: In patients with HFrEF in sinus rhythm (SR), digoxin may be considered to reduce recurrent hospitalization risk, although its action on those treated with beta-blockers has not been studied. Digoxin showed overall neutral effect on mortality in the Digitalis Investigation Group (DIG) trial. The outcomes of digoxin in patients with HFrEF and AF have not been studied in RCTs. Some trials have suggested very high risk of events in patients with AF and HF receiving digoxin, whereas another meta-analysis inferred, based on results of non-RCTs, that digoxin has no harmful consequences on mortality in patients with AF and HFrEF.
- *Ivabradine*: In the landmark trial SHIFT, ivabradine showed a decrease in the combined endpoint of CV mortality and HF hospitalization in patients with symptomatic HFrEF with an LVEF < 35%, with history of ≥1 hospitalization for HF in past 12 months, in SR and with a HR >70 beats/min who were on GDMT including an ACE-I (or ARB), a beta-blocker, and an MRA.[23] Ivabradine got approval from European Medicines Agency (EMA) for use in Europe in patients with HFrEF with LVEF ≤ 35% and in SR with a resting heart rate ≥75 beats/min, because in this group ivabradine demonstrated a mortality benefit based on a retrospective subgroup analysis.[24]

New Options

- *ARNI*: The landmark trial PARADIGM-HF showed sacubitril/valsartan (ARNI) to be superior to enalapril in decreasing hospitalizations for worsening HF, CV death, and all-cause mortality in patients with ambulatory HFrEF with LVEF ≤40%.[25] ARNI also improved symptoms and QOL, decreased the incidence of diabetes requiring insulin therapy, and reduced the decline in eGFR, as well as hyperkalemia. ARNI may also lessen loop diuretic requirement. So, an ARNI should replace an ACEI or ARB in ambulatory patients with HFrEF, who is symptomatic in spite of optimal medical therapy. An ARNI is recommended as de novo treatment in hospitalized patients with acute HF before discharge given improvement in health status, reduction in the prognostic biomarker NT-proBNP, and improvement of LV remodeling parameters compared with ACEI/ARB.
- *Sodium-glucose cotransporter-2 inhibitors (SGLT-2I)*: Dapagliflozin resulted in a 26% decrease in the primary endpoint—a composite of worsening HF or CV death in the landmark trial DAPA-HF. Also, the individual components were significantly reduced.[26] Additional benefits of dapagliflozin included reduction of all-cause mortality, lesser HF symptoms, improved physical function, and QOL in patients with symptomatic HFrEF. Benefits were noticed soon after the start of dapagliflozin,

and the absolute risk reduction was large. Mortality reduction was to the same extent in patients with HFrEF with and without diabetes, and across the whole spectrum of HbA1c values. Similar results were noted in the EMPEROR-REDUCED trial.[27] Therefore, dapagliflozin or empagliflozin is recommended, in addition to GDMT with an ACEI/ARNI, a beta-blocker, and an MRA, for patients with HFrEF regardless of diabetes status

- *Vericiguat*: The VICTORIA study assessed the efficacy and safety of the oral soluble guanylate cyclase stimulator, vericiguat, in patients with a reduced EF and recently decompensated congestive heart failure (CHF). The incidence of the primary endpoint of death from CV causes or hospitalization for HF was lower among those who received vericiguat than among those who received placebo. There was no reduction in either all-cause or CV mortality. Thus, vericiguat may be considered, in addition to standard therapy for HFrEF, to reduce the risk of CV mortality and hospitalizations for HF.[28] **Figure 1** shows the additional medical therapies for HFrEF.
- *Cardiac myosin activator*: The GALACTIC-HF study assessed the efficacy and safety of the cardiac myosin activator, OMECAMTIV MECARBIL, in HFrEF patients. The primary endpoint of a first HF event or CV death was reduced by 8%. There was no significant reduction in CV mortality.[29]

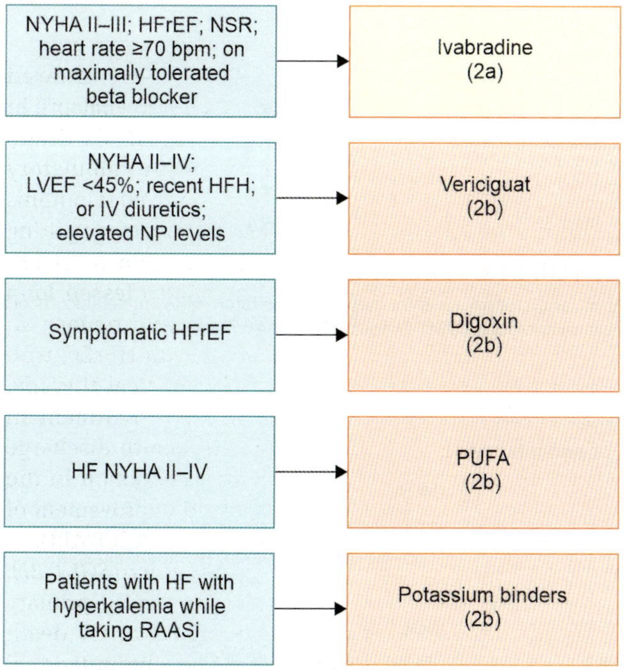

FIG. 1: Additional therapies for HF.

(HF: heart failure; HFrEF: HF with reduced ejection fraction; LVEF: left ventricular ejection fraction; NSR: normal sinus rhythm; NYHA: New York Heart Association; PUFA: polyunsaturated fatty acid; RAAS: renin–angiotensin–aldosterone system)

HOW TO START, SEQUENCE AND TITRATE THE AVAILABLE FOUR PILLARS OF PHARMACOTHERAPY FOR HFrEF

Conventional Sequencing

Flowchart 2 depicts the conventional sequencing of HF therapy. The conventional approach of achieving treatment with all four drug classes is to prescribe them in the precise sequence in which they were tested in clinical trials over the past 40 years. Physicians are asked to start with ACEI or ARBs, to be followed by a beta-blocker, then an MRA, then a neprilysin inhibitor, and, finally, a SGLT-2I. Prescribers are advised to titrate the dose of each drug class to the target dose used in large-scale trials before initiating the next recommended drug class. This approach recapitulates the sequence by which these agents were developed for the treatment of HF.

Limitations of Conventional Sequencing

- First, it presumes that the most effective and well-tolerated therapies were developed first. However, for making therapeutic recommendations, historical pattern is not a very good rationale in this era of evidence-based medicine; digitalis came in practice > 200 years ago but is no longer an important therapy
- Second, it assumes that foundational treatments are effective only when they reach target doses. Yet, low doses of drugs for HFrEF yield significant benefits to affect morbidity and mortality, and target doses are often only modestly more effective.
- Third, it presumes that the efficacy and safety of all classes of drugs were studied in clinical trials that needed patients to be getting all optimal therapy at target doses.

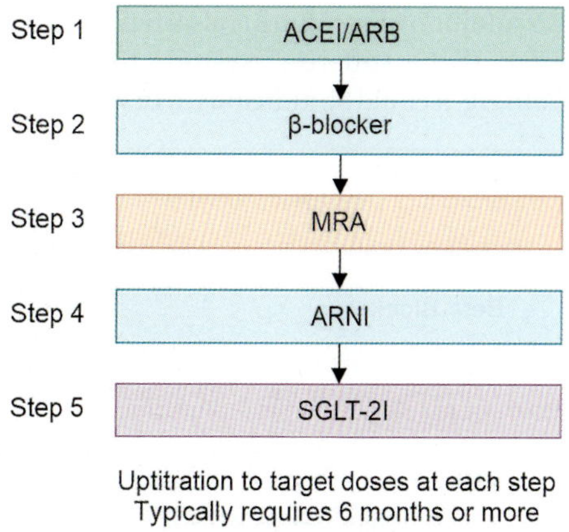

FLOWCHART 2: Conventional sequencing.

(ACEI: angiotensin-converting enzyme inhibitor; ARB: angiotensin receptor blocker; ARNI: angiotensin receptor–neprilysin inhibitor; MRA: mineralocorticoid receptor antagonist; SGLT-2I: sodium-glucose cotransporter-2 inhibitor)

However, in these trials, most patients were receiving subtarget doses of recommended drugs and still they were benefited.

- Quadruple therapy with an ARNI, evidence-based beta-blocker, MRA, and SGLT-2I may reduce risk of death by 73% over 2 years.[30] If physicians aim to achieve the target doses of each drug class before starting treatment with the next, it may take ≥6 months to prescribe all the foundational therapies. This estimate assumes that physicians and patients are fully dedicated to potentially adjusting treatment regimens at most visits. Such situations are very rare in clinical practice. Even if the current guideline-recommended approach was fully adopted, a delay of 6 months is unacceptable because each of the foundational drugs has been shown to reduce morbidity and mortality within 30 days of initiating treatment. With every passing visit, the absence of ≥1 therapy results in unnecessary hospitalizations and deaths. **Figure 2** demonstrates the risks of delaying or omitting GDMT.

Present Proposed Sequencing

To interrupt the culture of clinical inertia in HF care, the idea of simultaneous or fast sequence initiation and titration of GDMT for HFrEF has been proposed.[31] This proposed "new sequence" set of rules **(Flowchart 3)** involves three steps, to be started in a patient in whom diuretics has achieved clinical euvolemia.

1. Step 1 is simultaneous initiation of remedy with a beta-blocker and an SGLT-2I. Beta-blockers are (plausibly) the most beneficial drug for the treatment of HFrEF, specially with respect to the reduction of sudden cardiac death. SGLT-2Is have a strong impact to reduce the threat of hospitalizations for HF, and this advantage may additionally mitigate the short-term chance of worsening HF that may arise after a beta-blocker is initiated.
2. Step 2 is addition of sacubitril/valsartan, inside 1–2 weeks of step 1. If the sufferers' systolic blood pressure is < 100 mm Hg, it could be judicious to first assess tolerance, on the hypotensive patient, with an ARB before reverting to an ARNI.
3. Step 3 is the addition of an MRA, within 1–2 weeks of step 2, if serum potassium is within normal range and renal function is not significantly impaired. The favorable results of ARNI and SGLT-2I to improve renal function and potassium homeostasis might also increase the acceptability of MRAs. MRAs may be step 2 in a patient with symptomatic hypotension.

Used in appropriate patients, the approach outlined achieves treatment with all four foundational treatments within 4 weeks.

Principles behind Rapid Sequencing of Foundational Therapy[31]

- First, the extent of the benefit of each drug class is free of that gained from other agents. Specifically, the efficacy of ARNI remains unaltered with the use of MRAs, and also ARNI has no influence on the efficacy of an SGLT-2I.
- Second, low initiating doses of foundational drugs are potent in decreasing morbidity and mortality. Low doses of enalapril, carvedilol, and eplerenone exert significant effects on the risk of death or hospitalization for HF, as seen in large RCTs before protocol-wise increments in dose. For SGLT-2I, the target dose is same as the starting dose.

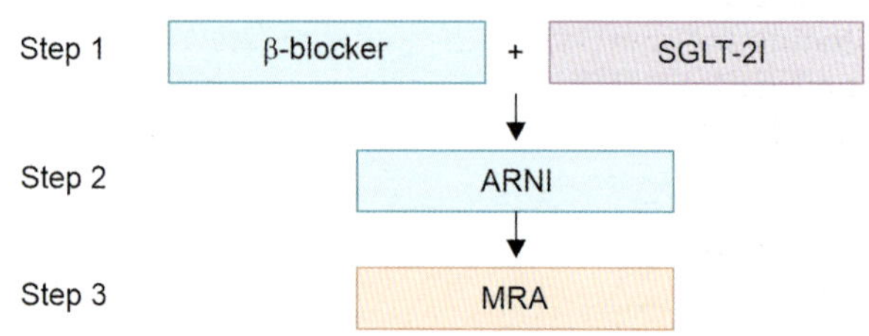

FLOWCHART 3: Proposed new sequencing.

(ARNI: angiotensin receptor–neprilysin inhibitor; MRA: mineralocorticoid receptor antagonist; SGLT-2I: sodium-glucose cotransporter-2 inhibitor)

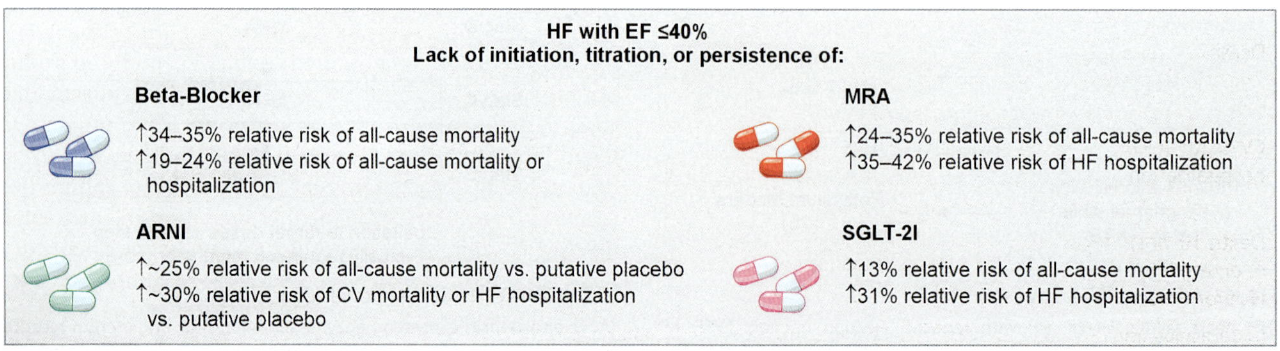

FIG. 2: Risks of delaying/omitting GDMT.

(ARNI: angiotensin receptor–neprilysin inhibitor; CV: cardiovascular; EF: ejection fraction; GDMT: guideline-directed medical therapy; HF: heart failure; MRA: mineralocorticoid receptor antagonist; SGLT-2I: sodium-glucose cotransporter-2 inhibitor)

- Third, the introduction of a new drug class yields greater benefits than up-titration of existing drug classes. Indeed, threefold to sevenfold increments in the dose of an ACEI or ARB show no mortality benefit as seen with the addition of a beta-blocker, ARNI, or SGLT-2I.
- Fourth, the proper sequencing of drug classes can improve safety and tolerability. Specifically, neprilysin inhibition can reduce the risk of renal insufficiency produced by an ACEI or ARB, and both ARNI and SGLT-2 inhibitors can minimize the risk of hyperkalemia with the use of MRAs.
- Fifth, as much of the advantages of foundational therapies are seen within 30 days of starting treatment, the protocol must achieve treatment with all Four classes of drugs within 4 weeks.

DISCUSSION

In spite of the strong evidence favoring the simultaneous or rapid sequence initiation of GDMT for HFrEF, some are in denial to accept this approach. Specifically, some have observed the lack of a dedicated RCT initiating multiple evidence-based HF medications all simultaneously or in rapid sequence. Additionally, some have doubted the ideal approach with initiating GDMT among patients with HF and LVEF > 40%.

To go with the preexisting evidence, the STRONG-HF (Safety, Tolerability and Efficacy of Uptitration of Guideline-directed Medical Therapies for Acute Heart Failure) study furnished direct RCT data which demonstrated that routinely initiating multiple HF medications together and quickly optimizing doses with close frequent follow-up is a safe and clinically effective approach to HF care when compared to the usual care group which improved minimally during follow-up.[32]

Recently, Pagnesi et al.[33] showed results grouped by LVEF phenotype. The strategy of rapid and intensive medical therapy plus close follow-up led to a large reduction in the primary endpoint of all-cause mortality or HF hospitalization over 180 days (relative risk reduction: 34%, absolute risk reduction: 8.1%, number-needed-to-treat: 12). The resulting advantages of high-intensity therapy were compatible independent of LVEF group, without any significant statistical interaction. Similarly, patient-reported QOL and symptoms showed significant improvement with high-intensity care, with no statistically significant separation in benefit among different LVEF groups. Irrespective of LVEF, serious adverse events were similar between high intensity and usual care.

In contemporary US outpatient practice, among patients with HFrEF who are eligible for therapy, one in three receives no beta-blocker and two in three receive no MRA. Only 14% are prescribed an ARNI. Primary prevention implantable cardioverter-defibrillators (ICDs) and other permanent devices continue to be implanted, often with suboptimal trials of guideline-directed medical therapies rather than the full complement of therapies for ventricular recovery.[34]

The PROVE-HF study showed that despite almost 100% use of beta-blockers and >75% of patients receiving ACEI or ARBs chronically, starting treatment with ARNI improved ejection fraction by a mean of 5.2% within 6 months, a result that would possibly decrease the need for ICD in practice.[35] **Table 1** shows the pattern of sequencing of the comprehensive disease modifying medical therapy (CDMMT) for HF.

TABLE 1: Pattern of sequencing of CDMMT for HF.

Simultaneous or rapid sequence initiation of comprehensive disease-modifying medical therapy (CDMMT) for heart failure (HF)							
Early relative risk reduction			Initiation and optimization of medication dosing				
Outcomes	Change %	CDMMT	Day 1	Days 7–14	Days 14–28	Days 21–42	After day 42
CV death or HF hospitalization	–42	ARNI	Initiate at low dose	Continue	Titrate, as tolerated	Titrate, as tolerated	Maintenance or additional titration of the four foundational therapies
Death	–25	β-Blocker	Initiate at low dose	Titrate, as tolerated	Titrate, as tolerated	Titrate, as tolerated	Consideration of EP device therapies or transcatheter mitral valve repair
CV death or HF hospitalization	–37	MRA	Initiate at low dose	Continue	Titrate, as tolerated	Continue	Consideration of add-on medications or advanced therapies, if refractory
Death, HF hospitalization, or emergency/urgent visit for worsening HF	–58	SGLT-2I	Initiate	Continue	Continue	Continue	Manage comorbidities

(ARNI: angiotensin receptor–neprilysin inhibitor; CV: cardiovascular; MRA: mineralocorticoid receptor antagonist; SGLT-2I: sodium-glucose cotransporter-2 inhibitor)

CONCLUSION

In order to make rapid improvement in patients with HFrEF simultaneous and rapid initiation of quadruple therapy is shown to have good tolerance among patients and there is no safety issue also. In properly indicated cases, rapid and simultaneous initiation will lead to therapeutic benefit in short period of time. For patients with HFrEF, this approach starts with simultaneous or rapid sequence initiation of four therapies (ARNI, beta-blocker, MRA, and SGLT-2I) among eligible patients at the time of HF diagnosis. For patients with HFpEF, the foundation is immediate initiation of SGLT-2I therapy, with additional consideration of ARNI and MRA. This sense of urgency should apply to both inpatients and outpatients, recognizing that every encounter with a HF patient (whether in-person or remote) is a critical opportunity to augment disease-modifying therapy as tolerated.

ONLINE REFERENCES

Please scan the QR code provided at the end of the table of contents for References of this chapter.

CHAPTER

48 Guideline-directed Medical Therapy for Heart Failure: The Other Side of the Story

Mrinal Kanti Das, Jayanta Sharma

ABSTRACT

Management of heart failure has evolved significantly over a long period of years. Various strategies have been formulated by various professional organizations of cardiologists and published in the journals in the form of guideline-directed medical therapy. The strategies have definitely yielded results by not only reducing recurrent hospitalizations, an important marker of overall prognosis, but also the mortality, especially with the advent of novel drugs and devices. But there have been some interesting stories as well on the flip side, which are rarely discussed in the forums. These are about therapeutic inertia, noncompliance, nonadherence even in the most advanced countries, and some unsung glories. The present chapter has attempted to unravel some of those issues with the primary aim of bettering our vigilance and implementation for better care of the patients.

Keywords: Heart failure, guideline-directed medical therapy (GDMT), pharmacotherapy, device therapy for heart failure.

INTRODUCTION

Heart failure (HF), a global health problem affecting >37.7 million people globally and 13–23 million people in Indian subcontinent, is a matter of concern for all healthcare stake holders. The disease is associated with increased mortality both over 1 year and 5 years period. Among Indians, HF presents 10 years earlier than in Western population and there is huge economic burden of about $1,186 per patient per year incurring almost 2% of total health budget.[1] The disease is projected to increase by 25% by 2030. The rehospitalization for HF is an important marker for further course of the disease and it needs to be evaluated thoroughly in appropriate time so that individualizing strategies for attenuating the different risk factors and unattended comorbidities and of HF-related rehospitalization can be done. Guideline-directed medical therapy (GDMT) based on various evidences and expert opinions is recommended for all patients everywhere. If required optimization of GDMT drugs and devices as additional therapy can be carried out depending on the country or region. This definitely reduces the morbidity, recurrent hospitalizations, and improved the survival of the patients of HF.[2] For this universalization we formulate, discuss, and publish with fun fare in major journals making lot of propaganda about the GDMT for HF like all other diseases. But do we know what is the other side of the story in this huge extravaganza? There is a huge therapeutic gap between GDMT recommendations and real-world scenario in the total management of patients with heart failure with reduced ejection fraction (HFrEF). There are multiple reasons for having this gap, which will be discussed in detail and attempts will be made to formulate many strategies to close this gap based on the available evidences following different trials and studies.

NATURAL HISTORY AND STANDARD CARE FOLLOWING GDMT IN HEART FAILURE

Heart failure is a relentlessly progressive disorder with waxing and waning. A normal heart over a period of time progresses to terminal state resulting to death. In between there are episodes of acute illness causing hospitalizations. More the hospitalizations, more will be the chance of catastrophe. **Figure 1** illustrates the progression of the disease.[3]

There is emphasis on the foundational therapy right from the beginning and initiate the induction therapy with the

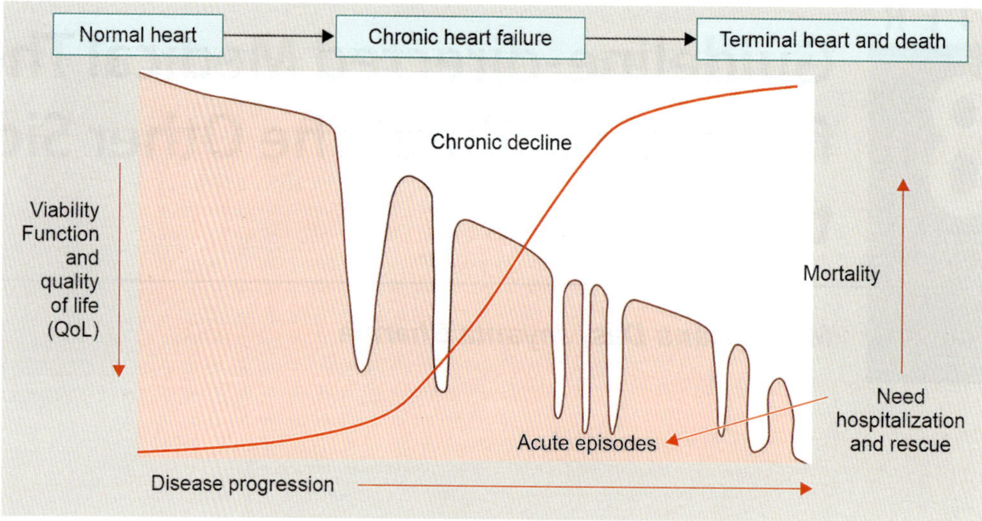

FIG. 1: Progressive nature of heart failure with hospitalizations and terminal state.

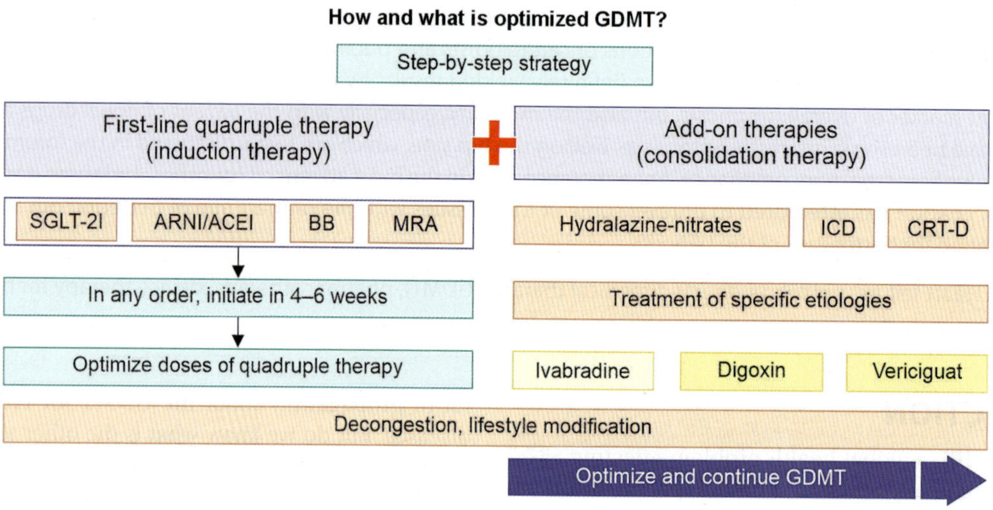

FIG. 2: GDMT and step-by-step strategy for HF.

(ACEI: angiotensin-converting enzyme inhibitor; ARNI: angiotensin receptor neprilysin inhibitor; BB: beta-blocker; CRT-D: cardiac resynchronization therapy-defibrillator; GDMT: guideline-directed medical therapy; HF: heart failure; ICD: implantable cardioverter-defibrillator; MRA: mineralocorticoid receptor antagonist; SGLT-2I: sodium-glucose cotransporter-2 inhibitor)

Source: With permission from Bozkurt (2022).[4]

quadruple drugs along with diuretic **(Fig. 2)**. The quadruple therapy includes angiotensin receptor neprilysin inhibitor/angiotensin-converting enzyme inhibitor/angiotensin receptor blocker (ARNI/ACEI/ARB) + beta blockers + mineralocorticoid receptor (MRA) + sodium-glucose cotransporter-2 inhibitors (SGLT-2Is). When they are also not showing salutary results, the add-on therapies should be considered. This may be device therapies like cardiac resynchronization therapy (CRT)/CRT-defibrillator (CRT-D) or implantable cardioverter-defibrillators (ICDs) or drugs as per the guideline. The use of GDMT in HF is undeniable and is effective in reducing sudden cardiac death as per the recent studies even in patients with ICDs or CRT/CRT-D.[4,5]

In case of advanced HF, the whole approach as recommended by the European Society of Cardiology[6] is depicted in **Flowchart 1** and is dependent on whether the goal is improve symptoms or palliation.

There is no denying the fact that newer HF therapies have proven efficacious when added to established therapies, significantly reducing the morbidity and mortality associated with HF. This is well demonstrated in different trial patients with HFrEF. High-level, randomized evidence has been incorporated into both European and American society recommendations for GDMT.[7,8]

One pertinent question is often asked, whether there has been any change in the practice pattern of implantation

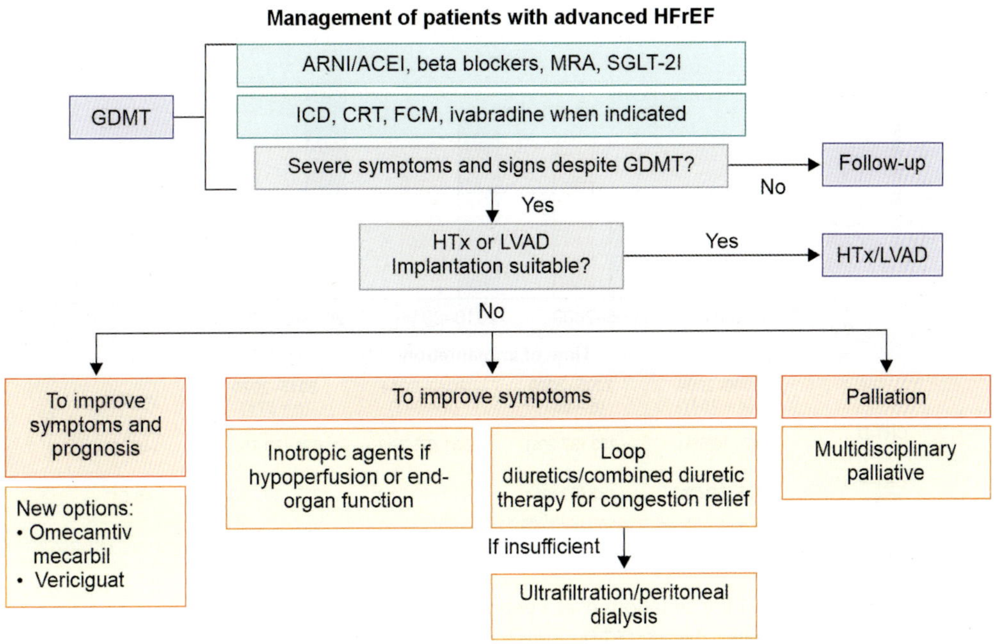

FLOWCHART 1: Algorithm for advanced HF.

(ACEI: angiotensin-converting enzyme inhibitor; ARNI: angiotensin receptor neprilysin inhibitor; CRT: cardiac resynchronization therapy; FCM: ferric carboxymaltose; GDMT: guideline-directed medical therapy; HF: heart failure; HFrEF: heart failure with reduced ejection fraction; HTx: heart transplant; ICD: implantable cardioverter-defibrillator; LVAD: left ventricular assist device; MRA: mineralocorticoid receptor antagonist; SGLT-2I: sodium-glucose cotransporter-2 inhibitor)

of the resynchronization therapy after the introduction of the novel drugs of HF and initiation of GDMT. The search of literatures could not unravel the data, though personal observations indicated about the lowering of number of implantations of CRT. Anett Behon et al. published a paper in 2023 at GeroScience (https://doi.org/10.1007/s11357-023-00739-z) on "long-term outcome of CRT patients in the elderly" and made comment on an observation that number of implantations significantly reduced in younger age group vis-à-vis older age group after the use of GDMT because of more preferences for the CRT by treating physicians for elderly patients.[9] This has been demonstrated in the **Figure 3**.

Having undoubted efficacy of the GDMT in treated patients, it is essential to know the real-world scenario happening behind the backs of guideline proponents, various national registries representative of the contemporary implementation of GDMT and also new studies like EVOLUTION-HF were studied and they demonstrate unacceptable and poor adoption, delayed initiation, and dose titration.[10]

Total 266,589 patients included showed mean times from hospitalization for heart failure (hHF) to GDMT initiation longer for novel GDMTs (dapagliflozin or sacubitril/valsartan) than for other GDMTs: 39 and 44 versus 12–13 days (Japan), 44 and 33 versus 22–31 days (Sweden), and 33 and 19 versus 18–24 days (United States). The pooled data revealed proportions of patients stopping treatment (excluding switches from ACEI or ARB to sacubitril/valsartan) within 12 months were 23.5% (dapagliflozin), 26.4% (sacubitril/valsartan), 38.4% (ACEI), 33.4% (ARBs), 25.2% (beta blockers), and 42.2% (MRAs). Corresponding target dose achievements were 75.7%, 28.2%, 20.1%, 6.7%, 7.2%, and 5.1%, respectively. The data demonstrates abysmal performance by the stakeholders.

Figure 4 shows the graphic representation of the follow-up even in the advanced countries.

Central illustration: Initiation, titration to target disease, and discontinuation of GDMTs among new users of GDMTs after hHF, in Japan, Sweden, and the United States.

Patient characteristics of hHF patients and percentage of patients on various GDMT drugs in Japan, Sweden, and USA are shown in **Table 1**. This is an eye-opener for all the strategists involved in the HF management.

The results of these failures are reflected in the form of increased mortality of HF even in the best of the countries with advanced economy. Conclusion by one study was: "In a real-world population of HFrEF patients, inadequate GDMT confers a 29% excess mortality risk over the 2-year follow-up". The study conducted revealed 14,880 HFrEF patients had 70% having a record of GDMT and 57% having a record of concurrent prescriptions. Patients without GDMT cohort had 29% increased risk of mortality versus GDMT [hazard ratio 1.29; 95% confidence interval (CI 1.19–1.40; $p < 0.0001$].[11]

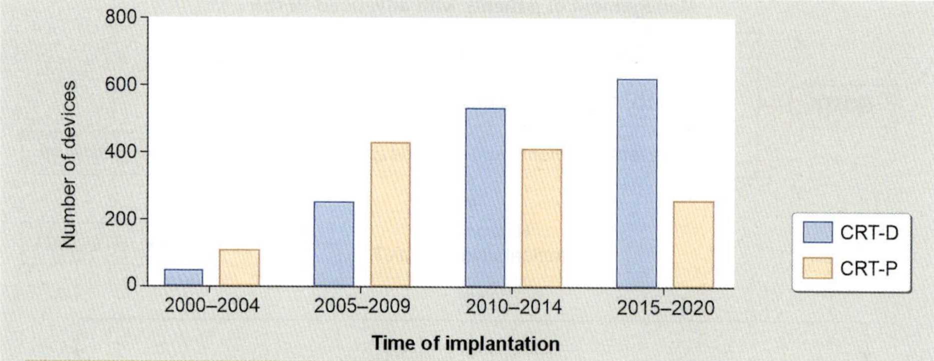

	2000–2004 (*n* = 154)	2005–2009 (*n* = 681)	2010–2014 (*n* = 943)	2015–2020 (*n* = 878)	*p*-value
CRT-D (n;%)	47 (30.5%)	253 (37.2%)	531 (56.3%)	621 (70.7%)	<0.01*
CRT-P (n;%)	107 (69.5%)	428 (62.8%)	412 (43.7%)	257 (29.3%)	<0.01*

* $p < 0.0001$

FIG. 3: Trend of the CRT implantations over a period of 20 years.
(CRT: cardiac resynchronization therapy; CRT-D: CRT-defibrillator; CRT-P: CRT-pacemaker)

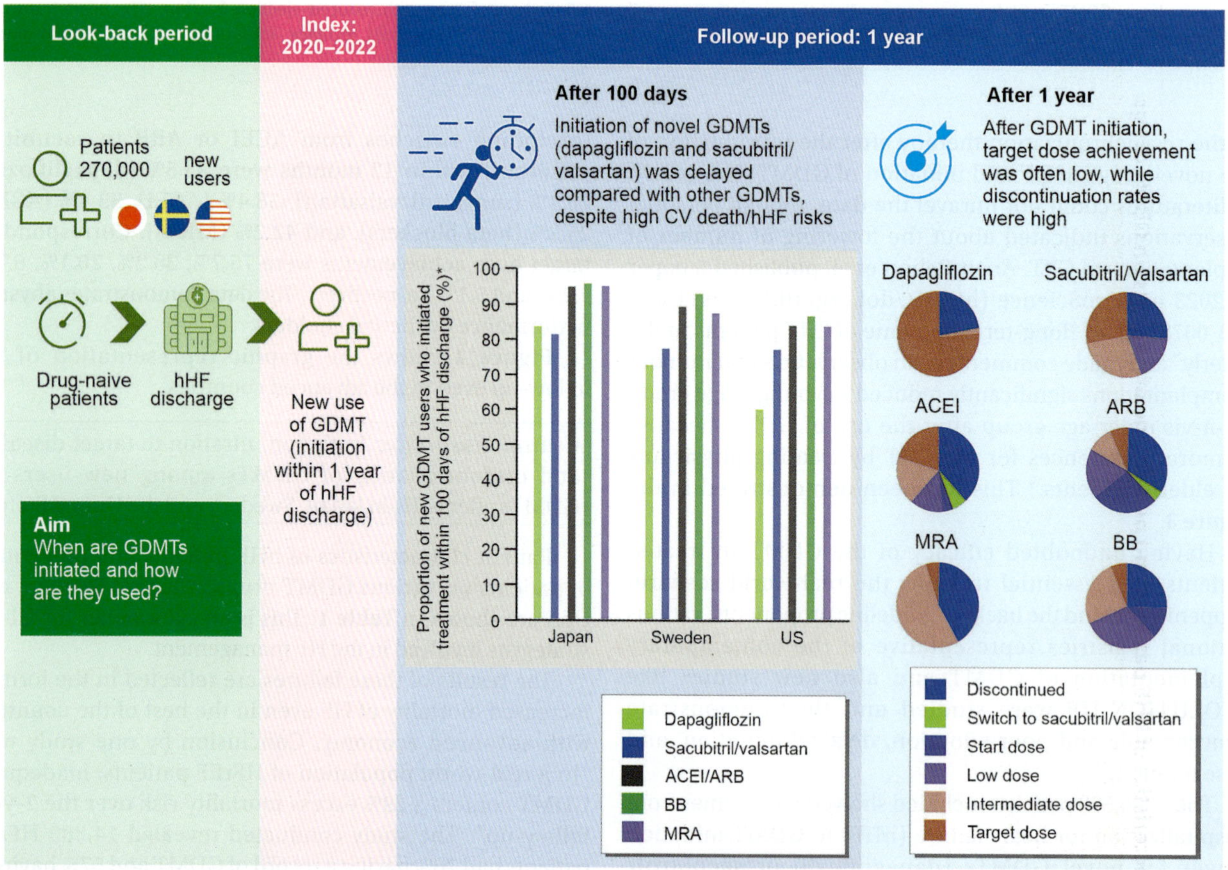

* By design, in each GDMT category, 100% of patients initiated treatment within 1 year of hHF discharge.

FIG. 4: Follow-up trends in the advanced countries.
(ACEI: angiotensin-converting enzyme inhibitor; ARB: angiotensin receptor blocker; BB: beta blocker; CV: cardiovascular; GDMT: guideline-directed medical therapy; hHF: hospitalization for heart failure; MRA: mineralocorticoid receptor antagonist)
Source: With permission from Savarese et al. (2023).[10]

TABLE 1: Characteristics of hHF patients and percentage of patients on GDMT drugs.

	Japan (n = 130,243)					Sweden (n = 26,394)					United States (n = 109,952)				
	Dapagliflozin (n = 7,443)	Sacubitril/Valsartan (n = 12,971)	ACEI/ARB (n = 64,831)	BB (n = 68,798)	MRA (n = 49,141)	Dapagliflozin (n = 5,443)	Sacubitril/Valsartan (n = 3,854)	ACEI/ARB (n = 8,511)	BB (n = 9,65S)	MRA (n = 14,315)	Dapagliflozin (n = 1,962)	Sacubitril/Valsartan (n = 12,200)	ACEI/ARB (n = 48,067)	BB (n = 63,335)	MRA (n = 30,350)
Age, y	75 ± 13	76 ± 13	78 ± 13	77± 13	80 ± 12	73 ± 12	70 ± 12	75 ± 14	74 ± 14	77 ± 12	61 ± 13	64 ± 14	68 ± 14	69 ± 14	66 ± 14
Female	2,515 (33.8)	4.919 (37.9)	28,829 (44.5)	30,324 (44.1)	24,786 (50.0)	1,590 (29.0)	999 (25.9)	3,554 (41.8)	3,775 (39.1)	6,163 (43.0)	635 (32.4)	4,146 (34.0)	21,504 (44.7)	29,043 (45.9)	13,095 (42.9)
Time from first HF diagnosis to GDMT initiation, d	229 (7–1,689)	352 (17–1,873)	13 (2–655)	14 (2–734)	34 (3–1,074)	347 (36–2,310)	212 (21–2,017)	14 (5–513)	11 (5–121)	71 (9–1,190)	938 (206–2,265)	679 (52–2,050)	506 (4–1,815)	521 (3–1,848)	658 (19–1,963)
Time from hHF to GDMT initiation, d	0 (0–32), 39 ± 79	0 (0–45), 44 ± 84	0 (0–0), 13 ± 48	0 (0–0), 12 ± 46	0 (0–0), 13 ± 46	20 (6–113), 44 ± 69	15 (6–87), 33 ± 56	7 (4–20), 30 ± 64	7 (4–15), 22 ± 50	10 (5–37), 31 ± 58	64 (7–178), 33 ± 64	6 (0–87), 19 ± 47	0 (0–22), 24 ± 62	0 (0–7), 19 ± 56	0 (0–36), 18 ± 50
Length of hHF stay, d	15 (9–25)	15 (9–25)	15 (9–26)	16 (9–27)	19 (11–31)	4 (2–7)	4 (2–7)	5 (3–8)	5 (3–8)	5 (3–8)	4 (2–7)	4 (2–7)	4 (2–8)	5 (2–8)	5 (2–8)
GDMT						GDMT									
BB	5,643 (75.8)	10.374 (80.0)	33,945 (52.4)	0 (0)	27,283 (55.5)	5,241 (95.6)	3,720 (96.5)	7,398 (86.9)	0 (0)	12,936 (90.4)	1,801 (91.8)	11,224 (92.0)	37,401 (77.8)	0 (0)	26,047 (85.3)
ACEI/ARB	5,326 (71.6)	10,418 (803)	0 (0)	34,865 (50.7)	25,052 (51.0)	4,385 (80.0)	3,152 (81.8)	0 (0)	7,615 (78.8)	11,789 (82.4)	1,327 (67.6)	7,700 (63.1)	0 (0)	27,945 (44.1)	19,556 (63.4)
MRA	3,588 (48.2)	5.908 (45.5)	15.983 (24.7)	17,594 (25.6)	0 (0)	3,956 (723)	2,876 (74.6)	3,013 (35.4)	3,683 (38.1)	0 (0)	1,152 (58.7)	5,380 (44.1)	7,304 (15.2)	7,678 (121)	0 (0)
Sacubitril/Valsartan	1,140 (15.3)	0 (0)	438 (0.7)	1,892 (2.8)	1,847 (3.8)	1,946 (35.5)	0 (0)	176 (2.1)	804 (8.3)	1,438 (10.0)	925 (47.1)	0 (0)	1,508 (3.1)	2,568 (4.1)	3,982 (13.0)
Dapagliflozin	0 (0)	4,920 (37.9)	6,270 (9.7)	7,133 (10.4)	5,777 (11.8)	0 (0)	1,528 (39.6)	922 (10.8)	1,366 (14.1)	2,575 (18.0)	0(0)	872 (7.1)	712 (1.5)	835 (1.3)	1,039 (3.4)

(ACEI: angiotensin-converting enzyme inhibitor; ARB: angiotensin receptor blocker; BB: beta blocker; GDMT: guideline-directed medical therapy; hHF: hospitalization for heart failure; MRA: mineralocorticoid receptor antagonist)

There have been many studies for improving the quality increasing the GDMT compliance carried out over a period of time. They are depicted in **Table 2**.

The factors responsible for such unwarranted gaps in the use and optimization of the therapeutic lines guided by GDMT are many. All these involving the provider and the healthcare system. Clinician competency, therapeutic inertia, low healthcare literacy, concerns for adverse events, inadequate access to multidisciplinary resources, uneven insurance coverage, and unwanted out-pocket costs are mostly sociobehavioral and are responsible for the slow uptake of GDMT.[12] These are enumerated here for easy reckoning.

The most important are *patient-related factors*. They could be:
- Increasing age and cognitive impairment
- Depression
- Frailty
- Financial burden due to huge cost of therapy
- Food security
- Home security
- Communication or language barriers
- Social isolation
- Transport

Second group of issues are treatment-related factors such as intolerance to drugs and adverse effects and healthcare-related factors that influence availability and accessibility of HF care.

The third one is *therapeutic inertia* which is caused by:
- Lack of awareness about the GDMT among the physicians
- Timidity to escalate or de-escalate the GDMT recommended drugs in suitable time frame
- Overwhelming consideration of the cost of therapy resulting in subtherapeutic drug schedules
- Failure to detect early the various adverse effects of the drugs and their correlation with symptoms

HOW TO INTEGRATE? ROLE OF DIGITAL TECHNOLOGY

In a review paper by Seferovic et al.,[12] workers highlighted evidence-based solutions, practical experience, and expert consensus on how to utilize appropriate procedures, newer medications, and cohorting patients to ensure and promote more acceptability of GDMT. The other essential factors are motivation, upgradation of knowledge, and continuous professional development. At the same time patients also need to be educated and empowered about self-care which increases GDMT implementation. The multidisciplinary care and involvement of the institutional care also add to the appropriate medicinal prescription rates and increase the adherence to GDMT as they become protocolized by the institution and thus improve the care for HF. The digital technology and digital therapeutics by various apps also definitely help in circumventing the overall care of the patients following GDMT as they facilitate modern technologies in advancing professional and patient education and facilitating patient-provider communication.[13,14] **Figure 5** depicts various measures for improving outcome of HF management.

The following approaches are mentioned for easy reckoning:
- Multidisciplinary team-based approaches. A pilot study (IMPLEMENT-HF) used cardiologists and pharmacists to virtually optimize HF therapies for HFrEF admitted in the hospital for noncardiac causes. 89 of the 118 total patients were included in the GDMT intervention group. Within this group, 46% experienced intensification of their GDMT during their hospitalization (compared to 31% in the usual care arm) and increased 30-day follow-up. IMPLEMENT-HF reasserted the concept of improved result by demonstrating the impact of a multidisciplinary team in the optimization of HF therapies during hospitalization.[15]
- Autopopulating HF registries that can measure integrated health system performance,
- Remote monitoring technologies including wearable,
- Nontraditional visits, and
- Electronic health record (EHR)-embedded tools including clinical alerts have tremendous potential to reduce implementation gaps and improve HF outcomes.

There are very many approaches utilizing the digital technology and digital therapeutics whereby the appropriate apps can be downloaded by the patients and health personnel and continuous online supports may be made available and used.

These apps have the ability to off-site monitoring and recommendation on:
- Blood pressure (BP), heart rate, and oxygen saturation (SpO_2) monitoring
- Type of food and quantity of fluid intake in a day-to-day basis
- Alarm for taking various GDMT drugs and nutrients at the right time
- Compliance with the recommended exercise schedule
- Sleep pattern
- Response to alarming electrocardiogram (ECG)
- Remote monitoring of some cardiac devices such as pacing, CRT, CRTD, ICDs, and CardioMEMS[16] for monitoring pulmonary artery pressure (PAP), etc. In the CHAMPION (CardioMEMS Heart Sensor Allows Monitoring of Pressure to Improve Outcomes in Class III Heart Failure) study, the monitored group had a higher frequency of optimization of medication comprising increases in the doses of neurohormonal blocking agents, upscaling of dose of diuretics, and vasodilators in patients with higher PAPs, with preservation of renal parameters despite increased diuretic use.
- Reminding the next follow-up of the patient by the physician
- Reminder for refilling the prescribed drugs
- Home delivery of many supports. Some of the health system approaches that can improve HF care are shown in following diagram.

Though there is chance of alert fatigue, multiple recent trials with tailored clinical alerts and patient-centered

TABLE 2: Notable clinical trials for HF quality improvement.

	Trail	Format	*n*	Primary findings	Strengths	Limitations	Implications
Multi-disciplinary	STRONG-HF [11]	Multinational, randomized, parallel group implementation trail	1,078	Rapid up-titration of GDMT after HF admission significant reduced all cause death or HF readmission at 180 days	Specific targets and timeline of intervention; similar rates of serious adverse events with usual care	Unblinded cause of readmission were not adjudicated; SGLT-2I not included	Four clinic visits within 2 weeks postdischarge in the intensive treatment arm requires significant patient, provider, and system commitment. Follow-up performed by HF experts
	CONNECT-HF [10]	Cluster-randomized, multicenter, implementation, postdischarge QI	5,647	No difference in composite of mortality or HF readmission; hospitals randomized to receive extensive HF-related education	Large, multicenter	Did not provide recommendation or automate orders/ referrals	No difference in outcomes detected with hospitals who were provided HF education and quality initiative information; limits buy in from health systems
	PACT-HF [26]	Stepped wedge cluster randomized single center	2,494	No difference in all cause readmission, ED visit, or death at 3 months patient-centered transitional care model vs. usual care	Significant resource commitment with transitional care; patients, providers and policy makers involved	Single healthcare system did not assess adherence to discharge (DC) recommendations	No difference in outcomes with transnational care model which included nurse lead self-care education, DC summary close follow-up ± home care visits
	Remote optimization Desai et al. [32]	Case-control study for algorithmic multidisciplinary GDMT optimization	1,028 (19% in optimization group)	Significant increases in dose or use of BB and RAAS antagonists (but not MRA) with navigator driven remote medication optimization vs. usual care	Clinical navigator driven algorithmic intervention, remote care, multidisciplinary approach	Nonrandomized short-term follow-up single-center	Potentially scalable would require dedicated navigator pharmacist and HF cardiologist efforts
EHR-based	PROMPT-HF [22]	Single center randomized pragmatic EHR-based, outpatient	100 providers; 1,310 patients	Increase in GDMT prescription (primarily with BB) at 30 days. Providers randomized to receive targeted prompts vs. usual care	Provides frameworks for rapid, lower cost EHR-based pragmatic randomized trails	Single-system detected changes quite modest (mostly beta blocker)	Relatively low cost and scalable requires integrated EHR average of 14 prompts per provider to prescribe 1 additional class of GDMT
	REVEAL-HF	Single center randomized pragmatic EHR-based	3,124	No difference in composite of all-cause mortality at 1 year and hHF within 30 days. Providers randomized to receive prognostic information vs. usual care	Easy to integrate within existing EHR	Did not provide recommendation or automate orders/ referrals	No benefit detected to providing 1 year mortality estimates

Continued

Continued

	Trail	Format	N	Primary findings	Strengths	Limitations	Implications
	IMPLEMENT-HF Pilot Study [44]	Prospective pilot study EHR-based	118	Increase in prescriptions at time of discharge for BB, ARNI, and MRA, primary team provided with algorithmic recommendations from pharmacist physician GDMT team	Increase in GDMT score in the intervention arm, proof-of-concept	Small, single-center pilot quality study	Requires dedicated HF cardiologist and pharmacist effort
	EPIC-HF [19]	Single-center, randomized patient centered	306	Increase in GDMT intensification at 30 days; 3 minutes video and 1 page checklist provided electronically to patients prior to clinic visit	Patient engagement readily scalable at centers with integrated EHR and patient messaging capability	Single system patients already scheduled with cardiology were enrolled	Relatively low cost and scalable for patients with technology literacy
Virtual RCT	CHIEF-HF [62]	Completely remote patient centered	476	Canagliflozin use improved KCCQ symptom score at 12 weeks	Similar QOL improvement with both HFrEF and HFpEF; all remote trail with no in-person interaction	Subjective symptom assessment and QOL measures	Virtual implementation of GDMT shown to be safe and effective, trail design efficient/cost effective. Fitbit devices to monitor activity level
Remote monitoring	CHAMPION [42]	Single blind randomized trial with CardioMEMS device	550	Reduction in HF hospitalization at 6 months with the addition of ambulatory PA pressure	Success with remote monitoring device	Single-blended; industry funded	Scalability has some limitations given invasive procedure that requires dedicated resources to

(ARNI: angiotensin receptor neprilysin inhibitor; BB: beta blocker; ED: emergency department; EHR: electronic health record; GDMT: guideline-directed medical therapy; HF: heart failure; hHF: hospitalization for heart failure; HFrEF: heart failure with reduced ejection fraction; HFpEF: heart failure with preserved ejection fraction; KCCQ: Kansas City Cardiomyopathy Questionnaire; MRA: mineralocorticoid receptor; QI: quality improvement; QOL: quality of life; RAAS: renin–angiotensin–aldosterone system; SGLT-2I: sodium-glucose cotransporter-2 inhibitor)

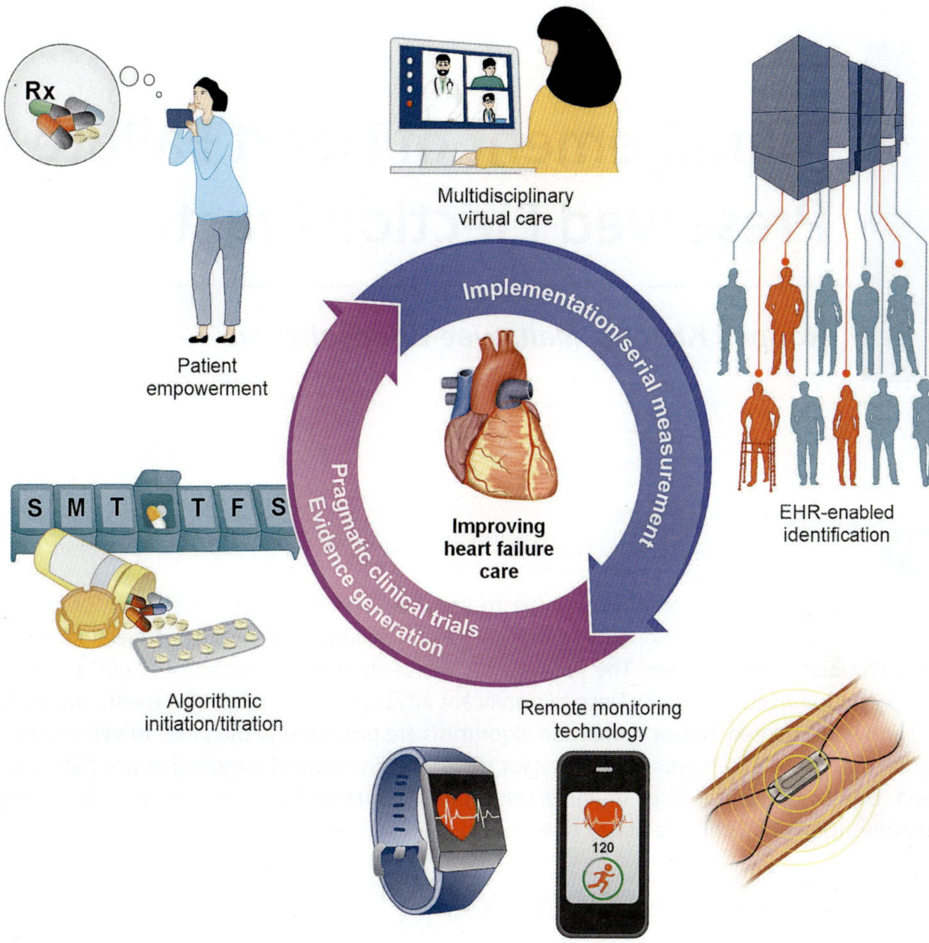

FIG. 5: Approaches to improve heart failure care.[13,14]
(EHR: electronic health record)

education initiatives have increased GDMT prescription. The Pragmatic trial Of Messaging to Providers about Treatment of Heart Failure (PROMPT-HF), an EHR-based cluster randomized trial that randomized 100 high-volume providers of HFrEF patients in the Yale-New Haven Health system to: (1) Usual care arm and (2) Care with electronic message arm. There was a demonstrable improvement in the primary outcome of an increase in the number of GDMT classes prescribed at 30 days and GDMT dose with targeted, integrated prompts within the EHR.[17]

CONCLUSION

There are many unanswered questions and unmet needs to improve the acceptability and implantation of GDMT. Mere development of the apps and electronic gadgets may not suffice. More studies are warranted to refine the clusters of HF for right kind of intervention and calibrate the right kind of resourcing of effective strategies for optimizing HF care. A multifaceted and motivated approach for HF therapy is the need of the hour. There should be generation of adequate evidences appropriate to a geographical location with heterogeneous economic background and available facilities. The quantum jump in the technological development may not necessarily be translated to higher level of HF care in its truest sense; however, our attempts should be always to walk with the time and use the technology to the level of maximum benefits to the patients of HF.

ONLINE REFERENCES

Please scan the QR code provided at the end of the table of contents for References of this chapter.

CHAPTER

49

Management of Heart Failure with Preserved Ejection Fraction

Roopali Khanna, Maitreyee Bhattacharyya

ABSTRACT

Heart failure is a complex clinical syndrome caused due to impaired ventricle filling or ejection of blood and is one of the major causes of morbidity and mortality worldwide. Heart failure with preserved ejection fraction (HFpEF) constitutes about 50% cause of heart failure. The survival and heart failure readmissions for HFpEF are as poor as heart failure with reduced ejection fraction (HFrEF). Despite significant advances in diagnosis and treatment, HFpEF is usually under-recognized and undertreated. Newer scores and algorithms are proposed to diagnose HFpEF and to differentiate it from other causes of dyspnea. The treatment options for HFpEF are limited and targeting newer pathways and newer drugs are required. Due to the presence of multiple comorbidities such as hypertension, diabetes mellitus, obesity, obstructive sleep apnea (OSA), and chronic kidney disease (CKD), the management of HFpEF requires a multidisciplinary approach.

Keywords: HFpEF, H_2FPEF score, HFA-PEFF score, SGLT-2I.

INTRODUCTION

Heart failure (HF) is a complex clinical syndrome caused due to impaired ventricle filling or ejection of blood resulting from structural and functional abnormality. As per the universal definition, HF is defined as symptoms and/or signs of HF caused by structural/functional cardiac abnormalities with at least one of (1) raised natriuretic peptides (NPs) or (2) objective evidence of cardiogenic pulmonary or systemic congestion.[1] HF has been classified as follows:

- *HF with reduced ejection fraction (HFrEF)*: Clinical diagnosis of HF and left ventricle ejection fraction (LVEF) ≤ 40%
- *HF with mildly reduced ejection fraction (HFmrEF)*: Clinical diagnosis of HF and LVEF 41–49%
- *HF with improved ejection fraction*: Previous LVEF ≤ 40% and a follow-up measurement >40%
- *HF with preserved ejection fraction (HFpEF)*: Clinical diagnosis of HF and LVEF ≥ 50% not explained due to an underlying cause such as infiltrative cardiomyopathy, valvular heart disease, pericardial disease, or high-output HF.[2]

Although the focus has been mostly on HFrEF, the incidence, prevalence, and lifetime risk of HFpEF have been steadily increasing over the last few years and are a major cause of morbidity and mortality, particularly in the elderly, obese, physically inactive, and those with cardiometabolic disorders.[3] The survival and HF readmissions for HFpEF are as poor as HFrEF.[3] The low threshold for diagnosing HFpEF in patients with dyspnea or effort intolerance will help in early diagnosis and treatment. Despite these facts, the diagnosis of HFpEF is often missed and hence needs special attention.

DIAGNOSIS OF HEART FAILURE WITH PRESERVED EJECTION FRACTION

Heart failure with preserved ejection fraction diagnosis is made on the basis of symptoms of dyspnea and fatigue along with objective evidence of congestion and LVEF ≥ 50%.[1,4,5] The clinical features of congestion on physical examination are often absent in ambulatory patients.[6] Plasma NPs are below the thresholds for HF diagnosis in nearly one-third of patients [ambulatory—brain natriuretic peptide (BNP) ≥ 35 pg/mL, N-terminal prohormone of brain natriuretic peptide (NT-proBNP) ≥ 125 pg/mL; hospitalized—BNP ≥ 100 pg/mL, NT-proBNP ≥ 300 pg/mL], especially in obesity-related HFpEF.[7-9] Besides obesity, relative NP deficiency is seen in African ancestry, insulin resistance, increased androgenicity in women, natriuretic peptide B (NPPB) polymorphisms, and lower LV diastolic wall stress for any given elevation in LV diastolic pressure.[10,11] This clearly shows that normal NP levels cannot be completely relied upon to exclude HFpEF in suspected cases. Objective evidence of congestion in the form of imaging and invasive hemodynamics can be used to make a diagnosis of HFpEF. The markers suggestive of chronic congestion in imaging include an increase in E/e′ ratio, left atrial enlargement, reduced left atrial reservoir strain, increases in estimated pulmonary artery pressures, and distention of the inferior vena cava.[12] Right heart catheterization to assess hemodynamics during rest and exercise is considered the gold standard diagnostic test for HFpEF.[1,4,13,14] An elevated pulmonary capillary wedge pressure (PCWP) of ≥15 mm Hg (at rest) or ≥25 mm Hg (with exercise) made at end-expiration during supine exercise is the hemodynamic definition for the diagnosis of HFpEF.[4,5,13,14] An increase in PCWP relative to the increase in cardiac output > 2 mm Hg/L/min during upright exercise can also be used to make a diagnosis of HFpEF.[15] An increase in PCWP ≥ 18 mm Hg with saline or ≥19 mm Hg with leg raise may also be helpful in identifying patients with HFpEF. Although invasive hemodynamics provide a more definitive diagnosis of HFpEF compared to imaging, greater cost and limited availability are the main drawbacks.[16,17]

In recent times, two diagnostic scoring systems for HFpEF, namely H_2FPEF and HFA-PEFF, have been developed to aid in the definitive diagnosis of HFpEF in a patient presenting with dyspnea.[13,18] The H_2FPEF score is a simpler scoring system comprising six components which include the following:

1. *H*eavy [body mass index (BMI) > 30 kg/m^2]: Score 2
2. *H*ypertension (on two or more antihypertensive medications): Score 1
3. Atrial *F*ibrillation (AF): Score 3
4. *P*ulmonary hypertension [estimated pulmonary artery systolic pressure > 35 mm Hg on Doppler echocardiography (echo)]: Score 1
5. *E*lder (age > 60 years): Score 1
6. *F*illing pressures (E/e′ > 9 on Doppler echo): Score 1

A score of 6 or more is highly suggestive of HFpEF.

A score of 2–5 is the intermediate probability for HFpEF and warrants a hemodynamic stress test.

A score of 0–1 makes a diagnosis of HFpEF unlikely.

In contrast, HFA-PEFF (Heart Failure Association Pretest assessment Echocardiography and natriuretic peptide, Functional testing, Final etiology) algorithm is a more complex scoring system that includes four steps in making a diagnosis of HFpEF:

Step 1: The pretest assessment using clinical parameters and standard diagnostic tests such as NPs, electrocardiogram (ECG), and echo

*P*retest assessment:

- Symptoms and/or signs of HF
- Comorbidities/risk factors
- Standard echo

Step 2: The echocardiographic and NP score

*E*cho and NP score **(Box 1)**:

- Comprehensive echo
- NPs

Step 3: Functional testing in doubtful cases which includes diastolic stress testing (exercise stress echo) followed by invasive hemodynamic measurements, if indicated.

*F*unctional testing in case of uncertainty:

- Diastolic stress test (exercise echo)
- Invasive hemodynamic measurements

BOX 1 **Components of echocardiography and natriuretic peptide score.**

- Functional
  - Major criteria:
    - Septal e′ <7 cm/s or
    - Lateral e′ <10 cm/s or
    - Average E/e′ ≥15 or
    - TR velocity >2.8 m/s
  - Minor criteria:
    - Average E/e′ 9–14 or GLS < 16%
- Morphological
  - Major criteria:
    - LAVI > 34 mL/m^2 or LVMI ≥ 149 (males), 122 (females) g/m^2 and RWT > 0.42
  - Minor criteria:
    - LAVI 29.34 or
    - LVMI > 115 (males), 95 (females) g/m^2 or RWT > 0.42 or LV wall thickness ≥ 12 mm
- Biomarker (sinus rhythm)
  - Major criteria:
    - NT-proBNP > 220 pg/mL or BNP > 80 pg/mL
  - Minor criteria:
    - NT-proBNP 125–220 pg/mL or BNP 35–80 pg/mL
- Biomarker (AF)
  - Major criteria:
    - NT-proBNP > 660 pg/mL or BNP > 240 pg/mL
  - Minor criteria:
    - NT-proBNP 365–660 pg/mL or BNP 105–240 pg/mL

(AF: atrial fibrillation; BNP: brain natriuretic peptide; GLS: global longitudinal strain; LAVI: left atrial volume index; LV: left ventricle; LVMI: left ventricle mass index; NT-proBNP: N-terminal prohormone of brain natriuretic peptide; RWT: relative wall thickness; TR: tricuspid regurgitation)

Step 4: Final etiology to exclude HF mimics.[13]
Final etiology:

- Special imaging [cardiac magnetic resonance (CMR), computed tomography (CT), positron emission tomography (PET), scintigraphy]
- Biopsies
- Genetic testing

Major criteria: 2 points each, minor criteria: 1 point each.

Score of ≥5 is diagnostic for HFpEF.

Score of 2–4 is an intermediate probability for HFpEF and warrants further hemodynamic stress test.

Score of 0–1 makes a diagnosis of HFpEF unlikely.

Overall, the H_2FPEF score was shown to be more sensitive, with greater accuracy and discrimination as compared to the HFA-PEFF algorithm.[19]

Heart Failure with Preserved Ejection Fraction Mimics (Table 1)

There are numerous conditions other than HFpEF that can present with symptoms of breathlessness and/or edema. These are collectively referred to as HFpEF mimics and can be subgrouped into noncardiovascular and cardiovascular entities.[20] The noncardiovascular entities which often mimic HFpEF include renal failure, nephrotic syndrome, liver dysfunction, anemia, obesity with peripheral edema, chronic venous insufficiency, lung disorders, primary pulmonary hypertension, and chronic respiratory failure hypoventilation syndrome.[20] These entities can be carefully ruled out using simple laboratory tests and basic imaging techniques. Once noncardiovascular entities mimicking HFpEF are ruled out, emphasis should be made on ruling out cardiac mimics. The most notable cardiac mimics include cardiac amyloidosis, hypertrophic cardiomyopathy, cardiac sarcoidosis, hemochromatosis, Fabry disease, high-output HF, myocarditis, pericardial diseases, and coronary artery disease (CAD).[20]

There are numerous clues to the possible presence of an HFpEF mimic; these include the following:[20]

- Clinically definite HFpEF as assessed by high NPs, high PCWP, and/or HF hospitalization with low H_2FPEF score
- *Presence of Kussmaul's sign*: On inspiration, there is a significant and persistent rise in jugular venous pressure (JVP).

TABLE 1: HFpEF mimics.[3,20]

HFpEF mimic	Clinical clues	Diagnostic evaluation
Cardiac amyloidosis	Progressively lower BP, orthostatic hypotension, bilateral carpal tunnel syndrome, lumbar spinal stenosis, biceps tendon rupture, neuropathy (sensory or autonomic), increased LV wall thickness with low voltage ECG	Monoclonal protein screen, technetium pyrophosphate scan, endomyocardial biopsy (if monoclonal protein screen is positive)
Hypertrophic cardiomyopathy	Positive family history, unexplained LV hypertrophy, LV outflow tract obstruction	Echocardiography with strain imaging, cardiac MRI
Cardiac sarcoidosis	High-grade AV blocks, ventricular arrhythmias despite preserved LVEF (especially if age <60 years), extracardiac disease (pulmonary, ocular, dermatologic)	Cardiac MRI, FDG-PET scan, tissue biopsy (cardiac/extracardiac)
Hemochromatosis	Family history, history of frequent blood transfusions, presence of hepatic dysfunction, diabetes, erectile dysfunction	Ferritin and transferrin, HFE genetic testing, CMR with T2* imaging
Fabry disease	Angiokeratomas, sensory neuropathy, significant proteinuria, echocardiogram with infiltrative appearance with increased voltages on ECG	Serum alpha-galactosidase level, GLA testing, biopsy of affected tissue
High-output HF	Echocardiogram with 4-chamber enlargement and/or increased LV outflow tract VTI	Evaluation of underlying cause of high output state (anemia, thiamine deficiency, cirrhosis, AV malformations, fistulas)
Myocarditis	History of antecedent viral infection, elevated troponin in the absence of CAD, heart blocks and/or ventricular arrhythmias	Cardiac MRI (epicardial or subepicardial late gadolinium enhancement), cardiac biopsy
Pericardial diseases	History of prior cardiac surgery, chest radiation or pericarditis, symptoms of right-sided HF	CMR, right and left heart catheterization to demonstrate RV/LV pressure discordance during inspiration
Coronary artery disease	All patients with symptoms/signs of HFpEF should be evaluated for CAD	Coronary CT angiography, stress testing, invasive coronary angiography

(AV: atrioventricular; BP: blood pressure; CAD: coronary artery disease; CMR: cardiac magnetic resonance; CT: computed tomography; ECG: electrocardiogram; FDG-PET: fluorodeoxyglucose positron emission tomography; HF: heart failure; HFpEF: heart failure with preserved ejection fraction; LV: left ventricle; LVEF: left ventricle ejection fraction; MRI: magnetic resonance imaging; RV: right ventricle; VTI: velocity-time integral)

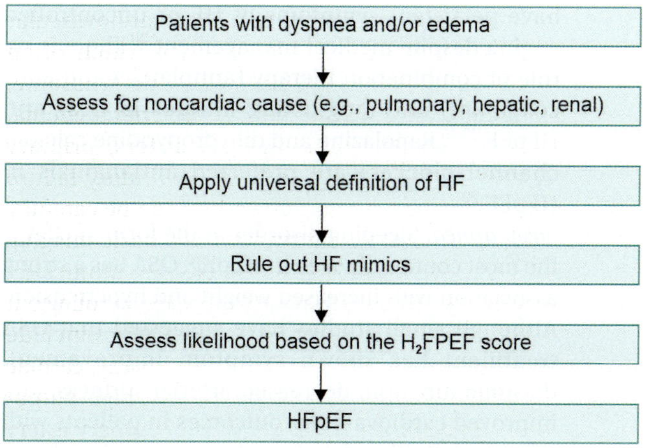

FLOWCHART 1: Diagnostic approach to HFpEF.[20]
(HF: heart failure; HFpEF: heart failure with preserved ejection fraction)

- Low-voltage ECG relative to increased LV wall thickness, LV hypertrophy without a history of hypertension
- Inability to up-titrate or initiate neurohormonal therapy
- History of recently coming off all antihypertensive therapy.
- Known risk factor for infiltrative/restrictive cardiomyopathy
- *Prominent musculoskeletal or neurologic features*: For example, bilateral carpal tunnel syndrome, lumbar spinal stenosis, biceps tendon rupture, significant peripheral neuropathy. The diagnosis of HFpEF should be done in a stepwise approach **(Flowchart 1)**.

TREATMENT OF HEART FAILURE WITH PRESERVED EJECTION FRACTION

Treatment of HFpEF includes nonpharmacological and pharmacological therapies and addressing underlying comorbidities:

- *Nonpharmacological treatment*: This plays a key role in improving functional capacity in HFpEF patients.
    - Exercise and calorie restriction: They have been suggested to facilitate weight loss and improve functional capacity along with exercise tolerance in patients with HFpEF.[21,22] Increase in physical activity, preferably in the form of aerobic activity, e.g., brisk walking for ≥150 min/week (≥30 min/day on most days of the week), is recommended to start with.[23] Aerobic exercise with or without caloric restriction has been shown to improve peak oxygen consumption in a randomized trial involving obese patients with HFpEF.[24]
    - Pulmonary artery pressure monitoring: Implantable devices to assess filling pressures and hence help in the titration of diuretics in HFpEF have been developed.[20] Although the use of device therapy has been associated with a reduction in HF hospitalizations, there have been no absolute reductions in mortality.[20]
- *Comorbidity management*:
    - Hypertension: It is an important comorbidity in patients with HFpEF, with a prevalence as high as 60–89%.[25] Hypertension has a strong association with HF outcomes; inverse with mortality and strong for HF hospitalization.[20] The blood pressure (BP) goal should be <130/80 mm Hg. In patients with labile BP or symptomatic orthostasis, a relatively higher BP should be targeted. The combination of diuretics, angiotensin receptor-neprilysin inhibitor (ARNI), angiotensin receptor blocker (ARB) or mineralocorticoid receptor antagonist (MRA) to be prescribed as per tolerability, comorbidities and recommendations. Beta-blockers due to their negative chronotropic effects often reduce tolerability in HFpEF and should be avoided.
    - Obesity: It is another comorbidity commonly seen in patients with HFpEF. It is strongly associated with hypertension, insulin resistance, dyslipidemia and sleep apnea, and increased risk of HF hospitalization.[26,27] Weight loss using a combination of exercise, caloric restriction, and bariatric surgery has been shown to improve hemodynamics, functional status, and quality of life in HFpEF.[20,28] Although, recently, there has been renewed interest in using glucagon-like peptide-1 receptor agonists (GLP-1 RAs),[29,30] namely semaglutide and tirzepatide, to augment weight loss, these drugs need further studies regarding their safety and potential benefits in HFpEF patients.[29,30]
    - Diabetes mellitus: The presence of diabetes mellitus increases the risk of HFpEF and is associated with an increased risk of adverse cardiovascular outcomes.[31,32] The target glycated hemoglobin (HbA1c) is <7–7.5% in patients with less severe HF or lower comorbidity burden, while in elderly with multiple comorbidities, polypharmacy, and risk of hypoglycemia the target HbA1c <8–8.5% is recommended.[33] Sodium-glucose cotransporter-2 inhibitor (SGLT-2I) is the first-line therapy for patients with HFpEF regardless of the presence of diabetes mellitus in view of improved outcomes (HF hospitalizations and cardiovascular mortality), functional status, and quality of life.[34-36] GLP-1RAs, namely semaglutide and tirzepatide, have shown benefit on cardiovascular outcomes and HF hospitalizations, as well as obesity.[37] These drugs should be considered in individuals with HFpEF and type 2 diabetes mellitus (T2DM) with preexisting atherosclerotic cardiovascular disease (ASCVD) or high risk for ASCVD.[38] Dipeptidyl peptidase-4 inhibitors and thiazolidinediones should be avoided in patients with

HFpEF as these have been associated with increased HF events.[2,39]

- *AF*: AF and HF coexist, and each predisposes to the development of the other. AF leads to pulmonary hypertension, right HF, tricuspid regurgitation, worsening functional status, HF hospitalization, and mortality in HFpEF.[40,41] Rate control should be the first objective in treating patients with HFpEF and AF, which can be achieved with beta-blockers and nondihydropyridine calcium channel blockers.[20] Aggressive rate control is best avoided. If rate control with beta-blockers and nondihydropyridine calcium channel blockers is not adequate or contraindicated, then digoxin may be added.[20] In those with continued symptoms despite adequate rate control or inability to achieve adequate rate control due to intolerance, a trial of pharmacological rhythm control is reasonable.[42] Anticoagulation is to be added to the rate control regimen as per the CHA_2DS_2-VASc score.[2,20]
- *CAD*: It has also been seen associated with HFpEF. Although epicardial obstructive disease is found in nearly half and microvascular dysfunction in over two-thirds of patients with HFpEF, there is very limited data on the impact of coronary revascularization on symptoms and outcomes in HFpEF.[43,44] Revascularization may be an option in patients with acute coronary syndrome (ACS) and HFpEF who have persistent symptoms of HF or uncontrolled angina despite medical management.[20] There is no role of combination therapy (antiplatelet and anticoagulant) and long-acting nitrates in CAD and HFpEF.[20,45] Ranolazine and dihydropyridine calcium channel blockers are preferred antianginals in HFpEF.[20]
- *Sleep apnea*: Sleeping disorder in the form of OSA is the most commonly seen in HFpEF. OSA has a strong association with increased weight and hypertension. Although small studies have suggested that OSA treatment has shown symptom improvement, diastolic function, decreased arterial stiffness, and improved cardiovascular outcomes in patients with HFpEF, definitive data from large clinical trials are lacking.[46,47]
- *CKD*: It is a strong risk factor for HFpEF.[48] CKD is strongly associated with the risk of HF hospitalization and mortality in HFpEF.[49] SGLT-2Is, renin–angiotensin–aldosterone system (RAAS) blockers, and finerenone have all been found to be beneficial in patients with CKD and HFpEF, particularly in T2DM.[50-54]

- *Pharmacological treatment*: Contemporary trials on initiation of guideline-directed medical therapy (GDMT) in patients with HFpEF failed to demonstrate any morbidity and mortality benefit **Table 2**. However, recent trials have demonstrated that few classes of drugs do

TABLE 2: Summary of major RCTs in individuals with HFpEF.

Trial name	Sample size (*n*)	Agent studied	EF entry criteria	Inference
DELIVER[35]	6,263	Dapagliflozin	>40%	18% relative reduction of worsening HF and CV death; 23% relative reduction of HF hospitalizations
EMPEROR-PRESERVED[36]	5,988	Empagliflozin	>40%	21% relative reduction worsening HF and CV death; 29% relative reduction of HF hospitalizations
TOPCAT[55]	3,445	Spironolactone	≥45%	Statistically insignificant reductions in HF hospitalizations, aborted cardiac arrest and CV death (except in North America); 17% relative reduction in HF hospitalizations
CHARM-PRESERVED[56]	3,023	Candesartan	>40%	14% relative reduction of worsening HF and CV death (borderline significant); 16% relative reduction of HF hospitalizations
I-PRESERVE[57]	4,128	Irbesartan	≥45%	Statistically insignificant reductions in HF hospitalizations and CV death
PARAGON-HF[58]	4,822	Sacubitril/Valsartan	≥45%	Statistically insignificant reductions in HF hospitalizations and CV death. A potential benefit observed in lower LVEF subgroup and in women
PARAGLIDE-HF[59]	466	Sacubitril/Valsartan	>40%	Statistically significant reductions in plasma NT-proBNP levels, reduced worsening renal function and increased symptomatic hypotension

(CV: cardiovascular; HF: heart failure; LVEF: left ventricle ejection fraction; NT-proBNP: N-terminal prohormone of brain natriuretic peptide; RCT: randomized controlled trial) improve symptoms, functional capacity, morbidity, and mortality in HFpEF. These include SGLT-2I, MRA, ARNI/ARB, and loop diuretics.[55-59]

RECOMMENDATIONS FOR GUIDELINE-DIRECTED MEDICAL THERAPY IN HEART FAILURE WITH PRESERVED EJECTION FRACTION[2]

- SGLT-2I can be beneficial in decreasing HF hospitalizations and cardiovascular mortality [class of recommendation (COR) 2a and level of evidence (LOE) B-R].[2]
- MRAs may be beneficial to decrease hospitalizations in selected patients with LVEF on the lower end of this spectrum (COR 2b, LOE B-R).
- ARBs may be considered to decrease hospitalizations, particularly among patients with LVEF on the lower end of this spectrum (COR 2b, LOE B-R).
- In selected patients with HFpEF, ARNi may be considered to decrease hospitalizations, particularly among patients with LVEF on the lower end of this spectrum (COR 2b, LOE B-R).

CONCLUSION

Heart failure with preserved ejection fraction is a systemic condition with multiorgan involvement. Although neglected for long, recent times have seen renewed interest and improved understanding of the pathophysiology and management options for HFpEF. Initially believed to be better than HFrEF in terms of morbidity and mortality outcomes, the course of HFpEF is as bad as HFrEF due to missed diagnosis and undertreatment. In current times, SGLT-2I forms the cornerstone of GDMT for HFpEF. However, with ongoing large-scale studies on HFpEF pathophysiology and treatment, we hope to have better diagnostic and therapeutic strategies in the future, which will improve outcomes in patients with HFpEF.

ONLINE REFERENCES

Please scan the QR code provided at the end of the table of contents for References of this chapter.

CHAPTER 50

Heart Failure with Preserved Left Ventricular Systolic Function in Valvular Heart Disease

Girish B Navasundi, Praneeth S, Moukthika KVN

ABSTRACT

The incidence and prevalence of heart failure with preserved ejection fraction (HFpEF) are on the rise with increasing comorbidities and life expectancy. HFpEF can be primary or secondary to valvular heart disease (VHD). Many times HFpEF secondary to VHD is amenable to transcatheter or surgical therapies. Increasing recognition of VHD coexisting with HFpEF confounds the management of primary HFpEF. Identifying cardiac amyloidosis is difficult in aortic stenosis due to common diagnostic features.

Keywords: HFpEF, valvular heart disease, diastolic dysfunction, aortic stenosis, amyloidosis.

INTRODUCTION

Heart failure is defined as the inability of the left ventricle to generate an adequate cardiac output at rest or during exercise while operating at a normal or enhanced filling pressures. The basic problem in diastolic dysfunction is the inability of the left ventricle to accommodate blood volume during diastole at low filling pressures. The result being inappropriate rise in left ventricular (LV) end-diastolic, left atrial, and pulmonary capillary wedge pressures with its associated clinical manifestations. The magnitude of the problem of heart failure has increased in recent years. The incidence and prevalence of heart failure with preserved ejection fraction (HFpEF) is more than that of heart failure with reduced ejection fraction (HFrEF).

According to the European Society of Cardiology (ESC) definition of HFpEF (2016), the diagnosis of HFpEF requires signs and symptoms of heart failure, preserved LV systolic function [defined by the ESC as an LV ejection fraction (LVEF) ≥50% and by the American College of Cardiology (ACC) as ≥40%], elevated cardiac biomarkers [B-type natriuretic peptide (BNP) and N-terminal pro-B-type natriuretic peptide (NT-proBNP)], and echocardiographic features (LV hypertrophy or left atrial enlargement and/or diastolic dysfunction). 1–1.5% of the population is affected with HFpEF with women affected more than men.

The pathophysiology of HFpEF has been understood better in recent years but its relation to valvular heart disease (VHD) is complex. HFpEF has a prognosis similar to or worse than HFrEF with poor quality of life.

PATHOPHYSIOLOGY

Heart failure with preserved ejection fraction is a clinical syndrome which is the result of multiple structural maladaptive remodeling mechanisms.[1] These maladaptive changes will progress over time leading to phenotypic expression of disease **(Flowchart 1 and Fig. 1)**.

HFpEF and Valvular Heart Disease

Background

- Valvular heart disease is associated with abnormal diastolic function of the left ventricle. The presence of diastolic dysfunction secondary to VHD affects clinical decision-making as it affects various diagnostic parameters.
- HFpEF contributes to around 50% of heart failure cases and it is classified into primary and secondary HFpEF based on the etiology **(Flowchart 2)**.
- In general, primary VHD with secondary HFpEF is amenable to surgery or transcatheter intervention. However, HFpEF following left-sided valve surgery is highly prevalent, associated with unfavorable outcomes, and is rarely recognized.

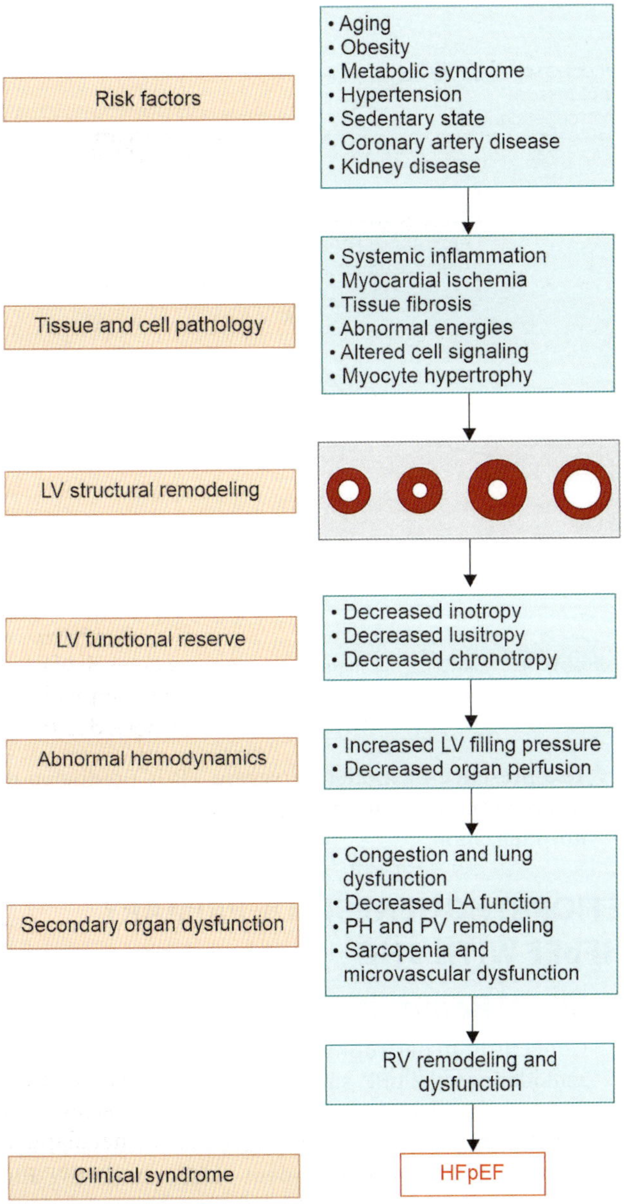

FLOWCHART 1: Pathophysiology of HFpEF.

(HFpEF: heart failure with preserved ejection fraction; LA: left atrial; LV: left ventricular; PH: pulmonary hypertension; PV: pulmonary vein; RV: right ventricular)

- There is an increasing recognition of the existence of secondary VHD complicating primary HFpEF. The mechanisms and best management approach remain to be defined.

Primary HFpEF

Heart failure is caused by impaired diastolic filling but not due to secondary cause, because of interaction with multiple risk factors such as hypertension, aging, systemic inflammatory state, or metabolic disorders without any specific underlying cause.

The primary HFpEF represents a specific phenotype which is usually a middle aged or older individual, mostly women, obese, with history of type 2 diabetes mellitus, hypertension, chronic kidney disease (CKD), and atrial fibrillation.

Secondary HFpEF

Syndrome of heart failure presents as HFpEF but with an identifiable cause. The list of secondary cause could be as follows:

- Hypertrophic cardiomyopathy
- Restrictive cardiomyopathy **(Table 1)**
- *Other forms of cardiomyopathy*:
  - Dilated cardiomyopathy with preserved EF (≥50%) (initial stage).
  - Ischemic cardiomyopathy with large areas of regional wall motion abnormalities and preserved global EF (≥50%).
- *Valvular heart disease*:
  - Aortic stenosis (AS) or insufficiency
  - Mitral regurgitation (MR) or stenosis
- *Pericardial disease*:
  - Constrictive pericarditis
  - Effusive-constrictive pericarditis
  - Pericardial effusion/tamponade
- Tachyarrhythmias (acute)
- *High-output HF*:
  - Anemia (severe)
  - Thyrotoxicosis

Primary HFpEF with VHD

Atrioventricular valve regurgitation with normal leaflet morphology secondary to diastolic dysfunction:

- The most common valves involved in this group are mitral and tricuspid valves.
- Mild-to-moderate MR or tricuspid regurgitation (TR) is frequently observed in HFpEF and is often considered a bystander rather than the cause of HF symptoms.
- Secondary MR and TR in HFpEF is less well defined and limited data exist unlike in HFrEF.

TABLE 1: Restrictive cardiomyopathy.

Increased LV wall thickness	Normal LV wall thickness
Infiltrative cardiomyopathies: • Amyloidosis • Sarcoidosis • Glycogen storage diseases	• Endomyocardial fibrosis • Radiation cardiomyopathy • Hemochromatosis • Idiopathic restrictive cardiomyopathy

(LV: left ventricular)

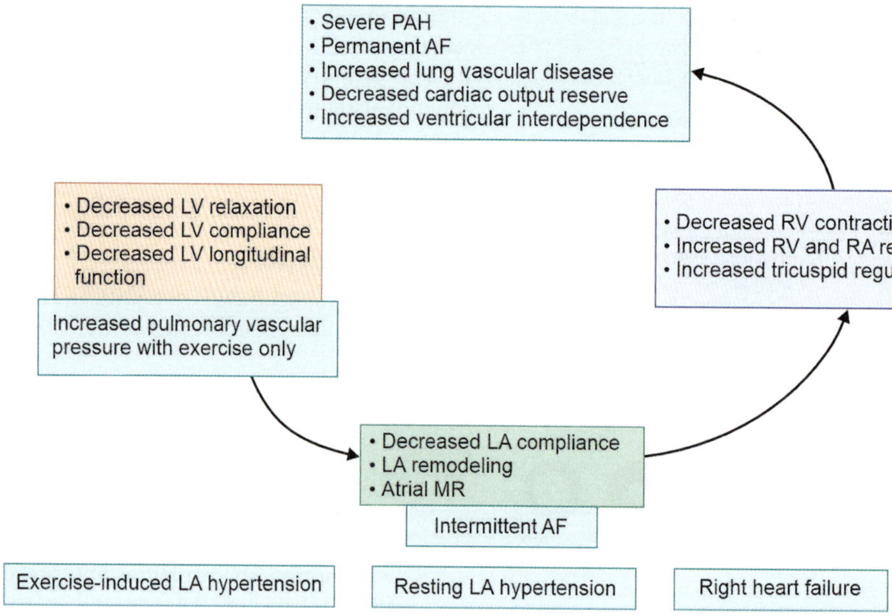

FIG. 1: Temporal progression of HFpEF (spectrum of HFpEF).

(AF: atrial fibrillation; HFpEF: heart failure with preserved ejection fraction; LA: left atrial; LV: left ventricular; MR: mitral regurgitation; PAH: pulmonary arterial hypertension; RA: right atrial; RV: right ventricular)

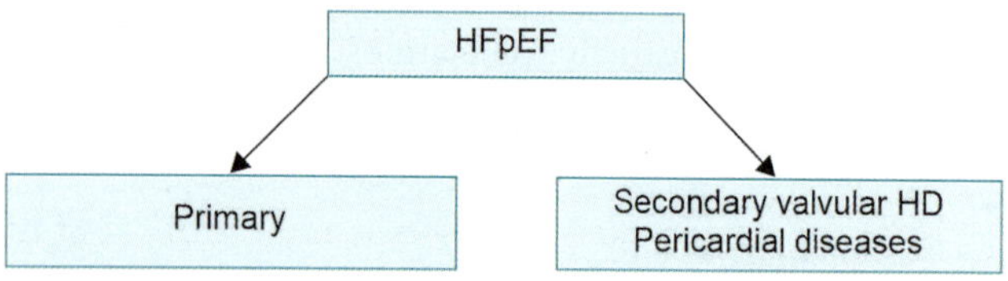

FLOWCHART 2: Types of HFpEF in valvular heart disease.

(HFpEF: heart failure with preserved ejection fraction; HD: heart disease)

EPIDEMIOLOGY

Mitral Regurgitation

- The prevalence of any MR is 60%, and moderate-to-severe MR is 10–15%, with women being more affected than men.
- The incidence and appearance of MR in HFpEF are dynamic. It depends on the hemodynamic status of the patient.[2] Studies have shown that residual MR at discharge was predictive of future cardiac death and/or HF readmission.
- The risk is 2.4 times with an increase in MR by 1 grade on follow-up.
- The risk of HF admission with HFpEF/AF with moderate MR was higher than that of HFrEF with mild MR.

Tricuspid Regurgitation

- The reported prevalence of moderate/severe TR in HFpEF is 9–51%.
- The presence of moderate/severe TR is predictive of worse outcomes such as higher risk of death and HF hospitalization.

ETIOPATHOGENESIS OF PRIMARY HFpEF WITH VHD

Mitral Regurgitation in HFpEF

- Concentric hypertrophy is the primary pattern of LV remodeling in HFpEF, subvalvular leaflet tethering being the major mechanism.
- A primary mechanism of functional MR is mitral annulus dilatation independent of LV remodeling and dysfunction.
- Atrial myopathy has been suggested because MR/atrial dysfunction in HFpEF can occur without atrial fibrillation.
- The longitudinal descent of the posterior portion of the mitral annulus along with the contraction of the longitudinal LV fibers normally has the function to fold the annulus into a deeper saddle shape. Loss of the systolic annular saddle shape is evident in patients with atrial functional MR.

Tricuspid Regurgitation in HFpEF

- The mechanisms of secondary TR in HFpEF most likely involve dilatation of the right atrium and right ventricle with dilation of the tricuspid annulus and subvalvular tethering of the tricuspid valve leaflets.

- Right ventricular dilatation, tricuspid annular dilatation, and tricuspid leaflet tethering may result from any underlying causes of HFpEF that also directly involves the right ventricle (e.g., cardiomyopathy and ischemia) or causes an elevation in right ventricular systolic pressure with pulmonary hypertension secondary to elevated LA pressure/MR associated with HFpEF.
- Whether the TR is the cause or effect of right atrial and ventricular dilation is unknown.

HFpEF Secondary to VHD

The most common VHDs presenting as HFpEF are lesions affecting the aortic and mitral valves and they respond to treatment of underlying cause with valve surgery or transcatheter interventions.

Aortic Valve Disease (Fig. 2)

Aortic Stenosis

- Chronic pressure overload on the LV → remodeling in the form of LV hypertrophy
- Concentric LV hypertrophy is associated with myocardial dysfunction due to abnormal calcium handling, disruption of cellular organization, loss of contractile elements, apoptosis, vascular rarefaction, titin isoenzyme shifts, and fibrosis.
- Four gradient patterns in severe AS with HFpEF are described.[3] They are:
  i. Normal-flow/normal-gradient AS
  ii. Low-flow/normal-gradient AS
  iii. Normal-flow/low-gradient (NF-LG) AS
  iv. Low-flow/low-gradient (LF-LG) AS
- The latter two patterns are classified as paradoxical low-gradient AS, which are present with the clinical syndrome of HFpEF.[4]
- Paradoxical low-gradient AS predominates in older patients and has a higher prevalence of comorbidities which are all characteristics of HFpEF.[5]
- A meta-analysis revealed that 30–50% of the AS population with HFpEF are LF-LG AS and 25–50% are NF-LG AS.[3,6-16] Most of the studies found that LF-LG AS had worse symptomatic status and an increased risk of mortality compared with other subtypes of AS, including moderate AS, NF-LG AS, and high-gradient AS.
- The outcomes of patients with NF-LG AS are similar to those with high-gradient AS and better than patients with LF-LG AS.
- Postaortic valve replacement myocardial mass will reduce due to a reduction in afterload but myocardial fibrosis will persist leading to myocardial stiffness.
- Based on the severity of baseline LV diastolic dysfunction, patients tolerate postprocedure aortic regurgitation (AR).

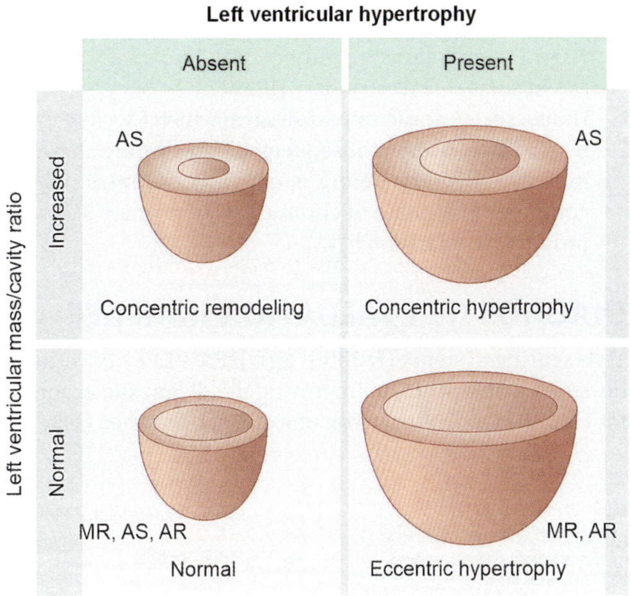

FIG. 2: Morphological changes in valvular heart disease.
(AR: aortic regurgitation; AS: aortic stenosis; MR: mitral regurgitation)

Aortic Regurgitation

- A recent study found that in a group of patients with HF hospitalized for acute HF, mild/moderate AR was associated with increased all-cause mortality in the subgroup of patients presenting with acute HFpEF.
- A possible explanation of the detrimental effect of no severe AR in patients with acute HFpEF is the small LV cavity and increased LV wall stiffness, even a small amount of AR can cause a disproportionately elevated end-diastolic pressure.
- In addition, new echocardiographic markers of early LV systolic dysfunction, including a decrease in the mitral annular plane excursion, systolic mitral annular velocity (s') measured by tissue Doppler, and global LV longitudinal strain measured by speckle tracking, may be helpful for detection of early LV dysfunction when EF is preserved.[17]

Mitral Stenosis

- Mitral stenosis (MS) is characterized by a chronic elevation in LA pressure and underfilling of LV leading to pulmonary hypertension and HF symptoms.
- Because of chronic reduction in preload, 84% of MS patients had an abnormal global longitudinal strain.[18]
- The cause of myocardial dysfunction in MS may be related to the underlying rheumatic inflammatory process, tethering effect by the rigid mitral apparatus, or lack of LV vortex formation.[19]

Mitral Regurgitation

- HFpEF secondary to primary MR (e.g., mitral valve prolapse) is called secondary HFpEF.[20]
- Unlike severe aortic valve disease in which LV concentric hypertrophy occurs consequentially to chronic afterload increase, LV remodeling is typically eccentric in the compensatory phase of chronic severe primary MR with progressive dilatation of LV.

DIAGNOSTIC EVALUATION IN HFpEF

Two scoring systems (H_2FPEF and HFA-PEFF) have been designed with the aim of improving the diagnostic accuracy for HFpEF in individuals with unexplained dyspnea **(Fig. 3)**.

H_2FPEF (Table 2)

This score is derived from invasive hemodynamic exercise testing. It includes:

- Comorbidities [obesity, hypertension (on at least two antihypertensive medications), and atrial fibrillation]
- Age > 60 years
- Measures of LV filling pressures (septal E/e' > 9 and estimated pulmonary artery systolic pressure > 35 mm Hg)

HFA-PEFF (Table 3)

It is an expert consensus algorithm, it includes:

- Biomarker levels
- Echocardiographic measures for diastolic dysfunction and structural abnormalities

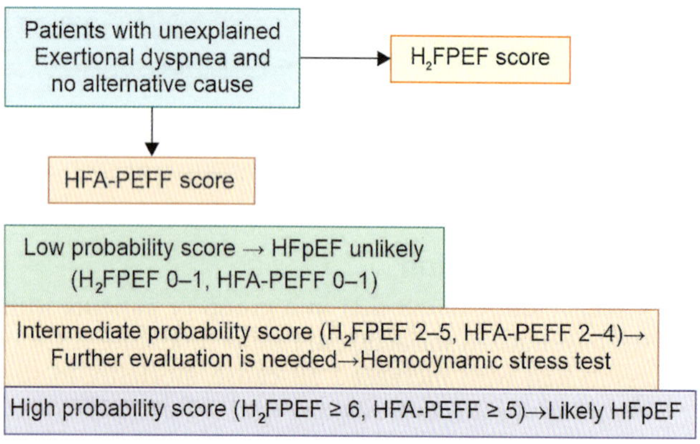

FIG. 3: Algorithm for Diagnosis of HFpEF.
(HFpEF: heart failure with preserved ejection fraction)

TABLE 2: H_2FPEF Score.

	Parameter	Definition	Points
H_2	*H*eavy	BMI > 30 kg/m²	2
	*H*ypertension	≥2 antihypertensive medications	1
F	Atrial *F*ibrillation	Persistent or paroxysmal	3
P	*P*ulmonary hypertension	PASP > 35 mm Hg by Doppler	1
E	*E*lderly	Age > 60 years	1
F	Elevated *F*illing pressure	E/e' ratio > 9 by Doppler	1

(BMI: body mass index; PASP: pulmonary artery systolic pressure)

TABLE 3: Diagnostic algorithm for HFpEF.

	Functional	Morphological	Biomarker (sinus rhythm)	Biomarker (AF)
Major	Septal e' < 7 cm/s or Lateral e' < 10 cm/s Or Average E/e' >15 or TR velocity > 2.8 m/s (PASP >35 mm Hg)	LAVI > 34 mL/m² Or LVMI > 149/122 g/m² (m/w) and RWT > 0.42	NT-ProBNP > 220 pg/mL Or BNP > 80 pg/mL	NT-proBNP > 660 pg/mL Or BNP > 240 pg/mL
Minor	Average E/e' 9–14 or GLS < 16%	LAVI 29–34 mL/m² or LVMI > 115/95 g/m² (m/w) or RWT > 0.42 or LV wall thickness >12 mm	NT-proBNP 125–220 pg/mL or BNP 35–80 pg/mL	NT-proBNP 365–660 pg/mL or BNP 105–240 pg/mL
Major criteria: 2 points		*>5 points*: HFpEF		
Minor criteria: 1 point		*2–4 points*: Diastolic stress test or invasive hemodynamic measurements		

(AF: atrial fibrillation; HFpEF: heart failure with preserved ejection fraction; LAVI: left atrial volume index; LVMI: left ventricular mass index; NT-proBNP: N-terminal pro-B-type natriuretic peptide; PASP: pulmonary artery systolic pressure; RWT: relative wall thickness; TR: tricuspid regurgitation)

MULTIMODALITY IMAGING IN HFpEF (FIG. 4)

Echocardiography is the most crucial and simple modality to identify LV filling pressure and to grade the extent of diastolic dysfunction **(Flowchart 3)**. After confirmation of elevated filling pressures, cardiac MRI is used to characterize tissue morphology, and nuclear scanning is used to identify amyloidosis.

Cardiac MRI provides detailed tissue characterization to differentiate between amyloidosis and other diseases. Characteristic features suggestive of amyloidosis are diffuse late gadolinium enhancement and expansion of the extracellular matrix. Myocardial biopsy will be needed in certain groups of patients for confirmation of diagnosis.

Assessment of LV-filling pressures in special populations **(Table 4)**.

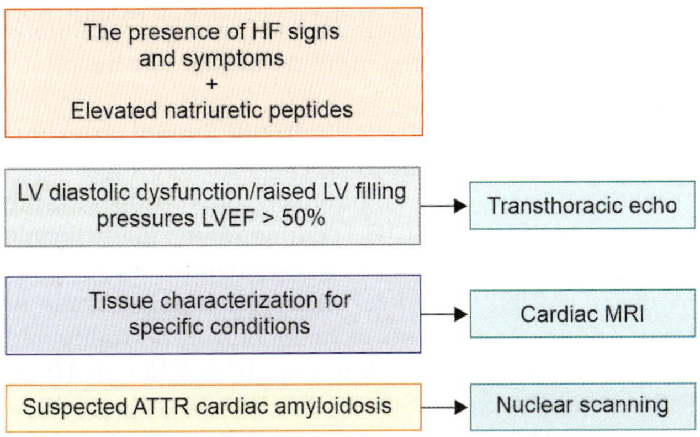

FIG. 4: Multimodality imaging in HFpEF.

(HFpEF: heart failure with preserved ejection fraction; LVEF: left ventricular ejection fraction; MRI: magnetic resonance imaging)

TABLE 4: Assessment of LV-filling pressures in special populations.

Disease	Echo measurement and cutoff
AF	• The peak acceleration rate of mitral E velocity (≥1,900 cm/s^2) • IVRT (≤65 ms) • DT of pulmonary venous diastolic velocity (≤220 ms) • E/Vp ratio (≥1.4) • Septal E/e' ratio (≥11)
Mitral stenosis	• IVRT (<60 ms has high specificity) • IVRT/TE2e' (<4.2) • Mitral A velocity (>1.5 m/s)
MR	• Ar-A (≥30 ms) • IVRT (<60 ms has high specificity) • IVRT/TE2e' (<5.6) may be applied for the prediction of LV filling pressures in patients with MR and normal EFs average E/e' (>14) may be considered only in patients with depressed EFs

(AF: atrial fibrillation; DT: deceleration time; EF: ejection fraction; IVRT: isovolumic relaxation time; LV: left ventricular; MR: mitral regurgitation)

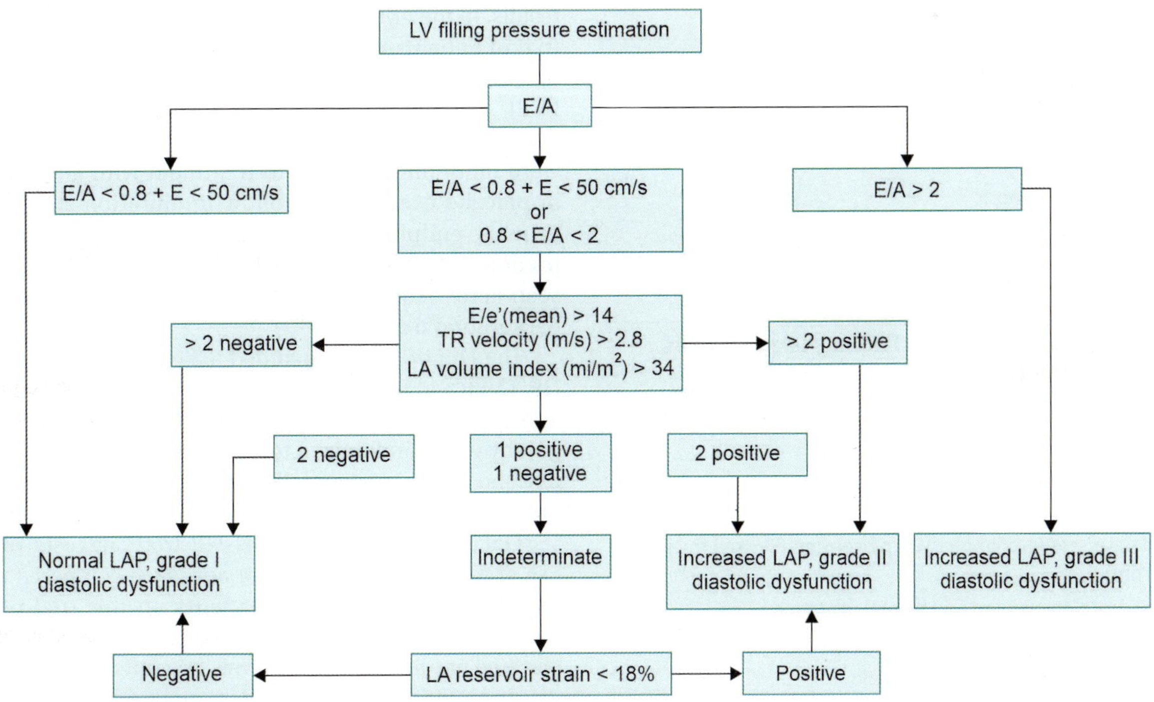

FLOWCHART 3: Echocardiographic assessment of LV-filling pressure.

(LA: left atrial; LAP: left atrial pressure; LV: left ventricular; TR: tricuspid regurgitation)

CARDIAC AMYLOIDOSIS WITH AORTIC STENOSIS

Cardiac amyloidosis is infiltrative cardiomyopathy which leads accumulation of amyloid fibrils in the extracellular matrix of the base of the heart spreading to other parts.

The diagnostic and screening protocols are like those associated with AS **(Box 1)**.

- Electrocardiogram findings suggestive of amyloidosis are low voltage QRS despite LV wall thickening, and abnormal Q waves **(Box 2)**.
- Disproportionate elevation of natriuretic peptide and troponin levels.

In the presence of co-existing amyloidosis, severity of AS is graded according to present guidelines but the high prevalence of low-flow gradient makes it difficult to grade severity.[21-23] Even dobutamine stress Echo fails to confirm the diagnosis, hence, noncontrast CT assessment of valvular calcium is the most practical approach. Thorough screening of amyloidosis is needed for patients with nonsevere AS with recurrent heart failure admissions.

Targeted therapies for TTR amyloidosis, higher heart rate maintenance, anticoagulation, and judicial use of beta-blockers and calcium channel blockers are crucial in pharmacological management.[24,25] Even though small studies outcomes of transcatheter aortic valve replacement (TAVR) were better than surgical aortic valve replacement (SAVR). Patients are at higher risk of complications, pacemaker implantation, and persistent poor quality of life after the procedure.

BOX 1 Red flags of amyloidosis.

- Disproportionate heart failure symptoms with right heart failure symptoms
- Bilateral/unilateral carpal tunnel syndrome
- Lumbar spinal stenosis
- Deafness

BOX 2 Echocardiographic findings suggestive of amyloidosis.

- Disproportionately elevated filling pressure (E/e' > 16) relative to the extent of LV hypertrophy
- Mitral S' < 6 cm/s
- Myocardial granular sparkling
- Moderate/severe pulmonary hypertension, RV wall thickening (>5 mm)
- Atrial septal thickening and biatrial dilatation
- Atrioventricular valve thickening (>2 mm)
- LV global longitudinal strain > –12%
- Apex/basal longitudinal strain ratio > 2
- Severe LV longitudinal systolic dysfunction with apical sparing

TREATMENT

Treatment of cardiac and noncardiac comorbidities is most important.

- Both diabetes and prediabetes have a high chance of hospitalizations in HFpEF, hence well-controlled diabetes preferably with sodium-glucose cotransporter-2 inhibitors (SGLT-2Is) is indicated.
- Screening and treatment of obstructive sleep apnea and obesity
- For patients with atrial fibrillation, a rhythm controlling strategy has to be tried first.
- Avoiding beta-blockers if not indicated because of chronotropic incompetence.
- Diuretics should be optimized according to natriuretic peptide values and symptoms to prevent hospitalizations.

Early randomized trials in HFpEF aimed to export the success of treatment in HFrEF with neurohormonal antagonists including angiotensin-converting enzyme inhibitors (ACEIs) [PEP-CHF (Perindopril in Elderly People with Chronic Heart Failure trial)], angiotensin receptor blockers (ARBs) [CHARM-Preserved (Candesartan in Heart Failure Assessment of Reduction in Mortality and Morbidity-Preserved], I Preserve (Irbesartan in Heart Failure With Preserved Systolic Function)], and mineralocorticoid receptor antagonists (MRAs) [TOPCAT (Treatment of Preserved Cardiac Function Heart Failure with an Aldosterone Antagonist)].

More recent randomized trials of angiotensin receptor-neprilysin inhibitor (ARNI) and SGLT-2Is showed promising results. In the EMPEROR-Preserved (EMPagliflozin outcome trial in Patients With chronic heart Failure with Preserved Ejection Fraction) trial, 5,988 patients with chronic HF, LVEF >40%, New York Heart Association (NYHA) class II–IV HF symptoms, and elevated natriuretic peptides were randomly assigned to treatment with empagliflozin or placebo over median follow-up duration 26.2 months. Primary endpoints showed a 21% reduction which was predominantly driven by HF hospitalizations which were seen across subgroups of diabetes mellitus, age, EF, and background treatment.[26]

The DELIVER trial included 6,263 patients with chronic HF, LVEF >40%, NYHA functional class II–IV HF symptoms, and evidence of structural heart disease by echocardiography were randomized to treatment with dapagliflozin or placebo over a median follow-up of 2.3 years. The primary outcome showed an 18% reduction in the treatment group.

Data from the PARAGON-HF trial suggests that the use of ARNI may be a superior approach compared to ARB monotherapy for selected patients. In this trial of 4,796 patients with NYHA functional class II–IV HF, LVEF 45%, and elevated natriuretic peptide levels, treatment with sacubitril/valsartan was associated with a modest reduction in the primary composite of HF hospitalizations without statistical significance with improvement in quality of life.

As many of the drugs studied in the treatment of HFpEF have resulted in equivocal results, new device-based therapies are studied in small, randomized trials, and preclinical studies. Although none of these devices are approved the testing results are promising. There are four groups of devices such as atrial shunts, LV expanders, electrical and neurostimulators, and MCS devices under evaluation and awaiting FDA approval.

CONCLUSION

With increasing prevalence of population with heart failure, HFpEF is recognized as a major contributor to the problem. The association of valvular lesions with heart failure syndrome especially in population with primary diastolic dysfunction of left ventricle is underrepresented in the clinical context. This association is found to have significant impact on the management of heart failure as there is no single test to diagnose HFpEF and presence of VHD further complicates the treatment. The success of various surgical and transcatheter valvular interventions in patients with HFpEF is reported; however, the appropriate usage of diagnostic modalities for diagnosis and characterization of disease process is necessary for best outcomes. Long-term data and studies are needed especially in special group of population with amyloidosis and multisystem dysfunction as they can impact the outcomes individually. An attempt is made in this article to give a glimpse of some of the confounders in the management of HFpEF spectrum which is challenging and a common presentation in the day-to-day practice.

ONLINE REFERENCES

Please scan the QR code provided at the end of the table of contents for References of this chapter.

CHAPTER

51

Diastology

Pankaj Harkut, Yogesh Kolamkar, Manish Chokhandre

ABSTRACT

Diagnosis of heart failure with preserved ejection fraction (HFpEF) and hemodynamics is evaluated by the assessment of left ventricular diastolic function (LVDF). LVDF can be evaluated by echocardiography. If clinical findings are not available, two-dimensional echocardiogram and specific Doppler indices of diastolic dysfunction, such as mitral annulus early diastolic velocity (E), left atrium (LA) maximum volume index, tricuspid regurgitation jet maximum velocity by continuous-wave Doppler, and the ratio of mitral inflow early diastolic velocity to e' velocity, can be employed to draw conclusions about LVDF. If diastolic dysfunction is present, mean LA pressure and grade of diastolic dysfunction should be assessed. If LA pressure is normal at rest, it is prudent to proceed with diastolic stress testing in an effort to identify patients with dyspnea due to diastolic dysfunction. Special algorithms are recommended for patients with atrial fibrillation, moderate or severe mitral annular calcification, and noncardiac pulmonary hypertension.

Keywords: Diastolic dysfunction, heart failure with preserved ejection fraction (HFpEF), left ventricular filling pressure (LVFP), left atrium (LA) volume index.

INTRODUCTION

Diastology refers to the evaluation of the diastolic function of the left ventricle (LV). In essence, it is just a question of "*how compliant the LV is*"? (evaluating dyspnea). LV filling during diastole ensures the delivery of a normal stroke volume.[1] However, when LV filling is accompanied by an abnormal rise in LV filling pressure (LVFP), diastolic heart failure results.[2] It is important to note that the term "LVFP" fails to distinguish LV end-diastolic pressure (LVEDP) from mean left atrial pressure (LAP) **(Figs. 1A to C)**.

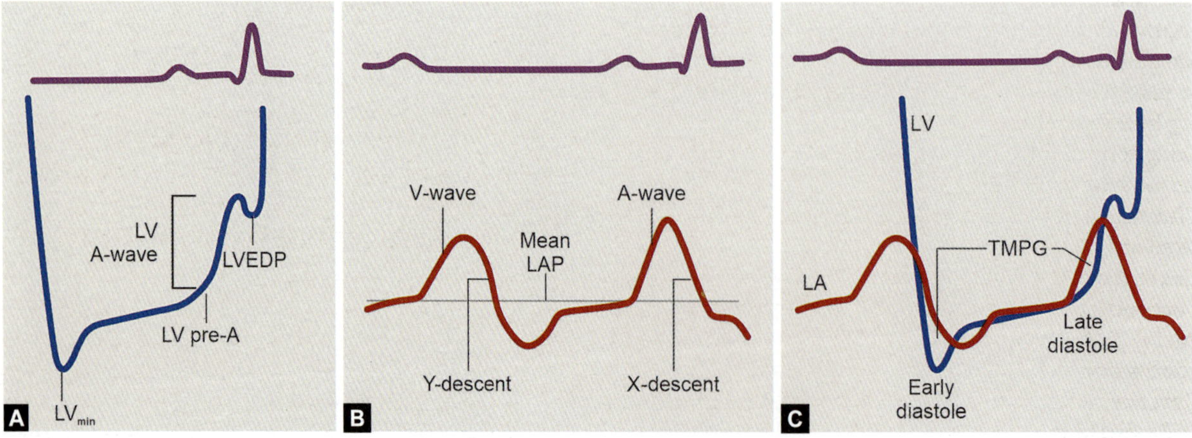

FIGS. 1A TO C: (A) Left ventricular (LV) pressure curve; (B) Left atrial pressure (LAP) curve; (C) Simultaneous LV and LAP curves. (LVEDP: left ventricular end-diastolic pressure; LV_{min}: left ventricular minimal pressure; TMPG: transmitral pressure gradient)

PHYSIOLOGY OF LEFT VENTRICULAR DIASTOLE

Isovolumic Relaxation Period

Between the closure of the aortic valve and the opening of the mitral valve comes the isovolumic relaxation phase. Tau (τ) is the amount of time needed for the LV pressure to drop by roughly one-third from its peak value (immediately after the aortic valve closes) when measured at the peak rate of LV pressure decay.[3] LV relaxation is almost complete by 3.5 times "τ" in a healthy heart, where τ lasts for about 30–40 ms. However, τ lengthens and complete relaxation might not be attained when LV relaxation is hindered. Extreme circumstances can lead to a state of contracture where relaxation may not fully occur at end-diastole.

Rapid Filling Period

The rapid LV filling process starts at the opening of the mitral valve. During this time, three physiological processes take place: Active relaxation, elastic recoil, and ventricular lengthening.

Diastasis

Diastasis is the period between the end of the rapid filling period (RFP) and the beginning of the onset of atrial systole. During this time, the left atrium (LA) and LV pressures remain in balance. As the heart rate increases, diastasis diminishes and disappears at a rate of 90–100 beats/min.

Atrial Systole

In young, healthy individuals with strong LV suction, atrial contraction contributes only 20% of the LV end-diastolic volume, while in elderly patients, it contributes up to 40%.

PATHOPHYSIOLOGY AND CAUSES OF DIASTOLIC DYSFUNCTION

It is not possible to provide a comprehensive analysis of the pathophysiology and underlying causes of heart failure with preserved ejection fraction (HFpEF) here; however, there are some potential comorbidities that may be relevant to their pathophysiology. These include:

- Long-term diabetes and hypertension, which can lead to an increase in LV stiffness
- Chronic kidney disease, which can cause chronic volume overload
- Grade II obesity (body mass index > 35 kg/m^2) leading to concentric remodeling and systemic inflammation
- Atrial fibrillation (AF), which can impede atrial contraction
- Coronary artery disease (CAD), constrictive pericarditis, and valvular heart disease

Patients with HFpEF tend to be older, are more likely to be female, and are likely to have a prior history of hypertension and AF compared to those with HFrEF.[3]

TRANSMITRAL FLOW DOPPLER

Transmitral flow Doppler is the first method applied in the echocardiographic study. Pulsed-wave (PW) Doppler is used to see the transmitral flow. Sample volume should be placed between the tips of the open mitral leaflets in the four-chamber view with alignment (not >20–30°) of the cursor (line of insonation) with the color Doppler LV inflow signal. Normally, E wave is more than A wave with E wave deceleration time (DT) of 160–200 ms.

Delayed Relaxation Filling Pattern (Grade 1)

Delayed relaxation is seen in the elderly with E wave DT >200 ms. The small transmitral gradient (decreased E) associated with delayed relaxation limits early diastolic filling, resulting in atrial residual volume, which is subsequently ejected into the LV during atrial systole. The combined effects of a decreased E wave and an increased A wave usually result in the reversal of the normal E/A ratio. Delayed relaxation is usually associated with normal LVFP (denoted as 1a). Sometimes, LVEDP may be elevated, in which case the designation grade 1b filling is used **(Fig. 2)**.

The steep rise in LV pressure that attends the reduced compliance seen in patients with 1b filling truncates atrial systole and, therefore, shortens the duration of the mitral A wave (A dur). An A-wave DT < 60 ms predicts an LVEDP >18 mm Hg. Lastly, it is important to appreciate that the LA does not usually enlarge, as the compensatory increase in atrial contractility can readily compensate for the increased LA load.[4]

Pseudonormal Filling Pattern (Grade 2)

Pseudonormal filling pattern occurs due to reduction in LV compliance. The reduction in early diastolic LV filling results in an atrial residual volume, which increases LAP. This causes an increase in peak mitral E-wave velocity. A concomitant increase in LVEDP produces shortening of A dur. The combined effects of a rise in E-wave velocity and a decrease in A-wave velocity result in an E/A ratio that is usually >1 (pseudonormalization) with decreased A-wave duration.

Restrictive Filling Pattern (Grade 3)

The transition from pseudonormal to restrictive filling is characterized by a further decrease in LV compliance, an additional increase in mean LAP, and the intercession of atrial failure. Worsening compliance causes additional shortening of mitral E-wave DT (to <160 ms). Continued rise in LAP further increases the peak E-wave velocity, and increased

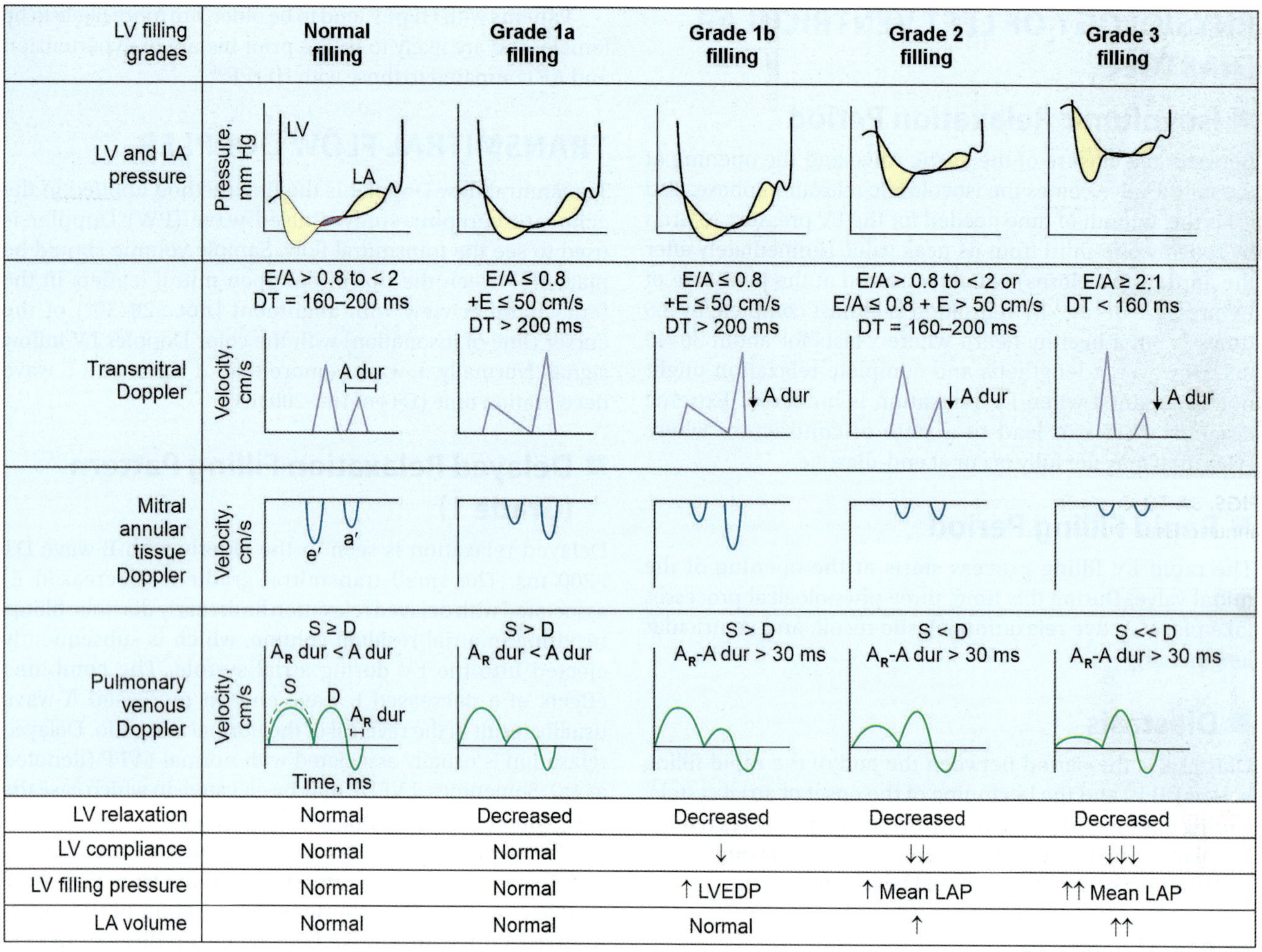

FIG. 2: Characteristic hemodynamic pressure and Doppler echocardiographic findings seen with different left ventricular (LV) filling patterns. (DT: deceleration time; LAP: left atrial pressure; LVEDP: left ventricular end-diastolic pressure)

LVEDP is reflected by a short A dur. The combined effects of the foregoing E- and A-wave changes further increase the E/A ratio. *It is important to note that the filling pattern normally found in healthy individuals < 40 years of age is similar to that found in patients with restrictive filling.* This is due to the large E wave produced by robust diastolic suction, which almost completely empties the atrium during rapid filling.

Grade 4 Diastolic Dysfunction

Grade 3 and grade 4 diastolic dysfunction differ from one another in that grade 3 is reversible. The Valsalva maneuver is employed to distinguish between them. In the strain phase of Valsalva, the intrathoracic pressure rises above the pressure in the great veins, creating a positive intrathoracic pressure that reduces venous return to the heart and, consequently, the preload.

To diagnose the pseudonormal transmitral inflow profile: In patients with a pseudonormal profile (*elevated LAP),* there is a *decrease* in the E/A ratio of ≥50%. Therefore, the Valsalva maneuver can unmask the underlying impaired relaxation pattern.

To differentiate reversible restrictive filling from an irreversible restrictive filling: Preload decrease will cause a reversal of this filling profile to either a pseudonormal filling profile or even an impaired relaxation filling profile when there is reversible restricted filling. The transmitral influx profile is unaffected by irreversible restrictive filling.

ADDITIONAL TRANSMITRAL DOPPLER FINDINGS: L WAVES AND ISOVOLUMIC RELAXATION TIME

L Waves

L waves occur due to abnormal mid-diastolic flow caused by markedly prolonged LV relaxation. They are best appreciated when there is adequate separation of E and A waves or when A waves are absent, as in AF. Those <20 cm/s are not clinically significant **(Figs. 3A to C)**.

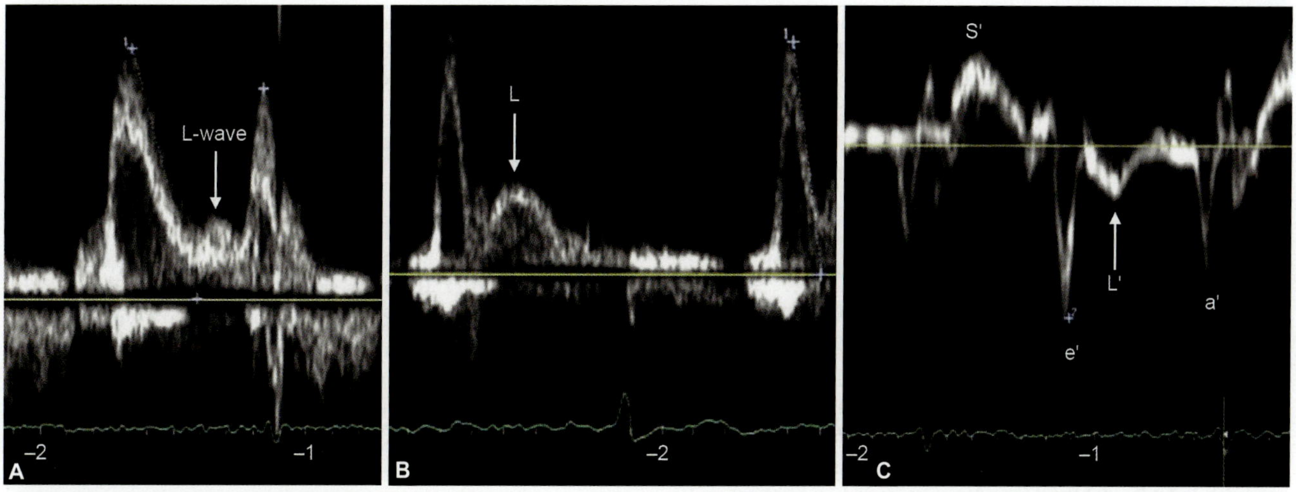

FIGS. 3A TO C: (A) Transmitral Doppler recording of an L wave. (B) Transmitral L wave in a patient with atrial fibrillation (AF). (C) Mitral annular tissue Doppler recording of an L' wave.

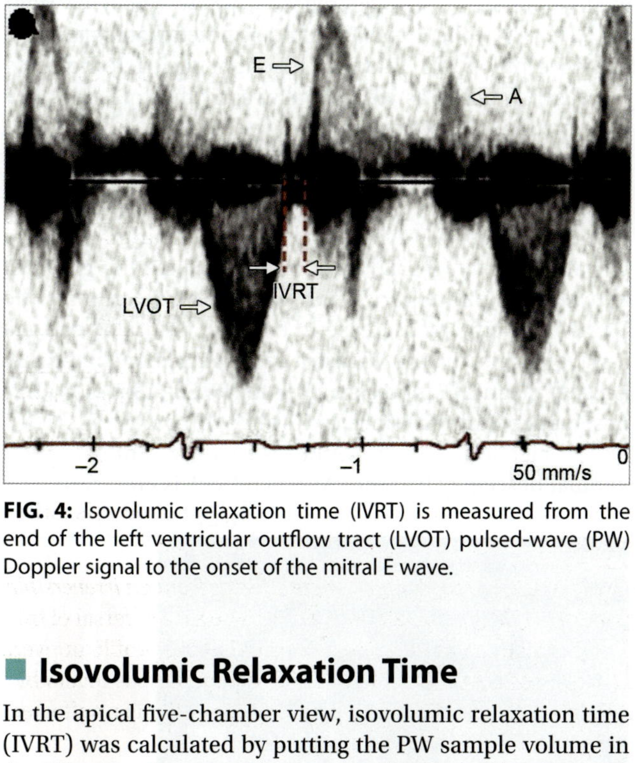

FIG. 4: Isovolumic relaxation time (IVRT) is measured from the end of the left ventricular outflow tract (LVOT) pulsed-wave (PW) Doppler signal to the onset of the mitral E wave.

Isovolumic Relaxation Time

In the apical five-chamber view, isovolumic relaxation time (IVRT) was calculated by putting the PW sample volume in the LV cavity between the aortic and mitral valves **(Fig. 4)**. IVRT prolongation (>110 ms) is the earliest Doppler sign of poor LV relaxation (prolongation of τ) and is observed in patients with grade 1 filling. Due to the longer time needed for LV pressure to reach atrial levels, increased systemic blood pressure can make IVRT longer. The mean LAP is raised if IVRT < 60 ms **(Figs. 5A to C)**. *It should be noted, nevertheless, that fast relaxation seen in young, healthy people can also cause a low IVRT.*

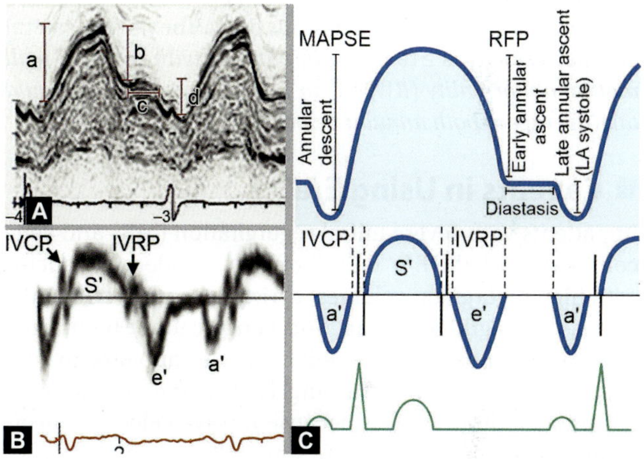

FIGS. 5A TO C: (A) M-mode recording of mitral annular motion. (a) Systolic descent of the annulus (ventricular systole); (b) early diastolic annular ascent; (c) diastasis; (d) late diastolic annular ascent (atrial systole). (B) Mitral annular tissue Doppler recording. (C) Illustration of simultaneous M-mode and tissue Doppler recordings of the mitral annulus.

(IVCP: isovolumic contraction period; IVRP: isovolumic relaxation period; LA: left atrium; MAPSE: mitral annular plane systolic excursion; RFP: rapid filling period)

MITRAL ANNULAR TISSUE DOPPLER

M-mode imaging can be used to track the annular motion by placing the line of insonation across the medial and lateral mitral annulus in the apical four-chamber view. By positioning a sample volume close to the hinge point at the base of the posterior mitral leaflet (lateral annulus) or the base of the anterior leaflet (medial annulus) in the four-chamber view, Doppler tissue imaging is used to assess the velocity of annular motion. This includes an S′ wave (ventricular systole), an e′ wave (early diastole), an a′ wave (atrial systole), as well as biphasic "spikes" before and after the S′ wave that correspond with isovolumic contraction and relaxation, respectively **(Figs. 5A to C)**. The hemodynamic determinants of e′ include LV relaxation, restoring forces, and filling pressure.

Mitral E to Annular e′ Ratio (E/e′)

The LA–LV pressure gradient may be represented by the numerator E as a proxy, and the degree to which ventricular suction is responsible for this gradient is represented by the denominator e′. Patients with low E/e′ ratios (≤9), sometimes known as "suckers," often have normal LAPs, whereas those with high ratios (≥14), also known as "pushers," typically have high LAPs. LAP cannot be measured in patients with E/E′ ratios between 9 and 14. Location affects how normal values for e′ change. Medial annular velocity is much lower than lateral annular velocity (≤7 cm/s), probably as a result of its attachment to the central fibrous body. The normal lateral annular velocity is ≥10 cm/s. *In patients with regional wall motion abnormality (RWMA) in basal segments, one should take average of both annular velocities.*

Caveats in Using E/e′

In patients with severe mitral regurgitation (MR) and vena contracta > 0.4, the E/e′ ratio should be avoided. In patients with high regurgitant volumes, e′ rises, probably due to the increased lengthening load, and hence cannot be utilized to "correct" peak E-wave velocity. E/e′ appears to lose predictive value for increasing LAP in individuals with rheumatic mitral stenosis because E-wave velocity reflects orifice narrowing rather than anomalies of relaxation or compliance. Furthermore, with mitral stenosis, annular e′ velocity decreases, probably due to diminished diastolic rebound of the posterobasal wall induced by the stiffness and tethering of the mitral apparatus. In individuals with considerable mitral annular calcification (MAC), E/e′ should not be employed because mitral E-wave velocity may rise due to diminished mitral inflow area. Furthermore, decreased e′ may represent the local consequences of tissue calcification rather than aberrant relaxation.

In patients with left bundle branch block and right ventricular (RV) or biventricular pacing, the E/e′ ratio fails to accurately predict mean LAP. This is owing to an underestimating of septal e′ as a result of insufficient (i.e., tangential) beam alignment with the septum as a result of paradoxical septal motion. An irregular rocking motion of the LV, documented in individuals with left bundle branch block, may produce an underestimate of lateral e′ for similar reasons in clockwise rotation. In patients with constrictive pericarditis, the E/e′ ratio should not be used to estimate mean LAP. In such cases, calcific pericardial adhesions may diminish lateral e′ velocity, while the velocity of the medial annulus (usually lower) may increase compensatory (annulus reversal). Last, the utility of E/e′ in estimating mean LAP in patients with acute decompensated systolic heart failure remains controversial.

PULMONARY VEIN FLOW DOPPLER

Interrogating the right upper pulmonary vein in the apical four-chamber view typically yields pulmonary vein (PV) Doppler flow data. The names of the PV waveforms are AR, S1, S2, and D. Blood is simultaneously pushed into the ventricle and returned into the pulmonary veins by LA contraction during late diastole. On the Doppler flow recording, the latter traces the AR (retrograde A wave). Early systole causes the LA to relax, which raises the PV–LA gradient. The ensuing PV inflow inscribes the S1 (early systolic) wave. LV contraction causes the plane of the mitral annulus to move apically later in the systole. The LA becomes more compliant as a result of the annulus lowering, which is a reflection of ventricular contractility. The ensuing decrease in atrial pressure also encourages PV inflow, which inscribes the S2 (late systolic) wave. It should be noted that the forward pressure pulse produced by the right ventricle helps to increase LA filling as well. Finally, early diastole (RFP) PV flow into the LA inscribes the D wave **(Fig. 6)**.

Pulmonary Vein S/D Ratio

Pulmonary vein S wave velocity is more than or equal to D wave velocity (S ≥ D) in normal LV. Since the gradient between the pulmonary veins and the LA determines the S-wave velocity, an increase in LAP will naturally lead the S-wave velocity to drop. In fact, it has been demonstrated that a higher mean LAP is present when the PV S/D ratio is <1. This observation is crucial since LAP estimation only works when the LV ejection fraction (LVEF) is reduced. Robust mitral annular descent will lower LAP when LVEF is preserved.

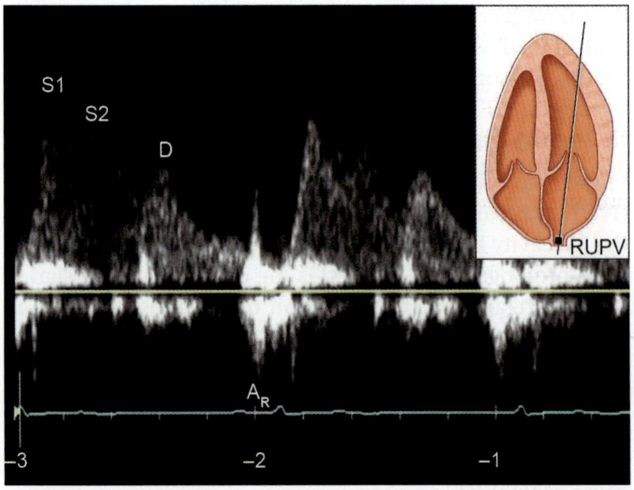

FIG. 6: Pulmonary vein (PV) Doppler recording demonstrating AR, S1, S2, and D waves. This recording is obtained by placing a pulsed-wave (PW) sample volume into the right upper pulmonary vein (RUPV), as shown in the inset.

Caveats in Using the PULMONARY VEIN S/D Ratio

A PV S/D ratio < 1 might not always be able to forecast an increase in mean LAP. As it was already established, it is useless in patients with preserved LVEFs. The relationship between PV systolic filling fraction and LAP has limited accuracy in patients with normal LVEF, AF, mitral valve disease, and hypertrophic cardiomyopathy (HCM).

Duration of PULMONARY VEIN A-wave Flow Reversal (AR dur)

Increase in LV pressure, driven by atrial contraction and LVEDP, is correlated with the interval between the duration of PV flow and mitral inflow during atrial contraction. It has been demonstrated that, independent of LVEF, A_R-A dur > 30 ms accurately reflects increasing LVEDP. It is also accurate in patients with MR and HCM. It can be difficult to interpret in patients with sinus tachycardia or first-degree atrioventricular (AV) block with E and A fusion and in patients with AF.

Diastolic Mitral Regurgitation

Significant elevations in LVEDP may be related to diastolic MR, as detected by transmitral PW recordings. When late diastolic LV operational compliance is severely diminished, blood entering the ventricle during atrial systole can cause LV pressure to exceed that in the LA, resulting in a "puff" of blood regurgitating (diastolic MR). In individuals with increased LVEDP, the B-bump detected on M-mode recordings most likely depicts the regurgitant orifice through which this blood flows.

TE – e′ Time Interval

The time between the QRS complex and the beginning of the mitral E velocity is deducted from the time between the peak of the R wave and the beginning of the e′ velocity. Both healthy persons and patients with mitral valve disease can have their LVFPs estimated using the ratio of IVRT to TE – e′. TE – e′ can be utilized to distinguish between patients with pericardial constriction, in whom the time interval is typically prolonged, and those with restrictive cardiomyopathy.[5]

THE 2016 AMERICAN SOCIETY OF ECHOCARDIOGRAPHY/EUROPEAN ASSOCIATION OF CARDIOVASCULAR IMAGING GUIDELINES

Estimating Mean Left Atrial Pressure

The guidelines advise taking into account both clinical and echocardiographic evidence of diastolic dysfunction. Dilated and infiltrative cardiomyopathy, hypertensive heart disease, and CAD are among the clinical conditions that point to the presence of diastolic dysfunction. Despite the fact that diastolic dysfunction is almost universal in HCM, the algorithm shown in **Flowchart 1** is not advised by the 2016 guidelines. Reduced LVEF, pathologic LV hypertrophy, A_R-A dur > 30 ms, prominent L waves, and decreased global longitudinal strain are all echocardiographic findings that point to the presence of diastolic dysfunction. Another relevant measure is increased LA volume since it accurately represents long-term LAP elevations. "LA volume is the HbA1c of LAP." Increased pulmonary artery systolic pressure (PASP) [tricuspid regurgitation (TR) velocity] is a similarly sensitive marker of LAP that also demonstrates a stepwise increase with worsening LV filling grade.

Finding the mitral E/A ratio is the initial step in using the approach. An elevated LAP (grade 3 filling) is indicated by an E/A ratio > 2. Normal LAP (grade 1 filling) is presumed to exist when the E/A ratio is <0.8 and the peak E-wave velocity is <50 cm/s. It is necessary to count how many of the following LA hypertension criteria are satisfied in order to evaluate

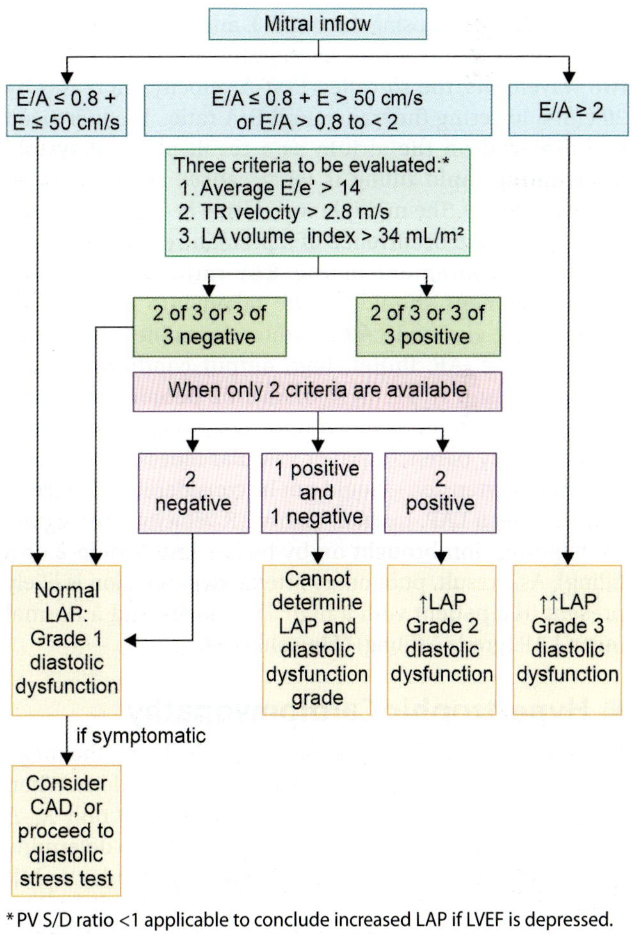

FLOWCHART 1: Algorithm for determining left ventricular (LV) filling grade and mean left atrial pressure (LAP) in patients with reduced left ventricular ejection fraction (LVEF), LV myocardial disease, or clinical evidence of diastolic dysfunction.

(CAD: coronary artery disease; PV: pulmonary vein)

whether people between these two extremes have normal or elevated LAP: E/e′ > 14, indexed LA volume > 34 mL/m², and peak TR velocity > 2.8 m/s (a proxy for elevated PASP) are the three requirements. If two or more requirements are satisfied, grade 2 filling and an elevated mean LAP are present. When there are just two possible criteria for analysis and they are incongruent, mean LAP cannot be calculated.[6]

In some cases, we need to be cautious. These include moderate-to-severe MAC, HCM, pericardial constriction, AF and atrial flutter, left bundle branch block, RV or biventricular pacing, and LV assist devices. More than moderate MR (effective regurgitant orifice area 0.30 cm²), mitral stenosis of any severity, prosthetic mitral valves, and annuloplasty rings are also included.

Caveats in Applying the 2016 Guidelines

Individuals with heart rates > 90–100 beats/min as well as those who have first-degree AV block should be carefully evaluated while determining LV filling grades. The diastasis in both narrows, causing the mitral E and A waves to merge. Peak A-wave velocity rises as the velocity "shared" by the two waveforms, the so-called E-at-A velocity, increases by 20 cm/s, lowering the transmitral E/A ratio. The increased strain placed on the atrium as a result of atrial systole interrupting rapid filling is what causes an increase in A-wave velocity. The multiple waveforms become separated by the fortunate occurrence of a premature beat, allowing precise measurement of the E/A ratio. Additionally, LA enlargement should not be taken into account for determining elevated LAP in athletes, people with mitral valve disease, AF, flutter, high output conditions (such as anemia and hyperthyroidism), or people who have bradycardia. Additionally, TR velocity > 2.8 m/s brought on by pulmonary parenchymal or vascular illness (pulmonary arterial hypertension) should not be considered evidence of elevated mean LAP. Instead, higher TR velocity must signify PV hypertension brought on by higher LAP (grade 2 or 3 filling). As a result, pulmonary arterial hypertension is likely present in a patient with a high TR velocity and a normal mean LAP (grade 1 filling) **(Flowchart 2)**.

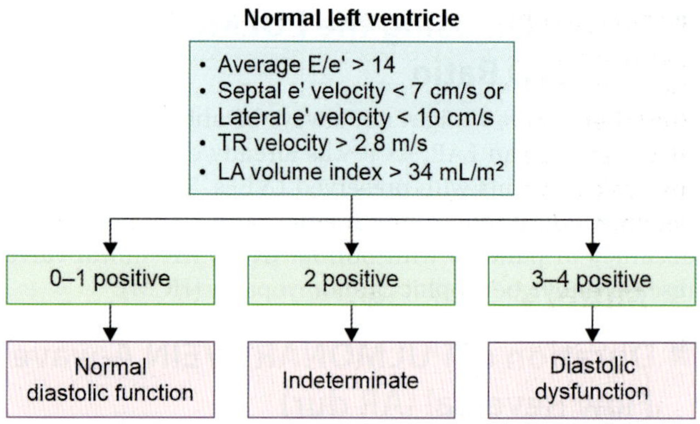

FLOWCHART 2: Algorithm for determining if left ventricular diastolic dysfunction is present in patients with normal left ventricular ejection fraction (LVEF) and no evidence of myocardial disease.
(LA: left atrium; TR: tricuspid regurgitation)

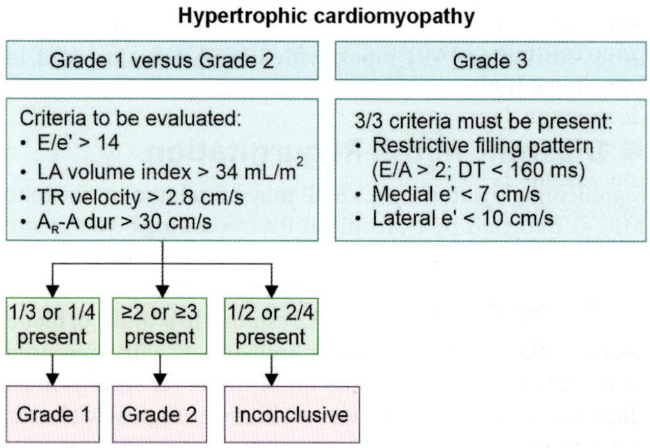

FLOWCHART 3: Algorithm for determining left ventricular (LV) filling grades in patients with hypertrophic cardiomyopathy (HCM). This algorithm may be applied whether or not LV outflow tract obstruction is present. If more than moderate mitral regurgitation (MR) is present, only tricuspid regurgitation (TR) velocity and A_R-A dur may be used to determine LV filling grade.
(DT: deceleration time; LA: left atrium)

Hypertrophic Cardiomyopathy

Flowchart 3 displays an approach for calculating the mean LAP in HCM patients using the 2016 recommendations. When using the method, it is crucial to remember that only A_R-A dur and peak TR velocity > 2.8 m/s can be used to determine the LV filling grade when there is more than moderate MR present.

Atrioventricular Block and Pacing

As long as there is no fusion of the mitral E and A velocities, the variables used to assess diastolic function and filling pressures in patients with first-degree AV block should still be accurate. In the presence of left bundle branch block, RV pacing, and in patients who have undergone cardiac resynchronization therapy, the accuracy of mitral annular velocities and E/e′ ratio is reduced. Only TR peak velocity (>2.8 m/s) can be used as an estimate of LVFPs if only mitral A velocity is present.[5]

Atrial Fibrillation

Peak TR velocities > 2.8 m/s are indicative of elevated LAP. When predicting elevated LV diastolic pressures and unfavorable clinical outcomes in patients with depressed LVEFs, mitral E DT (≤160 ms) has a respectable level of accuracy. Other Doppler measurements can be used in patients with incomplete TR jet, such as the peak acceleration rate of mitral E velocity of ≥1,900 cm/s^2, the IVRT of ≤65 ms, the DT of pulmonary venous diastolic velocity of ≤220 ms, the E/Vp ratio of ≥1.4, and the E/e′ ratio of ≥11. Lack of variation in peak E-wave velocity despite altering RR intervals is another indicator that there is a higher mean LAP in AF.

Mitral Valve Disease

In mitral stenosis, IVRT/TE – e′ < 4 has, however, been shown to predict pulmonary capillary wedge pressure (PCWP) > 15 mm Hg in these patients. In MR (VC > 0.3), parameters that do not reflect increased early diastolic flow resulting from MR are preferred. These include A_R-A dur > 30 ms (increased LVEDP), IVRT < 60 ms (increased mean LAP), and IVRT/TE – e′ < 3 (increased PCWP). If there is presence of moderate to severe MAC, which is characterized by calcification encroaching into mitral opening or covering more than one-third of the circumference of mitral annulus then the E/A ratio continues to be reliable indication of LAP at its extreme, much like traditional algorithm. As a result, a ratio of 0.8 or less denotes normal mean LAP, while a ratio of 1.8 or more denotes excessive mean LAP. Intermediate values (0.8–1.8) necessitate IVRT measurement for additional adjudication, with a value of 80 ms used to distinguish between normal and elevated mean LAP **(Flowchart 4)**.[7]

Noncardiac Pulmonary Hypertension

Peak E velocity, time velocity integral of diastolic flow through the mitral valve, and mitral E/A ratio are all decreased. The lateral E/e′ ratio is often 8 and is compatible with normal LA pressure. Lateral mitral annulus e′ velocity is typically preserved. Given the impact of RV function on septal and average E/e′ ratios in these patients, one should not depend on these measurements.

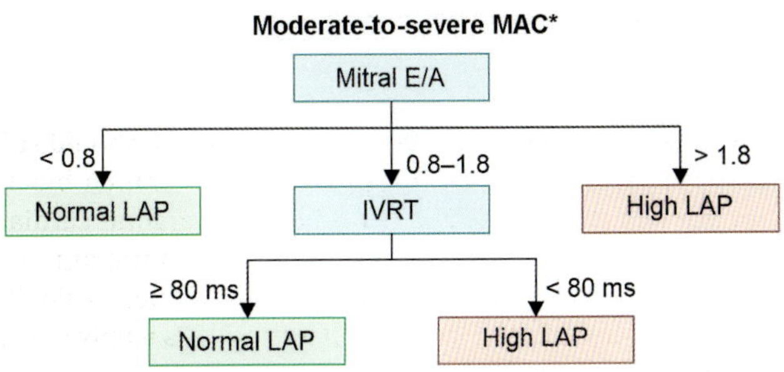

FLOWCHART 4: Algorithm for determining left atrial pressure (LAP) in patients with moderate-to-severe mitral annular calcification (MAC). The algorithm should not be applied when the transmitral gradient is ≥4 mm Hg.

(IVRT: isovolumic relaxation time)

Restrictive Cardiomyopathy

Patients with early disease typically exhibit grade 1 diastolic dysfunction, which develops to grade 2 as the disease progresses. Grade 3 diastolic dysfunction is observed in individuals with severe disease and is characterized by a mitral inflow E/A ratio >2.5, DT of E velocity <150 ms, IVRT < 50 ms, and decreased septal and lateral e′ velocities (3–4 cm/s). Patients with constrictive pericarditis typically exhibit higher septal e′ velocity than lateral e′ velocity, or annulus reversal, and the E/e′ ratio should not be utilized to predict LVFPs in these patients.

Aortic Stenosis and Regurgitation

The guidelines for patients without valvular heart disease can be applied to patients with aortic stenosis, regardless of valvular stenosis severity. Patients with severe MAC are not eligible. Premature mitral valve closure, diastolic MR, LA enlargement, average E/e′ ratio > 14, and TR peak velocity >2.8 m/s are all associated with higher LVFPs in patients with severe AR, whether acute or chronic.

Heart Transplantation

Because donor hearts are frequently sourced from healthy young people, a restricted-looking filling pattern in patients with maintained EFs is a common finding after heart transplantation. There appears to be no single diastolic characteristic that is dependable enough to predict graft rejection. In the absence of pulmonary illness, PASP estimation using the TR jet can be useful as a surrogate measurement of mean LAP.

Diastolic Stress Test

Diastolic stress testing is recommended in patients who have dyspnea and grade 1 diastolic dysfunction. Stress testing on a supine bike or a treadmill is used. At rest, the mitral E and annular e′ velocities, as well as the peak velocity of the TR jet from various windows, should be measured. Because elevated filling pressures frequently remain for a few minutes, the same data are recorded throughout exercise or 1–2 minutes after exercise cessation when E and A velocities are not blended. When all three of the following requirements are met during exercise, the test is considered positive: Average E/e′ > 14 or septal E/e′ ratio > 15, peak TR velocity > 2.8 m/s, and septal e′ velocity < 7 cm/s.[5]

NOVEL INDICES OF LEFT VENTRICULAR DIASTOLIC FUNCTION

Left Atrial Global Longitudinal Strain

Left atrial function, measured as LA reservoir strain, is an important metric in diagnosing LV diastolic dysfunction

(LVDD), grading its severity, and monitoring the effects of treatment. LA volume has been used as a surrogate of the chronicity and severity of LVDD. However, volume is an insensitive biomarker of the early phases of LVDD. LA phasic function can be assessed both by volumetric analysis, using three-dimensional echocardiography, and by strain/strain-rate analysis, using speckle tracking echocardiography. The latter is less affected by loading conditions. Measurement of LA function improves the diagnostic accuracy and prognostic value of both LVDD and HFpEF algorithms. LA strain provides a feasible biomarker of LA function.[8]

CONCLUSION

A comprehensive approach that integrates clinical data and echocardiographic findings is recommended to achieve higher accuracy in estimating LVFP and grading LV diastolic function. The present Euro-Filling study demonstrates that the new 2016 recommendations for assessing LVFP noninvasively are fairly reliable and clinically useful, as well as superior to the 2009 recommendations. Measurement of LA function metrics and exercise diastolic test may improve the diagnostic accuracy and prognostic value of both diastolic dysfunction and HFpEF algorithms.

ONLINE REFERENCES

Please scan the QR code provided at the end of the table of contents for References of this chapter.

CHAPTER

52

How SGLT-2I Changed the Paradigm in the Medical Management of HF?

Amal Kumar Khan, Amartya Khan, Indrani Mandal

ABSTRACT

Heart failure (HF) is a progressive disorder and comprises a broad range of left ventricular function and they are classified as:

- *HF with reduced ejection fraction (EF)*: <40%
- *HF with mildly reduced EF*: 41–49%
- *HF with preserved EF*: >50%
- *HF with improved EF*: Previous EF < 40% and follow-up EF > 40%

Recent guideline of ACC/AHA/HFSA, 2022 which is an update of 2013 and 2017 Focused Update for Management of Heart Failure gives us a 10-point guideline.[1] This new guideline also gives recommendations for select patients of HF with anemia, hypertension (HTN), type 2 diabetes mellitus (T2DM), obstructive sleep apnea (OSA), atrial fibrillation (AF), coronary artery disease (CAD), and malignancy.

Sodium-glucose cotransporter-2 inhibitors (SGLT-2Is) which were originally developed to treat patients of diabetes mellitus as a new class with entirely different mechanisms of action and have a vast range of cardiometabolic and renal effects which have contributed in a great way for management of HF of all classes.

Guideline-directed medical therapy (GDMT) of HF has included following four classes:

1. Renin–angiotensin system inhibitor (RASI) with angiotensin receptor–neprilysin inhibitors (ARNI), angiotensin-converting enzyme inhibitors (ACEIs), and on angiotensin receptor blocker (ARB) alone.
2. Beta-blockers such as metoprolol/carvedilol/bisoprolol
3. Mineralocorticoid receptor antagonist (MRA), i.e., spironolactone/eplerenone
4. Sodium-glucose cotransporter-2 inhibitors such as empagliflozin and dapagliflozin

In this article, we shall highlight the present role of SGLT-2I in management of HF and new terminology such as patients at risk (Stage A) on pre-HF (Stages) are also included.

Keywords: Sodium glucose cotransporter-2 inhibitor (SGLT-2I); heart failure with preserved ejection fraction (HFpEF); heart failure with reduced ejection fraction (HFrEF); heart failure with acute decompensation (HFADH); CVOT: cardiovascular outcome.

INTRODUCTION

Landmark well-conducted cardiovascular (CV) outcome trials have demonstrated that sodium-glucose cotransporter-2 inhibitors (SGLT-2Is) offer benefit in the composite endpoint of CV mortality/all-cause mortality and heart failure (HF) hospitalizations/urgent visits.

Diabetes mellitus (DM) is an established risk factor of cardiovascular diseases (CVDs) like HF. Nearly one in seven people suffering from diabetes mellitus (DM) and CVD come with HF as initial presentation. Others develop HF-related atherosclerotic syndromes.

A meta-analysis and systematic review of randomized placebo-controlled trials of SGLT-2Is in subjects with HF revealed important information.[2]

Fifteen randomized studies with 20,241 subjects were included, 10,594 (52.3%) received SGLT-2Is. All-cause mortality and CV mortality were found to be significantly lower in subjects treated with SGLT-2Is in comparison to placebo. The composite of CV mortality, HF hospitalizations, or urgent visits of HF was significantly reduced with SGLT-2Is in all the subgroups.

Figures 1A and B show the forest plot of all-cause mortality and CV mortality while **Figure 2** shows the forest plot of HF hospitalization. There was 14% risk reduction in

A

Study or subgroup	Log (hazard ratio)	SE	SGLT-2I Total	placebo Total	Weight	Hazard ratio IV, fixed, 95% CI
CANVAS, 2017	−0.3567	0.1612	803	658	7.8%	0.70 (0.51, 0.96)
CREDENCE 2019	−0.0747	0.2141	329	323	4.4%	0.93 (0.61, 1.41)
DAPA-HF 2019	−0.1863	0.0795	2,373	2,371	32.0%	0.83 (0.71, 0.97)
DECLARE–TIMI 58, 2019	−0.1393	0.1289	852	872	12.2%	0.87 (0.68, 1.12)
EMPA-REG OUTCOME, 2015	−0.2357	0.2133	462	244	4.4%	0.79 (0.52, 1.20)
EMPEROR-Reduced, 2020	−0.0834	0.0912	1,863	1,867	24.3%	0.92 (0.77, 1.10)
SOLOIST-WHF, 2020	−0.1985	0.1681	608	614	7.1%	0.82 (0.59, 1.14)
VERTIS CV 2020 EF < 45%	−0.0377	0.2362	319	159	3.6%	0.96 (0.61, 1.53)
VERTIS CV 2020 EF > 45%	0.0139	0.2191	680	327	4.2%	1.01 (0.66, 1.56)
Total (95% CI)			**8,289**	**7,435**	**100.0%**	**0.86 (0.79, 0.94)**

Heterogeneity: $Chi^2 = 3.54$, df = 8 ($p = 0.90$); $I^2 = 0\%$

Test for overall effect: Z = 3.41 ($p = 0.0007$)

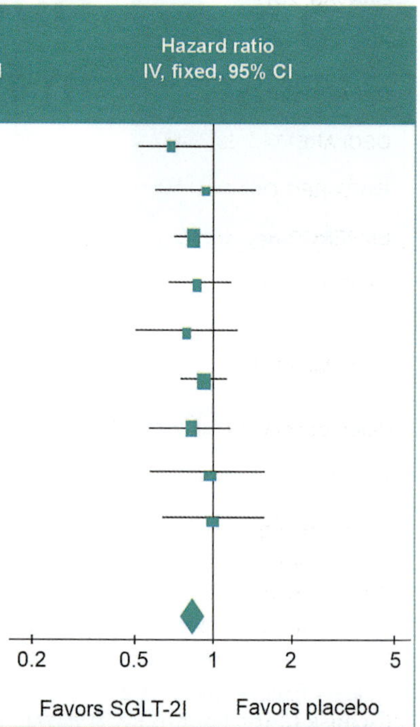

B

Study or subgroup	Log (hazard ratio)	SE	SGLT-2I Total	placebo Total	Weight	Hazard ratio IV, fixed, 95% CI
CANVAS, 2017	−0.3285	0.1777	803	658	8.9%	0.72 (0.51, 1.02)
DAPA-HF, 2019	−0.1985	0.0909	2,373	2,371	34.0%	0.82 (0.69, 0.98)
DECLARE–TIMI 58, 2019	0.01	0.1629	852	872	10.6%	1.01 (0.73, 1.39)
EMPA-REG OUTCOME, 2015	−0.3425	0.2505	462	244	4.5%	0.71 (0.43, 1.16)
EMPEROR-Reduced, 2020	−0.0856	0.1031	1,863	1,867	26.4%	0.92 (0.75, 1.12)
SOLOIST-WHF, 2020	−0.1744	0.1904	608	614	7.7%	0.84 (0.58, 1.22)
VERTIS CV 2020 EF < 45%	−0.0408	0.267	319	159	3.9%	0.96 (0.57, 1 62)
VERTIS CV 2020 EF > 45%	0.0724	0.2639	680	327	4.0%	1.08 (0.64, 1.80)
Total (95% CI)			**7,960**	**7,112**	**100.0%**	**0.86 (0.78, 0.96)**

Heterogeneity: $Chi^2 = 4.13$, df = 7 ($p = 0.77$); $I^2 = 0\%$

Test for overall effect: Z = 2.75 ($p = 0.006$)

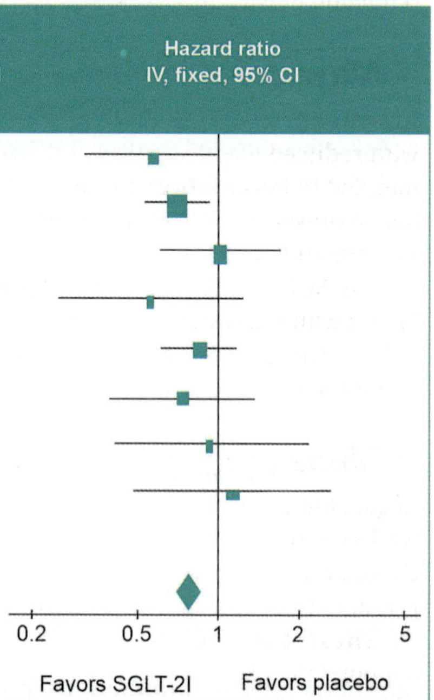

FIGS. 1A AND B: (A) All-cause mortality was significantly lower in the SGLT-2I group and (B) cardiovascular mortality was significantly lower in the SGLT-2I group.

Note: There was a significant 14% relative risk reduction in all-cause mortality among patients with HF treated with SGLT-2Is compared with placebo (OR 0.86; 95% CI 0.79–0.94). B Title: Cardiovascular mortality was significantly lower in the SGLT-2I group legend. There was a significant 14% relative risk reduction in cardiovascular mortality among patients with HF treated with SGLT-2Is compared with placebo (OR 0.86; 95% CI 0.78–0.96).

(CI: confidence interval; IV: intravenous; SGLT-2Is: sodium-glucose cotransporter-2 inhibitors)

Study or subgroup	Log (hazard ratio)	SE	SGLT-2I Total	placebo Total	Weight	Hazard ratio IV, fixed, 95% CI
CANVAS, 2017	−0.6733	0.2168	803	658	5.1%	0.51 (0.33, 0.78)
CREDENCE, 2019	−0.2771	0.2439	329	323	4.0%	0.76 (0.47, 1.22)
DAPA–HF, 2019	−0.3567	0.0869	2,373	2,371	31.7%	0.70 (0.59, 0.83)
DECLARE–TIMI 58, 2019	−0.3188	0.1424	852	872	11.8%	0.73 (0.55, 0.96)
EMPA-REG OUTCOME, 2015	−0.2824	0.2336	462	244	4.4%	0.75 (0.48, 1.19)
EMPEROR-Reduced, 2020	−0.3711	0.0818	1,863	1,867	35.8%	0.69 (0.59, 0.81)
VERTIS CV, 2020	−0.462	0.1831	1,286	672	7.1%	0.63 (0.44, 0.90)
Total (95% CI)			**7,968**	**7,007**	**100.0%**	**0.69 (0.62, 0.76)**

Heterogeneity: $Chi^2 = 2.64$, df = 6 ($p = 0.85$), $I^2 = 0\%$

Test for overall effect: Z = 7.65 ($p < 0.00001$)

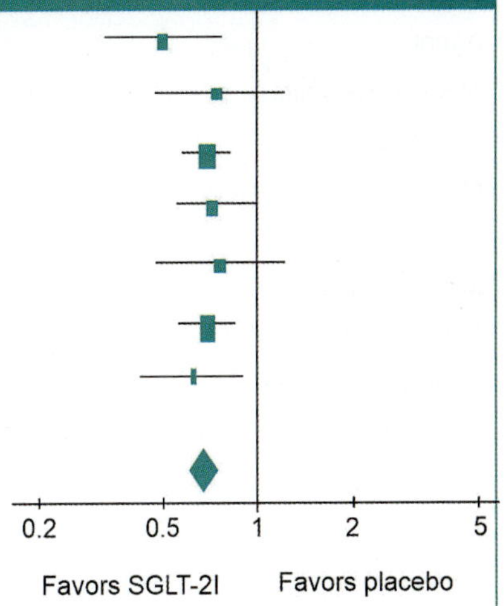

FIG. 2: Heart failure hospitalizations were significantly lower in the SGLT-2I group.

Note: There was a significant 31% relative risk reduction in heart failure hospitalizations among patients with HF treated with SGLT-2Is compared with placebo (OR 0.69; 95% CI 0.62–0.76).

(CI: confidence interval; IV: intravenous; SGLT-2Is: sodium-glucose cotransporter-2 inhibitors)

all-cause mortality and CV mortality and there was 31% risk reduction in HF hospitalization compared with placebo.[2]

Management of HFrEF

In symptomatic individuals with chronic heart failure with reduced ejection fraction (HFrEF), SGLT-2I is recommended to lower hospitalization and CV mortality irrespective of presence of type 2 diabetes mellitus (T2DM) (class of recommendation 1a).

The SGLT-2I also offer advantage in patients with heart failure with mid-range ejection fraction (HFmrEF) and heart failure with preserved ejection fraction (HFpEF) (class of recommendation 2a).

Management of HFpEF

Regarding management of HFpEF or mildly reduced EF, we have two trials such as EMPEROR-preserved[3] (NEJM, October 2021) and DAPA in HF with mildly reduced or preserved ejection fraction (DELIVER NEJM 22).[4]

These two studies provided further evidence that supports the use of SGLT-2I in subjects with HF irrespective of presence or absence of T2DM or left ventricular ejection fraction (LVEF). Both EMPA and DAPA resulted in lower risk of primary composite outcome, worsening HF or CV death, or HF hospitalization. In this clinical scenario, we have limited options and present recommendations of 2a, it is expected to further upgrade in near future.

These two randomized controlled trials in individuals with HFpEF are mentioned in twin table **(Table 1)**.

Green color identifies a Class 1 therapy from clinical practice guidelines, yellow color indicates a Class 2a therapy, and orange color denotes a Class 2b therapy **(Flowchart 1)**.

Another extension of indication of this group of drugs is their role in management of acute heart failure (AHF). AHF is known to be most common cause of hospitalization in individuals > 65 years of age and is associated with significant mortality and poor quality of life.

Management of Acute Heart Failure

A multicenter randomized double-blind 90-day superiority trial was conducted in 530 patients to assess the effect or clinical benefit. Safety and tolerability of once daily empagliflozin 10 mg, compared with placebo, initiated on patients hospitalized for AHF who have been stabilized (EMPULSE).[6] They revealed that starting SGLT-2I empagliflozin in subjects hospitalized for AHF was found to be associated with a statistically significant and clinically meaningful benefit in 90 days when initiated after clinical stabilization (median time 3 days after hospitalization).

These patients reached hospital with a primary diagnosis of acute de novo or decompensated chronic heart failure (CHF) regardless of LVEF or the presence or absence of diabetes.

TABLE 1: Randomized controlled trials in individuals with HFpEF.

	DELIVER[6]	EMPEROR-PRESERVED
Size	*n* = 6,263	*n* = 5,988
Agent	Dapagliflozin	Empagliflozin
Median age, years	72	72
Female sex	44%	45%
Median follow-up, years	2.3	2.2
EF entry criteria	>40%	>40%
Mean baseline LVEF	54%	54%
Proportion with T2DM	45%	49%
HF medical therapy		
Diuretic agent	77%	NR
ACEI or ARB	73%	81%
ARNI	5%	2%
Beta-blocker	83%	86%
MRA	43%	37%
Primary composite outcome, HR or rate ratio (95% CI)	Worsening HF and CV death: HR 0.82 (0.73–0.92)	Hospitalization for HF and CV death: HR 0.79 (0.69–0.90)
Hospitalization for HF, HR, or rate ratio (95% CI)	HR 0.77 (0.67–0.89)	HR 0.71 (0.60–0.83)
Urgent visit for HF, HR (95% CI)	0.76 (0.55–1.07)	NR
CV death, HR (95% CI)	0.88 (0.74–1.05)	0.91 (0.76–1.09)

(ACEI: angiotensin-converting enzyme inhibitor; ARB: angiotensin receptor blocker; ARNI: angiotensin receptor-neprilysin inhibitor; CV: cardiovascular; CI: confidence interval; EF: ejection fraction; HFpEF: heart failure with preserved ejection fraction; HR: heart rate; LVEF: left ventricular ejection fraction; T2DM: type 2 diabetes mellitus)

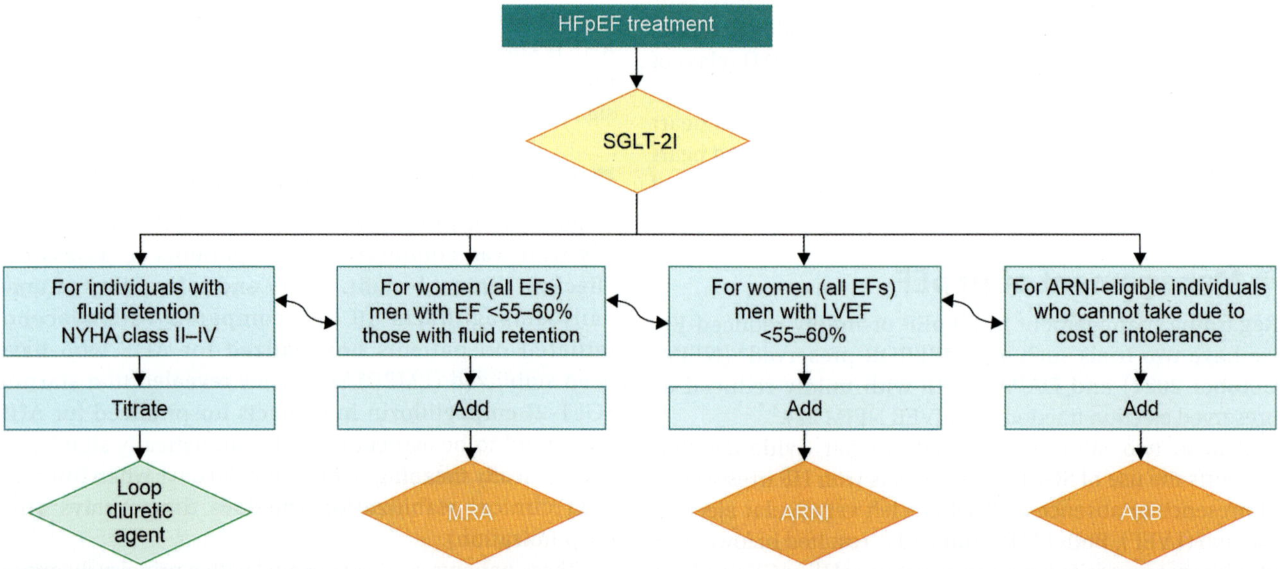

FLOWCHART 1: Proposed treatment algorithm for GDMT in HFpEF.[5]

(ARB: angiotensin receptor blocker; ARNI: angiotensin receptor-neprilysin inhibitor; GDMT: guideline-directed medical therapy; HFpEF: heart failure with preserved ejection fraction; LVEF: left ventricular ejection fraction; MRA: mineralocorticoid receptor antagonist; NYHA: New York Heart Association; SGLT-2I: sodium-glucose cotransporter-2 inhibitor)

CONCLUSION

In the light of recent publications of HF by robust clinical data in all forms such as HFrEF, HFpEF, and AHF, Expert Consensus statement and Guideline-directed Medical Therapy Recommendations have evolved. It is clear that this class of SGLT-2I drugs particularly empagliflozin and dapagliflozin has become the mainstay of treatment along the whole spectrum of HF, regardless of presence or absence of diabetes and without much safety concerns.

ONLINE REFERENCES

Please scan the QR code provided at the end of the table of contents for References of this chapter.

CHAPTER 53

Role of Iron Replacement Therapy in Heart Failure with Reduced Ejection Fraction

Umesh C Samal, Asmita Samal

ABSTRACT

As robustly evidenced in research and randomized trials, iron deficiency (ID) is extremely common[1] and endemic to the whole spectrum of heart failure (HF), i.e., HF with reduced ejection fraction/HF with mid-range ejection fraction (HFrEF/HFmrEF) with or without anemia. While its prevalence is 47–68% in HFrEF,[2] it is slightly higher in HFmrEF and more so in HF with preserved ejection fraction (HFpEF).[3,4] It is well stated in the European Society of Cardiology (ESC) guidelines 2021 that intravenous (IV) iron supplementation with ferric carboxymaltose (FCM) should be considered in all symptomatic patients with left ventricular ejection fraction (LVEF) < 45% and ID [defined as serum ferritin < 100 ng/mL or serum ferritin 100–299 ng/mL with transferrin saturation (TSAT) < 20%] to alleviate HF symptoms, improve exercise capacity, and quality of life (QOL) (Class IIa, Level A). It is recommended that all patients with HF be periodically screened for anemia and ID with a full blood count, serum ferritin concentration, and TSAT (Class I, Level C) and IV iron supplementation with FCM be considered in symptomatic HF patients recently hospitalized for HF and with LVEF < 50% and ID, to reduce the risk of HF hospitalization (Class IIa, Level B). FCM is the only recommended iron therapy at present. Ferric derisomaltose (in the ongoing IRONMAN trial) is evolving as an alternative as it has a reduced incidence of hypophosphatemia and downstream consequences[5] and may even be safer (PHOSPHATE trial) with fewer adverse reactions.[6]

IRONMAN (NCT02642562) trial, recently published in 2022, also complements to the previous randomized trials (with FCM) suggesting a reduced risk of the primary outcome, recurrent hospital admissions for HF and cardiovascular death, providing further evidence of the benefits of correcting Iron deficiency in this population.

Oral iron supplementation has several limitations due to its limited absorption due to gut edema and side effects such as metallic taste, nausea, diarrhea, constipation, and flatulence[8] and is moreover, ineffective, hence not recommended.

The exact mechanism of action of iron in HF is not only hemoglobinization and oxygen transport, but is also inclusive of erythropoiesis, mitochondrial function, electron transport redox reactions, myocardial and skeletal muscle metabolism as enzyme components, immune and nervous systems, inflammatory response, lipid metabolism, and many others.[1]

Keywords: IV iron therapy, outcome, oral iron.

INTRODUCTION

Iron has three functions in the body, principally oxygen carriage as component of the hemoglobin, electron transport in oxidative change reaction mitochondrial function, and deoxyribonucleic acid (DNA) synthesis mostly as prosthetic component of the various enzymes. Thus, iron is vital to the human body and organ system. However, free iron is toxic because of oxidative stress against other components of circulations such as lipid and protein; it always remains bound to protein called ferritin and as a matter-of-fact, ferritin reflects the iron store. Depletion of ferritin reflects the state of iron deficiency (ID). Iron can either exist intracellularly in its ferrous form (Fe^{2+}), where it is stored as ferritin or hemosiderin or extracellularly in its ferric form (Fe^{3+}), where it is circulated bound to transferrin.

As it emerges from different large, randomized trials and registries across, over the last decades, ID is very common in heart failure with reduced ejection fraction (HFrEF) almost nearly 50% or more. ID is recognized as ominous against heart failure (HF) outcome, with high morbidity and mortality and overall prognosis. We do not have large, randomized trials nor registry data in India to substantiate barring some consensus opinion about high prevalence of ID in general populations and HFrEF patients' populations. For study of intravenous (IV) iron in HFrEF, we have to score upon the source of randomized published trials as it is yet to be included in the regular text of cardiology books. More so, it is well illustrated in all the principal guidelines, such as European Society of Cardiology (ESC) guidelines 2021/ American College of Cardiology (ACC)/American Heart Association (AHA) guidelines 2022, without any difference as regard to the level of recommendation of IV iron is IIa in both the guidelines **(Tables 1 and 2)**.

At least four large, randomized trials, such as FAIR-HF (Ferinject Assessment in Patients with Iron Deficiency and Chronic Heart Failure), CONFIRM-HF (Study to Compare the Use of Ferric Carboxymaltose with Placebo in Patients with Chronic Heart Failure and Iron Deficiency), EFFECT-HF (Effect of Ferric Carboxymaltose on Exercise Capacity in Patients with Iron Deficiency and Chronic Heart Failure), and AFFIRM-AHF (Study to Compare Ferric Carboxymaltose with Placebo in Patients with Acute Heart Failure and Iron Deficiency), have shown that IV therapy with ferric carboxymaltose (FCM) reduces the composite risk of first hospitalization for the HF and cardiovascular (CV) mortality as well as the risk of first and recurrent hospitalization for HF, though not on all-cause mortality and CV mortality. It does reduce significantly the signs and symptoms of HF, exercise tolerance, and improvement in functional class and quality of life.

TABLE 1: Recommendations for the management of anemia and iron deficiency in patients with HF.

Recommendations	Class*	Level†
It is recommended that all patients with HF be periodically screened for anemia and iron deficiency with a full blood count, serum ferritin concentration, and TSAT	I	C
Intravenous iron supplementation with ferric carboxymaltose should be considered in symptomatic patients with LVEF < 45% and iron deficiency, defined as serum ferritin <100 ng/mL or serum ferritin 100–299 ng/mL with TSAT < 20%, to alleviate HF symptoms, improve exercise capacity, and QOL	IIa	A
Intravenous iron supplementation with ferric carboxymaltose should be considered in symptomatic HF patients recently hospitalized for HF and with LVEF < 50% and iron deficiency, defined as serum ferritin <100 ng/mL or serum ferritin 100–299 ng/mL with TSAT < 20%, to reduce the risk of HF hospitalization?	IIa	B

*Class of recommendation.

†Level of evidence.

(HF: heart failure; LVEF: left ventricular ejection fraction; QOL: quality of life; TSAT: transferrin saturation)

Source: With permission from McDonagh et al. (2021).[11]

TABLE 2: Recommendations for the management of comorbidities in patients with HF.

COR	LOE	Recommendations
		Management of anemia or iron deficiency
2a	B-R	1. In patients with HFrEF and iron deficiency with or without anemia, intravenous iron replacement is reasonable to improve functional status and QOL
3: Harm	B-R	2. In patients with HF and anemia, erythropoietin-stimulating agents should not be used to improve morbidity and mortality

Note: Referenced studies that support the recommendations are summarized in the Online Data Supplements.

(COR: class of recommendation; HF: heart failure; HFrEF: HF with reduced ejection fraction; LOE: level of evidence; QOL: quality of life)

Source: Adapted from Writing Committee Members; ACC/AHA Joint Committee Members. 2022 AHA/ACC/HFSA Guideline for the Management of Heart Failure. J Card Fail. 2022;28(5):e1-167.

TRANSFERRIN SATURATION CALCULATOR (TERMINOLOGY AND DEFINITION)

Transferrin saturation (TSAT) represents the percentage of iron-binding sites on serum transferrin that are bound by iron atoms. TSAT1 corresponds to the values calculated by the formula TSAT = (Fe/TIBC) × 100, while TSAT2 corresponds to the values resulted by the formula TSAT = (Fe/TF) × 70.9. Where: Fe is serum iron concentration, TIBC is total iron-binding capacity, and TF is serum transferrin concentration.

SERUM FERRITIN

Serum ferritin level is directly related to the amount of iron stored in the body, while ferritin is a protein bound to iron. Low levels of ferritin lead to ID anemia.

We realize in place of the classical calculation of iron requirement by Mentzer formula, it is real-world practice and pragmatic to calculate FCM dose as per kg of body weight as under:

Dosage of Ferric Carboxymaltose

- 50 mg/mL (in 2, 15, and 20 mL single-dose vials)
- Each mL contains 50 mg of elemental iron ≥50 kg

- 750 mg IV in two doses separated by at least 7 days; not to exceed the cumulative dose of 1,500 mg/course
- Alternatively, may administer 15 mg/kg IV as a single dose; not to exceed 1,000 mg <50 kg
- 15 mg/kg IV in two doses separated by at least 7 days

Dosage of Ferric Derisomaltose

- *<50 kg*: 20 mg/kg actual body weight IV infusion
- *≥50 kg*: 1,000 mg IV infusion

Repeat the dose if ID anemia reoccurs (dose expressed in mg of elemental iron; each mL containing 100 mg of elemental iron). IRONMAN and IRONMET (ongoing) trials.

Ferric derisomaltose (FDI) has been shown to be administered in very high doses rapidly and remains well tolerated, hence is an alternative to FCM, with reduced incidence of hypophosphatemia and deranged vitamin D metabolism, which would lead to reduced dietary calcium absorption.[5]

ETIOLOGY AND MECHANISM OF IRON DEFICIENCY

- Iron stores may be depleted due to nutritional deficiency and impaired absorption on account of gut edema or chronic blood loss, i.e., *absolute ID*.
- HF, being a chronic inflammatory state, could lead to an increased release of hepcidin, expressed by the liver as an acute phase reactant type II protein, which could play a major role in iron homeostasis,[9] i.e., hepcidin regulates the degradation of ferroportin, a transmembrane protein which transports iron absorbed after dietary intake from the inside of enterocytes in the small intestine to the bloodstream, and also mediates the release of recycled iron from macrophages in the spleen and liver, i.e., the reticuloendothelial system, thus causing *functional ID*[10] **(Figs. 1A and B)**. This cartoon has well demonstrated hepcidin, anemia, and iron interrelationship.

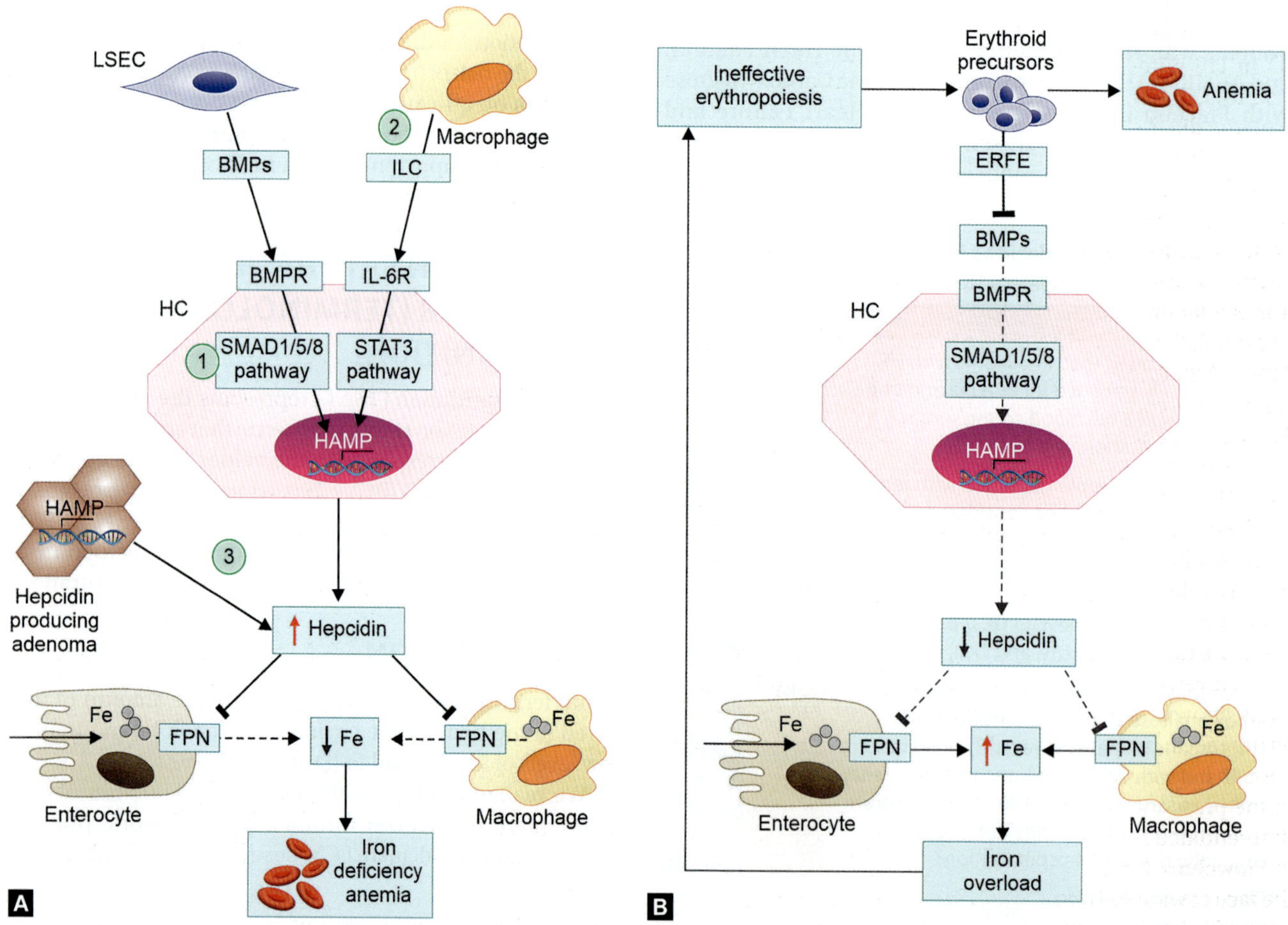

FIGS. 1A AND B: Mechanisms of anemias with (A) high and (B) low hepcidin. (A) Molecular pathogenesis of anemia associated with high hepcidin levels. LSEC produce BMPs. 1—IRIDA, 2—anemia of inflammation, and 3—hepcidin-producing adenoma. (B) Molecular pathogenesis of hepcidin variation in anemias due to ineffective erythropoiesis. ERFE sequester BMPs. Other mechanisms inhibiting hepcidin in this type of anemia, as decrease of transferrin saturation and hypoxia, are not shown.

(BMPs: bone morphogenetic proteins; BMPRs: BMP receptors; ERFE: erythroferrone; Fe: iron; FPN: ferroportin; HC: hepatocytes; IL-6: interleukin 6; LSEC: liver sinusoidal endothelial cells)

Source: Adapted from Pagani A, Nai A, Silvestri L, Camaschella C. Hepcidin and Anemia: A Tight Relationship. Front Physiol. 2019;10:1294.

PRINCIPAL GUIDELINES OF IRON DEFICIENCY AND HEART FAILURE WITH REDUCED EJECTION FRACTION

Needless to say, the definition of ID adopted in different trials is as per the ESC HF guideline **(Table 1)**. It is commonly used in the CV field and comes from the large, randomized controlled trials in HF, comprising to repeat a serum ferritin concentration <100 ng/mL or a ferritin concentration 100–299 ng/mL in combination with a TSAT < 20%. These cutoffs have been derived from the field of nephrology where they performed well as markers of sensitivity and specificity in diagnosing ID and also as targets for iron therapy.[12] Recent studies raise the question of whether this definition accurately reflects the presence of ID, as assessed by bone marrow histology, the "gold-standard" investigation for ID. Would it mean a positive diagnosis as per ferritin concentration, percentage of TSAT in patients who do not have ID, and/or the denial of an ID diagnosis in patients who are otherwise iron deficient.

Bone marrow iron status is not a point of reference of ID in HF guidelines. However, the positive results of IV iron trials in HF might suggest that a valuable proportion of patients diagnosed with ID by using the current definition, are genuinely iron deficient.

In HF patients, it is observed that serum concentrations of transferrin receptor (sTfR), which mediates the endocytosis of transferrin-iron complexes into cells, outperforms serum ferritin concentrations or TSAT in predicting bone marrow iron depletion.[13] Nonetheless, TSAT ≤ 19.8% and serum iron ≤13 µmoL/L both had a sensitivity of 94% and specificities of 84% and 88%, respectively, in predicting ID in bone marrow, whereas the common definition of ID only had a sensitivity of 82% and specificity of 72%.[14]

Serum ferritin may be a poor guide to ID in patients with HF or atherosclerotic heart disease. Indeed, both conditions are associated with chronic inflammation, which increases hepcidin secretion, thus reducing iron absorption but provoking the release of ferritin from cells, similar to troponin release from damaged cardiac myocytes, and therefore uncoupling ferritin from its usual relationship with ID.[15] However, it should also be recognized that the clinical trials showing the benefits of iron have included serum ferritin as an inclusion criteria; we should hence be cautious enough before questioning serum ferritin as a criteria as well. In the presence of very high hepcidin resulting in ID, can be differentiated from the true ID by using the algorithm shown in **Flowchart 1**. It further leads us to workable application in the face of wide ferritin range as per guideline: <100 ng/mL or serum ferritin 100–299 ng/mL with TSAT < 20%.

A point of reference to the EMPA-HEART (Effects of Empagliflozin on Cardiac Structure in Patients With Type 2 Diabetes)[17] trial that enrolled stable patients with type 2 diabetes mellitus (T2DM) and coronary artery disease (CAD) and reported that the rise in hemoglobin following treatment

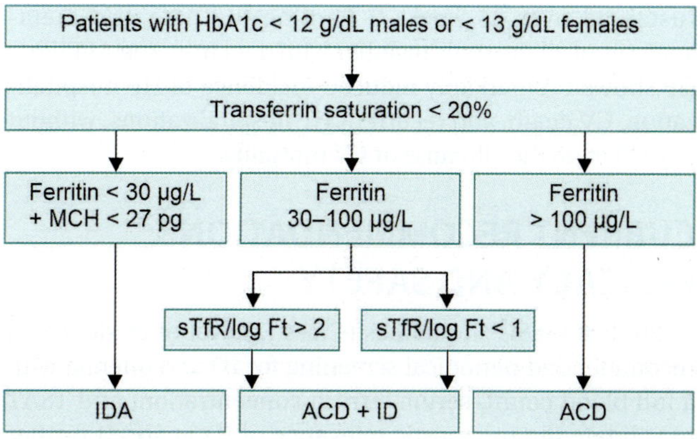

FLOWCHART 1: A simplified algorithm for the diagnosis of iron deficiency.[16]

(ACD: anemia of chronic inflammatory disease; Ft: ferritin; HbA1c: glycated hemoglobin; ID: iron deficiency; IDA: ID anemia; MCH: mean corpuscular hemoglobin; sTfR: serum transferrin receptor)

with empagliflozin was associated with an increase in erythropoietin and a reduction in serum ferritin but no change in TSAT. In a single center, randomized controlled trial enrolling 52 patients with obesity and T2DM, treatment with dapagliflozin for 12 weeks showed increased hemoglobin and erythropoietin (only at week 6) with a parallel reduction in ferritin and TSAT compared with placebo.[18] Whether the decline in ferritin reflects reduced iron availability due to increased red cell production or the anti-inflammatory properties of sodium-glucose cotransporter-2 inhibitor (SGLT-2I), however, is uncertain.[17]

ACUTE DECOMPENSATED HEART FAILURE AND INTRAVENOUS IRON SUPPLEMENTATION

In acute HF, IV FCM or placebo showed a negative result (PRACTICE-ASIA-HF trial), i.e., it did not show any difference across the trial arms in terms of 6-minute walk distance (6MWD) or quality of life at the end of 12 weeks.

Similarly, in the AFFIRM-AHF trial carried out on 1,132 patients with ID with decompensated HF seeking hospitalization with reduced ejection fraction (EF), FCM versus placebo did not show statistically significant difference even after 24 weeks. In terms of the composite of total hospitalization or HF-related CV death, total HF-related hospitalization, first hospitalization, and CV deaths were seen to be significantly reduced, i.e., the first hospitalization by 26% and CV death by 20% with IV FCM. The length of the stay was reduced with FCM as well. As a corollary, in coronavirus disease 2019 (COVID-19)-associated infections, FCM significantly reduced the primary outcome by 25%, CV hospitalization and CV death by 23%, and total HF by 30%.

The treatment with FCM has an early beneficial effect on heart-related quality of life measured by Kansas City Cardiomyopathy Questionnaire (KCCQ-12), which is sustained over 24 weeks.[19] Pooling the data and meta-analyses of all the trials together with data from the AFFIRM-HF showed remarkably reduced incidence of HF hospitalization, CV death, and recurrent HF hospitalizations, without any effect on the all-cause or CV mortality.

CURRENT RECOMMENDATIONS: EFFICACY AND SAFETY

In 2021, the ESC Guidelines (Class I, Level of evidence C) recommended periodical screening for ID and anemia with a full blood count, serum ferritin concentration, and TSAT to validate the prognostic relevance of ID in HF. It further provided a recommendation (Class IIa, Level of evidence A) for use of FCM in symptomatic HF patients with EF < 45% for alleviating patients' symptoms, improving exercise tolerance and quality of life (Class IIa, level of evidence B) and recommendation for FCM in patients with HF recently hospitalized for HF and EF < 50% to reduce the risk of further hospitalization.[11,20]

The ongoing trials consider FCM singularly important in the treatment of HF, regardless of anemia. The ongoing IRONMAN trial may highlight whether the beneficial effect with HF could be extended to FDI. As against iron dextran, nondextran IV treatment, i.e., with FDI seems to be better tolerated without hypersensitivity and anaphylaxis and has a better safety profile.[6] The FERWON program also supports the same, with FDI versus iron sucrose side effect profiles being 0.3% and 0.2%, respectively.[21] The PHOSPHATE (Pragmatic Randomized Trial of High Or Standard PHosphAte Targets in End-stage Kidney Disease) trial also confirms the safety profile of FDI and FCM, i.e., 0.8% versus 1.7%.[6]

Hypophosphatemia is a considerable side effect of FCM. FCM enhances fibroblast growth factor (FGF) production, which is the principal phosphaturic hormone, thus reducing serum phosphate levels, while also decreasing levels of 1,25-dihydroxyvitamin D. Nevertheless, HFrEF combined with chronic kidney disease (CKD) shows a transient increase in serum phosphate levels which normalize within 28 days of FCM infusion.[5] This may be due to HFrEF causing a lower increase in FGF-23 in the presence of kidney disease and assumed deficiency of Klotho protein, which causes an overall decreased tubular sensitivity to FGF-23.[22]

OBSERVATIONS ON IRON DEFICIENCY AND ITS CONSEQUENCES ON THE WHOLE SPECTRUM OF HEART FAILURE

Documented Registry Data

The prevalence of ID has been observed to range between 37–62% in chronic HFmrEF and HfrEF[14,23-25] mostly due to the flexibility of the definition of ID, i.e., ferritin 100–320 ng/mL range[14,23-25] and has been found to be higher in patients with concomitant anemia.[13,24] In the BIOSTAT-CHF (BIOlogy Study to TAilored Treatment in Chronic Heart Failure) trial, it was observed that patients with HF and EF ≤ 45%, 62% had ID, defined as a TSAT < 20%. Of these, 34% had a deficit in iron utilization (serum ferritin concentrations >128 ng/mL) and 66% had low iron stores (serum ferritin concentrations ≤128 ng/mL).[25]

Lower peak oxygen consumption, higher ratios of ventilation to carbon dioxide production, higher mortality and risk of HF hospitalization, and heart transplantation independently of anemia were seen in HFmrEF/HFrEF with ID.[23,24]

Exceptionally and notably, in 42 patients with HF and EF ≤ 45% undergoing coronary artery bypass grafting, 40% had bone marrow ID and a TSAT ≤ 19.8% or serum iron concentrations ≤ 13 μmoL/L, but no decrease in ferritin and were predictive of mortality.[18]

In a French cohort of ~2,800 HF patients, 38% women and 34% men had ID.[3] When observed in the spectrum of HF, i.e., HF with preserved ejection fraction (HFpEF), HFmrEF, and HFrEF, ID occurred in 23%, 24%, and 53% men, respectively, whereas ID was diagnosed in 36%, 30%, and 31% women, respectively.[3] Among those who were diagnosed with ID, 49% received iron supplementation and 80% of whom were treated with IV iron.[3]

In the Swedish HF Registry, ID was observed in 27% patients overall, out of which 29% were in HFrEF, 24% in HFmrEF, and 21% in HFpEF. Remarkably, those who were tested were more likely to have anemia, and in case of HFrEF with more severe HF, they needed specialized follow-up care.[26] Notably, the prevalence of ID was overall 49%; 56% in HFpEF, 50% in HFmrEF, and 48% in HFrEF. 20% had concomitant anemia and 36% had neither ID nor anemia. Iron supplementation with FCM was being given in 19% in the overall ID population and 24% in the HFrEF population.

The prevalence of ID was similar in HFrEF and HFpEF, i.e., 58%, in a longitudinal multicenter study in New Zealand and Singapore, and with higher coprevalence of anemia in HFpEF (56%) versus HFrEF (39%). Importantly, a TSAT < 20% independently predicted all-cause mortality and risk of death/HF hospitalization in HFrEF (EF < 50%) but not in HFpEF. In ~1,200 patients with HF across the EF spectrum, the overall prevalence was 53% (64% in HFpEF, 61% in HFmrEF, and 50% in HFrEF) and ID was associated with a lower VO_2 max, regardless of EF.[27]

In the French CARENFER study, the overall prevalence of ID was 49.6% with 57.5% in HFpEF, 47.4% in HFmrEF, and 44.3% in HFrEF.[28]

Cohorts of Acute Decompensated on Chronic Heart Failure

In ~850 patients hospitalized for acute decompensation of chronic HF, ID was observed in 69% of men and 75% of women. In nonanemic patients, the prevalence was higher in women versus men (79% vs. 57%). In 165 patients with acute

HF, concomitantly low hepcidin, and high sTfR, highlighting severe ID, were found in 37% of the population, associated with more severe HF and low hemoglobin, and with an overall 5% in-hospital mortality.[26]

In another cohort of ~600 patients hospitalized for HF, depleted iron stores but not low-circulating iron was associated with all-cause mortality or HF hospitalization.[29]

In patients with acute decompensated HF, ID was observed in 54% and 56% of patients with HFrEF and HFpEF, respectively, but only in the HFrEF population was it independently associated with longer hospital stay.[30]

INTRAVENOUS IRON THERAPY AND TRIAL HIGHLIGHTS

Table 3 shows randomized landmark trials in HFrEF and the content is self-explanatory.

TABLE 3: Design and results of the randomized controlled trials on iron deficiency in heart failure enrolling >100 patients.

	IRONOUT HF	FAIR-HF	CONFIRM-HF	EFFECT-HF (2017)	AFFIRM-AHF
Patients (*n*)	225	459	301	172	1,108
Duration (weeks)	16	24	52	24	52
Women	36%	53%	47%	25%	45%
Age, median (years)	63	67	69	63	71
Treatment vs. control	Oral IP vs. placebo	IV FCM vs. placebo	IV FCM vs. placebo	IV FCM vs. SoC	IV FCM vs. placebo
Key inclusion criteria					
Acute or chronic	Chronic	Chronic	Chronic	Chronic	Acute
NYHA class	II–IV	II–III	II–III	II–III	I–IV
LVEF	≤40%	≤45%	≤45%	≤45%	<50%
HbA1c (g/dL)	Female: 9–13.5; male: 9–15	9.5–13.5	<15	≤15	8–15
ID definition	Current ESC HF guidelines	Current ESC HF guidelines	Current ESC HF guidelines	Current ESC HF guidelines	Current ESC HF guidelines
Primary outcomes	= peak VO_2	↑ PGA ↓ NYHA	↑ 6MWD	↑ peak VO_2	= Recurrent HF hospitalization or CV death
Key secondary outcomes	= 6MWD	↑ 6MWD	↓ NYHA	= VE/VCO_2	↓ Recurrent CV hospitalization or CV death
	= VE/VCO_2	↑ EQ-5D	↑ PGA	↓ NYHA	= CV death
	= NT-proBNP	↑ KCCQ	↓ Fatigue score	↑ PGA	↓ Total HF hospitalization
	= KCCQ–CSS		↑ KCCQ	= NT–proBNP/BNP	↓ Time-to-first HF hospitalization or CV death
			= EQ–5D		↓ Days lost due to HF hospitalization or CV death
			Time to: = All-cause death = CV death = HF death		
			Risk of first/repeated = All-cause hospitalization = CV hospitalization ↓ HF hospitalization		

Note: aFerritin < 100 ng/mL or ferritin 100–299 ng/mL and TSAT < 20%.

(6MWD: 6-minute walking distance; BNP: B-type natriuretic peptide; CSS: clinical summary score; CV: cardiovascular; ESC: European Society of Cardiology; EQ-5D: European Quality of Life Five Dimension; FCM: ferric carboxymaltose; HbA1c: glycated hemoglobin; HF: heart failure; ID: iron deficiency; IP: iron polysaccharide; IV: intravenous; KCCQ: Kansas City Cardiomyopathy Questionnaire; LVEF: left ventricular ejection fraction; MLHFQ: Minnesota Living with Heart Failure Questionnaire; NT-proBNP: N-terminal pro-B-type natriuretic peptide; NYHA: New York Heart Association; PGA: patient global assessment; SoC: standard of care; TSAT: transferrin saturation; VE/VCO_2: ventilation/carbon dioxide production; VO_2: oxygen consumption; ↑: increase; ↓: decrease; =: no difference)

Source: Adapted from Savarese G, von Haehling S, Butler J, Cleland JGF, Ponikowski P, Anker SD. Iron deficiency and cardiovascular disease. Eur Heart J. 2023;44(1):14-27.

The FERRIC-HF trial is the first trial that randomized 35 patients with chronic HF and ID to IV iron sucrose versus no treatment in a single-blind design. This was a proof-of-concept study, i.e., it included patients without anemia (50%) and this study was the first to use the guideline recommendation-based definition of ID and finally proved an improved statistical trend peak toward VO_2, the gold standard of outcome.[31]

This study paved the path for the FAIR-HF trial, which recruited 459 subjects with HF, such that EF ≤ 40% if New York Heart Association (NYHA) Class II or EF ≤ 45% if NYHA Class III. This trial included patients with hemoglobin ranging 9.5–13.5 g/dL who were randomized 2:1 with FCM versus placebo in a thorough double-blind setting. At 24 weeks, when compared with placebo, FCM had improved PGA (patient global assessment), NYHA Class, 6MWD, and health-related quality of life (HRQOL). There was no difference noted in mortality and other adverse or serious events, regardless of anemia.[32-34] Despite no change in hemoglobin concentration, these benefits were strongly accorded. At 24 weeks, renal function improved, with no interaction between treatment effect and baseline renal function.[35] Body weight was reduced with an early reduction in estimated plasma volume status with FCM, suggesting a reduction in the congested state.[36]

The CONFIRM-HF trial was done on 304 patients with symptomatic HF with <45% and ID, randomizing them 1:1 with treatment with FCM versus placebo over the period of 52 weeks. After 24 weeks, FCM led to 6MWD, improved NYHA class, PGA, quality of life, and fatigue scores. HF hospitalization was reduced by 61% in the FCM arm and no difference was noted in adverse events across all trial arms.

The EFFECT-HF trial randomized 172 patients with EF < 45% and mild-to-moderate symptoms in spite of optimal HF therapy. While in the FCM group, peak VO_2 was preserved; it declined in the control group and FCM significantly improved patients' global assessment and NYHA class versus standard of care.[37] On the other hand, the FERWON-NEPHRO (Iron Isomaltoside/Ferric Derisomaltose vs. Iron Sucrose for Treatment of Iron Deficiency Anemia in Non-Dialysis-Dependent Chronic Kidney Disease) trial conducted in nondialysis-dependent CKD patients administered a single infusion of 1,000 mg of FDI versus up to five doses of iron sucrose was associated with a 41% lower risk of CV adverse events in all patients, with and without HF.[38]

In the IRON-CRT trial, 75 patients with ID and EF < 45% or more or after 6 months of cardiac resynchronization therapy (CRT) implantation were studied and FCM versus standard of care showed a greater improvement in EF and left ventricular end-systolic volume (LVESV) as well as an improvement in the cardiac contractility index slope during incremental biventricular pacing, functional status, exercise capacity, and peak VO_2 with FCM,[39] ID has been considered to be a negative predictor of effective CRT in terms of reverse modeling, clinical course, and response.[40]

A NEW FINDING

Intravenous iron therapy improves the hypercapnic ventilatory response and sleep-disordered breathing in HFrEF.[41] The mechanisms underlying this involve chemoreflex sensing and resetting nocturnal breathing patterns, resulting in improved oxygen delivery to exercising muscles which are likely to contribute to the effects of IV FCM in patients with ID and anemia with HF. It could be partially attributable to improvements in the hypercapnic ventilatory response and sleep-disordered breathing. This is a new finding. However, this is also reflected in ACC/AHA guideline 2022, largely untrodden arena.

ORAL IRON SUPPLEMENTATION

In the IRONOUT HF (Iron Repletion Effects on Oxygen Uptake in Heart Failure) trial, when 225 patients with HFrEF and ID were administered with oral iron polysaccharide versus placebo for 16 weeks, changes in peak VO_2 but no other benefits were observed.[42] This illusional finding could be due to: (1) a very short trial time,[43] (2) inclusion of more nonanemic patients than anemic patients, and (3) nonadherence to the guideline recommendation mentioned in the "criteria of inclusion."

However, as a proof of concept, a nonrandomized study, showed an increase in serum iron ferritin and hemoglobin along with quality-of-life measures such as KCCQ at 3 and 6 monthly follow-ups, suggesting that the potential use for oral iron in the setting would not be recommended.[44]

Interestingly, in a population of 15 patients with HFrEF and 15 with HFpEF, the increase in plasma iron 2 hours after supplementation with oral ferroglycine sulfate complex was almost twofold higher when compared with 12 control subjects without HF and ID, and no difference was observed across the EF spectrum,[45] which might lead to question if limited absorption has as a major role as a key mechanism for ID in HF. Alternatively, it might be hypothesized that ferroglycine, by having a good iron availability, could bypass the hepcidin block on iron absorption.

LONG-TERM SAFETY

However, the bottom line is that long-term safety with FCM is yet to be assured.

Four randomized controlled trials are ongoing and are being done on 839 patients with HFrEF and ID, 504 of whom were randomized to IV ferric carboxymaltose versus placebo. These, so far, suggest that short-term (mean follow-up at 32 weeks) treatment could also reduce HF hospitalizations when compared with placebo.

However, the analysis includes very few CV (n = 34) or other (n = 4) deaths. Even so, long-term safety is not ensured.[46] All upcoming trials are enlisted in **Table 4**,[7,47] which may throw light on this issue and would reveal new frontiers, while confirming to the randomized studies or otherwise.

TABLE 4: Upcoming randomized controlled trials on iron deficiency in HF.

Trials	Key selection criteria									
	n	Iron preparation	Placebo	NYHA	LVEF	Acute or chronic	HbA1c (g/dL)	Definition of ID	Other key selection criteria	Primary outcome
FAIR-HF2 (NCT03036462), phase 4, double blind	1,200	IV FCM	Yes	II–IV	≤45%	Chronic	9.5–14.0	Current ESC HF guidelines	–	Composite of recurrent HF hospitalization and CV death
IRONMAN (NCT02642562), phase 4, unblind	1,160	IV FDI	No	II–IV and recent HF hospitalization or raised NPs	≤45%	Chronic	Female: 9–13; male: 9–14	Ferritin < 100 or TSAT < 20%	–	Composite of CV mortality of HF hospitalization (first and recurrent)
FAIR-HFpEF (NCT03074591), phase 2	200	IV FCM	Yes	II–III	≥45%	Chronic	9–14	Current ESC HF guidelines	• HF hospitalization within 12 months or raised NPs • Diastolic dysfunction • Diuretic use • 6MWD < 450 m	Δ 6MWD
IRONMET-HFpEF (NCT04945707), phase 4, double blind	70	IV FDI	Yes	II–IV	≥50%	Chronic	Female: 9.0–13.5; male: 9.0–14.0	Current ESC HF guidelines	Raised NPs or PCWP ≥ 15 mm Hg or PCWP/CO ≥ 2.0 mm Hg/L/min	Δ peak VO_2
IV Iron in Acute Decompensated Heart Failure (NCT04063033), phase 4	200	IV FG	No	–	–	Acute	8–14	Current ESC HF guidelines	• Raised NPs • Signs of congestion • IV diuretics	6MWD at follow-up
HEART-FID (NCT03037931), phase 3	3,068	IV FCM	Yes	II–IV	≤40%	Chronic	Female: 9.0–13.5; male: 9.0–15.0	Current ESC HF guidelines	HF hospitalization within 12 months or raised NPs	Hierarchical composite of death and HF hosp and Δ 6MWD

Note: aFerritin < 100 ng/mL or ferritin 100–299 ng/mL and TSAT < 20%.

(6MWD: 6-minute walking distance; CO: cardiac output; CV: cardiovascular; EF: ejection fraction; ESC: European Society of Cardiology; FCM: ferric carboxymaltose; FDI: ferric derisomaltose; FG: ferri gluconate complex; HbA1c: glycated hemoglobin; HF: heart failure; ID: iron deficiency; IV: intravenous; LVEF: left ventricular ejection fraction; NP: natriuretic peptide; NYHA: New York Heart Association; PCWP: pulmonary capillary wedge pressure; TSAT: transferrin saturation; VO_2: oxygen consumption)

CONCLUSION

Up to 50% of patients with HF have ID with or without anemia. ID is associated with adverse outcomes, even in the absence of anemia, and is a potential target for treatment.[48] Due to the lack of large-scale use of IV iron, this is a missed opportunity, completely left out of sight. IV FCM in HFrEF improves signs and symptoms in NYHA class and has demonstrated statistically significant improvements in global health status, exercise status, and functional class. Contrarily, one has to realize that oral iron is cheap and widely available, but a very small amount of iron can be absorbed in a day (perhaps 2–10 mg/day compared with a total deficiency of >1,000 mg), thus making the therapy time-consuming. It may improve anemia but is highly unlikely to affect the iron status and compete with the benefits from IV iron.

Anemia and ID are two different entities, although ID with anemia is double trouble in terms of the outcome. In severe HFrEF, ID is singularly disastrous. In the context of randomized trials and recommendations from guidelines, FCM is ready for frontline application in terms of both safety and outcome.

The final word regarding FCM is yet to be said with respect to HFrEF, particularly on the aspects prolonged use and perhaps will surface in the outcome of HEART-FID (NCT03037931) and IRONMAN (UK) trial, currently in phase 3, involving 3,068 cases with chronic HFrEF, Classes II–IV, EF ≤ 40%, and anemia (9.0–13.5g/dL in women and 9.0–15.0 g/dL in men). This trial utilizes the definition of ID as per the ESC HF guidelines, while the key selection criteria is also inclusive of patients with HF hospitalizations within 12 months of hospitalization, and/or raised natriuretic peptide levels, thus finally aiming at primary outcomes such as the hierarchical composite of death and HF hospitalization and Δ6MWD.

Final Note

Risk for the CV outcomes with IV iron versus placebo is cited: Graham et al. (2021)[7] (pooling data from seven randomized controlled trials on intravenous iron supplementation in heart failure with iron deficiency) **(Fig. 2)**.

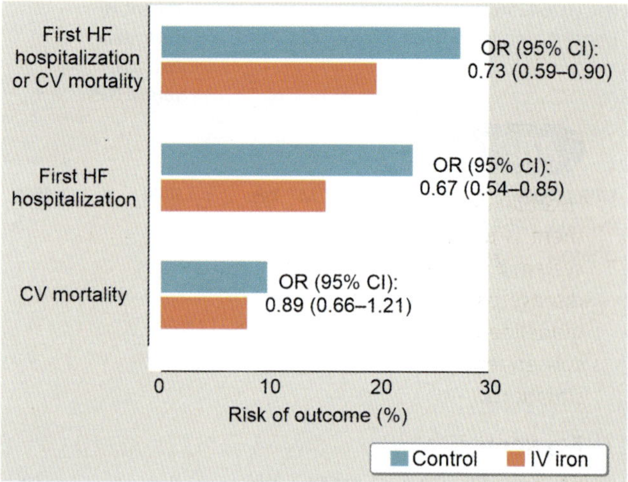

FIG. 2: Risk of CV outcomes with IV iron versus placebo.
(HF: heart failure; CI: confidence interval; CV: cardiovascular; IV: intravenous; OR: odds ratio)

ONLINE REFERENCES

Please scan the QR code provided at the end of the table of contents for References of this chapter.

CHAPTER

54

Managing Renal Dysfunction after Heart Failure Therapy Initiation

Asok Kumar Kar, Ayan Kar

ABSTRACT

Heart failure is a clinical syndrome dealing with impaired cardiac function where in order to preserve systemic perfusion, there is a maladaptive response of the renin–angiotensin–aldosterone system (RAAS) and the sympathetic nervous system (SNS). This often results in acute kidney impairment or further worsening of kidney function in established kidney disease patients. Although this is reversible in a majority of these patients, it often results in suboptimal initiation of guideline-directed medical therapy (GDMT), one of the most common causes for repeat heart failure hospitalizations and subsequent morbidity and mortality. This chapter attempts to review mechanisms and strategies to handle such clinical situations.

Keywords: Heart failure, renal dysfunction, optical guideline, directed medical therapy.

INTRODUCTION

As heart failure cardiologists, treating heart failure often entails walking that tightrope, managing cardiac and kidney functions despite all odds. The relationship between the heart and kidney is sacrosanct and intimately intertwined. Often, derangements in either cardiac or renal function have profound deleterious effects on the functioning of both organs.[1] Heart failure is a clinical syndrome described by symptoms or signs caused by a structural or functional cardiac abnormality, corroborated by elevated natriuretic peptide levels and objective signs and symptoms of pulmonary or systemic congestion.[2] Heart failure and kidney disease often coexist and happen to share common risk factors. This can present as acute kidney injury or worsening renal function. The onset of renal dysfunction in patients with heart failure results in significant challenges in initiation and optimization of guideline-directed medical therapy (GDMT), where many patients with moderate to advanced renal dysfunction are ineligible for life-saving therapies such as renin–angiotensin–aldosterone system (RAAS) blockade, mineralocorticoid receptor antagonist (MRA), and cardiac resynchronization therapy.[3,4] It is important to recognize the dynamic nature of changes in glomerular filtration rate (GFR) and the possibility of reversibility of such kidney dysfunction and to recognize treatable risk factors so that more patients become eligible for GDMT in optimal doses. However, it is also important to recognize patients in whom such therapies may be ineffective or undesirable, possibly due to the end-stage nature of the disease, and help them transition to advanced heart failure/transplant programs early.

HEART AND KIDNEY IN HEART FAILURE: THE PROBLEM AT HAND

The prevalence of chronic kidney disease (CKD) in the population is to the tune of 4.5%, but the prevalence of kidney disease in heart failure populations is almost 10-fold higher at 50%.[5] Hence, it is evident that worsening renal function, in the background of heart failure, portends an overall poorer prognosis compared to a reduction in left ventricular (LV) function alone.[6,7] When the heart fails, it provides inadequate renal perfusion. As a compensatory response, kidneys are bestowed with the ability to maintain transglomerular pressures by constriction of the efferent arteriole (EA) or by increasing blood flow in the afferent arterioles.[8] At the same time, cardiac preload is a direct outcome of solute and water handling by the kidney (glomerular + tubular function). More so, most of the traditional heart failure therapies have important direct effects on renal blood flow and solute handling. Thus, treatment of heart failure presents the following challenges:

- Hemodynamic-related kidney alterations (worsening renal function as an outcome of altered hemodynamics)
- Intrinsic disease-related kidney alterations (in patients with established kidney disease)
- Heart failure treatment-related kidney alterations (drug related)

Often, this is merely an appropriate renal response;[9,10] infrequently, it may be a sign of ongoing acute kidney injury. It is important to recognize the same and take cognizance of it.

Renal dysfunction in heart failure remains poorly defined in literature due to the dynamic nature of the disease, inhomogeneous patterns of reporting, different usage of biomarkers, and nonstandardized definitions **(Table 1)**. Most of it is extrapolated from nephrological definitions for worsening renal function and acute kidney injury as described by the Risk Injury Failure Loss End Stage (RIFLE), Acute Kidney Injury Network (AKIN), and Kidney Disease Improving Global Outcomes (KDIGO) criteria, as described in **Table 1**.[11,12]

However, in daily clinical practice, it is commonplace to see worsening renal function in the background of adequate urine output. Such cases of pseudo-worsening renal function[13] bear a good prognosis where the reduction in estimated glomerular filtration rate (eGFR) is purely a hemodynamic reflection of ongoing neurohormonal blockade. Paradoxically, similar worsening in glomerular function is also seen in patients with baseline CKD, where the benefits of neurohormonal blockade outweigh the acute risk of worsening glomerular function as long as the glomerular function stabilizes after the initial worsening and potassium remains within therapeutic range.[13]

Hence, after initiating GDMT in heart failure, it is recommended to do frequent and serial monitoring of renal function in order to:

- Establish a baseline
- Monitor effects of neurohormonal blockade and look at trends
- Risk-stratify patients (based on estimate renal reserve)
- Identify systemic diseases, pre-existing kidney disease, and end-organ function

CALCULATING RENAL FUNCTION

Renal function estimation comprises two parts: (1) Glomerular function and (2) tubular function.

Glomerular Function

Glomerular function is based on the filtration capacity of exogenous markers (which are not absorbed or secreted)

TABLE 1: Definitions of worsening renal function/acute kidney injury.

Definitions of worsening renal function		
GFR based	**Cystatin C based**	**Creatinine based**
• ≥20% decrease • >5 mL/min/1.73 m^2/year decrease	>0.3 mg/dL decrease	• ≥0.3 mg/dL • A+ >25% increase • >0.5 mg/dL increase • 1.5 × baseline • >25% increase + creatinine above 2.0 mg/dL

Definitions of acute kidney injury			
	Serum creatinine component		
Urine output component	**KDIGO**	**AKIN**	**RIFLE**
Grade I < 0.5 mL/kg/h for 6–12 hours	Serum creatinine 1.5–1.9× of baseline over 7 days or an absolute increase in creatinine ≥ 0.3 mg/dL over 48 hours	Serum creatinine 1.5–2.0× baseline or absolute increase > 0.3 mg/dL over 48 hours	Serum creatinine > 1.5× baseline within 7 days sustained for 24 hours
Grade II < 0.5 mL/kg/h for >12 hours	Serum creatinine 2.0–2.9× of baseline	Serum creatinine 2.0–3.0× of baseline	Serum creatinine > 2.0× of baseline
Grade III <0.3 mL/kg/h for >24 hours or anuric for 12 hours	Serum creatinine 3.0× baseline or an absolute increase >4.0 mg/day or requiring renal replacement therapy	Serum creatinine >3.0× baseline or creatinine >4.0 g/dL or an absolute increase >0.5 mg/dL or RRT	Serum creatinine > 3.0× baseline or creatinine > 4.0 g/dL or an absolute increase > 0.5 mg/dL or RRT

(AKIN: Acute Kidney Injury Network; GFR: glomerular filtration rate; KDIGO: Kidney Disease Improving Global Outcomes; RIFLE: Risk Injury Failure Loss End Stage; RRT: renal replacement therapy) such as inulin, which is both cumbersome and out of vogue; hence, we rely on endogenous markers such as creatinine or cystatin C, which replicate gold standard GFR or single nephron GFR (GFR divided by the number of nephrons based on cortical volume). It is more affected by renal venous hypertension due to congestion and often overestimates renal function in cachectic heart failure patients who have poor muscle mass.[14,15] Hence, cystatin C remains a more perfect and preferred marker for GFR estimation in patients of heart failure. Similarly, it is important to note that inflammation or obesity augments levels of cystatin C, and the relationship between creatinine and cystatin C is exponential (lower creatinine marked changes in cystatin C, higher creatinine less marked changes in cystatin C). Multiple formulas exist to estimate eGFR based on creatinine and cystatin C levels in the blood.[16] Of the available ones, the Cockcroft-Gault formula and the Modification of Diet in Renal Disease (MDRD) are commonly used. Despite the Cockcroft-Gault equation being grossly imprecise in estimating GFR, it seems to outperform MDRD equation in heart failure because of the element of body weight and cachexia involved in advanced heart failure **(Fig. 1)**.[17]

Tubular Function

Renal tubular function is extremely sensitive to hypoxia arising from reduced blood flow during episodes of renal hypoperfusion and congestion. This hypoxia can have profound changes in volume and electrolyte balance in the body. Given the differential function of the tubule over its entire length, it is almost impossible to have one biomarker to assess tubular dysfunction. Of the available[18,19] biomarkers, the most promising is neutrophil gelatinase-associated lipocalin (NGAL).[20] However, we have small studies which show that at present, it does not show any incremental benefit over the combination of GFR and N-terminal pro-B-type natriuretic peptide (NT-proBNP) to guide heart failure therapy. Thus, tubular function is often clinically assessed by:[21-23]

- The presence of natriuresis (urine spot sodium between 50 and 70 mEq/L) within 2 hours of diuretic administration
- Urine output of 100–150 mL/h in the first 6 hours
- Total diuresis of 3–4 liters in the first 24 hours of admissions

Biomarkers are often difficult to interpret in isolation. often, serial measurements are better to understand trends and differentiate between acute kidney injury and baseline CKD. In cases where this differentiation is not so clear, we rely on clinical history and renal imaging.

Renal imaging helps in evaluating the anatomic causes of acute renal injury, such as bladder outlet obstruction, unequal size of kidneys, corticomedullary differentiation, and evidence of renal artery stenosis. Renal venous Doppler flow patterns are often used to predict the response to diuretic therapy, with a continuous flow suggestive of lower venous hypertension and better diuretic response and a discontinuous flow more in favor of increased venous hypertension and poor diuretic response.[24]

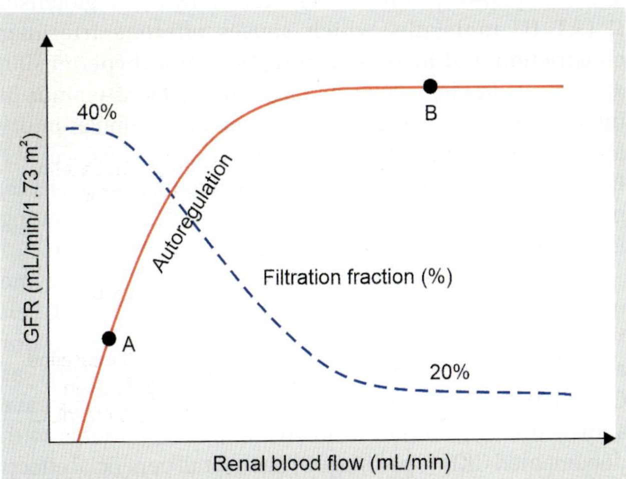

FIG. 1: Relationship of renal blood flow and glomerular filtration rate (GFR).

MANAGING RENAL FUNCTION IN ACUTE HEART FAILURE

The goal of therapy in acute congestive heart failure is to ensure adequate decongestion without compromising systemic perfusion, irrespective of the baseline LV function. Initiating loop diuretics early (door-to-furosemide time of <90 minutes) has been associated with lower in-hospital mortality.[25] Hence, renal function assessment as part of baseline labs is of utmost importance and establishes an estimate of renal reserve. A decreased GFR is one of the best predictors of acute kidney injury. Serial assessments of GFR using creatinine often show worsening renal function in close to 30–50% of cases, despite good urine output in the first 72 hours of therapy (often termed pseudo-worsening renal function).[9,10,26]

This is often the lag effect of the initial hemodynamic compromise and should not deter one from changing the course of therapy as long as the patient remains decongested and is passing adequate urine. In the background of good natriuresis and urine output, such worsening renal functions have always been associated with good overall outcomes.[27] During these initial acute stages, it is also important to maintain good perfusion pressures with mean arterial pressures preferably in excess of 65–70 mm Hg. However, abrupt and out-of-proportion rises in creatinine should warrant evaluation for ongoing renal injury, which may need early renal replacement therapy (often temporary if instituted early on), and rule out other reversible common causes such as urinary tract infection, bladder outlet obstruction, and renal artery stenosis. Other nonhemodynamic factors contributing to worsening renal function are RAAS blockade, activation of the sympathetic nervous system (SNS), inflammation, oxidative stress, and endothelial dysfunction.

Subsequently, in the course of their stay in the hospital, we start these patients on the four pillars of guideline-directed medical therapy (dictum: as many as possible in the lowest tolerable doses and then titrated upward).[28] This often results in worsening of renal function, which is acceptable (eGFR decline >30% from baseline worsening evaluation) as long as the patients remain decongested and maintain good perfusion pressure and stable serum potassium levels. There has been some interest in the early use of spot sodium to guide aggressive diuresis, as low spot sodium levels could suggest increasing diuretic therapy or adding MRAs and metolazone to break diuretic resistance.[27] The recently published rapid sequencing algorithm encourages early initiation of sodium-glucose cotransporter-2 inhibitors (SGLT-2Is) and beta-blockers followed by MRAs and RAAS blockers, possibly keeping in mind the wide range of GFR in which SGLT-2I and beta-blockers can be given and their relatively ease of administration.[28]

Thus, worsening renal function in acute heart failure is difficult to predict and must not be looked at in isolation; rather, it should always be interpreted in the larger context of the background clinical picture.[29] Meticulous use of simple clinical parameters such as input–output charts, daily body weight measurements, and biomarkers such as NT-proBNP, serum creatinine/cystatin C will preclude the premature withdrawal of life-saving heart failure therapy.

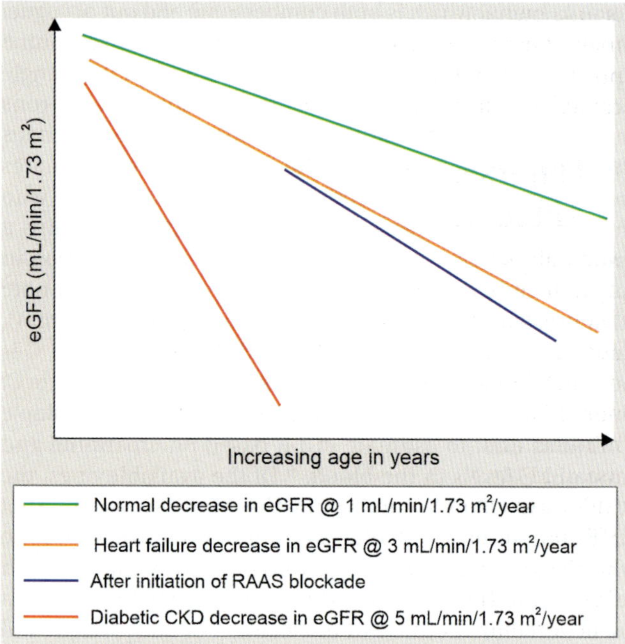

FIG. 2: Decline in glomerular function slope in health and disease: (1) Normal individuals (in green); (2) Heart failure individuals (in orange); (3) Heart failure individuals on RAASIs (in blue); (4) Patients with diabetic kidney disease (in red).

(CKD: chronic kidney disease; eGFR: estimated glomerular filtration rate; RAASIs: renin–angiotensin–aldosterone system inhibitors)

MANAGING RENAL FUNCTION IN CHRONIC HEART FAILURE

With aging, total GFR declines, with the number of functional nephrons declining (resulting in eGFR decline of) by 0.6–1 mL/min/1.73 m^2 after the age of 30–50 years. In heart failure patients, this decline is accelerated to 2.57 mL/min/1.73 m^2. Thus, heart failure patients inherently have almost twice the risk of developing CKD. The rapidity of decline in eGFR is almost 2.96 times higher in heart failure patients **(Fig. 2)**.[30]

Despite the ominous effect of heart failure on accelerated nephron loss, there have been few studies to show the improved benefit of RAAS blockers on improving the decline in GFR (as these trials were not designed that way and had short median follow-up). In fact, the benefit of RAAS blockade is largely extrapolated from nephrology trials of diabetic CKD. Fundamentally, diabetic CKD is a far more malignant disease where intraglomerular hyperfiltration is an outcome of the loss of glomerulus. Whereas in chronic heart failure, in order to preserve GFR in the background of renal hypoperfusion, we see intraglomerular hypertension, which results in a drop in GFR, which often manifests as an increase in creatinine. However, if this drop is unprecedented and in the absence of any trigger, it warrants further investigation.[31]

EFFECT OF STANDARD GUIDELINE THERAPIES ON RENAL FUNCTION

Angiotensin-converting Enzyme Inhibitors and Angiotensin Receptor Blockers

The final pathway of RAAS is mediated by the angiotensin II (AT II) molecule, which causes efferent arteriolar constriction and increased intraglomerular hypertension and results in glomerular damage. In clinical situations of intense EA constriction, it can result in acute tubular injury from hypoperfusion, which often takes longer to recover. AT II independently also causes increased glomerulosclerosis, platelet activation, and intrarenal atherosclerosis, resulting in worsening podocyte function and arterial obstruction.

Analysis of major angiotensin-converting enzyme inhibitor (ACEI) trials such as SOLVD (Studies Of Left Ventricular Dysfunction) and substudies of major angiotensin receptor blockers (ARBs) trials such as CONSENSUS, ValHeFT, CHARM Added, and ATLAS have shown that the initiation of ACEI/ARB in patients with documented CKD (up to stage 3) has overall beneficial effects despite the initial worsening of GFR. However, its long-term effect on prevention of progression of CKD in heart failure is unknown due to the short duration of follow-up in these trials. Presence of advanced CKD (stages 4 and 5) should not preclude the initiation of ACEI and ARB as long as there is careful monitoring of renal function.[32-34]

Mineralocorticoid Receptor Antagonists

Mineralocorticoid receptor antagonists are an established drug in heart failure and are given on the premise of "aldosterone escape," which has detrimental effects despite adequate RAAS blockade. Like RAAS blockade, initiation of MRA in patients with established CKD (eGFR < 60 mL/min/1.73 m^2) is associated with a drop of eGFR, which is minimal and persists and is not a reason to preclude the use of MRAs. In the EPHESUS trial, the acute mean drop in GFR was to the tune of 1.4 mL/min/1.73 m^2.[35] Additionally, MRA(s) did not influence the slope of GFR decline in the EPHESUS trial. Recently, with the advent of a molecule called finerenone (nonsteroidal MRA, selective), there has been seen a reduction in the slope of GFR decline (least square mean change in eGFR after 4 months -2.66 mg/dL vs. -3.97 g/dL/year). However, finerenone remains approved for diabetic proteinuria only at present. The use of MRA below a GFR of 30 mL/min/1.73 m^2 is currently not backed by safety and efficacy data.[36]

Beta-blockers

Overt activation of the SNS in heart failure results in alpha-adrenergic actions on both EA and afferent arteriole (AA), resulting in reduced renal blood flow and increased glomerular hypertension. Moreover, it also stimulates the granular cells to release renin and increase the tubular sodium reabsorption, worsening the already sodium-avid state that heart failure is pathologically.[37] Beta-blockers in heart failure are known to reduce mortality and morbidity, primarily by reducing arrhythmic deaths. However, in the CAPRICORN and COPERNICUS trials, the use of carvedilol is associated with minor reductions in eGFR because of its alpha-adrenergic blocking effect.[37] Other beta-blockers used in heart failure are metoprolol, nebivolol, and bisoprolol. Of the above-mentioned four, carvedilol is least dialyzable, followed by bisoprolol and nebivolol to some extent, and metoprolol is the most dialyzable because of its water-soluble property. Hence, dosing/time of administration of metoprolol needs to be adjusted in dialysis patients.[38,39]

EFFECT OF NOVEL HEART FAILURE THERAPIES ON RENAL FUNCTION

Angiotensin Receptor Blocker and Neprilysin Inhibition

Angiotensin receptor blocker and neprilysin inhibitions (ARNIs) have this novel mechanism of increasing levels of circulating natriuretic peptide, which potentiates natriuresis, increases GFR, and reduces SNS activation, plasma volume, and afterload to a failing heart. All the randomized controlled trials (RCTs) of ARNI, including PARADIGM, PARAMOUNT, and PARAGON-HF, have shown reduced risk of renal events (sustained 50% reduction in eGFR/progression to end-stage kidney disease). Additionally, it also reduces the GFR decline slope, preventing the progression of CKD. Specifically, diabetic CKD subsets seem to benefit particularly from the use of ARNI to reduce cardiac events and renal decline at the cost of a marginal increase in urinary ACR.[33,34,40]

Sodium-glucose Cotransporter-2 inhibitors

The SGLT-2 receptor is predominantly present in the S1 and S2 segments of the proximal convoluted tubule and is pathologically upregulated in diseased conditions such as diabetes, heart failure, and obesity. This being a cotransporter, along with increased glucose reabsorption, there is added sodium and chloride reabsorption too, resulting in reduced concentration of chloride to the macula densa, which in turn causes AA dilatation (tubuloglomerular feedback) and increased GFR or hyperfiltration commonly seen in early diabetes or heart failure. SGLT-2Is particularly reverse this process and are documented to reduce the rate of decline of GFR, irrespective of baseline GFR [most SGLT-2 trials in heart failure with reduced ejection fraction (HFrEF) have a cutoff of ≥20 mL/min/1.73 m^2]. Along with its potentially robust renal effects, it also causes osmotic diuresis, causing reduction in cardiac filling pressures and improving ventricular stiffness.[41,42]

Vericiguat

Another novel molecule available for heart failure therapy, now available in India, works on potentiating the role of soluble guanylate cyclase (sGC) independent of endothelium-derived nitric oxide. Although it currently remains indicated in worsening heart failure, it appears to have the potential to form the fifth pillar of heart failure therapy pending more regulatory data. It does not affect renal function and can be given in patients with advanced kidney dysfunction (eGFR up to 15 mL/min/1.73 m^2) **(Table 2)**.[43]

ROLE OF HEMODYNAMIC MONITORING IN HEART FAILURE AND ITS ROLE IN PATIENTS WITH WORSENING RENAL FUNCTION

Worsening renal function and the inability to decongest a heart failure patient often go hand in hand and are often the most difficult subset of patients in heart failure to treat. They generally tend to have a longer intensive care unit (ICU) stay and require increased invasive monitoring. In such

TABLE 2: Overview of standard available guideline-directed medical therapy (GDMT) backed by randomized controlled trials (in India) and its kidney interactions.

<table>
<tr><th>Drug class</th><th colspan="4">Evidence for initiation as per GFR strata in clinical trials</th><th>Acute drop in GFR after HF therapy</th><th>Effect on GFR slope</th></tr>
<tr><th></th><th>ESRD</th><th>15–30</th><th>30–60</th><th>>60</th><th></th><th></th></tr>
<tr><td>ACEIs/ARBs</td><td>Moderate (only in dialysis patients)</td><td>Moderate evidence</td><td colspan="2" rowspan="6">Strong evidence</td><td>Yes</td><td>No</td></tr>
<tr><td>Beta-blockers</td><td colspan="2"></td><td>No</td><td>No</td></tr>
<tr><td>MRA</td><td colspan="2" rowspan="2">Not indicated</td><td>Yes</td><td>No</td></tr>
<tr><td>ARNI</td><td>Yes</td><td>Yes</td></tr>
<tr><td>SGLT-2Is</td><td rowspan="2">No data</td><td rowspan="2"></td><td>Yes</td><td>Yes</td></tr>
<tr><td>Vericiguat</td><td>No</td><td>No</td></tr>
</table>

(ACEIs: angiotensin-converting enzyme inhibitors; ARBs: angiotensin receptor blockers; ARNI: angiotensin receptor and neprilysin inhibitor; ESRD: end-stage renal disease; GFR: glomerular filtration rate; HF: heart failure; MRA: mineralocorticoid receptor antagonists; SGLT-2Is: sodium-glucose cotransporter 2 inhibitors)

Source: Adapted from major HF trials.

situations, right heart catheterization can be more insightful. Based on the escape trial in 2005, which says pulmonary artery (PA) catheters being deployed in heart failure patients, it is largely considered a negative trial due to the higher levels of infection noted in patients who underwent PA catheterization. However, patients in cardiogenic shock who may have actually benefited from this intervention were largely excluded from this trial. Also, discussion and renal replacement are probably beyond the scope of this chapter.[44]

RECHALLENGING GUIDELINE-DIRECTED MEDICAL THERAPY AFTER WITHDRAWAL

Real-world patients are vastly different from the controlled realms of RCTs with oversight committees ensuring the implementation of uptitration strategies and ensuring patients receive standard of care in maximum tolerable doses. In the real-world setting, <1% of heart failure patients receive all four pillars in their target doses. There is a profound lack of physician inertia in understanding the difference between improvement in symptoms versus prolonging life. Thus, physicians experiencing early failures and intolerance to GDMT should never shy away from rechallenging with class I drugs whenever feasible or by adjusting other drug doses.[45]

CONCLUSION

The onset of kidney dysfunction during the treatment of heart failure is not uncommon. Its high incidence and prevalence are often associated with an overall poor prognosis in heart failure patients. Hence, it remains less reported and even less discussed and is often excluded from major heart failure trials. Identification of reversible causes of kidney dysfunction in the clinical context of heart failure is essential to initiate and maintain GDMT, often in the background of a fluctuating renal function. The use of biomarkers, a detailed clinical history, and renal imaging often helps in differentiating between acute kidney injury and CKD. The presence of worsening renal function in the background of adequate diuresis is generally associated with a good prognosis. The decision to withdraw or preclude GDMT should be done only if warranted and not merely to address a worsening GFR. Serial assessments of GFR, electrolytes, and clinical signs and symptoms as a part of close follow-up are often warranted. Thus, we propose a treatment pathway which could be useful and handy for clinicians **(Flowchart 1)**.

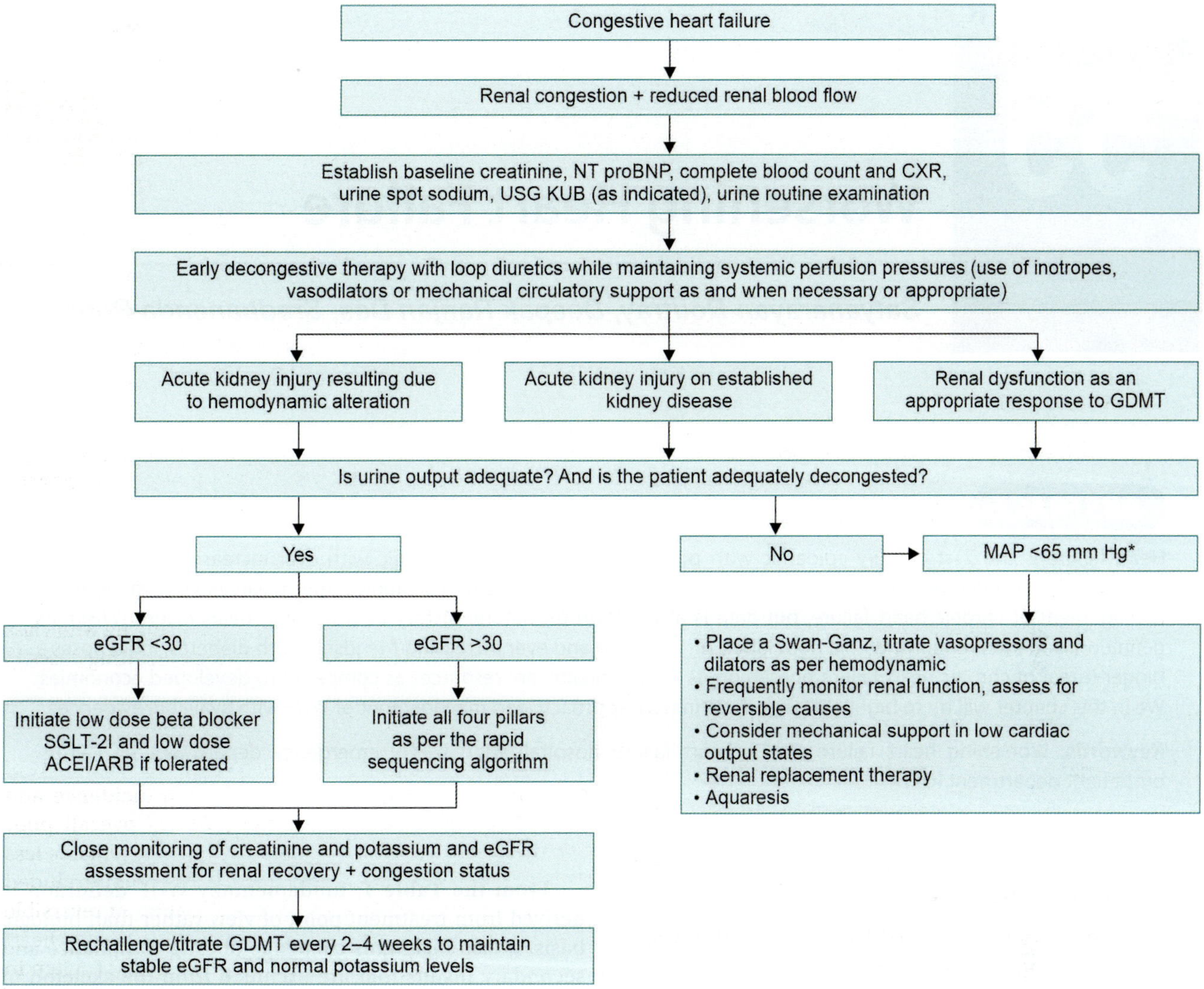

*Increasing level in lactates.

FLOWCHART 1: Treatment pathway.

(ACEI: angiotensin-converting enzyme inhibitor; ARB: angiotensin receptor blocker; CXR: chest X-ray; GDMT: guideline-directed medical therapy; MAP: mean arterial pressure; eGFR: estimated glomerular filtration rate; NT-proBNP: N-terminal pro-B-type natriuretic peptide; SGLT-2I: sodium-glucose cotransporter-2 inhibitor; USG KUB: ultrasonography of kidneys, ureters, and bladder)

ONLINE REFERENCES

Please scan the QR code provided at the end of the table of contents for References of this chapter.

CHAPTER

55

Worsening Heart Failure

Satyanarayan Routray, Deepak Ranjan Das, Sradhananda Rout

ABSTRACT

Heart failure is the 21st century epidemic with potential to become a pandemic with ever increasing life span and survival. With flooding of high-quality evidences, along with diuretics pharmacological four pillars have revolutionized management of chronic heart failure, but data is at its dawn on natural history of worsening heart failure (WHF), its definition, and interventions. With a population of 1.5 billion and ever increasing friendship with diabetes, India poses a bigger threat of chronic heart failure burden on its limited healthcare resources as compared to developed economies. We in this chapter will try to highlight present definition, approach, and management of WHF with available evidences.

Keywords: Worsening heart failure (WHF), heart failure hospitalization (HFH), emergency department (ED) visits, outpatient department (OPD).

INTRODUCTION

Worsening heart failure (WHF) is an inevitable traffic square on the journey of chronic heart failure (CHF). Its definition is still in infancy, which may be stated as per the recent clinical consensus statement by the Heart Failure Association of the European Society of Cardiology[1] as given in the **Table 1**.

From the **Table 1**, fundamentally WHF definition is derived from treatment point of view rather than biologic basis. It also highlights challenge of drug compliance and secondary insults that are excluded from the skeleton of definition. With multiple domains of pathophysiology associated with WHF involving different organ systems, inclusion of renal and pulmonary maladaptation into the definition of WHF is still a gray area.

TABLE 1: Worsening heart failure (WHF) definition as per clinical consensus statement by the Heart Failure Association of the European Society of Cardiology[1] June, 2023.

	Includes	Excludes
Definition	• Worsening symptoms and signs of heart failure (HF) • Requiring intensification of treatment, generally including diuretic therapy • Occurring in patients with preexisting HF	• New-onset HF • Episodes with concomitant factors, including comorbidities and/or poor compliance, as primary cause
Pathophysiology	• Disease progression • Congestion	Precipitating factors as main cause

Site of care	• Hospital
	• Emergency department
	• Ambulatory:
	  ○ With intravenous (IV) therapy
	  ○ With escalation of oral therapy
		Episodes requiring no changes in HF treatment

Once the patient with WHF comes for help, there are three primary points of care as where escalation/intensification of heart failure (HF) therapy normally undertaken as follows in **Table 2**.

TABLE 2: Point of care for escalation/intensification of heart failure (HF) therapy in worsening heart failure (WHF).

Point of care	Patient phenotype
Inhospital	Patients with WHF needing intravenous (IV) medications
Emergency department (ED) visit	Patients of WHF who are discharged without hospitalization
Outpatient department (OPD) visits	WHF outpatients treated with an escalation of their oral diuretic therapy

EPIDEMIOLOGY

Numerous trials and data exist on HF but specific data on WHF is limited. We are going to discuss on most recent trials/registries that specifically segregated WHF patients for analysis with adequate/acceptable power and sample size. From recent clinical trials and registries from 2016, we have considered four landmark trials and four registries as shown in **Table 3**.

From the **Table 3**, in PARADIGM-HF out of 8,399 study population, 1,107 (13.2%) hospitalized for WHF, which was significantly more than emergency department (ED) visits (1%) or outpatient department (OPD) visits (4.3%).[2] Similarly in DAPA HF trial, VICTORIA trial as well as PARAGON HF trial, the heart failure hospitalization (HFH) was significantly higher as compared to ED visits or OPD visits for index WHF.[3-5] This finding is corroborated by the National CV Data Registry PINNACLE,[6] by Madelaire et al.[7] study published

TABLE 3: Trials/registries that specifically segregated worsening heart failure (WHF) patients for analysis.

Author	Study/Registries	Year	Patients(n)	WHF phenotypes
Okumura et al.[2]	PARADIGM-HF	2016	8,399	• 1,107 patients (13.2%) were hospitalized • 78 (1.0%) had an emergency department (ED) visit • 361 (4.3%) outpatient intensification of therapy
Docherty et al.[3]	DAPA-HF	2020	4,744	Index episode of WHF: • 489 (10.3%) heart failure hospitalization (HFH) • 20 (0.4%) ED visit with intravenous (IV) therapy • 407 (8.6%) outpatient department (OPD) intensification of therapy
Lam et al.[4]	VICTORIA	2021	5,050	• 3,378 (67%) HFH for WHF—within 3 months of index presentation • 871—within 3–6 months of HFH • 801—within 3 months of outpatient WHF
Vaduganathan et al.[5]	PARAGON-HF	2021	4,796	884 patients suffered WHF, of 818 were hospitalized, and 66 were urgent HF visits only
Butler et al.[6]	The National CV Data Registry PINNACLE	2019	11,064	1,851 (17%) patients experienced WHF
Madelaire et al.[7]	Danish patients diagnosed with HF from 2001 to 2016	2020	74,790	Patients with WHF: • 4517 (6.0%) OPD event • 3160 (4.2%) hospitalized for WHF • 942 (1.6%) with both events
Shah et al.[8]	ASCEND-HF	2022	2,661	After 30-day follow-up: • 193 patients (7%) had ED visits • 459 patients (17%) had HFH
Ambrosy et al.[9]	Kaiser Permanente Northern California (KPNC) HF Registry (2010-2019)	2022	103,138	126,008 WHF episodes: • 34,758 (27.6%) OPD patients • 28,301 (22.5%) ED visits • 62,949 (50.0%) HFH

in 2020 on Danish patients diagnosed with HF from 2001 to 2016 and by Kaiser Permanente Northern California (KPNC) HF Registry (2010–2019).[6-8] In ASCEND-HF, from total 2,661 sample, after 30-day follow-up 193 patients (7%) had ED visits and 459 patients (17%) had HFH.[9] So from earlier mentioned epidemiological analysis, it is evident that in the natural history of WHF, HFH is the single most frequent morbidity indicator.

PATHOPHYSIOLOGY

There are many schools of thoughts on pathogenesis of WHF but fundamentally all leads to increased intracardiac pressure and systemic congestion.[10,11] **Flowchart 1** presents a schematic presentation of WHF. Fundamentally though the secondary causes significantly contribute to WHF, but was not considered in defining it. Congestion itself may decrease guideline-directed medical therapy (GDMT), especially oral drug absorption and further worsen HF in setting of WHF.[12] The various pathophysiological interplay is schematically presented in **Flowchart 1**.

DIAGNOSIS

Various available modalities for diagnosing WHF can be stratified as follows:

- Clinical risk scores
- Biomarkers
- Imaging
- Telemedicine devices and invasive modalities

Clinical Risk Scores

No clinical score or finding is affirmative of WHF till date. Compared to the New York Heart Association (NYHA) class alone, patient reported outcomes scores [e.g., Kansas City Cardiomyopathy Questionnaire (KCCQ)] or exercise tests (e.g., 6-minute walking test and cardiopulmonary exercise test) may be more accurate and objective for predicting WHF.[13,14] Alvarez-Garcia J et al., investigators of the Spanish Heart Failure Network (REDINSCOR), proposed a simple validated method for predicting the risk of hospitalization for worsening of HF in ambulatory patients,[15] the Redin-SCORE which had a sample size of 2,507 and followed up to 3.3 years. The Redin-SCORE had C-statistics for the models were 0.72 and 0.66, for predicting 1 month and 1 year HF readmission, respectively.

Biomarkers

Serial measurements of N-terminal pro-B-type natriuretic peptide (NT-proBNP) at predefined intervals may aid early identification of patients with WHF as most congestion are persistently subclinical.[16] Other potential biomarkers such as high-sensitivity cardiac troponin,[17] carbohydrate antigen 125 (CA-125),[18] biologically active adrenomedullin (bio-ADM)[19], soluble suppression of tumorigenicity 2 (sST2),[20] and accelerated decline in estimated glomerular filtration rate (eGFR) are some of the testing modalities at a HF specialist/cardiologists arsenal with variable sensitivity and specificity for predicting WHF.[17-20]

Imaging

Plane X-ray anterior and lateral views, echocardiographic estimates of inferior vena cava diameter, pulmonary artery pressure, and ventricular filling pressure provide good correlation with systemic congestion in WHF. Ultrasonographic measurement of pulmonary B-lines **(Fig. 1)** and magnetic resonance imaging provide immense

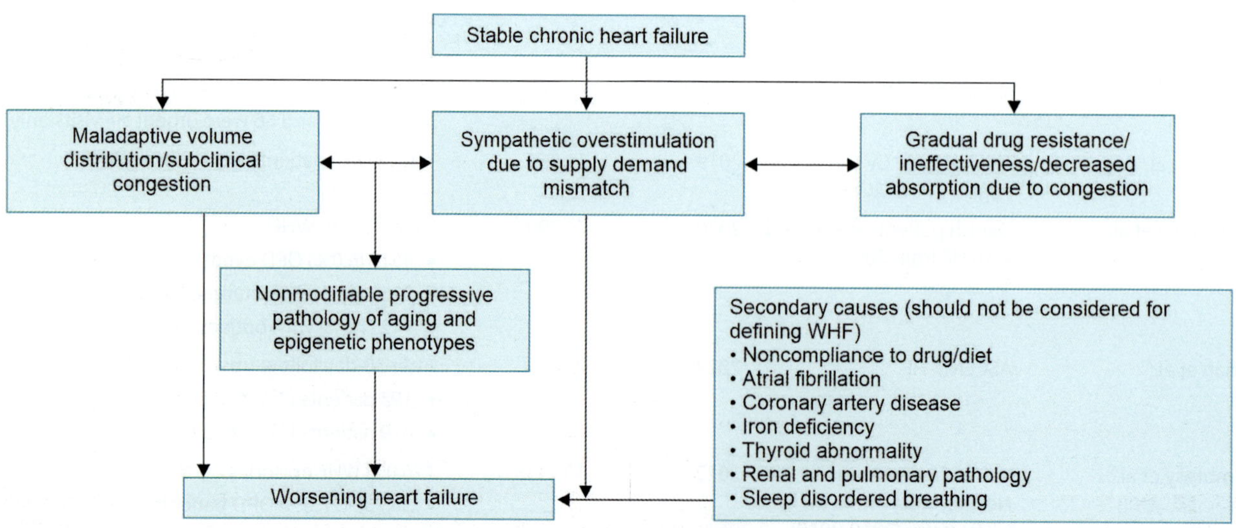

FLOWCHART 1: Pathophysiological interplay in worsening heart failure (WHF).

information about the hemodynamic parameters for early detection of WHF as well as therapeutic effectiveness monitoring.

Telemedicine Devices and Invasive Modalities

The CHAMPION (CardioMEMS Heart Sensor Allows Monitoring of Pressure to Improve Outcomes in NYHA Class III Heart Failure Patients) trial showed a significant reduction in HFHs for patients in NYHA class III who were managed with CardioMEMS, a wireless implantable pulmonary artery pressure sensor.[21] SIRONA a multicenter, open-label, first-in-human, and feasibility study to evaluate the usability of the comprehensive Cordella™ Heart Failure System (CHFS) showed that implantation of the Cordella sensor **(Figs. 2A and B)** was feasible and safe with excellent accuracy of the Cordella sensor pulmonary artery pressure measurements for predicting HF worsening.[22] Select population with cardiac resynchronization therapy and the implantable cardioverter-defibrillator offer diagnostic features for early detection of WHF.

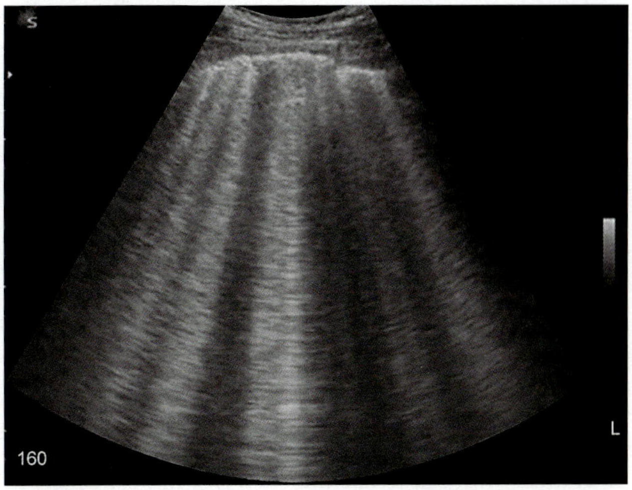

FIG. 1: Pulmonary B-lines in cardiogenic pulmonary edema.

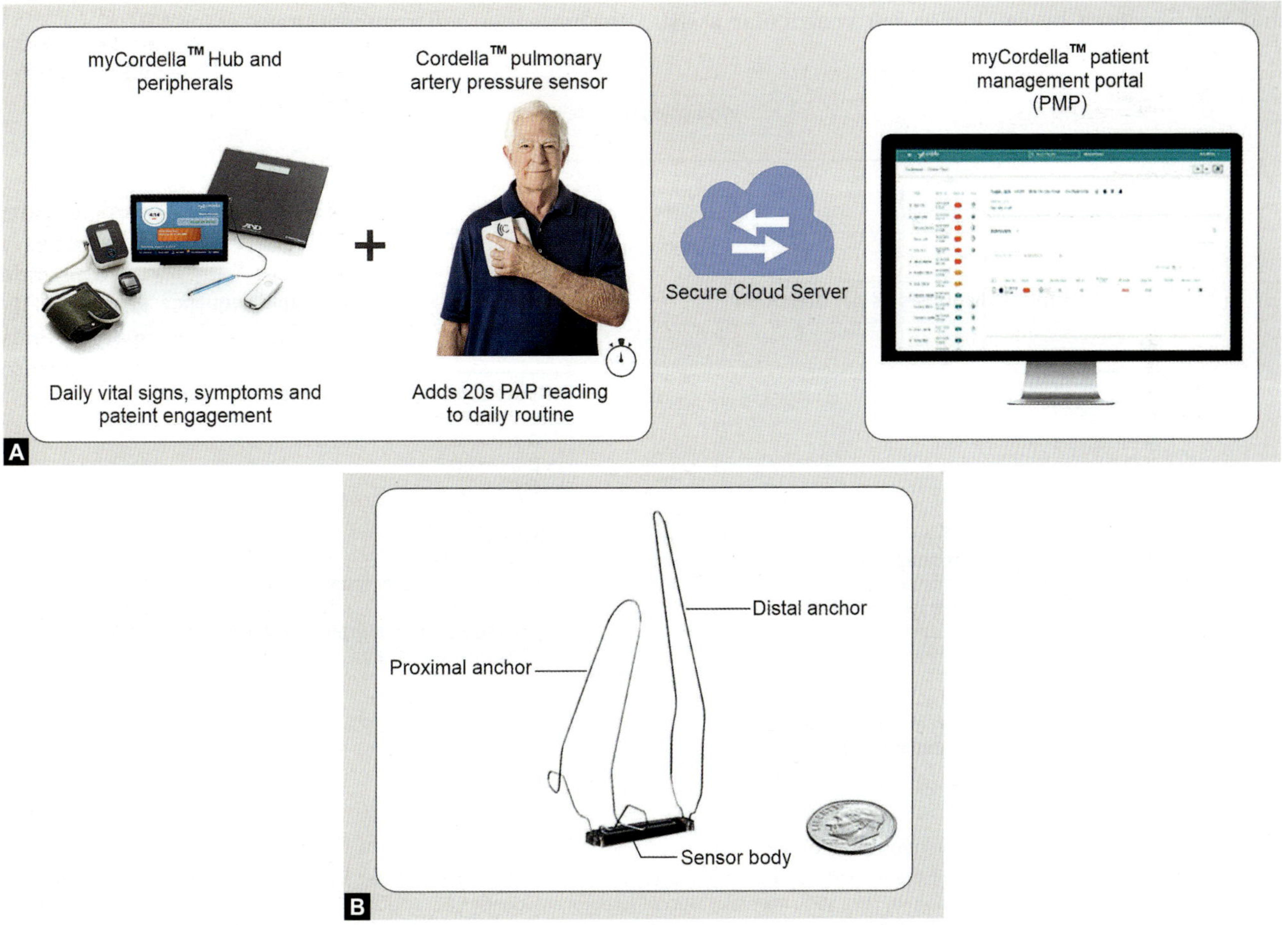

FIGS. 2A AND B: The Cordella™ Heart Failure System. (A) The Cordella™ System securely transmits daily health information (weight, blood pressure, saturations, and heart rate) as well as pulmonary artery pressure (PAP) data to clinicians from the patient's home; (B) The Cordella™ pulmonary artery pressure sensor.[22]

TREATMENT AND PREVENTION

The treatment and prevention of WHF is at its dawn as is its definition, waiting to see a bright morning. Besides the guideline directed four pharmacological pillars [angiotensin-converting enzyme inhibitor (ACEI) or an angiotensin receptor blocker (ARB) or an angiotensin receptor–neprilysin inhibitor (ARNI), a β-blocker, a mineralocorticoid receptor antagonist (MRA), and a sodium-glucose cotransporter-2 inhibitor (SGLT-2I)] of CHF treatment, ADVOR (Acetazolamide in Decompensated Heart Failure with Volume Overload) trial showed the benefit of intravenous (IV) acetazolamide compared to placebo in addition to furosemide in patients admitted with acute HF and volume overload.[23] The new concept of "door-to-furosemide time" must be shortened.[24] Thiazide-like diuretics, namely oral metolazone (2.5–5 mg) can be used in patients with advanced HF with diuretic resistance in a sequential nephron blockade or in those with eGFR < 30 mL/min/1.73 m^2, especially in OPD visits drug escalation strategy.[25]

A particular patients category that frequently need hospitalization (termed as frequent flyers by some authors) may get benefited by combining left ventricular assist device (LVAD) and medical management as shown by the ROADMAP (Risk Assessment and Comparative Effectiveness of Left Ventricular Assist Device and Medical Management) trial.[26]

Recently published PARAGLIDE HF trial ($n = 466$), among patients with ejection fraction (EF) > 40% stabilized after WHF, sacubitril/valsartan led to greater reduction in plasma NT-proBNP levels and was associated with clinical benefit compared with valsartan alone, despite more symptomatic hypotension.[27] Further adequately powered study will shed better light on suitability of ARNi over ACEi for managing WHF episodes. The VICTORIA (Vericiguat Global Study in Subjects with Heart Failure with Reduced Ejection Fraction) trial included patients with left ventricular ejection fraction (LVEF) < 45%, NYHA class II–IV, elevated natriuretic peptide concentrations and WHF, the primary endpoint of cardiovascular death or HFHs of 37.8 versus 33.6 events per 100 patient-years with placebo and vericiguat, respectively.[28] From the results, vericiguat may be included in upcoming guidelines for prevention strategies of WHF. Yoga and supervised exercise are well established interventions for all types of WHF prevention strategies. **Flowchart 2** summarizes the prevention and treatment strategies for WHF.

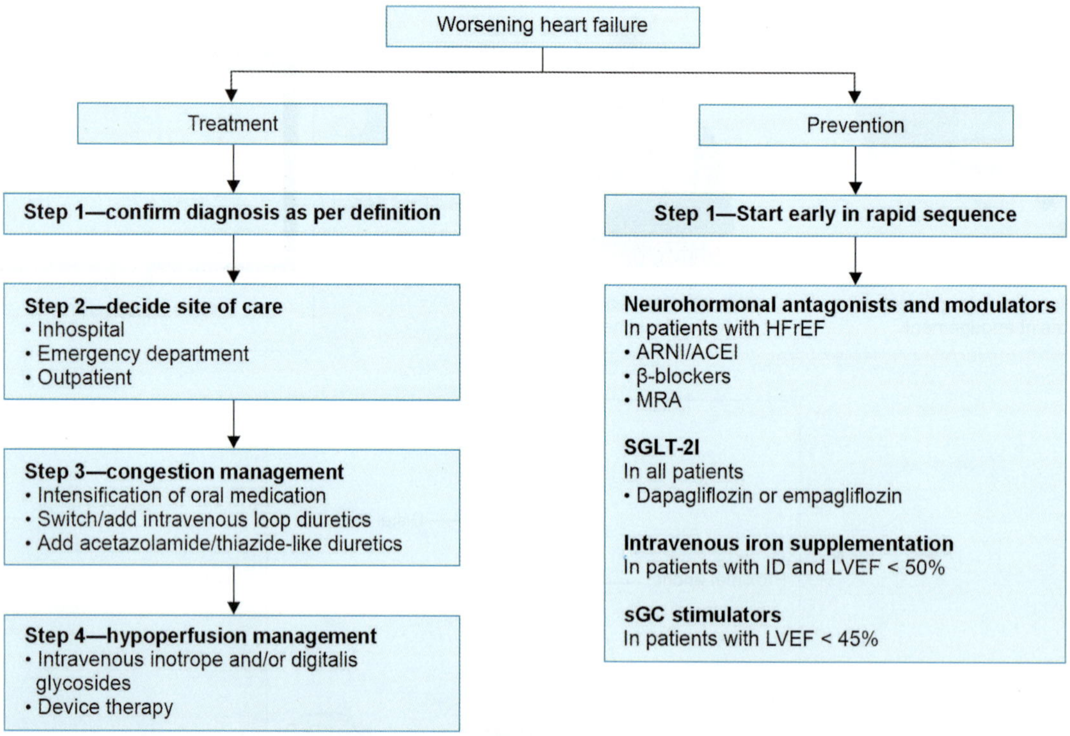

FLOWCHART 2: Treatment and prevention strategies for WHF.

(ACEI: angiotensin–converting enzyme inhibitor; ARNI: angiotensin receptor–neprilysin inhibitor; HFrEF: heart failure with reduced ejection fraction; ID: iron deficiency; LVEF: left ventricular ejection fraction; MRA: mineralocorticoid receptor antagonist; sGC: soluble guanylate cyclase; SGLT-2I: sodium-glucose cotransporter-2 inhibitor; WHF: worsening heart failure)

Source: With permission from clinical consensus statement by the Heart Failure Association of the European Society of Cardiology.[1]

CONCLUSION

Recognition of WHF as an event that marks the start of a new phase in the natural history of HF is essential to formulate treatment and prevention strategies. Future robust and adequately powered trials on novel biomarkers, implantable hemodynamic devices, yoga/patient tailored exercise protocols, and newer therapeutics will act as check point on the highway of HF progression and WHF prevention. With increasing average life span of world and India in particular, preventive interventions are sole of the HF epidemic mitigation strategies.

ONLINE REFERENCES

Please scan the QR code provided at the end of the table of contents for References of this chapter.

CHAPTER

56 Beyond ARNI: Upcoming Newer Pharmacotherapy in Heart Failure

Vidyut Jain, Avani Jain

ABSTRACT

In the last three decades, we have witnessed an increasing prevalence of patients suffering from chronic heart failure (HF) and its consequences. HF is a progressively worsening disease that significantly reduces both the patients' life expectancy and quality of life. This has resulted in major concern for global health and economic burden. Several advances have been made in understanding the mechanism of HF, paving the way for newer therapeutic options, including pharmacological treatments and innovative procedures. However, a large number of patients still remain ill and frequently require hospitalization due to the lack of effective therapies.

After implementing optimal therapy, many patients experience varying durations of clinical stability but still face residual risks of adverse outcomes, including sudden death. HF involves multiple additional cardiovascular and noncardiovascular pathophysiological abnormalities. There is likely widespread microvascular dysfunction affecting all cardiac chambers and other organs such as the lungs, kidneys, and skeletal muscles. Developing new drugs for HF therapy should therefore focus on novel approaches, including direct effects on cardiomyocytes, coronary microcirculation, myocardial interstitium, mitochondrial function, and inflammatory states. Equally important are the preservation of vital organ functions and the prevention of metabolic derangement and vascular events in distant areas. In this review, our aim is to understand current research in the HF management, particularly in identifying new pharmacological targets for the treatment of HF patients, with a focus on microcirculation, cardiomyocytes, anti-inflammatory therapy, and other pathways.

Keywords: Heart failure with reduced ejection fraction (HFrEF), heart failure with preserved ejection fraction (HFpEF).

INTRODUCTION

It is now widely accepted that a better understanding of heart failure pathophysiology, advanced diagnostic measures, early detection, and newer therapeutic options lead to improved outcomes, including reduced morbidity and cardiovascular mortality in the last three decades. However, need for recurrent hospitalization and high residual cardiovascular mortality remains a significant challenge in the heart failure management. This is primarily due to the suboptimal use of current therapeutic options, including under-dosing, failure to add or select available treatments, and the need for target and personalized therapies that address individual pathophysiological alterations.[1] Each patient may have a different etiology and comorbidities that influence the outcome. One of the most common cardiovascular risk factors for heart failure is diabetes mellitus, which affects over 500 million people worldwide. An analysis of UK data revealed that mortality and heart failure risk was nearly doubled in people with diabetes compared to those without it and females were more affected in this group.[2]

Incorporating various evidence-based therapeutic options for chronic heart failure, such as β-blockers, angiotensin-converting enzyme inhibitors (ACEIs)/angiotensin receptor blockers (ARBs)/angiotensin receptor-neprilysin inhibitors (ARNIs), mineralocorticoid receptor antagonists, and sodium-glucose cotransporter-2 inhibitors (SGLT-2Is) that offers benefits in terms of a reduced morbidity and a cardiovascular mortality. This approach has transformed the landscape of the heart failure management over the last three decades; however, it is recognized that the benefits of these drugs have reached a therapeutic plateau. Many patients remain symptomatic and experience worsening heart failure despite receiving optimal tolerable dosages. This enigma applies to both heart failure with reduced ejection fraction (HFrEF) and heart failure with preserved ejection fraction (HFpEF). There are many contributing factors which include comorbidities, such as diabetes, obesity, chronic kidney disease, anemia, chronic obstructive pulmonary diseases, and frailty. It should be acknowledged that these comorbidities often contribute to myocardial dysfunction through coronary microvascular endothelial inflammation in HFpEF **(Table 1)**.[3]

These comorbidities lead to a systemic proinflammatory state, causing inflammation of the coronary microvascular endothelium. Developing new drugs for heart failure therapy must focus on additional targets, both anatomical or structural (such as cardiomyocytes and myocardial interstitium) and physiological or functional (such as microcirculation and inflammation). It is essential to implement increasingly effective therapies at the appropriate time throughout the entire course of heart failure to prevent or improve prognosis and enhance the quality of life for the patients.

Implementing nanoscale technology in pharmacotherapy may prove highly beneficial. Nanotechnology plays a crucial role in cell signal transduction, enzyme action, and cell cycle, making it closely related to medical research. Its application in medicine provides an alternative and novel approach to the treatment of cardiovascular diseases and has shown promising results in targeted drug therapy and biomaterial development.[4] The aim of this review is to understand modern approaches, new perspectives, and future directions for the treatment of heart failure.

MITOCHONDRIAL PATHWAY

In the human body, the heart is the most active metabolic organ, producing a large amount of adenosine triphosphate (ATP)/day. There are about 6,000 mitochondria in each adult cardiomyocyte. Cardiac mitochondria regulate Ca^{2+} and reactive oxygen species (ROS) homeostatic pathways.[5] Mitochondria produce ATP to drive cardiomyocyte contraction. Mitochondrial biogenesis is regulated by transcriptional proliferator-activated receptor gamma coactivator-1 alpha (PGC-1α) which plays an important role in the development of the heart. Mitochondrial function can be affected by various factors such as oxidative stress, hypoxia, and hyperglycemia.[6] Similarly, transcription factor A, mitochondrial (Tfam) is also pivotal to intact cardiac function, and its targeted inactivation of Tfam in embryonic cardiomyocytes is lethal, which is the direct result of elevated ROS products, deoxyribonucleic acid (DNA) damage, and severely suppressed cardiomyocyte proliferation.[7] Cardiolipin, a phospholipid with multiple fatty acid side chains balances normal ATP generation by adjoining the proteins of the electron transport chain onto the inner mitochondrial membrane architecture and improves the coupling of the electron transport chain.[8] Stabilization of mitochondrial membrane and cytochrome can help mitochondrial function and ATP generation and thus opens new targets for heart failure treatment.[9]

Cytochrome C Enhancer

- *Elamipretide*: It is also known as MTP-131. It is a cell-permeable tetrapeptide that acts as a mitochondrial modulator. It is designed to rapidly enter cells and provide protective benefits to vulnerable or ischemic cells by improving mitochondrial energy and decreasing ROS levels. Elamipretide is believed to stabilize the mitochondrial membrane and cytochrome, thereby enhancing mitochondrial function and ATP generation.[10]

Research has shown the potential benefits of elamipretide in various cardiovascular conditions, including heart failure and mitochondrial sympathy. In a double-blind, placebo-controlled trial of elamipretide in patients with reduced left ventricular ejection fraction (LVEF), significant

TABLE 1: New targets in heart failure beyond four foundational therapies.

Pathway target	Target	Molecule	HF type
Mitochondrial	Cytochrome C	Elamipretide	HFrEF
	Partial adenosine A1 receptor	Neladenoson	HFrEF and HFpEF
Cardiomyocyte (calcium handling)	SERCA2a	Istaroxime	HFrEF
Cardiomyocyte (nitroxyl donors)	SERCA2a	BMS-986231	HFrEF and AHF
Myofibrillar pathway	Myosin	Omecamtiv mecarbil	HFrEF
Signaling pathways	sGC	Vericiguat	HFrEF
Inflammation	Interleukin-1 receptor	• Anakinra • Canakinumab	• HFrEF • HFrEF

(AHF: acute heart failure; HF: heart failure; HFpEF: heart failure with preserved ejection fraction; HFrEF: heart failure with reduced ejection fraction; SERCA2a: sarcoplasmic/endoplasmic reticulum calcium ATPase 2a; sGC: soluble guanylate cyclase)

improvements were observed.[11] Patients receiving elamipretide showed a significant decrease in the left ventricular end-diastolic volume and end-systolic volume compared to the placebo group.

The PROGRESS-HF Phase 2 trial, which included patients with LVEF of around 31%, also demonstrated some positive effects of elamipretide. Although left ventricular end-systolic volume was only marginally affected, no significant differences were observed in LVEF between the placebo and elamipretide groups[12] In the EMBRACE study, elamipretide was tested in patients with anterior wall ST-segment elevation myocardial infarction (MI) who received the drug before reperfusion.[13] Elamipretide has also been evaluated in other clinical trials, such as in patients with Barth syndrome (BTHS), a genetic disorder affecting the heart and the other organs. The results showed that elamipretide treatment led to an increased left ventricular volume and an improved cardiac stroke volume, which contributed to the better symptoms in BTHS patients. While there was no significant difference in infarct size between the elamipretide and placebo groups, it is important to note that clinical trial results may vary, and further research is needed to fully understand the efficacy and safety profile of elamipretide in different patient populations.[14]

Adenosine A1 Receptor Agonist

Neladenoson bialanate, a partial adenosine A1 receptor agonist in animal experiments, showed improvement in mitochondrial function, by enhancing sarco/endoplasmic reticulum 2a activity, and optimal energy substrate utilization. There was a reverse ventricular remodeling, which can extend anti-ischemic cardio protective effects without the adverse effects of full A1 receptor agonists.[15] Among patients with HFpEF, there was no significant dose-response relationship detected for neladenoson with regard to the change in exercise capacity from baseline to 20 weeks. In light of these findings, novel approaches will be needed in further development of neladenoson for the treatment of patients with HFpEF.[16]

CARDIOMYOCYTE HANDLING

Myocardial contractility is the most important aspect which defines cardiac output. Various intracellular chains of events establish a rhythmic untiring sequence of meaningful contractility. Any impairment in cellular ionic disturbance results in poor contractility. Multiple ionic changes across cell membranes in cardiomyocytes are vulnerable to cellular and mitochondrial dysfunction. One of the important ions is calcium and Ca^{2+} homeostasis in cardiac myocytes is regulated at ryanodine receptor and Ca-calmodulin kinase II delta level by istaroxime.[17]

Istaroxime is an important molecule that can augment Ca^{2+} handling by inhibiting Na^+/K^+-ATPase activity and increases cardiomyocyte contractility. Istaroxime has luso-inotropic properties and has an effective uncoupling of actin-myosin and upcoming ventricular relaxation. This is effected through sarcoplasmic/endoplasmic reticulum calcium ATPase2a (SERCA2a) which helps in sequestering cytosolic Ca^{2+} back to the sarcoplasmic reticulum (SR).[18] Istaroxime infusion in acute heart failure shows improvement in systolic and diastolic function without any significant adverse effects.[19]

The HORIZON-HF (Hemodynamic, Echocardiographic, and Neurohormonal Effects of Istaroxime, in Patients Hospitalized with Heart Failure) trial demonstrated that istaroxime lowers left ventricular (LV) filling pressure, improves cardiac output, decreases heart rate assessed by measuring the mitral deceleration time. It could not be used due to (1) short plasma half-life, (2) nonselective for SERCA2a, and (3) adverse gastrointestinal side effects.[20] Istaroxime infusion in acute heart failure shows improvement in systolic and diastolic function without any significant adverse effects.[21]

PST3093 a metabolite of istaroxime could be an excellent prototype to establish, a forthcoming pharmacodynamics class with robust ino-lusitropic nonselective effects to treat HF. PST3093 does not inhibit the Na^+/K^+-ATPase pump but only stimulates SERCA2a, thus qualifying PST3093 as a selective activator.[22] In addition, PST3093 acts by weakening the SERCA-PLN interaction, a mechanism that had been previously confirmed although not in an exclusive manner. Potential future directions include (1) investigating in detail the mechanisms underlying the lower toxicity of PST3093 compared with istaroxime and validating the hypothesis that this aspect depends on its different inhibitory capabilities and (2) evaluating the actions of PST3093 on other SERCA isoforms in another cell type.[23] Cariporide a NHE-1 inhibitor has shown its effect on reversing ventricular hypertrophy and preventing cell apoptosis by blocking calcium overload of the myocytes. It has some antiarrhythmic properties also.[24]

Nitroxyl Donors

Cimlanod (BMS-986231) has shown positive outcomes in terms of safety and hemodynamic profile in patients with advanced heart failure. The ongoing clinical trial, Stand-UP-AHF, is evaluating the efficacy and tolerability of cimlanod in patients with low LVEF. Nitroxyl (HNO) donors are compounds that can improve cardiomyocyte function by directly acting on SR Ca^{2+} cycling 6 HNO causes post-translational modification of thiol residues and, in particular, adenosine triphosphatase, ryanodine receptors, phospholamban, and myofilament proteins.[25] The nucleotide-binding oligomerization domain-containing protein 1 (NOD1) pathway is another potential target for heart failure therapy. NOD1 is implicated in cardiovascular diseases, and its overexpression may contribute to the intracellular calcium mishandling.[26] NOD1 receptor antagonists and specific signaling pathway inhibitors such as Noditinib-1 and receptor interacting protein-2 (RIP2) inhibitors like GSK'214 are mentioned as potential therapeutic options.[27]

MYOFIBRILLAR PATHWAY

Myofibril Myosin Activator

Omecamtiv mecarbil is a selective, small-molecule cardiac myosin activator that belongs to the class of drugs known as myotropes or myosin activators.[28] It directly targets the contractile mechanisms of the heart by binding to and recruiting more cardiac myosin heads to interact with acting during systole, thereby increasing the number and performance of active actin-myosin cross bridges during each cardiac cycle.[29]

The main purpose of omecamtiv mecarbil is to improve cardiac contractility without increasing intracellular myocyte calcium concentrations or myocardial oxygen demand. It facilitates the conversion of the actin-myosin complex from a weak to a strong bond, thus enhancing LV systolic function.[30]

Several clinical trials have evaluated the efficacy and safety of omecamtiv mecarbil. The ATOMIC-AHF trial, which included patients with symptomatic congestive heart failure (CHF) and a LVEF lower than 40%, demonstrated that omecamtiv mecarbil increased systolic function, decreased LV end-systolic diameter, and was well tolerated. It also significantly a decreased NT-pro-BNP levels compared to a placebo and was found to be safe for acute heart failure.[31] The GALACTIC-HF trial, a large Phase 3 study, compared omecamtiv mecarbil with a placebo in patients with HFrEF. The trial showed a significant relative risk reduction in a composite of heart failure events, cardiovascular death, and a primary-outcome event. The frequency of cardiac ischemic events and ventricular arrhythmias was similar or lower in the omecamtiv mecarbil group compared to the placebo group; additionally, N-terminal pro-B-type natriuretic peptide (NT-pro-BNP) levels were lower in the omecamtiv mecarbil group.[32] Omecamtiv mecarbil is also being assessed in the METEORIC-HF trial, a Phase 3 trial that aims to evaluate its effects on exercise capacity. It is important to note that aficamten is a cardiac myosin inhibitor, whereas omecamtiv mecarbil is a cardiac myosin activator. Aficamten is being studied in patients with symptomatic obstructive hypertrophic cardiomyopathy (HCM) in the SEQUOIA-HCM Phase 3 clinical trial and in nonobstructive HCM in the REDWOOD-HCM Phase 2 trial.[33]

SIGNALING PATHWAYS

Nitric oxide (NO) plays an important role in the preservation of vascular integrity and endothelial function. Low levels of NO are not an ideal situation for endothelium and cardiac myocyte.[34] The soluble guanylate cyclase (sGC)-mediated synthesis of cyclic guanosine monophosphate (CGMP) is needed for NO availability. NO is produced in the endocardium and endothelium. In conditions where there is a deficiency of NO, such as in HFrEF, the sGC-mediated synthesis of cGMP is impaired. Reduced sGC activity contributes to various cardiovascular abnormalities, including coronary microvascular dysfunction (CMD), cardiomyocyte stiffness, and interstitial fibrosis.

Currently, the available option for the therapy of heart failure does not address this pathway of NO deficiency. Soluble guanylate cyclase stimulators (riociguat and vericiguat) enhance sGC sensitivity to endogenous NO. Vericiguat has direct vasodilatory properties. It also has an effect on myocardial compliance, diastolic function, and endothelial function thus improving vasotonal regulation, ventricular–arterial coupling, and cardiac reserve in HF.[35] Vericiguat as an sGC stimulator, increases the production of cGMP, which helps to improve NO signaling and prevention of fibrosis.[36] Clinical trials have demonstrated the effectiveness and safety of vericiguat in patients with heart failure. The SOCRATES-PRESERVED study showed that vericiguat was well tolerated and associated with improvements in quality of life in patients with chronic heart failure.[37]

In the VICTORIA trial, which is a large-scale study with vericiguat in patients with worsening heart failure and reduced ejection fraction, the study group received a median dose of 9.2 mg and was followed for a median duration of 10.8 months. In this trial, patients who received vericiguat had a lower incidence (10%) of primary endpoint compared to placebo [35.5% vs. 38.5%, with low hazard ratio (HR) 0.90; 95% confidence interval (CI) 0.82–0.98; $p = 0.02$]. The secondary outcomes of death from any cause or first hospitalization for HF; and total hospitalization for HF were also remarkably lower in the vericiguat group. There were 414 (16.4) deaths from cardiovascular causes that occurred in the vericiguat group and in 441 patients (17.5%) in the placebo group (HR: 0.93; 95% CI 0.81–1.06). The composite of death from any cause or hospitalization for heart failure occurred in 957 patients (37.9%) in the vericiguat group and in 1,032 patients (40.9%) in the placebo group. In patients who received a higher dose of vericiguat, there was more reduction of NT-proBNP levels as compared with the placebo group. Improvement in LVEF was also noted in patients who received 10 mg of vericiguat. There was no intolerance to the drug and had no limitation in renal failure patients.[38] The ongoing VICTOR trial is evaluating the efficacy and safety of vericiguat in adults with chronic heart failure and reduced ejection fraction who have not experienced a recent worsening heart failure event. These studies indicate that vericiguat, as an sGC stimulator, has the potential to improve outcomes in heart failure by augmenting the cGMP pathway and increasing the availability of NO. However, the VITALITY trial done in HFpEF did not show any improvement.[33]

ANTI-INFLAMMATORY PATHWAY

In acute coronary syndrome, there is an enhanced inflammatory response, which further aggravates the myocardial injury leading to adverse ventricular remodeling, and systolic and diastolic dysfunction culminating in heart failure. The inflammatory response during ST-elevation myocardial infarction (STEMI) may modulate the response of the cardiomyocytes and other cells during the initial ischemic injury.[39]

It has been observed that there is a rise in the level of interleukin-1 (IL-1) which can induce upregulation of endothelial adhesion molecules, smooth cell proliferation, and cardiac remodeling, all these can affect the outcome of CV events. IL-1 interferes with the intrinsic property of cardiomyocytes to contract (inotropy) and to relax (lusitropy) leading to the impairment of systolic and diastolic cardiac reserve. It is presumed that IL-1 which is a key mediator of the inflammatory response, and its blockade can be a potential therapeutic strategy to prevent heart failure and other adverse events following.[40] Anakinra an IL-receptor antagonist, in three randomized trials of 139 patients of STEMI showed a significant reduction in the composite endpoint of all-cause mortality or new-onset HF at a 1-year of follow-up as compared to placebo. All these trials included patients who arrived in the first 12 hours of the onset of STEMI and were enrolled within 12 hours of reperfusion and randomized to anakinra 100 mg/day or placebo for 14 days. The composite endpoint of death or new-onset HF occurred in 23% of patients among those with anterior STEMI and in 13% of those who received Anakinra. Anakinra also reduced activation of macrophages 4 (13%) versus 7 (42%) in STEMI thus establishing its anti-inflammatory role.[41]

In the VCUART study, anakinra showed improvement in cardio respiratory fitness and prevention of HF hospitalizations irrespective of the infarct size, the severity of systolic dysfunction, STEMI location, and changes in LV volumes. Anakinra blunted the acute systemic inflammatory response without significant effects on the infarct size or cardiac remodeling. The benefit of IL-1 blockade may be therefore independent of the classic paradigm of infarct sparing for the prevention of adverse remodeling.[42] In the pilot REDHART trial, 60 patients with decompensated HFrEF were given anakinra (100 mg) or placebo for 4 and 12 weeks, the patients treated with anakinra showed an improvement in peak VO_2 compared with baseline as compared with placebo.[43]

Canakinumab is a fully human monoclonal antibody neutralizing interleukin-1 beta (IL-1β). Its mode of action is based on the neutralization of 1β signaling, resulting in the suppression of inflammation. In a large randomized trial of patients with atherosclerotic disease and increased inflammation, treatment with canakinumab led to a lower rate of recurrent cardiovascular events. In the CANTOS trial with canakinumab, it was observed that targeting inflammation can confer cardiovascular benefit in high-risk patients with established atherosclerotic disease who had already survived an MI and had residual inflammatory risk. Total cardiovascular events, defined as cardiovascular death, MI, stroke, and coronary revascularization, occurred in 8.4/100 person-years of the 50 mg group versus 8.3/100 person-years of the 150 mg group versus 8.2/100 person-years of the 300 mg group versus 10.4/100 person-years of the placebo group ($p = 0.004$ for 50 mg group, $p = 0.002$ for 150 mg group, $p = 0.001$ for 300 mg group vs. placebo). The greatest benefit was observed among those who achieved high-sensitivity C-reactive protein (hsCRP) <2 mg/L (HR 0.68; 95% CI 0.53–0.86; $p = 0.001$).[44]

Other promising therapeutic agents acting at different levels in controlling inflammatory states are in the development stages. Molecules like chemokine receptor antagonist and peroxisome proliferator-activated receptor activator—nuclear factor kappa B (NF-κB) which inhibits proinflammatory gene expressions and cellular proliferation of fibroblast may help in HFpEF.[45] Mesenchymal precursor cells (MPCs) have potent anti-inflammatory, proangiogenic, and prohealing effects. The MPCs effects were studied in the DREAM-HF (Double-Blind Randomized Assessment of Clinical Events with Allogeneic Mesenchymal Precursor Cells in Heart Failure) trial on 565 patients for 30 months with chronic heart failure already on standard-of-care heart failure treatment and symptomatic. These patients received a single intramyocardial injection of 150 million cells of rexlemestrocel-L, and the trial showed a reduction in HF-MACE; (hospitalization for decompensated HF, or cardiac death) in the study drug group (0/15, 0%) versus controls (5/15, 33%) HF-MACE ($p = 0.026$). It occurred only in patients with baseline left ventricular end-diastolic volume (LVEDV) > 100 mL—a surrogate for LV contractile state that is >3 SDs above the mean value for normal subjects.[46]

MICROCIRCULATION PATHWAY

Myocardial perfusion is dependent on the macrovascular and microvascular systems; the latter refers to the network of small blood vessels within the heart muscle, specifically the arterioles and capillaries that supply oxygen and nutrients to the cardiac tissue. Microcirculation plays a crucial role in maintaining the proper functioning of the heart. The arterioles may dilate or constrict in response to various factors, such as oxygen demand, metabolic needs, and hormonal signals. Impairment of this mechanism is defined as CMD.[47]

Microcirculatory anomalies can be often found in HF patients. CMD is associated with the development of HFpEF, due to perivascular fibrosis, and decreased bio-accessibility of NO, mainly in HF with (HFpEF).[48,49] In HFpEF models, coronary microvascular endothelial inflammation reduces NO bioavailability, cyclic guanosine monophosphate content, and protein kinase G (PKG) activity in adjacent cardiomyocytes.[50] Restoring a healthy microcirculation and endothelium could be another possible therapeutic approach to treat heart failure.[50] In the future emphasis will be to assess the new translational drugs on the microcirculation like growth factors and noncoding RNA therapeutics as well as the targeting of metabolites or metabolic signaling.[51]

CONCLUSION

Traditional treatments for heart failure still have a proven role, but many patients are still at high residual risk for recurrent hospitalization and high mortality. Research for newer modes of therapy for heart failure targeting molecular, cellular, biomaterial, and genetic pathways is ongoing. Apart from pharmacotherapy, the use of induced pluripotent stem cells (iPSCs), embryonic stem cells (ESCs), and skeletal muscle myogenic cells are also under trial for heart failure. Other newer pathways are the use of exosomes which are membrane-bound nanovesicles containing various biomolecules such as lipids, proteins, and nucleic acid for the repair of damaged myocardial tissue is also under investigation. Gene therapy is an attractive, but still far from being clinically applicable modality of treatment. Nanotechnology developed adenoviral S100A1, gene normalized S100A1 protein expression in a postinfarction model of heart failure have been tried in reversing contractile dysfunction of failing myocardium. This will take up a long time for future implications in heart failure therapy for a better outcome.

ONLINE REFERENCES

Please scan the QR code provided at the end of the table of contents for References of this chapter.

CHAPTER 57

Vericiguat in Heart Failure

AK Pancholia

ABSTRACT

Heart failure (HF) progression is associated with repeated worsening events and every event resulting in reduced cardiac function. Worsening HF (WHF) events are characterized by deterioration of signs and symptoms of HF for which medical treatment is warranted, despite the use of guideline-directed medical therapy (GDMT). At present, patients are categorized as having WHF if they require IV diuretics, HF hospitalization, or an emergency department visit. Each event is associated with a sharp drop in cardiac function, which only partially recovers after the event.

Currently, major pharmacological therapies used to treat HF target compensatory mechanisms in HF, such as the renin–angiotensin–aldosterone system (RAAS) inhibitor, sympathetic nervous system (SNS), or natriuretic peptide system (NPS). The nitric oxide-soluble guanylyl cyclase–cyclic guanosine monophosphate (NO–sGC–cGMP) pathway is essentially an untapped pathway in HF. However, oxidative stress and endothelial dysfunction in HF lead to reduced nitric oxide (NO) bioavailability, resulting in sGC deficiency and, therefore, reduction in cGMP synthesis. Vericiguat is a novel sGC stimulator and can act independently from or synergistically with NO. It can independently stimulate sGC even with low endogenous NO, and increases the sensitivity of sGC to NO, thereby having an increased effect on cGMP production. With this unique mechanism of action of vericiguat, it may be possible to decrease myocardial stiffening, hypertrophy, ventricular remodeling, fibrosis, and vasoconstriction, while increasing renal blood flow and endothelial function, thereby improving the pathophysiology of HF.

The VICTORIA (Vericiguat Global Study in Subjects with Heart Failure with Reduced Ejection Fraction) trial established the efficacy and safety of vericiguat on HF hospitalization and cardiovascular mortality in patients with heart failure with reduced ejection fraction (HFrEF) and a recent WHF event.

Keywords: Worsening heart failure, hospitalization, IV diuretics, emergency department (ED) visit, guideline directed medical therapy.

INTRODUCTION

The global number of patients with heart failure (HF) is roughly estimated to be 60 million, while in India, the estimates range widely from 1.3 to 23 million.[1,2] Over half of this population has heart failure with reduced ejection fraction (HFrEF).[1] HF progression is typically punctuated by repeated worsening events, each of which results in a reduced cardiac function.[3] Worsening HF (WHF) events are characterized by deterioration of signs and symptoms in a patient with chronic HF despite the use of previous guideline-directed medical therapy (GDMT).[4] WHF is regarded as a phase in the normal course of the disease, indicating its advancement, and it signifies a significantly poorer outlook.[5] Currently, WHF requires the need for a hospitalization for HF, treatment of HF in the emergency department (ED), or administration of intravenous (IV) diuretic therapy in the outpatient setting.[4,6]

According to a large US PINNACLE HF registry of 11,064 HFrEF patients, approximately 50% of the patients were rehospitalized within 30 days of a WHF event and more than one in five patients died within 2 years of their first WHF event.[5] Even according to the PARADIGM-HF trial, patients who had been hospitalized for HF within 6 months were 46% more likely to experience a primary event (CV death or HFH) than those without prior hospitalization.[7] Patients on quadruple therapy also remain at high risk of WHF and CV death.[1] According to the DAPA-HF, approximately 14.3% (1 in 7 patients) patients experienced a primary outcome event, despite confirmed use of quadruple therapy [angiotensin receptor-neprilysin inhibitor (ARNI), beta-blocker, mineralocorticoid receptor antagonist (MRA), and sodium-glucose cotransporter-2 inhibitor (SGLT-2I)].[8,9] With such a high unmet medical need, patients with WHF require newer therapeutic options to break their cycle of recurrent WHF events.

MECHANISM OF ACTION (FIG. 1)

All major pharmacological therapies used to manage and treat HF target compensatory mechanisms, such as the renin–angiotensin–aldosterone system (RAAS), sympathetic nervous system (SNS), or natriuretic peptide system (NPS).[10-13] Vericiguat is a novel soluble guanylate cyclase (sGC) stimulator and is the only therapy that targets and restores the impaired nitric oxide-soluble guanylyl cyclase–cyclic guanosine monophosphate (NO-sGC-cGMP) pathway.[14-16] The sGC acts as a receptor for NO and triggers the production of cGMP, which is crucial for maintaining the proper functioning of the heart and blood vessels.[17-20] In patients with HF, oxidative stress and endothelial dysfunction reduce NO bioavailability, resulting in sGC deficiency and, therefore, reduction in cGMP synthesis.[14,17-20] In case of vericiguat, the direct sGC stimulation, independent of NO availability, can restore this pathway.[16-21] This represents the unique mode of action of vericiguat.[16-21] Vericiguat can also act synergistically with NO and lead to

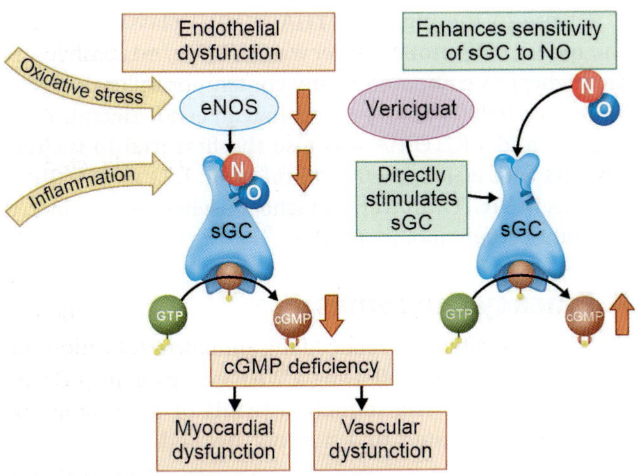

FIG. 1: Mechanism of action (MOA) of vericiguat.

(cGMP: cyclic guanosine monophosphate; eNOS: endothelial nitric oxide synthase; sGC: soluble guanylate cyclase)

Source: Armstrong PW, Roessig L, Patel MJ, Anstrom KJ, Butler J, Voors AA, et al.; VICTORIA study group. A Multicenter, Randomized, Double-Blind, Placebo-Controlled Trial of the Efficacy and Safety of the Oral Soluble Guanylate Cyclase Stimulator: The VICTORIA Trial. JACC Heart Fail. 2018;6(2): 96-104.

an increased effect on cGMP production.[22,23] By restoring the NO-sGC-cGMP pathway, through the mode of action for vericiguat, it may be possible to decrease myocardial stiffening, hypertrophy, ventricular remodeling, fibrosis, and vasoconstriction, while increasing renal blood flow and endothelial function, thereby improving the pathophysiology of HF.[14,17-21]

The VICTORIA (Vericiguat Global Study in Subjects with Heart Failure with Reduced Ejection Fraction) trial is backed by evidence from a phase IIb dose-finding study called SOCRATES REDUCED (SOluble guanylate Cyclase stimulator in heart failure) that involved participants with HFrEF.[24,25] In this study, standard treatment for patients with deteriorating chronic HF, who needed to be hospitalized or receive IV diuretic treatment, was supplemented with vericiguat.[25] This was done in cases where the levels of B-type natriuretic peptide (BNP) or N-terminal pro-B-type natriuretic peptide (NT-proBNP) had increased.[25] These patients were randomized at baseline to receive either 1 of 4 vericiguat dosage plans (1.25 mg, 2.5 mg, 5 mg, or 10 mg) or a placebo dose over 12 weeks.[25] The primary endpoint was change in NT-proBNP.[25] Safety and tolerability were also assessed as secondary endpoints.[25]

Although, in the primary endpoint analysis, vericiguat showed no significant benefit over placebo when pooling the change in NT-proBNP in the 2.5–10 mg dosage arms, the secondary exploratory analysis showed that the two higher dosage arms of vericiguat did yield significant differences in change in NT-proBNP compared with placebo, suggesting a dose-response relationship. Although this study was not powered for clinical events, the exploratory analysis suggested that the rates of CV mortality and HF hospitalizations were generally numerically lower among patients receiving vericiguat, compared with placebo, particularly among those randomized to the two highest-dose vericiguat groups.[25]

Overall, vericiguat was found to be safe and well tolerated when compared to the placebo. There was no significant difference between the vericiguat group versus placebo in terms of change in blood pressure or heart rate. The trajectories for glomerular filtration rate (GFR) and troponin were also similar in these study groups. This indicates that vericiguat is not associated with any deleterious effects on BP, HR, renal function, or troponin release.[25]

The positive findings, in terms of the efficacy and safety endpoints in this study, supported the decision to proceed with a large phase III study. The dosing regimen (2.5 mg to target 10 mg) was chosen based on the dose-finding data.[25]

PHASE-III TRIAL (VICTORIA TRIAL)

The VICTORIA was an international, randomized, placebo-controlled, parallel-group, multicenter, double-blind, event-driven trial to evaluate the effect of vericiguat in patients with symptomatic chronic HF following a WHF event.[14,16] A WHF event was defined as an HF hospitalization within

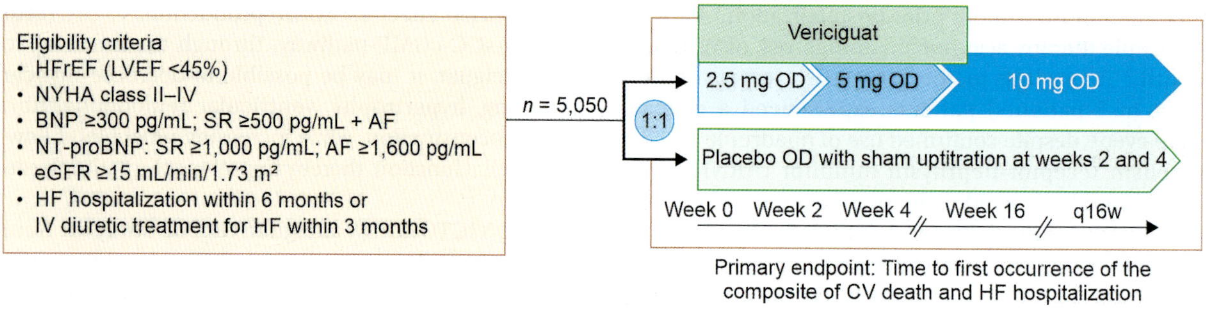

FIG. 2: VICTORIA study design.

(BNP: B-type natriuretic peptide; eGFR: estimated glomerular filtration rate; HF: heart failure; HFrEF: heart failure with reduced ejection fraction; IV: intravenous; LVEF: left ventricular ejection fraction; NT-proBNP: N-terminal pro-B-type natriuretic peptide; NYHA: New York Heart Association; SR: Sinus Rhythm)

Source: Armstrong PW, Pieske B, Anstrom KJ, Ezekowitz J, Hernandez AF, Butler J, et al. Vericiguat in patients with heart failure and reduced ejection fraction. N Engl J Med. 2020;382:1883-93.

6 months or outpatient IV diuretic use within 3 months.[16] VICTORIA is the only trial to specifically assess such HF patients following a WHF event.[9,16,26-28] All other contemporary HF trials enrolled patients with chronic symptomatic HF regardless of worsening events.[9,16,26-28]

The primary objective of the VICTORIA trial was to determine the efficacy of vericiguat in increasing the time to the first occurrence of the composite endpoint of cardiovascular (CV) death or HF hospitalization in patients with HFrEF following a recent WHF event as compared to placebo, on top of GDMT.[16]

VICTORIA Study Design (Fig. 2)

A total of 5,050 subjects were randomized in a 1:1 ratio and the enrolled patients were assigned to receive either vericiguat or placebo, on top of GDMT.

Inclusion Criteria

- Congestive heart failure (CHF); New York Heart Association (NYHA) class II–IV, left ventricular EF <45%, and guideline-directed HF therapy
- Recent HF hospitalization or IV diuretic use
- Elevated natriuretic peptides; NT-proBNP ≥1,000 pg/mL [≥1,600 pg/mL if atrial fibrillation (AF)] or BNP ≥300 pg/mL (≥500 pg/mL, if AF)
- Clinically stable [systolic blood pressure (SBP) ≥100 mm Hg and no IV diuretics for 24 hours]

Exclusion Criteria

- Use of long-acting nitrates, phosphodiesterase type 5 inhibitor, and riociguat
- Awaiting heart transplantation, continuous IV diuretics, or current/anticipated ventricular assist device
- Chronic kidney disease [estimated glomerular filtration rate (eGFR) 15 mL/min/1.73 m^2] or dialysis
- Severe pulmonary disease requiring continuous oxygen
- Severe hepatic insufficiency
- Correctable cardiac comorbidities

After a screening period of 30 days or less, without a run-in period, qualified individuals were treated until the desired number of CV deaths were recorded. The study participants were at least 18 years old and had chronic HF (NYHA functional classes II to IV) along with a reduced ejection fraction of <45%. They were receiving the standard treatment recommended by the European Society of Cardiology (ESC), American Heart Association/American College of Cardiology HF guidelines, and any country-specific guidelines that were applicable. The median follow-up duration was 10.8 months.[16]

Among these patients, 84% of patients were hospitalized within 6 months of randomization and the remaining patients required IV therapy in the outpatient setting.[17] 41% were in the highest NYHA (III/IV) classifications.[16] The median NT-proBNP level was 2,816 pg/mL, which was the highest as compared to any contemporary trial.[9,16,26-28] More than half (53%) of patients had an eGFR ≤60 mL/min/1.73 m^2 and VICTORIA was also the first trial to include patients with eGFR down to 15 mL/min/1.73 m^2.[16,29] Thus, patients in VICTORIA were at higher baseline risk compared with other contemporary HF trials.[9,16,26-28]

Efficacy Outcomes

Vericiguat significantly reduced the annualized absolute risk for HFH or CV death following a WHF event versus placebo, with an absolute risk reduction (ARR) of 4.2 events/100 PY, which translated to a number needed to treat of 24 **(Fig. 3)**.[16]

This ARR for the primary composite endpoint was comparable to the other Phase-III trials in HFrEF (PARADIGM-HF, DAPA-HF, and EMPEROR-Reduced) **(Table 1)**.[9,30,31]

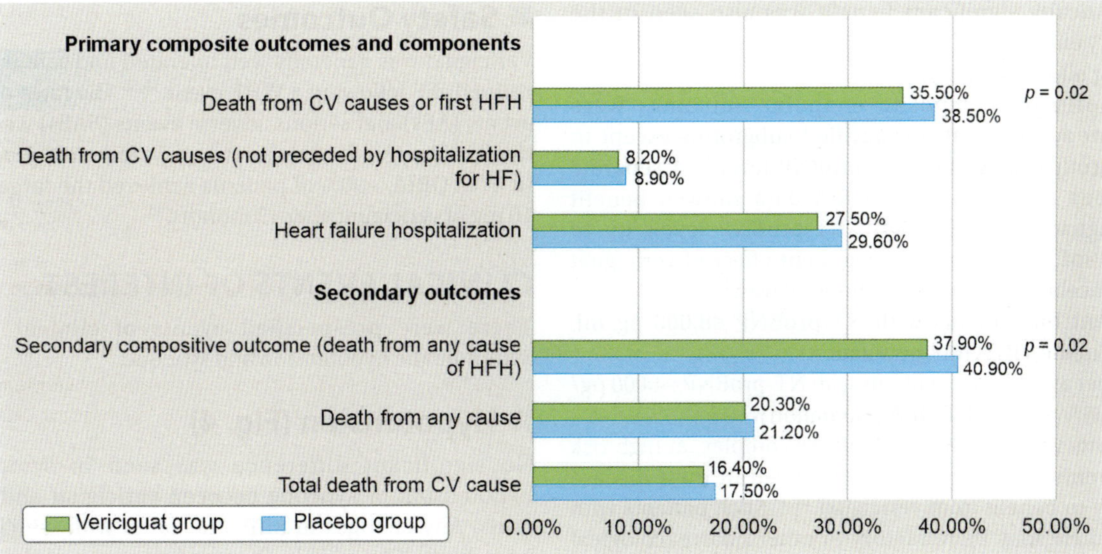

FIG. 3: Primary and secondary outcomes.

(CV: cardiovascular; HF: heart failure; HFH: heart failure hospitalization)

Source: Armstrong PW, Pieske B, Anstrom KJ, Ezekowitz J, Hernandez AF, Butler J, et al.; Victoria Study Group. Vericiguat in patients with heart failure and reduced ejection fraction. N Engl J Med. 2020;382:1883-93.

TABLE 1: Landmark clinical trials in HFrEF.

Key details	PARADIGM HF (*n* = 8,399)[1] Sacubitril/Valsartan	DAPA-HF (*n* = 4,744)[2] Dapagliflozin	EMPEROR-reduced (*n* = 3,730)[3] Empagliflozin	VICTORIA (*n* = 5,050)[4] Vericiguat
eGFR cut-off	>30 mL/min/1.73 m^2	>30 mL/min/1.73 m^2	>20 mL/min/1.73 m^2	>15 mL/min/1.73 m^2
Recent HF decompensation	Not required	Not required	Not required	HFH within 6 months or IV diuretic use for HF within 3 months
Median NT-proBNP	1,608	1,437	1,906	2,816
HFH <6 months	31%	16%	NA	84%
IV diuretic for HF (without hospitalization) within 3 months, n (%)	NR	NR	NR	15.9%
NYHA III–IV	25%	32%	25%	41%
eGFR <60 mL/min/1.73 m^2	37%	41%	48%	53%
Primary endpoint event rate (control arm)	13.2 events/100 PY	15.6 events/100 PY	21.0 events/100 PY	37.8 events/100 PY

(eGFR: estimated glomerular filtration rate; HF: heart failure; HFrEF: heart failure with reduced ejection fraction; HFH: heart failure hospitalization; IV: intravenous; NYHA: New York Heart Association; NT-proBNP: N-terminal pro-B-type natriuretic peptide; WHF: worsening heart failure)

Sources:

1. McMurray JJV, Packer M, Desai AS, Gong J, Lefkowitz MP, Rizkala AR, et al. Angiotensin-neprilysin inhibition versus enalapril in heart failure. N Engl J Med. 2014;371:993-1004.
2. McMurray JJV, Solomon SD, Inzucchi SE, Køber L, Kosiborod MN, Martinez FA, et al. Dapagliflozin in patients with heart failure and reduced ejection fraction. N Engl J Med. 2019;381:1995-2008.
3. Packer M, Anker SD, Butler J, Filippatos G, Pocock SJ, Carson P, et al. Cardiovascular and renal outcomes with empagliflozin in heart failure. N Engl J Med. 2020;383:1413-24.
4. Armstrong PW, Pieske B, Anstrom KJ, Ezekowitz J, Hernandez AF, Butler J, et al. Vericiguat in patients with heart failure and reduced ejection fraction. N Engl J Med. 2020;382:1883-93.

Statistically significant benefit was also seen in the secondary endpoints of total HFH and the composite of time to HFH or all-cause mortality.[16]

The primary composite endpoint outcomes were consistent across most prespecified subgroups except in the subgroups of age and NT-proBNP level.[16] A separate continuous analysis of VICTORIA data showed benefit of vericiguat in patients with NT-proBNP levels up to 8,000 pg/mL.[32] The positive treatment effect of vericiguat versus placebo on the primary endpoint was:[32]

- Evident for patients with NT-proBNP ≤8,000 pg/mL (86% of the VICTORIA population)
- Further amplified in patients with NT-proBNP ≤4,000 pg/mL (65% of the VICTORIA population)

Patients with high NT-proBNP are complex, at high risk of CV events, and may be too advanced in their disease trajectory to benefit from vericiguat.[14,33] Such patients with advanced HF may be refractory to other pharmacological therapies as well.[34] For instance, even in the LIFE trial, no benefit of sacubitril/valsartan over valsartan was seen in patients with advanced HFrEF with NYHA class IV symptoms.[34]

Overall, vericiguat demonstrated efficacy on the primary endpoint irrespective of background HF therapy in a well-treated population and concomitant use of ARNI did not alter vericiguat efficacy and safety. Vericiguat could benefit a wide range of patients following a WHF event, regardless of comorbidities such as AF and coronary artery disease (CAD). It also provided benefit in patients across eGFR categories.[16]

Safety Outcomes

Vericiguat was generally well tolerated and safe in patients with HFrEF following a WHF event.[16,35] The rates of adverse events (AEs) and serious adverse events (SAEs) were numerically lower with vericiguat compared with placebo.[16,35] In VICTORIA, ~90% of patients achieved the target dose of 10 mg of vericiguat after 12 months.[35]

CLINICAL EVENTS OF INTEREST

There were prespecified events of clinical interest: Symptomatic hypotension and syncope.

Hypotension (Fig. 4)

No significant difference was seen in symptomatic hypotension or syncope between vericiguat and placebo arms. Any changes in SBP associated with vericiguat use were limited to early in the titration phase and no further clinically relevant reductions in BP were observed throughout the remainder of the study.[16]

No excessive blood pressure reductions were observed with vericiguat even in potentially vulnerable patients.[16,35]

Renal Function

The VICTORIA trial evaluated "Vericiguat" which could be given upto eGFR of 15 mL/min/1.73 m^2.[9,16,26-28] Over half of patients had an eGFR ≤60 mL/min/1.73 m^2 in VICTORIA.[16]

Effect of vericiguat on renal function trajectories was similar to that of placebo. No difference in the incidence of

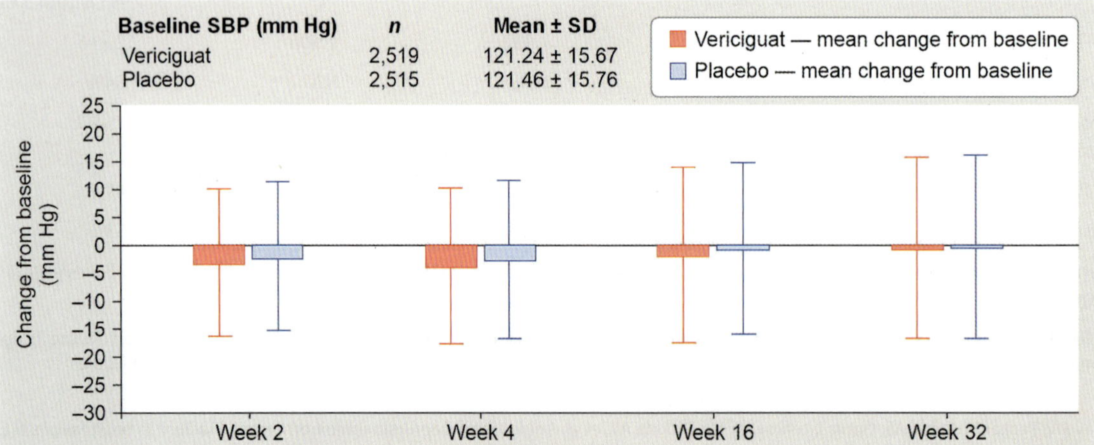

Patients with SBP assessment at each time point				
Vericiguat	2,516	2,388	2,147	1,769
Placbo	2,513	2,388	2,173	1,774

FIG. 4: Mean change in systolic blood pressure from baseline over time.

(SBP: systolic blood pressure)

Source: Armstrong PW, Pieske B, Anstrom KJ, Ezekowitz J, Hernandez AF, Butler J, et al. Vericiguat in patients with heart failure and reduced ejection fraction. N Engl J Med. 2020;382:1883-93.

worsening renal function was apparent between treatment arms. Although worsening renal function was more prevalent in patients with an eGFR ≤30 mL/min/1.73 m^2, no differences were apparent between patients on vericiguat versus placebo. Vericiguat provided benefit in patients across eGFR categories. No clinically significant differences in sodium or potassium levels were observed over time between treatment arms.[29]

Other Challenges

According to a recent Heart Failure Association (HFA) consensus document of ESC, various factors impact both the initiation and uptitration of GDMT in HFrEF.[36] Patients with HFrEF also often suffer from medication side effects, making adherence challenging.[36,37] Patient factors commonly associated with nonuse and subtarget dosing of GDMT include hypotension, hyperkalemia, worsening renal function, older age, and low body mass index.[36,37]

A multinational study (Sweden, UK, and US) also observed high discontinuation rates of newly initiated standard therapies among patients with recent HFH who were initially naive to therapy (n = 68,172).[38] Such patients not receiving standard therapies (nonuse or discontinuation) are at significantly increased risk of mortality (37%) versus those receiving standard therapies.[38,39]

Data from CHAMP-HF and PINNACLE also highlight the therapeutic gap in HFrEF, with up to one-third of patients not on individual components of background therapy.[40] According to an analysis from a large Swedish heart failure (SwedeHF) registry (n = 17,809), the incidence of CV death or heart failure hospitalization (HFH) according is much lower in patients receiving combination therapies than those receiving monotherapy.[41] Achieving 50–99% target dose of angiotensin-converting enzyme inhibitor (ACEI)/angiotensin receptor blocker (ARB)/ARNI and beta-blocker is more effective than monotherapy at 100% target dose.[41] Comprehensive therapy including vericiguat is, therefore, recommended.[41]

Thus, vericiguat owing to its strong safety profile would help to overcome these challenges and offer substantial benefits to patients.[41]

DRUG TITRATION SCHEMA AND DOSE MODIFICATION CRITERIA (FIG. 5)

Vericiguat is a once-daily treatment and has a straightforward dosing schedule. Vericiguat is initiated at a dose of 2.5 mg OD and doubled approximately every 2 weeks to a target dose of 10 mg OD.[16]

Guideline Recommendations (Table 2)

Vericiguat is consistently recommended for patients with HFrEF following a WHF event in various guidelines.[42-44]

ONGOING TRIALS

- *VICTOR trial*: This is an international, parallel-group, event-driven, randomized, double-blind, placebo-controlled, phase 3 trial designed to investigate the effect of vericiguat in chronic HFrEF patients without

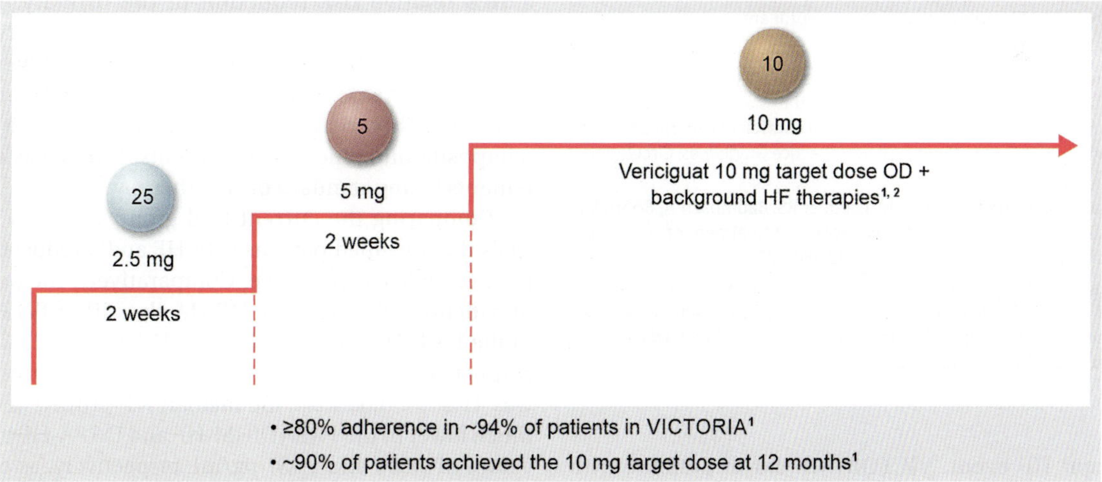

1. Bayer AG. Verquvo® (vericiguat) SmPC. https://www.ema.europa.eu/documents/product-information/verquvo-epar-product-information_en.pdf
2. Merck Sharp and Dohme Corp. VERQUVO™ (Vericiguat): Highlights of prescribing information. https://www.merck.com/product/usa/pi_circulars/v/verquvo/verquvo_pi.pdf

FIG. 5: Vericiguat dosing and titration schedule.

(HF: heart failure)

Source: Armstrong PW, Pieske B, Anstrom KJ, Ezekowitz J, Hernandez AF, Butler J, et al. Vericiguat in patients with heart failure and reduced ejection fraction. N Engl J Med. 2020;382:1883-93.

TABLE 2: Vericiguat guideline recommendations.

Recommendation	Class	Level
AHA/ACC/HFSA 2022 guidelines[1]		
In selected high-risk patients with HFrEF and recent worsening of HF already on GDMT, an oral sGC stimulator (vericiguat) may be considered to reduce HFH and CV death	2b	B-R[#]
ESC 2021 guidelines[2]		
Vericiguat may be considered in patients in NYHA class II–IV who have had worsening HF despite treatment with an ACEI (or ARNI), a beta-blocker and an MRA to reduce the risk of CV mortality or HFH	IIb	B
CCS/CHFS 2021 guidelines[3]		
We recommend that vericiguat, an oral sGC stimulator, be considered in addition to optimal HF therapies for HFrEF patients with worsening symptoms and HFH in the past 6 months to reduce the risk of subsequent HFH	Conditional*	Moderate quality

*A conditional recommendation is provided because vericiguat has not yet been approved for this indication in Canada.
#Level of evidence B from a randomized trial.

(ACEI: angiotensin-converting enzyme inhibitor; ARNI: angiotensin receptor-neprilysin inhibitor; AHA: American Heart Association; ACC: American College of Cardiology; HFSA: Heart Failure Society of America; CCS: Canadian Cardiovascular Society; CHFS: Canadian Heart Failure Society; CV: cardiovascular; ESC: European Society of Cardiology; HFrEF: heart failure with reduced ejection fraction; GDMT: guideline-directed medical therapy; MRA: mineralocorticoid receptor antagonist)

Source:

1. Heidenreich PA, Bozkurt B, Aguilar D, Allen LA, Byun JJ, Colvin MM, et al. 2022 AHA/ACC/HFSA Guideline for the Management of Heart Failure: A Report of the American College of Cardiology/American Heart Association Joint Committee on Clinical Practice Guidelines. Circulation. 2022;79:e263-421.
2. McDonagh TA, Metra M, Adamo M, Gardner RS, Baumbach A, Böhm M, et al. 2021 ESC Guidelines for the diagnosis and treatment of acute and chronic heart failure. Eur Heart J. 2021;42:3599-726.
3. McDonald M, Virani S, Chan M, Ducharme A, Ezekowitz JA, Giannetti N, et al. CCS/CHFS Heart Failure Guidelines Update: Defining a New Pharmacologic Standard of Care for Heart Failure With Reduced Ejection Fraction. Can J Cardiol. 2021;37:531-46.

a recent HF event. VICTOR will enroll patients with symptomatic chronic HFrEF receiving optimized GDMT. VICTORIA and VICTOR have complementary inclusion profiles. VICTOR and VICTORIA together will investigate the distinct MOA of vericiguat in >11,000 patients with HFrEF.[16,45]

- *Consensus statement*: Recently, a consensus given by the Indian experts on the definition, assessment, pharmacological management of WHF patients (both in hospitalized settings and in outpatient department) has also been published.[46]

DISCUSSION

Patients with HFrEF who need to be hospitalized or receive IV diuretics continue to experience significantly elevated rates of mortality.[15] Furthermore, temporary IV drug administration during hospitalization, in addition to the standard treatment for WHF, has proven ineffective in enhancing long-term results.[15]

The NO-sGC-cGMP pathway is an important and untapped pathway in the HF pathophysiology.[14,17-20] However, in HF, oxidative stress and endothelial dysfunction reduce NO bioavailability, resulting in sGC deficiency and, therefore, reduction in cGMP synthesis.[17-20] Vericiguat is a novel sGC stimulator and can act independently from or synergistically with NO, thereby restoring this impaired pathway.[16-21]

The VICTORIA trial is the only HF trial that was specifically designed to study patients who had chronic HF and a reduced ejection fraction and a WHF event.[16] Other contemporary HF trials enrolled patients with chronic symptomatic HF regardless of worsening events.[9,16,26-28]

VICTORIA specifically enrolled a higher-risk population in comparison with other HF trials.[9,16,26-28] The advantage in favor of vericiguat became noticeable after around 3 months of treatment and continued to exist throughout the entire trial.[16] In this high-risk population, there was a 10% relative risk reduction in the primary outcome, taking into account the context of the study lasting 10.8 months.[16] This translated to an ARR of 4.2 events per 100 patient-years.[16] Based on this, the number needed to treat with vericiguat for 1 year to prevent a primary composite outcome was 24 patients.[16] This was on top of patients taking standard of care therapy.[16]

Comparing the current trial group with two previous trials that included patients with HF and a reduced ejection fraction holds significance. Comparatively, the percentage of patients with severe HF (NYHA class III or IV) was lower in the PARADIGM-HF and DAPA-HF trials at 25% and 32% respectively, whereas in the VICTORIA trial, this number was 41%.[7,9,17] Likewise, the median NT-proBNP levels were much lower in the PARADIGM-HF and DAPA-HF trials, with values of 1,608 and 1,437 pg/mL respectively, as compared to 2,816 pg/mL in the VICTORIA trial.[7,9,17] The disparities mentioned may explain why the vericiguat group experienced a primary composite outcome at an annual rate of 33.6% in our study, which is more than double the rate observed in the two comparative trials.[7,9,17] While both trials demonstrated larger relative reductions in the primary composite outcome of VICTORIA (which includes death from CV causes or first hospitalization for HF), the annualized reductions in absolute risk were comparable.[7,9,16,26-28]

Vericiguat has a favorable safety profile and is well tolerated.[16,35] The rates of AEs and SAEs were numerically lower with vericiguat compared with placebo.[16,35] No significant difference was seen in symptomatic hypotension or syncope between vericiguat and placebo arms.[16,35] Effect of vericiguat on renal function trajectories was also similar to that of placebo and it is the only molecule which can be safely given till eGFR of 15 mL/min/1.73 m^2.[29]

It is also worth highlighting that there was >89% adherence to the target 10-mg dose of vericiguat after 12 months in VICTORIA trial.[16]

CONCLUSION

Vericiguat is a novel sGC stimulator designed toward meeting clinical needs of high-risk chronic HFrEF patients having WHF events despite being on optimized standard-of-care therapy.[16] Owing to its unique mechanism of action, its favorable efficacy, and safety profile, it will be a valuable addition to the armamentarium of such patients.

ONLINE REFERENCES

Please scan the QR code provided at the end of the table of contents for References of this chapter.

CHAPTER 58

Uncovering the Persistent Impact of Rheumatic Heart Disease on Heart Failure and Disease Burden in India

Rajeev Gupta, Manu Gupta, Anuj Gupta, Subroto Mandal

ABSTRACT

Patients with rheumatic heart disease (RHD) were associated with an increased risk of heart failure (HF). With an increase of life expectancy, the prevalence of older adults with RHD is likely to increase. In patients with and without RHD differences in outcomes are determined by the presence and severity of valvular disease. It is also possible that milder forms may progress at a disproportionately faster rate to more severe forms in those with RHD. Early and precise diagnosis of RHD with appropriate management can prevent or postpone the occurrence of congestive heart failure (CHF) and reduce both morbidity and mortality and the cost of repeated hospitalizations. Among community-dwelling older adults free of HF at baseline, despite the presence of mostly mild to moderate valvular disease, RHD has a significant association with incident HF.

Keywords: Rheumatic heart disease (RHD), congestive heart failure (CHF), heart failure (HF).

INTRODUCTION

Rheumatic heart disease (RHD) is the leading cause of cardiovascular morbidity including heart failure (HF). In community with older adults, the prevalence of RHD was relatively high and comprised mostly of a mild to moderate form of valvular disease. Patients with RHD were associated with an increased risk of HF. With an increase of life expectancy, the prevalence of older adults with RHD is likely to increase. In patients with and without RHD differences in outcomes are determined by the presence and severity of valvular disease.

Milder forms of RHD disease may progress to severe forms.[7] In RHD damage to the mitral subvalvular apparatus leads to the rapid progression of mild mitral regurgitation (MR) to a more severe form.[8] Damaged mitral subvalvular apparatus may also lead to diastolic and systolic left ventricular impairment.[9] Because of scarring and retraction of mitral valve leaflets and chordae may restrict leaflet motion, particularly during diastole.[10,11] Age-related dilatation of the aorta may accelerate the progression of aortic regurgitation (AR)[12-15] and vascular stiffness resulting in a more rapid progression to clinical HF. Manifestations of HF in RHD. Irrespective of which valve is involved, the first manifestation of congestive heart failure (CHF) is usually tachycardia. Invariably recent atrial fibrillation (AF) with fast ventricular rate precipitated CHF. Left-sided HF is generally associated with signs of pulmonary venous congestion and pulmonary edema, often seen in patients with multiple sclerosis (MS) and MR, whereas right-sided HF is associated with signs of systemic venous congestion as in cases with tricuspid stenosis (TS) and tricuspid regurgitation (TR) of severe pulmonary arterial hypertension (PAH). Later stages of CHF are characterized by signs and symptoms ot low cardiac output (CO). Generally, CHF with normal CO is called compensated CHF, and CHF with inadequate CO is considered decompensated.

Early and precise diagnosis of RHD with appropriate management can prevent or postpone the occurrence of CHF and reduce both morbidity and mortality and the cost of repeated hospitalizations. The importance of RHD as a major risk factor for incident HF among older adults who remained free of RHD-related complications for decades. HF in RHD is due to either systolic dysfunction as a result of aortic valve disease and or MR or diastolic dysfunction related to MS. Symptoms of HF and thromboembolism are aggravated by AF.

There is limited data about the association of RHD with HF. Current evidence of this association is mostly based on a few cross-sectional survey-based studies from developing nations.[6] A recent review of RHD reported a number of RHD-related incidents of cardiovascular morbidity and mortality but provided no data on RHD-related incident HF.[4] This may be due to the difficulty with the adjudication of HF in the setting of the Indian population.

Rheumatic heart disease is a major risk factor for cardiovascular morbidity and mortality. There is a risk of incident HF among symptom-free of RHD-related complications for decades.

PREVENTION AND PREVALENCE OF RHEUMATIC HEART DISEASE

For control of rheumatic fever (RF) and RHD renewed insight includes an approach toward tertiary interventions including medical management, anticoagulation, surgical, or endovascular approaches.

DECLINE OF RHEUMATIC HEART DISEASE IN INDIA

Epidemiological studies of RF/RHD by authors **(Table 1)**[16] and the Indian Council of Medical Research (ICMR) have suggested declining trends, especially after 2000 onward in multicentric survey studies **(Fig. 1)**. The improvement in

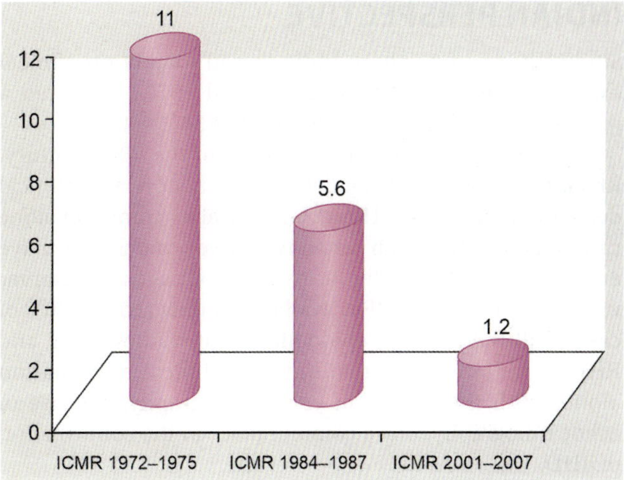

FIG. 1: Trends of change in prevalence of RF/RHD in ICMR-led multicentric survey studies across the country over the period of 40 years.

Note: From available data from RHD studies, the estimated average prevalence is 0.5/1,000 children in the age group of 5–15 years. There are expected to be >3.6 million patients of RHD estimated from the 2011 census.[31]

(ICMR: Indian Council of Medical Research; RF: rheumatic fever; RHD: rheumatic heart disease)

TABLE 1: School-based surveys on the prevalence of RHD based on clinical screening followed by echocardiography confirmation.

Author	Year of survey	Area	Methodology Clinical + echocardiography of suspected (C+ ES)	Population	Age group	Prevalence/1,000
Grover et al.[18]	1988–1991	Ambala (rural)	(C + ES)	31,200	5–15	2.1
Agarwal et al.[19]	1991	Aligarh (rural)	(C + ES)	3,760	5–15	1.3
Gupta et al.[20]	1992	Jammu	(C + ES)	10,263	5–15	1.3
Thakur et al.[21]	1992–1993	Shimla (rural + urban)	(C + ES)	10,805	5–16	• 4.8 (rural) • 1.98 (urban)
Vashistha et al.[22]	1993	Agra (urban)	(C + ES)	8,449	5–15	1.42
Kaul et al.[23]	1999–2000	Srinagar	(C + ES)	4,125	5–15	5.09
Jose et al.[24]	2001–2002	Vellore (rural)	(C + ES)	229,829	6–18	0.68
ICMR[25]	2002–2005	Kochi, Vellore, Chandigarh, Indore, Shimla, Dibrugarh, Wayanad, Jodhpur, Jammu, Mumbai (rural + urban)	(C + ES)	100,269	5–15	0.43–1.47
Kumar et al.[26]	2002–2009	Rupnagar	(C + ES)	813	5–14	1
Misra et al.[27]	2003–2006	Gorakhpur	(C + ES)	118,212	4–18	0.5
Periwal et al.[28]	2006	Bikaner (urban)	(C + ES)	3,292	5–14	0.67
Negi et al.[29]	2007–2008	Shimla (rural + urban)	(C + ES)	15,145	5–15	0.59 (95% CI 0.22–0.96/1,000)
Rama et al.[30]	2011	Prakasam; Andhra Pradesh	(C + ES)	4,213	5–16	0.7

(ICMR: Indian Council of Medical Research; RHD: rheumatic heart disease)

the socioeconomic state of our country,[17] could be the reason for declining trends.

INDIAN PERSPECTIVE

Studies done in northern India, based mainly on clinical examinations between the 1960s and 1970s, reported a prevalence of RF and RHD around 1.8–4.58/1,000.[18]

In the sixth and seventh decades of the 20th century, RF and RHD were mainly detected by history and clinical detection of murmurs. However, clinical examination alone cannot detect RHD with certainty. It is very much subjective and there is a lot of interobserver as well as intraobserver variability. History of RF is available in only around 30% of cases. Till the late 90s, epidemiological studies of RF and RHD in India were carried out with clinical examination alone. With the advent of echocardiography, the use of echocardiography took a commonplace in the confirmation of RHD.

MANAGEMENT

Advanced RHD is often associated with the onset of HF which may not be amenable to corrective surgery. With HF the risk of death is doubled independent of other prognostic variables,[32] and in patients with aortic stenosis or dominant regurgitant lesions indicate a poor prognosis.[33]

CONCLUSION

Rheumatic heart disease is still common in the developing world, where it is a major risk factor for cardiovascular morbidity and mortality. With increasing life expectancy due to economic prosperity and better management of other cardiovascular risk factors such as hypertension and coronary artery disease (CAD), and as such, the prevalence of older adults with RHD is likely to increase and is a major risk factor for incident HF among older adults who remained free of RHD-related complications for decades.

ONLINE REFERENCES

Please scan the QR code provided at the end of the table of contents for References of this chapter.

CHAPTER

59 Diabetes and Heart Failure: A Double Whammy!

Aditi Parimoo, Prafulla G Kerkar

ABSTRACT

Diabetes mellitus and heart failure (HF), when present concomitantly, present a unique clinical entity with specific treatment considerations. Diabetes is a major risk factor that predisposes to the development of HF and such patients tend to have a worse prognosis. HF as a complication of diabetes mellitus is underappreciated and could occur without epicardial coronary artery disease (CAD). Metabolic derangements and autoimmune mechanisms have been proposed to be the possible mechanisms for causing diabetic cardiomyopathy. Early detection of this entity by screening for biomarker levels may help in initiating HF therapy early in the course of the disease and slowing down disease progression. Management of HF in diabetic patients is like management of HF in nondiabetic patients. The four pillars of survival-enhancing HF therapy—angiotensin receptor/neprilysin inhibitors (ARNIs), sodium-glucose cotransporter-2 inhibitors (SGLT-2Is), β-blockers (BBs), and mineralocorticoid receptor antagonists (MRAs)—are to be initiated either simultaneously or sequentially (without waiting to achieve target doses, before initiating next drug), preferably in hospital, after achieving stability of hemodynamic parameters, laboratory values, and diuretic response. The dictum is to get all four on board within 4 weeks. However, antidiabetic drugs differ in their effects in patients with HF. Preference must be given to drugs that are both safe and reduce HF-related events, although hyperglycemia must be addressed promptly. SGLT-2I are the antidiabetic drug of choice in this group. The next choice of antidiabetic agents to be used is metformin, glucagon-like peptide-1 receptor agonists (GLP-1RAs), and insulin in that order. Due consideration must also be given to achieving iron repletion in patients with iron deficiency. A multidisciplinary approach must be adopted to optimize management in this patient population.

Keywords: Diabetes mellitus, heart failure, diabetic cardiomyopathy, SGLT-2Is, angiotensin receptor/neprilysin inhibitors, β-blockers, mineralocorticoid receptor antagonists.

INTRODUCTION

Diabetes mellitus and heart failure (HF) are among the most common comorbidities worldwide. When present concomitantly, their contribution to the socioeconomic burden of healthcare increases significantly. Diabetics tend to have a worse clinical outcome in HF and may respond differently than the rest of the population to HF therapy. Understanding the pathophysiology of both the comorbidities plays a key role in the optimum management of their clinical spectrum. Moreover, diabetes mellitus is known to cause HF even in the absence of coronary artery disease (CAD) and hypertension. This chapter aims to review the epidemiology, pathophysiology, disease progression, role of biomarkers, and finally the treatment modalities of diabetes and HF.

EPIDEMIOLOGY

Diabetes mellitus and HF are leading causes of morbidity and mortality worldwide. Data from the Indian subcontinent suggest that the prevalence of diabetes in the age group of 20–70 years is a whopping 8.8%.[1] Conversely, the estimated prevalence of HF in India is about 1%.[2] Concomitant burden of diabetes in patients with HF has been observed in various HF registries globally as well as in India. Diabetes was found to be the most common comorbidity in patients with HF.[3] The combination of diabetes and HF portends worse prognosis. The Framingham Heart Study was the first study to demonstrate an increased risk of developing HF in post-myocardial infarction patients among diabetic patients as compared to nondiabetic patients.[4] This was further corroborated in studies involving the subset of HF patients such as the Studies of Left Ventricular Dysfunction (SOLVD), the Heart Outcomes Prevention Evaluation (HOPE) study, and the Cardiovascular Health Study (CHS).[5-7] Various registries worldwide have demonstrated the relationship between diabetes and HF. As per the Scottish Registry, the risk of HF was increased twofold among individuals with diabetes than those who were nondiabetic.[8] The Reykjavik Study showed that any spectrum of hyperglycemia ranging from glucose intolerance to overt diabetes was associated with an increased incidence of HF.[9] The Swedish Registry showed that patients with diabetes, particularly type 1 diabetes mellitus (T1DM) admitted with acute decompensated HF, had worse outcomes than those without diabetes.[10] Furthermore, poor glycemic control and superadded renal dysfunction were associated with poorer outcomes in this subset.

PATHOPHYSIOLOGY

The diagnosis of diabetes mellitus-related cardiomyopathy requires exclusion of all other etiologies of HF, including coronary, valvular, hypertensive, and congenital heart disease, and of viral, toxic, familial, or infiltrative cardiomyopathy.[11] It must be remembered that HF in diabetes mellitus can occur independent of CAD.[12,13]

The clinical phenotypes of HF as seen in patients with diabetes mellitus are not unique to patients with diabetes and include the spectrum of exercise intolerance and diastolic and systolic dysfunction. Two clinical phenotypes of the disease have been described—a dilated phenotype and a restrictive phenotype.[11] These phenotypes are proposed to occur via distinct pathophysiological mechanisms. The dilated phenotype giving rise to HF with reduced ejection fraction (HFrEF) seems to be secondary to autoimmune mechanisms and hence is more prevalent in the subset of patients with T1DM. The restrictive phenotype is attributed to metabolic derangements such as hyperglycemia, lipotoxicity, and hyperinsulinemia, causing HF with preserved ejection fraction (HFpEF) **(Flowchart 1)**.

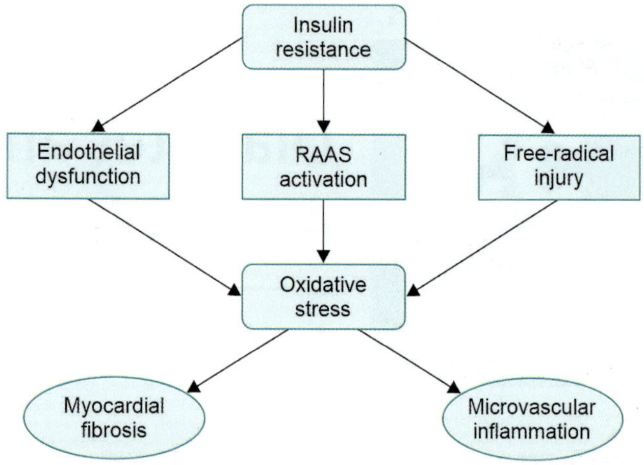

FLOWCHART 1: Mechanisms of cardiomyocyte injury in diabetes mellitus.

(RAAS: renin–angiotensin–aldosterone system)

Source: With permission from Naidoo (2016).[14]

Both diabetes mellitus and HF are associated with hyperactivity of the sympathetic system and the renin-angiotensin-aldosterone system (RAAS). This leads to increase in proinflammatory cytokines, which, in turn, gives rise to endothelial dysfunction and microangiopathic affection of vascular beds in the body.[15] This, in turn, exacerbates conventional cardiovascular (CV) risk factors such as hypertension and dyslipidemia, thereby accelerating the development of superadded CAD, which may be related to worse outcomes in patients with diabetes and HF. The fact that diabetes is associated with worse clinical outcomes in HF patients has also been studied in several patient subgroups. Diabetic patients may also respond differently to HF therapy than their nondiabetic counterparts, although the anti-HF drugs used are the same.[16] Additionally, diabetes seems to be an even more potent risk factor in females.[17]

ROLE OF BIOMARKERS IN EARLY DETECTION OF HEART FAILURE IN DIABETICS PATIENTS

Since the coexistence of diabetes and HF has a higher morbidity burden, the early detection of HF in diabetic patients is desirable. This will help in earlier initiation of measures to hamper disease progression. Higher values of three biomarkers, namely B-type natriuretic peptide (BNP), N-terminal pro-B-type natriuretic peptide (NT-proBNP), and high-sensitivity cardiac troponin, are associated with higher relative risk of HF onset.[13] BNP and NT-proBNP levels are sensitive markers of left ventricle (LV) dysfunction.[18,19] Furthermore, diabetic patients have been found to have higher levels of these biomarkers than nondiabetic patients. Various mechanisms have been postulated to explain this phenomenon, including increased production due to hyperglycemia, decreased degradation, and concomitant hyperactivity of the sympathetic system and the RAAS.[20,21] Whether these higher levels correlate with disease progression remains to be elicited. This also implies that the levels of these biomarkers must be interpreted carefully in diabetic patients.[16]

Recent guidelines recommend that rigorous and prompt screening, preferably annually, is essential in order to detect asymptomatic individuals with stages A and B HF so that the preventive and therapeutic measures can be instituted to hamper progression to overt HF (stages C and D).[13,22]

Several large population cohorts have been studied to ascertain optimal cutoff for biomarkers, i.e., BNP ≥ 50 pg/mL,

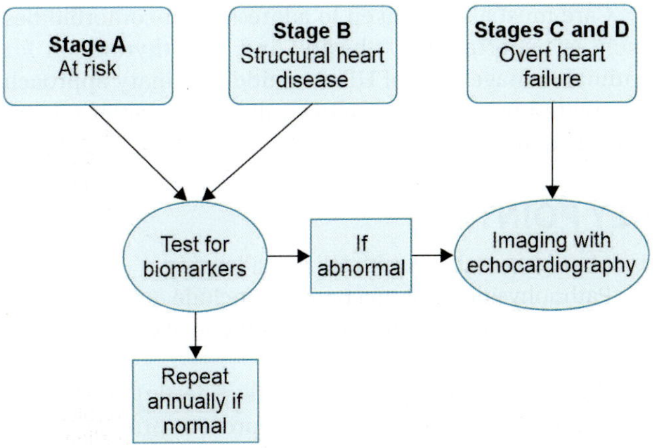

FLOWCHART 2: Approach for screening and diagnosis of heart failure in diabetes mellitus.

Source: With permission from Pop-Busui (2022).[13]

NT-proBNP ≥ 125 pg/mL, and high sensitivity troponin levels more than 99th percentile for the healthy patient population **(Flowchart 2)**.[23-25]

THERAPY

Addressing hyperglycemia and HF concomitantly is the current challenge in this patient subgroup. Diabetic patients may respond differently to HF therapies. It has been observed that poor glycemic control is associated with worse clinical outcomes in HF. Each 1% increase in glycated hemoglobin (HbA1c) level was associated with an 8% increase in the risk of HF.[26]

Treatment Considerations for Management of Hyperglycemia in Heart Failure

Different classes of antidiabetic drugs have different effects in patients with HF.[27] Thoughtful consideration should be given to the specific antidiabetic agents that are administered to each patient. Preference must be given to drugs that are both safe and reduce HF-related events.[27]

Sodium-glucose cotransporter-2 inhibitors (SGLT-2Is) have been proposed to be the antidiabetic agent of choice in this patient population. This is because of the beneficial effects of SGLT-2I demonstrated in several large patient cohorts.[25,28] This subgroup of drugs includes dapagliflozin, empagliflozin, and canagliflozin. This is the first class of antidiabetic agents to have shown benefit in the HF population, and their use is associated with significant reductions in the risk of CV death or hospitalization for HF and improvements in health status and quality of life.[13]

Since euglycemia is associated with better clinical outcomes, additional antidiabetic agents may be required for lowering blood glucose levels. The next choice of antidiabetic agents should be metformin, glucagon-like peptide-1 receptor agonists (GLP-1RAs), and insulin in that order, although insulin is also known to cause sodium retention and may aggravate congestion.

Metformin works by activation of 5′ adenosine monophosphate-activated protein kinase (AMPK), which was initially postulated to bring about regression of myocardial hypertrophy. However, this effect could not be substantiated in clinical trials. Initial concerns about metformin, leading to lactic acidosis and precipitating HF, have been subsequently dismissed.[29]

Dipeptidyl peptidase-4 (DPP-4) inhibitors and thiazolidinediones should be avoided in patients with HF. Use of DPP-4 inhibitors has been associated with an increased risk of HF hospitalizations.[30] In the TECOS (trial evaluating cardiovascular outcomes with sitagliptin), sitagliptin was not found to reduce hospitalization for HF as compared to the control group.[31] Although the CARMELINA (cardiovascular and renal microvascular outcome study with linagliptin) trial did not demonstrate an increase in the risk of CV events as compared to the control group, the sample size was not adequate to warrant the use of linagliptin in HF.[32] This seems to be a class effect of these drugs. DPP-4 inhibition potentiates the action of endogenous peptides such as stromal cell-derived factor 1 (SDF-1), substance P, and neuropeptide Y (NPY) which may precipitate HF.[33] Thiazolidinediones are associated with increased HF admissions, possibly due to increased fluid retention upon the use of these agents.[34]

The use of sulfonylureas must also be avoided in HF and should only be used when other therapies with proven benefits are contraindicated or are unavailable.[13]

Guideline-directed Medical Therapy in Diabetics with Heart Failure

Management of HF in diabetic patients is like management of HF in the general population. The four foundational pillars of therapy include angiotensin receptor/neprilysin inhibitors (ARNIs) [in preference to angiotensin-converting enzyme inhibitors/angiotensin-2 receptor blockers (ACEIs/ARBs)], β-blockers, mineralocorticoid receptor antagonists (MRAs), and SGLT-2Is **(Fig. 1)**.[35] Diuretics must be used at optimal dosage in this subset only for relief of congestion **(Fig. 1)**.[36]

Successful HF treatment is dependent on early initiation of all the four drugs during the initial HF admission itself once stability of hemodynamic parameters, key laboratory values, and the diuretic response for decongestion and euvolemia is achieved. The effects of these drug classes are additive, and they could be started either simultaneously at recommended low doses or sequentially without the need to achieve target dosing before initiating the next medication.[35] The modern-day mantra is to get all the four drugs on board in 4 weeks. In the recent STRONG HF trial, rapid up-titration

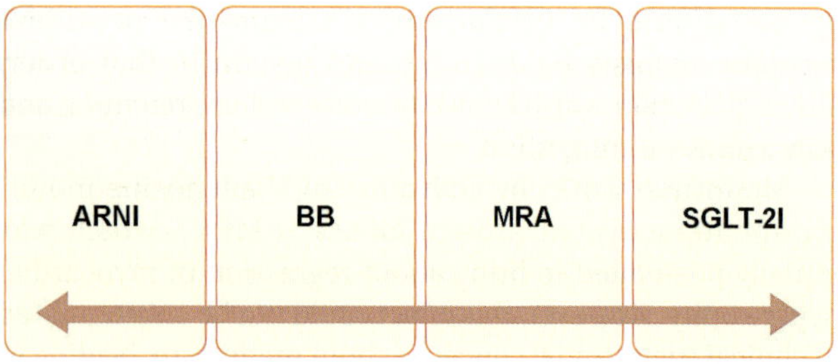

FIG. 1: Four foundational pillars of survival-enhancing HF therapy.
(ARNI: angiotensin receptor/neprilysin inhibitor; BB: β-blocker; HF: heart failure; MRA: mineralocorticoid receptor antagonist; SGLT-2I: sodium-glucose cotransporter-2 inhibitor)
Source: With permission from Kimmoun et al. (2019).[37]

of guideline-directed medical therapy (GDMT) with close follow-up after an acute HF admission was readily accepted by patients as it reduced symptoms, improved quality of life, and reduced risk of 180-day all-cause death or HF readmission compared with usual care.[37] Early initiation of the four pillars has been known to rapidly improve the patient's health status and left ventricular ejection fraction (LVEF) and reduce patient morbidity and mortality. It also improves patient compliance to treatment, leading to better patient outcomes both in the short term and in the long run.[38]

Sacubitril–Valsartan (S/V), a first-in-class ARNI, improves LVEF in diabetic patients as shown by the post-hoc analysis of PROVE HF trial which showed an 8.7% increase in LVEF in the diabetic subset at 12 months. It also has a favorable impact on CV death and reduces HF hospitalizations.[39] ARNIs also show significant reduction in HbA1c concentrations over 3 years in diabetic patients.[40] This could possibly be explained by an increase in insulin sensitivity after starting ARNIs in diabetic patients with HF. ARNIs were associated with decreased insulin requirement and decreased dose of oral hypoglycemic agents (OHAs). S/V is recommended as first-line therapy in diabetic patients with HF and is preferred over ACEI or ARB by the American Diabetes Association (ADA).[13]

Sodium-glucose cotransporter-2 inhibitors have been recommended for the treatment of diabetes in HF. This is because SGLT-2I have shown significant reductions in risk of CV death or hospitalization for HF and improvements in health status and quality of life in randomized controlled trials (RCTs), and this benefit is superadded on excellent background therapy.[13,41]

Beta-blockers (BBs) have also been shown to reduce remodeling and have mortality benefit in HF. The older belief that BBs may be detrimental in diabetics due to decreased sympathetic drive has not been proven as per current evidence.[42]

Testing for iron deficiency and treating with intravenous (IV) iron have been recommended in recent American College of Cardiology (ACC) 2022[35] and ADA 2022.[13]

Care must also be taken to address other comorbidities such as hypertension, obesity, and hypothyroidism for optimal management of HF. A multidisciplinary approach as adopted in western societies will help in better patient management in this large cohort.

KEY POINTS

- Managing diabetes with HF is challenging.
- Pathophysiological mechanisms include autoimmunity, metabolic derangements, sympathetic overactivity, and hyperactivity of RAAS.
- Rigorous screening with biomarkers testing in stages A and B HF may prove useful to prevent progression to symptomatic HF stages C and D.
- Hyperglycemia is a poor prognostic factor. Only those antidiabetics with proven CV safety and efficacy should be used to achieve euglycemia and improve disease outcomes.
- HF therapy in diabetic patients is like that of HF therapy in nondiabetic patients.
- The four pillars of survival-enhancing HF therapy, ARNIs, BBs, MRAs, and SGLT-2Is, must be initiated early and up-titrated to maximally tolerated doses used in trials to prevent readmissions and improve survival and quality of life.

CONCLUSION

Diabetes mellitus and HF when present together represent a formidable challenge to clinicians. Concomitantly addressing diabetes mellitus and HF is the key to better management of this cohort of patients. Various pathophysiological mechanisms including metabolic derangements, proinflammatory state, and hyperactivity of the sympathetic and the RAAS system have been proposed. Rigorous screening of individuals with stages A and B HF is recommended, including testing for biomarkers to detect and institute therapies early, so as to prevent their progression to symptomatic HF.

Treatment is directed at both addressing the HF and the hyperglycemic state. SGLT-2I are the first antidiabetic agents to have the additional benefit of significant reductions in risk of CV death or hospitalization for HF and improvements in health status and quality of life. Since hyperglycemia itself predicts poor outcomes in these patients, added treatment options may be required to achieve optimum control of blood sugar. Metformin, GLP-1RA, and insulin are the preferred agents of choice in this subset. DPP-4 inhibitors and thiazolidinediones are to be avoided in this group as they have been shown to possibly precipitate HF in large clinical trials. Also, sulfonylureas should be used judiciously only when therapies with proven benefits are not available.

The treatment for HF in diabetic patients is like that of HF due to other etiologies and includes administering the four foundational pillars of HF therapy, including ARNIs (preferred over ACEI or ARB), BBs, MRAs, and SGLT-2I. Renal effects of these drugs must be considered as renal insufficiency is a particularly poor prognostic factor in HF with diabetes.

A multidisciplinary approach is recommended for optimum management of this clinical entity. Care must also be taken to address other CV comorbidities such as hypertension, dyslipidemia, and obesity in this group. Cardiac rehabilitation also helps in improving quality of life in these patients. Only a comprehensive approach to this problem can help in combating this double whammy.

ONLINE REFERENCES

Please scan the QR code provided at the end of the table of contents for References of this chapter.

CHAPTER

60

Revascularization for Heart Failure

Vivekanand S Gajapati

ABSTRACT

Ischemic heart disease is estimated to account for over two-thirds of the heart failure (HF) patients and is associated with poor prognosis despite of optimal medical treatment. Coronary revascularization has been shown to improve myocardial function and prognosis in ischemic cardiomyopathy (ICM). In patients with ischemic HF, blood flow restoration of viable but ischemic myocardium might reverse the hibernation of the myocardium and prevents future spontaneous myocardial infarction (MI). Patients with ICM have been largely excluded from randomized trials of revascularization in stable coronary artery disease (CAD). Coronary artery bypass graft (CABG) surgery has been the main mode of revascularization in patents with extensive CAD and reduced ejection fraction (EF) based on the STICH (Surgical Treatment for Ischemic Heart Failure) trial. Recent development in the interventional cardiology has led to overall increase of percutaneous coronary intervention (PCI) procedures in the treatment of ischemic HF with reduced ejection fraction (HFrEF). The beneficial effect of PCI in ischemic cardiomyopathy has been challenged by recently published REVIVED-BCIS2 trial which demonstrated no added benefit of PCI over optimal medical therapy. A multidisciplinary approach is needed to tailor treatment strategy in these patients based on the ability to achieve complete revascularization.

Keywords: Coronary artery bypass surgery, ischemic cardiomyopathy, myocardial revascularization, myocardial viability, percutaneous coronary intervention.

INTRODUCTION

Coronary artery disease (CAD) remains the most common cause heart failure with reduced ejection fraction (HFrEF). Ischemic etiology is estimated to account for over two-thirds of all heart failure (HF) cases and is associated with impaired quality of life and poor prognosis.[1,2] Pharmacological and device therapy are the main modalities of the treatment of HFrEF. Revascularization should be offered to patients with impaired left ventricular (LV) function who present with angina or acute coronary syndrome.

There is a limited evidence to support revascularization in patients with stable ischemic HF and minimal symptoms. Separating true ischemic HF from bystander CAD in nonischemic HF is frequently challenging. The preferred choice of revascularization [percutaneous coronary intervention (PCI) or coronary artery bypass graft (CABG)] depend on age, sex, comorbidities, and coronary anatomy. Severe LV dysfunction is associated with an increased procedural mortality and morbidity following surgical or percutaneous revascularization. CABG surgery has been the important mode of revascularization in patients with multivessel CAD and HFrEF. However, recent advances in the interventional cardiology led to overall increase of PCI in the treatment of ischemic HFrEF. It is essential to understand the better modality for coronary revascularization in this unique and growing patient population to improve outcomes.

ROLE OF REVASCULARIZATION

Ischemic cardiomyopathy (ICM) is the LV dysfunction due to atherosclerotic CAD. It incorporates many clinical, imaging, and angiographic features. Revascularization, particularly CABG, is recommended for patients with ischemic HFrEF based on the assumption that blood flow restoration of viable but ischemic myocardium might reverse the LV dysfunction.[3] The potential mechanism of improving pumping function is the reversal of myocardial hibernation, an adaptive process triggered by repeated episodes of ischemia. Myocardial viability testing is the prospective identification of myocardium which is likely to be hibernating and it is one of the important considerations when adopting revascularization strategy. A large meta-analysis demonstrated a strong association between myocardial viability and improved survival after revascularization in patients with chronic CAD and LV dysfunction.[4]

TYPES OF REVASCULARIZATION

Coronary Artery Bypass Graft Surgery

Patients with ICM frequently presents with complex and extensive CAD, which often makes surgical revascularization, the preferred mode of invasive treatment. The contemporary evidence on the role of CABG comes from the results of the STICH (Surgical Treatment of Ischemic Heart Failure) trial which randomized 1,212 patients with ICM < 35% LV ejection fraction (LVEF) to either CABG or medical therapy.[5,6] At the first prespecified analysis at 5 years, there was no significant difference in primary outcomes of all-cause mortality between the groups. There was only borderline significance in the secondary endpoint of cardiovascular mortality. When followed up for 10 years, there was a significant reduction of all-cause mortality in CABG arm (7% absolute reduction), which translated into to 17 months median increase in the survival.

The STICH remains a landmark trial but there were several limitations which limits us to generalize its conclusions in routine clinical practice. Increasing age is known to be an important predictor of worse outcomes in patients with HF. Patients in STICH were younger than most contemporary registries of HF (the mean age was 60 years). Younger cohorts derived more beneficial outcomes than those over the age of 65. The use of medical and device therapy did not reflect contemporary practice with very low rates of implantable cardioverter-defibrillator (ICD) implantations and poor adherence to the medical therapy. Presence of three vessels disease, LVEF < 27% and LV end-systolic volume > 79 mL/m^2 were associated with greater benefit from CABG. Surprisingly the presence of angina, ischemia, viability, and diabetes did not appear to benefit more from CABG. Myocardial viability testing was not mandatory in STICH trial. Moreover, the evidence of viability was not associated with improved outcomes in the HF patients, undergoing CABG.[7,8] In conclusion, CABG is an effective mode of revascularization in selected cases and its modest benefit can be distinguished from the increased mortality due to the surgical procedure beyond 5 years.

Percutaneous Coronary Intervention

Percutaneous coronary intervention is now emerging as an important mode of revascularization in patients with ICM due to technological development and an advancing experience. The role of PCI have expanded to more complex cases such as left main disease, multivessel disease, and chronic total occlusions. The number of patients with ischemic HFs undergoing PCI has increased compared to those referred for CABG[9,10] even though most randomized clinical trials comparing CABG and PCI in stable patients have excluded patients with reduced LVEF.[11,12] The long-term outcomes are unknown in patients undergoing PCI for ischemic HF.[13] The theoretical advantage of PCI compared to CABG cannot be extrapolated as the mechanism of revascularization are substantially different. PCI may not achieve complete revascularization compared to CABG. Although PCI is considered to be associated with lesser mortality and morbidity than CABG, no robust comparisons has been made in patients with HF.

The US and European Society of Cardiology (ESC) guidelines recommend CABG as the preferred revascularization option in patients with ischemic HF.[14,15] CABG is superior to PCI according to ESC guidelines, while the US guidelines do not comment on PCI but recommends CABG. Still PCI is extensively performed in daily practice due preference of patients, refusal by surgeons and feasibility of PCI. More recently published large, randomized REVIVED (Revascularization for Ischemic Ventricular Dysfunction) trial provided critical evidence on the possible role of PCI in patients with ICM. It showed no significant prognostic impact of PCI over optimal medical therapy (OMT).[16] A total of 700 patients with LVEF ≤ 35% with extensive CAD suitable for PCI and confirmed myocardial viability were enrolled in the study. The primary outcome (composite of all-cause mortality and HF hospitalization) over a median of 41 months was comparable between the groups (PCI: 37.2% vs OMT: 38.0%). Furthermore, there was no difference in LVEF between the groups at 6 and 12 months. Longer term follow-up is planned, but late benefit is unlikely to emerge as 3.4 years follow-up did not show any discernible effect. However, the results need to be interpreted carefully as there are some major concerns. The trial included only patients with confirmed myocardial viability but previous studies did not demonstrate the benefit of revascularization guided by viability testing. Scar burden, but not viability predicts likelihood of LV function recovery. Therefore, based on myocardial viability alone, it is difficult to identify patients with HFrEF who might benefit from PCI.[17,18] Patients enrolled in REVIVED-BCIS2 were ten year older than those enrolled in STICH trial. Further analyses of REVIVED data are awaited, which will answer some of the questions, for example the extent of ischemia versus myocardial jeopardy (67% of patients had no angina). British Cardiovascular Intervention

Society (BCIS) Myocardial Jeopardy score which was used by investigators to define angiographic eligibility was not validated in HFrEF patients. It was hypothesized that PCI on top of optimal medical treatment would offer the benefits of revascularization without the early mortality associated with CABG.

In REVIVED trial, despite inclusion of patients with left main disease PCI was not associated with an increased early mortality. Periprocedural myocardial infarction (MI) constituted approximately 40% of all the MIs in PCI arm. There was twofold increase of spontaneous MI was observed in the optimal medical treatment group when compared to PCI (5.2% vs. 9.3%). Therefore, overall MI rates at the end were similar in both the groups (OMT: 10.8% vs. PCI: 10.7%). The concept of recovery of myocardial hibernation with revascularization has been challenged by this trial. The medical management of HF is evolving rapidly with the introduction of new therapies, such as sodium-glucose cotransporter-2 inhibitors (SGLT-2Is). The important role of OMT in HFrEF patients has been emerged as one of the significant findings of the REVIVED trial but role of SGLT-2Is has not been addressed by this trial.

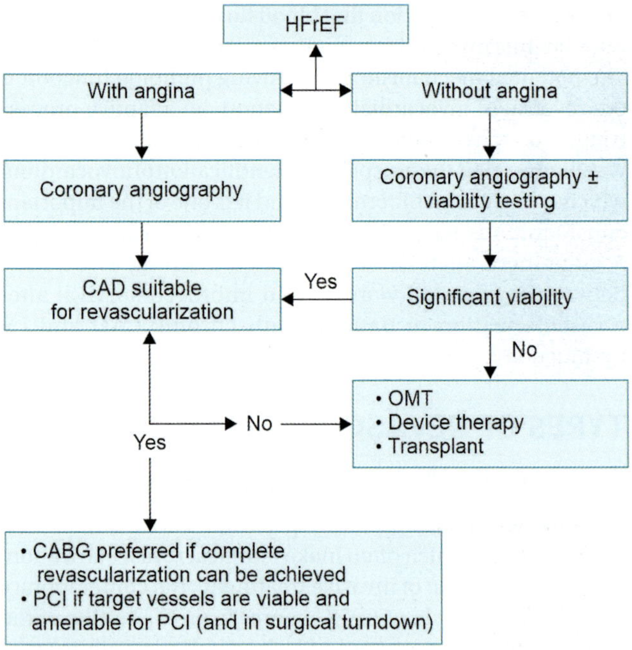

FLOWCHART 1: Tailored management algorithm for patients with ischemic HFrEF.

(CABG: coronary artery bypass graft; CAD: coronary artery disease; HFrEF: heart failure with reduced ejection fraction; OMT: optimal medical therapy; PCI: percutaneous coronary intervention)

CONCLUSION

Ischemic cardiomyopathy is associated with high morbidity and mortality and the identification of an ischemic substrate can help decision-making process and improve patient's outcomes. To date, the evidence base for coronary revascularization in ischemic LV dysfunction is largely informed by observational data. There is an absence of direct randomized controlled trial evidence comparing revascularization strategies in these patient population. This may illustrate why, despite the guidelines and the large body of observational evidence supporting CABG in favor of PCI, high PCI rates have been observed in this patient population in the real world. Better understanding this discrepancy between theory and practice will require direct randomized evidence of PCI vs. CABG in this specific patient population. Revascularization decisions in patients with reduced LVEF have so far been largely based on the STICH trial that showed a benefit of CABG over OMT alone. The beneficial effect of CABG is observed after extended observation (10 years), and therefore, it should be performed in carefully selected patients with acceptable perioperative risk. REVIVED trial confirmed the importance of contemporary pharmacological treatment in the HFrEF setting. But it demonstrated that in stable asymptomatic patients with confirmed myocardial viability PCI added no benefit in reduction of all-cause mortality or HF hospitalization rates, that is why, the extended follow-up and more detailed analyses of this study are crucial to confirm these results in the long-term observation and identify potential subgroups of patients in whom PCI might be beneficial. Both REVIVED-BCIS2 and STITCH trials challenge the hypothesis of hibernating myocardium amenable to functional improvement following successful revascularization that would ultimately improve prognosis. Assessment of myocardial viability does not aid the selection of patients who will benefit or not from the PCI for ICM. So REVIVED-BCIS2 also challenged long-held beliefs on myocardial viability prior to PCI. The decision on revascularization in ICM often cannot be made based on the guidelines, therefore, tailored treatment approach is essential with multidisciplinary approach **(Flowchart 1)**. These decisions should be based on ability to achieve complete revascularization which may not be accomplished in certain patients.

ONLINE REFERENCES

Please scan the QR code provided at the end of the table of contents for References of this chapter.

CHAPTER

61 Cardiac Rehabilitation in Heart Failure: High Expectations Unmet Applications

K Venugopal

ABSTRACT

Cardiac failure is one of the most important causes of morbidity and mortality in the world. The different types of heart failure depending on the ejection fraction have been well categorized and the treatment options for the different subsets have been well elucidated. Cardiac rehabilitation in a comprehensive manner involving physical activity, risk factor reduction, dietary advice, and psychosocial support has been shown to significantly reduce hospitalization and improve the quality of life of patients with heart failure with a modest reduction in mortality. Though there is enough data to support the role of cardiac rehabilitation, currently only 20% of eligible patients receive this treatment. The barriers to the adoption of this treatment in heart failure patients are physician-related, patient-related, and health system-related. A greater awareness and reduction of the barriers will enable more patients to receive this treatment option, which is a class 1 indication in the recent European Society of Cardiology (ESC) guidelines for acute and chronic heart failure.

Keywords: Cardiac failure, cardiac rehabilitation, benefits, protocols, underutilisation.

INTRODUCTION

Heart failure is emerging as a major health problem in developed and developing countries with almost an equal prevalence with cancer, 26 million versus 32 million, and accounts for 1–2% of total hospital admissions.[1] With an increase in longevity in most populations, the problem of heart failure is bound to increase all over the world. There have been remarkable advances in the management of heart failure, especially in heart failure with reduced ejection fraction (HFrEF), with less favorable advances in heart failure with preserved ejection fraction (HFpEF). While restriction of activities was earlier advised, the role of physical activity and rehabilitation has recently been recognized in various studies, especially with regard to improvement in quality of life as well as mortality benefit. There is a trend to include physical activity and rehabilitation as part of the treatment protocol in heart failure management, but this is still an underutilized therapeutic option in heart failure management.

DEFINITION

The World Health Organization (WHO) definition[2] states that "the sum of activities required to influence favorably the underlying cause of the disease as well as to provide best possible physical mental and social conditions so that patients may by their own effort preserve or resume when lost as normal a place as possible in the community."

BENEFITS OF EXERCISE IN HEART FAILURE AND MECHANISMS (FIG. 1)

The main aspects of treatment in heart failure are to decrease mortality, improve quality of life, and reduce hospitalizations. Initially, patients with heart failure were not advised to engage in physical activity for fear of worsening of heart failure, but multiple studies proved that monitored physical activity was beneficial in improving quality of life, reducing hospitalizations, and providing mild reductions in mortality. It also took away the disadvantages

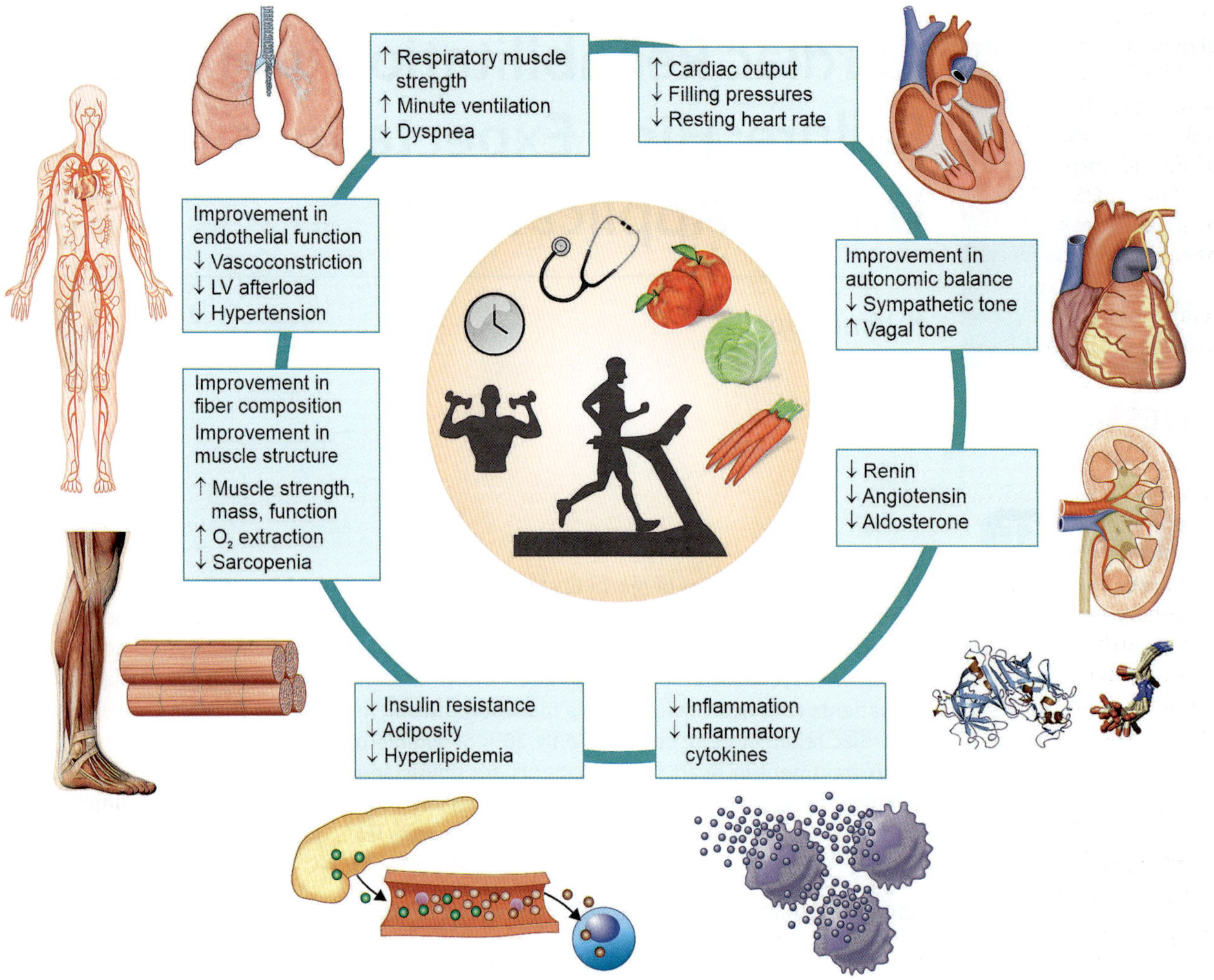

FIG. 1: Central illustration: Mechanisms of beneficial effects of exercise training and cardiac rehabilitation in patients with heart failure. (LV: left ventricular)

Source: With permission from Bozkurt et al. (2021).[3]

of immobilization such as sarcopenia and deep vein thrombosis.

The mechanisms by which cardiac rehabilitation improves a patient with heart failure are manifold.[3]

Exercise increases the cardiac output and decreases the filling pressures and the heart rate. There is reduction of sympathetic activity and increased parasympathetic activity. The renin–angiotensin system (RAS) is affected with reduction in the levels of renin, angiotensin, and aldosterone, which are therapeutic targets in heart failure. The inflammatory cytokines are reduced. Insulin resistance is reduced with concomitant reduction in lipids. Exercise leads to improvement in muscle fiber composition, O_2 extraction, and decrease in sarcopenia. Endothelial function is improved with reduction in blood pressure (BP), improved vasodilatation, and reduction in afterload. Respiratory muscle strength is improved and leads to reduction in dyspnea. Thus, by these multiple mechanisms, there is a definite improvement in the well-being of the patient. Along with the physical activity, there will be associated risk factor modifications, such as cessation of smoking and control of BP and blood sugars, which will go a long way in the primary endpoints of treatment. It is to be emphasized strongly that cardiac rehabilitation in heart failure is not only a physical exercise but also a combination of other modalities such as risk factor modification, dietary advice, psychosocial counseling, and assistance wherever needed.

The HF-ACTION (Heart Failure: A Controlled Trial Investigating Outcomes of Exercise Training) was a large trial in patients with HFrEF, which showed that regular exercise training was well tolerated, was safe, and improved quality of life.[4] The reductions in mortality were only modest and not statistically significant in the initial assessment, but post hoc analysis showed significant benefits in these parameters also. The benefits were seen irrespective of age, sex, severity of heart failure, and type of heart failure.

The Cochrane meta-analysis of 8,728 patients in 60 trials with 6-month follow-up also did not show a significant reduction in mortality but a definite improvement in quality of life and hospitalizations.[5]

The CROS-HF study analyzed different subgroups of heart failure based on ejection fraction (EF) but did not report benefits in endpoints, unlike the previous studies.[6]

The data from these trials is not clear regarding the reduction in mortality but unequivocal in the improvement in quality of life and reduction in hospitalizations.

ASSESSMENT OF PATIENTS

Ideally, patients before undergoing cardiac rehabilitation should be assessed for suitability of rehabilitation by cardiopulmonary exercise testing. The exercise protocol usually recommended is the Naughton protocol with a motorized treadmill. The parameters assessed include BP response, early ischemic changes, and development of cardiac arrhythmias. Another mode of assessment includes a bicycle ergometer. In centers that do not have a facility for cardiopulmonary testing, a 6-minute walk test can be used for the initial assessment of exercise capacity.

PROTOCOLS AND TYPES OF EXERCISE

HF-ACTION Protocol

The HF-ACTION trial used the heart rate reserve method using the peak heart rate from a recent test and the resting heart rate obtained after resting for 5 minutes. The heart rate reserve was calculated using the formula resting heart rate + 0.6 (peak HR - resting heart rate).[4] The exercise was started in the initial sessions to achieve 60% of the heart rate reserve. In those with advanced heart failure, 50% of the heart rate reserve was targeted. The duration was 15–30 minutes in the initial phase with one to two sessions, 3 times a week, which was then increased to 30–35 minutes in the ensuing weeks. Total sessions planned were for 36 weeks with 3 episodes per week. After 36 weeks, home exercises were recommended with 5 weekly sessions with 60–70% of heart rate reserve. For those with angina, the heart rate was kept at 10 beats/min, less than the heart rate at which angina occurred. Different rehabilitation centers may use their own protocols.

Types of Exercise Programs

The most important exercise programs involve endurance training or aerobic exercise program. The preferred mode of exercise is moderate continuous exercise or moderate continuous training (MCT), which is well tolerated by patients. It is shown to be safe and has been shown to reverse left ventricular (LV) remodeling in heart failure. Another mode of exercise program is endurance training, which involves muscle-strengthening exercises and increasing muscle mass. As older patients are likely to have loss of muscle, this type of exercise will be useful in patients who have sarcopenia. The usual resistance exercises involve resistance bands and lifting small weights such as dumbbells and barbells. The ideal method of exercise is a combination of both types of exercise, and resistance training is not a substitute for aerobic exercise. Resistance training involves more trainer-to-patient interaction than MCT. Another popular exercise program is high-intensity interval training (HIIT) program.[7] Studies have demonstrated superiority of HIIT over MCT in the reversal of LV remodeling. However, MCT is more familiar to patients, can be continued at home, and requires less supervisory effort compared to HIIT. Another exercise program adopted is inspiratory muscle training.

Inspiratory muscle training is beneficial in patients with heart failure who have exertional dyspnea by improving respiratory muscle weakness. It has been found to be useful in those with HFrEF as well as those with HFpEF and is currently being included as an addition to the existing exercise programs.[8]

COMPONENTS OF CARDIAC REHABILITATION PROGRAM

It is to be emphasized that physical conditioning is only one aspect of cardiac rehabilitation. The rehabilitation team should consist of physician, nurses, exercise specialists, dieticians, pharmacists, and behavioral health personnel. It is an integrated program to be implemented as a team with a physician interested in cardiac rehabilitation to guide and oversee the various aspects of rehabilitation along with his team members. Individualized decisions regarding patient management should be undertaken on a discussion basis as all patients with heart failure could not be put under one umbrella of care. Risk factor modification is an important aspect, and it is considered to be a major reason for improvement in quality of life. Smoking cessation, control of BP, diabetes, lipids, diet advice, weight reduction, and treatment of anxiety and depression are all important components of a comprehensive rehabilitation program.

The advantages of a comprehensive program are manifold. It involves the translation of risk factor modification in a better way as there is initially a closer interaction between the patient and the treating team. The program is currently recommended for all types of heart failure from HFrEF, heart failure with midrange ejection fraction (HFmrEF), and HFpEF.

The rehabilitation program ideally should be initiated in a dedicated rehabilitation unit and later can be transformed into a home-based activity program. This is likely to extend the utility of such a program in majority of the patients **(Fig. 2)**.

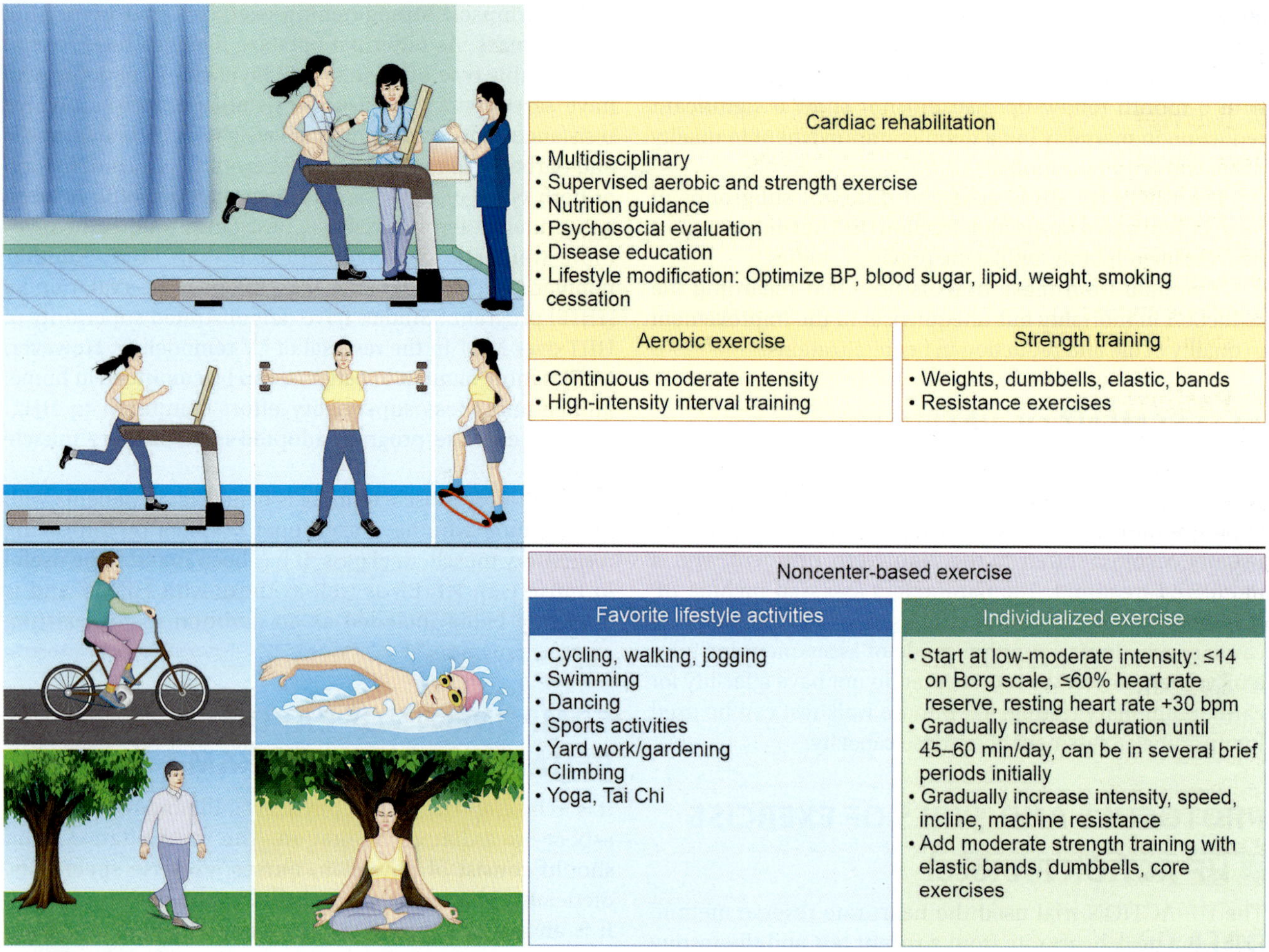

FIG. 2: Components of center-based rehabilitation program and noncenter-based exercise activities appropriate for patients with heart failure.

(BP: blood pressure)

Source: With permission from Bozkurt et al. (2021).[3]

CURRENT RECOMMENDATION OF EUROPEAN SOCIETY OF CARDIOLOGY GUIDELINES FOR ACUTE AND CHRONIC HEART FAILURE 2021[9]

Recommendations for exercise rehabilitation in patients with chronic heart failure are mentioned in **Table 1**.

TABLE 1: Recommendations for exercise rehabilitation in patients with chronic heart failure.

Recommendations	Class	Level
Exercise is recommended for all patients who are able to, in order to improve exercise capacity, QOL, and reduce HF hospitalization*	I	A
A supervised, exercise-based, cardiac rehabilitation program should be considered in patients with more severe disease, frailty, or with comorbidities	IIa	C

*In those who are able to adhere to the exercise program.

(HF: heart failure; QOL: quality of life)

WHY IS CARDIAC REHABILITATION UNDERUTILIZED?

While it is universally accepted that cardiac rehabilitation is definitely beneficial in improving quality of life, reducing hospitalizations, and modest improvement in mortality reduction, the use of this modality in established heart failure patients is very low in developed countries while it is used in negligible numbers in developing countries. Only 20–30% of patients in Europe and USA undergo rehabilitation.[10] There is no significant data from India. There are only few select centers in India that have a systematic rehabilitation program.

WHAT ARE THE BARRIERS TO CARDIAC REHABILITATION PROGRAM?

Barriers from Healthcare Professionals

Underestimation and lack of awareness of the benefits of cardiac rehabilitation are major factors. The reluctance to involve patients with heart failure in monitored physical activity is ingrained in majority of physicians as restriction of physical activity was advised earlier. The physician's inertia should be ameliorated through stressing the importance of rehabilitation through educational activities.

Patient-related Barriers

Psychosocial and economic factors, especially in large developing countries like India, are a major deterrent. Frequent visits to the rehabilitation center cause a significant economic burden. Ethnic and gender considerations are also important. Women, elderly patients, and ethnic minorities in all countries tend to be underrepresented in rehabilitation programs.

System-level Barriers

In countries where insurance is the major supporter of healthcare expenses, there are guidelines which prevent utilization of these services in certain groups of patients. While it is advocated for HFrEF, it is not recommended for those with HFpEF, though there is convincing data regarding benefits in this group of patients also.

DATA FROM INDIA

In a study by Babu et al.,[10] data from 17 centers that participated in the study was analyzed. Most programs accepted guidelines indicated patients and the expenditure was out of pocket. The programs were well coordinated and some programs also included yoga exercises. Barriers to the development of rehab program were felt to be a lack of patient referral and financial issues. Cardiac rehabilitation programs need to be developed systematically all over India, particularly in the northern parts.

SHOULD CARDIAC REHABILITATION BE ANOTHER PILLAR IN THE MANAGEMENT OF HEART FAILURE?

Now the management of heart failure rests on the four pillars of medications, i.e., angiotensin receptor-neprilysin inhibitor (ARNI)/angiotensin-converting enzyme inhibitor (ACEI)/angiotensin receptor blocker (ARB), beta-blockers, sodium-glucose cotransporter-2 (SGLT-2) inhibitors, and mineralocorticoid receptor antagonists (MRAs). There is a recommendation for including cardiac rehabilitation as another pillar in the management of heart failure irrespective of the type.[11] Once the barriers are overcome to a certain extent, more and more patients with heart failure should undergo cardiac rehabilitation and get the benefit of improvement in quality of life and reduction in hospitalizations. The review in European Heart Journal 2021 examining this aspect of heart failure treatment emphasizes the importance of cardiac rehabilitation and argues for its inclusion as the fifth pillar in the treatment of heart failure along with ACEI/ARB/ARNI, MRA, beta-blockers, and SGLT-2 inhibitors.

CONCLUSION

Heart failure is among the most important causes of morbidity and mortality in all populations. The problem is now assuming greater importance as the population is aging and the prevalence in the elderly population is increasing. There have been great advances in the pharmacotherapy in heart failure with the advent of RAAS inhibitors, beta-blockers, MRAs, and SGLT-2 inhibitors, yet the mortality and morbidity, especially in the quality of life, are very high. There have been various studies assessing the role of comprehensive cardiac rehabilitation in the management of heart failure irrespective of ejection fraction, which have demonstrated a clear-cut benefit in improving quality of life and reducing hospitalization with modest benefit in mortality reduction. Currently, though comprehensive rehabilitation is given class 1 indication in the management of heart failure, only 20% of eligible patients undergo this modality of treatment. Comprehensive cardiac rehabilitation involves not only physical activity but a teamwork involving physicians, nurses, pharmacists, physical medicine specialists, dieticians, and psychosocial healthcare experts. There are barriers in implementing from physician level, patient level, and system level, which need to be addressed properly to enable more patients with heart failure undergoing this treatment modality for improving quality of life and reducing hospitalizations and healthcare expenses. A greater awareness, improved access to rehabilitation, and reduced expenses in treatment will go a long way in the proper utilization of this greatly useful therapeutic strategy in heart failure.

ONLINE REFERENCES

Please scan the QR code provided at the end of the table of contents for References of this chapter.

SECTION 6

Lipids

CHAPTER

62

Genetics of Hypertriglyceridemia

Nitin K Kabra

ABSTRACT

Genetics of hypertriglyceridemia (HTG) are much more complex than that of familial hypercholesterolemia.

Inherited accumulation of multiple genetic variants (polygenic) exacerbated by lifestyle or other factors are the mechanism underlying HTG in most individuals. Many of these loci are also associated with other lipid traits and risk of coronary artery disease (CAD). Familial chylomicronemia syndrome (FCS) is a rare monogenic form of HTG associated with increased risk of recurrent acute pancreatitis. The knowledge of the genetic nature of HTG has also made it possible to identify targets for pharmacological treatments. As accessibility and affordability to genetic testing improves, the clinician needs to devise a strategy to deploy this powerful tool for patient care.

Keywords: Global Lipids Genetics Consortium, genome-wide association study, single-nucleotide polymorphisms, lipoprotein lipase, chylomicronemia, polygenic risk score.

INTRODUCTION

Plasma triglyceride (TG) concentration is the sum of the TG content of chylomicrons, very-low-density lipoprotein (VLDL), and their remnants together with small amounts of TG in low-density lipoprotein (LDL) and high-density lipoprotein (HDL) particles. It is dependent on both genetic (primary) and environmental (secondary) factors. About 50% of interindividual variability in plasma TG levels is determined by genetic factors. The molecular genetics of hypertriglyceridemia (HTG) have been elucidated with the help of rapid technological advancements in DNA analysis.

The Global Lipids Genetics Consortium (GLGC), a meta-analysis of >100,000 subjects of multiple ethnicity and lipid and cardiovascular disease (CVD) phenotypes identified 32 loci with common variants that contribute to variations in plasma TG concentrations.[1] Many of these loci are also associated with additional lipid traits such as HDL cholesterol, total cholesterol (TC), or LDL cholesterol. Seven TG-associated loci from GLGC studies were also associated with CAD, including apolipoprotein A5 (APOA5), lipoprotein lipase (LPL), TRIB1, APOE, CILP2, NAT2, and IRS1.[1,2]

Several methods are available to analyze the genotype of an individual **(Table 1)**, depending on whether the patient is suspected to have a rare mutation (monogenic HTG) or a collection of common small effect DNA variants (polygenic).

About 826 DNA variants associated with lipids have been identified across 400 genetic loci in a meta-analysis of >600,000 individuals.[3] Both common (allele frequency >5%) and rare (allele frequency <1%) variants in multiple genes collectively determine a person's plasma TG concentration along with lifestyle factors, medications, and other diseases **(Table 2)**.

Elevated levels of plasma TGs (levels >150 mg/dL) represent increased levels of TG-rich lipoproteins (chylomicrons and VLDL) and their remnants and are associated with increased risk of atherosclerotic cardiovascular disease (ASCVD) and pancreatitis. Almost all the same TG-raising alleles which determine the plasma TG concentration in healthy epidemiologic populations are also associated with HTG disease status. HTG may be categorized as mild-moderate (175–885 mg/dL) or severe (>885 mg/dL) or very severe (>1770 mg/dL).[4]

A genome-wide association study (GWAS) of HTG patients that tested for association with >2.1 million single-nucleotide polymorphisms (SNPs) using an additive multivariate logistic regression mode revealed that common variants in *APOA5, GCKR, LPL,* and *APOB* genes

TABLE 1: Genetic testing methods.[5]

Sanger sequencing	Single gene tests	Presence/absence of a known mutation in familial cascade testing
Targeted next-generation sequencing	Survey all DNA bases within coding regions of a single gene or several selected genes	For example, LipidSeq—a targeted resequencing panel for monogenic dyslipidemias
Whole exome sequencing	Simultaneous screen of all DNA bases within coding regions (exons)of all human genes	Condition suspected to have genetic basis which has not yet been identified
Whole genome sequencing	Simultaneous screen of all the DNA bases (coding and noncoding)	More comprehensive than whole exome sequencing
Genotyping	Rapid screen of entire genome using an array of common variant single nucleotide polymorphisms	• Whole genome examined • Cannot detect new variants
Polygenic risk score	Sum of minor effects of common variants	Complementary to traditional sequencing

TABLE 2: Genetic loci associated with triglyceride (TG) and other lipoproteins.

TGs	TG + HDL-C	TG + TC + LDL-C
MET	LPL	MIR148A
AKR1C4	LRP1	ANGPTL3
PDXDC1	IRS1	LRPAP1
MPP3	RSPO3	TIMD4
INSR	VEGFA	CILP2
MSL2L1	FTO	
KLHL8	MLXIPL	**TG + HDL-C + TC + LDL-C**
MAP3K1	GALNT2	CETP
PINX1		TRIB1
JMJD1C	**TG + HDL-C + LDL-C**	FADS1-2-3
CYP26A1	PIGV-NR0B2	APOA1
CAPN3		
FRMD5	**TG + HDL-C + TC**	
CTF1	LIPC	
PLA2G6		
TYW1B		

(HDL-C: high-density lipoprotein cholesterol; LDL-C: low-density lipoprotein cholesterol; TC: total cholesterol)

were associated with the HTG phenotype at genome-wide significance.[6] Additional HTG-associated genes, including *MLXIPL*, *TRIB1*, angiopoietin-like protein 3 (*ANGPTL3*), *GPIHBP1* or *LMF1*, *FADS1-2-3 cluster XKR6/PINX1*, *NCAN*, and *PLTP* further contribute to HTG phenotypes.

The majority of HTGs is usually multigenic or polygenic with DNA accumulation of common variants with small effect size or rare variants with large effect size in a spectrum of TG-associated genes. These variants include SNV (single-nucleotide variants), SNPs, and CNV (copy number variants). Small effect polygenic SNPs tend to cluster within families.[6] In a study of 563 patients with severe HTG, 1.1% of patients had monogenic HTG (defined as having two mutants, rare alleles in the same gene), 46.6% of patients had polygenic HTG [defined as either a heterozygous mutant rare allele or high polygenic risk score (PRS)], whereas the remaining 52.6% of patients had genetically uncharacterized HTG.[7]

An increased genetic burden of TG-raising alleles is characteristic of HTG. An individual SNP allele has a very small effect on plasma levels, but inherited accumulation of multiple genetic variants (polygenic) can add up and contribute to extreme lipid phenotypes, approximating that of a rare monogenic variant of large effect.[8]

The impact of such variants is quantified using a PRS. PRSs capture information on the aggregate burden of many small effect genetic variants. There is a significant increase in the mean score of risk alleles in HTG patients compared with those in population-based controls. In a meta-analysis of 46 lipid GWASs comprising of >100,000 individuals (>9,000 South Asians), calculation of risk scores summarizing the number of TG raising alleles weighted by effect size revealed that individuals in the top quartile of TG risk score were 44 times as likely to be HTG than individuals in the bottom quartile ($p = 4 \times 10^{-28}$).

Multiple PRSs have been described, with variable number of SNPs, which can be weighted or unweighted.

The TG risk scoring could help identify subjects at risk for developing HTG and who might benefit from early intervention **(Table 3)**.

Multifactorial Chylomicronemia Syndrome (Type V Hyperlipoproteinemia)[9,10]

It is the most common cause of not only mild-to-moderate but also severe HTG affecting about 1 in 400 individuals. Being polygenic in nature, it does not follow the mendelian inheritance pattern. GWASs have identified at least 400 loci across the human genome harboring common variants, which combine to contribute to extreme lipid phenotypes, widely across global populations. Some of these loci are associated not only with lipids but also with risk for CAD.

In patients with multifactorial chylomicronemia, chylomicronemia occurs later in life, typically in overweight adult patients with metabolic syndrome. Plasma TG levels in multifactorial chylomicronemia syndrome have more variability and are much more sensitive to dietary and/or fibrate treatment.

Monogenic HTG, which can result from large-effect mutations in six different genes, is quite rare.

Familial Chylomicronemia Syndrome (Type I Hyperlipoproteinemia)[10-13]

It is a rare (prevalence 1–2 per million) monogenic form of severe HTG with autosomal recessive inheritance and markedly increased risk of recurrent and potentially life-threatening acute pancreatitis.

It is characterized by the abnormal persistence of circulating chylomicrons in plasma beyond a fasting period of 12–14 hours because of impaired clearance of TG-rich lipoproteins (chylomicrons and VLDL) due to loss of LPL functionality.

The TGs in the TG-rich chylomicrons and VLDL are hydrolyzed by LPL present in the luminal surface of capillaries. LPL activity is regulated by APOC1, APOC2, APOC3, APOA5, ANGPTL3, ANGPTL4, and ANGPTL8. Lipase maturation factor and glycosylphosphatidylinositol-anchored high-density lipoprotein-binding protein 1 (GPIHBP1) is essential for movement of LPL to capillary endothelium. Loss of function mutations in LPL, APOC2, GPIHPB1, lipase maturation factor 1, and APOA5 can result in marked HTG (chylomicronemia). *APOC3* and *ANGPTL3* and *ANGPTL4* inhibit *LPL* activity and loss of function mutations in these genes is associated with increases in LPL activity and decreases in plasma TG levels.

More than 180 causative gene mutations have been found in *LPL* and its cofactors (*APOC2, GP1HBP1, APOA5,* and *LMF1*) genes. Mutations in the *LPL* gene account for >80% of the cases of familial chylomicronemia syndrome (FCS). Most of the subjects were homozygous for the p.P234L mutation of *LPL* gene (32%) or carried the p.G215E mutation of *LPL* gene (28%) or were compound heterozygotes for both (24%) **(Table 4)**.

Familial chylomicronemia syndrome often presents in childhood or adolescence with eruptive xanthomas, lipemia retinalis, hepatosplenomegaly, and acute or recurrent episodes of abdominal pain or pancreatitis.

Fasting plasma TG > 880 mg/dL on three consecutive samples, onset of symptoms at age <40 years, history of pancreatitis, TG/TC ratio >5 (mg/dL), plasma APOB <100 mg/dL and poor or absent response to therapy with traditional lipid-lowering agents are the features of FCS.

A clinical diagnostic scoring system (FCS score) proposed by a European expert panel has a sensitivity of 88% and a specificity of 85% for the diagnosis of FCS **(Table 5)**.[13]

Currently, full-gene sequencing of LPL and the four cofactor genes is the preferred method in establishing the diagnosis in patients with suspected FCS.

Patients with FCS show little or no response to TG-lowering pharmacotherapies, although novel therapies such as antisense oligonucleotides (ASOs) targeting APOC3 and ANGPTL3 mRNAs show promise as a future therapy. The backbone of the FCS therapy remains the adherence to an

TABLE 3: Single-nucleotide polymorphisms associated with hypertriglyceridemia.

Gene	Chromosome	TG raising allele
DOCK7, ANGPTL3	1	T
GALNT2	1	G
KLHL8, AFF1	4	T
MAP3K1, ANKRD55	5	T
MLXIPL	7	C
NAT2	8	G
LPL	8	A
TRIB1	8	A
JMJD1C	10	A
FADS1, FADS2, and *FADS3*	11	T
APOA1, APOC3, APOA4, and *APOA5*	11	G
CAPN3	15	A
FRMD5	15	T
CETP16	16	C
CSPG3, CILP2, and *PBX4*	19	T
PLTP	20	C

(TG: triglyceride)

TABLE 4: Genetic loci associated with familial chylomicronemia syndrome.

Disorder	Abnormality	Gene	Locus
Lipoprotein lipase deficiency	High chylomicrons	*LPL*	8p21
Familial APOC2 deficiency	High chylomicrons	*APOC2*	19q13
APOA5 deficiency	High VLDL and chylomicrons	*APOA5*	11q23
Combined lipase deficiency	High triglycerides	*LMF1*	16p13
GPIHBP1 deficiency	High chylomicrons	*GPIHBP1*	8q24.3

TABLE 5: Familial chylomicronemia syndrome (FCS) score.[13]

Feature	Points
Fasting triglycerides	
>10 mmol/L (three consecutive times)	+5
>20 mmol/L (at least once)	+1
Previous triglycerides <2 mmol/L	-5
No secondary factor except pregnancy and ethinylestradiol	+2
History of pancreatitis	+1
Unexplained recurrent abdominal pain	+1
No response to hypolipidemic drugs (TG decrease < 20%)	+1
No history of FCH (familial combined hyperlipidemia)	+1
Age at onset of symptoms	
<40 years	+1
<20 years	+2
<10 years	+3

Note: ≥10: FCS very likely/≥ 9: FCS unlikely/≥ 8: FCS very unlikely

extremely restrictive low-fat diet (15–25% of caloric intake, 10–20 g fat/day).

THERAPEUTIC APPROACHES

The knowledge of the genetic nature of HTG has also made it possible to identify targets for pharmacological treatments.

There are several approved or investigational agents whose origin can be traced to the identification of a human genetic defect, e.g., proprotein convertase subtilisin-kexin type 9 (PCSK9) inhibitors, cholesteryl ester transfer protein (CETP) inhibitors, microsomal triglyceride transfer protein (MTTP) inhibitors (lomitapide), APOB antisense RNA (mipomersen), and *LPL* gene therapy (Glybera), among others.

The SNP alterations may predict treatment efficacy. APOA5 SNPs and other variants have been shown to affect the plasma TG response to fibrates and niacin.

Gene Therapy

Gene Transfer

LPL gene therapy: *AAV1-LPLS447X* gene replacement therapy (alipogene tiparvovec) developed for treatment of familial chylomicronemia due to LPL deficiency (LPLD), promoting the synthesis and secretion of biologically active LPL which significantly lowers TG levels. Clinical trials showed reduction in pancreatitis up to 5 years after administration,[14] but potential tumorigenic effect and development of anti-AVV-1 antibodies led to its withdrawal.

Gene Editing[13,15]

Editing of genes regulating TG metabolism is an exciting new therapeutic approach for the treatment of HTG, promising a permanent effect. Introduction of nonsense or splice-site mutations or exon skipping are gene-editing tools which can be used for gene repair (limited to the treatment of monogenic diseases) or disruption (has broader applications). Among many gene-editing approaches, CRISPR/Cas9 system is the preferred method because of its simplicity and efficiency. These have showed promising results in preclinical studies. However, due to its permanent nature, use of gene editing requires careful ethical and safety considerations.

RNA-based Treatments[16]

Antisense oligonucleotides:

- *IONIS-ANGPTL3-LRx*: ANGPTL3 inhibits LPL and endothelial catalytic activity affecting TG hydrolysis, with the consequent increase in the TG-rich lipoproteins. A new ASO against ANGPTL3 reduces TG levels by 85%.
- *Volanesorsen*: APOC3 inhibits LPL and uptake of TGRL by their receptors. LOF mutations in APOC3 are associated with reduction in TG levels and CV risk. A second-generation ASO targeting of ApoC3 whose beneficial effects have been demonstrated in a study of genetically confirmed FCS patients giving rise to a 77% fall in TGs and an 84% fall in APOC3 at 3 months.

CONCLUSION

Even though there are no clinical guidelines or precise indications for genetic testing in dyslipidemias, declining costs should make it possible to consider genetic testing in selected dyslipidemic patients or their asymptomatic relatives based on clinical suspicion such as strong family history or syndromic features. Identifying a rare genetic disorder has implications for prognosis, treatment, and family counseling. As genetic testing becomes routinely available, the clinician needs to devise a strategy for its effective implantation in patient care. Inclusion of genetic variants in clinical trials will in future lead to prediction of therapeutic response based on individual's genetic score (precision medicine).

ONLINE REFERENCES

Please scan the QR code provided at the end of the table of contents for References of this chapter.

CHAPTER 63

Triglyceride-rich Lipoprotein as a Risk Factor for Atherosclerotic Cardiovascular Disease

Arijit Ghosh, Arup Dasbiswas

ABSTRACT

Atherosclerotic cardiovascular disease (ASCVD) is the leading cause of mortality and morbidity in the current era of medical practice. Low-density lipoprotein cholesterol (LDL-C) is a strong causal relationship with atherosclerotic disease burden. There is a considerable 30% residual risk of having a cardiovascular event even in patients who reach their recommended LDL targets with statin monotherapy, which is still considered the frontline LDL lowering agent. Hypertriglyceridemia as risk factor for ASCVD has always triggered controversy. Triglyceride-rich lipoproteins (TGRLs) and their metabolites can kindle the cascade of atherosclerosis by igniting inflammation, oxidative stress, and formation of foam cells. Contemporary genetic and epidemiological studies have substantiated that triglycerides and TGRLs are the main causal risk factors of the residual ASCVD. In this chapter, we will make a short review of TG and TGRL metabolism, display evidence of association between TG and ASCVD, and summarize the advances in TG-lowering therapies.

Keywords: Atherosclerotic cardiovascular disease, triglyceride-rich lipoprotein, residual risk, cardiovascular events, therapeutic targets.

INTRODUCTION

According to the World Health Organization (WHO) report in 2021, atherosclerotic cardiovascular disease (ASCVD) is the leading cause of death and disability across the globe. Cholesterol carried by lipoproteins in blood is the major inducer of ASCVD.[1] Among the lipoproteins, low-density lipoprotein (LDL) carries approximately 75% of total cholesterol (TC).[2] Elevated LDL cholesterol (LDL-C) has a linear correlation with increased ASCVD risk.[3] The lower the better concept of LDL lowering in terms of decreasing the risk of ASCVD events without any J-curve phenomenon has been proved beyond doubt in the various proprotein convertase subtilisin/kexin type 9 (PCSK9) trials. The first-line lipid lowering drug statins, can significantly reduce LDL-C levels, leading to a reduction in cardiovascular disease (CVD) events by 25–40%.[4] Moreover, the antibodies or siRNA of PCSK9 can decrease the LDL-C up to 75% from the baseline. However, patients treated with statins in combination with PCSK9 inhibitors still suffer ASCVD events despite their LDL-C level meeting recommended targets.[5] Therefore, researchers are impelled to find novel strategies for treatment of residual ASCVD risks.

Given a low high-density lipoprotein cholesterol (HDL-C) level is a string and independent risk factor associated with CVD events, enhancing HDL-C level has never been expected to prevent and/or recover CVD.[6] Cholesteryl ester transport protein (CETP) inhibitors can significantly improve HDL-C levels and reverse cholesterol transport. However, these inhibitors are found to be useless in prevention of CVD events.[7] Recent studies suggested that although HDL-C is a useful risk biomarker, accumulating evidence from Mendelian randomization studies and other research have demonstrated that HDL-C is not a casual risk factor for ASCVD.[8] Therefore, researchers turn their attention to other targets for treatment of ASCVD.

Clinical focus on whether to treat elevated triglyceride-rich lipoproteins (TGRLs) has fluctuated over the past many years. This fluctuation was driven by changes in the evidence base, suggesting that these lipoproteins either cause ASCVD or simply represent innocent bystanders to low HDL-C. There has not been a single, large, randomized trial aimed at reducing ASCVD by reducing TGRLs selectively in individuals with elevated levels. For mild-to-moderately elevated triglycerides (TGs) (2–10 mmol/L; 176–880 mg/dL), in the 1980s, advice was given in parallel to treat elevated TGs and cholesterol,[9-12] but from then on until 2011, most recommendations mainly focused on elevated LDL-C and largely ignored mild-to-moderately elevated TGs.[13,14] From 2011, some, but not all,[15,16] publications now advised on treating mild-to-moderately elevated TGs in high-risk individuals. These latter differences in recommendations were largely driven by whether only randomized, double-blind trial evidence for a benefit of TG lowering was evaluated, or whether the totality of evidence including randomized trials, epidemiology, genetics, and biology was evaluated. Many scientists and clinicians view the majority of fibrate trials as failed clinical trials for the TGs hypothesis; however, these trials did not examine the effect of reducing TGRL on ASCVD and all-cause mortality risk in individuals with elevated TGs. Finally, for severely elevated TGs (>10 mmol/L; >880 mg/dL), all publications from the 1980s to 2014 unanimously advise to reduce levels with the aim of reducing the risk of pancreatitis,[16,17] even in the lack of randomized trial evidence.

A SHORT REVIEW OF TRIGLYCERIDE AND TRIGLYCERIDE-RICH LIPOPROTEIN METABOLISM

In the circulation and in the cells the major storage form of fatty acids (FAs) are TG.[18,19] Liver plays the pivotal role in the metabolic process of FAs that are originated from the plasma and/or the hepatocytes **(Fig. 1)**. FA synthesis is precisely regulated by a cluster of enzymes including sterol regulatory element-binding protein (SREBP)-1c. With the abundance of glucose in the plasma, insulin activates the endoplasmic reticulum (ER) membrane-bound transcription factor SREBP-1c, which in turn upregulates genes responsible for FA biosynthesis.[18] However, only a small fraction of FA is stored as TG in lipid droplet because majority of the FAs are either oxidized in the mitochondrion or stored in the core of very LDL (VLDL) as TG and released into the blood. In the hepatocytes, a substantial proportion of TGs are assembled along with cholesterol, phospholipids, and apolipoprotein B100 (ApoB100) to form VLDL. In the small intestine, TG derived from diet is degraded into FA and monoglyceride or diglyceride before getting absorbed

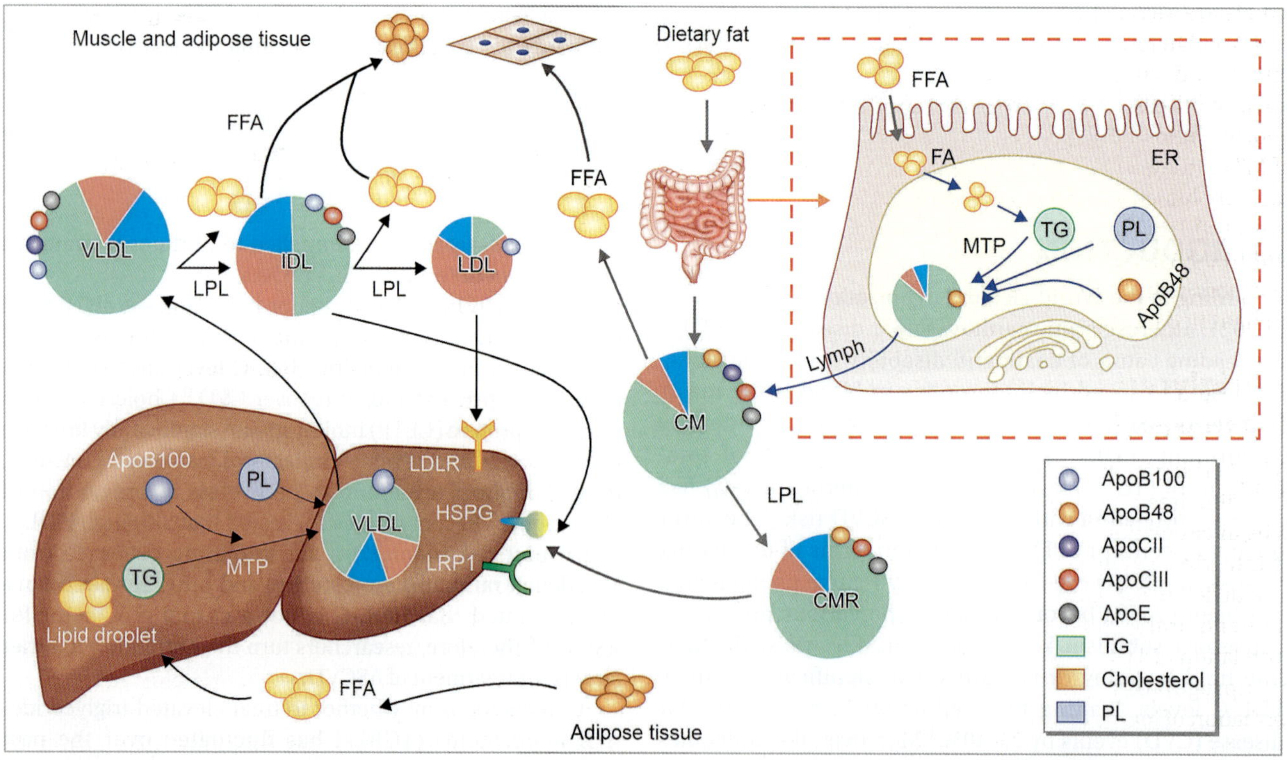

FIG. 1: TG and TGRL metabolism.

(Apo: apolipoprotein; CM: chylomicron; CMR: chylomicron residual; ER: endoplasmic reticulum; FA: fatty acid; FFA: free fatty acid; HSPG: heparan sulfate proteoglycan; IDL: intermediate-density lipoprotein; LDL: low-density lipoprotein; LDLR: low-density lipoprotein receptor; LPL: lipoprotein lipase; LRP1: LDLR-related protein 1; MTP: microsomal triglyceride transfer protein; PL: phospholipid; TG: triglyceride; TGRL: triglyceride-rich lipoprotein; VLDL: very low-density lipoprotein) by enterocytes. These breakdown products are reassembled into chylomicron (CM) along with cholesterol, phospholipids, and ApoB48.[20,21] Next, CMs are secreted into the lymphatic system and enter the circulation, where they bind with other apolipoproteins including ApoCII, ApoCIII, and ApoE.[22,23] Microsomal triglyceride transfer protein (MTP) significantly contributes in the assembly of VLDL and CM via transporting the related lipids to ApoB particles.[24] The secreted VLDL and CM particles transport FAs to muscle and adipose tissue for energy usage and/or storage via the blood flow.[19,25] In circulation, lipoprotein lipase (LPL) located at the surface of capillary lumen hydrolyzes TGs that are encapsulated in the core of CM and VLDL into FAs. Proteins such as ApoCII, ApoCIII, ApoE and angiopoietin-like protein 3 (ANGPTL3), ANGPTL4, and ANGPTL8 are the major regulatory proteins of LPL activity.[22,26] As TG gets hydrolyzed, CM gradually gets converted to smaller and cholesterol-rich CM remnant (CMR), and VLDL changes to intermediate-density lipoprotein (IDL), which is further catabolized to become LDL via hepatic TG lipase (HTGL) on the surface of hepatic sinusoidal endothelial cell cavity.[27] TGRL remnants in circulation are cleared by liver receptors including LDL receptor (LDLR), LDLR-related protein (LRP)-1, scavenger receptor B type 1 (SR-B1), and heparan sulfate proteoglycan (HSPG).[28-30]

Dietary fat is metabolized by intestinal cells into FAs, which are reassembled with cholesterol, phospholipids, and ApoB48 to form CMs **(Fig. 1)**. These CMs are released into blood via lymph. In the liver, exogenous and de novo synthesized FAs are assembled with cholesterol, phospholipids, and ApoB100 to form VLDL with the assistant of MTP. In the circulation, LPL located at the surface of the capillary lumen hydrolyzes the TG in the core of TGRL (CM and VLDL) and promotes the production of TGRL remnants and free FAs. TGRL remnants are cleared by liver through receptors including HSPG, LDLR, LRP1, and other potentially unidentified receptors.

Triglyceride-rich Lipoprotein and Atherosclerosis

Triglyceride-rich lipoprotein and the hydrolyzed derivatives including free FAs attach to the leukocytes and endothelial cells in circulation, and activate them leading to expression of integrins, generation of reactive oxygen species (ROS), production of cytokines along with complement activation.[31] Contemporary research has demonstrated the positive correlation of TGRL and their remnants with atherosclerosis by upregulating inflammation, oxidative stress, and formation of foam cells.

Triglyceride-rich Lipoproteins Activate Inflammation

Atherosclerosis is considered a chronic inflammatory process. Every mmol/L (39 mg/dL) elevation of TGRL cholesterol is related with a 37% increase of C-reactive protein level, and rise of other inflammatory markers such as interleukin-6 (IL-6) and tumor necrosis factor alpha (TNF-α), which are substantially higher in the postprandial state as compared to the fasting state, suggesting that elevation of postprandial TGRL cholesterol is strong correlates of inflammatory response, increasing the propensity for premature atherosclerosis. TGRLs with high TG content upregulates TNF-α mediated expression of vascular cell adhesion molecule-1 (VCAM-1) in human aortic endothelial cells and monocyte.[32-34] VLDL particles released in the circulation after meals have elevated levels of ApoCIII,[33,34] and activates inflammation in endothelial cells by stimulating the protein kinase C (PKC)/nuclear factor kappa B (NF-κB) signaling pathway.[35] Similarly, VLDL particles are also responsible for the NF-κB signaling pathway mediated endothelial cell inflammation.[36,37] Macrophage is a central link between lipid metabolism and inflammation. TG synthesis (lipid droplet formation) induces macrophage inflammation.[38] In vitro, VLDL enhances the expression of TNF-α, IL-1β, monocyte chemoattractant protein 1 (MCP-1), intercellular adhesion molecule-1 (ICAM-1), matrix metalloproteinase 3, and macrophage inflammatory protein 1-α.

The CMRs lead to the expression of IL-1β via activating caspase-1 and NF-κB in THP-1 cells.[39] In addition, CMRs also activate human monocytes and enhance their migration in vitro, contributing to an inflammatory milieu in the initial phases of atherosclerosis.[40]

Triglyceride-rich Lipoproteins Induce Oxidative Stress and Endothelial Cell Dysfunction

Oxidative stress is an important contributor of atherosclerosis progression by causing inflammation, endothelial dysfunction, and foam cell formation. Endothelial dysfunction is one of the initial events in the atherosclerotic process. Free FAs liberated during lipolysis of TGRL are a trigger to activate NADPH oxidase- and cytochrome P450-mediated ROS production within endothelial cells, leading to oxidative stress and malfunction of endothelial barrier.[41] TGRL remnants increase the vulnerability of coronary endothelium to oxidative stress, leading to inhibition of nitric oxide-induced vascular dilation causing vasomotor dysfunction.[42] Atherosclerosis progression even in normolipidemic individuals is seen to happen with postprandial elevation of TGRL cholesterol by promoting endothelial dysfunction, such as endothelium-dependent vasorelaxation.[43,44] TGRL lipolysis leads to endothelial dysfunction by production of ROS and alterations of lipid raft in morphology and protein components, such as LRP, nitric oxide synthase, and caveolin-1, leading to endothelial dysfunction.[45] Furthermore, TGRL and their lipolytic derivatives stimulate platelet aggregation, suppresses fibrinolysis, promotes the assembly of prothrombinase complex, and increases the expression of plasminogen activator inhibitor-1 and its antigen, endothelial expression of tissue factor contributing to increased thrombogenicity.[28,46,47] Furthermore, TGs promote atherosclerosis by increasing plasma viscosity, leading to impairment of microcirculatory flow and enhanced interactions amongst atherogenic lipoproteins and endothelium.[48]

Except for CM particles, TGRL and TGRL remnant particles can penetrate blood vessel due to their small size and are recognized and directly engulfed by macrophages through the ligand ApoE located at the surface of TGRL.[49,50] As it is oxidized LDL particles are known to be ingested by macrophages. TGRLs thus can cause rapid lipid accumulation in macrophages and smooth muscle cells, contributing to plaque formation and development of atherosclerosis.[51]

Triglyceride-rich Lipoproteins Promote Foam Cell Formation

Most of the ApoB proteins isolated from human atherosclerotic plaques are derived from VLDL and IDL, but not LDL, suggesting that VLDL and IDL have a significant contribution in the ongoing atherosclerotic process involving the intima of these arteries.[25,52,53] It appears that the remnant cholesterol, instead of TG, in TGRL particles is a causal agent of atherosclerosis.[54-56] In comparison to the VLDL particles isolated from people with normal TG levels, VLDL particles obtained from patients with elevated TG have a higher affinity for scavenger receptors, such as LDLR and VLDLR, that are selectively expressed by monocytes, macrophages, and endothelial cells.[57,58]

The CMRs also contribute to lipid accumulation in the atherosclerotic plaques. Independent of the ApoE-mediated pathway ApoB48 receptor is involved in CMR uptake and foam cell formation.

Cell death is triggered due to lysosomal instability resulting from rapid lysosomal accumulation of cholesterol due to CMR internalization, thereby promoting atherosclerosis deterioration.[59] Additionally, TG contained in TGRL particles can activate CETP-mediated exchange of TG in TGRL with cholesterol in LDL, and generate dense LDL particles that are more atherosclerotic than LDL particles.[57,60] In the same way, TGRLs are responsible HDL remodeling and the formation of smaller, low-cholesterol HDL particles that do not provide protection against atherosclerosis.[61]

EPIDEMIOLOGICAL ARGUMENTS

A considerable number of epidemiological studies and meta-analyses have substantiated that high concentrations of TGs (fasting and nonfasting) have a strong correlation with the risk of ASCVD.[62-64] In 2007, the twin prospective observational studies—the Copenhagen City Heart Study[63] and the Women's Health Study[62]—enlightened us in this regard. The Copenhagen City Heart Study demonstrated increased levels of nonfasting TGs to be related with an increased risk of myocardial infarction, ischemic heart disease, and death irrespective of gender.[63] The Women's Health Study (undertaken among a cohort of healthy women in the USA) could establish an association between nonfasting TGs and an increased risk of ASCVD, but failed to find any relationship with fasting TGs.[62] The point whether TGs are an independent risk factor was raised in 2009 by the Emerging Risk Factors Collaboration analysis.[65] On the basis of the analysis from 68 long-term prospective studies increased TGs was found to have a 37% increased risk of CHD after adjusting the nonlipid risk parameters. The significance of this association decreased on adjustment for HDL-C, and was completely abolished after adjusting non-HDL-C, which finally lead to the conclusions that the TG measurement does not further risk stratify patients. In fact, this finding is in tune with the concept that the cholesterol content of TGRLs is responsible for ASCVD rather than the raised TGs. In 2014, in studies taking together the Copenhagen City Heart Study and the Copenhagen General Population Study, with comparable statistical power to the Emerging Risk Factors Collaboration, nonfasting TGs were found to be associated with risk of ASCVD and all-cause mortality.[66] In these studies, when compared with individuals with plasma TG concentrations <89 mg/dL (<1 mmol/L), the multivariable adjusted hazard ratios for myocardial infarction were 1.6, 2.2, 3.2, 2.8, and 3.4 for individuals with TG 132–139 concentration of 1.00–1.99, 2.00–2.99, 3.00–3.99, 4.00–4.99 and ≥5.00 mmol/L, respectively.[67] Data from a complementary analysis from the Copenhagen General Population Study,[68] individuals in primary prevention with a TG concentration ≥ 3 mmol/L, but not candidates for statin therapy, had around a threefold higher susceptibility of myocardial infarction at 10 years as compared to the cohorts with a TG concentration < 3 mmol/L. In the Copenhagen studies,[61,69] high nonfasting residual lipoprotein cholesterol (RLP-C) (calculated as TC minus HDL-C minus LDL-C) had relation with ischemic heart disease risk, without any influence from reduced HDL-C,[10] and with all-cause mortality in patients with ischemic heart disease.[69] In some data from China, RLPC (measured by nuclear magnetic resonance spectroscopy) was also known to be associated with an increased risk of myocardial infarction and ischemic stroke.[70] However, in the ARIC (Atherosclerosis Risk in Communities) study,[71] although elevated TGs were associated with increased RLP-C, only the TG content in LDL particles was the predictors of ASCVD risk after adjustment for conventional risk factors. There might be one criticism of all these studies that they all had a cross-sectional design, especially when TGs are known to be highly variable. A recent study has evaluated the relation between multiple measurements of TGs overtime and future ASCVD, banking on the data from the ARIC study and the Framingham Offspring Study.[72] The investigators concluded, compared with a one-point TG measurement, average TGs overtime had a greater discriminating value for ASCVD risk, after adjusting for factors associated with both ASCVD and high TGs, such as diabetes, LDL-C, and HDL-C. However, the use of non-HDL-C weakened the association. This suggests that the risk associated with high levels TGs may be due to the elevations in RLP-C. This is also consistent with genetic studies showing that the risk associated with elevated TGRLs can be explained by their association with elevated concentrations of ApoB.[73]

Finally, majority of these observational epidemiological data were from the prestatin era. As statin therapy is considered as the first-line therapy for high-risk patients with elevated TGs,[63] it is important to investigate whether TGRLs and/or RLP-C elevation have any influence in statin-treated patients.

GENETIC ARGUMENTS

Several reviews have described the genetic association of TGs or TGRLSs and ASCVD risk.[8,74] To establish the causality of hypertriglyceridemia as a risk factor for ASCVD low HDL-C always comes in the way as a confounding variable on a population level. However, contemporary evidence has shown that TGRLs but not HDL-C are causally associated with ASCVD.[75-77] For instance, the Copenhagen study[75] found that a nonfasting RLP-C increase of 1 mmol/L (39 mg/dL) was associated with a 2.8-times higher risk of ischemic heart disease, irrespective of reduced HDL-C. Furthermore, several genes modulating TGRL metabolism, namely LPL and those controlling LPL function, are also associated with ASCVD: heterozygous carriers of LPL loss-of-function and missense pathogenic variants had elevated TG concentrations and an increased risk of CHD.[78] A genetic variant in ApoA5 that increased TG concentrations by 16% (0.25 mmol/L) was associated with an increased risk of CHD (odds ratio 1.18, 95% confidence interval 1.11–1.26).[79] A twofold rise in RLP-C concentrations due to mutations in ApoA5 was associated with a 2.2-fold increased risk of myocardial infarction.[54] Increased LPL activity ushered by ApoC3, ANGPTL3 and ANGPTL4 loss-of function genetic mutation, and consequently reduced plasma TGs, results in reduced ASCVD risk.[80,81] In one study, loss-of-function mutation of ApoC3 resulted in 39% lower TG levels and reduces CHD risk by 40%.[82] In another study, 17% lower level of TGs, a 12% fall in LDL-C and an overall 34% reduction in CHD risk was seen in individuals with heterozygous carriers of ANGPTL3 loss-of-function mutations.[83] In this evolving field of lipidology, we currently have several therapeutic targets (either monoclonal antibodies or antisense oligonucleotides) aiming at ApoC3 and ANGPTL3 for degreasing TGs and ASCVD risk. Loss-of-function mutation of ANGPTL4 is also related to the decrease in TG concentrations and consequent decrease in CHD risk.[84] However, the use of monoclonal antibodies to inhibit ANGPTL4 has not been proved to be safe in animal studies as it induces side effects in animals.[84]

TREATMENT OF HYPERTRIGLYCERIDEMIA TO REDUCE ASCVD RISK

Lifestyle modifications, including dietary changes, exercise, reduction of alcohol intake, and weight loss, are the most important principles for the management of hypertriglyceridemia. Beyond lifestyle interventions, and despite the association between TGs or RLP-C and cardiovascular risk observed in epidemiological and genetic studies, randomized controlled clinical trials focused on treatments that primarily lower TGs concentrations have not consistently shown a reduction in ASCVD events. However, with the exception of the recent REDUCE-IT trial,[85] these trials were not specifically conducted in patients with high TG concentrations on statin therapy. In addition to the modest (10–20%) TG-lowering effect of statins, if residual TG-associated risk for ASCVD is high, initiation of a specific TG-lowering drug may be justified. In a recent meta-regression analysis of the three classes of TG-lowering therapies (fibrates, niacin, and marine-derived omega-3 FAs), TG lowering does appear to be associated with a lower risk of major cardiovascular events, but to a lesser extent per absolute amount of reduction than for LDL-C.[86] Given that both the statin-era niacin trials failed to show a cardiovascular benefit, this drug is not currently available in Europe. Only one trial, ACCORD-Lipid,[87] has examined the effect of fenofibrate used in combination with statin therapy in patients with type 2 diabetes mellitus (T2DM). The authors found no further risk reduction, although subgroup analyses indicated that patients with high TGs and low HDL-C may benefit from this combination therapy. An ongoing outcome trial, PROMINENT, using a novel selective peroxisome proliferator-activated receptor alpha modulator called pemafibrate, will provide important insights for patients with T2DM on statin therapy and with moderate hypertriglyceridemia and low HDL-C.[88] In a meta-analysis of 10 trials involving >77,000 individuals, supplementation with low doses of omega-3 FAs was not associated with a cardiovascular benefit.[89] However, the REDUCE-IT trial[85] changed the perception of this class: a high dose (4 g/day) of icosapent ethyl, purified eicosapentaenoic acid, or placebo was added to background statin therapy in patients with elevated TGs (150–499 mg/dL) and either CVD or diabetes and an additional risk factor. A dramatic risk reduction was observed for ASCVD over a period of 4.9 years, with a 25% relative risk reduction and a 4.8% absolute benefit, concomitant with a 20% reduction in TGs and a 40% reduction in C-reactive protein concentrations.[85] It remains unclear whether the observed benefit relates to the particular omega-3 FA formulation or the high daily dose. Of note, another similar study (STRENGTH), with high doses of both eicosapentaenoic acid and docosahexaenoic acid, was stopped recently for futility.

CONCLUSION

Despite the reduction in ASCVD events seen with statins and additional LDL-lowering therapies, there is a substantial residual risk of recurrent events. Elevated TGs can be used to identify patients with higher residual risk as a result of the presence of potentially atherogenic TGRLs. Indeed, TGRLs have emerged as important contributors to residual risk on statin therapy, and genetic studies strongly support the hypothesis that remnants of TGRLs are a causal cardiovascular risk factor. Beyond lifestyle changes and statin therapy, a recent trial with high dose icosapent ethyl showed a significant cardiovascular benefit in high-risk patients with hypertriglyceridemia. Moreover, genetic studies have provided novel treatment targets to lower serum TGs, and clinical trials will be needed to test their impact on cardiovascular outcomes.

ONLINE REFERENCES

Please scan the QR code provided at the end of the table of contents for References of this chapter.

CHAPTER 64

Dyslipidemia in Women: An Update

Nagamani AC, Varun Marimuthu

ABSTRACT

The onset of dyslipidemia is an important milestone in the development of atherosclerotic vascular disease. Women and men are equally affected. Treatment of dyslipidemia more than any other therapy has led to a paradigm shift in the approach to primary prevention and is a major part of secondary prevention of cardiovascular diseases and stroke. Women were historically underrepresented in all the clinical trials, although the trend is changing. In this chapter, we will discuss lipid metabolism, its management, and some special scenarios pertaining to women.

Keywords: Dyslipidemia, women, pregnancy.

INTRODUCTION

The prevalence of cardiovascular (CV) disease is on the ascent, with equal distribution in men and women. It is aptly called an "epidemic" in India. CV disease continues to be the leading cause of death in India (25%[1] and, in many parts of the world, easily outnumbering deaths due to cancer, accidents, and lung disease. As populations age, the accrued risk factors—hypertension (HTN), diabetes mellitus (DM), dyslipidemia (DLP), smoking, obesity, and poor physical activity, often in combination, lead to CV disease and poor outcomes. CV disease in India is early in onset, progresses rapidly due to late presentation and poor initial and long-term care and has a high rate of mortality.[1] Over the last 20 years, there has been an epidemiological transition from infectious diseases, maternal, and childhood diseases to CV diseases. Prior to menopause during the childbearing years, women are protected from CV disease compared to matched male controls. Although more men succumb to CV disease compared to women, and the age of first myocardial infarction (MI) is 10 years later in women,[2] this trend is worryingly changing with more women developing CV disease sooner.

Surveys have shown the prevalence of DLP to be 20% among women and a larger number remain undiagnosed. Further, a significant population remain untreated despite diagnosis due to various sociocultural reasons. Medications work equally well in both the genders and reduce CV events significantly. There are several differences in the metabolism and management of lipids that are unique to women due in part to the circulating sex hormones.

In this chapter, we will discuss various caveats in dealing with DLP in women and offer a framework to reduce CV mortality and improve outcomes.

A BRIEF ON DYSLIPIDEMIA AND HOW IS IT DIFFERENT IN WOMEN?

Basic Lipid Metabolism

The important plasma lipids that have clinical relevance are cholesterol, cholesterol esters (CEs), and triglycerides (TGs). Cholesterol has multiple physiological roles including synthesis of steroids and other hormones, formation of the cell membrane and neuronal signaling. TGs are an important source of energy. These plasma lipids are insoluble, and they circulate as part of the lipoprotein particles—which include chylomicrons (CMs), very low-density lipoprotein (VLDL), intermediate density lipoprotein (IDL), low-density lipoprotein (LDL), and high-density lipoprotein (HDL). The lipoprotein particles have surface apolipoproteins and phospholipids which function as receptors and mediate their secretion and uptake to tissues.

Of the total plasma cholesterol, only 15–20% have a dietary source. The rest is endogenously synthesized from the liver. Dietary cholesterol is absorbed from the small intestine by the Niemann–Pick C1-like 1 (NPC1L1) transporter. Circulating cholesterol in the plasma is taken up by the liver, or Denovo synthesized via a multistep process which is rate limited by the 3-hydroxy-3-methylglutaryl-coenzyme A (HMG-CoA) reductase enzyme.

The TGs in the plasma are derived from the diet as well as by hepatic synthesis. Dietary TGs are attached to apolipoprotein B-48 (ApoB-48) and packaged into CM in the enterocytes and enter the circulation via lymphatics and the thoracic duct. CMs are cleared by lipoprotein lipases (LPLs), and the free fatty acids (FAs) are taken up by the cells for energy. The TG-depleted CMs are taken up by the liver.

The liver secretes VLDL, which contains TGs and cholesterol/CE in a 4:1 ratio and has an ApoB-100 molecule attached. The circulating VLDLs are hydrolyzed by the LPL, and FAs are liberated. The remaining remnant is the IDL, which now has TG and cholesterol in a 1:1 concentration.

Circulating HDLs exchange the TG in the IDLs for CE in the HDL, mediated via cholesterol ester transfer protein (CETP). This enriches the IDL and reduces its density. Further depletion of TGs in the IDL occurs via hepatic LPL. This process generates LDL. LDL is then taken up by the liver via LDL-receptors (LDL-R). Proprotein convertase subtilisin/kexin type 9 (PCSK9) targets the LDL-Rs for lysosomal degeneration. Inhibition of PCSK9 causes lack of LDL-R degeneration and its upregulation. This promotes LDL uptake by the liver, and thus PCSK9 inhibition is a major target for managing DLP. LDL can be classed into two patterns—(1) the more buoyant, larger LDL-A and (2) the smaller, denser, more atherogenic LDL-B.

Lipoprotein(a) [Lp(a)] is an important risk factor for atherosclerotic cardiovascular disease (ASCVD). Lp(a) contains an LDL molecule bound to apolipoprotein. Lp(a) promotes inflammation, thrombosis, and atherogenesis. It is attributed to the development of valvular aortic stenosis. Lp(a) is genetically determined and is high normal in people of South Asian ancestry.

To summarize, the ApoB-containing lipids—LDL, IDL, remnant lipoproteins, and Lp(a)—promote ASCVD.

Sex Difference in Lipid Metabolism and Cardiometabolic Disorders

The primary difference in women compared to men is the drive of the sex hormones during puberty, pregnancy, and childbirth all the way to menopause. The hormonal ebbs and surges promote a milieu of constant change in a woman's body. These changes alter lipoprotein levels. A newborn, independent of sex, will have the lowest total cholesterol levels naturally possible, at 65 mg/dL, and as they age, it rises to reach adult levels by 2 years.[3] Numerous studies have concluded the following on the differences in lipid levels between genders:

- Boys had a smaller LDL particle size compared to girls.[4]
- Low-density lipoprotein levels increase in both men and women after 20 years of age, but the increase is rapid and steeper in men.[5]
- High-density lipoprotein decreases in men, while it remains constant in women beyond puberty.
- High-density lipoprotein particle size decreases with age in men and the larger HDL levels stay constant in women.[6]
- Women have more LDL-B as they age and can cause more ASCVD risk in the later years, whereas men have more LDL-B even at younger ages.

Specific Situations in Women

Women, due to their gender-specific hormones, are at a lower risk for ASCVD. However, during specific times when hormonal imbalances occur, unfavourable changes in the lipid metabolism occurs, as follows.

Polycystic Ovary Syndrome, Childhood Obesity

Polycystic ovary syndrome (PCOS) is a condition seen commonly in young women due to elevations in the androgen hormone production. Metabolic disturbances and DLP are common in women with PCOS, with a prevalence of 70%.[7] In PCOS, the major abnormality is insulin resistance, and the DLP in PCOS is like that found in patients with DM, with high TG, ApoB, VLDL and low HDL, and ApoA1. Additionally, most of the women with PCOS have obesity, and have an abnormal lipid profile with high non-HDL cholesterol, and TG. Identifying this subgroup of women would help in mitigating long-term effects of DLP with good diet counseling and exercise. Childhood obesity and DLP are modifiable precursors for adult CV disease, and the risk is higher in women with hormonal imbalance.

Pregnancy and Postpartum

Pregnancy causes a wide flux in the hormonal levels. There is an increase in human chorionic gonadotropin (hcG), insulin, progesterone, and beta-estradiol. These perturbations cause elevations in the TC, LDL, HDL, and TG with the peak LDL occurring at 36 weeks. Lp(a) levels are also increased during pregnancy. These are essential for fetal growth and metabolism. Post pregnancy, the elevated HDL levels decline to lower than the prepregnancy levels, due to several reasons—(1) increase in androgen levels (like PCOS) and (2) insulin resistance and gestational DM.

Menopause

After physiological menopause, the circulating hormonal milieu changes compared to premenopausal women. This directly changes the lipid profile—leading to increased LDL, TC, and ApoB. An increase in cholesterol levels was attributed directly to menopause in the Framingham study.[8] Post menopause, there is a transition in the LDL to an atherogenic, denser LDL particle. This in combination with reduction in the HDL levels leads to higher risk in the postmenopausal period. Studies have detected increased Lp(a) levels after hysterectomy and oophorectomy.[9]

Hormone Replacement Therapy/Oral Contraception

Hormone replacement therapy (HRT) and oral contraception (OCP) can alter the lipoprotein levels based on the content of estrogen and progesterone. Estrogen increases the HDL fraction, TG, and reduces LDL levels. The increase in HDL is in part due to the estrogen-mediated reduction in the hepatic catabolism of HDL.[10] Progesterone produces opposite effects, causing elevations in the LDL and reduction in the TG levels. Once OCP is stopped, the lipoprotein levels return to normal. Various studies[11] have not entirely established the causal role of OCP use to CV diseases and ASCVD, but a link to venous thromboembolism (VTE) is well established. Women who develop ASCVD with OCP use were noted to have secondary traditional risk factors that would promote atherogenesis.

Hormone replacement therapy was conceived to reduce the adverse effects that women face after menopause. If the adverse change in lipid profile and the associated increase in ASCVD risk could be reversed with HRT, it would improve the long-term cardiac risk of an elderly woman. HRT also has additional antiplatelet and vasodilatory actions. So, various approaches were used.

- Hormone replacement therapy with unopposed estrogen causes elevations in HDL and reduces LDL and increases Apo-AI and -AII.
- Combination HRT (C-HRT) with estrogen and progesterone produced smaller increases in HDL and TG compared to pure estrogen formulations, as shown in the postmenopausal estrogen and progesterone interventions trial.[12]
- C-HRT causes reduction in the LDL particle size leading to the generation of smaller, more atherogenic LDL.[13]

Early studies on HRT showed some reduction in ASCVD risk in women on HRT. But later randomized studies did not show any benefit. In view of these conflicting studies, HRT was taken off the recommendations to prevent ASCVD in women.

- In the Nurse's health study, postmenopausal women on HRT have a relative risk reduction (RRR) of 37% compared to women not on HRT.[14]
- A meta-analysis of 32 studies between 1970 and 1992 showed a 35% RRR of ASCVD in women on HRT versus not on HRT, especially in women post hysterectomy or with a history of ASCVD.[15]
- In the Heart and Estrogen/Progestin Replacement Study (HERS), a randomized control study (RCT), a combination HRT showed a reduction in LDL and increase in HDL, but no benefit in ASCVD outcomes.[16]
- In the Women's Health Initiative (WHI), 10,739 postmenopausal women were started on estrogen. After 7 years, there was an increase in stroke and ASCVD, and the trial was stopped early.[17]

Dyslipidemia and ASCVD in Women

The presence of DLP and increased fraction of atherogenic lipids promotes ASCVD and increases risk of adverse events—MI, stroke, or peripheral vascular disease in both men and women. However, in women, the lipid abnormalities are different in their relative risk of causing disease. Various studies have found a 3% decrease in ASCVD risk for 1% reduction in TC.[18] Low HDL and elevated TG play a major role in enhancing risk in women, as revealed in the Lipid Research Clinics study.[19] The risk reduction differs among the sexes: a 1 mg/dL increase in HDL was associated with a 3% less risk of ASCVD in women and 2% in men.[20] Women have an HDL that is 10 mg/dL higher than men.

A large meta-analysis showed that the RR for TG to cause ASCVD was 1.32 in men and 1.76 in women, suggesting that the risk attributable to TG is twice in women,[21] and was correlated in another contemporary meta-analysis.[22] Excess LDL-B in younger age is associated with higher risk of vascular events. Additionally, the Framingham Heart Study (FHS) showed a correlation between high Lp(a) and risk of MI[23] and in HERS trial, postmenopausal women with elevated Lp(a) showed the highest CV risk, underscoring the importance of Lp(a) and the control of other lipid fractions, as there are no currently available therapies to reduce Lp(a) levels.

An analysis of 6,787 women included in the seminal INTERHEART study revealed the following sex-specific differences regarding the nine modifiable risk factors that were studied:[24]

- Median age of first MI was 9 years later in women (65 vs. 56 years)
- Hypertension, DM, physical activity, and moderate alcohol use were strongly associated with MI among women than men.
- Abnormal lipids, smoking, abdominal obesity, poor diet, and stress were equally contributory in women and men.

In the American Heart Association (AHA) ASCVD risk calculator, women-specific risk enhancers are preeclampsia and premature menopause. Calcium scoring in women was compared to men and was found to be more beneficial in women in a meta-analysis.

MANAGEMENT

Treating DLP in women is not different than men. However, in all the studies on DLP, the representation of women was dismal, with a few trials not representing women at all. This historical paternalization of women has persisted to this date, with trials having very low number of women. This is, however, changing, with newer studies being inclusive of women.

Lifestyle and Diet

A change in lifestyle is the most important initial strategy to reduce the abnormal lipid numbers. This includes moderate-intensity physical activity for 30 minutes a day for most days of the week, weight loss and reaching target body mass index (BMI), smoking, and alcohol cessation.

About 10–15% of the TC in the plasma can be attributed to dietary cholesterol, with the remainder being synthesized by the liver endogenously. Carbohydrate-rich diets promote intrinsic cholesterol synthesis. Still, dietary changes lead to reduction in the TC and TG levels. The AHA recommends the AHA step-1 diet for all women, with <30% of calories from fat (<10% of calories from saturated fat, <300 mg/day of cholesterol). For women with ASCVD, a step-II diet is recommended (<7% of daily calories from saturated fats, <200 mg cholesterol).[25]

Does lifestyle and dietary changes change the ASCVD risk? Improvement in plaque volumes and clinical ASCVD events has been noted in men on an intensive diet. Such data is as usual lacking in women.

- In the WHI Dietary Modification Study, 50,000 postmenopausal women were on a modified low-fat and high-fruit/vegetable diet versus control. However, after 8 years, there was no difference in both the groups.[26]
- A Mediterranean diet with nuts and olive oil reduced CV risk.
- The Nurses' Health Study II showed that in a 20-year follow-up of their 88,940 strong cohort of women, a healthy lifestyle and diet reduces the future ASCVD risk in those aged 27–44 years.[27]

Medications

Statins

Statins are often the first drug to be prescribed for patients with DLP. Statins are inhibitors of HMG-CoA, a rate-limiting step in the cholesterol synthesis pathway. They reduce the endogenous production of cellular cholesterol and increase the LDL receptors in the liver. This leads to uptake of circulating LDL, thereby reducing plasma LDL concentrations. They have additional pleiotropic effects, promoting vascular endothelial function. Meta-analysis of RCTs has found that a reduction of 39 mg/dL of LDL provides an RRR in ASCVD events by 22% and an all-cause mortality of 10%,[28] which is more significant than any other health promotion activity. This reduction shown by the Cholesterol Treatment Trialists (CTT) trial was equal in women and men.

Additionally, statins provide beneficial effects which accrue over many years, with a legacy effect. **Table 1** summarizes the RRR with the various statin trials in women. Women report more muscle symptoms compared to men, although this is attributed to be a nocebo effect, as shown in the SAMSON trial.

Ezetimibe

Ezetimibe acts on the NPC1L1 transfer protein in the liver and intestine, blocking it and causing impaired biliary and intestinal cholesterol absorption, thereby increasing the expression of LDL receptors, akin to statins. The IMPROVE-IT trial[29] conducted in patients with acute coronary syndrome (ACS) and elevated LDL showed that the addition of ezetimibe to simvastatin was associated with a 6% RRR in recurrent CV events over a 7-year period. It is often used as an add-on therapy after addition and optimization of statins and never in isolation. In this trial, 24% were women. In a prespecified analysis of sex differences in IMPROVE-IT, both men and women derived equal benefit with a similar side effect profile.

PCSK9 Inhibitors

Loss of function mutations of the *PCSK9* gene was associated with less degeneration of LDL receptors and low LDL levels in the plasma, leading to less ASCVD. This genetic aberrancy was harnessed into the design of PCSK9 inhibitors (PCSK9i). These monoclonal antibodies are subcutaneously injected, and they produce reductions of over 60% in the LDL levels, and over 27% in the Lp(a) levels. The two available molecules are evolocumab (FOURIER trial)[38] and alirocumab (ODESSEY OUTCOMES),[32] and both showed sustained reductions in LDL and in CV outcomes. However, PCSK9i has a sex-specific differential LDL reduction. Various studies, including a sex-specific analysis of FOURIER and the LIPID REAL registry,[39] have shown that the LDL reduction is less in women compared to men on PCSK9i, and could be due to compliance, less background therapy with statins and more importantly to a genetic, molecular, and hormonal mechanisms.[40]

N-3 Fatty Acids

N-3 polyunsaturated FAs are a mixture of eicosapentaenoic acid (EPA) and docosahexaenoic acid (DHA) or EPA in isolation. They reduce TG and VLDL levels production in the liver and increase VLDL clearance from the plasma. Although earlier trials such as GISSI[41] and JELIS[42] showed benefit of the N-3 FAs in CV risk reduction, there was no RCT showing benefit. In REDUCE-IT,[43] a proprietary purified EPA derivative—icosapent ethyl (IPE)—at a high dose of 4 g/day was used. This showed a 25% reduction in CV risk compared to a mineral oil placebo, in patients with DM and elevated TG. Due to the very high reduction in risk, additional benefits such as anti-inflammatory and antithrombotic were attributed to IPE. A subsequent trial, STRENGTH,[44] where EPA and DHA were used in combination failed to show benefit. Only 28% of the patients randomized in REDUCE-IT were women. However, there was no sex-specific subgroup differences noted.

TABLE 1: Relative risk reduction with statins in women—A summary.

Trial	Intervention type	Women (%)	Treatment	Primary endpoint	Relative risk in women (95% CI)
JUPITER[31]	Primary	6,801[32]	Rosuvastatin 20 mg/day versus placebo	MI, stroke, unstable angina, CHD death, revascularization	0.54 (0.37–0.80)
AFCAPS/TexCAPS[33]	Primary	997[15]	Lovastatin 20–40 mg/day vs. placebo	Sudden cardiac death, MI, unstable angina	0.54 (0.22–1.35)
4S[34]	Secondary	827[19]	Simvastatin 20–40 mg/day vs. placebo	All-cause mortality, CHD death	1.16 (0.68–1.99)
HPS[35]	Primary/secondary	5,082[25]	Simvastatin 40 mg/day vs. placebo	CHD death, MI, stroke, revascularization	0.80 (0.70–0.92)
CARE[36]	Secondary	576[14]	Pravastatin 40 mg/day vs. placebo	CHD death, MI	0.57 (0.34–0.96)
LIPID[37]	Secondary	1,516[17]	Pravastatin 40 mg/day vs. placebo	CHD death, MI	0.89 (0.67–1.18)

(JUPITER: Justification for the Use of Statins in Prevention, an Intervention Trial Evaluating Rosuvastatin; AFCAPS/TexCAPS: Air Force/Texas Coronary Atherosclerosis Prevention Study; 4S: Scandinavian Simvastatin Survival Study; CARE: Cholesterol and Recurrent Events trial; LIPID: Long-term Intervention with Pravastatin in Ischemic Disease Study; HPS: Heart Protection study; MI: myocardial infarction; CHD: coronary heart disease; CI: confidence interval)

Source: With permission from Phan (2014).[30]

Bempedoic Acid

Bempedoic acid (BA) is an inhibitor of ATP citrate lyase, upstream from the HMG-CoA step in endogenous cholesterol synthesis. It increases the LDL receptor genesis in the liver and promotes LDL lowering. The enzyme required for activation of BA is absent in the myocytes, and hence BA has no muscle-related side effects. In the CLEAR outcomes trial,[45] BA reduced LDL levels and improved CV outcomes compared to placebo, at a standard dose of 180 mg/day in nearly 14,000 statin intolerant patients. 48% of the trial participants were women, and there were no significant sex-specific differences.

TABLE 2: Drug category in pregnancy.

Drugs	FDA category in pregnancy
Statins	X (but hydrophilic statins—rosuva/pravastatin can be used in pregnancy)
Ezetimibe, fibrates, and niacin	C
EPA and DHA	C
Bile acid sequestrants	B

(FDA: Food and Drug Administration; EPA: eicosapentaenoic acid; DHA: docosahexaenoic acid)

Note on Management of Elevated Lipoprotein(a)

In patients with elevated Lp(a), it is currently unknown if reducing its levels reduces CV risk. However, as an important modifier of risk, if Lp(a) is elevated, LDL must be reduced to the lowest possible target level with statins and ezetimibe. PCSK9i modestly reduces Lp(a) levels. Additionally, niacin (2–4 g/day) can reduce Lp(a).

In women, estrogen replacement therapy (ERT) reduces Lp(a) levels. However, it is not recommended to start ERT for reduction of CV risk.

Management of Dyslipidemia in Pregnancy/Lactation

Derangements in lipids beyond what is normal in pregnancy occur in cases with gestational DM, HTN, preeclampsia, and after preterm birth. Preeclampsia causes a proatherogenic lipid milieu, with increased concentrations of LDL and Lp(a). In this current era, where obesity and elderly pregnancy in women with established CV risk factors such as DM and HTN are common, control of lipids is an important part of management during the gestational period. This is also important in women who have familial hypercholesterolemia. Women who develop DLP during pregnancy usually have elevated CV risk later in life.

There is a lack of data on treating DLP in pregnancy, and all trials have excluded pregnant women. Earlier, the Food and Drug Administration (FDA) had cautioned against the use of statins. However, now with newer data emerging, statins can be used cautiously. Hydrophilic statins such as rosuvastatin or pravastatin have no known teratogenic effect and can be used in pregnancy. Lipophilic statins such as atorvastatin should be avoided.

Other drugs with FDA category C and B are summarized in **Table 2**. The safest agents are the bile acid sequestrants, as they act locally in the gut. PCSK9i has no recommendation, and like statins, this is to be discontinued before planned pregnancy.

The only viable option for pregnant women with DLP is lifestyle and dietary changes, with the use of hydrophilic statins and bile acid sequestrants. In patients with severe LDL or TG elevations, apheresis can be considered.

During lactation, bile acid sequestrants and hydrophilic statins can be used.

CONCLUSION

Historically, women have been underprescribed, underdosed, and understudied with poor representation in the clinical trials, although this trend is changing. The penetrance of guideline-directed medical therapy is also less in women. Women are less likely to reach target drug doses. And additionally, women tend to discontinue therapy due to perceived side effects much more than men. But with education and awareness, the situation is improving.

Although women are physiologically different from men, the importance of early diagnosis, risk stratification, primary, and secondary prevention is equal in both the sexes. What works in men, works as well in women.

The care for a woman should be free of biases, less paternalistic, and more inclusive.

ONLINE REFERENCES

Please scan the QR code provided at the end of the table of contents for References of this chapter.

CHAPTER

65

Dyslipidemia in Diabetes

Yogesh Varma, Naima Parveen, Sachin Chittawar

ABSTRACT

Diabetic dyslipidemia, a collection of lipoprotein abnormalities, is characterized by elevated triglyceride levels, decreased high-density lipoprotein cholesterol levels, and a rise in small dense low-density lipoprotein (LDL) particles in diabetic patients. Diabetes is a key risk factor for atherosclerotic cardiovascular disease (ASCVD), which is the leading cause of mortality worldwide, and the primary predictor of ASCVD events in type 2 diabetes mellitus (T2DM) is low-density lipoprotein cholesterol (LDL-C). Since there is a link between ASCVD and serum cholesterol and triglyceride levels in type 1 diabetes mellitus (T1DM) and T2DM, patients with diabetes are more expected to die from ASCVD than nondiabetic patients. In this chapter, we have emphasized on the causes of dyslipidemia in diabetes, nonpharmacological treatment, including lifestyle modification, and pharmacological treatment, in which statin is the mainstay of treatment to minimize ASCVD by reducing LDL-C. In addition, the recommendation or guidelines of national or international associations to improve the condition of diabetic dyslipidemia are discussed in this chapter.

Keywords: Diabetes, dyslipidemia, ASCVD, low-density lipoprotein, high-density lipoprotein, triglycerides.

INTRODUCTION

Atherosclerotic cardiovascular disease (ASCVD) is the primary cause of death worldwide, and diabetes is a significant risk factor for ASCVD. A diabetic person is more likely to die from ASCVD as compared to a nondiabetic person.[1] As the number of individuals with diabetes increases, which is an estimated 536 million adults worldwide, the risk for ASCVD ultimately increases. There is high prevalence of diabetes in India also, and the numbers are increasing at an alarming rate. It is expected that in India alone, the cases of diabetes will increase from 74 million in 2021 to 125 million by 2045.[2,3] Diabetes can result in both microvascular effects (retinopathy, nephropathy, and neuropathy) and macrovascular problems (ASCVD), which appear as coronary artery disease, peripheral arterial disease, and stroke. Hence, it is stated that there is a link between ASCVD and serum cholesterol and triglyceride (TG) levels in type 1 diabetes mellitus (T1DM) and type 2 diabetes mellitus (T2DM).[3-5]

Disturbances in the synthesis and clearance of plasma lipoproteins are among the metabolic anomalies that frequently go with diabetes. Additionally, the emergence of dyslipidemia can be a sign of diabetes in the future. A defining pattern, termed diabetic dyslipidemia, is characterized by a decrease in high-density lipoprotein cholesterol (HDL-C), elevated TGs, apolipoprotein B (ApoB), and postprandial lipemia. The type 2 diabetic population is the one most likely to exhibit this pattern, which may be a manageable risk factor for developing cardiovascular disease (CVD) later on.[6] An evidence-based study suggests that low HDL-C is an autonomous aspect not only for CVD but also for the progression of diabetes. The abnormalities in lipid metabolism seen in diabetic patients may be caused by a variety of variables, such as insulin resistance or deficiency, adipocytokines, and hyperglycemia.[7] Although there are still many unanswered questions regarding the pathophysiology of diabetic dyslipidemia and its effects, the process by which hypertriglyceridemia develops is reasonably well recognized.[8,9] In the light of this, this chapter summarized the updates on the causes, available treatment, and recommendations for lipid anomalies, i.e., dyslipidemia in diabetic patients.

CAUSES OF DYSLIPIDEMIA IN DIABETES

Diabetes patients may experience changes in plasma lipoproteins as a result of insulin action defects and hyperglycemia. Alternately, particularly in the case of T2DM, the metabolic disorder brought on by obesity and insulin resistance that underlies this kind of diabetes may cause lipid abnormalities independent of hyperglycemia.

The link between diabetes, insulin insufficiency, and lipid/lipoprotein metabolism is more well understood with T1DM, formerly known as insulin-dependent diabetes mellitus. Hypertriglyceridemia and decreased HDL levels are frequently present in T1DM that is not well controlled, even in ketoacidosis. These irregularities may be corrected by insulin replacement in these patients, and diabetics with well-controlled blood sugar levels may have higher HDL and lower-than-average TG levels.[10]

Hypertriglyceridemia and decreased plasma HDL-C are two lipoprotein abnormalities that are frequently seen in T2DM, also known as noninsulin-dependent diabetes mellitus. Furthermore, low-density lipoprotein (LDL) is transformed into smaller, possibly more atherogenic lipoproteins known as small dense LDL.[11] This phenotype is typically not entirely corrected with glycemic management, unlike T1DM. Additionally, prediabetics patients with insulin resistance but normal plasma glucose indices often have this dyslipidemia. Therefore, this lipid anomaly is linked to anomalies in insulin function rather than hyperglycemia per se. This is supported by the fact that various thiazolidinediones enhance the effects of insulin on peripheral tissues and improve lipid profiles more than other glucose-reducing drugs.[12,13]

Diabetes-related dyslipidemia is most likely caused by a combination of mechanisms, including effects of insulin on apoprotein formation in liver, peripheral actions of insulin on adipose and muscle, lipoprotein lipase (LpL) regulation, and the effects of cholesteryl ester transfer protein (CETP).[14]

TREATMENT STRATEGIES FOR DIABETIC DYSLIPIDEMIA

Nonpharmacological

Lifestyle Modifications (Weight and Diet Management)

The first-line intervention for the management of diabetes dyslipidemia is the lifestyle modifications such as dietary changes, weight loss, and exercise.[15] Obesity can cause insulin resistance, an increase in TG and LDL levels, and a decrease in HDL level. Body weight reduction is thus associated with improvement in glycemic control, lipid profile, and insulin resistance. A decrease in TGs, increase in HDL-C, and improvement in blood pressure are the known outcomes of weight loss. Caloric restriction is the key to obtain sustainable weight loss. Physical activity and/or aerobic exercise may help to reduce body weight and thus help in improvement of glycemic control and lipid profile. Physical activity boosts the oxidation of fatty acids and enhances the hydrolysis of TGs in skeletal muscles. 11% of TG reduction has been observed by regular exercise, while 6% reduction has been observed by resistance exercise.[16]

Dietary changes are another approach for the management of diabetes dyslipidemia. Intake of food that is low in fat, specifically saturated fat, is encouraged. According to the American Diabetes Association (ADA), a diet which has low trans fat, saturated fat, and cholesterol is recommended. The ADA also recommends the Mediterranean diet and DASH (dietary approaches to stop hypertension) diet.[17] Diabetic patients are also recommended to consume fruits, vegetables, tree nuts, walnuts, and grains as they are good sources of unsaturated fats, which decreases blood pressure, cholesterol, and the risk of diabetes and ASCVD.[18]

Smoking and other tobacco use, including the use of e-cigarettes, should be absolutely avoided. Alcohol should be avoided because it hinders chylomicron hydrolysis, increases TG synthesis, and secretes VLDL that is rich in TGs. However, patients who drink should limit their intake to no more than two drinks per day for men and one drink per day for women. Ideally, patients with severe hypertriglyceridemia should not drink.[19]

Though weight loss, exercise, and proper diet help reduce the risk of diabetes and CVDs, the Look AHEAD study did not show any improvement in cardiovascular events (CVE) after long-term weight loss and following dietary changes,[20] signifying the requirement of pharmacological interventions along with these lifestyle changes to reduce ASCVD.

Pharmacological (Use of Lipid-lowering Agents)

Statins

A significant advancement in cardiovascular (CV) medicine is the discovery of statins. Statins inhibit 3-hydroxy-3-methylglutaryl-coenzyme A reductase, which is a rate-limiting enzyme of cholesterol biosynthesis in liver. Statins are used for the prevention of CVDs and strokes. Reduction in liver cholesterol levels results in upregulation of LDL receptors, which lowers plasma low-density lipoprotein cholesterol (LDL-C). Additionally, statins also decrease TG and increase HDL-C.[21] The statins such as rosuvastatin 20–40 mg and atorvastatin 40–80 mg, which can decrease LDL-C by around 50% or more, are called high-intensity statins. Similarly, statins, including rosuvastatin 5–10 mg, atorvastatin 10–20 mg, simvastatin 20–40 mg, pitavastatin 2–4 mg, pravastatin 40 mg, fluvastatin 80 mg, and lovastatin 40 mg, decrease LDL by approximately 30–50% and are called moderate-intensity statins. Lastly, low-intensity statins, including pitavastatin 1 mg, pravastatin 10–20 mg, simvastatin 10 mg, and fluvastatin 20–40 mg, decrease LDL by <30%.[22]

Several studies have demonstrated that statins may help reduce the CVE in diabetes patients, including the Heart Protection Study and the Collaborative Atorvastatin Diabetes Study, which have reported 22% and 37% reduction in primary endpoint of CVE, including ischemic stroke.[23,24] For every 39 mg/dL decrease in LDL-C over an average follow-up of 4.3 years, statin medication decreased CVE by 21% and vascular mortality by 13%, according to a meta-analysis of 14 randomized clinical studies involving >18,000 participants.[25]

Although statins might have side effects, they are generally well tolerated. The most frequent side effect, involving 5–10% of patients, is myalgia. Rhabdomyolysis, myositis, and elevation in liver enzymes are some other adverse effects associated with statins. Statins can also cause new-onset diabetes, but the basic mechanism is not clear.[26] In the study of JUPITER (Justification for the Use of Statins in Prevention: An Intervention Trial Evaluating Rosuvastatin), the risk of diabetes was 0.6% higher in the rosuvastatin group than in the placebo group. It was observed that the increased doses for patients with metabolic syndrome, BMI > 30 kg/m^2, and A1c > 6% have an increased risk of side effects. The advantages of lowering CVE outweigh the minor risk of diabetes, which can be avoided with a healthy diet and regular exercise.[27]

Niacin

Niacin is a highly effective medication for raising HDL-C levels. Additionally, niacin reduces TG and LDL-C. However, as compared to statin use alone, the statin and niacin combination did not provide any significant CV benefit. When niacin was added in high-risk patients who were already taking simvastatin and ezetimibe in the AIM-HIGH study, no CV benefit was observed.[28] Niacin/laropiprant was compared to a placebo in the HPS2-THRIVE (Heart Protection Study 2-Treatment of HDL to Reduce the Incidence of Vascular Events), which included 25,673 patients with atherosclerotic vascular disease. Although there was a large rise in new-onset diabetes, bleeding, and infections in the therapy group, there was no CV benefit. Since there is no chance of benefit, there are no recommendations for niacin-statin combination therapy in patients with diabetes and patients with ASCVD.[29]

Fibrates

Fibrates serve as a peroxisome proliferator-activated receptor alpha agonist, which decreases TG levels and increases LpL activity. Bezafibrate, gemfibrozil, ciprofibrate, and fenofibrate are the examples of fibrates. Fibrates can reduce postprandial lipemia by reducing the production of fatty acids and fasting plasma TG levels by 30–50%. Fibrates upregulate apoA-I and apoA-II, which increases HDL levels.[30] In some investigations, fibrates have also been demonstrated to lower the level of small dense LDL.[31]

According to the trial of Veterans Affairs High-Density Lipoprotein Cholesterol Intervention study, gemfibrozil reduced TG by 31%, decreased cholesterol by 4%, and increased HDL-C by 6% when compared to placebo. In patients with ASCVD and low HDL-C, 4.4% reduction in nonfatal myocardial infarction or mortality from coronary artery disease was observed. Nevertheless, these patients did not seem to be receiving statin medication and did not have a high-risk LDL-C.[32]

In 9,795 T2DM patients, the FIELD (Fenofibrate Intervention and Even Lowering in Diabetes) research assessed how well fenofibrate medication reduced macrovascular and microvascular problems. However, treatment with fenofibrate was not related to a substantial decline in the primary endpoint after a 5-year follow-up period.[33] Similarly, in ACCORD study, the rate of nonfatal myocardial infarction, nonfatal stroke, or fatal CVE did not reduce in 5,518 T2DM patients when treated with simvastatin and fenofibrate. Use of fibrates should be avoided, or it can be used with caution in a patient with chronic kidney disease as fibrates are metabolized in kidneys.[34]

Cholesterol Absorption Inhibitors (Ezetimibe)

By preventing intestinal cholesterol absorption, ezetimibe lowers cholesterol levels. It is used in people who cannot tolerate the prescribed dose of statins or in conjunction with statins to significantly lower LDL-C levels.

Simvastatin 40 mg with ezetimibe 10 mg or simvastatin 40 mg with placebo were the treatment options for 18,144 participants in the IMPROVE-IT study who had acute coronary syndrome (ACS) and LDL-C between 50 and 125 mg/dL. Patients who got simvastatin with ezetimibe had significantly lower LDL-C levels than those who received simvastatin alone, 54 mg/dL versus 70 mg/dL, during the course of a 6-year median follow-up.[35]

The key composite endpoint, which included myocardial infarction, CV death, coronary revascularization within 30 days, hospitalization for unstable angina, and stroke, decreased by 6.4%, suggesting the extra benefit of ezetimibe when combined with a statin.[35] More significantly, there was a higher improvement in the primary end objective with a 14% risk reduction in the individuals with diabetes (27% of patients). The importance of ezetimibe in diabetic patients with CVD has been highlighted by research showing that the combination of ezetimibe and simvastatin lowers the incidence of recurrent ischemic stroke when compared to simvastatin in people with T2DM.[36]

Bile Acid Sequestrants

Bile acids are the byproduct of cholesterol metabolism. Common bile acid sequestrants (BAS) include colesevelam, colestipol, and cholestyramine. These stimulate the generation of bile acid in the liver, which lowers cholesterol levels, by binding to bile acid in the intestinal lumen and reducing its enterohepatic circulation.

Bile acids are a useful adjunct to statins to reduce LDL-C. A study showed 13.4% and 20.3% reduction in total cholesterol and LDL-C, respectively, by the long-term use of cholestyramine. In addition to that, it also decreases coronary heart disease by 19% as compared to placebo.[37] There are numerous studies showing improved glycemic control with colesevelam in T2DM, which has the benefit of lowering both LDL-C and HbA1c levels. However, there is little evidence to support further reduction in CVE.[38]

Proprotein Convertase Subtilisin/Kexin Type 9 Inhibitor

Alirocumab and evolocumab are the types of proprotein convertase subtilisin/kexin type 9 (PCSK9) inhibitors. They are very effective when used as monotherapy as well as in combination with statins in lowering LDL-C significantly. By attaching to PCSK9, PCSK9 inhibitors stop PCSK9 from attaching to LDL receptors and selecting them for intrahepatic lysosomal degradation. This causes a decrease in LDL-C level by increasing the expression of LDL receptors. Every 2–4 weeks, they are injected subcutaneously in the patients with T2DM with dyslipidemia.[39]

Patients with ASCVD who are on maximum tolerated statin therapy with or without ezetimibe but have LDL-C 70 mg/dL or non HDL-C 100 mg/dL are permitted for PCSK9 inhibitors therapy. They are also recommended in patients with inherent homozygous familial hypercholesterolemia or heterozygous familial hypercholesterolemia as well as in patients with LDL 190 mg/dL.[39]

In 2015, 2,341 persons who were at high risk for CVE due to a history of the existence of heterozygous familial hypercholesterolemia, coronary artery disease, or coronary risk equivalent conditions including peripheral artery disease, ischemic stroke, diabetes mellitus, chronic kidney disease, etc., were enrolled in the ODYSSEY long-term experiment. Despite using the maximum tolerable dose of a statin, these participants' LDL-C levels were above 70 mg/dL, and they were randomly assigned to receive either alirocumab 150 mg or a placebo. At 48 months, alirocumab therapy reduced LDL-C from 122.8 to 53 mg/dL.[40]

The potency of alirocumab in ACS patients was investigated in the ODYSSEY outcome trial. The study was randomized, double blind, multicenter, placebo controlled, which involved 18,924 individuals who had an episode of ACS within the previous 1–12 months. These patients had non-HDL-C levels of at least 100 mg/dL, at least 80 mg/dL for apoB, and at least 70 mg/dL for LDL-C. These patients were randomized to receive alirocumab 75 mg subcutaneously or a placebo while already receiving the maximum tolerated dose of a statin or a high-intensity statin. After 2.8 years of follow-up, the primary endpoint had decreased by 15%.[41]

Evolocumab, a PCSK9 inhibitor other than alirocumab, was assessed by OSLER-1 and OSLER-2. A 2:1 ratio of 4,465 patients were randomly assigned to receive either conventional therapy alone or standard therapy plus evolocumab. When compared to conventional therapy alone, evolocumab reduced LDL-C from 120 to 48 mg/dL, i.e., 61% reduction.[42]

Inclisiran is a recently approved PCSK9 inhibitor, which is a small interfering ribonucleic acid (siRNA). The administration scheme of inclisiran is different from other PCSK9 inhibitors. It is subcutaneously administered initially at an interval of 3 months, i.e., at day 1, then day 90, then day 180, and afterward, it is administered once in every 6 months. The effectiveness of inclisiran was observed in the ORION studies. These studies revealed that when compared to placebo groups, LDL-C levels were lowered by almost 50%.[43] Although side effects are rare with inclisiran medication, upper respiratory tract symptoms, local reactions at the administration site, and muscular soreness are some of the common side effects observed.[44]

Omega-3 Fatty Acids

Purified omega-2 fatty acids can reduce TGs as much as fibrates, but they do not have much of an impact on HDL or LDL-C. Omega-3 fatty acids are mostly used as an add-on therapy. Formulations contain docosahexaenoic acid and eicosapentaenoic acid (EPA). A subanalysis of the Japan EPA Lipid Intervention trial revealed that the use of EPA reduced the risk of coronary artery disease by 22% in patients with hypercholesterolemia and impaired glucose metabolism when compared to those with normoglycemia.[45] However, in the ORIGIN trial, patients with impaired glucose tolerance, diabetes, or impaired fasting glucose did not experience any CV benefits from using omega-3 fatty acids compared to placebo.[46]

An interesting result of double-blind, randomized multicentered placebo-controlled trial study by REDUCE-IT (Cardiovascular Risk Reduction with Icosapent Ethyl for Hypertriglyceridemia) on 8,179 patients with diabetes dyslipidemia and other risk factors was published in 2019. Patients in this trial had fasting TG levels between 135 and 499 mg/dL and LDL-C levels between 41 and 100 mg/dL, and they were already receiving statin therapy. They were randomly assigned to receive either a placebo or a daily dose of 4 mg of icosapent ethyl. With a median follow-up of 4.9 years, the primary outcome was a composite of CV death, nonfatal stroke, nonfatal myocardial infarction, coronary revascularization, or unstable angina. Icosapent ethyl reduced the major endpoint by 25% compared to placebo.[47] Several other recent studies also demonstrated icosapent ethyl to be used for CV risk reduction.[48] A summary of lipid-lowering drugs with their mechanism of action and the side effects associated with them is represented in **Table 1**.

IMPACT OF HYPOGLYCEMIC AGENTS ON LIPOPROTEIN

Treatment with insulin and better blood glucose management can partially reverse diabetes dyslipidemia. In patients with poor glycemic control, insulin treatment improves

TABLE 1: Summary of lipid-lowering agents with their mechanism of action and adverse effects.

Lipid-lowering drug	Action mechanism	Efficacy	Adverse effects
Statins	Inhibits hydroxymethylglutaryl (HMG) coenzyme A reductase	Very highly effective	Rhabdomyolysis, myalgia, myositis, and elevation in liver enzymes
Niacin	Inhibits hepatocyte diacylglycerol acyltransferase-2, which is a key enzyme of triglyceride synthesis	Highly effective	Abdominal pain, nausea, vomiting, gout
Fibrates	Stimulate cellular fatty acids uptake, conversion to acyl-CoA derivatives, catabolism by beta oxidation pathways	Moderately effective	Constipation, abdominal pain, headaches, diarrhea
Omega-3 fatty acids	Inhibits acyl-CoA:1,2 diacylglycerol acyltransferase, increased beta oxidation in liver	Moderately effective	Vomiting, constipation, skin reactions
Proprotein convertase subtilisin/kexin type 9 (PCSK9) inhibitors	Inhibits proprotein convertase subtilisin/kexin type 9 (PCSK9)	Highly effective in combination with statins	Reactions including itching, swelling, pain, etc., at the site of injection
Ezetimibe	Binds to Niemann–Pick C1-like protein and inhibits cholesterol absorption in intestine	Moderately effective	Diarrhea, respiratory tract infection, disturbed liver function, myopathy, rhabdomyolysis
Bile acid sequestrants	Binds with bile acid in small intestine and avert reabsorption	Moderately effective	Abdominal pain, constipation, bloating

(CoA: coenzyme A)

TABLE 2: Impact of hypoglycemic agents on lipoprotein.

Hypoglycemic agents	Triglycerides	LDL-C	HDL-C	Total cholesterol	Reference
Metformin	0	–	+	–	Wulffele et al.[51]
Pioglitazone	–	0	+	+	Azimova et al.[52]
Sitagliptin	0	0	+	0	Lavalle-Gonzalez et al.[53]
Vildagliptin	0	0	+	0	Matikainen et al.[54]
Linagliptin	0	0	0	0	Zinman et al.[55]
Saxagliptin	0	0	0	0	Boland et al.[56]
Dapagliflozin	–	0	+	+	Bailey et al.[57]
Canagliflozin	+	+	+	+	Forst et al.[58]
Empagliflozin	0	+	+	+	Roden et al.[59]
Liraglutide	–	0	0	0	Hermansen et al.[60]
Exenatide	–	0	0	0	Schwartz et al.[61]
Gliclazide	–	0	0	–	Buse et al.[62]
Glimepiride	0	0	+	0	Araki et al.[63]

(0: no change; +: increased; –: decreased; HDL-C: high-density lipoprotein cholesterol; LDL-C: low-density lipoprotein cholesterol)

HDL-C and lowers blood TG levels.[49] Although metformin lowers serum TGs and improves insulin resistance, it is being ignored as a lipid-lowering drug and is exclusively used as a hypoglycemic agent in the treatment of diabetes.[50] Another diabetes medication may unintentionally affect lipoproteins in both favorable and unfavorable ways **(Table 2)**.

SCENARIO OF DIABETIC DYSLIPIDEMIA IN INDIA

The burden of diabetes in India has been rising gradually since 1990, but the rate picked up after the year 2000. As a result, the prevalence of diabetes increased from 7.1 to 8.9%

between 2009 and 2019. According to estimates, there will be more than 125 million people living with diabetes in India by 2045, rather than an estimated 74 million people today. This increase is mostly due to rising rates of elevated body mass index (BMI) and the metabolic syndrome associated with visceral adiposity.[3] It was estimated that the prevalence of risk factors for coronary artery diseases was significantly higher in Asian Indian patients with diabetes than patients with nondiabetes. According to carotid intima-media thickness (CIMT), two-thirds of South Asians with diabetes and around half of those without diabetes had subclinical CAD.[64]

There has been a three to fourfold higher risk of CVDs in Asian Indian people with T2DM than in white people, even after correcting for age, sex, smoking status, and obesity. This could be attributed to the increased prevalence of visceral adiposity, hypertriglyceridemia, insulin resistance, and low HDL-C that is associated with the atherogenic milieu among Asian Indian persons.[65] The data from the trial of chronic complications in newly diagnosed patients with T2DM in India (CINDI) showed that ASCVD risk factors are very high in young patients with T2DM, with nearly 83.2% overweight or obese, 62.4% having dyslipidemia, 27.6% having hypertension, and 25% being smokers.[66]

NATIONAL AND INTERNATIONAL RECOMMENDATIONS/GUIDELINES FOR THE MANAGEMENT OF DIABETIC DYSLIPIDEMIA: A GLANCE

In 2013, the American College of Cardiology (ACC)/ American Heart Association (AHA) released guidelines for the management of cholesterol to reduce ASCVD. Depending on the 10-year CV risk score and the presence or absence of ASCVD, these recommendations suggested using low-, moderate-, or high-intensity statins. These recommendations made no precise cholesterol targets. Any patient with T1DM or T2DM who is 40–75 years old should be treated with moderate-intensity statins with an aim to decrease LDL-C by 30–49%. According to the ACC/AHA, if the 10-year CV risk score is >7.5% or if ASCVD is present with a target LDL-C reduction of >50%, high-intensity statins are advised.[67]

According to the 2017 American Association of Clinical Endocrinologists (AACE) guidelines, diabetes patients can be classified as high, very high, or extremely high risk of developing CVD. It was advised that patients at high risk (10-year risk: 10–20%, CKD stage 3–4 with no other risk factor) should be treated for LDL targets of <100 mg/dL, those at very high risk (peripheral and coronary artery disease, ACS, carotid, heterozygous familial hypercholesterolemia, CKD stage 3–4 with more than one risk factor) should be treated for <70 mg/dL LDL target, and those at an extremely high risk (history of premature ASCVD in males and females of age <55 years and <65 years, respectively, coronary artery disease, progressive ASCVD, CKD stage 3–4, heterozygous familial hypercholesterolemia) should be treated for <55 mg/dL of LDL.[68]

According to the ADA's 2019 recommendations, in addition to making lifestyle changes, all diabetic patients with ASCVD or patients with a 10-year atherosclerotic CV risk of >20% should be treated with high-intensity statins (target of 50% decrease in LDL-C). Diabetes patients under the age of 40 years with additional atherosclerotic CV risk factors [LDL-C 100 mg/dL, hypertension, CKD, smoking, albuminuria, and familial hypercholesterolemia (FH) of premature ASCVD], diabetic patients between the ages of 40 and 75 years without ASCVD or with a 10-year ASCVD risk of <20%, and diabetic patients over the age of 75 years should all receive moderate-intensity statin therapy with 30–49% decrease in LDL-C.[69]

According to the Lipid Association of India (LAI) recommendation, 2022, the LDL-C goal recommended for patients without ASCVD who do not have target organ damage or more than one risk factor is 70 mg/dL, whereas the recommended LDL-C goal for patients with target organ damage or more than two risk factors is 50 mg/dL. With a recommended LDL-C target of <30 mg/dL, patients with diabetes and ASCVD who have zero to one other major ASCVD risk factors but no evidence of target organ damage are categorized as being at extreme risk category A, while those who have two to four major ASCVD risk factors or target organ damage are categorized as being at extreme risk category B.[70]

DYSLIPIDEMIA ASSOCIATED WITH METABOLIC SYNDROME

A frequent and significant risk factor for CVD and the development of T2DM is the metabolic syndrome. The metabolic syndrome includes dyslipidemia as a key component. Atherogenic mixed dyslipidemia, which is present in patients with metabolic syndrome, is characterized by low levels of HDL-C, higher TGs, and an increase in tiny, dense LDL particles. Atherogenic dyslipidemia present in patients with metabolic syndrome needs urgent treatment due to the extremely high risk of CVD and development of T2DM. It can be treated considerably by therapeutic lifestyle modification and pharmacological therapies as discussed above. Particularly in Southern Asia and the Middle East, the prevalence of T2DM, atherogenic dyslipidemia, and metabolic syndrome is rising globally. These disorders frequently coexist in a person, and their lipid profiles share a number of characteristics in common.[71]

CONCLUSION

Diabetes patients have a higher risk of developing ASCVD than patients without diabetes. Atherogenic dyslipidemia is prevalent in patients with T2DM and is an essential target for treatment. When diagnosed with diabetes, LDL-C, non-

HDL-C, and apoB lipid targets should be met based on the ASCVD risk group, if possible. Lifestyle modifications along with therapeutic strategies, including standardized dose of statin, niacin, PCSK9 inhibitors, ezetimibe, etc., can be used for the treatment of dyslipidemia in diabetes. Several guidelines and recommendations for the management of dyslipidemia in diabetes have been given time by various associations of national and international repute, including ADA, AHA, AACE, LAI, etc. It is expected that implementation of these recommendations in treatment will allow patients with diabetes to live longer, healthier lives and help reduce the burden of dyslipidemia in them.

ONLINE REFERENCES

Please scan the QR code provided at the end of the table of contents for References of this chapter.

CHAPTER 66

Elevated Lipoprotein(a) in Familial Hypercholesterolemia Patients: Double Heritable Risk for Atherosclerotic Cardiovascular Disease

Juhi Singh, JPS Sawhney

ABSTRACT

Lipoprotein(a) [Lp(a)] is an atherogenic lipoprotein produced in the liver in which the ApoB-100 component of low-density lipoprotein cholesterol (LDL-C) is covalently bound via disulfide bond to apolipoprotein(a) [Apo(a)] and plasma concentration is determined genetically by *LPA* gene. Elevated plasma Lp(a) (>50 mg/dL) is associated with an elevated risk for atherosclerotic cardiovascular disease (ASCVD) in the general population. Familial hypercholesterolemia (FH) is the most frequent genetically inherited disorder leading to increased levels of LDL-C from childhood and increased predisposition to ASCVD. Diagnosis of FH is based on genetic testing and clinical criteria using validated tools. An estimated prevalence for FH is about 1:200–300. The prevalence of elevated Lp(a) is 30–50% among FH patients as compared to 20% in general population. Cumulative pro-atherogenic effect of LDL-C and Lp(a) accelerates the risk of ASCVD in FH patients. Thus, plasma Lp(a) among patients with FH has been established as a significant cardiovascular risk factor, but the association between the two is debatable. Although statins are the mainstay of treatment in FH, they have no effect on the plasma levels of Lp(a). There are newer therapies for lowering Lp(a) levels that would provide additional reduction risk, thus reducing the cardiovascular morbidity and mortality among FH patients as compared to what is currently achieved with LDL-C lowering alone.

Keywords: Lipoprotein(a), familial hypercholesterolemia, atherosclerotic cardiovascular disease, Dutch Lipid Clinic Network.

INTRODUCTION

Familial hypercholesterolemia (FH) is a genetically inherited disorder that predisposes to premature coronary artery disease (CAD) (onset of CAD at a younger age before 55 years in men and 60 years in women). As per the World Health Organization, an estimated prevalence of heterozygous FH (HeFH) is 1 in 250 and that of homozygous FH (HoFH) is 1 in 10^6.[1] Elevated lipoprotein(a) [Lp(a)], defined as plasma levels of >50 mg/dL, is also an independent risk factor for premature CAD. Although both these conditions are independently inherited, elevated Lp(a) is more common in FH patients. Prevalence of elevated Lp(a) is 30–50% among FH patients as compared to 20% in the general population.[2] Unfortunately, there is limited data from Indian population regarding the prevalence of elevated Lp(a) in patients with FH.

FAMILIAL HYPERCHOLESTEROLEMIA

Familial hypercholesterolemia is inherited in an autosomal codominant manner and is identified by very high levels of low-density lipoprotein cholesterol (LDL-C) from childhood, predisposing to atherosclerotic cardiovascular disease (ASCVD) at an early age if not treated. FH is the most common monogenic cause leading to CAD at a younger age.

Genetics

Familial hypercholesterolemia is a highly penetrant disease with plasma LDL-C levels rarely below the 95th percentile of the general population. About 80–85% of mutations are seen with *LDLR* gene, resulting in deficiency or defect in LDL receptors. Mutations in other genes such as *APOB* gene missense mutation (5–10%), gain-of-function in proprotein convertase subtilisin/kexin type 9 (PCSK9) (1%), and *LDLRAP1* mutation is also seen in FH.[3] There are two types of FH based on:

1. HeFH, in which single mutant allele for FH is inherited
2. HoFH, in which the patient has two mutant alleles

Plasma Lp(a) levels are higher in homozygotes than in HeFH,[4] thus, demonstrating a gene dosage effect on Lp(a) plasma concentrations. Hence, cumulative exposure of LDL-C begins in fetal life in FH patients. Most of the untreated individuals with HoFH and HeFH develop symptomatic ASCVD before 20 and 60 years old, respectively.

Diagnosis

Diagnosis is based on genetic testing and clinically using validated tools.[5] Clinical tools include the US Make Early Diagnoses Prevent Early Deaths Program Diagnostic Criteria (US-MEDPED), Simon Broome Register Diagnostic Criteria, and Dutch Lipid Clinic Network (DLCN) diagnostic criteria. MEDPED assess LDL-C levels and family history. Both Simon Broome Register and DLCN criteria involve LDL-C levels, physical findings, family history of hypercholesterolemia and CAD, along with testing for the presence of mutant genes. The DLCN criterion **(Table 1)** is based on personal and family history of premature CAD, presence of arcus cornealis/tendon xanthomas, LDL-C levels, and genetic analysis. An individual is diagnosed as "definite" FH with a score of >8, score between 6 and 8 as "probable" FH, score between 3 and 5 as "possible" FH and if the score is <3, FH is "unlikely." Definite and probable FH patients are termed "potential" FH.[6]

TABLE 1: Dutch Lipid Clinic Network diagnostic criteria for familial hypercholesterolemia (FH).

Criteria	Points
Family history	
First-degree relative with known premature coronary and vascular disease, *or* First-degree relative with known LDL-C level above the 95th percentile	1
First-degree relative with tendinous xanthoma and/or arcus cornealis, *or* Children aged <18 years with LDL-C level above the 95th percentile	2
Clinical history	
Patient with premature coronary artery disease	2
Patient with premature cerebral or peripheral vascular disease	1
Physical examination	
Tendinous xanthoma	6
Arcus cornealis prior to age 45 years	4
Cholesterol levels mg/dL (mmol/L)	
LDL-C ≥ 330 mg/dL (≥8.5)	8
LDL-C 250–329 mg/dL (6.5–8.4)	5
LDL-C 190–249 mg/dL (5.0–6.4)	3
LDL-C 155–189 mg/dL (4.0–4.9)	1
DNA analysis	
Functional mutation in the *LDLR, ApoB*, or *PCSK9* gene	8
Diagnosis	**Total points**
Definite familial hypercholesterolemia	>8
Probable familial hypercholesterolemia	6–8
Possible familial hypercholesterolemia	3–5
Unlikely familial hypercholesterolemia	<3

(DNA: deoxyribonucleic acid; LDL-C: low-density lipoprotein cholesterol)

LIPOPROTEIN(A)

Lipoprotein(a) is a potent monogenetic risk factor for ASCVD irrespective of ethnicity. Plasma levels of Lp(a) are genetically determined by an autosomal dominantly inherited *LPA* gene, present on the long arm of chromosome 6 (6q26-27). There is heterogeneity in the size of apolipoprotein(a) [Apo(a)] isoforms, which is genetically determined. There is a reverse relation between Apo(a) isoforms size with Lp(a) density and plasma levels. An increased cardiovascular risk is seen in individuals with smaller Apo(a) due to ease of secretion by liver leading to elevated Lp(a) plasma concentration and vice-versa.[7]

Lipoprotein(a) Pathogenicity

The physiological role of Lp(a) is not known, but its pathogenic effect is mainly due to its two components: (1) ApoB-100 protein, which is an LDL binding ligand and is thus important for clearing LDL particles from liver and also plays a role in adherence of LDL to proteoglycan within the wall of vessels, leading to atherosclerotic lesions; (2) Apo(a), a highly polymorphic glycoprotein synthesized and secreted by the liver, which resembles plasminogen. Apo(a) and plasminogen contain a loop-like structure called kringles, which vary in type and number of copies. While plasminogen contains five different kringle structures (KI–KV), the Apo(a) has lost KI–KIII by deletion and harbors a single copy of KV and 10 types of KIV (KIV1–10). Increased Lp(a) levels and low LPA KIV2 repeat number are associated with an increased risk of mortality in the general population.[8]

The following mechanisms are responsible for its pathogenicity:[9]

- *Pro-inflammatory*: Increased macrophage interleukin-8 (IL-8) expression, monocyte cytokine release, oxidized phospholipids, and monocyte chemotaxis
- *Pro-thrombotic*: By reducing plasminogen activation and fibrin degradation and increasing endothelial cell plasminogen activator inhibitor type-1 (EC PAI-1)

expression, tissue factor pathway inhibitor (TFPI) activity, and platelet responsiveness

- *Pro-atherogenic*: Promoting EC binding, upregulation of adhesion molecules, smooth muscle cell proliferation, proteoglycan matrix binding, foam/cell formation, necrotic core formation, and calcification of lesion

Measurement of Lipoprotein(a)

Variation in the size of Apo(a) isoform poses difficulty for correct estimation of plasma Lp(a) levels. Sample containing Lp(a) with Apo(a) isoforms smaller than those in the calibrator are underestimated, whereas sample values with larger isoforms have limitations due to heterogenous size of Lp(a) particles. At present, assays for purpose of routine care that are linked to the World Health Organization and International Federation of Clinical Chemistry and Laboratory Medicine standards can identify individuals with Lp(a) levels >50 mg/dL. Also, accurate measurement is required to avoid misclassification of individuals with borderline Lp(a) (30–50 mg/dL). Sample handling and storage conditions are of utmost importance.

IS ELEVATED LIPOPROTEIN(A) MORE COMMON IN FAMILIAL HYPERCHOLESTEROLEMIA?

About 1.4 billion people worldwide have elevated plasma levels of Lp(a) (>50 mg/dL).[10] Considering that 1 in 250 individuals have HeFH, an estimate of 5 million patients with HeFH have an elevated plasma Lp(a). HeFH is considered as high-risk patients; even moderate elevation of Lp(a) further enhances their risk of ASCVD. ASCVD risk starts to increase already at plasma concentrations above 30 mg/dL.

Elevated plasma Lp(a) is associated with an increased risk for CAD, cerebrovascular accidents, peripheral vascular disease, calcified aortic valve, and retinal changes in diabetes mellitus. Elevated Lp(a) exerts a lifelong risk for ASCVD in FH patients.

The European Society of Cardiology/European Atherosclerosis Society (ESC/EAS) 2019 guideline recommends that adults should be tested for plasma Lp(a) at least once in lifetime. If Lp(a) levels are >180 mg/dL, then the ASCVD risk is like HeFH patients. Elevated Lp(a) should be used to reclassify considered in patients with a family history of premature CVD, and for reclassification of individuals who have an estimated 10-year risk of ASCVD and borderline between high and moderate risk.[11]

Khera et al. studied the prevalence of FH mutation among those with severe hypercholesterolemia and variation in CAD risk according to mutation status beyond the observed LDL-C levels based on 26,025 participants from seven case-control and 11,908 participants from five prospective cohort studies. About 7% participants had severe hypercholesterolemia (LDL-C ≥ 190 mg/dL), with only small proportion (<2%) carrying FH mutation. CAD risk was substantially high among patients carrying FH mutations as compared to those who did not, irrespective of LDL-C levels, with maximum risk, i.e., up to 22-folds in participants with LDL-C ≥ 190 mg/dL as well as a FH mutation [odds ratio (OR) 22.3; 95% confidence interval (CI) 10.7–53.2]. An increased CAD risk among carriers was partially explained by a greater cumulative exposure to LDL-C over a lifetime.[12]

In a study by Ellis et al., 316 patients with CAD were screened for FH using DLCN criteria and tested for plasma Lp(a) levels. Among CAD patients, 51.6% had premature CAD, 4.4% ($n = 14$) patients had both elevated plasma Lp(a) (>50 mg/dL) levels along with FH, only elevated Lp(a) was seen in 21.9% ($n = 69$), and 7.0% ($n = 22$) had phenotypic FH alone. The risk for premature CAD was increased to 5.3-fold in patients who had both elevated Lp(a) levels and FH as compared to those who had neither elevated Lp(a) nor FH ($p = 0.011$).[13]

In a study by Li et al., 8,050 patients undergoing coronary angiography were screened for FH using DLCN criteria. Mutational analysis was done in probable/definite FH. Plasma Lp(a) levels were elevated among clinically diagnosed FH patients (unlikely, possible, definite/probable FH) independent of the patient's status. The median Lp(a) levels were 51.7 versus 57.0 versus 60.4 mg/dL among patients with "no," "possible," and "potential" FH, respectively. The prevalence of premature CAD was higher in a patient with definite/probable FH with elevated Lp(a) than those without (6.1% vs. 2.4%; $p < 0.05$).[14] Trinder et al. enrolled clinically diagnosed 391 patients with HeFH using DLCN criteria, and plasma Lp(a) levels were estimated. About 35.8% (140 of 391) of individuals had elevated Lp(a) levels, which was 1.8 times more prevalent than among the general population in Europe (i.e., 20%). Elevated Lp(a) was associated with increased LDL-C, family history of cardiovascular disease, premature CAD, and FH.[15]

In a study by Chan et al., 907 patients attending lipid clinic were screened to diagnose FH patients using DLCN criteria. About 637 potential FH patients were diagnosed, and 36.1% had elevated Lp(a) levels. Elevated plasma Lp(a) was significantly related to premature CAD irrespective of the presence of genetic FH mutation.[16]

ELEVATED LIPOPROTEIN(A) IN FAMILIAL HYPERCHOLESTEROLEMIA: INDIAN POPULATION

Coronary artery disease is a leading cause of mortality worldwide, presenting at an earlier age and with increased severity among the South Asian population. Premature CAD is two to three times more prevalent in India. The prevalence of CAD risk in individuals living in India is 11% for nondiabetic patients and 21.4% for diabetic patients. Conventional risk factors for CAD include diabetes mellitus, hypertension, abdominal obesity, smoking, abnormal lipids, alcohol, psychosocial factors, physical inactivity, and diet. These conventional risk factors do not completely explain such a high prevalence of CAD among younger population.[17] Thus, the role of nonconventional risk factors such as Lp(a), homocysteine, and highly sensitive C-reactive protein has also been identified to aggravate the CAD risk, especially among the South Asian population.

In a study by Sawhney et al., 635 young CAD patients treated at a tertiary hospital in North India were screened with the help of the DLCN score. About 15% patients were diagnosed with potential FH (definite FH and probable FH). Thus, the prevalence of FH in young myocardial infarction (MI) in our country was estimated to be >15%.[18]

Sawhney et al. studied acute coronary syndrome (ACS) patients ($n = 1,021$) for prevalence of Lp(a) in ACS, association between elevated Lp(a) levels and severity of disease (Gensini score > 35). Lp(a) levels, coronary angiography, and screening for FH by DLCN criteria were done. Lp(a) levels of >50 mg/dL were considered as elevated. It was concluded that about 34% of ACS patients exhibited elevated Lp(a) levels (37% of young ACS vs. 32% elderly patients). Increased levels of Lp(a) were associated with severe disease (40% multivessel vs. 26% single vessel disease). 43% of FH patients had elevated Lp(a). There was a significant positive correlation of Lp(a) levels with Gensini score ($p = 0.002$).[19]

CASCADE TESTING FOR FAMILIAL HYPERCHOLESTEROLEMIA AND LIPOPROTEIN(A)

As per a global European Atherosclerosis Society-Familial Hypercholesterolemia Studies Collaboration (EAS-FHSC) registry, which includes adult patients from 70 countries, the rate of identification was found to be low for FH globally. This reinforces the importance of screening programs and appropriate implementation of health policies for early detection of FH. Cascade screening for elevated Lp(a) is recommended in the settings of FH, family history of elevated Lp(a), and personal or family history of ASCVD.[20]

Diagnostic tests are based on pathogenic mutation and is more accurate than using the phenotype alone because of greater overlap between normal and abnormal LDL-C levels. Cascade screening is done using age, gender, and plasma LDL-C levels if a genetic analysis is not available or cannot be done due to cost factors. Family pedigree has an important role in planning the screening process. Cascade screening starts with first-degree relatives followed by second- and third-degree relatives.

Therefore, cascade screening aids in identification of siblings and children with dyslipidemia, early diagnosis of FH, and early initiation of lipid-lowering therapy, thus reducing the morbidity and mortality due to premature CAD (up to threefold) not only for an index case but also for the family members.

As per the ESC/EAS 2019 dyslipidemia guidelines, FH is diagnosed in patients with CHD aged <55 years for men and <60 years for women, individuals with premature fatal or nonfatal CVD, tendon xanthomas, severely elevated LDL-C (adults >190 mg/dL, children >150 mg/dL), and in first-degree relatives of FH patients. Diagnosis of FH using clinical criteria and confirmation with genetic analysis is recommended. Once the identification of index case is done, cascade screening of family is must for FH and elevated Lp(a).[21]

FAMILIAL HYPERCHOLESTEROLEMIA TREATMENT

Lipid-lowering therapy should be initiated as early as possible once the individual is diagnosed as FH. ESC/EAS 2019 recommends LDL-C reduction of ≥50% from baseline and an LDL-C <1.4 mmol/L (<55 mg/dL). Patients with FH are considered as high risk in the absence of ASCVD or another major risk factor, and the recommended LDL-C goals are ≥50% reduction from baseline and an LDL-C <1.8 mmol/L (<70 mg/dL).

Initiation of high-intensity statins should be done with or without ezetimibe. PCSK9 inhibitors result in LDL-C level reduction by up to 60% on top of statins and are recommended in patients with very high-risk FH if the target goal is not achieved on maximal tolerated statin plus ezetimibe and statin-intolerant patients.

Homozygous FH is identified clinically by extensive xanthomas, premature and progressive CAD (before the age of 20 years), and/or positive genetic testing and total cholesterol >500 mg/dL. Prompt identification and timely referral to a specialized clinic are crucial. Intensive LDL-C lowering therapy and lipoprotein apheresis (LA) (every 12 weeks) can reduce plasma LDL-C levels by 55–70%. The frequency of procedure depends upon lipid level and symptoms. The goal in children >10 years of age is LDL-C <130 mg/dL (<3.5 mmol/L) and at younger age a ≥50% reduction of LDL-C. Healthy lifestyle and maximally tolerated pharmacological therapy are a mainstay of treatment.[21]

LIPOPROTEIN(A) MANAGEMENT (TABLE 2)

Plasma Lp(a) levels do not respond to dietary modifications. Nongenetic factors such as hormonal disorders (hypothyroidism—increases and hyperthyroidism—decreases), chronic kidney disease (three- to fivefold increase), pregnancy (twofold increase), inflammatory conditions (increases), and sepsis (decreases) influence Lp(a) concentration.[22] Although a significantly increased Lp(a) requires medical treatment, adherence to ideal cardiovascular risk behaviors, such as nonsmoking, maintenance of a desirable body weight, and regular physical activity, may reduce the Lp(a)-associated risk of ASCVD. Management of comorbid conditions such as control of blood sugar levels and blood pressure should be done.

TABLE 2: Lipid-lowering and lipoprotein(a) [Lp(a)] directed therapies.[27]

Therapeutic strategies to manage high lipoprotein(a)		
Drug	**Lp(a) lowering**	**LDL-C reduction**
Statins	No change	20–50%
Ezetimibe	0–7%	18–22%
Bempedoic acid	No change	17–21%
Niacin	–23%	–13%
CETP inhibitors	–20 to –40%	–20 to 40%
PCSK9 inhibitors	–15 to –30%	–50 to 60%
Apo(a) antisense oligonucleotides	–70 to –90%	–10 to 20%
Apheresis	–70% acutely, mean –35%	Up to 75%

[Apo(a): apolipoprotein(a); CETP: cholesteryl ester transfer protein; LDL-C: low-density lipoprotein cholesterol; PCSK9: proprotein convertase subtilisin/kexin type 9]

Statins

Statins only marginally affect Lp(a) plasma levels. Various studies have reported either no effect on or an increase of Lp(a) levels up to 21.9% after statin treatment. The mechanisms by which statins raise oxidized phospholipids on Lp(a) require further investigation.[23]

PCSK9 Inhibitors

Antibodies (evolocumab and alirocumab) bind to PCSK9 to recycle LDL-receptor, leading to a 60–70% decrease in LDL-C and Lp(a) by 20–30%. The FOURIER trial demonstrated a significant Lp(a) reduction with evolocumab and found that those with higher baseline Lp(a) had greater absolute cardiovascular disease risk reduction compared with their counterparts with lower Lp(a) levels.[24] The ODYSSEY OUTCOMES trial also demonstrated reduction of both Lp(a) levels and cardiovascular events by alirocumab.[25] However, it is difficult to conclude whether the PCSK9 inhibition-induced cardiovascular event reduction is related to the decrease of LDL-C or Lp(a). Thus, these agents are not currently licensed for lowering Lp(a).

Mipomersen

Mipomersen is an antisense oligonucleotide able to bind the messenger ribonucleic acid (mRNA) of ApoB-100, preventing the translation of ApoB protein and, consequently, reducing the production of atherogenic lipids and lipoproteins, including LDL and Lp(a). It is currently approved by the United States (US) Food and Drug Administration (FDA). Injection site reaction is the most common adverse effect observed with this drug. Another adverse effect is hepatic toxicity as it may lead to steatosis and increased transaminase levels. Its efficacy and long-term safety are currently under evaluation in patients with severe HeFH and in statin-"intolerant" patients.[26]

Pelacarsen

Pelacarsen is a potentially first-in-class treatment specifically targeting elevated Lp(a). A multicenter, double-blind, placebo-controlled pivotal phase 3 Lp(a) HORIZON cardiovascular outcomes study of pelacarsen, including 8,325 study participants, for evaluation of its safety and efficacy in reducing cardiovascular events in patients with cardiovascular disease and elevated levels of Lp(a) is being conducted. Results are expected in 2025 **(Box 1)**.[28]

Lipoprotein Apheresis

Lipoprotein apheresis is currently the most effective therapy available for reducing Lp(a) concentration. It was first introduced for the treatment of HoFH, it is based on the selective or nonselective removal of plasma/whole blood constituents. Several approaches can be used, including heparin-mediated extracorporeal LDL precipitation (HELP) and double filtration, to reduce both LDL-C and Lp(a) by >50% in one session. It is usually reserved for the most severe and refractory cases and is present in a limited number of tertiary centers. LA is approved for HoFH in the US, if LDL-C is persistently >12.9 mmol/L, for primary prevention in HeFH if LDL-C >7.8 mmol/L and secondary prevention if LDL-C >5.2 mmol/L.[29]

Small-interfering RNA

Inclisiran, a long-acting small-interfering RNA (siRNA) blocking PCSK9 synthesis, can lower Lp(a) by around 18–25%. It is not currently licensed for lowering Lp(a).[30]

Cholesteryl Ester Transfer Protein Inhibitor

Anacetrapib inhibits the transfer of cholesterol esters to increase high-density lipoprotein (HDL)-cholesterol and reduce LDL-C levels. It also decreases Lp(a) levels by around 35%.[31]

BOX 1 Emerging lipoprotein(a) [Lp(a)]-specific lowering therapies targeting synthesis of Lp(a).

Pelacarsen
- Antisense oligonucleotide therapy
- Monthly dosing
- Outcome results from phase 3 study are expected in 2025

Olpasiran
- siRNA technology
- Longer acting

(siRNA: small-interfering ribonucleic acid)

CONCLUSION

Familial hypercholesterolemia and Lp(a) are independent risk factors for cardiovascular disease. Both the risk factors are genetically predetermined. Despite evidence from clinical studies suggesting that lowering Lp(a) may reduce cardiovascular risk, there is no selective therapeutic management approved so far. The combined prevalence of FH and elevated Lp(a) in premature CAD patients is estimated to be higher as compared to individual prevalence of each factor among the general population, suggesting that elevated Lp(a) is more common in FH patients and has a synergistic role in the severity and early onset of CAD.

ONLINE REFERENCES

Please scan the QR code provided at the end of the table of contents for References of this chapter.

CHAPTER 67

Nonstatin Therapies

SN Narasingan, Aravind Duruvasal

ABSTRACT

Evidence clearly shows that by reducing low-density lipoprotein cholesterol (LDL-C), we get a substantial reduction in cardiovascular (CV) morbidity and mortality. Many primary and secondary prevention trials clearly demonstrated this important finding on the role played by LDL-C and the potency of statin in reducing CV risk. Research findings suggest that other lipoprotein classes beyond LDL-C also play important roles in atherosclerotic CV risk. The current efficacy of statin or other drugs comes short of providing the benefit that could be achieved from further reduction of LDL-C in high-risk and very high-risk patients. Hence, there is a need for newer nonstatin lipid-lowering agents to tackle residual risk.

Keywords: LDL-C, statins, residual risk, nonstatin drugs.

INTRODUCTION

Atherosclerotic cardiovascular disease is increasing in alarming proportion in India. Deaths occurring due to CVD are estimated to be around 24.8% when compared to other causes of death. Lipids and lipoproteins are considered as the main culprits in atherosclerosis. LDL-C plays a pivotal role in increasing the morbidity and mortality due to ASCVD. RCTs using statins in both primary and secondary prevention resulted in the reduction of CV risk by 20% and mortality reduction by 10%, with every 1 mmol/L (38.7 mg/dL) reduction in LDL-C as per Cholesterol Treatment Trialists' (CTT) Collaboration.[2] However, residual risk is seen in nearly 55–70% of individuals who received either high-dose statin or moderate tolerable dose of statins in trials. This residual risk is attributed to insufficient control of LDL-C. Other lipid abnormalities such as high triglyceride (TG) and low high-density lipoprotein cholesterol (HDL-C) and non-HDL-C are considered to be causal factors. Hence, there is a need for using nonstatin drugs with either high-dose or moderate-dose statin to reach the goal of LDL-C. This chapter is intended to cover the nonstatin drugs which are recommended in clinical practice either alone or with statins to reduce LDL-C and other lipid parameters. The role of LDL apheresis is also highlighted for its benefit.

NEED FOR NEWER LIPID-LOWERING AGENTS

Randomized controlled trials (RCTs) demonstrated that the efficacy of statin monotherapy is insufficient to achieve targets in all patients. Patients with familial hypercholesterolemia (FH) have very high low-density lipoprotein cholesterol (LDL-C), which may not respond even to high-dose statin therapy. There is also inhibition by physicians to start high-dose statins because of the fear of side effects. Patient's compliance and adherence to treatment may become suboptimal in many. Statin intolerance, side effects/adverse effects, or drug–drug interactions are not uncommon problems faced by Patients and Physicians. Evidence for ezetimibe as a secondary agent shows that it achieves 15–20% additional LDL-C lowering and a proportionately small augmentation of clinical benefit. Niacin has limited side effects with weak or poor outcome data. No data is available for resins as add-on to statins for cardiovascular (CV) benefit. CV outcome data with fibrates as an adjunct is variable and with limited effects on LDL-C. Lower LDL-C is better and safe in most patients in general and in high-risk and very high-risk patients in particular. Hence, there is a need for other lipid-lowering agents which may be considered as an add-on therapy to statins not only to reduce LDL-C but

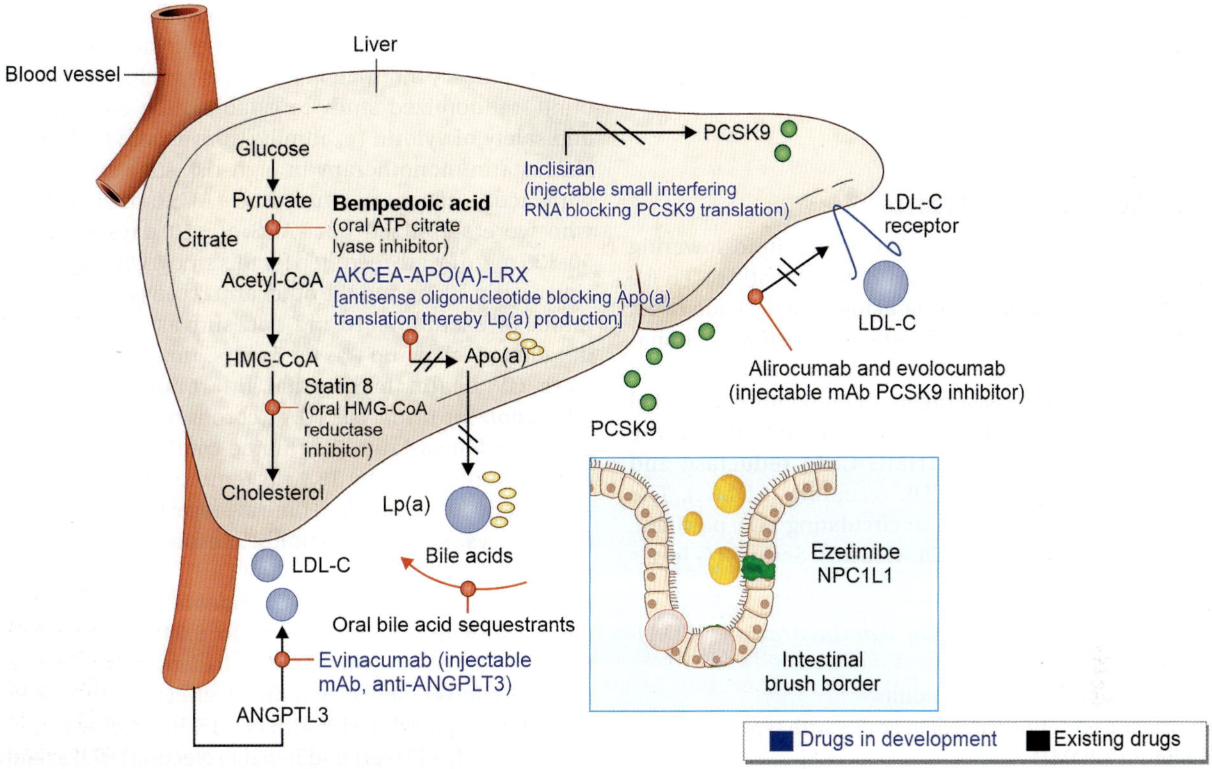

FIG. 1: Sites and action of statin and nonstatin drugs.

[ANGPTL3: angiopoietin-like protein 3; Apo(a): apolipoprotein (a); HMG-CoA: hydroxymethylglutaryl-CoA; LDL-C: low-density lipoprotein cholesterol; Lp(a): lipoprotein (a); NPC1L1: Niemann-Pick C1-Like 1; PCSK9: proprotein convertase subtilisin/kexin type 9]

also for further alterations in other lipid parameters with a focus on CV benefit. Under nonstatin therapies, the newly introduced proprotein convertase subtilisin/kexin type 9 (PCSK9) inhibitors, such as Evolocumab and Alirocumab, have shown marked reduction of LDL-C and enhance CV risk reduction. Inclisiran acts at the messenger ribonucleic acid (mRNA) level and blocks PCSK9 production. This drug is available in the United States and is yet to reach the Indian market. Oral PCSK9 inhibitor MK-0616 is undergoing trial for its efficacy. Phase II B study on oral PCSK9 inhibitor has shown promising results in LDL-C lowering equal to that of an injectable PCSK9 inhibitor.1 Bempedoic acid is now widely available, which has shown benefits in CV outcome with ezetimibe and statins. Icosapent ethyl (IPE) ester has shown CV benefits in patients with hypertriglyceridemia, with established atherosclerotic cardiovascular disease (ASCVD), and in people with diabetes after the LDL goal was achieved. ANGPTL3-(angiopoietin-like protein 3)-blocking drug Evinacumab was investigated in homozygous familial hypercholesterolemia (HoFH) patients and was found to be effective in lowering LDL-C when it was coadministered with statin and other nonstatin drugs such as ezetimibe and PCSK9 inhibitors **(Fig. 1)**. The drugs targeting lipoprotein(a) [Lp(a)] are undergoing investigation in phase 3 trials. Lipid apheresis is considered as the last resort in managing heterozygous familial hypercholesterolemia (HeFH) to reduce LDL-C levels to the goal. However, this procedure is considered as the first step also after starting high-dose statin in HoFH patients not only to reach the LDL-C goals but also to get protection from premature CVD and death.

CLASSIFICATION OF NONSTATIN DRUGS

- *Bile acid sequestrants (BAS)*:
  - Gastrointestinally active drugs
  - Bile acid resin (BAR)-anion exchange: Cholestyramine and colestipol
  - BAR-nonabsorbable polymer: Colesevelam
- *Cholesterol absorption inhibitor*: Ezetimibe
- *Fibrates*: Gemfibrozil, fenofibrate, bezafibrate, and fenofibric acid
- *Omega 3 fatty acids*: Docosahexaenoic acid (DHA) and eicosapentaenoic acid (EPA)—IPE ester is the purified form of EPA
- Niacin or nicotinic acid
- *PCSK9 inhibitors*: Monoclonal antibody—evolocumab and alirocumab and RNA interference drug—inclisiran
- Oral PCSK9 inhibitor
- *Acyl citrate lyase inhibitor*: Bempedoic acid
- *Monoclonal antibody targeting ANGPTL3*: Evinacumab

- *Antisense agents*: Lomitapide and mipomersen
- *Cholesteryl ester transfer protein (CETP) inhibitors*: Torcetrapib, anacetrapib, evacetrapib, and obicetrapib
- Targeted Lp(a)-lowering drugs
- LDL apheresis

Bile Acid Sequestrants[3,4]

Bile acid sequestrants are nonabsorbable, lipid-lowering polymers that bind bile acids in the intestine. These prevent the reabsorption of bile acids, which leads to an increase in the hepatic enzyme called cholesterol 7-alpha-hydroxylase. This results in the conversion of cholesterol to bile acids. This induces a higher demand for cholesterol in the liver. This leads to increased activity of the hydroxymethylglutaryl-CoA (HMG-CoA) reductase and higher numbers of hepatic LDL receptors (LDLRs). The combined effect is a decrease in circulating LDL particles, resulting in lowered serum LDL-C levels. Serum TG levels may also get altered.

Colesevelam—Food and Drug Administration (FDA)-approved indications:

- Primary hyperlipidemia in adults
- Improving glycemic control in adults with type 2 diabetes mellitus (T2DM)
- Lowering LDL-C in patients with HeFH who are unable to reach LDL-C targets.

Colesevelam can be taken as tablets or a suspension, with daily dosing ranging from 3.75 to 6 g tablets orally once daily. The mean LDL reduction with monotherapy is 15%. Combining colesevelam with low- to moderate-intensity statin therapy yields an additional 10–16% reduction in LDL-C.

Cholestyramine and colestipol: They lower LDL-C in patients with primary hyperlipidemia, as an adjunct to diet. The dosages and administration routes differ among the medications; Cholestyramine—oral dosing of 8–16 g/day divided into two doses; Colestipol—no specific dosage is mentioned in the prescribing information, but in a dose-ranging RCT, doses of 5, 10, and 15 g resulted in LDL-C reductions of 16.3%, 22.8%, and 27.2%, respectively.

Contraindications for Bile Acid Sequestrants

The contraindications are very high TG levels (>500 mg/dL), history of pancreatitis, and bowel obstruction. The common side effects include constipation, dyspepsia, and nausea. Colesevelam may lower glycated hemoglobin (HbA1c) by 0.5% in diabetic patients. CV outcome data are not available for all products.

Ezetimibe

Ezetimibe inhibits Niemann-Pick C1-Like 1 (NPC1L1) protein, reducing cholesterol absorption in the small intestine. It can achieve a mean LDL-C reduction of 18% in monotherapy and 25% when used in combination with statin therapy. IMPROVE-IT[5] (IMProved Reduction of Outcomes: Vytorin Efficacy International Trial) is a multicenter, double-blind, randomized study to establish the clinical benefit and safety of vytorin (ezetimibe/simvastatin tablet) versus simvastatin monotherapy in high-risk subjects presenting with acute coronary syndrome (ACS). 18,144 patients who were stabilized post-ACS of ≤10 days with LDL-C 50–125 mg/dLwere recruited for this study. One arm received simvastatin 40 mg and the other arm received a combination tablet of ezetimibe 10 mg and simvastatin 40 mg. The duration of follow-up was for 7 years. The primary endpoints were CV death, myocardial infarction (MI), hospital admission for urinalysis (UA), coronary revascularization, or stroke. Simvastatin + ezetimibe combination has shown reduction of LDL-C by 16.7 mg% more when compared to simvastatin alone (median time average: 69.9 vs. 53.2 mg/dL in simva vs. simva + ezetimibe, respectively). The study revealed absolute risk reduction (ARR) of 2% and relative risk reduction (RRR) of 6.64%. Patients with diabetes have shown RRR of 14% compared to 6.64% in nondiabetic patients. Moreover, patients with diabetes and polyvascular disease showed more beneficial effects with ezetimibe compared to placebo with ARR of 9.1% in another study. The SHARP (Study of Heart and Renal Protection) trial examined the clinical outcome benefit of ezetimibe/simvastatin 10/20 mg in patients with chronic kidney disease. After 5 years of therapy, 17% reduction was demonstrated in major atherosclerotic events and the risk reduction was proportional to LDL-C reduction.[6]

Indications

- Primary hyperlipidemia, either alone or in combination with statin therapy
- Patients with high risk and very high risk will derive more benefit in lowering LDL-C when combined with statin.
- Mixed hyperlipidemia in combination with fenofibrate
- HoFH in combination with statins

The recommended dose is 10 mg oral/daily.

Contraindications

Caution is advised in patients with moderate or severe hepatic impairment. Ezetimibe should be avoided during pregnancy and lactation.

The adverse effects are rare, either with monotherapy or in combination therapy.

Fibrates: Gemfibrozil, Fenofibrate, Bezafibrate, and Fenofibric Acid[7,8]

Fibrates should be used to treat severe hypertriglyceridemia (TG > 500 mg/dL). Peroxisome proliferator-activated receptor alpha (PPAR-α) agonists were used in various trials with disappointing CV benefits. In a meta-analysis of five landmark studies, such as ACCORD (Action to Control Cardiovascular Risk in Diabetes), FIELD (Fenofibrate Intervention and Event Lowering in Diabetes), BIP (Bezafibrate Infarction Prevention), HHS (Helsinki Heart Study), and VA-HIT (Veterans Affairs High-Density Cholesterol Intervention Trial) (n = 4,726), PPAR-α agonists reduced CV events significantly by 35% in patients with high TG ≥ 204 mg/dL and low HDL ≤ 34 mg/dL. In fact, more than five decades of their use resulted in failure to reduce CV risk and mortality. Combination therapy (statin and fibrate) is associated with an increased risk for abnormal transaminase levels, myositis, and rhabdomyolysis. The risk of rhabdomyolysis is more common with higher doses of statins and renal insufficiency and appears to be higher when statins are combined with gemfibrozil compared with fenofibrate.[9]

Omega 3 Fatty Acids: Docosahexaenoic Acid and Eicosapentaenoic Acid—[EPA] Icosapent Ethyl Ester is the Purified Form of EPA

Omega 3 is polyunsaturated fatty acid (PUFA), including EPA, DHA, and alpha linolenic acid, which is found in vegetable sources. EPA and DHA are present in marine organisms. Omega 3 fatty acids (FAs) are referred to as fish oil.

Mechanism of Action

- Decreased lipogenesis
- Increased β-oxidation
- Inhibition of phosphatidic acid phosphatase—an enzyme catalyzing the final step in the TG synthesis
- Increased degeneration of apolipoprotein B (ApoB)
- Increased lipoprotein lipase activity, an enzyme responsible for the conversion of very LDL (VLDL) to LDL particles

These five pathways result in decreased hepatic TG production and elevated TG clearance. They also possess anti-inflammatory, antithrombotic, and antiarrhythmic effects. In addition, they have effects on lowering BP and improving endothelial function. Though omega 3 FAs have the capacity to reduce TG levels among patients with hypertriglyceridemia, there is always an ongoing debate whether this therapy provides direct benefit in preventing CV events and deaths.

Adverse Drug Reactions

Omega 3 FAs have a good safety profile and are well tolerated. However, gastrointestinal (GI) side effects are reported. Arthralgia has been reported with IPE in APOLLO study. This product does not increase GI adverse drug reactions.

Reduction of Cardiovascular Events with Icosapent Ethyl Intervention Trial (REDUCE-IT)[10]

Icosapent ethyl is highly purified and stable EPA. Ethyl ester has been shown to lower TG levels. This study involved patients with established CVD or with diabetes and other risk factors who had been receiving statin therapy. These patients had fasting TG levels of 135–499 mg% and LDL-C levels of 41–100 mg/dL. The patients were randomly assigned to receive 2 g of IPE twice daily or placebo. The primary endpoint was a composite of CV death, nonfatal MI, nonfatal stroke, coronary revascularization, or unstable angina. The key secondary endpoint was a composite of CV death, nonfatal MI, or nonfatal stroke. 8,179 patients were recruited and were followed up for a median of 4.9 years.

Results: In REDUCE-IT, the addition of 4 g of IPE daily resulted in a 25% reduction in CV events beyond statins and other standard-of-care therapies. IPE is now the only therapy currently approved by the FDA to treat patients with elevated TGs (150–499 mg/dL) with CVD or T2DM and ≥2 CVD risk factors. The side effects are increased risk of atrial fibrillation and bleeding, although the risk of stroke was reduced and there were no cases of fatal bleeding **(Fig. 2 and Table 1)**.

Niacin (Nicotinic Acid)

Niacin decreases LDL-C and TG levels and increases HDL-C. It works by inhibiting the production of VLDL in the liver, which are precursors to LDL-C. It also reduces the breakdown of HDL-C, leading to increased HDL-C levels. RCTs conducted using niacin immediate release, extended

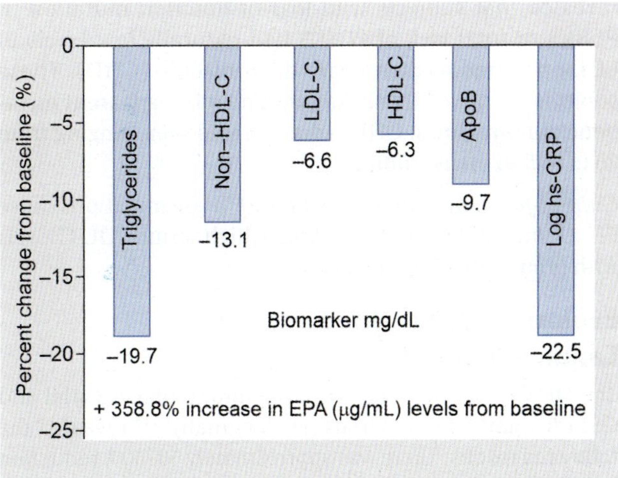

FIG. 2: Lipid parameters.

(ApoB: apolipoprotein B; CRP: C-reactive protein; HDL-C: high-density lipoprotein cholesterol; LDL-C: low-density lipoprotein cholesterol)

TABLE 1: Primary and secondary endpoints.

Endpoint	Hazard ratio (95% CI)	RRR (%)		*p* value
Primary composite (ITT)	0.75 (0.68, 0.83)	25	↓	<0.001
Key secondary composite (ITT)	0.74 (0.65, 0.83)	26	↓	<0.001
CV death or nonfatal MI	0.75 (0.66, 0.86)	25	↓	<0.001
Fatal or nonfatal MI	0.69 (0.58, 0.81)	31	↓	<0.001
Urgent or emergent revascularization	0.65 (0.55, 0.78)	35	↓	<0.001
CV death	0.80 (0.66, 0.98)	20	↓	0.03
Hospitalization for unstable angina	0.68 (0.53, 0.87)	32	↓	0.002
Fatal or nonfatal stroke	0.72 (0.55, 0.93)	28	↓	0.01

(CI: confidence interval; CV: cardiovascular; ITT: intention to treat; MI: myocardial infarction; RRR: relative risk reduction)

release, and with laropiprant did not show any benefit in CV outcome. In fact, many side effects were encountered such as GI, worsening of diabetes, and flushing and hepatic dysfunction. Hence, there is no recommendation to use niacin either alone or with statin.

PCSK9 Inhibitors: Monoclonal antibody—Evolocumab and Alirocumab, RNA Interference—Inclisiran

Proprotein convertase subtilisin/kexin type 9 plays an important role in LDL-C metabolism. It is a serine protease expressed by liver and intestine. This promotes intracellular degradation of LDLR and prevents its recycling to the hepatic cell surface. Hence, there is a reduction in the clearance of LDL from circulation.

Loss-of-function mutations in PCSK9:[11-14] Population studies revealed that subjects with loss-of-function mutation in PCSK9 or total lack of PCSK9 had naturally low levels of LDL-c and reduced coronary heart disease (CHD). These subjects are generally healthy with no other apparent metabolic abnormalities. CHD reduction was seen ranging from 30 to 88% in many studies.

Gain-of-function mutations in PCSK9: These mutations cause FH[15,16] including tendon xanthoma, high serum LDL-C levels with premature CHD and death.

Evolocumab and Alirocumab in Landmark Studies

The ODYSSEY LONG TERM (alirocumab) phase 3 trial and OSLER 1 and OSLER 2 trials (evolocumab)[17,18] revealed the following results: There was approximately 50–60% reduction in LDL-C from the baseline LDL-C of 120 mg/dL. The LDL-C achieved in these trials was approximately 50 mg/dL. This reduction was associated with 50% reduction in major adverse cardiovascular events (MACE), suggesting that lowering LDL-C to 50 mg/dL reduces MACE **(Fig. 3)**.

FOURIER Trial

About 27,564 high-risk, stable patients with established CVD, such as prior MI, prior stroke, or symptomatic peripheral artery disease (PAD), were recruited for this study after they fulfilled the criteria of receiving high- or moderate-intensity statin therapy ± ezetimibe and when their levels of LDL-C were ≥70 mg/dL or non-HDL-C ≥ 100 mg/dL. This trial was randomized double-blind, with one arm receiving injection evolocumab subcutaneously (SC) 140 mg once in 2 weeks or 420 mg once a month and the other arm receiving placebo injection in the same manner. Follow-up was done every 12 weeks till the end of the study.

Results: LDL-C levels came down to 30 mg/dL at 4 weeks and there was consistent reduction in LDL-C throughout the course of study for 3.2 years. 87% of the patients reached ≤70 mg/dL, 67% of the patients reached ≤40 mg/dL, and it was surprising to see the lowest level of ≤25 mg/dL in 42% of patients. The cumulative incidence of primary endpoints comprising major CV events, defined as the composite of CV death, MI, stroke, hospitalization for unstable angina, or coronary revascularization reduced by 15%. The key secondary efficacy endpoint of composite of CV death, MI, or stroke came down by 20%. There were no safety issues identified in this study except that there was an increase in injection site reactions in the active drug group. Adverse events (AEs) of the development of anti-evolocumab antibodies, both binding and neutralizing, were not seen in the evolocumab group. Clinical efficacy and safety of achieving very low LDL-C levels with the PCSK9 inhibitor evolocumab in the FOURIER outcomes trial were also presented in the European Society of Cardiology in 2017.

Highlights: LDL-C can now be reduced to unprecedented low levels with statin + PCSK9 inhibitor (< 1 mmol = << 38.7 mg%). A strong progressive relationship of achieved LDL-C and CV events was seen, down to LDL < 10 mg/dL. No excess in adverse events with very low achieved LDL-C < 20 mg/dL at 2.2 years. We should target considerably lower LDL-C

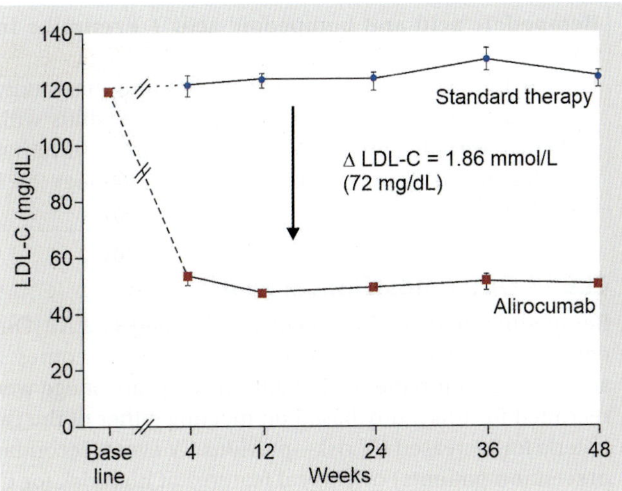

No. at risk						
Standard therapy	1,489	394	1,388	1,376	402	1,219
Alirocumab	2,976	864	2,871	2,828	841	2,508

Absolute reduction (mg/dL)	60.4	73.4	70.4	72.7	70.5
Percentage reduction	45.3	60.9	58.8	54.0	58.4
p value	<0.001	<0.001	<0.001	<0.001	<0.001

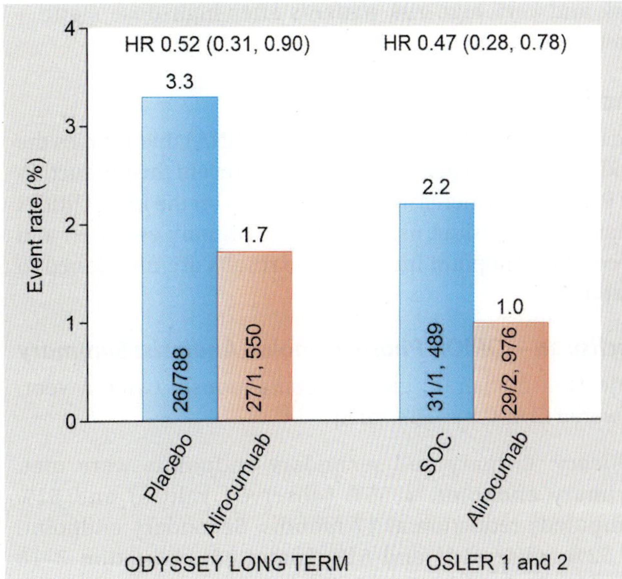

FIG. 3: Results of ODYSSEY LONG TERM and OSLER 1 and 2.
(HR: hazard ratio; LDL-C: low-density lipoprotein cholesterol; SOC: standard of care)

than what is currently recommended for our patients with ASCVD.[19]

Global Assessment of Plaque Regression with a PCSK9 Antibody as Measured by Intravascular Ultrasound (GLAGOV) Trial

Conclusion: Among patients with angiographic evidence of CAD on chronic statin therapy, the PCSK9 inhibitor evolocumab resulted in a greater change in percent atheroma volume and a greater proportion of patients with plaque regression.[20]

Odyssey Outcomes Trial[21]

The ODYSSEY OUTCOMES trial involved 18,924 patients in the post-ACS status who were randomized into two groups after a trial run-in period of 2–16 weeks on high intensity or maximum tolerated dose of atorvastatin or rosuvastatin and after meeting at least one lipid entry criterion. One arm received injection alirocumab (n = 9,462) 75 mg or 150 mg SC, once in 2 weeks compared with the other arm receiving injection placebo (n = 9,462). Patient and investigators remained blinded to treatment and lipid levels for the entire duration of the study. Investigators selected patients who had LDL-C > 70 mg, with an aim to bring it down to the target range between 25 and 50 mg. However, they allowed the patients to reach an acceptable range between 15 and 25 mg. In this process, an attempt was made to maximize the number of patients in the target range and minimize the number below target by blindly titrating alirocumab (75 or 150 mg SC Q2W) or blindly switching to placebo.

Primary efficacy endpoint: Pertaining to MACE, such as CHD death, nonfatal MI, ischemic stroke, or unstable angina, the Recurrence of hospitalization came down by 15% {hazard ratio (HR) 0.85 [95% confidence interval (CI) 0.78, 0.93]}. All-cause death was reduced by 15% [HR 0.85 (95% CI 0.73, 0.98)].

Who are the patients who can receive PCSK9 inhibitor therapy?[22]

The four groups of patients eligible to receive this therapy are:

1. Stable ASCVD + additional ASCVD risk factors. On-treatment LDL-C ≥ 70 mg/dL or non-HDL-C ≥ 100 mg/dL
2. Progressive ASCVD on-treatment LDL-C ≥ 70 mg/dL or non-HDL-C ≥ 100 mg/dL
3. LDL-C ≥ 190 mg/dL (including polygenic hypercholesterolemia, HeFH, and the HoFH phenotype) or those known to be LDLR defective LDL-C ≥ 70 mg/dL or non-HDL-C ≥ 100 mg/dL
4. Very high risk/statin intolerance

Dosage and administration by the SC route: HoFH—420 mg of evolocumab once monthly. Every 2 weeks—single-use, prefilled autoinjector. Primary hyperlipidemia with ASCVD or HeFH—140 mg every 2 weeks or 420 mg once a month.

PCSK9 inhibitors in specific populations: No dose adjustment is required in renally impaired patients in mild-to-moderate renal failure. No dose adjustment is necessary for hepatic impairment. However, the cost of treatment is prohibitive at this point of time to be used liberally. Healthcare providers are expected to use this drug for high-risk and very high-risk patients after high-dose statin ± ezetimibe therapy.

Inclisiran[23,24]

Inclisiran is a small interfering RNA (siRNA) that mimics the body's process of RNA interference to prevent the production of PCSK9, thus increasing LDL receptors on the liver. ORION trials with inclisiran usage depicting primary endpoint and secondary endpoint including the results are mentioned in **Table 2**.

Inclisiran—ORION Phase III Pooled Analysis: Summary

Injection inclisiran, given subcutaneously twice a year, lowered LDL-C by >50% safely.

Efficacy: Primary and secondary endpoints were met. Primary endpoint: ↓ 55% (observed values) and 51% (imputed) reduction at 17 months. Secondary endpoint: ↓ 52% (observed) and 51% (imputed) reduction 3–18 months. Reductions were consistent across subpopulations accompanied by substantial lowering of PCSK9, non-HDL-C, ApoB, and Lp(a).

Safety and tolerability: Inclisiran safety profile was similar to placebo. There were no adverse changes in laboratory markers. Exploratory basket of CV events less frequent in inclisiran group than in placebo.

Oral PCSK9 Inhibitor is Newer Therapy Under Trial

Results of a Phase 2b study of MK-0616 an oral PCSK9 inhibitor. All doses of MK-0616 demonstrated statistically superior reductions in LDL-C versus placebo with up to 60.9% placebo-adjusted reduction from baseline values. MK-0616 was well tolerated with no overall trends in AEs across treatment groups.

Acyl Citrate Lyase Inhibitor: Bempedoic Acid

Bempedoic acid is an adenosine triphosphate (ATP) citrate lyase inhibitor that targets cholesterol synthesis upstream of 3-hydroxy-3-methylglutaryl coenzyme A reductase, the enzyme inhibited by statins. Bempedoic acid is similar to statins in that it reduces cholesterol synthesis. It raises LDL receptor expression, thereby increasing clearance of LDL-C. However, bempedoic acid is a prodrug that is activated in the liver and not in most peripheral tissues including skeletal muscle. Hence, the drug may reduce adverse effects on muscles. Bempedoic acid reduced the level of LDL-C by 17–28%. In addition, C-reactive protein (CRP) levels were reduced between 18.7 and 22.4%. Based on this evidence, the FDA approved the following nonstatin drugs:

Bempedoic acid and bempedoic acid + Ezetimibe in 2020

Each is indicated as an adjunct to diet and maximally tolerated statin therapy for the treatment of adults with HeFH or established ASCVD who require additional lowering of LDL-C [American College of Cardiology 2021 (ACC 21)].

CLEAR Outcomes Clinical Trial[25]

Bempedoic acid in the recently published CLEAR Outcomes clinical trial shows benefits in CV outcomes in statin-intolerant patients. Patients 18–85 years of age were recruited for this study based on meeting either of the two criteria for increased CV risk—previous CV event (secondary prevention patients) or clinical features of high risk for CV events (primary prevention patients). A total of 13,970 patients underwent randomization; 6,992 were assigned to the bempedoic acid group and 6,978 to the placebo group. Patients were followed up for a median of 40.6 months. Patients for whom primary or secondary prevention of CVD was clinically indicated but who were unable or unwilling to take statins were included in the study. The risk of a primary endpoint event (death from CV causes, nonfatal MI, nonfatal stroke, or coronary revascularization) was significantly lower by 13% with bempedoic acid than with placebo. The first key secondary endpoint was 15% lower with bempedoic acid than with placebo. The mean percent reduction of LDL-C was 21.7% at the end of 6 months and 26.1% at 60 months. The median percent change of high-sensitivity CRP (hs-CRP) level was 22.2% at 6 months and 19.4% at the end of the trial. Few AEs that were noticed did not differ between the two trial groups. The incidence of cholelithiasis was higher with bempedoic acid than with placebo.

Monoclonal Antibody Targeting ANGPTL3: Evinacumab

Mechanism of Action

- Accelerated hydrolysis of VLDL particles by lipoprotein lipase enzyme
- Upregulation of VLDL-remnant clearance
- Increased ApoB-containing lipoprotein clearance

Evinacumab reduced LDL-C by 49%. This study was presented in the ACC Annual Scientific Session, 2020.

65 patients with HoFH, of whom about three quarters were on triple therapy (high-intensity statin, a PCSK9 inhibitor, and ezetimibe) and one-third was also on regular apheresis. On top of their usual lipid-lowering treatment regimen, 43 were randomized to evinacumab 15 mg/kg via intravenous infusion every 4 weeks for 24 weeks and 22 mg/kg to placebo infusions. Reductions in LDL-C with evinacumab were similar in HoFH patients with absent LDL receptor function and in those with some residual LDL receptor function.

TABLE 2: Summary of ORION trials with inclisiran.

Study	Phase/Patients enrolled	Primary endpoint	Secondary endpoint	Results
ORION-2	2/N = 4 (HoFH)	% change in LDL-C at 90/180 days	Absolute changes in LDL-C between day 1 and days 60, 90, and 180	3 points had substantial reductions in LDL-C maintained out to 180 days with maximum reduction of 43% in one point at 120 days
ORION-3	2/N = 490 (open-label extension study of ORION-1)	% change in LDL-C between 0 and 210 days	Proportion of points in inclisiran and evolocumab groups with >50% LDL-C reduction	Primary endpoint > 50% reduction in LDL-C
ORION-4	3/N = 1,500 (high ASCVD risk)	Occurrence of composite clinical endpoint of CHD death, MI, fatal/nonfatal ischemic stroke, or urgent coronary revascularization	Occurrence of composite clinical endpoint of CHD death, MI, or CV death	• Estimated primary completion date: 2024 • Estimated study completion date: 2029
ORION-5	3/N = 50–60 (HoFH)	Analysis of change in LDL-C during the course of treatment	N/a	Study completion date: 2021
ORION-7	1/N = 18 CKD vs. 6 normal persons	Analysis of safety, tolerability, pharmacodynamics, and pharmacokinetics in CKD	Changes in LDL-C and PCSK9 concentrations at 90 days	PCSK9 reduction at 60 days: • Normal renal function (68.1% ± 12.4%) • Mild RI (74.2% ± 12.3%) • Moderate RI group (79.8% ± 4.9%) • Severe RI group (67.9% ± 16.4%) *LDL-C reduction:* • Normal renal function (57.6% ± 10.7%) • Mild RI (35.1% ± 13.5%) • Moderate RI (53.1% ± 21.3%) • Severe RI (49.2% ± 26.6%)
ORION-9	3/N = 400 (HeFH)	• % change LDL-C at 510 days • Time adjusted % change between 90 and 540 days	• Absolute change in LDL-C at 510 days • Absolute change in LDL-C from baseline between 90 and 540 days	• *Primary endpoint*: 44.3% at 510 days • Time adjusted % change 53.8%
ORION-10	3/N = 1,500 (ASCVD)	• % change LDL-C at 510 days • Time adjusted % change between 90 and 540 days	• Absolute change in LDL-C at 510 days • Absolute change in LDL-C from baseline between 90 and 540 days	• *Primary endpoint:* 52.3% at 510 days • Time adjusted % change 53.8%
ORION-11	3/N = 1,500 (ASCVD or risk equivalent)	• % change LDL-C at 510 days • Time adjusted % change between 90 and 540 days	• Absolute change in LDL-C at 510 days • Absolute change in LDL-C from baseline between 90 and 540 days	• *Primary endpoint:* 49.9% at 510 days • Time adjusted % change 49.2%

(ASCVD: atherosclerotic cardiovascular disease; CHD: coronary heart disease; CKD: chronic kidney disease; CV: cardiovascular; HeFH: heterozygous familial hypercholesterolemia; HoFH: homozygous familial hypercholesterolemia; LDL-C: low-density lipoprotein cholesterol; MI: myocardial infarction; PCSK9: proprotein convertase subtilisin/kexin type 9; RI: renal impairment)

Antisense Agents: Lomitapide and Mipomersen

Lomitapide: It is used to treat HoFH. It inhibits the microsomal triglyceride transfer protein (MTP), which prevents the assembly of lipoproteins in enterocytes and hepatocytes, leading to reduced synthesis of chylomicrons and VLDL, resulting in lowered LDL-C levels. The FDA-approved indications for lomitapide include lowering LDL-C, total cholesterol, ApoB, and non-HDL-C in patients with HoFH as an adjunct to a low-fat diet and other lipid-lowering treatments, including LDL apheresis where available. The recommended dose of lomitapide is 5–60 mg orally once daily based on safety and tolerability. Lomitapide carries black box warnings due to its potential impact on the liver. Hepatic steatosis may occur.

Mipomersen: It is an antisense oligonucleotide (ASO), which blocks the creation of ApoB-100. Its efficacy, like that of lomitapide, is independent of the functionality of the LDLRs. LDL-C will drop by 25%. Injection site reaction and fatty liver are its side effects.

CETP Inhibitors: Torcetrapib, Anacetrapib, Evacetrapib, and Obicetrapib

Cholesteryl ester transfer protein inhibitors mediate the exchange of cholesteryl esters for TG between HDL and TG-rich remnant lipoproteins. This results in lower LDL-C and high HDL-C. Drugs to raise the HDL-C concentration have not shown reduction of ASCVD. The ILLUMINATE trial testing torcetrapib was stopped early due to increased mortality. Evacetrapib reduced LDL-C by 29 mg/dL. This ACCELERATE trial and large Dal-OUTCOMES study that tested dalcetrapib after ACS were terminated early after only 2 years of treatment because of a lack of efficacy in reducing ASCVD. The REVEAL study on anacetrapib was discontinued. Simmons et al. provided important efficacy results from an additional 2-year follow-up of these patients. The data shows increasing ASCVD risk reduction over time. The data clearly show that the absolute reduction in major coronary events in the anacetrapib group was about 50% larger at 6 years than it had been at the end of the 4-year treatment period.[26]

Obicetrapib:[27] 5 and 10 mg are an adjunct to high-intensity statins for effectively decreasing LDL-C, ApoB, non-HDL-C, and Lp(a) and increasing HDL-C and ApoA1 compared with placebo. The hypothesis that generates from this CEPT inhibitor-driven effects would be attenuated when used in combination with high-intensity statins. This trial supports the safety and tolerability of obicetrapib.

Targeted Lipoprotein-lowering Drugs on the HORIZONS

Currently, the two types of gene-silencing Lp(a)-lowering drugs in development are:

1. ASO
2. siRNA

Antisense Oligonucleotides[28]

The AKCEA-APO(a)-LRx20 was tried for dose finding in a trial, which reduced Lp(a) levels in a dose-dependent manner in patients with elevated Lp(a) and established CVD. Patients received 20, 40, or 60 mg every 4 weeks, 20 mg every 2 weeks, or 20 mg every 6–12 months. 20 mg every week reduced Lp(a) levels by 80%. Phase 2 trial results revealed significantly reduced levels of Lp(a), OxPL–ApoB, OxPL–APO (a), LDL-C, and ApoB levels. In fact, 98% of the patients achieved Lp(a) < 50 mg/dL. There were no safety concerns. The drug is now named as Pelacarsen which is in phase 3 Lp(a) HORIZON study. The results are expected in 2025.

Small interfering RNA reduces Lp(a) in CVD.[29] Olpasiran therapy significantly reduced Lp(a) in patients with ASCVD.

APOLLO Trial Using SLN 360

The APOLLO trial was presented by Steven Nissen as a late breaking clinical trial at ACC22. This trial used SLN 360 at 30, 100, 300, and 600 mg SC. The percentage changes in Lp(a) are nearly 90% at the end of 60 and 90 days with 300 and 600 mg doses.

Lipoprotein Apheresis[30]

Homozygous familial hypercholesterolemia patients will derive benefit if lipoprotein apheresis is performed every week. HeFH patients may require every other week. Observational studies indicated that ASCVD risk comes down by 72%. Apheresis is a procedure and/or therapy that should not be ignored in lipid lowering.

CONCLUSION

Statins are safe and efficacious in lipid lowering. Many patients who receive statin either high dose or moderate tolerable dose showed benefits in the reduction of LDL-C with reduced CV risk and mortality. However, there is always a residual risk which needs to be tackled. Nonstatin drugs with statin had shown benefits for further lowering of LDL-C not only in reaching the goal but also in reaching to the lowest level of <10 mg/dL, particularly with PCSK9 inhibitor. Nonstatin drugs enumerated in this chapter are potent and safe when added to statins in reducing LDL-C and decreasing CV risk. None of the nonstatin therapies introduced so far has shown any mortality benefit. In the view of strong evidence, we need to emphasize high lipid-lowering combination therapy than high-dose statins for the benefits that we had witnessed.

ONLINE REFERENCES

Please scan the QR code provided at the end of the table of contents for References of this chapter.

CHAPTER

68

Treatment of Dyslipidemia in Chronic Kidney Disease Patients

Manoranjan Mandal, Arshdeep Singh Sandhu, Aditi Rastogi

ABSTRACT

Patients with chronic kidney disease (CKD), including end-stage renal disease, patients on dialysis, or renal transplant recipients have an increased risk for cardiovascular disease (CVD) morbidity and mortality. Dyslipidemia, often present in this patient population, is an important risk factor for CVD development. Patients with CKD (dialysis-dependent and independent) have low high-density lipoproteins (HDLs), normal or low total cholesterol (TC) and low-density lipoprotein (LDL) cholesterol, increased triglycerides (TG), intermediate- and very low-density lipoprotein (IDL and VLDL; "remnant particles"), apolipoprotein B (apoB), and lipoprotein(a) [(Lp(a)]. In renal transplant recipients, TC, LDL, VLDL, and TG are elevated, whereas HDL is significantly reduced. Multiple factors including immunosuppressive agents contribute to the more atherogenic profile here. The European Society of Cardiology (ESC) 2019 guidelines on the management of dyslipidemia consider moderate-to-severe CKD [estimated glomerular filtration rate (eGFR) < 60 mL/min/1.73 m^2] as very high total cardiovascular risk and strongly recommend (Class I) initiation statins/statin–ezetimibe combination in non-dialysis-dependent stages 3–5 CKD. The KDIGO (Kidney Disease Improving Global Outcomes) guidelines also suggest statin treatment in adult kidney transplant recipients. Although various trials showed clear benefit of statins in non-dialysis-dependent CKD and postrenal transplant patients, the beneficial effects in patients on dialysis are uncertain.

Keywords: CKD, dyslipidemia, management.

INTRODUCTION

According to the Kidney Disease Outcomes Quality Initiative (K/DOQI), chronic kidney disease (CKD) is defined as renal impairment with reduced kidney glomerular filtration rate (GFR) of <60 mL/min/1.73 m^2 or the ratio of albumin/creatinine in urine >30 mg/g for at least 3 months.[1,2] CKD is classified into five stages based on the estimated GFR (eGFR) **(Table 1)**. The incidence and prevalence of CKD is rising worldwide with major contribution from hypertension and diabetes mellitus. The actual prevalence is underestimated due to asymptomatic early stages. End-stage renal disease (ESRD) is defined as needing dialysis or transplant, and the prevalence and incidence of ESRD have doubled over the past 10 years.[3]

Around 40–50% of all deaths in ESRD patients are attributed to cardiovascular disease (CVD), with CVD mortality risk approximating 15 times that seen in the normal population.[4] Apart from the traditional risk factors, such as age, male gender, diabetes, obesity, hypertension, and dyslipidemia, the novel markers such as proteinuria, inflammation, anemia, malnutrition, oxidative stress, and uremic toxins are postulated as the main risk factors for CVD.[5] Meta-analyses of studies in general as well as high-risk

TABLE 1: Staging of CKD.

CKD stages	GFR (mL/min/1.73 m^2)
CKD 1	≥90 (with renal damage or injury)
CKD 2 (mild)	60–89
CKD 3 (moderate)	30–59
CKD 4 (severe)	15–29
CKD 5 (end stage)	<15, dialysis or transplant

(CKD: chronic kidney disease; GFR: glomerular filtration rate)

population cohorts revealed that both lower eGFR (<60 mL/min/1.73 m^2) and higher albuminuria (>10 mg/g creatinine) are prognosticators of total as well as CVD mortality.[6] Evidence has clearly shown that lipid-lowering drugs have effectively reduced morbidity and mortality in patients with atherosclerotic cardiovascular disease (ASCVD). These medications may have the same beneficial effect in both CKD and renal transplant population.[7]

DYSLIPIDEMIA IN CHRONIC KIDNEY DISEASE

Dyslipidemia in nondialysis-dependent CKD and without nephrotic syndrome consists of elevated triglycerides (TG) with low high-density lipoprotein (HDL) cholesterol, while the levels of low-density lipoprotein (LDL) cholesterol and total cholesterol (TC) are generally not elevated. Hypertriglyceridemia occurs because of both—the delayed catabolism and the increased hepatic production of TG-rich lipoproteins [very low-density lipoprotein (VLDL) chylomicrons, and their remnants]. Decreased activity of hepatic TG lipase and peripheral lipoprotein lipase along with increased apolipoprotein C-III (apoC-III) (direct lipoprotein lipase inhibitor) contributes to hypertriglyceridemia. Insulin resistance, often associated with CKD, seems to be responsible for a hepatic VLDL overproduction.[8,9]

Although LDL is generally not elevated in patients with CKD, but the more atherogenic forms such as oxidized LDL and intermediate-density lipoprotein (IDL) are increased. Since these modified lipoproteins have low affinity for the classic LDL receptors and are thus engulfed by the macrophages through the scavenger receptors which are increased in uremia, they lead to the formation of foam cells in the vascular walls and evolve into atherosclerotic plaques.[8,10,11] Lipoprotein (a) [Lp(a)] is an LDL-like lipoprotein, which contains covalently bounded apo(a). It interferes with fibrinolysis, promotes endothelial dysfunction, and enhances foam cell formation. Recent evidences have shown that Lp(a) is highly associated with premature CVD incidence in the general population. Increased production and decreased catabolism of Lp(a) is found in CKD patients.[12]

High-density lipoprotein, which is a negative risk factor for atherosclerosis as well as inhibitor of inflammation, platelet adhesion, and LDL oxidation, is reduced in CKD due to the decreased levels of apo AI and AII, the main components of HDL, and decreased activity of lecithin-cholesterol acyltransferase, the enzyme required for the esterification of free cholesterol in HDL.[9,11,12]

In patients of CKD on dialysis, the profile is similar to that of early stages and with similar mechanisms. Additionally, low-molecular-weight heparin used for anticoagulation in this patients group may potentate TG elevation by releasing lipoprotein lipase from endothelial cells. Malnutrition and inflammation are usually present in this subgroup of patients and together with the impaired clearance of apo(a) may be responsible for increased Lp(a) and reduced TC. Observational studies have revealed the U-shaped curve between TC levels and risk of all-cause mortality. In other words, lower TC levels are associated with a higher mortality rate in CKD.[8]

Postrenal transplant patients have elevated plasma levels of TC, LDL, VLDL, and TG, while HDL is significantly reduced. Additional immunosuppressant drugs contribute additionally to dyslipidemia and may have negative impact on kidney graft function.[13] However, a recent study has shown an improvement in the lipid profile after kidney transplantation when compared with ESRD.[14]

MANAGEMENT OF DYSLIPIDEMIA

A study by Moorhead et al. in 1982 had shown the association between hyperlipidemia and worsening of renal function because of deposition of lipids in the kidney. Clinical trials have shown clearly that reduction of LDL decreases cardiovascular mortality, but in the CKD population, this association is not clear as CKD patients were excluded from major trials, although some physicians consider it as coronary artery disease (CAD) equivalent.[15,16] ESC 2019 guidelines on the management of dyslipidemia consider moderate to severe CKD (eGFR < 60 mL/min/1.73 m^2) as very high total cardiovascular risk and strongly recommend (Class I) initiation statins/statin-ezetimibe combination in nondialysis-dependent stages 3–5 CKD.[17] Also the American College of Cardiology/American Heart Association (ACC/AHA) 2018 guidelines consider CKD as a risk enhancer of ASCVD and give a class IIa recommendation for initiating statins/statin-ezetimibe combination in nondialysis-dependent stage 3–5 CKD.[18] KDIGO guidelines also recommend initiating statin or statin-ezetimibe combination in adults aged ≥50 years with eGFR < 60 mL/min/1.73 m^2 who are not treated with chronic dialysis or kidney transplantation (GFR categories G3a–G5).[19]

STATINS IN CHRONIC KIDNEY DISEASE STAGES 1–4

Statins effectively lower TC and LDL as they are in the general population, but their beneficial effect on cardiovascular morbidity and mortality in CKD patients seem to be severity-dependent. Moreover, statins do not have an effect on hypertriglyceridemia, elevated Lp(a), and decreased HDL levels, which are usually seen.[9,15] The Heart Protection Study (HPS), a subgroup of 1,329 CKD patients whose creatinine ranged from 1.3 to 2.3 mg/dL, was included and showed relative risk (RR) reduction of 28% [95% confidence interval (CI) 0.72–0.85; $p < 0.05$] in total mortality and fatal/nonfatal vascular events in the group that took simvastatin 40 mg/day.[15] In Cholesterol and Recurrent Events (CARE) study, the subgroup of 1,700 patients with mild CKD (creatinine clearance < 75 mL/min) who received 40 mg pravastatin/day, there was a 28% (95% CI 0.55–0.95; $p = 0.02$) RR reduction and a 4% absolute risk reduction in the primary endpoint, including death from coronary disease and symptomatic nonfatal myocardial infarction (MI).[20]

In the early stages of CKD, a majority of statins can be used safely. In stages 3–5, dose reduction is required. Atorvastatin is the safest among statins due to <2% renal excretion and can be used even in eGFR < 30 mL/min/1.73 m^2.[19]

Statins in Dialysis-dependent Chronic Kidney Disease

The SHARP (Study of Heart and Renal Protection) trial included 9,270 CKD patients [(nondialysis-dependent CKD patients ($n = 6{,}247$) and those receiving dialysis ($n = 3{,}023$)] who received simvastatin 20 mg plus ezetimibe 10 mg daily or placebo during the mean 4.9 years of follow-up period. These combined caused significant 17% RR reduction of the primary outcome of major atherosclerotic events (coronary death, MI, nonhemorrhagic stroke, or any revascularization) compared to placebo [hazard ratio (HR) 0.83; 95% CI 0.74–0.94; $p = 0.0021$]. But in the subgroup of dialysis-dependent patients, treatment with simvastatin–ezetimibe combination did not reduce the risk of the primary outcome significantly.[20]

The 4D Study (*D*ie *D*eutsche *D*iabetes *D*ialyse Studie) included 1,255 patients with type 2 diabetes mellitus undergoing hemodialysis (HD). At 4 weeks, atorvastatin treatment reduced the LDL levels by 42% compared to 1.3% reduction in the placebo group. Despite this significant reduction in LDL levels, atorvastatin had a nonsignificant 8% RR reduction (95% CI 0.77–1.10; $p = 0.37$) on the combined primary endpoint (a composite of cardiac death, nonfatal MI, and stroke).[21]

The AURORA (A Study to Evaluate the Use of Rosuvastatin in Subjects on Regular Dialysis: An Assessment of Survival and Cardiovascular Events) study included 2,776 HD patients, randomized to receive 10 mg of rosuvastatin per day or placebo. Despite this significant reduction in LDL levels, the combined primary endpoint (nonfatal MI, nonfatal stroke, and cardiovascular death) was not reduced after a median follow-up period of 3.8 years (HR 0.96; 95% CI 0.84–1.11; $p = 0.59$). Furthermore, there was no reduction in the risk of the individual components of the primary endpoint or reduction in all-cause mortality (HR 0.96; 95% CI 0.86–1.07; $p = 0.51$).[22] Combined data implied no significant ASCVD benefit in CKD patients on HD.

Statins in Postrenal Transplant

The ALERT (Assessment of Lescol in Renal Transplantation) study included 2,102 renal transplant recipients between 30 and 75 years and randomized to receive 40–80 mg/day fluvastatin therapy versus placebo and then followed up for 5–6 years. Compared with placebo, the RR reduction in cardiac death or definite nonfatal MI caused by fluvastatin therapy was significant (35%) (HR 0.65; 95% CI 0.48–0.88). Since the lipid-lowering and cardiovascular benefits observed here were comparable to those found in the general population, KDIGO guidelines suggest statin treatment in adult kidney transplant recipients **(Table 2)**.[11,16,19]

TRIGLYCERIDE-LOWERING AGENTS

The REDUCE-IT (Reduction of Cardiovascular Events with Icosapent Ethyl-Intervention Trial) randomly assigned 8,179 statin-treated patients with established CVD or diabetes to either 4 g daily of icosapent ethyl or placebo. In 1,816 patients of CKD, icosapent ethyl showed significant reductions in cardiovascular death or nonfatal MI in eGFR < 60 mL/min/1.73 m^2 [13.9% vs. 18.3%; HR 0.72 (95% CI 0.57–0.91); $p = 0.006$] and eGFR 60 to <90 mL/min/1.73 m^2 [8.8% vs. 11.4%; HR 0.76 (95% CI 0.63–0.92); $p = 0.004$] categories.[23] In contrast, fibric acid derivatives require dose reduction especially in combination with statins due to renal excretion.

TABLE 2: Statin dosing in chronic kidney disease (CKD).

Statin	Usual dose range (mg/day)	Clearance route	Dose range for CKD stages 1–3	Dose range for CKD stages 4–5	Use with cyclosporine
Atorvastatin	10–80	Liver	10–80	10–80	Avoid use with cyclosporine
Fluvastatin	20–80	Liver	20–80	20–40	Maximum dose 20 mg/day with cyclosporine
Lovastatin	10–80	Liver	10–80	10–20	Avoid use with cyclosporine
Pitavastatin	1–4	Liver/Kidney	1–2	1–2	Avoid use with cyclosporine
Pravastatin	10–80	Liver/Kidney	10–80	10–20	Maximum dose 20 mg/day when used with cyclosporine
Rosuvastatin	10–40	Liver/Kidney	5–40	5–10	Maximum dose 5 mg/day with cyclosporine
Simvastatin	5–40	Liver	5–40	5–40	Avoid use with cyclosporine

PCSK9 INHIBITORS IN CHRONIC KIDNEY DISEASE

The FOURIER (Further Cardiovascular Outcomes Research with PCSK9 Inhibition in Subjects with Elevated Risk) trial randomized 27,564 patients with atherosclerotic CVD and LDL > 70 mg/dL who were receiving statin therapy to receive evolocumab (either 140 mg every 2 weeks or 420 mg monthly) or matching placebo as subcutaneous injections. The primary efficacy endpoint was the composite of cardiovascular death, MI, stroke, hospitalization for unstable angina, or coronary revascularization. Relative to placebo, evolocumab treatment reduced Lp(a) by 26.9%. Also, it significantly reduced the risk of the primary endpoint [1,344 patients (9.8%) vs. 1,563 patients (11.3%); HR 0.85; 95% CI 0.79–0.92; $p < 0.001$]. The subgroup analysis confirmed efficacy and safety in CKD patients also.[24]

The ODYSSEY Outcomes (Evaluation of Cardiovascular Outcomes after an Acute Coronary Syndrome during Treatment with Alirocumab) trial which randomized acute coronary syndrome (ACS) patients with LDL > 70 mg/dL to maximally tolerated statin with placebo versus alirocumab showed that alirocumab had nearly twice the absolute reduction in cardiovascular events. However, patients with eGFR < 30 mL/min/m^2 were not included in the ODYSSEY Outcomes trial.[25]

CONCLUSION

As an ASCVD risk enhancer, CKD must be approached assertively with the screening of dyslipidemia and early initiation of lipid-lowering drugs. Although dyslipidemia differs quantitatively and qualitatively in nondialyses-dependent patients, ESRD patients, and renal transplant recipients, it significantly increases the risk of CVD development in all types. Thus, diagnosis and management of these patients are important to potentially improve their clinical outcome.

ONLINE REFERENCES

Please scan the QR code provided at the end of the table of contents for References of this chapter.

CHAPTER

69 Statin-induced Necrotizing Autoimmune Myopathy

M Chokkalingam, G Ashok, K Durga Devi

ABSTRACT

Statin-induced necrotizing autoimmune myopathy (SINAM) is a rare but potentially serious side effect associated with the use of statins. This chapter deals with the pathogenetic mechanism, genetic predisposition, clinical features, diagnosis, and treatment options of SINAM. It emphasizes the need to be aware of this uncommon side effect of a commonly used medication. Early recognition of this condition, stoppage of statin, and initiation of immunosuppressive treatment prevents morbidity and improves overall prognosis.

Keywords: Statins, necrotizing myopathy, anti-HMGCR antibody, muscle weakness, immunosuppression.

INTRODUCTION

Statins have long been used in cardiology for dyslipidemia and as a drug with pleotropic effects for the primary and secondary prevention of atherosclerotic cardiovascular disease (ASCVD). Statins are generally well tolerated; however, 10% of patients on statins can develop muscle-related side effects.[1] Statin-associated muscle symptoms (SAMS) can range from muscle pain, cramps, fatigue to a life-threatening myonecrosis and rhabdomyolysis.[2] Statins reduce cholesterol levels by inhibiting 3-hydroxy-3-methylglutaryl-coenzyme A (HMG-CoA) reductase, an enzyme in mevalonate pathway. Statin-induced muscle necrosis, that is associated with the presence of anti-3-hydroxy-3-methylglutaryl-coenzyme A reductase (HMGCR) antibodies is called as statin-induced necrotizing autoimmune myopathy (SINAM). SINAM is extremely rare but potentially life-threatening, occurring in 2 to 3 per 100,000 people exposed to statins.[3]

PATHOGENESIS

The pathogenesis of SINAM is unknown; it is most likely due to an immune-mediated damage to muscle fibers. An interplay of various proposed pathogenetic mechanisms may contribute to this rare myopathy.

- Patients who are prone to SINAM are genetically predisposed to overexpress HMGCR in muscle fibers when exposed to statins, resulting in autoantibody production.[4]
- The anti-HMGCR antibodies attaches itself to the HMG-CoA reductase in the surface of muscle fibers resulting in complement-mediated destruction of muscle fibers.[5] The regenerating muscle fibers also overexpress HMGCR in their surface leading on to further damage even after discontinuation of statins.
- *Genetic association with human leukocyte antigen (HLA) alleles*: *HLA-DRB1*11* is one gene that has the strongest association with SINAM. The risk is high in whites and African-American. The expression of earlier mentioned allele results in aberrant immune response when the person is exposed to statins.[6]
- *Mevalonate pathway and statins*: Along with cholesterol level, statins also alter the synthesis of coenzyme Q and isoprenoids both of which are needed for essential functioning of muscle fibers.[7] The reduction of isoprenoids might lead to immune dysregulation and activation of inflammatory pathway.
- Statins upregulate major histocompatibility complex (MHC) class I expression on muscle fibers, resulting in activation of cytotoxic T cells. The MHC class I expression can be focal or diffuse.[8,9]
- Statin exposure, infection, and vaccination can act as environmental trigger factors of SINAM as evidenced by case reports following coronavirus disease (COVID-19) infection or vaccination.[10]

CLINICAL PRESENTATION

The clinical features can vary from person to person and a high degree of suspicion is needed to identify SINAM at the earliest. The presentation can be acute to subacute in most patients. In some patients, SINAM can occur even after few years of statin exposure.[11]

- As like most inflammatory myositis, SINAM presents with proximal muscle weakness, often symmetrical. The weakness is progressive that patient finds it increasingly difficult to perform their activities of daily living such as getting up from chair, combing, and climbing up stairs. The onset of symptoms has a temporal relationship with the usage of statins. Dysphagia is present in a small group of patients with SINAM.[11] Truncal muscle weakness has been reported in some patients.[12] Hallmark of SINAM is that the symptoms and creatine phosphokinase (CPK) elevation may persist even after statin discontinuation.[13]

  Case reports are available where SINAM had progressed on to involve bulbar and respiratory muscles resulting in type 2 respiratory failure needing ventilatory support.[9] If not identified early, it can result in mortality.
- Muscle pain is the major differentiating feature between inflammatory myositis and SINAM; while the former is often painless, SINAMs often presents with pain in the group of muscles involved.[14] The pain can range from mild to severe and the involved group of muscles is tender to palpate **(Table 1)**.

  Rarely SINAMs can lead to rhabdomyolysis resulting in myoglobinuria and acute tubular injury leading to renal failure.

  Features such as arthritis, Raynaud's, interstitial lung disease, cardiomyopathy, and typical skin rashes which are often noted in other inflammatory myositis are not present in SINAM; this can be a differentiating feature.[13]

DIAGNOSIS

Creatine Phosphokinase Elevation

Creatine phosphokinase is a muscle enzyme that shows a rapid elevation when there is muscle damage. SINAM shows a marked elevation in CPK levels often >10,000 IU/L.[15]

TABLE 1: Comparison of inflammatory myositis, statin-induced myalgia, and statin-induced necrotizing autoimmune myopathy.

Variables	Inflammatory myositis	Statin-induced myalgia	Statin-induced necrotizing autoimmune myopathy
Onset	Subacute	Subacute	Acute to subacute
Age	Bimodal	Any age	>50
Muscle pain	Painless	• Pain + • Cramps +	Painful +++
Bulbar and respiratory muscle weakness	Present	None	Present
Other manifestations	Skin changes, interstitial lung disease, Raynaud's, arthritis, etc.	None	None
CPK elevation	>25–50 times the normal	<10 times the normal	>25–50 times the normal (usually >10,000 IU/L)
Rhabdomyolysis	Rare	None	Can be present
Antibodies	Anti-Mi-2, anti-Jo-1, anti-U1RNP, anti-SSA, anti-PM-Scl, anti-TIFγ, and many more	None	Anti-HMGCR
EMG	Insertional irritability	None	Insertional irritability
Muscle biopsy	• Marked inflammatory cell infiltration of muscle fibers, perimysial or perifascicular inflammation • Dominant membrane attack complex on sarcolemma	Normal	Muscle necrosis and regeneration is dominant. Scarce inflammatory infiltrate
Treatment	Steroids/IVIg/immunosuppression	None; if pain persistent statin discontinuation	• Discontinuation of statins • Steroids/IVIg/ immunosuppression

(CPK: creatine phosphokinase; EMG: electromyography; IVIg: intravenous immunoglobulin)

Autoantibodies Associated with SINAM

Anti-HMGCR antibody and anti-signal recognition protein (anti-SRP) antibodies had previously thought to be contributing to immune-mediated necrotizing myopathy (IMNM).[15] Necrotizing myopathy is a dominant feature in IMNM with little or no inflammation.[15] In recent times, SINAM has been defined as a separate entity due to its specific genetic association, statin as an environmental trigger, unique pathology, and its association with anti-HMGCR antibody, which is not only a diagnostic antibody but also pathogenetic.

Anti-HMGCR Antibodies

First identified in 2010, it is the hallmark of SINAM.[16] This antibody is usually not associated with other autoimmune myositis such as polymyositis and dermatomyositis. The presence of this antibody is an intermediate risk factor for malignancy in myositis.[17] Higher the levels of this antibody, higher the CPK levels in the patient affected and poorer the prognosis.[18] The commercial testing of this antibody has recently been made available in India. Anti-HMGCR antibodies have a high negative predictive value suggesting an absence of this antibody when done by enzyme-linked immunosorbent assay (ELISA) essentially rules out SINAM. The ELISA test has a reported sensitivity of 94.4% and specificity of 99.3%.[13]

Electromyography

Electromyography (EMG) in SINAM does not help to differentiate from other causes of inflammatory myositis. Insertional irritability, spontaneous activity, and fibrillations are noted, with low amplitude, small, and polyphasic complexes.[19]

Muscle Biopsy in SINAM

The histopathological hallmark of SINAM is necrosis and regeneration of muscle fibers with scant inflammatory cells in muscle biopsy.[20] The inflammatory cells are in perivascular regions and there is faint clustered MHC class I expression. Inflammatory cells though few, comprise of macrophages, in contrast to other inflammatory myositis where T cells are the predominant infiltrating inflammatory cell type.[9] In non-necrotic muscle fibers, C5b-9 membrane attack complex is expressed in the sarcolemma.[5] Complement-mediated damage to muscle fibers resulting in necrosis has been demonstrated in SINAM.[20]

IMAGING

Magnetic Resonance Imaging

Extensive edema in T1 and T2 short tau inversion recovery (STIR) sequence is noted in involved muscles.[21] MRI shows a trend toward fatty replacement. Limb girdle muscles are involved; in thighs the dorsal group and in leg, medial gastrocnemius seems to be the most common group affected. In upper limb, triceps and deltoid are the most affected muscle group. Since, SINAM has the tendency to progress to chronicity even after discontinuation of statins and immunosuppressive treatment, MRI can be a useful tool for follow-up or monitoring response.[22]

TREATMENT

The treatment of SINAM is aimed at alleviation of symptoms, reduce myonecrosis, preservation of muscle power, and prevent relapses. The rarity of the disease, limited awareness among treating physicians, and availability of anti-HMGCR commercial antibody kit are the major causes of diagnostic delay. This results in absence of proper treatment protocols in SINAM.

Statin Discontinuation

It forms the first line of treatment. Statins should not be restarted in patients with SINAM. In very few cases, statin discontinuation alone is enough to stop progression of disease. The unique pathogenesis in SINAM, in which a regenerating muscle fiber express HMGCR on its surface and acts as a positive feedback resulting in further destruction of muscle fibers necessitates use of further immunosuppression.[22] The mentioned reason is responsible for persistent CPK elevation and progressive symptoms in SINAM even after statin discontinuation.

Steroids

Steroids are the first line of immunosuppressive treatment. The dose—whether pulse methylprednisolone or oral steroids is used upfront depends on the severity of clinical features of patients. With high CPK levels, significant muscle weakness pulse steroids—intravenous (IV) methylprednisolone 500–1,000 mg IV for 3 days is started followed by 1 mg/kg of oral prednisolone.[23] Steroids are tapered based on the clinical response and the CPK levels.

Intravenous Immunoglobulin

In conditions where steroids are contraindicated or non-responsive, intravenous immunoglobulin (IVIg) that has immunomodulatory effect can be used in the treatment of SINAM. The dose of IVIg is 400 mg/kg body weight per day for 5 days.[24] The potential benefits of IVIg are:

- IVIg neutralizes pathogenetic anti-HMGCR antibodies, reduces proinflammatory cytokines, and promote anti-inflammatory state. It reduces muscle damage.[25]
- Can be used as a monotherapy when steroids are contraindicated or as combination/add-on to steroid therapy and other immunosuppressives.[26]

- Can be used for maintenance therapy.
- Refractory disease not responding to conventional treatment regimens.

Steroid-sparing Immunosuppressants

Methotrexate, mycophenolate mofetil, azathioprine, and rituximab are immunosuppressive agents used as steroid-sparing agents to achieve long-term maintenance and prevent relapse.[27]

For patients presenting with significant muscle weakness and a higher CPK elevation, induction regimen with dual therapy, steroid + steroid-sparing immunosuppression or triple therapy, steroids + IVIg + steroid-sparing immunosuppression regimen is preferred for achieving early remission.[26]

Physical Rehabilitation and Exercise

Physiotherapy plays a major role in regaining muscle strength in most myositis. A structured exercise program with a combination of stretches, aerobics, strength, and resistance training does help in achieving recovery.

CONCLUSION

Statin-induced necrotizing autoimmune myopathy is a rare life-threatening side effect of statin usage. Affected persons are genetically predisposed to develop this necrotizing myopathy. Acute or subacute onset of painful proximal muscle weakness is characteristic. High index of suspicion is needed in patients who have persistent symptoms and CPK elevation despite statin discontinuation. The hallmark of SINAM is the presence of anti-HMGCR antibodies. High levels of CPK, absence of other antibodies, MRI, and muscle biopsy contributes to the diagnosis. Statin stoppage alone does not change the course of the disease; most patients need steroids with add on IVIg and immunosuppressive treatment with methotrexate, azathioprine, mycophenolate mofetil, or rituximab.

ONLINE REFERENCES

Please scan the QR code provided at the end of the table of contents for References of this chapter.

CHAPTER

70 Management of Dyslipidemia in Young and Asymptomatic South Asians

Rajeev Garg, Vardhini Vijaykumar

ABSTRACT

Dyslipidemia is characterized by abnormal levels of lipids in the blood, is a major risk factor for cardiovascular diseases (CVDs), and a growing health concern among young and asymptomatic South Asians. This chapter aims to outline the dyslipidemic burden in South Asians and management strategies for dyslipidemia in this specific population, emphasizing the need for a comprehensive approach to reduce CVD morbidity and mortality.

Keywords: Dyslipidemia, South Asians, asymptomatic, coronary artery disease, LDL-C, statins.

INTRODUCTION

Dyslipidemia, a known risk factor for the onset and progression of atherosclerosis in coronary artery disease (CAD), is characterized by raised low-density lipoprotein cholesterol (LDL-C) and decreased high-density lipoprotein cholesterol (HDL-C). Raised LDL-C has a strong pathophysiological relationship with the development of coronary atherosclerosis. There is a strong evidence, that reducing its levels can slow and stabilize atherosclerotic vascular disease. Recent studies have also demonstrated a substantial correlation between increased lipoprotein(a) [Lp(a)] levels and the prevalence of CAD. The European Society of Cardiology (ESC) 2019 Guidelines advise measuring Lp(a) at least once over the patient's lifespan to identify very high atherosclerotic cardiovascular disease (ASCVD) risk patients.[1]

In contrast to other ethnic subgroups, South Asians have higher atherogenic particle burdens despite having comparable levels of LDL-C, elevated levels of triglycerides (TGs), low levels of HDL-C, and elevated levels of Lp(a). Also, in South Asians, HDL particles seem to be smaller, less functioning, and proatherogenic.

The Study of Health Assessment and Risk in Ethnic Groups assessed 985 participants of South Asian, Chinese, and European heritage living in Canada were evaluated for traditional and novel cardiovascular risk factors. In comparison to Caucasians, South Asians had higher levels of total cholesterol (TC), LDL-C, TG, and lower levels of HDL-C. They also had an increased prevalence of glucose intolerance. The elevated atherosclerosis load in this population, as determined by carotid atherosclerosis assessed with B-mode ultrasonography, was only partially explained by these abnormalities.[2] The elevated coronary heart disease (CHD) risk in South Asians may therefore be caused by other factors.

Despite these results, the INTERHEART study found that myocardial infarction (MI) was linked to smoking, diabetes or hypertension history, waist-to-hip ratio, dietary habits, physical activity, alcohol consumption, blood apolipoproteins, and psychosocial factors in nine ethnic populations, including South Asians. The INTERHEART South Asia study has revealed dyslipidemia as one of the most significant risk factors for CAD.[3]

In a recent cohort with 91,131 people (aged 20–100 years) from the Copenhagen General Population Study (CGPS) took subjects who neither used statins nor have diabetes or ASCVD at baseline. About 3,389 people had ASCVD, and 1,515 people had their first MI over the average 7 years of follow-up. 38 mg/dL increase in LDL-C, the risk of MI and ASCVD increased for the general population [hazard ratio (HR) 1.34; 95% confidence interval (CI)] and was magnified for all the age groups. LDL-C level (i.e., potential familial hypercholesterolemia) >193.35 mg/dL was also associated with an increased risk of MI compared to people with a cholesterol level of <116 mg/dL in individuals aged 80–100 years (HR 2.99; 95% CI) and in those aged 70–79 years (1.82, 1.20–2.77).

The risk of CHD among South Asian populations has been clearly linked to the conventional risk factors such as hypertension, hypercholesterolemia, diabetes mellitus, abdominal obesity, metabolic syndrome, and tobacco use.[4] With their natural genetic propensity for CHD, a diet with high in sugar, processed carbohydrates and the increasing sedentary lifestyle of South Asian population faces a significant risk for CHD.

DYSLIPIDEMIA IN SOUTH ASIANS

Low-density Lipoprotein Cholesterol

Low-density lipoprotein cholesterol is a recognized indicator of the onset, persistence, and severity of CHD. In accordance with the National Lipid Association's recommendations for managing cholesterol, it is the coprimary target for lipid lowering medication.[5] According to research, elevated LDL-C levels in the South Asian population accurately indicate the risk of CHD. However, CHD can also develop in South Asians with relatively low LDL-C levels as demonstrated in the INTERHEART study where the South Asians had LDL-C levels that were, on an average, 10 mg/dL lower than the other groups.[6]

Interesting results were seen in both sexes, with cases and control patients from Asia having LDL-C levels below 100 mg/dL in proportions of 25.5% and 32.3%, as opposed to 19.4% and 25.3% in non-Asians.[6] These findings suggest that whereas LDL-C is linked to an increased risk of acute myocardial infarction (AMI) among South Asians, this risk is higher than that of other ethnic groups even at considerably lower LDL-C levels.

There are population variations in atherogenic dyslipidemia, according to the prevalence studies from Heart SCORE and India SCORE, with Asian Indians having a higher prevalence of small-dense LDL and TG/HDL ratio >3.[7] Another study showed that compared to people of Hill ancestry, ethnic plains Madheshi were less likely to be overweight, although they were more likely to have dyslipidemia. Plasma hypertriglyceridemia (≥150 mg/dL) afflicted 8.5%, and 78% had low HDL-C concentrations [>40 mg/dL (male) and >50 mg/dL (female)]. Compared to men, women were overweight and had a higher risk of increasing blood pressure (OR 1.9; 95% CI 1.6–2.3), but a reduced risk of dyslipidemia.[8]

Indices are more effective than lipid profiles for assessing coronary risk in asymptomatic individuals. A cross-sectional research of 120 young, asymptomatic medical, and paramedical workers between the ages of 18 and 40 years old working in a tertiary care hospital was conducted to determine the prevalence of dyslipidemia using the lipid profile and Castelli's Risk Ratio I and II (CRR I and II). Those individuals who smoke, alcoholics, diabetic, hypertension, dyslipidemia, or undergoing treatment for any metabolic abnormalities, hypothyroidism, and any chronic sickness were prohibited. According to the World Health Organization (WHO) categorization and the results of Dr Chadha's anthropometric correlation study, anthropometric measurements such as height, weight, body mass index (BMI), and waist-to-hip ratio were determined. 43 (35.6%) men and 77 (64.1%) women made up the 120 participants. More than 50% of study subjects had the waist/hip (W/H) ratio >0.9, with men accounting for 34.1% (n = 41) which was greater than women for 17.5% (n = 21). About 50% of the population had low HDL-C. Most of the people showed a combined lipid derangement, although not for all four markers (TC, TG, LDL-C, and HDL-C) in the same person. It was discovered that the females had greater rates of hypertriglyceridemia and low HDL-C. Out of 120 participants, high risk for CRR-I and CRR-II was present in 41.5% (n = 51) and 16.3% (n = 16) of them, respectively.[9]

It has been noted that young, healthy South Asians aged (27.5 ± 3.2 years) are more susceptible to LDL aggregation than white Caucasians. This may be partially explained by South Asian's higher body fat percentage, which results in LDL that is more enriched in sphingomyelin. It is believed that young South Asians may accumulate more LDL in the artery wall due to the presence of sphingomyelin-rich and aggregation-prone LDL particles, which may raise their risk of developing ASCVD later in life.[10]

Triglycerides and High-density Lipoprotein Cholesterol

According to the recommendations of the Adult Treatment Panel III of the National Cholesterol Education Program, low HDL-C levels (<40 mg/dL) are a risk factor for CHD, however raised TG (>150 mg/dL) are linked to other lipid abnormalities (elevated non-HDL-C levels and increased LDL particle number) and nonlipid risk factors (diabetes mellitus and metabolic syndrome), increasing the risk of CHD.[11] Low HDL-C and high TG levels are among the dyslipidemias that affect South Asians most frequently.[12] In studies with high sample sizes, hypertriglyceridemia (>150 mg/dL) was found in up to 70% of South Asian populations[13] against 34% for Caucasians.[14] Up to one-third of the South Asians had low levels of HDL-C (<40 mg/dL).

A potential surrogate measure for this South Asian phenotype is the TG/HDL-C ratio. There is a lack of information regarding the usefulness of the TG/HDL-C ratio as a lipid marker in Indians. In a group of young and middle-aged Indian males who appeared to be in good health, abnormal TG/HDL-C ratio values were found in more than half of the subjects. Apart from its previously known specific link with small dense-LDL (sd-LDL) particles, the TG/HDL-C ratio was significantly correlated with other lipid markers and indices of adiposity, such as BMI and body fat. In the future, the TG/HDL-C ratio should be assessed for the risk of incident cardiovascular disease (CVD) among Indians.[15]

Lipoprotein(a)

Lipoprotein(a) levels are mostly genetically driven. South Asian immigrants have Lp(a) levels that are greater than those in Caucasians and comparable to those in their native countries.[16] When Indian immigrants in West London were compared to their relatives in Punjab, Lp(a) concentrations were found to be similar in both the Indian and Punjab populations, but significantly higher ($p = 0.01$) than those of a white European population in London, according to Bhatnagar et al. 1995 study.[17] Overall, these findings suggest that South Asians have a genetic predisposition to have increased Lp(a) levels. These raised Lp(a) levels are associated with CHD and may also help to explain why this population is at increased risk for having too many CHDs.

RISK FACTORS ASSOCIATED WITH DYSLIPIDEMIA

Gender Variation

Women have higher TG levels than men which is a major predictor of CAD. A study found that women are more likely than men to have hypertension, diabetes, and dyslipidemia in which only 11.5% of males had diabetes compared to 35.4% of females, which is statistically significant ($p < 0.001$). This demonstrates the need to promptly target diabetic women in order to stop CAD in the future. Only 15.9% of the women in this study had a normal BMI, whereas 69.5% were overweight and 14.6% were overtly obese.[18]

Genetic Variation

Another study looked at the relationship between genetic variation in the cholesteryl ester transfer protein (CETP) promoter region and HDL-C, CETP activity, CAD, CAD risk factors, and the interaction of genetic and environmental factors in a special cohort of Asian Indian Sikhs with diabetes. The connection between CETP activity and HDL-C levels was found to be strongly influenced by the interaction between rs3764261 and rs708272, and 'ATAA' haplotype was associated with increased HDL-C levels. These findings and past research demonstrate that a low level of CETP activity is linked to a higher risk of developing CAD.[19]

Although there have not been many direct comparisons between ethnic subgroups; it has been suggested that Asian populations need lower doses of statins for therapeutic effects similar to those in non-Asians.[20] This may be due to underlying genetic variations in genes related to the statin metabolism.

MANAGEMENT OF DYSLIPIDEMIA IN YOUNG SOUTH ASIANS

Despite the rapid expansion of the current literature with better understanding of the specific lipid abnormalities in this patient population, specific management goals and treatment thresholds do not exist for South Asians because of paucity of data. Most of the current therapy related management guidelines are drawn from Western standards. The management of dyslipidemia in South Asians often entails dietary and lifestyle modifications as well as medicines that can help reduce TG and LDL-C levels and raise HDL-C levels.

Risk Stratification

The SCORE system[20] calculates the probability of a first fatal atherosclerotic event over a 10-year period, such as a heart attack, stroke, and other occlusive artery disease, such as sudden cardiac death. Both TC and the TC:HDL-C ratio has SCORE charts available. However, following work on the SCORE database has demonstrated that entering HDL-C as a separate variable as opposed to the ratio can help risk estimate more; for instance, according to the estimates from the SCORE cholesterol charts, HDL-C modifies risk at all risk levels. This is crucial at risk levels just below the 5% cutoff for intensive risk modification since many of these people will be eligible for intensive counseling if their HDL-C is low.

Very high risk individuals are those who have diabetes mellitus (DM), target organ damage such proteinuria, or severe risk factors including smoking, hypertension, or dyslipidemia with an estimated SCORE 10% for a 10-year chance of fatal CVD. Subjects having one or more risk variables are markedly high such as blood pressure <180/110 mm Hg or cholesterol (>310 mg/dL) (for example, in familial hypercholesterolemia).

Most other diabetic patients with a computed SCORE of between 5 and 10% for a 10-year risk of fatal CVD are classified as high risk patients, while some young persons with type 1 diabetes mellitus (T1DM) may be at low or moderate risk. Although sd-LDL measurement is not now advised for risk calculation, it may be considered an emergent risk factor in the future and employed.[1]

Recent research has demonstrated that TC, LDL-C, and HDL-C findings from fasting and nonfasting sample are comparable. TGs are influenced by diet, with an average increase in the plasma levels of 27 mg/dL, depending on the makeup and timing of the last meal. Nonfasting lipid levels can be utilized for screening and general risk calculation since it has a similar predictive strength to fasting for risk estimation. However, it should be noted that the risk may be overestimated in diabetic individuals as they had LDL-C levels that were up to 0.6 mmol/L lower in nonfasting samples in one study.[21]

Detection of Subclinical Cardiovascular Disease

It is a new and developing discipline to employ computed tomography angiography to find high-risk patients in the South Asian community. An analysis of a US cohort of South Asians revealed smaller proximal left anterior descending artery luminal diameters. A larger mean percent stenosis and a higher proportion of patients with numerous diseased artery segments on computed tomography angiography were seen in South Asian cohort, indicating that their ASCVD was more severe.[22]

According to early results from the Mediators of Atherosclerosis in South Asians Living in America (MASALA) cohort compared to Multi-Ethnic Study of Atherosclerosis (MESA) cohort () participants who were matched, there was a greater internal/common carotid medial thickness. Furthermore, the comparison of the MASALA cohort and MESA cohort showed that South Asians had CAC scores that were greater than those of blacks and Latinos but comparable to those of Chinese Americans.[23]

A cross-sectional study was done at a hospital on 70 young ischemic heart disease (IHD) cases (males and females between the ages of 35 and 40 years old). TGs, TC, LDL-C, and TC/HDL-C increased in 38.6%, 41.4%, 32.9%, and 25.7% of patients, respectively. Homocysteine, plasma fibrinogen, and Lp(a), three more recent risk variables, were all increased in 61.4%, 77.3%, and 18.2% of patients, respectively. Serum TGs, TC/HDL-C, and LDL-C/HDL-C were substantially ($p = 0.05$) related with significant CAD compared to nonsignificant CAD, but no similar correlation was observed for newer risk variables. In conclusion, screening for risk factors should begin earlier in life for Indian boys in the South Asian community because they seem more susceptible to developing CAD. In this vulnerable population, it is crucial to promote physical activity, healthy eating habits, and the cessation of smoking and tobacco chewing.[24]

Lifestyle Modifications to Improve the Plasma Lipid Profile

Strong evidence suggests that dietary variables may affect atherogenesis directly or indirectly by having an impact on conventional risk factors like blood pressure, glucose levels, or plasma lipids. The reduction in LDL-C is greater if weight loss is accomplished with a low-fat diet. Body weight reduction also affects TC and LDL-C, but the magnitude of the effect is rather small. In severely obese subjects, a decrease in LDL-C concentration of 8 mg/dL is observed for every 10 kg of weight loss.[25,26]

Losing weight enhances insulin sensitivity and lowers TG levels. However, the positive benefits of losing weight and exercising on the CV risk profile go beyond lowering LDL-C and also affect other lipoprotein classes and other risk variables.

From 1995 through 2015, a multicentric prospective study was conducted at the Saaol Heart Centre in various Indian cities (Delhi, Kolkata, Bengaluru, Chennai, and Mumbai). A total of 5,000 CAD patients with obesity, hypertension, and diabetes were included in this study. Clinical evaluation was carried out utilizing Saaol safety wheel as a comprehensive tool, and yoga-based lifestyle modification counseling (consisting of the fundamental components; cardiac education, plant-based balanced diet, regular walk, yoga, and meditation) was administered to study subjects. Starting out, lifestyle adjustment counseling was offered once a month for a year. After that, it was repeated every 6 months with clinical assessments until the study's 5-year follow-up period.

The study's findings show a considerable improvement in angina with a drop in the New York Heart Association (NYHA) angina classification score from 3.08 ± 0.56 (mean ± SD) to 2.45 ± 0.70, as well as a decrease in the use of antianginal medications from 4.36 ± 1.35 to 3.82 ± 1.20. In this study, a significant improvement in heart attack protection score was also noted. Study participants demonstrated significant improvements in clinical outcomes (BMI, blood pressure, and lipid parameters), and cardiac patients experienced a decrease in their risk of heart attack and cardiac events. According to the findings of this study, yoga-based lifestyle interventions are a noninvasive, highly effective way to treat and manage cardiac risk factors in people with CAD.[27]

Statin in Young Adults

It may not be possible to avoid the onset of substantial atherosclerosis and consequent CHD by reducing exposure to LDL in young adulthood beginning at the age of 30 years old.[28] The onset of statin medication after three decades of exposure to suboptimal levels of LDL may only result in a minor improvement in atherosclerosis reduction and long-term CHD event prevention since the early signs of atherosclerotic alterations are obvious in a person's life.[29] A target LDL-C objective of 77 mg/dL was achieved in 81% of the patients in a study of 33 South Asians with hyperlipidemia after 4 weeks of treatment with 10 mg/day atorvastatin, without statin-related side effects being noted.[30]

Patients at high risk for atherosclerosis participated in the 12-week prospective, open-label ACTFAST (Achieve Cholesterol Targets Fast with Atorvastatin Stratified Titration) trial which compared the effects of atorvastatin on LDL-c in South Asians versus European origin. Atorvastatin reduced LDL-C to a similar extent in both groups after propensity matching (reduction in LDL-C from baseline was 34% in South Asians compared with 38% in Europeans, $p = 0.22$), with no variations in safety being noted.[31] Additionally, statins postmarketing data have not revealed any specific safety concerns in South Asians.[32] In adult Indian patients with dyslipidemia (mean LDL-C > 160 mg/dL and TG >400 mg/dL), Jayaram et al. 2004[33] compared the use of rosuvastatin 10 mg/day with atorvastatin 10 mg/day. The fall in the mean

LDL-C levels after 6 weeks of treatment in the rosuvastatin group was 40%, compared with 30% in the atorvastatin group.

In a pharmacokinetic study of rosuvastatin, Asian Indian residents of Singapore had greater peak plasma concentrations and longer serum half-lives than non-Asian Indian residents ($p < 0.0001$).[34] Given their lower statin metabolism, South Asians may experience more statin adverse effects, particularly at larger doses. The greatest statin doses that the United States Food and Drug Administration has permitted are, consequently, lower for Asians than for other groups,[35] and it may be wise to start Asian patients on a lower dose of a statin.

Statin Associated Side Effects

The high intensity statin medication frequently results in adverse effects linked with statins. The likelihood of myopathy and to a lesser extent of rhabdomyolysis appears to rise with increasing statin dose. This is true for lovastatin, simvastatin, pravastatin, rosuvastatin, pitavastatin, and cerivastatin, which was taken off the market in 2001. Neither atorvastatin[36] nor fluvastatin[37] have showed a clear dose-response relationship for myopathy.

Three studies[38]—HOPE-3 (Heart Outcomes Prevention Evaluation-3), JUPITER (Justification for the Use of Statins in Prevention: an Intervention Trial Evaluating Rosuvastatin), and ASPEN (Atorvastatin Study for Prevention of Coronary Heart Disease Endpoints)—reported marginal but statistically significant increases in muscle symptoms (up to 1.4% absolute difference) between statin- and placebo-treated groups. The 2018 American College of Cardiology (ACC)/American Heart Association (AHA) guidelines recommends that a moderate intensity statin should be initiated or continued with the aim to achieve 30–49% reduction in LDL-C levels in patients prone to statin-associated side effects.[39] It is also important to note that the majority of statin trials, including JUPITER, ASCOT-LLA, and PROVE-IT, increased the prevalence of diabetes. A large meta-analysis of the study-level data from 91,140 participants in 13 randomized trials (restricted to CVD outcome trials with >1,000 participants and a follow-up of >1 year) revealed that statin use was linked to a 9% proportional increase [odds ratio (OR) 1.09; 95% CI 1.02–1.17] in the risk of developing diabetes mellitus when compared to placebo or standard care.[40]

Dual PPAR-α/γ agonists

Dual peroxisome proliferator-activated receptor (PPAR)-α/γ agonists have significant PPAR-α and moderate PPAR-γ effects, where one enhances insulin sensitivity and the other enhances plasma lipid profile. The first member of the glitazar class of drugs to be approved as a treatment for diabetes and diabetic dyslipidemia is saroglitazar. Saroglitazar 4 mg demonstrated a 45% drop in serum TG levels compared to the baseline and pioglitazone 45 mg (15.5%), according to a phase III trial, PRESS V (Prospective Randomized Efficacy and Safety study of Saroglitazar) trial. By week 12, saroglitazar had its greatest impact on TG, which persisted through week 24.[41] Saroglitazar 2 mg and 4 mg significantly reduced TG levels by 45.5% and 46.7%, respectively, versus placebo and from baseline in patients who were uncontrolled on atorvastatin, according to results from the PRESS VI trials.[42] Another meta-analysis confirmed that saroglitazar significantly raised creatinine levels as compared to controls in type 2 diabetic patients with hypertriglyceridemia, but it also confirmed the medication's outstanding TG reducing effects.[43] In a real-world evidence research with 5,824 patients with diabetic dyslipidemia, saroglitazar 4 mg raised mean HDL cholesterol levels (up to 9%) from baseline at 12–58 weeks. In nonalcoholic fatty liver disease (NAFLD) patients with diabetic dyslipidemia, it reduced alanine aminotransferase levels and fatty liver (as measured by FibroScan™).[44]

Combination Lipid Lowering Drugs

Exons of NPC1L1 were sequenced by Stitziel et al.[45] in 7,364 CHD patients (844 South Asians) and 14,728 controls (1,107 South Asians). Natural mutations that impair NPC1L1 function have been linked to the lower plasma LDL-C levels and a lower risk of CHD in people of different racial and ethnic origins, including South Asians. This result showed that inhibitory medications like ezetimibe could lower LDL-C levels and CHD risk in South Asians much like in other ethnicities.

The INFINITY study looked at the effects of ezetimibe and statin combination therapy in 64 South Asian Canadians with CHD or diabetes and chronic hypercholesterolemia while taking statins. Patients were assigned to receive either a double dose of their existing statin medication or ezetimibe 10 mg/day coadministered with statin therapy. With an OR (95% CI) of 3.97, accounting for baseline LDL-C levels and adjusting for the age, the proportion of patients achieving target LDL-C (<77 mg/dL) was significantly higher among the ezetimibe plus statin treated patients compared with the statin-doubling group at 6 weeks (68% vs. 36%, respectively; $p = 0.031$). When compared to individuals whose statin dose was doubled, 76% of patients on ezetimibe plus a statin attained their target LDL-C at 12 weeks (adjusted OR 3.31; 95% CI 1.01–10.89; $p = 0.047$).[46] Despite these findings, it is important to note that the current cholesterol treatment guidelines recommend the use of maximum tolerated statin dose before adding a second LDL-C-lowering agent.

Newer Lipid Lowering Drugs

Bempedoic acid is used as an alternative when a statin is contraindicated or if a patient is statin-intolerant, either alone or in combination with other lipid-lowering treatments. It significantly reduced LDL-C levels by 26.5% compared to placebo, while the combination of bempedoic acid and ezetimibe at a fixed dose has reduced LDL-C by 39.2%. Meta-analysis on bempedoic acid show reduced new onset/worsening of diabetes mellitus, but there was an increase in gout incidence.[47] Moreover, results from the CLEAR Wisdom and CLEAR Harmony studies indicated lower levels of high-sensitivity C-reactive protein (hsCRP).[48]

According to CLEAR Outcome trials, over a median of 3.4 years, the risk of death from cardiovascular causes, nonfatal MI, nonfatal stroke, or coronary revascularization was 13% lower with bempedoic acid than with placebo. Bempedoic acid also had a 21% lower LDL-C level than placebo. It is interesting to note that the 30% of the patients in the main-prevention group and the 70% of patients in the secondary-prevention cohort experienced quantitatively higher effects of bempedoic acid on the primary endpoint.[49] Bempedoic acid should be used more frequently in patients with existing atherosclerotic vascular disease and in people at high risk for vascular disease who are unable or unwilling to take statins as a result of the CLEAR Outcomes trial's convincing findings.[50]

The FOURIER (Further Cardiovascular Outcomes Research With PCSK9 Inhibition in Patients With Elevated Risk) trial[51] was the first large-scale randomized controlled trial to demonstrate clear benefit in CVD outcomes with the addition of evolocumab in patients with preexisting CVD maintained on statins, despite the existence of ample data proving the efficacy and safety of evolocumab in LDL-C lowering.[52-56] LDL-C levels were found to be 60% lower from baseline to a median value of 30 mg/dL, and the key endpoint—a composite of MI, CVD mortality, stroke, coronary revascularization, or unstable angina requiring hospitalization—had decreased by 15% relative. The most current findings from the ODYSSEY Outcomes (Evaluation of Cardiovascular Outcomes After an Acute Coronary Syndrome During Treatment With Alirocumab) trial support these conclusions. The trial found a significant reduction (15%) in the primary endpoint of major CVD events in 18,924 patients on statins who had an acute coronary syndrome (ACS) in the year prior and an abnormal lipid profile. However, data on the use of proprotein convertase subtilisin/kexin type 9 (PCSK9) inhibitor in the South Asian population is scarce and requires further research.

Low-density Lipoprotein Cholesterol Targets

The recent ESC 2019 guidelines have recommended that in very high CV risk patients of SCORE ≥ 10% with DM and target organ damage: ≥3 major risk factors; or early onset of T1DM of long duration (>20 years), the target reduction of LDL-C level should be <55 mg/dL. Additionally, if in high CV risk patients with a SCORE ≥ 5% and < 10% with markedly elevated TC > 310 mg/dL or LDL-C > 190 mg/dL or BP ≥ 180/110 mm Hg, familial hypercholesterolemia without other major risk factors, DM without target organ damage, with DM duration ≥10 years or other additional risk factor, the target LDL-C levels should be <70 mg/dL. Also in very high and high CV risk categories, the target goals for LDL-C reduction must be ≥50% reduction from the baseline.[1]

CONCLUSION

The management of dyslipidemia in young and asymptomatic South Asians necessitates a multifaceted approach. It is important for South Asians to be aware of their risk of dyslipidemia and to take steps to manage their cholesterol levels. Firstly, screening for dyslipidemia should be performed regularly, starting at an early age, using lipid profile tests that measure TC, LDL-C, HDL-C, and TG levels. A risk assessment incorporating other CVD risk factors such as family history, diabetes, and hypertension should also be considered.

Once diagnosed, lifestyle modifications form the cornerstone of the management. South Asians should be educated on adopting a heart-healthy diet, which includes reducing saturated and transfats, increasing dietary fiber, and promoting consumption of fruits and vegetables. Regular physical activity such as aerobic exercises should be encouraged to improve lipid profiles and overall cardiovascular health.

Pharmacological interventions may be warranted in cases of persistently elevated lipid levels or high-risk individuals. However, large, prospective studies with outcomes data are needed to assess cardiovascular benefit associated with various combination therapies in this patient population. Although statins have been the gold standard for treating hypercholesterolemia for many years, many patients fail to meet their LDL-C objectives or are unable to tolerate cholesterol-lowering therapy because of adverse drug events (ADEs). In patients with clinical ASCVD, ezetimibe and PCSK9 inhibitors have demonstrated favorable outcomes in terms of major adverse cardiovascular events (MACE); nevertheless, multiple clinical outcomes trials for bempedoic acid and the investigational medication inclisiran are still ongoing. The ESC/EAS recommendations groups have stressed the significance of combination treatment, first with ezetimibe and subsequently a PCSK9 inhibitor to attain these targets, with the suggestion of these new lower LDL-C goals in very high-risk and high-risk patient categories. A PCSK9 inhibitor is advised in patients with ACS if the LDL-C objective is not met after 4–6 weeks of maximally tolerated statin treatment and ezetimibe. Although, the given available evidence and cost data for PCSK9 inhibitor are on the higher side for the South Asian population, these novel therapies tailored to the lipoprotein anomaly are currently undergoing phase III clinical trials in high- and very high-risk patients. Patients and clinicians now have nonstatin choices for significant LDL-C reductions and CV benefits as more innovative drugs for hypercholesterolemia gain Food and Drug Administration (FDA) approval. Furthermore, addressing comorbid conditions such as diabetes, hypertension, and obesity is crucial in managing dyslipidemia. An integrated approach involving multidisciplinary care teams, including physicians, dietitians, and exercise specialists, can provide personalized care and facilitate adherence to the treatment plans. Lastly, patient education and regular follow-up are paramount to ensure long-term success in managing dyslipidemia.

To summarize, the management of dyslipidemia in young and asymptomatic South Asians requires a comprehensive approach that combines early screening, lifestyle modifications, pharmacotherapy when necessary, and addressing associated comorbidities. By implementing these strategies, healthcare professionals can contribute to reducing the burden of CVD and improving the long-term health outcomes of South Asian populations.

ONLINE REFERENCES

Please scan the QR code provided at the end of the table of contents for References of this chapter.

CHAPTER

71

Familial Hypercholesterolemia: Diagnosis and Management

Sunil Modi, Ranjan Modi

ABSTRACT

Familial hypercholesterolemia (FH) is the most common genetically determined cardiovascular disease associated with markedly elevated lipids, particularly low-density lipoprotein (LDL) cholesterol which leads to premature cardiovascular disease and likely to be one of the most common reasons of young age coronary events. Most of the cases of FH remain asymptomatic, undiagnosed, and, therefore, untreated until an acute coronary event occurs. Prevalence of heterozygous FH (HeFH) is as high as 1 in 200–250 live births, with a wild guess of >5–6 million Indians having this disorder which makes them more prone for premature myocardial infarction (MI) and sudden cardiac death. Diagnosis of FH is easy but looking for this disease needs high level of suspicion, particularly if one has family history of young age MI or sudden cardiac death. The standard diagnosing criteria such as "Dutch Lipid Clinic Network Criterion" can be applied easily to diagnose FH and to start the treatment at the earliest stage. An attempt is required to educate the public and healthcare providers to be aware of this serious cardiovascular disorder. In this manuscript, we have attempted to give a brief outline to diagnose and treat FH.

Keywords: Familial hypercholesterolemia, genetic dyslipidemia, hereditary lipid disorder.

INTRODUCTION

Familial hypercholesterolemia (FH) is a hereditary condition characterized by the dominant inheritance pattern, resulting in substantial increases in total cholesterol and low-density lipoprotein cholesterol (LDL-C).[1-3] It is a common inherited lipid disorder that greatly increases the risk for cardiovascular (CV) diseases.

Worldwide, an estimated >10 million people have FH, of whom approximately 200,000 die prematurely each year.[4] Despite its high prevalence, approximately 80–85% of individuals with this disorder remain undiagnosed.[5-7] It is estimated that 84% of these individuals are not receiving any lipid-lowering treatment and, therefore, are at very high risk of CV events.

Familial hypercholesterolemia may be homozygous and heterozygous. Homozygous FH (HoFH) patients inherit *FH* genes from both parents and have total cholesterol in the range of 650–1,000 mg/dL with LDL well above 400 mg%. Patients with heterozygous FH (HeFH) inherit *FH* gene from one parent and have total cholesterol levels in the range of 350–550 mg/dL with LDL usually above 200 mg%. The levels of high density lipoprotein cholesterol (HDL-C) and triglycerides are relatively normal in most patients in both of these conditions.

The prevalence of heterozygous FH in the general population is estimated to be approximately 1 in 200–250 individuals, which is approximately twice as high as previously believed.[8] The prevalence of HoFH is around 1 in 1,000,000.

Due to its strong association with an increased susceptibility to premature coronary artery disease (CAD), it is imperative for healthcare practitioners to remain vigilant in identifying the clinical indicators observed during physical examinations, as well as the laboratory values that indicate FH.[9] Timely detection and proactive management aimed at reducing LDL-C levels are crucial in preventing or impeding the advancement of coronary atherosclerosis. Furthermore, by conducting screenings on the first-degree relatives of a patient diagnosed with FH, it is possible to identify and provide care for those individuals who carry the gene associated with this condition.[10]

PATHOPHYSIOLOGY

Genetic mutation leads to deficiency and significant dysfunction of LDL receptors influencing hepatic uptake of LDL particles, as liver is responsible for the processing of roughly 70% of circulating LDL.

The LDL receptor and its autosomal dominant mutation responsible for FH were initially found by Goldstein and Brown in 1985[11,12] who received Nobel prize for this discovery. Subsequently, over 1,700 mutations have been characterized, with approximately 79% of them likely resulting in a hypercholesterolemic phenotype. Approximately 5% and fewer than 1% of instances of FH can be attributed to genetic defects in the genes that encode apolipoprotein B (ApoB) and proprotein convertase subtilisin/kexin type 9 (PCSK9), respectively.[8] The functionality of LDL receptors can range from complete absence to approximately 25% of normal receptor activity.[13]

Elevated LDL results in an augmented uptake of cholesterol in nonhepatic cells, like in monocytes and macrophages, resulting in the production of foam cells which increase plaque built up in coronary arteries, in the skin, resulting in the formation of xanthelasmas, in the cornea leading to early corneal arcus and in the cardiac valves particularly in aortic valve causing aortic stenosis.

Race

There is an increased prevalence of FH observed among specific ethnicities, including those with Finnish, Lebanese, Ashkenazi Jewish, Afrikaner, or French Canadian ancestry. In a recent study of French population, the prevalence of FH was close to 1 in 120.[14]

Sex

The gene responsible for FH is located on chromosome 19, resulting in an inheritance pattern that is consistent across both males and females.

The clinical manifestation of severe hypercholesterolemia in individuals with HeFH occurs at an earlier stage in males compared to females due to the protective effects of hormones that benefit women until the postmenopausal period. While it is possible for a woman without significant risk factors for CAD to not experience symptoms of CAD throughout her lifetime, men are generally less likely to have the same outcome.

Both homozygous girls and boys exhibit an equal susceptibility to experiencing a CV event at a very early stage.

Age

The implications of a faulty LDL receptor and consequent increases in LDL-C levels are apparent from birth. However, the significance of age lies in the fact that individuals who live with persistently elevated LDL-C levels for a longer duration face a greater susceptibility to CAD.

CLINICAL PRESENTATION

Homozygous Familial Hypercholesterolemia

Children with HoFH may present with clinical features of ischemic heart disease, peripheral vascular disease, cerebrovascular disease, aortic stenosis, articular symptoms such as tendinitis or arthralgias and atypical skin lesions.

Young individuals are susceptible to experiencing premature coronary events, with the possibility of sudden mortality or acute myocardial infarction even as early as 1–2 years of age. Survival beyond young adulthood is improbable in the absence of extensive measures aimed at reducing blood cholesterol levels.

As in case of a child with HoFH, it is essential for both parents to have HeFH, they will exhibit significant elevations in LDL-C, with often evidence of premature CAD.

Various forms of xanthomas typically manifest during the initial decade of life. These include:

- Planar xanthomas, which are identifiable in the homozygous state and can be distinguished from other cutaneous xanthomas due to their yellow-to-orange hue, typically appearing on the hands, elbows, buttocks, or knees
- Tuberous xanthomas, which are observed on the hands, elbows, or knees
- Tendon xanthomas, which tend to occur at a later stage, particularly on the extensor tendons of the hands or the Achilles tendon

Corneal arcus, a condition occasionally observed in children and more infrequently even at birth, can manifest as a circumferential opacity in the cornea.

Although the clinical significance of cholesterol accumulation in nonvascular tissue (xanthelasma and corneal arcus) is quite low, with the exception of potential cosmetic concerns, the early identification and treatment of FH associated with these physical signs enable the prevention of potentially serious CV problems.[15,16]

Heterozygous Familial Hypercholesterolemia

The majority of children with HeFH do not exhibit the presence of tendon xanthomas or corneal arcus; however, by the age of 30, a significant proportion (exceeding 60%) will exhibit these manifestation. Similarly, clinical manifestations of CAD/atherosclerotic cardiovascular disease (ASCVD) are quite infrequent in pediatric age group.

Xanthomas are frequently observed on the Achilles tendons and extensor tendons of the metacarpophalangeal joints in the hands.

It is probable that untreated males will experience symptoms of CAD by the fourth decade. There is a delay of roughly 10–15 years in the manifestation of symptoms in women compared to men.

One of the parents is expected to exhibit severe hypercholesterolemia and is likely to have a personal or familial background of early CAD.

Due to the dominant nature of the gene responsible for FH, there is a 50% likelihood that the siblings of an affected patient will also possess heterozygous FH.

One or more first-degree relatives may exhibit premature CAD, significant hypercholesterolemia, or observable tendon xanthomas on their hands.

DIAGNOSIS

The primary method for diagnosing FH relies on the identification of significant elevations in LDL-C levels. The presence of a significant elevation in serum triglyceride levels should prompt consideration of an alternative lipid condition.[17,18]

The Dutch Lipid Clinic Network (DLCN) criteria produce scores leading to classification of either definite or probable FH. Numerical score definition of FH according to the DLCN is as below:

- *Family history*:
  - First-degree relative with known premature CAD or vascular disease (≤55 years for men; ≤60 years for women): 1 point
  - First-degree relative with known hypercholesterolemia: 1 point
  - First-degree relative with tendinous xanthomas: 2 points
  - Offspring(s)/children aged less than 18 years with known hypercholesterolemia: 2 point
- *Personal history:*
  - Of premature CAD (≤55 years for men; ≤60 years for women): 2 points
  - Of premature cerebral/peripheral vascular disease (PVD) (≤55 years for men; ≤60 years for women): 1 point
- *Physical examination:*
  - Tendinous xanthomas: 6 points
  - Arcus cornealis prior to age of 45 years: 4 points
- *Untreated LDL-C levels:*
  - >8.5 mmol/L or >325 mg%: 8 points
  - 6.5–8.4 mmol/L or 250–324 mg%: 5 points
  - 5.0–6.4 mmol/L or 190–249 mg%: 3 points
  - 4.0–4.9 mmol/L or 155–189 mg%: 1 point
- *DNA analysis:*
  - Functional mutation in the *LDLR, ApoB*, or *PCSK9* gene: 8 points
- *Diagnosis of FH (based on the total number of points obtained)*:
  - Definite familial hypercholesterolemia: >8 points
  - Probable familial hypercholesterolemia: 6–8 points
  - Possible familial hypercholesterolemia: 3–5 points
  - Unlikely: <3 points[19-22]

TREATMENT

The treatment guidelines outlined in the 2013 consensus statement by the European Atherosclerosis Society (EAS) for screening and treatment of FH are as follows:[22-25]

- The recommended LDL goal for children aged 8–10 years is <135 mg/dL, for adults <100 mg/dL, and for patients with CHD and or diabetes <70 mg/dL.
- The management of individuals with FH entails a multifaceted approach that includes implementing modifications to one's lifestyle, initiating statin as the primary intervention, and adding other proven LDL-lowering drugs on case-to-case basis.

Therapeutic Lifestyle Modifications

Lifestyle modifications as a primary intervention are to be emphasized and implicated in all cases. However, it is important to note that these modifications alone are unlikely to achieve desirable levels of LDL-C. Consequently, the use of cholesterol-lowering agents, typically multiple, becomes necessary in such cases.[26,27] It is also pertinent to note in the case of homozygous individuals, the effect of dietary modifications on LDL is minimal due to the absence of receptors to upregulate. Nevertheless, lifestyle adjustments can still provide additional CV advantages and should be vigorously advocated for.[26,27]

Substantial dietary modifications in these patients of FH can reduce cholesterol/LDL by around 15%. Minimizing the consumption of saturated fat, trans fat, and cholesterol outweighs the significance of limiting overall fat intake. Diets with significant reduction in overall fat content tend to be rich in carbs, potentially leading to elevated triglycerides and decreased levels of HDL-C. The replacement of carbohydrates with monounsaturated fats, such as olive and canola oils, avocados, and nuts, does not result in a rise in LDL-C, rather in the absence of weight gain, may lead to an increase in HDL and a decrease in triglyceride levels among those who have adhered to a low-fat diet. Carbohydrates should contribute not >50–60% of total energy intake and should comprise mainly of complex carbs, such as whole grains, legumes, as well as fruits and vegetables. These food items also possess a notable amount of soluble fiber, which has been observed to have a modest impact of reducing cholesterol levels by around 5%. Additionally, they exhibit significant levels of antioxidants and flavonoids, which have the potential to provide protection against CV diseases. Hydrogenated fats and trans fats, which are commonly included in a variety of food products, including margarines, cakes, cookies, crackers, should be avoided in one's diet as they have the propensity to elevate LDL-C and reduce HDL-C.

It is important to get a weight that is considered desirable. Substantial reduction in body weight is expected to improve many lipid markers, including LDL-C, HDL-C, and triglycerides.

Engaging in aerobic and toning workouts for durations exceeding 30 minutes, on at least four occasions each week, has been shown to improve blood lipid levels.

Drug Management in Familial Hypercholesterolemia

In addition to therapeutic lifestyle changes, almost all of the patients of FH will need high doses of statins to start with. Additionally, many other group of drugs such as ezetimibe, PCSK9 inhibitors, inclisiran, adenosine triphosphate-citrate lyase (ACL) inhibitors (bempedoic acid), angiopoietin-like 3 (ANGPTL3) inhibitor (evinacumab), probucol, bile acid sequestrants, and niacin have shown efficacy in managing the condition.[28] Estrogen replacement therapy has also demonstrated effectiveness in postmenopausal women; however, caution is advised due to the potential adverse effects in older women, and potential advantages may be balanced with associated hazards.

New medicines, such as lomitapide with or without apheresis, may be regarded as supplementary therapeutic options for individuals who fail to attain the recommended LDL-C levels and continue to face a heightened risk of CV events.

Nondrug Management of Familial Hypercholesterolemia

In cases when the LDL receptors are either absent or nonfunctional as is the case with HoFH, it is imperative to consider one of the following options as a necessary course of action.

Low-density Lipoprotein Apheresis

Lipoprotein apheresis may be required in many cases of HoFH with severely elevated LDL and should be initiated, if available, as early as possible, ideally at a minimum age of 5 years and should not be delayed beyond the age of 8 years.

Low-density lipoprotein apheresis entails the targeted elimination of lipoproteins containing ApoB using various methods such as heparin precipitation, dextran sulfate cellulose columns, or immunoadsorption columns. All approaches exhibit a reduction in LDL-C levels to the level exceeding 50%, while simultaneously decreasing lipoprotein(a), VLDL, and triglyceride levels. HDL is preserved. The operation typically requires a minimum of 3 hours to complete and is conducted at intervals of 1–2 weeks. A limited number of unfavorable incidents are encountered, the majority of which consist of noncritical occurrences of hypotension. LDL apheresis is a process that incurs significant costs and is not easily accessible.[29,30]

According to a study conducted by Drouin-Chartier et al., it was found that the efficacy of dextran sulfate adsorption in reducing LDL-C levels through LDL apheresis is inversely correlated with the initial blood triglyceride levels in individuals with HoFH, whereas LDL apheresis, facilitated by heparin-induced extracorporeal LDL precipitation, was not significantly influenced by the levels of serum triglycerides prior to apheresis.[31]

Surgical Options

Portacaval Anastomosis

It is a surgical procedure that involves creating a connection between the portal vein and the inferior vena cava. In contrast to liver transplantation, this particular surgery is characterized by a lower level of risk and does not necessitate the use of immunosuppressive medication. While the reduction in cholesterol levels may not be as significant as observed in transplantation or apheresis, the therapeutic advantages seem to be similar.

A reduction of 50% in LDL-C levels has been recorded, accompanied with verified regression of coronary lesions, aortic lesions, and xanthomas. The precise process through which LDL-C is reduced remains uncertain.

Liver Transplantation

Liver transplantation is a treatment option for individuals with HoFH. It results in the provision of functional LDL receptors, leading to significant reductions in LDL-C levels. The performance of liver transplantation is infrequent due to the significant dangers inherent in the surgical procedure and the need for prolonged immunosuppressive therapy.

Gene Therapy

It is a promising field of biomedical research that involves the manipulation and alteration of genes in order to treat or prevent genetic disorders.

Pharmacological Treatment of Familial Hypercholesterolemia

Patients with HeFH who possess up to 50% functioning LDL receptors do exhibit a favorable response to conventional cholesterol-lowering medications. This may not be the case in patients of HoFH because they have very few or no LDL receptors.

Statins

In order to achieve the desired LDL-C targets, it is advised to utilize high dosage of one of the three most potent statins: simvastatin, atorvastatin, or rosuvastatin, in conjunction with one or more additional medications that lower LDL levels, such as Ezetimibe. It is recommended to administer a statin dosage that is one level below the maximum dose to mitigate the risk of myopathy. Given that increasing the dosage of any statin results in a mere 6–7% further reduction in LDL-C, it is more efficacious to introduce additional agent such as Ezetimibe with lower dose of statins.[32] A comprehensive analysis of five clinical studies investigating statin medication demonstrated that the use of intensive-dose treatment was linked to a higher likelihood of developing diabetes in comparison to the use of moderate dosing.[33]

According to a study, it has been shown that rosuvastatin may exhibit a decelerating effect on the progression of atherosclerosis in children with heterozygous FH. In the CHARON trial, a randomized study involving 196 children and adolescents aged 6–17 years with heterozygous FH and 65 unaffected sibling controls, the administration of rosuvastatin to affected patients for a duration of 2 years demonstrated a deceleration in the progression of subclinical atherosclerosis (as evidenced by various sources).[34-36] Initially, individuals with heterozygous FH exhibited a significantly higher mean carotid intima-media thickness (IMT) of 0.398 mm compared to their healthy siblings with a mean IMT of 0.376 mm. However, after the 2-year treatment period with rosuvastatin, there was no discernible difference in the mean carotid IMT between the two groups. Furthermore, 38% of the individuals receiving rosuvastatin achieved the target LDL-C level of <110 mg/dL. It is worth noting that >85% of patients in the treatment group reported experiencing only mild adverse events, such as headaches, nasopharyngitis, and influenza-like symptoms.[34]

Bempedoic Acid: Inhibitor of the Adenosine Triphosphate Citrate Lyase

Bempedoic acid is a recent significant milestone in lipid-lowering therapy as it is the first inhibitor of ACL. The enzyme ACL is positioned upstream of HMG-CoA reductase in the cholesterol production pathway, hence playing a role in the reduction of hepatic synthesis of LDL-C.

Bempedoic acid is recommended for adult patients who have HeFH or have established ASCVD and require further reduction in LDL levels. It is used in conjunction with dietary modifications and the maximum dosage of statin medication that the patient can tolerate.

The approval of bempedoic acid was predicated on the results obtained from the phase-3 clinical studies known as CLEAR Harmony and CLEAR Wisdom. The inclusion of bempedoic acid in a treatment regimen consisting of the maximum tolerable dosage of statins led to an average reduction in LDL-C levels that was 18% greater than that observed in the placebo group, after accounting for the placebo effect.[37,38]

Bempedoic acid in combination with ezetimibe to maximally tolerated statins resulted in a significant reduction of 38% in LDL-C levels, as compared to the placebo group.[39]

PCSK9 Inhibitors

The PCSK9 inhibitors are recommended as a supplement to dietary changes and the maximum tolerated statin therapy for managing adults with HeFH or clinical ASCVD, who need further reduction of LDL.

Alirocumab

The ODYSSEY LONG TERM study assessed the efficacy and safety of administering alirocumab at a dosage of 150 mg subcutaneously every 2 weeks. In a study known as ODYSSEY COMBO I, the addition of alirocumab to the current standard of care, which includes maximally tolerated statins, resulted in a 58% reduction in LDL-C compared to a placebo after 24 weeks. Similarly, when 75 mg was used as an adjunct to statins, it led to an additional 45% reduction in LDL-C compared to a placebo after 12 weeks. Furthermore, at week 24 in the same trial, alirocumab led to an additional 44% reduction in LDL-C compared to a placebo. In the present investigation, if there was a need for further reduction of LDL-C as determined by predetermined criteria at week 8, the dosage of alirocumab was increased to 150 mg at week 12 throughout the duration of the trial. A total of 83% of patients maintained their initial dosage of 75 mg.

The approval of alirocumab as an adjunctive treatment, in combination with existing LDL lowering medicines for the management of HoFH was predicated on the findings of the ODYSSEY HoFH trial, which demonstrated a substantial drop in LDL-C levels among individuals afflicted with the condition.[40]

Evolocumab

Evolocumab has been granted approval for administration to both adult individuals and children between the ages of 10 and 17 who have been diagnosed with HoFH.

The approval of evolocumab was predicated on the findings of the OSLER (Open-Label trial of Long-term Evaluation Against LDL-C) trial. Over the course of approximately 1 year of therapy, the administration of evolocumab in conjunction with standard therapy demonstrated a significant reduction in LDL-C levels when compared to standard therapy alone.[41,42] Furthermore, analysis revealed that the evolocumab group experienced a decrease in the rate of CV events at 1 year as compared to the standard-therapy group.[41]

The HAUSER-RCT study provided confirmation of the effectiveness and safety of evolocumab in pediatric individuals between the ages of 10 and 17 who had HeFH. The study enrolled a total of 157 participants who were randomly assigned to receive either evolocumab (n = 104) or placebo (n = 53). At the 24th week, the evolocumab group exhibited a mean reduction of 44.5% in LDL levels, while the placebo group showed a mean decrease of 6.2%.[43]

The Trial Assessing Long Term Use of PCSK9 Inhibition in Subjects With Genetic LDL Disorders (TAUSSIG) conducted an interim subset analysis which demonstrated the efficacy of evolocumab in decreasing LDL-C in individuals with HoFH, even in the absence of apheresis treatment. The participants in the trial received subcutaneous therapy of evolocumab at a dosage of 420 mg either on a monthly basis or, if they were also having apheresis, every 2 weeks. Additionally, patients who were not undergoing apheresis had the opportunity to raise their dosage frequency to every 2 weeks after 12 weeks of treatment. The findings of the study revealed that over a 12-week period, there was a significant reduction of 20.6% in the mean LDL-C level, accompanied by a notable increase of 7.6% in the mean HDL-C level. Patients who were not undergoing apheresis and chose to extend their dose frequency to every 2 weeks observed an additional average reduction of 8.3% in LDL-C levels.[30,44,45]

Lomitapide (Microsomal Triglyceride Transfer Protein Inhibitor)

It belongs to the category of first-in-class inhibitors of microsomal triglyceride transfer protein (MTP). It has been granted approval for its use as a supplementary treatment, in conjunction with a low-fat diet and other lipid-lowering therapies, such as LDL apheresis when accessible. This approval was specifically for the purpose of reducing levels of LDL-C, triglycerides, ApoB, and non-HDL-C in individuals diagnosed with HoFH. Due to the heightened potential for hepatotoxicity associated with lomitapide, its dispensation is exclusively facilitated through a program that imposes restrictions on access. The approval decision was made following a limited trial including a cohort of 29 individuals who were administered lomitapide. Among these participants, 23 were exposed to the drug for a duration of 1 year, 15 were treated for 2 years, and 5 were exposed for 3 years. Initially, the average LDL-C level in individuals with HoFH was recorded as 336 mg/dL. Following a 26-week treatment period, there was a significant reduction of 50% in LDL-C levels ($p < 0.0001$).[46]

According to a literature review conducted by Liu et al., it was shown that lomitapide has the ability to lower LDL-C, total cholesterol, ApoB, and triglyceride levels in patients with HoFH, even in the absence of other lipid-lowering medications. However, it was also observed that lomitapide leads to a drop in HDL-C and ApoA1 values. This information was revealed in a study conducted by Liu et al.[47]

ANGPTL3 Inhibitor (Evinacumab)

It is a biotechnologically engineered human monoclonal antibody that effectively binds to and has inhibitory effects on ANGPTL3. The inhibition of lipoprotein lipase and endothelial lipase by ANGPTL3 leads to a decrease in lipid metabolism. The inhibition of ANGPTL3 through the administration of evinacumab results in enhanced lipid metabolism, hence causing a reduction in levels of LDL, HDL, and triglycerides.

It has been granted approval as a supplementary treatment for HoFH in individuals aged 12 years and above with the concurrent use of other LDL lowering medicines. The inclusion criteria were broadened in March 2023 to encompass individuals as young as 5 years old. The decision to widen the criteria was informed by the results of the phase-3 ELIPSE trial, which involved a sample size of 65 participants. According to the study, individuals who were receiving consistent lipid-lowering medication and were given a regular intravenous infusion of evinacumab every 4 weeks experienced a significant decrease in their LDL-C level by 47.1% at week 24. In contrast, patients who received a placebo treatment showed a minimal increase of 1.9% in their LDL-C level.

Probucol

Probucol, a pharmaceutical agent characterized by modest reductions in LDL and an unfavorable decrease in HDL, has demonstrated efficacy in inducing regression of cutaneous and tendon xanthomas in individuals affected by both homozygous and heterozygous FH. A study utilizing an animal model has exhibited a decrease in coronary atherosclerosis. There is a lack of evidence of long-term benefits of probucol for patients diagnosed with FH.

Inclisiran

Inclisiran in ORION-10 and ORION-11 trial reduced LDL by 52.3% and 49.9% respectively and was approved as an add on treatment for adults with clinical ASCVD, for those cases where further reduction of LDL-C was necessary.[48] However very recently, in July 2023, the scope of approval was broadened to encompass heterozygous FH.

PREVENTION OF CORONARY ARTERY DISEASE IN FAMILIAL HYPERCHOLESTEROLEMIA

The identification of relatives who possess the *FH* gene, enables the implementation of medicinal interventions aimed at averting the onset of CAD in individuals.

In addition to the management of hypercholesterolemia, it is imperative to identify and address other CV risk factors in a proactive and comprehensive manner. It is recommended that patients be advised diet modification, to initiate aerobic activity and, if deemed appropriate, to engage in a weight-loss regimen.

PROGNOSIS

The prognosis is significantly influenced by the degree to which LDL-C levels can be decreased. Individuals diagnosed with HoFH have a significantly restricted lifespan in the absence of substantial medical intervention.

The mitigation of additional modifiable risk factors, such as smoking, hypertension, and diabetes, has been shown to further reduce the likelihood of developing CAD.

Due to the absence of long-term prospective research involving individuals with FH, making accurate predictions regarding enhanced outcomes is challenging.

PATIENT INFORMATION AND COUNSELING

It is imperative for adult patients diagnosed with FH to possess a comprehensive understanding of their elevated susceptibility to premature CAD. It is crucial to underscore the significance of adhering to dietary and pharmacological interventions for the management of hypercholesterolemia.

It is imperative to identify additional risk variables that can be modified, and to elucidate their cumulative influence on the likelihood of experiencing a CV event. Provide support for individuals seeking to quit smoking. Elucidate the significance of exercise and adequate weight reduction in relation to the lipid and CV consequences, as well as the prevention or amelioration of diabetes and hypertension.

CONCLUSION

Familial hypercholesterolemia is a common genetic disorder, less known, less understood, underdiagnosed, and, therefore, neglected and undertreated. FH can be responsible for many of the young, premature myocardial infarctions and sudden cardiac deaths. Heterozygous form, which is the common variety of FH (>99.9% of total FH), is treatable to a great extent with use of standard LDL-lowering therapies but it is important that therapy should be started quite early in pediatric or adolescent life to gain maximum benefits. The newer lipid-lowering therapeutic agents are very effective and safe and are being gradually approved for add on uses in children and adolescents. The significance and method of early recognition of this potentially lethal disorder should be highlighted in all scientific meetings and knowledge should be distributed to all healthcare providers and public. Lipid profile, particularly LDL, should be checked as early as possible in one's lifetime, especially in those who have premature CAD event in their parents or in first blood relations.

ONLINE REFERENCES

Please scan the QR code provided at the end of the table of contents for References of this chapter.

CHAPTER 72

Overview of Data on How Low Low-density Lipoprotein is Optimal for Secondary Prevention of Cardiovascular Diseases

Gaurav Agarwal, Auriom Kar,
Rathindra Nath Karmakar, Sunandan Sikdar

ABSTRACT

Secondary prevention of cardiovascular events is of utmost importance to reduce mortality and morbidity. Successive guidelines have advocated further low-density lipoprotein cholesterol (LDL-C) lowering. However, some adverse effects of very low LDL-C have been described. This article reviews the benefits and risks of achieving very low LDL levels in order to explore the question how low should we go and in whom.

Keywords: Very low LDL-C, MACE, new onset diabetes, hemorrhagic stroke.

INTRODUCTION

Successive lipid guidelines have advocated lower and lower low-density lipoprotein (LDL) targets to reduce adverse cardiovascular (CV) events especially in secondary prevention. For secondary prevention in very high-risk patients, European Society of Cardiology has recommended a LDL cholesterol (LDL-C) reduction of >50% from baseline and an LDL-C goal of <1.4 mmol/L (<55 mg/dL).[1] For patients with atherosclerotic cardiovascular disease (ASCVD) who experience a second vascular event within 2 years (not necessarily of the same type as the first event) while taking maximally tolerated statin therapy, an LDL-C goal of <1.0 mmol/L (<40 mg/dL) is to be attained. The cut-off value of very low LDL has been kept at <40 mg/dL or <30 mg/dL in literature. Primary concerns in this approach are the safety and efficacy. Is there any relative benefit further reducing LDL to very low levels? Is there any adverse effect at these levels? This short overview is based on data concerning these aspects **(Table 1)**.

TABLE 1: Benefits and risks of lowering LDL-C to very low levels.

Benefits	Risks
Reduction of composite of: • Cardiovascular mortality • Myocardial infarction • Ischemic stroke • Coronary revascularization • Unstable angina • Peripheral arterial disease	• New-onset diabetes • Hemorrhagic stroke (inconclusive evidence) • Cataract (doubtful) • Cognitive decline (doubtful)
Coronary plaque regression	

(LDL-C: low-density lipoprotein cholesterol)

MEASUREMENT

An important aspect concerns the accuracy of measurement at low concentration of LDL.[2] The gold standard of measurement is beta quantification (ultracentrifugation). However, because of its cost and time required, it is seldom used. Direct measurement of LDL is by homogenous assays and is also increasing in popularity, but this method requires validation. Indirect methods of derivation are based on estimation of total cholesterol, high-density lipoprotein (HDL), and triglyceride and its application into an equation. Three equations are available. The most widely used is the Friedewald's equation. Its main limitation is that it cannot be used if—(1) the triglyceride level is >400 g/dL (2) in low LDL-C <70 mg/dL. Martin Hopkin's equation,[3] on the other hand, is useful in case of low LDL-C (<70 mg/dL) while Sampson's equation is useful in cases of high triglyceride levels (even up to 800 mg/dL). The importance of LDL measurement lies in the fact that using Martin Hopkin's equation may yield differing result from that of Friedewald's formula, thus reclassifying patients and lead to use of additional lipid-lowering drugs such as ezetimibe or proprotein convertase subtilisin/kexin type 9 (PCSK9) inhibitors.

Timing and Frequency of Measurement

Before starting lipid-lowering drug treatment, at least two measurements should be made, with an interval of 1–12 weeks, with the exception of conditions where prompt drug treatment is suggested, such as acute coronary syndrome (ACS) and very high-risk patients.[1] Measurement should be repeated after 2 months either after starting treatment or adjustment of dose. Once the target is achieved, annual measurement is enough. Measurement of liver enzymes [alanine transaminase (ALT)] should be done before initiation and after 2 months. Rise of enzyme more than three times upper limit of normal is an indication to discontinue therapy. Muscle enzyme creatinine phosphokinase (CPK) should be measured before initiation and if >4 times normal, statin initiation is withheld.

During the first day of ACS, LDL-C levels tend to decrease and, therefore, a lipid profile should be obtained as soon as possible after admission for ACS. Patients do not have to be fasting as this has little impact on LDL-C levels.[1] Lipid-lowering treatment should be initiated as early as possible to increase patient adherence after discharge. Lipid levels should be re-evaluated 4–6 weeks after ACS to determine whether treatment goals have been achieved.

BENEFIT

So, is very low LDL-C atheroprotective as levels continue to decrease? The GLAGOV study[4] used intracoronary intravascular ultrasound to evaluate atheroma volume while using evolocumab. Patients on evolocumab had lower LDL-C {36.6 vs. 93.0 mg/dL; difference—56.5 mg/dL [95% confidence interval (CI) –59.7 to –53.4]; $p < 0.001$}, slightly decreased percent atheroma volume (PAV) ($p < 0.001$), lower normalized total atheroma volume (TAV) ($p < 0.001$), and modest atherosclerotic plaques. A linear relationship between achieved LDL-C and PAV regression was found ranging from 110 mg/dL to as low as 20 mg/dL. There was significant reduction in the composite of CV death, myocardial infarction (MI), ischemic stroke, coronary revascularization, and unstable angina, in those with very low levels compared to patients with LDL-C values >30 mg/dL.

In FOURIER trial, which included 27,564 patients with atherosclerotic CV disease, the addition of evolocumab to statin therapy (69% under high intensity therapy) resulted in a 15% relative risk reduction of the composite primary endpoint throughout a 2.2-year follow-up. Results were similar in the subgroup of patients with a history of MI (81% of all patients). A subanalysis of the FOURIER trial showed that patients who achieved the lowest LDL-C values under PCSK9 treatment also had the lowest risk of future major adverse cardiac event (MACE).[5] An unexpected benefit was also noticed. A post hoc analysis of FOURIER showed that PCSK9 inhibition reduced venous thromboembolism (VTE) events by 46% [hazard ratio (HR) 0.54; 95% CI 0.33–0.88; $p = 0.014$] beyond 1 year.[6]

In a prespecified analysis of ODYSSEY OUTCOMES trial[7] in patients eligible for >3 years follow-up, alirocumab reduced all-cause death (HR 0.78; 95% CI 0.65–0.94; $p = 0.01$). A post hoc spline analysis from the above trial showed that in the alirocumab group all-cause mortality declines with lower achieved LDL-C levels, down to an LDL-C level of 30 mg/dL (adjusted p value for model = 0.017 for linear trend). Whether all-cause mortality continues to decrease for LDL-C below 30 mg/dL is still unclear.

In PROVE IT-TIMI 22, it was shown that achieving very low LDL < 40 mg/dL led to fewer cardiac events (death, MI, stroke, recurrent ischemia, and revascularization) compared to those having a higher level.[8]

The results of the SPARCL trial[9] among patients with recent stroke or transient ischemic attack (TIA) and no known coronary heart disease showed that atorvastatin reduced the first occurrence of stroke and of a composite of vascular events relative to placebo. Following ischemic stroke or TIA, patients are at risk not only of recurrent cerebrovascular events, but also of other major CV events, including MI. *Secondary prevention therapy with statins reduces the risk of recurrent stroke (by 12% per mmol/L reduction in LDL-C, MI, and vascular death).* So, there is a continuum of incrementally better outcomes as LDL goes down.

There are currently no available clinical trials on the reduction of CV risk with lipid-lowering therapy in patients affected by abdominal aneurysm or renal atherosclerosis. In patients with peripheral artery disease (PAD), lipid-lowering therapy, including a maximum tolerated dose of statin, plus ezetimibe, or a combination with a PCSK9 inhibitor if needed, is recommended to reduce the risk of ASCVD events.

Side Effect of LDL Reduction to Very Low Levels

Four conditions have been under consideration as side effect of statin-related extreme lipid lowering: (1) diabetes mellitus, (2) hemorrhagic stroke, (3) cognitive dysfunction, and (4) cataract. To understand whether lipid lowering per se causes these conditions, it is worth studying certain special population subsets who have very low LDL.

The very low (<30 mg/dL) LDL-C can be found in patients with genetic conditions characterized by hypocholesterolemia, in patients undergoing pharmacological treatment with lipid-lowering agents and transiently post LDL apheresis.

Low LDL-C Genetic Syndromes

The genetic conditions provide us with an idea about the prognosis and outcomes related to these levels—a peek into the future. Loss-of-function mutations in *PCSK9* gene, familial hypobetalipoproteinemia, abetalipoproteinemia, familial combined hypolipidemia, chylomicron retention disease, and Smith–Lemli–Opitz syndrome are genetic conditions characterized by congenital, lifelong, and very low LDL-C.[2]

The PCSK9 loss of function mutations and familial combined hypolipidemia (*ANGPTL3* mutation) does not lead to significant manifestations. Abetalipoproteinemia (*MTP* mutation) does have neurological deficits related to lack of lipid-soluble vitamins which can be treated by addition of vitamin E. However, nearly absent LDL-C does not seem to be the cause of these symptoms. Familial hypobetalipoproteinemia (*ApoB* mutation) may have hepatic steatosis and subsequent liver cirrhosis as presentation. Steatorrhea (fat malabsorption), decreased bone density, and demyelinating neuropathy which characterizes chylomicron retention disease (*SAR18* mutation) can have an LDL-C as low as 20 mg/dL but not the manifestations considered to be related to LDL lowering. Similar is the case with Smith–Lemli–Opitz syndrome (7DHC reductase mutation), which has syndromic features like growth and mental retardation and cardiac defects.[2]

Statin and Diabetes

Several meta-analyses have found 9% increased risk for diabetes over 4 years of statin therapy. Special attention should be paid to older patients or people with metabolic syndrome on statin therapy regarding potential development of new onset of diabetes.[10-12]

In individuals with normal glycemic control, statins increased HbA1c (mean difference 1.33%; 95% CI 1.31–1.35) in comparison with the placebo groups. The dose or type of statins did not modulate the diabetogenic effect. Statins slightly but significantly raise indices of diabetes in individuals with either adequate or altered glycemic control. This is in contrast to the PCSK9 inhibitors where these changes do not take place.

Several mechanistic hypotheses have been proposed to explain the link between statin treatment and new-onset diabetes (NOD), including changes in calcium channel function in pancreatic beta-cells, inhibition of GLUT4 translocation,[13] decreased cell signaling, and decreased adiponectin levels that may interact with insulin secretion and glucose homeostasis. No excess of NOD was observed with PCSK9 inhibitors even if patients in the active group achieved very low LDL-C level. In contrast, PCSK9 inhibitors only target circulating PCSK9 having limited impact on LDL receptor expression in pancreatic islet and hence does not cause cholesterol accumulation and β-cell dysfunction.

Low LDL-C and Intracranial Hemorrhage

Stroke Prevention by Aggressive Reduction in Cholesterol Levels (SPARCL) was a randomized trial of high-dose atorvastatin versus placebo in 4,731 patients with a recent stroke. It was found that although overall MI/stroke was reduced, intracranial hemorrhage (ICH) was observed in 55 patients for atorvastatin 80 mg versus 33 in the placebo group (0.011% vs. 0.006%; HR 1.66; $p = 0.02$). Despite this very low absolute number, this raised the possibility of harm.[9] A post hoc analysis of SPARCL showed that ICH was more frequent in patients with a history of hemorrhagic stroke at entry, but the small number of individuals did not allow definitive conclusions. On note, risk of ICH was neither related to the LDL-C levels at entry nor during follow-up.

On the other hand, IMPROVE-IT trial and Cholesterol Treatment Trialists (CTT) trial did not show any increase in ICH. Therefore, further studies are needed to confirm or refute whether ICH is indeed related to statins.

A meta-analysis of observational studies proposed a putative mechanism for ICH. Low LDL-C may play a role in promoting arterial medial layer smooth muscle cell necrosis increasing the risk of developing microaneurysms that are the chief pathological finding of intracranial hemorrhagic events.[14]

Although PCSK9 inhibitors lower LDL-C more than statins do, there was no excess hemorrhagic stroke risk with PCSK9 inhibitors ($p = 0.99$).

Low LDL-C and Cognition

The OSLER study showed that patients receiving evolocumab/statin treatment reported statistically more neurocognitive events (delirium, cognitive and attention disorders, dementia and amnestic conditions, disturbances in thinking and perception, and mental impairment disorders) compared to patients on statin monotherapy (0.9% vs. 0.3%); the risk of neurocognitive events did not significantly vary between patients achieving very low LDL-C and patients who did not.[15] However, brain cholesterol regulation is primarily dependent upon local de novo cholesterol synthesis in the brain rather than levels of circulating plasma cholesterol.[16] Therefore, lipid-lowering agents, which decrease peripheral LDL-C, are unlikely to have significant impact on brain cholesterol levels. Thus, EBBINGHAUS, a sub-study of FOURIER, investigated the effect of evolocumab on neurocognitive function and found no difference in cognitive function between the evolocumab/statin versus statin-only groups at a median of 19 months.

Low LDL-C and Cataract

In the HOPE-3 trial, individuals in the 10-mg rosuvastatin per day group had a statistically significant greater number of cataract surgeries than in the placebo group.[17] Pooled data from 14 alirocumab trials (though not including ODYSSEY OUTCOMES' data) showed that the rate of cataracts was higher in patients with LDL-C < 25 mg/dL (2.6%) versus > 25 mg/dL (HR 3.40; 95% CI 1.58–7.35). However, other studies in patients with very low LDL-C did not find any significant correlation between very low LDL-C and cataract development.

Low LDL-C and Cancer

With large numbers and significant patients/years of follow-up, no warning signal was ever observed regarding low LDL-C and cancer incidence with statins.[2]

CONCLUSION

Recent findings confirm that intensive decrease of LDL-C to *very low (<30 mg/dL) levels* is associated with *further* CV benefits by reducing ischemic events, which clearly contrast with the small possible increase in adverse effects, leading to a *major net* clinical benefit in *selected cases of high to extremely high-risk atherosclerotic patients.*

ONLINE REFERENCES

Please scan the QR code provided at the end of the table of contents for References of this chapter.

CHAPTER

73 Rare Treatment for Rare Dyslipidemia

Saumitra Ray, Srina Ray

ABSTRACT

Rare dyslipidemia is a group of diseases that occur very rarely in the population, typically with a prevalence of 5 per 10,000, and involves one or the other lipoprotein fraction in blood. Most common among these disorders is familial hypercholesterolemia (FH), both homozygous and heterozygous, but the latter is not really a rare disease. Apart from FH, rare dyslipidemia includes low levels of low-density lipoprotein (LDL), high and low levels of high-density lipoproteins (HDLs) and high and low levels of triglyceride (TG). Most of these disorders are genetic in origin, some being monogenic, and the rest are polygenic in nature. The inheritance may be very complex with autosomal recessive (AR), autosomal dominant (AD) or autosomal codominant (ACD) patterns with variable penetrance. All these make the clinical and pathological diagnosis rather complicated. The development of therapy is also slow due to few patients available for phase 3 trials, the slim chance of recovering the cost of a new drug development and the complicated pattern of clinical and biochemical abnormalities. Disorders with high LDL are treated in the usual line of hypercholesterolemia, but more aggressively, using high dose and early institution of statins, ezetimibe, proprotein convertase subtilisin/kexin type 9 inhibitor (PCSK9I), and inclisiran. Newer drugs like lomitapide and evinacumab and procedures like plasmapheresis and liver transplant are used in selected cases. Other rare diseases are treated symptomatically, with specific drugs available only for a few selected conditions.

Keywords: Rare diseases, dyslipidemia.

INTRODUCTION

Lipoprotein disorders causing dyslipidemia are very common conditions mainly manifesting as atherosclerotic cardiovascular disease (ASCVD). However, there are many lipoprotein disorders which are rare. Though to ascribe a disease as rare is somewhat arbitrary, there are some agreements regarding definition of rare disease between the American and the European authorities. The incidence of 5 or less per 10,000 populations generally qualifies a disease as rare, but usually it has to be life-threatening or chronically disabling. Interestingly, the US Food and Drug Administration also require a condition to be designated as rare if cost of development of the treatment of the disease is deemed not to be recoverable.

Most of the rare dyslipidemia are genetically determined, and genome sequencing and gene-based therapies are required for proper management of the patients. However, the diagnosis is often complicated due to varying phenotypical manifestation. The rare lipoprotein disorders usually involve either very high or very low blood levels of low-density lipoprotein cholesterol (LDL-C), high-density lipoprotein cholesterol (HDL-C), or triglyceride (TG).

Recently, the European Atherosclerosis Society (EAS) task force has published a consensus statement to help clinicians to manage patients with rare dyslipidemia.[1]

TYPES OF RARE DYSLIPIDEMIA

The EAS task force has identified at least 25 rare lipoprotein disorders, which are due to mutations in single genes and typically transmit as autosomal dominant (AD), autosomal codominant (ACD), or autosomal recessive (AR) pattern. Phenotypical manifestations are often confusing as same gene mutations may have varying features, and on the other hand, different gene mutations may have same manifestations.[1]

The conditions associated with extremely high levels of LDL-C (hyperbetalipoproteinemia) include familial hypercholesterolemia (FH) (ACD), familial defective apolipoprotein B-100 (ApoB-100) (ACD), AD hypercholesterolemia (ACD), AR hypercholesterolemia (AR), sitosterolemia (AR), and lysosomal acid lipase (LAL) deficiency (AR). The defective genes are located in chromosome numbers 1, 2, 10, and 19.

The hypobetalipoproteinemic conditions with very low levels of circulating LDL-C are abetalipoproteinemia (AR), homozygous hypobetalipoproteinemia (ACD), chylomicron retention disease/Andersen disease (AR), familial combined hypolipidemia (ACD), and proprotein convertase subtilisin/kexin type 9 (PCSK9) deficiency (ACD). The chromosomes involved are 1, 2, 4, and 5.

Very high TG levels are found in AR monogenic chylomicronemia which includes conditions such as lipoprotein lipase (LPL) deficiency, apolipoprotein C-II (ApoC-II) deficiency, lipase mutation factor 1 deficiency, and polygenic dysbetalipoproteinemia.

Conditions associated with low HDL-C (hypoalphalipoproteinemia) are all ACD and include Tangier disease, apolipoprotein A-I (ApoA1) deficiency and lecithin cholesterol acyltransferase (LCAT) deficiency (fish-eye disease). On the other hand, diseases with very high HDL-C (hyperalphalipoproteinemia) include cholesteryl ester transfer protein deficiency (ACD) and hepatic lipase deficiency (AR).

DISEASES WITH HIGH LOW-DENSITY LIPOPROTEIN CHOLESTEROL LEVELS

Familial Hypercholesterolemia

This is the most common of the rare dyslipidemia.[2]

Incidence and Pathology

Here due to impaired interaction between the LDL particles with the LDL receptors, plasma LDL-C levels are very high. This hypercholesterolemia manifests by physical signs such as arcus cornealis, xanthelasmas, and tendon xanthomas and leads to ASCVD in young persons. The more common form of FH, i.e., heterozygous FH (HeFH), is not a rare disease with prevalence of 1 in 200–250. The rare form is the homozygous variant (HoFH) with an occurrence rate of one in 160,000–300,000 of global population. As it is an ACD condition, one defective gene causes heterozygous FH whereas both the genes of LDL receptor (*LDLR*) if mutant, homozygous FH ensues, and circulating LDL particles are not at all cleared up by the liver. Some other genetic mutations involving *PCSK9* or *APOB* gene may produce similar conditions as HoFH.

Diagnosis

Traditionally a plasma level of LDL-C above 400 mg/dL (or >300 mg/dL, if on antilipidemic therapy) in a child aged below 10 years, along with skin or tendon xanthomata, is diagnostic of HoFH. But genetic heterogeneity considerably changes the classical features, and targeted DNA sequencing is recommended for final diagnosis. Clinical scoring system proves to be very useful, and there are several such scores.

Treatment

Treatment of HoFH involves lifestyle management, pharmacotherapy, and genetic counseling. Lifestyle management includes low-fat diet, and in case of sitosterolemia, dietary sterol restriction is very effective along with ezetimibe or bile acid sequestrants.

For pharmacotherapy, genetic testing is often helpful. In HoFH with two null *LDLR* mutations, PCSK9I is not effective, but effective in defective *LDLR* mutations. PCSK9 antibodies are useful in HoFH with biallelic gain-of-function *PCSK9* mutations. But given the very high baseline LDL-C and relatively ineffective pharmacotherapy, lipoprotein apheresis is the key treatment option, even though it is cumbersome, costly, and needs to be carried out for the rest of the life.

With very high baseline LDL-C level (>400 mg/dL in drug-naïve patients and >320 mg/dL in drug-treated patients), the secondary causes need to be excluded, e.g., nephrotic syndrome, primary biliary cirrhosis, hypothyroidism, and some medications. In pharmacotherapy, sequential treatment with highest tolerated dose of statin, ezetimibe, bile acid sequestrants, bempedoic acid, and PCSK9I is recommended.

Newer drugs are being investigated. The oral microsomal triglyceride transfer protein (MTTP) inhibitor lomitapide is used as an adjunctive therapy. It works best with low-fat diet with less than total calories coming from fat, and gastrointestinal symptoms are minimized by giving the drug on empty stomach. The most common side effect is fatty liver.

An ApoB antisense oligonucleotide, mipomersen, was withdrawn due to liver toxicity. Other potential therapies include monoclonal antibody to *ANGPTL3*, evinacumab, and *LDLR* gene therapy. If LAL deficiency is the cause, infusion of sebelipase alfa replaces the enzyme. Liver transplant is the last option in some selected cases.

Counseling is important and includes screening to identify HeFH among family members. Contraception and pregnancy counseling are other aspects. Detection of early ASCVD in the patients with HoFH is of paramount importance to prolong life.[3]

DISEASES WITH VERY LOW LOW-DENSITY LIPOPROTEIN CHOLESTEROL LEVELS

Very low levels of LDL-C and ApoB or even absent LDL-C in the blood occur in a group of conditions called primary hypobetalipoproteinemia. They are genetic diseases, and may be associated with abnormalities of other lipoproteins as well.[4]

Pathophysiology

Hypobetalipoproteinemia occurs either due to less production of ApoB or more catabolism of the same. Abetalipoproteinemia is an AR disease, and also known as Bassen–Kornzweig syndrome. Here the MTTP is not produced as the *MTTP* gene has loss-of-function mutation. This results in absence of very low-density lipoprotein (VLDL), chylomicron, LDL-C, and ApoB in plasma and very low blood levels of TGs and total cholesterol. This also is a heterozygous condition with many different types of mutations producing the same effect. The fundamental defect is to attach the lipid to the nascent lipoprotein particle.

Another similar condition is homozygous familial hypobetalipoproteinemia (FHBL), an ACD disease, where *APOB* gene is involved and is characterized by very low levels of LDL-C and ApoB. Anderson disease (AR), also called chylomicron retention disease, is a biallelic mutations of *SAR1B* gene, where chylomicron secretion from enterocytes is blocked.

Diagnosis

The EAS task force consensus statement has provided a diagnostic cum therapeutic algorithm.[1]

To begin with, the secondary causes of LDC below 40 mg/dL need to be addressed. They include statin treatment, dietary causes like strict vegan diet and malabsorption, cachectic illnesses, advanced hepatic, renal and pancreatic diseases, cystic fibrosis, hyperthyroidism, etc. Then, if the clinical and biochemical features are suggestive, targeted next generation sequencing (NGS) is indicated.

In these conditions, whatever little cholesterol present in the circulation is in the form of HDL-C. As the fat-soluble vitamins are dependent on the chylomicron for absorption and ApoB for transportation, severe deficiency of these vitamins occurs in the body.

Mild anemia with acanthocytosis, fat malabsorption, and growth failure from birth are characteristic. Later on, eye conditions like night blindness and atypical retinitis pigmentosa; bone diseases like osteomalacia or rickets; neurological conditions like posterior column disease, spinocerebellar ataxia, and peripheral neuropathy; and hematological conditions like prolonged prothrombin time, ensue. As abetalipoproteinemia is an AR condition, the parents of the patient have normal lipid profile, whereas, in homozygous FHBL, a condition, both parents have low levels of LDL-C. Interestingly, low LDL-C imparts a protection against ASCVD.

In the work up for patients with suspected hypobetalipoproteinemia, secondary causes of low ApoB such as chronic liver disease, chronic pancreatitis, malabsorption, cystic fibrosis, hyperthyroidism, end-stage renal disease and cachexia should be excluded.

Treatment

Early diagnosis is essential so that treatment can be initiated to restrict long-term eye and neurological complications. The basis of treatment is a fat-restricted diet, supplementation if essential fatty acids and high oral doses of vitamins A, D, E, and K. Apparently, the absorption occurs by the portal vein via the medium-chain triglyceride (MCT) pathways.

DISEASES WITH VERY HIGH TRIGLYCERIDE LEVELS

Mild hypertriglyceridemia with TG level above 180 mg/dL is common, especially in diabetic population. But levels above 885 mg/dL (10 mmol/L) are rare (prevalence 0.1–0.2%). This indicates the presence of chylomicronemia syndrome. Usually these conditions are polygenic. The even rarer monogenic form is more virulent in manifestations with TG levels often near 2,000 mg/dL, high rate of acute pancreatitis (60–70% cases), younger age of presentation, and frequent resistance to treatment.[5]

Pathology

Two basic pathological processes cause high TG in plasma, high VLDL production by the liver and defective LPL activity causing impaired lipolysis of chylomicrons carrying high amounts of TGs. Thus, the dietary fat when absorbed from intestine in chylomicron particles, is not cleared up.

Diagnosis and Clinical Features

When the serum TG level is above 885 mg/dL, the test should be repeated another two times to confirm the level. History of pancreatitis must be taken carefully. The secondary causes like uncontrolled diabetes, hypothyroidism, nephrotic syndrome, alcohol abuse, and drugs like estrogen and steroid should be excluded. If suggestive clinical features like abdominal pain, pancreatitis, hepatosplenomegaly, eruptive xanthoma, lipemia retinalis, and milky plasma are present, then NGS should be done to diagnose and characterize the exact condition.

The hypertriglyceridemia worsens with high-fat diet, alcohol, pregnancy, obesity, high blood sugar, hypothyroidism, or drugs like estrogen and steroid. Sibling screening is necessary with a 25% rate of affection.

Treatment

Fat-restricted food is the basis of treatment with ideally <10% of calorie coming from fat. This is often impractical. The essential fatty acids may be replenished with MCT. Fibrates increase LPL activity and help in polygenic form, but not in the monogenic variants. Omega 3 fatty acids in doses of 4 g/day help in polygenic diseases. Alcohol and food of high glycemic indices must be avoided.

Acute pancreatitis attack should be managed conservatively with complete fasting and intravenous fluid. Finding out the secondary or precipitating causes and controlling them are essential. Plasmapheresis is recommended only in selected cases of pregnancy with monogenic chylomicronemia.

Monogenic diseases have no good treatment as of now. Second anti-*APOC3* agents are being develop. The older version, volanesorsen, is still used, but has potential for thrombocytopenia. *LPL* gene therapy (alipogene tiparvovec) was available for a few years, but no longer.

Dysbetalipoproteinemia is a rare disease with prevalence of 1–2 per 20,000 population. Here, VLDL remnant or intermediate-density lipoprotein accumulates giving rise to high plasma levels of both TG and total cholesterol. ApoB-48 accumulates in blood and is diagnostic. The patients present with typical palmoplantar xanthoma and tuberoeruptive xanthoma on the elbows and knees. They are prone to premature ASCVD, especially peripheral vascular disease. Stain and fibrates are used for treatment.[3]

DISEASES WITH LOW TRIGLYCERIDE LEVELS

These are extremely rare and heterogeneous conditions with no specific gene mutation. Most of them are associated with low ApoB disorders. As they are clinically silent per se, no specific treatment is required.

DISEASES ASSOCIATED WITH ABNORMAL HIGH-DENSITY LIPOPROTEIN

The role of HDL in health and disease is still uncertain. It is traditionally considered as a negative risk factor for ASCVD, but epidemiological data are conflicting and pharmacological intervention to raise HDL has so far been proved to be futile, if not harmful. Physiologically, HDL causes reverse transport of cholesterol, meaning the transportation of cholesterol from the macrophages to the liver. But present understanding indicates a U-shaped relationship of HDL with ASCVD, chronic kidney disease, infection, and mortality, with the best results shown with HDL levels of 50–93 mg/dL. Following is a brief description of conditions with higher and lower HDL levels.[6]

DISEASES ASSOCIATED WITH LOW HIGH-DENSITY LIPOPROTEIN CHOLESTEROL

These conditions are generally called hypoalphalipoproteinemia. A low HDL is the most common lipid disorder as found in the Indian subcontinent, especially associated with diabetes mellitus and metabolic syndrome. However, extremely low levels like below 20 mg/dL are very rare and may be monogenic disorder by pathology. Many genes such as *APOA1*, *ABCA1*, *LCAT*, or *LPL* genes may be involved, and often the disorder is polygenic.[7]

Pathophysiology

Apolipoprotein A1 deficiency and Tangier disease are distinct clinical entities, though both have low HDL and ApoA1 levels. They involve *ABCA1* gene mutations.

Lecithin cholesterol acyltransferase deficiency and fish-eye disease are familial conditions with inactive LCAT. The fundamental defect of nonesterification of cholesterol where the unesterified cholesterol accumulates as an abnormal lipoprotein particle called lipoprotein X (LpX), which is cleared by the hepatic and splenic reticuloendothelial system. In fish-eye disease, the LDL-C is esterified, but HDL-C is not. The abnormal LpX is nephrotoxic, causing endothelial and vascular damage in the renal capillaries. As HDL function is normal in the familial LCAT deficiency, ASCVD is lower, whereas, in fish-eye disease, as HDL is defective, ASCVD prevails.

Diagnosis and Clinical Features

Secondary causes of low HDL should first be excluded. These include hypertriglyceridemia, diabetes, acute and chronic hepatic disorders, systemic inflammation, hematological malignancies, excess cortisol or growth hormone, smoking, physical inactivity, and drugs like probucol, thiazide diuretics, nonselective beta blockers, and retroviral agents. Once these are excluded and physical findings indicate certain specific diseases, targeted NGS tests should be done to clinch the specific diagnosis.

APOA1 mutations may cause hepatic and renal amyloidosis in certain mutations and cardiac, cutaneous, and laryngeal amyloidosis in some other mutations.

ABCA1 mutation causing Tangier disease presents with large yellow tonsils, hepatosplenomegaly and peripheral neuropathy, along with anemia and thrombocytopenia.

Familial LCAT deficiency and fish-eye disease present with corneal clouding and anemia and progressive renal failure.

Variable incidences of ASCVD are found in all these conditions.

Treatment

No specific treatment is available to improve the fundamental biochemical defects. Treatment is generally for the complications, like corneal transplant, hemodialysis or renal transplant, and management of ASCVD.

DISEASES ASSOCIATED WITH HIGH HIGH-DENSITY LIPOPROTEIN CHOLESTEROL

Hyperalphalipoproteinemia may be either due to loss-of-function mutations in cholesteryl ester transfer protein (*CETP*) gene, or loss-of-function mutations in scavenger receptor B-1 (*SRB1*) gene. In both these conditions plasma HDL level is typically above 100 mg/dL. Both are ACD conditions and are associated with premature ASCVD. Hepatic lipase deficiency may cause a generalized increase in LDL, HDL, and TG levels. No specific therapy is available for any of these conditions.[8]

FUTURE OF MANAGEMENT OF RARE DYSLIPIDEMIAS

As already elaborated, these rare dyslipidemias are not only rare in their occurrence, but also very heterogeneous and extremely variable in their mode of presentations. Progress in the field of genomic research holds promise for the future. Some drugs are licensed in some countries for some specific disorders, with variable results.

As already mentioned, volanesorsen, an anti-*APOC3* antisense oligonucleotide, is approved in the Europe for monogenic chylomicronemia. An anti-ANGPTL3 antibody, evinacumab, is being developed for HoFH and monogenic chylomicronemia. Lomitapide and mipomersen, an oral MTP inhibitor and anti-ApoB antisense oligonucleotide, respectively, are used for HoFH in various parts of the world. Sebelipase can be used in alfa LAL deficiency to replace the LAL.

CONCLUSION

The rare dyslipidemias pose a serious challenge to the clinicians for timely diagnosis and to detect and treat the complications. A team effort of experts of different fields is necessary. A timely referral to the expert center is needed by the physicians. A working knowledge of the typical presentations and biochemical abnormalities of some of the less rare disorders is required of the physicians. The updated guidelines from different appropriate bodies are necessary to achieve this end.

ONLINE REFERENCES

Please scan the QR code provided at the end of the table of contents for References of this chapter.

SECTION 7

Acute Coronary Syndrome

CHAPTER

74 ST-elevation Myocardial Infarction in Women—Challenges to Management

Madhuvanthi Rajendran, Thomas Alexander

ABSTRACT

ST-elevation myocardial infarction (STEMI) is a medical emergency that requires prompt diagnosis and early revascularization. Unfortunately, women have delayed presentation, more frequent missed diagnosis, and less revascularization as compared to men. This results in worse outcomes. Data from Indian studies show that these differences are magnified to a greater degree as compared to western data. Improved patient education, training medical personnel to recognize typical symptoms in women, understanding the difference in the pathological process of STEMI in women, and ensuring gender equity in healthcare delivery will help to reduce morbidity and mortality due to STEMI in women.

Keywords: Women, STEMI, CVD risk factors, MINOCA, SCAD.

INTRODUCTION

Worldwide, ischemic heart disease (IHD) has emerged as the leading cause of mortality in women.[1] Gender gap in cardiology is highlighted well in the western world; such awareness is lacking in India. The three most important characteristics of coronary artery disease (CAD) in women are as follows:

1. A lesser prevalence of "typical angina"
2. A lower burden of obstructive CAD on angiography
3. A poorer prognosis in comparison to men

In contrast to the prevailing notion that premenopausal women are protected from IHD, emerging data have shown that younger women hospitalized with acute myocardial infarction (AMI) are increasingly prevalent.

Women often report symptoms such as dyspnea, fatigue, light-headedness, or jaw pain leading to delays in presentation and diagnosis of acute coronary syndrome (ACS). Women presenting with ACS have less obstructive disease and more likely to have different pathophysiological mechanisms of CAD, such as spontaneous coronary artery dissection (SCAD) or coronary artery spasm (CAS) and myocardial infarction with nonobstructive coronary artery (MINOCA).

Women exhibit higher inhospital and 1-year mortality compared with men.[2-5] Additionally, women also experience a higher incidence of cardiogenic shock and heart failure (HF) compared with men.[6,7]

EPIDEMIOLOGY

Though the world is seeing a decline in the IHD mortality rates, it still remains the leading mortality and morbidity threat in women. The annual number of deaths from cardiovascular disease (CVD) in women is 2.2 million in Europe and 2.7 million in the United States (US). 20% of all deaths in women is due to CHD.[8]

The prevalence of IHD in Indian women can be estimated from the escalating IHD mortality trends. From the years 2000–2017, total IHD mortality in India has increased in both women and men. It has increased in women from 62.9/100,000 to 92.7/100,000; the increase is significantly greater in women 47.4% versus 32.8% in men ($p < 0.05$).[9]

The notable ST-elevation myocardial infarction (STEMI) registries in India, the Tamil Nadu-STEMI (TN-STEMI) and the North Indian-STEMI (NORIN-STEMI) show that ≈16% of the STEMI patients are women and mortality is significantly higher in female patients, both inhospital (10.4% vs. 4.8%)

and at 1 year (26.7% vs. 13%), compared with men.[4,5] Women were on average 7 years older than men at presentation with a greater risk factor burden, which majorly contributes to the increased mortality in women.[10,11] Women also experience a higher incidence of cardiogenic shock (8.5% vs. 7.6%) and HF (5.8% vs. 3.4%) compared with men.[12,13] Among all the risk factors, lack of revascularization with percutaneous coronary intervention (PCI) and being a female patient are the strongest predictors of in-patient and 30-day mortality.

RISK FACTORS

The INTERHEART study, a global case-control study shows that Asian Indians have a greater burden of cardiovascular risk factors, particularly at a younger age. For improved risk stratification of women, sex-specific traditional and novel risk factors for IHD should be considered.

Hypertension is more robustly associated with STEMI in women than in men. Even borderline elevation of blood pressure (BP) > 140/90 mm Hg causes significant endothelial dysfunction and cardiovascular complications in women than in men. Women with a systolic BP (SBP) > 185 mm Hg are reported to have a threefold increase in death versus women with a SBP < 135 mm Hg.[14]

Diabetes is also associated with a higher risk of coronary events in women than in men, especially in younger women, increasing their risk four- to fivefold. Women with type 2 diabetes mellitus (T2DM) have a higher adjusted hazard ratio (HR) of fatal CAD (HR 14.74; 95% confidence interval (CI) 6.16–35.27) compared with T2DM men (HR 3.77; 95% CI 2.52–5.65).[15]

Trends in the cardiometabolic risk factors in India from 2000 to 2015 showed greater increase in body mass index, diabetes, tobacco use, and periodontal infections among women than men.

Between second National Family Health Survey (NFHS-2) and NFHS-4 (three surveys, 20-year period), tobacco use among women increased from 3.0 to 10.8% and 6.8%, while overweight or obesity increased from 10.6 to 14.8% and 20.6%.[9] Female patients were more likely to present with lipid profiles diagnostic of dyslipidemia than male patients (89% vs. 76%; $p < 0.001$).[5]

Clearly, women in India are at a much higher cardiometabolic risk of CVD than men, especially after they lose their hormonal protection at menopause.

Certain risk factors are more potent for young women; for example, smoking is more strongly associated with STEMI incidence among women aged 18–49 years versus similarly aged men and older women.

Emerging, nontraditional atherosclerotic CVD (ASCVD) risk factors include early menarche, polycystic ovary syndrome (PCOS), preterm delivery, hypertensive pregnancy disorders, gestational diabetes mellitus, premature ovarian failure, breast cancer treatments, autoimmune disease status, and depression. In the INTERHEART study, an aggregate exposure to psychosocial risk factors, including depression, perceived home/work stress, low locus of control, and major life events, was significantly associated with AMI in women, with an adjusted odds ratio of 3.5.[16] Young women compared with young men presenting with AMI in the VIRGO study had significantly higher perceived stress scores.[17]

PATHOPHYSIOLOGY

Women have a unique phenotype of IHD with less calcified lesions, more nonobstructive plaques, and a higher prevalence of microvascular disease compared with men. Women have smaller epicardial coronary arteries than men which complicates accurate assessment of distal coronary arteries by coronary computed tomographic angiography, and women have thinner myocardial walls, which is challenging for noninvasive evaluation of nontransmural ischemia by cardiac magnetic resonance imaging.[18]

Myocardial Infarction—Coronary Artery Disease

Autopsy studies from the past have established that there are predominantly three major vascular events underlying thrombotic coronary occlusions responsible for AMI—plaque rupture, plaque erosion, and calcific nodule. Plaque rupture is by far the most common cause, responsible for 76% of men and 55% of women with fatal myocardial infarction (MI). Autopsy studies have shown an increased prevalence of plaque erosion in women compared with men, particularly in younger women. It has been shown that women have fewer calcified lesions, fewer calcific vessels, and lower coronary artery calcium (CAC) volumes.

The 5-year follow-up of the CONFIRM registry showed that, after adjustment, there was a strong association between increased major adverse cardiovascular event (MACE) risk and nonobstructive CAD (HR 2.16 for women, 2.56 for men; $p < 0.001$ for both) and nonobstructive plaque carries a higher relative risk in women than in men.[19]

Myocardial Infarction—Coronary Artery Spasm

The US VIRGO study has shown that 0.6% of MI in women is due to CAS versus 0.1% in men. It is a cause of MI in young patients (both women and men) but is often challenging to diagnose because it may not be apparent at initial angiography and may present as MINOCA.

The pathogenesis of CAS is multifactorial and includes vagal withdrawal, vascular smooth muscle hyperactivity, endothelial dysfunction, and an imbalance of the autonomic nervous system.

Patients with coronary spasm tend to be younger and it typically presents as rest angina occurring at night and early morning hours. Risk factors include smoking, cocaine, and methamphetamine use, as well as certain chemotherapy agents such as 5-fluorouracil and paclitaxel.

In patients with ACS from the CASPAR study, ≈25% had no obstructive culprit lesion on coronary angiography. CAS was present in almost 50% of the patients who underwent acetylcholine provocative testing.[20,21] Provoked CAS is an independent predictor of major adverse cardiac events.

Myocardial Infarction with Nonobstructive Coronary Arteries

Although the most frequent cause of AMI in women is obstructive CAD, up to 15% have unobstructed coronary arteries.[22] MINOCA can have multiple causes, including mild-to-moderate atherosclerosis with positive remodeling of the coronary artery, CAS, plaque microrupture and/or erosion, coronary embolism, and microthrombosis. An important association is coronary microvascular dysfunction (CMD), defined as impaired coronary flow reserve (CFR) and/or high index of microvascular resistance and/or endothelial dysfunction.

Myocardial Infarction—Spontaneous Coronary Artery Dissection

Spontaneous coronary artery dissection is an increasingly recognized cause of AMI and sudden cardiac death in young and middle-aged women and the most frequent cause of pregnancy-associated MI. Pregnancy-associated SCAD tends to be more severe, involving more proximal dissections, and resulting in larger infarctions, worse outcomes, and a high rate of maternal and fetal mortality.[23]

The etiologies of SCAD are largely unknown, although some may be associated with peripartum and postpartum status, oral contraceptive use, exercise, connective tissue disorders, and vasculitides (including fibromuscular dysplasia) arteriopathies such as fibromuscular dysplasia and extra-coronary aneurysms or dissections. Hypertension has been associated with both initial and recurrent SCAD. Recurrent SCAD is not uncommon, occurring in up to 30% of patients over 10 years.

CLINICAL PRESENTATION

Women who present with chest pain are at risk for underdiagnosis and potential cardiac causes should always be considered. In women presenting with chest pain, it is recommended to obtain a history that emphasizes accompanying symptoms that are more common in women with ACS. Associated symptoms such as shortness of breath, nausea or vomiting, light-headedness, confusion, presyncope or syncope, or vague abdominal symptoms are more frequent among women. A detailed assessment of cardiovascular risk factors, review of systems, past medical history, and family and social history should complement the assessment of presenting symptoms.

Young women are 50% more likely than similar-aged men to present without chest pain when they have STEMI.

MANAGEMENT

Delayed presentation due to "atypical symptoms" leads to delayed identification and increased mortality. The older age at presentation and the greater risk factor burden in women at presentation contribute to high inhospital and 30-day mortality. Underuse of cardiac procedures and medical therapies for women with STEMI is thought to be a significant contributor to the mortality differences for women with STEMI. This inequality in referral is more profound in younger women and might be explained by increased technical complexity related to smaller coronary arteries, less obstructive coronary plaque, and a higher rate of delayed/missed diagnosis in this population.

Thrombolytic Therapy

Women are at particular higher bleeding risks with antithrombotic agents and therefore, careful attention should be given to weight and renal calculation of doses. As per the GUSTO-1 multivariate model to predict hemorrhage,[24] the risk of moderate or severe bleeding was increased 1.43-fold in women. Female sex is an independent predictor of intracranial bleeding with thrombolytic therapy. This is a Class I, Level of Evidence B recommendation that also recommends consideration of weight and renal dosing of antiplatelet and anticoagulant agents because of the higher bleeding risks in women. There was no significant increase in severe bleeding in menstruating women compared with nonmenstruating women.

Worse outcomes in women is often due to other confounding risk factors. The GUSTO trial showed that women have more nonfatal complications such as shock, HF, reinfarction, recurrent ischemia, bleeding, and stroke compared with men.[25]

Primary Percutaneous Coronary Intervention

Because women have more complications from thrombolytic therapy, it would stand to reason that they benefit the most from primary PCI. The greater mortality benefit of primary PCI compared with thrombolytic therapy was confirmed in the GUSTO II-B angioplasty substudy,[26] with primary PCI preventing 56 deaths in women compared with 42 deaths in men per 1,000 treated.

A pooled analysis of 22 trials that randomized 6,763 STEMI patients to primary PCI versus thrombolytics found that women had lower 30-day mortality with primary PCI, regardless of whether they presented within the first 2 hours of symptom onset (7.7% vs. 9.6%) or after >2-hour delay (8.5% vs. 14.4%).[27] Of note was the extremely high mortality in women with delay in presentation treated with thrombolytic therapy.

Coronary interventions are much more challenging and less successful in the presence of SCAD. Those treated with conservative measures predominantly had favorable early outcomes, aside from a minority with SCAD progression within 7 days of presentation. Importantly, revascularization did not preclude the development of recurrent SCAD or late target vessel revascularization, so these patients need close follow-up over the long term.

Equally important for women after AMI is the discontinuation of harmful drugs or drugs that are of no benefit. Hormone therapy with estrogen plus progestin or estrogen alone should not be given de novo to postmenopausal women after AMI for secondary prevention of coronary events.

CLINICAL COURSE AND PROGNOSIS

The NORIN study showed women with a STEMI presented to hospital on an average 45 minutes later than men. The reasons for delay included lack of transport, patient unwillingness, misinterpretation of symptoms, and transient resolution of symptoms. One in five women perceive their symptoms as being related to anxiety or stress as opposed to AMI. In the VIRGO study, as compared to young men with STEMI, young women presented 6 hours after symptom onset (35% vs. 23%; $p = 0.002$).[28]

Delay in seeking treatment for a STEMI is often due to lack of awareness of risk, older age, lower education levels, living alone, fear, and embarrassment. It is possible that late presentation contributes to poorer outcomes for women.

CHALLENGES IN STEMI MANAGEMENT IN INDIA

Two important recent studies from India, one from North India and the other from South India, have looked at gender differences in presentation, risk factors, and outcomes in patients presenting with STEMI.

The first study was a subgroup analysis of the TN-STEMI program, a multicenter, prospective, observational study of a quality-improvement program studying patients with STEMI at four hub-and-spoke clusters in the southern state of Tamil Nadu, India.[4] In total, 2,420 patients were enrolled between 2012 and 2014 and the data from all four clusters, pre- and postimplementation of integrated STEMI systems, were combined for this analysis with a 1-year follow-up. The mean ± standard deviation (SD) age of presentation of female patients (16%) was significantly later (60.1 ± 10.9 years) compared with males (84%; 53.7 ± 12 years). Diabetes was more prevalent in women (35.2% vs. 23.8%; $p < 0.001$), as was hypertension (35.2% vs. 22.9%; $p < 0.001$). Symptom to first medical contact in female patients was significantly delayed compared with males (193 minutes vs. 170 minutes; $p \leq 0.009$). Women had higher mortality, both inhospital (10.4% vs. 4.8%; $p \leq 0.001$) and at 1-year (26.7% vs. 13%; $p \leq 0.001$). This pattern was persistent, even in the younger STEMI (<45 years) population [inhospital 9.1% vs. 3% ($p \leq 0.05$); at 1 year 18.2% vs. 3% ($p \leq 0.05$)]. In the regression model, females had a 1.8 times increased likelihood ($p < 0.04$) of mortality after adjusting for confounders.

The NORIN-STEMI registry is an investigator-initiated prospective cohort study of patients presenting with STEMI at tertiary medical centers in North India.[5] Of 3,635 participants, 16% were female patients. Compared with male patients, female patients were less likely to receive PCI (62% vs. 73%; $p < 0.0001$) and had a more than twofold greater 1-year mortality (22% vs. 9%; adjusted HR 2.1; 95% CI 1.7–2.7; $p < 0.001$).

The data from India clearly highlight the need for extra effort to address the gender disparity in access and care for STEMI patients. While these differences exist in the western world, it is exaggerated in India due to the various social, cultural, and economic disparities.

CONCLUSION

Women present with STEMI at an older age than the male counterparts. They have a higher prevalence of diabetes and hypertension but low levels of tobacco use. Delayed presentation due to various socioeconomic and gender discriminatory practices in society have a profound effect on outcomes in STEMI patients. Sensitization of emergency service healthcare personnel regarding "typical" symptoms of ACS/STEMI in women would aid in making timely identification, appropriate triage, and judicious use of testing and management in women patients.

Management of STEMI without obstructive CAD is a challenge and its increased frequency in women with STEMI adds to the challenge of managing STEMI in women. The lack of significant numbers of women in STEMI trials is a significant barrier that needs to be addressed and targeted research in managing STEMI in women should be a priority.

ONLINE REFERENCES

Please scan the QR code provided at the end of the table of contents for References of this chapter.

CHAPTER

75

Transdermal Troponin-I Sensor in Acute Myocardial Infarction

Shantanu P Sengupta

ABSTRACT

Early diagnosis of acute myocardial infarction is the key in the management of this disease as it is associated with high morbidity and mortality. Angina and electrocardiographic changes, supplemented with elevation of biomarker such as troponin, hold the key to diagnosis. Troponin testing requires blood sampling, and the time to get the results may vary depending on various factors. Noninvasive assessment of troponin is now possible. This brief review provides new insights about the assessment of troponin by a wrist-worn device by the process of spectroscopy.

Keywords: Troponin, acute myocardial infarction.

INTRODUCTION

Acute myocardial infarction (AMI) is the leading cause of mortality and morbidity worldwide.[1] For the diagnosis of AMI, two out of the following three are needed, that is, chest pain defined as angina, electrocardiogram abnormality, and elevation of biomarker demonstrating myocardial necrosis. Early diagnosis is the key for better outcome, and difficulties in early recognition of AMI and delays in initiating revascularization impact survival and quality of life.[2]

Assessment of cardiac troponin levels, as a marker of cardiac myocyte necrosis, is routinely recommended in patients presenting with acute coronary syndrome (ACS). It requires drawing of blood sample to have the report within minimal time. These turnover times for laboratory tests show wide variability and are challenging to implement in acute care settings confronted with staffing shortages and decreasing hospital resources.[3] Specifically, overcrowding in emergency rooms can be associated with delays in blood sampling, overall diagnostic workup, and increased costs for assessing patients presenting with ACS.

Advances in sensor and computing technologies have led to greater availability of smart wearable devices in cardiovascular medicine for disease prevention, diagnosis, and management. A potential solution to preventing delays in the diagnosis of AMI is to implement a point-of-care device that confirms and accurately risk stratifies patients with suspected AMI. There are many point-of-care solutions available to assess high-sensitivity cardiac troponin. However, there are no handheld devices approved for clinical use by the Food and Drug Administration (FDA). We have recently reported the development of a novel wrist-worn transdermal infrared spectrophotometric sensor (ISS) that can assess raised troponin-I levels based on infrared spectroscopy.[4] Infrared spectroscopy interrogates the material at the molecular level and is one of the cornerstones of analytical tools used to study structural and compositional chemistry.[5] The most significant advantage is that a sensitive sensor can produce results within 5 minutes, without collecting blood and transferring the sample to the testing device. The preliminary laboratory and benchtop translational studies have provided initial feasibility data; the device is being evaluated in real-life clinical settings.

We did a multicenter, observational study aimed to test the feasibility of implementing a remotely analyzable, transdermal-ISS with machine learning analytics in the clinical setting for predicting elevated circulating high-sensitivity cardiac troponin-I (hs-cTnI) levels during a single timepoint evaluation of patients hospitalized with AMI.[6] This was a prospective study involving five centers in India. For this, all patients who consented for the study had their simultaneous blood sampling done along with noninvasive troponin sensor. Serum troponin levels increase within 3–4 hours after the onset of symptoms and remain high for up to 4–7 days. We, therefore, sought a head-to-head comparison of hs-cTnI levels and transdermal-ISS recordings at a single random timepoint during the hospital stay after the patient was clinically stabilized to develop and validate deep learning models for predicting elevated troponin levels. The analysis of this important study was done by using a deep learning model with internal and external validation of the significant parameters.

A transdermal-ISS is a spectrophotometric device that functions based on an attenuated total internal reflection configuration.[5] It noninvasively measures the infrared absorption corresponding to the troponin concentration in the system through the dermis.[5] The detailed development of the device is outlined elsewhere.[4] Briefly, our previous study included four phases of development. First, in an ex vivo exploratory work, we tested blood samples of patients (n = 30) with various cTnI levels on a research-grade attenuated total reflectance-based infrared spectrometer. The optical readouts representing the signature cTnI absorbance peaks were investigated and showed a positive linear correlation of 0.71. Subsequently, we developed the transdermal-ISS device and tested its ability to fit on the wrist in two cohorts of patients ($n = 9$ and $n = 24$) to assess the potential to classify patients with elevated troponins. This exploratory analysis revealed an area under the receiver operator characteristic curve of 0.85 with a sensitivity of 100% and specificity of 70.59%.[4] We further tested a higher fidelity point-of-care device in a controlled clinical setting and observed a positive linear correlation of 0.77 over a wide range of hs-cTnI concentrations. These steps subsequently form the basis of testing the device further in real-life settings in the present study.

A transdermal-optical sensor device was used for patients to get an optical readout. First, the patient's volar aspect of the wrist has to be scrubbed with an alcohol wipe, following which the button is pressed on the optical device. After completion of the 45-second background, the device is strapped on the wrist with the sensor surface contacting the prepped portion of the wrist for 2 minutes. The device is then removed, while the data are wirelessly transmitted to the central cloud. Following this, blood gets drawn within 15 minutes of using the optical device to determine the ground truth troponin value with the Abbott-Architect STAT high-sensitivity assay. All optical data were further processed to segment and remove three electronic noise-related spikes occurring at the same locations in the time series that are common for all data. They occur due to the change in driving voltage states for the emitter/detector pair and are completely unrelated to the analyte measurement. Upon the unbiased removal of the spikes, the data are ingested by the machine learning algorithm without any further processing.

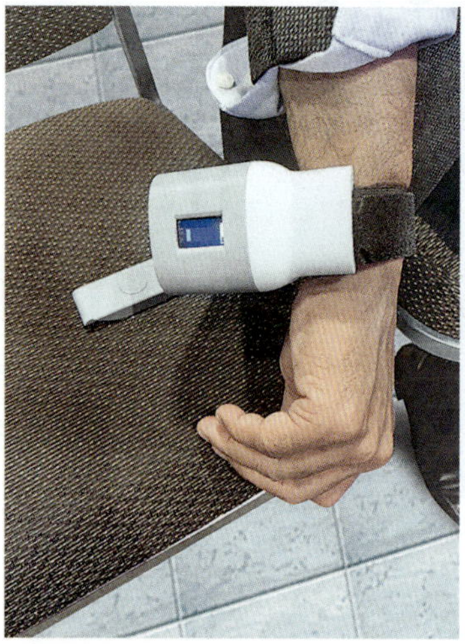

FIG. 1: Troponin sensor device for troponin measurement worn on the wrist.

This was the first time we demonstrated in a multicentric, real-world clinical evaluation of a wrist-worn device that is noninvasive to assess troponin in a setting of AMI. It utilizes infrared spectroscopy for transdermal assessment of elevated troponin levels in patients with AMI **(Fig. 1)**. We used deep learning models to show clinically significant correlation with blood troponin levels. The principal findings of our study were as follows: (1) the recording of transdermal-troponin assay waveforms and the transmission of data over the web is feasible and can be done accurately in clinical settings; (2) there is stability and high accuracy for detecting elevated troponin-I which differentiated patients with AMI from unstable angina and other causes; and (3) the model prediction was associated with the presence of significant coronary artery disease on coronary angiography and the presence of regional wall motion abnormalities on two-dimensional (2D) echocardiographic imaging. In this study, we used elevation of troponin of more than 99th percentile as the gold standard for diagnosis of AMI. The transdermal-troponin sensor device is designed to be sensitive to the wavelengths of interest for the detection of troponin. One of the limitations of the device is that the exact nature of the biomarker [troponin T-I-C, binary complexes (I-C), free submits (T and C), and fragments or related molecules thereof] tracked by the spectroscopy can be speculative. However, the values were correlated with central laboratory values of high-sensitive troponin in blood samples.

CONCLUSION

Future studies with a larger sample size will further address the diagnostic accuracy of the algorithm in chest pain units with a larger prevalence of borderline troponin levels. Also, the diagnosis of acute myocardial injury demands serial measurement of cardiac troponin. These all factors are being investigated in large multicentric studies.

ONLINE REFERENCES

Please scan the QR code provided at the end of the table of contents for References of this chapter.

CHAPTER

76

Pharmacoinvasive Strategy versus Primary Percutaneous Coronary Intervention in ST-segment Elevation Myocardial Infarction

Kajal Ganguly, Mainak Mukhopadhyay, Subhasis Roy Chowdhury, Arijit Ghosh

ABSTRACT

The difficulties presented by the geography and developing economy of India give rise to the need of developing alternative techniques to primary percutaneous coronary intervention (PPCI). In spite of the fact that acute myocardial infarction is the leading cause of mortality in India,[1] doing PPCI may be rather difficult since there are not as many facilities as there should be with the appropriate equipment. As a result, patients may have difficulty gaining access to the appropriate therapy and regaining the patency of their coronary arteries, which may result in an elevated risk of morbidity and death. In this context, pharmacoinvasive techniques provide a realistic option for the treatment of ST-segment elevation myocardial infarction (STEMI). This is particularly true in situations where it is not possible for the patient to reach a main percutaneous coronary intervention (PCI)-equipped hospital in time. Pharmacoinvasive therapy has the potential to be the principal treatment for STEMI in areas where PPCI is not commonly available.

Keywords: STEMI, pharmacoinvasive, primary-PCI, thrombolysis, CREATE registry.

INTRODUCTION

One in three fatalities worldwide is attributed to cardiovascular diseases, including ST-segment elevation myocardial infarction (STEMI). There is strong evidence tying primary percutaneous coronary intervention (PPCI) to better patient outcomes after an acute myocardial infarction (AMI).[2] Despite this, there is evidence to support the idea that alternate approaches, such as a pharmacological invasive strategy, may, in certain circumstances, be more advantageous for STEMI patients. This evaluation will assess the effectiveness and worth of the pharmacoinvasive strategy in addition to the advantages of main percutaneous coronary intervention (PCI) over competing approaches.

MYOCARDIAL VIABILITY AND TIME FRAME FOLLOWING INFARCTION

When it comes to treating a heart attack, time is of the essence. The obstruction of the coronary artery in STEMI leads to myocardial necrosis and cell death. Myocardial damage is directly proportional to total ischemic time (TIT). The most crucial factor in preventing future cardiac damage is prompt diagnosis and treatment. Even in developing countries, with an established STEMI network, there are still around 10–15% of late STEMI presenters (>12 hours after the onset of chest pain), whereas in developing countries like India, where we are yet to have a pan-India established STEMI network, the late STEMI presenters can be >50%. The ischemia event raises the patient's chance of acquiring irreversible myocardial cell death with each passing minute. The capacity of the heart muscle to operate in a manner that greatly benefits the heart in recovering from an infarction, known as myocardial viability, was originally defined in the 1960s.[3] Patients with STEMI may have varying amounts of viable myocardium, which may have a substantial impact on their response to therapy. Viability depends upon various factors, e.g., collaterals, ischemic preconditioning, and metabolic status of the perfused myocardium. Numerous techniques and tests may be used to detect the viability of the myocardium, including clinical evaluation (persisting ischemic pain) and imaging methods such as cardiac stress echo, positron emission tomography (PET), and magnetic resonance imaging (MRI) scans.[4] The patient's heart suffers less harm the sooner the blockage is removed. As per the "open-artery hypothesis," an optimally reperfused myocardial territory following acute coronary syndrome (ACS) leads to better scar and healing, less adverse remodeling, less fatal arrhythmia and event rate, and less infarct expansion. Therefore, it is crucial to make sure that every aspect of giving the proper therapy at the right time operates efficiently and securely.

Achieving reperfusion and recanalization are both essential in STEMI therapy and that is earlier the better since the chest pain onset. Reperfusion is restoration of the antegrade flow in the infarct-related artery (IRA) that can be done successfully in 75% of cases with early thrombolytic therapy (TLT) but more with PPCI. Recanalization is achievement of the original IRA vessel caliber with good thrombolysis in myocardial infarction (TIMI) flow using drug-eluting stents (DES). Although successful TLT can achieve reperfusion, in <60% of cases, it can ensure normal blood flow in IRA, hence the importance of recanalization. A major concern of TLT is a higher risk of hemorrhage.

The components of time are categorized as follows:

- *Chest pain to electrocardiogram (ECG) time*: The interval between the start of chest pain and the patient's first ECG diagnosis is known as the "chest pain to ECG time." The European Society of Cardiology (ESC) advises that this time should preferably *not go over 10 minutes.*
- *Chest pain to hospital time*: The interval between the start of chest discomfort and the patient's arrival at the hospital for treatment is known as the "hospital arrival time." Due to the urgency of the situation, the American College of Cardiology (ACC) advises a *90-minute door-to-door limit.*
- *Door-to-needle time*: The period between the patient's arrival at the hospital and the start of TLT is known as the "door-to-needle time."
- *Door-to-balloon time*: The period between the patient's arrival at the hospital and the start of wire crossing is known as the "door-to-balloon time."
- *Door-in door-out (DIDO) time*: Patients can self-present themselves in a noncardiac healthcare setup that can lead to substantial delay in the onset of proper therapy. Quick referral to a cardiac care-enabled healthcare setup with DIDO time of <30 minutes can ensure proper treatment within optimum time frame.

PRIMARY PERCUTANEOUS CORONARY INTERVENTION AND EVIDENCE

In the therapy of STEMI, PPCI is a therapeutic approach that is often used, and it may lower the risk of coronary artery reocclusions and death if it is done within the initial hours of STEMI.[5] Numerous clinical research and investigations lend credence to the idea of PPCI. Randomized trials such as STOPAMI 1, STOPAMI 2, DANAMI 2, PRAGUE 2, STAT, and AIR PAMI all have established the effectiveness of PPCI over TLT.[6-14] A meta-analysis by Keeley et al. has also proved the advantages of PPCI.[15] Edges of PPCI over TLT are:

- Higher TIMI 3 flow
- Lesser reinfarction
- Lesser intracranial bleeding
- Better survival outcome data

PHARMACOINVASIVE STRATEGY WITH EVIDENCE

Pharmacoinvasive techniques, commonly referred to as fibrinolytic therapy followed by PCI, have become a viable substitute to PPCI for STEMI.

The STREAM trial, a well-powered multicentered open labeled randomized clinical trial, was designed to test whether fibrinolytic therapy administered before arrival at the hospital or early after admission, coupled with early coronary angiography, provides outcomes like PPCI in patients presenting with acute STEMI.[15] At 30 days, the primary outcome was a composite of mortality from any cause, shock, congestive heart failure, or reinfarction. Ischemic stroke and intracranial and nonintracranial hemorrhagic bleeding were among the safety endpoints. The findings of this trial were as follows:

- At 30 days, the primary endpoint occurred in 12.4% in the pharmacoinvasive group and 14.3% in the PPCI group ($p = 0.21$).
- Up to 36% of patients in the pharmacoinvasive group required "rescue" PCI.
- Significantly more open vessels were found during coronary angiography (before PCI) in the pharmacoinvasive group compared to the PPCI group.
- Total stroke was, however, higher in the pharmacoinvasive arm than the PPCI arm.
- Hemorrhagic strokes were higher in the pharmacoinvasive arm.
- At 1-year follow-up, the all-cause mortality was 6.7% in pharmacoinvasive versus 5.9% in PPCI.
- Cardiac mortality was 4.0% in pharmacoinvasive versus 4.1% in PPCI.

The Canadian Vital Heart Response STEMI registry compared pharmacoinvasive treatment versus PPCI.[16] It has shown improved reperfusion and good clinical outcome within 1-year follow-up for those receiving pharmacoinvasive therapy.

EUROPEAN SOCIETY OF CARDIOLOGY AND AMERICAN COLLEGE OF CARDIOLOGY GUIDELINES ON THE STRATEGY

According to ACC/American Heart Association (AHA):[17]

- In a PCI-capable facility, all patients with STEMI and ischemic symptoms of <12 hours from presentation should undergo PCI.
- Latecomers (12–24 hours) with evidence of ongoing ischemia (symptomatic) are to be considered for PCI.
- If the patient is in cardiogenic shock, PCI is recommended regardless of the time of onset of symptoms.
- Delayed PCI (>24 hours) in asymptomatic stable patients with one or two diseased vessels and an occluded infarct artery without evidence of ischemia should not be performed because of the risk of harm (class III).
- In a non-PCI-capable facility (where delay from door to transfer to the balloon is >120 minutes), patients with early presentation (<12 hours) should be treated with fibrinolytic.
- In latecomers (12–24 hours) with evidence of ongoing ischemia, hemodynamic instability, or those with a large area of myocardium at risk, fibrinolytics are reasonable.
- After the administration of TLT, patients should be transferred to a PCI-capable facility.
- There is no indication for thrombolysis in asymptomatic latecomers or in patients with very late presentation beyond 24 hours from symptom onset.

The 2017 ESC guidelines[18] recommend PCI in late-presenting patients (>12 hours) with signs or symptoms of ischemia, hemodynamic instability, or life-threatening arrhythmias (class IC). In patients presenting days later, if symptoms are recurrent or silent ischemia is documented (on stress testing), revascularization may be considered. The European guidelines suggest consideration of routine PPCI in late presenters (12–48 hours). The ESC 2017 guideline emphasizes the maximum benefit of early lytic therapy (<2 hours) and routine transfer of patients for coronary angiography within 2–24 hours of lysis **(Fig. 1)**.

INDIAN REGISTRY

In the CREATE registry, 60% of patients had STEMI. Most patients were younger, belonging to poor socioeconomic strata, and late presenters (median time from symptom onset to hospital arrival was 300 minutes) in contrast to Western registry.[19] Although 60% of them received TLT, only 8% received PCI. The NORIN STEMI registry in India is another

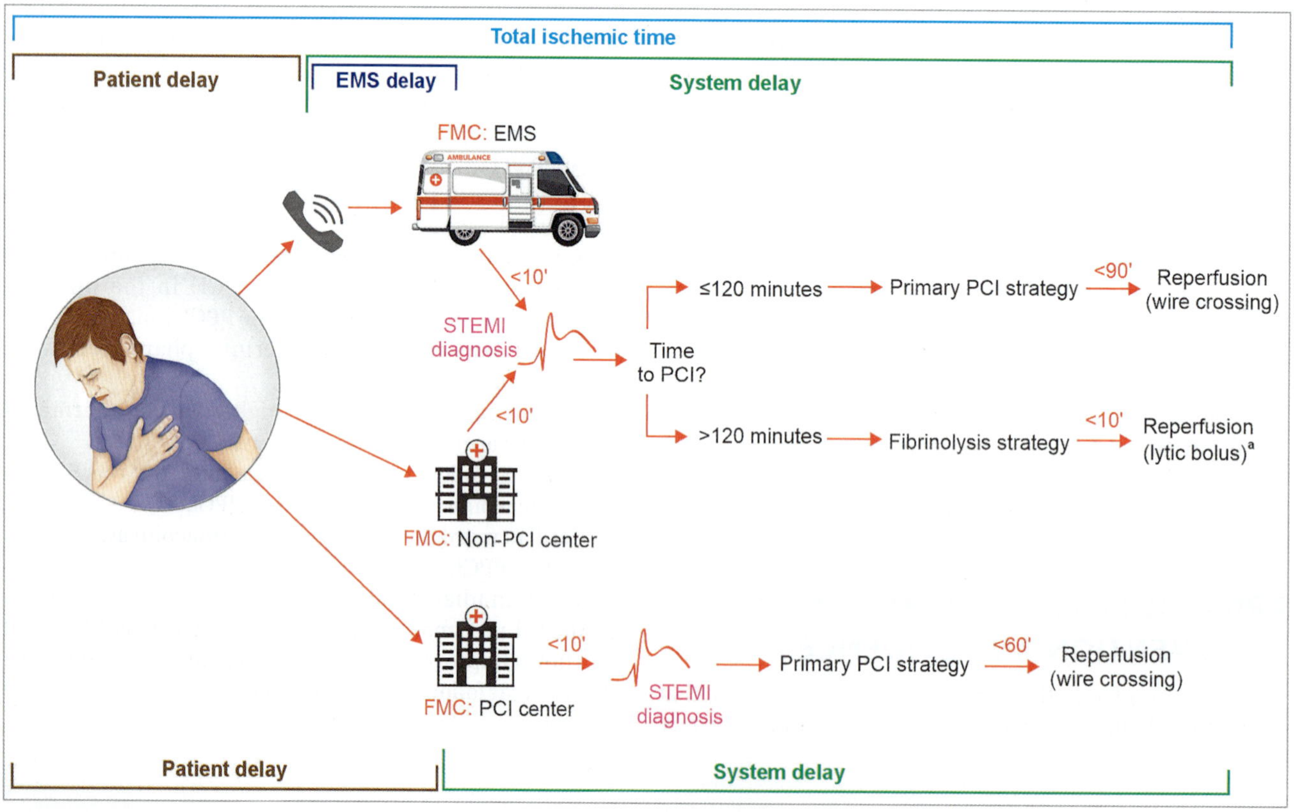

[a] Preferably with fibrin-specific agents in pre-hospital settings, but for elderly > 75 years, tenecteplase will be used in half-dose.

FIG. 1: European Society of Cardiology 2017 guideline on management of ST-segment elevation myocardial infarction (STEMI).
(EMS: emergency medical services; FMC: first medical contact; PCI: percutaneous coronary intervention)

observational cohort study of patients diagnosed with STEMI who were hospitalized in India.[20] This registry established that hospitalized STEMI patients who underwent PCI within the initial time frame had better outcome. Data from STEP PAMI and STREAM[21,22] have proved the feasibility of pharmacoinvasive strategy with respect to PPCI in the Indian context.

The Indian STEMI registry has also been essential in giving information on the accessibility and availability of PCI centers throughout India. The majority of hospitals in India lack cath labs, making it impossible for them to perform primary PCI on patients with STEMI. A significant portion of the population in India is still unable to access primary PCI centers for their treatment, despite attempts by the government and other groups to promote access to these facilities. Less than 10% of STEMI patients can reach a PCI-capable hospital within 120 minutes of the first medical contact (FMC). Hence, STEMI India has recommended that if patient can reach a PPCI-capable hospital within time, then PPCI should be the ideal treatment, whereas if there is no way to reach a PPCI-capable hospital within time, then a pharmacoinvasive strategy should be the ideal treatment strategy. The recommendation has emphasized on strengthening the "Hub and Spoke" model of an effective pharmacoinvasive strategy. Tamil Nadu STEMI program and Kovai Erode study have established the feasibility of this approach.[23,24]

CONCLUSION

To summarize, timely treatment of STEMI is critical to a full and speedy recovery. PPCI is the treatment of choice. But, in selected case, the pharmacoinvasive strategy is definitely an effective alternative.

ONLINE REFERENCES

Please scan the QR code provided at the end of the table of contents for References of this chapter.

CHAPTER

77

Recent Advances in Guideline-directed Management of Acute Coronary Syndrome

Lekha Adik Pathak, Ronak V Ruparelia

ABSTRACT

Coronary artery disease (CAD) remains the primary cause of death across India and the world. Acute coronary syndrome (ACS) remains the primary cause of death amongst patients with CAD. Several guidelines exist for the management of ACS. American College of Cardiology/American Heart Association (ACC/AHA) and European Society of Cardiology (ESC) guidelines are widely followed for management of ACS across the globe. Studies showed that management of ACS by guidelines in inpatient setting and at discharge along with timely reperfusion reduces 30-day mortality rate. Here, we will discuss salient points of management of ACS as per the guidelines.

Keywords: Acute coronary syndrome, guideline, recent advances, ESC, ACC/AHA.

INTRODUCTION

Acute coronary syndrome (ACS) remains the leading cause of death worldwide.[1] ACS comprises of three different clinical entities namely STEMI (ST-elevation myocardial infarction), NSTEMI (non-ST-elevation myocardial infarction) and unstable angina. In this chapter we will review major advances in guideline-directed management of ACS. We will try to focus on newer drugs for treatment of ACS, newer strategies to treat ACS in specific subgroup of patients and improvements in system of care for STEMI patients.

DIAGNOSIS OF ACUTE CORONARY SYNDROME

After publication of Universal Definition[2] of myocardial infarction (MI) in 2018, the classification of acute and chronic myocardial injury has increased among patients with elevated troponin biomarkers. This group has significantly higher rates of cardiovascular (CV) events. Adoption of high-sensitive troponin has also increased diagnosis of ACS. A negative troponin also has a potential role to rule out MI.

The 2015 European Society of Cardiology (ESC) guidelines[3] recommended using rapid rule out and rule in protocols. The ESC 0h/1h algorithm is based on blood sample at 0h and 1h thereafter, using validated thresholds for both baseline and variation levels of high-sensitivity troponin. The 2020 ESC, NSTEMI guidelines[4] have extended these recommendations to include validated 0h/2h algorithms based on multiple studies.[5-7]

Cardiac computed tomography angiogram (CCTA) has also emerged as an important diagnostic tool as an alternative to invasive coronary angiography in subset where electrocardiogram and troponin remain inconclusive.[4] VERDICT trial[8] has confirmed high negative predictive value of CCTA. In this study, CCTA was found to have high negative predictive value of 90.9% with sensitivity and specificity of 96.5% and 72.4%, respectively.

Primary Care for Acute Coronary Syndrome Patients

Relief of pain is of paramount importance because pain is associated with sympathetic activation that may lead to vasoconstriction and arrhythmia induction. Titrated use of intravenous (IV) opioids should be considered to relieve pain (Class IIa). A mild tranquilizer (benzodiazepine) can be considered in very anxious patients (Class IIa ESC 2017). Oxygen is indicated in patients with hypoxemia ($SaO_2 < 90\%$) (Class I).

REPERFUSION STRATEGIES

Multiple trials conducted between 1990 and 2010 have proven superiority of percutaneous coronary intervention (PCI) over fibrinolysis. 2017 ESC guideline for STEMI shortened time delay from diagnosis of STEMI to fibrinolysis from 30 minutes (as per ESC 2012 guideline) to 10 minutes. DANAMI-2 16-year follow-up[9] demonstrated a persistent benefit among patients treated with PCI. EXAMINATION trial[10] also showed lower rated of all-cause mortality, recurrent MI, and revascularization amongst patients treated with everolimus-eluting stents. Target vessel revascularization was also higher among patients receiving bare-metal stents (BMSs) in EXAMINATION trial. Even for patients with NSTEMI, PCI improved quality of life and mortality outcomes.

Primary PCI is preferred reperfusion strategy in patients with STEMI within 12 hours of symptom onset, provided it can be performed rapidly within 120 minutes from STEMI diagnosis. However, in certain cases, primary PCI is not an immediate option. Here, fibrinolysis could be initiated as early as possible. In absence of ST segment elevation, primary PCI is indicated in patients with suspected ongoing ischemic symptoms suggestive of MI and at least one of the following (hemodynamic instability or cardiogenic shock, recurrent chest pain refractory to medical treatment, life-threatening arrhythmias, mechanical complication of MI, acute heart failure, and recurrent dynamic ST-T changes). Early angiography (within 24 hours) is recommended if symptoms are completely relieved and ST segment elevation is normalized spontaneously or after nitroglycerin administration (Class I ESC 2017). In patients with time from symptom onset >12 hours, primary PCI is indicated in presence of ongoing symptoms suggestive of ischemia, hemodynamic instability, or life-threatening arrhythmias (Class I ESC 2017). In asymptomatic patients, routine PCI of an occluded IRA > 48 hours after onset of STEMI is not indicated (Class III ESC 2017).

INVASIVE MANAGEMENT OF ACUTE CORONARY SYNDROME

Vascular Access

Multiple trials have been conducted for evaluation of safety of femoral versus radial arterial access in primary PCI. Reduced bleeding and lower mortality in patients with radial access has made it a preferred route in patients with STEMI. The SAFARI STEMI trial[11] brings this into question. It was stopped prematurely due to futility with no difference in mortality or bleeding between radial versus femoral group. The possible controversial conclusion was secondary to less sick cohort of patients as well as adoption of low rate of glycoprotein IIb/IIIa (GPIIb/IIIa) use and high use of femoral closure devices. Overall, controversy about femoral versus radial access in STEMI remains.

Stenting in Percutaneous Coronary Intervention

Compared with balloon angioplasty alone, stenting with BMS was found to be associated with a lower risk of reinfarction and revascularization but was not associated with reduction in mortality. First-generation drug-eluting stent (DES) has reduced the risk of repeat target vessel revascularization. New-generation DES has shown superior safety and efficacy compared to first-generation DES in terms of lower stent thrombosis and recurrent MI. COMFORTABLE AMI[12] and EXAMINATION trial has proven superiority of newer generation stents over BMS.

Deferred stenting, which involved opening the artery and waiting 48 hours to implant a stent, is also not recommended any more. This recommendation is based upon DANAMI 3-DEFER trial, which found no effect on primary clinical outcome with deferred stenting. Routing deferred stenting was associated with higher need for target vessel revascularization.

Multivessel Disease

Many trials (PRAMI, VCLPRIT, and DANAMI-3-PRIMULTI) have shown benefit of PCI of nonculprit lesion in STEMI patients. The COMPLETE trial[13] demonstrated that complete revascularization was superior to culprit only PCI with reduced rate of CV death. Two meta-analysis[14,15] of 10 randomized trials of nonculprit PCI in STEMI were published in 2020. Both showed reduced CV mortality and subsequent MI without increased risk of vascular complications or bleeding. Furthermore, COMPARE ACUTE trial[16] demonstrated high major adverse cardiac event (MACE) rates in patients with lower fractional flow reserve (FFR) in nonculprit artery. Overall, the data supports the revascularization of noninfarction-related artery in patients with STEMI. Complete revascularization has been upgraded from Class III to Class IIa in ESC 2017 STEMI guideline. While thrombus aspiration is no longer recommended routinely in PCI for STEMI.

Less robust evidence is available for patients with multivessel disease and NSTEMI.

Facilitated Percutaneous Coronary Intervention/Pharmacoinvasive Approach

It is defined as the use of pharmacological treatment (thrombolysis) as soon as possible after the onset of STEMI in an attempt to establish early reperfusion, followed by transport to an interventional laboratory for emergent mechanical reperfusion, i.e., angioplasty. It is particularly useful for patients presenting to center where PCI facility is not available and it is not possible to transfer patient to PCI enabled center within window period of 120 minutes. Early studies of facilitated PCI showed improvement in coronary blood flow during angiogram, however, they failed to show improvement in clinical outcomes and major hemorrhagic complications were usually more frequent. More recent trials such as PACT, GRACIA-2, and BRAVE also showed improvement in infarct artery patency in facilitated PCI. Larger clinical trials such as ASSENT-4 and FINESSE evaluated tenecteplase and half dose reteplase + abciximab, respectively in facilitated PCI. ASSNET-4 and FINESS both showed improvement in primary endpoint of death, shock, and CHF at 90 days in facilitated PCI. CARESS-in-AMI, TRANSFER-AMI, and NORDISTEMI all three large, randomized trials noted no significant increase in major bleeding. A meta-analysis of these trials showed significant reduction in reinfarction, recurrent ischemia, and combined endpoint of death and reinfarction at 30 days. The clinician must choose the best reperfusion strategy in patients with STEMI presenting to noninterventional center based on an assessment of risk. This will include time from onset of symptom, time delay in transport for primary PCI, risk of fibrinolytic therapy, presence of cardiogenic shock, and cardiac arrhythmias.

Late Presenters

Late presentation is associated with increased mortality. In the treatment of late-presenting STEMI patients, clinical evaluation and risk stratification represent paramount factors helping in decision. As recommended by recent guidelines, patients who are still early in the course of STEMI (12–48 hours) should undergo PCI. Those beyond 48 hours should undergo myocardial viability studies such as cardiac magnetic resonance imaging (MRI), positron emission tomography (PET) scan, or single photon emission computed tomography (SPECT) scan. Patients presenting beyond 48 hours with evidence of silent ischemia or viability should also undergo PCI. Those with no evidence of silent ischemia or viability can safely be treated with medical therapy.

PHARMACOLOGICAL MANAGEMENT OF ACUTE CORONARY SYNDROME

Pretreatment with Antiplatelets

Aspirin and P2Y12 inhibitor remain the cornerstone of pretreatment medications, ensuring adequate platelet inhibition once ACS is diagnosed or suspected. Although pretreatment with potent antiplatelet may expose patients at times to unnecessary risk of bleeding if the diagnosis of ACS is disproved following coronary angiogram, which may happen in 35% of patients.[17] ACCOAST trial compared a strategy of systemic prasugrel pretreatment with 30 mg loading followed by 30 mg in case of PCI versus 60 mg loading dose of prasugrel. In this trial as well as ACCOAST PCI arm,[18] the pretreatment does not impact the rate of composite endpoint, but it significantly increased risk of TIMI life-threatening and major bleeding. Following ACCOAST trial, ESC guidelines have recommended against pretreatment, but only with prasugrel. While ticagrelor was compared against clopidogrel in PLATO trial, where ticagrelor was associated with reduced CV death, MI or stroke, and all-cause death without significant increase of major bleeding. ISAR-REACT 5[19] compared pretreatment with ticagrelor to prasugrel where loading dose was administered in case of PCI unless patients presenting with STEMI. ISAR REACT 5 demonstrated that ticagrelor was associated with significant increase of the risk of death, MI, or stroke at one year. This raised the question that "does more rapid-onset platelet inhibition really lead to long term clinical benefit?" More recently SCAAR study[20] evaluated 64,857 patients undergoing PCI for NSTEMI from 2010 to 2018. Majority of them were pretreated with ticagrelor. Here also, pretreatment did not result in improved survival at 1 month or 1 year, nor did it significantly reduce risk of stent thrombosis at 30 days. However, it increased risk of in-hospital bleeding. Following these evidences, the 2020 ESC NSTEMI guidelines have recommended against the routine administration of P2Y12 inhibitors in patients in whom coronary anatomy is unknown. However, the option is left open for pretreatment with P2Y12 inhibitors in patients who are not planned for early invasive strategy and are not at high risk of bleeding. Ticagrelor also possess risk of discontinuation as it provokes dyspnea in certain group of patients. According to the 2020 ESC NSTEMI guideline, prasugrel should be considered (Class IIa) in preference to ticagrelor for patients undergoing PCI for NSTEMI.

Cangrelor, a potent IV reversible P2Y12 inhibitor with rapid onset and offset of action has been assessed in three randomized controlled trial (RCT) with PCI for ACS. It reduced periprocedural ischemic complications at expense of increased risk of bleeding. As per ESC 2017 guideline, cangrelor may be considered in patients not pretreated with oral P2Y12 inhibitors at time of PCI or in those who are considered unable to absorb oral agents.

Prehospital routine use of GPIIb/IIIa inhibitors before PCI has not been demonstrated to offer any benefit. In fact, it increases risk compared with routine use in catheterization laboratory. GPIIb/IIIa inhibitor is recommended only as bailout therapy in the event of angiographic evidence of large thrombus, slow or no reflow phenomena, or other thrombotic complications. Overall, there is no evidence to use GPIIb/IIIa inhibitor as a routine.

ACS with High Bleeding Risk Patients

Personalized approach is recommended for patients with high bleeding risk (HBR). Scoring systems such as ARC-HBR and PRECISE dual antiplatelet therapy (DAPT) help to ascertain risk of bleeding. Clopidogrel should be the preferred choice with shorter DAPT duration in patients with HRB.

How Long to Continue DAPT?

Several RCT has been conducted to evaluate safety of early discontinuation of aspirin, after 1–3 months of DAPT. TWILIGHT trial[21] found ticagrelor monotherapy to be associated with a reduced major bleeding without any significant difference in ischemic events. De-escalation from ticagrelor or prasugrel to clopidogrel is also one of the options, but it should be guided with platelet function testing as in TROPICAL ACS trial.[22] The POPular Genetic trial[23] also reported a reduced risk of major bleeding with genotyping-guided strategy compared to standard DAPT with ticagrelor or prasugrel. Extended DAPT can be considered in patients with high ischemic risk without high risk of bleeding. Choice of regiment for such patients can be ascertained based on results of PEGASUS-TIMI 54 trial, COMPASS trial, and DAPT trials. DAPT trial proved that prolonged DAPT reduces stent thrombosis and MACE with increased risk of moderate or severe bleeding. PEGASUS TIMI 54 trial proved that ticagrelor 60 mg twice daily or 90 mg twice daily reduces risk of CV death, MI, or stroke with increased risk or TIMI major bleeding with 90 mg twice daily dosage. COMPASS trial proved that DAPT with rivaroxaban reduced CV death, MI, or stroke but not rivaroxaban alone. Both regimens increased risk of bleeding in COMPASS trial.

Lipid-lowering Drugs

Development and approval of proprotein convertase subtilisin/kexin type 9 (PCSK9) inhibitors (evolocumab and alirocumab) and success of bempedoic acid are the major breakthrough observed in lipid-lowering therapies in patients with ACS. FOURIER and ODYSSEY trials[24,25] have showed to significantly reduce low-density lipoprotein (LDL) level and adverse CV outcomes. 2019 ESC guideline was a major breakthrough in lipid lowering, as it targeted the LDL levels more aggressively. 2020 guidelines by Lipid Association of India have also adopted the similar targets as ESC.

- *For very high-risk patients (10-year risk of CV death ≥10%)*: Use an LDL-cholesterol (LDL-C) reduction of at least 50% from baseline and an LDL-C goal of <55 mg/dL.
- *For very high-risk patients who experience a second vascular event within 2 years (not necessarily of the same type as the first event) while taking maximally tolerated statin therapy*: An LDL-C goal of <40 mg/dL may be considered.
- *For patients at high risk (10-year risk for CV death of 5% to <10%)*: Use an LDL-C reduction of at least 50% from baseline and an LDL-C goal of < 70 mg/dL.
- *For individuals at moderate risk (10-year risk for CV death of 1% to <5%)*: Consider an LDL-C goal of <100 mg/dL.
- *For individuals at low risk (10-year risk for CV death <1%)*: Consider an LDL-C goal of <116 mg/dL.

Statin remained the primary drug for management of dyslipidemia followed by ezetimibe and PCSK9 inhibitors. Recently, published trials of bempedoic acid (CLEAR OUTCOME) may play a role of game changer in algorithm of lipid-lowering drugs in future guidelines.

CONCLUSION

Acute coronary syndrome is associated with high morbidity and mortality and is best managed by an expert team. Although invasive management plays a vital role to prevent mortality in early phase of the events, pharmacological therapies are equally important for long-term well-being of patients. Amongst pharmacological therapies, antiplatelet and lipid-lowering therapies remain cornerstone of the management of ACS. Beyond this, beta-blockers, blood pressure control, optimal control of diabetes mellitus, smoking cessation, and cardiac rehabilitation are also as important as antiplatelets and lipid-lowering agents.

ONLINE REFERENCES

Please scan the QR code provided at the end of the table of contents for References of this chapter.

CHAPTER

78

Managing Acute Coronary Syndrome in a Patient with Thrombocytopenia

Sudhir Chandra Sinha, G Venkateshwara Reddy

ABSTRACT

Antithrombotic agents, antiplatelets, thrombolytic agents, and percutaneous interventions form the backbone of the management of acute coronary syndrome (ACS). Of all these, antiplatelet therapy is ubiquitous. These therapies have an inherent risk of bleeding complications that may get exacerbated further by the presence of a low platelet count. Intravenous heparin remains the gold standard antithrombotic agent during percutaneous angioplasty which may lead to thrombocytopenia. Patients with thrombocytopenia are not immune to ACS. It becomes a daunting task to manage ACS in such patients. There are no studies specifically addressing such a clinical dilemma. This chapter discusses how to safely handle ACS in a patient who has preexisting thrombocytopenia or who has developed it after percutaneous intervention. This discussion focuses on the management of ACS in thrombocytopenic patients.

Keywords: Antiplatelets, thrombocytopenia, anticoagulants, acute coronary syndrome.

INTRODUCTION

Thrombocytopenia is defined as a platelet count that is $<150 \times 10^9$/L. It is further classified as mild, moderate, or severe[1] **(Table 1)**. In clinical practice, a drop in platelet count by >50% from baseline should alert the physician and be treated as potential thrombocytopenia.

The National Cancer Institute Common Terminology Criteria for Adverse Events[2] (NCI CTCAE) grades thrombocytopenia into four grades **(Table 2)**.

The risk of spontaneous bleeding occurs when the platelet count is $<10 \times 10^9$/L.

The CRUSADE (Can Rapid Risk Stratification of Unstable Angina Patients Suppress Adverse Outcomes with Early Implementation of the American College of Cardiology/American Heart Association Guidelines) quality improvement initiative evaluated 36,182 patients with non-ST-segment elevation acute coronary syndrome (ACS) enrolled in 379 hospitals in the United States between June 2004 and

TABLE 1: Grading of thrombocytopenia.

Clinical severity	Defining platelet count
Normal value	Platelet counts $>150 \times 10^9$/L
Mild thrombocytopenia	Platelet counts from 100×10^9/L to 150×10^9/L
Moderate thrombocytopenia	Platelet counts from 50×10^9/L to 100×10^9/L
Severe thrombocytopenia	Platelet counts $<50 \times 10^9$/L

TABLE 2: Grading of thrombocytopenia by the National Cancer Institute Common Terminology Criteria for Adverse Events (NCI CTCAE).

Grade	Platelet count ($\times 10^9$/L)	Platelet count (/mL)
Grade 1	<100–75	100,000–75,000
Grade 2	<75–50	<75,000–50,000
Grade 3	<50–25	<50,000–25,000
Grade 4	<25	<25,000

December 2006. New thrombocytopenia was noted in 13% of the patients. There were increased bleeding and mortality risks with each 10% drop in the platelet count. Adrop in the platelet count ≥50% from the baseline marked a higher risk of adverse events irrespective of nadir platelet count.[3]

TRUE THROMBOCYTOPENIA VERSUS ARTIFACTUAL THROMBOCYTOPENIA (PSEUDOTHROMBOCYTOPENIA)

Platelet clumping may occur in dipotassium ethylene-diaminetetraacetic acid (EDTA) samples, which is commonly used for sample collection for hemograms. It may lead to a falsely low platelet count, called pseudothrombocytopenia (PTCP). Platelet counts ranging from 10×10^9/L to 100×10^9/L have been reported in PCTP. Whenever thrombocytopenia is reported in a particular sample, it is prudent to have the sample collected in a heparin, citrate, or fluoride vial and have the sample be maintained and analyzed at room temperature (37°C). This step may prevent unnecessary panic and further testing. PTCP has been reported in 1:1,000 normal adults and is not associated with bleeding or thrombosis.[4]

A proper examination of peripheral blood smear is the simplest and the best test to evaluate thrombocytopenia. The presence of consistently large platelets suggests hereditary macrothrombocytopenia. These giant platelets are not counted as "platelets" in automated counters. The presence of large platelets along with normal-sized platelets indicates peripheral destruction of platelets like in heparin-induced thrombocytopenia (HIT). Smaller-sized platelets (micro-thrombocytopenia) are seen when there is decreased platelet production from the bone marrow. Fluid replacement or blood component replacement without platelets may lead to dilutional thrombocytopenia.

COMMONLY USED CARDIAC DRUGS CAUSING THROMBOCYTOPENIA

Apart from noncardiac drugs, some important cardiac prescription medicines can cause drug-induced immune thrombocytopenia (DITP). Unfractionated heparin (UFH) remains the most important cause of DITP, though its prevalence is very low. Other important agents include quinidine, amiodarone, glycoprotein (Gp) IIb/IIIa inhibitors (tirofiban, eptifibatide, and abciximab), thienopyridines, and protamine **(Table 3)**. Heparin and Gp IIb/IIIa inhibitors are commonly used in the management of ACS. Heparin is associated with two pathologically distinct thrombo-cytopenia, termed type 1 and type 2 HIT. Type 1 HIT is a nonimmune disorder, affecting platelets directly. It occurs in the first 2 days of heparin exposure and is self-limiting. It reverses even with the continued use of heparin. Type 2 HIT is an immune-related phenomenon, typically occurring 4–10 days after exposure. It can be fatal, mainly because of the difficulty in managing thrombotic complications. Tirofiban and eptifibatide react with Gp IIb/IIIa receptors and induce the formation of drug-dependent antibodies (DDAbs). In the case of abciximab, DDAbs recognize the murine component of the chimeric Fab fragment-specific for Gp IIIa. Gp IIb/IIIa-induced thrombocytopenia is relatively harmless and responds to discontinuation of the offending agent.[5]

Thienopyridines such as ticlopidine, clopidogrel, and prasugrel[6] have been found to cause thrombocytopenia. Ticlopidine was more commonly associated with DITP with a reported prevalence of 1:1,600–1:5,000. Thrombocytopenia is rare with clopidogrel, with a reported prevalence of 1:80,000. True thrombocytopenia with prasugrel has been limited to anecdotal case reports.

TABLE 3: Common drugs and therapies in ACS associated with thrombocytopenia.[9]

	Heparin	Gp IIb/IIIa inhibitors	Thienopyridines	IABP
Presentation	Mainly thrombotic events in type 2 HIT	Mucosal bleeding and petechiae	Mucosal bleeding and petechiae may cause TTP	• Usually mild • Bleeding may occur rarely
Onset of thrombo-cytopenia	• Type 1 HIT—first 2 days • Type 2 HIT—4–10 days	<12 hours	• Clopidogrel <2 weeks • Ticlopidine 2–12 weeks	Starts after the insertion of IABP and nadirs by day 3. Returns to the baseline in 2–3 days
Frequency	0.3% of the ACS population	• Abciximab—up to 9.2% • Eptifibatide and Tirofiban—up to 3.2%	• Clopidogrel: 1:80,000 • Ticlopidine:1:1,600	43–58%
Degree of thrombo-cytopenia	Severe with type 2 HIT	Moderate to severe if the drug is not discontinued	Moderate to severe and more severe with ticlopidine	• Mild thrombocytopenia in most of the cases • Severe thrombocytopenia in <10% of cases

(ACS: acute coronary syndrome; Gp: glycoprotein; HIT: heparin-induced thrombocytopenia; IABP: intra-aortic balloon pump; TTP: thrombotic thrombocytopenic purpura)

The mechanisms of thrombocytopenia involving these three thienopyridines are entirely different. Thrombocytopenia due to ticlopidine is linked with neutralizing ADAMTS-13 (antibodies to disintegrin and metalloproteinase with a thrombospondin type 1 motif, member 13). In >90% of cases, it occurred within 2–12 weeks from the initiation of therapy. The clinical picture mimics thrombotic thrombocytopenic purpura (TTP) with severe ADAMTS-13 deficiency. Thrombocytopenia has been reported within 2 weeks of initiation of clopidogrel and the mechanism is ADAMTS-13 independent.[6] The mechanism of thrombocytopenia due to prasugrel remains obscure. Thrombocytopenia has been reported with ticagrelor, though the exact prevalence is unknown. In one case report, it was linked to ADAMTS-13 deficiency.[7] In the pooled analysis of CHAMPION (Cangrelor Versus Standard Therapy to Achieve Optimal Management of Platelet Inhibition) trials, Cangrelor was not associated with an increased risk of acquired thrombocytopenia.[8]

THROMBOCYTOPENIA MAY CAUSE PARADOXICAL THROMBOSIS

Usually, thrombocytopenia causes excessive bleeding related to antiplatelets and antithrombotics, but HIT, antiphospholipid antibody syndrome, vaccine-induced thrombotic thrombocytopenia, hemolytic uremic syndrome, and TTP are all typically associated with very high thrombotic and ischemic risk. This risk increases with a further drop in platelet count.

The major complication of type 2 HIT is paradoxical thrombosis, especially venous thrombosis, pulmonary embolism, and sometimes arterial thrombosis causing ACS. Bleeding is unusual in type 2 HIT.

MANAGING ACUTE CORONARY SYNDROME IN A PATIENT WITH PREEXISTING THROMBOCYTOPENIA

Thrombocytopenia per se does not protect against thrombosis. Immune thrombocytopenia (ITP) increases the risk of the first arterial thrombotic event by 1.5%/year as compared to <1%/year for the general population. It is not related to any specific platelet-count threshold. The presence of thrombocytopenia is an independent risk factor for adverse outcomes in ACS. The chance of adverse events increases four- to fivefold due to inappropriate treatment decisions.

Loading Dose of Antiplatelets

The guidelines recommend the use of an initial loading dose of antiplatelets (aspirin, clopidogrel, prasugrel, and ticagrelor) in both non-ST-elevation and ST-elevation ACS. The safety of such a loading dose is not established in thrombocytopenic patients. A normal dose of antiplatelet therapy can be used safely if the platelet count is >50,000/mL. Ticagrelor and prasugrel should be avoided if the platelet count is below 50,000/mL. Cangrelor is not recommended in patients with platelet count < 50,000/mL.[10]

Use of Anticoagulants

The ACS guidelines are silent on dosage modification of parenteral anticoagulants [UFH or low-molecular-weight heparin (LMWH)] with platelet count. Guidelines on cancer and venous thromboembolism recommend a normal therapeutic dosage of parenteral anticoagulants in patients with grades 1–2 thrombocytopenia. LMWH should be preferred over UFH. For grade 3 thrombocytopenia, a 50% dose reduction is recommended. For grade 4 thrombocytopenia, avoid anticoagulation.[11]

Glycoprotein IIb/IIIa Inhibitors

The TARGET (Do Tirofiban and Reopro Give Similar Efficacy Trial) study compared tirofiban and abciximab in patients undergoing percutaneous coronary intervention (PCI). Thrombocytopenia occurred in 2.4% of patients treated with abciximab and in 0.5% treated with tirofiban. In this study, thrombocytopenia was associated with a higher risk of nonhemorrhagic death in 30-day follow-up, probably related to paradoxical platelet activation due to the formation of new platelets. The bleeding events were not higher in the Gp IIb/IIIa group as compared to the placebo. In the ESPRIT (Enhanced Suppression of the Platelet IIb/IIIa Receptor with Integrilin Therapy) trial, eptifibatide was associated with a 0.2% incidence of severe thrombocytopenia. Thrombocytopenia occurred in 2.8% of patients who received eptifibatide in the IMPACT-II (Integrilin to Minimize Platelet Aggregation and Coronary Thrombosis) trial.[12]

Gp IIb/IIIa inhibitors should be avoided in ACS complicated by thrombocytopenia. However, in high-risk ACS and PCI, a Gp IIb/IIIa inhibitor can be used if the platelet count is >50,000/mL.

Thrombolytic Therapy

The guidelines on the use of thrombolytic therapy in ACS do not mention thrombocytopenia as an absolute or a relative contraindication. However, ischemic stroke thrombolysis guidelines mention a platelet count of <100,000/mL as an absolute contraindication for thrombolysis with intravenous (IV) alteplase. Streptokinase-based thrombolysis has been used in patients with platelet counts of 50,000–100,000/mL without excess bleeding. Considering limited reports in the literature, it is difficult to draw a conclusion, and thrombolysis is best avoided in patients with platelet count <100,000/mL.[13]

Percutaneous Coronary Interventions

The following recommendations apply to PCI in ACS in a thrombocytopenic patient (primary PCI or elective PCI):[14-16]

- A diagnostic coronary angiogram can be performed irrespective of the platelet count. Radial access is preferred over femoral-arterial access.
- PCI can be performed if the platelet count is >30,000/mL. Ideally, PCI should be avoided if the platelet count is between 10,000 and 30,000/mL. A platelet count of <10,000/mL is an *absolute contraindication* for PCI. Avoid it unless it is a lifesaving procedure.
- A normal dose of UFH, 50–70 U/kg, is recommended for PCI if the platelet count is >50,000/mL. A UFH dose of 30–50 U/kg can be used if the platelet count is between 30,000 and 50,000/mL. It is important to monitor activated clotting time (ACT) and titrate the dose of UFH.
- Aspirin in low doses, 75 mg/day, can be used if the platelet count is above 10,000/mL.
- Clopidogrel, in addition to aspirin, can be used if the platelet count is >30,000/mL.
- Ticagrelor or prasugrel can be used in addition to aspirin if the platelet count is >50,000/mL.
- Gp IIb/IIIa inhibitors should preferably be avoided. However, if needed, Gp IIb/IIIa inhibitors can be used if the platelet count is >50,000/mL.
- The new-generation drug-eluting stent (DES) is preferred over bare-metal stents (BMS).
- Dual antiplatelet therapy (DAPT) should be in the form of aspirin plus clopidogrel for a duration of 2 weeks for plain old balloon angioplasty (POBA) 4 weeks after BMS implantation and 6 weeks after DES, if the platelet count is <50,000/mL.
- Avoid coronary artery bypass surgery (CABG) if the platelet count is <50,000/mL.
- Prophylactic platelet transfusion in the periprocedural PCI period is recommended if:
    - A rapid fall in platelet count noted
    - The platelet count is <10,000/mL
    - There is a high fever or leukocytosis
    - The platelet count is <20,000/mL in patients with ACS and solid tumors receiving treatment for bladder, gynecologic, colorectal tumors, melanoma, or necrotic tumors.

Table 4 summarizes the use of platelets during primary PCI in a thrombocytopenic patient.

TABLE 4: Antiplatelet therapy in a patient with ACS undergoing PCI.

Grade of thrombocytopenia	Antiplatelet therapy
Grade 1 thrombocytopenia (Platelet count 75,000–100,000/mL)	DAPT—aspirin plus clopidogrel for 6 months
Grade 2 thrombocytopenia (Platelet count 50,000–75,000/mL)	DAPT—aspirin plus clopidogrel for 6 months
Grade 3 thrombocytopenia (Platelet count 25,000–50,000/mL)	SAPT in the form of aspirin. Add clopidogrel if there are high thrombotic risk features
Grade 4 thrombocytopenia (Platelet count <25,000/mL)	Avoid PCI. If needed, use aspirin if the platelet count is >10,000/mL
Cardiogenic shock and grade 4 thrombocytopenia	Platelet transfusion to make aspirin administration safe

(ACS: acute coronary syndrome; DAPT: dual antiplatelet therapy; PCI: percutaneous coronary interventions; SAPT: single antiplatelet therapy)

Triple Therapy Post-percutaneous Coronary Interventions in Acute Coronary Syndrome

Triple therapy in the form of DAPT and an oral anticoagulant in the form of vitamin K antagonists (VKA) or a non-vitamin K antagonist oral anticoagulant (NOAC) may be required in patients with atrial fibrillation or left ventricular thrombus. NOAC is preferred over VKA. The European Heart Rhythm Association guidelines[17] on NOAC usage recommend caution while using NOAC in patients with platelet counts <100,000/mL. Patients with a platelet count >50,000/mL can receive a full dose of NOAC, a half dose of NOAC for those with a platelet count of 20,000–50,000/mL, and no NOAC for those who have a platelet count of <20,000/mL. In patients with normal platelet count, triple therapy in the form of aspirin clopidogrel and oral anticoagulant (VKA or NOAC) is recommended for 1 month post-PCI for ACS, followed by dual therapy including clopidogrel (discontinue aspirin) and oral anticoagulant for 12 months, and oral anticoagulants only after 12 months. In patients with grades 1–2 thrombocytopenia, triple therapy including aspirin, clopidogrel, and NOAC can be given for 1 week post-PCI for ACS, followed by clopidogrel and NOAC dual therapy for 6 months, and NOAC alone 6 months onward. In patients with grade 3 thrombocytopenia, dual therapy in the form of single antiplatelet therapy (SAPT) (aspirin) with NOAC (or VKA) is not recommended. It is preferable to use SAPT alone.

Platelet Transfusion and Thrombopoietin Receptor Agonists

Prophylactic platelet transfusion to achieve platelet count 40,000–50,000/mL may be used before PCI or to make a patient with ACS tolerate antiplatelet and anticoagulant therapies in grades 3–4 thrombocytopenia. However, it is preferable to use SAPT and half dose of LMWH instead of platelet transfusion. Low-dose aspirin SAPT can be used with platelet count >25,000/mL.

Thrombopoietin receptor agonists (romiplostin, avatrombopag, eltrombopag, and lusutrombopag) have been used in the treatment of ITP. These agents can be used in ACS patients with ITP where long-term management is contemplated.

THROMBOCYTOPENIA FOLLOWING PERCUTANEOUS CORONARY INTERVENTIONS

Almost the entire pharmacotherapy used in the management of ACS, such as all the antiplatelets, heparin, and Gp IIb/IIIa inhibitors, can cause ITP of varying degrees. Out of all these, thrombocytopenia caused by Gp IIb/IIIa inhibitors and heparin remains the most important. Gp IIb/IIIa inhibitor-induced thrombocytopenia can be managed by ceasing the offending medication. Heparin-induced thrombocytopenia needs special consideration.

Heparin-induced Thrombocytopenia

Heparin-induced thrombocytopenia can occur with exposure of any kind and any dose of heparin, including the bolus dose given in the cardiac catheterization laboratory for PCI. HIT has been reported in 1–2% of cases after CABG. It is of two types: Type 1 HIT and type 2 HIT.[18]

Type 1 HIT is a nonimmune phenomenon related to the direct action of heparin on platelet activation. It may occur within 24 hours up to 4 days after an exposure to heparin. It is also known as heparin-associated thrombocytopenia (HAT). There is a mild drop in the platelet count, which usually reverses itself even when heparin is continued.

Type 2 HIT is an immune-mediated thrombocytopenia and could prove lethal if not diagnosed and treated promptly. It occurs 4–10 days after exposure to heparin. The major complication of type 2 HIT is thrombosis, which ranges from venous thromboembolism to stent thrombosis; it is also called heparin-induced thrombocytopenia with thrombosis (HITT). The risk of a thromboembolic event is up to 50% and carries a mortality risk of >30%. It should always be suspected if platelet count drops >50% from the baseline, even if it is >150,000/mL.

Type 2 HIT is further divided into acute HIT, subacute HIT A, subacute HIT B, and remote HIT **(Table 5)**. *Acute HIT* is the period from a decline in platelet count to a recovery in platelet count. It is a period with the highest thrombotic risk. *Subacute HIT A* is the period from platelet count recovery to until functional assays become negative. It occurs around day 7 after heparin cessation. *Subacute HIT B* is the period after the functional assay becomes negative but before the immune assay becomes negative. Functional assays become negative with a median period of 50 days after stopping heparin. When antiplatelet factor 4 (anti-PF4)/heparin antibodies are no longer detectable by immune assays, it is called *remote HIT*. Once exposed to heparin, reexposure within 100 days can cause a serious recurrence of HIT.

Heparin-induced thrombocytopenia has been reported with LMWH, though less frequently. Fondaparinux has not been shown to cause HIT.

Platelet factor 4 is stored in alpha granules of the platelet and is released during platelet activation. Heparin binds to PF-4 which triggers the formation of immunoglobulin G (IgG) antibodies. This heparin PF4–IgG complex binds to the Fc receptor of platelets, causing further platelet activation. This activation causes enhanced thrombosis. This is also recognized by macrophages which engulf platelets, causing thrombocytopenia.

The diagnosis of type 2 HIT is based on clinical suspicion, '4T' score (thrombocytopenia, timing of thrombocytopenia relative to heparin exposure, thrombosis or other sequelae of HIT, and likelihood of other causes of thrombocytopenia), immune assays, and functional assays **(Table 6)**. A 4T score of 4–5 indicates intermediate probability and 6–8 a high probability. Heparin/PF-4 enzyme-linked immunosorbent assay (ELISA) is a commonly used immunoassay with a sensitivity of >99%. Serotonin release assay (SRA) and heparin-induced platelet aggregation assay (HIPA) are functional assays. Functional assays are more sensitive than PF4 ELISA. The SRA test is a gold standard test for HIT. A positive PF4 ELISA should be confirmed with SRA.

Management Principles of Heparin-induced Thrombocytopenia[19]

- Discontinue all heparin products including heparin flushes used to flush the IV cannula.
- Avoid platelet transfusion unless the patient has bleeding complications or the platelet count is <10,000/mL and the patient is to undergo emergency PCI.
- High-dose intravenous immunoglobulin (IVIG) 1 g/kg for 2 days is the treatment of choice for a rapid increase in platelet count in HIT patients.

TABLE 5: Classification of type 2 HIT.

Phases of HIT	Platelet count	Functional assay (SRA, HIPA)	Immunoassay (Heparin PF4 ELISA)
Acute	Low, >50% drop	Positive	Positive
Subacute A	Recovered	Positive	Positive
Subacute B	Recovered	Negative	Positive
Remote	Recovered	Negative	Negative

(HIPA: heparin-induced platelet aggregation assay; HIT: heparin-induced thrombocytopenia; PF-4 ELISA: platelet factor 4 enzyme-linked immunosorbent assay; SRA: serotonin release assay)

TABLE 6: 4T score.

Clinical features	2 points	1 point	0 point
Thrombocytopenia	>50% fall and platelet nadir 20–100 × 10^9/L	30–50% fall or platelet nadir 10–19 × 10^9/L	<30% fall or platelet nadir 10–19 × 10^9/L
Timing of platelet count fall	Clear onset on day 5–10 or ≤1 day, if heparin has been used within the last 30 days	Consistent with fall on day 5–10 but not clear (e.g., missing baseline platelet count); onset after day 10 or ≤1 day, if heparin has been used within last 30–100 days ago	Platelet counts fall ≤4 days, without recent heparin exposure
Thrombosis or other sequelae	New thrombosis (confirmed); skin necrosis at the heparin injection site; anaphylactoid reaction after intravenous (IV) heparin bolus; adrenal hemorrhage	Progressive or recurrent thrombosis; erythematous skin lesions; thrombosis suspected but not proven	None
Other causes of thrombocytopenia	None apparent	Possible	Definite
Score: *0–3*: Low probability *4–5*: Intermediate probability *6–8*: High probability			

- It has also been used to prevent acute HIT when reexposure to heparin is contemplated in antibody-positive cases.
- Avoid LMWH.
- Fondaparinux may be used as an anticoagulant. It is recommended in place of danaparoid in pregnant patients with HIT.
- It can be used as an alternative to danaparoid in pregnant patients with HIT.
- The direct thrombin inhibitor argatroban is recommended for treatment and prophylaxis of thrombosis in HIT.
- The direct thrombin inhibitor bivalirudin is recommended in place of heparin for PCI patients who either have or are at risk for HIT.
- The indirect factor Xa inhibitor danaparoid is recommended in pregnant patients with HIT.
- NOACs are not approved by the Food and Drug Administration (FDA) but can be used in HIT as alternate anticoagulation.
- Avoid warfarin in the long term because it may lead to skin necrosis. NOACs are a better long-term choice. If warfarin needs to be started, the platelet count should be >150,000/mL and it should be overlapped with fondaparinux for 5 days.
- For isolated HIT without thrombosis, anticoagulation for 1 month is recommended. In HITT patients, anticoagulation for 3 months is recommended. NOAC is preferred over warfarin.

The AT BAT (Anticoagulant Therapy with Bivalirudin in the Performance of Percutaneous Coronary Intervention in Patients With Heparin-Induced Thrombocytopenia) trial[19] was an open-label study of bivalirudin in HIT or HITT undergoing PCI. About 1 mg/kg bolus bivalirudin was given 5 minutes before PCI, followed by 2.5 mg/kg/h infusion for 4 hours (high-dose group), or 0.75 mg/kg bolus with 1.75 mg/kg/h infusion (low-dose group) in 52 patients. Procedural success was achieved in 98% and there was no drop in platelet count <50,000/mL.

CASE DISCUSSION

A 58-year-old gentleman was admitted with ST-elevation inferior myocardial infarction with a window period of 4 hours. He underwent primary PCI of right coronary artery requiring three stents (two stents for long lesion and one for edge dissection). He received intraprocedural IV UFH 100 U/kg. Post PCI, he was managed with standard oral antiplatelets (ticagrelor + aspirin). He did not receive any UFH or LMWH post procedure. Routine blood chemistry on day 6 revealed a platelet count of 63,000/mL which dropped to 4,000/mL on day 7. The 4T score was 6. Antiplatelet therapy was changed to clopidogrel monotherapy and IVIG 2 g/kg was given over 48 hours. The platelet count improved to 45,000/mL on day 12. He was discharged with clopidogrel + aspirin DAPT. The platelet count returned to 316,000/mL on day 30. Early recognition of HIT, continuation on SAPT, and institution of IVIG prevented acute stent thrombosis.

CONCLUSION

Thrombocytopenia poses an important therapeutic challenge in ACS management. It could preexist or could be the side effect of ACS pharmacotherapy. Either way, it is responsible for inappropriate management and adverse outcomes in ACS patients. Proper knowledge can help to treat such patients better. It is customary to exclude patients with thrombocytopenia in clinical trials evaluating

TABLE 7: Summary of the use of various therapies in ACS.

	Grade 1 thrombocytopenia	Grade 2 thrombocytopenia	Grade 3 thrombocytopenia	Grade 4 thrombo-cytopenia	Type 2 HIT
Platelet count	75×10^9/L to 100×10^9/L	50×10^9/L to 75×10^9/L	25×10^9/L to 50×10^9/L	<25×10^9/L	>50% fall in platelet count; 100×10^9/L to <10×10^9/L
Antiplatelets	• ASA • CLOP (DAPT can be used) Prasugrel ticagrelor	• ASA • CLOP (DAPT can be used) Prasugrel ticagrelor	• ASA • CLOP (SAPT only)	• ASA • CLOP (SAPT only)	• ASA • CLOP (SAPT only)
UFH for PCI	50–70 U/kg IV	50–70 U/kg IV	30–50 U/kg IV	Avoid	Avoid, including heparin flushes
LMWH	Normal dose/kg body weight	Normal dose/kg body weight	50% of normal dose	Avoid	Avoid, except fondaparinux
Gp IIb/IIIa inhibitors	Use with caution	Use with caution	Avoid	Avoid	Avoid
Thrombolytic therapy	Avoid	Avoid	Avoid	Avoid	Avoid
PCI	Safe	Safe	Caution	Avoid	Avoid PCI. Use bivalirudin in place of heparin
Platelet transfusion	Avoid (can be used if PCI is planned)	Avoid (can be used if PCI is planned)	Avoid (can be used if PCI is planned)	Avoid (can be used if PCI is planned)	Avoid, unless there is spontaneous bleeding
NOAC	Full dose	Full dose	Half dose		Can be used
Antiplatelet + OAC (NOAC)	Triple therapy in the form of ASA + CLOP + NOAC for 1 week, SAPT + NOAC for 6 months, and NOACs alone after 6 months	Triple therapy in the form of ASA + CLOP + NOAC for 1 week, SAPT + NOAC for 6 months, and NOACs alone after 6 months	• SAPT only • ASA or CLOP	• SAPT only • ASA or CLOP	SAPT + NOAC, step up with the rise in platelet count

(ACS: acute coronary syndrome; ASA: aspirin; CLOP: clopidogrel; DAPT: dual antiplatelet therapy; Gp: glycoprotein; HIT: heparin-induced thrombocytopenia; IV: intravenous; LMWH: low molecular weight heparin; NOAC: non-vitamin K oral anticoagulants; OAC: oral anticoagulant; PCI: percutaneous coronary interventions; SAPT: single antiplatelet therapy; UFH: unfractionated heparin)

antiplatelets and antithrombotics which prevents evidence-based recommendation. However, some generalizations for clinical practice can be made based on recommendations, are summarized in **Table 7**.

ACKNOWLEDGMENT

I sincerely thank Ms Shruti Sinha for helping with the review of the manuscript and preparation of the central illustration.

ONLINE REFERENCES

Please scan the QR code provided at the end of the table of contents for References of this chapter.

CHAPTER 79

The Late Show: Exploring the Consequences of Delayed Percutaneous Coronary Intervention in STEMI Patients

Manoj Chopda, Amit Patel, Rahul Shewale, Ganesh Jagdale, Kavish Chopda

ABSTRACT

Cardiovascular diseases (CVDs) is the leading cause of death globally, taking an estimated 17.9 million lives (32% of global deaths)[1] each year. Out of these, ST-segment elevation myocardial infarction (STEMI) alone is estimated to account for more than 2.5 million cases annually in India.

The key point for dealing with STEMI is early diagnosis and immediate reperfusion to limit myocardial ischemia and infarct size, and thereby reduce the risk of post-STEMI complications. Primary percutaneous coronary intervention (PCI) of the infarct-related artery within 12 hours of onset of the symptoms is the gold standard. But for many reasons, large number of patients reach the PCI-capable hospitals outside this window due to some reasons, such as delayed presentation, misdiagnosis, and lack of medical resources in remote areas. The clinical approach to the occluded infarct-related artery late after myocardial infarction remains variable and controversial.

Keywords: Delayed STEMI presenters.

INTRODUCTION

Patients who present late with an acute myocardial infarction (MI) are a heterogeneous population, and the clinical decision regarding percutaneous coronary intervention (PCI) should be individualized. As per current guidelines, patients with 12–48 hours of symptom onset can still be taken for primary PCI. Beyond 48 hours, those who have hemodynamic or electrical instability should be taken for primary PCI. Among clinically stable, late-presenting patients, myocardial viability assessment and functional testing can identify yet another subgroup that may benefit from late PCI.

CURRENT GUIDELINES OF PERCUTANEOUS CORONARY INTERVENTION[2]

- Reperfusion therapy is indicated in all patients with symptoms of ischemia of ≤12-hour duration and persistent ST-segment elevation—Class Ia
- In patients with time from symptom onset >12 hours, a primary PCI strategy is indicated in the presence of ongoing symptoms suggestive of ischemia, hemodynamic instability, or life-threatening arrhythmias—Class Ic
- A routine primary PCI strategy should be considered in patients presenting late (12–48 hours) after symptom onset—Class IIa
- In asymptomatic patients, routine PCI of an occluded infarct-related artery (IRA) >48 hours after onset of STEMI is not indicated—Class IIIa

Time to treatment is a crucial factor in patients with ST-segment elevation myocardial infarction (STEMI). With increase in duration of coronary occlusion, infarct size (IS) increases from endocardium to epicardium, the concept is known as the "wave front phenomenon." Hence, timely revascularization of IRA reduces IS and salvage viable hibernating myocardium. Delay in reperfusion causes prolonged ischemia and irreversible myocardial cell death ensues, leading to transmural infarct.[3]

Several imaging studies in humans have confirmed the wave-like expansion of irreversible myocardial damage with a markedly reduced myocardial salvage when coronary occlusion persists >90 minutes. However, a substantial amount of salvageable myocardium was found way beyond the observed time window in animal studies.

Busk et al.[4] did myocardial perfusion imaging (MPI) to assess area at risk (AAR) before angioplasty and repeated after 30 days to assess final IS (FIS) [% of left ventricular (LV) myocardium], salvage index (% of noninfarcted AAR), and left ventricular ejection fraction (LVEF); late presenters had a larger FIS, a lower salvage index and LVEF, and a higher LV end-diastolic volume (LVEDV) and LV end-systolic volume (LVESV) compared with early presenters.

Using cardiac magnetic resonance (CMR) imaging, Stiermaier et al.[5] showed a significantly decreased myocardial salvage in late presenters compared to early presenters. Still >25% of the AAR could be salvaged in delayed presenting patients of 12–48 hours **(Figs. 1 and 2)**.

Nepper-Christensen et al.[6] also analyzed CMR imaging of early presenting <12 hours and delayed presenting 12–72 hours, at index PCI and on follow-up 3 months later. Data showed that 65% of delayed PCI group had achieved substantial myocardial salvage ~0.50 **(Figs. 3A and B)**. Advances in CMR may help in better tissue characterization of the infarcted myocardium and better assessment for patient, to be benefited in delayed presenting cohort of patient in future, and lead toward personalized approach to treatment. Therefore, these results confirm the chance of achieving myocardial salvage in STEMI patients with a symptom duration of >12 hours using the reference standard of cardiac imaging. Several factors might explain the differences between clinical studies and experimental settings with fixed coronary occlusion in animal models.

Horie et al.[7] showed that LV remodeling in terms of LVEDV and LVESV indexes were significantly smaller in the percutaneous transluminal coronary angioplasty (PTCA) group than in the no-PTCA group ($p < 0.001$).

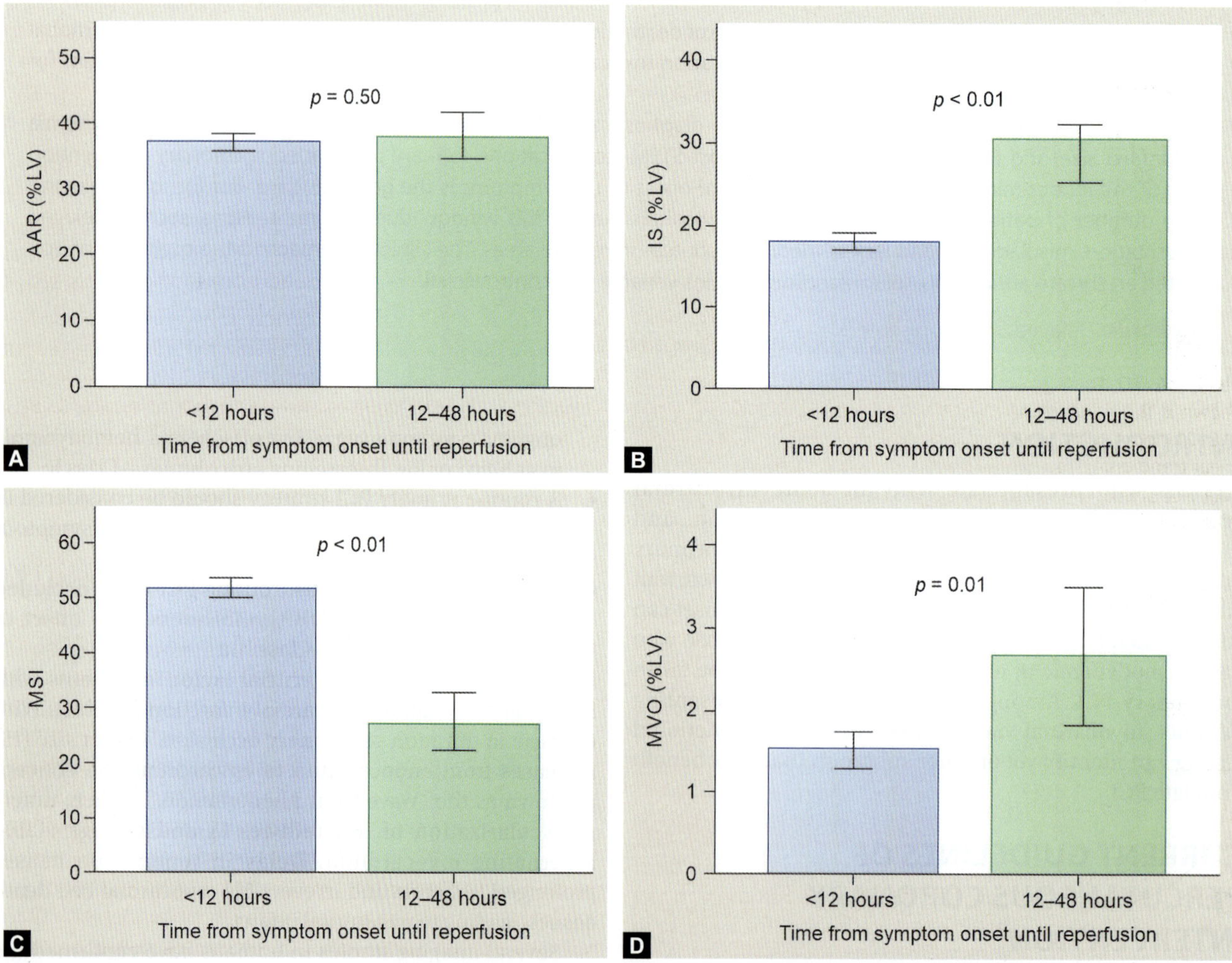

FIGS. 1A TO D: Cardiac magnetic resonance imaging parameters in STEMI patients with early and late reperfusion. Shown is the mean extent of AAR, IS, MSI, and MVO in STEMI patients with early and late reperfusion (<12 hours and 12–48 hours).[5]

(AAR: area at risk; IS: infarct size; LV: left ventricular; MSI: myocardial salvage index; MVO: microvascular obstruction; STEMI: ST-segment elevation myocardial infarction)

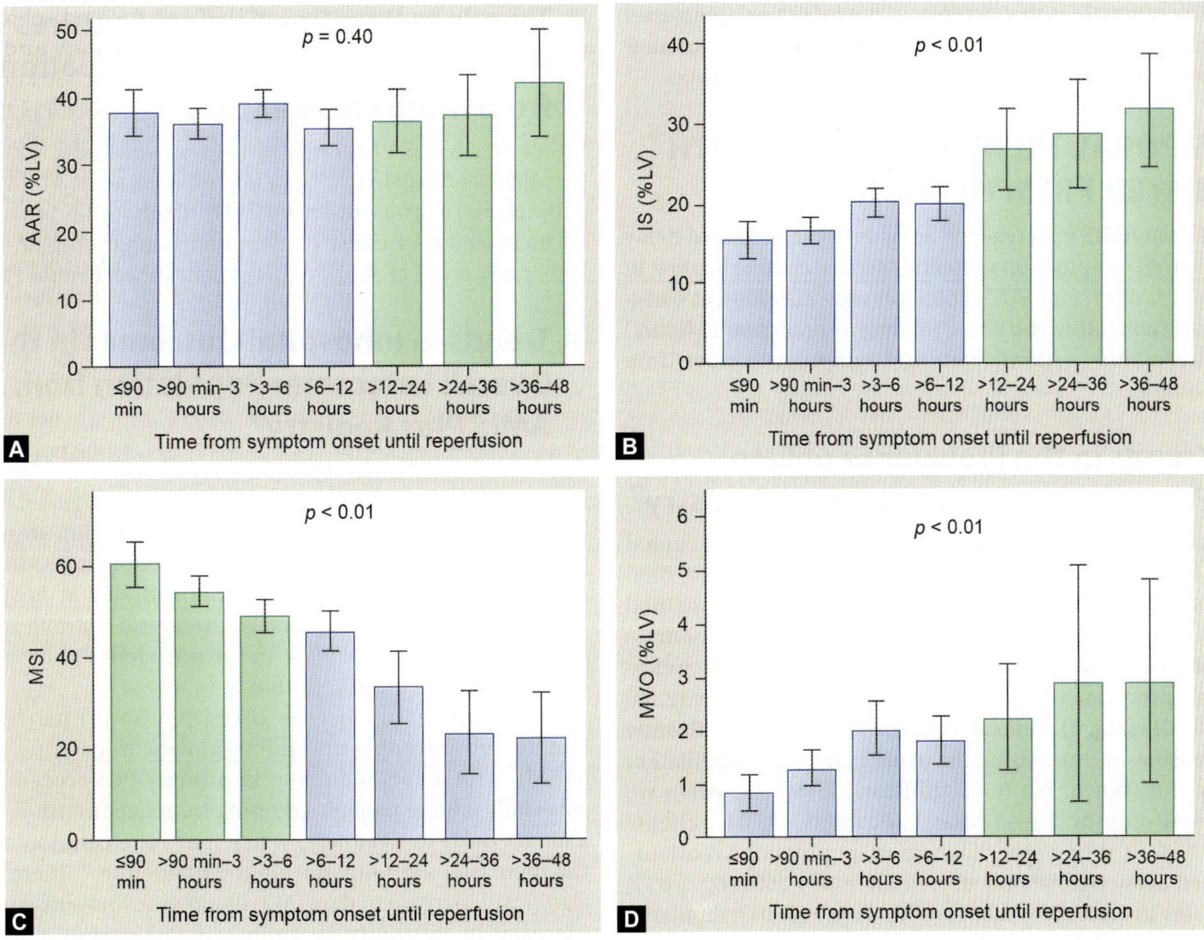

FIGS. 2A TO D: Cardiac magnetic resonance imaging parameters according to the time from symptom onset until reperfusion. Shown is the mean extent of AAR, IS, MSI, and MVO in STEMI patients (≤90 minutes, >90 minutes to 3 hours, >3–6 hours, >6–12 hours, >12–24 hours, >24–36 hours, and >36–48 hours). Error bars display 95% confidence intervals, *p* values were calculated with unadjusted linear trend analyses, and LV percentage of left ventricular mass.[5]

(AAR: area at risk; IS: infarct size; LV: left ventricular; MSI: myocardial salvage index; MVO: microvascular obstruction; STEMI: ST-segment elevation myocardial infarction)

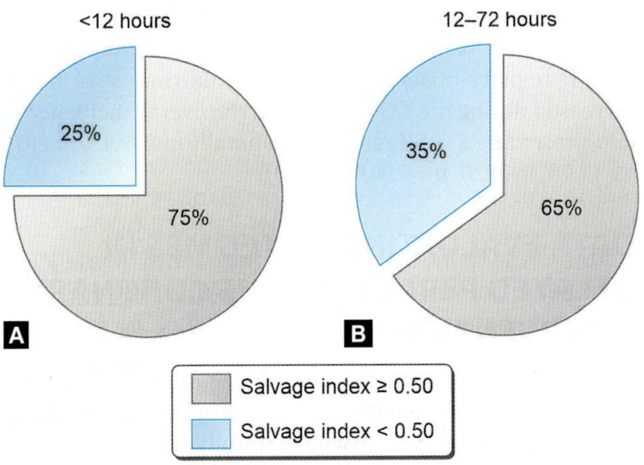

FIGS. 3A AND B: Percentage of patients achieving myocardial salvage index ≥ 0.50 stratified by duration from symptom onset to primary percutaneous coronary intervention. *p* value for the difference between groups was 0.146.[6]

POSSIBLE MECHANISM FOR BENEFIT IN DELAYED PERCUTANEOUS CORONARY INTERVENTION[8]

- A significant higher rate of apoptosis is evident in persisted-occluded artery and this apoptosis persists well beyond the acute phase of inflammation. Late revascularization of hibernating myocardium within the peri-infarct region tends to avoid this apoptosis and salvages significant myocardium.
- Thrombotic milieu during acute coronary syndrome results in a state of dynamic coronary occlusion, creates a state of ischemic preconditioning, and subsequent reperfusion results in delay of progression of irreversible myocardial damage.
- Reperfusion of IRA allows better early inflammatory phase and improvises healing of infarcted tissue and limits infarct expansion and helps ventricular remodeling.

- The rationale is that patency of the infarct-related vessel can improve LV systolic function and prevent ventricular remodeling and the late development of arrhythmias.

TEMPORAL TRENDS IN PATIENT WITH DELAYED PRESENTATION[9]

Data from AMIS Plus registry[9] assessed patient-related delay (time from symptom onset to first medical contact leading to hospitalization) and STEMI patients were classified as early-comers (patients with a first symptom-to-door time 12 hours) or latecomers (patients with first symptom-to-door time > 12 hours).

Trends in the Prevalence of Late Presentation from AMIS Plus Registry[9]

From 27,653 STEMI patients, 422 patients were excluded due to missing data on patient-related delay; hence, final analysis was done in 27,231 patients. Data were classified into early comers 22,928 patient (84%) and latecomers 4,303 (16%). Data showed overall significant decrease in the prevalence of late presentation from 22 to 12.3% ($p < 0.001$) **(Fig. 4)**. Patient-related delay did not significantly decrease over time within the overall latecomer population (data not shown; p = nonsignificant). However, when we focused only on 12–48-hour latecomers (3,704 patients and 85% of the overall latecomers population), patient-related delay significantly decreased from 1,260 (962–1,635) minutes to 1,103 (880–1,897) minutes ($p < 0.001$). Similarly, patient-related delay significantly decreased over time in the overall STEMI population from 210 (114–510) minutes to 158 (90–352) minutes ($p < 0.001$).[8]

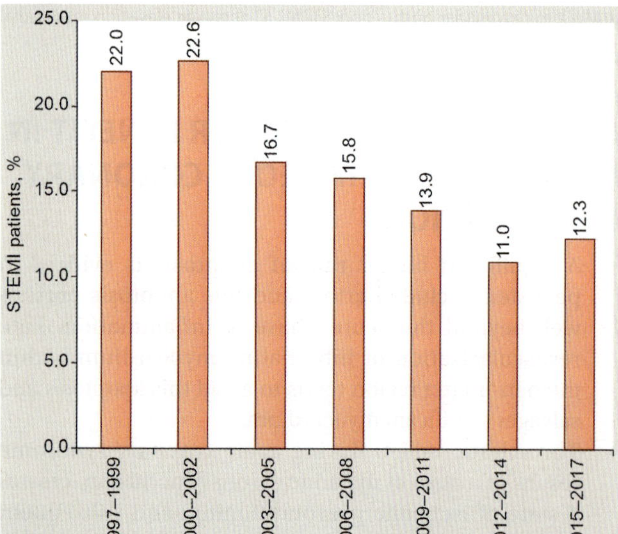

FIG. 4: Prevalence of late presentation during 20-year study period; data reported as percentage of ST-segment elevation myocardial infarction (STEMI).[9]

Trends in Baseline Clinical Features in the Overall Latecomer Population from AMIS Plus Registry[9]

Data from AMIS Plus registry shows overall decrease in prevalence of female sex, diabetes, previous acute MI (AMI), and coronary artery disease (CAD), likely to be linked to an increased awareness of symptoms, suggesting an AMI (especially atypical ones) in this patient subset **(Table 1)**.

Trends in Inhospital Outcomes in the Overall Latecomer Population from AMIS Plus Registry[9]

Data from AMIS registry shows significant reduction in mortality among late comers from 12.4 to 4.5% ($p < 0.001$). Similarly significant (p value < 0.001) reduction trend is seen in cardiogenic shock and reinfarction rates during index hospital admission and length of stay at hospital for index admission. Conversely, there was a strong trend toward a significant increase in the prevalence of bleeding complications (2.1–5.1%) **(Table 2)**.[9]

The coronavirus disease 2019 (COVID-19) pandemic had significant impact on the treatment of patients with STEMI, with a 19% reduction in primary PCI procedures, especially among patients suffering from hypertension, and a longer delay to treatment, which may have contributed to the increased mortality during the pandemic.[10] There was significant increase in door-to-balloon time and subsequent increase in mortality (p value < 0.003 and $p < 0.001$, respectively) **(Figs. 5A to F)**.

The KAMIR NIH (Korea Acute Myocardial Infarction Registry-National Institute of Health) STEMI registry[11] provides us with insights that may inform future guidelines. First, late-STEMI presentation is becoming increasingly rare; nearly 90% of patients present early. Even clear outliers for primary PCI (presentation >48 hours after symptom onset) have become quite rare, comprising <0.001 from 1997 to 2017. Second, a more recent large European multicenter STEMI registry observed total ischemia time > 12 hours increased during the COVID era, but the overall incidence of late-presenting STEMI remained generally low (9.1% in 2019 vs. 11.7% in 2020; $p < 0.001$) **(Fig. 6)**.

DATA EVALUATING OUTCOMES IN DELAYED PERCUTANEOUS CORONARY INTERVENTION

In BRAVE 2 trial,[13] which showed asymptomatic patients without persistent symptoms 12–48 hours after symptom onset, a small ($n = 347$) randomized study showed improved myocardial salvage and 4-year survival in patients treated with primary PCI compared with conservative treatment alone.

TABLE 1: Trends in baseline clinical features in latecomer population from AMIS Plus registry.[9]

	1997–1999 (n = 718)	2000–2002 (n = 690)	2003–2005 (n = 711)	2006–2008 (n = 657)	2009–2011 (n = 464)	2012–2014 (n = 533)	2015–2017 (n = 530)	p
Age, years	66.8 ± 13.0	66.1 ± 13.3	65.8 ± 13.0	65.5 ± 13.5	65.7 ± 13.3	65.9 ± 13.0	66.6 ± 12.0	0.495
Female sex	219/718 (30.5)	206/690 (29.9)	208/711 (29.3)	184/657 (28.0)	119/464 (25.6)	146/533 (27.4)	128/530 (24.2)	0.005
Resuscitation prior to admission	31/711 (4.4)	22/654 (3.4)	11/702 (1.6)	11/657 (1.7)	8/464 (1.7)	11/530 (2.1)	11/530 (2.1)	0.003
Killip class 3/4	60/682 (8.8)	62/687 (9.0)	38/710 (5.4)	30/654 (4.6)	38/459 (8.3)	27/533 (5.19)	27/528 (5.1)	0.002
Hypertension	373/702 (53.1)	363/659 (55.1)	380/666 (57.1)	377/630 (59.8)	268/442 (60.6)	297/514 (57.8)	308/498 (61.8)	0.001
Diabetes	176/703 (25.0)	158/674 (23.4)	153/687 (22.3)	121/636 (19.0)	101/449 (22.5)	107/502 (21.3)	93/503 (18.5)	0.006
Dyslipidemia	359/662 (54.2)	348/623 (55.9)	387/635 (60.9)	281/568 (49.5)	185/391 (47.3)	286/476 (60.1)	335/476 (70.4)	<0.001
Current smoker	258/688 (37.5)	272/637 (42.7)	269/672 (40.0)	224/607 (36.9)	186/425 (43.8)	188/472 (39.8)	212/463 (45.8)	0.051
Obesity (BMI > 30 kg/m^2)	78/432 (18.1)	123/625 (19.7)	117/605 (19.3)	118/566 (20.8)	94/413 (22.8)	114/501 (22.8)	107/513 (20.9)	0.071
CAD	132/376 (35.1)	232/687 (33.8)	204/707 (28.9)	194/657 (29.5)	98/451 (21.7)	80/495 (16.2)	87/498 (17.5)	<0.001
Previous AMI		38/282 (13.5)	95/699 (13.6)	71/648 (11.0)	43/457 (9.4)	36/528 (6.8)	53/511 (10.4)	0.001
Previous PCI			32/344 (9.3)	52/657 (7.9)	37/451 (8.2)	42/524 (8.0)	56/514 (10.9)	0.303
CCI > 1		70/282 (24.8)	142/699 (20.3)	139/648 (21.5)	88/457 (19.3)	84/475 (17.7)	110/494 (22.3)	0.357

Note: Unless otherwise indicated, values are expressed as proportion (%), or mean ± standard deviation.

(AMI: acute myocardial infarction; BMI: body mass index; CAD: coronary artery disease; CCI: Charlson comorbidity index; PCI: percutaneous coronary intervention)

TABLE 2: Trends in inhospital outcomes in the latecomer population from AMIS Plus registry.[9]

Temporal trends in inhospital outcomes in latecomer ST-segment elevation myocardial infarction (STEMI) patients between 1997 and 2017.

	1997–1999 (n = 718)	2000–2002 (n = 680)	2003–2005 (n = 711)	2006–2008 (n = 657)	2009–2011 (n = 464)	2012–2014 (n = 533)	2015–2017 (n = 530)	p
Length of stay, days	10 (6–14)	8 (4–13)	6 (2–10)	6 (2–10)	5 (2–8)	4 (2–7)	4 (1–7)	<0.001
Cardiogenic shock	104/710 (14.6)	80/630 (11.8)	44/699 (6.3)	34/657 (5.2)	19/464 (4.1)	11/480 (23)	22/514 (43)	<0.001
Reinfarction	38/706 (5.4)	22/631 (3.2)	15/699 (2.1)	4/657 (0.6)	10/464 (2.2)	3/533 (0.6)	1/530 (0.2)	<0.001
Bleeding event			7/336 (2.1)	19/657 (2.9)	21/464 (4.5)	17/533 (3.2)	27/530 (5.1)	0.025
Cerebrovascular event	5/708 (0.7)	11/652 (1.7)	1/696 (0.1)	4/657 (0.6)	2/464 (0.4)	5/533 (0.9)	9/530 (1.7)	0.42
Mortality	89/718 (12.4)	63/690 (9.1)	41/711 (5.8)	33/657 (5.0)	27/464 (5.8)	17/533 (4.5)	24/530 (4.5)	<0.001

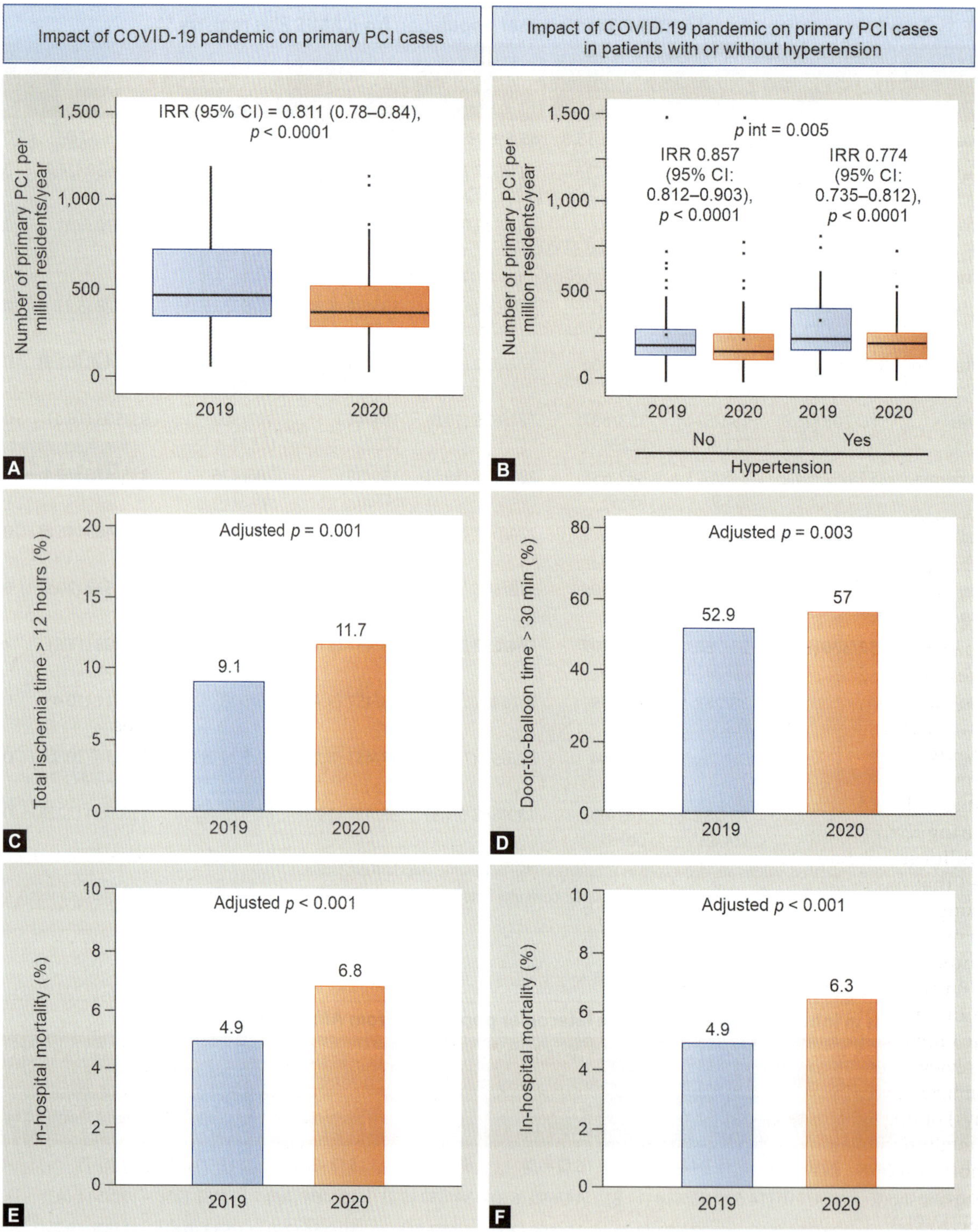

FIGS. 5A TO F: Impact of COVID-19 pandemic in PCI cases.[10]

(CI: confidence interval; COVID-19: coronavirus disease 2019; IRR: incidence rate ratio; PCI: percutaneous coronary intervention)

In stable patients with persistent occlusion of the IRA 3–28 days after MI, the large ($n = 2{,}166$) OAT (Occluded Artery Trial)[14] revealed no clinical benefit from routine coronary intervention with medical management, beyond that from medical management alone.

A meta-analysis[15] of trials testing whether late recanalization of an occluded IRA is beneficial showed no benefit of reperfusion. Therefore, routine PCI of an occluded IRA in asymptomatic patients >48 hours after onset of symptoms is not indicated. These patients should

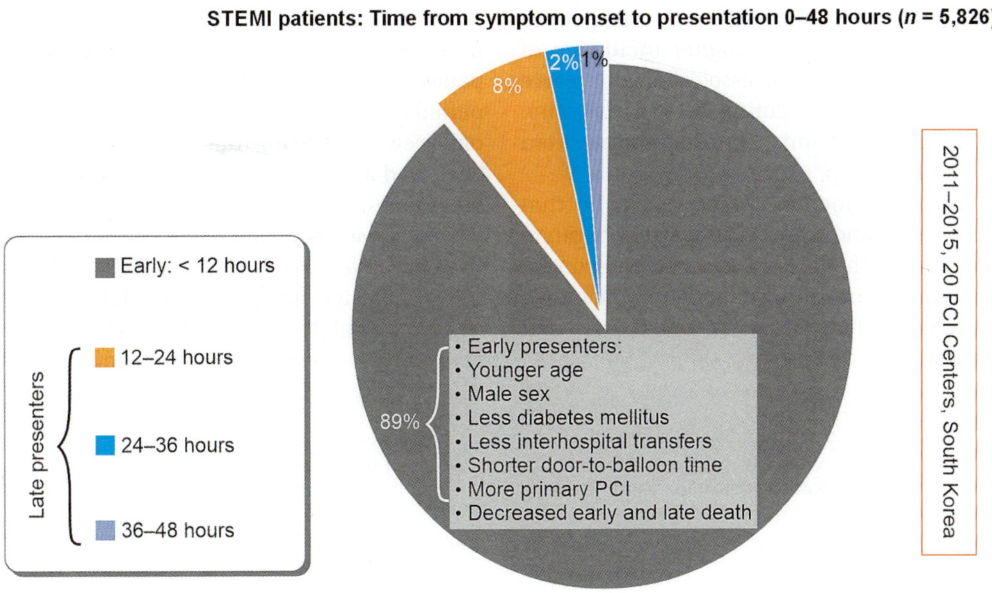

FIG. 6: Korean acute MI registry patient stratification in early <12 hours after symptom onset presenters and 24–48 hours late/delayed presenter.

(MI: myocardial infarction; PCI: percutaneous coronary intervention)

Source: Dauerman (2021).[12]

be managed like all patients with chronic total occlusion, in which revascularization should be considered in the presence of symptoms or objective evidence of viability/ischemia in the territory of the occluded artery.

Abbate et al.[16] published meta-analysis of 10 randomized controlled trials in 2008, including the OAT study, the SWISSI II study, and the BRAVE-2 study, comparing the efficacy of PCI and medication therapy (MT) following STEMI (12 hours–30 days). The results showed that mortality was significantly improved in the PCI group compared to that in the MT group [odds ratio (OR) 0.49; 95% CI 0.2–0.94; $p = 0.03$] **(Figs. 7A to D)**. PCI also outperformed MT in cardiac remodeling ($p = 0.009$) **(Figs. 8A to C)**.This meta-analysis showed that delayed reopening of the IRA (12 hours–60 days) could still improve cardiac function and survival.

A review presents a meta-analysis of data from five randomized controlled trials in which patients treated late (>3 days) during the course of AMI were randomized to PCI of the totally occluded IRA versus conservative management and shows a statistically significant improvement in cardiac function and a reduction in adverse remodeling, as measured by LVEF, LVEDV index (LVEDVI), and LVESV index (LVESVI), supporting the pathophysiologic value of the "open-artery hypothesis.[17]

Zheng et al.[18] investigated all STEMI patients who underwent delayed PCI (2–28 days after STEMI) during 2007–2010 in Beijing and excluded patients with hemodynamic instability. The study enrolled 5,417 STEMI patients and assigned them into three groups according to the presentation time—early group (day 2–7), 55.9%; medium group (day 8–14), 35.4%; and late group (day 15–28), 8.7%. The incidence of major adverse cardiovascular events (MACEs) were respectively 7.1%, 5.6%, and 6.7% among the three groups. The medium group had less recurrent MI plus cardiac death [hazard ratio (HR) 0.525; 95% CI 0.294–0.938; $p = 0.030$] than late group and less repeat revascularization (HR 0.640; 95% CI 0.463–0.883; $p = 0.007$) than early group in pairwise comparison **(Fig. 9)**.

Major adverse cardiovascular events **(Table 3)** were less in medium group probably because of reperfusion, helping in salvaging stunned or hibernating myocardium and also pathologic theory states that myocardial edema subsides and myocardial scar formation starts in the second week for better remodeling.[18]

Xiu et al.[19] analyzed retrospective data of STEMI patients from May 2012 to December 2015; a total of 1,072 STEMI patients received delayed PCI ($n = 594$) or standard MT ($n = 478$) more than 12 hours after the onset of symptoms. A less number of event in terms of all-cause death, cardiac death, and MACE in delayed PCI group versus medical therapy was found to be statistically significant (p value < 0.001).

Xue et al.[20] analyzed retrospective data of STEMI from 2014 to 2015 and divided them into early group (the period between STEMI onset and PCI was >3 days but <14 days) and the late group (the period between STEMI onset and PCI was more than 14 days).

No significant difference was found in primary and secondary end points of all-cause death and major adverse cardiac or cerebrovascular event (MACCE) between the two groups. However, they found early PCI group had three times higher recurrent MI event than the late group.

Coronary lesion were not analyzed from retrospective data, Xue et al. hypothesized that higher incidence of recurrent MI in early group might be associated with severe coronary lesion and complication during PCI in early group. However, they found more number of drug-eluting stent (DES) were used in early group.

The underlying pathological reason could be that myocardial edema faded, and myocardial scarring began to form in the second week. The higher incidence of recurrent MI in the early group requires further validation, including more retrospective data, randomized controlled trials, and translational studies.

Bouisset et al.[21] investigated the characteristics, prevalence, management, and outcomes of latecomer STEMI patients (i.e., admitted >12 hours after symptom onset) over a period of 10 years (2005–2015) in metropolitan France based on three registries conducted in a 1-month period [2005, 2010, and 2015 FAST-MI (French Registry of Acute Coronary Syndrome-MI) registries].

There was reduction of the latecomer patient proportion from 22.7% in 2005 to 16.1% in 2015, and an increase in the use of invasive strategy and evidence-based medications in this population. Also, Bouisset et al.[21] noticed that revascularization within 48 hours after hospital admission

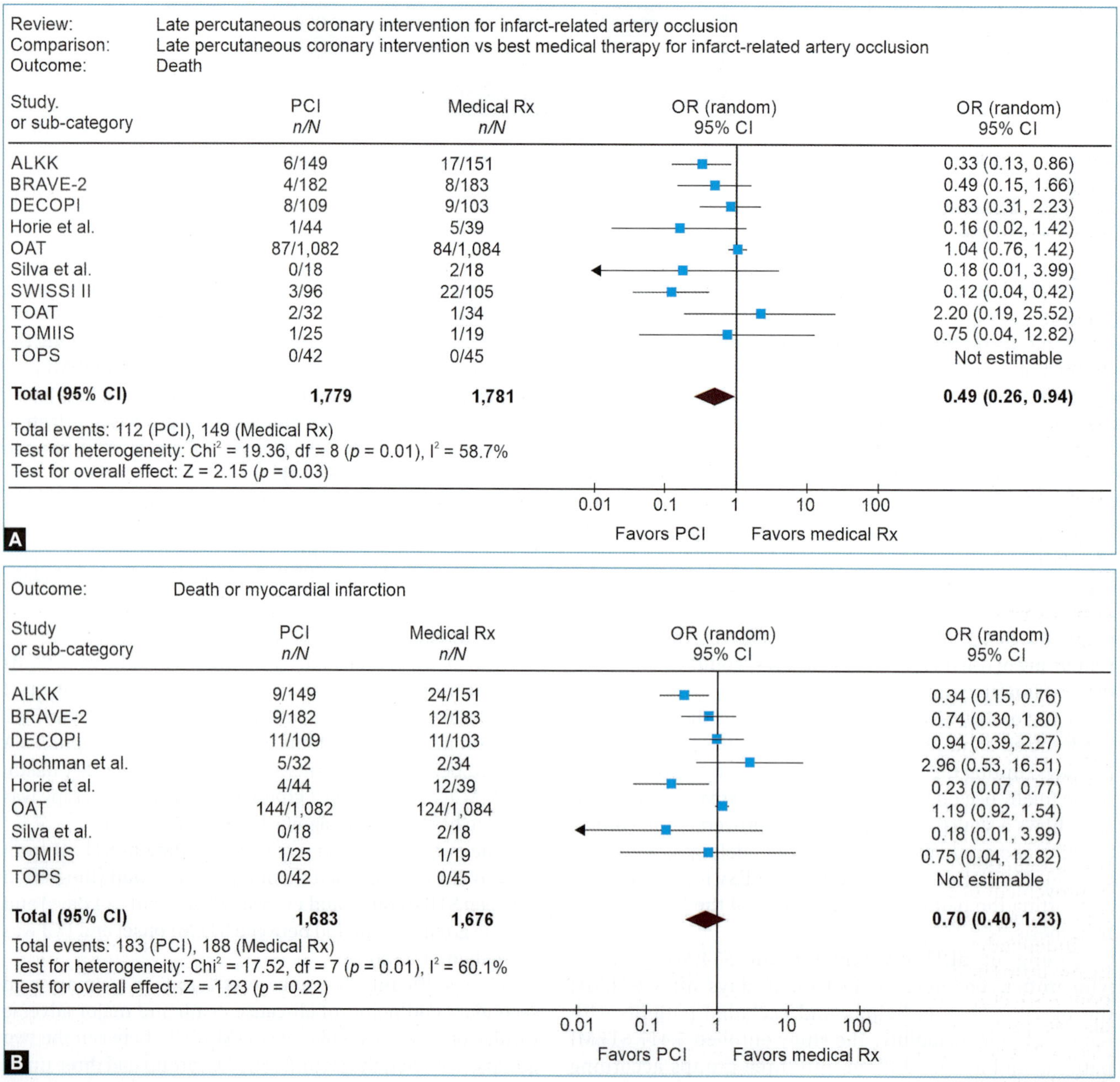

FIG. 7A TO D: *Continued*

Continued

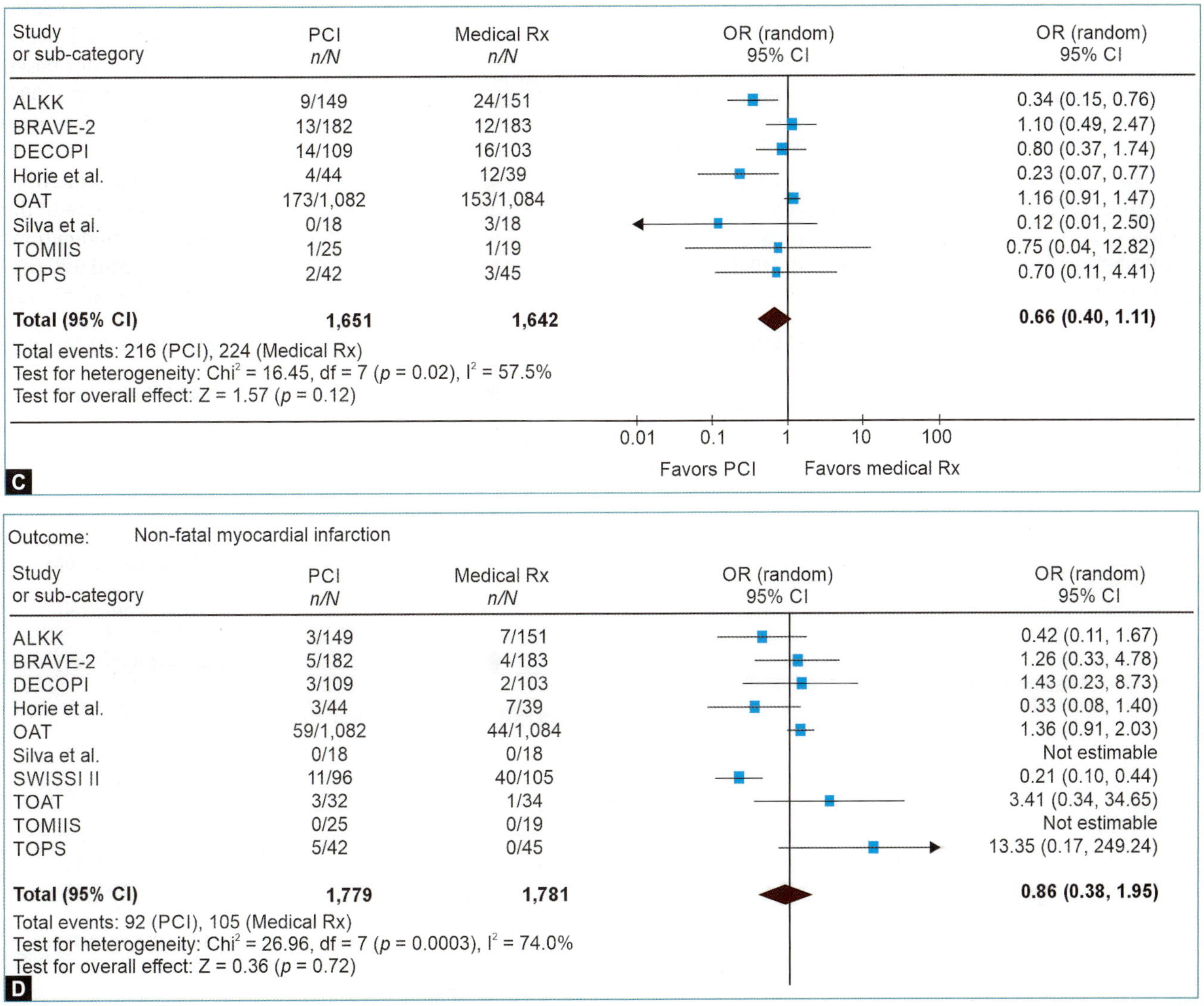

FIGS. 7A TO D: Forest plots showing individual and pooled risks of death. (A) Death and nonfatal recurrent myocardial infarction; (B) Death and nonfatal recurrent myocardial infarction or rehospitalization for angina/heart failure; (C) Nonfatal recurrent myocardial infarction; (D) Comparing late PCI versus best medical therapy (Rx) only for infarct-related artery occlusion late (>12 hours) in the course of acute myocardial infarction.[16]

(ALKK: Arbeitsgemeinschaft Leitende Kardiologische Krankenhausärzte; BRAVE-2: Beyond 12 Hours Reperfusion Alternative Evaluation Trial; CI: confidence interval; DECOPI: Randomized Trial of Occluded Artery Angioplasty after Acute Myocardial Infarction; OAT: Occluded Artery Trial; OR: odds ratio; PCI: percutaneous coronary intervention; SWISSI II: Swiss Interventional Study on Silent Ischemia Type II; TOAT: The Occluded Artery Trial; TOMIIS: Total Occlusion Post-Myocardial Infarction Intervention Study; TOPS: Treatment of Post-thrombolytic Stenoses)

was independently and significantly associated with an improvement of short- and long-term clinical outcomes in these patients **(Fig. 10)**.

Independent predictors of all-cause mortality during follow-up in late comers population are family history of AMI, prior AMI/PCI, chronic kidney disease, peripheral vascular disease, prior stroke/transient ischemic attack (TIA), Killip class > 2 at entry, LVEF < 40%, and revascularization within 48 hours of admission.

Although the relative proportion of latecomer STEMI patients decreased over the 10-year period of this study, they still constitute a significant proportion of STEMI patients who are more likely to present comorbidities and atypical presentation. Coronary revascularization of the infarct artery of latecomer STEMI patients admitted before 48 hours after symptom onset is associated with better long-term clinical outcomes on hard endpoints. Results from the FAST-MI strengthen the current European guidelines that recommend

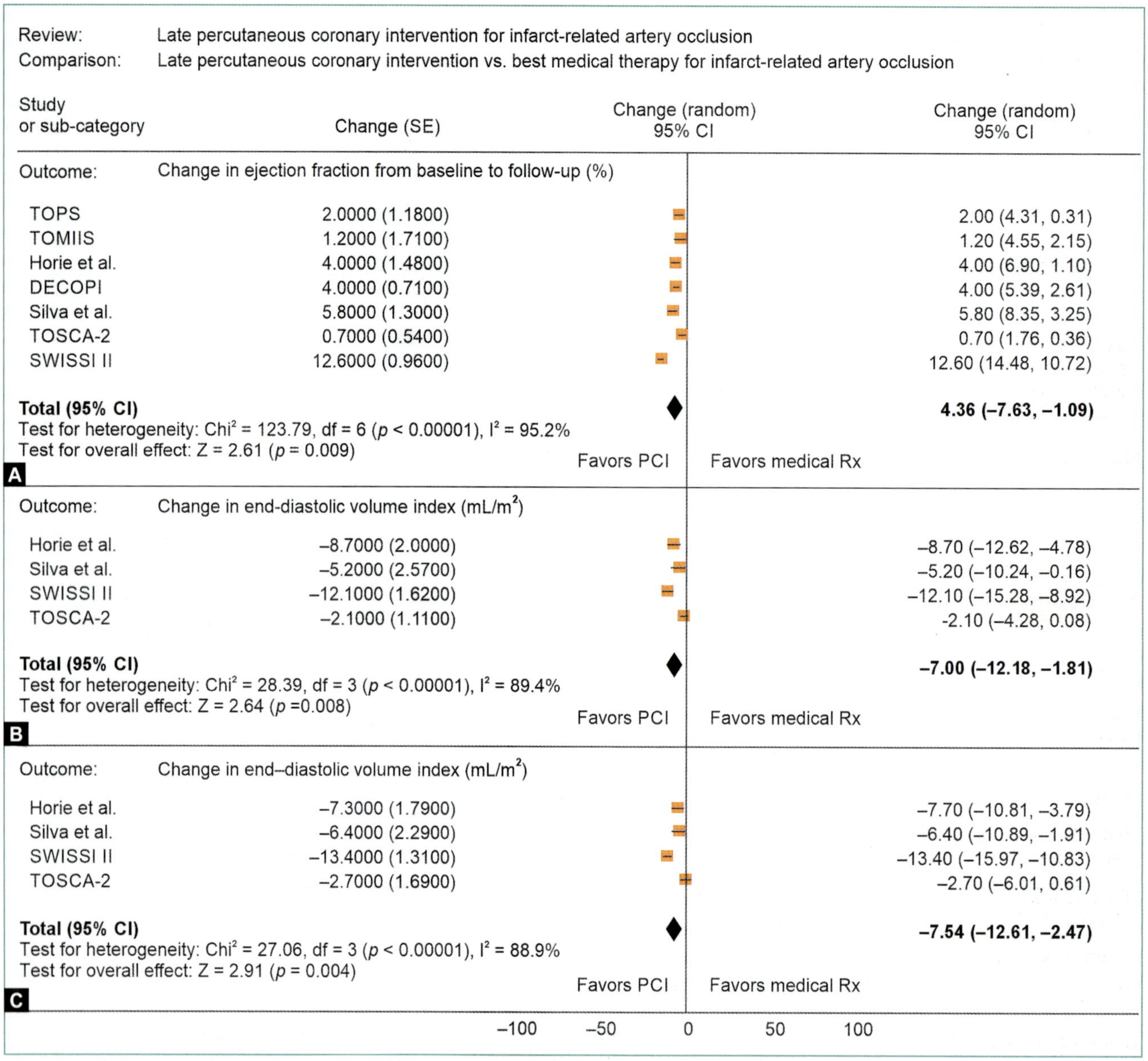

FIGS. 8A TO C: Individual and pooled group differences in changes in cardiac function and remodeling.[16] Forest plot showing individual and pooled changes in left ventricular ejection fraction, end-diastolic volume index, and end-systolic volume index at follow-up comparing late PCI versus best medical therapy only for infarct-related artery occlusion late (<12 hours) in the course of acute myocardial infarction. (A) Shows a +4% change in left ventricular ejection fraction favoring PCI. (B and C) Show a significant greater decrease in left ventricular end-diastolic volume index and left ventricular end-systolic volume index in the PCI, showing a more favorable remodeling pattern.[16]

(CI: confidence interval; DECOPI: Randomized Trial of Occluded Artery Angioplasty after Acute Myocardial Infarction; PCI: percutaneous coronary intervention; SWISSI II: Swiss Interventional Study on Silent Ischemia Type II; TOMIIS: Total Occlusion Post-Myocardial Infarction Intervention Study; TOPS: Treatment of Post-thrombolytic Stenoses; TOSCA-2: Total Occlusion Study of Canada-2)

performing a PCI on STEMI patients up to 48 hours after symptom onset.

Cho et al.[11] from the KAMIR NIH studied 13,707 patients from database, 5,826 consecutive patients diagnosed with STEMI within 48 hours of symptom onset during 2011–2015 were categorized as late (12–48 hours; n = 624) or early (<12 hours; n = 5,202) presenters.

Late presenters had remarkably worse clinical outcomes than early presenters (180-day mortality 10.7% vs. 6.8%; 3-year mortality 16.2% vs. 10.6%; both log-rank $p < 0.001$), whereas presentation at ≥12 hours of symptom onset was not independently associated with increased mortality after STEMI **(Figs. 11A to C)**. The use of invasive interventional procedures abruptly decreased from the first (less than 12 hours) to the

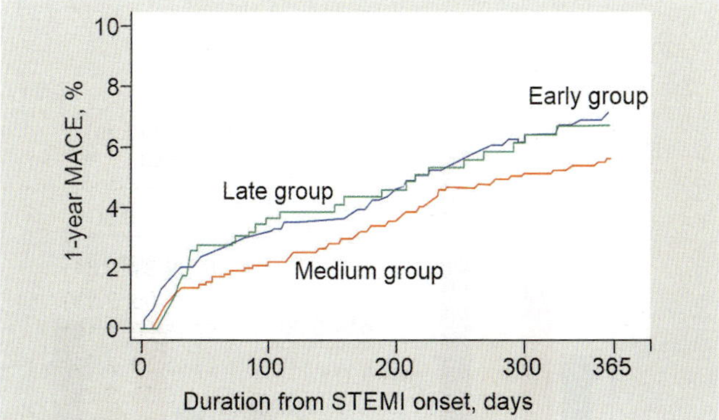

No. at risk					
Early group	3,030	2,726	2,501	2,236	2,069
Medium group	1,915	1,749	1,584	1,401	1,282
Late group	472	422	389	346	318

FIG. 9: MACCE at 1 year in early/medium/late group.

(MACCE: major adverse cardiac or cerebrovascular event; STEMI: ST-segment elevation myocardial infarction)

TABLE 3: Comparison of outcomes in different groups.[18]

Outcome	Early group (day 2–7)	Medium group (day 8–14)	Late group (day 15–28)
MACE	194 (7.1%) $p < 0.05$	96 (5.6%)	29 (6.7%)
Cardiac death	22 (0.8%)	14 (0.8%) $p < 0.05$	9 (2.1%)
Recurrent MI	57 (2.0%)	33 (1.8%)	13 (3.0%)
Repeat revascularization	146 (5.5%) $p < 0.05$	61 (3.7%)	12 (3.0%)
Cardiac death + recurrent MI	76 (2.5%)	45 (2.4%) $p < 0.05$	19 (4.0%)

(MACE: major adverse cardiovascular event; MI: myocardial infarction)

Note: *p* value is calculated between the highlighted green colored box.

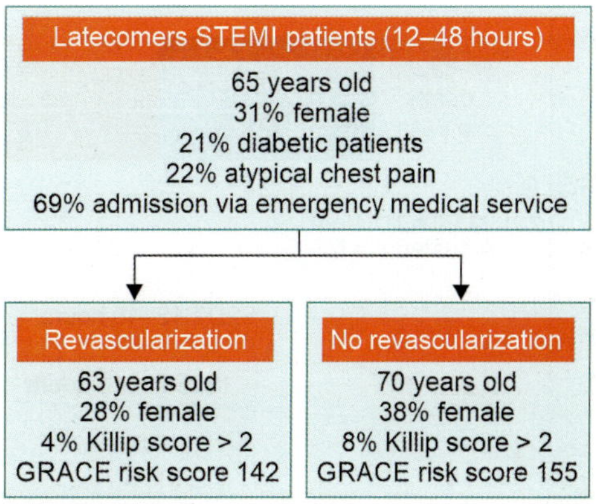

30-day mortality (%)	2.1%	7.2%	$p < 0.001$
Long-term mortality (for 1,000 patient-years)	30.4	78.7	$p < 0.001$

Long-term all-cause mortality

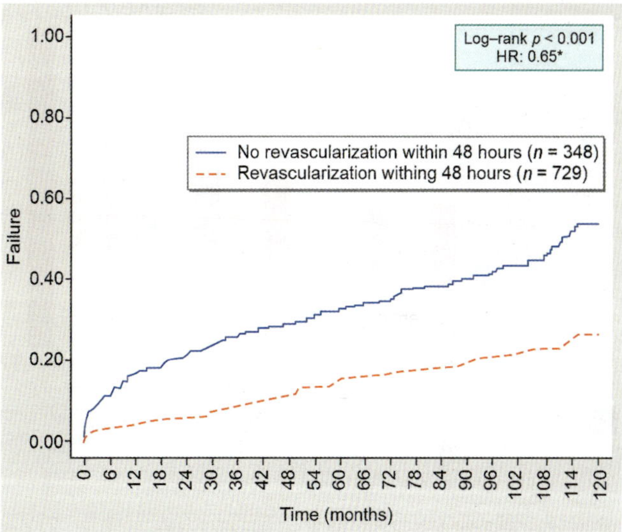

FIG. 10: Mortality comparison in the latecomer population according to revascularization status.[21]

(HR: hazard ratio; STEMI: ST-elevation myocardial infarction)

second (12–24 hours) 12-hour interval of symptom-to-door time ("no primary PCI strategy" increased from 4.9 to 12.4% and "no PCI" from 2.3 to 6.6%; both $p < 0.001$).

Late presenters (12–48 hours, $n = 624$) were older; more often women less likely to be admitted during off-hours; less often obese; and more likely to have a high heart rate, low LVEF, low hemoglobin level, and low cholesterol level than early presenters [<12 hours **(Fig. 12)**]. Additionally, they were more likely to have a history of diabetes and to present with Killip class II or III, but less likely to present with Killip class IV, suggesting that a considerable proportion of patients who were late presenters with Killip class IV died prior to hospital arrival. Similarly, mortality rates abruptly increased from the first 12-hour interval to the second 12-hour interval, but no significant difference or linear trend in mortality rates was noted from the second to the fourth 12-hour interval. These findings suggest that the clinical practice pattern of invasive interventional procedures might aggravate the clinical outcomes of STEMI late presenters, although the present study cannot appropriately address whether primary PCI is beneficial in all STEMI patients presenting late because of the lack of a control group.

Factors for Delayed Presentation and Percutaneous Coronary Intervention

Delayed presentation is the biggest global challenge for patients presenting with STEMI and this issue is far worse in developing countries for a variety of reasons. Traditional patient-related delays which are also seen in western developed countries include women, the elderly, and the diabetics patients. In low- and middle-income countries, there are additional and distinctive process delays, such as stoppages as a result of payment and consent issues.

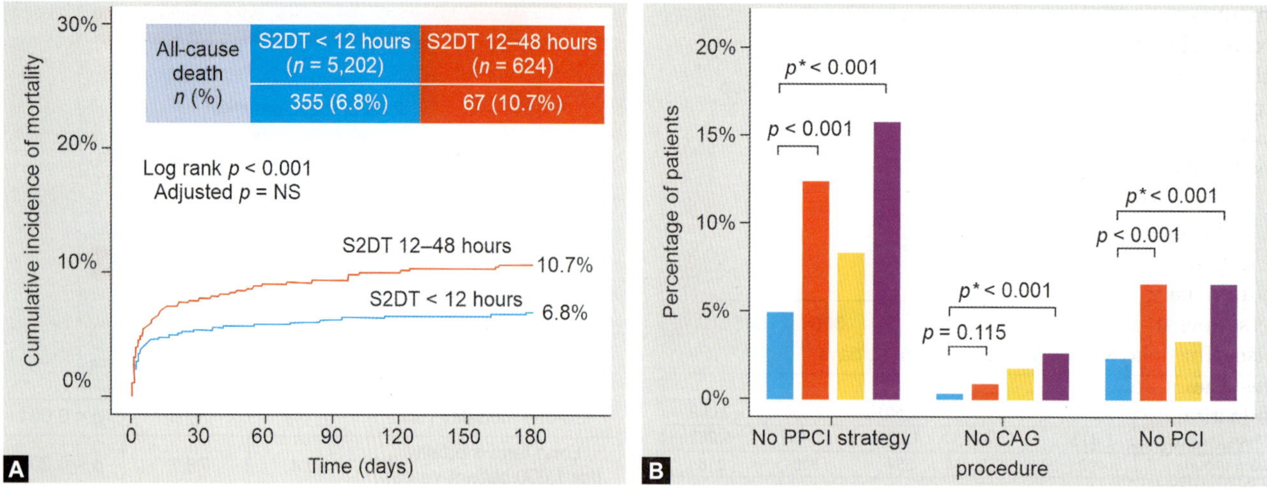

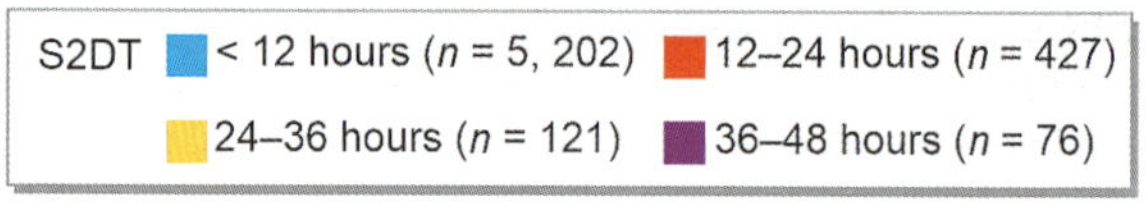

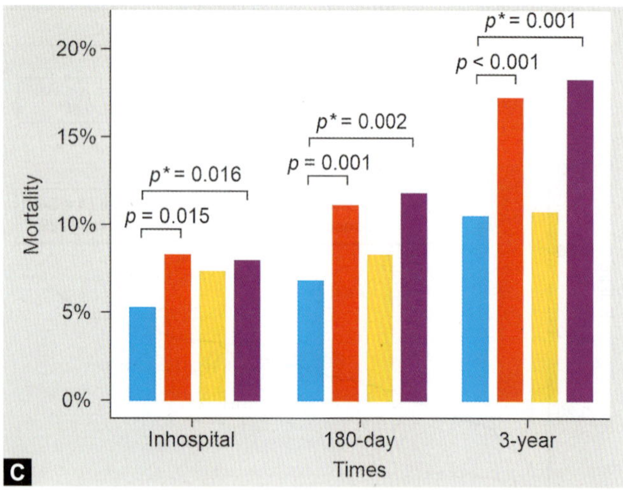

FIGS. 11A TO C: Real-world features of late presentation (12–48 hours of symptom onset) among patients with ST-segment elevation myocardial infarction in Korea.[11] (A) Cumulative incidence of mortality over 180 days for S2DT < 12 hours versus 12–48 hours. Use of invasive interventional procedures (B) and mortality rates during the 3-year follow-up (C) according to S2DT 12-hour intervals (<12, 12–24, 24–36, and 36–48 hours).

(CAG: coronary angiogram; PCI: percutaneous coronary intervention; PPCI: primary PCI; S2DT: symptom-to-door time)

	Hazard ratio (95% CI)	p value
Age, years	1.04 (1.03–1.05)	< 0.001
LVEF, %	0.96 (0.95–0.97)	< 0.001
Killip IV	45 (3.29–6.01)	< 0.001
Killip III	2.45 (1.78–3.38)	< 0.001
Killip II	1.43 (0.99–2.08)	0.059
SBP < 100	1.92 (1.47–2.52)	< 0.001
eGFR < 60	1.89 (1.53–2.34)	< 0.001
No PPCI strategy	1.82 (1.37–2.43)	< 0.001
Heart rate > 100 beats/min	1.74 (1.37–2.19)	< 0.001
Anemia	1.71 (1.39–2.12)	< 0.001
Anterior STE or LBBB	1.25 (1.03–1.53)	0.027
S2DT ≥ 12 hours	1.14 (0.87–1.48)	0.354

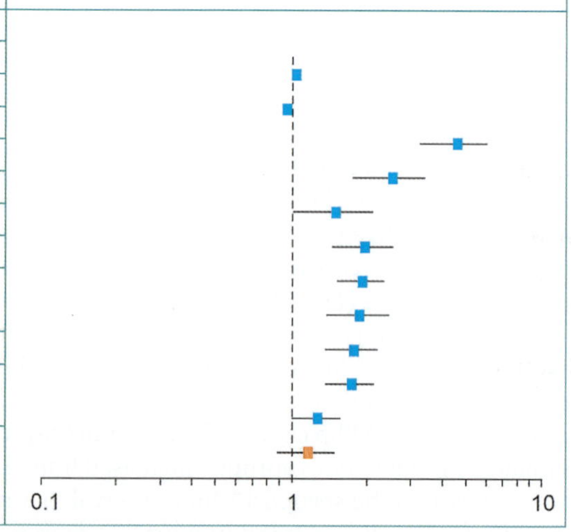

FIG. 12: Adjusted prognostic values of variables for 180-day mortality.[11]

(CI: confidence interval; eGFR: estimated glomerular filtration rate; LVEF: left ventricular ejection fraction; PCI: percutaneous coronary intervention; PPCI: primary PCI; S2DT: symptom-to-door time; SBP: systolic blood pressure; STE: ST-segment elevation; LBBB: left bundle branch block)

Emergency medical services and catheterization laboratories are poorly equipped and are more frequently found in urban areas. Therefore, patients living in rural areas have a higher risk of mortality from STEMI due to poorly equipped transportation systems and the lack of a prehospital care system making access to health facilities difficult.[22]

Alexander and Mullasari[23] reported a time to presentation in India of 300 minutes, in contrast to the Unites States where emergency telephone line 9-1-1 is available for prompt patient care, where emergency medical service (EMS) personnel arrive at patient site in <50 minutes after symptom onset. The delayed presentation in India (and in several other low- and middle-income countries) has critical implications for instituting pragmatic guidelines.

Delayed presentation is the Achilles' heel of STEMI care in low- and middle-income countries.

Specifically, the delayed presentation affects the STEMI pathways in three possible manners:

1. Delayed presentation fundamentally alters a fibrinolytic strategy as the door-to-needle (D2N) times are significantly prolonged and the benefits associated with early- and prehospital administration of thrombolytic therapy are reduced.
2. The longer time window of opportunity for primary PCI in patients with delayed presentation may be the most effective way to treat many patients with STEMI despite the lack of PCI facilities.
3. Delayed presentation requires a novel look at pharmacoinvasive strategies that may prolong the window of opportunity for reperfusion therapy.

To analyze this delayed presentation[24] **(Fig. 13 and Box 1)** which can be caused by:

- Patient delay as the time from symptom onset to contact with the EMS
- Prehospital system delay as the time from contact with the EMS to arrival at the PCI center
- System delay as the time from contact with the EMS to guiding-catheter insertion during primary PCI
- Door-to-balloon delay as the time from arrival at the PCI center to guiding-catheter insertion during primary PCI

Mehta et al.[22] suggested strategies to reduce system delays which are as follows:

- Treat STEMI interventions as a public health initiative in which there are numerous stakeholders that can be engaged to seek financial, logistic, structural, and medical support.
- Improve ambulance care, qualitatively and quantitatively, with the goal being to ensure a centralized, intelligent ambulance system, both for community emergency response and for interhospital transfer.

BOX 1 System delays.

- *Patient*: Barriers—social, personal, cultural, financial, and religious
- *Insurance*: Barrier—low penetration of insurance
- *Transport*: Barrier—lack of centralized ambulance system
- *Hospital*: Barriers—24/7 percutaneous coronary syndrome (PCI) capability; lack of transfer protocols and team-work
- *Physician*: Barriers—skills and 24/7 availability; ethics
- *Technology*: Barriers—devices and drugs

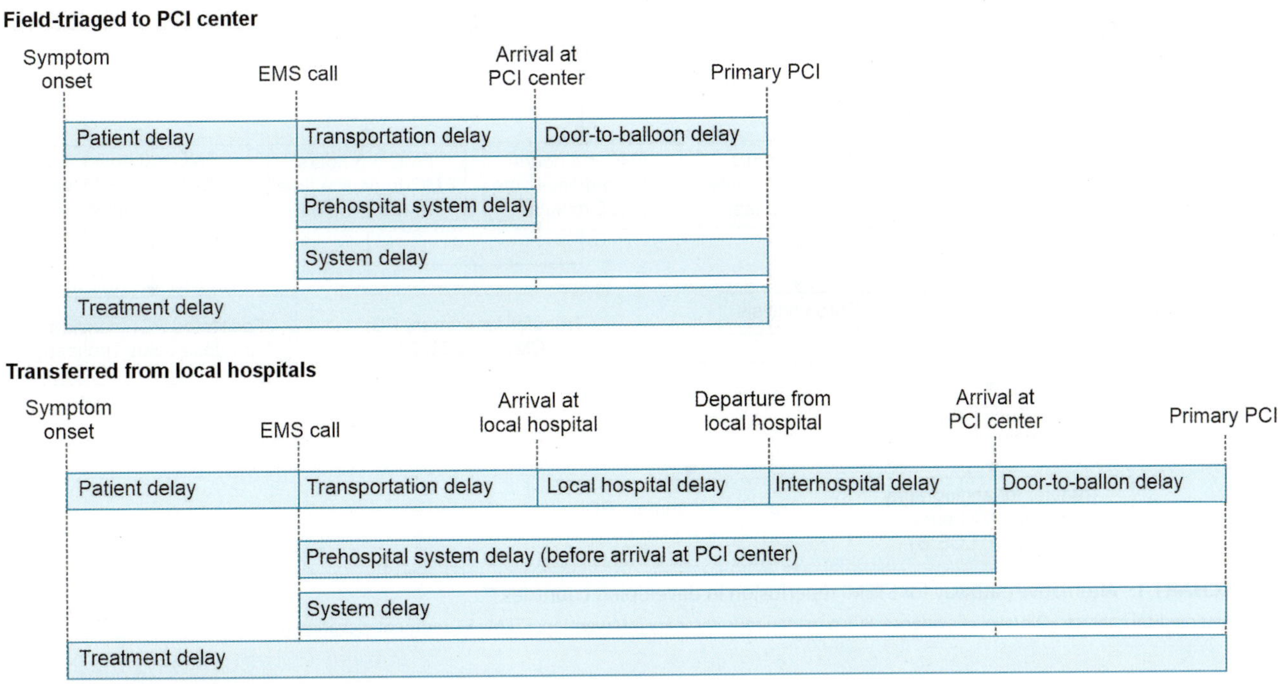

FIG. 13: Depicts various delay points in patient from symptom onset to primary PCI.[24]

Note: Stratified according to prehospital triage.

(EMS: emergency medical service; PCI: percutaneous coronary intervention)

- Increase 24/7 STEMI facilities, including the ability to perform primary PCI with or without the capability for on-site cardiac surgery.
- Create regional STEMI networks and systems of care for each community with a reperfusion protocol for every hospital.
- Develop prehospital alert whenever possible and electrocardiogram (ECG) transmission using internet, fax, or smartphone applications such as WhatsApp.
- Establish unambiguous payment policies and systems that are clearly understood by payers, hospital, and patient. Payment delays notoriously cause delays in obtaining consents. Penalize refusal to provide life-saving STEMI care.
- Use single-call activation to engage the catheterization laboratory, with teamwork and quality improvement (QI) feedback.
- Bypass the emergency department, when possible, relying on prehospital alert and single-call activation
- Consider telemedicine to increase access, accuracy, and remote guidance of comprehensive STEMI management.
- Educate the patient—this is the hardest assignment and it requires a multipronged approach, including empowering the general physician.

Alternative pathway for developing countries[22] **(Flowchart 1)** and integrating Hub and Spoke model for better patient outcome.

Development of Hub and Spoke model[23] **(Fig. 14)** is architecture for STEMI program, with timely and proper decision of primary PCI to pharmacoinvasive strategy with reduced morbidity and mortality among STEMI patients.

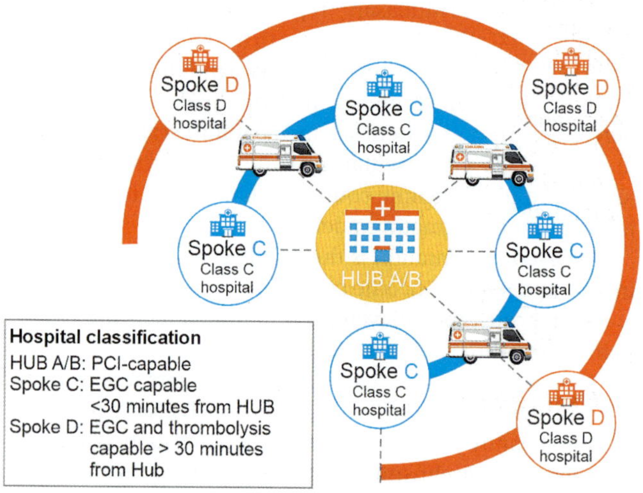

FIG. 14: Hub and Spoke model for effective STEMI program implementation.[23]

(ECG: electrocardiogram; PCI: percutaneous coronary intervention; STEMI: ST-segment elevation myocardial infarction)

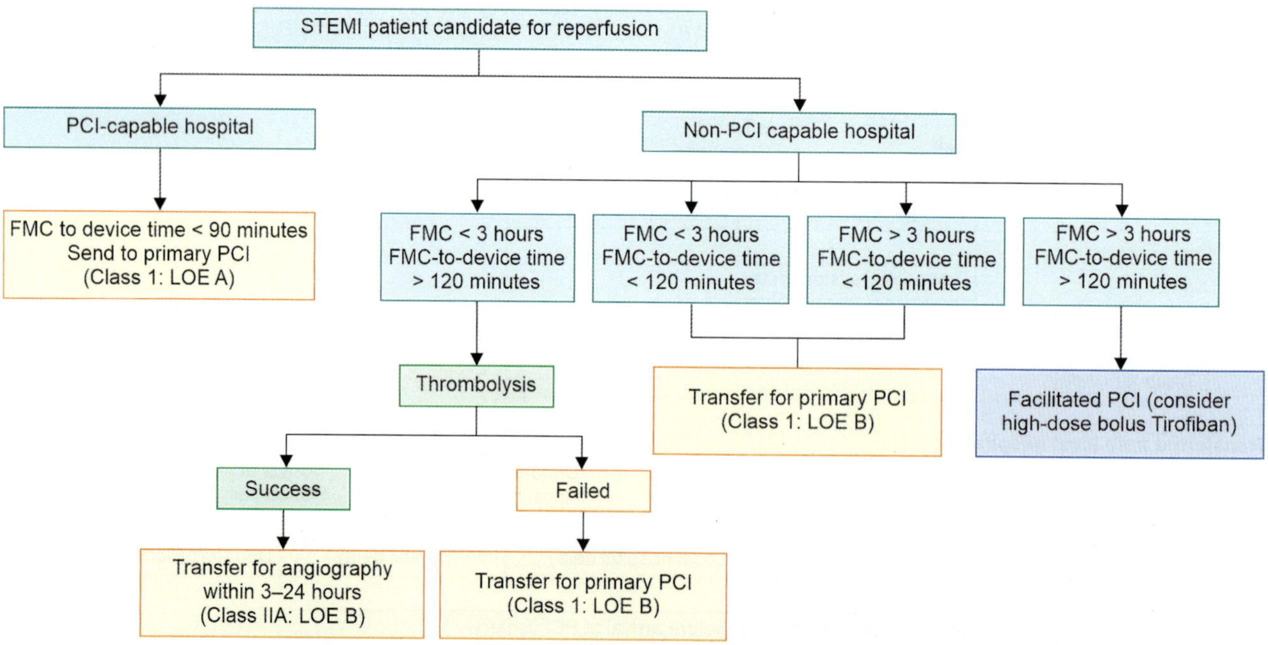

FLOWCHART 1: Alternative pathway for STEMI reperfusion in developing countries.[22]

(FMC: first medical contact; LOE: level of evidence; PCI: percutaneous coronary intervention; STEMI: ST-segment elevation myocardial infarction)

CONCLUSION

Patients who present late with an acute MI are a heterogeneous population and the clinical decision regarding PCI should be individualized. Late presentation is associated with increased death. Large number of late presenters are transferred from non-PCI centers and represent a high-risk group for death. Further, system-wide approaches might focus on bringing clarity to recommendations for best practices among late-presenting STEMI patients. In the treatment of latecomers with STEMI, clinical evaluation and risk stratification represent paramount factors helping in decision-making for the best therapeutic management. Crucial elements in decision making are the presence of hemodynamic or electrical instability and ongoing ischemic signs or symptoms guiding toward early-PCI. Among clinically stable, late-presenting patients, myocardial viability assessment and functional testing can identify yet another subgroup that may benefit from late-PCI.

Accordingly, as recommended and endorsed by the current guidelines, patients who are still early in the course of STEMI (12–48 hours) should undergo PCI. Those beyond 48 hours with evidence of silent ischemia or viability should also undergo PCI. Patients who are truly stable and asymptomatic beyond 48 hours from symptom onset, with no evidence of silent ischemia or viability, can safely be treated with medical therapy.

ONLINE REFERENCES

Please scan the QR code provided at the end of the table of contents for References of this chapter.

CHAPTER 80

Risk Stratification and Management Principles for Type 2 Myocardial Infarction

Prakas Chandra Mondal

ABSTRACT

Ischemic heart disease and diabetes mellitus are twin pandemic striking the Indian population at a younger age with relatively poorer outcomes in comparison to the western world. Obesity and metabolic syndrome in teenage group are increasing dramatically with nutritional transition without much rural–urban variations. Metabolic syndrome is the founder of future atherosclerotic cardiac events. There is a demographic shift in India with an increase in the life expectancy. Six major transitions can be considered largely responsible for high population level changes in risk of ischemic heart disease, namely epidemiological, demographic, nutritional, environmental, sociocultural, and economic. Multiple comorbid conditions are highly prevalent, increasing the susceptibility to both type 1 myocardial infarction (T1MI) and type 2 myocardial infarction (T2MI). Availability of high-sensitivity cardiac troponin (cTn) assays results in around 4% absolute and 20% relative reduction in the diagnosis of unstable angina and a corresponding increase in diagnosis of myocardial infarction as a consequence of atherothrombosis (T1MI). With this new assay, T2MI, i.e., myocardial infarction secondary to oxygen supply/demand mismatch in the absence of atherothrombosis, is also detected twice as much as with old assays.[1] Distinct pathogenesis of T1MI and T2MI needs relevant epidemiological, diagnostic, and clinical risk evaluations. Outcomes appear poorer and in-hospital complications are more frequent in T2MI and short- and long-term mortality rates are near threefold higher than T1MI.[2]

Keywords: Pandemic, metabolic syndrome, nutritional transition, atherosclerotic, cardiac troponin (cTn), atherothrombosis.

INTRODUCTION

According to the Fourth Universal Definition of Myocardial Infarction (UDMI), type 2 myocardial infarction (T2MI) is a clinical phenomenon of myocardial cell death due to an imbalance between myocardial oxygen supply and demand which is not related to acute coronary atherothrombosis.[3]

DEFINING CRITERIA OF TYPE-2 MYOCARDIAL INFARCTION

Detection of a rise and fall of high-sensitivity cardiac troponin (cTn) values with at least one value above the 99th percentile of upper limit[4] and at least one of the following:

- Symptoms of acute myocardial ischemia
- New ischemic electrocardiogram (ECG) changes
- Development of pathological Q waves
- Imaging evidence of new loss of viable myocardium or new regional wall motion abnormality in a pattern consistent with an ischemic etiology

ETIOLOGIES OF TYPE-2 MYOCARDIAL INFARCTION

Etiologies of T2MI are extremely variable:

- *T2MI as clinically presenting phenomena*: As in coronary artery dissection, sustained tachyarrhythmia, coronary embolism, and coronary vasospasm
- *T2MI as an epiphenomenon of another clinical illness*: As in pneumonia, sepsis, and noncardiogenic shock. Other main causes include renal failure, respiratory failure, anemia, and bleeding.

PATHOPHYSIOLOGY OF TYPE-2 MYOCARDIAL INFARCTION

As per criteria, acute atherothrombotic plaque disruption is not a feature of T2MI, but in patients with stable coronary artery disease (CAD), acute stressor such as hemorrhagic shock with precipitous fall in hemoglobin or a sustained tachyarrhythmia may result in myocardial injury with cell death and T2MI. Ischemic threshold of myocardial cell death varies substantially and depends on the magnitude of the stressors, presence of noncardiac comorbidities, extent of underlying CAD, and cardiac structural abnormalities. Coronary atherosclerosis is a common finding in T2MI and associated CAD carries worse prognosis than those without concomitant CAD.[4]

EPIDEMIOLOGY OF TYPE-2 MYOCARDIAL INFARCTION

Patients with T2MI have distinct pathogenesis and have relevant epidemiological differences compared to type 1 myocardial infarction (T1MI).[5]

- Patients with T2MI are older. Physiology of elderly people makes them more susceptible to imbalance between myocardial oxygen supply and demand.
- There is a lower prevalence of obesity, dyslipidemia, and smoking which are well known and more prevalent risk factors in T1MI.
- T2MI has a higher incidence in women. Women are more susceptible to coronary artery spasm, coronary microvascular dysfunction, and spontaneous coronary artery dissection.
- Prior history of myocardial infarction (MI), percutaneous coronary intervention, or coronary artery bypass graft surgery is less common in patients with T2MI.
- There is a higher prevalence of comorbidities such as atrial fibrillation, chronic kidney disease, chronic obstructive pulmonary disease, and peripheral vascular disease
- Concomitantly, patients with T2MI have a low functional status and higher GRACE (Global Registry of Acute Coronary Events) risk score at presentation.
- Higher mortality but with similar or lower rate of major adverse cardiovascular event (MACE). Associated ECG changes carry worse outcomes, though ischemic ECG changes, especially ST-segment elevation, are much lower in frequency than T1MI.
- ECG localization of myocardial injury and echocardiographic wall motion abnormalities are much less in T2MI.
- Atypical symptoms such as angina, breathlessness, and palpitations are more in T2MI.

Distinction of Type-1 and Type-2 Myocardial Infarction

As treatment differs substantially, distinction between T1MI and T2MI is very much important. Aggressive antithrombotic therapy and urgent revascularization are the mainstay of therapy in T1MI, whereas corrections of underlying triggers of the myocardial supply-demand mismatch are the cornerstone of management of T2MI.

Type 2 MI is usually associated with lower concentrations of biomarkers of cardiomyocyte damage such as high-sensitivity TnT, high-sensitivity TnI I, and cardiac myosin-binding protein C. On the other hand, T2MI is associated with higher levels of biomarkers of endothelial dysfunction, microvascular dysfunction, and/or hemodynamic stress. These include C-terminal prendothelin 1, midregional proadrenomedullin, midregional pro-A-type natriuretic peptide, and growth differentiation factor 15.

ASSESSMENT AND INVESTIGATION

The Fourth UDMI provides a framework of classification of myocardial injury by etiology. There are significant overlaps in risk factors, clinical presentations, laboratory parameters, and diagnostic criteria. No gold standard parameter or diagnostic criteria is there to accurately typify myocardial injury.

Symptom Analysis

As per UDMI, chest/upper extremity/mandibular/epigastric discomfort and dyspnea or fatigue during exertion or rest persisting for >10 minutes are consistent with MI. But these are not specific for myocardial ischemia and MI can occur with atypical symptoms or even without symptoms, especially in patients with diabetes mellitus, elderly, and women. So, the symptoms cannot differentiate types of myocardial injury.[6]

Electrocardiogram

- Dynamic ST segment and T-wave changes are indicative of significant ongoing acute myocardial ischemia and identify patients who can be benefited from urgent invasive evaluation and intervention.
- Dynamic ST segment and T-wave changes are seen only in fewer percentage of patients and cannot reliably discriminate T1MI from T2MI.

Cardiac Biomarkers

- T2MI is usually associated with lower concentrations of biomarkers of cardiomyocyte damage such as high-sensitivity Tn T and high-sensitivity Tn I. But overlapping ranges of troponin values limit the use of cTn levels to accurately differentiate between etiologies of myocardial injuries.

- Serial cTn estimation to demonstrate a rise or fall in cTn concentrations is needed to differentiate acute and chronic cTn elevation.
- A nonischemic ECG and stable pattern of cTn elevation are more consistent with chronic myocardial injury. Dynamic cTn elevation is consistent with acute myocardial injury.
- The UDMI suggests a 20% change in cTn to differentiate a stable versus a dynamic cTn pattern.

Noninvasive Imaging

Noninvasive imaging can help in differentiating T2MI from other causes of myocardial injury. Besides delineating coronary anatomy, myocardium can also be assessed for the presence of scar or inflamed area.

Echocardiography

Echocardiography can detect abnormalities in myocardial thickening and motion very early in myocardial ischemia. Regional wall motion abnormality in a specific coronary territory can be supportive of acute MI if documented to be new onset. But this cannot specify etiology. Echocardiography can detect stress cardiomyopathy, aortic stenosis, and other forms of cardiomyopathies.

Computed Tomography Coronary Angiography

- It can detect atherosclerotic plaque including plaque rupture and thus substantiate the presence or absence of T1MI.
- The presence of thrombus is difficult to be differentiated from noncalcified atherosclerotic plaque.
- Spontaneous coronary artery dissection is suspected to be the cause of acute MI in more than one-third of women in <50 years of age. Computed tomography (CT) angiography can reliably detect this entity.

Myocardial Perfusion Imaging

- Localized or generalized perfusion abnormalities can suggest types of injuries.
- Performed with contrast echocardiography, single-photon emission computerized tomography, positron emission tomography, CT, or magnetic resonance imaging (MRI).
- Delayed contrast enhancement on MRI can differentiate acute from chronic myocardial injury by detecting tissue edema.
- Ischemia-induced myocardial injury typically extends from subendocardium to the epicardium, whereas nonischemic myocardial injury can be seen at the epicardium, mid wall, or insertion points of right ventricle. All these are well demonstrable on MRI.
- Coronary arterial anatomy is not well evaluated by MRI. Cardiomyopathies, especially stress cardiomyopathy, are well characterized by MRI.
- T2MI and MI with nonobstructive coronary arteries (MINOCA) are strongly correlated in young patients with fewer comorbidities. The 2020 European Society of Cardiology (ESC) non-STE acute coronary syndrome (ACS) guidelines suggested for cardiac magnetic resonance (CMR) in all MINOCA patients in the absence of an obvious underlying cause.

Invasive Imaging

Coronary angiography is the gold standard for delineating coronary anatomy and the UDMI acknowledges the utility of coronary angiography in distinction between T1MI, T2MI, and acute nonischemic myocardial injury.

Advanced invasive coronary imaging such as intravascular ultrasound (IVUS) and optical coherence tomography (OCT) are also useful to demonstrate plaque disruption and intracoronary thrombus.

Arbab-Zadeh and Fuster V[7] had shown via pathology, OCT, angioscopy, and IVUS that up to 79% of plaque disruptions are clinically silent and heal without obstructive coronary thrombosis and resultant acute MI.

APPROACH TO THE ASSESSMENT AND TREATMENT OF PATIENTS WITH MYOCARDIAL INJURY[8]

- In the absence of a clear alternative diagnosis such as aortic dissection, pulmonary embolism, or pneumothorax, the initial working diagnosis for most patients in the emergency with evidence of acute myocardial injury and signs and symptoms of ischemia should be T1MI.
- Management should be started as per established guidelines for T1MI with antiplatelets, statins, and antithrombotics. Noninvasive and guided invasive evaluation should be done.
- When subsequent evaluation fails to confirm coronary atherothrombosis, then the alternative causes of acute nonischemic myocardial injury (such as myocarditis) or T2MI are to be considered.
- When acute myocardial injury occurs as an epiphenomenon of another acute illness or surgical procedure, T2MI is more likely though plaque disruption can occur with these stressors also.
- GRACE risk score is useful in risk stratification as significant differences in these parameters exist between T1MI and T2MI. Patients with T2MI rarely have a GRACE risk score <90. Patients with T2MI usually have higher heart rate, lower blood pressure, and increased Killip class. GRACE risk score is better than TORACCO score specifically designed for T2MI and T1MI risk score specific for ACS.[9]

SPECIFIC CLINICAL SCENARIOS WITH TYPE 2 MYOCARDIAL INFARCTION

- Congestive cardiac failure is a recognized entity with T2MI. Multiple causal relationships have been identified, namely increased transmural pressure, small vessel obstruction, endothelial dysfunction, wall stretch resulting in myocyte apoptosis, and autophagy. Inflammation can cause direct myotoxicity and neurohumoral toxicity.
- Majority of stress cardiomyopathy is thought to be secondary to direct catecholamine toxicity and categorized as acute nonischemic myocardial injury. A minority of cases are secondary to microvascular dysfunction, coronary artery spasm, or extracardiac stressor.
- Sepsis can cause myocardial injury in multiple ways. Inflammation is a strong driver for plaque disruption with resultant atherothrombosis and T1MI. Inflammation causes direct myotoxicity with nonischemic myocardial injury and septic shock can cause hypoperfusion, tachycardia, and tissue hypoxia which can culminate into T2MI.
- Postoperative inflammatory state causes nonischemic myocardial injury, and it bears a high short- and long-term mortality.

TREATMENT

Therapeutic strategies are well established for T1MI, but recommendations for non-T1MI categories are based on underlying clinical surrogates, resulting in T2MI or nonischemic myocardial injury. In the absence of contraindications (e.g., bradycardia, hypotension, and acute heart failure), early judicious use of β-blockers to control high myocardial demand should be considered.

The SWEDEHEART registry[10] data analysis results suggest judicious use of angiotensin-converting enzyme inhibitors (ACEIs) or angiotensin receptor blockers (ARBs), statins, and antiplatelets to have good in-hospital and short- and long-term outcomes. Dual antiplatelet therapy numerically reduces MACE incidences with a trend toward increasing bleeding risk.

Complete revascularization provides no clinical benefits to T2MI patients in the COMPLETE trial.[11] McCarthy et al. found a significantly lower in-hospital mortality with revascularization, but all-cause death and readmission for heart failure or MI at 30 days did not differ.

CONCLUSION

Myocardial injury can occur due to a wide variety of ischemic and nonischemic mechanisms. T2MI and nonischemic myocardial injury encompass heterogenous etiological groups. No definite study protocol or therapeutic recommendations exist for these clinical entities. Future epidemiological studies are in crying need. The Fourth UDMI provides an enhanced taxonomy for classifications of myocardial injury, and this will facilitate the studies for these common clinical entities.

ONLINE REFERENCES

Please scan the QR code provided at the end of the table of contents for References of this chapter.

SECTION

8

Chronic Coronary Syndromes

CHAPTER 81

Chronic Coronary Syndrome: Diagnosis and Management

Monotosh Panja, Madhumanti Panja

ABSTRACT

The chapter presents a comprehensive exploration of the intricacies involved in diagnosing and effectively managing chronic coronary syndrome (CCS). This chapter elucidates the multifaceted nature of CCS, encompassing stable angina, myocardial ischemia, and the underlying atherosclerotic processes. Through a meticulous examination of contemporary diagnostic methodologies, including cutting-edge imaging techniques, noninvasive stress tests, and coronary angiography, the chapter underscores their pivotal role in accurate disease assessment and risk stratification. Furthermore, it provides an in-depth analysis of the diverse management strategies available for CCS, ranging from lifestyle adjustments and pharmacological interventions to emerging therapeutic innovations. The chapter underscores the importance of a personalized, patient-centric approach to treatment, highlighting the significance of tailoring interventions based on individual patient characteristics.

Keywords: Angina, chronic coronary syndrome, coronary artery disease (CAD).

INTRODUCTION

The term "stable coronary artery disease (CAD)" has been replaced with "chronic coronary syndrome (CCS)." Clinical manifestations of CAD fall into two categories: acute coronary syndrome (ACS) and CCS. The CCS is a prevalent and complex medical condition that affects millions of individuals worldwide. It is characterized by the gradual narrowing and hardening of coronary arteries, which supply oxygen-rich blood to the heart muscle. This process, known as atherosclerosis, impedes blood flow, leading to persistent chest pain or angina and increasing the risk of heart attack and other cardiovascular events. CCS often develops over time due to various risk factors, including hypertension, high cholesterol levels, smoking, sedentary lifestyle, and family history of heart disease. As a chronic and potentially life-threatening condition, understanding the underlying mechanisms and adopting effective management strategies is crucial in providing optimal care and enhancing the quality of life for individuals living with CCS.

DIAGNOSIS OF CHRONIC CORONARY SYNDROME

Chronic CAD stems from the obstruction of a large epicardial coronary artery caused by the accumulation of atheromatous plaque. This plaque buildup hinders the flow of oxygen-rich blood to the heart muscle, resulting in a condition known as myocardial ischemia. The hallmark symptom of CAD is angina pectoris, which manifests as substernal discomfort or heaviness and may radiate to the jaw, shoulder, back, or arm. Typically lasting for a few minutes, angina is triggered by factors such as physical exertion, emotional stress, exposure to cold, or consuming a heavy meal. Thankfully, these symptoms are often alleviated with rest or the use of nitroglycerin, providing rapid relief. Some patients may experience anginal "equivalents," presenting as epigastric discomfort, dyspnea, fatigue, or faintness. These symptoms can be classified into three categories: typical angina, atypical angina, or noncardiac chest pain, each offering valuable insights into the nature and severity of the underlying CCS.

The clinical scenarios encountered in patients with suspected or established CCS encompass a range of presentations. Firstly, patients with suspected CAD and stable anginal symptoms and/or dyspnea constitute one group. Secondly, there are patients with new-onset heart failure (HF) or left ventricular (LV) dysfunction, where CAD is suspected. Thirdly, both asymptomatic and symptomatic patients with stabilized symptoms within 1 year after an ACS or recent revascularization fall under another category. Furthermore, there are asymptomatic and symptomatic patients with a history of >1 year after initial diagnosis or revascularization. Additionally, patients with angina and suspected vasospastic or microvascular disease form another distinct group. Lastly, asymptomatic individuals in whom CAD is detected during screening represent a unique scenario.

In the European Society of Cardiology (ESC) guidelines 2019,[1] there have been significant revisions in assessing the pretest probability (PTP) of CAD, which now consider age, gender, and the nature of symptoms, incorporating various risk factors associated with CAD. Furthermore, a novel term, "Clinical likelihood of CAD," has been introduced to incorporate these risk factors more effectively. The guidelines have also been updated to reflect the application of different diagnostic tests tailored to specific patient groups, aiming to either confirm or exclude the presence of CAD **(Tables 1 and 2)**.

TABLE 1: Recent guidelines of CCS.[1]

New major recommendations in 2019	Class
Basic testing, diagnosis, and risk assessment	
Noninvasive functional imaging for myocardial ischemia or coronary CTA is recommended as the initial test for diagnosing CAD in symptomatic patients in whom obstructive CAD cannot be excluded by clinical assessment alone	I
It is recommended that selection of the initial noninvasive diagnostic test be based on the clinical likelihood of CAD and other patient characteristics that influence test performance, local expertise, and the availability of tests	I
Functional imaging for myocardial ischemia is recommended if coronary CTA has shown CAD of uncertain functional significance or is not diagnostic	I
Invasive angiography is recommended as an alternative test to diagnose CAD in patients with a high clinical likelihood and severe symptoms refractory to medical therapy or typical angina at a low level of exercise and clinical evaluation that indicates high event risk. Invasive functional assessment must be available and used to evaluate stenosis before revascularization, unless very high grade (>90% diameter stenosis)	I
Invasive coronary angiography with the availability of invasive functional evaluation should be considered for confirmation of the diagnosis of CAD in patients with an uncertain diagnosis on noninvasive testing	IIa
Coronary CTA should be considered as an alternative to invasive angiography if another noninvasive test is equivocal or nondiagnostic	IIa
Coronary CTA is not recommended when extensive coronary calcification, irregular heart rate, significant obesity, inability to cooperate with breath-hold commands, or any other conditions make good image quality unlikely	II
Antithrombotic therapy in patients with CCS and sinus rhythm	
Addition of a second antithrombotic drug to aspirin for long-term secondary prevention should be considered in patients with a high risk of ischemic events and without high bleeding risk	IIa
Addition of a second antithrombotic drug to aspirin for long-term secondary prevention may be considered in patients with at least a moderately increased risk of ischemic events and without high bleeding risk	IIb
Antithrombotic therapy in patients with CCS and AF	
When oral anticoagulation is initiated in a patient with AF who is eligible for a NOAC, a NOAC is recommended in preference to a VKA	I
Long-term OAC therapy (a NOAC or VKA with time in therapeutic range >70%) is recommended in patients with AF and a CHA_2DS_2-VASc score ≥ 2 in males and ≥3 in females	I
Long-term OAC therapy (a NOAC or VKA with time in therapeutic range >70%) should be considered in patients with AF and a CHA_2DS_2-VASc score of 1 in males and 2 in females	IIa

Continued

Continued

New major recommendations in 2019	Class
Antithrombotic therapy in post-PCI patients with AF or another indication for OAC	
In patients who are eligible for a NOAC, it is recommended that a NOAC (apixaban 5 mg bid, dabigatran 150 mg bid, edoxaban 60 mg OD, or rivaroxaban 20 mg OD) is used in preference to a VKA in combination with antiplatelet therapy	I
When rivaroxaban is used and concerns about high bleeding risk prevail over concerns about stent thrombosis or ischemic stroke, rivaroxaban 15 mg OD should be considered in preference to rivaroxaban 20 mg OD for the duration of concomitant SAPT or DAPT	IIa
When dabigatran is used and concerns about high bleeding risk prevail over concerns about stent thrombosis or ischemic stroke, dabigatran 110 mg bid should be considered in preference to dabigatran 150 mg bid for the duration of concomitant SAPT or DAPT	IIa
After uncomplicated PCI, early cessation (≤1 week) of aspirin and continuation of dual therapy with OAC and clopidogrel should be considered if the risk of stent thrombosis is low or if concerns about bleeding risk prevail over concerns about risk of stent thrombosis, irrespective of the type of stent used	IIa
Triple therapy with aspirin, clopidogrel, and an OAC for ≥1 month should be considered when the risk of stent thrombosis outweighs the bleeding risk, with the total duration (≤6 months) decided upon according to the assessment of these risks and clearly specified at hospital discharge	IIa
In patients with an indication for a VKA in combination with aspirin and/or clopidogrel, the dose intensity of the VKA should be carefully regulated with a target international normalized ratio in the range of 2.0–2.5 and with time in therapeutic range >70%	IIa
Dual therapy with an OAC and either ticagrelor or prasugrel may be considered as an alternative to triple therapy with an OAC, aspirin, and clopidogrel in patients with a moderate or high risk of stent thrombosis, irrespective of the type of stent used	IIb
Other pharmacological therapies	
Concomitant use of a proton pump inhibitor is recommended in patients receiving aspirin monotherapy, DAPT, or OAC monotherapy who are at high risk of gastrointestinal bleeding	I
Lipid-lowering drugs: If goals are not achieved with the maximum-tolerated dose of statin, combination with ezetimibe is recommended	I
Lipid-lowering drugs: For patients at very high risk who do not achieve their goals on a maximum-tolerated dose of statin and ezetimibe, combination with a PCSK9 inhibitor is recommended	I
ACEIs should be considered in CCS patients at very high risk of cardiovascular adverse events	IIa
The sodium–glucose cotransporter 2 inhibitors empagliflozin, canagliflozin, or dapagliflozin are recommended in patients with diabetes mellitus and CVD	I
A glucagon-like peptide-1 receptor agonist (liraglutide or semaglutide) is recommended in patients with diabetes mellitus and CVD	I
Screening for CAD in asymptomatic subjects	
Carotid ultrasound IMT for cardiovascular risk assessment is not recommended	III
Recommendations for treatment options for refractory angina	
A reducer device for coronary sinus constriction may be considered to ameliorate symptoms of debilitating angina refractory to optimal medical and revascularization strategies	IIb

[ACEIs: angiotensin-converting enzyme inhibitors; ACS: acute coronary syndrome; AF: atrial fibrillation; bid: bis in die (twice a day); CAD: coronary artery disease; CCS: chronic coronary syndrome; CHA_2DS_2-VASc: cardiac failure, hypertension, age ≥ 75 years (doubled), diabetes, stroke (doubled), vascular disease, age 65–74 years, and sex category (female); CTA: computed tomography angiography; CVD: cardiovascular disease; DAPT: dual antiplatelet therapy; HF: heart failure; IMT: intima-media thickness; LV: left ventricular; NOAC: nonvitamin K antagonist oral anticoagulant; OAC: oral anticoagulant; OD: omni die (once a day); PCI: percutaneous coronary intervention; PCSK9: proprotein convertase subtilisin-kexin type 9; SAPT: single antiplatelet therapy; VKA: vitamin K antagonist]

TABLE 2: Changes in major recommendations.

<table>
<tr><th>2013</th><th>Class</th><th>2019</th><th>Class</th></tr>
<tr><td rowspan="2">Exercise ECG is recommended as the initial test to establish the diagnosis of stable CAD in patients with symptoms of angina and intermediate PTP of CAD (15–65%), free of anti-ischemic drugs, unless they cannot exercise or display ECG changes that make the ECG nonevaluable</td><td rowspan="2">I</td><td>Exercise ECG is recommended for the assessment of exercise tolerance, symptoms, arrhythmias, BP response, and event risk in selected patients</td><td>I</td></tr>
<tr><td>Exercise ECG may be considered as an alternative test to rule-in or rule-out CAD when other noninvasive or invasive imaging methods are not available</td><td>IIb</td></tr>
<tr><td>Exercise ECG should be considered in patients on treatment to evaluate control of symptoms and ischemia</td><td>IIa</td><td>Exercise ECG may be considered in patients on treatment to evaluate control of symptoms and ischemia</td><td>IIb</td></tr>
<tr><td>For second-line treatment, it is recommended that long-acting nitrates, ivabradine, nicorandil, or ranolazine are added according to heart rate, BP, and tolerance</td><td>IIa</td><td>Long-acting nitrates should be considered as a second-line treatment option when initial therapy with a beta-blocker and/or a non- DHP-CCB is contraindicated, poorly tolerated, or inadequate in controlling angina symptoms</td><td>IIa</td></tr>
<tr><td rowspan="2">For second-line treatment, trimetazidine may be considered</td><td rowspan="2">IIb</td><td>Nicorandil, ranolazine, ivabradine, or trimetazidine should be considered as a second-line treatment to reduce angina frequency and improve exercise tolerance in subjects who cannot tolerate, have contraindications to, or whose symptoms are not adequately controlled by beta-blockers, CCBs, and long-acting nitrates</td><td>IIa</td></tr>
<tr><td>In selected patients, the combination of a beta-blocker or a CCB with second-line drugs (ranolazine, nicorandil, ivabradine, and trimetazidine) may be considered for first-line treatment according to heart rate, BP, and tolerance</td><td>IIb</td></tr>
<tr><td rowspan="2">In patients with suspected coronary microvascular angina, intracoronary acetylcholine and adenosine with Doppler measurements may be considered during coronary arteriography, if the arteriogram is visually normal, to assess endothelium-dependent and non-endothelium-dependent CFR and detect microvascular/epicardial vasospasm</td><td rowspan="2">IIb</td><td>Guidewire-based CFR and/or microcirculatory resistance measurements should be considered in patients with persistent symptoms, but coronary arteries that are either angiographically normal or have moderate stenoses with preserved iwFR/FFR</td><td>IIa</td></tr>
<tr><td>Intracoronary acetylcholine with ECG monitoring may be considered during angiography, if coronary arteries are either angiographically normal or have moderate stenoses with preserved iwFR/FFR to assess microvascular vasospasm</td><td>IIb</td></tr>
<tr><td>In patients with suspected coronary microvascular angina, transthoracic Doppler echocardiography of the LAD, with measurement of diastolic coronary blood flow following intravenous adenosine and at rest, may be considered for noninvasive measurement of CFR</td><td>IIb</td><td>Transthoracic Doppler of the LAD, CMR, and PET may be considered for noninvasive assessment of CFR</td><td>IIb</td></tr>
</table>

[BP: blood pressure; CAD: coronary artery disease; CCB: calcium channel blocker; CFR: coronary flow reserve; CMR: cardiac magnetic resonance; DHP-CCB: dihydropyridine calcium channel blocker; ECG: electrocardiogram; FFR: fractional flow reserve; iwFR instantaneous wave-free ratio (instant flow reserve); LAD: left anterior descending; PET: positron emission tomography; PTP: pretest probability]

DIAGNOSTIC MANAGEMENT OF PATIENTS WITH ANGINA AND SUSPECTED CORONARY ARTERY DISEASE

A Detailed History Including Signs and Symptoms

To obtain a comprehensive understanding of the patient's condition, a thorough medical history is essential, encompassing various symptoms and risk factors, such as a family history of cardiovascular disease (CVD), dyslipidemia, diabetes, hypertension, smoking, and other lifestyle factors. The characteristics of chest pain can be classified into four main categories, including its location, character, duration, and its association with physical exertion, as well as other factors that may exacerbate or alleviate the symptoms. Classic features of angina include worsening of symptoms after a heavy meal or upon waking up in the morning. Interestingly, angina may sometimes show paradoxical improvement with further exercise (referred to as "walk-

TABLE 3: Classification of different angina symptoms.

Typical angina	Meets the following three characteristics: 1. Constricting discomfort in the front of the chest or in the neck, jaw, shoulder, or arm 2. Precipitated by physical exertion 3. Relieved by rest or nitrates within 5 minutes
Atypical angina	Meets two of these characteristics
Nonanginal chest pain	Meets only one or none of these characteristics

through angina") or on subsequent exertion (known as "warm-up angina"). Rapid relief from angina can often be achieved by administering sublingual nitrates **(Table 3)**.

The Canadian Cardiovascular Society classification remains a relevant grading system for angina, aiding in quantifying the level of physical activity at which symptoms manifest.[2] Conducting a thorough physical examination of patients with suspected CAD holds crucial importance in assessing the presence of various conditions, including anemia, hypertension, valvular heart disease, hypertrophic cardiomyopathy, and arrhythmias. Additionally, it is essential to evaluate for the presence of microvascular disease.

Various Comorbidities

It is necessary to assess the patient's general health, comorbidities, and quality of life. Noninvasive functional imaging for ischemia is an option to verify the diagnosis. If the pain is clearly nonanginal, other diagnostic tests should be indicated to diagnose gastrointestinal, pulmonary, or musculoskeletal causes of chest pain. Risk charts such as SCORE (Systematic COronary Risk Evaluation) can be used as a guideline for risk factor modification.[3]

Testing for Suspected Patients with Coronary Artery Disease

For patients with suspected CAD, basic testing typically comprises standard laboratory biochemical assessments, a resting electrocardiogram (ECG), potential ambulatory ECG monitoring, resting echocardiography, and a chest X-ray. These fundamental diagnostic tools aid in the initial evaluation and help healthcare providers gain insights into the patient's cardiac health and potential indications of CAD **(Table 4)**.

Resting ECG for Diagnosing Patients with Suspected Coronary Artery Disease

Table 5 outlines recommendations for diagnosis using ECG.

Ambulatory ECG for Diagnosing Patients with Suspected Coronary Artery Disease

Table 6 indicates ambulatory ECG monitoring in the initial diagnostic management of patients with suspected CAD.

TABLE 4: Basic tests in the initial diagnostic management of patients with suspected CAD.

Recommendations	Class*	Level†
If evaluation suggests clinical instability or ACS, repeated measurements of troponin, preferably using high-sensitivity or ultrasensitive assays, are recommended to rule-out myocardial injury associated with ACS	I	A
The following blood tests are recommended in all patients:		
• Full blood count (including hemoglobin)	I	B
• Creatinine measurement and estimation of renal function	I	A
• A lipid profile (including LDL-C)	I	A
It is recommended that screening for type 2 diabetes mellitus in patients with suspected and established CCS is implemented with HbA1c and fasting plasma glucose measurements, and that an oral glucose tolerance test is added if HbA1c and fasting plasma glucose results are inconclusive	I	B
Assessment of thyroid function is recommended in case of clinical suspicion of thyroid disorders	I	C

*Class of recommendation

†Level of evidence

(ACS: acute coronary syndrome; CAD: coronary artery disease; CCS: chronic coronary syndrome; HbA1c: glycated hemoglobin; LDL-C: low-density lipoprotein cholesterol)

TABLE 5: Resting ECG in the initial diagnostic management of patients with suspected CAD.

Recommendations	Class*	Level†
A resting 12-lead ECG is recommended in all patients with chest pain without an obvious noncardiac cause	I	C
A resting 12-lead ECG is recommended in all patients during or immediately after an episode of angina suspected to be indicative of clinical instability of CAD	I	C
ST-segment alterations recorded during supraventricular tachyarrhythmias should not be used as evidence of CAD	III	C

*Class of recommendation.

†Level of evidence.

(CAD: coronary artery disease; ECG: electrocardiogram)

Resting ECHO and Cardiac MRI in Diagnosing Patients with Suspected Coronary Artery Disease

Table 7 depicts recommendations for resting echocardiography and cardiac magnetic resonance in the initial diagnostic management of patients with suspected CAD.

TABLE 6: Ambulatory ECG monitoring in the initial diagnostic management of patients with suspected CAD.

Recommendations	Class*	Level†
Ambulatory ECG monitoring is recommended in patients with chest pain and suspected arrhythmias	I	C
Ambulatory ECG recording, preferably monitoring with 12-lead ECG, should be considered in patients with suspected vasospastic angina	IIa	C
Ambulatory ECG monitoring should not be used as a routine examination in patients with suspected CCS	III	C

*Class of recommendation
†Level of evidence
(CAD: coronary artery disease; CCS: chronic coronary syndromes; ECG: electrocardiogram)

TABLE 7: Resting echocardiography and CMR in the initial diagnostic management of patients with suspected CAD.

Recommendations	Class*	Level†
A resting transthoracic echocardiogram is recommended in all patients for: • Exclusion of alternative causes of angina • Identification of regional wall motion abnormalities suggestive of CAD • Measurement of LVEF for risk stratification • Evaluation of diastolic function	I	B
Ultrasound of the carotid arteries should be considered, and be performed by adequately trained clinicians, to detect plaque in patients with suspected CCS without known atherosclerotic disease	IIa	C
CMR may be considered in patients with an inconclusive echocardiographic test	IIb	C

*Class of recommendation
†Level of evidence
(CAD: coronary artery disease; CCS: chronic coronary syndrome; CMR: cardiac magnetic resonance; LVEF: left ventricular ejection fraction)

Assessment of Pretest Probability and Clinical Likelihood of Coronary Artery Disease

In cases where the likelihood of CAD is intermediate, diagnostic testing becomes especially valuable. It helps to clarify the diagnosis and guide appropriate management decisions. However, when the likelihood of CAD is high, performing extensive testing on many patients becomes less efficient. This is because many patients with high likelihood may indeed have the disease and a negative test result may not definitively rule out the presence of obstructive CAD.

To address this, a simple predictive model can be employed, estimating the PTP of obstructive CAD based on key factors such as age, sex, and the nature of symptoms. By utilizing this model, healthcare professionals can better stratify patients and determine the appropriate level of diagnostic testing needed, optimizing resources, and enhancing the diagnostic accuracy in patients with intermediate likelihood of CAD **(Box 1)**.[4]

BOX 1 Determinants of the clinical likelihood of CAD.

Decreases likelihood:
- Normal exercise ECG
- No coronary calcium by CT (Agatston score = 0)

Increases likelihood:
- Risk factors for CVD (dyslipedemia, diabetes, hypertension, smoking, and family history of CVD)
- Resting ECG changes (Q-wave or ST-segment/T-wave changes)
- LV dysfunction suggestive of CAD
- Abnormal exercise ECG
- Coronary calcium by CT

(CAD: coronary artery disease; CT: computed tomography; CVD: cardiovascular disease; ECG: electrocardiogram; LV: left ventricular)

Selection of Appropriate Testing

To make informed decisions regarding revascularization, comprehensive information about both the anatomy and ischemia of coronary arteries is essential. When evaluating patients at the higher end of the clinical likelihood range for revascularization or those with a prior CAD diagnosis, functional noninvasive tests are preferred **(Fig. 1)**. On the other hand, patients with suspected CAD but an extremely low clinical likelihood (<5%) should undergo an assessment of other potential cardiac causes of chest pain and adjustments based on their cardiovascular risk factors, utilizing a risk-score evaluation.

Incorporating stress echocardiography or single-photon emission computed tomography (SPECT) perfusion imaging in conjunction with dynamic exercise testing can provide additional valuable data, including exercise tolerance and heart rate response to exercise. A notable study, the SCOT-HEART (Scottish Computed Tomography of the HEART) trial, revealed that when coronary computed tomography angiography (CTA) was conducted alongside routine testing, predominantly using exercise ECG, patients experienced a lower rate of the combined endpoint of cardiovascular death or nonfatal myocardial infarction (MI) (2.3% vs. 3.9%) during a 5-year follow-up period.[5]

Risk Assessment

Definitions of high event risk for different modalities in patients with established CAD are given in **Table 8**.

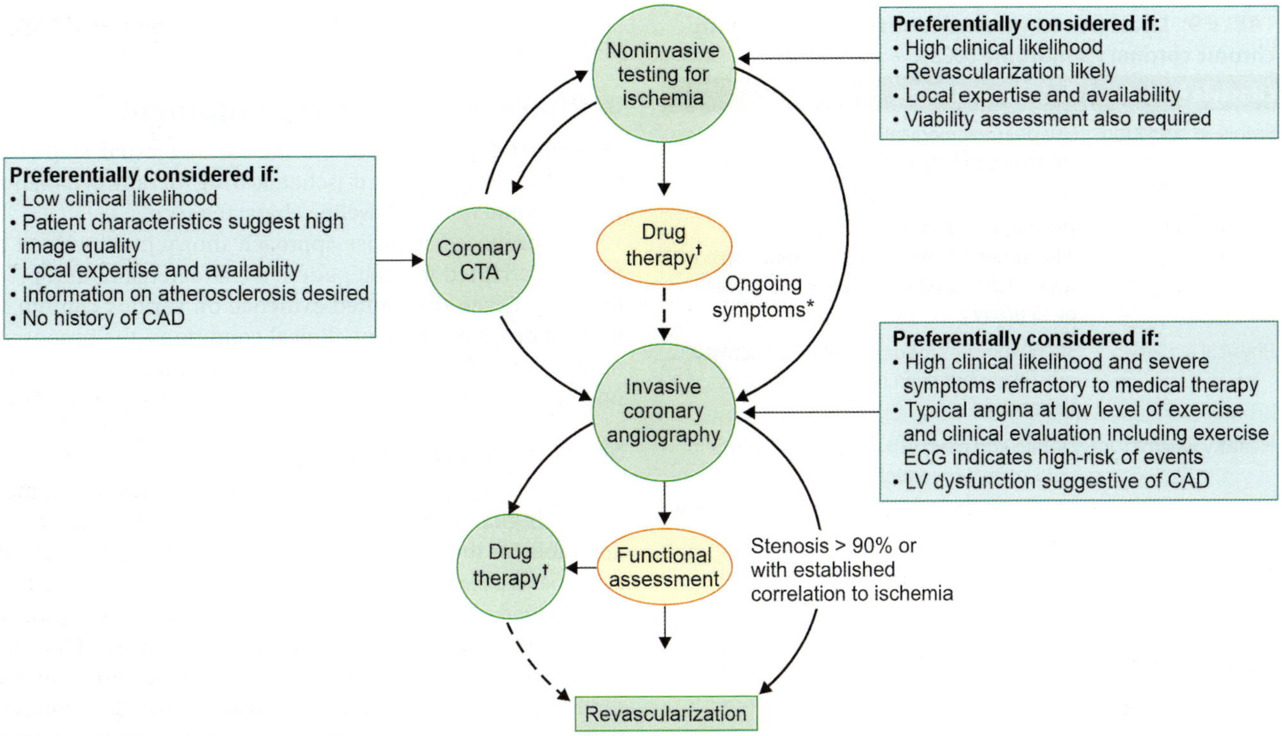

*Consider microvascular angina.
†Antianginal medications and/or risk-factor modification.

FIG. 1: Main diagnostic pathways in symptomatic patients with suspected obstructive CAD. Depending on clinical conditions and the healthcare environment, patient workup can start with either of the three options: noninvasive testing, coronary CTA, or invasive coronary angiography. Through each pathway, both functional and anatomical information is gathered to inform an appropriate diagnostic and therapeutic strategy. Risk-factor modification should be considered in all patients.

(CAD: coronary artery disease; CTA: computed tomography angiography; ECG: electrocardiogram; LV: left ventricular)

TABLE 8: Definitions of high event risk for different test modalities in patients with established chronic coronary syndrome.

Exercise ECG	Cardiovascular mortality > 3% per year according to Duke Treadmill Score
SPECT or PET perfusion imaging	Area of ischemia ≥10% of the left ventricle myocardium
Stress echocardiography	≥3 of 16 segments with stress-induced hypokinesia or akinesia
CMR	≥2 of 16 segments with stress perfusion defects or ≥3 dobutamine-induced dysfunctional segments
Coronary CTA or ICA	Three-vessel disease with proximal stenoses, LM disease, or proximal anterior descending disease
Invasive functional testing	FFR ≤ 0.8, iwFR ≤ 0.89

[CTA: computed tomography angiography; CMR: cardiac magnetic resonance; ECG: electrocardiogram; FFR: fractional flow reserve; ICA: invasive coronary angiography; iwFR: instantaneous wave-free ration (instant flow reserve); LM: left main; PET: positron emission tomography; SPECT: single-photon emission computed tomography]

Lifestyle Modification in Patients with Chronic Coronary Syndrome

The primary goal in managing CCS is to alleviate symptoms and enhance patients' long-term outlook by utilizing suitable medications and interventions while effectively controlling risk factors through lifestyle adjustments. The COURAGE (Clinical Outcomes Utilizing Revascularization and Aggressive Drug Evaluation) trial emphasized optimal medical therapy, which not only involved medication adherence promotion but also encompassed behavioral counseling and support for lifestyle risk factor management, administered by nurse case managers.[6]

Among the various lifestyle risk factors, smoking cessation holds particular significance, leading to a remarkable 36% reduction in mortality risk for those who successfully quit. By combining medical therapies, interventions, and lifestyle modifications, healthcare professionals aim to provide comprehensive and personalized management strategies to improve the quality of life and long-term prognosis for individuals living with CCS **(Table 9)**.[7]

TABLE 9: Lifestyle recommendations for patients with chronic coronary syndrome (CCS).

Lifestyle factors	Recommendations
Smoking cessation	Use pharmacological and behavioral strategies to help patients quit smoking. Avoid passive smoking
Healthy diet	Diet high in vegetables, fruit, and wholegrains. Limit saturated fat to <10% of total intake. Limit alcohol to <100 g/week or 15 g/day
Physical activity	30–60 minutes moderate physical activity most days, but even irregular activity is beneficial
Healthy weight	Obtain and maintain a healthy weight (<25 kg/m^2) or reduce weight through recommended energy intake and increased physical activity
Other	Take medications as prescribed. Sexual activity is low risk for stable patients not symptomatic at low-to-moderate activity levels

BOX 2 Healthy diet characteristics.

- Increase consumption of fruits and vegetables (≥200 g each per day)
- 35–45 g of fiber per day, preferably from wholegrains
- Moderate consumption of nuts (30 g/day, unsalted)
- 1–2 servings of fish per week (one to be oily fish)
- Limited lean meat, low-fat dairy products, and liquid vegetable oils
- Saturated fats to account for <10% of total energy intake; replace with polyunsaturated fats
- As little intake of trans-unsaturated fats as possible, preferably no intake from processed food, and <1% of total energy intake
- ≤5–6 g of salt per day
- If alcohol is consumed, limiting intake to ≤100 g/week or <15 g/day is recommended
- Avoid energy-dense foods such as sugar-sweetened soft drinks

Recommended Diet

Incorporating healthy lifestyle behaviors, such as quitting smoking, engaging in regular physical activity, adopting a balanced diet **(Box 2)**, and maintaining a healthy weight, play a crucial role in substantially reducing the risk of future cardiovascular events and mortality. Evidence from clinical trials demonstrates that psychological interventions, such as counseling and cognitive behavioral therapy, as well as pharmacological treatments, have proven to be beneficial in managing depression, anxiety, and stress. Moreover, these interventions have shown some evidence of reducing cardiovascular mortality, underscoring the significance of addressing both physical and psychological aspects in optimizing cardiovascular health and overall well-being.

Pharmacological Management

Flowchart 1 provides an outline for suggested stepwise strategy for long-term anti-ischemic drug therapy in patients with CCS and specific baseline characteristics.

The proposed stepwise approach shown in **Flowchart 1** must be adapted to each patient's characteristics and preferences. Given the limited evidence on various combinations of drugs in different clinical conditions, the proposed options are only indicative of potential combinations and do not represent formal recommendations.

Short-acting Nitrates

The rapidity of action of nitroglycerin spray surpasses that of sublingual nitroglycerin. When angina occurs, it is advisable for the patient to rest in a sitting position to avoid syncope associated with standing or increased venous return and preload while lying down. To alleviate the pain, the patient should administer nitroglycerin sublingually (0.3–0.6 mg tablet) without swallowing or as a spray (0.4 mg) directed to the tongue without inhalation or swallowing. This dose can be repeated every 5 minutes until the pain subsides or until a maximum of 1.2 mg has been taken within 15 minutes. In comparison, isosorbide dinitrate (5 mg sublingual) has a slightly slower onset of action compared to nitroglycerin due to hepatic conversion to mononitrate.

Long-acting Nitrates

When initial therapy with a beta-blocker or non-dihydropyridine (non-DHP) is not possible due to contraindications, long-acting nitrate formulations like nitroglycerin, isosorbide dinitrate, and isosorbide mononitrate may be considered as a second-line option for angina relief. However, it is important to be cautious with long-term use of these nitrates, as they can lead to tolerance and reduced efficacy over time. To counteract this, a nitrate-free or nitrate low interval of 10–14 hours should be prescribed.

Nitroglycerin can be administered orally or through slow-release transdermal patch systems. It is crucial to gradually taper nitrate usage to prevent a rebound increase in angina symptoms. Hypotension, headache, and flushing are common side effects associated with nitrate usage. Certain conditions, such as hypertrophic obstructive cardiomyopathy, severe aortic valvular stenosis, and coadministration of phosphodiesterase inhibitors (e.g., sildenafil, tadalafil, vardenafil, or riociguat), are contraindications for using nitrates and should be taken into consideration when prescribing these medications for angina relief.

Beta-blockers

A combination of beta-blockers and DHP calcium channel blockers (CCBs) can effectively reduce DHP-induced tachycardia. However, when considering a combination

	Standard therapy	High heart rate (e.g., >80 beats/min)	Low heart rate (e.g., <50 beats/min)	LV dysfunction or heart failure	Low blood pressure
1st step	BB or CCB*	BB or non-DHP-CCB	DHP-CCB	BB	Low-dose BB or low-dose non-DHP-CCB‡
2nd step	BB + DHP-CCB	BB + CCB†	Switch to LAN	BB + LAN or BB + ivabradine	Switch to ivabradine§, ranolazine, or trimetazidine‖
3rd step	Add second-line drug	BB + ivabradine§	DHP-CCB + LAN	Add another second-line drug	Combine two second-line drugs
4th step			Add nicorandil, ranolazine, or trimetazidine		

*The combination of a BB with a DHP-CCB should be considered as first step; the combination of a BB or a CCB with a second-line drug may be considered as a first step.

†The combination of a BB and non-DHP-CCB should initially use low doses of each drug under close monitoring of tolerance, particularly heart rate and blood pressure.

‡Low-dose BB or low-dose non-DHP-CCB should be used under close monitoring of tolerance, particularly heart rate and blood pressure.

§Ivabradine should not be combined with non-DHP-CCB.

‖Consider adding the drug chosen at step 2 to the drug tested at step 1 if blood pressure remains unchanged.

FLOWCHART 1: Suggested stepwise strategy for long-term anti-ischemic drug therapy in patients with CCS and specific baseline characteristics.

[BB: beta-blocker; CCB: (any class of) calcium channel blocker; CCS: chronic coronary syndrome; DHP-CCB: dihydropyridine CCB; HF: heart failure; LAN: long-acting nitrate; LV: left ventricular]

of beta-blockers with verapamil or diltiazem, caution is essential due to the potential risk of exacerbating HF, excessive bradycardia, and/or atrioventricular block. Combining a beta-blocker with a nitrate can help mitigate reflex tachycardia. It is important to be aware of the principal side effects of beta-blockers, which may include fatigue, depression, bradycardia, heart block, bronchospasm, peripheral vasoconstriction, postural hypotension, impotence, and masking of hypoglycemia symptoms. In patients with recent MI and those with chronic HF and reduced ejection fraction (EF), beta-blockers have demonstrated significant benefits, leading to a notable reduction in mortality and/or cardiovascular events. Therefore, their use in these patient populations is well-founded and clinically justified.

Non-dihydropyridine Agents

Verapamil: It boasts a broad spectrum of approved indications, encompassing various types of anginas (effort, vasospastic, and unstable), supraventricular tachycardias, and hypertension. However, its use carries certain risks, including the potential for heart block, bradycardia, and HF. When compared to metoprolol, verapamil exhibits similar antianginal activity. In hypertensive patients with CAD, verapamil shows advantages over atenolol as it is associated with a reduced risk of developing diabetes, fewer anginal attacks, and less psychological depression. However, caution is advised against combining beta-blockade with verapamil due to the risk of heart block.

Diltiazem: Similar to verapamil, diltiazem exerts its effects through peripheral vasodilation, alleviating exercise-induced coronary constriction, and has a modest negative inotropic effect, along with sinus node inhibition. However, the use of non-DHP CCBs in patients with LV dysfunction is not recommended.

Dihydropyridine Agents

In the ACTION (A Coronary disease Trial Investigating Outcome with Nifedipine gastrointestinal therapeutic system) trial, the addition of long-acting nifedipine (60 mg OD) to conventional angina treatment did not show any significant impact on major cardiovascular event-free survival.[8] However, long-acting nifedipine was deemed safe and led to a reduction in the need for coronary angiography and cardiovascular interventions. It is important to be cautious when using nifedipine in patients with severe aortic stenosis, hypertrophic obstructive cardiomyopathy, or HF. Combining nifedipine with beta-blockade is generally feasible and desirable. Vasodilatory side effects of nifedipine include headache and ankle edema.

Amlodipine, another CCB, may cause mainly ankle edema as a side effect. For patients with CCS and normal blood pressure, amlodipine at a daily dose of 10 mg has shown to reduce coronary revascularizations and hospitalizations for angina. It also leads to a reduction in exercise-induced ischemia.

Ivabradine, when added to atenolol therapy at a dosage of 7.5 mg bid, provides better control of heart rate and anginal symptoms.

Nicorandil, a nitrate derivative of nicotinamide, exhibits antianginal effects similar to nitrates or beta-blockers. However, it may cause side effects such as nausea, vomiting, and severe oral, intestinal, and mucosal ulcerations. In the IONA (Impact of Nicorandil in Angina) trial, nicorandil significantly reduced the composite of coronary heart disease (CHD) death, nonfatal MI, or unplanned hospital admission for suspected anginal symptoms in patients with CCS. However, it did not have an effect on death from ischemic heart disease or nonfatal MI.[9]

Ranolazine, a selective inhibitor of the late-inward sodium current, may cause side effects like dizziness, nausea, and constipation. It also increases QTc, so caution is advised in patients with QT prolongation or those on QT-prolonging drugs.

Trimetazidine, when added to beta-blockade (atenolol) at a dosage of 35 mg bid, improves effort-induced myocardial ischemia. However, it is contraindicated in patients with Parkinson's disease, motion disorders (such as tremor, muscle rigidity, and walking disorders), and restless leg syndrome.

The role of allopurinol in reducing clinical events in CVD remains unclear. An observational study suggested an association of allopurinol use with a reduced risk of incident MI in the elderly, especially when used for >2 years. However, more research is needed to establish its precise impact on CVD outcomes.

Recommendations for Event Prevention I

Table 10 represents recommendations for event prevention.

Treatment for Dual Antithrombotic Therapy with Aspirin in High- or Moderate-risk Patients Who do not have High Bleeding Risk

Treatment options for dual antithrombotic therapy in combination with aspirin 75–100 mg daily in patient who have a high or moderate risk of ischemic events and do not have a high bleeding risk **(Table 11)**.

Recommendations for Event Prevention II

Recommendations for event prevention are given in **Table 12**.

DYSLIPIDEMIA

The primary objective of treatment is to achieve a reduction of low-density lipoprotein cholesterol (LDL-C) by at least 50% from baseline and to reach a level below 1.4 mmol/L (55 mg/dL). In certain cases, a lower target of <1.0 mmol/L (<40 mg/dL) may be considered, especially for patients who have experienced a second vascular event within

TABLE 10: Recommendations for event prevention I.

Recommendations	Class*	Level†
Antithrombotic therapy in patients with CCS and in sinus rhythm		
Aspirin 75–100 mg daily is recommended in patients with a previous MI or revascularization	I	A
Clopidogrel 75 mg daily is recommended as an alternative to aspirin in patients with aspirin intolerance	I	B
Clopidogrel 75 mg daily may be considered in preference to aspirin in symptomatic or asymptomatic patients, with either PAD or a history of ischemic stroke or transient ischemic attack	IIb	B
Aspirin 75–100 mg daily may be considered in patients without a history of MI or revascularization but with definitive evidence of CAD on imaging	IIb	C
Adding a second antithrombotic drug to aspirin for long-term secondary prevention should be considered in patients with a high risk of ischemic events‡ and without high bleeding risk§	IIa	A
Adding a second antithrombotic drug to aspirin for long-term secondary prevention may be considered in patients with at least a moderately increased risk of ischemic events‖ and without high bleeding risk§	IIb	A

Continued

Continued

Recommendations	Class*	Level†
Antithrombotic therapy post-PCI in patients with CCS and in sinus rhythm		
Aspirin 75–100 mg daily is recommended following stenting	I	A
Clopidogrel 75 mg daily following appropriate loading (e.g., 600 mg or >5 days of maintenance therapy) is recommended, in addition to aspirin, for 6 months following coronary stenting, irrespective of stent type, unless a shorter duration (1–3 months) is indicated due to risk or the occurrence of life-threatening bleeding	I	A
Clopidogrel 75 mg daily following appropriate loading (e.g., 600 mg or >5 days of maintenance therapy) should be considered for 3 months in patients with a higher risk of life-threatening bleeding	IIa	A
Clopidogrel 75 mg daily following appropriate loading (e.g., 600 mg or >5 days of maintenance therapy) may be considered for 1 month in patients with very high risk of life-threatening bleeding	IIb	C
Prasugrel or ticagrelor may be considered, at least as initial therapy, in specific high-risk situations of elective stenting (e.g., suboptimal stent deployment or other procedural characteristics associated with high risk of stent thrombosis, complex left main stem, or multivessel stenting) or if DAPT cannot be used because of aspirin intolerance	IIb	C
Antithrombotic therapy in patients with CCS and AF		
When oral anticoagulation is initiated in a patient with AF who is eligible for a NOAC,¶ a NOAC is recommended in preference to VKA	I	A
Long-term OAC therapy (NOAC or VKA with time in therapeutic range >70%) is recommended in patients with AF and a CHA_2DS_2-VASc score** ≥2 in males and ≥3 in females	I	A
Long-term OAC therapy (NOAC or VKA with time in therapeutic range >70%) should be considered in patients with AF and a CHA_2DS_2-VASc score** of 1 in males and 2 in females	IIa	B
Aspirin 75–100 mg daily (or clopidogrel 75 mg daily) may be considered in addition to long-term OAC therapy in patients with AF, history of MI, and at high risk of recurrent ischemic events‡ who do not have a high bleeding risk§	IIb	B
Antithrombotic therapy in post-PCI patients with AF or another indication for an OAC		
It is recommended that periprocedural aspirin and clopidogrel are administered to patients undergoing coronary stent implantation	I	C
In patients who are eligible for a NOAC, it is recommended that a NOAC (apixaban 5 mg bid, dabigatran 150 mg bid, edoxaban 60 mg OD, or rivaroxaban 20 mg OD)¶ is used in preference to a VKA in combination with antiplatelet therapy	I	A
When rivaroxaban is used and concerns about high bleeding risk§ prevail over concerns about stent thrombosis†† or ischemic stroke,** rivaroxaban 15 mg OD should be considered in preference to rivaroxaban 20 mg OD for the duration of concomitant SAPT or DAPT	IIa	B
When dabigatran is used and concerns about high bleeding risk§ prevail over concerns about stent thrombosis†† or ischemic stroke,** dabigatran 110 mg bid should be considered in preference to dabigatran 150 mg bid for the duration of concomitant SAPT or DAPT	IIa	B
After uncomplicated PCI, early cessation (≤1 week) of aspirin and continuation of dual therapy with an OAC and clopidogrel should be considered if the risk of stent thrombosis†† is low, or if concerns about bleeding risk prevail over concerns about the risk of stent thrombosis,†† irrespective of the type of stent used	IIa	B
Triple therapy with aspirin, clopidogrel, and an OAC for ≥1 month should be considered when the risk of stent thrombosis†† outweighs the bleeding risk, with the total duration (≤6 months) decided according to assessment of these risks and clearly specified at hospital discharge	IIa	C
In patients with an indication for a VKA in combination with aspirin and/or clopidogrel, the dose intensity of the VKA should be carefully regulated with a target international normalized ratio in the range of 2.0–2.5 and with time in therapeutic range >70%	IIa	B
Dual therapy with an OAC and either ticagrelor or prasugrel may be considered as an alternative to triple therapy with an OAC, aspirin, and clopidogrel in patients with a moderate or high risk of stent thrombosis,†† irrespective of the type of stent used	IIb	C
The use of ticagrelor or prasugrel is not recommended as part of triple antithrombotic therapy with aspirin and an OAC	III	C

Continued

Continued

Recommendations	Class*	Level†
Use of proton pump inhibitors		
Concomitant use of a proton pump inhibitor is recommended in patients receiving aspirin monotherapy, DAPT, or OAC monotherapy who are at high risk of gastrointestinal bleeding	I	A

*Class of recommendation.

†Level of evidence.

‡Diffuse multivessel CAD with at least one of the following: Diabetes mellitus requiring medication, recurrent MI, PAD, or CKD with eGFR 15–59 mL/min/1.73 m^2.

§Prior history of intracerebral hemorrhage or ischemic stroke, history of other intracranial pathology, recent gastrointestinal bleeding, or anemia due to possible gastrointestinal blood loss, other gastrointestinal pathology associated with increased bleeding risk, liver failure, bleeding diathesis or coagulopathy, extreme old age or frailty, or renal failure requiring dialysis or with eGFR <15 mL/min/1.73 m^2.

||At least one of the following: Multivessel/diffuse CAD, diabetes mellitus requiring medication, recurrent MI, PAD, HF, or CKD with eGFR 15–59 mL/min/1.73 m^2.

¶See summary of product characteristics for reduced doses or contraindications for each NOAC in patients with CKD, body weight < 60 kg, age > 75–80 years, and/or drug interactions.

**Congestive HF, hypertension, age ≥75 years (two points), diabetes, prior stroke/transient ischemic attack/embolus (two points), vascular disease (CAD on imaging or angiography, prior MI, PAD, or aortic plaque), age 65–74 years, and female sex.

††Risk of stent thrombosis encompasses (1) the risk of thrombosis occurring and (2) the risk of death should stent thrombosis occur, both of which relate to anatomical, procedural, and clinical characteristics. Risk factors for CCS patients include stenting of left main stem, proximal LAD, or last remaining patent artery; suboptimal stent deployment; stent length >60 mm; diabetes mellitus; CKD; bifurcation with two stents implanted; treatment of chronic total occlusion; and previous stent thrombosis on adequate antithrombotic therapy.

[AF: atrial fibrillation; bid: bis in die (twice a day); CAD: coronary artery disease; CCS: chronic coronary syndrome; CHA_2DS_2-VASc: cardiac failure, hypertension, age ≥ 75 years (doubled), diabetes, stroke (doubled)-, vascular disease, age 65–74 years and sex category (female); CKD: chronic kidney disease; DAPT: dual antiplatelet therapy; eGFR: estimated glomerular filtration rate; HF: heart failure; LAD: left anterior descending; MI: myocardial infarction; NOAC: non-vitamin K antagonist oral anticoagulant; OAC: oral anticoagulant; OD: omni die (once a day); PAD: peripheral artery disease; PCI: percutaneous coronary intervention; SAPT: single antiplatelet therapy; VKA: vitamin K antagonist]

2 years. In situations where reaching these targets is challenging, the addition of ezetimibe has been shown to effectively decrease cholesterol levels and reduce cardiovascular events, particularly in post-ACS patients and those with diabetes.

For individuals who require further reduction in cholesterol levels, proprotein convertase subtilisin-kexin type 9 (PCSK9) inhibitors, such as evolocumab and alirocumab, have demonstrated remarkable efficacy. These inhibitors effectively and stably lower LDL-C to levels below 1.3 mmol/L (50 mg/dL), providing an advanced treatment option for individuals with persistent high cholesterol levels.

Renin–Angiotensin–System Blockers

Angiotensin-converting enzyme inhibitors (ACEIs) have shown significant benefits in reducing mortality, MI, stroke, and HF in patients with LV dysfunction, previous vascular disease, and high-risk diabetes. For patients with CCS who have coexisting hypertension, LV dysfunction with an EF of <40%, diabetes, or chronic kidney disease (CKD), it is recommended to use ACEIs or angiotensin receptor blockers (ARBs) as long as there are no contraindications (e.g., severe renal impairment, hyperkalemia).

Sacubitril/valsartan (LCZ696), a first-in-class medication, can be considered for patients with HF and an LVEF of <35% who remain symptomatic despite optimal treatment with an ACEI, a beta-blocker, and a mineralocorticoid receptor antagonist (MRA). In such cases, replacing the ACEI with sacubitril/valsartan is recommended to further reduce the risk of HF hospitalization and death in ambulatory patients. This advanced therapeutic option can provide significant benefits for patients with HF who have not achieved sufficient symptom relief with standard treatments.

Revascularization

Revascularization through percutaneous coronary intervention (PCI) or coronary artery bypass grafting (CABG) has proven to be an effective approach for relieving angina, reducing the need for antianginal medications, and enhancing exercise capacity and overall quality of life when compared to a strategy of medical therapy alone. In the long-term follow-up of the FAME 2 (Fractional Flow Reserve versus Angiography for Multivessel Evaluation 2) trial, revascularization demonstrated notable benefits by improving the quality of life, reducing the dependence on antianginal drugs, and minimizing associated side effects.[10]

On the other hand, the ORBITA (Objective Randomised Blinded Investigation with Optimal Medical Therapy or Angioplasty in Stable Angina) study, which involved a sham procedure in the control group, did not find a significant improvement in exercise capacity with PCI. This suggests that while revascularization can lead to several advantages in managing stable angina, the benefits may vary depending on the specific patient population and their individual clinical conditions.[11]

TABLE 11: Treatment options for DAPT in combination with aspirin 75–100 mg daily in patients who have a high* or moderate† risk of ischemic events, and do not have a high bleeding risk.‡

Drug options	Doses	Indications	Additional cautions
Clopidogrel	75 mg OD	Post-MI in patients who have tolerated DAPT for 1 year	
Prasugrel	10 mg OD or 5 mg OD; if body weight <60 kg or age >75 years	Post-PCI for MI in patients who have tolerated DAPT for 1 year	Age > 75 years
Rivaroxaban	2.5 mg BID	Post-MI > 1 year or multivessel CAD	Creatinine clearance 15–29 mL/min
Ticagrelor	60 mg BID	Post-MI in patients who have tolerated DAPT for 1 year	

*High risk of ischemic events is defined as diffuse multivessel CAD with at least one of the following: Diabetes mellitus requiring medication, recurrent MI, PAD, or CKD with eGFR 15–59 mL/min/1.73 m^2.

†Moderately increased risk of ischemic events is defined as at least one of the following: Multivessel/diffuse CAD, diabetes mellitus requiring medication, recurrent MI, PAD, HF, or CKD with eGFR 15–59 mL/min/1.73 m^2.

‡High bleeding risk is defined as history of intracerebral hemorrhage or ischemic stroke, history of other intracranial pathology, recent gastrointestinal bleeding, or anemia due to possible gastrointestinal blood loss, other gastrointestinal pathology associated with increased bleeding risk, liver failure, bleeding diathesis or coagulopathy, extreme old age or frailty, or renal failure requiring dialysis or with eGFR <15 mL/min/1.73 m^2.

Note: Treatment options are presented in alphabetical order.

[bid: bis in die (twice a day); CAD: coronary artery disease; CKD: chronic kidney disease; DAPT: dual antiplatelet therapy; eGFR: estimated glomerular filtration rate; HF: heart failure; MI: myocardial infarction; OD: omni die (once a day); PAD: peripheral artery disease; PCI: percutaneous coronary intervention]

TABLE 12: Recommendations for event prevention II.

Lipid-lowering drugs	Class*	Level†
Statins are recommended in all patients with CCS‡	I	A
If a patient's goal‡ is not achieved with the maximum-tolerated dose of statin, combination with ezetimibe is recommended	I	B
For patients at very high risk who do not achieve their goal‡ on a maximum-tolerated dose of statin and ezetimibe, combination with a PCSK9 inhibitor is recommended	I	A
ACEIs		
ACEIs (or ARBs) are recommended if a patient has other conditions (e.g., heart failure, hypertension, or diabetes)	I	A
ACEIs should be considered in CCS patients at very high risk of cardiovascular events	IIa	A
Other drugs		
Beta-blockers are recommended in patients with LV dysfunction or systolic HF.	I	A
In patients with a previous STEMI, long-term oral treatment with a beta-blocker should be considered	IIa	B

*Class of recommendation.

†Level of evidence.

‡The treatment goals are shown in the European Society of Cardiology/European Atherosclerosis Society Guidelines for the management of dyslipidemias.

(ACEIs: angiotensin-converting enzyme inhibitors; ARBs: angiotensin receptor blockers; CCS: chronic coronary syndrome; HF: heart failure; LV: left ventricular; PCSK9: proprotein convertase subtilisin-kexin type 9; STEMI: ST-elevation myocardial infarction)

Decision for Revascularization in Patients with Chronic Coronary Syndrome

Decisions for revascularization by PCI or CABG are based on clinical presentation (symptoms present or absent) and prior documentation of ischemia (present or absent) **(Flowchart 2)**.

MANAGEMENT OF PATIENTS WITH ISCHEMIC CARDIOMYOPATHY AND LEFT VENTRICULAR DYSFUNCTION

Recommendations for management of patients with ischemic cardiomyopathy and LV dysfunction are given in **Table 13**.

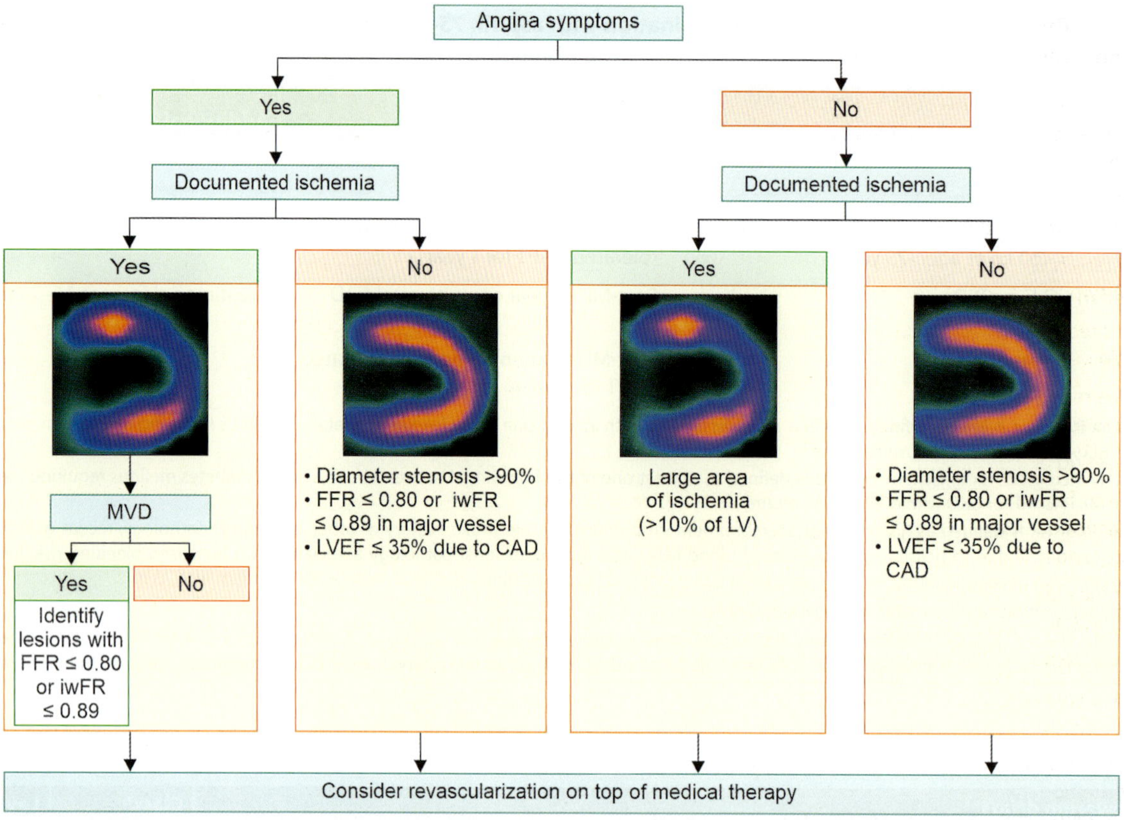

Note: In the absence of prior documentation of ischemia, indications for revascularization depend on invasive evaluation of stenosis severity or prognostic indications. Patients with no symptoms and ischemia include candidates for transcatheter aortic valve implantation, valve, and other surgery.

FLOWCHART 2: Decision tree for patients undergoing invasive coronary angiography.

(CAD: coronary artery disease; FFR: fractional flow reserve; iwFR: instantaneous wave-free ratio; LV: left ventricle; LVEF: left ventricular ejection fraction; MVD: multivessel disease)

RECOMMENDATIONS FOR PATIENTS WITH LONG-STANDING CHRONIC CORONARY SYNDROME

Recommendations for patients with long-standing chronic coronary syndrome are given in **Table 14**.

MICROVASCULAR ANGINA

Microvascular angina patients usually experience angina triggered by exercise and noninvasive tests reveal evidence of reduced blood flow to the heart muscle without significant blockages or with mild-to-moderate narrowing (40–60%) observed in invasive coronary angiography (ICA) or CTA. Secondary microvascular angina can occur when there are no obstructions in the large coronary arteries and it may be associated with cardiac or systemic conditions, such as hypertrophic cardiomyopathy, aortic stenosis, hypertensive heart disease, myocarditis, or vasculitis. To assess microcirculatory function, two essential parameters are considered: The index of microcirculatory resistance (IMR) should be >25 units and coronary flow reserve (CFR) should be <2.0. These measurements are typically obtained during intravenous vasodilator administration, such as adenosine or regadenoson. Treatment for patients with abnormal CFR (<2.0) or elevated IMR (>25 units), along with a negative acetylcholine provocation test, includes the use of beta-blockers, ACEIs, and statins **(Table 15)**. Lifestyle modifications, including weight loss, are also recommended to improve their condition. Additionally, patients who exhibit ECG changes and angina in response to acetylcholine testing but do not have severe epicardial vasoconstriction may be treated similarly to patients with vasospastic angina.

VASOSPASTIC ANGINA

Vasospastic angina should be suspected in patients with angina symptoms occurring predominantly at rest, with maintained effort tolerance. Attacks follow a circadian pattern, with more episodes at night and in the early morning hours. It is suspected in patients with patent coronary stents and persistent angina. The diagnosis is based on detecting transient ischemic ST-segment changes during an angina attack usually at rest. A provocation test for coronary spasm is considered positive when it triggers: (1) anginal symptoms,

TABLE 13: Recommendations for the management of patients with CCS and symptomatic HF due to ischemic cardiomyopathy and LV systolic dysfunction.

Recommendations for drug therapy	Class*	Level†
Diuretic therapy is recommended in symptomatic patients with signs of pulmonary or systemic congestion to relieve HF symptoms	I	B
Beta-blockers are recommended as essential components of treatment due to their efficacy in both relieving angina and reducing morbidity and mortality in HF	I	A
ACEI therapy is recommended in patients with symptomatic HF or asymptomatic LV dysfunction following MI, to improve symptoms and reduce morbidity and mortality	I	A
An ARB is recommended as an alternative in patients who do not tolerate ACE inhibition, or an angiotensin receptor/neprilysin inhibitor in patients with persistent symptoms despite optimal medical therapy	I	B
An MRA is recommended in patients who remain symptomatic despite adequate treatment with an ACEI and beta-blocker, to reduce morbidity and mortality	I	A
A short-acting oral or transcutaneous nitrate should be considered (effective antianginal treatment, safe in HF)	IIa	A
Ivabradine should be considered in patients with sinus rhythm, an LVEF ≤ 35% and a resting heart rate > 70 beats/min who remain symptomatic despite adequate treatment with a beta-blocker, ACEI, and MRA, to reduce morbidity and mortality	IIa	B
Amlodipine may be considered for relief of angina in patients with HF who do not tolerate beta-blockers and is considered safe in HF	IIb	B
For devices, comorbidities, and revascularization		
In patients with HF and bradycardia with high-degree atrioventricular block who require pacing, a CRT with a pacemaker rather than right ventricular pacing is recommended	I	A
An implantable cardioverter-defibrillator is recommended in patients with documented ventricular dysrhythmia causing hemodynamic instability (secondary prevention), as well as in patients with symptomatic HF and an LVEF ≤ 35%, to reduce the risk of sudden death and all-cause mortality	I	A
CRT is recommended for symptomatic patients with HF in sinus rhythm with a QRS duration ≥ 150 ms and LBBB QRS morphology, and with LVEF ≤ 35%, despite optimal medical therapy to improve symptoms, and reduce morbidity and mortality	I	A
CRT is recommended for symptomatic patients with HF in sinus rhythm with a QRS duration 130–149 ms and LBBB QRS morphology, and with LVEF ≤ 35%, despite optimal medical therapy to improve symptoms, and reduce morbidity and mortality	I	B
Comprehensive risk profiling and multidisciplinary management, including treatment of major comorbidities such as hypertension, hyperlipidemia, diabetes, anemia, and obesity, as well as smoking cessation and lifestyle modification, are recommended	I	A
Myocardial revascularization is recommended when angina persists despite treatment with antianginal drugs	I	A

*Class of recommendation.

†Level of evidence.

(ACE: angiotensin-converting enzyme; ARB: angiotensin receptor blocker; CRT: cardiac resynchronization therapy; HF: heart failure; LBBB: left bundle branch block; LV: left ventricular; LVEF: left ventricular ejection fraction; MI: myocardial infarction; MRA: mineralocorticoid receptor antagonist)

TABLE 14: Recommendations for long-standing chronic coronary syndrome.

Recommendations for asymptomatic patients	Class*	Level†
A periodic visit to a cardiovascular healthcare professional is recommended to reassess any potential change in the risk status of patients, entailing clinical evaluation of lifestyle-modification measures, adherence to targets of cardiovascular risk factors, and the development of comorbidities that may affect treatments and outcomes	I	C
In patients with mild or no symptoms receiving medical treatment in whom noninvasive risk stratification indicates a high risk, and for whom revascularization is considered for improvement of prognosis, invasive coronary angiography (with FFR when necessary) is recommended	I	C
Coronary CTA is not recommended as a routine follow-up test for patients with established CAD	III	C
Invasive coronary angiography is not recommended solely for risk stratification	III	C

Continued

Continued

Recommendations for asymptomatic patients	Class*	Level†
Symptomatic patients		
Reassessment of CAD status is recommended in patients with deteriorating LV systolic function that cannot be attributed to a reversible cause (e.g., long-standing tachycardia or myocarditis)	I	C
Risk stratification is recommended in patients with new or worsening symptom levels, preferably using stress imaging or, alternatively, exercise stress ECG	I	B
It is recommended to expeditiously refer patients with significant worsening of symptoms for evaluation	I	C
Invasive coronary angiography (with FFR/iwFR when necessary) is recommended for risk stratification in patients with severe CAD, particularly if the symptoms are refractory to medical treatment or if they have a high-risk clinical profile	I	C

*Class of recommendation.
†Level of evidence.
(CAD: coronary artery disease; CTA: computed tomography angiography; ECG: electrocardiogram; FFR: fractional flow reserve; iwFR: instantaneous wave-free ratio; LV: left ventricular)

TABLE 15: Investigations for diagnosis microvascular angina.

Recommendations	Class*	Level†
Guidewire-based CFR and/or microcirculatory resistance measurements should be considered in patients with persistent symptoms, but coronary arteries that are either angiographically normal or have moderate stenoses with preserved iwFR/FFR	IIa	B
Intracoronary acetylcholine with ECG monitoring may be considered during angiography, if coronary arteries are either angiographically normal or have moderate stenoses with preserved iwFR/FFR, to assess microvascular vasospasm	IIb	B
Transthoracic Doppler of the LAD, CMR, and PET may be considered for noninvasive assessment of CFR	IIb	B

*Class of recommendation.
†Level of evidence.
(CFR: coronary flow reserve; CMR: cardiac magnetic resonance; ECG: electrocardiogram; FFR: fractional flow reserve; iwFR: instantaneous wave-free ratio; LAD: left anterior descending; PET: positron emission tomography)

TABLE 16: Investigations for suspected vasospastic angina.

Recommendations	Class*	Level†
An ECG is recommended during angina if possible	I	C
Invasive angiography or coronary CTA is recommended in patients with characteristic episodic resting angina and ST-segment changes, which resolve with nitrates and/or calcium antagonists, to determine the extent of underlying coronary disease	I	C
Ambulatory ST-segment monitoring should be considered to identify ST-segment deviation in the absence of increased heart rate	IIa	C
An intracoronary provocation test should be considered to identify coronary spasm in patients with normal findings or nonobstructive lesions on coronary arteriography and a clinical picture of coronary spasm to diagnose the site and mode of spasm	IIa	B

*Class of recommendation.
†Level of evidence.
(CTA: computed tomography angiography; ECG: electrocardiogram)

(2) ischemic ECG changes, and (3) severe vasoconstriction of the epicardial vessel. CCBs and long-acting nitrates are the treatment of choice, control of cardiovascular risk factors, and lifestyle changes **(Table 16)**. Nifedipine has been shown to be effective in reducing coronary spasm associated with stent implantation.

RECOMMENDATIONS FOR SCREENING OF CORONARY ARTERY DISEASE IN ASYMPTOMATIC INDIVIDUALS

Recommendations for screening of CAD in asymptomatic individuals are given in **Table 17**.

TABLE 17: Recommendations for screening of CAD in asymptomatic individuals.

Recommendations	Class*	Level†
Total risk estimation using a risk-estimation system such as SCORE is recommended for asymptomatic adults >40 years of age without evidence of CVD, diabetes, CKD, or familial hypercholesterolemia	I	C
Assessment of family history of premature CVD (defined as a fatal or nonfatal CVD event or/and established diagnosis of CVD in first-degree male relatives before 55 years of age or female relatives before 65 years of age) is recommended as part of cardiovascular risk assessment	I	C
It is recommended that all individuals aged <50 years with a family history of premature CVD in a first-degree relative (<55 years of age in men or <65 years of age in women) or familial hypercholesterolemia are screened using a validated clinical score	I	B
Assessment of coronary artery calcium score with computed tomography may be considered as a risk modifier‡ in the cardiovascular risk assessment of asymptomatic subjects	IIb	B
Atherosclerotic plaque detection by carotid artery ultrasound may be considered as a risk modifier‡ in the cardiovascular risk assessment of asymptomatic subjects	IIb	B
ABI may be considered as a risk modifier‡ in cardiovascular risk assessment	IIb	B
In high-risk asymptomatic adults (with diabetes, a strong family history of CAD, or when previous risk-assessment tests suggest a high risk of CAD), functional imaging or coronary CTA may be considered for cardiovascular risk assessment	IIb	C
In asymptomatic adults (including sedentary adults considering starting a vigorous exercise program), an exercise ECG may be considered for cardiovascular risk assessment, particularly when attention is paid to non-ECG markers such as exercise capacity	IIb	C
Carotid ultrasound IMT for cardiovascular risk assessment is not recommended	III	A
In low-risk nondiabetic asymptomatic adults, coronary CTA or functional imaging for ischemia are not indicated for further diagnostic assessment	III	C
Routine assessment of circulating biomarkers is not recommended for cardiovascular risk stratification	III	B

*Class of recommendation.
†Level of evidence.
‡Reclassifies patients better into low- or high-risk groups
(ABI: ankle–brachial index; CAD: coronary artery disease; CKD: chronic kidney disease; CTA: computed tomography angiography; CVD: cardiovascular disease; ECG: electrocardiogram; IMT: intima-media thickness; SCORE: Systematic Coronary Risk Evaluation)

RECOMMENDATIONS FOR TREATMENT OF HYPERTENSION IN CHRONIC CORONARY SYNDROME

Recommendations for treatment of hypertension in CCS are given in **Table 18**.

TABLE 18: Recommendations for treatment of hypertension in chronic coronary syndrome.

Recommendations	Class*	Level†
It is recommended that office BP is controlled to target values: Systolic BP 120–130 mm Hg in general and systolic BP 130–140 mm Hg in older patients (aged >65 years)	I	A
In hypertensive patients with a recent MI, beta-blockers and RAS blockers are recommended	I	A
In patients with symptomatic angina, beta-blockers and/or CCBs are recommended	I	A
The combination of ACEIs and ARBs is not recommended	III	A

*Class of recommendation.
†Level of evidence.
(ACEIs: angiotensin-converting enzyme inhibitors; ARBs angiotensin receptor blockers; BP: blood pressure; CCBs: calcium channel blockers; MI: myocardial infarction; RAS: renin-angiotensin system)

MANAGEMENT OF VALVULAR HEART DISEASE IN CHRONIC CORONARY SYNDROME

Recommendations for management of valvular heart disease in chronic coronary syndrome are given in **Table 19**.

MANAGEMENT OF DIABETES MELLITUS

Recommendations for management of diabetes mellitus are given in **Table 20**.

TABLE 19: Recommendations for management of valvular heart disease in chronic coronary syndrome.

Recommendations	Class*	Level†
ICA is recommended before valve surgery and for any of the following: History of CVD, suspected myocardial ischemia, LV systolic dysfunction, in men >40 years of age and post-menopausal women, or one or more cardiovascular risk factors	I	C
ICA is recommended in the evaluation of moderate-to-severe functional mitral regurgitation	I	C
Coronary CTA should be considered as an alternative to coronary angiography before valve intervention in patients with severe valvular heart disease and low probability of CAD	IIa	C
PCI should be considered in patients undergoing transcatheter aortic valve implantation and coronary artery diameter stenosis > 70% in proximal segments	IIa	C
In severe valvular heart disease, stress testing should not be routinely used to detect CAD because of the low diagnostic yield and potential risks	III	C

*Class of recommendation.
†Level of evidence.
(CAD: coronary artery disease; CTA: computed tomography angiography; CVD: cardiovascular disease; ICA: invasive coronary angiography; LV: left ventricular; PCI: percutaneous coronary intervention)

TABLE 20: Recommendations for diabetes mellitus in chronic coronary syndromes.

Recommendations	Class*	Level†
Risk factor (BP, LDL-C, and HbA1c) control to targets is recommended in patients with CAD and diabetes mellitus	I	A
In asymptomatic patients with diabetes mellitus, a periodic resting ECG is recommended for cardiovascular detection of conduction abnormalities, AF, and silent MI	I	C
ACEI treatment is recommended in CCS patients with diabetes for event prevention	I	B
The sodium–glucose cotransporter 2 inhibitors—empagliflozin, canagliflozin, or dapagliflozin—are recommended in patients with diabetes and CVD‡	I	A
A glucagon-like peptide-1 receptor agonist (liraglutide or semaglutide) is recommended in patients with diabetes and CVD‡	I	A
In asymptomatic adults (age > 40 years) with diabetes, functional imaging or coronary CTA may be considered for advanced cardiovascular risk assessment	IIb	B

*Class of recommendation.
†Level of evidence.
‡Treatment algorithm is available in the 2019 European Society of Cardiology/European Association for the Study of Diabetes guidelines on diabetes mellitus, prediabetes, and cardiovascular diseases.
(ACEI: angiotensin-converting enzyme inhibitor; AF: atrial fibrillation; BP: blood pressure; CAD: coronary artery disease; CCS: chronic coronary syndrome; CTA: computed tomography angiography; CVD: cardiovascular disease; ECG: electrocardiogram; HbA1c: glycated hemoglobin; LDL-C: low-density lipoprotein cholesterol; MI: myocardial infarction)

RECOMMENDATIONS FOR ACTIVE CANCER IN CHRONIC CORONARY SYNDROME

Recommendations for active cancer in CCS are given in **Table 21**.

TABLE 21: Recommendations for active cancer in chronic coronary syndromes.

Recommendations	Class*	Level†
Treatment decisions should be based on life expectancy, additional comorbidities such as thrombocytopenia, increased thrombosis propensity, and potential interactions between drugs used in CCS management and antineoplastic agents	I	C
If revascularization is indicated in highly symptomatic patients with active cancer and increased frailty, the least invasive procedure is recommended	I	C

*Class of recommendation.
†Level of evidence.

RECOMMENDATIONS FOR ELDERLY PATIENTS WITH CHRONIC CORONARY SYNDROME

Recommendations for elderly patients with CCS are given in **Table 22**.

MANAGEMENT OF REFRACTORY ANGINA

For individuals with refractory angina, optimal care is provided within specialized "angina clinics" staffed by

TABLE 22: Recommendations for elderly patients with chronic coronary syndromes.

Recommendations	Class*	Level†
It is recommended that particular attention is paid to side effects of drugs, intolerance, and overdosing in elderly patients	I	C
The use of drug-eluting stents (DES) is recommended in elderly patients	I	A
Radial access is recommended in elderly patients to reduce access-site bleeding complications	I	B
It is recommended that diagnostic and revascularization decisions are based on symptoms, the extent of ischemia, frailty, life expectancy, and comorbidities	I	C

*Class of recommendation.
†Level of evidence.

TABLE 23: Potential treatment options for refractory angina and list of randomized clinical trials (RCTs).

Therapies	Types of therapies	RCTs
External counterpulsation	Enhanced external counterpulsation	MUST
Extracorporeal shockwave	Low-energy extracorporeal shockwave therapy	Not available
Coronary sinus constriction	Reducer device	COSIRA
Neuromodulation	Spinal cord stimulation	STARTSTIM
	Transcutaneous electrical neural stimulation	Not available
	Subcutaneous electrical neural stimulation	Not available
	Sympathectomy	Denby et al.
Gene therapy	Adenovirus fibroblast growth factor 5	Not available
Autologous cell therapy	Mononuclear bone marrow-derived hematopoietic progenitor cells	RENEW

skilled multidisciplinary teams. These teams leverage their expertise to tailor a precise treatment strategy for each patient, drawing from a thorough assessment of the underlying pain mechanisms. When standard anti-ischemic interventions have been thoroughly explored, encompassing enhancements in nutrient-rich blood flow and curbs in oxygen consumption, novel therapeutic options are systematically evaluated based on their mechanisms

TABLE 24: Recommendations for treatment options for refractory angina.

Recommendations	Class*	Level†
Enhanced external counterpulsation may be considered for symptom relief in patients with debilitating angina refractory to optimal medical and revascularization strategies	IIb	B
A reducer device for coronary sinus constriction may be considered to ameliorate symptoms of debilitating angina refractory to optimal medical and revascularization strategies	IIb	B
Spinal cord stimulation may be considered to ameliorate symptoms and quality of life in patients with debilitating angina refractory to optimal medical and revascularization strategies	IIb	B
Transmyocardial revascularization is not recommended in patients with debilitating angina refractory to optimal medical and revascularization strategies	III	A

*Class of recommendation.
†Level of evidence.

of action. These options include fostering collateral vessel growth, orchestrating transmural blood flow adjustments, and employing neuromodulation techniques to address the cardiac pain syndrome **(Table 23)**.

RECOMMENDATIONS FOR TREATMENT OPTIONS FOR REFRACTORY ANGINA

Recommendations for treatment options for refractory angina are given in **Table 24**.

CONCLUSION

A fundamental aspect of managing CCS involves commencing with medical therapy as the primary treatment. However, in cases where patients experience persistent symptoms, have a significant ischemic burden, or face challenges with drug tolerance, revascularization becomes necessary. Before proceeding to angiography, it is important to confirm the presence of ischemia through a noninvasive stress test. For patients who undergo angiography without prior noninvasive stress testing, utilizing fractional flow reserve (FFR) can assist in making informed decisions about the need for revascularization. Revascularization through PCI or CABG is highly effective in treating CAD, particularly when targeting specific culprit stenoses that are hemodynamically significant and causing ischemia. The appropriate choice of revascularization method depends on factors such as the angiographic characteristics of the ischemia-causing lesions, the presence of LV dysfunction, any existing comorbidities, and the patient's suitability for surgery. Ultimately, the physician's decisions regarding patient care must be based on the latest evidence-based medicine, while also taking into consideration the individual patient's preferences and expectations for their quality of life.

ONLINE REFERENCES

Please scan the QR code provided at the end of the table of contents for References of this chapter.

CHAPTER

82 Role of Invasive versus Medical Therapy in SIHD: What ISCHEMIA-EXTEND Says?

Sourabh Agstam, Rakesh Yadav

ABSTRACT

The evidence does not favor the initial invasive strategy in the stable ischemic heart disease (SIHD) excluding the left main disease. Invasive strategy over the failed guideline-directed medical therapy reduces the angina and improves quality of life in SIHD; however, it does not reduce the cardiovascular (CV) mortality. The ISCHEMIA (International Study of Comparative Health Effectiveness with Medical and Invasive Approaches) trial, one of the largest randomized controlled trial, after the median follow-up of 3.2 years found no statistical difference in the hard end points between invasive and conservative strategy in chronic coronary disease (previously SIHD) with moderate or severe ischemia on stress testing. The authors noticed that there was increase in periprocedural myocardial infarction (MI) but lower risk of spontaneous MI in invasive strategy and the reduction in spontaneous MI emerged over time. Additionally, the long-term effect of invasive strategy on CV mortality is not known. The ISCHEMIA-EXTEND trial was planned to look for long-term follow-up of surviving patients from the ISCHEMIA trial. An interim report of median 7-year follow-up for all-cause, CV, and non-CV mortality showed no difference in all-cause mortality, but with a lower risk of CV mortality and higher risk of non-CV mortality in invasive strategy.

Keywords: Stable ischemic heart disease, invasive strategy, conservative strategy.

INTRODUCTION

The optimal timing for revascularization in stable ischemic heart disease (SIHD) is still an enigma. The ISCHEMIA (International Study of Comparative Health Effectiveness with Medical and Invasive Approaches) trial helped us in decision making in the management of SIHD.[1] All the previous trails on routine invasive therapy in SIHD showed no mortality benefit over the guideline-directed medical therapy (GDMT). However, the long-term effect of invasive management strategy on mortality remains unclear. To answer the question, the ISCHEMIA-EXTEND has been planned.[2]

WHAT IS ISCHEMIA TRIAL: UNDERSTANDING THE ORIGINAL TRAIL

The aim of the ISCHEMIA trial was to determine whether routine cardiac catheterization and revascularization in patients with chronic coronary syndrome (CCS) (previously known as SIHD) reduce the likelihood of major adverse cardiac events when added to GDMT. It was a randomized controlled trial and after a median follow-up of 3.2 years, the trial found no statistical difference in the primary or major secondary clinical endpoints between initial invasive and conservative management of CCS patients with moderate-to-severe ischemia on stress testing (**Fig. 1**). An invasive strategy patient had more periprocedural myocardial infarction (MI) which is obvious relative to the medical strategy. On the other hand, a lower risk of spontaneous MI was noted in the invasive strategy.

ISCHEMIA-EXTEND: NOT A BAD NEWS FOR CARDIOLOGIST

The ISCHEMIA-EXTEND is an observational study to find the long-term effect of invasive strategy on mortality (**Fig. 2**). The surviving participants from the ISCHEMIA trial were followed for nearly 7 years (median follow-up of 5.7 years) to look for all-cause, cardiovascular (CV) and non-CV

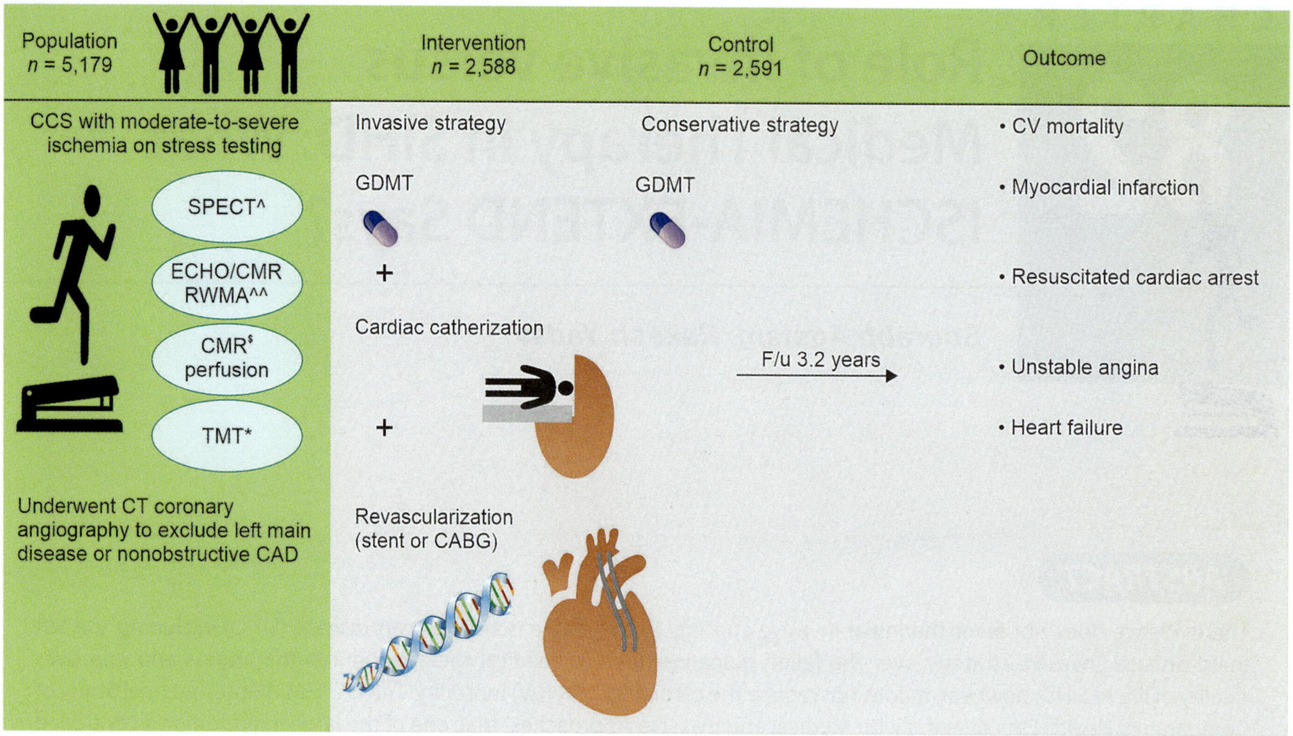

Moderate ischemia defined as:

^ SPECT: ≥10% LV.

^^ ECHO-CMR RWMA ≥3/16 segments or new/worse wall motion abnormality.

$ CMR perfusion >12% LV.

*TMT – ST ↓ ≥1.5 mm in 2 leads or >2.0 mm in ≥1 lead or ST ↑ ≥1.0 mm in non-infarct territory.

FIG. 1: Summary of ISCHEMIA trial.

(CABG: coronary artery bypass graft; CAD: coronary artery disease; CCS: chronic coronary syndrome; GDMT: guideline-directed medical therapy)

mortality. Out of the initial 5,179 patients in ISCHEMIA trial, 4,825 participants were included in the ISCHEMIA-EXTEND as few patients died by the end of the trial, some patients withdrew and few patients declined for further study. Although, there was no difference in the all-cause mortality in invasive versus medical therapy group; there was significant benefit in CV mortality over time in invasive strategy with an estimated 2.2% absolute reduction in CV mortality over 7 years. The CV mortality curves started to separate after 4 years and this benefit was offset by an estimated 1.2% absolute increase in the non-CV mortality (cancer or sepsis) in invasive strategy.

LIMITATIONS OF THE TRIAL

The use of all-cause mortality in the ISCHEMIA-EXTEND is controversial. From the cardiologist perceptive, CV mortality is of prime importance while managing the patient of SIHD. The non-CV mortality becomes amplified with a longer follow-up and hence keeping the all-cause mortality as primary outcome in long follow-up studies is dubious.

CONCLUSION

The routine initial invasive strategy in chronic coronary disease does not reduce all-cause mortality in CCS. There is benefit in CV mortality over time in invasive strategy, and henceforth, there should be shared decision-making while adding invasive strategy to guideline-directed medical management. The real question is "Can we identify high-risk patients of SIHD excluding left main disease who get benefit of initial invasive strategy?"

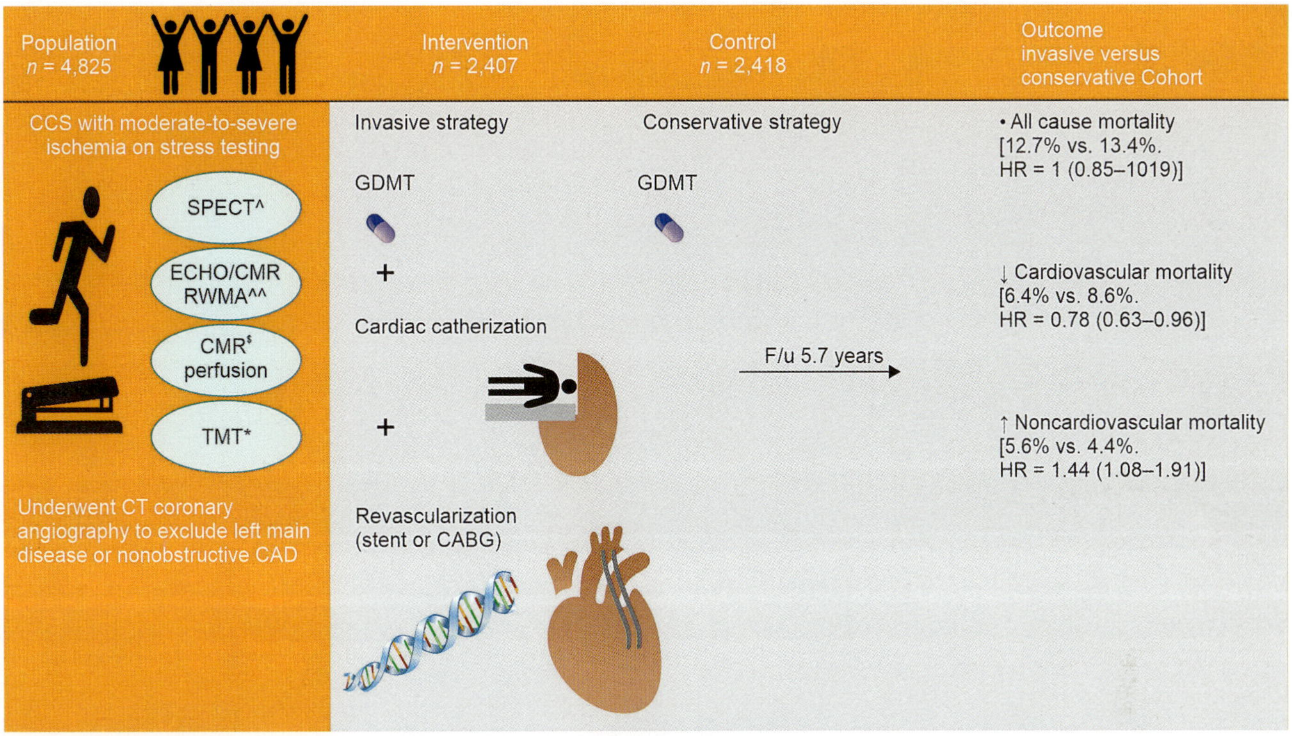

Moderate ischemia defined as:

^ SPECT: - ≥10% LV.

^^ ECHO-CMR RWMA ≥3/16 segments or new/worse wall motion abnormality.

$ CMR perfusion >12% LV.

*TMT – ST ↓ ≥ 1.5 mm in 2 leads or >2.0 mm in ≥1 lead or ST ↑ ≥1.0 mm in noninfarct territory.

FIG. 2: Summary of ISCHEMIA-EXTEND trial.

(CABG: coronary artery bypass graft; CAD: coronary artery disease; CCS: chronic coronary syndrome; GDMT: guideline-directed medical therapy)

ONLINE REFERENCES

Please scan the QR code provided at the end of the table of contents for References of this chapter.

SECTION

9

Cardiomyopathy

CHAPTER

83

Genetics in Cardiomyopathy

Devanu Ghosh Roy, Deepanjan Bhattacharya

ABSTRACT

Cardiomyopathy is a common cause of heart failure worldwide, and is most commonly genetic in etiology. Grossly, it can be classified into hypertrophic cardiomyopathy (HCM), dilated cardiomyopathy (DCM), restrictive cardiomyopathy (RCM), arrhythmogenic right ventricular cardiomyopathy (ARVC), cardiomyopathy with other extracardiac manifestations, and left ventricular noncompaction (LVNC).

Each disease is associated with a different set of genes, and has distinctive phenotypical characteristics. Early diagnosis is the key to successful management and proper genetic testing is essential. The prognosis also varies according to the gene involved and hence, is important in guiding the management of the patient.

There are several inherited genetic disorders which are associated with cardiomyopathy and myocardial disease. It is important to identify these associations as screening for cardiac disease is important for these disorders.

Moreover, it is also important to understand the role of genetic counseling and the need to identify the proper genetic tests for each disorder.

The data from India regarding the genetics of patients with cardiomyopathy is still evolving with a lot of research still underway.

In this article, we describe the various genetic mutations which are associated with cardiomyopathy and their clinical implications.

Keywords: Cardiomyopathy, genetics.

INTRODUCTION

Cardiomyopathy is defined by the structural or functional disorders of myocardium in the absence of secondary causes of heart failure (HF) such as hypertension, valvular heart disease, ischemic heart disease, and congenital heart disease that are sufficient to explain the observed myocardial abnormality.[1] They are a major cause of heart failure worldwide.

Broadly, it can be classified into hypertrophic cardiomyopathy (HCM), dilated cardiomyopathy (DCM), restrictive cardiomyopathy (RCM), arrhythmogenic right ventricular cardiomyopathy (ARVC), cardiomyopathy with other extracardiac manifestations, and left ventricular noncompaction (LVNC).

These patients usually present late with advanced disease and myriad of complications, such as arrhythmia, heart failure, and sudden cardiac death (SCD). Genetic testing thus helps to identify those at risk, and plan early intervention to reduce the complications.

GENETICS OF DILATED CARDIOMYOPATHY

Dilated cardiomyopathy is defined by the presence of left ventricular (LV) or biventricular dilatation (>112% of LV end-diastolic dimension predicted for age and body surface area) and systolic dysfunction [left ventricular ejection fraction (LVEF) < 45%)] after excluding abnormal loading conditions (hypertension and valve disease) or coronary artery disease sufficient to cause global systolic impairment.[2]

Approximately, 40% of DCM cases have a genetic etiology, and over 50 genes have been implicated **(Fig. 1)**. Majority

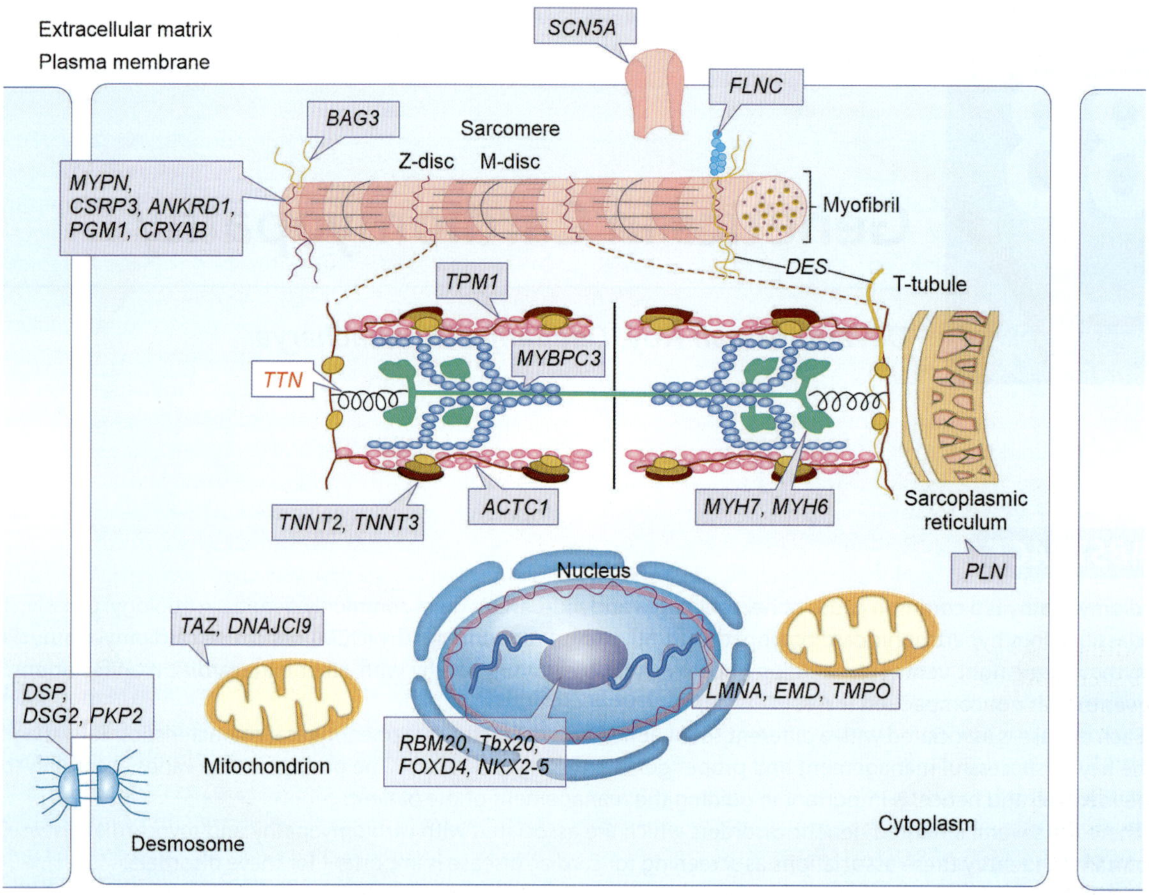

FIG. 1: Schematic diagram showing genes involved in dilated cardiomyopathy.

(ACTC1: cardiac α-actin 1; BAG3: BAG cochaperone 3; DES: desmin; DSG2: desmoglein-2; DSP: desmoplakin; EMD: emerin; FLNC: filamin C; LMNA: lamin A/C; MYBPC: myosin-binding protein C; MYH6: α-myosin heavy chain; MYH7: β-myosin heavy chain; MYPN: myopalladin; PKP2: plakophilin-2; PLN: phospholamban; RBM20: RNA-binding protein 20; SCN5A-sodium channel protein type 5 α-subunit; TMPO: trimethyl phosphate; TNNT: troponin T; TPM1: α-tropomyosin; TTN: titin)

are autosomal dominant with variable expression, while autosomal recessive, X-linked recessive and mitochondrial inheritance are infrequent.[3]

TTN is the most common gene associated with DCM, seen in 12–25%, with family clustering predominant.[4] It codes for titin, which is the largest known protein and serves as the major sarcomeric protein. It is associated with an overall good prognosis, less conduction defects and a tendency for ventricular reverse remodeling with optimal medical therapy.[5]

Lamin A/C (*LMNA*) is the second most common gene, accounting for 10–30%.[6] It is associated with conduction system defects, along with high arrhythmia burden and increased risk for SCD.[7] Onset is at young age, with high penetrance and poor response to medical therapy.

β-myosin heavy chain-7 (*MYH7*) and α-myosin heavy chain (*MYH6*) account for 4–6% of cases each, while myopalladin (*MYPN*) mutations are seen in 3–4%, and is associated with increased risk of SCD.[8]

Other affected genes include desmoplakin (*DSP*), ribonucleic acid (RNA)-binding protein 20 (*RBM20*), cardiac muscle troponin T (*TNNT2*), sodium channel protein type 5 α-subunit (*SCN5A*), and α-tropomyosin (*TPM1*).[8,9]

The American College of Cardiology (ACC)/American Heart Association (AHA) guidelines advocated for a detailed family history of at least three generations with a pedigree for all cases of DCM (class I), with clinical screening for cardiomyopathy in all first degree relatives (class I), variant specific cascade screening (class I), and comprehensive or LMNA/SCN5A targeted genetic sequencing in those with cardiac conduction disease or family history of SCD (class I).[10,11]

GENETICS OF HYPERTROPHIC CARDIOMYOPATHY

With a prevalence on 1 in 500, HCM is one of the most common cardiac disorders encountered.[12] A maximal

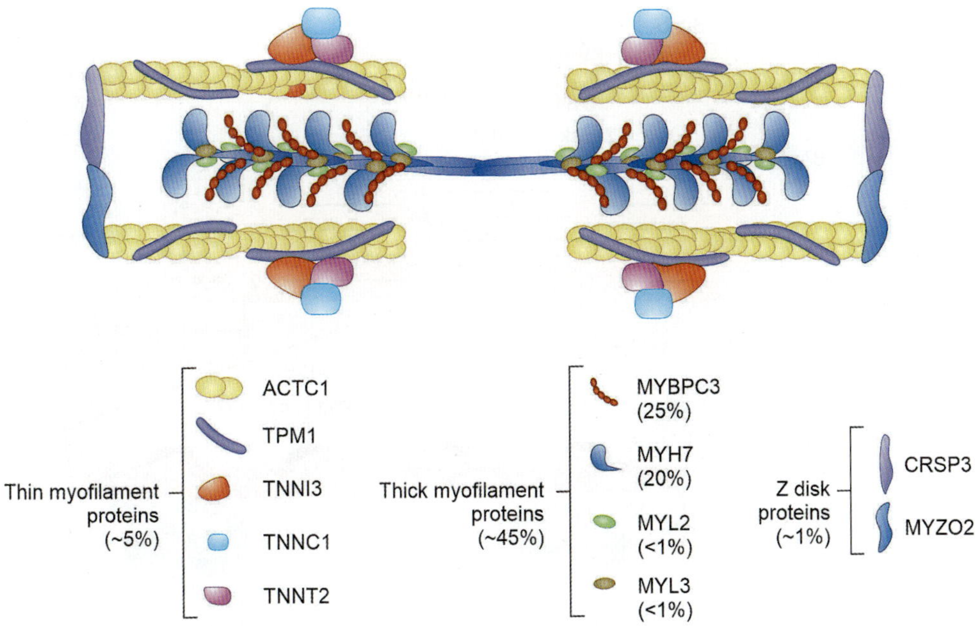

FIG. 2: Schematic diagram showing genes involved in hypertrophic cardiomyopathy.
(ACTC1: cardiac α-actin 1; MYBPC: myosin-binding protein C; MYH6: myosin heavy chain 6; MYH7: myosin heavy chain 7; MYL: myosin light chain; TNNI: troponin I; TNNT: troponin T; TPM1: α-tropomyosin; TTN: titin)

end-diastolic wall thickness of ≥15 mm anywhere in the left ventricle, in the absence of a confounding cause, or a wall thickness of ≥13 mm, with a positive family history or a positive genetic test, is diagnostic of HCM.[13]

Over 60% of cases are familial and the disorder is transmitted in an autosomal dominant manner, while nonsarcomeric mutations occur sporadically **(Fig. 2)**.[14]

Among thick filament proteins, myosin-binding protein C3 (*MYBPC3*) and (*MYH7*) are the two most common genes responsible for 25% and 20% of cases, respectively.[15] MYL2 and MYL3, which code for proteins in the myosin hexamer, account for <2% of cases.

Genes encoding thin filament proteins account for 5% of cases, and include troponin T (TNNT2), troponin I (TNNI3), TPM1, cardiac α-actin (ACTC1), and troponin C (TNNC1).[16-18]

A genetic diagnosis can be obtained in 60–70% of consecutive patients with familial HCM, though the yield is around 30% in sporadic cases.

Specific mutations in MYH7 (Arg403Gln, Arg453Cys, and Arg719Trp) and TNNT2 mutations are associated with adverse outcomes including increased risk of arrhythmia and SCD. Hence, these patients are kept at a lower threshold for automated implantable cardiac defibrillator.[19]

Phenocopies of HCM are seen in Fabry's disease, Danon's disease, Pompe's disease, and Noonan's syndrome, although histologically they are different.

The ACC/AHA 2020 guidelines give a class-IB recommendation for:[13]

- Genetic testing for patients with HCM
- Cascade testing for first degree relatives
- Postmortem genetic testing in families where unexplained death has occurred with a postmortem diagnosis of HCM
- Preconceptional and prenatal reproductive genetic counseling in affected families with HCM

They also do recommend against cascade genetic testing for patients with HCM but no pathogenic variants, and ongoing clinical screening for genotype-negative relative in families with genotype-positive HCM.

GENETICS OF RESTRICTIVE CARDIOMYOPATHY

Restrictive cardiomyopathy is characterized by increased biventricular stiffness, abnormal filling pattern, and increased end-diastolic pressures with biatrial enlargement.[20]

Genetic RCM is associated with a poor prognosis and is autosomal dominant in inheritance.

The genes which are involved **(Fig. 3)** can be classified into:[21-23]

- Sarcomeric proteins—*TNNI3, TNNT2, TNNC1, TPM1, TTN, MYH7*, and *MYBPC3*
- Myofibrillar proteins—desmin (*DES*), filamin C (*FLNC*), *MYPN, LMNA*, and crystallin αβ (*CRYAB*)

Storage disorders such as Gaucher disease, Fabry disease, glycogen storage disorders, Hurler syndrome, Hunter syndrome, and Niemann-Pick disease also manifest as RCM.[20]

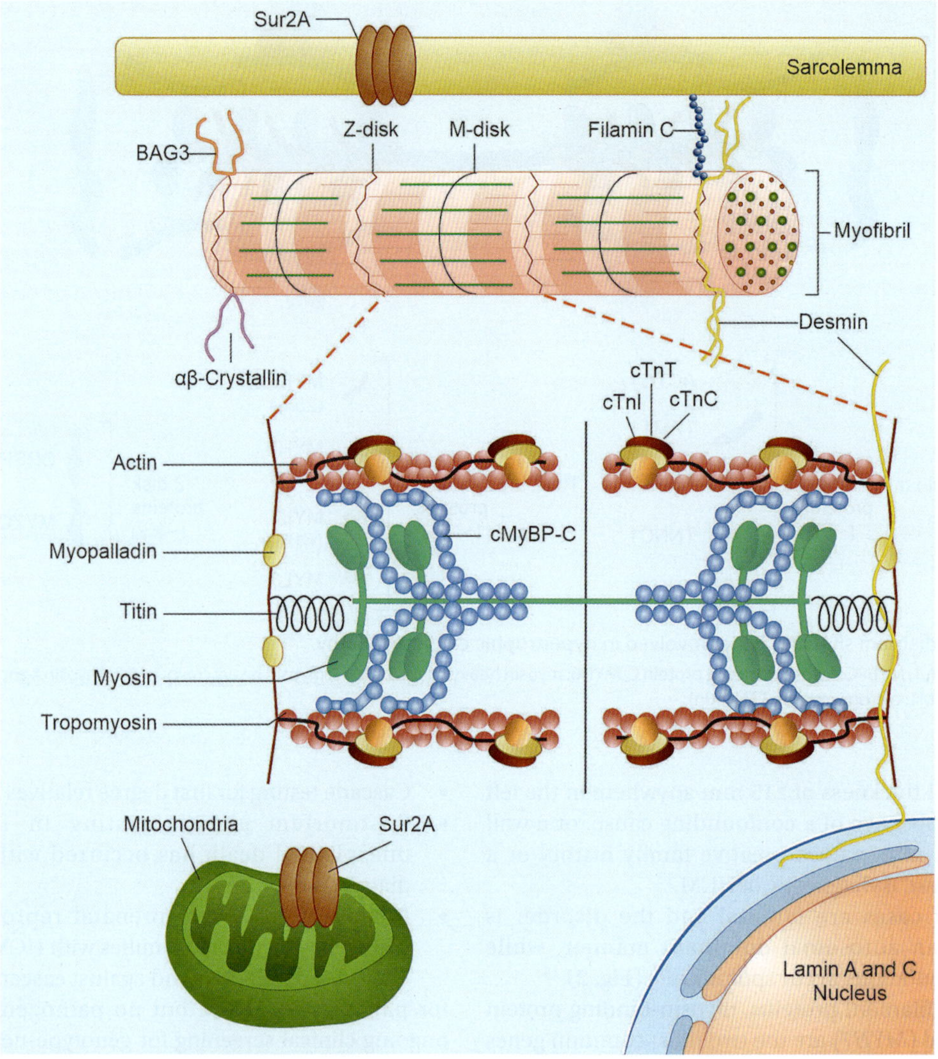

FIG. 3: Schematic diagram showing genes involved in restrictive cardiomyopathy.

(BAG3: BAG cochaperone 3; cMyBPC: cardiac myosin-binding protein C; cTnC: cardiac troponin C; cTnI: cardiac troponin I; cTnT: cardiac troponin T)

GENETICS OF LEFT VENTRICULAR NONCOMPACTION CARDIOMYOPATHY

Left ventricular noncompaction cardiomyopathy is characterized by prominent trabeculations of the left ventricle with deep intertrabecular recesses and thinned out compact epicardium.[24] It has a prevalence of 1 in 7,000 live births, and is characterized by noncompacted layer, i.e., compacted layer ration >2:1 in systole in the short-axis view.[25]

Autosomal dominant is the most common type of inheritance, followed by X-linked and maternal, while sporadic mutations are seen in about two-thirds of cases.

Sarcomeric gene mutations account for 35–60% of cases, with the most common ones being MYH7,[26] MYBPC3, ACTC1, TNNT2, and TPM1. Ion channel proteins (HCN4 and SCN5A) are implicated in rest of the cases.[27-29]

However, diagnostic yield of genetic test in LVNC is low, and genotype-phenotype correlation has not been well established.

ARRHYTHMOGENIC RIGHT VENTRICULAR CARDIOMYOPATHY

Arrhythmogenic right ventricular cardiomyopathy is characterized by progressive replacement of myocardial cells with fat and fibrosis, predominantly in the right ventricle, though the left ventricle is often involved.[30]

It is characterized by right ventricular dysfunction, malignant ventricular arrhythmias, and SCD. Criteria for diagnosis was first established in 1994,[31] which was then revised in 2010 by a Task Force.[32] Currently, the 2020 International Padua Criteria is being followed.[33]

Genetic abnormalities are seen in genes encoding desmosomal proteins, which link the cardiomyocytes. Plakophilin-2 (*PKP2*) is the most common gene involved, seen in 30–70%, followed by DSP in 10–15%, desmoglein-2 (DSG2) in 7–10%, and desmocollin-2 (DSC2) in 2%.[34,35] Inheritance is autosomal dominant in majority (30–50%), which syndromic ones (Naxos syndrome and Carvajal syndrome) exhibit autosomal recessive pattern.[36,37]

The Heart Rhythm Society (HRS)/European Heart Rhythm Association (EHRA)/American College of Medical Genetics and Genomics (ACMG) guidelines (2018) give a class-I recommendation for variant-specific cascade screening, and phenotyping screening for the first degree relatives.[36] Comprehensive or targeted testing is recommended for patients fulfilling task force criteria (Class IIA) and genetic testing for those fulfilling one major or two minor criteria (Class IIB).

INHERITED SYNDROMES ASSOCIATED WITH CARDIOMYOPATHY

There are multiple inherited genetic syndromes which are associated with cardiomyopathy. Mostly, they are diagnosed clinically with their myriad manifestations, but the cardiac involvement is often missed.

Hence, a patient with these disorders needs screening for cardiac involvement, which is important for prognostication **(Table 1)**.

TABLE 1: Inherited syndromes associated with cardiomyopathy.

Gene	Disease	Clinical features	Inheritance
DMD	• Duchenne muscular dystrophy • Becker muscular dystrophy	• DCM with muscular dystrophy (early onset) • DCM with muscular dystrophy (late onset)	X-linked, recessive
Mitochondria	• MERRF syndrome • MELAS syndrome • Kearns–Sayre syndrome	Myoclonic epilepsy, septal hypertrophy and DCM • Mitochondrial encephalopathy • Lactic acidosis • Stroke-like episodes • Heart failure • Symmetrical LVH	Maternal transmission/ autosomal dominant
		Ophthalmoplegia and DCM with conduction defects	
FRDA/FXN	Friedreich's ataxia	Cerebellar ataxia, dysarthria, HCM, diabetes, neurosensory hearing loss, and visual impairment supraventricular tachycardia	Autosomal recessive
PRKAG2	PRKAG2-related cardiomyopathy	• Left ventricular hypertrophy with diastolic dysfunction • Skeletal myopathy	Autosomal dominant
TTR	Amyloidosis	• Biventricular hypertrophy with diastolic dysfunction • Neuropathy, autonomic dysfunction, Carpal tunnel syndrome, renal failure, and proteinuria	Autosomal dominant
LAMP2	Danon disease	• Left ventricular hypertrophy with pre-excitation • Skeletal myopathy and intellectual disability	X-linked dominant
PTPN11-RAF1	Noonan syndrome	• Hypertrophic cardiomyopathy with pulmonary stenosis • Typical facies, short stature, webbed neck, pectus excavatum/carinatum, developmental delay, and bleeding disorders	Autosomal dominant
GLA	Fabry disease	• Left ventricular hypertrophy with pre-excitation • Sinus node dysfunction • Atrioventricular block • Tachyarrhythmias • Angiokeratoma, cornea verticillata, neuropathic pain, stroke/transient ischemic attack, vertigo, tinnitus, hearing impairment, renal failure and proteinuria, and GI symptoms	X-linked recessive

(DCM: dilated cardiomyopathy; GI: gastrointestinal; HCM: hypertrophic cardiomyopathy; LVH: left ventricular hypertrophy; MELAS: mitochondrial encephalomyopathy with lactic acidosis and stroke-like episodes; MERRF: myoclonic epilepsy with ragged red fibers)

COUNSELING BEFORE GENETIC TEST

Proper genetic counseling is recommended for all the patients with cardiomyopathy and their family members by an experienced physician or genetic counselor. Appropriate family history including multigenerational (at least three generations) history of cardiomyopathy and SCD events should be taken.

The patient and his family members should be explained about the pros and cons of genetic testing (including psychosocial, ethical, and financial implications).

CHOICE OF GENETIC TEST

Currently, next generation sequencing (NGS) for standard panel of cardiomyopathy genes is the choice for testing. It is superior to Sanger sequencing in terms of comprehensive exploration of genetic causes.

However, although a positive test helps in confirming the diagnosis, a negative test will not rule out the disease. In case of a positive test, cascade testing is to be performed in the family members.

If the phenotype is manifested in a relative, the diagnosis of cardiomyopathy is confirmed. Those of carry the genotype but are phenotypically negative, should undergo periodic clinical examination and appropriate evaluation.

INDIAN SCENARIO

Vaidya et al.,[38] analyzed 543 patients with cardiomyopathy, out of which HCM was the most common (47.3%), followed by DCM (36.5%) and RCM (2.6%). *MYH7, MYBPC3, TNNT2, GLA, TMP1, LMNA, TNNI3*, and *MYL2* were the most common genes identified, and 35.1% of the mutations were novel.

CONCLUSION

Genetic testing is of prime importance for patients with cardiomyopathy and helps in confirming the diagnosis. Moreover, identification of the proband helps in prognostication as well as cascade screening of family members.

ONLINE REFERENCES

Please scan the QR code provided at the end of the table of contents for References of this chapter.

CHAPTER

84 Hypertrophic Cardiomyopathy: Newer Therapeutic Modalities

Kashinath Ghosh Hazra

ABSTRACT

Hypertrophic cardiomyopathy is a relatively common primary myocardial disease of autosomal dominant inheritance with variable penetrance. The underlying pathology is unexplained left ventricular hypertrophy (LVH), hypercontractility, and impaired relaxation with myocyte hypertrophy, disarray, and myocardial fibrosis. Clinical presentation is diverse, varying from asymptomatic to severe effort intolerance due to left ventricular outflow tract obstruction (LVOTO). Appropriate use of implantable cardioverter-defibrillator (ICD) has reduced sudden cardiac death (SCD) in high-risk subjects. In many symptomatic patients with LVOTO despite standard medical therapy with negative inotropic agents such as nonvasodilating beta-blockers, nondihydropyridine calcium channel blockers and the antiarrhythmic disopyramide, septal reduction therapy (SRT) by means of septal myectomy (SM) or alcohol septal ablation (ASA) is the remaining option. Associated conditions such as anomalies of mitral valve apparatus, atrial fibrillation (AF), and heart failure are managed with special attention to the underlying substrate pathophysiology. Gene therapy is still an enigma but targeting the basic pathobiology, hyperactive actin myosin complex, remained a challenge till the advent of cardiac myosin inhibitors (CMIs) (mavacamten and aficamten) which unveiled a landscape of disease-specific pharmacotherapy with manipulation of myosin mechanochemistry having disease modifying potential.

Keywords: Hypertrophic cardiomyopathy, sarcomeric gene mutation, septal reduction therapy, septal myectomy, alcohol septal ablation, cardiac myosin inhibitors, mavacamten, aficamten.

INTRODUCTION

Hypertrophic cardiomyopathy (HCM) is a primary myocardial disorder characterized by unexplained left ventricular hypertrophy (LVH), hypercontractility, and impaired relaxation with a prevalence of 1:500 in the general population.[1] Diagnostic threshold is LV wall thickness ≥15 mm in adults and ≥13 mm for an individual with a family history of HCM or if the subject is a sarcomeric gene variant. The location and degree of hypertrophy are varied and LV cavity is small.[2] Histopathology shows myocyte hypertrophy, disarray, and myocardial fibrosis **(Figs. 1A and B)**. At the pathophysiological level, there is hyperactive actin-myosin complex in sarcomere. Many HCM subjects are asymptomatic, but some have disabling symptoms, mostly due to dynamic LV outflow tract (LVOT) obstruction.[3] With better mechanistic insights into the disease, many unmet therapeutic modalities are being explored to improve quality of life (QoL) and reduce mortality with cardiac myosin inhibitors (CMIs).[4,5]

HIGHLIGHTS OF THE UPDATE ON EXISTING MANAGEMENT

Prevention of Sudden Cardiac Death

Implantable cardioverter-defibrillator (ICD) in high-risk subjects has greatly reduced sudden cardiac death (SCD). Sarcomeric Human Cardiomyopathy Registry (SHaRe)[6] has shown that lifetime risk for ventricular arrhythmia is 32% in patients diagnosed below 40 years of age in contrast to 1% diagnosed above 60 years. The American College of Cardiology/American Heart Association (ACC/AHA) risk scoring[7] incorporates cardiac magnetic resonance (CMR) and includes LV apical aneurysm with scarring as a risk factor. The ACC/AHA risk scoring is more sensitive but less specific than

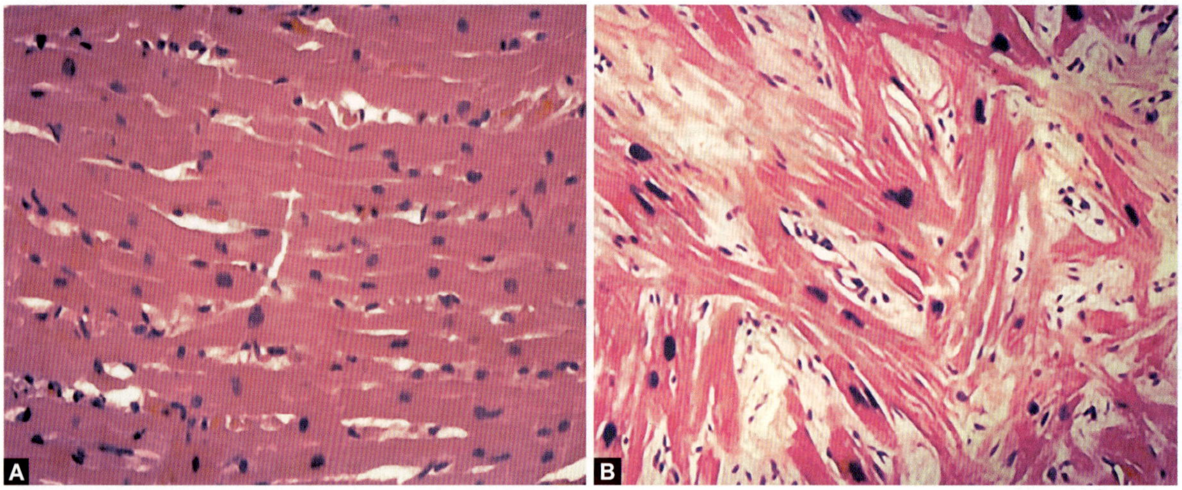

FIGS. 1A AND B: (A) Normal and (B) myofibrillar disarray.

European Society of Cardiology hypertrophic cardiomyopathy (ESC HCM) risk—SCD scoring, the latter may exclude ICD in some higher risk patients. According to ACC-AHA, the following parameters of nonsustained ventricular tachycardia (NSVT) on Holter monitoring are serious:

- More frequent (>3 runs)
- Longer (>10 beats)
- Faster (>200 beats/min)

There is a need for refined risk stratification for SCD in HCM in view of intercontinental differences in optimal utilization of ICDs. Single chamber ICD is preferred, subcutaneous ICD may be an evolving option particularly in the young, however, with limitations of absence of pacing function and inappropriate shock due to T-wave oversensing.

Left Ventricular Outflow Tract Obstruction

It is responsible for most heart failure symptoms with fourfold greater mortality than those without obstruction.

Standard medical therapy[7] includes:

- *Nonvasodilating beta-blockers (BB)*: Metoprolol causes symptomatic relief with improvement of both resting and exercise-induced LVOT gradient and reduces mitral regurgitation. Beta-blockers do not improve peak oxygen consumption (pVO_2) or N-terminal pro-b-type natriuretic peptide (NT-proBNP) level.
- *Nondihydropyridine calcium channel blocker (CCB)*: These are alternative to beta-blockers. However, they are avoided in patients with hypotension and very high resting gradients (>100 mm Hg) due to their vasodilatory properties.
- *Disopyramide*: It is a class Ia antiarrhythmic drug, as an adjunct to beta-blockers, CCB. In obstructive HCM (oHCM), its action is both sarcomere dependent and independent with improved calcium homeostasis and transmural homogenization of repolarization, side effects being QTc prolongation and anticholinergic action (dry mouth, blurred vision, urinary retention, etc.).

Septal Reduction Therapy

In drug refractory oHCM, septal reduction therapy (SRT) is next option with the following:.

- *Septal myectomy (SM)*: Nowadays transaortic extended Morrow's operation is carried out in specialized centers. It improves QoL and also probably survival (though no randomized study). Multiple anomalies of mitral valve apparatus such as anomalous papillary muscles, chordal slack, elongated mitral leaflets, and coronary artery bridging are also corrected during SM. "Chordal cutting"[8] (pioneered by Italian surgeons) involves cutting of thickened mitral valve secondary chordae, it moves the mitral valve apparatus away from LVOT relieving the obstruction. Mitral valve repair is preferred to mitral valve replacement. Concomitant atrial fibrillation (AF) is also addressed with biatrial maze type 4 operation with exclusion of left atrial (LA) appendage during SM. For mid-cavitary obstruction in apical HCM, transapical myectomy relieves obstruction and offers more spacious LV cavity with relief of symptoms. These are advances in newer surgical techniques.

Alcohol septal ablation (ASA): It is carried out where SM is contraindicated due to advanced age and other associated serious comorbidities.

Prerequisites are:

- Good septal perforator artery anatomy
- Interventricular septum (IVS) thickness <30 mm

Challenges:

- High need for permanent pacemaker
- Repeat procedure
- Concern for myocardial scar and ventricular tachycardia (though apprehension is not substantiated)
- Not applicable in children

There is no randomized trial comparing SM and ASA. Though short-term mortality is similar in both procedures, a recent study[9] showed all-cause 10-year mortality was 26.1% in ASA group and 8.2% in SM group irrespective of age, sex, and comorbidities (hazard ratio 1.68, *p* value < 0.001).

It has been highlighted that both SM and ASA should be carried out in HCM experienced centers. Due to lack of logistics, many septal reduction therapies are carried out at low volume centers with inherent mortality and complications of bleeding, infections, need for permanent pacemaker, and renal failure.

Limitation of SRTs: Though they offer symptomatic relief, long-term efficacy and disease-modifying properties are controversial.

Atrial Fibrillation

Anticoagulants[3] [vitamin K antagonist/direct oral anticoagulant (VKA/DOAC)] should be started after a documented AF episode. CHA_2DS_2-VASc Score is not applicable due to high-thromboembolic risk in HCM with AF. Rhythm control is preferred to rate control. AF is reduced by SRT, increases with age, and left atrial volume index (LAVI) is a prognostic marker for AF. AF ablation is performed in suitable cases.

Left Ventricular Systolic Dysfunction

Left ventricular systolic function is super normal in HCM and LV ejection fraction (LVEF) of <50% indicates severe LV systolic dysfunction. The four pillars of pharmacotherapy for heart failure with reduced ejection fraction—beta-blockers, angiotensin receptor/neprilysin inhibitors (ARNI), mineralocorticoid receptor antagonists (MRA), and sodium-glucose cotransporter-2 (SGLT-2) inhibitors have not been properly studied in systolic heart failure with HCM (obstructive and nonobstructive).

Cardiac resynchronization therapy (CRT) may delay need for LV assist devices (LVAD), which pose challenges due to small LV cavity, frequent biventricular involvement, and restrictive pathophysiology.[2] However, end-stage heart failure in HCM (obstructive and nonobstructive) may require cardiac transplantation.

Several experimental and clinical trials[10,11] have been published with unclear therapeutic applicability. These are as follows:

- Losartan and valsartan—transforming growth factor (TGF)-beta inhibitor
- Cyclosporin—calcineurin inhibitor
- Spironolactone—antifibrotic (replacement fibrosis)
- Microvascular ischemia—ranolazine

With variable response to these agents, newer disease-specific pharmacotherapy with CMIs opened up a new therapeutic vista.

Cardiac Myosin Inhibitors

Recently, there has been a paradigm shift in pharmacotherapeutics with modification of "myosin mechanochemistry". The actin-myosin interaction is fundamental for generating force in sarcomere.

Mavacamten is a selective allosteric inhibitor of myosin ATPase. It reduces actin-myosin cross-bridging and excess contractility. Under normal circumstances, unbound beta-myosin heavy chains are in equilibrium between super-relaxed (SRX) and disordered-relaxed (DRX) states. In resting SRX conformation, myosin heads are autoinhibited and do not form actin-myosin crossbridge with preservation of adenosine triphosphate (ATP). On the contrary, DRX state has 10-fold higher ATPase activity than SRX. In HCM, the balance of SRX/DRX is lost with DRX state predominating resulting in more actin-myosin complex and hypercontractility, albeit with more ATP expenditure **(Figs. 2A to C)**.

In experimental mice with pathogenic heterozygous major histocompatibility complex (MHC) mutation, it prevented LVH, myocyte disarray, and myocardial fibrosis.[12]

In phase 2, PIONEER-HCM study, mavacamten significantly reduced postexercise LVOT gradient and improved functional status in oHCM.

In **EXPLORER-HCM**,[13] a phase 3 randomized double-blind placebo-controlled trial, 251 symptomatic [New York Heart Association (NYHA) class II–III] oHCM patients with gradients ≥50 mm Hg were randomized to mavacamten or placebo along with beta-blockers or CCBs (dual therapy or disopyramide was not allowed) for evaluation of cardiopulmonary exercise test (CPET), functional status, and estimation of biomarkers.

At 30 weeks, functional capacity and symptoms (primary endpoint) improved >twice (37% vs. 17%) in the mavacamten group in contrast to placebo.

Primary endpoints were:

- Increase in pVO_2 ≥1.5mL/kg/min with ≥1 NYHA class improvement
- Increase in pVO_2 ≥3.0 mL/kg/min without worsening NYHA class

Secondary endpoints were also met:

- Greater mean reduction in postexercise LVOT gradient (–36 mm Hg)
- Greater increase in pVO_2 (+1.4 mL/kg/min)
- Improvement in symptoms score Kansas City Cardiomyopathy Questionnaire-Clinical Summary Score (KCCQ-CSS) +9.1
- Improvement in ≥1 NYHA functional class 34%

It was safe and well tolerated, only five patients on mavacamten had reduction of LVEF <50% requiring temporary discontinuation of the drug.

On the biochemical front, at 30 weeks in mavacamten group, there were reductions in NT-proBNP (80%) and

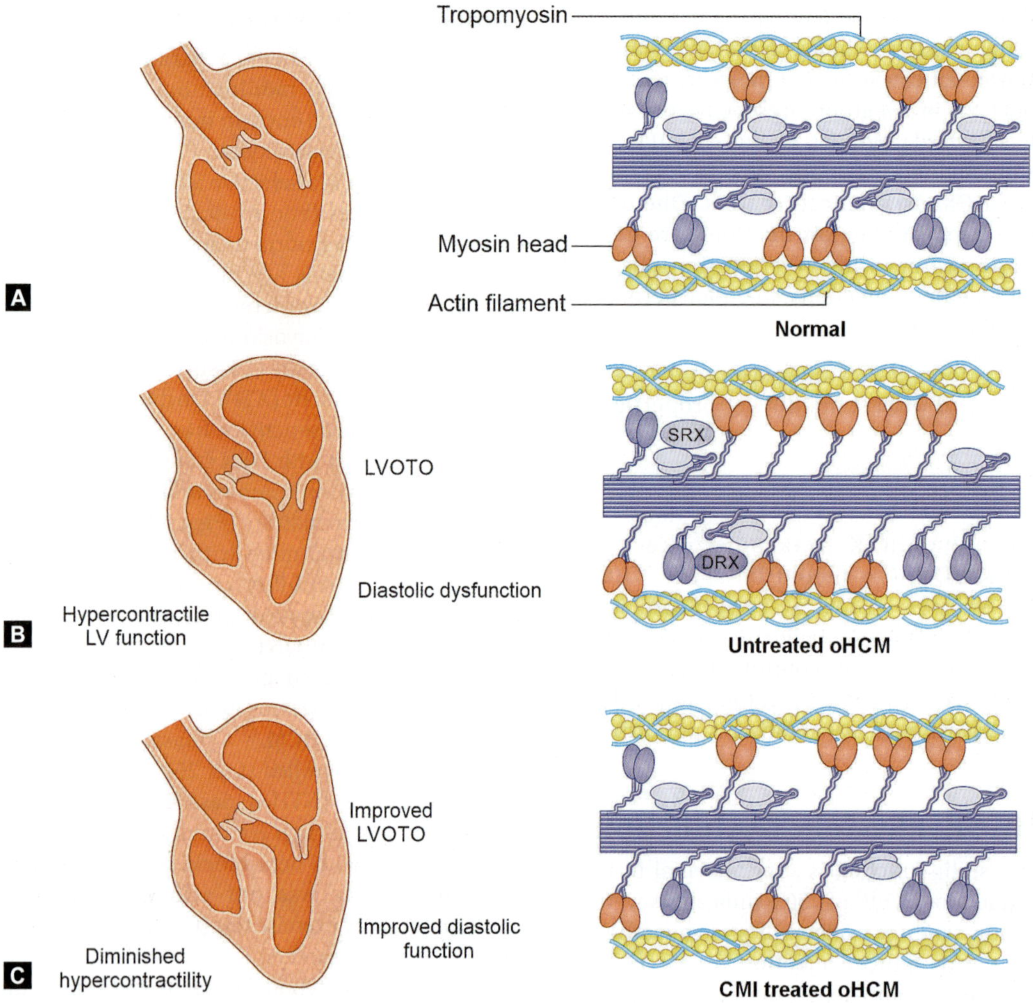

FIGS. 2A TO C: Mechanism of action of mavacamten.
(CMI: cardiac myosin inhibitor; LVOTO: left ventricular outflow tract obstruction; oHCM: obstructive hypertrophic cardiomyopathy)

high-sensitivity troponin I (hsTnI) (41%) which are predictors of long-term outcome in HCM.

Health status as judged by KCCQ-Overall Score (KCCQ-OS), at the end of 30 weeks improved ≥20 in 36% of patients on mavacamten versus 13% in placebo with absolute difference of 21% and number needed to treat (NNT) was only five.[14] The magnitude of benefit in KCCQ-OS was similar to that seen in transcatheter aortic valve implantation (TAVI).

In an echocardiographic substudy[15] of EXPLORER-HCM, 81% of patients in mavacamten group had disappearance of SAM versus 34% in placebo and there was also improvement in diastolic parameters, e.g., LAVI, septal and lateral E/e', and consistent with reduced NT-proBNP.

Left ventricular internal diameter in diastole (LVIDd) did not change, LV internal diameter in systole (LVIDs) marginally increased. IVS thickness did not change in mavacamten group, whereas placebo group demonstrated significant increase in IVS thickness. Reduced LAVI also correlated with diminished LVOT gradient, reduced MR severity and absence of SAM.

Cardiac magnetic resonance substudy[16] of EXPLORER-HCM showed that mavacamten favorably reduced the following at 30 weeks:

- LV mass index
- Maximum LV wall thickness
- Absolute intracellular myocardial mass index
- LAVI
- NT-proBNP and high-sensitivity cardiac troponin I (hsCTnI)

However, there was no change in fibrosis [late gadolinium enhancement (LGE)] and myocardial contractile fraction remained normal. These all indicate favorable cardiac remodeling with mavacamten.

After this landmark trial (EXPLORER-HCM) showing significant improvement in symptom relief and physical function, QoL and objective evidence of morphologic and hemodynamic benefits, Food and Drug Administration

(FDA) approved mavacamten in April, 2022,[17] however, with a boxed warning of monitoring of LVEF every 4 weeks.

Interim analysis of the 5-year long-term extension (MAVA-LTE)[18] also showed the results in consonance with the primary trial: Sustained improvement of LVOT gradient (resting and Valsalva), LV filling pressure, NT-proBNP, and NYHA functional class.

Beta-blocker treatment had chronotropic incompetence which affected heart rate-dependent measures [pVO_2, peak exercise time, and peak metabolic equivalents (METs)] and hence the endpoints in EXPLORER-HCM were more pronounced in patients without beta-blockers.

VALOR-HCM[19] a phase 3, double-blind, placebo-controlled trial evaluated the efficacy of mavacamten in oHCM in reducing the need for eligible SRT of 112 patients (56 each in each group of mavacamten and placebo). After 16 weeks of therapy, SRT requirement reduced to 17.9% in mavacamten group versus 76.8% in placebo. Moreover, the mean difference in postexercise LVOT gradient was 37.2 mm Hg with proportional reductions in NYHA functional Class, NT-proBNP and hsTnI, probably resultant of reduced LVOT obstruction or lusitropic effect of mavacamten.

In MAVERICK-HCM[20] a double-blind, placebo-controlled dose—ranging phase 2 trial in symptomatic (NYHA II–III) non-oHCM, NT-proBNP decreased by 53% in the pooled mavacamten group versus 1% in placebo, hsTnI decreased by 34% the pooled mavacamten group versus 4% in the placebo. These results suggest improvement in wall stress in non-oHCM patients also with mavacamten. More information from ongoing ODESSEY-HCM[20] phase 3 trial will be available.

Aficamten is the next-generation CMI. In comparison with mavacamten, it has a shorter half-life, shallow dose response curve, wide therapeutic window, and minimum drug-drug interaction. Aficamten is claimed to act via SRX-independent mechanism similar to blebbistatin (a nonspecific myosin inhibitor) preventing ATP binding of myosin. Thus, aficamten binds reversibly to cardiac myosin and reduces the actin-myosin cross bridges.

REDWOOD- HCM[21] is a phase 2, randomized, 2:1, (aficamten 28, 14 each in cohort 1 having dosage of 5–15 mg and cohort 2 of 10–30 mg, placebo group 13), multicenter placebo-controlled, double-blind, dose finding clinical trial in symptomatic oHCM patients on beta-blockers and CCBs. Primary endpoint was safety and tolerability, secondary endpoints were changes in LVOT gradients, NYHA functional class and biomarkers (NT-proBNP and hsTnI). Before each dose escalation, echocardiography was done to assess LVEF for safety reasons, as CMIs cause reduction of LVEF. After 10 weeks, aficamten reduced resting gradients –40 mm Hg and –43 mm Hg in cohorts 1 and 2, respectively and Valsalva gradients –36 mm Hg and –53 mm Hg in cohorts 1 and 2, respectively. Symptomatic improvement of ≥1 NYHA class was observed in 31% in placebo and 43% and 64% in cohorts 1 and 2, respectively. NT-proBNP was reduced significantly (62% relative to placebo). There was modest reduction in LVEF, however, there was no interruption of treatment as none had LVEF <40% which was the stopping criterion. Aficamten had no impact on blood pressure, heart rate, and other laboratory measures. Paradoxically beneficial effects were reversed after 2 weeks of stoppage of aficamten.

REDWOOD-HCM OLE (Open Label Extension), now FOREST HCM, was presented at ESC Heart Failure Congress 2022 for oHCM. Data (30 patients treated for 12 weeks and 19 patients treated for 24 weeks) showed substantial reduction in resting LVOT gradient (–32.6 mm Hg at 12 weeks and –32.8 mm Hg at 24 weeks) and Valsalva LVOT gradient (–42.7 mm Hg at 12 weeks and –51.1 mm Hg at 24 weeks). These reductions started at 2 weeks of initiation and was sustained through 24 weeks with only modest decrease in LVEF. At 12 weeks of NYHA functional class improved by one class in 72% and by two class in 7% whereas at 24 weeks by one class in 61% and by two class in 17%.

Limitations of REDWOOD-HCM: In contrast to EXPLORER-HCM, structural alterations (LA size LV wall thickness) were not studied with echocardiogram and MRI in REDWOOD-HCM. Similarly objective measures (CPET for pVO_2 and exercise induced LVOT gradient) were not included. Treatment effect was not correlated with genetic mutation.

However, to overcome these limitations in the background of positive results, SEQUOIA-HCM,[21] a phase 3 placebo-controlled, randomized, double-blind, international multicentric clinical trial has been designed with oHCM including disopyramide as the background medical therapy for 24 weeks. The primary outcome is improvement in pVO_2 at 24 weeks, secondary outcomes are Valsalva LVOT gradient, NYHA functional class and KCCQ-summary score. The planned enrolment is 270 patients and is likely to be completed in late 2023.

Thus, these CMIs (mavacamten and aficamten) offer disease-specific treatment targeting the pathobiological mechanism of contraction, i.e., actin-myosin cross-bridging of sarcomere. The existing therapeutic options alleviate only symptoms of HCM, while these CMIs have the promise of disease modification too.

CHALLENGES WITH CARDIAC MYOSIN INHIBITORS

Cardiac Myosin Inhibitors Nonresponders

Response to CMIs may be suboptimal in some cases of HCM. The probable explanations are:

- More advanced morphology and severe LVH and LVOT obstruction which are less amenable to CMIs at this short duration and dosage used in trials.
- Valvular and subvalvular abnormalities
- Myocardial ischemia
- Arrhythmia
- Severe diastolic dysfunction
- Autonomic dysfunction

Limitations of Cardiac Myosin Inhibitors Trials

These studies of CMIs were conducted in small cohorts and for a short duration. They have not been tried below 18 years. Minorities and Asian population had smaller representations in these studies. However, women had good representation in EXPLORER-HCM (41%) and VALOR-HCM (50%).

Long-term Safety and Efficacy of Cardiac Myosin Inhibitors

These issues are being studied in the long-term extension (LTE) studies of the existing and newer trials and controlled monitoring of LVEF at frequent intervals is mandated for possible deterioration of LV systolic function. Beta-blockers might have blunted the efficacy of CMIs and MAPLE-HCM (metoprolol succinate vs. aficamten) study will explore CMIs as the first-line therapy instead of beta-blockers.

Cost Concern

In spite of this "game changer" molecule (mavacamten) being approved by FDA, however, with boxed warning, Institute of Chemical and Economic Review (ICER),[22] USA, reported that SRT was superior to mavacamten for cost-effectiveness. In financially challenged nations, access to these costly but effective medicines may be limited to only a few in the backdrop of a large demand.

The trials of CMIs are shown in **Flowchart 1**.

FUTURE DIRECTION

Scope of Gene Therapy

Pathogenic sarcomeric gene mutation, mostly myosin-binding protein (MYBPC3) and myosin heavy chain (MYH7) are present in 60% of familial and 30% of sporadic HCM cases. These are often associated with earlier onset and greater disease burden with need for probable lifelong surveillance. Genetic testing and familial screening have now been accepted by the medical community and the public at large to identify high-risk population. In genotype—positive, phenotype—negative individuals with sarcomeric gene mutations, preventing development of phenotype is a basic demanding challenge. CRISPR/Cas9 technology has been applied for correction of heterozygous MYBPC3 mutation[23] in human preimplantation embryos using homologous wild type maternal gene template **(Fig. 3)**. A large number of wild type homozygous embryos were created without any "off target" effect. This is hypothesis generating and raises much hope for gene therapy of HCM, however, with many logistic, societal, and economic issues.

Stage-specific Therapy

Recently, four stages of HCM have been described **(Fig. 4)**.[24]

Stages 1 and 2 constitute nearly 75–80% of total HCM population. CMIs along with other therapeutic modalities have been proposed to be effective in this large group of HCM patients.

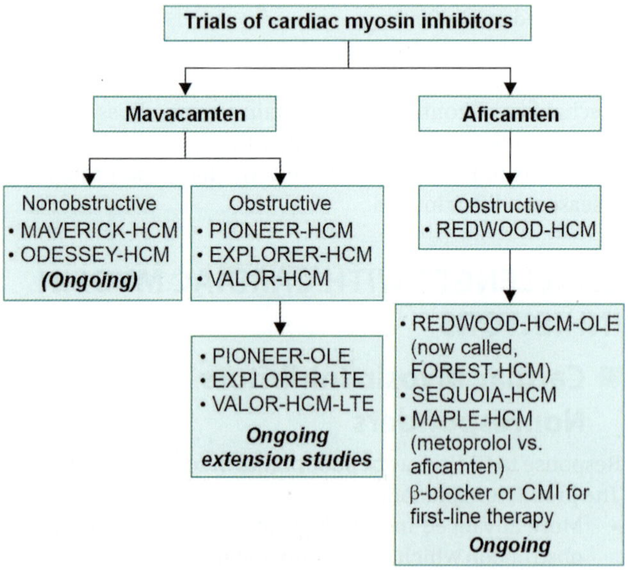

FLOWCHART 1: Trials of cardiac myosin inhibitors.

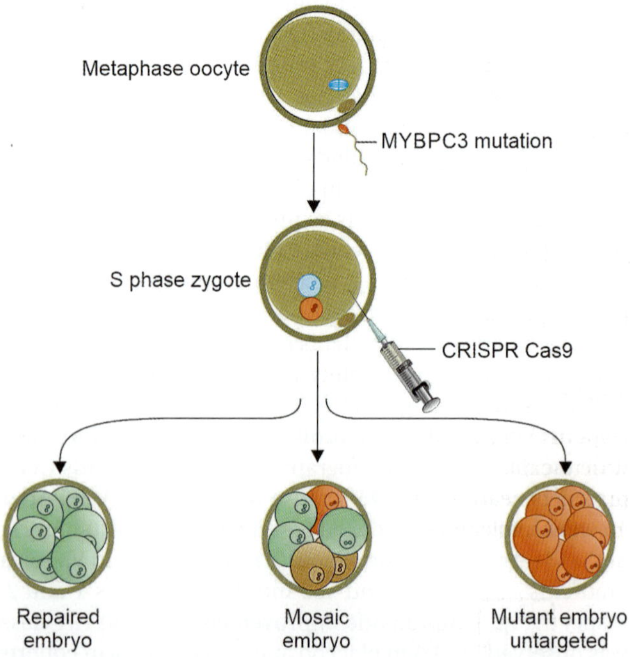

FIG. 3: CRISPR/Cas9 technology for gene therapy.

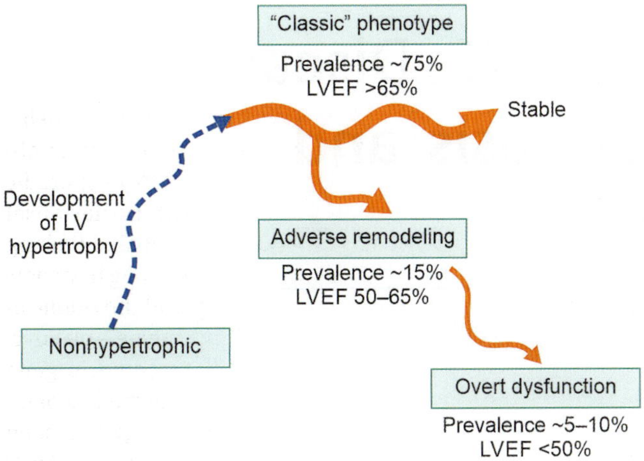

FIG. 4: Stages of hypertrophic cardiomyopathy.[24]
(LV: left ventricular; LVEF: LV ejection fraction)

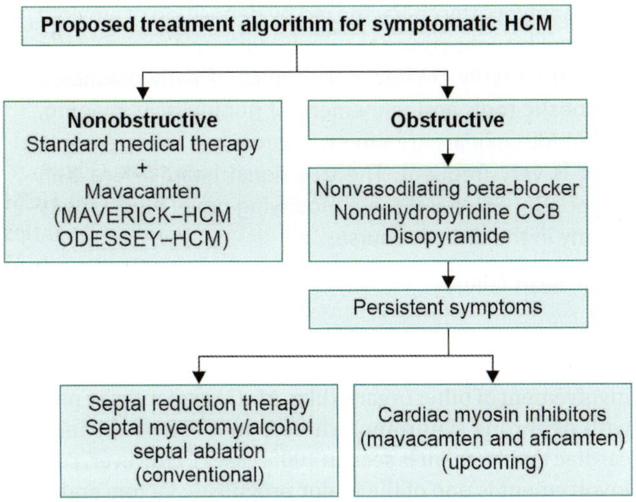

FLOWCHART 2: Proposed treatment algorithm for symptomatic hypertrophic cardiomyopathy (HCM).

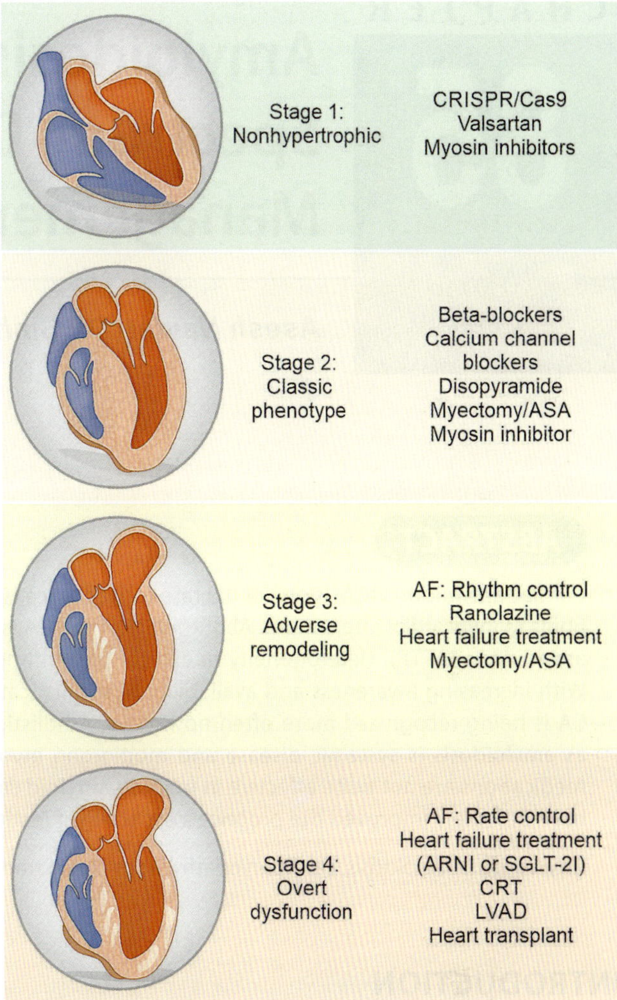

FIG. 5: Stage-specific therapy in hypertrophic cardiomyopathy.[24]
(AF: atrial fibrillation; ARNI: angiotensin receptor/neprilysin inhibitor; ASA: alcohol septal ablation; CRT: cardiac resynchronization therapy; LVAD: left ventricular assist devices; SGLT-2I: sodium-glucose cotransporter-2 inhibitor)

Stage-specific therapy for HCM[24] has been advocated as shown in **Figure 5**.

Proposed algorithm for management of symptomatic HCM is presented in **Flowchart 2**.

CONCLUSION

Hypertrophic cardiomyopathy is a genetic cardiomyopathy with unexplained LVH, hypercontractility. LVOT obstruction is present in nearly two-thirds of HCM patients and is responsible for effort intolerance. SRT by SM or ASA has relieved symptoms to a great extent in severely symptomatic patients despite optimal medical management with beta-blockers, CCBs, and dihydropyridine. The basic pathobiology of HCM, hyperactive actin myosin complex at sarcomere level, remains a challenging issue. CMIs (mavacamten and aficamten) have opened up a landscape of disease-specific pharmacotherapy with disease modifying potential. Apart from relief of symptoms and beneficial hemodynamic effects with alteration of myocardial morphology and biomarkers, they have the promise to alter the natural course of this disease to be confirmed by ongoing large scale multicenter randomized trials.

ONLINE REFERENCES

Please scan the QR code provided at the end of the table of contents for References of this chapter.

CHAPTER 85

Latest Concept of Cardiac Amyloidosis in 2023: Disease Spectrum, Diagnosis, and Management

Asesh Haldar, DP Sinha

ABSTRACT

Cardiac amyloidosis (CA) is one of the rare causes of restrictive cardiomyopathy characterized by deposition of amyloid fibrils in myocardial interstitium. About >95% of the CA is contributed by light chain (AL) amyloidosis and transthyretin amyloidosis (ATTR). Heterogeneity of clinical presentation has undoubtedly created a hindrance of early diagnosis. With increasing awareness and availability of sophisticated diagnostic tools and refinement of noninvasive imaging, CA is being recognized more often nowadays. A holistic and multidisciplinary treatment approach is indispensable as amyloidosis is systemic disease and multiorgan involvement is very frequent. The traditional heart failure (HF) medications are not quite effective in treating amyloid cardiomyopathy. Several disease modifying novel medications have definitely improved the prognosis especially if instituted early in the disease course.

Keywords: Amyloidosis, cardiomyopathy, light chain, transthyretin, heart failure.

INTRODUCTION

Cardiac amyloidosis (CA) is a kind of restrictive cardiomyopathy where there is a deposition of insoluble amyloid fibrils in the myocardial interstitium. Nomenclature of amyloidosis includes A (for amyloid) which is the abbreviated form of the misfolded protein.[1] Light chain (AL) amyloidosis and transthyretin (ATTR) amyloidosis are the two most common types of amyloidosis affecting heart.[2] Unfortunately the diagnosis is commonly made in the late stage of the diseases despite the availability of several diagnostic tools. The inception of disease modifying novel drugs and the tremendous improvement in the treatment strategy of amyloidosis over the last few years have made a remarkable impact on prognosis in the recent times. Once what was considered as a rare entity is now being increasingly recognized in different clinical scenario like, ATTR CA is seen in 16% patients with severe aortic stenosis undergoing transcatheter aortic valve replacement (TAVR),[3] autopsy study showed wild type ATTR (ATTRwt) CA in 25% of the patients above the age of 85 years old.[4] It is a systemic disease where heart may be involved in isolation or cardiac involvement may be seen with varying severity along with predominant involvement of other organs (like, AL-CA patient may present with nephrotic syndrome, whereas in ATTRwt amyloidosis cardiac involvement is seen in 100% cases). However, cardiac involvement is one of the major prognostic factors and early diagnosis is an important determinant of long-term survival.

PATHOGENESIS AND SPECTRUM OF DISEASE

- *Protein synthesis and its quality control:* Peptide chains after being synthesized in endoplasmic reticulum undergoes conformational modifications (folding) mediated by chaperons. Protein folding is an essential and critical step to produce its functionally viable three-dimensional stable conformation. Apart from regulating the generation of functionally normal "healthy" protein, proteostasis network is also responsible for the prevention of protein misfolding and aggregation (misfolded proteins are degraded by proteasome) and removal of misassembled protein. In short, this network ensures the quality control of protein from synthesis to its degradation, thus amyloidosis is a typical example of proteostasis failure.[5]

- *Precursor protein and amyloidosis*: Though there are >35 amyloidogenic precursor protein, only nine are intricately associated with CA. Light chain amyloidosis and ATTR amyloidosis constitute >95% of CA.[6]
- *Pathogenesis of AL amyloidosis*: In AL amyloidosis, there is a clonal proliferation of the plasma cells which produce amyloidogenic immunoglobulin light chains in abundance compared to heavy chains. Clonal proliferation of plasma cell secreting antibody or light chains has a potential of three possible outcomes which are (1) monoclonal gammopathy of undetermined significance (MGUS), (2) multiple myeloma (MM), or (3) AL amyloidosis. Germline gene mutation on λ light chain variable region and abnormal proteolysis has been implicated in the pathogenesis. λ light chain is seen in 80% of cases of AL amyloidosis. This misfolded free light chains or fragments aggregate to form insoluble amyloid fibrils. Though overproduction of free light chain is also seen in plasma cell disorders such as MM, MGUS, and Waldenström macroglobulinemia (WM), 1% patient with MGUS will develop AL amyloidosis and 10–15% patients with MM have AL amyloidosis concurrently. On the contrary, <10% patients with AL amyloidosis have clinically overt MM.
- *Pathogenesis of ATTR amyloidosis*: Transthyretin (TTR) is a homotetrameric protein, mainly synthesized in liver and choroid plexus of the brain and act as a transporter of the thyroid hormone and retinol (vitamin A). Hereditary transthyretin amyloidosis (hATTR) or variant ATTR amyloidosis (ATTRv), an autosomal dominant disease, occurs because of a single amino acid substitution in a 127-amino acid chain; it results from of one of the >130 mutations of *TTR* gene on chromosome 18. Like, Val122Ile (Pv142I according to new nomenclature) denotes valine is replaced by isoleucine at position 122 in TTR amino acid sequence. In contrast, wild type ATTR amyloidosis (ATTRwt and senile CA) occurs sporadically and misfolded proteins are formed because of proteostatic failure related to aging but having normal TTR genetic sequence. Irrespective of variety of ATTR amyloidosis, homotetramer is dissociated into monomer leading to formation of misfolded protein which aggregates to form fibrils.
- *Formation of amyloid fibrils*: The local concentration of misfolded protein should reach a critical value to form amyloid fibrils. Despite being originated from different precursor proteins, amyloid fibrils share some common characteristics, on electron microscope they appear as nonbranching protein structures of variable length with average diameter of 7.5–10 nm and cross-β-sheet, under polarized light fibrils show apple-green birefringence with Congo red.[2]
- *Components of amyloid deposit*: Apart from its core element of fibrils, amyloid deposit is also composed of components of extracellular matrix (such as collagen and lamin), glycosaminoglycans, and serum amyloid P-component (SAP) which imparts their resilience to degradation.
- *Organ tropism in amyloidosis*: Another important feature of the amyloidosis is their organ tropism. In AL amyloidosis, gene polymorphisms of variable region decide their organ tropism. The site of amino acid substitution and length of fibril (full length TTR fibrils or TTR fragments) dictate the predominant site of involvement (cardiac or nervous tissue) in TTR amyloidosis.[5]
- *Pathogenesis of CA*: Amyloidosis is a systemic disease involving multiple organs. CA, also known as "stiff heart syndrome" results in biventricular hypertrophy and increased ventricular stiffness which is the hallmark of restrictive cardiomyopathy. Interstitial amyloid deposition leading to architectural disorganization is responsible of diastolic dysfunction. Heart valves are commonly involved. In AL amyloidosis there is also amyloid deposition in the arteriolar wall leading to angina. Atrial infiltration increases the propensity of atrial fibrillation (AF). CA is "pan-heart disease" in true sense with involvement of myocardium, valves, vessels predominantly, and also endocardium and pericardium. Cardiac dysfunction is not correlated well with the amyloid fibril burden in myocardium because of direct cardiotoxicity contributed by free light chain, and it also explains the more aggressive disease expression in AL amyloidosis compared to ATTR amyloidosis. Tissue dysfunction in ATTR amyloidosis can precede the deposition of ATTR fibrils in myocardium explaining the importance of monomer and oligomer-induced cardiotoxicity. Intracardiac thrombus formation can also be seen irrespective of presence of AF specifically in AL-CA **(Flowchart 1)**.[2,7]

CLINICAL PRESENTATION (AL-CA VS. ATTR-CA)

In AL-amyloidosis cardiac (>75%) and kidney (>60%) are frequently involved organs, hepatomegaly is also seen in >50% cases. Other manifestations include autonomic neuropathy (20%), macroglossia (17%), periorbital purpura (15%), peripheral neuropathy (10–20%), and gastrointestinal (GI) involvement.[8,9]

The presentation of ATTR amyloidosis is myriad, cardiac involvement is invariably seen in ATTRwt, though orthopedic and soft tissue manifestations (lumber canal stenosis, biceps tendon rupture and carpal tunnel syndrome) are increasingly been recognized. In contrast, in ATTRv amyloidosis cardiomyopathy or neuropathy or both are seen. Predominant cardiac involvement is seen with Val122Ile (pV142I) and Leu111Met (pL131M) variant of ATTRv, whereas polyneuropathy and cardiomyopathy are characteristics of Val30Met (pV50M) variety of ATTRv. Val30Met variant presents with early onset neuropathy (third and

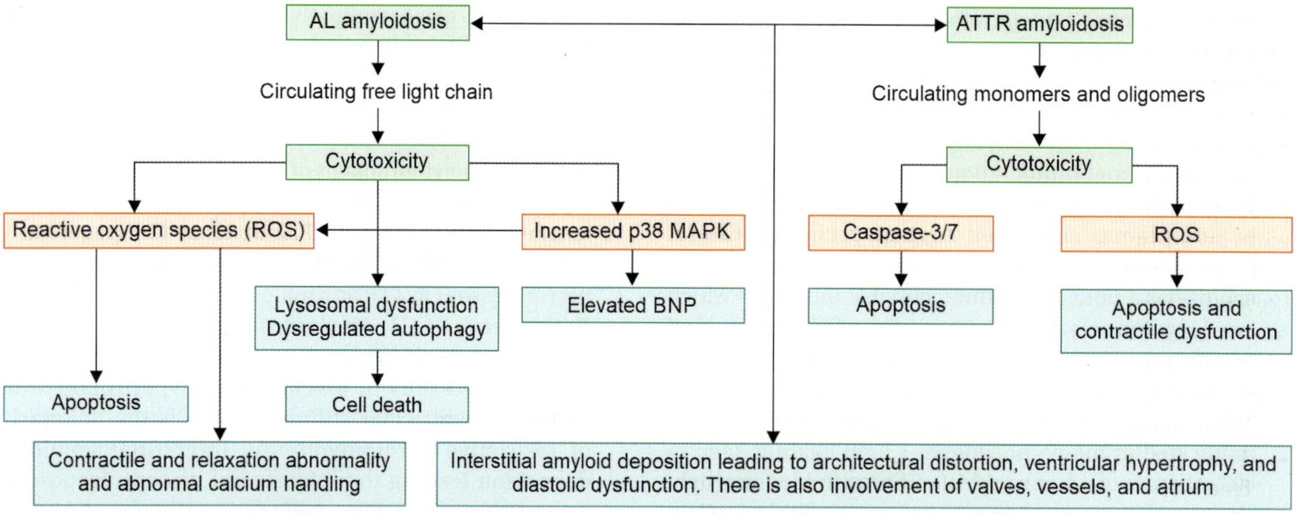

FLOWCHART 1: Pathogenesis of AL-CA and ATTR-CA.[2,5]

(AL: light chain; ATTR: transthyretin amyloidosis; BNP: B-type natriuretic peptide; p38 MAPK: p38 mitogen-activated protein kinase)

TABLE1: Clinical features of common types of CA.

	AL-amyloidosis	ATTRv Val122Ile (Pv142I)	ATTRv Val30Met (Pv50M)	ATTRwt
Average age (years)	63 (30–80)	• 72 (47–90) • 3.5% in black individual (USA) • Found worldwide	• *Early onset (30–50 years)*: Neuropathic, most common variant worldwide with >90% penetrance. Seen in Japan, Brazil, Portugal, and Sweden • *Late onset (>50)*: Mixed phenotype, seen worldwide	75 (50–100)
Sex	Male 50–60%	Male 70%	Male 50%	Male 90%
Fat pad biopsy	70–80%	<50%	<50%	<20%
Cardiac involvement	>75%	100%	Late onset >50 years and nonendemic areas—more common	100%
Other organ involvement	• Kidney (>60%) • Hepatomegaly >50% • Autonomic neuropathy (20%) • Macroglossia (17%), • Periorbital purpura (15%) • Peripheral neuropathy (10–20%) • GI involvement	Peripheral neuropathy and autonomic dysfunction rare	Peripheral neuropathy >80% by 50 years (Portugal-endemic)	• Carpal tunnel syndrome • Lumbar spinal stenosis • Biceps tendon rupture

(AL: light chain; ATTRv: hereditary amyloid transthyretin; ATTRwt: wild-type amyloid transthyretin; CA: cardiac amyloidosis; GI: gastrointestinal)

fourth decade, most common variant in the world) but mixed phenotype (cardiomyopathy and neuropathy) is a feature of later onset (sixth or seventh decade) disease **(Table 1)**.[1-3]

OTHER FORMS OF CARDIAC AMYLOIDOSIS

Some rare forms of CA include AA (serum amyloid A protein is the precursor protein seen in chronic infections and inflammatory diseases), AApoI (precursor protein apolipoprotein A-I), AApoAII (precursor protein apolipoprotein A-II), etc.

DIAGNOSIS

The diagnosis of CA essentially involves three steps (1) suspicion for CA—"red flags," definite diagnosis of CA and identifying the subtype precisely. Although, several scientific societies across the globe have different diagnostic framework but all of them are aiming for an early diagnosis.

Even after tremendous advancement and refinement of noninvasive diagnostic imaging and increasing awareness, delayed diagnosis is very commonly seen. Common occurrence of ATTR amyloidosis in hospitalized patients with heart failure with preserved ejection fraction (HFpEF) (13%), among patients undergoing TAVR (16%), in patients with carpal tunnel syndrome (10%), in patients with presumed hypertrophic cardiomyopathy (HCM) (5%), or in patients >80 years old with suspected HCM (26%) dictates us the clinical scenario where we need to have a high suspicion for CA.[2,3,10,11] Scientific societies have incorporated following diagnostic modalities in combination:

- When to suspect CA—"red flags?"
- Tests for monoclonal protein identification—serum free light chain (SFLC), serum immunofixation electrophoresis (SIFE) and urine immunofixation electrophoresis (UIFE).
- Electrocardiography (ECG) and imaging—echocardiography, cardiovascular magnetic resonance (CMR), and bone scintigraphy
- Tissue biopsy
- Genetic testing

Red Flags

- *Neurological*:
  - Sensorimotor polyneuropathy
  - Autonomic dysfunction
- *Cardiovascular*:
  - Hypotension or normotensive (if previously hypertensive), intolerance to antihypertensive medication
  - HF ≥65 years
  - Aortic stenosis ≥65 years
  - *ECG*: See later
  - *Echocardiogram*: See later
  - *CMR*: See later
  - *Laboratory parameters*:
    - Persistently elevated cardiac troponin T/I
    - Disproportionate rise of NT-proBNP to the degree of heart failure (HF)
- *Musculoskeletal*:
  - Bilateral carpal tunnel syndrome
  - Spinal canal stenosis → (unique to ATTR variety)
  - Atraumatic biceps tendon rupture → (unique to ATTR variety)
- *Renal*:
  - Proteinuria
  - Renal insufficiency
- *Eye*:
  - Vitreous opacity
- *Others*:
  - Skin bruising
  - Periorbital purpura (due to capillary fragility and acquired factor X deficiency, pathognomonic of AL-CA, seen in 15% patients)
  - Macroglossia (pathognomonic of AL-CA, seen in 17% patients)
  - Submandibular gland enlargement (pathognomonic of AL amyloidosis)
- *Family history*:
  - Cardiomyopathy
  - Polyneuropathy

Tests for Monoclonal Protein Indentification

Three tests, namely SFLC, SIFE, and UIFE in combination, can exclude the diagnosis of AL amyloidosis with a very high degree of precision (99% negative predictive value). Serum free light chain assesses the ratio of kappa (κ) and lambda (λ) light chain rather than their absolute value [clonality is represented by the abnormal ratio, normally κ:λ → 0.26–1.65 (Freelite), abnormal if <0.26 or >1.65].The production of κ is two times higher compared to λ from bone marrow, but kidney clears κ light chain preferentially, thus maintaining a balance. This balance is lost in renal failure leading to more accumulation of κ compared to λ (thus higher κ:λ ratio is found in renal failure, on the contrary lower κ:λ ratio is abnormal and indicates clonal production of λ), a ratio of 0.54–3.30 may be normal in situation where glomerular filtration rate (GFR) is <30 mL/min/1.73 m^2.

Serum immunofixation electrophoresis and UIFE assess the type of monoclonal protein, serum, and urine protein electrophoresis should always be done with immunofixation as it increases the sensitivity of detecting monoclonal protein. Abnormal SIFE and UIFE is seen in MGUS, MM, WM, AL amyloidosis, and B-cell lymphoma.[6]

Imaging[12,13]

Echocardiography

- Unexplained wall thickening of left ventricle (LV) (≥12 mm), thickening is more commonly seen in ATTR CA because of amyloid deposition for longer duration compared to AL CA.
- Thickening of right ventricular free wall, atrium, inter atrial septum, and valves
- Pericardial effusion
- Diastolic dysfunction
- Reduction in global longitudinal strain (GLS) with apical sparing
- Granular sparkling appearance—increased myocardial echogenicity is not specific for CA
- Biatrial enlargement
- European Society of Cardiology (ESC) document has suggested echocardiographic criteria to diagnose CA in presence of extracardiac biopsy proven amyloidosis. According to this:
  Unexplained left ventricular (LV) thickness of ≥12 mm with either ≥2 of the following three findings (grade ≥2 diastolic dysfunction; in TDI s′, e′, a′ <5 cm/s; GLS < –15%) should be present

Or,

Echocardiographic score (relative LV wall thickness >0.6, E/e'>11, TAPSE ≤ 19, LV-GLS ≤ –13% and systolic longitudinal strain apex to base ratio >2.9) should be ≥8.[6]

Cardiovascular Magnetic Resonance

It is helpful in differentiating CA from other hypertrophic phenocopies such as HCM and Fabry disease but it is not reliable in identifying the subtype of CA (like ATTR or AL CA). CMR might provide an important insight when bone scintigraphy is negative but monoclonal protein is found and a negative CMR makes CA very unlikely.

The following features are found in CA:[2,14]

- Global subendocardial or transmural (in advanced disease) late gadolinium enhancement (LGE) (sensitivity of 86% and specificity of 92%), LGE predicts mortality in CA
- Increased extracellular volume >0.4

Electrocardiography

Amyloid deposition disrupts the conduction system; cytotoxicity may also be implicated in the pathogenesis. Cardiac sympathetic denervation may also lead to arrhythmogenesis. Normal ECG in CA is seen in <10% patients.[15]

- Discordant QRS voltage in ECG (decreased) and increased wall thickness on imaging, low voltage QRS in ECG is seen in >50% of CA. ECG evidence of LVH can be found in ≤15% patients with ATTR-CA
- Pseudoinfarct pattern in anterior or inferior leads (>70% of AL-CA)
- *Conduction system disorders*—atrioventricular (AV) block, bundle branch block (BBB), intraventricular conduction delay (IVCD), and history of pacemaker implantation.
- *AF*: Most common arrhythmia is AF (10–69%) → atrial amyloid deposition and LA dilatation because of diastolic dysfunction are two responsible factors; (1) AF is more frequent in ATTRwt-CA compared to ATTRv-CA and AL-CA and (2) older age of presentation might have an impact on it.[15]
- Ventricular arrhythmia

Bone Scintigraphy

Imaging in myocardial infarction (MI) with bone avid radiotracer is not a new modality; it is there for >40 years. It was also being used to image CA for quite a long time but pyrophosphate ^{99m}Tc-PYP), diphosphono-1,2-propanodicarboxylic acid [^{99m}Tc-DPD], and hydroxymethylene diphosphonate [^{99m}Tc-HMDP]) have revolutionized the noninvasive diagnosis of CA only recently.[2,14]

Using a semiquantitative method (Perugini score) radiotracer uptake of myocardium can be compared with rib and graded accordingly into 0–3. Despite high sensitivity and specificity to diagnose ATTR-CA utilizing this technique, 10% patients with AL-CA may show grade 2,3 myocardial uptakes the importance of excluding the presence of monoclonal protein in urine and serum should not be ignored in such situation. The combination of grade 2 or 3 myocardial radiotracer uptake and absence of monoclonal protein in urine and serum in a patient with HF with typical echocardiogram or CMR evidence of amyloidosis is diagnostic of ATTR-CA with 100% specificity. Grade 1–3 uptake of any radiotracer (^{99m}Tc-PYP, ^{99m}Tc-DPD, or ^{99m}Tc-HMDP) detects ATTR-CA with a sensitivity of >99% and specificity of 86%.

Bone scintigraphy using ^{99m}Tc-PYP radiotracer (it is a quantitative uptake ratio of heart to contralateral lung) is helpful in differentiating ATTR-CA from AL-CA. The persistence of radiotracer inside ventricular blood pool may mimic the myocardial uptake. Single-photon emission computed tomography (SPECT) or SPECT/CT should be done concurrently to distinguish the myocardial uptake from the blood pool uptake.

Bone scintigraphy may be falsely positive in AL-CA, rare variety of amyloidosis (AApoAI, AApoAII, ApoAIV, and Aβ2M amyloidosis) or hydroxychloroquine cardiac toxicity. Result can be falsely negative in some ATTRv mutations (p.Phe84Leu and p.Ser97Tyr). The use of scintigraphy has replaced the need for tissue biopsy to diagnose ATTR-CA but simultaneous assessment of monoclonal protein is always required to avoid missing rare entities (ATTR-CA + MGUS and ATTR-CA + AL-CA). On the contrary, in AL-CA tissue biopsy is an essential part of the diagnostic algorithm.[2,10,14]

Tissue Biopsy

Histologic diagnosis is essential in AL-CA. It should also be done where bone scintigraphy is borderline positive (Perugini 1) in association with absent monoclonal protein. Biopsy is done from the involved organ (like heart) or from the surrogate sites. The gold standard is endomyocardial biopsy, sampling from ≥4 sites provides 100% sensitivity and specificity to diagnose CA. Alternative sites of biopsy are abdominal fat pad (sensitivity: 84% for AL-CM, lower sensitivity for ATTR-CA: 45% for ATTRv, and 15% for ATTRwt), kidney, bone marrow, skin, digestive tract, labial salivary gland, etc.

Cardiac amyloidosis is confirmed when EMB sample shows Congo red positivity. Precursor protein identification is must after this; though immunohistochemistry or immunogold immunoelectron microscopy are routinely done but mass spectrometry [liquid chromatography with tandem mass spectrometry (LC–MS/MS)] remains the gold standard with a sensitivity of 88% and specificity of 96%.[2,10]

Genetic Testing

Genetic testing is very crucial in ATTR-CA to identify the mutations in *TTR* gene and also to discriminate the ATTRwt from ATTRv. After identification of proband (index patient) asymptomatic carrier needs to identified in the family. One should also keep in mind the possibility of variable clinical penetrance. Non-TTR variant analysis is often required in CA with normal TTR sequence.[1]

BIOMARKER

NT-proBNP and high sensitivity troponin may be persistently elevated in CA. Retinol binding protein 4 which acts to stabilize the tetramer may be decreased in ATTRv.[2]

Summary of Diagnostic Approach (Flowchart 2)[10]

Several scientific societies like European Society of Cardiology, American Heart Association have their own diagnostic algorithm. Here we have given the algorithm as suggested by Canadian Cardiovascular Society/Canadian Heart Failure Society and American Heart Association.

PROGNOSIS

The prognosis of AL-CA and ATTR-CA is assessed by several scoring system based on biomarkers.[16-18] In general NT-proBNP and troponin are indicators of disease burden and prognosis in both types of CA.

Mayo 2004, Mayo 2004 with European modification, Mayo 2012 and Boston University scoring system are used to predict survival in AL-CA, for example, Troponin T/hs Trop-T and NT-proBNP/BNP and difference between involved and uninvolved free light chain are needed to assess the Mayo 2012 staging, in stage III disease the median survival is 14 months.

Mayo and UK staging system are there to prognosticate ATTRwt, ATTRwt, and ATTRv respectively; troponin T, NT-proBNP, and estimated glomerular filtration rate (eGFR) are taken into consideration to calculate the scores, for example, in UK staging system NT-proBNP and eGFR are used for disease staging, in stage III median survival is 24.1 months.[19,20]

Poor prognosis can also be predicted by lower GLS (by echocardiogram) or transmural LGE (by CMR), New York Heart Association (NYHA) III/IV functional status.

MANAGEMENT OF CARDIAC AMYLOIDOSIS[2,3,10]

Supportive Management of Cardiac Amyloidosis

Heart Failure Management

Alteration of pressure volume relationship, passive ventricular filling because of diastolic dysfunction/restrictive physiology, relatively fixed stroke volume, more dependency on heart rate to maintain cardiac output, inability to raise the cardiac output (CO) in response to vasodilation, concurrent autonomic dysfunction, all these have made it difficult to treat HF. Thus, they are very prone to volume overload leading to pulmonary edema, hepatic congestion, on the other hand with slight over diuresis there may be deterioration of organ function especially renal dysfunction. Therefore, the management of HF in CA is entirely different compared to what we usually do in other HF patients.[21,22]

- *Diuretics*: Goal is to relieve the congestion without compromising the preload as in restrictive physiology higher filling pressure is required to maintain cardiac output. Loop diuretic is preferred; bioavailability is a concern because of associated gut edema. Diuretic resistance in AL amyloidosis is expected to occur because of light chain deposition in kidney. Frequent dose adjustment is needed to avoid over diuresis. Furosemide is the first-line drug to be used, torsemide, and bumetanide are reserved for inadequate diuretic response as they have more potency and bioavailability.
- *Beta-blocker*: They are poorly tolerated as they reduce the heart rate which is the main factor responsible for maintaining the cardiac output in presence of restrictive filling, thus not recommended. Some scientific societies have commented on their cautious use with tolerated doses and in presence of AF for heart rate control.

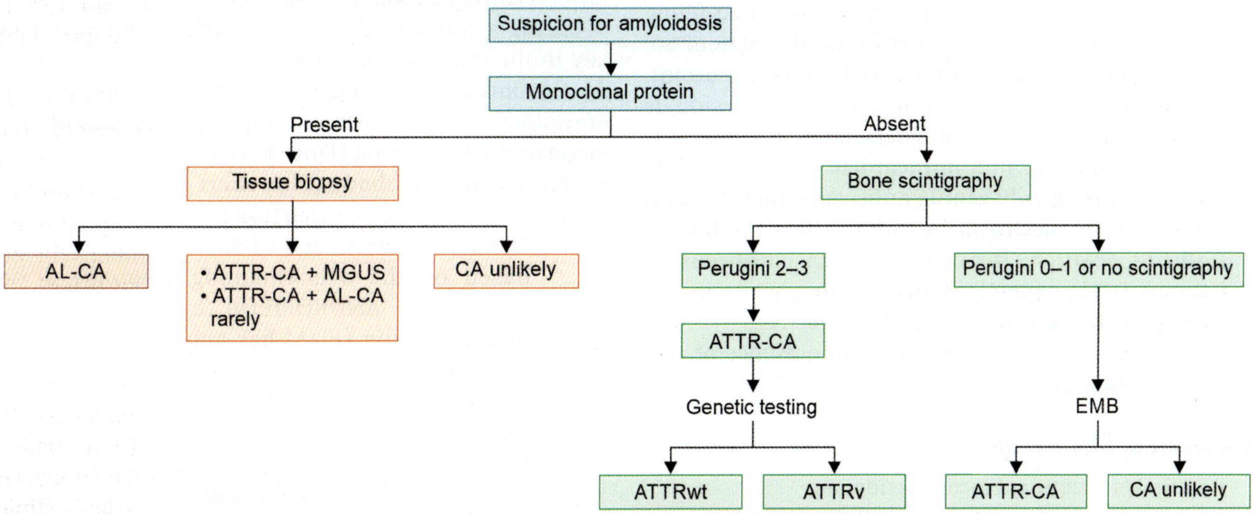

FLOWCHART 2: Summary of diagnostic approach.

(AL: light chain; ATTRv: hereditary amyloid transthyretin; ATTRwt: wild-type amyloid transthyretin; CA: cardiac amyloidosis; EMB: endomyocardial biopsy; MGUS: monoclonal gammopathy of undetermined significance)

- *ACEI/ARB/ARNI*: They are also not recommended as they potentiate hypotension related to autonomic dysfunction.
- *MRA*: It may be considered; in "TOPCAT" trial, among patients with echocardiographic features suggestive of amyloidosis showed benefit in respect to combined endpoint of cardiovascular disease (CVD), HF hospitalization or aborted cardiac arrest.
- *SGLT-2I*: Insufficient evidence
- Postural hypotension may be seen in ATTRv with autonomic neuropathy. Treatment options include midodrine, droxidopa, and stockings.[23,24]

Atrial Fibrillation/Atrial Flutter Management

- *Digoxin*: Though it binds with the amyloid fibril with high affinity, it can be used cautiously in low doses especially in patients prone to develop hypotension.
- *Amiodarone*: Might be considered as first choice.
- *Beta-blocker*: It might be considered to control heart rate in persistent AF, though some scientific societies have not recommended their use.
- *Non-DHP CCB*: Usually not recommended especially in presence of reduced LV function as they have negative inotropic action. Their heart rate slowing property might worsen heart failure. They can also bind to amyloid fibril as seen in AL-amyloidosis.
- *Anticoagulation*: All patients of AF/AFL need to be anticoagulated irrespective of CHA_2DS_2-VASc risk score. Anticoagulation might be considered even when in sinus rhythm as LAA and LA thrombus are not uncommonly seen even in sinus rhythm. Regarding the choice of anticoagulant, nonvitamin K antagonist oral anticoagulants (NOAC) is preferable in absence of contraindication but vitamin K antagonist (VKA) can also be given.
- *Cardioversion*: Atrial contribution to ventricular filling is reduced in CA because of poor atrial function. So, maintaining a sinus rhythm may be less important. TEE should be done routinely if cardioversion is required irrespective of anticoagulation status as it is not uncommon to find intracardiac thrombus while the patient is already getting anticoagulation. Rhythm control may be effective in the early course of the disease.
- *Catheter ablation*: It can be done in cavotricuspid isthmus (CTI)-dependent atrial flutter, while in AF, radiofrequency ablation (RFA) is less effective.
- *LAA closure*: It may be considered in presence of very high bleeding risk.

Device Therapy

- Pacemaker—standard recommendation
- Implantable cardioverter-defibrillator (ICD)—recommended for secondary prevention, should be avoided in primary prevention
- Chronic right ventricular (CRT)—might be considered in situation where high pacing burden is expected

Mechanical Circulatory Support

Limited data

Heart Transplantation

- ATTR-CA-orthotropic heart transplantation (OHT) can be done in absence of significant extracardiac disease.
- AL-CA-acceptable outcome in those who underwent OHT along with autologous stem cell transplantation (ASCT).

TREATMENT OF AL AMYLOIDOSIS (FLOWCHART 3)

About 10–15% patients of MM develop AL amyloidosis and 10% of the AL amyloidosis are associated with MM; most of the AL amyloidosis patients have <10% plasma cells in bone marrow. MGUS may progress to AL amyloidosis in 1% cases. In 10–40% of patients with ATTR-CA, monoclonal light chain is found in serum or urine without any evidence of AL amyloidosis or MM; prevalence of MGUS increases with age thus the coexistence of ATTR-CA and MGUS is also not uncommon. Meticulous follow-up and early diagnosis of AL-CA at the presymptomatic stage is possible in patients with MGUS who are screened at a regular interval to look for the biomarkers of target organ involvement (NT-proBNP, albuminuria, etc.), so that treatment can be initiated at the earliest in the presymptomatic stage. Disease has already progressed by the time patients with suspected AL amyloidosis present with symptoms pertaining to target organ involvement. In untreated patients the median survival is 8 months. It is not uncommon to be treated as unrelated cardiomyopathy before the accurate diagnosis is being made. Diagnostic delay beyond 6 months of symptom onset is correlated with poor survival.[7,25]

Being a systemic, disease multidisciplinary care is the key in the management of AL amyloidosis. Treatment of AL-CA aims at eliminating the plasma cell clone producing amyloidogenic light chain and supportive management for target organ dysfunction **(Flowchart 4)**.

- Monoclonal antibody **(Flowchart 5)**: They target the specific cell surface antigen (like CD38).
  - *Daratumumab*: An anti-CD38 monoclonal antibody. based on the overwhelming response of this molecule in "ANDROMEDA" trial, Food Drug and Administration (FDA) has approved this drug in newly diagnosed AL amyloidosis.[28]
- *Small molecule inhibitor*:
  - *Venetoclax*: It modulates the intrinsic apoptotic pathway by interacting with BCL-2.[29]
- *Inhibitors of amyloid fibril formation*:
  - *Doxycycline*: It acts as an inhibitor of matrix metalloproteinase (MMP) and prevents amyloid fibril formation.[30]

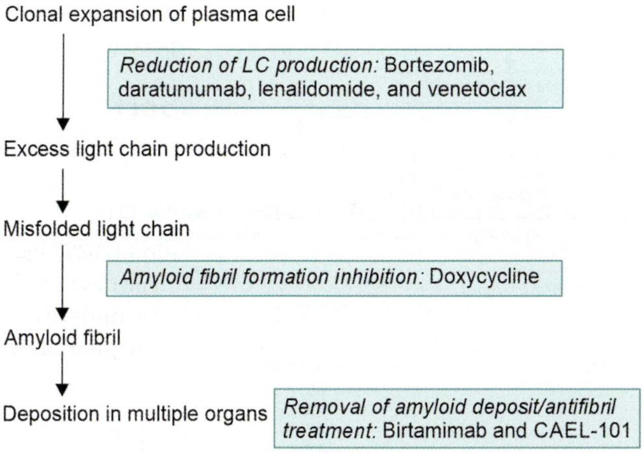

FLOWCHART 3: Treatment of AL amyloidosis.

(AL: light chain; LC: light chain)

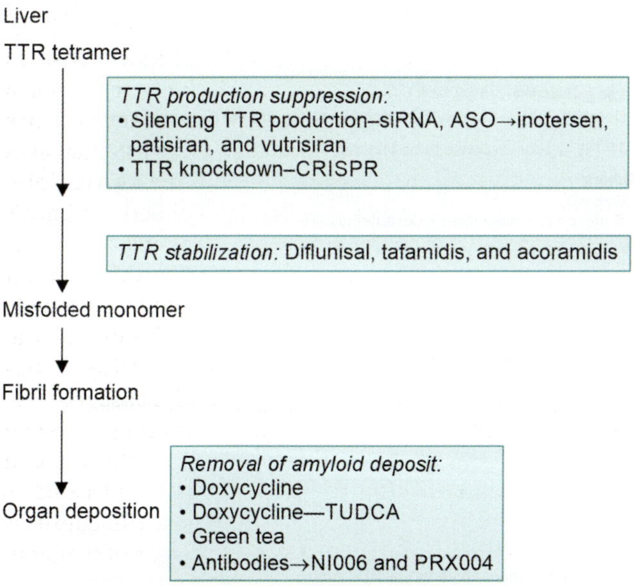

FLOWCHART 4: Treatment of ATTR-amyloidosis.

(ASO: antisense oligonucleotide; CRISPR: clusters of regularly interspaced short palindromic repeats; siRNA: small interfering ribonucleic acid; TTR: transthyretin; TUDCA: tauroursodeoxycholic acid)

- *Clearance of amyloid deposits/antifibril treatment*: This is one of the unmet needs of AL amyloidosis management. This emerging concept takes care of the deposited amyloid fibril in the target organ which could potentially reverse the organ dysfunction.[9]
- *CAEL-101*: It is a chimeric monoclonal antibody that targets the cryptic epitope of light chain when misfolded. According to the hypothesis, it opsonizes the misfolded light chain and amyloid fibrils which in turn attracts the macrophage leading to phagocytosis and degradation.
- *Birtamimab*: It binds to cryptic epitope of amyloid A protein when misfolded; it cross reacts with the amyloid light chain fibril and leads to macrophage-mediated degradation and clearance of amyloid fibril.

DISEASE MODIFYING TREATMENT OF ATTR-AMYLOIDOSIS (FLOWCHART 4)[1,3,6,9]

Currently there are two therapeutic targets, (1) TTR protein stabilization and (2) silencing the production of TTR protein.

Transthyretin Protein Stabilization

Transthyretin, a homotetrameric protein which acts as a transporter of retinol primarily and to a lesser extent thyroxine (<1% TTR binds with thyroid hormone in plasma because of alternate and higher affinity for other transporter like thyroid-binding globulin and albumin). This is in contrast to CSF where TTR serves as a principle transporter of thyroxine and interestingly amyloid fibril formation does not occur in CSF. The rate limiting step of TTR amyloidosis is the tetrameric dissociation leading to formation of amyloidogenic monomer and oligomers. Disease severity and penetrance depends on the specific mutation which in turn dictates the rapidity of dissociation. Like, L55P and V122I-mutant transthyretin are associated with rapid dissociation of TTR into amyloidogenic monomer leading to severe disease with 100% penetrance, on the other aspect milder disease expression (polyneuropathy) with 2% penetrance in seen in presence of the V30M mutant where dissociation is very slow.

- *Diflunisal*: It is a nonsteroidal anti-inflammatory drugs (NSAIDs) which binds to the T4-binding site on TTR tetramer thus preventing their dissociation into monomer and oligomer. Regular monitoring of renal function is required; GI hemorrhage, fluid retention, hypertension (HTN) are other adverse effects. Its use is associated with reduced rate of progression of amyloid polyneuropathy.
- *Tafamidis*: This benzoxazole derivative acts as a similar way like diflunisal but lacks the NSAIDs property. In the ATTR-ACT (Safety and Efficacy of tafamidis in patients with transthyretin cardiomyopathy) trial, tafamidis (20 mg or 80 mg) use in wild-type and hereditary ATTR-CA was associated with 13.4% absolute reduction of all-cause mortality and 32% lower risk of cardiovascular related hospitalization by 30 months among those who had NYHA I or II functional status compared to placebo.[31] Patients with NYHA III functional status had more cardiovascular-related hospitalization (patients with NYHA IV symptom status were excluded from the trial), thus suggested the need for early treatment. It certainly delays the progression of CA but does not help in regression. It is the only FDA approved drug in the treatment of ATTR-CA.
- *Acoramidis:* It is a synthetic small molecule which stabilizes the TTR tetramer. It is more potent and binds to TTR more selectively than tafamidis.

AL amyloidosis

Tissue biopsy of surrogate sites or affected organ
- Abdominal fat (sensitivity ~80%), bone marrow (sensitivity ~70%), and minor salivary gland (sensitivity ~80%)

Plasma cell dyscrasia

Blood tests for monoclonal protein
- sFLC and SIFE/UIFE

Bone marrow biopsy—mandatory
- Plasma cell population
- Exclude MM
- Exclude B cell lymphoproliferative disorders like WM, CLL, non-Hodgkin's lymphoma as they have different treatment strategy

Staging of the disease of a newly diagnosed AL amyloidosis:

- Mayo Clinic (2004) integrating European Collaborative Study 3B staging

Risk factors:
- cTnT >0.035 ng/mL
- NT-proBNP >332 pg/mL

Risk factors present	stage	Median overall survival (months)
0	1	86
1	2	43
2	3A	17
NT-proBNP ≥ 8,500	3B	4.6

- Revised Mayo clinic staging

Transplant eligible? (10–20%)

All must be met

Age/years	≤70
ECOG PS	0–2
Staging (revised Mayo 2004)	I–II
LVEF%	>45
NYHA	I–II
eGFR	≥30
SBP	≥90
DLCO%	>50

Autologous stem cell transplantation (ASCT):
- If bone marrow plasma cell is >10%: 2–4 cycles of Bortezomib based chemotherapy is given as induction therapy before transplantation
- High dose melphalan + ASCT
- CR and VGPR → 73%
- If CR is seen after ASCT → median survival 15 years
- Treatment related mortality → 3%

Not eligible for ASCT (80–90%)

Plasma cell directed therapy:

First choice: Cyclophosphamide, bortezomib, dexamethasone (CyBorD), and daratumumab (anti-CD38 monoclonal antibody)[7]
- CR and VGPR → 78% with this regimen
- Daratumumab is the only FDA approved drug to treat AL amyloidosis

t(11;14) → poor response to bortezomib

Others:
- CyBorD
- Bortezomib + melphalan + dexamethasone

Assess response to treatment: Organ response (improvement of organ function) may lag behind hematological response, so rescue therapy should be instituted looking at the hematological response

1. Hematological response—usually within 3–6 months[26]

CR	Both criteria must be fulfilled: • SIFE and UIFE negative for monoclonal protein • FLC ratio within the reference range Or, An uninvolved FLC concentration > involved FLC concentration with or without an abnormal FLC ratio
VGPR	Difference between involved and uninvolved FLC (dFLC) <40 mg/L
Partial response	dFLC decrease >50% from baseline
No response	All other patients

2. Organ response—separate criteria for cardiac, renal, hepatic, etc.[27]

Cardiac	
Improvement	NT-proBNP is reduced by >30% And >300 pg/mL reduction (if baseline NT-proBNP is >650 pg/mL) Or, ≥2 point reduction in NYHA functional class (if baseline NYHA functional class III or IV)

Irrespective of initially selected treatment option

Relapse or refractory to initial therapy?
- Daratumumab
- Immunomodulatory agents—lenalidomide, pomalidomide, and thalidomide
- Ixazomib, an oral proteasome inhibitor
- Venetoclax, which blocks the antiapoptotic B cell

Complete response
- Monitor
- No maintenance therapy

FLOWCHART 5: Management of AL-amyloidosis.

(AL: light chain; ASCT: autologous stem cell transplantation; CLL: chronic lymphocytic leukemia; CR: complete response; DLCO: diffusing capacity for carbon monoxide; ECOG PS: Eastern Cooperative Oncology Group Performance Status; eGFR: estimated glomerular filtration rate; FDA: Food and Drug Administration; LVEF: left ventricular ejection fraction; NYHA: New York Heart Association; MM: multiple myeloma; SBP: systolic blood pressure; sFLC: serum free light-chain; SIFE: serum immunofixation electrophoresis; UIFE: urine immunofixation electrophoresis; WM: Waldenström macroglobulinemia; VGPR: very good partial response)

Silencing TTR Production[32]

Transthyretin tetramer synthesis follows few steps.

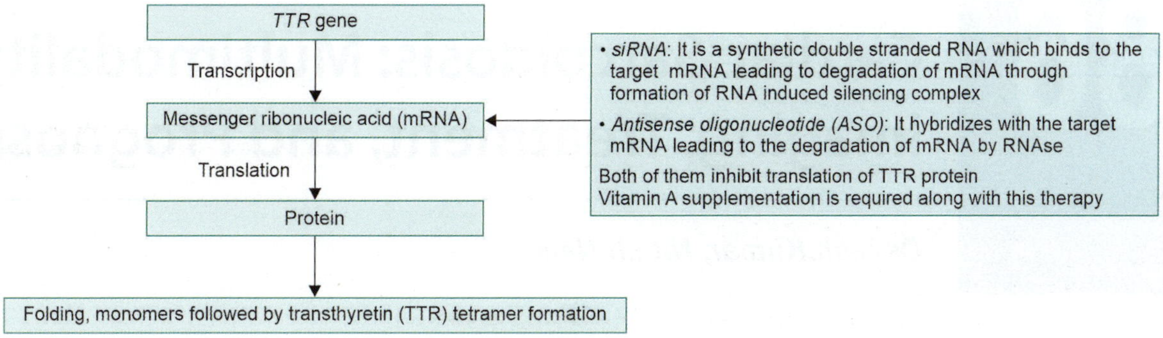

- *First-generation agent*:
    - Inotersen: Its limitations are glomerulonephritis and thrombocytopenia.
    - Patisiran: It is a small interfering ribonucleic acid (siRNA), formulated as lipid nanoparticle for a targeted delivery. It is approved by FDA for ATTRv amyloidosis with polyneuropathy with or without cardiomyopathy. In an open level extension of APOLLO-B study patisiran use is associated with favorable effect on functional capacity and quality of life compared to placebo in ATTR-CA (hereditary or wild type) at the end of 18 months.[3]
- *Second-generation agent*:
    - Vutrisiran: It is conjugated with N-acetylgalactosamine to facilitate its hepatic uptake.
    - *AKCEA-TTR-LRx*: It is conjugated antisense oligonucleotide (ASO) with a property of enhanced hepatic uptake

Novel Approach: Transthyretin Knockdown

- *NTLA-2001*: They are used as intravenous infusion and intended for in vivo gene editing. It has a lipid nanoparticle with liver tropism for the delivery of two components (1) mRNA encoding Cas9 protein and (2) single guide RNA (sgRNA) specific to *TTR* gene. After being taken up by hepatocyte, in the cytoplasm, translation of mRNA encoding Cas9 takes place producing Cas9 endonuclease enzyme. SgRNA specific to *TTR* gene interacts with the Cas9 endonuclease enzyme to form clusters of regularly interspaced short palindromic repeats (CRISPR)-Cas9 ribonucleoprotein complex. This complex enters into the nucleus and interacts with the deoxyribonucleic acid (DNA) through several intervening steps and engages endogenous DNA repair mechanism leading to reduced production functional target gene mRNA and thereby TTR protein. Animal data has shown >97% knockdown of mouse TTR protein after single administration.[33]

Others

- *Amyloid degradation/extraction:*[3]
    - PRX-004: It is a monoclonal antibody which binds to the misfolded TTR amyloid and clears the amyloid deposits from myocardium.
    - NI006: It is a recombinant monoclonal antibody targeting the misfolded and aggregated amyloid fibrils in ATTRwt and ATTRv.
- Doxycycline in combination tauroursodeoxycholic acid (TUDCA) may have some role in lowering nonfibrillar TTR
- Green tea contains epigallocatechin-3-gallate (EGCG) which was shown to inhibit fibril formation.

SUMMARY OF ATTR TREATMENT RECOMMENDATION[6]

- ATTRwt → cardiomyopathy → tafamidis
- ATTRv with cardiomyopathy only → tafamidis
- ATTRv with cardiomyopathy and polyneuropathy→
    - Tafamidis in polyneuropathy stage 1
    - Patisiran in polyneuropathy stage 1 and 2
- ATTRv with polyneuropathy only →
    - Tafamidis in polyneuropathy stage 1
    - Patisiran and inotersen in polyneuropathy stage 1 and 2

CONCLUSION

The diversity of clinical presentation in amyloidosis is certainly an impediment for early diagnosis. With increasing awareness and availability of newer diagnostic tools it is possible to pick up CA early in their disease course. The advent of novel disease modifying therapy is undoubtedly promising but the cost of treatment is an obstacle to their widespread use.

ONLINE REFERENCES

Please scan the QR code provided at the end of the table of contents for References of this chapter.

CHAPTER

86 Cardiac Sarcoidosis: Multimodality Imaging, Treatment, and Prognosis

Devesh Kumar, Nitish Naik

ABSTRACT

Cardiac sarcoidosis can have protean cardiac manifestations ranging from asymptomatic cardiac involvement to syncope, bradyarrhythmias, atrial and ventricular tachyarrhythmias, heart failure, or even sudden cardiac death. A definitive diagnosis requires histological evidence of noncaseating granulomatous inflammation along with supportive clinical and laboratory investigations. It should be considered in the differential diagnosis in patients presenting with heart block, ventricular tachyarrhythmias, and heart failure. Cardiac sarcoidosis may masquerade as a dilated/restrictive cardiomyopathy or even as an arrhythmogenic right ventricular cardiomyopathy. Imaging modalities such as cardiac magnetic resonance imaging (MRI) and Gallium-DOTA-NOC and ^{18}FDG–PET (^{18}F-fluorodeoxyglucose–positron emission tomography) scans, though not diagnostic, are useful in evaluating cardiac involvement and have high positive predictive values for cardiac sarcoidosis when index of suspicion is high. Endomyocardial biopsy, though diagnostic, has limited yield and is therefore not routinely performed. Medical management for cardiac sarcoidosis involves the use of immunosuppressive therapy, most often glucocorticoids. Steroid sparing therapy includes possible use of either methotrexate, azathioprine, leflunomide, and mycophenolate mofetil or infliximab. Cardiac implantable electronic devices including pacemakers or implantable defibrillators/cardiac resynchronization devices may be needed in some patients. Antiarrhythmic drugs or catheter ablation for ventricular arrhythmias may also be needed as per clinical course.

Keywords: Noncaseating granulomas, ventricular tachycardia, dotanoc scan, cardiac MRI.

INTRODUCTION

Sarcoidosis is a multisystemic, granulomatous disorder with a prevalence of 4.7–64.0 in 100,000 and a heterogenous distribution worldwide. The disease is reported with the highest frequency among European and African-American descent and is three times more prevalent in women.[1] The disease is seen to occur mainly in the age group of 25–60 years and is extremely rare under the age of 15 or above 70 years.[2] The etiology of sarcoidosis is poorly understood; however, it is thought to be due to an immunological reaction to an unknown antigen in a genetically susceptible individual.[3] The pathological hallmark of sarcoidosis is the presence of noncaseating granulomas with clusters of macrophages and epithelioid cells with abundant CD4 cells and few CD8 cells. The common antigenic triggers proposed to be causative are both infective [*Propionibacterium acnes* (*P. Acnes*) and *Mycobacterium tuberculosis*] and noninfective (molds).[4,5]

The clinical spectrum of sarcoid varies from asymptomatic (up to one-third) disease to severe disease, causing organ failure. The lungs are the most commonly involved organs with involvement in more than 90% of patients with sarcoidosis. Among the extrapulmonary involvement, the cutaneous and ocular manifestations are the most common, followed by gastrointestinal, neurological, and cardiac manifestations.[6]

Clinical cardiac involvement occurs in up to 5% of patients of sarcoidosis. Another 20–25% of patients with sarcoidosis have evidence of silent cardiac involvement as seen in autopsy studies. This finding has now been confirmed with newer imaging modalities which reveal cardiac involvement in an equal proportion of patients. In patients with clinical cardiac involvement, the cardiac symptoms usually dominate over the extracardiac symptoms as most patients with clinical sarcoid have minimal extracardiac disease and up to two-thirds have isolated cardiac sarcoid.[7-11]

Cardiac involvement is known to significantly worsen the prognosis of patients with sarcoidosis by increasing both morbidity and mortality. It is the most important cause of death in sarcoidosis patients, with a 5-year mortality rate between 25 and 66% despite immunosuppressive treatment. It is the leading cause of death in the Japanese population, accounting for up to 85% of all sarcoid-related deaths. It has also been shown in many studies that in patients with mild-to-moderate left ventricular (LV) systolic dysfunction, treatment with steroids leads to improvement in LV ejection fraction (LVEF), whereas in patients with severe decrease in EF, these benefits are not seen. Hence, early diagnosis and treatment are imperative to improve outcomes of this disorder.[12]

The underlying pathophysiology of cardiac sarcoidosis involves the formation of noncaseating granulomas, which may involve any part of the heart, but there is predisposition of the granulomas to involve the basal part of interventricular septum (IVS) and the left ventricle. There is a predisposition of the granulomas to involve the conduction system of the heart. The cardiac pathological features include three successive histological stages—edema, granulomatous inflammation, and fibrosis—leading to post inflammatory scarring.[13,14]

In India, some studies have been done to estimate the prevalence of cardiac sarcoidosis in patients with pulmonary sarcoid.[15] In one study done at All India Institute of Medical Sciences (AIIMS), New Delhi, by Sharma et al. on manifestations of sarcoidosis, cardiac involvement was seen in up to 15 patients out of 210 (7%) cases of diagnosed pulmonary sarcoidosis. In a subsequent study for rare manifestations of cardiac sarcoidosis done by Sharma et al. in 2012, cardiac sarcoidosis was found to be present in 5 out of 164 patients who were screened for cardiac involvement. However, neither of these utilized cardiac magnetic resonance imaging (MRI) or radionuclide scanning for the evaluation of cardiac involvement.

CLINICAL FEATURES

Cardiac sarcoidosis is known to have protean manifestations with granulomas which could lead to sudden cardiac death, ventricular arrythmias due to scar formed as sequelae of the chronic inflammation and fibrosis, or progressive heart failure either due to systolic dysfunction heart failure with reduced EF (HFrEF) or due to diastolic dysfunction.[16-18]

Cardiac sarcoidosis is considered a dreaded condition, with a 5-year survival limited to 60–75% 5-year among various published studies. The available outcome data are much more heterogeneous, although the reported prognosis varies from 73% 1-year mortality to 100% 10-year survival in the absence of LV dysfunction.[19]

Cardiac sarcoid may be the first manifestation of sarcoidosis in a variety of circumstances. In a study from Finland of 72 patients aged <55 years with new-onset, unexplained high-degree atrioventricular (AV) block, biopsy-proven cardiac sarcoidosis was found in 19% and probable CS was found in another 6%.[20] In a similar study from a Canadian center, CS was diagnosed in one-third of patients with unexplained Mobitz type II or third-degree AV block.[9] Similarly in a prospective study evaluating patients with ventricular tachycardia (VT) of unknown etiology, 4 out of 14 patients (29%) were subsequently diagnosed with cardiac sarcoidosis.[8] In another study done by Tung et al. in 103 patients with nonischemic cardiomyopathy and VT, 17 out of 103 (16.5%) had undiagnosed CS.[21] Similarly, cardiac sarcoidosis has been found to be present in 8 out of 130 patients who underwent cardiac transplant in a study of 130 heart transplants for nonischemic cardiomyopathy.[22]

DIAGNOSIS

Two-dimensional Echocardiography

There are no findings that are specific for the diagnosis of CS; however, thinning of the basal IVS is the most typical finding. Other findings are LV hypertrophy (LVH), regional wall motion abnormality (RWMA) typically seen in a noncoronary distribution, aneurysms, LV systolic dysfunction, and diastolic dysfunction. Thus, two-dimensional (2D) echo has a relatively good sensitivity (25–62%) for the screening of cardiac involvement in sarcoidosis but has lower specificity.[23] Both thinning of the basal septum and aneurysms are seen in up to 10% of the patients.[23]

Cardiac MRI

Cardiac MRI offers a multi-dimensional assessment of cardiac involvement, allowing for a noninvasive detection of scar, edema, biventricular function, and myocardial perfusion defects. There are no findings that are pathognomonic for CS. Cardiac involvement in sarcoidosis is typically patchy and multifocal in nature with sparing of the endocardial border.[24] The classical finding of sarcoidosis on MRI is late gadolinium enhancement (LGE) which is subepicardial or mid myocardial in location and is present mainly in the basal and lateral wall of left ventricle, although right ventricular (RV) involvement may also be seen.[25-27] It is also noteworthy that marked edema can also increase the interstitial space, thereby resulting in LGE. Therefore, the intensity of LGE may decrease with treatment.[28] Apart from utility in diagnosis, LGE on MRI has also been seen to be correlated with outcomes and a massively increased uptake on MRI correlates with poorer prognosis. LGE on MRI has been found to be associated with a ninefold increased hazard of combined adverse events and elevenfold increased hazard for cardiac death.[29]

Other MRI findings associated with cardiac involvement include thinning of ventricular wall, the presence of myocardial edema by T2-weighted sequences, and the identification of regional or global hypokinesia.[30] Another important role of cardiac MRI in diagnosis of CS is that it can facilitate endomyocardial biopsy (EMB) to be taken from site showing maximum LGE.[31]

Cardiac ^{18}F-fluorodeoxyglucose–Positron Emission Tomography

Macrophages in inflammatory regions tend to be more active metabolically than the surrounding myocytes, resulting in an increased uptake of glucose due to increased metabolism. This is the principle for using positron emission tomography (PET) in the diagnosis of cardiac sarcoidosis.[32] There are no patterns that have been classically described for diagnosis of cardiac PET; however, focal uptake and focal-on-diffuse uptake have been classically correlated with increased inflammation and are taken as findings suggestive of cardiac sarcoidosis.[33,34] Another important role of cardiac PET in the management of cardiac sarcoidosis is to map disease activity in patients on treatment. With the onset of immunosuppressive treatment, the activity of the macrophages decreases, leading to a fall in the inflammatory cells, and hence a decrease in the total inflammation consistent with a decreased fluorodeoxyglucose (FDG) uptake on PET. Hence, it can be used in the follow-up of cardiac sarcoidosis once therapy is initiated.[35] Apart from diagnosis and follow-up, increased cardiac uptake with profound FDG-avid lesions has been seen to correlate with poorer outcomes in patients with sarcoidosis.[36] Another role of PET in the management of patients with cardiac sarcoidosis, like an MRI, is to guide the site of biopsy in patients of cardiac sarcoidosis so as to increase the yield of EMB.[37] Lastly, it can also be used to see uptake of disease activity in other organs and hence can facilitate other amenable sites for biopsy. Earlier, Gallium-67 was used for sarcoidosis, but owing to its higher spatial resolution and higher sensitivity, ^{18}FDG–PET has now become the preferred nuclear imaging modality for CS.[38] To date, only one small study compared the diagnostic accuracy of FDG PET versus MRI, with the conclusion that PET may have a higher sensitivity than MRI (88% vs. 75%), although these estimates were based on Japanese Ministry of Health and Welfare (JMHW) criteria which itself suffers from a low sensitivity, and this difference was not statistically significant.[34]

A limitation of PET imaging as compared to MRI is that it involves patient preparation in order to facilitate the high uptake of glucose by inflammatory macrophages while suppressing the normal myocardial from uptake of glucose, and hence the patients have to generally adhere to a specific diet for a prolonged duration in accordance with various algorithms.[25]

A meta-analysis of 164 patients from 7 studies showed a pooled sensitivity of 89% and specificity of 78% for PET; however, it should be noted that the lower specificity was due to its comparison with the JMHW as the gold standard, which actually may have missed many of the patients due to a low sensitivity.[39] Similarly, Smedema et al. in a cohort of 58 patients evaluated the diagnostic accuracy of MRI against the JMHW for CS and found a sensitivity of 100% and a specificity of only 78%, which was consistent with the use of the JMHW criteria as the comparator criteria. The lower specificity of MRI was again due to the lower sensitivity of the JMHW criteria and also because MRI was able to pick up small areas of fibrosis before the presence of any symptoms or findings on any other imaging.[40] Another limitation to FDG PET is the heterogenous uptake seen even when myocardial suppression is achieved as some amount of glucose is generally taken up even by the normal myocardium.

Keeping this limitation of ^{18}FDG–PET in mind and the knowledge of increased expression of somatostatin receptors (SSTRs) on the inflammatory cells present in the granuloma in sarcoidosis, another scan that has been brought to the forefront as a potential diagnostic modality is the DOTA-NOC scan which uses SSTR-targeted radiotracers such as ^{68}Ga-DOTA-NaI octreotide.[41,42] The activated inflammatory cells found in sarcoid granulomas have abundant SSTR on their surface, in particular SSTR-2A, whereas normal myocytes lack such receptors.[43] The ^{68}Ga-DOTA-NOC has a high affinity for both SSTR-2A and SSTR-5 which are abundant on the inflammatory cells, and hence there is increased uptake at areas of active inflammation. This makes the imaging modality have a high signal-to-noise ratio as well as easily interpretable with lesser interobserver variability.[44]

As cardiovascular magnetic resonance (CMR) involves no ionizing radiation, is generally well tolerated, has a higher negative predictive value to exclude disease due to its higher spatial resolution, and can pick up the slightest of scar regions, it is generally the preferred imaging modality in most patients. However, some patients with cardiac devices and those with end-stage renal disease (ESRD) or with severe hypersensitivity to gadolinium (Gd) might be evaluated with PET scan upfront.[45]

Tissue Biopsy

A positive tissue diagnosis based on EMB confirms the diagnosis of CS. However, there are multiple limitations of EMB. Most importantly, the yield of EMB is around 20–25% due to the patchy and multifocal nature of the disease. Another factor limiting its yield is the high risk of complications associated with this procedure. Finally, the unavailability of EMB procedure readily in hospitals makes EMB of less clinical use as of today. Nowadays, imaging modalities are being used to guide the site of biopsy so as to increase the yield which has subsequently increased to as high as 50% in patients with image-guided biopsy.[45]

Diagnostic Criteria

Cardiac sarcoidosis is a disease with a low prevalence and myriad presentations. Hence, the diagnosis of cardiac sarcoid needs a high clinical suspicion. There are diagnostic criteria which have been proposed such as the JMHW diagnostic guidelines, 1993, and updated in 2006. These guidelines warranted a histological confirmation of cardiac sarcoidosis via EMB or clinical conformation via a combination of major and minor criteria. These criteria were subsequently found to be having many drawbacks due to undue reliance on EMB which has a sensitivity of only 25–30%.[45] Another limitation was the use of gallium as a major criterion, though it is no longer performed due to its limited diagnostic accuracy.[46] The modified criteria also have some limitations in that they included CMR but only as a minor criterion and totally ignored FDG-PET which has been shown to have high sensitivity.[36] Thus, the modified JMHW criteria for clinical diagnosis performed poorly when compared to diagnostic accuracy by advanced imaging techniques, reflecting the fact that newer imaging modalities have a higher sensitivity than these techniques.[27]

Heart Rhythm Society Consensus Statement for the Diagnosis of Cardiac Sarcoidosis

- *Histological diagnosis*: EMB specimens with noncaseating granulomas and no alternative cause identified
- *Clinical diagnosis of probable cardiac sarcoidosis*: Histological diagnosis of extracardiac sarcoidosis and one or more of the following is present, while reasonable alternative cardiac causes have been ruled out.
    - Steroid or immunosuppressive therapy-responsive cardiomyopathy or heart block
    - Unexplained, reduced LVEF (<40%)
    - Mobitz type II or third-degree heart block
    - Depressed LVEF < 50%
    - Patchy uptake on cardiac PET in a pattern consistent with CS
    - LGE on MRI in a pattern consistent with cardiac sarcoidosis
    - Positive gallium uptake in a pattern consistent with CS

(*Probable cardiac sarcoidosis*: >50% likelihood of sarcoidosis)

Japanese Ministry of Health and Welfare Criteria for Diagnosis of Cardiac Sarcoidosis (Revised 2006)

- *Histological diagnosis group*: Cardiac sarcoid is confirmed when EMB specimens suggestive of noncaseating granulomas with histological or clinical diagnosis of extracardiac sarcoidosis
- *Clinical diagnosis group*: Extracardiac sarcoidosis is diagnosed clinically or histologically and satisfies the following condition and more than one in six basic diagnostic criteria:
    1. Two or more from the four major criteria
    2. One of the four major criteria plus two from the five minor criteria
        a. Major criteria:
            i. Advanced AV block
            ii. Basal thinning of the IVS
            iii. Positive gallium uptake in heart
            iv. LVEF < 50%
        b. Minor criteria:
            1. Abnormal electrocardiogram (ECG): VT/axis deviation/abnormal Q waves/right bundle branch block (RBBB)
            2. Abnormal echo: Wall motion abnormality or morphological abnormality (aneurysm or wall thickening or ventricular dilation)
            3. Perfusion defects on nuclear imaging: Thallium/Technetium
            4. Delayed Gd enhancement on cardiac MRI
            5. Interstitial fibrosis or monocyte infiltration on cardiac biopsy

Another criterion for the diagnosis of cardiac sarcoidosis is proposed by the HRS (Heart Rhythm Society) which acknowledges the inherent uncertainty in diagnosis of cardiac sarcoidosis and states that it is probable that cardiac sarcoidosis is present (defined as >50% likelihood) if there is a histological diagnosis of extracardiac sarcoidosis and the patient meets one or more of the criteria. These criteria have a major limitation that they cannot diagnose isolated cardiac sarcoidosis.[47]

Given the aforementioned limitations of various criteria, there is a significant heterogeneity in the diagnostic and treatment algorithms for CS.[48]

MANAGEMENT

There are two cardinal features in the treatment of sarcoidosis. First, sarcoidosis undergoes spontaneous regression in up to 50% of cases without causing any permanent damage to the affected organs.[49] Secondly, use of steroids, the cornerstone for treatment of sarcoidosis, is associated with multiple side effects.[50,51] Hence, treatment is indicated only when inflammation is relentlessly progressive, causing life- or organ-threatening disease.[49]

Systemic steroids are the first line of treatment.[52] The optimal duration of immunosuppressive treatment to be given in patient with sarcoidosis is not known. However, treatment is given for at least 6 months and ideally for 1 year.[53] The rate of relapse is 14–74% for acute disease and 75% for chronic disease and the relapses usually respond to repeat corticosteroid course. A minority of patients may require lifelong treatment.[54]

The management of cardiac sarcoid is significant as it is one of the major causes of death in sarcoidosis and it has been seen that with earlier onset of therapy, further worsening of LV function and AV nodal disease can be prevented.[46] The highest quality of evidence for improvement with immunosuppression in CS is seen in the form of the improvement of LV function and improvement in the conduction in AV nodal disease.[46]

In a study by Sadek et al., 27 out of 57 patients treated with corticosteroids had improvement in AV node conduction, while among 16 patients not treated with steroids, none improved. Similarly for LV dysfunction in a total of 73 patients, 60 patients who received steroids and 13 who did not, it was seen that patients with normal LV function did not have a fall in LV function, whereas those with mild-to-moderate LV dysfunction had an improvement in LV function and no improvement was seen in LV function in those who were having severe LV dysfunction to start with or those who did not receive steroid therapy.[55]

Among other unknowns in the treatment of cardiac sarcoidosis is the optimal doses of corticosteroids. Most experts agree to start with a dose of 30–40 mg daily.[56] Response to treatment should be evaluated after 1–3 months and doses should be tapered gradually to 5–15 mg/day over a span of 6 months and then maintained for at least 1 year.[56]

In patients with no response to steroids or steroid intolerance, a switch to steroid-sparing agents such as methotrexate (MTX) or azathioprine should be made.[57] Azathioprine is a good alternative to MTX having similar efficacy as that of MTX in the management of CS but with a greater predilection of side effects and hence, MTX is preferred to azathioprine for CS as a second-line agent.[58] Leflunomide and mycophenolate mofetil have also been used in cardiac sarcoidosis to modify disease progression. Anti-tumor necrosis factor (TNF) drugs such as infliximab or adalimumab have also been used.[58] Infliximab should be used with caution in patients with overt heart failure. As infliximab increases risk of opportunistic infections, it should be used as a reserve drug when other therapies fail.

SCREENING STRATEGY FOR CARDIAC INVOLVEMENT

Cardiac involvement in sarcoidosis alters the natural history of the disease by worsening the prognosis significantly and hence, all patients with sarcoidosis should undergo screening for cardiac involvement. While advanced cardiac imaging is ideal, it is plagued with the problem of unavailability and high cost, which make it difficult to apply on all patients who need screening. To simplify the screening process, the HRS **(Flowchart 1)** proposed a novel screening algorithm comprising symptoms, electrocardiographic changes, and echocardiographic changes. Any patient who was positive for any one of these changes would subsequently undergo advanced cardiac imaging with cardiac MRI/cardiac PET.[35]

PROGNOSIS

The prognosis of sarcoidosis without cardiac involvement is good with a low risk of death or organ dysfunction. More than half the patients with systemic sarcoidosis have self-resolution within 2–5 years of diagnosis. Patients with pulmonary fibrosis, lupus pernio, bone cysts, cardiac or neurological disease, or renal stones are more likely to progress to a chronic stage.[53]

The prognosis for CS patients is generally worse than those without cardiac involvement with studies showing cardiac sarcoid to be one of the most common causes of death. Cardiac involvement is the most important cause of death in sarcoidosis patients, yielding a 5-year mortality between 25–66% despite immunosuppressive treatment. In a study from Japan, it has been seen that cardiac involvement accounted for more than 85% of all deaths among sarcoid patients.[43] Most deaths in CS today are due to arrythmias both VT and high-grade AV block rather than heart failure. The extent of LV dysfunction is commonly regarded as the most important predictor of survival.[49] Recent CMR studies have shown the presence and extent of myocardial LGE as an even more important prognostic factor than LV function with a ninefold increase in the risk

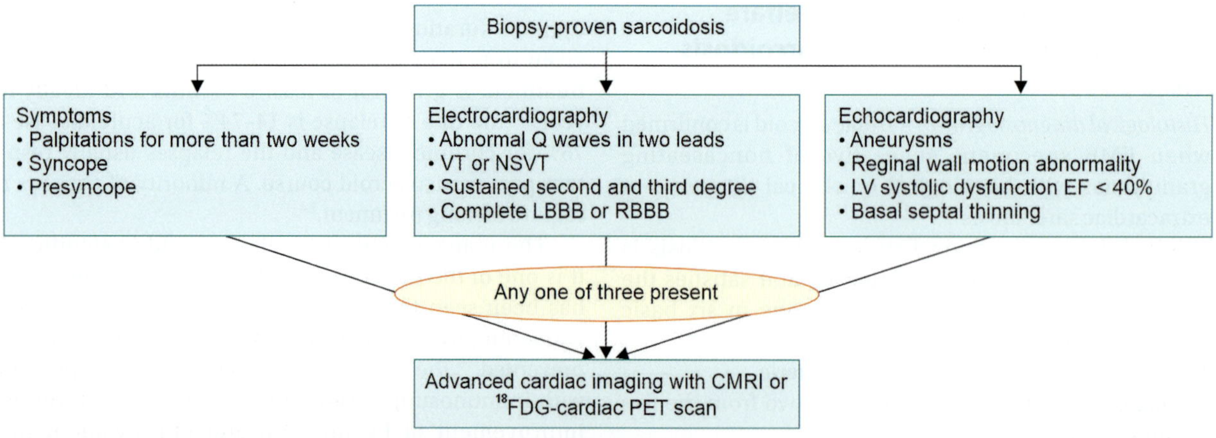

FLOWCHART 1: Screening algorithm as proposed by the Heart Rhythm Society.

(CMRI: cardiac magnetic resonance imaging; EF: ejection fraction; FDG: fluorodeoxyglucose; LBBB: left bundle branch block; LV: left ventricular; NSVT: nonsustained VT; PET: positron emission tomography; RBBB: right bundle branch block; VT: ventricular tachycardia)

of death or arrythmia events. In patients with extracardiac sarcoid and LGE or RV involvement on MRI, the patients are at high risk of death or ventricular arrythmias independent of LVEF.[29] Recent findings have also shown that amount of FDG uptake on PET has correlated with the overall prognosis.[36] Recent studies have also shown that RV involvement is also associated with worsened survival.[36]

CONCLUSION

Cardiac sarcoidosis is not an uncommon disorder in tertiary cardiac centers. It is believed to be present in at least a fifth or more of patients with systemic sarcoidosis. However, isolated cardiac sarcoidosis without any evidence of systemic sarcoidosis is frequently encountered in clinical practice. Establishing a definitive diagnosis in such patients is challenging as demonstration of noncaseating granulomas even on EMB has a very low yield. Use of multimodality imaging involving echocardiography, cardiac MRI, Gallium DOTA-NOC, and ^{18}FDG–PET scans combined with clinical presentation helps in arriving in a probable diagnosis of sarcoidosis. Clinical management is directed at addressing disease activity, conduction disturbance, and arrhythmias along with heart failure and risk of sudden death.

ONLINE REFERENCES

Please scan the QR code provided at the end of the table of contents for References of this chapter.

CHAPTER

87 Restrictive Cardiomyopathy: An Overview

Ajay Bahl

ABSTRACT

Restrictive cardiomyopathy is a rare cardiomyopathy associated with severe diastolic dysfunction (restrictive physiology) with normal or near-normal ventricular wall thickness without increase in ventricular volumes. Three common causes of restrictive cardiomyopathy in India include (1) idiopathic restrictive cardiomyopathy, (2) amyloidosis, and (3) endomyocardial disease which includes endomyocardial fibrosis and hypereosinophilia-associated disease. Idiopathic restrictive cardiomyopathy is the most common form of restrictive cardiomyopathy in young individuals and is often a genetic disorder caused by mutations in sarcomeric genes.

Keywords: Restrictive cardiomyopathy, genotyping, amyloidosis, endomyocardial fibrosis.

INTRODUCTION

Restrictive cardiomyopathies (RCMs) are disorders of diastolic function. Diastolic dysfunction may vary from mild to severe. Restrictive physiology is at the extreme end of the spectrum and indicates severe diastolic dysfunction. Higher filling (atrial) pressures are needed to overcome the increased ventricular stiffness. Thus, only small increases in ventricular volume result in marked rise in diastolic ventricular pressure. RCM is a rare cardiomyopathy associated with restrictive physiology and with normal or near-normal ventricular wall thickness with normal or reduced in ventricular volumes and relatively preserved systolic function.[1-3] In some types of RCM, systolic dysfunction may occur late in the course of the disease. Both ventricles are usually affected, though involvement of either right or left ventricle may dominate the clinical picture. There is increasing realization that many cardiomyopathies including several types of RCM are familial. These familial forms are commonly Mendelian disorders caused by a single mutation and transmitted in an autosomal dominant pattern. The common causes of RCM in India are idiopathic RCM, amyloidosis, and endomyocardial disease **(Box 1)**. Endomyocardial disease includes endomyocardial fibrosis (EMF) and hypereosinophilia-associated disease. Idiopathic RCM is the most common cause of RCM in young individuals whereas amyloidosis is usually found in older individuals. Other causes of RCM are rare and listed in **Box 2**.

IDIOPATHIC RESTRICTIVE CARDIOMYOPATHY

Idiopathic RCM is the most common form of RCM encountered in young individuals. As the genetic basis of this entity has been recognized, many of the patients have been reclassified as familial/genetic RCM.

So, what is idiopathic RCM? Idiopathic RCM is a disorder that overlaps with the hypertrophic cardiomyopathy (HCM) spectrum.[4,5] HCM is a disorder of diastolic function.

BOX 1 Common causes of RCM in India.

- Idiopathic RCM (often genetic and familial)
- Amyloidosis
- Endomyocardial disease:
  - Endomyocardial fibrosis
  - Hypereosinophilia

(RCM: restrictive cardiomyopathy)

The diastolic dysfunction may vary from mild to severe in patients with HCM. Approximately 1.5% patients with HCM have diastolic dysfunction severe enough to be classified as restrictive physiology.[5] Similarly, the HCM spectrum varies from no or mild hypertrophy to severe left ventricular hypertrophy. Patients with normal left ventricular wall thickness and restrictive physiology are said to have idiopathic RCM **(Fig. 1)**. Patients with restrictive physiology and left ventricular hypertrophy are diagnosed to have HCM with restrictive physiology. RCM and HCM with restrictive physiology are thus overlapping disorders with a similar pathophysiology and only a few millimeters difference in the left ventricular wall thickness **(Fig. 2)**.[6] Histologically also they are similar in having myocardial fibrosis and myocyte disarray. Etiologically idiopathic RCM and HCM are also similar. Like HCM, idiopathic RCM is also caused by mutations in cardiac sarcomere encoding genes in 33–66% cases. In idiopathic RCM, mutations are most commonly found in troponin I (*TNNI3*) and myosin heavy chain (*MYH7*) genes.[5-7] There is some difference in the spectrum of mutations in RCM and HCM. *TNNI3* mutations are far more common in RCM and HCM with restrictive physiology than in other more common forms of HCM. This indicates that mutations in *TNNI3* are disproportionately higher in RCM. However, mutations in other sarcomeric genes such as *MYH7* are common in both HCM and RCM. Mutations in the gene encoding desmin also cause RCM.

Even though RCM and HCM have similar etiopathogenesis, the clinical course is often very different. Patients with idiopathic RCM are more symptomatic and have much poorer long-term outcomes.[5] They have a high incidence of heart failure, atrial fibrillation, and a higher mortality. No specific treatment is available for idiopathic RCM. The aim of treatment is relief of heart failure symptoms using diuretics. These patients have biatrial enlargement and are at risk for developing atrial fibrillation. Any episode of atrial fibrillation warrants oral anticoagulation. Anticoagulation should be continued indefinitely even after a single episode of atrial

BOX 2 Etiology of RCM.

Familial:
- Sarcomeric protein mutations
  - Troponin I
  - β-myosin heavy chain
  - Others
- Desminopathy
- Familial amyloidosis
- Fabry disease
- Hemochromatosis
- Unknown mutation

Nonfamilial:
- Amyloidosis
- Endomyocardial disease
  - Endomyocardial fibrosis
  - Hypereosinophilia
- Radiation
- Metastatic cancer
- *Drugs:* Chloroquine, anthracyclines, busulfan, and ergotamine
- Carcinoid

(RCM: restrictive cardiomyopathy)

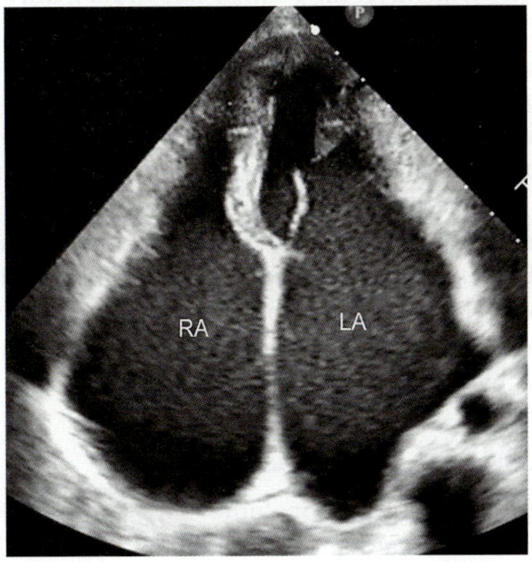

FIG. 1: Idiopathic restrictive cardiomyopathy. Normal ventricular size and wall thickness with marked biatrial enlargement.
(LA: left atrium; RA: right atrium)

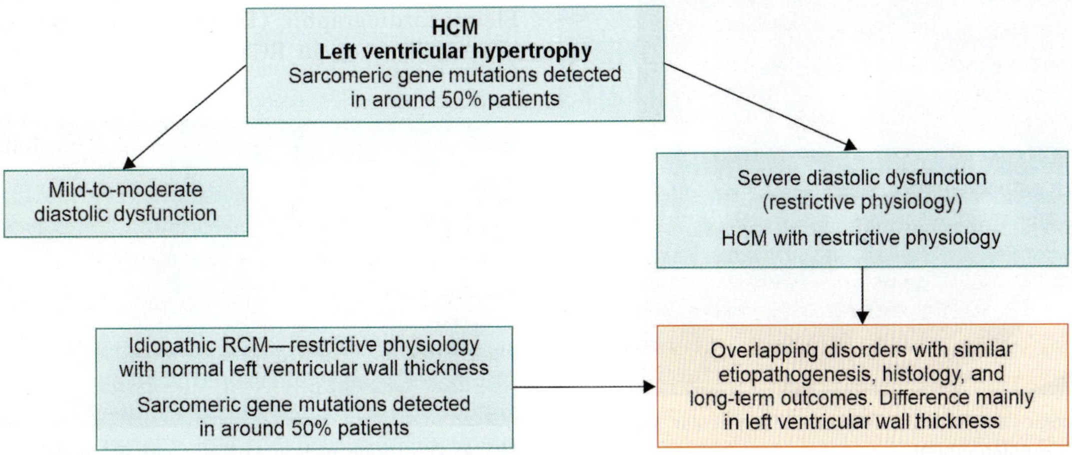

FIG. 2: The overlapping spectrum of idiopathic restrictive cardiomyopathy (RCM) and hypertrophic cardiomyopathy (HCM).

fibrillation. Oral anticoagulation is indicated even if the CHA_2DS_2-VASc score is zero. Patients with advanced heart failure should be considered for heart transplant.

AMYLOIDOSIS

Amyloidosis is caused by deposition of abnormal amyloid proteins in the interstitium. Primary amyloidosis (AL amyloidosis) and transthyretin amyloidosis cause RCM. Of these, AL amyloidosis is most commonly encountered. Transthyretin amyloidosis is being increasingly recognized especially in elderly patients with heart failure and preserved ejection fraction.[8] However, the prevalence of transthyretin amyloidosis in India is not known. Transthyretin is a transport protein synthesized in the liver, which was earlier called prealbumin. Transthyretin amyloidosis due to wild type transthyretin is called senile systemic amyloidosis. Familial transthyretin amyloidosis is caused by deposition of mutant transthyretin chains. Secondary amyloidosis rarely involves the heart. It is due to serum amyloid A protein deposition secondary to an underlying inflammatory disorder.

Primary amyloidosis is a multisystem disorder. Cardiac and renal involvements are the most important prognostic indicators. In addition to restrictive physiology, increased left ventricular wall thickness, conduction system abnormalities, and left ventricular systolic dysfunction may be present **(Fig. 3)**. AL amyloidosis is due to clonal plasma cell proliferation and the disease spectrum overlaps with multiple myeloma.

ENDOMYOCARDIAL DISEASE

Endomyocardial disease includes EMF and hypereosinophilia-associated cardiac involvement. Both these disorders are similar morphologically and may involve either or both ventricles. Biventricular or right ventricular involvement is more common. Isolated left ventricular involvement is uncommon. EMF is seen in the tropical regions. In India, EMF is most common in Kerala. The prevalence of EMF is decreasing.[9,10] Both EMF and hypereosinophilia initially have an inflammatory stage followed by a fibrotic phase. The fibrotic phase is characterized by dense EMF mainly involving the apices and inflow parts of the ventricles. In advanced cases, fibrosis may extend into the underlying myocardium. Ventricular thrombi may be seen especially in the inflammatory phase. Involvement of the mitral and tricuspid valvular apparatus is important and results in regurgitation. Imaging using echocardiography, MRI, or ventriculography typically shows obliteration and of ventricular apices and dilated atria.

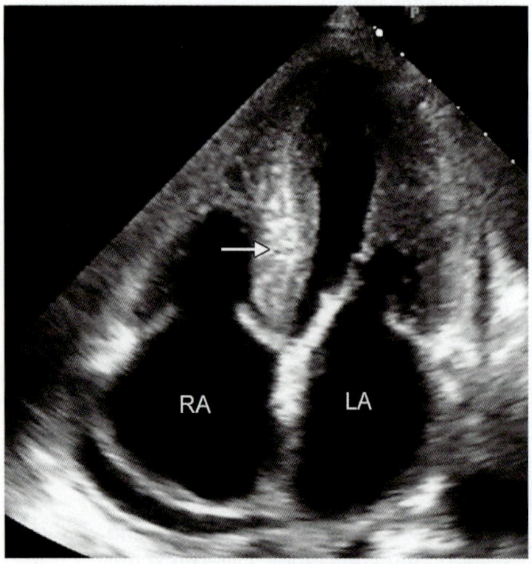

FIG. 3: Cardiac amyloidosis. Thickened ventricular walls with marked biatrial enlargement.

(LA: left atrium; RA: right atrium; arrow: thick ventricular septum)

CLINICAL PRESENTATION

Patients with RCM typically present with features of both left and right ventricular failure. Right-sided findings are often prominent, and RCM is an important differential diagnosis of right heart failure. Symptoms include exertional breathlessness, orthopnea, swelling of feet, abdominal distension, and palpitations. Atrial enlargement and raised atrial pressures predispose to atrial fibrillation.

Pulse is low or normal volume and the jugular venous pressure is raised with a positive Kussmaul sign. Right heart failure features such as tender hepatomegaly, pedal edema, ascites, and pleural effusion may be present. Carpel tunnel syndrome, macroglossia, dystrophic nails, and Raccoon's eye in a patient with RCM should raise suspicion of amyloidosis **(Fig. 4)**. The apical impulse is localized and normally located. Third and fourth heart sounds may be heard. Fourth heart sound is often absent in amyloidosis. This is due to amyloid infiltration causing atrial systolic dysfunction. Soft pansystolic murmurs of mitral and tricuspid regurgitation may be heard.

INVESTIGATIONS

Electrocardiographic (ECG) abnormalities are almost universally seen in RCM patients. Atrial enlargement

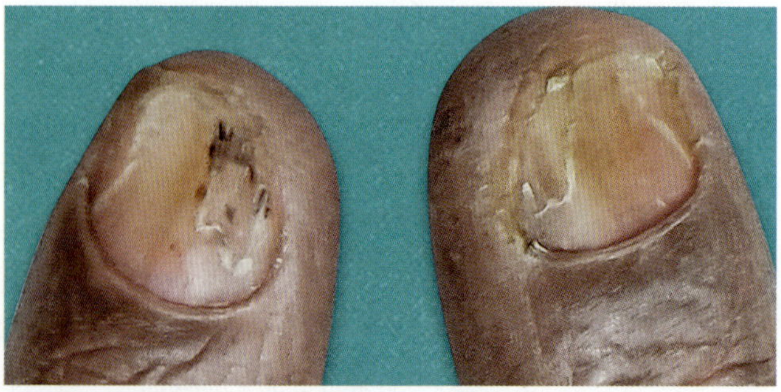

FIG. 4: Dystrophic nails in a patient with AL amyloidosis.

(AL: primary)

is commonly seen in patients with sinus rhythm. Atrial fibrillation may be present. In idiopathic RCM, the ECG findings are nonspecific and include intraventricular conduction defects, increased QRS voltage, and ST-T wave abnormalities. However, QRS voltage is usually normal in most patients. Typical ECG abnormality in amyloidosis is low voltage in limb leads **(Fig. 5)**. Precordial leads usually have normal voltage. Low limb lead voltage despite increased left ventricular wall thickness suggests amyloidosis. Chest X-ray typically shows cardiomegaly. Features of pulmonary venous hypertension are common. Pleural effusions may be seen in patients with heart failure. Cardiomegaly is due to atrial enlargement since the ventricular size is normal. Plasma brain natriuretic peptide levels are often raised and have prognostic importance. Imaging modality of choice is echocardiography. Presence of biatrial enlargement with normal sized ventricles is a typical finding and should immediately raise suspicion of RCM. Long-standing atrial fibrillation is a differential diagnosis and can also give rise to prominent biatrial enlargement. Restrictive filling pattern is seen on Doppler echocardiography. Patients with amyloidosis usually have increased ventricular wall thickness with a granular sparkling appearance, thickened interatrial septum, valvular thickening, and impaired left ventricular contractility in late stages. EMF patients typically have obliteration of ventricular apices. Involvement of valvular apparatus may cause mitral and tricuspid regurgitation. On catheterization, dip and plateau pattern is seen on both left and right ventricular pressure tracings. Cardiac MRI is useful in the evaluation of RCM. MRI findings include increased biventricular wall thickness, normal sized ventricular cavities, and late gadolinium subendocardial enhancement. Genotyping to detect underlying mutation is useful in patients with idiopathic RCM. Endomyocardial biopsy is useful in confirming the etiology especially in AL amyloidosis. Histologically idiopathic RCM and HCM are similar.

DIFFERENTIAL DIAGNOSIS

Constrictive pericarditis is the most important differential diagnosis. Constrictive pericarditis should not be missed since it is a treatable condition. Clinical findings of RCM and constrictive pericarditis are similar. Right heart failure is often prominent in both the conditions. There are, however, some differences. Prominent y descent in the jugular pulse is more common in constrictive pericarditis. Pulsus paradoxus occurs in one-third patients with constrictive pericarditis and is absent in RCM. A prominent apical impulse suggests RCM. Pericardial knock heard in constrictive pericarditis while third and fourth heart sounds may be present in RCM. Due to larger atrial size, plasma brain natriuretic peptide levels are higher in patients with RCM. Pericardial calcification may be seen on chest X-ray

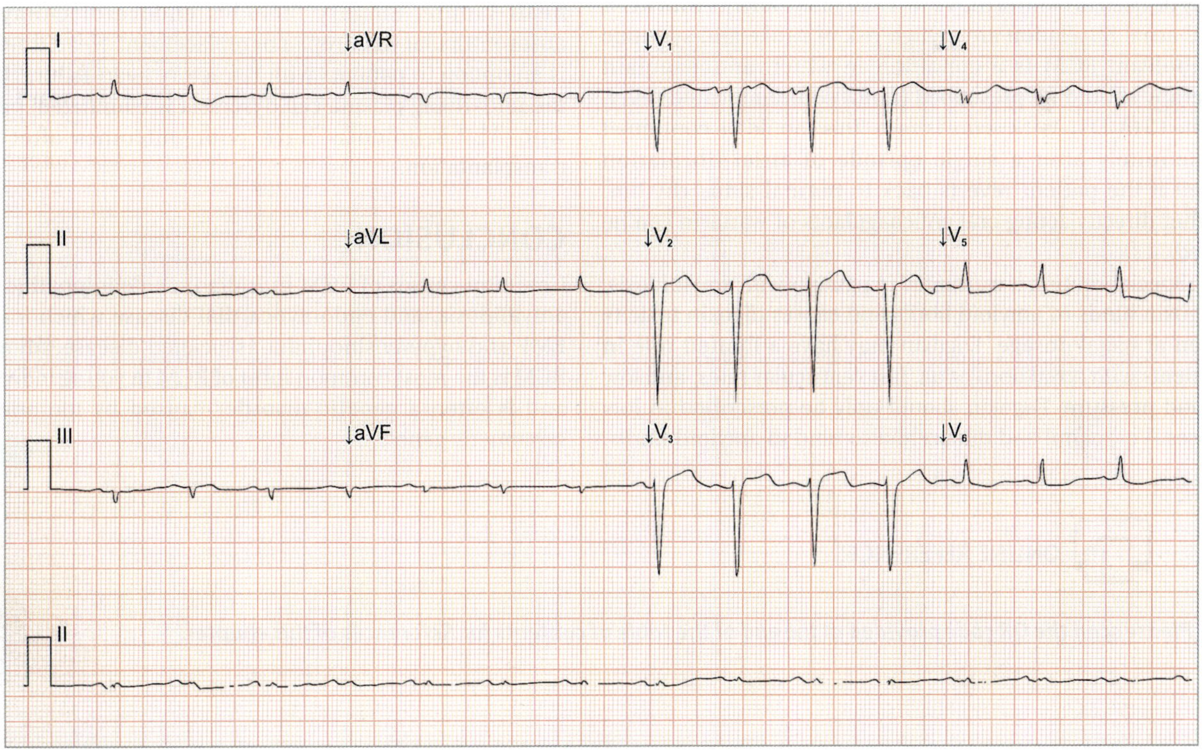

FIG. 5: ECG in a patient with AL amyloidosis shows low limb lead QRS voltages.
(AL: primary)

and especially in long-standing cases. Pericardial thickness is measured on CT scan or MRI. Pericardial thickening is not essential for diagnosis and is absent in 15% cases. The basic difference is that due to pericardial constraint, ventricular interdependence is seen in constrictive pericarditis but absent in RCM. Ventricular interdependence determines the difference in physiology between the two conditions. When the left ventricular volume increases in expiration, the right ventricular volume correspondingly decreases and vice versa. Ventricular interdependence results in septal bounce and increased respiratory variations in flow velocities on echocardiography. On cardiac catheterization, right and left ventricular end-diastolic pressures equalize. In addition, right ventricular end-diastolic pressure is usually greater than one-third of the right ventricular systolic pressure in patients with constrictive pericarditis. Patients with RCM are more likely to have pulmonary hypertension. Right ventricular systolic pressure ≥50 mm Hg favors RCM.

TREATMENT

Patients with RCM have systemic and pulmonary venous congestion. Loop diuretics are the drugs of choice for relief from breathlessness and systemic venous congestion. Atrial fibrillation is common and may cause marked aggravation of symptoms due to loss of atrial kick which is important for these patients. Conversion to sinus rhythm using electrical cardioversion or anti-arrhythmic drugs like amiodarone can be attempted. Beta-blockers or calcium channel blockers may be used to control the ventricular rate. Patients with RCM and atrial fibrillation are at high risk of stroke and systemic embolism. RCM is a condition in which anticoagulant therapy should be prescribed (if not contraindicated) even if the CHA_2DS_2-VASc score is zero. This should be continued indefinitely after a single episode of atrial fibrillation even if the patient reverts back to normal sinus rhythm. Either directly acting oral anticoagulants or warfarin can be used.

Special caution is warranted in patients with amyloidosis. Digoxin binds to amyloid fibrils and causes digoxin toxicity even at usual dosage. Digoxin may have a limited role in patients with atrial fibrillation, fast ventricular rates, and low blood pressure. Digoxin should only be prescribed in low doses. Verapamil and diltiazem also bind to amyloid fibrils. They can thus cause profound hypotension and should be avoided. Angiotensin-converting enzyme inhibitors and angiotensin receptor blockers may also cause hypotension. They may be considered in patients with reduced left ventricular ejection fraction and should only be initiated in low doses under close supervision.

Definitive treatment is not available for idiopathic RCM. In patients with AL amyloidosis, the underlying plasma cell dyscrasia is treated. Treatment typically involves combination of daratumumab, bortezomib, cyclophosphamide, and dexamethasone.[11] Melphalan-based regimens may also be used. Autologous stem cell transplant is usually not considered in patients with advanced cardiac involvement. Iron chelation therapy and phlebotomy may improve cardiac function in patients with hemochromatosis. Tafamidis, a transthyretin tetramer stabilizer, improves outcomes in patients with transthyretin amyloidosis.[12]

Patients with sarcoidosis and AL amyloidosis may develop high-grade heart blocks requiring pacemaker therapy. Cardioverter defibrillator may be implanted for prevention of sudden death in patients with extensive scarring or sustained ventricular tachyarrhythmias. Patients with familial/idiopathic RCM are also at risk of sudden death. Implantable cardioverter-defibrillator should be considered in patients with family history of premature sudden death, recurrent unexplained syncope, sustained ventricular arrhythmias, and extensive late gadolinium enhancement on cardiac MRI. Surgical treatment should be considered in patients with EMF with refractory heart failure. Surgery includes endocardiectomy with atrioventricular valve repair or replacement. Heart transplant is an option in patients with refractory heart failure. Unless the underlying plasma cell dyscrasia is eliminated, patients with AL amyloidosis have poor outcomes after heart transplantation.

CONCLUSION

Common causes of RCM in India include idiopathic RCM, amyloidosis, and endomyocardial disease which includes EMF and hypereosinophilia-associated disease. Idiopathic RCM is the most common form of RCM in young individuals and is often a genetic disorder caused by mutations in sarcomeric genes.

ONLINE REFERENCES

Please scan the QR code provided at the end of the table of contents for References of this chapter.

CHAPTER

88 An Overview of Takotsubo Cardiomyopathy

K Meenakshi, MS Ravi, R Rameshwar, SR Sharath Shanmugam

ABSTRACT

Takotsubo cardiomyopathy (TC) is one form of stress cardiomyopathy, with symptoms that mimic acute myocardial infarction, and characterized by typical wall-motion abnormalities, rapidly reversible heart failure, and absence of obstructive coronary artery disease (CAD). It occurs in 1–3% of people and 5–6% of women presenting with clinical features of ST-elevation myocardial infarction (STEMI). There are four types of TC based on the mode of ballooning but other types have been recently included. The exact pathophysiological mechanism is unknown. Catecholamine excess and hyperactivity of sympathetic nervous system are the most popular hypothesis, though transient coronary spasm or occlusion, microvascular dysfunction, and inflammatory mechanisms have been suggested. TC is most often precipitated by stress and occurs generally in postmenopausal women and is often associated with psychological and neurological disease. Clinical features, electrocardiography (ECG) changes with elevated troponin are often similar to acute coronary syndrome, which makes diagnosis of TC a challenge. The characteristic wall motion abnormalities with apical ballooning and basal hyperkinesis resembling a Japanese Octopus pot, seen in the classical variety clinches the diagnosis. Coronary arteries are generally normal, but rarely obstructed CAD can be a bystander disease. The management is as for acute STEMI. Although rapidly reversible in the majority, in-hospital mortality has been reported in 1.2–4.2% and recurrence is about 10%. Further research is needed to understand the pathophysiology and to devise more effective management strategies.

Keywords: Takotsubo cardiomyopathy, stress induced cardiomyopathy, apical ballooning syndrome, broken heart syndrome.

INTRODUCTION

Takotsubo cardiomyopathy (TC), broken heart syndrome, or apical ballooning syndrome is one form of stress cardiomyopathy, with symptoms that mimic acute myocardial infarction (MI), and characterized by typical regional wall-motion abnormalities, rapidly reversible heart failure and absence of obstructive coronary artery disease (CAD). Recent studies have claimed that patients with TC can continue to have subtle ongoing cardiac dysfunction, despite restoration of left ventricular ejection fraction (LVEF).

Sato et al. coined the term TC to describe a reversible acute heart failure syndrome, where the shape of the LV during systole, resembled a Japanese octopus trapping pot.

EPIDEMIOLOGY

Takotsubo cardiomyopathy occurs in 1–3% of people and 5–6% of women presenting with clinical features of ST-elevation myocardial infarction (STEMI).[1] 90% of TC patients are females >60 years.[2] Women > 55 years have a fivefold higher risk of developing TC than women <55 years and a 10-fold higher risk than men. TC has also been diagnosed in children and the youngest reported was a premature neonate born at 28 weeks of gestation.[3] It is common in Caucasians and is less often seen in African-Americans and Hispanics. TC prevalence in men is higher in Japan.

CLASSIFICATION

There are four types of TC based on the mode of ballooning **(Box 1 and Figs. 1A to D)**.[4]

Other types include[5] biventricular [apical type and right ventricular (RV)] involvement,[6] isolated RV (which has the worse outcome),[7] and global form.[5]

Global hypokinesia is often difficult to diagnose as TC because of the other causes of global hypokinesia such as tachycardia-induced cardiomyopathy and myocarditis.

BOX 1 Types of takotsubo cardiomyopathy.

Classification of takotsubo cardiomyopathy based on ballooning pattern:

- *Takotsubo type*: Apical akinesia and basal hypercontraction
- *Reverse takotsubo*: Basal akinesia and apical hypercontraction
- *Mid ventricular type*: Mid ventricular ballooning and basal/apical hypercontraction
- *Localized type*: Any other segmental ballooning when takotsubo-like left ventricular dysfunction is present

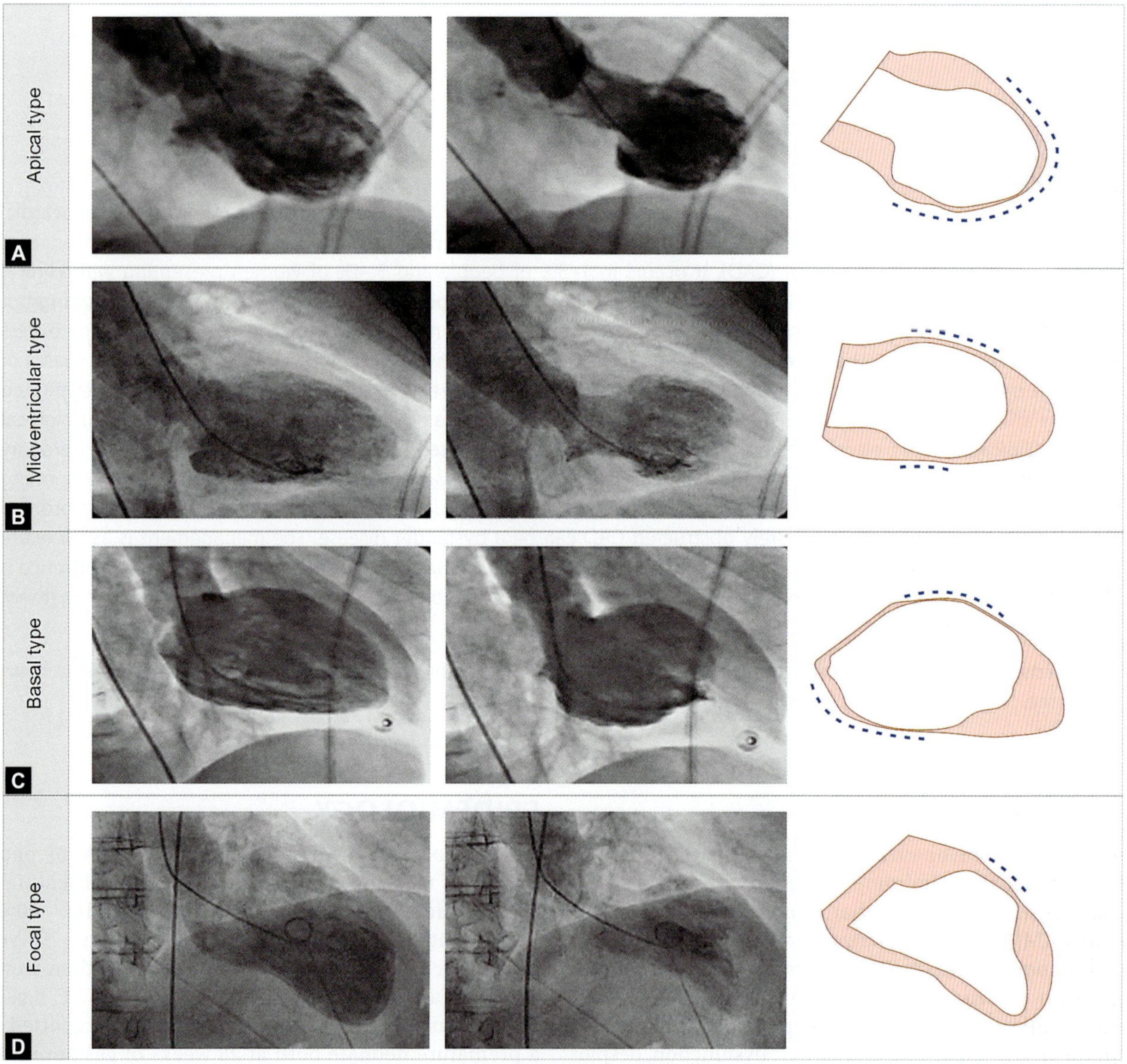

FIGS. 1A TO D: Left ventricular angiogram in different types of takotsubo cardiomyopathy.

Patients with recurrent TC can demonstrate different wall motion patterns at each event.

PATHOPHYSIOLOGY

The exact pathophysiological mechanism remains to be known, though several hypotheses have been put forth.

Catecholamine Excess and Hyperactivity of Sympathetic Nervous System

Endogenous adrenergic surge is the most established theory for the pathogenesis of TC.

That a brain-heart axis and interaction exists are shown by the observations that 20–30% with psychological stress, physical illness, which also has an element of psychological stress, preexisting, or acute psychiatric illness and acute neurological injury can develop transient LV systolic dysfunction.[6]

Current evidence indicates that TC is caused by an acute release of catecholamines in response to physical or psychological stress in subjects with increased susceptibility of the coronary microcirculation and cardiac myocytes to catecholamines. Serum catecholamine levels were reported to be 20 times higher in TC patients than in normal adults and two to three times higher than in MI patients.[7] Analyses of heart rate variability have also demonstrated sympathetic predominance and depression of parasympathetic activity during the acute phase. Endomyocardial biopsies revealed occasional contraction band necrosis, which is generally observed in clinical settings of extreme catecholamine production as in pheochromocytoma or subarachnoid hemorrhage. The severe wall motion abnormalities seen in TC are transient suggesting that protective mechanisms are likely to operate to preserve myocardial integrity.

Activation of myocardial survival or protective pathways: Studies have revealed that there is apical-basal gradients of β_2 adrenergic receptors (β_{2ARs}) and sympathetic innervation in mammalian LV, and the apex contains the highest β_{2ARs} and the lowest sympathetic nerve density. Normally an increased apical responsiveness to catecholamines occurs because of this ventricular β_{2ARS} gradient. With high levels of epinephrine, there is a molecular transition from Gs (stimulatory and positive inotropic) protein to Gi (inhibitory and negatively inotropic) protein signaling through the β_{2AR} resulting in a negative inotropic effect which is maximum in apex where the β_{ARs} density is highest.

The switch from Gs to Gi coupling, thus causing a negative inotropic response, which limits the myocardial response to the excess catecholamine.[6]

Paur et al. produced a rat model in which high intravenous epinephrine bolus resulted in a reversible apical ballooning followed with basal hypercontraction.

Oxidative stress response to excess catecholamine: Recent reports suggest that the underlying mechanism of LV dysfunction in TC is due to excess catecholamines-induced oxidative stress. However, it is unclear whether oxygen free radicals are due to excess catecholamines or due to microvascular changes or myocyte injury.

A surge of adrenoreceptor stimulation can dysregulate myocardial calcium handling or can cause myocellular hypoxia leading to reduced function.

Metabolic and energetic alterations: Derangements in the glucose metabolism and decrease in Krebs cycle substrates can cause metabolic stunning and may explain why patients continue to be symptomatic and have recurrent events despite apparent recovery of LVEF.[6]

Transient Multivessel Epicardial Coronary Artery Spasm

It can cause transient myocardial stunning without any lasting injury. However, provocative were able to provoke spasm in only 28% of these patients.[8]

Transient Coronary Artery Occlusion/Reperfusion Episodes Caused by Plaque Rupture that is not Visualized in the Coronary Angio

Animal models have, however, not supported this theory.[9] Intravascular ultrasound and optical coherence tomography have failed to identify ruptured plaques in the vast majority of TC patients.

Microvascular Spasm due to Excessive Catecholamine

Reduction of myocardial perfusion as assessed by thrombolysis in myocardial infarction (TIMI) frame count or myocardial perfusion imaging has been noticed in TC but studies are limited.[6]

Myocardial Stunning due to Microvascular Dysfunction

Local impairment of fatty acid metabolism can cause myocardial stunning. Kurisu et al. reported severe impairment of fatty acid metabolism than myocardial perfusion in the hypokinetic areas, during the early stages of TC using rest thallium-201 and single-photon emission computed tomography (SPECT) studies.[6]

Inflammatory Mechanisms

Presence of an inflammatory myocardial infiltrate rich in macrophage, changes in the distribution of monocyte subsets, and an increase in systemic proinflammatory cytokines could support that persistent subacute or chronic inflammation may contribute to long-term cardiac dysfunction.[10]

Persistent or Preexisting Syndrome

The HEROIC study's demonstration in TC patients, preserved ejection fraction (EF), limitation on exercise testing, reduced apical myocardial rotation during systole, microscopic fibrosis, and mild elevation of brain natriuretic peptide (BNP), raises the doubt whether there was a preexisting subtle and undiagnosed cardiomyopathy that is brought to light during an acute stressful event. If this were the case, then it would explain the cases with persistent cardiac symptoms or persistent cardiac dysfunction.[11]

Smaller LV Size Predisposing to Dynamic LV Outflow Tract Obstruction

Excess catecholamine may induce a dynamic left ventricular outflow tract (LVOT) obstruction causing dilatation of LV apex due to increase in intracavitary pressure.[12]

Infective Agent such as a Viral Illness

No infective agent has been isolated from TC patients till now.

Risk Factors

Possible risk factors for TC are reviewed here:

- *Hormonal factors*: Relative deficiency of estrogen TC occurs more in postmenopausal women hypothesizing that postmenopausal women lose the protective effect of estrogens which make them more prone to the excess of circulating catecholamines. Ueyama et al. showed that higher increase of the heart rate and reduction in LV function occurred in ovariectomized rats when compared to the rats that had estradiol supplementation.[13]
- *Genetic factors*: A report of five cases of familial TC, in combinations of mother daughters and sisters, suggests a genetic predisposition or a genetic-environmental interaction, or a polygenic etiology in TC.[14] However, no definite Mendelian inheritance pattern has been identified. Polymorphisms in adrenergic genes have been, however, identified.

Psychiatric and Neurologic Disorders

Psychiatric or neurologic disorders were substantially higher in TC than in acute coronary syndrome (ACS). 27% gave history of an acute, chronic, or former neurologic disorder such as stroke and seizures and 42% had a psychiatric disorder, 50% of which was depression. A few studies have found a high incidence of type-D-personality in TC patients which is characterized by negative emotions and social inhibition. Patients with depression, panic disorders, and anxiety have an exaggerated norepinephrine response to emotional stress, and decreased reuptake of norepinephrine and may facilitate myocardial stunning by increasing local levels of catecholamines.[6]

TABLE 1: Physical and psychological triggers.

Psychological triggers		Physical stressors
Traumatic emotions	**Positive emotions**	**Strenuous sport and heavy gardening**
Grief	Happy heart syndrome	Medical conditions and medical procedures
Interpersonal conflicts	Pleasant surprise	Acute respiratory failure, pneumothorax and thyrotoxicosis
Fear, panic, anger, and anxiety	Victory	Cholecystitis and pancreatitis
Assault and defeat	Gain	Trauma and sepsis
Public speaking	Winning a jackpot	Malignancy and chemotherapy
Financial or employment problems	Wedding	Pregnancy and cesarean section
Embarrassment	Birth of a child	Drowning and hypothermia
Natural disasters	Positive job interview	Alcohol and opiate withdrawal
		Pheochromocytoma

Triggers (Table 1)

Sharkey et al. reported that 89% with TC had experienced some form of extreme stress,[15,16] 12 hours prior to the onset of symptoms. Higher incidence of TC was noticed after earthquakes in Japan. The International Takotsubo Registry reported that reverse TC (rTC) presented more often with a neurological disorder and classical TC with an acute psychiatric episode.[17] Endogenous catecholamine spillover related to pheochromocytoma serves as a distinct physical trigger. Physical triggers are more common in males and emotional triggers in females. Sometimes both may be present.

DIAGNOSTIC CRITERIA

Similarities with ACS makes diagnosis of TC a challenge. Several criteria have been put forth, viz., the mayo clinic criteria in 2004 which was modified in 2008,[18] after which several criteria have been put forth **(Box 2)**. All have their limitations in atypical TC. Most of the criteria have excluded pheochromocytoma as a cause of TC. The Japanese criteria include the pheochromocytoma storm in TC.

BOX 2 International Takotsubo Diagnostic Criteria (Inter TAK Diagnostic Criteria).

1. Patients show transient[a] left ventricular dysfunction (hypokinesia, akinesia, or dyskinesia) presenting as apical ballooning or midventricular, basal, or focal wall motion abnormalities. Right ventricular involvement can be present. Besides these regional wall motion patterns, transitions between all types can exist. The regional wall motion abnormality usually extends beyond a single epicardial vascular distribution; however, rare cases can exist where the regional wall motion abnormality is present in the subtended myocardial territory of a single coronary artery (focal takotsubo syndrome)[b]
2. An emotional, physical, or combined trigger can precede the takotsubo syndrome event, but this is not obligatory
3. Neurologic disorders (e.g., subarachnoid hemorrhage, stroke/transient ischemic attack, or seizures) as well as pheochromocytoma may serve as triggers for takotsubo syndrome
4. New electrocardiographic (ECG) abnormalities are present (ST-segment elevation, ST-segment depression, T-wave inversion, and QTc prolongation); however, rare cases exist without any ECG changes
5. Levels of cardiac biomarkers (troponin and creatine kinase) are moderately elevated in most cases; significant elevation of brain natriuretic peptide is common
6. Significant coronary artery disease is not a contradiction in takotsubo syndrome
7. Patients have no evidence of infectious myocarditis[b]
8. Postmenopausal women are predominantly affected

Note:

[a]Wall motion abnormalities may remain for a prolonged period of time or documentation of recovery may not be possible. For example, death before evidence of recovery is captured.

[b]Cardiac magnetic resonance imaging is recommended to exclude infectious myocarditis and diagnosis confirmation of takotsubo syndrome.

Clinical Presentation

Clinical presentation is most often similar to ACS. Patients usually present with acute onset chest pain (68%) and breathlessness (17%) and mild-to-moderate heart failure. Syncope and out-of-hospital cardiac arrest are rare. Cardiogenic shock has been reported in 1.5%. Furthermore, it has been reported that patients of African-American descent have more in-hospital complications such as respiratory failure and stroke and require mechanical ventilation more frequently, compared to Caucasians and Hispanics.[8]

Electrocardiography

Electrocardiography (ECG) changes are similar to acute STEMI[6] with ST elevation in 70–80%, T wave changes in 64%, transient Q wave in 32%, and new bundle-branch block and QTc interval prolongation. A few have reported that the magnitude of the ST changes may not be as severe as STEMI atrial and ventricular arrhythmias, QT prolongation and torsades de pointes can occur.

Cardiac Enzymes

Troponin is elevated, which is less than with STEMI, BNP, NT-proBNP, and C-reactive protein were higher in TC than in STEMI. Several proinflammatory, interleukin- and anti-inflammatory cytokines can be raised at presentation and can continue to remain elevated for several months thereafter, reflecting the inflammatory pathophysiology.[19]

Coronary Angiography

Takotsubo cardiomyopathy is associated with absence of obstructive CAD in 75%. Spontaneous fibrinolysis of the clot and STEMI cannot be ruled out. Rarely, TC can, by chance, occur in the presence of obstructive CAD which is not the cause of the acute event.

Echocardiography

Distinct wall motion abnormality occurs in TC. The wall motion abnormality in typical TC is apical ballooning caused by akinesia/hypokinesia of the apical and mid ventricular LV and hyperkinesia of the basal LV. However, other combinations of akinesia and hyperkinesia can occur. The regional wall motion abnormality (RWMA), however, occurs beyond the distribution of a single coronary artery. There is also a reduction in global systolic function with an EF ranging from 25 to 50% in the initial ECHO which improves dramatically over days. RWMA corresponding to a single coronary artery can occur in focal TC. Global longitudinal strain by speckle tracking can be reduced even after the EF returns to normal. Approximately 20% have evidence of LVOT obstruction.[15]

The wall motion abnormality is also detected in the LV angiogram.

Cardiac Magnetic Resonance Imaging

Cardiac magnetic resonance imaging (MRI) is useful in differentiating TC from other conditions associated with chest pain, elevated troponin, and absent obstructive CAD, particularly MINOCA and myocarditis.[15] MRI in TC shows no late gadolinium enhancement as seen in STEMI or myocarditis. Absent gadolinium enhancement supports the myocardial stunning hypothesis in TC. A characteristic pattern of takotsubo syndrome rarely appears as a thin transmural band of fibrosis at the hinge points between the hyperkinetic base and dyskinetic apex. Intense myocardial edema is an important finding in TC.

Reverse takotsubo cardiomyopathy constitutes 1–23% of patients with TC. It seen at a younger age than classical TC, has less reduction of LVEF, higher incidence of neurological disease, and can be triggered by intracranial hemorrhage. Patients with rTC exhibited significantly higher levels of plasma epinephrine in comparison to the patients with TC. No significant differences were detected in plasma norepinephrine levels. The conclusion of the International Takotsubo Registry study is that ST-segment elevation, atrial fibrillation, and T-wave inversion were more common in typical TC while rTC presented more often with ST-segment depression and QTc prolongation.[16,17]

MANAGEMENT

The management at admission is as for acute STEMI, with continuous ECG monitoring and administration of aspirin, intravenous heparin, angiotensin-converting enzyme inhibitors (ACEIs) and β-blockers. Early diagnosis of TC is mandatory to avoid thrombolysis in nonpercutaneous coronary intervention (PCI) centers. Congestive heart failure occurs in 20% and diuretics should be given. Patients may present with hypotension at admission, either because of the LV dysfunction or because of the rare incidence of LVOT obstruction and intra-aortic balloon pump (IABP) rather than inotropes is recommended especially if hypotension occurs in the setting of the catecholamine-induced dynamic LVOT obstruction. When mechanical support is not available, low-dose levosimendan is licensed in some countries as a catecholamine-sparing positive inotrope. Peripheral vasoconstrictors such as phenylephrine may be advocated to increase afterload and LV cavity size and vasodilators, such as nitrates should be used with caution or not at all as the reduction in preload can worsen the dynamic LVOT obstruction. Arrhythmia can occur and magnesium sulfate is preferred to antiarrhythmics. Intracavity thrombus can occur due to the akinetic ventricular segments. Anticoagulation, with heparin and thereafter with warfarin for 3 months, is indicated irrespective of the heart rhythm. Anxiolytic drugs to reduce the stress can be use as supportive therapy. Renin–angiotensin drugs can usually be withdrawn once LV function has fully recovered. New treatments modalities in animals are underway such as estrogen treatment and use of adenosine and endothelin antagonist. Long-term beta-blockers to reduce recurrence is also being studied. Patients with concomitant CAD (bystander disease) should continue to receive preventative therapies including antiplatelet, statin, and ACEI therapies.[6]

PROGNOSIS

Although generally rapidly reversible, in-hospital mortality has been reported as 1.2–4.2%. Male patients had higher mortality compared to female (8% vs. 3.6%,). Complications, though rare are cardiac failure and thromboembolic strokes. In the majority who survive the acute phase, LV function starts improving by the first few days, and complete recovery is seen within months. Long-term survival is no different from the general age-matched population. Rate of in-hospital complications is comparable to that with ACS (21% vs. 19%). Recurrence rate is about 10%. Age < 50 years, male sex, LVEF < 45%, atrial fibrillation, physical triggers, and neurologic disease cardiac troponin concentration > 10-fold the upper normal limit were associated with increased 1-year mortality. Dyspnea, lethargy, and fleeting chest pains can persist for ≥2 years after the index of the event despite the normalization LVEF.[20]

CHRONOBIOLOGY

Evidence suggest that acute cardiac events can have chronobiological patterns. Two studies have reported a peak occurrence of TC in the morning and afternoon hours.[20] Two have observed the highest frequency on Monday and most studies reported a summer preference.[6]

PITFALLS IN DIAGNOSIS

Concomitant CAD can occur in 10–29% and patients with TC and bystander obstructive CAD are often wrongly diagnosed as ACS as differentiation can be challenging. Presence of obstructive CAD cannot be used as an exclusion criterion for TC. In TC wall motion, abnormalities extend beyond the territory of the obstructed coronary artery. Sometimes, ACS itself may trigger TCA ruptured plaque that can be missed in CAG and the need for intravascular imaging may be mandatory. Functional coronary vasculopathy as in MINCOA should be kept in mind before diagnosing TC.

FUTURE DIRECTIONS

International Takotsubo Registry which has launched a 10-year follow-up study in patients with takotsubo syndrome, the NACRAM trial on the early use of N-acetylcysteine and ramipril in TC (101) and BROKEN-SWEDE-HEART study to determine the possible treatment guidelines and interventions in TC are a few to name.[21]

CONCLUSION

Takotsubo cardiomyopathy is becoming more recognized, though diagnosis still remains challenging and it has to be distinguished from other causes of acute myocardial injury. Further research is needed to shed light on the pathophysiology and to devise more effective treatment and prevention strategies.

ONLINE REFERENCES

Please scan the QR code provided at the end of the table of contents for References of this chapter.

CHAPTER

89

Prediction of Sudden Cardiac Death in Hypertrophic Cardiomyopathy

Biswajit Majumder, Ratul Ghosh, Shibsankar Sarkar

ABSTRACT

Hypertrophic cardiomyopathy (HCM) is one of the most common cardiomyopathies detected worldwide. Incidence of sudden cardiac death (SCD) is very common in it. SCD can even be the very first manifestation of previously undetected HCM. Ventricular arrhythmias are the most common cause of SCD. Whereas it is impossible to accurately predict SCD in HCM, both American College of Cardiology (ACC)/American Heart Association (AHA) and European Society of Cardiology (ESC) have identified certain risk factors that can attribute to SCD. There are certain specific guidelines to use those risk factors cautiously to make preventive decisions. Implantable cardioverter defibrillator (ICD) implantation is the mainstay of primary prevention in HCM patients. More studies are required to find a balance between number of lives saved and the risks of ICD implantations complications. More consciousness among general population and even healthcare professionals is needed regarding risk factors of SCD in HCM and timely intervention.

Keywords: Hypertrophic cardiomyopathy, sudden cardiac death, implantable cardioverter defibrillator, risk predictor.

INTRODUCTION

Hypertrophic cardiomyopathy (HCM) is mostly inherited as an autosomal dominant genetic cardiomyopathy with estimated general population prevalence of approximately 1 in 500. HCM is one of the most common causes of sudden cardiac death (SCD) among young populations worldwide and it can even be the first manifestation of asymptomatic young patients with HCM. The estimated annual risk of SCD is 1%. SCD in HCM is caused mainly by ventricular arrhythmias. Appropriate utilization of implantable cardioverter defibrillators (ICDs) has resulted in significantly improved outcomes. The standard approach to the patient with HCM involves advice about family genetic screening and surveillance, risk stratification for SCD, and management of symptoms. Both American College of Cardiology/American Heart Association Joint Committee on Clinical Practice Guidelines and European Society of Cardiology (ESC) have laid down certain guidelines for risk stratification in HCM patients.

SUDDEN CARDIAC DEATH AND UNDERLYING MECHANISMS

In published series, SCD is the most common cause of death in young HCM patients.[1] SCD in HCM is caused mainly by ventricular fibrillation. The majority of ventricular arrhythmias occur while the patient is in normal sinus rhythm and are often preceded by premature ventricular complexes.[2] Ventricular fibrillation can also be precipitated by runs of ventricular tachycardia, atrial fibrillation with fast ventricular response, or accelerated atrioventricular (AV) nodal conduction.[3-6] In addition to ventricular fibrillation, asystole and pulseless electric activity have both been reported in association with SCD.[7] Advanced AV nodal block also has a role,[8] but its contribution to SCD is not properly known.

There are many possible mechanisms for ventricular arrhythmias. Intraventricular dispersion of conduction, attributed to myocyte hypertrophy, disarray, and fibrosis, provides alternative pathways for conduction and thus promotes re-entry.[9] Intercalated disks are disrupted hampering smooth conduction of action potentials and promoting anatomic re-entry. Increased myocyte calcium sensitivity causes shorter effective refractory periods and increased dispersion of repolarization capable of generating functional re-entry.[10] Abnormal intracellular calcium handling also leads to inhibition of physiological proteolytic pathways leading to accumulation of calcium handling proteins and may also give rise to after-depolarizations. A vicious cycle of increasing myocardial ischemia due to ventricular hypertrophy and less dense myocardial capillary network, left ventricular outflow tract obstruction (LVOTO), systemic hypotension, and decreased stroke volume may precipitate SCD both during exertion and rest even during sleep.[11]

RISK FACTORS OF SUDDEN CARDIAC DEATH IN HYPERTROPHIC CARDIOMYOPATHY

Various phenotypic characteristics have been conventionally linked with SCD. These risk factors were first recognized in small observational studies, and then they were re-examined in larger studies with multivariate analysis using the Cox proportional hazards model with SCD as the endpoint (composite of actual SCD, aborted SCD ± appropriate ICD shocks). Most HCM studies have used a modified cardiac arrhythmia suppression trial definition of SCD. It defines SCD as death of cardiac origin, occurring unexpectedly within 1 hour of the onset of new symptoms or a death that was unwitnessed and unexpected, unless a specific noncardiac cause of death is found.[12] *Among patients with HCM, younger patients are at higher risk for SCD than older patients.*

Proportion of SCD events in HCM patients from diagnosis was 8–10% for SCD events in childhood. There is no sex- or race-based differences in SCD risk.[13,14] Over several decades, multiple studies have focused on identification of major risk factors that identify high-risk patients who may be candidates for SCD prevention with ICD implantation. This risk identification and stratification and the use of ICDs into clinical practice have significantly decreased mortality.[15] The evolution of SCD risk assessment has resulted in the removal of abnormal blood pressure response to exercise as a routine part of the SCD risk evaluation. The current conventional SCD risk markers (AHA/ACCF 2020 guideline based) that are used to evaluate risk level in HCM patients and to identify those patients most likely to benefit from primary prevention ICD therapy are discussed **(Table 1)**.

TABLE 1: SCD estimation according to 2020 ACC/AHA HCM guideline.

COR	LOE	Recommendations
1	B-NR	1. In patients with HCM, a comprehensive, systematic noninvasive SCD risk assessment at initial evaluation and every 1–2 years thereafter is recommended and should include evaluation of these risk factors a. Personal history of cardiac arrest or sustained ventricular arrhythmias b. Personal history of syncope suspected by clinical history to be arrhythmic c. Family history in close relative of premature HCM-related sudden death, cardiac arrest, or sustained ventricular arrhythmias d. Maximal LV wall thickness, EF, LV, and apical aneurysm e. Nonsustained ventricular tachycardia episodes on continuous ambulatory electrocardiographic monitoring
1	B-NR	2. For patients with HCM who are not otherwise identified as high risk for SCD, or in whom a decision to proceed with ICD placement remains uncertain after clinical assessment that includes personal/family history, echocardiography, and ambulatory electrocardiographic monitoring, CMR imaging is beneficial to assess for maximum LV wall thickness, EF, LV apical aneurysm, and extent of myocardial fibrosis with late gadolinium enhancement
2a	B-NR	3. For patients who are ≥16 years of age with HCM, it is reasonable to obtain echocardiography-derived left atrial diameter and maximal left ventricular outflow tract gradient to aid in calculating an estimated 5-year sudden death risk that may be useful during shared decision-making for ICD placement

(ACC: American College of Cardiology; AHA: American Heart Association; COR: class of recommendation; HCM: hypertrophic cardiomyopathy; ICD: implantable cardioverter defibrillator; LOE: level of evidence; SCD: sudden cardiac death)

Source: Ommen S, Mital S, Burke M, Day SM, Deswal A, Elliott P, et al. 2020 AHA/ACC Guideline for the Diagnosis and Treatment of Patients With Hypertrophic Cardiomyopathy. J Am Coll Cardiol. 2020;76(25):e159-240.

Family History of Sudden Death from HCM

Sudden death judged definitively or likely attributable to HCM in more than one first-degree or close relative who are <50 years of age. Close relatives would generally be second-degree relatives; however, multiple SCDs in tertiary relatives should also be considered relevant. Aggregation of SCD in families of patients with HCM was noted by Donald Teare in his study of HCM in 1958.[16] The effect of family history of SCD is related to the *genetic nature* of the disease. Affected relatives share the same genetic defect and almost have similar environmental exposures.

Massive Left Ventricular Hypertrophy

Massive left ventricular hypertrophy (LVH) is defined as wall thickness ≥30 mm in any segment of left ventricle by echocardiography or cardiac magnetic resonance (CMR) imaging and consideration is also given to borderline values of ≥28 mm in individual patients at the discretion of the treating cardiologist. For pediatric patients, an absolute or z-score threshold for wall thickness has not been established; however, a maximal wall thickness that corresponds to a z-score ≥20 (and >10 in conjunction with other risk factors) is acceptable. Severe LVH may contribute to SCD because of its harmful effects on myocardial architecture, myocardial oxygen demand, coronary vascular resistance, and capillary density. LVH is associated with increasing prevalence of nonsustained ventricular tachycardia (NSVT) and exercise-induced ventricular arrhythmias.

Most studies have used *maximum wall thickness* (MWT), defined as the greatest thickness in any segment of the left ventricle as a marker of the severity of hypertrophy. The use of MWT has a number of limitations. All studies have included MWT as a binary or ordinal variable rather than a continuous variable. MWT ≥30 mm has been almost universally used to signify severe hypertrophy, but this cut-off is not based on any specific biological properties conferred by this particular wall thickness. MWT measurements are subject to observer variability, and poor echocardiographic windows may prevent adequate assessment of all myocardial segments. Furthermore, the thickness of a single myocardial segment may not adequately represent the true burden of hypertrophy. As, for example, a MWT of 20 mm in a patient with exclusively apical HCM is not prognostically equivalent of a MWT of 20 mm in a patient with hypertrophy involving all myocardial segments.[17]

Unexplained Syncope

Unexplained syncope is defined as more than one unexplained episodes involving acute transient loss of consciousness, judged by history unlikely to be of neurocardiogenic (vasovagal) etiology, nor attributable to LVOTO, and especially when occurring within 6 months of evaluation (events beyond 5 years in the past do not appear to have relevance). There are many causes of syncope in HCM such as atrial fibrillation, supraventricular tachycardias, bradyarrhythmias including AV nodal blocks, sustained ventricular arrhythmias, abnormal vascular responses to exercise and exertion, exercise-related LVOTO, mitral regurgitation, myocardial ischemia, neurally mediated syncope (vasovagal, situational, and carotid sinus syncope), and orthostatic hypotension.[18]

Hypertrophic Cardiomyopathy with LV Systolic Dysfunction

Systolic dysfunction with *ejection fraction (EF) < 50%* by echocardiography or cardiovascular magnetic resonance (CMR) imaging. Implantation of ICD in HCM patients with systolic dysfunction has been advised by some investigators. They also have suggested that systolic impairment should be considered as another independent risk factor for SCD. This is based on their observation that HCM patients with impaired systolic function received appropriate ICD therapies at a rate similar to previously reported HCM patients with aborted SCD.[19]

Left Ventricular Apical Aneurysm

Apical aneurysm is defined as a discrete thin-walled dyskinetic or akinetic segment of the most distal portion of the LV chamber independent of its size. It has been postulated that extensive myocyte fibrosis and disarray result in myocardial thinning and aneurysm formation giving rise to ventricular tachycardia and fibrillation.

Extensive Late Gadolinium Enhancement on CMR Imaging

Diffuse and extensive late gadolinium enhancement (LGE) on CMR, representing fibrosis, either quantified or estimated visually, comprising ≥15% of LV mass is one of the risk factors of SCD in HCM. LGE in CMR signifies the presence of extracellular myocardial collagen deposition. The presence of LGE is often associated with impaired systolic function and other risk factors for SCD, in particular NSVT.[20] In a recent study of 217 patients with HCM, the presence and extent of LGE were associated with increased cardiovascular morbidity and mortality.[21]

Nonsustained Ventricular Tachycardia on Ambulatory Monitor

Nonsustained ventricular tachycardia has been recognized and well-established as a risk factor for SCD in HCM patients. Higher importance is given to NSVT as a risk marker when runs are frequent (≥3), longer (≥10 beats), and faster (≥200 bpm) occurring usually over 24–48 hours of monitoring. For pediatric patients, a VT rate that exceeds the baseline sinus rate by >20% is considered significant. NSVT is more common with increasing LVH, which indicates increased myocardial fibrosis and disarray. In a recent systematic review, the average reported hazard ratio (HR) for NSVT (irrespective of definition) was 2.89 [95% confidence interval (CI) 2.2–3.6].[18] Even though the prevalence of NSVT increases with age, the risk of SCD associated with NSVT may be lower in older patients. Monserrat et al. showed that NSVT in patients aged ≤30 years was associated with a fourfold increase in the risk of SCD (univariable HR 4.35; 95% CI 1.54–12.28; $p = 0.006$), but there was no effect in older patients (univariable HR 2.16; 95% CI 0.82–5.69; $p = 0.1$).[22]

In 2014, the *ESC created an SCD-risk prediction model* that provides a 5-year SCD risk score for HCM patients. Several new risk factors, including age, left atrial diameter (LAD), and left ventricular outflow track obstruction (LVOTO), were added. The latest *2020AHA/ACCF guidelines* have added HCM with left ventricular systolic dysfunction, left ventricular apical aneurysm (LVAA), and extensive LGE on CMR imaging as established clinical risk factors for SCD in HCM patients. Some studies have also reported other risk factors associated with SCD risk, such as the B-type natriuretic peptide (BNP) level, atrial fibrillation, and the New York Heart Association (NYHA) functional class.

To calculate *estimated SCD 5-year risk* estimates for adults with HCM, another two echocardiographic parameters are needed—LAD and maximal instantaneous LVOT gradient.

Left Atrial Diameter or Left Atrial Volume

Left atrial size serves as a marker of chronic elevation in left atrial pressure. LA pressure may remain chronically elevated due to summation of impaired LV diastolic function, mitral regurgitation, and atrial arrhythmias which is very common among HCM patients. Among patients without documented atrial fibrillation, enlarged LAD was an independent determinant of SCD risk. But there was no significant difference in SCD risk between patients with and without enlarged LAD who had documented atrial fibrillation. This implies that the relationship between LAD and SCD is influenced by the presence or absence of atrial fibrillation in HCM patients.[23]

Left Ventricular Outflow Tract Obstruction

The LVOTO is defined as a peak instantaneous left ventricular outflow tract pressure gradient, measured by Doppler echocardiography, of at least 30 mm Hg either at rest or with provocation. Studies showed that a left ventricular outflow tract pressure gradient of at least 30 mm Hg have twofold risk for SCD.[24] LVOTO as a risk factor for SCD in HCM patients has certain limitations, because the left ventricular outflow pressure gradient is subjected to dynamic changes and can be influenced by many external environmental factors and routine daily activities.[25]

The ESC 2014 HCM risk-SCD formula is as follows:

$$\text{Probability}_{SCD\ at\ 5\ years} = 1 - 0.998^{\exp\ (\text{Prognostic index})}$$

Where prognostic index = [0.15939858 × maximal wall thickness (mm)] – [0.00294271 × maximal wall thickness^2 (mm^2)] + [0.0259082 × LAD (mm)] + [0.00446131 × maximal (rest/Valsalva) left ventricular outflow tract gradient (mm Hg)] + [0.4583082 × family history SCD] + [0.82639195 × NSVT] + [0.71650361 × unexplained syncope] – [0.01799934 × age at clinical evaluation (years)]

Risk Stratification Considerations in Pediatric Patients

Risk stratification for SCD in children has been based on risk markers derived from adult HCM studies. Adult risk factors have limited ability to predict SCD in pediatric patients. Lack of robust large-scale population-based studies caused lack of defined risk factors in pediatric age group. In a systematic review including all previous studies of pediatric HCM patients, four clinical factors have consistently came up. These are—previous aborted cardiac arrest or sustained VT, unexplained syncope, NSVT, and extreme LVH. Decision regarding ICD placement must be based on individual judgment, taking into account all age-appropriate risk markers, strength of the risk factors identified, the overall clinical profile of the patient, the level of risk acceptable to the patient and family, and the potential complications related to ICD, including psychological impact and inappropriate ICD shock. Recent studies suggest that LAD z-score is positively associated, while resting LVOT gradient is not associated with SCD risk in children.

Patient Selection for ICD Placement

With new studies and newer diagnostic methods including identification of novel risk markers and newer comprehensive scoring strategies, risk stratification and selection of patients for prophylactic ICD therapy continue to evolve. The proven efficacy of the ICD in aborting potentially life-threatening ventricular tachyarrhythmias and saving lives has placed increasing emphasis on the importance of timely identifying patients at risk of SCD. Patients with HCM are considered potential candidates for primary prevention ICDs who have more than one major risk markers which have a high sensitivity in predicting those patients at greatest risk for SCD.

Primary prevention ICD decision-making is often complex and challenging. In addition, the relatively young age of patients with HCM considered for SCD prevention means risk periods can often extend over many years of an individual patient's life. For these reasons, decisions regarding primary prevention ICD therapy should include a discussion with patients that includes risk for SCD and the benefit of ICD therapy in aborting life-threatening ventricular tachyarrhythmias along with the fact that long-term device therapy can be associated with complications.

Hypertrophic cardiomyopathy patients who have experienced a previous documented cardiac arrest or hemodynamically significant VT/VF remain at significantly increased risk for future life-threatening events and should, therefore, be strongly considered for ICD therapy as secondary prevention **(Flowchart 1; Tables 2 and 3)**.

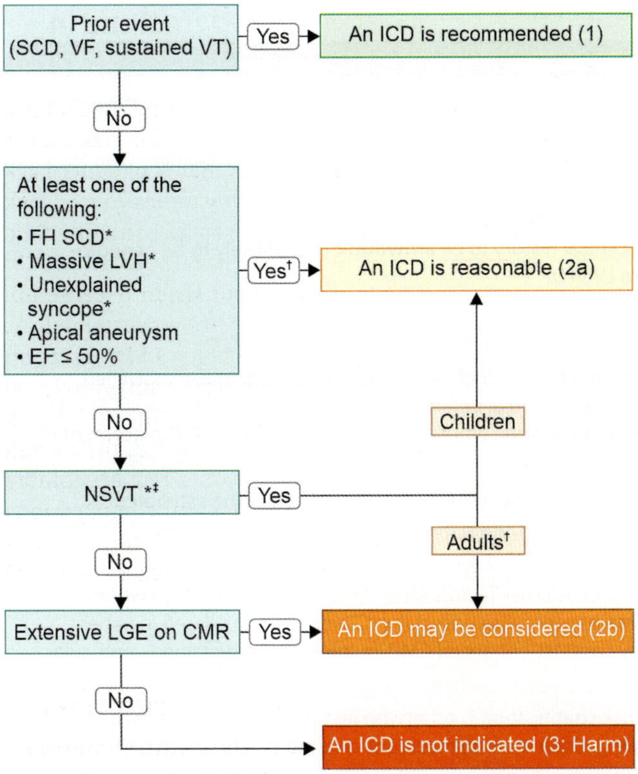

*ICD decisions in pediatric patients with HCM are based on ≥1 of these major risk factors: family history of HCM SCD, NSVT on ambulatory monitor, massive LVH, and unexplained syncope.

†In patients >16 years of age, 5-year risk estimates can be considered to fully inform patients during shared decision-making discussions.

‡It would seem most appropriate to place greater weight on frequent, longer, and faster runs of NSVT.

FLOWCHART 1: ACC/AHA 2020 algorithm for ICD implantation in HCM patients.

(ACC: American College of Cardiology; AHA: American Heart Association; CMR: cardiovascular magnetic resonance; EF: ejection fraction; FH: family history; HCM: hypertrophic cardiomyopathy; ICD: implantable cardioverter-defibrillator; LGE: late gadolinium enhancement; LVH: left ventricular hypertrophy; NSVT: nonsustained ventricular tachycardia; SCD: sudden cardiac death; VT: ventricular tachycardia)

Source: Ommen S, Mital S, Burke M, Day SM, Deswal A, Elliott P, et al. 2020 AHA/ACC Guideline for the Diagnosis and Treatment of Patients With Hypertrophic Cardiomyopathy. J Am Coll Cardiol. 2020;76(25):e159-240.

SUDDEN CARDIAC DEATH RISK PREDICTION: FUTURE DIRECTIONS

Genetic Factors

There are >50 genes and nearly 8,000 variants related to HCM in published studies. *MYBPC3* and *MYH7*, coding cardiac myosin-binding protein C and β-myosin heavy chain, respectively, are the two most common affected genes. A large meta-analysis reported 5% SCD in MYBPC3, 11% in MYH7, *17% in TNNT2*, and 0.4% in mutation-negative HCM. *Troponin T mutations have been associated with a high incidence of SCD, despite milder hypertrophy.* SCD rate was significantly higher in any mutation-positive group than in mutation-negative one.[26] Recently, Fahed et al. studied that the *TNNI3*p. Arg 21 Cys mutation can lead to extremely high rate of early onset SCD, sometimes accompanied by myocardial thinning and cardiac enlargement. It is sometimes called malignant HCM.[27] Other mutations associated with high SCD risk are—*MYL3*, *FLNC*, and *NXN* mutation. Several large-scale studies are required to ascertain significance of these genetic factors in routine SCD risk prediction.

Cardiac Biomarkers

Studies have found that an increase in B-type natriuretic peptide (BNP) and NT-proBNP, galectin-3, high-sensitive troponin T level is related to the occurrence of malignant ventricular arrhythmia and/or SCD.[28]

Other Factors

In some studies, *atrial fibrillation* (more importantly chronic atrial fibrillation) is associated with a high risk of SCD.[29]

Electrocardiogram Analysis

Several electrocardiogram (ECG) parameters such as T-wave amplitude in V2, pseudoinfarction pattern with ST elevation, QRS duration ≥120 ms and low QRS voltage, QRS fragmentation, QTc duration, Tpe (interval between the peak and the end of the electrocardiographic T wave) interval, and

TABLE 2: Recommendation regarding ICD in 2020 ACC/AHA guideline.

COR	LOE	Recommendations
1	C-EO	1. In patients with HCM, application of individual clinical judgment is recommended when assessing the prognostic strength of conventional risk marker(s) within the clinical profile of the individual patient, as well as a thorough and balanced discussion of the evidence, benefits, and estimated risks to engage the fully informed patient's active participation in ICD decision-making
1	B-NR	2. For patients with HCM and previous documented cardiac arrest or sustained ventricular tachycardia, ICD placement is recommended

Continued

Continued

COR	LOE	Recommendations
2a	B-NR	3. For adult patients with HCM with ≥1 major risk factors for SCD, it is reasonable to offer an ICD. These major risk factors include: a. Sudden death judged definitively or likely attributable to HCM in ≥1 first-degree or close relatives who are ≤50 years of age b. Massive left ventricular hypertrophy ≥30 mm in any left ventricular segment c. ≥1 recent episodes of syncope suspected by clinical history to be arrhythmic [i.e., unlikely to be of neuro-cardiogenic (vasovagal) etiology, or related to LVOTO] d. LV apical aneurysm, independent of size e. LV systolic dysfunction (EF < 50%)
2a	B-NR	4. For children with HCM who have ≥1 conventional risk factors, including unexplained syncope, massive left ventricular hypertrophy, nonsustained ventricular tachycardia, or family history of early HCM-related SCD, ICD placement is reasonable after considering the relatively high complication rates of long-term ICD placement in younger patients
2a	B-NR	5. For patients ≥16 years of age with HCM and with ≥1 major SCD risk factors, discussion of the estimated 5-year sudden death risk and mortality rates can be useful during the shared decision-making process for ICD placement
2b	B-NR	6. In select adult patients with HCM and without major SCD risk factors after clinical assessment, or in whom the decision to proceed with ICD placement remains otherwise uncertain, ICD may be considered in patients with extensive late gadolinium enhancement by contrast-enhanced CMR imaging or nonsustained ventricular tachycardia present on ambulatory monitoring
2b	C-LD	7. In select pediatric patients with HCM in whom risk stratification is otherwise less certain, it may be useful to consider additional factors such as extensive late gadolinium enhancement on contrast-enhanced CMR imaging and systolic dysfunction in risk stratification
3: Harm	B-NR	8. In patients with HCM without risk factors, ICD placement should not be performed
3: Harm	B-NR	9. In patients with HCM, ICD placement for the sole purpose of participation in competitive athletics should not be performed

(ACC: American College of Cardiology; AHA: American Heart Association; CMR: cardiovascular magnetic resonance; COR: class of recommendation; EF: ejection fraction; HCM: hypertrophic cardiomyopathy; ICD: implantable cardioverter-defibrillator; LOE: level of evidence; SCD: sudden cardiac death)

Source: Ommen S, Mital S, Burke M, Day SM, Deswal A, Elliott P, et al. 2020 AHA/ACC guideline for the diagnosis and treatment of patients with hypertrophic cardiomyopathy. J Am Coll Cardiol. 2020;76(25):e159-240.

TABLE 3: Recommendation regarding ICD type in ACC/AHA 2020 guideline.

COR	LOE	Recommendations
1	B-NR	1. In patients with HCM who are receiving an ICD, either a single-chamber transvenous ICD or a subcutaneous ICD is recommended after a shared decision-making discussion that takes into consideration patient preferences, lifestyle, and expected potential need for pacing for bradycardia or ventricular tachycardia termination
1	B-NR	2. In patients with HCM who are receiving an ICD, single-coil ICD leads are recommended in preference to dual coil leads
2a	B-NR	3. In patients with HCM who are receiving an ICD, dual-chamber ICDs are reasonable for patients with a need for atrial or atrioventricular sequential pacing for bradycardia/conduction abnormalities, or as an attempt to relieve symptoms of obstructive HCM (most commonly in patients >65 years of age)
2a	C-LD	4. In selected adult patients with nonobstructive HCM receiving an ICD who have NYHA class II to ambulatory class IV HF, left bundle branch black (LBBB), and LV ejection fraction (LVEF) <50%, cardiac resynchronization therapy for symptom reduction is reasonable
2b	C-LD	5. In patients with HCM in whom a decision has been made for ICD implantation and who have paroxysmal atrial tachycardias or AF, dual-chamber ICDs may be reasonable, but this decision must be balanced against higher complication rates of dual chamber devices

(ACC: American College of Cardiology; AHA: American Heart Association; AF: atrial fibrillation; COR: class of recommendation; HCM: hypertrophic cardiomyopathy; ICD: implantable cardioverter-defibrillator; LOE: level of evidence; LV: left ventricular)

Source: Ommen S, Mital S, Burke M, Day SM, Deswal A, Elliott P, et al. 2020 AHA/ACC Guideline for the Diagnosis and Treatment of Patients With Hypertrophic Cardiomyopathy. J Am Coll Cardiol. 2020;76(25):e159-240.

Tpe/QTc ratio were studied as predictors for SCD.[30] Both *QRS fragmentation in ≥ three territories* and a heart rate corrected QT *(QTc) duration ≥ 460 ms* were associated with ventricular tachyarrhythmia and SCD in HCM patients. The negativity of the *electromechanical window*, defined as the interval between the Q wave and aortic valve closure minus the QT interval, is an independent risk factor for life-threatening arrhythmic events.[31]

In a study by Higuchi et al., the results showed that *renal dysfunction* may be associated with increased risk of SCD in patients with HCM. However, the results are not conclusive.[32]

T1 Mapping and Entropy on CMR in the Evaluation of Fibrosis

Focal myocardial fibrosis can be identified by LGE. Diffuse fibrosis is not well measured by standard LGE-CMR imaging, but it can be seen using postcontrast T1 mapping. In adult patients with HCM, diffuse fibrosis is a predictor of nonsustained VT by providing pathways for anatomic and functional re-entry. Entropy measures the uncertainty of tissue composition as reflected by the uncertainty of CMR signal intensity. Recently, the measurement of entropy was applied to evaluate heterogeneity in fibrotic lesions. Scar heterogeneity was shown to be independent risk indicator of ventricular arrhythmias and SCD.

CONCLUSION

The evaluation of risk factors for SCD in HCM patients is continuously evolving with many new risk factors coming up and some traditional risk factors losing importance. In our country, lack of awareness about HCM and underdiagnosis of these risk factors remain one of main reason of SCD. Often, SCD is the very first presentation of previously undiagnosed HCM patient. Prompt diagnosis of HCM, risk stratification for SCD, timely follow-up, and re-evaluation remains the key to prevent this tragic consequence. However, no matter how precise the risk estimation becomes, there will always be conflicts in finding a balance between the number of lives saved and the risks of ICD implantation complications. More studies involving newer technologies such as machine learning and smart devices may open up newer avenues toward prevention of SCD in HCM patients.

ONLINE REFERENCES

Please scan the QR code provided at the end of the table of contents for References of this chapter.

SECTION 10

Cardio Diabetes

CHAPTER 90

Paradigm Shift in Diabetes Care: From Glucocentric Approach to a Cardiometabolic Approach

PC Manoria, Pankaj Manoria

ABSTRACT

During the last couple of years, there has been a paradigm shift in diabetes care. For several years, the treatment of diabetes was nearly restricted to glycemic control, which no doubt decreased microvascular disease but did not have any impact on atherosclerotic cardiovascular disease (ASCVD), particularly in patients with long-standing diabetes. Later on, attention was focused on avoiding weight gain and hypoglycemia, which adversely affect diabetes care. But the paradigm shift in diabetes care kicked off after 2015, when several trials of sodium-glucose cotransporter-2 inhibitors (SGLT-2Is) and glucagon-like peptide-1 receptor agonists (GLP-1 RAs) showed improved cardiorenal outcomes. This initiated the dawn of new era in diabetes care. The SGLT-2Is can be used across the spectrum of heart failure, irrespective of the ejection fraction, and they also slow down the trajectory of chronic kidney disease and postpone dialysis by 10–15 years. The GLP-1 RA improved ASCVD outcomes on top of standard care. Both of these agents have been recommended by all guidelines across the globe. Therefore, we are currently amidst a new era of diabetes care that is powered to improve the cardiorenal outcome of type 2 diabetes mellitus.

Keywords: SGLT-2 inhibitors, GLP-1 RA, diabetes care, Cardiometabolic approach.

INTRODUCTION

For several years, the treatment of diabetes was merely focused on a glucocentric approach. The management of diabetes has witnessed three revolutions **(Table 1)**.

Prior to 2008, the treatment of diabetes was nearly restricted to a glucocentric approach. This, no doubt, minimizes microvascular disease but has no impact on macrovascular disease. After 2008, in addition to good glycemic control, attention was also focused on minimizing hypoglycemia and preventing weight gain, which adversely affects diabetes. However, after 2015, with the availability of sodium-glucose cotransporter-2 inhibitors (SGLT-2Is) and glucagon-like peptide-1 receptor agonists (GLP-1 RAs), a new era of improving cardiorenal outcomes has erupted.

About 70% of diabetics die because of acute myocardial infarction, and interestingly, we now have GLP-1 RAs, which decrease atherosclerotic cardiovascular disease (ASCVD) events on top of standard of care. The SGLT-2Is are a panacea for heart failure, and they can be used across the spectrum of heart failure, irrespective of ejection fraction. They are a boon for chronic kidney disease (CKD). They slow down the trajectory of CKD and postpone dialysis for 10–15 years. Therefore, the current approach to the treatment of diabetes has shifted from a glucocentric approach to a cardiometabolic approach. This approach focuses on all three components of the cardiorenal metabolic continuum.

GLUCOCENTRIC ERA

Prior to 2008, the treatment of diabetes was merely focused on glycemic control and assessing glycated hemoglobin (HbA1c). Starting in the 1950s and continuing until 2008, glycemic control reduced microvascular complications but failed to reduce macrovascular outcomes. The glucose-lowering options were limited to insulin, sulfonylureas, and biguanides. The University Group Diabetes Program (UGDP) carried out with tolbutamide showed increased mortality with sulfonylureas, but this trial has limitations.[1] This was followed by UK Prospective Diabetes Study (UKPDS) trial.[2,3]

TABLE 1: Three revolutionary eras for the treatment of type 2 diabetes mellitus.

S. No.	Era	Year	Main target	Strategy	Recommendations
1	Glucocentric	Before 2008	• HbA1c • The lower, the better, but close to the normal	Sulfonylureas insulin	ADA/EASD
2	• Glucocentric w/o hypoglycemia • No weight gain	2008–2015	• HbA1c • But without hypoglycemia and weight gain	• Biguanides • Acarbose, DPP-4i	ADA/EASD 2015
3	Improving cardiorenal outcomes	After 2015	Decreasing cardiorenal and HF events	• SGLT-2I and/or GLP-1 RA • Thiazolidinediones	• ADA/EASD 2018 • ACC/AHA 2019 • ESC/EASD 2019

(ACC: American College of Cardiology; ADA: American Diabetes Association; AHA: American Heart Association; DPP-4i: dipeptidyl peptidase-4 inhibitor; EASD: European Association for the Study of Diabetes; ESC: European Society of Cardiology; GLP-1 RA: glucagon-like peptide-1 receptor agonist; HbA1c: glycated hemoglobin; SGLT-2I: sodium-glucose cotransporter-2 inhibitor)

The aim of the trial was to lower HbA1c close to normal. Metformin became the initial choice for the majority of patients with type 2 diabetes mellitus (T2DM) who require pharmacotherapy based on the results of a relatively small substudy on obese patients with newly detected diabetes in the UKPDS trial.[3] The UKPDS trial failed to show any significant reduction in cardiovascular (CV) disease, but microvascular disease, as expected, was improved. But the 10-year post-trial follow-up showed a reduction in myocardial infarction and all-cause mortality due to the so-called legacy effect.[4]

The three landmark trials, (1) Action to Control Cardiovascular Risk in Diabetes (ACCORD),[5] (2) Action in Diabetes and Vascular Disease: Preterax and Diamicron Modified Release Controlled Evaluation (ADVANCE),[6] and (3) Veterans Affairs Diabetes Trial (VADT)[7] in patients with long-standing diabetes showed that tight glycemic control failed to show any decrease in CV events. On the contrary, the ACCORD trial showed an increase in all-cause mortality due to hypoglycemia.[8] The treatment intensifications were associated with weight gain and hypoglycemia, which reduced the benefits of glycemic control.

GLUCOCENTRIC ERA WITHOUT HYPOGLYCEMIA AND NO WEIGHT GAIN

Weight gain and hypoglycemia are two important barriers in the treatment of diabetes. Compared to nonobese individuals, the likelihood of being diabetic is twice as high in overweight and obese individuals. With every one unit increase in body mass index (BMI), the probability of being diabetic increases by 1.5% among overweight and obese individuals, compared to a 0.5% increase among nonobese individuals.

Moreover, weight gain during treatment of T2DM is clinically dangerous because every 3 kg gain offsets the benefit of a 1% decrease in HbA1c. Moreover, every kilogram (kg) gained due to T2DM increases the relative risk of heart failure by 7.1%. Not only does this 1 unit increase in BMI in the first year of diabetes increase the mortality risk by 12%. The risk of coronary heart disease (CHD) is also higher with increasing BMI in these patients.

IMPROVING CARDIORENAL OUTCOMES

After the landmark Empagliflozin, Cardiovascular Outcomes, and Mortality in Type 2 Diabetes (EMPA-REG)[9] outcome trial in 2015 and thereafter many other CV outcome trials with SGLT-2I and GLP-1 RAs, a new era of improving cardiorenal outcome has erupted, and this has totally changed the face of diabetes care. These trials were mandated by the US Food and Drug Administration following the rosiglitazone controversy to document the safety of new antidiabetic medications.

Sodium-glucose Cotransporter-2 Inhibitors

The SGLT-2Is have emerged as a panacea for heart failure and a boon for CKD. They can be used across the spectrum of heart failure. They are a boon for CKD because they slow down the trajectory of the disease and postpone dialysis by 10–15 years. They also improve the cardiometabolic profile by decreasing weight and blood pressure. They are available in oral formulation, and dapagliflozin has become off-patent and is available at a cheap rate across the country. SGLT-2Is are therefore rightly designated as the molecule of the decade.

The EMPA-REG OUTCOME trial[9] carried out in patients with diabetes gave a big surprise in 2015 when it showed a statistically significant reduction in the primary endpoint of three-point major adverse cardiovascular events (MACE) by 14% **(Table 2)**. It also showed a decrease in hospitalization

TABLE 2: Trials of SGLT-2 inhibitors in the diabetic population.

	n	ASCVD	Primary outcome	HR (95% CI) *p* value
EMPA-REG OUTCOME	7,020	100%	MACE	0.86 (0.74–0.99); $p = 0.04$ for superiority
CANAVAS	10,142	71%	MACE	0.86 (0.75–0.97); $p = 0.02$ for superiority
DECLARE TIMI 58	17,160	40.5%	MACE	0.93 (0.84–1.03); $p = 0.17$
			Composite of CV death or hospitalization for HF	0.83 (0.73–0.95); $p = 0.005$
VERTIS CV	8,246	100%	MACE	0.97 (0.85–1.11); $p \leq 0.001$ for noninferiority

(ASCVD: atherosclerotic cardiovascular disease; CI: confidence interval; CV: cardiovascular; MACE: major adverse cardiovascular event; HF: heart failure; HR: hazard ratio; SGLT-2: sodium-glucose cotransporter-2)

for heart failure, a decrease in CV mortality, and all-cause mortality. The trial was carried out in patients with ASCVD. The Canagliflozin and Cardiovascular and Renal Events in Type 2 Diabetes (CANVAS) trial[10] also showed a similar reduction in three-point mortality by 14%, but CV mortality and all-cause mortality were not decreased because it was a mixed population of diabetic patients with 71% having ASCVD and 29% having only risk factors. However, it did show a decrease in hospitalizations for heart failure, like the above trial. The Dapagliflozin and Cardiovascular Outcomes in Type 2 Diabetes (DECLARE TIMI 58)[11] trials showed a decrease in hospitalization for heart failure, but the three-point MACE was not affected because only 40% of patients had ASCVD. However, the subgroup analysis of the CANVAS and DECLARE TIMI 58 trials showed that patients with ASCVD also showed a reduction in three-point MACE. Both of these trials gave the message that mortality benefit is seen only in the secondary prevention group, i.e., in patients with ASCVD, and not in the primary prevention group. Curiously enough, the Cardiovascular Outcomes with Ertugliflozin in Type 2 Diabetes (VERTIS CV) trials[12] which had 100% patients with ASCVD, failed to show a reduction in three-point MACE, but it did decrease hospitalization for heart failure.

The SGLT-2Is have improved outcomes in all subsets of patients with heart failure. The Dapagliflozin in Patients with Heart Failure and Reduced Ejection Fraction (DAPA-HF)[13] and Cardiovascular and Renal Outcomes with Empagliflozin in Heart Failure (EMPEROR Reduced) trial[14] in heart failure with reduced ejection fraction (HFrEF), the Empagliflozin in Heart Failure with a Preserved Ejection Fraction (EMPEROR Preserved),[15] and the DELIVER (Dapagliflozin Evaluation to Improve the Lives of Patients With Preserved Ejection Fraction Heart Failure) trial[16] in HFpEF showed improved outcome with SGLT-2Is. Patients with mildly reduced ejection fraction also showed benefit. Therapy with SGLT-2Is and other guideline-directed medications for HF should never be stopped even when the ejection fraction improves, the so-called subset of heart failure with improved ejection fraction. The SGLT-2I EMPULSE (EMPagliflozin in patients hospitalized with acUte heart faiLure who have been StabilizEd) trial[17] with empagliflozin in patients with acute decompensated heart failure and the SOLOIST-WHF (Effect of Sotagliflozin on Cardiovascular Events in Patients With Type 2 Diabetes Post Worsening Heart Failure) trial[18] with sotagliflozin in patients with worsening heart failure also showed improved outcomes.

Therefore, SGLT-2Is, unlike other guideline-directed drugs for heart failure, can be used across the spectrum of heart failure **(Table 3)**.

Mechanism of Action: SGLT-2 Inhibitors in Heart Failure

The SGLT-2Is have multifaceted actions, but their exact mechanism of action is not yet clear. But what is important is that they do act and produce multiple beneficial effects.

Data is also emerging on the use of SGLT-2Is in patients with acute myocardial infarction **(Table 4)**.[19]

SGLT-2 Inhibitors in Chronic Kidney Disease

The SGLT-2Is not only benefit heart failure, but they also improve CKD outcomes. The hint for their renoprotective effect came from the clinical trials of SGLT-2 in patients with T2DM and high CV risk and trials of SGLT-2Is in heart failure. Later on, dedicated trials were conducted to evaluate their renoprotective effects **(Table 5)**. All three trials of SGLT-2I, i.e., Canagliflozin and Renal Outcomes in Type 2 Diabetes and Nephropathy (CREDENCE),[20] Dapagliflozin in Patients with Chronic Kidney Disease (DAPA-CKD),[21] and Empagliflozin in Patients with Chronic Kidney Disease (EMPA-CKD)[22] were prematurely terminated because of the immense benefit in renal outcome. They slowed down the trajectory of CKD by slowing declining estimated glomerular filtration rate (eGFR) and postponing dialysis by 10–15 years. All trials also showed CV benefits. The Sotagliflozin in Patients with Diabetes and Chronic Kidney Disease (SCORED) trial[23] with sotagliflozin also showed renoprotective effects and CV benefits. SGLT-2 has become the standard of care on top of renin–angiotensin–aldosterone system (RAAS) blockers in

TABLE 3: Trials of SGLT-2 inhibitors for heart failure.

	n	T2DM	Primary outcome	HR (95% CI) *p* value	Remarks
HFrEF					
DAPA-HF	4,744	42%	Composite of CV death or worsening HF	0.74 (0.65–0.85)	Dapagliflozin improved HF outcomes in HFrEF on GDMT with or without T2DM
EMPEROR REDUCED	3,730	50%	Composite of CV death or HHF	0.75 (0.65–0.86)	Empagliflozin improved HF outcomes in HFrEF on GDMT, with or without T2DM
HFpEF					
EMPEROR PRESERVED	5,998	48.9%	Composite of cardiovascular death, or HHF	0.79 (0.69–0.90); $p < 0.001$	Empagliflozin reduced the combined risk of CV death and HF in patients with HFpEF, regardless of diabetes
DELIVER	6,263	44.7%	Composite of worsening HF and CV death	0.82 (0.73–0.92); $p < 0.001$	Dapagliflozin reduced the combined risk of WHF and CV death in patients with moderately reduced or preserved EF
ADHF					
EMPULSE trial	530	46.8%	Composite of death from any cause, number of HF events, and time to first HF events, or a five-point or greater difference in change from baseline in the KCCQ score at 90 days as assessed using a win ratio	Win ratio for empagliflozin 53.9% vs. placebo 39.7% HR yielding a win ratio of 1.36 in favor of empagliflozin 1.09–1.68; $p = 0.0054$	Initiation of empagliflozin in ADHF after stabilization results in significant clinical benefits at 90 days
Worsening HF					
SOLOIST WHF	122	100%	Total number of deaths from CV causes, hospitalizations, and urgent visits for HF	0.67 (0.52–0.85; $p < 0.001$)	In patients with diabetes and recent WHF, sotagliflozin decreased the total number of deaths from CV causes, hospitalizations, and urgent visits for HF

(ADHF: acute decompensated heart failure; CI: confidence interval; CV: cardiovascular; GDMT: guideline-directed medical therapy; HF: heart failure; HFpEF: heart failure with preserved ejection fraction; HFrEF: HF with reduced ejection fraction; HHF: hospitalization for heart failure; HR: hazard ratio; SGLT-2: sodium-glucose cotransporter-2; T2DM: type 2 diabetes mellitus)

TABLE 4: Trials of SGLT-2 inhibitors in AMI.

AMI					
EMMY trial[19]	476	63%	NT-proBNP) change over 26 weeks	Win ratio 1.36 (1.09–1.68); $p = 0.0054$	Empa produced a significantly greater reduction in NT-proBNP over 23 weeks, along with improvements in echo parameters

(AMI: acute myocardial infarction; NT-proBNP: N-terminal pro-B-type natriuretic peptide; SGLT-2: sodium-glucose cotransporter-2)

TABLE 5: Trials of SGLT-2 inhibitors in chronic kidney disease.

Study	Diabetic population	*n*	Drug	Inclusion criteria	Renal specific outcome	Hazard Ratio, 95% CI (*p* value)
CREDENCE	T2DM (100%)	4,401	Canagliflozin 100 mg daily	T2DM patients ≥30 years of age and CKD (eGFR 30 to <90 mL/min/1.73m^2 and UACR >300–5,000); on a stable dose of RAAS inhibitors for at least 4 weeks before randomization	Composite renal outcome of end-stage kidney disease (dialysis, transplantation, or a sustained estimated GFR of <15 mL/min/1.73m^2), a doubling of the serum creatinine level, or death from renal or cardiovascular causes	0.66 (0.53–0.81); ($p = 0.001$)

Continued

Continued

Study	Diabetic population	*n*	Drug	Inclusion criteria	Renal specific outcome	Hazard Ratio, 95% CI (*p* value)
DAPA-CKD	T2DM (67%) or without T2DM	4,304	Dapagliflozin 10 mg daily	Patients with or without T2DM and CKD (eGFR 25–75 mL/min/1.73m^2 and UACR 200–5,000); on a stable dose of RAAS inhibitors for at least 4 weeks before randomization	Composite renal outcome of decline in eGFR of ≥50%, ESKD, or death from renal causes	0.56 (0.45–0.68); ($p < 0.001$)
EMPA-CKD	T2DM (96.4%) or without T2DM	6,609	Empagliflozin 10 mg daily	Patient with and without T2DM and CKD (eGFR 20–45 mL/min/1.73m^2) and additional cardiovascular risk factors and UACR of at least 200 primary outcomes on stable dose RAAS inhibitors for at least 4 weeks before randomization	Composite renal outcome of end stage kidney disease, a sustained decrease in eGFR to <10 mL/min/1.73m^2, a sustained decrease in eGFR of ≥40% from baseline, or death from renal causes) or death from cardiovascular causes	0.72 (0.64–0.82) ($p < 0.001$)

(CI: confidence interval; CKD: chronic kidney disease; eGFR: estimated glomerular filtration rate; ESKD: end-stage kidney disease; RAAS: renin–angiotensin–aldosterone system; SGLT-2: sodium-glucose cotransporter-2; T2DM: type 2 diabetes mellitus; UACR: urine albumin-to-creatinine ratio)

TABLE 6: Cardiovascular outcomes trials of GLP-1 RAs.

Trial parameter	LEADER[24] liraglutide S/C	SUSTAIN-6[25] semaglutide S/C	PIONEER-6[26] semaglutide oral	REWIND[27] dulaglutide	HARMONY[28] outcomes albiglutide S/C
Number	9,340	3,297	3,183	9,901	9,463
Established ASCVD	81%	58%	84.9%	31%	100%
MACE (RRR)	13%	26%	21%	12%	22%
CV death (RRR)	22%	2%	51%	9%	7%
All-cause mortality (RRR)	15%	+5%	49%	10%	5%

(ASCVD: atherosclerotic cardiovascular disease; CV: cardiovascular; GLP-1 RA: glucagon-like peptide-1 receptor agonist; MACE: major adverse cardiovascular event; RRR: relative risk reduction)

all guidelines across the globe. SGLT-2Is act in diverse ways, but the important effect is due to afferent arteriolar constriction by decreasing intraglomerular pressure and thereby decreasing proteinuria.

Glucagon-like Peptide-1 Receptor Agonists

Glucagon-like peptide-1 receptor agonists are a class of new antidiabetic medications that have multifaceted actions. They increase glucose-dependent insulin secretion and suppress glucose-dependent glucagon secretion so hypoglycemia is minimal or absent with the use of these agents. They also decrease appetite through a central action that increases satiety and decreases food intake. They also slow gastric emptying so that less food is released into the blood stream. They also decrease hepatic glucose production and decrease steatosis. They increase insulin sensitivity in the liver and skeletal muscles. They also increase beta-cell function in the pancreas and have renoprotective effects. They decrease ASCVD events, as has been shown by several trials **(Table 6)**.[24-28]

Dipeptidyl Peptidase-4

Dipeptidyl peptidase-4 (DPP-4) inhibitors provide good glycemic control with minimal glycemic variability. They are CV neutral from the point of view of three-point MACE as has been shown by various trials.[29-33] Saxagliptin has shown an increase in hospitalizations for heart failure, while alogliptin only showed a numerical increase. Sitagliptin and linagliptin do not increase hospitalization for heart failure and are safe in patients with CV disease. The results of the various DPP-4 inhibitors are shown in **Table 7**.

TABLE 7: Completed cardiovascular outcome trials of DPP-4 inhibitors.

Study	Drug	Duration (weeks)	Intervention arms dosage and number	Patients with established CVD%	Hazard ratio, 95% CI (*p* value)	Risk of Hospitalization for HF (HR) 95% CI (*p* value)
SAVOR-TIMI 53[29]	Saxagliptin placebo	104	Saxagliptin 5 mg or 2.5 mg (8,280) placebo (8,212)	78.4	1.00, 0.89–1.12 (NS)	HR, 1.27; CI, 1.07–1.51; $p = 0.007$
EXAMINE[30]	Alogliptin placebo	160	Alogliptin 25/12.5/ 6.25 mg (2,701) placebo (2,679)	100	0.96, 1.16 (NS)	1.07 (NS)
TECOS[31]	Sitagliptin placebo	156	Sitagliptin 100 mg or 50 mg (7,332) placebo (7,339)	100	0.98, 0.88–1.09 (NS)	1.00 (NS)
CARMELINA[32]	Linagliptin	114	Linagliptin, 5 mg (3,494) placebo (3,485)	57	1.02, 0.89–1.17 (NS)	0.90 (NS)
CAROLINA[33]	• Linagliptin • Glimepiride	110	• Linagliptin 5 mg (3,023) • Glimepiride (3,010)	34.5	HR, 0.98, 0.84–1.14 (NS)	1.21 (NS)

(CI: confidence interval; CVD: cardiovascular disease; DPP-4: dipeptidyl peptidase-4; HF: heart failure; HR: hazard ratio; T2DM: type 2 diabetes mellitus; NS: not significant)

CONCLUSION

The treatment of diabetes has undergone a sea change from a glucocentric approach to a glucocentric approach without weight gain and hypoglycemia to a current approach of improving cardiorenal outcomes with two new antidiabetic medications, i.e., SGLT-2Is and GLP-1 RAs.

ONLINE REFERENCES

Please scan the QR code provided at the end of the table of contents for References of this chapter.

SECTION 11

Cardio-obstetrics

CHAPTER

91

Cardio-obstetrics as a Subspecialty: The Need of the Hour

G Justin Paul, S Anne Princy

ABSTRACT

The last few decades have seen an increasing number of women with heart disease (WWHD) going through pregnancy. About 1–4% of all pregnancies are complicated by cardiovascular disease (CVD). With the advancing medical care, there has been a steady improvement in the early diagnosis of heart diseases including antenatal diagnosis, leading to early appropriate management. With ongoing sociocultural changes, there is an increasing prevalence of delayed marriages and late conception and adverse lifestyle and cardiovascular risk factors in pregnant women. All these contribute to this increased proportion of WWHD going through pregnancy.

With medical advances, it is heartening to observe that maternal deaths during pregnancy are decreasing across the world and India. Along with this, it is also observed that CVD during pregnancy is becoming the leading cause of maternal mortality in developed nations. In India too, with the ongoing obstetric transition, the cardiac contribution to maternal mortality is increasing and is expected to increase further in the days to come. It has been shown that a high proportion of maternal mortality related to heart disease is preventable. Pregnancy outcomes have been shown to improve with the application of a cardio-obstetric team concept with well-written management protocols.

Data on pregnancy outcomes in WWHD is sparse in India, with no local risk scores or guidelines. The benefit of a cardio-obstetric team concept is yet to be realized in India. This chapter aims to give the reader a broad outlook on this newly developing subspecialty providing an Indian perspective.

Keywords: Pregnancy and heart disease, maternal mortality, preconception counseling.

INTRODUCTION

The number of women with heart disease (WWHD) going through pregnancy has been increasing in the last few decades. About 1–4% of all pregnancies are complicated by cardiovascular disease (CVD). Pregnancy is marked by the rapid onset of many hemodynamic and physiological changes to accommodate the physiological needs of the growing fetus. WWHD may not be able to cope with these greater demands imposed on the cardiovascular (CV) system by the physiological demands during pregnancy. Maternal cardiac dysfunction can impair the uteroplacental flow, and thereby a suboptimal fetal outcome. Further, pregnancy can exacerbate an already existing CV illness or can unmask a previously unrecognized disease.

INCREASING PREVALENCE OF HEART DISEASE IN PREGNANCY

The incidence of heart disease during pregnancy is on a steep rise and this could be related to multiple reasons. The widespread availability of echocardiography is now providing an opportunity for early diagnosis of cardiac illness. Further, school health and adolescent health programs lead to early diagnosis of congenital and rheumatic heart diseases. Advances in pediatric cardiac interventions and surgeries have led to more children with heart disease surviving to childbearing age. Apart from these, increased awareness and early diagnosis of genetic conditions, increasing prevalence of adverse lifestyle risk factors, delayed marriages, and advancing maternal age are all factors that result in more pregnant women presenting with CVD or risk factors.[1]

OBSTETRIC TRANSITION

The trend of nations gradually shifting from a pattern of high maternal mortality to low maternal mortality, from direct obstetric causes of maternal mortality (sepsis, bleeding, etc.), to indirect causes, ageing of maternal population, and institutionalization of maternity care is called obstetric transition. There are five stages in this epidemiological transition. Stage I describes nations, such as South Sudan, Chad, etc., where maternal mortality ratio (MMR) is >1,000 with the majority of deaths due to maternal obstetric causes, and where most women do not have access to appropriate healthcare. Stage V describes nations with MMR < 5, such as Iceland, Poland, Greece, etc., with almost no direct causes of maternal mortality. Most of the states in India are in stage III of obstetric transition with MMR between 50 and 299. Few such as Maharashtra and Kerala have entered stage IV and V with MMR < 50. In the developed nations, the most common cause of maternal deaths is CV and is responsible for 20–25% of all maternal deaths. As our country moves ahead in the obstetric transition, the number of maternal deaths complicated by heart disease is rising as the direct obstetric causes are slowly brought under control. Thus, one of the important steps forward to reduce maternal mortality will be improving the maternal care offered to pregnant WWHD (PWWHD).

PROFILE OF HEART DISEASE IN PREGNANCY

Although it has been considered for a long time that rheumatic heart disease is the predominant heart disease during pregnancy, it is becoming evident that there is a changing profile of heart disease in India. Congenital heart diseases, cardiac arrhythmia, cardiomyopathy, and acquired CVD and CV risk factors now account for an increasing proportion of heart diseases among pregnant women. This is due to improving medical care, sociocultural changes, and ongoing epidemiological transitions. In the western world, there are numerous studies and data suggesting the increasing prevalence of preexisting diabetes among pregnant women, gestational diabetes, and hypertensive disorders of pregnancy (HDP).[2,3] Peripartum cardiomyopathy (PPCM) has also been increasingly reported over the last 30 years with its morbidity and mortality related to its association with pre-eclampsia.[4] Since this data is not available from India, the need for research in these domains is increasing.

ADVERSE PREGNANCY OUTCOMES

Adverse pregnancy outcomes (APOs) refer to those pregnancy outcomes other than normal live births and include preterm birth, stillbirth, small for gestational age births, and HDP, encompassing gestational hypertension and pre-eclampsia and gestational diabetes mellitus. These represent a cluster of interrelated disorders sharing common-underlying disease pathways. Some of the factors that cumulate to APOs include inadequate trophoblastic invasion, impaired placentation, disturbances in uteroplacental blood flow leading to placental malperfusion, inflammation, ischemia, and development of antiangiogenic proteins.[5] Women who had an APO are more likely to develop hypertension and CVD and cerebrovascular disease in the future. The rise in CVD mortality associated with APOs is striking: 75% increase in preeclampsia, 67% increase in gestational hypertension, and 68% higher risk of gestational diabetes compared to those without APOs.[6,7]

While these associations are well-known globally, there is a lack of data on the long-term effects of APOs on CV health in India which highlights the need for more research and sustainable data in this area.

MATERNAL MORTALITY

Pregnancy complicated by cardiac disease is the most common cause of maternal mortality and morbidity in developed nations (20–30% of all maternal deaths),[8,9] and it is also becoming a significant contributor to maternal mortality in developing nations. In India too, heart disease is expected to be the major contributor to maternal mortality in the years to come.

The maternal mortality review in the United States furnished a comprehensive report that around 68% of maternal deaths linked to heart diseases were entirely preventable.[9] Although periodic maternal audit reviews are being conducted in India, there is no documented data on the preventable causes of maternal death PWWHD.

There are many preventable factors that could contribute to maternal mortality in India. These include a lack of data on PWWHD, risk stratification tools and guidelines, lack of coordination among the healthcare workers from different specialty involved in the care of these patients, suboptimal support to research in cardio-obstetrics (CO), inadequate administrative support, and a general lack of awareness about requirement of optimal care of PWWHD in the healthcare system. By focusing on developing the field of CO and working together to prevent causes of maternal deaths, we can help our country get closer to the United Nations' Sustainable Development goal of reducing maternal deaths to <70.

INDIAN DATA OF PREGNANT WOMEN WITH HEART DISEASE

There are a good number of publications addressing heart disease during pregnancy in India. However, they are often retrospective or from a single center with small sample sizes.

Unlike the western nations, where congenital heart disease predominates, valvular heart disease still continues to be the most common cause of heart disease in pregnancy in India.[1,10] The most common complication of PWWHD in India is heart failure similar to western data.[1,11]

We conducted the largest study ever done at a single medical center about pregnant women with heart problems, called the Madras Medical College Pregnancy And Cardiac (M-PAC) registry.[1,12] This study involved 1,005 women who had 1,029 pregnancies. Surprisingly, 60% of these women found out they had a heart problem for the first time while they were pregnant.

We identified that even patients with critical cardiac conditions such as severe mitral stenosis, left ventricular (LV) dysfunction, prosthetic heart valves, and pulmonary hypertension are diagnosed with heart disease only during pregnancy. We also found that only half of the women with congenital heart disease get counseling before getting pregnant. Risk factors for adverse maternal cardiac outcomes in our study included severe mitral stenosis, LV systolic dysfunction, mechanical prosthetic valve, pulmonary hypertension, the New York Heart Association (NYHA) class > II, modified World Health Organization (mWHO) grade > II, and a diagnosis during the current pregnancy.[1] We had also shown earlier that 50% of women with congenital heart disease do not get preconception counseling. It has been shown earlier that seeking medical attention late in pregnancy could lead to adverse maternal cardiac outcomes.[13,14]

Some of the lacunae noted in the Indian System of Healthcare include a lack of continuum of care from pediatric to childbearing age, lack of coordinated care among the involved specialties, counseling not appropriate for the disease or the person being counseled, the need for universal risk scores systems and guidelines and protocols, education programs, and field of CO.

Cardio-obstetrics Team or Pulmonary Hypertension Team or Maternal Cardiology Team

Cardio-obstetrics is an emerging subspecialty in the field of cardiology that focuses on the prevention, early detection, and appropriate management of PWWHD. It involves multidisciplinary team-based care dedicated to the management of PWWHD. It monitors PWWHD from preconception through the postpartum period. The goal is to better evaluate and counsel women of childbearing age with or at risk for CVD regarding maternal and fetal risks of pregnancy, to optimize medical intervention, and to provide appropriate contraception advice. A well-run multidisciplinary team has the potential to reduce adverse CV outcomes in high-risk pregnancies. The team usually includes cardiologists with expertise in CO, obstetricians, maternal–fetal medicine specialists, primary healthcare providers, obstetric anesthesiologists, neonatologists, geneticists, pharmacists, social workers, nurses, and other care team members. However, the obstetrician and the cardiologist take up the prime role in management and critical decision-making. Together, a good coordination between these specialists with sharing of knowledge will provide a unique perspective on the management of heart disease in pregnant women. An appropriate CO team-based approach has the potential to positively influence the outcome of PWWHD and improve the CV health and well-being of mothers during pregnancy and beyond.[15]

Role of the Cardio-obstetrics Team in Preconception Counseling

Prepregnancy counseling takes many different forms in our country with postconception counseling being more prevalent than preconception counseling. Although postconception counseling can educate a patient regarding the cardiac illness and its course during pregnancy, appropriate multidisciplinary preconception counseling can modify the medical, behavioral, and social risks to pregnancy outcome and improve the preparedness of a patient. The role of a trained CO team is of immense importance during this period since the dissemination of correct and medically sound information to the patient and her family by pertinent specialties will help them to pursue crucial decision-making that will positively influence the outcome of the pregnancy. Appropriate contraception and fertility advice are crucial in the risk management of WWHD. Many patients are diagnosed with heart disease only after marriage and during pregnancy. A good number of them are unaware of their cardiac condition because their parents either conceal or fail to pass on the information to them. In essence, the rate of preconception counseling is very low in our country.

Role of the Cardio-obstetrics Team in Antenatal Care

The frequency of follow-up must be decided by the CO team and must be individualized especially in high-risk patients. The need for optimization of medications, curtailing cardiac drugs prone to fetotoxicity, bridging therapy in patients on oral anticoagulants, evaluation of symptomatic patients who may require antenatal intervention, admissions for cardiac failure, symptomatology assessment of early detection of antepartum cardiomyopathy, and decisions regarding medical termination in mWHO intravenous (IV) patients are some of the important areas where the CO team can play a decisive role in management. Deciding on the mode of delivery, mode of analgesia, and anesthesia are important areas where the decision is better made by a CO team than one set of specialists.

Role of the Cardio-obstetrics Team in Postpartum Management

Postpartum care is the most essential part of CO management. The term "fourth trimester" refers to the period 12 weeks after delivery and it is the potential period for postpartum complications. It is also a critical period for addressing contraception and identifying CV risk factors. It is well established that most of the maternal complications including death in WWHD occur in the postpartum period. Efficient coordination between the various disciplines of the CO team can help in tiding over the anticipated complications in these cardiac patients. Further, an individualized approach with time- and need-based decisions can be achieved as a team approach, which can improve the outcomes of pregnancy. Included in this care is long-term CVD with high-risk patients receiving appropriate education and longitudinal follow-up. Optimization of medications and any interventions that may be needed should be a part of CO care. Advice for contraception should also be based on a multidisciplinary approach.

PRESENT SCENARIO OF CARDIO-OBSTETRICS IN INDIA

The present scenario of CO in India is not very encouraging. The importance of developing this field, in the light of the increasing cardiac contribution to maternal mortality is not yet fully recognized. Case record-auditing studies in developed nations have identified potential changes in therapy which could have produced changes in outcome in a high proportion of cases (24–68%).[8,16] The scenario in developing nations like ours is likely to be still worse. Failing to control seemingly minor preventable errors in the management may lead to grave complications. It is time for the involved specialists to recognize that additional focused expertise/training is necessary in managing pregnant women with serious heart disease.

Data has shown that 25–50% of counseling advice given to a high-risk patient with heart diseases has not been always appropriate.[12] This indicates the importance of giving specialized training for the healthcare personnel involved in counseling and care of these women.

The importance of the field of CO is not fully recognized by all the specialties (obstetrics, cardiology, anesthesia, and neonatology/pediatrics) involved in the management of PWWHD. Oftentimes, the specialties work independent of one another to the peril of the patient. The need for proper communication among the healthcare professionals involved in the care of WWHD to work as one team is not realized yet. It is important to remember that a lack of communication has the potential to result in gaps in management which could lead to serious complications including maternal deaths.

The amount of literature available in this field from our country is not yet adequate. As a result, there are no region/nation-specific guidelines for managing PWWHD in our country. Almost half of the WWHD come to know about their heart disease for the first time during pregnancy in our country.[12] As a result, the opportunity for medical/surgical optimization of the cardiac status before becoming pregnant is lost. Even among women with congenital heart disease, only half of them have some kind of preconception counseling. The expertise of the healthcare providers in offering appropriate preconception and contraception counseling needs improvement.

The good news is that the pockets of our country are involved in health research in PWWHD.[11,17] A large, multicenter research on PWWHD is ongoing in Tamil Nadu, with almost 2,500 participants being enrolled.[18]

Requirements for Cardio-obstetrics to Develop in India

Healthcare policies need to be designed to specifically address the needs of the WWHD from childhood, through adolescence and adulthood, and to marriage and pregnancy with enhanced CO care. The existing government school health program should continue to track and follow-up those detected with heart disease, providing an opportunity to offer health education and promotion counseling, risk assessment, preconceptional counseling, and if necessary, intervention before pregnancy to improve fetomaternal outcomes. There is a need for cardiologists to be more involved, seeking out collaborations with obstetricians, professional societies, patient support groups, healthcare institutions, and health policymakers.

Cardio-obstetric outpatient clinics, including all the specialties—cardiologists, obstetricians, providers, obstetric anesthesiologists, neonatologists, geneticists, pharmacists, and nurses, should be instituted so that once a patient with heart disease is registered, the progress of the patient should be available to all the members. The antenatal care should be decided by the team and the needs of the individual patient should be analyzed and addressed. Any decompensation and admissions needed should be managed by the team. The time of delivery and the mode of delivery should be decided by the team. A well-equipped CO intensive care unit (ICU) should be available to manage all complications that may be encountered during the peripartum period. Specific funding should be assigned for research in this area. Customized guidelines/position statements may be prepared based on the scientific information from the local database. Training and continuous medical education programs are to be organized for the dissemination of knowledge of CO. It is especially important to include more CO topics in general

CVD training programs and to organize dedicated CO programs.

Social media can be involved both in creating public awareness and increasing the dissemination of guidelines, best practices, and research publications. Ultimately, having a positive mindset among various specialties can affect health communication. There should be sufficient training for all medical professionals involved in the management of PWWHD so that guideline-based management can be provided to all patients. There should be healthy sharing of knowledge between specialties to eliminate the fear and reluctance. Changes in the logistics and existing policies and aid from policymakers and other stakeholders can improve the scope of CO.

Opportunities for Improvement of Cardio-obstetrics

- Creating an evidence-based plan of care to be in place for the management of PWWHD, both established CVD before pregnancy and for those who develop CVD during pregnancy
- Registries to source the indigenous data needed to develop region-specific guidelines and protocols for the management of PWWHD
- Formulation of Indian risk stratification tools and triaging systems
- Partnership between the various disciplines involved in the management of PWWHD
- Institution of professional societies to contribute to educational programs, continuing medical education (CME), and trainings in the field of CO

The following objectives should be implemented in a stepwise manner:

- Learning objectives and teaching content should be prepared.
- CO team with a predefined working pattern should be developed.
- Research in CO should be encouraged.
- Curriculum in CO should be developed and fellowship courses should be started.

CONCLUSION

There continues to be a growing need and interest in this newer field of CO in India because of the well-described manifestations of CVD during pregnancy and its contribution to maternal mortality and morbidity. It is the need of the hour to increase the number of practitioners in the field of CO and to increase training and knowledge sharing.

The time is now for CO to be developed as a specialized field in India. Awareness has to be created, academic fellowships have to be formed, the curriculum has to be developed, organizations and societies have to be formed, advocacy has to develop, and health policymakers and administrators have to be made aware of the need for this new field. Every institution with a large volume obstetric care units needs to have their own trained CO team to partner with the WWHD to ensure that they have a smooth sail through the pregnancy. This needs to be the main focus of our nation in reducing maternal mortality in the years to come. This will help us in achieving the United Nations' Sustainable Development Goal for India with regard to a maternal mortality rate of <70 by 2030.

ONLINE REFERENCES

Please scan the QR code provided at the end of the table of contents for References of this chapter.

CHAPTER

92

Pregnancy with Prosthetic Valve: Management

Chandrakanta Mishra

ABSTRACT

Prosthetic valve constitute high-risk pregnancy and has been classified by the World Health Organization (WHO) as risk category III with significant increase of maternal mortality and morbidity. Need for therapeutic anticoagulation during pregnancy adds an addictive burden of complications apart from the inherent thrombotic risk. Choice of anticoagulation strategy is challenging as there is *no ideal anticoagulant or strategy that is equally safe* for both mother and child. However, warfarin is associated with the lowest risk of valve thrombosis but can cause dose-dependent warfarin embryopathy when used in first trimester. *Warfarin* should be continued in all three trimesters, if dose is ≤5 mg/day. *Sequential therapy* [i.e., dose-adjusted low-molecular-weight heparin (LMWH)/continuous unfractionated heparin (UFH) for first trimester followed by warfarin in second and third trimester depending upon availability of monitoring of anti-Xa level] will be considered if required dose of warfarin is >5 mg/day to maintain therapeutic anticoagulation. Warfarin should be switched to continuous UFH or LMWH, at least 1 week before delivery. Subsequently all patients should be converted to continuous intravenous (IV) UFH from 36 to 6 hours before delivery and it should be resumed within 4–6 hours of delivery, provided no postpartum hemorrhage (PPH). Vitamin K antagonist (VKA) should be initiated postpartum as early as possible. Prosthetic valve thrombosis (PVT) is a life-threatening condition in pregnancy and should be treated with echo-guided low dose and slow infusion of tissue plasminogen activator (tPA) protocol with excellent thrombolytic success rate. Multidisciplinary prepregnancy counseling and maintenance of therapeutic anticoagulation throughout pregnancy are the paramount essential to prevent bleeding or thrombotic complications in patients with mechanical prosthetic valve (MPV) in pregnancy. These patients are best managed in tertiary care center with a multidisciplinary team to optimize maternal and fetal outcomes.

Keywords: Mechanical prosthetic heart valves, pregnancy, anticoagulation, thrombolysis, valve thrombosis, stuck valve, maternal outcomes, fetal outcomes.

INTRODUCTION

Prosthetic heart valves in pregnancy pose unique challenges and come with its own set of complications. Women within childbearing age, requiring prosthetic valve, should have a thorough discussion between the patient, cardiologist, and cardiac surgeon regarding plans for future pregnancy and the choice of valve: bioprosthetic versus mechanical. *Mechanical heart valves (MHVs)* offer excellent hemodynamic performance and long-term durability, but the need for therapeutic anticoagulation increases maternal and fetal mortality and morbidity.[1-3] *Bioprosthetic valves (BPVs)* does not require anticoagulation and have lower risk of thrombosis but are associated with a high-risk of structural valve deterioration resulting in the inevitable need for reoperation.[1,2] But long-term studies found no effect of pregnancy on BPV degeneration.[4] Although pregnancy experience is limited, women with a Ross procedure (pulmonary autograft and bioprosthetic pulmonary valve) also have good pregnancy outcomes.

CARDIOVASCULAR BURDEN AND OUTCOMES

Pregnancy is a hypercoagulable state, as the most of the clotting factors increase during pregnancy with decrease of several anticoagulant factors and fibrinolytic activity, which increases the risk of prosthetic valve thrombosis (PVT) and thromboembolic complications in patients with prosthetic valves and can be catastrophic for mother and child.[5] Normally in pregnancy, prosthetic aortic valve increases its peak and mean gradient by 50% in second trimester and prosthetic mitral valve increases its mean gradient by 35%.[6] In the women with MHV, maternal mortality rate remains >1% and in more than one-third cases are associated with serious maternal and fetal complications.[1,7,8] The risk is lower with adequate dosing of anticoagulant therapy and it depends upon the type, position of the mechanical valve, and patient-related risk factors such as pulmonary arterial hypertension (PAH) and left ventricular (LV) dsyfunctions.[9]

In the largest series to date *[Registry of Pregnancy And Cardiac disease (ROPAC) registry]*,[1] the maternal mortality rate in mechanical and BPV occurred in 1.4% and 1.5%, respectively in comparison to 0.2% with patient without prosthetic valve.[1] The chances of an event-free pregnancy with a live birth were 58% for women with a MHV compared with 79% for women with a bioprosthesis and 78% for women with heart disease without valve prosthesis.[1] The PVT occurred in 6.1% [more with mitral (4.4%) than aortic valve (2.6%)], heart failure (HF) 7.5%, and hemorrhagic events are significantly more common in mechanical valve (23.1%) than with BPVs (5.1%) or those without prosthetic valve (4.9%).[1]

The risk of PVT is relatively low with vitamin K antagonists (VKAs) throughout pregnancy (0–4%) and higher in older generation mechanical valve, mitral and tricuspid position, concomitant atrial fibrillation (AF), with history of thromboembolic events.[1] Warfarin is the most effective form of anticoagulant for mechanical valve and it provides the lowest risk of thromboembolic complication during pregnancy.

Infective endocarditis (IE) during pregnancy is not very common, and estimated rates are 3–12 per 1,000 with prosthetic valves.[10] The maternal and fetal mortality rates remain high at 33% and 29%, respectively with prosthetic valve endocarditis.

RISK STRATIFICATION

Risk stratification with prosthetic valves for cardiovascular complications in pregnancy depends on three factors: (1) disease-specific factors, (2) general pregnancy-related factors, and (3) patient-related specific variables. Prosthetic valves as a predictor of maternal cardiovascular events are risk stratified using CARPREG II and ZAHARA risk scores. The modified WHO maternal cardiovascular risk classifies BPV as Class II–III risk (maternal cardiac event rate of 10–19%) whereas mechanical valves are placed in Class III risk, i.e., significantly increased risk of maternal mortality or severe morbidity (maternal cardiac event rate of 19–27%).[10,11]

MATERNAL RISK VERSUS FETAL RISK

The maternal risk includes miscarriage, thromboembolic complications, obstetric hemorrhage, and maternal mortality.[5] Cardiac complications include HF, arrhythmia, PVT, and IE. Use of anticoagulation adds to peripartum bleeding, thrombocytopenia, and osteoporosis. The fetus or neonate risk includes intrauterine growth retardation, preterm birth, perinatal mortality, small for gestational age, and teratogenicity related to VKAs.

CHOICE OF ANTICOAGULANT AND ANTICOAGULANT STRATEGIES

For pregnant woman with mechanical valve, there is *no ideal anticoagulant or strategy that is equally safe* for both the mother and her child. There are three potential anticoagulant strategies: (1) continue warfarin throughout pregnancy; (2) use of heparin throughout pregnancy; and (3) use sequential therapy, with heparin during first trimester and warfarin during the second and third trimester **(Flowchart 1)**.

Warfarin is associated with the lowest risk of valve thrombosis and maternal mortality but it crosses placenta and can cause embryopathy (when used in first trimester) and fetopathy (when used in late pregnancy).[12] Warfarin embryopathy appears to be dose-dependent, no or least embryopathy (3%) with dose ≤5 mg/day in contrast to >30% in dose >5 mg/day.[8,9,13-18] Whereas unfractionated heparin (UFH) can cause fetopathy while used as the sole agent throughout. UFH is associated with high rate of valve thrombosis when given subcutaneously (s/c). Its use is recommended only when administered continuous intravenous (IV) infusion in the hospital setting. Low-molecular-weight heparins (LMWHs) have the lowest rate of adverse fetal outcomes but can have more maternal PVT events could be due to inadequate anti-Xa monitoring.

Use of anti-Xa direct oral anticoagulants (DOACs)[19,20] and antithrombin inhibitor (dabigatran)[21] are *not recommended* (Class III) during pregnancy with MHV. Use of *low-dose aspirin* is considered safe during pregnancy with MHV, if needed in other indication like prevention of preeclampsia.[22]

GENERAL PRINCIPLES OF MANAGEMENT

Prepartum Counseling

Preconception counseling is essential to discuss regarding risk benefits of anticoagulants and its strategy in pregnancy

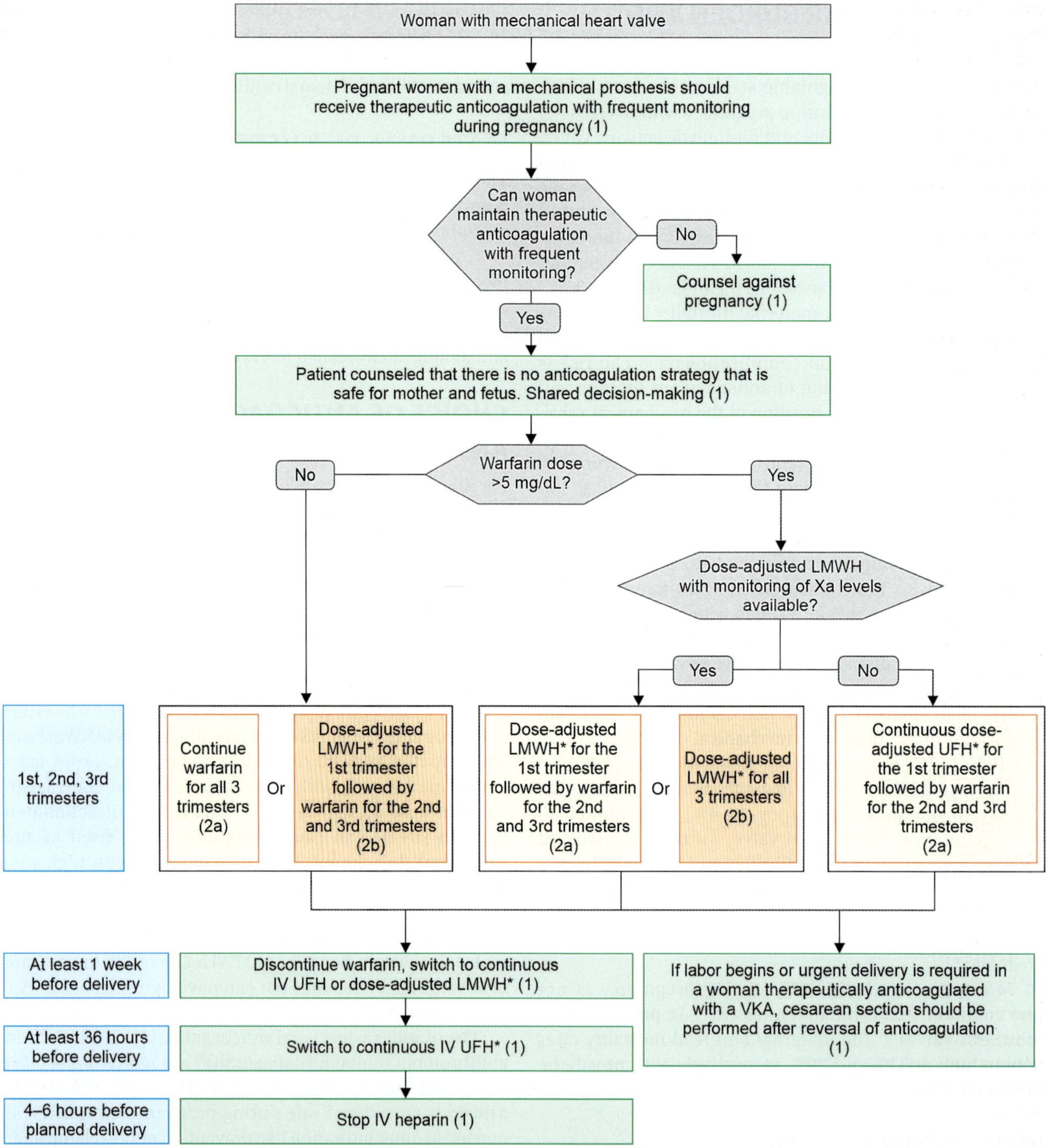

*Dose-adjusted LMWH should be given at least two times per day with close monitoring of anti-Xa levels. Target to Xa level of 0.8–1.2 U/mL, 4–6 hours after dose. Trough levels may aid in maintaining patient in therapeutic range. Continuous UFH should be adjusted to aPTT two times control.

FLOWCHART 1: Anticoagulation for prosthetic mechanical heart valves in women during pregnancy (2021 AHA/ACC guidelines). Colors indicating class of recommendation.

(ACC: American College of Cardiology; AHA: American Heart Association; aPTT: activated partial thromboplastin time; IV: intravenous; LMWH: low-molecular-weight heparin; UFH: unfractionated heparin; VKA: vitamin K antagonist) with MHV. Informed discussion about the risk of PVT, requirement for continuation of therapeutic anticoagulation with frequent monitoring throughout the pregnancy, and maternal and fetal risk involved with available anticoagulation strategy. The option of avoiding pregnancy should also be clearly discussed.

Baseline documentation of symptoms and echocardiographic parameters, such as prosthetic valve function, LV function, and pulmonary artery pressure, serves as a guide if the woman becomes pregnant. Patient should be counseled to monitor their menstrual cycle and frequent pregnancy test and contact cardiologist as soon as pregnancy is known.

Antepartum Phase

At the first antenatal visit, it is imperative to perform a full physical examination, electrocardiogram (ECG), 2D echocardiogram, and color Doppler study to assess valve hemodynamic such as valve gradient, regurgitant lesions LV function, and PAH. Detailed review of medical therapy to discontinue drugs that are contraindicated in pregnancy such as angiotensin-converting enzyme inhibitors (ACEI), angiotensin receptor blockers (ARBs), angiotensin receptor neprilysin inhibitor (ARNI), and aldosterone antagonists is also essential. Follow-up intervals of the patients will be depending upon the type of MHV and baseline valve functions. Good functioning BPV will be monitor at each trimester but poor functioning valve needs to be monitored more frequently. In MHV, frequent monitoring to maintain therapeutic anticoagulation fortnightly or preferably weekly is essential.

Discussion regarding various options for anticoagulation strategies in women with a MHV is shown in **Flowchart 1**. Any deterioration in clinical status warrants urgent attention of physician, with high index of suspicion for early detection of complications such as PVT, prosthetic valve IE, HF, and arrhythmia.

Delivery

In BPV, vaginal delivery is preferred. Women with MHV and in case of *elective delivery (vaginal or cesarean section)*, management of anticoagulation in peripartum period is of paramount importance. Patients on VKA need to be electively hospitalized at 36 weeks or 2 weeks prior to scheduled vaginal delivery for switching to long-acting heparin, i.e., LMWH. Dose-adjusted LMWH should be given twice daily till 36 hours prior to delivery with close weekly monitoring of anti-Xa activity (with a target anti-Xa level of 0.8–1.2 U/mL at 4–6 hours after dose). Those on LMWH needs to be discontinued with switching to IV continuous UFH 36 hours prior to delivery to keep aPTT more than two times of control levels, till 6 hours prior to delivery.[23-25] Stop IV UFH 4–6 hours before delivery. *Elective cesarean section* can also be considered in women on VKAs to minimize the interruption in anticoagulation and obstetric cause.

Emergency delivery, who present in active or preterm labor with therapeutic anticoagulation; patient on VKA, *cesarean section is the only choice*, appropriate reversal of anticoagulation, fresh frozen plasma (FFP) should be given to attain international normalized ratio (INR) <2 before surgery to reduce the risk of fetal intracranial hemorrhage.[8,21,26] Patients on LMWH or UFH, protamine should be used to reverse the effect of anticoagulation. Cesarean delivery is preferred to prevent intracranial bleed in anticoagulated foetus.[27]

Postpartum Phase

Parental heparin (UFH) should be resumed 4–6 hours after delivery provided there is no *postpartum hemorrhage (PPH)* or any bleeding and then switch to VKA as soon as possible. All the anticoagulants are safe during breastfeeding. Diuretics (except spironolactone), β-blockers (preferably and metoprolol), and digoxin can be given safely. ACEI and ARB are secreted in breast milk and are best to be avoided. If required, captopril, benazepril, and enalapril can be given.

Contraception

Estrogen-containing pills are contraindicated because of arterial and venous thrombosis. Barrier's methods and progesterone-based contraceptives can be used but failures rates are high. Intrauterine devices are preferable in extreme high-risk pregnancy like double mechanical valves, prior history of PVT, and prosthetic valve dysfunction. Permanent contraception should be considered in patients with already completed family.

MANAGEMENT OF COMPLICATIONS

Prosthetic Valve Thrombosis

Diagnosis

Prosthetic valve thrombosis during pregnancy is life-threatening for mother and fetus, require high index of suspicion for diagnosis. Clinical deterioration, embolic events, symptoms of HF, arrhythmia, or a significant increase of valve gradient by echo should alert the physician. Combination of clinical assessment, transthoracic and transesophageal echocardiography, and rarely, fluoroscopy should clinch the diagnosis.[28,29]

Management Options

These are similar to the nonpregnant setting and include: (1) parenteral anticoagulation, (2) surgery, and (3) fibrinolysis.

It depends upon the patient's clinical status, anatomical position, and size of thrombus. Guide the selection of management strategy.

- *Parenteral anticoagulation* (UFH or LMWH) is ideal for the patient who is hemodynamically stable in a noncritically ill patients with recent history of subtherapeutic anticoagulation, i.e., inadequate or interrupted anticoagulation.
- *Emergency surgery* is required when the patient is hemodynamically unstable with obstructive thrombus, large (>18 mm) nonobstructive thrombus, and when medical therapy fails in noncritically ill patients. However, the limitations of surgery include problem of availability in odd hours with higher rate of maternal and fetal mortality (6% and 30%, respectively) and morbidity (24% and 9%, respectively).[30]
- *Fibrinolysis* are indicated in hemodynamically stable and obstructive thrombus, valve thrombosis with embolic events, nonobstructive thrombus of size ≥10 mm,[31] right-sided PVT, high-risk surgery or nonavailability of surgery, and failure of parenteral heparin. In general, fibrinolytic agents do not cross the placenta because of their high-molecular weight, but are risk of placental bleeding and embolization to fetus.
    - Thrombolysis with an infusion of tissue plasminogen activator (tPA) under echo-guided low dose, slow infusion (25 mg of tPA infused over 6 hours with no bolus) protocol,[31] and can be repeated, once in every 24 hours up to six times to a maximum total dose of 150 mg in case of inadequate response.
    - UFH 70 IU/kg bolus with an infusion of 16 IU/h (up to 1,000 IU/h) with a target activated partial thromboplastin time (aPTT) of 1.5–2.0 times the mean reference range is administered after the termination of each tPA infusion. If repeat thrombolytic infusion is needed, heparin is held until the aPTT is <50 seconds, then tPA infusion is restarted.
    - This protocol of tPA is an effective and safest alternative to cardiac surgery or medical strategy published to date, with excellent thrombolytic success rate and can be considered first-line therapy of PVT in pregnant women (Class IIa).[31]
    - *In obstructive PVT*, in the absence of fatal or nonfatal major complications, *fibrinolytic complete success* is defined as attainment of all three criteria, i.e., (1) Doppler documentation of resolution of increased transvalvular gradient and decreased valve area; (2) Reduction by ≥75% in thrombus area or length; and (3) Improvement in symptoms. *Partial success* defined as fall short of three criteria.
    - *In nonobstructive PVT*, *fibrinolytic complete success* is defined as attainment of a ≥75% reduction in thrombus area or length. *Partial success* is defined as 50–75% reduction in thrombus area or length.
    - After resolution of valve thrombus, the therapy is shifted to VKA for rest period of pregnancy and switching to UFH before delivery as per protocol.

Prosthetic Valve Infective Endocarditis

Management of IE is as per the guidelines in nonpregnant situation. Antibiotics safe in pregnancy should be used such as penicillin, ampicillin, amoxicillin, erythromycin, and cephalosporins. Aminoglycosides and tetracyclines are harmful for the fetus at all times, and should be restricted as far as practicable. Surgery should be considered in refractory HF or cardiogenic shock, but it carries high fetal mortality.

Heart Failure

Guidelines for management of HF are same as nonpregnant women. ACEIs and ARB are avoided due to enhanced risk of fetal toxicity.[15,32] Hydralazine and nitrate are safer during pregnancy. Dopamine and levosimendan are preferred inotropes. Diuretics should be used judiciously as they can cause diminished placental flow. Spironolactone and eplerenone should be avoided. In view of inadequate data, ARNI should not be considered during pregnancy. β-blockers such as metoprolol should be preferred over atenolol.[33]

Supraventricular Arrhythmias

Supraventricular arrhythmias like paroxysmal supraventricular tachycardia (PSVT) should be treated as usual with adenosine for acute termination. β-blocking agents, except atenolol, are advised for prophylaxis. *Atrial flutter and AF* are managed as with nonpregnant cases. Direct current (DC) cardioversion is recommended in unstable patients, whereas ibutilide or flecainide should be considered in stable patients. β-blockers are used for rate control.

Ventricular Tachycardia

Direct current cardioversion for hemodynamic unstable patients, in stable patients IV sotalol or procainamide are preferred agents. Amiodarone should be reserved for refractory cases. An implantable cardioverter defibrillator (ICD) should be implanted before pregnancy in high-risk clinical situations, but it can be considered for therapy-resistant ventricular tachycardia (VT).

CONCLUSION

Prosthetic valves in pregnancy constitute a high-risk situation and are associated with increased maternal, fetal morbidity and mortality. Multidisciplinary prepregnancy counseling as well as vigilant cardiac and obstructive surveillance throughout the perinatal period remains warranted to prevent complications in women and their infants. *Tissue valves* are considered better with low thrombogenic risk without need for anticoagulation but suffer the risk of structural degeneration of valve. *Mechanical valves* have excellent durability, but need for therapeutic anticoagulation adds an additional burden of complications apart from the inherent thrombotic risk. A close monitoring is paramount essential to maintain therapeutic anticoagulation to avoid bleeding or thrombotic complications in mechanical prosthetic valve in pregnancy. These patients are best managed in tertiary care center with a team expert comprising of obstetrician, cardiologist, and neonatologist.

ONLINE REFERENCES

Please scan the QR code provided at the end of the table of contents for References of this chapter.

CHAPTER

93

Peripartum Cardiomyopathy: Diagnosis and Management

Chhabi Satpathy, Subhasish Singh, Hemant K Satpathy, Trinath K Mishra

ABSTRACT

Peripartum cardiomyopathy is an uncommon etiology of heart failure which manifests in late pregnancy and postpartum period. The symptomatology closely resembles features of normal pregnancy and requires a high index of suspicion for diagnosis. Workup includes B-type natriuretic peptide (BNP) and echocardiography in clinically suspected cases. The prognosis is diverse ranging from full normalization to long-standing heart failure to worsening disease requiring mechanical circulatory support and cardiac transplantation. Unique features of this condition in the Indian patient population include younger age at presentation and association with anemia.

Keywords: Peripartum, cardiomyopathy, heart failure.

INTRODUCTION

Peripartum cardiomyopathy (PPCM) is an idiopathic form of heart failure (HF) which occurs either in the last month of pregnancy or in the first 5 months postpartum.[1] Unlike maternal hemorrhage, which is the most common cause of maternal mortality (47%) in India, cardiomyopathy is a less common cause of pregnancy-related deaths.[2] With increases in disease awareness, rise in multiple pregnancies mostly from the use of artificial reproductive technology, multiparity, preeclampsia, maternal cardiovascular risk factors, and increases in maternal age, the incidence of PPCM and associated maternal mortality is likely to rise in the future.

A relationship between pregnancy and HF was noticed in the late 19th century. However, this entity was formally recognized in 1971 in a report of 27 peripartum patients who had cardiomegaly, an abnormal electrocardiogram (ECG), and congestive HF. The definition proposed by the Heart Failure Association of the European Society of Cardiology (ESC) in 2010 is most often used. It describes PPCM as an idiopathic cardiomyopathy occurring toward the end of pregnancy or in the 5 months following delivery, abortion, or miscarriage, without other causes for HF, and with a left ventricular (LV) ejection fraction (EF) <45% and/or LV end-diastolic dimension >2.7 cm/m^2 or fractional shortening (FS) <30% (**Box 1**).[3] The worldwide incidence has been stated to be 1:1,000 by the EURObservational Research Program (EORP), yet the actual number is likely higher given that mild disease would be indistinguishable from pregnancy-related symptoms. There is wide geographic variation from 1:100 in Nigeria to 1:20,000 in Japan, probably due to a combination of genetic predisposition and poor medical care. A higher incidence in Africans, African Americans, and

BOX 1 Definition of peripartum cardiomyopathy (PPCM) as per Heart Failure Association of European Society of Cardiology.

- Heart failure within 4 weeks prior to delivery or 5 months post-partum
- Absence of other sources of heart failure
- Absence of heart disease prior to 1 month before delivery
- Left ventricular dysfunction based on echocardiography—ejection fraction <45%

AND/OR

- Motion-mode fractional shortening <30%
- Left ventricular end-diastolic dimension >2.7 cm/m^2

Source: Modified from Hubbard JU, Lindheimer M, Lang RM. A modified definition for peripartum cardiomyopathy and prognosis based on echocardiography. Obstet Gynecol. 1999;94:311-6.

Haitians may represent a genetic susceptibility among those of African or Caribbean descent. Besides a higher incidence, African American women also have a more severe clinical presentation and greater likelihood of EF <30%.

RISK FACTORS

The average age at presentation is 30 years and thus, half of these cases are seen in women >30 years old. The chances of affliction in women over 40 years old are 10 times higher than in those <20 years old. Besides age, multiparity and multifetal pregnancy both increased the risk of PPCM. Around 7–15% of all PPCM patients have multifetal pregnancy in comparison to 3% of the general population. When pregnant patients develop gestational hypertension, preeclampsia, or HELLP (hemolysis, elevated liver enzymes, and low platelet count) syndrome, they are at a greater risk of developing PPCM. Bello et al., in 2013, reported a 22% prevalence of preeclampsia in women with PPCM—four times greater than the global prevalence. In comparison to Whites, African Americans are commonly known to be at a higher risk for PPCM.[4] In addition, socioeconomic status also has a direct influence on the incidence of PPCM. In a community-based study, Wolfe et al. found that low socioeconomic status was associated with a higher incidence of PPCM.

PATHOPHYSIOLOGY

Significant progress in the understanding of pathogenesis has occurred over the past decade. Although no unifying cause of etiology for PPCM has been recognized, a number of mechanisms have been proposed including infectious/environmental factors such as myocarditis, dietary inadequacy, angiogenic imbalance, altered prolactin processing, immunological factors, inflammation, genetic predisposition, and pregnancy-related hemodynamic changes. The most favored theory is the "double hit" hypothesis wherein vascular stress occurs on a background of genetic susceptibility **(Fig. 1)**.

CLINICAL FEATURES

Peripartum cardiomyopathy is usually diagnosed in the first 4 weeks postpartum and rarely presents prior to 36 weeks of gestation. The presenting symptoms are like those of any HF case including shortness of breath, orthopnea, paroxysmal nocturnal dyspnea, cough, and pedal edema. Almost half of the affected have hypertensive diseases of pregnancy such as preeclampsia. Since some of these symptoms can be found in normal pregnancies, the diagnosis is often delayed, thus leading to significant morbidity and mortality. As such, a high

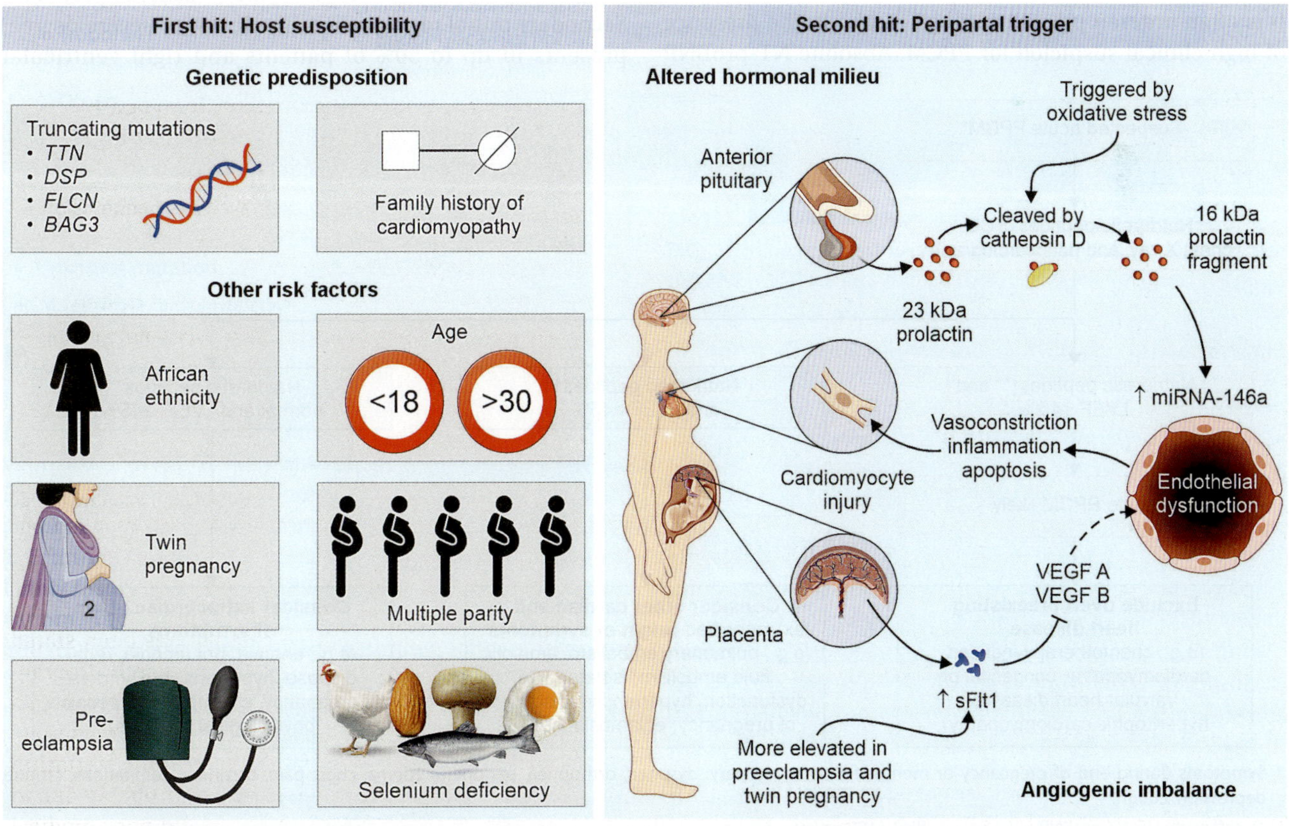

FIG. 1: A "two-hit" hypothesis has been proposed for the pathophysiology of peripartum cardiomyopathy.[9]
(miRNA: microribonucleic acid; VEGF: vascular endothelial growth factor)

clinical suspicion and low threshold for PPCM is warranted. The disease has a diverse presentation from a mild variety of HF with complete recovery to severe LV dysfunction and cardiogenic shock needing mechanical circulatory support (MCS). Clinical examination reveals typical findings of HF like edema, tachycardia, tachypnea, raised jugular venous pressure (JVP), third heart sound, and crepitations. Even in the absence of obvious signs of HF, a clinical suspicion should warrant further investigation for PPCM. Compared to HF from other causes, systemic and pulmonary thromboembolism is more common in PPCM, particularly with EF below 35%. Its incidence in PPCM patients has been reported to be 6.8%, a much higher rate than the 2.7% incidence noted in the overall congestive HF population.

INVESTIGATIONS

The workup of PPCM involves blood work including B-type natriuretic peptide (BNP), ECGs, and imaging studies such as chest X-rays, echocardiograms (echos), and cardiac magnetic resonance (MRs). HF may be excluded with reasonable certainty if BNP is <100 pg/mL and if N-terminal pro-B-type natriuretic peptide (NT-proBNP) is <300 pg/mL. Levels of both markers remain unchanged in uncomplicated pregnancies but are noted to be slightly elevated in the first few days after childbirth and in patients with preeclampsia. Raised BNP has been correlated with adverse cardiac events. It is often ordered prior to getting an echo in the presence of high clinical suspicion for PPCM. Absolute NT-proBNP value at the time of diagnosis (>900 pg/mL) predicts poor LV recovery. The 2019 ESC PPCM guidelines proposed an algorithm for the diagnosis of PPCM integrating X-ray, ECG, echo, and natriuretic peptide (NP) **(Flowcharts 1 and 2)**.[2] Of the blood tests ordered besides high NT-proBNP, raised troponin is a poor prognostic marker. **Table 1** shows the recommended tests at diagnosis and during follow-up.

Chest X-rays show features common to dilated cardiomyopathy such as cardiomegaly, pulmonary venous congestion, and interstitial edema. This helps rule out other causes of dyspnea from pulmonary pathology. The ECG, although not diagnostic, is abnormal in 95% of patients. ECG findings are mostly nonspecific and include atrial abnormality, ventricular hypertrophy, ST segment changes, and changes in T wave. Nonspecific T-wave changes, seen in 70% of PPCM patients, are the most common abnormality.[5] Severe LV dysfunction is indicated by T-wave inversion while upright T wave in aVR is a poor prognostic factor. Other ECG abnormalities include sinus tachycardia and prolonged QTc in 50%, ventricular arrhythmias in 5%, and left bundle branch block (LBBB) in <10%.

Echocardiography is diagnostic of PPCM and should be promptly utilized in any suspected case. The classical finding is a dilated LV with systolic dysfunction (EF < 45%). M-mode FS of LV < 30% and LV end-diastolic dimension > 2.7 cm/m^2 may also be present. Global longitudinal strain (GLS) and global circumferential strain (GCS) are considerably reduced. Secondary mitral regurgitation (moderate-to-severe degree) presents in up to 50% of patients and right ventricular

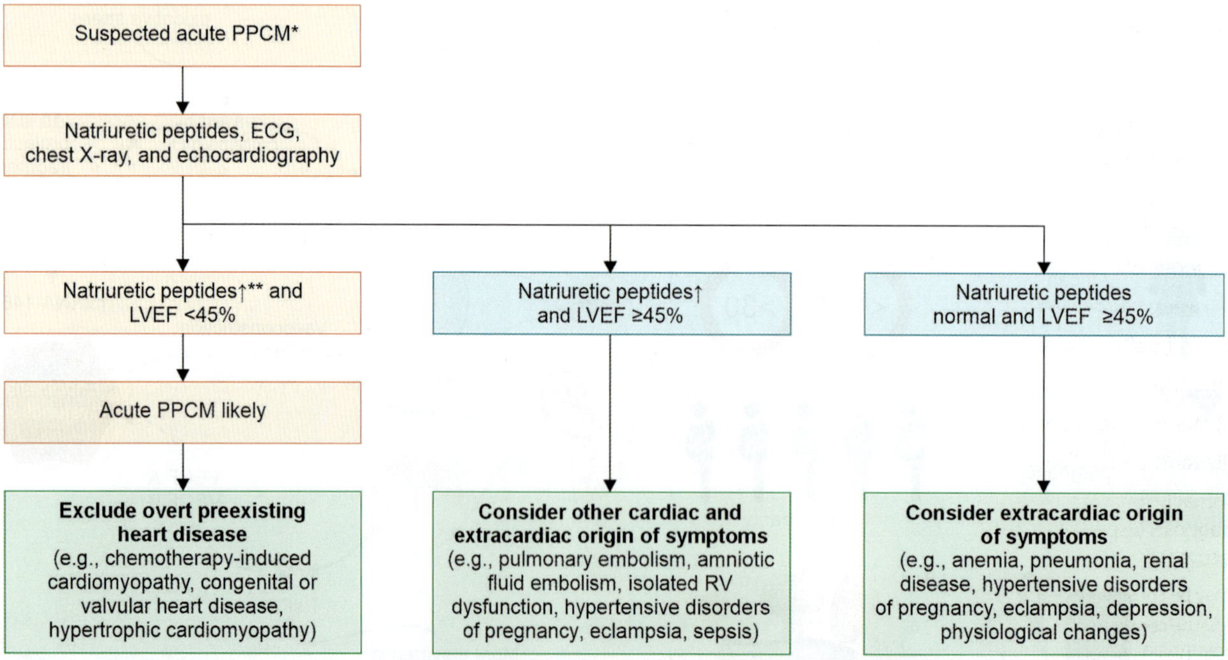

* Symptoms during end of pregnancy or months following delivery: dyspnea, orthopnea, peripheral edema, chest pain, dizziness, palpitations, fatigue, depression, cough.

** Cutoff acute HF: NT-proBNP >300 pg/mL, BNP >100 pg/mL.

FLOWCHART 1: Diagnostic pathway in patients with suspected peripartum cardiomyopathy (PPCM).[2]

(BNP: B-type natriuretic peptide; ECG: electrocardiogram; HF: heart failure; LVEF: left ventricular ejection fraction; NT-proBNP: N-terminal pro-B-type natriuretic peptide; RV: right ventricular)

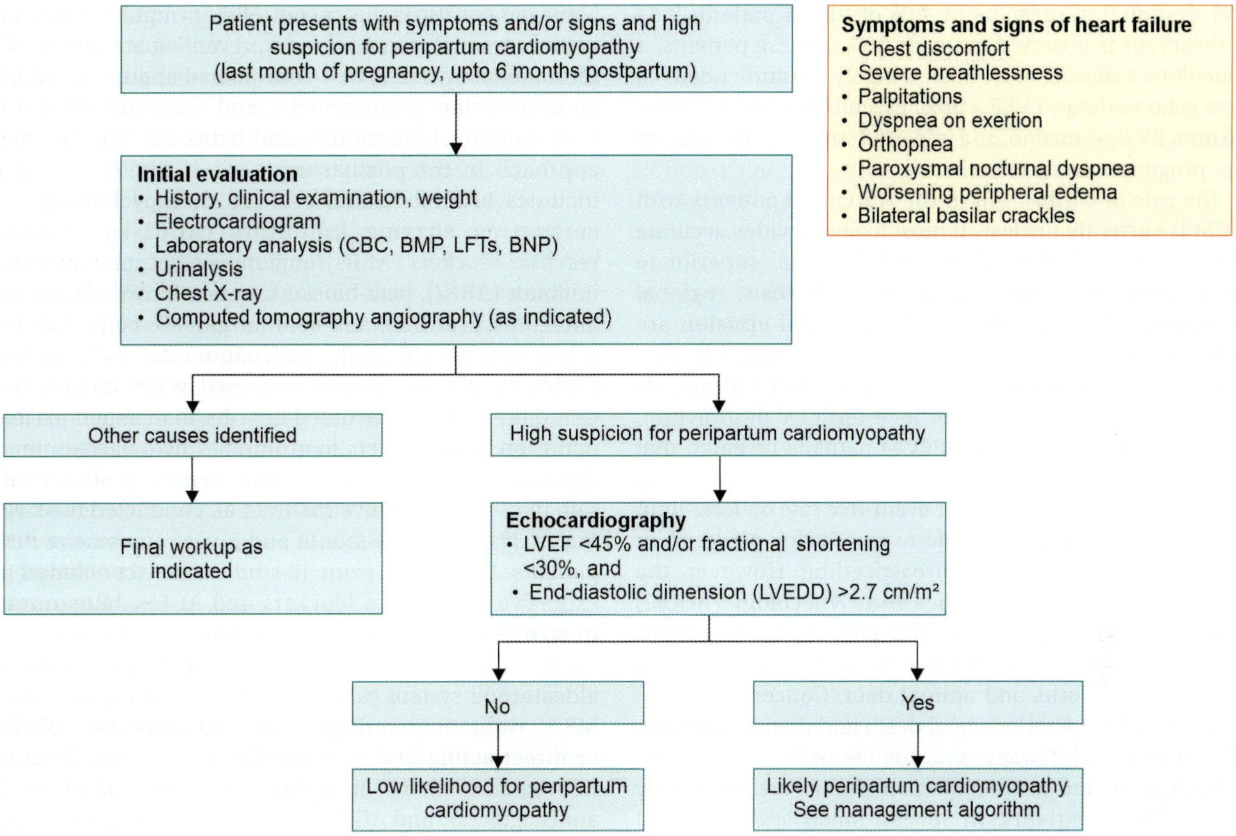

FLOWCHART 2: Evaluation of a woman with suspected peripartum cardiomyopathy.

(BMP: basic metabolic panel; BNP: B-type natriuretic peptide; CBC: complete blood count; LFT: liver function test; LVEDD: left ventricular end-diastolic diameter; LVEF: left ventricular ejection fraction)

Source: Cunningham FG, Byrne JJ, Nelson DB. Peripartum cardiomyopathy. Obstet Gynecol. 2019;133(1):167-79.

TABLE 1: Diagnostic tests that are recommended for the diagnosis of peripartum cardiomyopathy at initial diagnosis and at follow-up visits.

	Clinical examination	ECG	Natriuretic peptides	Echo-cardiography	Chest X-ray	Cardiac MRI	CT scan	Coronary angiography
Diagnosis of PPCM	X	X	X	X	X	(X)†	(X)†	(X)†
4–6 weeks after diagnosis	X	X	X	X				
3 months after diagnosis	X	X	X*	X				
6 months after diagnosis	X	X	X*	X		(X)†		
12 months after diagnosis	X	X	X*	X				
18 months after diagnosis	X	X	X*	X				
Annually for at least 5 years after diagnosis (especially if not fully recovered)	X	X	X*	X				

*May be considered depending on costs and local availability.

†May be considered depending on the clinical presentation and/or differential diagnoses.

Note: Generally, an individual approach is recommended depending on the severity of the disease and/or potential differential diagnoses.

(CT: computed tomography; ECG: electrocardiogram; MRI: magnetic resonance imaging; PPCM: peripartum cardiomyopathy)

(RV) dysfunction presents in 40% of PPCM patients.[6] As LV thrombus is observed in nearly 10% of these patients, a meticulous scanning of LV apex is highly recommended. Of these echo findings, LVEF < 30%, LV end-diastolic diameter >60 mm, RV dysfunction, and impaired strain parameters are poor prognostic factors.

The role of cardiac MR in the workup of patients with PPCM is currently unclear. It most likely provides accurate values for ventricular volume and function, superior to echocardiography. Myocardial edema, fibrosis, regional wall motion abnormalities, and pericardial effusion are common findings. Myocardial fibrosis identified by late gadolinium enhancement (LGE) is seen in 13–71% of patients and is possibly responsible for long-term LV dysfunction. A retrospective study of 121 PPCM patients revealed that LGE on magnetic resonance imaging (MRI) predicts poor prognosis and a lower 1-3-year event-free rate on long-term follow-up.[7] Gadolinium is safe to use during postpartum for mothers irrespective of breastfeeding. However, the American College of Obstetrics and Gynecology (ACOG) recommends limiting its use during pregnancy to situations where benefits clearly outweigh risks according to ongoing theoretical concerns and animal data. Concerns include increased risk for fetal/neonatal death and rheumatological, inflammatory, or infiltrative skin conditions.[8]

Both atrial and ventricular arrhythmias are commonly seen in these patients. In several small studies, atrial fibrillation (AF) was noted in 3–12% of patients with PPCM.[9] In one large study, ventricular arrhythmia was noted in 18.7% of patients. Of these, 4.2% had ventricular tachycardia (VT) and 2.2% had cardiac arrest. Because of a high incidence of arrhythmia, continuous telemetry during the early days of hospital stay is highly recommended. Extended ECG monitoring by 24-hour Holter ECG or implantable loop recorder (ILR) found both bradyarrhythmias and tachyarrhythmias to be common. In cases where a wearable cardioverter-defibrillator (WCD) is not an option, such monitoring should be liberally used in patients with severe LV dysfunction.

Patients with PPCM need genetic counseling and testing when available, particularly in the presence of a family history of dilated cardiomyopathy, sudden cardiac death, or PPCM. This is because 15–20% of patients with PPCM may carry the genetic mutations known to result in dilated cardiomyopathy. An endomyocardial biopsy is rarely suggested as it adds limited diagnostic or prognostic information. But it may be rarely considered to rule out viral myocarditis, autoimmune myocarditis, storage disease, metabolic disease, or in patients needing cardiac transplants.

TREATMENT

Management of PPCM is basically the same as that of systolic HF—it depends on the severity of clinical presentation and the time of presentation (before or after delivery). Management also includes controlling symptoms, repressing neurohormonal responses, and preventing arrhythmias and thromboembolism. A well-coordinated approach involving an obstetrician, perinatologist, and cardiologist offers the best result for both mother and baby. The recommended approach in the postpartum period (BROAD acronym) includes bromocriptine, oral HF therapy [angiotensin-converting enzyme inhibitors (ACEIs)/angiotensin receptor blockers (ARBs)/angiotensin receptor-neprilysin inhibitor (ARNI), beta-blockers, mineralocorticoid receptor antagonists (MRAs), and sodium-glucose cotransporter-2 inhibitors (SGLT-2Is)], anticoagulants, and diuretics **(Table 2)**. Of these, diuretics are used as per volume status. Overdiuresis is to be avoided in order to maintain placental perfusion. Beta-blockers, loop diuretics, hydralazine, nitrates, digoxin, and low-molecular-weight heparin (LMWH) are all safe in pregnancy. Hovelmann et al. conducted the largest metanalysis on the 6-month and 1-year outcome of PPCM patients. Using data from 47 studies, they concluded that extensive use of beta-blockers and ACEIs/ARBs resulted in significant mortality benefit at 6 and 12 months with better LV recovery at 12 months.[10] All renin-angiotensin-aldosterone system (RAAS) inhibitors (ACEI, ARB, ARNI, MRA), ivabradine, vericiguat, and anticoagulants (warfarin or direct-acting oral anticoagulants) are contraindicated in pregnancy. SGLT-2I, ivabradine, vericiguat, direct oral anticoagulants, and ACEIs/ARBs are also considered unsafe during lactation. As alternatives to ACEIs or ARBs, one can use vasodilators such as hydralazine, nitrates, or calcium channel blockers.

Inhibitors of prolactin, a culprit hormone incriminated in the pathogenesis of PPCM, are a potential therapeutic option. It is supposed to have beneficial effects on the immune system and prevent apoptosis. However, data on human use is still insufficient. A recent metanalysis of 10 studies concluded that bromocriptine significantly improved LVEF and chances of LVEF normalization but without mortality benefit. However, another metanalysis of eight studies concluded that it increased LVEF (53.3% vs. 41.8%; $p < 0.001$) as well as prolonged survival (91.6% vs. 83.9%; $p = 0.02$).[11] The ongoing REBIRTH trial will provide more clarity on its role. Use in the postpartum period is limited as bromocriptine is prothrombotic and suppresses milk production. Geographical heterogeneity in its use ranges from 87.5% in Europe to 20% in North America, Africa, and the Middle East. Cabergoline, a more selective and stronger D2 receptor agonist, has been found to be safe and effective in a small case series.[12] The convenience of weekly administration is likely to improve adherence. While ESC guidelines recommend the use of D2 agonists, ACC has not yet endorsed it since robust randomized controlled trial data remains unavailable.

Utility of digoxin is questionable. A heightened risk of ventricular arrhythmias is countered by the use of WCD for high-risk patients with an LVEF < 35% as a temporizing measure for the first 3–6 months. For women with persistent

TABLE 2: Chronic drug treatment in peripartum cardiomyopathy patients after delivery.

Drug	Persisting heart failure and absence of complete LV recovery	Complete and sustained recovery (LVEF > 55% and NYHA functional class I)
Beta-blocker	Essential for all patients in standard or maximally tolerated dosages	Continue all drugs (beta-blocker, ACEI/ARB/ARNI, MRA) for at least 12–24 months after full recovery, individual approach/ discuss with patient. Discontinue stepwise and monitor symptoms and LV function: • MRA • ACEI/ARB/ARNI • Beta-blocker
ACEI	Essential for all patients in standard or maximally tolerated dosages	
ARB	Recommended in patients who do not tolerate ACEI	
ARNI	Recommended in patients with LVEF < 40% who are symptomatic despite maximal dosages of beta-blocker, ACEI/ARB, and MRA	
MRA	Recommended in patients with LVEF < 40%, preferably eplerenone due to less hormonal side effects and less blood pressure reduction compared to spironolactone	
Ivabradine	Recommended in patients in sinus rhythm with a persisting heart rate > 70 bpm at rest despite maximal tolerated beta-blocker uptitration	Discontinue if heart rate < 50 bpm and/or in case of complete recovery
Diuretics	Recommended in patients with fluid overload	Taper dose/discontinue if no signs of fluid overload; maintain only if part of antihypertensive therapy

Note: Please note that initiation of all heart failure drugs is only possible in patients who do not breastfeed.

(ACEI: angiotensin-converting enzyme inhibitor; ARB: angiotensin receptor blocker; ARNI: angiotensin receptor-neprilysin inhibitor; LV: left ventricular; LVEF: left ventricular ejection fraction; MRA: mineralocorticoid receptor antagonist; NYHA: New York Heart Association)

LV dysfunction at or beyond 6 months from initial diagnosis, implantation of an implantable cardioverter-defibrillator (ICD) as well as cardiac resynchronization therapy (CRT) is recommended. Unfortunately, specific indications for the use of ICD and CRT therapy in these PPCM patients have not been defined. A study involving eight women who received a WCD in pregnancy found excellent arrhythmia detection but was inconclusive about the effectiveness as no shocks were delivered.[13] Duncker et al. noted several appropriate shocks for VT/ventricular fibrillation (VF) in 6 out of 49 patients on WCD. Where indicated, a subcutaneous ICD may be a better choice (in patients not needing a pacer) as it provides an option of easier removal if LV function recovers.

There is an increased risk for thromboembolism (2.2–6.6%) in patients with PPCM than other forms of cardiomyopathy.[14] Although controversial, most people recommend anticoagulation in the antepartum or postpartum period to patients with LVEF < 35%. Other indications include the presence of LV thrombus, systemic embolism, or AF. But it is unclear whether the dosage of anticoagulation should be therapeutic or prophylactic for the prevention of clot formation. While heparin is safely used both during pregnancy and lactation, vitamin K antagonists are used only during the postpartum period irrespective of breastfeeding. There is insufficient data regarding the safety of novel oral anticoagulants (NOACs) in pregnancy or breastfeeding. Of all available anticoagulants, LMWH is used most often.

Mechanical circulatory support has shown benefit in acute severe HF. It should be considered early in patients who are hemodynamically unstable and do not respond to inotropes. Extracorporeal membrane oxygenation (ECMO) and intra-aortic balloon pump (IABP) for short-term support or left ventricular assist devices (LVADs) for long-term support are both useful options. Such temporary devices should always be preferred as they are associated with high chances for complete recovery. They can be used either as "bridge to recovery," as "bridge to bridge" with implantation of more durable devices, or as "bridge to transplant." Heart transplant has been tried as a last resort in end-stage HF where MCS is not a viable option, especially for biventricular failure or profound RV failure. Transplantation rates of 4–23% have been reported in some studies.[15] It is delayed as long as possible since late recovery of LV function beyond 6–12 months is possible, and the outcome is worse following heart transplant in PPCM patients than in other cardiac cases. A greater likelihood of graft failure and death is observed in these patients possibly due to a higher incidence of allosensitization, acuity of illness, and more rejection.

Patients with persistent LV dysfunction should use HF medications indefinitely. Those with full recovery of LV function who show persistent normal LV function for at least 6 months can be offered gradual weaning off of HF medications with close clinical follow-up and 6-month interval echos up to at least 2 years. This is based on expert opinion.

DELIVERY

We have limited data for timing and mode of delivery. Input from perinatologists, anesthetists, neonatologists, and cardiologists is very important in this regard. Before delivery, the mother with PPCM must be hemodynamically stable. In stable patients without obstetric indications for cesarean delivery, vaginal delivery is recommended at term with, of course, close monitoring of maternal hemodynamics and under epidural analgesia. Some recommend using forceps or a vacuum to avoid Valsalva maneuver. On the contrary, in mothers with advanced HF, particularly when hemodynamically unstable, cesarean delivery is offered under regional anesthesia. If possible, delivery should be preferred at late preterm or early term gestation but when needed, it is typically done without further delay irrespective of the gestational age. However, PPCM when diagnosed in the antepartum period often occurs during the very last month of pregnancy. Thus, in most cases, there is little benefit in continuing the pregnancy. During delivery, regardless of the mode, the mother is placed in a lateral decubitus position to avoid aortocaval compression. Although regional block is preferred for cesarean delivery, general anesthesia is indicated for emergency cesarean section in patients with coagulopathy or severe HF. Endotracheal intubation during general anesthesia raises peripheral vascular resistance and should be countered with intravenous (IV) opioids. Positive end-expiratory pressure should also be kept at a minimum as it impedes venous return and raises RV afterload. The patient may deteriorate from rise in afterload (pain and intubation), rise in preload (increased venous return due to release of compression of IVC by the gravid uterus following childbirth), or bradycardia (anesthesia toxicity). It is important to maintain normal blood pressure levels as low BP compromises uterine blood flow and high BP raises LV afterload. In the presence of cardiogenic shock, pressors like ephedrine or norepinephrine are preferred over vasoconstrictors like phenylephrine. Most importantly, one needs to closely monitor IV fluid intake to reduce the risk of fluid overload and to follow the usual guidelines for oxytocin use. Those with extremely low EF consider continuous telemetry, and some do recommend invasive hemodynamic monitoring.

BREASTFEEDING

Opinion is divided about allowing breastfeeding in PPCM. According to the 2018 ESC guidelines for the management of cardiovascular disease in pregnancy, breastfeeding is discouraged in severely ill patients as lactation and breastfeeding involve substantial energy expenditure. Moreover, not breastfeeding allows the clinician extra leeway to administer all HF drugs including ACEIs and ARBs. In practice, however, most clinically stable patients without severe HF tolerate breastfeeding well. It also allows for the added advantage of psychological bonding between mother and child. In developing countries, limited access to potable water and high cost of infant food are practical considerations in support of breastfeeding. Findings of the IPAC study showed that breastfeeding women had higher levels of prolactin but with no impairment of myocardial recovery.[16] These reassuring results express that raised prolactin may not adversely affect the disease prognosis.

OBSTETRICS AND PERINATAL OUTCOME

Based on a small study, these mothers have a high cesarean rate of 40%. Most of these cesareans were for obstetrics indications.[17] An equally important aspect is the influence of the disease on the fetus and newborn. A metanalysis of 13 studies (involving more than 2 million pregnancies) found perinatal death to be more common in neonates born to women with cardiomyopathy (WC) as compared to women with noncardiomyopathy heart disease (NCHD) and those without heart disease (WHD).[18] Additionally, preterm delivery was six times more common than WHD and twice as common as NCHD. Similarly, being small for gestational age was six- and threefold more likely in the WC group than the other two groups, respectively.

PROGNOSIS

High potential for cardiac recovery (50–80%) mostly within the first 6 months is the hallmark of PPCM. But 20% progress to end-stage HF. Geographically, the recovery rate is highest in Asia-Pacific (62%) and lowest in the Middle East (25%).[19] Such deaths are due to refractory HF, pulmonary embolism, arrhythmia, or cardiac arrest. A considerable fraction of deaths occurred in the first week and about 90% were within 6 months of diagnosis. Overall mortality was reported to be 9% with significant geographic heterogeneity (14% in developing countries vs. 4% in developed countries).[20] Adverse prognostic factors include worse New York Heart Association (NYHA) functional class, EF < 25%, higher LV end-diastolic, poor socioeconomic status, African American race, multiparity, and age > 30–35 years.

Patients should be counseled about the possibility of PPCM recurrence in future pregnancies. The risk of recurrence in subsequent pregnancy is 30–50%, but the mortality risk is about 12%. Pregnancy is absolutely contraindicated if there is persistent LV dysfunction. As per Elkayam et al., the risk of recurrent HF and maternal mortality were better in women with normal LV function in comparison to those with persistent compromised LV function. This later group had a 44% risk of HF compared with 21%, and maternal mortality rate was 19% versus 0%, respectively.

Importantly, patients in both groups had a drop in EF following future pregnancies. For this reason, even in patients with normal LV function following PPCM, future pregnancy is also discouraged. If they plan for future pregnancies, preconception counseling with a perinatologist and cardiologist is highly recommended.[21] Preferably, all teratogenic drugs should be stopped nearly 3 months before planned pregnancy and an echo should be offered to confirm maintenance of normal LV function. Thereafter, conception may be planned against the background of pregnancy-compatible HF therapy. Stress echo and strain imaging may be useful to identify susceptible patients. Beta-blockers may be continued throughout the period of pregnancy even with normal LV function. Regular follow-up for 6 months following delivery is warranted to detect recurrence of the disease.

Counseling regarding appropriate contraception is a crucial part of the treatment plan. Safe methods include temporary options like progesterone-releasing subcutaneous implants, depot medroxyprogesterone, progesterone-only mini pills, and intrauterine devices as well as permanent measures like tubal ligation and vasectomy. Because of the increased risk of fluid retention and thromboembolism, estrogen–progesterone-containing combined contraceptives are undesirable.

INDIAN SCENARIO

Assessment of disease profile in India is handicapped by poor data compilation and nonexistent reporting mechanism. The incidence has been reported to be 1 per 1,541 live births from a tertiary care hospital but has been found to be 1 in 453 live births in a prospective study of a rural public hospital. While worldwide data show incidence rising after 30 years of age, Indian studies found the mean age to be 23 years with half of the patients being primigravida. Another retrospective, observational study also calculated the mean age as 25 years and 65% primigravida.[20] This profile is like the Haitian studies where multiparity and increased age are not critical risk factors. Chaitra et al. noted that 20% of the multigravida had a history of PPCM in the first pregnancy. Around 21% suffered from preeclampsia, whereas 8% had multiple pregnancies. Binu et al. found no significant association between PPCM and gestational hypertension, hypothyroidism, or diabetes.[22] On the other hand, smaller studies have found a strong association with preeclampsia (up to 66% prevalence). Joshi et al. noted that anemia, an easily treatable condition, is seen in 18% and is a strong risk factor for maternal as well as fetal death.[23] The majority of PPCM patients were diagnosed in early puerperium, which goes along with the trends worldwide. The most common symptom was breathlessness of which 60% were in NYHA class III and 26% in NYHA class IV. But cardiogenic shock was noted in 13%. This matches EORP registry data wherein NYHA class III or IV is the presentation in 70% of patients. The common ECG findings are sinus tachycardia and nonspecific ST-T changes. AF was found in 14% of patients, similar to the findings in other developing countries like Nigeria and Pakistan. Echocardiographic findings at diagnosis included an LV end-diastolic dimension of 5.8 cm and a mean LVEF of 25%. Cesarean delivery is recommended for decompensated HF or fetal distress. In various studies, 60–80% of patients were delivered by cesarean section, thus reflecting the severity of patient presentation. An additional 10% underwent operational vaginal delivery to shorten the second stage of labor and reduce maternal stress. Binu et al. reported maternal and fetal mortality to be about 10 and 25%, respectively. Small studies from tertiary care centers show low or even zero mortality rates, reflecting the role of optimum treatment in preventing death. Among the survivors, LV function recovery was complete with EF of 53% at 24 months of follow-up. A study from Madras Medical College found the predictors of complete recovery to be early diagnosis by periodic echocardiography as well as higher EF and FS at diagnosis. Cardiogenic shock was an adverse clinical prognostic factor (odds ratio of 16.9 for death).

CONCLUSION

A lot of progress has been made in the last several years in the understanding of PPCM. Unfortunately, we are missing disease-specific treatment as well as specific diagnostic and prognostic tests. Because this disease is so rare, we need multicenter collaborative studies along with higher enrollment in prospective registry, further support for research, and better-organized patient advocacy groups.

ONLINE REFERENCES

Please scan the QR code provided at the end of the table of contents for References of this chapter.

CHAPTER

94 Management Strategies of Pregnant Women with Congenital Heart Disease

Chandan Kumar Das

ABSTRACT

Impaired cardiac function in pregnant women represents the challenges to both the obstetrician and the cardiologist. The physiological changes during pregnancy at times submerge the symptoms of associated cardiac lesions. Detection of such cardiac lesions in the midterm pregnancy onward creates the nightmares for cardio-obstetrician team. Such lesions often prove to be fatal for both the mother and the fetus. Preconception counseling is the most ideal, but acceptance by many societies of such counseling is again a big question. Incorporation of a routine cardiac evaluation with echocardiography appears to be very promising in the antenatal clinics. Even after detection of adult congenital heart lesions in pregnant women, proper interventions by a multidisciplinary expert team or task force for antenatal, intrapartum, and postnatal should address the maternal and fetal morbidity and mortality.

Keywords: Adult congenital heart disease, multidisciplinary expert team, cardio-obstetrician, preconception counseling, atrial septal defect, ventricular septal defect, patent ductus arteriosus.

INTRODUCTION

The common belief which still persists in Indian culture today is that a woman is never complete without her motherhood part of life. In the earlier days women with congenital heart disease (CHD) rarely used to reach the age of reproduction. The growing modern medical technology and the improved living standard of the people of current era have brought some challenges to the field of cardio-obstetrics. Due to advance in early detection and proper management many female children born with CHD are reaching childbearing age. There occurs the real challenge for cardiologists to assist the concerned obstetrician for safe confinement of pregnant women with CHD. Most of these pregnant women carry moderate-to-high risk for both the mother and the fetus. In a recent study by Hiralal Konar et al., it was detected that out of 281 pregnant women with heart diseases 69% were rheumatic heart disease and 21% were CHD with ratio of 3.2:1.[1]

Many such women, however, do not have access to adult CHD tertiary centers with experts. Hence, it is essential for the clinicians to know the tips and guidelines and to get acquainted to manage such cases not only for preconception counseling and diagnostic evaluation to determine maternal and fetal risk but also to manage and to refer them to a regional center with expertise in pregnancy management.

INDIAN SCENARIO OF PREGNANCY WITH HEART DISEASES

Global maternal mortality rate (MMR) is 70/100,000 live births. Average Indian MMR is 97/100,000 and has been declined over the years to 97 in 2018–2020 from 103 in 2017–2019 and 130 in 2014–2016.[2]

Some Indian states are still in stage III of obstetric transition with a MMR as high as 215 per 100,000 live births, while few others have already moved into stage IV with a MMR as low as 43/100,000 live births.[3] States with lower MMR have to shift focus to target reduction of deaths due to heart diseases and other indirect causes, which needs a different set of interventions with multidisciplinary approach.[4]

Some common adult CHDs include:

- Atrial septal defect (ASD)
- Ventricular septal defect (VSD)
- Transposition of the great vessels
- Patent ductus arteriosus (PDA)

- Marfan syndrome
- Coarctation of aorta (CoA)
- Bicuspid aortic valve with stenosis
- Tetralogy of Fallot (TOF)
- Post-Fontan physiology

PREGNANCY AND CARDIOVASCULAR SYSTEM

Pregnancy brings remarkable hemodynamic changes in cardiovascular system. Sometime it is mistaken for an abnormal finding.

The plasma volume starts increasing from sixth week and goes up to second trimester by 50% increase of baseline. There occurs relative anemia. Hence, heart rate and cardiac output increases above 20% of baseline. Blood pressure decreases to some extent with increase in venous pressure leading to edematous legs.

During labor 500 mL blood is lost in vaginal delivery and 1,000 mL blood loss occurs in cesarean delivery of baby. After the delivery of the baby autotransfusion takes place from contracting uterus up to 72 hours. A chance of pulmonary edema remains during this period.

Examination of cardiovascular system of a pregnant lady near second trimester may lead to confusion:
- *Pulse*: Increased rate, high volume, and bounding character
- *Jugular venous pressure (JVP)*: Increased venous return in volume pulsation makes it more prominence
- *On auscultation*: S1 loud, S2 appear accentuated, and may have a systolic murmur (<3/6 grade) and S3.

All these findings may bring a confusion to diagnose an ASD. A cervical venous hum or a mammary soufflé may be confused with a continuous murmur. But there should not be any diastolic murmur. Presence of a diastolic murmur should bring a suspicion of a concomitant lesion.

APPROACH TO PLAN MANAGEMENT STRATEGY

- Risk stratification for individual case
- Preconception counseling
- Maternal and fetal risk during medical management of cardiovascular dysfunction
- Individual lesion concerned intervention

Risk Stratification

Before going for planning the management of a pregnant woman with CHD it is essential to look for the predictors of maternal cardiovascular complications. These predictions should be done on clinical and echocardiography assessment basis. **Table 1** shows the risk in mother and the fetus, **Table 2** shows the risk factors of the pregnant mother only.

TABLE 1: Maternal risk prediction at baseline evaluation.[5,6]

Baseline clinical assessment	Maternal risk	Fetal risk
Cardiac event before pregnancy	Present	
Cardiovascular drugs before pregnancy	Present	Present
NYHA Class III or IV	Present	Present
Anticoagulation	+/–	Present
Cyanosis	Present	Present
Smoking during pregnancy	Present	Present
Transthoracic echocardiography assessment		
Left ventricular dysfunction	Present	
Pulmonary hypertension	Present	
Severe AV valve regurgitation	Present	
Maternal cardiac lesion		
Cyanotic heart disease (corrected or uncorrected)	Present	Present
Pulmonary hypertension over a L to R shunt	Present	Present
Aortic coarctation	Present	

(AV: aortic valve; NYHA: New York Heart Association)

Heart failure and tachyarrhythmia have been found to be less fatal for maternal risk.

Preconception Counseling

The acceptability of preconception counseling in the present society certainly varies from a voluntary inclination to humble rejection under cultural influence. At the one end couples may welcome the advice of deferring pregnancy in view of safe life of woman partner and on the other hand, opportunity of motherhood for a woman is given priority over life risk. Preconception counseling should be done by a joint team of an obstetrician and a cardiologist. It should aim at empowering women to make informed choices. The team should explain the scopes and risks in a very simple and acceptable manner. Sometime, even after a safe confinement a woman may get severe deterioration of her cardiac malfunction and succumb to subsequent intervention leaving her child motherless at a very young age. All these factors should be well explained to the couples.

Importance of Cardiovascular Evaluation before and during Pregnancy

Females willing for pregnancy with various cardiac ailments coming to a cardiac clinic for counseling should be advised as per the following guidelines:
- *Should not go for pregnancy if suffering from*:
    - Pulmonary hypertension from any cause

TABLE 2: The WHO classification (modified version of 2018) of maternal risk.[7]

WHO (modified) class	Cardiac lesion	Maternal cardiac risk
Class I	Mild PS, PDA, and MVP	2.5–5%
	Successfully repaired ASD, VSD, PDA, and TAPVC	
Class II	Unrepaired ASD and VSD	5.7–10.5%
	Repaired TOF	
Class II or III	Mild LV dysfunction (EF >45%)	10–19%
	HCM	
	Repaired coarctation of aorta	
	Bicuspid aortic valve (aorta <45 mm)	
	Atrioventricular septal defect	
Class III	Moderate LV dysfunction (EF 30–45%)	19–27%
	Systemic RV with good or mildly impaired LV function	
	Unrepaired cyanotic heart disease	
	Mod aortic dilatation (40–45 mm in Marfan, 45–50 in bicuspid aortic valve, <50 mm in TOF)	
	Other complex congenital heart disease	
Class IV	Pulmonary arterial hypertension	40–100%
	Fontan with any complication	
	Severe (re)coarctation	
	Severe systemic ventricular dysfunction (EF <30%)	
	Severe aortic dilatation (>45 mm in Marfan, >50 in bicuspid aortic valve, >50 mm in TOF)	

(ASD: atrial septal defect; EF: ejection fraction; HCM: hypertrophic cardiomyopathy; LV: left ventricular; MVP: mitral valve prolapse; PDA: patent ductus arteriosus; PS: pulmonary stenosis; RV: right ventricular; TAPVC: total anomalous pulmonary venous connection; TOF: tetralogy of Fallot; VSD: ventricular septal defect; WHO: World Health Organization)

- Eisenmenger syndrome
- Dilated cardiomyopathy (DCM) with left ventricular ejection fraction (LVEF) <30%
- Peripartum cardiomyopathy with reduced ejection fraction (EF)
- Symptomatic severe aortic stenosis (AS)
- Severe mitral stenosis
- Marfan syndrome with aortic diameter >45 mm
- Chronic aortic dissection (AoD)

- *Can go for pregnancy with high risk if suffering from*:
  - Implanted with a mechano-prosthetic valve
  - DCM with mild-to-moderate LV dysfunction
  - Asymptomatic severe AS
  - Unrepaired CoA
  - Complex congenital cyanotic heart disease (non-Eisenmenger)

How to counsel those who want to undergo pregnancy with CHDs? Very careful preconception evaluation by experts needed to screen the followings:

Apart from the detail clinical examination to rule out any cardiac murmur, loud P2, raised JVP, and bibasal lung crepitations. Lung crepitations, one transesophageal echocardiography (TEE) should be considered if any information remains incomplete by transthoracic echocardiography (TTE). TEE may be done with precautions to avoid overstraining by the pregnant patient. Echocardiography remains the imaging of choice for cardiac evaluation of pregnant women.

Acyanotic Lesions

Shunt lesions such as ASD, VSD, and PDA with a small-sized communication and minimum hemodynamic derangements will tolerate well the pregnancy.

Stenotic lesions such as pulmonary valvular stenosis and CoA are also well tolerated.

All these cases should undergo a careful prepregnancy cardiac evaluation to check the stress capacity of the heart.

Cyanotic Lesions

Any surgically corrected congenital cyanotic heart disease with residual cyanosis should avoid pregnancy.

Tetralogy of Fallot cases that have undergone total internal correction and found to have good biventricular function may be allowed to undergo pregnancy.

Ebstein anomaly cases after surgical repair and replacement of tricuspid valve usually do well with pregnancy. Post-Fontan procedure patients are to be advised to avoid pregnancy in view of both maternal and fetal fatality.

Maternal and Fetal Risk during Medical Management of Cardiovascular Dysfunction

Certain commonly used cardiovascular drugs to be administered with caution if the recipient is pregnant. Some are contraindicated to avoid fetal complications.

Cardiovascular drugs in pregnancy:

- *Safe (commonly used) drugs*:
  - Aspirin—low dose
  - Clopidogrel

  - Digoxin
  - Heparin
  - Methyldopa
  - Sotalol
- *Partially safe with some cautions*:
  - Adenosine
  - Beta blockers
  - Calcium channel blockers
  - Hydralazine
  - Furosemide
  - Lidocaine
- *Contraindicated*:
  - Amiodarone
  - Aldosterone
  - Angiotensin-converting enzyme inhibitor (ACEI)
  - Angiotensin receptor blocker (ARB)
  - Statins
  - Warfarin

Individual Lesion Concerned Intervention

Most commonly come across congenital heart lesions in pregnant women are PDA, ASD, and VSD. This accounts almost 60% of all. Pregnant women with known CHD do have risk of 3–12% of having babies with CHD.[8] **Table 3** shows the possibilities of CHDs in fetus of affected pregnant women.

ACYANOTIC LESIONS

Atrioventricular Septal Defect (Atrioventricular Canal Defect)

Atrioventricular septal defect (AVSD) constitutes almost 3% of all CHDs. Pregnant women with this lesion do not tolerate well due to subsequent severe complications such as recurrent arrhythmia and heart failure due to dilated chambers. Optimum medical management for arrhythmia and heart failure may help in some cases if the left-sided atrioventricular valve is least affected. Maternal and fetal mortality is very high in this group.

TABLE 3: Congenital heart diseases in fetus.

Congenital defect in mother	% of chances of transmission in fetus
Atrioventricular septal defect (AVSD)	11.6
Aortic stenosis (AS)	8
Coarctation of aorta (CoA)	6.3
Atrial septal defect (ASD)	6.1
Ventricular septal defect (VSD)	6
Pulmonary stenosis (PS)	5.3
Patent ductus arteriosus (PDA)	4.1
Tetralogy of Fallot (TOF)	2
Total	5.8

Atrial Septal Defect

Compared to general population (pregnant women) and repaired ASD the unrepaired ASD group had 4.3% more chances of arrhythmia and 3% more chances of heart failure [deterioration in the New York Heart Association (NYHA) status]. Complications like prolapsed anterior mitral leaflet in to ASD and causing severe mitral regurgitation apart from occasions of paradoxical embolism have been reported. There is no usual requirement for closure of ASD during pregnancy unless it is complicated by cyanosis due to reversal of shunt (with no significant rise of pulmonary vascular resistance) or recurrent paradoxical thromboembolism.

Appropriate time to intervene is second trimester with minimum fluoroscopic exposure. Transesophageal or intracardiac echocardiography has been used to guide device closure of suitable ASDs without fluoroscopy. Surgical correction of ASDs has also been reported to be safe.[9,10]

Ventricular Septal Defect

Ventricular septal defect is usually well tolerated by pregnant women unless it is complicated by significant rise of pulmonary vascular resistance. VSD specific pregnancy data are limited. Incidences of preeclampsia are more in unrepaired VSD than in repaired VSD. But small for age fetus have been reported in mothers with repaired VSD.[11] A safe device VSD closure may be planned as long as the pulmonary vascular resistance is not raised.

Patent Ductus Arteriosus

Patent ductus arteriosus has incidence of 1 in 2,000 live births with female to male ratio of 2:1. The ductus serves as an important conduit in fetal circulation which usually closes by 72 hour of postnatal life. Small PDAs with pulmonary flow: systemic flow ratio is <1.5 and are usually tolerated well in pregnancy. Significant PDAs with ratio >2.2 cause volume overload with heart failure. As such pregnancy causes reduction of systemic vascular resistance enhancing right to left flow at large PDA level which precipitates heart failure.[12]

Device closure of smaller (<3 mm) PDAs may be deferred during pregnancy since chances of LV dysfunction is low compared to larger (>9 mm) PDAs where LV dysfunction is very likely to occur during pregnancy.[13] Suitable timing should be decided by the joint team of cardio-obstetrics for a safe device closure of large PDAs. Rare but significant complications of device closure of PDAs such as infective endocarditis, pinching of left pulmonary artery, and narrowing of descending aorta may be taken care of.

Pulmonary Arterial Hypertension

Pregnancy should be avoided in presence of significant pulmonary arterial hypertension (PAH) (>50 mm Hg). As per current guidelines if PAH is detected in pregnancy a therapeutic abortion may be advised in view of maternal and fetal mortality (30–56% and 11–28%, respectively).[14]

The presenting clinical features of PAH may be confused with that of pregnancy itself such as fatigue and swelling of legs (right heart failure). Such patients should avoid lying on their back to avoid compression of inferior vena cava. Injection low-molecular-weight heparin, judicious use of diuretics and calcium channel blockers may be tried. Early confinement should be planned to avoid complication of full term labor. Vitamin K antagonists should be avoided in view of fetal toxicity. Injection intravenous (IV) epoprostenol infusion may be initiated before inducing labor.

Pulmonary Stenosis

Isolated pulmonary stenosis (PS) is usually well tolerated in pregnancy. Rarely symptomatic patients of PS with peak gradient of 50 mm Hg or asymptomatic PS with peak gradient >60 mm Hg may require intervention. Balloon valvotomy can be safely performed during pregnancy (second trimester).

Marfan Syndrome

Most of the time the diagnosis of Marfan syndrome is missed before the conception. In common practice it goes unnoticed till the women attains reproductive age and even they remain asymptomatic. Once it is diagnosed by the specific clinical and echo criteria one has to ascertain the cardiovascular safety during pregnancy, since 80% of all Marfan syndrome cases do have cardiovascular involvement. Most dreaded complication is AoD apart from aortic regurgitation and mitral valve prolapse. Hence, screening by echocardiography is mandatory to assess the aortic root dimension.

Women with Marfan syndrome who has aortic root <4 cm has 1% chance of developing AoD. Dissection occurs mostly in the last trimester and postpartum period. Women with aortic root >4 cm or a strong family history of dissection or sudden death in absence of dilated aortic root also have risk of aortic rupture. If such patient comes for preconception counseling, the pregnancy may be delayed till surgical repair or replacement of aortic root. These patients need to be kept on cardioselective beta blockers as preventive measure.[15,16]

Aortic Stenosis

Pregnant women with bicuspid aortic valve with stenosis may remain asymptomatic for long time. But with a history of such lesion women are advised not to go for pregnancy if severe symptomatic AS or asymptomatic severe AS when associated with either impaired left ventricular systolic function with EF <50% or isolated bicuspid aortic valve when the ascending aorta is dilated >50 mm. Before pregnancy, the presence of pressure gradient of >50 mm Hg or AoV area <1 cm^2 may lead to aortopathy (dissection), arrhythmia, or heart failure. If detected during pregnancy, an optimum medical management with beta blocker, diuretic, and restricted activities with close echo monitoring on the earlier mentioned parameters may help for a safe confinement. If refractory to these, balloon valvotomy to be advised or plan for early cesarean section and go for valve replacement.[17]

Coarctation of Aorta

Most cases of CoA are usually corrected before the woman comes for pregnancy. Some missed cases may present with refractory hypertension in pregnancy. During pregnancy such cases are vulnerable for aneurysmal dilatation and dissection or rupture of aorta. Physical activities to be restricted in order to avoid cerebral arterial rupture and dissection of aorta. Beta blocker for control of hypertension should be started. Percutaneous approach with covered stent for re-CoA can be an alternative approach. Management to shorten the second stage of labor is necessary to avoid complication of CoA.[18]

CYANOTIC LESIONS

Tetralogy of Fallot

This is the most common lesion among the cyanotic heart diseases. Today, most of the cases of TOF are repaired at an early age and hence women are reaching up to reproductive age. Usually these women go with an uneventful pregnancy. But, in a country like India where awareness and modern medical facilities have not yet reached to rural areas many pregnant women with uncorrected TOF are reporting to cardiology outpatient department (OPD). They usually have history of recurrent abortions and small for date babies. Such patient may present with severe heart failure symptoms. They can also present with atrial and ventricular arrhythmias, infective endocarditis, and fatal complications such as pulmonary hemorrhage, brain abscess, and thromboembolism.[19,20] Close monitoring of both repaired and unrepaired cases of TOF during pregnancy is highly advisable. Cesarean section should be planned to cut short the second stage of labor. Right heart failure and arrhythmia should be treated according to the protocols.

Transposition of the Great Arteries

Pregnant women with dextro-transposition of the great arteries (d-TGA) have usually undergone repairs like atrial switch operation (Mustard or Senning) with redirection of systemic and pulmonary venous return in a systemic right ventricle (RV). During pregnancy this RV function determines the cardiovascular outcome. Some cases may need to address RV failure and arrhythmia.[21]

Post-Fontan Physiology

Children born with functionally single ventricle CHD such as hypoplastic left heart syndrome, tricuspid atresia, and double outlet RV survive further with surgical intervention like creation of a Fontan circulation. This has improved life expectancy for women who desire to go for pregnancy. But, the lack of a subpulmonary ventricle results in a chronic low cardiac output state with pulmonary blood flow dependent on adequate preload.[22] Patients often encounter complications in adulthood with a gradually declining functional capacity, atrial arrhythmias, myocardial dysfunction, thromboembolic events, and hepatic dysfunction.[23] A Mayo clinic study in 2015 found that Fontan physiology affected placental circulation like that of liver. Consequently fetal circulation and fetal growth apart from maternal low cardiac output are severely affected. Considering the data of fetal mortality and morbidity preconception counseling is strongly recommended for such cases.

SUMMARY OF MEDICAL, CARDIOLOGICAL INTERVENTION, AND INTRAPARTUM MANAGEMENT

Medical

Basically all pregnant women with CHD need special care to monitor the hemodynamics clinically as well as electro- and echocardiographically.

Heart Failure

Fluid management, diuretics, digoxin, and beta blockers are mainstay of treatment. Some cases may need hydralazine or oral isosorbide to reduce afterload. Despite paucity of data, infusion of dihydroxyphenylalanine (DOPA) or dobutamine may also be given in refractory cases.

Arrhythmia

- *Paroxysmal supraventricular tachycardia (PSVT)*: Adenosine, metoprolol, and digoxin can be given safely (atenolol to be avoid in view of fetal growth retardation).[24]
- *Atrial flutter or fibrillation*: Apart from metoprolol, a group B drug sotalol or group C drugs diltiazem, verapamil, and ibutilide are relatively safe. Antithrombotic drugs such as heparin and antiplatelets may be considered as per individualized case.[25]
- *Ventricular tachyarrhythmia*: Beta blocker may be required to continue throughout pregnancy if recurrent ventricular tachycardia appears. In emergency situations, injection lignocaine, amiodarone, or IV mexiletine can be used.
- *Heart blocks*: Atrioventricular block or sick sinus syndrome may occur during pregnancy with any CHD. Permanent pacemaker implantation (PPI) may be done after eighth week of pregnancy preferably under echocardiography guidance.
- *Cyanosis*: No definite treatment for cyanosis in pregnancy has been prescribed. Pregnancy should be terminated in cyanosis with congenital cyanotic heart disease.

Cardiological Intervention

Permanent pacemaker implantation, automatic implantable cardioverter defibrillator (AICD), and cardiac resynchronization therapy with defibrillator (CRT-D) in case of lifesaving situations may be done. Cardiovascular surgeries should be deferred till early delivery of the baby.

Intrapartum Management

Cardiological aspect of management of the case as a whole during labor should be very critical at times. Delivery should be conducted either in left or right lateral tilt position to avoid compression of inferior vena cava. In case of right to left shunt cases continuous pulse oximetry monitoring should be done. Prior to this individual risk stratification should be done. If needed, high-risk patient should be shifted to tertiary care hospital where cardio-obstetric team is active and experienced.

CONCLUSION

Continuous medical research and innovative mechanization have brought remarkable advancement in our clinical practice. The complex congenital heart lesions get corrected today and women with these lesions are coming up to reproductive age. Although the pregnancy itself is a challenge to the existing normal cardiovascular system, these complex lesions multiply the issues. However, the skilled clinicians have also updated themselves to tackle various complications of cardiovascular system in pregnant women with complex CHDs. Preconception counseling remains the gold standard for complex lesions. The social gesture is coming up today to welcome such healthy advices. It is recommended to have clinical and echocardiographic evaluation of pregnant women during their first visit in antenatal clinic. This will solve the majority of the issues. Once diagnosed to have CHD in pregnant women the treatment strategy should be jointly planned by cardiologist and the concerned obstetrician. Such patient should be counseled along with their husband or family members for choosing a suitable tertiary care center for safe confinement. Prevalence of uncorrected lesions of all CHDs are mostly found in rural health centers where specialty services like cardiac evaluation is lacking in the present healthcare system. At least all district hospitals should have cardiology unit with full team to support the treating obstetricians.

ONLINE REFERENCES

Please scan the QR code provided at the end of the table of contents for References of this chapter.

SECTION 12

Cardio-oncology

CHAPTER

95

Cardio-oncology in India: The Need, Scope, and Building Blocks

Sonu Abraham, Sumanth Khadke, Anju Nohria, Sarju Ganatra

ABSTRACT

Cardio-oncology focuses on the prevention, detection, monitoring, and treatment of cardiovascular issues in patients undergoing cancer treatment or in those with a history of cancer. Due to the increasing prevalence of cancer and cardiovascular disease in India, there is a growing necessity for a heightened understanding of cardio-oncology and specialists with expertise in the field. In this chapter, we discuss the cardiotoxic effects of antineoplastic agents and radiation therapy, cardiovascular risk stratification and prevention, and cardiac imaging in cancer patients. We also provide a framework encompassing clinical, educational, and research domains to help facilitate the establishment of cardio-oncology programs across the country.

Keywords: Cardio-oncology, immune checkpoint inhibitor myocarditis, anthracyclines, trastuzumab, cardiac MRI.

INTRODUCTION

Cardio-oncology refers to the cardiovascular (CV) subspecialty that focuses on the prevention, detection, monitoring, and treatment of CV issues in patients undergoing cancer treatment or in those with a history of cancer.[1] With cancer and cardiovascular diseases (CVDs) being the leading causes of global mortality, the field of cardio-oncology has gained significant attention in recent years. Improved cancer survivorship and an aging population have brought forth a convergence in CVD and cancer. Managing coexistent CV conditions that may influence cancer treatment decisions is becoming increasingly important. Furthermore, growing knowledge of CV adverse effects related to cancer therapeutics has highlighted the need for multidisciplinary expertise and collaboration between oncologists and cardiologists. The field of cardio-oncology aims to permit optimal cancer treatment while minimizing CV morbidity and mortality.

EMERGING NEED FOR CARDIO-ONCOLOGY IN INDIA

With the rising incidence of cancer and CVD in India, there is a need for increased awareness about cardio-oncology and for the development of integrated and country-wide cardio-oncology initiatives focused on the care of this patient population. One in nine people in India are likely to develop cancer during their lifetime.[2] Based on the National Cancer Registry Programme Report in 2020, the incidence of cancer in India is estimated to increase by 12.8% by the year 2025, with a crude rate of 100.4 per 100,000 persons in 2022.[2] India is ranked third, after China and the United States of America, in cancer incidence. The extensive utilization of established cancer therapies such as anthracyclines and trastuzumab, coupled with a rapid increase in the use of novel cancer therapeutics, has introduced a diverse range of potential CV toxic effects. Thus, expertise in cardio-oncology is needed to ensure that patients in India can safely navigate cancer treatment and transition to the survivorship phase.

The mortality risk due to CVD is more than doubled in individuals diagnosed with cancer as compared to the general population.[3] The impact on the Indian population is substantial. The age-standardized death rate from CVD in India (282 deaths per 100,000 persons) is higher than that in the rest of the world (233 deaths per 100,000 persons).[4] In India, the CVD burden is distinctively characterized by a higher risk factor burden, an earlier age of onset, higher rates of premature death, and greater overall mortality.[3] Therefore, identification of CVD and CV risk factors in cancer patients is central to their care, both with respect to appropriate risk stratification and to inform cancer treatment planning.

THE SCOPE OF CARDIO-ONCOLOGY

Cancer and CVD are interconnected due to shared risk factors such as obesity, malnutrition, smoking, alcohol abuse, hypertension, hyperlipidemia, and diabetes.[5] Common pathophysiological mechanisms including inflammation and oxidative stress drive this bidirectional relationship. In addition, the spectrum of cardiac toxicities related to antineoplastic therapies can include cancer therapy-related cardiac dysfunction (CTRCD), myocarditis [specifically immune checkpoint inhibitor (ICI) related], atherosclerosis, vascular toxicity, arterial hypertension, cardiac arrhythmias, and venous thromboembolism.[6]

RISK STRATIFICATION

In general, the presence of underlying CVD and CV risk factors is associated with an increased risk of cardiotoxicity in patients with cancer. Identifying individuals susceptible to CV toxicity prior to commencing cancer treatment, during therapy, and among survivors is a significant focus of cardio-oncology. Conventional CV risk prediction models like the Framingham risk score often underestimate risk in cancer patients because they fail to acknowledge cancer therapy as a distinct risk factor. The Heart Failure Association of the European Society of Cardiology (ESC) Cardio-Oncology Study Group in collaboration with the International Cardio-Oncology Society (ICOS) has attempted to overcome this limitation by developing a therapy-specific risk assessment tool (HFA-ICOS Risk Assessment tool) that classifies oncology patients into different risk categories—very high, high, moderate, and low—that enable physicians to predict the likelihood of CV toxicity prior to the initiation of cancer therapy. Older age, prior history of CVD, presence of CV risk factors, previous cardiotoxic treatments, and lifestyle risk factors contribute to increasing risk[7] in patients on anthracyclines, human epidermal growth factor receptor 2 (HER2) targeted therapies, vascular endothelial growth factor (VEGF) inhibitors, BRAF and MEK inhibitors, multitargeted kinase inhibitors, and certain multiple myeloma therapies.

In addition, further testing with an electrocardiogram (ECG), cardiac biomarkers, and a transthoracic echocardiogram (TTE) are recommended prior to the initiation of potentially cardiotoxic cancer therapies for risk stratification and to establish a baseline for comparison. A baseline ECG can help screen for arrhythmias, prolonged QTc, and ischemia. Cardiac troponins >99th percentile, brain natriuretic peptide (BNP) ≥35 pg/mL and N-terminal proBNP (NT-proBNP) ≥125 pg/mL confer a greater risk.[6] Increased cardiac biomarkers before initiation of cancer therapy can identify underlying myocardial injury and strain, allowing for early risk stratification and an opportunity to refine medical therapy prior to cancer treatment. Baseline TTE with accurate documentation of left ventricular (LV) systolic function (ideally using three-dimensional echocardiography) and global longitudinal strain (GLS) is recommended.[8] In the absence of availability of GLS, other markers like annular Doppler velocity can be utilized. Patients with a baseline left ventricular ejection fraction (LVEF) <50% or those in the low normal range (50–54%) are at increased risk of cardiotoxicity.[9] Cardiology referral is recommended for patients classified as high or very high risk.

CARDIOVASCULAR SURVEILLANCE DURING ANTINEOPLASTIC THERAPIES

The primary modalities of surveillance include cardiac biomarkers [troponin and natriuretic peptides (NPs)] and CV imaging including TTE with GLS and/or cardiac MRI. The frequency of monitoring depends on the cardiotoxic potential of the cancer therapy and the baseline risk of the patient. A change in NP levels during therapy may detect volume overload and congestion prior to changes in LVEF. Troponin elevation during treatment has been associated with a higher likelihood of overt LV dysfunction.

Cancer therapy-related cardiac dysfunction is considered mild when there is an asymptomatic reduction in LVEF to a value ≥50% or a relative reduction in GLS of ≥15% from baseline with a normal LVEF. It is considered moderate if there is an asymptomatic decline in LVEF by ≥10% points to a value <50% or a decline in LVEF of 10% to a value <50% with an accompanying change in GLS of ≥15% from baseline. It is considered severe if the EF falls below 40% or if the patient develops symptomatic heart failure (HF). The modalities for assessment of LVEF in descending order of preference include a 3D echocardiogram, cardiac MRI, Simpson's biplane 2D assessment, and multigated acquisition (MUGA) scanning. Cardiac MRI allows for accurate quantification of left and right ventricular function, valvular disease, pericardial disease, and evidence of cardiotoxicity, including ischemia, inflammation, and fibrosis. Cardiac CT is useful for the assessment of coronary artery disease (CAD) both prior to treatment initiation and after acute coronary syndrome (ACS)-like presentations. Functional macro- and microvascular ischemia can be well delineated with nuclear modalities.

Specific drug therapy-related surveillance recommendations are discussed here.

Common Cardiotoxicities

Traditional Chemotherapeutic Agents

Anthracyclines, including doxorubicin, daunorubicin, epirubicin, idarubicin, and mitoxantrone, have been used for the treatment of leukemias, lymphomas, sarcomas, and breast, stomach, uterine, ovarian, and lung cancers. Anthracyclines can cause dose-dependent myocardial damage that can be irreversible if not detected and treated early. Cardiac toxicity can range from acute arrhythmias and myopericarditis to LV dysfunction and HF, which can occur many years after treatment completion. CV risk factors, including blood pressure (BP), blood glucose, lipid profile, and glomerular filtration rate, should be evaluated and optimized before initiation of anthracyclines. In all patients receiving anthracycline therapy, a baseline TTE followed by a 12-month post-treatment TTE is recommended. In patients receiving a cumulative anthracycline dose ≥250 mg/m^2 of doxorubicin equivalence or in high/very high-risk patients, additional echocardiography should be considered during and after completion of therapy.[6] In addition to baseline and routine 12-month biomarker assessment in all patients, for patients at high and very high risk, it is advisable to monitor cardiac troponin and NPs before each cycle of anthracycline therapy and at 3- and 12-months following completion of therapy.[10] In patients with LVEF <40%, anthracyclines should be avoided unless there are no alternative treatments for their cancer. Cardioprotective agents such as angiotensin-converting enzyme inhibitors (ACEIs)/angiotensin receptor blockers (ARBs) and/or beta blockers should be considered for patients with borderline LVEF (50–55%). Dexrazoxane or liposomal anthracyclines should be considered in patients receiving high doses of anthracyclines. In patients who develop CTRCD during treatment with anthracyclines, anthracycline therapy should be continued with heightened echocardiographic monitoring in patients with elevated cardiac biomarkers or mild CTRCD. Treatment with ACEIs/ARBs and/or beta blockers can be considered to reduce the likelihood of overt LV dysfunction. Anthracyclines should be discontinued in all patients with moderate or severe CTRCD. If continued anthracycline use is deemed necessary despite CTRCD, concomitant dexrazoxane or substitution with liposomal doxorubicin should be considered. All patients with moderate or severe CTRCD should be treated with guideline-directed medical therapy (GDMT) as per the general HF management guidelines.

Pretherapy LVEF is considered as an important risk factor for the development of anthracycline-related CTRCD. Patients with preexisting cardiomyopathy are often excluded from receiving anthracycline-based chemotherapy, given the increased risk of worsening cardiomyopathy. This often results in inferior cancer outcomes or in cases where they receive anthracyclines and increased CV morbidity and mortality. While dexrazoxane is approved for use only in metastatic breast cancer patients who require an ongoing higher dose of anthracycline, the emerging evidence suggests that for patients with preexisting cardiomyopathy who requires anthracycline therapy for cancer, upfront concomitant dexrazoxane should be considered along with other GDMT and close monitoring.[11]

The *HER2 inhibitor*, trastuzumab, is widely used in the management of metastatic HER2-positive breast cancer and can be associated with LV dysfunction and HF. In contrast to anthracyclines, cardiotoxicity due to anti-HER2 therapies is not dose-dependent and is largely reversible. Other anti-HER2 agents, such as pertuzumab, trastuzumab emtansine, and trastuzumab deruxtecan also have cardiotoxic properties, albeit to a lesser extent. Risk factors include advanced age, diabetes mellitus, renal dysfunction, use of antihypertensives, and history of heart disease. The highest risk is in patients who have received prior anthracycline therapy. After a baseline TTE, repeat TTE is recommended every 3 months while on treatment. In patients treated with anthracyclines and trastuzumab, an additional TTE is recommended within 12 months of treatment completion. Based on the degree of risk and in patients with metastatic disease, the frequency of TTE can be adjusted. For high and very high-risk HER2-positive early breast cancer patients, NP and troponin monitoring every two to three treatment cycles and at 3- and 12-month post-therapy completion should be considered. Anti-HER2 therapies should be deferred in patients with an LVEF < 40% unless other options are not feasible. ACEIs/ARBs and/or beta blockers should be used in high-risk individuals. In patients who develop mild CTRCD during treatment with an HER2 antagonist, treatment with an HER2 agent can be continued on the background of maximally tolerated neurohormonal blockade and with close echocardiographic monitoring for further cardiac deterioration. In general, HER2-directed therapies should be interrupted in patients with moderate or severe CTRCD, and GDMT for HF should be initiated. However, HER2-directed therapy may be resumed with close monitoring if the patient remains asymptomatic and the LVEF improves to >40% with GDMT.

Fluoropyrimidines such as 5-fluorouracil (5-FU) and capecitabine, primarily used in the management of gastrointestinal malignancies, are associated with adverse CV consequences, including angina, myocardial infarction, hypertension, and stress-induced cardiomyopathy. Myocardial ischemia is precipitated by coronary vasospasm and endothelial dysfunction.[12] Infusional 5-FU is associated with a higher risk of cardiotoxicity. Patients at high risk should be preemptively screened for preexisting CAD (ECG and TTE). BP, lipids, and glycated hemoglobin (HbA1c) should be monitored and optimized before and during therapy. In patients with fluoropyrimidine-induced coronary vasospasm, the offending agent should be discontinued and an assessment for coronary ischemia should be performed. In general, vasospasm should be treated with non-dihydropyridine calcium channel blockers and/or nitrates. Reexposure to the offending agent is not recommended, given the high likelihood of recurrent cardiotoxicity. However, bolus 5-FU regimens with concomitant antivasospastic therapy are often well-tolerated.

Vascular Endothelial Growth Factor Inhibitors

Vascular endothelial growth factor inhibitor, commonly used in the treatment of renal, thyroid, and hepatocellular carcinomas, have been linked with CV complications, including hypertension, LV systolic dysfunction, HF, QTc prolongation, and arterial and venous thromboembolism. Patients with advanced age, CVD, preexisting hypertension, smoking history, obesity, and previous anthracycline therapy have a greater risk of developing VEGFi-associated adverse effects. Hypertension is dose-dependent, occurs early, and normalizes with discontinuation of the medication. BP monitoring at each ambulatory visit, supplemented by home BP monitoring during the first cycle, at the time of any dose escalation, and every 2–3 weeks thereafter, is recommended.[6] Regular ECG monitoring for QTc prolongation in the first 3 months, followed by repeat ECG every 3–6 months is advised.[13] A baseline TTE followed by risk-based repeat imaging is recommended for surveillance of LV dysfunction. Aggressive BP control is recommended in all patients. VEGFi-induced systolic dysfunction is not dose-dependent and is felt to be reversible with its withdrawal and initiation of GDMT.

Immune Checkpoint Inhibitors

There are currently 11 US Food and Drug Administration (FDA)-approved ICIs that inhibit four major classes of checkpoints including cytotoxic T-lymphocyte antigen 4 (CTLA-4) (ipilimumab and tremelimumab), programmed cell death protein-1 (PD-1) (nivolumab, pembrolizumab cemiplimab, dostarlimab, and retifanlimab), programmed death ligand-1 (PD-L-1) (atezolizumab, avelumab, and durvalumab), and lymphocyte-activation gene 3 (LAG-3) (relatlimab). ICI-associated myocarditis, while rare with an overall prevalence of 1.2–2.4%, can be associated with a high fatality rate (38–46%), highlighting the need for heightened clinical awareness. Combination therapy with two or more ICIs increases the likelihood of immune-related adverse events, including myocarditis. Preexisting conditions such as diabetes, hypertension, smoking, obesity, and autoimmune disorders are independent risk factors.[14] Baseline ECG, cardiac biomarkers, and echocardiography are recommended in high-risk patients. ICI myocarditis typically occurs within the first 3 months of exposure. Cardiac MRI is the definitive noninvasive imaging modality for the evaluation of ICI myocarditis, and identification of focal or diffuse myocardial edema and myocardial damage, including the presence of late gadolinium enhancement (LGE), are used to make the diagnosis.[9] Endomyocardial biopsy demonstrating lymphocytic infiltration with accompanying myocardial necrosis remains the gold standard. The ICOS has defined major and minor criteria to make the diagnosis.[15] Histologic evidence of myocarditis or the presence of an elevated troponin and MRI that fulfills both Lake Louis criteria meet major criteria for the diagnosis. In other patients, an elevated troponin plus two additional minor criteria (symptoms, new LV dysfunction, new high degree heart block or bundle branch block, new atrial or ventricular arrhythmias, other immune-related adverse events such as myositis or myasthenia gravis, and suggestive MRI) can be used to make the diagnosis. The ICOS has categorized ICI myocarditis severity into four groups **(Table 1)**.[15]

TABLE 1: Types of cancer therapy-associated myocarditis based on characteristics.

Types of myocarditis	Characteristics
Severe	Hemodynamic instability, heart failure requiring noninvasive or invasive ventilation, complete or high-grade heart block, and/or significant ventricular arrhythmia
Nonsevere (clinically significant)	Symptomatic but hemodynamically and electrically stable, may have reduced left ventricular ejection fraction (LVEF), no features of severe disease
Smoldering (subclinical)	Incidentally diagnosed myocarditis without any clinical signs or symptoms
Steroid refractory	Nonresolving or worsening myocarditis (clinical worsening or persistent troponin elevation after exclusion of other etiologies) despite high dose methylprednisolone

Treatment options include discontinuation of ICI therapy and prompt initiation of high-dose steroids. Usual dosing includes intravenous methylprednisolone 1,000 mg daily for 3 days, followed by oral prednisone 1 mg/kg/day. This is then followed by a gradual taper over a period of no <4–6 weeks following complete alleviation of symptoms, LVEF recovery, or stabilization of arrhythmias. In steroid nonresponders, immunosuppressive therapies such as tacrolimus, mycophenolate mofetil, antithymocyte globulin, intravenous gamma globulin, and plasmapheresis can be used. The current guidelines advocate for permanent discontinuation of ICIs in case of grade 3 or 4 immune-related adverse events. In milder cases, reintroduction of ICIs may be explored on an individual basis.

T-cell Antineoplastic Therapies

T-cell therapies, including chimeric antigen receptor (CAR) T-cell, bispecific T-cell engager/antibody (BiTE), and tumor-infiltrating lymphocyte (TIL) therapies, have revolutionized cancer therapy in patients with lymphoma, leukemia, melanoma, and multiple myeloma.[16] The immune response to T-cell therapies triggers a surge of cytokines and chemokines, which originate from the infused cells, are generated through the recruitment of nearby immune cells, and emerge due to tumor lysis. The ensuing systemic inflammatory response is referred to as cytokine release syndrome (CRS). Patients with CRS exhibit fevers accompanied by varying degrees of hypotension, hypoxia, and organ toxicity. This leads to immune-mediated cardiotoxic effects such as HF, arrhythmias, myocardial infarction, and capillary leak syndrome.[17] CRS usually occurs early with the greatest occurrence in the first 2 weeks. Predisposing risk factors include preexisting CVD, high cancer burden, greater infusion dose of T-cell therapies, and high-intensity pretreatment lymphocyte depletion regimens.

In patients with grade ≥2 CRS, close surveillance for cardiotoxicity with cardiac biomarkers and echocardiography should be considered since about 10% of patients develop cardiomyopathy. In addition to supportive management including intravenous fluids, oxygen supplementation and pressors, tocilizumab or siltuximab [interleukin 6 (IL-6) antagonists] should be considered in moderate-to-severe CRS.[17] In refractory cases or in cases with neurotoxicity, steroids are also recommended.

Multitargeted Tyrosine Kinase Inhibitors

BCR-ABL tyrosine kinase inhibitors (TKIs) (bosutinib, nilotinib, and ponatinib) are associated with accelerated atherosclerosis leading to CAD, stroke, and peripheral vascular disease. Other adverse effects include hypertension, hyperlipidemia, QTc prolongation, and to a lesser degree, LV dysfunction. Dasatinib is associated with pleural and pericardial effusions and group 1 pulmonary hypertension.[18] Baseline CV risk assessment is recommended for all patients on BCR-ABL TKI therapy. Reassessment every 3 months with echocardiography and QTc assessment on ECG in the first year and every 6–12 months thereafter is recommended, particularly in high-risk individuals. CV toxicity with bosutinib, nilotinib, and ponatinib is treated as per usual cardiology guidelines and the decision to continue or switch agents should be based on a multidisciplinary discussion. Dasatinib-induced pericardial effusions can be managed with dose reduction, with or without steroids. Dasatinib should be discontinued in patients who develop pulmonary hypertension since this can be irreversible and progressive.

Bruton Tyrosine Kinase Inhibitors

Bruton tyrosine kinase inhibitors (BTKIs), such as ibrutinib, acalabrutinib, and zanubrutinib, used for the treatment of chronic lymphoid leukemia and other B cell malignancies can cause hypertension, atrial fibrillation, ventricular arrhythmias, and HF. Strict BP control is key in the management of these patients and is associated with a lower incidence of major adverse CV events. Screening with an ECG during regular visits or in symptomatic patients is recommended for detection of atrial fibrillation. A baseline TTE is recommended in all patients. In those developing atrial fibrillation, repeat TTE should be performed.[15] BTKi also predispose patients to greater bleeding risk and therefore anticoagulation for atrial fibrillation, while recommended, may prove challenging.[6] There are significant interactions between BTKi and other drugs and these should be considered when treating patients for BTKi associated cardiotoxicity.

Radiation Cardiotoxicity

Radiation therapy (RT) for thoracic malignancies such as Hodgkin lymphoma, breast cancer, and lung cancer is associated with long-term CV complications including CAD, valvular heart disease, cardiomyopathy, pericarditis, myocardial fibrosis, dysautonomia, and conduction abnormalities.[19] Newer techniques such as intensity modulated RT and proton therapy have reduced radiation exposure to the heart and are felt to be associated with reduced cardiotoxicity. In general, the likelihood of radiation-related toxicities increases with younger age at diagnosis, use of concomitant cardiotoxic chemotherapy, chest radiation dose ≥15 Gy (greatest risk ≥35 Gy), mean cardiac dose, presence of CVD or CV risk factors, and time since RT.[19] The Childhood Cancer Survivor Study CV risk calculator identifies RT as one of the risk factors to predict the risk of HF, ischemic heart disease, and stroke by age 50 in survivors of childhood cancer.[20]

Annual risk factor assessment and aggressive modification, including strict BP control, lipid management, diabetes control, and healthy lifestyle interventions, is recommended in these patients. The use of statin therapy for primary prevention in patients with a high to very high CV toxicity risk from RT is a Class IIa recommendation according to the 2022 ESC guidelines on cardio-oncology.[6] Since established CV prevention guidelines do not include radiation exposure as a risk enhancer, patients with an atherosclerotic cardiovascular disease (ASCVD) risk score <7.5% should be further risk stratified with a coronary artery calcium (CAC) score with a consideration to initiate statins in those with a CAC score > 0.

It is recommended that asymptomatic RT survivors should be screened with a functional noninvasive stress test and echocardiogram 5–10 years after RT and every 5 years thereafter, unless there are noteworthy indications or symptoms that arise earlier. Coronary CT angiography or left heart catheterization is recommended if CAD is suspected. RT can cause restrictive cardiomyopathy due to myocardial fibrosis. Echo findings may include abnormal diastolic parameters, normal wall thickness, small LV dimensions, pericardial thickening, and evidence of constriction.[19] Valvular heart disease is a long-term complication that presents as late as 20 years after RT. The aortic and mitral valves are commonly involved with evidence of leaflet thickening, retraction, and late calcification leading to both regurgitant and stenotic lesions.

With respect to management, cardiac surgery is associated with unfavorable outcomes in survivors treated with RT. When possible, percutaneous options such as PCI and transcatheter aortic valve replacement should be considered. When patients need surgery, a thorough preoperative assessment should be performed, and any accompanying significant lesions should be addressed due to increased risks associated with reoperation.

PATHWAYS TO BUILDING A CARDIO-ONCOLOGY FRAMEWORK IN INDIA

We propose a three-pronged framework to help establish cardio-oncology programs in India, encompassing the clinical, educational, and research realms **(Fig. 1)**.

Clinical

The need for a cardiologist in a cancer center is now more apparent than ever before, both due to the rising incidence of cancer and due to the introduction of novel anticancer therapies in India. Cardiologists interested in a career in cardio-oncology may attend international cardio-oncology conferences, and review established guidelines and current evidence for the management of these patients. The establishment of a cardio-oncology program may pose several challenges including (1) a possible lack of institutional support driven by the novelty of the field and limited recognition among oncologists and cardiologists regarding the necessity for cardio-oncology services and (2) resource availability.[21] Lack of mentorship due to the nascency of the field poses an additional challenge. This can be overcome by seeking out faculty mentors in established cardio-oncology centers in the country and abroad and by approaching oncologists who have an interest in the CV toxicities of cancer therapy.

The initial step involves spreading awareness among other physicians and the hospital administration. This can be achieved by giving presentations on cardio-oncology at departmental grand rounds and in administrative committees to discuss the scope and impact of the field. This will also facilitate the establishment of a referral base from general medicine practitioners and oncologists within the hospital. Cardiologists may also attend oncology meetings like tumor board conferences fostering the beginnings of a multidisciplinary approach to the care of

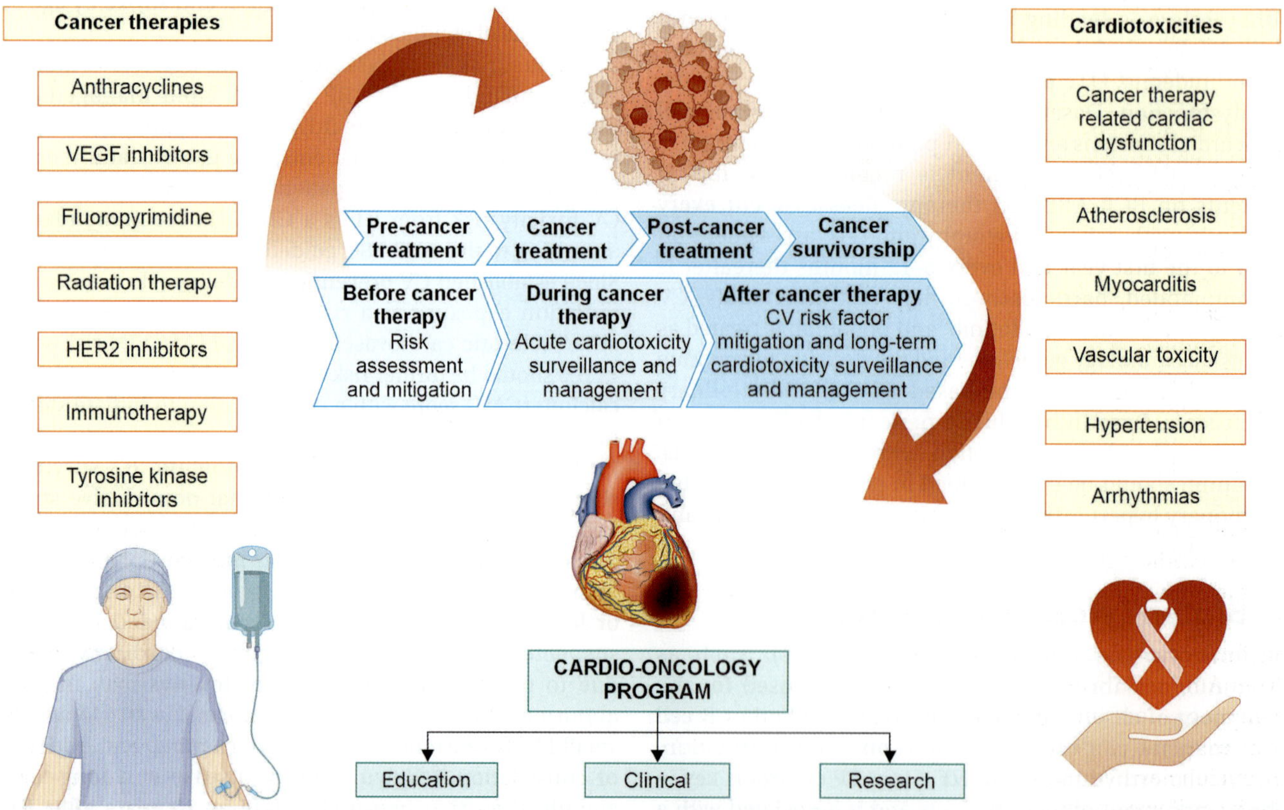

FIG. 1: The scope of cardio-oncology and building blocks of program development. It illustrates the potential cardiotoxic antineoplastic therapies, possible cardiovascular toxicities, and components of cardio-oncology program building.

(CV: cardiovascular; HER2: human epidermal growth factor receptor 2; VEGF: vascular endothelial growth factor)

patients requiring a cardio-oncology specialist. Formulation of institutional surveillance protocols for the commonly used anticancer therapies will further strengthen the collaborative approach with oncology in the care of these patients.

Once preliminary resources like support staff and medical services such as ECG and echocardiography are provided, a cardio-oncology clinic can be initiated. The clinic may be located either in the cancer center or in the CV department based on institutional preferences.[21] Logistically, it may be easier if it is located in the cancer center as this allows for spontaneous consultations from the oncology clinic. Internal metrics to objectively assess the growth of the clinic and benefits to the patients will then catalyze greater institutional support and a larger referral base. Ultimately, forming an internal database for the institution will enable generation of evidence suggestive of better patient outcomes. Monthly cardio-oncology conferences can be organized to include both cardiologists and oncologists to provide a forum to discuss challenging and interesting cases managed in collaboration.

Education

There is a need to train cardiology postgraduates in this area of growing need. As a primary competency, trainees will need to acquire the skills to recognize and screen for cardiac toxicity due to cancer treatments. Core lectures focused on CV risk stratification and prevention, cardiotoxic effects of antineoplastic agents and RT, cardiac imaging in cancer patients, arrhythmias, thromboembolism, and cardiomyopathy/HF management in cancer patients would lay the foundation.[22] Exposure to international practice guidelines and consensus documents including those from the ICOS,[15] ESC,[6] and the European Society for Medical Oncology[23] will allow trainees to stay updated. The formulation of a dedicated core curriculum in cardio-oncology with subsequent incorporation into both medical college and residency training will further increase awareness in early stages of medical training.

This knowledge can then be supplemented by clinical rotations both in oncology and cardio-oncology. Establishment of a cardio-oncology consultative service where cardiology postgraduates evaluate cancer patients admitted to the hospital with a focus on primary CV prevention and identification and treatment of cardiotoxicities will facilitate continued exposure to this patient population.[24] The American College of Cardiology (ACC) Cardio-Oncology Council published a statement[25] delineating the essential training prerequisites and fundamental proficiencies needed for training in cardio-oncology for both cardiologists and oncologists. It would be beneficial to utilize the recommendations outlined in this document as a framework to guide the training of cardiology postgraduates across a range of competencies, spanning from basic (Level I) to advanced (Level III) training. Away rotations at comprehensive cancer centers with established cardio-oncology clinics[26] may help fulfill the training requirements. The Asian Cardio-Oncology Society (ACOS) was established in India in 2020 which encourages the establishment of cardio-oncology clinics and has promoted increased awareness through national conferences. Attendance at such conferences and others internationally facilitates knowledge sharing and provides avenues for cardiologists to explore cardio-oncology as an area of interest. The ICOS also offers a certification examination in cardio-oncology for trainees who have at least 3–6 months of dedicated cardio-oncology training.[24]

Training in advanced imaging modalities remains a cornerstone of cardio-oncology. Trainees may pursue additional expertise in advanced echocardiography including strain imaging and cardiac MRI. However, the varied availability of advanced imaging modalities such as cardiac MRI and CT across the country and the related fiscal burden to patients cannot be overlooked. Regardless, acquiring the skills to identify the patients who would benefit most from advanced imaging is imperative.

The ultimate goal would be to establish cardio-oncology as a cardiology subspecialty fellowship. This would include inpatient consultative experience, outpatient continuity clinic, involvement in multidisciplinary meetings with oncology, rotations in advanced HF, and cardiac imaging. The main barriers include lack of dedicated time during general cardiology training, the variability across institutions in the availability of cardio-oncology inpatient and outpatient services, and reduced exposure to advanced cardiac imaging like cardiac MRI both due to availability and financial barriers.

Research

The exclusion of cancer patients in CV clinical trials and that of cardiac patients in oncology studies has led to a scarcity of data essential for guiding clinical decisions in cardio-oncology patients. Building a robust foundation for research in cardio-oncology in India is crucial. As the field gains prominence globally, increased efforts in India are encouraged, both to enhance the understanding of CV effects of cancer therapies in the Indian patient population and to develop tailored strategies for patient care. With the establishment of cardio-oncology clinics across the country, there arises an opportunity for the development of institutional and ultimately, national registries allowing for more granular analysis of outcomes in the Indian population using real world data. Distinct elements such as social determinants of health could be investigated specific to the Indian population, considering the differences in healthcare access and resource availability between urban and rural regions, as well as government and private healthcare settings. It is known that factors that influence social vulnerability (how external stressors adversely affect an individual's well-being and consequently impact broader communities) including socioeconomic status, minority status, household composition and disability and housing type and transportation lead to worse mortality rates in patients with comorbid cancer and CVD.[27,28] Health economics research may provide insights into outcomes based on the social background and income of patients, signaling the need for policy change at the state and national level to support and help bridge the gap in their care. Initiation of national clinical trials exploring the effectiveness of cardioprotective strategies and screening tools in India would inform and guide clinicians on management approaches unique to the Indian population.

CONCLUSION

The future of cardio-oncology in India holds promise as the field gains recognition and significance within the medical landscape. Tailored strategies can be developed to mitigate risks and optimize patient outcomes as collaboration between oncology and cardiology strengthens. As research in this domain flourishes, more data will become available to inform evidence-based practices and guidelines specific to the Indian population. By addressing the unique challenges and needs of patients, cardio-oncology is poised to make a significant impact on enhancing the quality of care for individuals navigating the intersection of cancer and CV health in India.

ONLINE REFERENCES

Please scan the QR code provided at the end of the table of contents for References of this chapter.

CHAPTER

96

Cardiac Toxicity of Oncology Drugs

Asha Moorthy, Jain T Kallarakkal

ABSTRACT

Considerable progress has been made in the field of cancer treatment with dramatic improvement in the prognosis of patients. However, cardiac toxicities resulting from these treatments represent a major hazard as they can compromise the success of the optimal treatment against the tumor. Such adverse events (AEs) are associated with older chemotherapy drugs such as anthracyclines as well as targeted therapies and immunotherapies.

Keywords: Cardiotoxicity, cardiac dysfunction, heart failure, cardio-oncology.

INTRODUCTION

Cardiovascular complications in patients with cancer represent a major challenge for cardiologists and oncologists with considerable advances in cancer treatment. As a result, there is a dramatic increase in the number of patients presenting with a combination of cancer and cancer treatment-related cardiovascular diseases.[1] Several international guidelines and position articles have been published on the cardiovascular monitoring and management of patients treated with cancer drugs.[2] A panel, from the French Working Group of Cardio-Oncology, analyzed and compared the key components of the pathways recommended by the most recent guidelines from the American and European societies of both oncology and cardiology. They then proposed pragmatic approaches based on harmonization of these guidelines and the most recent published studies.

The guidelines from the American Society of Clinical Oncology (ASCO-2017 and ASCO-2018), the European Society for Medical Oncology (ESMO-2017 and ESMO-2020), and the European Society of Cardiology (ESC-2016) give a clear-cut approach to these subset of patients. The ESMO-2017 and ASCO-2018 guidelines were specific to immune checkpoint inhibitor (ICI)-related toxicity. For cardiovascular monitoring strategies, only the cancer drugs associated with a high risk of cardiovascular toxicity were analyzed, including anthracyclines, human epidermal growth factor-2 inhibitors (HER2Is), vascular endothelial growth factor inhibitors (VEGFIs), Bcr-Abl kinase inhibitors, proteasome inhibitors (proteasomes), ICIs, and ibrutinib. Cardiovascular complications related to anticancer hormonotherapy and radiotherapy are not addressed. This work does not provide detailed information regarding the cardiovascular toxicities associated with each cancer treatment because these data are available in the existing guidelines; rather, it provides a more practical harmonization that can be useful in daily clinical practice for physicians who care for patients with cancer.

CARDIOVASCULAR MONITORING DURING CANCER TREATMENT

It is mandatory to identify patients with increased risk of developing cardiovascular toxicity. However, differences exist in the definition of high-risk patients and the recommended strategies for investigation. All of the definitions include patients with previous cardiovascular diseases or risk factors, high-dose anthracycline, and combination therapy based on several studies.[3] The pragmatic harmonized definition proposed by the working group is shown in **Box 1**.

BOX 1 Patients with increased risk of developing cardiovascular toxicity.

- High-dose anthracycline (e.g., doxorubicin ≥250 mg/m^2, epirubicin ≥600 mg/m^2)
- High-dose radiotherapy (≥30 Gy) where the heart is in the treatment field
- Lower-dose anthracycline (e.g., doxorubicin < 250 mg/m^2, epirubicin <600 mg/m^2) or HERIs or VEGFIs or proteasomes (proteasome inhibitors) or Bcr-Abl inhibitors and presence of any of the following factors:
  - Age ≥60 years
  - Lower-dose radiotherapy (<30 Gy) where the heart is in the treatment field
  - ≥2 risk factors, including smoking, hypertension, diabetes mellitus, dyslipidemia, chronic renal insufficiency, and obesity
- Previous heart disease
  - Elevated cardiac biomarkers before initiation of anticancer therapy
  - This parameter should be measured during the first evaluation but will be rechecked during follow-up only with cancer treatments that may modify them (e.g., Bcr-Abl inhibitors or mammalian target of rapamycin inhibitors)

(Bcr-Abl: Bcr-Abl kinase; HERIs: human epidermal growth factor-2 inhibitors; VEGFIs: vascular endothelial growth factor inhibitors)

BOX 2 Cardiovascular assessment included in the "cardio-oncological evaluation".

- Clinical consultation (including BP measurement)
- ECG
- Blood glucose, lipid profile, glomerular filtration rate calculation
- Cardiovascular global risk assessment using guidelines
- TTE including measurements of LVEF measurements (ideally three-dimensional but at least two-dimensional Simpson biplane method) and GLS; in the absence of GLS quantification of LV longitudinal function, use mitral annular displacement by M-mode echocardiography and/or peak systolic velocity of the mitral annulus by pulsed-wave DTI
- LV contrast agents could be potentially useful in two-dimensional echocardiography
- CMR is recommended if the quality of TTE is suboptimal
- Use the same imaging modality for monitoring
- Actively manage modifiable cardiovascular risk factors and diseases
- Encourage exercise on a regular basis and healthy dietary habits

(BP: blood pressure; CMR: cardiac magnetic resonance; DTI: Doppler tissue imaging; ECG: electrocardiogram; GLS: global longitudinal strain; LV: left ventricular; LVEF: left ventricular ejection fraction; TTE: transthoracic echocardiogram)

N-terminal Pro-B-type Natriuretic Peptide (or B-type Natriuretic Peptide) and/or Troponin

For a long time, cardiological assessment of patients receiving cancer therapy has been limited to the measurement of left ventricular ejection fraction (LVEF). It is now clearly established that this evaluation is insufficient and should include a more comprehensive cardiovascular risk evaluation allowing earlier detection of myocardial toxicities as well as other cardiovascular toxicities (e.g., hypertension, QTc interval prolongation, arrhythmias, and vascular diseases) **(Box 2)**.

Anthracyclines

Box 3 shows pragmatic approach for monitoring patients treated with anthracyclines and HER2Is.

Anthracyclines should not be used in patients with LVEF < 40% unless there is no effective alternative cancer treatment. In patients with LVEF < 50% but ≥40% and those exposed to multiple cardiotoxic cancer treatments who have a normal LVEF and associated cardiovascular risk factors, anthracyclines can be used with a cardioprotective strategy using angiotensin-converting enzyme inhibitors (ACEIs) [or angiotensin receptor blockers (ARBs)] and/or beta blockers (BBs). Regarding monitoring during therapy, the use of troponin to predict left ventricular systolic dysfunction (LVSD) is highly variable because of conflicting results.[4,5] Hence troponin assay is indicated in situations which it has most clearly demonstrated its value, namely, high-cumulative-dose anthracycline (doxorubicin ≥250 mg/m^2 or epirubicin ≥ 600 mg/m^2), lower-cumulative-dose anthracycline in association with other cardiotoxic therapy, or cardiovascular risk factors.

Human Epidermal Growth Factor-2 Inhibitors

A cardiological assessment before HER2I initiation is recommended, including physical examination, electrocardiogram (ECG), and cardiac imaging, preferably transthoracic echocardiogram. However, there are important differences regarding initial and subsequent

BOX 3 Pragmatic approach for monitoring patients treated with anthracyclines and human epidermal growth factor-2 inhibitors (HER2Is).

- The cardio-oncological evaluation will systematically include at least one visit with clinical consultation (including BP measurement)
- ECG
- Blood glucose, lipid profile, and glomerular filtration rate calculation should be evaluated before initiation of anthracyclines and HER2Is. Recheck at least at 1 year, 2 years, and periodically thereafter for patients who received anthracyclines
- TTE including measurements of LVEF measurements (ideally three-dimensional but at least two-dimensional Simpson biplane method) and GLS; In the absence of GLS quantification of LV longitudinal function, use mitral annular displacement by M-mode echocardiography and/or peak systolic velocity of the mitral annulus by pulsed-wave DTI
- LV contrast agents could be potentially useful in two-dimensional echocardiography
- CMR is recommended if the quality of TTE is suboptimal
- Use the same imaging modality for monitoring
- Actively manage modifiable cardiovascular risk factors and diseases
- Encourage exercise on a regular basis and healthy dietary habits
- For monitoring, assays should be performed by the same laboratory (same type of troponin, same method of measurement) and at the same time (before or within 24 hours after each cycle). Troponin+ if >99th percentile of the upper reference limit or significantly increased compared.

(BP: blood pressure; CMR: cardiac magnetic resonance; DTI: Doppler tissue imaging; ECG: electrocardiogram; GLS: global longitudinal strain; LV: left ventricular; LVEF: left ventricular ejection fraction; TTE: transthoracic echocardiogram)

evaluation of cardiac biomarkers and pretherapeutic introduction of ACEIs (or ARBs) and/or BBs in high-risk patients. While most guidelines recommend cardiac imaging monitoring every 3 months during treatment, the ASCO-2016 guidelines leave the choice of timing to the physician's discretion. No specific recommendations for HER2Is are proposed by the guidelines regarding the long-term follow-up in survivors.

These inhibitors should not be used in patients with LVEF < 40% unless there is no effective alternative cancer treatment. In patients with LVEF < 50% but ≥40% and those exposed to multiple cardiotoxic cancer treatments with a normal LVEF and associated cardiovascular risk factors, HER2Is can be used with a cardioprotective strategy using ACEIs (or ARBs) and/or BBs. A complete cardio-oncological evaluation is recommended every 3 months during HER2I treatment in all patients. The benefit of troponins to predict intravenous or subcutaneous HER2 is that cardiotoxicity is somewhat equivocal and appears to be more helpful, especially in patients with prior exposure to anthracyclines. Troponin evaluation may be used after each infusion in patients at higher risk of cardiotoxicity.

Vascular Endothelial Growth Factor Inhibitors

Initial cardiovascular evaluation includes screening and management of cardiovascular risk factors, baseline blood pressure (BP) value, and LVEF measurement. During VEGFI therapy, the guidelines recommend the same general rules as for other cancer treatments with potential cardiotoxicity but highlight the importance of performing appropriate and close BP monitoring and screening of early signs and symptoms of heart failure (HF). However, there is no consensus on the use of cardiac biomarkers or the timing of evaluations.

Bcr-Abl Kinase Inhibitors

The Bcr-Abl kinase inhibitors (imatinib, dasatinib, nilotinib, bosutinib, and ponatinib) are associated with accelerated atherosclerosis, peripheral artery disease development, acute coronary syndrome, stroke, hypertension, hyperglycemia, hypercholesterolemia, pericardial effusion, pulmonary arterial hypertension, QTc prolongation, and occasionally LVSD.

A monitoring strategy based on the specific risk of toxicity for each Bcr-Abl inhibitor drug and the individual global cardiovascular risk should be performed. Special attention should be paid to patients at very high or high individual cardiovascular risk and those treated with nilotinib and ponatinib. Indeed, previously unrecognized and severe peripheral atherosclerosis has emerged as a critical concern with nilotinib, along with serious arterial thrombotic events with ponatinib. The results of several studies support the utilization of the ankle-brachial index in this setting. An abnormal ankle-brachial index (<0.9) is sensitive and specific for peripheral artery disease and could indicate systemic atherosclerotic disease.

Proteasome Inhibitors

Proteasomes (carfilzomib, bortezomib, and ixazomib) are associated mainly with LVSD, HF, arterial hypertension, and myocardial ischemia.

All patients eligible for proteasomes and particularly for carfilzomib should have a baseline cardio-oncological evaluation before treatment begins. This initial evaluation should also contain a baseline measurement of natriuretic peptides and baseline home BP monitoring. This proposal is based on the fact that median time to first cardiovascular adverse event (AE) from proteasomes start was 31 days, with 86% of cardiovascular events occurring within the first 3 months, and that baseline natriuretic peptides were also predictive of cardiovascular events. After the baseline evaluation, it is suggested to repeat cardio-oncological evaluation, including natriuretic peptides, and home BP monitoring every 3 months in the first year, and every 6 months thereafter, throughout the course of proteasome therapy.[6]

Ibrutinib

Ibrutinib has been associated with atrial fibrillation (AF) since the early drug development phases. More recently, other cardiovascular toxicities were described, including hypertension, HF, ventricular arrhythmias, and conduction disorders.

All patients eligible for ibrutinib therapy should have a baseline cardio-oncological evaluation. After the baseline evaluation, asymptomatic patients should receive repeat cardio-oncological evaluation every 3 months in the first year (and every 6 months afterward) associated with home BP monitoring during all ibrutinib therapy. The decision to perform cardio-oncological evaluations every 3 months during the first year is based on the fact that conduction disorders mainly develop during the first 30 days, and AF, ventricular arrhythmias, and HF have a peak incidence at 2–3 months, whereas hypertension occurs mainly after 4–5 months. Overall, cardiac AEs steadily occur during the first year after ibrutinib initiation. In symptomatic patients, repeated Holter-ECG monitoring for AF screening is suggested.

Immune Checkpoint Inhibitors

Immune checkpoint inhibitors are associated with the occurrence of immune-related myocarditis, which has a high mortality of ≈50%. Pericarditis, supraventricular arrhythmias, acute coronary syndrome, and Takotsubo syndrome are other potential cardiovascular immune-related AEs.

Clinical suspicion of ICI–associated myocarditis is usually made by oncologists during patient monitoring. Hence, the proposed algorithm should be available in the oncology department, easy to perform, and easy for a noncardiologist to analyze. It is the proposal of the working group to consider two strategies that best reflect the entire possible clinical scenario. Strategy 1 considers baseline cardiovascular signs/symptoms, ECG, and troponin I or T for each patient deemed to receive ICI therapy. Strategy 2 considers that only cardiovascular signs/symptoms be checked before each ICI administration, and only patients with new cardiovascular signs/symptoms or noncardiovascular immune-related AEs be evaluated with ECG and troponin. Strategies 1 and 2 consider that asymptomatic patients with a rise in troponin or new ECG abnormalities or patients with new cardiovascular signs/symptoms who are rapidly referred to a cardio-oncology unit should be able to confirm or deny the diagnosis of ICI-related myocarditis.

CONCLUSION

Cancer therapy-related cardiac dysfunction (CTRCD) affects an increasing population of oncology patients. It can be classified as direct (dose-dependent vs. dose-independent) or indirect, either case being potentially permanent or reversible. Risk assessment, recognition, and prevention of CTRCD are crucial.

Traditional cardiac risk factors, as well as therapy-related risk factors, may be predictive of CTRCD. Anthracyclines, alkylating agents, HER2Is, taxanes, and fluoropyrimidines are traditional cancer therapies with the risk of cardiotoxicity, with more targeted therapies including tyrosine kinase inhibitors (TKIs) and immunotherapy more recently being described as culprits.

Troponin assessment has been shown to be of high negative and positive predictive values for CTRCD. Although cardiac magnetic resonance imaging (MRI) is the gold standard to evaluate cardiac function, echocardiography is the first-line screening tool and may be of greater value when global longitudinal strain (GLS) and three-dimensional echocardiography for ejection fraction (EF) are used.

We recommend screening all patients before starting cancer therapeutics with the potential for cardiac dysfunction with an ECG, troponin level, and left ventricular (LV) function assessment with an echocardiogram including GLS, echo contrast, and, if possible, three-dimensional EF.

Beta blockers, renin–angiotensin inhibitors, aldosterone antagonist therapy, and statins can preserve LV systolic function in patients at risk. Dexrazoxane in patients who are planned to exceed the recommended cumulative dose of anthracyclines and steroids in the event of immunotherapy-related cardiac dysfunction are important cancer therapy-specific considerations.

Results indicate that relative reduction of GLS > 15% from the baseline is a sensitive marker for predicting early anthracycline-related cardiotoxicity. GLS is superior to LVEF for the detection of CTRCD. Significant proportion of patients with cardiotoxicity were detected by GLS when compared to EF. Reduction in GLS precedes reduction in LVEF.

ONLINE REFERENCES

Please scan the QR code provided at the end of the table of contents for References of this chapter.

CHAPTER 97

Application of Strain by Speckle Tracking Echocardiography in Cardio-oncology

Jesu Krupa

ABSTRACT

Many therapies used in the treatment of cancer cause cardiotoxicity that manifests as left ventricular (LV) systolic dysfunction and heart failure (HF). Cardiotoxicity is detected mainly through echocardiography, which remains the main imaging modality with two-dimensional (2D) LV ejection fraction (LVEF) as the main measurement for evaluation. However, it lacks the sensitivity to detect early subclinical myocardial damage due to cardiotoxicity. Global longitudinal strain (GLS) measures the longitudinal function of the myocardium, which is reflective of a change in the length of the myocardial fiber compared to its initial length. GLS in various conditions is impaired even before a reduction in ejection fraction (EF) as it is less load dependent compared to EF. LV GLS values > 18% are normal and values between 16 and 18% are considered borderline abnormal. Cardiotoxicity is defined as a decrease in the LVEF by >10 absolute percentage points to a value of <50%. Probable cardiotoxicity is defined as a decrease in the LVEF by >10 absolute percentage points to a value of ≥50% with an accompanying decline in GLS by >15% from the baseline (if GLS measurement is available) and possible cardiotoxicity is recognized when the LVEF decreases by <10 absolute percentage points to a value of <50% or when the LVEF ≥ 50%, in the case of a relative percentage reduction in GLS by >15%. The SUCCOUR (Strain Surveillance of Chemotherapy for Improving Cardiovascular Outcomes) study, a multicenter prospective investigation involved patients undergoing cardiotoxic chemotherapy and regular LV function assessments using echocardiography. In this study, patients were randomly assigned to two groups, one guided by GLS assessment and the other by LVEF assessment. There was no significant statistical difference between LVEF values in the two groups, in the GLS-guided group (57% ± 6%) and in the LVEF-guided group, it was 55% ± 7%; $p = 0.05$. CardTox-Score is a recent novel scoring system proposed for predicting nonanthracycline chemotherapy-induced cardiotoxicity, which includes clinical, echocardiographic, and biomarkers.

Keywords: Left ventricular ejection fraction, global longitudinal strain, SUCCOUR study.

INTRODUCTION

Many therapies used in the treatment of cancer cause cardiotoxicity that manifests as left ventricular (LV) systolic dysfunction and heart failure (HF). Anthracyclines are the main agents but cardiotoxicity can also be caused by HER2-targeted therapies, tyrosine kinase inhibitors, multiple myeloma therapies, mitogen-activated protein kinase/rapidly accelerated fibrosarcoma (MAPK/RAF) inhibitors, immune checkpoint inhibitors (ICIs), and radiotherapy.

Cardiotoxicity is detected mainly through echocardiography which remains the main imaging modality with two-dimensional (2D) LV ejection fraction (LVEF) as the main measurement for evaluation. Echocardiography has great diagnostic value and prognostic power in various cardiovascular conditions. However, it lacks the sensitivity to detect early subclinical myocardial damage due to cardiotoxicity.[1]

Global longitudinal strain (GLS) measures the longitudinal function of the myocardium, which is reflective of a change in the length of the myocardial fiber compared to its initial length.[2] GLS in various conditions is impaired even before a reduction in ejection fraction (EF) as it is less load dependent compared to EF.[3] Many studies recommend GLS for management decisions due to its prognostic advantage.[4,5]

GLS is measured using speckle tracking which makes use of ultrasound backscatter from structures that are smaller than the wavelength of sound. This backscatter is called speckle, the position of which is tracked over time from frame to frame to give an estimate of strain. Optimal speckle tracking requires a frame rate of 40–90 frames/s.[6]

STEPS IN THE MEASUREMENT OF GLOBAL LONGITUDINAL STRAIN

1. Acquire the three apical views (apical 4-chamber, 2-chamber, and long-axis views) at similar heart rates and frame rates.
2. Adjust the depth such that the LV is seen up to the mitral valve but not the entire left atrium.
3. Optimize the sector size to just visualize LV walls including the interventricular septum in both phases of the cardiac cycle. Ensure proper depth and sector size to give the required frame rate of 40–90 frames/s. Also, adjust the gain so that there is just some gray in the LV blood pool. The endocardium should be visualized.
4. Avoid apical foreshortening of the LV because it may overestimate the strain. Moving the probe down and out and using respiratory maneuvers may be required. Breath holding may be required to avoid breathing artifacts.
5. A good quality electrocardiogram (ECG) tracing is a must and a minimum of three cardiac cycles should be acquired to ensure that at least one complete cycle is available for strain analysis.

Select the best images for analysis either manually or automatically based on the echo machine and the vendor. Endocardial border detection is either automated or semiautomated by marking the mitral annulus and apex. Care should be taken to ensure that the contour border should not extend into the left atrium. The quality of tracking should be visually assessed to ensure that the tracking moves with the myocardium and that the region of interest (ROI) is not too thin or too thick or reaching up to the pericardium. Endocardial strain values are usually higher than epicardial strain values and most current algorithms measure endocardial strain.[8] This highlights the importance of acquiring good quality images with a delineated endocardium. Manual repeated tracking revision should be avoided; instead, the aim should be to get better images. The strain values from the three apical views are then integrated to calculate the GLS as shown in **Figure 1**. End-diastole is defined by the beginning of the QRS complex or

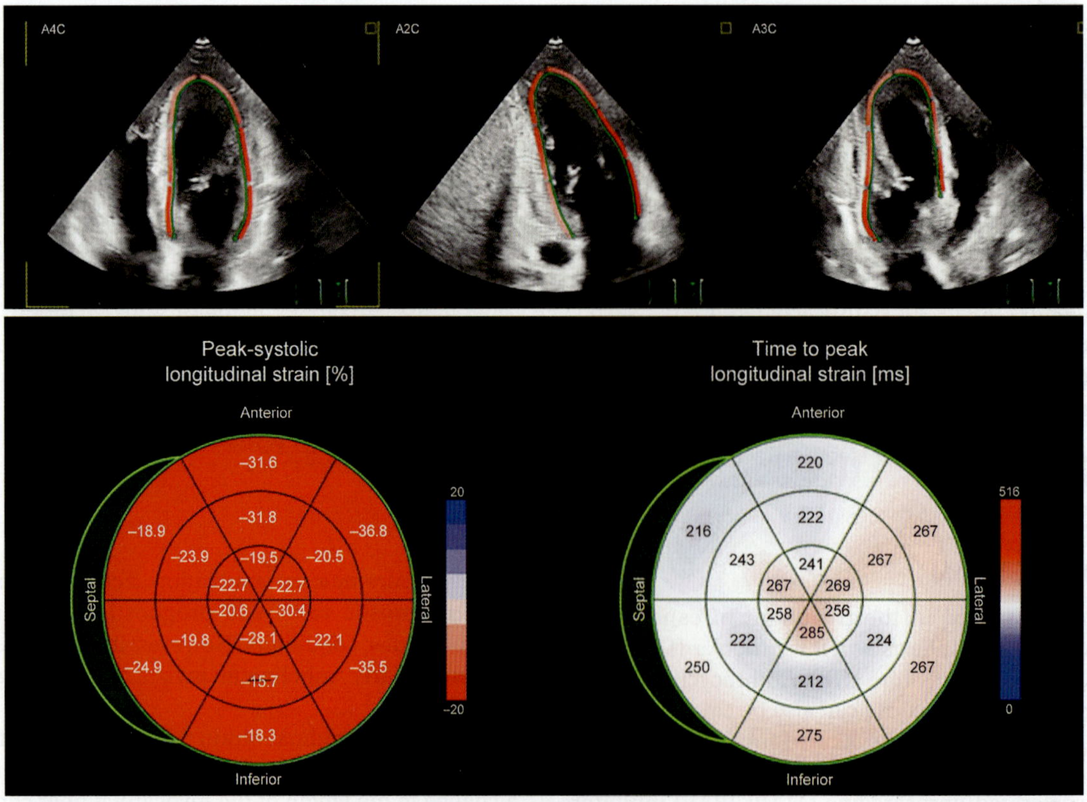

FIG. 1: Global longitudinal strain (GLS) by speckle tracking echocardiography. Assessment of GLS in a healthy, asymptomatic individual with a GLS of –25%. The top row displays a regional strain map superimposed on the grayscale two-dimensional echocardiographic images in apical four-chamber (A4C), apical two-chamber (A2C), and apical three-chamber (A3C) views. The bottom left bullseye displays regional longitudinal strain for each segment of a 16-segment model of the left ventricle. Bright red denotes to most negative normal values of GLS. The bottom right bullseye displays the time (ms) between aortic valve opening and peak longitudinal strain, a measure of dyssynchrony, for each segment.[7]

when the LV size is largest. End-systole is defined by the end of the spectral Doppler aortic flow tracing or visualization of the aortic valve closure in the apical long-axis view or the nadir of the LV volume curve. The European Association of Cardiovascular Imaging/American Society of Echocardiography (EACVI/ASE)/Industry Task Force recommendation is to report end-systolic strain.[9] A recent meta-analysis suggests that LV GLS values > 18% are normal and values between 16 and 18% are considered borderline abnormal.[10]

DEFINITION OF CARDIOTOXICITY

According to the 2014 ASE and EACVI, cardiotoxicity is defined as an absolute decrease in 2D LVEF by >10% from the baseline and up to <53%.[11] Subclinical LV dysfunction is diagnosed when there is a relative decrease in GLS of >15% from baseline.[11]

A more recent definition from the British Society of Echocardiography (BSE) and British Cardio-oncology Society (BCOS) defines cardiotoxicity as a decrease in the LVEF by >10 absolute percentage points to a value of <50%. Probable cardiotoxicity is defined as a decrease in the LVEF by >10 absolute percentage points to a value of ≥50% with an accompanying decline in GLS by >15% from the baseline (if GLS measurement is available) and possible cardiotoxicity is recognized when the LVEF decreases by <10 absolute percentage points to a value of <50% or when the LVEF ≥ 50% in the case of a relative percentage reduction in GLS by >15%.[12]

The 2022 European Society of Cardiology (ESC) guidelines on cardio-oncology define three degrees of cardiotoxicity.[13] Severe cardiotoxicity is when there is a new LVEF decline to <40%. Moderate cardiotoxicity is a new LVEF decrease by ≥10 percentage points to an LVEF of 40–49%, or a new LVEF decline by <10 percentage points to an LVEF of 40–49%, plus either a new relative decline in GLS by >15% from the baseline or a new increase in cardiac biomarkers. Mild cardiotoxicity is when the LVEF is ≥50% with a new relative decline in GLS by >15% from the baseline or a new increase in cardiac biomarkers.

GLOBAL LONGITUDINAL STRAIN FOR DETECTION OF CARDIOTOXICITY

A meta-analysis of 21 studies by Oikonomou et al. included patients treated with anthracyclines, with or without trastuzumab, showed absolute changes in GLS between 2 and 3% and relative changes between 10 and 15% as the cutoff for the diagnosis of subclinical cardiotoxicity, with a sensitivity of 80–90% and a specificity of 80%. However, studies done so far have shown significant statistical heterogeneity, and hence more data is required.[14]

Global longitudinal strain serves as an indicator for detecting subtle cardiac toxicity, however, it has not been definitively demonstrated to outperform LVEF monitoring in the context of cancer treatment. The SUCCOUR (Strain Surveillance of Chemotherapy for Improving Cardiovascular Outcomes) study, a multicenter prospective investigation, involved patients undergoing cardiotoxic chemotherapy and regular LV function assessments using echocardiography. In this study, patients were randomly assigned to two groups, one guided by GLS assessment and the other by LVEF assessment.[15] Patients on potentially cardiotoxic drugs such as anthracyclines, trastuzumab, and tyrosine kinase inhibitors were included and followed up for a period of 3 years. Therapy was initiated when cardiotoxicity was detected using a change in LVEF measured on three-dimensional (3D) echocardiography as the primary endpoint. A symptomatic LVEF reduction of >5% or an asymptomatic LVEF drop of >10% to LVEF <55% was considered abnormal in the traditional imaging group and in the GLS-guided group. This was defined by a relative decrease in GLS of around 12% compared to the baseline.[15] There was no significant statistical difference between LVEF values in the two groups, in the GLS-guided group, 57% ± 6%, and in the LVEF-guided group, it was 55% ± 7%; $p = 0.05$.[16]

GLOBAL LONGITUDINAL STRAIN AND CARDIAC BIOMARKERS

A study by Avila et al. showed that low GLS values < 17% and brain natriuretic peptide (BNP) serum concentrations > 17 pg/mL 2 months after chemotherapy is predictive of early-onset cardiotoxicity [100% sensitivity, 88% specificity, and area under the curve (AUC) = 0.94].[17] Other similar findings have been observed for N-terminal prohormone of BNP (NT-proBNP) and cardiac troponin.[18,19] This is a pointer to the fact that biomarkers indicating myocardial damage or overload may increase the significance of an abnormal strain finding.

CardTox-Score is a recent novel scoring system proposed for predicting nonanthracycline chemotherapy-induced cardiotoxicity. The variables in this risk model are GLS values < –20%, apart from clinical data such as age ≥60 years, body mass index (BMI) > 25 kg/m^2, and the presence of cardiovascular risk conditions such as arterial hypertension and diabetes. The model also includes laboratory markers such as highly sensitive troponin, NT-proBNP, and echocardiographic variables including LVEF ≤ 50% and LV diastolic dysfunction ≥ grade 1.[20] Development of cardiotoxicity is associated with a CardTox-Score > 6 points with a sensitivity of 100% and specificity of 84.2%.[20]

GLOBAL LONGITUDINAL STRAIN VERSUS REGIONAL STRAIN

Cardiotoxicity cannot be accurately diagnosed when only an echocardiographic view is used. Hence, a GLS assessment using three apical views should be the preferred method.[21]

Some studies have looked at regional heterogeneity in strain values,[22-24] but the LV segments involved were not uniform across these various studies. There is currently insufficient data for the use of global circumferential strain, LV systolic strain rate (SR), right ventricular (RV) GLS, and RV SR for detecting cardiotoxicity.[25]

GLOBAL LONGITUDINAL STRAIN ASSESSMENT IN VARIOUS CANCERS

Most studies on GLS for the diagnosis of subclinical cardiotoxicity have been conducted in patients with breast cancer treated with anthracyclines or HER2-targeted therapies (mainly trastuzumab). However, GLS detects cardiotoxicity in other malignancies as well, such as subclinical cardiac dysfunction in lymphoma patients in the early stages of anticancer therapy.[26] Oka et al. found that GLS before hematopoietic stem cell transplantation (HSCT) in patients with hematologic malignancies was predictive of a decrease in LVEF post-HSCT.[27] In patients with colorectal cancer, GLS was useful in the diagnosis of bevacizumab-induced cardiotoxicity.[28] Therapy with proteasome inhibitors such as carfilzomib for multiple myeloma may be cardiotoxic, as demonstrated by GLS changes and diastolic dysfunction occurrence.[29,30] The percentage change in GLS from baseline to 6 months after radiotherapy in patients with non-small cell lung cancer (NSCLC) is known to be an independent predictor of all-cause mortality. Hence, it might be of value to perform an echocardiography on these patients early after radiotherapy.[31] In patients with advanced light-chain (AL) amyloidosis, those with GLS values < –14.2% had a corresponding median overall survival (OS) and 5-year OS rates of 33.2 months and 39%, respectively, versus 7.7 months and 6% for those with GLS values ≥ –14.2%.[32]

GLOBAL LONGITUDINAL STRAIN IN VARIOUS METHODS OF ANTICANCER TREATMENT

Global longitudinal strain has value in detecting cardiotoxicity caused not only by drugs but also due to various other modalities for the treatment of cancer. In a recent meta-analysis, GLS was found to be useful in the early detection of radiation-induced heart disease in women with left breast cancer.[33] A decline in GLS was observed in patients with ICI-related myocarditis and was strongly associated with major adverse cardiac events (MACE), irrespective of the LVEF.[34] In melanoma patients, GLS can detect ICI-induced subclinical LV dysfunction even in the absence of myocarditis.[35]

RIGHT VENTRICULAR CARDIOTOXICITY

Keramida et al. proposed a cut-off value of –14.8% for the RV GLS percent change based on their study that predicted cardiotoxicity with a sensitivity of 66.7% and a specificity of 70.8% (AUC 0.68; 95% confidence interval 0.54–0.81).[36] Some studies report that cardiotoxicity after anthracyclines in the form of worsened RV GLS is more common than a decrease in LV GLS.[37]

CURRENT PERSPECTIVE

There is evidence that cancer therapy-related cardiac dysfunction (CTRCD) and "cardiac dysfunction" occurred in 27% of patients who received trastuzumab and an anthracycline, including New York Heart Association functional class III–IV HF in 16%.[38] This has formed the basis for monitoring patients receiving chemotherapy for LV dysfunction to enable early detection of cardiac dysfunction.

Echocardiography remains the most commonly used method for monitoring cardiac function in patients receiving cardiotoxic cancer therapy. LVEF estimation is routinely done and forms part of the definition for CTRCD. However, because of the large coefficient of variation inherent in the measurement of LVEF, it is not useful in the detection of small changes in LV function. Cardiac magnetic resonance (CMR) imaging is also being used and has many advantages; however, it is impractical and unlikely to become a regular tool for monitoring patients for CTRCD.

Hence, GLS will continue to have relevance in the early detection of cardiotoxicity, a significant change in GLS is known to occur without a significant change in LVEF.[39] A recent meta-analysis to assess the relevance of GLS in the detection of cardiotoxicity was limited in its conclusion as the overall patient numbers were small and most of the studies included had less than 100 patients each with different types of cancer, treatments, and definitions of CTRCD.[14] The SUCCOUR study compared patients that were started on cardioprotective therapy based on LVEF or GLS-guided monitoring strategy.[16] However, there was no benefit at 1-year or 3-year follow-up that could be a result of low event rates or due to the limitations of GLS.

The limitations of GLS in day-to-day practice are the requirements of trained personnel who follow the specifications for strain measurement and variability of software to ensure coherence of values between vendors. Very important causes of variability between studies are loading conditions and blood pressure as shown in an early meta-analysis.[38,40] Further, acquisition needs to be done at optimal heart rates. A prospective study showed that 48% of images were suboptimal and inadequate for GLS assessment in patients with breast cancer.[41]

There is recent evidence for improvement in the incidence and prognosis of CTCRD due to anthracyclines and trastuzumab. The mean decrease in LVEF was only 5.4% in the placebo arms in a meta-analysis of contemporary trials of cardioprotective medications in patients on anthracycline.[10] Hence, with improvements in cancer treatments making clinical decisions based solely on GLS could lead to unnecessary cessation of cancer therapy, and hence could be potentially harmful. Therefore, there is a need for a personalized approach that takes into account all aspects including the severity of the disease condition. For example, screening intervals recommended in the guidelines may not yield positive results in most cases given the low event rates and a very small proportion of patients may need frequent monitoring. Despite these issues, GLS monitoring is still a recommendation by many guidelines from major societies in the world **(Table 1)**. There is a need to refine monitoring using clinical risk factors, echo, and biomarkers, but more evidence is needed before adopting a widespread therapeutic approach. There is also a need for more research on the real-world use of GLS and the validity of treatment decisions made based on GLS measurements.

CONCLUSION

Cardiotoxicity is detected mainly through echocardiography which remains the main imaging modality with 2D LVEF as the main measurement for evaluation. GLS is more sensitive than LVEF in detecting subclinical LV dysfunction. LV GLS values > 18% are normal and values between 16 and 18% are considered borderline abnormal. Cardiotoxicity is defined as a decrease in the LVEF by >10 absolute percentage points to a value of <50%. However, there is no evidence currently to show that a GLS-guided approach for cardioprotection is better than an LVEF-guided one. We need to have a personalized approach based on risk versus benefit which takes into account clinical, echocardiographic, and biomarkers.

TABLE 1: Recommendations of scientific societies in recent years regarding the frequency of performing an echocardiographic examination with a global longitudinal strain (GLS) assessment.

Guidelines and years	Anthracyclines	HER2-targeted therapies
2022—The European Society of Cardiology (ESC) guidelines on cardio-oncology developed in collaboration with the European Hematology Association (EHA), the European Society for Therapeutic Radiology and Oncology (ESTRO), and the International Cardio-Oncology Society (IC-OS): Developed by the task force on cardio-oncology of the ESC[34]	• *Low baseline cardiotoxicity risk*: At baseline and 12 months post-treatment (may be also considered after the fourth cycle) • *Moderate risk*: At baseline and 12 months post-treatment (should be also considered after the fourth cycle) • *High and very high risk*: At baseline, after second, fourth, and sixth cycles and also 3 and 12 months after treatment	• *Low and moderate risk*: At baseline, after 3, 6, 9, and 12 months; and then 12 months post-treatment • *High and very high risk*: At baseline, after 3, 6, 9, and 12 months; and then 3- and 12-month post-treatment
2021—British Society for Echocardiography and British Cardio-Oncology Society guidelines for transthoracic echocardiographic assessment of adult cancer patients receiving anthracyclines and/or trastuzumab[12]	Every 3 months during chemotherapy and 3–12 months after its termination	Every 3 months during the therapy and 3–12 months after the end of therapy
2020—Management of cardiac disease in cancer patients throughout oncological treatment: ESMO consensus recommendations[42]	• After a cumulative dose of 250 mg/m^2 doxorubicin or equivalent • Next after each additional 100 mg/m^2	Every 3 months
2020—Role of cardiovascular (CV) imaging in cancer patients receiving cardiotoxic therapies: A position statement on behalf of the Heart Failure Association (HFA), the European Association of Cardiovascular Imaging (EACVI), and the Cardio-Oncology Council of the ESC[43]	Depending on the risk calculated according to the planned therapy and patient-related risk factors, including age, comorbidities, and CV risk factors	Risk is calculated according to the planned therapy and patient-related factors, including age, comorbidities, and CV risk factors (ranging from 6 to 12 weeks)
2016—Canadian Cardiovascular Society Guidelines for Evaluation and Management of Cardiovascular Complications of Cancer Therapy[44]	No recommendations	Every 3 months
2016—ESC Position Paper on cancer treatments and CV toxicity developed under the auspices of the ESC Committee for Practice Guidelines: The task force for cancer treatments and cardiovascular toxicity of the ESC[45]	After a cumulative dose of 200 mg/m^2 doxorubicin or equivalent	Every four cycles

ONLINE REFERENCES

Please scan the QR code provided at the end of the table of contents for References of this chapter.

SECTION

13

Echocardiography

CHAPTER 98

Usefulness and Limitations of Echocardiography in the Diagnosis and Assessment of Heart Failure with Preserved Ejection Fraction

Srijani Thannir, Donovon Allen, Vijayadithyan Jaganathan, Navin C Nanda

ABSTRACT

Heart failure with preserved ejection fraction (HFpEF) poses a growing clinical challenge in the context of an aging population and rising rates of cardiovascular risk factors. Echocardiography stands as a cornerstone in the diagnosis and assessment of HFpEF, offering valuable insights into cardiac structure, function, and hemodynamics. This review explores the usefulness of echocardiography in HFpEF diagnosis, risk stratification, and management, alongside various guidelines and scoring systems. Additionally, it addresses the limitations of echocardiography, especially in borderline cases where invasive measurements may be needed. Novel parameters like diastolic stress echocardiography and lung ultrasound are discussed, promising to enhance diagnostic accuracy. Furthermore, the role of artificial intelligence, global longitudinal strain, and invasive hemodynamic measurements in HFpEF evaluation is examined. Dyspnea clinics, integrating echocardiography into a multidisciplinary approach, offer a comprehensive strategy for the diagnosis and management of HFpEF. This review highlights the evolving landscape of HFpEF assessment, emphasizing the pivotal role of echocardiography alongside emerging diagnostic modalities.

Keywords: Heart failure with preserved ejection fraction (HFpEF), echocardiography, diastolic stress echocardiography, lung ultrasound, artificial intelligence, global longitudinal strain, invasive hemodynamic measurements, dyspnea clinics.

INTRODUCTION

Echocardiography is an excellent imaging modality for evaluation of patients with suspicion of cardiac disease. It provides many different parameters to evaluate cardiac function, anatomy, and pathology. The echocardiogram is also noninvasive, affordable, and easy to use. It is usually the first step of assessment and suggested by guidelines for heart failure.

Heart failure with preserved ejection fraction (HFpEF) is diagnostically challenging due to its heterogeneity related to phenotypes and predisposing diseases. As heart failure becomes more prevalent, ongoing techniques and parameters obtained via echocardiography are being discovered to assist in evaluation. These techniques have been reviewed and suggested by guidelines, which will be discussed in this chapter in addition to limitations of echocardiographic assessment and other examinations to augment the diagnostic workup of HFpEF.

Heart failure with preserved ejection fraction has emerged as the prominent description of heart failure on a global scale, driven by factors such as the aging population and rising rates of hypertension, diabetes mellitus, and obesity.[1] The understanding of HFpEF has shifted from being primarily based on exclusion criteria to the definitions focused on confirmation of increased left-sided filling pressures.[2]

When investigating unexplained dyspnea in patients suspected to have HFpEF, echocardiography provides significant insight about cardiac anatomy, functionality, and hemodynamics.[3] Demonstration of normal left ventricular ejection fraction (LVEF) by echocardiography excludes reduced left ventricular (LV) function as the cause of dyspnea in these patients. For HFpEF, echocardiography is often the first step of assessment, informing decisions for management, hemodynamic status, and conducting risk stratification for outcomes.[4]

Although echocardiography is a crucial tool in diagnosing HFpEF, it is important to appreciate the uncertainty in borderline cases. In such uncommon situations, obtaining invasive hemodynamic measurements can help definitively to characterize patients with HFpEF.[5]

Several guidelines and scoring strategies are designed to assist with the diagnosis of HFpEF, utilizing echocardiography findings alone or in combination with clinical characteristics or serum biomarkers. In this chapter, we will review four important guidelines:

1. American Society of Echocardiography (ASE) jointly with the European Association of Cardiovascular Imaging (EACVI, 2016)[3]
2. Mayo Clinic (2018)[6]
3. Heart Failure Association of the European Society of Cardiology (HFA-ESC, 2019)[7]
4. EACVI (2022)[8]

The role of diastolic stress echocardiography (DSE), role of lung ultrasound (LUS) and artificial intelligence (AI), need for invasive measurements, as well as limitations of echocardiography in the diagnosis of HFpEF will also be discussed.

TABLE 1: ASE–EACVI echocardiographic criteria and scoring.

1.	Ratio of maximum velocity of mitral flow in early diastole (E) by pulsed Doppler to average of maximum velocities from medial and lateral mitral annulus by tissue Doppler imaging during early diastole (e') more than 14 (E:e' > 14)
2.	e' of mitral valve (MV) septal annulus <7 cm/s or MV lateral annulus e' <10 cm/s
3.	Tricuspid valvular regurgitation (TVR) maximum velocity >2.8 m/s
4.	Left atrial chamber volume measured in apical views (in mL) in relation to body surface area >34 mL/m^2
Scoring:	
1 out of 4: Normal left-sided filling pressures	
2 out of 4: Indeterminate group	
≥3 out of 4: Increased left-sided filling pressures	

GUIDELINES

ASE–EACVI Guidelines (2016) (Table 1)[3]

Validation

Studies that compared the proposed echocardiogram ASE–EACVI guidelines to cardiac catheterization showed that the guidelines hold a lower sensitivity of 33–69% and higher specificity of 73–87%.[9-12] Many of the studies also revealed a significant number of patients with HFpEF could be in the indeterminate group presenting a limitation to the guidelines. In addition, these guidelines cannot be applied in certain conditions listed in **Table 2**.

Mayo Clinic Guidelines (H_2FPEF Score) (2018)[6]

The H_2FPEF score **(Table 3)** was developed from the Mayo Clinic in Rochester, Minnesota with retrospective analysis of patients being evaluated for unexplained dyspnea using invasive exercise testing for cardiac and noncardiac etiology. Noncardiac dyspnea was described as patients who had normal rest and exercise hemodynamics ruling out cardiac causes. Patients who had noncardiac causes of dyspnea served as controls to identify variables to evaluate.

During invasive testing, patients with HFpEF were defined as having increased pulmonary capillary wedge pressure (PCWP) at rest or during exercise at ≥15 mm Hg or ≥25 mm Hg, respectively. To determine variables for scoring, factors for HFpEF were included in simple logistic regression followed by multivariable logistic regression for those statistically significant on the univariate analysis. Atrial fibrillation (AF) and obesity were included a priori, given known association with development of HFpEF. Scores were assigned to the six variables creating a score range of 0–9. The acronym stands for the following:

- H_2 = Heavy and hypertension
- *F* = Atrial fibrillation
- *P* = Pulmonary hypertension
- *E* = Elderly
- *F* = Filling pressures of left heart chambers

TABLE 2: HFpEF guideline limitation categories.[3,6-8]

Valvular disease	Arrhythmia	Cardiomyopathy	Miscellaneous
Aortic valve (AV) disease: • AV regurgitation • AV stenosis *MV disease*: • MV stenosis • MV regurgitation • MV annular calcification (moderate or severe) • Mitral annuloplasty/mitral valve replacement	• AF or flutter • Atrioventricular (AV) nodal block • Sinus tachycardia cardiac resynchronization therapy • Right ventricular pacing	• Restrictive cardiomyopathy • Hypertrophic cardiomyopathy • High-output heart failure	• Normal individuals • Heart transplant • Noncardiac pulmonary hypertension • Left bundle branch block • Constrictive pericarditis

(AF: atrial fibrillation; HFpEF: heart failure with preserved ejection fraction; MV: mitral valve)

The H_2FPEF score can be utilized to assess the likelihood of HFpEF, enabling extremely low probability demonstrated by low scores (e.g., 0 or 1). Conversely, high scores (e.g., 6–9) provide a reasonably high level of confidence in establishing the diagnosis. In patients who have intermediate scores (e.g., 2–5), the H_2FPEF score helps to identify individuals who may require further testing to determine the presence of HFpEF. For every increase in 1-unit score, the odds of HFpEF doubled (odds ratio 1.98; 95% confidence interval (CI) 1.74–2.30; $p < 0.0001$). The scoring system incorporates solely two echocardiographic criteria, each assigned a low significance level (meriting only 1 point each) in comparison to AF and obesity, which are accorded greater weight. Additionally, unlike the ASE–EACVI criteria, the scoring system employed a lower threshold for the average mitral E/e′ ratio, set at >9 instead of >14. A study conducted within a population revealed a notable sensitivity of 89% in detecting HFpEF when utilizing a score >2. It exhibited a high specificity of 82% in excluding HFpEF when the score was <6.[13] In another study, H_2FPEF score was useful in determining all-cause mortality rates and readmission rates.[14] However, these guidelines were criticized because of their limitation of not incorporating specific HFpEF clinical phenotypes such as obesity, diabetes mellitus, and chronic kidney disease. It is worth mentioning that a significant proportion of patients fell into the indeterminate group when using these guidelines.[15] Similar to the ASE–EACVI guidelines, this scoring system is not applicable to patients with HF caused by other factors referred to in **Table 2**.

TABLE 3: H_2FPEF score.

Patient attributes	
AF (paroxysmal and persistent)	Score given 3
Obesity (BMI >30 kg/m^2)	Score given 2
Advanced age (>60)	Score given 1
Systemic hypertension (diagnosed as patient taking ≥2 antihypertensive medications)	Score given 1
Echocardiographic criteria	
Elevated pulmonary artery systolic pressure (PASP) >35 mm Hg	Score given 1
Increased left-sided filling pressure by Doppler (mitral average E/e′ >9)	Score given 1

(AF: atrial fibrillation; BMI: body mass index)

HFA-ESC Guidelines (2019)[7]

The HFA-ESC guidelines **(Table 4)** were developed in 2019. Compiling multiple diagnostic and risk factors for HFpEF,

TABLE 4: Criteria for HFA-PEFF.

Echocardiographic criteria	Major parameters	Minor parameters
Functional	Septal mitral valve (MV) annulus velocity (e′) < 7 cm/s or Lateral MV annulus velocity (e′) < 10 cm/s Or E: Average e′ ≥ 15 Or TVR velocity > 2.8 m/s (pulmonary arterial systolic pressure > 35 mm Hg)	Peak MV early diastolic flow velocity (E): Average e′ (average of septal and lateral MV annulus velocities) equals 9–14 Or Left ventricle (LV) global longitudinal strain <16%
Structural	Left atrial chamber volume to body surface area (BSA) > 34 mL/m^2 Or LV mass (in grams) to BSA (in m^2) ≥149/122 g/m^2 and LV relative wall thickness >0.42	Left atrial chamber volume to BSA equal to 29–34 mL/m^2 Or LV mass in grams to BSA >115/95 g/m^2 Or LV relative wall thickness >0.42 Or Thickness of LV wall ≥12 millimeters
Biomarker criteria	**Major parameters**	**Minor parameters**
Sinus rhythm biomarkers	N-terminal pro-brain natriuretic peptide (NT-proBNP) >220 pg/mL Or Brain natriuretic peptide (BNP) >80 pg/mL	NT-proBNP 125–220 pg/mL Or BNP 35–80 pg/mL
Atrial fibrillation biomarkers	NT-proBNP >660 pg/mL Or BNP >240 pg/mL	NT-proBNP 365–660 pg/mL Or BNP 105–240 pg/mL

the HFA-PEFF score was proffered to assist with diagnosis. The PEFF portion of the name stands for the stepwise fashion of the algorithm:

- *P*: Pretest assessment
- *E*: Echocardiogram and biomarkers
- *F*: Functional examination
- *F*: Final etiologic work-up

Score Significance

The three categories for scoring include—functional, structural, and biomarker. Each category has major and minor criteria with established scoring systems. Major criteria have a maximum assignment of 2 points in a single category regardless of the number of criteria identified. Minor criteria are assigned a point of 1 in the absence of any major criterion and regardless of the number of minor criteria met. It is important to note that points are not cumulative within a single category for major and minor criteria. The points are only combined if they come from different categories. A combined score of 5 or higher indicates HFpEF with greater accuracy. A score between 2 and 4 warrants further investigation such as diastolic stress echo or invasive hemodynamic measurements.

Subsequent validation studies involving a substantial number of patients ranging from 400–700 have shown that the HFA-PEFF criteria exhibit a high level of accuracy, ranging from 82 to 90%, in diagnosing HFpEF.

Stepwise Approach to Diagnose HFpEF According to HFA-ESC

Step 1: Pretest assessment (P)—

- *Assess clinical signs and symptoms of heart failure*: breathlessness, orthopnea, peripheral edema, decreased exertional tolerance, evaluate risk factors (e.g., age ≥ 70 years, obese, deconditioning, and diabetes mellitus), perform ECG.
- *Conduct basic echocardiography*: Look for increased volume of the left atrium, LV hypertrophy, AF, and to exclude valvular disorders, pericardial effusion, and pulmonary arterial hypertension.
- Measure biomarkers B-type natriuretic peptide (BNP)/N-terminal pro-BNP (NT-proBNP) <125 pg/mL or <35 pg/mL for BNP have high negative predictive value for exclusion of HFpEF.
- Perform ergometry/6-minute walking test (6MWT) for discovering coexisting coronary artery disease (CAD), assessing heart response as chronotropic incompetence is present in up to 70% of HFpEF patients. A 6-MWT of ≤300 meters is considered abnormal for elderly patients with suspicion of HFpEF

If there is a suspicion of HFpEF after the initial evaluation (Step 1), a targeted assessment can be performed to provide a more specific diagnosis confirmation or exclusion (Step 2).

Step 2: Diagnostic workup (E)—

- Perform comprehensive echocardiography (major and minor criteria mentioned in **Table 4**)
- Measure natriuretic peptide levels, if not measured in Step 1

Step 3: Functional testing if there is uncertainty after Step 2 (F1)—

- Conduct diastolic stress echocardiogram (DSE) (refer to the text below)
- Perform invasive hemodynamic measurements (refer to the text below)

Step 4: Final etiology workup (F2)—

- Cardiac magnetic resonance imaging (MRI) for ischemia workup or cardiomyopathy diagnosis

For cardiomyopathy workup:

- Consider cardiac and noncardiac biopsy samples, genetic tests depending on level of suspicion.
- Use scintigraphy/computed tomography (CT)/positron emission tomography

EACVI Algorithm for Elevated LV Filling Pressure (2022)[8]

The EACVI has introduced a novel algorithm, in 2022, for assessing filling pressures of left-sided chambers in the diagnosis of HFpEF (**Box 1**). The algorithm utilizes parameters identical to those published jointly by EACVI and ASE in 2016, apart from one parameter: tissue Doppler measurement of velocities of the mitral annulus at septal and lateral portions.

Validation

The guidelines have been recently published and have not been validated yet.

Guideline Comparison

All four of these guidelines are resources for making the challenging diagnosis of HFpEF. As their development

BOX 1 EACVI, 2022 criteria.

The criteria used are as follows:

1. Left atrial chamber volume index >34 mL/m^2
2. TVR velocity geared to patient BSA >2.8 m/s
3. E/average e′ >14
   - Two out of the three or all three criteria are positive: Elevated filling pressures can be diagnosed
   - Two out of the three or all three are negative: HFpEF can be ruled out
4. Left atrial strain (<18%) is used when two out of the above three criteria are available and one of them is positive and the other is negative

(EACVI: European Association of Cardiovascular Imaging; HFpEF: heart failure with preserved ejection fraction; TVR: tricuspid valvular regurgitation)

TABLE 5: Guideline comparison.

ASE-EACVI guidelines (2016)	Mayo clinic guidelines (H_2FPEF score) (2018)	HFA-ESC guidelines (HFA-PEFF) (2019)	EACVI algorithm for elevated LV filling pressure (2022)
• Lower sensitivity: 33–69% • Higher specificity: 73–87% • Purely echocardiographic criteria	• Introduces patient characteristics in addition to echocardiographic criteria • High sensitivity 89–90%, high specificity for ruling out HFpEF • Does not take into account the phenotypes such as obesity, diabetes, and chronic kidney disease	Stepwise algorithm with major and minor criteria focusing on patient characteristics, echocardiogram, BNP, invasive/exercise testing, ± biopsy	• Excludes septal and lateral MV velocities compared to 2016 ASE-EACVI • Takes into account speckle tracking echocardiography for LA reservoir strain assessment • Does not have patient attributes or measurement of BNP compared to H_2FPEF

(ASE-EACVI: American Society of Echocardiography-European Assoication of Cardiovascular Imaging; H2FPEF: H2—heavy and hypertension, F—atrial fibrillation, P—pulmonary hypertension, E—elderly, F—filling pressures of heart chambers; HFA-ESC: Heart Failure Association of the European Society of Cardiology; HFA-PEFF: Heart Failure Association-Pretest Echocardiogram and biomarkers Functional examination Final etiologic work-up; BNP: B-type natriuretic peptide; HFpEF: heart failure with preserved ejection fraction; LA: left atrial; LV: left ventricular)

occurred at different times, they each have unique emphasis on certain variables. **Table 5** illustrates a brief comparison summary of the guidelines.

Guideline Limitations

All four of the guidelines discussed have similar exclusion criteria of different categories that have been discussed in the literature. One of the limitations of importance is that of moderate-to-severe mitral valve calcification due to decreasing the accuracy of left ventricular filling pressures (LVFP) on echocardiography. One study demonstrated that mitral annular calcification could cause an inaccurate E/e′ secondary to increased mitral inflow velocities and decreased annular velocities.[16] This is of importance as E/e′ ratios are used as parameters in all of the guidelines. To bypass this, an algorithm was proposed using an early to late diastolic filling velocity (E/A) ratio and isovolumetric relaxation time (IVRT) to provide a better estimate of LVFP. The algorithm begins with measurement of E/A ratios, with <0.8 associated with normal LVFP and >1.8 associated with increased LVFP. In the case where the ratio was in between 0.8 and 1.8, it was suggested to measure IVRT. An IVRT time of <80 ms was associated with increased LVFP. The algorithm could not be applied to a small number of patients with AF, unavailable Doppler signals on echocardiogram, and fusion of E and A values linked to tachycardia. Although a small study with a total cohort of 71 patients, the algorithm was validated with 85% sensitivity and 95% specificity, and 89% diagnostic accuracy.[16]

Other listing of guideline limitations can be found in **Table 2**.

NEWER ECHOCARDIOGRAPHIC PARAMETERS

Newer echocardiographic parameters which could help with diagnosis of HFpEF are discussed here.

Diastolic Stress Echocardiography

Diastolic stress echocardiography is indicated when other tests such as resting echocardiography and natriuretic peptides fail to provide conclusive evidence of elevated filling pressures.[17] Patients who already show signs of elevated filling pressures based on established criteria do not require DSE due to the high probability of HFpEF.[3] Similarly, patients without any indications of HFpEF should not undergo DSE since a positive exercise test does not significantly improve the likelihood of making a conclusive diagnosis of HFpEF. Therefore, DSE is most appropriate for patients with an intermediate pretest probability (H_2FPEF score of 2–5 or HFA-PEFF score of 2–4).

Diastolic stress echocardiography involves evaluating the mitral E/average e′ ratio and peak velocity of tricuspid regurgitation (TR) during supine bike protocol or treadmill exercise. An abnormal DSE is defined as an E/average e′ ratio at peak stress of 15 or higher, with or without a peak TR velocity exceeding 3.4 m/s.[18]

Diagnostic Value of Lung Ultrasound in HFpEF

Lung ultrasound has become a propitious technique for screening and predicting outcomes in patients with heart failure, although more research is necessary to fully understand its predictive value.[19] In HFpEF, an elevated LVFP is a common abnormality that leads to increased left atrial (LA) pressures and outcome of pulmonary congestion.[20] Pulmonary congestion is consistently found in heart failure and has an association with increased risk of hospitalization and mortality in both acute and chronic HF cases.[21] LUS is simple, feasible, noninvasive, and radiation-free method to assess pulmonary congestion (also referred to as extravascular lung water) through the evaluation of B-lines.[22] The number of B-lines detected on LUS correlates with PCWP, NT-proBNP, and the E/average e′ ratio (indicative of LVFP) in patients with heart failure.[23-25] The quantity of B-lines is an autonomous risk factor for negative outcomes in HFpEF. It significantly enhances the value of commonly utilized diagnostic and risk stratification models.[19]

Left Atrial Strain

Using two-dimensional (2D) speckle tracking echocardiography (STE) to measure LA reservoir strain is becoming a superior clinical and prognostic tool compared to LV global longitudinal strain (GLS) and left atrial volume index (LAVI) in supporting the diagnosis of HFpEF.[26,27] LA relaxation and compliance strongly influence LA reservoir function, as it is significantly affected by disease progression due to myocardial fibrosis in HFpEF. Patients with elevated left-sided filling pressures exhibit reduced LA reservoir and pump strain.[28] LA strain has been incorporated into the new EACVI 2022 guidelines for HFpEF diagnosis, representing the sole addition to the 2016 ASE EACVI guidelines.[8]

Use of Machine Learning/Artificial Intelligence in Echo to Diagnose HFpEF

The use of AI in diagnosing HFpEF offers promising prospects for improved accuracy and personalized risk assessment. AI techniques such as logistic regression, random forest, gradient descent boosting, and support vector machine enable the analysis of complex patient data and uncover nonlinear relationships.[29] Through external validation steps, AI models have demonstrated their ability to predict invasive measures of LVFP, clinical outcomes, long-term outcomes, and assess biomarkers and exercise performance in patients with HFpEF.[30] Integrating AI-driven diagnostic tools into clinical practice has the potential to revolutionize HFpEF diagnosis, leading to more precise decision-making and improved patient management.[31] Further research and validation are needed to optimize and effectively implement AI-based approaches in HFpEF diagnosis.

Global Longitudinal Strain

There is increasing exploration into the presence of concomitant systolic dysfunction in HFpEF.[32] A promising method for evaluating this dysfunction is through GLS imaging, using 2D STE. This enables the quantitative assessment of LV deformation. GLS demonstrates activity of subendocardial longitudinally oriented fibers, which are vulnerable to wall stress. It has been observed that they can display abnormal contraction patterns in the setting of seemingly normal LVEF.[33] Based on a study involving approximately 4,000 patients, it was found that 84% of individuals diagnosed with HFpEF exhibited reduced GLS values <20%.[34]

Left Ventricular Untwisting Velocity

There is increased interest in LV untwisting rate as an alternative indicator of LV relaxation. In patients with abnormal LV relaxation, there is a decrease in untwisting rate which may hinder the required suction gradients for normal diastolic filling.[35] Peak LV untwisting velocity is measured using STE and is influenced by restoring forces and elevated LVFP apart from relaxation rate.[36] Currently, the routine clinical use of LV untwisting velocity is not advised, and further research is necessary to determine its potential clinical application.

INVASIVE HEMODYNAMIC MEASUREMENTS

To establish a diagnosis in patients exhibiting symptoms suggestive of HFpEF, the gold standard is the invasive measurement of left ventricular end-diastolic pressure (LVEDP) or wedge pressures at rest or during exercise if necessary.[37] This involves conducting right and/or left heart catheterization at rest. In cases where the results are inconclusive, exercise right heart catheterization utilizing cycle ergometry is recommended. A resting PCWP level of 15 mm Hg or higher serves as definitiveevidence of HFpEF. An increased PCWP of 25 mm Hg or higher during exercise is considered diagnostic for HFpEF.[7]

DYSPNEA CLINICS

Dyspnea clinics offer a systematic and comprehensive approach to evaluate patients with unexplained breathlessness on exertion for the diagnosis and management of HFpEF. They also aid in the diagnosis of pulmonary diseases. The integration of diagnostic scores, echocardiography, and exercise testing enables accurate diagnoses, prognostic information, and personalized treatment strategies for patients with HFpEF.[38]

The diagnostic process at a dyspnea clinic includes:[39]

- Conducting laboratory tests to assess blood count, serum iron levels, glycated hemoglobin (HbA1c), NT-proBNP, and more.
- Performing a spirometry test to evaluate lung function and capacity.
- Using transthoracic echocardiography and electrocardiogram to examine the structure and function of the heart at rest.

- Conducting a clinical evaluation and reviewing the patient's medical history with a cardiologist and pulmonologist.
- Undergoing a maximal bicycle test combined with echocardiography and respiratory gas analysis. Combining exercise testing with echocardiography offers insights into the dynamic changes that occur during exercise and can aid in confirming or ruling out HFpEF in patients with unexplained dyspnea or exertional symptoms. It provides prognostic information and aids in guiding appropriate treatment strategies for patients with HFpEF.
- Analyzing diagnostic findings as a multidisciplinary team and proposing further tests and treatment recommendations for shared decision-making with the patient and referring physician.

The step-by-step process aims to comprehensively evaluate patients, identify potential causes of dyspnea, and guide appropriate diagnostic and therapeutic interventions.

MULTIMODALITY IMAGING FOR HFpEF

In addition to echocardiography, cardiac MRI, cardiac CT, and nuclear imaging are resources for evaluation of HFpEF. The most established modality is cardiac MRI as it can help to assess ischemia and presence and extent of fibrosis in cardiac tissue with use of late gadolinium enhancement (LGE), and T1 mapping. LGE uses timing of contrast phases to help differentiate diseases based on enhancement patterns. T1 mapping has pre- and postcontrast utility with the precontrast phase defined as the native longitudinal relaxation time (also known as native T1). Postcontrast T1 is useful for further evaluation by calculating the extracellular volume (ECV).

Both native T1 and ECV are elevated in patients with amyloidosis and fibrosis. ECV has been connected to disease severity as these patients have worse outcomes.[40,41] Cardiac MRI can also be combined with nuclear imaging to assess cardiac energy utility by measuring the phosphocreatine/adenosine triphosphate ratio (PCr/ATP) via spectroscopy. A low PCr/ATP ratio is seen in patients with HFpEF, hypothesized to be due to inadequate use of energy contributing to decreased LV relaxation and exercise tolerance.[42] Limitations to MRI include its availability, cost, decreased reliability in the setting of arrhythmias, and patient comfort.

Nuclear imaging is well established for identifying myocardial ischemia using radionuclide dye. Different nuclear tests exist such as positron emission tomography with fluorodeoxyglucose (FDG-PET), scintigraphy, and single-photon emission computed tomography (SPECT). Scintigraphy and SPECT imaging are most useful for the diagnostic suspicion of cardiac amyloidosis using dye patterns to differentiate subtypes and in the context of autoimmune diseases such as sarcoid. In nuclear stress testing, the relaxation phase of diastole lengthens in patients with HFpEF.[43]

Cardiac CT shares similar utility to MRI but has limited studies to suggest use over MRI for evaluation of cardiac tissue. Some shared advantages of CT and MRI are evaluation of epicardial adipose tissue, opening of pulmonary arteries, chamber volumes, valvular calcification, and use calculated values to derive ECV.[40] The evaluation of epicardial adipose tissue has prognostic significance for obese patients with HFpEF as those with more have a worse prognosis if having more thickness and volume.[40,44] Cardiac CT is most established for evaluation of CAD with angiography. It can possibly rule out other diseases such as constrictive pericarditis and pulmonary hypertension unrelated to cardiac disease. In some studies, the measurement of LV GLS has been comparable to echocardiography; however, this was in the setting of patients with aortic stenosis of which the diagnostic criteria discussed above would not apply.[45] Some of the limitations for cardiac CT include prolonged exposure to radiation, less extensive tissue evaluation, contrast use for kidney disease, and patient comfort.

CONCLUSION

Echocardiography has a critical role in the diagnosis and assessment of HFpEF. It provides valuable information about cardiac structure, function, and hemodynamics, aiding in the evaluation, management, and risk stratification of HFpEF patients. However, it is important to acknowledge the limitations of echocardiography, particularly in borderline cases, where invasive hemodynamic measurements may be necessary for definitive characterization.

Various guidelines and scoring systems have been developed, but they have their own strengths and limitations. The incorporation of newer modalities such as DSE, AI, and LUS shows promise in enhancing the diagnostic accuracy and prognostic value of echocardiography in HFpEF. Dyspnea clinics incorporating echocardiography and multidisciplinary expertise have demonstrated promising outcomes in delivering personalized care for HFpEF patients.

ONLINE REFERENCES

Please scan the QR code provided at the end of the table of contents for References of this chapter.

CHAPTER 99

Role of Echocardiography in the Assessment of Pulmonary Embolism: Usefulness and Limitations

Debasish Roychoudhury, Navin C Nanda, Vijayadithyan Jaganathan, Nishank P Nooli, Yashaswi Koguru, Srijani Thannir

ABSTRACT

Pulmonary embolism is a sinister disease resulting in approximately 117 cases per 100,000 people in the United States causing 60,000–300,000 deaths annually. Diagnosis of pulmonary embolism rests on pretest probability, D-dimer levels, computed tomography (CT) angiogram, and echocardiography. Risk stratification of this disease relies heavily on echocardiographic assessment of right ventricular function, which is a strong predictor of mortality and morbidity. In addition, echocardiographic assessment of various parameters immensely help in deciding management strategy of using anticoagulant versus systemic or catheter based thrombolytic therapy. In this chapter, we describe the current role of echocardiography in the assessment of pulmonary embolism along with its limitations.

Keywords: Echocardiography, pulmonary embolism, thrombus, right ventricle, right ventricular longitudinal strain, interatrial shunt.

INTRODUCTION

Despite advancement in detection and management of venous thromboembolic disease and pulmonary embolism (PE), it still ranks as the third most common reason of cardiovascular death in the Western world.[1] According to the recent European Society of Cardiology (ESC) guidelines, echocardiography is useful in diagnosing and managing acute PE although computed tomography (CT) remains the prime noninvasive modality for detecting and assessing the extent of PE.[2]

DIAGNOSIS

When a patient presents to us with acute shortness of breath and with hemodynamic instability, we are faced with the dilemma to make a rapid bedside provisional diagnosis whether this is due to acute PE, pericardial tamponade, aortic dissection, or shock resulting from another etiology. In such a situation, echocardiography can play a very important role in the identification and subsequent management of PE. Important echocardiographic features, which may point to PE, are given in **Box 1 (Figs. 1 to 5)**.

Both three-dimensional (3D) transthoracic echocardiography (TTE) and 3D transesophageal echocardiography (TEE) may complement 2D TTE by providing more

BOX 1 Two-dimensional transthoracic echocardiography (2D TTE) features of pulmonary embolism.

- Right ventricular (RV) dysfunction with mild, moderate, or severe wall motion abnormalities. RV fractional shortening <36%, tricuspid annular plane systolic excursion (TAPSE) by M-mode echocardiography 1.6 cm or less, RV systolic excursion peak velocity by tissue Doppler <10 cm/s
- Dilated RV with RV/left ventricle (LV) diameter ratio >0.9
- Ventricular septal flattening with D-shaped LV
- McConnell's sign which is RV hypokinesis with apical sparing[3]
- The "60/60" sign which is defined as pulmonary artery flow acceleration time <60 ms in the presence of tricuspid regurgitation pressure gradient <60 mm Hg
- Dilated inferior vena cava (IVC, measuring 21 mm or more) with <50% collapse with inspiration, sniff, or abdominal pressure suggestive of significantly elevated right atrial pressure
- Decreased RV free wall longitudinal strain by speckle tracking echocardiography which may further help in the diagnosis but more importantly in intermediate to high risk cases shows substantial reversal as pulmonary embolism resolves following thrombolytic therapy[4]
- Thrombus or thrombi, especially mobile may be detected in the right atrium, RV, or in the main pulmonary artery or left/right pulmonary artery branches. Thrombi wedged in a patent foramen ovale or atrial septal defect with potential for left sided embolism have also been noted by echocardiography[5,6]

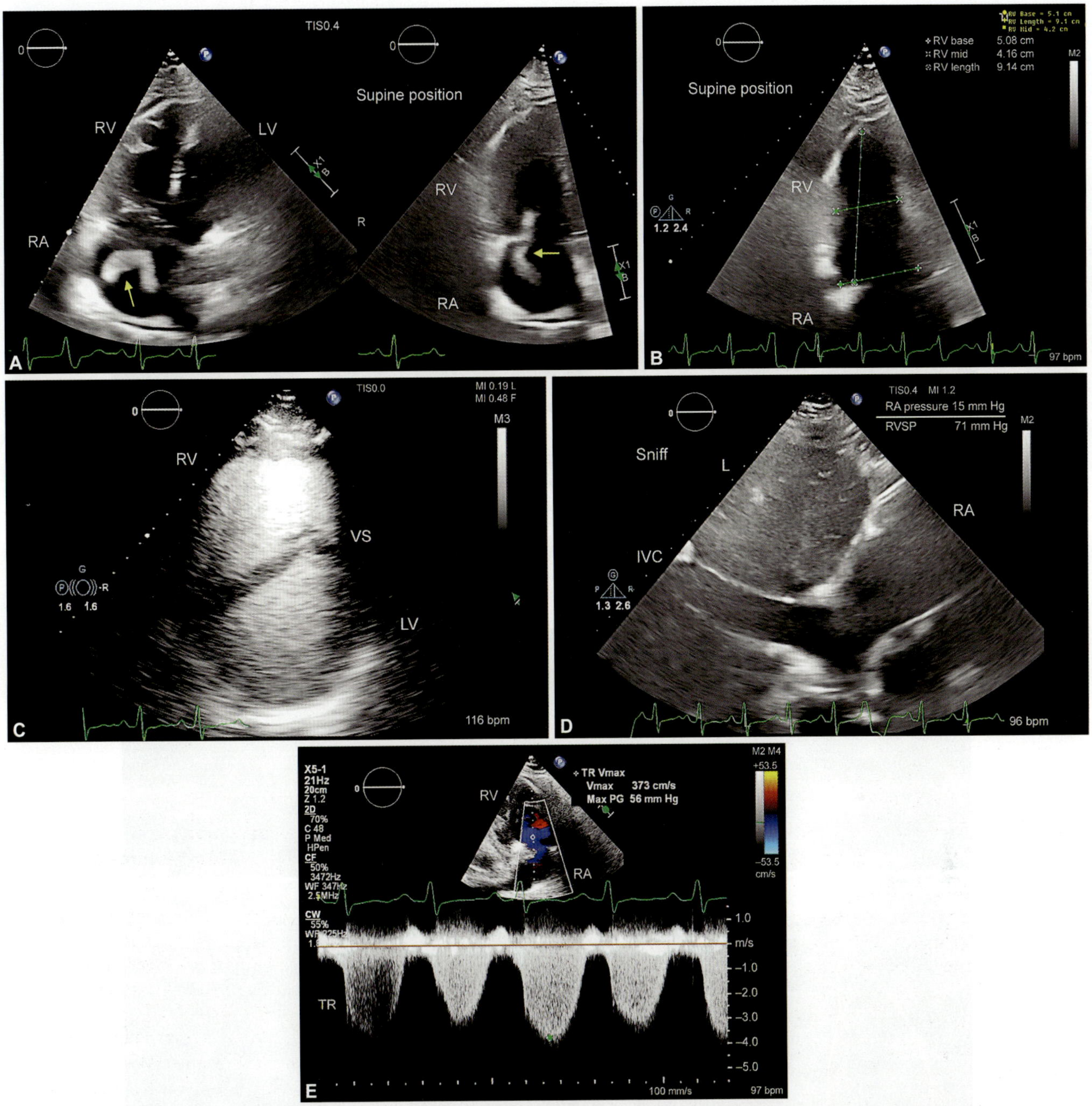

FIGS. 1A TO E: Two-dimensional transthoracic echocardiography. A 56-year-old male with pulmonary embolism. (A) Apical view. Arrows in both right and left panels point to a thrombus in the right atrium (RA) which prolapsed into the right ventricle (RV) in diastole. The thrombus is tubular in shape suggesting it may have originated from a peripheral vein. (B) Apical view. RV base, mid, and RV base to apex measurements are increased consistent with RV enlargement. (C) Short-axis view of left ventricle (LV) demonstrates enlargement of RV and a D-shaped ventricular septum (VS). (D) Subcostal view shows a dilated inferior vena cava (IVC) which did not collapse with sniff indicative of increased RA pressure. (E) Continuous wave Doppler interrogation of the tricuspid regurgitation (TR) jet shows a maximum peak gradient (PG) of 56 mm Hg consistent with very significant pulmonary hypertension.

(L: liver)

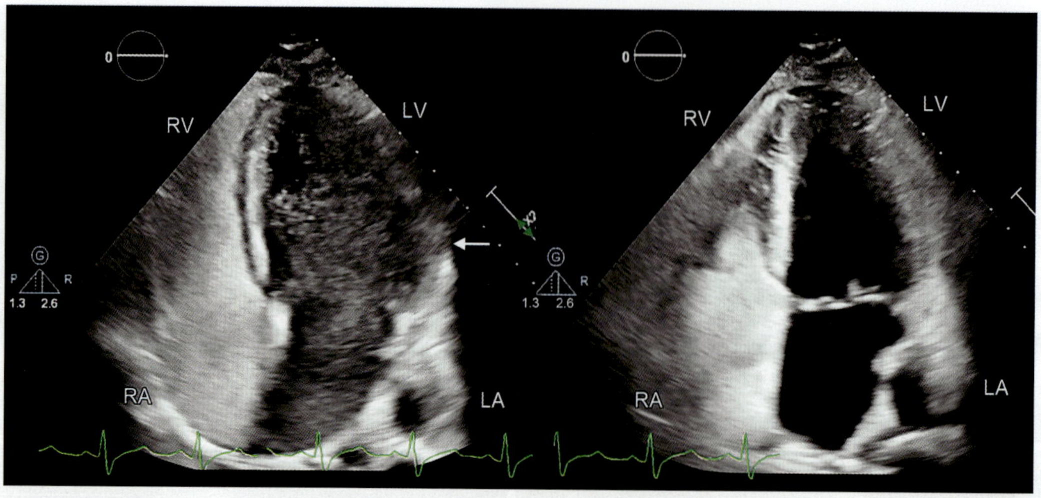

FIG. 2: Two-dimensional transthoracic echocardiography. A 34-year-old male with liver cirrhosis. Bubble study. Injection of normal saline through a line in the right internal jugular vein (IJV) showed appearance of contrast echoes in the LA and then into LV (arrow, left panel) within two beats indicative of interatrial shunt. Right panel shows no contrast echo in the LA or LV immediately after contrast appeared in the right cardiac chambers. Presence of interatrial shunt may result in a RA thrombus transiting into the LA and systematic circulation resulting in vascular obstruction.

(LA: left atrium; LV: left ventricle; RA: right atrium; RV: right ventricle)

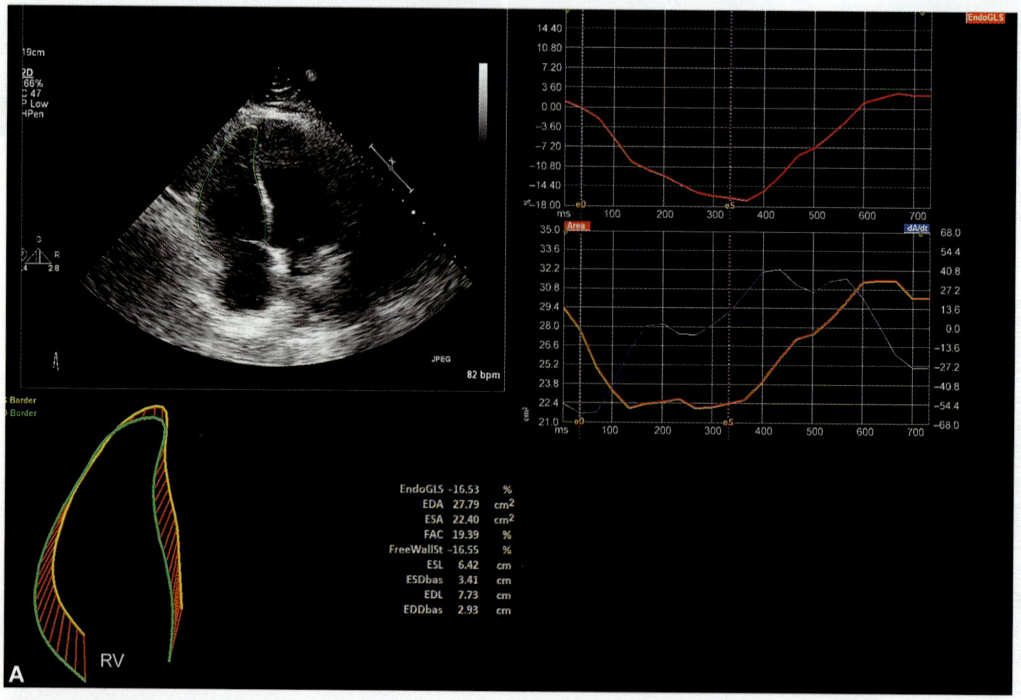

FIGS. 3A AND B: *Continued*

Continued

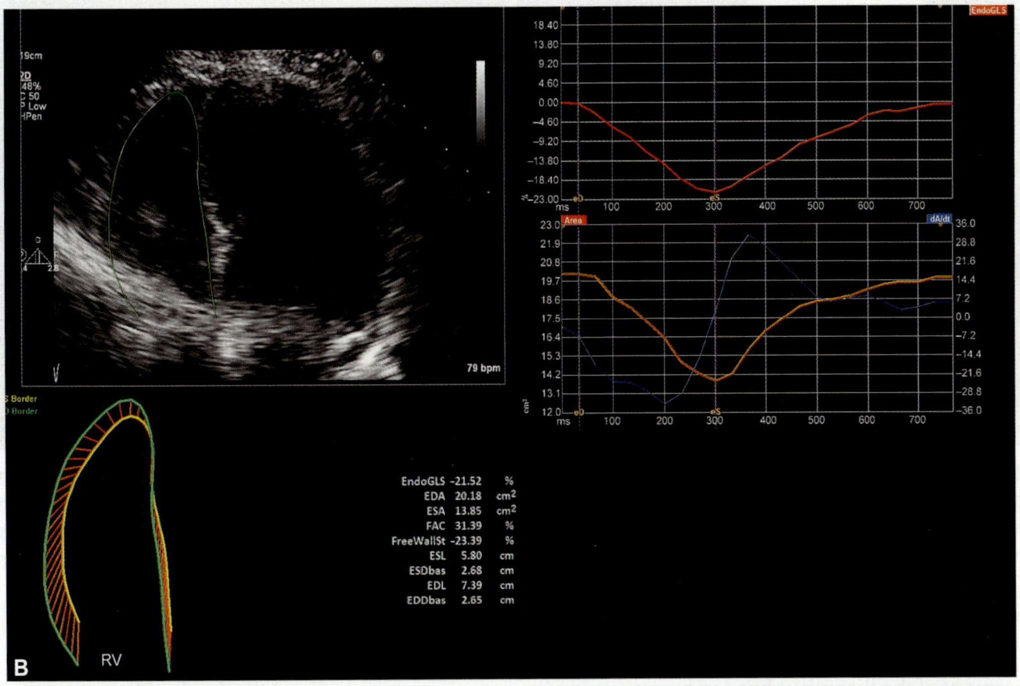

FIGS. 3A AND B: Two-dimensional speckle tracking echocardiography in a 64-year-old female with history of hypertension presenting to the emergency department with 1 week history of shortness of breath and left-sided chest pain. Computed tomographic scan revealed bilateral submassive pulmonary embolism. Before ultrasound facilitated thrombolysis: (A) Reduced RV peak endocardial global longitudinal as well as free wall longitudinal strain. Following ultrasound facilitated thrombolysis: (B) Both strain parameters and other two-dimensional measurements show improvement.

(EDA: end-diastolic area; EDDbas: end-diastolic dimension at base; EDL: end-diastolic length; EndoGLS: peak endocardial global longitudinal strain; ESA: end-systolic area; ESDbas: end-systolic dimension at base; ESL: end-systolic length; FAC: fractional area change; St: strain)

Source: With permission from Dod et al. (2019).[4]

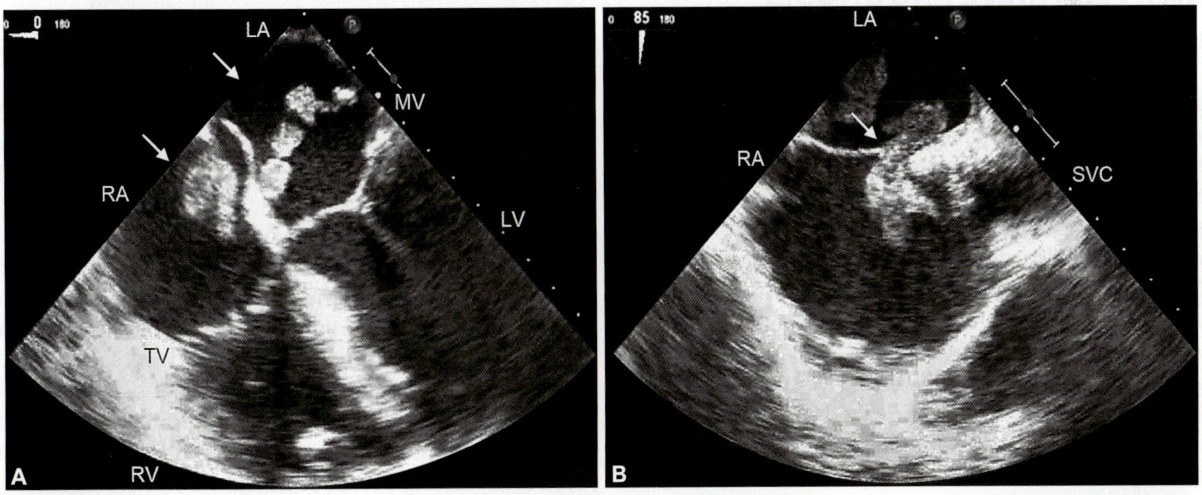

FIGS. 4A AND B: Two-dimensional transesophageal echocardiography of a right atrium (RA) thrombus in transit through a patent foramen ovale in a 68-year-old female with chest pain and progressive shortness of breath. (A) Arrows show a thrombus in the RA and multiple thrombi in the left atrium (LA). The tricuspid valve (TV), right ventricle (RV), mitral valve (MV), and left ventricle (LV) are seen. (B) Arrow shows the point where the thrombus is stretching open patent foramen ovale (PFO) when transiting from the RA to the LA. The superior vena cava (SVC) is also visualized.

Source: With permission from Thind et al. (2015).[5]

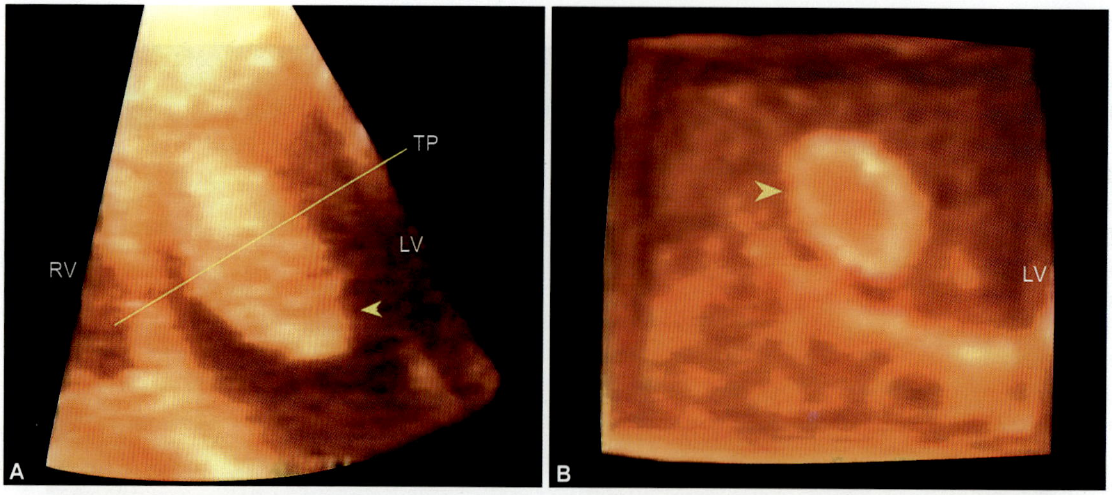

FIGS. 5A AND B: Peripartum cardiomyopathy. Morphological assessment of left ventricle (LV) thrombus by live/real-time three-dimensional transthoracic echocardiography. (A) Arrowhead points to the thrombus in the LV apex with no obvious evidence of lysis. (B) Site of transverse plane (TP) cropping of the thrombus (arrowhead), which demonstrates practically complete resolution of thrombus from lysis with only an intact outer shell (arrowhead). Lysis may occur in a thrombus in any location including the right atrium (RA), right ventricle (RV), or pulmonary arteries.

Source: With permission from Sinha et al. (2004).[7]

accurate assessment of the thrombus burden by measuring its size more accurately, identifying ongoing lysis or liquefaction within the thrombus, and by excluding thrombi in other cardiac chambers.[6,7] In patients on anticoagulant therapy, the first step in thrombus dissolution is development of lysis, which may progress over time resulting in complete resolution and disappearance of the thrombus. Echocardiography is thus useful in the follow-up of these patients.[7]

RIGHT VENTRICLE PROGNOSIS

Right ventricular (RV) longitudinal strain measured by 2D speckle-tracking echocardiography can assess RV longitudinal myocardial systolic base to apex shortening which provides another parameter of assessing RV function. RV strain value closely correlates with prognosis in patients with acute PE with stable hemodynamics. In a small prospective study, it was noted that RV ejection fraction based on 3D echocardiography and longitudinal strain in midportion of RV free wall had independent association with 6-month detrimental consequences in acute submassive PE.[8] Thus, RV mid-free wall strain is an independent parameter of prognosis such as inhospital PE-related mortality.

In another study, authors showed the usefulness of RV free wall strain imaging in submassive pulmonary embolus and therapeutic thrombolytic therapy thereafter with good outcome.[4]

In a retrospective study of 21 normotensive patients with PE, our group found that RV/left ventricular (LV) end-diastolic diameter (EDD) ratio >1 in four chamber view, ventricular septal flattening with or without paradoxical motion, and McConnell's sign seen in almost three-fourths of the patients by echocardiography were associated with worse outcomes including four deaths. Thus, we concluded that the normotensive patient with a cluster of such findings would probably benefit from institution of thrombolytic therapy or some other form of intervention.[9]

In an article slated for publication this year in the Journal of the American Society of Echocardiography, RV fractional area shortening <14–16% in severe cases, tricuspid annular plane systolic excursion (TAPSE) <1.7 cm, and RV systolic velocity by tissue Doppler (S' wave) <10 cm/s were indicators of RV dysfunction in PE. Both LV outflow tract (LVOT) velocity time integral (VTI) ≤ 15 cm and RV outflow tract (RVOT) VTI < 9.5 cm were closely related to adverse outcomes. Abnormal pulmonary artery systolic pressure (PASP)/LV stroke volume (SV) >1 mm Hg/mL, TAPSE/PASP < 0.4 and early systolic notching (ESN) of RVOT pulse wave Doppler were also predictors of adverse outcomes in these patients.[1]

Registro Informatizado de Enfermedad Trombo-Embólica (RIETE) represents a large registry of patients with venous thromboembolism comprising of 179 centers in Asia, Europe, and the Americas. The study included 35,935 patients who had acute PE and were symptomatic. Early 2D TTE was performed in 42.8% of patients, who had risk for cardiovascular disease and clinically recognizable indicators of PE severity such as hypotension, hypoxemia, and tachycardia. Presence of right atrial enlargement, RV hypokinesis, and thrombi in the right atrium or ventricle were good predictors of 30-day PE-related mortality in this high-risk subgroup.[10]

In a manuscript published in the Journal of the American Society of Echocardiography, Bernard and colleagues[11] explored the implication of characteristic ESN in the RVOT spectral Doppler tracing. In patients with pulmonary hypertension, this notching of RVOT tracing was noted to be related to abrupt systolic closure of pulmonic valve leaflets visualized on M-mode echocardiography. This resulted in an abrupt diminution in the systolic flow velocity in the pulmonary artery.[11] Afonso et al.[12] studied ESN as an echocardiographic parameter to detect and categorize PE. The basis of their study was a large group of 5,152 patients referred for CT angiography for suspected PE in an academic institution. Inclusion criteria for this study included patients with massive, submassive, or subsegmental PE undergoing echocardiography within 48 hours of such presentations. Of these, 187 patients with PE and 90 controls with no PE by CT angiography were included in the study. Over 90% of patients with massive PE or submassive PE were found to have ESN in contrast to only 2% of patients with subsegmental PE and none in the control group. Both the sensitivity and specificity of ESN for PE were much higher in the range of 92% and 99%, respectively, in this selected group of patients in comparison to other traditional findings of PE such as McConnell's sign, the "60/60" sign, and RVOT acceleration time (AT).

In another very recently published study by Bigdelu et al.,[13] between years 2020 and 2022, 30 patients with acute or subacute PE as was evidenced by CT angiography were compared with 30 controls without PE in regards to the following echocardiographic features: ESN, McConnell's sign, RVOT VTI, RV EDD, tricuspid regurgitation (TR) peak pressure gradient, pulmonary artery pressure (PAP), and AT or RV ejection time (ET). ESN was found in as many as in 96.6% of PE patients and none in the control group ($p < 0.001$). Also, when compared to the control group, RVOT VTI, RV ET, and AT values were lower in patients with PE with highly significant p values while RV EDD, TR gradient, PAP, ESN, McConnell's sign, and D-shaped LV were higher with high statistical significance. Both presence of ESN and AT/ET ratio < 0.4 predicted massive and submassive PE with a sensitivity of 97.0% and 100%, specificity of 99.0% and 97%, and confidence interval (CI) = 0.844–1.0, respectively.

In another recently published multicenter study[14] conducted in the emergency departments of four academic centers, echocardiographic feature of ESN in patients presenting with suspected PE undergoing CT angiography was evaluated in 201 patients. In all emergency department patients, the sensitivity of ESN was 34% and specificity was 97% whereas it was found to be 69% sensitive in high or intermediate-high risk patients with a specificity of 90%. The authors concluded that in the emergency department setting, ESN had moderate-to-high specificity but relatively low sensitivity for detecting PE. These findings are in contrast to the more favorable results reported in the other studies. Thus, the usefulness of ESN may be limited in certain clinical settings. Further work is needed to ascertain the exact role of ESN in PE.

In an abstract published in the Journal Circulation in the year 2000,[15] the role of echocardiography in diagnosing of RV dysfunction and its implication on clinical outcome of PE patients with normotension was studied in 209 patients with documented PE. The criteria used for diagnosing acute RV dysfunction echocardiographically were one or more of the following: Dilatation of RV with no RV wall hypertrophy, paradoxical systolic motion of the ventricular septum, and presence of pulmonary hypertension. It was found in this study that patients with acute PE presenting with normal hemodynamics but signs of RV dysfunction on the echocardiogram had a high rate of PE-related shock (10%) and inhospital mortality (5%) and thus may need more aggressive management. On the other hand, patients with PE and stable hemodynamics without signs of RV dysfunction on echocardiogram had good short-term prognosis. The results of this study highlight the importance of performing echocardiography for early identification of RV dysfunction with its implication in the risk stratification of patients with acute PE with normal blood pressure.

In a paper published recently in the Journal of the American Society of Echocardiography, authors performed a retrospective analysis of 150 patients with acute PE with an endpoint of all-cause mortality or clinical deterioration requiring intubation, vasopressor use, and systemic or catheter-based thrombolysis. Patients meeting primary endpoints showed significantly more severe RV dysfunction demonstrated by various echocardiographic criteria such as greater reduction in the velocity of the RV annulus during systole, and greater reduction in both RV global and free longitudinal strain. The ratio of TAPSE to RV systolic pressure indicative of RV pulmonary artery uncoupling was also lower in this group of patients. In addition, the RV was larger with D-shaped ventricular septum in these patients.[16] This study highlights the importance of RV dysfunction detected by echocardiography in patients with PE.

As we can see through numerous studies published so far that echocardiography plays a significant role in helping establishing a provisional diagnosis of PE and eliminating other possibilities of dyspnea with hemodynamic compromise such as cardiogenic shock, pericardial tamponade, and acute aortic dissection to name a few differential diagnoses.

Echocardiography also helps in management decision of thrombolytic or other interventional therapies particularly in patients presenting with acute PE but stable hemodynamics.

LIMITATIONS

However, echocardiography has limitations too in the assessment of PE. The main limitation is the very low sensitivity in the diagnosis of PE at an early stage and the mainstay for diagnosis of PE is CT angiogram. The predictive value of echocardiographic signs is low and hence it cannot be used to exclude PE except for visualization of thrombus in the right heart. Echocardiography is not indicated for patients who have low probability for PE. Also, in patients with suboptimal acoustic windows, echocardiography does not provide adequate visualization of RV and other structures.

CONCLUSION

Pulmonary embolism and venous thromboembolism still remain sinister disease entities all over the world with significant morbidity and mortality despite advances in management strategies. Although the standard modality for the diagnosis of PE is CT angiography, echocardiography can immensely complement by its easy ability and cost-effectiveness to identify not only RV dilatation but also RV dysfunction using many parameters. It is also effective in assessing the right atrial pressure as well as presence and severity of pulmonary hypertension. In addition, it can detect thrombi in right heart chambers and pulmonary artery and diagnose interatrial communications using bubble studies. Besides these, echocardiography is useful in assessing prognosis and can be helpful in making treatment decision regarding anticoagulant versus thrombolytic therapy in patients with acute PE who are hemodynamically stable. It can be also useful in follow-up of dissolution of thrombus in patients with acute PE receiving anticoagulation.

ONLINE REFERENCES

Please scan the QR code provided at the end of the table of contents for References of this chapter.

CHAPTER

100 Three-dimensional Echocardiography: Past, Present, and Future

V Amuthan, RVA Ananth

ABSTRACT

The ever-increasing use and the literature on three-dimensional (3D) echocardiography are proof of the acceptance of this technique in the real world. However, with more and more development of techniques and transducer technology, the spatial and temporal resolutions of the 3D datasets are increased and there is single-beat acquisition possible with software beam formers, suggesting and complementing authors' belief that 3D examination should be routine in all patients. Major advantages of 3D echocardiography compared to traditional two-dimensional (2D) echocardiography are the following: (1) Left ventricular (LV) function assessment: Improved accuracy of evaluation of the LV chamber volumes (by eliminating the need for geometric modeling as well as a reduction in errors caused by foreshortened views). The principal reasons for requesting an echocardiogram in clinical practice include the assessment of LV chamber size and systolic function. (2) Realistic visualization of cardiac valves and congenital abnormalities: Volume-rendered 3D displays of transthoracic or transesophageal images enable improved evaluation of the anatomy of the heart valves and their supporting structures. Accordingly, 3D imaging is particularly helpful to the cardiac surgeon or interventional cardiologist to provide the most detailed anatomic and functional information. (3) Right ventricular (RV) volume assessment: 3D echocardiography permits evaluation of regional LV function and objective detection of wall motion abnormalities. (4) Data from 3D echocardiography can provide objective evidence of LV systolic dyssynchrony, which may serve as an additional criterion for referral for cardiac resynchronization therapy. (5) Interventional echocardiography: The improved echo–fluoroscopic fusion images, transillumination, and transparency modes are very useful for the interventional cardiologist during structural heart interventions involving transseptal puncture, mitral, aortic interventions, and left atrial (LA) appendage occlusion. This chapter uses the current standard new format in which figures are arranged as Tables instead of random placement in the manuscript.

Keywords: Three-dimensional echocardiography, echo–fluoro fusion echocardiography, interventional echocardiography.

INTRODUCTION

Echocardiography has been the marvel of the 20th century. This ultrasound technique, since its inception from the days of Elder, has revolutionized the diagnosis and treatment in the management of cardiac patients. From the days of single-crystal probe to M-mode, two dimensional (2D), color flow mapping, the advancement has reached the stage of three-dimensional (3D) echocardiogram with added fourth dimension of time [four-dimensional (4D) echocardiography—the real-time 3D echocardiography]. The cumbersome big mechanical probes are now replaced with smaller Matrix probes with more than 3,000 elements, which can acquire images from a single cardiac cycle.[1-3] The introduction of the first-phased array real-time volumetric 3D imaging system (Duke University, Durham, North Carolina) enabled transthoracic real-time acquisition of 3D echocardiographic datasets.[4,5] In addition to transthoracic real-time acquisition, simultaneous presentation of perspective images became possible; the spatial and temporal image resolutions were considerably improved with developments in software technology.

PRESENT DAY 3D ECHOCARDIOGRAPHY

The newer 3D Matrix array transducers have more uniform atomic structure, larger bands, and have efficient electromechanical coupling. They have >2,500 crystals arranged as 50 rows and 50 columns. The performance of the 3D echocardiogram has the same methodology as standard 2D echocardiography.[6-8] The image dataset is essentially acquired from the same parasternal and apical windows.[9-13] The acquisition of optimized 2D images along with routine electrocardiogram (ECG) connection is the most important prerequisite. These images can be viewed in multiple newer formats: (1) Multiplane view, (2) real-time, zoom view, (3) full volume view, and (4) 3D color full volume or color zoom view.[14-26] The advantages and disadvantages of the different formats are given in **Table 1**.

TABLE 1: Acquisition of 3D echocardiographic images.

Acquisition modalities	Descriptions	Images
Multiplane view: By using the cursor in the primary image shown on the left, the secondary orthogonally opposite image in any cut plane can be obtained	• *Biplane*: Simultaneously orthogonally two opposite planes of two-dimensional echocardiograms can be viewed in biplane • *Triplane*: It can also be seen in triplane view with slices 60° apart. The accompanying figure shows the images in apical four-chamber, two-chamber, and three-chamber views simultaneously	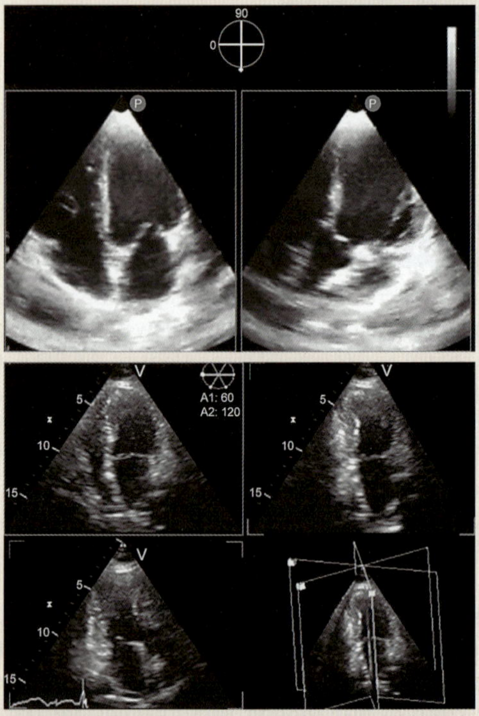
Real-time zoom modality	For example, (A) acquisition boxes may be applied in azimuthal plane and elevation plane and (B) zoomed 3D en face view of mitral valve can be obtained	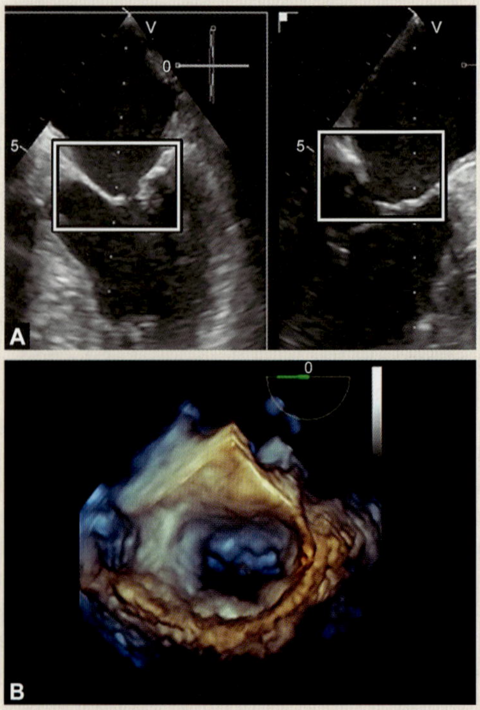

TOOLS FOR 3D ECHOCARDIOGRAPHY: CROPPING

Cropping is an important tool in 3D echocardiography. Just like the surgeon or the anatomist has to view the internal structures after cutting through the superficial structures, cropping is used in 3D echocardiography. By cropping, the unwanted elements in the images can be removed. **Table 2** shows how to crop from this pyramidal dataset and display cross-sectional views and en face views. In modern machines, the cropping has been simplified to use the 2D-guided selection of region of interest (ROI). For example, 2 Click Crop is used. Any two points can be clicked and a rectangular area in between them can be cropped. We can also select the direction to view the cropped images. Dual cropping technique displays the view from both sides of the ROI.

3D DISPLAY FORMATS

The 3D images can be viewed in six different formats as follows:

1. *Volume rendering*: The echo machine can display the 3D images in a stereoscopic fashion or 3D-rendered image **(Table 3)**.

TABLE 2: Cropping techniques of 3D echocardiography.

Cropping modalities	Images
Standard 3D crop: The cropping planes in the X, Y, and Z axes can be selected and cropped. This has been largely replaced by the 2D-guided 2 click crop	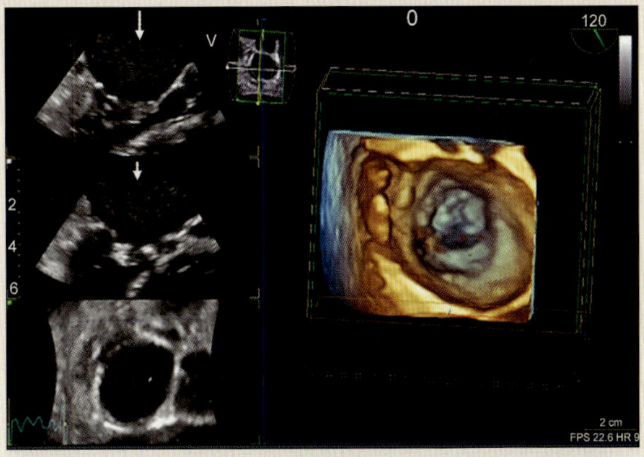
2 click crop: This is also called focused crop where the 2D images are used to select the area of interest. The first region of interest is selected in the left atrial side of mitral valve and clicked, followed by the second region of interest (ROI) in the left ventricular side. This also selects the view from left atrial side (surgeon's view) in this patient with mitral stenosis	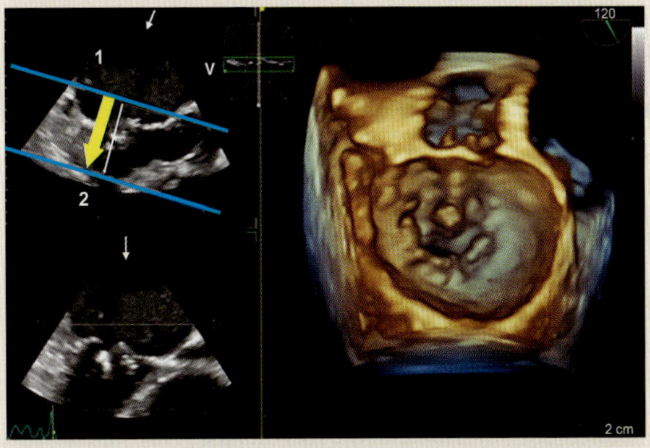
Dual crop: In the dual crop mode, the cropped images from the left atrial side and the left ventricular side are displayed simultaneously, while ROI is selected for mitral valve	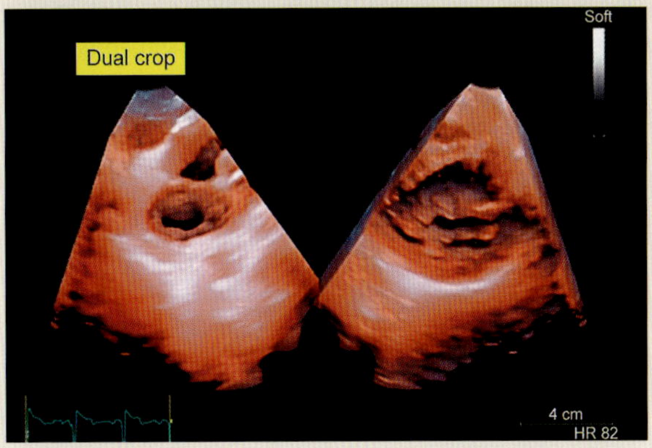

TABLE 3: Modality of display of 3D echocardiography.

Modalities of display	Images
Volume rendering: These are 3D rendered images *Example*: On the right the 3D images of aortic valve are displayed in stereoscopic fashion or 3D-rendered image	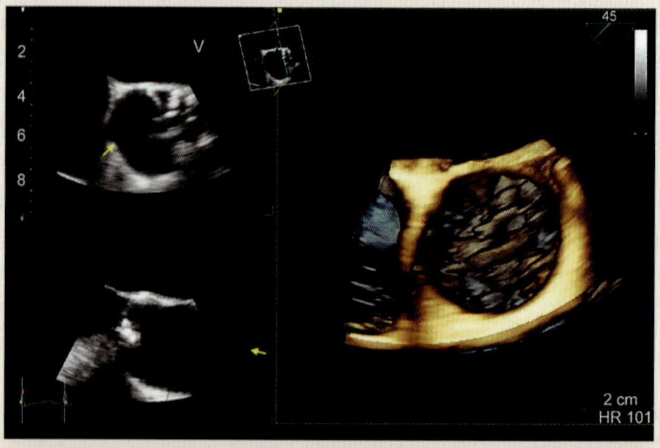
Surface rendering: In this modality the surfaces are shown as solid structures. The surface-rendered images of left ventricle is shown on the right and mitral valve is shown on the right	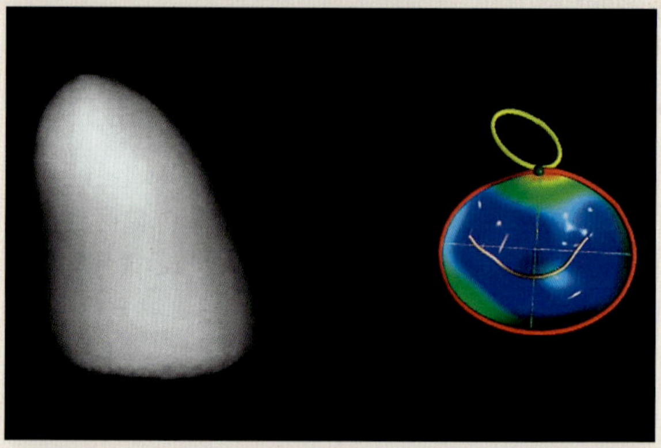
Tomographic slices: 3–12 tomographic slices of the images can be made. The image on the right-hand side shows 12 tomographic slices. The apical four-chamber, two-chamber, and three-chamber views are seen on the left-hand side and nine serial cuts from the apex to the base on the right-hand side	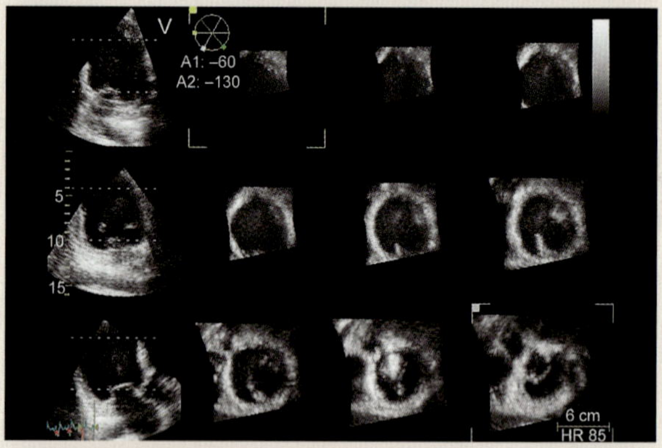
Photorealistic transillumination: This tool uses Flexi light or virtual light to create shadowing and the perception of depth. The picture on the right depicts the P2 prolapse from the surgeon's view	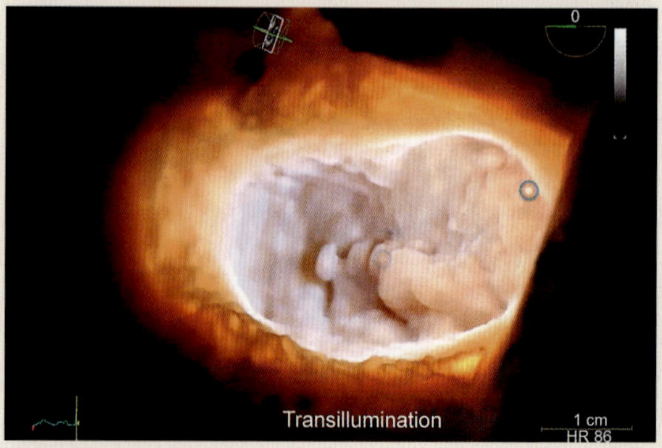

Continued

Continued

Modalities of display	Images
Glass view (transparency): • By increasing the light intensity and adding light with sunset silhouette features, glass view can be created • The accompanying picture of calcific mitral stenosis reveals regions of calcifications beautifully	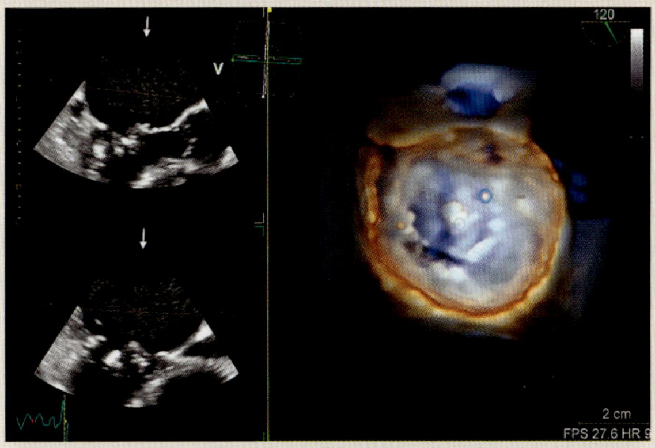
Flexi slice (multiplanar reconstruction): This tool allows to cut 3D dataset at any orthogonal plane and rotate. This makes real-time measurements in any 2D or 3D planes and thus avoids the parallax error associated with direct 3D measurements	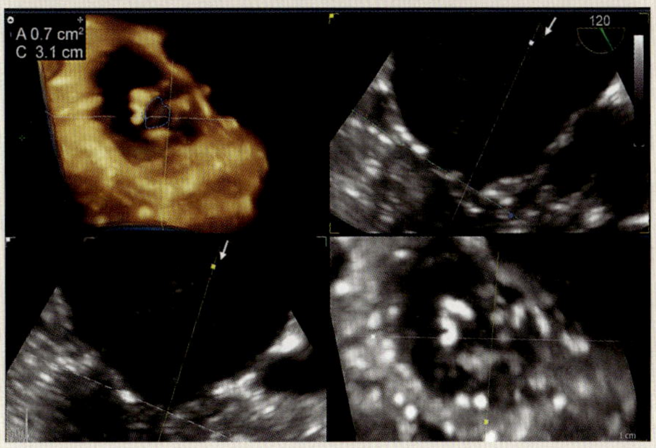

2. *Surface rendering*: It is a visualization technique that shows the surfaces of structures or organs in a solid appearance. The left ventricular (LV) shape, regional function, and the degree of each scallop in mitral valve prolapse can be viewed.
3. *Tomographic slices*: After acquiring the images in the full volume, 3–12 tomographic slices of the images can be made.
4. *Photorealistic transillumination*: This tool uses flexi light or virtual light to create shadowing and the perception of depth.
5. *Glass view (transparency)*: By increasing the light intensity and adding light with sunset silhouette features, glass view can be created. The accompanying picture of calcific mitral stenosis reveals regions of calcifications beautifully.
6. *Flexi slice (multiplanar reconstruction)*: This tool allows to cut at any orthogonal plane and rotate. This makes real-time measurements in any 2D or 3D planes and thus avoiding the parallax error associated with direct 3D measurements.

CLINICAL APPLICATIONS OF 3D ECHOCARDIOGRAPHY IN PRACTICE

Examination of Left Ventricle and Left Ventricular Function Assessment

Left ventricular ejection fraction (LVEF): The cornerstone of the prognostication and treatment schedule for echocardiographic evaluation starts with the evaluation of LVEF. Despite its limitations, EF has become part of the lingua franca of cardiology.[13] The evidence base for modern cardiology is so heavily based on this simple measurement that it is unlikely to disappear. The problems in calculating EF as the ratio between stroke volume and end-diastolic volume and their solutions are enumerated in **Table 4**. 3D imaging is available with echocardiography, magnetic resonance imaging (MRI), and computed tomography (CT). The main attraction and advantage of 3D imaging is to avoid geometric assumptions when calculations of LV volumes are being obtained and to avoid errors created by cutting a 3D structure in two dimensions. The current software for 3D evaluation of

TABLE 4: Applications of 3D echocardiography for LV function.

Clinical applications	Images
LV function: The main advantages of 3D LV function are– • It avoids geometric assumptions of LV volumes calculated from 2D • It avoids errors created by cutting a 3D structure in two dimensions • The current software for 3D evaluation of LVEF is much easier and can be performed within minutes in the setting of the emergency room On the right is the technique of calculation of LVEF from the heart model	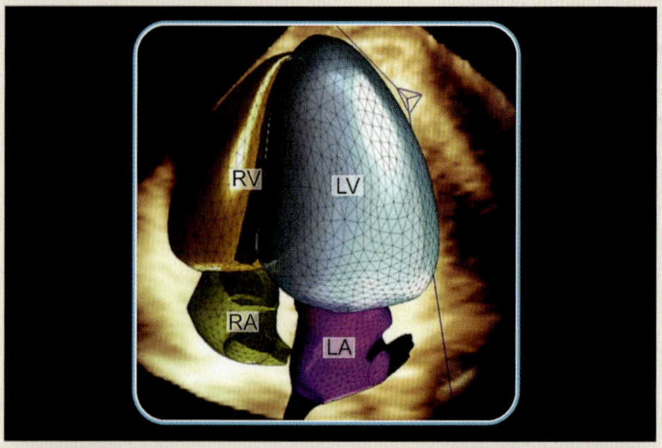
4D LV strain: The advantages of 4D strain are– • Out of plane-speckle motion is avoided • The bull's-eye map is dynamic • The global strain calculation is simultaneous in all segments • Area strain and LV twist can be calculated with ease • At present, their use is limited to patients with HFpEF and selection of patients for CRT	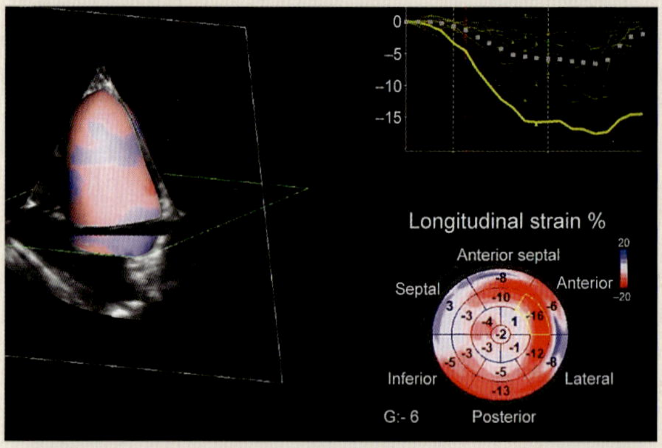
LV regional function and stress echo • 3D echocardiography has the advantage of acquiring triplane images from LV apex, before and after treadmill exercise from single-beat acquisition. From these triplane images, the AFI bull's-eye plot can be plotted easily • In this 75-year-old diabetic patient, treadmill exercise ECG was normal. However, the postexercise bull's-eye plot clearly demonstrates the new strain abnormality in the anterior septum, post stress. The coronary angiogram revealed a 99% tight, mid-LAD lesion	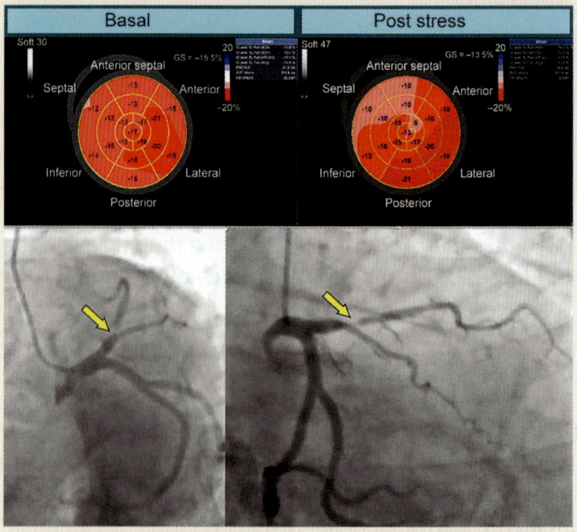

(AFI: automated functional imaging; CRT: cardiac resynchronization therapy; ECG: electrocardiogram; HFpEF: heart failure with preserved ejection fraction; LAD: left anterior descending; LV: left ventricular; LVEF: left ventricular ejection fraction; RV: right ventricular)

LVEF is much easier and can be performed within minutes in the setting of an emergency room.[27]

4D Left Ventricular Strain

Shortening and lengthening, which are the basic functions of the myocardial fibers, result in a systolic twist followed by a diastolic untwisting of the left ventricle due to helical orientation of the fibers. In systole, the LV apex undergoes a counterclockwise rotation about its longitudinal axis as viewed from the apex, preceded by a brief clockwise rotation due to the earlier shortening of the subendocardial fibers during isovolumic contraction. Rotation of the LV base in systole is opposite in direction compared to apical rotation, with a brief counterclockwise rotation during isovolumic contraction followed by a clockwise rotation during LV ejection. This motion has been compared with that used to squeeze water out of a wet towel.[28] The main determinant of the LV twist is the apical rotation. A recent study by Ashraf et al. to compute LV twist from 3D echocardiography concluded that LV twist and torsion can be computed accurately.[29,30] 3D speckle tracking has improved the accuracy of LV deformation imaging and torsion dynamics. To date, no prognostic information exists on the role of rotational parameters of LV function. The areas most likely to benefit are heart failure with preserved ejection fraction (HFpEF) and cardiac dyssynchrony resynchronization therapy.[31-33]

Global longitudinal strain (GLS) has evolved as one of the most robust parameters, and this has been shown to identify subclinical LV dysfunction. GLS is calculated using a variety of proprietary software (EchoPAC, GE Medical Systems, Milwaukee, Wisconsin, USA; Syngo velocity vector imaging, Siemens, Mountain View, California, USA; and LV analysis, TOMTEC GmbH, Unterschleißheim, Germany). GLS is well validated as a marker for the measurement of LV longitudinal deformation, which has emerged as a sensitive and specific marker to detect early and subtle myocardial dysfunction. In one of the recent meta-analyses, Kalam et al. have shown the independent prognostic significance of GLS in patients with mild LV global impairment. The prognostic value of this information seems likely to be superior to that provided by LVEF.[34] LV GLS before discharge after ST-segment elevation myocardial infarction (STEMI) is independently associated with LV dilatation at follow-up.[35] In another study of 576 patients who underwent echocardiography ≤24 hours after primary percutaneous coronary intervention for STEMI, GLS, and wall motion score index (WMSI) were comparable and both superior for early risk assessment compared with volume-based LV function indicators, such as LVEF and end-systolic volume index (ESVI). Compared with WMSI, the advantage of GLS is the provision of a semiautomated quantitative measure.[36]

3D Evaluation of Left Ventricular Regional Function

The American Society of Echocardiography has recently recommended a 17-segment model for this.[37,38] In a 17-segment model, beginning at the anterior junction of the interventricular septum and the right ventricular (RV) free wall and continuing counterclockwise, basal- and midventricular segments should be labeled as anteroseptal, inferoseptal, inferior, inferolateral, anterolateral, and anterior. The apex is divided into five segments including septal, inferior, lateral, and anterior segments, as well as the "apical cap," which is defined as the myocardium beyond the end of the LV cavity. A bull's-eye plot can be constructed where the outer ring represents the basal segments, the middle ring represents the segments at midpapillary muscle level, and the inner ring represents the distal level. The fact is that some manufacturers and many echocardiography laboratories never adopted these guidelines.[39] The severity of contractile dysfunction is scored visually in each segment as 1 for normal contraction or hyperkinesia, 2 for hypokinesia, 3 for akinesia, and 4 for dyskinesia. The global wall motion score is there, calculated by averaging the readings in all the segments. A score of 5 for aneurysmal segments has been deleted from the recent guidelines statement from American Society of Echocardiography.[38] A normal LV has a WMSI of 1, and the index increases as wall motion abnormalities increase in severity. A WMSI of 1.1–1.9 can predict a small infarct size, and an index ≥ 2.0 can predict a larger infarct size. However, this approach is subjective and operator dependent, demands complete visualization of the endocardium, and is subject to the vicissitudes of cardiac loading and heart rate. The ability of 3D echocardiography in providing tomographic slicing of left ventricle to nine short-axis tomographic slices with simultaneous display of left ventricle in apical two-chamber, three-chamber, and four-chamber views greatly enhances the diagnostic accuracy. 4D strain analysis would help in this in depicting the bull's-eye plot or the automated functional imaging of the longitudinal and circumferential area and radial strain on a scale of –20 to +20 instead of the four-grade regional wall motion score analysis. Further myocardial deformation analysis by speckle-tracking echocardiography has been shown to accurately predict viability in patients with chronic ischemic LV dysfunction.[40]

3D Evaluation of Right Ventricular Function

Echocardiographic assessment of the right ventricle is difficult because of its complex shape. RV performance is known to be a major determinant of clinical status and long-term outcomes in patients with pulmonary hypertension, cardiomyopathies, and congenital heart disease. Apical acquisition of volumes is recommended in the adult population. The modified RV apical four-chamber view is used. One way (medial approach) is to move the transducer medially to get the RV-modified apical four-chamber view and then tilt the transducer cranially and anteriorly and even rotate to include the pulmonary valve in the guidance images. Because of the complicated structure and geometry of the right ventricle, conventional 2D echocardiography is unable to correctly estimate RV volume using reasonable geometric assumptions. From the echocardiographer's perspective, the right ventricle is divided into four segments: The infundibulum (or outflow tract), anterior free wall, lateral wall, and inferior wall.[41-43] The dual blood supply [right coronary artery (RCA) and left anterior descending (LAD)] of the infundibulum and the anterior wall makes these segments most resistant to ischemia, while the inferior wall is the most susceptible, and the lateral wall has an intermediate level of susceptibility to ischemia. The steps involved in 3D evaluation of RV are shown in **Table 5**.

3D Evaluation of Left Atrium

Although 2D assessment remains the current standard for left atrial (LA) volume assessment in clinical practice, the visualization of the left atrium in 3D shape, independent of geometric assumptions, favors its use, and it may be the preferred method for LA volume assessment.[44-46] The 3D LA quantification software has the advantage in that it can be used for calculation of LA volume as well as LA strain as shown in **Table 5**. For assessing the 3D LA function,

TABLE 5: Clinical applications of 3D echocardiography for RV and LA function.

Clinical applications	Images
RV function: 3D echocardiographic RV functional analysis correlates with CMR because of the inclusion of RV inlet, trabecular body, and outlet. On the right, the RV function analysis in a patient with Brugada syndrome is shown. The RVEF of 59% correlated with CMR-derived RVEF	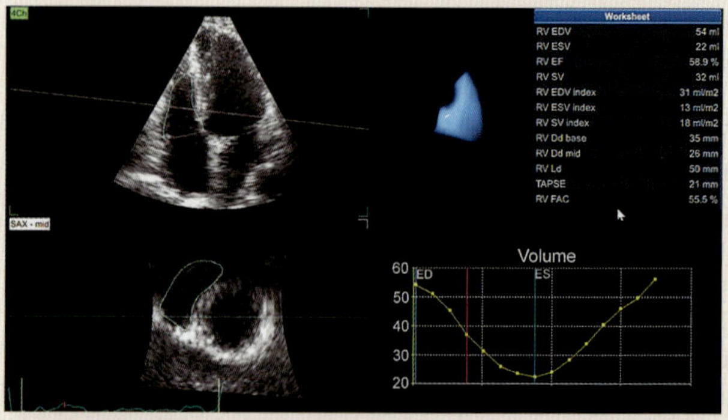
LA function: A. For assessing the 3D LA function, LA focused apical four-chamber view is acquired and the image is optimized for alignment and temporal resolution. The mitral valve coaptation center point is land marked and the LV end-diastolic, end-systolic, and preatrial contraction phases are set. The results of 3D LA function analysis are displayed as LA volumetric data (LA Vmax and LA EF) and LA strain values [(LA reservoir strain (LASr), LA conduit strain (LAScd), and LA contraction strain (LASct)]. B. Normal LA strain curve is displayed (the normal LA reservoir strain is around 40%) C. LA strain curve in the patient with Brugada syndrome referred above—shows abnormally reduced LASr to 14%	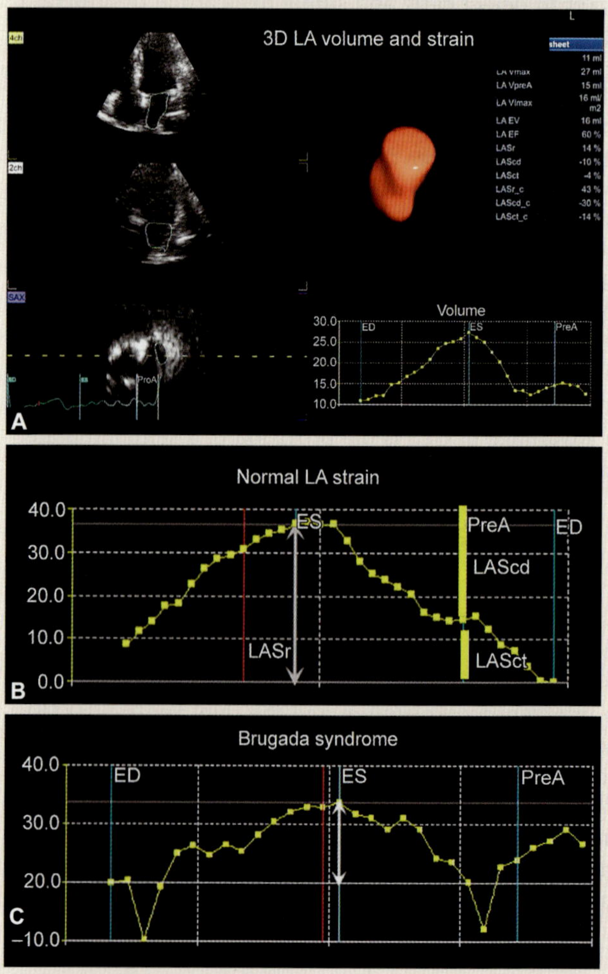

(CMR: cardiovascular magnetic resonance; EF: ejection fraction; LA: left atrial; RVEF: right ventricular ejection fraction)

LA-focused apical four-chamber view is acquired and the image is optimized for alignment and temporal resolution. The mitral valve coaptation center point is land marked and the LV end-diastolic, end-systolic, and preatrial contraction phases are set. The results of 3D LA function analysis are displayed as LA volumetric data (LA Vmax and LA EF) and LA strain values [(LA reservoir strain (LASr), LA conduit strain (LAScd), and LA contraction strain (LASct)].

3D Evaluation for Structural Heart Disease Intervention: Interatrial Septum

Interatrial septum (IAS) is a 3D structure, which is very important in structural and interventional cardiology **(Table 6)**. The landmarks on the left and right side of the IAS are very well studied using 3D transthoracic and

TABLE 6: 3D echocardiography in structural interventions of IAS.

Structural interventions	Images
3D viewing of IAS: A. After obtaining a good 2D TEE image in the 90° plane, region of interest is selected by using the acquisition box of the zoom view and image size is adjusted in the elevation plane to select the potential area of atrial septal defect in the IAS involving a segment of inferior vena cava B. Now, 3D zoom is again selected to have a good view of IAS from left atrial perspective C. At this point Saric et al. have used the TUPLE (tilt up and left rotation for Philips users) maneuver.[49] Left or counterclockwise rotation is done at this point and the left superior pulmonary vein could be viewed to enter the left superior aspect of the left atrium D. 180° rotation in the Y axis at this point can bring about the view of the IAS from the right atrial perspective *Brockenbrough puncture*: E. Use of fusion echocardiography with fusion of fluoroscopy and 3D echocardiography gives the added advantage of viewing the soft tissue of IAS in the fluoroscopic screen.[52,53] The placement of septal puncture in the specific areas of IAS is made possible with this technique F. For example, puncture in foramen ovale area for balloon mitral valvuloplasty, superioposterior aspect of foramen ovale for MitraClip application and prosthetic mitral paravalvular leak interventions and inferoposterior aspect for left atrial appendage interventions are possible with this technique[54,55]	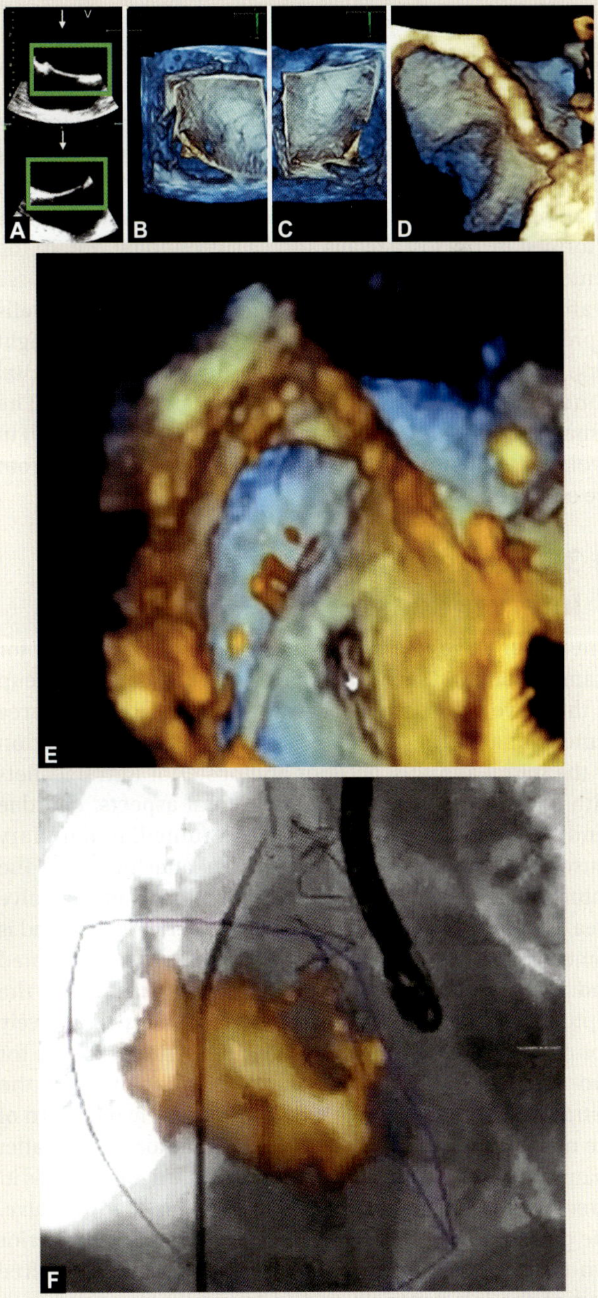

Continued

Continued

Structural interventions	Images
ASD device closure	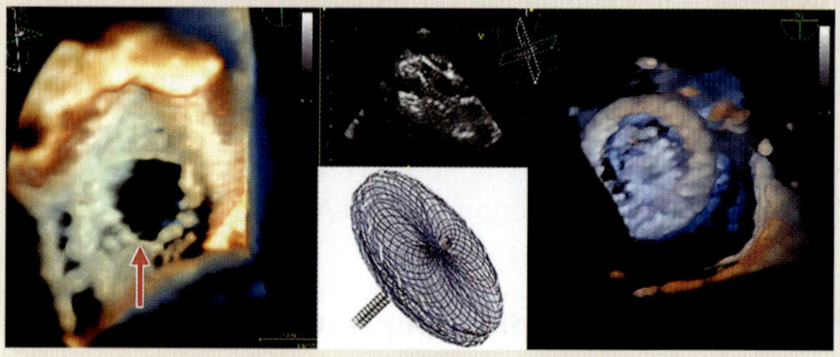

(ASD: atrial septal defect; IAS: interatrial septum; TEE: transesophageal echocardiogram)

transesophageal echocardiography (TEE).[47-50] Now more recent advancements have led to fusion echocardiography and techniques of integration of 3D transesophageal images over the fluoroscopic screen. 3D imaging of the LA side is characterized by a homogeneous, flat surface showing only small pits and dents. From the right atrial perspective, IAS is formed by the fossa ovalis and its surrounding rim. In the center of the IAS from the right atrial perspective, the fossa ovalis can be visualized as a depression. The fossa ovalis represents the true IAS as it directly separates left and right atria and hence is an important landmark for transseptal puncture for all the interventional procedures. The remaining areas of IAS contain a portion of the atrial wall in folding into the IAS with fibro-fatty tissue that extends from the epicardium.[51]

3D Evaluation for Mitral Valve Interventions

The mitral valve is a complex structure ideally suited for examination by 3D echocardiography as the mental makeup of the valve when 2D echocardiography is difficult. Three dimensionally, it consists of an atrioventricular junction or the mitral annulus, anterior and posterior mitral leaflets with commissures in medial and lateral aspects, chordae tendineae, anterolateral and posteromedial papillary muscles, and the ventricular myocardial attachments.[56] The anterior leaflet comprises roughly two-thirds of the valve area, is about twofold longer than the posterior leaflet, and is somewhat triangular. The posterior leaflet is more elongated and rectangular. The anterior leaflet is attached to the septum and fibrous annulus of the heart, and it is relatively nondistensible. Although the anterior leaflet accounts for two-thirds of the mitral valve area, its attachment to the mitral annulus accounts for only approximately one-third of the mitral annular circumference. The anterior mitral leaflet spans the distance between the two fibrous trigones and is in direct continuity with the noncoronary cusp of aortic valve. The posterior mitral valve leaflet is attached to the posterior two-thirds of the mitral annulus, which runs along the free wall of the left ventricle and is primarily muscular with little fibrous tissue (explaining its tendency to distend and elongate).[56]

Edge-to-edge Repair of Mitral Valve Regurgitation

Percutaneous edge-to-edge repair of mitral valve regurgitation using MitraClip system mimics the surgical mitral repair introduced by Otavio Alfieri in the year 1991. The EVEREST I (Endovascular Valve Edge-to-Edge Repair Study) showed the safety and efficacy of the MitraClip system (Evalve Inc, Menlo Park, California). The mortality was low and the severity of the mitral regurgitation was reduced remarkably **(Table 7)**.[39,40] Dual crop with simultaneous 2D quad view layout can be very valuable in MitraClip procedures. In fact, one can see the orientation of the catheter and the clip in 4D from both the ventricular and atrial view while monitoring the grasping of the leaflets in the 2D planes. This may avoid the need to switch from 2D to 4D in this very critical step potentially reducing.

3D Evaluation of the Aortic Valve for Transcatheter Aortic Valve Replacement

Three-dimensional echocardiography has been used for anatomic assessment of the aortic valve and root morphology and to calculate the valve area in aortic stenosis (AS). The technique has been used to delineate aortic flow patterns and has demonstrated feasibility and accuracy in quantifying aortic regurgitation.[57] Other applications have included the detection and localization of aortic valve vegetations, assessment of congenital outflow obstruction abnormalities, and demonstration of morphological changes in the valve after balloon dilation. The aortic surgical annulus is a complex, 3D, crown-shaped structure. The diameter at the base of the aortic root, the basal ring, is also called the "aortic annulus." The basal ring is not a true anatomical entity but is defined as a virtual ring with three anchors at the nadir of each of the attachments of the aortic cusps.[58]

TABLE 7: Mitral valve interventions.

Mitral interventions	Images
From the biplane view, zoom acquisition window is applied and the elevation plane width is adjusted and clicked. Both from TTE and TEE, the 3D dataset is rotated to bring the aorta to 12 O'clock position. By selecting the dual crop, simultaneous viewing of mitral valve from both left atrial and left ventricular side is possible. The anterior leaflet has three scallops: A1—anterolateral, A2—middle, and A3—posteromedial. Similarly, the posterior leaflet has three scallops: P1—anterolateral, P2—middle, and P3—posteromedial. The left atrial appendage is also seen at 9 O'clock position in this view	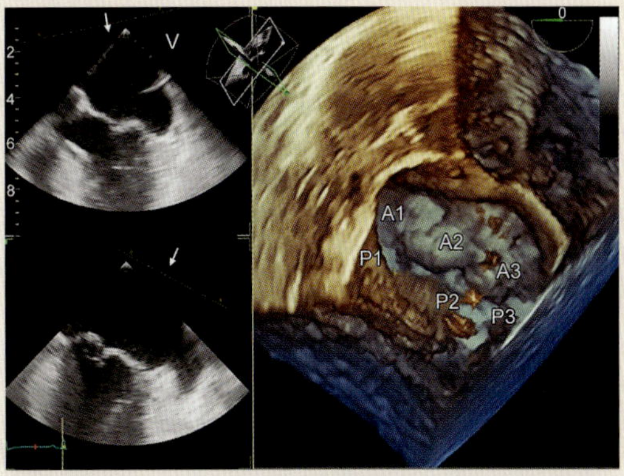
Dual crop with simultaneous 2D: This quad view layout can be very valuable in MitraClip procedures. In fact, one can see the orientation of the catheter and the clip in 4D from both the ventricular and atrial view while monitoring the grasping of the leaflets in the 2D planes	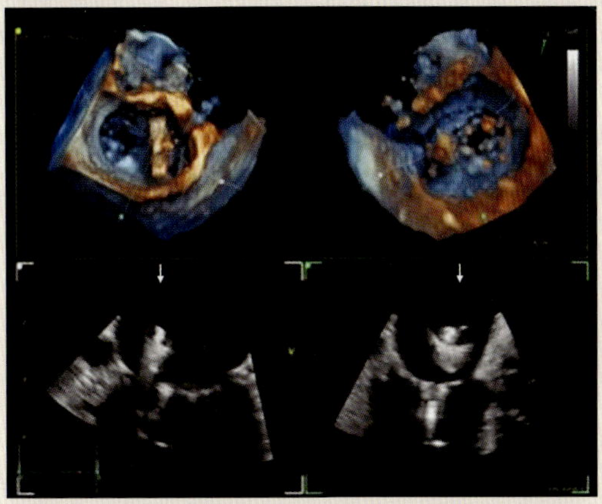
Typical owl's-eye view: After the deployment of successful MitraClip, the typical owl's-eye view can be seen in this dual crop on adding color flow	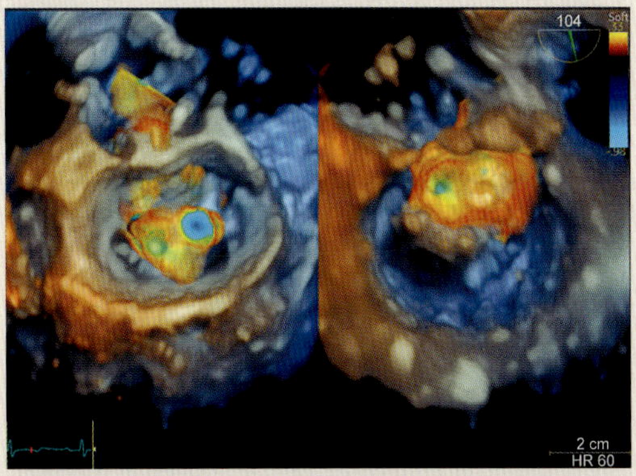
Paravalvular leak closure: • Using dual crop with 4D color allows simultaneous visualization of the location of the paravalvular leak enface • At the end of the procedure, the image on the right visualizes the successful closure of both paravalvular leaks on both the enface view and ventricular view as identified by the 4D markers	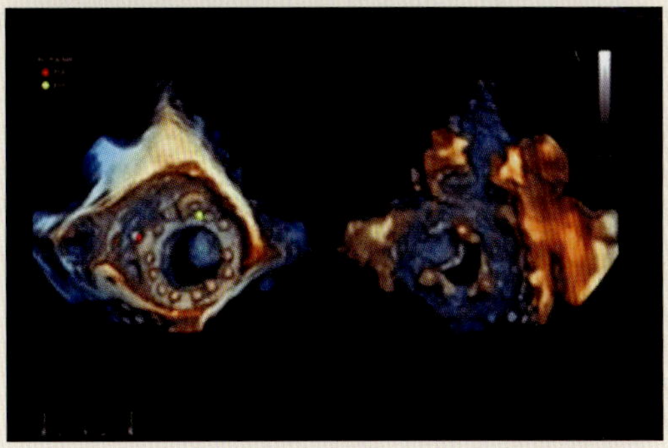

(TEE: transesophageal echocardiogram; TTE: transthoracic echocardiogram)

Aortic stenosis is either congenital (usually bicuspid) or acquired (degenerative calcific valve). The normal aortic valve area is 3–4 cm^2. 3D echocardiography greatly aids in quantification of aortic area.[53,54] Echocardiography has become the standard means for evaluation of AS severity. Cardiac catheterization is no longer recommended **(Table 8)**.

Left ventricular outflow tract (LVOT) diameter is measured in 3D parasternal long-axis view from inner edge to inner edge by using the zoom mode in mid-systole after adjusting the gain to optimize the blood tissue interface, parallel and adjacent to the aortic valve or at the site of velocity measurement. This diameter is used to calculate a circular cross-sectional area. The most common errors in aortic valve area calculations occur in 2D echocardiography in measuring the LVOT diameter.

LVOT velocity: Pulsed-wave Doppler maximum velocity is obtained from peak of dense velocity curve in apical long-axis or five-chamber view. Velocity time integral (VTI) is traced from modal velocity. Sample volume is positioned just on LV side of the valve and moved carefully into the LVOT if required to obtain laminar flow curve. The velocity baseline

TABLE 8: Aortic valve interventions.

<table>
<tr><th>Aortic interventions</th><th>Images</th></tr>
<tr><td>3D zoom view: The 3D zoom acquisition boxes are placed in the long axis 120° and are adjusted in the elevation plane to include the whole of aortic valve. Now choosing the long axis or short axis from the touch panel, it will display the long axis and short axis planes, respectively. The aortic annulus is measured from the inner-to-inner borders</td><td>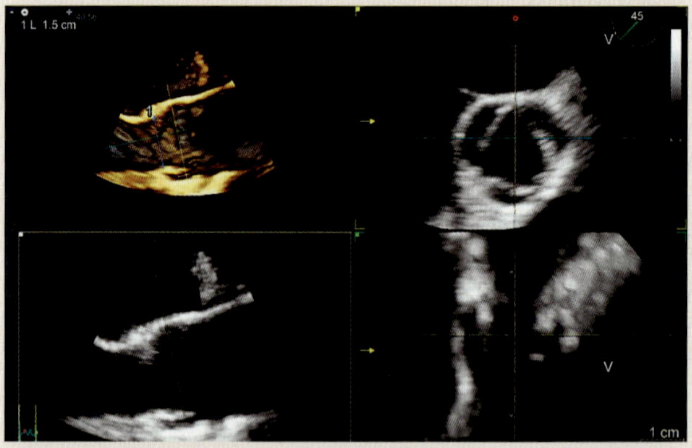
</td></tr>
<tr><td>The LM height or distance from the virtual annulus plane to the coronary ostium (yellow arrow) is measured from the coronal plane (blue box). The left coronary leaflet (LCC; blue curved line) is seen on the 3D-rendered view and the coronal plane (blue box), and its length is measured from the 2D image. An LCC length that is <2–3 mm shorter than the LM height, or an LM height <10–11 mm (particularly in the setting of a short root), poses a risk for possible coronary artery obstruction with transcatheter valve implantation</td><td>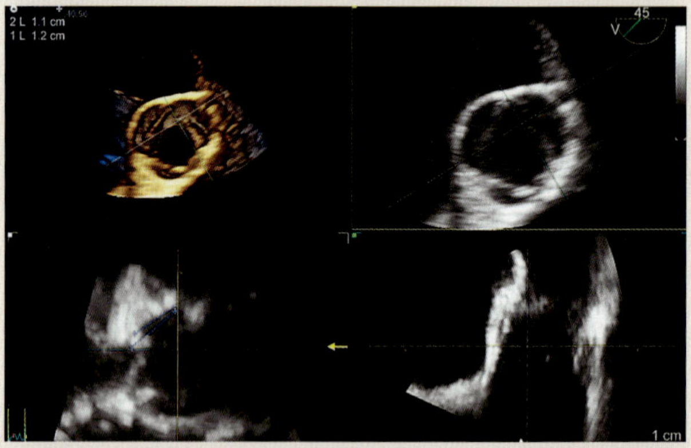
</td></tr>
<tr><td>Aortic valve quantification software can be applied at this point. Initially, the aortic valve is displayed in coronal and sagittal plane with cursors. The center point of the cursor is to be aligned exactly over the center point of the aorta. The corrections in the contours are made. Usually, the aortic annular maximal diameter, minimal diameter, aortic annular circumference and aortic annular area are displayed from which the prosthetic valve annular diameter size can be calculated</td><td>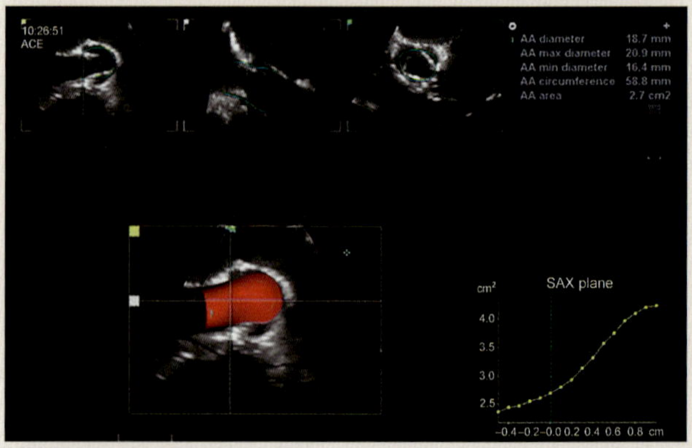
</td></tr>
</table>

(LCC: left coronary cusp; LM: left main)

and scale are adjusted to maximize the size of the velocity curve. The sweep speed of 100 mm/s is selected with a low wall filter setting and the VTI is measured.

AS jet velocity: Continuous wave (CW) Doppler is used to obtain VTI and maximum velocity at peak of dense velocity curve. Multiple acoustic windows can be used. From these measurements, simplified continuity equation formula for aortic valve area is used as follows: AVA = Cross-sectional area (LVOT) × VTI (LVOT)/VTI (aortic valve). When adequate window is not obtainable by transthoracic echocardiography, the aortic valve is acquired by 3D TEE as per the details mentioned earlier. Planimetry of aortic valve can be made during mid-systole from the coronal plane image. This correlates very well with transcatheter measurements.[59-63]

3D Evaluation of Left Atrial Appendage

The left atrial appendage (LAA) is a finger-like projection from the left atrium and has different sizes and shapes and three regions: Ostium, neck, and body, which is of considerable importance in these days of interventional closure of LAA in patients with atrial fibrillation **(Table 9)**.[64,65] The LAA ostium is the opening from the left atrium into the LAA. The ostium is generally oval in shape. The wall around the ostium can be very thin. The ostium opens to the neck region that constitutes a tubular junction between the ostium and the lobar region. The left circumflex coronary artery is in close proximity. The lobar region is the largest and the most variable distal part of the LAA and may have one to five lobes. The four different LAA morphologies have been described by TEE, cine angiography, and 3D CT and are as follows:[66-68]

- *Chicken wing*: The most common type of LAA morphology is chicken wing and occurs in 48% of individuals. The chicken wing LAA morphology has an obvious bend in the proximal or middle part of the dominant lobe or folding back of the LAA anatomy on itself at some distance from the perceived LAA ostium
- *Cactus morphology*: This is the second most common morphology and occurs in 30% of individuals and has a dominant central lobe with secondary lobes extending from the central lobe in both superior and inferior directions.
- *Windsock*: This morphology has one dominant lobe of sufficient length as the primary structure and occurs in 19% of individuals. Variations may occur with secondary and even tertiary lobes arising from the main lobe.
- *Cauliflower* type of LAA morphology has limited overall length with more complex internal characteristics and occurs in 3% of individuals. The Cauliflower morphology is associated with the highest number of embolic events due to its complex shape and number of lobes.

TABLE 9: Interventions of left atrial appendage.

Left atrial appendage interventions	Images
• Left atrial appendage is best viewed from transesophageal echocardiography from the midesophageal level. 2D acquisition is shown in (A) 0°, (B) 45°, (C) 90°, and (D) 120° • Biplane acquisition is done from 45°. Zoom acquisition boxes are placed over the left atrial appendage and elevation plane adjustments are made and zoom view is acquired. Full volume acquisition can be made at the juncture. The area of the ostium of the left atrial appendage can be planimetered during atrial diastole and systole (E)	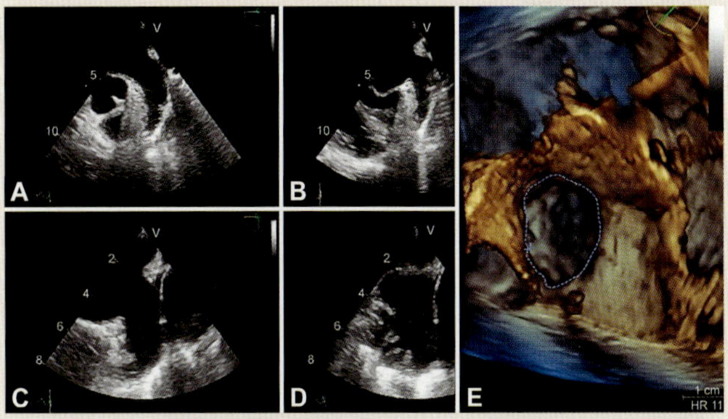
Echo fluoroscopic fusion can be of use during the accurate placement of the device in the left atrial appendage A. Echo fluroscopic fusion of two dimensional images B. Echo fluroscopic fusion of 3D images of Left atrial appendage	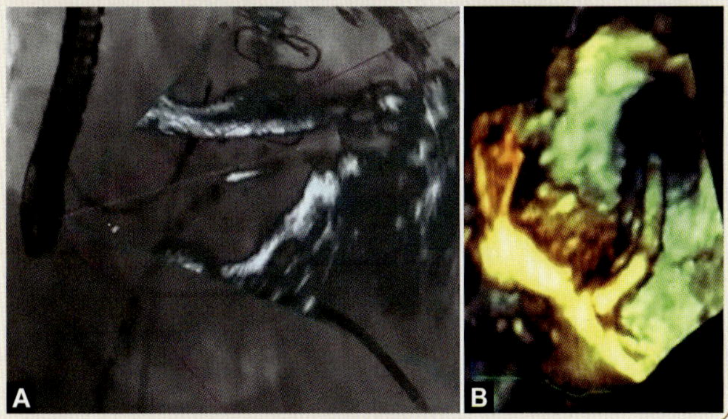

CONCLUSION

At present the following are the areas where 3D echocardiography has demonstrated the usefulness:[69]

- *LV function assessment*: By eliminating the need for geometric modeling and avoiding errors caused by foreshortened views, 3D echocardiography remains the choice of methods for determination of left ventricular function. Its results are comparable to cardiac MRI and are economically cheaper.
- By the current photorealistic en face views of cardiac valves, congenital abnormalities and their supporting structures, 3D imaging is particularly helpful to the cardiac surgeon and the interventional cardiologist.
- *RV volume assessment*: 3D echocardiography is the only economically viable alternative to cardiac MRI in evaluation of RV function permits evaluation of regional LV function and objective detection of wall motion abnormalities.
- Regional wall motion abnormality and LV systolic dyssynchrony assessment by 3D echocardiography serve as an additional referral criterion for cardiac resynchronization therapy.
- CT-echo fusion and echo fluoroscopic fusion are two new techniques which helps the structural interventional cardiologist during transseptal puncture, mitral, aortic interventions and LA appendage occlusion.

ONLINE REFERENCES

Please scan the QR code provided at the end of the table of contents for References of this chapter.

CHAPTER 101

Cardiac Amyloidosis and the Role of Echocardiography and Noninvasive Imaging Modalities in the Diagnosis and Prognosis

Nitin J Burkule

ABSTRACT

Cardiac amyloid cardiomyopathy is both delayed and underdiagnosed disease in a significant proportion of patients with heart failure. The misfolded precursor proteins such as transthyretin, light chain immunoglobulin, and ApoAI-IV cause cardiac amyloid infiltration leading to myocardial hypertrophy and restrictive cardiomyopathy. The characteristic features on echocardiography, cardiac magnetic resonance, and bone avid radiotracer scintigraphy help in reliable diagnosis of cardiac amyloidosis in majority of patients while cardiac or extracardiac biopsy is required in specific clinical situations. There is growing interest in cardiac amyloidosis firstly, due to validation of imaging techniques to accurately diagnose transthyretin cardiac amyloidosis without endomyocardial biopsy and secondly, due to discovery of pathobiology of amyloid formation leading to new targeted therapies for transthyretin cardiac amyloidosis.

Keywords: Cardiac amyloidosis, echocardiography, cardiac magnetic resonance, transthyretin amyloidosis, light chain amyloidosis.

INTRODUCTION

Cardiac amyloidosis is an extracellular deposition of insoluble, beta-pleated sheets of fibrils which are aggregates of misfolded precursor proteins such as transthyretin (TTR) or light chains (L) of monoclonal gamma globulins along with nonfibrillar components made of serum amyloid P (glycoprotein), proteoglycans, and other proteins.[1-3]

Although systemic amyloidosis is caused by over 30 different precursor proteins, cardiac amyloid infiltration-related cardiomyopathy (CM) occurs mainly either due to liver generated transthyretin (ATTR) or plasma cell generated (Kappa or Lambda) immunoglobulin light chain (AL) precursor proteins.[4] Apolipoprotein AI amyloidosis (AApoAI) and Apo AIV amyloidosis (AApoAIV) are other rare causes of cardiac amyloidosis[5].

TYPES OF CARDIAC AMYLOIDOSIS

Different types of cardiac amyloidosis are as follows:

- Hereditary transthyretin cardiac amyloidosis (hATTR-CM)
- Nonhereditary or wild type form of transthyretin cardiac amyloidosis of elderly (wATTR-CM)
- Apo AI cardiac amyloidosis (AApoAI-CM)
- Apo AIV cardiac amyloidosis (AApoAIV-CM)

PATHOGENESIS OF CARDIAC AMYLOIDOSIS

The TTR tetramer is secreted mainly from the liver, and a small amount is secreted by the choroid plexus (for cerebral spinal fluid) and retinal pigmented epithelial cells (for the vitreous of the eye).[2] It functions as a carrier protein for thyroxine hormone and holoretinol. The unstable TTR tetramer dissociates into monomers, which get partially denatured and get misassembled as amyloid fibrils.[2]

Systemic AL amyloidosis is due to proliferation of clonal plasma cells, resulting in production of clonal antibodies (e.g., IgG-Kappa or IgG-lambda), clonal light chains (e.g., Kappa or lambda light chain), or both. The high kappa or lambda light chains circulating in the bloodstream get deposited extracellularly.[6]

The ApoAI is a 28 kDa plasma protein component of high-density lipoprotein particles synthesized by the liver and small intestine.[5] Wild-type ApoAI-amyloid is present in atherosclerotic plaques due to the atherosclerotic inflammatory process and is not associated with systemic disease. The pathogenic mutations in the *ApoAI* gene cause misfolding of ApoAI protein leading to amyloid deposition in various organs (liver, spleen, kidney, and larynx) and the heart (systemic AApoAI).[5]

The ApoAIV is a 46 kDa protein synthesized in the small intestine and is utilized for the absorption, transportation, and metabolism of lipids. The systemic AApoAIV is not a hereditary disease and its etiopathogenesis is still not understood.[5]

GENETICS OF HEREDITARY HATTR AND AAPOAI

There are > 120 mutations in the *TTR* gene that are associated with hATTR-CM. The common genotypes in hereditary ATTR-CM are Val30Met (V30M) or pV50M in Portuguese, Swedish, and Japanese, Val122Ile (V122I) or pV142I in Afro-Americans, Afro-Caribbeans, Thr60Ala (T60A) or pT80A in Irish, Leu111Met in Denmark, and Ile68Leu in Italy[1,2].

The elderly patients with wATTR do not show any pathogenic genotype. The AApoAI is a strongly hereditary disease. Arg173Pro variant of ApoAI protein universally causes cardiac and laryngeal involvement.[5]

INCIDENCE AND PREVALENCE OF CARDIAC AMYLOIDOSIS

The ATTR-CM is identified by bone tracer imaging in approximately 16–18% of patients with calcific aortic stenosis (AS) undergoing transcatheter aortic valve replacement (TAVR) with 62% of them having low-flow, low-gradient (LFLG) severe AS.[2] ATTR-CM is also identified in 13–17% of elderly patients presenting with heart failure with preserved ejection fraction (HFpEF) and in 10% of patients with carpal tunnel syndrome.[1,3,7] Autopsy data reveals that 25% of patients above 80 years of age have significant myocardial TTR amyloid deposits.[6]

The hATTR prevalence in Europe is <1 in 100,000 population.[6] The TTR mutation allele of valine 122 isoleucine substitution is prevalent in 3–4% of African-American population. In male Caucasian patients with LV thickness ≥ 15 mm, hATTR-CM was found in 1.6% of patients aged between 55 and 64 years, 11.1% of patients aged between 65 and 74 years, and 11.3% of patients aged between 75 and 84 years.[6]

Systemic AL amyloidosis is relatively a rare disease affecting approximately 8–12 per million person years.[7] Unlike multiple myeloma, patients with AL amyloidosis have ≤ 20% of plasma cells in the bone marrow. However, 5–10% of patients with AL amyloidosis show evidence of multiple myeloma, and 5–10% of multiple myeloma patients show AL amyloidosis.[8]

A monoclonal gammopathy of uncertain significance (MGUS) is a premalignant, plasma cell disorder, with small monoclonal (M) protein band, and <10% clonal plasma cell in the bone marrow in the absence of multiple myeloma or lymphoplasmacytic malignancies.[9]

The AApoAI-CM and AApoAIV-CM are very rare forms of cardiac amyloidosis. Both these forms of cardiac amyloidosis made up to 1.0% of cases assessed at the United Kingdom (UK) National Amyloidosis Centre during a study period of 21 years.[5]

MECHANISM OF HEART FAILURE IN AMYLOID CARDIOMYOPATHY

Although ATTR-CM is purely infiltrative CM causing noncompliant cardiac structural changes, AL amyloidosis may be considered as both myotoxic and infiltrative CM.[8] The structural changes caused by TTR or light chain amyloid deposition leads to:[8]

- Increased cardiac and vascular stiffness
- Impaired contraction and relaxation
- Abnormal electrical conduction

In addition, the proteotoxicity caused by light chain amyloid leads to:[8]

- Stress kinase activation
- Lysosomal dysfunction
- Defective autophagy
- Reactive oxygen species
- Cellular dysfunction
- Impaired calcium homeostasis
- Mitochondrial dysfunction
- Cell death

Perivascular amyloid deposits and autonomic dysfunction results in coronary microvascular dysfunction, which is further aggravated by high left ventricular (LV) filling pressure due to noncompliant LV hypertrophy (LVH).[3]

WHAT ARE THE CLINICAL RED FLAGS?

Cardiac amyloid should be suspected when echocardiography or cardiac magnetic resonance (CMR) shows biventricular increased wall thickening (IWT of >12 mm), noncompliant ventricles in the absence of abnormal afterload.[4]

- Unexplained LV wall thickness (LVWT) > 12 mm
- LVWT and electrocardiogram (ECG) QRS voltage mismatch
- LVH with thickened valves, interatrial septum (IAS), and right ventricular (RV) free wall
- Reduced global longitudinal strain (GLS) with apical sparing
- Very low mitral tissue Doppler imaging (TDI) E' /S' /A' < 5 cm/s
- Lone atrial fibrillation (AF) or complete heart block (CHB) with LVH (more common in wATTR-CM, CHB in one-third, AF in 40–60% of patients at diagnosis)
- Unexplained HFpEF
- LFLG AS
- Intolerance to beta-blockers, angiotensin-converting enzyme inhibitors (ACEIs), and diuresis in HF

- "Natural cure" of hypertension (HTN)
- Persistent rise in troponin I (Trop I) and N-terminal pro-brain natriuretic peptides (BNP or NT-proBNP)
- History of carpal tunnel syndrome or spinal canal stenosis (thickening of the ligamentum flavum), spontaneous biceps tendon rupture (ATTR-CM). Carpal tunnel syndrome is seen in approximately 50% of wATTR-CM often preceding by an average of 5–10 years.[2] Biceps tendon rupture is reported in 33% of patients with wATTR-CM.[2]
- Unexplained symmetric, predominantly sensory peripheral neuropathy beginning in the lower limbs and following an ascending pattern (in AL-CM and mutation-specific hATTR-CM) with HF
- Unexplained proteinuria (AL-CM) with HF
- HFpEF with macroglossia, periorbital bruising, and autonomic nervous system dysfunction (10% of AL-CM)[8]
- LVH with autonomic dysfunction causing orthostatic hypotension, diarrhea or constipation, and erectile dysfunction (more common in hATTR-CM compared to wATTR-CM and less in AL-CM)[6,7]
- LVH with microvascular angina, jaw, buttock, and leg claudications (perivascular amyloid deposition) especially in AL amyloidosis[3]
- LVH with eye disease such as glaucoma, intravitreal deposition, and scalloped pupils (hATTR-CM)
- Family history of amyloidosis, laryngeal involvement causing dysphonia, and right-sided cardiac disease on cardiac imaging (AApo AI)[5]

WHAT ARE THE INVESTIGATIONS AND THE CHARACTERISTIC FINDINGS IN CARDIAC AMYLOIDOSIS?

Electrocardiogram

The mismatch of low ECG voltages and the hypertrophy on echocardiography (voltage: mass ratio) should raise the suspicion of infiltrative CM **(Fig. 1)**. A classical low-voltage

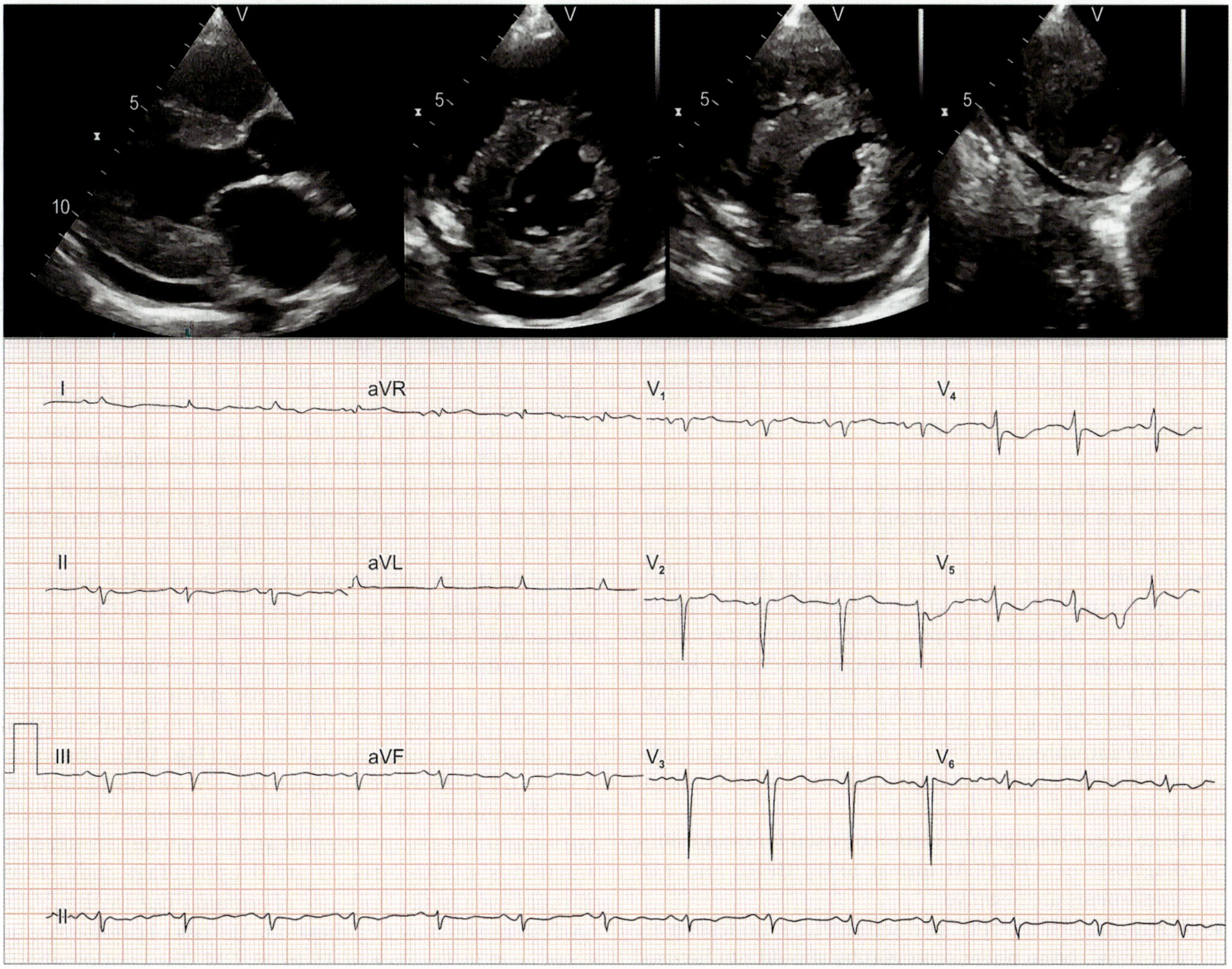

FIG. 1: A case of transthyretin amyloid cardiomyopathy (ATTR-CM) showing severe left ventricular hypertrophy and low-voltage QRS amplitudes in the ECG (<0.5 mV QRS in limb leads, <1 mV QRS in V_5 and V_6).

ECG (<0.5 mV QRS amplitudes for limb leads and <1.0 mV for precordial leads) is described in advanced stage of cardiac amyloidosis. However, only 40% of cardiac amyloid patients show low-voltage ECG and approximately 60% show poor R wave progression. The AF is seen in approximately 20% patients and is associated with very high risk of cardioembolic stroke.[10]

Biomarkers

The almost ubiquitous rise in NT-proBNP, troponin, and frequent reduction in estimated glomerular filtration rate (eGFR) is sensitive tests for determining the progression of the disease and prognosis and has been utilized for staging systems.[1]

Serum and Urine Protein Immunofixation and Free Light Chain Assay

All suspected cases should have serum protein immunofixation electrophoresis (SPIE) and urine protein immunofixation electrophoresis (UPIE) to prove the monoclonal origin of the light chains.[11]

The clonal antibodies are at higher concentration in the serum than the clonal light chains. These clonal antibodies are identified by SPIE. The light chains are concentrated in the urine, hence the UPIE is used to identify clonal light chains.[11] The serum free light chain (FLC) assay proves relative increase in one form of light chain immunoglobulin (kappa or lambda) by change in their ratio in either direction but does not prove clonal origin.

The sensitivity of only serum protein electrophoresis for AL amyloidosis is approximately 70%. The sensitivity of SPIE is >90% and the measurement of SPIE, UPIE, and FLC assay together increases the sensitivity >99% for the diagnosis of AL amyloidosis.[1]

The bone marrow produces Kappa light chains twice more than lambda light chains. Although the reticuloendothelial system clears both light chains at equal rate, the kidney excretes the Kappa much more efficiently than Lambda keeping the ratio 0.26–1.65 at normal eGFR.[11] The patients with lower eGFR excrete Kappa at lower rate and the normal limits of Kappa/Lambda ratio are different in chronic kidney disease (CKD). The normal limits of Kappa/Lambda ratio[11] are 0.5–2 for eGFR 40–60 and 0.72–2.25 for eGFR < 40.

While interpreting SPIE, UPIE, and FLC ratio in the context of bone tracer scintigraphy following facts should be considered:[11]

- Bone tracer scintigraphy cannot be used for establishing diagnosis of ATTR-CM unless SPIE, UPIE, and FLC assessments are negative.
- If any of the SPIE, UPIE, and serum FLC ratio testing are abnormal, bone tracer scintigraphy should not be used but to proceed for cardiac or extracardiac (bone marrow, abdominal fat pad, and rectal) biopsy to rule out systemic AL amyloidosis.
- Normal ranges of FLC ratio should be interpreted in the context of eGFR to avoid false-negative and false-positive results.

Echocardiography

Echocardiography is the primary modality to raise suspicion of cardiac amyloid in patients with unexplained LVH and is the gatekeeper for referral to bone tracer scintigraphy **(Figs. 2 and 3)**.[12] The LVH is more symmetrical in AL-CM compared with more asymmetrical septal thickening [interventricular septum (IVS)/posterior wall (PW) thickness > 1.3] seen in 20–25% of wATTR-CM. The septum in ATTR-CM may be either sigmoid shape (70% of cases) or with reverse septal curvature (30% of cases).[4] The LVH is usually concentric with high relative wall thickness (RWT) **(Fig. 4)**. The RV free wall may show thickening (>3 mm) due to amyloid infiltration. A thin layer of pericardial effusion is often seen in both AL-CM and ATTR-CM.

There is almost universal presence of high-grade LV diastolic dysfunction (restrictive LV filling pattern) in cardiac amyloidosis. The mitral annular TDI shows very low E', A', and S' often < 5 cm/s **(Fig. 5)**. The mitral flow on pulse wave Doppler shows high E/A wave ratio and very high E/E' ratio **(Fig. 6)**. The mitral annular plane systolic excursion (MAPSE) and tricuspid annular plane systolic excursion (TAPSE) are invariably low **(Fig. 7)**.

Cardiac amyloid shows a characteristic pattern of severely reduced longitudinal shortening with relatively preserved LV ejection fraction (LVEF) due to preserved radial shortening. A typical pattern of distribution of GLS is seen on Bull's eye map in cardiac amyloidosis (cherry-on-top) in which basal and mid LV segmental strain is severely reduced while apical segmental strain is relatively spared **(Fig. 8)**.[7] In other causes of LVH (AS and hypertrophic CM), the reduced LV longitudinal strain (LS) is generally encountered in the regions of maximal hypertrophy. For a given level of LVH, the AL-CM shows lower strain values compared with ATTR-CM, supporting the concept of light chain myocyte toxicity.[3] The LV twist and torsion function governed by the epicardial helical myocardial fibers are relatively well preserved in cardiac amyloidosis **(Fig. 9)**.

In cardiac amyloidosis, left atrial (LA) and right atrial (RA) reservoir strain and contractile strain are significantly reduced, irrespective of LA size, due to atrial amyloid deposition and restrictive LV filling **(Fig. 10)**.[7] The atrial A wave on pulse wave Doppler flow, A' on mitral annular TDI, LA emptying fraction, and LA contractile strain are characteristically significantly reduced in cardiac amyloidosis. The atria or atrial appendage may show thrombi even in the presence of normal sinus rhythm.[7] The LA dysfunction may be a marker of the risk of cardioembolic event even in absence of AF in AL-CM. The cardioembolic risk increases multifold with advent of AF.

Different echocardiographic parameters and their ratios and scoring systems have been evaluated to differentiate the cardiac amyloidosis from other common causes of cardiac hypertrophy such as hypertrophic cardiomyopathy (HCM) and hypertensive heart disease (HTHD).

- EF to strain ratio (EFSR) = LV EF/GLS **(Fig. 11)**
- Relative apical sparing (RELAPS) index = Average apical segments LS/Sum of average of middle and basal segments LS **(Fig. 12)**
- Septal apical-basal strain ratio (SAB) = Apical septal LS in 4CH/Basal septal LS in 4CH **(Fig. 13)**
- Myocardial contraction fraction (MCF) = Stroke volume (SV)/Myocardial volume
- Mass to strain ratio (MSR) = LV mass/GLS **(Fig. 11)**

The sensitivity, specificity, and area under curve (AUC) of the various echocardiographic parameters[12,13] for diagnosing cardiac amyloidosis in patients with WT ≤ 16 mm and normal EF > 55% are shown in the **Table 1**.

The simple combination of LV inferolateral WT ≥ 14 mm, average basal LS ≤ 8% has been shown to be a robust predictors of ATTR-CM performing as good as the more complex scoring systems and ratio indices.[12]

Increased wall thickness (IWT) score ***(Table 2)****:*[14]

- <2 points cardiac amyloid unlikely (sensitivity 98%)
- 8 points cardiac amyloid highly likely (specificity 98%)
- With IWT score diagnosis or exclusion of cardiac amyloidosis is obtained in 31% and 15%, respectively.

If IWT with systemic AL amyloid present ***(Table 3)****:*[14]

- <1 point cardiac amyloid unlikely (sensitivity 100%)
- ≥5 points cardiac amyloid highly likely (specificity 98%)
- With IWT AL score diagnosis or exclusion of cardiac amyloidosis in systemic AL amyloidosis is obtained in 35% and 15%, respectively.

Transthyretin cardiac amyloid score (TCAS) ***(Table 4)****:*[12] TCAS ≥ 6 sensitivity 93.7%, TCAS ≥ 9 specificity 93.3% for ATTR-CM

T-Amylo score ***(Table 5)****:*[15]

- 0–2 point ATTR-CM unlikely (sensitivity 99%)
- 7–11 points TTR-CM highly likely (specificity 94%)

Compared to AL-CM, the patients with ATTR-CM show more myocardial hypertrophy and more reduction in GLS. A study[16] of 126 patients of cardiac amyloid (52 with ATTR and 74 with AL) MSR was significantly higher in ATTR -CM versus AL-CM (19 ± 9 vs. 9 ± 6) and was the best discriminator in differentiating ATTR from AL.

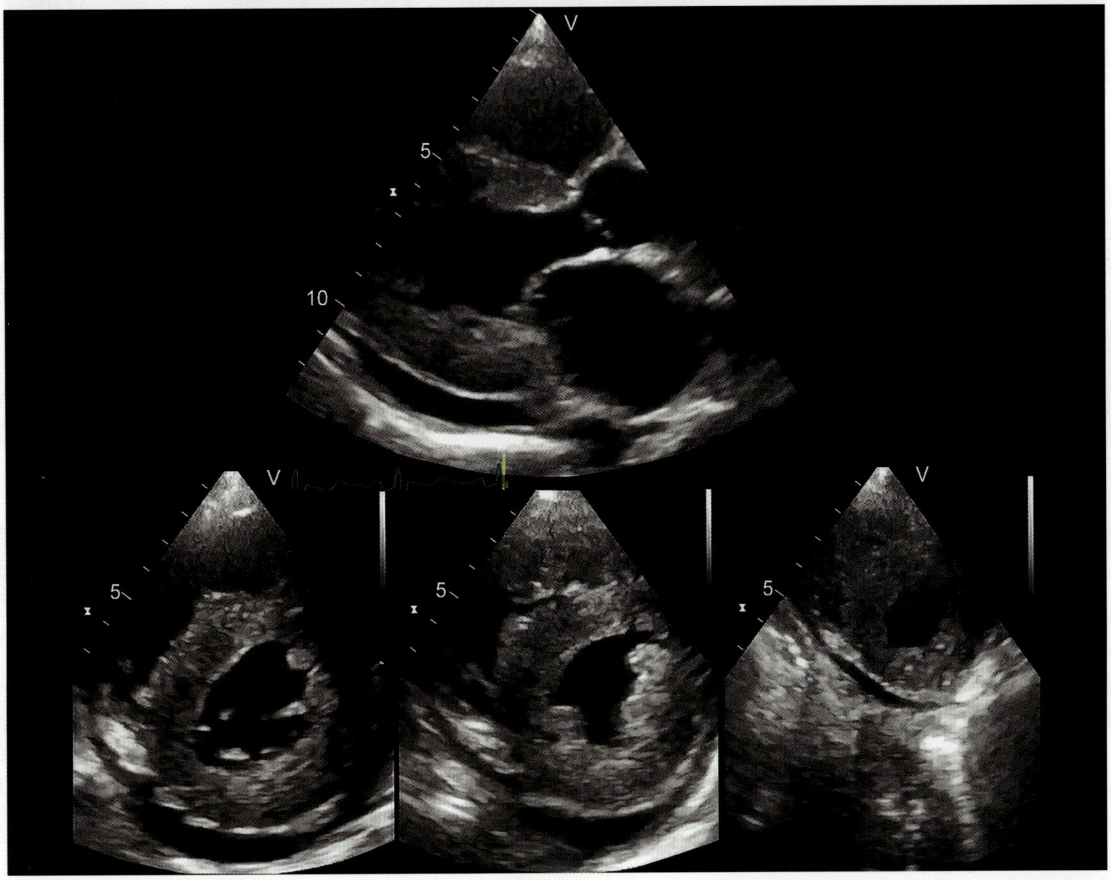

FIG. 2: A case of transthyretin amyloid cardiomyopathy (ATTR-CM) showing severe concentric left ventricular hypertrophy with small pericardial effusion.

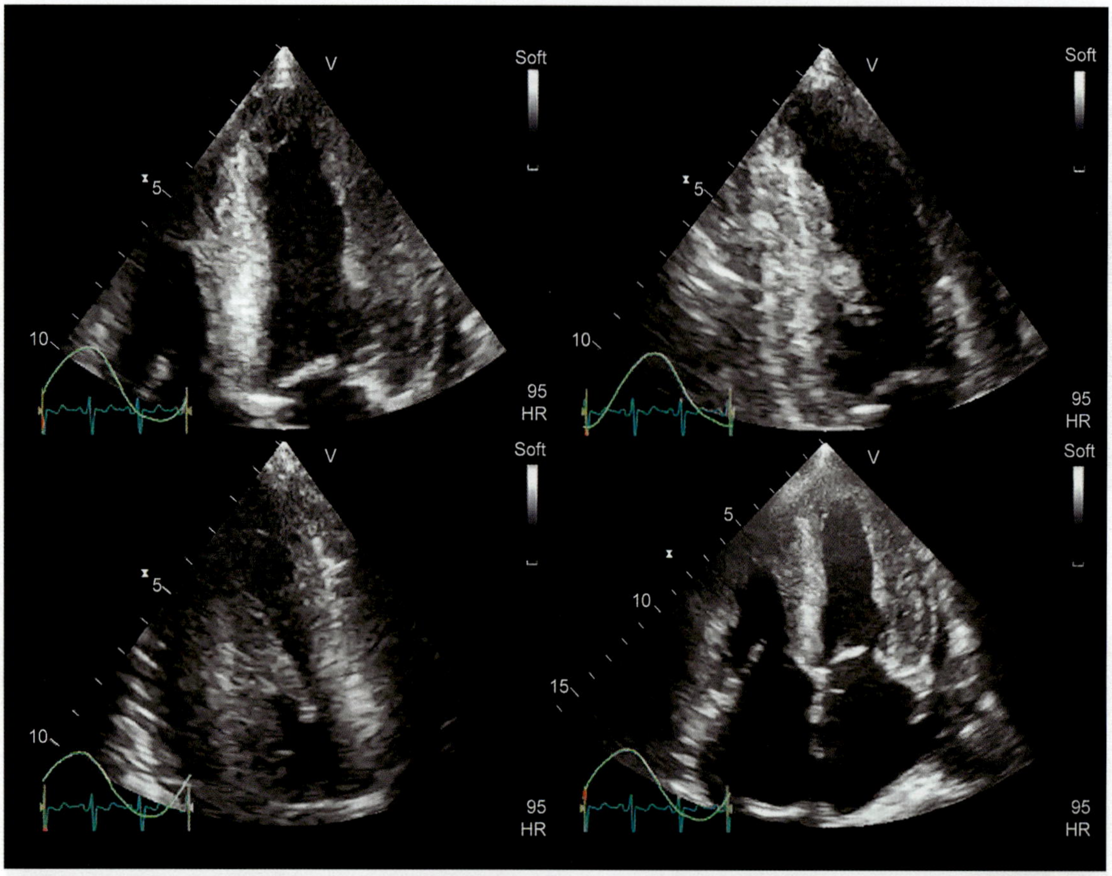

FIG. 3: A case of transthyretin amyloid cardiomyopathy (ATTR-CM) showing severe left ventricular hypertrophy and biatrial dilatation.

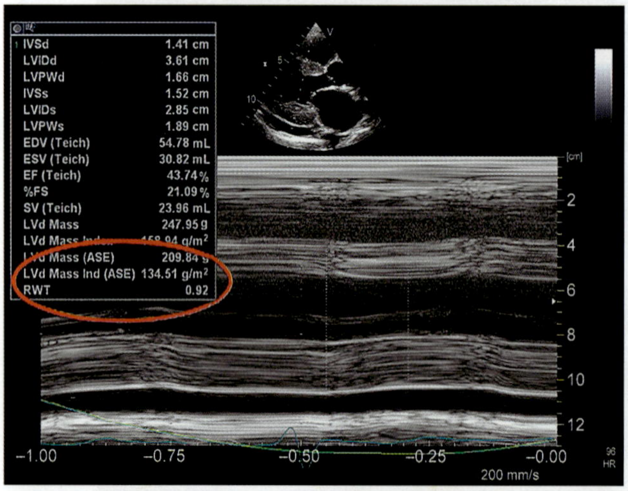

FIG. 4: A case of transthyretin amyloid cardiomyopathy (ATTR-CM) showing severe increase in left ventricular (LV) mass (134.5 g/m^2) and increased relative wall thickness (RWT = 0.92).

The AApoAI-CM presents with greater incidence of right heart involvement such as RV free wall hypertrophy, tricuspid stenosis and tricuspid regurgitation, and lesser incidence of classical LV apical sparing pattern on strain imaging.[5] The AApoAIV-CA patients show classical cardiac amyloid features on echocardiography including apical-sparing strain pattern.

Cardiac Magnetic Resonance

The native global T1 value on the T1 map is a composite signal from both myocytes and interstitial amyloid deposits. The T1 values are very high in cardiac amyloid and have a high sensitivity (92%) and specificity (91%) to detect cardiac amyloid **(Fig. 14)**.[4]

The cardiac amyloid infiltration has a high affinity for gadolinium and shows characteristic kinetics with nulling of the myocardium before the LV cavity blood pool on Look-Locker (TI scout) sequence **(Figs. 15A and B)**. The late gadolinium enhancement (LGE) imaging shows initially

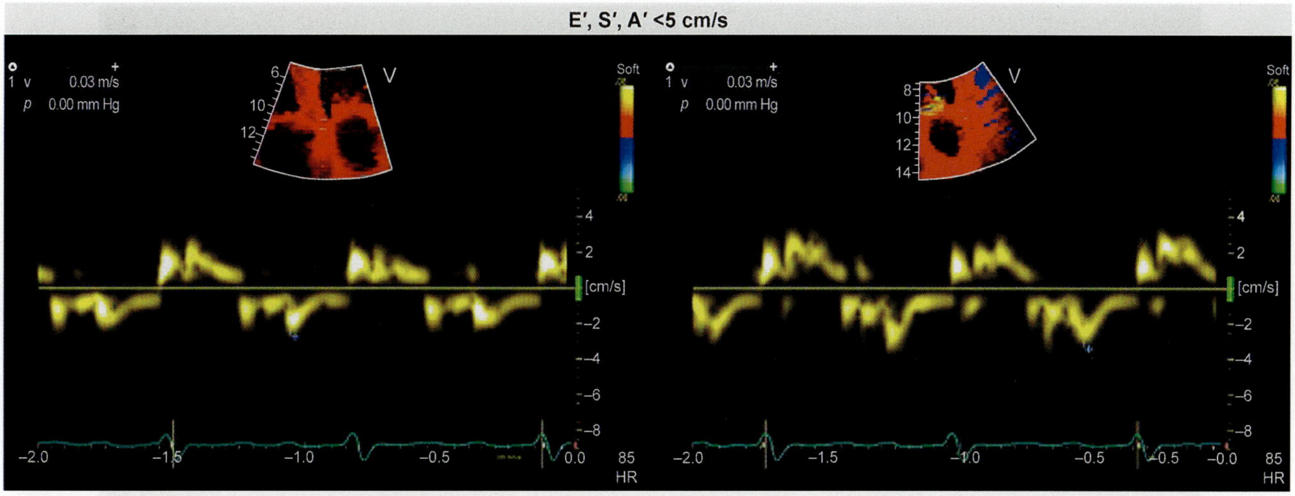

FIG. 5: A case of AL-CM showing severely reduced left ventricular (LV) longitudinal function as assessed by tissue Doppler imaging (E', A', and S' all < 5 cm/s)

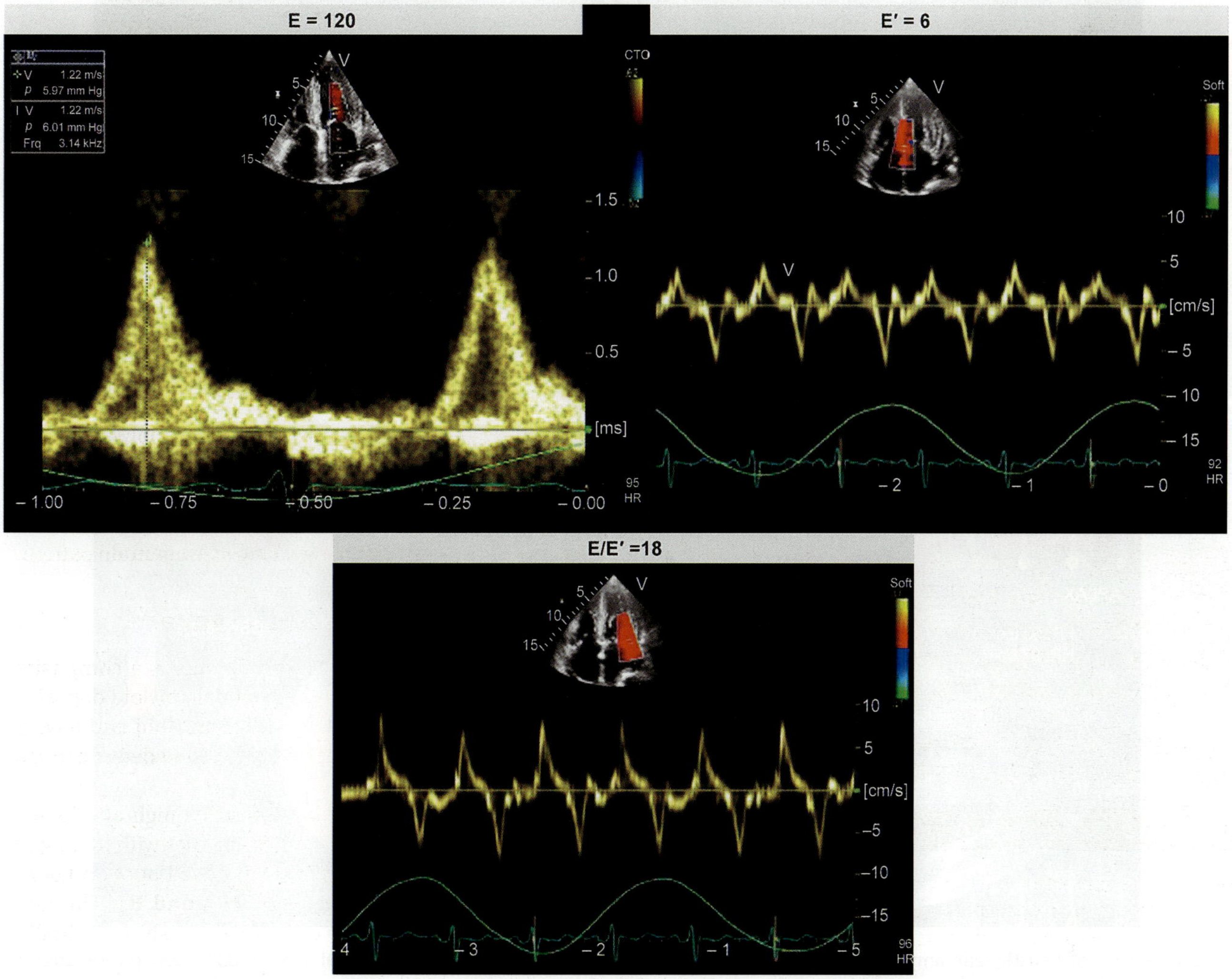

FIG. 6: A case of transthyretin amyloid cardiomyopathy (ATTR-CM) showing grade III left ventricular (LV) diastolic dysfunction. E/A >> 2, E/E' = 18.

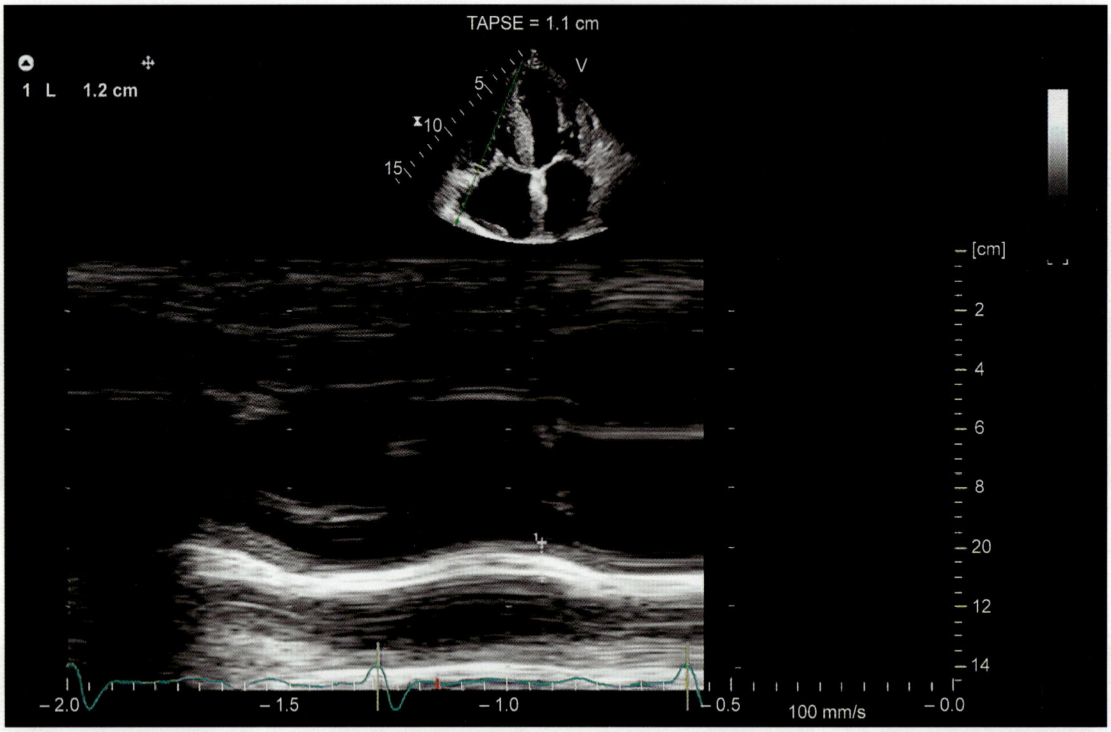

FIG. 7: A case of AL-CM showing severely reduced tricuspid annular plane systolic excursion (TAPSE = 1.1 cm).

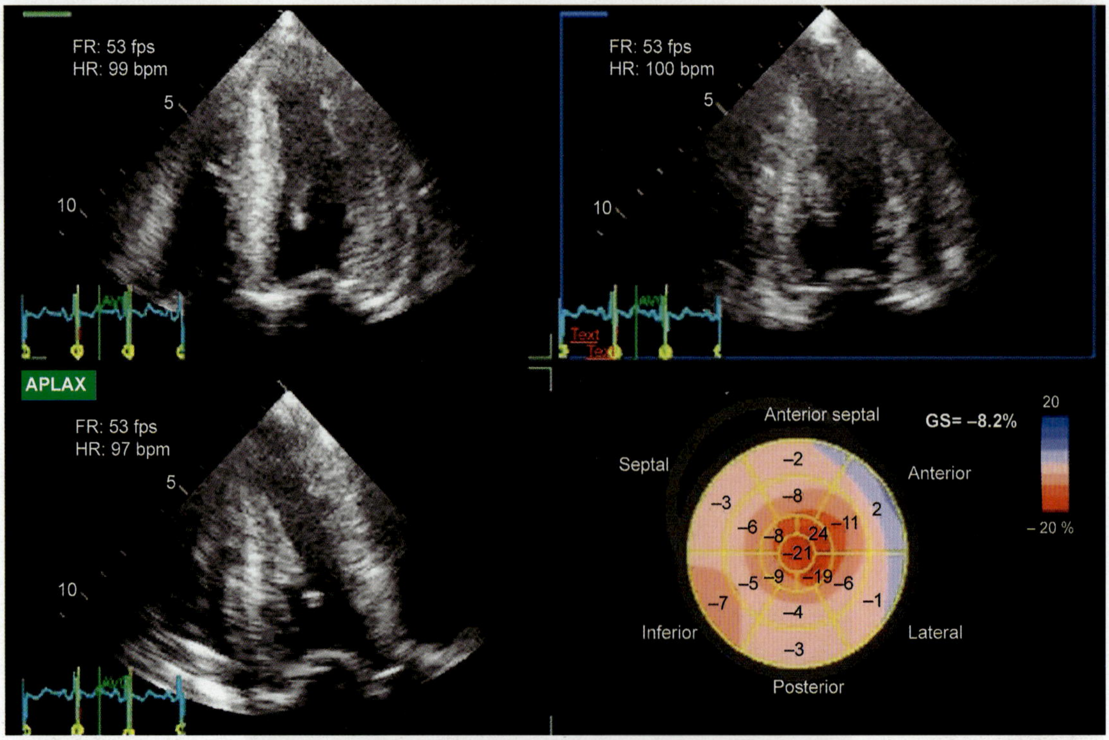

FIG. 8: A case of transthyretin amyloid cardiomyopathy (ATTR-CM) showing low global longitudinal strain (–8.2%) and preservation of strain in apical segments causing typical "cherry-on-top" pattern on the Bull's eye strain map.

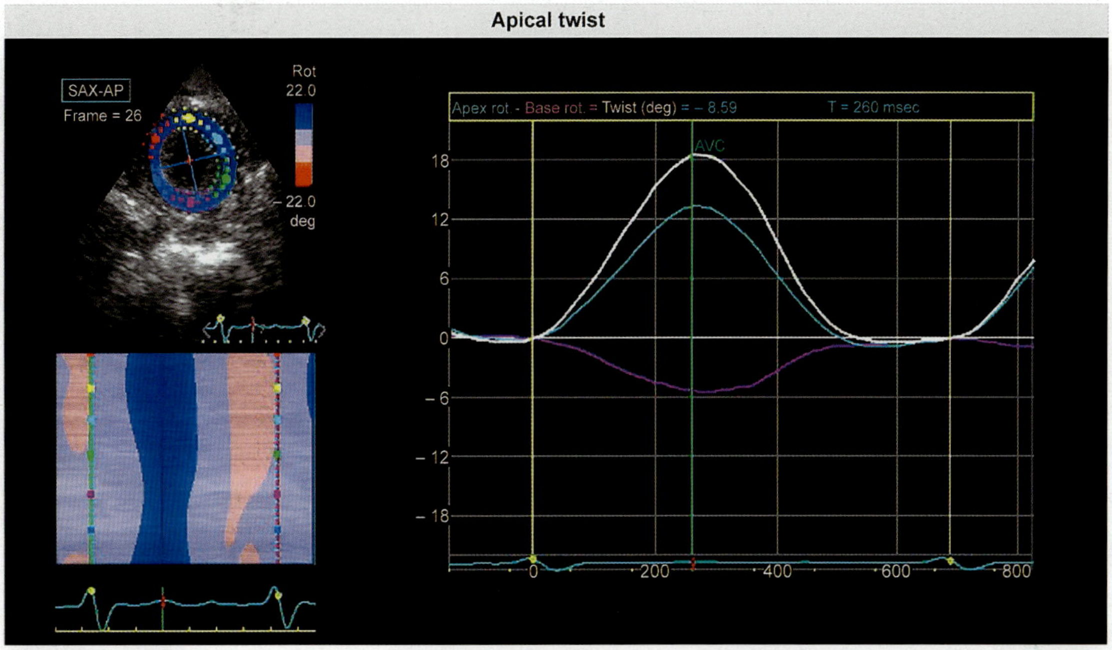

FIG. 9: A case of AL-CM showing preserved torsional motion of the heart. Basal clockwise rotation = 8°, apical anticlockwise rotation = 12° and LV twist = 18°.

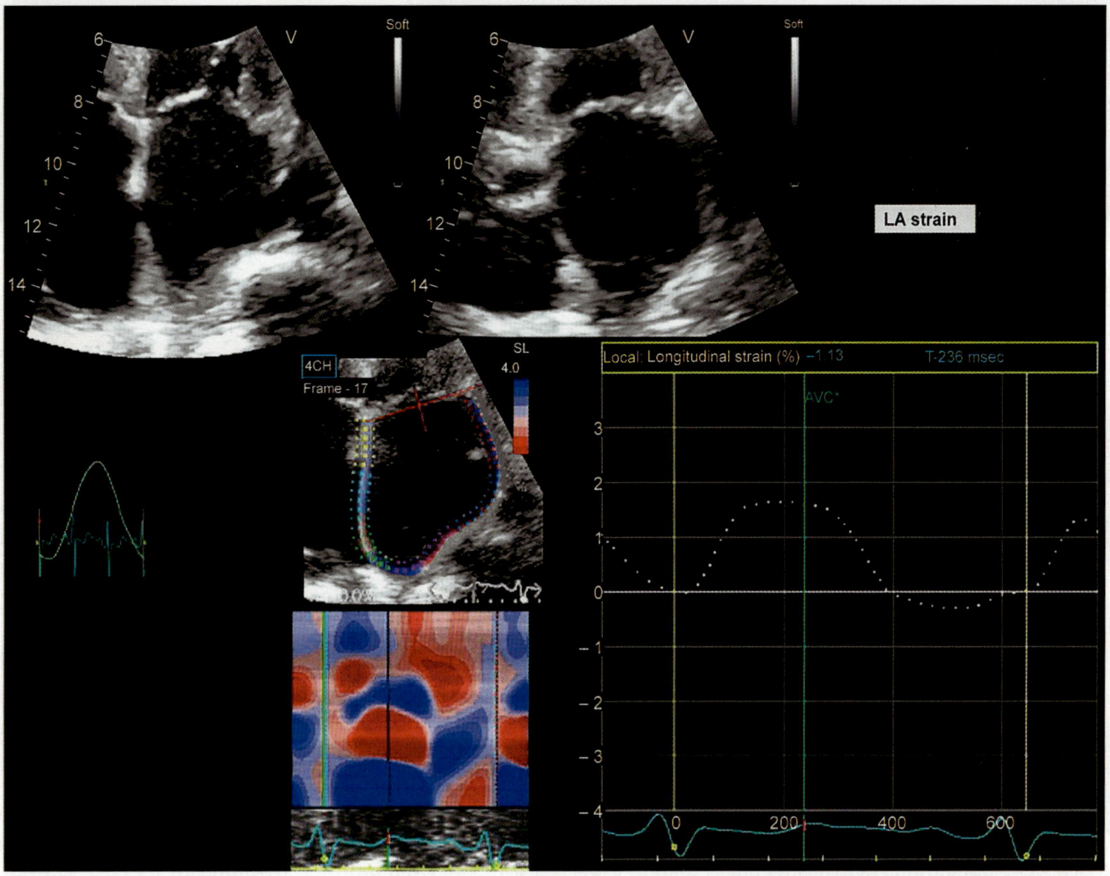

FIG. 10: A case of transthyretin amyloid cardiomyopathy (ATTR-CM) showing severely depressed left atrial (LA) reservoir strain (<5%) and absent LA contractile strain suggesting atrial amyloid infiltration.

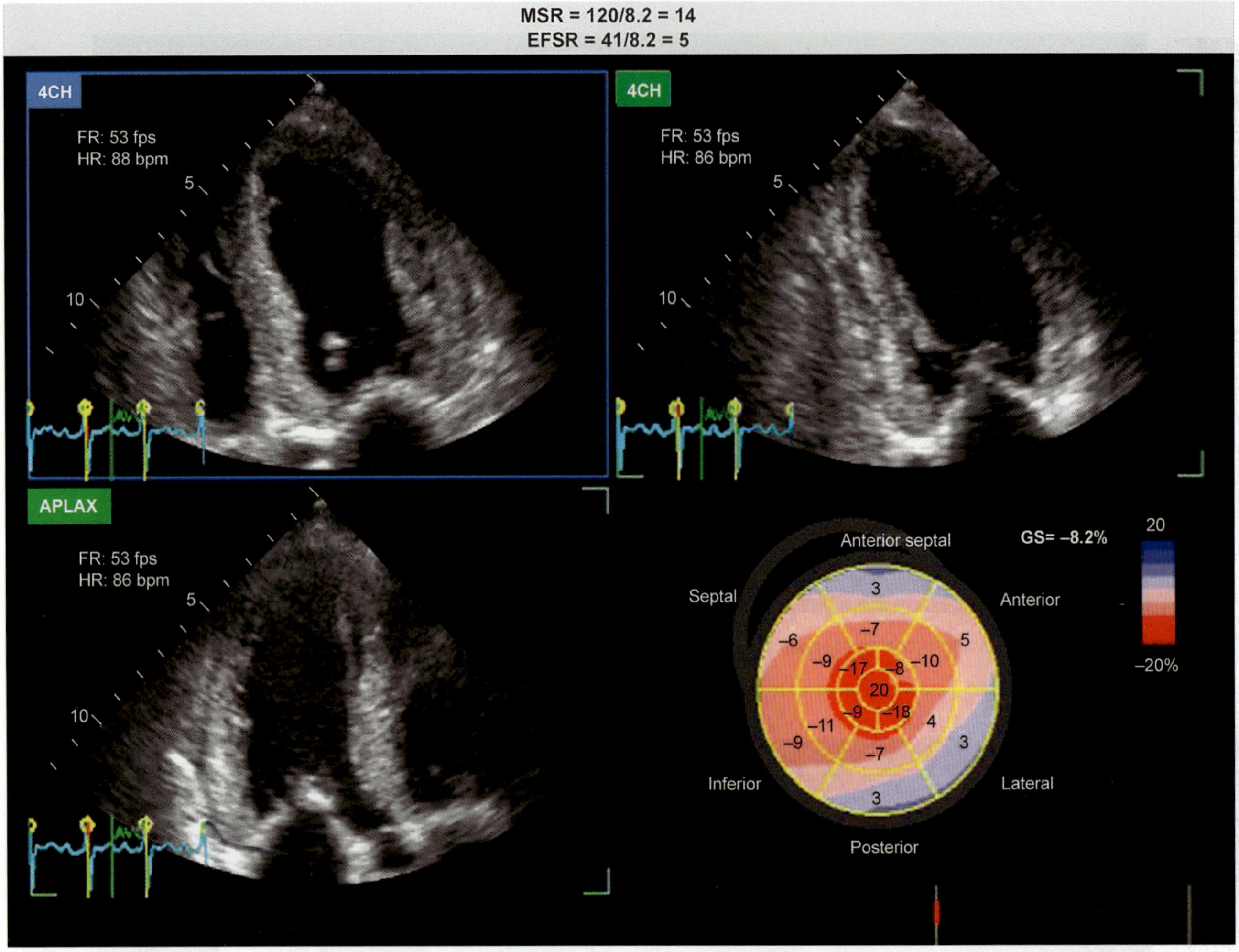

FIG. 11: A case of AL-CM showing high left ventricular (LV) mass to strain ratio = 14 and high left ventricular ejection fraction (LVEF) to strain ratio = 5.

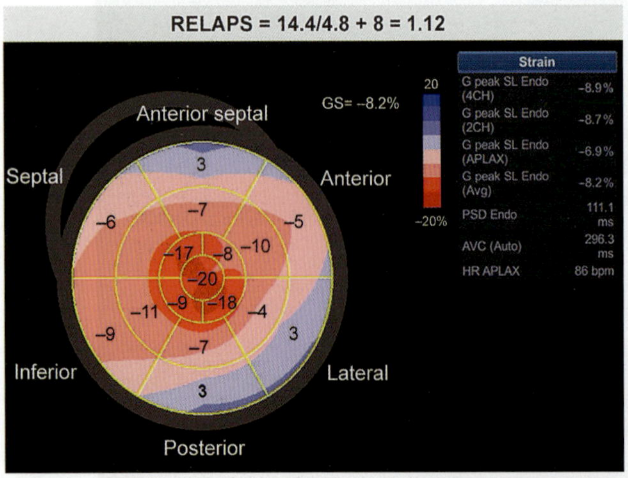

FIG. 12: A case of AL-CM showing high relative apical sparing score (RELAPS = 1.12).

circumferential subendocardial enhancement (not confined to any coronary territory), followed by transmural LGE as the amyloid disease progresses **(Fig. 16)**. The subendocardial LGE is more prevalent in AL and transmural LGE is more prevalent in ATTR cardiac amyloidosis.[7] The characteristic LGE pattern has sensitivity (86%) and specificity (92%) to detect cardiac amyloidosis.[4]

The extracellular volume fraction (ECV) in healthy subjects is about 20–25% and in conditions with interstitial fibrosis such as AS, HF, and hypertrophic CM is about 25–35%. There is severe expansion of ECV in cardiac amyloidosis **(Fig. 14)**.The ECV elevation in the patients with cardiac amyloidosis (generally >40%, average ECV 54% in ATTR-CM and 51% in AL-CM) is highly sensitive (92%) and specific (82%) for diagnosing cardiac amyloidosis.[17] The myocyte cell volume calculated by subtracting ECV from indexed total LV myocardial volume, is higher in ATTR-CM than AL-CM, suggesting compensatory myocyte hypertrophy.[3]

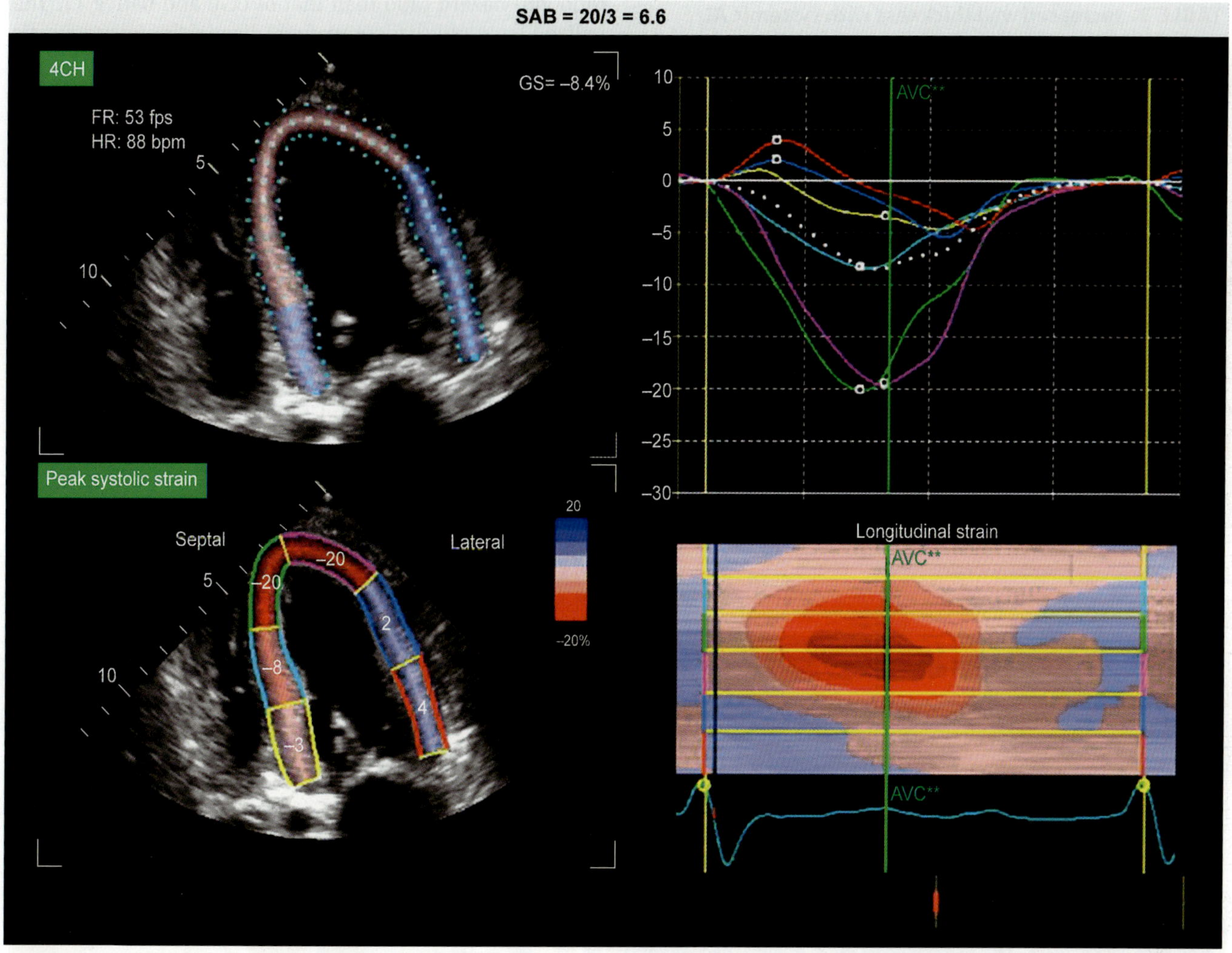

FIG. 13: A case of AL-CM showing high septal apical to base strain ratio (SAB = 6.6) suggesting apical sparing characteristic of amyloid infiltration.

TABLE 1: The echocardiographic parameters for diagnosis of cardiac amyloidosis (in patients with wall thickness ≤16 mm and normal EF > 55%).[12,13]

Parameter	Cut off	Sensitivity %	Specificity %	AUC
EFSR	>4.1	89.7	91.7	0.95
RELAPS	>0.87	62.5	85	0.78
	>1	73	99	
SAB	>2.1	74.2	63.7	
	>3.1	47.5	86.7	0.67
MCF	<0.24	56.4	96.7	0.8
IVS/PW	<1.38	93	57	0.77
E/E'	>9.6	50	100	0.69

(AUC: area under curve; EF: ejection fraction; EFSR: EF to strain ratio; IVS/PW: interventricular septum/posterior wall; MCF: myocardial contraction fraction; RELAPS: relative apical sparing; SAB: septal apical-basal ratio)

TABLE 2: Increased wall thickness (IWT) score.[14]

Parameter cut off	Points
RWT > 0.6	3
E/e' > 11	1
TAPSE ≤ 19 mm	2
LA strain ≤ 13%	1
SAB > 2.9	3
Total	10

(LA: left atrium; RWT: relative wall thickness; SAB: septal apical-basal ratio; TAPSE: tricuspid annular plane systolic excursion)

A meta-analysis[17] of 18 diagnostic (n = 2,015) and 13 prognostic studies (n = 1,483) of diagnostic and prognostic performance of native T1, ECV mapping, and LGE imaging showed that ECV had a significantly higher diagnostic odds

TABLE 3: Increased wall thickness with systemic AL score.[14]

Parameter cut off	Points
RWT > 0.52	2
E/e' > 10	2
TAPSE ≤ 19 mm	1
LA strain ≤ 14%	1
Total	6

(LA: left atrium; RWT: relative wall thickness; TAPSE: tricuspid annular plane systolic excursion)

TABLE 4: Transthyretin cardiac amyloid score (TCAS).[12]

Parameter cutoff	Points
Age:	
• 60–69	+2
• 70–79	+3
• 80 and above	+4
Sex male	+2
RWT > 0.57	+2
Inferolateral wall ≥ 12 mm	+1
LVEF < 60%	+1
HT present	–1

(HT: hypertension; RWT: relative wall thickness; LVEF: left ventricular ejection fraction)

ratio and hazard ratio than that of LGE and native T1. The native T1 mapping has comparable diagnostic and prognostic performance with that of LGE.

The CMR examination may be particularly considered in younger (age < 60 years) HF patients, without a family history of TTR variant, where other myocardial diseases are to be ruled out such as HCM, HTHD, inflammatory myopathies, lysosomal storage diseases, or hemochromatosis.[4] CMR is also useful in detection of early cardiac involvement in patients with evidence of systemic AL amyloidosis.[7]

The probability of different cardiac structural and functional variables being abnormal as the cardiac amyloid burden progressively increases are shown in **Box 1** grouped together for low burden (ECV of 40–50%), intermediate burden (ECV 51–70%), and high burden (ECV > 70%) of cardiac amyloid infiltration **(Fig. 17)**.[14,18]

TABLE 5: T-Amylo score.[15]

Parameter cut off	Points
History of carpal tunnel	3
Age > 80 years	1
Male gender	3
Hypertrophy IVS > 16 mm	2
Low-voltage QRS	2
Total	11

(IVS: interventricular septum)

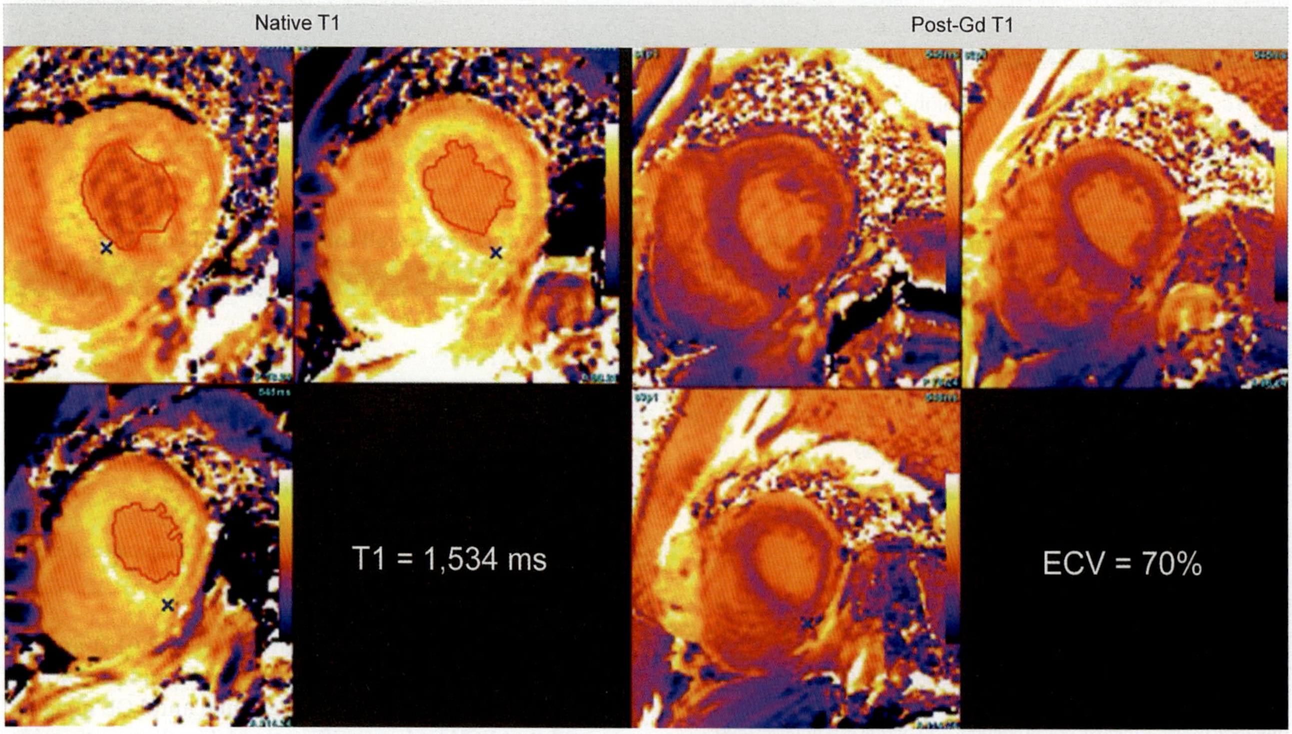

FIG. 14: A case of transthyretin amyloid cardiomyopathy ATTR-CM showing high native T1 values (1,534 ms) and high extracellular volume fraction (ECV = 70%) on cardiac magnetic resonance imaging.

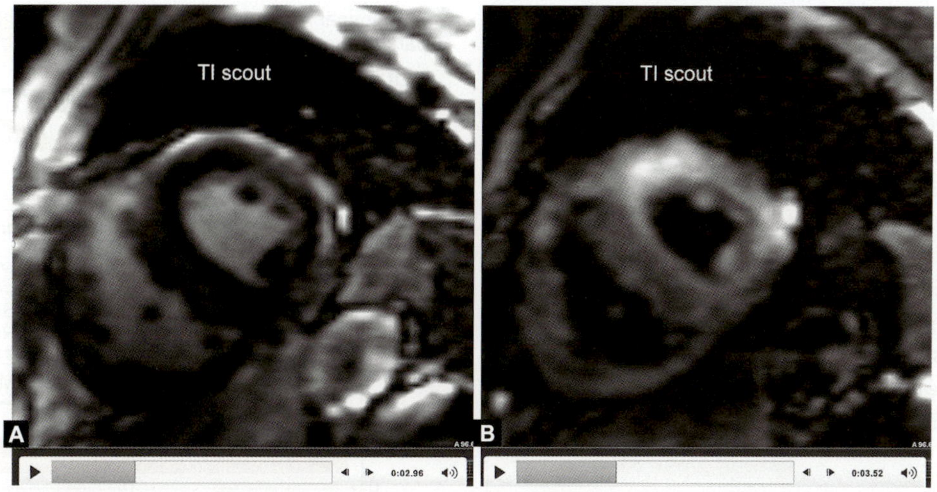

FIG. 15A AND B: A case of transthyretin amyloid cardiomyopathy (ATTR-CM) showing abnormal gadolinium kinetics—(A) nulling of the myocardium before the left ventricular (LV) cavity blood pool on Look-Locker (TI scout) sequence and (B) nulling of the LV cavity blood pool after the myocardium on Look-Locker (TI scout) sequence. Note the timer on the video playing bar.

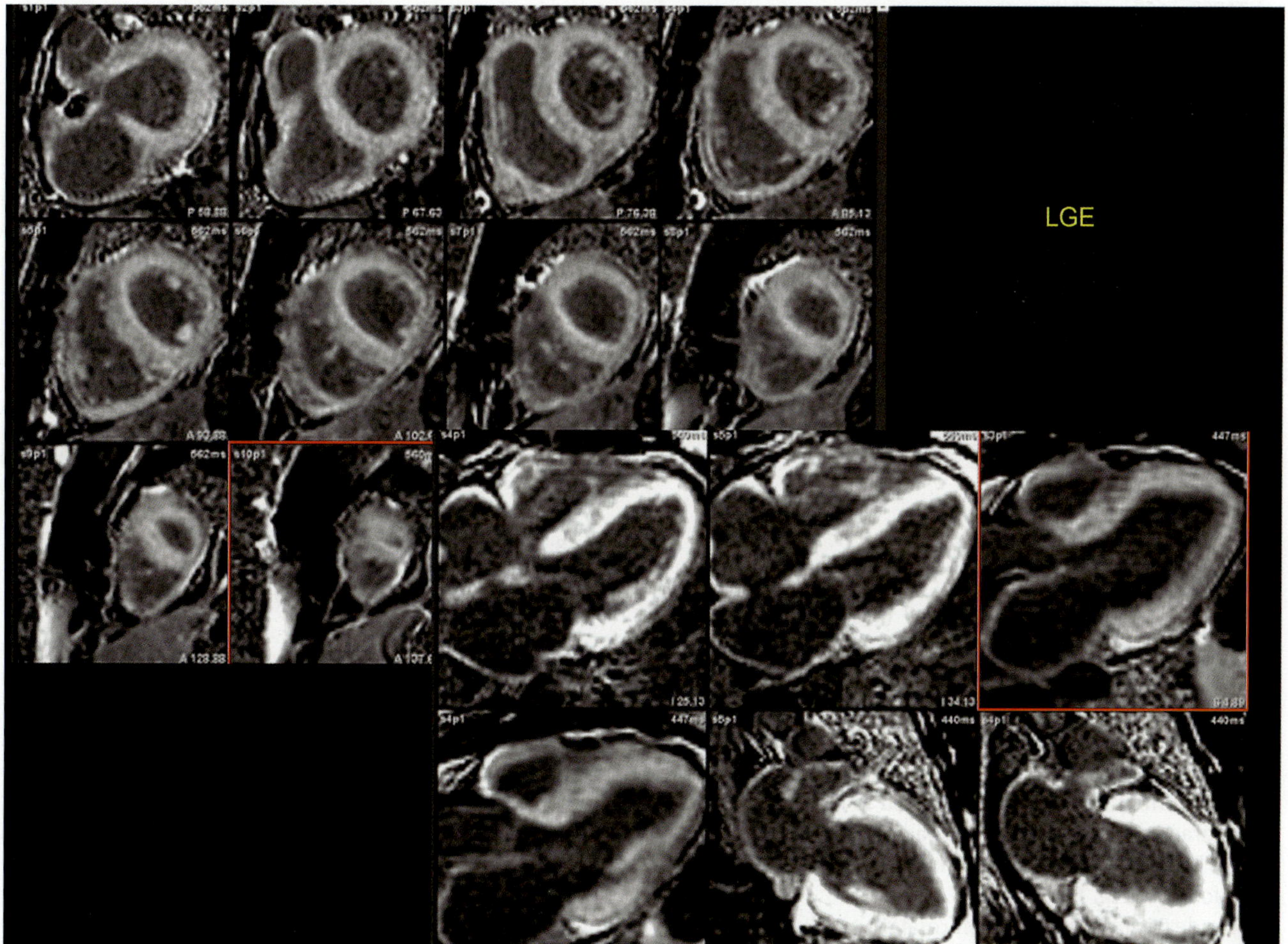

FIG. 16: A case of transthyretin amyloid cardiomyopathy (ATTR-CM) showing transmural late gadolinium enhancement with low left ventricular (LV) cavity blood pool signals.

BOX 1 Probability of echocardiographic and CMR variables being abnormal as per the ECV measured amyloid burden.[14,18]

Low burden (ECV of 40–50%) variables (affected first):
- GLS < 20% (Echo)
- Average E/e' > 8 (Echo)
- IVS, PW thickness ≥ 12 mm (Echo)
- RWT > 0.42 (Echo)
- MCF < 23.4% (Echo)
- MAPSE < 11 mm (CMR)
- Indexed LV mass > 81 g/m^2 (CMR)

Intermediate burden (ECV 51–70%) variables:
- LAA > 20 cm^2 (Echo)
- E/A >2 (Echo)
- SAB >2.1 (Echo)
- RELAPS >1 (Echo)
- EFSR > 4.1 (Echo)
- MAPSE <11 (Echo)
- Indexed SV < 42 mL/m^2 (CMR)
- TAPSE < 16 mm (CMR)
- MCF < 38% (CMR)

High burden (ECV > 70%) variables (affected late):
- TAPSE < 16 (Echo)
- LVEF < 55% (Echo), <57% (CMR)
- RVEF < 52% (CMR)
- Indexed LA area > 15 cm^2/m^2 (CMR)
- Indexed RA area >16 cm^2/m^2 (CMR)

(CMR: cardiac magnetic resonance; ECV: extracellular volume fraction; EFSR: ejection fraction to strain ratio; GLS: global longitudinal strain; IVS/PW: interventricular septum/posterior wall; LAA: left atrium area; LVEF: left ventricular ejection fraction; MAPSE: mitral annular plane systolic excursion; MCF: myocardial contraction fraction; SAB: septal apical-basal ratio; SV: stroke volume; RA: right atrium; RELAPS: relative apical sparing; RVEF: right ventricular ejection fraction; RWT: relative wall thickness; TAPSE: tricuspid annular plane systolic excursion)

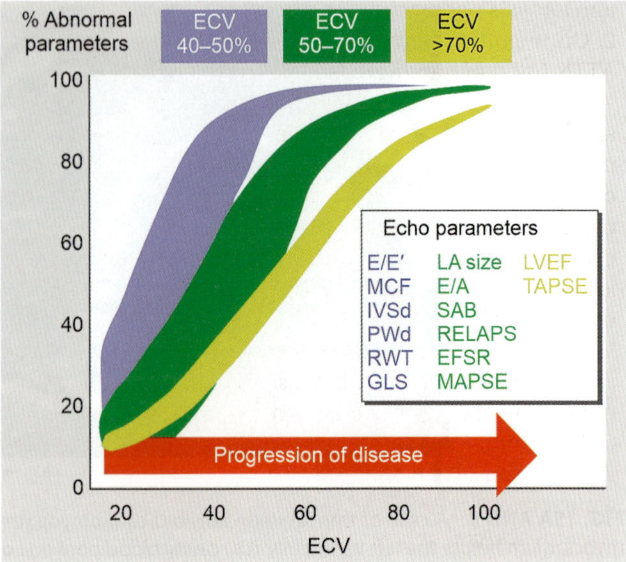

FIG. 17: Probability of echocardiographic and cardiac magnetic resonance variables being abnormal as per the progression of amyloid burden measured by extracellular volume fraction.

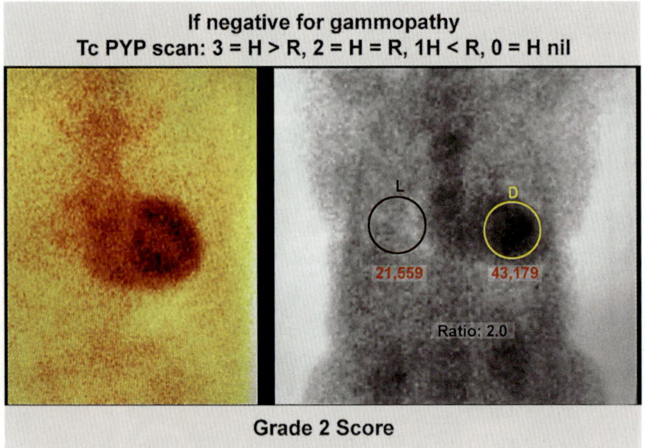

FIG. 18: A case of transthyretin amyloid cardiomyopathy (ATTR-CM) showing grade III abnormality on Tc pyrophosphate bone tracer scan (heart uptake > rib uptake) and the ratio of H/CL uptake > 1.5.

Nuclear Scan

Bone Scintigraphy

The planar and single photon emission computed tomography (SPECT) with ^{99m}Tc bone avid tracers such as ^{99m}Tc-pyrophosphate (^{99m}Tc-PYP), ^{99m}Tc-3,3-diphosphono-1,2-propanodicarboxylic acid (^{99m}Tc-DPD), and ^{99m}Tc hydroxymethylene-diphosphonate (^{99m}Tc-HMDP) are used for the diagnosis of ATTR-CM.[1] The microcalcification in the myocardium in ATTR-CM is supposed to be responsible for the characteristic uptake of these radiotracers.

The Tc PYP/DPD cardiac uptake is semiquantitatively graded by as follows **(Fig. 18)**:[7]

- Grade 0 is no cardiac and normal rib uptake.
- Grade 1 is cardiac uptake less than rib uptake.
- Grade 2 is cardiac uptake equal to rib uptake.
- Grade 3 is cardiac uptake greater than rib uptake with mild/absent rib uptake.

The grade 2 or 3 cardiac uptake or the heart to contralateral lung (H/CL) ratio of tracer uptake > 1.5 at 1 hour and >1.3 at 3 hours are specific for ATTR-CM only if the monoclonal gammopathy is ruled out. SPECT imaging is required in positive or equivocal cases to differentiate myocardial tracer uptake from the blood pool signal and to detect myocardial regional heterogeneity.[7]

In a landmark study[19] 1,217 patients of ATTR-CM, who underwent bone scintigraphy and laboratory testing for SPIE, UPIE, and serum FLC, the combination of a positive scan and a negative monoclonal protein assessment correctly diagnosed 391 out of 391 patients (100% specificity for ATTR-CM). However, in the same study, 22% of patients with AL amyloidosis had positive bone scintigraphy scans of grade 2. On the other hand, approximately 20% of patients with ATTR-CM may have unrelated MGUS.[8,20]

False positives Tc PYP or DPD uptake may occur in AL amyloidosis (22% of cases), old myocardial infarction, diffuse myocardial fibrosis in CKD, mitral annular calcification, overlying healed rib facture, the blood pool signal on planar imaging, hydroxychloroquine toxicity, and in rare ApoA1 type of cardiac amyloidosis.[1] Cardiac uptake on bone scintigraphy is less common in AApoAIV-CM than AApoAI-CM (grade 1 uptake14% vs. 82%).[5]

A negative Tc PYP/DPD scan does not exclude cardiac amyloid infiltration since bone scintigraphy can be negative in majority of cases of AL-CM and in rare variants of ATTR-CM (rare non-V30M mutations and in some V30M mutations with early onset and only full-length TTR fibrils).[4,7] Following a negative Tc PYP/DPD scan, a CMR examination or endomyocardial biopsy are required if the clinical suspicion of cardiac amyloid remains high on echocardiography.

The quantitative evaluation of Tc DPD scan is done by measuring cardiac peak standardized uptake value (SUV) and composite SUV retention index = (cardiac peak SUV/vertebral peak SUV) × (paraspinal muscle peak SUV) with excellent diagnostic accuracy.[21] Cardiac SUVpeak increases from grade 0 to grade 2 and then remains constant between grade 2 and 3. The paraspinal muscle SUVpeak increases and vertebral SUVpeak decreases with grade 0–3.

Bone scintigraphy can be particularly considered following echocardiography in older (age> 60 years) HF patients with LVH and clinical history suggestive of ATTR-CM.[4] Bone-scintigraphy is also sensitive in the early identification of hATTR-CM in genotype carriers without apparent cardiac involvement.[7]

Cardiac Positron Emission Tomography Imaging

Cardiac positron emission tomography (PET) has the promise of directly imaging amyloid deposits, before morphological and clinical manifestations of the disease. The radiotracers 18F-florbetapir, 18F-flutemetamol, and 18F-florbetaben are all derivatives of thioflavin-T, a dye used for staining tissue amyloid deposition.[22]

The PET indices of target to background (LV myocardium to blood pool) ratio > 1.5 and retention index (tracer uptake between the early and late stages) of >0.025 min^{-1} with 18F-florbetapir and 18F-florbetaben are used to differentiate patients with cardiac amyloidosis from controls.[7] The cardiac PET has sensitivity of 95% and specificity of 98% for detection of cardiac amyloid. By injecting amyloid-binding PET tracers such as 18F-florbetapir, 18F-florbetaben, 11-C-Pittsburgh compound B, and 18F-flutemetamol, the amyloid deposits in other systemic organs apart from the heart can also be detected and the systemic load of amyloidosis can be quantified.[7]

There is evidence to suggest that PET amyloid radiotracers can detect early cardiac amyloid deposition in both AL and ATTR before echocardiographic evidence of IWT or increase in serum biomarkers.[23] Patients with active or 1 year in-remission AL-CM showed similar degree of myocardial 18F-florbetapir uptake. The patients with active AL amyloid but no evidence of cardiac amyloid by current criteria (normal LVWT and normal cardiac serum biomarkers) showed lower median value of 18F-florbetapir uptake.[24] The therapeutic implications of early detection of myocardial PET amyloid tracer uptake in the at-risk patients are unclear. In future, it may be possible to start the therapy before cardiac structural or functional damage sets in or cardiac serum biomarkers starts rising.[22]

The ratio of heart to mediastinum uptake (HMR) of iodine-123-metaiodobenzylguanidine (^{123}I-MIBG) can indicate sympathetic nervous system involvement by amyloid infiltration. Decreased HMR at 4 hours post-^{123}I-MIBG administration indicates sympathetic dysfunction and is an independent prognostic factor for ventricular arrhythmia.[7]

Cardiac Computed Tomography Imaging

The cardiac CT is the mainstay of TAVR planning in elderly patients with degenerative AS and creates an opportunity to evaluate cardiac amyloid in this group of patients.[4] The CT contrast imaging with dual-energy equilibrium CT to measure the myocardial iodine concentration can differentiate cardiac amyloid from other cardiomyopathies with sensitivity of 100% and specificity of 92%.

Endomyocardial and Extracardiac Biopsy

The amyloid deposits in the tissue are identified by the affinity for Congo red staining and with apple green birefringence under polarized light. The type of amyloid is confirmed by immunohistochemistry and/or proteomic evaluation by mass spectroscopy at specialized centers.[9]

Approximately, one in four to five patients with ATTR have coincidentally MGUS,[20] or an abnormal FLC ratio[25] and may need cardiac or extracardiac biopsy for confirmation. The definitive diagnosis of AL-CM in the presence of monoclonal gammopathy requires a tissue biopsy for showing amyloid deposits, either from the heart (sensitivity 100%) or abdominal fat (sensitivity 70%) or rectum (sensitivity 70–85%) or bone marrow (sensitivity 50–55%).[26]

When monoclonal gammopathy is suspected on SPIE, UPIE, and FLC, initial bone marrow biopsy is required to determine percentage of plasma cells in the marrow and to rule out multiple myeloma and less common diseases such as Waldenström macroglobulinemia and lymphomas.[8]

Endomyocardial biopsy is required in the following circumstances to establish the diagnosis:[1,8]

- A positive PYP/DPD scan suggesting ATTR-CM and monoclonal gammopathy of unknown significance on SPIE, UPIE, and FLC to exclude AL-CM (ATTR-CM and AL-CM may rarely coexist in elderly).
- The echocardiography or CMR showing high likelihood of infiltrative CM with SPIE, UPIE, and FLC suggesting monoclonal gammopathy and negative extracardiac biopsy for AL amyloid.
- A negative or Gr 1 PYP/DPD scan in presence of high clinical and imaging suspicion of ATTR-CM
- Equivocal results or unavailability of Tc PYP/DPD scan

WHAT ARE THE DIAGNOSTIC CRITERIA?

In the "Expert Consensus Recommendations" for diagnosis of cardiac amyloidosis the typical imaging features of cardiac amyloidosis are described in **Table 6.**[9]

The "Expert Consensus Recommendations" has suggested three criteria for clinical diagnosis of ATTR cardiac amyloidosis **(Box 2)**.[9] The same consensus recommendations also suggest the criteria for histological diagnosis of ATTR and AL cardiac amyloidosis **(Table 7)**.[9]

WHAT IS THE DIAGNOSTIC ALGORITHM?

The diagnostic algorithm[3] for diagnosis of cardiac amyloidosis and its types involves stepwise utilization of diagnostic imaging and laboratory tests as shown in **Flowchart 1**.

The diagnostic algorithm[3] for detecting early cardiac amyloidosis in the patients at-risk of cardiac amyloid infiltration (pathological TTR genotypes and systemic AL amyloidosis) also involves stepwise utilization of diagnostic imaging and laboratory tests as shown in **Flowchart 2**.

WHAT ARE THE PROGNOSTIC FACTORS?

Cardiac amyloid once diagnosed has poor outcome with median survival in untreated patients is 6 months for AL, 2.5 years for hereditary ATTR (*TTR* Val122Ile or pV142I) mutations and 3.6 years for wide type ATTR.[1]

Among different types of hereditary ATTR mutations, the prognosis varies significantly. There is 16% 4-year survival in valine to isoleucine at position 122 (Val122Ile) mutations, compared with 40% 4-year survival in threonine to alanine at position 60 (Thr60Ala) and 79% 4-year survival in valine to methionine at position 30 (Val30Met) mutations.[2]

Patients with AApoAI-CM have median survival > 172 months and AApoAIV-CM have median survival > 30 months.[5]

The cardiac biomarkers (NT-proBNP and troponin) and eGFR are used for prognostic staging[1,27] of cardiac amyloid (Mayo staging system and UK staging system) and for assessing the response to treatment **(Tables 8 and 9)**.

TABLE 6: Typical imaging features of cardiac amyloidosis.[9]

Modality	Typical findings
Echocardiography	• LV wall thickness > 12 mm • RELAPS > 1 • ≥ grade 2 LV diastolic dysfunction
Cardiac MRI	• LV wall thickness > 7 mm/9 mm (long axis) and 7 mm/8 mm (short axis) on cine CMR at midcavity level for women/men, respectively • Global ECV > 0.40 • Diffuse LGE • Abnormal gadolinium kinetics (myocardial nulling before blood pool nulling)
• Positron emission tomography (PET) • 18F-florbetapir or 18F-florbetaben PET	• Target to background ratio > 1.5 • Retention index >0.030 min–1

(CMR: cardiac magnetic resonance; ECV: extracellular volume fraction; LGE: late gadolinium enhancement; LV: left ventricular; MRI: magnetic resonance imaging; RELAPS: relative apical sparing)

BOX 2 Criteria for clinical diagnosis of ATTR-CM.[9]

- ^{99m}Tc-PYP, DPD, and HMDP grade 2 or 3 myocardial uptake of radiotracer
- Absence of a monoclonal gammopathy as assessed by serum FLCs and SPIE and UPIE
- Typical cardiac imaging features

(CM: cardiomyopathy; FLC: free light chain; ^{99m}Tc-DPD: ^{99m}Tc-3,3-diphosphono-1,2-propanodicarboxylic acid; ^{99m}Tc-HMDP: ^{99m}Tc hydroxymethylene-diphosphonate; ^{99m}Tc-PYP: ^{99m}Tc-pyrophosphate; SPIE: serum protein immunofixation electrophoresis; UPIE: urine protein immunofixation electrophoresis)

TABLE 7: Criteria for the histological diagnosis of ATTR-CM and AL-CM.[9]

Histological diagnosis of cardiac amyloidosis: Endomyocardial biopsy	
ATTR and AL	• Endomyocardial biopsy positive for cardiac amyloidosis with Congo red staining with apple-green birefringence under polarized light • Typing by immunohistochemistry and/or mass spectrometry at specialized centers
Histological diagnosis of cardiac amyloidosis: Extracardiac biopsy	
ATTR	• Extracardiac biopsy proven ATTR amyloidosis • Typical cardiac imaging features
AL	• Extracardiac biopsy proven AL amyloidosis • Typical cardiac imaging features • Abnormal cardiac biomarkers: Abnormal NT-proBNP, troponin

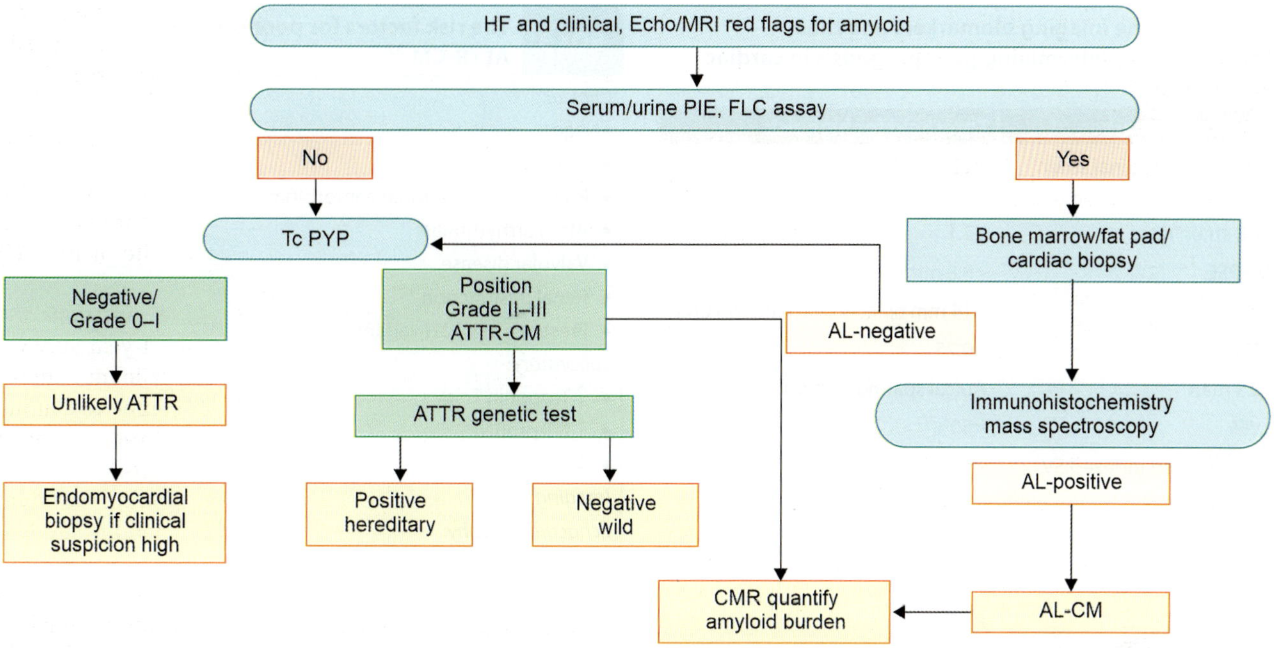

FLOWCHART 1: A diagnostic algorithm for cardiac amyloidosis and its transthyretin amyloid (ATTR) and AL subtypes.
Source: With permission from Dorbala et al. (2020).[3]

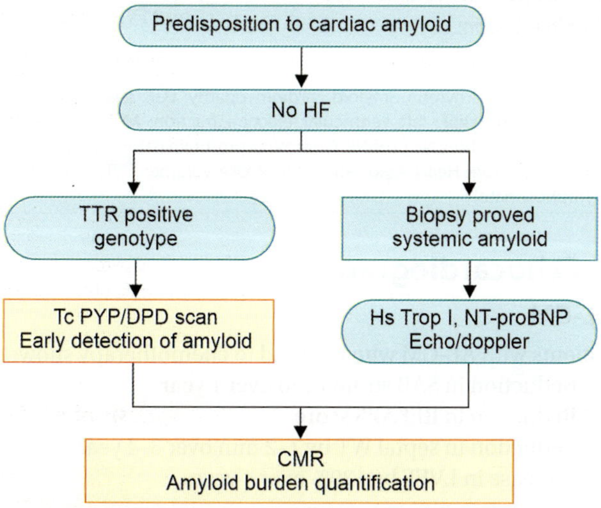

FLOWCHART 2: A diagnostic algorithm for cardiac amyloidosis in the evaluation of "at-risk" patients.
Source: With permission from Dorbala et al. (2020).[3]

The imaging biomarkers and their thresholds[4,18] evaluated for determining prognosis of cardiac amyloidosis in general are shown in **Table 10**. The risk factors for worse prognosis specifically in ATTR-CM are shown in **Box 3**. More the number of risk factors aggregation worser is the prognosis.[27]

A study of 109 patients with cardiac amyloidosis, the lower LS values of all the four chambers were significantly

TABLE 8: Mayo prognostic staging system of cardiac amyloidosis.[1,27]

Parameter	Stage	Median survival
Troponin T ≤ 0.05 ng/mL NT-proBNP ≤ 3,000 pg/mL	I	66 months
Troponin T ≤ 0.05 ng/mL NT-proBNP > 3,000 pg/mL OR Troponin T > 0.05 ng/mL NT-proBNP ≤ 3,000 pg/mL	II	40 months
Troponin T > 0.05 ng/mL NT-proBNP > 3,000 pg/mL	III	20 months

TABLE 9: UK prognostic staging system of cardiac amyloidosis.[1,27]

Parameter	Stage	Survival
NT-proBNP ≤ 3,000 pg/mL eGFR ≥ 45 mL/min	I	69.2 months
NT-proBNP ≤ 3,000 pg/mL eGFR < 45 mL/min NT-proBNP > 3,000 pg/mL eGFR ≥ 45 mL/min	II	46.7 months
NT-proBNP > 3,000 pg/mL eGFR < 45 mL/min	III	24.1 months

(eGFR: estimated glomerular filtration rate; NT-proBNP: N-terminal pro-brain natriuretic peptides)

TABLE 10: The imaging biomarkers and their thresholds for determining poor prognosis in cardiac amyloidosis.[4,18]

Imaging biomarker	Threshold for high risk
Global longitudinal strain (GLS)	<12%
SAB strain ratio	>2.1
MAPSE	<8.8 mm
TAPSE	<14 mm on echo, <16 mm on CMR
MCF	<0.25
GLS map	Apical sparing pattern
LVEF	<50%
CMR-derived indexed SV	<42 mL/m^2
T1 values	>1,044 on 1.5-T CMR
ECV measurement	>0.45
LGE	Transmural
RV LGE	Present
Markers of myocardial edema on CMR	Elevated native T1 and T2 values in AL-CM
Scintigraphy myocardial uptake of Tc PYP	Grade 3

(CMR: cardiac magnetic resonance; ECV: extracellular volume fraction; LGE: late gadolinium enhancement; LVEF: left ventricular ejection fraction; MAPSE: mitral annular plane systolic excursion; MCF: myocardial contraction fraction; SAB: septal apical-basal ratio; TAPSE: tricuspid annular plane systolic excursion; Tc PYP: Tc-pyrophosphate)

associated with survival. The patients having strain values below the median (LV GLS < 10.4%, LA strain < 13.2%, RV free wall strain < 17.0%, and RA strain < 12.4%) had significantly lower survival than patients having strain values above the median.[28]

How to Monitor Cardiac Amyloid Regression on Treatment?

The progression or regression of cardiac amyloid infiltration on pharmacotherapy can be monitored effectively by serial biomarkers, echocardiography and CMR imaging.

Biomarkers

The serum levels of NT-proBNP or BNP are monitored in cardiac amyloidosis patients on definitive therapy. >30% reduction of these biomarkers from the baseline indicates a cardiac response.[4] In ATTR-CM, change in prealbumin concentration from baseline is being investigated as a biomarker for treatment benefit. In AL-CM, reduction in the serum FLC and normalization of the plasma cell count in the bone marrow are markers of efficacy of chemotherapy.[4]

BOX 3 The risk factors for poor prognosis in ATTR-CM.[27]

Clinical:
- Age
- NYHA class
- Presence of additional comorbidities
- Atrial arrhythmias
- Valvular disease
- Renal dysfunction
- Presence of V122I variant

Laboratory:
- ↑ Troponin T
- ↑ NT-proBNP
- ↓ eGFR

Imaging:

Echocardiography:
- ↓ LVEF < 50%
- ↓ MCF < 25%
- ↓ Longitudinal strain apical < 14.5%, basal < 8%
- ↓ SV index < 33 mL/m^2

Cardiac magnetic resonance:
- ↑ LGE subendocardial vs. transmural
- ↑ Extracellular volume > 0.4

99mTc-PYP scan:
- ↑ H/CL ratio > 1.6

(ATTR-CM: transthyretin amyloid cardiomyopathy; LGE: late gadolinium enhancement; LVEF: left ventricular ejection fraction; MCF: myocardial contraction fraction; NT-proBNP: N-terminal pro-brain natriuretic peptides; NYHA: New York Heart Association; SV: stroke volume; ^{99m}Tc-PYP: ^{99m}Tc-pyrophosphate)

Echocardiography

AL-CM

Patients with AL-CM who respond to chemotherapy show:[4]
- Reduction in SAB strain ratio over 1 year
- Reduction in RELAPS score
- Reduction in septal WT by 1–2 mm over 3–4 years
- Increase in LVEF by >20% over 4 years

Patients with AL-CM who do not respond to chemotherapy show:[4]
- Decrease in LV cavity size
- Decrease in LV SV index by 10 mL/m^2
- Reduction in LV diastolic strain
- Increased mitral E/e' > 20
- Reduction in GLS

ATTR-CM

In APOLLO trial, Patisiran treatment improved LV GLS (by 1.4 ± 0.6%) and reduced LVWT (by –0.9 ± 0.4 mm) after 18 months of treatment compared with placebo. In ATTR-ACT trial, Tafamidis treatment reduced the rate of decline of

LV SV after 30 months of treatment compared with placebo. The trial with diflunisal reduced the rate of decline in LV GLS in wild type ATTR-CM.[4]

Cardiac Magnetic Resonance

Patients with AL-CM who respond to chemotherapy show:[4]

- Reductions in LVWT
- Reduction in LV mass
- Reduction in LA size
- Reduction in native T1 values
- Reduction in LGE extent
- Reduction in ECV > 5%

After 12 months of therapy with TTR-specific small interfering RNA (siRNA) patisiran in ATTR patients, there was reduction in ECV (by mean of 6.2%), reduction in cardiac uptake of bone tracer (by mean of 19.6%), reduction in NT-proBNP (by mean of 1,342 ng/L), and increase in 6-minute walking distance (by mean of 169 m).[29]

Scintigraphy/Positron Emission Tomography

The studies in ATTR patients have shown 19.6% reduction in cardiac tracer uptake on DPD scintigraphy on treatment with Patisiran.[4] However, currently scintigraphy is not recommended to track disease progression or response to therapy.[7] The reduction in retention index of tracer uptake correlates with successful chemotherapy in AL-CM.

Time Course of Changes in Imaging Biomarkers on Treatment of Cardiac Amyloidosis

Treatment nonresponders can be identified, as early as 6 months, with rapid decrease in LV dimensions, SV, cardiac index, GLS and increase in mitral E/e', and ECV.

Treatment responders (chemotherapy benefit in AL-CM) can be identified, as early as 12 months, with slow increase in GLS and reduction in SAB strain ratio, reduction in LV mass, reduction in ECV and as late as 3–4 years with reduction in IVS-WT and improvement in EF over the period of 3–4 years.[4]

CONCLUSION

Cardiac amyloid CM is caused by deposition of amyloid fibrils of misfolded precursor proteins such as TTR, light chain immunoglobulin, and ApoAI-IV leading to restrictive CM. The characteristic findings on echocardiography (GLS mapping and scoring systems), CMR (ECV and LGE), and bone avid radiotracer uptake on scintigraphy (ATTR-CM) help in diagnosis of cardiac amyloidosis and to monitor the disease progression or regression on treatment.

ONLINE REFERENCES

Please scan the QR code provided at the end of the table of contents for References of this chapter.

CHAPTER

102 Transcatheter Edge-to-edge Repair with MitraClip System

Vijayakumar Subban, Sai Satish, Krishnaswamy Chandrasekaran

ABSTRACT

Mitral regurgitation (MR) is the most prevalent heart valve disease in the elderly population. Surgical intervention improves outcomes in patients with symptomatic moderately severe or severe MR or asymptomatic patients with underlying left ventricular (LV) dysfunction. However, a significant number of patients are ineligible for surgery despite suitable anatomy due to comorbidities. Transcatheter edge-to-edge repair (TEER) with MitraClip (Abbott Vascular, Menlo Park, California, US), the transcatheter version of the surgical Alfieri stitch, transformed the treatment of these patients. TEER with MitraClip improves outcomes in both primary and secondary MR. This review provides an overview of the clinical evidence and indications, followed step-by-step approach to the procedure, and finally complications and troubleshooting.

Keywords: Mitral regurgitation, transcatheter edge-to-edge repair, MitraClip.

INTRODUCTION

Mitral regurgitation (MR) is the most prevalent heart valve disease in the elderly population.[1] It results from the structural abnormalities of the mitral valve (MV) apparatus (papillary muscles, chordae tendinae, or leaflets)—primary MR or from the abnormalities of left ventricle (LV) or left atrium (LA) and the mitral annulus—secondary MR.[2] MR causes LV volume overload that results in progressive LV dilatation and dysfunction, leading to heart failure (HF) and increased mortality.[3] Surgical intervention improves outcomes in moderately severe or severe MR in symptomatic patients or asymptomatic patients with underlying LV dysfunction.[4] However, a significant number of patients do not receive surgery despite suitable anatomy due to comorbidities. Transcatheter edge-to-edge repair (TEER) with MitraClip (Abbott Vascular, Menlo Park, California, US), the transcatheter version of the surgical Alfieri stitch, transformed the treatment of these patients.[5] The current chapter provides an overview of the clinical evidence and indications, followed step-by-step approach to the procedure, and finally complications and troubleshooting.

CLINICAL EVIDENCE AND INDICATIONS

Since its first human implantation in 2003, the MitraClip device has been evaluated in a series of clinical studies.

The Phase 1 *EVEREST* (*Endovascular Valve Edge-to-Edge Repair*) study assessed the safety and feasibility of TEER with MitraClip in a population of 27 patients with symptomatic moderate-to-severe MR or severe MR or asymptomatic moderate-to-severe (grade 3+) or severe MR (grade 4+) with LV dysfunction and are candidates for MV surgery. The device was successfully implanted in 24 patients, remaining three patients underwent surgery. The primary endpoint of freedom from major adverse events (death, myocardial infarction, cardiac tamponade, cardiac surgery for failed clip, clip detachment, stroke, or septicemia) at 30 days was achieved in 85% of the participants. Clip detachment occurred in three patients and there were no procedural deaths or emergency surgery.[5]

The *EVEREST II trial* randomly allocated 279 patients with grade 3+ or 4+ MR in a 2:1 ratio to either TEER with

MitraClip or surgical repair or replacement. The primary composite efficacy endpoint of freedom from death, MV surgery and no residual grade 3+ or 4+ MR at 12 months occurred in 55% of the patients in MitraClip arm and 73% in surgical arm ($p = 0.007$). The safety outcomes of major adverse events occurred in 15% of the patients in MitraClip group and 48% in the surgical group ($p < 0.001$). There was greater reduction in MR severity in the surgical group compared to the device group. 23 patients in the device arm underwent surgery for persistent 3+ or 4+ MR. These promising outcomes led to the Food and Drug Administration (FDA) approval of the device in selected patients with primary MR.[6]

Secondary Mitral Regurgitation

Two randomized trials evaluated the superiority of TEER with MitraClip in addition to guideline-directed medical treatment (GDMT) compared to GDMT alone in patients with secondary MR.

The *COAPT* [Cardiovascular Outcomes Assessment of the MitraClip Percutaneous Therapy for heart failure patients with functional (secondary) mitral regurgitation] trial randomly assigned 614 patients with moderate-to-severe or severe secondary MR with the New York Heart Association (NYHA) class III or IV symptoms despite maximum tolerated GDMT and/or cardiac resynchronization therapy when indicated between TEER with MitraClip in addition to GDMT (no = 302) and GDMT alone (no = 312). The device was successfully implanted in 98% of the patients and MR was ≤2+ in 95% of them at the time of discharge. The 30-day mortality and stroke rates were 2.3% and 0.7%, respectively. The primary efficacy endpoint of hospitalizations for HF within the 24 months follow-up was significantly lower in the device group [35.8% vs. 67.9% per patient year, hazard ratio (HR) 0.53; 95% confidence interval (CI) 0.40–0.70; $p < 0.001$]. Death from any cause within 24 months was significantly lower in the device arm (29.1% vs. 46.1%, HR, 0.62; 95% CI, 0.46–0.72; $p < 0.001$). The device-related adverse events occurred in 1.4% of the patients and all occurred within the first 30 days.[7] At 5-year follow-up, the annualized HF-related hospitalization rate remained lower in the device group (33.1% vs. 57.2%, HR 0.53; 95% CI 0.41–0.68). All-cause mortality was significantly lower in the device group (57.3% vs. 67.2%, HR 0.72; 95% CI 0.58–0.89). There were no additional device-related events during this period.[8]

The *MITRA-FR* (Percutaneous Repair with the MitraClip Device for Severe Functional/Secondary Mitral Regurgitation) trial randomly assigned 304 patients with HF with reduced ejection fraction [left ventricular ejection fraction (LVEF) between 15 and 40%] and severe secondary MR [effective regurgitant orifice area (EROA) > 20 mm^2 or regurgitant volume (RV) > 30 mL] between TEER with MitraClip in addition to medical treatment (intervention group, $n = 152$) and medical treatment alone (control group, $n = 152$). The primary composite outcome of death from any cause or unplanned hospitalization for HF was not significantly different between the intervention and the control groups (54.6% vs. 51.3%, odds ratio 1.16; 95% CI 0.73–1.84; $p = 0.53$). Similarly, there was no difference in individual endpoints of the rate of death from any cause (24.3% vs. 22.4%, HR 1.11; 95% CI 0.69–1.77) and unplanned hospitalization for HF (48.7% vs. 47.4%, HR 1.13; 95% CI 0.81–1.56).[9]

The difference in the outcomes between the earlier mentioned trials were attributed to inclusion of patients in the MITRA-FR trial with advanced LV damage (LVEDV–MITRA-FR: 135 ± 35 mL/m^2 vs. COAPT: 101 ± 34 mL/m^2 and EF–MITRA-FR: 15–40% vs. COAPT: 20–50%) and less severe MR (EROA–MITRA-FR: EROA: 31 ± 10 mm^2 vs. COAPT: 41 ± 15 mm^2) compared to COAPT.[10]

The earlier mentioned observations reinforce the necessity to provide TEER at an early stage in patients with secondary MR to prevent advanced myocardial damage and poor outcomes. Based on the outcomes of these trials, FDA approved MitraClip for patients with secondary MR meeting COAPT criteria.

Newer-generation Devices

Newer-generation devices were introduced recently that expanded TEER to more complex anatomies. Two registries evaluated the outcomes of TEER with these devices.

EXPAND: The EXPAND study is a contemporary, real world, prospective, single arm registry of TEER with *third-generation MitraClip NTR/XTR* system. It enrolled 1,040 patients with primary and secondary MR and 18% of them had complex MV anatomy (non-EVEREST). The device was successfully implanted in 98.9% of the patients and the procedural success was achieved in 95.8% of the patients. There was significant reduction in MR severity compared to the baseline, with 97.5% and 87.2% of the patients achieving ≤2+ and ≤1+ MR, respectively at 1 year. There was substantial improvement in the functional capacity and quality of life compared to baseline, with 80.3% of patients were in NYHA class I or II functional status and +21.6-point improvement in Kansas City Cardiomyopathy Questionnaire summary scores, at 1 year. All-cause mortality and HF admissions occurred in 14.9% and 18.9% of the patients, respectively at 1 year.[11]

EXPAND G4: EXPAND G4 is a prospective, multicenter, single arm, postapproval real-world registry with MitraClip G4 device. 1,141 patients with primary and secondary MR were included in the study. MitraClip was implanted in 98% of the participants and the procedural success rate was 96%. More than one clip was implanted in 35% of the patients. There was significant reduction in MR severity compared to the baseline, with 98% and 91% of the patients achieving MR ≤ 2+ and ≤ 1+ MR, respectively at 30 days.

There was substantial improvement in the functional capacity and quality of life compared to baseline, with 83% of patients were in NYHA class I or II functional status and 18-point improvement in Kansas City Cardiomyopathy Questionnaire summary scores, respectively at 30 days. The major adverse cardiovascular event and all cause death rates were 2.7% and 1.3%, respectively at 30 days.[12]

MitraClip G4 System

The following discussion addresses the important components of the MitraClip device **(Fig. 1)**. *Steerable guide catheter (SGC)* is 80 cm in length and 25 Fr at the proximal end that tapers to 23 Fr at the distal end. It has a handle at the proximal end with a (+/–) knob. Rotation of the knob in the "+" direction increases the distal curve and "–" direction straightens the distal curve. Counter-clockwise direction of the handle moves the catheter anteriorly and clockwise rotation moves it posteriorly.

Clip delivery system (CDS) is made up of two components: (1) steerable sleeve (SS) and (2) delivery catheter (DC).

- *SS*: It has two knobs mounted on the handle—the "M" knob and "A/P" Knob. "M" knob helps in deflecting the clip toward the MV to achieve perpendicularity. "A/P" knob rotation in "A" direction moves the catheter anterior and lateral and "P" direction moves the catheter posterior and medial.
- *DC*: Advancing and retracting the DC handle helps in advancing the clip below the MV leaflets and grasping the leaflets, respectively. Handle rotation helps in orienting the clip to the mitral leaflets. The gripper lever helps in raising and lowering the gripper. Gripper lever in G4 allows simultaneous and independent leaflet grasping. One of the gripper levers is indicated with a tactile marker to facilitate its easy identification during the procedure.
- *Clip*: The clip is mounted at the distal end of the DC. It is a cobalt chromium device with two arms and covered with Dacron. The clip in the G4 system comes in four sizes with two clip arm lengths (9 mm for NT/NTW and 12 mm for XT/XTW) and two widths (4 mm for NT/XT and 6 mm for NTW/XTW).[13,14]

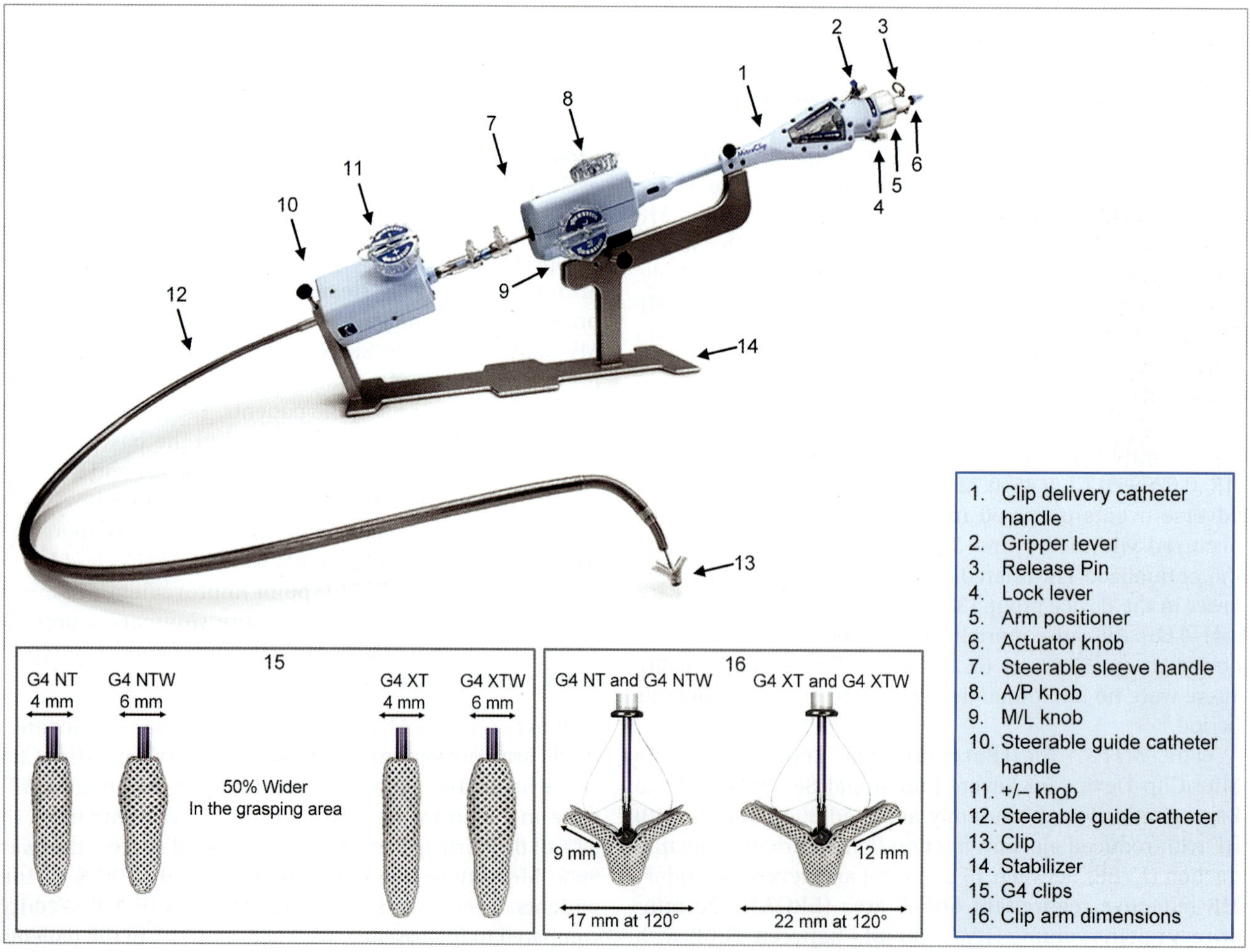

FIG. 1: MitraClip G4 system with components.
Courtesy: Abbott Vascular.

MitraClip PROCEDURE

Transesophageal echocardiographic (TEE) assessment of the MV is crucial prior to, during and post deployment of MitraClip. Although, TEE imaging could be performed only during device deployment, it is useful to know the details of the MV morphology and mechanism of regurgitation, MV mean gradient, MV area, atrial septal morphology, and pericardial effusion prior to making the decision **(Figs. 2A and B)**. Once the patient is under anesthesia, reconfirming the findings that were noticed in the preprocedure TEE and the underlying mechanism of regurgitation is very important.

The lift is positioned 80 cm from the center of the heart and then sterile preparation is performed.

MitraClip is a transfemoral venous procedure. The right femoral venous access is accomplished under the guidance of both fluoroscopy and ultrasound using a 4 Fr micro-puncture system. It is then preclosed using single ProGlide suture. Once vascular access is established, half or full dose of heparin is administered to prevent thrombus formation.

Transseptal Access

Transcatheter edge-to-edge repair mandates a pathology specific transseptal puncture (TSP). The TSP is obtained with TEE and fluoroscopic guidance. An ideal TSP is one that positions CDS above the valve ensuring optimal trajectory and height for leaflet grasping. There are three basic TEE views that guide TSP. The bicaval view provides information on the position of transseptal sheath/needle assembly (TSA) in superior-inferior direction. Under real-time TEE imaging, TSA is brought into right atrium (RA) till it arrives at mid fossa level. The TEE probe is rotated to aortic short-axis view to delineate the location of the TSA in the anterior-posterior dimension. The catheter is rotated clockwise in this view to obtain a more posterior position in the fossa. The next step is to assess the transseptal height above the mitral annular plane in the four-chamber view. A height of 4–4.5 cm and 3.5–4 cm is recommended for primary and secondary MR, respectively **(Figs. 3A to C)**. Once the position is confirmed in all the three views, the needle is advanced across the septum in the aortic short-axis view, and the dilator/sheath assembly is then advanced over the needle into LA. The patient is fully heparinized and activated clotting time is maintained at 250–300 seconds throughout the procedure.[15]

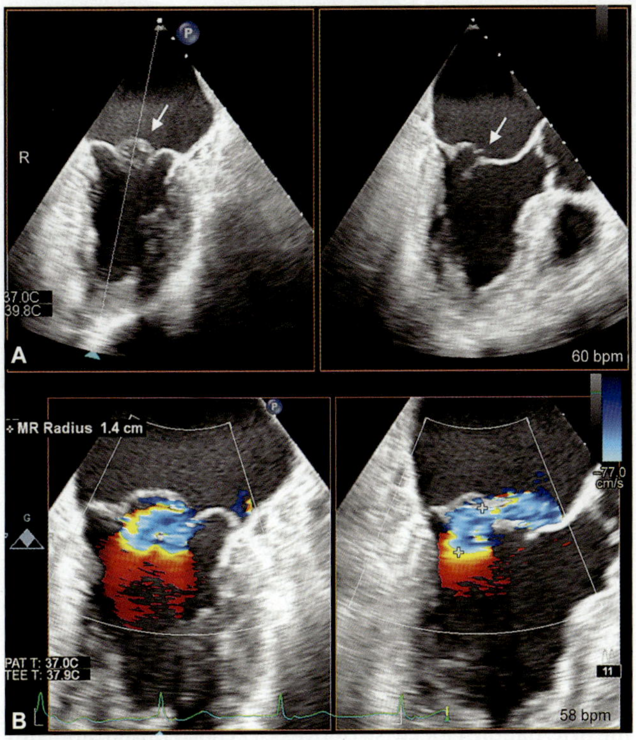

FIGS. 2A AND B: Simultaneous biplane transesophageal echocardiographic image showing flail P2 segment (arrow) of the posterior mitral leaflet (A) with severe mitral regurgitation (B).

Introducing Steerable Guide Catheter into Left Atrium

Once TSP is accomplished, the needle and dilator are removed. Two 0.035" Amplatz Super Stiff wires are advanced through the transseptal sheath into LA and positioned inside the left upper pulmonary vein. A 4 Fr pig tail is positioned in LA over one of the wires for continuous monitoring of LA pressure. The femoral access is then predilated over the other wire with a 22 Fr Cook dilator. The SGC tip is straightened by applying "–" to "+/–" knob and advanced over the second wire into RA. Once SGC enters the RA, SGC tip curve is brought back to neutral position. The SCG is then advanced across the septum into LA for 2–3 cm under continuous TEE guidance **(Fig. 4A)**. After placing the SGC in the LA, the silicone pad is positioned on the lift over the sterile drape and stabilizer is placed onto it. The SCG is then secured in the stabilizer using the fastener. The dilator and guidewire are then removed together while maintaining continuous aspiration to the side arm with a 50 cc syringe.

Clip Delivery System Insertion into the Steerable Guide Catheter

Once the SGC is in optimal position in the LA, the preloaded clip introducer is advanced into the hemostasis valve of the SCG in a continuous motion while the second operator freely and continuously irrigates the hemostasis valve with heparinized saline. The CDS is advanced till the clip is visualized distal to the hemostasis valve and the blue alignment marker on the SGC is then lined up with the corresponding one on the CDS sleeve (keying). The CDS is advanced to the tip of the SCG under fluoroscopy and then into LA under fluoroscopic and TEE guidance till the RO markers on the CDS are aligned on either side of the SGC tip RO marker (straddling) while keeping the clip away from the LA wall all the time. When the space in the LA

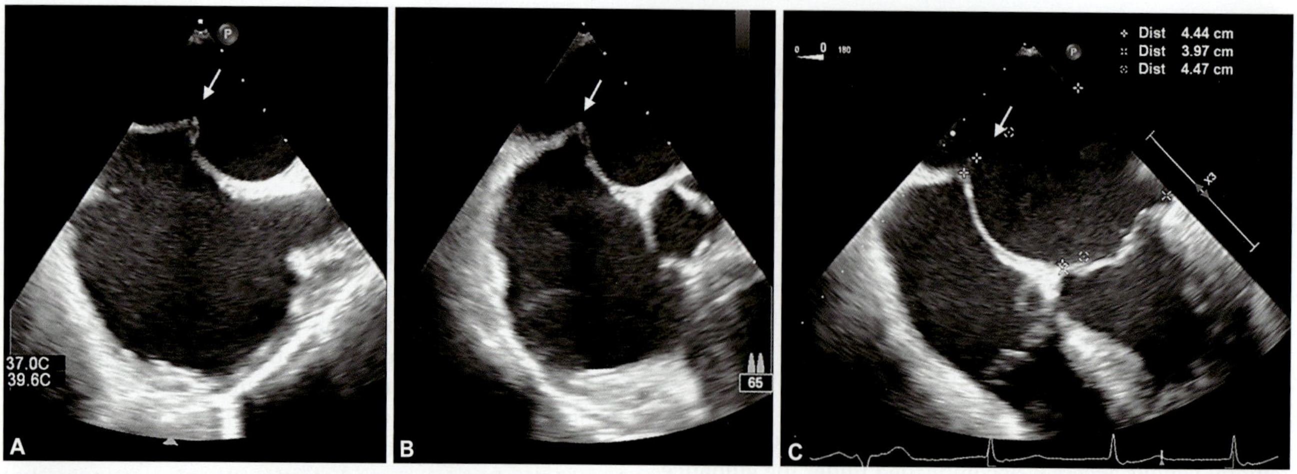

FIGS. 3A TO C: Transesophageal echocardiographic images showing position of the transseptal needle (arrow) in bicaval (A), aortic short axis (B), and four-chamber views (C) in a mid-posterior position at optimal height above the annulus.

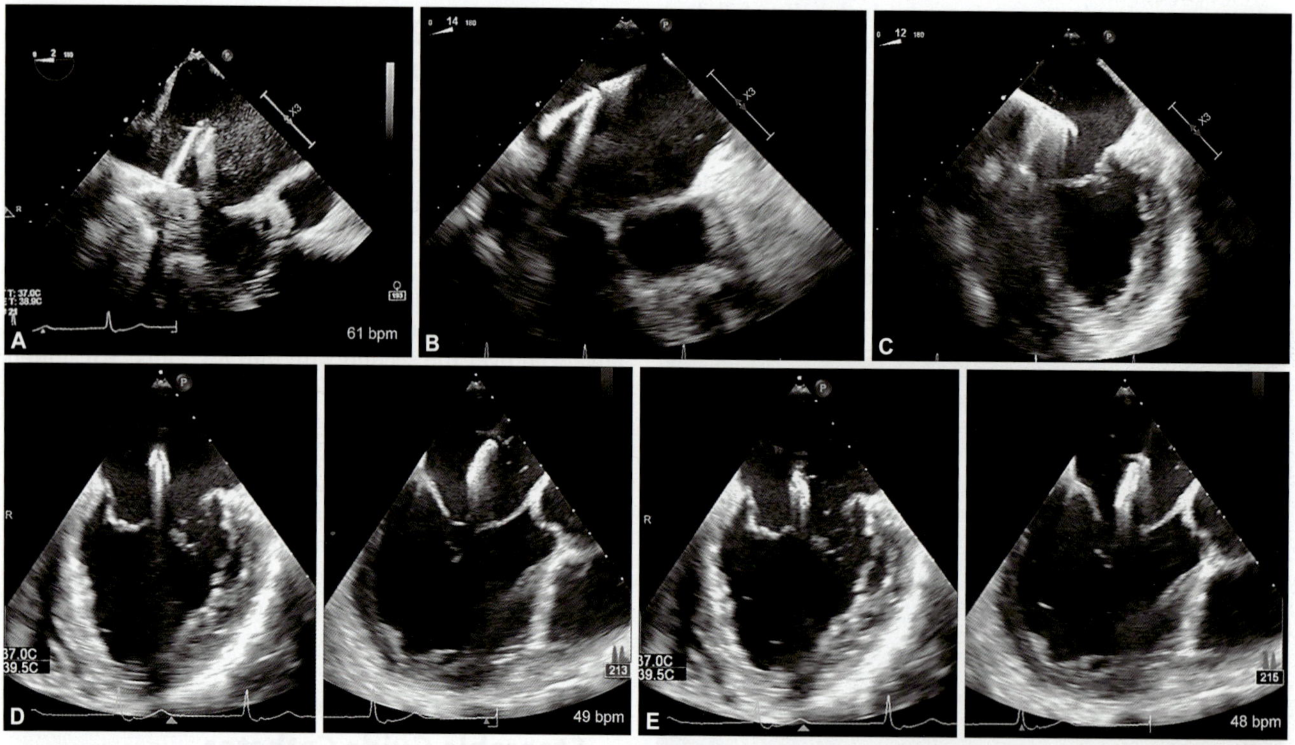

FIGS. 4A TO E: Transesophageal echocardiographic images showing (A) steerable guide catheter in left atrium (LA); (B to E) maneuvering of the clip to a perpendicular position above the mitral valve.

is limited to achieve optimal straddling, additional space can be created by withdrawing the SCG, counterclockwise rotation of the SGC handle, by applying "+" to "+/–" knob and by applying "M" before straddling **(Fig. 4B)**. Once the CDS is in the straddled position, the "M" knob is applied to deflect the clip toward the MV.

Left Atrial Steering

The aim of LA steering is to achieve optimal clip position, trajectory, and orientation above the valve before entering the LV **(Figs. 4C to E)**. The position should be perpendicular to the annular plane and the trajectory toward the apex in both anteroposterior and medial-lateral directions. Advanced steering maneuvers are necessary when the position or trajectory is suboptimal. When the clip is at or below the valve after applying the medical deflection (inadequate height), additional height is gained by torquing the SGC handle clockwise (moves CDS posteriorly), applying A knob (moves CDS anteriorly and laterally) and adding M knob (corrects the lateral movement). When the CDS length is inadequate to advance below the valve (excessive height), height is eased by torquing the SGC handle counterclockwise (moves CDS anteriorly), applying P knob (moves CDS posteriorly and medially) and releasing M knob (corrects the medial movement). When there is loss of perpendicularity in anteroposterior direction and the trajectory is anterior to posterior (aorta hugger), it is corrected by adding "+" knob (moves CDS posteriorly and medially), torquing the SCG counterclockwise (corrects posterior movement) and releasing "M" (corrects lateral movement).[16]

After achieving optimal trajectory, the next step is orienting the clip arms perpendicular to coaptation line at the site of the pathology in 3D enface view from LA perspective. The clip arms are opened to 180°, and the DC handle is rotated to align the arms perpendicular to coaptation line at the site of the pathology. The orientation is 12 o'clock–6 o'clock, 1 o'clock–7 o'clock, and 11 o'clock–5 o'clock in central, lateral, and medial pathologies, respectively. The optimal clip alignment is confirmed by clip arms superimposed on one another in the bicommissural view and visible at equal lengths in the left ventricular outflow tract (LVOT) view. The gripper with tactile marker is then identified on TEE by unlatching the gripper levers and lowering the gripper with tactile marker. The grippers are raised and latched back. Finally, the clip arms are closed, and the clip arm parallax is removed in right anterior oblique with caudal or cranial C-arm angulation.[17]

Left Ventricular Entry and Leaflet Grasping

The CDS is then advanced slowly into the LV while continuously monitoring the trajectory, and orientation with both TEE (simultaneous LVOT and bicommissural views) and fluoroscopy. Once the clip is under the leaflets, the arms are opened to 120° and the orientation is reassessed using 3D enface view on TEE. The DC handle is gradually retracted until both the leaflets rest on the clip arms during both systole and diastole. The grippers are then lowered and the clip arms are closed to 60° and locked. Adequacy of leaflet insertion is carefully assessed by live TEE in simultaneous bicommissural and LVOT views as well as gradual panning of the leaflets medial to lateral **(Figs. 5A to D)**.

Assessment of Leaflet Insertion

Leaflet insertion must be assessed in multiple TEE views. In the bicommissural view, leaflet segments should enter at the same level on either side of the clip. In the LVOT biplane view through the clip, the leaflets should be inserted to the base of the "V" between the gripper and clip arms with

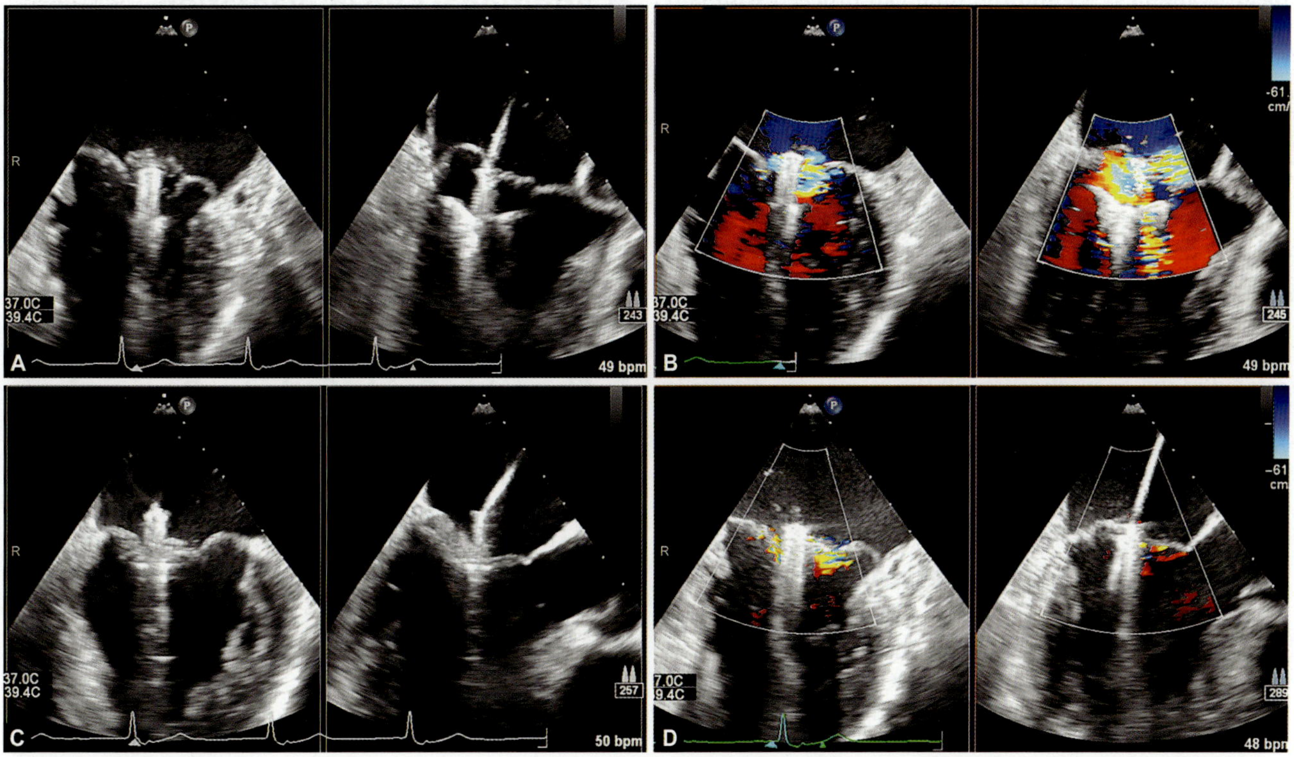

FIGS. 5A TO D: Transesophageal echocardiographic images showing maneuvers into the left ventricle (LV) leading to leaflet capture.

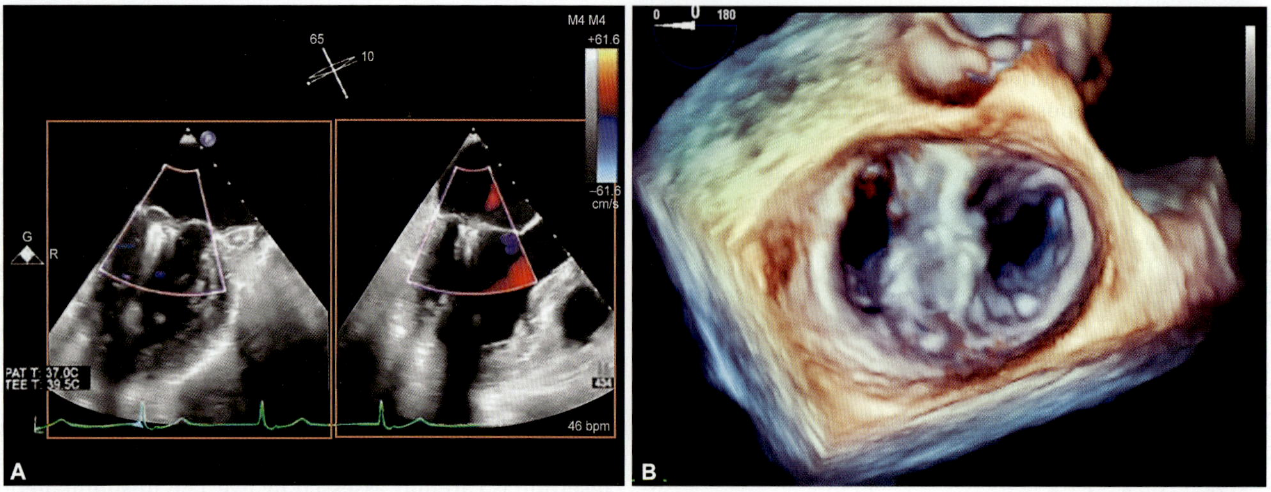

FIGS. 6A AND B: Transesophageal echocardiographic images post clip deployment showing mild residual mitral regurgitation (A). 3D echocardiography showing the double orifice and tissue bridge (B).

minimal leaflet motion. In the 3D enface view, the clip should be perpendicular to the line of coaptation and not rotated or biased toward one of the leaflets. In addition, there should be a "good tissue bridge" **(Figs. 6A and B)**. Once the leaflet insertion is satisfactory, the clip is fully closed and then Doppler assessment is performed for residual MR and MV gradient. If the residual MR grade is ≤1+ and MV mean gradient is <5 mm Hg, then can proceed with clip deployment. MR reduction may be further evidenced by normalization of pulmonary vein flow and reduction in V wave height and mean LA pressure.

Clip Deployment

The clip deployment in G4 system involves a five-step process: (1) *Establishing final arm angle:* An attempt is made to open the clip when it is locked. The clip should remain stable and should not open >5°; (2) *Removing the lock line;* (3) *Re-establishing the final arm angle*; (4) *Removing the release pin;* (5) *Clip deployment:* The arm positioner is rotated in the open direction till the release pin groove is fully exposed. The actuator knob is then unthreaded by rotating it in counterclockwise direction for approximately eight turns and pulled back for approximately 0.5 cm. Finally, gripper levers are fully retracted, and the clip is deployed.

Removing the Clip Delivery System

After the clip deployment, the DC fastener is released, and the DC handle is slowly retracted until the RO ring approximates the RO ring of the SS. The DC fastener is secured again. Under continuous TEE monitoring, the CDS is slowly retracted back into the SGC while releasing the deflections on the "M" the "+/–" knobs. The CDS is then removed from the SGC while gently aspirating the side port with a 50 cc syringe. The removal of CDS is continuously monitored by TEE with bicommissural and LVOT views to make sure that the tip is in the body of the LA to avoid inadvertent injury to the LA or aortic root until it is safely secured within the SGC.

Additional Clip Implantation

The choice of the second clip is based on the width of the residual MR, the MV gradient, and the intended location of the second clip. A wide clip is favored in case of larger valve area, smaller MV gradient, and a wider residual jet. A narrow clip is implanted otherwise. The second clip is implanted closer to the first clip to prevent residual jet in between the clips, and for optimal valve gradient. The second clip should be in a closed position before advancing it into the LV and the trajectory should be continuously monitored under both fluoroscopy and TEE.

Steerable Guide Catheter Removal and Access Closure

Once the procedure is completed, SGC is retracted into the RA. The distal curve is straightened applying "–" to the "+/–" knob. The SGC is then removed from the femoral vein and hemostasis achieved by tightening the sutures of the ProGlide deployed at the beginning the procedure or by figure of "8" suture.

COMPLICATIONS

MitraClip is a transvenous procedure performed under continuous TEE monitoring and complications are relatively uncommon compared to arterial procedures, such as transcatheter aortic valve implantation. The adverse events may be related to either the transseptal access (perforation/tamponade, air embolism, and thrombosis) or specific to the MitraClip procedure.[18] The following discussion focuses on the complications specific to the MitraClip procedure.

Single-leaflet Device Detachment

Detachment of one of the leaflets from the device occurs in 1.5–4.8% of TEER procedures. It often occurs either during the procedure or in the first few days after the procedure and late detachment is uncommon. It commonly results from inadequate leaflet insertion or device related leaflet injury. It is recognized on echocardiography by complete detachment of the device from one of the leaflets, new excessive leaflet mobility, MR through the device-leaflet interface and absence of diastolic tissue bridge. Single-leaflet detachment (SLD) is treated by implanting additional clips alongside the detached clip. In case of severe leaflet injury, it requires surgical removal of the clip followed by MV replacement.[19,20]

Device Embolization

Device embolization is a very rare complication and often occurs during the procedure. The embolized device either remains inside the left heart chambers or lodges in one of the major peripheral arteries. It often occurs due to SLD with unstable device or failure of the locking mechanism.[21] The management depends on the location of the embolized device. Device retrieval requires large bore access (16 Fr) and larger sized snare catheters (25–30 mm). Two snare techniques with first snare capturing the device and the second snare favorably orienting it for retrieving it into the sheath is more efficient than the one snare technique. If the embolization is into the LA, retrieval may be attempted through the SCG. In rare instances where percutaneous retrieval is unsuccessful, surgical removal may be considered.[19]

Chordal Entanglement

Chordal entrapment is an uncommon complication of the MitraClip procedure, resulting from excessive manipulation of the clip inside the ventricle, particularly in the commissural position. It is recognized by the lack of transmission of the CDS handle manipulations to the device on TEE and fluoroscopy. Once recognized, further manipulations should be stopped and the maneuvers that preceded the entanglement are reversed to release the clip. If unsuccessful, the clip arms are everted, and the clip is slowly retracted to the LA. If there is resistance to this movement, the device is readvanced, gently rotated, jiggled, grippers are raised and lowered, and retracted back again. If all these maneuvers fail, the clip may be deployed in the subvalvular apparatus.[19]

Iatrogenic Atrial Septal Defect

Persistent atrial septal defect (ASD) is common following TEER and occurs in about one-fourth of the patients. ASD closure may be considered in the presence of large defect (>10 mm), predominant right to left shunt with hypoxemia, severe right ventricular dysfunction, severe tricuspid regurgitation, and severe pulmonary arterial hypertension. Device closure can be performed through the SGC by using Amplatzer septal occluder. Device is sized 1–2 mm larger than the maximum color flow Doppler width.[22]

CONCLUSION

Transcatheter edge-to-edge repair is a breakthrough in the treatment of high-risk patients with moderate-to-severe or severe MR both primary and secondary MR. It reduces HF hospitalizations and mortality in patients with secondary MR that is sustained over 5 years. Newer device iterations have extended TEER to more complex anatomies. Understanding the device technology, adapting optimal procedure techniques, and timely recognition and treatment of complications improve procedure outcomes.

ONLINE REFERENCES

Please scan the QR code provided at the end of the table of contents for References of this chapter.

CHAPTER

103

Global Longitudinal Strain Assessment by Speckle Tracking Echocardiography in Clinical Practice: How Much Hype? Technical and Acoustic Window Limitations

Manish Bansal, Ravi R Kasliwal, HK Chopra

ABSTRACT

Left ventricular (LV) global longitudinal strain (GLS) measured using speckle-tracking echocardiography has emerged as a useful parameter for assessing LV systolic function. Compared with LV ejection fraction (LVEF), LVGLS offers several advantages. It has much better reproducibility, can detect early myocardial dysfunction when LVEF is still within the normal limits, and has a strong prognostic value which is independent of and superior to that of LVEF. For these reasons, LVGLS has been proposed as a tool for guiding management in many cardiac conditions, especially for patients receiving potentially cardiotoxic cancer chemotherapy and those with valvular heart diseases. However, despite robust data showing the utility of LVGLS, there are important limitations. Accurate LVGLS estimation is dependent on grayscale image quality and careful attention to technical aspects during image analysis. Like LVEF, LVGLS is also dependent on loading conditions. The GLS measurements also vary according to the software used for image analysis, although this measurement variability has now decreased substantially. And most importantly, outcome studies showing the benefit of GLS-guided management are currently lacking.

Keywords: Left ventricular systolic function, myocardial deformation, subclinical left ventricular systolic dysfunction.

INTRODUCTION

Accurate assessment of myocardial contractile function, especially, that of the left ventricle, has been one of the important goals of echocardiography since the inception of this modality. Several different tools/parameters have been developed to achieve this objective, including fractional shortening, centerline approach, acoustic quantification, mitral annular plane systolic excursion, left ventricular ejection fraction (LVEF), and tissue Doppler imaging. Of these, LVEF, estimated using the biplane Simpson's method, is the most validated and used parameter for this purpose and is the one recommended by the guidelines.[1] Extensive clinical and research experience has established LVEF as the preferred echocardiographic measure of left ventricular (LV) systolic function.

Despite the well-established clinical utility of LVEF, it has several limitations which are also well recognized.[2] First, LVEF only represents fractional LV volume change during systole and is not a true measure of myocardial contractility. Second, being a global parameter, it is not sensitive enough to detect subtle changes in the LV contractile performance which may have significant prognostic implications. Third, LV myocardial contraction is a complex, multi-directional deformation process. LVEF, unfortunately, represents an oversimplification of the same. Lastly, LVEF estimation by echocardiography has significant measurement variability.[3,4] Three-dimensional (3D) echocardiography minimizes this variability but requires considerable technical expertise and very good quality images.

Over the last two decades, strain imaging using speckle-tracking echocardiography has emerged as a useful modality for the assessment of myocardial contractile function. Strain represents the percent change in the length of a myocardial segment during a given phase of the cardiac cycle. For the left ventricle, myocardial deformation can be quantified in different directions as longitudinal strain, circumferential strain, radial strain, rotation, twist, and torsion.[5] Of these, longitudinal strain is clinically the most useful. Since the left ventricle shortens during systole, longitudinal strain is denoted with a negative sign. The average longitudinal strain of all the LV myocardial segments is known as LV global longitudinal strain (GLS) and is the one most used in clinical practice. This chapter provides an overview of its clinical utility while also discussing the challenges in its use.

ADVANTAGES OF LEFT VENTRICULAR GLOBAL LONGITUDINAL STRAIN

As a measure of LV contractile function, LVGLS has three main advantages over LVEF.

Sensitive to Subtle Changes in Contractile Function

Left ventricular myocardium is composed of multiple layers of myofibers. The fibers arranged in the subendocardial layer are aligned relatively parallel to the LV long-axis and govern mainly the long-axis shortening of the left ventricle. In contrast, the fibers in the middle and subepicardial layers are arranged more horizontally and obliquely and thus govern mainly the short-axis deformation (circumferential shortening, radial thickening, and rotation).[5,6]

The subendocardial layer of the LV myocardium is the most susceptible to injury because of its poorer blood supply and exposure to high intracavitary pressures. As a result, in most of the LV myocardial diseases, the subendocardial layer is affected first resulting in impairment of LV longitudinal deformation. During the initial stages, LV short-axis deformation remains unaffected or may even be exaggerated to compensate for the loss of longitudinal deformation. As a result, the LVEF remains preserved despite significant LV myocardial injury. LVGLS is able to detect this subclinical LV systolic dysfunction and can also track subtle changes in the LV contractile function **(Figs. 1 and 2)**. This represents the greatest advantage of strain imaging at present. Notably, LVGLS has been shown to correlate well with the extent of LV myocardial fibrosis as assessed using cardiac magnetic resonance (CMR) imaging or histopathology.[7,8]

Excellent Reproducibility

Since LVGLS is the average of the longitudinal strain of all the different LV myocardial segments, any measurement variability at the segmental level gets nullified to a great extent, rendering LVGLS a reproducible measure of LV contraction. Several studies have shown that LVGLS is currently the most reproducible measurement of LV systolic function and has the best correlation with LEVF estimated using CMR.[4] 3D LVEF also has good reproducibility but is technically challenging compared to LVGLS estimation. Estimation of LVGLS is easy to perform, quick, and easy to learn.

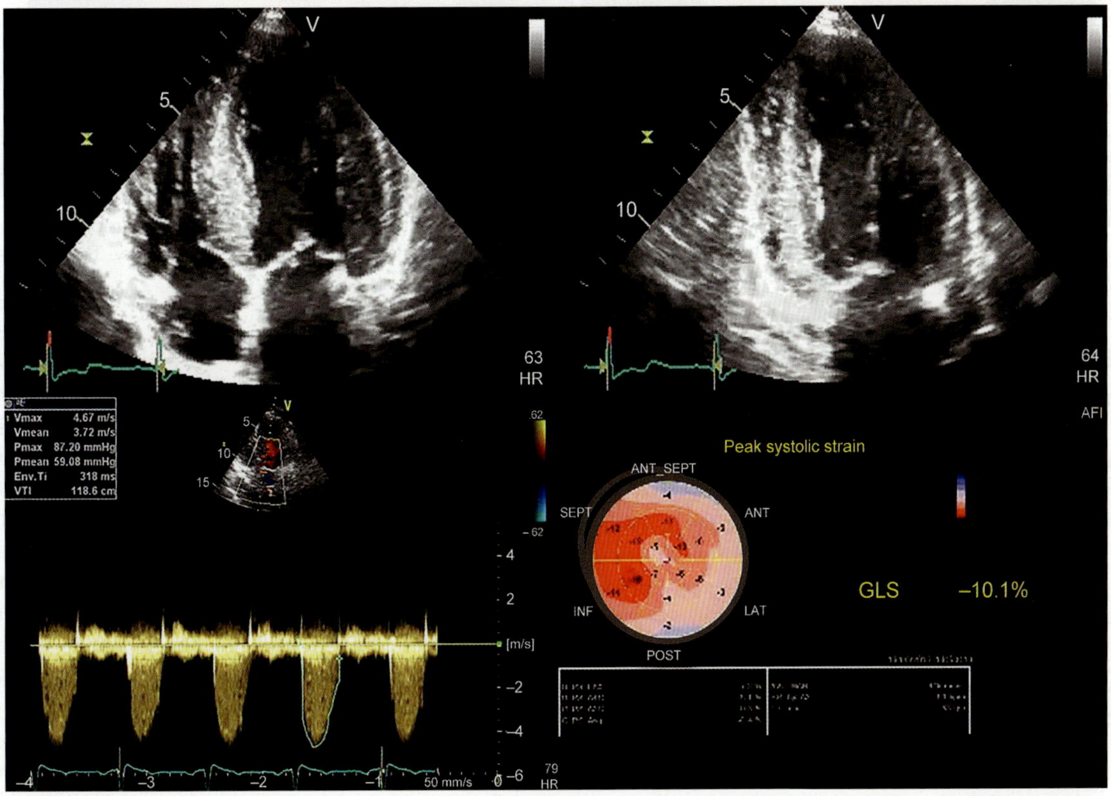

FIG. 1: Role of left ventricular global longitudinal strain (GLS) for detecting subclinical left ventricular systolic dysfunction in aortic stenosis. The images in the upper panel show hypertrophied left ventricle in a patient with severe aortic stenosis. The lower left panel shows significantly increased transaortic gradients (mean 59 mm Hg and peak 87 mm Hg). The lower right panel shows markedly reduced (–10.1%) left ventricular GLS even though the estimated left ventricular ejection fraction was 72%.

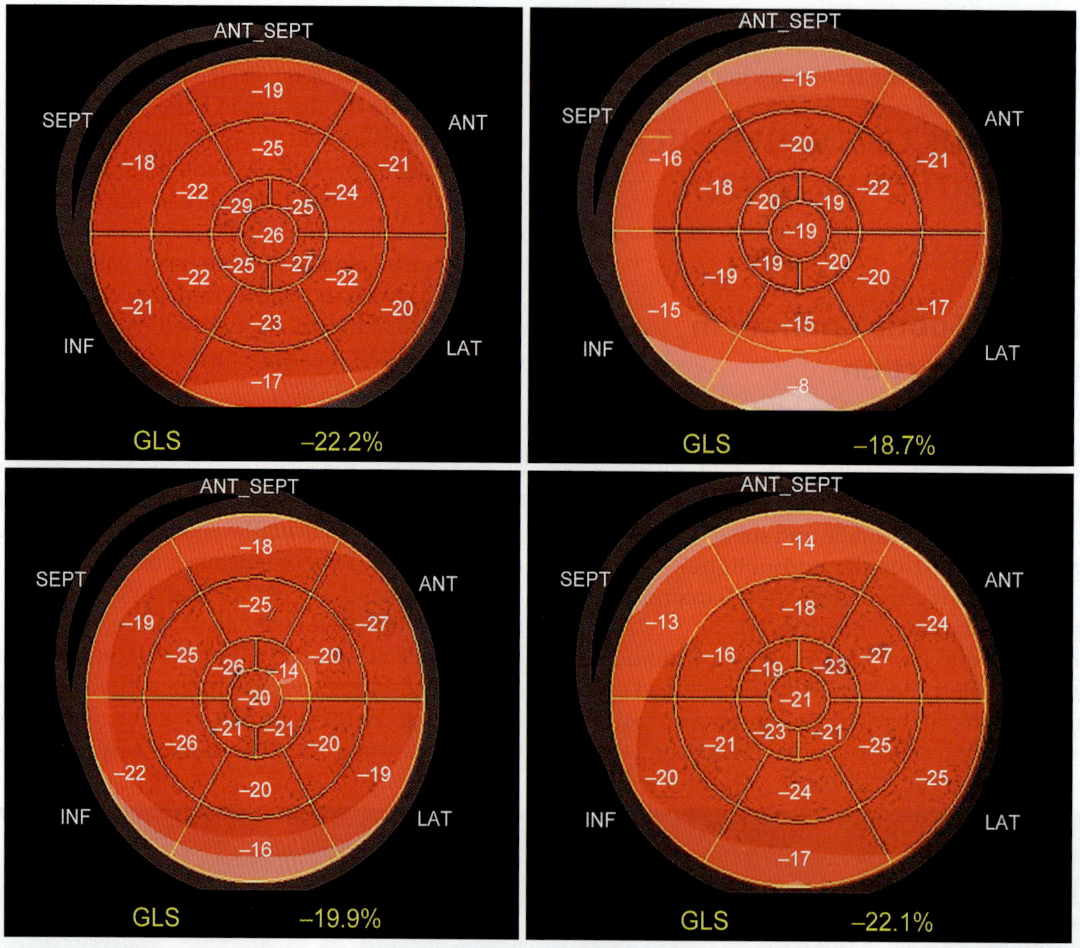

FIG. 2: The utility of left ventricular global longitudinal strain (GLS) in following up patients receiving potentially cardiotoxic cancer chemotherapies. Upper left-baseline image in a patient with breast cancer previously treated with epirubicin and now starting trastuzumab; upper right—3 months after initiation of trastuzumab. There is already a 15.8% relative reduction in GLS; lower left—3 months after addition of a beta-blocker while trastuzumab was also continued; lower right—at the completion of trastuzumab therapy. The left ventricular ejection fraction remained in the range of 60–62% throughout the course of therapy.

Excellent Prognostic Value

A large number of studies, as discussed subsequently, in different clinical settings have demonstrated that LVGLS is an excellent predictor of overall prognosis, regardless of the underlying disease entity. The prognostic value of LVGLS is incremental and often superior to LVEF. The ability of LVGLS to detect subclinical LV systolic dysfunction coupled with its excellent prognostic value renders LVGLS an excellent tool for clinical application.

CLINICAL UTILITY OF LEFT VENTRICULAR GLOBAL LONGITUDINAL STRAIN

Valvular Heart Diseases

Aortic stenosis (AS), aortic regurgitation (AR), and mitral regurgitation (MR) are valve lesions that are associated with increased LV pressure and/or volume overload. When sustained for long periods, such pressure/volume overload results in chronic myocardial injury with progressive myocardial fibrosis. The presence of LV myocardial fibrosis is associated with adverse prognosis over the long term. Once replacement fibrosis occurs, it is usually not reversible and leads to permanently impaired LV contractile function and an increased risk for heart failure and overall mortality.

Currently, there are mainly two indications for surgical intervention in AS, AR, and MR-development of symptoms and a fall in LVEF. For AS and AR, a threshold of LVEF <50% is recommended for surgical intervention, whereas for MR, the cut-off value is <60%. However, it is well-recognized that the development of symptoms or a reduction in LVEF are very late events in the natural history of these valve lesions and occur when a significant amount of LV myocardial fibrosis has already occurred **(Fig. 1)**. Intervening at this stage is already too late and is associated with worse clinical outcomes compared to when intervened at an earlier stage.[9]

Left ventricular GLS, given its ability to detect subclinical LV systolic dysfunction, has emerged as an excellent tool to indicate the appropriate timing for intervention in these valve lesions. Preoperative LVGLS has been shown to correlate with the extent of LV myocardial fibrosis, postoperative LVEF and LV remodeling, and clinical outcomes (with or without surgical intervention) in these patients.[7,10-14]

Ng et al. studied 294 patients with severe AS, who were followed up for all-cause mortality. It was found that the patients with reduced LVGLS but preserved LVEF (LVEF >55%) had the same mortality risk as those with reduced LVEF.[10] A similar finding has been reported in many other studies showing the value of LVGLS in predicting mortality in patients with severe AS. A meta-analysis of 10 such studies was performed.[11] Overall, 1,067 patients with severe asymptomatic AS with preserved LVEF (LVEF >50%) were included. The mean indexed aortic valve area was 0.49 ± 0.17 cm^2/m^2 and the mean LVEF was 63.5 ± 8% with 65% of the subjects having LVEF above 60%. The median LVGLS was –16.2%. All-cause mortality was the primary endpoint. It was found that LVGLS, and not LVEF, was a predictor of all-cause mortality over a 2-year follow-up. An LVGLS value below –14.7% (i.e., less negative than –14.7%) had the best ability to predict the increased mortality risk.[11]

Similar data is available for AR and MR also. LVGLS predicts postoperative LVEF in these patients and also correlates with the clinical outcomes. Alashi et al. studied 1,063 asymptomatic patients with 3–4+ chronic AR, preserved LVEF (>50%), and indexed LV end-systolic diameter <2.5 cm/m^2. Of these, 671 patients (63%) underwent aortic valve replacement at a median of 42 days after the initial evaluation. A baseline LVGLS cut-off value of –19% identified the individuals at increased risk of mortality during the follow-up. The patients with LVGLS above the median value had similar clinical outcomes regardless of whether they were treated medically or surgically. However, among those with LVGLS below the median, the outcomes were much worse if surgery was not performed.[14] Identical findings were reported in another study which included 737 consecutive asymptomatic patients with >3+ primary myxomatous MR, indexed LV end-diastolic dimension <3.3 cm/m^2, absolute LV end-systolic dimension <4 cm, and LVEF >60%. However, in this study, the LVGLS cut-off associated with a worse prognosis was comparatively higher (–21%), reflecting the effect of reduced LV afterload in MR.[13]

Left ventricular GLS is also helpful in gaining insights into the pathophysiology of various valve diseases. For example, reduced LVGLS implying subclinical LV dysfunction could be one of the mechanisms explaining low transvalvular gradients in patients with paradoxical low-flow, low-gradient severe AS.[15]

Patients Receiving Potentially Cardiotoxic Cancer Chemotherapies

Several chemotherapeutic agents such as anthracyclines, trastuzumab, and alkylating agents are associated with the risk of causing LV myocardial dysfunction, which is known as cancer therapy-related cardiac dysfunction (CTRCD). CTRCD is one of the most dreaded complications of cancer chemotherapy and is a major contributor to heart failure and mortality during and after chemotherapy. Hence, early recognition and prevention of CTRCD is an important goal of management in patients who are receiving chemotherapeutic agents with the potential to cause CTRCD. Timely intervention can prevent or reverse CTRCD, whereas delayed management can lead to irreversible myocardial injury.[16]

Left ventricular ejection fraction, for the reasons mentioned above, may not be the best method for early detection of CTRCD as the fall in LVEF occurs only when significant LV myocardial injury has already occurred. LVGLS could be a useful tool in this setting **(Fig. 2)**. In a study of 81 consecutive women receiving trastuzumab (37 were on anthracyclines also), the change in LVGLS during serial follow-up was the strongest predictor of CTRCD occurring subsequently. An 11% fall in GLS had 65% sensitivity and 94% specificity for predicting CTRCD.[17] Based on this and other similar studies, a 15% reduction in LVGLS from the baseline has been proposed as a predictor of subsequent CTRCD.[16] It has also been shown that among patients developing subclinical LV systolic dysfunction, treatment with cardioprotective agents such as beta-blockers may lead to functional recovery, highlighting the importance of timely identification of such individuals.[18]

Heart Failure

Left ventricular GLS has several important applications in heart failure (HF). Among patients with risk factors for developing HF, such as those with hypertension and/or diabetes, LVGLS is a good parameter to recognize stage B heart failure and predict adverse outcomes. It may also be a target for interventions aimed at the prevention of HF.[19-21]

Left ventricular GLS has special utility in patients with HF with preserved EF (HFpEF). A varying degree of impairment of LV diastolic dysfunction is the dominant pathological abnormality in HFpEF. However, nearly half of all patients with HFpEF have also been reported to have evidence of LV systolic dysfunction in the form of reduced LVGLS.[22] Recognition of this finding has led to the transition from the term "diastolic heart failure" to HFpEF. For the same reason, LVGLS has also been included as one of the echocardiographic criteria for diagnosing HFpEF.[23] Apart from the diagnostic value, LVGLS also has prognostic and therapeutic implications in HFpEF. It has been shown that reduced LVGLS in HFpEF is an independent predictor of HF hospitalization, cardiovascular death, and the composite of the two.[22] In another study that followed up 4,312 patients with acute HF (1,969 with LVEF ≥40%), treatment with beta-blockers was associated with a lower risk of 5-year all-cause mortality if the LVGLS was impaired (below –14%). This benefit was seen regardless of whether LVEF was between 40 to 50% or >50%.[24]

Left ventricular GLS is also useful in HF with reduced EF (HFrEF). It is an independent predictor of clinical outcomes in HFrEF with prognostic value even superior to that of LVEF.[25,26] In the aforementioned study involving acute HF patients, LVGLS was a stronger predictor of 5-year all-cause mortality than LVEF. It was associated with all-cause mortality in all three major EF subgroups, namely <40%, ≥40–<50%, and ≥50%.[26]

Cardiomyopathies

Cardiomyopathies are the primary diseases of the myocardium, excluding myocardial dysfunction due to ischemia, chronic valvular disease, hypertensive heart disease, and pulmonary heart disease. The major forms of cardiomyopathy include dilated cardiomyopathy, hypertrophic cardiomyopathy (HCM), restrictive cardiomyopathy (RCM), and arrhythmogenic cardiomyopathy.

Since cardiomyopathies are inherently diseases of the LV myocardium, LV myocardial dysfunction is a common finding in these conditions even if LVEF is normal (as in HCM and RCM). Thus, the presence of LV myocardial dysfunction is an important finding to differentiate these entities from conditions that could be phenotypically similar (e.g., hypertensive heart disease and athletes' heart mimicking HCM and constrictive pericarditis mimicking RCM). LVGLS is a useful parameter for this purpose.[2,27] Apart from its role in the differential diagnosis of cardiomyopathies, LVGLS can also help in identifying the underlying etiology in some of these conditions **(Fig. 3)**. For example, relative LV apical sparing or the so-called "cherry-on-top" appearance of the LVGLS bull's eye plot points toward the underlying possibility of cardiac amyloidosis.[28] In addition, just like other cardiac diseases, LVGLS is also a strong predictor of clinical outcomes in all forms of cardiomyopathy.[2,27]

Apart from the above, there are many other conditions in which LVGLS can be helpful in recognizing subclinical LV systolic dysfunction and assessing prognosis.[29] These include a wide variety of systemic diseases such as obesity, hypertension, diabetes, obstructive sleep apnea, viral infections such as dengue fever, and coronavirus disease 2019, connective tissue diseases such as systemic lupus erythematosus, hematological diseases such as thalassemia and sickle cell anemia, chronic liver disease, and chronic kidney disease.

LIMITATIONS OF LEFT VENTRICULAR GLOBAL LONGITUDINAL STRAIN

Despite several studies showing the clinical utility of LVGLS, there are some important limitations that need to be recognized.

Lack of Outcome Data

Although there are numerous studies that have shown that LVGLS is an excellent predictor of clinical outcomes and can help in selecting patients for various cardiac interventions, currently there is only one randomized clinical trial that has evaluated the merits of strain-guided management. This study—the Strain Surveillance of Chemotherapy for Improving Cardiovascular Outcomes (SUCCOUR)—compared the impact of strain-guided versus LVEF-guided management on the risk of developing CTRCD in patients receiving cancer chemotherapy.[30] Overall, 331 patients were enrolled, of whom 255 (77%, age 54 ± 12 years, 95% women) completed 3-year follow-up. Breast cancer was the most common cancer (93% of subjects) and anthracycline followed by trastuzumab was the most common chemotherapy regimen (84%). A greater number of patients in the GLS-guided arm received cardioprotective therapy (a beta-blocker with or without an angiotensin-converting enzyme inhibitor). However, at the end of the 3-year follow-up, there was no difference between the two groups in the delta LVEF or the overall incidence of CTRCD. This study has thus been a major disappointment but the overall low incidence of CTRCD in the study group appeared to be the major reason underlying the lack of benefit with the strain-guided management.

In patients with valvular heart disease, data from the observational studies is quite robust to suggest that impaired LVGLS could be used as an indication for referring patients for valvular intervention. However, validation in randomized studies is currently lacking, which is limiting the incorporation of LVGLS in the management guidelines. Similarly, LVGLS could also be helpful in guiding the pharmacological management of heart failure, cardiomyopathies, and some other cardiac conditions but this would also require evaluation in randomized clinical trials.

Image Quality Issues

Speckle-tracking echocardiography is a grayscale-based technique and hence, dependent on good image quality. It is essential to acquire good quality apical views (apical four-, two-, and three-chamber) with electrocardiographic gating for accurate estimation of LVGLS. The frame rate should be proper (preferably 40–80 frames per second), the endocardium should be clearly visible and there should not be any foreshortening or rib artifacts.

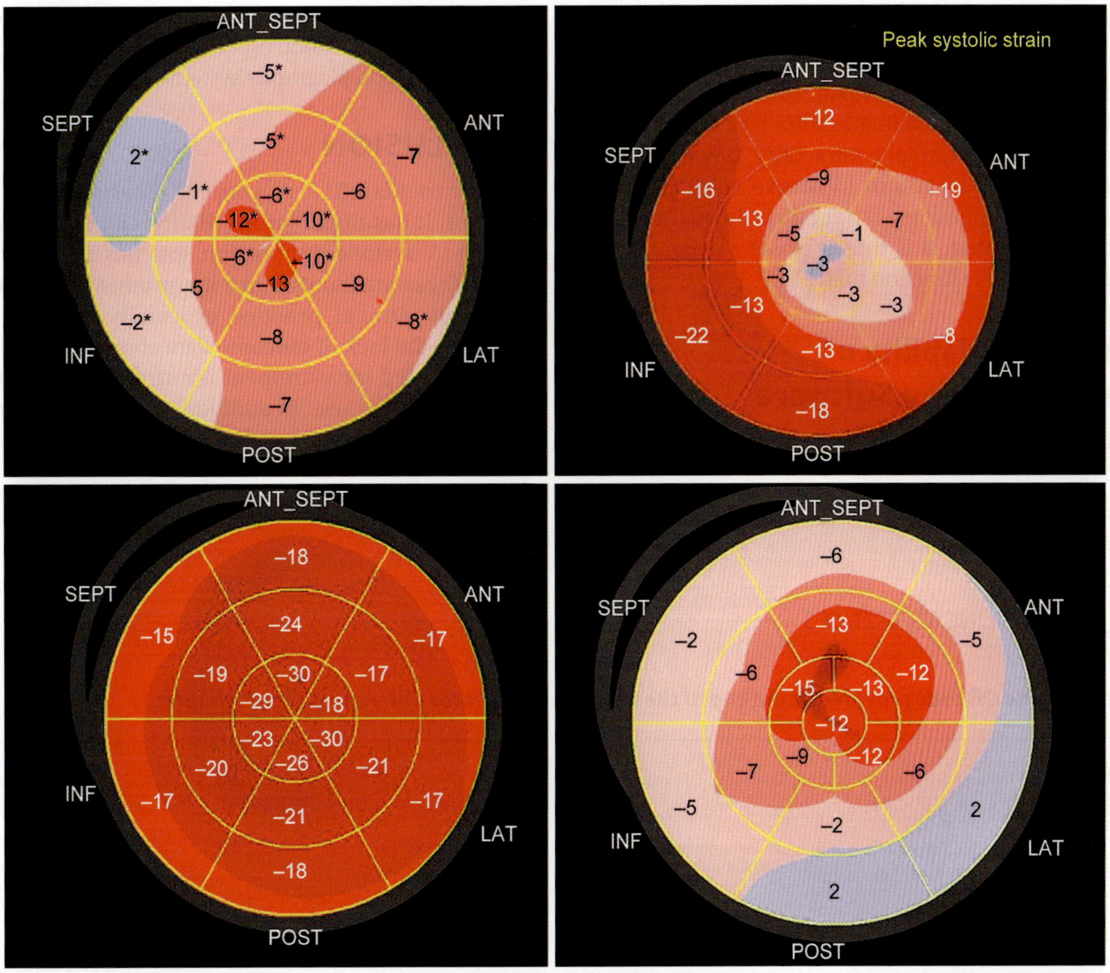

FIG. 3: Left ventricular global longitudinal strain (GLS) bull's eye plots in different conditions associated with left ventricular hypertrophy. Upper left—a patient with hypertrophic obstructive cardiomyopathy with significantly reduced longitudinal strain in disproportionately thickened basal and mid-septal segments; Upper right—a patient with apical hypertrophic cardiomyopathy; Lower left—normal GLS in an athlete with echocardiographic features of athlete's heart; Lower right—the typical apical sparing pattern in cardiac amyloidosis.

The tracking and image analysis also require careful attention to detail. The region-of-interest created for strain analysis should follow the LV myocardial contour, avoiding the papillary muscles or the muscle bundles present in the LV cavity. It should neither be too wide nor too narrow and should not be extending into the LV outflow tract or the left atrium. Also, the region-of-interest should move in sync with the LV myocardium.

Through-plane Motion

The speckle-tracking software tracks acoustic speckles within the LV myocardium frame-by-frame throughout the cardiac cycle. However, during the cardiac cycle, the acoustic speckles may move in and out of the imaging plane because of myocardial motion or breathing. As a result, the same speckles may not be available for tracking during the different phases of the cardiac cycle, thus compromising the measurement accuracy. However, the problem of through-plane motion is much greater for short-axis deformation than for longitudinal deformation and does not seem to have a significant impact on the accuracy of LVGLS. 3D speckle-tracking echocardiography overcomes this challenge but is limited by a greater dependence on the image quality.

Vendor Variability

Different speckle tracking software developed by different vendors has important differences in the image processing algorithms employed for strain quantification. This results in intervendor variability in the strain measurement for the same echocardiographic images. Measurement variability is seen even between the different versions of the same software. However, this variability has now become much less due to the collective effort of the leading echocardiography societies and the various industry partners.[31] Still, it is recommended to use the same software with the same version for serially following up the patients.

Load Dependency

As mentioned above, a major limitation of LVEF is that it is dependent on preload and afterload. Unfortunately, LVGLS is also dependent on the loading conditions and is not really a true measure of myocardial contractility. However, unlike LVEF, which is only a ratio of LV stroke volume to end-diastolic volume, longitudinal strain directly quantifies the myocardial shortening. It is thus a closer surrogate of LV myocardial contractile function than LVEF.

Limited Availability of Speckle-tracking Software

Although all the high-end echocardiography systems nowadays have speckle-tracking software available onboard, most of the lower-end and even the mid-level systems are currently lacking it. This limits the availability of strain imaging to a great extent, especially in India where the cost of high-end echocardiography systems is prohibitive.

CONCLUSION

Left ventricular GLS is a useful measure of LV systolic function. It has high reproducibility, can detect early, sub-clinical LV systolic dysfunction, and has strong prognostic value. These attributes make it a promising tool for application in clinical practice especially in heart failure. However, the lack of outcome data showing the superiority of GLS-guided measurement is currently the main reason limiting its wider use. In addition, there are some technical and logistic challenges also, including the need for good-quality images and the necessary expertise for accurate strain measurement.

ONLINE REFERENCES

Please scan the QR code provided at the end of the table of contents for References of this chapter.

CHAPTER

104

Left Atrial Strain in Clinical Practice

V Jacob Jose, Jesu Krupa

ABSTRACT

The left atrium (LA) modulates left ventricular (LV) filling by its reservoir function in systole, as a conduit during diastole and pump function during atrial contraction. LA strain analysis using speckle tracking can be used for the assessment of this phasic LA function. The normal value for left atrium reservoir strain (LARS) is >24%. It is usually determined in a LA-focused apical four chamber view or in combination with an apical two chamber view, keeping the zero reference as the R wave on electrocardiogram (ECG) and tracking the LA endocardium. LARS may be helpful in assessing diastolic dysfunction and LA pressure especially when it is indeterminate by the existing algorithms. It is useful in predicting the risk of recurrence of atrial fibrillation and stroke. It also correlates with outcomes in chronic kidney disease (CKD), hypertrophic cardiomyopathy (HCM), and cardiac amyloidosis. It has been studied to a limited extent in a variety of other cardiac conditions including valvular heart diseases, such as mitral regurgitation and aortic stenosis. It is also found to be low in diabetic patients as compared to controls. Patients with hypertension show improvement in LARS with better blood pressure control, hence, this simple tool is likely to be of great clinical value in the days ahead.

Keywords: Left atrium (LA), speckle tracking echocardiography (STE), left atrial reservoir strain (LARS), left atrial volume index (LAVI).

INTRODUCTION

Left atrium (LA) modulates the left ventricular (LV) filling by its reservoir function in systole and as a conduit during diastole and pump function during atrial contraction. LA dysfunction is a major contributing factor for elevated LA pressure. Usually, LA function is assessed by volumetric methods such as LA volume, LA expansion index or by Doppler methods using mitral flow pattern. More recently, LA strain analysis has been used for the assessment of LA function. LA strain measurements can be done using tissue Doppler, velocity vector imaging or by 2D speckle tracking echocardiography (STE). With the speckle tracking method, LA phasic function can be easily assessed. The reservoir strain component is easy to obtain, and it is the single index that we can use for the estimation of LA pressure as well. In this article we summarize the methodology and clinical applications.

METHODOLOGY

Though LA strain can be studied using tissue Doppler or STE, the latter method has now become the most acceptable measurement of LA strain. LA strain is quantified as a global longitudinal strain (GLS) of the entire LA wall. Segmental LA strain is not measured or clinically relevant. Given the limited thickness of the LA wall and the minimum thickness of any region of interest, a distinction of endocardial strain and full wall strain is not done.

Our zero reference is end-diastole which can be marked by the electrocardiogram (ECG) trigger for R wave or nadir of the atrial strain if the QRS is wide. Some studies have used zero reference at the beginning of atrial contraction. This causes confusion by giving a different curve and is hence not recommended.

The morphology of the strain curve is characterized by a monophasic systolic part where the LA fills and stretches prior to opening of the mitral valve. When the mitral valve opens, LA emptying starts and there is a decline in the strain, and it reaches a plateau. With atrial contraction, there is another dip.

The European Association of Cardiovascular Imaging/American Society of Echocardiography[1] recommends LA strain analysis by tracing the LA endocardial border, starting at the medial mitral annulus excluding the pulmonary veins and going up to the lateral mitral annulus, using the *apical four chamber view*. Biplane LA strain (from four and two chamber views) could also be considered as an option. The left atrial appendage (LAA) orifice is excluded in the apical two chamber view. The myocardial region of interest of the LA is defined by the endocardial border and the epicardial border, like LV strain measurement. If the tracking software requires the definition of the region of interest, a default width of 3 mm is recommended. The region of interest size and shape should be adjusted in order to include the thickness of LA wall and to avoid including the pericardium. If the tracking software uses endocardial tracking only, the *endocardial contour* is delineated. The user should visually assess the tracking to the motion of the underlying LA wall in order to judge the accuracy of the LA strain estimate.

LEFT ATRIUM STRAIN WAVE FORMS

There are three strain values that can be obtained but the one that is clinically most useful is the reservoir strain **(Fig. 1)**. *Left atrium reservoir strain (LARS)* or LASr is the peak atrial longitudinal strain which is positive and occurs due to atrial filling during ventricular systole against a closed mitral valve. *Conduit strain* is calculated as the strain value at the onset of atrial contraction minus the peak atrial longitudinal strain and it is always negative. *Left atrium contraction strain (LASc)* is calculated as the difference of the strain value at end-diastole and the value at the onset of atrial contraction. This is always a negative value since it occurs during late diastole as a result of atrial contraction and emptying. In short, the value is positive during LA filling and negative during emptying.

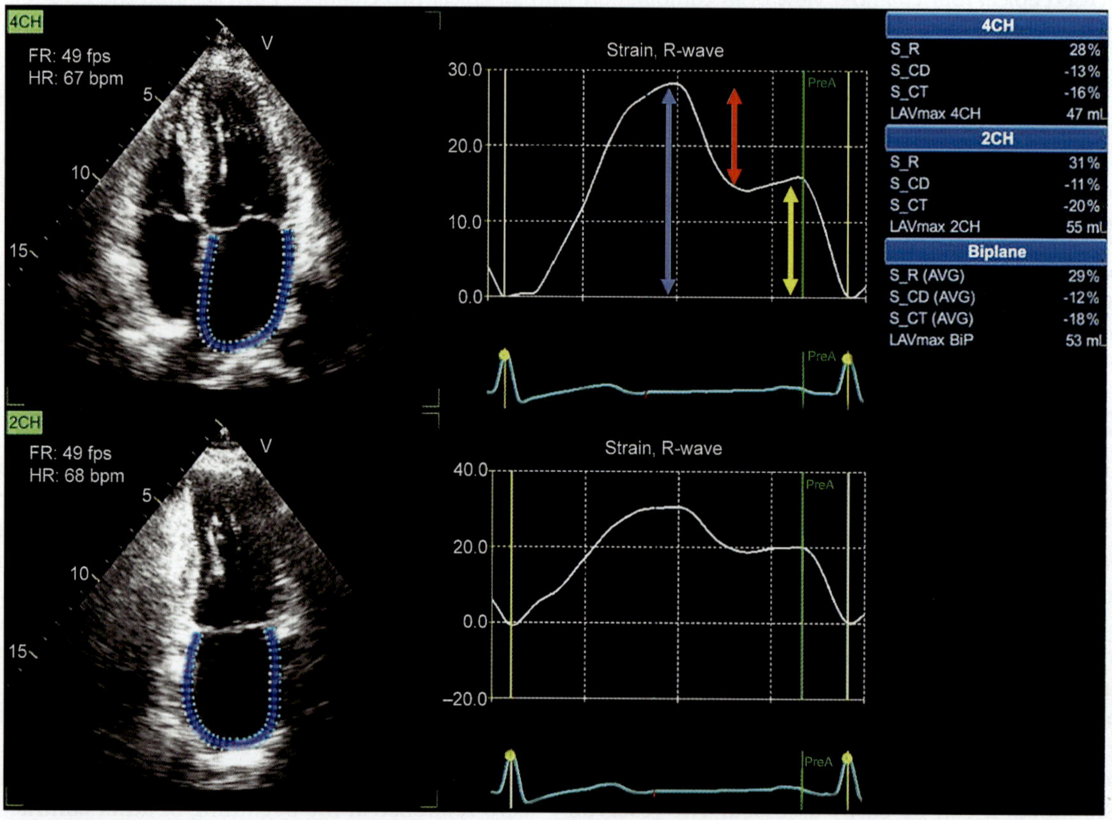

FIG. 1: A 53-year-old, asymptomatic diabetic and hypertensive with normal LVEF, abnormal LV GLS of –15.3%, grade 1 LV diastolic dysfunction with normal LV filling pressure at rest. LA strain in four chamber and two chamber views showing reduction in LARS but still > 20–24%. The blue arrow shows the peak LA strain or reservoir strain, the red arrow shows the conduit strain and the yellow arrow shows the atrial booster pump strain.

(GLS: global longitudinal strain; LA: left atrial; LARS: left atrial reservoir strain; LV: left ventricle; LVEF: left ventricular ejection fraction)

NORMAL STRAIN VALUES

The strain values differ based on the age and gender of the person. In the study by Morris et al. of 393 normal persons, the LARS was 45.5 + 11.4% and the lowest expected value was 23%.[2] In the study by Singh et al., they used a vendor independent software and did include individuals from several countries. The normal value for LARS is >24%.

HEMODYNAMIC DETERMINANTS OF LEFT ATRIUM RESERVOIR STRAIN

As the LA reservoir strain in systole, it should reflect the systolic function of the ventricle. Mitral annulus descent that occurs in systole is directly related to LV systolic function. LARSs also affected by LA chamber stiffness. The stiffer the LA, the lower will be the pressure gradient between the pulmonary veins and LA and hence LARS will be reduced. The main determinants of LARS as invasively studied in patients undergoing transcatheter mitral valve edge to edge repair were LV relaxation, LV GLS and LA chamber stiffness.[3]

Left Atrium Reservoir Strain for Diastolic Dysfunction

Five parameters have been suggested for the assessment of diastolic dysfunction.[4] Of the five, E/e′ ratio is the one that correlates reasonably well with the left atrial pressure (LAP). In the study by Singh et al., when E/e′ ratio is compared with LARS with simultaneous pulmonary artery wedge pressure, LARS was better than the E/e′ ratio, hence many authors have tried to use LARS in the diagnosis of diastolic dysfunction. As per the diastolic dysfunction algorithm, a subset will be called *indeterminate*. It is in this group of patients we can use LARS. In the study by Potter et al.,[5] they used LARS instead of left atrial volume index (LAVI), and they could reduce the indeterminate cases by 75%. In another study, they looked at these intermediate groups with exercise. Left atrial reservoir strain has been used for the assessment of LAP with exercise in patients with heart failure with preserved ejection fraction (HFpEF). The addition of LARS improved the diagnostic value of HFpEF score with area under the curve from 0.7 to 0.8.[6] LARS has been most accurate for the estimation of LA pressure in patients with depressed LVEF, rather than with preserved ejection fraction. In patients with preserved EF, a LARS < 18% has high specificity for increased LV filling pressure.[7] A comparison of LARS versus LAVI is enumerated in **Table 1**.[8]

TABLE 1: LA volume versus LA strain.

	LAVI	LARS
Abnormal cut off	>34 mL/m^2	<23%
Feasibility	90–93%	89–97%
Correlation with wedge pressure	Mild	Modest
Reflection of diastolic function	Chronicity	Early
Marker of LA fibrosis	May not be	May be
Prognostic value	Weak	Strong

(LA: left atrium; LARS: left atrial reservoir strain; LAVI: left atrium volume index)

LEFT ATRIUM STRAIN FOR PROGNOSIS

The addition of LARS can be useful for not only identifying patients with diastolic dysfunction, but also for prognostication. Risk of heart failure hospitalization was increased at an odds ratio of 6.6 (CI 2.6–16.6) in a group of patients with normal LAVI, but abnormal LA strain. The absolute increase in the prognostic value was 9.9% when LARS was added to LAVI.[9]

Prediction of Atrial Fibrillation

Left atrium strain parameters have been shown to predict atrial fibrillation (AF) in many studies. In the fifth Copenhagen City Heart Study which had 4,466 participants who were followed up for a median of 5.3 years, 4.3% of them had developed AF. For patients with LA strain of <23%, there was a 6.8-fold increased risk of developing AF, thus integrating LA strain into an echo study for the general population will be useful for risk stratification.[10]

Left atrium strain has been useful for predicting recurrence of AF following AF ablation. In a study of 172 patients undergoing cryoablation, 50 of them had recurrence. A LARS of <17% the highest incremental predictive value for AF recurrence (HR 9.45; 95% CI 3.17–28.13; $p < 0.001$). Even in patients with nondilated LA, the predictive value for recurrence was HR 5.39; 95% CI 1.66–17.52.[11]

RISK OF STROKE AND LEFT ATRIUM STRAIN

In a study cohort of 806 adults without stroke or AF were followed for 10.9 years. New onset stroke occurred in 53 participants (7%). Reduced LA strain was independently associated with new stroke even after control of other factors, such as LA volume, AF, and LV strain. Thus, in the elderly population, adding the LA strain may risk stratify patients who may develop stroke in the future.[12]

ROLE OF LEFT ATRIUM STRAIN IN POSTMYOCARDIAL INFARCTION PATIENTS

Left atrial reservoir strain is noted to be a good predictor for AF in patients following myocardial infarction. In a study of 392 patients of ST elevation myocardial infarction treated with primary angioplasty who were followed for 5.6 years,

6.3% of patients were noted to have AF. The LA strain was 24.1% or less in patients with incident AF.[13]

ROLE OF LEFT ATRIUM STRAIN IN CHRONIC KIDNEY DISEASE PATIENTS

Chronic kidney disease (CKD) patients are known to have higher cardiovascular risk. In a study of 243 patients with CKD and no previous heart disease were followed up over 5 years, LA peak strain was the only predictor for the primary endpoint for death.[14] In another study of 280 patients with CKD stage 3 or 4, reduced LA reservoir strain was associated with a 2.5-fold higher risk of composite outcomes (HR 2.51; 95% CI: 1.19–5.30; $p = 0.02$) and was the only echocardiographic parameter that predicted progressive renal failure independent of established clinical risk factors for end-stage renal failure.[15] In a systematic review of LA strain in CKD patients that included six studies, it was noted that this is a promising marker for cardiovascular events.[16]

Left Atrium Strain in Hypertrophic Cardiomyopathy

Hypertrophic cardiomyopathy is expected to have diastolic dysfunction. LA strain has been studied in this group as a prognostic marker for the development of heart failure, stroke, and death in a small study. In this study, lower event-free survival in patients with reservoir strain ≤23.8% or conduit strain ≤10.2%.[17]

Left Atrium Strain in Hypertension

In hypertensives, LA strain was abnormal despite normal volumetric measures of LA, suggesting that LA strain becomes abnormal earlier than LA dilatation.[18] It has also been shown that strain improves with blood pressure control. This improvement is not dependent on the class of drugs but on the level of blood pressure control. In a study of 160 patients of mild to moderate hypertension, nebivolol was compared with irbesartan and there was no significant difference between these two drugs for LA strain reduction.[19]

Left Atrium Strain in Diabetes

Diabetes is usually associated with strain abnormalities of the LV and they also have diastolic dysfunction. Impairment of LA reservoir and conduit function by STE strain has been shown even in the absence of LV hypertrophy or hypertension. In a systematic review of and meta-analysis of 41 studies with 6,668 asymptomatic patients with diabetes mellitus (DM) compared to 7,218 healthy controls, it was shown that LA reservoir strain was significantly lower in individuals with diabetes compared to healthy controls [28.0% (23.9, 32.1) vs. 36.5 (34.2, 38.9)] with a large mean difference of –8.41 (–11.5, –5.33).[20]

Left Atrium Strain in Other Diseases

Left atrial strain has been studied in a variety of other cardiac conditions and the practical utilities of this need to be studied further. In a study of 65 patients of *mitral regurgitation* who were followed up after surgery for the development of heart failure and mortality, it was noted that a peak atrial strain <21% was the best discriminator for the development of these endpoints.[21] LA strain has been shown a better marker than natriuretic peptides in patients with *aortic stenosis* and preserved ejection fraction to identify patients who are likely to worsen their NYHA class or hospitalization heart failure. In this study of 173 patients, LARS of <20% was the best cutoff.[22] LA function has been shown to be abnormal in *obese individuals* and LA strain in obese individuals between the age of 35–55 was studied in Asklepios Study. As the body mass index (BMI) increased, the LARS decreased significantly from 35% in BMI < 25–30% in those with BMI of 30 or more. This suggests that with increasing obesity, LA function is important for diastolic function and loss of this compensatory function may contribute to the AF and heart failure in these patients.[23] LA strain has been studied in patients with *cardiac amyloidosis* and it has been shown that LARS < 13.2% was associated with less survival **(Figs. 2A to D)**.[24]

CONCLUSION

Left atrial strain has become easy to measure with the newer echo machines due to in built software for speckle tracking. Many of the machines have automatic measurement of the same. LA reservoir strain maybe particularly useful in the large group of patients with indeterminate diastolic function assessment. In addition, it plays a major role in the risk stratification of various patients and in the prediction of AF. In the coming years this will be another robust measure in our echo armamentarium.

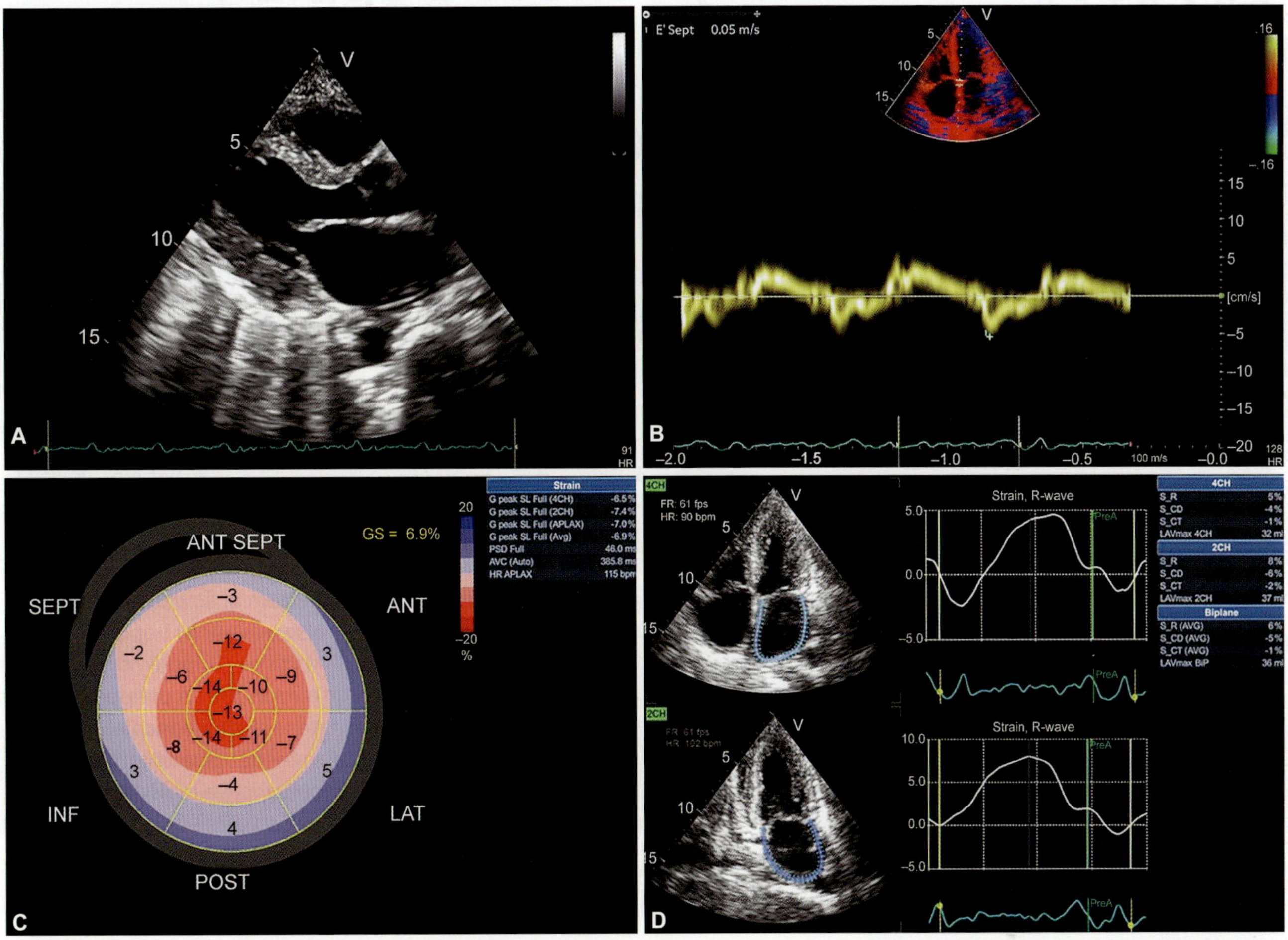

FIGS. 2A TO D: A 43-year-old female with heart failure symptoms and low voltage QRS complexes on ECG. (A) LV with thick walls and a dilated LA; (B) Reduced mitral annular tissue Doppler velocities; medial e′ = 5 cm/s; (C) "Cherry on top" appearance of LV GLS; and (D) Markedly reduced four chamber and two chamber LA strain, biplane LARS = 6%.

Note: These findings are typical of cardiac amyloidosis. The markedly reduced LA strain is indicative of severe LA dysfunction and could predispose to LA clot and thromboembolic phenomena even though the patient is in sinus rhythm.

(ECG: electrocardiogram; GLS: global longitudinal strain; LA: left atrial; LARS: left atrial reservoir strain; LV: left ventricle)

ONLINE REFERENCES

Please scan the QR code provided at the end of the table of contents for References of this chapter.

CHAPTER 105

Pulmonary Venous Doppler: An Easy and Accurate but Underutilized Estimate of LA Pressure and Function

Biswaranjan Mishra, Shishu Shankar Mishra

ABSTRACT

Pulmonary veins (PVs) are conduits that join the pulmonary circulation to the left atrium (LA). Pattern of flow from the PVs to LA reflects LA and left ventricular (LV) mechanics and pressure changes. Assessment of PV pulse wave (PW) Doppler flow is relatively easy from transthoracic window without requiring advanced technologies such as tissue Doppler, strain, or 3D imaging. This easier modality can be performed routinely. The advantage is that it exactly mirrors the LA pressure and LV end-diastolic pressure (LVEDP) during the cardiac cycle making it an additional and accurate tool for diagnosing heart failure both with preserved and reduced LV ejection fraction (EF). Further, it has immense diagnostic value in estimating severity of mitral regurgitation (MR). It plays a very important role in differentiating between constrictive pericarditis and restrictive cardiomyopathy. It has also the potential for diagnosing different conduction blocks and cardiac arrhythmias.

Keywords: Pulmonary venous flow, left atrial pressure, left ventricular end-diastolic pressure.

INTRODUCTION

Pulmonary veins (PVs) are conduits from the lungs to the left atrium (LA) that carry the right ventricular (RV) output through lungs to the LA. In spite of only systolic flow to the lungs from the RV with considerable respiratory variation, pulmonary venous flow to LA occurs throughout the cardiac cycle with minimal respiratory variation. Flow from these thin-walled vessels which are highly compliant reflect exactly the hemodynamics of LA.[1] Assessment of pulmonary venous flow by pulse wave (PW) Doppler gives an unique opportunity to know the LA hemodynamics in physiological as well as pathological states. The advantage of the noninvasive assessment by transthoracic echocardiography (TTE) and not-so-difficult interpretation makes it an easy way to estimate LA pressure in different disease states. Routine assessment of PV PW Doppler spectrum will greatly add to assessment of LA pressure throughout the cardiac cycle and left ventricular (LV) filling pressure in diastole. This is of immense importance particularly in the current epidemic of heart failure where LA filling pressure assessment has become essential.[2] It uses the conventional spectral Doppler technology which is universally available without requirement of high-end machines with strain, tissue Doppler or 3D facilities. In addition, it is of immense help in assessing severity of mitral regurgitation (MR) and differentiating between constrictive and restrictive physiology.[3] The characteristic flow profile of PV Doppler spectrum in certain congenital disease, conduction disorders, and arrhythmias further increases the utility of this imaging modality.

IMAGING OF PULMONARY VEINS

There are four separate PVs: right upper pulmonary vein (RUPV) and right lower pulmonary vein (RLPV), left upper pulmonary vein (LUPV), and left lower pulmonary vein (LLPV). Each of the PV has a distinct ostial opening to the LA. The right PVs come from behind the superior vena cava and right atrium to open in the posterosuperior aspect of LA medially adjacent to atrial septum. The left PVs run anterior to descending aorta and enter the lateral wall of the LA. The typical anatomy is not always present, and in 30% of cases both PVs from one side may join making a single PV; alternatively there are multiple PVs joining the LA.[4]

The apical four-chamber view is most useful as Doppler flow alignment is best obtained from this view for both RUPV and RLPV. The RUPV is imaged in the apical four-chamber with a slight anterior tilt to partly see the aorta **(Fig. 1A)** and the RLPV is imaged with a slight posterior tilt of the four-chamber view **(Fig. 1B)**.[5] In infant and children, classically

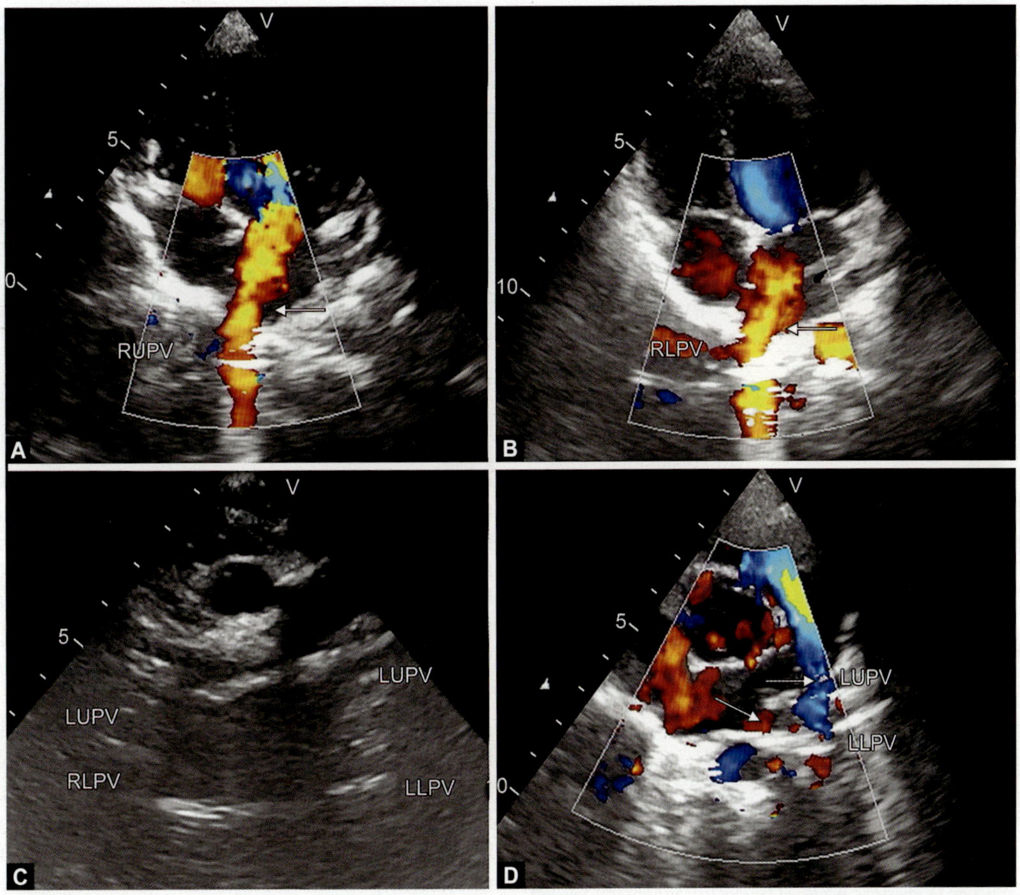

FIGS. 1A TO D: 2D Transthoracic echocardiographic imaging of pulmonary veins with color flow. (A) Right upper pulmonary vein (RUPV) (arrow) seen by upward tilting of the probe, toward five chamber view or partially seeing the aorta. (B) Right lower pulmonary vein (RLPV) seen in posterior tilt of the apical four-chamber view (arrow). (C) Suprasternal crab view in an infant showing all pulmonary veins entering left atrium (LA). (D) Parasternal short axis showing left upper and lower pulmonary veins entering the LA near the appendage and descending aorta respectively (arrows).

(LLPV: left lower pulmonary vein; LUPV: left upper pulmonary vein)

the crab view **(Fig. 1C)** from the suprasternal window visualizes all the PVs, but this window is not useful in adults.

Left-sided PVs are best imaged in parasternal short-axis view, but the flow direction away from the Doppler beam precludes its usefulness for PV flow assessment. The LUPV is seen entering the left side of the LA wall below the left atrial appendage and the LLPV is seen adjacent to the descending aorta in short-axis view **(Fig. 1D)**. Transesophageal echocardiography (TEE) images in midesophageal window provide more precise and clear views and also better flow profile for Doppler beam alignment than TTE images because of the close proximity of the transducer to the PVs, but the semi-invasive nature of the test makes it less useful than TTE for routine assessment of PV flow.[6]

NORMAL PULMONARY VENOUS FLOW

Color flow interrogation of the posteromedial portion of the LA in apical four-chamber view is first required to identify PV flow and its direction in relation to the Doppler beam. A good flow is often seen with right alignment of the flow with lowering the set Nyquist limit of the color flow spectrum. The PW sample volume is placed 1–2 cm inside the PV to obtain the spectral Doppler waves which reflect the pressure gradient between PVs and LA depending on the LA, mitral annular and LV mechanics.[7] PV Doppler flow is a phasic bidirectional flow, but predominantly there occur a forward flow from PVs to LA resembling LA pressure wave.[8] The timing and identification of the waves are done by a gated electrocardiogram (ECG).

There are two antegrade or forward flows in systole (S1 and S2) which are recorded as positive spectrums, another forward or positive spectral flow is recorded in diastole (D), and one retrograde or negative spectral flow is recorded during atrial contraction called the atrial reversal (AR) wave **(Fig. 2)**.[9] The S1 and S2-waves are fused in approximately 80% of cases particularly in TTE giving rise to one systolic antegrade flow (S) where as in TEE two distinct S1 and S2 are visible.[8] S-waves represent the X-descent on LA pressure tracing occurring in the reservoir phase.

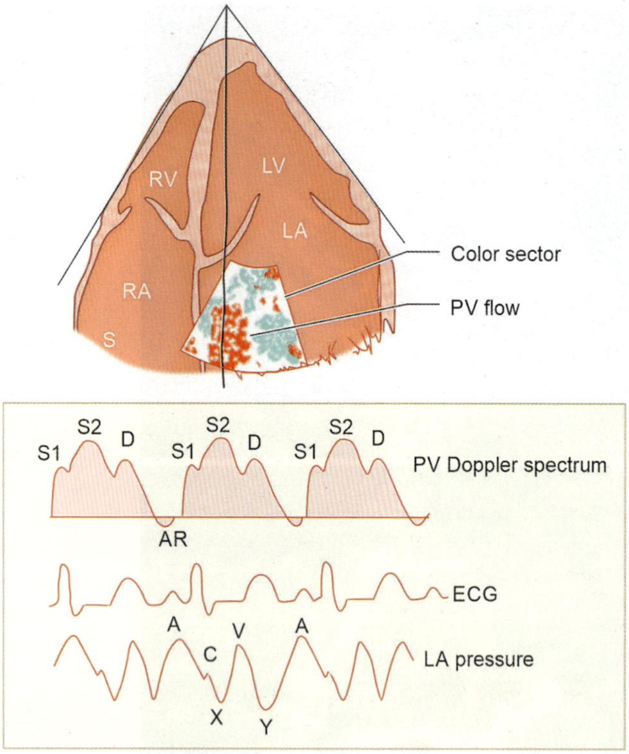

FIG. 2: Schematic presentation of transthoracic echocardiography of pulmonary venous Doppler spectrum corresponding to 2D and color sector image, simultaneous ECG and left atrial pressure tracing.

(AR: atrial reversal wave; D: diastolic wave; ECG: electrocardiogram; LA: left atrium; LV: left ventricle; PV: pulmonary vein; RA: right atrium; RV: right ventricle; S1: first systolic wave; S2: second systolic wave; A, C, and V are positive waves and X- and Y-descent are negative waves in left atrial pressure tracing)

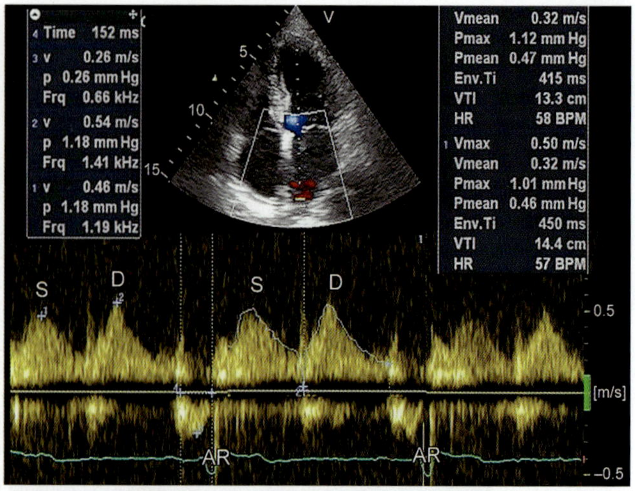

FIG. 3: Transthoracic echocardiography of pulmonary venous Doppler spectrum. The typical measurements, S velocity 0.46 m/sec, D velocity 0.54 m/sec, S/D <1, S VTI 415 msec, D VTI 450 msec, systolic fraction 47%, AR velocity 0.26 m/sec, AR duration 152 msec.

(AR: atrial reversal wave; D: diastolic wave; S: systolic wave; VTI: velocity–time integral)

Left atrium relaxation following LA contraction causes suction of blood to LA causing the S1-wave representing LA contractile function. S2 results from both a forward push and a suction effect. Forward push comes from RV systole, the ejection wave which comes across the lungs helps in LA filling. The suction effect is due to downward displacement of mitral annulus during systole, the LV longitudinal function. S2 is also dependent on LA compliance and RV stroke volume.[8] In highly compliant LA, the forward flow velocities are less whereas in a less compliant LA the velocities are high.

D-waves represent the Y-descent on LA pressure tracing that occur during the LA conduit phase. As the mitral valve (MV) opens, blood flows from LA to LV, the ensuing negative pressure in LA draws blood from PVs to LA. Therefore, the D-wave is a reflection of mitral inflow PW Doppler E-wave. LV relaxation and compliance both influence D-wave similar to their effects on the mitral inflow E-wave.

The AR-wave or the atrial reversal wave represents atrial contraction. During atrial contraction the pressure in LA exceeds that of PVs causing backward flow which is responsible for inscribing a retrograde spectral wave. AR-wave represents *a*-wave in LA pressure tracing occurring in late diastole during the LA pump phase and also the mitral inflow PW Doppler A-wave. Therefore, AR-wave is influenced by the contractile function and stiffness of LV which is also influenced by the cardiac rhythm, PR interval, and the P-QRS relationship. But a distinct AR-wave is very often difficult to obtain particularly in TTE.[8]

The following measurements are made in the PV spectral Doppler **(Fig. 3)**.[10]

- The peak velocities of the S, D, and AR-waves are measured.
- Ratio of the peak velocity of S to peak velocity of the D-wave (S/D)
- The AR-wave velocity
- The AR-wave duration
- The D-wave deceleration time
- Velocity–time integral (VTI) of S and D-waves
- *Systolic fraction of PV flow*: VTI of S-wave/VTI of S-wave + VTI of D-wave

PULMONARY VENOUS FLOW IN ADOLESCENTS AND YOUNG ADULTS

Blood flow in the PVs reflects LV mechanics. Normal adolescents and young adults have very good and rapid early relaxation of LV causing rapid early diastolic filling and less flow during atrial contraction which represents the large early diastolic E-wave and a shorter A-wave in mitral inflow Doppler. In PV flow the D-wave represents early diastolic flow. In synchrony with the mitral inflow Doppler, the PV D-wave is prominent with a small AR-wave. The ratio S/D is <1 **(Fig. 4)**.

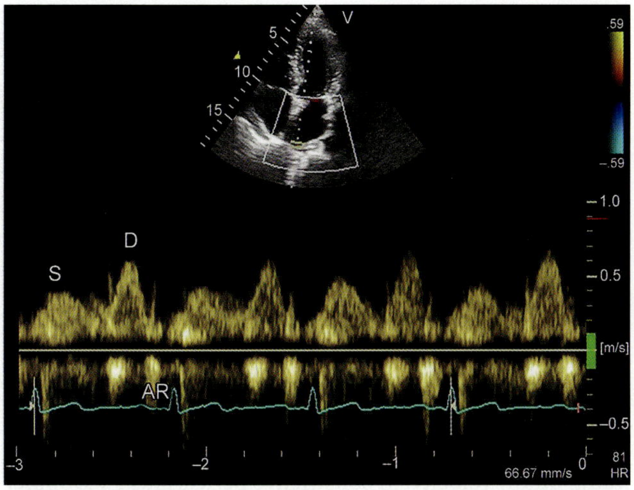

FIG. 4: Pulmonary venous Doppler spectrum in a young healthy individual, D-wave is larger corresponding to rapid early diastolic filling, the S/D ratio is <1.

(AR: atrial reversal wave; D: diastolic wave; S: systolic wave)

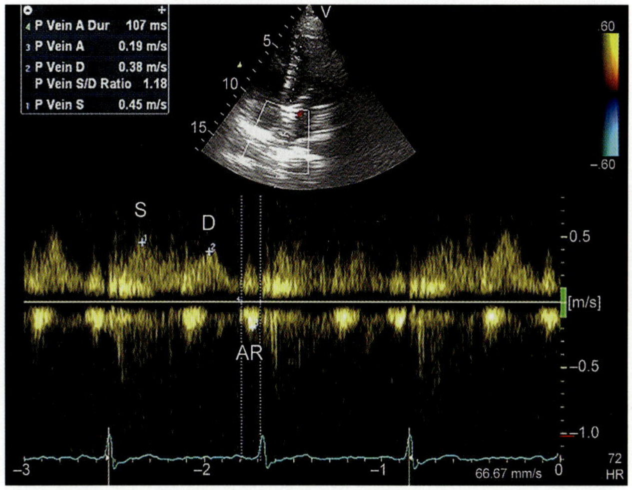

FIG. 5: Pulmonary venous Doppler spectrum in an older healthy individual, S-wave is larger. Smaller D-wave corresponding to slower early diastolic filling (grade I diastolic dysfunction), the S/D ratio is >1.

(AR: atrial reversal wave; D: diastolic wave; S: systolic wave)

PULMONARY VENOUS FLOW IN OLDER ADULTS

With aging the rate of early diastolic relaxation decreases, consequently the early diastolic filling becomes less, the mitral inflow Doppler E-velocity becomes less with increased deceleration time. The early diastolic reduced filling is compensated by more vigorous atrial contraction with increased A-wave velocity representing grade I diastolic dysfunction. The pattern of mitral inflow Doppler is also reflected in PV Doppler, PV Doppler D-wave becomes smaller making S/D >1. The AR-wave becomes more prominent but in grade I diastolic dysfunction the AR velocity does not exceed 3.5 m/sec **(Fig. 5)**.[8]

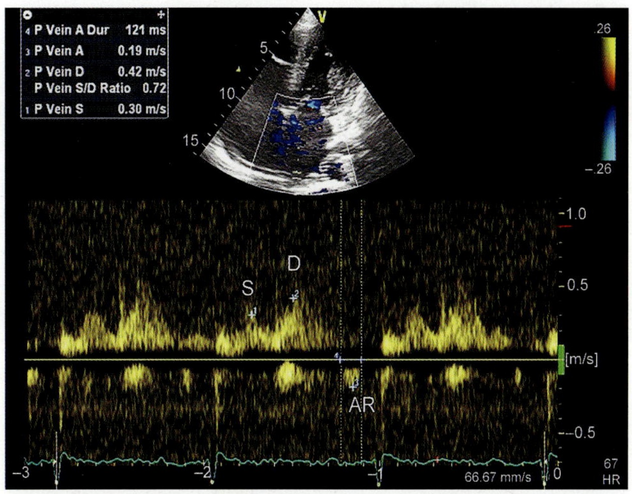

FIG. 6: Pulmonary venous Doppler in high left atrial pressure, the S/D ratio is <1, there is increased duration and velocity of AR-wave.

(AR: atrial reversal wave; D: diastolic wave; S: systolic wave)

PULMONARY VENOUS FLOW IN HIGH LEFT ATRIAL PRESSURE

After fourth decade, normally the S/D ratio is >1. Increased LA pressure produces a high gradient between LA and LV. As the MV opens the high gradient in early diastole will result in greater LV filling as reflected in high velocity E-wave in mitral inflow Doppler. Greater LV filling causes more negative pressure in LA driving in more blood from the PVs causing a larger D-wave, the ratio of S/D reverses **(Fig. 6)**. *The S/D ratio is inversely proportional to LA pressure.*[11]

Synchronous with the deceleration time of mitral inflow Doppler E-wave, the deceleration time of the PV D-wave decreases.[12] In patients with reduced LV ejection fraction (EF), S2 is less because of the less longitudinal motion of the mitral annulus, and less RV output in low cardiac output states also reduce S2 velocity. Therefore, the S/D ratio is significantly less in low LVEF and in low cardiac output states. When LV contraction is normal with high LA pressure, the low S2 velocity is negated by a good downward motion of the mitral annulus drawing blood from the PVs. Therefore, the sensitivity S/D ratio is decreases in preserved EF. In spite of decreased sensitivity, S/D ratio is a strong prognostic marker independent of grade of diastolic function and is a predictor of survival and future cardiovascular events in heart failure with preserved EF (HFpEF).[13] Using the systolic fraction <55% calculated as the VTI of S-wave/VTI of S-wave + VTI of D-wave, the sensitivity of predicting LA pressure in HFpEF increases significantly to 91% and 87%, respectively.[14]

The S/D ratio should not be used to assess LA pressure in patients with atrial fibrillation (AF), hypertrophic cardiomyopathy, and when there is significant MR. In young healthy individuals <40 years of age as described above, the S/D ratio is <1, but the AR-wave is of low velocity and duration, which should not be confused as high LA pressure.

Pulmonary vein AR-wave may be small and short in atrial mechanical failure even though the rhythm is sinus, a state of atrial cardiomyopathy in long-standing atrial stretching of various etiologies, and due to atrial myocardial infiltration such as cardiac amyloidosis.[15]

PULMONARY VENOUS FLOW IN HIGH END-DIASTOLIC PRESSURE

Left ventricular end-diastolic pressure (LVEDP) increases early in progression of diastolic dysfunction before the mean LA pressure is raised. The mitral inflow Doppler A-wave and the PV AR-wave are due to atrial contraction occurring simultaneously. Normally the duration of both are near equal or the mitral inflow A is slightly longer.[16] When the LVEDP is raised, the MV closes prematurely before the LA contraction is complete. Continuing LA contraction in face of a closed MV increases the PV–AR velocity and duration **(Fig. 7)**. Duration of AR-wave exceeding 30 msec from the duration of mitral inflow A-wave is a highly accurate and independent predictor of raised LVEDP, it is 82% sensitive 92% specific to predict LVEDP >20 mm Hg. For accurate estimation of duration of both waves, the R-wave in ECG is referred as a marker of the end of both waves. Increase in velocity of PV–AR velocity to >3.5 m/sec is also an indicator of increased LVEDP, but the accuracy is less than the increased duration.

Unlike the S/D ratio the increased duration of PV–AR wave >30 msec indicates high LA pressure irrespective of LVEF. It is useful in separating pseudonormalization of mitral inflow from that of normal and importantly it helps to identify patients with high LVEDP in spite of normal mean LA pressure. This parameter is particularly useful in assessing LVEDP in cases of hypertrophic cardiomyopathy.[17] It has been seen to well correlate with hospitalization in heart failure.[18] **Figure 8** shows comparisons of various echocardiographic parameters in worsening diastolic function and increasing LA pressure. In AF, the PV–AR and mitral inflow A-velocities cannot be measured due to loss of atrial contraction.

PULMONARY VENOUS FLOW IN CONSTRICTIVE/RESTRICTIVE PHYSIOLOGY

Constrictive pericarditis is characterized by marked respiratory variation of mitral inflow. Synchronous to the mitral inflow velocity, in constrictive pericarditis PV Doppler profile shows an exaggerated respiratory variation. Forward flow velocities in PV Doppler are markedly decreased during inspiration with a reciprocal increase in expiration, the effect are particularly prominent in the D-wave which is the counterpart of mitral inflow E-wave.[19] The variation is more marked in the first inspiratory and expiratory beats. S/D ratio 65% or more combined with a 40% or more decrease in D-wave velocity in inspiration than that of expiration is useful in differentiating constrictive pericarditis from restrictive cardiomyopathy.[20]

Exaggerated respiratory variation is also noted in cardiac tamponade, however respiratory variation of PV Doppler flow is neither sensitive nor specific for diagnosis of pericardial pathology and should not be taken in isolation as a marker of constrictive pericarditis or cardiac tamponade.[21] Respiratory variation may occur due to fluctuation in intrathoracic pressure in obesity and also in chronic obstructive pulmonary disease (COPD).

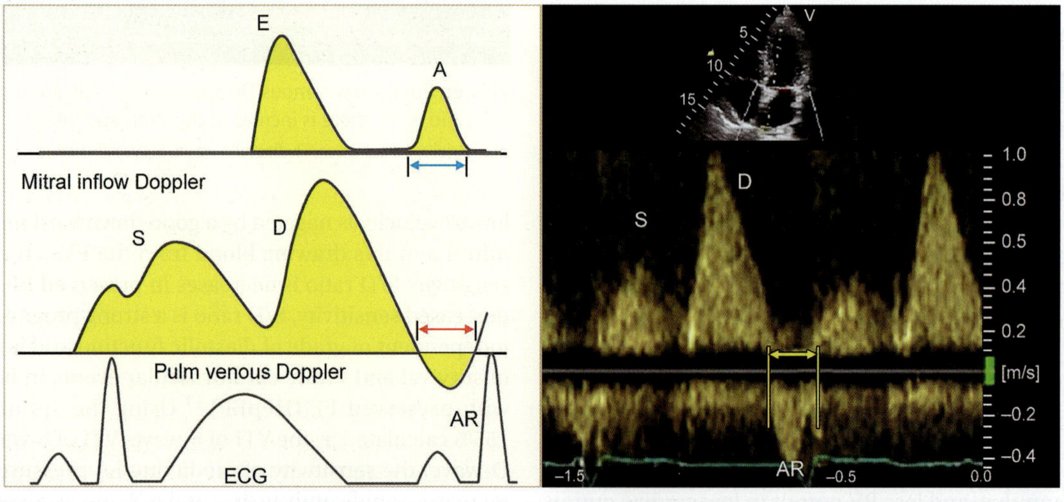

FIG. 7: Pulmonary venous flow in high end-diastolic pressure; the left panel shows the schematic presentation and right panel shows the actual recording. The S/D ratio is <1 and the AR-wave duration and velocity are increased. In the left panel, blue double-headed arrow shows the duration of mitral inflow Doppler A and red double-headed arrow shows the duration of AR-wave.

(A: mitral inflow atrial contraction wave; AR: atrial reversal wave; D: diastolic wave; E: mitral inflow early diastolic wave; ECG: electrocardiogram; S: systolic wave)

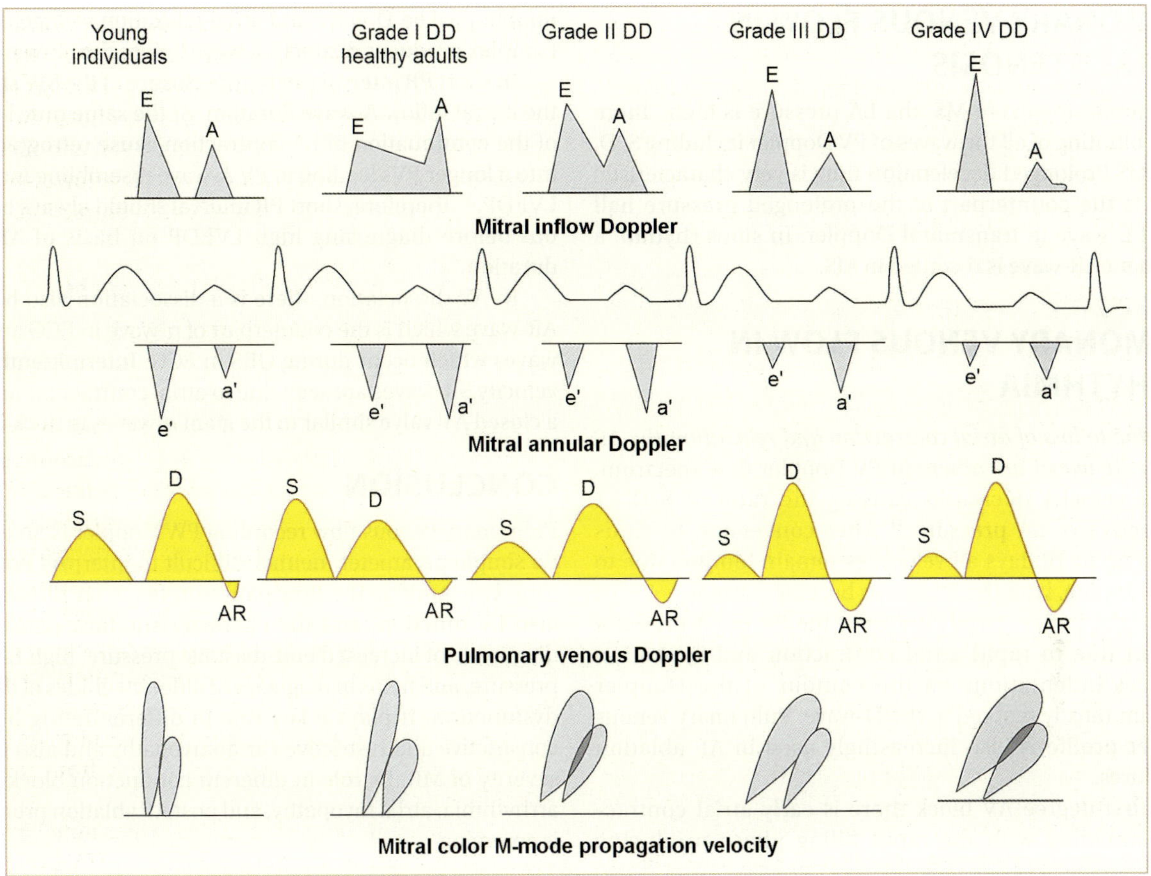

FIG. 8: Comparisons various echocardiographic parameters in worsening diastolic dysfunction and increasing left atrial pressure.
(A: mitral inflow atrial contraction wave; a': mitral annular atrial contraction wave; AR: pulmonary venous atrial reversal wave; D: pulmonary venous diastolic wave; E: mitral inflow early diastolic wave; e': mitral annular early diastolic wave; S: pulmonary venous systolic wave)

In restrictive cardiomyopathy, the PV Doppler spectrum also reflects the mitral inflow pattern of restrictive flow with decrease in S-wave velocity due to high LA pressure, decreased longitudinal function of LV, and due to AF which is sometimes associated. At the same time, the velocity is high with a S/D ratio <1, the deceleration time of D-wave becomes short and respiratory variation is minimal.[22]

PULMONARY VENOUS FLOW IN MITRAL REGURGITATION

Pulmonary vein Doppler aids in the determination of the severity of MR. As severity of MR increases, there occurs proportionate decrease in S-wave velocity, at the same time the velocity of the D-wave increases progressively.[23] Severe MR is characterized by systolic reversal (SR)-wave, which is a retrograde wave in place of the forward S-wave.[24] The SR-wave may occur in mid or late systole with a forward or absent S1, or the reversal may be pansystolic including both S1 and S2 indicating a very severe MR. The SR-wave is the counterpart of the *v*-wave in LA/pulmonary artery wedge pressure tracing due to systolic transmission of the LV pressure to the LA.[25]

Sensitivity and specificity of SR-wave is less in grading severity of MR,[26] as its velocity is dependent on LA compliance. An equal regurgitant volume will produce a large SR-wave in acute MR but not in chronic severe MR due to increased compliance of LA in chronic MR as opposed to acute MR. However, with worsening of chronic severe MR.[26] LA compliance decreases with blunting and even reversal of the S-wave.[27] Blunting of the S-wave or SR-wave is more common when there is associated mitral stenosis (MS), LV systolic dysfunction, AF or when MR is primary. Recording of SR-wave is also influenced by the MR jet direction which may selectively enter one or more PVs. In such cases TEE is more useful where individual PVs can be assessed. Therefore, SR-wave is highly specific but less sensitive for severe MR.[28] It should also be noted that SR-wave may also be present in junctional or idioventricular rhythm or intermittently in atrioventricular (AV) dissociation. Contamination of MR jet while recording PV flow can give rise to false-positive SR-wave, which should be avoided by placing the sample volume well inside the PVs. Recently, PV flow profile has also been shown to have prognostic value in MV repair procedures.[29]

PULMONARY VENOUS FLOW IN MITRAL STENOSIS

In moderate-to-severe MS, the LA pressure is high. There occurs blunting of all the waves of PV Doppler including S, D, and AR.[30] Prolonged deceleration time is very characteristic which is the counterpart of the prolonged pressure half time of E-wave in transmitral Doppler. In sinus rhythm, a prominent AR-wave is recorded in MS.

PULMONARY VENOUS FLOW IN ARRHYTHMIA

In AF due to loss of atrial contraction and relaxation the AR and the S1-waves are absent in PV Doppler flow spectrum. The S2 velocity decreases causing the ratio of S/D <1 irrespective of LA pressure.[31] After conversion to sinus rhythm up to 10 days all velocities remain blunted due to atrial stunning, later the PV-waves become normal.

In atrial flutter, rapid change in the PV to LA pressure gradient due to rapid atrial contraction and relaxation produces indentations on the contour of the Doppler spectrum mostly marked in the D-wave. Pulmonary venous Doppler profile is also increasingly used in AF ablation procedures.

In first-degree AV block there is early atrial contraction coinciding with the rapid filling phase producing double-peaked D-wave and atrial relaxation well before QRS complex produces distinct S1-wave before the S2-wave.[32]

In short PR interval premature closure of the MV shortens the mitral inflow A-wave duration. At the same time because of the continuation of LA contraction cause retrograde flow into a longer PVs leading to PV A-wave resembling increased LVEDP.[33] Therefore, short PR interval should always be ruled out before diagnosing high LVEDP on basis of AR-wave duration.

In AV dissociation, there is a dissociation also between AR-wave which is the counterpart of p-wave in ECG and S/D-waves which occur during QRS in ECG. Intermittently high-velocity SR-waves are seen due to atrial contraction in face of a closed AV valve similar to the giant *a*-waves in neck veins.[34]

CONCLUSION

Pulmonary venous flow recording PW Doppler is an easy-to-do simple parameter, neither difficult to interpret nor much time-consuming. The flow pattern reflects LA pressure and also LV function, and the characteristic flow patterns are diagnostic of increased end-diastolic pressure, high LA mean pressure, and helps in diagnosis of different grades of diastolic dysfunction. It plays a key role in differentiating between constrictive and restrictive cardiomyopathy and also grading severity of MR. Its role in different conduction blocks, atrial arrhythmia, atrial myopathy, and post AF ablation procedures is emerging.

ONLINE REFERENCES

Please scan the QR code provided at the end of the table of contents for References of this chapter.

CHAPTER

106 Echo Assessment of Prosthetic Valve Dysfunction

Debika Chatterjee

ABSTRACT

Prosthetic valve dysfunction is a rare but life-threatening complication. Therefore, its early detection is of paramount importance, which requires not only transthoracic echocardiography but also transesophageal echocardiography. Three-dimensional (3D) transesophageal echocardiography is required in some special situations.

Keywords: Prosthetic heart valve, mechanical heart valve, bioprosthetic heart valve, transthoracic echocardiography, transesophageal echocardiography, two-dimensional echo, three-dimensional echo, transvalvular regurgitation, paravalvular regurgitation.

INTRODUCTION

Introduction of valve replacement either by surgical or transcatheter implantation of a prosthetic heart valve (PHV) has dramatically improved the outcome of the patients with valvular heart disease. Though PHVs are designed to replicate the function of normal valves, but from time to time, a large number of these patients suffer from PHV dysfunction despite significant improvement in valve implantation techniques and prosthetic valve design including better hemodynamics, more durability and less thrombogenicity. Some of these complications are serious and even life threatening requiring urgent intervention. So, early diagnosis of PHV dysfunction is crucial to reduce the morbidity and mortality. Echocardiographic evaluation of prosthetic valves is more complex compared to native valve. A special knowledge about types of PHVs along with their normal and abnormal function is necessary for echocardiographic examination and correct interpretation of the prosthetic valve dysfunction. Echocardiography allows to identify various causes of prosthetic valve dysfunction by demonstrating degenerative changes in bioprosthetic valve, presence of thrombus, pannus, vegetation, or other complications of infective endocarditis, such as ring abscess and dehiscence. Doppler echocardiography can identify presence and assess the severity of stenosis or regurgitation in the prosthetic valve due to various causes of dysfunction in prosthetic valve.

ECHO ASSESSMENT OF PROSTHETIC VALVE DYSFUNCTION

Dysfunction of PHV is a specific pathology, which needs special knowledge regarding their function, method of examination and the causes of dysfunction. Echocardiography, being the main imaging modality for assessment of PHV, plays a great role for evaluation of proper function as well as dysfunction of PHV. As there is a large variety of PHVs and there are many causes of their dysfunction, detection of exact cause dysfunction by echocardiography is often challenging. So, a careful systematic approach with transthoracic echocardiography (TTE) and transesophageal echocardiography (TEE) using two dimensional (2D), three-dimensional (3D), and Doppler echocardiography is crucial to find out the exact cause of PHV dysfunction and thus, to determine the appropriate treatment strategy.

Depending on the valve type and patient related factors, various early and late complications can arise with PHV resulting in its dysfunction. The complications are as follows:

- Structural valve deterioration (bioprosthetic valves)
- Thrombus formation and thromboembolism
- Pannus formation
- Regurgitation (transvalvular and paravalvular)
- Endocarditis

Structural valve deterioration is an acquired intrinsic valve abnormality occurring in bioprosthetic heart valves

(BHVs) due to progressive spontaneous tissue degeneration resulting in thickening, calcification, tearing, or disruption of the prosthesis. This results in stenosis, regurgitation, or a combination of both.[1,2] Mitral bioprosthetic valves are at higher risk of degeneration possibly due to higher mechanical stress on closed mitral leaflets during ventricular systole.[3,4] Structural deterioration does not happen overnight. It takes few years to happen. So, echocardiographic findings also vary depending on the progress of the degenerative process.

The key 2D echocardiographic findings in structural deterioration of bioprosthetic valve are leaflet thickening, calcification **(Fig. 1A)**, perforation, tear, or prolapse. There is reduced mobility of the leaflets. Color flow Doppler shows turbulent flow across the valve due to stenosis **(Fig. 1B)**. Continuous wave (CW) Doppler shows with elevated trans-prosthetic pressure gradient. There may be pathological transvalvular regurgitation or a combined picture of stenosis and regurgitation on echocardiography.

Thrombus formation is a rare but potentially life-threatening complication of PHV characterized by thrombus formation on the prosthetic structures. Formation of thrombus subsequently results in dysfunction of prosthesis with or without incidence of thromboembolism.[5] Risk of thrombus formation is related to the type of valve, position of the valve and also adequacy of anticoagulation. Mechanical heart valves (MHVs) are more thrombogenic than BHVs.[6] Risk of thrombus formation is higher in mitral position than aortic position and also higher for right sided than left sided PHVs.[5] BHV is increasingly being recognized as a cause of prosthetic valve thrombosis occurring in 6–11% of cases in surgically implanted valves.[7] The risk of thrombus formation after transcatheter aortic valve replacement is highest in the first 3 months after the implantation and thereafter decreases.[8] To prevent thrombus formation and subsequent thromboembolism, all patients are given short- or long-term anticoagulation after implantation of PHV. Risk and possibility of thrombus formation is high in patients with subtherapeutic international normalized ratio (INR). Thrombosis may result in hemodynamically severe stenosis or regurgitation. Clinical presentation of PHV thrombosis is usually subacute or chronic although it may present acutely with a fresh thrombus. When thrombosis is suspected, a careful physical examination should be done with particular attention to muffling or absence of prosthetic sound and appearance of a new stenotic or regurgitant murmur on auscultation.

Irrespective of the location or type of prosthesis, the initial diagnostic work-up in suspected PHV thrombosis starts with a TTE.[9,10] A standard complete TTE examination of the PHV along with other cardiac structures is done using multiple conventional and unconventional views. PHV should be inspected by 2D echocardiography with particular attention to the opening and closing motion of the moving parts of the prosthesis. Limited opening or complete immobility of disks/leaflets is a sign of prosthetic valve thrombosis **(Fig. 2A)**. Thrombus may be visualized as soft, homogeneous, mobile, or sessile mass in relation to the sewing ring and disks/leaflets **(Fig. 2B)**. Thrombi tend to start in the sewing ring area and then spread to the disks/leaflets leading to malcoaptation. Location of thrombus is usually on the atrial side of the mitral and aortic side of the aortic prosthesis. If a thrombus is visualized, its size should be measured and location should also be identified in order to determine the adverse hemodynamic consequences of thrombus. A large thrombus extending beyond the valve is a risk factor for complication of thrombolytic therapy. A thrombus area <0.85 cm^2 on TEE anticipates a low risk for embolism or death associated with thrombolytic therapy. Vegetation in PHV endocarditis may look similar to a thrombus and difficult to differentiate by echocardiography.

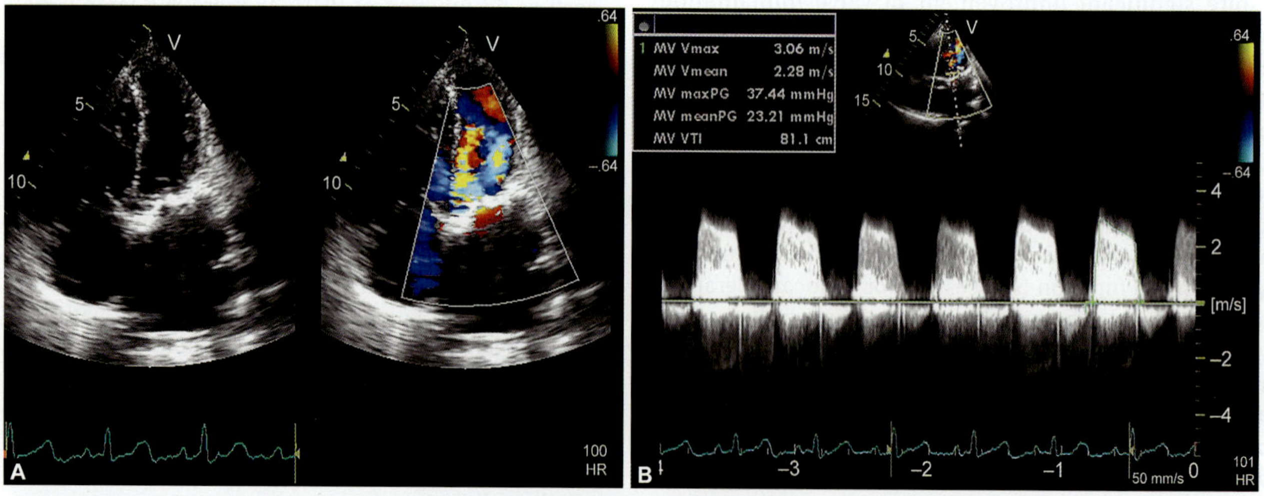

FIGS. 1A AND B: (A) Apical four-chamber view showing degenerative changes (dense calcification) in the leaflets of a mitral bioprosthetic valve (a 2D image) resulting in severe obstruction to mitral inflow. (B) Color flow shows turbulent flow across mitral prosthesis (a color flow across mitral prosthesis) with a mean pressure gradient of 23 mm Hg on continuous wave (CW) Doppler.

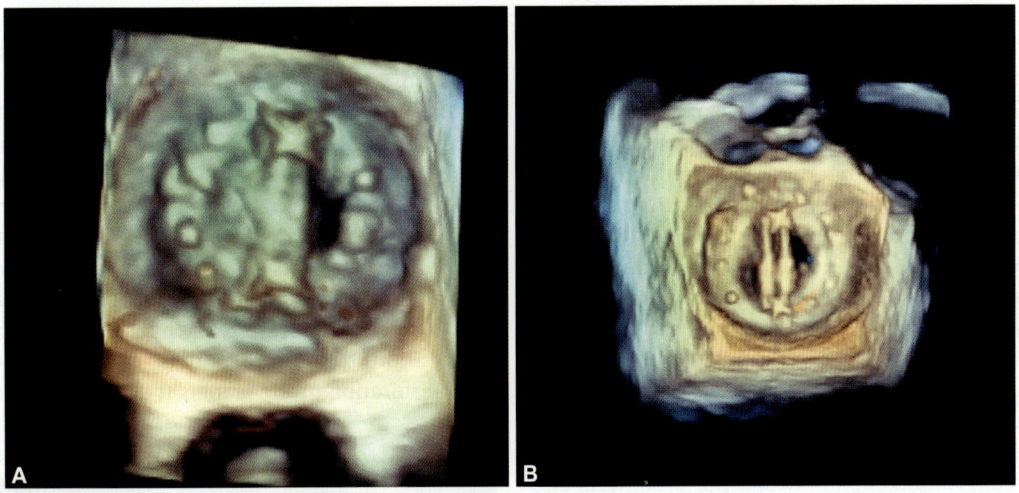

FIGS. 2A AND B: A 3D TEE image of bileaflet MPV in mitral position before (A) and after (B) thrombolysis in a case of stuck mitral prosthesis due to formation of thrombus.

(3D: three dimensional; MPV: mitral prosthetic valve; TEE: transesophageal echocardiography)

In such situations, diagnosis is to be made combining of clinical and imaging criteria.

Color flow Doppler echocardiography shows abnormal turbulent flow across the prosthesis if the thrombus is causing obstruction and CW Doppler shows a high transvalvular gradient. There may be a transvalvular regurgitation **(Box 1)**. Echocardiographic signs of pulmonary hypertension may be present in PHV thrombosis with obstruction in mitral or aortic position. Obstruction due to thrombus in a PHV is associated with catastrophic hemodynamic consequences and needs urgent diagnosis and management with thrombolytic therapy or surgical intervention.

It is often difficult to visualize clearly the mobility of the disks and presence of thrombus by TTE because of acoustic shadowing caused by mean platelet volume (MPV).[9,10] Moreover, quality of TTE images becomes suboptimal due to presence of various other conditions, such as obesity, emphysematous lung, sternotomy from previous surgery, and pericardial effusion.[10] TEE solves this problem by providing better quality image for both mechanical and bioprosthetic valves with greater diagnostic accuracy for detection of mechanical PHV dysfunction.[10] TEE has a higher sensitivity for identification of thrombus and is also able to assess leaflet motion better. TEE as a complementary tool to TTE allows better visualization and has a higher sensitivity for identification of structural valve degeneration (SVD), presence of thrombus, pannus, or vegetations and is also able to assess leaflet motion better, especially in the mitral and to a lesser degree in the aortic position.

Therefore, after initial screening by TTE, TEE should be done in all cases of suspected prosthetic valve dysfunction for confirmation of findings obtained by TTE and also for additional echocardiographic findings of thrombosis.

BOX 1 Echocardiographic signs of PHV thrombosis with obstruction.

- Limited opening or complete immobility of disks/leaflets
- Presence of a thrombus in the sewing ring/disk/leaflet
- Abnormal turbulent flow across the prosthesis
- New onset transvalvular regurgitation
- Stenosis with elevated transprosthetic pressure gradient
- Mixed findings of stenosis and regurgitation

Five risk factors are associated with BHV thrombosis which are (1) thickened leaflets, (2) abnormal mobility of leaflets, (3) about >50% increase in transprosthetic mean pressure gradient from baseline within 5 years, (4) atrial fibrillation, and (5) subtherapeutic INR.[7] The presence of all five risk factors is associated with a specificity of 93%, a positive predictive value of 85%, and a negative predictive value of 89% for thrombosis.

However, 2D TEE cannot differentiate a thrombus from pannus. It is 3D TEE that can identify and differentiate pannus from thrombus.[10]

With MHV, fluoroscopy or computed tomography (CT) can be done to see the excursion of the disks. Fluoroscopy cannot be used in BHV as it is radiolucent.[10]

Pannus Formation

Pannus related prosthetic valve dysfunction is an uncommon but serious complication.[11] Pannus is a slow overgrowth of fibroelastic tissue and collagen over the years along the suture line of sewing ring and spreads to the prosthesis in a centripetal direction.[12] Although thrombosis remains the most common cause of obstruction of PHV, protrusion of pannus into the valve orifice may disturb the blood flow through prosthesis resulting in its obstruction with increased transprosthetic pressure gradient.[11,13] This is a serious issue, which needs to be identified, as surgery is the only treatment option in patients with PHV obstruction by pannus formation. But, imaging of a pannus by standard echocardiography is a problem as it is almost impossible to visualize pannus by 2D TEE, which is the method of choice for diagnosis of PHV obstruction. On the other hand, differentiation of thrombus and pannus is extremely important for deciding the line of management, as thrombolysis is done for thrombus formation, whereas pannus needs surgical intervention **(Table 1)**. Real time 3D TEE imaging plays a great role in this situation as this sophisticated technology can visualize the pannus.[10] Real-time 3D TEE is a milestone in the era of cardiovascular imaging of prosthetic valve and their dysfunction. This novel tool provides unique "en face" views which allows better understanding of the pathology and anatomical relationships between the prosthesis and intracardiac structures. Diagnosis of pannus can be made by visualizing the fixed, bright, high echo density mass with a semicircular configuration along the sewing ring on "en face" view **(Fig. 3)**. With its high resolution, it provides better visualization of the atrial and ventricular sides of mitral prostheses and can differentiate thrombus from pannus formation.[14,15] Pannus and thrombus may coexist because pannus may induce thrombus formation. Pannus formation with obstruction can happen both in BPV and MPV with similar incidence.[16]

Prosthetic Valve Regurgitation

Like stenosis, prosthetic valve dysfunction can also result in regurgitation. When color Doppler examination reveals regurgitation in a PHV, next important step is to distinguish whether it is physiological or pathological regurgitation. Mild physiological transvalvular regurgitation is normally observed both in mechanical and 10% of bioprosthetic valves. These washing jets occur at the hinges by motion of the disks **(Fig. 4)**. Physiological regurgitation is laminar nonturbulent, early in onset and persists for a brief duration **(Box 2)**. There is a characteristic pattern of physiological regurgitation for each valve type. In bileaflet PHV there are three jets, on the other hand there are two jets of in monoleaflet prosthesis. Physiological regurgitation jets are intended to reduce risk of thrombosis in PHVs.

But *pathological regurgitation* can occur in PHV dysfunction. Pathological regurgitation can be transvalvular or paravalvular.

Pathological transvalvular regurgitation in BHV is associated with chronic structural degenerative changes in the valve leaflets or with endocarditis leading leaflet destruction. 2D echocardiography can detect the different finding of degenerative changes, such as calcification, perforation, tear in the leaflets or presence of vegetation, and perforation in the leaflets if there is endocarditis. Color

TABLE 1: Difference between a pannus and thrombus.

Pannus	Thrombus
INR—normal	INR—low
Slow onset of symptoms	Sudden onset of symptoms
Mass grows along suture line	Mass projects from valve disk
Echogenic	Less echogenic
Stable pressure gradient	Sudden increase of pressure gradient
Not visualized by 2D TEE. Needs 3D TEE to visualize	Visualized by TTE, 2D TEE

(2D: two-dimensional; 3D: three-dimensional; INR: international normalized ratio; TEE: transesophageal echocardiography)

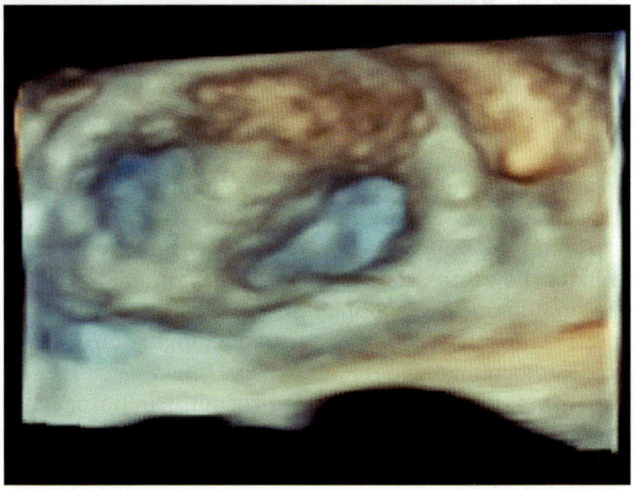

FIG. 3: A 3D TEE image of pannus over the sewing ring extending to the hinges in a bileaflet MPV in mitral position.

(3D: three-dimensional; MPV: mean platelet volume; TEE: transesophageal echocardiography)

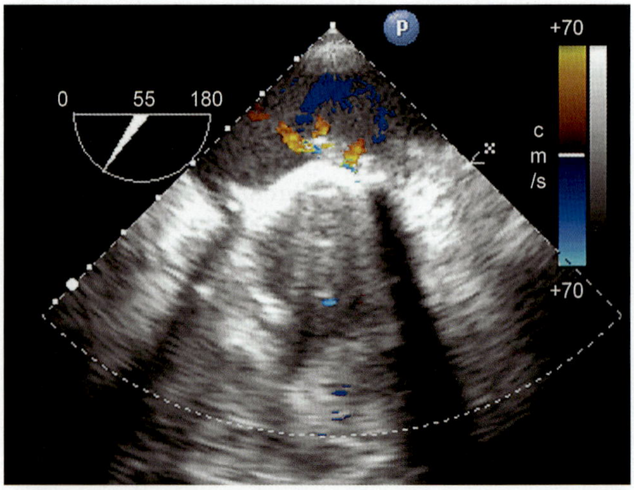

FIG. 4: Transesophageal echo of a bileaflet mechanical prosthetic valve in mitral position showing three small jets of physiological transvalvular regurgitation.

BOX 2 Echocardiographic signs of physiological transvalvular regurgitation.

- Laminar nonturbulent flow
- Early in onset and persists for a brief duration
- Symmetric
- Characteristic pattern for each valve
- Normal looking valve disks/leaflets

BOX 3 Echocardiographic signs of pathological transvalvular regurgitation.

- Nonlaminar turbulent flow
- Greater flow duration
- Does not maintain any characteristic pattern
- Presence of thrombus, pannus, or vegetation
- Associated findings, such as chamber dilatation and pulmonary hypertension

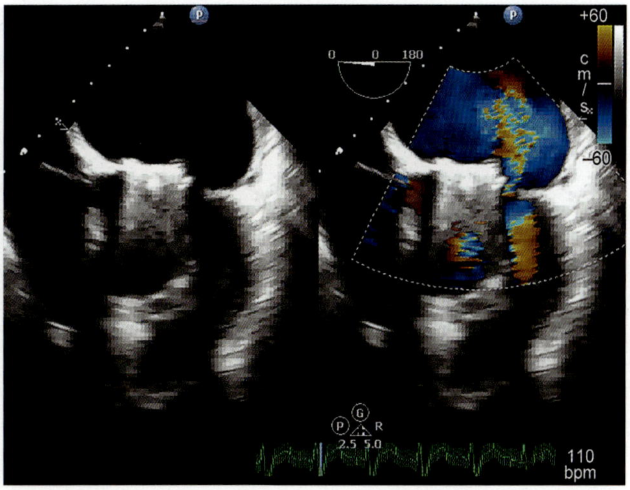

FIG. 5: Transesophageal echocardiography (TEE) image showing dehiscence in mitral prosthesis with paravalvular regurgitation across the dehiscence on the color flow mapping.

flow Doppler shows presence of transvalvular regurgitation, which may be moderate to, severe.

Pathological transvalvular regurgitation in MHV is associated with formation of thrombus, pannus, or vegetation, which prevent complete closure of the occluder. TTE, TEE, and 3D TEE can demonstrate presence of thrombus, pannus or vegetation impinging the motion of the disks or trapping the disk in open position. Color flow shows transvalvular regurgitation. Pathological transvalvular regurgitation jet is nonlaminar, turbulent having greater flow duration unlike physiological regurgitation, which persists only for a brief period **(Box 3)**. There may be associated findings such as chamber dilatation and pulmonary hypertension depending on the severity and duration of regurgitation.

Regurgitation jets are often difficult to demonstrate by color Doppler in mechanical prosthesis due to presence of acoustic shadowing and reverberation artifacts produced on the back of the prosthesis. Because of this, sensitivity for the detection of mitral prosthetic regurgitation is lower as regurgitation jets are hidden by acoustic shadowing and reverberation artifacts in left atrium (LA) in apical four-chamber view of TTE. It is more difficult to distinguish physiological from pathologic regurgitation. TEE solves this problem by keeping the LA clear of artifacts and is indicated when the diagnosis is suspected on clinical ground. TEE can differentiate transvalvular from paravalvular regurgitation. So TEE is invaluable in this regard. Aortic MPVs are less susceptible to the acoustic shadowing. Parasternal long and short axis, apical long axis, four chambers, and five chambers views of TTE are used to assess presence and severity of regurgitation from MPVs. When there is a double valve replacement with mechanical prosthesis, left ventricular (LV) outflow region may be obscured during TEE by the artifacts produced by mitral prosthesis making the assessment of aortic prosthesis difficult.

Paravalvular regurgitation or leak (PVL) is a pathological complication commonly due to dehiscence from disruption or avulsion of sutures in sewing ring precipitated by infective endocarditis with abscess formation or presence of significant calcification and fibrotic scar of the native annulus. Incomplete fixation of sewing ring to the native annulus due to the suture technique during surgery may also play a role. This will result in a gap between the sewing ring of prosthesis and native cardiac tissue resulting in leak of blood through that gap. PVL may result in severe hemolysis. PVL may occur both in MPV and BPV but incidence is more in MPV.[17-20] PVL is more common in mitral than aortic PHV. PVL may be single or multiple in number.[18,21] The leak can appear early when it is due to surgical procedural technique, or late, when caused by suture dehiscence or infection.[19] In transcatheter aortic valve replacement (TAVR), PVL is due to under sizing of prosthesis. Aortic PVL is a common finding following TAVR occurs in 65–96% of TAVR cases.[22,26] In most of the cases, PVL is mild. Moderate to severe PVL occurs in 2–24% of patients.[22-26]

Echocardiography of PVL is challenging due to presence of artifacts especially in MPV.TTE often cannot identify PVL and also can not differentiate PVL from transvalvular regurgitation. TEE is invaluable in this regard. However, if the quality of image is good, it is possible to locate the gap outside the sewing ring in 2D TTE. Color flow confirms presence of PVL by demonstrating regurgitation flow through the gap. Multiple and atypical views are needed to demonstrate PVL. TEE provides superior quality of image than TTE and can identify and confirm the presence of PVL **(Fig. 5)**.

But 2D TEE cannot define the exact size, shape, and location of PVL in relation to cardiac structures, which are crucial information for percutaneous device closure of PVL. Three dimensional TEE has emerged as the preferred imaging modality to evaluate the morphology and extent of

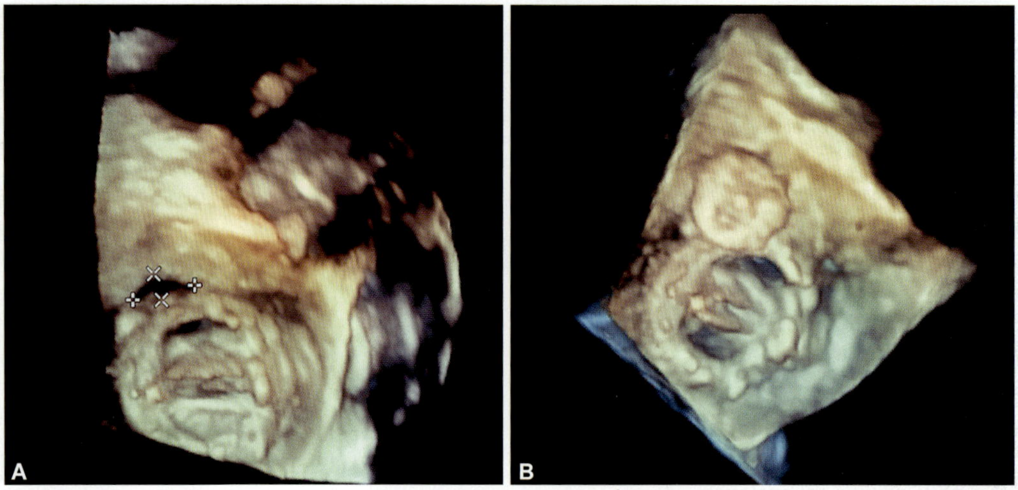

FIGS. 6A AND B: A 3D TEE "en face" view of bileaflet mitral prosthesis showing paravalvular leak at 11 o'clock position (A) before and (B) after transcatheter device closure.

PVL, as it better demonstrates, compared with 2D echo, the shapes and sizes of the leaks. 2D TEE measurement of PVL is a single dimensional measurement, which is true if the PVL is cylindrical in shape, but PVL is not cylindrical, rather it is a crescent shaped having a minor and a major dimension. Measuring and sizing of the PVL is crucial in order to choose the correct size of the percutaneous closure device, which can be done precisely by measuring the areas of echo dropout in 3D TEE image that represent the presence of a leak **(Figs. 6A and B)**. Successful percutaneous device closure of PVL depends not only on the accurate sizing, but also on accurate localization of the site of regurgitation in relation to the surrounding cardiac structure. With the help of 3D TEE it is possible to get "en face" view of the prosthesis, which accurately localizes the leak in relation to surrounding cardiac structures.[27,28]

Prosthetic Valve Endocarditis

Prosthetic valve endocarditis (PVE) is a nightmare to the patient as well as to the physician as it is an extremely serious and potentially fatal complication after valve replacement, associated with a high mortality risk of about 20–30%[29,30] which is higher than native valve endocarditis. Bioprosthetic and mechanical valves are equally affected. Mitral PVE is less affected than aortic, with an incidence of 0.49% versus 0.91% per patient per year in bioprosthetic valves and 0.18% versus 0.27% per patient per year in mechanical valves.[31,32]

Lower incidence of vegetation is noted in PVE than native valve endocarditis but PVE is characterized by more incidence of devastating paravalvular complications resulting in the formation of ring abscess, intercavitary fistula communicating two neighboring chambers, pseudo-aneurysm, and dehiscence of prosthesis due to spread of infection to the periannular tissue **(Fig. 7)**.

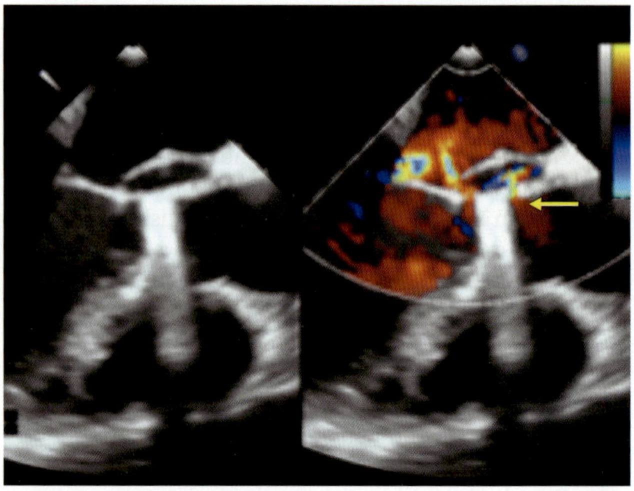

FIG. 7: A 2D TEE image of a mechanical prosthetic valve in aortic position showing a periannular abscess, which has ruptured into the left ventricle. A fistulous communication is seen between aortic root and the abscess demarcated by the yellow arrow.

(2D: two-dimensional; TEE: transesophageal echocardiography)

Echocardiography is considered the basic diagnostic tool for PVE.[33,34] However, findings of infective endocarditis are more difficult to detect by TTE in prosthetic valves than in native valves because of acoustic shadowing and reverberation artifacts in PHV. Hence, TEE is the mandatory diagnostic imaging technique in a suspected case of PVE as TEE has got a high sensitivity for detection of various findings of PVE with precise anatomic information, which are needed for planning of surgery[29,33] Attention should be paid to detect periannular complications while doing echocardiography in a suspected PVE. Abnormal rocking motion of a sewing ring seen in TTE/TEE is a clue to

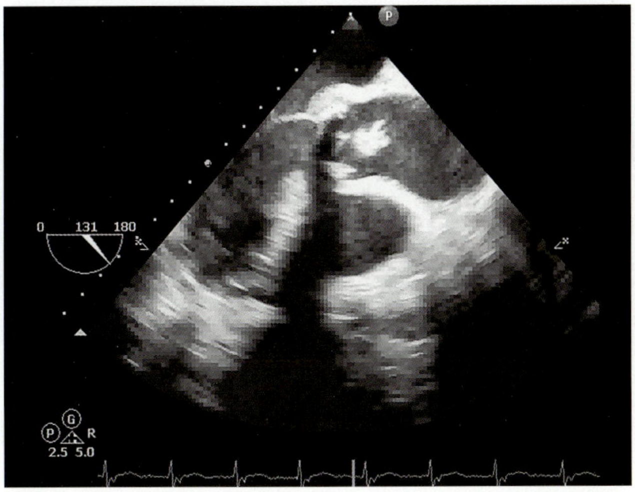

FIG. 8: A 2D TEE image showing a large vegetation in aortic prosthetic valve.

(2D: two-dimensional; TEE: transesophageal echocardiography)

dehiscence of the prosthesis. Vegetation in PVE is a linear or nonlinear mobile mass with irregular margin and low echogenicity. It shows chaotic motion especially when the vegetation is linear **(Fig. 8)**. Like thrombus, vegetation also starts in the ring and then spread to the leaflets, which may cause valve malcoaptation leading to transvalvular regurgitation **(Box 4)**. As discussed earlier, it is often difficult to differentiate vegetation from thrombus by echocardiography as both look similar. In such situations, both clinical and imaging criteria are combined to come to a diagnosis. A large vegetation may cause obstruction to blood flow resulting in increased transprosthetic pressure gradient.

BOX 4 Echocardiographic signs of prosthetic valve endocarditis.

- Vegetation (lower incidence than native valve IE)
- Perforation in leaflet in BPV
- Ring abscess
- Fistulous communication between neighboring chambers
- Rocking motion of the sewing ring—a clue for dehiscence
- Dehiscence outside the sewing ring with paravalvular regurgitation
- Pseudoaneurysm
- Transvalvular regurgitation from malcoaptation of leaflets caused by vegetation

(BPV: bioprosthetic valve; IE: infectious endocarditis)

CONCLUSION

Prosthetic valve dysfunction may introduce a new disease process in a patient who has undergone valve replacement. Though rare, but prosthetic valve dysfunction is potentially life threatening associated with significant morbidity and mortality. So, it is important to identify these dysfunctions as early as possible so that appropriate treatment can be initiated promptly to reduce morbidity and mortality and improve the patient outcome. On suspicion of prosthetic valve dysfunction, work is started initially with routine transthoracic echocardiogram. Use of transesophageal echo is mandatory for identification of the exact cause of prosthetic valve dysfunction as it provides better visualization of the prosthetic valve structure and function. Use of 3D transesophageal echo is necessary in some situations like paravalvular leak as it shows accurate location, size, and shape of the paravalvular leak which are necessary information for percutaneous device closure of paravalvular leak.

ONLINE REFERENCES

Please scan the QR code provided at the end of the table of contents for References of this chapter.

CHAPTER

107 Subcostal Window in Pediatric Echocardiogram

S Gnansambandam, S Kumaran

ABSTRACT

Subcostal windows provide an alternative view to visualize the heart at multiple planes, especially when transthoracic windows are suboptimal. In newborns and pediatric patients, better resolution can be obtained due to the lack of interference from the lungs and thoracic cage. However, the disadvantage is that the chambers may appear foreshortened, which can underestimate their dimensions. Doppler assessment may also be inaccurate due to suboptimal alignment of the cursors. Additional nomograms are required to improve the diagnostic value of subcostal views.

Three-dimensional echocardiography subcostal views can be used to analyze cardiac structures from the surgeon's point of view, mostly in preprocedural, periprocedural, and postprocedural assessment.

Keywords: Subcostal window, tetralogy of Fallot, left ventricle, inferior vena cava.

INTRODUCTION

Early reports on subcostal window were from 80's of 20th century.[1,2] Substernal angle **(Fig. 1)** is formed in front of thoracic cage by the cartilages of 7th, 8th, 9th, and 10th ribs which ascend toward sternum and join at the xiphoid process.[3] Normal subcostal angle is 90° and more acute in males. The subcostal plane **(Fig. 2)** bisects the thorax at the level of 10th costal margin and L3 vertebra.

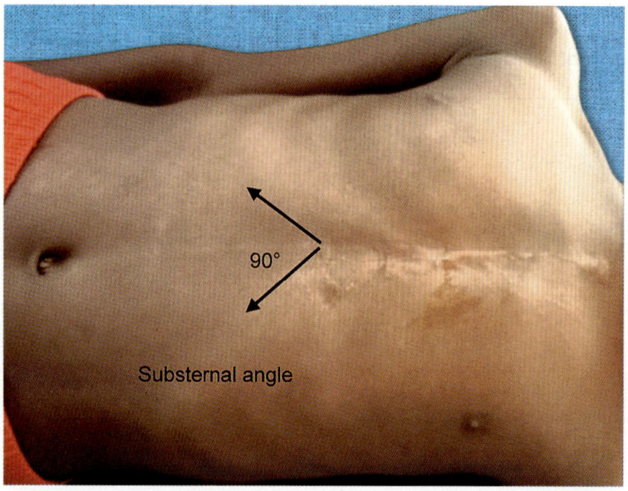

FIG. 1: Subcostal angle.

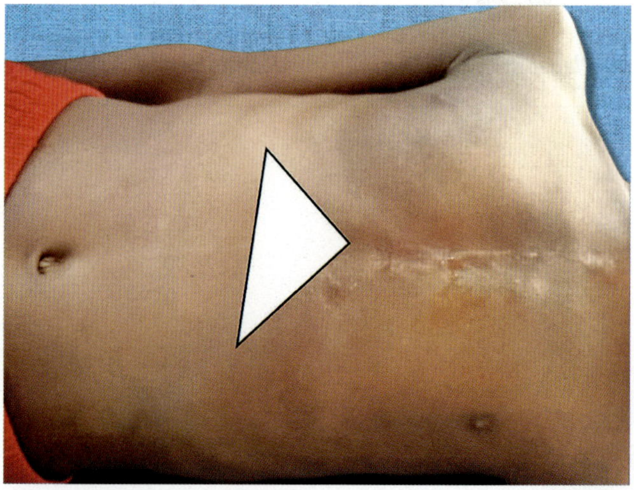

FIG. 2: Subcostal plane.

ADVANTAGES

- Subcostal window gives good spatial appreciation of cardiac anatomy, more often used in congenital heart disease and providing good imaging quality when thoracic window is suboptimal as in pneumothorax, postsurgical states and when chest wound and surgical dressing limit transthoracic imaging.
- In newborn, toddlers and subcostal windows provide good imaging quality.
- No lung or bone tissue to interfere in cardiac imaging with liver providing a good window.
- Echo using subcostal window can be done in supine position.
- Useful in rescue cardiac ultrasonogram when the patient is hemodynamically unstable.

DISADVANTAGES

- Suboptimal in obese patients and adolescents due to altered spatial orientation.
- In postoperative state with mediastinal and pericardial drainage, subcostal viewing is challenging.
- *Assessment of great arteries*: Proximal portion can be assessed as they are closer to probe but the distal vessels are far away in the field, limiting the proper assessment.
    - Anatomy of patent ductus arteriosus and its hemodynamics is poorly assessed by subcostal window.
    - Aortic isthmus is inadequately visualized in coarctation of aorta and interrupted aortic arch.[4,5]
- The angle at which cardiac chambers are viewed is foreshortened leading to underestimation of dimension, and overestimation of its function and inaccurate Doppler assessment.

PROCEDURE

Optimal Probe Selection

Use low-frequency probes (ranging from 4 to 12 MHz) to achieve desired penetration depths based on specific requirements. High-frequency probes offer superior resolution but less penetration, while lower frequency probes provide better penetration but lower resolution. In neonates and infants, high-frequency probes are preferred. Zoom mode is used to increase the resolution whenever required. In neonates and infants, these views can be readily obtained unlike adult patients. Subcostal approach may be the best option in children suffering from lung disease and in intensive care units.[5]

Breath Holding and Inhalation

In children and adolescents, optimal images can be obtained by instructing the patient to hold their breath or take a deep inhalation during the procedure.

Patient Positioning

Positioned in supine with folded legs and relaxed abdomen.

ANATOMICAL ORIENTATION OF IMAGE

Inverting the images corresponds to anatomical view of cardiac structures (surgeon's view of anatomy) **(Figs. 3A and B)**.

Probe placed 2–3 cm below the xiphoid process with marker pointing toward 6 o'clock position. In situs solitus, inferior vena cava (IVC) **(Fig. 4)** and aorta **(Fig. 5)**, liver is on the right and stomach on the left, both hemidiaphragms are visualized with spine visualized posteriorly.

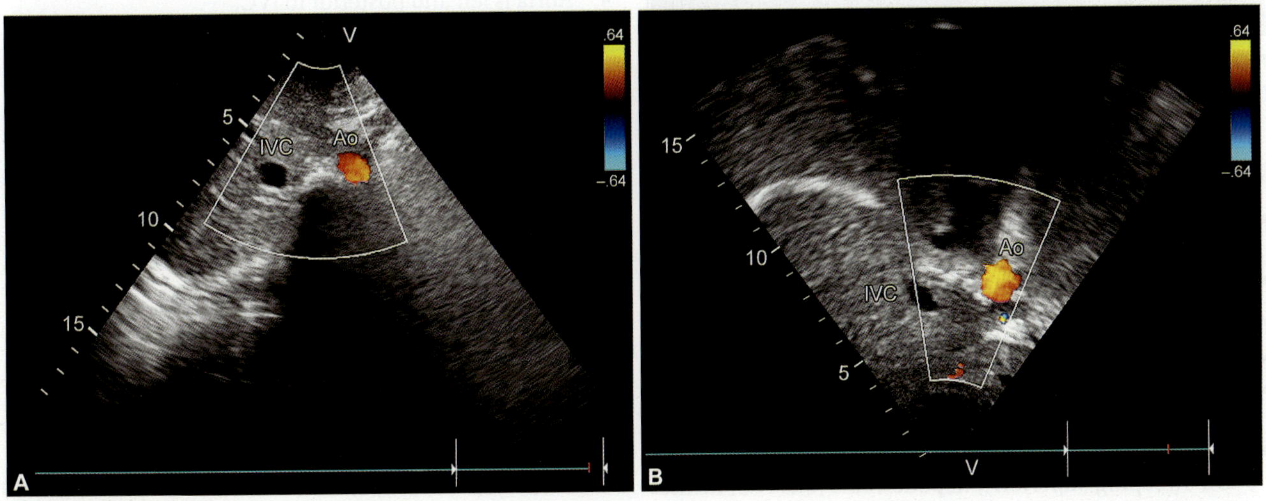

FIGS. 3A AND B: (A) Normal projection and (B) anatomical projection.
(Ao: aorta; IVC: inferior vena cava)

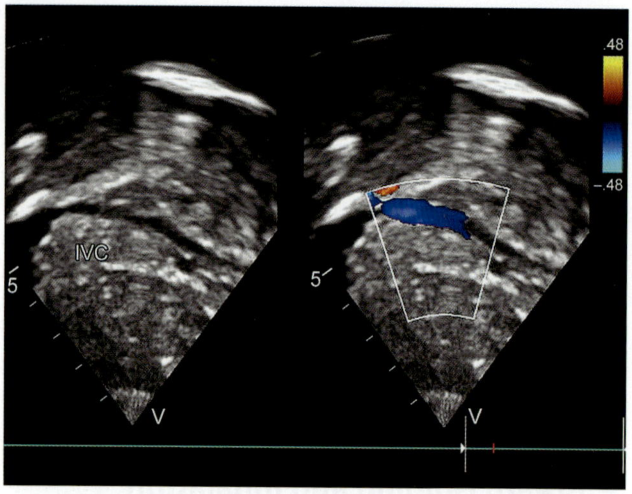

FIG. 4: Subxiphoid abdominal inferior vena cava (IVC) long-axis view.

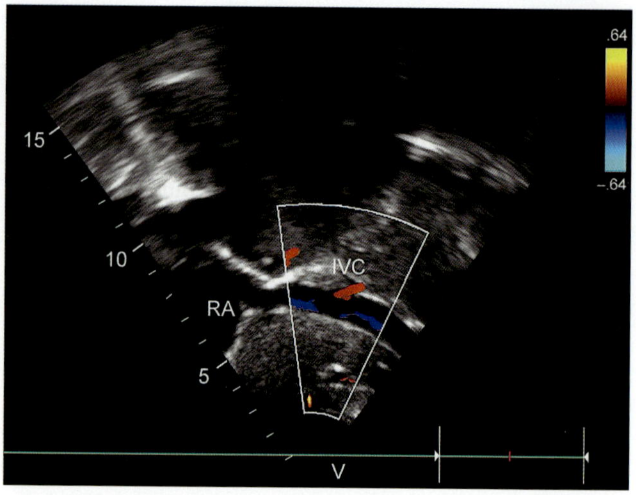

FIG. 6: Subxiphoid abdominal long-axis inferior vena cava (IVC) view.

(RA: right atrium)

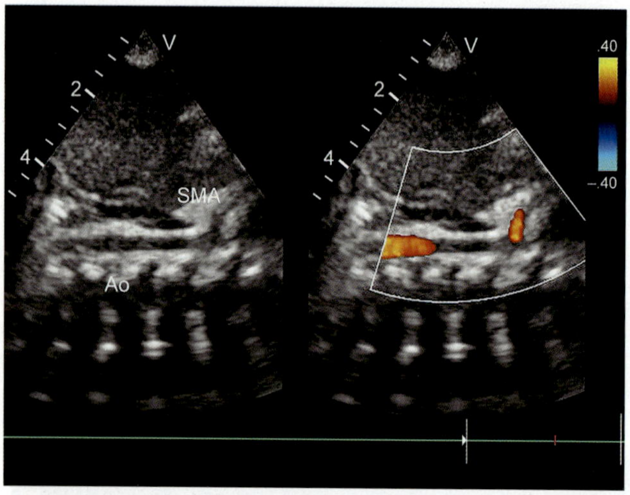

FIG. 5: Aorta (Ao) long-axis view.

(SMA: superior mesenteric artery)

Aorta

- Circular structure on the left of IVC, posterior to IVC, and overlying the spine posteriorly
- *Color Doppler*: Pulsatile flow toward thorax

IVC visualization:

- Ash-leaf shaped, right, anterior, and left to aorta
- *Color Doppler*: Nonpulsatile flow with respiratory variation
- *Flow direction*: Away from thorax

On sweeping superiorly, hepatic veins join IVC, further sweep visualizes both atrium, interatrial septum (IAS), and pulmonary veins into posterior wall of left atrium (LA), and further superior sweep finally superior vena cava (SVC) is joining into right atrium (RA).

SUBXIPHOID ABDOMINAL LONG-AXIS IVC VIEW DRAINING INTO RIGHT ATRIUM

Inferior vena cava would be visualized along the long axis **(Fig. 6)**. Probe may be tilted to visualize its entry into RA.

Situs Solitus Abdominus

- Aorta is left and posterior to IVC.
- IVC is on the right side and anterior to aorta.[6]

Situs Inversus Abdominus

- Aorta is right and posterior to IVC.
- IVC is on the left and anterior to aorta.

SITUS AMBIGUOUS: LEFT-SIDED ISOMERISM OR RIGHT-SIDED ISOMERISM

Right-sided Isomerism (Asplenia Syndrome)

Both aorta and IVC are juxtaposed (same side of spine) in parasternal gutter.

Left-sided Isomerism (Polysplenia Syndrome)

Interrupted IVC continues as azygos and hemiazygos seen posterior to descending aorta to drain into SVC.[6]

SUBXIPHOID CORONAL LONG-AXIS VIEWS (FIG. 7)

Subcostal Coronal Long-axis Four-chamber View (Reference View for Subcostal Long-axis View) (Fig. 8)

- *Probe positioning*: The ultrasound probe is placed on the upper abdomen utilizing the liver as an acoustic window to the heart with the *marker to the patient's left side at 3 o'clock*, and it is tilted horizontally against the anterior abdominal wall **(Fig. 9)**.
- *Cardiac apex and IAS*: In the subcostal four-chamber view, the apex of the heart is located more to the patient's left side compared to the traditional apical four-chamber view and the IAS appear more oblique.
- *Right heart chambers*: In this view, the right heart chambers (RA and right ventricle) are situated in the near field, below the liver. The ultrasound beam passes perpendicular to the IAS, enabling clear visualization of the entire septum using both color flow and B-mode imaging.
- *Pathology assessment*: This view is particularly useful for assessing certain cardiac pathologies, such as myxomas (benign tumors) and thrombi (blood clots) within the heart chambers.
- *Pericardial sac*: Global visualization of the pericardial sac from multiple angles, which is beneficial for assessing conditions such as pericardial effusion or cardiac tamponade.

Subxiphoid Coronal Long-axis Five-chamber View (Fig. 10)

Probe position is optimized and tilted anteriorly opening the left ventricular (LV) outflow tract and aorta **(Fig. 11)**.

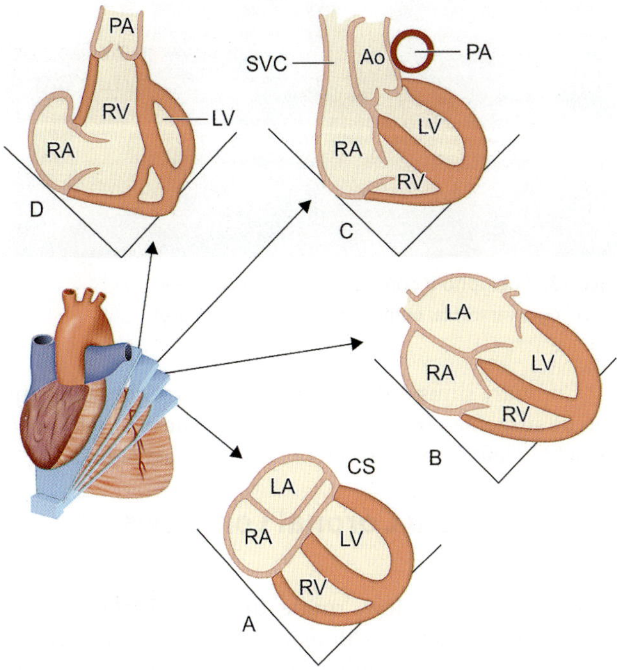

A. Four chamber coronary sinus view; B. Four chamber view; C. LVOT view; D. RVOT (right heart view)

FIG. 7: Subxiphoid coronal long-axis views.

(Ao: aorta; CS: coronary sinus; LA: left atrium; LV: left ventricular; LVOT: left ventricular outflow tract; PA: pulmonary artery; RA: right atrium; RV: right ventricular; RVOT: right ventricular outflow tract; SVC: superior vena cava)

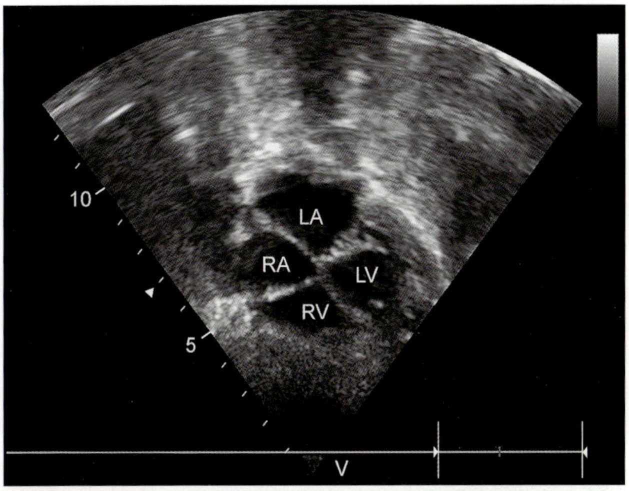

FIG. 8: Subcostal coronal long-axis four-chamber view.

(LA: left atrium; LV: left ventricular; RA: right atrium; RV: right ventricular)

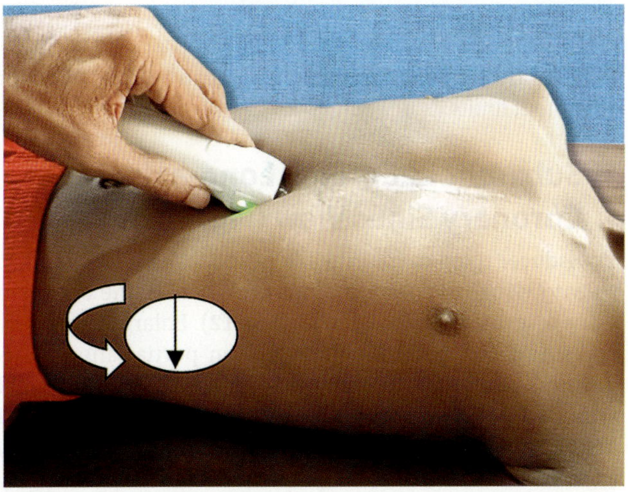

FIG. 9: Probe position in four chamber view.

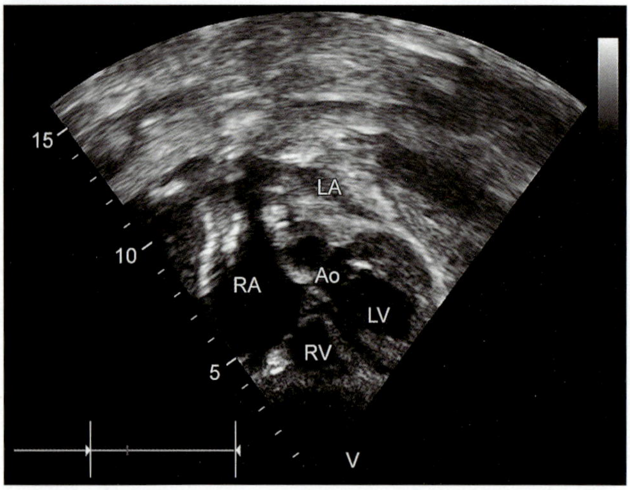

FIG. 10: Subxiphoid coronal long-axis five-chamber view.
(Ao: aorta; LA: left atrium; LV: left ventricular; RA: right atrium; RV: right ventricular)

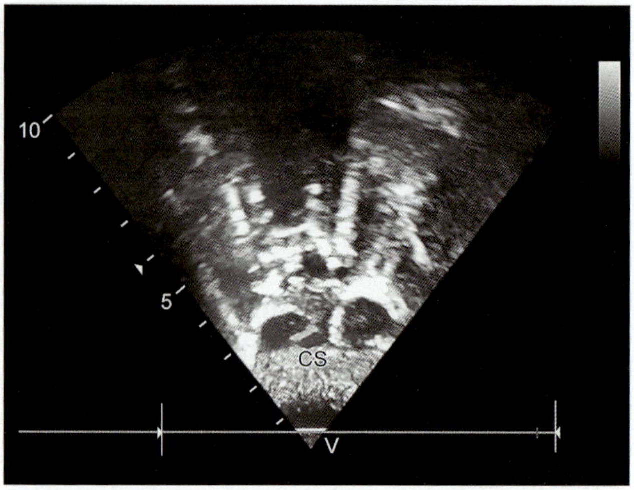

FIG. 12: Subxiphoid coronal long-axis coronary sinus (CS) view.

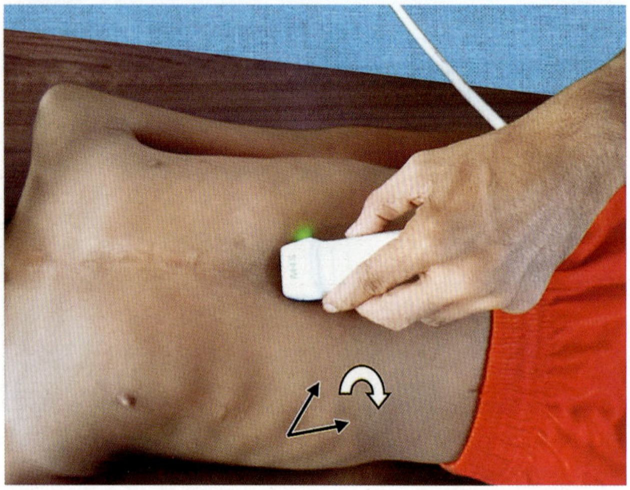

FIG. 11: Probe position.

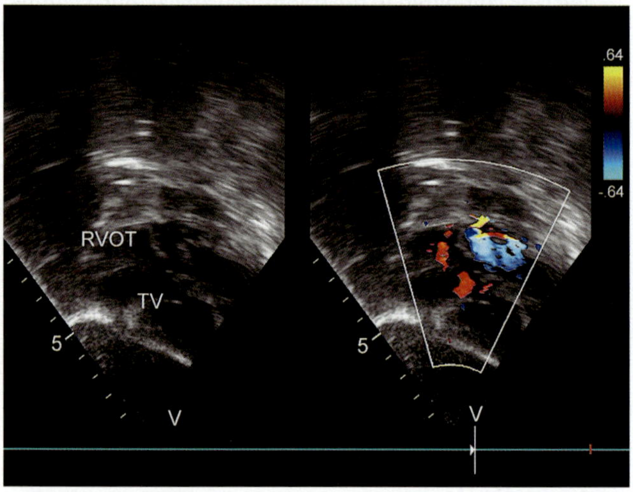

FIG. 13: Subxiphoid coronal long-axis RVOT view.
(RVOT: right ventricular outflow tract; TV: tricuspid valve)

Doppler assessment of LV outflow tract can be done but poor alignment limits its utility.

Subxiphoid Coronal Long-axis Coronary Sinus View (Fig. 12)

Transducer tilted caudally while in subcostal four-chamber view to visualize coronary sinus and flow in the coronary sinus assessed by color Doppler **(Fig. 12)**. Enlarged coronary sinus and increased flow are seen in partial anomalous pulmonary venous communication (PAPVC) and total anomalous pulmonary venous (TAPVC), coronary sinus atrial septal defect (ASD), persistent left-sided SVC, and elevated right atrial pressure such as pulmonary hypertension.[7]

Coronary sinus ASD due to unroofing of coronary sinus can be suspected by color flow Doppler showing right to left or right to left shunt between LA and coronary sinus.

Subxiphoid Coronal Long-axis RVOT View

In four-chamber view, rotate the transducer counter-clockwise, transducer with marker at 2 o'clock to visualize tricuspid valve, right ventricle, right ventricular (RV) outflow tract, and pulmonary valve **(Fig. 13)**. This view is best for visualizing pulmonary stenosis.

Tilting more cranially to progressively visualize pulmonary artery branches and patent ductus arteriosus. Though subcostal window is not recommended for PDA

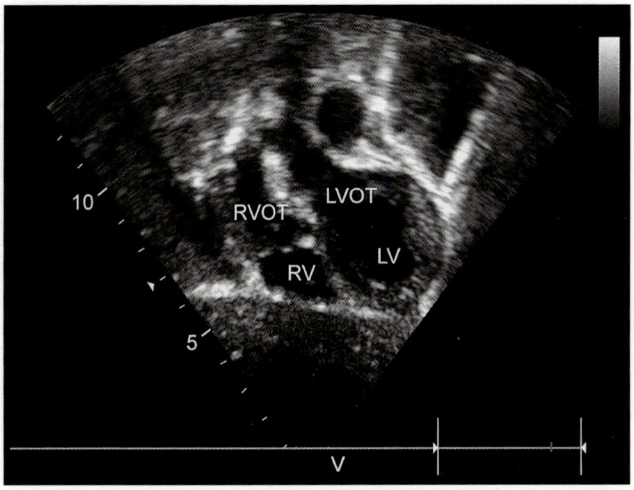

FIG. 14: Subxiphoid coronal long-axis LVOT view.
(LV: left ventricular; LVOT: left ventricular outflow tract; RV: right ventricular; RVOT: right ventricular outflow tract)

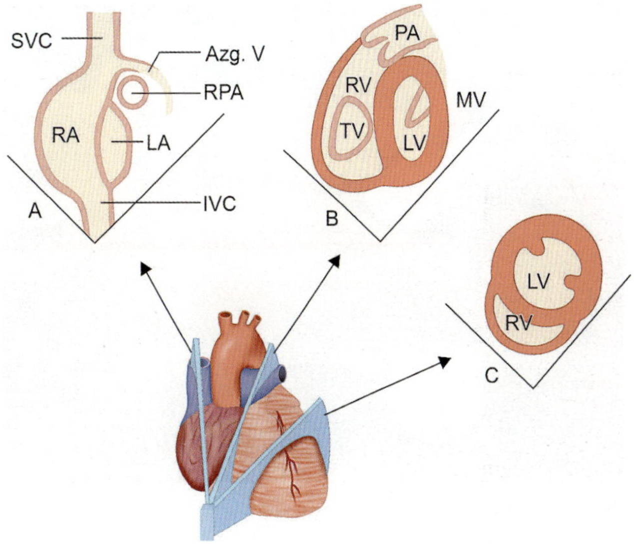

A. Bicaval view; B. RVOT view; C. RV/LV view

FIG. 15: Subxiphoid sagittal short-axis views.
(IVC: inferior vena cava; LA: left atrium; LV: left ventricular; RA: right atrium; RPA: right pulmonary artery; RV; right ventricular; RVOT; RV outflow tract; SVC: superior vena cava)

assessment. This right heart view is of particular value in infants and newborns with Ebstein's anomaly.

Subxiphoid Coronal Long-axis Left Ventricular Outflow Tract View

Probe tilted cranially to visualize LV outflow tract and aortic valve. In this view, interventricular septum (IVS), SVC, tricuspid valve (TV), pulmonary artery (PA), RV, LV aortic valve, and ascending aorta are visualized **(Fig. 14)**. Muscular and subaortic ventricular septal defect (VSD) can be evaluated in this view. Goose neck deformity of AV canal defect can be better seen this view. LV outflow tract obstruction and Doppler study can be assessed accurately.

SUBXIPHOID SAGITTAL SHORT-AXIS VIEWS (FIG. 15)

Subxiphoid Sagittal Short-axis Bicaval View (Fig. 16)

This *"reference view" with transducer notch positioned inferiorly (6 O'clock) views* **(Fig. 17)** the atria, RA appendage, IAS, SVC and IVC, cross section of right pulmonary artery (RPA) seen posterior to SVC and above roof of LA, and right upper pulmonary vein (RUPV) lateral and posterior to SVC. Azygos is seen arching above RPA joining SVC.

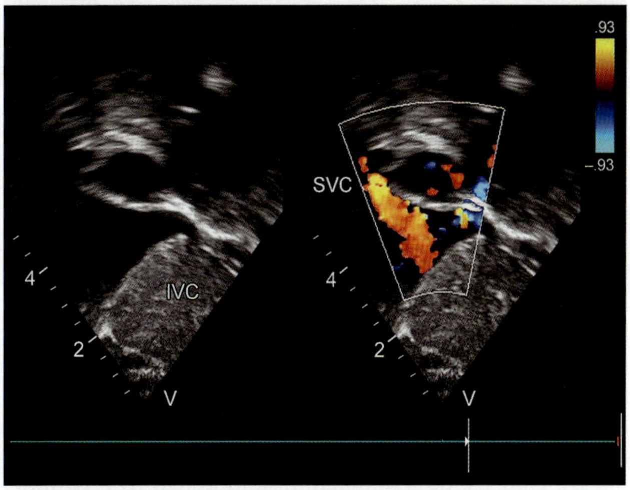

FIG. 16: Subxiphoid sagittal short-axis bicaval view.
(IVC: inferior vena cava; SVC: superior vena cava)

Subcostal Sagittal Short-axis View at the Level of Mitral Valve and Papillary Muscles

- *Cleft mitral valve in Down syndrome patients with atrioventricular (AV) canal defect*: Down syndrome patients with AV canal defects are associated cleft mitral valve and this view is ideal for identifying clefts.
- *Parachute mitral valve with single papillary muscle*: Mitral valve has a single papillary muscle instead of the normal two.
- *Assessment of LV function using M-mode echocardiogram*: When the transthoracic window is suboptimal and other imaging views are challenging to obtain, M-mode echocardiogram in the subcostal view can be used to assess LV function to measure LV dimensions and wall motion analysis.
- *Short-axis view at the level of LV apex*: This specific short-axis view at the level of the LV apex is useful for

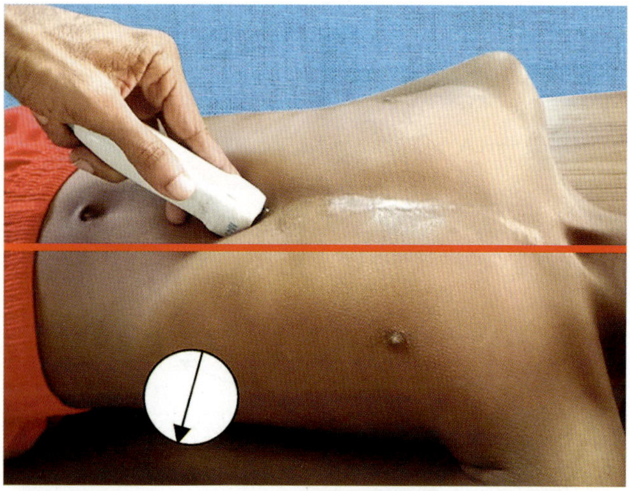

FIG. 17: Probe in short-axis bicaval view.

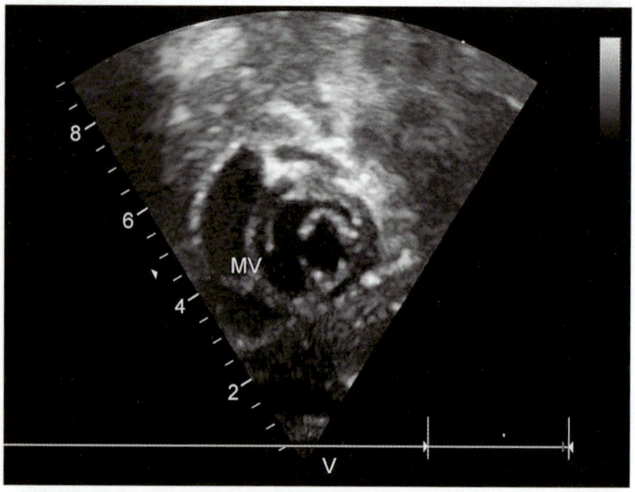

FIG. 19: Short-axis [mitral valve (MV)].

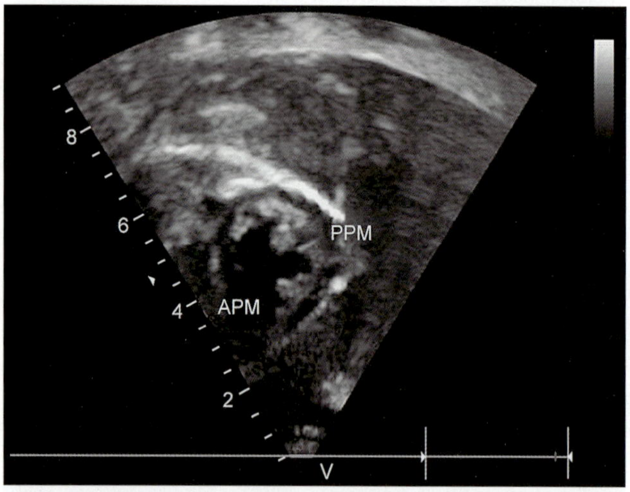

FIG. 18: Subcostal sagittal short-axis view (papillary muscle).
(APM: anterior papillary muscle; PPM: posterior papillary muscle)

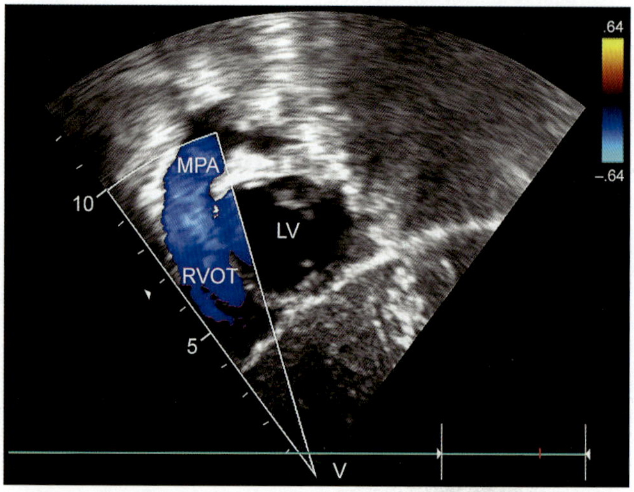

FIG. 20: Subcostal sagittal short-axis RVOT sweep view.
(LV: left ventricular; MPA: main pulmonary artery; RVOT: right ventricular outflow tract)

LV clot, LV noncompaction, and apical hypertrophic cardiomyopathy:

- "Bread loafing" technique also known as the "stack of disks" technique, performed to obtain short-axis images at multiple levels of the heart **(Figs. 18 and 19)**. It involves systematically adjusting the position of the ultrasound probe to acquire sequential short-axis views from the base to the apex of the heart. This technique is particularly helpful for assessing the shape, size, and function of the left ventricle.

Subcostal Sagittal Short-axis Right Ventricular Outflow Tract Sweep

Pulmonary regurgitation and pulmonary stenosis can be assessed well in this view **(Fig. 20)**. Using color Doppler muscular VSD especially LV to RVOT shunt as well as pulmonic, subvalvular, and valvular stenosis can be evaluated.

Subxiphoid Short-axis LV/RV View

The short-axis view obtained by rotating the ultrasound transducer clockwise with pointer of probe at around 6 o'clock position from the subcostal four-chamber view with the LV cavity appearing as circular as possible **(Fig. 21)**. Useful in detecting muscular VSD, elevated RV pressure in pulmonary hypertension or pulmonary stenosis results in D-shaped septum and LV hypertrophy (LVH).[8]

Subcostal Sagittal Short-axis View at Aortic Level (Fig. 22)

Probe is positioned with the pointer at the 5 to 6 o'clock position **(Fig. 23)**, with aorta at the center with LA, RA, right

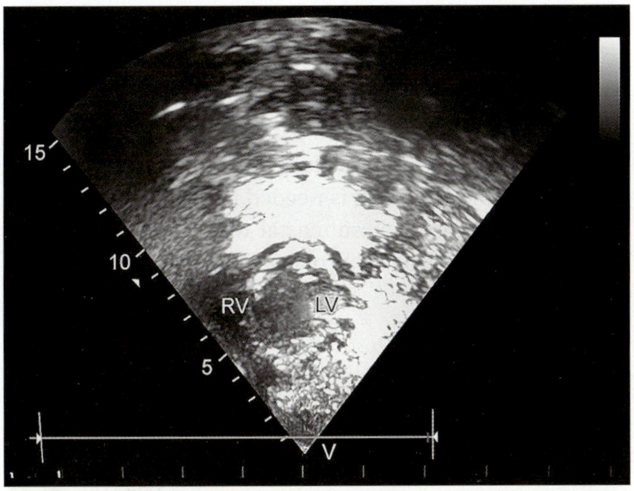

FIG. 21: Subxiphoid short-axis LV/RV view.
(LV: left ventricular; RV: right ventricular)

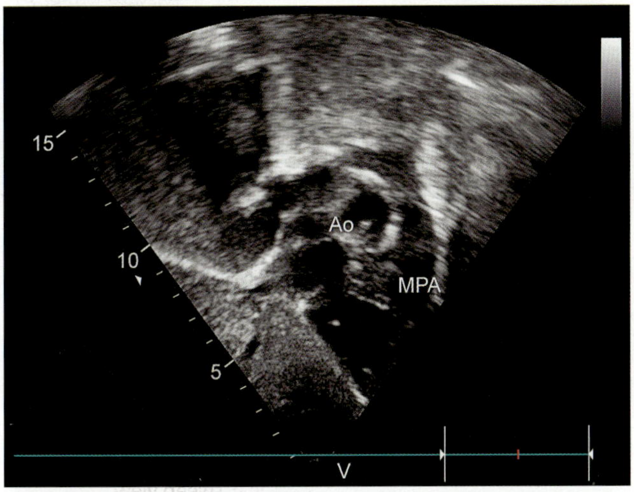

FIG. 22: Subcostal sagittal short-axis view (aortic level).
(Ao: aorta; MPA: main pulmonary artery)

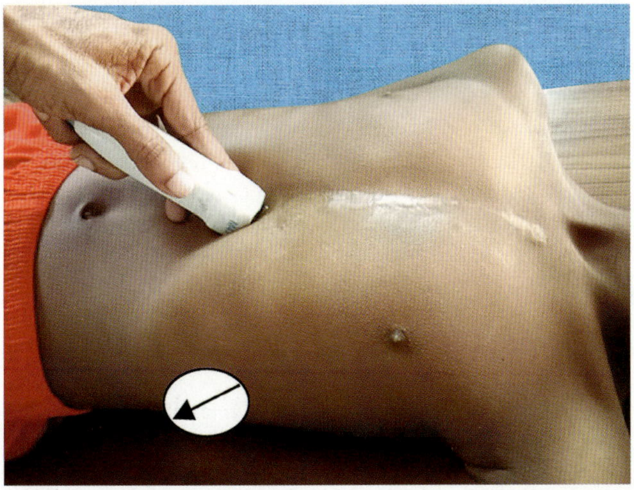

FIG. 23: Probe position.

ventricle, RVOT, pulmonary valve, and main pulmonary artery are visualized sequentially (similar to parasternal short axis at aortic valve).

THREE-DIMENSIONAL SUBCOSTAL ECHOCARDIOGRAM

Three-dimensional (3D) echocardiography offers valuable insights as it allows visualization of cardiac structures from a surgeon's perspective, capturing the heart in motion. Realtime 3D echocardiography provides even more detailed information compared to simple cross-sectional echo. In ASD, 3D reconstruction of defects within the fossa ovalis, crucial information about their location, size, and integrity of rims can be obtained.

In cases of sinus venosus defect associated with partial anomalous pulmonary venous drainage, 3D reconstruction proves invaluable in understanding the relationship between interatrial communication, the orifice of the SVC, and the connection of the RUPV. This aids in avoiding the risk of inappropriate closure of the defect by mistakenly suturing the hyperplastic Eustachian valve to the atrial wall.

For coronary sinus defects, 3D echocardiography offers an enface view of the entire coronary sinus roof, revealing circular defects that communicate with the LA.

In ASD device closure, subcostal 3D views (subcostal four-chamber view and bicaval view) supplemented by two-dimensional (2D) Doppler color flow mapping are highly beneficial **(Fig. 24)**. These views help accurately position the device within the atrial septum, especially the inferior margin, which may not be well defined by transesophageal echocardiography traversing between the two septa.

When dealing with children, it is crucial to account for the thin structure of the atrial septum, which is susceptible to dropout artifacts. In older children and adults, the IAS can be cropped up to visualize it "en face."

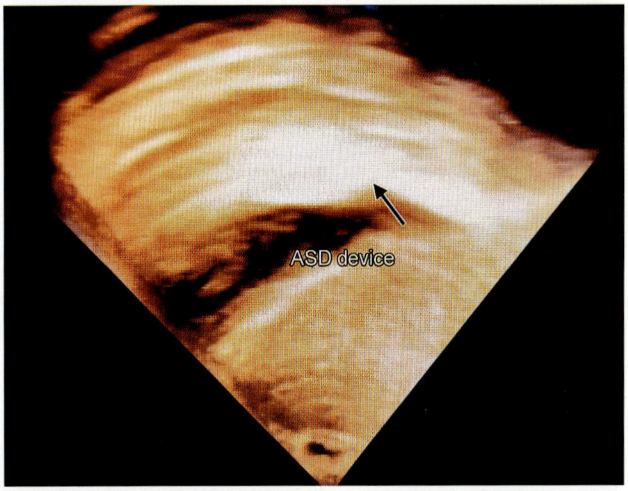

FIG. 24: Three-dimensional echo view of atrial septal defect (ASD) device.

Three-dimensional subcostal echocardiogram is also a viable option for assessing RV volume in pediatric patients, comparable to cardiac magnetic resonance imaging (MRI),[9] but is not superior to 3D apical or parasternal views for assessing cardiac function, dimension, and volumetric assessment.[10] Real-time 3D subcostal short-axis views provide additional information for assessment of septum defects and AV valves in congenital heart disease.

CONCLUSION

In critical care and perioperative patients, transthoracic echo imaging can be challenging, particularly for parasternal and apical windows. In these patients, subcostal windows can be used to assess cardiac function from multiple planes. However, further research is needed to establish normative values and Z-scores for subcostal windows which would improve the diagnostic value of these views.

ONLINE REFERENCES

Please scan the QR code provided at the end of the table of contents for References of this chapter.

CHAPTER 108

Fetal Cardiac Echocardiography and Obstetrics Counseling

IB Vijayalakshmi

ABSTRACT

Fetal echocardiography (Echo) is a complete two-dimensional and Doppler ultrasound evaluation of the fetal heart which is completely noninvasive and harmless. It has become the only means that allows a complete evaluation of cardiac structure and function of the fetus. Fetal Echo also serves as the electrocardiogram for the fetus and helps in monitoring during fetal life. Hence, it is the most useful tool to detect, diagnose, and monitor arrhythmia in utero, which are now manageable with transplacental therapy. Fetal Echo is recommended between 18 and 22 weeks, mean gestational age. Three-fourths of the patients with complex congental heart diseases (CHDs) are referred only after 22 weeks. This may be due to late performance of anomaly scans or inability to diagnose lesions like conotruncal lesions by first level of fetal echocardiographic examination is carried out by obstetrician or generic ultrasonographer who screens routinely all normal and abnormal pregnancies. The specificity is 99% and the sensitivity is over 80% depending on the expertise of the examiner. Early fetal Echo can effectively identify abnormal hearts and guide the obstetrician to take the concern in Indian scenario is late referrals, low utilization of tertiary care services despite diagnosis and high rates of nonsurvival in the fetuses.

Keywords: Electrocardiogram, abnormal pregnancies, indications, vaginal probes.

INTRODUCTION

Fetal echocardiography (FE) is a complete two-dimensional and Doppler ultrasound evaluation of the human fetal cardiovascular system. It is completely noninvasive and harmless for the fetus. Hence, it has become the only means that allows a complete evaluation of cardiac structure and function of the fetus. Fetal Echo also serves as the electrocardiogram for the fetus and helps in monitoring during fetal life. Hence, it is the most useful tool to detect, diagnose, and monitor arrhythmia in utero, which are now manageable with transplacental therapy.

BACKGROUND

The earliest experience with 2D Echo detection of congenital heart disease (CHD) in fetus was reported in 1972 by Winsberg.[1] Since then, widespread use of general fetal ultrasound examination among women receiving prenatal care has resulted in increased referral for specific cardiac analysis.[2] Definition of fetal cardiac structure is currently possible at 10–12 weeks of gestation with the use of vaginal probes with high-resolution transducers. By 16–18 weeks, accurate segmental analysis of cardiac structure is possible with a conventional transabdominal approach.[3,4] The specificity is 99% and the sensitivity is over 80% depending on the expertise of the examiner. The first level of fetal echocardiographic examination is carried out by obstetrician or generic ultrasonographer who screens routinely all normal and abnormal pregnancies. A second level fetal echocardiographic examination must be done for all expectant women who present with any conditions listed below are indications for fetal echocardiography.

INDICATIONS FOR FE

The various indications for FE are given in **Table 1**.

TABLE 1: Various indications for fetal echocardiography (FE).

Fetal	Maternal	Familial
• Abnormal cardiac screening examination • Fetal chromosomal anomaly • Extracardiac anomaly • Increased nuchal translucency >3.5 mm • Nonimmune hydrops • Fetal arrhythmia • Monochorionic twins	• Maternal congenital heart disease (CHD) • Metabolic disorders [e.g., diabetes, phenylketonuria (PKU)] • Autoimmune disease [e.g., systemic lupus erythematosus (SLE), Sjögren's] • Exposure to teratogens • Rubella infection • In vitro fertilization	• Family H/O of CHD–paternal or sibling • Mendelian syndromes (DiGeorge syndrome, Tuberous sclerosis, William syndrome, Ellis–Van Creveld syndrome, Marfan, Noonan's, etc.)

	Class
1. Abnormal appearing heart on general fetal ultrasound examination	I
2. Fetal tachycardia, bradycardia, or persistent irregular rhythm on clinical or screening ultrasound examination	I
3. Maternal/family risk factors for cardiovascular disease such as a parent, sibling, or first degree relative with congenital heart disease	I
4. Maternal diabetes	I
5. Maternal systemic lupus erythematosus	I
6. Teratogen exposure during vulnerable period	I
7. Other fetal system abnormalities (including chromosomal)	I
8. Performance of transplacental therapy or presence of a history of significant but intermittent arrhythmia. Re-evaluation examinations are required in these conditions	I
9. Fetal distress or dysfunction of unclear etiology	IIa
10. Previous history of multiple fetal losses	IIb
11. Multiple gestation	IIb
12. Low-risk pregnancies with normal anatomic findings on ultrasound examination	III
13. Occasional premature contractions without sustained tachycardia or signs of dysfunction or distress	III
14. Presence of a noncardiovascular system abnormality when evaluation of the cardiovascular system will not alter either management decisions or fetal outcome	III

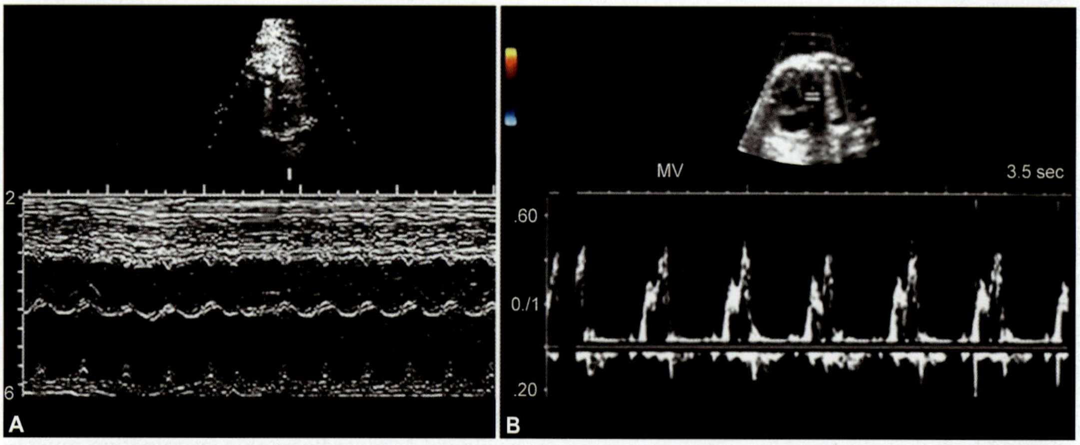

FIGS. 1A AND B: (A) M-mode in FE shows sinus rhythm. (B) Doppler interrogation of mitral valve shows sinus rhythm. (FE: fetal echocardiography)

The FE has unique features like:

1. It serves as the *ECG for the fetus*. Since we cannot obtain routine ECG for the fetus, we rely on ECHO demonstration of atrial and ventricular wall motion simultaneously in M-mode and use the temporal relationship of the motions to determine rate and rhythm, i.e., when atrial contraction precedes ventricular contraction and the contractions are in one-to-one relationship at a normal rate—the fetus is in sinus rhythm **(Figs. 1A and B)**.

2. The FE can be used to assess fetal well-being in a more global sense. Umbilical and cerebral arterial and umbilical venous flow patterns change with altered fetal and placental vascular resistance and provide important clues to fetal status, cerebral vessels dilate in the distressed fetus while peripheral and placental vessels generally constrict **(Fig. 2)**. Serous cavities can accumulate effusions **(Figs. 3A and B)** pericardial, pleural effusion/ascites in a fetus with infection, or low cardiac output. Advanced level obstetric (OB) ultrasound is capable of this type of assessment as well and is more frequently used for this purpose. However fetal *"well-being"* should be routinely assessed and commented upon as a part of a complete FE.

How accurate is FE?

Most published reports describe a 10–15% rate of detecting structurally abnormal fetal hearts (when using the high risk referral indications mentioned above). In these published series, false negative rates have been very low (1–2%). False positive occurs at similar rates. Because of the small size of the structures being examined, limitations exist. Pulmonary veins can be difficult to image. Thus, anomalies of pulmonary venous drainage are one major cardiac lesion not likely to be imaged reliably. Also, because of the fetal flow patterns, coarctation of the aorta can be difficult to diagnose reliably, although interruption of the aortic arch can usually be distinguished. Also, very small ventricular septal defect (VSD), any secundum atrial septal defect (ASD), and mild forms of pulmonary and aortic stenosis are difficult to detect. Therefore, FE reports tend to contain much greater percentage of complex anomalies than we expect to see in the general newborn population. As a result, most common fetal diagnoses are AV canal defects, tetralogy of Fallot (TOF) **(Fig. 4)**, single ventricle **(Fig. 5)**, Ebstein's anomaly, transposition of great arteries, tricuspid atresia, and hypoplastic left heart syndrome, while the most

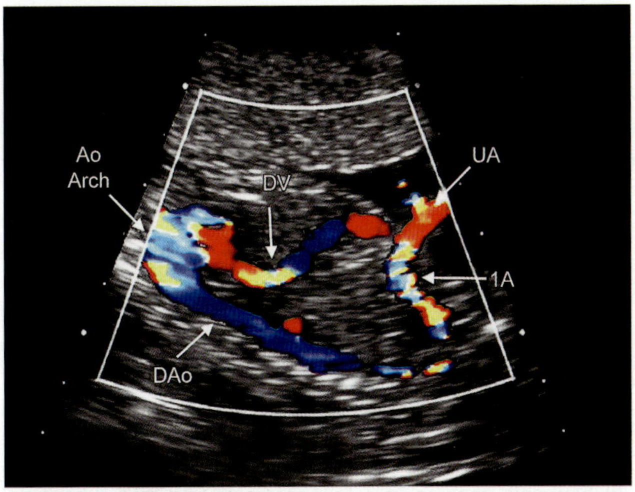

FIG. 2: Normal fetal circulation.

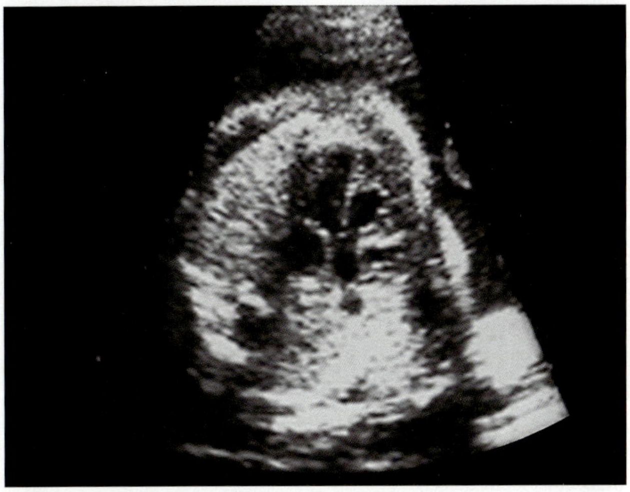

FIG. 4: Tetralogy of Fallot in 24 weeks fetus.

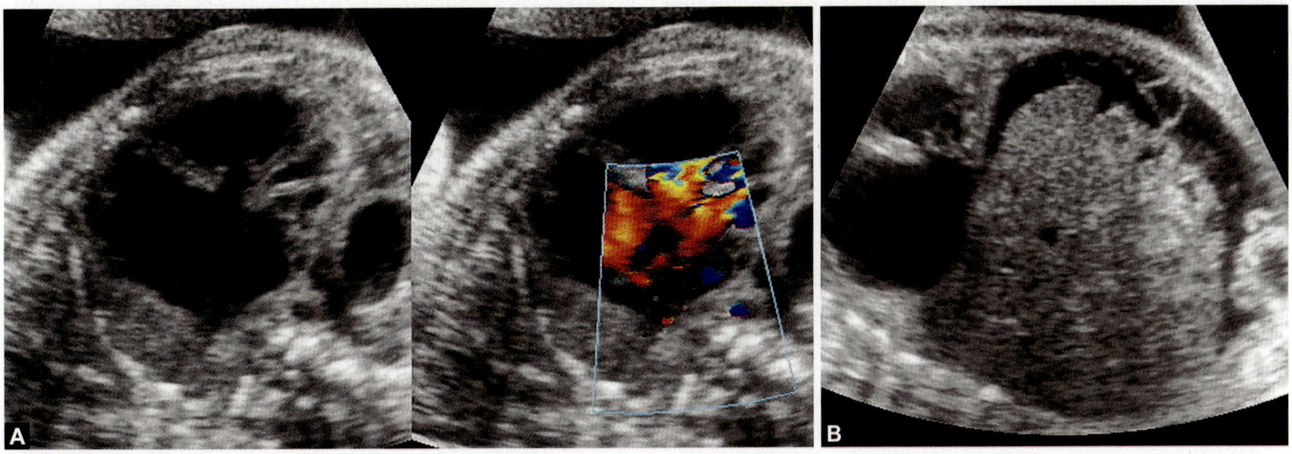

FIGS. 3A AND B: (A) Pericardial effusion and pleural effusion. (B) FE shows ascites in a case of hydrops fetalis.

(FE: fetal echocardiography)

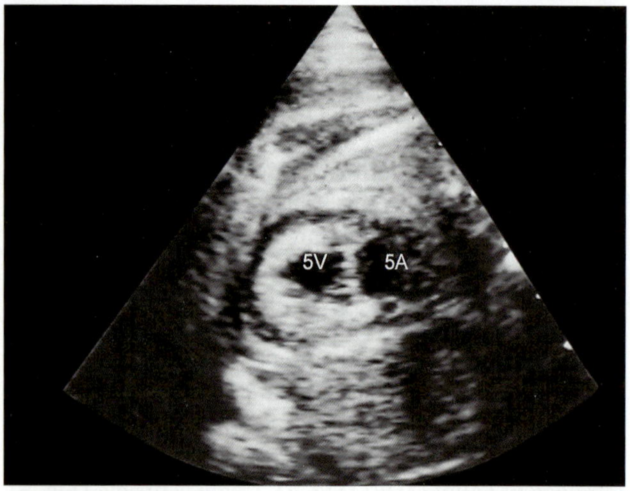

FIG. 5: Single ventricle.

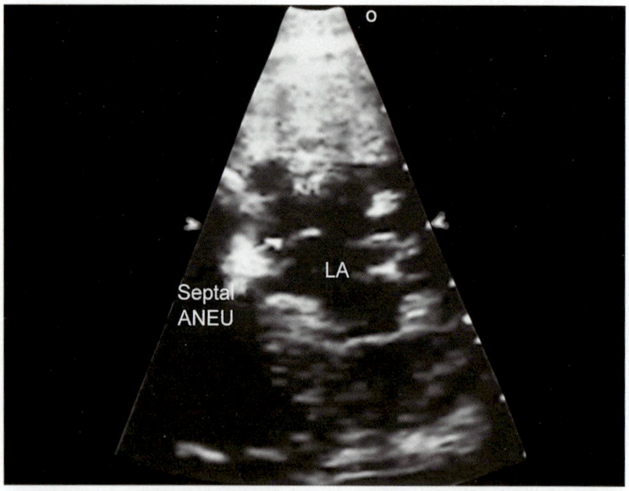

FIG. 6: ASD with septal aneurysm.
(ASD: atrial septal defect)

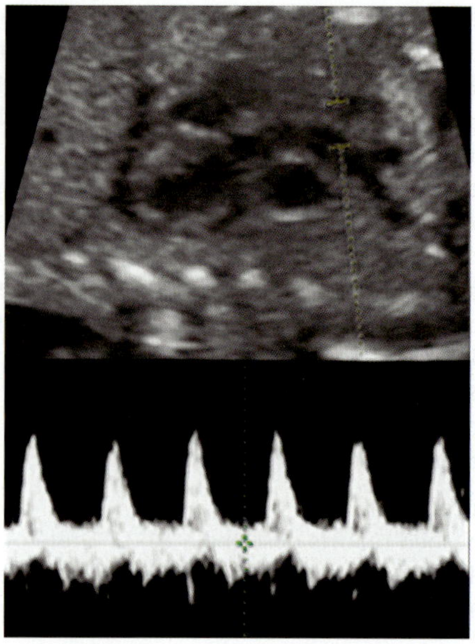

FIG. 7: Doppler study.

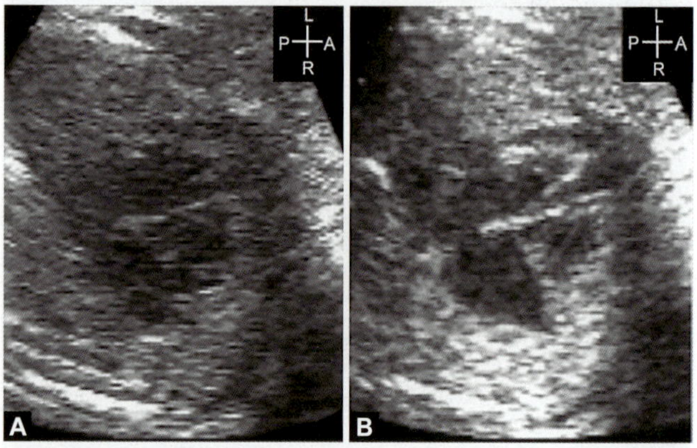

FIGS. 8A AND B: Comparison of (A) fundamental imaging and (B) harmonic imaging in a four-chamber view in a suboptimal echocardiographic windows.

common postnatal diagnoses tend to be ASD, VSD, PS, and patent ductus arteriosus (PDA).[5] The PDA is a normal finding prenatally and cannot be diagnosed by FE. There is a similar problem with ostium secundum ASD, since foramen ovale is patent in utero **(Fig. 6)**.

EQUIPMENT

The requirements of machine for FE are more stringent as there is increased demand for both spatial and temporal resolution. The axial resolution of 1 mm or less is particularly important, due to small size of critical fetal cardiac structures. Frames rates of 80–100 Hz are frequently needed to view structures at heart rates of >140 beats per minute. The machine should have 2-D, M-mode, Doppler including color, pulse, high pulse repetition frequency, and continuous wave should be available **(Fig. 7)**. The tissue Doppler imaging is recently applied for assessment of fetal arrhythmia.[6] Compared to fundamental imaging, harmonic imaging improves image quality and visualization of cardiac structures in fetuses with suboptimal echocardiographic windows **(Fig. 8)**. Harmonic imaging is useful when acoustic penetration is difficult such as in the presence of maternal obesity, scar tissue, polyhydramnios, or other problems.[7] Further phased array transducers with fundamental frequencies between 4 and 12 MHz are generally used to improve the image.

EXAMINATION TECHNIQUE

The goal is to visualize every essential components. But many a time everything cannot be visualized in every fetus during interrogation. The position of the fetus in the uterus or increased fetal activity often changing the position may limit the proper visualization of components of the heart.

The number of vessels in the umbilical cord is counted by Doppler sampling of the umbilical artery and vein. Once the position of the fetus is established, the right/left and anterior/posterior orientation, then initial survey of fetus is done to estimate the gestational age, establish abdominal situs, and cardiac position. The presence or absence of fluid in pericardial/pleural/peritoneal space is looked for carefully. The position of inferior vena cava and descending aorta at the level of the diaphragm are also noted carefully. A systematic uniform method must be followed. All studies begin with a wide-angle format to permit the determination of fetal orientation heart within the thorax. The diagrams demonstrate the anatomical correlates to the tomographic imaging planes used for the views may be utilized to image the various structures of the fetal heart and accomplish a comprehensive fetal echocardiogram.

The four-chamber view is the most useful view for the FE. Though it does detect all defects, it detects more serious defects. Before other parts of heart can be examined, a good four-chamber view is a must **(Figs. 9 and 10)** as it helps to examine the atrioventricular valves, atrial septum, and inlet portion of the ventricular septum. The septum primum is seen moving within the left atrium because of flow across the foramen ovale. The septum primum, which is always in the left atrium, helps as a marker to identify the left atrium, even in presence of atrioventricular discordance.

Next, the tricuspid and mitral valve can be distinguished because the mitral valve attaches to the crux of the heart slightly more cephalad than the tricuspid valve. Because the mitral valve is always within the morphologic left ventricle, atrioventricular concordance or discordance can be determined. Finally, abnormalities of the atrioventricular

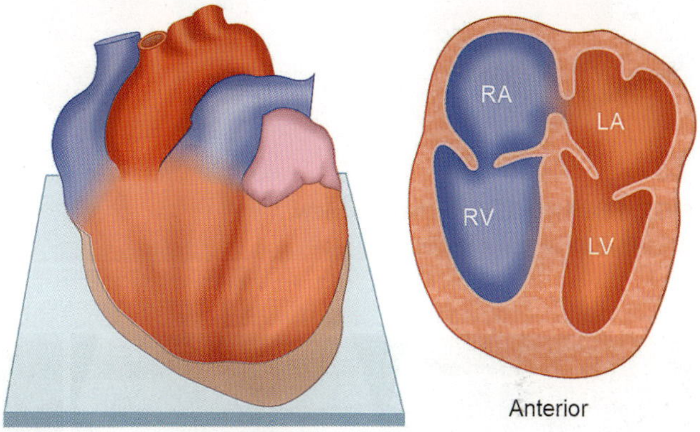

FIG. 9: Four-chamber view.

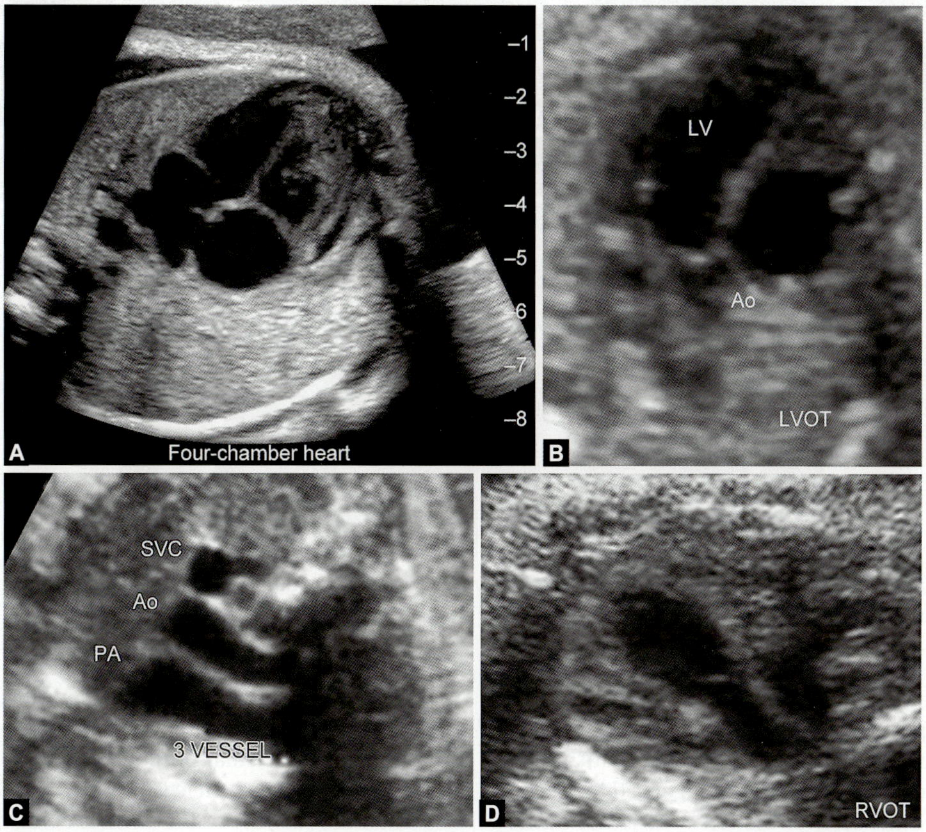

FIGS. 10A TO D : (A) Apical four-chamber view; (B) Left ventricular outflow tract (LVOT) view; (C) Three vessels view; (D) Right ventricular out flow tract (RVOT) view.

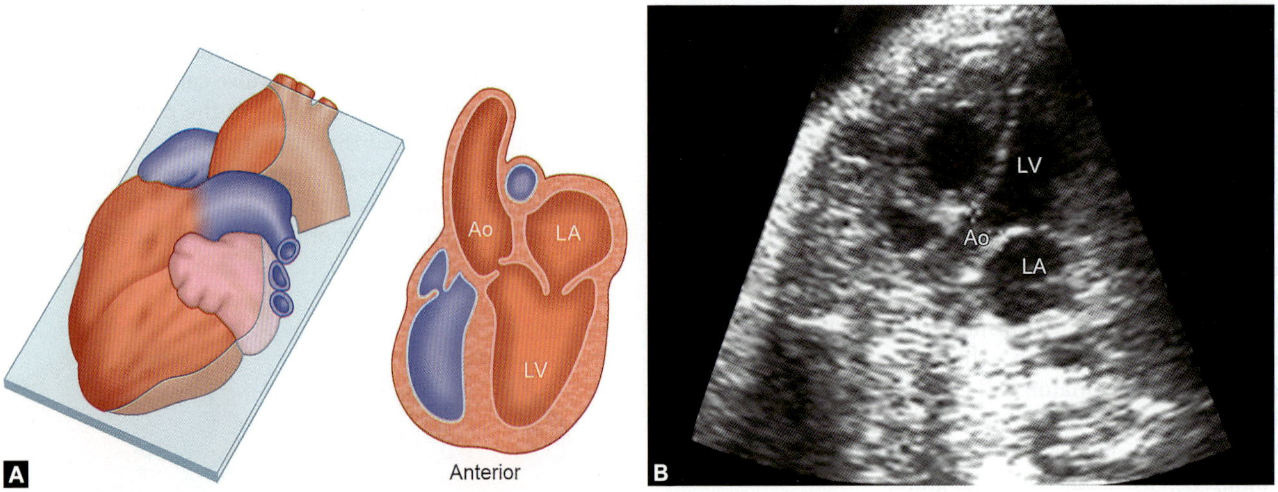

FIGS. 11A AND B: Five-chamber view.
(LA: left atrial; LV: left ventricle)

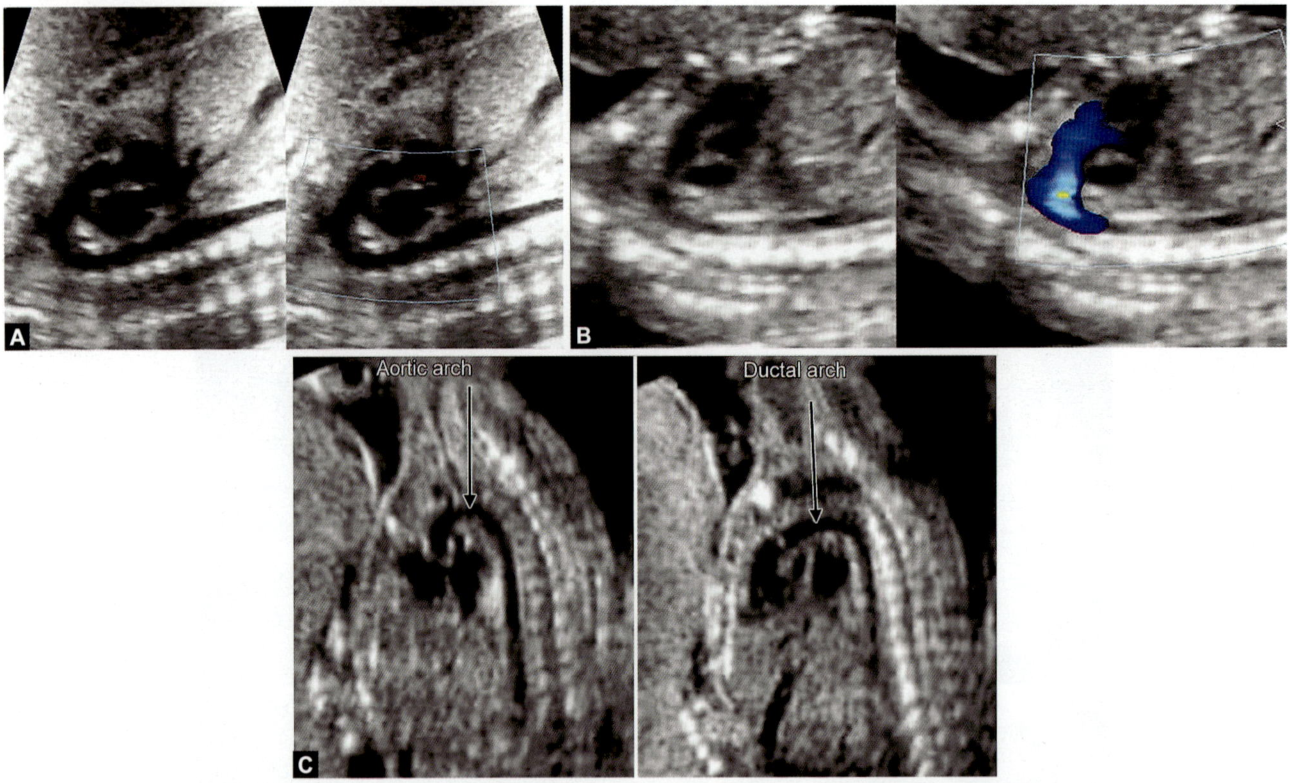

FIGS. 12A TO C: (A) Aortic arch with cephalic vessels; (B) Ductal view; (C) FE shows the difference between aortic arch and ductal arch.
(FE: fetal echocardiography)

junction resulting in atrioventricular septal defects can be evaluated. Of particular importance is the diagnosis of hypoplastic left heart syndrome in utero because of the extremely poor prognosis. This is best diagnosed in the four-chamber view and the view of the left ventricular outflow tract where measurements of the aortic annulus can be made and compared with normal. From the four-chamber view, progressive angulation of the scan plane in a ventral direction results in imaging the outlet portion of the heart beginning with the left ventricular outflow region. The aorta is seen to arise from the left ventricle **(Figs. 11A and B)**.

Then the identity of the aorta is confirmed by following its course and imaging the origin of the arch vessels **(Fig. 12)**. The ascending aorta and arch vessels are easily seen by following the aortic arch as it arcs cephalad to the heart. The transition between the proximal arch and the descending aorta may be small, because the flow through this region is low. It may be difficult to distinguish a normal small transverse arch and a true coarctation. The systemic veins should be imaged next. Entrance of the hepatic veins and the inferior vena cava into the right atrium can be imaged **(Figs. 13 and 14)**. The position of the inferior vena cava and descending aorta at the level of the diaphragm are established.

Parasternal long-axis view with left ventricular outflow tract **(Figs. 15A and B)**, short-axis sweep [cephalad angling includes "3-vessel" view **(Figs. 16A and B)**]. Caval long-axis view, ductal arch view, aortic arch view, Doppler examination of inferior and superior vena cava, pulmonary veins, hepatic veins, ductus venosus, foramen ovale, atrioventricular valves, semilunar valves, ductus arteriosus, transverse aortic arch, umbilical artery, umbilical vein, measurement of atrioventricular valve, semilunar valve, diameter of main pulmonary artery (MPA), ascending aorta (AO), and branch pulmonary arteries should be noted. The various conditions that have poor prognosis in utero include atrioventricular septal defect with complete heart block and pulmonary atresia with intact ventricular septum. The lesions such as tetralogy of Fallot and hypoplastic left heart syndrome, as well as the cardiomyopathy associated with infants of mothers with diabetes mellites, may progress in utero. Serial fetal echo examinations should thus be performed to detect complex CHDs like hypoplastic left heart syndrome (HLHS), hypoplastic right heart syndrome, tricuspid atresia, double-inlet left ventricle, truncus arteriosus, single atrium, double-chambered right ventricle (DCRV) with pericardial effusion, etc. as shown in **Figures 17A to G**.

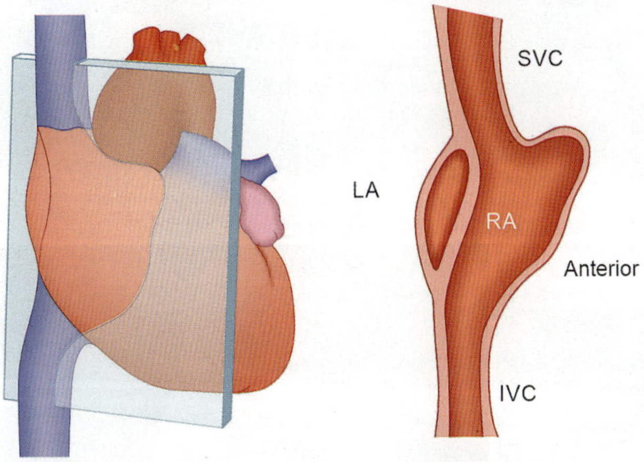

FIG. 13: The diagramatic imaging of systemic veins (SVC and IVC).

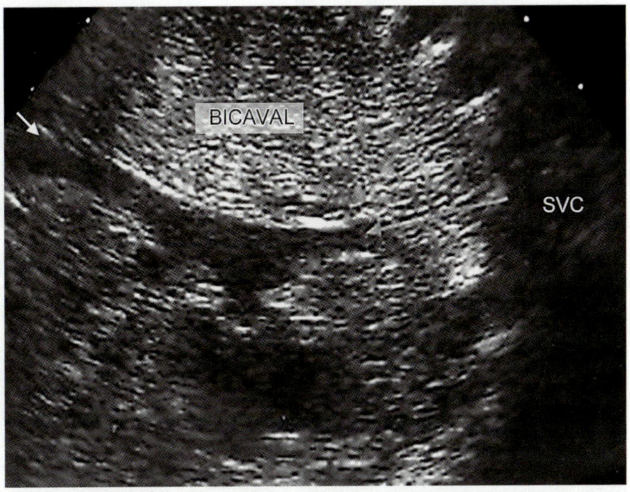

FIG. 14: Bicaval view shows SVC and entrance of the hepatic veins and the inferior vena cava into the right atrium.

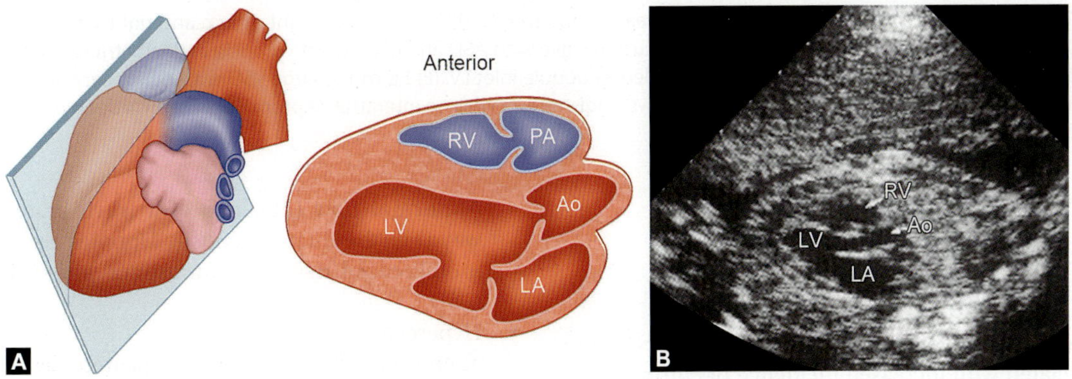

FIGS. 15A AND B: Parasternal long-axis view.
(LA: left atrial; LV: left ventricle; PA: pulmonary artery; RV: right ventricle)

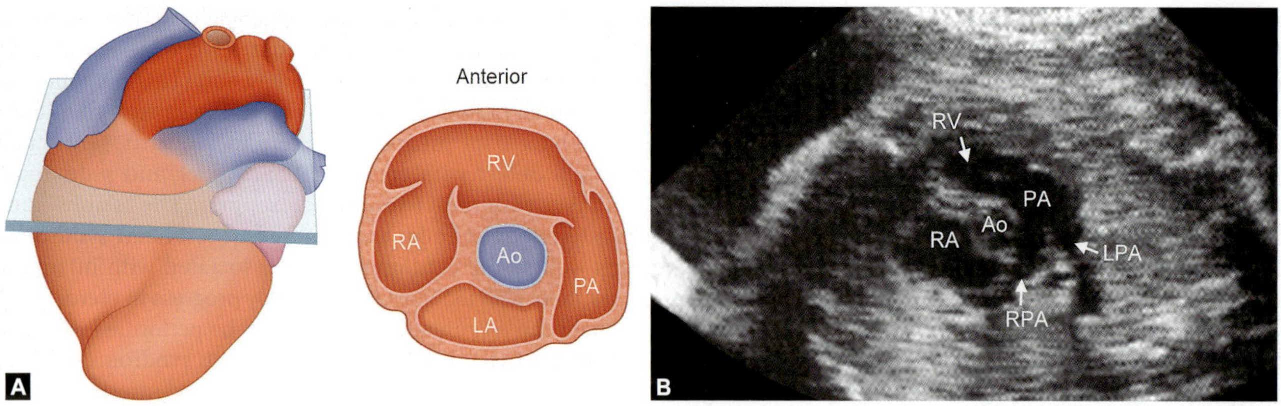

FIGS. 16A AND B: Short-axis view.
(LA: left atrial; PA: pulmonary artery; RA: right atrial; RV: right ventricle)

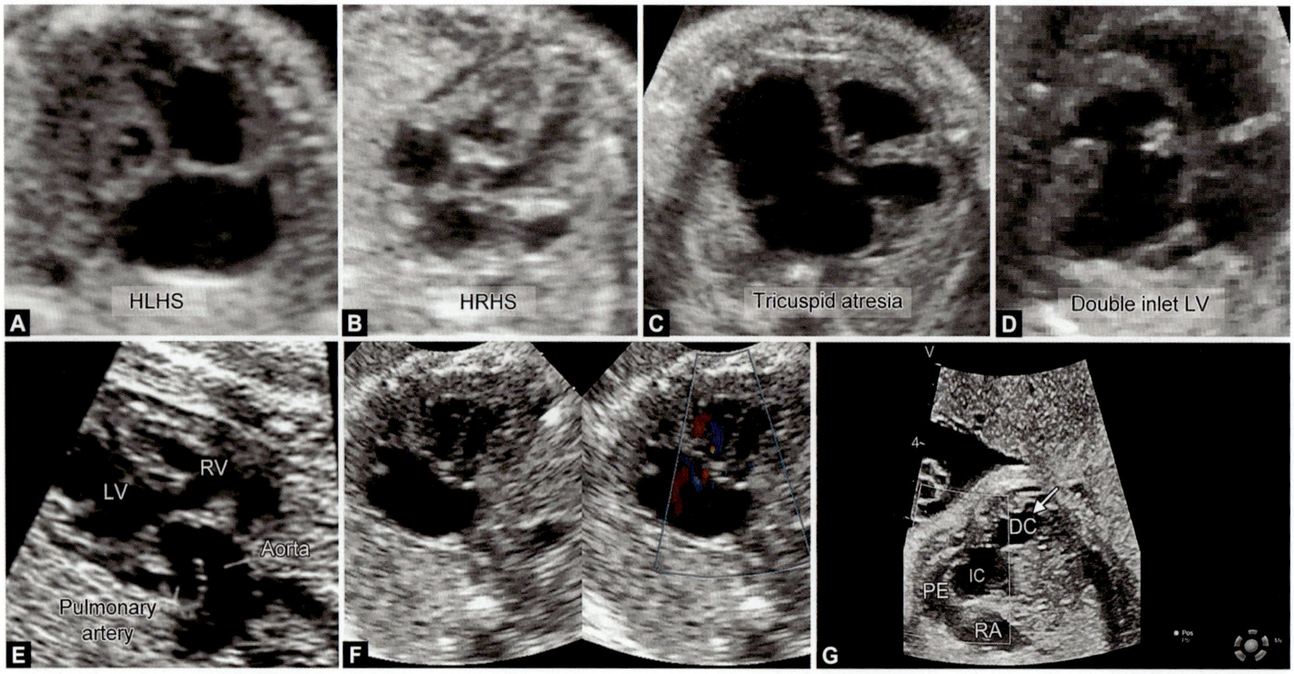

FIGS. 17A TO G: (A) Fetal echo shows hypoplastic left heart syndrome (HLHS) with dilated right atrium and right ventricle. (B) FE shows hypoplastic right heart syndrome. (C) FE shows atretic tricuspid valve with ASD and dilated left ventricle and left atrium. (D) FE shows both mitral and tricuspid valves opening into lent ventricle called as double inlet LV. (E) FE shows large VSD with pulmonary artery arising from LV and aorta arising from RV in a case of DTGA. (F) FE shows single atrium with no interatrial septum. (G) FE shows double chambered right ventricle with pericardial effusion (PE).

FIRST-TRIMESTER MARKERS OF CONGENITAL HEART DISEASE (11–14 WEEKS)

- If in the first trimester, the nuchal fold thickness > 3.5 mm is associated with increased incidence of chromosomal anomalies and CHD.
- The presence of tricuspid regurgitation (TR) determined by pulsed wave Doppler has been shown to be a marker for trisomy 21 and CHD.
- Abnormal flow (absence of a wave or reversal of a wave) in the ductus venosus Doppler associated with an increased risk of chromosomal abnormalities and CHD
- Hyperechogenic spot in LV

Then detailed FE should be repeated in such targeted high-risk group.

Echogenic foci within the left ventricle of the fetal heart **(Figs. 18A to C)** represent papillary muscle mineralization. Until more data are available to investigate any possible

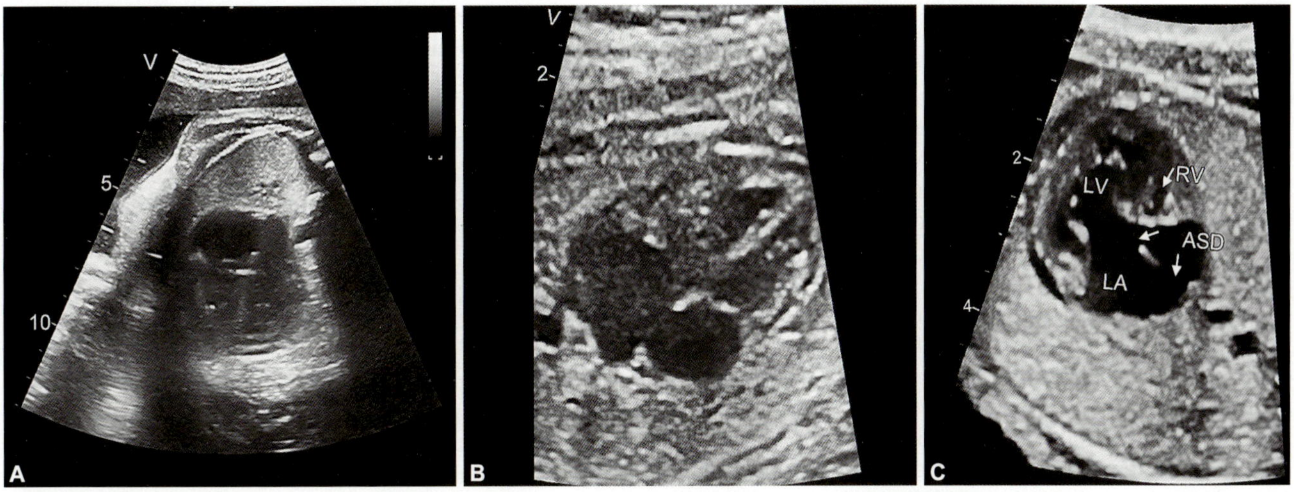

FIGS. 18A TO C: (A) Single hyperechogenic focus in LV. (B) Multiple hyperechogenic focus in both LV and RV in a case of large VSD. (C) FE shows multiple hyperechogeic focus in single ventricle with ostium primum ASD.

association with aneuploidy, a hyperechogenic focus in the left ventricle should still be considered a normal variant. Sometimes multiple hyperechogenic spots could indicate healed vegetations due to intrauterine infection **(Figs. 18A and B)** which invariably leads to fetal wastage or still birth or neonatal sepsis and death. We see the vegetations along the fetal circulation, e.g., hyperechogenic spots indicating vegetations at inferior vena cava (IVC) and right atrial junction, at foramen ovale on left atrial side, on coumadin ridge or warfarin ridge, mitral valve, aortic valve, tricuspid valve, pulmonary valve, and more interestingly at the junction of pulmonary ductus arteriosus with aorta. This can be confirmed by Echo after birth **(Fig. 18)**. If treated in time, neonatal mortality can be reduced.[8]

FETAL ARRHYTHMIAS

In recent years, FE has become the most useful modality to detect, diagnose, monitor fetal arrhythmias, and manage the pregnancies complicated by fetal arrhythmias.[9-12] This application of FE is particularly successful for several reasons. Fetal ECGs are very difficult to record and when they are recorded only the ventricular depolarization is seen. FE provides information concerning the atrial rate and the sequence of atrioventricular activation. The FE also provides information on the atrial rate, ventricular rate, and the atrial-ventricular relationship and thus allows a precise determination of the type of arrhythmia. Secondly, FE provides a tool to assess the hemodynamic consequences of the arrhythmia. Thirdly, the FE provides a method to detect associated structural cardiac anomalies. This information is particularly useful since 15% of all fetus with a persistent arrhythmia have a structural cardiac defect. From such a recording, the atrial rate, the ventricular rate, and the relationship between the atrioventricular contractions can be determined in the same way an ECG can be analyzed.

BRADYARRHYTHMIAS

The slow fetal heart rates are often the reason for referral for an echo. The most common cause is complete heart block; this must be distinguished from sinus bradycardia, which has a much worse prognosis. Sinus bradycardias, defined as rates below 100/min, are uncommon; when they occur, they usually indicate fetal compromise. In the presence of complete heart block or sinus bradycardia, careful inspection of the anatomy is necessary as well as evaluation for signs of in utero heart failure. Heart rate in an older fetus is normally somewhat slower but should remain above 100/min. Complete heart block, manifest as a slow ventricular rate with a faster atrial rate, can be noted at any stage of gestation but is not necessarily present from the time of conception. The heart block often becomes manifest after 20 weeks. The fetus must be observed for the development of heart block when predisposing factors, such as the presence of maternal collagen vascular disease, are present.[13] This does not have to take the form of overt clinical disease in the mother but may be present only as a positive serologic test. In addition, complete heart block can be associated with certain structural diseases in the fetus, such as L-transposition of the great arteries, atrioventricular septal defects, and any anomaly of the tricuspid valve. Fetuses with heart block should be monitored closely with repeat echoes for development of congestive heart failure. There is no proven in utero therapy, and premature delivery must be considered when signs of significant heart failure develop. The consequences of a premature birth must be weighed against the possibility of in utero fetal death, especially in patients with multiple risk factors are present.

TACHYARRHYTHMIAS

Any arrhythmias in fetus with fast heart rate of >200 beats/min are pathologic. Most often detected tachyarrhythmias in utero are supraventricular tachycardia (SVT), atrial flutter (AF), and ventricular tachycardia (VT). Of these, SVT is the most common and can be recognized by FE when heart rate is >200 beats/min with 1:1 atrioventricular conduction. Although SVT is not often associated with structural disease, a careful examination of the heart is needed, because the hemodynamic effects tend to be worse in those fetuses with heart diseases. When anomalies of the tricuspid valve are present, the presence of Wolff-Parkinson-White (WPW) syndrome is more likely and may change the method of treatment. Finally, the examiner should find out whether the tachycardia is incessant or intermittent. There are less serious hemodynamic effects in cases with intermittent tachycardia compared to incessant tachycardia. The fetus must be examined for hydrops, signs of heart failure by frequent serial examinations to detect onset of heart failure.

Atrial flutter (AF) can be recognized by detecting rapid atrial rate compared to slower ventricular rate. When atrial rate is greater than 400/min, that distinguishes atrial flutter from SVT with atrioventricular block. Although AF is usually not associated with structural disease, still one should rule out structural anomalies. Apart from presence or absence of heart failure, look for the ventricular rate and also degree of effect of the arrhythmia on ventricular filling. More chaotic atrial rhythms worse the effect. It is unknown if any other factors contribute or it is entirely by altered filling in a less compliant ventricle **(Fig. 19)**.

It is difficult to recognize VT. The diagnostic feature is atrioventricular (AV) dissociation with the ventricular rate faster than the atrial rate. Usually, ventricular rate is around 160–200/min, although it can be quite variable. When retrograde conduction is present, resulting in a 1:1 atrioventricular relationship, the VT can be suspected. One should suspect VT is the presence of variability in the fetal heart rate. In the presence of VT, the fetal heart rate is quite stable with loss of the normal variability; especially true in late gestation. And it can be detected as a lack of heart rate variability on a nonstress test. Left ventricular ejection fraction (LVEF) must be assessed in presence of VT and viral myocarditis. Effects of this arrhythmia upon cardiac hemodynamics are quite variable. The presence of AV synchrony leads to less hemodynamic compromise. Thus, even if the arrhythmia cannot be completely corrected, slowing of the heart rate is enough to restore atrioventricular synchrony, leading to significant improvement.

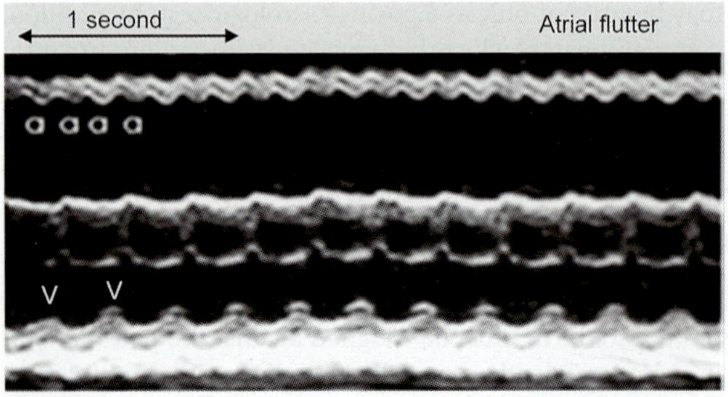

FIG. 19: M mode echo shows dilated RV with tachycardia in a case of fetal atrial flutter.

EXTRACARDIAC ANOMALIES

The incidence of structural cardiac anomalies in the presence of other extracardiac anomalies is variable. The incidence can range from as low as 2–5% when central nervous system (CNS) malformations are present to as high as 50% when there are anomalies of kidney.

In addition, one should be aware of some extracardiac anomalies that have a high association with specific congenital heart defects (CHDs). The most common association is that of omphalocele and either a VSD or TOF. The presence can range from 10% if the caudal fold is involved to nearly 100% if cephalic fold is involved. Abnormalities of splenic formation (asplenia or polysplenia) are commonly associated with AV canal defects as in Down's syndrome. The right atrial isomerism may be present in the case of asplenia, along with abnormalities of pulmonary venous drainage. The left atrial isomerism may be seen in presence of polysplenia, along with systemic venous anomalies. In addition, an increased incidence of arrhythmias presumed to be caused by altered sinoatrial node development. Whenever a chromosomal anomaly is detected by amniocentesis, FE should and must be done, because the association with CHDs is very high.[14] Nearly 40% of Down's syndrome have AV canal defect. Therefore, whenever FE shows AV canal defect **(Fig. 20)**, Karyotype study should be done **(Fig. 21)** to confirm the

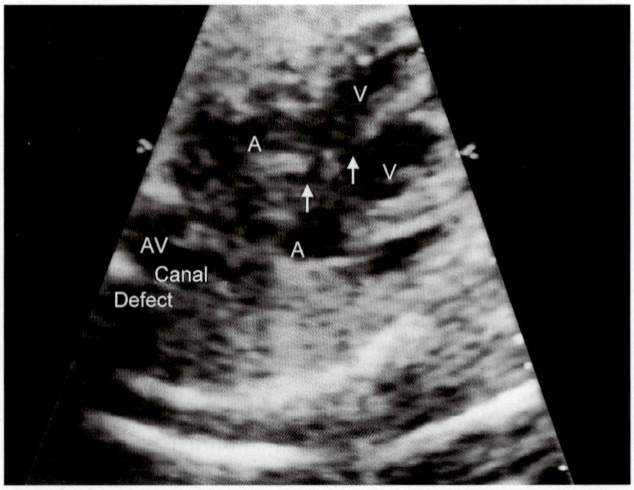

FIG. 20: Complete AV canal defect.
(AV: atrioventricular)

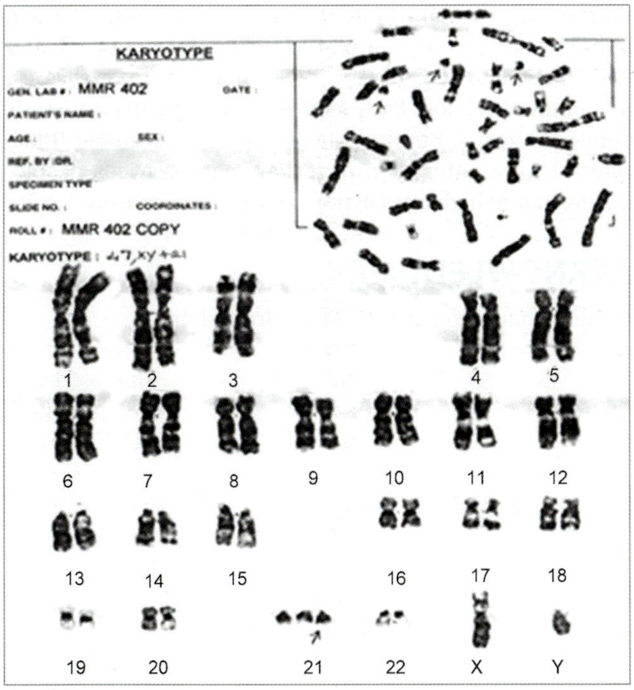

FIG. 21: Karyotype—47,xy,+21 in Down's Syndrome.

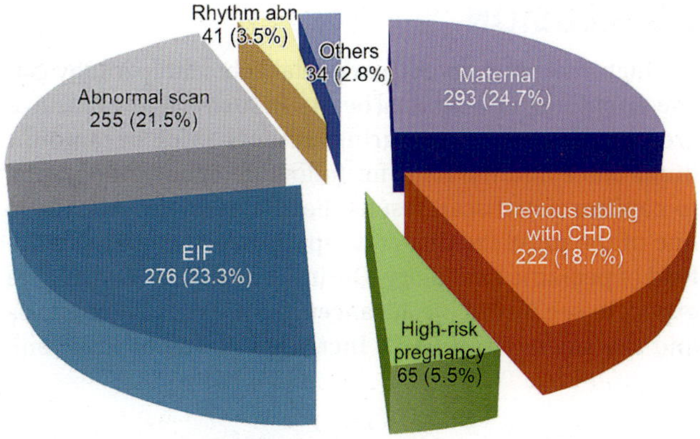

FIG. 22: Reasons for referring for fetal Echo.

diagnosis, before genetic counseling or contemplating on medical termination of pregnancy. There is a dictum which states that if an anomaly is detected, one must look for a second; if one finds a second, one must search for a third. This is particularly true for congenital heart defects, as they often occur in the context of aneuploidy. Even in the absence of chromosomal abnormalities or genetic syndrome complexes, certain extracardiac anomalies such as cleft lip/palate, spina bifida, tracheoesophageal fistula, duodenal atresia, omphalocele, diaphragmatic hernia, nuchal edema, or a single umbilical artery should make one suspicious for a possible associated cardiac defect.[15]

In our study, total of 478 cases of fetal echocardiograms performed over a period of 5.5 years. The data was systematically compiled and analyzed. The various details of gestational age, maternal, family history, exposure to teratogens, and reason for referral were recorded systematically. In this study, average gestational age at referral was 24.8 ± 4.6 weeks and maternal age was 24.7 ± 4.3 years. Usually referred for abnormal fetal cardiac scan in 128 (26.8%), the presence of CHD in previous sibling was in 99 (20.7%) of cases and, maternal indications was in 87 (18.2%), echogenic intracardiac focus (EIF) was in 87 (18.2%), high risk in 50 (10.5%), rhythm problems in 21 (4.4%), and others (extracardiac malformations) in 6 (1.2%). In the 87 CHD cases diagnosed, nearly 70% had complex CHD and 66.7% were referred only after 22 weeks of gestation. A further 103 cases had EIF, 17 cases had fetal arrhythmia, whereas three cases had cardiac masses, and the remaining 268 cases had normal fetal echocardiograms. Three fourth of the patients who had complex CHDs were referred only after 22 weeks. This may be due to late performance of anomaly scans or inability to diagnose lesions like conotruncal lesions.[16] Various reasons for referrals 478 cases are given in **Figure 22**.

What to do with the information gained from FE?

Obstetrics counseling is very important. In general, parents should be counseled shortly after the fetal echocardiogram. Counselors may use diagrams of the diagnosed CHD, hand drawings, models, or online material to explain the heart disease and therapeutic options. Accordingly, a truthful picture of the prognosis, including long-term issues and reoperation rates needs to be provided. If FE is normal, reassure high-risk families that major cardiac anomalies are absent and the baby is probably normal from cardiovascular standpoint. If FE detects major defect, then counseling and preparation of the family for expected congenital heart disease is done. In complicated cases, this will usually involve a multidisciplinary team (e.g., obstetrician, neonatologist, pediatric cardiologist, and genetician).

- High-risk lesions delivery in the center where definitive care of the newborn can be provided is advised. Because it is always safer to transport a healthy pregnant mother than a sick neonate.
- Low-risk lesions (i.e., not duct dependent)—delivery can occur locally with foreknowledge of how the child is likely to "behave" in the neonatal period.
- High-risk lesions with limited long-term prognosis—usually multiple congenital anomalies (Trisomy 13,18). Offer counseling, amniocentesis, and explore all therapeutic options such as intervention, comfort care, and termination of pregnancy.
- Can monitor fetal "well-being" in selected situation such as fetal heart block, diaphragmatic hernia, and chronic indomethacin tocolysis.

Future impact of FE:

- May reduce the frequency of newborns with severe CHD
- Increasing frequency of prenatal interventions
- Increased prenatal "patient" transfer to centre of excellence
- Uncertain impact on the prevalence of complex CHD

CONCLUSION

For high-risk pregnancies, early fetal echocardiography can effectively identify abnormal hearts. In such a highly sensitive area of diagnosis, reassuring parents is of paramount importance and the need for follow-up echocardiography to confirm initial scan results. Fetal cardiology represents one of the most exciting and rapidly evolving areas in the field of pediatric cardiology. During the next 10–20 years, we expect to see incredible advances in the prenatal diagnosis and management of CHD. Increased ability to intervene medically, percutaneously and perhaps surgically on the fetus has enhanced the importance of prenatal detection of CHD. Fetal Echo has opened a new horizon and is the best tool in this direction. Early fetal Echo can effectively identify abnormal hearts. But the concern in Indian scenario is late referrals, low utilization of tertiary care services despite diagnosis and high rates of nonsurvival in the fetuses.

ACKNOWLEDGMENT

Grateful thanks to late Dr Chitra Narasimhan .

ONLINE REFERENCES

Please scan the QR code provided at the end of the table of contents for References of this chapter.

CHAPTER

109 Echocardiographic Evaluation of Mitral Regurgitation

Shanmugasundaram S, Ilayaraja U, Rajeswari K

ABSTRACT

Assessing the severity of mitral regurgitation (MR) is important for optimal timing of surgical or catheter intervention. Stepwise approach is required to get an accurate estimate of its severity. 2D echo provides information about the etiology and mechanism of MR, its effects on left atrium (LA) and left ventricle (LV), and is useful in diagnosing severe MR if failure of coaptation is demonstrable. Color Doppler echo offers a qualitative method of assessment in the form of jet area and semi-quantitative methods such as vena contracta and proximal isovelocity surface mapping. Using inflow and outflow dimensions and velocity time integral in the respective sites, regurgitant volume, and fraction can be calculated, which are quantitative measures. Each method has advantages and pitfalls and a comprehensive integrative method may be needed for accurate estimation of severity.

Keywords: Mitral regurgitation, primary MR, secondary MR, estimation of severity, echocardiography, vena contracta, PISA, volumetric, timing for intervention.

INTRODUCTION

Mitral regurgitation (MR) is a common valvular heart disease (VHD) encountered in practice. In a retrospective analysis of 13,289 patients with primary VHD done in a tertiary center in Southern India, MR was seen in 25.6%. Rheumatic heart disease (RHD) was the commonest cause (40.8%) with mitral valve prolapse (MVP)/myxomatous valve contributing to another 40.8%.[1] In USA, MR is the commonest VHD, occurring in 1.7% of the population further increasing to 9.3% in those beyond 75 years.[2] In Euro Heart survey of moderate to severe VHD, MR was the second common valve disease (24.8%), next to aortic stenosis (AS) (33.9%). 61% had degenerative MR (DMR) while 14% had rheumatic MR.[3] In addition, secondary MR (SMR) occurs in about 25–50% after acute myocardial infarction (MI) and 10% of all MI have severe MR. SMR is seen in 50% of patients with heart failure with reduced ejection fraction (HFrEF) which is severe in 20%. Both types of MR lead to reduced survival and result in morbid events such as heart failure, arrhythmias mainly atrial fibrillation (AF), and embolic events. Timely intervention, either surgical or catheter based, improves the survival and reduces complications. Estimation of severity of MR is essential for optimal timing of intervention, particularly in asymptomatic individuals. Echocardiography plays a crucial role in determining the severity of MR and additional tests like cardiac MR (CMR) are rarely required.

ETIOPATHOGENESIS

Mitral regurgitation refers to the retrograde flow of blood from left ventricle (LV) into left atrium (LA) in systole, due to defective apposition of leaflets. It may manifest because of defective structure and function of one or more of the components of mitral valve apparatus, that include the valve leaflets, chordae, papillary muscles, annulus, a part of LA and LV (primary or organic or structural MR) or secondary to left ventricular enlargement ± dysfunction [SMR or functional MR (FMR)] that derange the functional integrity of the mitral apparatus. It is well said that in primary MR it is the leaky valve that makes the ventricle sick and in SMR it is the sick ventricle that makes the valve leaky.

Secondary MR typically occurs in idiopathic dilated cardiomyopathy (IDCM) or ischemic heart failure [post MI or chronic coronary artery disease (CAD)]. In IDCM and after a large anterior wall MI, global (often spherical) remodeling of LV and LV dysfunction are present which result in increased tethering force (due to outward enlargement of LV with resultant lateral and apical displacement of papillary muscles) and decreased closing force (due to decreased contractile power of LV) on mitral leaflets as a result of which MR occurs. Mechanical dyssynchrony of LV and dilatation and dysfunction of mitral annulus may additionally contribute to MR. MR jet is typically central in such situations. In contrast, MR occurring in inferolateral myocardial infarction (ILMI) is characterized by regional remodeling of LV leading to asymmetric tethering of posterior mitral leaflet (PML) and eccentric (posterolateral) MR. Variable degree of remodeling of mitral leaflets seems to influence the severity of MR in these conditions. Atrial FMR (AFMR) is a subtype of FMR caused by dilatation of annulus due to LA enlargement and it occurs in the setting of chronic AF or heart failure with preserved ejection fraction. SMR may also occur secondary to aortic valve disease. In aortic regurgitation (AR), marked dilatation of LV with or without LV dysfunction may lead to MR. In AS, MR is often due to concomitant mitral pathology such as mitral annulus calcification (MAC), MVP or flail mitral leaflet. Dilatation of annulus either due to pressure overload or dilated LA or LV dysfunction could also play a role. In hypertrophic cardiomyopathy (HCM), MR which is often eccentric (posterolateral jet), results from systolic anterior motion (SAM) of anterior mitral leaflet (AML). Structural changes in mitral leaflets and papillary muscles may also variably contribute to MR in this condition.

Primary MR may be acute in onset, which is invariably severe and life threatening, often caused by rupture of chordae (spontaneous, traumatic, infective, and inflammatory) or papillary muscle (infarction) or avulsion (trauma) or perforation/destruction of valve leaflets [infective endocarditis (IE)]. Rapid onset cardiomyopathy (myocarditis, takotsubo cardiomyopathy and peripartum cardiomyopathy) may also cause acute MR. Regurgitation of large volume of blood into an unprepared noncompliant LA results in marked elevation of pressures in LA, pulmonary veins, and capillary bed resulting in pulmonary edema. Pulmonary hypertension (PH) sets in rapidly and is often severe leading to right ventricular (RV) dysfunction. In contrast, chronic MR has an insidious onset and slow progression with slow progression with no or mild elevation of pressures in LA and pulmonary venous/capillary bed. PH occurs late if at all.

Chronic MR may be caused by structural abnormality of the leaflets or any of the components of mitral apparatus.

- *Degenerative MR*: (a) Myxomatous degeneration or fibroelastic deficiency (FED) leading to prolapse or flail leaflets, manifesting as nonsyndromic or syndromic (Marfan syndrome, Ehlers-Danlos syndrome or pseudoxanthoma elasticum); (b) Mitral Annulus Calcification (MAC).
- Inflammatory (RHD, connective tissue disorders such as systemic lupus erythematosus and scleroderma)
- Infective endocarditis
- Hyper eosinophilic syndrome and endomyocardial fibrosis (EMF)
- Carcinoid syndrome
- Mucopolysaccharidosis (MPS)
- Drugs such as ergot, methysergide, pergolide, cabergoline, fenfluramine, dexfenfluramine, and methylenedioxymethamphetamine (MDMA)
- Irradiation
- Congenital (cleft or fenestration of leaflets, anomalous origin of left coronary artery from pulmonary artery).

In developed countries, the commonest cause of FMR is ischemic and the commonest cause of primary MR is degenerative. In developing countries like India, RHD is the dominant cause of primary MR. It is also possible to encounter patients with mixed variety, for example, fibrocalcific degeneration of annulus and leaflets with FMR due to DCM or CAD; LV enlargement and geometry change due to primary MR may cause displacement of papillary muscle and variable tethering of leaflets and AFMR superimposed on another cause of MR when AF supervenes.

ROLE OF ECHOCARDIOGRAPHY IN EVALUATION OF MITRAL REGURGITATION

Echocardiography is the initial and often the only diagnostic tool required for evaluation of MR. It helps in identifying the etiology and mechanism of MR, assessing its severity, its impact on LV function, effect on chambers upstream and pulmonary vasculature as well as in guiding therapeutic strategies. Echo assessment of MR should be methodical and stepwise, with an initial evaluation of the morphology and function of mitral valve leaflets and the other components of mitral apparatus by 2D Echo (2DE). Once the structural details are obtained, qualitative assessment of MR severity may be done by eyeballing or measuring the jet size. Then the semi-quantitative measures such as vena contracta (VC) and proximal isovelocity surface area (PISA) are done. Finally, the quantitative measures namely regurgitant volume (RVol) and regurgitant fraction (RF) are measured. Subsequently, the impact of MR on the size and function of LV and LA, the pulmonary artery pressures, and RV function should be assessed. The temptation to begin the study with color Doppler imaging should be avoided. The best strategy is to switch off the color Doppler and delineate the anatomy of the entire mitral valve apparatus in multiple views, which include parasternal long and short-axis views, apical long axis view, A4C and A2C views, at a high frame rate (>50 Hz). The overlay of color may mask important information about the mechanism of MR.

IDENTIFYING THE MECHANISM AND ETIOLOGY OF MITRAL REGURGITATION

Carpentier's classification of MR based on the leaflet mobility is an ideal framework based on which the mechanism and etiology of MR can be studied by echo **(Fig. 1)**. In Type I, MR occurs with normal mobility of leaflets as in congenital clefts or fenestrations in mitral valve, perforations caused by IE and AFMR causing dilatation and flattening of mitral annulus with atriogenic tethering of posterior leaflet. In Type II, the leaflet mobility is excessive as it occurs in MVP due to FED or Barlow's syndrome, flail leaflets due to chordal rupture, IE and papillary muscle dysfunction. In Type IIIa, the leaflet mobility is restricted both in systole and diastole as in rheumatic MR, carcinoid, hypereosinophilic syndrome, EMF, drugs, radiation, lupus and MPS. Type IIIb is characterized restricted leaflet motion in systole which is a feature of DCM and ischemic heart failure.

MORPHOLOGY OF MITRAL APPARATUS AS A CLUE TO THE ETIOLOGY OF MITRAL REGURGITATION

- Rheumatic MR is characterized by diffuse thickening of both the leaflets with or without commissural fusion, minimal or no calcification, rolled up margins and chordal thickening and shortening. Because of postinflammatory scarring that causes shrinkage of margins, the coaptation length is almost zero with the leaflets apposing at the free margins **(Fig 2)**. Typically, the posterior leaflet is predominantly affected exhibiting no or limited excursions. Commissural fusion if present is usually mild in predominant MR but is virtually diagnostic of rheumatic etiology.
- There are two distinct subtypes of DMR namely Fibroelastic deficiency and Myxomatous (Barlow's)

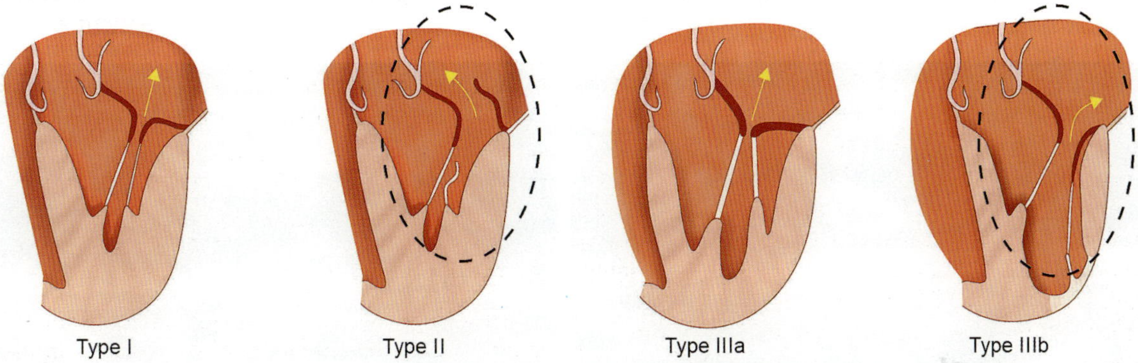

Normal	Excessive	Restricted in systole and diastole	Restricted in systole
• Endocarditis • Cleft MV • AFMR	• Prolapse • Flail • PM rupture • Rheumatic carditis	• Rheumatic, SLE • EMF, eosinophilic • Drugs, radiation • APLAS	• Ischemic DCM • Idiopathic DCM

FIG. 1: Carpentier classification of mechanism of mitral regurgitation.

(AFMR: atrial functional mitral regurgitation; APLAS: antiphospholipid antibody syndrome; DCM: dilated cardiomyopathy; MV: mitral valve; PM: papillary muscle; SLE: systemic lupus erythematosus)

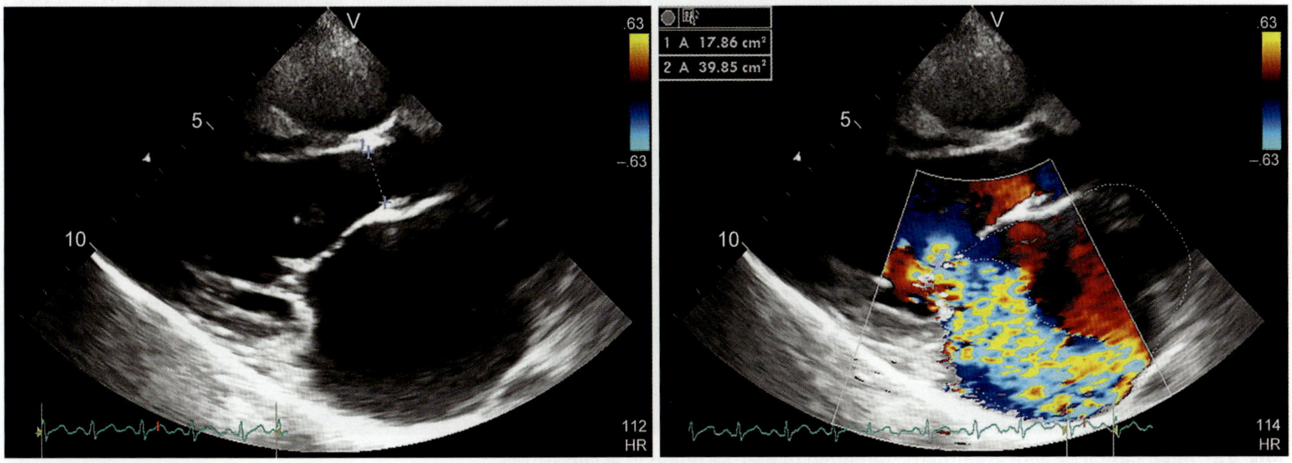

FIG. 2: Rheumatic mitral regurgitation (MR). Thickened leaflets and chorade, coaptation length 0 with nonapposition leading to severe MR.

valve. The former is characterized by preserved leaflet thickness with at the most focal thickening of prolapsing scallop. The prolapse is often segmental involving one or more scallops **(Fig. 3A)**. Leaflet surface area is normal and annulus is often normal in dimension and function. In contrast, myxomatous valve is characterized by marked and uniform thickening with redundancy of both leaflets **(Fig. 3B)**. Annulus is often dilated and may exhibit dysfunction. Chordae may lengthen, get thinner and rupture in both conditions.

- Ischemic MR in a patient with ILMI with regional LV remodeling (LV inferolateral wall) may result in tethering of PML (usually the P3 segment) with its tip facing LV apex and not fulling moving toward annulus in systole. In this situation, AML overrides and comes behind PML trying to appose with the atrial aspect of tethered PML. This creates an apparent appearance of AML prolapse but can be recognized by the fact that AML does not go beyond annulus superiorly (pseudo prolapse) **(Fig. 4A)**. AML may also exhibit a classical bent knee (sea gull or hockey stick) appearance caused by the tethering of the basal strut chordae. MR is eccentric resulting in a posterolateral jet. In 3D echo, the regurgitant orifice is larger at P3 segment and irregularly shaped with asymmetric tethering. LV is only mildly dilated and global systolic function may be normal or only slightly reduced. In contrast, patients with FMR due to large anterior wall MI or IDCM exhibit apical and lateral displacement of both papillary muscles with symmetrical tethering of both leaflets, resulting in increased tenting height and area **(Fig. 4B)**. LV is significantly dilated with global (spherical) remodeling and dysfunction. MR jet is typically central in this situation.
- It is easy to recognize annulus calcification, wherein the annulus, predominantly the posterior part, is densely calcified with extension into the posterior leaflet interfering with its mobility. MR is often mild to moderate.

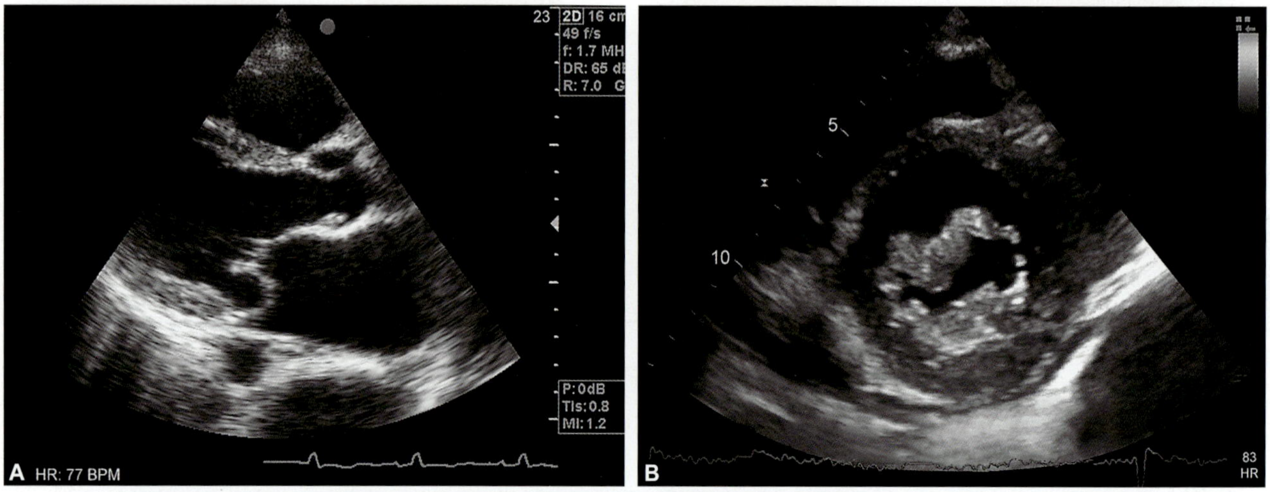

FIGS. 3A AND B: (A) Fibroelastic degeneration with segmental prolapse (left) and (B) Barlow's valve (right).

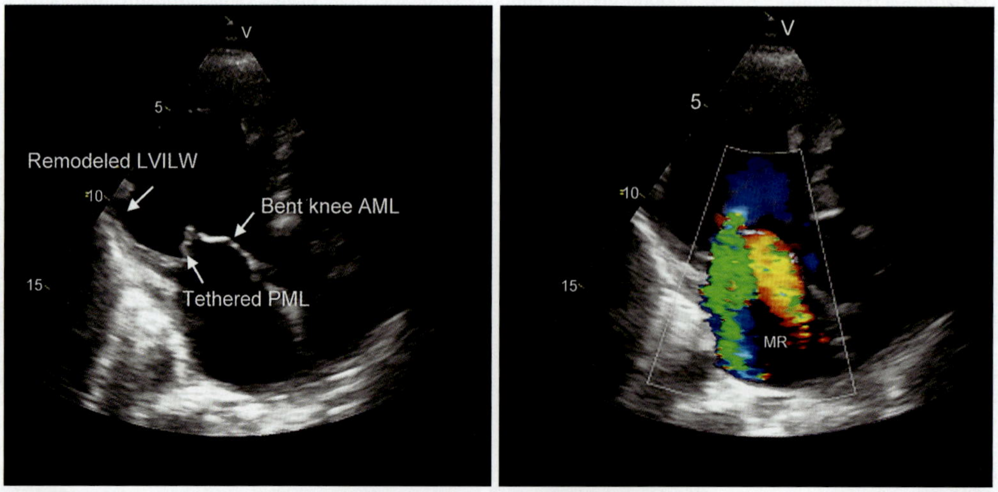

FIG. 4A: Inferolateral MI with asymmetric tethering of PML resulting in eccentric MR.

(AML: anterior mitral leaflet; LVILW: left ventricular inferolateral wall; MI: myocardial infarction; MR: mitral regurgitation; PML: posterior mitral leaflet)

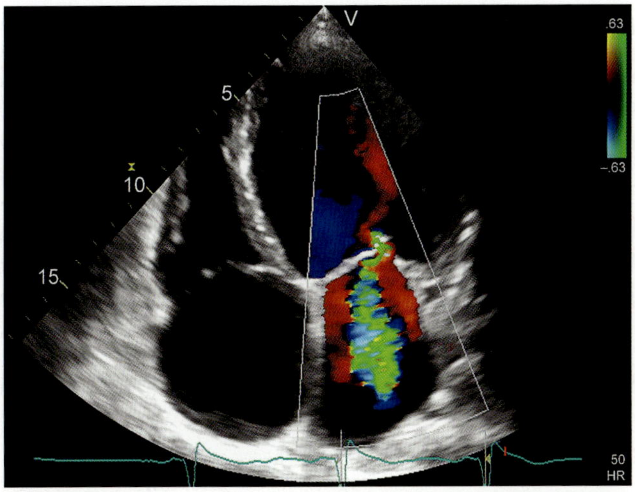

FIG. 4B: Symmetric tethering in functional mitral regurgitation (FMR).

- In hypereosinophilic syndromes and EMF, the PML is characteristically plastered down to the ventricle not allowing its apposition with AML. Apart from this finding, the apex of LV and RV may be obliterated with thrombus and fibrotic tissue.
- In carcinoid and drug valvulopathies the leaflets and chordae are encased by glistening fibrotic tissue with plastering down of leaflets.
- In radiation valvulopathy and in MPS, the leaflets may show uniform thickening of leaflets with restricted mobility but no commissural fusion.
- Recognition of SAM of AML in HCM, vegetations and leaflet aneurysms of IE, congenital clefts, and fenestrations is usually straightforward.
- Atrial functional MR is usually encountered in chronic AF and the patients are likely to be much older and more often females. Echocardiographic features include grade II-III MR, normal ventricular dimensions and function, significant LA enlargement, dilated annulus which is less elliptical than in ventricular FMR or primary MR. The ratio of A3C annulus/A2C annulus is likely to be nearly one and is due to selective dilatation of annulus in the anteroposterior direction. PML may be tethered from upward.

ESTIMATION OF THE SEVERITY OF MITRAL REGURGITATION

An accurate assessment of severity of MR is essential (i) to choose the optimal time for valve intervention, (ii) to prognosticate the patients, and (iii) to decide about the time interval at which reassessment is required in asymptomatic individuals. The hemodynamic determinants of severity of MR can be understood by rearranging Gorlin hydraulic orifice equation. $RVol = ROA \times C_d \times MPG \times T$, where ROA is regurgitant orifice area, C_d is the discharge coefficient, MPG is the square root of the systolic mean pressure gradient between LA and LV and T denotes the duration of MR. Echocardiographic evaluation of MR severity should start with acquisition of 2D data followed by color and spectral Doppler studies. While the jet area offers qualitative information, VC width and PISA-derived Effective Regurgitant Orifice Area (EROA) provide semi-quantitative measures of severity, RVol and RF are the quantitative methods of volume overload caused by MR. Though it may be impractical to use all the available methods of severity assessment in all patients, at least few methods which are appropriate for the jet direction and morphology should be employed.[4,5] An integrative approach combining all the variables is recommended for estimation of severity of MR as each individual method has its own fallacies and limitations **(Table 1)**. Finally, and most importantly, the interpretation should be done with the clinical context in mind (symptomatic status, etiology, acute versus chronic, compensated or decompensated, loading conditions, heart rate and rhythm etc.). During conscious sedation for transesophageal echocardiography (TEE) or during intraoperative period, MR may be underestimated because of reduced driving pressure. Rhythm disturbances may influence estimation of severity of MR. In AF with rapid ventricular response, the jet may be underestimated. On the other hand, chronic AF may induce MR by itself or may aggravate preexisting MR due to other causes. Atrial contraction induces flow vortices around the valve leaflets initiating valve closure. Prolonged PR may lead to loss of appropriately timed atrial contraction and cause mild MR. RV pacing or left bundle branch block (LBBB) may result in dyssynchrony which may contribute to MR.

- *2D Echo*:
  - Valve morphology: Demonstration of coaptation failure indicates that MR is severe. Normally the coaptation occurs not at the free margin but a few mm proximally—the "clapping hands" appearance. The coaptation length is 8–10 mm in a normal mitral valve. Coaptation length (or height) refers to the length of apposed leaflet margins and is different from coaptation depth or tethering distance which refers to the distance from the coaptation point to mitral annulus. When the leaflet is flail due to chordal rupture, a large coaptation gap is demonstrable and MR is invariably severe **(Fig. 5)**. Exception is minor chordal rupture resulting in a limited flail segment of the leaflet. Coaptation failure may also be demonstrated when the leaflet margins get rolled up and shrunk as in rheumatic MR resulting in apposition at the free margin with a demonstrable gap. Whenever PML is tethered and AML apposes on the atrial aspect of PML, the resultant MR is likely severe. Acute MR after MI is usually due to papillary muscle rupture (PMR) and rarely to chordal rupture. Though both conditions result in flail leaflets, a mobile mass attached to

TABLE 1: Assessment of severity of MR by various echocardiographic techniques.

MR severity	Mild	Moderate	Severe
Valve morphology	None or mild abnormality	Moderate leaflet abnormality	Apposition failure, flail, PM rupture
LV and LA size	Normal	N or mildly dilated	Dilated
Color flow jet area cm^2	<4	4–8	>8
Jet area/LA area %	<20	20–40	>40
Flow convergence	Not seen or small	Intermediate size	Large and throughout systole
CWD waveform	Faint, partial	Dense, parabolic	Dense parabolic or triangular
Vena contracta mm	<3	3–7	>7
Pulmonary vein PWD	Systolic dominance	N/systolic blunting	Systolic reversal
Mitral inflow PWD	N/"A" dominant	Variable	E dominant >1.2 m/s
EROA cm^2	<0.20	0.20–0.39	≥0.40
Regurgitant volume mL	<30	30–59	≥60
Regurgitant fraction %	<30	30–49	≥50

(CWD: continuous wave Doppler; EROA: effective regurgitant orifice area; LA: left atrium; LV: left ventricle; MR: mitral regurgitation)

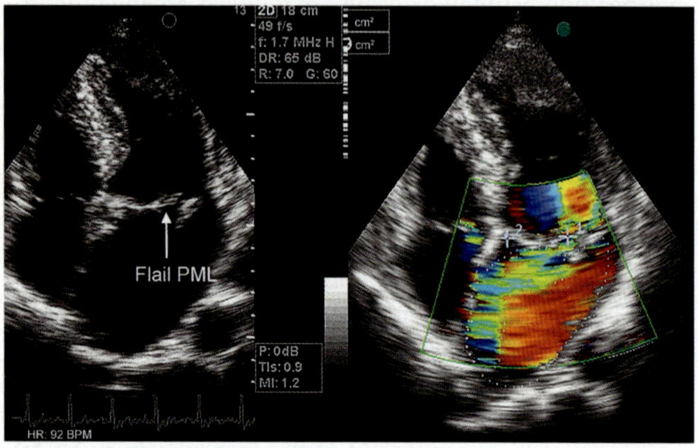

FIG. 5: Flail PML with severe eccentric mitral regurgitation (MR).
(PML: posterior mitral leaflet)

chordae moving back and forth is diagnostic of PMR. MR is invariably severe, but an apparently smaller jet area and normal chamber dimensions may be misleading in this condition. Hyperdynamic LV in a patient with post MI cardiogenic shock should alert to this possibility. TEE may be required to diagnose this condition with precision.

- Dimensions of LV and LA: In chronic primary MR of ≥ moderate severity significant dilatation of LV and LA occur which is roughly proportional to the severity (and the chronicity) of MR. But this finding is of no value in assessing the severity of secondary chronic MR and acute MR for obvious reasons. Similarly, LA size has limited value for assessing severity of MR in the presence of long-standing AF. Moreover, when the preregurgitant chamber dimensions were smaller (often unknown), as in short statured females, the absolute values of chamber dimensions may falsely underestimate the severity of MR. Measurement of volumes rather than linear dimensions would be more reliable, as the pattern of LA and LV remodeling may differ from one patient to the other. 2D echo has inherent limitations in accurately estimating LV volumes because of foreshortening, difficulties in endocardial delineation, presence of trabeculations, etc. Hence 3D volumes or contrast enhanced 2D volume measurements should be used in preference. Left ventricular end diastolic volume (LVEDV) >100 mL/m^2 (M)/>80 mL/m^2 and LA volume >48 mL/m^2 indicate severe lesion provided it is primary and chronic MR.

- *Color Doppler imaging*: When there is an abnormal flow from a high pressure chamber (LV) to a low pressure chamber (LA), through a narrow regurgitant orifice, the velocity is increased and turbulence sets in. This leads to formation of three successive components of abnormal flow as visualized by color Doppler—(1) flow convergence proximal to the orifice (usually seen in moderate to severe MR) in the form of converging flow with increasing velocity and aliasing, (2) high velocity flow across the orifice, the VC, and (3) the flow disturbance (turbulence) caused by the regurgitant jet in LA, the jet area. Analysis of all the three components is capable of providing measures of severity of MR **(Fig. 6)**. For an optimal visualization and quantification of the components of MR jet, high frame rate should be achieved by decreasing the depth of imaging and narrowing the color sector width, just enough to include all the components. Nyquist limit should be kept at 50–60 cm/s and the color gain is adjusted just enough to eliminate random color speckles from nonmoving objects.

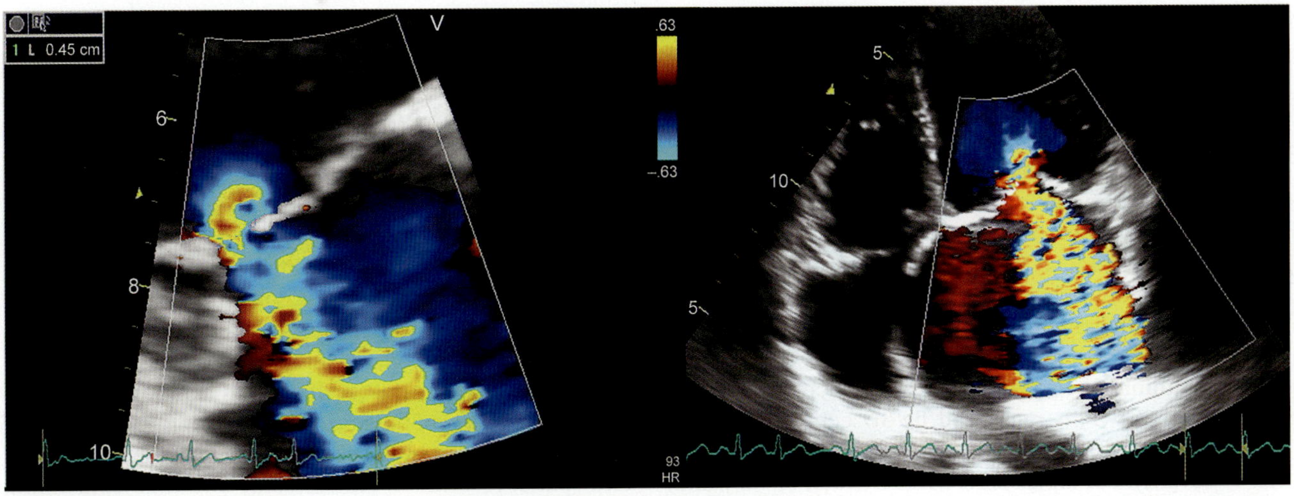

FIG. 6: Color flow imaging of mitral regurgitation (MR) in PS LAX and apical four chamber (A4C) views demonstrating all the three components of MR jet, proximal flow convergence, vena contracta, and MR jet.
(PS LAX: parasternal long-axis)

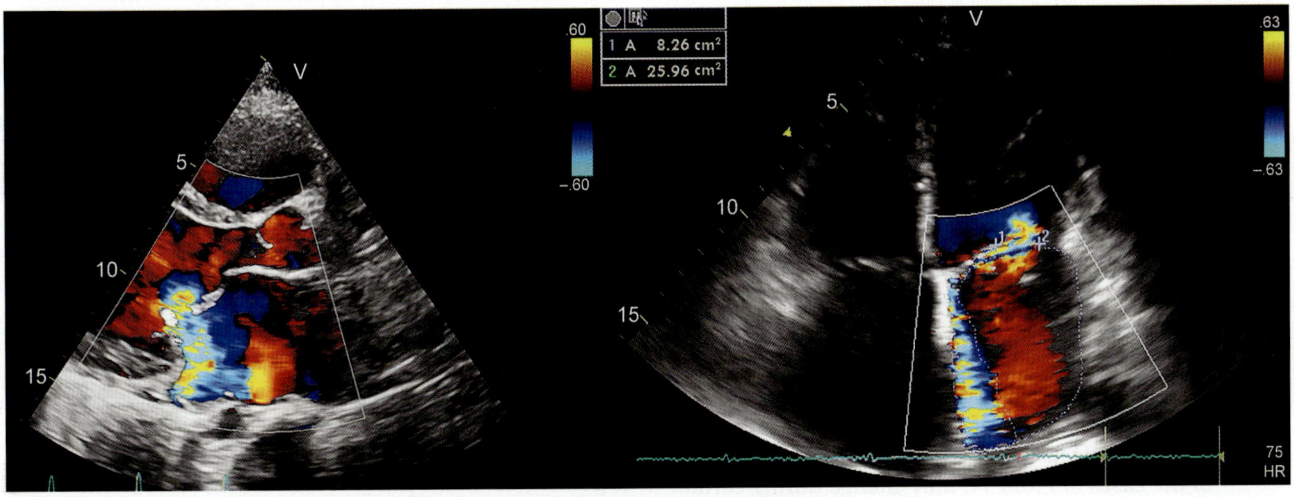

FIG. 7: Eccentric jets of mitral regurgitation (MR)—posterolateral and anteromedial.

- Mitral regurgitation jet area: Though this method was the first one to be used as a measure of severity of MR, it has numerous fallacies. The jet area in LA, the receiving chamber, depicts the flow disturbance caused by the momentum of regurgitant flow. The momentum of the regurgitant flow is determined by orifice area and velocity ($A \times v^2$) and modified by the contractile force of LV. Jet area depicts flow disturbance in LA and not a measure of volume of regurgitant flow. The jet area may be modified by the receiving chamber constraints. A compliant LA may make the jet size larger and a noncompliant LA with an elevated pressure may make it smaller. When an eccentric jet hugs the left atrial wall, the momentum decreases quickly and hence the jet area may be deceptively smaller **(Fig. 7)**. Slit like orifice when imaged along its long axis and multiple separate orifices lead to larger jets than single jets through round orifices. Apart from such disease-related factors, the following instrumental variables may also alter the size of the jet. Increased Doppler gain, decreasing the Nyquist limit and decreasing the pulse repetition frequency may exaggerate the jet size. Attenuation in far field due to large body habitus and interposed reflective structures such as calcium or prosthesis may decrease the jet area. If tissue priority in imaging is set high the structures may encroach on the color signals. If the angle of interrogation is increased (obliquely directed beam) the jet may appear smaller. Transducer frequency may alter the jet in two ways. Higher frequency results in significant Doppler shift at lower velocities making the jet appear larger in TEE. On the other hand, such higher frequencies get attenuated in far field in TTE making the jet smaller in size. Because of so many confounding factors, visualization of jet in LA is useful to identify the mere presence of MR and the direction of jet and to a certain extent helps in differentiating mild MR from severe MR. Jet area of <4 cm^2 and the ratio of jet area/LA area of <20% is considered to indicate mild MR and a jet area of >8 cm^2 with jet area/LA area ratio of >40% severe MR.

- Vena Contracta: It is the narrowest portion of the regurgitant flow that occurs at or just downstream the regurgitant orifice. It will be evident in the form of high velocity laminar flow that is slightly smaller than anatomical regurgitant orifice. The cross-sectional area of VC (as measured by 3D echo) represents EROA, which is true measure of hemodynamic severity. For an accurate measurement of VC width, zoomed image is required and the ultrasonic beam has to be perpendicular to the flow for an accurate axial measurement **(Fig. 8)**. Thus, parasternal long-axis view is ideal for measuring VC of MR flow. A4C view is undesirable because of poor lateral resolution resulting in measurement errors. Similarly, A2C view (commissural view) is also not recommended as the MR jet is visualized in its long axis resulting in an apparently a wider VC. Frame by frame analysis should be done to get the largest and best visualized VC. It is mandatory to have all the three components of regurgitant flow visualized in order to get a proper VC. VC width of <3 mm suggests mild MR and a value of ≥7 mm indicates severe MR. It is a reliable semi-quantitative method of assessing the severity of MR and is independent of flow rate and driving pressure. It is not affected by technical factors. It is valid in eccentric jets, but not reliable when multiple jets are present **(Fig. 9)**. When MR is dynamic as in most of the cases of FMR, VC may change during cardiac cycle, appearing bigger in early and late systole and smaller in mid systole. VC is also unreliable in nonholosystolic MR which is unlikely to be severe despite a larger VC size.

3D VC area (VCA) offers a better estimate of severity of MR, particularly when there are multiple jets and in FMR where the turbulent flow across the crescentic orifice is optimally imaged. From 3D volume set, 2D long axis (systolic phase) images are created and adjusted so as to bisect the jet in both images. Each frame is examined to get the largest and best VC. Then a short-axis image is obtained to get the en face image at the valve orifice or just on the atrial side of orifice. VCA is then measured by planimetry to get the VCA. During offline analysis of the images, B mode image may be removed to get a clear view of the narrowest neck of the jet. Pitfalls of VCA measurement by 3D echo include the limited temporal and spatial resolution, cumbersome and time-consuming technique and over estimation when MR is not holosystolic. Moreover, 3D VC may overestimate MR severity due to the color blooming effect, inclusion of low velocity eddies in measurement, and nonplanarity of the orifice. VCA of ≥0.4 cm^2 is diagnostic of severe MR.

Proximal Isovelocity Surface Area Method: Concept and Methodology

In MR, the blood flow converges toward the regurgitant orifice on the ventricular side of mitral valve forming concentric hemispherical shells of increasing velocity and decreasing surface area. PISA method of estimation of severity of MR is based upon the principle of conservation of mass according to which the flow through any of the hemispheric shells is equal to the flow through the regurgitant orifice. The flow rate is obtained by multiplying the surface area of the shell with the corresponding aliasing velocity (Va). In order to reduce measurement errors, the Nyquist limit is decreased in order to get a bigger hemisphere of aliasing. The first aliasing zone is used for measurement of radius. Imaging is ideally done

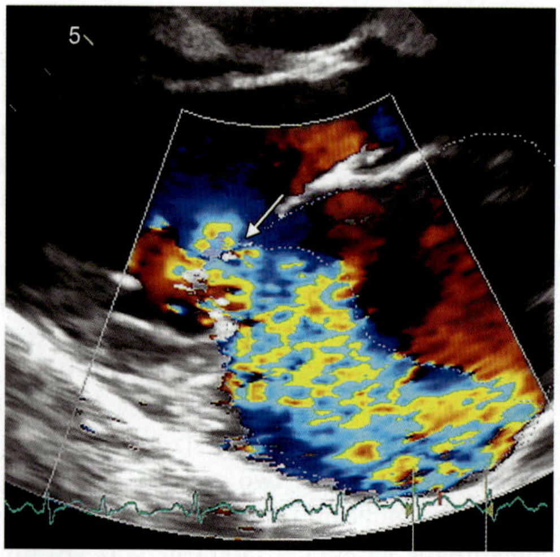

FIG. 8: Vena contracta.

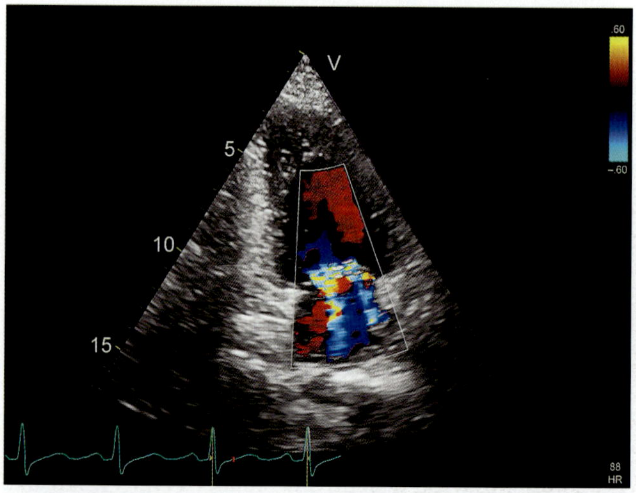

FIG. 9: Multiple jets of mitral regurgitation (MR).

from a zoomed four chamber view as the ultrasound beam can be aligned parallel to the jet and interrogation could be done at the centerline of flow convergence. Then the color baseline is shifted toward the direction of regurgitant jet—downward in TTE and upward in TEE, which may enhance the formation of larger flow convergence. Nyquist limit is often set in the range of 20–40 cm/s. The Pulse repetition frequencey (PRF) may also be decreased to achieve this. Moreover, the aliasing contour is better detected if variance color mapping is switched off. The wall filter may be kept at the factory default setting "high" in order to get the best color Doppler PISA with least suppression and least oversaturation of color Doppler.

The first Va is the one at which the flow convergence changes from blue to yellow in TTE or red to yellow in TEE. To obtain the regurgitant flow rate, Va is multiplied by the surface area of the hemispheric shell which is obtained by using the formula $2\pi r^2$, r being the radius of PISA, measured from the maximum curvature (zenith of PISA) to the regurgitant orifice **(Fig. 10)**. Identifying the first aliasing point is easily done but it may be difficult to locate the regurgitant orifice. The midpoint in the neck of the hemisphere where the color velocities converging into the orifice become low and not registered thus appearing black (perpendicular to the ultrasound Doppler), may be taken as the other end of the radius of PISA. Regurgitant Flow = Va × $2\pi r^2$. From this value, EROA and RVol can be derived. EROA = regurgitant flow/peak velocity of MR. Regurgitant volume = EROA × Velocity time integral (VTI) of MR Doppler signal. RF, radius, Va, and MR peak velocity are all measured or expressed in "cm" in these formulae.

Application: Qualitatively, MR may be considered severe if PISA radius is >0.9 cm and mild if <0.3 cm, when imaging is done at a Nyquist limit of 30 cm/s.[6] Quantitatively, MR is considered mild when EROA is <0.2 cm^2 and severe when it is >0.4 cm^2. Apart from being useful in severity assessment, this technique is helpful in identifying the origin and direction of jets, the mechanism of MR and repairability. The parasternal SAX and A2C views in TTE and bicommissural view in TEE (around 60°) provide information about where along the commissural line the jet arises. Localization is better done with the proximal convergence zone on the LV side than on where the jet is seen in LA, because the later might have come from out of plane.

Limitations of PISA method:

a. Accuracy is less in eccentric jets and when jets are multiple.
b. Small errors in measurement of PISA radius may result in gross errors of severity assessment. For example, EROA is roughly 30% higher at a radius of 8 versus 7 mm.
c. PISA radius is conventionally measured at mid-systole to coincide with the timing of peak of MR velocity, in order to get the maximal instantaneous (single point estimate) flow rate. ECG may be used to make sure that PISA radius and peak MR velocity are obtained at similar time. Obviously, a single point estimate of MR flow rate obtained from mid systolic PISA radius and peak velocity of MR, may not indicate the average regurgitant flow and hence the average regurgitant volume. But practically this single point estimate provides a close approximation of average flow rate and volume, provided the orifice does not change in size.
d. It is assumed that the orifice maintains the same size throughout systole which may not be true all the time. In DMR and rheumatic MR, the PISA radius (and by extrapolation the orifice size) tends to be uniform throughout systole in most of the patients. In some patients with DMR, the PISA radius may increase in mid systole. In considerable number of patients with FMR, the PISA radius and hence the orifice size tends to be minimal in mid systole and larger in early and late systole. Because of such dynamic variations of orifice size, single point

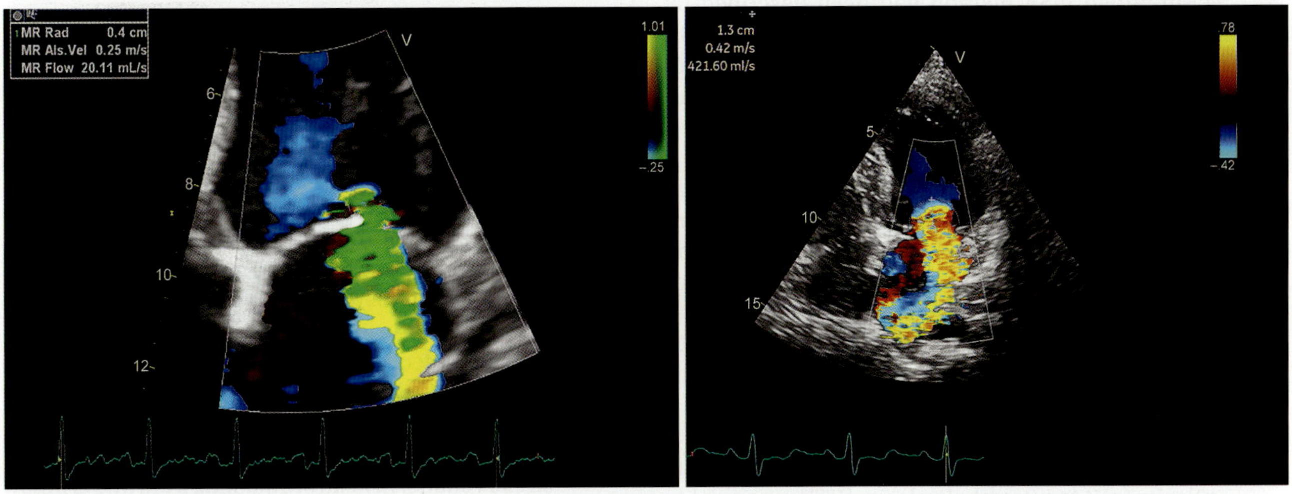

FIG. 10: Proximal isovelocity surface area (PISA)—smaller radius (left), larger radius (right).

estimate of RVol may be misleading and often the values are underestimated. If an average of multiple-point PISA radius with simultaneous MR velocity is obtained, the magnitude of underestimation is minimized. It may be obtained from color Doppler imaging or M-mode color Doppler imaging. However, the method is complex and time consuming.[7]

e. Other limitations of this technique include assumption that the regurgitant orifice is circular and the ventricular side of closed mitral valve is flat (180°). Either or both the conditions are not met in most valvular pathologies causing MR, particularly so in SMR in which the orifice is elongated, slit like, and crescentic (smiley face). PISA derived EROA is underestimated in FMR with a slit like orifice, particularly when the long axis dimension/short-axis dimension of the elliptical orifice exceeds 1.5. In such cases, 3D color Doppler-derived EROA provides a better method of estimating the severity of MR as the regurgitant orifice is directly measured.[8] When the mitral leaflets are tethered the closure plane is more obtuse (>180°) and in such circumstances, angle correction may be done by using the formula—corrected RVol = RVol × (α°/180°). If the regurgitation is close LV wall the wall constraint may make the PISA hemielliptical rather than hemispherical. In this case, PISA may overestimate MR and angle correction may be needed. However, in such difficult scenarios, it is better to use volumetric measurements like RVol and RF rather than PISA-derived EROA.

f. In MVP with late systolic MR, EROA calculated by the PISA method may overestimate the severity of MR as it measures the orifice size but not the duration of regurgitation. It is very unlikely for the RVol to be larger when MR confined to late systole. In this situation, PISA-derived RVol may provide a better estimate of MR because only the densest part of VTI caused by late systolic MR is measured. Alternatively, volumetric method of measuring RVol may be adopted.

   Simplified methods of PISA:

   i. A simplified PISA method had been described by Chaliki who evaluated the product of $r^2 \times Va$ (PISA flow rate) in estimating the severity of MR in a group of 41 patients. All patients with a value of <10 cm^3/s had grade 1–2 MR in LV angiography, while those with a value of 20 cm^3/s had grade 3–4 MR.[9]

   ii. Another simplified PISA method is to assume that MR jet peak velocity is 5 m/s (100 mm Hg pressure difference between LA and LA in systole) as most of the patients have MR velocity in the range of 4–6 m/s. With that assumption, if Va is kept at or close to 40 cm/s, EROA is simply obtained by using the formula $r^2/2$. With such settings, PISA radius of >8 mm indicates severe MR, provided the MR velocity is not >6 m/s.[10]

   iii. In another study of 272 patients with isolated MR, it was found that the ratio of maximal velocity or peak velocity (pV) to integral of velocity (VTI) was roughly 3.25 with a narrow range of variation and hence suggested omission of continuous wave Doppler (CWD)-derived MR VTI for calculation of regurgitant volume. Instead of using the conventional formula of MR flow rate × peak velocity of MR/MR VTI, simplified formula of MR flow rate divided by 3.25 was used in this study (RVol = Va × $2\pi r^2/3.25$). It was shown that MR flow rate obtained by this method correlated well with conventional method (r 0.96 with a point error estimate of 11 mL).[11]

- *Volumetric method*: Regurgitant volume may be calculated by either using PISA method (EROA × MR VTI) or VC method (MR VTI × VCA from 3D or derived from VC width, assuming it is circular). Alternatively, RVol may be calculated by subtracting forward stroke volume (FSV) (LVOT VTI × LVOT CSA) from total stroke volume (TSV) [calculated from 2D volumes obtained Simpson's method (end diastolic volume – end systolic volume) or from mitral flow volume (CSA of MVA annulus × MV VTI obtained from keeping the sample volume at mitral annuls level)]. This method, called as volumetric method, is valid in the absence of regurgitation of other valves.

  Methodology of volumetric method: For measuring the TSV or the mitral stroke volume, zoomed focused A4C view may be obtained without foreshortening LA and LV and the annulus is measured by leading edge to leading edge technique, from the septal attachment of anterior leaflet to the lateral attachment of posterior leaflet, in early to mid-diastole. MVA area may be obtained from this dimension assuming that the annulus is circular (πr^2) or the orthogonal dimension may be obtained from A2C view and incorporated in the formula ($\pi \times r_1 \times r_2$). Pulsed Doppler sample volume (1–3 mm) may be placed at the mid annulus to get a smooth transmitral Doppler. Doppler gain should be appropriate, recordings obtained at 50–100 mm/s speed and the modal (densest part) velocity is traced. An average of VTI obtained from 3–5 cycles (sinus rhythm) or 5–10 cycles (AF) is obtained with the breath held in mid expiration. Mitral stroke volume = MVA CSA × Mitral VTI. To get the FSV, LVOT is measured in mid systole by leading edge to leading edge method from a zoomed parasternal long axis (PLAX) view in mid systole just below the hinge point of aortic leaflets. LVOT area is calculated by using the formula πr^2. LVOT VTI is obtained by keeping the pulsed Doppler sample volume (3–5 mm) in A5C or A3C view at the center of LVOT a few mm below the aortic leaflets. Aortic valve closing click is often recorded when it is recorded at the right place. FSV = LVOT CSA × LVOT VTI. RVol is obtained by subtracting forward stroke from mitral stroke volume; RF is calculated by using the formula RVol/mitral stroke volume. Instead of obtaining from mitral inflow method, TSV may be calculated by the formula TSV = EDV – ESV, obtained by modified Simpson method.

Then RF is calculated by using the formula RF = RVol/TSV. EROA may then be calculated by dividing RVol with MR VTI. EROA = RVol/MR VTI. It is shown that RVol is dependent on EDV of LV which is variable from individual to individual and may depend on the chronicity of MR. Thus at least theoretically, RF appears to be better method of quantification of MR.

Limitations of volumetric method: This method may conceptually look simple but tends to be inaccurate because of multiple anatomic measurements. Errors are likely to be more unless the operator is well trained in this method who is expected to have done numerous trial measurements in normal individuals and proven that mitral and aortic stroke volumes are equal in them. Quite often MR severity is overestimated by this method. Small errors in measurement of annuli may result in large errors as the annulus radii are squared. It is assumed that mitral annulus and LVOT are circular which is not anatomically true. Failure to place the sample volume in the appropriate site at the annulus and properly align to flow may introduce errors. VTI values are likely to be erroneous if modal velocities are not traced. Despite the limitations, this method may be a better option if there are multiple jets of MR or if MR is nonholosystolic or in the presence of wall constraints in eccentric MR.

ROLE OF CONTINUOUS WAVE DOPPLER EVALUATION

Evaluation of MR by echo is incomplete if CWD interrogation is not performed. It might provide qualitative or semi-quantitative estimates of severity and also would be helpful in differentiating holosystolic from non-holosystolic MR.

- The intensity (amplitude) of the Doppler signal is proportional to the number of RBCs interrogated. While mild MR may result in faint and often incomplete CWD signals, severe MR is characterized by uniformly dense Doppler signals, but this method is at the best a qualitative assessment. It may not differentiate between moderate and severe MR. Direction of the jet may also influence the density of CWD signal. In a central jet interrogated from A4C view, the signals are dense even in mild MR and may be faint and incomplete if the regurgitant jet is eccentric.
- A simplified extrapolation of LV volumetric assessment of MR is to use the ratio of E of transmitral velocity to the LVOT VTI [LV early inflow to outflow index (LVEIO)]. In a study of 550 patients with MR, the LVEIO ratio was 9.3 ± 3.9, 7.0 ± 3.2, and 4.2 ± 1.7 for those with severe, moderate, and mild MR respectively.[12] A value of ≥8 indicates severe MR with a likelihood ratio of 26.5. LVEIO ratio of ≤4 implies nonsevere MR with a likelihood ratio of 0.11. This index performed better in those with preserved EF when compared to those with reduced EF (<50%), the area under the curve was 0.92 versus 0.80 in this study.

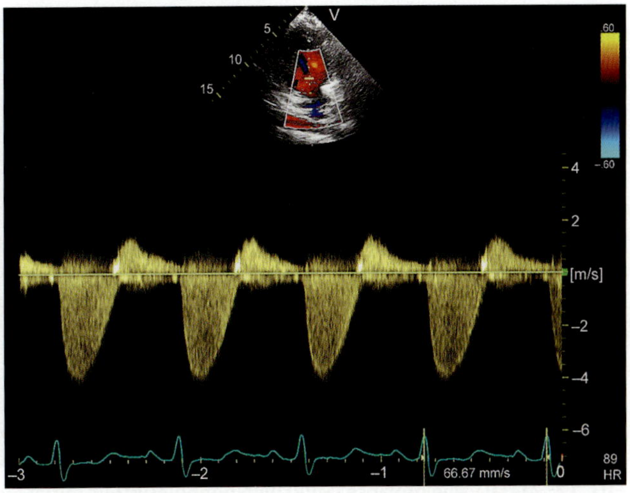

FIG. 11: Acute severe ischemic mitral regurgitation (MR) with v cut off sign.

High LA pressure may increase E amplitude and reduced ejection may lead to decreased LVOT VTO resulting in a higher LVIEO in patients with FMR despite the lesion being mild to moderate. LVEIO index was validated in an Indian study of 500 patients with MR, 52% of whom had rheumatic etiology. The index was 9.91 ± 3.70, 6.56 ± 1.52, and 4.65 ± 1.45 in patients with severe, moderate, and mild MR. LVEIO index of ≥8 had 93.25% specificity for diagnosing severe MR with a positive predictive value of 86.36%.[13] This finding may lose its validity in the presence of mixed or multiple valve diseases.

- A triangular blunted CWD waveform with early peaking and rapid deceleration in late systole, the so-called v cut-off sign, indicates rapid equalization of pressures in LV and LA in late systole and is a feature of acute severe MR **(Fig. 11)**.
- An approximate value of LA pressure may be obtained by subtracting MR pressure gradient from brachial systolic pressure (surrogate of LV systolic pressure).
- Chronic MR commonly results in holosystolic CWD signals with a smooth parabolic configuration. In MVP caused by Barlow's phenotype late systolic MR may occur which is documented by either CWD or M-mode color Doppler **(Fig. 12)**. MVP caused by FED of MV is often holosystolic. Though ERO measured by PISA may look larger, late systolic MR implies that MR is unlikely to be severe.
- Biphasic MR jet with dense early and late systolic signal with faint or no mid systolic signals is characteristic of FMR.
- MR occurring in hypertrophic obstructive cardiomyopathy (HOCM) caused by SAM of mitral valve is also likely to be mid-late systolic, starting at the time of onset of SAM. Holosystolic MR in HOCM should alert the echocardiographer toward the presence of abnormal mitral apparatus. SAM may also occur in some patients with anterior MI or Takotsubo cardiomyopathy when the basal segments are hyperkinetic and in some patients after mitral repair with a ring annuloplasty.

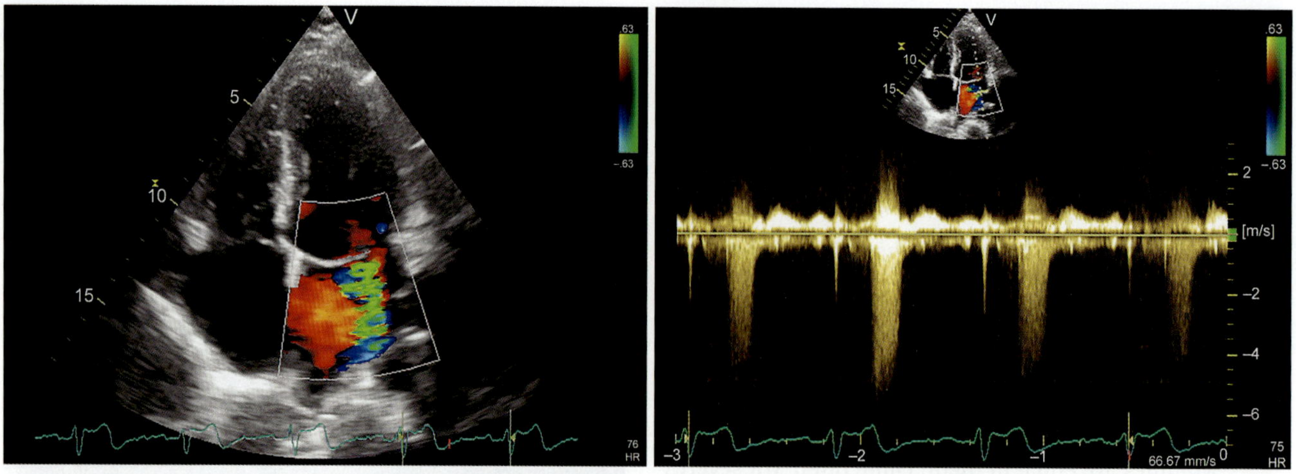

FIG. 12: Mitral valve prolapse (MVP) with nonholosystolic mitral regurgitation (MR).

- CWD estimation of pulmonary artery systolic pressure (PASP) is important as significant elevation may indirectly imply severe MR. Moreover, PASP of >60 mm Hg is an indication for intervention in asymptomatic patients with chronic severe MR.

ROLE OF PULSED DOPPLER MEASUREMENTS

- Mitral Doppler E velocity of ≥1.2 m/s, often with a shorter deceleration time is a supportive finding for severe MR **(Fig. 13)**. On the contrary, dominant A wave inflow pattern excludes severe MR. However, this parameter is invalid in SMR which may be associated with restrictive filling pattern, in AF and in the presence of mitral stenosis, MAC or mitral ring. It is affected by LV relaxation and filling pressures.
- A dimensionless index of the ratio mitral to aortic VTI was found to predict severity of MR of primary etiology. Calculating this ratio is very simple and less time consuming. It also avoids the fallacies involved in calculating the LVOT or mitral orifice areas. Normally transmitral VTI is smaller than LVOT VTI resulting in a mitral aortic VTI ratio of <0.8, which gets reversed in moderate to severe MR. A ratio of >1.3 could predict grade III–IV MR with a sensitivity of 87% and a specificity of 91%. It also correlated with the RF. A ratio of >1.3 identified an RF of >40% with a sensitivity of 90% and a specificity of 85%.[14]
- Systolic flow reversal in more than one pulmonary vein is specific for severe MR and normal pulmonary vein flow pattern excludes severe MR. Eccentric MR directed into one pulmonary vein may falsely suggest severe MR. Systolic blunting is however not specific for severe MR as it may occur in SMR, AF and when LA pressure is high.

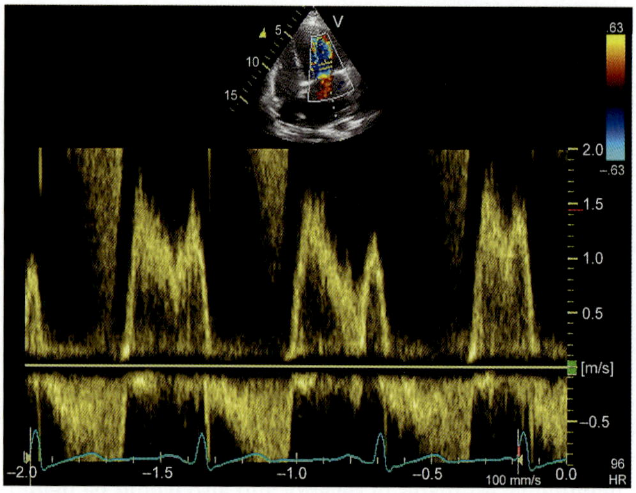

FIG. 13: Mitral E of >1.7 cm/s in severe mitral regurgitation (MR).

GENERAL PRINCIPLES

- It is generally not difficult to differentiate mild from severe MR based on clinical status, LV and LA dimensions and the qualitative and semi-quantitative color Doppler data that include jet size and VC size. If MR is deemed mild, multiple measurements or quantitative methods are not needed. In moderate and severe MR one may have to use multiple methods, at least one semi-quantitative and one quantitative method to differentiate moderate from severe MR. If values are discrepant, the remaining quantitative method needs to be performed as a cross-check. A comprehensive, integrative approach using multiple measurements with wisdom to ignore the outliers, needs to be adopted to avoid over or underestimation.[15] Concordance between different methods is poor and in a study of 159 patients, concordance of all parameters was present in only 6%. Concordance was poor as the severity of MR increased.[16] The operator should be conversant with all the techniques, though he may prefer to develop expertise in few. If challenges are met, one may have to resort to CMR evaluation of MR.

- Since the regurgitant volume is load dependent, determination of cuff systolic pressure (surrogate of afterload) at the time of imaging is mandatory. In serial studies, it is important to make sure that the studies are performed at similar hemodynamic situations—similar systolic blood pressure and heart rate.
- Estimation of severity of SMR is reliable only when the heart failure is controlled, the patient is in compensated state and off vasopressors, preferably after sinus rhythm is restored. When the patient is in a state of acute decompensation, increased LV volumes and depressed contractility may be responsible for apparently more severe MR than in compensated state. Presence of AF with rapid rate and the use of vasopressors may also confound measurement. If intervention is planned, reassessment should be done after 3 months of optimal medical therapy, revascularization if coronary anatomy dictates and/or cardiac resynchronization therapy if appropriate.
- Though it is controversial and remains to be proven, it is better to understand and apply the concept of proportionate versus disproportionate MR in FMR. When the ratio of EROA (mm^2)/LVEDV (mL) is below 0.15, it is called as proportionate MR meaning that MR is proportionate to the degree of LV remodeling and management should be in terms of improving heart failure. Valve-directed procedures may be ineffective. If >0.15 it is disproportionate MR which will respond to MR directed therapies such as transcatheter edge-to-edge repair (TEER).[17]
- Acute MR is almost always severe but because of rapid onset, LV and LA may be normal or only mildly dilated, the jet is often small (due to rapid equalization of LV-LA pressures and the receiving chamber constraints) and eccentric thereby resulting in potential under estimation of severity of MR. Demonstration of the flail scallop or leaflet or papillary muscle may reveal the true severity for which TEE is often required. Hyperkinetic LV in the presence of lower stroke volume (LVOT VTI) or in a sick patient with hypotension/shock is an indirect clue toward the presence of acute MR. Flow reversal in pulmonary veins may also be demonstrable in acute MR.

Transesophageal echocardiography: TEE, particularly 3D TEE, offers excellent visualization of mitral valve and the subvalvular apparatus because of the proximity of transducer to mitral valve. MR jet is often overestimated because of the transducer frequency chosen. Valve pathologies causing primary MR such as MVP, chordal or PMR with flail leaflets, fenestrations, vegetations, etc., are better delineated in TEE. Enface (surgeon's view) imaging of mitral valve has a distinct advantage in studying individual scallops or segments which helps in planning the suitability and type of mitral repair. The leaflets that are imaged in mid-esophageal four-chamber view at 0° are A2 and P2. If the probe is withdrawn slightly bringing the aortic valve in view, A1 and P1 leaflets are seen. When probe is advanced deeper, A3 and P3 would be imaged. In mid-esophageal view at 60°, P1/A2/P3 scallops are seen and with clockwise medial rotation A1/A2/A3 would be imaged and with counterclockwise rotation, P1/P2/P3 can be visualized. Tethering of leaflets in FMR, symmetrical or asymmetrical, tethering distance and area in FMR, leaflet angles (α and β), interpapillary distance, papillary muscle to intervalvular fibrosa distance, annular size, shape and dynamics, the jet origin and direction, etc., are imaged and measured with precision. VC measurements are better done in TEE with the probe at mid-esophageal level at an angle of 120° (perpendicular to mitral commissural plane). 3D PISA measurements can be done from mid-esophageal long-axis view. 3D TEE obtained en face view of mitral valve may be used to measure the anatomical valve area which is slightly larger than EROA.

PERIPROCEDURAL EVALUATION FOR PERCUTANEOUS MITRAL REPAIR

Transcatheter edge-to-edge repair using MitraClip (Abbott) has become an acceptable option for those with DMR and FMR occurring in ischemic or IDCMs, who are not surgical candidates. The procedure is indicated in those with symptomatic severe MR despite guideline directed therapy that includes cardiac resynchronization therapy/conduction system pacing and revascularization when indicated. Heart team of the hospital including a clinical cardiologist, an echocardiographer with expertise in 3D TEE, an interventional cardiologist trained in the procedure and cardiac surgeon should evaluate in detail regarding the candidacy of the individual and the suitability of mitral anatomy for the procedure.

Though a central mitral valve pathology with involvement of A2/P2 leaflets is an ideal situation, segmental prolapse involving other segments may be considered depending on the expertise of the team. Suitable anatomy in DMR (Barlow's syndrome and FED) includes a mitral orifice area of >4 cm^2, MV gradient of <4 mm Hg, leaflets of normal thickness and mobility, no or minimal calcification (at least sparing a 5-mm free margin), no or mild annulus calcification and posterior leaflet mobile length of >10 mm. In flail valve, the flail width should be <15 mm and the flail gap <10 mm. In SMR, coaptation depth of <11 mm and coaptation length of >2 mm are considered favorable for TEER. Presence of cleft or perforation in leaflets and asymmetrical tethering may reduce the success of the procedure. Rheumatic or IE valve, moderate to severe calcification of leaflets or annulus, grasp zone <7 mm, MV area <3.5 cm^2, MV gradient of

>5 mm Hg, length of PML <7 mm, immobile leaflet, MA annulus of >50 mm, and EROA >70 mm^2 are considered as unfavorable anatomy for TEER.[18,19]

During the procedure, TEE would be immensely useful for choosing the ideal site for septal puncture, >4 cm from annulus for DMR and 3–4 cm for FMR measured at mid-systole. Tenting of the atrial septum with simultaneous biplane imaging, four chambers at 0° including aortic valve in cross-section and the bi-caval view at 110° to determine superior height should be performed before puncture. TEE may also guide safe guidewire placement in pulmonary vein, avoiding left atrial appendage. Imaging is also useful in advancing the device across mitral valve, grasping the leaflets, assessing residual MR, need for additional clips, detection of mitral obstruction (mean gradient >5 mm Hg), and procedure-related complications.

Secondary effects of MR: Progressive LV enlargement, LA enlargement, and LV dysfunction occur in long standing MR. Presence of LV dysfunction (EF <60%), left ventricular internal dimension in diastole (LVIDd) >40 mm (25 mm/m^2), marked LA enlargement (dimension >55 mm or volume >50 mL/m^2), occurrence of AF or PH (PA systolic pressure >50 mm Hg) predict events in asymptomatic individuals with chronic primary MR and hence considered as indications for surgery. Since reduced afterload due to MR may mask the onset of LV dysfunction, calculation of forward (effective) EF is considered as an alternative. It is calculated by dividing FSV (LVOT area × LVOT VTI) by EDV. A value of <50% is considered to indicate LV dysfunction. 2D strain imaging is believed to identify early decline in LV function. In early stages of MR, global longitudinal strain (GLS) is increased when compared to normal (median value of -21.6%). Though a definite cut off remains to be determined, decline in values particularly during serial imaging should be given importance.

Exercise echo: Apart from unmasking symptoms in primary MR, exercise echo may be useful in identifying patients at risk of developing events when the grade of MR increases by at least one grade, EF fails to increase by >4% or GLS drops by >2%. Exercise-induced increase of EROA by >13 mm^2 predicts death in patients with SMR.

Multimodality imaging: Cardiac magnetic resonance (CMR) derived RVol and RF might prove to be reliable and dependable when there are multiple jets of MR, the MR jet is eccentric, there is a discrepancy between clinical judgement and echo severity and when there is multivalvular disease. Sequential short axis images are obtained from mitral valve level to apex in diastole and systole to calculate LVEDV and LV end systolic volumes (LVESVs). TSV is obtained by subtracting LVESV from LVEDV. Forward stroke volume is calculated by phase contrast imaging at left ventricular outflow. RVol and RF can then be calculated by usual methods. In addition CMR may be useful in assessing the extent of myocardial scarring and viability.

CONCLUSION

Though it may look apparently a complex time-consuming process, if MR severity assessment is done methodically, a reliable estimate can be obtained most of the time. Ideally the echocardiographer should possess the knowledge of underlying concepts, methodologies, and interpretation of different methods available, though he may prefer to develop expertise in some. Experience will teach the echocardiographer which method is more reliable in a given pathoanatomy of MR, based on the etiology, jet origin, and direction. Meticulously done study which is interpreted in the clinical context may avoid the need for additional imaging.

ONLINE REFERENCES

Please scan the QR code provided at the end of the table of contents for References of this chapter.

SECTION 14

Imaging

CHAPTER 110

Advanced Cardiac Imaging Update: Role of Computed Tomography and Cardiac Magnetic Resonance

Soma Sen, Y Chandrashekhar

ABSTRACT

Advanced cardiac imaging is enhancing our diagnostic, therapeutic, and prognostic capabilities. Cardiac computed tomographic angiography (CTA) is now a first-line test for diagnosis of coronary artery disease (CAD), especially symptomatic patients <65 years of age; it is best suited for ruling out flow-limiting CAD since it has high sensitivity and high negative predictive value. Lower positive predictive accuracy (60–70%) makes it less useful in patients with moderate stenosis and this might need a second test to assess functional significance of the lesion [CT-derived fractional flow reserve (CT-FFR), computed tomography perfusion (CTP), or stress imaging]. CTA, especially coronary calcium evaluation, provides excellent risk stratification in asymptomatic subjects without history of CAD. Plaque imaging allows prognostication but needs more robust data before clinical use. Cardiac magnetic resonance (CMR) provides a "one-stop shop" for evaluating structure, function, myocardial perfusion, valve physiology, vascular flows, and, most importantly, tissue characterization—this is a unique strength which allows for phenotyping the failing heart. Stress CMR is excellent at identifying inducible ischemia and is the gold standard for myocardial viability. In future, we will be measuring tissue oxygenation and 4D flow as biomarkers. Lastly, artificial intelligence (AI) and machine learning (ML) will optimize both cardiac CT and CMR all the way from acquisition to reporting.

Keywords: Cardiac computed tomographic angiography, cardiac magnetic resonance imaging, myocardial tissue perfusion, coronary artery disease, heart failure and myocardial viability.

INTRODUCTION

Advanced cardiac imaging is being used increasingly in clinical practice and recent advances in imaging speed, coverage, resolution along with new hardware technologies are likely to further enhance our diagnostic and prognostic capabilities. We will, therefore, summarize the current evidence in this focused update regarding of the current role of cardiac computed tomography (CT) and cardiac magnetic resonance (CMR) in managing cardiovascular disease.

CARDIAC CT ANGIOGRAPHY

Cardiac computed tomographic angiography (CTA)—a technique to noninvasively image the cardiac structure and function—has gained well-deserved recognition as an important modality in the diagnoses of heart disease, especially in evaluation of the presence and anatomical as well as physiological significance of atherosclerotic coronary artery disease (CAD), prognostication, and for formulating optimal medical or interventional therapy for CAD.[1,2] Apart from its obvious advantages in showing cardiac structure and function with high spatial and temporal resolution, it excels in two important areas: understanding as well as optimally managing subclinical CAD and evaluation of obstructive CAD.

Evaluation of Obstructive CAD

Computed tomographic angiography has extremely high sensitivity (95%) for detecting flow-limiting stenosis with even better negative predictive value (>98%) for excluding significant lesions in stable patients with chest pain. CTA, however, has suboptimal positive predictive accuracy (60–70%) which makes it less useful in patients with moderate stenosis (50–70% lesions) where an additional test might be needed to assess the significance of the stenosis—current guidelines recommend functional stress testing in this situation. However, additional strategies that can be used in the same patient encounter [like fractional flow reserve derived from CT (CT-FFR) and computed tomography perfusion (CTP)] overcome most of these limitations bringing the specificity equivalent to MRI and positron emission tomography (PET) without significant loss of sensitivity. Additional emerging methods can also allow some degree of tissue characterization like scar through late enhancement [something akin to late gadolinium enhancement (LGE) on CMR though with lesser validation so far].

Computed tomographic angiography provides excellent prognostic valve across the entire spectrum of risk—in asymptomatic subjects without history of CAD but at risk of developing it, in those with subclinical CAD as well as in patients with flow-limiting disease. Presence of subclinical atheroma confers major risk for future events and CT is excellent for detecting this with its ability to identify coronary calcification with a noncontrast CT (reported as a CAC score) and nonobstructive plaque using a contrast CT. CAC has been shown to risk classify patients better than predicting future risk using the presence of risk factors or using scores like the pooled cohort equation.

Robust evidence exists that atherosclerosis identified on a CTA is associated with worse prognosis in a graded fashion depending on the number of vessels affected and degree of stenosis.[3,4] A normal CTA identifies subjects with good outcomes including an annual event rate of <1% and very low long-term mortality[5] and offers an approximately 2-year warranty. Recent data have shown that this low event-free survival associated with a normal CTA persists even over a decade.[6]

Nonobstructive CAD

Cardiac CTA is unique in revealing subclinical CAD, in the form of either coronary calcification (CAC) or nonobstructive coronary plaque, both of which are of immense value in identification of individuals at a high risk of future events. A CAC score of zero has a longer warranty (>10 year) against events and is more predictive than a normal stress myocardial perfusion imaging (MPI).[7] Detecting subclinical atheroma, therefore, allows for deploying optimally targeted primary and secondary preventive efforts—early data indeed signal that this might improve long-term outcomes[8] including a reduced risk of myocardial infarction.[9] Nonobstructive plaque is turning out to be an important marker of worse outcomes despite not being severe enough to cause ischemia, limiting coronary flow, and CAC may be better than functional testing for predicting flow-limiting CAD.[10]

Plaque Morphology Imaging

Plaque extent and its composition might be the main reason for future events and could explain why nonobstructive CAD is predictive of future events despite absence of ischemia. CTA allows detailed assessment of plaque including vulnerable plaque characteristics and comprehensively identifying these features is becoming important for patient management. Total atheromatous plaque volume (PAV) predicts CAD progression and events better than stenosis or ischemia alone while extent of noncalcified plaque or plaque with low attenuation (indicating a necrotic core) may also predict vessel perfusion,[11] modulating FFR,[12] stenosis progression,[13] and acute events in patients with prior acute coronary syndrome (ACS)[14] as well as in those with chest pain but no known CAD[15] and indeed might allow better risk stratification in patients with stable CAD.[16]

Computed tomographic angiography can identify other high-risk indicators such as positive remodeling, or spotty calcification, or the rather rare napkin-ring sign that are considered a part of adverse coronary artery plaque characteristics—these are clearly associated with an increase in future events,[14,15] but there is still some uncertainty about how much these plaque characteristics add value over and above extent of atheroma alone and its progression.

In summary, randomized controlled clinical trials and robust observational studies have clarified the utility of CTA in clinical practice. It is best indicated in younger patients with chronic stable angina (<65 years of age), low-to-intermediate pretest probability of obstructive CAD where it has the best power to rule out flow-limiting CAD or guide further testing as appropriate. CTA accelerates the diagnosis of CAD in the emergency room (ER) without affecting hard outcomes compared to traditional testing strategies. In patients with stable coronary syndromes, CTA and functional testing seem to provide similar outcomes but CTA seems to provide greater diagnostic certainty about confirming or excluding flow-limiting CAD. CTA has had a variable effect on frequency of downstream invasive angiography and possibly results in a more optimal rate of medical therapy and revascularization; this may have been associated with possible reduction in future myocardial infarctions.[9] CTA also allows optimal referral for downstream testing including identifying those who do not need invasive angiography[17] and those who need a functional test as a second-line investigation.[1] Using CTA to guide further management instead of proceeding directly to invasive coronary angiography in patients with stable CAD with an indication for invasive angiography seems to be as effective and probably safer as compared to our usual strategy of using invasive angiography.[17] A comprehensive reporting of CTA findings as recommended in the CAD reporting and data systems (RADs) 2.0 is necessary to harness the full potential of cardiac CT.[18]

Coronary Artery Stenosis Physiology

Computed tomographic angiography can provide functional information regarding the physiological significance of a stenosis in the epicardial coronary arteries using techniques that can mathematically calculate pressure drop across the stenosis (a surrogate for reduced blood flow post stenosis)—CT-FFR, that is like invasively measured FFR, or measure myocardial perfusion (CT perfusion or CTP).

CARDIAC CT-DERIVED FRACTIONAL FLOW RESERVE

Computed tomography-derived FFR uses the anatomic information available in the CT scan together with computational flow dynamics methodology (or more recently, machine learning strategies) to accurately provide FFR values along the length of the three major coronary arteries. It can thus provide lesion-specific FFR and match it to the myocardial territory at risk of ischemia. FFR-CT has high sensitivity (90%) and may be one of the best tests for detecting flow-limiting stenosis, especially when the study quality is good, being better than single-photon emission computed tomography (SPECT) imaging and even reaching the diagnostic accuracy of PET.[19] Adding FFR-CT to CTA significantly improves test accuracy.[19] In addition, it acts as a useful gatekeeper for appropriate downstream angiography.[20] There have, however, been concerns about its accuracy in the borderline stenosis zone (FFR of 0.7–0.8).[21]

Computed tomography-derived FFR clearly improves the diagnosis and management of CAD even in real-world settings[22] over and above CTA alone, guides revascularization,[23] and could influence outcomes.[24] Not surprisingly, this technique is now endorsed by the NICE guidelines[25] since it can be cost-effective by optimizing the use of subsequent invasive angiography and revascularization.

The FFR-CT may not be needed in all patients and is best reserved for cases where there is uncertainty about a stenosis in CTA, e.g., 40–90% stenosis per recent guidelines[26] or more rationally in the 50–69% range as practiced previously,[2] which could be approximately 20–30% of patients in real-world practice.[27] Some technical issues need to be considered. For one, the degree of FFR abnormality is strongly dependent on the location of the stenosis, the size of the coronary arteries, as well as the bed it subtends and the ventricular mass in that area of risk; thus, a stenosis in the left circumflex (LCX) might have a different FFR and significance compared to an equivalent stenosis in the LAD. Similarly, the location of the measurement distal to the stenosis might influence the results. It needs good-quality images and is affected by extent of calcification, albeit less than that for CTA. 20–25% of the studies done in real-world practice may not be suitable for FFR-CT evaluation. The studies are currently read at a vendor location resulting in some delay in getting the results. On-site CT-FFR methods are available but have not found widespread utility beyond research centers. CT-FFR is not feasible in chronic total occlusions (CTOs). More recent real-world data in UK shows a less encouraging utility for CT-FFR: 60% of patients were referred for FFR-CT for inappropriate indications, the positive predictive value was lower (33–50%) than reported in clinical trials (71%) and the procedure had a high cost of utilization.[28]

COMPUTED TOMOGRAPHY PERFUSION

Much of our diagnostic armamentarium for detecting functionally significant CAD relies on identifying differences in myocardial perfusion between various myocardial territories, and myocardial CTP testing is showing promising results.[29]

The ability to detect time-dependent, regional changes in myocardial contrast enhancement allows CTA to measure myocardial blood flow (MBF) and is the basis of CT MPI. Current machines have the required temporal resolution as well as wide detector arrays to allow scanning over the entire heart rapidly, either in a static perfusion imaging mode (the entire heart is imaged once at maximal myocardial enhancement after vasodilatation providing a qualitative or semiquantitative estimate of MBF) or more recently in a dynamic perfusion imaging mode (quantitating MBF via high-resolution serial sampling as contrast medium transits the myocardium).

Stress CTP improves specificity as well as the accuracy to detect flow-limiting CAD over and above information from CTA alone[30] has accuracy similar to perfusion imaging with PET or CMR imaging[31] and has good performance compared to CT-FFR; it also allows one to localize the perfusion defect to detailed coronary anatomy obtained via CTA in a single examination whether localized to a single obstructive lesion or in diffuse disease including cardiac allograft vasculopathy.[32] In addition, it has shown strong prognostic value in CAD.[33] It compares well with CT-FFR for identification of functionally significant CAD.[34] CTP has been tested in randomized controlled trials (RCTs) and found to be an excellent gatekeeper for optimal downstream testing in chronic CAD[35] as well as in patients coming with acute chest pain.[36]

The CTP has clear advantages but has not taken off for several reasons including a feeling that it is difficult to do or analyze compared to MBF measurements with PET or CMR (since resting images are not often recorded to limit radiation and instead, stress flow values are normalized to areas without stenosis or to global MBF). In addition, the need to use more dye and relatively longer acquisitions needed to sample dynamic flow could introduce artifacts. CTP competes in an arena full of other methods to assess myocardial stenosis including CT-FFR. In summary, CTP is valued for its positive predictive value and is best indicated for evaluating coronary lesions of uncertain significant or when CTA is difficult to evaluate as with severe calcification, in patients after bypass graft surgery with extensive native or graft disease where anatomic localization of perfusion abnormalities may be useful in further management or with multiple or small coronary stents or in patients with suspected coronary disease after heart transplantation where

CTP may detect early CAV and reduce need for repeated invasive angiography. Two ongoing RCTs [PERFUSERCT (Prospective Evaluation of MyocaRdial PerFUSion ComputEd Tomography) and the CTP-PRO (Impact of Stress CT Myocardial Perfusion on Downstream Resources and Prognosis)] will help us to understand the exact role of CTP very soon.

The CT-FFR and CTP have comparable performance when added to CTA,[34] so the choice of the next test after detecting an intermediate range stenosis depends on local expertise and the influence of some procedural differences. CT-FFR has the advantage of not needing an extra imaging step that incurs some additional radiation, and avoids the need for vasodilation and dye exposure. However, it needs high-quality images and may be suboptimal in the presence of a CTO, stents or significant calcification, and prior bypass grafts. CTP is not affected by any of these but needs more radiation, vasodilatation, and contrast administration.

What is coming in the future?

There have been exciting improvements in CT hardware in 2022. Photon-counting detectors (using semiconductors rather than scintillation detectors) providing ultrahigh spatial and temporal resolution with lower radiation as well as fewer artifacts are likely to change cardiac imaging in a major way. This might allow imaging vessels that are currently suboptimal studies with CT including small stents and severely calcified arteries. Adding AI to image analysis will automate CT acquisition and interpretation and early studies seem to show its effectiveness. Lastly, Radiomics is likely to revolutionize plaque information leading to better decision making but we await robust studies to show its utility.

CARDIAC MAGNETIC RESONANCE

Cardiac MR provides a "one-stop shop" for evaluating heart disease including structure **(Fig. 1)**, function, myocardial perfusion **(Fig. 2)**, valve physiology, vascular flows, and, most importantly, tissue characterization **(Figs. 3A to D)**. The latter not possible with any other imaging modality and is thus a unique strength of CMR.

While CMR is informative in many cardiac conditions, there are two major roles for CMR in current practice. One is the evaluation of structure and function of the heart including infiltrating disease and phenotyping the failing heart. The other major indication of CMR is diagnosing coronary heart disease and coronary physiology.

Although CMR can image the coronary arteries, it is inferior to cardiac CT and has a minor role at present (e.g., identifying coronary anomalies in children). It, however, has a prominent role in two other areas—(1) demonstrating regional and global myocardial ischemia[37,38] and (2) assessment of myocardial viability.[39]

Myocardial ischemia is detected through identifying gadolinium in the myocardium (qualitatively or now quantitatively) pre and post a vasodilator like Regadenoson. It has a steep learning curve but information from LGE in the same study helps to exclude scar and artifacts while improving predictive accuracy. Stress CMR studies are accurate (89% sensitivity along with a 76% specificity), better than SPECT MPI[37] for diagnosing flow-limiting CAD and is great at prognostication (a positive CMR is a marker for high event rates while a negative CMR is associated with a <1% event rate), and can guide therapy giving outcomes similar to that obtained with invasive FFR-guided revascularization.[38]

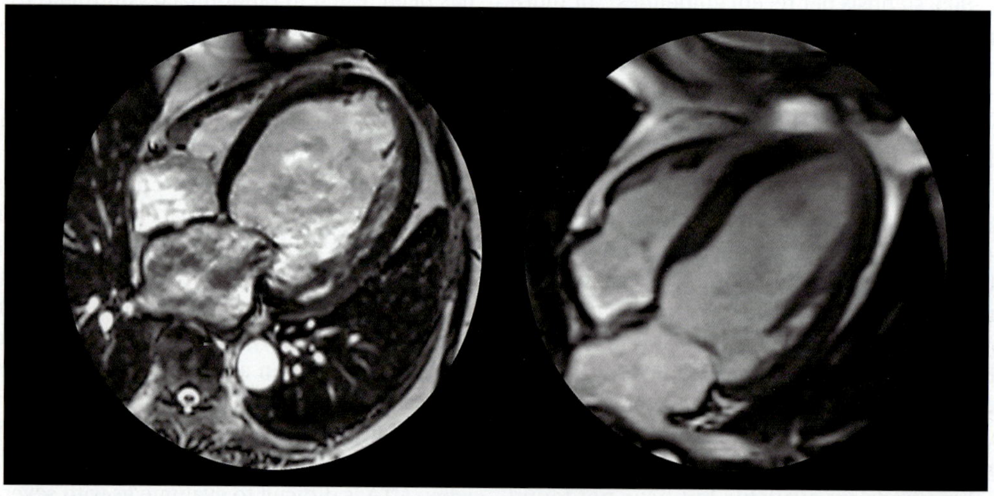

FIG. 1: CMR can show chamber morphology with great clarity. Left panel—HFrEF and right panel—HFpEF. (HFpEF: heart failure with preserved ejection fraction; HFrEF: heart failure with reduced ejection fraction; CMR: cardiac magnetic resonance)

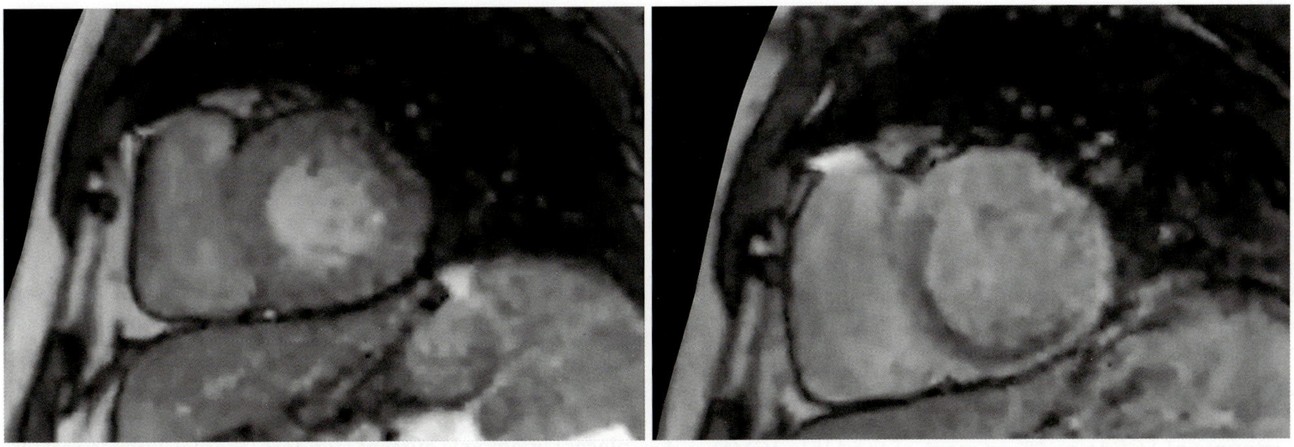

FIG. 2: Stress CMR to localize and quantitate ischemia. Left panel—rest study and right panel—stress study showing a dark band, subendocardial in location consistent with inducible ischemia in the RCA territory.
(CMR: cardiac magnetic resonance; RCA: right coronary artery)

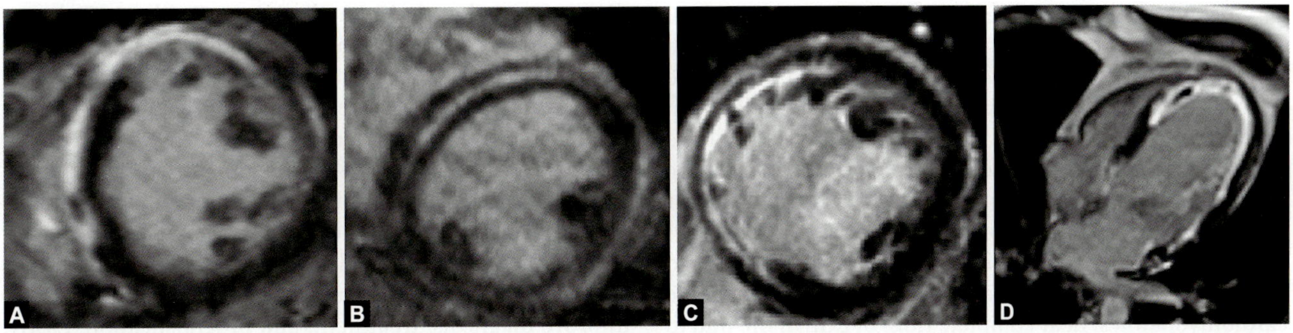

FIGS. 3A TO D: LGE to identify various etiologies of cardiomyopathy. (A) Sarcoidosis with LGE in a typical noncoronary distribution in the septum and lateral wall. (B) A mid myocardial stripe of LGE can be seen in any DCM but the presence of subepicardial lateral wall LGE makes it consistent with acute myocarditis. (C) LGE in a typical coronary distribution suggestive of an old, partial thickness myocardial infarction scar. (D) LGE in a typical coronary distribution suggestive of an old, full-thickness myocardial infarction scar with MVO. This myocardium is unlikely to recover with revascularization.
(DCM: dilated cardiomyopathy; LGE: late gadolinium enhancement; MVO: microvascular obstruction)

The CMR can accurately detect dead tissues (scar) and thus might be the gold-standard myocardial viability with scar thickness being a potent marker of improved left ventricular (LV) function after revascularization (predictive values > 95%).[40]

Cardiac MR is pivotal in evaluation patients with heart failure, especially for etiologic phenotyping in nonischemic cardiomyopathies since this allows for targeted therapies. Patients are often referred with multiple questions including determining the cause of a hypertrophic or an arrhythmic heart. Ischemic cardiomyopathy (ICM) needs to be differentiated from dilated cardiomyopathy (DCM) and CMR has excellent ability to do this, but this technique is now also revealing situations where a DCM can coexist with ischemic heart disease.[41] CMR provides high-definition imaging of structure and function, inducible ischemia, but its major strength is the ability to provide precise tissue signatures of disease[42] [inferred from a combination of macroscopic scarring (LGE), tissue changes including edema (T2 mapping), and microscopic interstitial fibrosis and hypertrophy (T1 mapping) and changes in the interstitium (ECV)]. Severe LVH underlies many serious conditions such as hypertrophic cardiomyopathy (HCM), cardiac amyloid (CA), and Fabry's disease, and using a combination of structure, function, LGE, T1 mapping, and ECV helps in differentiating between them.

The location, pattern, and extent of LGE expressed as % of myocardium have robust diagnostic and prognostic significance[43,44] in most cardiac conditions. LGE shows a typical pattern in ICM (significant congruent gadolinium uptake in the subendocardial region that follows a coronary artery distribution). DCM, on the other hand, has a multitude of patterns, some of which are strong pointers to the etiology of DCM. LGE is particularly useful in infiltrative diseases, where it follows a noncoronary distribution, and is mainly seen in the mid and epicardial myocardium; while no pattern is specific for a diagnosis, location in mid septum and lateral subepicardial wall points toward sarcoid and diffuse LGE suggests amyloidosis (especially if there is also very high T1 and ECV values). On the other hand, Fabry's disease or conditions with high iron overload shows low T1. Finally, abnormalities in all three parameters (LGE, T1, and ECV) strongly predict future events in nearly every cardiac condition. CMR plays a central role in identifying underlying cause of high-grade arrhythmia and LGE location, pattern and burden can guide diagnosis, help in management, triage for ICD implantation, and finely estimate prognosis.[45] Once again, a combination of structure, function, LGE, and mapping is used to stratify the risk.

Risk of future events strongly correlates with increasing amounts of LGE (e.g., 5% or more of the LV in ICM[46] and 15% or more in HCM[47] are useable thresholds for events) even after accounting for ejection fraction (EF). In fact, EF is a poor predictor of sudden cardiac death (SCD) with more events happening patients with EF > 35%; CMR is thus very useful since events are rare in patients without LGE (100% sensitivity compared to 57% with EF) and presence of gray zone areas of LGE which represent an admixture of scar and partially surviving myocytes have the highest predictive value for events.[48] Metabolically active scars have more events than inactive scars in sarcoidosis and adding scar inflammation (FDG uptake on PET-MR) data to scar burden improves prediction and response to therapy.[49] Lastly, while there is no definitive pattern on CMR to identify genetic mutations responsible for arrhythmogenic cardiomyopathies, near complete rings of LGE in the mid to epicardial LV walls[50] should prompt a deeper look for high-risk genetically mediated arrhythmic conditions. While CMR is valuable for early diagnosis and identifying underlying etiology accurately, it should be used judiciously to answer targeted questions since it is expensive and needs significant expertise. A CMR first strategy leads to earlier diagnosis but has not yet been shown to improve outcomes compared to conventional diagnostic paradigms.[51]

CONCLUSION

Cardiac MR technology is changing rapidly in both speed and resolution and, in future, may provide continuous real-time 3D information. Current CMR studies take 30–45 minutes but some recent data show ability to complete a full basic study in just a few minutes. While 1.5T (and 3T in some places) imaging is current standard, there is intense interest in tweaking the strength to improve signal to noise ratio (SNR), spatiotemporal resolution, reducing artifacts and speeding up acquisitions. Imaging at 7.0T provides some of these benefits but needs further studies to minimize patient discomfort and optimize methodology. Fields <1.5T do not need the heavy duty cooling as in traditional magnets and could allow low-cost scanning with reasonable images, less artifacts, and probably more safety. Tissue characterization is likely to improve and provide richer data on myocardial tissue properties in newer ways. Advancements in quantitative CMR will enhance our ability to measure flow, volumes, microvascular function, and tissue oxygenation. This along with 4D flow methods will provide new biomarkers (e.g., ascending aorta risk in patients with bicuspid valves) to improve diagnosis, treatment, and prognostication. Lastly, AI and ML are already starting to optimize cardiac MR all the way from acquisition to reporting.

ONLINE REFERENCES

Please scan the QR code provided at the end of the table of contents for References of this chapter.

CHAPTER 111

Role of CMR in Nonischemic Cardiomyopathies

Mona Bhatia, Parveen Kumar, Amit Garg, Prasit Maity, Natisha Arora, Sachin Raiya, Akash

ABSTRACT

Cardiac magnetic resonance (CMR) is considered the most reliable method for assessing ventricular mass, volumes, and ejection fraction due to its superior spatial resolution. It plays a crucial role in accurately diagnosing and managing nonischemic cardiomyopathies. In this chapter, we provide a comprehensive review of the utility of CMR in the diagnosis and management of both common and rare types of nonischemic cardiomyopathies. We highlight specific CMR findings associated with each type of cardiomyopathy. CMR not only helps differentiate nonischemic from ischemic cardiomyopathy, but also assists in accurately diagnosing and managing different subtypes of nonischemic cardiomyopathy. Incorporating CMR into the routine diagnostic evaluation of various cardiomyopathies is highly recommended.

Keywords: Non-ischemic cardiomyopathy, cardiovascular magnetic resonance, cardiomyopathy, dilated cardiomyopathy, and myocarditis.

INTRODUCTION

Nonischemic cardiomyopathy is defined as a myocardial disorder in the absence of other identifiable causes such as systemic hypertension, valvular disease, coronary artery disease (CAD), and congenital heart disease. Cardiac magnetic resonance (CMR) is a valuable tool and provides insight into the etiology, prognosis, and treatment response of various nonischemic cardiomyopathies. CMR is the reference standard for quantifying cardiac chamber volumes and ejection fraction.[1] The CMR-based tissue characterization techniques such as late gadolinium enhancement (LGE), parametric mapping, and extracellular volume (ECV) calculation have been validated against histological findings. Various recommendations, expert opinions, and consensus statements from different societies include CMR as a primary imaging technique for cardiomyopathies.[2-4] The present chapter outlines the role of CMR imaging in diagnosing various nonischemic cardiomyopathies and illustrates the spectrum of their appearances on CMR imaging.

CLASSIFICATION

The American Heart Association classifies cardiomyopathies into primary and secondary types. Primary cardiomyopathies are further divided into genetic, acquired, or mixed subtypes.[5] The European Society of Cardiology classifies cardiomyopathies into specific morphological and functional phenotypes, i.e., dilated cardiomyopathy (DCM) and hypertrophic cardiomyopathy (HCM).[6]

CARDIAC MAGNETIC RESONANCE PROTOCOLS

There are three standard cardiac planes which include a short axis, a horizontal long axis, and a vertical long axis. A broad range of CMR sequences is available for functional and tissue characterization.[7,8] The various CMR sequences can be divided into two groups—dark (black) blood and bright (white) blood sequences. Black blood sequences are primarily used for cardiac morphology. Examples of dark blood sequences include spin echo and fast spin echo. Bright blood sequences are primarily used to evaluate cardiac function. Examples of bright blood sequences include gradient echo and refocused steady-state free precession.[9] After the routine black and bright blood imaging, LGE images are acquired. Phase-sensitive inversion recovery (PSIR) is the best sequence that produces consistent image quality with minimal artefacts.[10,11] Modified Look-Locker inversion recovery (MOLLI) and shortened MOLLI (ShMOLLI) are primarily used for T1 mapping.[12-14] Myocardial tagging is used to evaluate the dynamic deformation of the myocardium during the cardiac cycle. Tagging allows quantification of myocardial rotation, torsion, as well as orthogonal components of myocardial motion.[15-17]

CLINICAL APPLICATIONS OF CMR IN VARIOUS NONISCHEMIC CARDIOMYOPATHIES

Hypertrophic Cardiomyopathy

Hypertrophic cardiomyopathy is the most common primary genetic disease of the heart, transmitted in an autosomal manner with variable penetrance and clinical expression. HCM exhibits various morphological expressions including sigmoid septal contour, reversed septal contour, mid-ventricular obstruction, apical HCM, symmetric HCM, and focal HCM.[18]

The typical imaging features of HCM include a left ventricular (LV) wall thickness ≥15 mm at end-diastole or septal to lateral wall thickness ratio of >1.3 in the absence of any loading condition **(Fig. 1)**. CMR can also assess HCM-associated dynamic left ventricular outflow tract (LVOT) obstruction and systolic anterior mitral valvular motion. Myocardial tagging provides a detailed assessment of myocardial contractility and relaxation.[18,19] T1 mapping can identify myocardial fibrosis outside the diagnostic zones of LGE.[20,21] ECV calculation is another helpful tool. The mapping techniques are also helpful stratification of risk for adverse cardiac events by longitudinal follow-up of the degree of fibrosis.[20,21] LGE is also an invaluable tool in the assessment of HCM. Studies have shown a strong association between the presence of LGE and adverse myocardial events even in asymptomatic patients **(Fig. 2)**.[22]

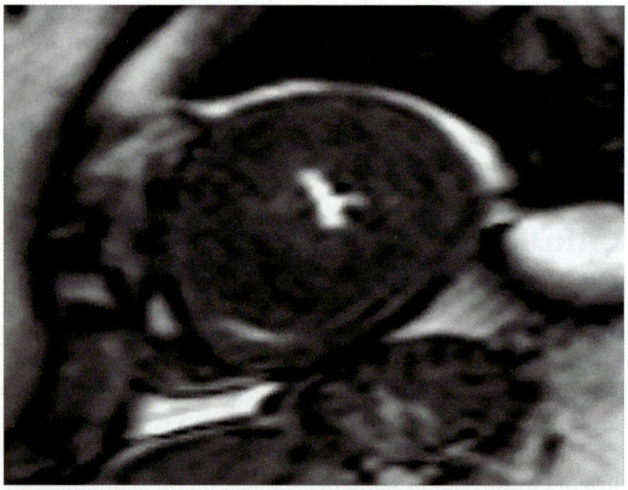

FIG. 1: Short-axis, balanced turbo-field-echo (BTFE) cardiac magnetic resonance (CMR) image at mid left ventricular (LV) cavity level demonstrating typical imaging features of hypertrophic cardiomyopathy (HCM) include an LV wall thickness ≥15 mm at end-diastole.

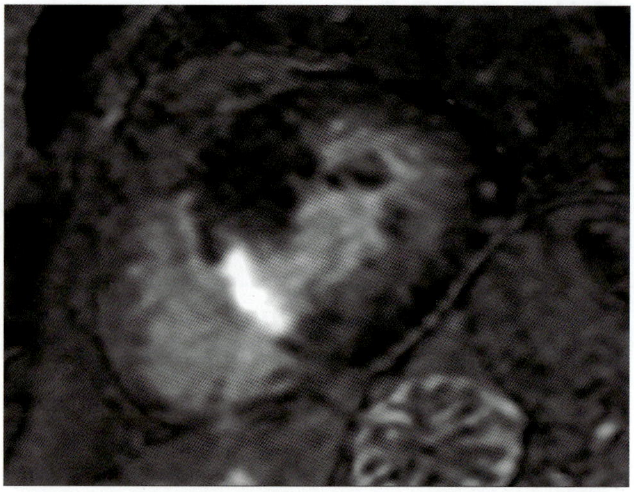

FIG. 2: Short-axis, post-gadolinium enhancement phase-sensitive inversion recovery (PSIR) image demonstrating scar in a patient with hypertrophic cardiomyopathy (HCM).

Various conditions increasing myocardial afterload such as hypertension and aortic stenosis can mimic HCM phenotypes. The common mimicker is athlete's heart, in which physiological cardiac remodeling leads to LV hypertrophy (LVH) with LV wall thickness measuring up to 15 mm. The most useful distinguishing parameter is ratio of end-diastolic wall thickness to end-diastolic volume. A cut-off value of 0.15 mm/mL/m^2 has 80% sensitivity and 99% specificity.[23]

Arrhythmogenic Right Ventricular Cardiomyopathy

Arrhythmogenic right ventricular cardiomyopathy (ARVC) is a genetic disease characterized by the replacement of fibrofatty tissue in the right ventricle, leading to right ventricular (RV) dysfunction and ventricular arrhythmias.[24] The initial diagnostic criteria for ARVC were established by the task force of the European Society of Cardiology and the Scientific Council on Cardiomyopathy of the World Heart Federation in 1994. These criteria considered structural, histological, genetic, electrocardiographic, and arrhythmic factors. Diagnosis of ARVC requires the fulfilment of either two major criteria, one major and two minor criteria, or four minor criteria.[25] In 2010, the task force revised these criteria, placing greater emphasis on volume, ejection fraction, and wall motion, while eliminating fatty infiltration as a diagnostic factor.[26]

Common CMR findings in ARVC include RV enlargement and RV wall motion abnormalities such as akinesia, dyskinesia, and segmental dilatation. Although LGE is a validated technique for assessing myocardial fibrosis, it is not included in the diagnostic criteria due to certain limitations. These include the thin wall of the RV, which hampers LGE detection, and the nonspecific nature of LGE, which can be present in conditions mimicking ARVC such as right-sided myocarditis, sarcoidosis, and DCM. It is crucial to note that fatty infiltration of the RV is not specific to ARVC and can be observed in healthy individuals, obese individuals, elderly patients, chronic steroid abusers, and idiopathic RV outflow tract tachycardia.[27] Similarly, RV LGE is also not a specific feature and can be present in conditions such as DCM, Chagas disease, right-sided myocarditis, and sarcoidosis.[28]

Left Ventricular Noncompaction

Left ventricular noncompaction (LVNC) is a genetic cardiomyopathy characterized by thick noncompacted lining of the left ventricle, prominent trabecular outpouchings, and impaired LV systolic function **(Fig. 3)**. The clinical manifestations of LVNC can vary from asymptomatic individuals to heart failure, ventricular arrhythmias, sudden cardiac death, and thromboembolic events.[29]

The standard diagnostic criterion for LVNC is a ratio of noncompacted to compacted myocardium >2.3.[30] However, this criterion may not be reliable for assessing LV apical noncompaction due to the thinness of the apical compact myocardium. Alternative quantitative methods have been proposed, such as calculating the trabeculated LV mass or measuring the trabeculated LV myocardial volume as a percentage of the total LV myocardial volume.[31,32] When assessing prominent trabeculations, it is important to exclude the papillary muscles. The noncompacted segments may exhibit hypokinesia compared to normal adjacent segments. Furthermore, the trabecular layer may show perfusion defects after gadolinium administration, indicating microvascular abnormalities. LGE images may reveal delayed enhancement in the trabeculae, which correlates with disease progression.[33]

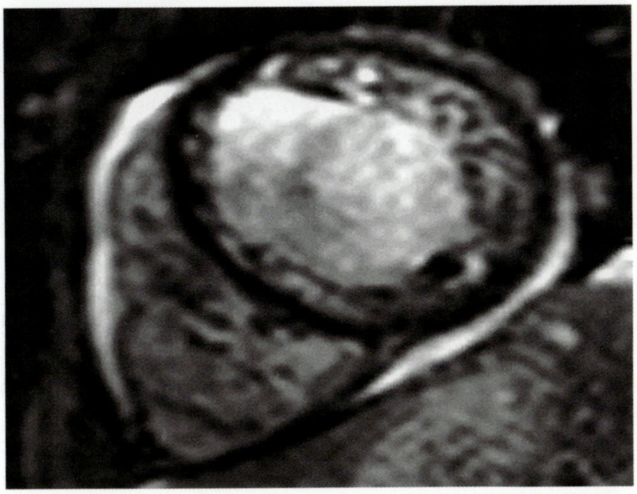

FIG. 3: Short-axis, balanced turbo-field-echo (BTFE) cardiac magnetic resonance (CMR) image at mid left ventricular (LV) cavity level demonstrating typical imaging features of noncompaction with hypertrabeculation of the LV myocardium.

Dilated Cardiomyopathy

Dilated cardiomyopathy is characterized by the dilatation of the left ventricle or both ventricles, along with systolic dysfunction, in the absence of systemic hypertension, valvular disease, CAD, and congenital heart disease. Common presenting complaints include progressive dyspnea and orthopnea.[34]

Cardiac magnetic resonance imaging is another valuable modality for DCM evaluation. It provides precise measurements of cardiac chamber volumes due to its high spatial resolution and improved visualization of the blood-endocardium interface. CMR myocardial tagging is particularly useful in identifying subtle abnormalities in contractile function, enabling early detection of DCM. Left atrial (LA) dilatation is commonly observed and is primarily attributed to diastolic dysfunction, functional mitral regurgitation, and LV enlargement. The measurement of LA volume holds independent predictive value for adverse outcomes in DCM.[35] Additionally, DCM frequently involves RV remodeling, often leading to secondary pulmonary hypertension. As the LV enlarges, the mitral annulus dilates, resulting in defective coaptation of the mitral leaflets and functional mitral regurgitation. Functional mitral regurgitation serves as an independent risk factor for adverse outcomes in DCM. Mitigating its severity has been associated with improved survival without the need for heart transplantation.[36,37] In advanced DCM, focal myocardial fibrosis is a common finding resulting from myocardial injury and subsequent repair processes. LGE imaging can identify these fibrotic areas. The presence and extent of myocardial fibrosis have prognostic implications and can help determine the likelihood of myocardial remodeling following medical management or cardiac resynchronization therapy.[38-40] T1 myocardial mapping techniques provide quantitative measurements of myocardial T1 relaxation time. Increased native T1 values are observed not only in areas showing LGE but also in regions without LGE, indicating that T1 mapping has the ability to detect fibrosis beyond the diagnostic range of LGE.[21] These advanced imaging techniques provide valuable information about the presence, extent, and prognostic implications of fibrosis in DCM, helping guide treatment decisions and risk stratification **(Fig. 4)**.

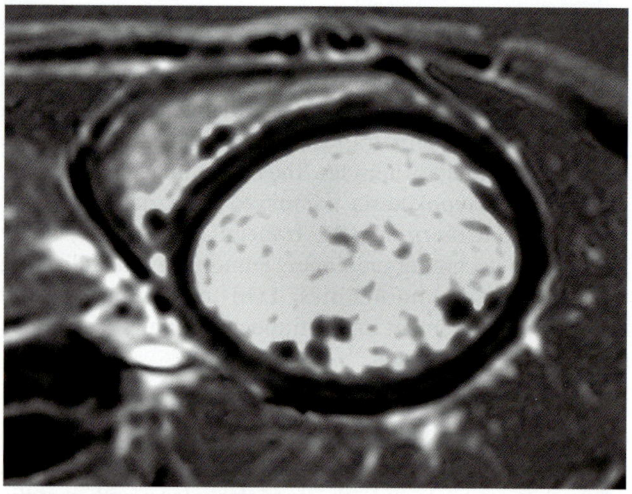

FIG. 4: Short-axis, post-gadolinium enhancement phase-sensitive inversion recovery (PSIR) image demonstrating dilated cardiomyopathy with global wall thinning and a mid-wall scar in a patient with dilated cardiomyopathy (DCM).

Restrictive Cardiomyopathy

Restrictive cardiomyopathy (RCM) is characterized by increased myocardial stiffness, resulting in impaired ventricular filling and diastolic dysfunction. The size and systolic functions of both ventricles are typically normal in RCM. The etiology of RCM can be inherited, acquired, or a combination of both, and it is broadly classified into infiltrative, noninfiltrative, storage disorders, and endomyocardial types. Patients with RCM may present with signs and symptoms of either RV or LV failure, depending on the involvement of the respective ventricle. Conduction disturbances and arrhythmias are also not uncommon in RCM.[41]

Cardiac magnetic resonance plays a fundamental role in diagnosing RCM. The imaging features common to all types of RCM include normal ventricular size and biatrial enlargement, which distinguish RCM from other types of cardiomyopathies where ventricular enlargement is typically observed. Assessing diastolic function is an important aspect of RCM evaluation, and CMR provides various indices for this purpose. Parameters such as peak filling rate and early diastolic filling time can be measured to evaluate diastolic function.[42-44] Myocardial tagging is another useful CMR sequence that provides detailed analysis of myocardial strain and deformation. It can help assess myocardial function and identify abnormal patterns of strain in RCM. Differentiating RCM from constrictive pericarditis is crucial, as their management approaches differ. In constrictive pericarditis, pericardial thickening and persistent concordance of tagged signals between the myocardium and pericardium throughout the cardiac cycle are characteristic findings.

Cardiac Amyloidosis

Cardiac amyloidosis is characterized by the deposition of amyloid proteins in the heart's extracellular space. The two most common types seen in cardiac amyloidosis are AL amyloidosis and ATTR amyloidosis, which can both lead to RCM. Patients with cardiac amyloidosis often experience symptoms such as reduced exercise tolerance, fatigue, and lower limb edema. Conduction system involvement can lead to heart blocks and arrhythmias.[45]

Cardiac magnetic resonance imaging is an important tool for diagnosing and characterizing cardiac amyloidosis. The characteristic findings on CMR, such as diffusely decreased signal intensity on T1-weighted images and thickening of the right atrial posterior wall and interatrial septum, can be indicative of cardiac amyloidosis. LGE sequences are particularly useful in visualizing the distribution of contrast material in the myocardium **(Fig. 5)**.[44,46] CMR provides valuable information about the structural and functional changes in the myocardium associated with cardiac amyloidosis. By assessing myocardial tissue characteristics and visualizing the patterns of involvement, CMR complements other clinical and laboratory findings, contributing to a comprehensive evaluation of the disease. T1 mapping is a valuable technique in CMR imaging for quantifying T1 relaxation times in the myocardium. ECV is another important marker in cardiac amyloidosis. It represents the fraction of the myocardium occupied by extracellular space, including interstitial fluid and amyloid deposits. Elevated native T1 and ECV values have been found to precede the appearance of LGE, making them valuable in detecting early cardiac involvement in amyloidosis.[47-49]

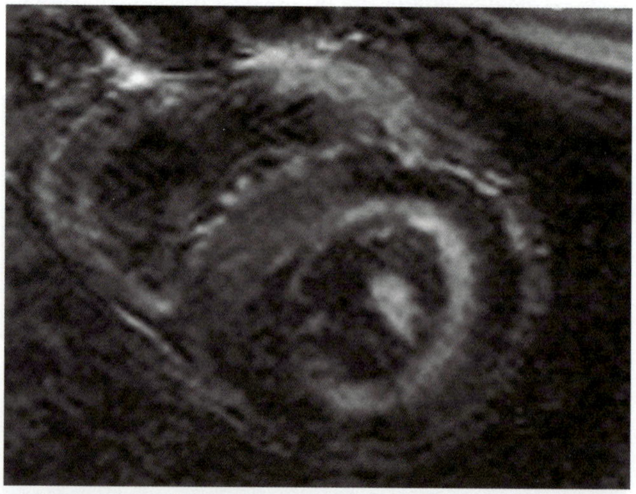

FIG. 5: Short-axis, post-gadolinium enhancement phase-sensitive inversion recovery (PSIR) image demonstrating the typical feature of circumferential subendocardial enhancement in a patient with amyloidosis.

Cardiac Sarcoidosis

Cardiac sarcoidosis is a significant cause of mortality in patients with systemic sarcoidosis. The clinical manifestations of cardiac sarcoidosis can vary and include congestive heart failure, cor pulmonale, ventricular and supraventricular arrhythmias, valvular dysfunction, pericardial effusion, and ventricular aneurysm formation.[50]

Endomyocardial biopsy is considered the gold standard for diagnosing cardiac sarcoidosis; however, it has limitations such as low sensitivity and invasiveness, which may hinder its routine use. As a result, the diagnosis of cardiac sarcoidosis often relies on a combination of clinical symptoms and specific findings on imaging modalities. CMR has emerged as a powerful noninvasive tool for the diagnosis of cardiac sarcoidosis. T2-weighted images can reveal patchy areas of myocardial hyperintensity, representing inflammatory lesions commonly associated with sarcoidosis. LGE imaging is particularly informative in cardiac sarcoidosis. It can demonstrate myocardial scarring, which can involve any layer of the myocardium. The most commonly affected regions are the subepicardium and mid-wall regions **(Fig. 6)**. CMR plays a crucial role in risk stratification for cardiac sarcoidosis as well. LGE has been identified as an independent risk predictor in both symptomatic and asymptomatic patients. LGE is considered a minor criterion in the Japanese Ministry of Health and Welfare (JMHW) criteria and a major criterion in the Heart Rhythm Society (HRS) criteria for the diagnosis of cardiac sarcoidosis.[51-55] These criteria provide guidelines for the diagnosis of cardiac sarcoidosis based on a combination of clinical, imaging, and histopathological findings. Both T1 and T2 mapping have shown potential as predictors of survival and heart failure in patients with cardiac sarcoidosis. Elevated T1 values have been associated with worse outcomes and increased risk of adverse cardiac events. These mapping techniques can also be utilized to monitor the response to anti-inflammatory treatment, as changes in T1 and T2 indexes can reflect the effectiveness of therapy in reducing inflammation and tissue remodeling.[56]

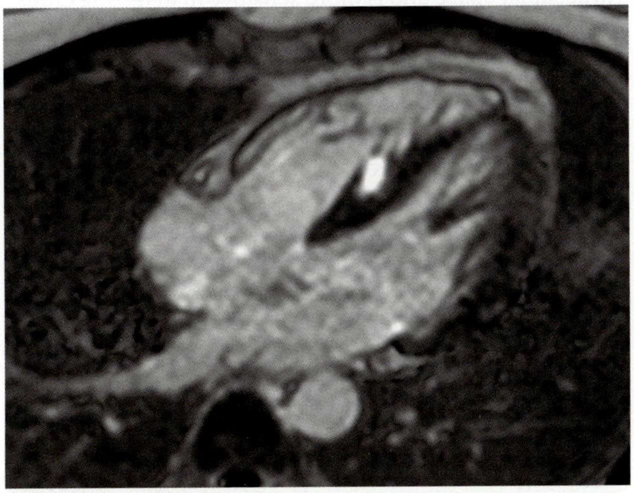

FIG. 6: Four-chamber post-gadolinium enhancement phase-sensitive inversion recovery (PSIR) image demonstrating the typical focal nodular enhancement along the right ventricular (RV) aspect of the septum in a patient with sarcoidosis.

Iron Overload Cardiomyopathy

Iron overload cardiomyopathy (IOC) is a condition characterized by the excessive accumulation of iron in the myocardium, which can lead to the development of cardiomyopathy. The clinical presentation of IOC can vary, but common complaints include exertional dyspnea due to restrictive physiology caused by impaired diastolic function. Supraventricular arrhythmias and first-degree atrioventricular block are not uncommon findings.[57]

Cardiac magnetic resonance imaging plays a crucial role in the noninvasive evaluation of IOC. Unlike other infiltrative cardiomyopathies, IOC does not typically present with increased LV wall thickness. On functional evaluation, IOC often demonstrates restrictive filling patterns, with or without LA enlargement. As the disease progresses it may lead to dilated phenotype or a restrictive phenotype. Iron is a paramagnetic substance that affects the relaxation time of magnetic resonance imaging sequences. T2-weighted sequences, specifically T2*-weighted imaging, have proven to be useful in the noninvasive quantification of myocardial iron. T2* values reflect the decay of the magnetic resonance signal and are typically <20 ms in cases of RCM due to iron overload. A T2* value of <10 ms indicates profound iron overload and has been shown to predict the risk of heart failure.[58]

Endomyocardial Diseases

Endomyocardial Fibrosis

Endomyocardial fibrosis (EMF) is a form of RCM that primarily affects young adults and demonstrates a bimodal age distribution, with peaks around 10 and 30 years.[59] On CMR imaging, EMF typically presents with normal ventricular wall thickness, small ventricles, and dilated atria. LGE imaging in EMF typically demonstrates a characteristic three-layered appearance known as the "V sign".[60] It is important to note that EMF on LGE can resemble CAD with apical infarction and intracavitary thrombus. However, these two entities can be differentiated by the presence of preserved inward apical systolic motion in EMF and its absence in CAD.[61]

Endocardial Fibroelastosis

Endocardial fibroelastosis (EFE) is characterized by diffuse thickening of the endocardium due to the proliferation of fibroelastic tissue. This may lead to dilated and restricted phenotypes.[62]

Hypereosinophilic Syndrome

It was previously referred to as Loeffler's endocarditis. In hypereosinophilic syndrome (HES), the release of active mediators from eosinophils leads to damage to the endomyocardium, resulting in eosinophilic myocarditis. CMR is a reliable modality for visualizing and evaluating all three stages of cardiac involvement in HES. CMR can demonstrate characteristic findings such as intracardiac thrombi and endocardial fibrosis.[63] While CMR provides valuable diagnostic information, endomyocardial biopsy is considered the gold standard for confirming the diagnosis, particularly in cases where the diagnosis is uncertain.

Anderson–Fabry Disease

Anderson–Fabry disease (AFD) is a rare metabolic disorder caused by a deficiency of the enzyme alpha-galactosidase A. Cardiac involvement in AFD can result in several manifestations, including LVH, myocardial inflammation, and myocardial fibrosis. RV involvement can also occur, although it is not sex-specific, unlike LVH. The presence of LVH and RV hypertrophy (RVH) can contribute to the development of various cardiac symptoms, including arrhythmias, angina, and heart failure.[64] CMR can provide valuable information regarding the extent and severity of cardiac involvement, aiding in risk stratification and treatment planning.[65,66]

Radiation-induced Heart Disease

Radiation-induced heart disease (RIHD) has become a significant concern as the use of radiotherapy has increased and cancer patients are experiencing improved survival rates. The latent period for RIHD is typically 10–15 years, during which time various manifestations can arise.[67-69] These include accelerated CAD, aortopathy (abnormalities of the aorta), constrictive pericarditis, RCM, and valvular dysfunction. By utilizing CMR, clinicians can noninvasively evaluate the impact of radiation on the heart, assess the presence and extent of fibrosis, and monitor disease progression over time. This information is crucial for risk stratification, treatment planning, and ongoing surveillance of cancer patients who have undergone radiotherapy.[70]

Myocarditis

Myocarditis is characterized by inflammation of the myocardium and can have various etiological factors including toxins, ischemia, drugs, transplant rejection, and immune reactions. Patients with myocarditis typically present with symptoms such as chest pain, dyspnea, fatigue, and arrhythmias. Electrocardiogram (ECG) findings may resemble those of acute myocardial infarction, with ST segment changes.[71-73] The diagnosis of myocarditis has been refined with the updated Lake Louise criteria, which incorporates CMR imaging findings. According to these criteria, myocarditis is diagnosed if there is at least one T2-based criterion (regional or global increase in signal intensity on T2-weighted images or an increase in T2 relaxation time) and at least one T1-based criterion (increased myocardial T1 relaxation time, ECV, or LGE).

Cardiac magnetic resonance allows for the assessment of myocardial edema, which is a common finding in myocarditis. Hyperemia, another characteristic feature of myocarditis, can be targeted with gadolinium administration. Its presence increases the accuracy of CMR for diagnosing myocarditis and is one of the Lake Louise criteria. Necrosis or scarring is frequently observed in myocarditis, indicating irreversible myocardial injury. On LGE imaging, necrosis appears as bright signal intensity areas, suggesting acute necrosis or chronic scarring.[74-77] The presence of necrosis or scarring is associated with high cardiovascular and overall mortality. T2 mapping is more accurate in identifying myocardial edema compared to traditional T2-weighted imaging. T1 relaxation time is sensitive in detecting intra- and extracellular changes in free water content but cannot differentiate between acute and chronic processes. It is considered a marker of disease presence rather than disease activity. ECV mapping can detect the expansion of the extracellular space and is more sensitive in detecting diffuse and milder edema or fibrosis.[78-82]

Takotsubo Cardiomyopathy

Takotsubo cardiomyopathy (TC), also known as stress cardiomyopathy, broken heart syndrome, or transient apical ballooning syndrome, is characterized by acute temporary stunning of the apical myocardium in the absence of CAD. The exact underlying mechanisms of TC are not fully understood, but various hypotheses have been proposed. These include abnormal coronary microvascular reactivity, catecholamine surges, abnormalities of the central or peripheral nervous system, estrogen deficiency, and other endocrine factors.[83] CMR plays a valuable role in the diagnosis and assessment of TC. It allows for the accurate quantification of cardiac function, evaluation of regional wall motion abnormalities, and the exclusion of other cardiac pathologies such as CAD. The absence of edema and LGE on CMR images is a characteristic feature of TC.[84]

CONCLUSION

Cardiac magnetic resonance is an excellent modality for evaluating the morphological and functional features of nonischemic cardiomyopathies. It allows reliable and precise assessment of various aspects of the disease and helps in differentiating them. The ability of CMR to accurately measure the size, wall thickness, and function forms the basis of clinical diagnosis. The latest methodologies like parametric mapping are robust techniques for tissue characterization and have shown growing body of evidence regarding the clinical utility of this maturing field. Therefore, CMR should routinely be integrated in the diagnostic workup of various cardiomyopathies.

ONLINE REFERENCES

Please scan the QR code provided at the end of the table of contents for References of this chapter.

CHAPTER 112

Myocardial Perfusion Imaging with Cardiac Positron Emission Tomography and Single-photon Emission Computed Tomography

GN Mahapatra

ABSTRACT

Coronary artery disease (CAD) remains the leading cause of mortality and morbidity across the world. Invasive coronary angiography is currently the gold standard for diagnosis and treatment of CAD. However, it is an invasive procedure associated with risk and complications. Moreover, it is reported that around 30–40% of all diagnostic invasive coronary angiography procedures are performed usually for diagnostic purposes without any interventional procedures being applied. Thus, investigation of less invasive rather noninvasive imaging modalities is important for reducing or avoiding the use of invasive coronary angiography examination. Myocardial perfusion imaging with single-photon emission computed tomography (SPECT) is an established method and widely applied for noninvasive evaluation of coronary artery stenosis. However, the most important applications of SPECT are in the diagnosis of CAD, prediction of disease prognosis, selection of patient for revascularization, and assessment of acute coronary syndrome. Moreover, SPECT holds special value in so many patients of subgroup and the sensitivity is consistently above 80% but in the better designed studies, it is within the range of 85–95%. Positron emission tomography (PET) has contributed significantly where the diagnostic accuracy of myocardial perfusion by PET in the assessment of CAD has been reported to be superior to SPECT. PET with stress myocardial perfusion imaging is regarded as an exact imaging modality for diagnosing and managing patients with CAD. Moreover, the combined modality of PET/CT further increases the diagnostic accuracy in CAD.

Keywords: Positron emission tomography (PET), single-photon emission computed tomography (SPECT), myocardial perfusion imaging (MPI).

INTRODUCTION

Coronary artery disease (CAD) is one of the main causes of mortality worldwide which is mainly attributed to coronary artery atherosclerosis. Invasive coronary angiography is currently the gold standard for diagnosis of CAD pertaining to intraluminal coronary narrowing. Moreover, it is reported that around 40–50% of coronary angiographies are performed for diagnostic procedures in all asymptomatic and with symptomatic comorbid conditions leading to subjecting the suspected patients unnecessarily for invasive interventional procedures. Additionally, catheter-based fractional flow reserve (FFR), which is an invasive approach, has been regarded as a precise approach to evaluate the hemodynamic relevance of coronary artery stenosis though stress single-photon emission computed tomography (SPECT) myocardial perfusion scan can pinpoint this problem. Noninvasive myocardial perfusion imaging (MPI) tagged with short-lived radioisotope Tc-99m sestamibi/Tc-99m-labeled tetrofosmin or using SPECT and PET myocardial tracers such as N-13 ammonia, O-15-labeled water (O5-H2O) or generator produced PET tracers such as rubidium-82 (Rb-82) and shortly going to be introduced new F-18-labeled tracers, F-18 flurpiridaz, a game changer are being used in clinical day-to-day practice. Apart from the information of MPI, one can estimate myocardial flow reserve/coronary flow reserve (CFR) using PET tracers to detect microvascular disease, culprit coronary artery lesion in the subset of patients having balanced ischemia. SPECT MPI study is also very commonly applied to all type of detection and extent of myocardial involvement including estimation of myocardial viability following intraluminal narrowing in coronary arteries. So far as PET MPI is concerned, it is widely used MPI modality having increased sensitivity and specificity for the detection of CAD in all clinical subset of CAD patients. It offers better diagnostic performance, improved resolution of images, and inherent attenuation correction (AC). Furthermore compared with SPECT protocol, PET imaging provides lower radiation exposure to patients due to the physical property of radiotracers including Rb-82, N-13 ammonia, and O-15 H_2O.

Although a normal or mildly abnormal SPECT MPI does not exclude the presence of subclinical nonobstructive CAD (rendering the patient prone to more aggressive cardiovascular risk modifications), it is associated with an annual major adverse cardiac event rate of about 1%. This risk varies from a low of 0.3% for women to a high of nearly 2% for patients undergoing pharmacologic stress imaging. MPI is cost-effective as a gatekeeper to invasive coronary angiography in patients with stable chest pain. It has also been shown that patients with less reversible ischemia on SPECT MPI have a survival advantage with medical therapy rather than revascularization, while those with more severe ischemia are more likely to benefit from invasive procedure. In addition, in patients with apparently "false-positive results in MPI," endothelial dysfunction can often be demonstrated which is linked to adverse cardiovascular outcomes regardless of invasive coronary angiography in cardiac risk associated with abnormal findings. SPECT MPI in patients with normal invasive coronary angiography further emphasizes the prognostic power of the technique.[1-4]

CLINICAL APPLICATION OF SPECT MYOCARDIAL PERFUSION IMAGING

The following are the important clinical subset of patients having suspected or proved CAD with or without history of heart attack in the past to diagnose and advocate further treatment planning including future risk stratification.

- *Suspected patients having strong family history of having one/two risk factors (hypertension, diabetes, smoking, etc.)*: In this particular subset of patients, if thallium/Tc-99m-labeled sestamibi stress test shows normal stress perfusion pattern with normal washout/reperfusion with Tc-99m sestamibi perfusion pattern in the 4 hours rest image with reinjection of Tc-99m sestamibi (thallium has got a property to redistribute into the myocardium as compared to Tc-99m sestamibi). If there is normal stress perfusion pattern in all the defined myocardial segments indicates that the suspected patient does not have any evidence of CAD which would save him or her to go for further invasive test such as coronary angiography and the nuclear imaging is cost-effective as the thallium/Tc-99m sestamibi stress test is approximately one-third that of the cost of angiography.
- *Known case of CAD to evaluate ischemia/infarction stratifying impending ischemia for future coronary events*: Patient having a known history of previous myocardial infarction (MI) or recovering from acute MI from the hospital, stress thallium/stress sestamibi-gated myocardial scintigraphy delineates the area of ischemia/infarcted myocardium by revealing a stress perfusion defect in the part of the myocardium with evidence of redistribution (filling of the perfusion defect) in 4 hours or reperfusion pattern with resting reinjection of Tc-99m sestamibi image indicates viable myocardium, where revascularization procedure would convert completely the affected myocardium to its normal status/pattern. In an another group of patients, fixed perfusion defect at stress and rest and even with the resting reinjection of thallium-201(Tl-201)/Tc-99m sestamibi is likely to have scarred myocardium (dead) where further angiography/revascularization procedure would not help the patient as the dead myocardium cannot be recovered even if the circulation is reestablished by angioplasty/coronary artery bypass graft (CABG) procedure. Tl-201 has got a unique property of not only evaluating the extent and viability of the affected segments resulting from MI, it can also detect the other impending ischemic zones in the myocardium for future coronary events (future myocardial infarct) which warn the patient for the future and also give a clear-cut guideline to the cardiologist to advocate his/her treatment planning **(Figs. 1A and B)**.
- *To assess borderline lesions in coronary angiography*: Most of the coronary artery lesions are eccentric, unless and until it is viewed in multiple projections during angiography, one cannot assess the lesions correctly **(Figs. 2A and B)**. In true sense, these lesions are originally borderline where cardiologists very commonly underestimate or overestimate the same lesions. The borderline lesions are 40% or 50% or 60% on coronary angiography, which needs the stress thallium myocardial scintigraphy to assess to have whether hemodynamic significant perfusion defect exists on the myocardial segments. In our experience, we always routinely give this information whether the coronary intervention is necessary for these borderline lesions or by seeing a significant perfusion defect/normal on stress thallium test. This is considered to be an important subset of patients which cardiologists are aware of.
- *To assess myocardial blood flow (MBF) in significant multi- or single-vessel lesion on coronary angiography*: This is an important subset of patients where coronary angiography and stress thallium test do not match and it is called "mismatch pattern" **(Figs. 3A and B)**. In our experience of more than a decade on stress thallium studies, we have found normal stress thallium pattern in the myocardium, where multiple significant lesions are there in coronary angiography. This situation is due to the establishment of sufficient collaterals, which has been opened up as a result of significant lesion in coronary artery. The establishment of these collaterals is resulted due to the change in the lifestyle of the patient pertaining to the regular exercise including yoga or pranayama, diet restriction, and control of risk factors (diabetes, hypertension, etc.).

- *Equivocal or false positive treadmill stress test results*: Suspected patients having false positive ST-T depression <3 mm or borderline ST-T changes or patients having left bundle branch block (LBBB) or female patients not able to perform the treadmill quite effectively, all these types of patients can be subjected for a stress thallium test which clearly delineates, whether a stress perfusion defect is existing in any part of the myocardium or not. Depending on the stress thallium findings, patient should be subjected for further invasive test or else, the normal stress thallium/stress sestamibi test does not indicate need for any further test such as angiography, etc. **(Figs. 4A and B)**.
- *Normal treadmill stress test with no significant ST-T depression*: Suspected patients having no significant ST-T depression in any of the chest leads are subjected for a stress sestamibi myocardial perfusion scan showing a clear-cut area of stress-induced perfusion defect involving anteroseptal segment with evidence of significant reversible ischemia **(Figs. 4C and D)**.
- *Follow-up of patients of CABG/balloon angioplasty/ thrombolytic therapy*: Cardiac patients who have undergone triple/four-vessel bypass graft surgery or following post-balloon angioplasty procedure complaints of shortness of breath, heaviness in the chest, and transient short angina pain may be subjected to a stress thallium test to find out any significant perfusion defect at stress with evidence of reversible ischemia that would definitely warrant redo CABG/redo angioplasty procedure as the

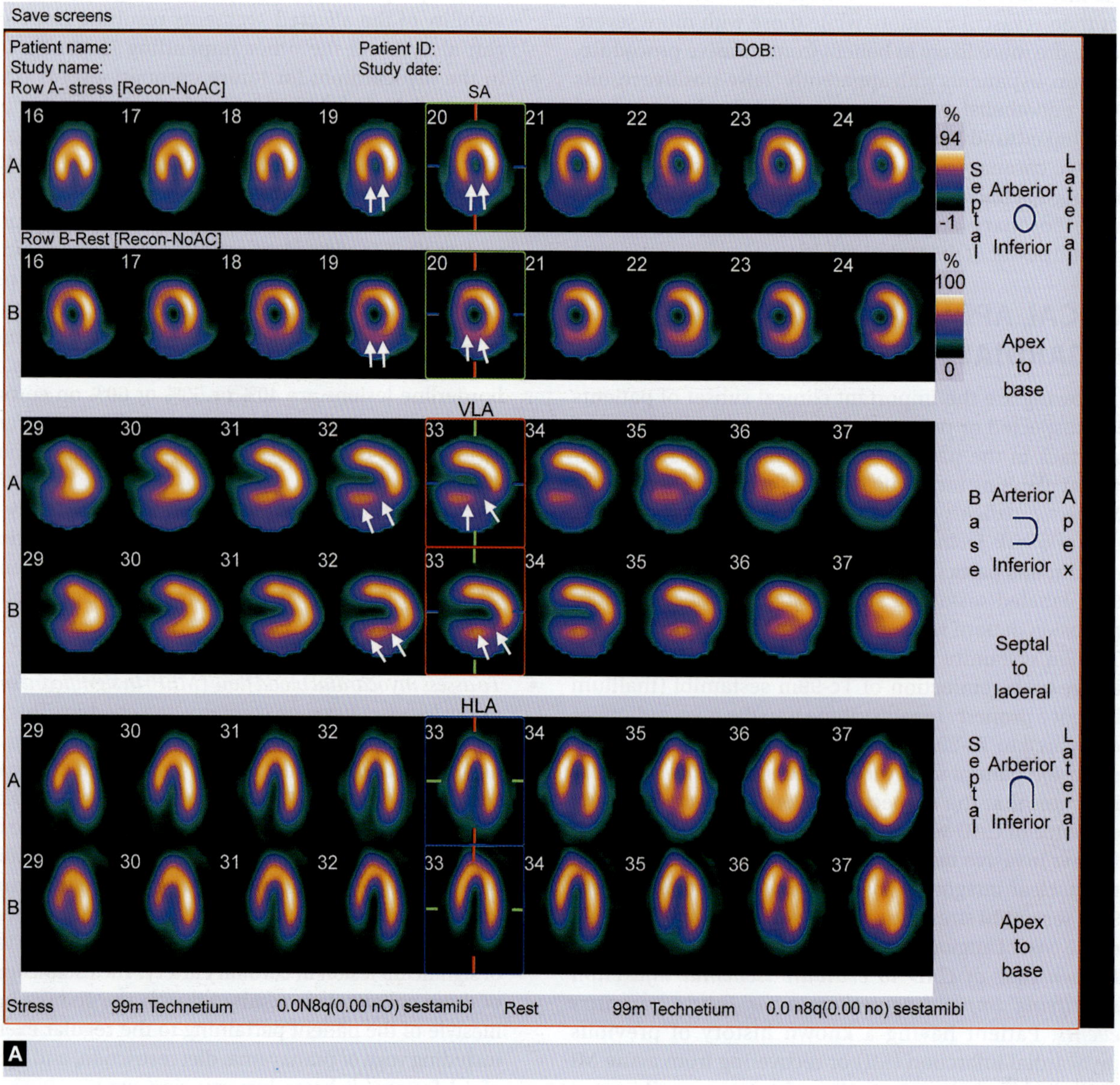

A

FIGS. 1A AND B: *Continued*

Continued

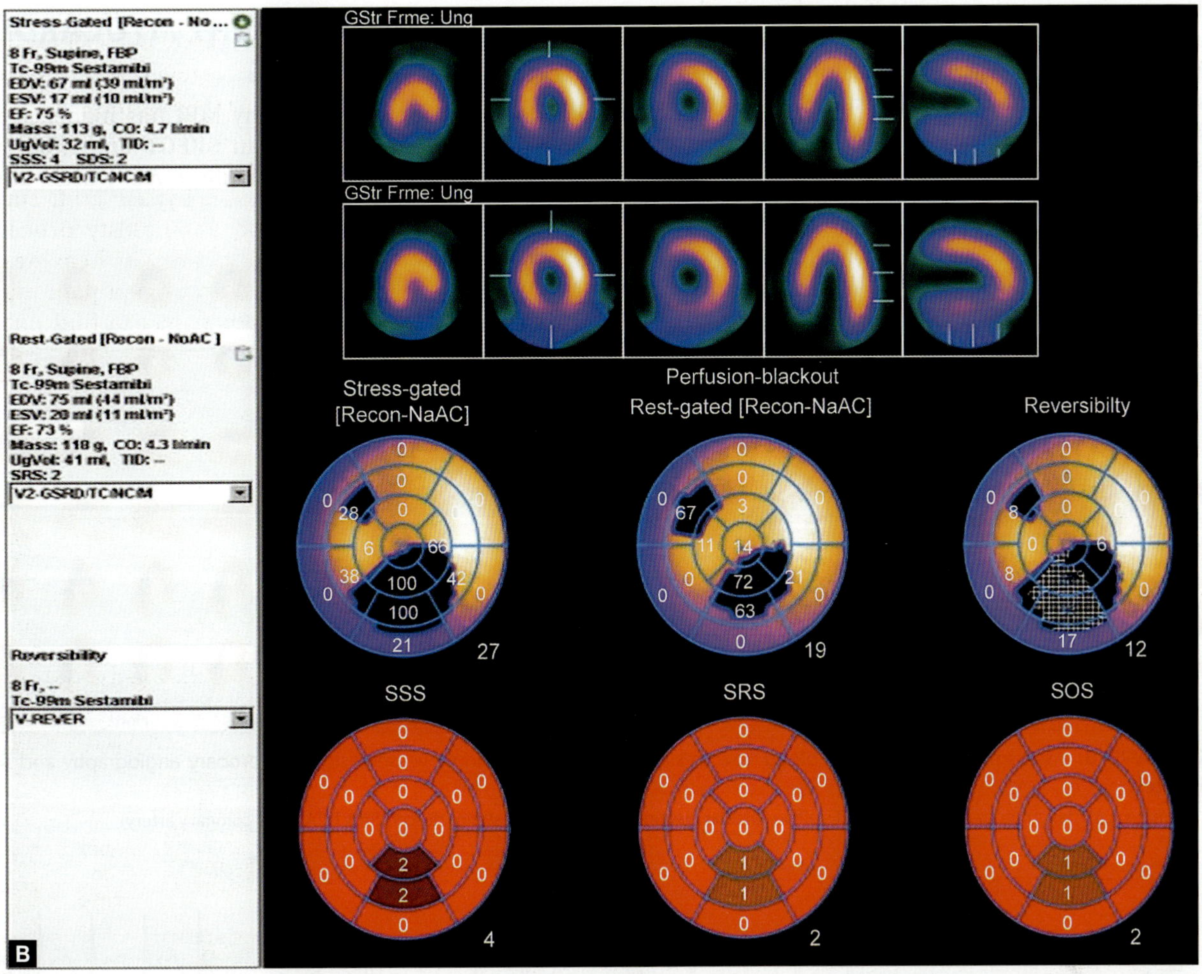

FIGS. 1A AND B: (A) Showing a definite area of stress perfusion defect involving inferior segment of the myocardium with reversible ischemia. (B) Image quantitation showing stress-gated blackout as well as summed stress score having 4 has reduced to as well as resting gated blackout image size of the quantitation suggestive of reversible ischemia in inferior segment.

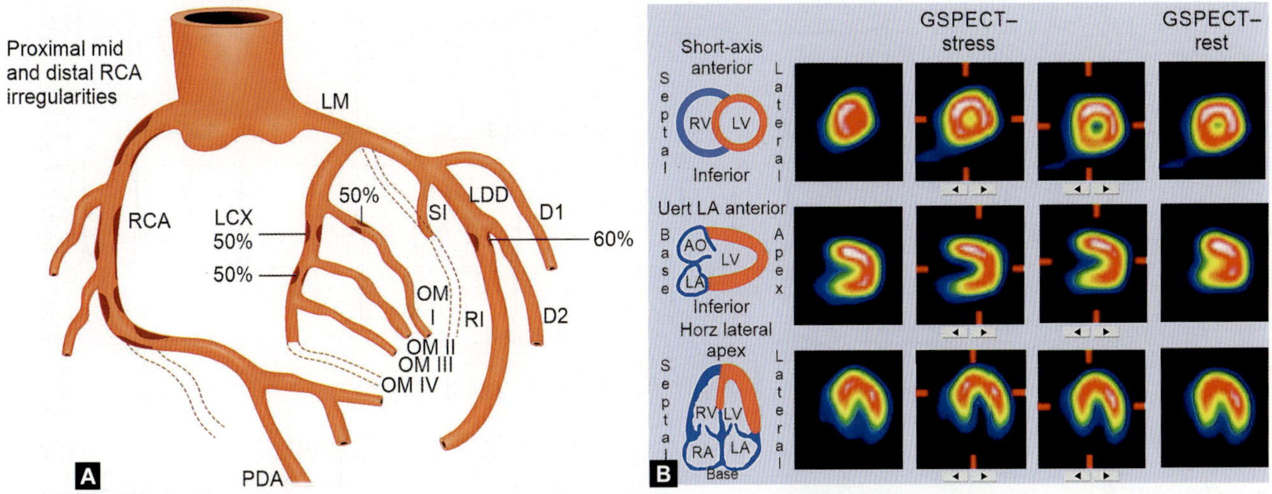

FIGS. 2A AND B: Assessment of borderline lesions in coronary angiography, multiple projections.

(GSPECT: gated single-photon emission computed tomography; LCX: left circumflex; LM: left main; PDA: posterior descending artery; RCA: right coronary artery) restenosis of the arterial/venous graft has occurred. These types of patients even if they have undergone a routine treadmill stress test, literature review says if all the grafts are closed, stress test does not show any significant positive changes. Certainly stress thallium myocardial perfusion scan has an upper hand in this subset of patients.

CLINICAL APPLICATIONS OF POSITRON EMISSION TOMOGRAPHY MYOCARDIAL PERFUSION IMAGING

Positron emission tomography MPI has higher spatial and temporal resolution than SPECT and inherently uses accurate depth independent AC which allows

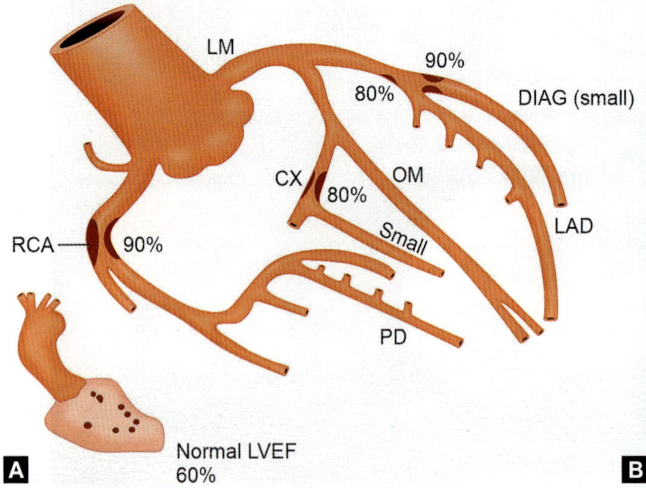

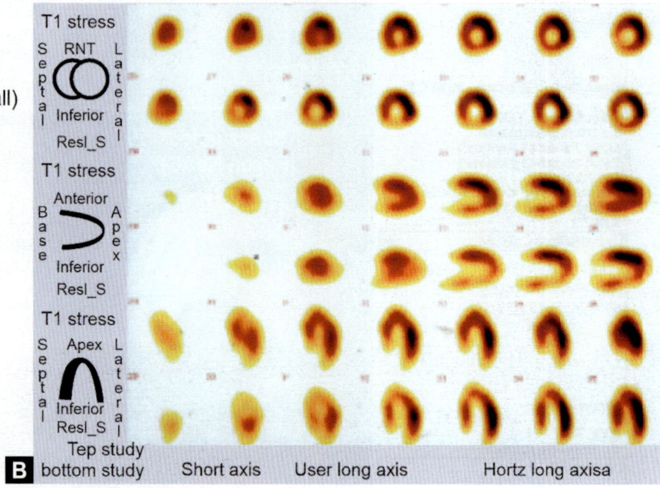

FIGS. 3A AND B: Assessment of myocardial blood flow in significant multi- or single-vessel lesion on coronary angiography and stress thallium test.

(CX: circumflex; LAD: left anterior descending; LVEF: left ventricular ejection fraction; PD: posterior descending; RCA: right coronary artery)

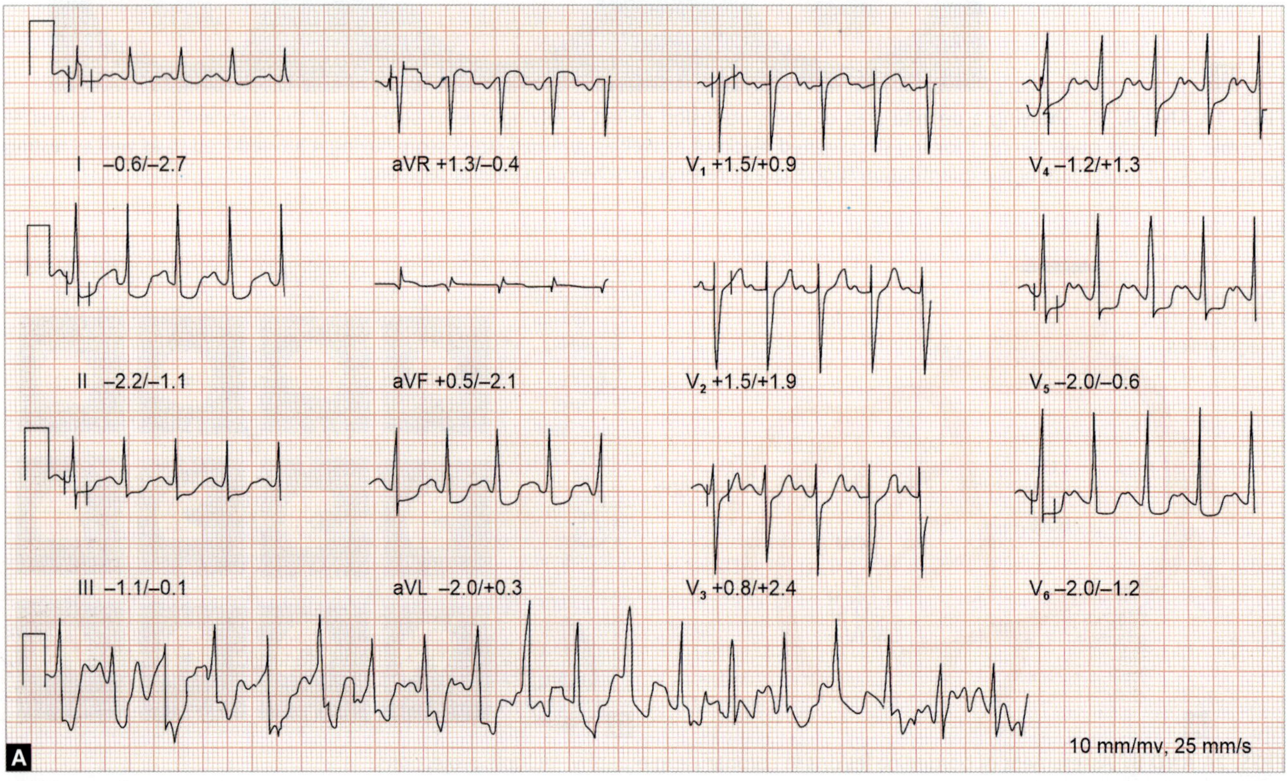

FIGS. 4A AND B: *Continued*

Continued

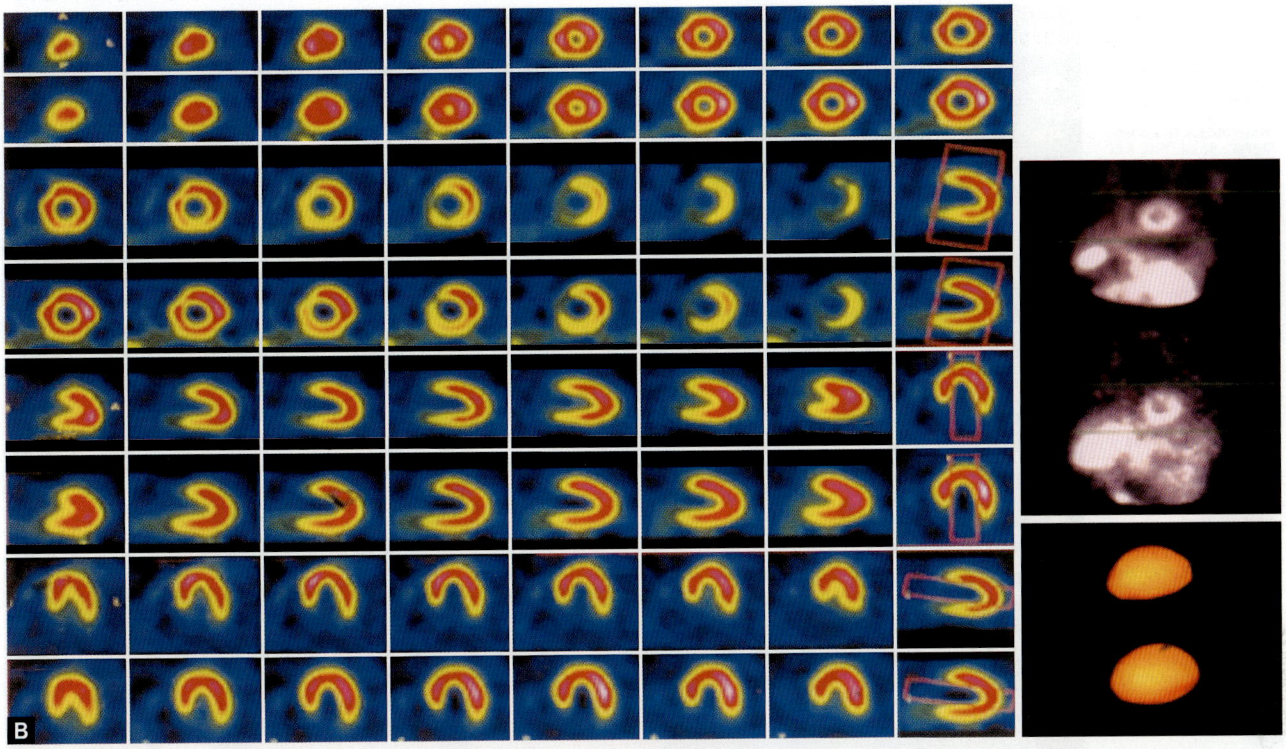

FIGS. 4A AND B: (A) Treadmill stress test showing significant ST-T depression in all chest leads. (B) Stress sestamibi myocardial perfusion scan showing uniform stress perfusion pattern in all the defined myocardial segments.

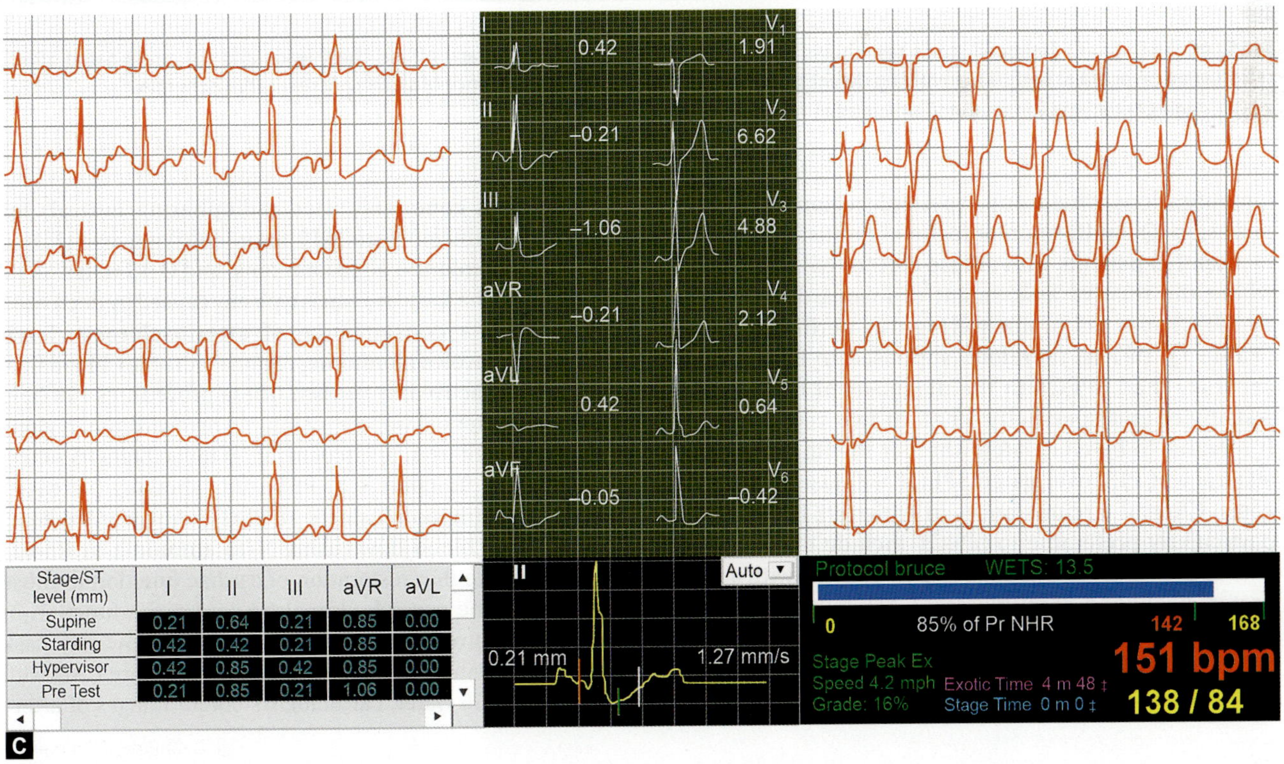

FIGS. 4C AND D: *Continued*

Continued

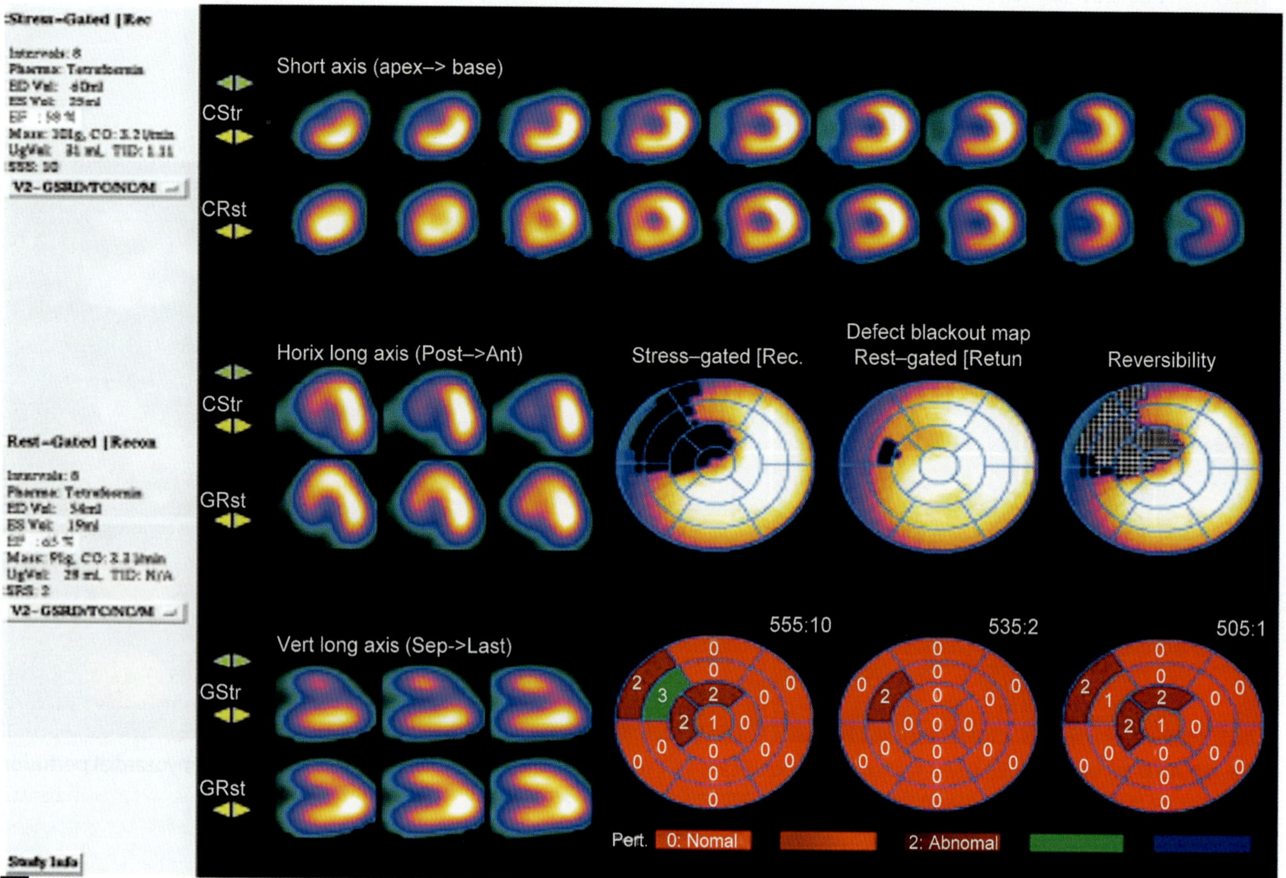

D

FIGS. 4C AND D: (C) Treadmill stress test shows no significant ST-T depression in any of the chest leads and (D) stress-gated SPECT tetrofosmin myocardial perfusion involving defect in anteroseptal segment with evidence of significant reversible ischemia.
(SPECT: single-photon emission computed tomography)

quantifications of basal and hyperemic regional myocardial perfusion. Quantification of regional perfusion appears to be useful in patients with diffuse CAD or balanced disease where the relative assessment of myocardial perfusion by SPECT may fail in uncovering true perfusion changes **(Table 1)**. PET is, therefore, supposed to have a higher accuracy than SPECT in the diagnosis of CAD showing sensitivity and specificity >90% in two recent reviews. It remains to be elucidated whether the improvement of accuracy of PET over gated SPECT will justify the higher costs. Clinical circumstances in which PET MPI may be particularly preferable to SPECT include obese patients with high soft tissue attenuation and patients with a higher pretest likelihood of multivessel CAD. Furthermore, MPI may be more difficult to interpret in patients with heart failure or cardiomyopathy, who usually have reduced and heterogeneous perfusion.

The most commonly used radiopharmaceuticals for cardiac PET imaging are F-18 fluorodeoxyglucose (FDG), rubidium-82 chloride, N-13 ammonia, and O-15 water.

Injury to the myocardium is typically caused by decreased blood flow, a consequence of arteriosclerosis. Such evaluations involve monitoring regional coronary blood flow and ongoing active metabolism. These procedures can help to identify potential viability of injured myocardium, regions likely to benefit from revascularization to facilitate its return to its normal function, e.g., PET study showing increased glucose consumption (using F-18 FDG) in myocardial areas of decreased blood flow (using N-13 ammonia or Rb-82) would indicate that restoration of cardiac function in those areas would be possible. Impaired contractile function in response to chronic reduction of resting blood flow may mask myocardial viability in some patients with severe CAD with the use of O-15 water; cardiologists obtain images of artery

TABLE 1: Positron emitting isotopes used in cardiac positron emission tomography (PET).

Category/Compounds	Function (mechanism)
Tracers of blood flow:	
13-N ammonia	Metabolic trapping
82 Rb	Sodium-potassium pump
15 O-water	Diffusion
62-Copper PT SM	Lipophilicity
11-C (gallium 68) albumin microsphere	Capillary blockage
18-F-flurpiridaz	Metabolic trapping
Tracers of metabolism:	
11C-palmitate	Fatty acid metabolism
18-F-FDG	Exogenous glucose metabolism
11C-acetate	Oxidative metabolism
150-oxygen	Oxygen consumption
11C (13N) amino acid synthesis	Amino acid and protein metabolism
Other tracers:	
18F-misonidazole	Hypoxic and ischemic tissue
11C-carbon monoxide	Blood pool

walls, where live tissue is designated by areas of illumination caused by high oxygen consumption.

Tracers of Myocardial Perfusion

Positron-emitting radionuclides used for assessment of regional perfusion can be classified into two groups:

1. Tracers that are only partly extracted by the myocardium (Rb-82 chloride and N-13 ammonia)
2. Tracers that are freely diffusible (O-15 water)

Rubidium-82 PET Myocardial Perfusion Study

Myocardial perfusion imaging with positron emitter can be done without onsite cyclotron which is relatively complicated with an onsite source of generator produced tracer, i.e., rubidium-82.

Rubidium-82 is a monovalent cation and has an ultra-short half-life of 75 seconds. Sr-82 decays to an elution column. Rb-82 is eluted with 25–50 mL of normal saline by a computer-controlled elution pump, connected by intravenous (IV) tubing to the patient. This generator has almost no breakthrough of strontium and has useful life of 4–6 weeks. Serial evaluations of regional myocardial perfusion can be made at intervals as short as 5 minutes. The short half-life of Rb-82 taxes the performance limits of PET scanners; it facilitates the rapid completion of a series of resting and stress myocardial perfusion studies. Rb-82 is a very efficient imaging agent for routine clinical usage. Although the cost per patient at a low volume of studies per day is high, the cost with 6–10 studies per day is competitive with SPECT tracers.

The first-pass extraction of Rb-82 at rest is approximately 50–60% and it is via Na^+/K^+-ATPase pump. Myocardial extraction of Rb-82 is similar to thallium-201 and slightly less than N-13 ammonia, decreasing during hyperemia. Rb-82 extractions can be altered by severe acidotic hypoxia and ischemia. Thus, uptake of Rb-82 is a function of both blood flow and of myocardial cell integrity. Rb-82 perfusion imaging is usually performed before and after vasodilator stress rather than with exercise. Infarcted myocardium does not retain intravenously administered Rb-82. After administration, it washes out rapidly from damaged myocardial cells following the initial uptake phase. A mixture of reversible and irreversible myocardial tissue in the field of view results in an intermediate level of Rb-82 wash out that is proportional to the percentage of viable or infarcted tissue.

Imaging of Rb-82

Patient preparation for stress and rest myocardial PET perfusion imaging is identical to SPECT perfusion imaging. Despite the short half-life of Rb-82, modern PET gamma cameras are able to obtain good quality images. The usual protocol takes approximately 15 minutes with a bismuth germinate ($Bi_4Ge_3O_{12}$) or BGO crystal PET scanner and 35 minutes with lutetium oxyorthosilicate (Lu_2SiO_5) or LSO crystals PET scanner. The proper positioning is done with a low dose (20 mCi) injection of Rb-82 and short 3 minutes scout acquisition and quick reconstruction. Subsequently, rest transmission imaging, rest perfusion two-dimensional (2D) imaging, and rest gated three-dimensional (3D) imaging were done sequentially. Stress imaging is also done in similar manner. Transmission imaging is usually done with a germanium-68 pin or rod source, which takes about 8 minutes.[6]

Tomographic data from Rb-82 images can be displayed using polar maps utilizing the bulls eye approach with the apex located at the center and the base at the rim. Both relative and absolute flow reserve can be depicted on quantitative polar maps on Rb-82 activity. In this manner, the rest and stress images are functionally interrelated. 3D topographic displays of Rb-82 cardiac activity are more quantitative with respect to the polar maps. An automated quantitative analysis programed may enhance accuracy and reproducibility of cardiac PET flow studies.[7]

The sensitivity and specificity of PET MPI are superior to other noninvasive tests. Four studies involving a total of 342 patients have made direct comparisons of Tl-201 SPECT and PET MPI. In addition, a survey of numerous studies of PET MPI in 1,391 patients found excellent sensitivity [92%; confidence interval (CI) 90–94%] and specificity (90%; CI 88–92%). Though all patients with intermediate risk of CAD can undergo PET MPI, it is preferable to SPECT MPI in a subgroup of patients with attenuation problems, i.e., large patients, women, breast implants or left mastectomy, chest wall deformity, and left pleural or pericardial effusion.[5] However, it must be emphasized that attenuation problems in SPECT cannot be predicted with confidence from examination of body habitus. There is an incremental benefit caused by greater specificity and sensitivity which gives rise to incremental economic benefit caused by more accurate tests such as Rb-82 PET MPI **(Figs. 5A and B)**.

During the last 10–15 years, both SPECT and PET imaging have undergone significant improvements. A recent comparison between Tc-99m sestamibi SPECT and Rb-82 PET MPI revealed a significant margin of improvement for CAD detection accuracy with Rb-82 PET compared to SPECT. Given the proven value of PET MPI in the diagnosis of CAD, it is expected that the prognostic value of gated PET is also high, similar to SPECT imaging.

Positron emission tomography-computed tomography unit has become the preferred approach for PET imaging in oncology. The potential benefit of PET-CT in cardiac imaging is reduction in acquisition time by 10–12 minutes in comparison to a dedicated PET system. PET-CT imaging holds challenges and solution for the AC problem.

N-13 Ammonia/O-15-labeled Water PET Myocardial Perfusion Imaging

N-13 ammonia has been used for most of the scientific investigation in cardiac PET imaging for the past two decades. Its 10 minutes half-life requires an onsite cyclotron and radiochemistry synthesis capability. Imaging protocol from scout position to stress imaging takes 100–120 minutes. Pharmacologic stress imaging usually follows resting injection and imaging, after the initial activity has been allowed to decay by staggering patients or using differential dose for rest and stress. Both rest and stress images can be gated. A dynamic acquisition is acquired for the quantification of blood flow. This can be accomplished by performing separate dynamic and gated acquisition with the same injection, or included list mode acquisitions. A third injection may be included for cold pressor testing. 13-N ammonia imaging is time cumbersome, needs logistic and coordination.[8]

N-13 ammonia allows good-quality gated and ungated images, taking full advantage of the superior resolution of PET imaging **(Fig. 6A)**. Interestingly, normal volunteers show mild heterogeneity or mild defect of N-13 ammonia retention in the lateral wall of the left ventricle compared with other segments **(Fig. 6B)**. The mechanism of this is not known. This must be taken into account for both visual activity and increased lung activity in patient with lung congestion.[9]

Stress F-18-FDG PET Myocardial Ischemia Imaging

Direct myocardial ischemia imaging using FDG radionuclide MPI during exercise or pharmacological stress and at rest is the most widely used noninvasive test for evaluation of known or suspected CAD. This technique relies on the demonstration of perfusion abnormalities on stress images which normalize on rest images in the presence of myocardial ischemia, but persist in the presence of scar due to prior MI.

Myocardial ischemia results in a dramatic and sustained switch to glucose uptake. At myocellular level, hypoxia results in an upregulation and translocation of glucose transporters from cytosol to the cell membrane. Once activated, these transporters remain upregulated for several hours. The differential uptake of glucose in ischemic and normal myocardium can help to develop "hot spot" imaging agent for myocardial ischemia. Fluorine-18

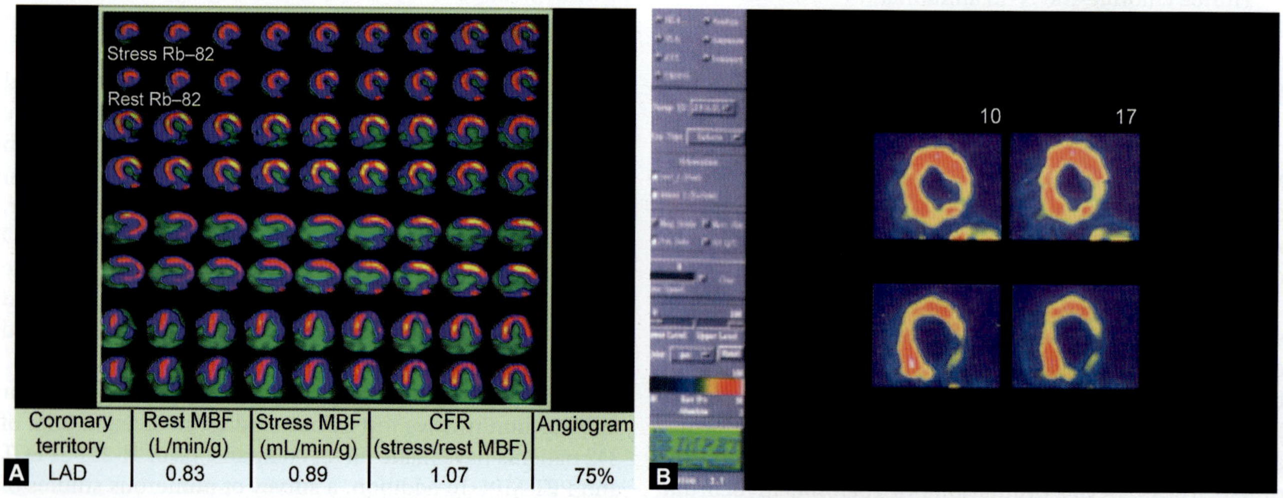

FIGS. 5A AND B: (A) Rubidium-82 positron emission tomography (PET) myocardial perfusion image showing a fixed defect involving inferolateral segments and (B) rubidium-82 PET myocardial perfusion image showing a reversible perfusion defect involving small part of anterior and inferolateral myocardial segments.

(18F)-labeled 2-deoxyglucose (18FDG) is a glucose analog, which tracks the initial steps of glucose transport and uptake across the cell membrane. Once, in the cell, this is phosporylated by hexokinase to 18FDG-6-phosphate similar to glucose. However, unlike glucose-6-phosphate cannot be phosphorylated further and because of its strong negative charge, 18FDG-6-phosphate is trapped intracellularly.

The feasibility and accuracy of exercise 18FDG imaging for hot spot imaging of exercise-induced myocardial ischemia was studied by performing simultaneous exercise perfusion and 18FDG imaging in patient scheduled to undergo exercise and rest MPI for suspected CAD. All patients underwent a symptom-limited exercise after an overnight fast. 99mTc-sestamibi (25 mCi) and 18FDG (8–10 mCi) were injected intravenously at peak exercise. The patients underwent imaging using a dual-head large field of view single—crystal SPECT imaging camera (Varicam, GE, Milwaukee, USA) equipped with ultra-high energy parallel hole collimators and 5/8" thick sodium iodide crystal to optimize the detection of high-energy (511 KeV) 18F photons. Use of separate energy window of 99m-Tc (140 KeV + 20%) and 18F (511 KeV + 30%) allowed simultaneous imaging of 99mTc-sestamibi and 18FDG. The results of exercise 18FDG imaging were compared with those of standard exercise and rest MPI and coronary angiography.

Stress F-18 FDG ischemia imaging showing intense F-18 FDG uptake in the inferior and lateral walls of the myocardium which was showing a fixed defect in the regular stress and rest MPI **(Figs. 7A and B)**.

Myocardial Metabolism

A fundamental characteristic of the myocardium is its continuous requirement for oxygen and metabolic substrates to meet its energy demands. This process largely occurs by oxidizing fatty acids and glucose. Under normal conditions, fatty acids are the preferred energy source for overall oxidative metabolism. When blood flow is reduced to the heart muscle and ischemia ensues, fatty acids can no longer be oxidized and glucose becomes the preferred energy source. This metabolic phenomenon is useful for the identification of myocardium that is underperfused but still viable. Such tissue is often hypokinetic or akinetic but returns to normal or near-normal function if blood flow is restored. Consequently, in patients with severely impaired ventricular function, combined measurements of myocardial perfusion

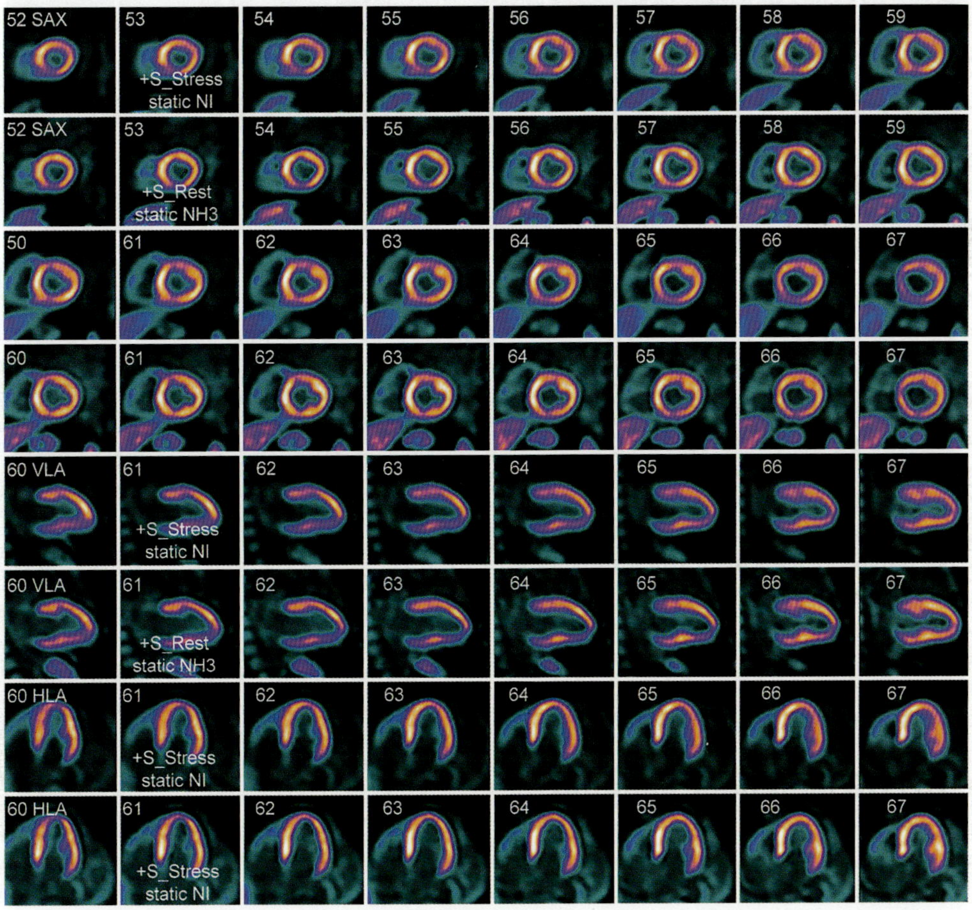

FIG. 6A: Nitrogen-13 positron emission tomography (PET) myocardial perfusion image showing uniform stress perfusion pattern involving all the defined myocardial segments such as anteroseptal, anterolateral, posterolateral, and infero-apical myocardial segments.

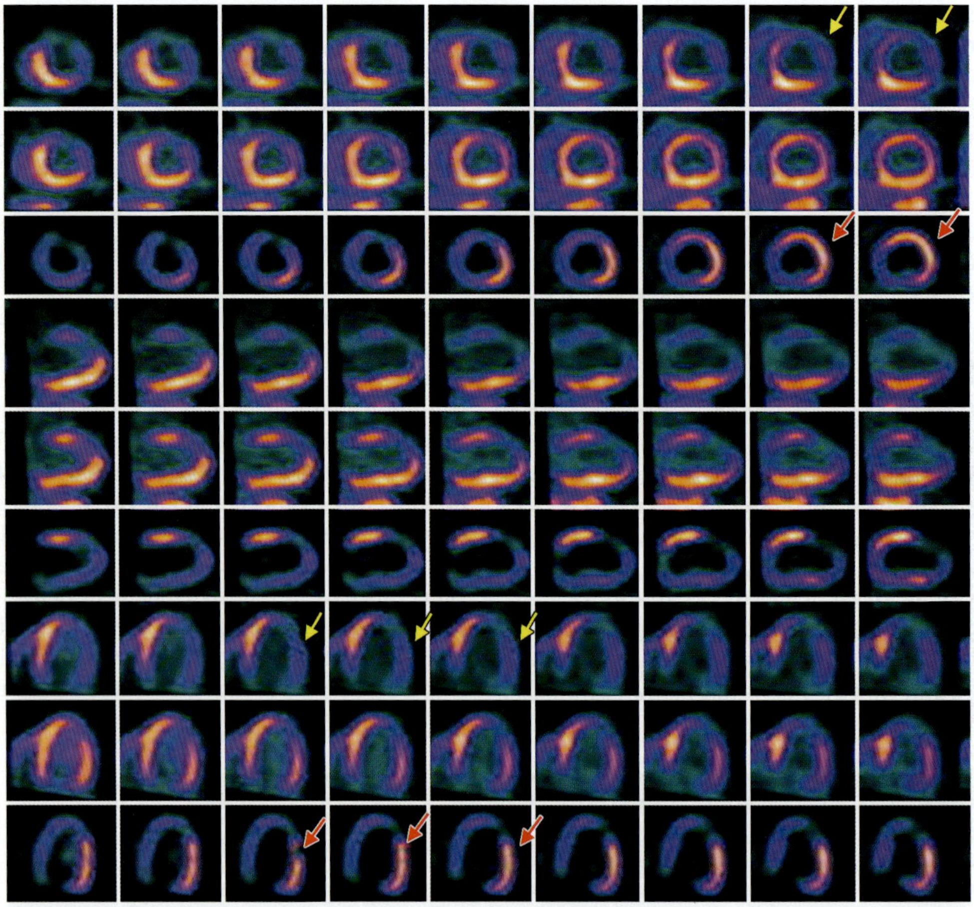

FIG. 6B: Nitrogen-13 positron emission tomography (PET) myocardial perfusion image showing a reversible stress perfusion defect involving anterolateral myocardial segments.

and glucose metabolism have been advocated. It may be noteworthy to mention that eating fat and protein shifts the heart away from using glucose as an energy source.[11]

Metabolic Tracers

Positron emission tomography radiopharmaceuticals are used for metabolic cardiac studies. "Deoxyglucose" is an analog of glucose that can be labeled with F-18, a cyclotron produced radionuclide, to form F18-FDG. Its myocardial uptake reflects overall myocardial utilization of glucose. Palmitate is a naturally occurring fatty acid that can be chemically synthesized and labeled with C-11, a cyclotron-produced radionuclide with a physical half-life of approximately 20.4 minutes. Its myocardial uptake and clearance reflect the myocardial utilization of fatty acids.[10]

Fluorine-18 FDG Metabolic Imaging

18F-FDG is a glucose analog which crosses the capillary and sarcolemmal membrane at a rate proportional to that of glucose. Following myocardial uptake, FDG is phosphorylated to FDG phosphate and is then trapped in the myocardium unlike phosphorylated glucose. Regional myocardial uptake of FDG, therefore, reflects relative distribution of regional rates of exogenous glucose utilization, unlike the brain which mainly depends upon glucose metabolism. The myocardium is an omnivore. There are three major circulating substances which affect the myocardial metabolism: (1) blood glucose, (2) free fatty acids (FFAs), and (3) insulin. Many other factors, such as the fasting period and age, also affect the FDG uptake. Even hospitalization status (in patient or outpatient) has an influence on the myocardial FDG uptake.

This complexity interferes with the interpretation of data obtained from FDG-PET imaging. To accommodate this complexity of metabolism, there are several different protocols for myocardial FDG-PET imaging. These protocols can be divided into two major categories:

1. One is imaging under low myocardial glucose metabolism which includes imaging under fasting conditions.

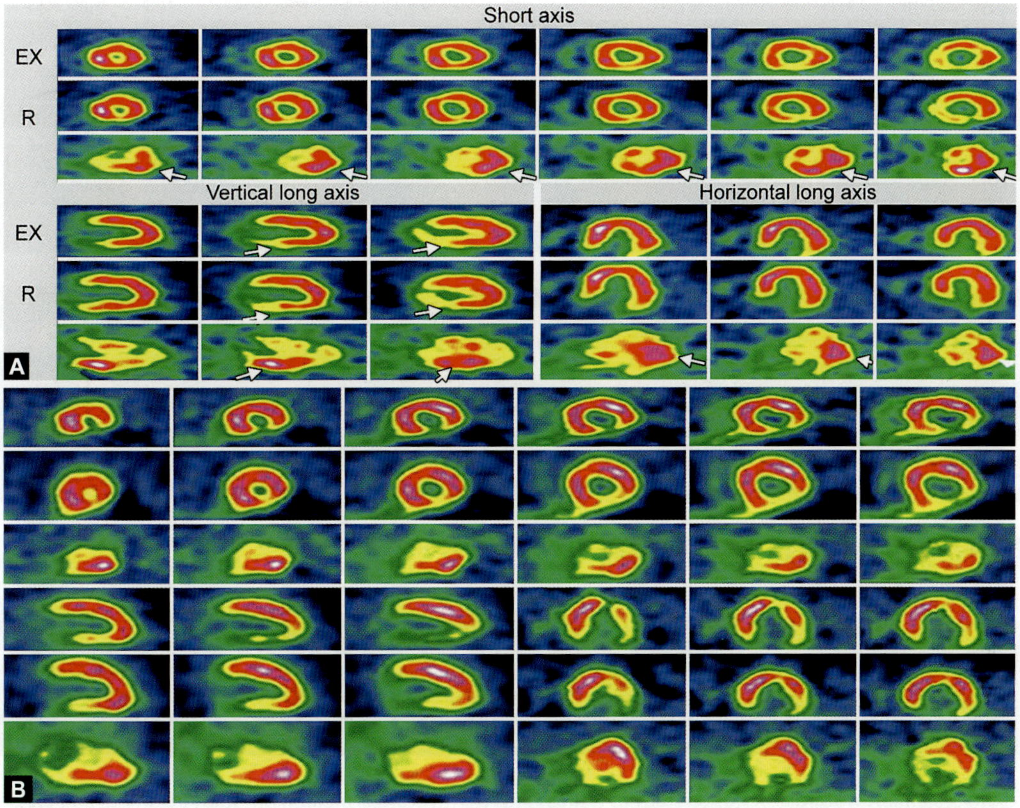

FIGS. 7A AND B: (A) Intense F-18 FDG uptake in the lateral wall of the myocardium in the stress ischemia imaging which is showing as a fixed defect in the regular stress and rest myocardial perfusion imaging and (B) intense F-18 FDG uptake in inferior and lateral walls with a small fixed defect in regular stress and rest myocardial perfusion imaging.

(FDG: fluorodeoxyglucose)

2. The other protocol images the myocardium under high to maximum myocardial glucose metabolism which includes oral glucose loading and the euglycemic insulin clamp technique.

Under fasting conditions, the normal myocardium primarily utilizes fatty acids while glucose utilization and thus FDG uptake becomes minimal. Under this condition, ischemic myocardium with enhanced glucose metabolism markedly takes up FDG, which is displayed on PET images as hot spots. The problem of imaging under fasting conditions is the heterogeneous distribution of FDG into normal myocardium. Usually, the lateral wall of the left ventricle tends to show higher FDG uptake than the septum. High background activity with low tissue FDG uptake also leads to poor image quality. For these reasons, FDG PET under fasting condition has recently not been recommended for clinical viability assessment.

The most commonly used protocols are either of oral glucose loading or overnight fasting which stimulates insulin secretion and increases the FDG uptake or no significant FDG uptake into normal myocardium. This enhances the image quality. Euglycemic insulin clamping is an alternative technique to oral glucose loading and is slightly more complex but guarantees more stable and controlled metabolic conditions. FDG uptake into normal and ischemic but viable myocardium is enhanced or increased FDG uptake as compared to no significant FDG uptake which is considered to be a match pattern indicating scar tissue. Thus, hibernating myocardium, therefore, would demonstrate increased FDG uptake in the overnight fasting state protocol unlike the surrounding normal myocardium. But in the postprandial state (with oral glucose loading), hibernating myocardium would show enhanced FDG uptake as compared to normal FDG myocardial uptake. Therefore, either preserved or even enhanced FDG uptake in dysfunctional myocardial regions represent presence of myocardial viability by the help of most popular criterion of flow-metabolism mismatch methods. However, using this criterion requires a perfusion image preferably acquired either with PET or SPECT perfusion study **(Figs. 8A and B)**.

Regional dysfunction is due to stunned myocardium and may be manifested by normal blood flow and normal, enhanced, or reduced glucose utilization using FDG and flow images. Only criterion to diagnose this myocardium is the presence of regional myocardial wall motion abnormalities.

Perfusion-metabolism mismatch using N-13 ammonia and F-18-FDG PET imaging tracer suggests decreased perfusion with adequate metabolism involving septal and apical myocardial segments **(Fig. 9A)**. Match defect involves anterior and apical segments of the myocardium **(Fig. 9B)**.

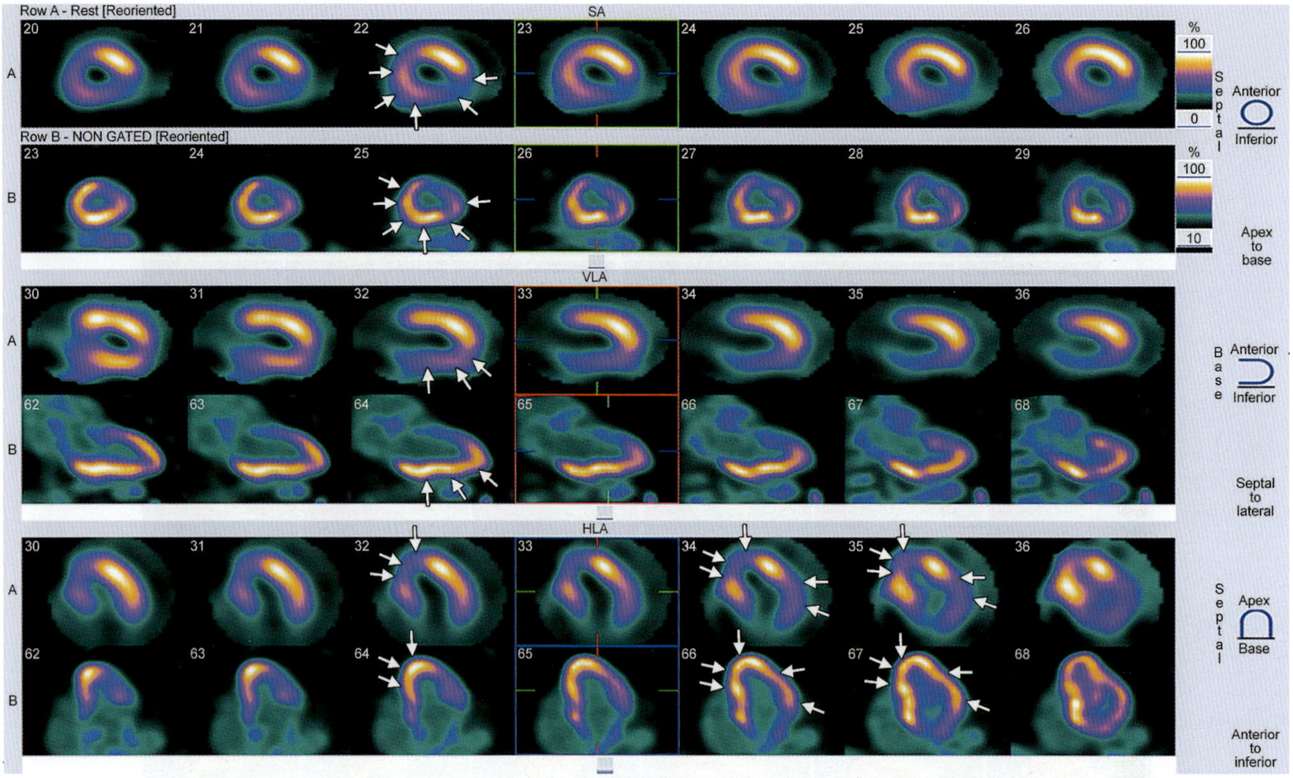

FIG. 8A: Rest Tc99m-sestamibi myocardial perfusion study as well as F-18 FDG myocardial metabolism study involving multiple perfusion defects in septal, inferior, and lateral myocardial segments with adequate metabolism suggestive of hibernating ischemic myocardium (mismatch pattern). (FDG: fluorodeoxyglucose)

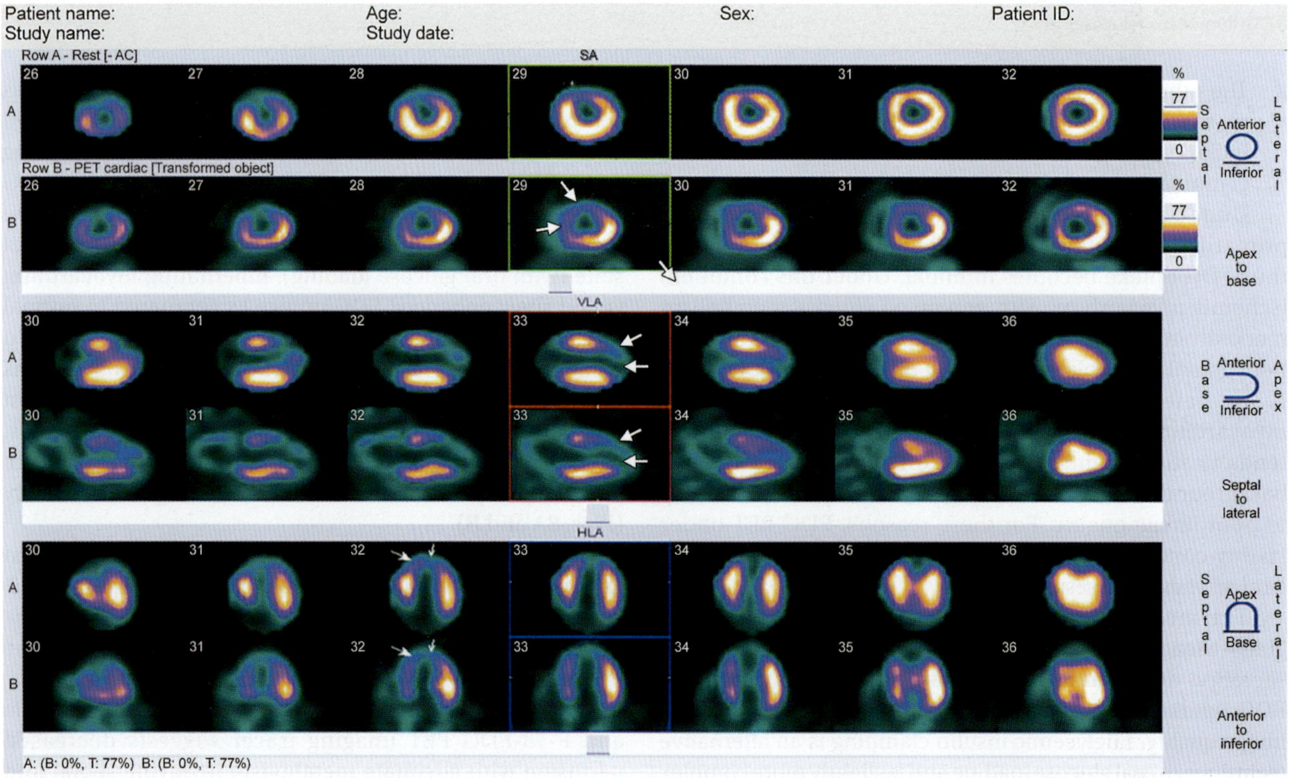

FIG. 8B: Rest Tc99m-sestamibi myocardial perfusion study as well as F-18 FDG myocardial metabolism study showing multiple perfusion defects in anterior, septal, and apical myocardial segments having no significant FDG uptake suggestive of (match pattern) dead scarred myocardium. (FDG: fluorodeoxyglucose)

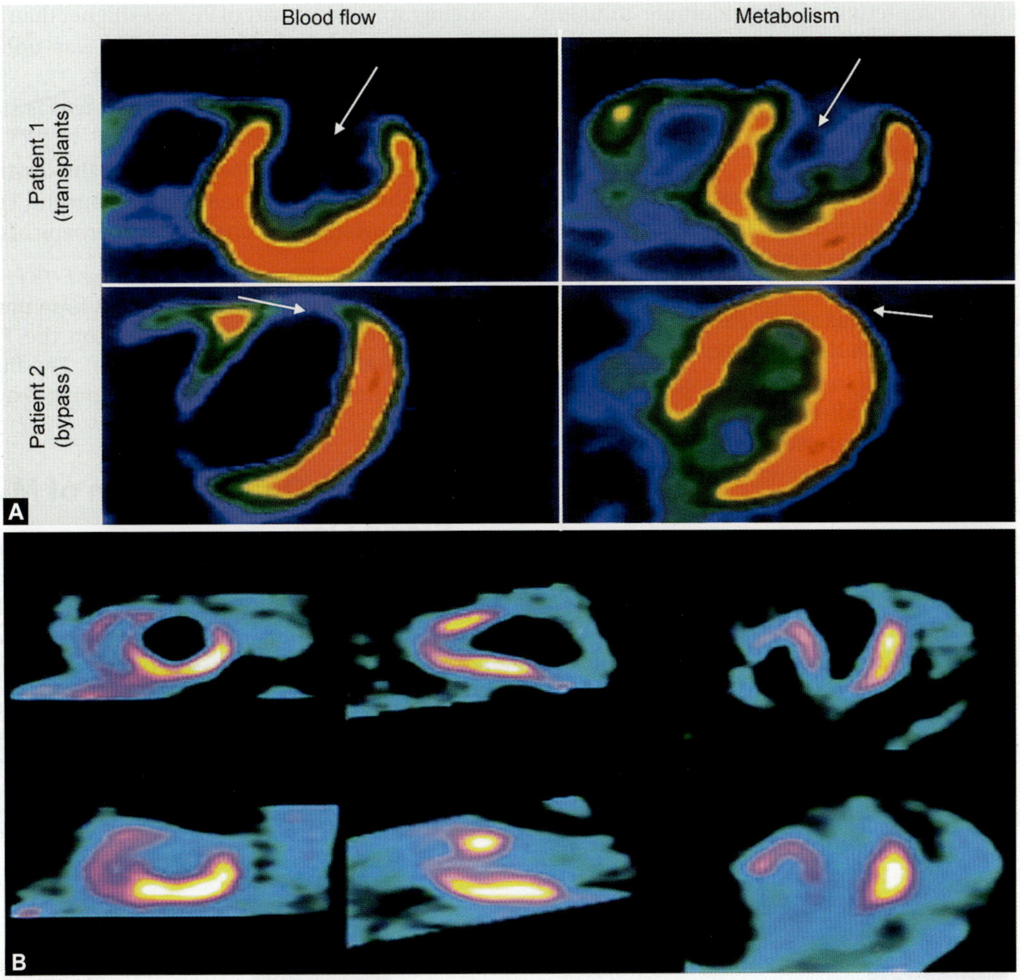

FIGS. 9A AND B: (A) Perfusion–metabolism mismatch using N-13 ammonia and F-18-FDG PET imaging tracer suggesting decreased perfusion with adequate metabolism of involving septal and apical segments of the myocardium. (B) Presence of scarred myocardium as evidenced by fixed perfusion defect involving anterior, apical, and anterolateral segments which do not show any significant F-18 FDG metabolism.

(FDG: fluorodeoxyglucose; PET: positron emission tomography)

EMERGING CONCEPTS IN CLINICAL APPLICATIONS

Quantitation of Myocardial Blood Flow

Quantitation is particularly helpful in patient suffering from severe CAD having balanced ischemia. It is also helpful in patient having subclinical CAD where diagnosis is more important particularly in subset of patient having microvascular dysfunction. It is also helpful in monitoring the response to therapy, i.e., progression or regression of CAD. Here, standard MPI may underestimate the extent of disease in three-vessel coronary atherosclerosis. PET quantification of perfusion reserve (CFR) by use of Rb-82 net retention suggests a greater extent of the disease than the standard approach in patients with three-vessel disease.

Protocol

Initially a scout scan is performed by administering a small dose of Rb-82 (10–20 mCi). Next, the AC image is acquired by using CT. List mode acquisition allows summed gated and dynamic image reconstruction is available from one injection. Most often rest scan is performed first followed by the stress scan. A single injection of Rb-82 (40–60 mCi) is injected followed by emission scanning after permitting a prescan delay. This delay is important to allow for Rb-82 myocardial extraction from the blood pool and is usually 70–90 seconds. This will give highly accurate peak stress-gated imaging reflecting wall motion, ejection fraction (EF) at peak stress. IV dipyridamole is given as a weight-based infusion over 4 minutes (0.56 mg/kg). Imaging is started as a list mode acquisition starting with the time of radiotracer injection

(3 minutes after completion of dipyridamole infusion). Usually, 40–60 mCi of Rb-82 is given into the infusion.

Stress Myocardial Perfusion Scan using F-18 Flurpiridaz

Flurpiridaz F-18 is a new PET MPI radiopharmaceutical in phase-III clinical trial for detection of CAD. It is a structural analog of pyridaben and binds to mitochondrion complex I with high affinity. Preclinical studies show that the extraction fraction of flurpiridaz F-18 was >90%. The positron range of F-18 is approximately seven times shorter than that of Rb-82, so it would be accepted to produce images with higher resolution. With a longer half-life, 18F-labeled flurpiridaz may be produced at regional cyclotron and delivered to imaging centers in much the same way as F-18-labeled FDG thus, obviating need for an onsite cyclotron. The longer half-life of F-18 also ensures that the radiotracer is present long enough to allow a patient injected at peak treadmill exercise to move to the camera and still be effectively imaged. Higher myocardial extraction facilitates detection of milder perfusion defects and allows more accurate quantification of MBF.[12-15]

A higher percentage of images where rated as excellent/good on PET versus SPECT on stress (99.2% vs. 88.5%) and rest (96.9% vs. 66.4%) images diagnostic certainty of interpretation is higher for PET versus SPECT (90.8% vs. 70.9%). In 86 patients who underwent invasive coronary angiography, sensitivity of PET was higher than SPECT (78.8% vs. 61.5% respectively). Specificity was not significantly different (PET 76.5% vs. SPECT 73.5%).

The overall quality of the PET images is superior to the Tc-99m SPECT images. Flurpiridaz F-18 PET images show severe anterior and apical defects in the distribution of the diseases of CAD in coronary artery, but the Tc-99m SPECT images showed only a small mild anteroapical defect.

The TC-99m SPECT images and flurpiridaz F-18 PET images from patients with a low likelihood of CAD: A false positive partially reversible inferior defect is present on the Tc-99m SPECT images due to soft-tissue attenuation. The flurpiridaz F-18 PET study, however, provides superior images quality and was normal.

Absolute Quantification of Myocardial Blood Flow

The preliminary results of absolute quantification of MBF with flurpiridaz F-18 PET represent a major advantage over SPECT MPI and is potential game-changer in the noninvasive evaluation of CAD. Studies with $13NH_3$, H_215O, and Rb-82 have shown that absolute quantification of MBF allows better identification of multivessel diseases, assessment of the severity of microvascular disease, allows evaluation of endothelial dysfunction, and responses to treatment and has incremental value in prognostication in patients with suspected or known CAD **(Figs. 10 to 12)**.

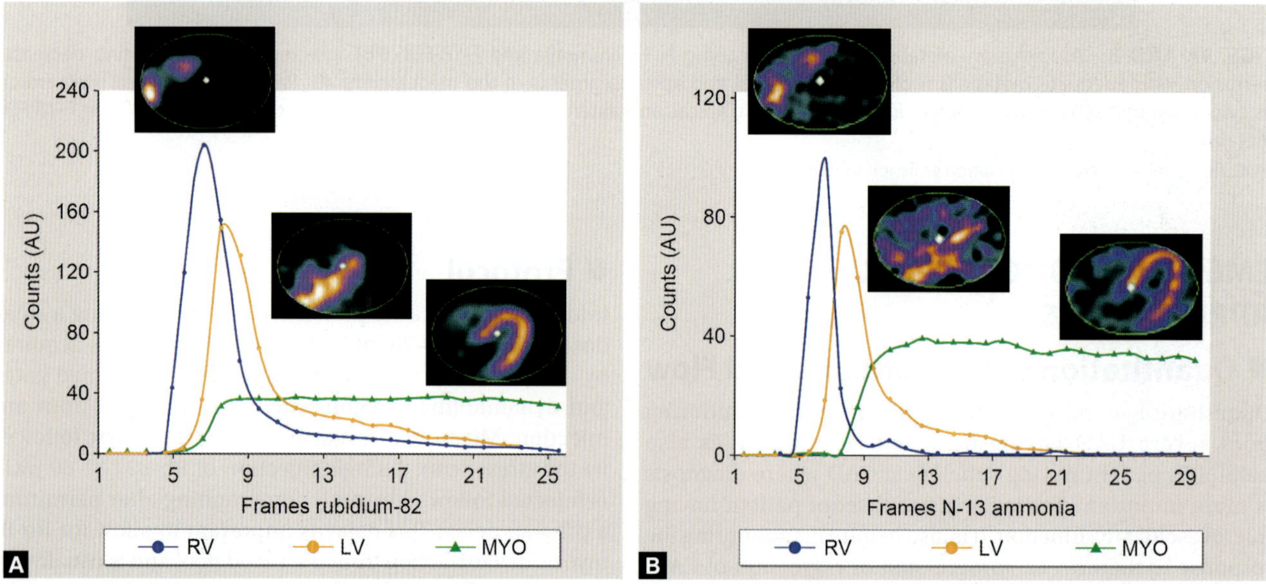

FIGS. 10A AND B: Computation of myocardial blood flow with rubidium-82 and comparison to N-13 ammonia.
(LV: left ventricle; RV: right ventricle)

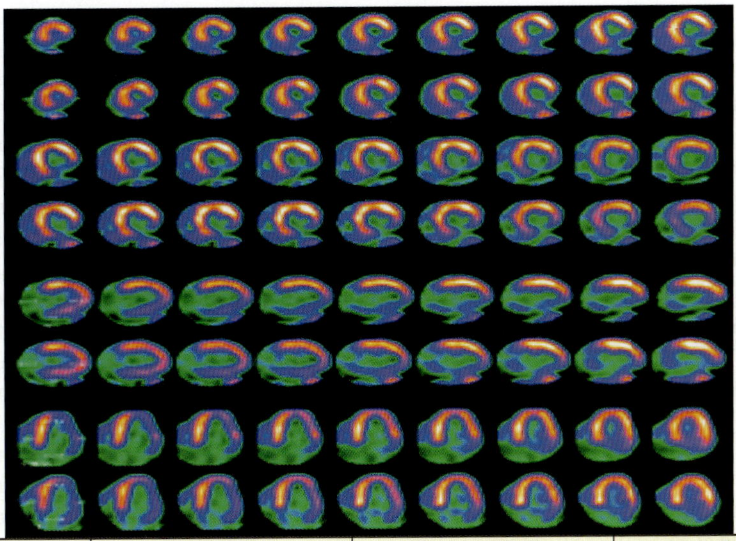

Coronary territory	Rest MBF (mL/min/g)	Stress MBF (mL/min/g)	CFR (stess/rest)
LAD	0.86	0.89	1.07
LCX	0.64	0.66	1.03
RCA	0.86	1.00	1.16

FIG. 11: Rubidium-82 stress and rest PET myocardial perfusion study showing fixed perfusion defects seen in inferior, posterolateral myocardial segments with slightly reduced perfusion pattern seen in anterior segment. CFR of stress/rest reveals reduced CFR value involving left anterior descending (LAD), left circumflex (LCX), and right coronary artery (RCA) territory.

(CFR: coronary flow reserve; MBF: myocardial blood flow; PET: positron emission tomography)

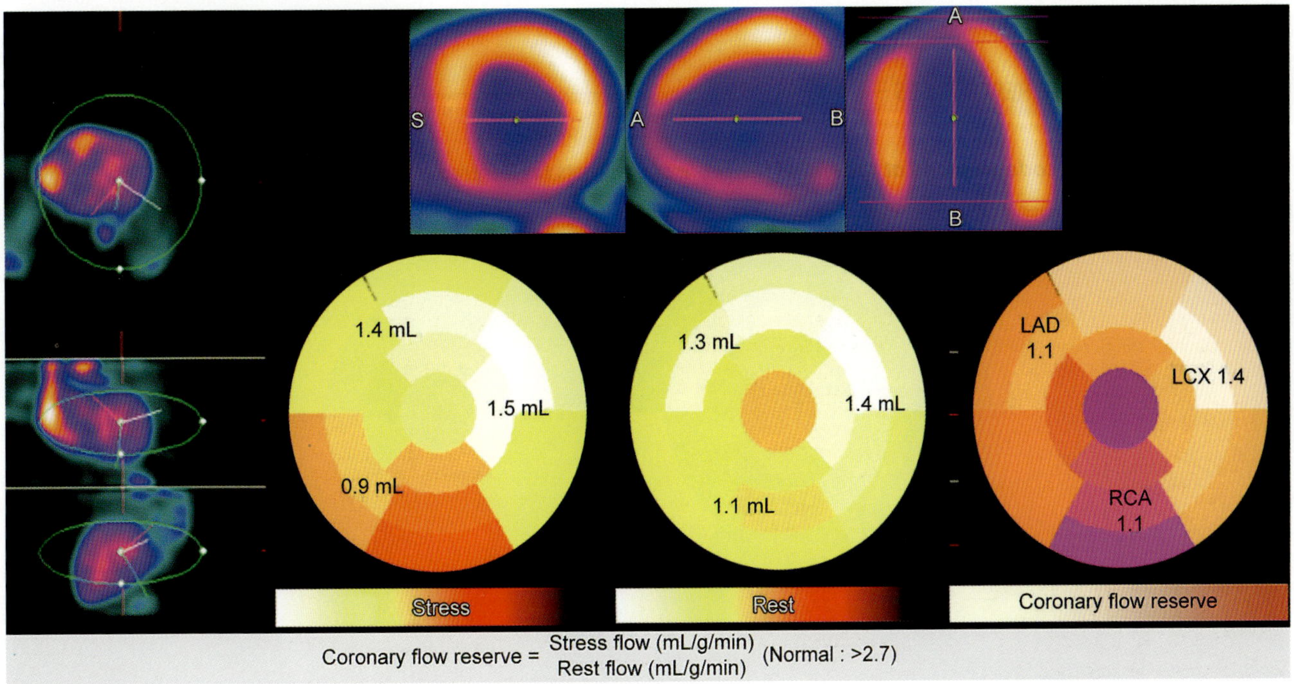

FIG. 12: Rubidium-82 myocardial perfusion scan showing global reduction of flow to the myocardium with CFR values LAD = 1.1 mL, LCX = 1.4 mL, and RCA = 0.9 mL. Overall myocardial perfusion pattern looks to be almost normal in patients with significant CAD and coronary steal.

(CAD: coronary artery disease; CFR: coronary flow reserve; LAD: left anterior descending; LCX: left circumflex; RCA: right coronary artery)

CONCLUSION

Nuclear cardiology using radioisotope is an important noninvasive diagnostic procedure which is utilized in the clinical practice. Various nuclear techniques have proved their superiority over other available diagnostic procedures such as 2D echocardiography, multidetector computed tomography (MDCT), MRI, and contrast echocardiography in the detection and further evaluation in patients suffering from CAD. In this context, Tl-201/Tc-99 sestamibi has been proved to be the patients having CAD for more than four decades. Subsequently, the advent of various TC-99m-labeled perfusion agents, particularly Tc-99m sestamibi (cardiolite) or Tc-99 tetrofosmin (Myoview), has improved their incurred sensitivity and specificity in the detection of CADs. In addition to the information regarding myocardial perfusion, one can obtain information on global EF, wall motion, and wall thickening at rest/stress study.

Pharmacological Tl-201 stress perfusion imaging is useful for patients who cannot exercise for various reasons including physical limitations, medications, lung diseases, peripheral vascular disease, severe osteoarthritis, elderly aged persons, aortic aneurysms, etc. It has also been developed to provide a unique opportunity to evaluate myocardial perfusion during maximal coronary vasodilatation in the early days of the origin of MI and to substitute submaximal predischarge exercise testing as a method for evaluating the extent of CAD and risk of future cardiac events in patients who are admitted with acute MI and in patients who are unable to do exercise. Scientists have also found out that dobutamine has demonstrated comparable sensitivity and specificity in detecting abnormality in myocardial imaging than that of dipyridamole or adenosine in patients with asthma or severe chronic constrictive pulmonary diseases.[16]

Improvements in software and hardware have recently enabled the integration of different imaging modalities into hybrid imaging producing important changes in the study of patients with known or suspected CAD. New innovation such as PET/CT offers the opportunity for a comprehensive noninvasive evaluation of the quantitative information about absolute myocardial perfusion through individual coronary artery and cardiac metabolism and the evaluation of the consequences atherosclerosis in the coronary artery. This integrated platform assessing anatomy and biology offers a great potential for translating advances in molecular targeted imaging into humans.

However, hybrid cardiac imaging combining SPECT and PET with MDCT data is an externally promising noninvasive cardiac imaging tool, allowing detection and quantification of the burden of the extent of calcified and noncalcified plaques [coronary artery calcification (CAC) and coronary angiography], quantification of vascular reactivity and endothelial dysfunction identification of flow/limiting coronary stenoses, and assessment of myocardial viability.

This integration of MDCT with PET will play an important role in molecular diagnostic and therapeutics.

ONLINE REFERENCES

Please scan the QR code provided at the end of the table of contents for References of this chapter.

CHAPTER

113 Role of Cardiac Magnetic Resonance in Heart Failure

Johann Christopher

ABSTRACT

Heart failure is a complex syndrome characterized by the inability of the heart to pump blood commensurate with the metabolic requirements of the body. Heart failure imaging involves a multimodality approach ranging from electrocardiogram (ECG), echocardiogram (ECHO), computed tomography angiogram (CTA), cardiac magnetic resonance (CMR), and invasive catheterization study. However, the prime position in imaging is truly reserved for CMR. CMR is a radiation free, window free, and interobserver free technique with a tissue characterization that is unmatched. CMR has evolved from a unidimensional tool to a multidimensional tool which has a diagnostic, prognostic and management role in the care of heart failure patients.

Keywords: Heart failure, cardiac magnetic resonance.

INTRODUCTION

Heart failure (chronic heart failure—CHF) is a complex syndrome and causes a major impact on the healthcare system. CHF prototypes are classified according to the left ventricular ejection fraction (LVEF). Current guidelines base recommendations on the following designations: heart failure with preserved ejection fraction (HFpEF: EF >50%), heart failure with mildly reduced EF (HFmrEF: EF 41–49%); heart failure with improved EF (HFimpEF; history of HFrEF with 10% EF improvement); heart failure with reduced EF (HFrEF: EF <40%). An important assessment in patients with CHF is whether left ventricular (LV) dysfunction is due to coronary artery disease (CAD) or due to noncoronary etiology. This differentiation is clinically important as ischemic cardiomyopathy (ICM) patients are associated with a shorter mean survival than patients with idiopathic dilated cardiomyopathy (DCM). In addition, the management plan is altered as patients with ICM may benefit from revascularization and secondary preventive pharmacotherapy, whereas patients with DCM may have better response to the standard heart failure medication including beta blockers, sodium-glucose cotransporter-2 inhibitors (SGLT-2Is), ngiotensin receptor/neprilysin (ARN), magnetic resonance angiography (MRA) **(Fig. 1)**. Determining the exact etiology in this group can be challenging using the currently available imaging techniques such as echocardiogram (ECHO), radionuclide imaging or coronary angiography, especially if history of CAD is lacking.

Over the last decade, cardiac magnetic resonance (CMR) imaging has become a well-established noninvasive modality for visualizing myocardial diseases. The delayed contrast enhancement (DCE) technique using gadolinium-based contrast media is a newly developed technique that allows direct visualization of myocardial necrosis or fibrosis as regions of bright signal (hyperenhancement) compared with normal myocardium. The pattern of hyperenhancement may favor one diagnosis over the other. CMR is used for the noninvasive assessment of the function and structure of the cardiovascular system. CMR has a few limitations especially if there are non-compatible permanent pacemakers or defibrillator, intracerebral clips or severe patient claustrophobia.[1] Routine MRI sequences are adapted for cardiac imaging using electrocardiogram (ECG) gating and high temporal resolution protocols. The development of CMR imaging is an ongoing area of research and continues to see a slew of emerging applications. Limited access to scanners, lack of technologists and skilled clinicians, relatively high costs, and competing diagnostic modalities continue to be major obstacles in its growth.[2] The CMR

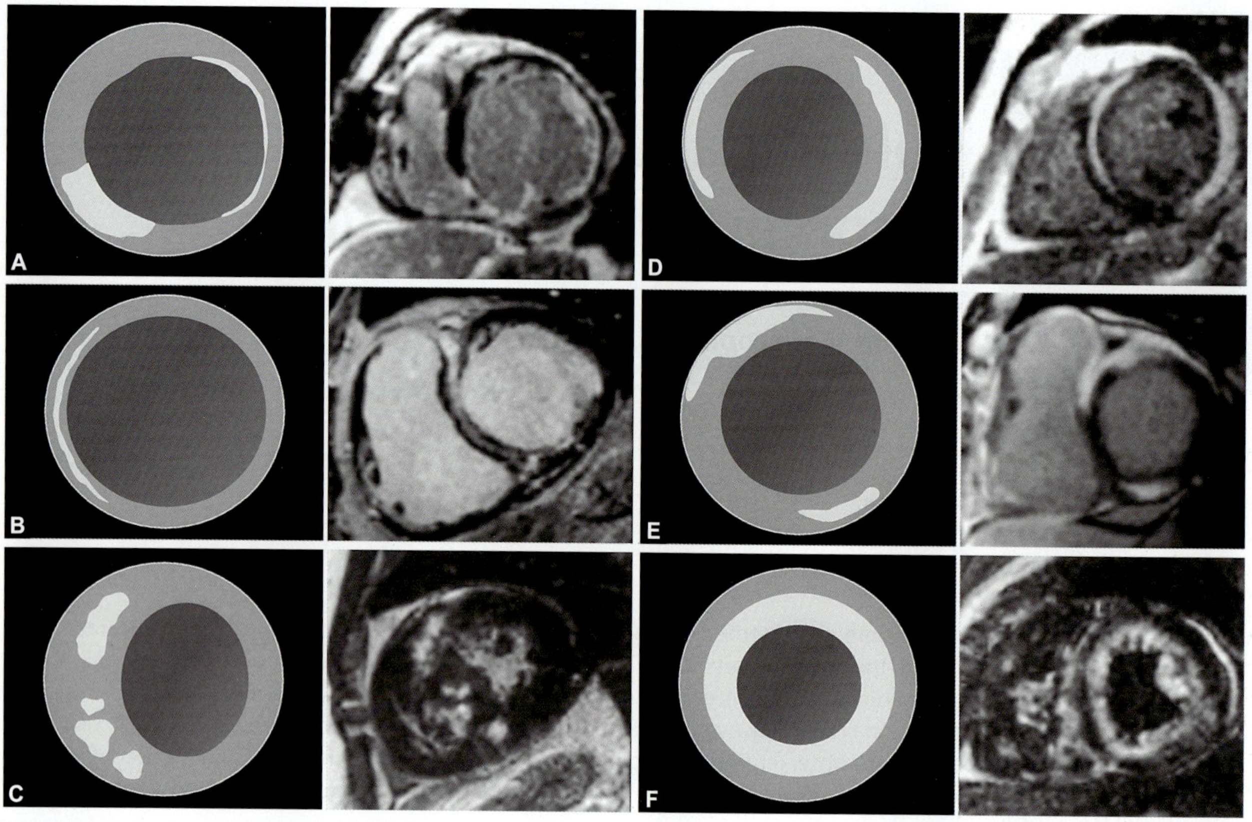

FIGS. 1A TO F: Patterns of delayed enhancement.

community is working on solutions to reduce these obstacles so that more clinics can adopt CMR into their clinical workflow.[3] These solutions are often software platforms that provide clinical decision support and improve the efficiency of the procedures. A CMR study typically comprises a set of sequences in a protocol tailored to the specific indication for the examination.[4] The study begins with localizers to assist with image planning, and then a set of retrospectively gated cine sequences to assess biventricular function in standard orientation. Functional and structural information is acquired using balanced steady-state free precession (bSSFP) cine sequences which have a good temporal resolution and intrinsic image contrast. These are usually retrospectively gated and have intrinsically high contrast in cardiac imaging due to the relatively high T2:T1 ratio of blood compared to myocardium. Images are typically planned sequentially to achieve the standard cardiac planes used for assessment. The LV short axis cines are acquired from base to apex and are used for quantifying end-diastolic and end-systolic volumes, as well as myocardial mass. T1-weighted sequences are used to visualize anatomy and detect the presence of intramyocardial fat. T1 mapping has also been developed to quantify diffuse myocardial fibrosis.[5] T2-weighted imaging is mainly used to detect myocardial edema especially seen in acute myocarditis or infarction. Turbulent flow causes dephasing and signal loss allowing valvular disease to be qualitatively appreciated. Phase-contrast imaging uses bipolar gradients to encode velocity in a given direction. It may be used to quantify valvular regurgitant fraction and shunt volume. Tagging sequences excite a grid pattern that deforms with cardiac contraction allowing strain to be assessed. Gadolinium-based contrast agents are administered intravenously, and delayed imaging is performed at least 10 minutes later to achieve optimum contrast between normal and infarcted myocardium. An inversion recovery (IR) sequence is used to null the signal from normal myocardium. Myocardial viability can be assessed by the degree of transmural enhancement. Genetic, inflammatory, and infiltrative diseases may also have distinctive patterns of nonischemic late gadolinium enhancement (LGE). Stress imaging is performed with adenosine which is a vasodilator, via the A_{2A} receptor, to accentuate the heterogeneity in perfusion between myocardial territories supplied by normal and stenosed coronary arteries. A continuous intravenous infusion is administered for a few minutes until there are hemodynamic signs of vasodilatation, a bolus of contrast medium is then administered via a separate IV line while acquiring saturation recovery images of the heart with a high temporal resolution readout. A positive result is evident from an inducible myocardial perfusion defect. Cost and availability mean that its use is often confined to patients with intermediate pre-test probability; however, it has been shown to reduce unnecessary coronary angiography compared with guideline-directed care. Conventional phase contrast imaging can be extended by applying flow-sensitive gradients in three orthogonal planes within a 3D volume throughout the cardiac cycle. 4D imaging encodes the velocity of flowing blood at each voxel in the volume enabling fluid dynamics to be visualized using specialist software. Applications are in complex congenital heart disease and for research into cardiovascular flow characteristics—however it is not in routine clinical use due to the complexity of post-processing and relatively long acquisition times. The majority of CMR is performed on conventional superconducting MRI systems at either 1.5T or 3T.[6] Imaging at 3T field strength offers greater signal to noise ratio which is of greatest value in first-pass perfusion studies.[7] However, greater capital costs and effects of off-resonance artefact on image quality mean that many studies are routinely performed at 1.5T.[8]

CORONARY ARTERY DISEASE

In CAD the role of CMR has great importance. The first objective is the reliable and reproducible evaluation of EF. It can do this in a consummate easy manner with the available software with a fair degree of low inter and intraobserver reproducibility.[9] EF evaluation by CMR is the gold standard in comparison to competing technologies. The second objective is evaluation of regional wall motion abnormalities (RWMAs) in a reliable and accurate fashion especially in patients with previous LV dysfunction, multivessel disease, and thinned out segments. This will enable the referral doctor to target the artery of interest for subsequent revascularization. This is possible through the windowless ability of CMR to orient the acquisition slices despite limitations of body habitus. The third objective is to assess the myocardial perfusion at stress followed by rest to assess myocardial ischemia.[10] Myocardial perfusion is carried out at rest and stress. Previously dobutamine stress was in vogue but due to its inherent risk most laboratories have switched to adenosine. Adenosine is a 6-minute infusion with gadolinium injected at the 3rd minute of the infusion at the time of maximal vasodilatation via a separate IV line. It is safe, short acting, side effects are minimal, and the sensitivity and specificity are in the high 90s. This is followed by a stack of short axis to measure EF followed by delayed enhancement imaging by the end of 10 minutes. In a case where there are no stress perfusion defects and no delayed enhancement it denotes no ischemia. In a case where is a stress perfusion defect and no gadolinium enhancement it denotes ischemia. In a case where there are perfusion defects and gadolinium enhancement, it denotes an infarction and necrosis.[11]

Adenosine CMR is an effective method to risk stratify patients of CAD in a safe, radiation free, timely and accurate manner with no limitation of balanced ischemia such as the nuclear techniques. The fourth objective is to look for viability in the territory of the occluded artery to assess the success of revascularization. The scar visualization capability of CMR is as good as a histopathological evaluation of the specimen **(Fig. 2)**.[12]

VALVULAR HEART DISEASE

The role of CMR in valvular heart disease (VHD) is steadily increasing. It is based on the fact that the ASE 2017 guidelines have been written in association with the Society of Cardiovascular Magnetic Resonance (SCMR). In valvular aortic stenosis **(Fig. 3)** the primary modality for the evaluation of the valve and the outflow gradient is the transthoracic echocardiogram (TTE). Mitral stenosis is also best evaluated by TTE. In select cases of borderline aortic stenosis and mitral stenosis, inconsistency between clinical features and gradients, obese patients with poor ECHO window, severely deformed and stenotic valves CMR can be employed as a third umpire in this situation for its ability for accurate planimetry. The regurgitant valves on the other hand are most suitable for evaluation by CMR. Using the physics of the velocity encoded imaging tool an accurate assessment of the flow can be made by using a perpendicular plane above the aortic valve to assess the regurgitation across the valve by a simple and independent technique not related to the LV stroke volume **(Fig. 4)**. Similarly, the pulmonary regurgitation can be

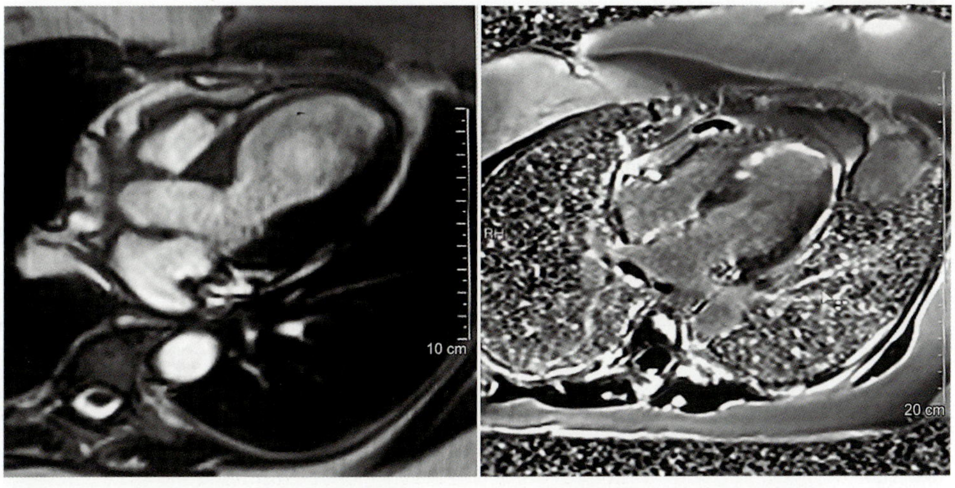

FIG. 2: Left anterior descending (LAD) territory infarct [ischemic cardiomyopathy (ICM)].

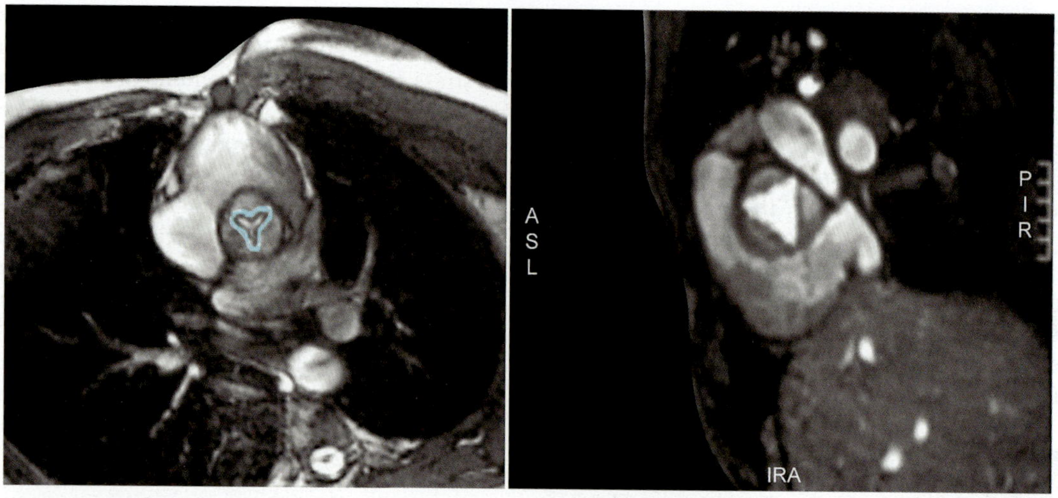

FIG. 3: Aortic valve planimetry (VHD).

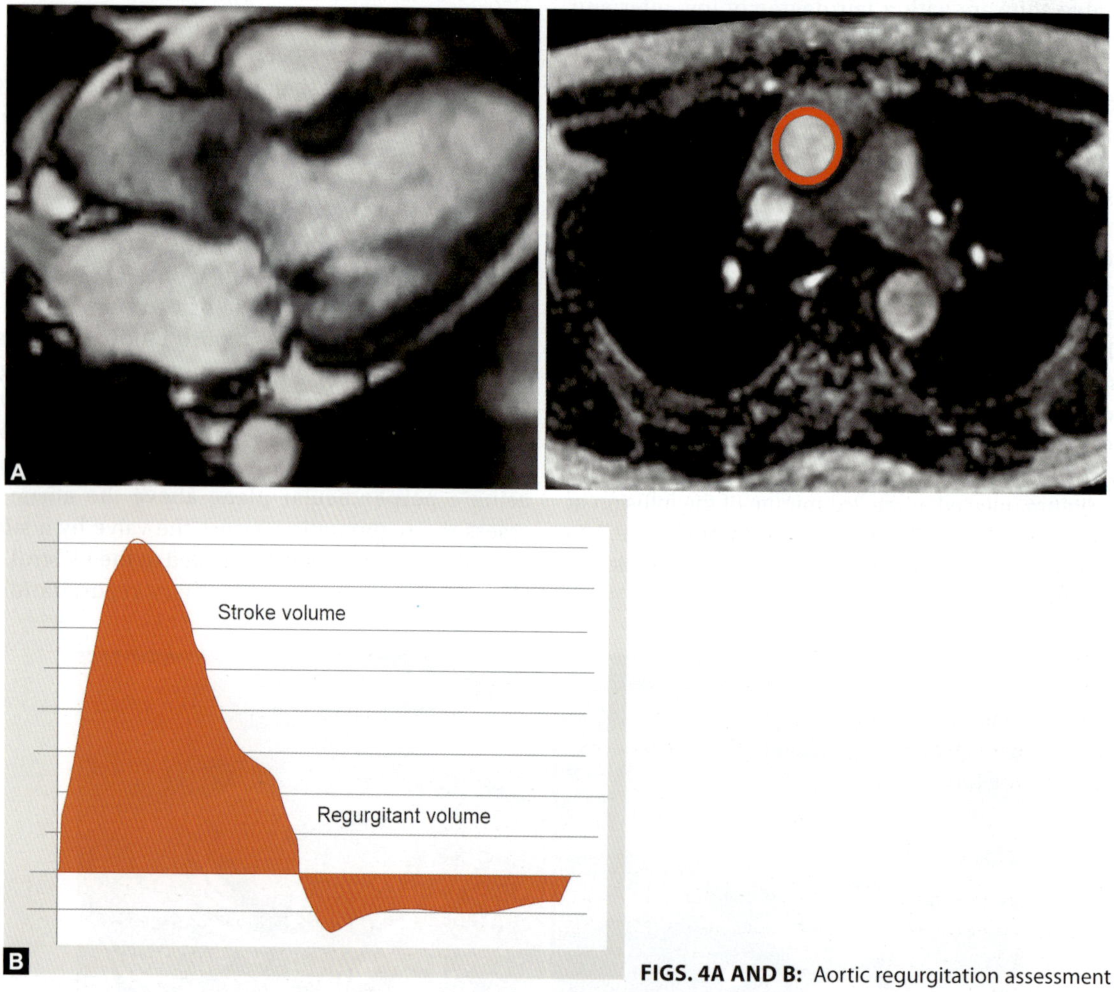

FIGS. 4A AND B: Aortic regurgitation assessment (VHD).

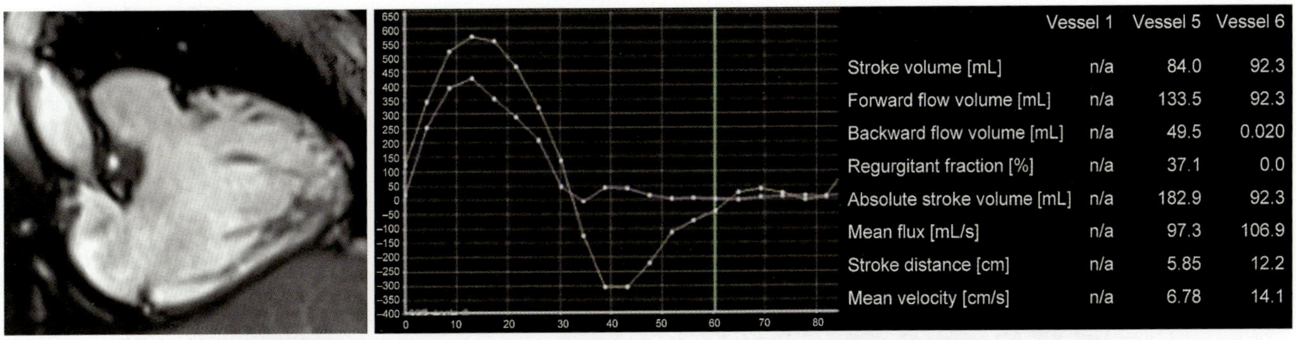

FIG. 5: Pulmonary regurgitation assessment (VHD).

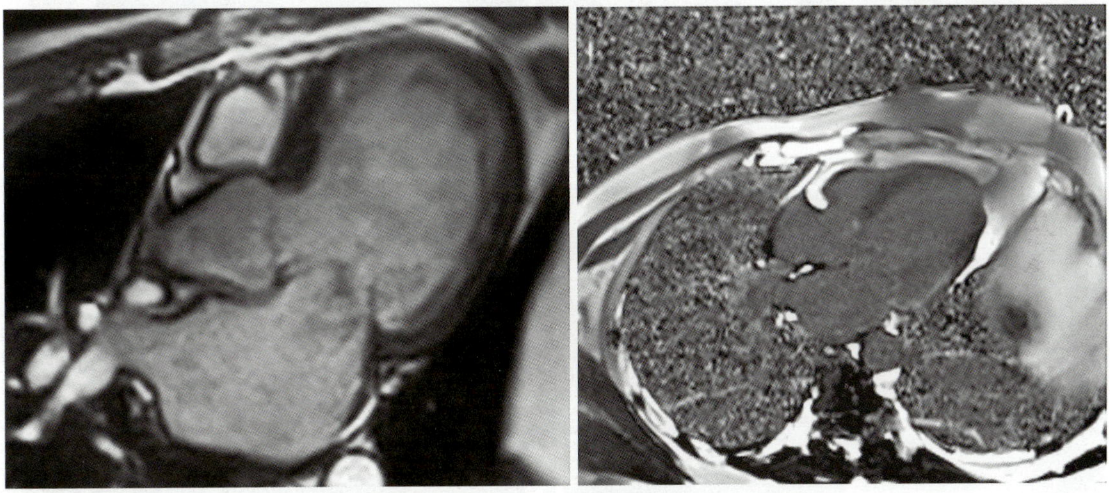

FIG. 6: Mitral regurgitation assessment (VHD).

assessed by a perpendicular plane above the pulmonary valve and using the velocity encoded cine (VEC) to assess pulmonary regurgitation **(Fig. 5)**. CMR is an accurate third umpire especially when there is discrepancy between clinical evaluation and ECHO results. Evaluation of mitral regurgitation and tricuspid regurgitation is a little more complex as it involves evaluation of the LV/RV stroke volume followed by the subtraction of the aortic/pulmonary flow by VEC imaging to derive the mitral/tricuspid regurgitation **(Fig. 6)**. Direct evaluation of the mitral and tricuspid valves is fraught with inconsistent results due to the movement of the annulus during the cardiac cycle.[13]

PERICARDIAL DISEASES

The role of CMR in pericardial diseases is primarily to assess the pericardial thickness, hemodynamics of constriction (including septal bounce, lateral wall hypokinesia, systemic venous dilatation, and biatrial dilatation), mediastinal nodes and more importantly pericardial enhancement post gadolinium administration suggesting an inflamed pericardium more amenable to anti-inflammatory therapy as opposed to a pericardium not enhancing, more suitable for pericardial surgical stripping **(Fig. 7)**. Localized versus generalized pericardial constriction can be assessed. Pericardial effusion analysis (exudate versus transudate) can be done by CMR without resorting to an invasive analysis. The syndrome of effusive constrictive pericarditis is also well characterized by CMR. Pericardial tumors (malignant versus benign) can also be reliably distinguished based on their morphology, edema, and gadolinium characteristics.[14]

CARDIAC MASSES

The role of CMR in cardiac masses is unique due to the tissue characteristics intrinsic to CMR imaging. Based on their T1, T2, first pass perfusion and post-gadolinium features a broad reliable differential diagnosis can be ascertained which may be specific and accurate in certain cases akin to a biopsy such as myxoma, lipoma, fibroma, thrombi **(Fig. 8)**, rhabdomyoma, hydatid cyst, **(Fig. 9)** and hemorrhagic cyst **(Fig. 10)**. The anatomic location is the first criteria, T1/T2 characteristics,

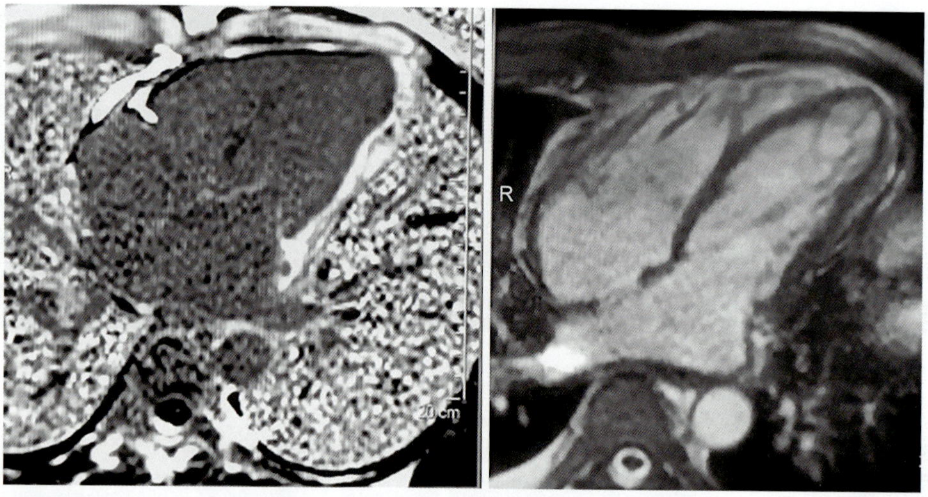

FIG. 7: Constrictive pericarditis.

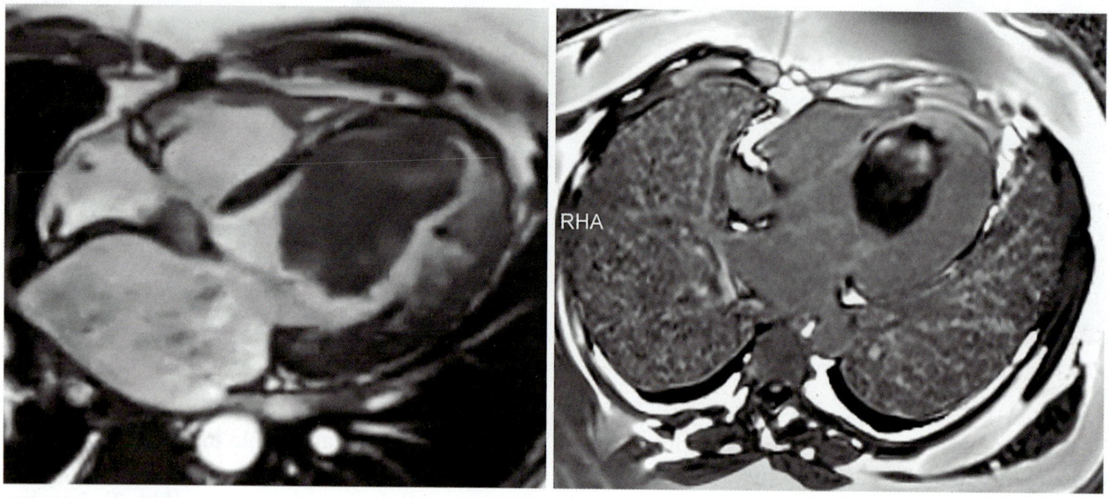

FIG. 8: LV thrombus.

first pass perfusion, delayed enhancement with routine T1, and delayed enhancement using an extended T1 preferably 600 to rule out a thrombus. However, in the other tumors an accurate directed differential diagnosis can be suspected on CMR imaging and specific invasive tools employed to further ascertain the diagnosis. The origin and spread of the tumor can also be ascertained due to the large field of vision which is intrinsic to CMR.[15]

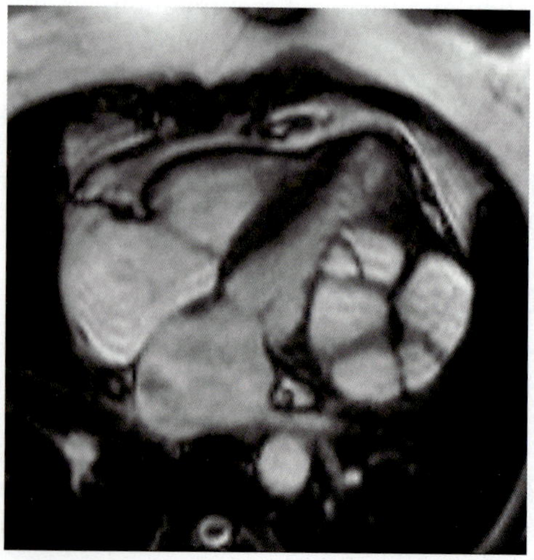

FIG. 9: Hydatid cyst.

NONISCHEMIC CARDIOMYOPATHIES

The role of CMR in non-ICM is the most relevant role of CMR in cardiology practice as there is no clear competitor in this space. The features of volumetry, tissue characterization, and scar quantification are important diagnostic and prognostic features in the overall assessment.

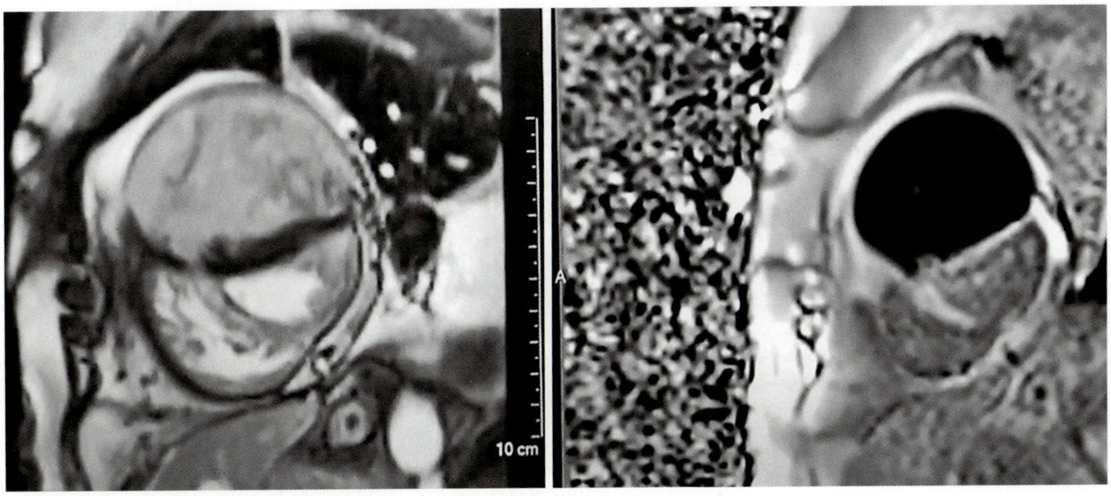

FIG. 10: Coronary Pseudoaneurysm.

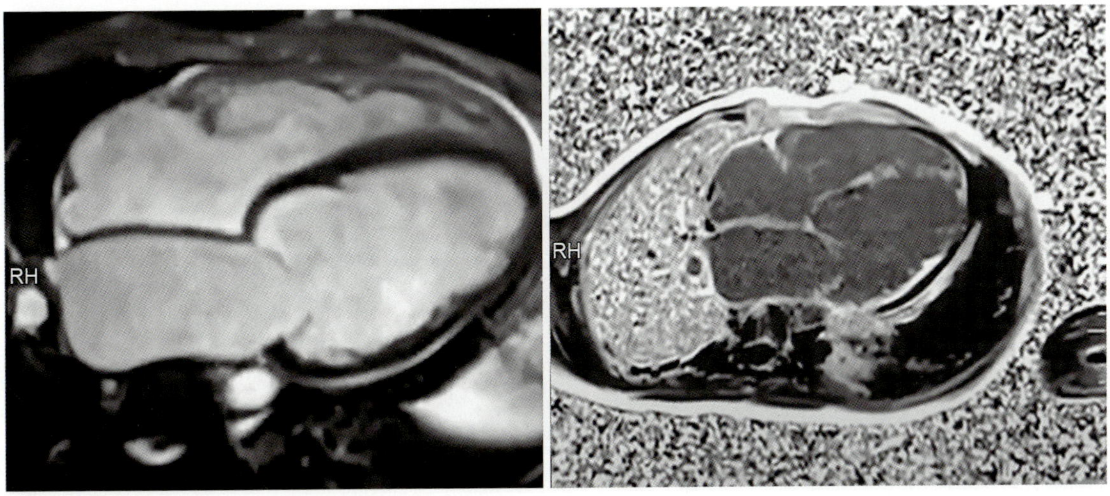

FIG. 11: Dilated cardiomyopathy (DCM).

Dilated cardiomyopathy is characterized by dilated atria and ventricles with thinned out walls (eccentric hypertrophy) with a varying EF ranging from 50% downward. CMR plays an important role in characterizing the phenotype, quantifying the volumes and EF, scar quantification, MR and TR quantification, pulmonary artery sizes and pressures, mediastinal nodes presence and pericardial effusion **(Fig. 11)**.[16]

Hypertrophic cardiomyopathy (HCM) is characterized by dilated atria and normal-sized ventricles with concentric hypertrophy with a supranormal EF. CMR plays an important role in characterizing the phenotype of hypertrophy, varying hypertrophy distribution especially the apical variant **(Fig. 12)**, which is missed on a cursory ECHO examination. The degree of hypertrophy, the location of obstruction, papillary muscle arrangement, mitral valve leaflet motion in systole, mitral regurgitation, degree of obstruction and most importantly the presence of scar and quantification which is significant if >15% **(Fig. 13)**.[17]

Restrictive cardiomyopathy (RCM) is characterized by dilated atria and normal-sized ventricles with concentric hypertrophy with a subnormal EF. CMR plays an important role in characterizing the phenotype, especially the septum and lateral wall hypertrophy. The presence of dilated systemic veins, concentric hypertrophy, biatrial dilatation with thickened walls and scarring, the presence of global subendocardial scarring and its quantification, the evaluation of amyloid kinetics on the T1 scout sequence are the key features on CMR.[18] Amyloidosis is a typical restrictive cardiomyopathy characterized by biatrial dilatation, normal-sized ventricles, mildly reduced EF, restrictive LV filling pattern and clinical features of heart failure **(Fig. 14)**. CMR plays an important role in characterizing the phenotype, distinguishing it from HCM or constrictive pericarditis,

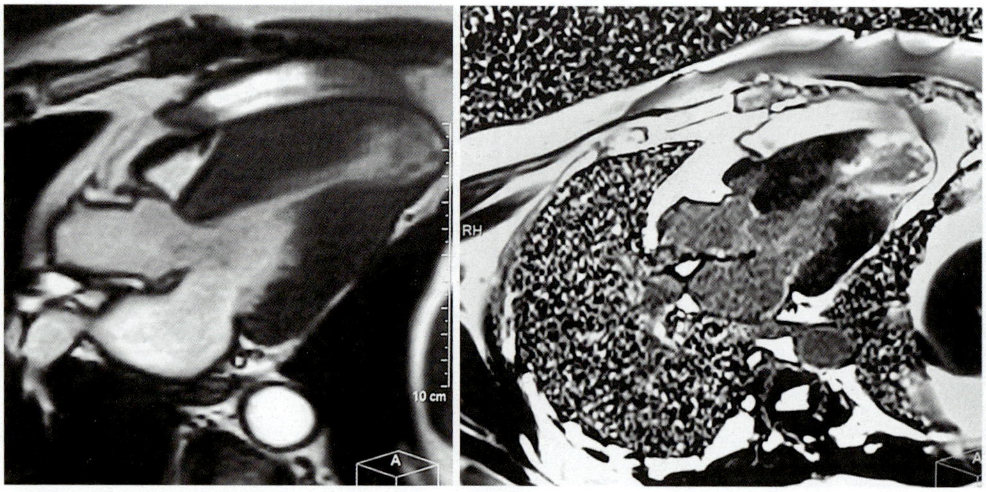

FIG. 12: Hypertrophic cardiomyopathy with apical aneurysm.

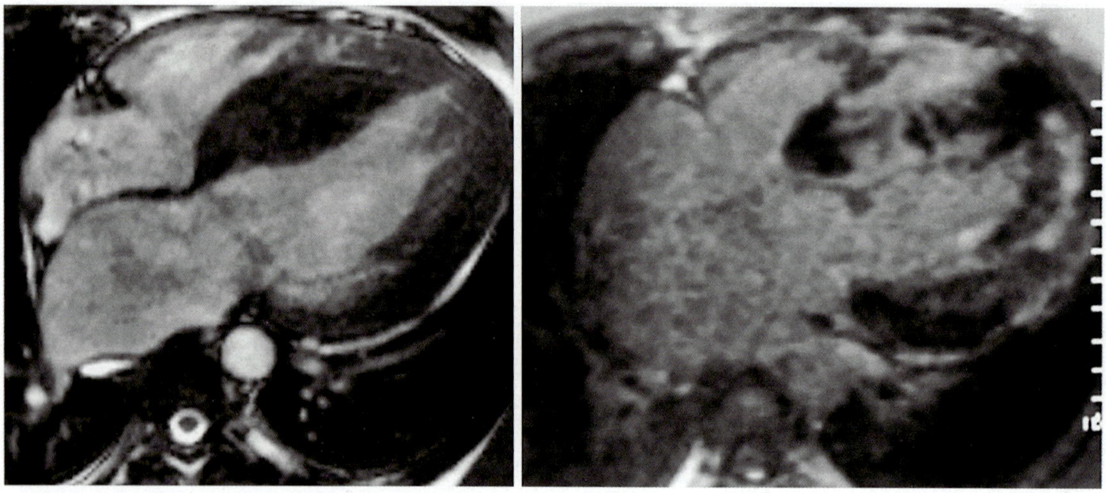

FIG. 13: Hypertrophic cardiomyopathy.

assessing gadolinium kinetics using the T1 scout sequence, establishing the typical subendocardial global delayed enhancement, elucidating the restrictive filling pattern (systemic vein dilatation, pericardial effusion, pleural effusion, dilated atria, etc.). The T1 mapping sequence is very characteristic as the T1 values are extremely high with corresponding high extracellular volume (ECV) values. This is not only good for diagnosis but also for sequential follow-up of the patient to assess the response of immunomodulator medication that is in vogue today.

Left ventricular noncompaction (LVNC) is characterized by the presence of dilated cardiac chambers with eccentric hypertrophy, trabeculation, and significant spongy to compact layer of myocardium. CMR plays an important role in characterizing the phenotype, more importantly quantifying the extent of spongy myocardium, i.e., 2.3:1 of spongy to compact myocardium in end diastole, presence of thrombus, and extent of fibrosis.[19]

Sarcoidosis is a multisystem disease which in a small proportion of cases present as pure cardiac sarcoidosis. It is characterized by basal septal thinning, RWMA not consistent with coronary territory, LV dysfunction, patchy myocardial edema, mid myocardial septal predominant scarring, and mediastinal lymphadenopathy. CMR plays a stellar role in that all these attributes discussed above are picked up if done in a careful protocolized manner. CMR is exquisite for edema and scar identification **(Fig. 15)** and quantification which immediately helps in risk stratification of the patient in terms of whether immunosuppressive therapy predominates or implantable cardioverter-defibrillator (ICD) with antiarrhythmics if there is dominant scar.[20] However, for follow-up if an ICD is implanted then a PET/CT

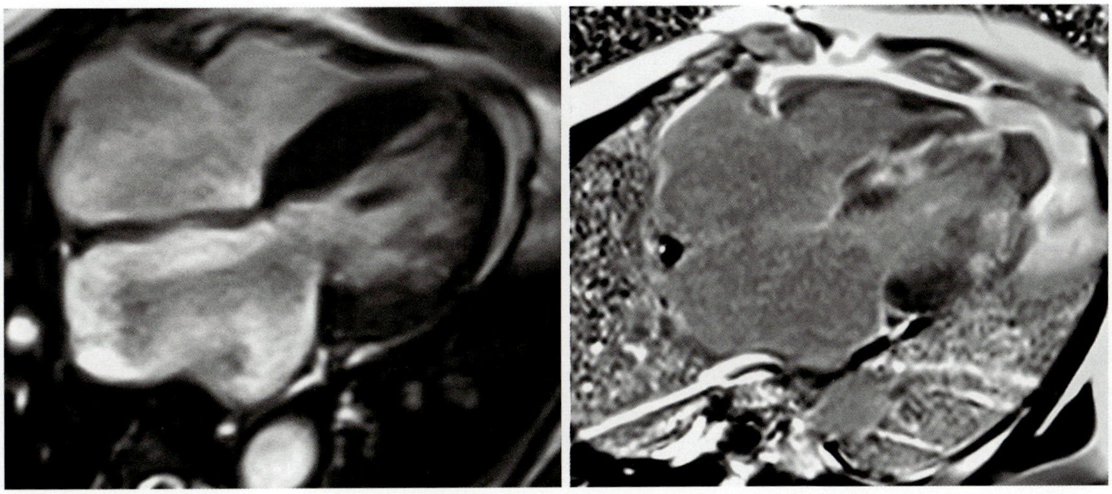

FIG. 14: Amyloidosis.

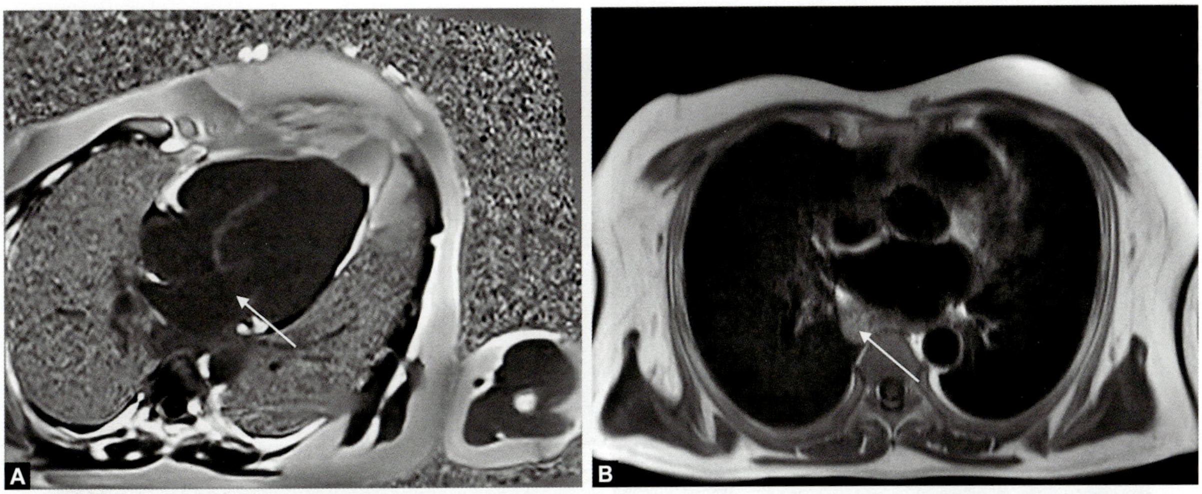

FIGS. 15A AND B: (A) Sarcoidosis (scar). (B) Sarcoidosis (nodes).

(low carbohydrate diet protocol) is a preferred modality for follow-up **(Fig. 16)**.

Iron overload syndromes including thalassemia and hemochromatosis are perfectly suited for visualization by CMR due to its iron affinity. The T2* sequence employed prior to the administration of contrast is extremely sensitive to the pickup of iron and its quantification. The lower the T2* the more the iron content and this can be used for sequential follow-up after the administration of iron therapy. The location of iron, heart predominant versus liver predominant for the same level of ferritin can also be ascertained **(Fig. 17)**.[21]

Endomyocardial fibrosis is a degenerative disease characterized by HFpEF. It is rare nowadays and is seen in patients with near normal EF with heart failure syndromes with obliterated apices, involving the LV/RV or both. CMR is excellent in characterizing these patients and elucidating the thrombus, fibrous, and muscle components in the apical mass and thereby fine tuning the management **(Fig. 18)**.[22]

Arrhythmogenic right ventricular dysplasia (ARVD) is a developmental genetic disease with late expression in young adults presenting with syncope and sudden cardiac death. Risk stratification is based on clinical, ECG, ECHO, CMR, and Holter data. CMR is an objective technique which contributes one out of two major criteria and two out of six minor criteria to confirm the diagnosis. CMR is excellent for volumetry and EF assessment which is a major criterion and establishes fat replacement of the wall and scar deposition which are by themselves high risk features, however, not in the revised guidelines **(Fig. 19)**.[23]

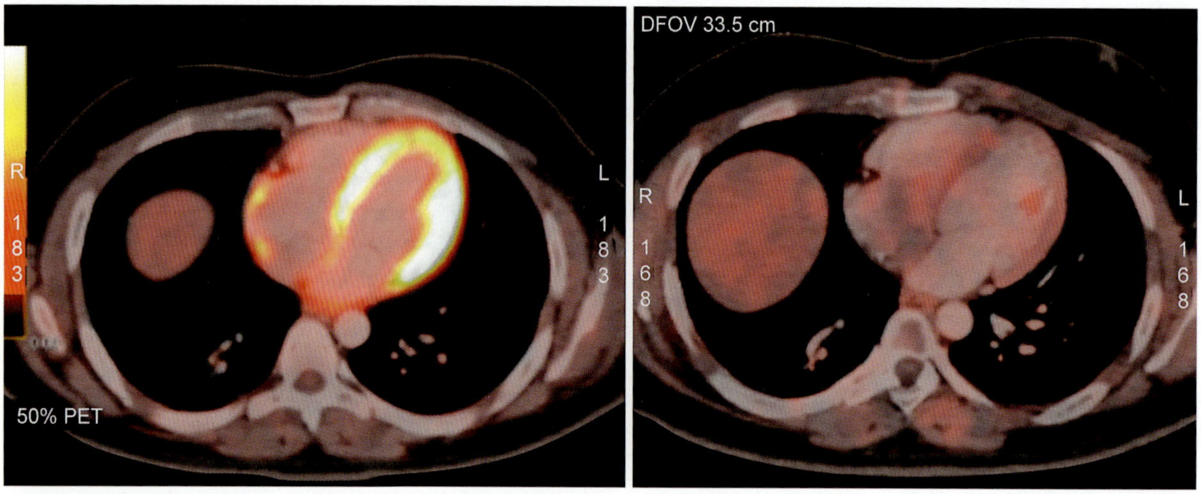

FIG. 16: PET/CT follow-up in sarcoidosis.
(PET/CT: positron emission tomography/computed tomography)

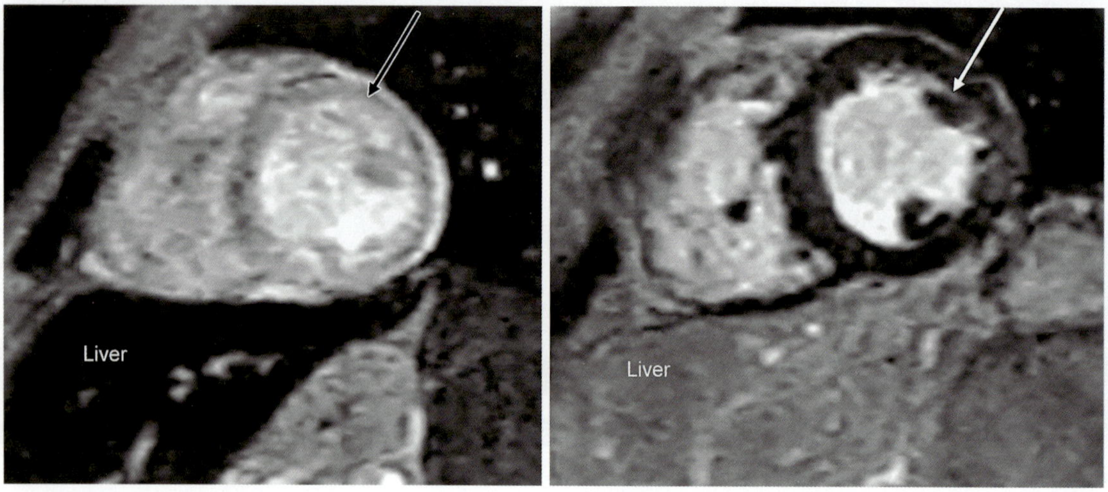

FIG. 17: Iron overload.

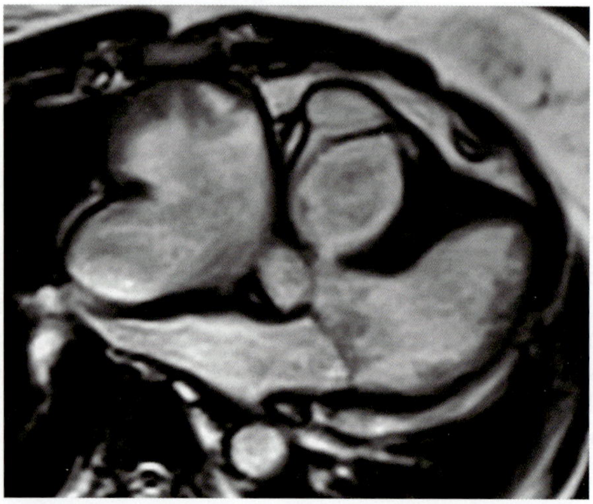

FIG. 18: Right ventricular endomyocardial fibrosis (RVEMF).

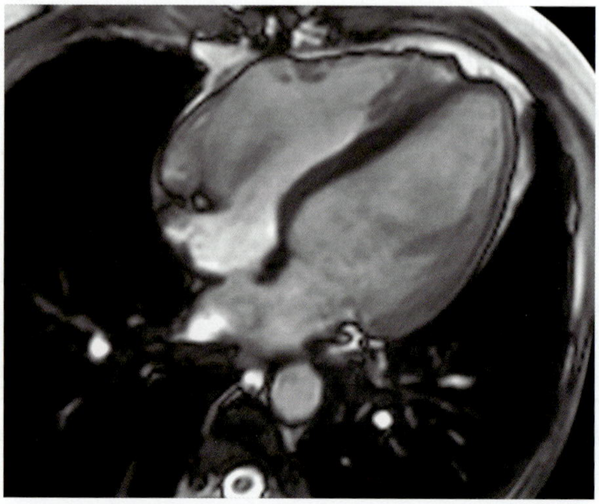

FIG. 19: Arrhythmogenic right ventricular dysplasia (ARVD).

CONCLUSION

In conclusion CMR is a one-stop shop technique to image a wide variety of myocardial pathology. It does so in an accurate, quick, efficient, radiation free, cost effective, and comprehensive manner.[24] CMR is available freely in most tier I and tier II cities in India. The number of CMR technicians is adequate and the relative paucity of CMR trained physicians is being corrected by many imaging societies through online and offline training sessions. CMR is certainly not a standalone tool. It, however, adds value to a well-done clinical examination by adding information which helps in the diagnosis, prognosis, and formulating a management strategy for a particular clinical situation.

ONLINE REFERENCES

Please scan the QR code provided at the end of the table of contents for References of this chapter.

CHAPTER 114

Role of CT Calcium Score in Current Day Practice

Marsha Barreto, Rajesh Thachathodiyl

ABSTRACT

The association of coronary artery calcification (CAC) with cardiovascular disease is a well-known concept for the last 30 years. CAC occurs and progresses hand in hand with the atherosclerotic plaque and hence, it is a useful marker of atherosclerosis rather than the severity of coronary artery disease. It should be considered in asymptomatic individuals >40 years of age with an intermediate to high risk as per the 10-year atherosclerotic cardiovascular disease (ASCVD) risk stratification system as well as those with a significant family history of cardiovascular disease. The absolute CAC score is representative of the short-term risk for the patient. Calcium plaques with a low density, spotty areas of calcification, positive remodeling, and the napkin ring sign are "unstable plaques" and more likely to have acute coronary events. Plaques with a higher density are associated with a lower number of events as they are less prone to erosions/ruptures. Hence both the area and volume of the calcium with its density should be taken into consideration. The current recommendations require measuring the plaque volume and peak/mean density as two separate variables and then analyzing them individually to determine ASCVD risk. The absence of CAC or a score of 0 is the "strongest negative risk factor" in asymptomatic patients. Aggressive modification of lifestyle and risk factors in all individuals with CAC, along with appropriate timely initiation of therapy in those requiring it, is the cornerstone of CAC scanning.

Keywords: Coronary artery calcification, agatston scoring, atherosclerosis, ASCVD risk score, coronary artery disease.

INTRODUCTION

Coronary artery calcification (CAC) and its association with cardiovascular disease (CVD) is a well-known concept for the last 30 years, since it was first described by Agatston et al. in 1990. It allows for prompt and aggressive lifestyle and risk factor modifications for the primary prevention of cardiovascular events.

PATHOPHYSIOLOGY

Atherosclerosis is characterized by the presence of smooth muscle apoptosis resulting in the formation of an atherosclerotic plaque. CAC occurs and progresses hand in hand with this atherosclerotic plaque. It begins as microscopic calcifications of 0.5–15 µm and can grow into large sheets of calcium of >3 µm. Usually, it involves only the coronary artery intima but in some cases, such as chronic kidney disease and hyperparathyroidism, it may also involve the tunica media.[1] Hence, in the early stages it may only appear as intimal thickening, when examined microscopically and progresses later to cluster deep within the plaque lipid core. Younger patients have more of a noncalcified plaque as compared to the elderly. However, the size of the plaque does not have a direct correlation with the extent and pattern of CACs. Although the severity of CAC can predict the presence of coronary artery stenosis it is more useful as a marker of atherosclerosis than severity of coronary artery disease (CAD).[1]

WHOM DO WE SCAN?

Asymptomatic individuals >40 years of age with an intermediate to high risk as per the 10-year atherosclerotic cardiovascular disease (ASCVD) risk stratification system are the ideal candidates. However, in such patients already requiring lipid-lowering therapy, there is no indication for CAC estimation. The CVD risk restratification is most beneficial in those at a borderline or intermediate risk. In the Heinz Nixdorf Recall Study, nearly 22% of intermediate risk patients were reclassified into a higher or lower risk group after CAC estimation.[1]

Screening may also be considered in those patients with a significant family history where CAC scoring may result in life changing alterations to risk factors and therapies.

Coronary artery calcification scoring is strongly advised against, in patients with symptoms of angina, effort intolerance, and dyspnea which may be suggestive of myocardial ischemia, as it does not carry the same negative predictive value as compared to asymptomatic patients.[1] In such patients, if they are already undergoing a CT coronary angiogram, a CAC scoring may be done in adjunction, in which case, it may have a prognostic value.

Repeat scans for assessing the efficacy of therapy and risk factor modification are not recommended.[1] However, additional large scale studies are yet required for in-depth analysis of the effects of statins and other medications on the nature of the plaque and the benefits, and improvements on the future risk of ASCVD.

HOW DO WE SCAN?

The CAC scan is a rapidly acquired noncontrast CT image of the heart. The ease of obtaining a CT scan as compared to an invasive angiography, as well as the minimal requirements in terms of preparation, no iodinated IV contrast, and most notably, the relative lower effective radiation doses are few of the striking benefits of CAC. These reductions in radiation doses are now enabled by the presence of dual source CT scanners with prospective high-pitch helical acquisition at low doses, and even lower doses may be used when iterative reconstruction techniques are employed.[1]

Most commonly, the Agatston method for CAC quantification is used. CAC is given as a product of the plaque area and the "peak plaque density" which is then summed across plaques in all the coronary arteries.[2]

On an electrocardiogram (ECG)-gated CT scan, an area of 1 mm^2 or more with a density of >130 HU when multiplied with a density weighting factor gives us the area of calcified atherosclerosis. This is then added up for the entire coronary tree, allowing prediction of the severity of disease based on the presence of proximal vessel involvement and the number of vessels involved.

The score is then given as:

- 0: No disease
- 1–99: Mild disease
- 100–399: Moderate disease
- ≥400: Severe disease

Coronary artery calcification may also be incidentally detected on CT scans done for other purposes. The Society of Cardiovascular Computed Tomography hence recommends that CAC be reported in all noncontrast CT chest imaging studies.[1] In these cases, Agatston scoring may not be possible; nonetheless, it has a high prognostic importance. Other methods of estimation including a visual estimation method or the ordinal scoring method may be applied in these cases.

In angiographic lesions having >50% stenosis, it is a highly sensitive tool but is only moderately specific, especially in older individuals. The sensitivity and specificity vary with the extent of CAC with a fall in the sensitivity and a rise in the specificity with rising CAC scores **(Figs. 1A to C)**.

It should also be kept in mind that the absolute CAC score is representative of the short-term risk for the patient and so a low score for a younger age and sex may not necessarily indicate low lifetime CVD risk.[1]

CORONARY ARTERY CALCIFICATION PLAQUE CHARACTERISTICS

Calcium plaques with a low density, spotty areas of calcification, positive remodeling, and the napkin ring sign (low attenuation plaque surrounded by a hyperattenuating ring) are indicative of plaque vulnerability and these patients are more likely to have acute coronary events.[4]

When we consider the risk association between calcium density and cardiovascular risk alone, it is seen that a higher calcium density is seen in older individuals, long duration of coronary heart disease (CHD), and a larger plaque area. However, these plaques with a higher density are associated with a lower number of events as they are less prone to erosions/ruptures. Hence the area and volume should also be accounted for in conjunction with the calcium density.

One of the biggest drawbacks of the Agatston scoring system is the notion that a higher score directly correlates with a higher ASCVD risk. Newer data suggests that an improved risk prediction is obtained by using CAC volume with CAC density in which volume is directly proportional whereas density is inversely proportional.[2]

This is consistent with the observation that the use of statins increases the Agatston score despite its protective effect against CVD. Further, it has also been seen that physical activity results in faster CAC progression and hence endurance athletes are seen to have a higher CAC.[2] These patients, however, do not have an increased risk of ASCVD mortality which may be attributable to the higher proportion of purely calcified plaques, which is a more stable plaque and hence less prone to acute coronary events.[4]

Thus, came about the question whether a new method of scoring was the need of the hour. The CAC consortium 2022, proposed that the use of mean density instead of peak density may be a better measure as well as a better indicator of the diversity of the plaque.[2] The calcium density is given by the concentration of calcium within a plaque. Subsequently this study showed that the mean density was a better predictor. However, this study also showed that plaque density may only be relevant in those patients with mild CAC that is with scores of 1–99. Further, the maximum difference between mean and peak density was seen in those with small plaques

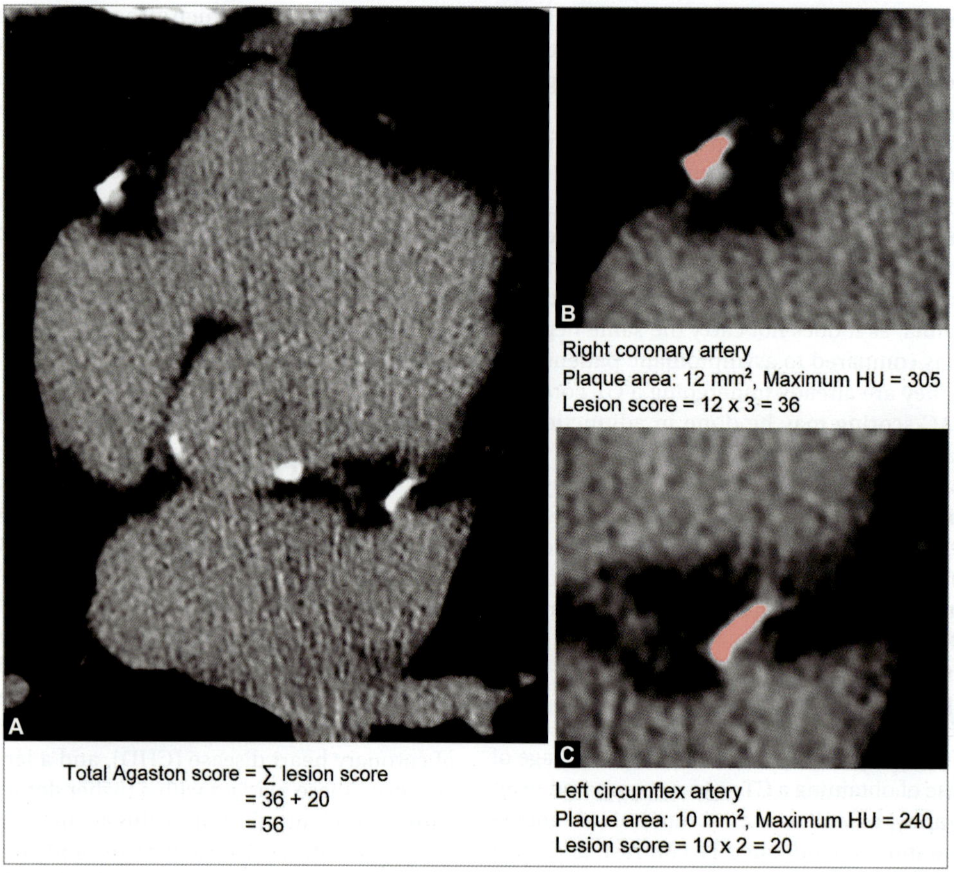

FIGS. 1A TO C: Measurement of coronary artery calcium using Agatston scoring.[3]

and at a younger age group. Keeping this in mind, the current recommendations state that measuring the plaque volume and peak/mean density as two separate variables and then analyzing them individually to determine ASCVD risk would be a better option.[2]

The remodeling index is given as the ratio between the vessel diameter, at the lesion and proximal to the lesion. Studies show that this index, along with a low plaque density, has the highest predictive value for a future ASCVD event and hence provides better prognostic information than only CAC estimation.[4]

Other methods that can be used to assess the calcium density include the standard deviation method in which the variation of the density in a given lesion is calculated and the range method in which the minimum and the maximum density within a given lesion is estimated.[4]

In doing so, we are able to fine tune the models used for stratifying patients for CVD risk reduction. This then allows the patient to understand the importance of making drastic lifestyle changes as well as the role of preventive therapies **(Table 1)**.

TABLE 1: Various method of coronary artery calcium quantification.

Metric	Description
Peak calcium density	Maximum plaque attenuation (HU) within a given lesion
Mean calcium density	Average plaque attenuation (HU) within a given lesion
Standard deviation	Variation in calcium density/attenuation within a given lesion
Range	Minimum and maximum calcium density/attenuation within a given lesion

BENEFITS OVER OTHER MODALITIES

The two most important uses of CAC as a screening tool are in the prediction of patients with ASCVD and then deciding which of these patients warrant treatment apart from aggressive lifestyle modifications.

Being a widespread and easily reproducible tool, CAC is hence used to increase the value of already existing validated risk calculators such as the Framingham risk score and the American College of Cardiology/American Heart Association (ACC/AHA) pooled cohort equation. In the Multi-Ethnic Study of Atherosclerosis (MESA), it was demonstrated that CAC scores of 101–300 had a hazard ratio of 7.7 for coronary events and those with scores of >300 a ratio of 9.7 and higher CVD-related mortality, thus unequivocally establishing the prognostic benefit of CAC estimation.[1]

As compared to other risk enhancers, such as high-sensitivity C reactive protein, high-sensitivity cardiac troponin T, absence of carotid plaque, carotid intima-medial thickness, B type natriuretic peptide, ankle-brachial pressure index, and others, the absence of CAC or a score of 0 is the "strongest negative risk factor" in asymptomatic patients. Although each of the earlier mentioned markers brought about an increase in the C-statistic over Framingham risk score, CAC had the highest rise. That is, the absence of coronary calcium allows for the "de-risking" of patients to a very high level of accuracy.[1]

On the other hand, many patients who would have been considered as low or intermediate risk may have a high CAC and hence may require active intervention and therapy. This was demonstrated in the MESA study, which showed that 6.8% of patients in the intermediate risk category had CAC scores of >400. These patients may have otherwise never have been considered as possible candidates for lipid-lowering therapy and other measures. The MESA study showed that patients with a score of >100 had an ASCVD risk of >7.5% and warranted preventive therapy.[1]

EPIDEMIOLOGICAL VARIATIONS IN CORONARY ARTERY CALCIFICATION

In terms of its prognostic value, it is equal for both the sexes; however, data suggests that in males and those with diabetes, age of the first scanning should be earlier. Recent studies show the occurrence of CAC in males, precedes that in women by almost 15 years on an average.[4] It has also been seen that women, although having larger and higher density plaques, have fewer plaques and fewer vessels involved. It has been proposed that this occurs secondary to a well-preserved estrogen status of the females.[4] The lower calcium density of CAC in men predisposes them to four times higher ASCVD risk. A 1.8% lower calcium density score was seen in diabetics and a 1% lower score with every 5 kg/m^2 increase in body mass index (BMI).[4] Diabetes and obesity were seen to have the maximal negative association with calcium density. Chronic kidney disease patients have a high degree of vascular calcification predisposing them to a higher cardiovascular morbidity and mortality, but if there exists any additional predictive value for the same has not been established.

The prevalence as well as the amount of CAC was found to be higher in the white population, but the predictive value remains the same across all ethnic groups. Inversely, people of Chinese descent were found to have 10.3% higher calcium density than the Caucasian population, leading to the conclusion that people of Chinese descent as well as the Hispanic and African American population have more stable and calcified plaques.[4] This suggests a difference in the pathophysiology of atherosclerosis and calcification among the various ethnicities.[4]

THE INDIAN SCENARIO

The South Asian population including Indians are at an especially high risk for CVD and with a higher mortality from ischemic heart disease. The onset of CAD occurs almost one decade before the rest of the world population with twice as much severity.[5] Although most of the larger studies looking at CAC have been done in the West, a few small studies give us an insight into the role of CAC in the South Asian population. In the Mediators of Atherosclerosis in South Asians Living in America (MASALA) trial, the CAC was studied in the South Asian population in two centers in the United States of America and then followed up.

As compared to other studies, the population in the MASALA study were younger, males, with the highest diabetes prevalence, lower number of smokers, and lower exercise levels. The South Asian men on the other hand were found to have a CAC prevalence similar to white men and higher than the other ethnicities studied in the MESA trial. Along with prevalence, the progression of CAC in South Asian men was also seen to be at a faster rate. Among the 290 patients who had detectable CAC at the onset, a median annual CAC progression of 26 in men versus 13 in women was seen.[6] The change in CAC showed significant association with only older age, males, smoking, diabetes mellitus, and use of statins and antihypertensives. As this study had a higher proportion of younger and healthier individuals, with no evidence of CAD, it is proposed that if these results are generalized to the South Asian population at large, the results would be much more alarming.[6]

The incidence and progression of CAC was much higher in the South Asian men as compared to the women. There was no difference in the CAC progression and incidence among women across all the ethnicities studied.[6]

It was also found that in those individuals who had been living in the United States for a longer duration of time, smokers, and high levels of alcohol consumption were associated with higher rates of CAC progression while higher incomes were associated with lower changes in the CAC.[6]

A higher amount of visceral and pericardial fat was associated with a higher rate of CAC change while exercise and number of calories consumed had no effect.

In another study, which looked at the CAC score and Framingham risk score in symptomatic Indian population and its correlation with CAD severity, a higher coronary calcium score was associated with a higher extent and severity of CAD. Plaques were more commonly seen in the proximal portion of the left anterior descending artery.[5]

HOW DOES IT AFFECT THE MANAGEMENT OF PATIENTS?

In patients <70 years of age with a CAC ≥100, aspirin was found to have a net clinical benefit regardless of the ASCVD risk category. Whereas in patients with no CAC, it caused more harm than benefit.[1]

Similar findings were also reported for statins with better long-term outcomes. Furthermore, one study also showed that patients with any detectable CAC that were treated with statins had reduced ASCVD outcomes as compared to patients not on therapy. It is interesting to note at this point that patients with no CAC derived no benefit from statin therapy unless they already had a high baseline risk for ASCVD **(Table 2)**.[1]

Other lipid-lowering therapies, such as icosapent ethyl and 5-lipoxygenase inhibitors also have been found to reduce the low-attenuation plaques as compared to their placebo counterparts.[5]

FOLLOW-UP SCANNING FOR CORONARY ARTERY CALCIFICATION

It is recommended that in patients with a low 10-year ASCVD risk CAC scanning should be repeated after 5–7 years, in those with an intermediate risk at 3–5 years, and those with diabetes in 3 years.[1]

When CAC scoring was followed up in patients with calcific plaques, patients on various modalities of therapy showed changes in the composition of the plaque density along with a difference in the progression of disease. Statin use was found to decrease the size and volume of the necrotic core which leads to an increase in calcium plaque attenuation and density. This acceleration of calcification may be due to the macrophage Rac1-interleukin 1B signaling axis. It confers stability and is one of the factors by which statins are protective against future ASCVD events.[5]

Although repeat scanning for progression of CAC has no proven benefit in patients with an already elevated CAC score at baseline, further studies may be required to study the progression of not only calcium area but also density. This may be especially important in patients on therapy to further estimate the decrease in the future risk of ASCVD.

CONCLUSION

Coronary artery calcium is an easily reproducible and accessible tool as a marker for atherosclerosis and future CVD. It should be considered in all asymptomatic individuals >40 years of age with an intermediate to high 10-year ASCVD risk as well as those patients with a strong family history of CVD.

The absolute CAC score is representative of the short-term risk for the patient. Calcium plaques with a low density, spotty areas of calcification, positive remodeling, and the napkin ring sign are "unstable plaques" and more likely to have acute coronary events. Plaques with a higher density are associated with a lower number of events as they are less prone to erosions/ruptures. Hence both the area and volume of the calcium with its density should be taken into consideration. Mean density is a better predictor; however, plaque density is relevant in those patients with mild CAC. The current recommendations require measuring the plaque volume and peak/mean density as two separate variables and then analyzing them individually to determine ASCVD risk. The absence of CAC or a score of 0 is the "strongest negative risk factor" in asymptomatic patients.

Coronary artery calcification in males precedes that in women by almost 15 years, with fewer plaques and fewer vessels involved in women. The lower calcium density of CAC in men predisposes them to a four times higher ASCVD risk. South Asian men have a CAC prevalence similar to white men. The progression of CAC was also faster. Diabetes and obesity were seen to have the maximal negative association with calcium density.

TABLE 2: Statin therapy guidelines based on 10 year ASCVD risk + CAC scores.[3]

	10-year ASCVD risk			
Medical scenario	**Low risk (<5%)**	**Borderline risk (5.0–7.5%)**	**Intermediate risk (>7.5–20.0%)**	**High risk (>20%)**
Considering ASCVD risk estimate alone	Statin therapy not recommended	Consider statin therapy	Stalin therapy recommended	Statin therapy recommended
Considering ASCVD risk estimate + CAC score If CAC score = 0 If CAC score > 0	• Stalin therapy not recommended • Statin therapy not recommended	• Statin therapy not recommended • Consider statin therapy	• Statin therapy not recommended • Statin therapy recommended	• Statin therapy recommended • Statin therapy recommended
CAC score has role in modifying treatment plan	No	Yes: Reclassification up or down based on CAC score	Yes: Reclassification up or down based on CAC score	No

(ASCVD: atherosclerotic cardiovascular disease; CAC: coronary artery calcification)

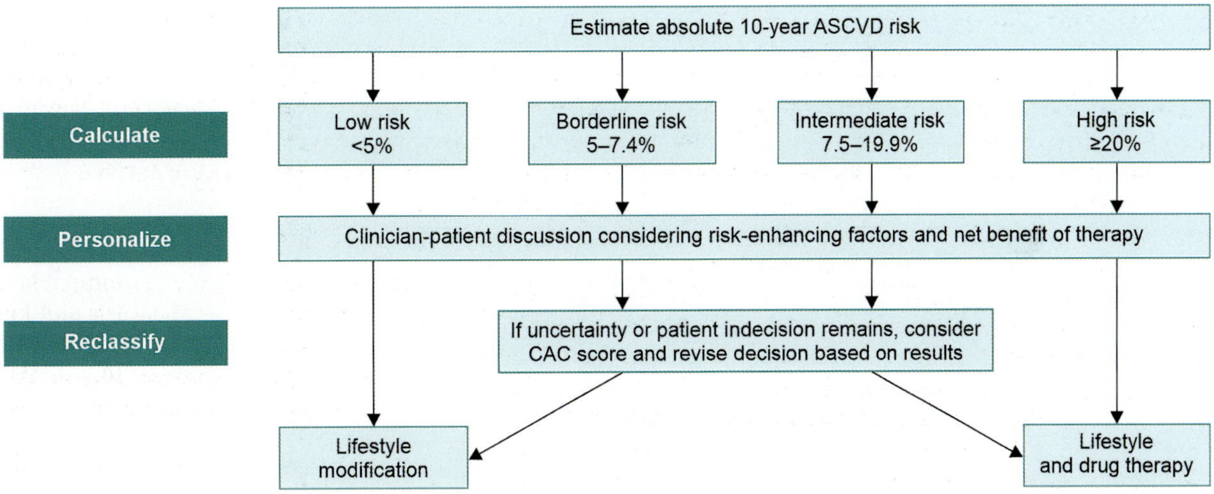

FLOWCHART 1: Approach to risk assessment in primary prevention of atherosclerotic cardiovascular disease (ASCVD) in the 2018 guideline on the management of blood cholesterol and the 2019 American College of Cardiology/American Heart Association (ACC/AHA) guideline on the primary prevention of cardiovascular disease.

Aggressive modification of lifestyle and risk factors in all individuals with CAC, along with appropriate timely initiation of therapy in those requiring it, is the cornerstone of CAC scanning. Although a CAC scan in all individuals after the age of 40 years would allow for the earlier and more thorough detection of a larger set of individuals with a higher risk for CVD. A more judicious method that has been proposed is given in **Flowchart 1**.[7]

ONLINE REFERENCES

Please scan the QR code provided at the end of the table of contents for References of this chapter.

SECTION 15 Preventive Cardiology

CHAPTER 115

Metabolic Risk Factors for Atherosclerotic Cardiovascular Disease: A Modern Lifestyle Disease Entity

Vijay Bang, Ashish Deshpande

ABSTRACT

Despite vast efforts being taken to reduce atherosclerotic cardiovascular disease (ASCVD) burden with conventional risk factor control, there remains significant residual risk. Recent evidence on nontraditional determinant factors of cardiometabolic health has advanced our understanding of modern lifestyle-related risk factors and their disease interactions. Chronic exposure to environmental stressors such as poor diet quality, ambient air pollution and noise, sedentarism, sleep deprivation, and psychosocial stress affects numerous intermediary pathways related to ASCVD, with a significant interplay with the conventional risk factors. These include body composition, cardiorespiratory fitness, and muscle strength and functionality which are increasingly recognized as major determinants of cardiovascular health. Collectively, low-risk lifestyle factors cause phenotypic adaptations, which shift the proinflammatory milieu conducive for high-risk atherosclerosis to an antiatherogenic milieu. By inhibiting the NLRP3 inflammasome, the ketone body β-hydroxybutyrate is likely to be an intermediary for many of these observed benefits. Adhering to low-risk lifestyle factors adds to the prognostic value of optimal conventional risk factor management. The aims of this chapter are (1) to discuss these novel lifestyle risk factors and their underlying biochemical principles and (2) to provide new perspectives on potential recommendations to improve long-term adherence to these low-risk lifestyle factors.

Keywords: ASCVD, metabolic risk factors, lifestyle risk factors, public health awareness.

INTRODUCTION

The global burden of obesity, type 2 diabetes mellitus (T2DM) and metabolic syndrome (MetS) is on the rise **(Fig. 1)** and may be the largest noninfectious pandemic known till date, subsequently leading to an enormous increase of atherosclerotic cardiovascular diseases (ASCVDs).[1] ASCVD heavily depends on modifiable factors,[2] but despite major efforts to manage conventional risk factors, significant residual risk remains which is found to vary across studies and methods of statistical analysis.[3]

Lifestyle modification has failed to show a significant impact on the burden caused by the twin epidemics of metabolic disease and ASCVD till present date. Rising healthcare costs highlight the need for new strategies that have the potential to improve long-term adherence to these low-risk lifestyle factors.

This chapter will (1) discuss the new lifestyle risk factors and potential public heath interventions that can reduce the burden from ASCVD and (2) provide novel perspectives on feasible recommendations to improve long-term adherence to low-risk lifestyle risk factors.

Of particular relevance in cardiovascular (CV) prevention is the effect of lifestyle risk factors on plaque phenotype and vulnerability, which is depicted in **Figure 2** and discussed below.[4]

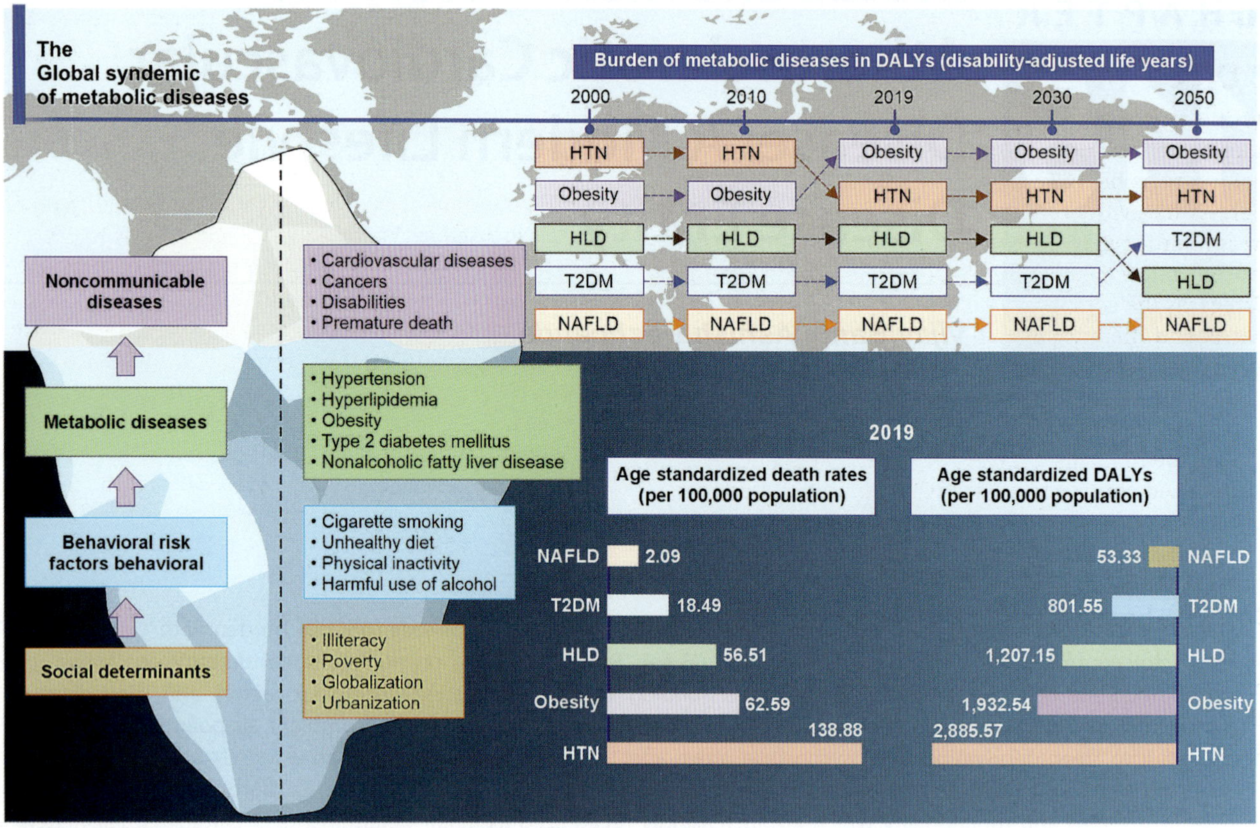

FIG. 1: Global burden of metabolic diseases.

(HLD: hyperlipidemia; HTN: hypertension; NAFLD: nonalcoholic fatty liver disease; T2DM: type 2 diabetes mellitus)

Courtesy: Professor Mamas A Mamas, Keele University, Keele, UK.

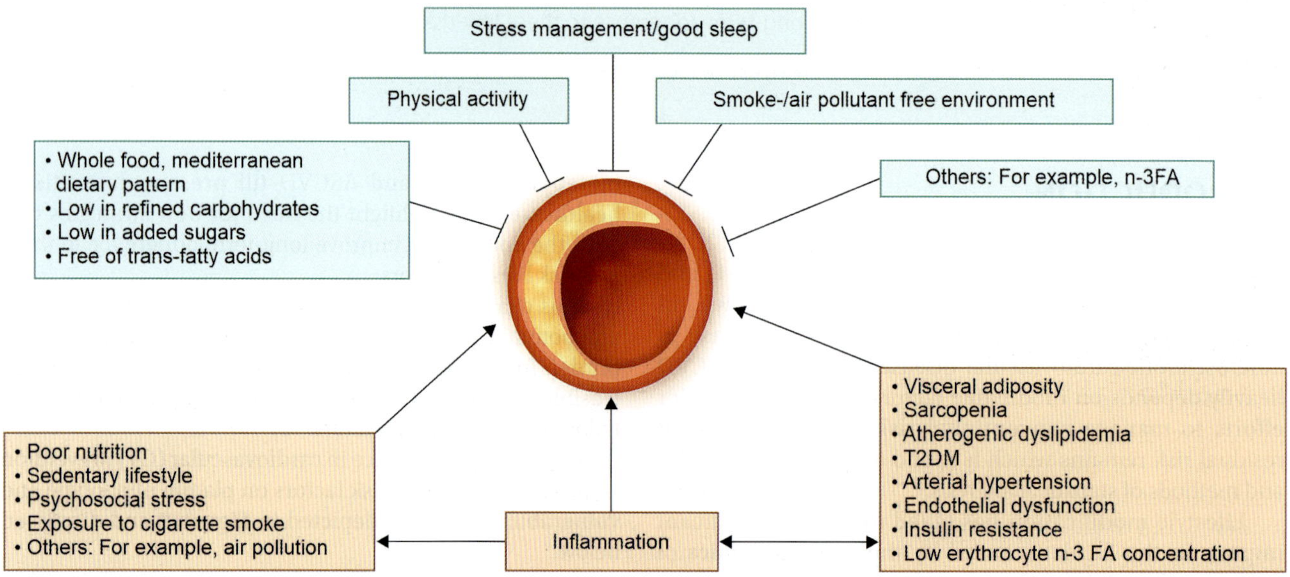

FIG. 2: Lifestyle and high-risk atherosclerosis. Lifestyle risk factors influence plaque composition by modulating traditional and novel pathways associated with CV risk. Red color indicates initiation of high-risk atherosclerosis and green color indicates inhibition of high-risk atherosclerosis.[4]

(FA: fatty acids; T2DM: type 2 diabetes mellitus)

LIFESTYLE RISK FACTORS

Diet

During the past decades, dietary advice has focused on calorie- and nutrient-based approaches, with one of the major targets being restriction of saturated fat.[5] However, there is no evidence that this has substantially reduced overall burden of cardiovascular disease (CVD). The calorie- and nutrient-centric model has a major limitation that it disregards the complex, weight-independent effects of food matrix and dietary patterns on metabolic and hormonal responses relevant to cardiovascular (CV) health.[5-8] Memory-based assessment methods such as food frequency questionnaires often produce data that is physiologically implausible.[9,10] This chapter will focus on evidence from randomized controlled trials (RCTs) on surrogate markers for cardiometabolic health and the clinical endpoints.

Food Based Recommendations versus Nutrient-based Recommendations

Judging a food's health effects by its individual nutrients and not considering the overall food matrix does not convey meaningful information.[2] Evidence from RCTs on clinical endpoints provides good support for the superiority of food-based recommendations without specific guidance regarding calories, as against nutrient- and calorie-based recommendations.[8] Two large dietary intervention trials with CV endpoints support this concept. The PREDIMED trial showed that a calorie-unrestricted Mediterranean-style dietary pattern adherence supplemented with four tablespoons of extravirgin olive oil or 30 g mixed nuts per day over 4.9 years in high-risk patients reduced inflammation[11] and the incidence of major CV events by 31% and 28%, respectively.[12] These effects were independent of body weight and lipid lowering.[12] This stands out in stark contrast to the Women's Health Initiative (WHI), the largest dietary RCT ever performed, in which a fat-restricted dietary pattern involving specific guidance on caloric intake failed to significantly reduce CV endpoints after 8 years despite achieving a substantial reduction in total fat intake (37.8–28.8%).[13]

Diet, Cardiovascular Disease, and Mortality

Unhealthy diets have been ranked as a major global factor for death and CVD.[14,15] Contemporary nutritional recommendations are based on studies on individual foods, nutrients, and dietary patterns in many prospective cohort studies conducted in North America, Europe, and East Asia, many short-term randomized intervention trials of physiologic risk factors and a few RCTs of dietary patterns on clinical outcomes which were conducted mainly in Western countries.[16]

Previous diet patterns [Dietary Approaches to Stop Hypertension (DASH), Mediterranean, Healthy Eating Index (HEI), and the recent EAT-Lancet Planetary diet] and their relationship to CVD and mortality have been tested almost exclusively in Western countries.[17] These diet scores have combined foods that are believed to be protective with foods or nutrients considered to be harmful and thus no diet score is focused exclusively on protective foods but there is an increased focus recently on higher intakes of protective foods for CVD prevention.[16] Additionally, all these previous diet scores have in common an emphasis on increased fruits, vegetables, legumes, nuts, and fish.

The PURE (Prospective Urban Rural Epidemiology) study was carried out replicated in five independent studies on a total of 245,000 people from 80 countries. The aim was to develop a healthy diet score that is associated with good health outcomes and which could be applied globally. In the PURE study, a healthy diet score was developed in 147,642 persons, from 21 countries, and the consistency of the diet score with events was examined in five large independent studies involving 70 countries. The healthy diet score was developed based on six foods each of which has been since long associated with a significantly lower risk of mortality, namely fruits, vegetables, nuts, legumes, fish, and dairy (mainly whole-fat). The range of scores was 0–6. The main outcome measures were all-cause mortality and major CV events. A higher diet score was associated with a significantly lower risk of death or CVD in regions with lower gross national incomes ($p < 0.0001$) than with high gross national incomes. The PURE score showed slightly stronger association with death or CVD than several other commonly used diet scores ($p < 0.001$ for comparison).[18]

Acknowledging that there is no one-size-fits-all approach to healthy eating across cultures, the PURE healthy diet generally translates to an eating pattern including **(Fig. 3)**:[18]

- *Fruits and vegetables*: 4–5 servings daily
- *Legumes*: 3–4 servings weekly
- *Nuts*: 7 servings weekly
- *Fish*: 2–3 servings weekly
- *Dairy*: 14 servings weekly

Body Composition versus Body Weight

The effects of diet on health seem to be more closely related to body composition rather than body weight and total fat mass per se, suggesting that body mass index (BMI) is not a sufficient indicator for assessing the effects of diet on health.[19] In the CENTRAL-MRI trial, a Mediterranean low-carbohydrate dietary pattern was superior to a low-fat diet in mobilizing atherogenic and diabetogenic fat depots in liver, pericardium, and pancreas. Changes in lipid traits related to MetS [triglycerides (TGs) and TG/high-density lipoprotein (HDL) cholesterol ratio] did not correlate well with BMI but correlated with reductions in visceral/hepatic fat.[20] This supports the notion that visceral fat, intraorgan

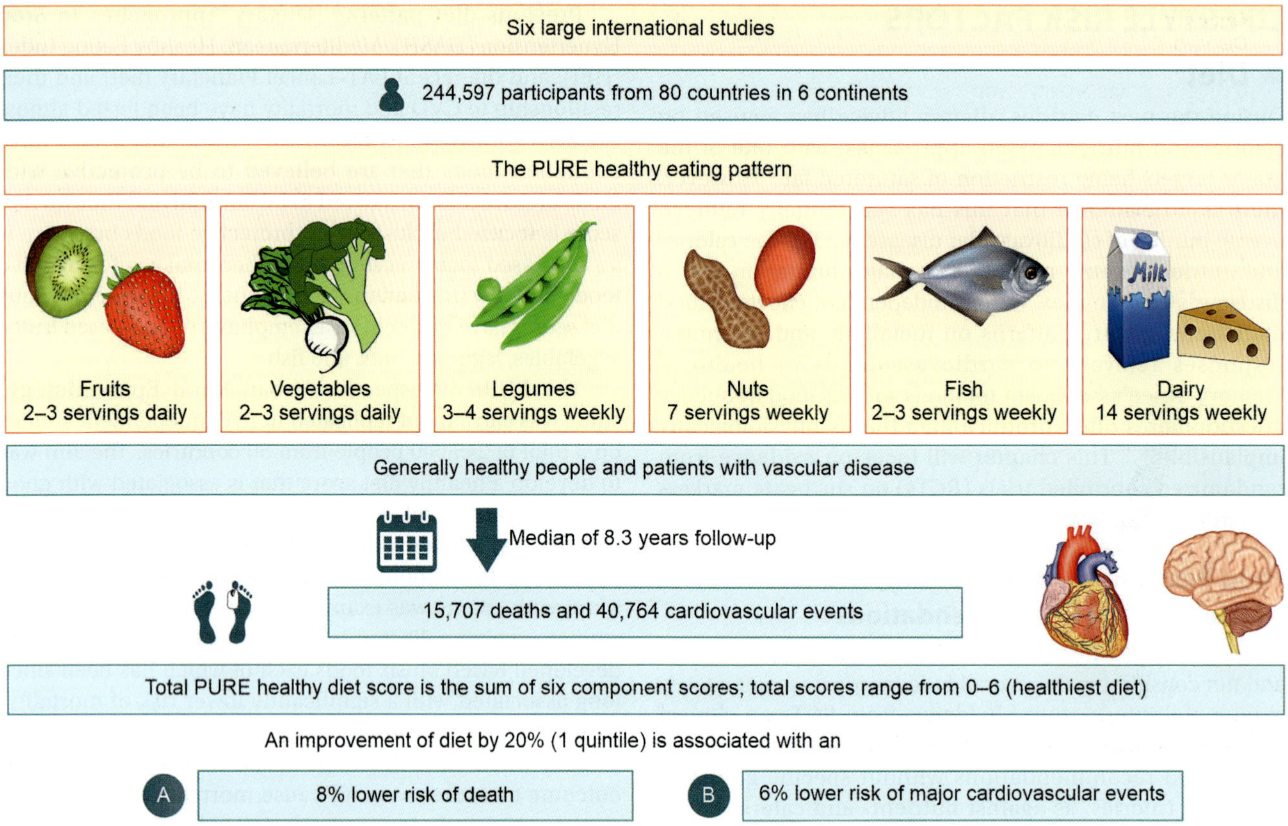

FIG. 3: The PURE (Prospective Urban Rural Epidemiology) study.[18]

fat, and subcutaneous adipose tissue depots have distinct correlation with cardiometabolic health,[21,22] and selective mobilization of visceral/ectopic fat is a fundamental mechanism which underlies improved metabolic function. Thus, the combination of anthropometric and laboratory markers which are indicative of visceral adiposity (e.g., waist circumference and TGs) appears more indicative of adipose tissue distribution than BMI.[23] Hypertriglyceridemic waist, a visceral adiposity marker combining elevated waist circumference (≥90 cm) and elevated fasting plasma TGs (≥2 mmol/L), is indicative of the high-risk metabolic phenotype[24] and/or high-risk atherosclerosis.[16] Waist-to-height-ratio is another inexpensive metric for better CV risk stratification than BMI and/or waist circumference alone; the suggested general cutoff being 0.5.[22,25]

Carbohydrate Restriction

Insulin resistance alters the metabolic responses to dietary signals. Insulin resistance clinically manifests itself as an intolerance to dietary carbohydrate wherein glycogen synthesis is impaired and dietary carbohydrate is diverted into de novo hepatic lipogenesis.[26] This is clinically relevant for dietary recommendations in MetS and T2DM and it provides a reasonable explanation in support of use of dietary carbohydrate restriction and (intermittent) caloric restriction in the dyslipidemic, insulin-resistant patient, where favorable metabolic changes are observed even in the absence of weight loss.[27-29]

Carbohydrate restriction is not a new concept and it was successfully applied to treat diabetes mellitus prior to the discovery of insulin.[30] With the discovery of insulin in 1923, which allowed acute diabetic control even with high carbohydrate diets, this potent therapy has largely been forgotten.

With more clarity in the delineation of the various cellular and metabolic responses to carbohydrate restriction, these dietary regimens have recently regained significant scientific interest. In the insulin-resistant phenotype, very low-carbohydrate dietary patterns resulting in nutritional ketosis have been shown to reduce systemic inflammation and most biomarkers of ASCVD risk **(Figs. 4A to C)**.[31]

Intermittent Calorie Restriction

Caloric restriction is a broad term which summarizes a set of dietary interventions involving chronically or periodically reduced energy intake without causing malnutrition.[32] It has consistently been found to extend healthy life span across a wide variety of species. However, the major limitation in humans is to sustain it for long-term. The fact that intermittent fasting regimens evoke similar cellular and

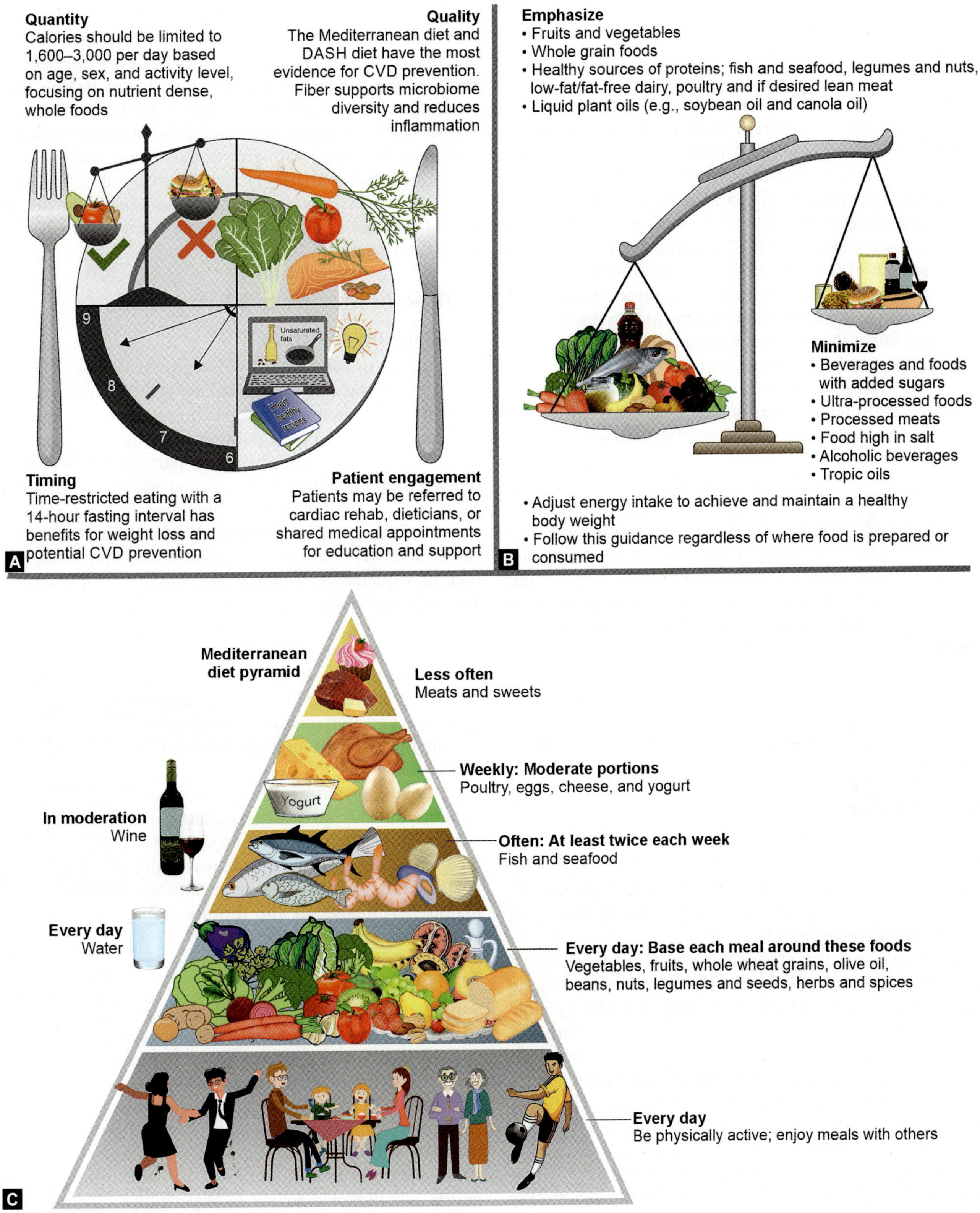

FIGS. 4A TO C: (A) Dietary pattern and intermittent calorie restriction.[2,34] (B) 2021 dietary guidance to improve cardiovascular health: A scientific statement from the American Heart Association. (C) Mediterranean diet pyramid.

metabolic adaptations to chronic caloric restriction is very encouraging. Time-restricted food intake has been linked to good cardiometabolic health in animals[33] as well as in humans.[28]

Intermittent states of negative energy balance activate a set of mechanisms wherein metabolism switches from lipid synthesis and fat storage to fat mobilization as free fatty acids and fatty acid-derived ketones. This has been linked to improvement in markers for cardiometabolic health (e.g., weight loss) and consequently beneficial effects on body composition such as visceral fat mobilization and retention of lean mass.[28] In people who have insulin resistance, metabolic outcomes are more favorable when the consumption of the daily dietary allotment is in the first half of the day rather than when the same caloric intake divided into multiple meals throughout the day.[34]

In a controlled feeding trial in men who had prediabetes, those who consumed their meals in a 6-hour window period in the morning showed a greater amelioration of metabolic markers than those on a control schedule (12-hour window period) within 5 weeks, which was independent of body weight.[35] Another study which compared two isocaloric weight-loss interventions showed greater improvement in metabolic markers in those consuming a bigger breakfast and a smaller dinner than in those doing vice versa.[36] The overall evidence supports the notion that the amount of time spent eating during each day[32] and the time at which food is consumed relative to the circadian rhythm (chrono-nutrition)[37] both modulate the effects of diet on cardiometabolic health. To date, no adverse signa such as electrolyte imbalance, nausea and vomiting, and hyperuricemia have been reported in intermittent fasting regimens.[38]

Dietary Patterns

To maintain good CV and overall health, strong evidence exists and the broad consensus is to minimize consumption of added sugars and refined grains and avoid industrial trans-fatty acids. These should be replaced with plant-based and animal-based whole foods.[2]

In the insulin-resistant phenotype, there is an large body of scientific literature which has convincingly documented the superiority of low-carbohydrate dietary patterns for glycemic control and weight control in T2DM.[27,39] It is therefore that the recently published Consensus Report of the American Diabetes Association and the European Association for the Study of Diabetes endorsed low carbohydrate diets (<26% of total energy) as one of the strategies to manage both hyperglycemia and hyperinsulinemia in T2DM.[40]

The "Mediterranean diet" supplemented by extravirgin olive oil and nuts is one of the most established dietary pattern with regard to reducing CV endpoints[12] and lowering apolipoprotein B (ApoB).[41] However, (1) the Mediterranean diet is very heterogeneous, (2) it has mostly been tested in a Mediterranean country, and (3) it might not be a feasible option for the global populations.

Emerging evidence from both animal and human studies suggests the utility of time restricted eating in cardio-metabolic disease. Ketogenic diets seem to phenocopy some of the biochemical characteristics of fasting that are associated with longevity and CV health. Nutritional ketosis has been linked to an inhibition of major signaling pathways associated with growth like insulin and insulin-like growth factor 1 (IGF-1) and induction of antioxidant genes. β-hydroxybutyrate (BHB) is also likely to be one of the intermediaries for many of the benefits observed with nutritional ketosis and caloric restriction.[42]

Role of Marine n-3 Fatty Acids

Mechanisms of Action

The marine n-3 fatty acids eicosapentaenoic acid (EPA) and docosahexaenoic acid (DHA) are essential to tissue cell membrane health, thereby modulating a variety of humoral, metabolic and structural parameters, **(Fig. 5)** which are related to cardiometabolic risk—in part due to their anti-inflammatory properties.[4] Of particular relevance to ASCVD is the beneficial effect of EPA on lipid metabolism, oxidative stress/inflammation, and endothelial function, which may delay the onset of atherosclerosis and may ameliorate the clinical sequelae associated with acute plaque disruption. The relevant associated mechanisms are inhibition of inflammation-related pathways and reduced leukocyte-endothelial adhesive interactions which include reduced circulating plasma levels of interleukin-6 (IL-6), tumor necrosis factor alpha (TNF-α), monocyte chemoattractant protein-1, and asymmetric dimethylarginine.[4]

The most consistent and significant CV benefit of DHA and EPA is protection from sudden cardiac death. This has been linked, in part, to their membrane stabilizing and antiarrhythmic properties in the setting of ischemia-induced ventricular tachycardia and ventricular fibrillation.[43]

It has also been linked to increased plaque stability and protection from the clinical sequelae associated with acute plaque destabilization and rupture, namely occlusion of arterial blood flow and infarction.[43,44]

Trial Evidence

Supplementation trials with high doses of both EPA[45] and DHA[46] have shown to affect surrogate markers relevant to ASCVD. EPA at a dose of 4 g/day, reduced oxidized-low density lipoprotein, lipoprotein-associated phospholipase A2 (Lp-PLA2) and high-sensitivity C-reactive protein (hsCRP) levels as compared to placebo.[45] DHA at 3 g/day reduced levels of IL-6, hsCRP, and granulocyte monocyte-colony stimulating factor and increased the anti-inflammatory matrix-metalloproteinase-2 in hypertriglyceridemic men after 3 months in various studies.[46]

Despite biological plausibility and favorable short-term effects on surrogate markers of cardiometabolic health, results of large trials assessing EPA and/or DHA supplementation on CV endpoints have been mixed, with

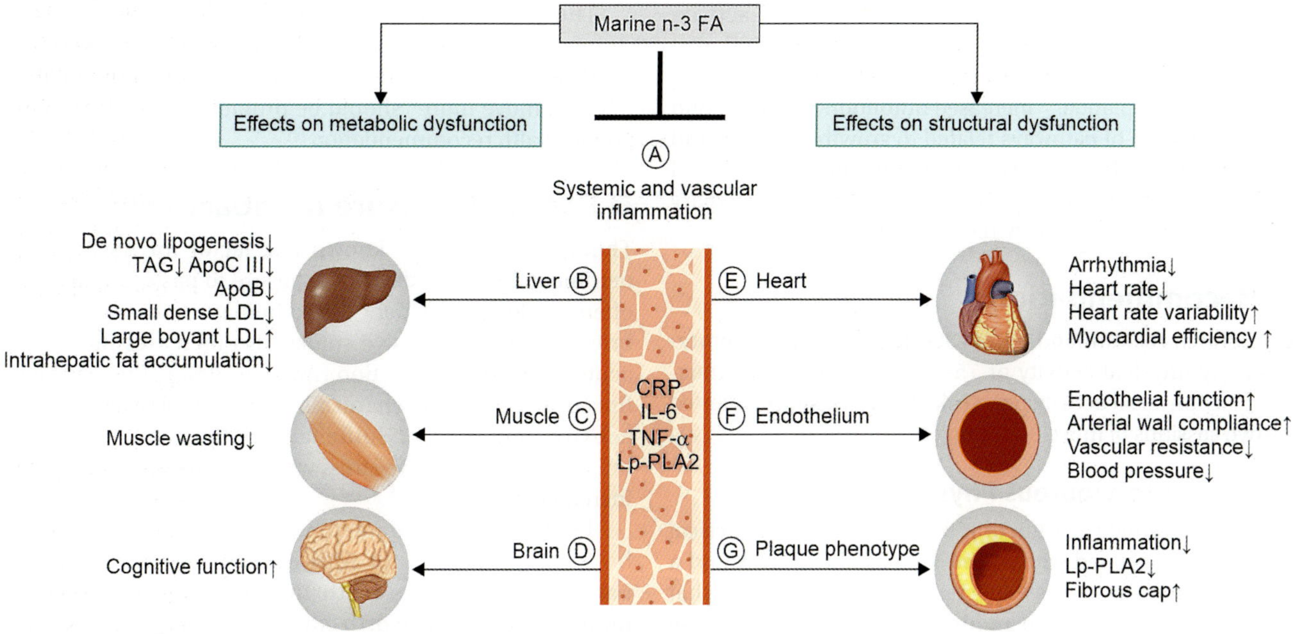

FIG. 5: Effects of marine n-3 FA, as demonstrated in mechanistic studies in human. Marine n-3 fatty acids and mechanisms related to cardiovascular risk. Mechanistic studies in humans have demonstrated that the marine n-3 fatty acids eicosapentaenoic acid (EPA) and/or docosahexaenoic acid (DHA) reduce serum triglycerides, shift low-density lipoprotein subfractions and reduce ApoB (B), favorably change body composition (B and C), have direct effects on cardiac electrophysiology, and mitigate adverse remodeling of the left ventricle after myocardial infarction (E), improve endothelial function and lower systolic and diastolic blood pressure (F), and increase plaque stability (G)—in part due to their inflammatory resolving properties (A). Furthermore, EPA/DHA improve cognitive function across different age groups (D).

(Apo: apolipoprotein; CRP: C-reactive protein; FA: fatty acids; IL-6: interleukin-6; LDL: low-density lipoprotein; Lp-PLA2: lipoprotein-associated phospholipase A2; TAG: triglycerides; TNF-α: tumor necrosis factor α)

few trials definitely showing a beneficial effect and others showing no significant effect. In ASCEND trial, 1 g n-3 fatty acids/day did not reduce adverse vascular events in patients with T2DM.[47] Conversely, in REDUCE-IT trial, treatment of patients at high CV risk (due to elevated TG levels and previous CV event or T2DM) with 4 g of EPA/day resulted in a 25% relative risk reduction in the primary composite endpoint of CV death, nonfatal myocardial infarction (MI), nonfatal stroke, coronary revascularization, or unstable angina compared with the placebo group.[48] These results were achieved on top of statin therapy, suggesting additive value of EPA.[48]

Collectively, the overall cumulative evidence from controlled studies on risk factors and recent clinical trials with CV endpoints, combined with the low-risk profile of n-3 polyunsaturated fatty acids, justifies their supplementation as a reasonable option to lower ASCVD risk in individuals who are infrequent fish consumers or are at high risk of ASCVD.[8]

PHYSICAL ACTIVITY

Physical inactivity and low cardiorespiratory fitness (CRF) are under-recognized cardiometabolic risk factors but which are strong independent predictors of CV outcomes in primary and secondary prevention of ASCVD across groups with different BMI.[49-52] High levels of physical activity and CRF in large part neutralize the adverse effects of adiposity and other traditional CVD risk factors, including the MetS.[49] Furthermore, there is clinically relevant evidence that a sedentary lifestyle independent of physical activity and loss of muscle strength and functionality might independently contribute to ASCVD risk.[53-55] Importantly, these factors can be improved, also in the middle age and elderly population.[56,57] Even if started late in life, physical activity improves functional independence and reduces mortality, maintaining a strong effect even after controlling for confounders like smoking, hypertension, diabetes, and obesity.[55] Thus, sedentary behavior reduction should be targeted as an independent therapeutic objective for overall CVD prevention and management.

Mechanism of Action

Physical activity evokes a complex endocrine and paracrine response linked to cardiometabolic health. Physical activity, especially resistance training, affects body composition in such a way that it promotes an overall anti-inflammatory and an antiatherogenic milieu.[57] There is a particular interest currently in skeletal muscle maintenance as a way of attenuating immunosenescence and inflammation, which is a hallmark of chronic, age-related diseases.[58]

Additional mechanisms of action of physical activity relevant to CV health include improvement in endothelial function, preservation of the stable phenotype of pre-existing atherosclerotic plaque,[57] increased autonomic balance, and downregulation of pathways related to growth signaling and inflammation.[57] There is also a mild antidepressant effect of physical activity which may constitute another intermediary pathway that can potentially reduce CV risk.

Recommendations

Guidelines recommend a 150–300 minutes of moderate-intensity physical activity or 75–150 minutes of vigorous-intensity physical activity per week for adults, supplemented by two sessions of muscle-building exercise.[59]

Moderate-to-vigorous Physical Activity

The recommended amount of 150–300 min/week of physical activity is associated with a 15% decreased CVD risk and a 4.5 year increase in life expectancy.[60] Given the fact that long-term adherence to moderate-to-vigorous exercise is difficult, it is encouraging to note that even 15 min/day of moderate-intensity exercise has been shown to confer significant health benefits and has been associated with a 14% reduction in all-cause mortality and increased life expectancy of 3.5 years.[61]

Sedentary Time

Sedentary time is very common and it accumulates while commuting, in schools and colleges, in the workplace, at home and in leisure settings.[62] Objective measurements from US adults show that they are exposed to an average of 6–8 hours of prolonged sitting time, and adults > 60 years old to an average of 8.5–9.6 hours sedentary time per day. The metabolic consequences of this sedentary behavior are obviously deleterious.

Epidemiological evidence implies that greater the time spent in sedentary behavior, greater is the all-cause and CV morbidity and mortality, suggesting prolonged sitting time as a population-wide, universal health risk. Evidence from preclinical and short-term studies in humans has identified various potential biological mechanisms, including decreased insulin sensitivity and impaired vascular endothelial-dependent dilation which are the key antecedents of age-related ASCVD risk. These factors can be reversed by having several short bouts of exercise as compared to uninterrupted sitting,[53] also including in the elderly population, which is very encouraging.[63]

This underscores the importance of working on population-wide initiatives to reduce sedentary behavior and to increase exercise time.[62] This can be implemented by workplace-based interventions that offer activity-permissive workstations wherein office workers are allowed to stand, walk, or pedal while doing desk-based tasks and the use of certain other activities to interrupt sedentary time.[53,59]

Thus, exercise training can be an effective and safe strategy for primary and secondary prevention of ASCVD across all age and weight groups. Thus, it is appropriate that "sit less, move more" should be promoted as an important public health recommendation.[59]

Passive Exposure to Tobacco Smoke

Though smoking is a known risk factor for ASCVD, the detrimental health effects of exposure to passive smoke are often overlooked. Evidence from human studies shows that brief exposure to passive smoke also increases the risk of acute myocardial infarction (AMI) by 30%.[64] This has been linked to various mechanisms such as increased platelet activity, impaired endothelial function, and increased inflammation/oxidative stress which are the mechanisms for increased risk of AMI.[64]

Epidemiological data shows an overall reduction in hospital admissions for AMI by 17% following smoking bans in public areas, with the greatest effect seen in nonsmokers.[65] It is worth noting that Helena, Montana experienced a decline in hospital admissions for AMI of 40% within 6 months after smoke-free legislation was, which was temporary, with admission rates returning to baseline (+46%) after the ban was suspended.[65] On the basis of all available evidence, smoke-free legislation, thus appears to be a prudent public health action in countries that have not already endorsed this yet.

Alternative Modes of Nicotine Delivery

Electronic nicotine delivery systems (ENDSs) such as e-cigarettes are increasingly used as they are supposed to be potentially less harmful, alternative modes of nicotine delivery.[66] Although results are mixed, there is some evidence to suggest that smokers switching to ENDS improve lung function[67] and disease symptoms which are attributable to asthma and chronic obstructive pulmonary disease.[67,68] However, considering the use of ENDS relative to absolute no use of nicotine, the best advisory is complete abstinence from smoking.

NOVEL LIFESTYLE RISK FACTORS

Chronic exposure to environmental stressors such as ambient air pollution and nocturnal and diurnal noise pollution,[69] sleep deprivation, both quantitative and qualitative, and psychosocial stress factors such as loneliness and depression are increasingly being recognized as independent risk factors for ASCVD. Evidence points to overlapping disease mechanisms which are closely related to sympathoadrenergic activation, upregulation of the hypothalamic–pituitary–adrenal (HPA) axis and systemic and cerebral chronic low-grade inflammation with resultant endocrine signaling and downstream ill effects on vascular health.[60,70]

Exposure to Ambient Air Pollution

Epidemiological and toxicological studies have long since established the fact that ambient air pollution is an independent risk factor for ASCVD.[69] Ambient particulate matter (PM), which is a principal component of air pollutants, has both acute and chronic effects on the CV system. The acute toxic effects (from seconds–hours) of exposure to ambient PM are mediated by oxidative stress, sympathoadrenergic activation, endothelial dysfunction, and effects on blood coagulability.[69] The highest risk for acute toxicity occurs within the framework of chronic exposure in susceptible patients characterized by preexisting "vulnerable plaque", "vulnerable, proarrhythmic myocardium", and "vulnerable, prothrombotic circulation".[69] These associations are strongest for fine particulate air pollutants [PM < 2.5 µm in diameter ($PM_{2.5}$)], which are a principal component of the combustion-derived nanoparticulate in diesel exhaust.[69] Public health interventions targeting reduced burden from ambient PM from air pollution, particularly $PM_{2.5}$, if targeted properly in a concerted manner have the potential to globally reduce morbidity and mortality from ASCVD on a large scale.[71]

- *Exposure to noise*: Exposure to noise exerts its detrimental effects on CV health through mechanisms which are similar to those of exposure to ambient air pollution.[69] To cite examples, exposure to nocturnal aircraft noise dose-dependently impaired endothelial function and caused sympathoadrenergic activation in a cohort of healthy adults previously free from ASCVD. Thus, chronic nonresolving inflammation appears to be a biologically plausible explanation for the observed association between chronic noise exposure and ASCVD, rendering it an important public health target, similar to air pollution.[72,73]
- *Sleep deprivation*: Chronic disruption of circadian rhythms, through adipose tissue dysfunction and associated high-risk metabolic traits, creates a milieu conducive for ASCVD.[74] A scientific statement from the American Heart Association argues that a sleep duration of ≥7 h/night for adults is conducive for good CV health.[70] This is in agreement with epidemiological data and evidence that total sleep duration of 6–8 h/day was associated with the lowest risk of deaths and major CV events in a large cohort of 116,632 people from 21 countries.[75] One common cause for sleep disturbance in adults is obstructive sleep apnea syndrome (OSAS), which calls for a broader screening for OSAS in CV prevention.[70]
- *Psychosocial stress*: The upregulation of the HPA axis is one of the principal mechanisms which translates chronic stress into adverse cardiometabolic outcomes. Chronic elevation of the stress hormone cortisol activates and enhances a set of phenotypic adaptations which promote a proinflammatory and proatherogenic milieu. This causes multiple changes such as visceral fat accumulation, increased peripheral protein/muscle catabolism, and insulin resistance.[76] These observations provide a biologically plausible concept for the increased risk for ASCVD with chronic stress in humans and would justify the implementation of stress management programs like meditation or physical activity to prevent and manage ASCVD. This is particularly important given the fact that psychosocial distress serves as a barrier to adoption of a healthy lifestyle on the one hand and, on the other hand, behavioral compensations (e.g., smoking and increased alcohol consumption) exacerbate novel and traditional risk factors, thus causing an additive detrimental effect.[77]

Circadian Rhythm and Cardiovascular Disease

A growing body of clinical and experimental evidence suggests a significant link between CV dysfunction and the intrinsic human circadian biology. There is now substantial evidence that diurnal changes in the normal daily 12-hour light and 12-hour dark cycle significantly influence the physiology and the pathophysiology of the CV system **(Fig. 6)**. One of the most profound effects of the circadian rhythm on CV function is its influence on heart rate (HR) and blood pressure (BP). These parameters exhibit diurnal rhythms with BP higher in the morning and lower in the evening. Endothelial cellular function, platelet aggregation, and thrombus formation also exhibit normal circadian rhythms that follow 24-hour cycle. It is noteworthy that the onset of many cardiac events, such as MI, arrhythmias, stroke, heart failure, and sudden cardiac death, exhibits diurnal variation with higher incidence of events occurring in the early morning.[78]

Effects of the Circadian System and Lifestyle on CV Function

The CV responses to all common behaviors (e.g., sleep and exercise) across day and night have been well-established. These CV responses are superimposed on the basal circadian

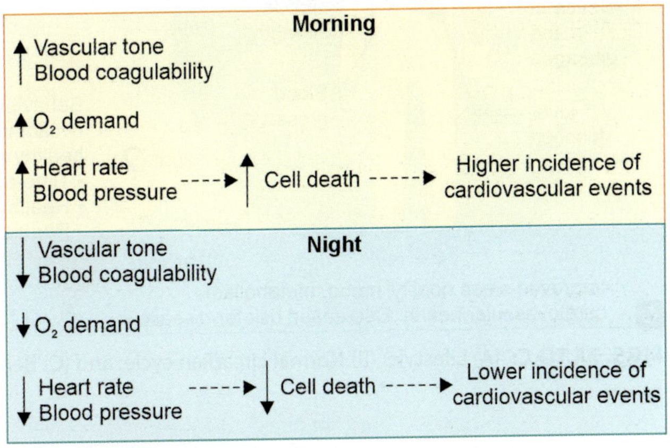

FIG. 6: Circadian rhythm regulates the physiological and pathological function of the heart.[79]

rhythms in CV physiology. These behaviors can occur at any circadian phase; for example, emergency workers such as healthcare workers or firefighters or law enforcement officers may be exposed to stresses at any time of day or night. It is thus important to determine the nature of these interacting effects. It is important to see whether the behavioral and circadian CV effects are simply additive, or are there more complex interactions (e.g., multiplicative). For example, common daily behaviors such as arousal from sleep, a sudden postural change, and a sudden increase in physical activity during the morning could trigger adverse events at specific circadian phases, especially in vulnerable individuals **(Figs. 7A to C)**.[80]

INTERPLAY BETWEEN METABOLIC RISK FACTORS AND LIFESTYLE RISK FACTORS

Five CV risk factors accompany the MetS—atherogenic dyslipidemia comprising of [elevated ApoB, elevated TG, small low-density lipoprotein (LDL) particles, and low HDL cholesterol], high BP, elevated glucose levels, a prothrombotic state, and a proinflammatory state. The likelihood of a person developing MetS is increased by underlying risk factors such as obesity, insulin resistance, sedentary habits, and advancing age. Besides being at a higher risk for ASCVD,

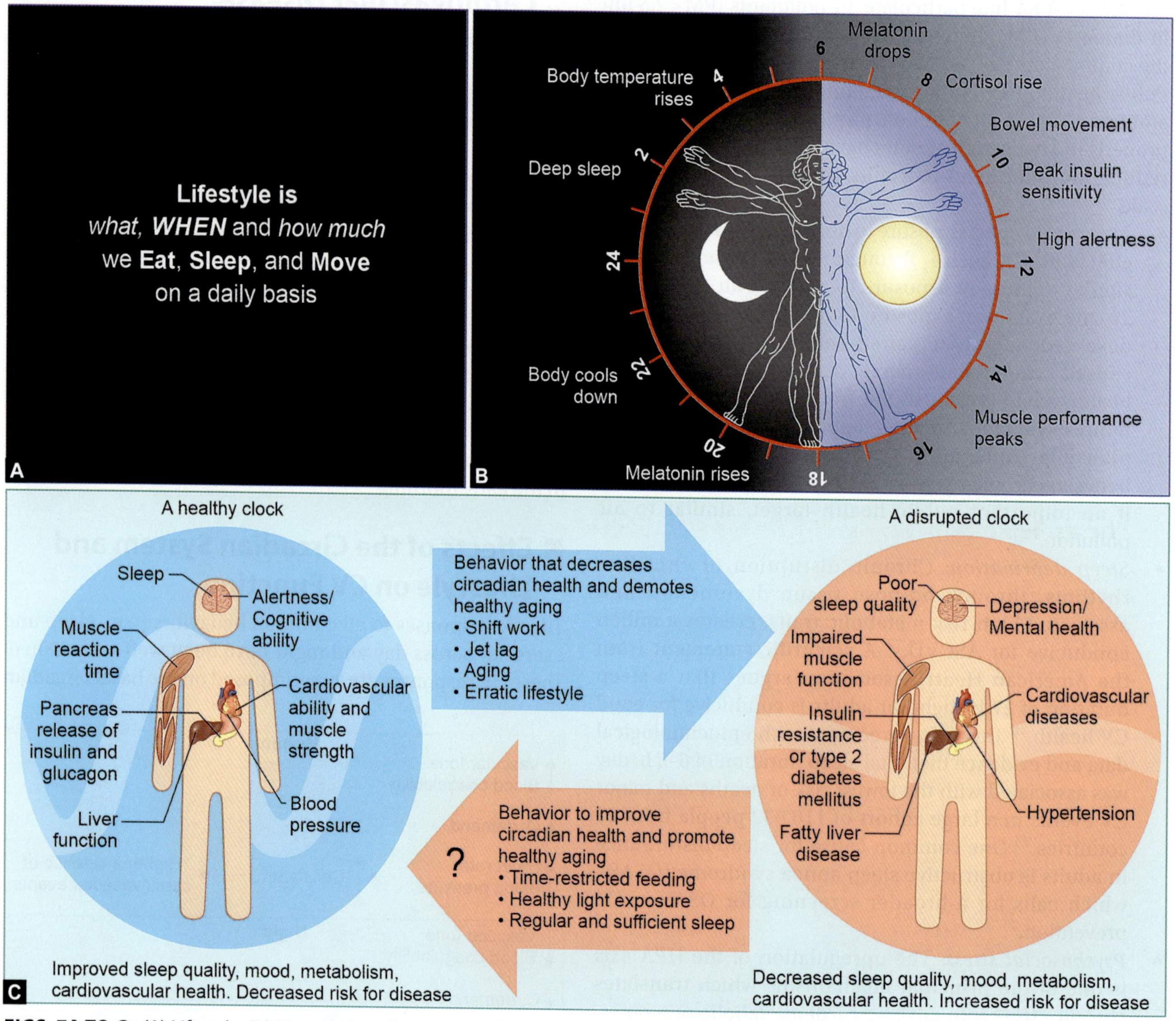

FIGS. 7A TO C: (A) Lifestyle; (B) Normal circadian cycle; and (C) Behaviors to improve circadian health.[80]

persons with the MetS are also at increased risk for T2DM and deserve management to reduce the risk for both T2DM and ASCVD.

The two major strategies for treatment of affected persons are modification of the underlying risk factors and drug treatment of the particular metabolic risk factors wherever appropriate. For the underlying risk factors, the first-line therapy is therapeutic lifestyle changes, which include weight loss in obese persons, increased physical activity, and antiatherogenic diet. These changes when implemented together will improve all of the metabolic risk factors. Considering individual risk components, drug therapies that promote lowering of ApoB and raise HDL cholesterol will be needed for atherogenic dyslipidemia in high-risk patients. Hypertension will require requisite treatment with drugs. When hyperglycemia reaches diabetic levels, glucose-lowering agents will be required when dietary control is no longer effective. Thus, ASCVD can very well be considered a modern lifestyle disease entity in today's era.[81]

FUTURE DIRECTIONS

Shifting the focus (1) from BMI to body composition and CRF, (2) from nutrient- and calorie-based approaches to food-based, dietary recommendations,[82] and (3) addressing the issues novel lifestyle risk factors through public health interventions might lead to more feasible and sustainable lifestyle guidance, improve the long-term adherence to risk factor control, and enhance prognosis,[80] with a multipronged approach achieving a better cumulative benefit.[83]

Several approaches have been proposed to encourage lifestyle modification; (1) peer group-based interventions have already been shown to be effective for global CV risk factor modification and it has been well documented in tobacco cessation in particular, (2) use of e-health devices, (3) rehabilitation programs, (4) motivational interviews, and (5) the use of positive messages rather than negative ones which stress upon the positive impact of lifestyle modification.[82]

CONCLUSION

Cardiovascular disease risk factors such as obesity, diabetes, hypertension, and dyslipidemia are in part consequences of high-risk lifestyle risk factors such as poor diet quality, sedentary behavior habits, high exposure to ambient air pollution/noise, sleep deprivation, and psychosocial stress. Adhering to a low-risk lifestyle reduces CVD risk in a multifactorial and multipronged manner. It adds significantly to the prognostic benefit of conventional risk factor control in CVD prevention. Collectively, these low-risk lifestyle factors cause a set of phenotypic adaptations that shift the proinflammatory milieu conducive for high-risk atherosclerosis, to an antiatherogenic milieu which has tremendous CV benefits. This serves as a powerful public health message for both clinicians and patients globally.

ONLINE REFERENCES

Please scan the QR code provided at the end of the table of contents for References of this chapter.

CHAPTER 116

Meditation and Yoga for Cardiac Rehabilitation after Myocardial Infarction

Mohit D Gupta, Dixit Goyal, Girish MP

ABSTRACT

Despite recent advances in pharmacological and interventional therapies, coronary artery disease carries a high morbidity and mortality, and exercise-based cardiac rehabilitation (CR) programs have shown to reduce cardiovascular mortality and hospitalization and improve physiological and psychological well-being in patients with cardiovascular disease. Such programs are expensive and limited to resource-limited countries such as India. Yoga is a traditional Indian mind–body practice that combines gentle physical exercises (physical functioning) with breathing and meditation (psychological functioning) and promotes healthy lifestyles (secondary prevention), thereby inherently addressing the key objectives of CR. It has been shown in different trials and meta-analysis to act through multiple pathways such as downregulating hypothalamic–pituitary–adrenal (HPA) axis, modulating neurotransmitters, decreasing sympathetic overactivity, improving metabolic parameters and leading to reduced cardiac risk factors, improvement in physical (functioning, quality of life) and psychological (decreased anxiety and depression) health, and reduction in cardiac events. A recent trial has shown improved self-rated health and early return to preinfarct activities after acute myocardial infarction. However, based on existing literature, yogic and meditation interventions are not proven superior to exercise-based CR and still can be used as a suitable alternative, especially in a country such as India.

Keywords: Cardiovascular diseases, cardiac rehabilitation, yoga, meditation.

INTRODUCTION

Cardiovascular diseases (CVDs) are the most common cause of death across the globe, with every one in four deaths in India attributed to it. Coronary artery disease (CAD) and stroke are major contributors of CVD mortality in India (83%), with CAD being predominant.[1] The number of cases of ischemic heart disease increased from 10.2 million in 1990 to 23.8 million in 2016, and its rising prevalence is an alarming concern.[2] Despite improvements in pharmacological and interventional therapies, these patients still carry high mortality and risk of further events. Risk factor modification plays a crucial role in secondary prevention. Hypertension, diabetes mellitus, dyslipidemia, obesity, smoking, physical inactivity, unhealthy diet, and psychosocial stress are the common risk factors for CVD.

Exercise-based cardiac rehabilitation (CR) is an established evidence-based program that has been shown to reduce cardiovascular mortality and hospitalization and improve physiological and psychological well-being in patients with CVD.[3] It is a comprehensive recovery program involving multidisciplinary teams to deliver exercise training, stress management, promote healthy eating, smoking cessation, medication adherence, psychosocial support, and secondary prevention. It is a Class I recommendation for use in patients with myocardial infarction (MI) by the European Society of Cardiology, American Heart Association, and American College of Cardiology guidelines.[4,5] Such rehabilitation programs are quite expensive and need large infrastructure, so they are limited in low- and middle-income countries such as India. Potentially, low-cost models of CR based on traditional mind–body practices (e.g., *raja*-yoga, tai chi) could improve availability of CR in low- to middle-income countries and increase options of exercise training in high-income countries.[6]

Meditation and yoga have been known since medieval times. The word "yoga" is derived from a Sanskrit word that is symbolically described as the association of inner self with the universe with a main purpose to achieve consonance between the mind, soul, and body. Its aim is to attain salvation of the soul. Yoga can be defined as a holistic approach to mind–body interaction and is an incorporation of various gentle physical exercises (physical working) with respiratory training and meditation practices (psychological functioning). Yoga also includes lifestyle modifications such as smoking and alcohol cessation and promotes a healthy diet intake.[7,8]

POTENTIAL MECHANISMS OF ACTION OF YOGA AND MEDITATION

Several risk factors are often responsible for triggering the chain of pathophysiological processes that underly the clinical continuum of CVD manifesting with various symptoms.[9] Risk factors such as elevated cholesterol, hypertension, diabetes mellitus, smoking, and obesity induce oxidative stress and hence endothelial dysfunction leading to target organ damage. The target organ damage is preceded by numerous mediating events, including vasoactive mediators, inflammatory response, and vascular remodeling. Yogic interventions are known to have *various physical and psychological effects* that interrupt this chain of events by several mechanisms **(Flowcharts 1A and B)**.

- *Affecting autonomic nervous system (ANS)*: It affects the ANS by downregulating the hypothalamus–pituitary–adrenal axis and sympathetic stimulation. It mainly enhances the parasympathetic supply through vagus and maintains sympathovagal balance. It helps psychologically by reducing the perceived stress

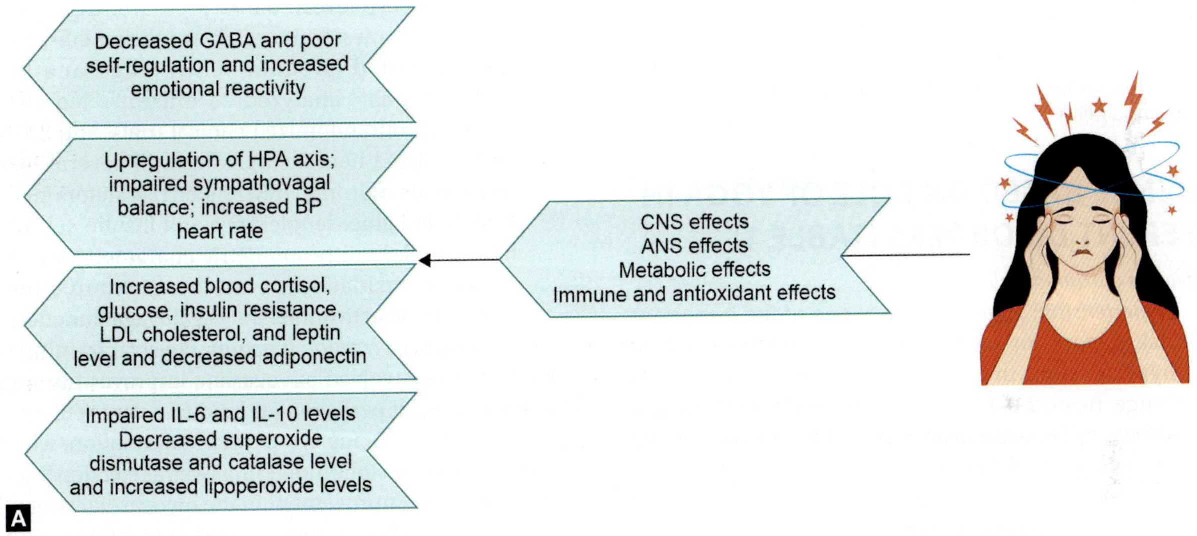

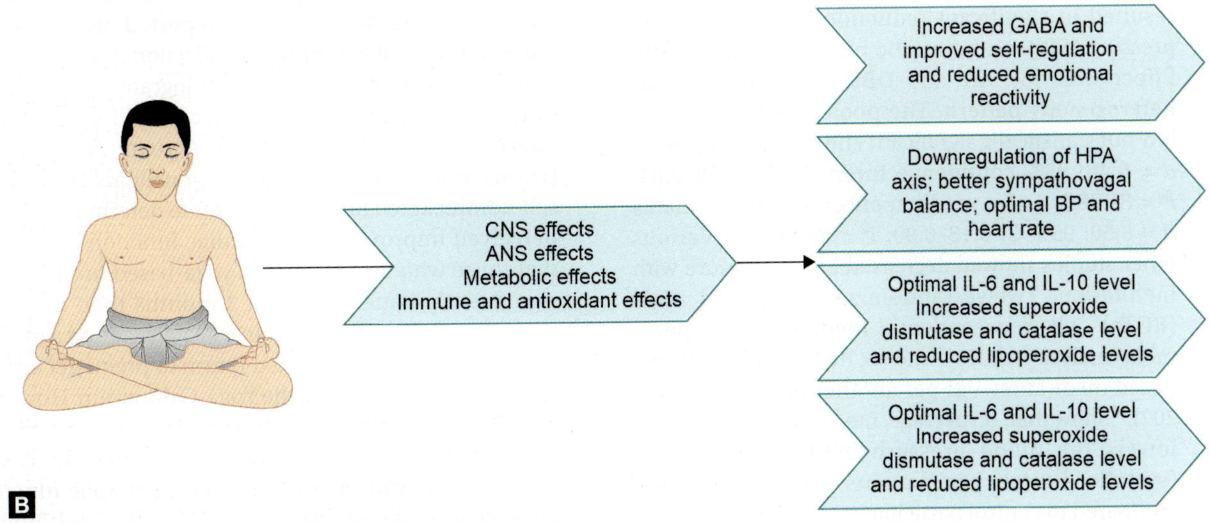

FLOWCHARTS 1A AND B: Different pathways of action of meditation and yoga.

(ANS: autonomic nervous system; BP: blood pressure; CNS: central nervous system; GABA: gamma-aminobutyric acid; HPA: hypothalamic–pituitary–adrenal; IL: interleukin; LDL: low-density lipoprotein) and physiologically by decreasing cardiac workload through optimal heart rate, blood pressure, heart rate variability, and other inflammatory mediators. This twofold psychophysiological effect improves the metabolic profile (insulin resistance, high cholesterol, glucose tolerance, etc.), and hence combats the risk factors (oxidative stress, endothelial dysfunction, and deranged coagulation profile) leading to reduction in cardiovascular events.

- Normalization of endocrinal function (lower cortisol and reduced renin activity) and gastrointestinal function
- Improved musculoskeletal fitness and posture
- Enhanced energy levels
- Normalization of body weight
- Better sleep and immunity
- Reduced pain and better quality of life
- Enhanced mood
- Feeling of subjective well-being and self-acceptance
- Reduced anxiety and depression
- Improved biochemical profile in terms of antioxidant effects of yoga such as reduced cholesterol, triglycerides, and glucose levels, increased lymphocyte count, and many more[10,11]

EVIDENCE BASED ON ROLE OF YOGA IN DIFFERENT DISORDERS (TABLE 1)

- *Effect on cardiovascular risk factors*:
  - *Hypertension*: Hypertension is one of the important risk factors for CVD. Depending on the stage of hypertension, the mean odds of developing CVD range from 2.0 to 3.6.[12] Yogic interventions are known to decrease heart rate and blood pressure by modulating ANS. In a recent meta-analysis, eight trials comprising 1,035 participants reported resting blood pressure. The results show that yogic interventions resulted in significant reduction in systolic blood pressure (SBP) and diastolic blood pressure (DBP). Effect sizes for SBP and DBP depicted a similar heterogeneity pattern. The pooled results depict a low but statistically significant effect on SBP [Cohen's d = 0.46; 95% confidence interval (CI) 0.08–0.84; I^2 = 81.86%] and a medium effect on DBP (Cohen's d = 0.56; 95% CI 0.13–0.99; I^2 = 84.84%).[13] Various other studies showed decreased blood pressure with meditation. Twelve randomized controlled trials (RCTs)—all transcendental meditation—as per a meta-analysis in 2015[14] and six RCTsall mindfulness-based meditation—as per another meta-analysis in 2021[15] show that, on average, meditation intervention lowers the blood pressure by 4–5/2–3 mm/Hg (systolic/diastolic) in patients with hypertension compared to control participants.
  - *Metabolic syndrome*: This is characterized by hypertension, dyslipidemia, elevated fasting blood glucose, and abdominal obesity and is a significant risk factor for CVD.[16] Yogasana and meditation intervention have been extensively studied in the context of metabolic syndrome in different trials. In a recent meta-analysis comprising a total of 15 trials, 4 trials comprising 700 participants reported lipid profiles and showed reduction in total cholesterol, low-density lipoproteins, and triglyceride levels and increase in high-density lipoprotein (HDL) levels.[13] Another two studies that included meditation intervention, one with 103 coronary heart disease (CHD) patients, showed significant improvement in insulin resistance, blood pressure, and glucose tolerance with transcendental meditation intervention.[17] The other study showed significant improvement in waist circumference, blood glucose levels, blood pressure, triglycerides, and HDL cholesterol level.[18] Another meta-analysis that included predominantly yogasana-based interventions[19] analyzed 26 uncontrolled clinical trials, 21 nonrandomized clinical trials, and 22 RCTs and reported beneficial changes in several insulin resistance syndrome (IRS) related risk factors for CVD. It included glucose tolerance and insulin sensitivity, lipid profiles, anthropometric characteristics, blood pressure, oxidative stress, coagulation profiles, sympathetic activation, and cardiovagal function.
- *Improvement in cardiac function*: Physical training such as stretching involved in yogasana improves fibrinolysis and myocardial perfusion and reduces ventricular filling pressures by reducing sympathetic stimulation, which in turn improves systolic function, as well as ejection fraction, because of an improvement in the myocardial strength.[20] In different studies, changes in cardiac function have been looked at using clinical patient-reported measures and measurements of left ventricular ejection fraction (LVEF) and diastolic function on echocardiogram. Three studies evaluated cardiac function using clinical improvement. Sharma et al.[21] used the Duke Activity Status Index (DASI) and derived metabolic equivalents from these self-administered functional scores to determine patient-perceived improvement in cardiac function and found that those who underwent the yoga-based program had significantly better scores at 3 months than a control group ($p < 0.001$). Prabhakaran et al.[8] also found a modest improvement in self-reported return to preinfarct activity (88.3 vs. 87.0; $p = 0.039$) in the Yoga-CaRe group. However, a similar questionnaire administered by Tillin et al.[22] (The International Physical Activity Questionnaire) showed no subjective improvement in perceived cardiac function between groups ($p = 0.8$).

TABLE 1: Randomized controlled trials looking at yoga-based cardiac rehabilitation (CR).

Study	Place	Presentation	Number of patients (I:C)	Intervention	Control	Follow-up	Outcomes	Results
Raghuram et al.[23]	India single center	CABG	250 (129:121)	12-month yoga program	12-month exercise-based CR	6 weeks, 6 months, 6 years	LVEF, BMI, lipid profile, FBS physiological scoring, HADS-anxiety, HADS-depression, PSS, PANAS	• Overall improvement in LVEF with no difference with groups • At 12 months, LVEF improved in yoga group ($p = 0.001$) in those with LVEF < 53%, LVEF 47–53% at 1 year versus 49% in control • Significant difference in weight loss in those with BMI > 23 kg/m^2 ($p = 0.038$), total cholesterol ($p = 0.61$), total triglycerides ($p = 0.03$), total HDL ($p = 0.003$), total LDL ($p = 0.75$), total VLDL ($p = 0.03$), PSS ($p = 0.12$), PANAS-positive ($p = 0.02$), PANAS-negative ($p = 0.97$), HADS-anxiety ($p = 0.42$), HADS-depression ($p = 0.07$)
Yadav et al.[27]	India single center	Stable CAD	80 (40:40)	60 minutes daily yoga regimen for 3 months + educational sessions	Conventional medical treatment	3 months	Pulmonary function, HR, SBP, and DBP	Statistical improvement in pulmonary function reduction in HR, SBP, and DBP (all $p < 0.05$)
Christa et al.[28]	India multicenter	ACS-MI	79 (39:40)	12-week yoga-based cardiac rehab as adjunct	Standard care (not exercise based)	ECG at 3 weeks, 13 weeks	Heart rate variability	No deference in time domain indices, high frequency power (ms2) $p = 0.005$, total power (nu) $p = 0.10$
Tillin et al.[22]	UK multicenter	ACS	60 (25:35)	Addition of at least 18 yoga classes to standard program control-standard UK NHS cardiac rehab program	Exercise-based CR	3 months	Filling pressures (E/e'), 6MWT, BP, HR, blood profile, QOL	E/e' $p = 0.4$, 6MWT $p = 0.7$, resting SBP $p = 0.5$, resting DBP $p = 0.6$, resting HR $p = 0.8$, international physical activity score $p = 0.8$, EQ-5D health status $p = 0.10$, EQ-5D self-rated thermometer $p = 0.6$, PSS $p = 0.11$
Prabhakaran et al.[8]	India multicenter	ACS	3,959 (1,970:1,989)	Yoga-CaRe 12-week program	Enhanced standard care (dependent on site, but not all exercised based)	Minimum 6 months; median 21.6 months	• MACE, QOL using EQ-5D-5L at 12 weeks • Self-reported return to preinfarct activity	• MACE $p = 0.41$ • EQ-5D-5L $p = 0.002$ • Return to preinfarct activity $p = 0.039$
Sharma et al.[21]	India single center	CAD-medically managed MI with LVSD	66 (33:33)	12-week yoga-based cardiac rehab as adjunct	Standard care (not exercise based)	3 months	LVEF biochemical, total triglycerides, cholesterol, LDL, HDL, QOL, DASI and MET, anxiety and depression; HAM-A CDS	• No difference in LVEF ($p = 0.218$) • No difference in biochemical measures • Statistically significant improvement in QOL ($p < 0.001$) and anxiety and depression ($p < 0.001$)

(ACS: acute coronary syndrome; BMI: body mass index; BP: blood pressure; CABG: coronary artery bypass graft; CAD: coronary artery disease; CDS: cardiac depression scale; DASI: Duke Activity Status Index; DBP: diastolic blood pressure; ECG: electrocardiogram; EQ-5D: EuroQol-5 Dimension; FBS: fasting blood sugar; HADS: Hospital Anxiety and Depression Scale; HAM-A: Hamilton Anxiety Rating Scale; HDL: high-density lipoprotein; HR: heart rate; LDL: low-density lipoprotein; LVEF: left ventricular ejection fraction; LVSD: left ventricular systolic dysfunction; MACE: major adverse cardiovascular events; MET: metabolic equivalent of task; MI: myocardial infarction; 6MWT: 6-minute walk test; PANAS: positive and negative affect schedule; PSS: Perceived Stress Scale; QOL: quality of life; SBP: systolic blood pressure; VLDL: very-low-density lipoprotein)

Two studies looked at LVEF after yoga-based rehabilitation. Raghuram et al.[23] found that in patients with reduced systolic function at baseline (<53%), significant improvement in LVEF was seen in the yoga group at 1 year, whereas Sharma et al.[21] did not find a statistically significant difference between the groups, which could be due to shorter follow-up being limited to only 3 months.

- *Improvement in psychological health*: Psychosocial variables such as stress, depression, and anxiety are always linked to CVDs at different stages, causing arteriosclerosis and severe cardiac symptoms that may progress to chronic diseases.[24] Yoga and meditation have been shown to modulate neurotransmitters where increase in melatonin, aminobutyric acid, endorphins, and a variety of other neurotransmitters and a drop in stress markers such as 8-hydroxydeoxyguanosine can help in reducing stress.[25] In a meta-analysis, 4,138 participants from 5 trials were assessed for quality of life using 3 different questionnaires [Minnesota Living with Heart Failure Questionnaire (MLWHFQ), The Kansas City Cardiomyopathy Questionnaire (KCCQ), and EuroQol-5 Dimension (EQ-5D)]. Stress was measured in two studies using perceived stress scale and anxiety was assessed with "The Hospital Anxiety and Depression Scale (HADS)" in two studies and depression in three studies with two scales, HADS and "Beck's Depression Inventory. Significant decrease in depression and anxiety was seen with improved quality of life with yoga.[13]
- *Reduction in major adverse cardiovascular events (MACE)*: Prabhakaran et al. conducted a large RCT in India (Yoga-CaRe) to evaluate the effects of yoga-based CR on MACE (composite of all-cause mortality, MI, stroke, or emergency cardiovascular hospitalization) and self-rated health on the EQ-5D level visual analog scale at 12 weeks. The study enrolled 3,959 patients with acute myocardial infarction (AMI) with a median and minimum follow-up of 22 and 6 months, respectively. Patients were individually randomized to receive either a Yoga-CaRe program (n = 1,970) or enhanced standard care involving educational advice (n = 1,989). No statistically significant difference was seen in MACE events between both the groups (6.7% vs 7.4%, $p = 0.41$), whereas the Yoga-CaRe group had greater return to preinfarct activities with significantly improved self-rated health. No difference in MACE could be due to lack of statistical power to show a difference in MACE.

In another small trial from India (n = 42), a CR program that included yoga was associated with greater reductions in cardiovascular risk factors, need for revascularization procedures, and size of atherosclerotic lesions on coronary angiography at 1 year, when compared with controls.[26]

CONCLUSION

In low- and middle-income countries, such as India, conventional exercise-based CR programs are lacking as most hospitals cannot afford the infrastructure, and recruiting large multidisciplinary teams is challenging. Each year approximately 1.5 million people suffer from MI in India, further highlighting the need for more accessible and easier to afford options. Different studies have shown effectiveness of yogic and meditation interventions in improving cardiac risk factors and psychological parameters such as blood pressure, metabolic variables, depression, stress, anxiety, and quality of life of patients in CAD patients. Patients who underwent yoga-based CR showed improvement from baseline in multiple domains, and while not proven to be superior to comprehensive exercise-based CR, yoga-based CR might be a suitable alternative option, especially in countries such as India. Furthermore, in future, RCTs with larger sample size and better designs are needed to improve our understanding of yogic and meditation interventions on cardiac parameters such as MACE.

ONLINE REFERENCES

Please scan the QR code provided at the end of the table of contents for References of this chapter.

CHAPTER

117 Reversibility of Atherosclerosis is a Fact Not a Myth

Shishu Shankar Mishra, Biswaranjan Mishra, Satyanarayan Routray

ABSTRACT

Atherosclerosis is the most common cardiovascular disease due to lipid accumulation and resulting inflammation of the arteries thereby leading to clinical complications like myocardial infarction and stroke. In recent times there have been advances in understanding of molecular and cellular level of pathogenesis of atherosclerosis. In past decade with use of exploring strategies, it has been well established that the process of atherosclerosis can be prevented and treated as well as reversed with both pharmacological as well as nonpharmacological modalities. This chapter encompasses the pathophysiology of atherosclerosis along with strategies to reverse the process. Measures such as early screening, precise imaging, and molecular probes help repair the atherosclerotic arteries, thereby reducing the cardiovascular events and morbidities.

Keywords: Atherosclerosis, reversing, plaque progression.

INTRODUCTION

Atherosclerosis is the most common form of cardiovascular disease arising due to lipid accumulation and resulting inflammation of the large arteries leading to clinical complications such as myocardial infarction and stroke.[1] Although the pathogenesis traces back to 19th century, the understanding of its cure traces back to 20th century. Fewer animal studies and human studies described reduction of the atherosclerosis and reversal of partially blocked arteries with controlling the circulating level of lipoproteins.[2] With advancement in imaging and advances in treatment modalities it has been well established that atherosclerotic plaque can be regressed.

PATHOGENESIS OF ATHEROSCLEROSIS

Sustained exposure of pathogenic factors such as diabetes, hypertension, tobacco-smoking, stress, and air and nanoplastic pollution lead to endothelial dysfunction and formation of atherosclerotic plaque. The permeability of endothelium increases and allows the movement of lipoproteins such as low-density lipoprotein cholesterol (LDL-C) into intima, recruitment of inflammatory cells ingest LDL-C to form foam cells, and there occurs proliferation of vascular smooth muscle cell.[3] Consequently, plaque is formed with a fibrous cap, thus establishing atherosclerosis which gradually progresses.[4,5]

Progression of atherosclerosis may be complicated by rupture or erosion of plaque.

Stages of plaque progression: These include asymptomatic intimal thickening, intimal xanthoma and thickened cap of fibroatheroma, unstable lesions resulting in myocardial infarction of thin fibrous cap atheroma and calcified nodules, and finally the stenosis by fibrocalcific plaque **(Fig. 1)**.[6,7]

Earlier it was believed that acute coronary syndromes (ACSs) were due to rupture of small plaque volume producing mild stenosis. However, present scientific data suggests that plaque enlarges in few months of acute event and progresses prior to its rupture.[8] Carotid intima media thickness (CIMT) is a surrogate marker of coronary atherosclerosis, progression of atherosclerosis, and nature of plaque can be well assessed by ultrasonic measurement of CIMT.[9]

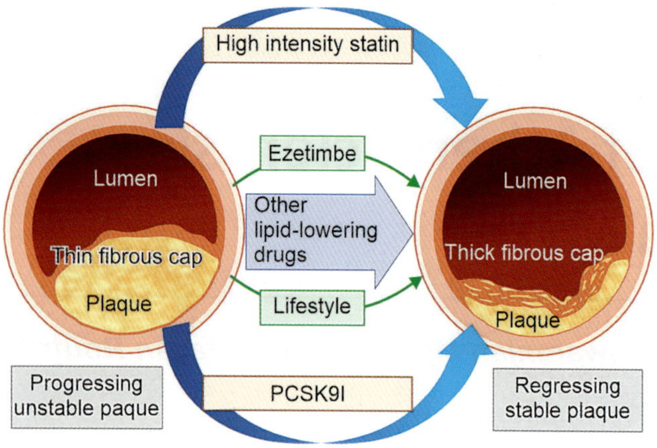

FIG. 1: Schematic presentation of plaque regression and stabilization inside the vascular lumen by various means projected in arrows.

(PCSK9I: proprotein convertase subtilisin/kexin type 9 inhibitors)

Glagov phenomenon is in which coronary arteries enlarge in parallel with size of plaque by positive remodeling, till the plaque area in relation to internal elastic lamina increases above 40%, after which it starts encroaching lumen causing stenosis.[10] Studies have shown that in patient with ACS approximately 10–20% of nonculprit lesion often progress within 8–12 months of initial presentation.[11]

In case of larger plaque or high-risk features such as thin cap atheroma, lower attenuation, and positive-vessel remodeling, they are more likely to progress. With plaque progression almost 15–20% of patients presents with coronary events at 10–12 months, as compared to <1% patient without plaque progression.[12,13] The available data suggests that identifying and preventing the progression of plaque and development of high-risk plaque at early stage can well reduce the risk of cardiovascular events.

PLAQUE REGRESSION

Plaque regression can be defined as the increase in luminal diameter as measured by coronary angiography as a secondary estimate of reducing size of plaque. It has been suggested that reducing lipid content, macrophage content, and controlling state of inflammation can lead to plaque regression.[14]

Advances in imaging techniques, however, can aid in estimating both the volume and composition of plaque. Thus serial measurement of total atheroma volume can reflect plaque regression. Volume of necrotic core, fibrous cap thickness, and positive remodeling are risk predictors of cardiovascular events and the reductions in these values also reflect clinically reduction of such risk.[15] Assessment of CIMT by ultrasound provides an easy and noninvasive way to measure the plaque which may also be used to estimate plaque regression.[16]

Thus, plaque regression can be defined as "changes in plaque morphology that reduces the subsequent risk of cardiovascular events." This can be attained with reduction in plaque volume, high-risk features and changing of unstable noncalcified plaque to stable calcified plaque **(Fig. 1)**. Plaque regression as prevention strategy thus includes both the reduction on total volume of plaque as well as modification of components to reduce the risk of rupture. As all the plaque is not modifiable, thus it becomes imperative to identify and address the changes early in patient.[17]

PLAQUE REGRESSION MODALITIES

Plaque regression can be achieved by the following treatment modalities **(Figs. 2A and B)**. They are broadly categorized into two groups namely:

1. Diet and lifestyle changes
2. Pharmacological methods

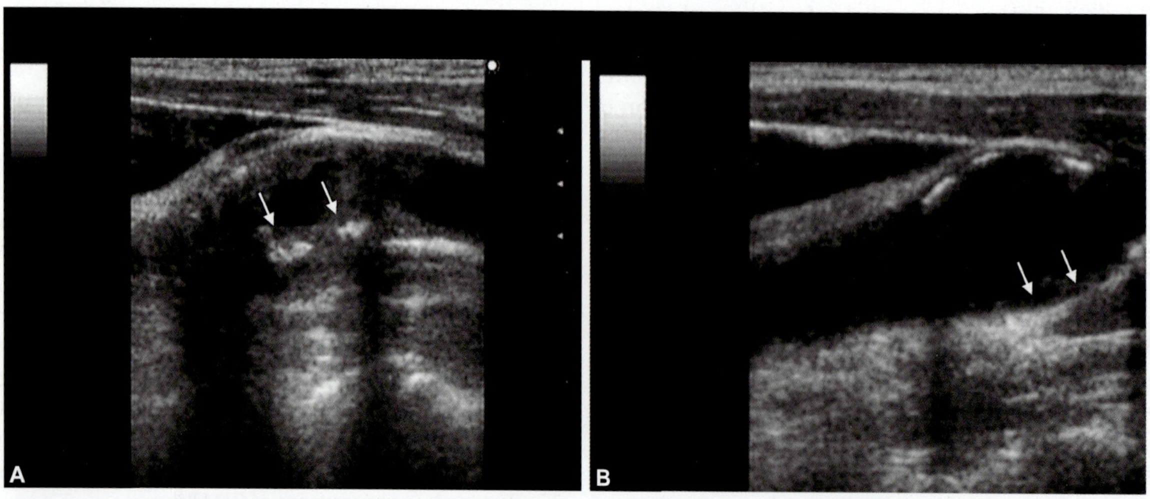

FIGS. 2A AND B: Regression of atherosclerosis demonstrated in a 55-year-old male on optimal medical management. (A) Carotid ultrasound shows atherosclerotic plaque (arrows). (B) Regression of the plaque in a repeat ultrasound of the same vessel with optimal medical management (arrows).

Changes in Diet and Lifestyle

Excessive caloric intake added with specific diet pattern includes processed meat and sweetened beverages. However, modification of diet alone has not proven to demonstrate plaque regression.[16,18] Ornish et al. in 1998 conducted trial on 48 patients with intensive changes in diet and lifestyle (10% whole food, vegetarian diet, aerobic, cessation of smoking, and group support) and showed plaque regression with coronary angiography.

Another trial, DISCO-CT, evaluated 92 randomized patients, in addition to dietician along with follow-up with strict adherence to "Dietary approach to stop Hypertension Nutrition model" and compared with optimal medical therapy only. Computed tomography (CT) evaluation showed greater regression in volumes of noncalcified plaque in experimental group.[19]

Various other trials conducted along with medical therapy concluded that most dietary modified patients undergoing statin therapy showed regression. Thus, it was concluded that mere diet changes will not significantly regress the plaque volume.[20,21]

Exercise/Physical Activity

A Cochrane review of 63 studies concluded that cardiac rehabilitation based on exercise model showed 26% of reduction in cardiovascular mortality and 18% reduction in hospitalization. However, it showed no significant difference in total mortality, myocardial infarction, or revascularization.[22,23] Madssen et al. and Nishitani-Yokoyama et al. also evaluated the effect of intensive exercise on regression of plaque. In each trial, there was plaque regression in exercise arm, however, no study showed any significant difference in treatment groups.[24,25]

Tani et al. identified reduction in total atheroma over 6 months as measured by intravascular ultrasound. It was associated with modification in lifestyle comprising exercise frequency, body mass index and smoking cessation.[26] Other studies evaluated plaque among athletes and showed higher calcific volume of plaque as compared to sedentary participants who presented mixed morphologies and higher risk of coronary events.[27,28] Thus with available scientific data it can be concluded that incorporating exercise offers only modest benefits in regression of plaque.

Smoking and Alcohol Cessation

Cigarette smoking is well-established risk factor for subclinical atherosclerosis, ischemic episodes, and coronary calcification. It is also known that the atherosclerotic indexes reduce with smoking cessation.[29] Various studies have demonstrated high volumes of necrotic core, burden of plaque and fibro-fatty volume with lower amount of fibrous plaque volume, and no difference observed in calcification or thickness of atheroma cap.[30]

Limited data is available on effect of alcohol on progression of plaque. Gisbertz et al. demonstrated alcohol to be inversely proportional with lipid core volume and degree of infiltration of macrophages in patients for femoral endarterectomy. Longitudinal studies to explain relation of smoking with coronary plaque volume still remain lacking in available literature.[31]

Pharmacological Therapy

Statins

Statins are among the backbone of lipid control since 1990s as supported by numerous trials and meta-analyses proving reduced risk of coronary events and death in patients with high-risk group or with established cardiovascular diseases.[32] Statins inhibit hydroxymethyl coenzyme A (HMG CoA) reductase enzyme thereby reducing levels of LDL-C by 30–50%. The relative risk of ischemic events is thus reduced and thus levels of LDL-C has been used widely to monitor response to the treatment.[33] Scattered studies have shown statins can induce regression of plaque, reduce the total atheroma volume by 0–20% in comparison to control subjects showing up to 10% progression.[34] Pleotropic effect of statins plays a significant role in addition to its cholesterol lowering property in overall improvement of cardiovascular outcome including reducing incidence of heart failure.[35]

Takagi et al. in 1997 was first to conduct randomized controlled trial to assess plaque response to treatment with statin using intravenous ultrasound. It showed significant reduction in total volume of atheroma in 36 months when treated with pravastatin 10 mg.[36]

Similar results were shown by various other authors as well, however, statistically significant difference was not reached.[37]

In a study to evaluate the effect of rosuvastatin in 2006, it demonstrated reduction of 6.1% in atheroma volume in 24 months in 507 subjects taking rosuvastatin 40 mg as assessed using intravascular ultrasound imaging.[38] Similar results were also reported in 2009 in Japanese subjects and in 2015 when assessed using integrated Biomarkers and imaging study.[39,40]

In diabetic patients it was seen that greater increase in volume of plaque occurs suggesting the blunting of effectiveness of statin therapy in plaque regression when patient presents with comorbidities.[41] Trials with high-intensity statin showed plaque regression as compared to low-intensity statin with significant reduction in plaque volume assessment using intravascular ultrasound imaging.[42] In 2004, trial REVERSAL (Reversal of Atherosclerosis with Aggressive Lipid Lowering) compared 80 mg atorvastatin in comparison to 40 mg pravastatin and showed greater reduction in 18 months.[43]

Similar study SATURN (The Study of Coronary Atheroma by intravascular Ultrasound: the effect of Rosuvastatin vs. atorvastatin) demonstrated significant decrease in atheroma volume in patient with 40 mg rosuvastatin in 24 months.[44]

Hiro et al. in 2009 conducted a trial named JAPAN-ACS (Japan Assessment of Pitavastatin and Atorvastatin in Acute

Coronary Syndrome) with 30 patients and showed 18.1% greater regression of plaque in patient with 20 mg atorvastatin in 12 months.[45]

Another trial STABLE (Statin and Atheroma Vulnerability Evaluation) in 2016 demonstrated higher reduction in 10 mg rosuvastatin as compared to 40 mg rosuvastatin as evaluated by ultrasound in 12 months. Multivariate analysis showed significant regression at follow-up in terms of baseline plaque burden and presence of thin cap atheroma. This study also concluded in contrary to other trials that no significant difference exists between low- and high-intensity statin therapy.[46] In response to statin therapy, it has demonstrated increase in volume of fibrous plaque and reduction in fibro-fatty component, necrotic core, and noncalcified plaque. As evaluated by optical coherence tomography (OCT), patient with statin therapy showed increase in fibroatheroma capping.[47] In 2013, a trial named YELLOW (Reduction in Yellow Plaque by Aggressive Lipid-Lowering Therapy) showed reduction of lipid content in patient with 40 mg rosuvastatin therapy as compared to other statins as assessed using near-infrared spectroscopy (NIRS).[48]

Similarly, another study in 2018 used OCT to evaluate Effect of Early Pitavastatin Therapy on Coronary Fibrous Cap Thickness in Patients with Acute Coronary Syndrome (ESCORT), and showed early or late pitavastatin showed greater increase in fibroatheroma thickness of cap by almost 20 mm when started early and decrease of 5 mm among late group at 36 weeks.[49]

A study by Komukai et al. in 2014, the EASY-FIT (Effect of Atorvastatin Therapy on the Fibrous Cap Thickness in Coronary Atherosclerotic Plaque) showed increase in thickness of fibrous cap and reduction in lipid content in subjects with more intensive therapy of statins.[50]

Lee et al. in 2018 conducted trial PARADIGM (Progression of AtheRosclerotic PlAque Determined by Computed TomoGraphic Angiography Imaging) which demonstrated reduction in high-risk atherosclerotic plaque features as low plaque attenuation and positive arterial remodeling.[41]

Based on available scientific literature, it can be well suggested that therapy with statins induces plaque regression with a direct relation to dose and proportionate reduction in level of LDL.

Ezetimibe

Studies have shown improved regression of plaque by using 10 mg ezetimibe in addition to medical therapy in 6 months.[51] Trials such as HEAVEN (Virtual Histology Evaluation of Atherosclerosis Regression During Atorvastatin and Ezetimibe Administration) in 2012, ZEUS (eZEtimibe Ultrasound Study) in 2014, PRECISE-IVUS (Plaque Regression with Cholesterol Absorption Inhibitor or Synthesis Inhibitor Evaluated by Intravascular Ultrasound) in 2015, OCTIVUS (Ezetimibe in Addition to Atorvastatin Therapy on the Plaque Composition in Patients with Acute Myocardial Infarction) in 2017, and ZIPANGU (ezetimibe clinical investigation for regression of intracoronary plaque evaluated by angioscopy and ultrasound) in 2017 showed significant plaque regression when ezetimibe is used along with medical therapy as compared when medical therapy is used alone.[52-55] Hibi et al. in 2018 assessed effect on plaque composition using intravascular ultrasound. Using ezetimibe reduced LDL-C and lesser cardiovascular events were reported in patients.[56]

Proprotein Convertase Subtilisin/Kexin Type 9 Inhibitors

Proprotein convertase subtilisin/kexin type 9 (PCSK9) enzyme has been identify to work in plaque remodeling by reducing clearance of LDL from plasma. Randomized controlled trials of PCSK9 inhibitors has resulted in increased clearance of LDL-C by liver.[57]

In 2016, The GLAGOV (Global Assessment of Plaque Regression with PCSK9 Antibody as Measured by Intravascular Ultrasound) trial involving 968 patients showed plaque volume reduction by using evolocumab after 76 weeks.[58] Evaluating effect of alirocumab on coronary volume of atheroma in Japanese patients with comorbidities showed using 75 mg alirocumab reduces slightly the total volume in 206 patients after 36 weeks.[59]

Cholesteryl Ester Transfer Protein Inhibitors

Cholesteryl ester transfer protein (CETP) inhibitors prevent transfer of cholesterol from HDL to LDL. Though it showed favorable changes in cholesterol levels, these did not show significant improvement in clinical trials and thus were stopped due to futility. In 2007 ILLUSTRATE trial evaluated effect of torcetrapib on total atheroma volume as assessed by intravascular ultrasound in 24 months. It showed increased mortality and morbidity and thus not used further.[60]

Eicosapentaenoic Acid

In recent years novel strategies have been tried such as omega-3 fatty acids like eicosapentaenoic acid (EPA). They mediate the process to stabilize endothelial dysfunction.[61] In 2017, a trial abbreviated as CHERRY (Combination Therapy of Eicosapentaenoic Acid and Pitavastatin for Coronary Plaque Regression) evaluated the plaque regression in 6 months using backscatter ultrasonography in patients taking 1,800 mg/day of EPA.[62] However, no significant changes were seen in other studies by Niki et al. in 2016.[63]

Alfaddagh et al. in 2019 reported that plaque progression is reduced among patients using EPA in 18 months and also showed reduced attenuation of plaque, fibro-fatty volume, and volume of fibrous component.[64] As initial reported data prove to be promising, inclusion of EPA-based strategies can form important part of future regression strategies in managing plaque.

Lipoprotein and Triglyceride-lowering Therapy

Various studies have proved lipoprotein to be associated with plaque volume and as features of high risk. However, very minimal data suggests its impact on volume as well as composition of plaque.[65] Niacin has shown lowering of lipoprotein by almost 25% but no difference was observed in volume of atheroma percentage in saphenous vein grafts. But owing to its lack of efficacy and side effects, it is not widely used in clinical practice.[66]

Antihypertensive Medications

Various studies have been conducted to assess effect of antihypertensive medications on plaque volumes and most of them showed no improvement in regression except CAMELOT trial in 2004. This trial compared effect of amlodipine and enalapril in limiting thrombosis events, in 274 patients for period of 24 months. Amlodipine demonstrated minimal reduction in plaque progression and enalapril arm showed similar plaque progression.[67] Hirohata et al. studied effect of olmesartan on progression of atherosclerosis (OLIVUS) in 2010 among 247 patients. In a period of 14 months, it showed reduced plaque progression as compared to control group patient.[68] Contrary to other trials like AQUARIOUS in 2013, Han et al. in 2012, and PERSPECTIVE in 2007, did not show significant drop in plaque regression with antihypertensives such as aliskiren, ramipril, and perindopril, respectively.[69-71]

Colchicine

The anti-inflammatory medication acts by inhibiting formation of microtubule and tubulin polymerization thereby reducing the inflammatory response.[72]

In 2017 Vaidya et al. conducted a trial on 80 patients to evaluate effect of colchicine 0.5 mg/day. After 12 months it showed significant reduction in plaque volume and noncalcified atheroma.[73]

Anticoagulants

Several studies have reported regression of plaque by usage of oral anticoagulants and warfarin. In 2018, Lee et al. conducted trial with 97 patients using either rivaroxaban or warfarin and showed reduced plaque volumes in period of 12 months.[74] In 2018, Win et al. studied effect of apixaban and warfarin in patients with *atrial fibrillation* and reported increase in low plaque attenuation in 12 months.[75] In another observational cohort study among 161 patients by Beyer et al. in 2019, warfarin showed reduced plaque burden in 38 months.[76]

Contrary to these, in 2018 Andrews et al. showed when used independently warfarin produces increased calcification without increasing plaque volumes in post hoc analysis of eight trials.[77] As the data are either from small cohort studies or observational studies, further elaborated controlled trials are needed to form conclusions.

The Compass trial has also highlighted the role of low-dose rivaroxaban with aspirin in showing reversal of atherosclerosis resulting in cardiovascular benefit.

Oral Hypoglycemic Therapy

Some studies among diabetic patients have shown enhanced plaque regression when on thiazolidinedione treatment. Nissen SE et al. and Yang et al. have shown greater regression of plaque as well as reduced rates of thin cap fibroatheroma in patient on pioglitazone as compared to placebo in period of 18 months and 6 months respectively.[78,79] Another study in using rosiglitazone showed reduced in total plaque as compared with glipizide. However, rosiglitazone showing cardiovascular morbidity and thus not being used.[80]

MISCELLANEOUS

Various other novel treatments have been proposed to reduce plaque burden.

- LACMART (Low Density Lipoprotein Apheresis Coronary Morphology and Reserve Trial) in 2002 evaluated LDL apheresis in comparison to usual therapy for period of 12 months and proved to be efficacious in regression of plaque area. However, limited availability and complexity of treatment makes it difficult for wide clinical practice.[81]
- Apolipoprotein A1 (ApoA-1)-based HDL mimetics. ApoA-1 Milano trial in 2003 and CHISQUARE trial in 2014 showed enhanced plaque regression.[82,83]
- ACAT trial in 2006 using pactimibe, STRADIVARIUS trial in 2008, reconstituted HDL infusions, LS-001 trial by HDL delipidation, SECURE trial using combination of cilostazol and probucol, succinobucol, and ASSURE trial using bromodomain and extraterminal (BET) protein inhibitor, have also assessed using intravascular ultrasound but none of them showed profound regression.[84]
- Testosterone has been also assessed for limiting coronary plaque regression in patients with hypogonadism and proved efficacious in reducing plaque volume.[85]
- Garlic extract have been evaluated in two small randomized trials with coronary artery calcification and progression of low attenuated plaque.[86]

CONCLUSION

Various studies have been conducted and strategies have been tried to cause reduction on plaque volumes as well as altering plaque composition. This has further been aided by improved understanding of pathophysiology and advances in imaging modalities making precise monitoring possible with higher efficacy. Studies so far have strongly reaffirmed the reversal of atherosclerosis with plaque regression by different strategies. Newer agents like Inclisiran act by interfering RNA through inhibition of PCSK9 enzyme, and Apo A1 trials are ongoing and produces promising results.

Advancements in imaging modalities for plaque characterization, multimodal imaging, using molecular probes can well facilitate better understanding of response of treatment.

Development of precision medicine with specifically targeting the mechanism provides direction for further research. Better treatment strategies with predictable outcome provides for strong rationale to be used in clinical practice. Identifying risk factors and detection of subclinical plaque can facilitate early diagnosis and predictable reversal in larger population, thereby reducing cardiac morbidity and mortality.

ACKNOWLEDGMENT

We are grateful to Dr Antarmayee Panigrahi, Associate Professor Orthodentics and Research Associate, SOA University for her immense help and cooperation in preparation of the manuscript.

ONLINE REFERENCES

Please scan the QR code provided at the end of the table of contents for References of this chapter.

CHAPTER 118

Environmental Pollutants, Climate Change, and Cardiovascular Diseases

Suganthi Jaganathan, Dorairaj Prabhakaran

ABSTRACT

Climate change is multifaceted global emergency with enhanced greenhouse gas emissions leading to ambient air pollution, extremes of temperature, both heat and cold coupled with extreme weather events such as cyclones, floods, hurricanes, and droughts. All of these can have severe impact on human health. As of 2023, the effects of climate change have been experienced by almost every country in the world. However, research on health effects of climate change, and mitigation strategies have been limited to specific parts of the world. There is a need to amplify the mitigation strategies across the world and especially to the climate susceptible population groups. In this chapter we discuss about the various climate change-related exposures, the state of health research with focus on cardiovascular diseases (CVDs), globally and in India. We are also discussing about the various mitigation strategies undertaken so far.

Keywords: Environmental exposures, cardiovascular diseases, climate change, air pollution, extremes of temperature.

INTRODUCTION

Globally, human activities have resulted in emissions of greenhouse gases (GHGs) causing global warming, with 1.1°C increase in global temperature in 2011–2020 above what was observed in 1850–1900.[1] GHG emissions have continued to increase globally resulting from fossil fuel use, deforestation, expansion of human habitats, changing patterns of land-use, lifestyles and patterns of consumption and production across regions, between and within countries, and among individuals. The emerging environmental threats affect the health of populations, especially vulnerable communities causing increased mortality, and worsening morbidities. Across the world, researchers are cognizant of threats posed by environmental risk factors, and they have included environmental risk factors in the traditional framework of social determinants of health. Among the top 15 risk factors for cardiovascular diseases (CVDs), five of them are environmental risk factors such as ambient particulate matter air pollution (rank 4), household air pollution (rank 9), lead exposure (rank 10), low temperature (rank 11), and high temperature (rank 15) respectively.[2-4] In this chapter, we will briefly discuss air pollution, both ambient and household; extremes of temperature and extreme weather events, and how it impacts CVDs globally and in India.

OVERVIEW OF ENVIRONMENTAL POLLUTANTS AND CLIMATE CHANGE

Last year marked the 30th anniversary of the signing of the UN Framework Convention on Climate Change (UNFCCC), in which countries agreed to prevent dangerous anthropogenic climate change and its deleterious effects on human health and welfare. Meaningful actions are yet to happen; we have been witnessing extreme temperatures, extreme weather events, and wildfires irrespective of the country. Ambient and household air pollution has been disproportionately increasing in low- and middle-income countries. These environmental challenges have a vast impact on the human health and other species and on the infrastructure. Analyses of daily death rates have shown that both low and high temperatures are associated with increases in CVD mortality. Power generation is still dominated by fossil fuels, which not only produces GHG emissions and causing air pollution but creates a perfect storm for extremes of temperature. The rising temperature combined with droughts catalyze for rampant wildfires, incessant rains and flooding leading mortality and other health effects among vulnerable communities. Health-centered development goals are essential to braze for the impacts that climate change have blown at us. The changes caused by climate change are also driving rise in infectious diseases, old and new, affecting food and water security, worsening air quality across the regions, and damaging socioeconomic systems, coupled with wide range of health impacts.[1,5,6]

Ambient air pollution alongside household air pollution has been on the rise in India. Indo-Gangetic plains have largely been the focus of the topic of air pollution in India.[7,8] India being a tropical country literally faces the heat and the climate change has only exacerbated the effects of the heat. The studies assessed the exposure-response relationship between extreme temperatures and mortality, and have described higher mortality risks at variable temperature thresholds. Extreme heat conditions adversely affect the functioning of the human body by placing undue load on the cardiovascular (CV) system and other organ systems. Rising sea levels, cyclones, flooding, and droughts have become frequent in India which affects human life in more than one way **(Fig. 1)**.

MECHANISMS

Air Pollution and Cardiovascular Diseases

To date, many studies have evaluated the mechanisms underlying the effects of air pollution on CVDs. Air pollutants such as particulate matter, nitrogen dioxide, and ozone **(Fig. 2)** all have similar pathways in which they affect the functioning in CVDs—most common initial pathways are (1) oxidative stress and inflammation, (2) autonomic nervous imbalance, and (3) direct particle translocation which cascade to endothelial dysfunction, thrombotic pathways, activation of a hypothalamic-pituitary-adrenal axis, and epigenomic changes. The pathogenesis and temporality of these pathways are distinct; however, they are highly interrelated leading to the common outcome of increased risk of CVD. In addition, intermediate outcomes of CVDs also share similar pathways, leading to arrhythmogenesis, increased blood pressure, atherosclerosis development, heart rate variability, and increased arterial stiffness. These increase the risk of developing distinct cardiovascular clinical events, including cardiac arrest, ischemic heart disease (IHD), heart failure, stroke, and finally, CVD mortality. The duration of air pollution exposure and type of air pollutant may activate different pathways at various stages. Overall, the influence on the pathways will depend on the type of pollutant, dose, and duration of exposure, specific cardiovascular endpoints, and individual health status.[10,11] Fine particulate matter < 2.5 μm ($PM_{2.5}$) air pollution is the most important environmental risk factor contributing to the global cardiovascular mortality and disability.[12]

Extremes of Temperature and Cardiovascular Diseases

Thermal stress from extreme temperature triggers physiological responses to changes in central body temperature, leading to increased sweating, elevated heart and breathing rates, vasodilatation, and increased or decreased coagulation. These changes can cause imbalances in the autonomic control of the heart, increase local arterial pressures, induce systemic inflammation, and impair clotting responses. With increasing temperature, there is an increased risk of acute-onset IHD, given the

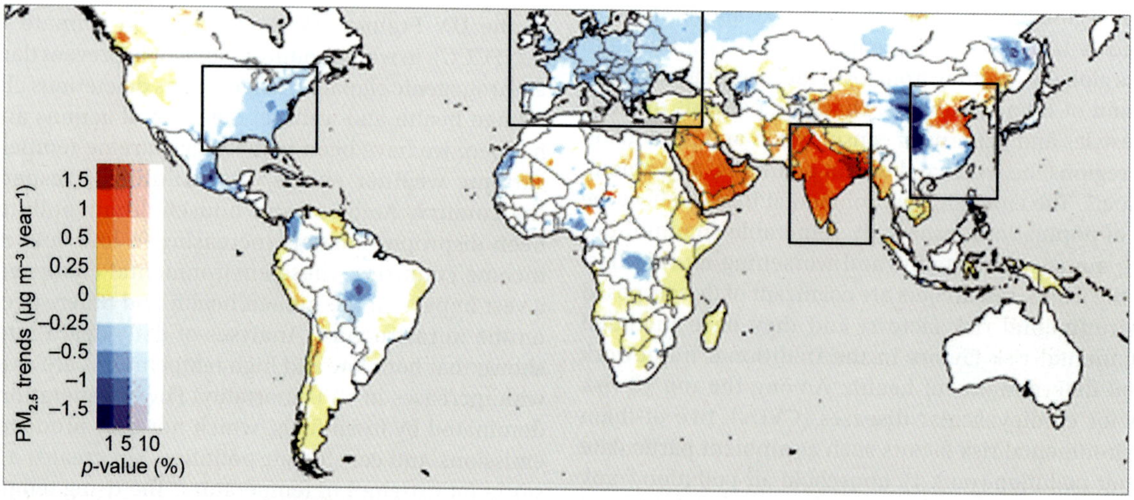

FIG. 1: Trends in $PM_{2.5}$ from 1998 to 2018. It can be noted that India has exceeded trend by 1 μg/m³/year and an increasing trend can also be noticed in parts of China, the Middle East, Central and Southern Africa, and Canada, whereas negative trends could be noted in Eastern United States of America, Europe, Central South America, and Australia.[9]

pathophysiological implications of increased heat exposure. The physiological responses predispose vulnerable individuals to hemodynamic compromise and subsequent acute cardiovascular events such as atherosclerotic plaque rupture and subsequent myocardial infarctions (MIs). Similarly, individuals with heart failure and reduced left ventricular ejection fraction are likely to be unable to compensate for the increased circulatory demand induced by heat exposure.[14]

Extreme Weather Events and Cardiovascular Diseases

Extreme weather events such as cyclone, floods, droughts, and hurricanes may not directly affect the CVDs, but indirectly affect the delivery of health services for vulnerable individuals and exacerbate the existing health condition. They may also trigger cardiovascular events in susceptible communities. These events can also strain the food supply

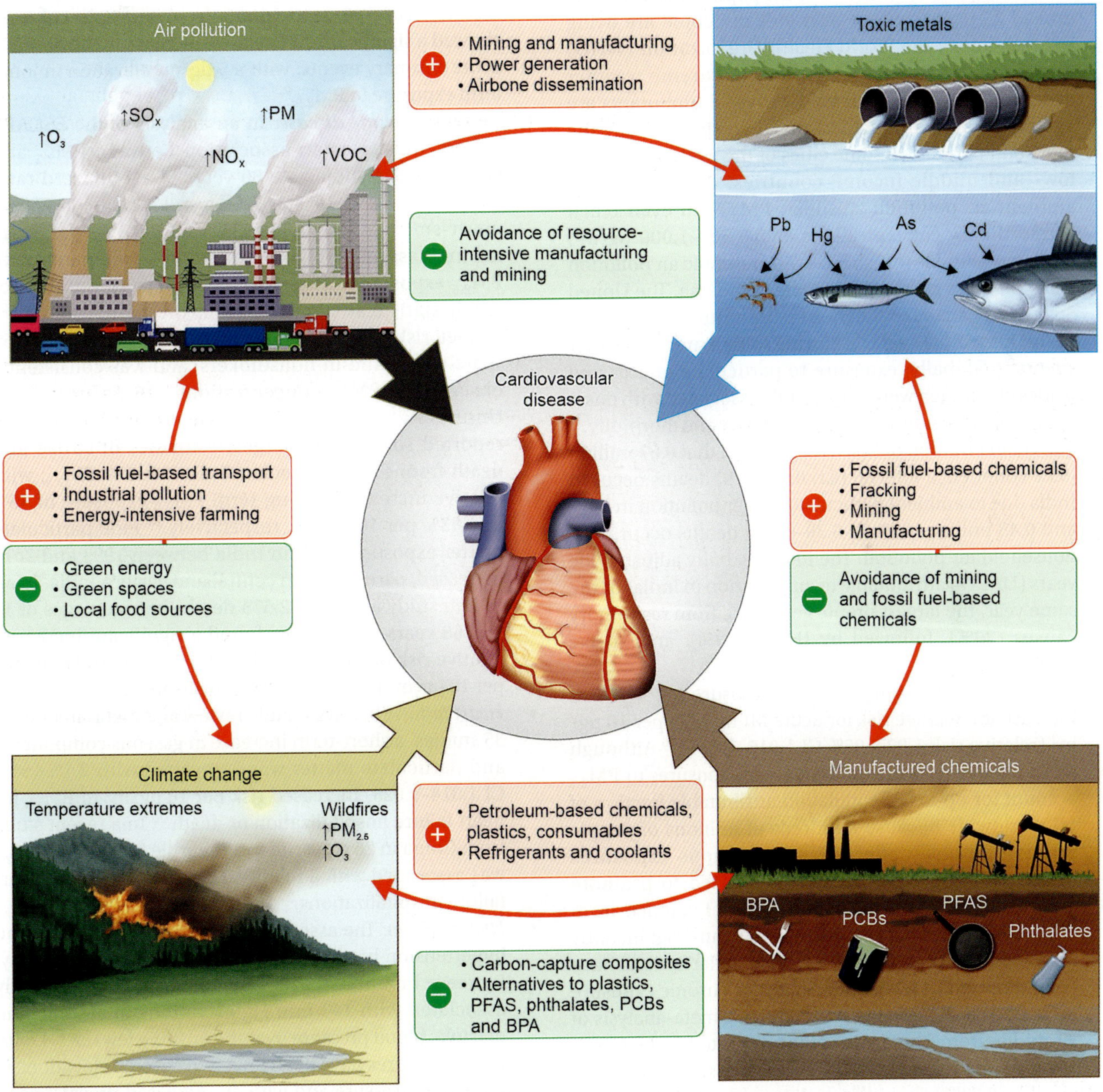

FIG. 2: Pollution, climate change, and cardiovascular disease.[13]

(BPA: bisphenol A; NO_x: nitrogen oxides; PCBs: polychlorinated biphenyls; PFAS: per-and polyfluoroalkyl substances; SO: sulfur monoxide; O_3: ozone)

and may affect the nutritional availability, albeit short-term. Long-term effects of these extreme weather events are yet to be studied in detail, with increasing frequency it makes an important case for the study.

AIR POLLUTION AND CARDIOVASCULAR DISEASES: GLOBAL CONTEXT, INDIAN CONTEXT

- *Ambient air pollution*: The levels of fine particulate matter over many parts of Asia (70% of the population) routinely exceed 35 μg/m^3, where over 99% of people are living in areas above the World Health Organization (WHO) recommended annual levels. Unlike extreme weather events and heat waves or cold waves, air pollutants are at similar levels throughout the year, sparing only the monsoon periods. In some cities of the world, especially low- and middle-income countries, during extreme ambient air pollution episodes, $PM_{2.5}$ can even reach extraordinary concentrations above 500–1,000 μg/m^3, levels comparable to high levels of household air pollution using biomass for cooking or active smoking. The United States and Canada routinely measure around average < 12 μg/m^3 for annual average, barring some extreme weather events.[11] Globally, exposure to particulate matter and oxides of nitrogen were consistently associated with onset of MI, hypertension, and stroke mortality and morbidity.[10] The Global Burden of Disease estimated that 0.67 million [95% confidence interval (CI) 0.55–0.79] deaths occur in India due to ambient particulate matter pollution in 2017 and 0.48 million (95% CI 0.39–0.58)] deaths occur from household air pollution. The total disability adjusted life years (DALYs) attributable to air pollution in India for the same year, the largest proportions were from respiratory causes (29%), followed by IHD (23.8%), and stroke (7.5%).[15]
- *Cardiovascular mortality*: Acute exposure to $PM_{2.5}$ can increase the relative risk for acute MI by 2.5% per 10 μg/m^3 (relative risk 1.025; 95% CI 1.015–1.036).[16] Although these relative risks are modest, acute exposures to $PM_{2.5}$ account for up to 5% population attributable fraction of MI worldwide because hundreds of millions of people are continuously affected.[17] Continuous exposures to air pollution have been hypothesized to promote atherosclerosis and recurrent events. Evidence from Canadian studies suggests risk of IHD deaths significantly increased with exposure to $PM_{2.5}$.[18,19] Similar findings have been reported in the United States for chronic exposure increased cardiovascular mortality. In a meta-analysis of 59 studies from China, the authors reported that for each 10 μg/m^3 increment in $PM_{2.5}$ there was associated with an absolute 0.63% increase in cardiovascular mortality, even though $PM_{2.5}$ ranged from 39 to 177 μg/m^3.[20] An important recent study in China confirmed that the increased risk for morbidity and mortality persists, even at very high air pollution exposure (average $PM_{2.5}$ levels of 43.7 μg/m^3). The relative risk for cardiovascular mortality increased by 9% per 10 μg/m^3 elevation in $PM_{2.5}$.[21]
- *MI*: Short-term changes in air pollution and daily changes in MI have been explored with time-series and case-crossover studies across the globe. A systematic review and meta-analysis of studies of short-term air pollution exposures and MI showed that $PM_{2.5}$, along with nitrogen dioxide (NO_2), and sulfur dioxide and carbon monoxide were associated with increased risk of MI.[16] The ESCAPE study (European Study of Cohorts for Air Pollution Effects) (100,166 participants from multiple cohorts) showed a significant 13% relative increase in the nonfatal acute coronary events, with a 5 μg/m^3 elevation in long-term exposure to $PM_{2.5}$.[22]
- *Cerebrovascular disease*: In an analysis of the ESCAPE cohort, there was an association between $PM_{2.5}$ and stroke among subjects ≥ 60 years of age [hazard ratio (HR) 1.40; 95% CI 1.05–1.87/5 μg/m^3] increase in $PM_{2.5}$), never-smokers (HR 1.74; 95% CI 1.06–2.88 per 5 μg/m^3 increase in $PM_{2.5}$), and among participants with $PM_{2.5}$ exposure < 25 μg/m^3 higher hazard but did not reach statistical significance in the main analysis.[23] Higher risk was especially seen in subjects above 60 years of age and in nonsmokers, and was consistently observed at $PM_{2.5}$ concentrations <25 μg/m^3. In the United States, the Women's Health Initiative study reported some of the largest estimates of stroke and death from cerebrovascular disease due to $PM_{2.5}$, with relative increases in long-term $PM_{2.5}$ exposure of 35% and 83% per 10 μg/m^3, respectively.[24] Fine particulate matter exposure levels in India between 1999 and 2014 increased, particularly in central and eastern India. In an Indian study among 212,573 deaths between ages of 15 and 69 years, the authors found a significant increased relative risk of 1.09 (95% CI 1.04–1.14) for stroke deaths per 10 μg/m^3 increase in $PM_{2.5}$ exposure.[25]
- *Heart failure*: In a systematic review and meta-analysis of 35 studies, a short-term increase in gaseous components and particulate matter was associated with 2.1% (95% CI 1.014–1.028) increased risk per 10 μg/m^3 in $PM_{2.5}$ for heart failure hospitalization or death.[26] In a recent study from China in 26 cities, an interquartile increase in $PM_{2.5}$ was associated with a relative 1.3% increase in the heart failure hospitalizations.[27]
- *Hypertension*: The association between air pollution and hypertension has been previously reviewed extensively. Increase in ambient $PM_{2.5}$ by 10 μg/m^3 is consistently associated with 1–3 mm Hg elevations in systolic and diastolic blood pressure over the ensuing few days. Long-term exposures have been linked to chronic elevations in the blood pressure and with an increased prevalence or incidence of hypertension in many studies as well. Robust associations have been noted at extreme levels of the exposure response relationship in a Chinese megacity.[28]

This body of evidence strongly supports inclusion of higher blood pressure levels and hypertension-related morbidity in air pollution global burden estimates. In a study published by GEOHealth investigators in New Delhi, the authors investigated the association between exposure to ambient particulate matter with blood pressure and incident hypertension in a cohort of ~5,300 individuals and followed for 7 years (2010–2016). The authors found strong effects of long- and short-term exposure on systolic and diastolic blood pressure (BP) as well as risk of developing hypertension. It was also observed higher average systolic BP (1.8 and 3.3 mm Hg per interquartile range differences (~9–15 μg/m^3 of $PM_{2.5}$) in monthly and annual exposures, respectively. Average $PM_{2.5}$ over durations of 1, 1.5, and 2 years increased the risk of developing hypertension by 1.5 × (50% higher risk) 1.6 × (60% higher risk), and 1.2 × (20% higher risk), respectively. These results were also found to be stronger in study participants with higher waist-to-hip ratios, which is an indicator of central obesity.[29]

Household Air Pollution

The levels of household air pollution typically encountered in low- and middle-income countries can be an order of magnitude higher than ambient outdoor levels in the same geographic location, contributing to steep indoor-outdoor gradients. The sources of household air pollution can be from unclean cooking fuel, such as biomass burning, and use of agricultural waste for cooking. A study reported that mean indoor 24-hour PM_{10} levels ranged between 200 and 2,000 μg/m^3 while peak exposures of >30,000 μg/m^3 were observed during periods of cooking with exposure to low-efficiency combustion of biomass fuels. Compared with a decade ago, there is a decrease in the contribution of household air pollution to global morbidity/mortality. However, the trend is not uniform and consistent.[30,31]

Components of Air Pollution

Evidence from a recently published umbrella review shows that short-term exposures to particulate matter measuring < 2.5 μm ($PM_{2.5}$), < 10 μm (PM_{10}), and nitrogen oxides (NO_x) were consistently associated with increased risks of hypertension and triggering of MI, and stroke (fatal and nonfatal). Long-term exposures of $PM_{2.5}$ were largely associated with increased risk of atherosclerosis, incident MI, hypertension, and incident stroke and stroke mortality. Very few reviews evaluated other CVD outcomes including arrhythmias, atrial fibrillation, or heart failure but they generally reported positive statistical associations. Stronger associations were found in Asian countries and vulnerable subpopulations, especially among the elderly, cardiac patients, and people with higher weight status. Consistent with experimental data, the umbrella review found strong evidence that higher levels of ambient air pollution increase the risk of CVDs, especially all-cause CVD mortality, stroke, and IHD.[10] A study examining short-term $PM_{2.5}$ exposures and nonaccidental mortality in New Delhi, India reported that for each 25 μg/m^3 increment in exposure was associated with a 0.8% (95% CI 0.3–1.3%) increase in daily nonaccidental mortality and a 1.5% (95% CI 0.8–2.2%) increase among those aged 60 years and above.[32]

EXTREMES TEMPERATURE AND CARDIOVASCULAR DISEASES: GLOBAL CONTEXT AND INDIAN CONTEXT

Rising Temperature

In an analysis of 74 million deaths that occurred between 1985 and 2012, 7.71% (95% CI 7.43–7.91) of mortality was attributable to non-optimum temperature, with substantial differences between countries, ranging from 3.37% (95% CI 3.06–3.63) in Thailand to 11.00% (95% CI 9.29–12.47) in China.[33] In a study conducted in England on the effect of heat on cause-specific mortality reported that per 1°C rise above the regional heat threshold caused deaths due to cardiovascular causes by 1.8% (95% CI 1.2–2.5%) and MI by 1.1% (95% CI 0.7–1.5%), but increased noticeably for arrhythmias by 5.0% (95% CI 3.2–6.9%) and pulmonary heart disease by 8.3% (95% CI 2.7–14.3%).[34]

Heat Waves

There is an increased risk for CVD due to ambient heat exposures in different climate zones. The widespread prevalence of exposure to hot temperatures, in conjunction with an increase in the proportion of the older people in the population, might result in a rise in poor CVD health outcomes associated with a warming climate. Evidence-based prevention measures are needed to attenuate peaks in cardiovascular events during hot spells, thereby lowering the worldwide total heat-related burden of CVD-related morbidity and death. The overall risk of CVD-related mortality due to heat waves increased by 2.1% [relative risk 1.021 (95% CI 1.020–1.023)], with the highest specific disease risk being for stroke and coronary heart disease. A 1°C temperature rise was also associated with a significant increase in morbidity due to arrhythmias, cardiac arrest, and coronary heart disease. The findings suggest heat exposure leads to elevated risk of morbidity and mortality for women, people 65 years and older, individuals living in tropical climates, and those in countries of lower-middle income.[35]

A study conducted in Spain has assessed trends in temperature-related CVD mortality by sex and age, and we investigated the association between climate warming and changes in the risk of mortality. Between 1980 and 2016, 4.5 million cardiovascular deaths were recorded in Spain. In the warm temperatures, the increase in relative risk of death from CVDs was higher for women than men and higher for older individuals (aged ≥ 90 years) than younger individuals (aged 60–74 years), whereas in the cold temperatures, RRs were higher for men than women, with no clear pattern by age group. The heat-attributable fraction of cardiovascular deaths was higher for women in all age groups, and the cold-attributable fraction was larger in men. The heat-attributable fraction increased with age for both sexes, whereas the cold-attributable fraction increased with age for men and decreased for women.[36]

A study conducted in Puducherry used in-hospital CVD mortality data and climate data from the Indian Meteorological Department, the authors analyzed the association between apparent temperature and in-hospital CVD mortalities between 2011 and 2020. Using a case-crossover model with a distributed lag nonlinear model the authors captured the delayed and nonlinear trends over a 21-day-lag period to identify the optimal temperature range for Puducherry. The optimal temperature range for Puducherry was between 30 and 36°C with respect to CVDs. Both cold and hot nonoptimal temperatures were associated with an increased risk of overall in-hospital CVD mortalities, resulting in a U-shaped association curve. Cumulatively, up to 17% of the CVD deaths could be attributable to nonoptimal temperatures, with a slightly higher burden attributable to heat (9.1%) than cold (8.3%). Males were more vulnerable to the colder temperatures; females above 60 years were more vulnerable to the heat while females below 60 years were affected by both heat and cold. Mortality with cerebrovascular accidents was associated more with heat compared to cold, while IHDs did not seem to be affected by temperature.[37]

Cold Spells

The findings from a study conducted in Czech Republic between 1994 and 2009 show that while excess deaths due to IHD during hot spells are mainly of persons with chronic diseases whose health had already been compromised, cardiovascular changes induced by cold stress may result in deaths from acute coronary events rather than chronic IHD, and this effect is important also in the younger population.[38] A population-based retrospective study from Catalonia in Spain has concluded that cold spells for over 7 days led to an increased incidence of emergency cardiovascular hospitalizations.[39]

EXTREME WEATHER EVENTS AND CARDIOVASCULAR DISEASES: GLOBAL CONTEXT AND INDIAN CONTEXT

The effects of floods, cyclones, and hurricanes are more noticeable in terms of the destruction caused to infrastructure and deaths caused droughts on the other hand, affect the supply chain which is more apparent. The direct impact on the human health, especially on CVDs is not very well evaluated to date. In general, cyclone, flood, and storm-related disasters impact on the treatment management and care for people with noncommunicable diseases. Possible consequences include exacerbation of illness, complications or even death. There is a need to expand traditional disaster approaches by public health to include management of noncommunicable diseases. This includes understanding all the factors that influence both direct and indirect (preventable) morbidity and mortality related to noncommunicable diseases during and after disasters.[40]

Floods, Cyclones, Hurricanes, and Droughts

There are concerns that certain racial/ethnic groups, older individuals, and residents of socioeconomically disadvantaged neighborhoods are at increased risk after hurricanes of cardiovascular-related morbidity and death in comparison with other segments of the population. This may be due to predisaster factors such as insurance coverage and postdisaster factors such as access to healthcare and financial resources that would otherwise insulate vulnerable individuals from short- and long-term harm. Furthermore, evidence suggests threat perception among vulnerable subgroups is different from the general population and lack of ability to leave, forcing them to endure the hurricanes' effects while sheltering in place. Several research papers reported evaluations of extreme weather events and short-term adverse CVD outcomes.[41] Although droughts are not directly responsible for increased CVDs and mortality, they are responsible for food insecurity and through malnutrition can influence CVDs.[42]

MITIGATION STRATEGIES: GLOBAL CONTEXT AND INDIAN CONTEXT

Achieving a zero-carbon emission economy is essential for dealing with climate change. Countries must invest in developing low-carbon public transport systems and safe walking paths and cycling networks to promote low-carbon dependence. These measures decrease GHG emissions and reduce air pollution, while also promoting physical activity and offering benefits for cardiovascular health. These much-needed political changes will reduce the CVD burden for the future generations, but we must also consider the immediate implications for preventing and treating CVDs.

Air Pollution

Interventions to reduce air pollution must be multipronged such as shifting to clean cooking fuel, working toward cleaner transport options, and reducing emissions and personal strategies to lower air pollution using face mask and air purifiers among vulnerable communities. The personal strategies have demonstrated a reduction in blood pressure.[43-45] Evidence on the effectiveness of reducing air pollution and improving health effects were mixed or no clear pattern emerged.[46] Educating about the adverse effects of air pollution using air quality index can also prove to be effective.

National Clean Air Programme

In India, one of the most recent policies launched to tackle air pollution is the National Clean Air Programme (NCAP) launched in early 2019. The NCAP identified 132 cities across India to develop city-level Clean Air Plans to implement mitigation strategies for ambient PM concentrations.[47] The NCAP is envisioned as a comprehensive strategy to provide the State and Union governments with a blueprint to combat air pollution. The program sets a target of reducing key air pollutants PM_{10} and $PM_{2.5}$ by 20–30% by 2024, with 2017 as the base year. This 5-year action plan intends to create a pan-India air quality monitoring network and generate citizen awareness.

Interventional Studies in India

Indian researchers are also doing experimental studies in the air pollution space, with the use of air purifier and assessing the health outcomes. One of the notable studies funded by National Institutes of Health (NIH) and Indian Council of Medical Research (ICMR) is the PURI-HF trial, a 5-year-long trial to test out the effectiveness of a novel low-cost air purifier intervention on heart failure outcomes. The study aims to evaluate the effectiveness of indoor air purifiers on heart failure functional capacity (6-minute walk test) among patients with reduced ejection fraction < 40% heart failure with reduced ejection fraction (HFrEF) in three cities: (1) New Delhi, (2) Ludhiana, and (3) Thiruvananthapuram compared to the control group receiving a bacterial filter. The results from this study will be helpful to understand the effect of low-cost air purifiers on the heart failure outcomes but can also present an opportunity to understand the impact of usage of air purifiers on various health outcomes.

Temperature

Heat warning systems have been implemented in many countries, regions, or cities. Increasing awareness and enabling the patients with CVDs to take preventive measures about the heat warnings. Physicians are encouraged to raise awareness and potentially to adjust treatment regimens owing to the climate change-related extremes of the temperature. In order to develop guidelines, further research on health status monitoring during climate change-related events via wearable devices and ambulatory measurements of blood pressure, arrhythmia or dysglycemia and potential interactions with specific medications and accompanying comorbidities is needed.

Heat Action Plans

Heat action plans (HAPs) are guidance documents prepared by state, district, and city governments to help prepare for, respond to, and recover and learn from heatwaves. One of their most important functions is to direct scarce healthcare, financial, information, and infrastructural resources to those most vulnerable to extreme heat in that jurisdiction. There are currently around 37 HAPs at the city (9), district (13), and state (15) levels across 18 states in India. HAPs regularly include a heatwave warning system (sharing alerts with vulnerable populations); means of coordination between several government departments; an awareness, training, and behavior change component to reduce heat exposure; a list of short-term actions (focused on healthcare or changing work hours); and longer-term solutions such as investing in infrastructure (e.g., cool roofs and water harvesting bodies), changes in agricultural practice, or adjusting urban planning (e.g., green corridors). HAPs prescribe a balanced mix of short and long-term actions (those that have an impact over more than one heat season) though it is unclear to what extent these actions are being implemented. Cardiologists should be aware of the consequences of extreme heat and advice their patients accordingly (e.g., to sit indoors, adequate hydration and recognize early warning with regard to worsening of heart failure, MI, or stroke). Long-term transformational actions, such as climate-sensitive urban planning and changing cropping patterns, will likely come with higher implementation costs than immediate responses but could significantly reduce the heat exposure and ease HAP implementation in the long run. The risks of extreme heat are experienced disproportionately—some workers are disproportionately affected by the impacts of extreme heat due to personal risk factors (e.g., age, living in poorly ventilated or cooled housing), occupational risk factors (e.g., working outdoors) and societal risk factors (e.g., urban planning). Well-designed and effectively implemented HAPs could reduce negative impacts on productivity and health.[48]

Extreme Weather Events

Disruption of healthcare infrastructure, due to events such as wildfires, floods, and hurricanes is already affecting a substantial amount of healthcare delivery. Health systems should invest in disaster planning and early warning systems to prepare for waves of the patients in extreme weather events or climate refugees. Plans to access and provide nutritious food should also be developed.[49] Steps to eliminating GHG production in the healthcare sector include reducing demand through preventive care, use of clean energy, choosing medical supplies and equipment with lower carbon footprints, and employing telemedicine where possible.[50,51]

CONCLUSION

The incidence of CVDs due to environmental risk factors is on the rise. With rampant climate change, it is imperative to step up the appropriate prevention strategies to reduce the effect on human health. This can be accomplished through implementing changes in clinical guidelines, societal changes, public health interventions and evidence-based health policies. As a society, we must take on a large-scale transition from fossil fuels to clean, renewable energy that will not only reduce CVD and associated deaths but also slow the pace of climate change and thus benefit all humanity. In addition, the medical community has a role to play. We should advice our patients regarding the adverse consequences of $PM_{2.5}$ particularly on the days when air quality is poor. Patients should be advised to wear N95 masks which can filter $PM_{2.5}$ particularly if they need to go outdoors. At a system level it has been estimated that the health system in the US contributes to around 5% of the GHGs. We do not have such data from India, but we should attempt reduce this by addressing issues such as waste disposal, avoiding food wastage, and paying attention to supply chain issues in our hospitals.

ONLINE REFERENCES

Please scan the QR code provided at the end of the table of contents for References of this chapter.

SECTION 16

Pulmonary Arterial Hypertension

CHAPTER

119 Pulmonary Hypertension: Diagnosis and Management

Goutam Datta, Anirban Das, Amritesh Biswas

ABSTRACT

Globally, 1% of the population is suffering from pulmonary hypertension (PH). PH is a disease with a grim prognosis. Although early initiation of treatment prolongs survival, early diagnosis requires a high degree of suspicion. The nonspecific nature of symptoms makes this entity difficult to diagnose. Because right heart catheterization is the gold standard of diagnosis of PH and it also plays a vital role in management, therefore, specialized centers are required for proper patient management. Patients with pulmonary arterial hypertension (PAH) are categorized into three groups—low, intermediate, and high—depending on several risk factors, and therapy is initialized accordingly. Patients of PH with cardiopulmonary comorbidities require individualized treatment. Recently in 2022, the European Society of Cardiology/European Respiratory Society (ESC/ERS) have published their guidelines on PH, which provide valuable information in different aspects of diagnosis and management of this disease entity. However, due to lack of adequate specialized centers and high cost of therapy, in a resource-limited country like ours, only a handful of patients receive adequate care.

Keywords: Pulmonary hypertension, pulmonary arterial hypertension, chronic thromboembolic pulmonary hypertension, left heart disease, lung disease, connective tissue disease, endothelin receptor antagonist, phosphodiesterase-5 inhibitors, prostacyclin analogues, soluble guanylate cyclase stimulators, pulmonary endarterectomy, atrial septostomy, lung transplantation.

INTRODUCTION

Normal pulmonary vasculature is a low-pressure system, with less than one tenth of the resistances provided by systemic vasculature. Pulmonary hypertension (PH) refers to the hemodynamic state where the pressure in the pulmonary artery (PA) is elevated above a mean of 20 mm Hg. Several studies have shown that each increase of 10 mm Hg is associated with a 2.7-fold greater risk for mortality. Presently, approximately 1% of the global population is suffering from PH.

DIAGNOSIS OF PULMONARY HYPERTENSION

The diagnosis of PH is often overlooked because the symptoms are nonspecific, gradual in onset, and overlapped with many common disease conditions. Therefore, a high index of suspicion is required for diagnosis. Additionally, there is a misconception that in patients with comorbid cardiopulmonary conditions (interstitial lung disease (ILD) and mitral valve disease), PH is merely an extension of the underlying disease rather than a specific disease entity **(Flowchart 1)**.

Clinical Features

Dyspnea, easy fatigability, bendopnea, palpitations, and hemoptysis are the presentations of most of the patients. *On the other hand, ankle edema and weight gain (due to fluid retention), chest pain, and presyncope/syncope are the presentations of more advanced diseases and carry poor prognoses.* Rarely, due to huge dilation of the PA, dynamic compression of the left main coronary artery (LMCA) may lead to exertional chest pain; compression of left recurrent laryngeal nerve may lead to hoarseness of voice (cardiovocal or Ortner's syndrome); or compression of the bronchi may lead to wheezing, cough, or recurrent lower respiratory tract

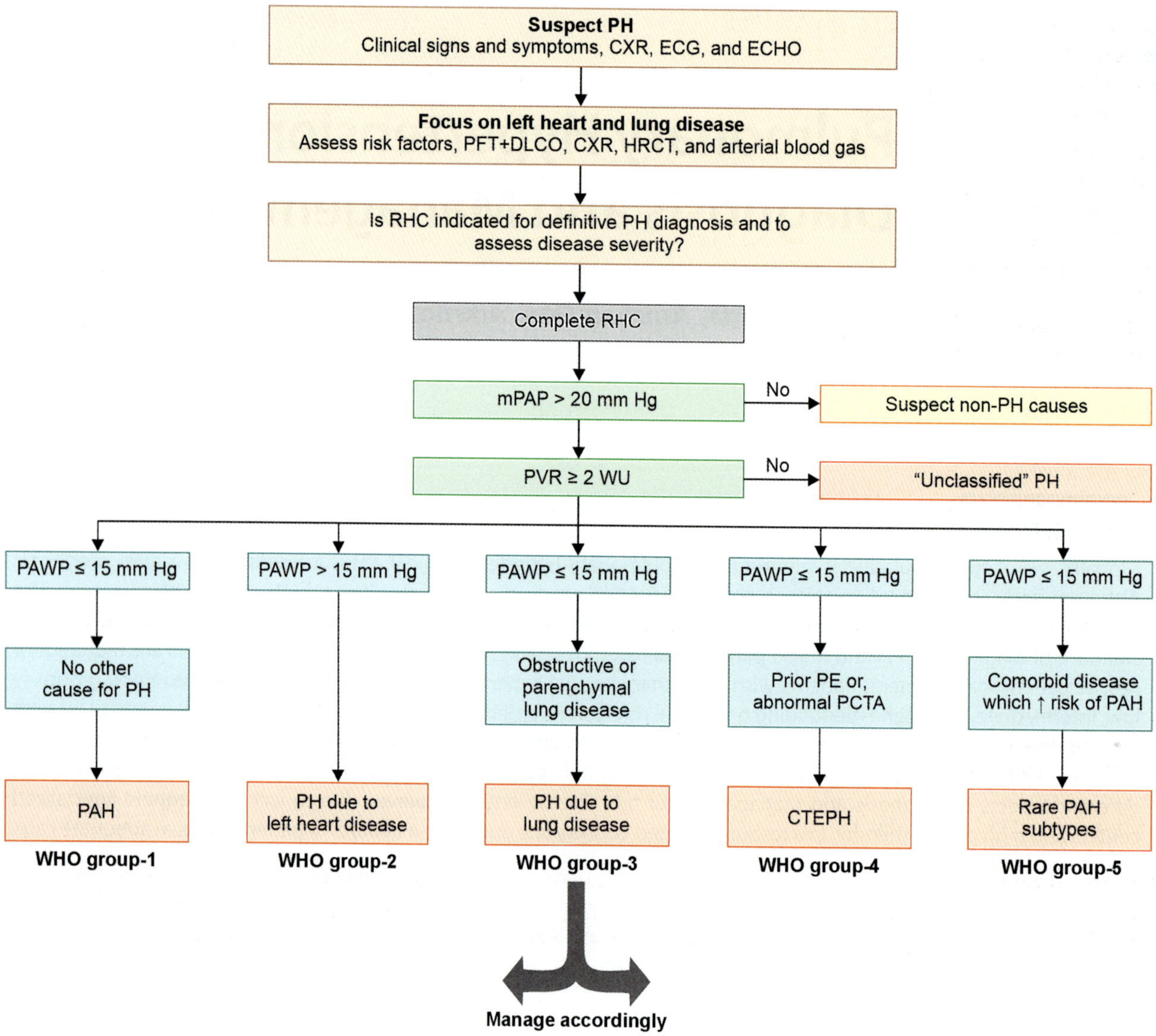

FLOWCHART 1: A simplified and practical approach to diagnose PH.

(CTEPH: chronic thromboembolic pulmonary hypertension; CXR: chest X-ray; DLCO: diffusing capacity of lung for carbon monoxide; ECG: electrocardiogram; ECHO: echocardiogram; HRCT: high-resolution computed tomography; mPAP: mean pulmonary artery pressure; PAH: pulmonary arterial hypertension; PAWP: pulmonary artery wedge pressure; PCTA: pulmonary CT-angiography; PE: pulmonary embolism; PFT: pulmonary function test; PVR: pulmonary vascular resistance; PH: pulmonary hypertension; RHC: right heart catheterization; WHO: World Health Organization; WU: Wood unit)

infection (LRTI). *Physical examination* in the early phase of pulmonary arterial hypertension (PAH) is often unrevealing. As the disease progresses evidence of right ventricular (RV) failure such as raised jugular venous pressure (JVP), lower extremity edema and ascites appear. *Cardiovascular examination* may reveal accentuated P2, a right-sided S3 or S4 and a holosystolic tricuspid regurgitation murmur. *Additional clinical features* of underlying disease that lead to PH may be found occasionally, e.g., clubbing and crackles in some chronic lung diseases, tightening of skin, sclerodactyly, and telangiectasia in scleroderma.

Diagnostic Evaluation

Once clinical suspicion is raised, a systemic approach should be followed for diagnostic confirmation and etiological evaluation of PH.

Electrocardiogram (ECG): It may show P-pulmonale (height of $P > 2.5$ mm in lead II), right axis deviation, RV hypertrophy ($R/S > 1$ with height of $R > 5$ mm in V_1), right bundle branch block (RBBB) at V_1, or RV strain pattern [ST-depression/T-wave inversion at right precordial (V_1–V_4) and inferior leads (II, III, and aVF)].

Chest radiography: Enlargement of PAs and obliteration of the retrosternal space sometimes with pruning of the peripheral vessels may be revealed by chest X-ray (CXR). However, a normal CXR does not exclude PH.

Echocardiography: It is the first line of investigation in a suspected case of PH. Important echo-parameters for assessment of PH are given in **Table 1**. Apart from this, transthoracic echocardiogram (TTE) is also helpful to find out the underlying etiologies such as valvular heart disease (VHD), intra-cardiac shunt, and left ventricular (LV) systolic/diastolic dysfunction. A *bubble contrast echocardiography* helps to identify a suspected intracardiac [atrial septal defect (ASD) and ventricular septal defect (VSD)] or extracardiac [patent ductus arteriosus (PDA) and pulmonary arteriovenous fistula (AV-fistula)] shunt lesions and it is often the most valuable initial screening test. Patients with echocardiographic evidence of PH or in whom unexplained dyspnea or hypoxemia is evident despite a near-normal echo finding require further evaluation.

6-minute walking distance (6MWD): It is the most widely used measure to assess the functional capacity of PH patients. 6MWD is influenced by several factors such as age, sex, height, weight, need for oxygen during comorbidities, and motivation. Change in 6MWD is one of the most commonly used parameters in clinical trials as primary endpoint or component of clinical worsening. For example, a 6MWD >440 meters along with a World Health Organization functional class I or II (WHO FC-I/II) and normal N-terminal prohormone of brain natriuretic peptide (NT-proBNP) level is associated with >95% 1-year survival; on the other hand, a 6MWD of <165 meters is associated with 10–15% risk of mortality at 1 year.

Cardiopulmonary exercise testing (CPET): It differentiates cardiac and pulmonary causes of dyspnea. It measures peak volume of oxygen consumption (VO_2), end-tidal partial pressure of carbon dioxide ($P_{ET}CO_2$), and oxygen pulse [VO_2/heart rate (HR)]. In patients with PAH, all these parameters are reduced. The *presence of normal CPET excludes further invasive testing.*

Right heart catheterization (RHC): It is the gold standard of diagnosis of PH and severity assessment. Diagnosis requires a mean pulmonary artery pressure (mPAP) > 20 mm Hg. Precapillary and postcapillary PH are then differentiated by measuring pulmonary artery wedge pressure (PAWP) or LV end-diastolic pressure (LVEDP). PAWP ≤ 15 mm Hg defines precapillary PH and PAWP > 15 mm Hg as postcapillary PH. The next step is the measurement of pulmonary vascular resistance (PVR). PVR is the afterload imposed on right ventricle. Quantification of afterload on right ventricle is measured by using transpulmonary gradient (TPG), which forms the numerator of the equation of PVR:

$$PVR = (mPAP - PAWP)/CO = TPG/CO$$

Cardiac output (CO) is measured by either thermodilution technique or Fick's method. *As per available data, the upper limit of normal PVR should be <2 Wood units (WU).*[1,2] For this reason, the cutoff of PVR was recently reduced from 3 to 2 WU in the current European Society of Cardiology/European Respiratory Society (ESC/ERS)-2022 guidelines of PH. Patients with isolated precapillary PH have PVR ≥2 WU, whereas postcapillary PVR is present when PVR <2 WU. Nowadays, combined pre- and postcapillary PH is increasingly recognized. It is defined as mPAP >20 mm Hg, along with increased PAWP (>15 mm Hg) and PVR (≥2 WU). There is also a small group of patients who has an elevated mPAP (>20 mm Hg), but normal PAWP (<15 mm Hg) and PVR (<2 WU). This group is termed "unclassified" PH and is found in patients with congenital heart disease (CHD), liver disease, or hyperthyroidism. Clinical and RHC follow-up is recommended for this group.

TABLE 1: Echocardiographic assessment of PH.

Four-chamber view	Dilated RV with basal RV/LV ratio >1	Enlarged right atrial area (>18 cm^2)		Pericardial effusion
Parasternal short-axis view	Flattened interventricular septum, leading to D-shaped septum			
Subcostal view	Distended IVC with decreased inspiratory collapsibility	IVC	Collapse	eRAP
		<21 mm	>50%	3 mm Hg
		>21 mm	>50%	8 mm Hg
		>21 mm	<50%	15 mm Hg
M-mode	Decreased TAPSE; TAPSE < 18 mm			
CW Doppler	Peak TRV >2.8 m/s*			
PW Doppler	RVOT acceleration time of pulmonary ejection < 105 ms. The pattern of RVOT blood flow ("midsystolic notch") is indicative of precapillary PH			

*As per updated hemodynamic definition, peak TRV >2.8 m/s, which was previously >3.4 m/s.

Note: Estimation of systolic pulmonary artery pressure (sPAP) = TR pressure gradient + estimated right atrial pressure (eRAP).

(CW: continuous wave; IVC: inferior vena cava; LV: left ventricular; PW: pulsed-wave; RV: right ventricular; RVOT: RV outflow tract; TAPSE: tricuspid annular plane systolic excursion; TRV: tricuspid regurgitation velocity)

Vasoreactivity testing during RHC involves inhalation of short-acting vasodilators such as inhaled nitric oxide or inhaled epoprostenol and simultaneous measurement of mPAP. A decrease in mPAP ≥10 mm Hg to an absolute value of ≤40 mm Hg without a decrease in CO is defined as positive vasodilator response. Persons with a positive vasodilator response have favorable prognosis and this group responds to long-term treatment with calcium channel blockers (CCBs). Unfortunately, among patients with PAH, only <5% are vasoreactive.

Pulmonary function test: Restrictive or obstructive lung disease can be detected by pulmonary function test (PFT) as a cause of PH. Isolated reduction of diffusing capacity of lung for carbon monoxide (DLCO) is a classic finding of PAH.

Pulmonary computed tomography (CT): It is a valuable tool for distinguishing comorbid ILD, emphysema, or overlap syndromes which include fibrosis and obstructive pulmonary disease. High-resolution CT (HRCT) may reveal enlargement of main PA (a PA to aorta ratio > 0.9), right heart enlargement, as well as peripheral pruning of small arteries. A combination of *three parameters* [PA diameter ≥ 30 mm, RV outflow tract (RVOT) wall thickness ≥ 6 mm, and RV/LV ratio ≥1] is highly predictive of PH.[3] Signs of venous congestion such as centrilobular ground glass infiltrate and thickened septa can also be detected by HRCT and in the absence of left heart disease (LHD), these findings are indicative of pulmonary venous disease, a rare cause of PAH which is quite challenging to diagnose.

Ventilation-perfusion (V/Q) scan: In patients with unexplained dyspnea and evidence of PH in echocardiography, chronic thromboembolic PH (CTEPH) must be excluded. V/Q scan is the study of choice in this situation, which often shows multiple perfusion defects that are not matched with ventilation. Although spiral CT is an excellent tool for the assessment of acute pulmonary embolus, it sometimes fails to detect surgically accessible chronic thromboembolic disease. If either of these studies detects an abnormality, further evaluation with CT pulmonary angiography is required.

CT pulmonary angiography (CTPA): It is usually used to diagnose CTEPH, which is a widely underdiagnosed cause of PH. *Importantly, 25% of patients with CTEPH have no history of clinical venous thromboembolism.* Currently, CTPA is commonly used for diagnostic confirmation of CTEPH. Contrast enhancement in this study provides detailed information on webbing, stricture, and vascular tapering patterns pathognomonic for CTEPH.

Other ancillary tests: Serological testing for human immunodeficiency virus (HIV) and hepatitis C virus (HCV) should be done when suspected. Scleroderma, rheumatoid arthritis, and systemic lupus erythematosus (SLE) are the most common rheumatologic conditions associated with PH. Therefore, screening of anti-Scl-70 antibodies, rheumatoid factor, and antinuclear antibodies is necessary when clinically indicated. Liver function test (LFT) and thyroid functions should be screened in all patients with underlying PH. BNP and NT-proBNP are two valuable biomarkers which correlate with disease severity, RV dysfunction, as well as prognostication of the patients. A successful treatment reduces these markers and so their measurement is often carried out to assess the impact of therapy in clinical practice.

MANAGEMENT

Pulmonary hypertension patients require multidisciplinary care for their disease.

Management of WHO Pulmonary Hypertension Group-1 (PAH)

Physical Activity

Pulmonary arterial hypertension patients should remain active up to their highest extent.[4] They should be encouraged to engage in low-level-graded aerobic exercises such as walking and slow cycling. Patients should avoid heavy physical exertion or isometric exercise as both of them may provoke exertional syncope. Recently a large randomized controlled trial (RCT) showed significant benefit in 6MWD, World Health Organization functional class (WHO-FC), and peak VO_2 compared with standard care.[5] However, before initiation of rehabilitation program, patients must be stable with guideline-directed medical therapy (GDMT). Exposure to high altitude may contribute to hypoxic pulmonary vasoconstriction and may not be well tolerated.

Anticoagulation

Logically, patients with PAH should receive anticoagulation as histopathological specimens from PAH patients showed in situ thrombosis of pulmonary vessels. The largest registry analysis suggested a potential survival benefit with anticoagulation in patients with idiopathic PAH (IPAH),[6] but this fact was not established by other RCTs.[7] Therefore, individual decision-making is required.

Diuretics

Right heart failure (RHF) is associated with reduced renal blood flow and renin–angiotensin–aldosterone system (RAAS) activation. Once patients develop features of fluid retention such as edema or ascites, fluid restriction and diuretics are recommended. Renal function tests should be monitored regularly to avoid intravascular volume depletion as it may further decrease CO and blood pressure.

Oxygen

Although oxygen administration is associated with reduced PVR and improved functional capacity, studies failed to show any sustained benefit from oxygen therapy.

Anemia and Iron Deficiency

Iron deficiency is common in patients with PAH, which is defined as a serum ferritin value of <100 μg/L or a transferrin saturation < 20%. Iron deficiency is associated with poor WHO-FC and increased mortality. Therefore, regular checking of serum iron profile is an important part of the management of PAH and in patients with severe iron deficiency anemia (Hb <7–8 g/dL), intravenous iron supplementation is recommended.

Vaccination

Vaccination against influenza, *Streptococcus pneumoniae*, and severe acute respiratory syndrome coronavirus 2 (SARS-CoV-2) is recommended in all patients with PAH.

Pharmacological Management

Prior to the availability of disease-specific therapy, the 1- and 3-year survival rates for IPAH/hereditary PAH were 52% and 32%, respectively. In the modern era, with the availability of disease-specific agents, 1- and 3-year survival rates have improved to 91% and 69%, respectively.

Calcium Channel Blockers

Patients with positive vasoreactivity tests respond favorably to CCBs. Nifedipine, amlodipine, felodipine, and diltiazem are the CCBs that are used predominantly. The daily doses that are used in PAH are considerably higher (such as the target dose for amlodipine is 15–30 mg/day) than used for systemic hypertension. Because a positive vasoreactivity response does not predict a long-term response to CCBs, therefore, their efficacy should be assessed for at least after 6 months by RHC. As per ESC/ERS-2022 PH guidelines, a satisfactory chronic response is defined as WHO-FC I/II, mPAP <30 mm Hg and PVR <4 WU while on CCB therapy. In the absence of a satisfactory response, additional PAH therapy should be added. *Persons who did not undergo vasoreactivity testing or who are negative responders should not be put on CCBs as it may precipitate severe hypotension, syncope, and RHF.*[8]

Phosphodiesterase-5 Inhibitors and Guanylate Cyclase Stimulators

Nitric oxide is generated by endothelial nitric oxide synthase in endothelial cells and activates soluble guanylyl cyclase (sGC) to generate cGMP (cyclic guanosine monophosphate) in vascular smooth muscle cells and platelets. cGMP acts as a second messenger that induces vasodilation through relaxation of arterial smooth muscle cells and inhibits platelet activation. The enzyme phosphodiesterase-5 (PDE-5) is expressed in high concentration in pulmonary vascular tissue which hydrolyzes cGMP and terminates its action. The PDE-5 inhibitors (PDE-5is), by inactivating PDE-5, increase the concentration of cGMP and thereby augment NO-mediated vasodilation. Two PDE-5is used in PAH are *sildenafil* and *tadalafil*. Both the agents have shown to improve hemodynamics and 6MWD but failed to demonstrate any mortality benefit.

Riociguat is the first in-class sGC stimulator, which directly stimulates sGC independent of NO. In an RCT that included patients previously treated with endothelin receptor antagonists (ERAs) or nonparenteral prostanoids, riociguat (at a dose of 1–2.5 mg three times daily) significantly improved pulmonary hemodynamics, WHO-FC, and time to clinical worsening.[9] *Riociguat should not be used concurrently with PDE-5is.*

Prostanoids

Prostacyclin (PGI_2) activates cyclic adenosine monophosphate (cAMP)-dependent pathways that mediate pulmonary vasodilation. In clinical trials, intravenous *epoprostenol* improves functional class, exercise endurance, hemodynamics, and survival in patients with IPAH. *It also improves exercise tolerance and hemodynamics in patients with PAH related to scleroderma.* Each patient must learn the techniques of sterile preparations, operation of the ambulatory infusion pump, and care of the central venous catheter. Infections and interruptions can be life-threatening.

Subcutaneous treprostinil can provide a modest but statistically significant improvement in exercise tolerance. The main drawback of this agent is pain and erythema at the site of administration that may be found in up to 85% of patients. Oral treprostinil is also modestly effective as monotherapy.[10]

Inhaled iloprost is *approved for patients with PAH and severe heart failure symptoms*. However, cough is an additional side effect of this method of administration.

Selexipag is a recent addition in the armament of PAH medication, which acts orally and is a selective PGI_2 receptor agonist. In two RCTs,[11,12] it has been shown that selexipag monotherapy or adding selexipag on top of monotherapy (ERAs or PDE-5is) or double therapy (ERAs + PDE-5is) in patients with PAH reduces the relative risk of composite morbidity and/or mortality by 40%.

Endothelin Receptor Antagonists

Endothelin receptor antagonists inhibit the detrimental effect of endothelin-1 (ET-1), the strongest endogenous vasoconstrictor. In PAH, ET-1 is directly associated with PVR and mPAP and inversely associated with CO and 6MWD. Bosentan improves pulmonary hemodynamics and exercise capacity and delays clinical worsening. The BREATHE-1 trial, which compared Bosentan to placebo, demonstrated symptomatic improvement and WHO-FC in patients with bosentan.[13] The EARLY trial, which compared bosentan to placebo in WHO-FC-II PAH patients, also demonstrated improvement in PVR and 6MWD in bosentan group.[14] *Ambrisentan* in the ARIES-1 trial showed improvement in exercise tolerance, WHO-FC, hemodynamics, and quality of life in patients with PAH.[15] SERAPHIN (Study with an Endothelin Receptor Antagonist in Pulmonary Arterial Hypertension to Improve Clinical Outcome) trial which included 742 PAH patients with some form of background PAH treatment demonstrated that adding *macitentan*, a dual ERA, (10 mg/day for 85 weeks) is associated with 45% reduction in death or disease progression.[16] Macitentan is associated with headache, nasopharyngitis, and anemia. Anemia (Hb < 8 g/dL) is found in up to 4.3% of patients.

Interventional Therapy

Balloon Atrial Septostomy and Potts Shunt

Both of these procedures are aimed to decompress the right heart and increase systemic blood flow, and thereby improving systemic oxygen transport at the cost of arterial oxygen desaturation. In balloon atrial septostomy, a balloon is used to create an interatrial shunt, and on the other hand, Potts shunt is created by connecting the left PA and the descending aorta. Because of the procedural complexity and high mortality, they are only performed at high volume and at dedicated centers.

Pulmonary Artery Denervation

Sympathetic overdrive leads to pulmonary vasoconstriction and vascular remodeling through a stretch receptor-mediated baroreflex. These stretch receptors are situated at the bifurcation of the PAs. It has been shown that radiofrequency ablation of these stretch receptors is associated with acute and long-term improvement of pulmonary hemodynamics in patients with PAH who are still symptomatic despite on recommended medical therapy.[17] Although promising, PADN is still in experimental stage during writing of this chapter.

Lung and Heart–lung Transplantation

Lung transplantation is considered in intermediate-high- to high-risk PAH patients with refractory symptoms despite orally received optimal medical management. High-risk patients[18] receiving subcutaneous/intravenous PGI_2 analogues are also the candidates for lung transplantation. Combined heart–lung transplantation is usually reserved for those with underlying noncorrectable cardiac conditions.[19] In transplant recipients who survive the early post-transplant period, long-term outcomes are good.

Risk Assessment and Assessment of Response to Therapy in Pulmonary Arterial Hypertension

World Health Organization functional class is considered as the strongest predictor of survival in patients with PAH. In 2015, ESC/ERS PH guidelines classify patients into low-, intermediate-, or high-risk groups based on estimated 1-year mortality rates of <5%, 5–10%, and >10%, respectively. This model is updated in ESC/ERS PH guideline-2022 **(Table 2)** and serves as a valuable tool for initial patient assessment as well as to assess response to therapy in patients with PAH.

Approach to Pulmonary Arterial Hypertension Treatment

There is a paradigm shift in the treatment approach of PAH. Previously, treatment success was defined by delaying death in an end-stage disease patient. But nowadays, identifying the disease in an early stage and early initiation of treatment is the target. From a pharmacological standpoint, combination therapy is preferred over single-agent therapy **(Flowchart 2)**. AMBITION (A Study of First-Line Ambrisentan and Tadalafil Combination Therapy in Subjects with Pulmonary Arterial Hypertension) trial is a landmark trial[20] that explores the role of early aggressive treatment with ambrisentan and tadalafil in treatment-naïve PAH patients. This trial included 500 patients randomized into three groups—a combination of ambrisentan + tadalafil, ambrisentan alone, and tadalafil alone. At the end of the trial, 50% lower incidence of composite of death, lung transplantation, PAH-related hospitalization, and worsening PAH was found in the combination arm compared to the monotherapy arms. Importantly, combination therapy was not associated with increase in drug-related adverse events. Registry data suggest patients with combination therapy with PDE-5i plus ERA alternative to the drugs studied in AMBITION trial also have better outcome compared to patients on monotherapy, suggesting *benefit from combination therapy is not drug specific.* Several small prospective clinical trials on selective high-risk PAH patients have shown 100% survival in 3 years with combination regimen of intravenous epoprostenol + bosentan + sildenafil.

Management of Pulmonary Arterial Hypertension-associated Complications

Arrhythmias

Atrial fibrillation (AF) is the most common arrhythmia in PAH population. PAH patients are highly sensitive to arrhythmias and loss of atrioventricular synchrony puts a heavy burden on pulmonary hemodynamics. Therefore, whenever possible, maintenance of sinus rhythm should be the main target of therapy. Electrical cardioversion is safe and sometimes lifesaving in AF with hemodynamic compromise. To achieve and maintain a stable sinus rhythm, prophylactic use of oral amiodarone may be considered. Low-dose beta-blocker or digoxin may also be used on individual case basis. The role of catheter ablation in this population is less well established.

Hemoptysis

Massive hemoptysis is particularly common in patients with heritable PAH and PAH associated with congenital heart disease. They usually originate from bronchial arteries and contrast-enhanced CT is the diagnostic modality of choice. In the absence of localization of the culprit vessel, embolization of enlarged bronchial arteries is recommended. In patients with massive or recurrent hemoptysis despite embolization, lung transplantation is the last resort.

TABLE 2: Comprehensive risk assessment in pulmonary arterial hypertension (PAH).

Determinants of prognosis (estimated 1-year mortality)	Low risk (<5%)	Intermediate risk (5–10%)	High risk (>10%)
Signs of right heart failure	Absent	Absent	Present
Progression of disease symptoms and clinical manifestations	No	Slow	Rapid
Syncope	No	Occasional	Repeated
WHO-FC	I and II	III	IV
6MWD	>440 m	165–440 m	<165 m
CPET	Peak VO_2 >65% predicted	Peak VO_2 35–65% predicted	Peak VO_2 <35% predicted
BNP and NT-proBNP (ng/L)	• BNP <50 • NT-proBNP <300	• BNP 50–800 • NT-proBNP 300–1,100	• BNP >800 • NT-proBNP >1,100
Echocardiography	• RA area <18 cm^2 • TAPSE/sPAP >0.32 • No pericardial effusion	• RA area 18–26 cm^2 • TAPSE/sPAP 0.19–0.32 • Minimal pericardial effusion	• RA area <18 cm^2 • TAPSE/sPAP <0.19 • Moderate-to-large pericardial effusion
Cardiac MRI	• RVEF >54% • SVI >40 mL/m^2 • RVESVI <42 mL/m^2	• RVEF 37–54% • SVI 26–40 mL/m^2 • RVESVI 42–54 mL/m^2	• RVEF <37% • SVI <26 mL/m^2 • RVESVI >54 mL/m^2
Hemodynamics	• RAP <8 mm Hg • CI ≥2.5 • SVI >38 mL/m^2 • SvO_2 >65%	• RAP 8–14 mm Hg • CI = 2–2.4 • SVI = 31–38 mL/m^2 • SvO_2 = 60–65%	• RAP <8 mm Hg • CI <2 • SVI <31 mL/m^2 • SvO_2 <60%

(6MWD: 6-minute walking distance; BNP: brain natriuretic peptide; CI: confidence interval; CPET: cardiopulmonary exercise testing; MRI: magnetic resonance imaging; NT-proBNP: N-terminal prohormone of BNP; RA: right atrial; RAP: right atrial pressure; RVEF: right ventricular ejection fraction; RVESVI: right ventricular end-systolic volume index; sPAP: systolic pulmonary artery pressure; SVI: stroke volume index; SvO_2: mixed venous oxygen saturation; TAPSE: tricuspid annular plane systolic excursion; WHO-FC: World Health Organization functional class)

Left Main Coronary Artery Compression

Compression of LMCA by enlarged PA is an increasingly common complication which is associated with angina, arrhythmia, heart failure, and sudden cardiac death. Studies suggest that at least 6% of patients with PAH have significant LMCA compression. Hugely dilated PA (>40 mm) and a narrow LMCA take-off angle (<60°) are important risk factors. Percutaneous coronary stenting is a safe and effective treatment.[21]

Right Heart Failure

Infections, arrhythmias, and anemia are the major precipitants of RHF. A negative fluid balance to reduce RV preload by diuretics improves RV function.[22] The key objective of treatment is maintaining mean blood pressure >60 mm Hg. Patients who are persistently hypotensive, pressure agents such as dobutamine or noradrenalin are valuable.

Management of WHO Pulmonary Hypertension Group 2 (PH Associated with Left Heart Disease)

Pulmonary hypertension related to LHD is the most prevalent form of PH, contributing 65–80% cases. PH-LHD is defined by mPAP >20 mm Hg and PAWP >15 mm Hg. Confined by this hemodynamic condition, isolated postcapillary PH is defined by PVR ≤2 WU and combined pre- and postcapillary PH is defined by PVR >2 WU. Patients with suspected PH-LHD will have an established diagnosis of LHD, like heart failure with preserved ejection fraction/heart failure with midrange ejection fraction (HFpEF/HFmrEF) or heart failure with reduced ejection fraction (HFrEF), VHD, or congenital heart disease. The distinction between PH associated with HFpEF and other forms of PH (e.g., PAH and CTEPH) is often difficult in clinical practice because of the increased cardiovascular burden in PAH population. In such situations, validated clinical scores for diagnosing HFpEF (e.g., HFA-PEFF and H_2FPEF) are helpful. *Treatment of the underlying left-sided heart disease is the mainstay of management.* Drugs approved for PAH have variable and potentially detrimental effect in PH-LHD and therefore are not recommended.

HFpEF: Apart from managing the precipitating factors, e.g., obesity, hypertension, and sleep apnea, studies have shown that the sodium-glucose cotransporter-2 inhibitors (SGLT-2Is) (dapagliflozin and empagliflozin) improve LV function in HFpEF. *In patients with predominantly combined pre- and postcapillary PH profile, sildenafil improves hemodynamics,*

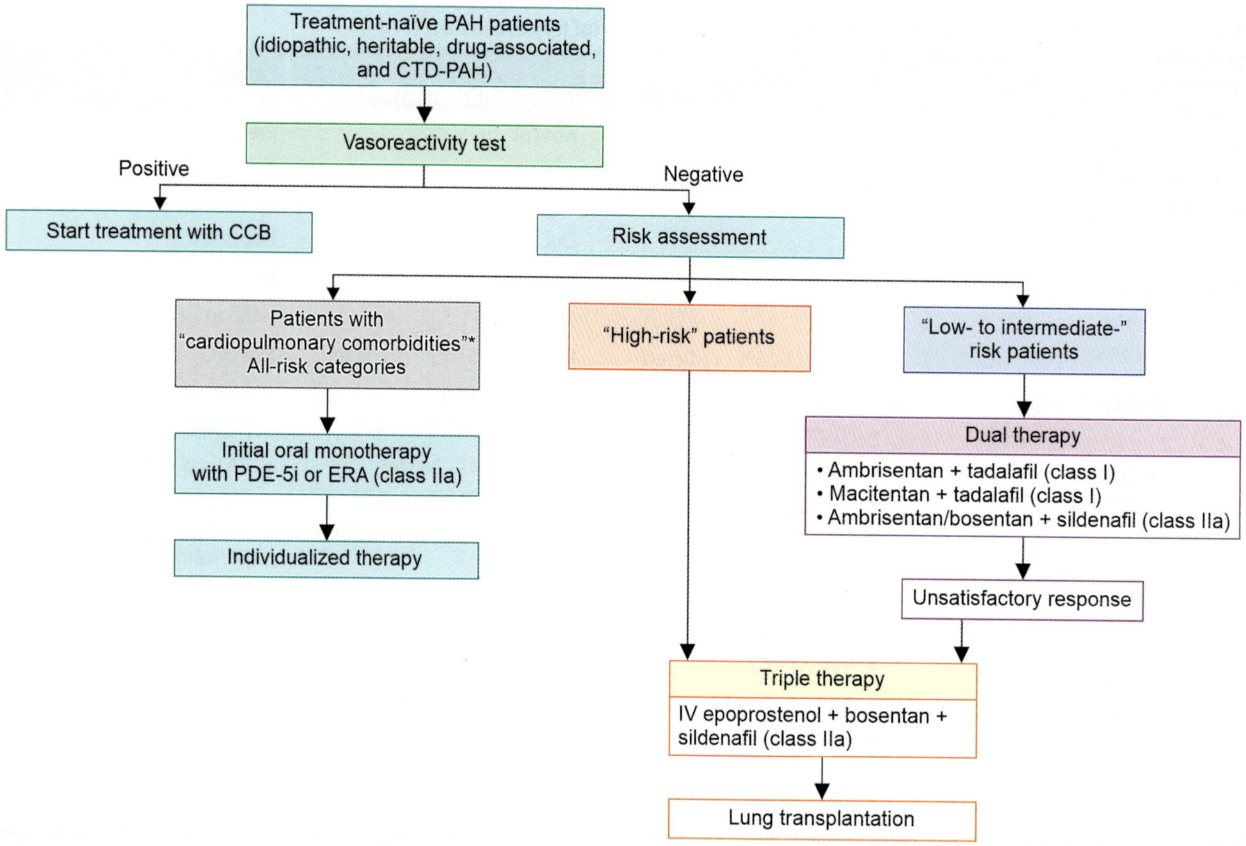

*Cardiopulmonary comorbidities = cardiac comorbidities + pulmonary comorbidities. Cardiac comorbidities include = left ventricular systolic or diastolic dysfunction, hypertension, diabetes mellitus, and coronary artery disease; and pulmonary comorbidities include: parenchymal lung disease that is often associated with a low DLCO (<45% of the predictive value).

FLOWCHART 2: Treatment algorithm for PAH as proposed by 2022 ESC/ERS pulmonary hypertension guideline.

(CCB: calcium channel blocker; CTD: connective tissue disease; ERA: endothelin receptor antagonists; PAH: pulmonary arterial hypertension; PDE-5i: phosphodiesterase-5 inhibitor)

RV function, and quality of life at 6 and 12 months versus placebo. However, in patients with predominantly isolated precapillary PH profile, sildenafil is of no value.

HFrEF: GDMT with angiotensin-converting enzyme inhibitors (ACEIs)/angiotensin receptor blocker (ARB)/ angiotensin receptor-neprilysin inhibitor (ARNI), beta-blocker, SGLT-2I, and Aldactone receptor antagonist is the first-line management. In selected patient population, implantation of left ventricular assist device (LVAD) significantly reduces mPAP.[23] Few studies have suggested that sildenafil improves pulmonary hemodynamics and functional capacity in HFrEF, but large RCTs are required to make a definite recommendation.[24,25]

VHD: Correction of underlying VHD often improves PH, *but in some cases, it may persist and be associated with adverse outcome.* Treating persistent PH after repairing VHD with drugs such as sildenafil is associated with worse outcome and is not recommended.[26]

Management of WHO Pulmonary Hypertension Group 3 (PH due to Lung Disease)

Intrinsic lung disease [chronic obstructive pulmonary disease (COPD) and ILD] is the second most common cause of PH in patients with lung disease; PH is categorized by "severe" or "nonsevere" depending on hemodynamic parameter. Previously, severe PH was defined by mPAP >35 mm Hg. As two recent studies have shown that PVR >5 WU is a better threshold to predict grim prognosis in COPD- and ILD-associated PH, therefore, recent guidelines use PVR to distinguish between the two.[27,28] Usually group 3 PH is moderate in severity. *Severe PH (PVR > 5WU)* is observed only in ~5% cases.

PH associated with COPD or emphysema: Optimizing treatment of underlying lung disease is of primary importance. *Supplemental oxygen therapy* is indicated in patients with COPD when PaO_2 <60 mm Hg or SaO_2 <92%.[29] Medicines approved for the treatment of PAH are *not recommended* in WHO PH group 3 patients with "nonsevere" PH as they may precipitate V/Q mismatch and worsen pulmonary hemodynamics, exercise capacity, and outcome in this population. However, in patients with severe PH, registry data showed improvement in WHO FC, 6MWD, and PVR when treated with PDE-5is.

PH associated with ILD: PDE-5is, ERAs, and riociguat are associated with negative clinical outcome in PH associated with ILD. As per INCREASE trial,[30] there is a ray of hope for *inhaled treprostinil*. In this RCT, which included 326 ILD patients with PH, it was shown that inhaled treprostinil at the dose of 72 μg four times daily had 31 meters improvement in 6MWD and also in NT-proBNP levels at 16 weeks compared to placebo. But further data are required to assess the long-term outcome. Eligible candidates should be referred for lung transplantation evaluation.

Management of WHO Pulmonary Hypertension Group 4 (CTEPH)

A multimodal treatment is required for management of CTEPH. This includes: Pulmonary endarterectomy (PEA), balloon pulmonary angioplasty (BPA), and medical therapies to address the anatomical location of lesions—proximal, distal, and at microvascular level, respectively.

Anticoagulation: As recurrent pulmonary thromboembolism accompanied by insufficient clot resolution is the key pathological feature of this disease, therefore, *lifelong therapeutic anticoagulation* is recommended in CTEPH patients. Although both vitamin K antagonists (VKAs) and direct oral anticoagulants (DOACs) can be used for therapeutic anticoagulation, but as per EXPERT (EXamining PErsonalised Radiation Therapy for Low-risk Early Breast Cancer) trial, comparable bleeding rates for both the agents with higher number of recurrent venous thromboembolic events was found with DOACs.[31] *In patients with antiphospholipid antibody (APLA) syndrome, VKAs are recommended.*

PEA: It is the treatment of choice for proximal PA thrombus. In European CTEPH centers, the surgical outcome is excellent with <2.5% periprocedural mortality rate. The long-term survival after PEA is 90% at 3 years and 83% at 5 years. On the other hand, patients who refused surgery had a 5-year survival rate of 53%.[32,33]

BPA: It is recommended for patients with inoperable CTEPH or persistent or recurrent PH after PEA. Although this is an effective procedure, the rate of procedural complications is high and includes wire-related vascular injury and lung injury with hemoptysis and hypoxia. In patients with PVR >4 WU, preprocedural medical therapy is indicated.

Medical therapy: *Riociguat*, which decreases PVR by 31% and improves 6MWD compared to placebo, is recommended for medical therapy. Among other drugs, *subcutaneous treprostinil* also showed improved 6MWD in inoperable CTEPH cases and in those with persistent/recurrent PH after PEA.[34] Another study conducted among inoperable CTEPH subjects, showed *macitentan* at the dose of 10 mg/day, is associated with improved 6MWD and PVR versus placebo.[35] Although other drugs such as PDE-5is and ERAs are often used in CTEPH, their efficacy was not proven by RCTs.

Management of WHO Pulmonary Hypertension Group 5 (PH with Multifactorial Mechanisms)

Group 5 encompasses varied conditions ranging from hematological disorders to systemic diseases (sarcoidosis and neurofibromatosis type-1) to chronic kidney disease. In the absence of positive RCTs, use of PAH drugs for treating group 5 PH is not advised and treating the underlying disorder remains the standard of care.

Hematological Disorders

Sickle cell disease (SCD) is the major contributor of group 5. Thrombotic lesions are the key feature of PH related to SCD. Management of anemia is the cornerstone of management. There is lack of data to support the use of PAH drugs in patients with SCD-associated PH.

Chronic myeloproliferative disorders, particularly chronic myelogenous leukemia (CML), is associated with PH in 8–10% cases. Importantly, drugs such as dasatinib, bosutinib, and ponatinib, which are used to treat this condition, are associated with reversible drug-related PH. Unfortunately, no PAH drugs are specifically recommended to treat PH associated with this disorder.

CONCLUSION

Pulmonary hypertension encompasses a diverse group of diseases with significant morbidity and mortality and it is often difficult to diagnose unless suspected. After the diagnosis is made, response to therapy is highly variable and the cost of therapy is also high. **Table 3** highlights the do's and don'ts in diagnosis and management of PH. Due to lack of awareness of patients as well as physicians, limited number of specialized PH centers, and high cost of therapy, in a resource-limited country like ours, only handful of patients receive adequate care.

TABLE 3: Do's and don'ts from ESC/ERS PH guidelines-2022.

Recommended	Not recommended
RHC to establish diagnosis of PAH/CTEPH or in diagnostic dilemma	Vasoreactivity testing in patients with PAH other than I/H/D PAH* and in PH groups 2, 3, 4, and 5
Echocardiography as first-line test in suspected PH. TRV >2.8 m/s should be taken as the probability threshold of PH	Use of ACEis, ARBs, ARNI, SGLT-2Is, beta blockers, or ivabradine in PAH unless required by comorbidities
Risk stratification at the time of diagnosis and during follow-ups using three strata model	Calcium channel blockers without vasoreactivity testing
Supervised exercise training after clinical stabilization	Initial combination therapy with macitentan, tadalafil, and selexipag
Lifelong therapeutic anticoagulation patients with CTEPH	Addition of riociguat to PDE-5is
VKAs for patients with APLA	Pregnancy is contraindicated in PH
Initial combination therapy with ambrisentan and tadalafil or macitentan and tadalafil	Combining bosentan and sildenafil to reduce morbidity/mortality
In patients with ASD, VSD, or PDA and a PVR <3 WU, go for shunt closure	In patients with ASD and a PVR >5 WU, despite PAH treatment, shunt closure is contraindicated
Bosentan in symptomatic Eisenmenger syndrome	Use of PAH medications in unclassified PH
Inhaled treprostinil in patients with PH associated with ILD irrespective of PH-severity	Use of PAH medications in patients with lung disease with nonsevere PH

*D PAH: Drug- or toxin-associated PAH.

(ACEis: angiotensin-converting enzyme inhibitors; APLA: antiphospholipid antibody; ARBs: angiotensin receptor blockers; ARNI: angiotensin receptor-neprilysin inhibitor; ASD: atrial septal defect; CTEPH: chronic thromboembolic pulmonary hypertension; ESC/ERS: European Society of Cardiology/European Respiratory Society; I/H/D PAH: idiopathic, heritable, drug-associated pulmonary arterial hypertension; ILD: interstitial lung disease; PAH: pulmonary arterial hypertension; PDA: patent ductus arteriosus; PDE-5is: phosphodiesterase-5 inhibitors; PH: pulmonary hypertension; PVR: pulmonary vascular resistance; SGLT-2Is: sodium-glucose cotransporter-2 inhibitors; TRV: tricuspid regurgitation velocity; VKAs: vitamin K antagonists)

ONLINE REFERENCES

Please scan the QR code provided at the end of the table of contents for References of this chapter.

CHAPTER

120 Therapeutic Options for Pulmonary Hypertension

BKS Sastry

ABSTRACT

Pulmonary hypertension (PH) defined as pulmonary artery mean pressure >20 mm Hg is seen in different diseases. It is classified into five groups based on underlying pathophysiology and response to treatment. Pulmonary vasodilators that include phosphodiesterase-5 (PDE5) inhibitors, endothelin receptor antagonists, and prostaglandins are specifically studied in group 1 PH with favorable effect on clinical outcomes. Calcium channel blockers are reserved for those with positive vasodilator challenge. Sotatercept is a new drug with proven efficacy that is awaiting regulatory approval. Balloon atrial septostomy and Potts shunt are palliative procedures useful in select patients. Patients with refractory symptoms should be considered for bilateral lung transplantation. PH patients due to left heart diseases (group 2) and those due to pulmonary diseases (group 3) should be treated aggressively for the underlying diseases. Specific pulmonary vasodilators have limited role and may even be harmful. They should be used under close medical supervision. Group 4 PH patients due to chronic pulmonary thromboembolism should be considered for pulmonary endarterectomy or balloon angioplasty. Pulmonary vasodilators are used in those who are not candidates for either of these procedures. Oral anticoagulants are used in all group 4 patients and those with idiopathic pulmonary arterial hypertension (PAH). Treatment for group 5 PH is individualized based on the underlying specific disease. General measures such as oxygen, vaccination, rehabilitation, and contraception must be advised to all patients.

Keywords: Pulmonary hypertension, pulmonary vasodilators.

INTRODUCTION

Pulmonary hypertension (PH) is a hemodynamic abnormality seen in different diseases. As per the 2022 ESC/ERS guidelines on PH, it is defined as pulmonary artery (PA) mean pressure of >20 mm Hg and pulmonary vascular resistance (PVR) <2 Wood units as measured by right heart catheterization (RHC).[1] The presence of PH indicates poor prognosis of the underlying disease. It tends to be a progressive disease eventually leading to ventriculoarterial uncoupling and right heart failure.

Based on underlying etiology, pathophysiology, natural history, and response to treatment, it is divided into five categories as can be seen in **Table 1**.

PATHOPHYSIOLOGY

It is essential to understand underlying pathophysiology to treat the disease effectively. Pathophysiological mechanisms vary depending upon the underlying etiology.

In group 1 disorders, due to different abnormalities in molecular mechanisms, vasoconstriction occurs. Endothelial proliferation and smooth muscle cell hypertrophy and proliferation follow. Vascular remodeling ensues. Vascular lumen gets narrowed, thrombotic, and fibrotic occlusion of small vessels is followed by development of plexiform lesions. Arterioles are obliterated and lost. In patients with pulmonary venoocclusive disease, similar involvement of venules and capillaries is seen.

In group 2 disorders, which are secondary to left heart disease, the main abnormality is elevated PA wedge pressure (PAWP). An increased wedge pressure passively elevates PA diastolic pressure, then PA mean pressure and PA systolic pressure. Initially, PVR remains normal. This condition is called isolated postcapillary PH (IPcPH). However, with time pulmonary arterial constriction and later remodeling ensues. This leads to elevated PVR which further raises PA pressures. PH with elevated PAWP and PVR is called combined pre- and postcapillary pulmonary hypertension (CpcPH). PH

TABLE 1: Classification of pulmonary hypertension.

Group		Diseases
Group 1	Pulmonary arterial hypertension	• Idiopathic • Heritable • Connective tissue associated • Toxin or drug related • Human immunodeficiency virus infection associated • Portopulmonary hypertension associated • Congenital heart disease associated • Pulmonary veno-occlusive disease • Persistent pulmonary hypertension of newborn
Group 2	Due to left heart diseases	• Left ventricular systolic and diastolic dysfunction • Congenital and acquired valvular heart disease
Group 3	Due to pulmonary diseases	• Hypoventilation syndromes • High altitude • Chronic obstructive airway diseases • Restrictive lung diseases • Obstructive sleep apnea • Chronic pulmonary fibrosis with emphysema
Group 4	Obstruction in pulmonary vasculature	• Chronic pulmonary thromboembolism • Tumor embolization and obstruction
Group 5	Miscellaneous or multiple etiologies	• Sarcoidosis • Hemolytic anemia, hereditary spherocytosis, and sickle cell anemia • Pulmonary Langerhans's cell histiocytosis • Chronic renal failure • Glycogen storage and Gaucher disease • Mediastinal tumors or fibrosing mediastinitis

(HIV: human immunodeficiency virus)

is disproportionate to the elevated PAWP and it may not respond to measures to decrease PAWP alone.

In PH due to group 3 diseases, predominant mechanism is reflex vasoconstriction secondary to hypoxia. However, in some patients, arteriolar vasoconstriction and vascular remodeling occur leading to disproportionate PH.

In group 4 disorders, thromboembolism or in situ tumors or tumor emboli occlude vessels and thereby increase PA pressures. Localization of the occlusions within vascular compartments is important in deciding the treatment.

In group 5 disorders, more than one pathophysiological mechanism is involved. There may be varying degrees of vasoconstriction, remodeling, and extrinsic or intrinsic vascular obstruction of pulmonary arterial tree. In situ thrombosis or emboli may be seen. Sometimes, in sarcoidosis elevated PAWP may be contributing to PH.

Treatment depends on the underlying pathophysiological mechanism.

MANAGEMENT OF PULMONARY HYPERTENSION: DIFFERENT GROUPS

Management of PH depends upon the class to which it belongs since the treatment targets the underlying pathophysiology.

Group 1 Pulmonary Hypertension

Various drugs that target different molecular mechanisms involved in the pathophysiology are used to treat pulmonary arterial hypertension (PAH). These pathways include nitric oxide pathway, endothelin pathway, and prostacyclin pathway. Calcium channel blockers may be effective only in a few patients. All these drugs improve symptoms, functional class, 6-minute walk distance, quality of life, and mortality **(Flowchart 1)**.

Acute Vasodilator Challenge and Calcium Channel Blockers

Calcium channel blockers should be used only in idiopathic PAH (IPAH), heritable PAH, and drug-induced PAH patients who respond to acute vasodilator challenge. They should not be used without doing acute vasodilator challenge testing. Approximately, 10% of adults and 35% of children may respond to acute vasodilator challenge. During this test, patients are given short-acting vasodilator medication such as intravenous epoprostenol, inhaled iloprost, or nitric oxide for short duration in cardiac catheterization laboratory while monitoring PA pressures, systemic pressures, and cardiac output. A positive response is when the PA mean pressure decreases by >10 mm Hg to a value <40 mm Hg without decrease in cardiac output.[2] Such patients may benefit from regular use of oral calcium channel blockers in the long run. Patients should have a repeat RHC after 3 months. CCB should be continued only when the patient continues to respond with PA mean pressure <30 mm Hg and PVR >4 Wood units. In chronic nonresponders, CCB may be withdrawn, and other pulmonary vasodilators given. Amlodipine and felodipine are the most often drugs and at higher doses than used to treat systemic hypertension.

Phosphodiesterase-5 Inhibitors

Cyclic guanosine monophosphate (cGMP) is a potent smooth muscle dilator, and it is metabolized by phosphodiesterase-5 (PDE5) in pulmonary vascular smooth muscle cells. PDE-5

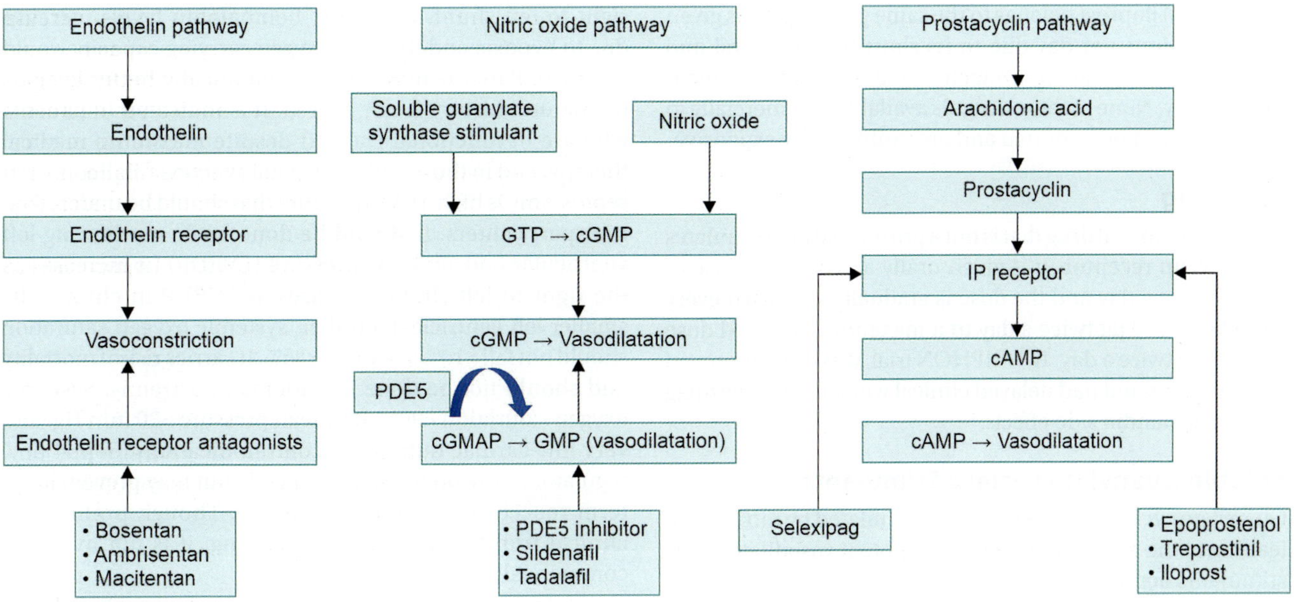

FLOWCHART 1: Targeted molecular pathways. Molecular pathways that are targeted to treat pulmonary hypertension are depicted. These include endothelin pathway, nitric oxide pathway, and prostaglandin pathway. Endothelin receptor antagonists counter the vasoconstriction and proliferation signals caused by increased levels of endothelin in PAH patients. Nitric oxide stimulates guanylate cyclase that generates cyclic guanosine monophosphate (cGMP) from guanosine triphosphate (GTP). cGMP is a vasodilator and is antiproliferative. Its levels are also increased by riociguat, a stimulant of guanylate cyclase. Phosphodiesterase-5 (PDE5) inhibitors inhibit degradation of cGMP to guanosine monophosphate (GMP). Prostacyclin and its analogs generate cyclic adenosine monophosphate (cAMP), a vasodilator, and an antiproliferative molecule by stimulating IP receptor. Selexipag also stimulates IP receptor.

inhibitors such as sildenafil and tadalafil cause pulmonary vascular smooth muscles by inhibiting its degradation. In randomized controlled trials (RCTs), these drugs were proven to show clinical benefit.[3] Recommended dose of sildenafil is 20 mg three times a day and that of tadalafil 40 mg once a day. These drugs should not be used in combination with nitrates or soluble guanylate cyclase (sGC) stimulants since that can lead to hypotension. Common side effects include nasal congestion and frequent nasopharyngitis. Rarely, sudden blindness (ischemic optic neuropathy) and sudden loss of hearing are reported with sildenafil.

Endothelin Receptor Antagonists

Endothelin is a potent vasoconstrictor whose levels are increased in pulmonary vessels of PAH patients. Endothelin receptor antagonists (ERA) improve clinical condition of patients with PAH. Bosentan started at a dose of 62.5 mg twice a day and increased to 125 mg twice a day after 1 month. Frequent monitoring of liver function tests, at least every month for the first 6 months is mandatory. Bosentan has multiple drug interactions. Ambrisentan given at a dose of 10 mg once a day is devoid of any hepatotoxicity but can produce pedal edema in a few patients. In SERAPHIN trial macitentan given at a dose of 10 mg once a day improves clinical status and delays clinical worsening.[4] Anemia with hemoglobin less than 8 gm% is seen in about 4% of patients. All these drugs are teratogenic.

Prostanoids

Prostacyclin is a potent vasodilator, and it inhibits smooth muscle cell proliferation and platelet aggregation. Prostacyclin expression is impaired in PAH patients. Prostacyclin analogs and prostacyclin receptor stimulants are useful in these patients. These drugs by way of systemic vasodilatation can cause headache, flushing, jaw pain and diarrhea. Side effects are common, and some patients get used to them overtime. Constant encouragement and symptomatic treatment may help tolerate the side effects. Each patient should be encouraged to take the maximum tolerated dose. Different dosages of the drugs seem to be equally effective provided patient is taking his or her maximum tolerated dose.

The first drug to be studied in this class was epoprostenol, which must be given as a continuous intravenous infusion due to its very short half-life. Dose is slowly up titrated to the maximum tolerated dose. Drug is administered through a subcutaneously implanted pump and a tunneled indwelling catheter. Patient and the family should get trained to constitute the drug and administer it. Adverse events include pump malfunction, obstruction, local infection, and systemic sepsis. Treprostinil is a similar drug that can be given by continuous subcutaneous or intravenous infusion. Infusion site pain can be an adverse effect. It was studied as an oral drug also but does not appear to be very effective. Oral treprostinil was shown to be effective in drug naïve patients but not as an add on therapy to PDE5 inhibitors and ERAs.

Inhalational iloprost belongs to the same group and it is given 6–9 inhalations per day due to its short half-life. Oral and inhalational drugs are less effective that those administered parenterally. None of these drugs is available commercially in India and must be imported and are prohibitively expensive.

Selexipag

Selexipag is an oral drug that is not a prostanoid but stimulates prostacyclin receptor. It is given orally at a starting dose of 200 µg twice a day and the dose is gradually increased every 2 weeks by 200 µg twice a day to a maximum tolerated dose or 1,600 µg twice a day. In GRIPHON trial, this drug improved clinical status and had delayed clinical worsening.[5] Selexipag has prostaglandin side effects.

Soluble Guanylate Cyclase Stimulants

Guanylate cyclase (GC) is normally stimulated by nitric oxide leading to the generation of cGMP, a potent vasodilator. sGC stimulants act directly on GC. They are effective even when the nitric oxide synthesis in the endothelium is deficient as seen in advanced disease. While PDE5 inhibitors increase the available cGMP by inhibiting its degradation, these drugs increase the production of cGMP. Combining these drugs can lead to hypotension and hence should not be given in combination. Riociguat is a drug widely studied and found to be effective in PAH patients and chronic thromboembolic PH (CTEPH) patients.[6] It is started at a dose of 0.5 mg three times a day. Dose is increased every 2 weeks by 0.5 mg per dose to a maximum dose of 2.5 mg three times a day. if the patient can tolerate it without hypotension. Common side effects include gastritis, hypotension, syncope, and hemoptysis. Also, this drug is effective when substituted for sildenafil or tadalafil as the patient worsens on these drugs.

Sotatercept

It is a fusion molecule of Fc domain of immunoglobulin G1 and extracellular domain of activin receptor type IIA. This molecule traps the circulating activin ligands and decreases the signal for smooth muscle cell proliferation. The drug given at a dose of 0.3 and 0.7 mg/kg dose by subcutaneous injection once in three weeks has shown significant improvement in clinical status, PVR, 6-minute walk distance, and N-terminal pro-B-type natriuretic peptide (NT-proBNP) levels.[7] The drug has tolerable side effects of increased hemoglobin levels and decreased platelet counts. This drug is yet to be approved by regulatory agencies.

Balloon Atrial Septostomy

Advanced PAH is characterized by low cardiac reserve due to very high PVR. During exercise cardiac output will not rise and blood pressure falls leading to syncope. PAH patients often have right atrial (RA) pressures more than left atrial pressures. Creation of communication between right and left atria will decompress the right heart. This would improve cardiac output at the cost of systemic desaturation due to right to left shunt. Overtime, hemoglobin levels increase due to hypoxia and the total oxygen carrying capacity would improve. Patients may be symptomatically better even as the natural history is not altered. It is indicated in patients who are in functional class III despite maximum medical therapy, and in those with exertional syncope.[8] Balloon atrial septostomy is high-risk procedure that should be undertaken in expert centers. It should be done while monitoring left ventricular end-diastolic pressure (LVEDP) (it increases as the right-to-left shunt increases as LVEDP in chronically smaller left ventricles). Further, systemic oxygen saturation should not fall >10% to a value <80%. It carries risk of mortality and should not be done in patients in extremis. Systemic oxygen saturation <90%, RA mean pressure >20 mm Hg, and very low cardiac output are contraindications. Septal flow regulators work on the same principle but may prevent long-term reocclusion of the septostomy. Though preliminary clinical trial findings are encouraging, it is not available commercially.

Potts Shunt

Creating a shunt between the left PA to descending aorta in patients with suprasystemic PH can decompress the pulmonary circulation. Cardiac output improves at the cost of systemic desaturation in the territory supplied by descending aorta. This spares perfusion of desaturated blood into coronary and cerebral circulation that is seen with balloon atrial septostomy. The shunt can be done either surgically or percutaneously. It is more suitable in children where the left PA and descending thoracic aorta are close to each other. In adults, it can be challenging. In a retrospective international registry of 110 children, the operative mortality was 15%. 5-year survival was 68% for those discharged home. There was significant clinical improvement and >50% of the children could be free from prostaglandin infusion. Preoperatively, very sick patients had higher operative mortality.[9]

Pulmonary Artery Denervation

Sympathetic nervous system overactivity may play an important role in PAH. Oral beta-blockers are not effective and can be detrimental. However, localized targeted denervation of proximal pulmonary arteries was shown to be safe and effective in the treatment of PAH in a small phase 2 multicenter study using a proprietary therapeutic intravascular ultrasound (TIVUS).[10] It would avoid systemic adverse effects. Further studies are needed.

Heart Lung Transplantation

Medical management for PAH is not curative. Patients continue to deteriorate and die. Close monitoring of these patients is needed to assess the functional status and assess prognostic factors. Several risk stratification criteria like REVEAL scores are available to estimate one year mortality risk. Patients with progressive PAH and estimated 1-year mortality >10% calculated from any of the risk stratification tools, should be offered bilateral lung transplantation. Patients with severe right ventricular dysfunction and uncorrectable congenital cardiac abnormalities should undergo heart lung transplantation. Patients not responding adequately to maximum medical therapy, those who may not respond well to medication such as severe hypoxemia due to pulmonary veno-occlusive disease and pulmonary capillary hemangiomatous and patients with recurrent hemoptysis, PA aneurysms, and liver and renal dysfunction due to PAH are also candidates for lung transplantation. Post-transplant, median survival is 10 years in those who survive the first year. In India, a few centers have been doing bilateral lung transplantation for IPAH and other pulmonary diseases. The overall experience in IPAH is limited and long-term survival reports are awaited.[11]

Pulmonary Arterial Hypertension with Cardiopulmonary Comorbidities

Many elderly PAH patients have cardiopulmonary comorbidities. Two phenotypes can be identified in them. Left heart phenotype consists of elderly female patients with heart failure with preserved ejection fraction (HFpEF), precapillary PH and history of atrial fibrillation. Cardiopulmonary phenotype consists of elderly male patients with history of smoking and hypoxemia, risk factors for left heart disease, and low DLCO. These patients respond poorly to pulmonary vasodilators, cannot tolerate them, and have higher mortality. Cautious administration of PDE5 inhibitors as monotherapy may be started.[12] Close monitoring is needed since they can have worsening of their left heart failure or respiratory failure. Additional therapy may be guided by clinical status as there are no clear guidelines.

Treatment Strategies

Patients diagnosed with PAH should undergo RHC and acute vasodilator challenge test unless they are in right heart failure. Responders may be prescribed CCB and a repeat RHC done after 3 months. Thos who continue to show favorable response will continue with CCB. Nonresponders to acute vasodilator challenge, those who are at low or intermediate risk should be started on combination therapy with a PED5 inhibitor and ERA.[13] Upfront treatment strategy of initiating triple drug therapy combing PDE5 inhibitor, ERA, and selexipag in a low-risk patient is not supported in a clinical trial.[14] High-risk patients in functional class IV should receive intravenous prostaglandins. Patients should be monitored frequently at least every 3 months. In each visit, functional class is assessed, NT-proBNP levels and 6-minute walk test are done, and patients are risk stratified. Objective of treatment is to achieve low-risk status. Patients who are deteriorating or move to high risk should be considered for additional therapies including selexipag, riociguat,[15] prostaglandin infusion, balloon atrial septostomy, Potts shunt, or heart lung transplantation. Patients with PAH and cardiopulmonary comorbidities will be started on either PDE5 inhibitors or ERA and are closely monitored.

Group 2 Pulmonary Hypertension

The mainstay of the treatment is to treat the underlying valvular heart disease or systolic or diastolic dysfunction as per guidelines. Effective treatment of LV dysfunction very often corrects the PH. If PH persists after the adequate treatment of the LV dysfunction additional mechanisms for PH such as pulmonary thromboembolism, obstructive sleep apnea (OSA), or chronic obstructive airway disease should be considered and treated.

In general, pulmonary vasodilators are not used to treat PH in patients with heart failure. Intravenous prostanoids increase mortality. Oral ERAs have increased heart failure readmissions. Hence, both these classes of drugs are contraindicated in treatment of PH in left heart failure. Small single center clinical trials have shown mixed results with PDE5 inhibitors. Sildenafil has improved hemodynamics and functional capacity in patients with LV dysfunction both in systolic and diastolic heart failure. However, there does not seem to be any significant difference in heart failure admissions or mortality. Probably, a select group of patients with CpcPH may benefit from PDE5 inhibitors. As a rule, these drugs should be given only after adequate treatment of underlying LV dysfunction and achieving euvolemic status. Close medical supervision is needed when this treatment is initiated. Ideally, these patients may be referred to expert centers. Referral to expert centers is indicated.

Onset of PH is often an indication for the repair or replacement of underlying left-sided valvular heart diseases. There is no role for pulmonary vasodilators in treatment of unrepaired left-sided valve diseases. Valve repair or replacement should normalize PA pressures. Sometimes, it may take a few months for the PH to regress. In one trial, treatment with sildenafil was ineffective in treatment of residual PH after valve replacement patients. In this study, the pathophysiology of the cohort was not well defined. MitraClip is useful in treating patients with heart failure, severe mitral regurgitation, and PH. Following successful MitraClip PH regresses in majority of these patients. Implantable MEMS is another device used in the management of heart failure patients. With this device PA pressures can be monitored remotely, and continuously. It helps in optimizing the treatment of left heart dysfunction and thus helps in the management of PH due to heart failure.

Patients with long-standing PH due to heart failure develop vascular remodeling and fixed PH. PVR >5 Wood units portends poor prognosis. This becomes an important issue in selecting patients with HFrEF for heart transplantation. Patients with pretransplant PVR of >3 Wood units do not do well after heart transplantation and it is a relative contraindication. Heart transplant may be performed if PVR can be brought down to >3 Wood units with acute vasodilator testing during RHC. Aggressive treatment with inotropes, vasodilators, and diuretics under hemodynamic monitoring may bring down PVR. If this fails, LVAD implantation is an option. Some patients require additional treatment with sildenafil. Patients may be considered for heart transplantation if the PVR can be brought down with these aggressive measures.

Group 3 Pulmonary Hypertension

Generally, PH due to lung disease is mild. Pulmonary pressures are marginally elevated even in the presence of severe pulmonary disease. Treatment is directed toward underlying lung disease. Often, the onset of PH in these patients indicates advanced lung disease and need for consideration of lung transplantation. A few patients with pulmonary vascular phenotype, probably due to genetic predisposition, have disproportionate PH with PVR >5 Wood units. In such select patients, cautious administration of pulmonary vasodilators may be tried. Though there is no data from RCTs, registry data suggests widespread usage of sildenafil in patients with chronic obstructive pulmonary disease (COPD) and interstitial lung disease (ILD). In COPD, these drugs can cause adverse effect on gas exchange. ERA have shown adverse impact on outcome in patients with ILD. However, there is no data to either support or refute its usage in patients with ILD. Again, the emphasis is on close medical supervision, preferably in expert centers. Magnitude of benefit with these drugs is uncertain. Patients with ILD have higher mortality with ERA. However, treprostinil inhalations were shown to be beneficial in INCREASE trial. Patients with OSA have only mild PH and presence of severe PH suggests associated PAH. Patients with combined pulmonary fibrosis and emphysema have a particularly poor prognosis due to PH.

Group 4 Pulmonary Hypertension

Thromboembolic PH is a disease that can be treated very effectively. All patients presenting with PH should mandatorily be investigated to rule out CTEPH. Patients with imaging evidence of CTEPH should be referred to expert centers that can offer pulmonary endarterectomy. After successful surgery PA pressures get normalized and the patient will be free of symptoms and can lead a normal life. Pulmonary endarterectomy is a complex surgery and competence, and results of different centers vary substantially. When a patient is refused surgery in any center, such patient should be referred to another expert center before condemning the patient for medical management. On medical management alone, patients deteriorate overtime. Such patients who are refused surgery due to inoperable disease or patient's comorbid conditions or when the severity of PH is disproportionately more than extent of pulmonary thromboembolism, must be considered for balloon angioplasty or medical management. Decisions should be made in an expert center with a team approach. At present, balloon angioplasty in CTEPH is being done only in a few expert centers. This requires multiple sessions in which four to five arteries are dilated in each session.[16] Even dilatation of a few vessels will offer significant symptom relief. Prior treatment with medication seems beneficial if PVR is >4 Wood units. Riociguat, subcutaneous treprostinil infusion, and macitentan have been proven in clinical trials to improve exercise tolerance in these patients. Other pulmonary vasodilators are often used off label in this disease. All patients including those who underwent successful surgery or angioplasty should be prescribed lifelong oral anticoagulants. There is no RCT evidence for either vitamin K antagonist (VKA) or non-VKA oral anticoagulants (NOACs). Patients with antiphospholipid antibodies, who constitute about 10% of this patient group should receive VKA only. Though some patients require multimodality treatment, no patient should be condemned to medical management alone without offering surgery or angioplasty. Long-term follow-up is mandatory since recurrence is a possibility in a few patients after surgery and balloon angioplasty.

Group 5 Pulmonary Hypertension

Group 5 PH includes different diseases with different and unknown pathophysiological mechanisms. Sometimes PH may be due to more than one mechanism. Treatment in such patients should be directed to the underlying mechanisms. In patients with sarcoidosis, PH may be due to arterial vasculitis, granulomas, LV dysfunction, extrinsic compression of mediastinal nodes, or pulmonary thromboembolism. Hence, it is important to do diligent evaluation prior to proceeding with specific therapies. There are no guidelines for treatments and treatment has to be individualized based on clinical condition.

GENERAL MEASURES

Diuretics

Diuretics should be given as per clinical assessment. Sometimes these patients require higher doses.

Oral Anticoagulants

There are no specific guidelines regarding routine use of oral anticoagulants. Small uncontrolled studies and registry data have given conflicting results. To date there are no RCTs. Recent large registry data from Europe has suggested marginal benefit with VKA in IPAH patients, while in large American registry REVEAL, such benefit was not shown.[17,18] Both registries have shown that VKA can be harmful in connective tissue disease associated PAH. Patients with PA aneurysm and class IV patients with severe right heart failure, patients with indwelling venous catheters may benefit from oral anticoagulants.

Oxygen Therapy

Routine oxygen therapy is not indicated, and it may be supplemented if the oxygen saturation gets below 92%. Air travel is often a concern. Modern aircraft are pressurized, and air travel may be permitted if the room air saturation is >90%. Patients should be mindful of unaccustomed exertion in large airports during travel. Prolonged air travel may indicate prophylaxis against venous thrombosis. Patients should avoid traveling at high altitudes above 1,500 m.

Cardiovascular Drugs

Drugs used to treat left heart failure and hypertension such as angiotensin system inhibitors, beta-blockers, sodium-glucose cotransporter-2 inhibitors (SGLT-2Is) , and ivabradine have no role in the treatment of PAH and right heart failure. They should not be used.

Anemia and Iron Deficiency

Anemia and iron deficiency should be identified and corrected. Oral drugs are poorly tolerated and intravenous supplementation is recommended in patients with iron deficiency.

Pregnancy and Contraception

Pregnancy carries high mortality and female patients of reproductive age group should be advised against it. ERAs have teratogenic potential and it includes male patients taking ERAs. In case, a patient does not want to terminate pregnancy, the patient should be monitored closely through pregnancy, delivery, and postpartum period. During pregnancy, ERAs, selexipag, and riociguat should be avoided due to their teratogenic potential. PDE5 inhibitors, calcium channel blockers, and inhaled, subcutaneous, and intravenous prostacyclin analogs may be given. Patients should be advised about contraception and progesterone alone or low estrogen contraceptive pills are preferred. Intrauterine implants are preferred.

Vaccinations

Patients should routinely be advised of annual influenza and periodic pneumonia vaccinations.

Diet

No specific dietary restrictions are advised. Patients with heart failure should restrict salt and water. Patients receiving warfarin type oral anticoagulants (VKA) should take an appropriate diet.

Physical Activity

Patients should avoid unaccustomed physical exertion. Supervised physical rehabilitation by an expert physio-therapist can improve their exercise tolerance and quality of life. When adequately treated and stable, all patients with PH should be considered for cardiopulmonary physical rehabilitation program.

Psychosocial Support

Diagnosis of PAH can be devastating to patients and their families. A compassionate attitude, tact sympathy, and sufficient time are expected from the physician. Patients support groups, trained social workers, and clinical psychologists can be helpful.

CONCLUSION

Pulmonary hypertension is not a single disease, it is a manifestation of underlying disease. Treatment varies depending upon the underlying disease. Proper diagnosis is essential before embarking on therapy. Pulmonary vasodilators are useful in group 1 PAH. They should be used very cautiously in other groups of PH.

ONLINE REFERENCES

Please scan the QR code provided at the end of the table of contents for References of this chapter.

CHAPTER

121 Advances in Management of Chronic Thromboembolic Pulmonary Hypertension

Sanjay Tyagi, Vishal Batra, Ankur Gautam

ABSTRACT

Chronic thromboembolic pulmonary hypertension (CTEPH) is a rare, underdiagnosed form of pulmonary hypertension. It is caused by intravascular obstruction of pulmonary arteries due to fibrotic transformation of thromboembolic material and microvasculopathy. It is important to diagnose this variant as potentially curative treatment in the form of pulmonary endarterectomy (PEA) is available. The last two decades have seen rapid advances in targeted medical management and refinement in balloon pulmonary angioplasty (BPA) technique, which has provided a viable therapeutic option for patients who are deemed to be inoperable.

Keywords: Chronic thromboembolic pulmonary hypertension, pulmonary embolism (PE), balloon pulmonary angioplasty, ventilation/perfusion scan (V/Q) scan, pulmonary endarterectomy, right heart catheterization (RHC), pulmonary artery pressure (PAP).

INTRODUCTION

Chronic thromboembolic pulmonary hypertension (CTEPH) is a rare, progressive pulmonary vascular disease that belongs to group 4 of pulmonary hypertension (PH) classification.[1] CTEPH is caused by obstruction of pulmonary artery vasculature, secondary to pulmonary embolism (PE), with combination of incomplete resolution of thrombus, ineffective fibrinolysis, and endothelial dysfunction, which lead to high pulmonary vasculature resistance and right ventricular pressure overload and ultimately develop right ventricular failure.[2-4] Early diagnosis requires a high index of suspicion. CTEPH usually develops within 1 year after an episode of PE.[1] The exact incidence of CTEPH is difficult to quantify, and it is largely underestimated because of nonspecific and variable presenting symptoms and the underutilization of lung ventilation/perfusion (V/Q) scintigraphy scan.[2-4] The incidence of CTEPH confirmed by right heart catheterization (RHC) is around 0.5–5% after a symptomatic episode of PE, and it is reported to be more frequent in the history of recurrent PE.[4]

DIAGNOSTIC EVALUATION OF CHRONIC THROMBOEMBOLIC PULMONARY HYPERTENSION

The diagnosis of CTEPH requires at least 3 months of effective anticoagulation and hemodynamic parameters for PH along with evidence of proximal or distal thromboembolic occlusion of the pulmonary vasculature.[5] The diagnostic algorithm of CTEPH is shown in **Flowchart 1**. Echocardiography is often used as the first modality to detect PH for screening symptomatic patients at risk for developing CTEPH. Tricuspid regurgitation (TR) velocity max > 3.4 m/s is considered high probability of PH. A significant number of patients with severe PH may not have an accurate TR signal on Doppler; other parameters such as right atrial enlargement, right ventricular systolic function, and leftward displacement of the interventricular septum can be used in patients with CTEPH.[6] Chest radiography may show enlargement of right heart chambers with areas of hypo- or hyperperfusion in the lung fields. An isolated out-of-proportion decrease in

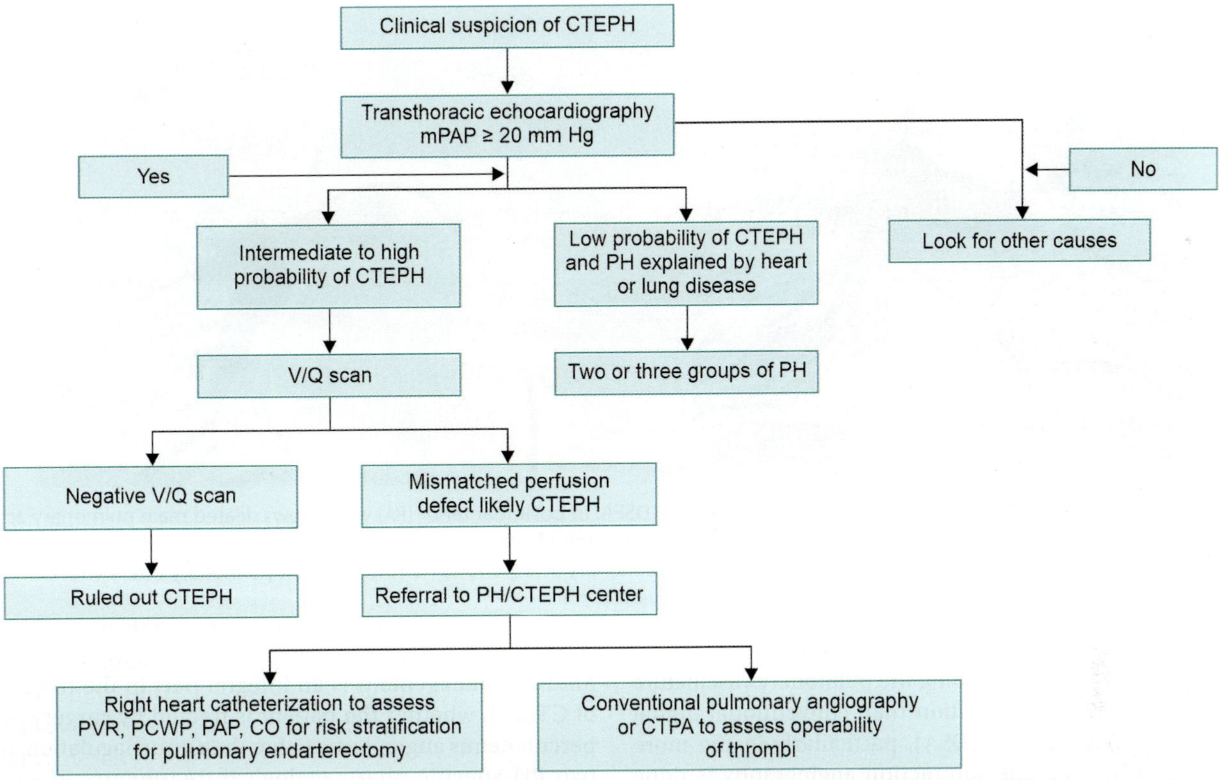

FLOWCHART 1: Diagnostic algorithm of chronic thromboembolic pulmonary hypertension (CTEPH).

(CO: cardiac output; CTPA: computed tomography pulmonary angiography; mPAP: mean pulmonary artery pressure; PAP: pulmonary artery pressure; PCWP: pulmonary capillary wedge pressure; PH: pulmonary hypertension; PVR: pulmonary vascular resistance; V/Q: ventilation/perfusion)

diffusing capacity for carbon monoxide (DLCO) hints toward a probable underlying pulmonary vascular defect. Arterial blood gas may show an increased alveolar-arterial (A–a) gradient with a low partial pressure of oxygen, especially with exertion.[7]

A V/Q scan is preferred over computed tomography pulmonary angiography (CTPA) as the initial imaging of choice because of its greater sensitivity and ability to differentiate CTEPH from more distal small-vessel involvement in group 1 PH.[8] Group 1 PH shows smaller subsegmental defects, whereas in CTEPH, large mismatches are seen on the V/Q scan. In the disease of distal pulmonary vascular bed, perfusion scans either are normal or exhibit a "mottled" appearance characterized by nonsegmental defect. A normal V/Q scan effectively excludes CTEPH with a sensitivity of 90–100% and a specificity of 94–100%.[7] A study done in confirmed cases of CTEPH by Tunariu et al. found that the V/Q scan was superior to CTPA with a sensitivity of 97.4% versus 51%.[9] A recent study has shown that both V/Q scan and CTPA are accurate methods for the detection of CTEPH with excellent diagnostic efficacy (100% sensitivity, 93.7% specificity, and 96.5% accuracy for V/Q scan; 96.1% sensitivity, 95.2% specificity, and 95.6% accuracy for CTPA).[10] Although VQ scan is not available in majority of centres, CTPA is the investigation of choice due to its widespread availability.

Magnetic resonance angiography (MRA) with lung perfusion magnetic resonance imaging (MRI) is an upcoming tool in the diagnostic evaluation of CTEPH, which needs further validation. MRI also assesses right ventricular disease and pulmonary hemodynamics. Lung perfusion MRI had sensitivity of 96% compared to 96% of V/Q scan and 94% of CTPA in a study done by Rajaram et al. in the United Kingdom.[11,12]

Pulmonary Angiography and Right Heart Catheterization

Pulmonary angiography with RHC is the gold standard imaging in patients of CTEPH. It is used for the confirmation of diagnosis as well as to assess whether the thrombotic occlusions are surgically amenable.[13] Furthermore, it also confirms that the increased pulmonary vascular resistance (PVR) is not secondary to distal vessel disease, arteriopathy, or pulmonary venous hypertension.[7] Conventional pulmonary angiography may not be able to provide fine details of distal vasculature in patients where the disease burden is more in distal vasculature. Advanced computed tomography (CT) technologies, including dual-energy CT (DECT), electrocardiogram (ECG)-gated area detector CT (ADCT), cone-beam CT (CBCT), and contrast-enhanced magnetic resonance pulmonary angiography, are emerging as

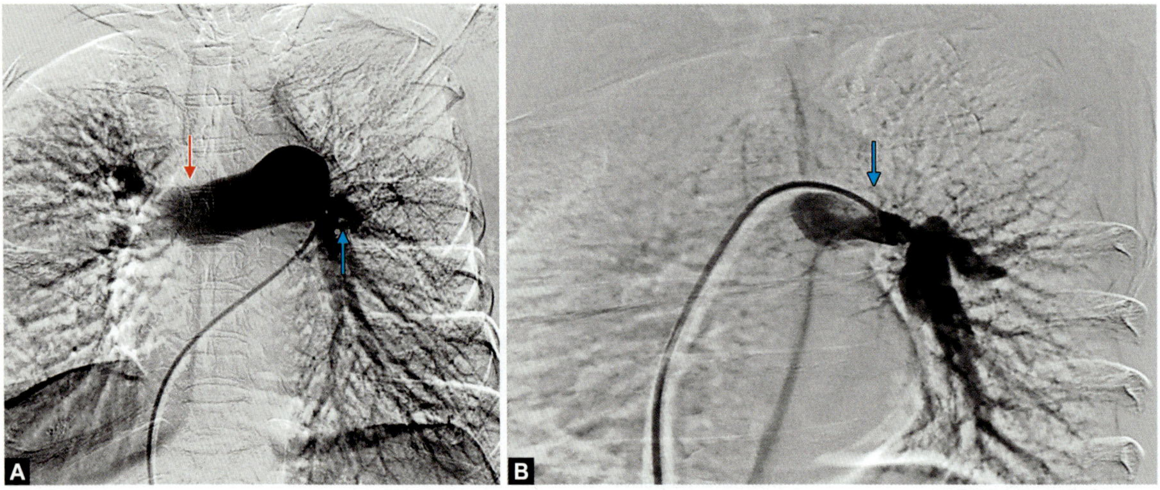

FIGS. 1A AND B: (A) Digital subtraction pulmonary angiogram (DSPA) in posteroanterior (PA) view shows dilated main pulmonary artery, occlusion of right lower lobe pulmonary artery (up arrow), and narrowing of left pulmonary artery with complete occlusion of left upper lobe pulmonary artery (down arrow). (B) Selective DSPA of left pulmonary artery shows narrowing of left pulmonary artery with complete occlusion of left upper lobe pulmonary artery (down arrow).

valuable modalities for detailing the pulmonary vasculature by providing greater resolution than conventional digital subtraction angiography (DSA), particularly in the more distal vessels.[14] Biplane subtraction angiography is done for right pulmonary artery; the frontal and lateral flat detectors are kept in anterior-posterior and left lateral views, respectively. Left pulmonary angiograms are performed in anterior-posterior and left lateral views to avoid the overlap of lung fields and mediastinum. Angiograms are acquired at 4 frames/s during contrast injection and reduced to 1 frame/s during the levophase. Imaging during levophase is necessary to rule out pulmonary vein stenosis and other venous anomalies. Angiographic findings suggestive of CTEPH are webs or bands, intimal irregularities, pouch defects, abrupt vascular narrowing, and complete obstruction **(Figs. 1A and B)**.[15]

MANAGEMENT OF CHRONIC THROMBOEMBOLIC PULMONARY HYPERTENSION

The management depends on whether the disease is operable or inoperable, which can be decided by the level of obstruction, functional status, and comorbidities **(Flowchart 2)**. CTEPH is the only type of PH that is potentially curable and amenable to surgical treatment, but almost half of the patients are technically inoperable. Pulmonary endarterectomy (PEA) is the surgical treatment of choice. All eligible patients with CTEPH should be offered PEA regardless of hemodynamic parameters and clinical symptoms.[16,17] Balloon pulmonary angioplasty (BPA), which has been there for decades, has been recently refined to give therapeutic options to patients deemed inoperable. Medical management is an integral part in the treatment of CTEPH, whether the patient is treated by surgery or by percutaneous angioplasty. Other than anticoagulation, only two PH-specific pharmacological treatments—riociguat and subcutaneous treprostinil—are currently approved for CTEPH.

Pulmonary Enarterctomy

Bilateral pulmonary enarterctomy offers the best survival advantage in patients of CTEPH. The technique was introduced in University of California (UC) San Diego in 1970. The perioperative mortality has come down drastically from 20 to 2% over the last five decades.

The decision to choose PEA depends on comorbidities complicating peri- and postoperative outcomes, surgical accessibility of thrombotic occlusions, imbalance between peripheral vascular resistance, and the accessibility of occlusions and patient's preference.[18] Thrombotic occlusions located in the proximal pulmonary vasculature, including main, lobar, and segmental arteries, are more easily amenable to PEA and can be expected to have lower PVR postsurgery.[16,17]

Nevertheless, around 50% of the patients are ineligible for PEA **(Box 1)**, either because of associated comorbidity or involvement of distal (sub-segmental) vessels, which are not surgically accessible.[19] Furthermore, almost one-third of patients who undergo PEA may have persistent or residual PH despite having undergone a successful procedure, and this complication was associated with higher early mortality. Complications of PEA are summarized in **Table 1**. Postoperative persistent PH can be due to distal inoperable disease or incomplete removal of distal thrombi during the surgery.[19-21]

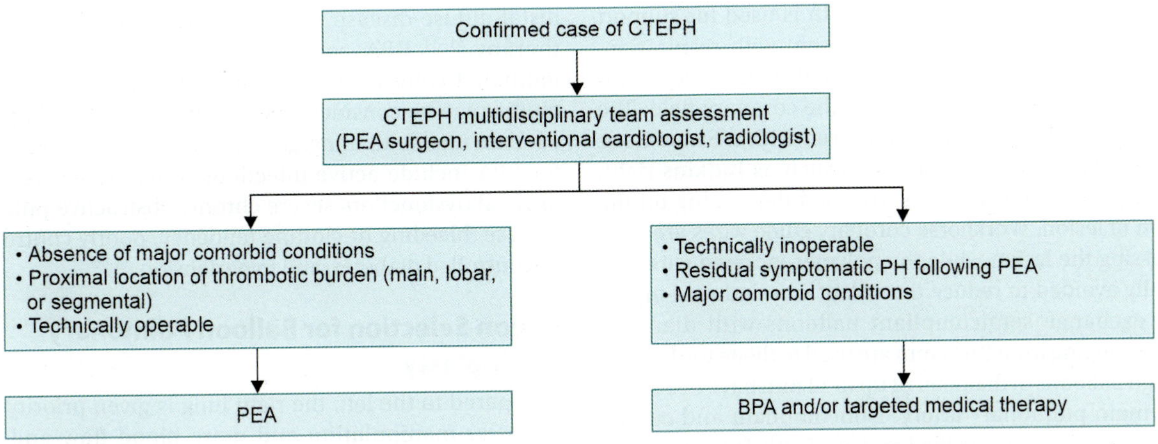

FLOWCHART 2: Treatment algorithm for chronic thromboembolic pulmonary hypertension (CTEPH).
(BPA: balloon pulmonary angioplasty; PEA: pulmonary endarterectomy; PH: pulmonary hypertension)

BOX 1 Factors determining noneligibility for pulmonary endarterectomy (PEA).

Comorbidities:
- Advanced age
- Coronary artery disease
- Left ventricular dysfunction
- Severe lung disease
- Diabetes
- Chronic kidney disease

Disease involvement:
- Distal vessel thrombus
- Inaccessible thrombus
- Small vessel disease

Hemodynamic factor:
- Imbalance between PVR and volume of accessible occlusions

(PVR: pulmonary vascular resistance)

TABLE 1: Complications of pulmonary endarterectomy (PEA).

Complication	Mechanism
Neurological complications	Brain ischemia due to deep hypothermic circulatory arrest
Persistent pulmonary artery hypertension	Inadequate or incomplete endarterectomy
Pulmonary hemorrhage	Pulmonary vessels injury
Reperfusion lung injury (RPE)	Abrupt normalization of extracellular osmotic pressure in endarterectomized parts of lungs (up to 10% of cases)
Arrhythmias, atelectasis, wound infection, and delirium are the other complications	

Technique of Pulmonary Endarterectomy

This procedure is done via median sternotomy and requires cardiopulmonary bypass and deep hypothermia (core temperature 18–20°C). Pulmonary artery is exposed, and the plane of dissection is identified. The plane of dissection is between the intimal and medial layers, but it is usually distorted. The endarterectomy is continued into the lobar, segmental, and subsegmental branches, which require a bloodless field. The circulatory arrest time is usually 20 minutes, but the cooling and rewarming time each may take 30–75 minutes.[22,23] Operating for distal disease is more challenging than the proximal disease. Surgery also has the theoretical advantage of halting the progression of disease and irreversible changes in small vessels. There is also improvement in functional class and right ventricular remodeling during the follow-up.[24] There is no cutoff for PVR, which is a contraindication for surgery, although very high values (above 1,000 dynes/s/cm^5) are associated with higher perioperative mortality. Two important exceptions to this are advanced pulmonary emphysema and severe left ventricular (LV) systolic dysfunction.[25] The 5- and 10-year survival rates are 82% and 75%, respectively, as reported by the UC San Diego group.[26,27]

Balloon Pulmonary Angioplasty

Balloon pulmonary angioplasty is an old technique for the treatment of CTEPH, which has been redefined recently. The first case of BPA was reported in 1988, and the first series of 18 patients was published by Feinstein et al. in 2001. In 2015, the European Society of Cardiology recommended BPA for inoperable patients of CTEPH with a class 2b recommendation.[28]

Procedural Details

The procedure is done under mild sedation. Venous access is taken through either femoral vein (preferred) or internal jugular vein. A long sheath is used for support and minimizing the catheter movement with respiration. There is no dedicated hardware for this procedure and most of the hardware is taken from the coronary field. The baseline hemodynamics are measured with a Swan-Ganz catheter. Coronary guide catheters such as Judkins right, multipurpose, or hockey stick are used depending on the location of lesion. Workhorse coronary guide wires are used for crossing the lesion while the polymer-jacketed wires are generally avoided to reduce the risk of wire-induced injury. Rapid exchange semicompliant balloons with diameter typically ranging from 2 to 5 mm are used to dilate the lesions, although balloons of diameter of up to 14 mm have been used in the main pulmonary artery. Noncompliant and cutting balloons are generally avoided and used only for recalcitrant lesions.[29-31] BPA mainly targets distal lesions in segmental and subsegmental vasculature down to distal pulmonary arteries of 3–5 mm diameter. Navvus microcatheter or pressure wire can be used for pressure measurement distal to lesion to achieve a distal pressure of 0.75–0.80 of proximal pressure where mean pulmonary artery pressure (mPAP) is <35 mm Hg. Anticoagulation is done with heparin to achieve the activated clotting time (ACT) of around 200–250 seconds. Angiography is done with diluted saline (50:50), and the lesions are identified.

Ventilation/perfusion scan assessment will guide to prioritize the underperfused areas. The lower lobe vessels (right lung > left lung) are prioritized as this will have greater physiological impact. On an average, two to six sessions are required for each patient, with two to five segments being treated per session (one BPA procedure for each lung as per the UC San Diego protocol). The procedure is also concluded if the total contrast volume exceeds 400 mL or radiation dose of 2 Gy is reached. Patients are monitored for 24 hours after the procedure and started on heparin to provide a bridge for oral anticoagulation. The interval between two sessions can vary from 1 week to a month. In severe pulmonary arterial hypertension (PAH), during the initial sessions, simpler nonocclusive lesions are targeted to optimize the hemodynamics and reduce the risk of complications.[29,30]

Patient Selection for Balloon Pulmonary Angioplasty

There have not been any fixed criteria for patient selection undergoing BPA, and the selection for this procedure is complex and multifactorial. Most of the patients who underwent BPA had severe vascular disease, comorbidities, and rejection for PEA. Anatomically, subsegmental disease (level 4) is more amenable to BPA. Assessment is made on the degree and level of vascular obstruction, hemodynamics, and symptoms. A new ongoing registry is comparing BPA versus PEA in proximal disease. Another role of BPA will be for bridging sick patients for PEA in whom the initial surgical risk is very high. BPA is also effective in post-PEA patients who have recurrence of disease. The subset of patients with distal diffuse disease will have only the option of medical therapy.[31-34] BPA contraindications include history of iodinated contrast allergy, although gadolinium contrast media may be considered as an alternative and in patients who are unable to undergo RHC. Relative contraindications for BPA include active infectious diseases, severe hepatic or renal dysfunction, severe chronic obstructive pulmonary disease, bleeding or clotting tendency, poorly controlled or uncontrolled diabetes, and hypertension.[34-36]

Lesion Selection for Balloon Pulmonary Angioplasty

Compared to the left, the right lung is given priority owing to easier manipulation and more blood flow and lesion distribution. Because of gravity, the blood flow in the inferior lobe is physiologically larger than in the superior and middle lungs; therefore, targeting lesions in the lower lobes may enable more prevalent improvements in pulmonary hemodynamics.[29,37] The complication rates are highest for total occlusions and tortuous lesions and lowest for webs or bands. The success rate is highest for webs or bands and lowest for total occlusions and tortuous lesions. Moreover, high mPAP before BPA is an independent predictor of the need for mechanical ventilation once lung injury occurs after BPA. Thus, priority selection of target lesions is as follows: Right lung > left lung, inferior lobe > superior or middle lobes, webs or bands > subtotal occlusion > chronic total occlusion > tortuous lesions.[37,38]

Imaging in Balloon Pulmonary Angioplasty

Optical coherence tomography (OCT) is a promising diagnostic method that can help characterize lesion morphology, enabling better lesion selection and treatment. OCT characterizes lesions into lesion with septum, multihole with thin wall, multihole with thick wall, and monohole types, which can help identify lesions more amenable to BPA. Although dye, radiation, and cost constraint limit their use, studies have shown that patient with thin wall respond better to BPA.[39]

Intravascular ultrasound (IVUS) can provide useful information regarding vessel diameter for selection of appropriate balloon sizing, while virtual histology IVUS can characterize lesion composition in stenotic lesions amenable to BPA.[40]

Complications of Balloon Pulmonary Angioplasty

Two major complications of BPA leading to periprocedural mortality are reperfusion pulmonary edema (RPE) and vascular injury, rarely perforation/rupture.[29] Complications of BPA can be either vascular access related, contrast or radiation related, or procedure related. Procedural complications such as wire perforations, rupture, dissection, or reperfusion injury, may occur. Ogo et al. proposed methods to avoid vascular injury, which include proper wire positioning, knuckle wire technique, avoiding pouch lesions without distal runoff, and under- or proportionate balloon sizing.[14]

Outcomes

Inoperable CTEPH patients can benefit from BPA. A multidisciplinary team approach considering PEA, medical therapy, and BPA is required for best outcomes in CTEPH. Experienced centers have shown 50–60% reduction in PVR after BPA, which is maintained at 1 year. Long-term survival is reported up to 7 years after a mean follow-up of 51 months. Despite the procedure, up to one-fourth of patients had persistent symptoms. There are no endpoints or universal definition of procedural success after BPA.[41,42] Riociguat versus BPA in nonoperable CTEPH (RACE) trial included 124 patients randomized 1:1 to BPA versus riociguat. After 6 months, PVR fell by 60% in BPA patients and 32% in the medical therapy group ($p < 0.001$) although the adverse events were significantly more common in BPA group (50% vs. 26%).[43] Long-term results after BPA are available up to 8 years after the procedure. The safety and efficacy of BPA correlate with center experience. Vascular injury rather than RPE is the likely cause of any severity of lung injury after BPA. Like PEA, proper training in a high-volume center is critical for BPA.

MEDICAL MANAGEMENT

Chronic thromboembolic pulmonary hypertension represents consequence of at least one or more unresolved episodes of acute PE. Early initiation of anticoagulation is strongly recommended. Previously, vitamin K antagonists have been widely used as these were only available. However, recent data indicate a shift toward direct oral anticoagulants (DOACs) due to lower bleeding risk with these drugs as seen in patients of venous thrombosis, despite lack of data on the safety and efficacy in this patient population. Therapeutic anticoagulation must be continued for long term, regardless of whether patients are treated surgically or medically.

Most of the PAH targeted therapies have been tried in CTEPH, but till now riociguat, a soluble guanylate cyclase stimulator, was only approved. Recently, subcutaneous treprostinil has been approved by the European Medicines Agency. The CHEST-1 trial was a multicenter double blind randomized trial of 261 patients with either inoperable CTEPH or persistent symptoms following thromboembolism. There was significant improvement in a 6-minute walk distance of 39 m in the riociguat group, reduction in PVR, NT-Pro BNP levels, and improvement in functional class.[44] Subcutaneous treprostinil was found useful in the CTREPH trial, which showed significant improvement in 6-minute walk test and functional class.[45]

Recently, endothelin receptor antagonist macitentan was also studied in phase 2 trial (MERIT trial) in 80 patients with inoperable CTEPH. There was reduction of PVR in the macitentan-treated group and increase in 6-minute walk distance. However, this trial was smaller in size, and many patients were on background phosphodiesterase-5 (PDE-5) inhibitors or prostanoids.[46] Bosentan was used in BENEFIT trial (bosentan effects in inoperable forms of chronic thromboembolic pulmonary hypertension), which also showed a slight decrease in PVR but no improvement in 6-minute walk distance. The subgroups of patients treated with PAH therapies had no advantage but a significant delay in referral for surgery.[47]

Selexipag, an oral selective IP prostacyclin-receptor agonist, got approved for PAH. In a recent study, selexipag significantly improved PVR and other hemodynamic variables in patients with CTEPH, although exercise capacity remained unchanged **(Table 2)**.[48]

TABLE 2: Randomized clinical trials of pharmacotherapy in patients with chronic thromboembolic pulmonary hypertension (CTEPH).

Medication	Approval for CTEPH	Medication class	Study	Participants	Outcome
Riociguat	Yes (FDA)	Soluble guanylate cyclase stimulator	• CHEST-1[44] • CHEST-2 (open label extension of CHEST-1)	261	Significant improvement in PVR and 6-MWD at 16 weeks
Bosentan	No	Dual endothelin receptor antagonist	BENEFiT[47]	157	Significant improvement in PVR, no significant improvement in 6-MWD at 16 weeks
Macitentan	No	Dual endothelin receptor antagonist	MERIT-1[46]	80	Significant improvement in PVR and 6-MWD at 16 weeks
Ambrisentan	No	Selective endothelin receptor antagonist	AMBER-1[49]	33	Trend toward improvement in 6-MWD and PVR at 16 weeks
Sildenafil	No	Phosphodiesterase-5 inhibitor	Suntharalingam et al.[50]	19	Significant improvement in PVR, no significant improvement in 6-MWD at 12 weeks

Continued

Continued

Medication	Approval for CTEPH	Medication class	Study	Participants	Outcome
Treprostinil (subcutaneous)	Yes (EMA)	Prostacyclin analog	CTREPH[45]	105	Significant improvement in PVR and 6-MWD at 24 weeks
Inhaled iloprost	No	Prostacyclin analog	AIR trial[51]	203	Significant improvement in PVR and 6-MWD at 12 weeks
Selexipag	No	Oral selective IP prostacyclin-receptor agonist	Ogo et al.[48]	39	Significant improvement in PVR and hemodynamics

(6-MWD: 6-minute walk distance; EMA: European Medicines Agency; FDA: Food and Drug Administration; PVR: pulmonary vascular resistance)

Intervention versus Medical Management in Inoperable Treatment

Balloon pulmonary angioplasty and riociguat have both been used in inoperable CTEPH. MR BPA is an open randomized trial comparing BPA and riociguat in inoperable CTEPH patients in World Health Organization (WHO) functional classes 2 and 3. A total of 61 patients were enrolled, out of which 32 were randomized to the BPA group. Patients in the BPA group underwent a total of 147 procedures (4.7 procedures per patient) over a period of 4 months.[52] Patients in the riociguat group were started on a dose of 1 mg thrice daily, and increment of dose was done by 0.5 mg every 2 weeks to a maximum of 2.5 mg thrice daily in 4 months. Over the next year, mPAP improved by 16.3 mm Hg in BPA group versus 7 mm Hg in riociguat group, although there were some procedure-related complications in the intervention group.

CONCLUSION

Chronic thromboembolic pulmonary hypertension is the only curable form of PH with PEA, although all the patients of CTEPH are not amenable to PEA. A hybrid or a bridging approach might be beneficial for patients who are not amenable to PEA. One-third of the patients who have persistent symptoms after PEA can be benefitted by BPA or medical management. Few patients who are not amenable to PEA initially can be bridged with BPA or medical therapy to undergo PEA. Most of the patients who have undergone BPA were surgical reject for PEA, so there is a need for larger data comparing these two treatment modalities. In future, we need to characterize patients who can benefit with either BPA or medical therapy or a hybrid approach for the best outcome.

ONLINE REFERENCES

Please scan the QR code provided at the end of the table of contents for References of this chapter.

SECTION 17

Pediatric Cardiology

CHAPTER

122

Breaching the Realms of Cardiac Surgery: Sinus Venosus ASD and RVOT Stenting

Anil Sivadasan Radha, Jenu Rose Jose E

ABSTRACT

Sinus venosus atrial septal defect (SV-ASD) is located high in the atrial septum where the right superior vena cava (RSVC) enters the right atrium (RA) and is commonly associated with partial anomalous pulmonary venous return of right upper pulmonary vein (RUPV) into RSVC.

Anomalous connection of the right-sided pulmonary veins is universal but is not limited to the right upper lobe, and not all individuals have overriding of superior caval vein, and the defect can have a significant caudal extension.

The SV-ASD is traditionally corrected by a surgical patch that routes the anomalously draining RUPV to the left atrium. The recent interest in nonsurgical correction of these defects by using a covered stent has to be tempered with the understanding of the complex anatomy. It often necessitates the use of multiple imaging modalities.

The conventional method of palliation in tetralogy of Fallot (TOF) physiology has been Blalock–Taussig (BT) shunt, but right ventricular outflow tract (RVOT) stenting is being increasingly preferred now as institutes are gaining more experience. It is suited in babies who are at high risk for complete repair and in those with hypoplastic pulmonary arteries. Though it has a significant learning curve, it has fewer complications and causes physiological growth of pulmonary arteries. By sparing the infundibulum, it can also avoid future transannular patches.

Keywords: Anomalous pulmonary vein drainage, balloon occlusion, covered stent, nonsurgical closure, superior vena cava, RVOT stenting, hypoplastic pulmonary arteries, palliation in TOF.

SINUS VENOSUS ATRIAL SEPTAL DEFECT: TRANSCATHETER CLOSURE

INTRODUCTION

The superior sinus venosus (SV) defect is the most common interatrial communication outside the oval fossa region, accounting for 10% of all atrial septal defects (ASDs).[1,2] It is characterized by an anomalous connection of one or more of the right-sided pulmonary veins (PVs). The orifice of the superior caval vein usually overrides the atrial septum but is not universal.[3] Surgical repair is the standard of care. More recently, transcatheter closure has been introduced as an option for correction by placing a covered stent in the superior caval vein with its lower end in the right atrium (RA) flared to close the defect, simultaneously redirecting the right-sided PV into the left atrium (LA).[4-6] This review discusses patient selection, hardware, procedure, follow-up evaluation, and a critical appraisal of the possible complications. This new interventional technique, reported initially from India, attempts to create a shared common wall between right superior vena cava (RSVC) and right upper pulmonary vein (RUPV) by placing a covered stent in RSVC.[2] This simultaneously covers the lower end of ASD by opposing the lower end of the stent to the inter-atrial septum (IAS) and redirects RUPV to LA **(Figs. 1A and B)**.

PATIENT SELECTION

The diagnosis of SV-ASD is confirmed on transthoracic or transesophageal echocardiography when the defect identified near the SVC orifice is posterosuperior to the oval fossa and is accompanied by anomalous drainage of the RUPV. All patients for the procedure should have a

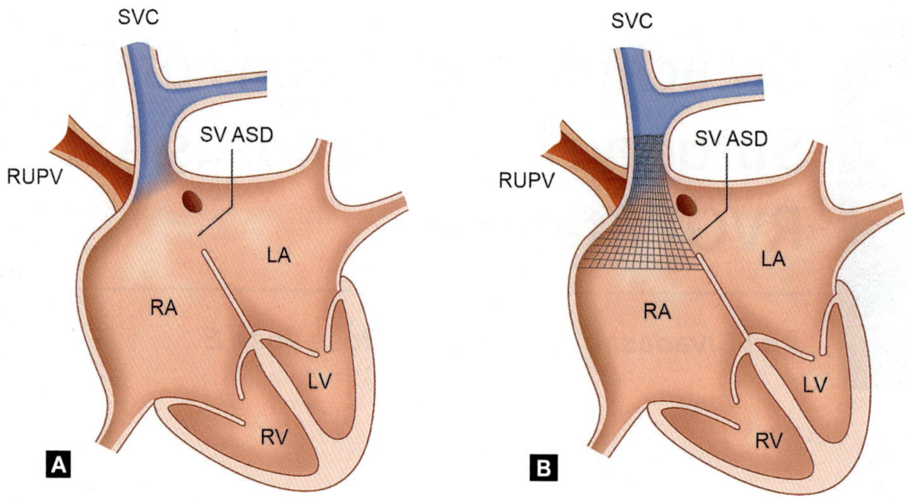

FIGS. 1A AND B: (A) Diagrammatic representation of sinus venosus (SV) ASD, with anomalously draining RUPV overriding the defect. (B) Diagrammatic representation of the sinus venosus defect closed with a covered stent, with RUPV draining unobstructed into the left atrium (LA).

(ASD: atrial septal defect; LV: left ventricle; RA: right atrium; RV: right ventricle; RUPV: right upper pulmonary vein)

clinical, radiographic, and electrocardiographic evaluation, including pulse oximetry, to demonstrate a significant left-to-right shunt of >1.5:1 without evidence of pulmonary vascular disease. Computed tomography (CT) and magnetic resonance imaging (MRI) may sometimes be needed to assess the complex anatomy, as the PV drainage is often variable.

Echocardiography

The initial assessment is for the inferior extension of the defect toward the oval fossa on a bicaval view. Suppose the vertical distance of the SV-ASD is >2.5–3 cm from the cavoatrial junction to the upper end of the defect at the fossa ovalis area; then in that case, the flared portion of the covered stent may not completely cover the lower part of the defect, and closing these defects can be challenging. This is mainly limited by the length of the stents (<8 cm) available, the shortening of the stent on expansion and the need for at least 50% of the stent to clasp onto superior vena cava (SVC) to prevent it from dislodging into RA.[7] The site of drainage of the RUPV in either the SVC or the RA is the next variable to be assessed. RUPV that drains in cavoatrial junction is ideally suited. If they drain in the RA or high in SVC, these defects are not routed to LA after covered stents. It may be challenging to obtain the precise anatomical detail of the site of drainage of the RUPV, sometimes by echocardiography alone and may warrant additional imaging **(Figs. 2A to D)**.

Acquisition and Analysis of the Computed Tomography Datasets

The CT angiograms were acquired with retrospective electrocardiographic gating on either a 256-slice or 384-slice dual-source scanner (Siemens Healthcare, Germany), using an intravenous injection of 1.5 mL/kg iodinated contrast followed by a half-saline chase. The recirculation phase was assessed to delineate venous anatomy.

A contrast multislice computed tomographic nongated study has become the routine investigative tool for assessing a defect for nonsurgical closure. When the posterior wall of the RUPV is seen in direct anatomic continuity to the posterior wall of LA, these defects are ideally suited for SVD stent exclusion **(Figs. 3A and B)**. Serial axial sections identify RUPVs that drain too high or too low from the cavoatrial junction and are excluded. Medical grade printing with elastic models is expensive and reliable methods to understand the complex anatomy and aid in better planning for this procedure.

CATHETER PROCEDURE TECHNIQUE

All procedures were performed under general anesthesia with transesophageal echocardiographic (TEE) guidance. Vascular access was obtained in the right internal jugular vein (RIJV), the left and right femoral veins (RFVs), and the left femoral artery. Heparin (100 u/kg)was given to maintain an activated clotting time of >250 s. Antibiotic prophylaxis with cefuroxime was administered at the start of the procedure.

A 5F angiographic catheter was placed in the RUPV to allow serial venography and pressure monitoring. The RUPV can be entered directly across the defect, retrogradely from the left ventricle, or by a transseptal puncture using a Brockenbrough transseptal needle (St Jude Medical, St Paul, Minnesota), allowing simultaneous LA and RUPV monitoring. A venovenous guidewire circuit was established, with a 0.035-inch Amplatz Extra Stiff wire (Cook Medical) from the RFV to the RIJV.[6,7]

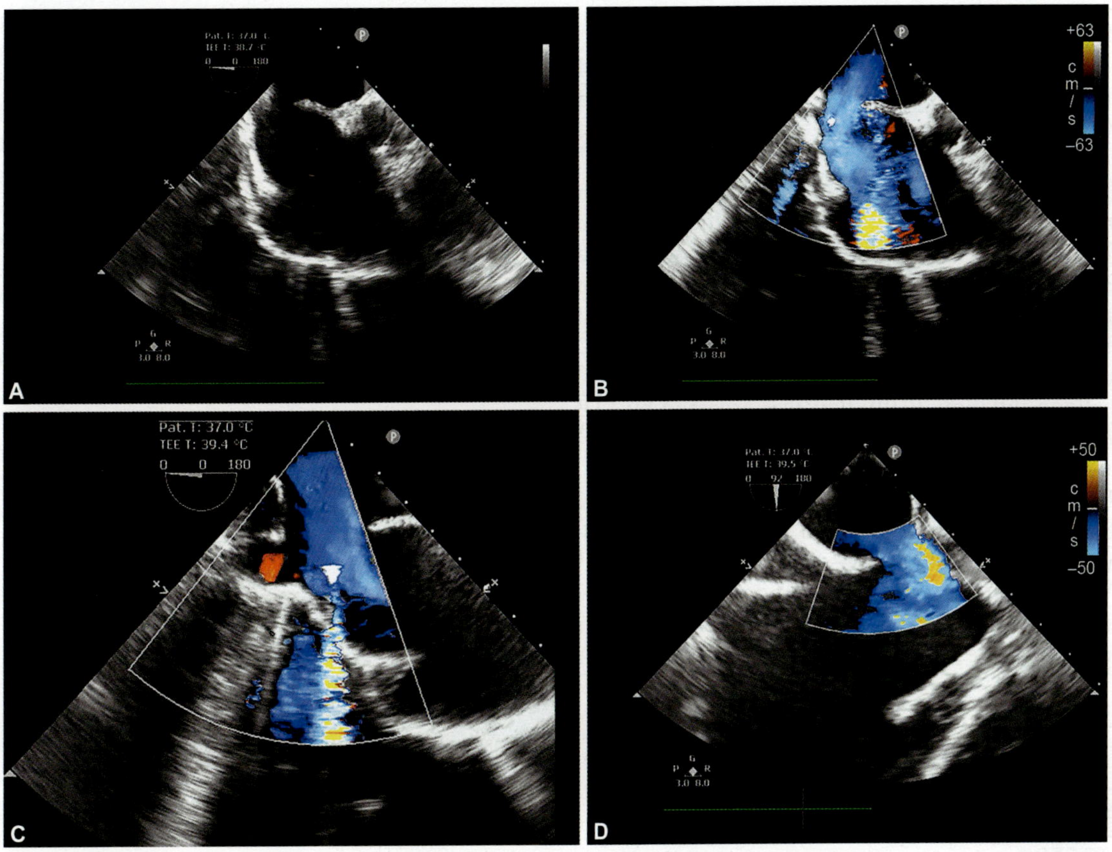

FIGS. 2A TO D: TEE evaluation of sinus venosus ASD. (A) TEE at 0° midesophageal view showing sinus venosus defect. (B) Color flow showing left to right shunt. (C) The red color indicates the RUPV draining at the cavoatrial junction. The posterior wall of RUPV continues with posterior wall of left atrium (D) TEE at 90° shows left-to-right shunt across sinus venosus defect.

(ASD: atrial septal defect; RUPV: right upper pulmonary vein; TEE: transesophageal echocardiographic)

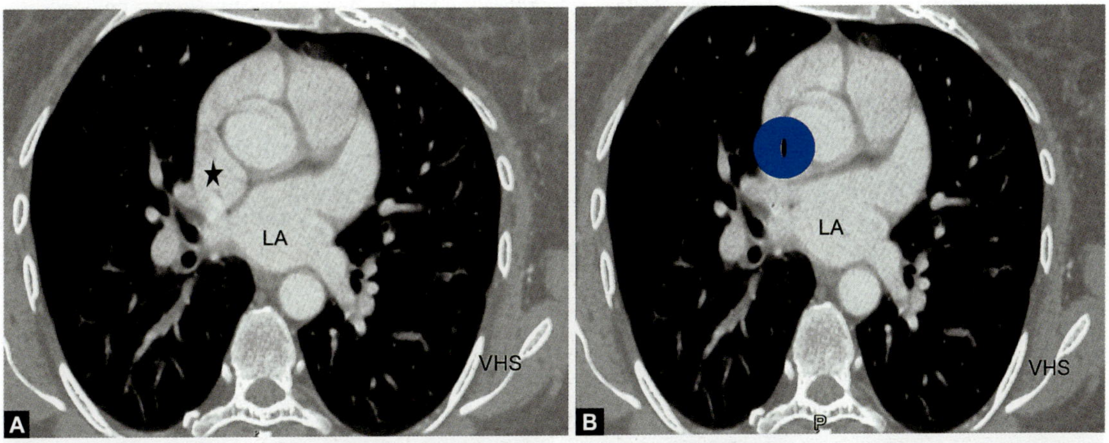

FIGS. 3A AND B: Axial CT images. (A) The asterisk represents the sinus venosus ASD. The RUPV drainage at cavoatrial junction is also seen. The posterior wall of the RUPV is in continuity with posterior wall of left atrium. (B) The blue circle represents how the covered stent is deployed closing the defect and the RUPV drains normally into left atrium (LA).

(ASD: atrial septal defect; CT: computed tomography; RUPV: right upper pulmonary vein; VHS: vertebral heart size)

BALLOON OCCLUSION TEST

The SV-ASD correction aims to close the interatrial communication and redirect the anomalous RUPV toward the LA with a covered stent in SVC. Balloon occlusion of the defect is the first step in selecting the ideal patient. A long (4–6 cm) semicompliant, noncompliant balloon or a 24-mm or 34-mm Amplatzer Sizing Balloon (St Jude Medical) is used. The initial balloon size was chosen to be at least 2–4 mm larger than the SVC diameter. The balloon was inflated in the anticipated stent landing zone, until TEE confirmed elimination of the interatrial shunt. An SVC angiogram was obtained to document SVC flow occlusion.[3] During balloon inflation, RUPV flow was assessed by TTE **(Figs. 4A and B)**, angiography from the RUPV catheter, and simultaneous RUPV and LA pressure measurements. A simultaneous angiography from the RUPV should demonstrate unobstructed flow toward the LA. On occlusion, if the lower end of the balloon stops the interatrial flows and the RUPV flow is unobstructed on TEE and angiographically with no significant elevation of PV pressure, then correction of the SV-ASD can be done with a covered stent **(Figs. 5A to D)**.

COVERED STENT/STENT GRAFT SELECTION

Diameter

Once the balloon test is completed, the diameter of the chosen covered stent should be equal to the diameter of the balloon, which completely occludes the interatrial flow. The covered Cheatham Platinum (CP) (NuMed Corporation, Hopkinton, NY) stents in 5–8 cm lengths mounted on balloon-in-balloon (BiB) catheters with outer balloon diameters between 18 and 30 mm (NuMED, Hopkinton, New York) or appropriate-sized numed balloons are used. The stents were introduced through a long delivery sheath (18F Check-Flo, Cook Medical, Bloomington, Indiana, or 20F DrySeal, Gore, Flagstaff, Arizona) from the RFV. The stents were deployed using simultaneous TEE imaging and angiography from the RIJV and RUPV. The cranial end was intended to sit sufficiently high in the SVC to allow secure anchoring, while the caudal end of the stent was well below the inferior rim of the defect on TEE. Flaring of the RA portion of the stent to ensure complete coverage of the interatrial communication was performed with the outer balloon of the BiB or with an additional numed balloon introduced from the opposite groin.

An aortic stent graft—Endurant II stent graft of diameter 28–32 mm with length 49–69 mm can also be used and has clips that hold onto the SVC and prevent migration.

All stents foreshorten on larger diameters as specified by the vendors.

Length

The stent should have a sufficient length to anchor onto the SVC to avoid embolization. The junction of the innominate veins ensures a secure anchor of the stent in the SVC. Maintenance of patency of the azygos vein is not too vital in these patients as SVC obstruction is unlikely after large stent placement. The lower end of the stent (or inferior landmark) should extend to the inferior edge of the ASD. The distance between the superior and the inferior landmarks is measured with a marker pigtail to estimate the length of the covered stent. The longest commercially available CP stent is 60 mm, while they can be custom-ordered up to 80 mm. The longest commercially available Andrastent XXL and Optimus CVS is 57 mm, while the longest Endurant II is 69 mm.

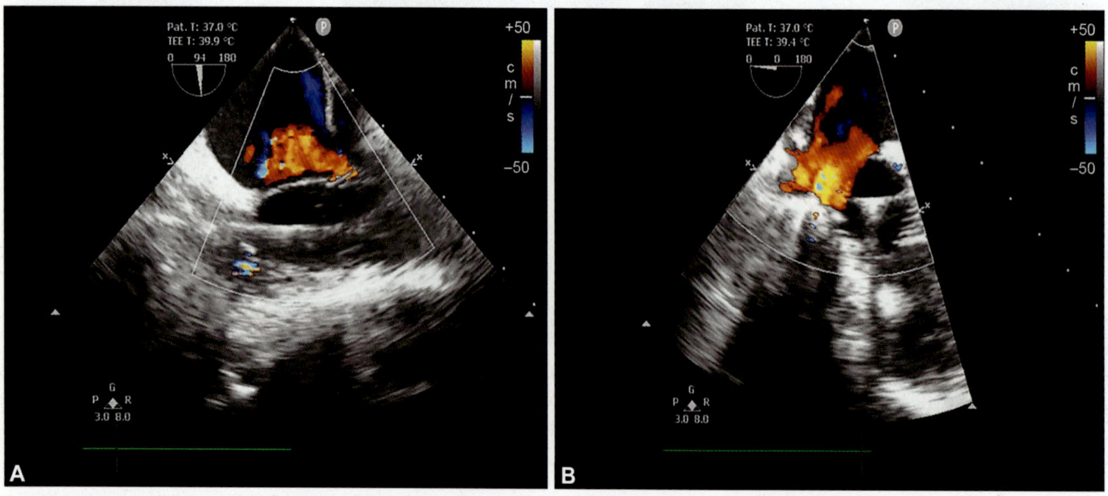

FIGS. 4A AND B: TEE at balloon occlusion test. (A) There is no residual flow across the defect when the balloon is inflated. (B) There is unobstructed flow in the RUPV to LA when the balloon is inflated.

(LA: left atrium; RUPV: right upper pulmonary vein; TEE: transesophageal echocardiographic)

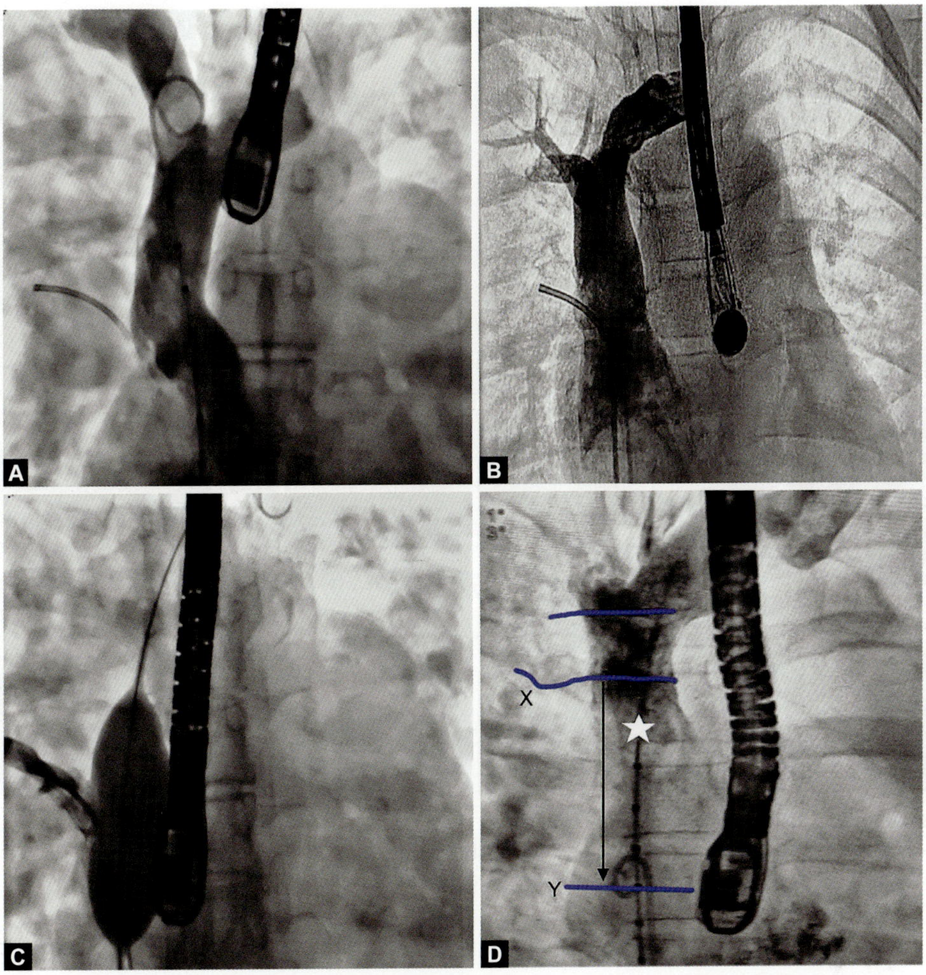

FIGS. 5A TO D: Balloon occlusion testing. (A) SVC angiogram in AP view with second catheter in RUPV shows negative clearing of the RUPV draining into the SVC at cavoatrial junction. (B) SVC angiogram with second catheter in the RUPV shows an anomalously draining right pulmonary vein draining high into the SVC just below the innominate vein. This patient subsequently underwent surgical closure. (C) RUPV angiogram during balloon occlusion shows unobstructed drainage. (D) The measurements to select the stent length are marked on the fluoroscopy screen.

(AP: anteroposterior; ASD: atrial septal defect; RUPV: right upper pulmonary vein; SVC: superior vena cava; TEE: transesophageal echocardiographic)

Deployment

Covered Stent

Fluoroscopic cine images and TEE were used to decide the length of the stent. Fluoroscopy images done in anteroposterior (AP) projection were used for measurements, and the table is frozen once the implantation is planned. The SVC injection was done, and the maximum diameter of SVC was measured at the SVC-RA junction. The maximum diameter between the lateral wall of RA and the atrial septum just below the defect was measured by TEE and by fluoroscopy **(Figs. 6A to D)**. This would be the maximum diameter. The stent has to be flared distally.

The upper end of the stent is marked in relation to the tracheal bifurcation and the intervertebral disk using a marker pen. Using a 5 F marker pigtail placed in SVC, the lower edge of the defect was determined with the help of TEE with the balloon manipulated so that the lower edge of the balloon is at the distal edge of the defect. This would be the final desired position of the stent, and the marker pigtail gives the desired length of the proposed stent. The femoral vein access is upsized to an 18 F/20 F sheath (Cook Medical, Bloomington, IN) or Sentrant (Medtronic) to allow large profile-covered stents mounted on large balloons. After obtaining a 6 F right jugular venous sheath, a venovenous circuit is made between the femoral and jugular veins. The covered stent is mounted on an appropriate balloon whose diameter is equal to that of the balloon used for occlusion test. The stent should straddle across the RUPV catheter and should satisfy the superior and inferior landmarks before it is expanded fully. A check angiogram from the side arm of the jugular and femoral sheath as well as a check angiogram from

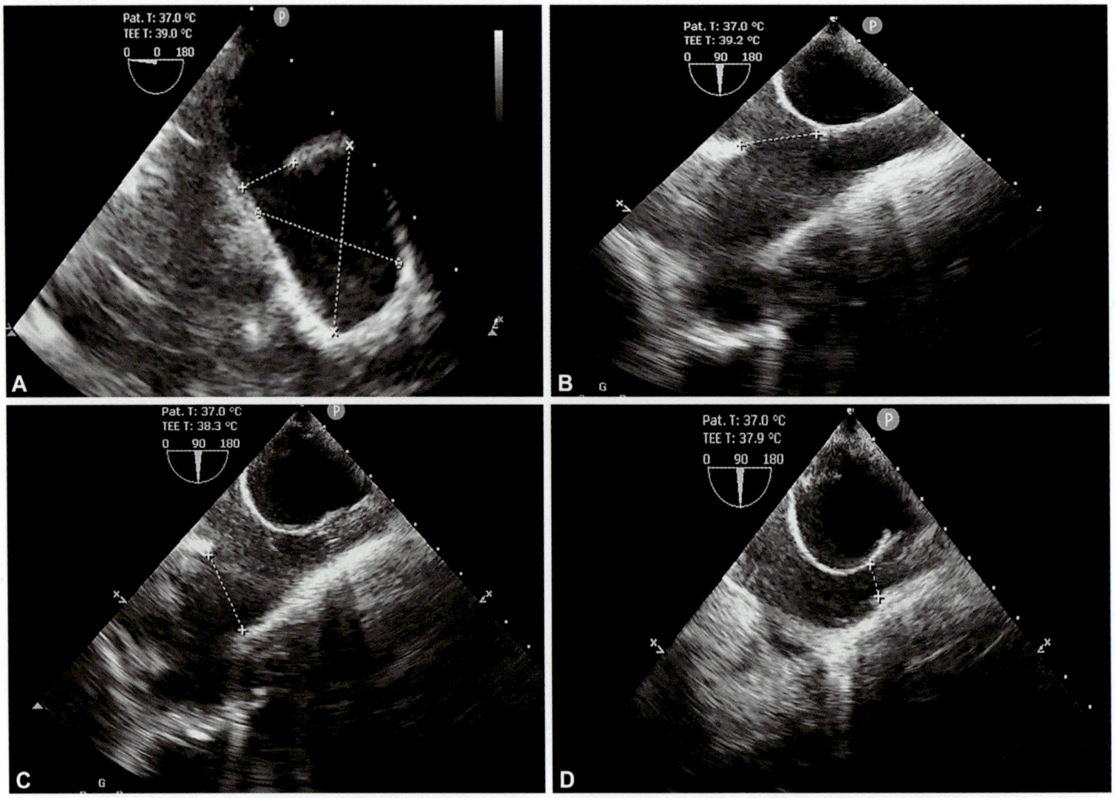

FIGS. 6A TO D: Measurements taken at TEE for selection of stent. (A) TEE at 0° shows the size of the sinus venosus defect and the SVC dimensions at the cavoatrial junction. (B) The size of the defect can also be measured at 90°. (C) The distance between the lateral wall of the RA and the lower edge of the defect at 90°. (D) The diameter of SVC at cavoatrial junction at 90°.

(SVC: superior vena cava; TEE: transesophageal echocardiographic)

the RUPV catheter can guide slow-controlled inflation of the balloon-stent assembly till the stent is anchored well in the SVC. The lower end of the stent can be flared using the same balloon moved inferiorly and reinflated at higher pressures.

Stent Graft

The maximum diameter between the lateral wall of RA and the atrial septum just below the defect was measured by TEE and by fluoroscopy. When using the stent graft, 4 mm is added to the measured diameter to determine the stent diameter.

Right femoral vein sheath was further upgraded to 18 F Sentrant (Medtronic)/20 F short sheath (Cook medical, USA) over the Amplatz Super Stiff wire. Over this wire, the desired Endurant IITM stent (Medtronic) graft system was taken and positioned with previous fluoroscopy markings and TEE guidance. The stent was placed with check angiograms to reconfirm the position. We slowly deployed the stent and made sure that the lower portion hinged on with the inferior margin of the defect we drew on the fluoroscopy screen **(Figs. 7A to C)**. Poststent deployment RUPV angiogram was done to show unobstructed flow into LA without any residual shunts. The RUPV pressure is also recorded to rule out obstruction.[6]

Any residual flow is managed by flaring the lower end of the stent using a larger balloon. Hemostasis is obtained using a figure-of-eight stitch after removing the 20 F large venous sheath. The postprocedural antiplatelet regimen includes aspirin and clopidogrel for 6 months.[6,7]

The primary anticipated complication for this procedure would be stent migration, which may need surgery but sometimes can be prevented and salvaged by an overlapping stent. Occlusion of the RUPV is unlikely if we stick to a proper balloon occlusion test. In case, this is anticipated, balloon inflation with a noncompliant (8 mm × 2 cm) Mustang balloon (Boston Scientific, Boston, MA) would create sufficient deformation in the covered stent so that it protrudes less into the PV to allow free flow in the RUPV.

RIGHT VENTRICULAR OUTFLOW TRACT STENTING

INTRODUCTION

In a cyanotic infant with tetralogy of Fallot physiology, the treatment options include early complete anatomic repair or some method of palliation that can help to delay the complete

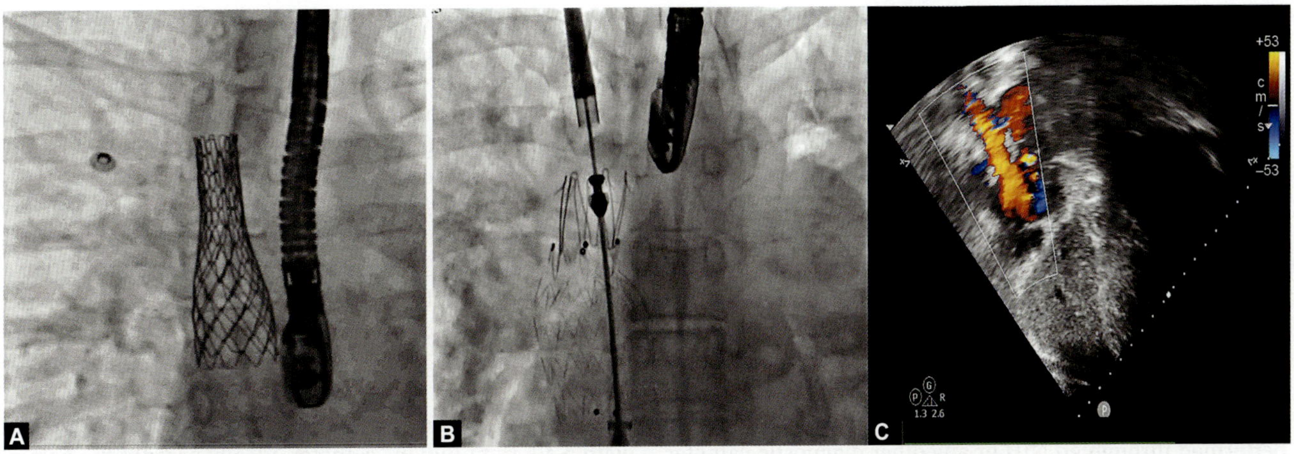

FIGS. 7A TO C: Stent deployment. (A) Covered stent deployed across the sinus venosus defect. (B) 32 x 49-mm stent graft deployed across the sinus venosus defect. (C) Subcostal view showing the stent graft in situ with no residual defect.

repair till an appropriate time. The various techniques of palliation include (1) surgical systemic to pulmonary artery (PA) shunt, e.g., Blalock-Taussig (BT) shunt, (2) patent ductus arteriosus (PDA) stent, (3) percutaneous pulmonary balloon valvuloplasty, and (4) right ventricular outflow tract (RVOT) stent.

An ideal palliative procedure should:[8]

- Provide a balanced yet stable source of pulmonary blood flow
- Aid in the growth and adequate development of PAs
- Give sufficient time so that surgery can be delayed till the ideal time for complete repair
- Facilitate complete repair without the need for further reinterventions

The ideal treatment of the child needs to be individualized. Those without early cyanosis can have primary repair electively at an optimal age, usually between 3 and 11 months. Early direct repair, <3 months, depends on institution preference and can avoid the progressive right ventricular hypertrophy that can occur in the unrepaired form, complicating repair. There is concern about increased early mortality and the universal need for transannular patch in this age group.

Among the palliative surgeries, BT shunt remains the procedure of choice at most centers; however, it is associated with significant morbidity and mortality. There are also concerns about its effects on the growth of the pulmonary valve and PAs. It is associated with unpredictable postoperative course, such as pulmonary overcirculation and distortion of PA anatomy.

Transcatheter techniques in the initial palliation of these patients have previously been attempted but did not gain widespread acceptance. Palliative balloon pulmonary valvuloplasty has been used with reasonable success, although issues related to durability and limited efficacy in patients with significant dynamic subvalvular obstruction limit its use. Qureshi et al. attempted balloon dilatation[9] as initial palliation in 15 infants with modest results, with 10 requiring more than one dilatation.

Patent ductus arteriosus stenting is also a favored palliative option with encouraging effects on PA growth. However, it is a technically challenging procedure, and the establishment of pulmonary blood flow is unpredictable and sometimes leads to flooding of pulmonary circulation.

Gibbs first described RVOT stenting in 1997[10] as a palliative procedure in four patients with associated comorbidities, but the initial results were not encouraging, it was reintroduced from 2010 onward as a mode of palliation.

INDICATIONS FOR RIGHT VENTRICULAR OUTFLOW TRACT STENTING

Cyanosed infants especially those who are duct-dependent or with refractory cyanotic spells but with:

- *Comorbidities which preclude primary complete anatomic repair*: Prematurity, low birth weight, infection (sepsis), necrotizing enterocolitis, and other conditions requiring emergency noncardiac surgery such as tracheoesophageal fistula and complex intracardiac anatomy
- Poor anatomy of the RVOT like small pulmonary valve annulus, ideally z score <–5
- Hypoplastic branch PAs, especially with Nakata index $\le 100\ mm^2/m$.[2,11]

PROCEDURE

Quandt and Stumper et al. in 2017[12] have detailed the preprocedure work up and techniques employed. It is usually performed under general anesthesia and mechanical ventilation since these children are generally hypoxic and sick. Ambient temperature should be maintained using a warming system (Bair Hugger, 3 M, Minnesota, USA) to prevent hypothermia. Prostaglandin infusions are usually continued. Emergency drugs prepared before the procedure were propranolol 0.1 mg/kg in 10 mL and phenylephrine solutions 1 in 10,000. High-inspired oxygen concentrations were used in all.

The child is positioned on the table with the arms elevated to allow for biplane angiography. Access is usually via the RFV in babies > 2.5 kg. Sometimes, an internal jugular venous approach is preferred if crossing of RVOT is difficult, especially in smaller children. A right femoral artery cannula is inserted for continuous blood pressure monitoring and for blood gas analysis. Once, the right femoral venous sheath (usually 5 F) is inserted, 50–100 IU/kg of heparin is given. The child also receives a prophylactic antibiotic dose.

A right ventricular cineangiogram **(Figs. 8A and B)** is performed through an NIH or any other diagnostic catheter placed within the apex of the right ventricle; 30° right anterior oblique (RAO) with 20° cranial tilt and a straight lateral projection are commonly used. Some centers prefer to do angiograms in left anterior oblique (LAO) 60/90° view instead of lateral view. The intent is to delineate the RVOT, its length and diameter, the diameter of pulmonary valve annulus, and the size of branch PAs, which is compared with echocardiographic measurements. Angiographic reference images would be selected and displayed.

Selection of the size and the type of stent to be implanted are guided by the patient's size, the dimensions of the outflow tract, and the anticipated length of palliation. It was preferred to avoid crossing the pulmonary valve annulus with the stent. For smaller children and neonates with short-term palliation (3–6 months), coronary stent is preferred. For older children or those who require medium to longer-term palliation, a bare metal peripheral vascular stent, preferably Cook Formula premounted 414 or 418 stent (Cook Europe, Bjaeverskov, Denmark), which does not foreshorten may be used.

Another advantage of Cook Formula stent is that it can be redilated if required and provides long-term palliation. If availability is an issue, any peripheral stent may be used though balloon-mounted stents are preferred.

All the hardware should be well prepared, before any attempt to cross the RVOT is made.

After the selection of the stent, the appropriate delivery sheath or guide catheter is selected. For coronary stents, a 4 F Flexor sheath (Cook Europe, Bjaeverskov, Denmark) or a 60 cm 6 F right Judkins guide catheter (Cordis Corp, Miami Lakes FL) may be used. Cook Formula stents are implanted through either 5 F or 6 F Flexor sheaths or at times Mullins sheath.

The delivery sheath is placed in the RA. RVOT is crossed with a 4 F right Judkins catheter, ideally without the help of a guidewire. A 0.014″ coronary wire is advanced through the catheter and a stable position is achieved by placing the wire in distal branch PAs. Then the delivery sheath or guide catheter was advanced over the diagnostic catheter into the distal branch PA. Then the diagnostic catheter was removed over the coronary wire and the sheath was aspirated and flushed. A rotating hemostatic valve is placed on the hub of the Judkins catheter, connected to the pressure line and side arm contrast syringe. If there is difficulty in tracking the catheter across the wire into distal branch PAs, another option is to cross the ductus arteriosus into the descending aorta which provides better stability.

In older children where a stiff wire is required,[13] first, a softer catheter such as a Glide catheter is passed over 0.032 Terumo wire into the distal branch PAs and then a Judkins right (JR) or multipurpose catheter may be used for replacing the Terumo wire with the Amplatz Super Stiff wire. This is done due to the hypertrophied infundibular area which may not allow the diagnostic catheter to pass over the coronary wire.

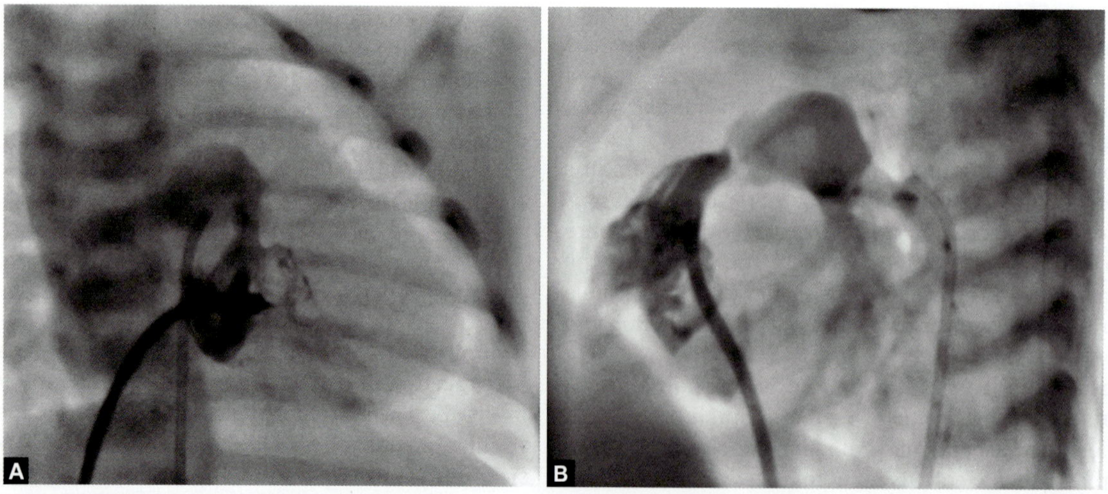

FIGS. 8A AND B: RVOT stenting. (A) RV angiogram in AP view showing narrow RVOT. (B) RV angiogram in lateral view showing infundibular and valvar pulmonary stenosis. The second catheter is placed in the descending aorta.

(AP: anteroposterior; RVOT: right ventricular outflow tract)

The premounted stent is placed over the wire but within the delivery sheath and advanced to the intended position within the RVOT. The stent is fully uncovered only after the position of the stent appears satisfactory, after repeated test angiograms and echocardiographic assessment. The delivery balloon would be inflated manually with one hand whilst the other hand controls the position of the stent system. Following placement of the stent, the balloon is slowly deflated whilst the delivery sheath was advanced over the balloon, so as to resheath it.

In all cases, the balloon was then advanced across the pulmonary valve for valvuloplasty. The final position of the stent, opacification of the branch PAs and pulmonary valve movements are confirmed on the check angiogram via the side arm of the sheath **(Figs. 9A and B)**. Echocardiography is performed for confirmation of the position of the stent, ventricular function, any interference with tricuspid valve function, and evidence of effusion. A repeat blood gas analysis is obtained and improvement in PO_2 is recorded. If satisfactory, the coronary wire and the delivery sheath are removed under fluoroscopic monitoring and manual hemostasis is achieved.

If the stiff sheath does not easily cross the infundibular area, especially in older children who present late and have very hypertrophied RVOT, it is placed just below the infundibular area and the stent is negotiated across the RVOT avoiding the annulus. However, if the annulus is small or if there is supravalvular PA narrowing, the stent may be placed across the pulmonary valve achieving a two-point fixation, one at infundibular, and another at valve annulus level.

The infant/child is transferred back to the ICU and vital signs are monitored. Patients who experience an increased oxygen saturation in excess of 20% are commenced on twice-daily diuretics. Chest X-ray is performed for any evidence of flooding of the lungs. Heparin infusion is continued and replaced with aspirin (3–5 mg/kg) once the child starts to take orally and the aspirin is continued till the child undergoes complete repair. RVOT stenting usually leads to a uniform growth of branch PAs.

In the study by Quandt and Stumper et al. in 2017,[12] 72 patients underwent RVOT stent implantation at a median age of 57 (4–406) days. Median weight was 3.4 (range 1.7–12.2) kilograms. The median procedure time was 53 (23–260) minutes. Median stent diameter was 5 (4–7) mm and median stent length was 16 (12–24) mm. Oxygen saturations increased from a median of 70 to 93%. There was also significant growth of branch PAs over time. There was one death due to perforation of branch PA and pericardial effusion. The other complications included RVOT perforation, early BT shunt due to persistent desaturation, early complete repair due to tricuspid valve injury, and aortic valve repair due to injury after embolization. The rate of catheter reintervention after RVOT stenting was high 37.5%. The majority of patients required redilatation of the stent or a second stent to provide longer-term palliation by augmenting pulmonary arterial blood flow.

The use of a long sheath as described by Quandt et al.[12] is mainly performed to minimize the tricuspid valve or conduction system injury by covering the stiff wire at all times and to achieve a stable stent position by repeated test angiograms to prevent slippage. However, the use of a long delivery sheath may be associated with hemodynamic instability, particularly in smaller and sicker patients due to tricuspid valve splinting open leading to compromised cardiac output and extreme cyanosis.

Linnane et al. have used periventricular approach in four patients weighing ≤2 kg through a small subxiphoid incision.[14] This approach provided a more direct route to

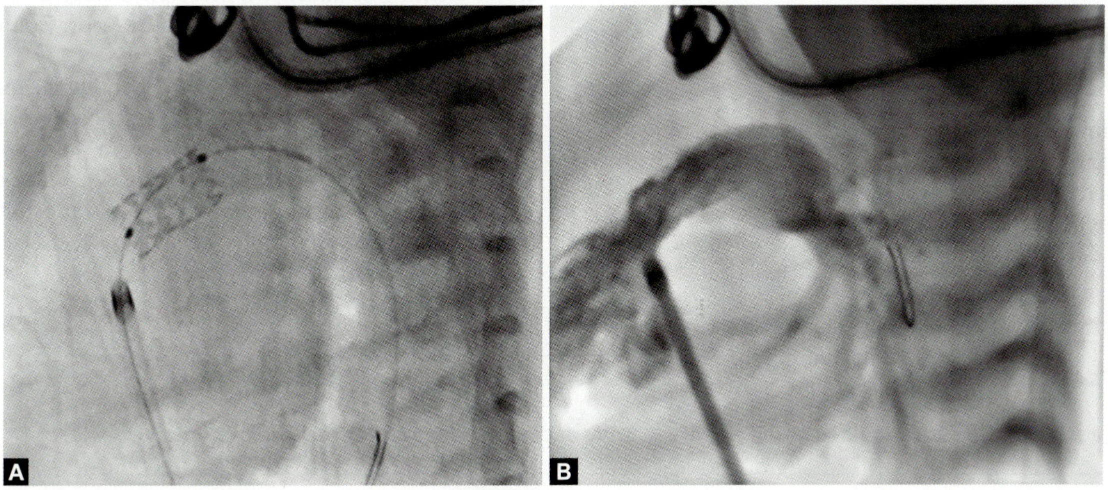

FIGS. 9A AND B: Deployment of the RVOT stent. (A) Here the Amplatzer Super Stiff wire through a 5 F Mullins sheath is across the PDA into the descending aorta which helped to track the stent. (B) Final angiogram showing well-placed RVOT stent (6 × 12 mm formula).

(PDA: patent ductus arteriosus; RVOT: right ventricular outflow tract)

the RVOT and the stent was deployed under transthoracic echocardiography (TTE) guidance rather than angiography.

Angiographic measurements usually underestimate the length of the RVOT and covering the proximal portion of RVOT is crucial.

In those with associated atrioventricular septal defect (AVSD), the stent should avoid the chordal attachments of the superior bridging leaflet and increase in AV valve regurgitation should be monitored. In those with double outlet right ventricle (DORV), the RVOT is more horizontal and the entire length has to be covered. In those with comorbidities requiring long-term palliation, the stent selected should be amenable to be overdilated without shortening. In those Fallot patients presenting late, RVOT stenting helps in gradually increasing pulmonary blood flow so as to reduce the risk of reperfusion injury of the lungs during late one-stage repair.

COMPLICATIONS

Malposition or migration of the stent may occur due to more proximal deployment of the stent. If the stent does not achieve two-point fixation, it remains unstable. The most common site of embolization is descending aorta. The use of a long delivery sheath for confirming the position and preventing the slippage of the stent minimizes the risk. Sometimes, distal deployment of the stent can lead to migration of stent into branch PAs.

Other complications include inadvertent RVOT perforation with tamponade, dissection, stent-induced pulmonary edema, arrhythmias, injury to adjoining structures such as tricuspid valve leading to tricuspid regurgitation, or to aortic valve. There could be hypotension and hemodynamic instability during the procedure.

Early BT shunt or complete repair could be needed if there is persistent desaturation or valve injury.

ADVANTAGES OF RIGHT VENTRICULAR OUTFLOW TRACT STENTING

- The immediate outcome in children undergoing RVOT stenting is quite favorable with saturations improving immediately after the procedure.
- Fewer postprocedural complications
- More physiological growth of PAs encourages equal growth of small PAs providing a better surgical substrate for subsequent repair.

DISADVANTAGES

- It is a technically difficult procedure with a significant learning curve.
- There is risk of complications especially in the learning curve period.
- There is significant burden of reinterventions, especially if performed in early neonatal period with very hypoplastic PAs.
- The initial methods of RVOT stenting prevented consideration for a valve-sparing anatomic repair. But the newer techniques of sparing the valve and covering the infundibular area alone can protect the child from future transannular patches.
- Presence of RVOT stent may complicate the subsequent anatomic repair. The cardiopulmonary bypass (CPB) time was significantly longer in the stent group, which could be related to the time needed for stent removal. Other concerns related to the incomplete removal of stent material include difficulty sewing the ventricular septal defect patch and concerns of injury to adjoining structures such as aortic and tricuspid valve.
- Long-term data on RVOT stenting is lacking, especially RV dilatation, function, and future reinterventions.

CONCLUSION

Transcatheter RVOT stenting is being increasingly preferred over other palliative procedures especially neonatal BT shunts. The risks of shunt thrombosis or pulmonary overcirculation can influence the postoperative recovery, shunt leads to disruption and distortion of the PAs which can significantly impact the definitive repair at a later date. RVOT stenting establishes a more physiological flow to PAs and encourages equal growth of small PAs providing a better surgical substrate for subsequent repair.

With increasing expertise RVOT stenting is emerging as a safer alternative to other palliative procedures. It should be considered the first-line palliation in patients who are not suitable or considered high risk for one-stage complete repair and short-term palliation for late presenters with markedly reduced pulmonary blood flow.

ONLINE REFERENCES

Please scan the QR code provided at the end of the table of contents for References of this chapter.

CHAPTER

123 Recent Developments in Adult Congenital Heart Diseases

Rishika Mehta, Amitabha Chattopadhyay

ABSTRACT

Children with congenital heart disease (CHD) now reach adulthood in >95% of industrialized countries because of better medical care in the last three decades. The number of adults with congenital heart disease (ACHD) is estimated at 50 million worldwide which will steadily rise in the upcoming years. Interventions in ACHD focus on surgical and percutaneous interventions which keep on changing from time to time. In this update, we have provided with timing and type of interventions related to right and left ventricular outflow obstruction, tetralogy of Fallot, coarctation, aortopathy associated with bicuspid aortic valve (BAV), atrioventricular canal defects, Ebstein anomaly, complete and congenitally corrected transposition, and patients with the Fontan operation which are helpful in clinical decision-making.

Keywords: ACHD, PA pressure, arrhythmias, heart failure.

INTRODUCTION

Congenital heart diseases (CHDs) with complete surgical/physiologic corrections or those repaired with palliative surgeries/interventions may have anatomic and functional residual and sequelae. Heart failure, arrhythmias, pulmonary vascular disease, aortopathies, infective endocarditis, concomitant acquired organ disease, and other residual complications affect the quality of life, work capacity, and psychology of adults with congenital heart disease (ACHD) with advancing age. If treated appropriately, further development of heart failure, arrhythmias, and possible premature death can be prevented. Hence, most patients with CHD require lifelong follow-up in a multidisciplinary approach.

Congenital heart diseases may be considered as a lifelong journey. If the lesions are corrected in infancy or early childhood, either by surgical or interventional techniques, mortality and morbidity rates tend to be low with most of them enjoying a good quality of life afterward. The teenage period may be utilized best in training and motivating them for a better and healthy lifestyle. The young adults may be receptive in discussions on healthy lifestyles, diet and exercises, family planning, and life trajectories with emphasis on professional and vocational options. The elderly population with repaired CHDs are projected to be higher in numbers gradually, where a holistic care may be needed with reinterventions required in some of them along with drug therapies for the heart disease along with prevention of other age-related disorders.

LESION-SPECIFIC GUIDELINES

Atrial Septal Defect

Atrial septal defect (ASD) is the most common type of congenital heart lesion presenting in the adult. Patients whose interatrial communications are unrepaired, or repaired at a late age, have increased morbidity and mortality compared with an age-matched population.

Closure of an ASD [secundum ASD, partial atrioventricular septal defect (AVSD), sinus venosus defect, or unroofed coronary sinus] is recommended in a symptomatic patient with a net left-to-right hemodynamically significant shunt (RV enlargement and/or Qp:Qs > 1.5) when the pulmonary arterial pressure (PAP) is <50% of systemic pressure, and/or pulmonary vascular resistance (PVR) is less than one-third systemic vascular resistance (SVR) and is reasonable in an asymptomatic patient with similar hemodynamics. Percutaneous closure of ASD is the method of choice if the defect is amenable to device closure, presently limited to secundum ASDs with acceptable rims of tissues around the defect and selected cases of sinus venosus ASDs with a covered stent. Surgical closure of a partial AVSD, sinus venosus defect, or unroofed coronary sinus defect is advisable.

The ASD closure may be done in high pulmonary pressures, in presence of a left-to-right shunt, PAP and PVR index (PVRI) are less than two-thirds of systemic pressure, and SVR index (SVRI), respectively. These patients should be assessed at a center with experts in pulmonary arterial hypertension (PAH). If the PAP and PVRI are more than two-thirds of systemic pressures respectively with a right-to-left shunt, ASD closure will be detrimental. Certain other indications of a hemodynamic insignificant ASD are unexplained stroke, transient ischemic attack (TIA), suspected paradoxical embolism, and orthodeoxia-platypnea syndrome.

Ventricular Septal Defect

Ventricular septal defect (VSD) is the most common CHD. Symptoms and signs of a large VSD and the absence of irreversible pulmonary vascular disease decide the shunt closure. VSD closure is recommended if there LV volume overload and Qp:Qs are > 1.5 with no PAH which is determined by PAP and PVRI < 50% systemic and less than one-third of SVRI, respectively. If there is significant, i.e., PAP > 50% systemic and/or PVR more than one-third SVR but Qp:Qs > 1.5 at baseline and a positive vasodilator response, VSD closure is advisable.

If pulmonary artery (PA) pressure is more than two-thirds of the systemic pressure and PVRI more than two-thirds of the SVRI with a right-to-left shunt, such VSD should not be closed and be referred to a center expert in PAH. If there is constant infective endocarditis with hemodynamically significant VSD, its closure can be considered.

In presence of a hemodynamically insignificant perimembranous or supracristal VSD and in absence of PAH VSD closure may be considered if there is serial aortic regurgitation secondary to aortic cusp prolapse in echocardiogram. Surgical closure of VSD is gold standard, but device closure may be an alternative in some cases.

Patent Ductus Arteriosus

One per 1,000 adults is the incidence of persistent ductus arteriosus. In 1939 first surgical ligation of patent ductus arteriosus (PDA) was performed, but in the current era percutaneous procedure is the choice of PDA closure and is recommended in presence of left ventricular (LV) volume overload with a significant left-to-right shunt, and PA pressure less than half of the systemic pressure and PVRI less than one-third of SVRI.

If there is left-to-right shunt even in the presence of PA pressure more than half systemic, and PVRI between one-third and two-thirds of SVRI, PDA closure may be considered. In presence of a right-to-left shunt or PA pressure and PVRI more than two-thirds systemic or SVRI, respectively, PDA closure is detrimental and should be referred to a center expert in PAH. Closure of a silent PDA though controversial but is recommended after an episode of endarteritis.

Atrioventricular Septal Defect

Prevalence of AVSD in adults is nearly 0.21/1,000. Most adults with a complete AVSD undergo a childhood surgical repair as they become symptomatic and most of them who are unrepaired develop pulmonary vascular obstructive disease. Adults with partial or intermediate AVSD are the ones who have unrepaired defects. Postsurgical repair complications include LV outflow tract (LVOT) obstruction, left atrioventricular valve regurgitation (AVVR), AV block, and atrial arrhythmias.

Surgery in adults with AVSD is recommended primarily when the PAP is less than half systemic, and PVRI is less than one-third SVRI or a residual defect with Qp:Qs > 1.5. In patients with AVSD who have severe left-sided AVVR should undergo valve surgery as per valve guidelines for mitral valve regurgitation.

In AVSD patients with LVOT obstruction, surgical correction is advised if the mean Doppler gradient is >40 mm Hg and or if there are symptoms of heart failure, moderate-to-severe left AV valve or aortic regurgitation, even if the gradient is less than that. Surgery should be considered for primary repair or for a significant residual left-to-right shunt, if the PA pressure is more than half systemic, PVRI is one-third to two-thirds of SVRI. However, surgery is detrimental in an AVSD or a residual shunt if the shunt is right to left with the PA pressure and PVRI are more than two-thirds of the systemic pressure or SVRI, respectively.

Bicuspid Aortic Valve and Aortopathy

In more than half of patients with BAV, there is presence of aortopathy in the form of aortic dilatation which generally occurs at the level of the mid ascending and unusually at the level of the sinuses of Valsalva. In patients with BAV aortopathy, medical management with beta-blockers, angiotensin-converting enzyme inhibitors, or statins has not been proven to be totally effective. Repair or replacement of either a stenotic or a regurgitant BAV should be according to the valve guidelines.

If the widest ascending aorta diameter is >55 mm in a patient with BAV; aortic replacement is recommended. Aortic replacement is also reasonable if the widest diameter of ascending aorta > 50 mm in the presence of high-risk features which include family history of dissection, rapid progression (>3–5 mm/year) on serial echocardiograms and maximum cross-sectional area/height ratio > 10 cm^2/m. Aortic replacement is advisable in patients with Turner syndrome, if widest aortic diameter measures > 2.5 cm/m^2. Prophylactic aortic valve replacement is advised in patients with severe aortic stenosis or regurgitation if the widest aortic diameter measures >45 mm.

Coarctation of Aorta

In an adult patient significant upper body hypertension, differential systolic arm-leg blood pressure (highest arm blood pressure 20 mm more leg blood pressure), angina, dyspnea, faint femoral pulses, murmur, leg fatigue on exertion, and rarely intracerebral hemorrhage are the signs and symptoms of significant CoA with death due to heart failure, aortic rupture/dissection, endocarditis, cerebral hemorrhage, along with coronary artery disease if this condition remains untreated. During catheterization, if simultaneous peak-to-peak gradient is > 20 mm Hg or there is more than half the narrowing of the aorta compared with the diaphragmatic aorta on magnetic resonance images along with systemic hypertension, patients with native or recoarctation should undergo correction. Stenting is the method of choice in patients weighing > 25 kg with a discrete coarctation, however, in cases of long-segment coarctation of aorta (CoA) surgery is the method of choice. Presently, with the advent of redilatable stents, coarctation stenting is feasible in younger children as well.

Right Ventricular Outflow Tract Obstruction: Valvar, Supravalvar and Subvalvar Pulmonary Stenosis

According to the natural history, patients with mild pulmonary stenosis might never require an intervention. Those with severe stenosis mostly would have undergone a childhood intervention. Ones with moderate obstruction have varied presentation. Undiagnosed right ventricular outflow tract obstruction (RVOTO) in the adults presents with right heart failure and ventricular arrhythmias. Percutaneous balloon valvuloplasty is the method of choice to relieve severe and symptomatic moderate pulmonary valvar stenosis. In severe pulmonary valve (PV), stenosis with RV dysfunction percutaneous or surgical intervention is reasonable even in absence of symptoms. Symptomatic adults with severe pulmonary regurgitation (PR) and RV dilation with or without dysfunction should be referred for PV replacement, which may be surgical or transcatheter.

Tetralogy of Fallot

Tetralogy of Fallot (TOF) if remains untreated in adulthood presents with severe dyspnea on exertion, right- or left-sided heart failure, ventricular arrhythmias, or sudden death. In adults, following total correction for TOF in childhood most common residual lesion is severe PR resulting from transannular patch repair or a nonvalved conduit and which causes RV dilation with dysfunction, ventricular arrhythmias, and exercise intolerance. The most common reintervention in repaired adult TOF is PV replacement. Other interventions include residual VSDs valvar or peripheral PA stenosis, tricuspid valve surgery, or electrophysiology procedure.

The PV replacement is guideline directed and is recommended if patients are severely symptomatic. It is also recommended in asymptomatic patients with who have severe PR and RV enlargement with or without RV systolic dysfunction, significant RVOTO and in patients with severe PR who require intervention for other hemodynamic significant residual lesions and in sustained ventricular tachyarrhythmias. Severe PR seen on echocardiography is substantiated with a regurgitation fraction > 25% on cardiac magnetic resonance (CMR), RV end-diastolic volume index (RVEDVI) > 160 mL/m^2 or RV end-systolic volume index (RVESVI) > 80 mL/m^2 on CMR.

Significant RVOTO is defined as an RV systolic pressure more than two-thirds of systemic pressure. Symptoms attributable to PR with RV enlargement ± right ventricular dysfunction are decrease in objective exercise capacity and require correction along with residual cardiac lesions if any.

Ebstein Anomaly

Milder form of Ebstein anomaly is asymptomatic and is an incidental diagnosis. In an asymptomatic adult, it might just present with an accessory pathway-mediated supraventricular tachycardia. The presentation of severe form of the disease is due to severe low-pressure tricuspid regurgitation (TR) leading to fatigue, exercise intolerance, and features of heart failure. The other presentation might be cyanosis due to right-to-left shunting across an ASD. Hemodynamic worsening is caused due to progressive TR, ventricular dysfunction and increased right-to-left shunt across the ASD which is reflected by increasing cyanosis and atrial tachyarrhythmias and are ominous signs.

Symptomatic adults in functional class >2 with severe TR must undergo tricuspid valve surgery. Even asymptomatic patients with severe TR with progressive RV dilation and RV systolic dysfunction on MRI, along with exercise intolerance, cyanosis (<90%), paradoxical embolism, or incessant atrial arrhythmias should undergo tricuspid valve surgery.

A bidirectional Glenn shunt [superior vena cava (SVC) to PA] might be added at the time of tricuspid valve surgery if the RV does not seem to accommodate the total systemic venous return of the SVC and inferior vena cava (IVC). An ASD closure may be done after careful hemodynamic evaluation using test occlusion if there is no increase in filling pressures and decrease in cardiac output. Indications of ASD closure are progressive desaturation (<90%) or paradoxical emboli.

Transposition of Great Arteries

Three types of adult with dextro-transposition of great arteries (d-TGA) are encountered. Those who underwent an atrial switch in the form of Mustard or Senning operations before 1985, those who underwent arterial switch operation, and some with a VSD and LVOTO who underwent a Rastelli operation, Rev, Nikaidoh or other ventricular repair surgeries.

Long-term mortality and morbidity is increased due to heart failure, development of PAH, and arrhythmias after the atrial switch surgeries. In about 65% of patients, there are interatrial baffle leaks.

Long-term complications after an arterial switch operation include coronary kinking (seen in almost 7% of patients), RVOTO, and significant progressive AR. RVOTO is the most common reason for reintervention which occurs mostly due to scarring at the anastomotic site between the PA and the neopulmonary root. After 25 years of surgery in almost 20% of patients with simple d-TGA and in 40% of patients with complex d-TGA, significant AR is seen.

After Atrial Switch

Surgical replacement of the tricuspid valve is recommended in symptomatic patients with severe TR and RV ejection fraction > 45%. Symptomatic patients with obstruction or narrowing of the pulmonary venous or systemic venous baffle are advised to undergo repair, either percutaneous or surgical. In patients requiring transvenous pacemaker/defibrillator implantation with baffle narrowing or baffle leak, stenosis correction and percutaneous correction of baffle leak should be done before lead implantation to prevent paradoxical emboli even if they are asymptomatic. Percutaneous intervention is recommended both in symptomatic and asymptomatic patients with significant baffle leak (Qp:QS > 1.5). Referral to a heart transplant unit is recommended in severely symptomatic patients due to systemic ventricular failure nonresponsive to maximal medical therapy.

After Arterial Switch

Patients should undergo revascularization, if they have ischemic symptoms due to coronary kinking. Intervention is recommended in symptomatic and asymptomatic patients with severe RVOT obstruction defined by peak Doppler gradient of >64 mm Hg or RVSP more than two-thirds of systemic pressure and ones with severe right ventricular dysfunction where gradients are underestimated. In symptomatic aortic regurgitation, asymptomatic patients of aortic regurgitation with LV ejection fraction < 50%, or LVESD > 50 mm and LVEDD > 65 mm—aortic valve repair or replacement is recommended, if the ascending aortic diameter is >45 mm and the aortic root is dilated, repair of the aorta is reasonable. If the patient is undergoing an aortic valve surgery, the aortic diameter is >55, simultaneous aortic root replacement is advisable.

Congenitally Corrected Transposition

Due to the lack of signs and symptoms, patients of simple congenitally corrected TGA (cTGA) remain unidentified till they reach adult life and are not intervened till the late third decade. They become symptomatic in the fourth decade when the systemic RV fails and there is systemic AV valve regurgitation or there is a setting of complete heart block. If the patients are symptomatic due to severe TR even without any RV dysfunction they should underdo tricuspid valve replacement. Tricuspid valve replacement is also indicated in asymptomatic adults with severe TR with RV dilatation.

In patients repaired with LV to PA conduit, if the patient becomes symptomatic due to conduit failure, conduit repair should be done. Conduit failure means a peak Doppler gradient >64 mm Hg, a peak velocity >4 m/s, pulmonary ventricle pressure more than two-thirds of systemic blood pressure, and severe PR. Patients should be considered for transplant if they develop symptoms secondary to severe systemic RV dysfunction not managed by medical and interventional therapy. If there is significant systemic RV dysfunction (RVEF < 40%) with AVVR, there might be postoperative RV failure after valve replacement. There might be worsening of TR after conduit replacement for LV to PA conduit failure.

Fontan Circulation

Dysfunction over years following a Fontan surgery presents in varied symptoms such as progressive exercise intolerance, increasing cyanosis, heart failure, protein-losing enteropathy, liver cirrhosis, and other extracardiac organ dysfunction.

If there is any obstruction to systemic or pulmonary venous return or any of the branch pulmonary arteries obstruction, percutaneous intervention is recommended. Presence of a residual shunt following any previous surgery causing significant volume overload, Fontan fenestration causing significant desaturation in presence of normal PVRI and presence of venovenous collaterals or pulmonary arteriovenous malformation further warrants percutaneous intervention.

Surgical intervention may be considered in patients with Fontan circulation dysfunction and one or more of the following, in the absence of significant ventricular dysfunction:

- Significant TR
- LVOTO with a significant gradient

In patients with recurrent atrial tachyarrhythmias refractory to pharmacological therapy and catheter ablations, epicardial pacemaker, Fontan conversion surgery, or arrhythmia corrective surgery is reasonable. If the patient is having refractory protein losing enteropathy or liver cirrhosis with failing Fontan, there should be early referral for heart or heart liver transplant.

CONCLUSION

Adults with CHDs are a unique and heterogenous group of population with special needs. It is an unexplored area and needs a multidisciplinary team approach between pediatric and adult interventional cardiologists, surgeons, and reproductive physicians to make complex decisions related to ACHD interventions. The gap in knowledge continues to persist in ACHD care. The guidelines related to ACHD interventions keep on updating from time to time with incorporation of latest developments in the field of pediatric and congenital cardiology and surgery, along with the advancement of newer technologies for diagnostic and treatment purposes.[1-3]

ONLINE REFERENCES

Please scan the QR code provided at the end of the table of contents for References of this chapter.

CHAPTER

124 Approach to Adult Person with Cyanotic Congenital Heart Disease

Srinivasa Rao Malladi

ABSTRACT

Adult cyanotic heart disease cases constitute a heterogeneous population. With the improved medical care and palliative procedures, the survival into adulthood is increasing in cyanotic congenital heart disease patients. Due to the right-to-left shunt, these patients are more prone to paradoxical embolism. Hypoxia and its compensation by increased erythropoiesis affect various systems of the body causing multisystem dysfunction. A variety of surgical intervention options are available for those without severe obstructive pulmonary arterial hypertension (PAH) with variable success. For those with severe obstructive PAH, pulmonary vasodilator drugs such as endothelin receptor antagonists and phosphodiesterase-5 (PDE-5) inhibitors. All these patients have a very delicate, balanced circulation and any perturbations will have an adverse and sometimes catastrophic consequence. Prevention of these issues by taking appropriate measures and patient education constitute the important components of the management of cyanotic patients.

Keywords: Cyanosis, congenital heart disease, pulmonary blood flow, pulmonary stenosis, pulmonary hypertension, right-to-left shunt, hyperviscosity, tetralogy of Fallot, Eisenmenger syndrome.

INTRODUCTION

Cyanosis means bluish discoloration of skin and mucous membranes resulting from inadequate oxygenation of blood. For cyanosis to be visible 5 g/dL of deoxygenated hemoglobin (Hb) in tissues is needed.[1] Severely anemic persons cannot develop cyanosis even in the situation of significant hypoxemia. Cyanotic congenital heart diseases are characterized by the presence of right-to-left shunts at various levels leading to desaturated blood entering the systemic circulation causing hypoxia and cyanosis.

Adult cyanotic heart disease cases constitute a heterogeneous population. In the Euro Heart Survey on adult congenital heart diseases (ACHDs), 9.48% are cyanotic with 60% of them having Eisenmenger syndrome.[2] Bhardwaj et al.[3] reported a prevalence of 2.4/1,000 in adults of which 26% are cyanotic diseases with tetralogy of Fallot (TOF) being common in 16%. Mathur et al.[4] from West Rajasthan reported a prevalence of 7.7/1,000 adults, of which 19.14% were cyanotic and TOF was seen in 10.4%.With the improved medical care and palliative procedures, the survival into adulthood is increasing in cyanotic congenital heart disease patients.

CLASSIFICATIONS OF CYANOTIC CONGENITAL HEART DISEASE[5,6]

Anatomical and Physiological Classification

According to congenital heart diseases anatomical and physiological (AP) classification, cyanotic heart disease falls into great complexity (class III) and physiological stage C or D.[7]

Clinical Classification (Perloff)

- *Increased pulmonary blood flow*:
  - Dextro-transposition of the great arteries (d-TGA)
  - Taussig–Bing anomaly
  - Truncus arteriosus
  - Total anomalous pulmonary venous connection (TAPVC)

- Univentricular heart with no pulmonary stenosis (PS)
- Common atrium
- Fallots tetralogy with pulmonary atresia with increased collateral flow
- Tricuspid atresia (TA) with nonrestrictive ventricular septal defect (VSD)

- *Normal or decreased pulmonary blood flow*:
  - Dominant left ventricle:
    - TA
    - Pulmonary atresia with intact ventricular septum (IVS)
    - Ebstein's anomaly
    - Single ventricle left ventricular (LV) type with PS
    - Vena cava to left atrium (LA) communication
  - Dominant right ventricle:
    - No pulmonary arterial hypertension (PAH):
      - VSD + PS/pulmonary atresia
      - Atrial septal defect (ASD) + PS
      - d-TGA, VSD + PS
      - Double-outlet right ventricle (DORV), VSD + PS
    - PAH present:
      - ASD with reversal
      - VSD with reversal
      - Patent ductus arteriosus (PDA) with reversal
      - DORV with PAH, reversal
      - d-TGA PAH
      - TAPVC with PAH
      - Hypoplastic left heart syndrome (HLHS)
  - Near normal ventricles:
    - Pulmonary arteriovenous (AV) fistula (AVF)
    - Vena cava to LA communication

Cyanotic Congenital Heart Diseases

Cyanotic congenital heart diseases can be broadly grouped into three categories depending on the pulmonary blood flow as shown in **Flowchart 1**.

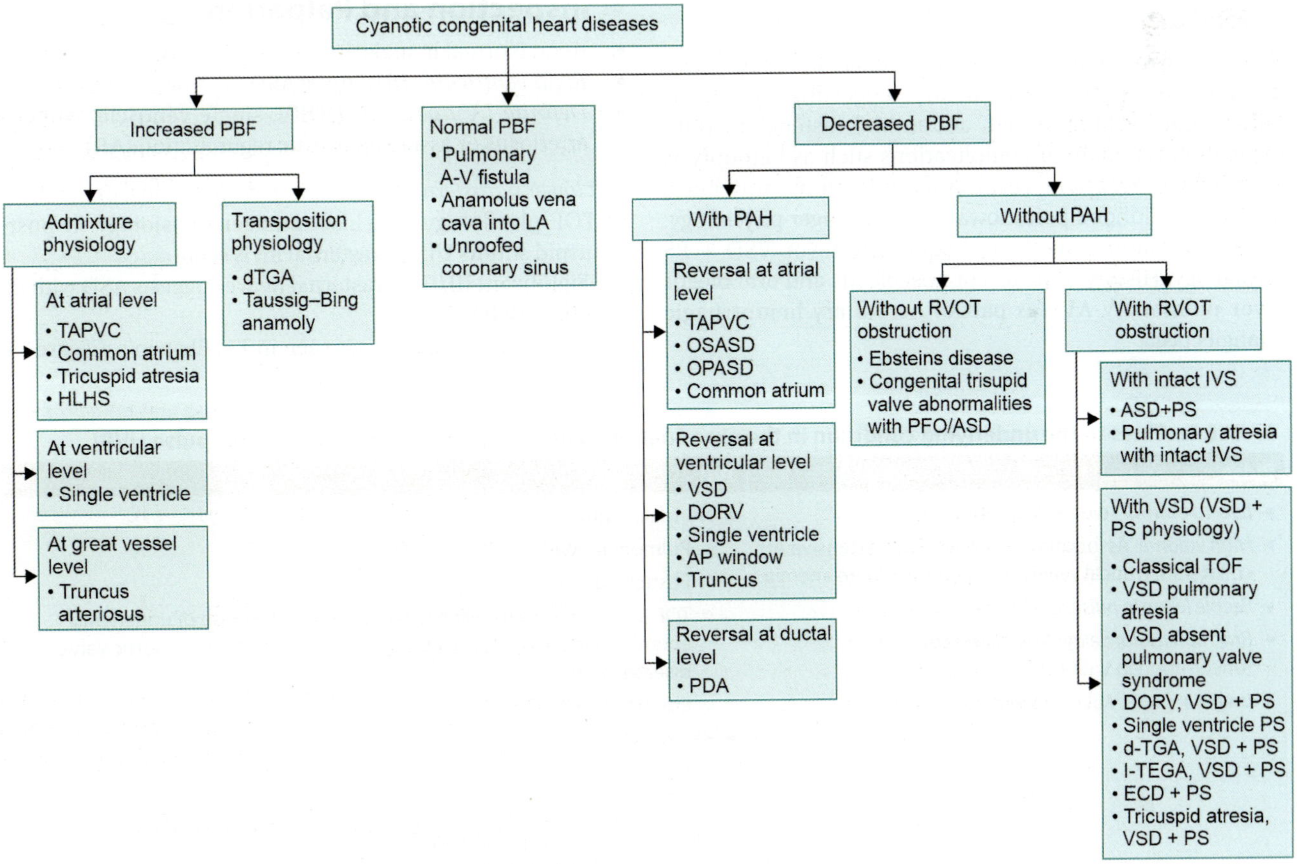

FLOWCHART 1: Classification of cyanotic congenital heart diseases based on pulmonary blood flow (PBF).

(AP: aortopulmonary; AV: arteriovenous; ASD: atrial septal defect; DORV: double-outlet right ventricle; d-TGA: dextro-transposition of the great arteries; ECD: endocardial cushion defect; HLHS: hypoplastic left heart syndrome; l-TGA: levo-TGA; LA: left atrium; IVS: intact ventricular septum; OPASD: ostium primum atrial septal defect; OSASD: ostium secundum atrial septal defect; PAH: pulmonary arterial hypertension; PDA: patent ductus arteriosus; PFO: patent foramen ovale; PS: pulmonary stenosis; RVOT: right ventricular outflow tract; TAPVC: total anomalous pulmonary venous connection; TOF: tetralogy of Fallot; VSD: ventricular septal defect)

Adult cyanotic patients can also be classified into the following subsets:

- Those without palliative procedures (classification given earlier)
- Those who underwent palliative procedures earlier
  - Post-aortopulmonary (AP) shunts with obstruction: Blocked Blalock–Taussig (BT) shunt, etc.
  - Post-AP shunts with segmental PAH
  - Post Fontan procedure with fenestration
  - Post bidirectional Glenn shunt with pulmonary AVF

Most of the adult patients with cyanotic congenital heart diseases have either TOF or Eisenmenger syndrome. Other conditions are seen in small numbers.

CLINICAL APPROACH[5,6,8,9]

Along with the history, physical examination, examination of chest X-ray, and electrocardiogram (ECG) are crucial to arrive at reasonable diagnosis. Examination of previous medical records is essential.

History

Common symptoms are effort intolerance, breathlessness, palpitations, and syncope; history suggesting right heart failure like swelling of feet, abdominal distension, right hypochondrial pain; or complications such as hemoptysis and stroke. Frequent respiratory infections and heart failure in childhood point toward Eisenmenger physiology. Previous cyanotic spells and squatting favor VSD + PS physiology. History of recurrent nosebleeds and oral bleeds favor pulmonary AVF as part of hereditary hemorrhagic telangiectasia.

Physical Examination

It is important to keep in mind that physical findings may be altered in adult patients because of associated conditions such as hypertension, aortic valve disease, and musculoskeletal deformities and previous surgeries.

Specific syndromic features should be noted which point toward particular conditions such as DiGeorge syndrome and Down's syndrome.

Central cyanosis unless there are significant anemia and clubbing of digits is seen in all cases. Differential cyanosis indicates underlying duct with reversal and reverse differential cyanosis in d-TGA or Taussig–Bing anomaly (DORV, subpulmonic VSD, No PS) with duct and reversal.

Examination of Pulse and Jugular Venous Pulse

The points mentioned in **Table 1** give a clue to the underlying condition.

Inspection and Palpation

- *Apex*: Normal in majority
- *Right ventricular (RV) apex*: ASD
- *Definite LV apex*: TA, DORV, single ventricle, truncus arteriosus or associated aortic regurgitation (AR)

Left lower parasternal pulsations and lift: In most of the cases of TOF physiology and Eisenmenger physiology in post-tricuspid shunts I/III parasternal lift is seen.

Significant III/III parasternal heave suggests ASD with PS or ASD with PAH.

Quiet parasternal area is seen in TA, Ebstein's disease.

TABLE 1: Clues to the underlying condition in the examination of arterial pulse and jugular venous pulse (JVP).

Pulse	JVP
• *Low to normal volume*: Majority • *High volume*: Associated severe AR, PDA, extensive AP collaterals, truncal valve regurgitation, severe anemia • *Feeble left arm pulse*: Classical BT shunt • *Brachiofemoral delay*: Associated coarctation (uncommon in VSD + PS) • *Irregular pulse*: ASD, previous atriotomy	• Normal height: ○ Pulmonary AVF ○ Ebstein's disease ○ TOF (but many adults will have elevated JVP because of underlying anemia, myocardial dysfunction, systemic hypertension, aortic valve disease, or restrictive VSD) ○ Eisenmenger VSD, PDA • Raised JVP: ○ ASD + PS ○ ASD + PAH • *Giant a waves*: Tricuspid atresia, TS • *Cannon waves*: l-TGA, ECD, single ventricle • *Nonpulsatile and raised JVP*: Cavopulmonary shunt (Glenn shunt) • *Elevated JVP on left side*: LSVC

(AP: aortopulmonary; AR: aortic regurgitation; ASD: atrial septal defect; AVF: arteriovenous fistula; BT: Blalock–Taussig; ECD: endocardial cushion defect; LSVC: left superior vena cava; l-TGA: levo-TGA; PAH: pulmonary arterial hypertension; PDA: patent ductus arteriosus; PS: pulmonary stenosis; TOF: tetralogy of Fallot; TS: tricuspid stenosis; VSD: ventricular septal defect)

In double-chambered right ventricle (DCRV), right ventricle may be palpable lower down or only at epigastrium.

Pulsations in the left second space favor PAH; pulsations in this area due to aorta may be seen in levo-TGA (l-TGA).

Thrills: Parasternal systolic thrill is uncommon in VSD + PS physiology, Eisenmenger syndrome secondary to post tricuspid shunts.

Prominent systolic thrill is seen in ASD + PS, ASD + PAH, or DORV.

Systolic thrill at apex may be seen in endocardial cushion defect (ECD) and at left lower sternal border (LLSB) in Ebstein's disease or due to tricuspid regurgitation (TR).

Diastolic thrill at left second intercostal space (ICS) may be seen in Eisenmenger syndrome.

Diastolic thrill at LLSB may be seen in Ebstein's disease.

Systolodiastolic thrills may be noted in TOF with absent pulmonary valve, postoperative BT shunts, etc.

Auscultation: S1—wide split—Ebstein's disease

S2—single: VSD + PS physiology, ASD + PS, VSD + PAH, associated malpositions

Fixed split: TAPVC, ASD + PAH, ASD with prominent Eustachian valve

Normal split S2 with normal pulmonary component (A2 > P2): Pulmonary AVF, unroofed coronary sinus, left superior vena cava (LSVC) to LA

Normal split S2 with loud pulmonary component (P2 > A2): - PDA + PAH

RVS3 and RVS4: ASD + PS, ASD + PAH, TAPVC, Ebstein's disease, RV dysfunction

LVS3: LV dysfunction, associated severe AR, ECD with severe mitral regurgitation (MR)

Ejection systolic murmur (ESM) in left second and third ICS: ASD + PS, TOF physiology or in ASD Eisenmenger syndrome

Pansystolic murmur (PSM) in LLSB: DORV, Ebstein's disease, hypertensive TR

Pansystolic murmur at apex: ECD with MR

Early diastolic murmur (EDM): Hypertensive pulmonary regurgitation (PR)—Eisenmenger syndrome, AR in TOF physiology with severe AR, Eisenmenger VSD/PDA with severe AR, truncal regurgitation in truncus arteriosus.

To and fro murmur with gap between S2 and diastolic murmur: TOF with absent pulmonary valve syndrome.

Continuous murmurs indicate TOF pulmonary atresia or associated PDA or post-shunt status.

Soft prolonged systolic murmurs or continuous murmurs widely audible over chest indicate pulmonary AVF.

VSD + PS and ASD + PS physiology can be differentiated based on physical examination and chest X-ray as mentioned in **Table 2**.

VSD + PS physiology can be differentiated from PAH physiology (Eisenmenger syndrome) as mentioned in the **Table 3**.

Lesion causing severe PAH (Eisenmenger syndrome) can be identified to some extent as shown in the **Table 4**.

TABLE 2: Differentiating points between ventricular septal defect (VSD) + pulmonary stenosis (PS) physiology and atrial septal defect (ASD) + PS physiology.

	VSD + PS	ASD + PS
History of cyanotic spells, squatting	Common	Not seen
Features of right heart failure	Rare	Common
Irregular pulse (AF)	Uncommon	Common
JVP	Normal	Raised
Cardiomegaly	Uncommon	Common
Parasternal heave	1/3	2/3 or 3/3
Systolic thrill	Uncommon in classic TOF, may be seen in DORV, single ventricle, tricuspid atresia	Common
RVS3 and S4	Rare	Common
RVOT ESM	Up to 3/6	Loud ≥3/6
PSM of TR	Rare	Common
Chest X-ray	• Pulmonary oligemia • No cardiomegaly • Concave pulmonary bay	• Pulmonary oligemia • Cardiomegaly + convex pulmonary bay due to dilated MPA

(AF: atrial fibrillation; DORV: double-outlet right ventricle; ESM: ejection systolic murmur; JVP: jugular venous pulse; MPA: main pulmonary artery; PSM: pansystolic murmur; RVOT: right ventricular outflow tract; TOF: tetralogy of Fallot; TR: tricuspid regurgitation)

TABLE 3: Differences between ventricular septal defect (VSD) + pulmonary stenosis (PS) and pulmonary arterial hypertension (PAH) (Eisenmenger) physiology.

	VSD + PS physiology	Eisenmenger physiology
History of (H/o) recurrent LRTI and heart failure in infancy	Not seen	Common
H/o cyanotic spells and squatting	Common	Not seen (7–10% of VSD Eisenmenger can give H/o squatting)
Pulse	Normal	Normal (irregular in ASD)
JVP	Not raised	Not raised except in ASD
Cardiomegaly	Not seen	Not seen except in ASD
Parasternal lift	1/3	1/3 to 3/3 in ASD
Systolic pulsations and increased dullness on percussion in pulmonary area	Not seen	Seen
Palpable second sound	May be seen (A2)	Seen
Systolic thrill	+	Uncommon except in ASD
Second sound	single	Single (VSD), fixed split (ASD) normal split (PDA with loud P2
EC (Ejection click)	+/– Constant (aortic)	+/– Constant (pulmonary vascular)
ESM	3/6	Uncommon except in ASD
EDM	Not seen (systolodiastolic murmur seen in TOF absent pulmonary valve syndrome)	May be seen hypertensive PR
PSM of TR	Uncommon	May be seen
Continuous murmurs	May be seen	Not seen except over back in associated coarctation
Chest X-ray	Concave pulmonary bay with pulmonary oligemia	• Dilated pulmonary arteries • Pruning of peripheral pulmonary arteries

(ASD: atrial septal defect; EDM: early diastolic murmur; ESM: ejection systolic murmur; JVP: jugular venous pulse; LRTI: lower respiratory tract infection; PDA: patent ductus arteriosus; PR: pulmonary regurgitation; PSM: pansystolic murmur; TOF: tetralogy of Fallot; TR: tricuspid regurgitation)

TABLE 4: Differences between various subsets of Eisenmenger syndrome.

	ASD	VSD	PDA
Cyanosis	Uniform	Uniform	Differential
JVP	Elevated	Normal	Normal
Irregular pulse	May be seen	Not seen	Not seen
Cardiomegaly	Present	Absent	Absent
Parasternal lift	3/5	1/5	1/5
Second sound	Fixed split	Single	Normal split
RVS3	May be seen	Not seen	Not seen
ESM	May be seen	Rare	Rare
PSM of TR	May be seen	Not seen	Not seen
Ascending aorta in chest X-ray	Inconspicuous	Normal/Right arch	Dilated

(ASD: atrial septal defect; ESM: ejection systolic murmur; JVP: jugular venous pulse; PDA: patent ductus arteriosus; PSM: pansystolic murmur; TR: tricuspid regurgitation; VSD: ventricular septal defect)

CHEST X-RAY[6,10,11]

Chest X-ray is an important tool in the assessment and follow-up. Systemic evaluation of thoracic cage, cardiac chambers, great vessels, and pulmonary vasculature is needed. In some cases chest X-ray have characteristic appearance. Main chest X-ray findings in various conditions are summarized in **Table 5**.

ELECTROCARDIOGRAM[6]

Systematic analysis of ECG in detail is useful in the identification of the condition. Some of the important ECG abnormalities which help in the diagnosis are mentioned in the **Box 1**.

In the subdifferentiation for various causes of VSD + PS physiology, ECG will be helpful as mentioned in **Table 6**.

CARDIAC IMAGING[12]

Multimodality imaging approach is needed in the evaluation and management.

Echo[13]

Echo is the primary investigation in the management of ACHDs. Detailed analysis of all structures using different standards as well as unconventional views is necessary. 3D gives better anatomical details. Strain imaging is useful in functional assessment of ventricle.

Cardiac Computed Tomography and Cardiovascular Magnetic Resonance

Cardiac computed tomography (CT) and cardiovascular magnetic resonance (CMR) are needed for quantification

TABLE 5: Chest X-ray in cyanotic congenital heart diseases.

Condition	X-ray features
Pulmonary arteriovenous fistula	No cardiomegaly; lobulated or round masses looking like nodules connected to hila by dilated vessels
LSVC with unroofed coronary sinus	No cardiomegaly; left upper border may be convex extending into neck
ASD + PS	Cardiomegaly, prominent right border; pulmonary bay convex (due to enlarged MPA and LPA) with pulmonary oligemia
Ebstein's disease	Cardiomegaly, water bottle/box-like silhouette, narrow pedicle, pulmonary oligemia
VSD + PS physiology	• Common features are (1) absence of cardiomegaly (unless associated with severe anemia, IE, aortic valve disease, hypertension, myocardial dysfunction), (2) concave pulmonary bay, and (3) pulmonary oligemia • *RV apex*: Classic TOF, DORV, VSD + PS, d-TGA, VSD + PS, l-TGA VSD + PS • *LV apex*: Tricuspid atresia, VSD, PS, single ventricle + PS • *TOF + pulmonary atresia*: In addition may have collateral vessels forming reticular pattern • *TOF with absent pulmonary valve syndrome*: Cardiomegaly +/–; dilated and aneurysmal MPA, LPA, and RPA with peripheral oligemia • *TOF with absent pulmonary artery*: Narrow hemithorax (opposite side of arch) • *Convex left upper border*: l-TGA, (DILV with inverted infundibular chamber)
Supracardiac TAPVC	Snowman/Figure of 8 appearances; PVH +

Eisenmenger syndrome	• Dilated MPA, LPA, RPA
	• Right descending PA diameter >17 mm peripheral pruning
	• In addition, special features indifferent subsets:
	  ○ Atrial level: Cardiomegaly, pulmonary artery and branches are very much dilated, aorta inconspicuous
	  ○ Ventricular level: No cardiomegaly, right aortic arch can be seen
	  ○ Ductal level: Ascending aorta prominent

Truncus arteriosus	• Cardiomegaly with LV apex, pulmonary bay may be concave or pulmonary artery at higher level • Pulmonary plethora or pruning • Right aortic arch, enlarged ascending aorta • *Absent pulmonary artery*: Small hemithorax, reduced pulmonary vascularity (same side of aortic arch)

(ASD: atrial septal defect; DILV: double-inlet left ventricle; DORV: double-outlet right ventricle; d-TGA: dextro-transposition of the great arteries; IE: infective endocarditis; LPA: left pulmonary artery; LSVC: left superior vena cava; L-TGA: levo-TGA; LV: left ventricular; MPA: main pulmonary artery; PA: pulmonary artery; PS: pulmonary stenosis; PVH: pulmonary arterial hypertension; RPA: right pulmonary artery; RV: right ventricular; TAPVC: total anomalous pulmonary venous connection; TOF: tetralogy of Fallot; VSD: ventricular septal defect)

BOX 1 Important electrocardiogram (ECG) finding in various subsets of cyanotic congenital heart diseases (CCHDs).

ECG abnormalities in CCHD

- Rhythm:
    - Ectopic atrial rhythm: Sinus venous ASD, heterotaxy syndromes, atriotomy
    - Complete heart block: l-TGA, ECD, single ventricle
    - Preexcitation: Ebstein's disease
- Axis:
    - Right axis: ASD + PS, Eisenmenger syndrome
    - Left axis: Tricuspid atresia, DORV, single ventricle (SV)
- Loop:
    - Clockwise loop (q in II, III, AVF with rS in 1, AVL): TOF, Eisenmenger syndrome, d-TGA, l-TGA, Ebstein's
    - Counterclockwise loop (q in I, AVL with rS in II, III, AVF): tricuspid atresia, DORV, ECD
- Himalayan P waves: Ebstein's disease, tricuspid atresia
- Polyphasic QRS complexes: Ebstein's disease
- Sudden QRS transition from V_1 to V_2: Classic TOF
- Right axis deviation with counter clockwise loop DORV, VSD + PS
- Stereotyped QRS in precordial leads: SV
- Absence of q in left lateral leads: l-TGA
- Biventricular hypertrophy: Truncus, single ventricle, some cases of DORV

(ASD: atrial septal defect; AVF: arteriovenous fistula; DORV: double-outlet right ventricle; d-TGA: dextro-transposition of the great arteries; ECD: endocardial cushion defect; l-TGA: levo-TGA; TOF: tetralogy of Fallot)

TABLE 6: Electrocardiogram (ECG) findings in ventricular septal defect (VSD) + pulmonary stenosis (PS) physiology.

Right axis + RVH: • TOF • d-TGA, VSD + PS • DORV, VSD + PS	*Left axis + RVH:* • ECD + PS • Single ventricle + PS • l-TGA, VSD + PS • DORV, VSD + PS
Right axis + LVH: • Single ventricle + PS • Pulmonary atresia with intact IVS	Left axis + LVH: Tricuspid atresia, VSD + PS

(DORV: double-outlet right ventricle; d-TGA: dextro-transposition of the great arteries; ECD: endocardial cushion defect; IVS: intact ventricular septum; l-TGA: levo-TGA; LVH: left ventricular hypertrophy; RVH: right ventricular hypertrophy; TOF: tetralogy of Fallot)

of RV size and function, evaluation of the right ventricular outflow tract (RVOT), evaluation of pulmonary arteries and the aorta, evaluation of systemic and pulmonary veins, evaluation of collaterals and arteriovenous malformations, coronaries, quantification of myocardial mass and identification of myocardial fibrosis/scar.

Computed tomography is superior to CMR in the setting of critically ill, or claustrophobic patients, presence of noncompatible implants for magnetic resonance imaging (MRI), and for evaluation of lung parenchyma or airways, when there is calcification and detailed evaluation of coronaries is needed.

Catheterization and Angiography

Recommended for intracavity and vascular pressure measurements. Cardiac catheterization is the gold standard for the diagnosis of pulmonary vascular disease. Cardiac catheterization is mainly employed when a percutaneous therapeutic procedure is contemplated.

Cardiac 3D Printing[14-17]

Cardiac 3D printing produces a replica of the patient's heart anatomy and is a powerful application that offers several advantages to patient care particularly in the ACHD population. In complex cardiac anatomy, 3D models allow precise understanding of the patient's anatomy and enabling detailed presurgical planning, and for patient counseling, trainee education, and simulation.

6-Minute Walk Test[18,19]

This test is useful in the assessment of functional capacity, prognostication, and assessment of response to treatment.

Holter monitoring and loop recorders when arrhythmias suspected.

Hematology

Packed cell volume (PCV), Hb%, red blood cell (RBC), white blood cell (WBC) count, platelet counts, Red cell indices [mean corpuscular volume (MCV), mean corpuscular hemoglobin (MCH), mean corpuscular hemoglobin concentration (MCHC)]; hematocrit should be calculated by automated electronic particle counter.

When hematocrit is above 55%, standard amount of citrate given in the sampling tubes may become excessive to the low plasma volume. So citrate amount must be adjusted.

Iron Studies

Ferritin, transferrin, transferrin saturation, and iron saturation are needed for the diagnosis and management of iron deficiency.

Others

Glucose, creatinine, electrolytes, uric acid; to avoid false reading of hypoglycemia, sodium fluoride tubes should be used for blood glucose sample collection.

Brain natriuretic peptide (BNP)/proBNP levels are useful in the follow-up of Eisenmenger syndrome and patients with ventricular dysfunction.[20,21]

MANAGEMENT[18,19,22]

Management of cyanotic congenital heart diseases patients requires team of medical and paramedical staff with expertise in ACHD care. Regular follow-up is necessary.

Broadly, management can be grouped into definitive management and general management.

Definitive Management[9]

This includes surgical correction, palliative procedures, or special medical management in various subsets. Surgical correction or interventional correction is indicated whenever feasible. Palliative procedures may be needed in some cases. Studies showed that surgery when done by pediatric cardiac surgeons gives better results.[23]

Definitive Management Options in Various Subsets

- *ASD + PS*: Ostium secundum atrial septal defect (OSASD) + PS can be treated with balloon pulmonary valvotomy and device closure of ASD. When device closure is not possible like in sinus venous ASDs, ostium primum atrial septal defects (OPASDs) surgical closure of the defect after pulmonary valvotomy needed. Post-procedure beta blockers to prevent infundibular spasm are required.
- *LSVC + unroofed coronary sinus*: Surgical closure or device closure
- *Classic TOF*: Intracardiac repair (ICR) with VSD patch closure and RVOT enlargement; in cases where anomalous coronary artery crosses RVOT, right ventricle to pulmonary artery (PA) conduit may be needed. Associated DCRV must be identified and muscle bundles need to be resected, before surgery identification of AP collaterals should be identified and closed percutaneously or rarely by surgery.
- *TOF pulmonary atresia*: Pulmonary arterial confluence and size of the pulmonary arteries determine the management. If confluence is present with adequate size pulmonary arteries, ICR is possible. Collaterals and palliative shunts done earlier should be closed. When pulmonary arteries are nonconfluent, surgical reconstruction by staged unifocalization is possible in some cases.[24,25] When it is not possible, palliative measures like stenting of collateral may be required.[26]
- *TOF absent pulmonary valve syndrome*: Surgical correction with enlargement of annulus with homograft implantation along with VSD patch closure or VSD patch closure with valve conduit from right ventricle to PA may be necessary.
- *DORV, VSD+PS*: Creating a tunnel from left ventricle to aorta through VSD using Dacron patch and RVOT repair or placement of right ventricle to PA conduit
- *ECD + PS*: Surgical repair with defect closure, AV valve repair and RVOT repair
- *Single ventricle + PS*:[27,28] Many patients will have an earlier palliative surgery like Glenn shunt or BT shunt. Some form of Fontan surgery is required after careful assessment.
- *TA, VSD + PS*: Fontan type surgery
- *Ebstein's disease*:[29-31] Tricuspid valve repair (cone procedure)/replacement with bioprosthetic valve plus ASD closure; in addition Glen shunt may be needed (one and a half ventricle repair) if the adequacy of pulmonary flow is questionable. When right ventricle is very much hypoplastic, Fontan procedure may be necessary. Preoperatively, these cases need to be assed for accessory pathways by electrophysiology (EP) study and radioablation may be required or surgical ablation at the time of surgery. In rare cases where cyanosis alone is the problem, ASD device closure may be needed after careful assessment.
- *Pulmonary arteriovenous fistula*: If localized, surgical resection by segmentectomy or lobectomy may be useful. Transcatheter closure with coils or vascular plugs is one option.
- *TAPVC*: Surgical repair with routing of common pulmonary vein into LA and ASD closure
- *Transposition cases* rarely survive till adulthood and develop severe pulmonary hypertension by then.
- *Palliative procedures*: In cases where definite surgery is not possible, palliative options like creation of AV shunts or venovenous shunts or stenting of collaterals can be done.
- *Eisenmenger syndrome*:[18,19,32] Once obstructive PAH with Eisenmenger syndrome with resting hypoxia sets in, surgical correction is contraindicated. Definitive therapy for Eisenmenger syndrome includes (1) endothelin receptor antagonist like baseman, (2) phosphodiesterase-5 (PDE-5) inhibitors like sildenafil and tadalafil, and (3) prostacyclins. Oral agents may be initiated alone or in combination and addition of subcutaneous prostacyclins may be necessary in some. There are case reports of so-called treat and repair strategy where patients are initially treated with pulmonary vasodilators and followed and once significant fall in pulmonary vascular resistance occurs, attempt surgical closure.[33] Anticoagulants are not useful and indicated only in cases with PA thrombosis or atrial arrhythmias. Prognosis in Eisenmenger syndrome when compared to idiopathic PAH is better. Predictors of worse outcome are:[32,34-36] World Health Organization functional class (WHO FC) III and IV, exercise intolerance assessed by 6-minute walk test, hospitalizations for right heart failure, biomarkers [N-terminal pro-B-type

natriuretic peptide (NTproBNP) 500 pg/mL, CRP 10 mg/mL, high creatinine, low albumin] iron deficiency, echo indices of RV dysfunction, pretricuspid shunt, advanced age, low oxygen saturation, absence of sinus rhythm, and presence of pericardial effusion.

CARDIAC COMPLICATIONS

Arrhythmias[37]

Patients with ASD, postoperative scars, post-Fontan status, and Ebstein's disease are more prone for atrial arrhythmias. Antiarrhythmic medications such as beta blocker and amiodarone are useful. Those with atrial arrhythmias need long-term oral anticoagulation. Electrophysiological interventions may be needed in some cases. Ebstein's diseases cases may need presurgical evaluation by EP studies and radioablation or surgical ablation of accessory pathways.

Patient with complete heart block need permanent pacing preferably by epicardial route as endocardial leads are associated with paradoxical systemic embolism.

Patients with ventricular dysfunction and ventricular arrhythmias need implantable cardioverter-defibrillators (ICDs), and subcutaneous and epicardial routes are preferable.

Infective Endocarditis

These patients are at high risk of developing infective endocarditis. Appropriate prophylaxis is needed in all situations associated with transient bacteremia. Suspected infective endocarditis must be promptly treated with appropriate antibiotics.

Heart Failure[38]

Earlier studies describe heart failure as uncommon entity in many cyanotic diseases such as VSD + PS, Eisenmenger VSD where RV pressure will not increase beyond systemic pressure. With increased survival of patients, heart failure is becoming the leading cause of hospitalization and death in adult cyanosis heart diseases.

Causes of heart failure in adult cyanotic congenital heart disease can be divided into the following:

- Systolic dysfunction of the systemic morphological left ventricle
  - Pressure overload [associated aortic stenosis (AS), coarctation of the aorta]
  - Volume overload (AR, multiple collaterals, MR in ECD)
  - Myocardial injury due to prior surgery
- Systolic dysfunction of the subpulmonary morphological right ventricle
  - Volume overload (PR in absent pulmonary valve syndrome, ASD)
  - Pressure overloads (severe RVOT obstruction)
- Systolic dysfunction of the morphological systemic right ventricle—l-TGA.
- Systolic dysfunction of the systemic single ventricle—post-Fontan repair
- Systolic dysfunction of the cyanotic systemic and/or subpulmonary ventricle with or without pulmonary hypertension—myocardial injury by chronic hypoxia (VSD with PS) or pressure overload (Eisenmenger syndrome)
- Acquired ischemic heart disease and ventricular dysfunction
- Systolic dysfunction of the systemic ventricle due to tachyarrhythmias

Systolic heart failure is managed with renin-angiotensin-aldosterone system (RAAS) blockers, beta blockers, aldosterone antagonists, diuretics, and digoxin. Diastolic heart failure is managed with diuretics treatment of arrhythmias, etc.

There are no guidelines regarding the management of acute heart failure. Treatment is individualized and same as management of acute heart failure in other situations such as oxygen, diuretics, vasodilators/inotropes, and correction of precipitating factors.

GENERAL MANAGEMENT

Chronic cyanosis and hypoxemia causes multisystem dysfunction and measures are necessary to address them.[18,19,22,39]

Hyperviscosity Syndrome

Chronic cyanosis and hypoxemia stimulate erythropoietic system with production of more number of red cells which in turn increases increased hematocrit which increases blood viscosity. If there is associated iron deficiency blood viscosity is further increased as the microspherocytes are less deformable. Patients present with history of headache, dizziness, visual blurring, myalgia, and weakness. Common reasons are dehydration and iron deficiency. The first step in the management is adequate hydration, if necessary by intravenous (IV) fluids (with air filters) and correction of iron deficiency with oral iron. If symptoms persist despite these measures, isovolemic phlebotomy with removal of minimal volume and simultaneous replacement with saline, to alleviate symptoms, is needed. It is only a temporary measure.

Iron Deficiency

Common causes of iron deficiency are inappropriate phlebotomy, nutritional deficiency, and menorrhagia in women. It is associated with hyperviscosity and poor exercise tolerance. Serum iron studies are needed for accurate assessment. Treatment of iron deficiency by low-dose oral iron supplementation is preferable. Care should be taken to prevent side effects like gastric irritation which may cause vomitings and diarrhea leading to dehydration and exacerbation of symptoms. Hematological parameters must be monitored frequently as sometimes sudden increase in counts and hematocrit may be seen in which case iron replacement should be slowed. Replacement should be done slowly over months. Simultaneous supplementation of folic acid and vitamin B12 may be needed.

Bleeding Manifestations

These patients have dysregulated hemostasis with increased tendency for bleeding as well thrombosis; these patients have thrombocytopenia, deficiency in the von Willebrand factor multimers, and other coagulation factor abnormalities. Superficial mucosal bleeds such as epistaxis, easy bruising, and oral bleeds are common. Most of these can be managed conservatively with rest and local measures.

Hemoptysis is a frequent problem. Most of the times it can be managed with rest, adequate hydration, centrally acting cough suppressants like codeine. Blood pressure should be maintained at low normal levels, especially in patients with Eisenmenger syndrome with post-tricuspid shunts as systemic pressure and pulmonary pressure are same in these cases and hypertension is associated with increased bleeding. It needs evaluation with chest X-ray, CT scan, or angio. Bronchoscopy should be avoided. If not controlled by local measures, selective therapeutic embolization of collaterals or limited resection, if lung is involved, may be necessary. Diffuse pulmonary AVF following bidirectional Glenn shunt may require surgical inclusion of hepatic venous flow into lungs.

Pulmonary Thromboembolism

In situ thrombosis of pulmonary arteries is seen in cases of Eisenmenger syndrome. Though anticoagulants are contraindicated in general, these patients need anticoagulation initially with heparin and later with vitamin K antagonists with careful monitoring. In situ pulmonary thrombosis is associated with poor prognosis and terminal event most of the times with high mortality.

Hyperuricemia and Gout

Hyperuricemia is common because of increased RBC turnover and decreased uric acid excretion by the kidneys. But attacks of gouty arthritis are uncommon. Asymptomatic cases do not require treatment. Symptomatic cases need colchicine and narcotic analgesics for acute cases and allopurinol for maintenance.

Arthralgias secondary to pulmonary osteoarthropathy need oral paracetamol or agents like salsalate. Salicylate and other nonsteroidal anti-inflammatory drugs (NSAIDS) should be avoided. Bisphosphonates are effective for relieving pain when it is refractory to conventional analgesics.

Gallstones

Due to excessive unconjugated bilirubin levels, which is a by-product of heme metabolism, which is increased due to increased erythrocyte turnover, pigment gallstones consisting of calcium bilirubinate are common. Many are asymptomatic. Symptomatic cases with biliary colic and cholecystitis need cholecystectomy or endoscopic procedures.

Renal Dysfunction

Many have tubular abnormalities, hyperplasia of juxtaglomerular cells, and activation of RAAS system. Kidney reserve is decreased and more prone for acute kidney injury. Preventive measures such as avoidance of dehydration, inappropriate use of diuretics, and avoidance of nephrotoxic drugs is essential. Conservative management is indicated mostly. Dialysis is required in selective cases but is poorly tolerated due to associated hemodynamic perturbations and needs special care and monitoring.

Neurological

Stroke can occur due to paradoxical embolism or intracerebral hemorrhage secondary to abnormal coagulation. Venous thrombosis and brain abscess are also common. Any cyanotic heart disease patient with headache, altered sensorium should undergo CT/MRI promptly to detect the etiology. Anticoagulation and antiplatelet usage is associated with increased bleeding risk. Seizure disorders are increased and need long-term anticonvulsants.

Cerebral Abscess

Cerebral abscess should be suspected in patients with fever, vomiting, and change in mental status, headache, seizures, etc. High index of suspicion is essential and prompt CT/MRI of head is needed. Brain abscess should be treated with appropriated antibiotics and surgical evacuation.

Lung Problems

Lung function abnormalities are common. Majority have restrictive pattern. Chest wall abnormalities, kyphoscoliosis, prior thoracotomies, collaterals, and in situ thrombus formation contribute to the problem. Incidence of respiratory infections is increased and should be recognized and treated early.

Psychosocial Issues

There is increased incidence of anxiety and depressions in these people which should be addressed appropriately.

Exercise and Work

Regular low-intensity exercise like walking is encouraged. Competitive sports, isometric exercises should be avoided. They should avoid dehydration and extremities of weather. Most people are productive and able to do sedentary work for limited hours.

Noncardiac Procedures

These should not be undertaken unless there are clear indications. In patients with high hematocrit preoperative phlebotomy with removal of blood is needed to decrease postoperative bleeding. Air filters in IV lines is essential. Avoidance of dehydration and prompt volume replacement is essential. Cases should be managed by experienced team with careful monitoring. Postoperative management in intensive care is essential.

Menstrual Problems

Menorrhagia is very common and needs iron supplementation. Measures like estrogen + progesterone combination are contraindicated. Low-dose progesterone containing pills may be used carefully. Local causes like fibroids may need therapeutic embolization.

Pregnancy and Delivery[40]

Unrepaired cyanotic congenital heart diseases and Eisenmenger syndrome come under modified WHO III (mWHO III) and mWHO IV classes, respectively and are associated with very high risk of maternal and fetal mortality and morbidity. These patients must be counseled against pregnancy. Termination also carries increased risk. Endothelin receptor antagonists cause embryopathy and are contraindicated and PDE-5 inhibitors like sildenafil, and prostacyclins can be given.

Maternal complications are seen in 19–27% of mWHO III and 40–100% of mWHO IV cases. Worsening of clinical status, sudden death, thromboembolism, and paradoxical embolism can occur.

Fetal Complications

Early fetal loss, preterm labor, intrauterine growth restriction (IUGR); fetal echo is indicated whenever there is risk of fetal anomalies.

If a women wishes to continue pregnancy, she should be managed by an experienced multidisciplinary team with regular follow-up and prompt admission well before expected date of delivery. Supplemental oxygenation, avoidance of bearing down, and shortening of second stage by vacuum extraction/outlet forceps is needed. Lower segment Cesarean section (LSCS) is indicated for obstetric reasons or in Eisenmenger syndrome (class IIa). Regional anesthesia is better than general anesthesia. Avoidance of hypovolemia is crucial. Postpartum monitoring in intensive care unit is needed. As thrombotic risk is very high, necessary precautions like elastic stockings and heparin may be considered; these patients remain at high risk of events for many months after delivery and should be counseled appropriately.

Contraception

Estrogen-containing contraceptives are contraindicated as they are associated with increased thrombotic risk. Barrier methods plus progestin depot injection or progestin eluting intrauterine devices (IUDs) are preferable. IUD insertion must be done in the hospital under careful monitoring as it can cause vasovagal attacks which may be fatal in these cases.

Travel

Travel in commercial flights is safe and does not require supplemental oxygen. Avoidance of dehydration with frequent intake of water and fluids is essential. Journeys should be carefully planned to avoid exertion and stress, high-altitude travel should be avoided.

Vaccination against influenza and pneumococcal is advised.

Cigarette smoking, tobacco use, use of recreational drugs, and alcohol are strictly prohibited.

Heart Transplantation[41]

Heart transplantation in patients with ACHD is a complicated issue and associated with early morbidity and mortality but has better long-term survival.

CONCLUSION

With the improved medical care and palliative procedures, the survival of cyanotic congenital heart disease patients is increasing into adulthood. These patients need regular follow-up at the centers for ACHDs. All these patients have a very delicate balanced circulation and any perturbations will have an adverse and sometimes catastrophic consequence. Prevention of these issues by taking appropriate measures and patient education constitutes an important component of the management of cyanotic patients. These patients and their families must be educated not only about current treatment options and plans, but also about anticipated advanced medical care and palliative care which may be required in the future. They should be told about the need to make necessary arrangements, like insurance plans and will.

ONLINE REFERENCES

Please scan the QR code provided at the end of the table of contents for References of this chapter.

SECTION

18

Miscellaneous

CHAPTER

125 Late Cardiovascular Manifestation of COVID-19 Infection

Tripti Deb

ABSTRACT

Late cardiovascular manifestations of coronavirus disease (COVID) refer to the cardiovascular symptoms and complications that persist after the acute phase of COVID-19 has resolved. These symptoms and complications can include chest pain, heart palpitations, shortness of breath, myocarditis, pericarditis, and arrhythmias among others. The mechanism of cardiovascular injury following COVID-19 is complex and involves several factors, including direct viral invasion, immune-mediated response, inflammation, endothelial dysfunction, and dysregulation of the renin-angiotensin system. Diagnostic tools for the late cardiovascular manifestations of COVID-19 include advanced cardiac imaging, echocardiography, and cardiac magnetic resonance (CMR) imaging. High-sensitive cardiac troponin (hs-cTn) and N-terminal pro-B-type natriuretic peptide (NT-proBNP) are the most notable cardiac biomarkers associated with COVID-19-related cardiovascular disease. There is no specific treatment for cardiovascular complications in late COVID-19 syndrome. The recommended treatments involve managing risk factors for the cardiovascular disease, monitoring for more severe cardiac involvement, and attention to cardiovascular health and disease. Further research is essential to establish the relation between different variants of virus, vaccination, and cardiac complication, mechanism of cardiac injury and potential therapy targeted to prevent cardiac complications.

Keywords: COVID-19, cardiovascular, complications, myocarditis, pericarditis, arrhythmias, cardiomyopathy, heart failure, biomarkers.

INTRODUCTION

Coronavirus disease 2019 (COVID-19) is a viral infection that has affected millions of people worldwide. Although the respiratory symptoms of the disease are well-known, there is a mounting evidence that the virus can also lead to long-term cardiovascular complications. This article delves into the delayed cardiovascular effects of COVID-19 infection, which include the increased risk of developing cardiovascular disease, myocardial injury, arrhythmias, and cardiomyopathies. Additionally, it examines the potential mechanisms of myocardial injury, such as direct viral infiltration and autoimmune dysregulation. Lastly, the article underscores the critical importance of managing cardiovascular health and disease in individuals who have survived COVID-19.[1-3]

Studying the late cardiovascular manifestations of COVID-19 is essential for several reasons. Firstly, it helps us comprehend the virus's long-term impact on the cardiovascular system and identifies potential risk factors for developing cardiovascular complications. This knowledge can inform the development of effective prevention and treatment strategies and improving the health outcomes of COVID-19 survivors.

Secondly, studying the late cardiovascular manifestations of COVID-19 can help healthcare providers to better manage the care of COVID-19 survivors. By understanding the potential long-term cardiovascular complications of the virus, healthcare providers can monitor the patients for these complications and provide timely interventions to prevent further harm. This can also help mitigate the burden on healthcare systems and reduce costs associated with the long-term care.

Finally, studying the late cardiovascular manifestations of COVID-19 can inform public health policies and resource allocation. By comprehending the long-term impact of the virus on the cardiovascular system, policymakers can make informed decisions about how to allocate resources to support COVID-19 survivors and prevent further complications. This can also help prepare for future pandemics by improving our understanding of the potential long-term impacts of viral infections on cardiovascular health **(Fig. 1)**.

OVERVIEW OF STUDIES ON LATE CARDIOVASCULAR MANIFESTATIONS

Numerous studies have been conducted to investigate the late cardiovascular manifestations of COVID-19. One study, showed that the individuals with COVID-19 face an elevated risk of developing various types of cardiovascular diseases, including cerebrovascular disorders, dysrhythmias, ischemic and nonischemic heart disease, pericarditis, myocarditis, heart failure, and thromboembolic disease, even if they were not hospitalized during the acute phase of the infection.[4]

Another study highlights the cardiovascular sequelae in COVID-19 survivors and proposes essential questions that need to be addressed through prospective studies to understand and manage these persistent cardiovascular consequences. This study emphasizes the need for prospective studies to begin now, with adequate resources made available to monitor and research this population in the coming years.[5]

PREVALENCE AND RISK OF LATE CARDIOVASCULAR MANIFESTATIONS OF COVID-19

The prevalence of cardiovascular complications among COVID-19 survivors is alarming and has not been extensively studied. In a study published in Nature,[4] it was revealed that individuals with COVID-19 have an increased risk of developing incident cardiovascular disease across multiple categories. These include cerebrovascular disorders, dysrhythmias, ischemic and nonischemic heart disease, pericarditis, myocarditis, heart failure, and thromboembolic disease. It is worth noting that the risk of incident cardiovascular disease persists even after the acute phase of COVID-19 has passed. Another study published in COVID-19 survivors are at a higher risk of cerebrovascular diseases, arrhythmia-related disorders, and inflammatory heart disease.[6] Additionally, the study revealed that the risk and 1-year burden of cardiovascular disease in survivors of acute COVID-19 are substantial.

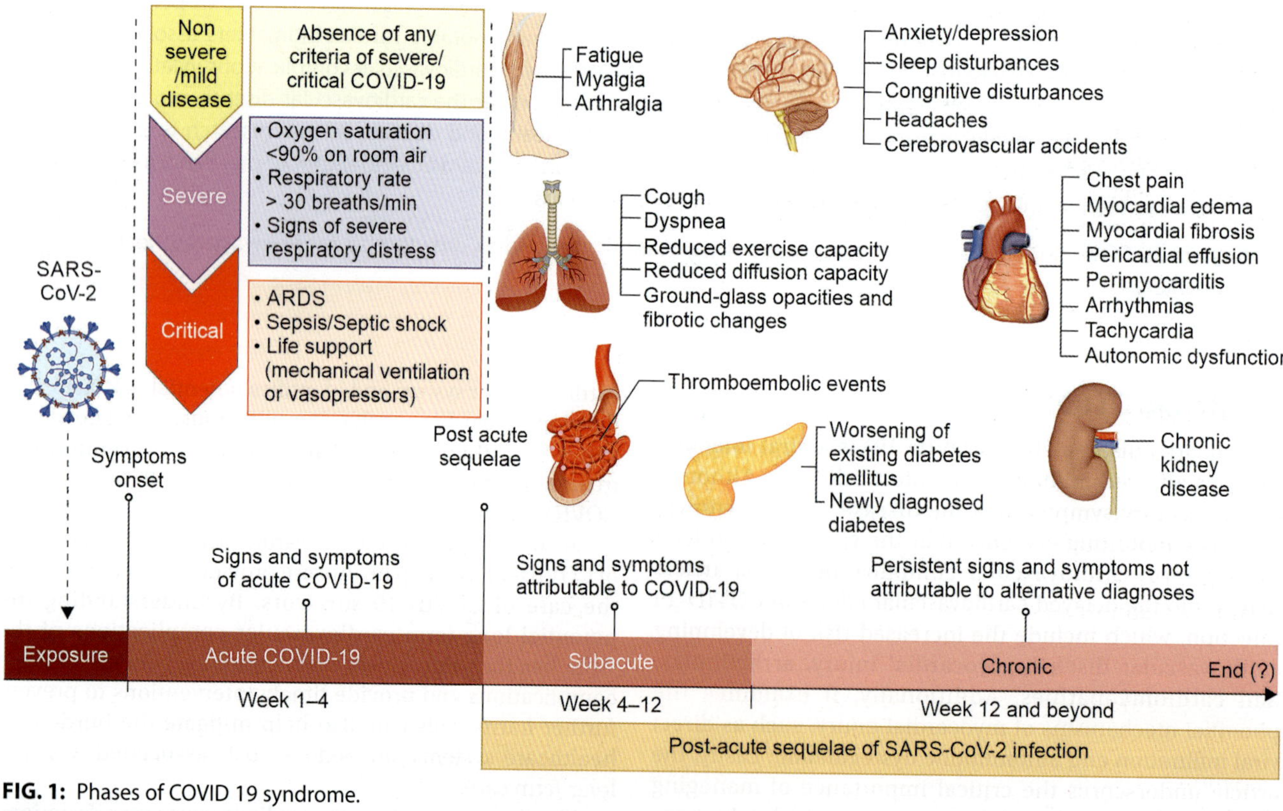

FIG. 1: Phases of COVID 19 syndrome.

(ARDS: acute respiratory distress syndrome; COVID-19: coronavirus 2019; SARS-CoV-2: severe acute respiratory syndrome coronavirus 2)

Source: Cenko E, Badimon L, Bugiardini R, Claeys MJ, De Luca G, de Wit C, et al. Cardiovascular disease and COVID-19: a consensus paper from the ESC Working Group on Coronary Pathophysiology & Microcirculation, ESC Working Group on Thrombosis and the Association for Acute CardioVascular Care (ACVC), in collaboration with the European Heart Rhythm Association (EHRA). Cardiovasc Res. 2021;117(14):2705-29.

Therefore, it is crucial to prioritize cardiovascular health and disease management in the care pathways of COVID-19 survivors. This will require a multidisciplinary approach that includes regular monitoring for potential cardiovascular complications and timely interventions to prevent further harm. It is also important for healthcare providers to recognize and address the potential psychological impact of cardiovascular complications on COVID-19 survivors, as this can have a significant impact on their overall well-being and recovery.[4]

TYPES OF LATE CARDIOVASCULAR MANIFESTATIONS (BOX 1)

Myocardial Injury

Myocardial injury is common and starts from the acute phase and subclinically persists over the chronic phase of disease. The evidence of myocardial injury, defined as an elevated troponin level, is common among patients hospitalized with COVID-19. Putative causes of this injury include stress cardiomyopathy, hypoxic injury, ischemic injury caused by cardiac microvascular damage or epicardial coronary artery disease, and systemic inflammatory response syndrome.[7]

The mechanism of myocardial injury is still under investigation, but hypotheses include direct viral infiltration and autoimmune dysregulation. Furthermore, research suggests that severe acute respiratory syndrome coronavirus-2 (SARS-CoV-2) can affect the cardiovascular system, leading to a wide range of complications, including acute myocardial injury.[8]

Taken together, these findings demonstrate that COVID-19 can cause myocardial injury and other cardiovascular complications. It is crucial for healthcare providers to monitor COVID-19 patients for potential cardiovascular complications and provide timely interventions to prevent further harm.

Arrhythmias

Coronavirus disease 2019 can lead to cardiac arrhythmias **(Box 2)**, which are a common late manifestation of the disease. The COVID-19-related arrhythmic manifestations include atrial arrhythmias (such as atrial fibrillation and atrial flutter), sinus node dysfunction, atrioventricular conduction abnormalities, ventricular tachyarrhythmias, sudden cardiac arrest, and cardiovascular dysautonomia including the so-called long COVID syndrome.[9] These arrhythmias can occur in any phase of the disease, including the infective, recovery, or postrecovery phase.

A study suggests that cardiac arrhythmias may persist even after recovery from COVID-19. Therefore, healthcare providers should be vigilant in monitoring for cardiac arrhythmias in COVID-19 patients and survivors, and timely interventions should be provided to prevent further harm.[10]

Thromboembolic Events (Box 3)

Thromboembolic complications are a well-known and potentially serious late manifestation of COVID-19 infection. COVID-19 patients have an increased risk of serious thrombotic complications, including pulmonary embolism and deep vein thrombosis, which can be life-threatening.[11] COVID-19-induced coagulopathy, an immunothrombotic state, has been linked to thromboembolic and hemorrhagic events.[12,13]

Given the potential severity of thromboembolic complications, it is important for individuals who have recovered from COVID-19 to be aware of the risk and seek medical attention if they experience symptoms such as chest pain, shortness of breath, or swelling in the legs. It may be necessary for the patients to undergo medical testing and treatment to prevent or address thromboembolic complications associated with COVID-19.[11-13]

Vasculitis

Recent studies have shown that vasculitis can manifest as a cardiovascular complication of COVID-19 infection. There is evidence showing that COVID-19 can cause vasculitis, including *coronary artery vasculitis*, as a late complication of the infection.[14] Additionally, COVID-19 can cause endothelial alterations, including vasculitis, which can promote *pulmonary infiltration, edema,* and later *pulmonary*

BOX 1 Types of late cardiovascular manifestations.

- Myocardial injury
- Arrhythmias
- Thromboembolic events
- Vasculitis
- Cardiomyopathies
- Heart failure

BOX 2 Cardiac arrhythmias.

- Atrial flutter and fibrillation
- Sinus node dysfunction
- Atrioventricular conduction defects
- Ventricular arrhythmias
- Sudden cardiac arrest
- Dysautonomia

BOX 3 Thromboembolic events.

- Cerebrovascular disease
- Pulmonary embolism
- Deep venous thrombosis
- Retinal artery thrombosis

fibrosis in the affected patients.[15] Vasculitis is a potential cardiovascular complication of COVID-19 infection.[16]

While the evidence for COVID-19-induced vasculitis is still limited, it is important to monitor patients who have recovered from the virus for any signs of vasculitis, especially those who have had severe or prolonged infections. Early recognition and management of vasculitis can help prevent long-term complications and improve patient outcomes.[14-16]

BOX 4 Risk factors for late cardiovascular manifestations of COVID-19.

- Severe illness
- Old age
- Female
- Comorbidity
- Unvaccinated

Cardiomyopathy

Cardiomyopathy can occur as a chronic complication following COVID-19 infection. Even a mild case of COVID-19 can lead to long-term; sometimes permanent, heart damage. Viral infections like COVID-19 can worsen preexisting cardiomyopathy. Some researchers have even suggested that cardiomyopathy and heart failure may be the natural result of COVID-19 rather than a rare complication. In severe COVID-19 infections, sepsis and cardiogenic shock are common complications. There also has been evidence that some people who become severely ill with COVID-19 go on to develop *takotsubo syndrome or stress cardiomyopathy.*[17]

Cardiomyopathies were discovered in 21.47% of the patients with a raised troponin and a raised D-dimer in most of the patients. Echocardiography shows mild-to-severe left ventricular dysfunction.[18]

Heart Failure

Heart failure is a serious complication that can arise in COVID-19 patients. Heart failure was defined as the presence of typical symptoms in addition to the signs of structural and/or functional cardiac abnormalities. The study found that 19.8% of the COVID-19 patients had an acute cardiac injury and 18.1% had an acute heart failure, making an acute cardiac injury the most common complication among the COVID-19 patients.[19]

The long COVID can result in persistent cardiac ischemia, atrial and ventricular arrhythmias, and new-onset heart failure in previously healthy patients. This highlights the importance of monitoring COVID-19 patients for signs of heart failure, even after their acute illness has resolved. Effective management of heart failure in COVID-19 survivors can help improve their long-term outcomes and quality of life.[8]

RISK FACTORS FOR LATE CARDIOVASCULAR MANIFESTATIONS OF COVID-19 (BOX 4)

Research suggests that the severity of COVID-19 infection is correlated with an increased risk of late cardiovascular complication. Patients with preexisting cardiovascular disease have a higher prevalence of severe forms of COVID-19, intensive care unit (ICU) admission, and higher mortality rates.[4] Even mild COVID-19 cases can result in cardiac abnormalities, which are mostly self-limiting but may require cardiac surveillance using electrocardiogram (ECG) and/or serum biomarkers to detect more severe cardiac involvement, including atrial fibrillation and left ventricular dysfunction.[20]

Taking evidence from post-COVID syndrome data conditions can affect anyone with a history of SARS-CoV-2 infection, including those who had clinically presumptive or polymerase chain reaction (PCR)-confirmed acute infection, mild, moderate, or severe acute infection, and even those who were initially asymptomatic. It can affect all the demographics, regardless of age, sex, or race including previously healthy individuals without underlying illness. However, certain groups appear to be disproportionately affected, such as those who had severe initial illness, females, older adults, and individuals with preexisting conditions. Additionally, people who have not been vaccinated against COVID-19 may be at higher risk of developing long COVID compared to those who have received the vaccine.[21-24]

MECHANISMS OF CARDIOVASCULAR INJURY

The mechanism of cardiovascular injury following COVID-19 infection is complex and involves several factors. Coronavirus disease 2019-associated cardiac injury can result from a multitude of mechanisms, including myocardial oxygen supply–demand imbalance, direct viral invasion, and indirect mechanisms sustained by systemic inflammation, immune-mediated response, and dysregulation of the renin-angiotensin system.[25] Cytokine-mediated inflammation can cause myositis and cardiomyocyte death, chronic inflammation and cellular damage may result in fibrosis, and autonomic dysfunction can lead to the postural orthostatic tachycardia syndrome (POTS).[26,27]

Coronavirus disease 2019 patients may experience cardiovascular manifestations due to a profound disturbance of endothelial homeostasis. Furthermore, there are hypotheses that direct viral infiltration and autoimmune dysregulation may also contribute to the mechanism of myocardial injury.[28]

Coronavirus disease 2019 infection can cause myocardial injury, affecting about one-quarter of the patients, and may manifest even in the absence of previous cardiovascular disease. This injury is associated with higher mortality rates and long-term sequelae. Therefore, the mechanism of cardiovascular injury following COVID-19 infection is multifactorial and involves direct and indirect mechanisms, including viral invasion, inflammation, and endothelial dysfunction. It is important to continue investigating the mechanisms underlying COVID-19-associated cardiac injury to better understand its impact on the patient outcomes and develop effective treatments **(Fig. 2)**.[29,2]

DIAGNOSIS AND MANAGEMENT OF LATE CARDIOVASCULAR MANIFESTATIONS

Clinical Evaluation (Table 1 and Box 5)

Any patient with cardiac symptoms such as chest pain, irregular, and rapid heart rate breathlessness following COVID should be thoroughly evaluated for other manifestations of post-COVID-19 syndrome such as fatigue, symptoms that get worse after physical or mental effort, fever, lung (respiratory) symptoms, including difficulty breathing or shortness of breath and cough.[30]

Neurological manifestations, for example, difficulty in thinking or concentrating (also referred to as "brain fog"), headache, sleep problems, dizziness when standing up

TABLE 1: Clinical evaluation of late cardiovascular manifestations.

Symptoms	History
Chest pain	Severity of acute disease
Breathlessness	Timeline for evolution
Palpitation	Need for respiratory and circulatory support
Syncope	Existing cardiac disease
Exercise intolerance	Diabetes
Fatigue	Hypertension
Review of system	Medication

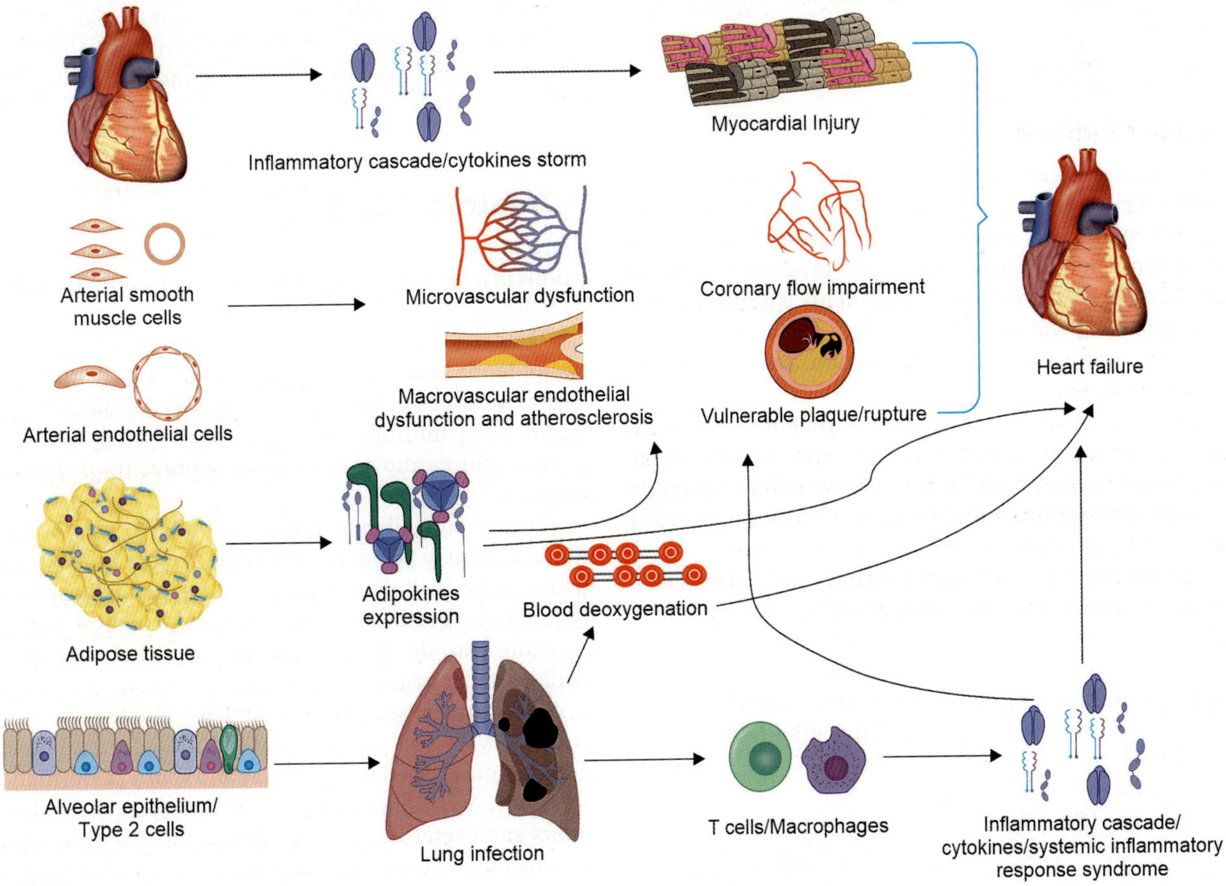

FIG. 2: Mechanism of cardiovascular injury.

Source: Cenko E, Badimon L, Bugiardini R, Claeys MJ, De Luca G, de Wit C, et al. Cardiovascular disease and COVID-19: a consensus paper from the ESC Working Group on Coronary Pathophysiology & Microcirculation, ESC Working Group on Thrombosis and the Association for Acute CardioVascular Care (ACVC), in collaboration with the European Heart Rhythm Association (EHRA). Cardiovasc Res. 2021;117(14):2705-29.

BOX 5 Examination for late cardiovascular manifestations.

- Heart rate, blood pressure (BP) sitting and standing
- Pulse oximetry
- Peripheral artery and veins for occlusion
- Signs of volume overload
- Cardiac examination

BOX 6 Diagnostic tools.

- Echocardiogram
- Cardiac magnetic resonance imaging (CMR)
- Computed tomography (CT) of chest

(lightheadedness), pins-and-needles sensation, changes in smell or taste, and depression or anxiety.[31,21]

Delayed thromboembolic complications are also a risk in patients with COVID-19 infection.[32] A new perspective on post-COVID syndromes suggests that mast cell activation syndrome (MCAS) is a primary manifestation of post-COVID syndromes.[33,34]

Diagnostic Tools

Imaging Studies (Box 6)

Diagnostic tools for late cardiovascular manifestations of COVID-19 include advanced cardiac imaging, *echocardiography, and CMR imaging*. Cardiac imaging is a gold standard in the diagnosis of cardiac involvement during acute COVID-19. On follow-up of patients with significant cardiovascular involvement, echocardiography and CMR can be used to assess cardiac function and detect late cardiovascular complications.[35-37]

Cardiac magnetic resonance is a reliable diagnostic tool for detecting both acute and long-term cardiovascular sequelae of COVID-19 infection due to its unique capability of detecting myocardial injury and characterizing myocardial tissue properties in vivo.[38]

Echocardiography is often the first imaging modality used in patients with suspected cardiovascular involvement in COVID-19 as it is widely available and can provide real-time information on cardiac function. Therefore, advanced cardiac imaging, echocardiography, and CMR are reliable diagnostic tools for detecting late cardiovascular manifestations of COVID-19.[39]

Biomarkers (Box 7)

Several cardiac biomarkers have emerged as valuable predictors of prognosis in patients with late cardiovascular manifestations of COVID-19. Creatine kinase (CK), CK-MB, high-sensitive cardiac troponin (hs-cTn) and N-terminal pro-B-type natriuretic peptide (NT-proBNP) are the most notable cardiac biomarkers associated with COVID-19-related cardiovascular disease.[40,41]

TABLE 2: Risk factor management.

Risk factor management	Education
Dyslipidemia	Lifestyle modification
Diabetes	Diet and nutrition
Hypertension	Exercise
Obesity	Medications
Tobacco and alcohol	Resources
Depression	Reassurance

BOX 7 Biomarkers.

- High sensitivity cardiac troponin
- Creatine kinase [CK, CK-myocardial band (MB)]
- N-terminal pro B-type natriuretic peptide

Furthermore, a study found that cardiac injury, manifested by cardiac biomarker elevation, is detected in a sizable number of COVID-19 patients and is associated with increased mortality.[42] Therefore, hs-cTn, NT-proBNP, CK, CK-MB, and plasma TnT levels are some of the biomarkers associated with late cardiovascular manifestations of COVID-19.

Treatment Strategies

There is no specific treatment for cardiovascular complications in late COVID-19 syndrome. According to the Centers for Disease Control and Prevention (CDC), managing risk factors **(Table 2)** for cardiovascular disease, such as dyslipidemia and diabetes, is essential in individuals with cardiovascular symptoms following COVID-19.[31] Lifestyle modification, nutrition, diet, exercise, and other established practices for cardiovascular disease prevention should be followed.[31]

Cardiac surveillance in the form of ECG and/or serum biomarkers may be advisable to detect more severe cardiac involvement, including atrial fibrillation and left ventricular dysfunction.[4] Furthermore, care pathways of those surviving the acute episode of COVID-19 should include attention to cardiovascular health and disease.[20]

To ensure the safe return of athletes who have recovered from COVID-19, proper evaluation, counseling, and guidance on a staged return to play and sports performance is necessary. According to the American College of Cardiology Sports and Exercise Cardiology Leadership Council, athletes may resume exercise training when the following criteria have been met:

- Asymptomatic athletes with recent SARS-CoV-2 infection who have abstained from exercise for three days during self-isolation.

- Athletes with recent SARS-CoV-2 infection, who experienced mild or moderate noncardiopulmonary symptoms, have resolved.
- Athletes with remote infection (>3 months ago) without ongoing cardiopulmonary symptoms and require no additional testing.

It is important to note that athletes with severe COVID-19 infection, those with ongoing cardiopulmonary symptoms, or those with cardiovascular involvement during the acute phase of the disease require more extensive evaluation before returning to sports.[43,44]

Therefore, the recommended treatments for cardiovascular complications in late COVID-19 syndrome involve managing risk factors for cardiovascular disease, monitoring for more severe cardiac involvement, and attention to cardiovascular health and disease.[4,20,31]

CONCLUSION

Late cardiological manifestations of COVID-19 can occur in both hospitalized and nonhospitalized patients, with an estimated prevalence ranging from 10 to 30% of patients who have had COVID-19.

Clinical manifestations include dysrhythmias, myocarditis, heart failure, thromboembolic disease, pericarditis, and ischemic and nonischemic heart disease.

The pathogenesis is not yet fully understood, but it is thought to involve a combination of direct viral damage, systemic inflammation, and hypercoagulability.

Diagnosis typically involves a combination of clinical assessment, laboratory testing, electrocardiography, echocardiography, and CMR imaging.

Treatment depends on the specific manifestation and severity of the disease. It may include medications such as anticoagulants, antiarrhythmics, and heart failure medications as well as lifestyle modifications and follow-up monitoring.

The prognosis varies depending on the severity of the disease and the specific manifestation. However, early recognition and management of these manifestations can improve outcomes. To investigate whether controlling cardiovascular risk factors improves outcomes in late COVID syndrome, and to identify the relationship between late cardiovascular complications and specific COVID-19 variants and vaccination status, needs further research.[31]

The management of late cardiovascular manifestations of COVID-19 requires a deeper understanding of the complex association between the disease and cardiovascular health. Future research should focus on understanding the mechanisms of COVID-19-mediated cardiovascular disease to improve the treatment and management of these patients.[45]

Moreover, endothelial-targeted therapies such as statins, nitric oxide donors, and angiotensin-converting enzyme (ACE) inhibitors may be beneficial in treating COVID-19-related cardiovascular injury.[46] In addition, it recommended cardiac surveillance in the form of ECG and/or serum biomarkers to detect more severe cardiac involvement, including atrial fibrillation and left ventricular dysfunction.[47]

Therefore, future research should aim to develop targeted therapies to manage late cardiovascular manifestations of COVID-19 based on a better understanding of the disease mechanisms.

ONLINE REFERENCES

Please scan the QR code provided at the end of the table of contents for References of this chapter.

CHAPTER

126

Factors Impacting Survival and Neuroprognostication after Out-of-hospital Cardiac Arrest

Srinivas Ramaka, Vemuri S Murthy, Vasudeva Murthy Sindgi, Anirudda Deshpande

ABSTRACT

Out-of-hospital cardiac arrest (OHCA) is a global public health problem. The Utstein data elements impact the survival of OHCA subjects. A strong chain of survival involving early recognition of OHCA, early activation of the emergency medical services (EMS), early cardiopulmonary resuscitation (CPR) with high-quality chest compressions, rapid defibrillation, advanced resuscitation by EMS, expert postresuscitation care, and recovery influence OHCA outcomes.

In postcardiac arrest comatose survivors, after attaining return of spontaneous circulation (ROSC), survival to discharge and prognosis is impacted by the severity of hypoxic-ischemic brain injury (HIBI). Accurate neuroprognostication in postcardiac arrest survivors is essential in decision-making to prevent early withdrawal of life-sustaining therapy (WLST).

Neuroprognostication is recommended 72 hours after attaining ROSC, after excluding significant confounders.

The most critical modalities in neuroprognostication are clinical neurological examination, electrophysiology, biochemical markers, and brain imaging.

Findings that indicate a poor neurological outcome are:

- Bilateral absence of pupillary light reflexes (PLRs) and corneal reflexes
- Presence of an early postanoxic status myoclonus
- Bilateral absence of the N20 cortical wave of somatosensory evoked potential (SSEP) at 72 hours from ROSC

Biomarkers which include neuron-specific enolase (NSE), S100B protein, tau protein, neurofilament light chain (NFL), and glial fibrillary acidic protein (GFAP) are useful in neuroprognostication.

Brain imaging studies such as computed tomography (CT) scans and magnetic resonance imaging (MRI) are also helpful in neuroprognostication in combination with other predictors.

While no single modality is 100% accurate, a multimodal neuroprognostication is employed in decision-making in a postcardiac arrest comatose survivor.

Keywords: Chain of survival, out-of-hospital cardiac arrest, cardiopulmonary resuscitation, bystander CPR, automated external defibrillator (AED), return of spontaneous circulation, neuroprognostication, withdrawal of life-sustaining therapy (WLST), survival.

INTRODUCTION

Out-of-hospital cardiac arrest (OHCA) is a leading cause of death worldwide. Various factors affect the survival of a subject of OHCA. Even after timely resuscitation, the extent of neurological damage impacts the recovery of subjects of OHCA. Prognostication of neurological outcome following OHCA is based on various criteria. The goal of neuroprognostication is to provide patients and their families with information about the patient's likely outcome so that they can make informed decisions about their care. In this context, it is pertinent to review the factors impacting the survival of OHCA and also neuroprognostication after OHCA.

FACTORS IMPACTING THE SURVIVAL OF OUT-OF-HOSPITAL CARDIAC ARREST

Out-of-hospital cardiac arrest is a global public health problem with variations in reported survival outcomes of OHCA. The Utstein data elements impact the survival of OHCA subjects. They include system factors, dispatch factors, patient factors, event factors, process factors, and outcome factors.[1]

Out-of-hospital cardiac arrest is a time-sensitive emergency wherein chances of survival decrease with every minute of treatment delay.

A strong chain of survival involving early recognition of OHCA, early activation of the emergency medical services (EMS) by calling for help, early cardiopulmonary resuscitation (CPR) with high-quality chest compressions, rapid defibrillation, advanced resuscitation by EMS, expert postresuscitation care, and recovery (including additional treatment, observation, rehabilitation, and psychological support) influence OHCA outcomes.[2]

Successful outcomes involve coordinating the "chain of survival"—a complex relationship between lay people, emergency dispatchers, first responders, EMS, and hospital providers.

Observational studies suggest that survival from cardiac arrest can be increased from twofold to fourfold with bystander CPR. The time it takes to initiate CPR has the most significant impact on survival. It, therefore, falls to the community to start CPR and maintain viability while emergency services arrive. Differences in bystander CPR response are associated with significant variability in OHCA survival. Bystander CPR nearly doubles an individual's likelihood of survival compared to no-bystander CPR, according to a meta-analysis of 19 trials involving 232,703 patients.[3]

Bystander use of an automated external defibrillator (AED) is known to improve the survival rate of OHCA. Each minute of delay in defibrillation decreases the chances of survival by 10%. Early defibrillation within 3–5 minutes can produce survival rates as high as 50–70%.[4] Optimization of the provision of CPR and AED use in all communities helps improve survival outcomes.

Emergency medical services-witnessed OHCA has better survival than a bystander-witnessed OHCA.[5]

Most published literature indicates that individuals with EMS-witnessed OHCA have better survival outcomes than bystander-witnessed or unwitnessed OHCAs. Various registries have pointed out that different EMS systems account for the variation in OHCA survival rates worldwide.[6]

Utstein survival is defined as the rate of survival among those persons whose arrests were witnessed by a bystander and who had an initial rhythm of ventricular fibrillation or pulseless ventricular tachycardia.[7] These cases have the highest rate of survival, responding to CPR and defibrillation.

Prehospital efforts such as early recognition of cardiac arrest, high-quality CPR performance, and AED use impact the early return of spontaneous circulation (ROSC). Subsequently, early transfer to a cardiac care center, provision of postcardiac care, and evidence-based management of postcardiac arrest syndrome (PCAS) impact the survival of the OHCA subject.

The overall survival rate of OHCA can be improved by strengthening the weak links in the chain of survival and evidence-based and quality postcardiac care. An optimized chain of survival is proven to result in ROSC in 49% of the cases and a 1-year survival rate of 27%.[8]

Disparities in OHCA survival are due to disparities in bystander CPR, accessibility to AEDs, EMS arrival, and postcardiac arrest care. There is a need to address these disparities and overcome barriers along the continuum of OHCA care to improve survival outcomes from OHCA.

NEUROPROGNOSTICATION AFTER OUT-OF-HOSPITAL CARDIAC ARREST

Background

Following OHCA, only 25–30% of subjects initially achieve a ROSC and are admitted to the hospital. Despite advances in postresuscitation care management, about 50% of resuscitated patients from cardiac arrest die or have a poor neurological prognosis.[9] Postanoxic brain injury leading to severe neurological damage is a leading cause of mortality following cardiac arrest. About 80% of postcardiac arrest resuscitation patients are comatose.[10] Half will remain comatose for 72 hours following ROSC or 72 hours from rewarming when hypothermia is used. Two-thirds of them will die because of hypoxic-ischemic brain injury (HIBI).[11]

A minority of deaths in comatose cardiac arrest survivors are due to extensive neuronal injury.[12] Most deaths are due to withdrawal of life-sustaining therapy (WLST), which usually occurs on the first day of treatment.[13,14]

Comatose ROSC patients have varied natural courses. Various factors impact prognosis. Prognostication by the emergency department (ED) physician is of concern to the family, to avoid suffering to the patient and unnecessary costs and prolonged hospital stay.

While prognostication is comparably easy at the extremes of the clinical range (i.e., at the very good and the very bad ends), a neurological consultation is strongly recommended in cases from the "gray area," where a significant proportion of unresponsive patients can make a good recovery despite unclear initial examination results and even after a long period of management.

To avoid premature withdrawal, accurate prediction of neurological outcomes is needed. While no predictor is 100% accurate, a multimodal prognostication is recommended for accurate prognostication and decision-making.[15]

In this context, a review of neuroprognostication after OHCA and factors impacting the survival of OHCA subjects is of immense practical importance.

Hypoxic-ischemic Brain Injury after Out-of-hospital Cardiac Arrest

Hypoxic-ischemic brain injury is the leading cause of death in comatose patients after cardiac arrest.[16] HIBI can lead to delayed neuronal death and diffuse cerebral edema, which can cause severe morbidity and mortality. The severity of HIBI can be used to predict the prognosis of patients after cardiac arrest. A poor neurological outcome is a death from neurological causes, persistent vegetative state, or severe neurological disability.

Prognostication of a poor neurological outcome often leads to WLST.

The International Liaison Committee on Resuscitation (ILCOR) recommends that health-related quality of life (HRQOL) be assessed at 3 months after cardiac arrest.[17] HRQOL, as a goal of resuscitation, should be included as an outcome measure in future neuroprognostication studies.

Key Principles of Managing a Comatose Return of Spontaneous Circulation Survivor

The fundamental principles to follow are: (1) early communication with the family, (2) delay prognostication, and (3) multimodal evaluation.

- Establish rapport with the family and give them meaningful information about the patient's condition. Understand their expectations and goals.
- The current evidence supports assessing the patient's prognosis after 24 or 72 hours, depending on whether they received or not received targeted temperature management (TTM). Neuroprognostication is typically performed after 72 hours of ROSC. However, in some cases, it may be necessary to wait longer, such as if the patient is sedated or other confounding factors could affect the accuracy of the prognostic tests.
- A detailed knowledge of the clinical trajectories of consciousness recovery and the ability to correctly interpret the results of multimodal investigations are essential for accurate prognostication.

The clinical trajectories in postcardiac arrest patients vary from coma to unresponsive wakefulness syndrome (UWS), minimally conscious state (MCS), and a fully conscious state.[18] Some patients initially thought to have poor prognosis may eventually have late recovery, while others may have varied levels of residual consciousness.

The optimal time to predict outcomes with neurological examination is after 72 hours of ROSC. However, some experts recommend waiting until 5 days after ROSC or 3 days after normothermia in patients treated with therapeutic hypothermia.[19] When counseling surrogates of comatose ROSC survivors, age, initial cardiac rhythm, and time to ROSC alone should not be considered reliable predictors of poor functional outcomes assessed 3 months or later.[3]

One of the primary sources of bias in neuroprognostication is a self-fulfilling prophecy. This occurs when the treating team is aware of the results of prognostic tests and uses them to make decisions that affect patient outcomes, such as withdrawal of life-sustaining therapy (WLST). To avoid a self-fulfilling prophecy, the results of prognostic tests need to be blinded to the treating team, though this is not practically possible.

Another source of bias is the absence of an active WLST policy. If there is no clear policy on when to withdraw life support, then the treating team may be more likely to interpret prognostic tests in a way that supports their own biases.

In addition to the severity of brain injury, several other factors can influence neuroprognostication, including the patient's age, preexisting medical conditions, cardiac status, and acute complications. The patient's wishes and the family's expectations should also be considered.

Here are some good practice recommendations in neuroprognostication:

- Wait 72 hours after ROSC before making any definitive prognostication.
- Avoid sedation or other confounders.
- Use multimodal assessment, including neurological examination, neuroimaging, and electroencephalography (EEG).
- Allow an extended observation period for awakening in patients with an indeterminate prognosis.
- Use validated prognostic predictors.
- Neuroprognostication is a complex and challenging task. However, following good practice recommendations makes it possible to make more accurate predictions about the long-term outcome of patients who have suffered a cardiac arrest.

COMA SCALES OR CATEGORIES FOLLOWING CARDIAC ARREST

Following OHCA, poor neurological outcomes are assessed and classified by cerebral performance categories (CPC). The spectrum of CPC includes the best possible outcome with no or minor disabilities (CPC 1) at one end and death (CPC 5) at the other end. CPC was adapted from the Glasgow Outcome Scale (GOS) for traumatic head injury. Interestingly, GOS scores correspond to those of the CPCs in the reverse order. So, GOS 1 corresponds to CPC 5 and vice versa. These scales have their limitations, and none has been explicitly designed for prognosticating global outcome post HIBI.[20]

NEUROPROGNOSTICATION

Neuroprognostication predicts the long-term neurological outcome of a patient who has suffered a cardiac arrest. The most critical components in neuroprognostication are the clinical neurological examination, electrophysiology, biochemical markers, and brain imaging.[21]

The clinical neurological examination is the foundation of neuroprognostication. It includes assessment of wakefulness, ability to verbalize and follow commands, brainstem reflexes, response to pain, and motor responses.

Electrophysiology is another essential tool in neuroprognostication. It can be used to assess the activity of the brain and to identify abnormalities that may be associated with poor neurological outcomes.

Biochemical markers are also used in neuroprognostication. These markers can measure brain damage and predict the likelihood of a good neurological outcome.

Brain imaging is the final tool in neuroprognostication. It can visualize the brain and identify abnormalities associated with poor neurological outcomes.

The most valuable outcome indicators are brainstem reflexes and motor response to pain. An extensor or absent pain response is associated with poor outcomes. However, it is essential to note that not all patients with an extensor or absent pain response will have a poor outcome.

Neuroprognostication is a complex and challenging task. However, using the tools described above makes it possible to make more accurate predictions about the long-term neurological outcome of patients who have suffered a cardiac arrest.

Clinical Exam Features for Neuroprognostication

The absence of pupillary light reflex (PLR) and corneal reflex, presence of myoclonus, extensor pain response, or absent pain response are clinical examination tools used for neuroprognostication.

Pupillary Light Reflex

An intact PLR indicates proper midbrain function. The absence of PLR 3 days after the ROSC in patients with PCAS who did not receive TTM strongly predicts poor outcomes (false-positive rate 0–3%). On the other hand, in PCAS patients who received TTM, the absence of PLR at 3 days after normothermia or 5 days after ROSC remains predictive for poor outcomes with a 2.1% false-positive rate. Therefore, early absent PLR after ROSC before initiating TTM may not always predict poor outcomes.[22]

Corneal Reflex

The corneal reflex indicates the degree of intactness of the pathway from the ophthalmic branch of the fifth cranial nerve through the pons to the seventh cranial nerve and facial muscles. The absence of bilateral corneal reflex 3 days after ROSC in PCAS patients who did not receive TTM strongly predicts poor outcomes (false-positive rate 0–3%).[23]

Other Clinical Examination Features

Bilateral absence of PLRs and of corneal reflexes indicate a poor prognosis (specificity 99% and 95%, sensitivity 20–30%).

Quantitative automated infrared pupillometry is a more accurate measure of PLR. It is an emerging test in bedside critically ill patients.[24] Abnormal neurological pupil index and PLR quantitative measurements by pupillometry early after ROSC increase accuracy to predict poor outcomes.

Absent motor and extensor responses are unreliable indicators. Patients with localizing movements within 72 hours tend to have an excellent functional outcome (sensitivity 76%).

Physicians usually use the lack of oculocephalic reflex and the absence of other brainstem reflexes to indicate poor outcomes for withdrawal of life support in PCAS patients.

The absence of vestibular-ocular reflex at >24 hours after ROSC in PCAS patients who did not receive TTM usually predicts poor outcomes with a false-positive rate of 14%.

MYOCLONUS

Myoclonus is a clinical phenomenon of sudden, brief, involuntary jerks caused by muscular contractions or inhibitions. It can occur in up to 20% of patients after cardiac arrest and is cortical or subcortical.

Postanoxic Myoclonus

Postanoxic myoclonus is a type of myoclonus that occurs within 48 hours of cardiac arrest. It is characterized by continuous and generalized myoclonus that persists for at least 30 minutes. It is almost invariably associated with poor neurological outcomes.[25]

Lance–Adams Syndrome

Lance–Adams syndrome is a benign condition in some patients with postanoxic myoclonus. It is characterized by involuntary movements that persist after recovery of consciousness. However, patients with Lance–Adams syndrome can still have an excellent long-term outcome if treated with antimyoclonic medications.[26]

Electroencephalography

Electroencephalography can help diagnose postanoxic myoclonus and rule out other conditions that can cause similar symptoms. It typically shows a continuous activity background with superimposed myoclonic discharges in patients with postanoxic myoclonus.

Prognosis

The prognosis for patients with postanoxic myoclonus is generally poor. However, some patients can still have an excellent long-term outcome if treated with antimyoclonic medications if they are diagnosed with Lance-Adams syndrome.

Recommendations

Myoclonus should be assessed within 96 hours of ROSC. EEG should be performed to rule out other conditions that can cause similar symptoms. Patients with postanoxic myoclonus should be treated with antimyoclonic medications.

The clinical examination is prone to interference from body temperature, sedatives, and neuromuscular blocking drugs, which can confound the results. Additionally, the clinical examination results cannot be concealed from the training team, which can lead to a self-fulfilling prophecy.

Electroencephalography is a noninvasive and relatively inexpensive test used to identify and treat seizures, monitor response to treatment, and evaluate postcardiac arrest encephalopathy. EEG is performed in all patients who are comatose survivors of ROSC.

Electroencephalography can be performed 48–72 hours after cardiac arrest. Continuous long-term video EEG monitoring is more sensitive for seizure detection than spot EEG assessments. Postanoxic status epilepticus generalized periodic discharges, and other malignant EEG patterns, such as generalized background suppression and burst suppression, occur in up to 40% of cardiac arrest patients and are often associated with poor outcomes.

Highly malignant EEG patterns (suppressed background with or without periodic discharges and burst suppression) at the end of TTM and after sedation are indicators of a poor prognosis.[27] The presence of unequivocal seizures on EEG during the first 72 hours after ROSC also indicates a poor prognosis. The absence of background reactivity on EEG indicates a poor prognosis. Burst suppression on EEG at ≥24 hours from ROSC, in combination with other indices, predicts poor outcomes.

However, postanoxic status epilepticus is not an absolute criterion for a poor neurologic prognosis. Repeating the investigations helps to identify favorable and unfavorable trajectories. In selected cases, aggressive and prolonged treatment of status epilepticus can result in strikingly positive outcomes.

Amplitude-integrated EEG provides a simplified and more suitable method for monitoring the EEG. The bispectral index (BIS), an automated analysis of the EEG signal designed to monitor the depth of anesthesia, is also a prognostic tool after cardiac arrest. BIS values range from 100 (awake) to 0 (flat EEG).[28,29]

EVOKED POTENTIALS

Evoked potentials are noninvasive tests used to assess the function of the nervous system. They are beneficial in prognosticating the outcome of patients who have suffered a HIBI after cardiac arrest.

The most well-studied evoked potential is the somatosensory evoked potential (SSEP). The SSEP is a small electrical signal recorded from the scalp after a peripheral stimulus is applied, usually one exciting the median nerve in the wrist. The N20 potential, which is recorded in the contralateral postcentral gyrus, is the most diagnostically useful SSEP.[30]

The bilateral absence of the N20 cortical wave of SSEP at 72 hours from ROSC predicts a poor neurological outcome.[31] SSEPs are relatively insensitive to the effects of sedation and cooling, making them a valuable prognostic tool in patients treated with these interventions. In addition, SSEPs are less affected by patient movement than other imaging techniques, such as computed tomography (CT) and magnetic resonance imaging (MRI).

BIOMARKERS

Hypoxic-ischemic brain injury results in the release of several chemicals from the brain into the blood and cerebrospinal fluid. These chemicals, known as biomarkers, can be measured in the blood or cerebrospinal fluid to assess the injury's severity and predict the outcome.

The most well-studied biomarker for this purpose is neuron-specific enolase (NSE). NSE is an enzyme that is released from damaged neurons. Elevated levels of NSE in the blood or cerebrospinal fluid are associated with a poor prognosis after cardiac arrest.

Other biomarkers studied for prognostication after cardiac arrest include S100B protein, tau protein, neurofilament light chain (NFL), and glial fibrillary acidic protein (GFAP). In some studies, these biomarkers are also released from damaged neurons and are predictive of poor outcomes.

NEURON-SPECIFIC ENOLASE

Neuron-specific enolase is an isoenzyme of the glycolytic pathway in neurons. Hypoxic ischemic injury anaerobically upregulates glycolysis, producing and releasing NSE from damaged neurons into the bloodstream. Serum NSE levels were correlated with the severity of HIBI and the most helpful biomarker for cardiac arrest prognostication. NSE levels correlate with the severity. Sampling at multiple time points, 24, 48, and 72 hours, is recommended by current guidelines to assess reproducibility and reduce false-positive results. Elevated NSE levels of 60 μg/L at 48 or 72 hours post arrest are consistently associated with poor neurological outcomes. Increasing NSE values between 24 and 48 hours or 72 hours, and high values at 48 and 72 hours indicate a poor prognosis.[32]

Neuron-specific enolase, the most widely available biomarker, is limited by origin from extracerebral sources such as red blood cells (RBCs), neuroendocrine tumors, and small cell carcinoma.

S100, a glial derived protein, >0.2 μg/L in serum within 72 hours after ROSC may predict poor outcomes. Serial serum S100 at 24, 48 and 72 hours after ROSC did not add any predictive accuracy to serial serum NSE levels. The serum level of NSE alone, measured ≤72 hours from the ROSC, is not considered a reliable predictor of poor functional outcome assessed at 3 months or later until a consistent threshold is validated.

The accuracy of tau protein, a marker of axonal injury, and a neuron-derived protein at 24, 48, and 72 hours after ROSC is comparable with serial serum NSE for predicting poor outcomes. Its use is limited to special laboratories.

Neurofilament light chain is associated with axonal damage, a key determinant of long-term outcomes in various brain injuries, including neurodegenerative disorders. A recent systematic review and meta-analysis of 10,000 patients suggest that NFL is likely the most robust predictor of outcome.[33]

Serial plasma NFL at 24, 48, and 72 hours after ROSC with cutoff values of 127, 263, and 344 pg/mL predicts poor outcomes.

Glial fibrillary acidic protein is released into the bloodstream only in pathologic conditions and is more specific for acute brain damage than NSE or S100. Elevated GFAP of >0.8 μg/L at 48 hours after ROSC predicts poor outcomes.

MicroRNAs (microribonucleic acid), RNA molecules 20–22 nucleotides long, regulate gene expression and provide information on the severity of brain injury and neuronal cell function. miR-124-3p is an independent predictor of both survival and neurological outcome.

Current guidelines do not recommend any particular biomarker threshold to predict poor outcomes with 100% specificity. Extracerebral sources may result in false-positive results.

Other tools such as near-infrared spectroscopy (NIRS), ultrasound, and lab testing have been used to prognosticate the outcome of patients who have suffered a HIBI.

Near-infrared spectroscopy is a noninvasive technique for monitoring regional cerebral tissue oxygen saturation ($SctO_2$) at the microvascular level. Decreased $SctO_2$ is associated with a poor prognosis after cardiac arrest.

ULTRASOUND

Ultrasound has been studied as an adjunct to the clinical examination by measuring the optic nerve sheath diameter as a correlate for neurologic outcome. A larger optic nerve diameter may indicate increased intracranial pressure from cerebral edema and, thus, a worse neurologic outcome.

LABORATORY TESTING

The initial arterial pH is not a reliable prognostic tool for patients who have suffered a cardiac arrest. However, other laboratory tests such as lactate, procalcitonin, troponin, D-dimer, and C-reactive protein are associated with worse patient outcomes.

IMAGING

Computed tomography (CT) scans and MRIs can identify signs of hypoxic-ischemic encephalopathy in patients with cardiac arrest. A marked reduction in gray matter/white matter (GM/WM) ratio or sulcal effacement on brain CT within 24 hours after ROSC, or extensive reduction in diffusion on brain MRI at 2–5 days later ROSC, predicts poor outcome.[34]

COMPUTED TOMOGRAPHY SCANS

The main CT finding of HIBI following cardiac arrest is cerebral edema, which appears as an attenuation of the GM/WM interface. This has been measured as the ratio [gray–white matter ratio (GWR)] between the GM and the WM densities, usually sampled at three levels: Basal ganglia, centrum semiovale, and high convexity. The loss of GWR attenuation indicative of cerebral edema correlates with hypoxic-ischemic changes and predicts poor outcomes.[35]

MAGNETIC RESONANCE IMAGING

Magnetic resonance imaging is a more sensitive and specific tool for identifying HIBI than CT. A diffuse pattern of loss of gray–white differentiation with sulcal effacement on noncontrast CT brain imaging performed at least 48 hours from the ROSC is considered a moderately reliable predictor of poor functional outcome assessed at 3 months or later.

Magnetic resonance imaging findings in comatose ROSC survivors include hyperintense areas on diffusion-weighted imaging (DWI), which can be quantified using the apparent diffusion coefficient (ADC).[36]

These changes are a result of cytotoxic edema due to hypoxic-ischemic encephalopathy.

The timing of MRI is an essential factor in its prognostic value. MRI DWI imaging is practical for picking up anoxic changes when performed beyond 48 hours after the ROSC. Hence, guidelines recommend DWI imaging 2–6 days postcardiac arrest.

Though MRI can predict changes as early as 3 hours after ROSC, it is ideally done 2–5 days after ROSC. Diffusion tensor imaging (DTI) may become increasingly important as WM tract injury detected on DTI appears to be an even more robust neuroimaging predictor of postcardiac arrest outcome.

A diffuse pattern of restricted diffusion on MRI of the brain performed between 2 and 7 days from ROSC is considered a moderately reliable predictor of poor functional outcome assessed at 3 months or later.

Current guidelines suggest using brain imaging in experienced centers with other predictors.

Magnetic resonance imaging is a valuable tool for prognosticating the outcome of patients who have suffered a cardiac arrest. It can be used to identify ischemic changes in the brain and to predict the likelihood of a poor outcome. However, the timing of MRI is essential, and experienced radiologists need to interpret the results.

PREDICTION MODELS

There is insufficient evidence for the OHCA and cardiac arrest hospital prognosis (CAHP) prediction models. The Good Outcome Following Attempted Resuscitation (GO-FAR) clinical prediction model is not a reliable predictor.[37]

POOR NEUROLOGICAL OUTCOME

In the past, there was no definite consensus on what would ultimately amount to a poor neurological outcome. Most neuroprognostication literature mentions poor outcomes as CPC 4–5 (vegetative state or death) and good outcomes as CPC 1–3 (good neurological outcome and moderate-to-severe neurological disability). However, in the last 10 years, most studies have included CPC 3 in the bracket of poor outcomes. As per the latest version of Utstein guidelines, CPC 3–5 should be used for defining poor outcomes.

- The Glasgow Coma Scale (GCS) motor scores <3 at 3 days after ROSC in PCAS patients not treated with TTM strongly predict poor outcomes (false-positive rate 0–3%). On the other hand, in PCAS patients treated with TTM, the GCS motor scores <3 at 3 days after normothermia or 5 days after ROSC may not always predict poor outcomes (false-positive rate 19%). The GCS motor scores of >3 before initiation of TTM strongly predict good outcomes.
- GCS ≤ 2, although low in specificity and high in sensitivity, is a reliable method of identifying the most severe HIBI. The absence of PLR bilaterally at or after 72 hours from ROSC is more specific but less sensitive in predicting poor prognosis. Absent corneal reflex bilaterally at 72 hours after ROSC is another poor outcome indicator in postcardiac arrest resuscitation patients.

Indicators of Poor Outcome

Poor outcome is likely when two or more of the following predictors are present:[34]

- No pupillary and corneal reflexes at ≥72 hours
- Bilaterally absent N20 SSEP wave at ≥24 hours
- Highly malignant EEG at >24 hours
- NSE > 60 µg/L—one at 48 and/or 72 hours
- Status myoclonus ≤72 hours
- A diffuse and extensive anoxic injury on brain CT/MRI

PREDICTORS OF GOOD NEUROLOGICAL OUTCOME

Though significant evidence suggests studies on poor neurological outcomes, despite their absence in guidelines, specific predictors of good outcomes are known.[38]

- Continuous or nearly continuous EEG within 12 hours from ROSC
- Presence of early EEG reactivity and improvement of auditory discrimination (an analysis of EEG responses to auditory stimuli) from the first to the second day after ROSC
- Absence of DWI abnormalities on MRI within 1 week of ROSC is also highly suggestive of a good neurological outcome.

DELAYED AWAKENING

Patients with renal insufficiency, older age, or postresuscitation shock have an increased risk of delayed awakening. Prehospital ROSC, extracorporeal CPR, therapeutic hypothermia, and male sex were associated with delayed awakening.[39]

FUTURE DIRECTIONS

Three factors are prone to influencing efforts to improve neuroprognostication after cardiac arrest in the future:

1. The types of data that will become available to characterize different brain states along the spectrum of postanoxic disorders of consciousness, e.g., cognitive motor dissociation (CMD)
2. The modeling paradigms used for data analysis
3. The ability to implement classification schemes in the clinical setting

ARTIFICIAL INTELLIGENCE

Artificial intelligence (AI) will undoubtedly enable the refinement of neuroprognostication soon. In one recent study, deep learning algorithms based on interpretable features such as neural synchrony and complexity of EEG responses, modulated by independent clinical evaluations such as motor responses and brain CT, improved the accuracy of prognostication in comatose patients after cardiac arrest.[40]

CONCLUSION

Utstein data elements, along with a strong chain of survival, impact the survival of OHCA subjects.

Neuroprognostication requires a profound knowledge of clinical trajectories across the spectrum of disorders of consciousness and solid expertise in interpreting a range of clinical modalities and laboratory techniques. The latter should be utilized in parallel and multimodal to avoid premature decision-making based on isolated tests.

ONLINE REFERENCES

Please scan the QR code provided at the end of the table of contents for References of this chapter.

CHAPTER

127

Mental Health of Doctors: Issues and Solutions

Vitull K Gupta, Meghna Gupta, Varun Gupta

ABSTRACT

Mental health encompasses psychological, emotional, and social well-being, influencing cognition, perception, and behavior. State of mental health is determined by several social, individual, structural, genetic, psychological, and biological factors including the risk factors which can manifest at all stages of life. The medical profession is considered to be one of the most demanding and stressful professions and the global data suggests high prevalence rates of mental health problems among healthcare professionals (HCPs) of all the ages, genders, specialties, and institutions as compared to other professional groups and general population. Risk factors predisposing to mental health issue are occupational and individual risk factors associated with the nature of the job, clinical, structural and individual characteristics. Management strategies include detailed assessment, risk factor management, early initiation of preventive strategies, self-management measures, and specific psychiatric management of mental disorders.

Keywords: Mental health, doctors, healthcare professionals, mental health issues.

"Being a doctor does not exclude you from being a human being."

—Eleanor James, a consultant oncologist

INTRODUCTION

Mental health encompasses psychological, emotional, and social well-being, influencing cognition, perception, and behavior. Mental health determines how one handles stress, interpersonal relationships, and makes healthy choices or decision-making.[1] Mental health also includes perceived self-efficacy, subjective well-being, competence, autonomy, intergenerational dependence, and self-actualization of one's emotional and intellectual potential among others.[2] Mental health from the perspectives of holism or positive psychology may include one's ability to create a balance between efforts to achieve psychological resilience and life activities and to enjoy life. But how one defines "mental health" is influenced by cultural differences, conflicting or competing professional ideas, or theories and subjective assessments.[3] Mental health is a state of mental well-being, an integral component of health, and is a basic human right. Mental health is crucial to community, personal, and socioeconomic development. It is more than just absence of mental disorders, existing in complex continuum, experienced differently from person to person, with varying degrees of distress and difficulty with a potential for very different clinical and social outcomes.[1]

DETERMINANTS OF MENTAL HEALTH

During one's lifetime several social, individual, and structural determinants may combine to influence one's mental health with variable mental state on the mental health continuum. Individual genetics, psychological, and biological factors can make people more vulnerable to mental health problems including the risk factors such as exposure to unfavorable economic, social, environmental, and geopolitical circumstances. Similarly, the protective factors such as one's family support, social and emotional skills, positive social interactions, decent work, quality education, community cohesion, and safe neighborhoods may be present throughout one's life and serve to strengthen resilience. Mental health's protective as well as risk factors are present at different scales in an individual or society and each single protective as well as risk factor has limited predictive strength as one may or may not develop a mental health condition in spite of exposure to a risk factor and vice versa.[1]

MENTAL HEALTH DISORDERS

Mental health disorders are health-related conditions affecting or altering emotional responses, cognitive functioning, and behavior associated with impaired functioning and/or distress.[4] Conceptualized in the 19th century, the latest International Classification of Diseases (ICD)-11 has been the global standard for diagnosis, treatment, research, and reporting of various diseases including mental disorders.[5] The Diagnostic and Statistical Manual of Mental Disorders, Fifth Edition (DSM-5), published by the American Psychiatric Association (APA) is also widely used as the authority for classification and diagnoses of mental disorders.[6]

India's National Institute of Mental Health and Neurosciences (NIMHANS) recent survey documented that over 10% of Indian population is suffering from diagnosable mental health or substance use disorders and about 150 million people are in need of mental healthcare services, but <30 million are seeking care. The prevalence of mental disorders in India accounts for about 15% of the global mental health burden.[7] Since medical practice has peculiar challenges as compared to any other professions, so it is associated with a high degree of mental health issues and occupational burnout which is defined as a pathological syndrome due to occupational stress incorporating three characteristic sequentially occurring dimensions of emotional exhaustion, depersonalization, and reduced personal accomplishment among professionals. Burnout is neither depression nor anxiety and affects women healthcare professionals (HCPs) more than a male HCPs.[8,9]

MENTAL HEALTH OF DOCTORS

The medical profession is considered to be one of the most demanding and stressful professions and stress starts form medical college entrance exams and continues throughout professional life. The association of mental disorders and stress is well known so medical students and HCPs have higher incidence of mental disorders. Presently, the data on the psychological or mental health problems among HCPs is limited and the worldwide data suggests high prevalence rates of mental health problems among HCPs in all age groups, genders, and specialties than other professional groups as well as the general population.[9,10] About three times more prevalence of mental health problems were reported among HCPs as compared to general population in New Zealand.[11] Studies reported existence of stress in three-fourth of the subjects and about 91.1% prevalence of stress among interns. Studies have reported 51.3% depression, 66.9% anxiety, and 53% stress among undergraduate medical students.[8] Data from UK suggested that 10–20% of doctors at some point in their career become depressed and have a higher risk of suicide as compared to general population.[12] A survey among UK-based Doctors Support Network members showed 68% had depression and others reported of anxiety, bipolar disorder, eating disorders, and addictions.[13]

Depression

Studies from different countries evaluating depression among doctors have documented 8.2–27% prevalence of depression.[14,15] A meta-analysis of studies including medical students documented 27.2% prevalence of depression and 13.5% increase in depressive symptoms when assessed before joining the medical college and during the medical course.[16] A meta-analysis of studies on resident doctors showed 28.8% estimated pooled prevalence of depressive symptoms or depression and also showed 15.8% increase in depressive symptoms after starting the residency.[17] Meta-analysis from Australia showed 27% prevalence of depression among medical students, 29% in registrars, and 60% in practicing doctors.[18] A large survey documented 73.7% prevalence of depression including 71.7% among nonmedicos and 74.7% among medicos, and the survey observed that most subjects had minimal depression among the study population including medicos and nonmedicos.[19] A meta-analysis of 28 research articles from India on medical students estimates a 40% pooled prevalence of depression with girls at higher risk than boys.[20] A study from North India found that 30.1% resident doctors had depression, 16.7% had suicidal ideations, and up to 90% reported some burnout.[8]

Burnout

A study from Canada reported that 80% of physicians were suffering from burnout.[21] Data suggest that depending on the specialty among residents, the prevalence of burnout varies between 50 and 76%.[22,23] Indian Medical Association (IMA) reported 82.7% doctors felt stressed-out in their profession.[24] A study conducted to explore violence against doctors and its effect on psychosocial health documented that 52.2% doctors who faced work place violence (WPV) reported feeling of shame and loss of self-esteem, 51.2% reported stress/anxiety/depression/ideas of persecution, and 41.7% felt a sense of defeat.[25] A number of studies showed 16–80% prevalence of burnout in medical students, 27.13–90% in residents, registrars, and physicians.[26] A meta-analysis of 15 studies from India estimated 24% prevalence of emotional exhaustion, 27% depersonalization, and 23% for burnout related to personal accomplishment among HCPs.[27] Among medical students and residents the incidence of burnout has been shown to be between 40 and 76%.[28] A meta-analysis of 24 studies showed 44.2% prevalence of burnout including 40.8% prevalence of emotional exhaustion, 35.1% depersonalization, and 27.4%

prevalence of personal accomplishment.[29] A systematic review of 182 studies published between 1991 and 2018 including 109,628 subjects in 45 countries reported 0–80.5% prevalence of burnout, 0–86.2% prevalence of emotional exhaustion, 0–89.9% depersonalization, and 0–87.1% for low personal accomplishment.[30]

Alcohol and Substance Abuse

Studies from USA reported high rate of suicide, prescription drug use, especially opiates and benzodiazepines among doctors.[31,32] Global data shows 10–15% prevalence of substance use among physicians that is almost similar to the general population.[26] A meta-analysis from India showed 40.3% prevalence of substance abuse in medical students.[33] A study showed 72.4% HCPs making weekly use of alcohol and an abusive pattern was observed in 30% HCPs. Another study documented 7.3% were hazardous drinkers and 23% were moderate drinkers. Substance abuses of self-prescription drugs such as lorazepam and alprazolam is common. Presently, medical students may indulge in cannabis more often than alcohol, which is agonizing.[9]

Suicidal Ideation and Suicide

Data shows 1.8–53.6% risk of suicidal ideation among medical students.[34] There is severe paucity of data on suicide among HCPs in India. A study from India documented 30 suicides by doctors in between March 2016 and March 2019 including 18 females, 12 males, 80% were <40 years of age.[34] Data from UK between 2011 and 2015 documented suicide by 430 doctors, and from China between 2008 and 2016, 51 doctors committed suicide.[35,36] A systematic review and meta-analysis documented 11.1% prevalence of suicidal ideation among medical students[16] and 17% among physicians.[37] A study from India estimated the prevalence of suicidal ideations among medical students to be 53.6%.[38] A study among resident doctors and faculty members showed 16.7% prevalence of suicidal ideations.[39] An Australian survey reported significantly higher prevalence of suicidal ideation in doctors (24.8%) than the general population (13.3%) and other professionals (12.8%).[9] A study estimated the suicide rate for doctors varied between two and five times the general population rate.[40] A systematic review including 183 studies from 43 nations documented 27.2% crude prevalence of depression in medical students and prevalence of suicidal ideation was 11.1%.[16]

Anxiety

About 9% of doctors in the National Mental Health Survey from Australia reported anxiety disorder as compared to 5.9% Australian population.[41] A large survey including 4,333 subjects documented 80.5% prevalence of anxiety including 81.9% among nonmedicos and 79.3% among medicos, and survey observed that most subjects had mild anxiety.[19]

RISK FACTORS FOR MENTAL HEALTH DISORDERS[9,10]

Risk factors can be discussed under two categories:

1. *Occupational risk factors*: These are associated with the nature of the job, clinical, or structural.
2. *Individual risk factors*: These are related to individual characteristics and personality traits.

Occupational Risk Factors (Clinical)

Medical Specialty

Every medical specialty has a unique stress levels, some having long working hours, unpredictable night duties, and stress of emergencies especially agitated caregivers and breaking bad news. Data suggests that burnout is more prevalent among department of emergency medicine, trauma, and surgical specialities, frequent traveling, and neglecting sleep lead to early exhaustion, monotony, and decreased recreational activities.

Psychosocial Work Environment

This is an important risk factor for developing a psychological or mental health disorder because of long working hours, increased workload, unpredictable shifts, lack of team work, relationships issues, and conflicts with junior or seniors colleagues and workplace bullying.

Stress of Breaking Bad News

Many stressors are unique to HCPs like breaking bad news, anxiety, suffering of patients, and death, so the HCPs are faced to patient's emotional reaction, caregiver's stress and anxiety, listen to their emotional let-out and distress, and to comfort and soothe them.

High Expectations from HCPs

Emotional demands and high expectations of favorable clinical results from HCPs put unrealistically high pressure and sometimes lead to both verbal and physical aggression from patients in event of death and disease.

Easy Access to Prescription Drugs

Abuse of prescription drugs is common among HCPs because of easy access, availability, and knowledge about drugs.

Occupational Risk Factors (Structural)

Work Place Violence

Work place violence is an important risk factor for mental health disorders among HCPs. Doctors facing WPV reported feeling of shame, loss of self-esteem and stress, and depression, anxiety, and ideas of persecution adversely affecting their professional capabilities.[25]

Administrative Environment

Manpower deficiencies, budgetary constraints, heavy workload, inconvenient and unpredictable working hours, long shifts, lack of cohesive team work, lack of social support, problematic relationships, and conflicts with colleagues are important risk factors. Other risk factors may be poor work environment or organization, comprehensive electronic documentation, poor financial remuneration, risk of malpractice suits, limited interpersonal collaboration, and limited opportunities for career advancement.[39]

Individual Risk Factors

Age: Evidence suggests high prevalence of mental health issues among young doctors and interns.

Gender: Most of the studies report significant prevalence of depression, anxiety, and burnout among female doctors than men, but men are more into substance use and prescription drug abuse as compared to female doctors.

Personality traits: Some personality traits such as being a perfectionist, increasingly self-critical, nature to please everyone, extreme sense of responsibility, self-guilt, self-doubt, and obsessive–compulsive traits are risk factors and in combination, individual personality traits, can create mental health disorders.[9]

BARRIERS TO SEEKING MENTAL HEALTHCARE BY HCPS[10,26]

Healthcare professionals work culture expects them to project themselves as good doctors, not to complain or express pain, not to shirk work, and not to disclose any signs or symptoms of mental disorders and if at all some HCP express stress perception or mental problems are considered to be weak-minded, unfit for the job, so much so that the work environment compels them to pretend to be infallible, supernaturally, and omnipotent.[42] That is why HCPs generally avoid seeking treatment. Barriers can be broadly classified as individual-level barriers and system-level barriers.

Individual-level Barriers

Barriers can be different for medical students and medical professionals and interns.

Barriers for Medical Students

A review of 33 papers identified that the most common barriers by medical students were fear of the negative effect on career opportunities/residency, apprehension about stigma, breach in confidentiality, lack of perceived seriousness/normalization of symptoms, and fear of shaming from peers. Students also preferred outside of their institution consultation for fear of disclosure of their mental disorder to their colleagues[43] and those who sought help in their own institution suggests being negatively judged by their seniors and peers, revealing their mental health issues to others.[44] A study from India reported barriers as 61.2% lack of confidentiality, 56.4% fear of unwanted interventions, 50.3% unsure about where to seek help, 45.8% stigma, 40.1% lack of time, 38.8% fear of the impact on the academic performance, 30.2% fear of side effects, and 11.5% cost of treatment. Other barriers included fear of mental healthcare being noted on academic record, fears of decreased career opportunities, fear of discrimination or judgment, a belief of self-resolving issue or not severe enough to seek care, lack of experience with mental illness in close contacts, preference for mental support from family, friends, peers, competition with peers, self-diagnosis, and lack of positive mentorship.[26]

Barriers for Medical Professionals and Interns

Commonly identified barriers to seeking help include perceived structural stigma of not be accepted onto a specific training program, perceived stigma of what others might think of them, self-stigma, lack of prioritizations, and time, recognition and knowledge of mental disorders, treatment attitudes and expectations, preference for self-management, and the belief that treatment does not work. A study identified common barriers to seeking help like fear of being labeled as "weak" and stigmatized of having a mental disorder, fear of adverse impact on the attitude of faculty toward them, fear of being accused of shrugging work, and time constraints to seek help.[8]

System-level Barriers

System-related barriers to seek mental healthcare include lack of access to mental healthcare, lack of access to anonymous and convenient services, concerns regarding confidentiality, fear of negative impact on career, affiliation of treating practitioner with the same institution, access issues, limited number of sessions, mandatory reporting by law, lack of education on resources, lack of available resources, and more importantly cultural stigma.[26]

MENTAL HEALTH OF FAMILIES OF HCPs[9]

There is paucity of research about health of families of HCPs, still generally doctors cherish the success of treating patients and get upset with adverse outcomes. Doctors spend most of the time on duty and spend less time with family. Situation is worse when both husband and wife are doctors, still much worse if both are in surgical field. Doctors because of their professional commitments might spend less time with children, give less attention to their studies, or miss several memorable events, etc., and may have to miss pleasure trips or other social obligations. Sometimes many children develop a personality disorder, fall to substance abuse or some mental health issue and cause an embarrassment to parents and HCPs feel guilty and helpless thinking about what is more important, profession compulsions or proper attention to family, such a situation may lead to adverse mental health issues for whole of the family.

SOLUTIONS FOR PREVENTION AND INTERVENTION STRATEGIES[9,26]

Effective solution to mental health disorders of HCPs lays in prevention and immediate effective intervention strategies. Prevention should start very early and continue through professional life practising soft skills, life skills, learning to deal with a patient in various situations and personality development programs will prepare them to face the difficulties of medical profession.

Assessment[26]

Before any intervention, assessment of mental health issues is an important step especially specific for evaluating HCPs. Like any other patient, HCP as a patient may be anxious and frightened so friendly environment is important. History should include current symptoms, onset of problem, risk and precipitating factors, duration, course and severity of illness, psychiatric symptoms, suicidal ideations or attempts. Past as well as family history of mental disorders and substance abuse is important. History of comorbid chronic medical disorders needs to be asked. Disorders specific to age or gender, sexual history, gender orientation, sexual harassment may have implications on mental health. Detailed medication history, medication adherence, self-medication must be integral part of assessment protocol. History of work place stress, interpersonal relationship issues, academic pressure, sleep deprivation, financial remuneration, risk of malpractice suits, and level of autonomy at the workplace may affect mental health. History about work-related behavior, studies-related stress, patient and caregiver-related behaviors, pending medicolegal issues, violence against the doctors, level of social support, marital status, personality issues, personal stressors, coping mechanisms, hobbies, socialization, social support may have adverse mental health consequences. Preintervention assessment should include detailed physical and mental status examination and disorder specific assessment and laboratory investigations.

Issues Specific to HCPs Confronting Mental Health Problems[26]

Many HCPs are uncomfortable in taking treatment from a fellow HCP especially for mental health issues. Issues like stigma, poor help-seeking behavior, VIP syndrome, fear of loss of privacy and confidentiality, habit of self-diagnosis and treatment, reluctant about full-disclosure, unable to adjust in patient role, poor adherence to medication, sessions and follow-up, hesitation to disclose the mental health issues has to be taken into consideration while managing a HCP having mental health issues.

Self-improvement Strategies[26]

Self-prevention and improvement strategies help HCPs to imbibe these qualities and strategies which are helpful in preventing, managing as well as improving mental health issues. Strategies to improve self-efficacy include celebrating success, encourage positive feedback and avoid people with negative feedback, counter negative thoughts with positive thoughts. Strategies to improve empowerment include cultivating positive attitude, focus on self-care, keep achievable and reasonable goals, be assertive and keep company of positive thinking people. Strategies to improve self-compassion may include being not being harsh and belittling to others and yourself, to understand that everyone has some deficiencies and no one is perfect, keep broader perspective of life and should be aware of own negative thoughts.

MANAGEMENT[9,10,26,39]

It is important to understand that assessment and management should go hand in hand and the follow-up with both nonpharmacological and pharmacological management would be influenced by the attitude of HCP toward mental illnesses, psychotropics, and psychosocial interventions.

Advocacy

Advocacy is important to sensitize HCPs to come out openly and seek help for their mental health issues. Various professional organizations like IMA, specialty associations like Cardiological Society of India and the Indian Psychiatric Society should form a special joint task force to address the mental health issues of HCPs and evolve a feasible strategy. Promotion of telepsychiatry may be the path-breaker. Advocacy through social and mass media is already creating awareness and helping in destigmatizing mental illness so much so that leading personalities including bollywood stars are coming out in public to create awareness about mental health. Several advocacy nongovernmental organizations (NGOs) are formed to reach out to silent sufferers and motivate them to seek treatment.

Interventions at Hospital Level

At hospital level team work is always associated with less stress, mental issues, and burnout. Working environment should be created with a team leader who empathizes with juniors and senior colleagues, listens to their problems, facilitates effective communication, identifies the risk factors, makes efforts to resolve the issues, acts promptly, and allows ventilation. Hospital administration should provide a safe and enjoyable work environment, protect doctors from litigation, facilities for proper individual and professional risk coverage, rotation of high stress to lower stress jobs, appropriate shift breaks and holidays to distress HCPs. Frequent discussion on common mental health problems, debrief on events of unfortunate outcomes, early identification of mental health problems and early referral to confidential and specialized psychiatric intervention.

At Individual Level

Interventions at individual level by HCPs are very effective in prevention as well as management of mental health issues and burnout. At individual level HCPs should balance profession and household work and manage leisure time, maintain good relationship with friends and family. Do not compromise on health and family in a bid to earn more money, participate in religious or spiritual activities, practice meditation and relaxation exercises, adopt some social activities and hobbies. Physical health influences mental health and vice versa so ensuring work breaks, adequate sleep, avoiding self-medications for insomnia, moderation of alcohol intake and cessation of tobacco or nicotine use will help both for good physical and mental health. At individual level HCPs should not stigmatize the problem and if needed seek professional psychiatry help and follow recommended therapy, learning to enhance the resilience will help resolving mental health issues.

INDICATIONS FOR INPATIENT CARE

A few indications if present suggest that HCP may need inpatient care. Indications may be current history of suicidal ideations and/or plans of any recent suicide attempt, HCP has threatened or physically hurt someone, impairment of poor insight, reality testing and poor judgment, rapidly increasing mental health problem or deteriorating course, severe illness, violent or aggressive behavior of HCP, psychosis and mania, severe emotional breakdown, substance abuse, intoxication or severe withdrawal or when HCP needs special therapy.

Management of specific psychiatric illness should be done according to the clinical practice guidelines and treating psychiatrists should follow the guideline recommendations and modify the treatment to suit the requirement of the patient that is HCP.

CONCLUSION

The prevalence of mental health issues is high among HCPs and there are several risk factors which predispose HCPs including medical students to mental disorders. There are several barriers to seeking mental healthcare by HCPs including individual- and system-level barriers. Solution to mental health disorders of HCPs lies in careful assessment, initiating preventive strategies, and both nonpharmacological and pharmacological management of specific psychiatric illness according to the clinical practice guidelines. Issues specific to HCPs confronting mental health problems must be studied and self-improvement strategies should help HCPs in preventing, managing as well as improving mental health issues. Health, especially mental health, is everyone's right more importantly the HCPs as the health of all depends on health of HCPs. So slogan should be "mental health to all". Let us invest in the mental health, increase access to mental healthcare, let us talk about mental health, and remove stigma to talk about mental health. The phrase, "there is no health without mental health" expresses the fact stressing that mental health especially of HCPs is an essential and integral component of individual health as well as the health of society cannot and should not be ignored at any cost.

"We as physicians can only look after our patients, if we look after ourself, first."

ACKNOWLEDGMENT

We thank Dr Aniket V Inamdar, and several CSI members and HCPs for anonymous inputs helping writing this chapter.

ONLINE REFERENCES

Please scan the QR code provided at the end of the table of contents for References of this chapter.

CHAPTER

128

Stem Cell Therapy for the Regeneration of Cardiomyocytes: Myth or Reality!

Subroto Mandal, W Sunil, Chan KS Mike, U Ankur, Anil J, Rajeev Gupta

ABSTRACT

Cardiovascular disease is the leading cause of death across the globe. Worldwide rise in the number of ischemic heart diseases are due to limited treatment option for chronic and advanced heart failure, and it progresses to more complicated due to progressive nature of the disease. After myocardial infarction, cardiomyocytes sustain irreversible loss in addition to adverse remodeling and different stages of heart failure. A need for newer technologies to manage the issues with the bioregenerative capacity of the cardiovascular system is desired.

The presently available therapies are focused on and limited to lessening the symptoms of heart failure. There are no options available to reverse the disease. To reverse myocardial injury and improve cardiac function, the use of stem cells has the potential to regenerate cardiac cells.

The goal of a research scholar is focused on identifying new tracts of cardiomyocytes and organizing cell formation. Many studies testify that cardiac stem cells (CSCs) have the ability to repair and regenerate myocardial injury with effectiveness at the therapeutic level. The effectiveness of stem cell therapy depends on individual patient factors.

Fundamental biology and mechanisms of action are one of the important questions raising serious concerns about the potency of CSCs by scientists. The study should focus on target populations, delivery approach, dosing pattern, and watchful scrutiny of the results, which are critical to evaluating even relatively small clinical trials to receive pivotal information.

Safety issues have been carefully observed by nearly 200 studies since the last two decades, and these translate that most of the cell types are relatively safe. Serious concerns have been raised by many scholars about their efficacy and practice guidelines. Trustworthiness is needed in procedures such as the regularization of conditions, isolation techniques, techniques of measurement, and calculation by standard methods for the usefulness of stem cells. Many bigger studies have started to testify to these questions raised by scholars.

In this chapter, we focused on the analysis and updates since the last few decades about the types of CSCs and their potential roles of CSCs in myocyte regeneration. Special observation is to be given to the research approach and technical aspect. Basics understanding of myocardial regeneration is related to the boundaries and rewards of clinical studies with different research approaches. Discussed about futuristic newer technological advancements and methodological progress and downfall in the field of cardiac regeneration.

Keywords: Embryonic stem cell (ESC), bone marrow-derived cell (BMC), coronary artery bypass graft (CABG), ESC-derived cardiomyocyte (ESC-CM), hematopoietic stem cell (HSC), induced pluripotent stem cell (iPSC), left ventricular ejection fraction (LVEF), myocardial infarction (MI), mesenchymal stem cell (MSC), cardiomyocytes, stem cell, myocardium, endocardium, cardiomyoblast.

INTRODUCTION

Cardiovascular diseases have the highest death rates, with an estimated 17 million people dying of heart and related diseases. Cardiovascular disease is one of the important factors associated with disabilities for life and the loss of productive life, along with physical, social, psychological, and financial loss.

Nearly one-third of deaths, with principle causes are due to cardiovascular disease (CVD) with 32.3% of all deaths in the United States in 2009. Reduction in early mortality and survival rates are improved by upgraded optimum medical care and better management of myocardial infarction (MI), which leads to an increased number of chronic heart failure patients resultant of scarring followed by ventricular remodeling.[1-3]

Till now, with the present available pharmacological, interventional, or operative therapies, we have been unable to counterbalance the irreversible loss of myocardial cells. An ischemic insult to cardiomyocyte results into a serious protective and deleterious effect.

Production of cytokines, inflammatory mediators, such as tumor necrosis factor (TNF)-α, monocyte chemoattractant protein-1, and interleukin (IL)-1β, IL-6, and IL-8, etc., is released. At the site of myocardial injury, an acute penetration of monocytes, leukocytes, and macrophages leads to scars tissue formation.[2-4]

A 33% reduction in the mortality rate may be achieved by primary angioplasty in myocardial infarction (PAMI). Along with all surgical interventions, the pharmacoinvasive approach improves the recovery of myocytes and decreases the chances of developing heart failure.[5]

With any of the standard available therapy surgical or medical, lost myocytes cannot be compensated, progressed to chronic heart failure, which has managed by heart failure management. Elementary loss of myocytes may be addressed by only transplantation, which is in present situation depends mainly an appropriate donors.[6,9,10]

To overcome these current issues, future cardiovascular management will be targeted toward cell-based therapy, the regeneration of myocytes with futuristic approaches in tissue engineering, and reprogramming of scar tissue and fibroblasts.[5-8]

REGENERATION IN AMPHIBIANS AND FISH

Many animals have the capacity to regrow their organs after the loss of the organ during predator escape. Specifically, the tails regrow very fast. Salamanders and newts have the special capacity to regenerate their limbs, jaws, spinal cord, and hearts, other than the tail. Even after removing one-eighth of the cardiac ventricle, within 30 days, regeneration of ventricle was noticed. Becker and others reported the high regenerative potential of the salamander heart.

Few fish have the ability to regenerate their heart; for example, after resection of up to 20% of the ventricle of zebrafish heart, it can regenerate completely. There are difference of opinion regarding the regenerative capacity of fish or animals, after external injury and other type of injury like cellular injury by ischemia.

Scientists have induced heart injury in two additional ways: Genetic ablation of cardiomyocytes and cardiac cryoinjury to aggravate heart injury in zebrafish. A nitrogen cooled probe is used for cryoinjury to the heart, about 20–30% of the ventricle, including injury to all the layers of heart, endocardium, myocardium and epicardium. Studied and result were analysed in 30, 60 and 120 days. In case of resection of ventricle full regeneration undertaken in 60 days, while 120 days needed for complete regeneration from cryoinjury **(Fig. 1)**.[82-85]

After MI in mammals, there is a sequence of cell death followed by the development of an irreversible scar. Myofibroblasts are responsible for the formation of the scar, which further became rigid and acellular and replace the lost myocardium and fibrosis.

STEM CELL TYPES AND SOURCES

For the regeneration of cardiomyocytes, different types of cells are used with their different developmental stages. These cell types and stages are mainly embryonic, fetal, and adult

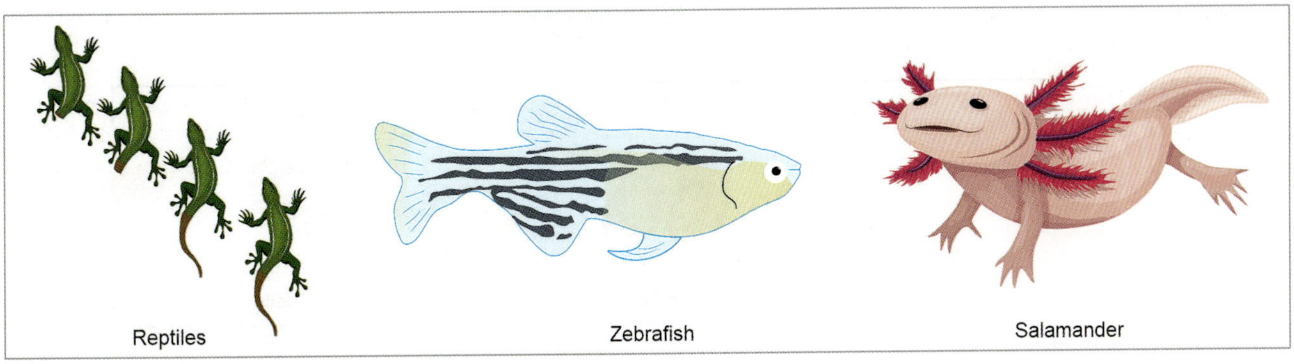

FIG. 1: Regeneration capacity of fish, amphibians, and reptiles.

cells. Each cell type has its own properties, characteristics, and mode of action during transplantation into the heart by any route, intramuscular, intravenous, or direct injection to the site, or any other methods **(Fig. 2)**.

Human Embryonic Stem Cell

Embryonic stem cells (ESCs) carry very unique characteristics and properties. These can be obtained from blastocyst, especially from the inner mass area.[11-13] "The capacity to divide indefinitely and differentiate into any cell type" is a special property of ESCs. ESCs may propagate indefinitely in their undifferentiated state while maintaining karyotype. These cells can be grown in vitro while maintaining multilineage character; therefore, in vitro, over time, they can differentiate into all cell types present in an organism.[14-17]

But ESCs are unable to differentiate spontaneously into cardiomyocytes, although they may be guided to cardiac progenitor cells or differentiated into cardiomyocytes by different methods of induction.[18] Human ESCs have immense potential, with a huge probability of successful application in therapeutic options for patients **(Fig. 3)**.[19-21]

Along with the massive probability, there are controversies raised due to the therapeutic relevance of ESCs and autologous adult progenitor cells. One of the benefits of ESCs is the capability of ESC-derived cardiomyocytes (ESC-CMs) to electrically integrate with the cardiac muscle. A study with model of swine that created an atrioventricular block, treated with transplanted human ESC-CMs, showed reversal of the block with electrical coupling.[22]

Attaining high purity of ESCs and yielding differentiated cells of a single lineage type are the technical challenges faced by initial research scholars.[23] To achieve purified, homogeneous, and functionally integrated ESC-CMs that originated from heterogeneous ESCs, various methods, namely specialized culture methods, genetic modification, and treatment with chemical and biological factors, are used.[24-26]

Embryonic stem cell-derived cardiomyocytes, generated by Chong and colleagues were able to engraft and repair myocardial injury after MI in a primate model. Although the clinical use of ESCs is hindered despite the evidence of ESCs' efficacy in bigger animal models, this is due to the limitations, including their genetic instability and tumorigenic and immunogenic character. Ethical issues of source and the origin of these cells are important considerations in ESCs. Regarding the use of stem cells, laws are different in different countries. In the United States, the use of embryos that have been discarded after in vitro fertilization may be permitted for research by federal laws. But many European countries, there are stringent laws that disallow destructive embryo research.[27-29]

Skeletal Myoblast

Skeletal myoblasts are abundantly expressed in the human body; they are progenitor cells with myogenic capability. These cells can be made to proliferate and expand in vitro.

Skeletal myoblasts have the capacity to withstand ischemic insult because of their contractile ability. SMCs, these cells are also called as satellite cells of skeletal muscle, in which one of the initial few cell types first considered for cardiac regeneration.[30-32]

The first randomized placebo-controlled trial with myoblast transplantation was done in the *"Myoblast Autologous Grafting in Ischemic Cardiomyopathy"* (MAGIC)

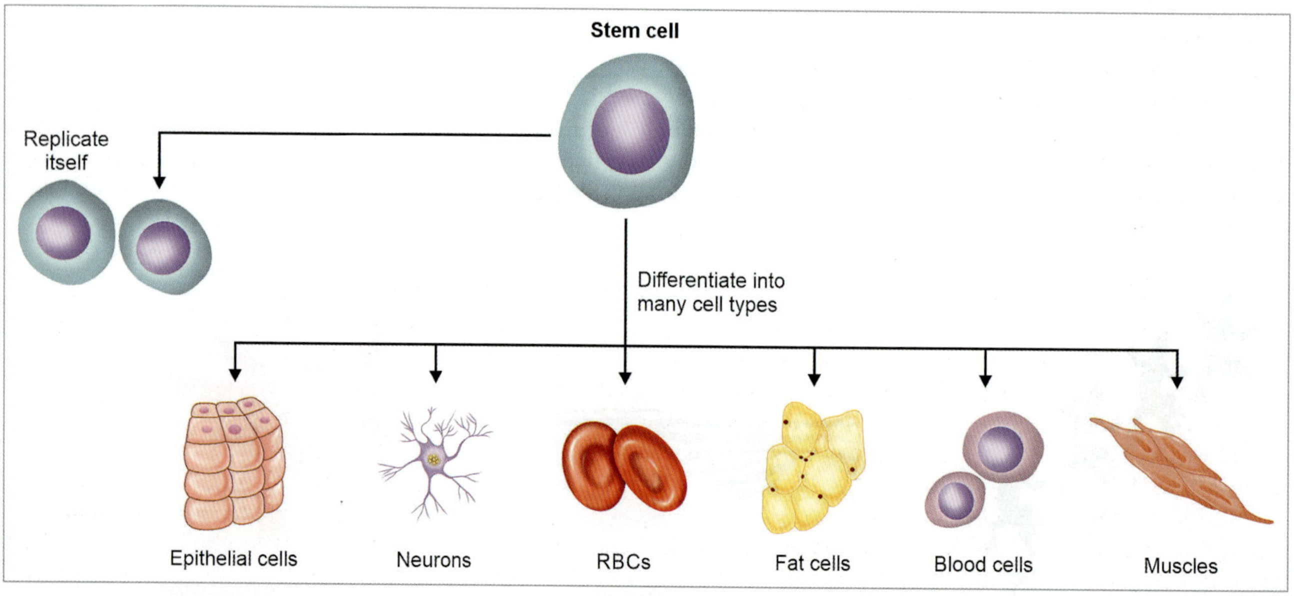

FIG. 2: Stem cell and differentiation.
(RBCs: red blood cells)

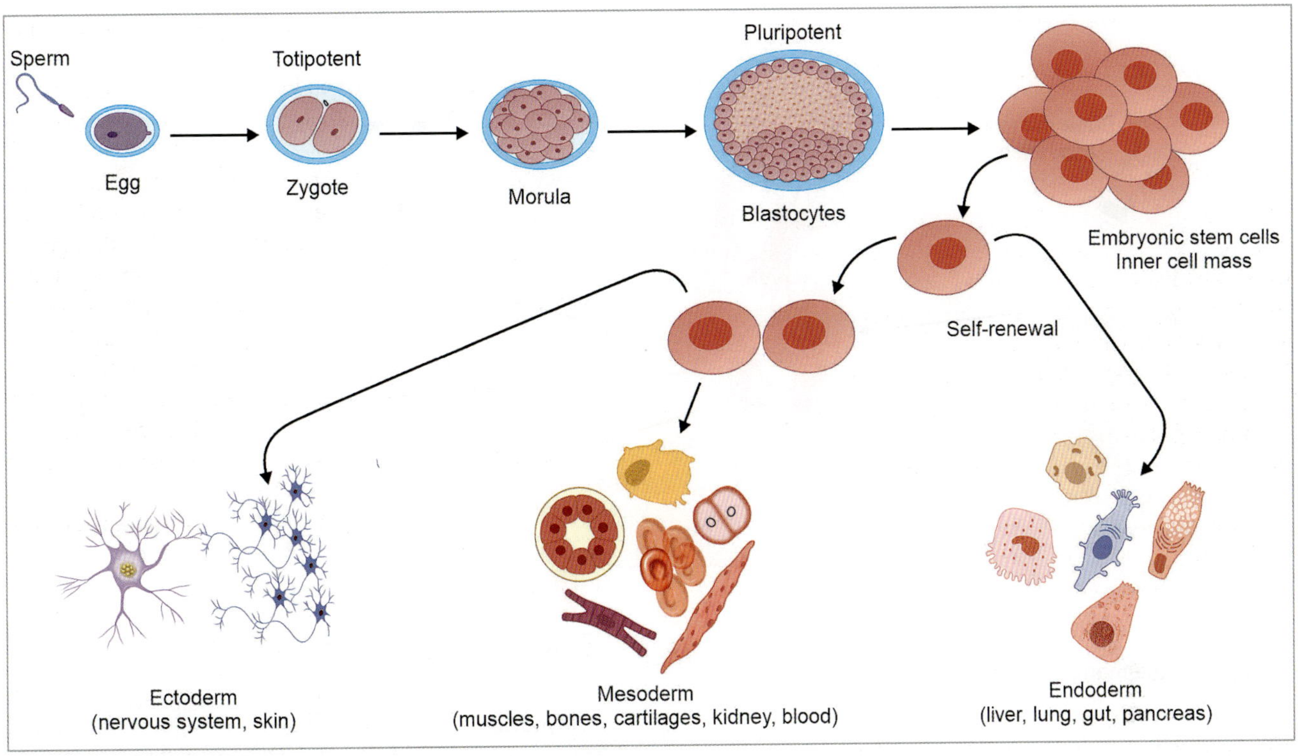

FIG. 3: Types of embryonic stem cell and regeneration pattern.

study. It found the effectiveness of skeletal myoblasts studied in animal models, along with some comments regarding the improvement of left ventricle (LV) function over time. Further, many attempts were made to prove the efficacy of skeletal myoblasts, which failed.[18,20]

Important factors of failure were skeletal myoblasts unable to connect electromechanically with the myocardium of the host due to a lack of adhesion proteins. Initial eagerness was further reduced when they found frequent multiple events of ventricular arrhythmias in transplanted patients. Myofibers also has arrhythmogenic property. To overcome the limitations, genetic modification and expression of connexin 43 was done. Later study reported that this genetic modification was not capable to manage the arrhythmogenic character of these cells.[21,22]

Bone Marrow Stem Cell

The study on bone marrow was initiated as early as 1950 and reported a minimum of two kinds of stem cells present, i.e., hematopoietic stem cells (HSCs) and mesenchymal stem cells (MSCs). In 2001 researcher found that marrow-derived cells (BMCs) has a capacity to regenerate the infarcted related myocardium.[23]

Murine model with MI was used to demonstrate that HSCs (observed by the surface protein c-kit) were responsible for the differentiation of BMCs into cardiomyocytes maturity, smooth muscle, and endothelial cells development. They injected isolated c-kit$^+$ cells into the infarcted area.[23] The important point to observe is that the efficacy of c-kit$^+$ HSCs, when compared with other types of cells, has never been clinically justified.

Later, many scientists have questioned their claim of the capability of HSCs to transdifferentiate into cardiovascular myocytes in many other studies. Körbling and colleagues observed that these cells are not only present in bone marrow but also in the peripheral blood.[34-38]

Study revealed that CD34 also express by EPCs and differentiated endothelial cells. And bone marrow and peripheral blood-derived CD34+ cells have the angiogenic capability. Post-transplantation into an infracted related area, it has capability to differentiate into cardiomyocytes, smooth muscle, and endothelial cells.[39]

Interestingly, Norol et al. have mistrusted their approach and reported that they did not find any cardiac phenotype post transplantation of CD34+ cells into nonhuman primates.[40] In spite of these questionable results, most of the studies were conducted using (HSCs, MSCs, and monocytes) bone marrow mononuclear cells **(Fig. 4)**.[41,42]

The effectiveness of BMCs for cardiac regeneration after acute MI has been meta-analyzed by the Cochrane Heart Group. Out of 33 clinical trials (1,765 patients) that were reported, an improvement was noted in the mortality and morbidity of the patients receiving BMCs. After 12 to 61 months follow-up claimed an improvement in left ventricular ejection fraction (LVEF), which was significant and sustained for long period.[50]

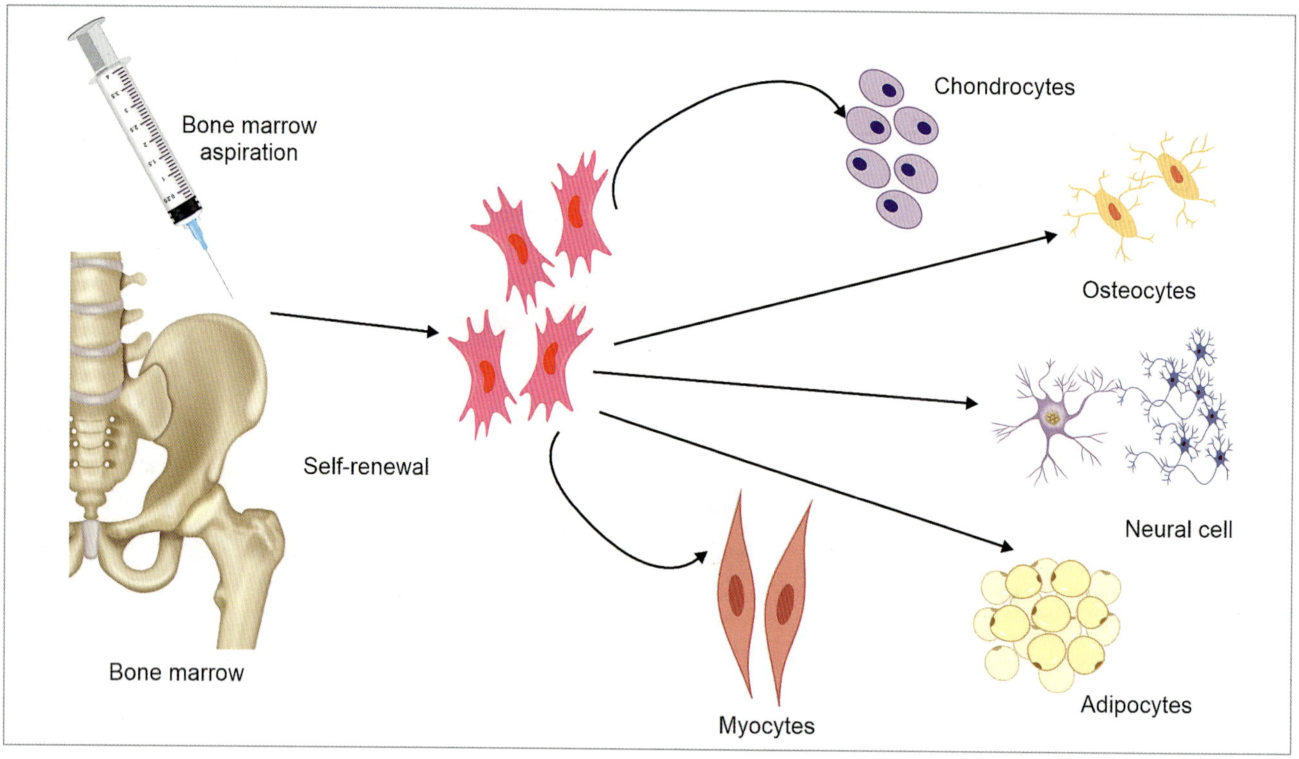

FIG. 4: Bone marrow stem cell and differentiation.

A similar meta-analysis was done by the Cochrane Heart Group again, with 23 clinical trials and 1,255 patients, and it was reported that BMCs have not only the capacity to increase ejection fraction but also the ability to improve morbidity and mortality in chronic ischemic heart disease (IHD) and congestive heart failure patients.[43]

Even after these encouraging results, arguments arise regarding the potential therapeutic ability to improve LVEF by BMCs, and it is claimed that paracrine effects might be responsible for the improvement. Enthusiastic results of the Cochrane Heart Group were limited by the heterogeneity observed in the results.[44]

Recently, a meta-analysis was done from 49 trials using BMCs for cardiac regeneration to compare the results and discrepancies. The study utilized weighted regression and identified 600 discrepancies in 133 reports from these trials. The largest discrepancies were observed in the increment in LVEF in patients, while on the other hand, it failed to reveal any advantage from BMCs, with the lowest number of discrepancies.[45] With these findings, it was concluded that it is extremely difficult to draw assumptions on the efficacy of BMCs.[46]

Mesenchymal Stem Cell

Mesenchymal stem cells are those cells with the ability to self-renew and differentiate into mesenchymal lineages, which mostly include skeletal myoblasts, chondrocytes, and adipose tissue.[47] This classical view is now challenged as they have been shown to differentiate into neural (nonmesenchymal) tissues as well.[47,48] Surface markers of the MSC population are mainly CD73, CD105, CD29, CD44, and CD90 and lack CD34 and CD45, which are mainly expressed by HSCs.[49] As MSCs may be obtained and isolated from different kinds of tissues such as cord blood, adipose tissue, and bone marrow, this provides more therapeutic options for bioregenerative medicine.

Another important benefits of MSCs are their capacity of an innate ability to overcome the rejection by immune responses. This advantages of MSCs is due to the lack of major histo-compatibility complex II and B7 co-stimulatory molecule expression; which gives the chance for patients with non-autologous transplantation.[47,50]

In vitro, MSCs have the ability to differentiate into cardiomyocytes and vascular endothelial cells. When MSCs are transplanted in an experimental model in vivo, MSCs activate paracrine factors and participate in neovascularization and cardiomyocyte protection. In vivo, their ability to differentiate into phenotype myocardial cells is still under consideration.[47,51]

Induced Pluripotent Stem Cell

Many study has concluded that induced pluripotent stem cells (iPSCs) has the potential capacity of differentiating cells, including capability to differentiate into cell types from any of the three germ layers. Initially the experimental efficiency was poor with iPSCs because lack of successful induction of pluripotency to somatic cells **(Fig. 5)**.

Takahashi and Yamanaka reported that self-renewal of ESCs has been achieved by inducing pluripotency in somatic cells through retroviral transduction of several factors. They faced many challenge due to cellular differentiation process to be an irreversible process.[52,53]

Induced pluripotent stem cells have been found to differentiate into cardiomyocytes, endothelial cells, and smooth muscle cells in vitro. When injected into the infarcted heart of mice, iPSCs can differentiate into the cardiac phenotype.[54,55]

Rais and colleagues reported successful synchronisation of all cells to attain pluripotency by depleting the Mbd3 gene by the Mbd3/NuRD (*Nucleosome remodelling and de-acetylation repressor complex*). Mbd3/NuRD is the predominant molecular block preventing the deterministic induction of ground-state pluripotency.[56] With this may overcome a prime barrier of the for the therapeutic and clinical use.[56]

Induced pluripotent stem cells also have ESC-like properties to be tumorigenic. Martens and colleagues, hence, differentiated iPSCs into cardiomyocytes in vitro upfront before transplanting them into the infarct-related myocardium to overcome the issues of tumorigenesis. They found that transplanted cells localized to the myocardium and convalesced the myocardial functions.[54,57] Another important step taken is that cardiac cells derived from iPSCs are also used to create biosynthetic tissues.[58]

Endogenous Cardiac Stem Cell

Till the last decade, researchers' dogma was that the only response of myocardial cells to stress was considered to be either hypertrophy or death. Scientist has the belief that the heart is a lastly differentiated organ and unable to of generating new parenchymal cells. But recent study showed that myocardial cell have the ability to undergo replication, mitotic division, and spontaneous regeneration in the myocardium.[59]

Research has been conducted which revealed that a large pool of cardiac progenitor cells and resident cardiac stem cells (CSCs) are present while expressing the stem cell surface marker c-kit in the human heart and adult rat heart.[60]

New opinions and considerations have cleared that the homeostasis of the myocardial organ is maintained by cell death and cell restoration, although with a very minimum rate of renewal/turnover of myocardial cells in comparison to other organs and tissues. Another important characteristic of cardiac progenitor cells is immaturity and committed myocardial cells, which mature into precursor cells and further differentiate into cardiac cell types.[61]

Cardiac stem cells are present in special areas of the heart, such as the atria or pericardium, where they are present in concentrated and large numbers of cells.[61] With this finding, CSC research is rapidly emerging, and many stem cell-like populations are being newly uncovered in the myocardium.

Chong et al.[62] isolated adult epicardial-resident cardiac colony-forming unit fibroblasts with a property by displaying broad trans-germ layer potency in vitro and in vivo.

Recent studies support the use of CSCs than BMCs because CSCs may be preferable over cells from other lineages as they reach functional competence and obtain the structural characteristics of mature myocytes and vessels faster than other cell lineages.[63]

In the CADUCEUS (Cardiosphere-Derived Autologous Stem Cells to Reverse Ventricular Dysfunction) study, 31 patients were enrolled who had undergone successful coronary angioplasty after post-acute MI with reduced

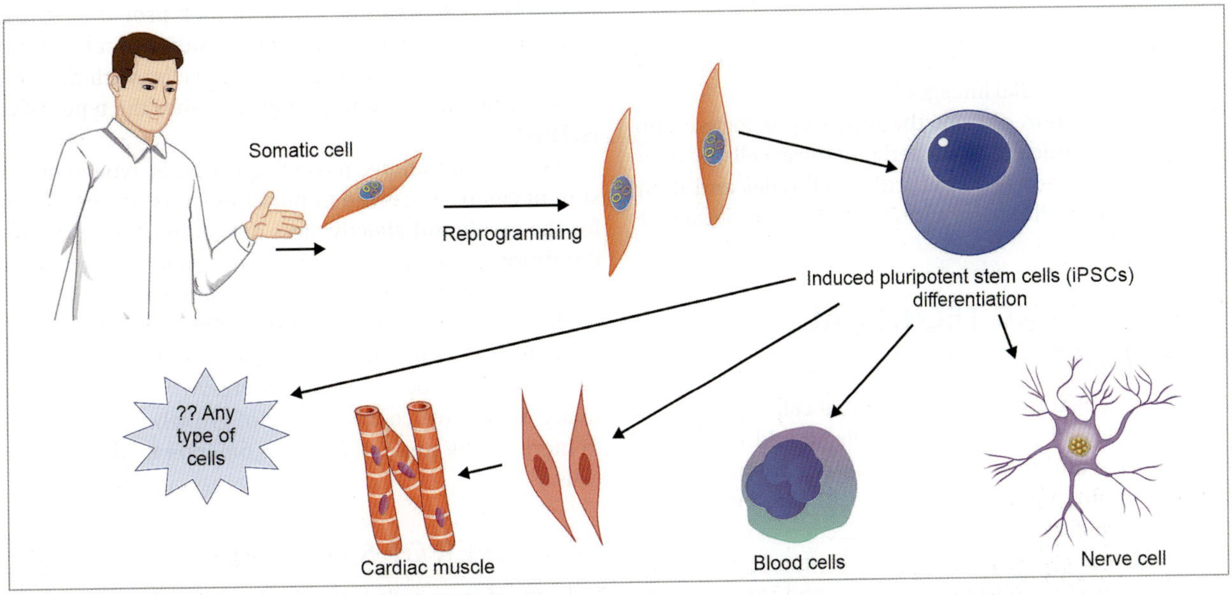

(?? any type of cells = ? may differentiate into any type of cells)

FIG. 5: Induced pluripotent stem cells (iPSCs) and differentiation.

cardiac function. They were randomized, with one group treated with autologous cardiosphere-derived cells (CDCs) and another to receive standard care.[65] CDCs-treated patients had better results with a reduction in scar tissue mass, increased viable heart mass, and better regional wall motion and contractility.[65]

Gene expression and functional efficacy of atrial and ventricular cardiomyocytes are different. It is difficult to know whether the stem cells from atria and ventricles have the same efficacy, characteristics, and functions.[66]

ISOLATION OF BEST SOURCES OF STEM CELL FOR CARDIAC REGENERATION

With the appreciating results of recent trials on stem cell therapy, it is now concluded that this therapy can be safely performed clinically for the treatment of cardiac regeneration. One of the important issues now is the selection of the best sources of stem cells for the target organ for the best and optimum results, especially during preclinical, clinical, and first-in-human studies **(Fig. 3)**.

Evidence-based therapy is the first need to obtain a clear result from the previous study to perform a successful therapy. The mechanism of the action of stem cells is also important to get the best results and avoid criticism.

The difference between other stem cell to CSC therapy is that CSC need to differentiate cardiomyocyte and regenerating ability of blood vessels to improve the blood supply to the infarcted area, along with incorporating mechanical and electrical activity with native myocytes. An important aspect to improve myocardial function is the paracrine factors secreted by the stem cells, which play a more important role. This gives us insight and modifies our view that stem cells need to differentiate into cardiac cell types to improve cardiac function. Therefore, stem cells that are not multipotent may still improve cardiac function, and comparable results may be obtained with stem cells committed to myocardial lineages.[65]

After the selection of cells, the next step is focused on technically and clinically characterizing these cells by their capability to differentiate into cardiac cell types and their capacity to restore heart condition by different paracrine mechanisms.[33]

PRAGMATIC AND TECHNICAL CHALLENGES

One of the essential factors for myocardial cell regeneration is that the selected population of cells should have high cardioselective ability. There is a risk of carcinogenicity with noncommitted pluripotent stem cells with injection of exceedingly proliferative characters. Selection of committed myocardial lineage stem cells can be made by using different systems linked to the activation and expression of cardioselective genes. A huge number of heterogeneity with total numbers and quality of adult stem cells are presenting organ are seen in the stem cells. To achieve safe and effective stem cell therapy, it is crucial to isolate and inject the purified form of cell population with a cardiac lineage and committed stem cells.[68]

Factors such as age, gender, pre-existing conditions, and procedural therapy are responsible for the effectiveness and number of stem cells. This finding was reported by Sanada and colleagues; they found a significant reduction in the c-kit$^+$ numbers with advanced age. This finding supported by other research, which noted that the cardioprotective property is less with stem cell collected from elderly patients.

Similar results are also seen in individuals with comorbid conditions such as diabetes, hypertension, or stage four heart disease, along with gene expression differentiation, cell longevity, and cardiac functional capability compared with healthy individuals. Severity of the disease condition, duration of acute or chronic events, and the extent of pre-existing diseases such as diabetes and hypertension are also important issues to be answered **(Fig. 6)**.[69-72]

Sources and the location of the organ for stem cell collection are also important issues for efficacy and results. Atria and the ventricles source may have different gene expression and functional capacity with similar with cardiomyocytes from these different sources.[66]

In stem cell therapy, isolation and expansion are crucial and challenging tasks for the preclinical and clinical settings for therapeutic use. The most easy process of collection is through peripheral blood samples, even though the expansion capabilities of the EPCs are limited.[71]

In the case of endomyocardial samples, which are difficult to obtain and very small (nearly 5 mg), CSCs isolated and expanded from the endomyocardium are more effective in cardiac regeneration with complex procure.[73] Studies advocate that stem cell culture conditions also carry a challenging task in the expansion of cells. Variation in the intensity of enzymatic digestion may alter the types of cells isolated.[74]

Growth conditions, passaging methods, type of cell, and sum of cell passages are important factors of consideration for the result and effectiveness of therapy. Suitable culture conditions and the use of growth factors might be the important role in the efficacy of functional properties.[75,76]

Studies suggest that the use of fibroblast growth factor for culture of the cell may extend the doubling of these cells up to 80 population doublings.[76,77] In many studies, many distinctive combinations of growth factors are used to increase the proliferation and functional efficacy of stem cells.[78]

TRANSFER OF STEM CELL

Delivery of stem cells is the final step for the patient, where consideration of the type and nature of the injury, timing of

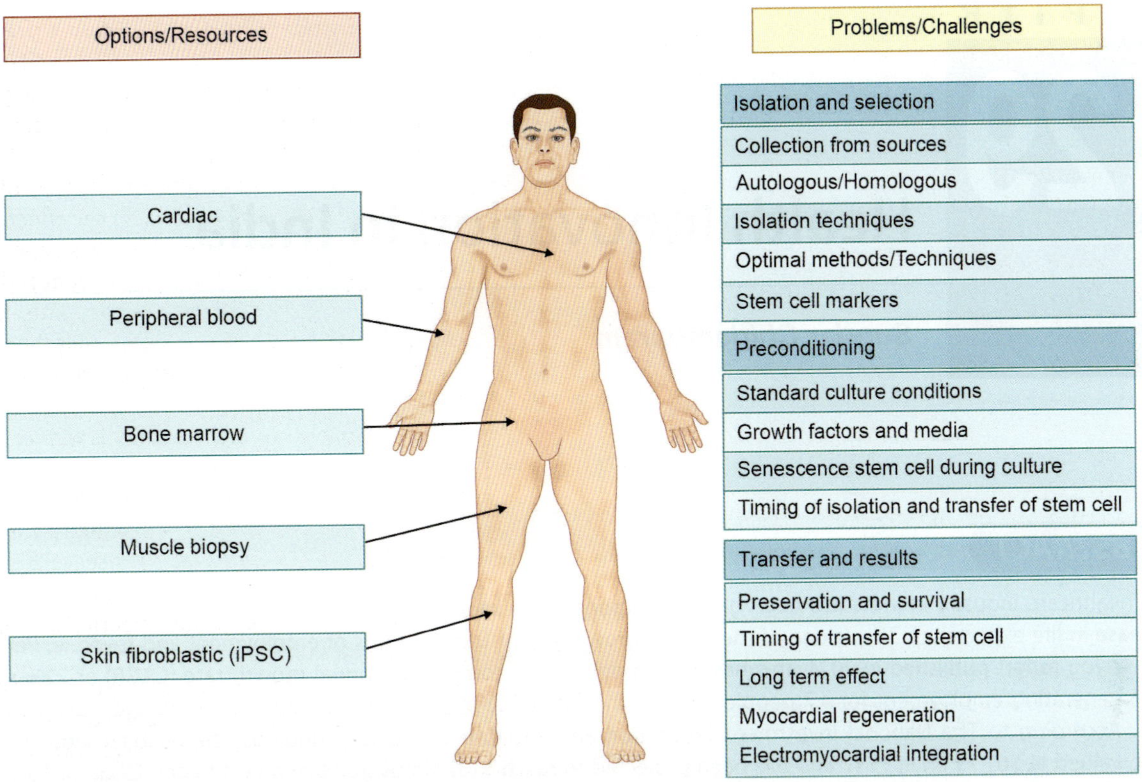

FIG. 6: Potential challenges and options in stem cell delivery.
(iPSC: induced pluripotent stem cell)

the therapy, and the engrafting ability to the host myocardium are the most important factors to be managed. In the case of long-term angina due to ischemia with intact functional myocardium, the purpose of stem cell therapy is to improve the blood supply to ischemic myocardial tissue. To achieve the optimum result, it is necessary to use a cell type that secretes proangiogenic factors, for example, BMCs, EPCs, or cells that increase vascular regeneration.

Conversely, progenitor cell types, such as CSCs with cardiac and vascular regeneration capability, can be used if the target is to regenerate an infarcted heart with non-functional (MI) tissue.[79] Decision-making for the best time for stem cell therapy to patients is very important for the optimum result. Timing of stem cell therapy was studied in two trials [LateTIME and REPAIR-AMI (Reinfusion of Enriched Progenitor Cells and Infarct Remodelling in Acute Myocardial Infarction)] and compared the results. In (REPAIR-AMI) intra-coronary infusion done in 3 to 5 days, whereas in (LateTIME) BMCs infused during 2 to 3 weeks.

Patients who received BMCs within 5 days after the acute event showed considerable improvement in LV ejection fraction. But the procurement of CSCs in the case of autologous transplantation is extremely difficult.[80,81] SCIPIO and CADUCEUS trials have shown an advantage in patients where cell transplantation was performed 4 months and 2–4 weeks, respectively, after an acute event.[64,65]

CONCLUSION

Primary focus of present therapy is to minimize the symptoms only due to nonavailability of therapy that can potentially reverse the disease. Stem cell therapy has the potential to reverse myocardial injury, improve cardiac function, and regenerate the infarcted myocardium. Many myths are still present in the scientific community, but in reality, to make stem cell therapy a next-generation treatment, there is a need to overcome several barriers for the routine management strategy for cardiovascular regeneration. It is necessary to design clinical trials and studies that may focus on different cell types at the similar time frame with less variability in the type of disease, age, gender, pre-existing disease, and comorbid conditions.

ONLINE REFERENCES

Please scan the QR code provided at the end of the table of contents for References of this chapter.

CHAPTER

129

Health Innovation in India

Sundar Chidambaram

ABSTRACT

The healthcare industry in India has been growing exponentially keeping pace with the growing population and the increase in life expectancy. This is one of the fastest-growing industries in terms of employment and revenue. Per the NITI Aayog report published in 2021, this has been growing at a compound annual growth rate (CAGR) of 22% since 2016 generating employment for 4.7 people and has the capability of generating an additional 500,000 new jobs per year. According to The National Investment Promotion and Facilitation Agency's findings, the hospital industry has been valued at $61.79 Bn in FY17 and has been projected to reach $132 Bn by 2023, at an estimated CAGR of 16–17%. Statistics have proven that >75% of Indians pay for their healthcare needs from their pocket. Data proves that among those with insurance, government-sponsored insurance schemes stood first followed by employer-sponsored insurance and individual insurance schemes took the last place.[1]

Central- and state-budgeted health expenditure has been increasing steadily and has touched 2.1% of the gross domestic product (GDP) in the year 2023 and this stood at 1.6% of GDP in the year 2022 as per the information released by the government of India (https://pib.gov.in/PressReleasePage.aspx?PRID=1894902). This is much less when compared to the average expenditure of the world stood which at 10.89 in 2020 per the data provided by the World Bank. Innovations which are low-cost, scalable, and replicable and those which provide quick solutions are the need of the hour.

Keywords: Innovations, healthcare, medical device.

INTRODUCTION

Villages are the backbone of India and there is a deep divide in the quality of healthcare available to the urban and rural population. Healthcare innovations should be focused on lessening this divide and be made economically feasible for the rural population. The healthcare system is burdened due to factors such as lifestyle changes, urban migration, an aging population, white-collar jobs which promote a sedentary lifestyle, and increased globalization which has resulted in the consumption of fast food. A sedentary lifestyle and unhealthy changes in food habits have resulted in a phenomenal increase in noncommunicable diseases (NCDs). The high population density has resulted in the rapid spread of communicable diseases (CDs) as proven by the COVID-19 pandemic and the recent outbreak of the Nipah virus in Kerala.[2]

The saying "necessity is the mother of invention" is well known and this can be modified to state that "necessity is the mother of innovation". India is a land of "*jugaad*" which refers to frugal innovation where people are famous for finding workarounds and solutions through innovative ideas. The use of IV lines and disposable water bottles in the place of urinary catheters during health camps by a doctor for draining distended bladders in the absence of urinary catheters is one such example. The high cost of hospitalization due to NCDs in private hospitals can be afforded only by the rich. It is well known that prevention is better than cure. Prevention, diagnosis, treatment, and continuous follow-up are part of the progression of disease. The opportunities for innovation at all these stages are immense. Out-of-box thinking for providing affordable, accessible, and available healthcare to all citizens should be the driving force behind innovation.

HEALTHCARE INNOVATION IN THE INDIAN SCENARIO

The four P's method is used for organizing and focusing the innovation efforts. The four P's encompass (1) *p*roduct, (2) *p*rocess, (3) *p*osition, and (4) *p*aradigm. Ministry of Health and Family Welfare, Government of India as part of the National Health Mission has been encouraging and scaling up of innovations in the healthcare industry. The Ministry of Health and National Innovation Council encourages and supports innovations which focus on providing quality healthcare at an affordable cost. The success of an innovation can be attributed to its affordability, accessibility, financial feasibility, and ability to scale the product up. The technological know-how and medical expertise make India a hub of medical product innovation. These include diagnostic tools, medical devices, and assistive tools. Lower pricing, efficient scaling of production, availability of skilled manpower, and targeting emerging markets who are willing to purchase in bulk would help in making this a profitable venture.[3]

The Aatmanirbhar Bharat Abhiyaan packages provide several short-term and longer-term measures for the health system, including production-linked incentive (PLI) schemes for boosting domestic manufacturing of pharmaceuticals and medical devices.

As India celebrated the Azadi ka Amrit Mahotsav—75th Year of Independence, NITI Aayog launched a digi-book on the "Innovations for You series by Atal Innovation Mission" with emphasis on the healthcare sector. This digi-book has a compilation of 45 health tech startups. These startups use technology including artificial intelligence (AI), the internet of things (IOT), and information of communication (ICT) to find innovative solutions to problems like anemia, malaria, dental care, and mental health and some of these innovations focus on neonatal and childcare and monitoring.

Jaipur foot is one of the best examples of cost-effective innovations of international repute which was developed in 1968. SS Innovations International, Inc a healthcare startup in India is the developer of innovative surgical robotic technologies which is cost-effective with broad-spectrum surgical applications, including cardiovascular, thoracic, head and neck surgery, gynecology, urology, and general surgery.

Swasth Bharat Mobile Application has been designed to provide detailed information regarding healthy lifestyle, disease conditions (A–Z), symptoms, treatment options, first aid, and public health alerts. The government under the "National Tobacco Control Program" has developed and deployed mobile-based strategy called m-Cessation, this helps those who are keen on quitting tobacco use and smoking. This can be availed by calling a toll-free number from the mobile phone number of those interested in quitting smoking for good.

The CoWIN platform and the Aarogya Sethu mobile app were used by the government of India during the COVID-19 pandemic. The CoWIN platform was used to effectively manage the testing and vaccination of the population. The Aarogya Sethu mobile app helped in intimating the users when they were in close proximity of COVID-positive individuals and this app was used by the government to identify and isolate COVID-19 clusters. Both these innovations were linked to another technology-driven unique identification number-based (UID) system called Aadhaar. The COVID-19 detection, vaccination, and tracking in a country like India with a population which has crossed 1.4 billion would have been an impossibility.[4]

The government of Andhra Pradesh (AP) has introduced mobile medical units (MMU) for the rural population who have limited medical facilities. It has also introduced the Thalli-Bidda Express (mother-child express), these vehicles are used for transporting the mother and child after delivery to their place of residence. This is a boon to people who are not able to afford the cost of transportation. "Akha Boat" clinics have been promoted by the government of Assam to cover the healthcare need of remote villages which are only accessible through rivers.

Telemedicine services in India fall under the combined jurisdiction of the Ministry of Health and Family Welfare and the Department of Information Technology (MoHFW). National Medical College Network (NMCN) had been established for e-education and a National Rural Telemedicine Network for e-healthcare delivery. Indian Space Research Organization's (ISRO) telemedicine network has made inroads in connecting remote regions including Andaman and Nicobar and Lakshadweep islands, the hilly remote regions of Jammu and Kashmir, Medical College hospitals in Odisha, and some of the rural/district hospitals throughout the country which have poor access by road.

The social security schemes provided by the state and central government speak volumes of the innovative reforms which are carried out by the government. The Ayushman Bharat Programme provides holistic and integrated health care. AB-Pradhan Mantri Jan Arogya Yojana (AB-PMJAY) provides free and cashless care to about 500 million poor and deprived people for secondary and tertiary hospitalization care. AP government also provides subsidized health coverage under the Arogya Sri scheme which caters to the population below the poverty line.

Facilitated by the National Rural Health Mission, nongovernmental organizations (NGO) have spearheaded a number of innovations in the delivery of public health services in India. One example is Jaipur-based Khushi Baby, which has developed wearables that can monitor the health of babies and pregnant women and this has been possible with the support of NGO Seva Mandir. Kushi Baby team adapted to the need of the hour during the COVID-19 pandemic by creating a new version of the platform which was used by 58,0000 health workers and facilitated door-to-door screening, referral, and follow-up, this platform helped in screening 1.2 crore people across Rajasthan between July and October of 2020.

COST-EFFECTIVE INNOVATION IN THE INDIAN CONTEXT

Low cost and quality which meet international standards and those which are applicable to Indian conditions are the ones which can scaled and provide an effective and sustainable in the long run with a feasible and profitable business model. Healthcare-related industries have been setting up production units where equipment and test kits are assembled with imported raw materials. The materials and processes designed for specific countries might not be able to withstand the Indian conditions where power cuts, voltage fluctuations, and pollution are prevalent in India. The government has been promoting the Make in India label. Innovations which are made from scratch would stand a greater chance of being effective in the Indian context.[5,6]

The innovation arm of the pioneering medical device manufacturing ecosystem, the Andhra Pradesh MedTech Zone (AMTZ), Medi Valley Atal Incubation Centre was set up with the help of funding from NITI Aayog under the Atal Innovation Mission. This provides a conducive environment for innovation and state of the art laboratory where innovators can transform their ideas into reality. Other state governments should follow the lead taken by Andhra Pradesh in setting up MedTech incubation Centers to promote innovation. There is no dearth of talent and India is a land of *Jugaad* where workable fixes, workarounds, problem-solving, and unique fixes using limited resources lead to innovation. This exemplifies the resourcefulness, enterprise, resilience, and ingenuity of the Indians.

GOVERNMENT HEALTH INITIATIVES

Centrally Sponsored Ayushman Bharat-National Health Protection Mission (AB-NHPM) is the largest funded government health initiative across the world. AB-NHPM includes the Rashtriya Swasthya Bima Yojana (RSBY) and the Senior Citizen Health Insurance Scheme (SCHIS). This targets 10 crore families belonging to poor and vulnerable populations based on the latest SECC (Socio-Economic and Caste Census) data, covering both rural and urban areas. This scheme would provide a coverage of ₹ 5 lakh per family per year. This is provided as a cashless, paperless transaction through an IT-enabled platform in partnership with NITI Aayog. The mission of AB-NHPM is to integrate the private and public healthcare institutions under a common network to enable the beneficiaries to avail the cashless and paperless health insurance provided by this scheme in a smooth and hassle-free manner. The Ayushman Bharat Digital Mission (ABDM) aims to develop the necessary digitally enabled platform for integrating the digital health infrastructure of the country. Ayushman Bharat Health Account (ABHA) is an essential constituent of the larger ABDM which paves the way for improved transparency, efficiency, and accessibility in healthcare insurance.[7]

The innovation of the future should be a biometric-enabled smart health card which would be like an electronic medical record which could be accessed by healthcare providers when a patient approaches them for treatment it would contain the past medical history, details from birth including immunization, doctor visits, hospitalizations, discharge summaries, medication taken by the patient, and the allergies. This would help the medical provider come to an accurate diagnosis and provide the correct treatment when the patient does not provide the proper history. The medical insurance detail also could be integrated in the smart card for seamless healthcare delivery.

REGULATION OF HEALTHCARE INNOVATION

Regulatory frameworks which are on par with international regulatory standards like the US Food and Drug Administration (FDA) and European Medicines Agency (EMA) should be in place for innovations which have the potential for phenomenal growth. The Central Drugs Standard Control Organisation (CDSCO) under the Directorate General of Health Services, Ministry of Health and Family Welfare, Government of India is the National Regulatory Authority (NRA) of India. CDSCO is India's regulatory body for pharmaceuticals and medical equipment. Some of the electronic components/accessories included in medical devices (medical electronic equipment), including batteries, monitors, and power adaptors require certification from the Bureau of Indian Standards (BIS). Reduction in turnaround times and transparency for certification by the regulatory authorities would be beneficial for the medical device and the pharmaceutical industry. A conducive environment should be provided by the regulatory authorities which encourages both process and product innovation.[8]

ROLE OF TRAINING AND COLLABORATION IN HEALTHCARE INNOVATION

Healthcare providers are instrumental in bringing the innovations to fruition. They should be open to continuous training and development and should be up to date on the latest developments in medical technology and medical devices. They should be promoting innovation and seek to use it for the benefit of the most vulnerable population. Collaboration between experts in technology and healthcare providers leads to new innovative ideas. Stanford-India Biodesign was launched in 2007 and this is a collaboration between Stanford University, the All India Institute of Medical Sciences (AIIMS), and the Indian Institute of Technology (IIT) Delhi. This was instrumental in creating innovation leaders who would promote the growth of the Medtech industry in India. This resulted in the development of 14 technologies and in the establishment of 13 new companies[9] (https://biodesign.stanford.edu/programs/global-initiatives/stanford-india-biodesign.html). The Healthcare Hackathon was conducted at the Indian Institute of Information Technology and promoted the participation of students from the leading technical institutions in India which included the IIT and the National Institute of Technology (NIT), this was conducted in November of 2022 by the Indian Institute of Information Technology Sri City, Andhra Pradesh. Indian Council of Medical Research (ICMR) collaborated with IIT Kharagpur and candidates were recruited for ICMR Medtech Biodesign CLiMB Fellowship in October 2021.[10,11]

CONCLUSION

Healthcare innovations are here to stay. There is a definite shift from product to process innovations. Frugal innovation, increased use of technology, collaboration between healthcare providers and experts in technology and medical device industry, encouragement by the government and partnership between educational institutions both national and international, and the healthcare authorities are paving the way for an exponential growth of healthcare innovations.

ONLINE REFERENCES

Please scan the QR code provided at the end of the table of contents for References of this chapter.

CHAPTER

130

Recent Trials in Cardiology

Vineet Bhatia, Meetu Arora, VK Bahl

ABSTRACT

Several landmark trials were published in the year gone. They helped us in answering simple questions such as deciding about the use of newer oral anticoagulants (NOACS) or vitamin K antagonists (VKAs) in mitral stenosis while others put forward groundbreaking technologies such as the use of transcatheter tricuspid valve edge-to-edge repair. Newer technologies such as use of RNA interference agents in hypertension have opened up a new chapter in the pharmacological treatment of hypertension.

Keywords: Clinical trials, cardiology.

INTRODUCTION

Well-designed and meticulously executed clinical trials go a long way in shaping the future of modern medicine. Their results help pave the path for further research in real world settings and formulation of practice guidelines. Despite the global pandemic of COVID-19 over the past couple of years the quest for medical excellence has not dampened the spirits of researchers from all over the world. Several landmark trials have been completed while others are in the pipeline. This article shall discuss some of the important recent clinical trials published in the year gone by.

TRILUMINATE PIVOTAL[1]

It is a landmark randomized clinical trial of transcatheter tricuspid valve (TV) edge-to-edge repair (EER) for tricuspid regurgitation (TR).

Isolated surgical management of symptomatic severe TR poses significant challenges due to high periprocedural mortality. In order to deal with this issue, transcatheter interventions have been developed with good success. The largest experience, so far, has been with the tricuspid transcatheter EER (T-TEER).

Results of pioneering work in the unblinded, single-arm TRILUMINATE study and data from the TriValve registry, have proven the safety and efficacy of T-TEER. However, so far, no randomized data comparing T-TEER with optimized medical therapy alone was available. To address this, the TRILUMINATE Pivotal trial, randomizing T-TEER against guideline-directed medical therapy (GDMT), was designed.

The study enrolled 450 patients (mean age 78 years with more than half being females) across two continents (North America and Europe) at 75 sites and 12-month follow-up data on 350 patients is available at the present time. The trial is a multicenter randomized controlled trial that randomized patients in a 1:1 manner to either T-TEER with the TriClip device (Abbott Medical) or medical therapy alone. All patients suffered from symptomatic significant TR (severe/massive/torrential: 97.7% in device arm, 98.8% in control arm) and were at intermediate or greater risk for mortality or morbidity with TV surgery.

The clinical trial primary and secondary endpoints are given in **Box 1**.

BOX 1 Endpoints of the clinical trial.

Primary endpoint: Composite of all-cause mortality or tricuspid valve (TV) surgery, heart failure hospitalizations, and assessment of quality-of-life improvement using the Kansas City Cardiomyopathy Questionnaire (KCCQ) (at 12 months)

Secondary endpoint: Freedom from MAE after procedure (at 30 days), change in TR from severe to ≤ moderate (at 30-day), change in QoL by KCCQ and 6-minute-walk-test (at 12 months)

(MAE: major adverse events; QoL: quality of life; TR: tricuspid regurgitation)

The results revealed that at 12 months, the primary endpoints were superior for the device group as compared to the medical therapy group. The favorable results were largely driven by the improvements in the Kansas City Cardiomyopathy Questionnaire (KCCQ) score in the device group (improved by ≥ 15 KCCQ points in 49.7% patients compared to only 26.4% in the medical group and the degree of improvement in quality of life was directly related to degree of TR reduction).

Freedom from all cause death, TV surgery need and heart failure (HF) hospitalization were more or less similar at the end of 12 months in both the groups.

At 30 days, freedom from major adverse events (MAE) in the device group was 98.3%, and TR grade was ≤ moderate in 87.0% (vs. 4.8% in control group, $p > 0.001$).

This is being hailed as a landmark trial and may go a long way in the shaping the clinical outcomes of patients with severe TR in the future.

SAFETY, TOLERABILITY, AND EFFICACY OF UPTITRATION OF GUIDELINE-DIRECTED MEDICAL THERAPIES FOR ACUTE HEART FAILURE (STRONG-HF): A MULTINATIONAL, OPEN-LABEL, RANDOMIZED TRIAL[2]

Total 87 hospitals in 14 countries enrolled 1,078 patients aged 18–85 years who were admitted to hospital with acute heart failure. Prior to discharge, they were assigned in a 1:1 fashion to usual care or high-intensity care (the drugs were administered in accordance to guideline-directed medical treatment), were up titrated to the maximum recommended doses over a period of 2 weeks. For outpatient department visits were planned over the next 2 months wherein patients were closely followed up clinically and using laboratory parameters. Rehospitalization for HF at 180 days was the primary endpoint.

The study was terminated prematurely as the interim results showed marked benefits in the high-intensity group as compared to the usual care group. In the former group, patients were up titrated to recommended doses in an easier fashion and blood pressure, pulse, New York Heart Association class, bodyweight, and NT-pro-B-type natriuretic peptide (BNP) concentration had decreased more than in the usual care group. Readmission for HF and all-cause mortality were lower in the high intensity group.

Patients accepted the intensive treatment strategy guided by GDMT upgradation well as it rapidly alleviated symptoms, improved the quality of life, and reduced the risk of 180-day all-cause mortality and HF readmission when compared to usual care.

TORSEMIDE COMPARISON WITH FUROSEMIDE FOR MANAGEMENT OF HEART FAILURE (TRANSFORM-HF)[3]

This was a randomized, parallel design open label trial which compared outcomes associated with the use of torsemide with furosemide after hospitalization for HF regardless of ejection fraction. A total of 2,859 patients (mean age 64 years; 37% females) were enrolled and randomized in a 1:1 fashion and followed up for a period of 17.4 months. The primary outcome, all-cause mortality, occurred in 26.2% of the furosemide group versus 26.1% of the torsemide group (p = 0.76). Secondary outcomes: all-cause mortality or hospitalization: 49.3% of the furosemide group versus 47.3% of the torsemide group (p = 0.11). Also, at 12 months no differences were noted in the KCCQ-Clinical Summary Score (CSS) scores in the two groups.

The authors concluded that for patients admitted with decompensated heart failure, postdischarge management with torsemide was not superior to furosemide. All-cause mortality and patient-reported quality of life were similar between treatment groups. Either furosemide or torsemide is acceptable options for diuresis among patients with heart failure.

MAVACAMTEN IN ADULTS WITH SYMPTOMATIC OBSTRUCTIVE HCM WHO ARE ELIGIBLE FOR SEPTAL REDUCTION THERAPY-VALOR-HCM[4]

Apart from drug therapy (disopyramide/beta-blockers), alcohol septal ablation has been used often to treat hypertrophic cardiomyopathy (HCM). There has been an ongoing search for newer oral agents. Recently, mavacamten has been shown to be beneficial in the treatment of HOCM in the EXPLORER-HCM trial. The drug acts by inhibiting the actin-myosin cross-bridge formation and thereby the cardiac contractility. In the VALOR-HCM trial, the drug use was associated with a reduced need for septal ablation in patients who otherwise were on optimal medical therapy but continued to be symptomatic. A total number of 108 patients were enrolled, randomized in a 1:1 fashion and followed up for a period of 16 weeks. The drug was initiated at a dose of 5 mg and then adjusted as per left ventricular ejection fraction (LVEF), left ventricular outflow tract (LVOT) gradient estimations at rest and after Valsalva maneuver. The patients in the placebo group were at the end of 16 weeks crossed over to receive 5 mg mavacamten daily. The need to procced with septal reduction therapy at the end of 16 weeks was 17.9% versus 76.8 % in the mavacamten and placebo groups, respectively ($p < 0.0001$).

The secondary endpoints were significantly better in the mavacamten group which included improvement in NYHA class, change from baseline in resting LVOT gradient, change from baseline in Valsalva LVOT gradient at 16 weeks, and change from baseline in KCCQ. Safety outcomes [nonsustained ventricular tachycardia (NSVT), congestive heart failure (CHF), syncope, and sudden cardiac death] were also favorable for the study drug group.

The trial establishes the ability of the drug in bringing about symptomatic improvement, reducing the need for septal reduction procedures in symptomatic patients.

INVESTIGATION OF RHEUMATIC ATRIAL FIBRILLATION TREATMENT USING VITAMIN K ANTAGONISTS, RIVAROXABAN, OR ASPIRIN STUDIES (INVICTUS)[5]

Maintaining patients with rheumatic heart disease (RHD) with atrial fibrillation (AF) in the therapeutic range with VKAs has several challenges and majority patients do spend the desirable time in therapeutic range (TTR). To overcome this hurdle, newer oral anticoagulants (NOACS) have been tried in such clinical settings. This trial was a randomized, parallel, and open-label study in which patients with RHD who were at least 18 years of age and had AF/flutter and had at least one the following—mitral valve area below 2 cm^2, evidence of spontaneous contrast to thrombus in the left atrium or CHA_2DS_2-VASc score > 1. The patients were randomized into two groups one which received 20 mg of rivaroxaban daily versus the other where VKA was administered with a target international normalized ratio (INR) of 2–3. A total of 4,531 enrollees were followed up for a duration of follow-up: 3.1 years. Patients with mechanical heart valve were excluded. The primary outcomes studied included death from vascular or unknown cause, stroke, systemic embolism, or myocardial infarction (MI). The primary endpoint occurred at a rate of 8.2% and 6.5% in the rivaroxaban and VKA group respectively ($p < 0.001$). Vascular death and ischemic stroke were the secondary outcomes studied. Vascular death rates were 4.8% in the vitamin K antagonist group versus 6.3% in the rivaroxaban group ($p < 0.05$). The rates of ischemic stroke were higher in the rivaroxaban group at 1.1% versus 0.7% of the VKA group ($p < 0.05$). Thus, in RHD and AF, rivaroxaban does not prevent adverse cardiovascular events compared with a VKA. Also, the NOAC compared with a vitamin K is associated with higher rates of ischemic stroke and vascular death. This trial reiterated the guidelines which advocate the use of VKA rather than NOACS for stroke prevention among patients with RHD (moderate/severe mitral stenosis) and AF.

EFFECTS OF THE PCSK9 ANTIBODY ALIROCUMAB ON CORONARY ATHEROSCLEROSIS IN PATIENTS WITH ACUTE MYOCARDIAL INFARCTION (PACMAN-AMI)[6]

In patients presenting with acute MI (AMI) while carrying out primary angioplasty, visualization of plaques in proximal portions of nonculprit vessels is always a matter of concern to the treating cardiologist and patients as far as future events are concerned. PCSK9 antibodies have shown promise in treating such patients. Patients who underwent primary PCI to the infarct-related vessel following ACS [ST-elevation MI/non-STEMI (STEMI/NSTEMI)] with findings > 20% but <50% stenosis in the proximal portion of the other two noninfarct-related arteries along with either low-density lipoprotein cholesterol (LDL-C) at baseline ≥ 125 mg/dL and no statin treatment for 4 weeks, or ≥70 mg/dL in those who have been on stable dose of statin for 4 weeks were randomized in this trial in a 1:1 ratio to receive either 150 mg alirocumab ($n = 148$) or placebo ($n = 152$), administered biweekly via subcutaneous injection for 52 weeks. The first dose of the study drug was administered to the patient within 24 hours after PCI, without dose adjustment during the study period. Patients in both the groups received same statin in fixed dose during the whole course of the study, i.e., rosuvastatin 20 mg once daily.

A total of 300 patients aged 18 years and above were enrolled and followed up for 1 year. Patients with left main disease, prior coronary artery bypass graft (CABG), severe chronic kidney disease (CKD) or chronic liver disease (CLD), or statin intolerance were excluded. The primary endpoint was the change in mean percent atheroma volume (PAV) from baseline. In the alirocumab group versus placebo, the change was −2.13% versus −0.92% ($p < 0.001$). Secondary endpoints were favorable in the alirocumab group versus placebo group in the form that PAV regression was seen in 84.6% in alirocumab group versus 65.9% in the placebo group ($p < 0.001$). The total lipid core burden index that was evaluated on near-infrared spectroscopy imaging was also 29.3 versus −12.38 ($p = 0.004$), change in LDL-C from baseline was 131.2 versus −76.5 mg/dL ($p < 0.001$), change in HDL-C from baseline was 7% versus 3.7% ($p < 0.001$), clinical events in the form of all-cause mortality—1.4% versus 0.7% ($p > 0.05$); ischemia driven coronary revascularization—8.2% in the drug arm versus 18 5% in the placebo arm.

These beneficial results are comparable to findings of trials like the ODYSSEY OUTCOMES trial in which alirocumab when initiated 1–12 months (median 2.6 months) after an ACS presentation, a similar reduction in LDL-C was noted along with a significant reduction in major adverse cardiovascular events.

This trial also highlights the fact that early initiation must be considered in high-risk patients so as to be benefitted the most.

FRACTIONAL FLOW RESERVE AND INTRAVASCULAR ULTRASOUND-GUIDED INTERVENTION STRATEGY FOR CLINICAL OUTCOMES IN PATIENTS WITH INTERMEDIATE STENOSIS (FLAVOR)[7]

The debate as to what would be the optimal strategy [fractional flow reserve or intravascular ultrasound (FFR or IVUS)] while evaluating patients with intermediate grade coronary lesions (40–70%) in favor of revascularization has been looked at and settled by this trial. 1,682 patients were randomized to IVUS or FFR-guided strategy to decide regarding revascularization of such intermediate lesions. In the FFR group, percutaneous coronary intervention (PCI) was indicated if FFR $\leq$ 0.8 and considered optimized if post-PCI FFR $\geq$ 0.88. In the IVUS group, PCI was indicated if minimal luminal area (MLA) was $\leq$ 3 mm^2, or >3–4 mm^2 with plaque burden > 70% and considered optimized if post-PCI MLA was $\geq$5.5 mm^2 and plaque burden at stent edge was $\leq$55%. The patients were followed up for 24 months. In the FFR group, the mean FFR was 0.83 and 50% had optimized PCI. In the IVUS group, the mean MLA was 3.4 mm^2 and 55% had optimized PCI. The primary outcomes revealed no significant differences in the two groups. The rates of all cause death, MI, or revascularization at 24 months were 8.15 in the FFR-guided group and 8.5% in the IVUS group (p for noninferiority = 0.015). Secondary outcomes were also similar. This trial shows that both coronary physiology or anatomy act as equally efficient modalities when intervention is being contemplated in patients with intermediate grade coronary lesions.

EARLY AGGRESSIVE INVASIVE INTERVENTION FOR ATRIAL FIBRILLATION (EARLY-AF)[8]

Paroxysmal AF may be treated using drug therapy or cryoablation. This trial was undertaken with the aim to look at the response to the two modes of therapy available as regards to subsequent persistent AF. The study was a randomized parallel design study in which 303 patients above the age of 18 years who had symptomatic paroxysmal AF in the past 24 months underwent cryoballoon ablation (n = 154) or received antiarrhythmic drug therapy (n = 149). All patients had an implantable loop recorder placed. Two primary outcomes were studied: persistent AF and recurrent atrial tachyarrhythmias. The incidence of the former was 1.9% in the ablation group versus 7.4% in the drug group (<0.05). Recurrent atrial arrhythmias occurred in 56.5% in the ablation group versus 77.2% in the drug group. Secondary outcomes which included hospitalization and serious events were lower in the ablation group, though the latter did not reach statistical significance. The trial results favor cryoablation.

ZILEBESIRAN, AN RNA INTERFERENCE AGENT FOR HYPERTENSION[9]

Zilebesiran is the latest and much promising innovation in hypertension management. Its mRNA interference inhibits the production of angiotensinogen, the precursor of angiotensin, eventually targeting one of the main pathways in the pathogenesis of hypertension.

In the 107 patients enrolled in the trial, minimal side effects were reported (mainly of mild discomfort at the injection site were reported and no significant adverse effects like worsening of kidney functions, hyperkalemia, or episodes of hypotension) as compared what we commonly observe in conventional oral hypertensive drugs.

Significant dose-dependent efficacy was noted at 8 weeks with a 10 mm Hg drop in the blood pressure readings when zilebesiran was administered at a dose of 200 mg every 6 months and a more significant reduction of over 20 mm Hg was over the 24-week period when administered at a higher dose of 800 mg. Another two subsets were chosen—one which assessed the effect of the 800-mg dose of zilebesiran on blood pressure under low- or high-salt diet conditions, and another which looked at the effect of that dose when coadministered with irbesartan. Results from these two subsets were consistent with attenuation of the effect on blood pressure by a high-salt diet and with an augmented effect through coadministration with irbesartan, respectively.

One of the most promising aspects of zilebesiran is the convenience of its administration and dosing. Unlike the traditional oral hypertensives that need to be taken daily, this drug is administered subcutaneously and at regular intervals of approximately 6 months. This drug has the potential of significantly improving the most common challenge i.e., patient compliance, reach guideline recommended blood pressure targets, reducing the risk of cardiovascular and cerebrovascular events and leading to better health outcomes.

CHRONIC HYPERTENSION AND PREGNANCY[10]

The Chronic Hypertension and Pregnancy (CHAP) trial was undertaken to evaluate antihypertensive therapy versus control in pregnant women (gestational age < 23 weeks) with chronic hypertension and whether this strategy improves clinical outcomes. The study was a randomized, parallel, open labeled study and 2,408 women (mean age 32 years) were enrolled and followed up for a period of 34 weeks. 15.8% of participants were diabetic. In the drug therapy arm the goal of blood pressure was to achieve a blood pressure below 140/90 mm Hg. In the other group, all antihypertensive medications were withheld unless the blood pressure was ≥160/105 mm Hg.

In the active treatment group, standard medications used in first line such as labetalol and extended release nifedipine were used. The doses were up titrated as per standard recommendations and a second agent was only added once maximal dose of the first agent had been used.

The exclusion criteria included need of more than one antihypertensive medication for adequate BP control, secondary hypertension, pregnancy with more than one fetus, any obstetric conditions that might increase fetal risk, any known contraindications to the first-line antihypertensive drugs in pregnancy, or presence of any high-risk illness or complications that could warrant treatment at a lower blood pressure level. The primary outcome, composite of preeclampsia with severe features, medically indicated preterm birth at <35 weeks gestation, placental abruption, or fetal/neonatal death, occurred in 30.2% in the active treatment group versus 37.0% of the control group ($p < 0.001$).

Secondary outcomes included data on safety outcome, small for gestational age, birth weight below the 10th percentile for gestational age which was 11.2% in the active treatment group versus 10.4% in the control group ($p = 0.56$), rates of preeclampsia with severe features were 23.3% in the active treatment group versus 29.1% in the control group while fatal neonatal deaths were 3.5% in the active treatment group versus 4.3% in the control group.

This trial restates the benefits of treating chronic mild hypertension among pregnant patients.

Antihypertensive therapy to target a blood pressure <140/90 mm Hg reduced the incidence of adverse pregnancy outcomes compared with usual care. Active treatment improved overall outcomes without increasing the risk for low birth weight.

INTRAVENOUS FERRIC DERISOMALTOSE IN PATIENTS WITH HEART FAILURE AND IRON DEFICIENCY IN THE UK (IRONMAN): AN INVESTIGATOR-INITIATED, PROSPECTIVE, RANDOMIZED, OPEN-LABEL, BLINDED-ENDPOINT TRIAL[11]

Iron deficiency is not only commonly seen in patients with chronic heart failure, but it is also associated with more severe symptoms, poorer exercise capacity, and an increased risk of hospitalization and death regardless of the LVEF or hemoglobin concentrations. Improved quality of life and exercise capacity assessed at 24 weeks for ambulatory patients with heart failure and a reduced ejection fraction after treatment with intravenous ferric carboxymaltose was reported in placebo-controlled trials. Inspired by these trials, IRONMAN (Effectiveness of Intravenous Iron Treatment versus Standard Care in Patients with Heart Failure and Iron Deficiency trial was undertaken in 70 centers in the UK to look into the fact that whether repeated doses of IV iron have any effect on the CV death and hospitalization for heart failure in subset of patients with HF and iron deficiency anemia.

Patients aged 18 years or older with heart failure, and transferrin saturation < 20% or serum ferritin < 100 µg/L with LVEF ≤ 45% in the preceding 24 months were eligible. Patients were required either to have a hospital admission due to heart failure within 6 months or have NT-proBNP > 250 ng/L if patient was in sinus rhythm. The cut off values for diagnosis were a NT proBNP level > 1,000 ng/L if patient was in AF, or BNP > 75 ng/L in sinus rhythm or >300 ng/L in AF. Patients were excluded from the study if they had serum ferritin levels in excess of 400 µg/L or hemoglobin concentration was below 9 g/dL and also men and women with hemoglobin concentration >14 g/dL and >13 g/dL, respectively were excluded. 1,137 patients were randomly assigned of whom 569 received intravenous ferric derisomaltose and 568 patients were given usual care. The median duration of follow-up was 2.7 years.

Dose of ferric derisomaltose was determined on the basis of hemoglobin value and bodyweight **(Table 1)**.

Trial visits were planned at 4 weeks after the random assignment and every 4 months thereafter until the trial was completed. The dose ferric derisomaltose in the drug group was repeated if ferritin was <100 µg/L irrespective of transferrin saturation or if ferritin was 400 µg/L or less with transferrin saturation < 25%.

At 4 months, those randomized to ferric derisomaltose had a better overall quality of life score and physical domain score on the Minnesota living with heart failure questionnaire compared with those in the usual care group, however, there were no differences between the groups in these scores at 20 months or in the 6-minute walk test distance at 4 months.

No serious adverse events were noted in the iron replacement group. The usual care group on the other hand

TABLE 1: Dose of ferric derisomaltose was determined on the basis of hemoglobin value and bodyweight.

Body weight	Dose of intravenous ferric derisomaltose
<50 kg	20 mg/kg, irrespective of hemoglobin
50–70 kg	1,000 mg if hemoglobin was 10 g/dL or more and dose was 20 mg/kg if hemoglobin was <10 g/dL
>70 kg	20 mg/kg up to a maximum of 1,500 mg if hemoglobin was 10 g/dL or more, or 2,000 mg if hemoglobin was <10 g/dL

reported increased incidence of adverse events such as heart failure, acute coronary events, and cardiac arrest. Blood transfusions, hemorrhages, hospital admissions, and deaths for infections were in a similar number of for those assigned to ferric derisomaltose and usual care.

This trial highlights the basis for IV iron replacement when needed and the fact that it leads to multiple clinical benefits.

REVIVED BALLOON PUMP-ASSISTED CORONARY INTERVENTION STUDY (BCIS) TRIAL[12]

Optimal medical therapy has proved to beneficial in many clinical scenarios. One such setting is severe ischemic LV systolic dysfunction—the question is whether such patients should be subject to revascularization by PCI or medical therapy (i.e., individually adjusted pharmacologic and device therapy for heart failure) and as to what would be the outcomes of the two strategies as far as event-free survival and LV function in such patients is concerned.

About 700 patients with severe LV dysfunction and demonstrable myocardial viability were assigned to revascularization with PCI along with optimal medical management or optimal medical management group.

Death from any cause or hospitalization for heart failure was the primary endpoints. Major secondary outcomes were LVEF at 6 months and at the end of the first year and quality-of-life scores.

About 347 patients were assigned to the PCI group and 353 patients to the optimal-medical therapy group. When followed up over a median of 41 months, 37.2% ($n = 129$) and 38.0% ($n = 134$) patients in the PCI and optimal-medical-therapy group [hazard ratio 0.99; 95% confidence interval (CI) 0.78–1.27; $p = 0.96$] has a primary event. The LVEF was also similar in the two groups at 6 months and at 12 months. Quality-of-life scores at 6 and 12 months appeared to favor the PCI group, but the difference had diminished at 24 months.

The authors concluded that in patients with severe ischemic LV systolic dysfunction who received optimal medical therapy, revascularization by PCI did not result in a lower incidence of death from any cause or hospitalization for heart failure.

TABLE 2: Secondary outcome in immediate and delayed revascularization groups.

Outcome	Immediate complete revascularization group	Delayed complete revascularization group
All-cause death rates	1.9%	1.2% ($p = 0.30$)
MI	1.9%	4.5% ($p = 0.0045$)
Unplanned revascularization	4.2%	6.7% ($p = 0.030$)

IMMEDIATE VERSUS STAGED COMPLETE REVASCULARIZATION IN PATIENTS PRESENTING WITH ACUTE CORONARY SYNDROME AND MULTIVESSEL CORONARY DISEASE (BIOVASC): A PROSPECTIVE, OPEN-LABEL, NONINFERIORITY, RANDOMIZED TRIAL[13]

There is always a dilemma as to whether in acute coronary syndromes the patients should be subject to immediate complete revascularization or delayed revascularization (around 6 weeks). This has been addressed to in the present trial. A total of 1,525 patients with ACS (NSTEMI 53.0% and STEMI 40%) were included in this randomized, parallel design, open-labeled trial. 764 patients were assigned to the immediate revascularization group and 761 to the delayed revascularization group. The duration of follow-up was 12 months.

All-cause mortality, MI, and unplanned revascularization were the primary outcomes and occurred at rates of 7.6% and 9.4% in the immediate and delayed revascularization groups.

Secondary outcomes are given in **Table 2**.

CONCLUSION

Constant perseverance on the part of the doctors, scientists, and industry brings about exciting advances each year opening up greater avenues for medical care of human mankind. The above discussion is an apt example of the same. Well-designed clinical trials shall continue to guide us in the coming years and help the medical fraternity in providing rational medical care to the community at large.

ONLINE REFERENCES

Please scan the QR code provided at the end of the table of contents for References of this chapter.

INDEX

Page numbers followed by *b* refer to box, *f* refer to figure, *fc* refer to flowchart, and *t* refer to table.

A

B

C

D

E

F

G

H

I

J

K

L

M

Q

R

S

T

U

V

W

X

Y

Z

Cardiological Society of India

CARDIOLOGY

UPDATE 2023

Cardiological Society of India

CARDIOLOGY

UPDATE 2023

Volume 2

Editor-in-Chief

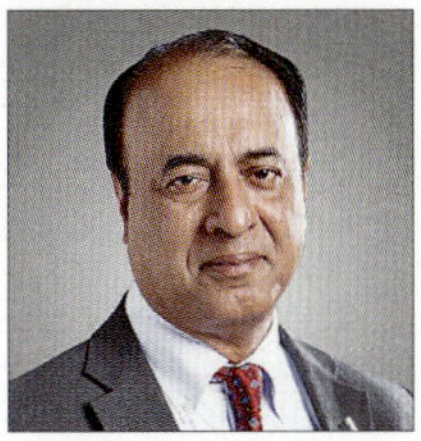

Pratap Chandra Rath
MD DM FICC FESC FACC FRCP (London) FRCP (Edinburgh)
Senior Consultant Cardiologist and HOD
Department of Cardiology
Apollo Hospital, Jubilee Hills
Hyderabad, Telangana
Apollo Hospital
Bhubaneshwar, Odisha, India

Co-Editors

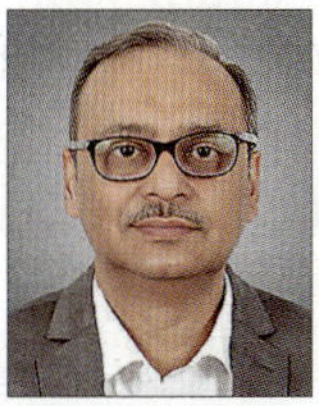

Manoj Kumar Agarwala
MD (PGI) DM (PGI) FACC
Consultant Cardiologist
Department of Cardiology
Apollo Hospital, Jubilee Hills
Hyderabad, Telangana, India

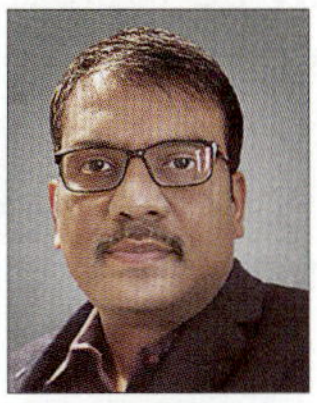

Sundar Chidambaram
MD DNB DM FNB
Senior Consultant Interventional Cardiologist
Kauvery Hospital
Chennai, Tamil Nadu, India

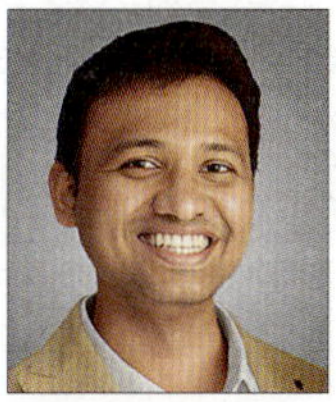

Shabbir Ali Shaik
MD DM FNB
Fellow Interventional Cardiologist
Department of Cardiology
Apollo Hospital, Jubilee Hills
Hyderabad, Telangana, India

Foreword

Alain Cribier

JAYPEE

JAYPEE BROTHERS MEDICAL PUBLISHERS
The Health Sciences Publisher
New Delhi | London

Jaypee Brothers Medical Publishers (P) Ltd

Headquarters
EMCA House
23/23-B, Ansari Road, Daryaganj
New Delhi 110 002, India
Landline: +91-11-23272143, +91-11-23272703
+91-11-23282021, +91-11-23245672
E-mail: jaypee@jaypeebrothers.com

Corporate Office
Jaypee Brothers Medical Publishers (P) Ltd.
4838/24, Ansari Road, Daryaganj
New Delhi 110 002, India
Phone: +91-11-43574357
Fax: +91-11-43574314
E-mail: jaypee@jaypeebrothers.com

Overseas Office
JP Medical Ltd.
83, Victoria Street, London
SW1H 0HW (UK)
Phone: +44-20 3170 8910
Fax: +44(0)20 3008 6180
E-mail: info@jpmedpub.com

Website: www.jaypeebrothers.com
Website: www.jaypeedigital.com

Inquiries for bulk sales may be solicited at: jaypee@jaypeebrothers.com

***CSI Cardiology Update 2023 (Volume 2)* / Pratap Chandra Rath**

First Edition: **2024**

ISBN: 978-93-5696-437-2

Printed at: Samrat Offset Pvt. Ltd.

DEDICATION

The CSI Update Book 2023 is dedicated to all cardiologists and students in particular

Pratap Chandra Rath

CONTRIBUTORS

Editor-in-Chief

Pratap Chandra Rath MD DM FICC FESC FACC FRCP (London) FRCP (Edinburgh)
Senior Consultant Cardiologist and HOD
Department of Cardiology
Apollo Hospital, Jubilee Hills
Hyderabad, Telangana
Apollo Hospital
Bhubaneshwar, Odisha, India

Co-Editors

Manoj Kumar Agarwala MD (PGI) DM (PGI) FACC
Consultant Cardiologist
Department of Cardiology
Apollo Hospital, Jubilee Hills
Hyderabad, Telangana, India

Sundar Chidambaram MD DNB DM FNB
Senior Consultant Interventional Cardiologist
Kauvery Hospital
Chennai, Tamil Nadu, India

Shabbir Ali Shaik MD DM FNB
Fellow Interventional Cardiologist
Department of Cardiology
Apollo Hospital, Jubilee Hills
Hyderabad, Telangana, India

Contributing Authors

Aarya Naik MBBS
Research Assistant
Marengo CIMS Hospital
Ahmedabad, Gujarat, India

Abdul S Talpur MD
Research Student
Department of Cardiology
West Virginia University School of Medicine
Morgantown, WV, USA

Abha Bajaj Nee Sheth MS
Associate Professor
Department of Anatomy
Dr Harvansh Singh Judge Institute of Dental Sciences and Hospital
Panjab University
Chandigarh, India

Abhinav Shrivastava MD DM
Consultant
Maharaja Agrasen Hospital
Punjabi Bagh, New Delhi, India

Abhishek MD DM
Resident, Department of Cardiology
Dayanand Medical College and Hospital
Unit Hero DMC Heart Institute
Ludhiana, Punjab, India

Abraham Oomman MD DM (Cardiology)
Senior Consultant Interventional Cardiologist
Department of Cardiology
Apollo Main Hospital
Chennai, Tamil Nadu, India

Aditi Parimoo MD
Senior Resident
Department of Cardiology
KEM Hospital, Parel
Mumbai, Maharashtra, India

Aditi Rastogi DNB (Medicine) DM-PDT
Postdoctoral Trainee
Department of Cardiology
Medical College
Kolkata, West Bengal, India

Aditi Singhvi MBBS Fellowship in Cardiovascular Medicine (USA)
Consultant – Heart Failure and Transplant Cardiology
Narayana Institute of Cardiac Sciences
Narayana Health City
Bengaluru, Karnataka, India

Aditya Goyal MD (Medicine)
DM Cardiology Resident 2nd Year
Mahatma Gandhi Medical College and Hospital
Jaipur, Rajasthan, India

Aftab Khan MD (Medicine) DM (Cardiology) DNB (Cardiology)
Consultant Interventional Cardiologist
Director Electrophysiology Services
Apollo Multispeciality Hospitals
Kolkata, West Bengal, India

Ajay Bahl DM FRCP
Professor
Department of Cardiology
Postgraduate Institute of Medical Education and Research
Chandigarh, India

Ajay Naik MD DM DNB FACC FHRS
Cardiac Electrophysiologist
Room 1, CIMS East
Marengo CIMS Hospital
Ahmedabad, Gujarat, India

Ajit Desai MD (Medicine) DM DNB (Cardiology)
Additional Director
Jaslok Hospital
Consultant Cardiologist
HN Reliance, Breach Candy, Nanavati, Asian Heart Hospitals
Mumbai, Maharashtra, India

Ajit S Mullasari MD DM
Director
Department of Cardiology
Institute of Cardio Vascular Diseases
The Madras Medical Mission Hospital
Professor of Practice
Indian Institute of Technology – Madras
Chennai, Tamil Nadu, India

Ajoe John Kattoor MD
Staff Cardiologist
Division of Cardiovascular Medicine
Northwest Health
La Porte and Porter, IN, USA

Akash MD (Radiodiagnosis)
Senior Resident
Department of Imaging
Fortis Escort Heart Institute
New Delhi, India

AK Pancholia MD FACC FESC FCSI FISH FIMSA MAMS
Head
Department of Medicine, Clinical and Preventive Cardiology
Arihant Hospital
Indore, Madhya Pradesh, India
BC Roy and Charak Awardee of MPIMA

Alain Cribier MD FACC FESC
Emeritus Professor of Medicine
Former Head
Department of Cardiology
University Hospital Charles Nicolle
Rouen, France
Adviser for Cardiology Programs
Rouen Normandy Medical Training Center

Alla Gopala Krishna Gokhale MS MCh DNB SMP (IIM-C) DSc (Hon)
Cardiothoracic and Transplant Surgeon, Apollo Hospitals, Jubilee Hills
Hyderabad, Telangana, India

Amal Kumar Khan MD MNAMS DM
Former Professor of Cardiology
WBMES
Visiting Consultant
AMRI Hospital, Salt Lake
Kolkata, West Bengal, India

Aman Makhija MD DM
Senior Consultant Cardiologist
Sir Ganga Ram Hospital
New Delhi, India

Aman T Patel MD DM
Consultant Interventional Cardiologist, Apex Heart Institute
Ahmedabad, Gujarat, India

Amartya Khan MD
RMO Clinical Tutor
JNM Medical College, Kalyani
Kolkata, West Bengal, India

Amitabha Chattopadhyay DCH DNB Fellowship in Pediatric Cardiology (Australia)
Chief Pediatric Cardiologist and Clinical Lead Eastern India
Department of Pediatric Cardiology
Narayana Superspeciality Hospital
Howrah, West Bengal, India

Amit Garg MD (Radiodiagnosis)
Senior Consultant
Department of Imaging
Fortis Escort Heart Institute
New Delhi, India

Amit Kumar Chaurasia MD DM FESC FAPSIC
Unit Chief (1), Chief Cath Lab, Chief TAVR and Structural Heart Disease
Artemis Hospital
Gurugram, Haryana, India

Amit Patel MD
Cardiologist
Magnum Heart Institute
Nashik, Maharashtra, India

Amritesh Biswas MD
Postdoctoral Trainee
Institute of Postgraduate Medical Education and Research
Kolkata, West Bengal, India

Anand M MD DM (Cardiology) Fellowship in EP
Associate Professor
Christian Medical College Hospital
Vellore, Tamil Nadu, India

Anantharaman Rajaram MRCP FRCP CCT (Cardiology)
Senior Consultant Interventional Cardiologist
Clinical Lead
Advanced Heart Failure, Cardiomyopathy and Transplantation, Transcatheter Valve Therapy
Kauvery Hospital
Chennai, Tamil Nadu, India

(Col) Anil Dhall Sena Medal MD (Medicine) DM (Cradiology) FACC FESC FAHA FRCP (Edinburgh) FSCAI FHRS FCSI
Professor and Head
Department of Cardiology
Janakpuri Super Speciality Hospital
New Delhi, India

Anil J MD DNB (Cardiology)
Former Professor and Head
Deaprtment of Cardiology
Dutta Meghe Institute of Medical Sciences
Wardha, Maharashtra, India

Anil Sharma MD (Medicine) DM (Cardiology) FAPSC (Taiwan), DSc FWSIM FSCAI (USA) FACC (USA) Advanced Fellowship in Complex Angioplasty (Italy)
Professor, Head and Senior Consultant and Interventional Cardiologist
Department of Cardiology
Bombay Hospital and Medical Research Centre
Mumbai, Maharashtra, India

Anil Sivadasan Radha MD DCH DNB (Pediatrics) DNB (Cardiology)
Senior Consultant and Head
Department of Pediatric Cardiology
Lisie Hospital
Kochi, Kerala, India

Anirban Das MD DM
Senior Resident
Burdwan Medical College
Burdwan, West Bengal, India

Anirudda Deshpande MD (Internal Medicine) DM (Neurology) FRCP (London) FRCP (Edinburgh) DNB Neurology Fellowship in Stroke (Canada)
Consultant Neurologist
Vinayaka Neuro Multispecialty Centre
Warangal, Telangana, India

Anita Saxena MD DM FACC
Vice Chancellor
Pt BD Sharma University of Health Sciences
Rohtak, Haryana, India

Anju Nohria MD
Director
Cardio-Oncology and Cancer Survivorship Program
Dana Farber Cancer Institute
Cardiovascular Division
Brigham and Women's Hospital
Harvard Medical School
Boston, MA, USA

Ankit Gulia DNB
Senior Resident
Department of Cardiology
Dayanand Medical College and Hospital
Ludhiana, Punjab, India

Ankur Gautam MD DM (Cardiology)
Assistant Professor
Department of Cardiology
GB Pant Institute of Postgraduate Medical Education and Research
New Delhi, India

Ankush Gupta MD DM FACC
Professor of Medicine and Interventional Cardiologist
Department of Cardiology
Army Institute of Cardio Thoracic Sciences (AICTS)
Pune, Maharashtra, India

Anoop Agrawal MBBS MD FACC
American Board Certified in Internal Medicine, Cardiovascular Diseases, and Interventional Cardiology
Consultant Cardiologist
Krishna Institute of Medical Sciences
Secunderabad, Telangana, India

Anuj Gupta MBBS
All India Institute of Medical Sciences
Bhopal, Madhya Pradesh, India

Anuradha D MD DNB (Cardiology)
Junior Consultant
Apollo Hospital
Visakhapatnam, Andhra Pradesh, India

Anushree D Kumbhalkar MD (Medicine)
Senior Resident
Department of Cardiology
Bombay Hospital and Medical Research Centre
Mumbai, Maharashtra, India

Aqdas Mumtaz MD
Senior Resident
Department of Cardiology
Institute of Medical Sciences
Banaras Hindu University
Varanasi, Uttar Pradesh, India

Aravind Duruvasal MD DM
Consultant Interventional Cardiologist
SNN Specialities Clinic and SNN Diagnostic Centre
Chennai, Tamil Nadu, India

Aravind MS MPH
Research Associate
Department of Public Health
Amrita Institute of Medical Science
Kochi, Kerala, India

Arijit Ghosh MD DM
Consultant Interventional Cardiologist
Department of Cardiology
AMRI Hospital, Salt Lake
Kolkata, West Bengal, India

Arijit Kumar Ghosh MD DM FACC FESC FSCAI FAPSIC FAPVS FICC
Professor and Head
Department of Cardiology
All India Institute of Medical Sciences
Nagpur, Maharashtra, India

Arijt Ghosh MD DM (Cardiology)
In-charge, Cath Lab
AMRI Hospital
Kolkata, West Bengal, India

Arshdeep Singh Sandhu MD (Medicine) DM-PDT
Postdoctoral Trainee
Department of Cardiology
Medical College
Kolkata, West Bengal, India

Arun Kumar MD DM (Cardiology)
Fellow Peripheral Vascular and Aortic Intervention
Christian Medical College
Vellore, Tamil Nadu, India

Arun Mohanty MD DM
Professor, Sir Ganga Ram Hospital
New Delhi, India

Arup Dasbiswas MD DM (Cardiology) FACC FESC FSCAI
Director, Cath Lab
BMRC Hospital
Ex-Director, ICVS, IPGME&R
Ex-Professor and Head
Department of Cardiology
IPGME&R and SSKM Hospital
Kolkata, West Bengal, India

Asesh Haldar MD DM
Consultant, Medica Institute of Cardiology Sciences
Kolkata, West Bengal, India

Asha Mahilmaran MD DNB DM FCSI FACC FESC FSCAI
Senior Interventional Consultant Cardiologist, Apollo Hospitals
Chennai, Tamil Nadu, India

Asha Moorthy MD DM FCCP FIACM FICP FIMSA FICC
Professor and Head
Sri Ramachandra Medical College and Saveetha Medical College (Former)
Chennai, Tamil Nadu, India

Ashesh Halder MD (Medicine, Gold Medalist) DM (Cardiology) Fellowship in Electrophysiology
Consultant – Medica Institute of Cardiology Services
Medica Institute of Cardiac Science
Kolkata, West Bengal, India

Ashish Deshpande MD DM (Cardiology) FACC
Consultant Interventional Cardiologist
Oriion Citicare Superspeciality Hospital
Ex-Professor and Head
MGM Medical College and Hospital
Aurangabad, Maharashtra, India

Ashish Jai Kishan MD DNB
Senior Consultant Interventional Cardiology
Fortis Escorts Heart Institute
New Delhi, India

Ashish Kumar MD DM
Associate Consultant
Division of Interventional Cardiology
Medanta Heart Institute
Medanta – The Medicity
Gurugram, Haryana, India

Ashish Kumar Jain MD DNB (Cardiology)
Associate Consultant Cardiologist
Sir Ganga Ram Hospital
New Delhi, India

Ashok Seth FRCP FACC MSCAI FAPSIC DSc
Chairman
Fortis Escorts Heart Institute
New Delhi, India

Ashraf SM MD DM FACC
Professor and Head
Department of Cardiology
GMC Kannur, Hrudayalaya
Kannur, Kerala, India

Ashwin B Mehta MD FACC FCCP FISE FICP
Interventional Cardiologist
Director of Cardiology
Jaslok Hospital and Research Centre
Mumbai, Maharashtra, India

Ashwin Mahesh MD
Cardiovascular Disease Fellow
UPMC Harrisburg
Harrisburg, PA, USA

Asit Das MD DM (Cardiology)
Associate Professor
IPGME&R and SSKM Hospital
Kolkata, West Bengal, India

Asmita Samal MD DNB (Medicine)
Senior Resident
DY Patil Medical College
Pune, Maharashtra, India

Asok Kumar Kar MD DM FACC
Senior Interventional Cardiologist
Peerless Hospitals
Kolkata, West Bengal, India

Atul Mathur MD DM
Executive Director Interventional Cardiology and Chief of Cardiac Cath Labs
Fortis Escorts Heart Institute
New Delhi, India

Auriom Kar MD DM
Consultant
Department of Cardiology
Narayana Multispeciality Hospital
Kolkata, West Bengal, India

Avani Jain MD
Medical Officer
DNS Hospital
Indore, Madhya Pradesh, India

Ayan Kar DNB (General Medicine) DNB (Cardiology)
Interventional Cardiologist and Clinical Lead in Heart Failure Services
Narayana Health-Rabindranath Tagore
International Institute of Cardiac Sciences
Kolkata, West Bengal, India

Babu Reddy MD DM (Cardiology)
Associate Professor
Department of Cardiology
Sri Jayadeva Institute of Cardiovascular Sciences and Research
Bengaluru, Karnataka, India

Badrinarayana Tumula MD DM FICC FESC FIAMS LICC
Senior Consultant Cardiologist
Apollo Hospital, Jubilee Hills
Hyderabad, Telangana, India

Bagirath Raghuraman MD DNB DM (Cardiology) FESC FSCAI FHFA
Senior Consultant Cardiologist and Program Director
Heart Transplant
Narayana Institute of Cardiac Sciences
Narayana Health City
Bengaluru, Karnataka, India

Bahuleyan CG MD DM FRCP FSCAI
Chairman
Cardiovascular Centre
Ananthapuri Hospitals and Research Institute
Thiruvananthapuram, Kerala, India

Baruah DK DM FACC FSCAI FICC FCSI
Senior Consultant and Director
Catheterization Laboratory
Apollo Hospital, Health City
Visakhapatnam, Andhra Pradesh, India

BC Srinivas MD DM (Cardiology)
Professor
Department of Cardiology
Sri Jayadeva Institute of Cardiovascular Sciences and Research
Bengaluru, Karnataka, India

Bharat Vijay Purohit MD DM
Senior Consultant and Director of Cathlab
Department of Cardiology
Yashoda Hospital Hitech City
Hyderabad, Telangana, India

B Hygriv Rao MD DM FACC FESC
Senior Consultant Cardiologist and Director
Division of Pacing and Electrophysiology
KIMS Group of Hospitals,
Hyderabad, Telangana, India

Biswajit Majumder MD DM FACC
Professor and Head
Department of Cardiology
RG Kar Medical College and Hospital
Kolkata, West Bengal, India

Biswaranjan Mishra MD DM FCSI FIAE FICC
Senior Consultant Cardiologist
Max Diagnostic
Cuttack, Odisha, India

BKS Sastry MD DM FACC
Head
Department of Cardiology
CARE Hospital
Hyderabad, Telangana, India

Blessvin Jino MD DM
Consultant Cardiologist
Meditrina Hospital
Kollam, Kerala, India

Brian Pinto MD DM FACC FSCAI
Director and Consultant Interventional Cardiologist
Holy Family Hospital, Breach Candy, Khar Hinduja, Saifee, Nanavati
Mumbai, Maharashtra, India

B Srinivas MD DM
Professor and Head
Department of Cardiology
NIMS
Hyderabad, Telangana, India

BVA Ranga Reddy MD DM
Consultant Cardiologist
Apollo Hospital, Jubilee Hills
Hyderabad, Telangana, India

Byomakesh Dikshit MD DM (Cardiology)
Senior Consultant
Apollo Hospitals
Bhubaneswar, Odisha, India

Chhabi Satpathy MD DM
Professor and Head
Division of Cardiology
MKCG Medical College
Berhampur, Odisha, India

Chaitanya Gupta MBBS
Final Year Student
Santosh University
Ghaziabad, Uttar Pradesh, India

Chakradhar P MD DM
Consultant, Apollo Hospital
Visakhapatnam, Andhra Pradesh, India

Chandan Kumar Das MD (Medicine) DNB (Cardiology)
Assistant Professor
Advance Cardiology Institute
Pt JNM Medical College
Raipur, Chhattisgarh, India

Chandrakanta Mishra MD (Medicine) DM (Cardiology) FACC FCSI FICC FESC
Associate Professor
Department of Cardiology
SCB Medical College and Hospital
Cuttack, Odisha, India

Chandrashekhar K Ponde MD DM (Medicine) DNB (Cardiology)
Consultant Cardiologist
Head
Department of Cardiology
PD Hinduja National Hospital and MRC
Mumbai, Maharashtra, India

Chan KS Mike BSc (Science) Researcher Stem Cell
Professor, Researcher and Author
Founder
European Wellness Biomedical Group
Germany

Chinmay Gupta MBBS FICC MBA (Hospital Administration)
Clinical Associate (Cardiology)
Indraprastha Apollo Hospitals
New Delhi, India

CM Nagesh MD DM (Cardiology)
Professor
Department of Cardiology
Sri Jayadeva Institute of Cardiovascular Sciences and Research
Bengaluru, Karnataka, India

C Narasimhan MD DM
Head
Department of Cardiac Electrophysiology
AIG Hospital
Hyderabad, Telangana, India

C Venkata S Ram MD MACP FACC FASH
Director
Apollo Institute for Blood Pressure Management
Apollo Group of Hospitals
Hyderabad, Telangana, India
Professor of Internal Medicine
University of Texas Southwestern Medical Center
Dallas, TX, USA

Darshan Krishnappa MD DM FACC
Assistant Professor
Sri Jayadeva Institute of Cardiac Sciences and Research
Bengaluru, Karnataka, India

Dayasagar Rao V DM FRCP (Canada) FRCP (Edinburgh)
Consultant Cardiologist
KIMS Hospital
Secunderabad, Telangana, India

Debabrata Dash MD DM FICC FAPSC FCCP FSCAI FACC FESC
Director and Consultant Interventional Cardiologist
Department of Cardiology
Aster Hospital Mankhool
Dubai, Al Quasis, UAE

Debabrata Roy MD DM (Cardiology) FACC FESC FSCAI FAHA
Senior Consultant Interventional Cardiologist and Academic Co-ordinator
NH-RTIICS
Kolkata, West Bengal, India

Debasish Roychoudhury MD FACC FASE
Clinical Associate Professor
Department of Medicine
Weill Cornell University
New York, NY, USA

Debdatta Bhattacharyya MD MRCP CCST (Cardiology)
Senior Interventional Cardiologist
Clinical Director and Chief of Cathlab Services
Narayana Health RN Tagore Hospital
Kolkata, West Bengal, India

Debika Chatterjee MD
Senior Consultant and Head
Department of Noninvasive Cardiology
NH RTIICS
Kolkata, West Bengal, India

Debopriyo Mondal MD (Internal Medicine, Gold Medalist) DM (Cardiology)
Consultant Interventional Cardiologist
Medica Institute of Cardiac Science
Kolkata, West Bengal, India

Deepak Padmanabhan DM (Cardiology) Fellowship in Electrophysiology and Advanced Adult Cardiology (USA)
Assistant Professor
Department of Electrophysiology
Sri Jayadeva Institute of Cardiac Sciences and Research
Bengaluru, Karnataka, India

Deepak Ranjan Das MD DM (Cardiology)
Associate Professor
SCB Medical College and Hospital
Cuttack, Odisha, India

Deepanjan Bhattacharya MD DM
Senior Consultant
Advanced Cardiac Centre
BR Singh Hospital and Centre for Medical Education and Research
Eastern Railways
Kolkata, West Bengal, India

Deepesh Agarwal MD (Medicine) DM (Cardiology)
Professor, Department of Cardiology
Mahatma Gandhi Medical College and Hospital
Jaipur, Rajasthan, India

Devanu Ghosh Roy MD DM MRCP (UK) FRCP (London)
Senior Consultant
Advanced Cardiac Centre
BR Singh Hospital and Centre for Medical Education and Research
Eastern Railways
Kolkata, West Bengal, India

Devesh Kumar MD DM
Senior Resident
Department of Cardiology
All India Institute of Medical Sciences
New Delhi, India

Dev Pahlajani MD FACC FSCAI
Head
Department of Cardiology
Breach Candy Hospital
Mumbai, Maharashtra, India

Devyani Dogra MBBS
Student
American International College of Arts and Science
Antigua

Dheeraj Kela MD
Senior Resident
Department of Cardiology
Institute of Medical Sciences
Banaras Hindu University
Varanasi, Uttar Pradesh, India

Dhiman Kahali MD Dip (Cardiology) DM (Cardiology)
Senior Consultant and Director
BM Birla Heart Research Centre
Kolkata, West Bengal, India

Dibya Kumar Baruah MD DM (CMC, Vellore) FACC FSCAI FAPSC FCSI
Senior Consultant Cardiologist and Director
Interventional Cardiology and Cardiac Catheterization Laboratory
Apollo Hospitals, Health City
Visakhapatnam, Andhra Pradesh, India

Dilip Kumar MD DM FACC FRCP (Glasgow) FSCAI FESC FICC FHRS FHFA Certified Cardiac Device Specialist (CCDS, HRS, USA)
Director – Cardiac Cath Lab Services
Senior Consultant Interventional Cardiologist and Electrophylogist
Chief Academic Co-ordinator
Medica Institute of Cardiac Science
Kolkata, West Bengal, India

Dipanjan Chatterjee MD FNB (Cardiac Anaesthesia)
Head, Department of Cardiopulmonary Critical Care
Director
ECMO and Transplant Programme (Heart and Lungs)
Medica Institute of Cardiac Science
Kolkata, West Bengal, India

Dipankar Ghosh Dastidar DCH MD (Medicine) DM (Cardiology) FESC FACC FICP FCSI FSCAI
Associate Professor and Head
Department of Cardiology
Burdwan Medical College
Burdwan, West Bengal, India

Dixit Goyal MD
Senior Resident
Department of Cardiology
GB Pant Hospital
New Delhi, India

Donovon Allen MD
Internal Medicine Resident
Department of Medicine
University of Alabama
Birmingham, AL, USA

Dorairaj Prabhakaran MD DM (Cardiology) MSc FRCP FNASc FNA DSc (Honoris Causa)
Executive Director, Centre for Chronic Disease Control (CCDC)
Distinguished Professor – Public Health Foundation of India (PHFI)
New Delhi, India
Professor, Department of Epidemiology
London School of Hygiene and Tropical Medicine, UK
Adjunct Professor, Rollins School of Public Health, Emory University, USA

DP Sinha MD DM
Head, Department of Cardiology
ILS Hospital
Dumdum, West Bengal, India

DS Gambhir MD DM FAMS FCSI FICC FCAPSC FSCAI FACC (USA)
Padma Shri Awardee
Group Director, Cardiology
Kailash Health Care Ltd
Director
Kailash Hospital and Heart Institute
Noida, Uttar Pradesh, India

Evgeniya V Shalaeva MD MPH CHES
Dean, School of Medicine, Central Asian University
Tashkent, Uzbekistan

Filippo Crea MD
Department of Cardiovascular Medicine
Fondazione Policlinico Universitario Agostino Gemelli IRCCS
Department of Cardiovascular and Pulmonary Sciences, Catholic University of the Sacred Heart
Rome, Italy

Florian A Wenzl MD
Research Assistant
Center for Molecular Cardiology
University of Zurich
Switzerland and Zurich Heart House
Zürich, Switzerland

Franz H Messerli MD HonD FACC FESC
Department of BioMedical Research
University of Bern, Switzerland
Jagiellonian University Krakow, Poland

G Ashok MD DM
Associate Professor and Senior Interventional Cardiologist
Chettinad Academy of Research and Education
Chettinad Super Speciality Hospital
Chennai, Tamil Nadu, India

Ganesh Jagdale MD
Cardiologist
Magnum Heart Institute
Nashik, Maharashtra, India

Gaurav Agarwal MD DM
Consultant
Department of Cardiology
Narayana Multispeciality Hospital
Kolkata, West Bengal, India

Gaurav Kumar Arora MD DM
Assistant Professor
Department of Cardiology
Vardhman Mahavir Medical College and Safdarjung Hospital
New Delhi, India

George Wuni MD
Postgraduate Year 3 Resident
Department of Internal Medicine
Harlem Hospital Center in affiliation with Columbia University
New York, NY, USA

Girish B Navasundi MD DNB
Senior Consultant Cardiologist
Director, Cath Lab
Apollo Hospital
Bengaluru, Karnataka, India

Girish MP MD DM
Professor
Department of Cardiology
GB Pant Hospital
New Delhi, India

Giuseppe Mancia MD PhD
Emeritus Professor of Medicine
University of Milano-Bicocca
Milan, Italy

G Justin Paul MD DNB (Medicine) DM DNB (Cardiology) FACC FESC
Director and Head (i/c)
Department of Cardiology
Madras Medical College
Chennai, Tamil Nadu, India

GN Mahapatra FRCP (Glasgow) DRM (Delhi University) FCSI (India) FCCP (USA) FRSH (UK) Spl Train Nucl Med (University of Texas, MD Anderson, Houston)
Consultant and Head
Department of Nuclear Medicine and PET-CT
SPECT–CT Seven Hills Hospital (JCI, USA Accredited)
Mumbai, Maharashtra
Director
Department of Nuclear Medicine and PET-CT
Sri Aurobindo Institute of Medical Sciences (SAIMS)
Indore, Madhya Pradesh, India
President – World Federation of Cardiac Imaging and Clinical Cardiology

Gopala Krishna Koduru MD DM
Consultant Cardiologist
Aayush Hospitals
Vijayawada and Eluru,
Andhra Pradesh, India

Gopal Chandra Ghosh DM (Cardiology) FACC FESC FSCAI
Consultant Interventional Cardiologist
Director, Cath Lab
Rabindranath Thakur Diagnostic and Medical Care Center
Berhampore, West Bengal, India

Gourav Bhattacharya MD DM (Cardiology)
Senior Resident
Department of Cardiology
Burdwan Medical College and Hospital
Burdwan, West Bengal, India

Goutam Datta MD DNB DM MRCP (UK) FESC FSCAI
Professor
Institute of Postgraduate Medical Education and Research
Kolkata, West Bengal, India

Guido Grassi MD
Clinica Medica
University of Milano-Bicocca
Milan, Italy

Gunjan Ghodeshwar DM (Cardiology)
Assistant Professor
Department of Cardiology
All India Institute of Medical Sciences
Nagpur, Maharashtra, India

Gurpreet Singh Wander MD DM FACC FAMS
Professor
Department of Cardiology
Dayanand Medical College and Hospital
Unit Hero DMC Heart Institute
Ludhiana, Punjab, India

G Venkateshwara Reddy MD DM
Head
Department of Cardiology
Star Pinnacle Heart Centre
Visakhapatnam, Andhra Pradesh, India

Harendra Kumar MD (Medicine) PhD (Medicine) FICP FIAE FCSI FICC
National Professor of Medicine, Senior Consultant Cardiologist, Ex-Director
Indira Gandhi Institute of Cardiology
Patna Medical College Campus
Visiting Senior Consultant Cardiologist
Jeevak Heart Hospital
Patna, Bihar, India

Haresh G Mehta MD (Medicine) DNB (Cardiology) FACC FESC FSCAI
Director of Cardiology
Healing Hearts
Mumbai, Maharashtra, India

Harikrishnan S DM FACC FRCP FAMS
Head and Professor
Department of Cardiology
SCTIMST
Thiruvananthapuram, Kerala, India

Harshit Khare MD DM (Cardiology)
Assistant Professor
Department of Cardiology
Sanjay Gandhi Postgraduate Institute of Medical Sciences
Lucknow, Uttar Pradesh, India

Hemant K Satpathy MD
Maternal-Foetal- Medicine (MFN) Specialist
Methodist Women's Hospital
Omaha, NE, USA

Himanshu Dabral MD DM
Director
Division of Interventional Cardiology
Medanta Heart Institute
Medanta – The Medicity
Gurugram, Haryana, India

Himanshu Jain MD
Senior Resident
Department of Gastroenterology
Superspeciality Hospital
MGM Medical College
Indore, Madhya Pradesh, India

HK Chopra MD DM FRCP FACC FISC FISCU FASE FCSI FIAE FIMSA
Senior Consultant Cardiologist
Medanta Moolchand Heart Institute
New Delhi, India
Past President – National CSI
Past Editor – IHJ, JIAE
Past President – National IAE
Country Head, AHA
President, WHA, WWF

Ilayaraja U MD DM
Cardiologist
Billroth Hospital
Chennai, Tamil Nadu, India

Indrani Mandal MD
Consultant Pediatrician
WBHS
Midnapore, West Bengal, India

I Sathyamurthy MD DM FACC FRCP DSc (Honoris Causa)
Senior Interventional Cardiologist
Department of Cardiology
Apollo Main Hospitals
Chennai, Tamil Nadu, India

IB Vijayalakshmi MD DM DSc FICC FIAE FICP FCSI FIAMS FAMS FISH FRCP (London)
Professor Emeritus
Former Professor and Head
Department of Pediatric Cardiology
Sri Jayadeva Institute of Cardiovascular Sciences and Research
Bengaluru, Karnataka, India

Jagdish C Mohan MD DM
Interventional Cardiologist
Department of Cardiology
Institute of Heart and Vascular Diseases
Jaipur Golden Hospital
Rohini, Delhi, India

Jaideep C Menon DM (Cardiology)
Professor
Department of Adult Cardiology
Amrita Institute of Medical Science
Kochi, Kerala, India

Jain T Kallarakkal MD DM FRCP
Senior Interventional Cardiologist
Sree Narayana Institute of Medical Sciences
Eranakulam, Kerala, India

Jasneet Singh MBBS
Senior Resident
Department of Cardiology
Janakpuri Super Speciality Hospital
New Delhi, India

Jasur B Babadjanov C MD MScPHS
Division of Public Health Science
Westminster International University
Tashkent, Uzbekistan

Jayagopal PB MD DM DNB FACC FICC FCSI FESC FSCAI FRCP(E)
Director, Head and Senior Interventional Cardiologist
Lakshmi Hospital,
Palakkad, Kerala, India

Jayanta Sharma MD FCSI
Consultant Cardiologist
Apollo Gleneagles Hospital
Kolkata, West Bengal, India

Jenu Rose Jose E MD (Pediatrics) DNB (Pediatrics) DM (Cardiology) PDF (Pediatric Cardiology)
Junior Consultant
Department of Pediatric Cardiology
Lisie Hospital
Kochi, Kerala, India

Jesu Krupa MD DM (Cardiology)
Faculty
Department of Cardiology
Christian Medical College
Vellore, Tamil Nadu, India

Johann Christopher MD DNB FACC
Director of Cardiac Imaging
Care Hospital
Hyderabad, Telangana, India

John Jose MD DM Fellowship in Interventional Cardiology (Germany)
Professor and Head
TAVI and Structural Heart Interventions
Department of Cardiology Unit-2
Christian Medical College Hospital
Vellore, Tamil Nadu, India

John Roshan Jacob MD DM (Cardiology) CEPS CCDS Fellowships in Adult and Pediatric EP
Professor
Christian Medical College Hospital
Vellore, Tamil Nadu, India

Jo Joseph MD DM
Senior Consultant Cardiologist
Department of Cardiology and Vascular Medicine
Lisie Heart Institute, Lisie Hospital
Kochi, Kerala, India

JPS Sawhney DM FESC FACC FRCP
Chairperson
Department of Cardiology
Dharma Vira Heart Center
Sir Ganga Ram Hospital
New Delhi, India

Juhi Singh MD DNB (Medicine)
Senior Resident
Department of Cardiology
Dharma Vira Heart Center
Sir Ganga Ram Hospital
New Delhi, India

Kabir Sethi MD DM
Consultant, Department of Cardiology
Delhi Heart and Lung Institute
New Delhi, India

Kajal Ganguly MD DM FACC
Consultant Interventional Cardiologist
Department of Cardiology
AMRI Hospital, Salt Lake
Kolkata, West Bengal, India

Kamal K Sethi MD DM FACC FHRS FCSI FISE
Director of Cardiology
Chairman and Managing Director
Delhi Heart and Lung Institute
New Delhi, India

Karthikeyan Balakrishnan MD DM
Consultant Cardiologist
Hindu Mission Hospital
Chennai, Tamil Nadu, India

Karunakar Rapolu MD DM
Consultant Cardiologist
Apollo Hospital, Jubillee Hills
Hyderabad, Telangana, India

Kashinath Ghosh Hazra MD DM DNB (Cardiology) MNAMS FNB (Interventional Cardiology)
Senior Consultant Interventional Cardiologist
NH-Rabindranath Tagore International Institute of Cardiac Sciences
Kolkata, West Bengal, India

Kavish Chopda MD
Physician
Magnum Heart Institute
Nashik, Maharashtra, India

Kayan Siodia DNB (Medicine) DNB (Cardiology)
Consultant Cardiologist
Healing Hearts
Mumbai, Maharashtra, India

K Durga Devi MD DM
Assistant Professor and Senior Interventional Cardiologist
Chettinad Academy of Research and Education
Chettinad Super Speciality Hospital
Chennai, Tamil Nadu, India

Kesavamoorthy MD DM
Consultant
Department of Interventional Cardiology
Meenakshi Hospital
Thanjavur, Tamil Nadu, India

Kiran Gaur MSc PhD
Associate Professor and Head
Department of Statistics, Mathematics and Computer Science
Government SKN Agriculture University
Jaipur, Rajasthan, India

Kiran Gopinath MD DM
Senior Consultant Cardiologist
NIMS Heart Foundation
Thiruvananthapuram, Kerala, India

Kiran Kumar G MD DM
Interventional Cardiologist
Care Hospitals
Hyderabad, Telangana, India

K Meenakshi MD (General Medicine) DM (Cardiology)
Professor and Head
Department of Cardiology
Saveetha Medical College
Chennai, Tamil Nadu, India

KN Srinivasan MD DNB (Cardiology) FCSI FESC FSCAI
Senior Interventional Cardiologist
Department of Cardiology
Apollo Main Hospitals
Chennai, Tamil Nadu, India

Kousalya Gopalsamy MBBS
DMO, Department of Cardiology
Meenakshi Hospital
Thanjavur, Tamil Nadu, India

Krishnaswamy Chandrasekaran MD FACC FASE
Senior Consultant
Department of Cardiovascular Diseases, Apollo Hospitals
Chennai, Tamil Nadu, India
Professor of Medicine, Mayo Clinic
Rochester, MN, USA

K Sivakumar MD DCH DNB (Pediatrics) DM DNB (Cardiology)
Head
Department of Pediatric Cardiology
Institute of Cardio Vascular Diseases
The Madras Medical Mission Hospital
Chennai, Tamil Nadu, India

Kunal Patankar MD (Medicine)
Senior Resident
Department of Cardiology
PD Hinduja National Hospital and MRC
Mumbai, Maharashtra, India

K Venugopal MD DM FCSI FICC FACC FESC
Senior Consultant Cardiologist
SP Fort Hospital, Thiruvananthapuram
Former Professor and Head
Department of Cardiology
Government Medical College
Kozhikode, Kerala, India

Lekha Adik Pathak MD (Medicine) DM (Cardiology) FRCP (Edinburgh)
Director and Head
Department of Cardiology
Nanavati Max Super Speciality Hospital
Mumbai, Maharashtra, India

Madhumanti Panja MD DNB (Cardiology)
Consultant Interventional Cardiologist
Belle Vue Clinic, AMRI Hospital
Kolkata, West Bengal, India

Madhu Shukla MBBS PhD
Head of Noninvasive Cardiology
Department of Cardiology
Institute of Heart and Vascular Diseases
Jaipur Golden Hospital
Rohini, New Delhi, India

Madhu Sreedharan MD DM MRCP (UK) FRCP FACC
Director
NIMS Heart Foundation
Thiruvananthapuram, Kerala, India

Madhuvanthi Rajendran DNB
Registrar in Cardiology
Kovai Medical Center and Hospital
Coimbatore, Tamil Nadu, India

Mahendra Chouhan DNB (Medicine) DrNB
Senior Resident
Department of Cardiology
Janakpuri Super Speciality Hospital
New Delhi, India

Mahesh Nalin Kumar MD DrNB FACC FESC
Head and Senior Consultant Cardiology
St Gregorios Medical Mission Hospital
Parumala, Kerala, India

Mainak Mukhopadhyay MD MRCP DM FESC CCDS
Consultant Interventional Cardiologist
Department of Cardiology
AMRI Hospital, Salt Lake
Kolkata, West Bengal, India

Maitreyee Bhattacharyya MD DM
Assistant Professor
LPS Institute of Cardiology
Kanpur, Uttar Pradesh, India

Mandava Satya Sahitya MD
Fellow
Department of Cardiology
Advanced Cardiac Centre
Postgraduate Institute of Medical Education and Research
Chandigarh, India

Manik Chopra MD DM
Clinical Lead – Structural Heart Disease Interventions
Department of Cardiology
Narayana Multispeciality Hospital
Ahmedabad, Gujarat, India

Manish Bansal MD DNB (Cardiology) FACC FASE
Senior Director
Department of Clinical and Preventive Cardiology
Medanta Heart Institute
Medanta – The Medicity
Gurugram, Haryana, India

Manish Chokhandre MD
Consultant Pediatric Cardiologist
Swasthyam Superspeciality Hospital
Nagpur, Maharashtra, India

Manoj Chopda MD DM (Cardiology)
Consultant Interventional Cardiologist
Director
Magnum Heart Institute
Nashik, Maharashtra, India

Manoj Kumar Agarwala MD (PGI) DM (PGI) FACC
Consultant Cardiologist
Department of Cardiology
Apollo Hospital, Jubilee Hills
Hyderabad, Telangana, India

Manoranjan Mandal MD Dip Card DM (Cardiology)
Professor and Head
Department of Cardiology
Medical College
Kolkata, West Bengal, India

Mansi Kaushik MBBS PGDCC FNIC
Consultant
Department of Clinical and Preventive Cardiology
Medanta Heart Institute
Medanta – The Medicity
Gurugram, Haryana, India

Manu Gupta MBBS
JR (Academic)
Department of Medicine
Peoples College of Medical Sciences
Bhopal, Madhya Pradesh, India

Manu Rajendran MD DM
Consultant Cardiologist
Meditrina Hospital
Kollam, Kerala, India

Marsha Barreto MD DM
Cardiology Resident
Department of Cardiology
Amrita Institute of Medical Sciences
Kochi, Kerala, India

Mayuri Mhatre MD DNB (Emergency Medicine)
Senior Clinical Associate
Department of Cardiology
PD Hinduja National Hospital and MRC
Mumbai, Maharashtra, India

M Chokkalingam MD DNB FACC FESC
Professor and Senior Interventional Cardiologist
Chettinad Academy of Research and Education
Chettinad Super Speciality Hospital
Chennai, Tamil Nadu, India

Meeraji Rao MD DM (Cardiology)
Senior Conultant and Head
Cardiology
Continental Hospital
Hyderabad, Telangana, India

Meetu Arora MBBS PGDCC (Cardiology) CCEBDM (Diabetes)
Consultant
Department of Cardiac Sciences
Max Super Speciality Hospital
Patparganj, New Delhi, India

Meghna Gupta MD (Psychiatry)
Senior Resident
Department of Psychiatry
All India Institute of Medical Sciences (AIIMS)
Bathinda, Punjab, India

Mohammed Abdul Azeez Asad MD DNB FNB
Consultant Cardiologist
Bahrain Specialist Hospital – Apollo Heart Centre
Juffair, Manama, Bahrain

Mohit D Gupta MD DM
Professor, Department of Cardiology
GB Pant Hospital
New Delhi, India

Mohsin Wali MD FACC
Professor and Senior Consultant
Department of Internal Medicine
Sir Ganga Ram Hospital
New Delhi, India

Mona Bhatia MD FRCR (UK) FSCCT (USA) FSCMR (USA)
Principal Director and Head
Department of Radiodiagnosis and Imaging
Fortis Escorts Heart Institute
New Delhi, India
Convener, Multimodality Imaging, Cardiological Society of India
Chair, International Regional Committee, India Chapter
Society of Cardiovascular CT, USA

Monotosh Panja MD FACC (USA) FCSI FICP DM (Cardiology)
Senior Consultant Interventional Cardiologist
Belle Vue Clinic
BM Birla Heart Institute
Ex-Director, ICVS, IPGME&R and SSKM Hospital
Kolkata, West Bengal, India

Moukthika KVN MD DM PDF (Electrophysiology)
Consultant Cardiologist and Electrophysiologist
Apollo Hospital
Bengaluru, Karnataka, India

Mrinalini Alla MD
Resident
Department of General Surgery
Flushing Hospital Medical Center
Queens, NY, USA

Mrinal Kanti Das MD DM FICP FICC FCSI FACC FESC
Consultant Cardiologist
CK Birla Hospitals (BMB/CMRI)
Kolkata, West Bengal, India

MS Ravi MD DM (Cardiology)
Former Director of Cardiology
Madras Medical College and Rajiv Ghandhi Government General Hospital
Chennai, Tamil Nadu, India

Mufaddal Lunawadawala DNB (Medicine) DrNB Cardiology
Senior Clinical Associate
Department of Cardiology
PD Hinduja National Hospital and MRC
Mumbai, Maharashtra, India

Musna PJ MD DM
Consultant Cardiologist
Department of Cardiology
St Mary's Hospital
Thodupuzha, Kerala, India

Mustafa Sajjad Cheema MBBS
Research Fellow
Department of Cardiology
West Virginia University School of Medicine
Morgantown, WV, USA

Nagamani AC MD DM
Professor
Department of Cardiology
Sri Jayadeva Institute of Cardiovascular Sciences and Research
Bengaluru, Karnataka, India

Nagaraj Desai MD (Medicine) DM (Cardiology)
Adjunct Professor
Department of Cardiology
JSSAHER, Mysuru
Director
Namana Medical Centre
Bengaluru, Karnataka, India

Nagendra Boopathy Senguttuvan MD DM FACC FSCAI
Professor of Cardiology and Senior Consultant Interventional Cardiologist
Sri Ramachandra Institute of Higher Education and Research
Chennai, Tamil Nadu, India

Nagendra Singh Chouhan MD DNB FNB
Senior Director
Division of Interventional Cardiology
Medanta – The Medicity
Gurugram, Haryana, India

Naima Parveen PhD
Research Coordinator
Harmony – Dr Sachin's 360 Degree Diabetes Care
Bhopal, Madhya Pradesh, India

Nandhakumar Vasu MD DNB (Cardiology) FNB (Interventional Cardiology)
Consultant, Department of Cardiology
Institute of Cardio Vascular Diseases
The Madras Medical Mission Hospital
Chennai, Tamil Nadu, India

Narra Lavanya MD (General Medicine) DrNB (Cardiology)
Cardiologist
Department of Cardiology
Apollo Main Hospital
Chennai, Tamil Nadu, India

Natisha Arora MD DNB
Senior Resident
Department of Imaging
Fortis Escort Heart Institute
New Delhi, India

Navanil Biswas MD (General Medicine) DrNB (Cardiology)
Consultant Interventional Cardiologist
Apollo Multispeciality Hospital
Kolkata, West Bengal, India

Navanil Biswas MD DNB (Cardiology)
Senior Resident
Department of Cardiology, NH-RTIICS
Kolkata, West Bengal, India

Naveen Garg MD DM DNB MNAMS FACC FSCAI FCSI
Professor, Department of Cardiology
Sanjay Gandhi Postgraduate Institute of Medical Sciences
Lucknow, Uttar Pradesh, India

Navin C Nanda MD DSc (Hon) DSc (Medicine) (Hon) FACC FAHA FASE FISCU (D)
Distinguished Professor of Medicine and Cardiovascular Disease
University of Alabama
Birmingham, AL, USA

Neusha Gopal MD DNB (Cardiology)
Associate Consultant Cardiologist
Remedy Hospital
Hyderabad, Telangana, India

Nihar Mehta MD DNB (Medicine) DNB (Cardiology)
Consultant Cardiologist
Jaslok, HN Reliance, Breach Candy Hospitals
Mumbai, Maharashtra, India

Nihar P Mehta MD (Medicine) DNB (Medicine) DNB (Cardiology) FICP FRCP (London)
Consultant Cardiologist, TAVI Specialist
Jaslok Hospital and Research Centre
Mumbai, Maharashtra, India

Nishad Chitnis MD MRCP DNB
Interventional Cardiologist
Heart Care Clinic
Kolhapur, Maharashtra, India

Nishank P Nooli MBBS
Assistant Professor
Department of Anesthesia
University of Alabama
Birmingham, Alabama, USA

Nishit Chandra MD DM
Director Cardiology
Fortis Escorts Heart Institute
New Delhi, India

Nitin Bajaj DM (Cardiology)
Associate Professor
Department of Cardiology
AICTS/AFMC
Pune, Maharashtra, India

Nitin J Burkule MD DM DNB FACC FASE FSCMR
Director, Department of Cardiology
Jupiter Hospital
Thane, Maharashtra, India

Nitin K Kabra MD DM FACC
Professor and Head
Department of Cardiology
Gandhi Medical College Hospital
Secunderabad, Telangana, India

Nitin Kumar Parashar MD DM
Consultant Cardiology
Artemis Hospital
Gurugram, Haryana, India

Nitish Naik MD DM
Professor
Department of Cardiology
All India Institute of Medical Sciences
New Delhi, India

NN Khanna MD DM FRCP (London, Glasgow, Edinburgh) FACC FSCAI FESC FAPSIC FCCP FEISI FICC FCSI
Senior Consultant Cardiologist
Indraprastha Apollo Hospital
New Delhi, India
Chairman – Asia Pacific Vascular Society
Advisor – Apollo Group of Hospitals in India

Panagiotis I Georgianos MD PhD
Assistant Professor
Department of Nephrology
School of Medicine
Aristotle University of Thessaloniki
Thessaloniki, Greece

Panchanan Sahoo MD (Medicine) DM (Cardiology) FACC FESC FICC FISE
Professor, Senior Consultant and Electrophysiologist
Department of Cardiology
Kalinga Institute of Medical Sciences
Bhubaneshwar, Odisha, India

Panigrahi NK MD DM FACC FSCAI FICC FCSI
Senior Consultant and Director
Interventional Cardiology
Head, Division of Cardiology
Apollo Hospital, Health City
Visakhapatnam, Andhra Pradesh, India

Pankaj Harkut MD DM (Cardiology) FACC FESC
Consultant Interventional Cardiologist
Swasthyam Superspeciality Hospital
Nagpur, Maharashtra, India

Pankaj Lakhwan MSc CEPS
Lead Clinical Scientist
Nference Labs Pvt Ltd
Bengaluru, Karnataka, India

Pankaj Manoria MD DM FACC FESC
Director
Manoria Heart and Critical Care Hospital
Bhopal, Madhya Pradesh, India

Parayaru Kottayil Asokan MD DM FRCP FACC FESC FSCAI FICC
Chief Consultant Interventional Cardiologist
Fathima Hospital
Kozhikode, Kerala, India

Parth Mashru MD (Medicine)
DM Cardiology Resident 2nd Year
Mahatma Gandhi Medical College and Hospital
Jaipur, Rajasthan, India

Parveen Kumar MD EDiR DICRI FRCR
Ex-Attending Consultant
Department of Radiodiagnosis and Imaging
Fortis Escort Heart Institute
New Delhi, India

Paul V George MD DM
Senior Professor
Department of Cardiology Unit-2
Christian Medical College Hospital
Vellore, Tamil Nadu, India

PC Manoria MD DM FACC FESC FCAPSC
Director
Manoria Heart and Critical Care Hospital
Bhopal, Madhya Pradesh, India

PLN Kapardhi MD DM
Senior Interventional Cardiologist
Care Hospitals
Hyderabad, Telangana, India

Prabhakar Koregol MD DM (Cardiology)
Senior Consultant Cardiologist
Fortis Hospitals
Bengaluru, Karnataka, India

Pradeep Kumar MD DNB
Associate Consultant Cardiologist
Apollo hospital, Jubilee Hills
Hyderabad, Telangana, India

Prafulla G Kerkar MD DM FCSI FACC FESC
Professor Emeritus
Department of Cardiology
KEM Hospital, Parel
Mumbai, Maharashtra, India

Prakas Chandra Mondal MD MRCP (UK, Ireland) MRRCPS (Glasgow) DM (Cardilogy) DNB (Cardiology) FACC (USA)
Consultant Interventional Cardiologist and Head
Department of Cardiology
Apolo Multispeciality Hospital
Kolkata, West Bengal, India

Praneeth S MD DM
Consultant Cardiologist
Apollo Hospital
Bengaluru, Karnataka, India

Prasant Kumar Sahoo MD DM FRCP (London and Glasgow) FACC FESC FSCAI FAPSIC FCSI FICC
Senior Consultant and Director
Interventional Cardiology
Apollo Hospitals
Bhubaneswar, Odisha, India

Prasit Maity DNB
Attending Consultant
Department of Imaging
Fortis Escort Heart Institute
New Delhi, India

Pratap Chandra Rath MD DM FICC FESC FACC FRCP (London) FRCP (Edinburgh)
Senior Consultant Cardiologist and HOD
Department of Cardiology
Apollo Hospital, Jubilee Hills
Hyderabad, Telangana
Apollo Hospital
Bhubaneshwar, Odisha, India

Prathap Kumar MD DM
Chief Interventional Cardiologist
Meditrina Hospital
Kollam, Kerala, India

Pratibha Misra MD (Biochemistry)
Molecular Biologist and Head
Department of Laboratory Sciences
Base Hospital
Guwahati, Assam, India

Praveen Chandra MD DM FACC FESC FSCAI FAPSIC
Chairman
Department of Cardiology
Medanta – The Medicity
Gurugram, Haryana, India

Prayaag Kini MD (Medicine) DNB (Cardiology) Fellow (Interventional Cardiology) FSCAI
Additional Senior Consultant
Department of Cardiology
Sri Sathya Sai Institute of Higher Medical Sciences
Bengaluru, Karnataka, India

Preetish Rath PhD
Candidate (Computer Science)
Tufts University, Medford
Massachusetts, USA

PS Banerjee MD DM (Cardiology) FACC
Chief Interventional Cardiologist
Manipal Hospital
Former Head
Department of Cardiology
Medical College
Kolkata, West Bengal, India
Immediate Past President
Cardiological Society of India

Purneshwar Kumar Pandey MD DM
Associate Consultant
Max Super Specialty Hospital
Saket, New Delhi, India

P Vijay Shekar MD DM
Consultant Cardiologist and Electrophysiologist
Division of Cardiac Pacing and Electrophysiology
Department of Cardiology
Apollo Speciality Hospitals
Tiruchirappalli, Tamil Nadu, India

Raghuram Palaparti MD DM
Consultant Cardiologist
Aayush Hospitals
Vijayawada and Eluru
Andhra Pradesh, India

Rahul Shewale MD
Cardiologist
Magnum Heart Institute
Nashik, Maharashtra, India

Rajan Joseph Manjuran MD DM PGDHRM FICC FIAE FISE FCSI FACC
Emeritus Professor of Cardiology
Pushpagiri Medical College
Thiruvalla, Kerala, India

Rajeev Garg MD (Medicine) Dip Card (NIMS) DNB (Cardiology) MNAMS FSCAI FESC FACC Diplomate National Board
Senior Consultant Interventional Cardiologist
Aware Gleneagles Global Hospital
Hyderabad, Telangana, India

Rajeev Gupta MD DM (Cardiology)
Professor and Head
Department of Cardiology
Gandhi Medical College
Bhopal, Madhya Pradesh, India

Rajeev Gupta MD PhD
Chairman
Department of Preventive Cardiology and Medicine
Eternal Heart Care Centre and Research Institute
Jaipur, Rajasthan, India

Rajendra Kumar Jain MD DM DIU (Paris)
Founder Director
KIMS Group of Hospitals
Hyderabad, Telangana, India

Rajesh Natuva MD DrNB (Cardiology)
Consultant Interventional Cardiologist
Star Hospital, Jubilee Hills
Hyderabad, Telangana, India

Rajesh Thachathodiyl MD DM FACC
Senior Interventional Cardiologist
Professor and Head
Department of Cardiology
Amrita Institute of Medical Sciences
Kochi, Kerala, India

Rajesh Vijayvergiya MD DM FSCAI FACC FESC FISES
Professor
Department of Cardiology
Advanced Cardiac Centre
Postgraduate Institute of Medical Education and Research
Chandigarh, India

Rajeswari K Dip Echo MBA
Echo Technologist
Billroth Hospital
Chennai, Tamil Nadu, India

Rajiv Agarwal MD MS
Professor
Department of Medicine
Division of Nephrology
Indiana University School of Medicine and Richard L Roudebush Veterans Administration Medical Center
Indianapolis, IN, USA

Rajneesh Kapoor MD DNB FACC
Chairman
Division of Interventional Cardiology
Medanta Heart Institute
Medanta – The Medicity
Gurugram, Haryana, India

Rakesh Yadav MD DM
Professor
Department of Cardiology
All India Institute of Medical Sciences
New Delhi, India

Ramakrishna Janapati MD DM
Consultant Cardiologist
Apollo Hospital, Jubilee Hills
Hyderabad, Telangana, India

Ramesh Daggubati MD
Vice Chair and Chief of Interventional Cardiology
Department of Cardiology,
West Virginia University School of Medicine
Morgantown, WV, USA

Rana Rathor Roy MD (General Medicine) DM (Cardiology)
Senior Consultant Interventional Cardiologist
Medica Institute of Cardiac Science
Kolkata, West Bengal, India

Ranjan Modi MD DM (Cardiology)
Senior Consultant and Unit Head
Department of Cardiology
Sarvodaya Healthcare
Faridabad, Haryana, India

Rathindra Nath Karmakar MD DM
Consultant
Department of Cardiology
Narayana Multispeciality Hospital
Kolkata, West Bengal, India

Ratul Ghosh MD
Postdoctoral Trainee
Department of Cardiology
RG Kar Medical College and Hospital
Kolkata, West Bengal, India

Ravi Kant T MD DM
Consultant, Apollo Hospital
Visakhapatnam, Andhra Pradesh, India

Ravinder Singh Rao MD DM FACC FSCAI
Chairman and Managing Director
Department of Cardiology
Rajasthan Hospital Limited
Jaipur, Rajasthan, India

Ravi R Kasliwal MD DM FASE FIMSA MNAMS
Chairman
Department of Clinical and Preventive Cardiology
Medanta Heart Institute
Medanta – The Medicity
Gurugram, Haryana, India

Raymond R Townsend MD FAHA
Professor of Medicine
University of Pennsylvania
Philadelphia, PA, USA

Reeta Varyani MD (Medicine) DNB (Cardiology) Fellow (Interventional Cardiology) FSCAI
Senior Consultant and In-Charge
Department of Cardiology
Sri Sathya Sai Institute of Higher Medical Sciences
Bengaluru, Karnataka, India

Reinhold Kreutz MD PhD
Charité - Universitaetsmedizin Berlin
Corporate Member of Freie Universitaet Berlin and Humboldt-Universitaet zu Berlin
Institute of Clinical Pharmacology and Toxicology
Berlin, Germany

Riccardo Rinaldi MD
Department of Cardiovascular and Pulmonary Sciences
Catholic University of the Sacred Heart
Rome, Italy

Rishika Mehta MD (Pediatrics) DrNB (Pediatric Cardiology)
Pediatric Cardiologist
Department of Pediatric Cardiology
Narayana Superspeciality Hospital
Howrah, West Bengal, India

Ritesh Acharya MD (Medicine) DM (Cardiology)
Assistant Professor
Department of Cardiology
Pursuing Fellowship in Electrophysiology
Kalinga Institute of Medical Sciences
Bhubaneshwar, Odisha, India

Ritwik Ghosal MBBS
Resident
Department of Cardiology
IPGME&R and SSKM Hospital
Kolkata, West Bengal, India

Rocco A Montone MD PhD
Department of Cardiovascular Medicine
Fondazione Policlinico Universitario Agostino Gemelli IRCCS
Rome, Italy

Rohit Mody MD DM
Director of Cardiology
Department of Cardiology
Max Super Specialty Hospital
Bathinda, Punjab, India

Ronak V Ruparelia DNB (Medicine) DNB (Cardiology)
Interventional Cardiologist
Bankers Super Speciality Hospital
Vadodara, Gujarat, India

Rony Mathew MD DM DNB (Medicine) DrNB (Cardiology) FACC FESC FCSI FRCP (London)
Head, Department of Cardiology and Vascular Medicine
Lisie Heart Institute, Lisie Hospital
Kochi, Kerala, India

Roopali Khanna MD DM
Professor, Sanjay Gandhi Postgraduate Institute of Medical Sciences
Lucknow, Uttar Pradesh, India

R Rameshwar MD (General Medicine)
PG in DM Cardiology
Saveetha Medical College
Chennai, Tamil Nadu, India

R Ravi Kumar MD DM
Senior Consultant and Clinical Lead – Heart Failure and Heart Transplantation
MGM Healthcare
Chennai, Tamil Nadu, India

Rufus Demel X MD DNB (Cardiology) FNB (Interventional Cardiology)
Chief Consultant Cardiologist
Devaki Heart Center
Madurai, Tamil Nadu, India

RVA Ananth MD (General Medicine) PGDCC
Department of Cardiology
Government Medical College, Virudhunagar
Consultant Cardiologist
Jeyalakshmi Heart Center
Madurai, Tamil Nadu, India

Sabari Krishnan MD DM
Consultant, Department of Interventional Cardiology
Meenakshi Hospital
Thanjavur, Tamil Nadu, India

Sabyasachi Rout MD DM (Cardiology)
Consultant Cardiologist
Apollo Hospitals
Bhubaneswar, Odisha, India

Sachin Chittawar MD DM (Endocrinology)
Former Associate Professor
Gandhi Medical College
Director, Harmony – Dr Sachin's 360 Degree Diabetes Care
Bhopal, Madhya Pradesh, India

Sachin Raiya MD
Senior Resident
Department of Imaging
Fortis Escort Heart Institute
New Delhi, India

Sagar R Makode DM (Cardiology)
Assistant Professor
Department of Cardiology
All India Institute of Medical Sciences
Nagpur, Maharashtra, India

Saibal Kar MD DM FACC FSCAI
Program Director, Cardiology
Los Robles Regional Medical Center
National Physician Director
Interventional Cardiology
HCA Healthcare
Thousand Oaks, CA, USA

Sai Satish MD DM
Senior Interventional Cardiologist
Clinical Lead – Transcatheter Heart Valve Therapeutics
Apollo Hospitals
Chennai, Tamil Nadu, India

Sajan Narayanan MD DM FESC
Consultant and Interventional Cardiologist
Little Flower Heart Institute, Angamaly
Kochi, Kerala, India

Sameer S Ambar MD DM
Associate Professor
Department of Cardiology
JN Medical College, KAHER
Belgavi, Karnataka, India

Samir B Pancholy MD FAHA FACC MSCAI
Professor of Medicine
Geisinger Commonwealth School of Medicine
Program Director, Fellowship in Cardiovascular Diseases
The Wright Center for Graduate Medical Education
Scranton, PA, USA

Sandeep Bansal MD DM DNB MNAMS FESC FSCAI
Professor and Head
Department of Cardiology
Vardhman Mahavir Medical College and Safdarjung Hospital
New Delhi, India

Sanjay C Shah MD DM
Director
Department of Cardiology
Apex Heart Institute
Ahmedabad, Gujarat, India

Sanjay Kumar Chugh MD DM (Cardiology) FACC FSCAI FIMSA FCSI
Associate Director and Senior Consultant
Cardiology and Interventional Cardiology
Narayana Healthcare Superspeciality Hospital
Gurugram, Haryana, India

Sanjay Mehrotra MD DM
Consultant and Interventional Cardiologist
NH Institute of Cardiac Sciences
Bengaluru, Karnataka, India

Sanjay Tyagi MD DM (Cardiology) FAMS FESC FSCAI FRCP FACC (USA)
Clinical Director
Department of Cardiology
Apollo Hospital Groups - North
Ex-Director Professor and Head
Department of Cardiology
GB Pant PGI and Dean MAMC
New Delhi, India

Sanjeeb Roy MD DM
Director Cardiology
CK Birla Hospital
Jaipur, Rajasthan, India

S Anne Princy MD DM
Assistant Professor,
Department of Cardiology
Tamil Nadu Government Multi Super Speciality Hospital
Chennai, Tamil Nadu, India

Santosh Kumar Singh MD DNB
Associate Consultant
Max Super Specialty Hospital
Saket, New Delhi, India

Santosh Palled MD DM
Interventional Cardiologist
Care Hospitals
Hyderabad, Telangana, India

Sarju Ganatra MD
Director
Cardio-Oncology Program
Division of Cardiovascular Medicine
Vice Chair, Department of Medicine
Lahey Hospital and Medical Center
Beth Israel Lahey Health
Burlington, MA, USA

Saro Avedikian MD MPH
Resident Physician, Internal Medicine
Los Robles Regional Medical Center
HCA Healthcare
Thousand Oaks, CA, USA

Sarumathi Thangavel MD FACC
Consultant
Advanced Heart Failure and Transplant Cardiology
MGM Healthcare
Chennai, Tamil Nadu, India

Satyanarayan Routray MD DM FICC FCSI FACC FSCAI
Professor
SCB Medical College and Hospital
Cuttack, Odisha, India

Satyendra Tewari MD DM (Cardiology) FACC FSCAI FCAPSC FESC FCSI FICC
Professor
Department of Cardiology
Sanjay Gandhi Postgraduate Institute of Medical Sciences
Lucknow, Uttar Pradesh, India

Saumitra Ray MD FRCP FCSI FICP FESC FACC FSCAI
Ex-Professor, Vivekananda Institute of Medical Sciences
Director – Invasive Cardiology
Advanced Medical Research Institute(S)
Kolkata, West Bengal, India

Saurabh Dhumale MD DrNB (Cardiology)
Consultant Interventional Cardiologist
Narayana Health RN Tagore Hospital
Kolkata, West Bengal, India

SB Gupta MD FCSI FICP FISE FACC
Ex-Consultant Physician Cardiologist
Asian Heart Institute Mumbai
Former Head
Department of Medicine and Cardiology
Central Railway Headquarters Hospital
Mumbai, Maharashtra, India

Selvamani S DNB (Cardiology)
Senior Consultant and Interventional Cardiologist
Meenakshi Mission Hospital and Research Centre
Madurai, Tamil Nadu, India

Sengottuvelu G MD (General Medicine) DM (Cardiology) DNB (Cardiology) FRCP (Glasgow, London) Fellowship in Interventional Cardiology (France) FMMC FSCAI FCSI
Clinical Lead
Structural Heart Disease Program
Apollo Hospitals Group
Chennai, Tamil Nadu, India

Senthilraj Thangasami MD (General Medicine), DM (Cardiology)
Interventional Cardiologist
Apollo Hospitals
Chennai, Tamil Nadu, India

S Gnansambandam MD (Pediatrics) DCH DM (Cardiology)
Professor of Cardiology
Head
Department of Pediatric Cardiology
Institute of Child Health and Hospital for Children, Egmore
Chennai, Tamil Nadu, India

Shabbir Ali Shaik MD DM FNB
Fellow Interventional Cardiologist
Department of Cardiology
Apollo Hospital, Jubilee Hills
Hyderabad, Telangana, India

Shanmugam K MD DM (Cardiology)
Assistant Professor
Department of Cardiology
Sri Jayadeva Institute of Cardiovascular Sciences and Research
Bengaluru, Karnataka, India

Shanmugasundaram S MD DM
Cardiologist
Billroth Hospital
Chennai, Tamil Nadu, India

Shantanu P Sengupta MD DNB PhD FACC FASE
Heart Failure Specialist
Director, Sengupta Hospital and Research Institute
Nagpur, Maharashtra, India

Shashank C MD DM
Consultant
Apollo Hospital
Visakhapatnam, Andhra Pradesh, India

Shibba Takkar Chhabra MD DM
Professor
Department of Cardiology
Hero DMC Heart Institute
Dayanand Medical College and Hospital
Ludhiana, Punjab, India

Shibsankar Sarkar MD
Postdoctoral Trainee
Department of Cardiology
RG Kar Medical College and Hospital
Kolkata, West Bengal, India

Shifas Babu M MD DM DNB MNAMS
Senior Consultant Cardiologist
Cardiovascular Centre
Ananthapuri Hospitals and Research Institute
Thiruvananthapuram, Kerala, India

Shirisha Reddy Kommareddy MD DrNB (Cardiology)
Junior Consultant Cardiologist
KIMS
Hyderabad, Telangana, India

Shirley Adivi MD
Research Student, Department of Cardiology, West Virginia University School of Medicine
Morgantown, WV, USA

Shishu Shankar Mishra MD FAIMS MCAM DoCM FCCP FIAE FICC FCSI
Professor and Director
SOA University, Bhubaneswar
Professor and Director
Dreams Health Sciences and Padmini Care Hospital
Director Med-n-Heart Clinic
Cuttack, Odisha, India

Shivangi Tiwari MBBS
Resident Doctor Final Year (Medicine)
Department of Medicine
RD Gardi Medical College
Ujjain, Madhya Pradesh, India

Shunmuga Sundaram Ponnusamy MD DM CEPS
Associate Professor
Department of Cardiology
Velammal Medical College Hospital and Research Institute
Madurai, Tamil Nadu, India

Shyam Prasad Sahoo MBBS
Medical Officer, SRM Medical College Hospital and Research Centre
Chennai, Tamil Nadu, India

Sibaram Panda MD (Medicine) DM (Cardiology)
Assistant Professor
Department of Cardiology
Veer Surendra Sai Institute of Medical Science and Research
Burla Sambalpur, Odisha, India

Siddhartha Mani MD DM FSCAI
Consultant
Department of Adult Cardiology
RN Tagore Hospital
Kolkata, West Bengal, India

Siddharth Bajaj MD DM
Consultant Cardiologist
Apollo Hospital, Jubillee Hills
Hyderabad, Telangana, India

Siddharth Chinta MD
Research Fellow
Division of Cardiac Imaging/Cardiology
Tufts Medical Center
Boston, USA

Siddhant Gupta MBBS
Resident Doctor Final Year (Medicine)
Department of Medicine
RD Gardi Medical College
Ujjain, Madhya Pradesh, India

Siddarth Varshney MD DM
Associate Consultant
Division of Interventional Cardiology
Medanta – The Medicity
Gurugram, Haryana, India

S Kumaran MD (General Medicine) DCH DM (Cardiology)
Associate Professor
Department of Cardiology
Institute of Child Health and Hospital for Children, Egmore,
Chennai, Tamil Nadu, India

Smit Shrivastava MD PGDHHM DM (Cardiology) FACC FSCAI FESC FICP FIMSA FICN FISE
Professor and Head
Advance Cardiac Institute
Pt JNM Medical College and Dr BRAM Hospital
Raipur, Chhattisgarh, India

Sneha Karekar MD (Medicine) DrNB
Cardiology Resident, Manipal Hospital
Bengaluru, Karnataka, India

SN Narasingan MD FRCP (Edinburgh and Glasgow) FACP FICP FCCP (USA)
Managing Director
SNN Specialities Clinic and SNN Diagnostic Centre
Chennai, Tamil Nadu, India
Vice Chairman, Lipid Association of India
Vice President, World Hypertension League

Soma Sen MD FACC
Consultant Cardiologist and Director of Nuclear Imaging
Park Nicollet Health Partners Care Group and Methodist Hospital
Bloomington, MN, USA

Sonu Abraham MD
Clinical and Research Fellow
Cardio-Oncology Program
Division of Cardiovascular Medicine
Department of Medicine
Lahey Hospital and Medical Center
Beth Israel Lahey Health
Burlington, MA, USA

Soumen Devidutta MD DM PDF
Consultant Cardiologist and Electrophysiologist
Apollo Hospitals
Hyderabad, Telangana, India

Soumen Prasad Behera MD DM (Cardiology)
Consultant Cardiologist
Hitech Medical College and Hospital
Rourkela, Odisha, India

Sourabh Agstam MD DM
Assistant Professor
Department of Cardiology
All India Institute of Medical Sciences
New Delhi, India

Sourav Das MD
PDT Cardiology
Medica Superspecialty Hospital
Kolkata, West Bengal, India

Sradhananda Rout MD DM (Cardiology)
Senior Resident
SCB Medical College and Hospital
Cuttack, Odisha, India

Sreenivas Kumar A MD DM FACC
Senior Consultant Cardiologist and Director
Department of Cardiology and Clinical Research
Apollo Hospital, Jubilee Hills
Hyderabad, Telangana, India

Sridhar Kasturi MD DM FACC FESC FSCAI FICC
Head
Department of Cardiology and Cardiothoracic Surgery
KIMS – Sunshine Hospitals
Secunderabad, Telangana, India

Srijani Thannir MBBS
Research Fellow
Division of Cardiology
University of Alabama
Birmingham, AL, USA

Srina Ray MBBS (Cal)
Clinical Assistant
Heart Clinic
Kolkata, West Bengal, India

Srinivasa Rao Malladi MD (General Medicine) DM (Cardiology) DNB (Cardiology)
Professor
Department of Cardiology
Andhra Medical College/King George Hospital
Visakhapatnam, Andhra Pradesh, India

Srinivas Kudva MD (Medicine) DNB (Cardiology)
Consultant Cardiologist
Healing Hearts
Mumbai, Maharashtra, India

Srinivas Ramaka MD DM FIAE FACC FAHA FCSI
Honorary Professor IMA
Consultant Cardiologist
Srinivasa Heart Centre
Chairman and Managing Trustee
Srinivasa Heart Foundation
Warangal, Telangana, India

SR Sharath Shanmugam MD (General Medicine)
PG in DM Cardiology
Sri Ramachandra Medical College
Chennai, Tamil Nadu, India

SS Binu MD (Medicine) DNB (Medicine) DM (Cardiology) FSCAI FESC
Senior Consultant Cardiologist
Sree Gokulam Medical College and Research Foundation
Thiruvananthapuram, Kerala, India

SS Iyengar DM (Cardiology)
Consultant Cardiologist
Manipal Hospital
Bengaluru, Karnataka, India

S Sunilkumar MD DM (Cardiology)
Professor and Head
Department of Cardiology
JSSMC, JSSAHER
Mysuru, Karnataka, India

Subasis Dash DNB (Medicine) DNB (Cardiology) MNAMS
Consultant Cardiologist
Apollo Hospitals
Bhubaneswar, Odisha, India

Subhasish Singh MD DM
Associate Professor
Division of Cardiology
MKCG Medical College
Berhampur, Odisha, India

Subhasis Roy Chowdhury MD DM
Consultant Interventional Cardiologist
Department of Cardiology
AMRI Hospital, Salt Lake
Kolkata, West Bengal, India

Subroto Mandal MD DM DC FACC FICC FCPCI FSCAI
Professor and Head
Department of Cardiology
Director, Cath Lab
Ubuntu Heart and Super Specialty Hospital
Bhopal, Madhya Pradesh, India

Sudhir Chandra Sinha MD DM FACC
Senior Consultant Cardiologist
Star Pinnacle Heart Centre
Visakhapatnam, Andhra Pradesh, India

Sudhir Lakamsani MD (General Medicine) DrNB (Cardiology)
Cardiology Registrar
Department of Cardiology
Apollo Main Hospital
Chennai, Tamil Nadu, India

Suganthi Jaganathan BDS MPH PhD (Pursuing)
Senior Research Associate
Centre for Health Analytics Research and Trends (CHART)
Trivedi School of Biosciences, Ashoka University
Institute of Environmental Medicine, Karolinska Institute
Stockholm, Sweden
Centre for Chronic Disease Control
New Delhi, India

Suman Bhandari MD DM FACC FESC FSCAI FIMSA
Director
Department of Cardiology
Fortis Escorts Heart Institute
New Delhi, India

Sumanth Khadke MD
Research Fellow
Cardio-Oncology Program
Division of Cardiovascular Medicine
Department of Medicine
Lahey Hospital and Medical Center
Beth Israel Lahey Health
Burlington, MA, USA

Sunandan Sikdar MD DM FACC
Consultant
Department of Cardiology
Narayana Multispeciality Hospital
Kolkata, West Bengal, India

Sundar Chidambaram MD DNB DM FNB
Senior Consultant Interventional Cardiologist
Kauvery Hospital
Chennai, Tamil Nadu, India

Sunil Kumar Sharma MD (Medicine) DM (Cardiology) FACC
Professor and Head
Department of Cardiology
Veer Surendra Sai Institute of Medical Science and Research
Burla Sambalpur, Odisha, India

Sunil Modi MD DM FACC FICC FCSI
Senior Consultant
Department of Cardiology
Indraprastha Apollo Hospital
New Delhi, India

Surendra Poonia DM (Cardiology)
Senior Consultant Interventional Cardiology
Apex Hospital
Bikaner, Rajasthan
Consultant Interventional Cardiologist
Holy Family Hospital
Mumbai, Maharashtra, India

Suresh V Patted MD DM FACC FCSI FAPSIC
Professor and Head
Department of Cardiology
JN Medical College, KAHER
Belgavi, Karnataka, India

Sushant Mishra MD DM (Cardiology)
Consultant Cardiology
Meditrina Hospitals
Gurugram, Haryana, India

Suvro Banerjee MD MRCP (UK) FRCP (London) FRCP (Edinburgh) FCSI FICC FSCAI FESC FACC
Senior Consultant Cardiologist
Apollo Multispeciality Hospitals
Kolkata, West Bengal, India

Swasthi S Kumar MD
Senior Resident, Department of Cardiology, SCTIMST
Thiruvananthapuram, Kerala, India

Swati Singh MD DM (Cardiology)
Consultant Cardiology
Meditrina Hospitals
Gurugram, Haryana, India

Syed Imamuddin MD DM FACC FESC FSCAI FCSI
Professor and Head
Department of Cardiology
Osmania Medical College/Osmania General Hospital
Director
Heart Beat
Hyderabad, Telangana, India

Tanmay Mukhopadhyay MD DM (Cardiology) FESC FSCAI
Associate Professor
Department of Cardiology
Burdwan Medical College and Hospital
Burdwan, West Bengal, India

Tejas M Patel MD DM FCSI FACC FESC FSCAI
Chairman and Chief Interventional Cardiologist
Apex Heart Institute
Ahmedabad, Gujarat, India

T Govindan Unni MD DM
Professor
Department of Cardiology
Jubilee Mission Medical College and Research Institute
Thrissur, Kerala, India

Thajfeer UM MD
Senior Resident
Department of Cardiology
GMC Kannur, Hrudayalaya
Kannur, Kerala, India

Thomas Alexander MD DM
Head of Cardiology
Kovai Medical Center and Hospital
Coimbatore, Tamil Nadu, India

Thomas F Lüscher MD FRCP FESC
Director of Research, Education and Development
Royal Brompton and Harefield Clinical Group,
Guy's and St Thomas' NHS Foundation Trust
Professor of Cardiology
Imperial College and King's College London
London, United Kingdom

Thomas Xavier Paulsingh JS DM FNB (Interventional Cardiology)
Associate Consultant and Interventional Cardiologist
Meenakshi Mission Hospital and Research Centre
Madurai, Tamil Nadu, India

Tiny Nair MD DM FACC FRCP
Head, Department of Cardiology
PRS Hospital
Thiruvananthapuram, Kerala, India

Trinath K Mishra MD DM
Professor, Division of Cardiology
MKCG Medical College
Berhampur, Odisha, India

Tripti Deb MD DNB
Senior Consultant Cardiologist
Apollo Health City, Jubilee Hills
Hyderabad, Telangana, India

U Ankur B Pharma M Pharma Toxicology
Senior Safety Scientist, Project Coordinator, Safety Science Specialist
Department of Pharmacology and Toxicology
Durham College
Oshawa, Canada

Umesh C Samal MD FACC FIACM FICC FIAE FISE FISC FAPVS FEAC
Former Professor of Cardiology and Head
Department of Medicine
Patna Medical College
Patna, Bihar, India

V Amuthan MD DM FACC FASE FEACVI FCSI FIAE
Emeritus Professor of Cardiology
The Tamil Nadu Dr MGR Medical University
Formerly Professor and Head
Department of Cardiology
Madurai Medical College
Director
4D Echo Lab, Jeyalakshmi Heart Center
Senior Interventional Cardiologist
Vadamalayan Hospital
Madurai, Tamil Nadu, India

Vaibhav Bandil MD (Medicine) DrNB (Cardiology)
Associate Consultant
Department of Cardiology
Fortis Escorts Heart Institute
New Delhi, India

Vardhini Vijaykumar BDS MDS
Hyderabad, Telangana, India

Varsha Kiron MD DM (Cardiology) DNB (Cardiology) FSCAI FESCC
Consultant Cardiologist
Apollo Health City
Hyderabad, Telangana, India

Varun Bhatia MD DM
Consultant – Structural Heart Interventions
Department of Cardiology
Aster Medicity Hospital
Kochi, Kerala, India

Varun Gupta MD (Thoracic Surgery)
Resident – Thoracic Surgery
Lungenklinik Hemer
Hemer, Germany

Varun Marimuthu MD DM
Assistant Professor
Department of Cardiology
Sri Jayadeva Institute of Cardiovascular Sciences and Research
Bengaluru, Karnataka, India

Vasudeva Murthy Sindgi M Pharm PhD
Principal and Professor
Department of Phamacology
Jayamukhi College of Pharmacy
Narsampet, Telangana, India

Vemuri S Murthy MD MS FAHA FICS
Associate Professor (Adjunct)
Department of Emergency Medicine
University of Illinois College of Medicine
Chicago, IL, USA

Venkata RS Subrahmanya Sarma MD DM
Consultant Cardiologist
Aayush Hospitals
Vijayawada and Eluru
Andhra Pradesh, India

Venkatesh CR MD (Medicine)
Assistant Professor
Department of Medicine
JSSMC, JSSAHER,
Mysuru, Karnataka, India

Vidyut Jain MD FSCAI FACC FESC
Consultant Cardiologist
Choithram Hospital
Indore, Madhya Pradesh, India

Vigyan Vijay Bang MD FACC
Interventional and Structural Cardiologist
Freeman Heart and Vascular Institute
Joplin, MO, USA

Vijay Garg MD FIAE FICP FCSI FICA (USA) FISE FACC (USA) FACP (USA) FIMSA FISC FESC (EUROPE)
Professor, Department of Medicine
RD Gardi Medical College
Ujjain, Madhya Pradesh, India

Vijayadithyan Jaganathan MD
Research Fellow, Division of Cardiology
University of Alabama
Birmingham, AL, USA

Vijayakumar Subban MD DM FNB
Senior Consultant
Interventional Cardiologist
Clinical Lead – Cardiac Imaging Services
Apollo Hospitals
Chennai, Tamil Nadu, India

Vijayanand B Metgudmath MD DNB (Cardiology)
Associate Professor
Department of Cardiology
JN Medical College, KAHER
Belgavi, Karnataka, India

Vijay Bang MD DM FCSI FESC FSCAI FACC
Senior Interventional Cardiologist
Lilavati Hospital and Research Center
Honorable Professor and Head
Grant Medical College and
Sir JJ Group of Hospitals (Former)
Mumbai, Maharashtra, India

Vijay Iyer MD PhD FACC FSCAI
Chief
Division of Cardiovascular Medicine
Department of Medicine
Jacobs School of Medicine and Biomedical Sciences
University at Buffalo
Buffalo, NY, USA

Vijay Kumar MD DNB (Cardiology)
Director, Interventional Cardiology
Fortis Escorts Heart Institute
New Delhi, India

Vijaykumar JR MD DM DNB (Cardiology)
Associate Professor
Department of Cardiology
Sri Jayadeva Institute of Cardiovascular Sciences and Research
Bengaluru, Karnataka, India

Vikas Agrawal MD DNB (Cardiology)
Professor
Department of Cardiology
Institute of Medical Sciences
Banaras Hindu University
Varanasi, Uttar Pradesh, India

Vinay Wasan
Business Major
James Madison University
Harrisonburg, VA, USA

Vineet Bhatia MD DM DNB (Cardiology) MNAMS
Director
Department of Cardiac Sciences
Max Super Specialty Hospital
Patparganj, New Delhi, India

Vishal Batra MD DM (Cardiology)
Associate Professor
Department of Cardiology
GB Pant Institute of Postgraduate Medical Education and Research
New Delhi, India

Vishal Rastogi MD DM (Cardiology)
Director Interventional Cardiology
Fortis Escorts Heart Institute
New Delhi, India

Vitull K Gupta MD (Medicine) FICP FCSI FACP FIACM
Health and Human Rights Activist
Consultant, Kishori Ram Hospital and Diabetes Care Centre
Honorary Teaching Faculty
All India Institute of Medical Sciences (AIIMS)
Bathinda, Punjab, India

Viveka Kumar MD DM FSCAI FACC FECS FAPSIC FRCP (Edinburgh)
Principal Director and Chief of Cath Labs
Max Super Specialty Hospital
Saket, New Delhi, India

Vivekanand S Gajapati MD DM
Consultant Cardiologist
SDM Naryana Heart Centre
Dharwad, Karnataka, India

Vivek Gupta MD DM FACC FESC FSCAI FAPSIC FEAPCI FIEIC FCSI FICC FIC (France)
Senior Interventional Cardiologist
Indraprastha Apollo Hospitals
New Delhi, India
Scientific Course Chairman, Indo European Course on Revascularization (IECR)

V Jacob Jose MD DM (Cardiology) FACC FASE FCCP MS
Consultant Cardiologist
Naruvi Hospitals
Vellore, Tamil Nadu, India

VK Bahl MD DM (Cardiology)
Director, Cardiac Sciences
MS Ramaiah Medical College
Bengaluru, Karnataka, India

VS Ramchandra MD DM FACC
Electrophysiologist
Sri Sri Holistic Hospitals
Hyderabad, Telangana, India

V Suryaprakasa Rao MD DM FACC FSCAI
Senior Interventional Cardiologist
Care Hospitals
Hyderabad, Telangana, India

W Sunil MD DNB (Cardiology)
Associate Professor
Department of Cardiology
Super Speciality Hospital, GMC
Nagpur, Maharashtra, India

Yasar Satar MD
Fellow in Cardiovascular Disease
Department of Cardiology
West Virginia University School of Medicine
Morgantown, WV, USA

Yashaswi Koguru MBBS
Observer, Clinical Electrophysiology
University of Alabama
Birmingham, Alabama, USA

Y Chandrashekhar MD FACC
Professor, Department of Medicine
University of Minnesota/VAMC
Minneapolis, MN, USA

Yogesh Kolamkar MD DrNB (Cardiology)
Consultant Interventional Cardiologist
Swasthyam Superspeciality Hospital
Nagpur, Maharashtra, India

Yogesh Om Sharma MD DM
Consultant Cardiologist
Artemis Hospital
Gurugram, Haryana, India

Yogesh Varma MD DM (CMCH Vellore)
Former Professor and Head
Director Cardiac Science Centre
Department of Cardiology
Dean, Gandhi Medical College
Bhopal, Madhya Pradesh, India

Zoofi Shan MBBS
Resident, Department of Cardiology
Dayanand Medical College and Hospital
Unit Hero DMC Heart Institute
Ludhiana, Punjab, India

FOREWORD

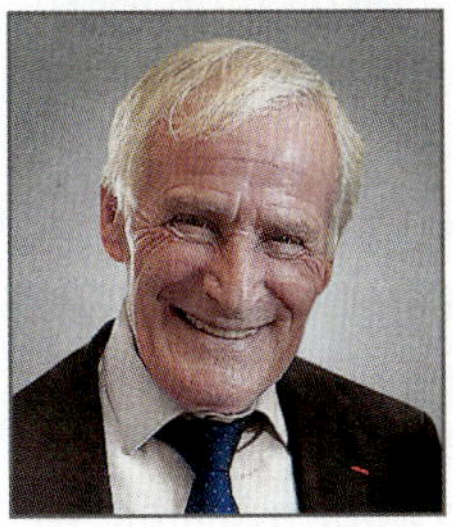

Alain Cribier MD
Emeritus Professor of Medicine
Past-Chief of the Department of Cardiology
Consultant for the Rouen Normandy Medical Training Center
Charles Nicolle Hospital, University of Rouen, France

It is an honor and a pleasure for me to preface this 2023 edition of the CSI Update Book. This is an outstanding edition, covering in no less than 2 volumes and 217 chapters the current state and most advanced aspects of general cardiology and interventional cardiology worldwide and particularly in India.

In over 20 years, accelerating technological, therapeutic, and organizational advances have changed the face of cardiology. Thanks to scientific discoveries in recent years, new gains in life expectancy can be achieved. Decisive victories have been won in cases of myocardial infarction, stroke, rhythm disorders, valvular diseases, and heart failure. Nevertheless, it should be remembered that cardiovascular disease (CVD) remains the world's leading cause of mortality and is set to grow exponentially as the population ages. Over the past 10 years, cardiovascular deaths have soared worldwide, rising from 12.1 million in 1990 to 29.5 million in 2021, according to the report of the World Heart Association, with 4 out of 5 deaths occurring in low- or mid-income countries. These are also the countries where the coronavirus disease 2019 (COVID-19) has had the most devastating impact.

The challenges of the future must include progresses in primary and secondary prevention methods and the fight against risk factors, such as smoking, alcohol, sedentary lifestyle, hyperlipidemia, diabetes, and high blood pressure, and adapt them to the considerable disparity of medical and social situations around the world. In countries with limited economic resources the challenge is particularly high due to the often-insurmountable difficulties of acceding to preventive and therapeutic measures.

These subjects are superbly covered in the first volume of the book in which the current state of prevention and treatment of CVD in India is fully documented.

The second volume of the book is dedicated to "Interventional Cardiology" which includes a special overview of the situation in India. The history of interventional medicine is short with an explosion of innovative treatments emerging at the end of the 20th century and dramatically expanding in the 21st century. For the newer generation of interventional specialists, with the armamentarium of these strategies at their fingertips, it is intellectually impossible to imagine what it was like treating CVD less than 50 years ago. Conceptually described by Dotter and Judkins in 1964, the crucial milestone has been the first coronary angioplasty performed by Andreas Gruentzig in September 1977 (who initiated at the same time the specialty of "interventional cardiology"), a great source of inspiration for many others. Coronary stent implantation was launched 10 years later by Jacques Puel in France who performed the first case. This technique has been dramatically expanding to become a routine daily procedure in the whole world and particularly in India.

"Structural Heart diseases" covers all noncoronary heart diseases and their dedicated interventional techniques and valve replacement and repair that have been the fastest developing areas. Following the footsteps of trans-catheter treatment of congenital pulmonic (1979) and aortic valvular stenosis (1983), mitral valvuloplasty (1984) and aortic valvuloplasty in adults by our group (1985), and then pulmonic valve replacement in degenerated conduits (2000), the technique of transcatheter aortic valve implantation (TAVI) for the transcatheter treatment of degenerative aortic stenosis, initiated by us after 15 years of research, emerged in 2002 to profoundly alter the landscape of cardiovascular medicine. Helene Eltchaninoff and I have the pleasure of describing the amazing odyssey of TAVI development in one of the chapters of this volume. Over the last 20 years, this breakthrough lifesaving procedure has been constantly improved and used in about 3 million of patients worldwide, with expanding indications. Since 2011, the year of the first case performed in India, the number of cases has been steadily but rather slowly increasing due to several obstacles including high cost and lack of coverage by insurance companies. However, thousands of patients have benefited from TAVI in the country to date. TAVI, in turn, became a strong source of inspiration for the development of new interventional techniques aimed at treating other valvular diseases, such as mitral and tricuspid insufficiency by repairing or replacing the diseased valve.

The most recent technical and procedural advances, the issues of patient's selection, procedural techniques, prevention and treatment of complications, and the latest scientific results obtained in all aspects of interventional cardiology are fully overviewed in the book.

The sum of information provided in this edition of the CSI Update Book 2023 is a real achievement, thanks to the Editor and the outstanding contribution of all expert authors. There is no doubt that having this book available will immensely benefit anyone working in the field of healthcare in India and far beyond.

PREFACE

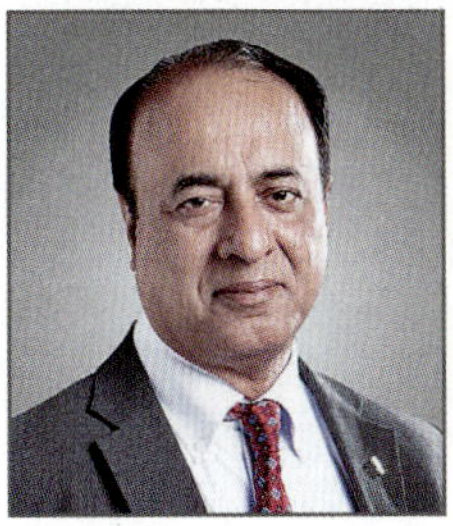

Pratap Chandra Rath MD DM FICC FESC FACC FRCP (London) FRCP (Edinburgh)
Senior Consultant Cardiologist and HOD
Department of Cardiology
Apollo Hospital, Jubilee Hills
Hyderabad, Telangana
Apollo Hospital
Bhubaneshwar, Odisha, India

As a President Elect of the Cardiology Society of India (CSI), it is my immense pleasure and privilege to introduce the book *Cardiology Update 2023* which aims to provide a comprehensive and up-to-date overview of the entire cardiology field. Our goal is to produce a clinically oriented book including all the major cardiovascular advances.

Over the years, interventional and preventive cardiology has revolutionized the management of cardiovascular diseases, offering different prevention strategies, new medical management guidelines, and minimally invasive procedures that have transformed the lives of countless patients. The development of wearable devices, smartphone applications, and telemedicine platforms has made remote monitoring and management of cardiovascular conditions a reality. Patients can now actively participate in their own care. From the early days of balloon angioplasty to the more recent advancements in percutaneous coronary interventions, the field has witnessed remarkable progress. There has been an explosion of structural interventions such as transcatheter aortic valve replacement (TAVR), transcatheter mitral valve replacement (TMVR), MitraClip, and left atrial appendage (LAA) occluder in the last decade. These recent trends are reflected in the book and are covered in great detail.

This book serves as a valuable resource for both aspiring and experienced interventional cardiologists, clinical cardiologists, and other healthcare professionals. The book is divided into sections that deal with specific themes involving various topics.

The chapters in this book are written by pioneers in the field who have dedicated their careers to advancing the practice of cardiology. We have recruited young cardiologists as authors of many key topics with an eye on the future. Each chapter provides a concise yet comprehensive overview of a specific aspect of interventional cardiology, supported by evidence-based research and clinical experience. We hope that this edition of *Cardiology Update 2023* will provide guidance and education to cardiologists of various disciplines and primarily students. Please enjoy reading the update and adopt this as a resource in your daily practice.

CONTENTS

VOLUME 1

SECTION 1: ARTIFICIAL INTELLIGENCE IN CARDIOLOGY

SECTION 2: GENERAL CARDIOLOGY

SECTION 4: HYPERTENSION

SECTION 5: HEART FAILURE

SECTION 6: LIPIDS

SECTION 8: CHRONIC CORONARY SYNDROMES

SECTION 9: CARDIOMYOPATHY

SECTION 10: CARDIO DIABETES

SECTION 11: CARDIO-OBSTETRICS

SECTION 12: CARDIO-ONCOLOGY

SECTION 13: ECHOCARDIOGRAPHY

SECTION 18: MISCELLANEOUS

VOLUME 2

SECTION 19: CORONARY INTERVENTION

SECTION 21: ENDOVASCULAR AND PERIPHERAL

Scan the QR code to access references of all the chapters.

SECTION 19

Coronary Intervention

CHAPTER

131 Plaque Rupture versus Erosion: Common Consensus in ST-segment Elevation Myocardial Infarction

Dhiman Kahali, Ritwik Ghosal, Asit Das

ABSTRACT

Plaque rupture (PR) causing ST-segment elevation myocardial infarction (STEMI) is a well-established event. Owing to the development of intracoronary imaging, the incidence of plaque erosion (PE) is increasingly recognized phenomena. With recent studies, the difference between PR and PE in pathophysiological mechanisms, biomarkers, and clinical outcomes is getting evident. So, accurate diagnosis and specific management is the need of the hour in patients of STEMI. In this chapter, we have portrayed recent studies showing distinct contrast between PR and PE from clinicopathological and radiological aspect to guide us for further management.

Keywords: Plaque rupture, ST-segment elevation myocardial infarction (STEMI), pathophysiological mechanisms.

INTRODUCTION

The ST-segment elevation myocardial infarction (STEMI) is a significant health problem in industrialized countries and is becoming an increasingly significant problem in developing countries. It is familiar that atherosclerotic plaque rupture (PR) is the primary pathological cause of STEMI.[1] Progress has been made in the uncovering of the etiopathogenesis and progression of preventive procedures against "vulnerable plaques."[2,3] By using intraluminal imaging, specifically optical coherence tomography (OCT), it was distinguished that plaque erosion (PE) is likewise a vital mechanism underlying STEMI.[4] Evidences are presenting that those with eroded plaques are unlike the ones having traditional ruptured plaques in the pathophysiological mechanisms, prognostic biomarkers, and prognosis.[5,6] Atherosclerosis is universally the foremost reason of death at the current time and infirmity with the majority of disease in the emerging world.[7]

CAUSES

An increased blood level of apolipoprotein B-containing lipoproteins, especially low-density lipoprotein (LDL) typically most prevalent, is a constant factor for atherosclerosis, such as in familial hypercholesterolemia (FH) and other hereditary hyperlipidemias (monogenic disease). Nevertheless, the ailment progresses at lesser levels of LDL in amalgamation with other risk elements that enable atherosclerosis (multifactorial disease).[8,9] These consist of smoking, diabetes mellitus, hypertension, male gender, and an intricate heritable predilection to the disease.

MECHANISM OF FORMATION OF PLAQUE

Low-density lipoprotein and the additional influential factors are multifaceted as concerning lipoprotein retaining, inflammatory cell recruitment, production of foam cells, natural cell death (apoptosis) and pathological cell death (necrosis), creation of smooth muscle cell (SMC) and matrix, deposition of calcium salts leading to calcification, formation of new blood vessels, arterial makeover, fibrous cap rupture, thrombosis, etc. Most plaques are symptomless (subclinical ailment), some become obstructive (stable angina), and some incite acute thrombosis and may give rise to an acute coronary syndrome (ACS).

PREDILECTION SITE

Atherosclerosis is a multifactorial disease that targets the reproducible areas of the arterial hierarchy. Sites having less or oscillatory endothelial shear stress, positioned adjoining the division points and along internal curvatures, are utmost predisposed areas[10] and the abdominal aorta, coronary arteries, iliofemoral arteries, and carotid bifurcations are classically the majorly affected. Preceding to the development of atherosclerosis, these proclivity sites are demonstrated by vagaries in endothelial turnover and manifestation of genetic characteristics,[10] occurrence of subendothelial dendritic cells,[11] and, in humans, by the existence of adaptive intimal thickening.[12] Adaptive intimal thickenings develop extemporaneously after birth and may grow to be as broad as the underlying media. They may offer a soil for preliminary lesion progression,[12] and the rate of development remains astronomical here than at other arterial sites. Nevertheless, with time, the disease stretches to adjoining intima[13] and in aged patients having myocardial infarction (MI) as cause of death, most of the epicardial coronary arteries are distressed by plaques.[14]

MECHANISMS OF PLAQUE RUPTURE

Rupture of plaque transpires at the thinnest cap area and frequently insinuated by foam cells (macrophages)[15] and fibrous caps are at vulnerability of breaking. Discovered by microscopic investigation in a postmortem study of abrupt cardiac death, the average thickness of ruptured caps was found to be only 23 μm and 95% of ruptured fibrous caps (RFCs) were under 65 μm.[16] Based on these annotations, Virmani et al.[17] presented the term thin-cap fibroatheromas (TCFAs) meant for coronary fibroatheromas with a fibrous cap thickness of <65 μm, which can thus be presumed to incorporate the majority of plaques at risk for rupture.[17]

Diminishing or thinning of the fibrous cap undoubtedly comprises two contemporaneous mechanisms. First being the slow loss of SMCs from the fibrous cap. Ruptured caps comprehend fewer SMCs and reduced collagen than the intact caps[18] and SMCs are typically not present at the real site of rupture;[18,19] infiltrating macrophages destroy the collagen-rich cap matrix. Ruptured caps that were scrutinized at postmortem are generally profoundly insinuated by macrophage foam cells[19] which produce proteolytic enzymes such as plasminogen activators, cathepsins, and matrix metalloproteinases (MMPs). The MMPs are released as latent zymogens that necessitate extracellular initiation, following which they are competent of disintegrating fundamentally all components of the extracellular matrix. Whether thinning of the fibrous cap takes years to grow or is much more dynamic is yet unknown. Yet, the fact that fibroatheromas are frequently noticed from 30 years of age,[20] where ACS is exceptionally sporadic, seems to designate that it is a sluggish, smoldering process.

The rupture of a thin cap and consequent thrombosis may take place suddenly, but in few cases, a momentary upsurge in emotional or physical stress delivers the ultimate trigger of the event. Documented triggers are physical and sexual activity, anger, anxiety, work stress, earthquakes, war and terror attacks, temperature changes, infections, and cocaine use.[21] Likewise, elementary daily activities or the quotidian rhythm of biological pathways may regulate the onset of ACS, which are most common in the morning.[22] The activating pathways may include initiation of the sympathetic nervous system with augmented heart rate and blood pressure, leading to PR, or amplified coagulability and platelet responsiveness, leading to an emphasized thrombotic response on already ruptured plaques.[23]

MECHANISMS OF PLAQUE EROSION

The mechanism leading to thrombus without rupture is one of the most imperative, unanswered questions within atherosclerosis research. The surface endothelium under the thrombus is typically not present; nonetheless, no diverse morphological features of the underlying plaque have been recognized. Eroded and thrombosed plaques instigating sudden cardiac death are often barely calcified, frequently allied with negative remodeling, and less inflamed than ruptured plaques.[17,24] Some, but not all, have reported focused inflammation proximately underneath the overlaid thrombus.[17] Vasospasm has been proposed as origin of the endothelial damage and succeeding thrombosis.[25] Unswerving with this theory, PE lesions archetypally show unbroken internal and external elastic laminas and a mature media with contractile SMCs, contrasting to lesions of PR, where the whole internal lamina is often disrupted and the underlying media is thin and muddled.[26]

Remarkably, morphology matching to that of PE (endothelial stripping over pathological intimal thickening and fibroatheromas with thick cap) can frequently be found in segments up- or downstream of PR with a lethal superimposed thrombus.[17] This exemplifies the prerequisite for tightly spaced sectioning to diagnose erosion (by exclusion of rupture). It might also propose that injury or loss of endothelium can occasionally happen secondarily to thrombus creation on condition that one assumes that the bordering rupture in these cases is the solitary-triggering cause. Autopsy studies direct that only a smaller number of ruptures lead to clinical symptoms, although the others heal silently with only mural thrombus.[27-29] Putatively, loss of the antithrombotic characteristics of the plaque surface, which in its extremity may present as PE, could be an influential factor among these results, concurrently with circulating thrombogenic factors **(Fig. 1)**.

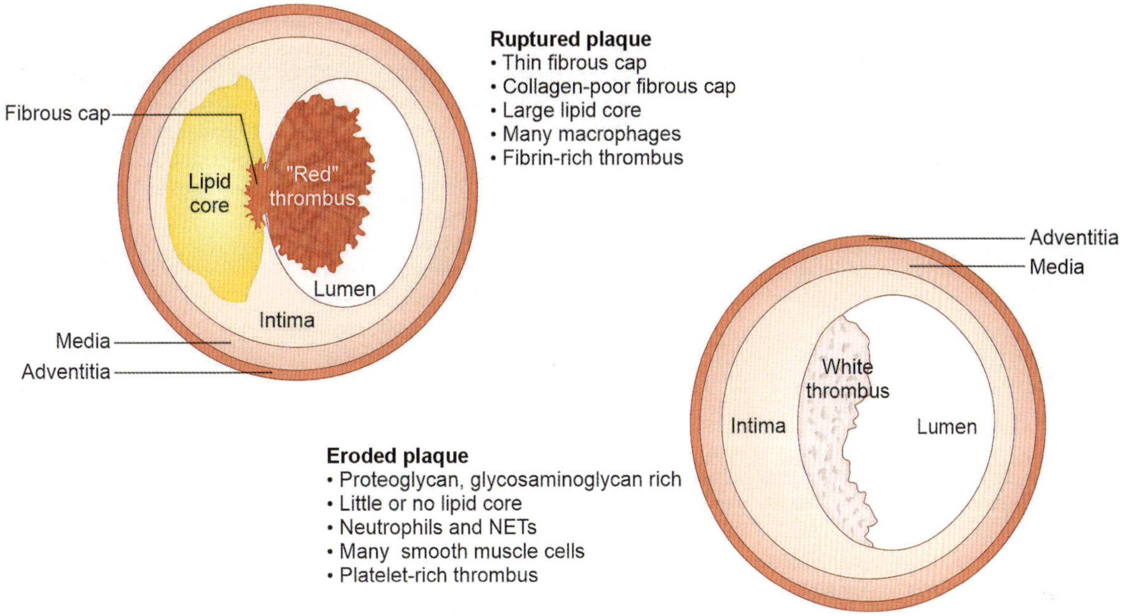

FIG. 1: Comparison of the characteristics of human atheromata complicated by thrombosis because of plaque rupture (top) or superficial erosion (bottom). The text highlights some of the characteristics demonstrated by analyses of human coronary arterial lesions that have undergone thrombosis by these two diverse mechanisms. Neutrophil extracellular traps (NETs) indicate neutrophil extracellular traps.[30]

CLINICAL STRATEGIES AND OUTCOMES IN PATIENTS WITH PLAQUE EROSION

The introduction of OCT immensely guides us to appraise the clinical treatment approaches and consequences in patients with PE. The current standard of care dictates instantaneous stenting for STEMI, and usually an early invasive strategy with stenting for many cases of non-STEMI, which is called "one-size-fits-all" clinical strategy.[31] Though, bearing in mind the distinct demographic features and pathologies of PE and PR, customized treatment strategies are of utmost importance.

An evaluation of the angiographic features of patients with PE and PR revealed that patients with PE had scarcer multivessel lesions, lesser Gensini Risk Scores, more preserved vascular structure and a greater lumen.[32] All of these discoveries suggest that PE may not unavoidably require stent implantation **(Table 1)**. A single-center, unrestrained, prospective, proof-of-concept study was completed to gauge the practicability and safety of long-term antithrombotic therapy without stenting in patients with ACS caused by PE. Patients with residual diameter stenosis <70% on coronary angiography and identified with PE by OCT were treated with antithrombotic therapy without stent implantation.[33] Thrombus volume decreased from 3.7 (range 1.3–10.9) to 0.2 (range 0.0–2.0) mm^3.[33] At 1-year follow-up, OCT confirmed that the median residual thrombus volume lessened meaningfully from 1 month to 1 year (0.3 vs. 0.1 mm^3).[34] The majority 92.5% of patients with ACS caused by PE managed with antithrombotic therapy without stent implantation continued free of major adverse cardiovascular events for up to 1 year.[34] Sugiyama et al. estimated whether tirofiban, a glycoprotein IIb/IIIa inhibitor, had supplementary benefits in ACS patients with PE treated with antiplatelet therapy without stent implantation. The tirofiban group had lesser residual thrombus volume, thrombus burden, and superior reduction of thrombus volume at the 1-month follow-up. These differences were maintained for up to 1 year. There was no difference in the 1-year major adverse cardiovascular event rate between the two groups.[35] Above all, the results proposed that antithrombotic as an alternative of stent implantation maybe innocuous and effective for partial patients with PE.

Prati et al. executed OCT after aspiration thrombectomy and recognized 31 PE patients presenting with STEMI. 40% of the patients with nonobstructive lesions were treated with antiplatelet strategy alone and the remaining 60% underwent angioplasty and stenting. At a median follow-up of 753 days, all patients were symptomless, regardless of stent implantation. They have confidence in that if intracoronary imaging can authenticate intact fibrous cap (IFC) or PE with nonobstructive lesions precisely, the safety and efficiency of these substitute methods could be considered, unswerving with the EROSION study.[36] Souteyrand et al. showed a two-step strategy of invasive management without stenting in ACS patients, guided by OCT. 46 patients were treated with antithrombotic therapy and completed delayed angiography and OCT in a median period of 6 (3–10) days. PE was noticed

TABLE 1: Representative studies of the clinical strategies and prognosis of the patients caused by plaque erosion.

References	Number in study	Strategy	Follow-up time	End point	Key observations
Jia et al.	55 patients with ACS caused by PE	Residual diameter stenosis <70% on coronary angiogram were treated with antithrombotic therapy without stenting	1 month	The primary end point was >50% reduction of thrombus volume at 1 month compared with baseline. The secondary end point was a composite of cardiac death, recurrent ischemia requiring revascularization, stroke, and major bleeding	47 patients met the primary end point, and 22 patients had no visible thrombus at 1 month
Prati et al.	31 patients with STEMI	40% of patients with subcritically occlusive plaque were treated with dual antiplatelet therapy without PCI, and the remaining 60% of patients underwent angioplasty and stenting	753 days	Myocardial infarction, heart failure, or deaths	All patients were asymptomatic, regardless of stent implantation
Souteyand et al.	46 patients with ACS, 39.1% of PR and 54.3% of PE	Medical therapy treatment alone without stenting in case of absence of vulnerable plaque rupture and <70% stenosis	12 months	MACE	23 patients benefited from systematic delayed OCT over a median period of 171 days, showing an increase in minimal lumen area
Hu et al.	141 patients with ACS, 79 of PR and 62 of PE	Stent implantation was performed in 77 (97.5%) patients with PA vs. 49 (79.0%) in those with PE	12 months	MACE	OCT showed a higher incidence of malposition (37.5% vs. 7.3%, $p < 0.001$), thrombus (59.4% vs. 14.6%, $p < 0.001$) and protrusion (93.8% vs. 73.2%. $p = 0.008$) in the rupture group compared with the erosion group
Saia et al.	32 plaques (33.0%) with an IFC, 63 (64.9%) plaques with a RFC	Primary PCI with everolimus-eluting stent implantation	2 years	MACE	At the 9-month OCT, IFC, and RFC had similar high rates of stent strut coverage (92.5% vs. 91.2%; *p* ¼ 0.15) and similar percentage of volume obstruction (12.6% vs. 10.2%: *p* ¼ 0.27). No significant differences in clinical outcomes were observed up to 2 years
Higuma et al.	112 patients with STEMI, 64.3% of PR and 26.8 of PE	Primary PCI	No follow-up visits	–	PE had a lower incidence of no-reflow phenomenon after PCI than PR and associated with less microvascular damage after PCI
Niccoli et al.	139 patients with ACS, 82 of PR and 57 of IFC	Primary PCI	31.58 + 4.69 months	MACE	Major adverse cardiac events occurred more frequently in patients with PR when compared with those having IFC (39.0% vs. 14.0% *p* ¼ 0.001)

(ACS: acute coronary syndrome; STEMI: ST-segment elevation myocardial infarction; PCI: percutaneous coronary intervention; PE: plaque erosion; PR: plaque rupture; MACE: major adverse cardiac events; OCT: optical coherence tomography; IFC: intact fibrous cap; RFC: ruptured fibrous cap) in 54.3% of patients, PR in 39.1%, and calcified nodule in 6.5%. 23 patients, who had a rise in minimal lumen area, profited from methodically delayed OCT over a median period of 171 days. They believed that it might be a steadfast option to choose conventional treatment without stenting in a designated population (PE or nonvulnerable PR without significant stenosis).[37] It might be an unfailing option to choose conventional treatment without stenting in a nominated population.

In contrast, a prospective multicenter study demonstrated that STEMI patients who underwent primary percutaneous coronary intervention (PCI) and received everolimus-eluting stent (EES) were separated into IFC and RFC groups. Saia et al. exhibited that IFC and RFC unveiled analogous degrees of stenosis and an elevated occurrence of residual endoluminal thrombus after manual thrombectomy, and that the vascular response to the EES was admirable and comparable in the two groups.[38] Roule et al. equated the characteristics of plaques and thrombi between PR and PE in STEMI patients, efficaciously treated with fibrinolysis by intracoronary optical frequency domain imaging. PE had a lesser thrombus volume and burden equated to PR at baseline, while there was no noteworthy variance in thrombotic volume, burden, and its dispersal, as well as angiographic estimators of myocardial reperfusion between the two groups after stenting.[39] Of note, 52 patients in EROSION (Effective Antithrombotic Therapy without Stenting: Intravascular Optical Coherence Tomography-Based Management in Plaque Erosion) study completed 4-year follow-up. All patients were free from hard endpoints, while 11 patients underwent elective target lesion revascularization (TLR) due to a lesser amount of enhancement in diameter stenosis.[40] Consequently, whether plaque morphology underlying STEMI should lead to a diverse therapeutic method remains hypothetical. Future studies are needed to corroborate this therapeutic tactic.

Plaque erosion equated with PR had quite dissimilar pathological features that may lead to unlike consequences. Hu et al. retrospectively appraised 141 patients with ACS who underwent OCT of the culprit lesion prior to stent implantation. Compared with PR, patients with PE had a lesser frequency of distal embolization, higher baseline thrombolysis in myocardial infarction (TIMI) flow grade, and lesser incidence of TIMI flow grade ≤ 2 after stenting. Besides, the rate of revascularization in patients with PE was arithmetically lesser than that in patients with PR, even though no statistical difference was found. OCT analysis revealed a higher occurrence of malapposition, thrombus, and protrusion in the rupture group equated to the erosion group.[41]

Previous studies have revealed that patients with PE have scarcer lipid plaques, heavier fibrous caps, slighter lipid arcs, and petite lipid lengths than those with PR.[1,4,42] Besides, ruptured plaques release highly thrombogenic substrates, encouraging repeated local thrombosis and distal embolization. These discoveries suggest that PE may be related with more promising outcomes. Higuma et al. compared the postprocedure results of PR and PE. The study unveiled that PE had a superior plaque eccentricity index and a lesser occurrence of the no-reflow phenomenon after PCI than PR. In addition, PE was allied with less microvascular injury after PCI.[43] Dai et al. described that STEMI patients with PE were linked with improved myocardial perfusion than those with PR.[44] Recently, Niccoli et al. assessed the prognostic value of PR and IFC in patients with ACS. Equated to patients with IFC, major adverse cardiac events happened more often in patients with PR. Patients with PR as offender lesions by OCT have a worse prognosis after a 3-year follow-up compared to those with IFC.[45] However, White et al. conjectured that a higher frequency of the residual incidence of MI and stroke was the outcome of erosion.[46] These conflicting verdicts divulge that more clinical trials were desired to reconnoiter the connotation among clinical outcome and criminal plaque morphology.

Hayashi et al. studied 107 patients with acute MI (PR 44; PE 28; and unclassified 35) by means of coronary angiography and intravascular ultrasound instantly before PCI. Patients with eroded plaques had additional preinfarction angina, less STEMI, lesser peak creatine kinase level, less distal embolization after PCI, and less Q-wave MI 1 month after the onset of MI than those with ruptured plaques. Patients with eroded plaque lesions had reduced infarctions than those with ruptured plaque lesions, demonstrating that eroded lesions were less thrombogenic than ruptured lesions.[47] A three-vessel OCT study was accomplished to examine the nonculprit plaque phenotype in patients with ACS based on culprit lesion pathology (PE 17 and PR 34). None of the PE patients had nonculprit PR, whereas 26% of PR patients had nonculprit PR. The culprit PE group had a lesser number of nonculprit plaques per patient and a reduced prevalence of PR, macrophage gathering, microvessels, and spotty calcium in the nonculprit lesions compared with the culprit PR group, which established that PR and PE had dissimilar pathophysiological mechanisms.[3,30] Several reports propose more extensive inflammation and unsteadiness in culprit PR patients versus PE patients.[5,48,49] Sugiyama et al. endorsed that PE might involve local endothelial damage rather than prevalent coronary arterial inflammation, leading to ACS.[50] These consequences help us to better understand the phenomenon that patients with PE are characteristic with better clinical outcomes compared with PR **(Fig. 2)**.

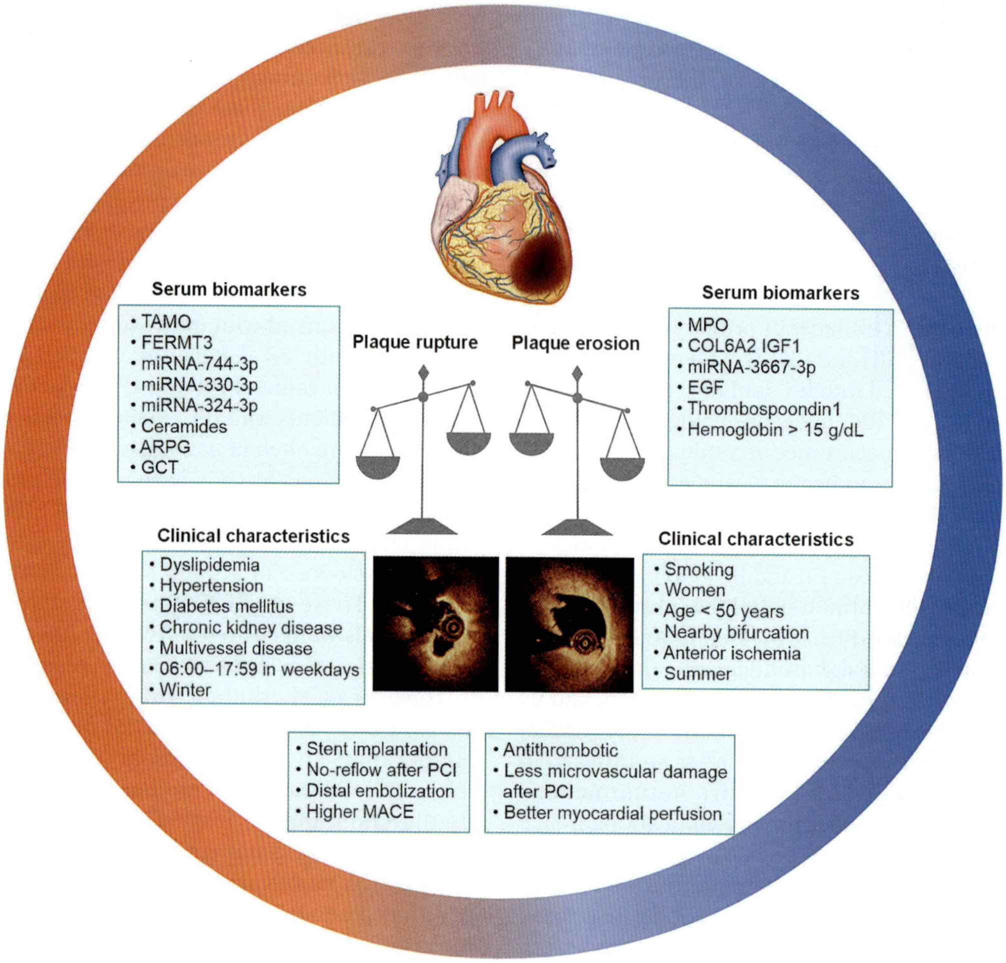

FIG. 2: The prediction and clinical outcome of plaque erosion and plaque rupture.

(ARPG: random plasma glucose on admission; MACE: major adverse cardiac events; miRNA: micro ribonucleic acid; MPO: myeloperoxidase; PCI: percutaneous coronary intervention)

Source: Adapted from Luo X, Lv Y, Bai X, Qi J, Weng X, Liu S, et al. Plaque Erosion: A Distinctive Pathological Mechanism of Acute Coronary Syndrome. Front Cardiovasc Med. 2021;8:711453.

CONCLUSION

Plaque erosion is a common and vital pathological mechanism of ACS and its pathological features and mechanisms are quite diverse from those of PR. The mechanism of eroded plaque is still abstruse and requires further study. PE is a foreseeable clinical entity different from PR in STEMI patients. Antithrombotic therapy alone may be safe and effective for some patients with eroded plaques, but then needs more clinical trials to sustenance this concept. The long-term prognosis of patients with eroded plaques might be improved than that of patients with ruptured plaque.

ONLINE REFERENCES

Please scan the QR code provided at the end of the table of contents for References of this chapter.

CHAPTER

132 Diagnostic Criteria for Microvascular Angina

Filippo Crea, Riccardo Rinaldi, Rocco A Montone

ABSTRACT

Microvascular angina (MVA) is a frequent and often underdiagnosed cause of myocardial ischemia. MVA is caused by an alteration of coronary microcirculation, including prearterioles, arterioles, capillaries, and venules. Diagnosing MVA is complex due to the inability to directly visualize coronary microcirculation, thus necessitating a systematic approach.

The use of standardized diagnostic criteria for MVA, as provided by the Coronary Vasomotor Disorder International Study (COVADIS) group, is of utmost importance in clinical practice. Indeed, such an approach can help in distinguishing MVA from other causes of chest pain, leading to appropriate management strategies. Moreover, an accurate diagnosis allows for risk stratification and identification of patients who may benefit from more aggressive interventions. Finally, it helps in improving patient outcomes and quality of life by tailoring treatment to address the specific mechanisms underlying MVA.

In this chapter, we discuss the diagnostic criteria and the various invasive and noninvasive modalities used for the diagnosis of MVA.

Keywords: Diagnosis, microvascular angina, microvascular spasm, coronary microvascular dysfunction.

INTRODUCTION

Angina pectoris, the typical symptom resulting from myocardial ischemia, is estimated to affect about 112 million people worldwide.[1] Notably, up to 50% of patients undergoing invasive coronary angiography due to angina and/or demonstrable myocardial ischemia do not have obstructive coronary artery disease (CAD) explaining their symptoms.[2]

Microvascular angina (MVA) is the most prevalent and often underdiagnosed cause of myocardial ischemia in the absence of obstructive CAD. MVA is caused by an alteration of coronary microcirculation (cross-sectional diameter <500 μm), including prearterioles, arterioles, capillaries, and venules.[3] Diagnosing MVA can be complex due to the inability to directly visualize the coronary microcirculation, thus necessitating a systematic approach.[4,5] Nonetheless, a timely and accurate diagnosis of MVA is crucial for optimal patient management.[6-8]

The diagnostic criteria for MVA provide a standardized framework that helps to reduce misdiagnosis and guide clinicians in providing optimal care. By comprehensively understanding the diagnostic criteria and the various modalities used for diagnosis, clinicians can effectively identify and manage MVA patients, ultimately improving their quality of life and clinical outcomes.[9]

COVADIS DIAGNOSTIC CRITERIA

The Coronary Vasomotor Disorder International Study (COVADIS) group is a multidisciplinary team comprising researchers, clinicians, and experts dedicated to improving the understanding, diagnosis, and management of coronary vasomotor disorders, including MVA. A key objective of COVADIS is to establish and promote standardized diagnostic criteria for MVA, ensuring consistent identification and classification of patients with this condition.[10] By employing these criteria, clinicians can systematically evaluate patients who present with symptoms indicative of MVA, leading to enhanced diagnostic accuracy.

The diagnostic criteria provided by COVADIS are: (1) Symptoms of myocardial ischemia, (2) absence of obstructive CAD, (3) objective evidence of myocardial ischemia, and

(4) evidence of impaired coronary microvascular function **(Flowchart 1)**. Definitive MVA is diagnosed only if all four criteria are present. Suspected MVA is diagnosed if symptoms of ischemia are present (criteria 1) with no obstructive CAD (criteria 2), but only objective evidence of myocardial ischemia (criteria 3) or evidence of impaired coronary microvascular function (criteria 4) alone.[10]

Symptoms of Myocardial Ischemia

The presence of symptoms consistent with myocardial ischemia is a fundamental criterion for diagnosing MVA. These symptoms typically include chest pain or discomfort, commonly referred to as angina pectoris. However, patients may also experience atypical symptoms such as shortness of breath, fatigue, or pain radiating to the neck, jaw, or arms.[11] Notably, patients with MVA show a comparatively less notable response to the use of sublingual or oral nitrates, in contrast to patients with angina resulting from obstructive CAD.[12] A higher prevalence of coronary microvascular dysfunction (CMD) among women, especially postmenopausal women, has been reported, despite the clinical presentation being similar between men and women.[13,14]

Absence of Obstructive Coronary Artery Disease

A distinctive feature of MVA is the absence of obstructive CAD. This implies the absence of significant narrowing (stenosis) in any major epicardial coronary artery [i.e., <50% diameter stenosis or fractional flow reserve (FFR) >0.80] assessed by computed tomography (CT) coronary angiography or invasive coronary angiography.[9] CT-FFR is an attractive and emerging noninvasive technology for evaluating flow-limiting stenoses, even if it may preclude the implementation of functional vasomotor testing.[15]

Objective Evidence of Myocardial Ischemia

The objective evidence of myocardial ischemia strengthens the diagnosis of MVA. This evidence can be obtained through noninvasive testing, such as stress tests (exercise or pharmacological) using the electrocardiogram (ECG) to detect ischemic ST changes, myocardial perfusion imaging or cardiac magnetic resonance (CMR) to detect regional hypoperfusion, or echocardiography to detect regional wall motion abnormalities.[16] A distinctive feature of MVA is the dissociation between the presence of clinical and ECG indicators of ischemia during stress and the lack of regional wall motion abnormalities. This dissociation likely results from the patchy distribution of small ischemic regions throughout the myocardium caused by CMD, which are not confluent enough to generate detectable regional wall motion abnormalities although they frequently cause transient diastolic dysfunction. This contrasts sharply with the presence of regional wall motion abnormalities, which typically precede ischemic ECG changes in patients with obstructive CAD.[17]

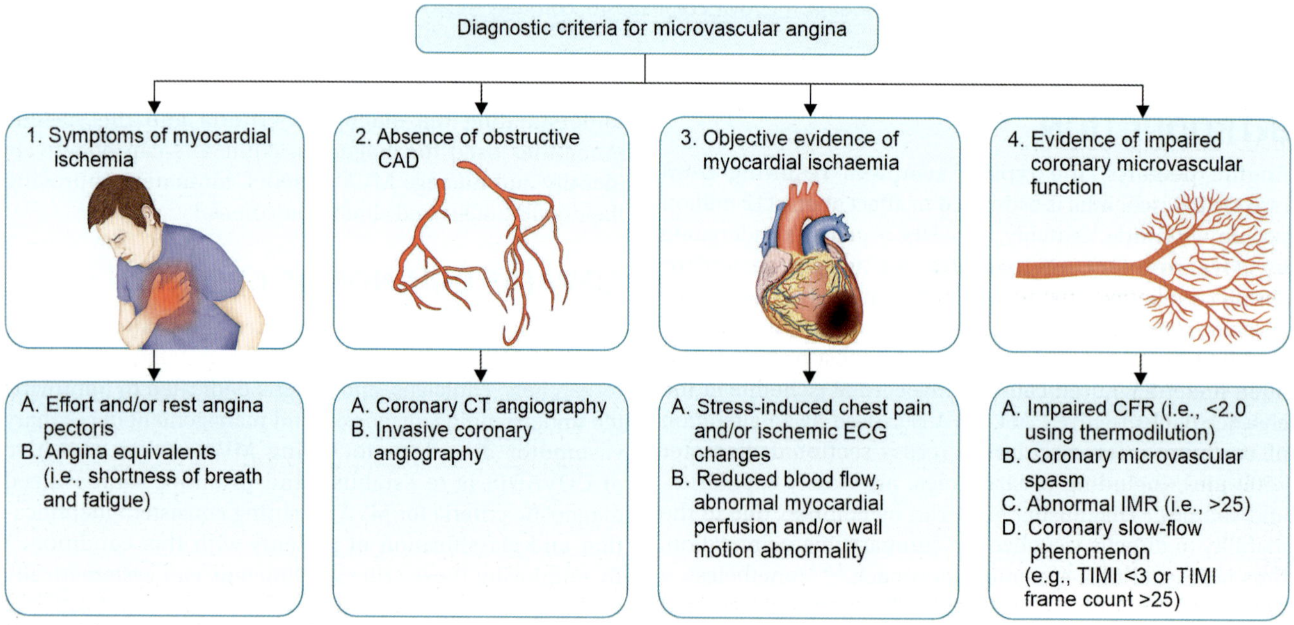

FLOWCHART 1: Diagnostic criteria for microvascular angina.

(CAD: coronary artery disease; CFR: coronary flow reserve; CT: computed tomography; ECG: electrocardiogram; IMR: index of microvascular resistance; TIMI: thrombolysis in myocardial infarction)

Source: With permission from Boden et al. (2023).[59]

Evidence of Impaired Coronary Microvascular Function

Microvascular angina is the clinical manifestation of CMD, which can arise from structural (e.g., adverse arteriolar remodeling, capillary rarefaction, and perivascular fibrosis, leading to impaired vasodilation and/or elevated microvascular resistance) or functional alterations (e.g., reduced metabolic vasodilation and/or hyperreactivity of smooth muscle cells to constrictor stimuli, resulting in microvascular spasms) of the coronary microcirculation.[3] Such alterations, on the one hand, limit the ability of the coronary microcirculation to adequately supply coronary blood flow (CBF) to meet the metabolic demands of the myocardium, ultimately resulting in a reduction of coronary flow reserve (CFR) and stress-induced angina.[18] On the other hand, they can cause rest angina caused by microvascular spasm. Various techniques, such as invasive coronary reactivity testing, intracoronary Doppler wire, intracoronary thermodilution-derived methods, noninvasive cardiac positron emission tomography (PET), cardiac CT, or CMR imaging, can be employed to evaluate coronary microvascular function and confirm the presence of CMD.[19]

Invasive Diagnostic Methods for Impaired Coronary Microvascular Function in MVA

The invasive approach remains the gold standard for the assessment of coronary microvascular function.[9,16] Indeed, such an approach allows for the simultaneous exclusion of functionally significant epicardial CAD and enables the infusion of intracoronary vasoactive agents such as acetylcholine (ACh). Additionally, a comprehensive invasive functional assessment, which also includes measurements of CFR, microvascular resistance, and intracoronary provocation testing allows to identify the specific mechanism(s) of CMD in the individual patient.[20,21]

Interestingly, the transit of the contrast medium through epicardial arteries can provide a semiquantitative assessment of coronary microcirculation. Indeed, the “coronary slow-flow phenomenon” refers to the delayed opacification of the distal coronary vasculature in the absence of obstructive CAD and is considered an angiographic marker, indicating the presence of CMD.[22] The criteria used to define the coronary slow-flow vary among studies, such as a thrombolysis in myocardial infarction (TIMI) flow grade ≤2 or a corrected TIMI frame count >25 frames (with images acquired at 30 frames/s).[10]

Coronary Functional Testing to Assess Impaired Microvascular Vasodilation

Coronary function testing is performed advancing a specific diagnostic guidewire into a coronary artery. The left anterior descending coronary artery is usually chosen as the prespecified target vessel due to its large-subtended myocardial mass.[9] There are two main diagnostic options, coronary thermodilution using a pressure-temperature sensor guidewire or Doppler techniques using a specialized wire with a Doppler ultrasound probe. To induce a steady-state maximal hyperemia, intravenous adenosine (140 μg/kg/min) is typically infused in order to achieve maximal vasodilation.[23]

Fractional flow reserve represents the ratio of mean distal coronary pressure to mean aortic pressure at maximal hyperemia.[24] In patients with suspected MVA, normal FFR values (>0.80) are required to confirm the absence of flow-limiting obstructive CAD.

Coronary flow reserve is a measurement that assesses the vasodilator capacity of the entire coronary bed, including both epicardial vessels and microcirculation. It is calculated as the ratio of maximum hyperemic CBF to basal CBF. In other words, CFR indicates how much myocardial coronary flow can increase above its baseline value in response to increased demand through the dynamic reduction of vascular resistance.[25,26] CFR can be calculated using thermodilution (resting mean transit time divided by hyperemic mean transit time) or Doppler flow velocity (hyperemic flow velocity divided by resting flow velocity).[27,28] An impaired CFR, defined as a value <2.0 using thermodilution and <2.5 using the Doppler technique, in the absence of obstructive CAD, provides the diagnosis of CMD. A novel method utilizing continuous thermodilution has been introduced as an alternative approach to directly quantify absolute CBF and microvascular resistance. This method offers potential advantages such as high reproducibility, operator independence, and the avoidance of adenosine administration.[29] However, further research is needed before implementing absolute CBF measurement in daily clinical practice.

The index of microvascular resistance (IMR) is a dimensionless parameter obtained through thermodilution. It is calculated by measuring the product of distal coronary pressure and mean transit time of a saline bolus during maximal hyperemia and reflects the resistance to blood flow in the coronary microvasculature.[30,31] Currently, a value of <25 is considered normal, while values ≥ 25 indicate CMD due to increased microvascular resistance. Combining CFR and IMR can provide a better understanding of microcirculatory function as, owing to coronary autoregulation, CFR may remain within normal limits despite increased microvascular resistance.[32]

Finally, the hyperemic microvascular resistance (HMR) is a Doppler-based index that reflects the resistance to blood flow in the microvasculature during maximum vasodilation. HMR is calculated by dividing intracoronary pressure by hyperemic flow velocity and values ≥1.9 are considered indicative of CMD.[32] However, the role of HMR in the diagnosis of CMD is less well established, as most studies have primarily focused on the thermodilution-derived parameters, such as CFR and IMR.

Coronary Functional Testing to Assess Microvascular Spasm

The diagnosis of coronary vasomotor disorders requires performing an intracoronary provocation testing using pharmacologic vasoconstrictor agents. These agents can induce an intense vasoconstrictive response at the epicardial and/or microvascular level in individuals with hyperreactive smooth muscle cells.[33,34] The most used agent in clinical practice to this end is ACh. ACh, by binding muscarinic-3 (M3) receptors, stimulates nitric oxide (NO) release from endothelium to vasodilate and directly induces vascular smooth muscle cells contractility. Therefore, the net effect of intracoronary ACh administration is either vasodilatation (healthy endothelium) or coronary spasm (increased vascular smooth muscle cells reactivity with or without associated endothelial dysfunction).[35] Epicardial coronary spasm is diagnosed when the reproduction of typical anginal symptoms (e.g., chest pain) and ischemic changes in the ECG are accompanied by a ≥90% reduction in the diameter of any epicardial coronary artery segment compared to baseline.[36] On the other hand, microvascular spasm is diagnosed in the presence of ischemic ECG changes and typical anginal symptoms without angiographic evidence of epicardial spasm.[10] In cases where continuous measures of flow are available (e.g., by Doppler flow velocity), the diagnosis of microvascular spasm can also be based on physiological responses. Indeed, in the absence of any change in the diameter of the epicardial artery, isolated microvascular spasm can cause a decrease in CBF compared to the resting state. Therefore, the demonstration of a flow reduction in response to ACh confirms microvascular spasm.[37]

Noninvasive Diagnostic Methods for Impaired Coronary Microvascular Function in MVA

Noninvasive methods such as echocardiography, cardiac PET or single-photon emission computed tomography (SPECT), CMR, and cardiac CT offer valuable approaches for the assessment of coronary microvascular function and the diagnosis of MVA. These imaging modalities can provide information about myocardial blood flow (MBF) as well as other valuable parameters, aiding in the detection and characterization of CMD. However, it should be noted that the diagnosis of CMD should be made only after the exclusion of obstructive CAD using coronary CT angiography or invasive coronary angiography. Furthermore, these techniques do not allow to exclude the presence of epicardial or microvascular spasm. Finally, each technique has its advantages and limitations, and the selection of the appropriate method depends on factors such as availability, patient suitability, and clinical context.[38] In some cases, a multimodal approach combining invasive and noninvasive methods may be warranted to enhance diagnostic accuracy. Indeed, combining different modalities can provide complementary information and improve the overall assessment of coronary microvascular function **(Table 1)**.

TABLE 1: Noninvasive and invasive diagnostic techniques for the assessment of coronary microvascular function.

Modalities	Techniques	Agents	Parameters	Diagnostic thresholds	Pros	Cons
A. Noninvasive diagnostic techniques						
TTDE	Pulsed-wave Doppler on the proximal LAD artery	Adenosine Dipyridamole	CFRV	CFRV < 2	• Cheap and readily available • No radiation exposure • Safe with minimal risk	• Limited to LAD artery region • Operator dependent • Technical pitfalls (poor acoustic window in obese and in lung diseases) • Need to exclude obstructive CAD • Assesses vasodilatory microvascular function only
PET	Dynamic first-pass vasodilator stress and rest perfusion images	Adenosine ^{15}O-H2O ^{13}N-ammonia ^{82}Rb ^{18}F-flurpiridaz	• MPR* • MBF	MPR < 2	• Gold standard for non-invasive assessment of microvascular function • Global evaluation of all coronary territories simultaneously	• Limited availability and expensive • Radiation exposure • Limited spatial resolution • Time-consuming • Need to exclude obstructive CAD

Continued

Continued

Modalities	Techniques	Agents	Parameters	Diagnostic thresholds	Pros	Cons
CMR	Dynamic first-pass vasodilator stress and rest perfusion images	Adenosine Regadenoson Gadolinium-based contrast agents	MPR MBF CMR-derived MPR index	MPR index <2	• No radiation exposure • Evaluation of all coronary territories simultaneously • Image quality independent of individual characteristic (e.g., obesity) • Identification of underlying structural heart disease and CMD	• Limited availability and expensive • Time-consuming • Limited ability for absolute quantification of MBF • Need to exclude obstructive CAD • Contraindicated in patients with severe renal disease, claustrophobia, arrhythmias, and implanted devices
CT scan	Dynamic first-pass vasodilator stress and rest perfusion imaging	Adenosine Regadenoson Iodine-based contrast agent	MPR	MPR <2	• Combined assessment of epicardial and microvascular disease • Evaluation of all coronary territories simultaneously • CTA-derived FFR (FFRCT)	• Radiation exposure • Risk of contrast-induced nephropathy • Overestimation of MBF (due to the vasodilatory effect of iodinated contrast) • Limited ability for absolute quantification of MBF • Still needs validation in CMD
B. Invasive diagnostic techniques						
Coronary angiography	Dynamic passage of angiographic contrast	Iodine-based contrast agent	TIMI flow TFC	TIMI ≤2 TFC >25 frames	• Simple and readily available • No additional costs or radiation	• Semiquantitative assessment • Do not provide information regarding the mechanism of MVA (impaired dilation vs. microvascular spasm)
Intracoronary temperature–pressure wire	Estimate of CBF using bolus or continuous thermodilution techniques	Adenosine Papaverine Saline solution	CFR IMR	CFR <2.0 IMR ≥25	• Combined assessment of impaired vasodilation and microvascular hyper constrictive response • IMR is specific to microcirculation and unaffected by resting hemodynamic	• CFR does not distinguish between microvascular and epicardial disease • Cutoff values for IMR still debated
Intracoronary Doppler flow-pressure wire	Direct measurement of coronary peak flow velocity	Adenosine	CFR HMR	CFR <2.5 HMR ≥1.9	• HMR is independent of resting coronary flow • Better reproducibility and correlation with PET than IMR	• Technical complexity • Cutoff values for HMR still debated
Intracoronary provocative testing	Intracoronary infusion of vasoactive agents	Acetylcholine Ergonovine	–	–	• Easy to assess • Simple and safe • No need for additional equipment	• Additional contrast and radiation • Do not provide direct evidence of microvascular spasm

*MPR is preferred to CFR when it is not calculated invasively.

(CAD: coronary artery disease; CFR: coronary flow reserve; CFRV: coronary flow reserve velocity; CMR: cardiac magnetic resonance; CMD: coronary microvascular dysfunction; CT: computed tomography; CTA: computed tomography angiography; FFR: fractional flow reserve; HMR: hyperemic microvascular resistance; IMR: index of microvascular resistance; LAD: left anterior descending; MBF: myocardial blood flow; MPR: myocardial perfusion reserve; MVA: microvascular angina; PET: positron emission tomography; TFC: TIMI frame count; TIMI: thrombolysis in myocardial infarction; TTDE: transthoracic Doppler echocardiography)

Echocardiography

Echocardiography is a widely used noninvasive imaging modality that offers various techniques for assessing MBF and evaluating the presence of CMD.

Transthoracic Doppler echocardiography is a commonly employed technique for evaluating the flow in the middle left anterior descending coronary artery. It utilizes color Doppler imaging to visualize blood flow and pulsed Doppler wave to assess maximal diastolic CBF velocity. Abnormally reduced CBF velocity may suggest impaired microvascular vasodilation due to CMD. Furthermore, CBF velocity can be evaluated at baseline and during hyperemia and, therefore, coronary flow velocity ratio (CFVR) can be obtained.[39,40] CFVR is a reliable measure of coronary microvascular function in absence of any epicardial flow limitation, and cutoff values ≤2–2.5 are commonly used as indicative of impaired coronary vasodilatory function.[18,25,26,41] Notably, this technique is readily available and can be performed during a routine echocardiographic examination. One advantage of transthoracic Doppler echocardiography is its widespread availability in clinical practice, as it can be easily performed by trained echocardiography technicians or physicians. However, it is important to note that the quality of the Doppler signal and the accuracy of the measurements can be operator dependent. Additionally, some patients may have suboptimal echocardiographic windows, limiting the visualization and assessment of CBF velocity.

Myocardial contrast echocardiography is a technique that utilizes the distribution of an echocardiographic contrast medium to evaluate MBF. Echogenic, gas-filled microbubbles of the contrast agent that are similar in size and rheological properties to red blood cells are injected intravenously, and their distribution within the myocardium is detected by high-intensity ultrasound pulses. Myocardial perfusion abnormalities during dipyridamole infusion in patients with otherwise normal wall motion seems to be a marker of CMD.[42] Although myocardial contrast echocardiography shows promise for assessing MBF, its reliability and clinical utility have been investigated in only a limited number of studies.[43,44] Further research is needed to establish its efficacy, sensitivity, and specificity in diagnosing MVA and detecting CMD.

Cardiac Positron Emission Tomography

Cardiac PET imaging is a noninvasive diagnostic technique that has been extensively used to assess coronary microvascular function in patients with suspected MVA. This imaging modality allows for the quantitative measurement of MBF by administering radiotracers such as ^{13}N-ammonia, ^{82}Rubidium, $^{15}O\text{-}H_2O$, or ^{18}F-flurpiridaz. These tracers are taken up by myocardial cells in proportion to the blood flow and can be detected by the PET scanner.[45-48] By analyzing the distribution of the radiotracer in the myocardium, the relative blood flow to different regions of the heart can be assessed, aiding in the evaluation of coronary microvascular function.[49] Furthermore, myocardial perfusion reserve (MPR) and myocardial flow reserve (MFR) are other important parameters for the evaluation of coronary microvascular function that can be measured by cardiac PET. MPR represents the ratio of MBF during stress (induced by pharmacological agents or exercise) to blood flow at rest. MFR, on the other hand, is the ratio of maximal blood flow during coronary vasodilation to blood flow at rest.[50] A decreased MFR has been associated with impaired microvascular function and is considered indicative of CMD. A threshold value of MFR <1.5 is commonly used to diagnose CMD in patients with symptoms suggestive of MVA.[51] However, the limitations such as radiation exposure, high costs, and limited availability should be considered.

Cardiac Computed Tomography

Cardiac CT can assess both coronary anatomy (excluding the presence of obstructive CAD) as well as coronary microvascular function by evaluating CT perfusion (CTP). This technique involves the intravenous injection of contrast medium followed by serial CT imaging of the heart, capturing the passage of contrast medium through the coronary circulation and myocardium. By analyzing the dynamic changes in contrast enhancement, both at rest and during vasodilation induced by adenosine or other pharmacological agents, CT can provide insights into the presence of CMD. Indeed, cardiac CT allows for both static and dynamic evaluation of CTP.[52] Static CTP provides a qualitative and semiquantitative assessment of myocardial perfusion, offering information about the relative distribution of blood flow within the myocardium.[53] On the other hand, dynamic CTP enables the quantification of MBF and the calculation of parameters such as MPR.[54] However, cardiac CT has certain limitations that should be considered. Firstly, radiation exposure associated with CT imaging remains a concern, particularly when repeated examinations are required. Additionally, the availability of cardiac CT scanners and the expertise required to perform and interpret the imaging results may be limited in certain healthcare settings. Furthermore, patient-related factors such as renal function and the presence of contraindications to iodinated contrast agents should be considered.

Cardiac Magnetic Resonance Imaging

Cardiac magnetic resonance with the use of contrast agents, such as gadolinium, has emerged as a promising noninvasive modality for the evaluation of myocardial perfusion. The contrast medium, diffusing from the microvasculature into the interstitial space, results in an increase in signal intensity that is proportional to the perfusion and blood volume of the tissue, the extravascular compartment size, and capillary permeability. A delayed signal increase and persistently hypointense regions are indicative of reduced perfusion, indicating potential CMD.[55,56] Interpretation of the data can be semiquantitative using the signal intensity index and/or the upslope rate or fully quantitative.[57] CMR can also quantify blood flow in the coronary arteries and myocardium using advanced techniques such as phase-contrast imaging. This approach allows for the measurement of blood flow velocities and volumes, providing additional information about the function of the coronary microcirculation.[56] Recently, an automated pixel-wise perfusion mapping technique has been successfully employed to detect physiologically significant CAD as defined by FFR and CMD as defined by IMR and to differentiate CMD from multivessel coronary disease. However, further clinical validation is required for such an approach.[57] CMR offers several advantages, such as being noninvasive, offering excellent spatial resolution, and providing valuable information about both myocardial structure and function without requiring ionizing radiation. However, the availability of CMR is more limited compared to other imaging methods, and factors such as patient motion or metallic implants can restrict its use in certain cases. As a result, the evaluation of MBF using CMR is primarily conducted in research settings and its clinical application is currently limited.

A COMPREHENSIVE DIAGNOSTIC APPROACH TO PATIENTS WITH SUSPECTED ANGINA

The immediate consequence of not considering the multiple mechanisms of stable myocardial ischemia is that patients with true angina pectoris but without stenoses are typically dismissed without a diagnosis. Indeed, cardiologists tend to lose interest in patients without stenoses. Thus, in a patient with suspected angina, a diagnostic workup, which comprehensively assesses both anatomic and functional alterations of coronary circulation, is needed to convincingly exclude or confirm the diagnosis of angina.[58,59]

A possible algorithm for a comprehensive assessment of the multiple causes of angina is shown in **Flowchart 2**. It shows a pragmatic approach which stems from the recent ISCHEMIA (International Study of Comparative Health Effectiveness with Medical and Invasive Approaches) trial showing that in patients with stable angina and without left main stem (LMS) disease, myocardial revascularization does not improve the outcome, in keeping with several previous studies.[60]

In patients with a very low angina threshold and/or with a large area of myocardium at risk of ischemia at

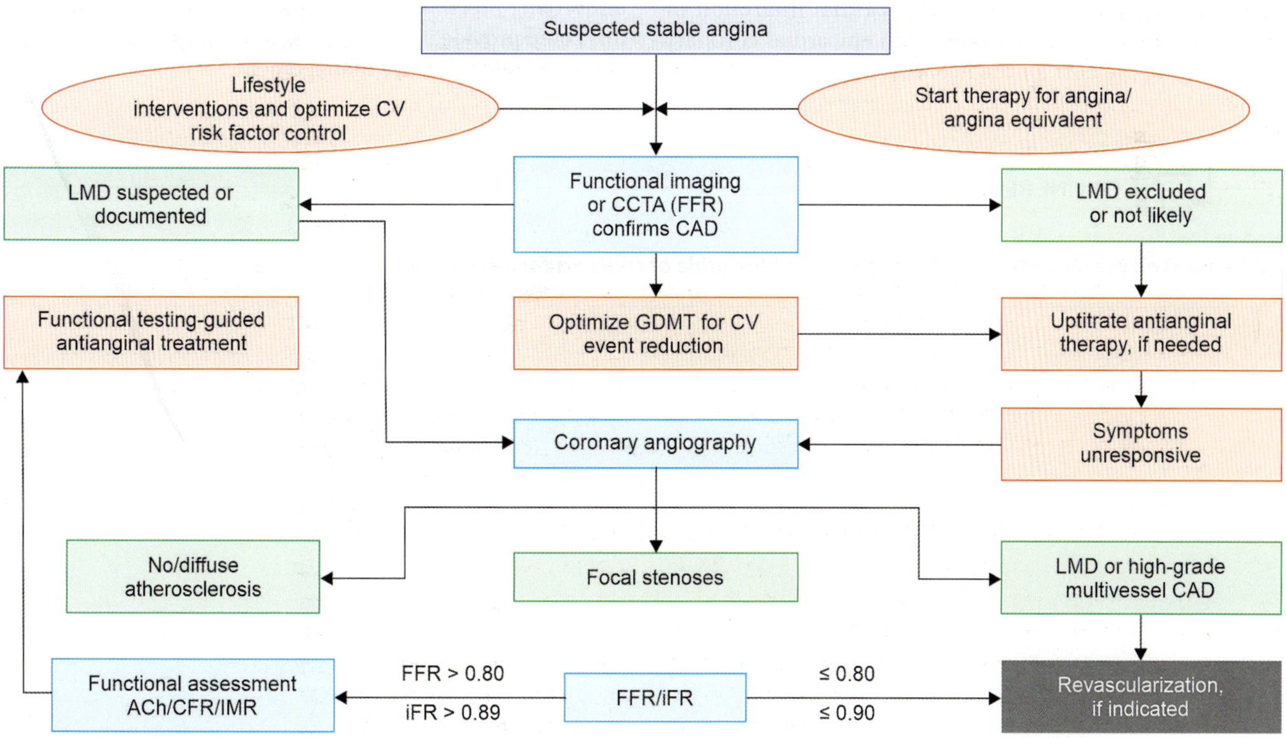

FLOWCHART 2: Diagnostic flowchart in patients with suspected angina.

[ACh: acetylcholine; CAD: coronary artery disease; CCTA: coronary computed tomography angiography; CFR: coronary flow reserve; CV: cardiovascular; FFR: fractional flow reserve (a hyperemic pressure ratio); GDMT guideline-directed medical therapy; iFR: instantaneous wave-free ratio; IMR: index of microvascular resistance; LMD: left main disease] noninvasive stress testing, CT coronary angiography or invasive coronary angiography may be useful to exclude LMS disease. In the remaining patients, a trial of empirical antianginal treatment is a useful initial step. In the presence of symptom persistence, coronary angiography is indicated to identify patients with obstructive stenoses who might get symptomatic benefit from myocardial revascularization. In patients without obstructive stenoses, the functional assessment of coronary circulation including ACh testing and measurement of CFR and of intramyocardial vascular resistance is needed in order to guide treatment. This algorithm puts less emphasis on CT coronary angiography which, in its currently used form, is unable to identify functional coronary alterations responsible for ischemia. Accordingly, in the SCOT-HEART (Scottish Computed Tomography of the Heart) trial, a strategy guided by CT coronary angiography in patients with suspected angina was associated with a worse symptomatic control as compared to a strategy guided by functional testing, probably because the former failed to identify the large proportion of anginal patients in whom the symptoms were caused by functional alterations of coronary circulation.[61]

The detrimental consequences of missing the diagnosis of angina caused by functional alterations of coronary circulation are multiple. First, patients frequently keep living a miserable life limited by invalidating symptoms. Second, they are exposed to the risk of myocardial infarction or sudden death, in particular those with epicardial coronary spasm. Third, the cost for the health system is considerable as the rate of recurrent hospitalizations and repeat coronary angiography is rather high. Last but not least, the origin of chest pain in some of the patients with suspected angina may be of noncardiac origin. Thus, the exclusion of structural and functional alterations of the coronary circulation based on hard evidence opens the way to the investigation of other noncardiac causes of chest pain.

CONCLUSION

The use of standardized diagnostic criteria for MVA, as provided by COVADIS, is of utmost importance in clinical practice. Firstly, such an approach helps in distinguishing MVA from other causes of chest pain, leading to appropriate management strategies. Secondly, an accurate diagnosis allows for risk stratification and identification of patients who may benefit from more aggressive interventions. Lastly, it helps in improving the quality of life by tailoring treatment plans to address the specific mechanisms underlying MVA. Nonetheless, the field of MVA diagnosis is continuously evolving, and several areas warrant further exploration. Continued research in the field of noninvasive diagnostic techniques for the assessment of coronary microvascular function may lead to the refinement of existing methods and the development of novel approaches. Furthermore, research efforts should focus on better understanding the underlying mechanisms and pathophysiology of MVA, as this could provide insights into novel therapeutic targets and approaches for effective management.

ONLINE REFERENCES

Please scan the QR code provided at the end of the table of contents for References of this chapter.

CHAPTER

133 MINOCA and INOCA: A Contemporary Review

Asha Mahilmaran

ABSTRACT

Myocardial infarction with nonobstructive coronary artery disease (MINOCA) and ischemia with nonobstructive coronary artery disease (INOCA) are representations of acute coronary syndrome (ACS) and chronic coronary syndrome (CCS), respectively. They are oftentimes treated by clinicians as mild form of coronary artery disease (CAD) and treated less aggressively. Both MINOCA and INOCA are more common in women but involve men as well. They are not benign conditions and cause future major adverse cardiovascular events (MACE) and contribute to heart failure, both reduced and preserved types. They may be associated with conventional cardiac risk factors and the prognosis is related to the number of risk factors.[1]

The causative mechanism in MINOCA can be atherosclerotic plaque rupture erosion or calcific nodule and non-atherosclerotic causes such as spontaneous coronary artery dissection (SCAD) or coronary thrombus in hypercoagulable disorders or emboli from cardiac tumors, vegetation or left ventricular thrombus which needs intravascular imaging such as intravascular ultrasound (IVUS) or optical coherence tomography (OCT), transthoracic echocardiography (TTE), and transesophageal echocardiography (TEE). The MINOCA mimics such as myocarditis and takotsubo cardiomyopathy need to be differentiated in unclear cases by cardiac magnetic resonance imaging (MRI).

The three major subtypes of INOCA are (1) coronary microvascular dysfunction (CMD), (2) vasospastic angina, and (3) mixed type. The diagnosis of INOCA needs noninvasive tests such as stress imaging, cardiac MRI, positron emission tomography (PET) scan, and single-photon emission computed tomography (SPECT). The subtype quantification needs coronary functional testing such as coronary flow reserve (CFR), index of microcirculatory resistance (IMR), hypermyocardial resistance (HMR), and vasoreactivity testing. The INOCA diagnosis needs to be differentiated from noncardiac causes.

The major limitation in understanding, diagnosis, and appropriate treatment of MINOCA and INOCA is the extensive, exhaustive, and expensive diagnostic pathways and lack of clearcut randomized trials and guidelines in the management. Further research, understanding and simplification of diagnostic and treatment pathways and specific guidelines are the need of the hour in unravelling the enigma of MINOCA and INOCA.

Keywords: MINOCA, INOCA, MI, ACS, SCAD, ischemia, coronary vasospasm, nonobstructive CAD, CMR, CFR, IMR, HMR, PET scan, cardiac MRI.

INTRODUCTION

Myocardial infarction with nonobstructive coronary artery disease (MINOCA) is defined as acute myocardial infarction (AMI) with normal or nonobstructive coronary arteries diagnosed by invasive coronary angiography. This entity was first described by Miller et al. in 1951. MINOCA constitutes 6–15% of acute coronary syndrome (ACS) presentation. There can be multiple etiologies for this presentation such as plaque erosion, vasospasm, recanalized thrombus by spontaneous fibrinolysis, coronary microvascular dysfunction (CMD), or spontaneous coronary artery dissection (SCAD) and often needs invasive imaging by intravascular ultrasound (IVUS) or optical coherence tomography (OCT), vasoreactivity testing, and measurement of coronary vascular reserve (CFR) and coronary microvascular resistance (CMR) for accurate characterization. A combination of etiologic factors can also be contributing to MINOCA in an individual patient. This makes it challenging to accurately categorize and appropriately treat these patients.

DEFINITION AND CRITERIA

The diagnosis of MINOCA needs two important criteria.

1. Diagnosis of AMI as per fourth universal definition of myocardial infarction (MI)
2. Absence of obstructive coronary artery disease (CAD), lesions <50% stenosis on invasive coronary angiogram

Conditions with raised troponin due to myocarditis, sepsis, takotsubo cardiomyopathy, and pulmonary thromboembolism are not considered to be MINOCA.

CLINICAL PRESENTATION

The MINOCA has greater prevalence in women as compared to men, almost twofold. MINOCA involved younger age <55 years more commonly and had lesser dyslipidemia as compared to patients with obstructive CAD. There are lesser degrees of ST changes on electrocardiogram (ECG), there is lower magnitude of increase in troponin levels.

ETIOLOGY OF MINOCA

Coronary Atherosclerosis

Coronary atherosclerosis is the most common underlying cause in most patients with plaque erosion, rupture, or calcific nodule. Plaque erosion occurs with intact fibrous cap with overlying thrombus and is more common in females. It is seen only on imaging by IVUS or OCT and cannot be diagnosed angiographically.

Coronary Vasospasm

Coronary vasospasm causing significant epicardial artery constriction can cause reduced myocardial flow and necrosis. There is a case report of coronary spasm causing inferior wall MI with cardiac rupture and pseudoaneurysm formation by Mahilmaran et al.[2] Vasospasm is more common in smokers and substance abuse such as cocaine and amphetamine. Vasospasm can coexist with atherosclerotic CAD.

Coronary Thromboembolism

Coronary emboli can occur from vegetations, tumors-like myxoma, left ventricular or left atrial, left atrial appendage thrombi in patients with atrial fibrillation, or dilated cardiomyopathy. In situ thrombosis has been known to occur in patients with hypercoagulable disorders.

Spontaneous Coronary Artery Dissection

Spontaneous coronary artery dissection occurs almost exclusively in women in 80–90% of cases. There is an intimal tear extending into media and causing intramural hematoma and compromise of lumen. It is predominantly occurring in younger women where it is the cause of spontaneous MI in 35% of MI in women <50 years of age. The overall incidence of SCAD is 2–4% of all ACS. There is an increased incidence during pregnancy and postpartum, Danhof's syndrome, Marfan's, and fibromuscular dysplasia. The diagnosis is confirmed by imaging with IVUS or OCT.

DIAGNOSIS IN MINOCA

Myocardial infarction with nonobstructive coronary artery disease can present with chest pain and ECG changes of ST-segment elevation myocardial infarction (STEMI) or non-STEMI.

It constitutes 5–15% of ACS presentations and diagnosis needs to be established by absence of >50% stenosis on invasive coronary angiogram.

Transthoracic echocardiogram may show regional wall motion abnormality and is useful to exclude alternative diagnosis like takotsubo cardiomyopathy.

The underlying etiology and management need intravascular imaging by IVUS or OCT. An IVUS-based study revealed atherosclerotic plaques with erosion or rupture in 40% of cases of MINOCA. Coronary function testing is done by fractional flow reserve (FFR) in borderline lesions and index of microvascular dysfunction by coronary flow reserve (CFR) and index of microcirculatory resistance (IMR). CFR <2 after vasodilator adenosine, IMR >25, and TIMI frame count >3 beats to fill a vessel indicate CMD. FFR is not reliable in ACS in culprit arteries. Coronary vasospasm is diagnosed by spontaneous >90% coronary constriction with angina and ischemic changes or testing is done by acetylcholine infusion given during coronary angiography. Patients with normal angiogram need imaging with cardiac magnetic resonance imaging (MRI) which may show scar related to MI, myocarditis or takotsubo cardiomyopathy and differentiate MINOCA from other disorders mimicking MINOCA. Cardiac MRI when done in the first week after ACS, the yield is 90%, if done later within 3 months diagnostic yield is 70–80%. Establishing the diagnosis and underlying mechanism is crucial to appropriate management and follow-up and can avoid wrongly categorizing myocarditis and takotsubo cardiomyopathy with MINOCA. A combination of OCT with CMR has been shown to unravel the etiology in as much as 85% of cases with the vast majority of 64% being due to atherosclerotic ischemic etiology.

Cardiac Magnetic Resonance Imaging Patterns and Diagnosis

- Subendocardial enhancement or transmural enhancement-ischemic etiology
- Subepicardial enhancement—myocarditis and cardiomyopathy

- Mid-wall enhancement—dilated cardiomyopathy, hypertrophic cardiomyopathy, and sarcoidosis
- Global enhancement—cardiac amyloidosis and hypereosinophilic syndrome

Coronary artery embolism is suspected with valvular disease, prosthetic valve, vegetations, cardiac tumors, atrial fibrillation, left ventricular thrombi, malignancy, systemic lupus, and thrombophilic disorders. Transesophageal echocardiogram (TEE) is needed to evaluate the source of thrombus.

MANAGEMENT

- *Statins*: The most important underlying pathogenesis is atherosclerosis and statin use has been shown to improve outcomes.
- Renin–angiotensin system (RAS) blockers help in stabilizing plaque, improve endothelial function, and prevent left ventricular remodeling and heart failure occurrence.
- Beta-blockers are useful to prevent angina and heart failure.
- Calcium channel blockers are beneficial in subset of patients with vasospasm. In the KAMIR-NIH registry, about 20% of patients with MINOCA had vasospasm as the underlying mechanism.
- Long-acting nitrates, ranolazine, and ivabradine may play a role in angina relief.

Patients with SCAD should receive beta-blockers, aspirin and angiotensin-converting enzyme inhibitor/angiotensin receptor blocker (ACEI/ARB), statins, and clopidogrel may be used but evidence is scarce.

Patients with vasospasm benefit from calcium channel blockers in addition to statins, dual antiplatelet therapy (DAPT), and ACEI/ARB. Vasospasm may coexist with atherosclerotic CAD. The Swede-heart registry showed better outcomes of MINOCA patients on statins, RAS blockers, and beta blockers and DAPT was beneficial up to 1 year and beyond that had no significant benefits.

The MINOCA-BAT is an ongoing trial comparing beta-blockers with ACE/ARB in outcomes, mortality, or readmission due to MI, stroke, or heart failure in MINOCA.

PROGNOSIS

The MINOCA has better outcomes with lower major adverse cardiovascular event (MACE) rates than AMI with obstructive CAD, but it is not benign and carries risk of reinfarction, heart failure, and mortality. In a large study of 55,369 MINOCA cases, all-cause mortality at 1 year was 3.4%, MACE was 9.6%, reinfarction was 2.6%, and hospitalization for heart failure was 2.6%. A meta-analysis of 1,924 patients with MINOCA had a 12-month mortality rate of 4.7%. In the Korean study by KAMIR-NIH investigators 2-year mortality of MINOCA was like patients with obstructive CAD (9.1% vs. 8.8%), but repeat revascularization was lower. Patients who were not treated with RAS blockers, statins had a higher mortality.[3] MINOCA patients were less likely to receive statins and RAS blockers. An OCT-based study of 190 patients of MINOCA, an atherosclerotic etiology such as plaque erosion, rupture, or calcific nodule had long-term higher MACE as compared to nonatherosclerotic etiology such as SCAD and vasospasm.[4] The important prognostic factors in MINOCA include presence of multiple risk factors for atherosclerosis, an atherosclerotic etiology, presence of nonobstructive plaques in all three coronaries, and markers of inflammation such as raised CRP levels.[2-8]

ISCHEMIA WITH NONOBSTRUCTIVE CORONARY ARTERY DISEASE

Ischemia with nonobstructive coronary artery disease (INOCA)[9] is a syndrome characterized by symptoms of angina with objective evidence of ischemia and on invasive coronary angiogram shows no evidence of obstruction (<50% stenosis). As per the WISE data 3–4 million men and women suffer from INOCA. Women are more likely to suffer from INOCA. Nearly 50% of women with angina undergoing angiogram have no obstructive stenosis (>50% stenosis) as compared to 7–17% of men. The disease is not benign and carries higher MACE, repeat hospitalization for angina and heart failure **(Fig. 1)**.

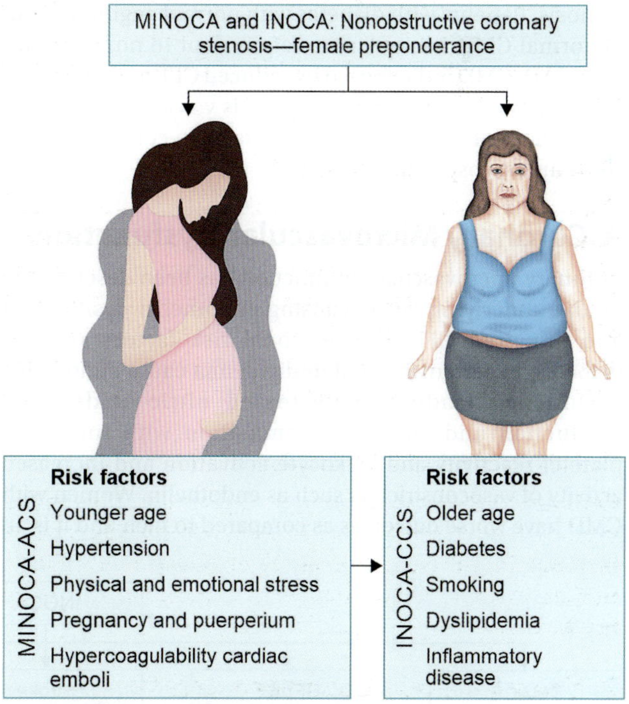

FIG. 1: MINOCA and INOCA—a comparison.

(ACS: acute coronary syndrome; CCS: chronic coronary syndrome; MINOCA: myocardial infarction with nonobstructive coronary artery disease; INOCA: ischemia with nonobstructive coronary artery disease)

Prognosis in INOCA

Patients with diagnosis of INOCA have an intermediate risk of MACE—mortality, no fatal MI, stroke and hospitalization, or angina, at a rate of 2.5% per year. Women, older age, diabetes, hypertension, and smoking are predictors of adverse outcomes. Increased C-reactive protein has been correlated with increased CMD and angina episodes and INOCA is increased in patients with systemic lupus and rheumatoid arthritis.

In the Women with Ischemia Syndrome Evaluation (WISE) cohort at 10 years, the incidence of cardiovascular death or mortality was 6.7% in individuals with INOCA and normal coronaries and 12.8 % in those with nonobstructive CAD. Women with INOCA were fourfold higher risk of readmission for angina within 180 days as compared to men.[8] The number of vessels involved and extent of disease are also correlating with poorer prognosis and the pattern of diffuse nonobstructive CAD in women also forms a higher risk subset. CFR was a predictor of adverse outcomes and in the WISE cohort, patients with CFR <2.32 had a 5-year MACE incidence of 27% as compared to 9.3% in patients with CFR >2.32 **(Fig. 2)**.

Pathophysiological Mechanism

The most important mechanism underlying INOCA is CMD. It can occur with angiographically normal coronaries, nonobstructive CAD, diffuse CAD, or with obstructive CAD. The severity does not correlate with angiographic stenosis. Patients with diabetes with normal angiogram but abnormal CMD has outcomes equivalent to nondiabetics with CAD. CMD is diagnosed by reduced CFR and increased IMR. The second major mechanism is vasospasm of major epicardial artery, and some patients have combination of CMD and vasospasm.[12.]

Coronary Microvascular Dysfunction

Coronary microvascular dysfunction has been described to be the underlying defect causing endothelial dysfunction and impaired CFR. Conventional risk factors such as diabetes, hypertension, and dyslipidemia cause endothelial dysfunction leading to decreased nitric oxide (NO) production and chronic inflammation with increased platelet reactivity and leukocyte activation and increased activity of vasoconstrictors such as endothelin. Women with CMD have worse outcomes as compared to men and it is an important precursor to heart failure with preserved ejection fraction (HFpEF).

Epicardial Vasospasm

Epicardial spasm is related to smoking, enhanced sympathetic tone, and substance abuse such as cocaine. Epicardial spasm can occur due to vasoactive agents such as acetylcholine and serotonin, which normally cause vasodilatation and in patients with endothelial damage act on vascular smooth muscle cells (VSMC) and cause paradoxical vasoconstriction.[10]

Diagnosis of INOCA

The diagnosis of INOCA is challenging and often underreported as not all patients undergo invasive angiogram or coronary CT angiogram (CCTA). The diagnosis is suspected with symptoms of angina or angina equivalent with nonobstructive coronary stenosis. The appropriate tailoring of therapy needs a functional coronary procedure to stratify the type of INOCA, which can be established in up to 80% of patients. But in real world practice, it is not routinely done and results in empirical therapy which leads to reduced quality of life, repeated hospitalization, recurrent testing, increased health burden costs, and future MACE and heart failure admissions.[11] The presence of nonobstructive stenosis is not equivalent to absence of CAD and a huge plaque burden has been found on IVUS in these patients and positive remodeling results in less lumen compromise and an apparent mild CAD.

The various endotypes of INOCA have been described by the Coronary Vasomotor Disorders International Study (COVADIS) group.

The three major endotypes include:

1. *Coronary microvascular angina*: Coronary microvascular angina is due to abnormalities in the coronary microvascular system which may be functional affecting vascular spasm and resistance or structural due to inflammation, reduced capillary density, or vascular remodeling.
2. *Vasospastic angina*: Vasospastic angina occurs due to spontaneous or induced epicardial coronary constriction >90% with angina and or ischemic changes. This was described as Prinzmetal or variant angina for the first time in 1959. It is precipitated often by emotional stress and occurs in rest but may also occur with exercise and is more common in men and smokers.

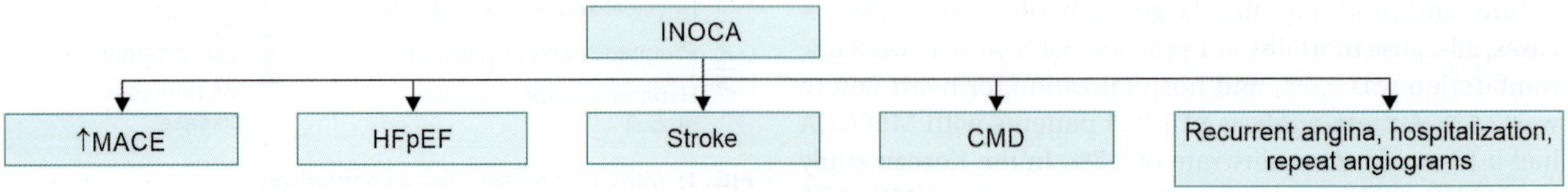

FIG. 2: Outcomes in INOCA.

(CMD: coronary microvascular dysfunction; HFpEF: heart failure with preserved ejection fraction; INOCA: ischemia with nonobstructive coronary artery disease; MACE: major adverse cardiovascular event)

3. *Mixed microvascular and vasospastic disorder*: Mixed disorders have a combination of epicardial spasm with microvascular dysfunction.

Noninvasive Tests

The INOCA needs demonstration of objective ischemia and nonobstructive CAD. CMD can be evaluated by noninvasive tests and invasive tests.

Stress Transthoracic Doppler ECHO

Doppler evaluation of mid-left anterior descending (LAD) at rest and induced hyperemia using dipyridamole is used to calculate CFR. CFR <2.5 has been shown to predict CMD evaluation can be done with either physical stress such as treadmill or pharmacological stress such as dobutamine or adenosine can be used.

Cardiac Magnetic Resonance Imaging

Coronary microvascular resistance is emerging as a useful tool to calculate myocardial perfusion reserve index (MPRI) on exercise or pharmacological stress but is not yet in widespread use.

Cardiac Positron Emission Tomography

It is highly accurate and by use of tracers such as 15 O-Water, N-ammonia can be used to study CMD but is limited by lack of widespread availability and expenditure.

Single-photon Emission Computed Tomography with Myocardial Perfusion Imaging

It shows areas of impaired myocardial perfusion and has prognostic value. It is useful in the measurement of CFR and CMD.

Coronary Computed Tomography Angiogram

It can reveal anatomical nonobstructive lesions and CT-derived FFR has been found to have good correlation with invasive FFR values to diagnose obstructive stenosis.

Coronary Functional Tests (Fig. 3)

Interventional diagnostic procedures include assessment of FFR in borderline lesion, a value of <0.8 after a hyperemic stimulus considered to be significant for obstructive stenosis. INOCA patients have an FFR >0.8.

Invasive tests for CMD include.

- *Coronary flow reserve*: It can be measured by thermodilution pressure wire following a 3 mL saline bolus to measure resting flow and repeat measurement following adenosine for hyperemic stimulus, coronary resting transit time divided by hyperemic transit time in thermodilution method gives CFR value. A value of <2 is impaired CFR and correlates with future MACE. CFR is a sum of epicardial and microcirculatory flow and is a less specific index for microcirculatory function.
- *IMR:* It is measured by distal coronary pressure multiplied by hyperemic transit time and a value >25 indicates CMD.
- *HMR*: It is measured by intracoronary pressure divided by hyperemic flow velocity and a value >1.9 indicates CMD.
- *A TIMI frame count >27* in coronary angiogram taken at 30 frames/s indicates coronary slow flow.[12-16]

Invasive Vasoreactivity Test

Invasive vasoreactivity tests are done after 24 hours abstinence from vasoactive agents and caffeine and during radial catheterization, vasodilator drugs are avoided in cocktail except short-acting nitrates. During testing, intracoronary acetylcholine is given as infusion at 10^{-6}, 10^{-5}, and 10^{-4} in increasing concentrations for 2 minutes at 1 mL/min followed by 100 μg bolus and epicardial spasm is detected in a view without foreshortening of the major epicardial artery with positive for vasospasm showing >90% epicardial artery constriction. Acetylcholine can produce prolonged coronary spasm, bradycardia, or atrial fibrillation. Nitrates should be used for significant coronary spasm. Atropine and isoprenaline may be required but pacing is

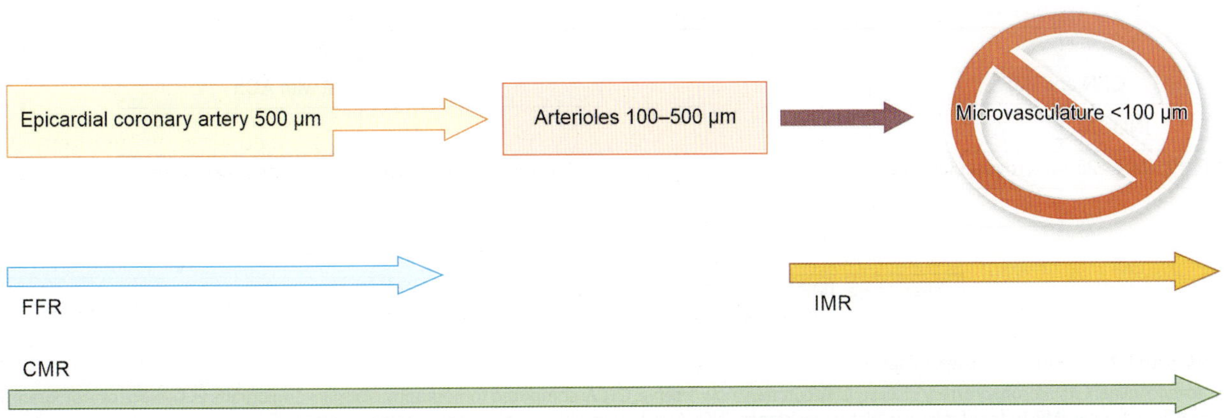

FIG. 3: Coronary function tests and site of measurements.

(CMR: coronary microvascular resistance; FFR: fractional flow reserve; IMR: index of microcirculatory resistance)

seldom required as the action of acetylcholine lasts only for 15 seconds. A coughing maneuver by patient is usually sufficient for heart rate recovery. Pacing is seldom required. A TIMI flow rate <2 indicates microvascular spasm. The test has been found to be safe with zero deaths in a study of 1,500 patients and a complication rate of <1% **(Boxes 1 and 2, and Flowchart 1)**.[8]

Heart Failure and INOCA

Patients with INOCA and CMD are prone for future heart failure, the predominant type being HFpEF. On the reverse, 75% of HFpEF patients have underlying CMD. A low CFR is a powerful risk factor and Taqueti et al. reported an association of HFpEF with impaired myocardial flow reserve <1.5 on cardiac MRI. Microvascular dysfunction can lead to endothelial dysfunction and myocardial fibrosis which is potentiated by the associated inflammation and the coupling of these factors lead to diastolic dysfunction and precipitate HFpEF.[1] The myocardial perfusion is dependent on coronary microcirculation and myocardial contraction

BOX 1 Protocol for vasoreactivity testing with ACh.

Protocol for vasoreactivity test:

- Withhold long-acting CCB >48 hours
- Withhold nitrates, caffeine for 24 hours
- Avoid radial cocktail during angiogram
- Confirm nonobstructive stenosis by FFR
- Heparin 50–70 IU/kg—ACT of 250 to be maintained
- Use 5-F or 6-F guide catheter
- Check LVEDP
- Introduce flow wire proximal—mid-third of LAD
- Measure resting flow and hyperemic flow
- Initiate ACh infusion at increasing doses of 0.364, 36.4, and 108 µm for 2 minutes
- Measure average peak velocity (APV)
- Measure coronary artery diameter distal to flow wire in the same projection after infusion

(ACh: acetylcholine; ACT: activated clotting time; CCB: calcium channel blocker; FFR: fractional flow reserve; LAD: left anterior descending artery; LVEDP: left ventricular end-diastolic pressure)

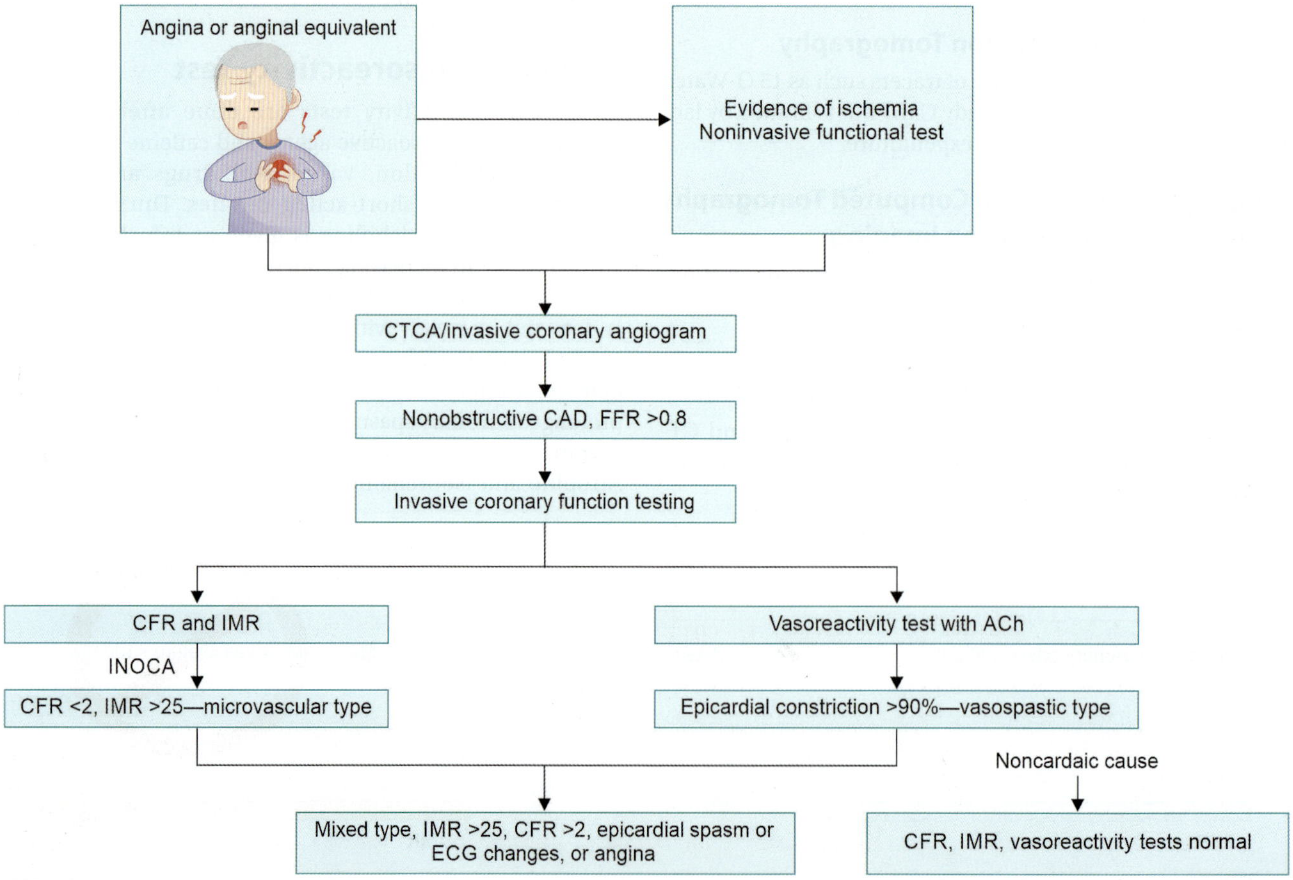

FLOWCHART 1: Diagnostic flow of INOCA.

(ACh: acetylcholine; CAD: coronary artery disease; CFR: coronary flow reserve; CTCA: computed tomography coronary angiogram; ECG: electrocardiogram; FFR: fractional flow reserve; IMR: index of microcirculatory resistance; INOCA: ischemia with nonobstructive coronary artery disease)

BOX 2 Diagnostic differentiation of endotypes of INOCA.

Coronary microvascular angina:
- FFR >0.8
- CFR <2
- IMR >25

Vasospastic angina:
- FFR >0.8
- CFR >2
- IMR <25
- Acetyl choline test > 90% epicardial coronary constriction + ECG changes + angina

Mixed type:
- FFR >0.8
- CFR >2
- IMR >25
- Acetylcholine test—ECG changes + angina/no epicardial coronary spasm

(CFR: coronary flow reserve; ECG: electrocardiogram; FFR: fractional flow reserve; IMR: index of microcirculatory resistance; INOCA: ischemia with nonobstructive coronary artery disease)

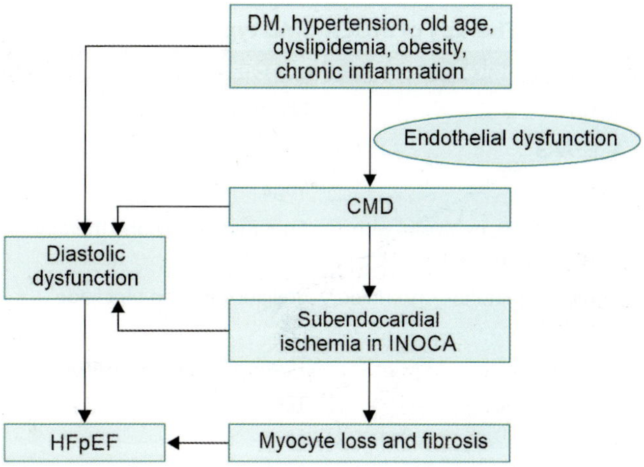

FLOWCHART 2: Pathways to CMD, INOCA, and HFpEF.

(CMD: coronary microvascular dysfunction; DM: diabetes mellitus; HFpEF: heart failure with preserved ejection fraction; INOCA: ischemia with nonobstructive coronary artery disease)

and relaxation which can compress the coronary arteries and affect coronary perfusion and this link is referred to as coronary-cardiac coupling. A WISE cohort study of 6-year follow-up of 493 patients, 3.7% developed heart failure. Diabetes, tobacco use, elevated IL-6, multiparty, poor functional status, tachycardia, and low CFR were associated with enhanced risk **(Flowchart 2)**.[17,18]

Pharmacological Management

- Statins—to prevent future MACE and improve endothelial function
- ACEI/ARB—to improve endothelial function and stabilize plaques
- The question as to if statins and ACEI reduce MACE in INOCA is being studied in women in the Women's IschemiA TRial to Reduce Events In Non-Obstructive CAD (WARRIOR) trial.
- The CORMICA trial in150 patients randomized to a tailored therapy based on functional testing versus conventional strategy showed better angina relief in the guided strategy and it is advised to stratify the patients into vasospastic angina or CMD type or mixed type for better outcomes.
- Beta-blockers—to decrease myocardial oxygen demand and decrease angina, should be avoided in patients with isolated major epicardial vasospastic angina.
- Calcium channel blockers—nondihydropyridine and dihydropyridine drugs such as diltiazem, amlodipine can be used in patients with vasospastic angina, and it is found to be extremely useful in high doses such as diltiazem 200 mg twice daily or amlodipine 10 mg.
- Long-acting nitrates—beneficial in both vasospasm and CMD
- Nicorandil acts by NO donor action and vasodilatation, useful in angina relief in both vasospastic, microvascular angina, and mixed types.
- Ivabradine—sinus node inhibitor controls heart rate and helps in angina relief.
- Trimetazidine helps by shifting metabolism from fatty acid to glucose metabolism, conserves cardiac energy, and assists in ischemia control.
- Ranolazine acts by inhibiting late sodium channel preventing calcium overload in cells and causes vasodilation by acting on VSMC contraction in arterioles.
- Phosphodiesterase inhibitors—cilostazol and sildenafil cause VSMC relaxation and cause vasodilatation but sildenafil should be avoided in combination with nitrate therapy.
- Rho kinase inhibitor—fasudil inhibits VSMC Rho kinase acting on myosin light chain and causing vasodilatation.
- Methylxanthines act by increasing adenosine levels and cause vasodilation in VSMC.
- Ticagrelor also acts by inhibiting adenosine uptake and its role is being studied in patients with coronary slow flow states. A meta-analysis of seven randomized control trials showed that compared to clopidogrel, ticagrelor had better microcirculation blood flow and myocardial perfusion.[19]
- Metformin has vasodilator properties and has been tried.
- L-arginine has been used to improve endothelial function with variable results.
- Endothelin receptor antagonist—endothelin is a powerful vasoconstrictor and its blocker zibotentan

TABLE 1: Therapy of INOCA-CMD type.

Pharmacological therapy	Nonpharmacological therapy
Statins	Lifestyle measures
ACEI/ARB	Exercise
CCB	Yoga
Beta-blockers, nebivolol with alpha-blocking action	Cognitive behavioral therapy
Single antiplatelet—aspirin or clopidogrel	Stellate ganglion blockade
Ranolazine	Thoracic sympathectomy
Trimetazidine	TENS
Ivabradine	EECP
Nitrates	Experimental therapies
Nicorandil	Coronary sinus flow reducer
PDE5 inhibitors—cilostazol and sildenafil	
Aminophylline	
Fasudil—Rho kinase inhibitor	
Experimental drugs: • Ticagrelor • Metformin • L-arginine • Zibotentan • Rhodiola rosea • Rho kinase inhibitor—fasudil • Autologous CD34 stem cells • Nociceptive agents • Tricyclic antidepressants	

(ACEI: angiotensin-converting enzyme inhibitor; ARB: angiotensin receptor blocker; CCB: calcium channel blocker; CMD: coronary microvascular dysfunction; EECP: enhanced external counterpulsation; INOCA: ischemia with nonobstructive coronary artery disease; PDE5: phosphodiesterase-5 inhibitor; TENS: transcutaneous nerve stimulation)

10 mg daily is evaluated in ongoing PRIZE trial in microvascular angina.
- Rhodiola rosea is an herbal medicine with active ingredient salidroside with antioxidant, anti-inflammatory, and ability to inhibit calcium in VSMC and is being evaluated in a randomized control trial in INOCA patients.
- Autologous CD34 stem cells which promote angiogenesis ARE being studied for angina relief in INOCA.
- Antidepressants—serotonin inhibitors like imipramine to reduce pain perception and stress.

TABLE 2: Therapy of INOCA-vasospastic type.

Pharmacological therapy	Nonpharmacological therapy
CCB—diltiazem and amlodipine	Avoid smoking and beta-blockers
Nicorandil	Avoid stress
Nitrates	

(CCB: calcium channel blocker; INOCA: ischemia with nonobstructive coronary artery disease)

Nonpharmacological Measures

- Diet and exercise to reduce weight and risk factor modification have been found to be beneficial.
- Yoga can improve risk parameters and response to pain is improved.
- Stellate ganglion blockade to remove the sympathetic overflow causing vasospasm.
- Thoracic sympathectomy works on a similar principle.
- Transcutaneous electrical nerve stimulation (TENS) has been used for refractory angina.
- External extended counter pulsation (EECP) has been used to increase coronary diastolic pressure and thereby improving coronary perfusion.
- Coronary sinus flow reducer—a percutaneous method to implant an hourglass stainless-steel device placed in coronary sinus increases venous pressure and improves coronary microcirculatory perfusion **(Tables 1 and 2)**.[1,8-14]

CONCLUSION

The MINOCA and INOCA represent nonobstructive coronary stenosis in the ACS and CCS situations and both are more common in women and have different underlying mechanisms with common overlap being atherosclerosis and vasospasm. They are both underdiagnosed and undertreated and mistreated as well. The diagnosis is even though laborious and needs invasive imaging or pressure wire measurements and vasoreactivity testing, the additional cost and time is justified in rendering the appropriate treatment tailored to the underlying path physiological mechanisms and recent trials have shown that a tailored approach improves long-term outcomes.[17] They are not benign diseases and carry risk of future MACE, HFpEF, reduced quality of life, recurrent testing, recurrent angina, and hospitalizations and needs to be addressed and given due importance.

ONLINE REFERENCES

Please scan the QR code provided at the end of the table of contents for References of this chapter.

CHAPTER 134

Management of Nonculprit Lesions in ST-elevation Myocardial Infarction

Parayaru Kottayil Asokan

ABSTRACT

Complete revascularization (CR) is superior to culprit-only revascularization in reducing the risk of reinfarction and urgent revascularization in patients with ST-segment elevation myocardial infarction (STEMI) and multivessel disease (MVD). Percutaneous coronary intervention (PCI) of nonculprit lesions (NCLs) can be performed during the index primary PCI or as a staged procedure and can be guided by angiography, functional assessment, or intracoronary imaging. The optimal timing of CR remains disputed, but there is some evidence that staged CR may be associated with lower risks of bleeding and stroke. Although there is robust evidence that revascularization of NCLs should be pursued in patients presenting with STEMI and MVD, the optimal timing of CR remains disputed.

Keywords: Complete revascularization, nonculprit lesions, STEMI, multivessel coronary artery disease, primary PCI, angiography, functional assessment, FFR, intracoronary imaging, OCT, cardiogenic shock, staged procedure, myocardial infarction, cardiovascular events, revascularization strategies, patient selection, risk assessment.

INTRODUCTION

Multivessel disease (MVD) is common in patients with ST-elevation myocardial infarction (STEMI), affecting approximately 30–50% of patients. MVD in the setting of STEMI is associated with worse outcomes, including a higher risk of death, reinfarction, and repeat revascularization.[1-3] Whether to routinely revascularize these nonculprit lesions (NCLs) or to manage them conservatively with guideline-based medical therapy alone is a common dilemma.[4-6] The decision of whether to revascularize NCLs in STEMI patients with MVD is a complex one. The 2017 European Society of Cardiology (ESC) guidelines recommended considering routine revascularization of NCLs in STEMI patients with MVD before hospital discharge (Class II, level of evidence A),[7] while the 2021 American College of Cardiology/American Heart Association/Society for Cardiovascular Angiography and Interventions (ACC/AHA/SCAI) guidelines for coronary artery revascularization recommended considering percutaneous coronary intervention (PCI) of NCLs as a planned staged procedure after successful primary PCI in selected patients with STEMI and MVD who are hemodynamically stable (Class I, level of evidence A).[8]

The recommendation in the STEMI guidelines to consider routine revascularization of NCLs in STEMI patients with MVD was based on several randomized controlled trials (RCT),[9-12] which demonstrated that complete revascularization (CR) is superior to a culprit only strategy in terms of major adverse cardiovascular events (MACE), but the beneficial effect was driven by the need for revascularization and reduction in angina.[9-12] The recently published COMPLETE trial was the first to demonstrate the superiority of CR with respect to the primary endpoint of myocardial infarction (MI) or cardiovascular mortality.[13] However, the optimal timing and approach to revascularization of NCLs in STEMI patients with MVD are still being debated.[14-16] Several clinical strategies can be considered when NCLs are present. These include when it is best to treat NCLs (immediately during the index procedure or as a staged procedure) and whether revascularization should be guided by angiographic, functional, or imaging lesion assessment. Each strategy presents pros and cons because angiographic assessment may be overestimated by approximately 10% during the acute STEMI setting,[14] whereas changes in the coronary tone and physiology during STEMI may also impact the assessment of NCL severity.[15,16]

The prevailing uncertainty regarding optimal management has persisted despite the recent trials, which demonstrated benefit from CR during the index procedure.

ANGIOGRAPHY-GUIDED COMPLETE REVASCULARIZATION

Angiography-guided CR, the landmark trials contributing to the evidence of an angiography-based approach to CR have been the PRAMI[9] (Preventive Angioplasty in Acute Myocardial Infarction), CvLPRIT[11] (Complete Versus Lesion-Only Primary PCI Trial), and COMPLETE.[13] The PRAMI trial randomized patients with STEMI and MVD to undergo either preventive PCI of all NCLs with a diameter stenosis ≥ 50% (CR group) or PCI of the culprit lesion only (culprit-only group).[17] The CR group had a significantly lower risk of the primary composite endpoint of cardiac death, nonfatal MI, or refractory angina at 2 years [35.2% vs. 51.4%; hazard ratio (HR) 0.65; 95% confidence interval (CI) 0.47–0.90; $p = 0.005$] and a lower risk of MI (20.4% vs. 33.3%; HR 0.59; 95% CI 0.41–0.85; $p = 0.003$). CvLPRIT trial randomized patients with STEMI and MVD to undergo either CR or culprit-only PCI. The CR group had a significantly lower risk of the primary endpoint of cardiovascular death, MI, or urgent revascularization at 1 year (10.0% vs. 21.2%; HR 0.45; 95% CI 0.24–0.84; $p = 0.009$). COMPLETE trial randomized patients with STEMI and MVD to undergo either CR or culprit-only PCI. The CR group had a significantly lower risk of the primary endpoint of cardiovascular death or MI at 3 years (7.4% vs. 9.1%; HR 0.74; 95% CI 0.60–0.91; $p = 0.004$). All three trials found that CR was superior to culprit-only PCI in terms of reducing the risk of death, MI, and revascularization. The CR group also had a lower risk of angina and heart failure. The results of these trials have led to the recommendation that CR should be considered the standard of care for patients with STEMI and MVD. The optimal timing of CR is still being debated, but the landmark trials suggest that it can be performed safely and effectively during the index procedure.

FUNCTION-GUIDED COMPLETE REVASCULARIZATION

Coronary angiography is not reliable in evaluating the functional criticality of NCLs in acute STEMI. Two trials involving patients with STEMI and MVD that evaluated a fractional flow reserve (FFR)-based approach to guide NCL PCI did not show a reduction in the risk of cardiovascular death or MI.[10,12] However, neither trial was powered for this outcome. The decision as to which NCLs to treat with PCI rather than conservative treatment is controversial randomized clinical trials.[10,12] RCTs on culprit lesion-only PCI versus multivessel PCI clinical trials have shown that the use of FFR to guide decisions related to the percutaneous treatment of NCLs in acute STEMI is safe and effective as shown in **Table 1**.

The use of FFR to guide decisions related to the percutaneous treatment of NCLs in acute STEMI is safe and effective. The DANAMI3-PRIMULTI and COMPARE-ACUTE[10,12] trials have shown that CR guided by FFR reduces the rate of ischemic recurrence with a median follow-up of 12 and 27 months, respectively, compared to PCI of culprit lesion alone. Specifically, the difference between the two groups was due to a lower rate of urgent revascularization procedures, while cardiac death and recurrence of acute myocardial infarction (AMI) did not differ significantly. However, there are some limitations to the use of FFR in STEMI. First, the FFR measurement requires the

TABLE 1: Randomized controlled trials on culprit-lesion-only PCI versus multivessel PCI.

DANAMI-3 PRIMULTI	COMPARE-ACUTE	FLOWER-MI	FRAME AMI
$n = 627$	$n = 885$	$n = 1,163$	$n = 562$
314 patients with CR during staged procedure in index admission	295 patients with CR during index procedure or index admission	586 patients with CR. FFR-guided during index procedure or index admission	284 patients with CR FFR-guided PCI
313 patients with culprit-only revascularization	590 patients with CR angio-guided during index procedure or index admission	577 patients with CR angio-guided during index procedure or index admission	278 patients with CR angio-guided PCI
Angiography > 90% or angiography > 50% and FFR < 0.80	Angiography > 50% and FFR < 0.80	Angiography > 50% in the control group and angiography > 50% and FFR < 0.80 in the intervention group	Angiography > 50% and FFR < 0.80 in the intervention group
MACE: Death, reinfarction, ischemia driven revascularization at 27-month FU	MACE: Death, nonfatal MI, revascularization, cerebrovascular events at 1-year FU	Composite of death for any cause, nonfatal MI and unplanned hospitalization leading to urgent revascularization at 1-year FU	Composite of time to death, MI, or RR at 3.5-year FU
13% vs. 22%	8% vs. 21%	5.5% vs. 4.2%	7.4% vs. 19.7%

(CR: complete revascularization; FFR: fractional flow reserve; FU: follow-up; MACE: major adverse cardiovascular events; MI: myocardial infarction; PCI: percutaneous coronary intervention; RR: relative risk)

achievement of maximal hyperemia, which may not be possible in patients with STEMI due to microvascular dysfunction. Second, the FFR can underestimate the severity of an NCL in the acute phase of STEMI. Furthermore, the NCL can be associated with plaque rupture and distal embolization, which hinders the vasodilator response of the microcirculation.[18] Evaluation with instantaneous wave-free ratio (iFR) is performed in the absence of hyperemic stimulation, thus avoiding any limitations regarding the incomplete response to adenosine.[19] In a study by van der Hoeven et al.,[15] iFR, FFR, coronary flow reserve (CFR), and index of microcirculatory resistance (IMR) were evaluated in the NCLs of patients with STEMI in the acute phase and at 1-month follow-up. The results showed that nonhyperemic indices, such as iFR, can overestimate the severity of an NCL in the acute phase of STEMI, while FFR can underestimate it.

A meta-analysis of ten trials, including >7,000 patients, showed that CR was associated with a reduced risk of CV death compared with culprit lesion-only PCI, with no difference whether it was achieved using FFR assessment or not.[20,21] The FLOWER-MI trial[22] did not show a benefit of FFR-guided PCI over angiography-guided PCI in patients with STEMI and MVD. The FRAME-AMI trial randomized patients with STEMI and MVD to either FFR-guided PCI or angiography-guided PCI for NCLs. The results showed that there was no significant difference in the risk of death, MI, or urgent revascularization at 1 year between the two groups. However, a longer-term follow-up study of the FRAME-AMI trial showed that FFR-guided PCI was associated with a significantly reduced risk of death, MI, or repeat revascularization (7.4% vs. 19.7%; HR 0.43; 95% CI 0.25–0.75; $p = 0.003$) at the 3.5-year follow-up.[23] Overall, the evidence suggests that FFR-guided CR may be beneficial in patients with STEMI and MVD, but more research is needed to confirm these findings.

ROLE OF INTRACORONARY IMAGING

The natural history of coronary lesions is different from their stable counterpart and the presence of vulnerable nonculprit plaques may have a role in determining the higher risk of ischemic recurrence. Coronary angiography does not allow identifying plaque vulnerability features that could suggest an increased probability of ischemic recurrence.

In this context, intracoronary imaging can facilitate the identification of high-risk patients who could benefit from the revascularization of NCLs. The PROSPECT study showed that the simultaneous presence of three vulnerable plaque characteristics such as TFCA, the high atherosclerotic burden (70%), and a minimal luminal area (MLA 4 mm^2) were associated with an increase in the combined endpoint including cardiac death, target vessel AMI, and hospitalization due to myocardial ischemia.[24] The Massachusetts General Hospital optical coherence tomography (OCT) registry showed that the rate of MACE related to NCLs was higher in patients with plaques rich in lipids (defined as plaque with lipid arc > 1 quadrant) compared to those without lipid-rich plaques.[25] The lipid-rich plaque study showed an 18% increase in MACE related to NCLs for each 100-unit increase in the lipid core maximum load index.[26]

The CLIMA study showed that the presence of MLA < 3.5 mm^2, the thickness of the fibrous cap < 75 mm, the circumferential extension of the lipid arch > 180, and the presence of macrophages were associated with an increased risk of the primary endpoint, a compound of cardiac death and IMA of the target lesion.[27] The CLIMA study also showed that the simultaneous presence of these four OCT criteria in the same plaque was an independent predictor of event. Intracoronary imaging techniques can facilitate the identification of patients with high-risk NCLs [e.g., presence of thin-cap fibroatheroma (TCFA), large lipid pool with a high atherosclerotic load, MLA < 3.5–4 mm^2, and macrophages defined by the OCT]. In a substudy of the COMPLETE trial, OCT of at least two coronary arteries before NCL PCI was performed in 93 patients. TCFA was detected in the NCLs of about half of the patients and were more commonly found in obstructive lesions, defined as >70% visual diameter stenosis, than in nonobstructive lesion.[28] The FORZA trial compared OCT guidance and FFR guidance in patients with angiographically intermediate coronary lesions and showed that an OCT-guided approach may reduce the risk of adverse events, at the expense of higher costs.[29]

COMPLETE REVASCULARIZATION IN CARDIOGENIC SHOCK

The current ACC/AHA and ESC guidelines do not recommend PCI of noninfarct-related artery (IRA) at the time of primary PCI during AMI in patients with cardiogenic shock (CS) because of the higher risk of death or renal failure (Class III, level of evidence B).[8,30] The CULPRIT-SHOCK trial showed superior outcomes for culprit lesion-only versus immediate multivessel revascularization in patients presenting with AMI, MVD, and CS.[31] A meta-analysis by Khan et al. showed that multivessel PCI was not associated with increased mortality when compared with culprit lesion-only PCI but showed higher rates of acute kidney injury (AKI).[32]

TREATMENT ALGORITHM

Nonculprit lesions may be stable plaques, for which revascularization could not give any benefit, or unstable plaques, which confer a higher risk of rupture and then of future cardiovascular events, thus routine NCL PCI could be beneficial.[10] The question of whether the hemodynamic relevance of NCLs may be determined by invasive physiological assessments or by noninvasive ischemia imaging remains unresolved, but irrespective of the employed method, the general purpose should be to treat only hemodynamically relevant lesions.[33,34] The optimal timing for staged procedures also remains uncertain. Current STEMI guidelines recommend CR before discharge, but they were written before the COMPLETE trial results. The decision of whether to perform PCI on NCLs in patients with STEMI is a complex one. There is no clear consensus on the best approach, and the optimal strategy is likely to vary depending on individual patient factors. Some of the factors that may be considered when making this decision include the severity of the NCLs, the patient's overall risk of complications from PCI, and the patient's preferences.

The BIOVASC trial found that immediate CR was noninferior to staged CR for the primary composite outcome of death, MI, or unplanned revascularization at 12 months. The trial also found that immediate CR was associated with a reduction in MI and unplanned ischemia-driven revascularization.[35] The optimal timing for staged procedures is also uncertain. Some experts recommend that staged procedures should be performed within 2 weeks of the index procedure, while others recommend that they can be performed up to 3 months later.

CONCLUSION

The results of the ongoing trials iMODERN, FULLREVASC, and SAFE-STEMI are awaited to establish the optimal strategy in patients with STEMI and MVD.

The decision of whether or not to treat NCLs in patients with STEMI is a complex one that should be made on a case-by-case basis. There is no one-size-fits-all answer, and the best approach will vary depending on the individual patient's characteristics and anatomy.[36] In general, the first goal of primary PCI is to restore blood flow to the culprit artery as quickly as possible. If the culprit lesion is successfully treated, then multivessel primary PCI may be considered for patients with low-to-moderate complexity lesions, after low-to-moderate contrast volume load, and in the presence of high-degree stenoses with high probability of functional relevance. In patients without CS, decision-making should be related to patient and anatomic characteristics. A pragmatic algorithm for the management of these patients is given in **Flowcharts 1 and 2**. This algorithm involves considering patient and anatomic characteristics when making the decision of whether to perform immediate or staged CR.

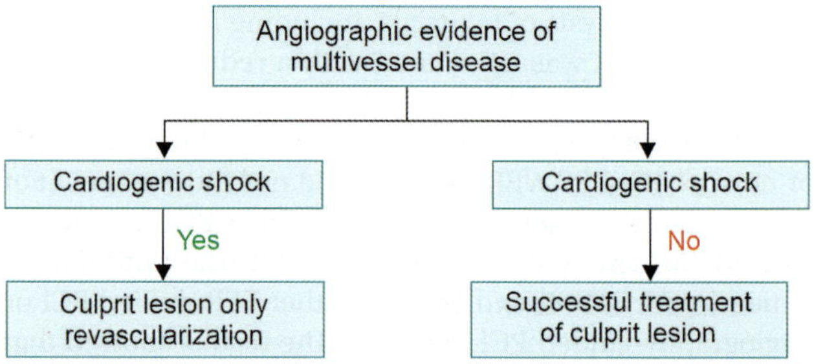

FLOWCHART 1: Angiographic evidence of multivessel disease.

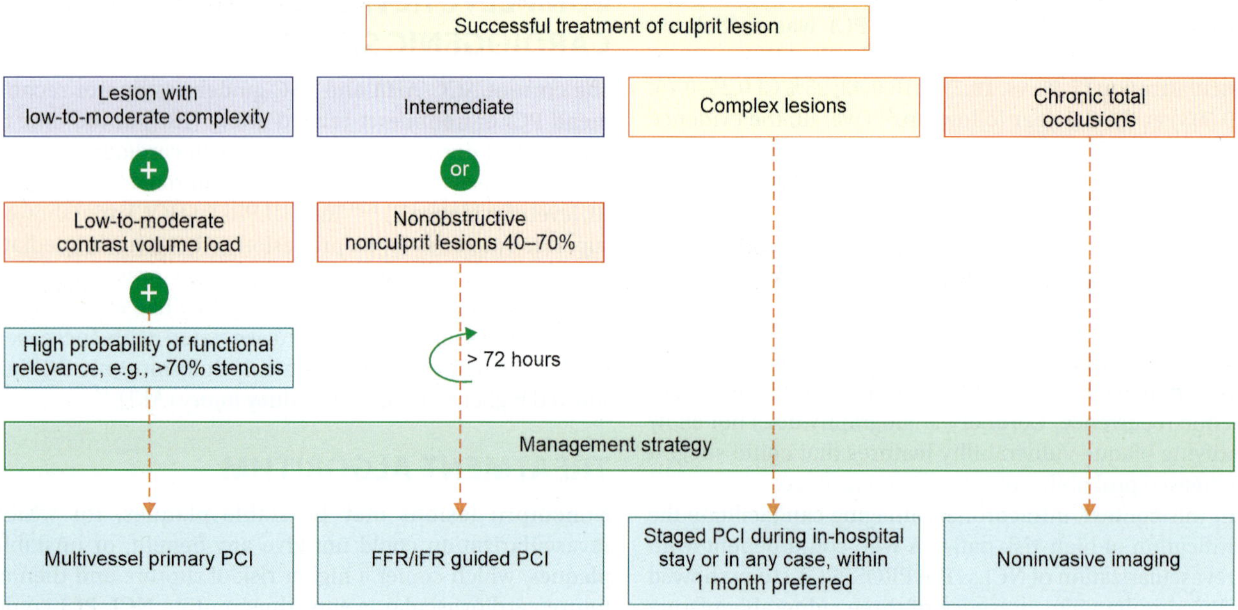

FLOWCHART 2: Successful treatment of culprit lesion.

(FFR: fractional flow reserve; iFR: instantaneous wave-Free Ratio; PCI: percutaneous coronary intervention)

ONLINE REFERENCES

Please scan the QR code provided at the end of the table of contents for References of this chapter.

CHAPTER

135 Management of Thrombus-containing Coronary Lesions

Ajit Desai, Nihar Mehta

ABSTRACT

Thrombus-containing lesions are seen in over 90% of patients presenting with ST elevation myocardial infarction (STEMI) and massive intracoronary thrombus is seen in about 16% of patients. Thrombus is a major deterrent to successful outcomes due to distal embolization, slow flow and no reflow, as well as increased infarct size. Antiplatelets and anticoagulation including use of GP IIb/IIIa inhibitors form the cornerstone of therapy. Interventionists must be well versed with various strategies to manage intracoronary thrombus including use of manual and mechanical aspiration catheters as well as embolic protection devices. Advanced therapies to manage thrombus like excimer laser coronary angioplasty (ELCA) are also available to combat thrombotic lesions. Recent studies also show the efficacy of intracoronary thrombolysis. Drug-eluting stents are currently the standard of care but the option of deferred stenting should be considered in case of large thrombus burden and ectatic vessels. We present a modified algorithm in conclusion to individualize therapy for management of thrombus burden.

Keywords: Coronary thrombus, aspiration catheter, excimer laser, Angiojet, Penumbra.

INTRODUCTION

Thrombus is the hallmark of unstable atherosclerotic plaques which leads to acute coronary syndrome. Angiographic evidence of thrombus can be seen in 91.6% of patients presenting with an ST elevation myocardial infarction (STEMI) whereas massive intracoronary thrombus has been reported in 16.4% of patients.[1,2] Despite the advancements in antiplatelet medications, anticoagulant regimens, and percutaneous coronary intervention (PCI), massive thrombus remains a formidable obstacle to successful revascularization. It can lead to increased rates of major adverse cardiovascular events (MACEs), no reflow, stent thrombosis, recurrent MI, and death.[3]

PATHOPHYSIOLOGY OF THROMBUS

A thrombus-containing lesion develops when the fibrous cap of an atherosclerotic plaque undergoes structural defects such as disruption or erosion. Plaques vulnerable to disruption or erosion have thin fibrous caps and large lipid cores which are infiltrated with lipid-filled macrophages (foam cells).[4] The shoulder region of a plaque is more prone to disruption. The contact of the disrupted, exposed, and highly thrombogenic subendothelial matrix with the circulating platelets and white blood cells activates the coagulation cascade. The resultant platelet adhesion and aggregation lead to white (platelet-rich) thrombus formation.

The concomitant release of tissue factor from the arterial injury site activates the extrinsic coagulation cascade which leads to generation of thrombin, which converts fibrinogen to fibrin. This leads to formation of red (erythrocyte-rich) thrombus which contains erythrocytes, platelets, fibrin, and inflammatory cells and is denser and progressively tougher to disrupt.[5] These constituents determine the level of stability and "aggressiveness" of the thrombus encountered during intervention.

Furthermore, activated platelets release agents which promote vasoconstriction and aggregation such as serotonin, adenosine diphosphate, thromboxane A2, oxygen-derived free radicals, endothelin, and platelet-activating factor. As the thrombus accumulates, the distal vessel is often accompanied with dynamic vasoconstriction which contributes to the clinical ischemic events.[6]

DETECTION OF THROMBUS-CONTAINING LESIONS

Various modalities are available to diagnose coronary thrombus. Coronary angiography remains the practical "gold standard" for the recognition of thrombus, which shows the classic findings of haziness or reduced contrast density, persistent staining, irregular lesion contour, "filling defect," or a smooth convex meniscus at the site of a total thrombotic occlusion **(Figs. 1A and B)**.

When a thrombus is suspected but not apparent angiographically, the more sensitive techniques for its detection may be utilized, including angioscopy, intravascular ultrasound, or optical coherence tomography **(Figs. 2A and B)**.

GRADING OF THROMBOTIC LESIONS

Angiographically, thrombotic lesions are graded using the thrombolysis in myocardial infarction (TIMI) scale which uses a score ranging from grade 0 (no thrombus) to grade 5 (large thrombus with complete occlusion). Additional classifications have been suggested as outlined in **Box 1**. The factors favoring the formation of large thrombus burden are listed in **Table 1**.

MANAGEMENT OF INTRACORONARY THROMBUS

In the presence of a small thrombus burden (grade 1–2), the recommended PCI strategy includes standard

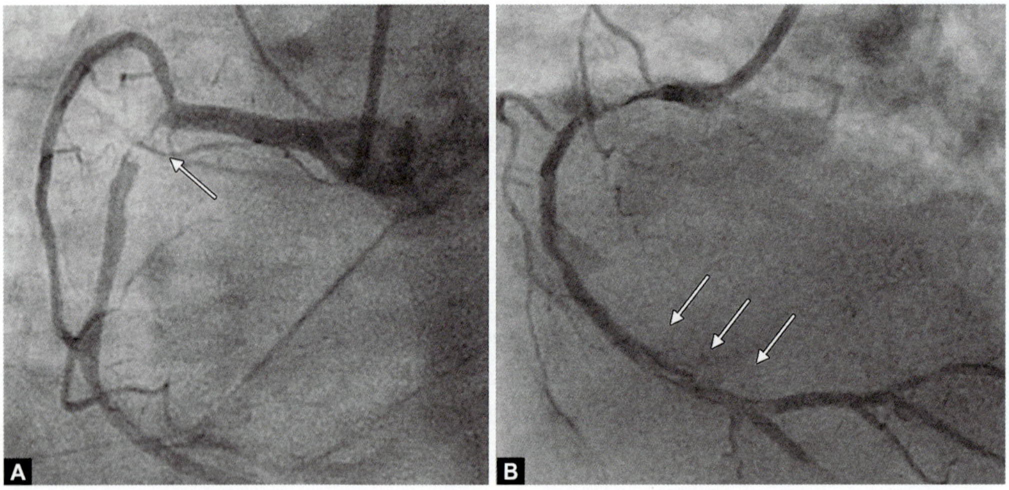

FIGS. 1A AND B: Images from left to right: Angiography of right coronary artery showing haziness with irregular filling defect in the proximal vessel representing a thrombotic lesion (arrow); angiography of RCA with a long linear thrombus in the distal RCA (arrows).
(RCA: right coronary artery)

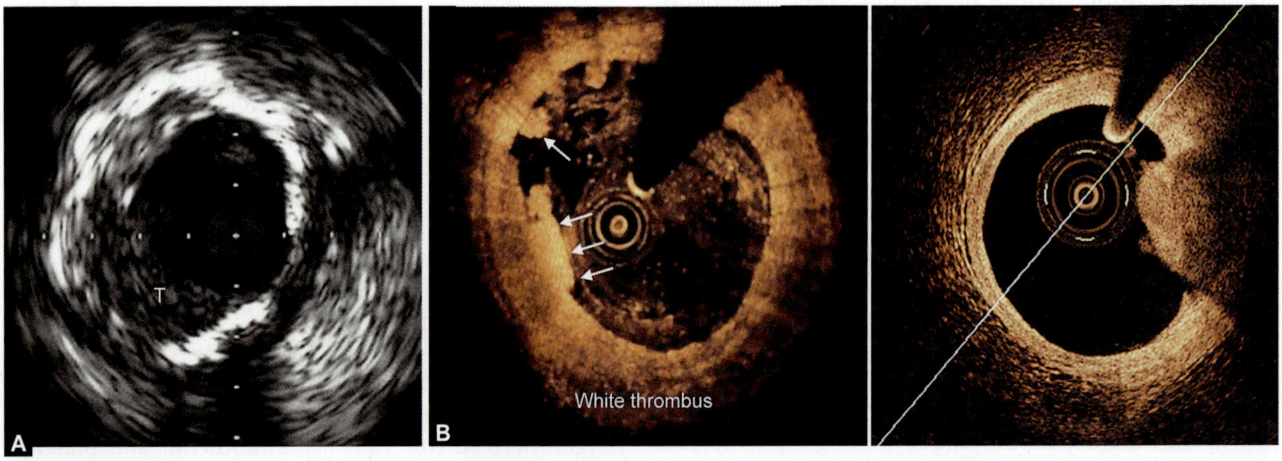

FIGS. 2A AND B: Images from left to right: IVUS image showing a calcified, thrombotic lesion (marked T); OCT image showing white thrombus (arrows); OCT image showing a red thrombus (arrows).
(IVUS: intravascular ultrasound; OCT: optical coherence tomography)

BOX 1 Grading of thrombotic lesions.

TIMI scale:[7]

- *Grade 0*: No angiographic characteristics of thrombus
- *Grade 1*: Possible thrombus—angiographic features include decreased density of contrast, haziness, irregular lesion contour, or a smooth, convex meniscus at the site of total occlusion suggestive but not diagnostic of thrombus
- *Grade 2*: Definite thrombus present in multiple angiographic views—m irregular lesion contour with a significant filling defect. The thrombus's greatest dimension is <1/2 vessel diameter
- *Grade 3*: Definite thrombus in multiple views with greatest dimension >1/2 but <2 vessel diameters
- *Grade 4*: Definite large thrombus with greatest dimension >2 vessel diameters
- *Grade 5*: Complete thrombotic occlusion of the vessel—a convex margin that stains with contrast and persists for several cardiac cycles

Grade 5 reclassification:[1]

Intervention-based: The occlusion is crossed with a guidewire or small balloon. Once antegrade flow is restored, the culprit thrombus undergoes restratification:

- Small thrombus, grade 1–3
- Large thrombus, grade 4

Thrombus grading by a two-category scale:[8]

- Low thrombus grade corresponds to TIMI thrombus grades 1–3
- High thrombus grade corresponds to TIMI thrombus grades 4–5

(TIMI: thrombolysis in myocardial infarction)

TABLE 1: Factors favoring large thrombus burden.

Patient-related factors	Myocardial infarction-related factors
• Hypercoagulability • Hyperglycemia • Hyperhomocysteinemia • Heparin-induced thrombocytopenia and thrombosis (HITT) • Vasculitis • Increased WBCs • Prothrombotic states • Smoking • *Substance abuse*: Cocaine and methamphetamine • Male sex	• Late presentation (>12 hours) after onset of chest pain • Established Q-wave MI with continuous chest pain and ischemia • Cardiogenic shock • Failed thrombolytics
Vessel-related factors	**PCI-related factors**
• Slow or stagnant antegrade coronary or SVG flow • Large anatomical size increases thrombus formation and accumulation in native coronary vessels and SVG • *Morphology*: Ectasia and aneurysm	• Triggering of the plaque and thrombus with guidewire, balloon, or stent—the "angry clot" phenomenon • Inadequate anticoagulation during intervention • Inadequate stent apposition to the vessel wall • Lack of or premature cessation or abrupt termination of antiplatelet therapy
Lesion-related factors	
Acute plaque rupture and complex morphology	

(MI: myocardial infarction; PCI: percutaneous coronary intervention; SVG: saphenous vein graft; WBC: white blood cell)

pharmacotherapy and stenting. In the presence of significant thrombus burden (grade 3-5), the managements strategies are significantly challenging including pharmacotherapy and mechanical approaches.

Pharmacotherapy

The mainstay of pharmacotherapy includes antiplatelets agents which include aspirin, glycoprotein IIb/IIIa platelet receptor antagonists, P2Y12 inhibitors (clopidogrel, prasugrel, ticagrelor, and cangrelor), as well as heparin and anticoagulants. A beneficial reduction in the thrombotic burden can be achieved with the mainstay agents even before the initiation of PCI, with resultant improved results and reduced risk of distal thrombotic embolization.

- Chronic aspirin therapy has been shown to decrease the thrombotic burden before stent deployment.
- Heparin reduces fibrin formation and abolishes platelet contractile forces.[9]
- Glycoprotein IIb/IIIa receptor antagonists dramatically reduce platelet aggregate size as well as improve access to the platelet-rich clot's fibrin **(Table 2)**.[10]

However, these agents are less useful in the presence of well-formed, active, unstable, or high-grade thrombus, for example, revascularization of old degenerated saphenous vein grafts (SVGs) with large thrombus burden.

Slow-flow and no-reflow phenomenon occurs due to severe microvascular obstruction due to thrombus. While this is best prevented, the strategies used to treat it include manual aspiration catheters (given below), autohemoperfusion, and intracoronary pharmacological agents **(Table 3)**.[11]

Intracoronary Thrombolysis

Intracoronary thrombolytic therapy results in a higher concentration of the thrombolytic agent delivered to the site of the thrombus and has been proven effective. Small studies of using of thrombolytic agents as an adjunct to primary PCI showed good results with large thrombus burdens, with improved myocardial blood flow and no increase in major bleeding.[12] The randomized control study DISSOLUTION Study[13] studied use of intracoronary urokinase versus saline

TABLE 2: GP IIb/IIIa inhibitors.[10]

	Abciximab	Eptifibatide	Tirofiban
Trade name	ReoPro	Integrilin	Aggrastat
Molecule	Fragment antigen binding (Fab) 7E3	Synthetic peptide	Nonpeptide mimetic
Molecular weight (Da)	~50,000	~800	~500
Stoichiometry (drug to glycoprotein IIb/IIIa)	~1.5:1	>>100:1	>>100:1
Binding	Noncompetitive	Competitive	Competitive
Half-life (h)	*Plasma*: 10–15	*Plasma*: 2.0–2.5	*Plasma*: 2.0–2.5
	Biologic: 12–24	Biologic = plasma	Biologic = plasma
PCI dosing	*Bolus*: 250 μg/kg	*Bolus*: 180 μg/kg plus 180 μg/kg (after 10 min)	*Bolus*: 25 μg/kg
	Infusion: 0.125 μg/kg/min (12 h)	*Infusion*: 2 μg/kg/min (12–24 h)	*Infusion*: 0.15 μg/kg/min (up to 18 h)
Renal adjustment	No	*Bolus*: 180 μg/kg	*Bolus*: 25 μg/kg
		Infusion: 1 μg/kg/min (12–24 h)	*Infusion*: 0.075 μg/kg/min (up to 18 h)

(GP IIb/IIIa: glycoprotein IIb/IIIa; PCI: percutaneous coronary intervention)

TABLE 3: Pharmacological management of slow flow and reflow.[11]

Drug	Route	Dose	Side effects
Adenosine	IC, IV	• IV: 70 μg/kg/min × 3 h • IC: 48–200 μg bolus	Transient heart block, hypotension, and bronchospasm
Nicorandil	IC, IV	• IV: 8 mg/h infusion • IC: 2 mg bolus	–
Sodium nitroprusside	IC	50–200 μg bolus	Hypotension
Calcium channel drugs:			
(a) Verapamil	IC	100–250 μg bolus or 100 μg/min up to 1,000 μg	Hypotension, heart block
(b) Diltiazem	IC	400 μg	-do-
(c) Nicardipine	IC	50–200 μg bolus (up to 500 μg)	-do-
• Abciximab • Eptifibatide • Tirofiban	IC IV IV IV	• IC: 0.25 mg/kg bolus • IV: 0.25 mg/kg bolus followed 0.125 mg/kg/h • 2 μg/kg/min • IV: 10 μg/kg	Bleeding
Epinephrine	IC	50–200 μg	Arrhythmias

(IV: intravenous; IC: intracerebral)

solution via a microcatheter and showed that the urokinase group had a high incidence of TIMI grade-III flow, myocardial blush grade, and ST segment resolution. However, McCartney et al.[14] showed that use of alteplase in dose of 10 or 20 mg did not reduce the microvascular obstruction or the major adverse cardiac events compared to a placebo group.

Studies have shown that intracoronary Tenecteplase[15] or alteplase can improve the TIMI flow and myocardial blush grade with reduced in-hospital mortality and no increase in bleeding risks. The use of intracoronary Tenecteplase was evaluated in a study of 9 patients with STEMI and a large thrombus burden where one-fifth of the dose of Tenecteplase was given intracoronary and four-fifths was given intravenously followed by a heparin infusion for 24 hours to maintain activated partial thromboplastin time (APTT) 1.5–2 times normal. Check angiography was done in all patients at 4 hours and showed all patients showed recanalized coronary artery except one patient who needed stenting for a residual lesion. No patients had in-hospital mortality, stroke, or major bleeding. This study showed the feasibility of use of intracoronary thrombolysis as a means to obviate stenting in patients with large thrombus burdens or ectatic vessels.[15]

When a huge thrombus burden is documented on coronary angiogram, lytic therapy by intracoronary routes could be administered through the guiding catheter or via a microcatheter or using the thrombus aspiration catheter. A Clear Way (Atrium Medical, Hudson, NH) is a low-profile, rapid-exchange therapeutic infusion catheter which can be used for localized delivery of thrombolytic agents into the thrombus via a microporous balloon.

Thrombectomy Devices

Thrombectomy devices aim at reducing the intracoronary thrombus burden. They are classified into mechanical or manual devices.

Manual Thrombus Aspiration Devices

Manual thrombus aspiration of the infarct-related vessel is a useful method of reducing the thrombus burden and improving the microvascular flow rapidly. The catheters are usually 5–7 F in size, user-friendly, flexible, with a hydrophilic coating and have a low crossing profiles. They are advanced over the guidewire. The distal end is passed up to or across the thrombus and the proximal end is attached to a continued suction. The catheter is passed through the thrombus in order to retrieve as much as possible. Commonly used devices are Export AP (Medtronic) or Thrombuster (Kaneka Corp, Japan) **(Figs. 3A to C)**.

The REMEDIA (Randomized Evaluation of the Effect of Mechanical Reduction of Distal Embolization by Thrombus Aspiration in Primary and Rescue Angioplasty) trial showed that manual aspiration was associated with higher rates of ST resolution, better myocardial blush grade, decreased no reflow, and distal embolization, although it did not lead to clinical benefit.[16] The TAPAS (thrombus aspiration during percutaneous coronary intervention in acute myocardial infarction study) trial in 1,071 patients showed decreased in MACE rate in the thrombus aspiration arm.[17] However, the TASTE (Thrombus Aspiration during ST-segment Elevation Myocardial Infarction)[18] and TOTAL (ThrOmbecTomy with PCI versus PCI Alone)[19] study did not show the benefit of routine thrombus aspiration in all patients with STEMI. These trials did not improve the myocardial salvage or MACE rates and could lead to increase in infarct size.

Based on the above studies, the European Society of Cardiology (ESC) guidelines 2017 do not recommend routine use of thrombus aspiration in primary PCI [Class III recommendation, level of evidence (LOE) A], but in patients with a large residual thrombus burden after opening a vessel with a guidewire or balloon, a bailout thrombus aspiration may be considered (Class IIb, LOE C).[20]

The manual aspiration catheters have some limitations including difficult delivery to tortuous vessels and distal coronary vessels, risk of dissection/perforation in case guidewire is not in the true lumen, requirement of multiple runs in large thrombus burdens, inadequate clot extraction due to small holes and low aspiration negative pressure and distal embolization.

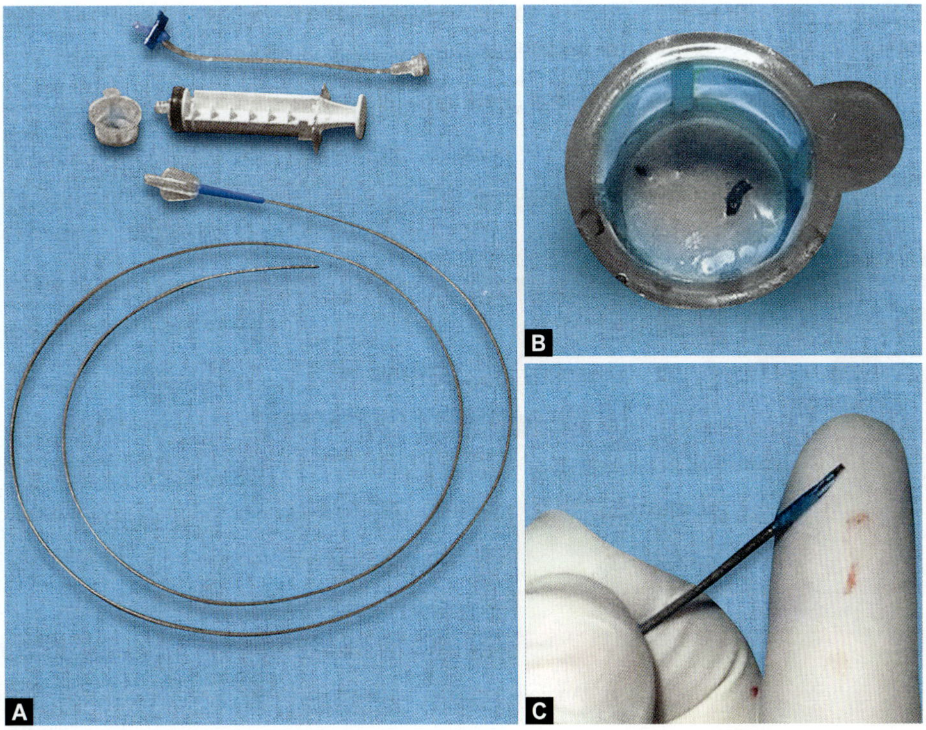

FIGS. 3A TO C: Manual thrombus aspiration catheter.

Mechanical Thrombectomy Devices

- The Angiojet Rheolytic thrombectomy (AngioJet, Possis/Medrad, Minneapolis, Minnesota, United States) uses high-velocity saline jets which dissolve the thrombus and travel backwards at high speed to create a negative pressure zone (venturi effect) leading to suction of the thrombus. The JETSTENT (Comparison of AngioJet Rheolytic Thrombectomy Before Direct Infarct Artery Stenting With Direct Stenting Alone in Patients with Acute Myocardial Infarction) trial evaluated 501 patients with STEMI and did not find significant differences between mechanical thrombectomy and direct stenting in terms of ST segment resolution, TIMI-3 flow, TIMI blush grade 3, or infarct size. However, the mechanical thrombectomy group had reduced MACE at 1 month and 6 months (3.1% vs. 6.9% and 12% vs. 21% respectively in Angiojet vs. direct stenting groups) and improved 1-year event-free survival rates.[21] There are risks of hemolytic anemia with prolonged use and bradyarrhythmias due to adenosine release. In conclusion, the Angiojet may be beneficial in cases with large thrombus burden **(Figs. 4A and B)**.
- X-sizer (eV3, Plymouth, Minnesota, United States) consists of a helical cutter enclosed within a protective housing, attached to a dual-bore catheter shaft containing guidewire and vacuum extraction lumens. Activation of the handheld controller rotates the helical cutter at 2,100 rpm, which entraps and macerates the thrombus and extracts it into a vacuum collection bottle. The X-TRACT-AMI[22] (X-Sizer for Treatment of Thrombus and Atherosclerosis in Coronary Interventions Trial in Acute Myocardial Infarction) study showed improvement in TIMI-3 flow and MBG post procedure. The X-sizer in Acute MI for Negligible Embolization and Optimal ST Resolution (X AMINE ST) trial included 201 patients with STEMI and showed an improved ST segment resolution and reduced distal embolization and no reflow rates, but it did not demonstrate any significant clinical benefit at 1 and 6 months **(Figs. 5A and B)**.[23]
- *Excimer laser coronary atherectomy (ELCA)*: The pulsed-wave ultraviolet-wavelength excimer laser (Spectranetics, Colorado Springs, Colorado, United States) has been successfully applied in patients with acute myocardial infarction (AMI). The excimer laser light interacts favorably with several components of the occluding thrombus. Laser-generated acoustic shock waves can separate thrombus from the vessel wall, dissolve clot, vaporize procoagulant mediators, dissolve fibrin fibers, and suppress platelet aggregation **(Figs. 6A and B)**.

  The Cohort of Acute Revascularization of Myocardial infarction with Excimer Laser (CARMEL) multicenter registry[24] enrolled 151 patients and showed TIMI flow grade was significantly increased after ELCA, with an improvement in angiographic stenosis. The maximal effect was observed in arteries with a large angiographic thrombus burden.
- CAT RX mechanical thrombectomy system (Penumbra)[25] delivers consistent suction for increasing efficacy of thrombus aspiration. The catheter in the coronary artery has a physician-controlled flow switch. The catheter is connected to the Penumbra Engine which uses vacuum to aspirate thrombus **(Fig. 7)**.

Embolic Protection Devices

Embolic protection devices (EPDs) aim at capturing the debris liberated during PCI and decrease distal embolization. EPDs can be divided into three distinct types based on their mechanism of operation: distal occlusion aspiration devices, distal filters, and proximal occlusion aspiration devices **(Table 4)**.

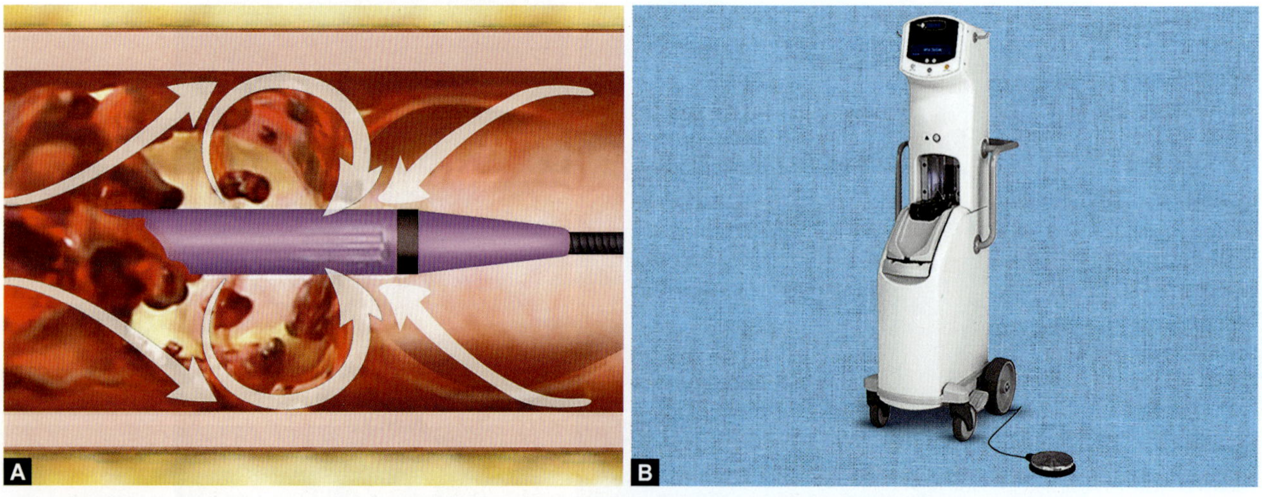

FIGS. 4A AND B: Angiojet rheolytic thrombectomy. (A) Angiojet catheter with venturi effect for thrombosuction. (B) Angiojet console.

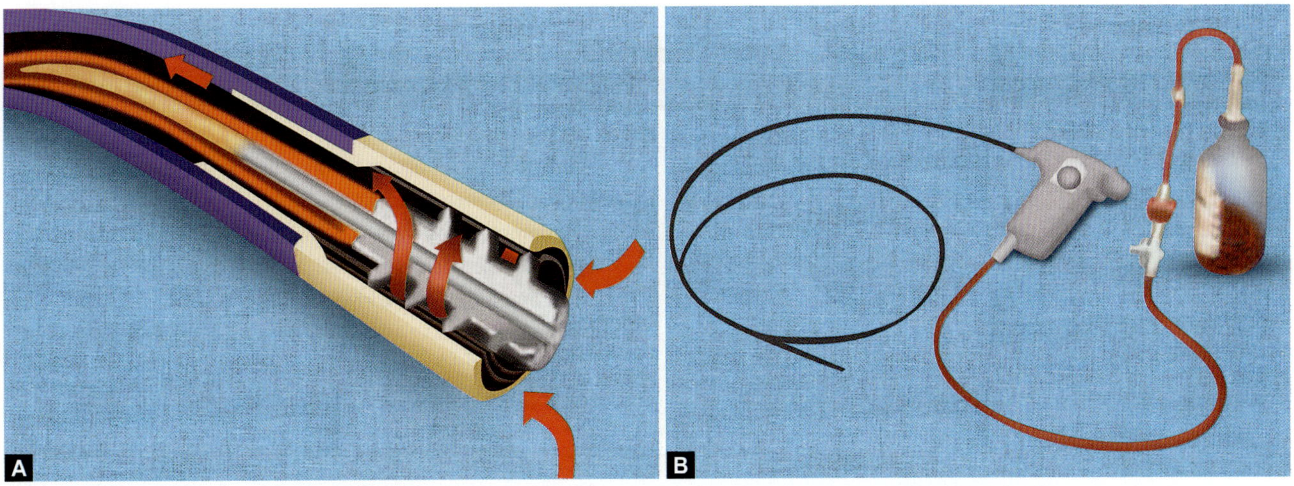

FIGS. 5A AND B: X-sizer system. (A) Helical cutter inside the inner lumen of the catheter. (B) Handheld module.

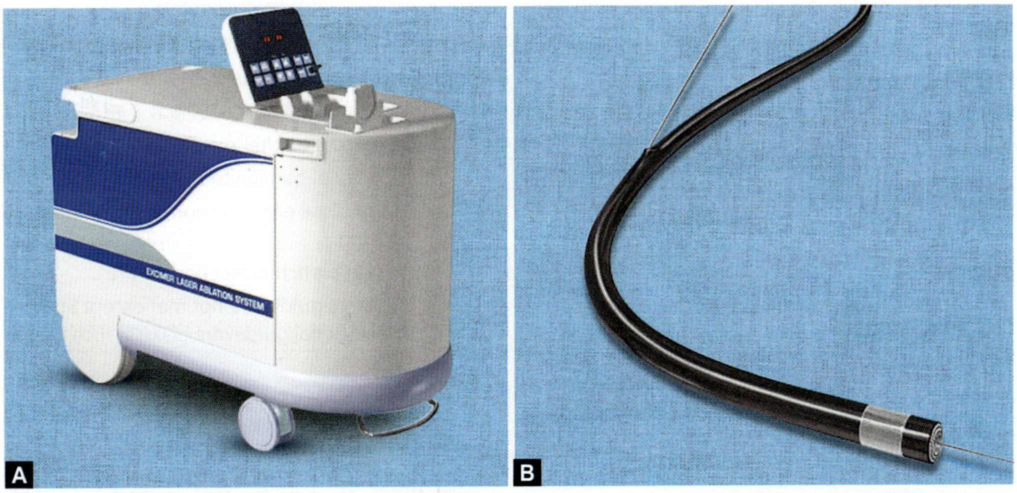

FIGS. 6A AND B: Excimer laser coronary atherectomy.

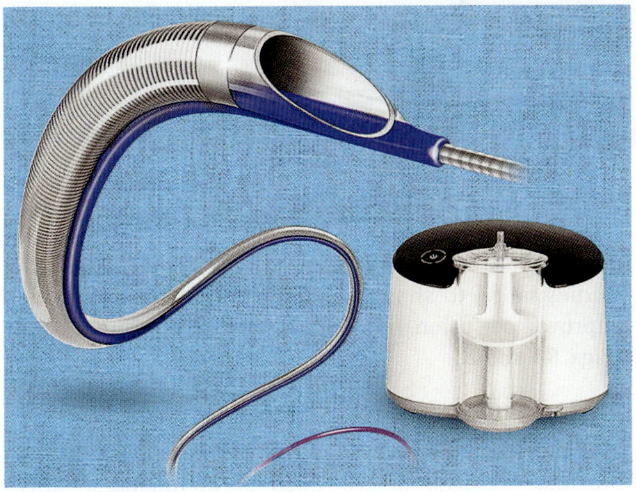

FIG. 7: CAT RX Penumbra system.

Distal Occlusion Aspiration Devices

These contain an inflatable balloon which is passed several centimeters distal to the lesion and is inflated to obstruct antegrade flow. The balloon traps the debris released during PCI which is subsequently removed using an aspiration catheter. The limitation of this device is the total occlusion of the flow with a risk of thrombus formation distally. The EMERALD[26] and ASPARAGUS[27] trials compared use of PercoSurge to conventional primary PCI and demonstrated safety of the device but did not show benefit in terms of infarct size.

Distal Embolic Filters

Distal embolic filters have a filter bag mounted at the distal part of a coronary guidewire. The device is advanced through the guide catheter with the filter bag in a collapsed state in a delivery sheath (3.2F) and is deployed 2.5–3.0 cm distal to

TABLE 4: Embolic protection devices (EPDs).[30]

EPD	Used in vessel size	Guide catheter	Crossing profile	Comments
Proximal balloon: Proxis (Velocimed, Maple Grove, MN, USA)	3–5 mm	7F'	None	*Advantage*: • Establish protection before crossing the lesion • Side branch protection • Complete recovery of debris and vasoactive mediators • Unlimited debris removal • Compatible with conventional guidewire *Disadvantage:* • Myocardial ischemia during balloon occlusion
Distal occlusion balloon: • PercuSurge guidewire (Medtronic) • TriActiv (Kensey Nash Corp)	3–6 mm	• 6F' • 7F'	• 2.1F' • 2.8F'	• Can capture debris <100 µm and soluble vasoactive mediators with unlimited debris capture *Disadvantage:* • Aspiration may not remove all particles • Risk of embolization in side branch • Choice of guidewire limited • Risk of myocardial ischemia during balloon occlusion
Distal embolic filters: • FilterWire EZ (Boston Scientific) • Spider RX (Abbott) • Interceptor PLUS (Medtronic)	• 2.5–5.5 mm • 3–6 mm • 2.5–5.5 mm	• 6F' • 6F' • 6F'	• 3.2F' • 3.2F' • 2.7F'	• Maintain antegrade perfusion • Can capture debris >100 µm • But unable to filter mediators • Capacity of bag limited • Risk of distal embolization during wiring and lesion crossing • No side branch protection • Choice of guidewire not met except Spider RX for which conventional guidewire of 0.014 inch can be used

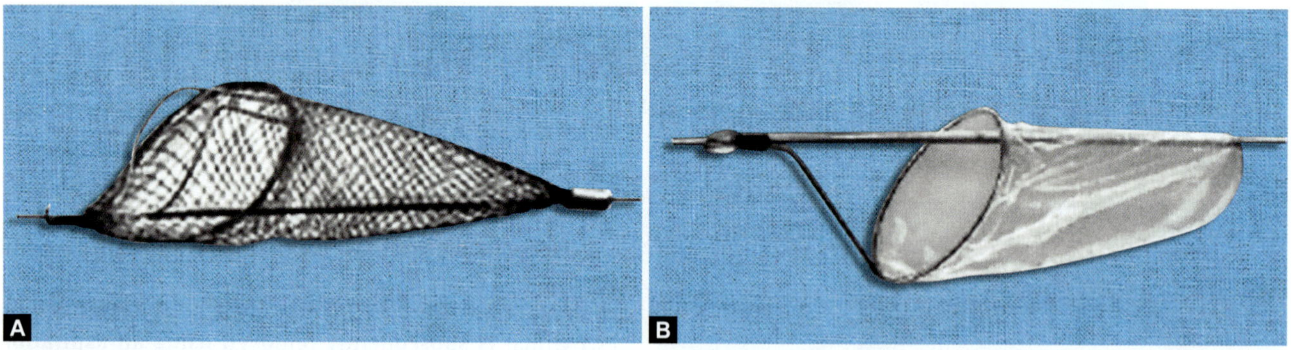

FIGS. 8A AND B: Distal embolic filters. (A) Spider Rx; (B) FilterWire.

the lesion. The filter bag with the accumulated plaque debris is later retrieved with a retrieval catheter (4.2–4.9F) after the procedure. The devices are effective at filtering particles >100–110 µm with maintaining antegrade perfusion. The limitations of this device include the passage of small particles, limited capture efficiency and complications related to advancement, and deployment and recovery of the filters. The Spider Rx (eV3; MedNova, Abbott, Abbott Park, IL), the FilterWire (Boston Scientific), and the Interceptor Plus Coronary Filter System (Medtronic Vascular, Santa Rosa, CA) are examples of distal embolic filters. Randomized studies failed to show a benefit of their use in terms of improved perfusion, limit infarct size, or reduced MACCE[28] **(Figs. 8A and B)**.

Proximal Occlusion Aspiration Devices

Proxis system (St Jude Medical, Minneapolis, MN) is a proximal occlusion device which has an inflatable balloon which is inflated proximally, occluding antegrade flow, and creating a stagnant column of blood containing debris which is aspirated. The limitation is that it cannot be used in small vessels <2.5 mm or in ostial or proximal target lesions due to lack of a landing zone for the balloon **(Fig. 9)**. It has not shown clinical benefit in trials.[29]

Stenting Strategies

- *Direct stenting*: A direct stenting approach reduces the incidence of distal embolization by reducing the manipulation and hardware across the thrombus and by trapping the thrombus behind the stent. The disadvantages include underestimation of vessel size, inadequate stent expansion, late stent malapposition, and failure to cross the lesion or inadequate stent expansion in calcified or tortuous vessels. A meta-analysis of five small single-center trials showed improved outcomes with direct stenting as evidenced by a significant improvement of ST-resolution and reduction of in-hospital cardiac death.[31] Direct stenting with or without thrombus aspiration might be applied safely in selected patients with AMI with low thrombus grade.
- *Covered stent*: Covered stents are made up of bare metal stent (BMS) platform covered with a fine mesh that can trap the thrombus and prevent distal embolization. There are two types of stents which have been evaluated in the past: MGuard (InspireMD) and STENTYS (STENTYS SA).
  - The MGuard stent consists of a BMS with a polyethylene terephthalate microfiber sleeve attached to its outer surface. It is compatible with a 6F system but has the limitation of increased risk of side branch occlusion due to its bulky double-layer design and high rate of stent dislodgement. Although MASTER I trial[32] demonstrated benefit of MGuard in terms of complete ST-segment resolution and lower 1-year mortality, but MASTER II trial[33] that aimed to recruit 1,114 patients was terminated early due to a high rate of stent dislodgement (3.87%).
  - The STENTYS is a self-apposing and self-expanding nitinol stent coated with a drug (Rapamycin) containing durable polymer and covered with fine mesh, which allows retention of the thrombus against the vessel wall. The APPOSITION V trial was stopped prematurely because the noninferiority standard was not met.[34]
  - At present, there is no sufficient data for routine use of covered stents in thrombus-containing lesions.
- *Deferred stenting*: This strategy potentially limits the risk of distal coronary embolization in presence of high thrombus burden. Antithrombotic therapy including prolonged GP IIb/IIIa inhibitors and heparin intravenously can be given for 24–48 hours followed by angiography and PCI in case thrombus burden reduces.
  - The DEFER STEMI trial[35] showed significantly lower rates of no-reflow/slow-flow and higher TIMI flow grade in deferred stenting group. The DANAMI 3-DEFER trial[36] deferred stenting for 48 hours but did not reduce the outcome of all-cause death, heart failure, myocardial infarction, or repeat revascularization compared to conventional PCI over 42 months follow-up.

In conclusion, deferred stenting is not recommended as the routine strategy in primary PCI.[20]

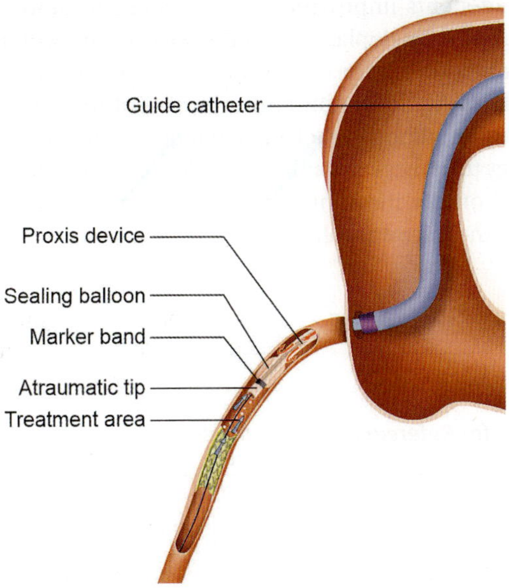

FIG. 9: Proxis proximal occlusion device.

SPECIAL CLINICAL SITUATIONS

- *Stent thrombosis*: Early (<30 days after PCI), late (>30 days after PCI), and very late (>12 months after PCI) stent thromboses are devastating clinical conditions which significantly impact outcomes. Stent thrombosis presents as nonfatal and fatal acute MI, often with marked hemodynamic instability. The key to a favorable outcome is expedient thrombus management. Primary PCI, including imaging, additional stenting with or without thrombectomy, is effective in restoring vessel patency, but reocclusion and restenosis are frequent. Usually, pharmacotherapy and manual thrombus aspiration catheters are sufficient for small or medium thrombus burdens but mechanical thrombectomy may be required in case of large thrombus burdens. Nevertheless, even successful PCI for stent thrombosis is associated with a larger infarct and poorer outcomes.[37]
- *Multivessel coronary thrombosis*: Patients with simultaneous multivessel thrombosis is an uncommon occurrence but frequently presents as acute coronary syndrome with hemodynamic compromise. The mechanisms include thrombotic embolization from left heart clots or tumors or acute thrombosis of a single vessel leading to cardiogenic shock, reduced coronary perfusion pressure, and thrombus formation on other

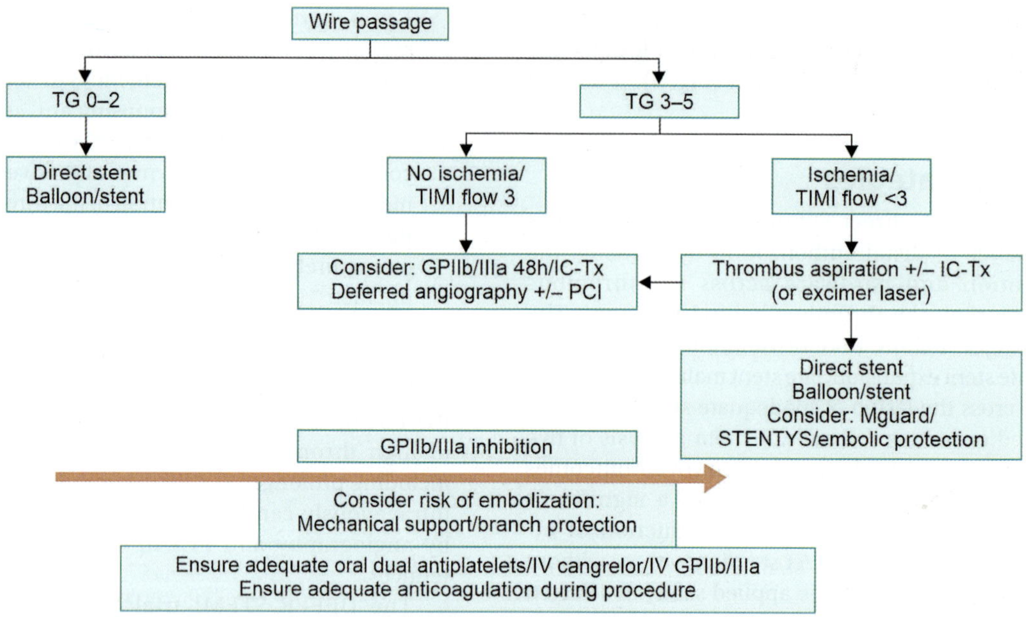

FLOWCHART 1: Algorithm for primary PCI in presence of large thrombus burden.[39]
(GP: glycoprotein; IC-Tx: intracoronary thrombolysis; PCI: percutaneous coronary intervention; TG: thrombus grade; TIMI: thrombolysis in myocardial infarction)

pre-existing lesions.[38] Optimal treatment is unknown with options of multivessel PCI or coronary artery bypass graft (CABG) surgery.

- *Bypass grafts*: Early after CABG, graft thrombosis can occur due to surgery-related mechanical issues. Late ischemic events are caused by progression of soft atheromatous plaques in grafts, the thrombotic content being much higher in venous grafts. Venous graft revascularization should be done with use of adjunctive pharmacotherapy and distal protection devices and subsequent stenting, trying to minimize the distal embolization.

CONCLUSION

Large thrombus burdens can be a significant deterrent to successful primary PCI in STEMIs due to distal embolization, no-reflow, slow-flow, or poor myocardial blush grade and increased infarct size. The therapy includes potent dual antiplatelet agents and effective anticoagulation including use of GP IIb/IIIa inhibitors. In case of small thrombus burden, direct stenting can be considered. When there is a larger thrombus burden, the use of manual aspiration catheters or ELCA should be considered. In case of no antegrade flow and persistent or extensive thrombus, mechanical thrombectomy using Angiojet, CAT RX, or Excimer Laser should be considered. In spite of these maneuvers, if the thrombus persists, stenting should be deferred with use of intracoronary thrombolysis, intravenous heparin, and/or GP IIb/IIIa inhibitors for 24–48 hours **(Flowchart 1)**. Drug-eluting stents are the stents of choice at present. Larger clinic studies are needed to determine if covered stents improve outcomes. Stent thrombosis and venous graft angioplasties require special care with regards to thrombotic burden. Distal protection devices can be used based on the discretion and expertise of the operator. In conclusion, although each patient requires an individualized strategy to manage thrombotic burden, but the outcomes are hinged on the thrombus management and restoration of flow to the microvasculature.

ONLINE REFERENCES

Please scan the QR code provided at the end of the table of contents for References of this chapter.

CHAPTER 136

Percutaneous Coronary Intervention in Chronic Stable Coronary Artery Disease

Vivek Gupta, Chinmay Gupta, Chaitanya Gupta, Devyani Dogra

ABSTRACT

Percutaneous coronary intervention (PCI) is a nonsurgical, minimally invasive procedure that aims to relieve the narrowing or occlusion of the coronary artery and improve blood supply to the ischemic tissue in patients with chronic stable coronary artery disease (CAD). PCI is an important tool for symptomatic improvement in patients with stable CAD who have refractory angina despite maximal medical therapy. It has been found to reduce all-cause mortality, cardiovascular mortality, and myocardial infarction (MI) in stable CAD subsets. The present chapter gives comprehensive overview of PCI in chronic stable CAD, emphasizing its role in relieving angina, improving blood supply, and reducing adverse cardiovascular events. The exploration of clinical outcomes and future directions sheds light on the continuous efforts to enhance the efficacy and safety of PCI, ultimately benefiting patients with chronic stable CAD.

Keywords: Percutaneous coronary intervention, stable chronic coronary artery disease, interventional cardiology, revascularization, coronary angioplasty, coronary stenting, ischemia, myocardial revascularization, coronary artery bypass surgery.

INTRODUCTION

In recent decades, cardiovascular diseases have emerged as a significant global health challenge, affecting millions of individuals worldwide. Among these conditions, chronic stable coronary artery disease (chronic stable CAD) stands out as a prevalent and complex condition with potentially life-threatening implications. According to the 2021 American College of Cardiology/American Heart Association/Society for Cardiovascular Angiography and Interventions (ACC/AHA/SCAI) guideline for coronary artery revascularization, CAD is a complex cardiovascular condition characterized by the formation of atherosclerotic plaques within the coronary arteries that limit oxygenated blood to reach to heart.[1] CAD stands as the leading cause of cardiovascular-related deaths worldwide, accounting for 16% of the world's total deaths.[2] From 2000 to 2019, this disease experienced the most substantial surge in mortality, witnessing a staggering increase of over 2 million deaths, resulting in a total of 8.9 million fatalities in the later year.[2] In India, CAD prevalence is 3.5% with men have a higher definite CAD prevalence (5.8%) than women (4.2%).[3] Urban areas show higher rates, and angina prevalence decreased from 27.8 to 11.2% over 5 years.[4] CAD can present as stable ischemic heart disease (SIHD) or acute coronary syndrome (ACS), which can further progress into congestive heart failure (CHF) if left uncontrolled. ACS encompasses a spectrum of conditions, including unstable angina, non-ST-elevation myocardial infarction (NSTEMI), and ST-elevation myocardial infarction (STEMI), each representing varying degrees of severity based on the level of arterial obstruction and tissue damage.[5]

Coronary artery disease is influenced by modifiable lifestyle factors such as smoking, dyslipidemia, obesity, sedentary lifestyle, diabetes, and alcohol consumption.[6,7] Arterial hypertension is a critical modifiable risk factor significantly impacting ischemic diseases and cerebral circulation disorders. Reducing blood pressure has shown a 30% decrease in cerebral circulatory disorder risk and a 23% decrease in cardiovascular events.[8] Nonmodifiable characteristics such as age, sex, and family history also play a role in CAD susceptibility. Addressing these risk factors is essential in CAD prevention and management for better heart health and overall well-being.[6] The present chapter highlights emerging trends, advancements, and potential challenges in the field of percutaneous coronary intervention (PCI) for stable CAD, providing clinicians and researchers with valuable insights to enhance patient outcomes and shape future directions in CAD management.

UNDERSTANDING THE PATHOPHYSIOLOGY OF CHRONIC STABLE CAD

The pathophysiology of chronic stable CAD involves the development of atherosclerotic plaque, narrows the vessel lumen, and impedes blood flow. The development of atherosclerosis begins with the accumulation of low-density lipoprotein (LDL) cholesterol in the arterial wall, triggering an immune response that activates T cells and B cells. This immune response leads to the recruitment of macrophages and the release of inflammatory cytokines such as interleukin 1 (IL-1), IL-6, and tumor necrosis factor alpha (TNF-α). These cells engulf the lipids, forming foam cells, and together with smooth muscle cells, they contribute to the formation of fatty streaks that progress into advanced plaques called atheromas. Vulnerable plaques with a thin fibrous cap and a large lipid core are prone to rupture, potentially leading to the enlargement of the plaque through blood deposition. Disrupted plaques can trigger thrombosis by activating platelets and exposing the subendothelial matrix to blood coagulation factors.[9,10] In chronic stable CAD, the narrowing or blockage of coronary arteries due to plaque buildup can lead to reduce blood flow to the myocardium.[11] This can result in symptoms such as angina pectoris, fatigue, hyperhidrosis, shortness of breath, and nausea.[12-14] The presence of obstructive CAD secondary to atherosclerosis or functional disorders such as coronary artery spasm or myocardial bridging can contribute to macrovascular disease. Additionally, abnormalities in the coronary microvasculature, either anatomical or functional, can also play a role in the pathophysiology of CAD.

WHAT CONSTITUTES OPTIMAL MANAGEMENT FOR CHRONIC STABLE CAD?

Managing CAD requires a comprehensive approach encompassing lifestyle modifications, risk factor control, medical therapy (MT), and revascularization strategies. MT is the cornerstone of CAD treatment, usually comprising a combination of anti-ischemic drugs such as beta-blockers or calcium-channel blockers, antiplatelet agents, and lipid-lowering agents.[15] Revascularization, which aims to restore blood flow to the cardiac muscle, involves two main procedures—(1) PCI and (2) coronary artery bypass grafting (CABG).[1] PCI, also known as angioplasty, utilizes a balloon and stent to open narrowed coronary arteries and improve blood flow. On the other hand, CABG is a surgical procedure that creates new paths for blood circulation to bypass blocked arteries. The choice between these approaches should be based on individual patient characteristics and risk factors.[1,16]

OPTIMAL MEDICAL THERAPY WITH OR WITHOUT PCI FOR CAD: LESSONS LEARNED FROM CLINICAL TRIALS

For patients with stable CAD and peripheral artery disease (PAD), the standard therapy involves treatment with a single antiplatelet agent, such as aspirin or clopidogrel.[17] Aspirin remains the drug of choice for preventing secondary events in CAD and is recommended in most guidelines for secondary prevention.[18] Intravenous antiplatelet agents such as abciximab, eptifibatide, and tirofiban are not suitable for stable CAD patients.[19] Antiplatelet medications continue to play a vital role in treating atherosclerotic cardiovascular and cerebrovascular diseases. Studies indicate that 3- to 6-month dual antiplatelet therapy (DAPT) is feasible for the general population undergoing PCI with contemporary drug-eluting stents (DESs).[20] Precision medicine trends are shifting toward patient-centered approaches in antiplatelet therapy, aiming to select the appropriate agent, optimal dose, and therapy duration based on each patient's unique clinical characteristics and circumstances.[21]

Antithrombotic therapy also plays a crucial role in the management of patients undergoing PCI. Recent clinical trials have focused on optimizing antithrombotic therapy in various patient populations to improve outcomes. The TROPICAL-ACS randomized trial found that platelet function testing-guided de-escalation of antiplatelet therapy in patients with ACS undergoing PCI did not lead to worse outcomes.[22] The Popular AGE trial investigated antithrombotic therapy in elderly patients undergoing PCI and found that oral anticoagulation plus a P2Y12 inhibitor was noninferior to triple therapy in reducing bleeding events.[23] However, the ISAR-TRIPLE trial revealed that triple therapy with aspirin, clopidogrel, and a vitamin K antagonist was associated with a higher risk of bleeding compared to dual therapy with aspirin and clopidogrel.[24] In contrast, the TWILIGHT trial showed that ticagrelor monotherapy was associated with a lower risk of bleeding without an increased risk of ischemic events in patients undergoing PCI.[25] These findings offer valuable insights into tailoring optimal MT for specific patient groups, ensuring better outcomes while minimizing bleeding risks during PCI procedures **(Table 1)**.

WHAT IS PERCUTANEOUS CORONARY INTERVENTION AND ASSOCIATED INDICATION?

Percutaneous coronary intervention is a minimally invasive, nonsurgical procedure designed to address coronary artery narrowing or blockage, thereby enhancing blood flow to the ischemic tissue. PCI has demonstrated its potential

TABLE 1: List of novel antiplatelet and antithrombotic agents with their mode of action and clinical trial.

Agent	Mode of action	Reference
Cangrelor	P2Y12-receptor inhibitor	• CHAMPION PCI trial[26] • CHAMPION PHOENIX trial[27]
Bivalirudin	Glycoprotein IIb/IIIa inhibitors	• EARLY ACS trial[28] • ACUITY trial[29]
Prasugrel	P2Y12 receptor inhibitor	HOST-REDUCE-POLYTECH-ACS RCT[6]
Ticagrelor	P2Y12 receptor inhibitor	• TWILIGHT trial[30] • TAPER-S trial[31]
Vorapaxar	Protease-activated receptor-1 (PAR-1) inhibitor	• TRA-2P-TIMI 50 trial[32] • TRA 2°P-TIMI 50 trial[33]
Cilostazol	Phosphodiesterase type 3 (PDE-3) inhibitor	Zhao et al., 2022[34]

to provide a survival advantage in individuals with ACSs and cardiac arrest patients who may experience ischemia-induced arrhythmia due to significant stenosis (≥70%) in one of the coronary arteries on the heart's surface. Moreover, for patients with chronic stable CAD, who continue to experience symptoms despite being on the highest tolerable goal-directed MT, PCI is recommended as an intervention to improve their symptoms by addressing significant stenosis in the coronary vessels.[35]

Percutaneous coronary intervention plays a crucial role in addressing various clinical scenarios associated with coronary artery stenosis, leading to improved patient outcomes. In the case of STEMI, primary PCI is the recommended reperfusion method, particularly when promptly performed by experienced operators. Beneficial results are observed when PCI is administered to STEMI patients experiencing ischemic symptoms for <12 hours. Furthermore, for STEMI patients who develop ischemic symptoms within 12 hours and have contraindications to fibrinolytic therapy, PCI becomes the preferred treatment approach.[36] For non-ST-elevation ACS (NSTE-ACS) cases, early invasive therapy is recommended within 2 hours of symptom onset for patients exhibiting refractory angina, recurrent angina, symptoms of heart failure, new or worsening mitral regurgitation, hemodynamic instability, or sustained ventricular tachycardia/fibrillation. Additionally, an elevation in troponin levels should prompt early therapy within 24 hours for NSTE-ACS patients.[36]

In the context of stable angina, PCI may be considered for patients who remain symptomatic despite optimal MT. This procedure is also appropriate for individuals with stable angina exhibiting high-risk stress test findings. Similarly, in cases of anginal equivalents such as dyspnea, arrhythmia, dizziness, or syncope, PCI may be warranted. Moreover, for patients with critical coronary artery stenosis ineligible for coronary artery bypass surgery (CABG), PCI offers a viable alternative treatment option. Overall, these diverse clinical scenarios highlight the significance of PCI in managing CAD and its potential to optimize patient care and outcomes.

WHAT ARE THE CONTRADICTION ASSOCIATED WITH PERCUTANEOUS CORONARY INTERVENTION?

Percutaneous coronary intervention is a widely employed and effective procedure for managing CAD. However, it is crucial for healthcare professionals to recognize both absolute and relative contraindications to ensure the safety and success of the intervention. Absolute contraindications for PCI include patients who are noncompliant with the procedure or unable to adhere to DAPT, individuals with a high risk of bleeding due to conditions such as thrombocytopenia, peptic ulcers, or severe coagulopathy, and those with a history of multiple PCI restenosis.[36] On the other hand, relative contraindications warrant careful consideration, as PCI may still be performed under certain circumstances. Patients' intolerance to long-term oral antiplatelet therapy, those lacking immediate access to cardiac surgery backup, and individuals with hypercoagulable states are among the group with relative contraindications. Furthermore, patients with high-grade chronic kidney disease, chronic total occlusion (CTO) of saphenous vein grafts, an artery with a diameter of <1.5 mm, and stenosis below 50% are also considered to have relative contraindications. Additionally, individuals with critical left main stenosis, especially if there is no collateral flow or patent bypass graft, require careful evaluation before considering PCI.[36] Recognizing these contraindications and carefully assessing individual patient factors is essential in guiding the appropriate selection of treatment options and ensuring the best possible outcomes for patients with CAD.

PERCUTANEOUS CORONARY INTERVENTION TECHNIQUES AND RECENT ADVANCEMENT IN CHRONIC STABLE CAD

Percutaneous coronary intervention offers several techniques to address chronic stable CAD.

Balloon Angioplasty

This form of PCI involves inflating a balloon inside a narrowed coronary artery to disrupt plaque and open up the vessel. While it is no longer the primary intervention due to the risk of restenosis, it is performed when stent placement is not possible or could be harmful. It can also serve as a bridge to future PCI or CABG.[37]

Stent Implantation

Stent implantation is a crucial component of PCI used to address coronary artery stenosis and restore blood flow to the heart muscle. During stent implantation, a catheter containing a stent is carefully guided over a guidewire and positioned at the site of the narrowed coronary artery segment. Once in place, the balloon is inflated, causing the stent to expand and deploy against the artery walls, effectively relieving the stenosis and allowing for improved blood flow.

Two main methods of stent placement are employed—direct stenting and predilation with stenting. In predilation, the balloon is first inflated to widen the narrowed segment, and then the stent is deployed at the expanded site. On the other hand, direct stenting involves using a low-profile stent delivery system, which is introduced directly to the lesion without prior predilation, and the stent is deployed immediately.[38] The efficacy of direct stenting was evaluated in a randomized trial of 206 patients with acute STEMI undergoing primary stenting. The study found that direct stenting showed favorable outcomes compared to predilation, with a significantly lower incidence of the composite angiographic endpoint (slow and no-reflow or distal embolization) and more frequent ST-segment resolution. Stent implantation has become a standard and effective technique in managing CAD, providing relief to patients with ischemic heart conditions.[39]

Coronary Atherectomy

Atherectomy is an invasive procedure utilized to physically remove obstructive material (atheroma, calcium, or cellular debris) from coronary arteries. It involves using specialized instruments, such as a burr or crown, to cut through the lesions. There are following types of atherectomy—directional coronary atherectomy, orbital atherectomy, rotational atherectomy, and laser atherectomy.

Following atherectomy, balloon angioplasty, and stent placement are often performed to optimize vessel patency and restore blood flow. While atherectomy can be beneficial in cases where a calcified segment impedes stent delivery, routine use of atherectomy before stenting has not demonstrated consistent improvement in outcomes and should be employed judiciously based on specific clinical indications.[40] Rotational atherectomy may be infrequently necessary for internal mammary artery graft stenosis, although angioplasty is more commonly practiced.[41] Atherectomy is generally less favored for treating saphenous vein graft lesions. Potential complications of atherectomy include arterial dissection, coronary artery perforation, and particle embolization.[42]

Brachytherapy

In-stent restenosis (ISR) remains a significant concern, even with DESs. It carries a high risk of recurrence. Brachytherapy is emerging as an alternative treatment for resistant ISR. It is feasible and effective for treating resistant ISR in patients with DES and shows high immediate procedural success. Brachytherapy proves promising in complex patient populations.[24,43]

Intravascular Ultrasound

Intravascular ultrasound (IVUS) is a medical imaging technique that allows for the visualization of the coronary artery wall using a small ultrasound transducer positioned at the tip of a flexible catheter. IVUS helps in assessing plaque morphology and distribution within the artery, aiding in the decision-making process for PCI. The advantage of IVUS lies in its ability to provide accurate intraluminal measurements, which are not feasible with conventional coronary angiography. Unlike angiography, which provides a two-dimensional view of the vessel lumen and may not represent the true diameter accurately, IVUS offers more precise information, especially in cases of complex and asymmetric narrowing.[35] A study evaluating the routine use of IVUS in 1,563 patients with suspected CAD found that the incidence of adverse events related to the procedure was low. Additionally, IVUS identified nonobstructive lesions that carried an increased risk of future cardiovascular events.[44] This highlights the utility of IVUS in identifying patients and arterial segments at higher risk. In the ADAPT-DES study, involving 813 patients with STEMI, the use of IVUS was associated with improved outcomes in STEMI patients. The study demonstrated the clinical benefits of incorporating IVUS in the management of STEMI cases.[45] The 3-Year Outcomes of the ULTIMATE trial comparing IVUS versus angiography-guided DESs implantation showed that IVUS guidance improved 3-year clinical outcomes among all-comer patients who underwent DESs implantation.[46] Overall, IVUS is a valuable tool in assessing CAD, providing detailed information on plaque characteristics and guiding treatment decisions for better patient outcomes. Its ability to identify high-risk lesions contributes to more effective interventions and management strategies.

Shockwave Intravascular Lithotripsy

Shockwave intravascular lithotripsy (IVL) is a novel and minimally invasive approach to treating severely calcified plaques in the coronary and peripheral vessels. It utilizes a percutaneous device to produce acoustic pressure waves, breaking superficial, and deep calcium deposits. It has been used in the treatment of coronary artery calcification and complex lesions.[47] It has shown promise in improving clinical outcomes and reducing complications associated with calcified cardiovascular disease.[48]

COMMON COMPLICATIONS AND HOW TO MINIMIZE RISKS

- *Stent thrombosis*: It is a potentially serious complication of PCI. It occurs when a blood clot forms inside the stent, leading to vessel occlusion and potentially causing a heart attack. The risk of stent thrombosis can be minimized by appropriate antiplatelet therapy and adherence to DAPT guidelines.[49]

- *Bleeding*: Bleeding is a common complication of PCI, which can occur at the access site or as a result of anticoagulant and antiplatelet medications used during the procedure. Strategies to minimize bleeding risk include using radial access instead of femoral access, careful management of anticoagulant and antiplatelet therapy, and close monitoring of the patient's hemostasis status.[50]
- *Vascular complications*: Vascular complications can occur during or after PCI, including arterial dissection, perforation, or pseudoaneurysm formation. These complications can lead to bleeding, hematoma formation, or vessel occlusion. Proper technique, meticulous guidewire manipulation, and the use of closure devices can help minimize the risk of vascular complications.[51]
- *Coronary artery dissection*: Coronary artery dissection is a rare but potentially serious complication of PCI. It occurs when the inner layers of the coronary artery separate, leading to reduced blood flow to the heart muscle. Careful lesion preparation, appropriate sizing of balloons and stents, and cautious wire manipulation can help minimize the risk of dissection.[52]
- *Acute kidney injury*: Acute kidney injury can occur as a result of contrast-induced nephropathy during PCI. Measures to minimize the risk include using low-osmolar or iso-osmolar contrast agents, adequate hydration before and after the procedure, and avoiding unnecessary contrast administration.[53]

SHORT-TERM AND LONG-TERM EFFECTS OF PCI IN CHRONIC STABLE CAD: INSIGHTS FROM CLINICAL TRIALS

Several clinical trials have investigated the short-term and long-term results of PCI in CAD. In stable CAD, PCI does not appear to reduce mortality, but it does lower spontaneous myocardial infarction (MI) rates at the expense of causing some periprocedural MI.[54] The primary purpose of PCI in stable CAD is to relieve angina, though its effectiveness in achieving this outcome remains uncertain. Patients and physicians often opt for PCI instead of initially trying antianginal medications, as per the NICE (National Institute for Health and Care Excellence) guideline.[55] Comparing PCI outcomes between hospitals with and without cardiac surgery on-site (SOS hospitals), a clinical trial found similar results between the two settings, but SOS hospitals had a higher in-hospital mortality rate.[56] In a meta-analysis of 12 randomized clinical trials, PCI was not found to reduce the risk of death, MI, or other major cardiovascular events compared to optimal MT in patients with stable CAD.[57] In patients with left main CAD, a randomized trial revealed that PCI with DES led to a higher occurrence of the composite outcome of death, stroke, or MI at 5 years compared to CABG.[58]

Various clinical trials have demonstrated clinical improvement and symptom relief through PCI in patients with CAD. The ISCHEMIA (International Study of Comparative Health Effectiveness With Medical and Invasive Approaches) trial, focusing on patients with stable CAD/CCS and severe angina pectoris, revealed relevant symptomatic improvement, aiming to reduce disease burden and enhance quality of life.[59] Another randomized trial, the randomized trial of PCI Choice Decision Aid, compared the effect of a PCI decision aid with usual care in patients facing a choice between PCI and MT for stable CAD, examining its impact on patient decision-making and outcomes.[60] In addition to these trials, the COURAGE trial investigated PCI plus optimal MT versus MT alone in stable CAD patients, showing no significant difference in major cardiovascular events but highlighting greater symptom relief and improved quality of life with PCI.[15] The FAME 2 trial assessed PCI guided by fractional flow reserve (FFR) versus MT alone, finding that PCI with FFR guidance reduced the risk of major adverse cardiovascular events and improved symptom relief and quality of life.[61] The ORBITA trial compared PCI with a sham procedure instable angina patients, showing no significant difference in exercise time but indicating greater symptom relief and improved quality of life with PCI.[62] Collectively, these clinical trials provide robust evidence supporting the effectiveness of PCI in improving symptoms and clinical outcomes in patients with stable CAD.

NAVIGATING TREATMENT CHOICES: LESSONS LEARNED FROM CLINICAL TRIALS ON PCI VERSUS CABG

In recent years, PCI has been widely utilized, with approximately 80% of procedures involving stent placement. Notably, over the past two decades, PCI has demonstrated significant improvements in short-term mortality, MI rates, and the need for target vessel revascularization.[54] When comparing outcomes from various trials involving PCI, CABG, and MT, specific treatment preferences emerge for different patient categories. The SYNTAX score, a tool assessing the complexity of coronary lesions, plays a crucial role in the decision-making process between PCI and CABG.[63] The 2023 AHA/ACC/ACCP/ASPC/NLA/PCNA guideline for the management of patients with chronic coronary disease has shared recommendation on revascularization in chronic stable CAD that has been listed in **Table 2**.

TABLE 2: Recommendations for revascularization: PCI versus CABG.[16]

Indication	Recommendation
CCD patient	Require revascularization for significant left main involvement associated with high-complexity CAD, CABG is recommended in preference to PCI to improve survival
	Require revascularization for multivessel CAD with complex and diffuse CAD (e.g., SYNTAX score > 33), it is reasonable to choose CABG over PCI to improve survival
CCD patients at high surgical risk	Appropriate for revascularization but poor candidates for surgery, it is reasonable to choose PCI over CABG to improve symptoms and reduce MACE
CCD patient with diabetes	Multivessel CAD with involvement of the left anterior descending artery, CABG (with a left internal mammary artery to the left anterior descending artery) is recommended in preference to PCI to reduce mortality and repeat revascularizations
	Left main stenosis and low- or intermediate-complexity CAD (e.g., SYNTAX score ≤ 33), PCI may be considered as an alternative to CABG to reduce MACE

(CABG: coronary artery bypass grafting; CCD: chronic coronary disease; MACE: major adverse cardiovascular events; PCI: percutaneous coronary intervention)

OPTIMAL MANAGEMENT OF STABLE CAD: INSIGHTS FROM CLINICAL TRIALS COMPARING PCI AND MEDICAL THERAPY

A recent review of clinical trials comparing MT with PCI for the management of stable CAD provides valuable insights into the efficacy and effectiveness of these treatment strategies. One study focused on meta-analysis included 11 randomized controlled trials (RCTs) involving 9,629 patients and evaluated PCI versus MT for stable CAD. The results indicated that PCI reduced the overall risk of the composite outcome, encompassing all-cause mortality, MI, revascularizations, rehospitalizations, or stroke. Additionally, PCI was associated with a decreased risk of unplanned revascularization and fatal MI. However, there were no significant differences in overall risk of all-cause mortality and other cardiovascular events between PCI and MT.[64] The ISCHEMIA trial investigated routine invasive therapy, including PCI, compared with optimal MT in patients with SIHD and moderate-to-severe myocardial ischemia. This trial enrolled 5,179 patients and had a follow-up duration of 3.3 years, potentially offering additional insights into the comparison between invasive therapy (including PCI) and MT for stable CAD. The study did not show any evidence supporting the superiority of an initial invasive strategy over an initial conservative strategy in reducing the risk of ischemic cardiovascular events or all-cause mortality during a median follow-up of 3.2 years. Notably, the trial findings were influenced by the specific definition of MI employed in the study.[59]

Available evidence from clinical trials suggests that PCI may reduce the risk of certain outcomes compared to medical treatment in stable CAD, including the composite outcome of all-cause mortality, MI, revascularizations, rehospitalizations, or stroke. Decisions regarding treatment for stable CAD should consider individual patient characteristics and preferences. Continued research and updated meta-analyses will contribute to a better understanding of the efficacy and effectiveness of different treatment approaches for CAD.

EMERGING TECHNOLOGIES IN PERCUTANEOUS CORONARY INTERVENTION FOR BETTER PATIENT OUTCOME

Recent advancements in PCI techniques and tools have revolutionized the management of stable CAD. One notable improvement has been in device technology, with the development of DES and bioresorbable scaffolds, leading to better outcomes for PCI procedures.[65] Furthermore, PCI techniques have evolved significantly, encompassing rotational atherectomy, IVL, and CTO interventions, allowing for the successful treatment of complex lesions and enhancing procedural success rates.[66] In conjunction with the advancements in PCI techniques, there have been remarkable strides in adjunctive pharmacotherapy for PCI. The utilization of newer antiplatelet agents, such as ticagrelor and prasugrel, has contributed to reduced risks of stent thrombosis and major adverse cardiovascular events.[66] Moreover, the integration of intracoronary imaging techniques such as IVUS and optical coherence tomography (OCT) has become more widespread, enabling detailed visualization of coronary arteries for better lesion assessment, stent optimization, and procedural guidance. The integration of invasive coronary physiology techniques, such as FFR and instantaneous wave-free ratio (iFR), has also become crucial in guiding PCI procedures.[67] These techniques aid in assessing the functional significance of coronary lesions, enabling targeted and appropriate interventions. Overall, these advancements in PCI techniques and tools have significantly enhanced the outcomes of CAD management.

CONCLUSION

Percutaneous coronary intervention has become a widely used and highly effective treatment for stable CAD. Advancements in the past two decades have led to improved short-term survival rates, reduced heart attack occurrences, and decreased need for repeat procedures. The choice between PCI, CABG, and MT depends on patient characteristics and the complexity of the CAD lesions, evaluated using the SYNTAX score. PCI may be more suitable for single-vessel CAD, less complex left main CAD in diabetic patients, and those at high surgical risk. Moreover, PCI has shown potential in lowering the risk of certain outcomes compared to MT, such as the combined risk of all-cause mortality, MI, revascularizations, hospital readmissions, or stroke. Future directions in PCI for managing stable CAD offer promising opportunities for improving patient outcomes. These include prioritizing patient-centered health status outcomes, advancements in PCI techniques, innovations in device technology, personalized medicine through genetic testing, exploring combination therapies, and comparative effectiveness research. These future directions require a commitment to evidence-based practices and continuous research to achieve the best possible patient outcomes.

ONLINE REFERENCES

Please scan the QR code provided at the end of the table of contents for References of this chapter.

CHAPTER 137

Hyperemic and Nonhyperemic Pressure Assessment of Coronary Artery Disease

Madhu Sreedharan, Kiran Gopinath

ABSTRACT

The advent of the pressure wire has ushered in a paradigm shift in the management of patients with chronic coronary syndrome with focus changing from anatomy to physiology. It is a class IA recommendation prior to percutaneous coronary intervention (PCI) in borderline lesions. Fractional flow reserve (FFR) or instantaneous wave-free ratio (iFR) and other nonhyperemic indices determine the functional significance of the lesion. Revascularization can be safely deferred if FFR is >0.8 or iFR > 0.89. Revascularization of lesions with FFR < 0.8 (or iFR < 0.89) results in lower event rates compared to medical treatment. Standardized measurement of these indices is of utmost importance to get accurate values which impact management of the individual. The clinical data in support of physiological assessment and recommendations for performing and interpreting the procedure is summarized in this chapter.

Keywords: Coronary artery disease, physiology, fractional flow reserve, Nonhyperemic indices.

INTRODUCTION

Significance of coronary artery disease (CAD) lesions of moderate severity is often difficult to determine. Revascularization of significant lesions provide symptomatic relief while revascularization of nonsignificant lesions may not be of any benefit and often harmful. Fractional flow reserve (FFR) is a tool to determine the functional significance of these lesions.

In a pilot study of 21 patients, the sensitivity of FFR in identification of reversible ischemia was 88%, specificity 100%, the positive predictive value was 100%, negative predictive value was 88%, and the accuracy 93%.[1] Since then numerous trials[2-4] have firmly established the use of physiology as a class IA recommendation to guide decision to proceed with revascularization in patients with angina or anginal equivalent, undocumented ischemia and angiographically intermediate stenoses.[5]

WHY PHYSIOLOGY RATHER THAN ANATOMY?

Angiography has limitations in assessment of the severity of the lesions. There is significant interobserver variations in the assessment of the severity of the lesion even amongst experienced cardiologists.[6] There may be overlap, foreshortening of vessels, changes in angulation all of which may affect assessment of lesion severity. Physiological assessment provides an objective evidence of the functional significance of the lesion taking into account the size of the perfusion territory, viability of myocardium, microvascular disease, collateral flow, and the length and number of lesions. Routine use of physiology in percutaneous coronary intervention (PCI) has been shown to reduce major adverse cardiac events (MACE), improve procedure outcome as well as lower the cost.[7,8]

FRACTIONAL FLOW RESERVE

Pijls et al. published the first study of assessment of coronary pressures to assess the physiological significance of coronary stenoses during hyperemia.[9] FFR is defined as the maximum achievable flow in the presence of a stenosis divided by the maximum flow in the same distribution in the absence of a stenosis. The principle of Ohm's law (V = IR) was used to rationalize that when resistance is minimal and stable, as happens with maximal arteriolar vasodilatation, coronary pressure and flow are directly related.[10] FFR is calculated as distal coronary pressure (Pd)/aortic pressure (Pa) during hyperemia. FFR of a normal vessel would be 1.0 and an FFR of 0.7 means that the maximum flow to the distal myocardium is only 70% of what it would have been, if the vessel was normal.

Measurement of Fractional Flow Reserve

A standardized method of measurement of FFR is essential as these values are important for the patients' outcome and a high technical quality is desirable.[11]

- *Guiding catheter*: Any guiding catheter can be used. Avoid guide catheter with side holes as pressure signal with them reflects a mix of the pressure signals through the distal end and the Pa through the side holes. Large-bore catheter can cause damping of pressures especially when ostial lesions are present. Dicrotic notch should be seen in the aortic waveform. Diagnostic catheters should not be used as the waveform may be unreliable.
- *Hyperemic agent*: Adenosine is the most commonly used though nitroprusside or nicorandil may also be considered.

Intravenous (IV) adenosine: For ostial or serial lesions, IV adenosine has to be used as it provides reliable and stable maximal hyperemia which is sustained. Dose recommended is 140 µg/kg/min. There is no benefit in further increasing the dose. There is no clinically relevant difference between central venous versus cubital venous administration of adenosine **(Fig. 1)**.

Intracoronary adenosine: Vasodilatation is similar and FFR values comparable to those obtained with IV adenosine. 100 µg for the right coronary artery and 200 µg for the left coronary artery achieves >95% of maximal hyperemia without significant side effects **(Fig. 2)**. Higher doses do not increase the hyperemic effects but may be associated with atrioventricular block.

Practicalities of Fractional Flow Reserve Measurements[12]

- *Calibration of pressure systems*: Before pressure wire insertion, atmospheric pressure has to be set as zero reference for the fluid-filled pressure transducer and for the coronary pressure measuring system. Fluid-filled pressure lines should be flushed with saline.
- *Equalizing the pressures*: The pressure sensor should be advanced and positioned 1–2 mm distal to the guiding catheter. The guide catheter should be flushed with saline to remove any residual contrast inside. Here the two pressures should be identical, if not the pressures have to be equalized electronically. If aorto-ostial lesion is present, equalization can be done with wire in the aorta after disengaging the guide. The introducer needle may be used if it is thin and there is no leak, else it has to be removed.
- *Position of the wire*: The sensor (at the proximal opaque part of the wire) should be at least 2–3 cm distal to the lesion. It should not be in a small branch or in contact with the vessel wall, which may cause whipping artifact. In tortuous vessels, keeping the sensor distally may cause accordion effect which might lead to falsely low FFR values.
- Intracoronary nitroglycerine 100–200 µg to be given to avoid vasospasm with the guide wire.
- *Inducing hyperemia and recording*: Recording should be started at least 30 seconds after contrast injection to ensure stable baseline condition. At least 10 heart cycles are to be recorded before induction of hyperemia. With IV

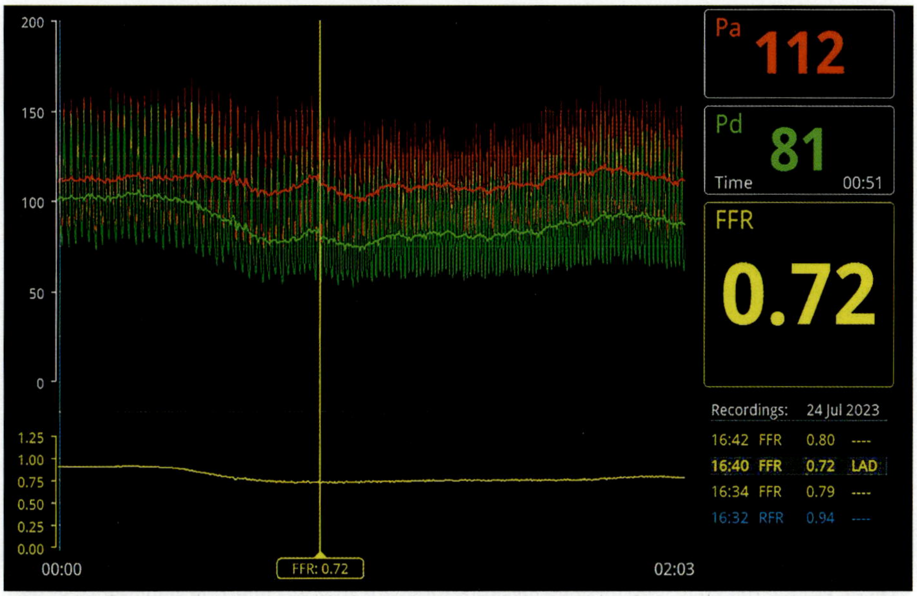

FIG. 1: Fractional flow reserve (FFR) with intravenous (IV) adenosine.

adenosine, start recording after 45–60 seconds of infusion for steady state hyperemia to be achieved.

- *FFR value*: FFR is the lowest value of Pd/Pa tracing. It is indicated automatically by the system. Manual control may be used to avoid artifacts.
- *Pullback*: Pullback of the wire preferably with angiographic co-registration is absolutely essential to identify other lesions which may be causing significant obstruction, particularly in serial lesions or diffusely diseased vessels. In case of manual pullback, do it at a constant rate over 15–20 seconds **(Fig. 3)**.
- *Signal drift*: After measurement of the FFR, the wire has to be pulled back to 1–2 mm of the guide catheter tip and pressures measured again. The two pressures (pressure wire and the aortic pressure) should be identical or within 1–2 mm Hg of each other. If more, the measurement is not correct and the FFR measurement would have to be repeated again.

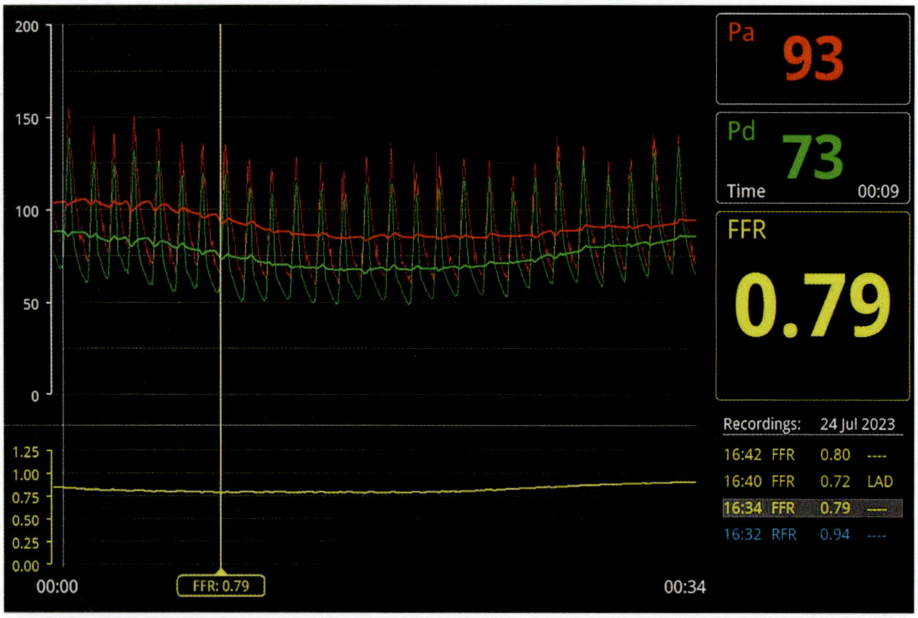

FIG. 2: Fractional flow reserve (FFR) with intracoronary (IC) adenosine showing the decline in pressure after IC bolus.

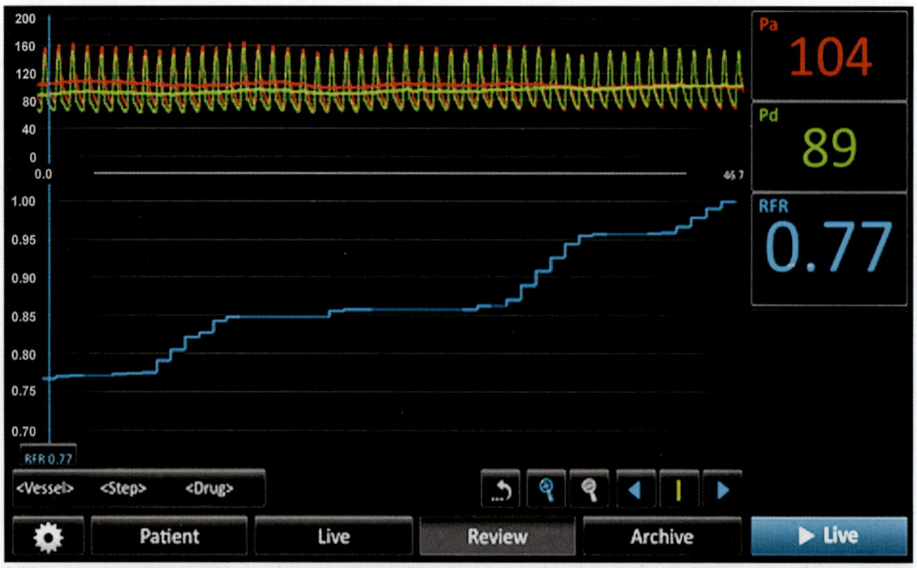

FIG. 3: Resting full-cycle ratio (RFR) pullback showing two step-ups implying significance of both lesions.

Precautions for accurate measurement of FFR/iFR:

- Transducer to be kept at level of aortic root
- Pressure wire to be completely flushed with saline
- Zeroing of the aortic pressures
- Avoid guide catheters with side holes
- Flush the guide catheter with saline before equalization
- Remove the introducer needle from the Y connector
- Avoid excessive intubation of the guide catheter to prevent damping/disengage guide before measurements particularly when aorto-ostial lesions are present.
- Check for drift at the end of any FFR measurement; if drift >2 mm Hg, the measurement has to be repeated.

Fractional Flow Reserve and Clinical Outcome Studies

DEFER Trial

Deferral versus performance of PTCA in patients without documented ischemia Study was conducted to define the role of FFR as a tool for clinical decision-making in planning revascularization strategy.[2] A total of 325 patients with stable CAD and intermediate lesions for percutaneous transluminal coronary angioplasty (PTCA) underwent FFR and subsequent randomization to three groups. If FFR > 0.75, patients were randomly assigned to deferral (deferral group; $n = 91$) or performance (performance group; $n = 90$) of PTCA. If FFR was < 0.75, PTCA was performed as planned (reference group; $n = 144$). The primary endpoint was the absence of adverse cardiac events on 24 months follow-up. Follow-up of this group of patients is available at 5 years[13] and 15 years[14] all of which showed that deferral of stenoses with FFR > 0.75 is safe and revascularization of stenoses with FFR > 0.75 gives no additional benefit.

FAME Trial

The FAME (Fractional Flow Reserve versus Angiography for Multivessel Evaluation) was done to assess the efficacy of FFR-guided approach to revascularization in patients with multivessel coronary disease.[15] 1,005 patients with at least 50% stenosis in at least two of the three epicardial vessels were included. FFR cutoff was chosen as 0.8 as this was shown to exclude ischemia in 90% of cases[16] and so the number of ischemic lesions left untreated would be less. The primary endpoint of death, nonfatal myocardial infarction (MI) and repeat revascularization at 1 year was less in the FFR group versus angiography alone group ($p = 0.02$) and the difference was maintained at 2 years.[3]

FAME 2 Trial

Fractional Flow Reserve Guided PCI versus Medical Therapy in Stable Coronary Disease—FAME 2 study tested the hypothesis that FFR-guided PCI plus optimal medical therapy (OMT) would be superior to OMT alone.[4] FFR was performed in all lesions and if at least one stenosis was <0.8, patients were assigned to either PCI with OMT or OMT alone. The primary endpoint was a composite of death, MI, or urgent revascularization. The study was halted prematurely due to a significant reduction in the primary endpoint in the PCI group [hazard ratio (HR) 0.32; 95% confidence interval (CI) 0.19–0.53; $p < 0.001$] driven by reduction in fewer urgent revascularization.

The various trials of FFR are shown in **Table 1**.

NONHYPEREMIC PRESSURE RATIO—INSTANTANEOUS WAVE-FREE RATIO

Resting flow remains stable over a wide range of stenoses' severity while hyperemic flow declines significantly beyond approximately 50% reduction in lumen diameter.[17] The stable flow conditions in this state provides provide an ideal environment for the application of pressure-based index of stenosis severity. As per the principles of coronary autoregulation, for a stenosis to have a physiological impact on the blood flow to the myocardium, it should have a gradient that is detectable at rest.[18] Instantaneous wave-free ratio (iFR) measures the physiological impact of the coronary

TABLE 1: Summary of patient outcome fractional flow reserve (FFR) trials.

Study	Size/Year	Clinical presentation	FFR cutoff	Outcome
DEFER	325 patients (2001)	SIHD—SVD with intermediate lesion	0.75	No benefit in PCI of nonischemic stenosis
FAME	1,005 patients (2009)	Multivessel	0.8	Routine FFR reduces MACE at 1 year
FAME 2	888 patients (2012)	Stable CAD	0.8	FFR-guided PCI + OMT versus OMT: ↓ TLR
DANAMI-3 PRIMULTI	627 patients (2015)	STEMI and MVD—S/P PPCI	0.8	FFR-guided staged complete revascularization of nonculprit vessels in same admission: ↓ MACE (TLR)
Compare–Acute	885 patients (2017)	STEMI and MVD—S/P PPCI	0.8	FFR-guided PCI of nonculprit vessel in same setting: ↓ MACE (TLR)

(CAD: coronary artery disease; MACE: major adverse cardiac events; MVD: multivessel disease; OMT: optimal medical therapy; PCI: percutaneous coronary intervention; PPCI: primary PCI; SIHD: stable ischemic heart disease; SVD: single-vessel disease; STEMI: ST-segment elevation myocardial infarction; TLR: target lesion revascularization)

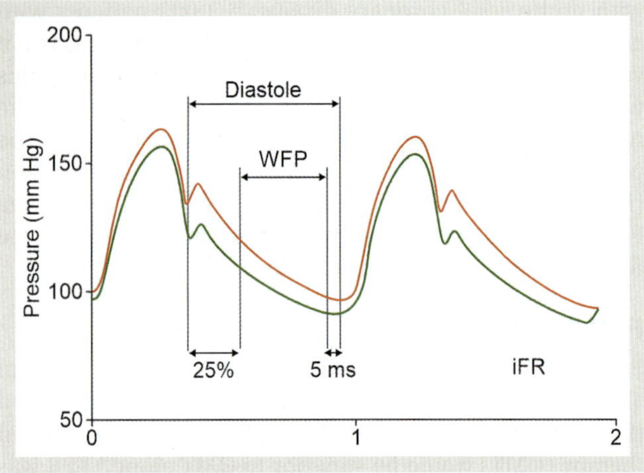

FIG. 4: Wave-free period (WFP) for assessment of instantaneous wave-free ratio (iFR).

stenosis by measuring the distal pressure during the "wave-free period" which was the period from 25% into diastole (identified from dicrotic notch on the waveform) and 5 ms before systole **(Fig. 4)**.

The ADVISE registry was the first to assess the accuracy of iFR against FFR as the reference standard.[19] The CLARIFY study compared iFR and FFR to the hyperemic stenosis resistance (HSR) index[20] and found that iFR, FFR, and iFR with adenosine had equal diagnostic efficacy to match an ischemic classification with HSR. In the JUSTIFY-CFR study of 216 patients looking at FFR and iFR with regards to coronary flow reserve (CFR), iFR showed stronger correlation with CFR.[21]

Patient Outcome Data with Instantaneous Wave-free Ratio

DEFINE FLAIR trial: Functional lesion Assessment of Intermediate Stenosis to Guide Revascularization[22] showed that coronary revascularization guided by iFR was noninferior to that guided by FFR with respect to MACE at 1 year. Among 2,492 patients, the primary endpoint occurred in 78 of 1,148 patients (6.8%) in the iFR group and in 83 of 118 patients (7%) in the FFR group $p < 0.001$ for noninferiority. Patients who had adverse procedural symptoms were significantly lower in the iFR group (3.1% vs. 30.8%) and mean procedural time was shorter.

iFR SWEDEHEART trial: Evaluation of iFR versus FFR in Stable Angina or Acute Coronary Syndrome[23] showed concordant results with those of DEFINE FLAIR trial. Among 2,037 patients randomized to undergo revascularization guided by iFR or FFR, the primary endpoint occurred in 68 of 1,012 patients (6.7%) in iFR and 61 of 1,007 (6.1%) in the FFR group $p = 0.007$ for noninferiority. 5-year follow-up date of the iFR SWEDEHEART trial showed no difference in the outcome of death, MI, or unplanned revascularization between an iFR versus FFR guided revascularization strategy.[24]

The pooled data of 4,529 patients provide outcome data of those with intermediate lesions guided by physiology. It showed noninferiority of iFR versus FFR-guided revascularization. Further, deferral of revascularization was more with iFR and yet the patient outcome remained the same.

The potential advantages of the resting indices are better comfort as it avoids adenosine, does not require a specific vascular access for adenosine, and reduces procedure time and radiation. Further large outcome data shows that it is comparable to FFR. Resting indices are better than FFR in interrogating tandem lesions and "virtual stenting" by co-registration with angiogram. Since iFR, multiple other resting indices have come into the market, all of which are comparable.[25] The summary of the non-hyperemic indices available are given in **Table 2**.

HOW DOES PHYSIOLOGICAL ASSESSMENT HELP IN REAL WORLD?

Examples of the use of physiology in managing cases on a routine basis are shown in **Figures 5 to 10**.

- Defer lesions which are not significant **(Figs. 5A and B)**
- Avoid missing significant lesions **(Figs. 6A and B)**
- Reclassify disease **(Figs. 7A to C)**
- Safety of deferred lesions **(Figs. 8A and B)**
- LMCA disease **(Figs. 9A to C)**
- Serial lesions **(Figs. 10A to C)**

FRACTIONAL FLOW RESERVE OR INSTANTANEOUS WAVE-FREE RATIO?

The question should not be whether one uses FFR or iFR, it should be whether physiology is used or not. We have a large amount of data which shows that the use of physiology improves outcomes and so adoption of physiology should be the cornerstone. The use of nonhyperemic indices has the advantage of avoidance of adenosine. This is particularly useful in the assessment of nonculprit lesions in the setting of acute coronary syndrome (ACS) patients with hemodynamic instability. However, there are some subsets of patients where one is preferred over the other.

In LMCA disease FFR has more robust data[26] though iFR has been shown to be safe for deferral of left main stenosis in the DEFINE-LM registry.[27] In the Instantaneous Wave-Free Ratio for the Assessment of Intermediate Left Main Coronary Artery Stenosis: Correlations with Fractional Flow Reserve/Intravascular Ultrasound and Prognostic Implications: The iLITRO-EPICO7 study, iFR and FFR were used to assess intermediate LMCA stenoses and in case of discordance, IVUS-MLA (intravascular ultrasound-minimal lumen area) was measured. Both indices had agreement of 80%. 8.7% of FFR + and 14.6% of iFR + had MLA > 6 mm^2. At median follow-up of 20 months, MACE was 8.3% in the defer group and 13.3% in the revascularization group showing that deferral based of iFR is safe in intermediate LMCA disease.[28]

TABLE 2: Summary of nonhyperemic pressure indices.

Resting index	Calculation	Cutoff indication ischemia	Number of cycles for calculation	Comments
iFR	Pd/Pa during wave-free interval—25% of way into diastole till 5 ms before systole	<0.89	• 1 beat • Average multiple beats in irregular rhythm	RCT noninferiority to FFR for outcome *PHILIPS*
Diastolic hyperemia-free ratio (DFR)	Pd/Pa when Pa is less than the average Pa, and Pa downsloping	<0.89	Average of 5 cycles	High correlation with iFR *Boston Scientific*
Diastolic pressure ratio (dPR)	Pd/Pa over the entire diastolic period	<0.89	Average of 5 cycles	Excellent correlation with iFR and FFR *OPSENS*
Pd/Pa	Pd/Pa over the whole cardiac cycle	<0.92	Average of 5 cycles	Good correlation with iFR. Increased susceptibility to hemodynamic conditions and drift
Resting full-cycle ratio (RFR)	Lowest Pd/Pa at any point in the entire cardiac cycle	<0.89	Single lowest value from 5 cycles	Excellent correlation with iFR and FFR *ABBOTT*

(FFR: fractional flow reserve; iFR: instantaneous wave-free ratio; Pa: aortic pressure; Pd: distal coronary pressure; RCT: randomized controlled trial)

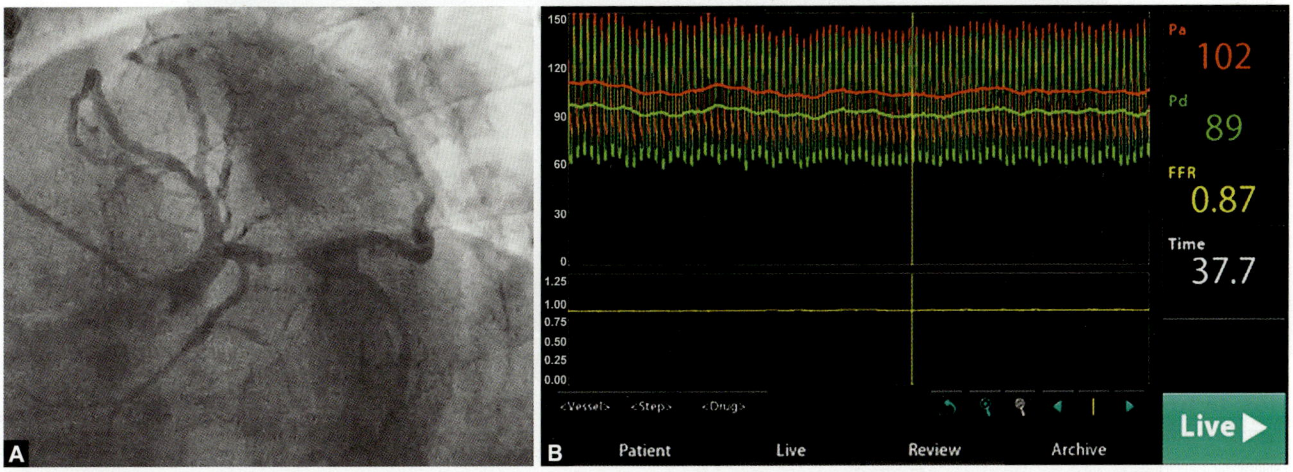

FIGS. 5A AND B: A 60-year-old doctor referred with a positive treadmill test (TMT). He was asymptomatic at 5-year follow-up.

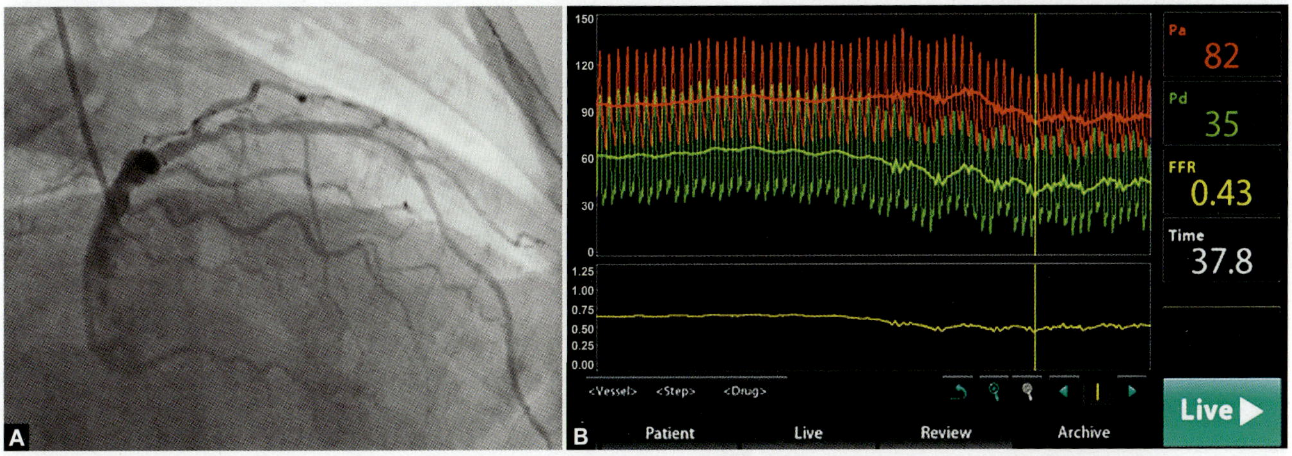

FIGS. 6A AND B: Irregular lesion in mid-left anterior descending (LAD)—highly significant fractional flow reserve (FFR).

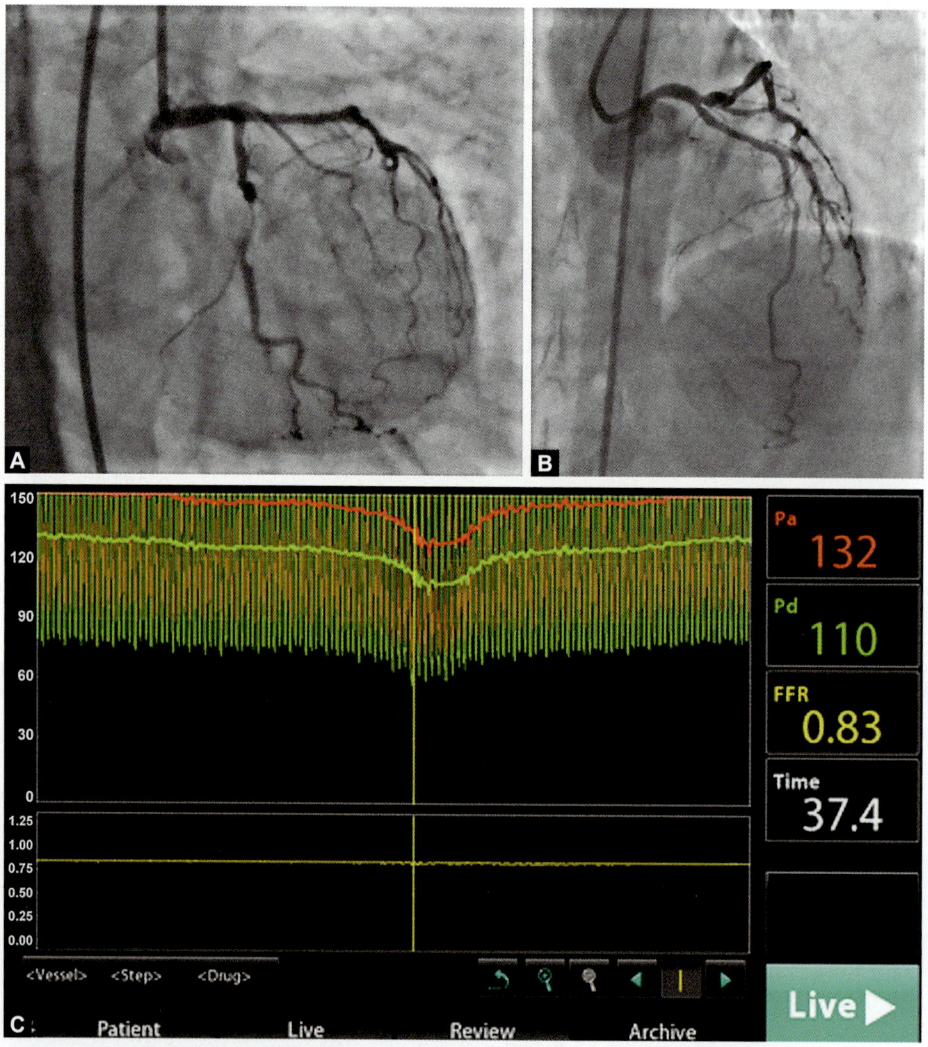

FIGS. 7A TO C: Two-vessel disease of left anterior descending (LAD) and left circumflex (LCX) is converted to single vessel disease of LCX; fractional flow reserve (FFR) of LAD being nonsignificant.

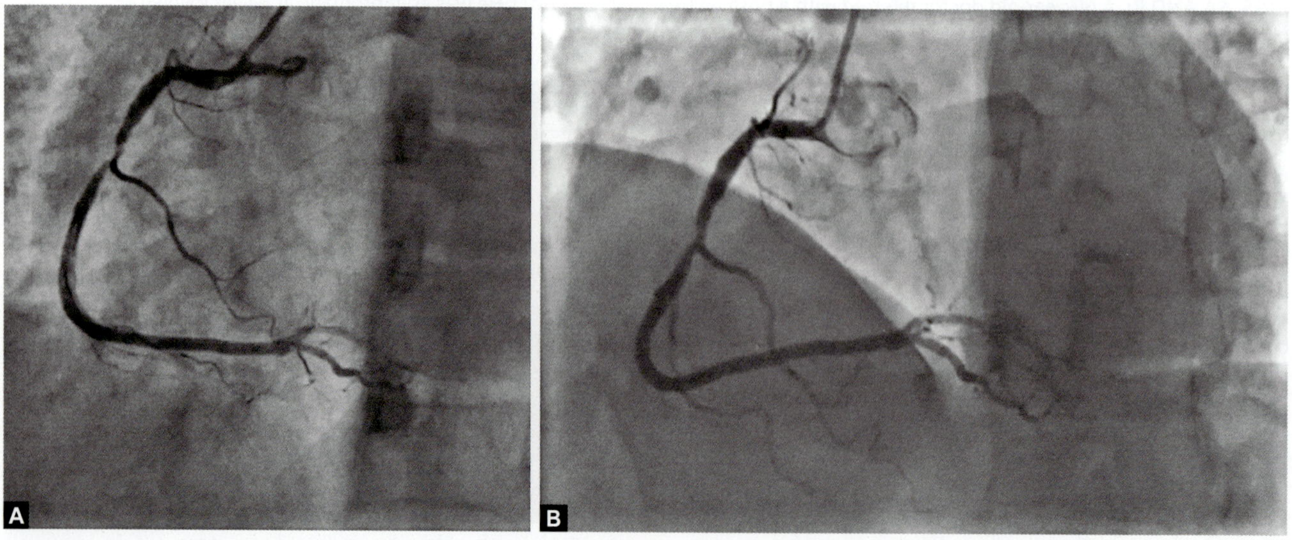

FIGS. 8A AND B: (A) Fractional flow reserve (FFR) of right coronary artery (RCA): 0.92 in 2013; (B) remains the same in 2020.

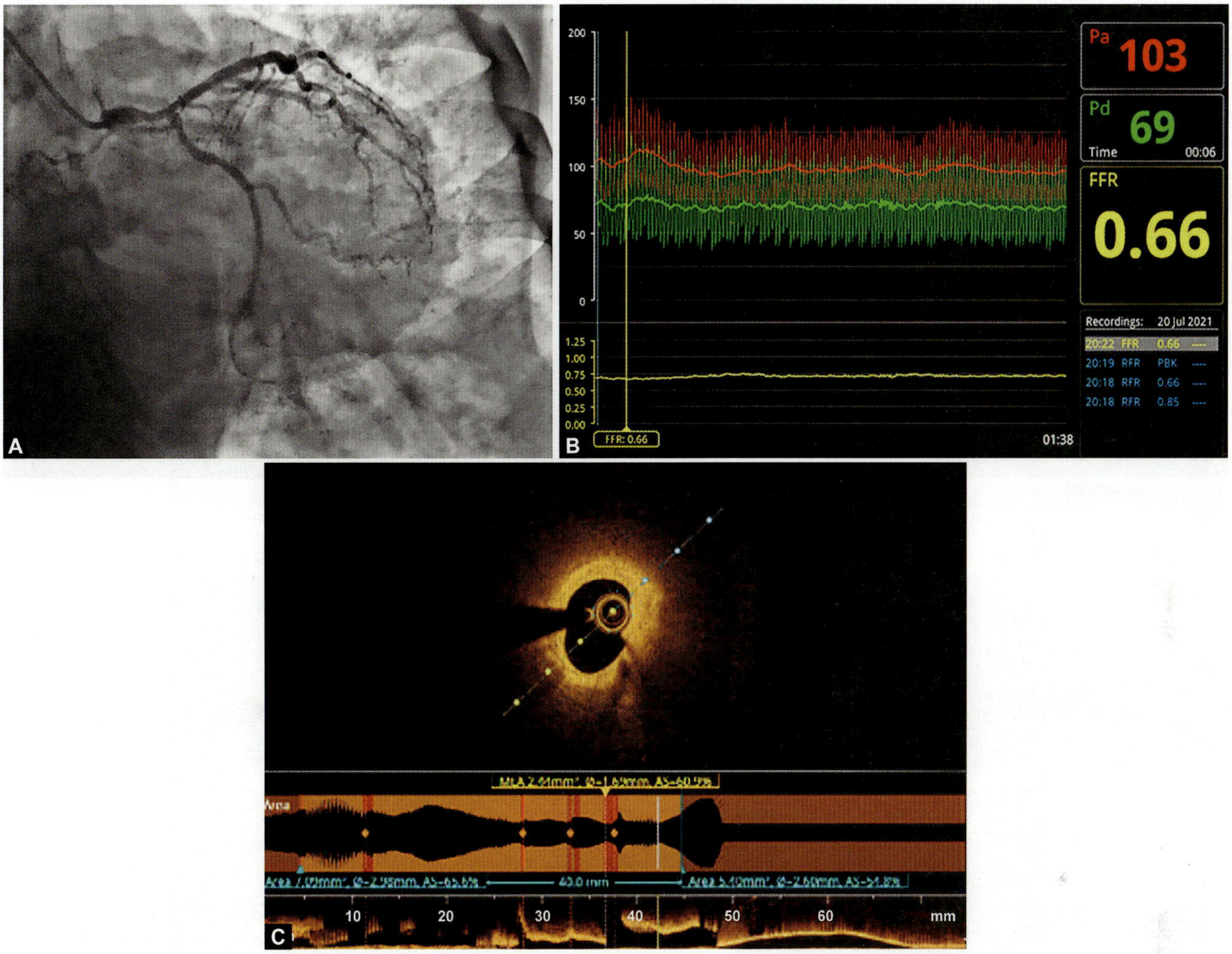

FIGS. 9A TO C: (A) Distal left main coronary artery (LMCA) ~70%; (B) fractional flow reserve (FFR) significant; (C) minimal lumen area (MLA) in OCT: 2.4 mm^2 confirms significance.

In tandem and serial lesions iFR has a significant advantage. It is not possible to assess the significance of individual lesions in the presence of tandem lesions under hyperemic conditions. Hyperemic flow decreases significantly when there is >50% reduction in diameter and so the flow through one stenosis would be affected by the second stenosis and vice versa. Resting flow is more consistent and there is less cross talk between the lesions. It was shown that iFR pullback can predict the hemodynamic impact of each stenosis and thus facilitate intervention and stenting strategy.[29]

FRACTIONAL FLOW RESERVE/ INSTANTANEOUS WAVE-FREE RATIO DISCORDANCE

Discordance between FFR and iFR is found in approximately 20% of patients.[30] Discordance is frequently found immediately on either side of the FFR cutoff of 0.8. Warisawa et al. found that pattern of disease was more likely to result in FFR–/iFR+ discordance. Pressure loss across a stenosis is related to separation and frictional components. For diffuse disease, frictional component predominates and results in iFR positivity. For focal lesions, separation forces (where flow is squared) dominates and hyperemic index (FFR) is more likely to be positive.[31]

The questions to be considered when faced with FFR/iFR discordance are: (1) physiological difference for the discordance, (2) prognostic difference among patients deferred in the two groups, and (3) what should be the treatment strategy when faced with discordance.[32] These were addressed in this trial of 840 vessels from 596 patients looking at discordant lesions between iFR and FFR and prognosis at 5 years.[32] iFR correlated better with CFR than FFR. There was no difference in the patient-oriented composite outcome (POCO) among patients with deferred lesions and high FFR irrespective of the iFR values. Similarly, there was no difference in the outcomes among those deferred due to high iFR with low or high FFR. Neither of

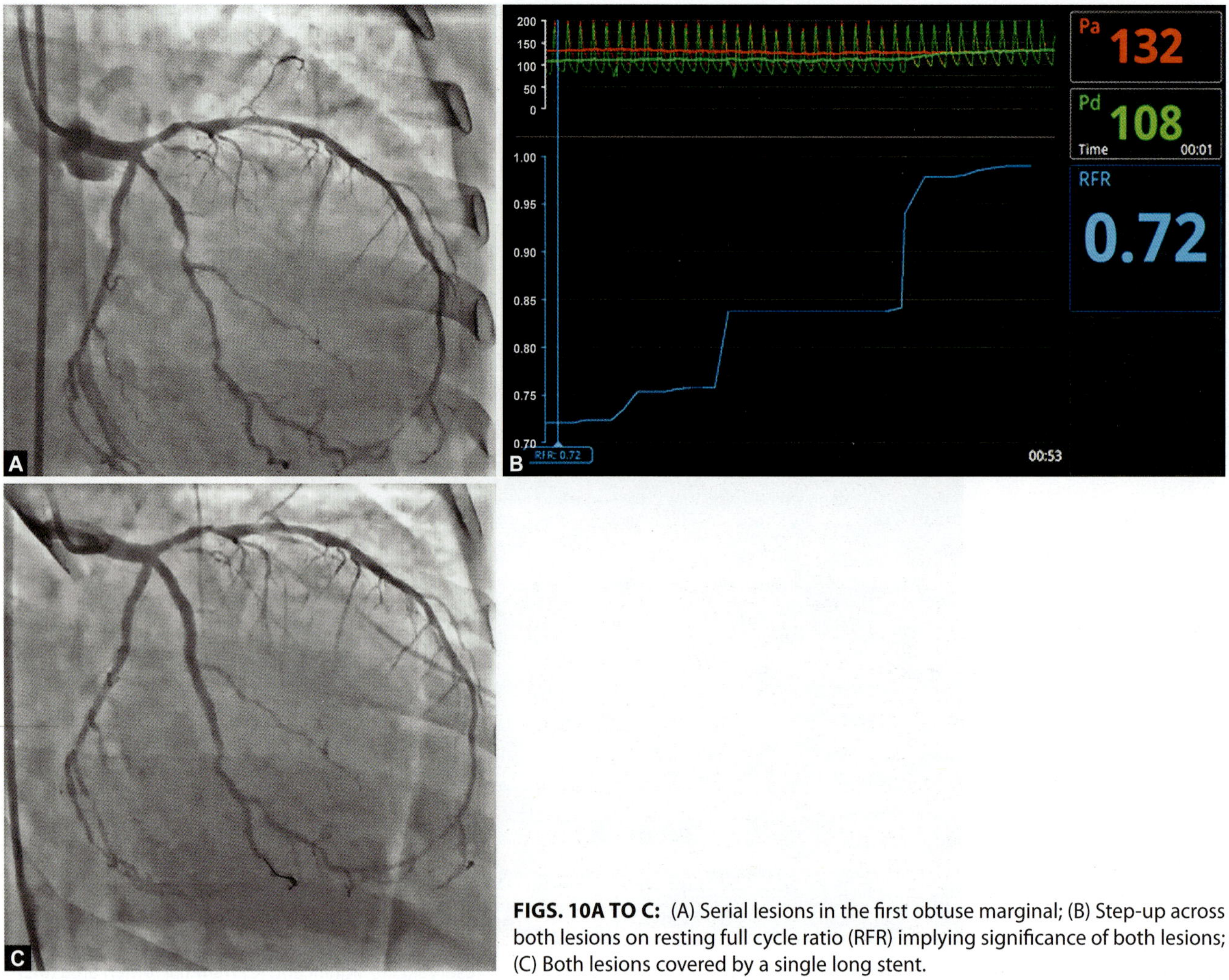

FIGS. 10A TO C: (A) Serial lesions in the first obtuse marginal; (B) Step-up across both lesions on resting full cycle ratio (RFR) implying significance of both lesions; (C) Both lesions covered by a single long stent.

the two discordant groups was associated with an increase in POCO compared with the high FFR-high iFR group. The results were similar to that from another study with a shorter follow-up of 2 years.[33]

There is no evidence regarding the ideal treatment strategy for discordant lesions. Considering data from DEFINE FLAIR and iFR SWEDEHEART where iFR guidance resulted in fewer revascularization but similar clinical outcome to FFR, not all patients with high iFR-low FFR need revascularization. Those with low iFR-high FFR may be due to microvascular dysfunction and not by epicardial coronary stenosis. Hence decision to revascularize must be made on an individual basis among those with discordant results—deferral being relatively safe.

DOES FFR-GUIDED PCI REDUCE MORTALITY?

Data from the SCAAR (Swedish Coronary Angiography and Angioplasty Registry) registry on all patients undergoing PCI with or without FFR guidance for stable angina pectoris in Sweden from January 2005 to March 2016 was analyzed. The primary endpoint was all-cause mortality. Secondary endpoints were stent thrombosis or restenosis and periprocedural complications.[34] Of 23,860 patients, FFR guidance was used in 3,367. At a median follow-up of 4.7 years, FFR group had a significant reduction in mortality, stent thrombosis, and restenosis. Periprocedural complications did not differ.

The findings of this trial complement the pooled analysis of three randomized trials FAME 2,[4] DANAMI-3-PRIMULTI[35] and COMPARE ACUTE[36] which showed that FFR-guided PCI reduces the combined outcome of death and MI.[37] The difference in these was driven by reduction in MI, no difference in mortality was detected. Neither the individual trials nor the pooled data had adequate statistical power to evaluate whether FFR resulted in reduction of mortality. This trial was four times larger than the pooled cohort.

The mortality curves did not diverge till the second year of follow-up and was similar to the timeline of the DEFER trial where deferral was associated with a lower incidence of MI after 5 years of randomization,[13,14] possibly related to neoatherosclerosis developing in hemodynamically insignificant lesions treated with stents.

Sensitivity analysis showed that survival was improved even after excluding patients with in-stent restenosis or stent thrombosis. This may be due to undertreatment of functionally significant lesions with increased residual ischemia and mortality. Treatment of high-risk plaques with stents followed by optimal medical treatment leads to stabilization of these lesions preventing plaque rupture and future events. This would explain the delay in the beneficial effects of FFR-guided PCI on survival. In summary, FFR-guided PCI results in a reduction in mortality by preventing stenting of insignificant lesions and detecting functionally significant lesions particularly vulnerable plaques in proximal coronaries which may be missed by coronary angiography alone.

WHAT ABOUT THE "NEGATIVE TRIALS" ON FRACTIONAL FLOW RESERVE?

No discussion about the physiological indices would be complete without looking into the negative trials of FFR which came out in the last couple of years. FAME 3 was a randomized trial comparing multivessel PCI guided by FFR and using contemporary drug-eluting stents (DES) with coronary artery bypass graft (CABG). Patients having >50% stenosis in all three coronaries deemed suitable for both modes of revascularization were randomized to FFR-directed PCI (n = 757) or to CABG (n = 743). The primary endpoint of death, MI, stroke, and repeat revascularization at 1 year occurred in 10.6% of PCI patients versus 6.9% in CABG (p = 0.35 for noninferiority).[38]

In FLOWER-MI (Flow Evaluation to Guide Revascularization in Multivessel ST-Elevation Myocardial Infarction), 1,171 patients with ST-segment elevation myocardial infarction (STEMI) in whom primary PCI was done, were randomized to have FFR-guided PCI versus angiogram-guided PCI for nonculprit lesions. There was no difference in the composite primary endpoint (death, nonfatal MI, urgent revascularization) between the two arms at 1 year.[39] Routine FFR assessment of all vessels did not shown any difference in quality of life at 1 year or change in resource utilization in RIPCORD 2 trial.[40] The FUTURE (Functional Testing Underlying Coronary Revascularization) trial was stopped prematurely at 1 year due to increased mortality in treatment of multivessel CAD using an FFR-guided strategy.[41]

The FLOWER-MI and FUTURE showed the fallacy of FFR in ACS. Physiology has limitations in ACS setting with events being higher due to vulnerable plaques, missing culprit lesions, etc. In chronic coronary syndrome physiologic assessment does play a significant role. In FAME 3, only 24% lesions were deferred. It is not failure of FFR, but essentially a trial of PCI versus CABG for multivessel disease and shows that CABG is better than PCI in complex cases. The biggest advantage of FFR is as a means to defer a stent in functionally nonsignificant lesions.

POST-PCI PHYSIOLOGICAL ASSESSMENT

A higher post PCI FFR is associated with better outcomes. Post-PCI FFR of >0.9 was associated with a lower risk of repeat PCI and MACE in >7,000 patients.[42] A post-PCI iFR of >0.95 was associated with better outcomes in the DEFINE PCI study.[43] Suboptimal post-PCI FFR/iFR values are seen in 24–38%[43,44] Post-PCI FFR was <0.9 in 68.1% of patients in the Target-FFR trial[45] This could be due to stent-related problems (underexpansion, plaque protrusion, edge dissection, inadequate lesion coverage, etc.), or due to vessel-related factors (diffuse disease or untreated focal lesion). However, post-PCI FFR optimization with IVUS[46] or with postdilatation/additional stent implantation[45] did not have a significant impact on improvement of post-PCI FFR or reducing target vessel failure at 1 year follow-up.

CONCLUSION

Optimal medical therapy is the mainstay of treatment of chronic coronary syndrome as shown in the COURAGE[47] and ISCHEMIA[48] trials. Revascularization of borderline lesions is not going to provide symptomatic relief let alone mortality benefit. Identifying such lesions by angiography has limitations. Physiological assessment by FFR/non-hyperemic indices provide a method to identify those that are significant and to safely defer those that are not. Large-outcome trials show benefit of this approach with reduction in hard endpoints including death, MI, and urgent revascularization. An overview of physiological assessment, recording, and interpretation of results, use in special subsets, FFR/iFR discordance, fallacy in ACS, and its use in post-PCI assessment has been covered in this section.

ONLINE REFERENCES

Please scan the QR code provided at the end of the table of contents for References of this chapter.

CHAPTER 138

Evaluation of Intermediate Coronary Lesions—Beyond Physiology

Bahuleyan CG, Shifas Babu M

ABSTRACT

Coronary physiology assessment has been considered as the standard method to determine the functional significance of intermediate lesions. The approach of doing percutaneous coronary intervention (PCI) for coronary physiology positive cases and medical management for negative cases has been well established in patients with stable coronary artery disease (SCAD) with superior clinical outcomes than angiography-based decisions. However, in acute coronary syndrome (ACS), the role of physiology-based decision is less clear. Non-culprit lesions (NCLs), which are PCI-deferred on the basis of negative physiology, are found to be associated with more future cardiac events. More than half of these NCLS showed the presence of vulnerable plaque (VP) characteristics such as thin cap fibroatheroma (TCFA), lipid-rich plaque (LRP), and signs of inflammation making them more prone to plaque rapture. High-risk morphological features of NCLs are likely to be more predictive of future events than ischemic potential. Intravascular imaging (IVI) with the capability of detecting VP characteristics and other vessel details is likely to assume more importance either alone or in combination with physiology in deciding treatment options for these lesions. Several outcome trials addressing the issue of PCI or optimal medical therapy for physiology-negative lesions with high-risk plaque characteristics (HRPC) are ongoing.

Keywords: Intermediate coronary lesion evaluation, the role of physiology in NCLs, role of imaging in intermediate coronary lesions, vulnerable plaques.

INTRODUCTION

Coronary lesions with angiographic diameter stenosis of 40–70% have been considered intermediate lesions in American guidelines[1] and 50–90% as per the European guidelines.[2] Various clinical trials have revealed that up to 25% of patients undergoing coronary angiography have intermediate lesions which pose a challenge in decision-making for revascularization.[3] Coronary angiography has several limitations in deciding the ischemic potential of intermediate lesions and roughly about 30% of lesions undergoing angioplasty have doubtful functional significance.[4] Inadvertent placement of stent for insignificant lesions will lead to adverse events such as stent thrombosis and stent restenosis while deferring treatment for ischemic lesions will necessitate future revascularization. Improved techniques like quantitative coronary angiography (QCA) or three-dimensional QCA could not overcome the limitations of angiography in detecting the severity of intermediate lesions.[5,6] Invasive physiological evaluation has been considered the gold standard for determining the severity of these lesions with clinical superiority over angiography-based decisions for intervention.[7-9] However, there are several limitations recognized in undertaking the physiology testing as well as interpretation of the results. Intravascular imaging (IVI) such as intravascular ultrasound (IVUS) and optical coherence tomography (OCT) has also been utilized in evaluating the need for intervention in intermediate lesions. This article intends to discuss the limitations of physiology and what would be the possible role of IVI alone or in combination with physiological data in the evaluation of intermediate coronary lesions.

PHYSIOLOGY IN INTERMEDIATE LESIONS

Fractional flow reserve (FFR) has been established as the method of choice to decide the ischemic potential of non-left main (LM) intermediate lesions based on pivotal clinical trials such as DEFER [Deferral Versus Performance of Percutaneous Transluminal Coronary Angioplasty (PTCA) in Patients Without Documented Ischemia], FAME (Fractional Flow Reserve Versus Angiography for Multivessel Evaluation), and FAME 2.[9-11] Similarly, non-hyperemic pressure ratios (NHPRs) like instantaneous wave-free ratio (iFR) have also been accepted for the same purpose based on randomized controlled trials (RCTs) such as DEFINE-FLAIR (Functional Lesion Assessment of Intermediate Stenosis to Guide Revascularisation)[12] and iFR-SWEDEHEART (Instantaneous Wave-free Ratio versus Fractional Flow Reserve to Guide PCI).[13] Use of FFR or iFR is recommended by guidelines to assess the hemodynamic significance of intermediate coronary stenoses in the catheterization laboratory.[2] All other NHPRs could be used to determine the functional significance of intermediate lesions like iFR with a cutoff value of ≤0.89.[14] Image-based physiology from invasive coronary angiogram, QFR (quantitative flow ratio), vFFR (vessel fractional flow reserve), FFR-angio (FFR derived from coronary angiography) and CT-FFR (computed tomography derived fractional flow reserve) has shown good correlation with pressure wire-based FFR.[15-17] Longitudinal vessel analysis which allows a physiological mapping of the vessel thereby classifying disease into focal, diffuse, or mixed is possible with image-based physiology. FAVOR III China, an RCT of QFR versus angiography-based percutaneous coronary intervention (PCI) of intermediate lesions (50–90%) revealed a 2-year major adverse cardiac event (MACE) rate of 8.5% and 12.5% respectively ($p < 0.0001$).[18] These advances may enhance faster diagnosis of the functional significance of intermediate lesions but with many technical challenges and pitfalls.[19]

LIMITATIONS OF PHYSIOLOGY: ACUTE CORONARY SYNDROME

In patients presenting with acute coronary syndrome (ACS), an FFR-based deferral of PCI of intermediate non-culprit lesions (NCLs) was associated with more than twofold increase of combined endpoint of myocardial infarction (MI) or target vessel revascularization (TVR) at 3.4 years of follow-up [ACS 23% vs. stable coronary artery disease (SCAD) 11%].[20] In RCTs such as DANAMI3-PRIMULTI (Complete Revascularisation versus Treatment of the Culprit Lesion Only in Patients with ST-Segment Elevation Myocardial Infarction and Multivessel Disease) and Compare-Acute, FFR-guided complete revascularization in ST-segment elevation myocardial infarction (STEMI) patients with multivessel disease (MVD) resulted in lower MACE rate mainly due to a reduction in repeat revascularization compared to angiography guidance.[21,22] However, in these trials FFR-guided PCI has not been compared to angio-guided PCI directly. FFR-based deferral of PCI in a pooled analysis of 8,579 ACS patients from three large registries and two RCTs has shown a higher rate of MACE at 1 year compared to SCAD, mainly contributed by unplanned revascularization in the first months after FFR interrogation.[23] In a meta-analysis of seven randomized studies comparing culprit-only PCI and complete revascularization in STEMI patients, angiography-based PCI resulted in significant benefit compared to FFR-guided PCI.[24] Furthermore, the FLOWER-MI (Flow Evaluation to Guide Revascularization in Multivessel ST-Elevation Myocardial Infarction) trial revealed no significant benefit of reduction in the risk of death, MI, or urgent revascularization for FFR-guided complete revascularization compared to angiographic guidance in patients with STEMI during 1-year follow-up (5.5% vs. 4.2% HR 1.32). The Kaplan–Meier curves appeared to separate late in favor of an angiography-guided strategy.[25] FRAME-AMI (Fractional Flow Reserve vs. Angiography-Guided Strategy for Management of Non-Infarction Related Artery Stenosis in Patients with Acute Myocardial Infarction) trial showed a MACE rate of 7.4% versus 19.7% ($p = 0.003$) with FFR-guided versus angiography-guided complete revascularization in patients with ACS over a median follow-up of 3.5 years.[26] The strategy of physiology-based PCI in patients with ACS has not shown convincing superiority over angiography-based strategy, especially for the reduction of hard endpoints, such as death and MI. The microvascular dysfunction and altered epicardial coronary flow dynamics seen in ACS can lead to an underestimation of the severity of NCLs by FFR and an overestimation by non-hyperemic indices like iFR when measured in the acute phase of STEMI. Moreover, nearly half of all lesions in ACS are having high-risk features such as lipid-rich plaque (LRP), thin cap fibroatheroma (TCFA), and other vulnerable features, which will lead to future plaque rupture and cardiovascular events.[27] What could be the safe and effective strategy to identify the lesions associated with increased cardiovascular events: physiology, morphology, or both?

ROLE OF IMAGING IN THE EVALUATION OF INTERMEDIATE LESION: IVUS

Intravascular ultrasound has also been used in the catheterization laboratory for assessing intermediate coronary lesions. The correlation between FFR and IVUS-derived minimal luminal area (MLA), minimal lumen diameter (MLD) and percent stenosis area have been investigated earlier. An MLA of 3 mm^2 has been identified as correlating with an FFR value of ≤0.75 with a sensitivity of 83% and specificity of 92.3%.[28] An MLA cutoff of 2.6 mm^2 correlated with FFR of ≤0.8 with sensitivity 0.79 and specificity 0.65.[29] However, the correlation of IVUS-derived MLA with

FFR <0.8 has been found to be low in intermediate lesions.[30] Similarly IVUS MLA, when correlated with NHPRs such as iFR, diastolic pressure ratio (dPR), and resting full-cycle ratio (RFR), provided limited diagnostic accuracy of the functional significance of the intermediate lesion.[31] FIRST (Fractional Flow Reserve and Intravascular Ultrasound Relationship Study), a multicenter registry of patients with intermediate coronary lesions (40–80% stenosis by angiography), observed that an MLA of 3.07 was the best threshold value for identifying FFR ≤0.8 [64.0% sensitivity, 64.9% specificity, the area under curve (AUC) 0.65]. The accuracy improved when reference vessel-specific analyses were performed. An MLA of <2.4 mm^2 was best for reference vessel diameters <3.0 mm (AUC = 0.66), an MLA of <2.7 mm^2 for reference vessel diameters of 3.0–3.5 mm (AUC = 0.71), and an MLA of <3.6 mm^2 for reference vessel diameters >3.5 mm (AUC = 0.68).[32] The thresholds were smaller in Asians, most probably due to lower body mass index and the common cutoff value was approximately 3.0 mm^2.[33] A meta-analysis of 14 prospective studies, a mean MLA of 2.68 mm^2 in Asian populations, and 3.03 mm^2 in Western populations predict significant non-LM stenosis.[34]

In clinical practice, generally, IVUS-derived MLA has been used to defer PCI because of its better negative predictive value (75–96%) and low positive predictive value (28–67%). Furthermore, PCI based on IVUS-determined lesion severity results in more stent use and subsequent stent-related adverse events.[35] In a recent multicenter trial [FLAVOUR (Fractional Flow Reserve and Intravascular Ultrasound-Guided Intervention Strategy for Clinical Outcomes in Patients with Intermediate Stenosis)], 1,682 patients with stenosis of 40–70% on angiography was randomized to undergo PCI based on either FFR (≤0.80) or IVUS [MLA ≤3 mm^2, or 3–4 mm^2 with plaque burden (PB) > 70%]. The composite primary outcomes of death, MI, or revascularization at 24 months were similar in the FFR and IVUS groups (8.1% vs. 8.5%, respectively). This study concluded that in patients with intermediate coronary lesions, FFR guidance is noninferior to IVUS guidance with respect to composite endpoints over a period of 2 years after the index procedure.[36]

ROLE OF IMAGING IN INTERMEDIATE LESIONS: OPTICAL COHERENCE TOMOGRAPHY

Optical coherence tomography-derived MLA has been correlated with functional ischemia and compared with IVUS in a study from Japan involving 203 intermediate coronary lesions of 186 patients. OCT-MLA had significantly better diagnostic efficacy than IVUS-MLA in identifying ischemia (FFR <0.75) with the best MLA cutoff values of 1.39 mm^2 for OCT and 2.57 mm^2 for IVUS. There was no significant difference between OCT and IVUS-MLA for the prediction of FFR ≤0.80 ($p = 0.13$). A smaller MLA, greater percent stenosis area, and higher maximum lipid arc are seen in patients with ischemia by OCT whereas IVUS revealed a smaller MLA and greater percent PB.[37] Pooled analysis from a recent meta-analysis including a total of 33 studies revealed similar sensitivity for OCT- and IVUS-derived MLA to predict the functional significance of intermediate lesions; however, OCT-MLA had a higher specificity and better accuracy than IVUS-MLA.[38] The FORZA trial randomized patients with angiographically intermediate coronary lesions in a 1:1 fashion to FFR-guided and OCT-guided PCI groups. In the FFR arm, PCI was performed if FFR was ≤0.80. In the OCT arm, PCI was performed when at least one of the following criteria was present: (1) percent area stenosis (AS) >75%; (2) AS between 50 and 75% and MLA <2.5 mm^2; and (3) AS between 50 and 75% and plaque rupture. The primary endpoint of MACEs or significant angina at 13 months occurred in 14.8% of patients in the FFR arm and in 8.0% in the OCT imaging arm ($p = 0.048$).[39]

COMBINING MORPHOLOGY AND PHYSIOLOGY

There are clinical situations and lesion subsets where physiological data alone may result in inaccurate treatment decisions. ACS, serial lesions, or diffuse disease, LM stenosis with downstream lesions in left anterior descending artery (LAD) or left circumflex artery (LCX), and coronary artery disease (CAD) in patients with severe aortic stenosis are some of them. In the SWEDEHEART trial, MACE occurred in 19% of patients at 5 years after deferral by FFR or iFR.[40] Long-term follow-up in RCT has shown the occurrence of clinical events in PCI deferred patients with FFR >0.80 and iFR >0.89. The presence of high-risk plaque characteristics (HRPC) which are not detected by physiology interrogation has been cited as responsible for these events. In a study evaluating the association between physiological stenosis severity and coronary computed tomography angiography (CTA)-defined HRPC (seven quantitative and four qualitative parameters), the presence of ≥3 coronary CTA-defined HRPC showed a significantly higher risk of vessel-oriented composite outcome (VOCO) compared to those with <3 HRPC in the group with FFR >0.80. By multivariate analysis, the presence of ≥3 HRPC was independently associated with the risk of VOCO.[41] Physiological severity along with the degree of HRPC may predict the possibility of future events in intermediate lesions, especially in the group with FFR >0.80.

Assessment of intermediate lesions by IVI may be of prognostic value in patients with ACS. In the PROSPECT study (a prospective natural history study of coronary atherosclerosis) lesions with the presence of TCFA, PB ≥70% or MLA ≤4 mm^2 were associated with significantly more events than lesions without these features. At 3 years, it was found that nearly half of the events were associated with angiographically mild NCLs. A large PB, a small luminal area, and TCFA were found predictive of MACE.[42] In the

PROSPECT natural history II study, vulnerable plaques (VPs) detected by near-infrared spectroscopy (NIRS)-IVUS imaging showed that a combination of lipid rich plaque [maximum 4 mm Lipid Core Burden Index ($maxLCBI_{4mm}$) ≥324.7] and PB (≥70%) led to a higher future MACE rate.[43] In the LRP study, maximum LCBI (≥ 250 $maxLCBI_{4mm}$) in non-culprit segments predicted MACE at patient and segmental levels.[44] The influence of HRPC detected by OCT on the clinical outcomes at the end of 1 year was investigated in patients with proximal LAD lesions in the CLIMA study. Lesions with an MLA of <3.5 mm^2 TCFA, lipid arc circumferential extension >180°, and OCT-detected macrophages were found to be associated with a composite primary endpoint of cardiac death and target segment MI.[45] A recent study using three-vessel OCT revealed that the detection of HRPC are associated with a higher incidence of cardiovascular events at follow-up.[46] Presence of TCFA was identified as a strong predictor of MACE in diabetic patients despite nonischemic FFR (>0.80) in intermediate coronary lesions with angiographic stenosis of 40–80%.[47] Several studies using IVI have shown the impact of aggressive pharmacological treatment on regression and stabilization of HRPC with beneficial clinical outcomes. Mechanical stabilization of the VPs by stenting is still debated. PROSPECT ABSORB study showed that in angiographically mild lesions with large PB, PCI with bioresorbable vascular scaffold substantially enlarged the follow-up MLA, and was associated with favorable long-term clinical outcomes.[48] A few other clinical trials are progressing in this direction. The COMBINE-INTERVENE (COMBINEd Ischemia and Vulnerable Plaque Percutaneous INTERVENtion to Reduce Cardiovascular Events) trial[49] investigates, whether a PCI revascularization strategy based on combined FFR and OCT assessment is superior to PCI revascularization strategy based on FFR alone in patients with MVD with any presentation. In the group with FFR >0.75, PCI is undertaken for those lesions with OCT-detected VP. VP is defined as TCFA (cap thickness ≤75 microns); ruptured plaque; or plaque erosion with >70% AS or MLA <2.5 mm. This will be the first trial investigating the outcome of stenting for lesions with VP without ischemia. The VULNERABLE Trial[50] randomizes lesions with FFR >0.80 and OCT-detected TCFA in patients with multivessel STEMI to PCI or optimal medical therapy. The COMPLETE-2,[51] an ongoing trial, is comparing a physiology-guided PCI strategy using RFR or FFR to an angiography-guided strategy for NCL in a trial of >5,100 patients with STEMI and non-STEMI (NSTEMI). In this ongoing study, OCT imaging is used in 1,510 patients to define the predictive potential of plaque morphology (LRP and TCFA) for future cardiac events.

CONCLUSION

Physiology-guided PCI has been associated with significant reduction in MACE and use of lesser number of stents compared to angiography-based strategy in stable CAD. In ACS the role of physiology is less clear. Deferring PCI for angiographically intermediate NCLs in ACS based on either hyperemic or NHPRs is associated with increased cardiac events. HRPC in these functionally negative NCLs are found to be more predictive of future cardiac events. Multimodality imaging with potential to detect HRPC, PB, and vessel details will establish its role in evaluating these lesions. The strategy of PCI or optimal medical therapy for physiology-negative, HRPC-positive lesions is being investigated in several ongoing clinical trials.

ONLINE REFERENCES

Please scan the QR code provided at the end of the table of contents for References of this chapter.

CHAPTER

139 Intravascular Imaging and Physiology Coregistration: How Best is the Combination

Rohit Mody, Abha Bajaj Nee Sheth, Debabrata Dash

ABSTRACT

Plaque morphology characterization and percutaneous coronary intervention (PCI) performance can be optimized by the use of emerging contemporary intravascular imaging technologies. Intravascular imaging technologies such as intravascular ultrasound (IVUS) and optical coherence tomography (OCT) can be used for vessel assessment, stent deployment, lesion preparation, and postintervention assessment of clinical endpoints. Furthermore, in comparison to the use of angiography alone, marked improvements in clinical outcomes have been achieved with the use of coronary physiology assessment by using the fractional flow reserve (FFR) parameter. In the efficient management of stable coronary heart disease, invasive coronary physiology has become established in contemporary guidelines. Assessment of coronary artery disease (CAD) functional severity can be done by using a new validated parameter known as the instantaneous wave-free ratio (iFR). iFR pullback investigation not only provides the guidance for PCI, but also facilitates the mapping of ischemia contribution of the same artery. However, considering certain drawbacks associated with continuous iFR measurements, real-time iFR coregistration concept has been introduced. In the last few years, for IVUS and coronary angiography (CAG), the coregistration concept has also been started.

Keywords: Percutaneous coronary intervention, intravascular ultrasound, optical coherence tomography, fractional flow reserve, coronary angiography.

INTRODUCTION

Coronary artery disease (CAD) can be assessed by using coronary angiography (CAG) as a gold standard which can also be used to make a decision regarding the selection of percutaneous coronary intervention (PCI) as a therapeutic approach. However, it has limitations, such as providing only two-dimensional luminogram images, lacking detailed information about atherosclerotic plaque, and vessel wall morphology. To overcome these limitations, several intravascular imaging modalities have been developed, including intravascular ultrasound (IVUS), optical coherence tomography (OCT), angioscopy, and near-infrared spectroscopy (NIRS).[1] These techniques offer high-resolution cross-sectional imaging of coronary arteries and play a crucial role in understanding CAD's pathophysiological mechanisms.

Intravascular ultrasound and OCT are particularly significant in improving clinical outcomes for CAD patients undergoing medical therapy or interventions. They provide incremental value in PCI by enabling the identification of major plaque components such as fibrotic tissue, thrombus, calcium, and lipid pools. Ischemia-guided revascularization with invasive coronary physiology has revolutionized the management of stable CAD. It helps to identify patients who would benefit from revascularization and allows real-time investigation of the significance of epicardial stenosis and assessment of hemodynamically significant lesions.

However, recent data has shown a complex link between ischemia and symptoms, challenging the paradigm of using ischemia as the sole criterion for therapeutic intervention. Even physiologically and angiographically nonsignificant lesions can be responsible for cardiovascular events.[2] Invasive coronary physiology helps to investigate lesion and vessel-specific ischemia, but optimal medical therapy remains crucial after physiological investigations.

Criticism has been directed at using angiography alone to make decisions about revascularization, particularly when suboptimal functional results are achieved with PCI. Invasive coronary physiology can improve PCI outcomes through preprocedural simulation and planning, enhancing PCI precision in identifying flow-limiting disease, and guiding the optimization of clinical outcomes in cases of suboptimal PCI. Physiology applications in guiding and planning of procedures of PCI are shown in **Figures 1A to C**.

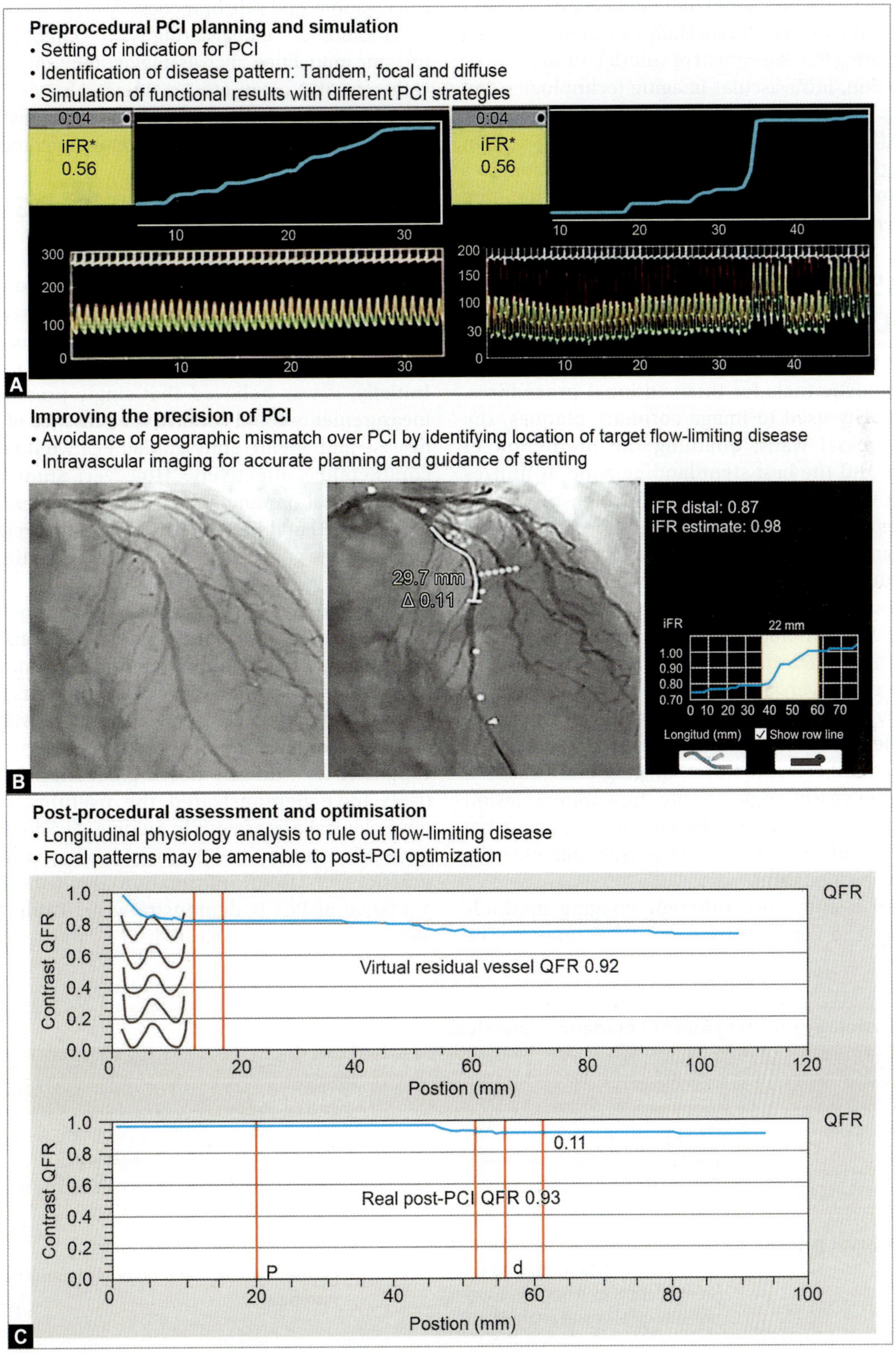

FIGS. 1A TO C: Physiology applications in guiding and planning of procedures of PCI.
(iFR: instantaneous wave-free ratio; PCI: percutaneous coronary intervention; QFR: quantitative flow ratio)

Recently, an advanced IVUS system has been introduced, allowing coregistration with other imaging modalities such as angiography, fractional flow reserve (FFR), or instantaneous wave-free ratio (iFR) assessment in a physiological manner. This coregistered view provides a more detailed description of the lesion and its severity, especially in heavily diseased arteries, facilitating the assessment of culprit lesions.

In conclusion, intravascular imaging technologies and intracoronary physiological assessment have significantly improved CAD diagnosis and PCI outcomes. Coregistration of IVUS with physiological measurements further enhances the understanding and treatment of CAD, ensuring more effective patient management.

INTRAVASCULAR ULTRASOUND TECHNOLOGIES

Over the last three decades, IVUS and OCT have become efficient diagnostic tools for interventional procedures. IVUS is primarily used to image coronary plaques, the lumen, and vessel walls, enabling the prediction of lesion length and the best stent landing zone. It utilizes miniaturized ultrasound transducers for high-resolution vessel images.[3] In contrast, OCT offers superior imaging of the coronary vessel wall, but this diagnostic method is challenging due to the need for saline to clear the blood pool in the vessel segment.[4]

While both technologies share similar advantages, deciding which intravascular diagnostic method to use remains controversial due to the risks and costs of multimodality invasive imaging investigations.[5] Operators must consider the positive effects and drawbacks of each modality and select the best imaging tool based on factors such as vessel angiographic appearance, lesion characteristics, and clinical need. Recent surveys suggest that specific patient and anatomical characteristics influence the choice of imaging modality.[6]

In a serial fashion, two different imaging methods have been used to combine OCT and IVUS images. The multimodality imaging system shows significant synergistic efficiency in assessing plaque composition, but the need for separate pullbacks to acquire strict coregistration images is a limitation, especially for identifying landmarks such as calcifications and side branches.[7,8]

Additionally, coregistering IVUS technologies with other imaging modalities, such as angiography and hybrid imaging catheters, offer a new efficient method for visualizing plaque lesions. These advancements enhance diagnostic capabilities and improve interventional outcomes for clinicians.

INTRACORONARY PHYSIOLOGICAL ASSESSMENT

In patients with acute coronary syndrome (ACS), intracoronary physiological assessment is recommended as the most effective strategy for evaluating flow-limiting epicardial stenosis and determining the need for PCI.[9] Initially, it was believed that single pressure guidewire measurements could confirm the presence of flow-limiting disease and angiography-guided PCI would restore vessel conductance effectively. However, studies evaluating physiological parameters such as nonhyperemic pressure ratio (NHPR) and FFR after PCI found that relying solely on angiographic guidance could lead to suboptimal functional results.[10]

Physiological investigations are routinely performed in the catheter laboratory to guide decisions about PCI,[11] often using a binary approach to determine the need for intervention.[12] The limitations of CAG in characterizing flow-limiting coronary stenosis can be overcome with noninvasive and/or adjunctive invasive physiological assessments, as supported by evidence-based guidelines. Several clinical trials have demonstrated the usefulness of invasive physiological assessment in guiding decisions on coronary revascularization, leading to an increased use in clinical practice.[13,14] Useful information about the physiological guidance of PCI is demonstrated in **Table 1**. Dedicated software provides stable FFR, iFR, and resting full-cycle

TABLE 1: Physiology planning and PCI guidance objectives.

Pre-PCI physiological assessment		
Objective	**Technique**	**Advantages**
PCI clinical indication determination	Determination of flow-limiting disease presence by using the pressure wire or FCA	• Prognostic or symptomatic benefit is achieved by significant stenosis management • Risk of unnecessary PCI is reduced by the deferral of non-flow-limiting disease
Flow-limiting disease patterns investigation	Various patterns of low-limiting disease such as diffuse, tandem, and local identification by using longitudinal physiological vessel analysis	• Facilitates the PCI effectiveness • Potentiates the planning of stent length and stent numbers

Continued

Continued

Pre-PCI physiological assessment		
Objective	**Technique**	**Advantages**
In specific areas simulating of stenting impact	Simulation of stenosis relief virtually by using imaging-based and NHPR-based functional investigations	• Before deployment of stent, PCI planning in an effective manner • Before PCI, facilitates various simulations
Potentiation of precision deployment of stent	Use of coregistration technologies or virtual assessment to correlate angiography and physiology	• During stenting, reducing the risk of geographical miss, missing flow-limiting lesions • Balloons and stents sizing in an accurate manner
Post-PCI physiological assessment		
Objective	**Technique**	**Advantages**
Ensuring the PCI functional result in an optimum way	After achieving the angiographic results quite satisfactory, PCI target vessel physiological investigations, jailed side-branch interrogation	After the intervention, in the PCI target vessel, residual flow-limiting disease early determination
PCI functional optimization potential targets prediction	Post-PCI longitudinal vessel analysis	• Suboptimal functional PCI results cause development • PCI optimization and feasibility method development
PCI optimization impact assessment	After physiology-based optimization, physiological measurements in repeat manner	Directed medical therapy or surgical revascularization is needed in case if residual disease is not amenable to PCI

(FCA: functional coronary angiography; NHPR: nonhyperemic pressure ratio; PCI: percutaneous coronary intervention)

ratio (RFR), which helps to assess coronary stenosis hemodynamic significance.[15,16] Longitudinal vessel assessment enables differentiation between focal and diffuse patterns of flow-limiting disease, providing valuable information on pressure loss distributions along the epicardial vessel which is demonstrated in **Figure 2**.

The commonly used index for determining coronary stenosis severity is FFR, which calculates hyperemic pressure investigations directly. iFR, on the other hand, assesses stenosis severity and demonstrates the hemodynamic role of individual lesions without requiring adenosine, making it faster to perform than FFR.

However, in patients with severe aortic stenosis (AS), investigating coronary plaque-induced ischemic burden becomes challenging as valve hemodynamics can affect pressure wire indices such as iFR and FFR. Complex interactions between elevated left ventricular end-diastolic pressure, left ventricular hypertrophy, and coronary microcirculation remodeling can reduce FFR's reliability in AS and underestimate the ischemic significance of coronary obstruction.[17]

To simulate PCI functional results, longitudinal vessel analysis is used, helping in accurate localization of flow-limiting atherosclerotic disease and facilitating procedural planning. Functional PCI results simulation can be achieved by using various approaches from baseline longitudinal vessel analysis demonstrated in **Figure 3**.

Coregistering physiological data with the coronary angiogram provides benefits such as optimal target lesion localization and clear distribution of pressure loss regions that may benefit from PCI.[18] Pitfalls and challenges related to physiological assessment are demonstrated in **Table 2**.

In summary, intracoronary physiological assessment plays a crucial role in guiding decisions for PCI in ACS patients. By combining physiological indices such as FFR and iFR with imaging modalities and CAG, clinicians can make well-informed decisions for more successful interventions. However, in AS patients, certain considerations are needed to ensure accurate assessments of coronary stenosis and ischemic burden.

FRACTIONAL FLOW RESERVE

Coronary stenosis severity can be assessed by using FFR as a crucial invasive parameter and to guide myocardial revascularization decisions. Clinical studies and guidelines have demonstrated the clinical benefits of using FFR, as it accurately identifies ischemia-producing lesions and improves outcomes in patients with stable coronary disease undergoing PCI.

The predictive value of FFR was first tested in the DEFR trial, where patients were randomized to PCI deferral or PCI groups based on FFR values. The study showed that a large group of patients referred for PCI had nonsignificant lesions when assessed with FFR, indicating that FFR can help avoid unnecessary interventions.[19] The FAME (Fractional Flow Reserve Versus Angiography for Multivessel Evaluation) trial compared FFR-guided and angiography-guided approaches in stable CAD patients, and the FFR-guided group showed significantly reduced primary endpoints, including

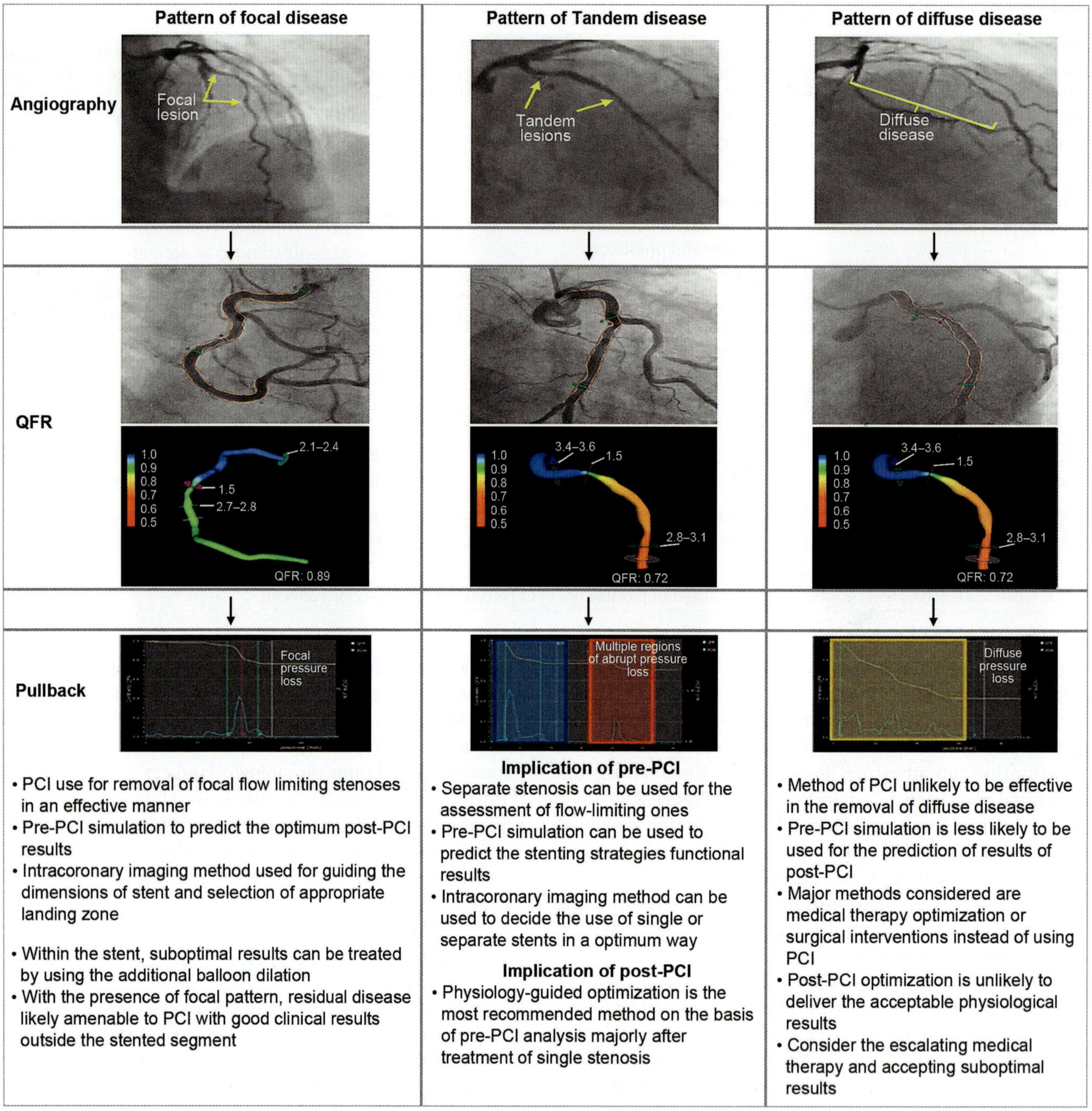

FIG. 2: Before and after PCI, use of longitudinal vessel analysis to assess the flow-limiting disease patterns.
(PCI: percutaneous coronary intervention; QFR: quantitative flow ratio)

myocardial infarction (MI) and repeat revascularization, at the 1-year follow-up.[14]

Fractional flow reserve has also been shown to diagnose coronary stenosis with the potential to induce reversible myocardial ischemia. The FAME-2 trial further demonstrated the independence of FFR from anatomical features, making it a major predictor of clinical outcomes related to lesion severity.[13,20]

Fractional flow reserve has been instrumental in reclassifying the revascularization decision for patients recommended for CAG, with more than half of the patients showing a change in the decision based on FFR measurements.[21] In ST-elevation myocardial infarction (STEMI) patients with multivessel disease, FFR-guided complete revascularization was linked with a reduced risk of adverse cardiovascular events compared to treatment of the infarct-related artery only.[22]

New FFR technologies have been developed, providing functional and anatomical information through an invasive coronary angiogram or noninvasive computed tomography coronary angiography (CTCA). FFR-CT obtained by merging 3D vessel reconstruction from CTCA with computational fluid dynamics shows good correlation with wire-based FFR. It allows reliable estimation of invasive FFR, making it a valuable tool in assessing functional stenosis severity.[23]

In conclusion, FFR has revolutionized the assessment of coronary stenosis severity and guided revascularization decisions. Its success has led to the development of new imaging technologies like FFR-CT, providing additional options for evaluating CAD in a more comprehensive and efficient manner.

INSTANTANEOUS WAVE-FREE RATIO

The adoption of FFR has been limited due to various issues, including added time, lack of familiarity, and cost. As an alternative, iFR was emerged as an adenosine-free resting index[24,25] for functional evaluation of coronary stenosis. iFR has shown promise in investigating left main coronary artery (LMCA) disease, such as bifurcation stenosis, where multiple measurements in daughter branches are required.

Studies have compared iFR with FFR for guiding coronary revascularization decisions, and iFR has been found to be noninferior to FFR in terms of clinical outcomes.[26] The safety and accuracy of deferring treatment based on iFR or FFR were compared, with iFR-guided deferral appearing to

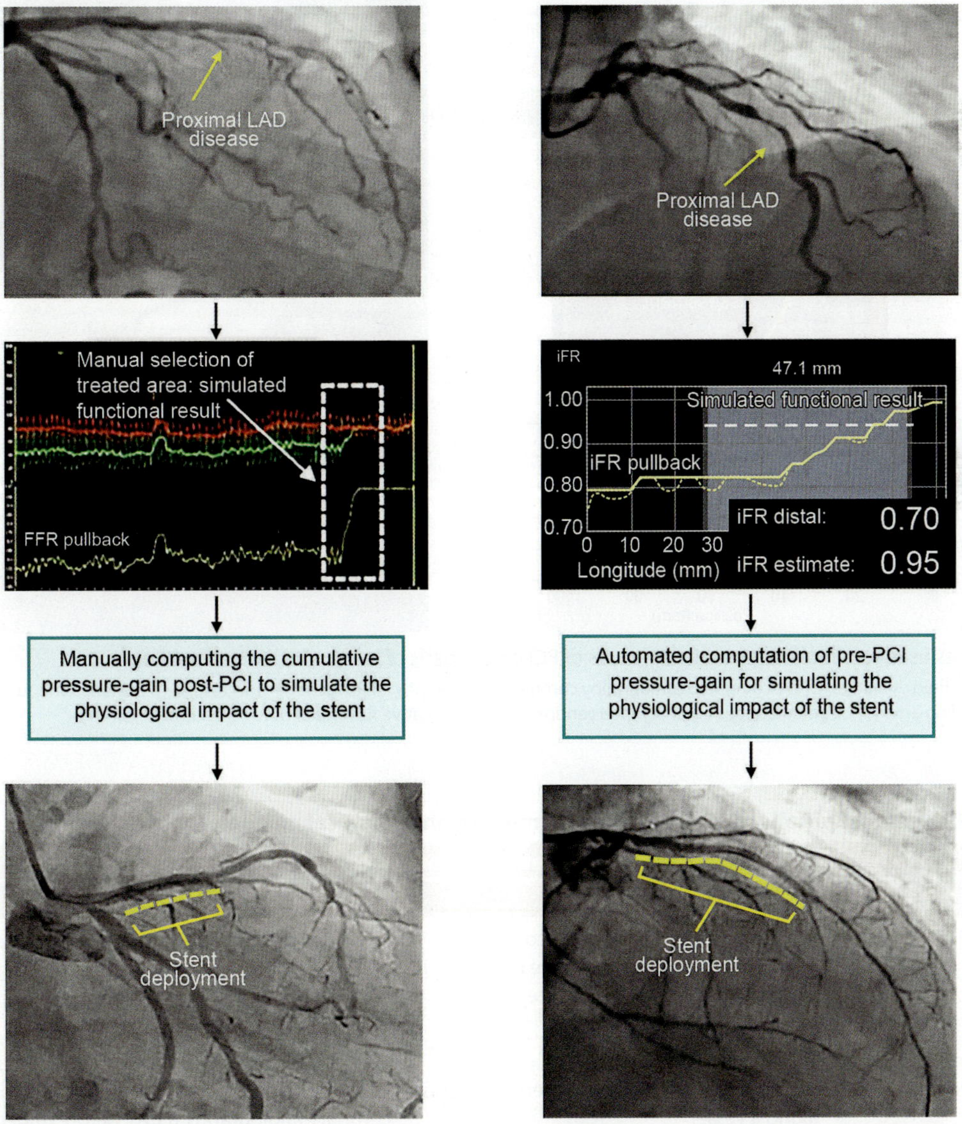

FIG. 3: *Continued*

Continued

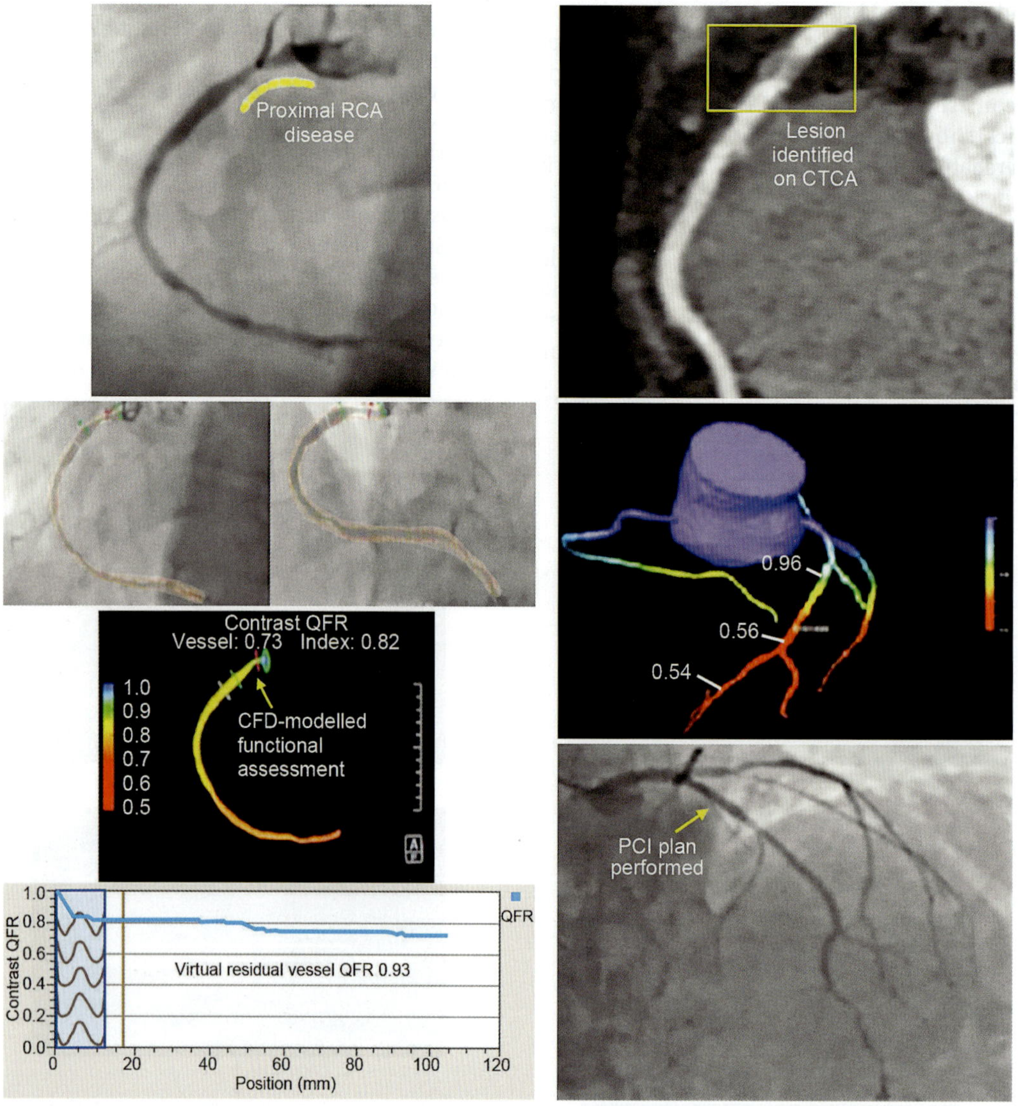

FIG. 3: Approaches used for simulating functional results of PCI on the basis of longitudinal vessel analysis.

(CFD: computational fluid dynamics; CTCA: computed tomography coronary angiography; FFR: fractional flow reserve; iFR: instantaneous wave-free ratio; LAD: left anterior descending artery; PCI: percutaneous coronary intervention; QFR: quantitative flow ratio; RCA: right coronary artery)

TABLE 2: Challenges and pitfalls related to the assessment in physiological manner.

Patient factors		
Objective	**Comment**	**Solution**
Significant ostial CAD presence	If FCA modalities are not able to assess, using damping pressure or ventricularization to investigate it modalities	To a more proximal position, guide catheter repositioning, ensure coaxiality, guide catheter downsizing consideration, controlling catheter tip position by using an additional guidewire or septal wire
In the presence of tandem lesions, hemodynamic crosstalk	Other lesions in the vessel are affected in physiological manner by sequential lesions along a vessel	On the basis of longitudinal vessel analysis obtained with various imaging methods such as NHPR, or FFR, functional coronary angiography (FCA), before undertaking PCI on one or two stenoses, considering simulated planning

Continued

Continued

Procedural factors		
Objective	**Comment**	**Solution**
Pressure wire drift	During the procedure, offset of pressure reading	Repeat procedure by using the imaging-based methods or drift correction/renormalize
Intracoronary wires induced pseudostenosis	Introsusceptions may be generated by intracoronary wire used for tortuous vessels straightening	As an alternative option to the intracoronary pressure guidewire, FCA can be considered
Aortic pressure damping/ ventricularization	In significant ostial lesions or during the abutting of vascular lumen, guiding catheter was engaged	Guide catheter repositioning, guide catheter downsizing consideration, pressure guidewire equalization
Using the guide catheter presence with two holes	At the guiding catheter tip, Pa false estimation	Intracoronary assessment should not done with using catheter with two side holes. Even after that, it is required for clinical reasons, ensure the usage of IV adenosine and catheter disengagement
Guide catheter extension usage	Pa ventricularization can occurred, if it is introduced after equalization of pressure	Use extension present within guide catheter with the objective to perform pressure equalization, further during the physiological assessment, withdraw guide extension
Coronary microcatheters usage	Measurements can be affected and Pa can be modified, if after pressure equalization it is used	Microcatheter within guide catheter can be used to achieve pressure equalization before measurements
Wire whipping	Through the contact with vascular lumen, degradation of pressure wire signal	This issue can be resolved by pressure wire repositioning
Procedure-induced transient microvascular dysfunctioning	Microparticles generated by PCI tools and rotational atherectomy may induce transient microvascular dysfunctioning which further influence pressure indices	If there is risk of transient microvascular dysfunctioning, consider FCA as an alternative approach for intracoronary assessment
Without stable hyperemia, investigation of FFR in region	While lowest physiological reporting are demonstrate by software, in stable hyperemia, these might not be stable and therefore severity of lesions overestimation can occur	In stable hyperemia, measure FRR and if required, adopt manual adjustments of points

(CAD: coronary artery disease; FFR: fractional flow reserve; IV: intravenous; NHPR: nonhyperemic pressure ratio; PCI: percutaneous coronary intervention)

be safe for patients with LMCA lesions and showing lower cardiovascular event rates than FFR-guided deferral.[27]

Instantaneous wave-free ratio has also been used to perform entire vessel hemodynamic mapping, providing physiological maps of coronary vessels to predict stenosis intensity, severity, and length. It helps in selecting stenting and intervention strategies and predicts poststenting iFR and residual ischemia patterns in patients with coronary vessel disease after PCI.

Furthermore, iFR has been evaluated for its usefulness in predicting the severity of coronary lesions and assessing individual lesion hemodynamic contribution. By coregistering iFR with other imaging modalities such as IVUS and angiography, a more precise assessment of lesion morphology, length, and vessel width can be achieved.

Overall, iFR offers a valuable and efficient alternative to FFR for assessing coronary stenosis severity and guiding revascularization decisions. Its noninferiority to FFR in various clinical scenarios and its ability to predict long-term clinical outcomes make it a promising tool for intracoronary physiological assessment. iFR and coregistration were used to perform the pullback curve analysis, including simulated stenting at a specific region which is demonstrated in **Figures 4A to C**.

NOVEL NONHYPEREMIC PRESSURE RATIOS

Various alternative NHPRs such as diastolic hyperemia-free ratio (DFR), diastolic pressure ratio (DPR), and RFR have emerged in clinical practice following the successful adoption of iFR. These ratios measure the ratio of distal coronary to proximal aortic pressure without the need for vasodilators such as adenosine, making them easier and safer to use compared to pharmacological hyperemia.[28] FFR, iFR, and RFR pullback curves are provided by dedicated software which are free of fluctuations induced by Venturi effect **(Fig. 5)**. Over a vessel with stenosis, intracoronary

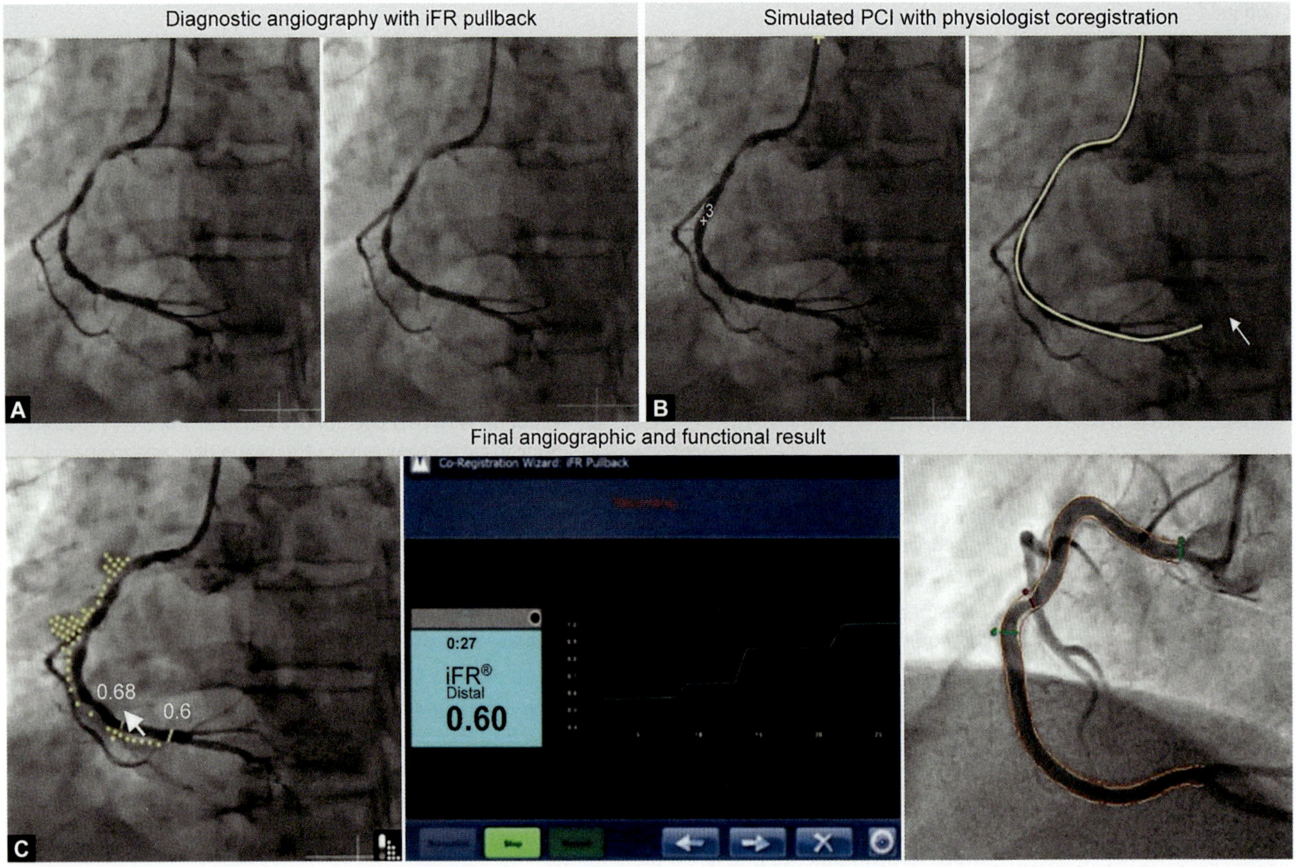

FIGS. 4A TO C: Functional percutaneous coronary intervention (PCI) results simulated using coronary angiogram and physiology coregistration. (A) Longitudinal vessel assessment use for the left circumflex artery angiography. (B) Distal instantaneous wave-free ratio (iFR) of 0.57 use to demonstrate the presence of flow-limiting disease in the vessel. Focal disease phenotype is revealed by longitudinal vessel analysis. In the coronary anatomy, flow-limiting disease localization is facilitated by iFR coregistration with angiography in an accurate manner. Intervention adequate functional results are suggested by the PCI simulation, with a predicted 0.94 post-PCI iFR. (C) Final results with final 0.90 iFR are demonstrated by final coregistred angiography physiology.

guidewires are used to acquire the pressure pullback curve which demonstrates pressure-induced ups and downs flow velocity relationships (Venturi effect). Over the pullback, within the reference segment, intraluminal pressure distal to a stenosis reduced when it is reaching to a high-flow velocity intrastenotic location which is translated into a translational pressure ratios iFR, FFR, and others dip. Software-based correction of pullback curve omits like reduction in iFR values is demonstrated by the **Figure 5** which facilitate longitudinal vessel analysis interpretation.

Nonhyperemic pressure ratios show a close association with iFR and have been favorably used in clinical practice due to their lower cost and time of procedure. Studies have demonstrated the noninferiority of NPHR-guided revascularization to FFR-guided revascularization for major adverse cardiovascular events (MACE) at both 5-year[29] and 1-year follow-ups.[24]

SEVERITY OF LEFT MAIN AND NON-LEFT MAIN LESIONS

Unprotected LMCA intervention is associated with a huge clinical challenge which is reported in 3–10% of patients undergoing CAG. However, with the introduction of drug-eluting stents, skilled operators, and rise in the use of IVUS, the huge rise in the intervention strategies for the effective management of LMCA was seen which ultimately led to the change in guidelines recommended for LMCA procedures in patients present with stable angina. Further, marked correlation was seen between minimum lumen area (MLA) and ischemia. In the assessment of LMCA, the combination of various parameters (MLA plus plaque burden or lesion length), or incorporating tissue characterization, is not quite better than MLA. Furthermore, FFR was recommended as a class-I indication for the prediction of severity of non-LMCA

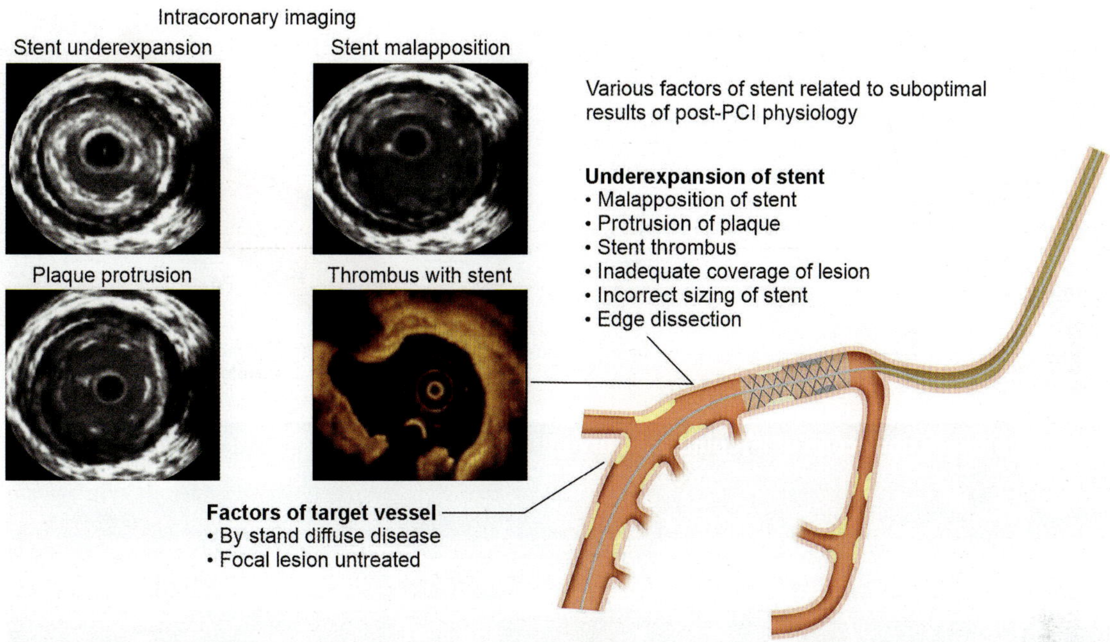

FIG. 5: Dedicated software used for intracoronary pressure pullback curves correction which address the Venturi effect-induced fluctuations. (PCI: percutaneous coronary intervention)

lesions by the findings of three randomized clinical trials named DEFER, FAME, and FAME-2. However, the use of FFR as the class-I indication method is challenged by the findings of recently conducted negative trials FLOWER-MI, FUTURE, and FAME-3.

Further, in patients present with angiographically intermediate coronary lesions (AICL), the decision to perform PCI is associated with a huge clinical challenge. Physiological assessment using FFR is recommended by international clinical guidelines to guide the decision of revascularization. Yet, a huge rise in interest of the use of various intracoronary imaging methods, such as OCT was seen. Considering this, in the patients present with at least one AICL, to compare the clinical outcomes and cost in patients randomized to FFR versus OCT guidance, a single-center open-label prospective FORZA trial was conducted in which a total of 350 patients were enrolled. At the follow-up of 13 months, the occurrence of MACE after observation was considered as the primary endpoint of the study. A huge rate of medical management or lower cost was reported in patients of FFR-guided group while a lower incidence of MACE or significant angina was reported in patients of OCT guided group.[30] Considering the findings, it was concluded that OCT use for guidance is quite safe which is associated with a lower incidence of MACE or significant angina, while a high rate of medically managed patients was seen in the FFR-guided group of patients at the follow-up of 13 months.

POST-PERCUTANEOUS CORONARY INTERVENTION PHYSIOLOGY ASSESSMENT AND IMAGING

Even after the significant improvement in clinical outcomes after PCI, the failure of the target vessel is of huge concern. Considering this, various physiological tools and intravascular imaging methods have been introduced with the objective to facilitate the post-PCI investigation. Major key reasons responsible for the suboptimal PCI are revealed by the post-PCI imaging tools (IVUS and OCT) and physiological assessment parameters (FFR and iFR). Findings of recent studies suggested that clinical outcomes can be improved in patients after stenting by using coronary physiology and intravascular imaging methods for stent optimization. Every technology is associated with certain advantages and drawbacks, and requires dedicated training with the objective to assess vessel-related and stent-related issues which can occur after the post-PCI.[31] In **Figure 6**, potential mechanisms to achieve suboptimal post-PCI physiology results are demonstrated. **Flowchart 1** demonstrates malapposition, which needs correction by postdilatation.

Furthermore, findings of various studies suggested that after performing PCI successfully, in certain patients, residual ischemia (characterized as FFR $\leq$ 0.80) can occur which is associated with a worse prognosis. Even after that, there are

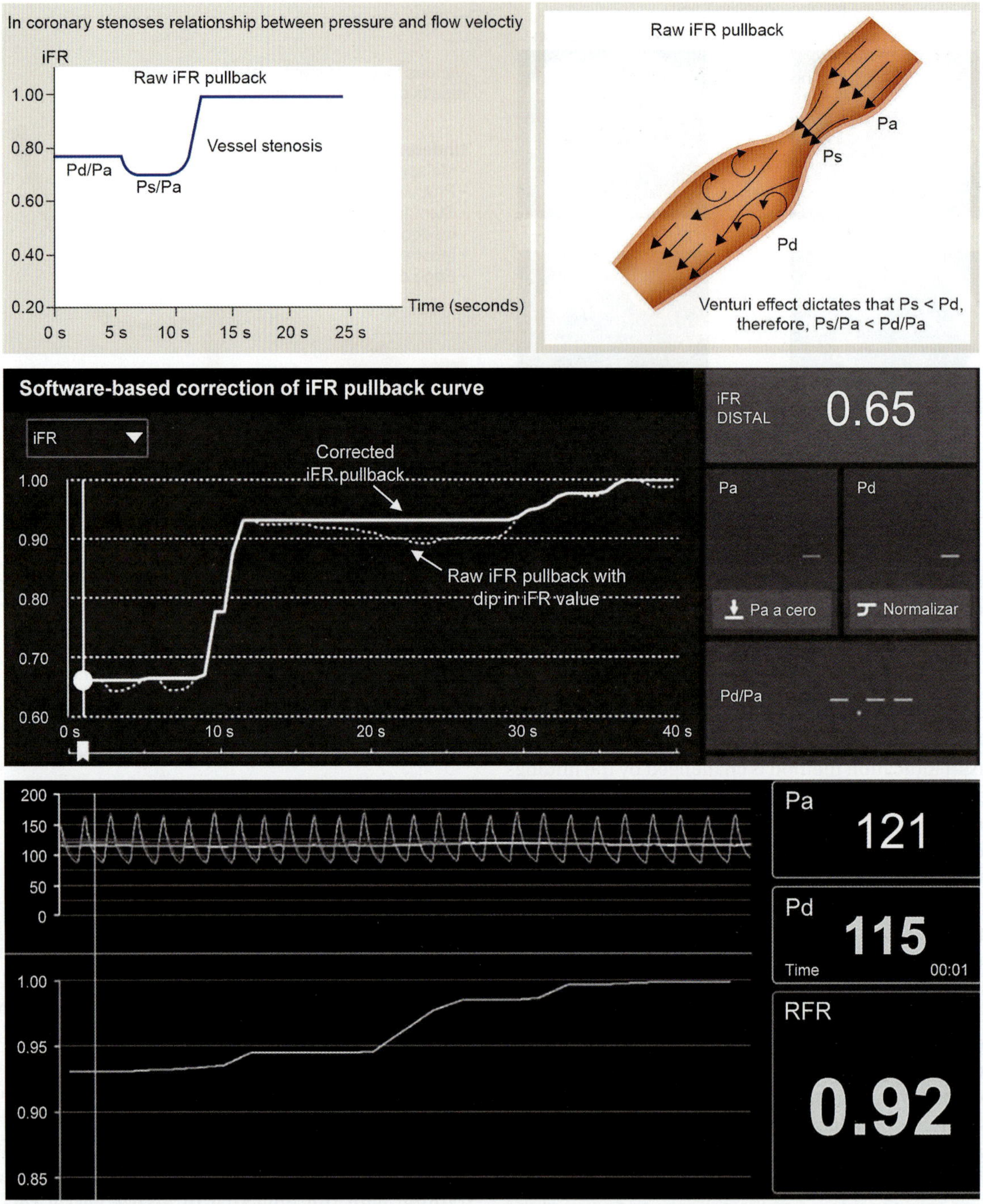

FIG. 6: Suboptimal post-PCI physiological results mechanisms.
(iFR: instantaneous wave-free ratio; PCI: percutaneous coronary intervention)

no specific clinical guidelines recommended for the routine use of post-PCI FFR assessment. Recently, iFR, a resting physiological index a marked correlation was seen with noninvasive ischemia testing which is also quite noninferior to FFR in guiding revascularization decisions in patients as demonstrated by the findings of two large randomized clinical trials. However, the causes and occurrence of abnormal iFR after PCI is not known. To assess the causes and occurrence of an abnormal iFR after performing PCI successfully in patients, DEFINE PCI, a prospective, observational study was conducted in 562 vessels in 500 patients. Findings of the study suggested that instead of the operator assessing successfully angiographic results after coronary stenting, residual ischemia was evaluated in one out of four patients

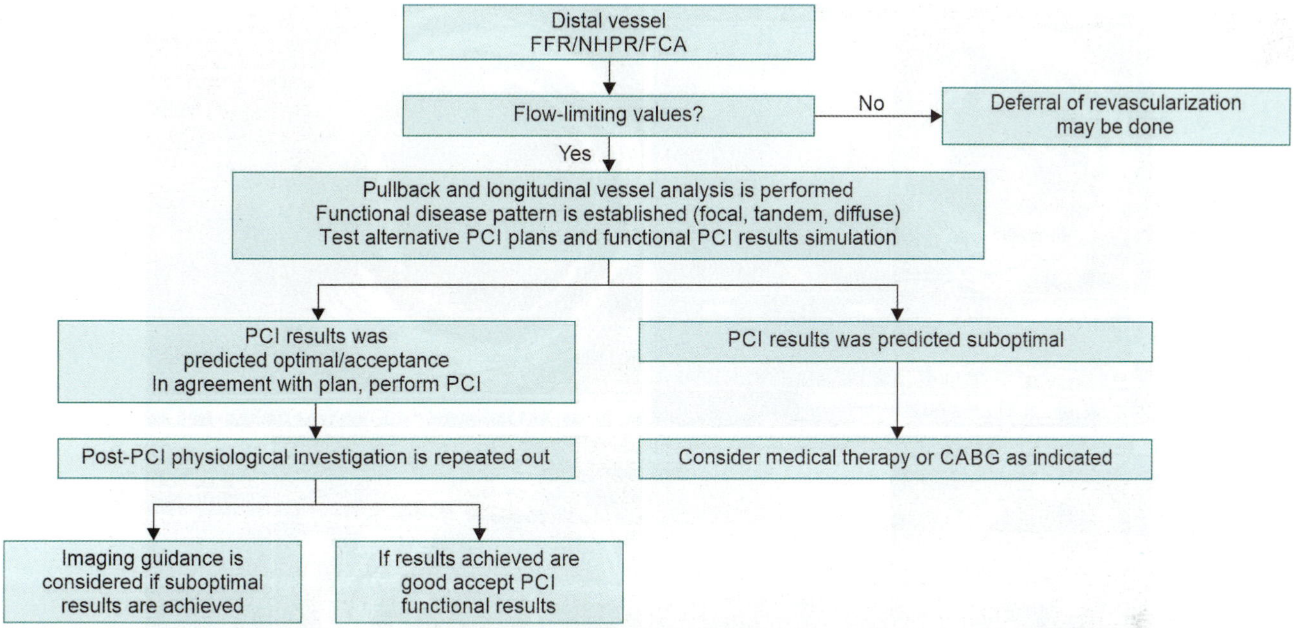

FLOWCHART 1: Poststenting malapposition detected by IVUS and correction thereof.

(CABG: coronary artery bypass grafting; FCA: functional coronary angiography; FFR: fractional flow reserve; IVUS: intravascular ultrasound; NHPR: nonhyperemic pressure ratio; PCI: percutaneous coronary intervention)

by blinded post-PCI physiological assessment.[32] Inapparent focal lesions were observed as the potential reason behind the maximum cases of residual ischemia. It also proposed algorithm for using the post-PCI and pre-PCI physiology for assessment of lesion in a comprehensive manner **(Fig. 7)**. Further, various findings demonstrated in comparison to the non-left anterior descending artery (LAD) vessels, FFR values post-PCI is quite less in LAD, considering that it might require vessel-specific optimization. Various factors such as intramuscular coronary tracts higher incidence seen in the lead might be the reason behind the lower LAD value.

INSTANTANEOUS WAVE-FREE RATIO WITH VIRTUAL STENTING

In most of the catheterization laboratories, an FFR-based intervention strategy has been developed as a physiological standard to guide PCI. However, evaluation of FFR is associated with huge challenges in serial coronary lesions present with multiple stenoses. Considering this, by using the angiographic reconstruction and fluid dynamics algorithms, an angiographically derived FFR parameter, quantitative flow ratio (QFR) has been developed. Pressure wire and hyperemic induction is not required in the QFR assessment. Side branch's automatic detection is facilitated by recently upgraded QFR analysis software which could potentiate reference vessel reconstruction by using a step-down reference diameter function.

With the objective to assess the murray law-based quantitative flow ratio derived virtual stenting techniques assessment potential in guiding the decision of intervention in patients present with serial coronary lesions, a study was planned in 54 patients by using FFR as the reference standard. Results of the study demonstrated that murray law-based quantitative flow ratio derived virtual stenting technique can assess the primary flow limiting lesions for revascularization in vessels with serial coronary lesions.[33] **Figure 8** shows how virtual stenting can depict poststenting results.

FRACTIONAL FLOW RESERVE VERSUS ANGIOGRAPHY FOR MULTIVESSEL CORONARY ARTERY DISEASE EVALUATION

In the patients present with the multivessel CAD, coronary artery bypass graft surgery is recommended for the treatment by the guidelines. Furthermore, better clinical outcomes are also produced by PCI of ischemia-causing lesions; however, it is difficult to assess the exact lesion causing ischemia in patients present with multiple stenoses. Considering this, in the patients present with the multivessel disease, to assess the FFR-guided PCI clinical outcomes, FAME trial was conducted in which 1,005 patients were enrolled. 496 patients were randomized to angiography-guided PCI and 509 to FFR-guided PCI. At the follow-up of 5 years, quality of life, cost-effectiveness, and individual adverse events were considered

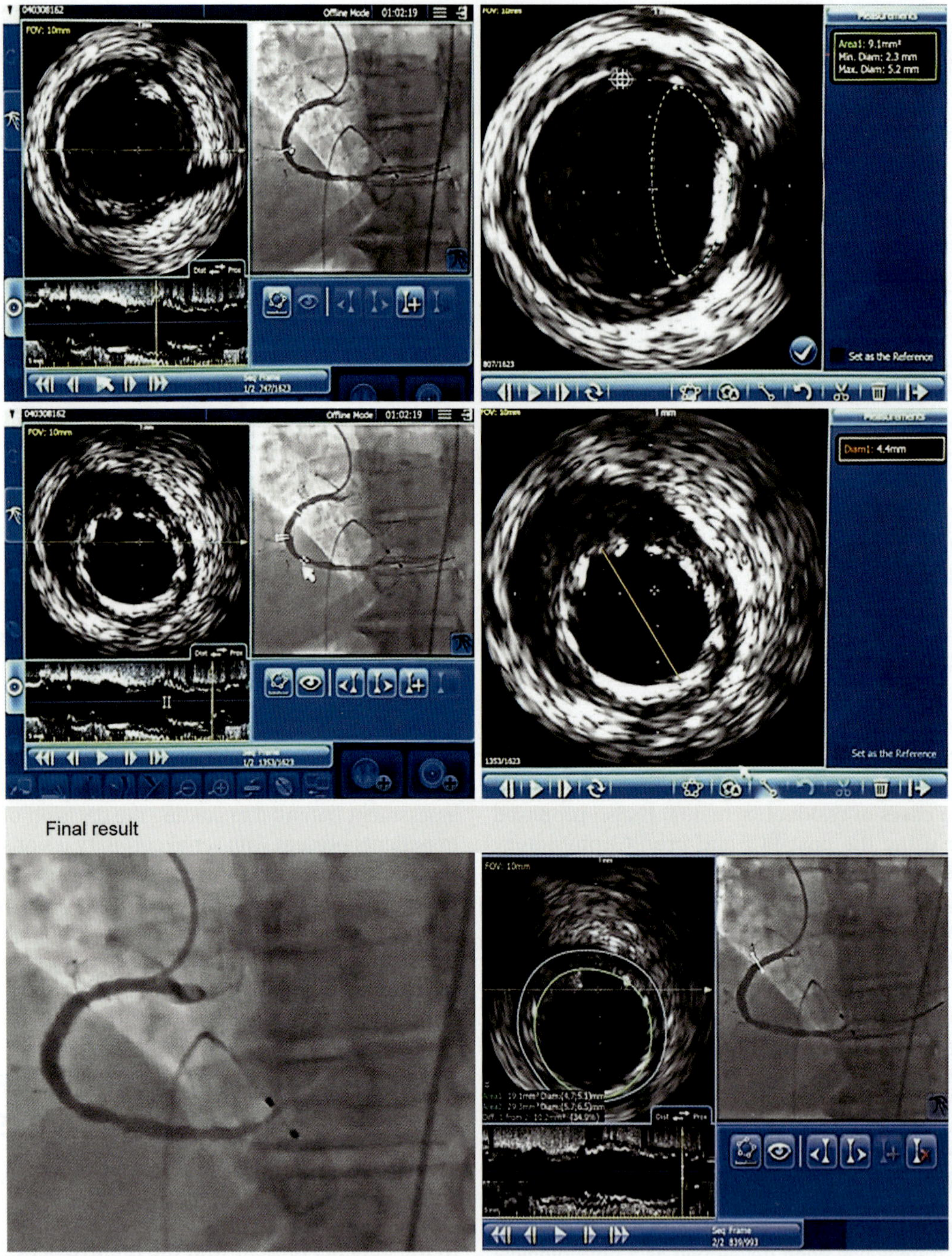

FIG. 7: Pre-percutaneous coronary intervention (PCI) physiology planning and assessment proposed algorithm based on physiological interrogation.

as the secondary endpoint of the study. Results of the study demonstrated that in comparison to the angiography-guided PCI, a lower incidence of MACE was reported in the FFR-guided PCI patients' group, with a marked reduction in procedure time, reduced cost and utilization of resource.[34] More clinical trials are further required to consider the clinical use of FFR in patients undergoing multivessel PCI on a routine basis.

LEFT MAIN CORONARY ARTERY DISEASE ASSESSMENT BY FFR AND IFR

Coronary angiography used for the investigation of LMCA is associated with various limitations. Considering this, for the precise assessment of left main (LM) disease, IVUS and FFR methods have been established as an adjunctive diagnostic method. Furthermore, iFR have also been established

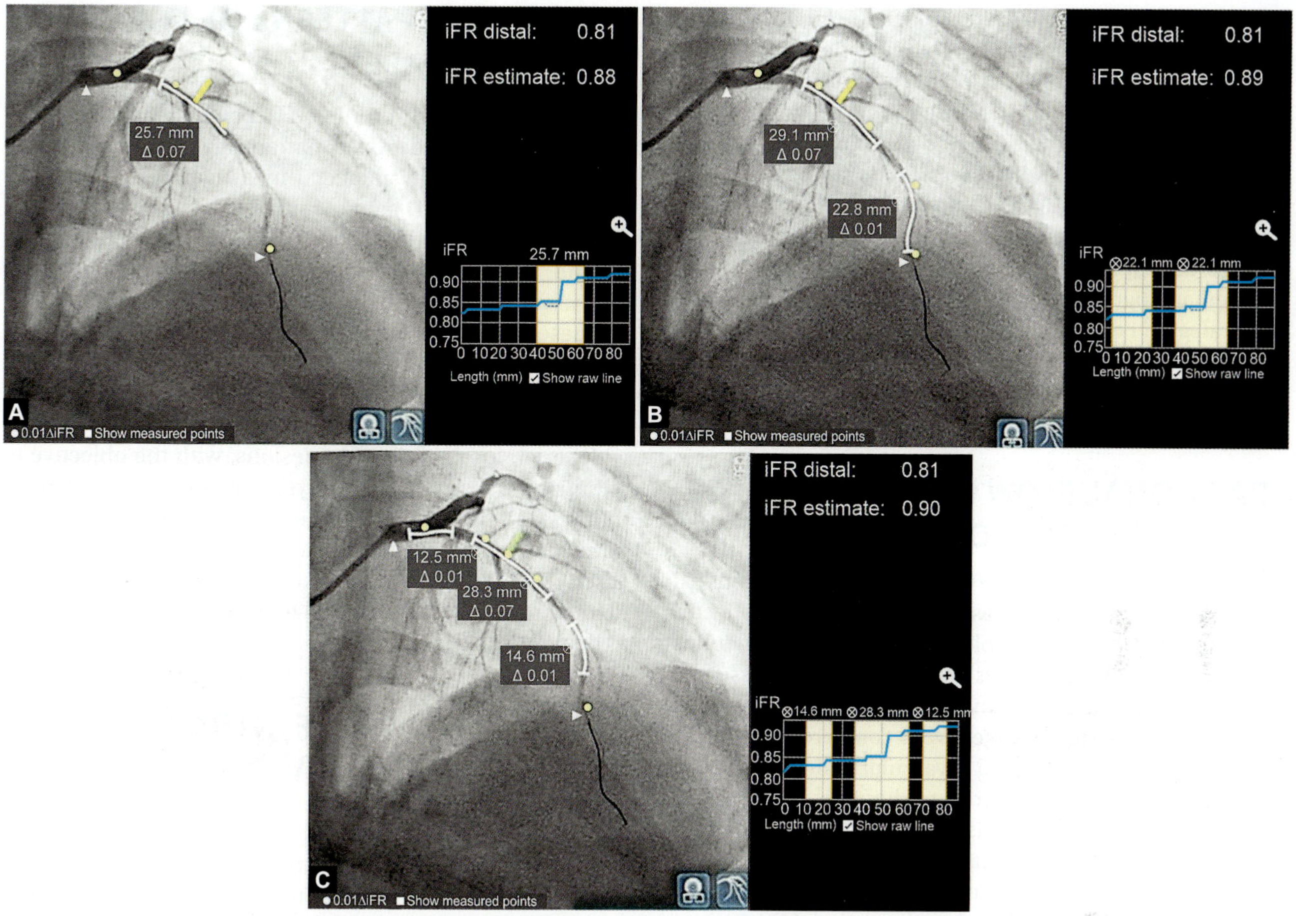

FIGS. 8A TO C: Virtual stenting showing presumable results after stenting. (A) Virtual stenting in proximal LAD showing estimated iFR of 0.88. (B) Virtual stenting in proximal and distal LAD showing estimated iFR of 0.89. (C) Virtual stenting in Ostial LED, proximal LAD and distal LAD showing estimated iFR of 0.90, which is the ideal result.

with the objective to simplify the functional assessment of coronary arteries. However, the iFR use for the assessment of LMCA has not been well explored. Considering this, with the objective to clarify that if iFR can be used to reach out a decision, various clinical studies were conducted.[35,36] In the patients present with LMCA stenosis, for the assessment of long-term clinical outcomes, multicenter observational study was conducted in 314 patients. In this study, iFR was used to reach a decision about the treatment strategy. All-cause death, ischemia-driven target revascularization, and nonfatal MI were considered as the major primary endpoint of the study. Findings of study proposed that use of iFR for the revascularization deferral of LM stenosis was appear to be quite safer method; with presence of similar long-term clinical outcomes in comparison to patients in iFR value was used to perform LM revascularization.[37] Furthermore, another retrospective, observational, and multicenter study was conducted in 125 presents with angiographically intermediated LMCA. In the evaluation of intermediate LMCD, findings of current study demonstrate the use of iFR. Other than this, correlation of IVUS MLA < 6 mm^2 with iFR of ≤0.89 was seen.[38] Considering the positive findings in both studies, it is concluded that iFR measurements is quite promising method for the assessment of severity of LMCA stenosis.

FRACTIONAL FLOW RESERVE VERSUS ANGIOGRAPHY IN THE SETTING OF ACUTE MYOCARDIAL INFARCTION

In the patients present with acute ST-segment elevation, infarct-related coronary artery PCI can be used for the effective management of MI. Further, ischemia-producing lesions are identified in an accurate manner by FFR.[39] Identification of functional assessment of nonculprit lesions in patients present with STEMI is the major clinical application associated with use of FFR. In addition to this, in comparison to the angiography-guided PCI or conservative treatment, serious adverse events risk was less in FFR-guided PCI patients present with stable CAD.

Considering this, with the objective to compare the clinical outcomes of FFR-guided PCI decision versus angiography-guided PCI in patients present with multivessel disease and STEMI, randomized, multicenter, and open-label FLOWER-MI (Flow Evaluation to Guide Revascularization in Multivessel ST-Elevation Myocardial Infarction) clinical trial was conducted. At the follow-up of 1 year, no marked difference was seen in various parameters such as urgent revascularization, death, and MI risk in between angiography-guided PCI strategy and FFR-guided PCI strategy.[22] Furthermore, two other clinical studies FAME and FAMOUS-STEMI also suggested that no strong evidence is present to demonstrate that clinical outcomes in patients present with ACS are improved by FFR-based guidance.

FRACTIONAL FLOW RESERVE IN ACUTE CORONARY SYNDROME

Functional significance of intermediate coronary lesions can be determined by using FFR as the well-established effective technique. Use of FFR in stable CAD is supported by robust data, however, in the ACS, its use is not properly assessed. Considering this, a pooled analysis of the seven published studies was done with the objective to compare FFR used for prognosis of lesions deferred revascularization in patients present with ACS in compared to the non-ACS patients. Findings of pooled analysis demonstrates no marked difference in various parameters such as target vessel revascularization (TVR) and cardiovascular disease (CVD) mortality in between non-ACS patients and ACS patients after revascularization deferral was done by using FFR. In stable patients, FFR prognostic value in patients present with ACS is not good. Furthermore, low risk of mortality, CV mortality and TVR, and huge risk of MI were reported in ACS patients.[40]

MACHINE LEARNING

The association between morphological features of plaque, myocardial ischemia, and luminal stenosis, and their collective influence on clinical outcomes has not been explored in clinical studies. With the objective to predict the association of plaque features and stenosis with myocardial ischemia and their association with myocardial ischemia investigated by FFR, patients present with suspected CAD were enrolled in the study. Machine learning was used to study the relevant anatomical features associated with low value of FFR. In the findings of the study, six clusters for low FFR were investigated by machine learning interrogation and most relevant features identified from each cluster was plaque volume, necrotic core volume, percent atheroma volume, necrotic core and fibrofatty volume, remodeling index, and proximal LAD coronary artery lesion. Presence of myocardial ischemia is defined by these clusters which are also associated with marked prognostication in patients present with CAD.[41]

FUNCTIONAL PATTERNS OF CORONARY ARTERY DISEASE

Pattern and distribution of CAD, including serial lesions, diffuse disease, and mixed pattern significant effect the coronary lesions physiological investigation. In everyday clinical practice, CAD patterns such as mixed patterns, serial lesions, and diffuse disease are commonly seen and require careful investigation. Angiography-derived physiology indexes and pressure wire accuracy is strongly influenced by these major CAD patterns. Considering this, relevant information about the therapeutic management of CAD and procedural planning of PCI is provided by investigation of disease physiological pattern. In the patients present with serial, focal, and diffuse lesions, with the objective to optimize the use of coronary physiology angiography-derived indexes and pressure wire indexes, a practical algorithm is developed with the use of intracoronary imaging in specific cases.[42] Focal, pattern, and tandem patterns of CAD can be defined by using criteria based on physiological assessment as demonstrated in **Table 3**.

COREGISTRATION OF INTRAVASCULAR IMAGING METHODS WITH ANGIOGRAPHY

Interventional X-ray imaging methods such as fluoroscopy and angiography are majorly used for the investigation of lumen of coronary arteries while, on the other hand, IVUS demonstrates marked intravascular information of stent expansion and composition of vessel wall. Considering the fact that these two diagnostic methods are quite complementary to each other, with the aim to acquire coronary arteries comprehensive pictures, these two imaging modalities can be coregistered. Various clinical studies have demonstrated the efficiency of coregistration of angiography and IVUS. A novel image-based device-tracking solution in which additional software such as electromagnetic sensors is not required has been developed initially for the coregistration of angiography and IVUS in an efficient manner. In a reference angiography image, coronary branch is majorly detected by this system. Both electrocardiogram (ECG)-triggered fluoroscopy and IVUS images are acquired by this system during the IVUS transducers pullback by which it automatically track medical devices positioning in fluoroscopy. Convenient integration of this image-based solution can be done into existing cardiology workflow. Furthermore, with the objective to exchange and communicate information for coregistration of IVUS/OCT and angiography, two commercially available software packages were modified. This newly developed method is based upon catheter path angiographic reconstruction which does not need landmark identification of operator to developed image synchronization.[43]

TABLE 3: Criteria used to characterize the various patterns of obstructive coronary disease such as focal, tandem, and diffuse patterns.

Pre-PCI physiology measurements			
Pattern	**FFR**	**NHPR**	**FCA**
Focal	Abrupt the pressure loss single point, if FFR is ≤0.80 at the distal segment	Over ≤15 mm segment, abrupt single point of ≥0.03 index units if iFR/RFR/DFR is measured ≤0.89 at distal segment	In <10 mm segments pressure loss single region of >0.05 with QFR/vFFR/FFRCT measured is ≤0.80 at distal segment
Tandem	FFR ≤0.80 at distal segment, presence of ≥2 abrupt change of FFR values.		
Post-PCI physiology measurements			
Pattern	**FFR**	**NHPR**	**FCA**
Focal	At the stented site or at certain other site within the treated vessel, loss of FFR with abrupt pressure	At the stented site or at certain other site within the treated vessel abrupt loss of iFR/RFR/DFR values	At the stented site or at certain other site within the treated vessel abrupt loss of QFR/FFR values
Tandem	At the level of an untreated tandem stenosis, drop of FFR values abruptly	At the level of an untreated tandem stenosis, drop of iFR/RFR/DFR values abruptly	At the level of an untreated tandem stenosis, drop of QFR/FFR values abruptly
Diffuse	During pullback, over length of stented vessel loss in FFR values in progressive and linear manner	During pullback, over length of stented vessel loss in iFR/RFR/DFR values in progressive and linear manner	During pullback, over length of stented vessel loss in QFR/FFR values in progressive and linear manner

(DFR: diastolic hyperemia-free ratio; FCA: functional coronary angiography; FFR: fractional flow reserve; iFR: instantaneous wave-free ratio; NHPR: nonhyperemic pressure ratio; PCI: percutaneous coronary intervention; QFR: quantitative flow ratio; RFR: resting full-cycle ratio; vFFR: vessel fractional flow reserve)

COREGISTRATION WITH ANGIOGRAPHY

Coregistration of coronary angiogram with the longitudinal vessel physiology facilitates the flow-limiting atherosclerotic disease localization in an accurate manner and also helps in preprocedural planning. The coregistered map further also facilitates specific target lesions optimal localization and pressure loss regions clear distributions. In conjunction with iFR, this technology can be used specifically in forming strategies for therapeutic interventions on tandem lesions and diffuse disease.[44]

COREGISTRATION OF INSTANTANEOUS WAVE-FREE RATIO AND INTRAVASCULAR ULTRASOUND

Instantaneous wave-free ratio, a validated method used for CAD functional severity assessment, can be associated with certain drawbacks specifically during the matching of values of iFR with angiographic coronary lesions. Considering this, concept of iFR calculations coregistration with their anatomical location has been established, which is associated with marked potential to simplify the overall measurements and marked increase in accuracy. SyncVision Volcano system is introduced which provided both iFR and IVUS angiographic coregistration which demonstrates the functional compromise of each lesion. With the objective to assess the efficacy of iFR and SyncVision software to guide the decision regarding the use of PCI in long, diffuse coronary lesions, randomized, open label, and multicenter clinical trial was planned. In this clinical trial, angiography-guided revascularization was compared with SyncVision/iFR-guided revascularization in patients present with angiographic coronary lesions which are long, sequential, or diffused. Results of this clinical study are still pending.

TRI-REGISTRATION OF IMAGING, PHYSIOLOGY, AND ANGIOGRAPHY

Tri-registration joint facilitates the easy navigation between the three imaging modalities; angiography, physiological values, and IVUS images. In tri-registration, the roadmap for IVUS and physiology coregistrations should be the same which can be achieved by same zoom, table, and C-arm position for IVUS and physiology pullback.

FUTURE DIRECTIONS

- CAD patterns and distribution, such as diffuse disease, mixed patterns, focal lesions, and serial lesions, significantly impact physiological investigation of coronary lesions.
- The accuracy of angiography-derived physiology indexes and pressure wire measurements is influenced by CAD patterns.

- Assessing the physiological pattern of disease provides relevant information for CAD management and PCI procedural planning.
- A practical algorithm has been developed to optimize the clinical applicability of angiography-derived and pressure wire indexes in patients with serial, focal, and diffuse diseases.
- Recent advancements in coronary lesions physiology assessment include the introduction of physiology coregistration in the catheter laboratory.
- OCT-derived FFR (OFR) is an exciting coregistration tool that improves the assessment of thermodynamically significant lesions compared to using OCT alone.
- Another developing tool, "iFR and IVUS tri-registration" by Philips, enables the coregistration of IVUS and iFR pullback with the angiogram, providing precise measurements in cases like ostial LMCA in-stent re-stenosis where FFR investigation might be misleading.

CONCLUSION

Various diagnostic modalities real-time coregistration has emerged as the quite useful approach in coronary interventions. Specifically, diagnostic and therapeutic accuracy significantly increased by the combination of functional and imaging techniques. Exact assessment of focal pressure lost after PCI can be achieved by synergistic usage of intracoronary imaging and post-PCI longitudinal vessel pullback. In the era of precision PCI, intravascular imaging and physiology coregistration with the angiogram will be quite common and with the marked modifications in pressure wire technology, it will be quite easier for the clinicians to optimize their PCI outcomes by physiological assessment.

ACKNOWLEDGMENT

I thank Ms Nikita and Mr Rohit for assisting me to finalize the chapter. Figures are edited by Jiwan Singh.

ONLINE REFERENCES

Please scan the QR code provided at the end of the table of contents for References of this chapter.

CHAPTER 140

Comparison and Limitations of Invasive Fractional Flow Reserve with Resting Full-cycle Ratio and CT-derived Fractional Flow Reserve for Ischemia Detection

Arun Mohanty, Ashish Kumar Jain, Aman Makhija

ABSTRACT

Fractional flow reserve (FFR) is the current invasive gold standard for assessing the ischemic potential of an angiographically intermediate coronary stenosis. Other nonhyperemic indices to assess functional coronary stenosis, such as resting full-cycle ratio (RFR), instantaneous wave-free ratio (iFR), and noninvasive modality computed tomography-derived FFR (CT FFR), have been introduced. This chapter focuses on the utility of these physiological indices used for the assessment of coronary stenosis and pitfalls.

Keywords: FFR, iFR, RFR, CT FFR, adenosine.

INTRODUCTION

Coronary angiography has become the standard method of evaluation of the extent and severity of coronary artery disease (CAD), with significant interobserver variability. Intracoronary physiological assessment is a strategy to identify the presence of flow-limiting epicardial stenosis in patients with CAD to determine an indication for revascularization. Fractional flow reserve (FFR) is a pressure-derived estimate of coronary flow impairment and one of the most established invasive physiological tests. Recently, resting coronary pressure indices, such as instantaneous wave-free ratio (iFR), resting full-cycle ratio (RFR), and computed tomography-derived FFR (CT FFR), have been shown to have comparable diagnostic performance to FFR. This chapter addresses the use of coronary physiology to plan and guide percutaneous coronary intervention (PCI) using physiological tools, providing evidence from the literature and expert opinion from operators.

FRACTIONAL FLOW RESERVE

Fractional flow reserve is defined as the ratio of the pressure distal to a stenosis (P_d) relative to the pressure proximal to the stenosis (P_a) during hyperemia induced by a vasodilating agent. During maximal hyperemia, coronary resistance is at its lowest and remains constant. In this condition, coronary blood flow is pressure-dependent (Ohm's law).[1]

Requirement of Fractional Flow Reserve

When there is an intermediate stenosis (between 50 and 70%) of the coronary artery, coronary angiogram is not an exclusively reliable marker to determine revascularization. Coronary angiography produces two-dimensional luminograms; it does not give an idea about the characteristic or physiological significance of an intermediate coronary artery stenosis.[2]

Fractional flow reserve is calculated at maximal hyperemia; because of this, it is independent of heart rate, blood pressure, and other hemodynamic parameters.[3] Various agents have been studied for the induction of hyperemia; continuous intravenous (IV) infusion of adenosine (140 μg/kg/min) is the most commonly studied and used drug. Intracoronary bolus injection of adenosine [40 μg for right coronary artery (RCA) and 80 μg for left coronary artery (LCA)] provides equivalent diagnostic accuracy compared to IV administration.[4] Other drugs that are used in clinical practice are regadenoson, intracoronary nicorandil (2 mg), and papaverine (8 mg for RCA and 12 mg for LCA). Administration of intracoronary nitroglycerine (100–200 μg) is recommended before doing FFR to reduce vascular resistance. Flushing of contrast in the coronary should be done while measurement, as it will influence the P_d and FFR value. Based on studies, an FFR cutoff value of 0.75 was considered significant that means distal coronary pressure was reduced by 25% from the normal value. The range between 0.75 and 0.80 is considered a gray zone; however, in this range, major adverse cardiovascular event (MACE) rates are higher without revascularization. The cutoff value was increased to 0.80 later on to increase the sensitivity of FFR.[5]

Trial-based Evidence of Invasive Fractional Flow Reserve (Table 1)

Based on these studies, the American Heart Association (AHA) and the European Society of Cardiology (ESC) have recommended the use of invasive FFR in patients with angina or anginal equivalent symptoms, undocumented ischemia, and angiographically intermediate stenosis to guide the decision to proceed with PCI (class 1A).[12]

POST PERCUTANEOUS CORONARY INTERVENTION FRACTIONAL FLOW RESERVE

Post PCI, despite high residual gradients, angiographic results may look adequate. The FFR SEARCH (Fractional Flow Reserve–Stent Evaluated at Rotterdam Cardiology Hospital) registry showed that 56% of patients treated in routine practice had ≥1 lesion with post PCI FFR ≤ 0.90.[13] A meta-analysis by Johnson et al. revealed an inverse continuous relationship with post-PCI FFR and subsequent events.[14] The optimal cutoff for post-PCI FFR with regard to cardiovascular events is ≥0.90.

Fractional Flow Reserve and Intravascular Ultrasound Relationship

The "FIRST STUDY" showed that a minimum lumen area (MLA) on intravascular ultrasound (IVUS) < 3.07 mm^2 (64.0% sensitivity, 64.9% specificity) was the best threshold value for identifying FFR < 0.80. FFR correlated with plaque burden but not with other plaque morphology. An MLA < 2.4 mm^2 was best for reference vessel diameters < 3.0 mm, an MLA <2.7 mm^2 for reference vessel diameters of 3.0–3.5 mm, and an MLA < 3.6 mm^2 for reference vessel diameters > 3.5 mm.[15]

Limitations of Invasive Fractional Flow Reserve

Fractional flow reserve can assess only the functional significance of a stenosis and cannot assess limitations in myocardial perfusion that arise due to abnormal microcirculatory flow reserve in coronary resistance vessel. FFR measurements are dependent on achieving maximal pharmacologic vasodilation (underestimating stenosis

TABLE 1: Trial-based evidence of invasive fractional flow reserve (FFR).

Study name	Year and number of patients	Trial design	Clinical setting	Cutoff	Outcome
DEFER[6]	2001 325	Prospective randomized	• Stable CAD, intermediate lesion without objective ischemia • PCI versus FFR-guided referral	<0.75	No additional survival benefit in stenting nonischemic lesions
FAME[7]	2009 1,005	Prospective randomized	• Multivessel CAD • Angiography versus FFR-guided PCI	≤0.80	FFR-guided PCI reduces MACE at 1 year
FAME 2[8]	2012 1,220	Prospective randomized	Stable CAD hemodynamically significant stenosis FFR-guided PCI + OMT versus OMT	≤0.80	Significant reduction in the rate of urgent revascularization. In FFR-negative lesions, OMT has a good outcome
DANAMAI-3 PRIMULTI[9]	2015 627	Prospective randomized	• STEMI and multivessel CAD patients who had undergone primary PCI of an infarct-related artery • Further invasive treatment versus FFR-guided revascularization	≤0.80	FFR-guided complete revascularization decreases the risk of future events (less repeat revascularization)
Compare-acute[10]	2017 885	Prospective randomized	STEMI and multivessel CAD patients who had undergone primary PCI of infarct-related artery, FFR-guided revascularization versus no revascularization	≤0.80	FFR-guided complete revascularization decreases MACE
IRIS-FFR[11]	2017	Prospective registry	Patients with at least one coronary lesion	≤0.75	FFR ≤ 0.75, significant reduction in MACE for revascularized lesions than deferred lesions

(CAD: coronary artery disease; MACE: major adverse cardiovascular events; OMT: optimal medical therapy; PCI: percutaneous coronary intervention; STEMI: ST-segment elevation myocardial infarction)

severity if vasodilation is submaximal at the time of measurement). In addition, ignoring the backpressure to coronary flow by assuming that it is equal to zero and ignoring curvilinearity of the pressure–flow relation lead to underestimation of the FFR. This is particularly problematic at low coronary pressures and in determining the functional significance of coronary collaterals, where venous pressure needs to be considered. Inserting the pressure wire across a severe stenosis can lead to overestimation of stenosis severity in the presence of diffuse disease or small branch vessels. Both the DANAMI-3 PRIMULTI and COMPARE ACUTE trials demonstrated the applicability and general safety of FFR to guide complete revascularization in ST-elevation myocardial infarction (STEMI). However, due to the lack of a physiological comparator arm, the full potential of coronary physiology applied to acute coronary syndrome (ACS) cannot be elucidated from these data. In contrast to stable angina, ACS can unpredictably upset the microvascular milieu by a variety of mechanisms, including intramyocardial hemorrhage and microvascular obstruction. These factors have been demonstrated to limit the attainment of "maximal" hyperemia. In such situations, the true hemodynamic significance of a stenosis may be underestimated by FFR. Administration of adenosine for hyperemia is associated with side effects such as atrioventricular (AV) block, flushing, chest pain, and breathlessness.[16]

RESTING FULL-CYCLE RATIO

Resting full-cycle ratio is a nonhyperemic pressure ratio used to determine the physiologic significance of intermediate coronary stenosis. RFR can be calculated by determining the lowest instantaneous P_d/P_a ratio in the entire cardiac cycle length. A minimum of five consecutive heart cycles are required to calculate RFR. A major advantage of RFR over iFR is that RFR does not require the identification of a specific landmark or the selection of a specific time point during diastole. By calculating the minimum P_d/P_a over the entire cardiac cycle, RFR calculates the maximum pressure gradient across the stenosis during resting status. The cutoff value of RFR is 0.89. When RFR ≤ 0.89, coronary revascularization may be beneficial. When RFR > 0.89, deferral of revascularization should be considered.

Resting full-cycle ratio has been studied in over 3,500 lesions and 2,500 patients, showing clinical accuracy and outcomes **(Table 2)**.

TABLE 2: Clinical accuracy and outcome studies of RFR.

Study	Study type	Lesion	Patients
ILUMIEN I + PREDICT[17]	Clinical accuracy	313	299
VALIDATE RFR[18]	Clinical accuracy	672	504
RE-VALIDATE RFR[19]	Diagnostic equivalence	501	431
IRIS FFR[11]	Outcome	1,102	926
3V FFR FRIENDS[20]	Outcome	1,024	435

Comparison between Resting Full-cycle Ratio and Invasive Fractional Flow Reserve in Intermediate Coronary Artery Stenosis

Resting full-cycle ratio is free of side effects of hyperemic agents, and it is comparable to FFR in the assessment of physiologic significance of intermediate coronary stenosis. A study by Wienemann et al.[17] compared RFR with FFR in a real-world cohort. It included 617 patients with stable angina having 712 coronary lesions with intermediate stenosis. In this study, RFR showed a significant correlation with FFR ($r = 0.766$; $p < 0.01$). Diagnostic accuracy, sensitivity, specificity, positive predictive value, and negative predictive value of RFR were 78% (95% confidence interval = 75; 81), 72% (65; 78), 81% (77; 84), 63% (57; 69), and 86% (83; 89), respectively. A study also determined certain predictors affecting concordance and discordance between RFR and FFR. Relevant predictors for discordance of RFR ≤ 0.89/FFR > 0.8 were left anterior descending artery (LAD) lesions, peripheral artery disease, female gender, and diffuse stenoses. Predictors for discordance of RFR > 0.89/FFR ≤ 0.8 were nonleft circumflex artery (LCX) lesions, percent diameter stenosis, and previous PCI in the target vessel. The overall discordance was around 20% between RFR and FFR.[17] The RECOPA study also showed significant correlation between FFR and RFR in evaluating physiologic significance of intermediate coronary artery stenosis, with 79% agreement between RFR ≤ 0.89 and FFR ≤ 0.80.[21]

Limitations of Resting Full-cycle Ratio

Resting full-cycle ratio has smaller gradients, making it more sensitive to noise, hydrostatic effect, and wire drift during pullback. It could be more sensitive to variations in hemodynamic conditions, such as heart rate and systolic blood pressure (SBP) as these parameters can affect basal coronary flow.[22]

CT-derived Fractional Flow Reserve

Computed tomography-derived FFR is a physiological simulation method. It is based on computational fluid dynamics principle. It uses routine computed tomography coronary angiography (CTCA) to model coronary flow, pressure, and resistance mathematically. During CT FFR, a patient-specific three-dimensional anatomic model is obtained, followed by the development of a patient-specific physiologic model depending on inflow–outflow hemodynamic conditions, resting or hyperemic myocardial blood flow, and microvascular resistance **(Fig. 1)**.[23]

Utilization of CT-derived Fractional Flow Reserve in Stable Ischemic Heart Disease

The PLATFORM study included patients with new-onset chest pain and randomized patients to usual invasive coronary angiography versus CT FFR-guided coronary angiography.

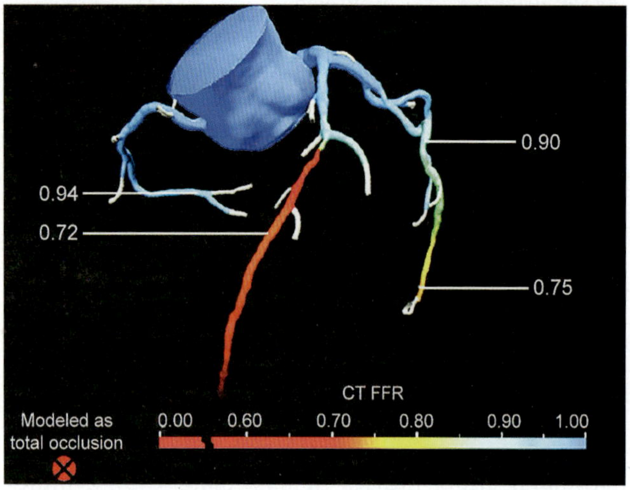

FIG. 1: CT-derived fractional flow reserve (CT FFR) results.

Patients in whom revascularization was deferred based on an fractional flow reserve computed tomography (FFRCT) > 0.80 showed no significant difference in cardiovascular mortality, myocardial infarction, or urgent revascularization **(Flowchart 1)**.[24]

Comparison between CT-derived Fractional Flow Reserve and Invasive Fractional Flow Reserve

A study by Röther et al. enrolled 71 patients with stable ischemic heart disease and calculated CT FFR and FFR in 91 vessels. For both CT FFR and FFR, a cutoff of ≤0.80 was used to indicate a hemodynamically significant stenosis. There was a very close correlation between CT FFR and FFR ($r = 0.85$; $p < 0.0001$) with mild systematic overestimation of FFR values in CT [mean difference 0.0049, 95% limits of agreement ±2 standard deviation (SD) –0.007 to 0.008]. Compared to invasive FFR, the sensitivity of CT FFR to detect hemodynamically significant lesions was 91% [19/21; 95% CI 70–99%], specificity was 96% (67/70; 95% CI 88–99%), positive predictive value was 86% (95% CI 65–97%), and negative predictive value was 97% (95% CI 90–100%).[25]

A meta-analysis of a total of 2,191 vessels in 1,294 patients revealed pooled sensitivity and specificity, with corresponding 95% CI at the per-patient level being 83% (79–87)

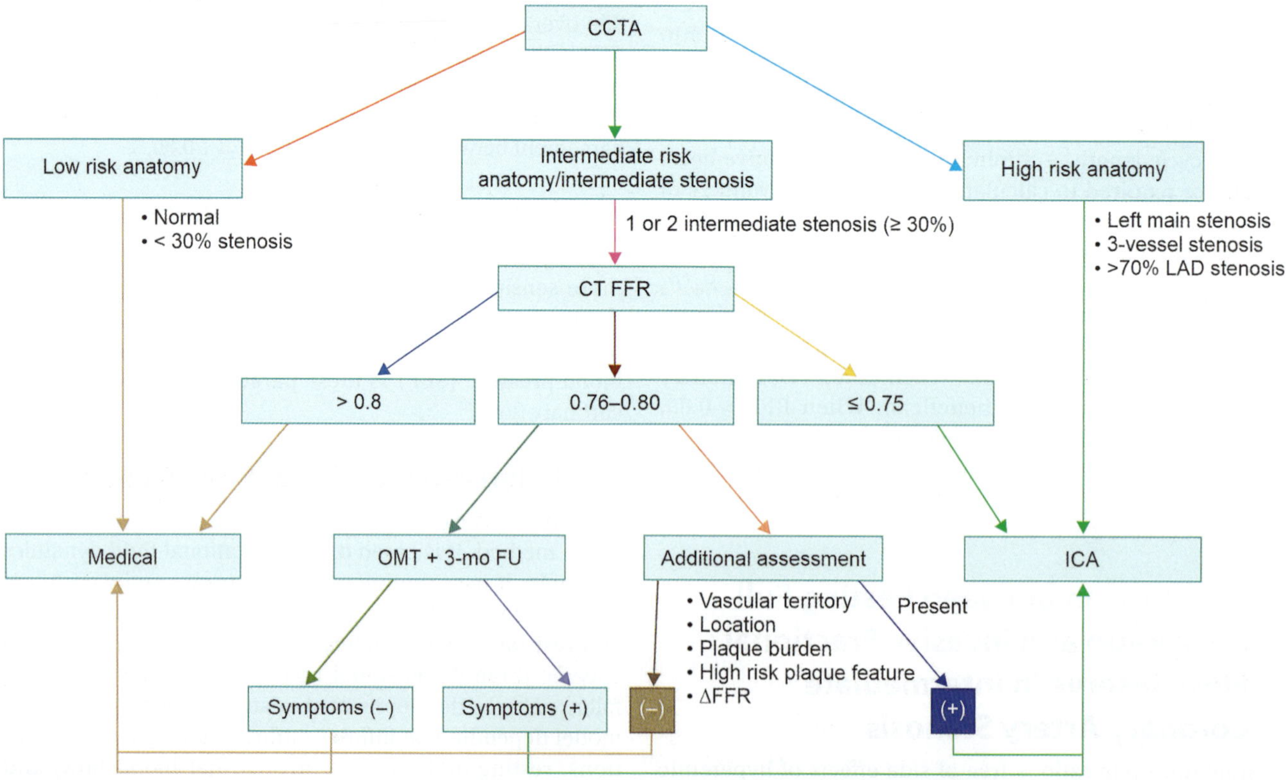

FLOWCHART 1: Utilization of CT-derived fractional flow reserve (CT FFR) in patients with stable ischemic heart disease.[23]
(CCTA: coronary computed tomography angiography; ICA: invasive coronary angiography; LAD: left anterior descending artery; OMT: optimal medical therapy)

and 72% (68–76), respectively. In this study, CT FFR had a good diagnostic performance in identifying functionally significant coronary artery stenosis when compared with invasive FFR.[26]

Computed tomography-derived FFR has low diagnostic cost when compared to invasive FFR. Moreover, invasive FFR is calculated within 2 cm distal to the stenosis, whereas CT FFR gives the FFR value of the whole coronary tree. Being a noninvasive test, it is free of the side effects of invasive coronary assessment, such as pain and bleeding.[23]

Limitations of CT-derived Fractional Flow Reserve

There are no sufficient randomized controlled trials utilizing CT FFR to guide coronary intervention in patients with stable coronary heart disease. CT FFR relies on accurate anatomic and physiologic modeling. Any factors affecting modeling, such as misalignment, metallic artifact, blooming, noise, suboptimal contrast, and motion artifact, may give false results. The specificity of CT FFR is decreased when sufficient nitroglycerine or beta-blockers are not used leading to suboptimal image quality.[23]

TABLE 3: Comparison of utility of FFR versus RFR in various clinical situations and angiographic lesions.[26]

	Nonhyperemic index	FFR
Uses of FFR		
Left main coronary artery	–	+++
Post-PCI side branch interrogation	–	+++
Post PCI assessment	–	+++
Equivalent assessment		
Multivessel disease	+++	+++
Diabetes	+++	+++
Uses of nonhyperemic index (RFR)		
Tandem lesions	+++	+
Diffuse lesions	+++	+
Acute coronary syndrome	+++	++

(FFR: fractional flow reserve; PCI: percutaneous coronary intervention; RFR: resting full-cycle ratio)

CONCLUSION

Invasive FFR is the gold standard in determining the physiologic significance of intermediate coronary artery stenosis in patients with stable ischemic heart disease. However, newer invasive physiologic indices such as RFR and noninvasive modalities such as CT FFR are comparable to invasive FFR in determining the physiological significance of intermediate coronary stenosis. More randomized data is required for CT FFR to increase its utility **(Table 3)**.

ONLINE REFERENCES

Please scan the QR code provided at the end of the table of contents for References of this chapter.

CHAPTER

141 Complex High-risk Transradial Interventions

Sanjay Kumar Chugh

ABSTRACT

Complex high-risk interventions also called complex high-risk indicated procedures (CHIP) are now frequently performed. Although the definition of CHIP is ambiguous and the procedural risk as well as risk of major adverse cardiovascular and cerebrovascular events (MACCE) may be higher, successful revascularization could mitigate angina and also concomitantly improve impaired left ventricular (LV) function, quality of life, and even survival in some. The seven patient-related complex high-risk or CHIP factors have been described as elderly aged ≥80 years, female gender, previous stroke, previous myocardial infarction (MI), peripheral vascular disease, poor LV function with left ventricular ejection fraction (LVEF) <30%, and chronic kidney disease (CKD); while the six procedural complex high-risks or CHIP factors described are needed for use of rotablation, percutaneous coronary intervention (PCI) for left main coronary artery (LMCA), three-vessel PCI; dual arterial access, as in chronic total occlusion (CTO) PCI; and hemodynamic compromise with poor LV function requiring mechanical circulatory support (MCS), and long coronary lesions >60 mm. With newer developments and miniaturization of hardware for PCI, complex high-risk procedures are being done successfully transradially with enhanced patient safety and lower risk of bleeding and vascular complications, which often translates into lower morbidity and mortality especially in the higher risk and acute cases. Data on transradial complex high-risk procedures along with interesting illustrative cases are presented. To conclude, successful transradial complex high-risk PCI is feasible. In view of current recommendations, a default radial-first approach is recommended over transfemoral access (TFA), for PCI in all patients, and should be adapted in the interest of patient safety and survival because of reduced risk of bleeding, vascular complications, and mortality especially in acute- and high-risk patients.

Keywords: Complex high-risk indicated procedures, complex high-risk transradial interventions, percutaneous coronary interventions, mechanical circulatory support, chronic total occlusion, bifurcation lesion, provisional stenting, 2-stent strategy, Medina classification, double kissing (DK) crush, Society for Thoracic Surgeons Cardiac Surgery Risk Models (STS) score, European System for Cardiac Operative Risk Evaluation II (EuroSCORE II), SYNTAX (SYNergy between PCI with TAXUS™ and Cardiac Surgery), simultaneous kissing stent (SKS), kissing balloon (KB), left main coronary artery disease, unprotected left main PCI.

INTRODUCTION

The definition of complex high-risk indicated procedures (CHIP) is still ambiguous and arbitrary. While SYNTAX score is used to assess the complexity of coronary artery disease; it is inadequate for assessing the risk of percutaneous coronary interventional procedures in patients. One group[1] identified seven patient-related and six procedure-related high-risk factors and referred to by them as CHIP factors. The seven patient-related complex high-risk or CHIP factors have been described as elderly aged ≥80 years, female gender, previous stroke, previous myocardial infarction (MI), peripheral vascular disease, poor LV function with left ventricular ejection fraction (LVEF) <30%, and chronic kidney disease (CKD). The six procedural complex high-risks or CHIP factors described are needed for use of rotablation, percutaneous coronary intervention (PCI) for left main coronary artery (LMCA), three-vessel PCI; dual arterial access, as in chronic total occlusion (CTO) PCI, to look for retrograde filling of distal stump; hemodynamic compromise with poor LV function or cardiogenic shock requiring LV mechanical support, and long coronary lesions with total lesion length exceeding 60 mm.[1]

The American Heart Association (AHA)/American College of Cardiology (ACC) Type B2 and C complex lesions are known to have a higher failure rate over 5 years compared to type A or B1 lesions.[2] The target lesion failure over 5 years follow-up increased from 6.8 and 9.9% for types A, B1 to 11.2%, and 13.7% for type B2 and C lesions, respectively. With CHIP score of zero, overall major adverse cardiovascular and cerebrovascular event (MACCE) in-hospital was 0.6 versus 1.2% if a CHIP factor was present ($p < 0.001$). An exponential increase in inhospital MACCE was observed with increasing CHIP factors.[1,3]

Nevertheless, data from the PROTECT II,[4] BCIS-1 (British Cardiovascular Intervention Society 1),[5] and the Roma-Verona Registry[6] uniequivocally found a significant increase in LVEF and a significant improvement in functional status after revascularization, thus supporting the practice of interventions in complex high-risk indicated cases.

SURGICAL TURNDOWN CHIP CASES

Current guidelines fail to provide clear recommendations for revascularization for patients found unsuitable for coronary artery bypass surgery; such patients, though symptomatic, are routinely excluded from clinical trials. Further, there is limited data on outcomes following CHIP-PCI in these surgical turndown patients. It is not clear if the benefits of PCI outweigh the risks in this group of high-risk surgical turndown patients which often have poor LV function, New York Heart Association (NYHA) class III–IV heart failure, left main (LM) stenosis, prior coronary artery bypass grafting (CABG), recent acute coronary syndrome (ACS), recent stroke, CKD with severe valvular disease, and life expectancy <5 years.

Successful revascularization could improve both survival and quality of life in the above category of high-risk patients, as was suggested by the OPTIMUM registry[7] (clinicaltrials.gov identifier: NCT02996877) which enrolled similar patients, mostly octogenarians, with multiple comorbidities; fragile patients with reduced mobility; and some with history of neoplastic disease and expected survival of less than a year.

MECHANICAL CIRCULATORY SUPPORT FOR COMPLEX HIGH-RISK INTERVENTIONS

Although guidelines support the use of mechanical circulatory support (MCS) during high-risk PCI,[8,9] the observed low rate of planned mechanical LV support use in large CHIP registries[2] probably is a consequence of increasing operator comfort in CHIP, with experience, a lack of supporting clinical data for their use, in addition to implications for cost, and last but not the least, concerns regarding the risks and complications associated with the devices themselves.

TRANSRADIAL COMPLEX HIGH-RISK INTERVENTIONS

Transradial PCI in CTO have been performed now for over two decades by the author in India, since his return from North America in 2002, when the author performed the country's first transradial rotablation at Escorts Heart Institute, New Delhi, and also has been doing PCI in CTOs, bifurcation lesions, and PCI in cardiogenic shock following acute MI, with intra-aortic balloon pump support since then. But it is only recently that the term CHIP transradial interventions (CHIP-TRI) has been coined for transradial complex high-risk interventions.

Radial CHIP Factors Adding to Complexity of Complex High-risk Interventions

The radial factors that add to the complexity and risk of a CHIP-TRI are small-diameter radial arteries (1.6 mm or smaller); radial artery to sheath mismatch and anatomical challenges such as a cubital loop, retroesophageal right subclavian artery; and type 3 bifurcation with high origin of radial artery which often has a narrowing at its origin allowing an angiography guidewire or a 4F catheter to pass but not allowing a 5F diagnostic or 5/6F guiding catheter to pass. So the question that naturally arises is why go radial and why add radial factors to the CHIP factors and increase difficulty? That is so because transradial access (TRA) is currently recommended over transfemoral access (TFA) as default, for PCI in all patients, by the European and American guidelines because of reduced risk of bleeding, vascular complications, and mortality especially in acute- and high-risk patients.[10,11]

In the MATRIX (Minimising Adverse Haemorrhagic Events by Transradial Access Site and Systemic Implementation of AngioX)/ACCESS study, in ACS, PCI complexity did not affect the comparative efficacy and safety of (TRA versus TFA; but compared with TFA, TRA was associated with lower access-site major [Bleeding Academic Research Consortium (BARC) 3–5] bleeding in both complex and noncomplex PCI. Interestingly, the reduction in major access-site bleeding (BARC 3–5) was greater with TRA in complex PCI; with an absolute risk reduction of (1.7%) as opposed to in noncomplex PCI.[12] In a study on octogenarians (mean age 81 years), *non-radial access* (RA) was reported to be a CHIP factor for 1 year MACCE,[13] with adjusted hazard ratio (HR) confidence interval (CI) 95% 0 of 1.57 (1.19–1,85), $p = 0.002$, along with the other CHIP factors as described above.[14]

"As happens to anything new and different, such as Werner Forssman's first cardiac catheterization in humans or Copernicus' theory about the sun being the center of the universe, transradial interventions too were opposed two decades ago, by those unwilling or unable to do radials."[15] "It needed guts to do radials in those days because it had to be better than a femoral; so the authors started sizing radials in all patients."[15] Using their sheath sizing protocol[16] **(Fig. 1)**, not only did the author perform *the country's first* transradial rotablation using 7F sheath and guiding catheter **(Figs. 2A to E)**, but they also performed the *country's first* 4 French TRI[15] and the *country's first slender 5 French CTO series*[17] **(Figs. 3A to D)**.

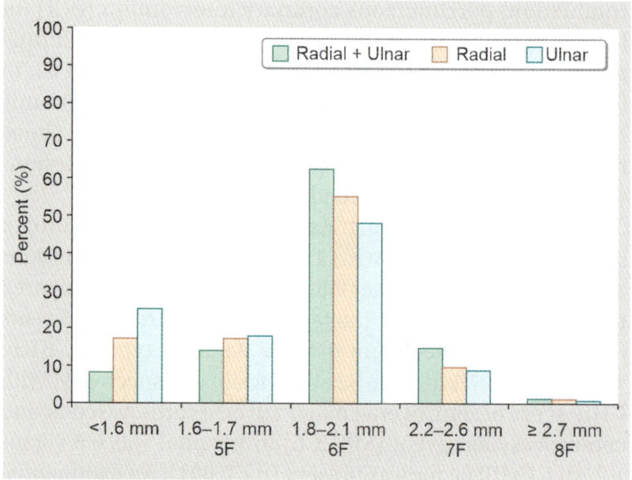

FIG. 1: Sheath sizing protocol.

Source: With permission from Chugh SK et al. (2013).[16]

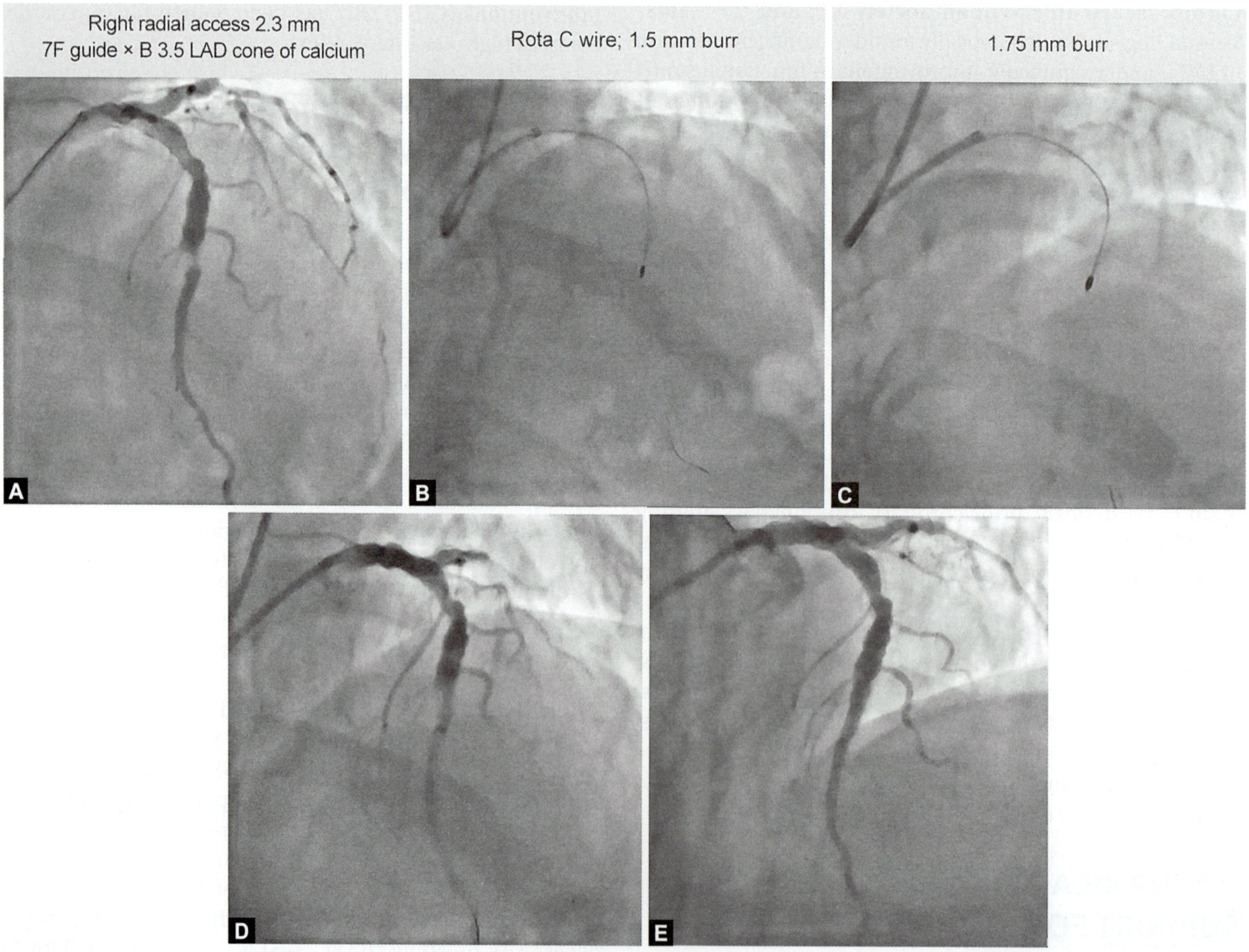

FIGS. 2A TO E: (A) Fibrocacific lesion with cone of calcium in left anterior descending (LAD) coronary artery; (B) 1.5 mm rotational atherectomy burr in use over a Rota C wire through a 7F × B 3.5 guide catheter through a 7F sheath in right radial artery (RRA); RRA diameter 2.3 mm; (C) a rotational atherectomy burr of 1.75 mm burr in use as 1.5 mm burr was unsuccessful in achieving desired plaque modification; (D) a Rotational atherectomy 4.0 × 15 mm stent being positioned in the lesion after successful predilatation with balloon; (E) final good result, thrombolysis in myocardial infarction (TIMI) 3 flow in LAD.

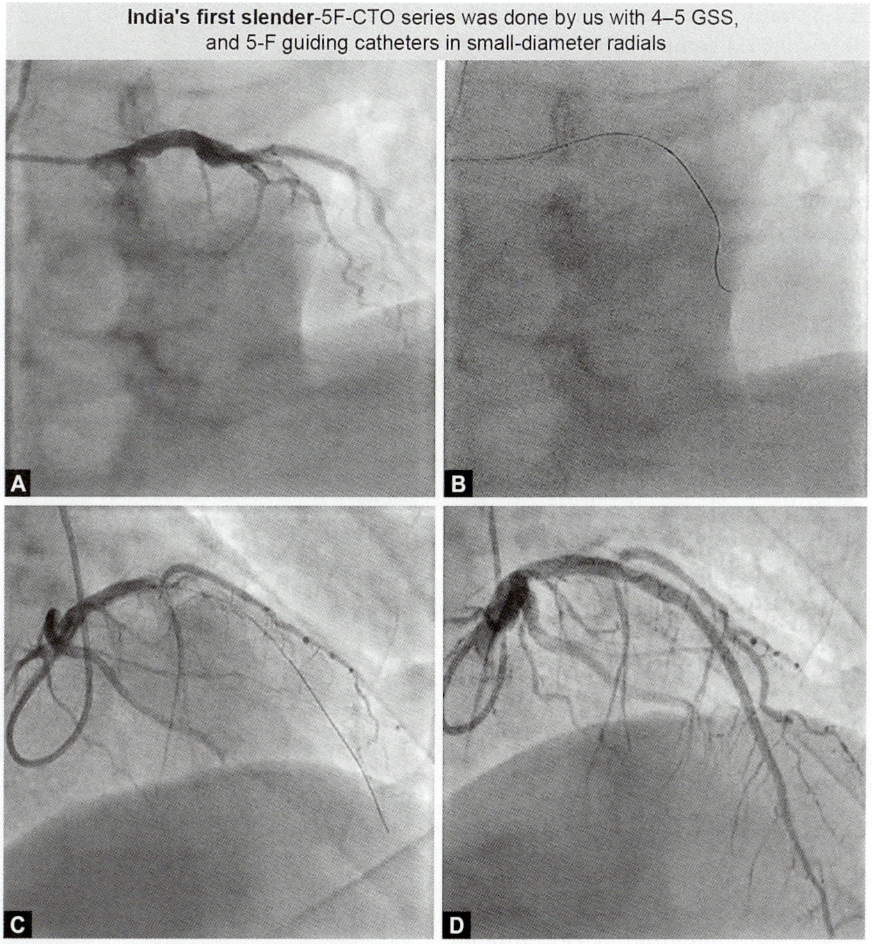

FIGS. 3A TO D: (A and B) Use of 5F JL 3.5 guide catheter used for successfully crossing a left anterior descending (LAD) chronic total occlusion (CTO) with wire, transradially using a 5F glide slender sheaths (GSS); (C and D) successful completion of LAD CTO percutaneous coronary intervention (PCI).

Technical Tips on Compatibility of Device and Techniques with Catheter Size and Wide-bore Access

- 5F is compatible with intravascular ultrasound (IVUS), microcatheter, balloon <5 mm, stent <4.5 mm, rotational atherectomy burr 1.25 mm; but not for kissing balloon (KB).
- 6F is compatible with all balloons, all stents, Tornus, all protection devices, rotational atherectomy burr 1.5 mm, cutting balloon and angiosculpt balloon; KB, one monorail balloon, with microcatheter or two microcatheters, anchor balloon.
- 7F is compatible with Angioguard protection device, rotational atherectomy burr ≥1.75 mm; kissing stents [two stents together as in simultaneous kissing stent (SKS)], IVUS with microcatheter.
- For 7F access, one can use either a 7F sheath; alternatively, if the radial artery diameter is <2.2 mm or palpably small, then options are to either use a 6–7 glide slender sheaths (GSS) or the sheathless Railway system from Cordis. Alternatively, one can choose a bigger alternate forearm access. The choice of femoral access adds a 3% risk of vascular and bleeding complications.[18]

Transradial Chronic Total Occlusion–Percutaneous Coronary Intervention

A recently published Multicenter PROGRESS CTO (Prospective Global Registry for the Study of Chronic Total Occlusion Intervention) registry found RA to be associated with a lower sheath size (6.6 ± 0.7 vs. 7.3 ± 0.8 $p < 0.0001$), lower number of post-CABG (18% vs. 35%, $p < 0.001$), and post-PCI cases (60% vs. 66% $p < 0.005$), lower J-CTO score

(2.1 ± 1.4 vs. 2.5 ± 1.3) and lower complication rate (2.3 ± 1.9 vs. 3.2 ± 1.9; $p < 0.001$) compared to TFA group. Further, retrograde techniques and antegrade dissection reentry (20% vs. 32%; $p < 0.001$) were less commonly used with RA versus TFA. The overall rates of technical success (89% vs. 86%; $p = 0.061$), procedural success (86% vs. 85%; $p = 0.528$), and inhospital major complications (2.47% vs. 3.40% vs. 2.18%; $p = 0.830$) were similar in both groups, whereas major bleeding was lower in the RA group (0.55% vs. 0.88%; $p = 0.013$).[19]

Transradial CTO-PCI is safer, with lower bleeding and vascular complications compared to TFA, when procedures are performed by experienced operators at high-volume specialized interventional cardiology centers. It behoves the operators to be facile with both TFA and TRA techniques as well as with the various techniques for CTO-PCI to achieve the best results; of course, physician preferences and experience also play an important role in achievement of successful outcomes and most operators prefer to combine TFA with TRA for CTO-PCI. TRA is restricted to 6F or 7F guide catheter, limiting the use of relatively bulky equipment or techniques requiring several devices simultaneously. Recent developments with miniaturization of equipment, availability of glide "slender sheaths" (GSS, Terumo, Japan), and sheathless Railway system (Cordis, USA) guide catheter extensions (Guideliners) that can enhance guide support, as well as a host of new revascularization strategies, have all made it increasingly possible to perform CTO-PCI via TRA with lower complication rates but comparable success rates compared to TFA; though the latter is often preferred with increased complexity of anatomy such as with high J-CTO scores, long occlusions, heavily calcified arteries.[20-22]

The author has successfully performed PCI for CHIP transradially, over the last two decades, including CTO-PCI. **Figures 4A to F** illustrate a successful CTO-PCI of proximal left circumflex (LCX) with J-CTO score of 3 and bridging collaterals via TRA using a 6F catheter, in a post-CABG patient, performed live by the author at Radial Live from Apollo Hospital, New Delhi in February 2008. This patient had a double bifurcation of LCX with two major obtuse marginal (OM) branches which were managed with provisional stenting strategy **(Figs. 4A to F)**.

J-CTO scoring is done as follows, with 1 score for each:

- Blunt entry stump
- Calcification
- Bend >45°
- Occlusion length >20 mm
- Previous failed attempt

The J-CTO score has been well correlated to successful wire crossing within 30 minutes with success rates of 88, 67, 42, and 10% with increasing J-CTO scores.[23]

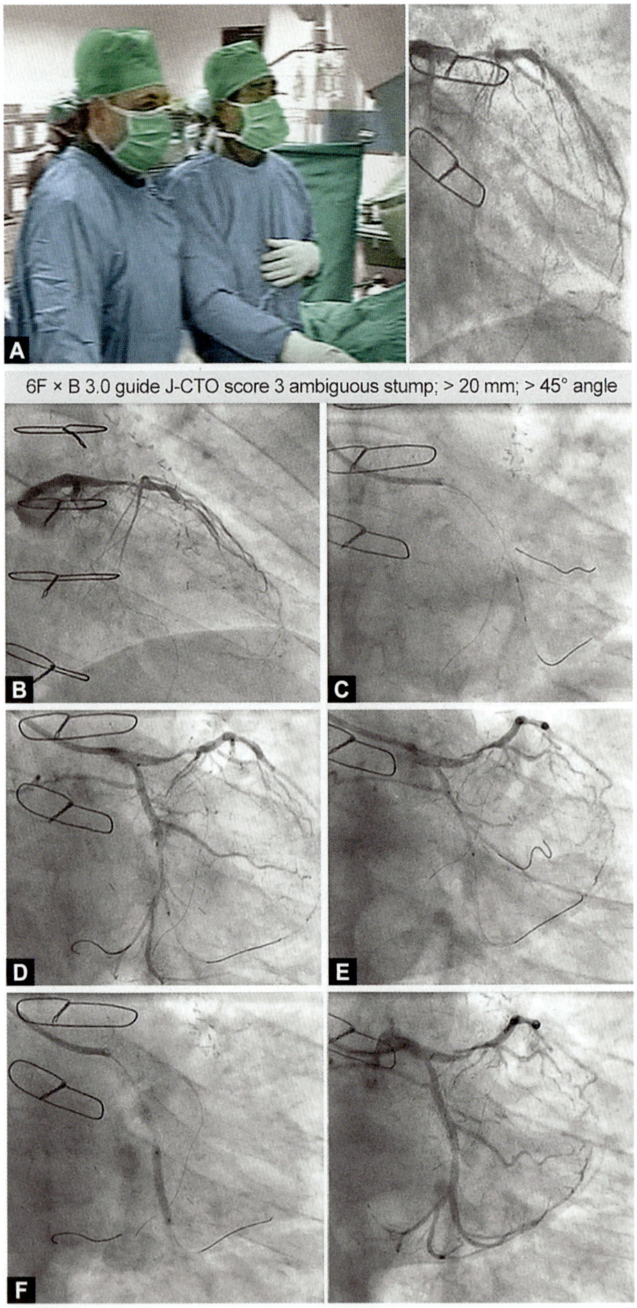

FIGS. 4A TO F: (A) Chronic total occlusion (CTO) of ungrafted left circumflex (LCX) J-CTO score 3 with bridging collaterals was disobliterated transradially, live at RADIAL LIVE, on February 10, 2007, from Apollo Hospital, N. Delhi; (B) LCX CTO crossed with CROSS-IT 300 wire; revealed underlying LCX–second obtuse marginal (OM2) bifurcation; (C) balloon in position to predil LCX–OM2 lesion and stent positioned from LCX to OM2 branch; (D) a Xience V stent being deployed from LCX to OM2 (bifurcation); (E) a second Xience V stent being positioned in the LCX across the first obtuse marginal (OM1) branch; (F) final result after deployment of two stents.

Transradial Bifurcation Including Left Main Coronary Artery Percutaneous Coronary Intervention

Radial arterial access has previously been shown to be associated with improved outcomes with unprotected left main PCI (uLMS-PCI).[24,25] In hospital major adverse cardiovascular events (MACE), major bleeding, and access-site arterial complications were reported to be lower with use of RA, after propensity matching. While mortality after bifurcation-PCI increased with age, diabetes, smoking and preexisting kidney disease, mortality and target lesion revascularization did not differ between provisional and 2-stent strategies. Further, with increased use of imaging for LM and other bifurcation interventions, most PCI could be performed successfully via TRA ($p < 0.01$), with reduction in use of a 2-stent strategy ($p < 0.01$), as cutting balloons, intravascular lithotripsy, and drug-eluting balloon use increased.[26]

The author has performed bifurcation CHIP cases transradially or using distal TRA with preference for provisional stenting strategy followed by KB; while using the 2-stent strategy in selected cases, where indicated.

An example of using the former provisional stent strategy is illustrated by **Figures 5A to G**. A post-bypass patient who presented with ACS, congestive heart failure (CHF) with severe aortic regurgitation and severe mitral regurgitation (MR), severe LV dysfunction with LVEF of 35% was found on coronary angiogram to have a 90% proximal LCX and a bifurcation lesion of ungrafted LCX with 90% ostial stenosis of a major second obtuse marginal (OM2) branch. Using a 6F Amplatz left-2 (AL2) guide, to hook the left coronary in a dilated ascending aorta, the OM2 lesion was stented and a KB done successfully for the bifurcation, followed by stenting of the proximal LCX stenosis, with good result **(Figs. 5A to G)**, The MR disappeared as heart failure and angina improved following the successful CHIP-TRI.

The latter, 2-stent strategy, is illustrated in the following two cases **(Figs. 6 and 7)**, which were also performed transradially (CHIP-TRI) for bifurcation lesions. While **Figures 6A to E** illustrate a simultaneous kissing stent strategy followed by KB performed using a 7F guide catheter via distal RA with a 6–7 GSS, in a patient of ACS, anteroseptal (AS) MI; **Figures 7A to H** illustrate a successful double kissing crush (DK crush) in a patient with ACS done transradially using a 7F, JL 3.0 guide catheter, through a 6–7 GSS in a patient with radial artery diameter of 1.6 mm only.

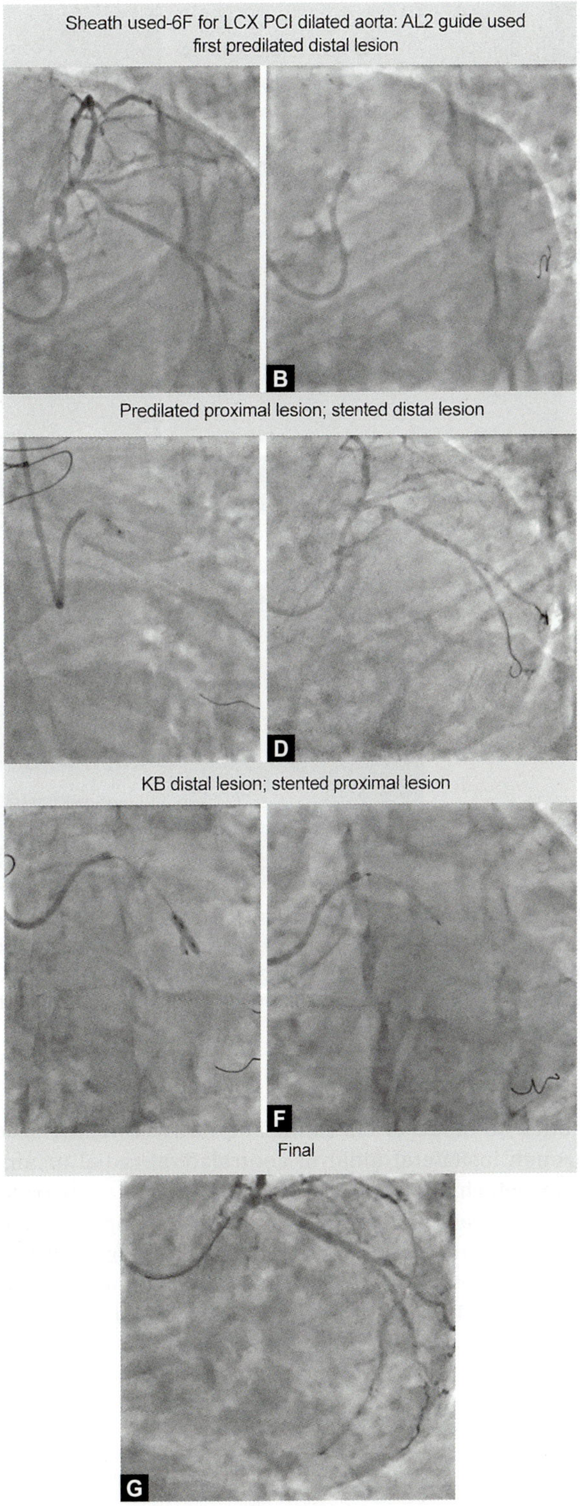

FIGS. 5A TO G: (A) an 6F, Amplatz left-2 (AL2) guide used to engage the left coronary artery; left circumflex (LCX) has 90% proximal stenosis; second obtuse marginal (OM2) has 90% ostial stenosis; (B) balloon pre-dilatation of OM2 lesion; (C) balloon predilating proximal LCX lesion; (D) a stent is positioned in LCX–OM2 after predilating the OM2 lesion; (E) kissing balloon (KB) to LCX–OM2 bifurcation; (F) stent being positioned in proximal lesion; (G) final result. (PCI: percutaneous coronary intervention)

CONCLUSION

Transradial access can be used for all kinds of complex high-risk interventions successfully. In view of current recommendations, a default radial-first approach should be adapted in the interest of patient safety and survival. In situations where an RA is not considered feasible, an attempt

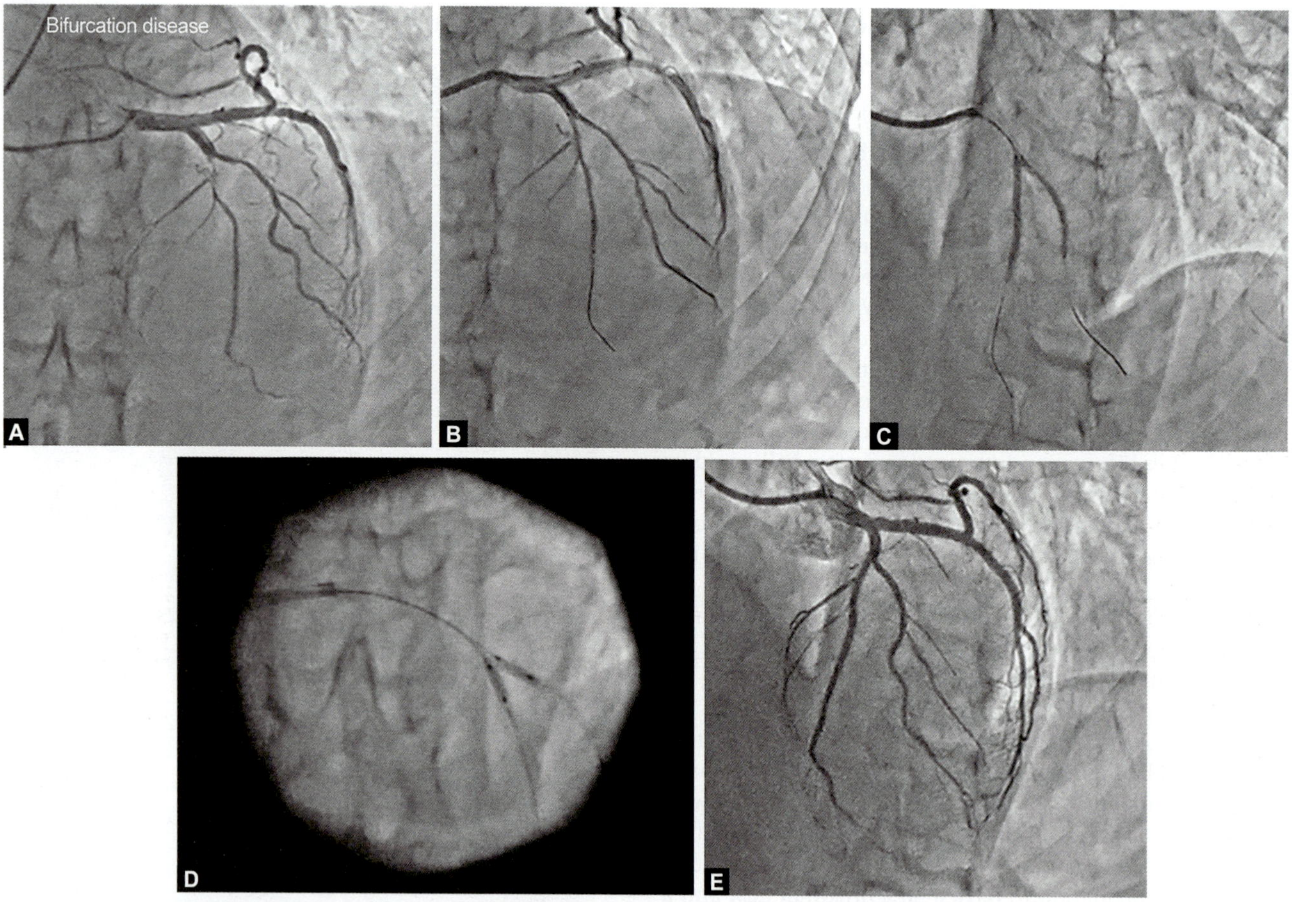

FIGS. 6A TO E: (A) Left anterior descending (LAD)-large D1 Medina 0,1,1 bifurcation disease; (B) two stents simultaneously positioned in both LAD and large D1 for simultaneous kissing stent (SKS) through a 7F × B 3.0 guide catheter; right radial access using 6–7 glide slender sheaths (GSS); (C) LAD-D1 stents deployed simultaneously for SKS; (D) final kissing balloon (KB) with noncompliant balloons; (E) final result, thrombolysis in myocardial infarction (TIMI) 3 flow, no residual stenosis in both LAD and D1.

should be made to check for alternative forearm access through ipsilateral ulnar or contralateral radial or ulnar, failing which a femoral access is chosen with an associated 3% risk of vascular complication and bleeding.[18] CTO-PCI operators often prefer to use biradial access or at least one secondary access as TRA, where TFA is deemed necessary for the PCI. The use of MCS has decreased for PCI in CHIP cases. Even if MCS is necessary via TFA, the PCI can still be performed via TRA to reduce risk of vascular complication and bleeding because the MCS is withdrawn later usually when most anticoagulant effect has weaned off. For further details on transradial interventions, the reader is advised to look up the Handbook of Transradial Interventions, Chugh SK (Ed). Oxford University Press, 2023 (in Press).

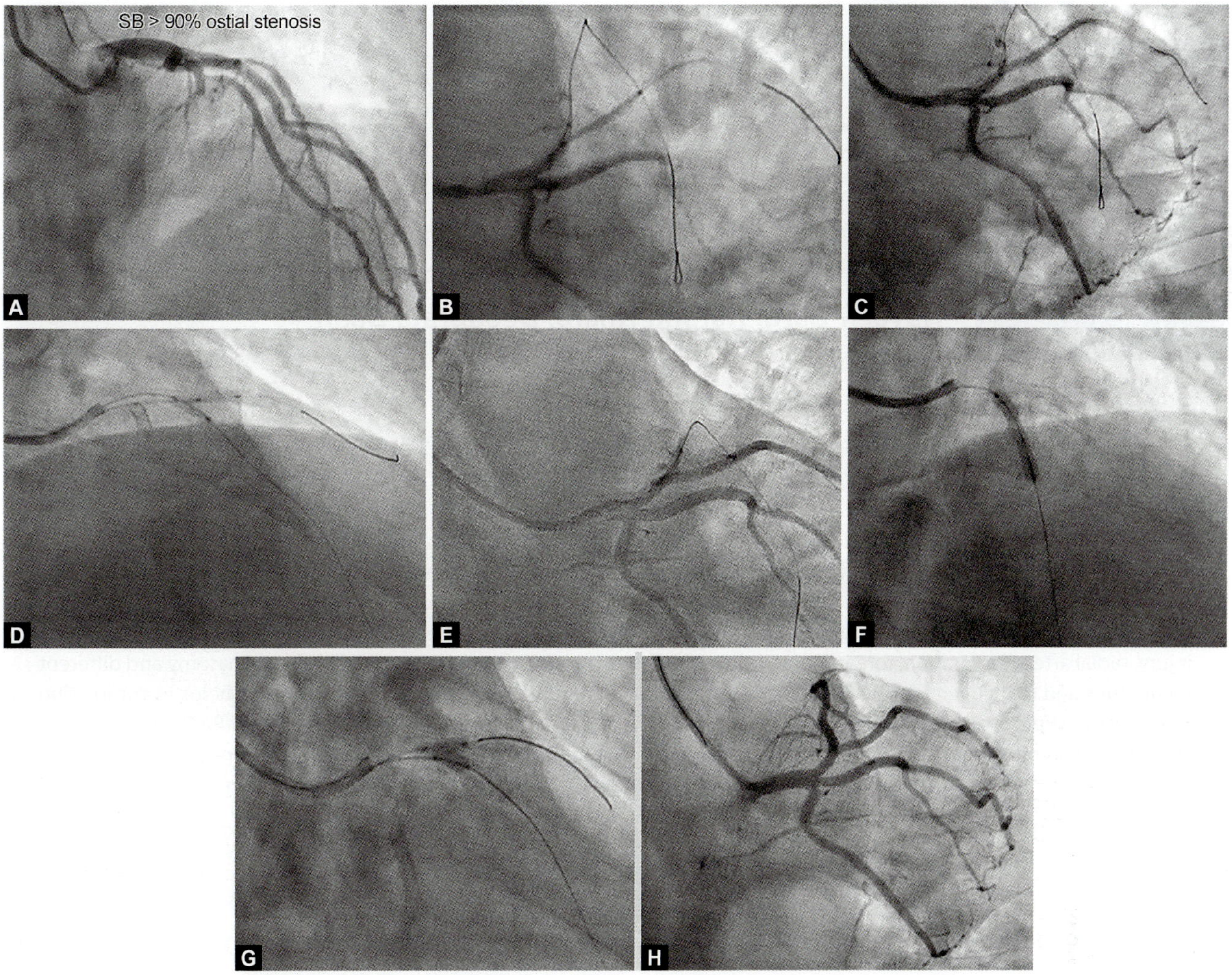

FIGS. 7A TO H: (A) Left anterior descending (LAD) 100% mid, D1 large with ostio-proximal 95% stenosis, Medina 0,1,1 bifurcation stenosis appropriate for 2-stent double kissing (DK) crush]; (B) a stent positioned in D1 at the lesion, with a balloon simultaneously positioned in the LAD lesion after predilatation; (C) result after stent is deployed in D1; LAD balloon is in place; result of D1 stent deployment is satisfactory; (D) first kissing balloon (KB) after crushing D1 stent with LAD balloon after removing D1 wire and balloon post-confirmation of satisfactory stent deployment in D1; (E) stent in LAD; Please note that the side branch (SB) (D1) wire is out; (F) LAD stent being deployed; SB (D1) wire is out; (G) second KB of LAD, D1; (H) final good result.

ONLINE REFERENCES

Please scan the QR code provided at the end of the table of contents for References of this chapter.

CHAPTER

142 Stepwise Approach for Navigating the Difficult Radial

Naveen Garg, Harshit Khare, Debabrata Dash

ABSTRACT

Transradial access (TRA) navigation failure is the most common cause of access site switchover. It is mostly related to the small size of the radial artery, radial spasm, radial tortuosity and loops, and radial artery atherosclerosis, etc. Many times, in these situations, navigating the radial artery becomes difficult and could induce a severe spasm, radial artery injury, radial artery perforation, forearm hematoma, etc. A thorough understanding of radial artery anatomy and different techniques and maneuvers can help radial operators in navigating through such complexities and helps in completing the transradial procedures. Pigtail-assisted tracking (PAT) technique and balloon-assisted tracking (BAT) technique are helpful even in most difficult radial navigation situations. The following review highlights the potential challenges and suggests several tips to assist transradial operators in recognizing and overcoming these challenges in a stepwise manner.

Keywords: Transradial access, transradial navigation, radial artery loop, pigtail-assisted tracking, balloon-assisted tracking.

INTRODUCTION

Transradial access (TRA) for coronary angiography and percutaneous coronary interventions (PCIs) has now become the method of choice worldwide, offering greater patient comfort and early mobilization, having lesser hospital stay, lesser vascular complications when compared to femoral access.[1] The major limitations of TRA navigation are mostly related to the small size of the radial artery, radial spasm, radial tortuosity and loops, and radial artery atherosclerosis.[2] Many times, in these situations, navigating the radial artery becomes difficult and could induce a severe spasm, vascular complication, and access site crossover or abandoning radial procedure all together leading to switching to femoral access.[3] A thorough understanding of radial artery anatomy and stepwise approach in these situations can help radial operators in navigating through such complexities and help in completing the transradial procedures. Operator should also have thorough knowledge of variety of wires, catheters, and techniques to navigate forearm vasculature. The following review highlights the potential challenges and suggests several tips to assist transradial operators with recognizing and overcoming these challenges in a stepwise manner.

STEPWISE APPROACH FOR NAVIGATING THE DIFFICULT RADIAL

Step I: Radial Roadmapping to Identify the Cause

Whenever operator feels any difficulty in navigating the forearm vasculature, operator should not exert any force in pushing the guidewire/catheter. Different causes of transradial navigating difficulties and potential navigation failure are enumerated in **Box 1**. Radial roadmapping by

BOX 1 Different causes of transradial navigating difficulties and potential navigation failure.

- Radial artery spasm
- Anatomical variations:
  - Tortuosity
  - Loops
  - High origin of radial artery
  - Aberrant radial artery
- Acquired abnormalities:
  - Atherosclerotic lesions (stenosis)
  - Calcification of radial artery
  - Perforation

contrast injection through the side port of radial sheath identifies the cause of navigation difficulty **(Figs. 1A to H)**.

Step II: Rule Out Radial Artery Spasm

Radial artery spasm is the most common cause of difficult radial navigation. It should be suspected whenever patient complains of forearm pain, which increases with guidewire/catheter manipulation, with marked resistance in catheter manipulation. Pressure waves obtained through the side port of radial sheath become damp and contrast injection can clearly show the area and degree of spasm. Radial spasmolytic cocktail of diltiazem/verapamil, nitroglycerin mixed with Xylocaine has been shown to be most effective as a spasmolytic. Spasmolytic "cocktails" used judiciously after sheath insertion, with each catheter exchange and prior to sheath removal, are of paramount importance in preventing spasm. If clinically severe spasm is encountered, analgesia and sedation, local infiltration of cocktail at the spasm site apart from intra-arterial spasmolytic agents must be initiated. After initiating these measures, one should give adequate time for spasm to be relieved before proceeding. Detailed algorithm dealing with radial artery spasm is outlined in **Flowchart 1**.

Step III: Hydrophilic Guidewire Navigation

After the radial artery course is laid out by radial roadmapping, maneuvering the hydrophilic guidewire (Terumo) under fluoroscopy is often successful. In case of any difficulty, pathway assistance can be taken using contrast injection through the side port of radial sheath to navigate in the correct direction. After successful navigation of guidewire, diagnostic catheter usually navigates over the guidewire

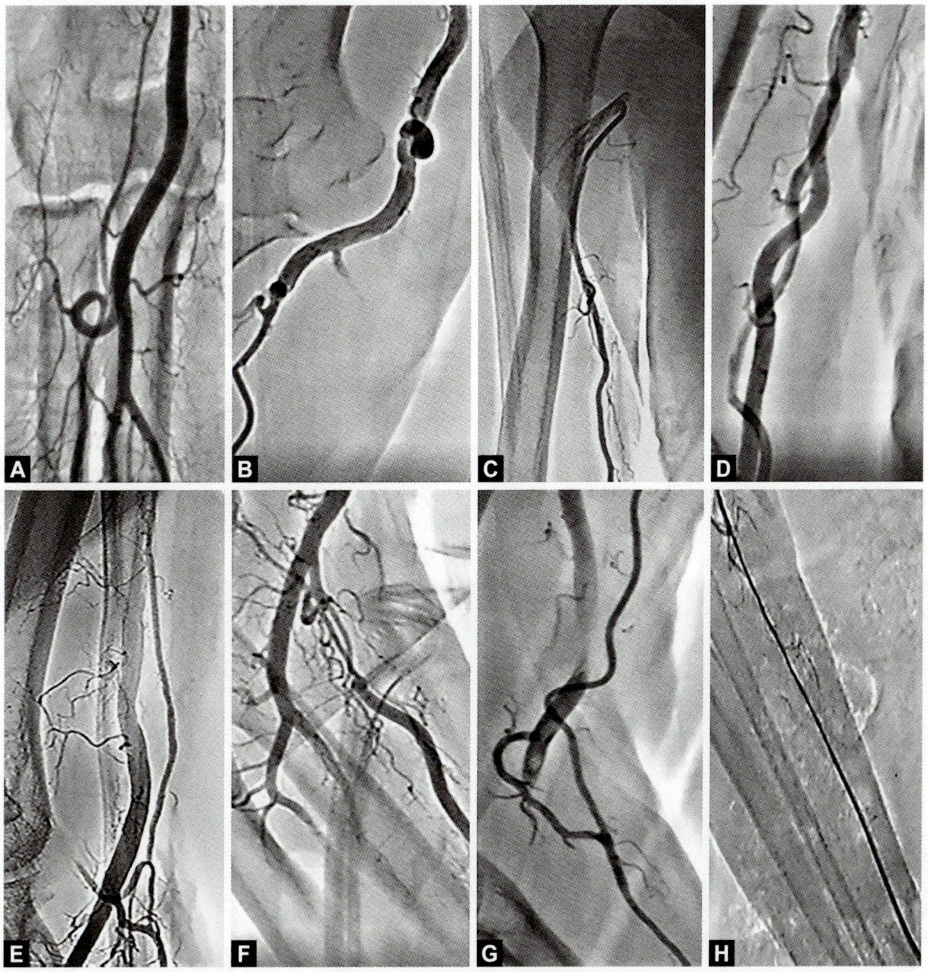

FIGS. 1A TO H: Different causes of radial navigation difficulty as documented by radial roadmapping: (A) Radial artery loop; (B) Brachial artery loop; (C) High origin of radial artery from axillary artery; (D) High origin of radial artery with extreme tortuosity; (E) Aberrant radial artery; (F) Dual radial artery; (G) High origin of radial artery with radiobrachial anastomotic sling; (H) Diffuse radial artery spasm.

(Figs. 2A to C). Manipulation of hydrophilic wires sometimes can induce subintimal dissection and vessel perforation, especially in small muscular radial artery side branches. It must be prevented with gentle wire manipulation.

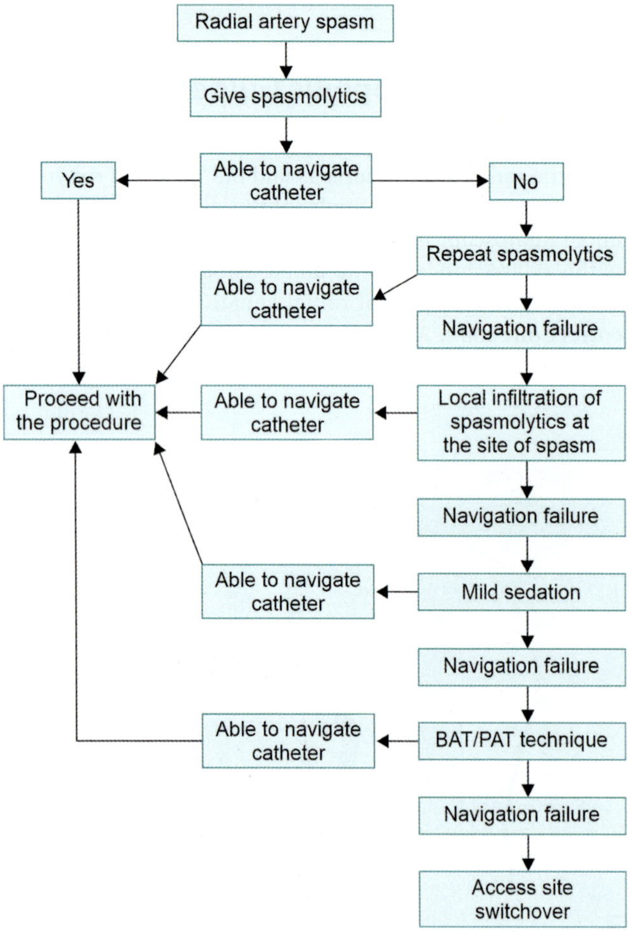

FLOWCHART 1: Algorithm for management of radial artery spasm.
(BAT: balloon-assisted tracking; PAT: pigtail-assisted tracking)

Step IV: Angioplasty Wire Navigation

In cases of navigation failure of hydrophilic Terumo guidewire, which is usually the case in radial loops and severe radial artery tortuosity, one should switch to regular 0.014″ angioplasty wire for navigation. The tip of a guidewire can be shaped to the angle of the loop/tortuosity to facilitate crossing. When the guidewire crosses the loop, its tip is parked as high as possible in the subclavian region. Then the diagnostic catheter usually navigates over the angioplasty wire **(Figs. 3A to D)**. When a single angioplasty wire provides inadequate support for a catheter, use of additional one or two angioplasty wires as "buddy wire" may facilitate the advancement of the catheter by adding an additional support.

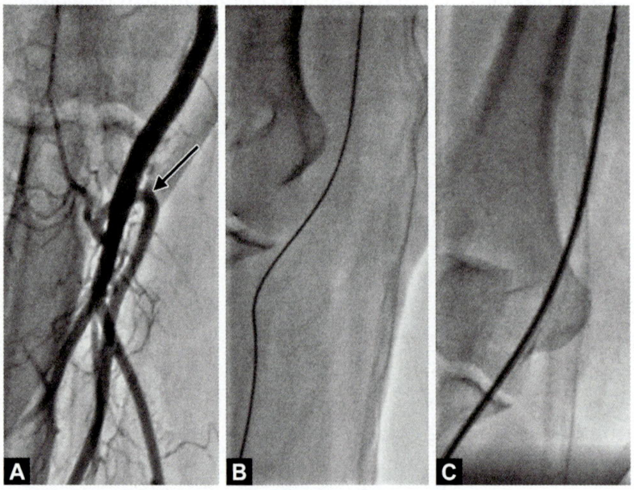

FIGS. 2A TO C: Radial artery loop crossing using hydrophilic guidewire followed by easy catheter navigation. (A) Radial angiogram revealing 360° loop in the proximal segment of the radial artery (black arrow). (B) Loop was easily crossed with 0.035″ hydrophilic J-tip guidewire. Note the straightening of the radial loop by the guidewire. (C) Easy navigation of guide catheter.

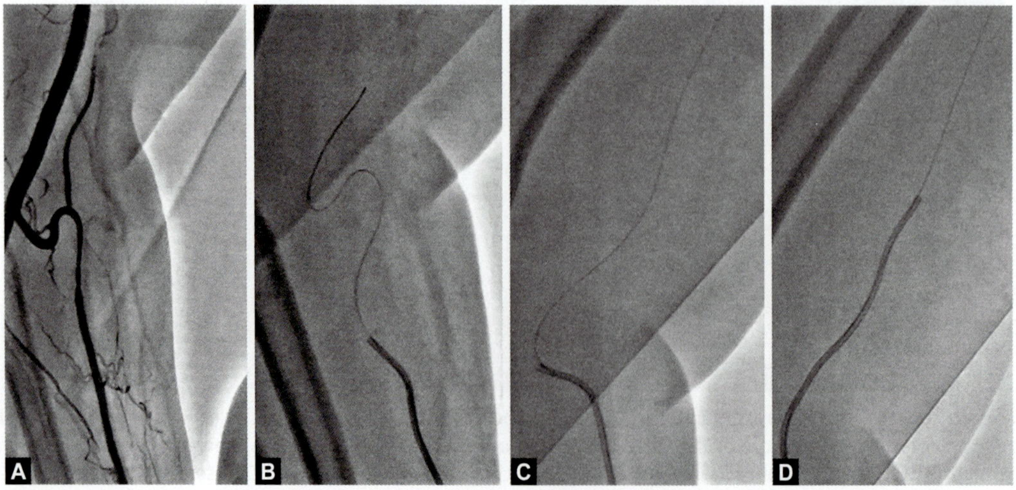

FIGS. 3A TO D: Radial artery loop crossing with coronary angioplasty wire followed by easy catheter navigation.

Step V: Straightening the Loop/Tortuosity

If unable to advance the catheter over the angioplasty wire, straightening maneuver should be performed. This involves advancing the angioplasty wire as far as possible and the catheter also as far as possible. Pulling the entire assembly back with slight rotation opens the tortuosity/loop and may straightens the segment. Rotation of arm leaving the 0.035 guidewire in the catheter while torquing is also sometimes helpful. Giving "cork-screw movement" to the catheter while advancing may reduce the friction and is sometimes helpful.

Step VI: Balloon-assisted Tracking

If the diagnostic catheter cannot be navigated over the angioplasty wire, balloon-assisted tracking (BAT) technique is often helpful. It is a well-described technique to overcome the "razor effect" of catheter tip causing the navigation failure and arterial inner wall injury.[4] In this technique, coronary angioplasty balloon of size 2–2.5 × 12–15 mm is positioned at distal part of diagnostic/guide catheter in such a way that two-thirds of the balloon remains outside the catheter. Balloon is then inflated at 8–10 atmospheric pressure. Then, the whole assembly (balloon with catheter) is advanced over the percutaneous transluminal coronary angioplasty (PTCA) wire. Once advanced till the subclavian level, angioplasty wire and balloon are taken out and a regular 0.35 J guidewire is passed through the catheter and the procedure can be proceeded in the usual manner **(Figs. 4A to E)**.

Identification and Navigation of Radial Loop

Radial loop should be suspected, whenever after getting the clear radial access, 0.035″ J wire cannot be navigated through the forearm course of radial artery or wire takes curvy course in the forearm. Sometime in cases of radial artery loop, guidewire passes easily and straight through the forearm but cannot be navigated through the arm. This phenomenon usually happens due to passage of guidewire into the aberrant radial artery which usually originates from the top of the radial loop and goes straight in the arm. In all cases of suspected radial artery loop, radial roadmapping is a must to define the anatomy of radial loop and aberrant radial artery and can be done by contrast injection either through radial sheath or through brachial catheter itself, if it is stuck halfway somewhere in the forearm **(Figs. 5A to E)**.

Once radial loop is diagnosed and its complete anatomy is documented, loop should be navigated carefully in a stepwise manner **(Figs. 5A to E)**. Otherwise, one may end-up with the complication of radial artery perforation and forearm hematoma. Sometime, guidewire or diagnostic catheter may navigate through the loop, but may not straighten the loop. Rotating the forearm in either extension or laterally can eliminate the loop. BAT technique and pigtail-assisted tracking (PAT) techniques are especially helpful in cases of radial artery loop navigation.

Step VII: Pigtail-assisted Tracking

Sometimes, even after successful completion of transradial diagnostic coronary angiogram, navigation of guiding catheter over the 0.035 J exchange wire is not possible due to extreme resistance. This situation usually occurs due to radial loop or tortuosity, radial artery spasm, or high origin of radial artery which is usually of small caliber tortuous vessel having an acute angulation at the site of origin. Guide catheter when loaded over 0.035 guidewire has got a wide free space between the inner lumen of guide catheter and guidewire **(Figs. 6A and B)** leading to

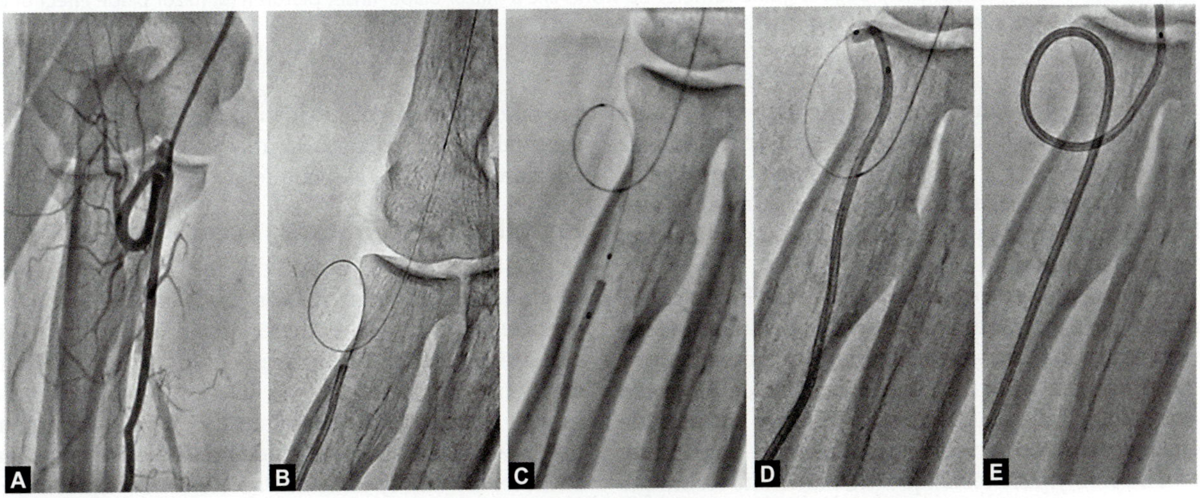

FIGS. 4A TO E: Balloon-assisted tracking (BAT) navigation of radial loop.

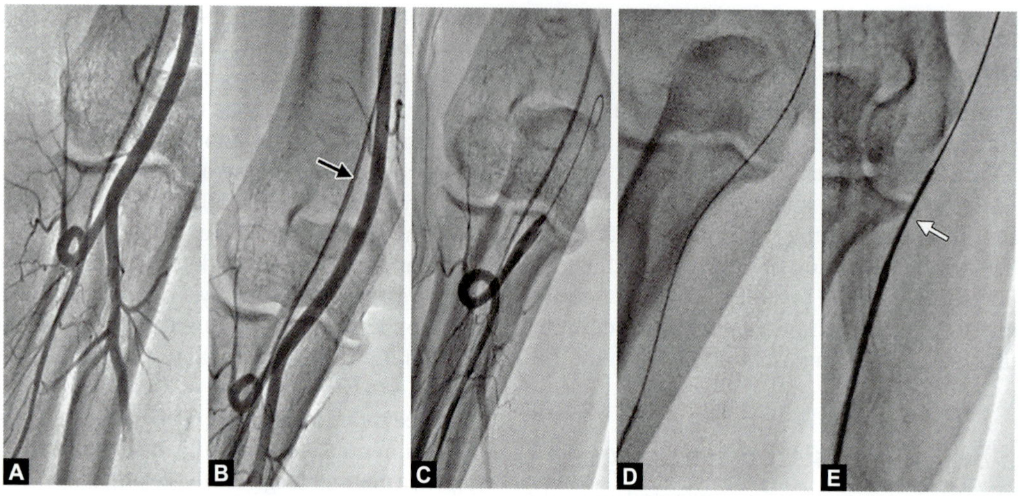

FIGS. 5A TO E: Pigtail-assisted tracking (PAT) technique (white arrow) of 360° radial artery loop with overdeveloped aberrant radial artery (black arrow).

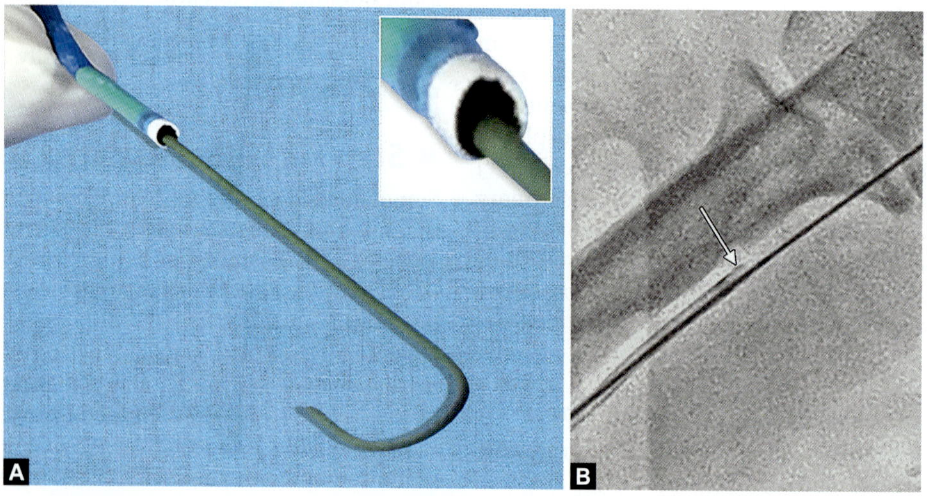

FIGS. 6A AND B: Razor blade effect. (A) Guide catheter loaded over 0.035" guidewire. Note the wide free space between the inner lumen of guide catheter and guidewire. Sharp edge at guide catheter tip works like a "Razor Blade" (inset picture). (B) Razor blade effect of guide catheter tip during procedure (arrow).

a direct contact of the unopposed sharp edge of the guide catheter tip with the inner surface of radial artery leading to a "razor blade effect".[5] This not only prevents the catheter navigation through the radial artery but sometimes can also lead to radial artery injury/perforation leading to forearm hematoma formation.

This situation can be tackled by either BAT or PAT techniques. BAT technique is performed as described in Step VI after exchanging exchange guidewire with the angioplasty wire and using a 2.5 × 12 mm balloon inside 6F guide catheter. Many times, angioplasty wire does not provide adequate support for navigating guide catheter–angioplasty balloon assembly. PAT technique is an alternate technique to overcome this hurdle and is very easy to perform and provide nontraumatic navigation of guide catheter through the challenging radial artery anatomy.[5] It also has multiple advantages over BAT technique.

Pigtail-assisted Tracking Technique

In this technique, 5F pigtail catheter is introduced inside 6F guide catheter in such a way that both the proximal and distal ends of pigtail catheter remain outside the guide catheter **(Fig. 7)**. This pigtail guide catheter assembly easily navigates through the challenging radial anatomy as well as through the radial artery spasm by overcoming the "razor blade effect" of guide tip. Once the pigtail guide catheter assembly is at the aortic root, pigtail catheter and guidewire can be fully removed, and the procedure

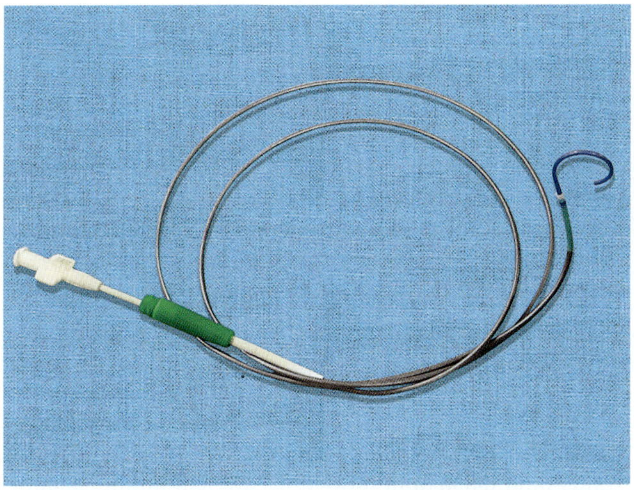

FIG. 7: Pigtail catheter-EBU guide catheter assembly: 5-Fr pigtail catheter inside the 6-Fr EBU guide catheter with both ends of pigtail catheter outside the guide catheter. This assembly resembles and works like any single guide catheter for PAT technique.
(EBU: extra-backup; PAT: pigtail-assisted tracking)

can be completed in the usual way **(Figs. 5 and 8)**. Care should be taken to ensure that the catheter assembly does not separate during advancement, otherwise one my encounter radial artery injury from the guide catheter tip. Pigtail catheter basically fills the free space between the lumen of guide catheter and guidewire leading to a smooth tapering transition from guidewire to the pigtail catheter and then from pigtail catheter to the guide catheter **(Figs. 9A and B)**. So, the unopposed guide catheter tip (working as sharp razor blade) will no longer be directly exposed to the radial artery lumen and abolishes the "razor blade effect". Pigtail catheter serves like a dilator of the guide catheter in the same way as any dilator works for any introducer sheath. A 5-Fr pigtail catheter is an ideal catheter to track the 6-Fr guide catheter because it passes very easily inside the 6-Fr guide catheter, and it is always longer (110 cm) than all the standard guide catheters (100 cm) and it is almost always available in all the cardiac catheterization laboratories. PAT technique has several advantages over the BAT technique. Firstly,

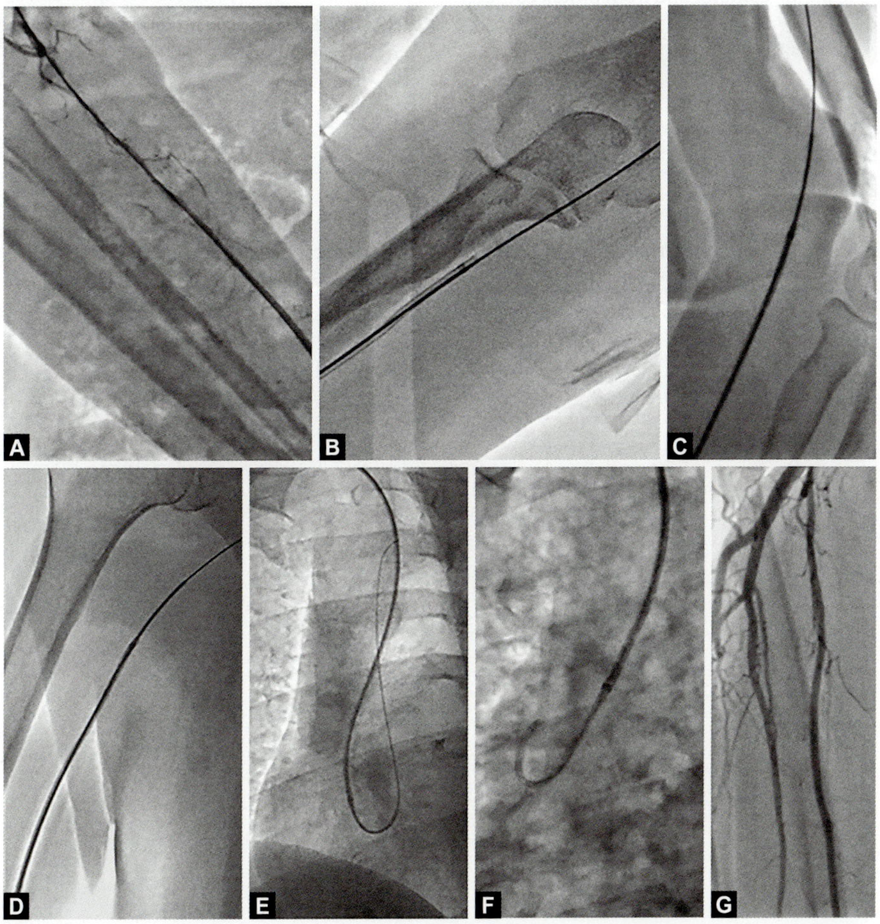

FIGS. 8A TO G: Steps of pigtail-assisted tracking (PAT) technique: Severe radial artery spasm persisting despite the multiple doses of spasmolytic cocktail. A 6-Fr EBU guide catheter was successfully navigated through the radial artery spasm segment using PAT technique. Postprocedure radial angiogram showed a total relief in the radial artery spasm and no damage to the radial artery.
(EBU: extra-backup)

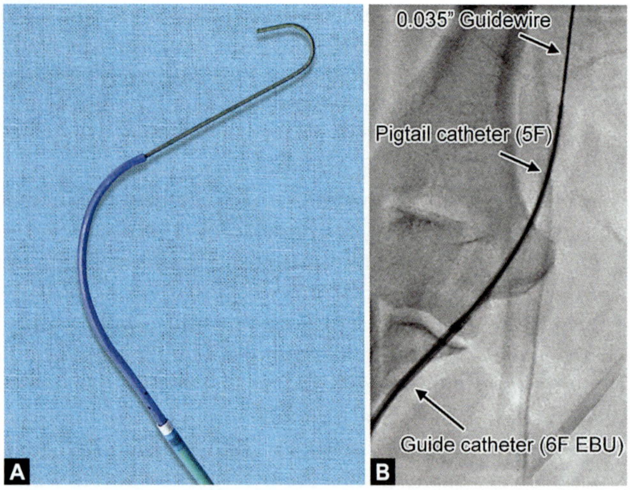

FIGS. 9A AND B: (A) Pigtail catheter-EBU guide catheter assembly: Pigtail catheter fills free space between the inner lumen of guide catheter and guidewire. It helps in abolishing the "razor-blade" effect. Additionally, it works like the dilator of EBU guide catheter and helps in navigating the complex forearm vasculature. (B) EBU-pigtail assembly across the radial loop. Note the smooth tapering from guide catheter to the pigtail catheter and from pigtail catheter to 0.035" guidewire.

(EBU: extra-backup)

costly hardware such as angioplasty wire and balloon is not required. Secondly, 0.035 guidewire provides stronger support than angioplasty wire. Finally, in cases of BAT failure, PAT technique is usually successful.

Microcatheter assistance, sheath less guide catheters, 4-Fr or 5-Fr guide catheters and long sheath introducers can also be used in such a situation.[6] These are not always available and add substantially to the cost of the procedure.

Step VIII: Switch the Access Site

With the failure of all these steps, operator should switch to the contralateral side or to the femoral approach.

CONCLUSION

Transradial navigation difficulties are commonly encountered in daily practice. Management of a vast majority of important vascular challenges can be accomplished following simple algorithms. A thorough understanding of radial artery anatomy and suggested step-wise approach in these situations can help radial operators in navigating through such complexities in most of the cases and helps in successful easy completion of transradial procedures.

ONLINE REFERENCES

Please scan the QR code provided at the end of the table of contents for References of this chapter.

CHAPTER

143 Complications of Transradial Interventions: How to Manage!

Tejas M Patel, Sanjay C Shah, Aman T Patel, Samir B Pancholy

ABSTRACT

Transradial access (TRA) lowers the risk of access site complications compared to transfemoral access (TFA), although several complications unique to the radial artery need to be considered. In view of the structural and functional characteristics of the radial artery, which are different compared to other large arteries such as femoral artery, these complications are unique to the radial access site. Characteristics such as higher density of sympathetic receptor expression, smaller lumen with a bulkier wall, and the dual arterial circulation in the forearm are likely responsible for some of these unique complications associated with radial access. In view of these differences, prevention and treatment of these complications are also fairly unique to this access site. Over the past two decades, due to better understanding of the occurrence of these complications, several highly effective and low-risk treatment strategies have evolved. In this chapter, we describe the complications and their prevalence, followed by strategies for prevention and treatment in an itemized fashion.

Keywords: Transradial access, access site-related complications, prevention and treatment.

INTRODUCTION

In comparison to transfemoral access (TFA), transradial access (TRA) has been shown to significantly decrease the incidence of access site-related complications, enhance patient comfort, reduce procedural cost, and, in certain subsets, improve hard outcomes.[1-5] However infrequent, several complications specific to TRA occur. In this chapter, we will discuss the prevalence, the possible mechanism of causation of these complications, and strategies for prevention and treatment of these complications.

RADIAL ARTERY SPASM

Radial artery spasm (RAS) is the most common functional complication of TRA. High density of alpha receptors in the muscular radial artery (RA) wall,[6] and tactile stimulation due to hardware transit in the setting of a hyperadrenergic state generated in an anxious patient, usually leads to RAS.

Puncture-related Spasm

There is a definite learning curve of RA puncture in view of the small caliber as well as a significantly higher wall thickness to lumen diameter ratio.[7] As the RA lumen is significantly smaller than the other arterial access locations, successful advancement of guidewire is at times difficult. Failed cannulation after needle puncture may lead to loss of radial pulse. Severe spasm of the distal RA because of multiple failed punctures is frequently observed during the operator's initial learning curve. Insistence on the anterior puncture should be resisted due to a small diameter lumen of RA. After puncturing the anterior wall and entering the lumen, stabilization of the cannula is difficult, and frequently, due to the antegrade flow of blood, the cannula is pushed back out of the lumen; hence, wire advancement is at times difficult. Development of RAS leads to a resultant loss of pulsatile sensation, making further attempts more difficult.

Prevention

The best strategy to prevent failed puncture-related RAS is to aim for a first-attempt successful access. As the two-point discrimination of the human fingertip is roughly in the same vicinity as the diameter of the RA, early in the learning process, first-attempt puncture could be difficult. Some centers use ultrasonography to maximize first-attempt success in cannulation.[8] The counterpuncture technique, by the way of transfixation of RA, has proven to be simpler and reliable for first-attempt successful cannulation.[9]

Treatment

If the RA at puncture site has developed spasm and the pulsation is either very faint or nonpalpable, several strategies could be used to relieve the spasm. Although several methods have been described, local subcutaneous injection of 200 µg nitroglycerin in the vicinity of the failed attempted puncture has been shown to provide rapid resolution of RAS and has not been associated with systemic side effects.[10]

Radial Artery Spasm after Obtaining Transradial Access

Radial artery spasm may occur after obtaining successful TRA, beyond the introducer sheath. In majority of the cases, some spasm occurs although it is not perceived by the operator or the patient, and the procedure remains uninterrupted as a result of minor spasm. Significant spasm is noted in younger patients, more in women compared to men, and in those patients who are anxious. Nonhydrophilic introducer sheaths, as well as multiple catheter exchanges, also increase the incidence of RAS.[11] Due to lack of consensus on the definition of RAS, its incidence in the literature varies from 0.3 to 14%. RAS leading to inability to advance hardware across the RA occurs in roughly 0.7% of patients.[12] In general, treatment with additional intra-arterial vasodilators is successful in relieving spasm. Focal spasm is more forgiving both from the standpoint of resolution after treatment and its ability to obstruct hardware movement. Long segments of spasm usually require dedicated treatment and lead to prolongation of procedure duration.

Prevention

In view of different mechanistic influences, the best strategy for the prevention of RAS should include the following:

- A calm and quiet catheterization laboratory environment with a confident team, including the operator as well as the ancillary professionals
- Administration of anxiolytics and sedation before the procedure in a few vulnerable patients
- Use of a hydrophilic introducer sheath has been shown to lower the incidence of RAS.
- Limiting the number of catheter/guidewire exchanges might reduce the incidence of RAS.

Treatment

Once RAS has occurred, the best strategies to address it include the following:

- Administration of intra-arterial vasodilators, either nitroglycerine or diltiazem **(Figs. 1 and 2)**
- Administration of additional sedation in a very anxious patient
- If spasm is not improving despite the above interventions, an adverse anatomic substrate should be suspected, as frequently these instances of "RAS" are not spasm but aberrant anatomy leading to impediment in hardware transit through the RA.

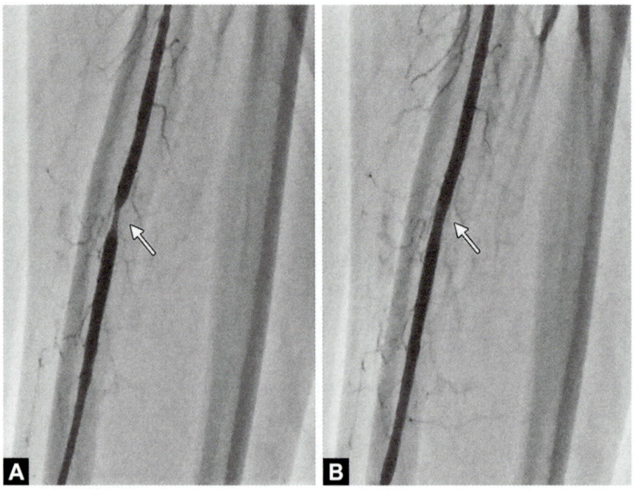

FIGS. 1A AND B: (A) An example of focal RA spasm (arrow); (B) RA spasm was relieved after intra-arterial injection of 200 µg nitroglycerin.
(RA: radial artery)

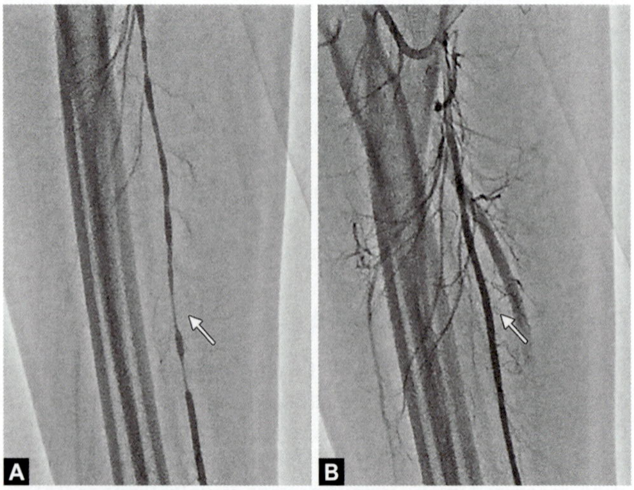

FIGS. 2A AND B: (A) An example of diffuse RA spasm (arrow); (B) RA spasm was relieved after intra-arterial injection of 5 mg diltiazem.
(RA: radial artery)

PERFORATION AND HEMATOMAS

Radial artery perforation occurs because of several mechanisms. The most common mechanism of a small perforation is inadvertent advancement of the tip of a J-tipped guidewire into a small muscular branch while traversing through the RA. Entry of this metallic or hydrophilic guidewire into a small muscular side branch leads to injury and extravasation. In most instances, the patient reports transient severe localized pain that subsequently quickly resolves and frequently goes unattended. A high index of suspicion with attention to any discomfort in the forearm, no matter how trivial and transient it may be, may lead to immediate detection and subsequent management of this complication with optimal outcomes.

The other mechanism of perforation is forceful advancement of a guidewire and/or a catheter through abnormal lumen as a result of either spasm or aberrant anatomy. Due to large transitions, "razor effect" is frequently operational and leads to deep medial dissections and subsequent perforation if undue force is used **(Fig. 3)**. Perforations, if not attended promptly, lead to extravasation and accumulation in the interosseous compartment, resulting in increase in compartmental pressure and injury to the nerves as well as the other components of the compartment, with catastrophic long-term consequences if untreated **(Fig. 4)**.

Prevention

The most important routine to follow while traversing the forearm arterial vasculature is to have a low threshold to perform RA angiogram if any resistance is felt or if the patient reports discomfort or pain in the forearm. If difficult anatomy is encountered, using techniques that decrease wire to catheter transition, such as combo technique or balloon-assisted tracking,[13-15] leads to a near total elimination of the razor effect and hence atraumatic transit of hardware through a hostile segment without causing vessel trauma **(Figs. 5 and 6)**.

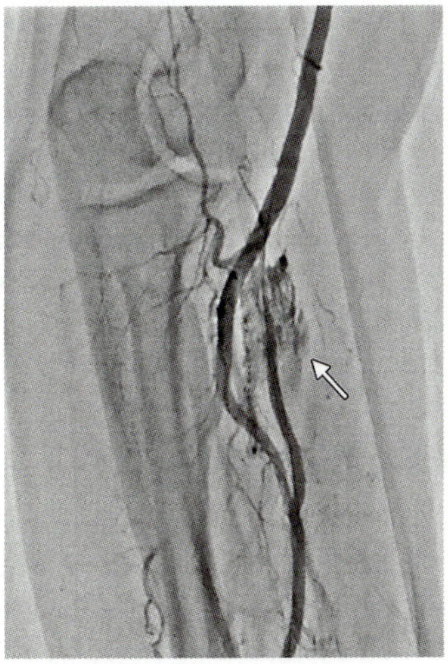

FIG. 3: An example of RA perforation (arrow).
(RA: radial artery)

Treatment

- If RA angiography is performed, perforation will be detected before arterial access is abandoned. In most instances, the best modality of treatment for RA perforation is to maintain guidewire access and advance a catheter proximal to the perforated segment, allowing enough dwell time for the artery to tamponade itself from the inside, leading to adequate closure of the perforated segment and cessation of extravasation in most cases. Reversal of anticoagulation is usually not necessary, and in most instances, a diagnostic or interventional procedure could be performed without interruption as long as the catheter remains across the perforated segment. In our experience, a dwell time of 20–30 minutes has proven to be adequate in sealing the perforations successfully in most cases.
- Perforations detected after removal of introducer sheath from the RA pose a more difficult challenge in view

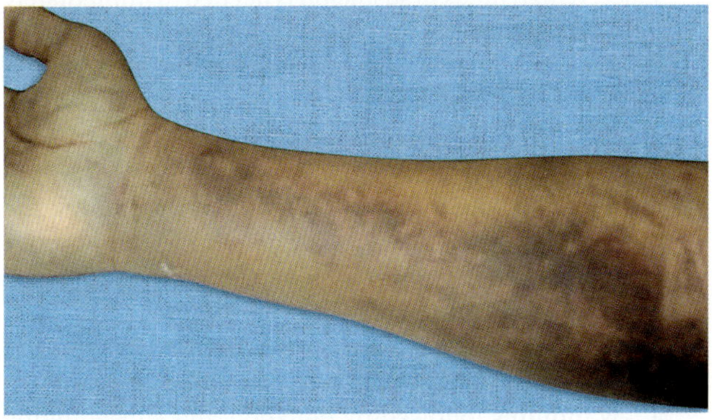

FIG. 4: An example of forearm hematoma.

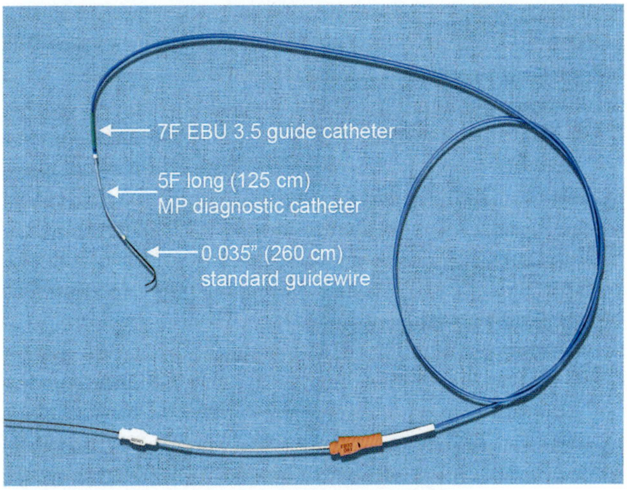

FIG. 5: In vitro demonstration of "combo" technique.
(EBU: extra backup guide catheter; MP: multipurpose guide catheter)

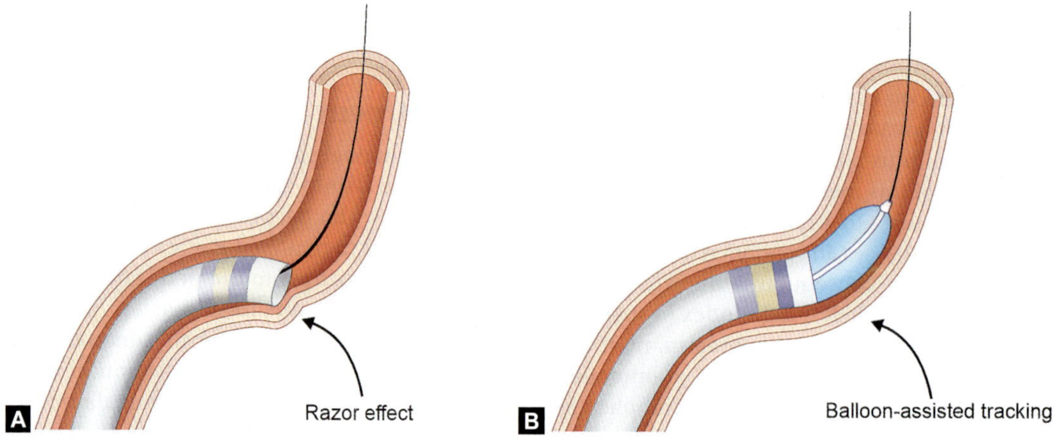

FIGS. 6A AND B: Schematic representation of "razor" effect and its elimination using "balloon-assisted tracking."

of the lack of clarity of the mechanism and location of vessel wall injury. In this instance, the only option for treatment is extrinsic compression of the potential perforation site with the aim to prevent extravasation and hence increase in pressure in the interosseous space. A high index of suspicion is needed to immediately treat this possibility. Any pain in the forearm reported by the patient after the procedure should be taken very seriously, and a presumed perforation should be treated with extrinsic compression of the RA, especially if the forearm appears to be swollen. A preprocedural inspection of the forearm is very helpful in aiding the operator in detection of postprocedural hematomas. In our institute, the forearm hematoma is addressed by encircling the sphygmomanometer cuff and inflating it at a systolic pressure 5–10 mm Hg higher as compared to the patient's systolic blood pressure for a few minutes followed by deflation and subsequently several such repetitions **(Fig. 7)**. In most cases, the hematoma disperses, leading to elimination of the compression effect in the affected area. Any significant delay in immediate recognition and treatment of this perforation-related hematoma formation could lead to a catastrophic complication of compartment syndrome, frequently leading to irreversible damage to the forearm nerves with loss of function of the hand if not treated promptly. In the event of occurrence of forearm hematoma, neurologic function as well as perfusion of the digits should be very closely monitored. This is one complication of TRA where vascular surgery consultation should be obtained on an emergent basis. Any decrease in neurologic function of the digits should lead to immediate operative decompression of a forearm hematoma using either fasciotomy or other means.

Brachial artery (BA) perforation is certainly possible, although the majority of BA perforations are avulsed, accessory, or high-insertion radial arteries due to forceful catheter advancement. Once again, these could be prevented by attending to any tactile feeling of resistance to advancement of hardware. Perforations in the subclavian and innominate artery sectors are caused by hydrophilic guidewire-related perforations of smaller branches due to inadvertent forceful entry and need to be treated at times with covered stent placement, as these sites are frequently noncompressible.

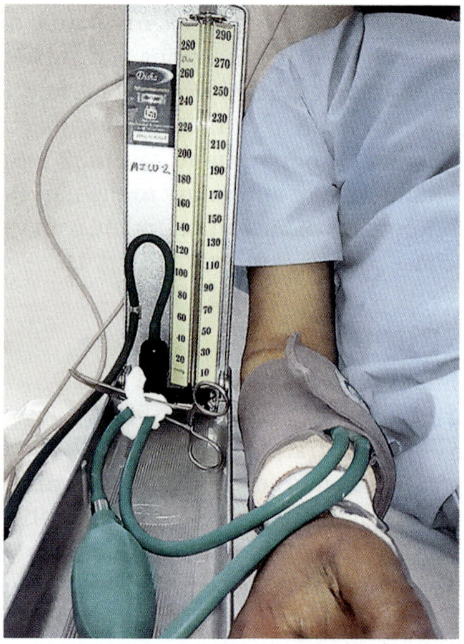

FIG. 7: Use of sphygmomanometer cuff to disperse the forearm hematoma.

HARDWARE ENTRAPMENT

Although very infrequent, one of the most painful instances in the catheterization laboratory is the inability to remove catheters and introducers from the RA access site at the end of the procedure. This is usually caused by spasm, although once again, focal spasm does not cause impediment of hardware transit both when entering and upon removal.

Long areas of spasm are usually present when entrapment happens. In addition to spasm, in most instances, an abnormal anatomic substrate is identified. Entrapment should be suspected when, during attempted withdrawal of a catheter or an introducer, the patient experiences pain, and a linear indentation is observed on the skin overlying the path taken by a superficial artery.

Prevention

Minimization of tactile stimulation of the arterial wall by limiting the number of catheter exchanges, avoiding forceful hardware movement, and paying careful attention to the catheter-to-artery ratio lowers the incidence of catheter entrapment. Using hydrophilic equipment, especially introducers, is also essential in preventing entrapment. Careful attention to tactile feel while advancing the guidewire, in order to detect abnormal anatomy upfront, eliminates inadvertent placement of hardware through aberrant anatomy and hence eliminates the subsequent problem of entrapment. Shorter procedure durations would also help in decreasing the likelihood of entrapment.

Treatment

In view of the fact that RAS is the likely culprit mechanism, all measures known to reduce radial spasm are effective in relieving entrapment. These include the following:

- Administration of one or more doses of intra-arterial vasodilators such as nitroglycerin or diltiazem
- If these initial simple treatments are not effective, utilizing local physiology to cause profound local vasodilatation is an attractive option. A technique described earlier,[16] using the principle of ischemia and flow-mediated vasodilatation, has been shown to be effective in relieving entrapment with high success rates. In this technique, a sphygmomanometer cuff is applied to the proximal upper arm with an intent to occlude flow in the axillary or BA, by inflating the cuff to pressures exceeding the systolic blood pressure. The cuff is left inflated at this pressure for approximately 5 minutes, leading to mild ischemia of the distal extremity. It is usually well tolerated for this duration. Upon relieving the pressure from the cuff and re-establishing antegrade flow in the arterial circuit, a profound wave of vasodilatation in the distal arterial circulation is observed with frequent release of the entrapped hardware. This technique has several benefits, including its high success rate as well as total lack of systemic adverse effects.
- In the event of failure of the above-mentioned maneuvers in relieving entrapment, administration of deep sedation using propofol in the setting of monitored anesthesia care or administration of general anesthesia may be necessary to relieve entrapment. Although local nerve blocks such as brachial plexus block have been described in isolated instances to be effective, in an anticoagulated patient, these are usually not advisable.

It is very important to not apply excessive force to remove the entrapped hardware. Application of excessive force could lead to a serious complication of total avulsion of the arterial wall, which has very serious consequences.[17]

CATHETER KINKING

In patients with significant tortuosity of the upper extremity and central vasculature, catheter manipulation, especially rotational torque application, is difficult; hence, operators may frequently apply torsion that may not be transmitted to the proximal catheter, resulting in kinking of the catheter. Kinking not only results in interruption of the continuity of the lumen of the catheter, making the catheter lose its utility as a conduit for transit of contrast or other hardware, but in many instances, it folds upon itself, developing a larger profile that leads to inability to advance or remove the catheter from the artery. Forceful movement of a kinked catheter could lead to severe luminal and deeper injury to the artery and should be avoided.

Prevention

While navigating with a catheter through tortuous anatomy, caution should be advised when applying rotational torque, with careful attention paid to the amount of torque applied in one direction and systematic offsetting by rotating the catheter in the opposite direction. Frequently, leaving a guidewire in the catheter lumen while applying torque may be necessary to both increase the efficacy of torque transmission and prevent catheter kinking.

Treatment

- If the catheter proximal to the kink segment is in a superficial location (e.g., upper arm or forearm), external compression of the proximal segment of the catheter, either using manual pressure or application of a sphygmomanometer cuff inflated to supra-systemic pressures, may lead to immobilization of the proximal segment of the catheter, after which if opposite torque is applied, the kink could be "undone," and the catheter successfully removed without further arterial trauma **(Figs. 8A to C)**.
- Similar immobilization of the proximal shaft of the catheter could be achieved by using a snare advanced to the proximal portion of the catheter from an alternative access site. Once the proximal portion of the catheter is anchored by the snare and immobilized, opposite torque is applied once again to "undo" the kink, after which the proximal portion of the catheter is released from the snare, and the catheter is successfully removed from the artery.

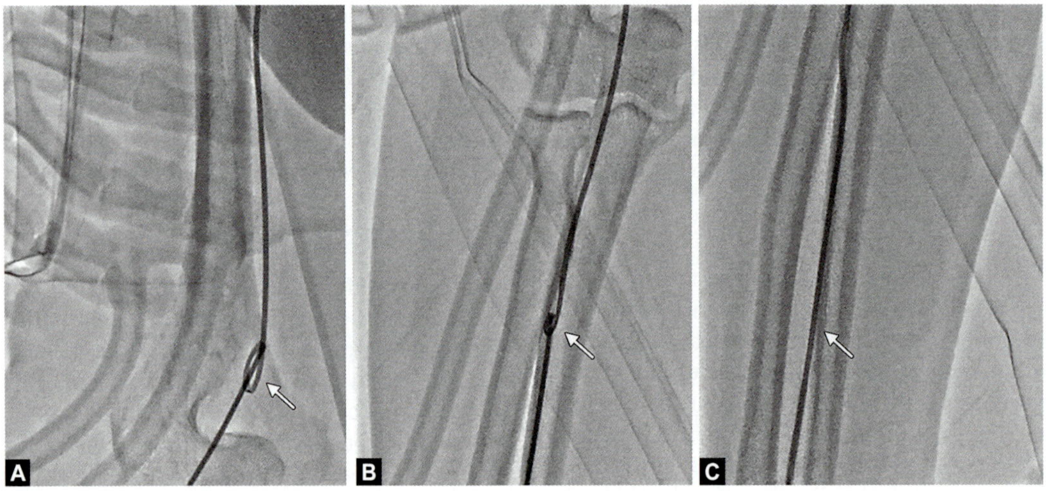

FIGS. 8A TO C: Use of sphygmomanometer cuff to remove the catheter kink (arrow).

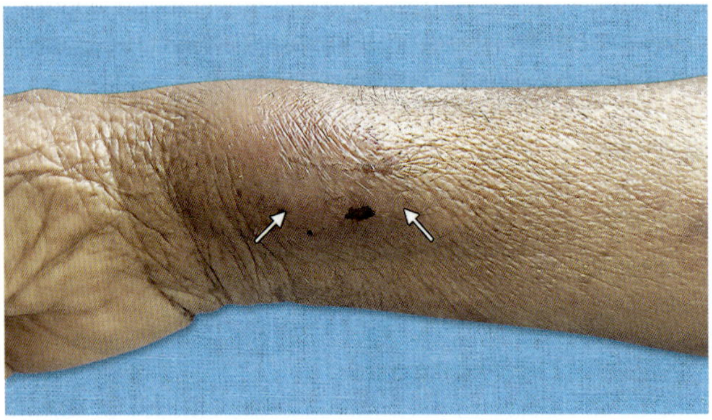

FIG. 9: An example of radial artery pseudoaneurysm (arrow).

RADIAL ARTERY PSEUDOANEURYSM

Pseudoaneurysm (PA) occurs in 0.03% of patients undergoing TRA.[18] They are mostly observed in patients with diseased RA such as elderly patients with high atherosclerotic burden, chronic kidney disease patients, in the setting of continued long-term systemic anticoagulant therapy. They usually occur a few days after the procedure with the usual presentation of a painless or tender pulsatile swelling at the puncture site with a palpable thrill or audible bruit **(Fig. 9)**. Ecchymoses to a varying degree are noted surrounding the PA. In view of the risk of dehiscence and subsequent massive bleeding, despite their apparent tolerance, they need to be treated with an intent to definitively eliminate flow in the PA sac and seal the rent in the RA.

Prevention

Careful attention to hemostasis, with adequate duration of compression allowing for stabilization of the occlusive thrombus plug, is essential in decreasing the probability of subsequent PA formation.

A localized swelling at the puncture site should be carefully examined with palpation for a thrill and auscultation to assess for the presence of a bruit with a very low threshold to perform ultrasonography to evaluate the swelling. Documentation of flow in the PA sac with a rent in the RA wall is essential for the diagnosis of PA. Definitive treatment is needed once the diagnosis is made.

Treatment

- Application of extrinsic pressure using a hemostatic compression device with an intent to interrupt flow from the radial artery into the PA sac is frequently effective in thrombosing the PA.
- Larger PA not responding to compression either manually or using a band, with or without ultrasound guidance, may need ultrasound-guided thrombin injection. Due to its superficial location, visualization of the neck as well as the contents of the PA is very easily accomplished using duplex ultrasound. Using a micropuncture needle, the PA sac is entered, and the needle tip is directed away from the neck of the aneurysm. After a test injection of saline under ultrasound guidance, 50 µg of thrombin is injected as 1 mL solution in the aneurysm sac while compressing the neck of the aneurysm. Within 5–10 minutes, the echogenicity of the contents of the PA sac is noted to increase, with the ultrasound signature of the PA sac changing from a deep black appearance to a gray appearance. This is a morphologic marker of thrombosis of the PA sac. At this point, with gradual release in pressure on the neck of the PA, complete lack of flow is frequently observed. Thrombin should not be injected without compression of the neck and cessation of flow to prevent distal ischemic complications due to thrombin.

- PA with a wide neck may pose a particular challenge with failure of the abovementioned treatments. Surgical excision of the PA with subsequent repair of the rent in the RA is highly effective and could be usually performed under local anesthesia.

RADIAL ARTERY OCCLUSION

Radial artery occlusion (RAO) is the most common structural complication of TRA. It occurs in 2–10% of patients undergoing TRA. RAO is likely caused by intimal injury caused by the hardware at the puncture site and beyond, in conjunction with stasis created by placement of the hardware as well as subsequent hemostatic compression leading to thrombus formation and subsequent rapid organization with obliteration of the lumen. Due to extensive macro as well as microcollateralization in the forearm, acute ischemia due to the RAO is usually not observed. The isolated reports of digital ischemia published in the literature are presumed to be embolic in etiology. Despite its lack of potential to cause ischemic complications, it is of paramount importance to prevent RAO in order to preserve the RA for future access as well as prevention of other unmeasurable consequences of RAO.

Prevention

Several strategies have been shown to be effective in lowering the incidence of RAO.

- In an effort to reduce intimal trauma, the lowest profile hardware necessary to achieve the goal of the endovascular procedure should be used. The caliber of the hardware should be preferably smaller than the lumen diameter of the RA.
- Use of intraprocedural parenteral anticoagulation administered at adequate doses is essential in preventing RAO. Several datasets have demonstrated excellent efficacy of unfractionated heparin (UFH), with a dose–response relationship with higher efficacy noted with higher doses.[19,20] Other anticoagulants such as enoxaparin and bivalirudin[21] have also been shown to be effective. The currently recommended dose based on available evidence is 5,000 or 50 units/kg of UFH in patients at the extremes of weight, administered as a bolus, either intra-arterially or intravenously during the procedure.
- The most effective strategy for prevention of RAO is careful attention to avoid interruption of RA flow during hemostatic compression of the RA.[22] This method termed "patent hemostasis," has been proposed as a "best practice," and is highly effective in significantly lowering the incidence of RAO without any adverse effects.[23] Hemostatic compression is initiated by any methodology preferred by the operator, and after establishment of initial hemostasis, the hemostatic compression pressure is titrated to the least necessary pressure applied to achieve dry hemostasis. If using a compression device, the device is left in place at this level of compression pressure, with frequent observation of the puncture site as well as the distal digits for adequacy of hemostasis as well as presence of antegrade RA flow, respectively.
- Longer duration of compression is associated with a higher rate of RAO; hence, excessively long compression durations should be avoided.[24,25] Very short duration of compression may be associated with rebound bleeding. Rebound bleeding is the strongest predictor of RAO as demonstrated in the recent randomized trial[26] and should be avoided.
- The arterial circulation in the forearm comprises two large arterial conduits, the radial and the ulnar artery, with both macroscopic and microcommunications between these two arteries. In view of these communications and hence interdependence, flow dynamics in one of these vessels affect the flow dynamics in the other vessel. This anatomic and physiologic substrate could be exploited to maximize the probability of RA patency while performing radial hemostatic compression. Compression of the ipsilateral ulnar artery has been shown to increase the RA velocity time integral by nearly 40%.[27] As flow increase is associated with a lower probability of thrombosis, this increase in RA flow could be recruited to further prevent RAO. Recent observational[28] and randomized studies[29] have demonstrated the efficacy of ipsilateral ulnar artery compression in further lowering the incidence of RAO compared to the standard patent hemostasis protocol.

Treatment

- Patients with RAO frequently complain of nonspecific local symptoms such as pain likely caused by inflammation as a result of instrumentation and/or presence of thrombus. Local therapeutic measures such as application of cold or hot compresses, and, if necessary, a short course of anti-inflammatory agents are usually sufficient in providing relief.
- Local exercises such as opening and closing of the hand, exercising the palmar apparatus, and flexing and extending the wrist joint as well as the elbow and the shoulder joints are frequently effective in relieving the nonspecific symptoms.
- Recanalization of RA that has been occluded as a result of TRA should not be performed as a default strategy. RAO typically does not cause ischemia in view of extensive collateralization of forearm arterial circulation, and instrumentation is associated with the risk of distal embolization; hence, the potential minor benefit does not justify the risk of distal embolization-related irreversible ischemic consequences.

- If prophylactic ipsilateral ulnar artery compression was not used during radial hemostatic compression, upon detection of RAO after removal of the radial hemostatic compression device, ipsilateral ulnar compression could be applied to improve the probability of recanalization of RAO before discharge.[19]
- Systemic anticoagulant therapy could be used in patients who develop RAO to promote recanalization, although careful weighing of risk versus benefit of systemic anticoagulation, especially keeping major bleeding in mind, is necessary before prescribing such treatment.[30]

RADIAL ARTERITIS

Tenderness along the course of the RA with associated localized pain in the absence of RAO is reported by a minority of patients after TRA. This is presumed to be from local inflammation of the RA architecture due to instrumentation. It frequently responds to local symptomatically driven treatments such as cold or warm compresses, and if necessary, anti-inflammatory therapy including nonsteroidal agents or a short course of corticosteroids. In most instances, it is self-limiting and does not require dedicated treatment.

NONINCLUSIVE RADIAL ARTERY INJURY

Injury to the RA wall is very common as shown by elegant studies performed using microscopy,[31] optical coherence tomography, and high-resolution ultrasound,[32-34] although it appears to be well tolerated with the majority of the patients undergoing TRA not developing any major adverse consequence. Intimal thickening, hypertrophy of the media, and increased fibrous burden have been reported. Although not impeding reaccess or hand function, these changes might be of relevance, especially if multiple entries are made in the same RA over the patient's lifetime.

CONCLUSION

Although infrequent, several TRA site-related complications occur in clinical practice. Understanding the mechanisms responsible for these complications may aid in devising prevention and treatment strategies to prevent adverse outcomes.

ACKNOWLEDGMENTS

The authors thank Yash Soni and Chidambaram Iyer for assistance with manuscript preparation.

ONLINE REFERENCES

Please scan the QR code provided at the end of the table of contents for References of this chapter.

CHAPTER 144

Distal Radial Access versus Standard Radial Access versus Transulnar Access in Percutaneous Coronary Intervention

Rufus Demel X

ABSTRACT

Ischemic heart disease is managed by percutaneous intervention or surgically or medically. Percutaneous coronary intervention starts with good arterial access. Historically, femoral access was the only route through which all the interventions were carried out. Femoral access complications made the cardiologist to look out for other routes. Later, radial access became familiar. Radial artery occlusion during arterial access prevents the radial artery from being used as a conduit for coronary artery bypass grafting (CABG). Distal radial access prevented radial artery occlusion; hence, it became popular, but it is technically difficult. Ulnar access is similar to radial access, but it has a high crossover rate.

Keywords: Percutaneous coronary intervention, arterial access.

INTRODUCTION

Arterial access is the first and foremost for any intervention. Percutaneous revascularization is the basic of ischemic heart disease management. Common femoral artery is the predominant choice for every cardiologist historically. However, 1.5–9.0% of the procedure develops some form of complications; the most common is bleeding at the femoral access site.[1] The incidence of major femoral bleeding complications reduced drastically during 1994–2005 from 8.4 to 3.5%,[2] which was due to reduction in the size of interventional devices and the introduction of vascular closure devices. However, these major complications remain important. Later, radial, ulnar, and distal radial routes were introduced.

STANDARD TRANSRADIAL ACCESS

Campeau in 1989 reported the first radial coronary angiogram. Kiemeneij et al. in 1993 reported the first radial percutaneous coronary intervention (PCI). After that, the usage of transradial access (TRA) around the world increased drastically.

Advantages of Transradial Access

- Early ambulation
- Reduction in incidence of bleeding/hematoma
- Reduction in hospital stay
- Reduction in costs

These advantages made the cardiologist perform interventions in an outpatient care regimen. The dual blood supply of the hand limits the potential for limb-threatening ischemia;[3] therefore, assessment of dual hand circulation is considered essential before performing TRA. Allen or Barbeau tests are done noninvasively for testing collateral hand circulation, which does not predict adverse outcomes and should not be used for access site triage. Right radial access (RRA) versus left radial access (LRA) is based on the discretion of the operator.

The radial artery should be punctured at 30–45° to the horizontal and 2 cm proximal to the radial styloid process to minimize the risk of introducing the sheath into a smaller diameter distal radial artery (DRA). Radial artery anomalies were associated with a significant incidence of procedural failure (14.2 vs. 0.9% in nonanomalous radial arteries). Despite this, the overall procedural success was found to be 96.8%, with only 1% having vascular complications.

Radial artery spasm is found to be around 1.7%. The usage of verapamil 5 mg showed no significant difference in access site conversion, radial artery spasm, or subjective pain, compared with placebo.[4] Simpler anomalies such as radial tortuosity can be overcome by simple maneuver. Radial tortuosity, spasm, or loops may be overcome by balloon-assisted tracking. The advantages of the radial artery are its superficial location, which allows safe and effective hemostasis by compression. Radial artery occlusion (RAO) is the most frequent complication of radial procedures. It can be significantly reduced by the technique of patent hemostasis at 30 days. Ulnar-palmar collateralization of the hand prevents RAO.

The RIVAL (Radial Versus Femoral Access for Coronary Angiography and Intervention in Patients with Acute Coronary Syndromes) study was done to determine whether radial access was superior to femoral access in patients with acute coronary syndrome (ACS) undergoing coronary angiography and angioplasty.[5] This large randomized study, a multicenter trial of 7,021 patients, demonstrated a 60% reduction in vascular complications in transradial procedures when compared with the femoral approach. There was no significant difference in rates of death, myocardial infarction (MI), stroke, or major bleed. But sub-analysis of RIVAL primary PCI in ST-elevation myocardial infarction (STEMI) found that the radial artery approach was associated with a significant reduction in the rate of 30-day all-cause mortality.[6]

The MATRIX (Minimizing Adverse hemorrhagic events by TRansradial access site and systemic Implementation of AngioX) trial is a large randomized, multicenter trial. This trial compared transradial versus transfemoral approach in 8,404 patients with ACS.[7] The rate of MI, stroke, or noncoronary artery bypass graft-related major bleeding at 30 days showed no reduction in this trial, but vascular-access complications were reduced by 63% in the transradial group. The net adverse clinical events, all-cause mortality, and major bleeding rates were lower in the transradial group. This reduction in the rates of all-cause mortality and bleeding was not limited to patients with STEMI, and it occurred in all patients with ACS.

The European Society of Cardiology guidelines for the management of ACS in 2015 gave class I recommendation for TRA for any PCI, irrespective of clinical presentation.[8]

DISTAL RADIAL ACCESS

A new approach was proposed to overcome the limitations of TRA and also to give advantage over the transfemoral approach. This approach was known as "distal transradial approach" (dTRA). The first publication was proposed in 2017 by Kiemeneij.

Radial pulse can be found in two sites. These are the anatomic snuffbox and the first intermetacarpal space. These two sites represent alternative puncture points for TRA.[9] Flow interruption in radial artery is avoided as it has already given rise to some branches when the radial artery has reached the anatomic snuffbox. Flow interruption appears to play a significant role in artery occlusion.

Distal radial artery diameter is 80% less than the proximal. This may affect suitable French sheath that can be used, and it varies according to sex, race, and other factors. The mean internal diameter of radial artery in India is 2.325 ± 0.4 mm.[10] The risk of tendon damage is increased in blind puncture. The double-wall technique can irritate the underlying periosteum and increase the risk of hematoma formation. The utilization of ultrasound (US) allows identification of anatomical landmarks and enables accurate vessel access, especially in impalpable DRA.

The dTRA technique seems to have more advantages.

The patient is more comfortable during the distal radial procedure than the conventional radial approach as he does not have to expose the palmar side of the arm while flexing the upper arm toward the operator.

Since antegrade flow through the superficial palmar arch is still maintained, the radial artery does not thrombose in case of occlusion of the radial artery in the snuffbox; there is a low rate of DRA obstruction.

Advantages

- Early hemostasis
- Low risk for hematoma formation
- Reduced risk of compartment syndrome
- Keeping the radial artery for possible future coronary artery bypass graft
- The ability of the operator to work at a safe distance from the radiation source
- It might be a potential site for retrograde recanalization of RAO.

Disadvantages

- dTRA puncture is technically more demanding and time-consuming.
- The radiation time was more.
- There is a higher risk of puncture-mediated vasospasm than TRA as the DRA is smaller in diameter than the radial in anatomical snuffbox.
- The short length of a typical radial catheter is a significant drawback to the snuffbox technique as the snuffbox artery is 5 cm below the common radial entry site; these catheters may, therefore, be too short, especially in taller patients.

The DORA (Dorsal Radial Artery Access Versus Classical Radial Artery Access for Percutaneous Coronary Angiography) trial randomized 970 patients undergoing coronary angiography at three Indian centers.[11] The rate of forearm RAO at 12 hours was 2% in the DRA group and 13% in the conventional TRA group ($p < 0.0001$). The DRA group showed a lesser incidence of radial artery spasm. There is no difference in the rate of hematoma between the two groups. Hemostasis was achieved with an elastic hemostatic bandage in the DRA group and an air-filled compression device in the conventional TRA group.

The DAPRAO (Distal Radial Approach to Prevent Radial Artery Occlusion) trial was a single-center, prospective, randomized Mexican study in which patients undergoing a percutaneous coronary procedure were randomly assigned (1:1) to conventional TRA or DRA.[12] The primary outcome of the study was forearm RAO assessed by vascular US at 24 hours. RAO occurred in 1 (0.7%) of 140 patients in the DRA group compared to 12 (8.4%) of 142 patients in the conventional TRA group. Importantly, there is a high crossover rate from DRA to TRA (13.3%) than from TRA to DRA (0.7%) ($p < 0.001$). The incidence of forearm and hand hematoma and radial artery spasm did not show significant differences.

A meta-analysis by Talha in 2022 compared six randomized clinical trials comprising 3,240 patients.[13] The dTRA group had a lower risk of RAO and a shorter hemostasis time. This group had a higher crossover rate and a longer access time. This group also had a higher rate of unsuccessful cannulation. There was no significant sdifference between the groups for radial artery spasm and hematomas.

TRANSULNAR ACCESS

Trashima and his colleagues were the first to report the feasibility of transulnar approach for diagnostic catheterization of coronary arteries. The ulnar artery has a larger diameter than the radial artery, and men have larger arteries than women. Ulnar artery diameter was proportional to body mass index (BMI), and the ulnar artery has different morphologic characteristics as compared to the radial artery.

The advantages of doing a transulnar approach are to avoid vascular trauma to radial artery and keep it intact for subsequent coronary artery bypass grafting (CABG).[14] The ulnar artery may serve as an alternative access site for repeated angiographies and PCI in patients with an abnormal Allen's test. In cases of poor radial pulse or as a crossover strategy after radial approach failure, the transulnar access (TUA) is a patient-friendly angiographic strategy for minimizing transfemoral use.

The complications associated with ulnar approaches are nerve injury causing paresthesia, hematoma formation resulting in nerve compression, digital ischemia, pseudoaneurysm formation, arteriovenous fistula, arterial dissection, arterial occlusion (symptomatic or asymptomatic), arterial spasm, arterial perforation, and access site pain.[15] Vasospasm is less likely to happen than in radial procedures given less alpha receptors in the ulnar artery.[16]

A regression-matched meta-analysis by Faisaluddin in 2023 compared a total of 4,796 patients in eight studies for cardiovascular outcomes of transulnar versus transradial percutaneous coronary angiography and intervention.[17] The study had more males compared to females. TUA had lower rates of local access site bleeding but higher crossover than TRA. There was no difference in in-hospital mortality, all-cause major adverse cardiovascular events, arterial spasm, and large hematoma between both cohorts. Furthermore, there was no difference in procedural time, fluoroscopy time, and contrast volume used between TUA and TRA. TUA has higher crossover rates than TRA, but it is a safer approach, associated with lower access site bleeding.

CONCLUSION

Arterial access has evolved over time, yet it is debatable which is the best access. Currently, the transradial approach is the preferred arterial access because of its easy access, lower complication, and crossover rates.

ONLINE REFERENCES

Please scan the QR code provided at the end of the table of contents for References of this chapter.

CHAPTER

145 LMCA PCI Stenting Techniques—with Tips and Tricks

Vijay Bang, Manoj Chopda, Ashish Deshpande

ABSTRACT

In left main coronary artery (LMCA) disease, a large area of myocardium is jeopardized which increases the risk of major adverse cardiovascular events significantly. LMCA disease is found in around 5–7% of all diagnostic coronary angiographies, and >80% of the patients enrolled in various large randomized controlled trials (RCTs) had distal left main (LM) bifurcation or trifurcation disease. Prospective registries and RCTs have proven that there is a solid basis for percutaneous coronary intervention (PCI) as a treatment option in selected patients with unprotected LMCA disease. Despite improvement in stent technology and operator experience, management of LMCA disease can be challenging especially in bifurcation lesions. Therefore, an integrated approach combining together advanced devices, tailored techniques, adjunctive physiologic evaluation, and imaging tools should be reinforced to improve clinical outcomes.

Keywords: Left main, bifurcation, provisional stenting, 2-stent technique.

INTRODUCTION

More than 80% of the patients enrolled in recent large randomized controlled trials (RCTs) on left main coronary artery (LMCA) disease had distal left main (LM) disease.[1] Clinical evidence from prospective registries and randomized trials has provided a strong basis for percutaneous coronary intervention (PCI) as a valuable treatment option in unprotected LMCA disease.[2,3] Yet, no uniform recommendations as to the optimal stenting strategy for LM bifurcation lesions exist. The conventional dictum of a single stent for all bifurcation lesions has been recently challenged, especially for LMCA lesions.[4,5]

Continued improvements in drug-eluting stent (DES) platforms, widespread use of intracoronary imaging, and tailored antiplatelet therapy may potentially lead to improved clinical outcomes. Operator experience (defined as 15 LM PCIs per year; mean 25 per year) may also affect procedural and clinical outcomes in LM PCI.[6] A single stent should ideally suffice in isolated ostial or midshaft LMCA disease while true LMCA bifurcation lesions are more challenging in terms of stenting strategy selection.

Recent RCTs support an elective two-stent techniques or a stepwise approach for true bifurcation LMCA disease.[4,5] This chapter summarizes the provisional LMCA PCI technique and the determinants of escalation to a two-stent strategy.

IMPORTANCE OF LEFT MAIN CORONARY ARTERY STENOSIS

The LMCA supplies 75% of the left ventricular (LV) cardiac mass in patients with right dominant circulation and almost 100% of cardiac mass in the case of left dominant circulation. Thus, severe LMCA stenosis reduces flow to a large portion of the myocardium, and places the patient at jeopardy for life-threatening arrhythmias and LV dysfunction.[7] The LM is anatomically divided into three regions: ostium, midshaft, and distal portion.[8] The distal LMCA, by definition, always ends in a bifurcation, or even trifurcation, giving rise to the left anterior descending artery (LAD) and left circumflex artery (LCx), and sometimes a ramus intermedius artery. The high elastic recoil and high restenosis following balloon angioplasty is explained by the greater elastic content of LMCA.[9] About 70% of significant LMCA lesions are found to involve the distal bifurcation.

There are quite a few unresolved issues to optimally treat bifurcation lesions as PCI procedures continue to evolve for complex lesions:

- Are increased rates of repeat revascularization at bifurcation versus shaft/ostial lesions due to anatomical or technical factors or both?
- Which strategy be used routinely for bifurcations—single-stent or double-stent strategy?
- Which technique should be preferred among the various double-stent strategies?
- Whether intravascular ultrasound (IVUS) is to be routinely used for these procedures?
- What would be the optimal duration of antiplatelet therapy for patients undergoing LMCA stenting, especially distal LM stenting?

This chapter reviews the evidence supporting PCI for LMCA stenosis as compared with coronary artery bypass grafting (CABG), and discusses the various interventional techniques as well as imaging tools and pharmacotherapy required for these complex cases.

PROVISIONAL LMCA PCI IN REGISTRIES AND PCI VERSUS CORONARY ARTERY BYPASS GRAFTING TRIALS (TABLES 1 AND 2)

Trends in the long-term outcomes of unprotected LMCA disease using "real-world" clinical experience from the IRIS-MAIN (Interventional Research Incorporation Society-Left MAIN Revascularization) registry showed an increased rate of the simple one-stent crossover technique over time.[10] In the DELTA-2 (Drug-Eluting Stent for Left Main Coronary Artery 2) study, the largest "all-comers" LMCA PCI registry with second-generation DES (n = 3,986) covering a period from 2006 to 2015, a single-stent strategy was chosen in almost 80% of the cases, with 84% of the lesions located at the distal LMCA. Combined data from the KOMATE (Korean Multicenter Angioplasty Team) multicenter registry and the COBIS (Coronary Bifurcation Stenting) II registry examined 1,353 distal bifurcation LMCA lesions. A single-stent strategy was adopted in 71.4% of the patients, and up to 83.0% received current-generation DES.[11] PCI has been compared with CABG in the setting of LMCA disease in six RCTs, but only two of these—the EXCEL (Evaluation of XIENCE versus Coronary Artery Bypass Surgery for Effectiveness of Left Main Revascularization) and the NOBLE (Nordic-Baltic-British Left Main Revascularization Study) trials—were conducted in the era of second-generation DES.[10-12] Distal LMCA lesion rates ranged from 58% in LE MANS (Left Main Coronary Artery Stenting) trial to 81% in the EXCEL and NOBLE trials.[12] Provisional stenting was reported in 30%, 46.3%, 61.5%, 65%, and 63.2% in the study from Boudriot et al.[13] in the PRECOMBAT (Premier of Randomized Comparison of Bypass Surgery versus Angioplasty Using

TABLE 1: Registries of left main (LM) intervention.[17]

Registry	Year	LM PCI patients (*n*)	Follow-up (years)	Stents used	Main outcome
MAIN-Compare	2008	1,102	2.7	BMS (28.9%); DES–SES and PES (71.1%)	Death and composite outcome similar, TVR higher in the PCI group
DELFT	2008	358	3	SES and PES	MACE at 30 days 11.4%, at 3 years 32.1%
FRIEND	2009	151	1.2	PES	MACE 10.6%
CUSTOMIZE	2011	342	2	DES	8.1% mortality in the SYNTAX score <34; 32.7% in the SYNTAX score >34
CREDO-KYOTO	2012	365	3	DES (68.3%)	Adjusted death/MI/stroke similar to CABG, repeat revascularization 43.4%
DELTA	2012	1,874	3.5	SES (44.7%) and PES (47.6%)	MACCE 34.9% and TVR 15.5%
IRIS-MAIN 3	2016	2,866	9.7, 5.6, and 3	BMS, first- and second-generation DES	Rate of repeat revascularization decreased over time
MILAN-NEW TOKYO (MITO registry)	2016	1,026	4.3	DES	MACE 31.8%, TLR 19.2%
ZHENG	2016	1,442	3	DES	All-cause mortality 3.8%, TVR 9.9%

(BMS: bare metal stent; CABG: coronary artery bypass grafting; DELTA: Drug-Eluting Stent for Left Main Coronary Artery; DES: drug-eluting stent; IRIS-MAIN: Interventional Research Incorporation Society-Left MAIN Revascularization; LM: left main; MACE: major adverse cardiovascular event; MACCE: major adverse cardiac and cerebrovascular event; MI: myocardial infarction; PCI: percutaneous coronary intervention; PES: paclitaxel-eluting stent; SES: sirolimus-eluting stent; SYNTAX: Synergy Between Percutaneous Coronary Intervention with Taxus and Cardiac Surgery; TVR: target vessel revascularization)

TABLE 2: Randomized controlled trials (RCTs) of left main coronary artery (LMCA) intervention compared with coronary artery bypass grafting (CABG).[17]

RCT	Year	Patients (*n*)		Follow-up (years)	Stents used	Main outcome
		PCI	CABG			
LE MANS	2008	52	53	2	BMS, DES (35%)	PCI group had improved ejection fraction
SYNTAX-LM	2010	357	348	1	PES	MACCE 13.7%, similar to CABG patients
Boudriot et al.[13]	2011	100	101	1	SES	MACCE 19%, noninferior to CABG
PRECOM BAT	2011	300	300	2	SES	MACCE 8.7%, noninferior to CABG
EXCEL[1]	2016	948	957	3	EES	Primary outcome 15.4% in PCI arm
NOBLE[16]	2016	598	603	5	SES, BES	MACCE 28% for PCI

(BMS: bare metal stent; DES: drug-eluting stent; EXCEL: Evaluation of XIENCE versus Coronary Artery Bypass Surgery for Effectiveness of Left Main Revascularization; LE MANS: Left Main Coronary Artery Stenting; MACCE: major adverse cardiac and cerebrovascular event; NOBLE: Nordic–Baltic–British Left Main Revascularization Study; PCI: percutaneous coronary intervention; PRECOMBAT: Premier of Randomized Comparison of Bypass Surgery versus Angioplasty Using Sirolimus-Eluting Stent in Patients with Left Main Coronary Artery Disease; RCT: randomized controlled trial; SYNTAX: Synergy Between Percutaneous Coronary Intervention with Taxus and Cardiac Surgery)

Sirolimus-Eluting Stent in Patients with Left Main Coronary Artery Disease), SYNTAX (Synergy Between Percutaneous Coronary Intervention with Taxus and Cardiac Surgery), EXCEL, and NOBLE trials, respectively.[14-16]

WHO IS A GOOD CANDIDATE FOR LEFT MAIN STENTING?

The first step in the safe performance of any LM PCI is careful patient selection. The choice to subject a patient for PCI or CABG for treatment of unprotected LMCA stenosis depends on several clinical and anatomical coronary features.

Left main coronary artery disease (CAD) is often associated with lesions in the other territories. These lesions need to be taken into consideration while deciding on the treatment strategy in this subset of patients. Following are the different groups of patients with unprotected LMCA disease who are likely to have favorable clinical outcomes with PCI as compared to that of CABG.[18]

- Ostial and/or midshaft LMCA disease
- Isolated LMCA disease
- LMCA disease plus single-vessel disease
- LMCA bifurcation disease treatable by single-stent approach
- Low SYNTAX score or intermediate SYNTAX score (SYNTAX score < 33)

STENTING STRATEGIES AND TECHNIQUES

Ostial and Midshaft Lesions

Ostial and midshaft lesions can be stented like any other artery and with a single-stent strategy and have good immediate and long-term outcomes **(Figs. 1 and 2)**.[19]

In ostial lesions, careful angiographic views must be taken to ensure adequate visualization of the ostium and the adjacent aorta. Usually anterior-posterior cranial and (or) slightly left anterior oblique cranial projections are used to have a good visualization. The guide catheter may occlude the artery with severe ostial stenosis. After the coronary wire is in position in the distal vessel, the guide should be disengaged slightly from the ostium, to minimize coronary ischemia. The guide catheter should preferably be short-tipped and with side holes. Ostial lesions are often predilated. The stent needs to be placed carefully with 1–2 mm of the stent protruding into the aorta. After deployment, the balloon is withdrawn slightly into the aorta and the proximal part of the stent is postdilated and flared which ensures good stent apposition at the LM ostium. IVUS may be used to ensure a satisfactory end result.[20]

Left Main Coronary Artery Bifurcation Lesions

Distal LMCA lesions are mostly treated as true bifurcation lesions, except in cases where one branch is either very small (usually the LCX), or is chronically occluded or protected by a patent surgical graft. In such cases, the distal LMCA lesion may be treated with a single-stent technique by stenting across the ostium of the other vessel. True bifurcation lesions can be addressed either by a single-stent or by a two-stent strategy. The choice of strategy depends on various factors such as plaque distribution, the diameter of the side branches (SBs), and the angle between the branches. The provisional stenting is a single-stent strategy, although it allows the placement of a second stent [T, T and protrusion (TAP), culotte technique] if required. More complex lesions may require an upfront double-stent strategy like T stenting, TAP, double-kiss (DK) crush, culotte, or V stenting.[18]

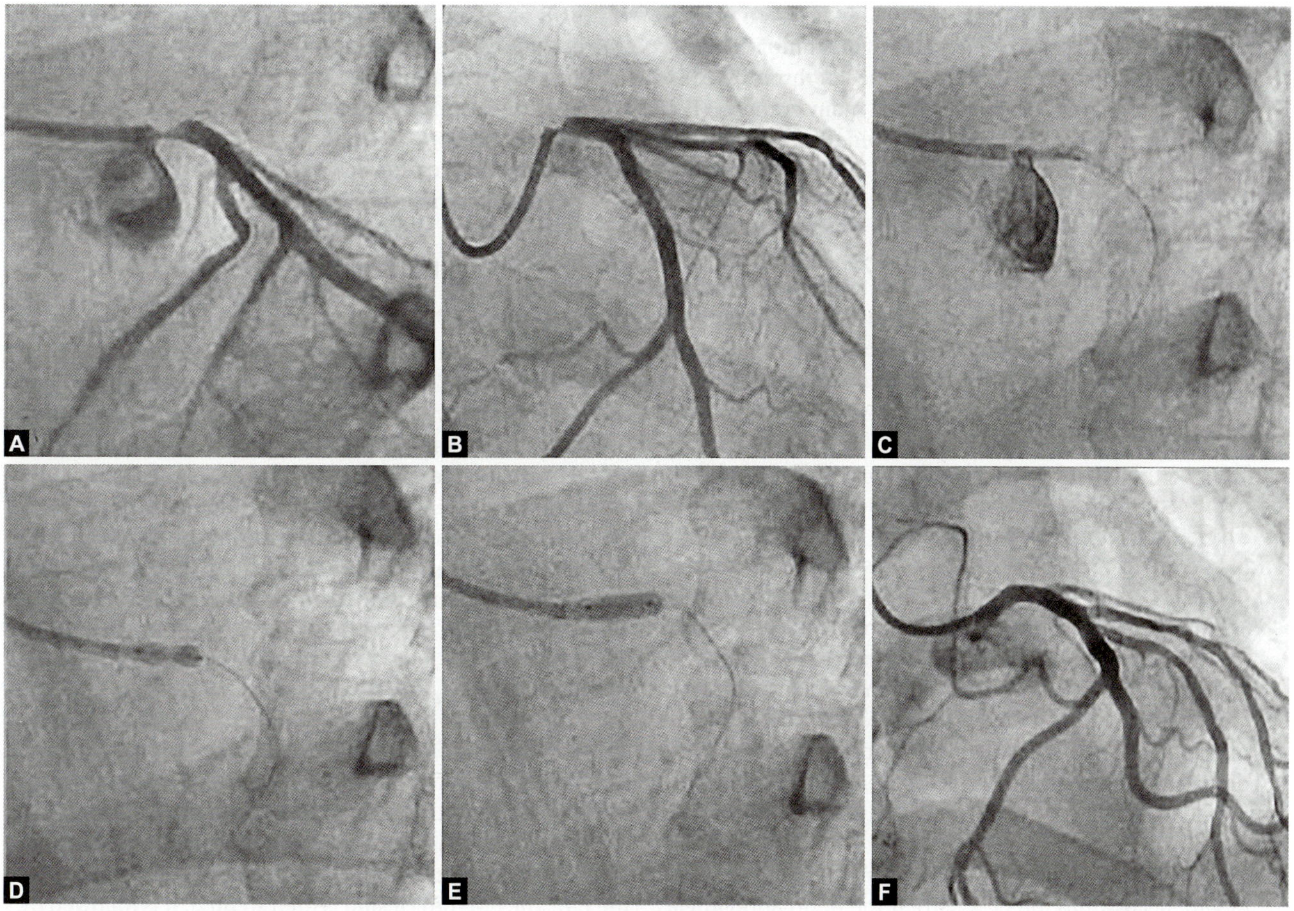

FIGS. 1A TO F: Stenting of isolated ostial left main stenosis. (A and B) initial appearance; (C) positioning of stent; (D) stent deployment with proximal stent slightly protruding into the aorta; (E) postdilatation; (F) final result.

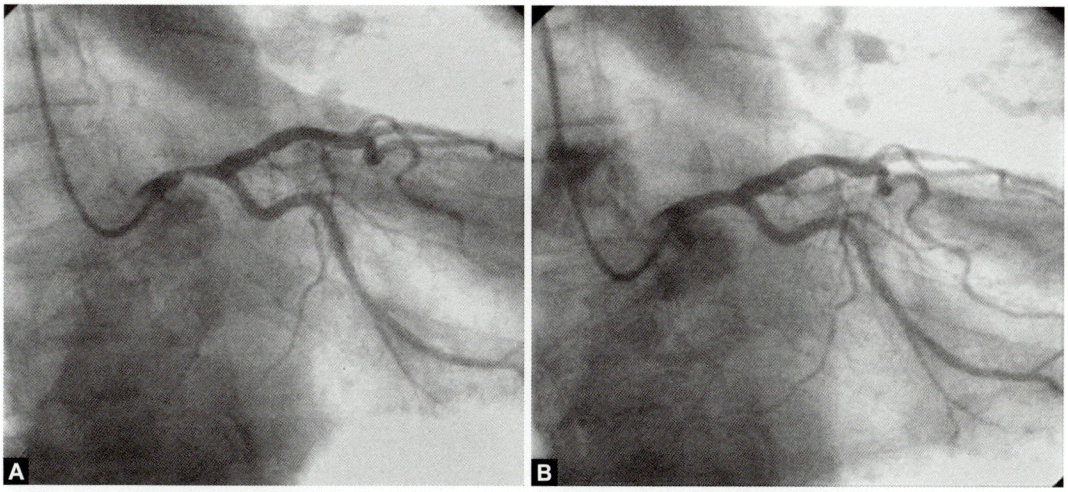

FIGS. 2A AND B: Direct stenting of isolated midshaft left main stenosis. (A) Baseline angiography: Short, lesion of mid-left main treated by direct stenting. (B) final angiographic result.

Bifurcation PCI is associated with a higher risk of procedural complications, lower angiographic success rates, and restenosis as compared to nonbifurcation PCI as seen in various trials.[21]

Left main bifurcation lesions can be classified as: simple or complex.[22]

- *Simple*: SB diameter stenosis <70% and LCX lesion length <10 mm (major criteria)

- *Complex*: SB diameter stenosis >70%, LCX lesion length >10 mm plus presence of any two of six minor criteria: (1) bifurcation angle >70°, (2) presence of thrombus, (3) moderate-to-severe calcification, (4) main branch (MB) diameter <2.5 mm, (5) MB lesion length >25 mm, (6) multiple lesions

Bifurcation Percutaneous Coronary Intervention Principles[23,24]

- *Bifurcation anatomy*: The plaque burden at the bifurcation, and plaque location (ostial or beyond the ostium) in the LCX and LM, the LCX diameter, and lesion length (≥10 mm), and the bifurcation angle should be carefully assessed.
- The potential mechanisms leading to compromised flow in the ostial LCX should be recognized: (1) plaque shift or carina shift, (2) elliptical deformation of ostial SB, and (3) dissection or protrusion of LM stent struts on SB arterial flow.
- The predictors of compromised coronary flow in the LCX SB after LM-to-LAD stenting should be borne in mind: (1) LM stent length, (2) plaque burden in LCX, and (3) ostial LCX MLA (minimal lumen area) on IVUS.[25]
- *Bifurcation angle*: The angle between the LCX and LAD determines the risk of SB (LCX) occlusion during LM PCI. Similarly, it also determines the choice of bifurcation stent technique.
- The angle between the LM and LCX determines the ease of wire access into the LCX (SB). If the bifurcation angle is <70° wiring is easier and difficult when the angle is >90°.
- The bifurcation angle is independently associated with restenosis.[26]
- IVUS plays an important role in stent optimization and reduction of adverse cardiac events leading to better long-term outcomes.[27]
- True bifurcation lesions are, Medina 1,1,1 and Medina 0,1,1, where both SB show >50 % stenosis.
- Nontrue bifurcation lesions should ideally be treated with a one-stent technique.

Single-stent Strategy

Provisional Stenting

This is a single-stent strategy but it allows the use of a second stent if required. The main vessel (which is almost always the LAD) is first wired. A second wire is then placed in the SB. The stent in the LM–LAD is deployed and postdilated. The LCX may be left untouched if there is no significant SB compromise or treated by a kissing balloon inflation (KBI) if required. If necessary, a second stent may be deployed into the ostial LCX using the "T" or the "TAP" technique. A KBI should be done mandatorily if two stents have been used **(Figs. 3A to D)**.[19]

Double-stent Strategies

T Stenting

The T stent strategy is used when a two-stent strategy is required but the angulation between LAD and LCX approaches 90°. A stent is deployed in the SB, making sure that the ostium is covered with only marginal protrusion into the LM. The LM–LAD lesion is then stented. It is followed by a KBI. This technique provides a good reconstruction of distal LM bifurcation T shape. However, there is a risk of leaving either the SB ostium uncovered or of the SB stent protruding too much inside the LM stent. The "T" technique can also be

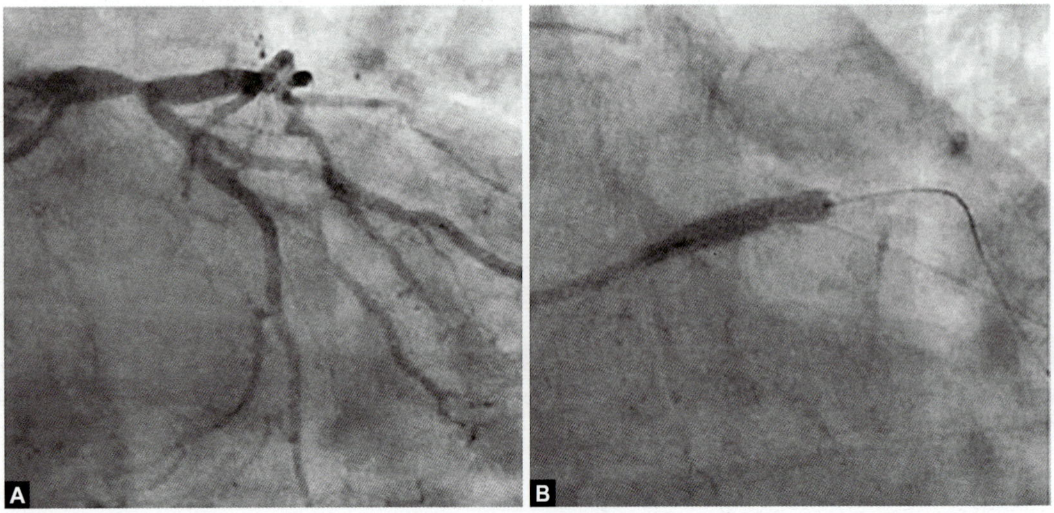

FIGS. 3A TO D: *Continued*

Continued

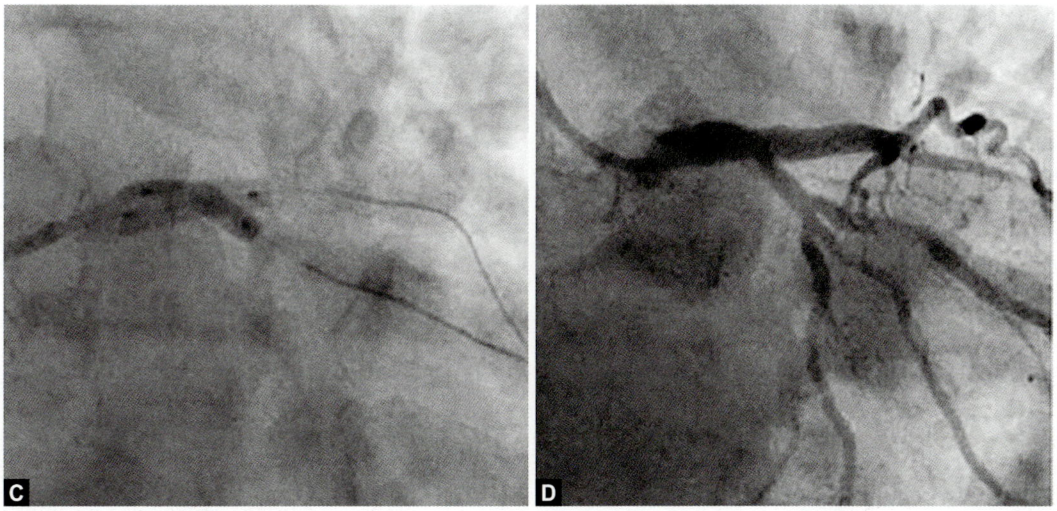

FIGS. 3A TO D: Provisional stenting. (A) Initial picture; (B) stent to left main–left anterior descending (LM–LAD); (C) kissing balloon post-stenting; (D) final result.

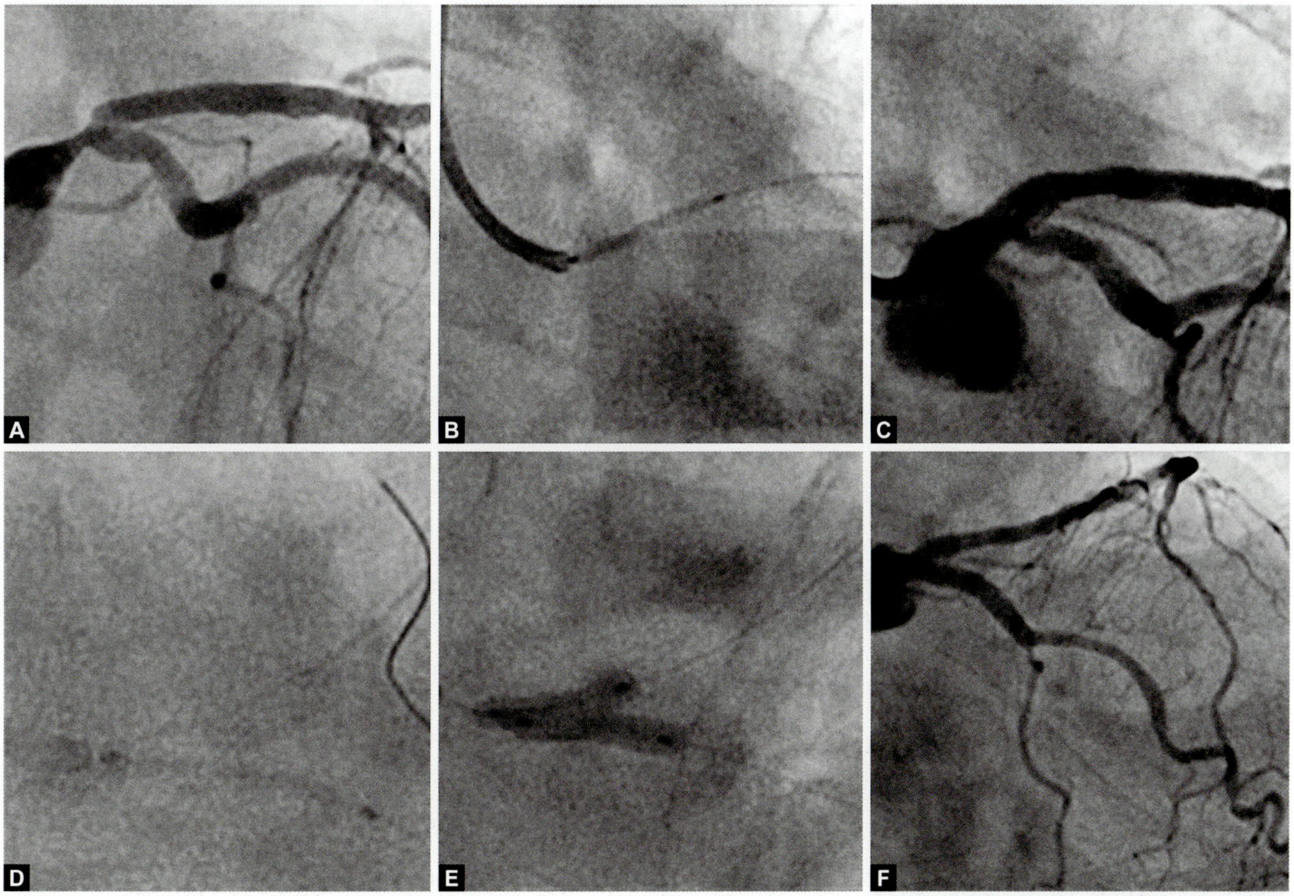

FIGS. 4A TO F: T stenting. (A) Initial picture; (B) stent from left main–left anterior descending (LM–LAD); (C) dissection of ostial left circumflex artery (LCX); (D) advancement of stent into LCX; (E) kissing balloon; (F) final result.

performed by placing the first stent in the main vessel and the second stent in the SB afterwards **(Figs. 4A to F)**.[19]

T and Protrusion (TAP) Technique

This technique can be used in the vast majority of LMCA bifurcation lesions. This technique provides a good reconstruction of distal LM bifurcation with minimal stent overlap. The main vessel (LM–LAD) is first stented. Then, after dilating the stent strut, another stent is placed at the ostium of the SB (LCX) with a balloon positioned in the main stent. The proximal edge of the SB stent is positioned 1–2 mm inside the main stent and the SB stent is deployed while a deflated balloon is there in the main stent. Then, a final kissing balloon inflation (FKI) is performed so that the carina is properly reshaped **(Figs. 5A to G)**.[18]

Culotte Stenting

This is a strategy suitable for lesions in cases where the ostium of the LCX shows disease, the angulation between the vessels is around 60° leading to a higher risk of plaque shift, and the two vessels are nearly same in diameter. The main vessel, usually the LM–LAD, is first stented. A wire is passed

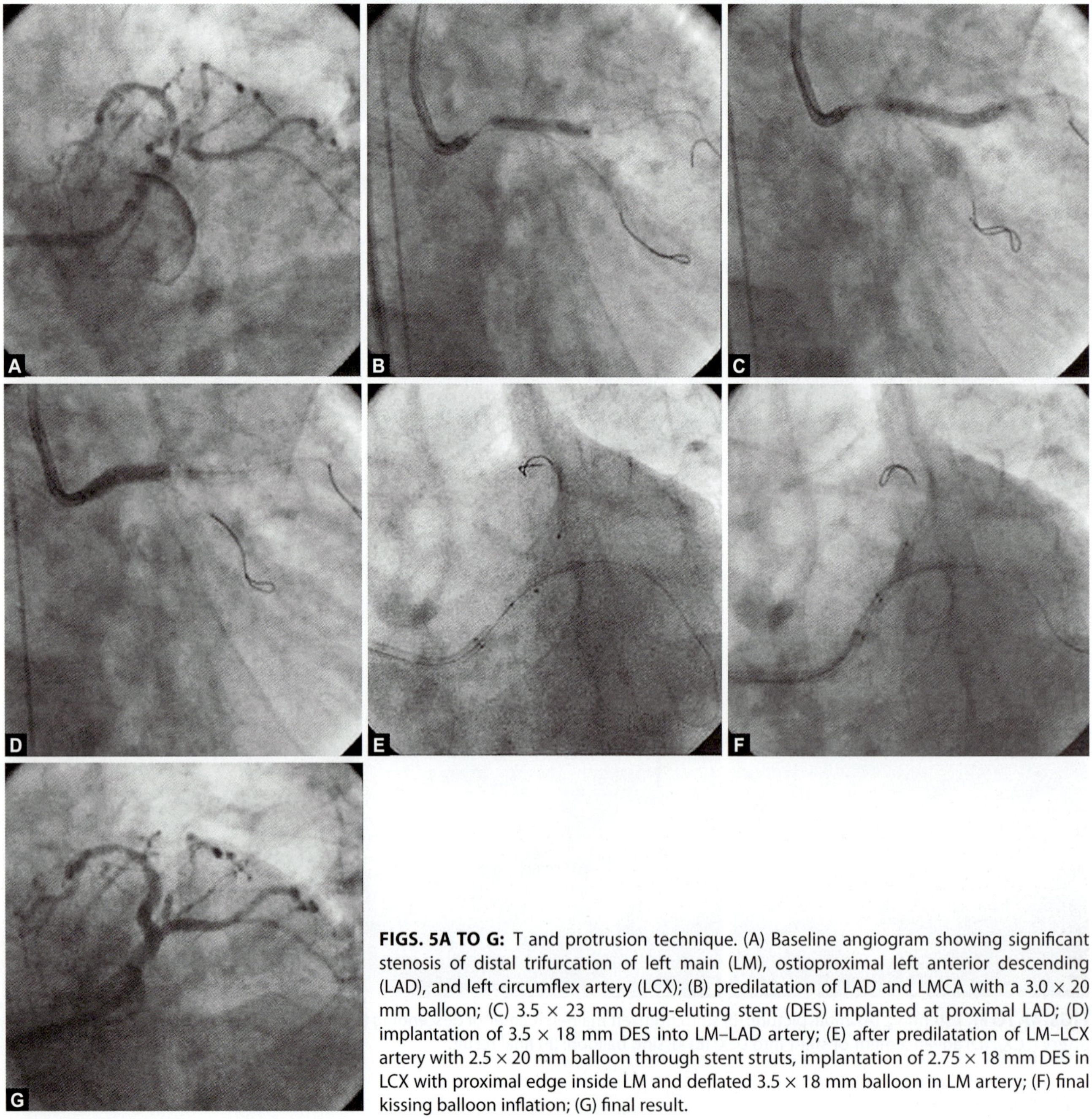

FIGS. 5A TO G: T and protrusion technique. (A) Baseline angiogram showing significant stenosis of distal trifurcation of left main (LM), ostioproximal left anterior descending (LAD), and left circumflex artery (LCX); (B) predilatation of LAD and LMCA with a 3.0 × 20 mm balloon; (C) 3.5 × 23 mm drug-eluting stent (DES) implanted at proximal LAD; (D) implantation of 3.5 × 18 mm DES into LM–LAD artery; (E) after predilatation of LM–LCX artery with 2.5 × 20 mm balloon through stent struts, implantation of 2.75 × 18 mm DES in LCX with proximal edge inside LM and deflated 3.5 × 18 mm balloon in LM artery; (F) final kissing balloon inflation; (G) final result.

in the SB through the stent struts and the struts dilated with a balloon. A second stent is then passed through the struts of the first stent into the side vessel, which leaves an overlap of both stents in the LM. The LM-LCX stent is then deployed. The wires are then recrossed and a mandatory final KBI is done. This technique provides an optimal reconstruction of distal LM bifurcation but with a significant area of stent overlap leading to more metal in the LM **(Figs. 6A to F)**.[19]

Mini-crush Stenting

The mini-crush technique is suitable for LM bifurcations in patients in whom the diameter of LAD is greater than LCX and the angle between LAD and LCX is <60°. This technique provides excellent coverage of the SB ostium. This technique is suitable for almost all true bifurcation lesions but should be avoided in wide angle bifurcation lesions.

The SB stent is first positioned in the SB after adequate predilatation, followed by advancement of MB stent. The SB stent is pulled back into the MB about 1–2 mm and is deployed. The MB is then stented at high pressure, usually above 12 atm which crushes the proximal SB stent against the LMCA wall. The SB (LCX) is then rewired through the stent struts of LAD and crushed LCX stent to perform the mandatory FKI. The disadvantage of this technique is that in order to perform FKI, multiple struts need to be recrossed with a wire and a balloon, which may be cumbersome **(Figs. 7A to G)**.[19]

Double-kiss Crush Stenting

Double-kiss crush is superior to culotte and provisional T-techniques for LM bifurcation in terms of target lesion failure (TLF), target vessel MI, and stent thrombosis. This has been clearly demonstrated in the DK-CRUSH III and DK-CRUSH V studies.[5]

The DK-crush technique begins with predilatation of LAD and LCX lesions. After placing an uninflated balloon in the LM, a stent (1:1 for the LCX) is deployed in the LCX protruding 1–2 mm into the LM. After confirming an optimal result in the circumflex and after removal of the stent balloon, the part of the LCX stent protruding in the LM is crushed by inflating the LM-LAD balloon. The LCX is then rewired through the crushed stent preferably through

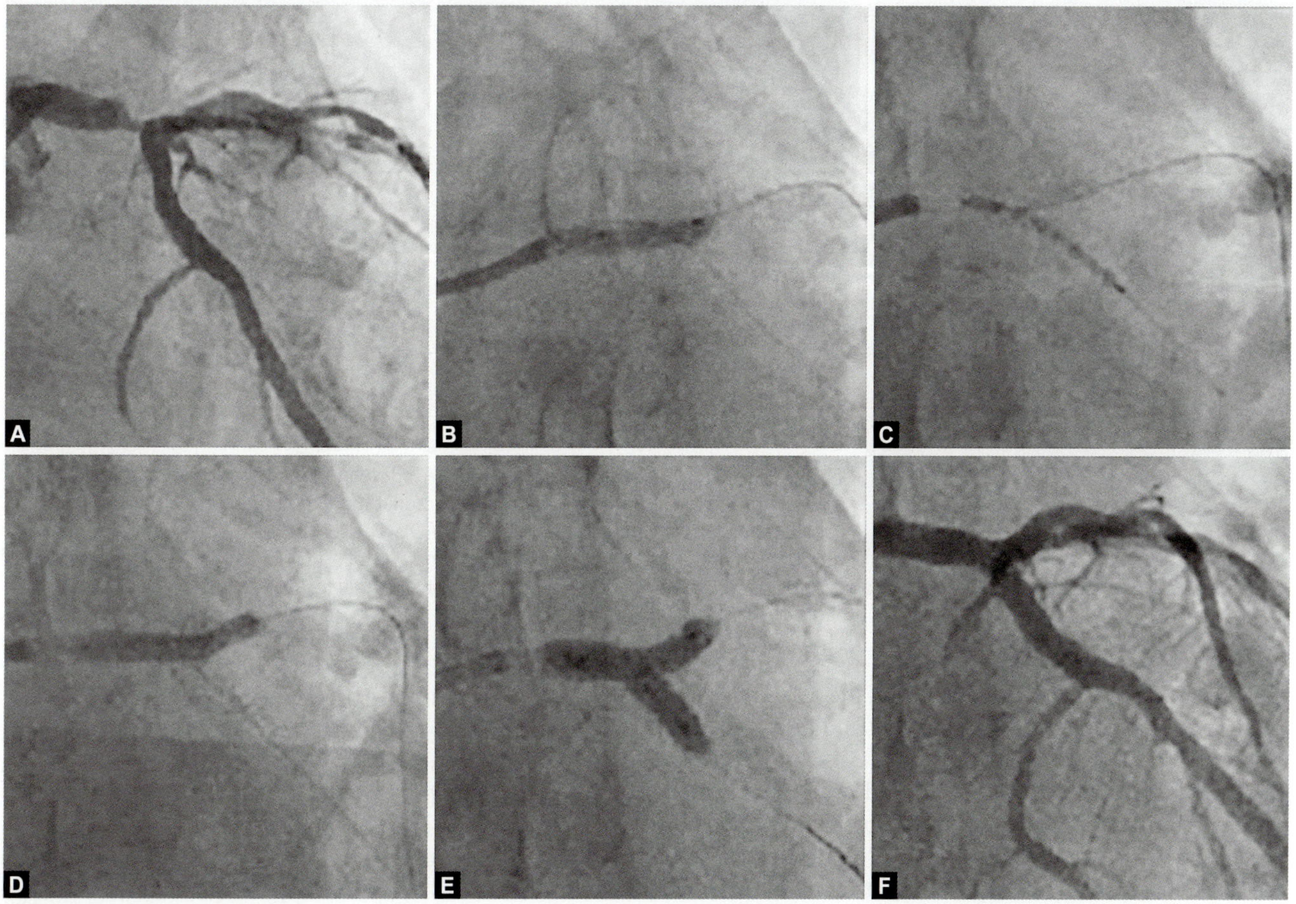

FIGS. 6A TO F: Culotte stenting. (A) Initial picture; (B) predilatation of the left anterior descending; (C) first stent deployed in the left circumflex; (D) second stent deployed in the left anterior descending after recrossing with wire and predilatation of stent strut; (E) kissing balloon postdilatation; (F) final result.

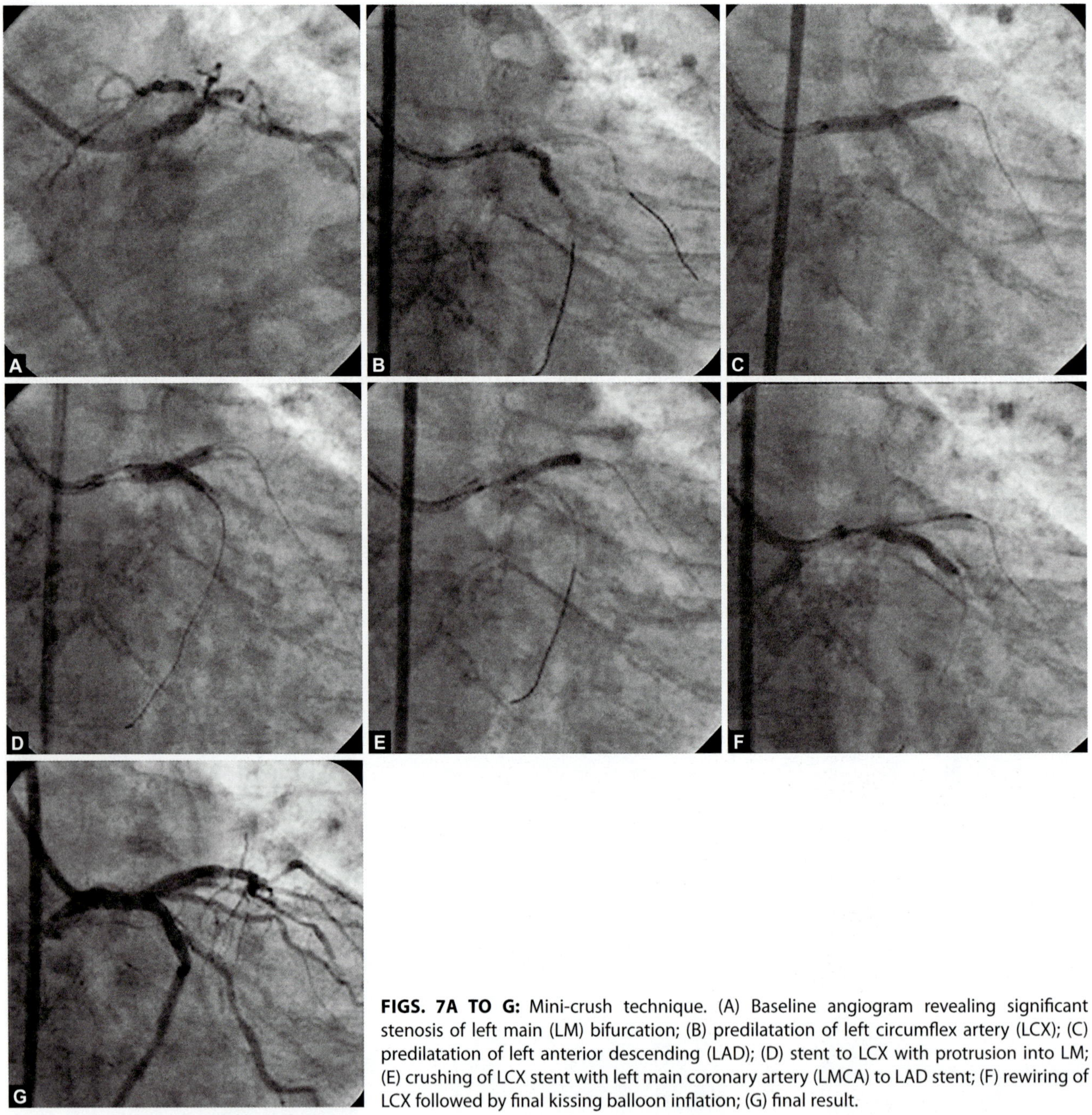

FIGS. 7A TO G: Mini-crush technique. (A) Baseline angiogram revealing significant stenosis of left main (LM) bifurcation; (B) predilatation of left circumflex artery (LCX); (C) predilatation of left anterior descending (LAD); (D) stent to LCX with protrusion into LM; (E) crushing of LCX stent with left main coronary artery (LMCA) to LAD stent; (F) rewiring of LCX followed by final kissing balloon inflation; (G) final result.

the proximal strut. Simultaneous KBI of the LCX and LM is performed (balloons sized 1:1 with LCX and LAD—the first kiss). A stent is then deployed in the LM extending into the LAD (sized 1:1 with the LAD), followed by proximal optimization technique (POT) of LM portion of the stent (balloon sized 1:1 with LM), then the LCX is rewired through the LM stent (crossing proximal stent strut), and simultaneous KBI is repeated (the second kiss), and then final re-POT of LM stent is performed **(Figs. 8A to H)**.[18,28]

V and the Simultaneous Kissing Stent

The V and simultaneous kissing stent (SKS) techniques are performed by placing and deploying two stents simultaneously. Wires are placed in LAD and LCX and the two stents are then placed into the LMCA extending into the respective branches and deployed by simultaneous inflation. If a variable amount of protrusion is allowed in the LM, it creates a long, double barrel; this technique is called SKS. The main advantage of this technique is that future

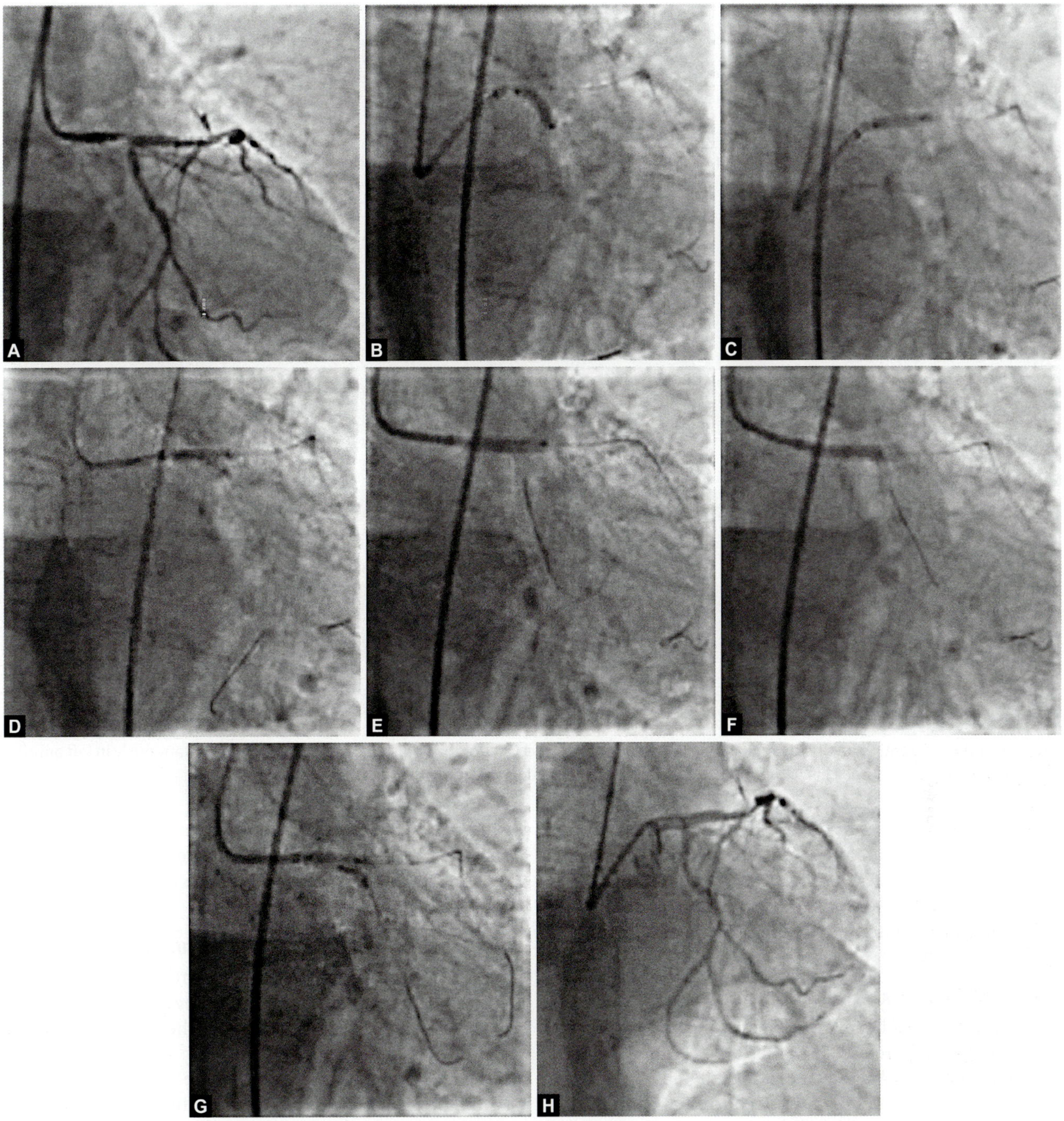

FIGS. 8A TO H: Double-kiss (DK) crush technique. (A) Baseline coronary angiography (CAG) revealing significant left main (LM) bifurcation lesion (Medina 1, 1, 1); (B) stenting of left circumflex artery (LCX); (C) crushing of LCX stent with noncompliant balloon placed in LM–LAD; (D) first kissing balloon inflation after first side branch (LCX) recross; (E) deployment of stent in LM–LAD; (F) proximal optimization technique in LM; (G) second kissing balloon inflation after high-pressure sequential dilatation of LAD and LCX; (H) final result.

access to both branches is well preserved with no need for rewiring as in other techniques. V stenting is relatively easy and quick and thus ideal for emergency situations. It is indicated in patients with a short LMCA-free disease and critical disease involving the ostia of LAD and LCX **(Figs. 9A to F)**.[19]

Double-kiss Culotte Technique

Contemporary stenting techniques for coronary bifurcation lesions have evolved to minimize stent layers at the SB ostium and to avoid incomplete vessel coverage to reduce restenosis at the SB origin.[29] DK culotte technique is an alternative to DK crush for appropriate lesions. This

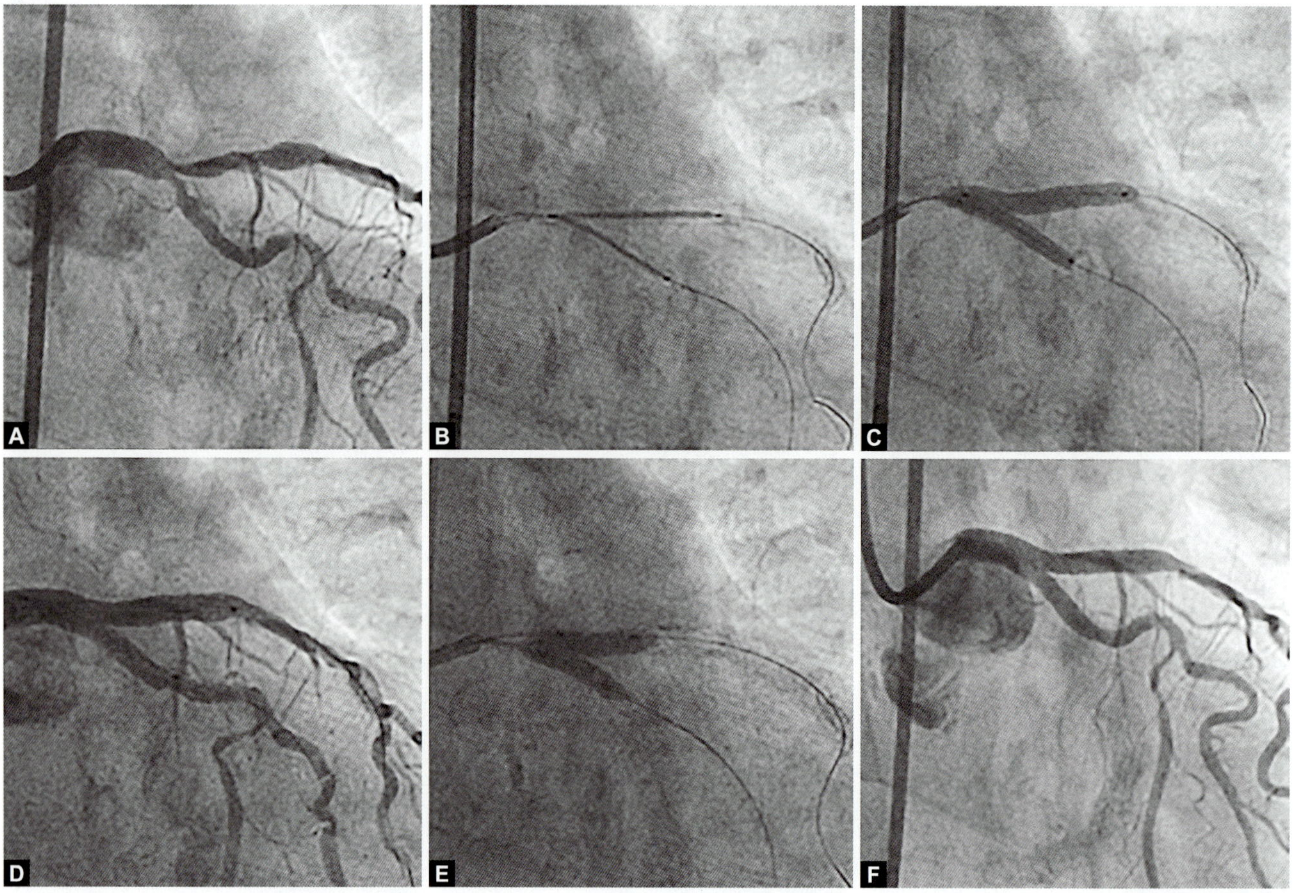

FIGS. 9A TO F: V stenting. (A) Initial appearance (Medina 0,1,1); (B and C) two drug-eluting stents implanted simultaneously in left anterior descending and left circumflex; (D) intermediate result; (E) postdilatation (kissing); (F) final angiographic result.

technique differs from conventional culotte by having an additional kissing balloon dilation performed after SB stenting and before MB stenting, which reduces stent malapposition.[30] The two variations of this technique are the standard DK culotte and the other is single-cell DK culotte technique.

Standard Double-kiss Culotte Technique

This technique has the following steps **(Figs. 10A to N)**: two guidewires (GWs) are used, i.e., the "MB-GW" and the "SB-GW" (A), the SB-GW is advanced into the SB (B), and the stent is deployed from MB to SB (C). Proximal optimization is done in the proximal MB (D). The MB-GW is removed and reintroduced into the distal MB, crossing the stent at the most distal cell (E). The cell can be first dilated with a small balloon for easy access (F). The first kissing dilation is performed next using balloons according to the diameter of the distal branches. Deflation is done simultaneously (G). The SB-GW is removed next and a stent deployed from the proximal to distal MB (H). POT is then performed (I). The SB-GW is then introduced into the SB, crossing the previously implanted stent at the most distal cell (J). The cell can be first dilated with a small balloon for easy access (K). Next, the second kissing balloon dilation is performed, using balloons according to the distal branch diameters. First, the MB balloon is inflated followed by the SB balloon. Deflation is done simultaneously (L). As a final step, proximal optimization is again performed.[30]

Single-cell Double-kiss Culotte Technique

After insertion of guidewires into each branch and performing IVUS for appropriate sizing, the following steps are done for single-cell DK culotte technique (the first four steps are performed outside the body):

1. The SB stent is prepared outside the guide catheter. The proximal few millimeters of the stent are partially uncovered and the stent is slowly inflated to 2–3 atm. Once the proximal struts open, the stent balloon is deflated **(Fig. 11A)**.
2. Distal part of the MB guidewire is inserted through the single proximal open strut **(Fig. 11B)**.
3. MB balloon [noncompliant (NC) sized 1:1] is loaded on the MB guidewire and advanced through the open stent strut **(Fig. 11C)**.
4. The stent is loaded onto the SB guidewire and then carefully crimped back for deployment **(Figs. 11D and E)**.
5. Entire unit (MB-NC balloon and SB stent) is advanced together into the coronary artery **(Figs. 11F to H)**. The

SB stent is now in position (with one cell strut covering the SB ostium) and the MB-NC balloon is in position to perform the first KB inflation after SB stent deployment **(Fig. 11I)**.

6. SB stent is first deployed **(Fig. 11J)**.
7. SB stent balloon and MB balloon are then simultaneously inflated to perform the first kissing **(Fig. 11K)**.
8. Both SB and MB balloons are removed. SB wire is also removed.
9. MB stent is now deployed **(Fig. 11L)**.
10. POT in the LM done **(Fig. 11M)**.
11. The SB is rewired through distal-most cell.
12. SB and MB NC balloons sized 1:1 used to perform second KBI **(Fig. 11N)**, followed by a final POT **(Figs. 11A to N)**.[31]

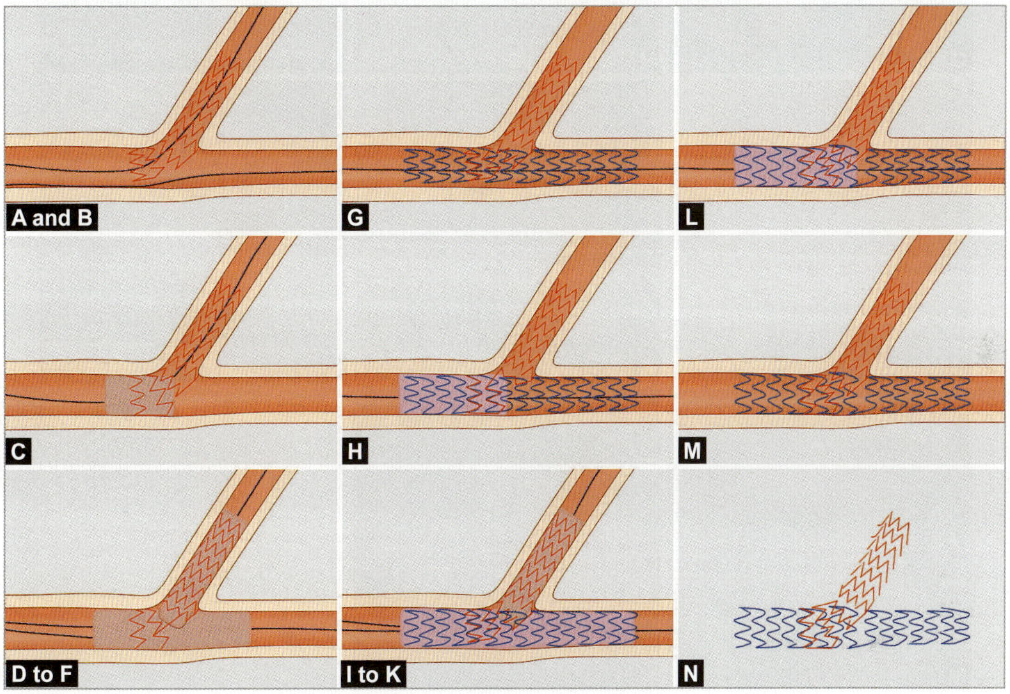

FIGS. 10A TO N: Steps of the double kiss (DK) culotte technique. Details are given in text.

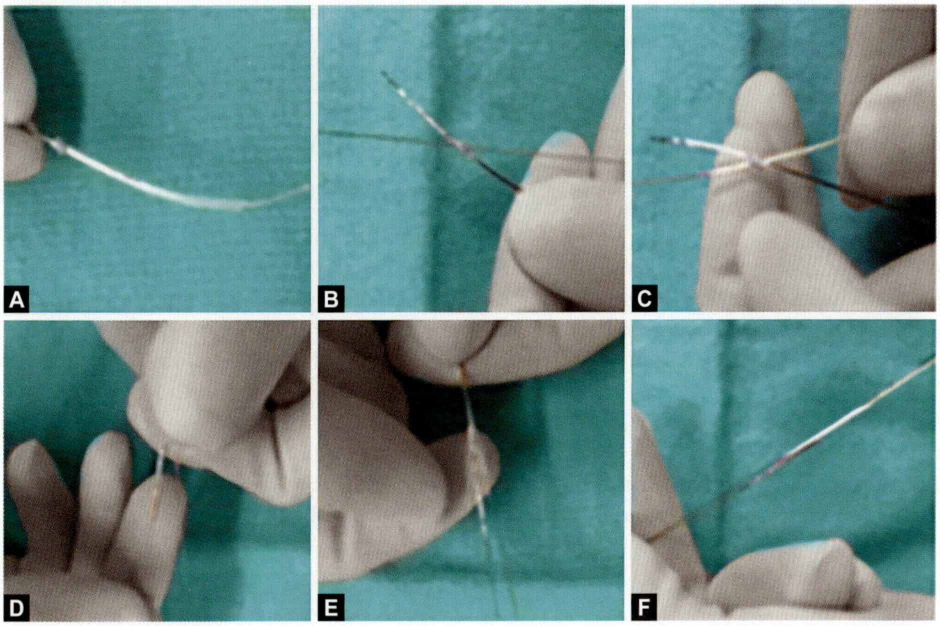

FIGS. 11A TO N: *Continued*

Continued

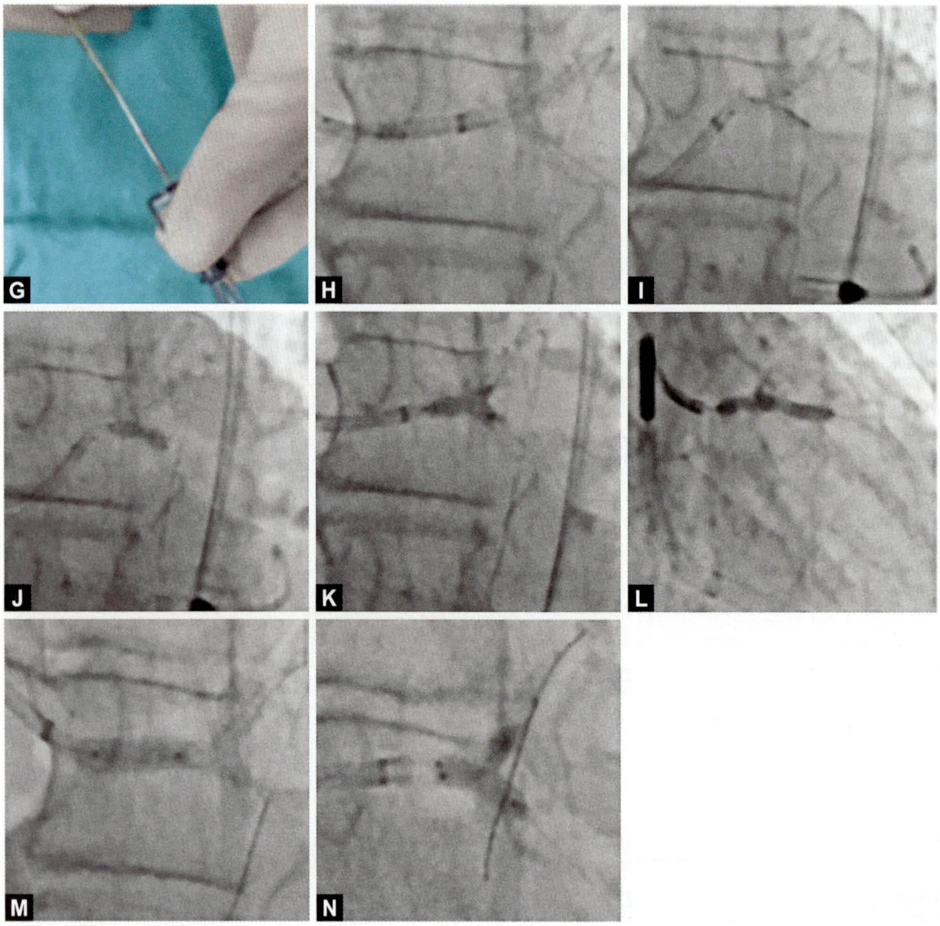

FIGS. 11A TO N: Double-kiss (DK) culotte technique. (A) The proximal few millimeters of stent struts are uncovered; (B) the distal MB guidewire is inserted through a single-stent strut; (C) the MB balloon is loaded on the MB guidewire and advanced through the stent struts; (D and E) the stent is loaded on the SB wire and crimped back; (F to I) the MB balloon and SB stent are advanced as a unit in position in the coronary artery; (J) SB stent deployment; (K) first KBI; (L) MB stent deployed; (M) proximal optimization technique; (N) second KBI.
(KBI: kissing balloon inflation; MB: main branch; SB: side branch).

Advantages of the DK culotte technique:[31]

- Wire access is maintained in the MB throughout the procedure. The SB wire is only removed once the SB stent is deployed.
- Insertion of the MB guidewire through stent struts and premounting the MB balloon outside the guide catheter eliminate the initial guidewire crossing and delivering the balloon through stent struts which are already deployed.
- Accurate positioning of the SB stent with good carinal coverage is ensured.
- This technique minimizes steps within the coronary arteries as the first few steps are performed outside the body.

INTRACORONARY IMAGING AND PHYSIOLOGY FOR LMCA DISEASE

Evaluation of the LMCA lesion by coronary angiography (CAG) is sometimes hampered due to various factors such as lack of a reference segment, lesion eccentricity, varying angulations, overlapping branches, and foreshortening.

A more detailed evaluation of the severity and hemodynamic significance of borderline LMCA lesions can be obtained by invasive intracoronary imaging with IVUS or physiologically with pressure wire assessment of the fractional flow reserve (FFR) to improve and guide the appropriate PCI strategy and PCI optimization in LM PCI practice.[32]

Intravascular Ultrasound Guidance

Intravascular ultrasound is useful to determine the vessel size, lumen area, and plaque extent and distribution within the LMCA and its MB, the LAD and LCX.[33] The IVUS-derived MLA provides information on the ischemic burden due to LMCA stenosis. An old US study suggested an MLA cutoff value of 5.9 mm^2 with a sensitivity and specificity of 93% and 94%, respectively, for an FFR of <0.75.[34] Since then, many studies evaluating the use of IVUS in intermediate LMCA disease demonstrated that an MLA of ≥6 mm^2 on IVUS is safe for deferring revascularization for intermediate LMCA stenoses. Currently, an MLA of ≥6 mm^2 is generally accepted as the safe and optimal cutoff value for deferring treatment for LMCA disease.

Intravascular ultrasound also provides additional information on distal LMCA and bifurcation stenoses extending into LAD and LCX. Ideally, pullbacks from both LAD and LCX should be used to obtain complete information on LMCA bifurcation to avoid overestimation of the MLA within the LCX ostium which can happen if only an LAD pullback is taken.[35]

The other important role of IVUS is ensuring stent optimization in LMCA PCI. IVUS imaging can identify stent underexpansion or malapposition, edge dissection, or significant residual disease, which is difficult to be detected on CAG. Thus, the use of IVUS guidance is naturally associated with improved clinical outcomes, particularly in patients with LMCA bifurcation treated with a two-stent strategy as the malapposition or underexpansion can be duly corrected.[36,37] The proposed IVUS-derived minimal stent area is the best criteria that predicted angiographic restenosis were 5.0 mm^2 for the LCX ostium, 6.3 mm^2 for the LAD ostium, 7.2 mm^2 for the polygon of confluence, and 8.2 mm^2 for the distal LMCA (the so-called 5-6-7-8 rule).[29]

Thus, use of IVUS may be clinically relevant in reducing event rates and improving long-term outcomes **(Figs. 12A to I)**.

Optical Coherence Tomography

Optical coherence tomography (OCT) requires selective, coaxial LMCA guide catheter engagement and it makes comprehensive LMCA assessment challenging. The prospective, multicenter LEMON (LEft Main Octguided iNterventions) trial showed adequate expansion in 86% of the patients with mid/distal LMCA stenosis in enrolled patients.[39] OCT has inherent limitations in ostial LM lesions due to inadequate blood clearance. The imaging determinants of escalation from the provisional to two-stent strategy on OCT are plaque distribution and plaque morphology. OCT imaging also confirms proper LM stent expansion, apposition, and geometry like IVUS **(Fig. 13)**.[39]

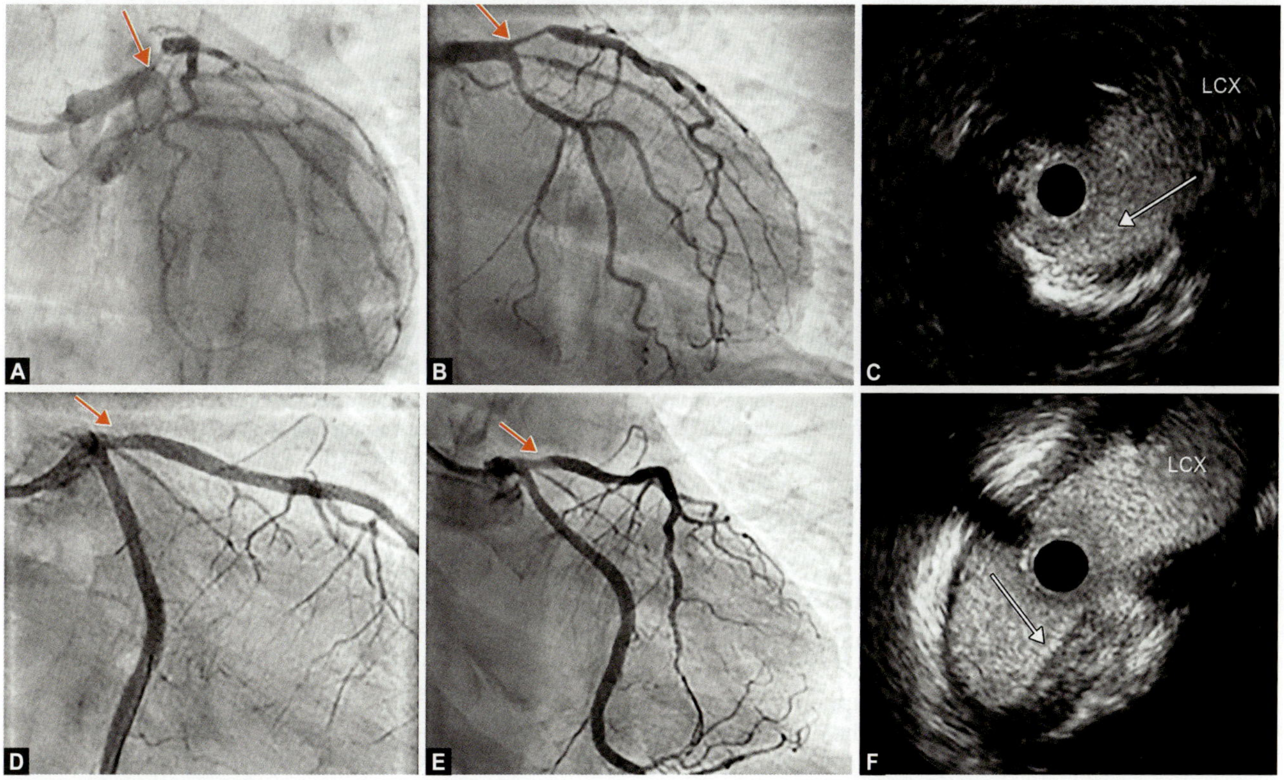

FIGS. 12A TO I: *Continued*

Continued

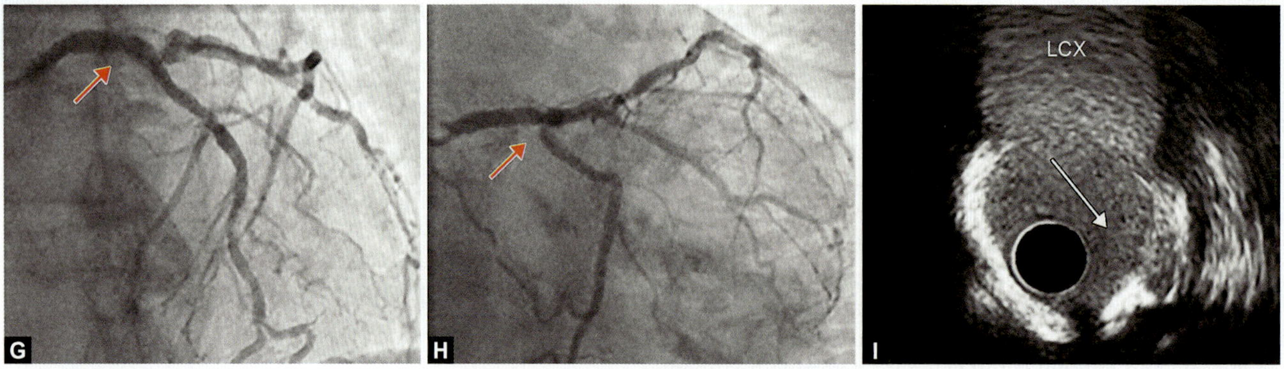

FIGS. 12A TO I: Representative cases of intravascular ultrasound (IVUS) guidance in evaluation and treatment of left main coronary artery (LMCA) bifurcation lesions.[38] (A and B) Angiographic images of ostial left anterior descending (LAD) stenosis suggesting no LMCA involvement (red arrows). (C) Cross-sectional IVUS showing ostial LAD fibrocalcific plaque extending into LMCA distal bifurcation (white arrow). (D and E) Angiographic images of ostial LAD hazy plaque with intermediate narrowing (red arrows). (F) Cross-sectional IVUS shows soft plaque at the LAD ostium with severe stenosis extending into LMCA (MLA: 4.88 mm^2) (white arrow). (G and H) Angiographic images of mildly diseased LMCA bifurcation. (I) Cross-sectional IVUS shows critical and severely calcified LMCA bifurcation (MLA: 4.35 mm^2) (white arrow).

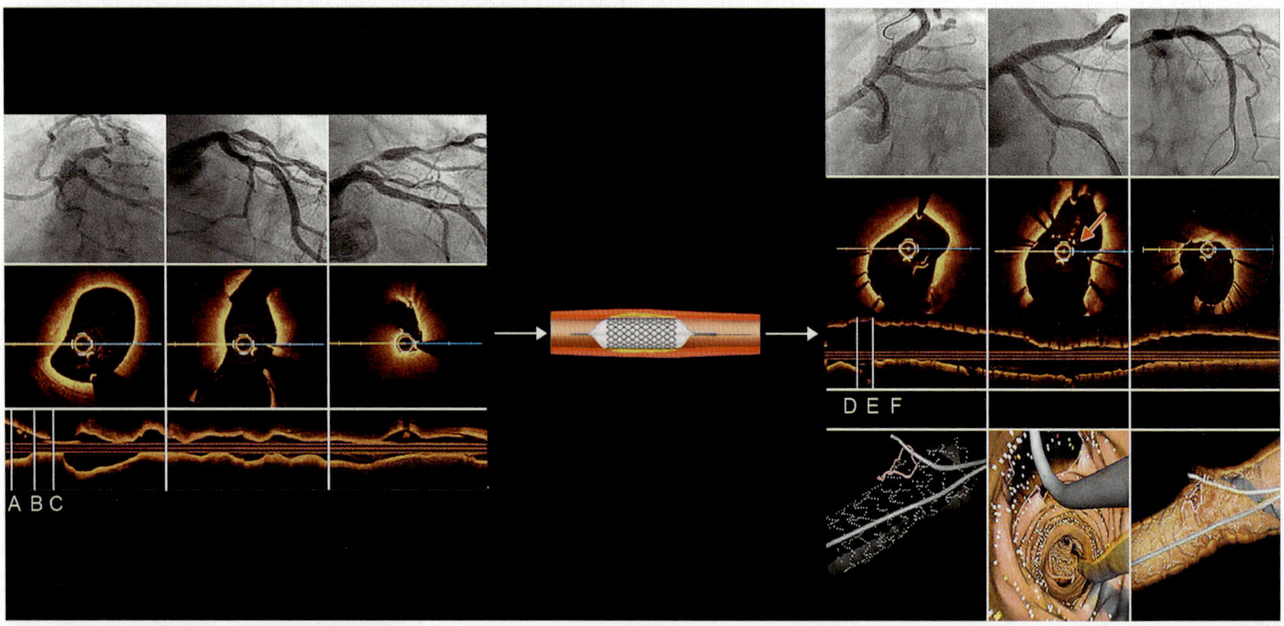

FIG. 13: Representative cases of optical coherence tomography (OCT) guidance in evaluation and treatment of ostial LAD disease involving left main coronary artery (LMCA) bifurcation. (Left) Cross-section A: thin-cap fibroatheroma at LMCA shaft; cross-section B: LMCA bifurcation stenosis minimal lumen area (MLA); cross-section C: ostial left anterior descending artery (LAD) with image of intimal dissection after predilatation. (Right) Cross-section D: strut apposition at LMCA shaft; cross-section E: strut apposition at LMCA bifurcation toward LAD with overhanging struts in front of right coronary artery ostium (red arrow); cross-section F: strut apposition at LAD ostium.

Fractional Flow Reserve Assessment

The functional significance of angiographically challenging LMCA lesions should be further evaluated. As angiography alone has inherent limitations in accurate evaluation of functionally significant LMCA disease, there are significant interobserver variations and poor correlation between the severity of angiographic stenosis and functional significance.[40,41] Various trials showed a 30–40% visual-functional mismatch in intermediate LMCA disease with functional assessment,[40,42] and such intermediate LMCA lesions with FFR values of >0.75 or 0.80 were safely deferred.[40,43] Of late, the instantaneous wave-free ratio (iFR) which was introduced as a resting index of functional coronary stenosis showed that deferring the revascularization of non-LMCA obstructive CAD with an iFR of >0.89 is safe and is supported by compelling clinical data.[44,45] Furthermore, the FFR interpretation in LMCA lesions should be done carefully in cases with the presence of downstream LAD and LCX stenoses, which may underestimate the hemodynamic significance of LMCA disease.[46]

An observational study in Korea evaluated the long-term impact of FFR in jailed LCX branch after simple LMCA–LAD crossover stenting.[47] The patients with a high FFR in the jailed LCX had better 5-year TLF than those patients with a low FFR. TLF was defined in this study as a composite of cardiac death, target vessel MI, or target lesion revascularization. This suggests that FFR measurement in the jailed LCX after LM crossover stenting can be helpful in selecting a proper treatment strategy and may reduce unnecessary escalation to a two-stent strategy. Among patients with concomitant multivessel disease, the use of physiology-guided revascularization significantly reduced the rate of major adverse cardiac and cerebrovascular events (MACCEs) as shown in the FAME (Fractional Flow Reserve versus Angiography for Multivessel Evaluation) trial. The FAME trial showed that physiology-guided PCI for multivessel CAD resulted in a significant reduction of a composite of death or MI as compared to angiography-guided PCI.[48]

DUAL ANTIPLATELET THERAPY

Coronary bifurcation lesions may act as focus of turbulent flow with an enhanced propensity for platelet aggregation, plaque rupture, and thrombosis. The geometry of vascular bifurcations carries an intrinsic higher risk of periprocedural strut malapposition and stent underexpansion. This translates into a stent thrombosis incidence rate of 1.5–2% in bifurcation PCIs, which is almost twice as high as compared with nonbifurcation PCIs.[49]

European guidelines recommend a longer dual antiplatelet therapy (DAPT) duration for both acute coronary syndrome (ACS) and stable CAD complex PCI (class IIb, level of evidence: B).

A patient-level pooled analysis of five nationwide multicenter registries on LMCA PCI, showed the risks for TLF and thrombotic adverse cardiovascular events to be significantly higher in the two-stent group than in the one-stent group when DAPT was interrupted <1 year [hazard ratio (HR) 2.78; 95% confidence interval (CI) 1.25–6.19], while it was similar in those maintaining DAPT > 1 year (HR 0.51; 95% CI 0.15–1.69).[50]

Risk stratification for antiplatelet therapy is based on clinical presentation, baseline bleeding risk, stenting strategy, and systematic use of intracoronary imaging and should be meticulously followed according to the European Bifurcation Club (EBC) consensus on antithrombotic therapy after PCI of bifurcation lesions.[51,52]

MECHANICAL CIRCULATORY SUPPORT

In patients with ACS, severe LV dysfunction, and hemodynamic instability undergoing LMCA intervention, mechanical circulatory support may often be required. These devices provide cardiac output sufficient to maintain myocardial flow and end-organ perfusion, and help unload the left ventricle during the procedure. Currently, the percutaneous mechanical circulatory devices available are: intra-aortic balloon pump (IABP), Impella, extracorporeal membrane oxygenator, and the TandemHeart. IABP is the most commonly available device but is associated with low efficacy. Impella provides a higher cardiac output and may be considered in high-risk LM PCI or during severe shock.[53] It is very important to plan the device strategy prior to the commencement of LM intervention, rather than doing a crash insertion.

LEFT MAIN BIFURCATION STENTING: TIPS AND TRICKS

Left Circumflex Artery Wiring Techniques[31,54-56]

- A workhorse/polymer-jacketed guidewire should be used for jailing the wire.
- The more difficult vessel should always be wired first—to reduce the risk of wire twisting around a previously placed guidewire (wire wrap).
- *Guidewire tip*: Four basic curves are commonly used—single bend with short tip (2–3 mm); single bend with long tip (4–6 mm); single wide bend (if the main artery wire is to be used for LCX rewiring); and double-bend shape.
- For wide carinal angles, a wide smooth bend or double-bend tip should be used.
- *Antegrade wiring*: Here, the wire is advanced directly from the proximal LM into the LCX ostium, without going into LAD.
- *Pullback wiring*: The wire is withdrawn from the distal LM–LAD into the bifurcation and redirected into the ostial LCX. A broad smooth distal tip curve (fish hook-like bend) helps the guidewire to easily engage the LCX during the pullback.
- *Reverse wire technique*: This is used for extreme angles (>150°). A hairpin bend is created about 3–5 cm from the wire tip. The guidewire with the hairpin bend is advanced into the distal MB (LAD) vessel. Once the guidewire is in the LAD, it is pulled back toward the bifurcation and once the tip of the guidewire enters the LCX, gentle counterclockwise rotation will advance the wire in the LCX.
- *Deflectable tip/microcatheter guidewire technique*: The guidewire is loaded onto a microcatheter with a deflectable tip. The microcatheter is advanced just distal to the origin of the SB (LCX). The guidewire is then retracted into the microcatheter and the catheter's tip is deflected toward the LCX and the wire advanced through the deflected catheter into the LCX.
- *Last resort for difficult LCX wiring*: Perform LM predilatation. This causes plaque or carina shift and

helps to wire the LCX. Alternatively, perform debulking techniques such as rotational atherectomy.

- *Balloon block and support technique*: A balloon is inflated about 1–2 mm from the carina in the distal main branch (LAD). It helps advance the guidewire into the LCX. Balloon to LAD diameter ratio should be 1:1 and the balloon inflation should be at low pressure around 8–10 atm. The balloon is deflated once guidewire reaches the mid-LCX.

Left Circumflex Rewiring after LM Stent Implant[55]

- The goal in this case is to recross from a distal stent strut of the LM–LAD stent as this is associated with improved ostial scaffolding and good short- and long-term outcomes.
- The LCX can be rewired with the LM–LAD guidewire before removing the jailed LCX wire and then the jailed SB wire can be retracted from the LCX and redirected into the LM–LAD vessel. A third wire can be used if it is important to keep the MB wire in situ.
- Pullback rewiring technique is usually preferred to access the distal stent strut.
- A guidewire with a wide curve allows the wire to slide across the LM–LAD stent struts during pullback and protrude into the LCX once the LCX ostium is reached.
- To avoid using a third wire, the distal tip of the LM–LAD wire can be preshaped to match the angulation of the LCX and the diameter of the LM, i.e., primary and secondary curves.
- An underexpanded stent in the LM can provide difficulties in recrossing into the LCX. Hence, POT should be routinely performed to aid LCX rewiring.

SUMMARY

Figure 14 summarizes the algorithmic approach for LMCA bifurcation lesions in a stepwise manner.[43]

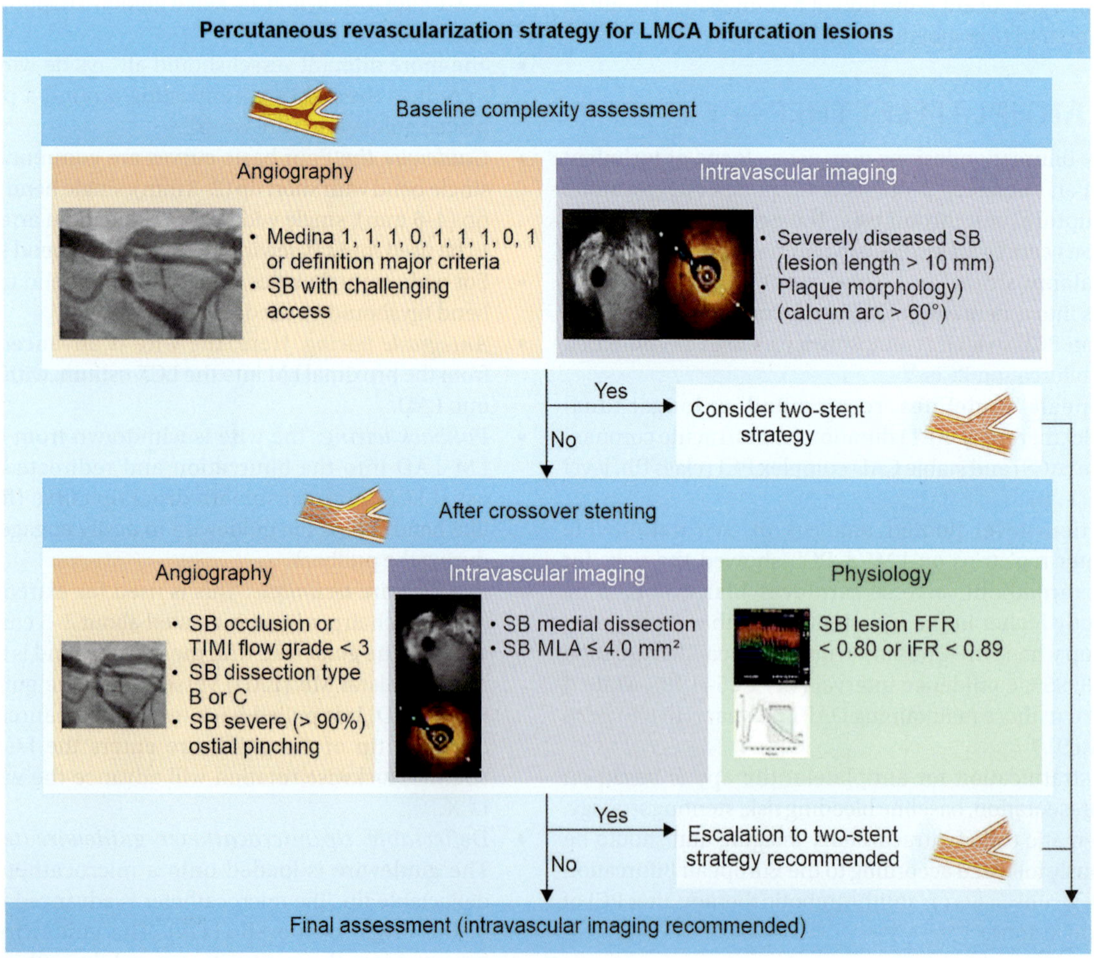

FIG. 14: Algorithm for LMCA bifurcation lesion treatment.

(FFR: fractional flow reserve; iFR: instantaneous wave-free ratio; LMCA: left main coronary artery; MLA: minimal lumen area; SB: side branch; TIMI: thrombolysis in myocardial infarction)

CONCLUSION

Over the past few decades, there have been remarkable advancements in stent technology and PCI techniques. There have been tremendous advances in intracoronary imaging, physiologic guidance, and adjunctive pharmacotherapy which have helped to progressively improve clinical outcomes of LMCA PCI. The heart team approach can play an important role in tailored decision-making in individual patients as there is no single appropriate approach for LMCA revascularization. Further efforts are required to optimize procedural outcomes and to improve adjunctive medical management in different LMCA revascularization strategies.

ONLINE REFERENCES

Please scan the QR code provided at the end of the table of contents for References of this chapter.

CHAPTER 146

Two-stent Strategy for Bifurcation: Current Best Practices

Vaibhav Bandil, Suman Bhandari

ABSTRACT

Bifurcation lesions are common and associated with higher risks of major cardiac events and restenosis after percutaneous coronary intervention (PCI). Treatment requires understanding of lesion characteristics, stent design, and therapeutic options. We review the evidence for provisional versus two-stent techniques. We conclude that provisional stenting is suitable for most bifurcation lesions. We detail situations where a two-stent technique should be considered and the steps for performing each of the two-step techniques. We review the importance of lesion preparation, intracoronary imaging, proximal optimization technique (POT), and kissing balloon inflation.

Keywords: Bifurcation, two stent techniques, POT.

INTRODUCTION

For anatomical reasons and because of the distributive function of the coronary tree, bifurcation sites are prone to the development of atherosclerotic lesions, as a result of flow turbulence generating proatherogenic low-wall shear stress. Bifurcation lesions account for up to 30% of lesions in patients with multivessel coronary artery disease. The treatment of bifurcation lesions remains a controversial problem in terms of therapeutic indications, interventional strategy, and technical considerations.

FUNDAMENTAL ASPECTS (FIG. 1)

In the coronary tree, there is a linear relationship between the diameter of the vessel, flow, and perfused myocardial mass. Coronary artery branching complies with the fractal geometry pattern and its self-similarity principle.[1]

The asymmetric branching is repeated throughout the coronary tree following the branching law described in 1923 as Murray's law:[2] D^3mother = D^3daughter1 + D^3daughter2.

This law was recently modified by Kassab:[3] D2/^{3}mother = D2/^{3}daughter1 + D2/^{3}daughter2.

The Finet's formula,[4] as validated in the coronary arteries by intravascular ultrasound (IVUS), is easier to use: Dmother = (Ddaughter1 + Ddaughter2) × 0.678.

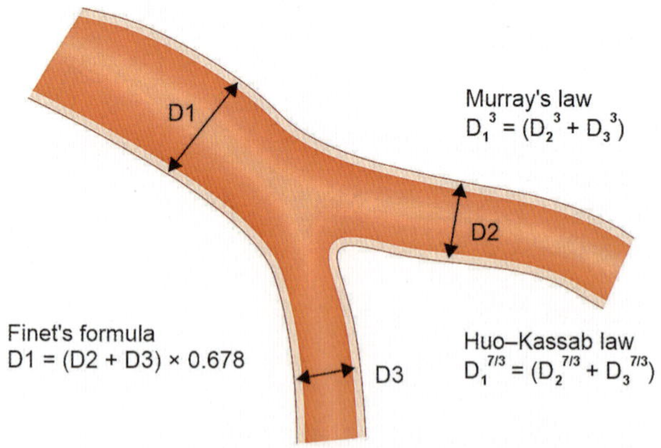

FIG. 1: The relationship between the diameter of the proximal segment of the main branch and the two distal segments.

DEFINITION OF BIFURCATIONS AND ANATOMIC CONSIDERATIONS (FIG. 2)

The most common classification system for bifurcation lesions is the Medina classification. This is a three-digit binary code which defines a bifurcation by the presence of disease proximal and distal to the bifurcation in the main vessel (MV) and presence/absence of disease in the side branch (SB).[5]

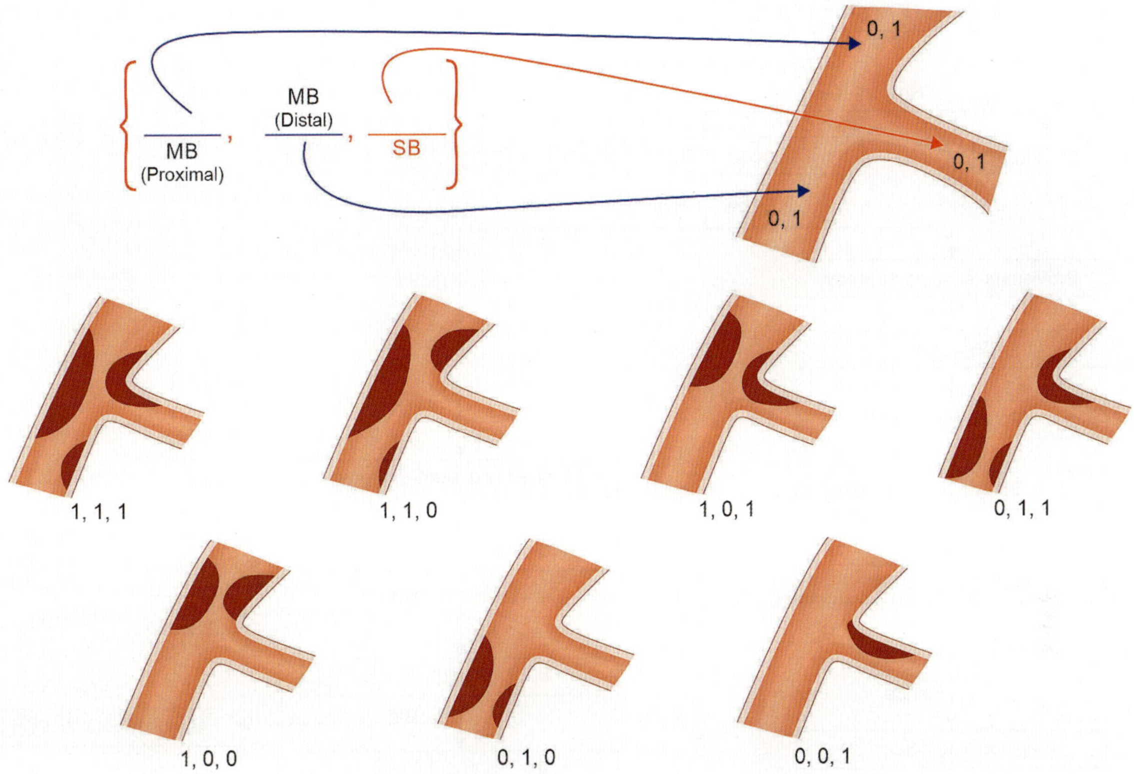

FIG. 2: Modified Medina classification. An anatomical-based description of the three components of a bifurcation lesion. Before the first comma, 1 or 0 depending on the presence or not of >50% stenosis in the proximal main vessel, between the two commas the same for distal main vessel, after the second comma the same for SB.

(MB: main branch; SB: side branch)

CHOOSING A STRATEGY FOR BIFURCATION TREATMENT

The choice of approach for treatment of bifurcations depends on the lesion characteristics and complexity.[6] The current European Bifurcation Club (EBC) guidelines[7] suggest that PS may be the preferred option for most lesions, while an upfront two-stent strategy may be considered for more complex lesions with a large SB supplying a significant myocardial territory.

LESION PREPARATION AND USE OF INTRACORONARY IMAGING

The lesion must be adequately prepared to ensure full-stent expansion. There should be a low threshold for intracoronary imaging as this will guide lesion preparation and size of stent(s). Cutting and scoring balloons are helpful for fibrotic and mild/moderately calcified lesions, while severely calcified lesions may require rotablation. More recently, intravascular lithoplasty using the Shockwave balloon (Shockwave Medical, Santa Clara) has emerged as a promising treatment for circumferential calcification.[8]

During bifurcation stenting, optical coherence tomography (OCT) allows identification of whether wire cross is through a proximal or distal strut.[9,10] Following stent implantation, IVUS and OCT may be used to ensure optimal stent expansion.

GUIDING CATHETER SELECTION

Most bifurcation lesions can be approached with a 6-Fr guiding catheter because a provisional strategy will be utilized most of the times. When the operator needs to make a decision following predilatation, we suggest usage of a 7- or 8-Fr guiding catheter. If 6-Fr guiding catheter is employed, the two stents can only be inserted and deployed sequentially. The standard crush technique and the V or kissing stents technique cannot be performed unless a guiding catheter of 7 or 8 Fr is utilized.

GENERAL OUTLINE WHEN TREATING A BIFURCATION LESION

Flowchart 1 summarizes a proposed approach to bifurcation lesions with an attempt to give directions regarding SB stenting as intention-to-treat only in cases where disease on the SB extends beyond the ostium and the SB has a significant area of distribution.

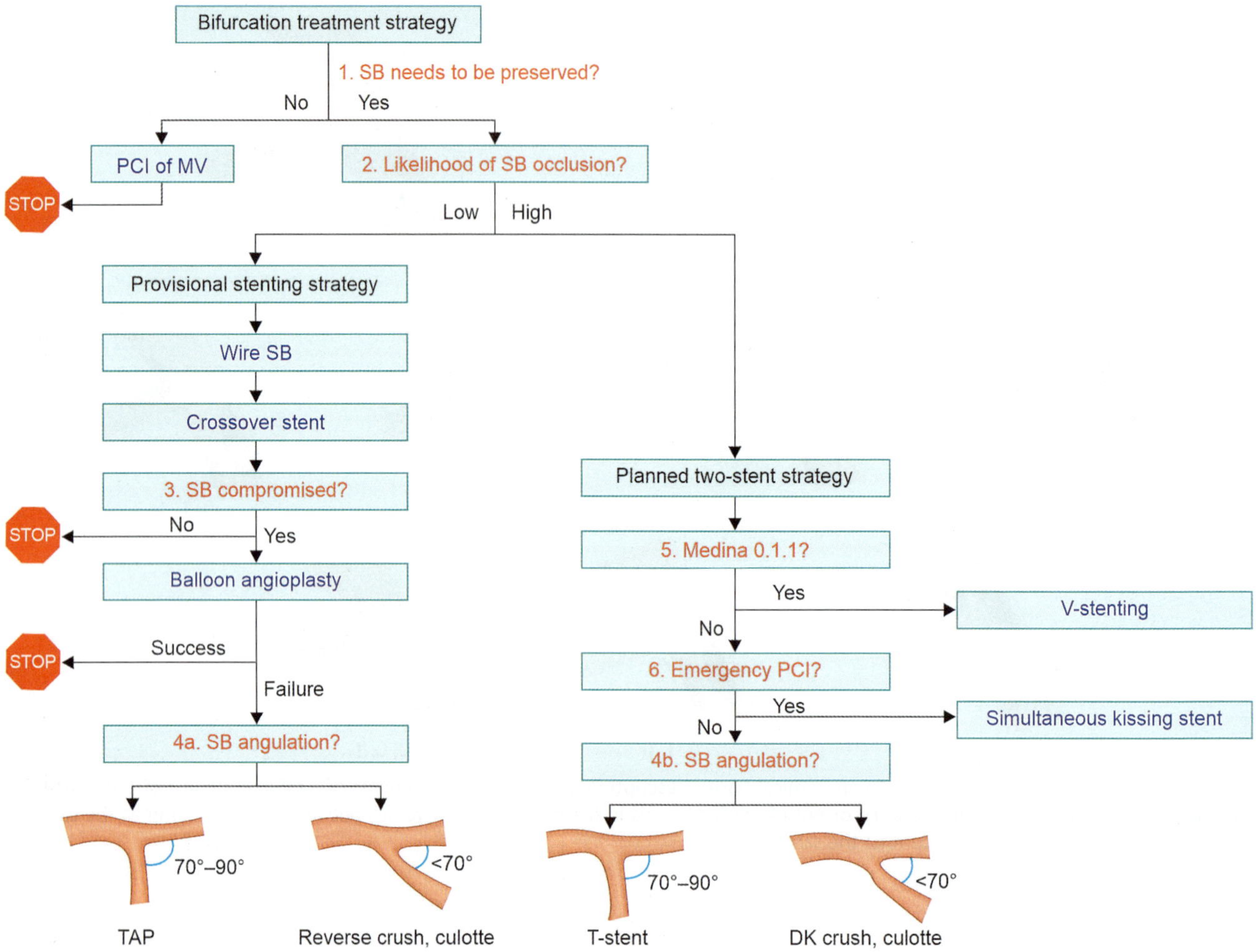

FLOWCHART 1: Algorithm for approaching coronary bifurcation lesions.
(MV: main vessel; SB: side branch; PCI: percutaneous coronary intervention; TAP: T and protrusion; DK crush: double kissing crush)

PROVISIONAL SB STENTING[11]

Steps

1. Placement of two wires (MB and SB)
2. Predilatation of MB or both branches, when needed[12]
3. Stenting of the MB
4. Stent optimization with proximal optimization technique (POT)
5. Recrossing with a wire into the SB
6. Crossing with a balloon into the SB
7. Performance of final kissing balloon inflation (FKBI), with moderate pressure (8 atm) in the SB, until the balloon is fully expanded
8. Final POT, if result in the SB is adequate after FKBI[11]
9. Placement of a second stent in the SB when the result is unsatisfactory [>75% residual stenosis, dissection, thrombolysis in myocardial infarction (TIMI) flow grade <3 in a SB ≥2.5 mm or fractional flow reserve (FFR) <0.80]

In the provisional technique, wire crosses through the distal strut (the "carina strut") following MB stenting is strongly suggested because it creates better SB scaffolding than proximal crossing.[10] If the result remains unsatisfactory after MB stenting, SB stenting should be performed with T stenting or T stent and protrusion (TAP)-stenting, reverse/internal crush or culotte, followed by kissing balloon inflation.[10]

TWO-STENT STRATEGIES

Second Stent in Side Branch Following Provisional Approach

When we are not satisfied with the result obtained with balloon dilatation of the SB, we implant a second stent using one of the following strategies: T, TAP, culotte, or reverse/internal crush configuration.

T Technique

This technique is the one most frequently utilized to transition from provisional stenting to stenting the SB.[13,14] The T technique consists in advancing a second stent into the SB (following adequate dilation of the MB stent struts). The stent

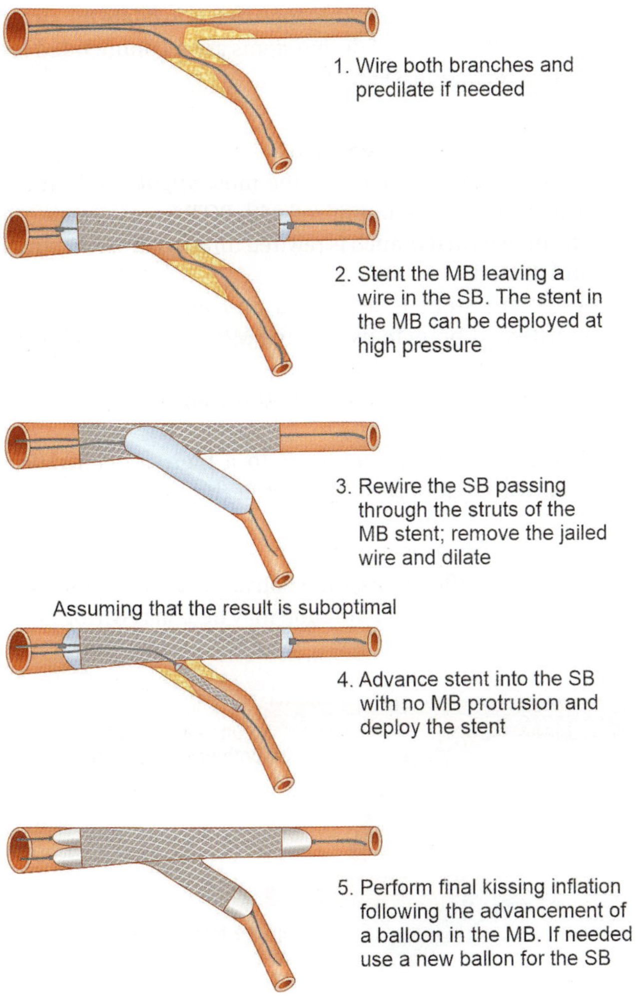

FIG. 3: A schematic representation of the T technique.
(MB: main branch; SB: side branch)

is positioned at the ostium of the SB trying to minimize any possible gap. A second kissing balloon inflation is also performed.

The T technique is associated with the risk of leaving a small gap between the stents implanted in the MB and the SB which may be a factor contributing to ostial restenosis at the SB **(Fig. 3)**.

T Stenting and Small Protrusion

The TAP technique is a modification of the T stenting technique and is based on an intentional minimal protrusion of the SB stent within the MB.[15,16]

Steps:
1. A second stent is advanced in the SB in a way to minimally protrude (1or 2 mm) into the MB.
2. A balloon is advanced in the MB.
3. The SB stent is deployed as usual (12 atm or more), and the MB balloon is simultaneously inflated at 12 atm or more.
4. Both balloons are deflated and removed.

Reverse/Internal Crush[17,18]

The main purpose in performing a reverse crush is to allow an opportunity for provisional SB stenting. This technique was developed with the intent to minimize any possible gap between the MB and SB stents **(Fig. 4)**.

Steps:
1. After stenting the MB, a second stent is advanced into the SB and left in position without being deployed.
2. A balloon sized according to the diameter of the MB, and shorter than the stent already deployed, is advanced in the MB and positioned at the level of the bifurcation, taking care to stay inside the stent previously deployed in the MB.
3. The stent in the SB is retracted about 3 mm or less into the MB and deployed.
4. The SB struts are recrossed with a wire and a balloon. The balloon is sized to the SB reference diameter and inflated at high pressure (12–20 atm).
5. The final kissing balloon is performed.

Nowadays, this technique has been completely superseded by the TAP.

Two Stents as Intention-to-treat

The two-stent approach will be reserved only for selected "true" bifurcations following the evaluation of additional parameters:

- *The size and the territory of distribution of the SB*: There are various anatomical conditions in which the SB is as important as the MB, regarding both the size and territory of distribution. A left main coronary artery (LMCA) that bifurcates into left anterior descending (LAD) and left circumflex (LCX), a right coronary artery (RCA) that bifurcates in a posterior descending artery and a number of posterolateral branches, a dominant LCX that bifurcates into a distal circumflex, and a large obtuse marginal branch are all examples in which the SBs are important vessels that may lead to ischemia if left with a critical stenosis.
- *The length of the lesion at the ostium of the SB*: While most of the studies found that a focal lesion at the ostium of the SB does not prevent a provisional approach, the situation may be different when the stenosis extends for several mm into the SB.
- *The angle between the MB and the SB and the narrowing at the ostium of the SB*: The narrower the angle between the two branches, the higher the risk of plaque prolapse and compromise of the ostium of the SB.[19]

Two-stent Techniques

Culotte Technique

The culotte technique uses two stents and leads to full coverage of the bifurcation with excess of metal covering of the proximal end.[20,21]

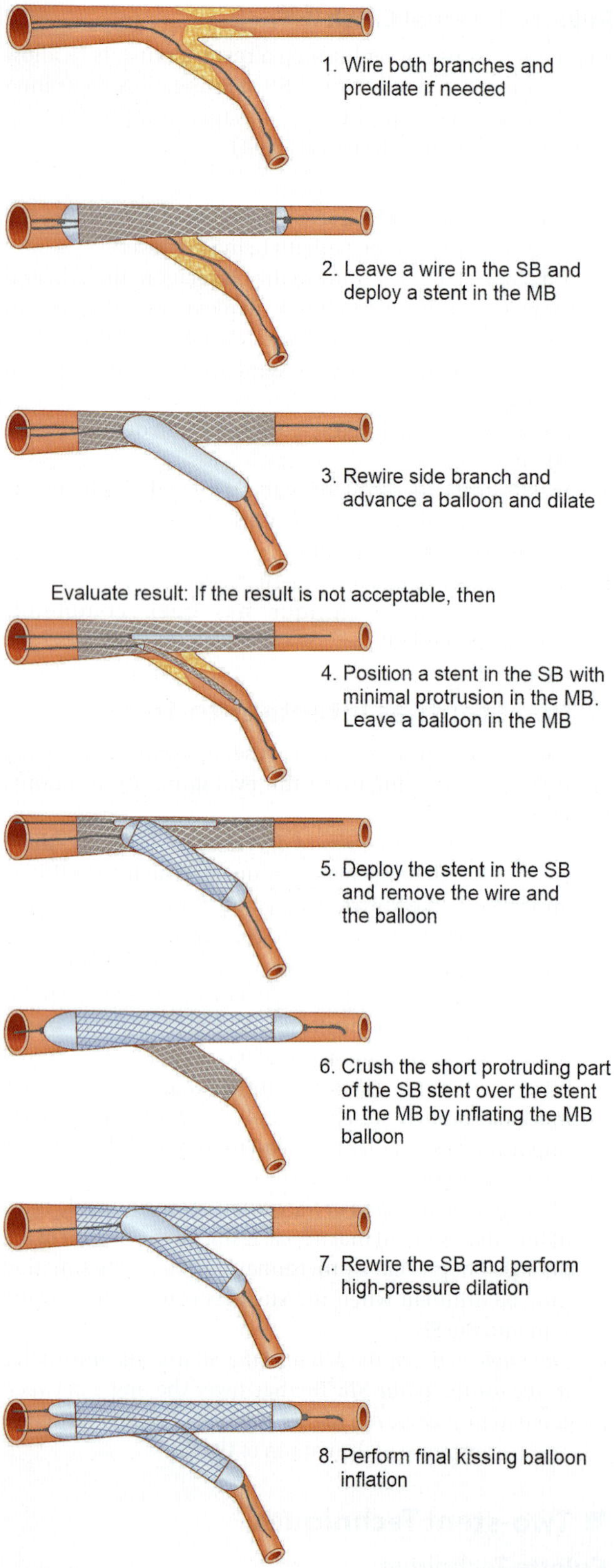

FIG. 4: A schematic representation of the reverse/internal crush technique.
(MB: main branch; SB: side branch)

An important caveat to this approach is to dilate the struts toward the SB. Open-cell design stents are recommended for the culotte technique **(Fig. 5)**.

Steps:

1. Both branches are predilated.
2. A stent is deployed across the most angulated branch, usually the SB and optimized with POT.
3. The nonstented branch is rewired through the stent struts and dilated.
4. A second stent is advanced and expanded into the nonstented branch, usually the MB and optimized with POT.
5. Finally, kissing balloon inflation and final POT are performed.

The culotte technique leads to a high concentration of metal with a double-stent layer at the carina and in the proximal part of the bifurcation. Other disadvantages of the technique are that rewiring both branches through the stent struts can be difficult and time consuming. Performing the POT after each stent implantation may help in rewiring.

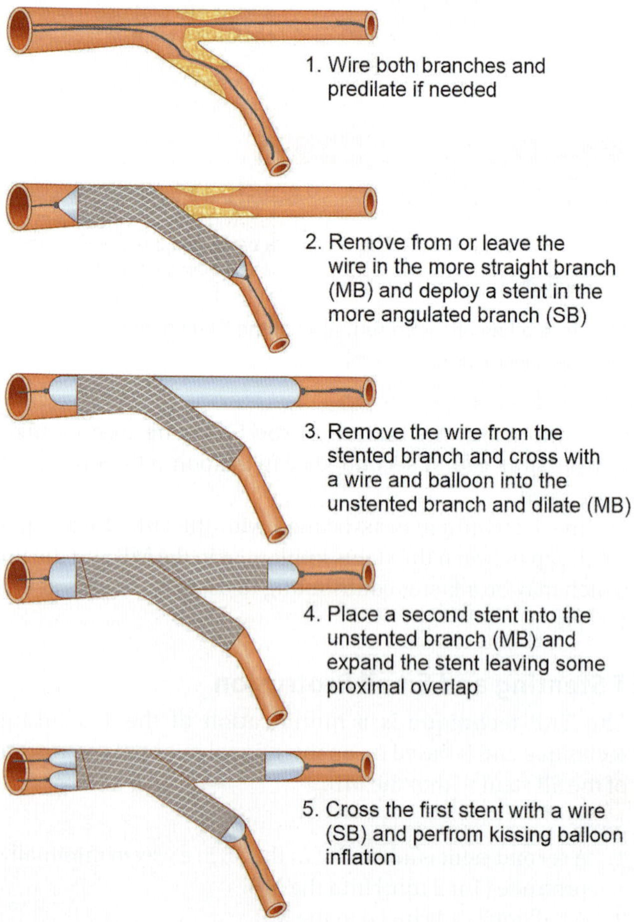

FIG. 5: A schematic representation of the culotte technique.
(MB: main branch; SB: side branch)

Mini-crush Technique (Side-branch Stent Crushed by the Main Branch Stent) (Fig. 6)

The crush technique originated with the availability of drug-eluting stent (DES).[22] It highlights the need to decrease as much as possible the amount of stent overlap between the SB and MB.[23,24] Since routine performance of the FKBI was adopted, restenosis at the ostium of the SB appears to be declining.[25]

The main advantage of the crush technique is that immediate patency of both branches is ensured.

The performance of the crush technique requires a 7- or 8-Fr guiding catheter, and the technique commits the operator to implant two stents.

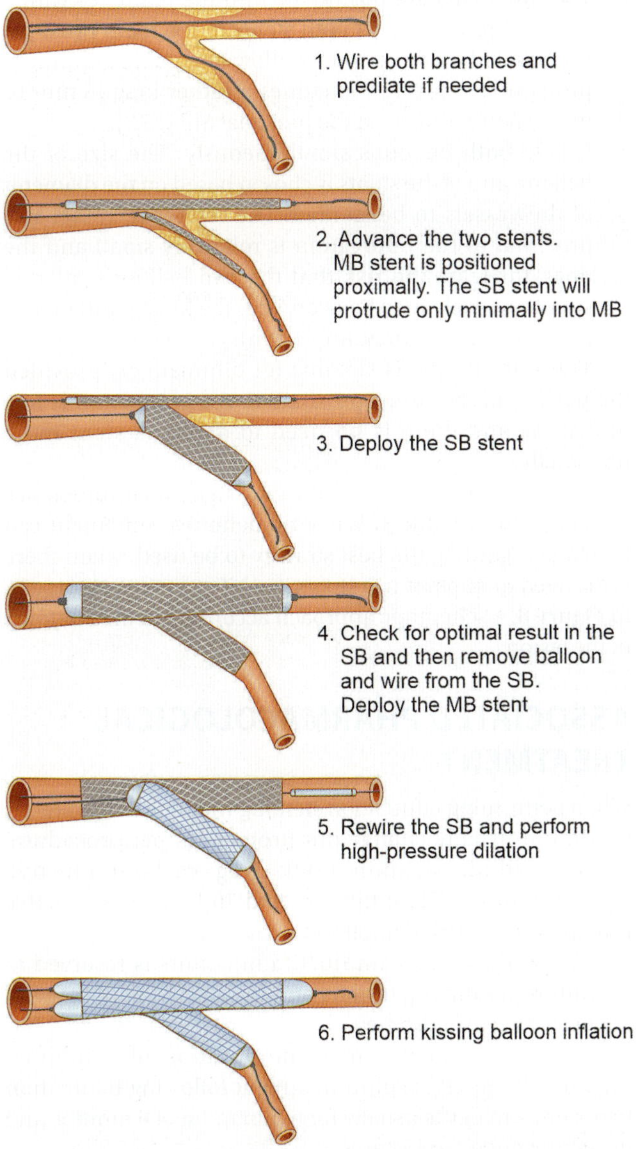

FIG. 6: A schematic representation of the mini-crush technique. (MB: main branch; SB: side branch)

Steps:

1. Both branches are wired and fully dilated. Particular attention is paid to dilate the SB, and we often utilize a 6-mm long cutting balloon if there is evidence that the predilating balloon does not fully expand at the ostium of the SB.
2. The stent for the SB is positioned in the SB, and then the MB stent is advanced.
3. The SB stent is pulled back into the MB for about 2–3 mm. This step is verified in at least two projections.
4. The stent in the SB is deployed at least at 12 atm. The balloon is deflated and removed from the guiding catheter. An angiogram is taken to verify that the SB has an appropriate lumen, normal flow, and that no distal dissection or residual lesions are present. If an additional stent is needed in the SB, this is the time to perform the implant. Following this check, the wire is removed from the SB and the stent in the MB is fully deployed at high pressure, usually above 12 atm and optimized with POT. An angiogram is taken following removal of the balloon from the MB.
5. A wire is advanced in the SB aiming to cross through the central or proximal strut.[26] This maneuver may be challenging. In addition to trying with the initial floppy wire, first try to cross through the stent struts into the SB with a 1.5- to 1.25-mm diameter balloon. If this very small balloon cannot cross, then consider repositioning of the wire traversing the stent struts. It is important to perform a final dilatation on the stent toward the SB with a balloon appropriately sized to the diameter of this branch and inflated at high pressure (12 atm or more).
6. A second balloon is advanced over the wire which was left in place in the MB, and kissing balloon inflation is performed at 8 atm or more.

Step Crush and Double-kissing Crush

When there is the need to perform a two-stent technique as intention-to-treat and a 6-Fr guiding catheter is the only available approach (radial approach), the "step crush" or "the modified balloon crush" techniques can be used.[27]

The final result is basically similar to that obtained with the standard crush technique, with the only difference that each stent is advanced and deployed separately.

The techniques named DK-crush and sleeve techniques are other variants of the crush technique, which may optimize stent deployment and apposition.[28,29] In a randomized study, the 12-month rate of target vessel revascularization (TVR) using the DK-crush technique was decreased compared with a provisional SB stenting strategy[30] and was recently shown to reduce TLF when compared with provisional SB stenting in patients with distal LM true bifurcation lesions.[31]

Steps:

1. Same as the standard crush technique.
2. A stent is advanced in the SB protruding a few millimeters into the MB. A balloon is advanced in the MB across the bifurcation.

3. The stent in the SB is deployed, the balloon is removed, an angiogram is performed, and if the result is adequate, the wire is also removed. The MB balloon is then inflated (to crush the protruding SB stent) and removed. Optionally, kissing balloon inflation can be performed at that time (double-kissing crush technique).[28,30]
4. A second stent is advanced in the MB and deployed (usually at 12 atm or more).

The next steps are similar to those of the crush technique and involve recrossing into the SB, SB stent dilatation, and FKBI.

The V and the Simultaneous Kissing Stent Techniques (Fig. 7)

The V and the simultaneous kissing stent (SKS) techniques are performed by delivering and implanting two stents together.[32,33] One stent is advanced in the SB; the other one is advanced in the MB. Both stents are pulled back to create a new carina as close as possible to the original one. The main advantage of the V technique is that the operator will never lose access to any of the two branches. In addition, when an FKBI is performed, there is no need to recross any stent. When the two stents protrude into the MB with the creation of a double barrel and a very proximal carina, the technique is called SKS.[33] We prefer the V technique for selected bifurcation lesions where the lesions are distal to the bifurcation (Medina 0,1,1); if there is a proximal stenosis in the MB, we prefer a different approach rather than creating an overlap with the SKS.

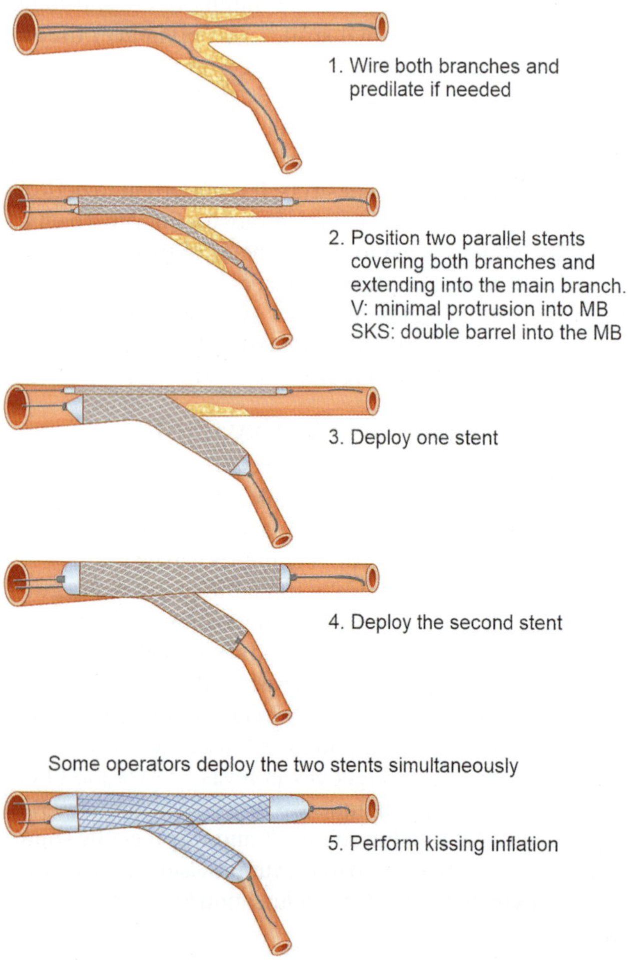

FIG. 7: A schematic representation of the V technique.
(MB: main branch; SKS: simultaneous kissing stent)

Steps:
1. Both branches are wired and fully predilated. It is important to perform an adequate predilatation in order to allow full-stent expansion.
2. The two stents are positioned into the branches with a minimal protrusion of both stents in the main proximal branch. Different operators allow a variable amount of protrusion creating sometimes a rather long (5 mm or more) double barrel in the proximal MB (SKS).
3. Inflate both balloons simultaneously. The size of the balloon and of the stents is chosen based on the diameter of the vessels to be stented. The reference vessel size proximal to the bifurcation is relatively small and the operator fears the risk that the two balloons inflated simultaneously may be oversized, the kissing inflation is performed at low pressure (4 atm).

The V technique is suitable for bifurcations, provided the portion of the vessel proximal to the bifurcation is free of disease and there is no need to deploy a stent more proximally.

The most frequently used two-stent techniques are summarized in **Table 1**. While no definitive statement can be made regarding the best strategy to be used, when there is the need to implant two stents in a bifurcation, we present, in **Figure 8**, a schematic approach according to the anatomy of the lesion.

ASSOCIATED PHARMACOLOGICAL TREATMENT

When performing bifurcation stenting with one or two stents, we do not usually change our protocol of periprocedural heparin administration (100 U/kg without elective glycoprotein IIb/IIIa inhibitors and 70 U/kg with elective glycoprotein IIb/IIIa inhibitors).

Usage of glycoprotein IIb/IIIa inhibitors is reserved to thrombus-containing lesions and in selected patients with acute coronary syndromes.

In our current practice, the duration of combined thienopyridine and aspirin treatment following bifurcation two-stent strategy is usually for a minimum of 6 months and usually extended to 1 year.

TABLE 1: Main characteristics of two-stent techniques.

	T/TAP	Mini-crush	Culotte	SKS
Guiding catheter (Fr)	6	7[a]	6	7
Provisional SB stenting	Yes	No	Possible	No
Preserved GW access MB	Yes	Yes	No	Yes
Preserved GW access SB	No	No	No	Yes
Bifurcation angle				
• <70° • >70°	• Not ideal • Ideal	• Ideal • Not ideal	• Suitable • Not ideal	• Suitable • Not ideal
MB and SB diameters				
• Similar diameters • Discrepancy in diameters	• Suitable • Suitable	• Suitable • Ideal	• Ideal • Not ideal	• Ideal • Not ideal

Note: [a]6 Fr could be used for balloon "Step-Crush" and "Double-Kissing Crush."
(GW: guidewire; MB: main branch; SB: side branch; SKS: simultaneous kissing stent; TAP: T and protrusion)

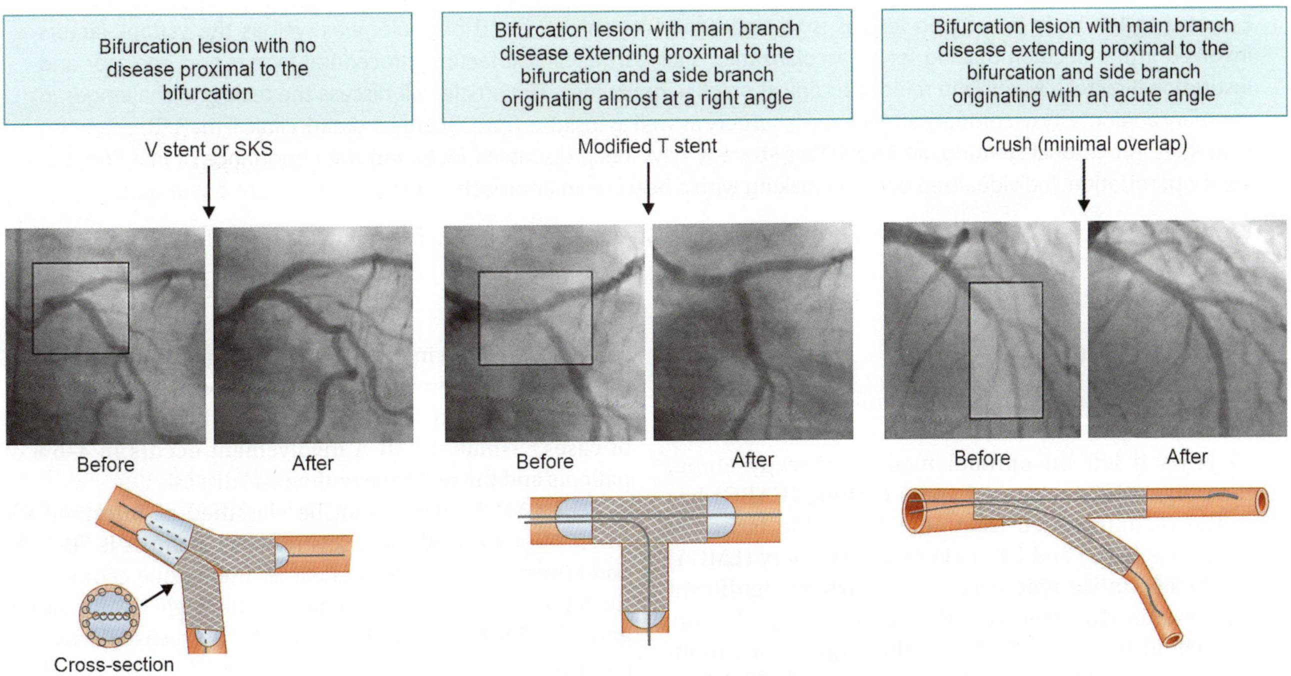

FIG. 8: Proposed approach when implanting two stents on a bifurcation as intention-to-treat.
(SKS: Simultaneous kissing stents)

CONCLUSION

Bifurcation lesions are common and associated with increased risks of restenosis. While a provisional stent approach may be suitable in many cases, an upfront two-stent approach should be considered in patients with complex anatomy or a large myocardial area supplied by the SB. In this case, choice of bifurcation technique should be determined by the specific anatomy and operator experience. It is, therefore, important that percutaneous coronary intervention (PCI) operators remain competent in two-stent techniques.

ONLINE REFERENCES

Please scan the QR code provided at the end of the table of contents for References of this chapter.

CHAPTER 147

Left Main Bifurcation Stenting: What we have learnt from Recent Bifurcation Trials

Ashwin B Mehta, Nihar P Mehta

ABSTRACT

Essential to left main bifurcation lesions is to understand its anatomy and physiology as well as the various factors involved in the decision making for revascularization such as the clinical factors, procedural factors and operator and institutional factors, keeping in mind the clinical practice guidelines. The article will discuss the technical challenges in coronary angioplasty or coronary artery bypass surgery as well as insights from recent landmark clinical trials. The stenting strategies, provisional stenting, and two-stent strategy have been discussed including the importance of imaging and stent optimization. Individualized decision making with a heart team approach optimizes the patient outcomes.

Keywords: Left main bifurcation, provisional stenting, two-stent strategy, NOBLE, Excel, EBC Main, DKCRUSH.

INTRODUCTION

Left main bifurcation lesions are a complex subset of coronary artery disease with a natural history of 73% mortality at 15 years if left on optimal medical therapy alone. Historically, coronary artery bypass grafting (CABG) has been the recommended treatment for stable ischemic heart disease (IHD) and left main coronary artery (LMCA) involvement. Unlike epicardial arteries where significant stenosis is defined as stenosis >70%, in case of LMCA disease, the threshold is set at 50% due to the large myocardium subtended as well as survival benefit after CABG.[1] Due to the strategic location of the LMCA bifurcation, various management options have evolved including stenting techniques to address its unique anatomical and physiological characteristics, requiring a maintaining blood flow to both branches and preventing complications such as side branch (SB) closure, dissection, restenosis, thrombosis, and reduced coronary flow.

ANATOMY AND PHYSIOLOGY

The LMCA arises from the aorta, branches into the left anterior descending artery (LAD) and left circumflex (LCx) coronary arteries. It supplies a large part (70–100%) of the left ventricular myocardium and a myocardial infarction (MI) after LMCA plaque rupture can affect the entire left ventricle (LV) and inferior wall of the right ventricle in a left dominant circulation. LMCA stenosis occurs at the ostium in 23%, mid shaft in 15%, and distal bifurcation in 61% of cases.[2] Isolated LMCA involvement occurs in 4–6% of patients and the rest have multivessel disease.

The LMCA disease can be classified as intermediate when stenosis is 60–70%, severe when stenosis is 70–90%, and critical when stenosis is >90%. The unique geometry of the left main bifurcation, including the angle of bifurcation and distribution of plaques, affects the revascularization strategy.

Assessing angles in LMCA bifurcation lesions involves measuring two key angles:

1. The "Take-off Angle" or Proximal Angle (Angle A), which is the angle between the Proximal LMCA and the LCx.
2. The "Carina Angle" (Angle B) between the LAD and the SB (LCx) **(Fig. 1)**.

Angle A provides valuable information about the ease of accessing the SB. Meanwhile, the sharpness of Angle B increases the likelihood of carina displacement and SB occlusion following stent placement. These angles between the LAD and SB (Angle B) have a significant impact on the outcome of PCI, influencing aspects such as wire access, stent deliverability, plaque shift, the "snow-ploughing" effect, and complete coverage of the ostium of the SB.[3]

- When Angle B measures <70°, it is referred to as "Y-angulation," facilitating easier wire access to the SB. However, there may be a higher likelihood of plaque shifting, making precise stent placement with complete ostial coverage challenging or even geometrically impossible.
- Conversely, when Angle B exceeds 70°, it is termed "T-angulation," and achieving wire access to the SB is typically more challenging. Nevertheless, plaque shifting occurs less frequently, making precise stent placement with complete ostial coverage technically easier and more likely.

In bifurcation lesions, plaque distribution is primarily concentrated on the outer wall of one or both daughter vessels, particularly in regions with low wall shear stress (WSS). WSS refers to the stress on the arterial wall caused by friction from the flowing viscous fluid **(Fig. 2)**. Atherosclerosis tends to develop early in areas characterized by non-uniform, low WSS, while areas with uniform, high WSS tend to remain protected. Consequently, the carina usually remains unscathed, and plaques tend to form in both branches opposite to the carina. Intravascular ultrasound (IVUS) studies have supported this theory by demonstrating the preservation of the carina.

Relation Between Sizes of Vessels: Murray's Law and Finet's Law

In the bifurcation anatomy, it is important to understand the relationship between the sizes of the vessels. The fact that the MV is larger than the MB is frequently forgotten during procedures.

There is an important mother-daughter mathematical relationship first described by Murray,[4] based on the principle of minimum work. Murray's Law states that the size of the proximal MV (D_{MV}) and the size of the daughter vessels (D_{MB} and D_{SB}) are represented by the following formula:

$$D_{MV}^3 = D_{MB}^3 + D_{SB}^3$$

This formula has been proven in normal and diseased vessels by IVUS study.[5] It, however, was incorrect in calcified vessels and in the culprit lesions of acute coronary syndrome. The following implications can be derived from this formula.

- The difference in the diameter (size discrepancy) between the proximal main vessel (MV) and distal main branch (MB) is dependent on the size of the SB. The larger the SB, the more is the size discrepancy. Therefore, it is imperative to perform the proximal optimization technique (POT) in bifurcation lesions with a large SB.
- When kissing balloon inflation (KBI) is performed with balloons sized according to the two branches—MB and SB, the balloons would always be oversized for the proximal MV. According to Murray's law, the sum of the cross-sectional areas of the balloons of the two branches would be larger than the cross-sectional area of the proximal MV. Therefore, it would be advisable to be conservative in balloon inflation pressures, going up to only moderate pressures during KBI.

  Finet et al. modified this to derive the simple formula:[5]

$$D_{MV} = 0.678\,(D_{MB} + D_{SB})$$

This formula can be used to calculate the size of one vessel if the sizes of the other two vessels in the bifurcation are known. However, this relationship can be quite variable according to the vessel size. For example, if the SB is small, the calculated value of the MV is smaller than the MB, which cannot be true!

To summarize, the relationship between the size of the MV, MB, and SB is the key to select the optimal strategy of POT and KBI. Considering the variation in the size of the branches and the inadequacy of the Murray's and Finet's laws, imaging with IVUS or optical coherence tomography

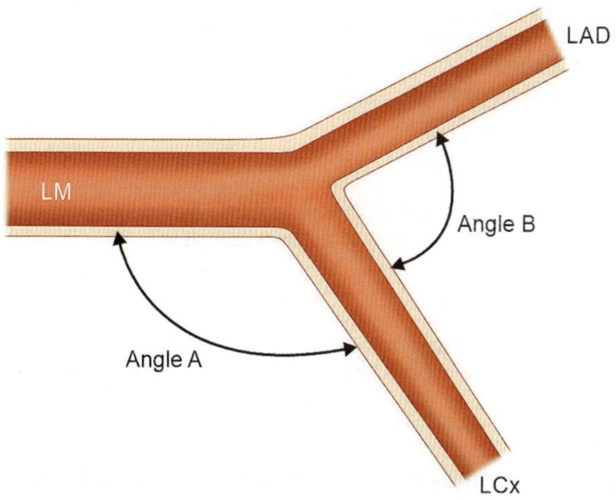

FIG. 1: Anatomy of the bifurcation angle.
(LAD: left anterior descending; LCx: left circumflex; LM: left main)

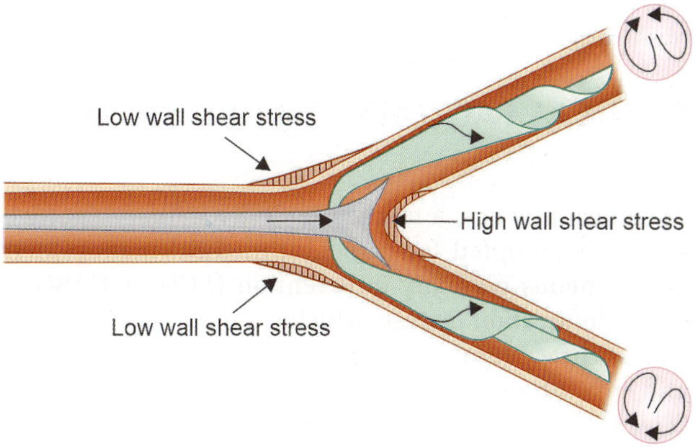

FIG. 2: Illustration of flow patterns and resulting wall shear stress in the region of a bifurcation (Murray, et al.).[4]

(OCT) should be used for optimal sizing and improved cardiovascular outcomes.

CLINICAL FACTORS FOR DECISION MAKING[1]

In clinical practice, a tailored multidisciplinary approach should be adopted for choice of medical management, percutaneous coronary intervention (PCI) or CABG for LMCA bifurcation disease, which should integrate clinical factors, procedural considerations, operator experience, and institution issues and guideline recommendations **(Fig. 3)**. The team should ideally involve the interventional cardiologist, cardiac surgeon, anesthetist, physician, and the patient or family members. It is important to highlight that a single approach cannot be adopted of this heterogenous disease complex.

Factors favoring CABG surgery include diabetes mellitus, complex multivessel disease, contraindication to dual antiplatelet therapy, severe LV systolic dysfunction, and concomitant valvular pathology with an independent indication for surgery.

Factors that favor PCI include frailty or comorbidities which hamper the patients ability to recover from CABG such as chronic obstructive pulmonary disease, severe chest deformity, redo-surgery, lack of conduits or appropriate targets, prior chest radiation, porcelain aorta, advanced chronic kidney disease, immunosuppression, ST elevation MI, or cardiogenic shock.

Medical therapy alone may be the preferred option in case of severe comorbidities, low life expectancy, or patients preference.

Age, frailty, and comorbidity burdens are often underrepresented in trials and often coexist. They increase the risk for CABG as well as PCI. Especially for octogenarians or nonagenarians, short-term risks such as acute kidney injury, risk of stroke, atrial fibrillation, physical disability, and dependence may favor a less invasive approach.

Similarly, LV systolic dysfunction and decompensated heart failure increase the short-term risks of both CABG or PCI; however, in observational studies, CABG is superior to PCI in case of severe LV dysfunction.[6] In case mechanical support is required to perform PCI in this subset, the risks of vascular complications and bleeding should be factored into the decision-making process. In certain patients, advanced therapies such as left ventricular assist device as destination therapy or a transplant should be considered when appropriate.

TECHNICAL CHALLENGES FOR PCI IN LMCA BIFURCATION

Majority of LMCA stenoses involve the bifurcation and also have multivessel involvement. Imaging and functional testing form an integral part of PCI: Imaging is used to assess the lesion length, lesion severity and morphology, lesion preparation and debulking strategy, stenting strategy, the size of the stents, stent apposition, and complications. Functional testing can be used to test the hemodynamic significance of the stenosis as well as SB compromise in case of provisional stenting strategy, with fractional flow reserve (FFR) >0.80, an acceptable cutoff to defer PCI. IVUS can also be used to defer stenting in case the minimal lumen area is >6 mm^2 or >4.5 mm^2 in Asians.[7,8]

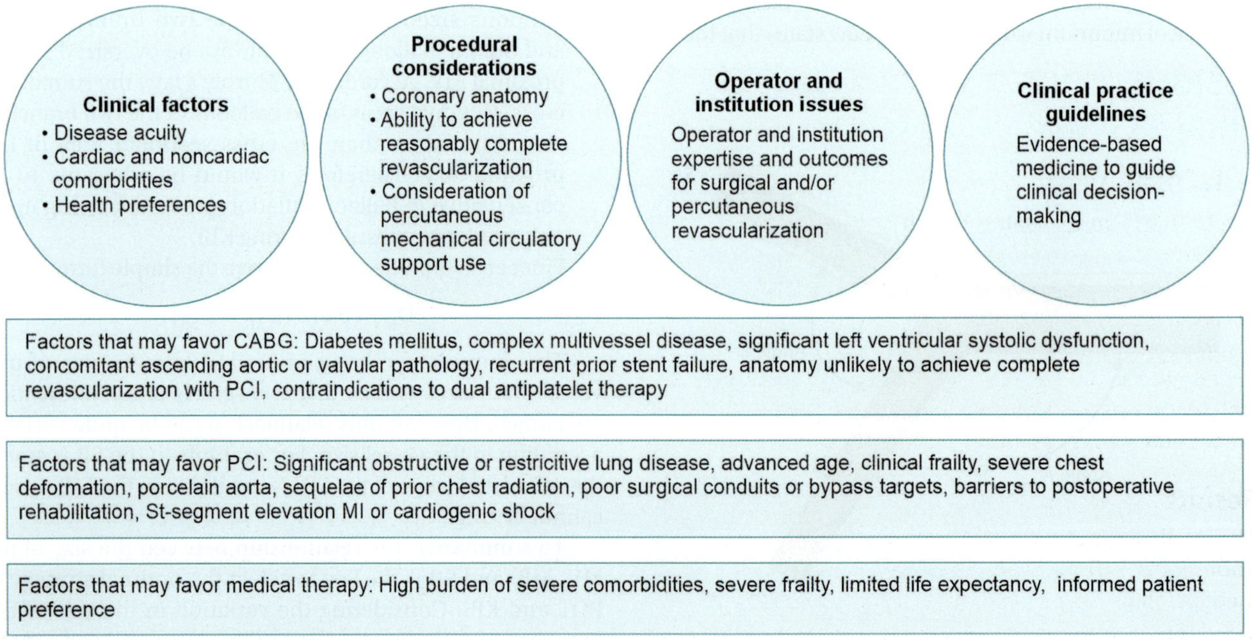

FIG. 3: Heart team approach to LMCA bifurcation.[1]

(CABG: coronary artery bypass grafting; LMCA: left main coronary artery; MI: myocardial infarction; PCI: percutaneous coronary intervention)

Lesion complexity and technical challenges play an important role in determining the stenting strategy, provisional single stent strategy or a dedicated two-stent strategy. This is discussed in the subsequent section.

For patients with unstable hemodynamics, reduced ejection fraction, and unable to tolerate ischemia (left dominant system or right coronary totally occluded), mechanical circulatory devices can be used such as intra-aortic balloon pump, Impella (Abiomed), or ECMO to provide essential hemodynamic support. The appropriate arterial access site should be considered.

TECHNICAL CHALLENGES FOR CABG IN LMCA BIFURCATION

In patients with isolated LMCA disease or LMCA with multivessel disease, complete revascularization is achievable as long as adequate (minimum 1.5 mm) distal target vessels are available. CABG is challenging in cases with diffuse distal disease, calcified walls at target arteries, or intramyocardial course of vessels.

Technical considerations also include the hemodynamic instability that may be encountered during induction of anesthesia in patients with critical LMCA disease, therefore, less cardio depressive agents should be selected and upfront mechanical support with intra-aortic balloon pump should be used. Antegrade cardioplegic arrest of the heart may be hampered by LMCA stenosis resulting in poor distribution of cardioplegia and inadequate myocardial protection. This may be mitigated by addition of retrograde cardioplegia to facilitate adequate myocardial protection. In Porcelain aortas or aortic atheromas, off-pump CABG is necessary to avoid aortic cannulation, cross-clamping, and graft anastomosis to the aorta.

INSIGHTS FROM LANDMARK CLINICAL TRIALS COMPARING CABG VERSUS PCI

NOBLE Trial[9]

The NOBLE (Nordic-Baltic-British Left Main Revascularization) trial conducted a randomized study involving 1,201 patients to assess whether PCI was noninferior to CABG in treating LMCA disease and reported the outcomes over a span of 5 years. The primary endpoint was defined as major adverse cardiac or cerebrovascular events (MACCE), which comprised a composite of all-cause mortality, nonprocedural MI, repeat revascularization, and stroke.

Results

The analysis included 592 patients in each group, one undergoing PCI and the other undergoing CABG. After a median follow-up period of 4.9 years, the MACCE rates were 28% (165 events) for the PCI group and 19% (110 events) for the CABG group, with a hazard ratio of 1.58 [95% confidence interval (CI) 1.24–2.01]. This indicated that CABG was superior to PCI for the primary composite endpoint. All-cause mortality was comparable between both groups, but the PCI group exhibited significantly higher rates of nonprocedural MI and repeat revascularization **(Fig. 4)**.

Interpretation

When it comes to revascularization of LMCA disease, PCI demonstrated an inferior clinical outcome at the 5-year mark compared to CABG. PCI was associated with higher rates of nonprocedural MI and repeat revascularization.

EXCEL Trial[10]

The EXCEL (Evaluation of XIENCE Versus Coronary Artery Bypass Surgery for Effectiveness of Left Main Revascularization) trial conducted a random assignment of 1,905 patients who had LMCA disease with low or intermediate anatomical complexity (as determined by a Syntax Score of <32). These patients were divided into two groups: (1) one undergoing PCI with everolimus-eluting stents (PCI group, consisting of 948 patients) and (2) the other undergoing CABG (CABG group, consisting of 957 patients). The primary outcome of interest was a composite endpoint comprising death, stroke, or MI.

Results

After a 5-year follow-up, the occurrence of a primary outcome event was observed in 22.0% of the patients in the PCI group and 19.2% of the patients in the CABG group (with a 95% CI –0.9 to 6.5; $p = 0.13$). It is worth noting that the incidences of definite cardiovascular death and MI were similar in both the PCI and CABG groups. However, cerebrovascular events were less frequent following PCI compared to CABG. Additionally, ischemia-driven revascularization occurred more frequently after PCI than after CABG.

Interpretation

For patients with LMCA disease of low or intermediate anatomical complexity, no statistically significant difference was observed between PCI and CABG concerning the rate of the composite outcome, which includes death, stroke, or MI at the 5-year mark **(Figs. 5A and B)**.

STENTING STRATEGIES FOR LMCA BIFURCATION

Insights from Landmark Trials Regarding Stenting Strategies

European Bifurcation Club (EBC) Main[11]

A total of 467 patients who presented with true left main stem bifurcation lesions were randomly assigned to one of two strategies: (1) the stepwise layered provisional strategy (PS)

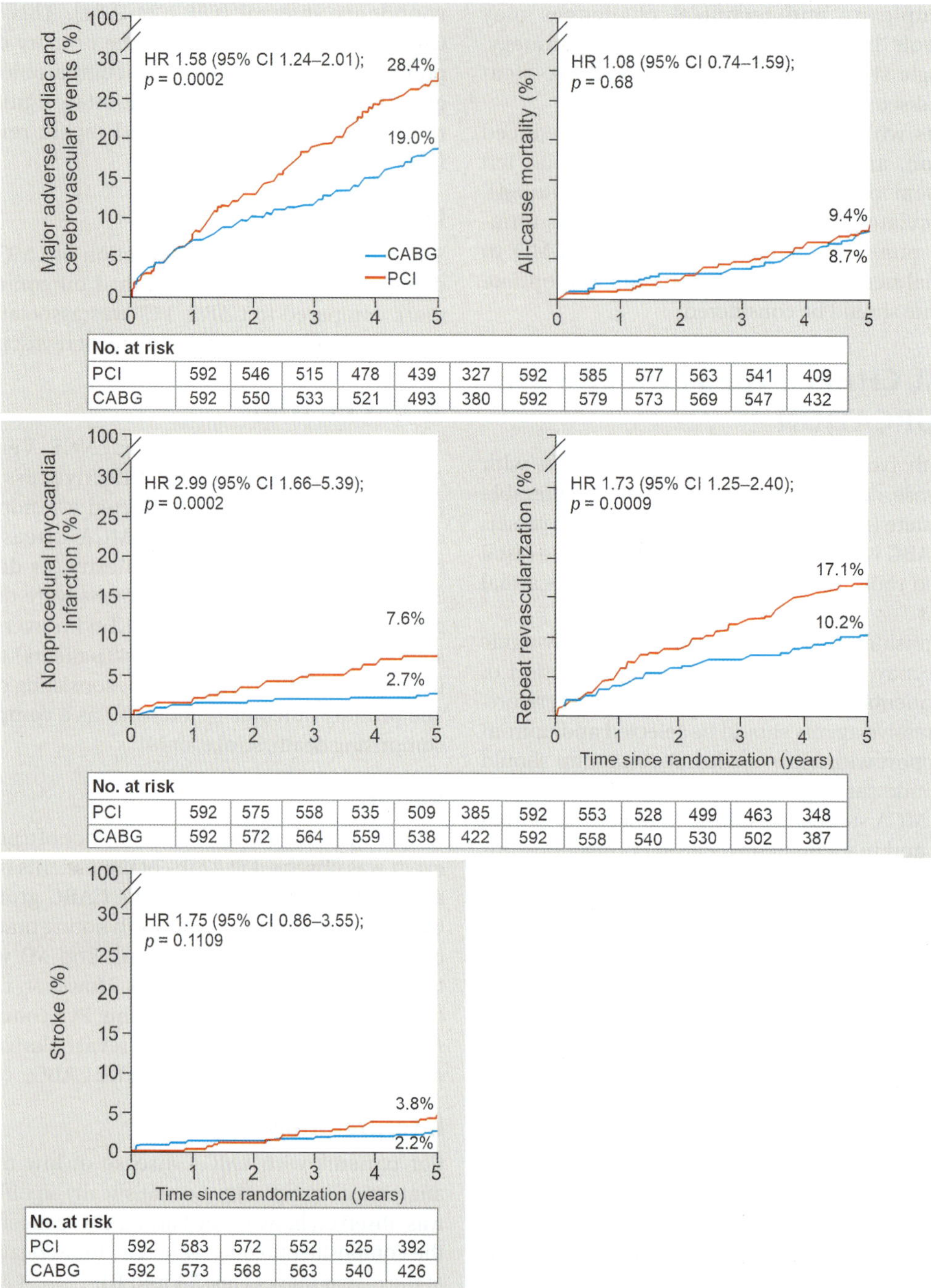

FIG. 4: Primary outcomes of NOBLE trial at 5 years.
(CABG: coronary artery bypass graft; CI: confidence interval; HR: hazard ratio; PCI: percutaneous coronary intervention)

(comprising 230 patients) or (2) the systematic dual-stent approach (comprising 237 patients).

Results

The primary endpoint, defined as a composite of death, MI, and target lesion revascularization at the 12-month mark, occurred in 14.7% of the patients in the stepwise provisional group and 17.7% of the patients in the systematic dual-stent group. Secondary endpoints, including death, MI, target lesion revascularization, and ST, exhibited similar rates in both groups **(Fig. 6)**.

Interpretation

For patients with LMCA bifurcation lesions, a stepwise layered provisional approach demonstrated numerically fewer major adverse cardiac events compared to the planned

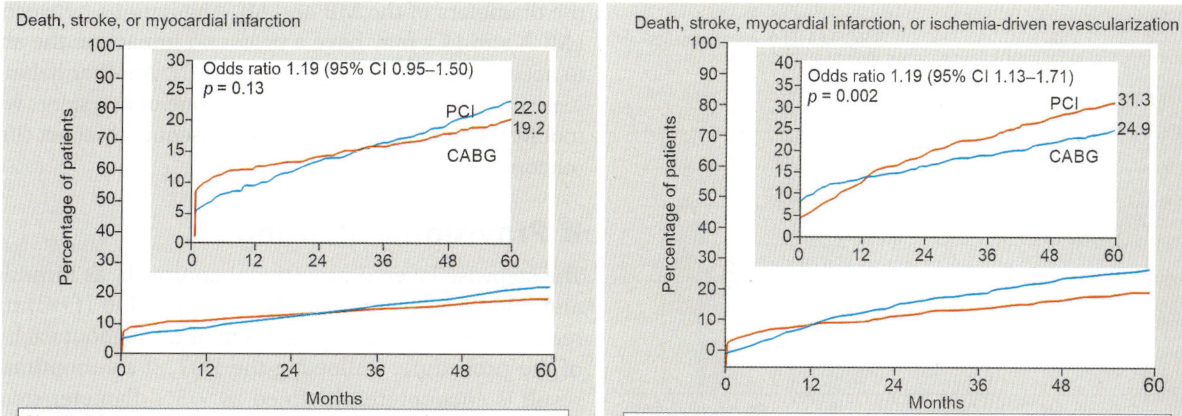

Death, stroke, or myocardial infarction

No. at risk						
PCI	947	854	809	778	738	486
CABG	957	818	789	763	734	532

Death, stroke, myocardial infarction, or ischemia-driven revascularization

No. at risk						
PCI	948	813	746	706	653	428
CABG	957	895	757	725	686	494

FIG. 5A: Composite primary and secondary outcomes of Excel trial at 5 years.
(CABG: coronary artery bypass graft; CI: confidence interval; PCI: percutaneous coronary intervention)

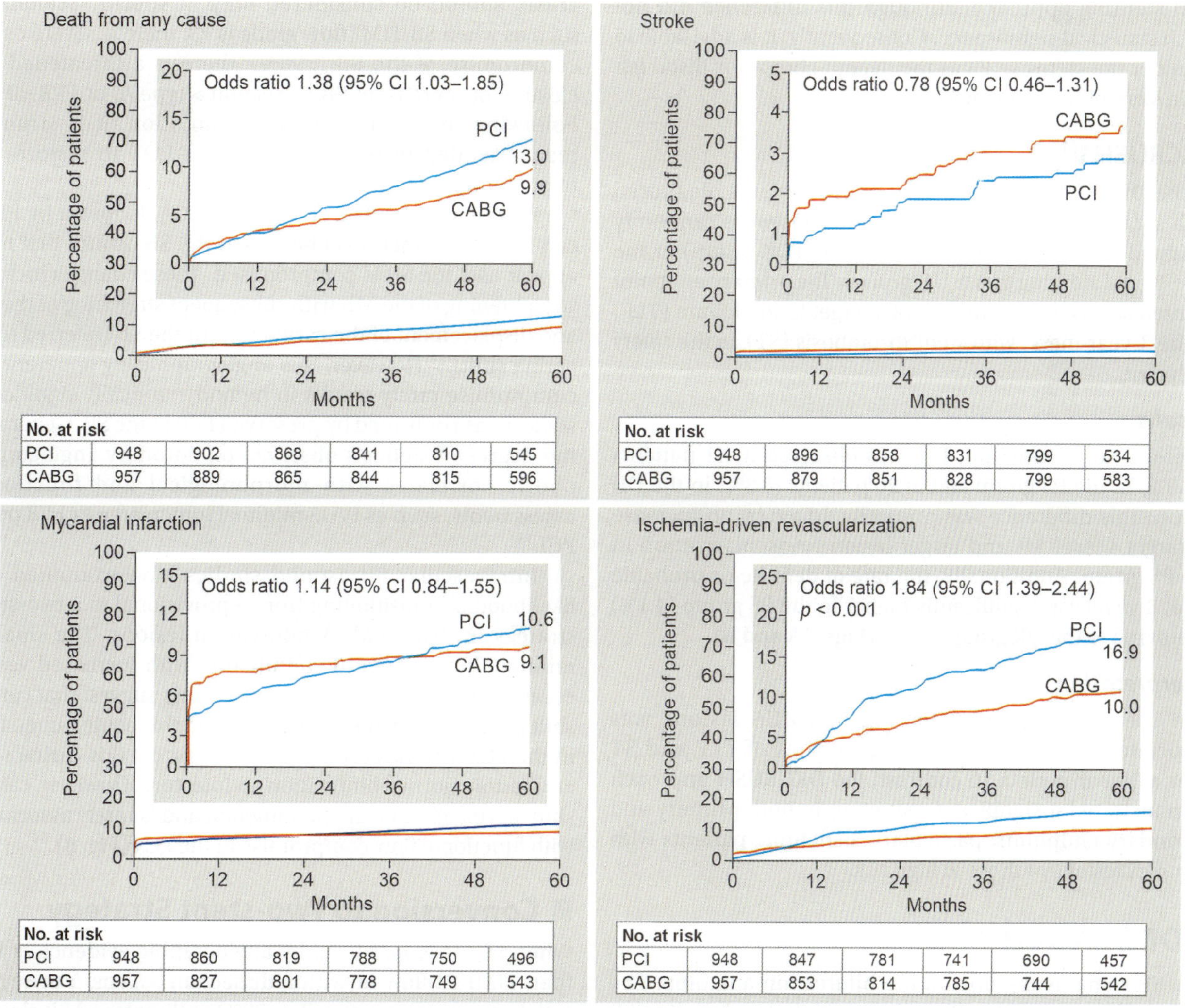

Death from any cause

No. at risk						
PCI	948	902	868	841	810	545
CABG	957	889	865	844	815	596

Stroke

No. at risk						
PCI	948	896	858	831	799	534
CABG	957	879	851	828	799	583

Mycardial infarction

No. at risk						
PCI	948	860	819	788	750	496
CABG	957	827	801	778	749	543

Ischemia-driven revascularization

No. at risk						
PCI	948	847	781	741	690	457
CABG	957	853	814	785	744	542

FIG. 5B: Components of primary and secondary outcomes of Excel trial at 5 years.
(CABG: coronary artery bypass graft; CI: confidence interval; PCI: percutaneous coronary intervention)

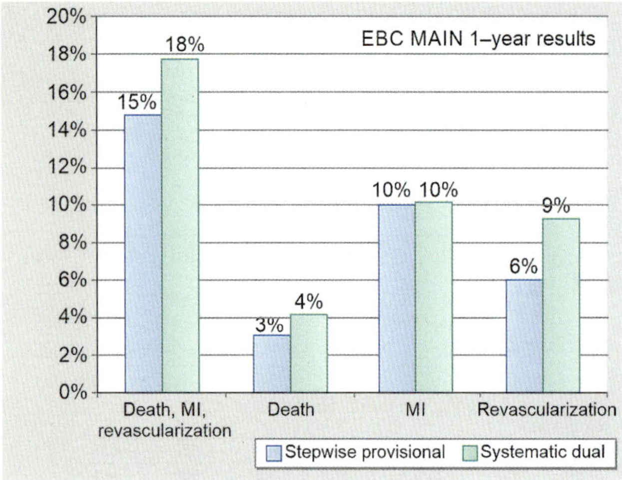

FIG. 6: Outcomes of EBC main.

(EBC: European Bifurcation Club; MI: myocardial infarction)

dual stenting approach, although this difference did not reach statistical significance. Consequently, it is advisable to consider the stepwise PS as the default choice for distal left main stem bifurcation interventions.

DKCRUSH V[12]

In the DKCRUSH V trial, a total of 482 patients diagnosed with significant LMCA bifurcation lesions were randomly assigned to either the DKCRUSH group (DK group) or the provisional stenting group (PS group). The primary endpoint of interest was the occurrence of a target lesion failure (TLF) at the 3-year mark, with stent thrombosis (ST) as the safety endpoint.

Results

After a 3-year follow-up, TLF was observed in 41 patients (16.9%) in the PS group and in 20 patients (8.3%) in the DK group. This difference was primarily driven by an increase in target vessel MI and target lesion revascularization in the PS group. Additionally, the rate of definite or probable ST at 3 years was significantly higher in the PS group (4.1%) compared to the DK group (0.4%) **(Figs. 7A and B)**.

Interpretation

The use of provisional stenting in LMCA lesions was associated with significantly higher rates of TLF and ST over a 3-year period. In contrast, the DKCRUSH approach demonstrated a significant reduction in both primary and secondary endpoints, particularly benefiting patients with complex lesions or those at high risk.

SIDE BRANCH

The SB remains the crux of the bifurcation anatomy. The factors influencing the SB occlusion include a baseline SB diameter stenosis, angulation of the SB, and the ratio of the diameters of the MB and SB. Angulations between the LMCA and LCx may have a profound impact on the ability to access and maintain patency of LCx. Another debatable issue is whether the implantation of one or two stents would modify the bifurcation angle and consequently affect clinical outcomes.[13]

Provisional Stenting

The stepwise layered provisional approach, as formulated and adopted by European Bifurcation Club (EBC) main, recommends continuous assessment throughout each step of the procedure. Following the POT, if a suboptimal SB result is encountered [defined as >75% diameter stenosis or thrombolysis in myocardial infarction (TIMI) flow grade <3], the SB should be rewired, and KBI should be performed using noncompliant balloons. At this stage, re-POT is advised to reduce the eccentricity index.

Further stent implantation, using techniques such as T stenting, T and small protrusion, culotte, or reverse (mini-) crush, should be considered only in specific scenarios, such as when SB TIMI flow grade is <3, there is severe ostial compromise of the SB (>90%), there is a threatened SB closure, or there is an SB dissection > type A, or FFR <0.80. Following the second stent implantation, it is strongly recommended to repeat KBI and re-POT to restore the bifurcation geometry.

Provisional stenting of a distal LMCA, followed by POT, can lead to geometrical changes at the SB ostium that may appear as if the SB is compromised. These changes include straightening of the MB with subsequent stretching of the SB and displacement of the carina toward the SB (referred to as carina shift).[14] However, this angiographically apparent SB compromise rarely results in hemodynamically significant stenosis, as confirmed by preserved FFR in the SB. Generally, the degree of stenosis observed on coronary angiography poorly correlates with morphological and functional assessments, such as IVUS minimal lumen area or FFR post-PCI.[15]

Intravascular ultrasound studies have examined the likelihood of transitioning from a provisional to a two-stent strategy in distal LMCA bifurcation lesions. The smaller minimal lumen area in conjunction with increased vessel eccentricity and unchanged plaque mass suggest that carina shift is the primary mechanism behind this acute lumen loss in the LCx. KBI has the potential to correct this carina shift and restore normal bifurcation architecture. However, carina shift is typically a focal phenomenon and is rarely associated with functional flow compromise in the LCx **(Fig. 8)**.[14]

Conversion to Two-stent Strategy

When LCx is jeopardized by angiographic evidence of less than TIMI III flow or with a dissection > Type A or severe ostial compromise of the SB (>90%) or threatened SB closure or hemodynamically significant stenosis (FFR < 0.80), a second stent should be placed. Upgrade from provisional to a two-stent strategy may include T stenting, T and small protrusion stenting, culotte, or reverse crush techniques.

- T stenting or T and small protrusion stenting may arguably be the easiest stepwise two-stent strategy especially if the angle is close to 90°. LCx stent implantation should be performed with minimal LMCA protrusion balancing between neocarina formation and incomplete ostial coverage.
- Culotte technique may be attractive in case LCx and LAD have similar sizes and there is an acute bifurcation angle but requires several steps, wire recrossing, and creates double-stent layers in the LMCA.
- The reverse (mini-) crush technique has advantages of ensuring coverage of bifurcation anatomy, suitable to all angles and to arteries with a size mismatch between the LMCA and LCx.[16]

INTRAVASCULAR IMAGING

Intravascular ultrasound has received a Class IIa recommendation for evaluating the severity of LMCA lesions.[17]

Intravascular imaging offers distinct insights into various aspects of coronary atherosclerosis, including the extent and distribution of plaques, plaque composition, lesion morphology, and complications related to stent placement in LMCA bifurcations. It is noteworthy that calcified lesions, as opposed to fibrotic ones, tend to create an elliptical lumen cross-section with a smaller lumen area. Therefore, initial imaging assessments that gauge the thickness and extension

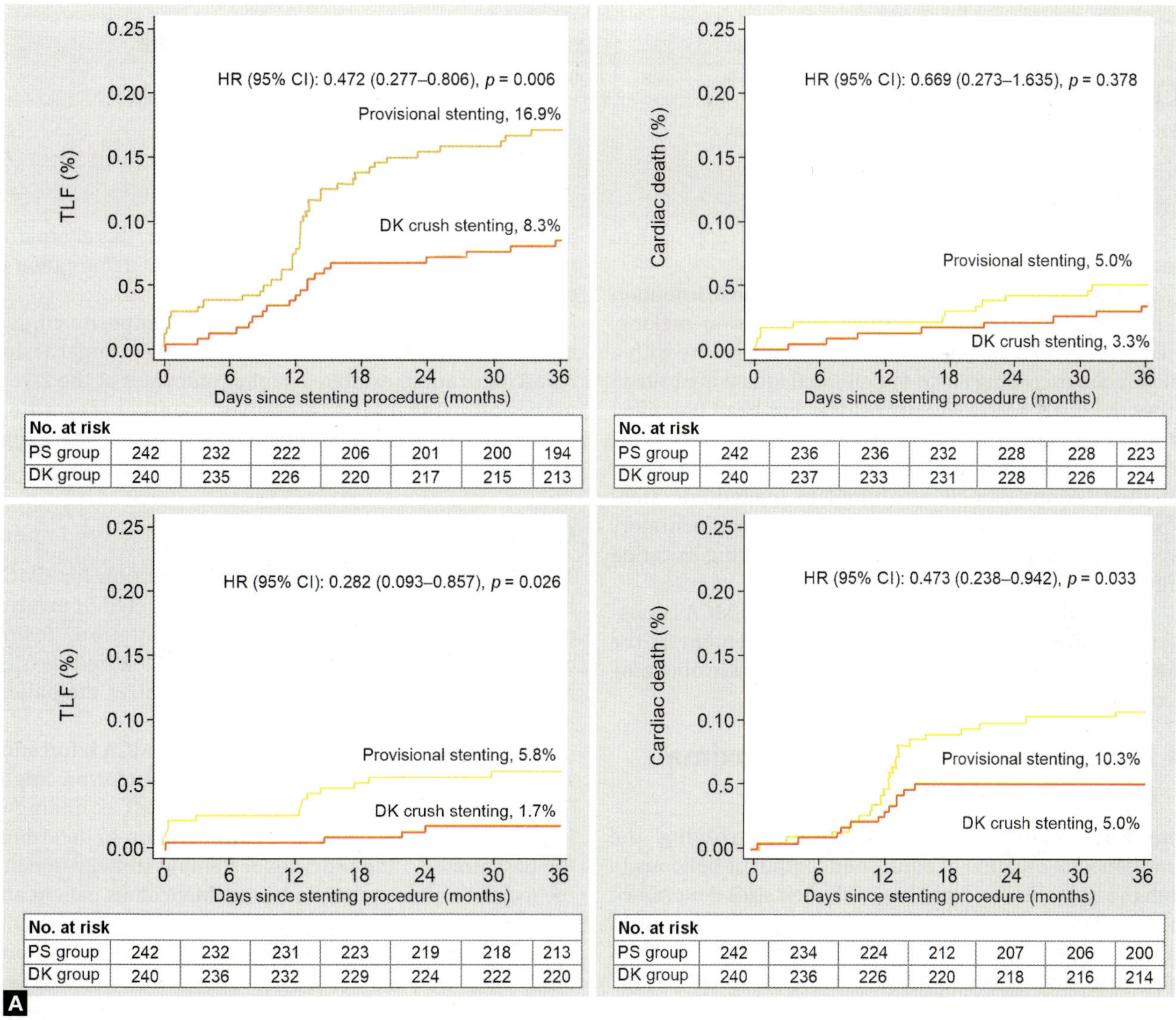

FIGS. 7A AND B: *Continued*

Continued

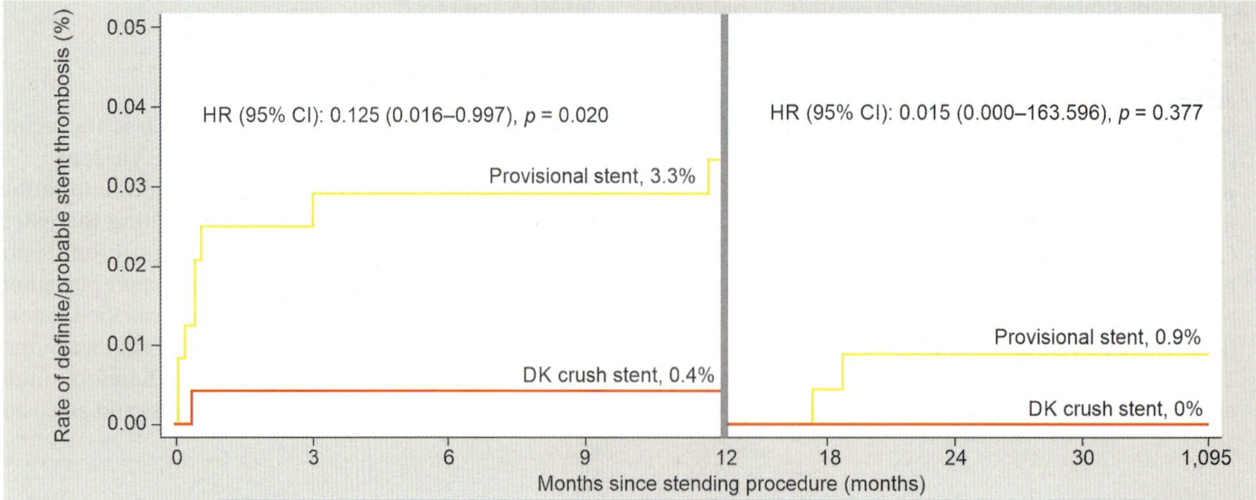

No. at risk									
PS group	242	236	234	234	234	231	226	221	216
DK group	240	239	238	238	237	232	230	227	222

B

FIGS. 7A AND B: Outcomes of the DKCRUSH V trial.

of calcium play a pivotal role in determining the approach to plaque modification and stenting strategies.[18]

Intravascular ultrasound analysis of plaque distribution at the LMCA bifurcation is crucial for decision-making. The presence of a calcified plaque, particularly one with a calcium arc exceeding 60° at the minimal lumen area site in either the distal LMCA or LAD ostium, has been identified as an independent predictor of post stenting narrowing in the LCx. This phenomenon of SB compromise in highly calcified lesions can be attributed to inadequate stent expansion at the calcification site, leading to compensatory overexpansion at the carina, ultimately resulting in carina shift.

It is worth noting that the use of OCT for LMCA assessment requires selective and coaxial engagement of the LMCA guide catheter, which can pose challenges in obtaining a comprehensive evaluation.

Final Kissing Inflation and Proximal Optimization Technique

The EBC recommends a procedure involving the simultaneous inflation of short, noncompliant balloons in both the LAD and LCx branches, with their sizes determined in accordance with Murray's law. Subsequently, a re-POT should be performed. An alternative technique involves sequential single-balloon dilation in the proximal MB, SB, and proximal MB (POT-side-POT). However, this alternative method may lead to a higher degree of stent deformation in the MB when compared to KBI.

It is crucial to emphasize that the composite clinical endpoints, including death, MI, and LMCA target lesion revascularization, exhibited similar outcomes at the 2-year mark following LMCA crossover stenting, regardless of whether the final step involved KBI or an alternative technique.[19]

CONCLUSION

The choice between surgery and intervention for LMCA bifurcation lesions is complex and multifaceted. It involves patient characteristics, clinical presentation, lesion complexity, and operator experience. Individualized decision making with a heart team approach optimizes the patient outcomes.

There is no single optimal strategy for LMCA bifurcation stenting. Angiographic features like bifurcation angle, SB plaque morphology and severity as well as finding of imaging need to be taken into consideration to determine the best strategy. The provisional stenting strategy remains the most common strategy adopted. Meticulous patient and strategy selection including intravascular imaging and stent optimization are keys for successful short- and long-term outcomes.

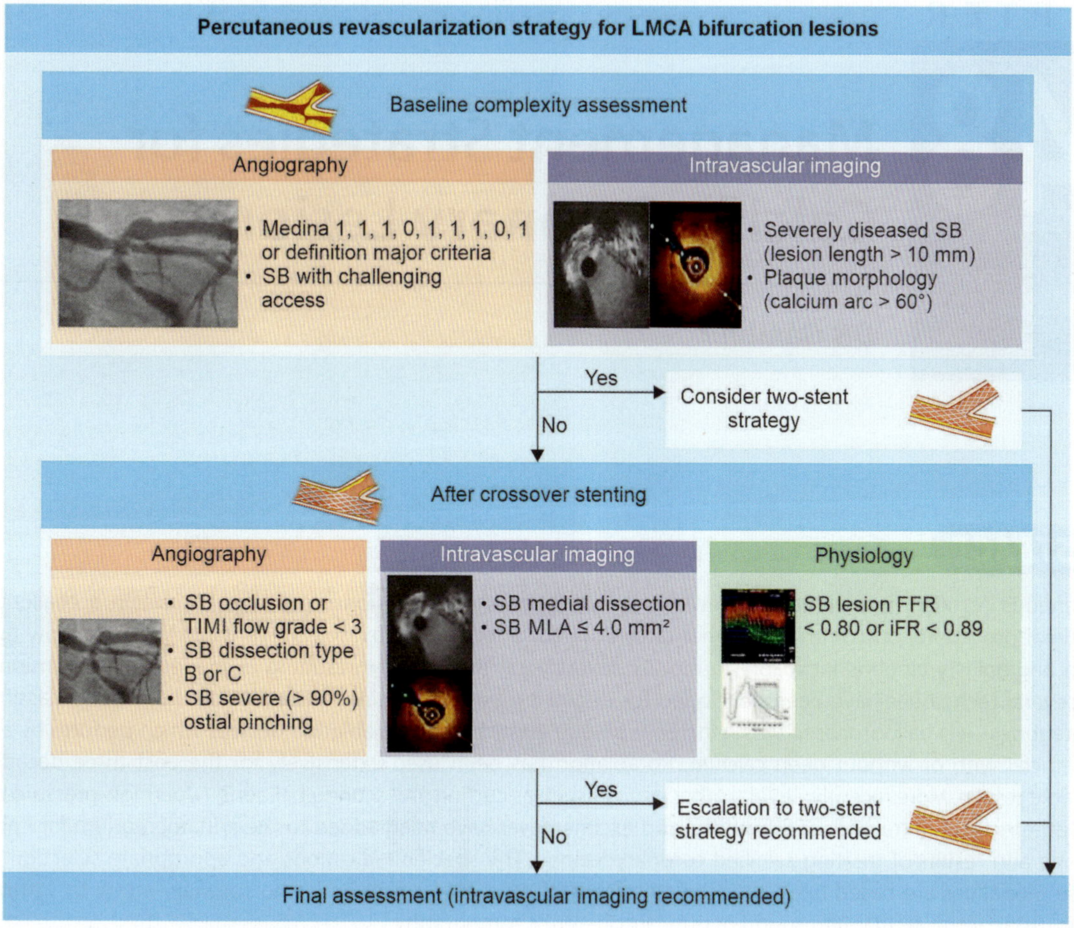

FIG. 8: Approach to LMCA bifurcation stenting.

(FFR: fractional flow reserve; iFR: instantaneous wave-free ratio; LMCA: left main coronary artery; SB: side branch; TIMI: thrombolysis in myocardial infarction)

Source: With permission from Paradies et al. (2023).[13]

ONLINE REFERENCES

Please scan the QR code provided at the end of the table of contents for References of this chapter.

CHAPTER

148 Management Strategies for Calcific Coronary Lesions

DS Gambhir

ABSTRACT

Percutaneous coronary intervention of severely calcified and stenotic lesions continues to remain a challenge with suboptimal procedural outcomes and higher rates of major adverse cardiovascular events (MACE) on follow-up. Since balloon angioplasty alone is incapable to modify severely calcified plaque resulting in inadequate expansion of the stent, several techniques have been developed for debulking before stenting. These devices have been classified into two categories—(1) balloon-based which increase plaque elasticity and (2) ablation devices which perform by abrasion of superficial with or without deep calcium. Rotablation has been used extensively for the past three decades with acceptable results. More recently, several other devices such as cutting and scoring balloons, superhigh-pressure balloon, orbital atherectomy, intravascular lithotripsy, and excimer laser have been added to the armamentarium for enhancing the scope and results of treating calcified coronary lesions. The specific indications and appropriate selection of each of these modalities are based upon precise assessment of type of calcification in the coronary artery by intravascular imaging, using intravascular ultrasound or optical coherence tomography.

This chapter deals with various debulking devices in brief, followed by calcium scoring systems. At the end, the author has attempted to develop an algorithmic approach for selection of the most appropriate device for specific lesion on the basis of intravascular imaging.

Keywords: Coronary, calcification, imaging, debulking.

INTRODUCTION

Severe calcified lesions are associated with higher rates of failure, procedural complications, and worst short and long-term outcomes after percutaneous coronary intervention (PCI) compared to noncalcified lesions,[1] by impairing the crossability of stent at the target site. During implantations, severe calcification may lead to disruption of drug polymer from the stent surface[2] affecting delivery of drug in the vessel wall[3] and inadequate expansion and apposition of the stent.[4] Patients with highly calcified coronary stenosis undergoing PCI are less likely to receive complete revascularization (48% vs. 55.6%; $p < 0.001$) and more likely to die after procedure from target lesion failure (10.8% vs, 1.4%; $p < 0.001$).[5] Optimization of results of PCI in calcified lesions is of paramount importance and modification of calcified plaque is therefore the first step for adequate deployment and expansion of stent.

Several modalities have evolved during the past three decades and have been successfully used for modification of calcified plaque before stenting the coronary arteries. The role of each of these and their appropriate application, based upon assessment of lesion by intracoronary imaging, has been highlighted in this chapter. Finally, an algorithmic approach has been suggested considering the review of literature and the author's experience.

STRATEGIES FOR MODIFICATION OF CALCIUM

A number of calcium modification techniques are now available to achieve an optimal result of stenting. These modalities can be classified into two categories[1]—(1) balloon-based and (2) ablation techniques.[2] Balloon-based techniques do not remove calcium but aim to increase plaque elasticity and thereby allow adequate stent expansion by cracking the calcified component in one or more quadrants. Most ablation techniques perform by abrasing the superficial calcified plaque, resulting in its fracture and thereby facilitating balloon to dilatate the stenosed segment.

Balloon-based Modalities

These include[1] superhigh-pressure balloon (OPN),[2] cutting and scoring balloons, and[3] shockwave balloon [(intravascular lithotripsy (IVL)].

Superhigh-pressure Balloon

This is a dual-layer, rapid exchange, noncompliant (NC) balloon allowing high-pressure inflation up to 35–45 atmospheres with uniform expansion without causing rupture of the balloon. It has been reported successful for unexpandable stents due to underlying calcification, in-stent restenosis (ISR), and de-novo, moderately severe calcified stenosis where conventional noncomplaints balloons have failed.

Cutting and Scoring Balloons

These balloons improve vessel compliance by causing incisions in the calcified plaque, enabling more vessel expansion, and reducing recoil while preventing large, uncontrolled dissections.

The cutting balloon consists of a set of three microsurgical blades bonded to the surface of a NC balloon. On inflation at low pressure (6–8 atm), the cutting blades produce controlled incisions on the plaque, which may then become amenable to dilatation by NC balloon. Use of cutting balloon is limited to ISR and mild-to-moderate calcified plaque. These balloons have shown low rates of target lesion revascularization (TLR) and stent thrombosis when used alone or in combination with rotational atherectomy (RA) in severely calcified lesions.[6,7]

Scoring balloon is a low profile, semicompliant balloon with scoring element on its surface. During inflation, a radial force is exerted mainly on the scoring element which is transmitted to the vessel wall causing incisions in the atheromatous calcified plaque. The presence of internal element ensures anchoring of the balloon, and low risk of melon-seeding and/or balloon slippage when compared to RA. Scoring balloon has similar clinical outcome with 83.3% success versus 92.5% with rotablation.[8] Predilatation with a scoring balloon has been demonstrated to enhance stent expansion.[9] These devices might be helpful in calcified lesions where other modalities are unavailable or may be used in combination.[10]

Both scoring and cutting balloons are limited by their bulkier profile and difficulty in delivery through calcified and tortuous vessels with critical stenosis.

Intravascular Lithotripsy

Lithotripsy consists of a rechargeable generator which is connected to a balloon that contains two emitters. These create sonic pressure waves equivalent to approximately 50 atm for a circumferential field effect. The energy thus generated interacts with calcification in the atheromatous plaque, causing vibrations which crack and fracture the calcium, both in the superficial as well as deeper layer of vessel wall. The preferential effect on the deeper calcification is a major advantage over other modalities. The efficacy of this technique is proportional to the calcium burden in the plaque with a higher rate of calcium fracture (77%) with greater degree of coronary calcification.[11]

The IVL is preferred for plaque modification in relatively larger size vessels with heavy calcification, both superficial and deep. The lesion should be reachable and crossable by IVL balloon because of its bigger size and crossing profile. The complication rates such as slow flow, dissections, and perforations are also low. The more appropriate indications for IVL are acute coronary syndrome (ACS), unprotected left main coronary artery (LMCA) stenosis, and underexpanded stent due to insufficient modification of underlying calcified plaque.

- *Acute coronary syndrome*: Calcific lesions in the culprit vessel presenting as non-ST-elevation myocardial infarction (STEMI) or STEMI are not uncommon. In one study,[12] moderate calcification was found in 26.1% and severe calcification in 5.9% of cases undergoing PCI for ACS. Primary PCI using IVL for underlying calcific atherothrombotic plaque has shown favorable results.[13,14]
- *Underexpanded stent*: Patients with suboptimal expansion of the stent in a heavily calcified coronary stenosis are at a higher risk of stent thrombosis and adverse cardiac events. Expansion with superhigh-pressure balloon, cutting balloon, and debulking devices is either unsuccessful or associated with high risk of procedural complications and stent damage.[15-19] Delivery of sonic waves by the coronary IVL system has the advantage of transmitting pressure beyond struts and fracture the deep layers of calcium. The success has been reported in several reports.[17,19,20]
- *Unprotected LM calcific stenosis*: Calcification of LM stenosis increases the complexity of the procedure and risk of complications. Since LM is a relatively large vessel, severe stenosis with moderate-to-heavy calcification may not be a suitable subgroup for PCI using ablation techniques. The coronary IVL system using sonic pulses under low pressure might be potentially successful for plaque modification with low risk of complications. There are several reports with acceptable results.[21,22]

Rotational Atherectomy

This modality consists of elliptical-shaped diamond—studded burr which works on the principle of differential cutting. The diamond coating on the distal half of the burr, when rotated at a high speed, and advanced through the calcified coronary stenosis, results in ablation of superficial calcium, thereby facilitating delivery, deployment, and adequate expansion of the stent. The advised burr size to artery ratio is 0.5–0.6 and a safe range of burr revolution speed is 135,000–180,000 RPM. The ideal coronary stenosis which provides an optimal luminal gain after rotablation should have concentric and superficial calcification with a minimal lumen area smaller than the burr size.

Rotational atherectomy is indicated in moderate-to-severe calcific stenosis, which cannot be crossed with the smallest size balloon. It should be avoided in highly tortuous vessels with sharp angulation in the lesion, long and diffusely calcified disease, and the presence of thrombus or an unstable/ulcerated plaque in the clinical setting of ACS.

Orbital Atherectomy

Orbital atherectomy (OA) is a relatively newer modality for treatment of calcified coronary disease. It consists of an eccentrically mounted diamond coated 1.25-mm crown, connected through a drive shift to a controller, powered by pneumatic console. Compared with rotablation burr, the crown of OA is provided with diamond chips both on the front and back, allowing circumferential ablation during antegrade and retrograde motion in the target vessel.

Orbital atherectomy, because of its increase in orbit with increasing speed of rotation, allows ablation of calcium in vessels up to 3.5-mm diameter using the same device (1.25-mm crown). It has distinct advantages over rotablation in releasing smaller-sized particles, without interruption in blood flow during orbiting of crown and less vascular heating.[23]

Rotational versus Orbital Atherectomy

Although both the modalities are based upon the principle of abrasion of calcific plaque using diamond coating on the surface of burr for rotablation and eccentrically mounted crown for OA, there are definite differences between the two technologies **(Table 1)**. In a retrospective analysis of 55 consecutive patients who underwent LM PCI using either OA (n = 25) or rotablation (n = 30), there was no significant difference in major adverse cardiovascular and cerebrovascular events (MACCE), both in-hospital as well as one month follow-up, between the two devices.[24] It was concluded that OA and rotablation are both safe and effective modalities for lesion preparation in high-risk population with calcific LM disease.

In a prospective randomized trial called DIRO, 100 patients with e-novo, heavily calcified coronary lesions were randomized to optical coherence tomography (OCT)-guided PCI with RA versus OA.[25] The stent expansion was significantly greater with RA versus OA (p = 0.02). Similarly, the maximum atherectomy area was larger after RA compared to OA (p = 0.004). However, there was no significant difference in the procedural outcomes and clinical events at 8 months follow-up. The study thus showed that, although RA could produce more favorable plaque modification leading to larger stent expansion, it does not translate into better clinical outcome, when compared to OA.

TABLE 1: Differences between rotational and orbital atherectomy.

Feature	Rotational atherectomy	Orbital atherectomy
Distal cutting or crossing profile	0.3 mm (0.012") (cutting at tip)	0.66 mm (0.026") (crossing profile)
Cutting mechanism	• Unidirectional • Front cutting	• Bidirectional • Circumferential
Need for stepping the device size	Larger vessels require more than one size burr (stepped burr)	Single size crown can treat vessels up to 4.0 mm by creating centrifugal force
Particle size	5–10 µ	1–3
Blood flow in distal vessel	Restricted during rotation of burr	Allows continuous flow during orbiting
Entrapment of device during abrasion	May occur	Rare
Lumen gain (mm)	1.25–2.5	1.25–1.84

Excimer Laser

This technique is based upon the principle of photoablation of atherosclerotic plaque. Clinical use of coronary laser system is limited to treatment of lesions uncrossable and undilatable with balloon. The procedural success is reported to be 93%.[26] Unfortunately, increasing proportion of calcification reduces the efficacy of laser; therefore, laser is rarely used as the first line of debulking strategy

Laser technique does seem to have a role in calcific, undilatable ISR, especially due to an initially underexpanded stent.[16] It is the only option when either the microcatheter or the rotawire/viper wire cannot be deployed. The feasibility and efficacy of combining laser to facilitate rotablation have been described and referred to as the RASER technique.[26]

ASSESSMENT OF CORONARY ARTERY CALCIFICATION

There are four important modalities for assessment and quantification of coronary calcium—(1) computed tomography (CT), (2) coronary angiography, (3) intravascular ultrasound (IVUS), and (4) OCT. Both fluoroscopy and angiography lack sensitivity in detection of coronary artery calcification, hence not useful in quantification. Intravascular imaging is essential before PCI, to delineate precisely the distribution, extent, length, and degree of calcification before PCI.

Intravascular Imaging

Intracoronary imaging using either IVUS or OCT has become essential procedures to provide in-depth analysis of coronary artery calcification and then select the most appropriate modality for plaque modification before stenting.

Based upon intracoronary imaging, the distribution of coronary artery calcification can be divided into three morphological subtypes—(1) eccentric, (2) concentric, and (3) nodular. When calcification is confined to two quadrants or less (<180°), it is defined as eccentric and >180° distribution is classified as concentric. Nodular calcification is visualized as an eruptive calcific protrusion into the lumen. Besides distribution, the length and depth of calcium in the atherosclerotic plaque are also important in predicting the results and, therefore, taken into consideration before decision-making of modality for debulking during PCI. OCT provides better assessment of calcium depth due to the ability of light to penetrate calcium. Thickness of coronary calcification can be assessed on IVUS, by the presence of posterior reverberations which correlate with thinner calcium (<0.5 mm), and significant shadowing, suggestive of thicker calcium (>1 mm).

SCORING FOR CORONARY CALCIFICATION BY INTRAVASCULAR IMAGING

Optical coherence tomography provides additional information on calcium burden by quantifying calcium thickness and volume.[27,28] Based upon maximum calcium angle (degree), thickness (mm), and calcium length (mm), the total score ranges from 0 to 4 points **(Table 2)**.[29] The authors postulated that there will be a stepwise decrease in stent expansion with progressively increasing score.

Recently, an IVUS-specific scoring system was found to be useful in predicting underexpansion of stent using the following four criteria—(1) calcium arc > 270° for a length of 5 mm, (2) presence of 360° calcification, (3) presence of calcified nodule, and (4) an adjacent vessel diameter of <3.5 mm **(Table 3)**. The authors suggested plaque modification by atherectomy if the calculated calcium score is 2–4.[30]

TABLE 2: Optical coherence tomography-based calcium scoring system.

Variable	Score
Maximum calcium angle	
• <180	0
• >180	2
Maximum calcium thickness (mm):	
• <0.5 mm	0
• >0.5 mm	1
Calcium length (mm):	
• <5 mm	0
• >5 mm	1
Total score	0–4

SELECTION OF MODALITY FOR PLAQUE MODIFICATION

Several algorithms have been described but primarily all are based upon assessment of coronary calcification by intravascular imaging. The interventionist should make selection based upon the following observations—(1) distribution of calcification: eccentric, concentric, or nodular, (2) arc of calcification: <180° or >270°, (3) calcium thickness, (4) length of calcified diseased segment, (5) depth of calcification, and (6) diameter of the target vessel. Based upon the personal experience, the author has suggested a stepwise approach, taking into consideration the findings of intracoronary imaging **(Flowchart 1)**.

CONCLUSION

Calcified coronary artery disease continues to remain a challenge for successful PCI. Stent underexpansion resulting in short-term and long-term adverse clinical outcomes is the most frequent hazard with calcified stenosis. Therefore, better understanding of calcium distribution, length, extent, and thickness is extremely important in planning and selection of appropriate debulking modality for achieving an optimal result. The role of intravascular imaging before and after calcium modification is mandatory for assessment of appropriate deployment of stent and satisfactory outcome.

A number of technologies with different mechanisms of action are available for coronary calcified plaque modification, but using the most appropriate modality for a particular stenosis is highly essential and should be based upon the various morphological features assessed by intravascular imaging. It is also important to understand that a combination of devices may be required for optimization of result. Although all techniques have potential complications, but most have demonstrated good safety profile when used appropriately by an experienced operator.

TABLE 3: Calculation of calcium score on intravascular ultrasound.

Variable	Point	
	Yes	NO
Calcium arc >270° for a length of >5 mm	1	0
Calcification 360°	1	0
Calcified nodule	1	0
Vessel diameter <3.5 mm	1	0
Consider atherectomy if calcium score: 2–4		

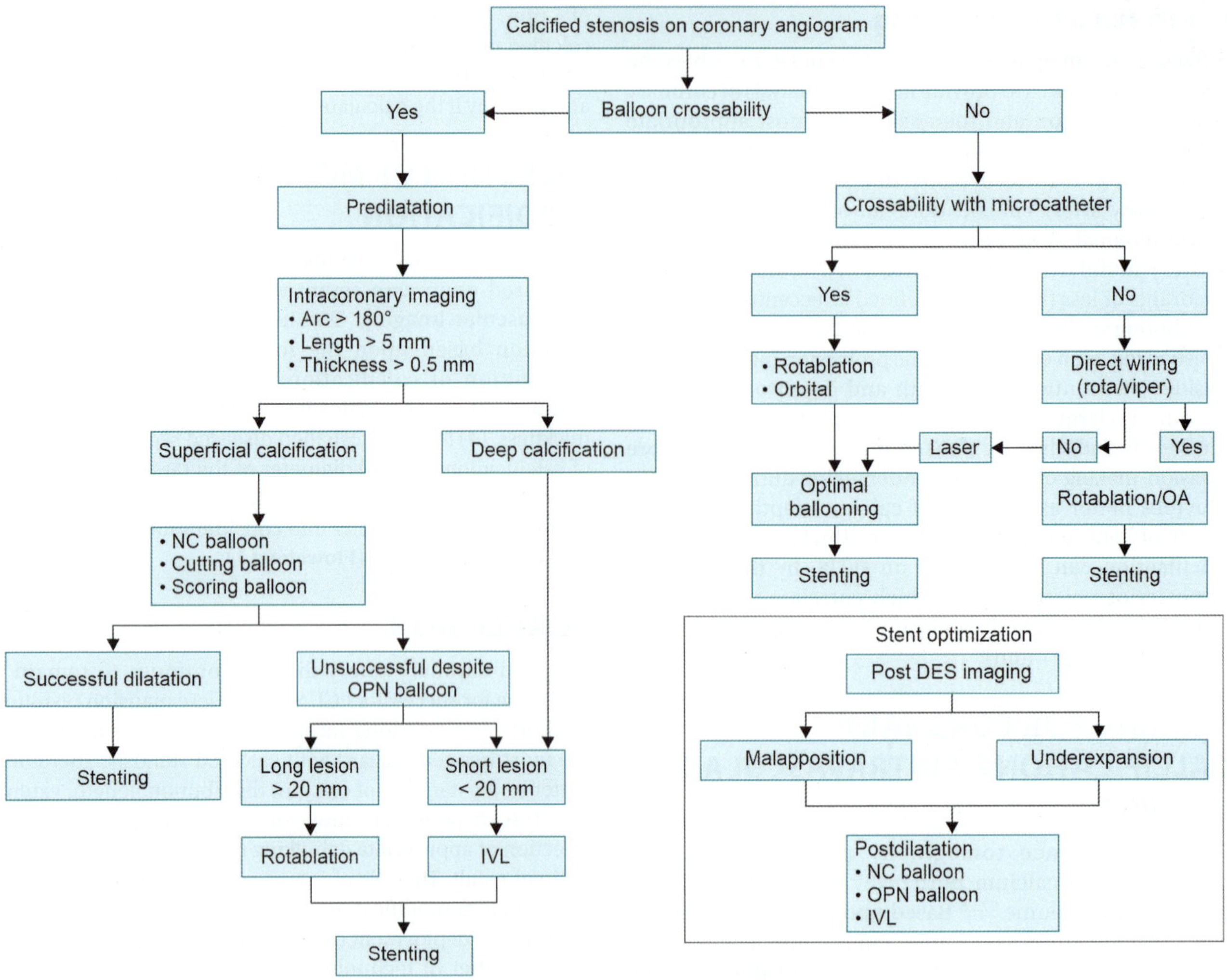

FLOWCHART 1: Algorithm for PCI of calcified lesions visible on coronary angiogram.
(DES: drug-eluting stent; IVL: intravascular lithotripsy; NC: noncompliant; PCI: percutaneous coronary intervention)

More studies are needed to compare the efficacy and safety of various modalities, and follow an algorithmic approach for the treatment of calcific coronary artery disease, based upon clinical profile of the patient, plaque characteristics, availability of various modalities, and most importantly, the experience of the operator.

ONLINE REFERENCES

Please scan the QR code provided at the end of the table of contents for References of this chapter.

CHAPTER

149 Calcific Nodule—A Tough Nut to Crack

I Sathyamurthy, KN Srinivasan, Sengottuvelu G

ABSTRACT

Coronary artery calcification is inevitable with the progression of atherosclerosis. It starts as microcalcification and progresses to calcified nodule (CN). Most often, CN is silent. When it ruptures, it can present as acute coronary syndrome (ACS). CN gives challenges in diagnosis and management if not handled properly. Newer intravascular imaging and calcium-modifying techniques have been made to achieve satisfactory results with percutaneous coronary intervention (PCI) in patients with CN.

Keywords: Calcific nodule, acute coronary syndrome, coronary angiogram, intravascular ultrasound (IVUS), optical coherence tomography (OCT), rotational atherectomy (RA), orbital atherectomy (OA), intravascular lithotripsy (IVL), excimer laser coronary angioplasty (ELCA).

INTRODUCTION

Dense calcification protruding as a nodule inside the coronary lumen is defined as calcified nodule (CN). When CN is associated with acute coronary syndrome (ACS), there is fibrous cap disruption with luminal thrombus over it, and it becomes an eruptive calcified nodule (ECN).

PREVALENCE

The prevalence of culprit CN ranged between 2 and 8% in various series.[1] It varied according to the diagnostic modality used such as coronary angiogram (CAG), intravascular ultrasound (IVUS), or optical coherence tomography (OCT). What was thought to be thrombus (intraluminal filling defects) by CAG turned out to be CN by IVUS. Maximum calcium arc > 180° in OCT was associated with CN, irrespective of clinical presentation.

Among the three etiologies for ACS, namely coronary plaque erosion, plaque rupture, and calcified nodule, the latter seems to be the least frequent cause of luminal thrombosis.

In Lee et al.'s series,[2] 4.2% of all culprit lesions were CN irrespective of clinical presentation and were noted more frequently in elderly (>65 years of age), renal dysfunction and hemodialysis patients, ostial or mid right coronary artery (RCA) segments, and lesions with a large systolic-diastolic angle. The prevalence of CN jumped to 30% once culprit lesion with severe calcification presenting as ACS was included.

Using OCT, Jia et al. reported 10% prevalence of CN culprit lesions, presenting as non-ST-elevation myocardial infarction (NSTEMI) ACS.[3] In other OCT studies, with ST-elevation myocardial infarction (STEMI) ACS patients, the prevalence of CN varied between 3.1 and 8%.[4-6] The prevalence of nonculprit CN lesion was assessed by three-vessel PROSPECT IVUS imaging study and found to be 17% per artery.[7]

Though CN seems more frequent in women, there is no gender difference in the prevalence, once corrected for age, renal dysfunction, and coronary calcium artery arc in multivariate analysis.

Smaller minimum lumen area (MLA) with thrombus was the significant differentiating feature between CN with ACS and CN without ACS.

PRESENTATION

A CN can be silent in nonculprit lesions. In the culprit lesions, it predominantly presents as NSTEMI than STEMI.

DIAGNOSIS

Coronary Angiogram

Identification of coronary calcification by CAG **(Fig. 1A)** is suboptimal, and CNs can present as intraluminal filling defects and be mistaken as thrombus. Hence, intravascular imaging (IVI) modalities such as IVUS and OCT will be useful in diagnosing this entity.

Intravascular Ultrasound

Calcium appears as echo dense in IVUS **(Fig. 1B)**. Parameters such as calcified nodule, 360° of superficial calcium, vessel diameter <3.5 mm, superficial calcium angle >270° larger than 5 mm were associated with stent underexpansion and needed plaque modification by rotablation.[3,8] Though IVUS detected the radial and longitudinal extent of the calcium, it failed to measure the thickness of the calcium due to acoustic shadowing. Deep calcium hidden behind necrotic core and microcalcifications, irregular or corroded surface, and thin fibrous cap were also missed by IVUS.

Optical Coherence Tomography

Calcium appears as low signal intensity with sharply demarcated borders in OCT **(Fig. 1C)**. CN is seen as a small calcium deposit with disruption of fibrous cap on the calcified plate. Culprit lesion containing CN shows more calcium, less lipid, and fewer thin cap fibroatheroma.

Though OCT is less sensitive than IVUS in detecting coronary calcium, it addresses several limitations encountered with IVUS in quantification of calcium. Detection of deep calcium, especially underneath the lipidic or necrotic core, is challenging with OCT.

With OCT, parameters such as calcium arc, calcium thickness, calcium length, and three-dimensional volume can be measured. Fujino et al. have given a score that predicts stent underexpansion when the score is 4. This score comprises >0.5-mm calcium depth (1 point), >5-mm calcium

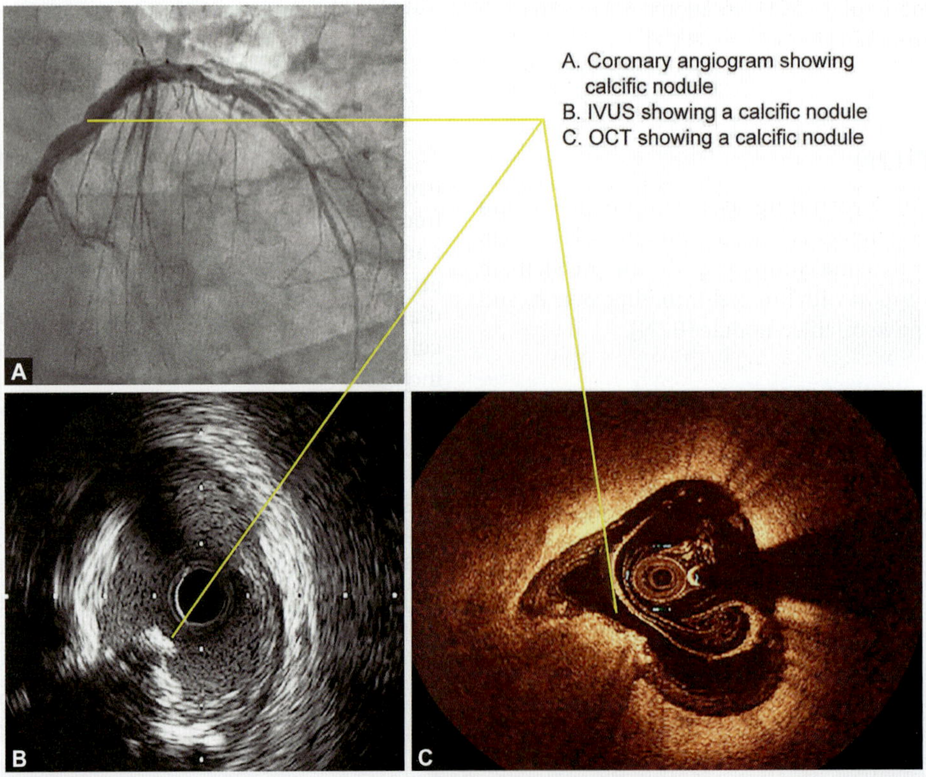

FIGS. 1A TO C: (A) Coronary angiogram showing a calcific nodule; (B) Intravascular ultrasound (IVUS) showing an echo dense calcific nodule at 7–8 o'clock position; (C) Optical coherence tomography (OCT) showing a protruding nodular calcium with disruption of fibrous cap at 7–8 o'clock position.

longitudinal length (1 point), and >180° calcium width (calcium arc) (2 points).[9]

TREATMENT

Treatment modalities available are balloon-based techniques such as high-pressure balloon, scoring balloon and cutting balloon, rotational atherectomy (RA), intravascular lithotripsy (IVL), orbital atherectomy (OA), and excimer laser coronary angioplasty (ELCA). The treatment modality depends upon the morphology of calcium (eccentric vs. concentric, short vs. long).

Balloon-based Technique

Balloon-based technique includes cutting balloon, scoring balloon, and high-pressure balloon. The former two will create cracks in the calcium and facilitate vessel dilation. This can be used alone or can be combined with other modalities such as RA to get maximal luminal gain.

Very-high-pressure balloons are used in both eccentric and concentric calcifications. OPN high-pressure balloons can be dilated to 50 atm. This plays a crucial role in undilatable lesions. ISAR-CALC trial has compared high-pressure balloon versus scoring balloon in lesions with residual stenosis >30% after standard balloon dilatation.[10] This is an OCT-based study, and there was no difference in OCT-defined stent expansion index between the groups. Similarly, there is no difference in angiographic, procedural, strategic success between the groups. However, with the OPN balloon group, there was larger angiographically assessed minimal lumen diameter, less residual stenosis, and less need for poststent noncompliant (NC) balloon dilatation compared to scoring balloon group.

Rotational Atherectomy

Rotational atherectomy creates differential ablation of calcified tissue without disturbing the healthy elastic tissue. The end result of RA depends upon the eccentricity of the calcium, minimal luminal area, burr size, and degree of guidewire bias. Selection of proper rota burr will facilitate optimal wire contact with the CN. CN with concentric calcification gives favorable ablation with RA. Eccentric CN has got favorable outcomes after RA if the wire is biased towards CN.

Orbital Atherectomy

Orbital atherectomy consists of a 1.25-mm, eccentrically mounted, diamond-coated crown that can be ablated in both forward and backward motion unlike RA. Safety and efficacy of the OA were studied in the Orbit I and II trials.[11,12] In >98% of the lesions, OA could achieve diameter stenosis to <50%. There was only 2.3% significant dissection in the study. This device is slided over a 0.014″ dedicated wire, which allows better maneuverability, unlike RA, which uses a 0.009″ rota wire. OA produces more deeper and longer cuts than RA. Whether this translates to better clinical outcomes needs to be ascertained in future trials. A real-world, multicenter, single-arm, retrospective study was done by Lee et al.[13] It included 458 consecutive patients with heavily calcified coronary lesions (HCCL) treated with OA. The primary endpoint of 30-day major cardiac and cerebrovascular events was 1.7%. Dissection, perforation, and no reflow were 0.9%, 0.7%, and 0.7%, respectively. The 30-day all-cause mortality was 1.3%, myocardial infarction (MI) 1.1%, stroke 0.2%, and stent thrombosis 0.9%.

Unlike RA, there is continuous coronary perfusion both during the rest period and during atherectomy treatment in OA. Similarly, a microvascular resistance index was lower with OA than RA. A meta-analysis of observational studies shows no difference in procedural complication, 30-day events including death, MI, and target vessel revascularization (TVR) between OA and RA.[14]

Lithotripsy

Intravascular lithotripsy uses acoustic energy that propagates through the vessel wall and creates cracks in both superficial and deep calcium. The Ali et al. series show efficacy proportionately increased with calcium burden.[15] There were no serious safety issues. There was >90% procedural success (≤30% residual angiographic stenosis) in pooled analysis of DISRUPT CAD series.[16]

Though IVL is predominantly recommended in concentric calcium, it is used off label in eccentric calcium, stent underexpansion and calcified neo-atherosclerosis. It can be combined with RA in uncrossable lesions, and IVI will help in optimizing the end result.

There is a risk of proarrhythmia with IVL because of electrical interference causing VOO mode pacing. Hence, special caution should be taken in pacemaker patients while using IVL.

Excimer Laser

Excimer laser disrupts plaques through three mechanisms, namely photochemical, photomechanical, and photothermal. It mixes a rare gas and halogen to generate brief pulses of high-frequency short wavelength ultraviolet (UV) light. Evidence of use of ELCA in calcified lesion is limited and is rarely used as a first-line strategy for calcium modification. However, this is the only option available in uncrossable and undilatable lesions. ELCA when combined will facilitate RA (RASER technique).[17] In patients with calcific undilatable in-stent restenosis, ELCA was found to be superior to high-pressure balloon dilatation.

CONCLUSION

Dense calcified CAD is no more a nightmare with the availability of better IVI techniques (IVUS, OCT) and high-level calcium-modifying techniques such as RA, OA, IVL, and ELCA, in addition to cutting balloon, scoring balloon, and high-pressure balloon. With the increase in life expectancy, aged population is increasing with a proportionate increase in severe calcific CAD. Choosing the right mode of calcium-modifying technique with IVI assistance is the key to the success of the procedure.

ONLINE REFERENCES

Please scan the QR code provided at the end of the table of contents for References of this chapter.

CHAPTER

150 Coronary Orbital Atherectomy System: Case Selection and Procedural Challenges

Dibya Kumar Baruah

ABSTRACT

Calcified coronary artery requires adequate lesion preparation before stent implantation. Strategy of stent implantation without appropriate lesion preparation may lead to suboptimal result and more complications. Therefore, an upfront calcium modification strategy has become a primary step in the treatment of a moderate-to-severe calcified coronary artery lesion. The rotational atherectomy device has been a useful tool for decades in the treatment of a severely calcified lesion and its efficacy has been proved in different clinical trials. However, due to the complexity of the procedure and a relatively long learning curve, its adaptation rate has been low among interventional cardiologists and a less complex, user-friendly device has been a long due for interventionalists. Finally, after decades of wait, a new atherectomy device, orbital atherectomy system, has been launched with new promises. Powered with a different mechanism of action, its 1.25-mm diamond-coated eccentrically mounted crown orbits rather than spins concentrically on a dedicated guidewire allowing differential sanding of the fibrotic and calcified lesions. Based on the speed of the crown, the same burr can treat arteries of different diameters obviating the need for changing the burr. Moreover, differential and incomplete contact of the crown allows intermittent distal blood flow enabling flushing of the microdebris and facilitating cooling effect resulting in less thermal injury and low incidence of slow flow or no reflow. The device has been evaluated for the treatment of calcified coronary lesions in ORBIT I and ORBIT II trials and found to be effective in crossing majority of the lesions with successful stent implantation.

Keywords: Calcified coronary lesion, atherectomy, PCI.

INTRODUCTION

Percutaneous coronary intervention (PCI) has evolved leaps and bounds in the past two decades, enabling it to treat more complex, diffuse, and calcified coronary artery lesions. Since the early days of coronary intervention, calcified coronary artery lesions have been considered as a difficult subset and posed as a predictor of worst clinical outcomes. From the plain balloon angioplasty era to the bare-metal stent era, calcified lesions have met with various challenges such as procedural failures, stent failures, and high incidence of target lesion failures.[1] Introduction of drug-eluting stents (DES) has revolutionized PCI with a high success rate, less in-stent restenosis rate, and reduced target lesion revascularization.[2] As a result, the landscape of contemporary PCI has changed and more complex and calcified interventions have come into its fold. Parallel to this development, new challenges have emerged. Preparation of the calcified coronary bed for laying DES has become a necessity and, at the same time, become a challenging task. Lesion preparation prior to stent implantation allows easy deployment of stent with its adequate expansion, which are important prerequisites for optimal result and good long-term outcomes. Calcified lesions are encountered more frequently in present-day practice, and in real-world scenarios, one-third of present-day PCI consists of these lesions.[3] Calcification transforms compliant coronary artery into a rigid vessel, which prohibits stent delivery and impedes stent expansion, leading to higher rates of serious complications such as stent thrombosis and stent restenosis.[4] Therefore, prior lesion preparation is of paramount importance for smooth delivery of stents, their expansion, and the desired result with adequate final lumen diameter. To treat these rocky-hard lesions, routine balloon therapy is not enough for which various advanced coronary tools have been introduced in the last few decades, e.g., cutting balloon, scoring balloon, ultra-high-pressure balloon, atherectomy devices, and recent addition of intravascular lithotripsy device.[5] Nevertheless, challenges still remain as no particular device is fully effective in the treatment of all calcified lesions encountered in different clinical scenarios; therefore, the search for newer and more efficient tool is always on.

A relatively recent advancement in the field of atheroablation is orbital atherectomy system (OAS) (Diamondback 360®, Cardiovascular Systems Inc) **(Figs. 1A to C)**, gaining Food and Drug Administration approval in 2013 based on the results of the ORBIT II (Evaluate the Safety and Efficacy of OAS in Treating Severely Calcified Coronary Lesions) trial.[6] The system consists of a 1.25-mm diamond-studded crown, which can be advanced over a dedicated 012″ guidewire with 014″ tip (ViperWire, Advance Coronary Guide Wire, Cardiovascular Systems Inc), and is compatible with a 6F guide catheter. The crown orbits in two speeds, 80,000 and 120,000 rpm, which can be controlled by a hand-held electric power handle mounted on the system. A readymade lubricant used during the procedure is ViperSlide (Cardiovascular System Inc). Orbital atherectomy (OA) treats calcified plaques by the mechanism of differential sanding along with calcium rupture. Based on the rotational speed, it can adjust to the diameter of the target vessel without the need of changing the burr multiple times as required in rotational atherectomy. A distinguishing feature of OA is its ability to ablate bidirectionally, potentially decreasing the likelihood for burr entrapment, which is a feared complication seen during rotational atherectomy. Owing to the elliptical mechanism of action, OA is contraindicated in vessels < 2.5 mm in diameter due to increased risk of vessel perforation.

Compared to rotational atherectomy, OA produces more tissue dissection and allows better stent expansion resulting in less stent malaposition.[7] The ablative process produces smaller particles (<2 µm), and unlike rotational atherectomy, allowing continuous blood flow during ablation. These features potentially reduce the likelihood of slow flow/no reflow, decrease thermal injury during the procedure, and obviate the need for the routine use of a temporary pace-

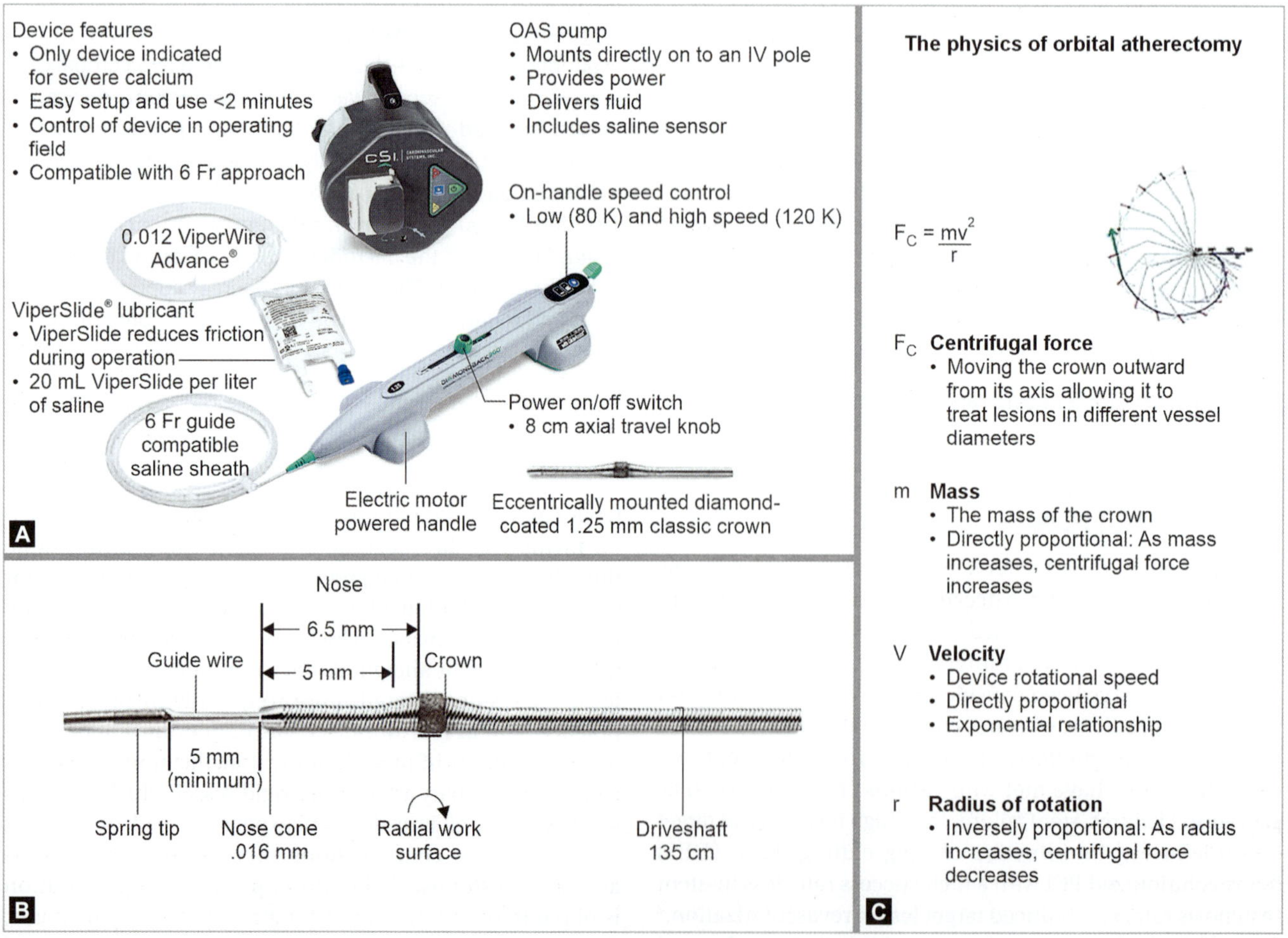

FIGS. 1A TO C: (A) Diamondback 360® Coronary Orbital Atherectomy System; (B) 1.25 mm coronary classic crown; (C) Orbital motion and principle.

(IV: intravenous; OAS: orbital atherectomy system)

maker during OA. The orbital motion of the crown is based on the formula for centrifugal force: $F_c = mv^2/r$. If F_c (force) was not present, object (m) would move along its velocity vector (v). F_c can be produced by gravitational attraction (as the earth is moving around the sun) or a string as in this case **(Figs. 1A to C)**. It is evident from this formula that the radius of rotation (R) can vary according to the velocity of the crown **(Fig. 2)**.

PROCEDURAL CONSIDERATIONS AND CASE SELECTION FOR ORBITAL ATHERECTOMY

Though atherectomy has been a bailout tool for undilatable and uncrossable calcified lesions, a better approach to a calcified lesion is a planned strategy with prior evaluation of severity and type of coronary calcification with the help of coronary imaging.[8] The strategy of planned atherectomy has multiple advantages of high success rate, less contrast, and shortened procedural time. **Flowchart 1** demonstrates the systematic approach while treating a calcified lesion.[9]

Orbital atherectomy is indicated to facilitate stent delivery in patients with known severely calcified coronary artery de novo lesions who are candidates for percutaneous transluminal coronary angioplasty or stenting (case example, **Figs. 3A to F**). Though the clinical trial did not include all cases of calcified lesions like ostial and left main disease, procedural simplification of OA, and adjustable ablation diameter with the same crown size with the rotational speed control, its application can be extended to various other potential situations as follows.

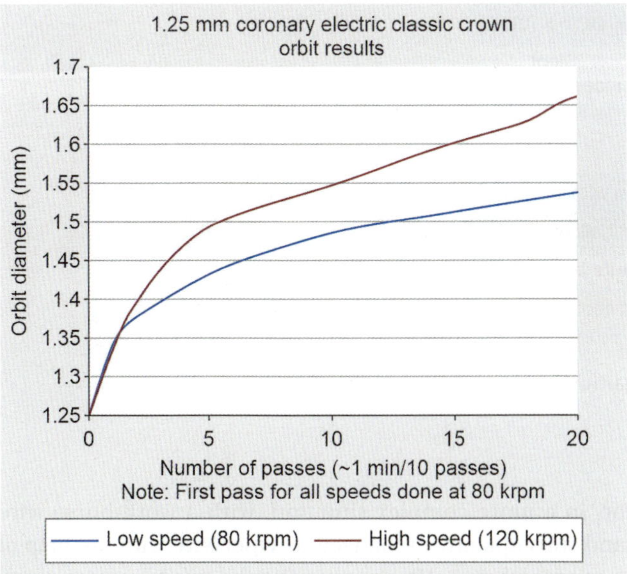

FIG. 2: Maximum lumen diameters after orbital atherectomy with a 1.25-mm classic crown. It demonstrates typical orbit diameter versus duration of operation (as measured in simulated calcified lesions); it is for reference only. Actual orbit performance may vary.
Courtesy: CSI IFU.

MULTIVESSEL DISEASE WITH SEVERE CALCIFICATION

The biggest challenge in the treatment of severely calcific multivessel disease is to achieve complete revascularization. A higher residual SYNTAX score is an indicator for incomplete revascularization after treatment of multivessel disease and a powerful determinant of prognosis.[10] OA helps in lesion modification, facilitates stent delivery, and subsequent complete revascularization resulting in a lower residual SYNTAX score. Whether this could translate into improved clinical outcome is yet to be established.[11]

OSTIAL LESIONS, UNPROTECTED LEFT MAIN DISEASE, CHRONIC TOTAL OCCLUSIONS

Ostial and left main lesions require more aggressive ablation similar to chronic total occlusion. Though not studied in the clinical trial, OA can be potentially a safe tool to prepare these lesions by applying optimal precautions.

LESION PREPARATION FOR IMPLANTATION OF BIORESORBABLE SCAFFOLDS

Bioresorbable scaffold implantation requires more extensive lesion preparation, especially in calcified lesions due to its relatively bulkier size and limited mechanical strength. Atherectomy device like OA has a great role in lesion preparation before implantation of the scaffolds.

CONTRAINDICATIONS OF ORBITAL ATHERECTOMY

Orbital atherectomy is contraindicated in the following conditions:

- Uncrossable lesion: Guidewire fails to cross.
- Lesion is within a graft or stent (in-stent restenosis).
- Patient is not a suitable candidate for atherectomy, coronary angioplasty, or bypass surgery.
- Angiographic presence of thrombus in the target lesion
- Multivessel disease with only a single functional coronary artery
- Evidence of coronary dissection on angiogram
- Pregnant women
- Children

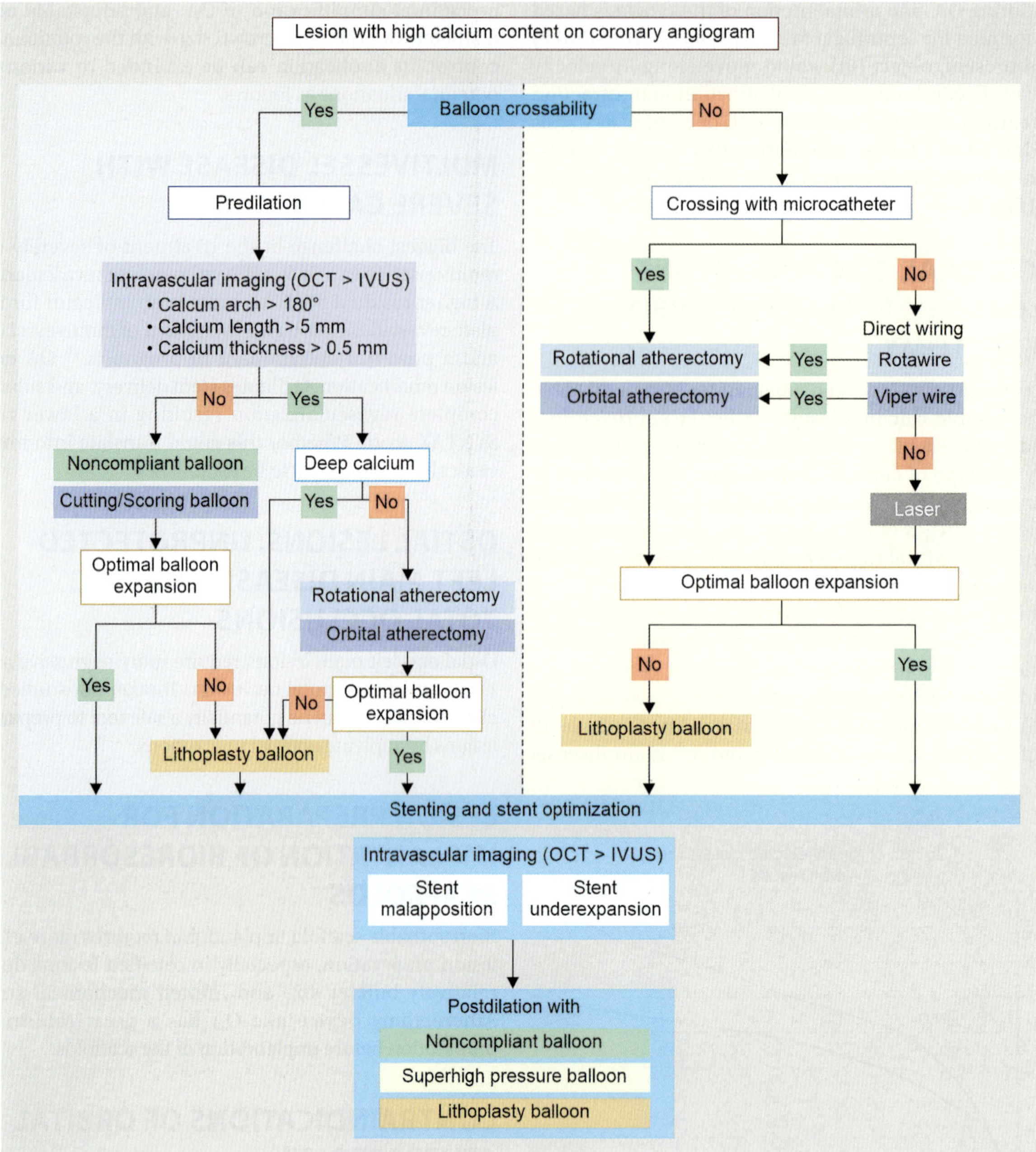

FLOWCHART 1: Algorithm for the optimal management of coronary calcium.
(IVUS: intravascular ultrasound; OCT: optical coherence tomography)

TECHNIQUE

Necessary equipment should be arranged before starting the procedure [coronary OAS, guide catheter, intravenous (IV) pole, normal saline, and fluoroscopy imaging equipment]. After obtaining vascular access, engage the selected coronary artery to be treated with a 6F guide catheter and use angiography, intravascular ultrasound (IVUS), or optical coherence tomography (OCT) to localize and evaluate the target lesion. The lesion can be crossed with the ViperWire or, in a more complex situation, with a work-horse wire and subsequently exchanged to ViperWire with the help of a microcatheter. After connecting the orbital atherectomy device (OAD) to the OAS, the pump should be primed. Prior testing should be performed to ensure appropriate crown advancement and rotation using the on and off button. Under fluoroscopic guidance, the OAD can be advanced carefully over the guidewire till about 10 mm proximal to the lesion ensuring that the distal tip is beyond the lesion. Now

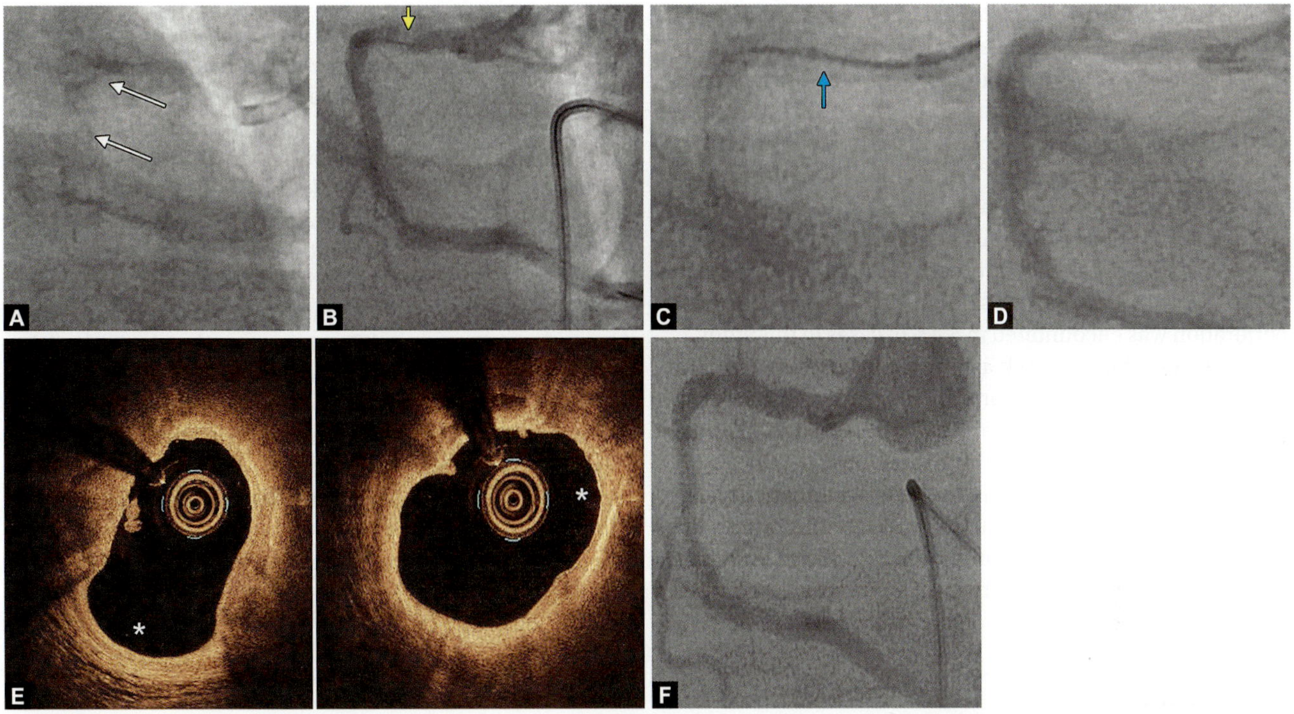

FIGS. 3A TO F: Typical case example of angiography and optical coherence tomography images after orbital atherectomy. A 78-year-old man presents with stable angina. A heavily calcified right coronary artery (OCT catheter could not be crossed prior to OA due to heavy calcification) was successfully treated by orbital atherectomy (1.25-mm classic crown) followed by drug-eluting stent implantation. Total orbital atherectomy system (OAS) run time was 90 seconds (three passes at 80,000 rpm). (A) Calcification by fluoroscopy (white arrow); (B) Eccentric calcified lesion (yellow arrow); (C) OA crown (blue arrow); (D) Post-OA angiogram; (E) Post-OA OCT shows the typical scooped-out ablated area of the calcified lesions (star); (F) Final result after stenting.

(OA: orbital atherectomy; OCT: optical coherence tomography)

the device can be activated for atherectomy with an initial speed of 80,000 rpm and the crown should be advanced using the advancer knob at a slow speed, not faster than 1 mm/s. It should be mentioned that the crown needs to move continuously as the static position of the crown with rotation in the same segment can result in vascular damage. After a series of careful ablation utilizing back and forth movement of the crown, with an intermittent interval of rest in between, the result can be checked with an angiogram. The usual recommended treatment interval is 25 seconds and can be extended to a maximum of 30 seconds. The OAS pump emits a beep after 25 seconds of treatment, which can be used as a guide for treatment time. If the angiographic result is not adequate with low speed, high speed (120,000 rpm) can be considered and should be performed if there is no high-risk angiographic feature such as significant tortuosity, and the vessel size is big. Once the result is satisfactory, OAD can be removed safely after locking the control. Further preparation of the coronary bed can be performed with balloon dilatation prior to stent implantation.

COMPLICATIONS AND CHALLENGES

The safety and effectiveness of OA have been demonstrated in clinical studies and all-comer real-world registries.[12,13] Complications have been reported to be low even in high-risk group of patients such as elderly, diabetics, female, ostial and aorto-ostial lesions, subtotal occlusion, bifurcation lesions, post-coronary artery bypass graft (CABG), and patients with low left ventricular (LV) ejection fraction.[14-16] Common complications reported during OA are dissection, slow-flow, and coronary perforation. Data related to the treatment of ostial and aorto-ostial lesions with OA are less, and challenges can be mitigated by adapting the optimal OA ostial technique.[17] The recommended technique for ostial lesion is retrograde ablation, in which after crossing the lesion with the crown, ablation can be activated from distal to proximal direction. In a situation where the lesion is too tight to cross, a guide can be advanced for better coaxial position and more support. Once it is done, the crown should be placed more closer to the lesion (5 mm proximal to the lesion than the normal position of 10 mm), and it can be slowly and steadily advanced across the lesion. After the initial success, further ablation can be carried out in the retrograde direction. Important technical considerations during ostial or aorto-ostial ablation are coaxial guide position and its proper engagement to achieve maximum support. The same principle should be applied before escalation of crown speed to a higher level. This strategy of OA discussed above, while treating ostial and aorto-ostial lesions, might be of help to reduce the possibility of vessel perforation as well as damage to the aorta.

Complications have been reported in the form of coronary dissection, and perforation in the ORBIT I and the ORBIT II trials with low incidences of slow flow and no reflow due to distal emboli.[18] Nevertheless, perforation of the coronary artery has been reported as the most serious complication of OA in various studies. In the largest real-world experience in calcified ostial lesions by Chambers et al., OA was found to be safe and effective.[19] Coronary perforation was encountered in 5.4% of cases in this study.

Transient heart block is uncommon with OA, but bradycardia has been reported. In a study by Lee et al. involving 50 patients, bradycardia was observed in 4%, none of which required pacemaker implantation.[20]

Other rare complications include pseudoaneurysm[21] and dislodged microtip,[22] and device malfunctions like detachment and separation of pieces and device structural damage that can involve various components like crown, body, guidewire tip, driveshaft tip, and driveshaft body.[23]

CONCLUSION

Percutaneous coronary intervention has been increasingly undertaken in high-risk subsets of coronary artery disease, including elderly population. High prevalence of diabetes and chronic kidney disease has further increased the number of these complex calcified lesions in the present-day practice, significantly limiting the success rate of PCI. In this scenario, upfront treatment of calcified lesions is a prerequisite for adequate stent expansion and deployment to achieve good result. Though various tools have been in use for calcium modification, none has been found to be perfect in this respect. Recent addition of OA into this tool basket has added an extra strength to the calcium management with new promises. At present, this novel device allows lesion preparation of severely calcified plaque in a limited clinical situation prior to stent implantation. However, more experiences and randomized data are in the queue for further strengthening its efficacy and extending its horizon to embrace more complex lesions in different clinical situations.

ONLINE REFERENCES

Please scan the QR code provided at the end of the table of contents for References of this chapter.

CHAPTER

151 Application of Excimer Laser in Cardiovascular Interventions

Smit Shrivastava

ABSTRACT

The excimer laser has evolved to be a very safe percutaneous coronary intervention tool that compliments and supplements other tools to achieve greater success in balloon uncrossable or undilatable stenosis, in-stent restenosis, and high thrombus burden coronary and peripheral vascular lesions. The LASER ablation is finding newer applications that are extending beyond coronary vasculature into LASER pacemaker lead extraction, saphenous vein graft angioplasty. The laser has been recently introduced to India and is growing fast across the country. This chapter illustrates the various applications of excimer laser in the field of cardiovascular interventions and explores the evolution of each indication and application with the status in India.

Keywords: Excimer laser coronary angioplasty (ELCA) Tripsy, laser lead extraction, in-stent restenosis, chronic total occlusion, RASER PCI, primary percutaneous coronary intervention, saphenous vein graft.

INTRODUCTION

Excimer laser coronary angioplasty (ELCA) in cardiovascular interventions has evolved as an effective and safe accoutrement to the percutaneous coronary and vascular intervention tools. The ELCA was introduced in early 1980 for critical limb ischemia and later evolved application for coronary interventions as an alternative to balloon angioplasty.[1] The Cedar Sinai Medical Center, Los Angeles in 1988 is credited to have done the first successful human ELCA,[2] and in India, the official first case outside license trial study was done at Advanced Cardiac Institute, Pt J N M Medical College, Raipur **(Fig. 1)**. The ELCA however proved to be an expensive, cumbersome, and nonsuperior to balloon angioplasty and therefore, its application became recessed to some niche indications including balloon uncrossable or undilatable stenosis, in-stent restenosis, stent underexpansion, saphenous vein graft (SVG) restenosis, and large thrombus burden percutaneous coronary intervention (PCI). This chapter aims to explore and exemplify the various applications of excimer laser in the field of cardiovascular interventions.

PLAQUE MODIFICATION TOOLS

The best suited solution to achieve plaque modification is plaque annihilation rather than plastic deformation

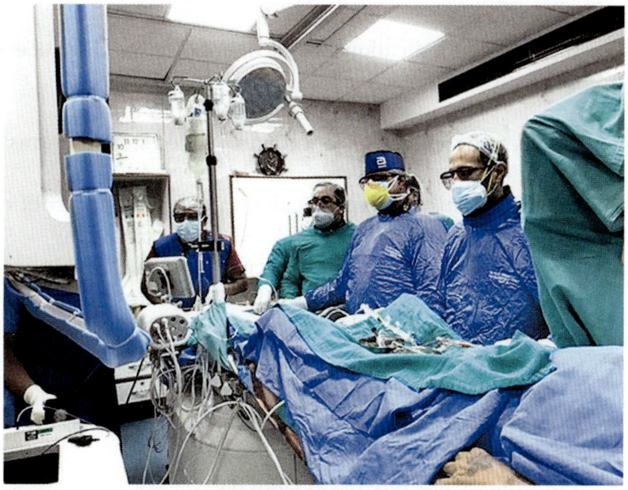

FIG. 1: Introduction of excimer laser therapy to India.

of obstructive plaque accompanied by intimal tears and dissections risking abrupt vessel closure and slow flow phenomenon. Among the routine plaque modification tools, excimer laser stands out as the only ablation tool that avoids violent plaque abruption, platelet activation experienced with all other plaque modification tools including percutaneous transluminal coronary angioplasty (PTCA) balloon, and directional or rotational atherectomy. Excimer laser energy has been shown to ablate inorganic material by photochemical mechanisms that break molecular bonds by a photochemical–thermomechanical effect without generation of excessive heat. The inorganic material ablation happens by vapor formation and accompanies thrombus dissolution and platelet inactivation. The ELCA therefore is devoid of immediate elastic recoil and platelet activation witnessed in PTCA and rotablative techniques.[2]

APPLICATIONS OF EXCIMER LASER IN CARDIOVASCULAR INTERVENTIONS

The frequent indications for ELCA with approval from the Food and Drug Administration (FDA) are:[3]

- Undilatable lesion
- Uncrossable lesion—chronic total occlusions (CTOs) and Takayasu aortoarteritis
- Long and diffuse atherosclerotic lesions
- Moderately calcified lesions
- In-stent restenosis (due to excessive neointimal proliferation)
- Ostial or bifurcation lesions requiring ablative plaque modification
- Primary PCI with large thrombus burden
- Pacemaker lead extraction
- Thrombus annihilation/restenosis in SVG
- Ostial or bifurcation lesions requiring ablative plaque modification

The off-label indications for excimer laser that have been applied with success are:

- Ancillary to routine PCI in heavy thrombus burden
- Auxiliary to routine PCI in underexpanded stent (contrast grenadoplasty)
- Modification of proximal calcium cap after unprolific tracking of rotablation wire

The ELCA bears no absolute contraindications unlike other plaque addressing tools. The relative contraindications include:

- Coronary dissection
- Acute vessel angulation (>45°)
- Unprotected left main coronary artery
- Heavily calcified vessel
- Vessel sizes <0.9 mm ELCA catheter

Undilatable Lesion: ELCA-Tripsy

There are only two cases in the world reported for the use of excimer laser and subsequent intravascular lithotripsy (IVL) for PCI. Alfonso Jurado-Román reported the first use of excimer laser to allow passage of an IVL balloon for PCI of the right coronary artery in a 61-year-old patient.[4] The second case is demonstrated here by the author at Advanced Cardiac Institute, Pt J N M Medical College, Raipur, India.

Application

The patient was a male in 70s with diabetes and hypertension with chronic angina and ejection fraction of 35% and regional wall motion abnormalities in the left anterior descending artery and left circumflex artery territories. He underwent radial percutaneous intervention while the guidewire could track across the lid left anterior descending artery diffuse calcified lesion, a balloon of 1.2 × 12 mm failed to cross. The ELCA was used from the proximal end of the calcified lesion at increasing ablative power from 45 mJ/mm × 25 Hz to 30 mJ/mm × 30 Hz followed by subsequent balloon dilatation with 1.2 × 12 mm, 2.0 × 10 mm, and 2.5 × 12 mm and IVL with 2.75 × 12 mm balloon. This represents the first use of these two disruptive technologies together in a patient in Asia and second in the world ***(Figs. 2A to D).***

Undilatable Lesion: ELCA-OPN

The prospective multicenter study compared the standard laser therapy and the increased laser therapy to demonstrate a successful 89% safe ablation of balloon undilatable lesions. This subgroup is amenable to limited choice of PCI tools, all other tools like rotational or orbital atherectomy bear complications like no reflow or slow flow due to downstream embolization and platelet activation. However, excimer laser stands out as the only alternative that promotes platelet deactivation. The study had eight lesions that were not tracked by laser in full length yet it modified the proximal lesion enough to permeate balloon tip crossing and successful stent implantation. The study observed no pertinent complications such as perforations, spasm, or no-reflow phenomenon in the group.[5] In the study on veterans, the second most common indication for ELCA was balloon undilatable after balloon uncrossable lesions (40.8%) with 94.3 and 93.8%, technical and procedural success rates, respectively.[6]

Application

This female in mid-40s presented with anterior wall myocardial infarction and ejection fraction of 45% and postmyocardial angina. The balloon failed to track the mid-left anterior descending fibrotic lesion and the patient was planned 4 days later for a intravascular ultrasound

(IVUS)-guided ELCA and OPN-NC PCI to left anterior descending artery with 1.4 mm × 60 mJ/mm × 40 Hz lasing followed by OPN-NC dilatation at 30 and 40 mm Hg inflation pressures. The final stents of 3.0 × 48 and 2.5 mm × 32 mm were deployed in the left anterior descending artery. This case was the first application of ELCA in India outside a license trial study and it was followed by establishment and growth of laser therapy at other centers in India ***(Figs. 3A to D)****.*

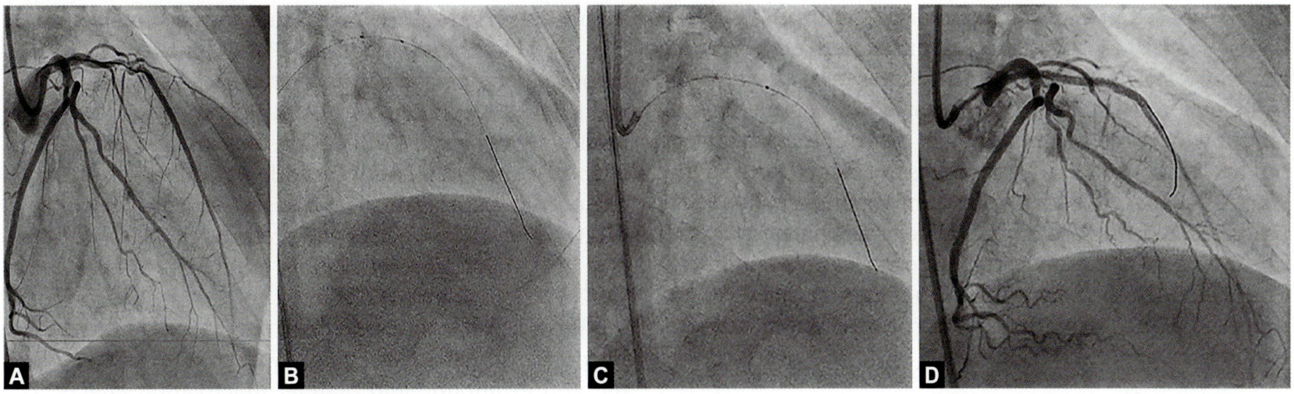

FIGS. 2A TO D: Undilatable lesion—excimer laser coronary angioplasty (ELCA)-Tripsy.

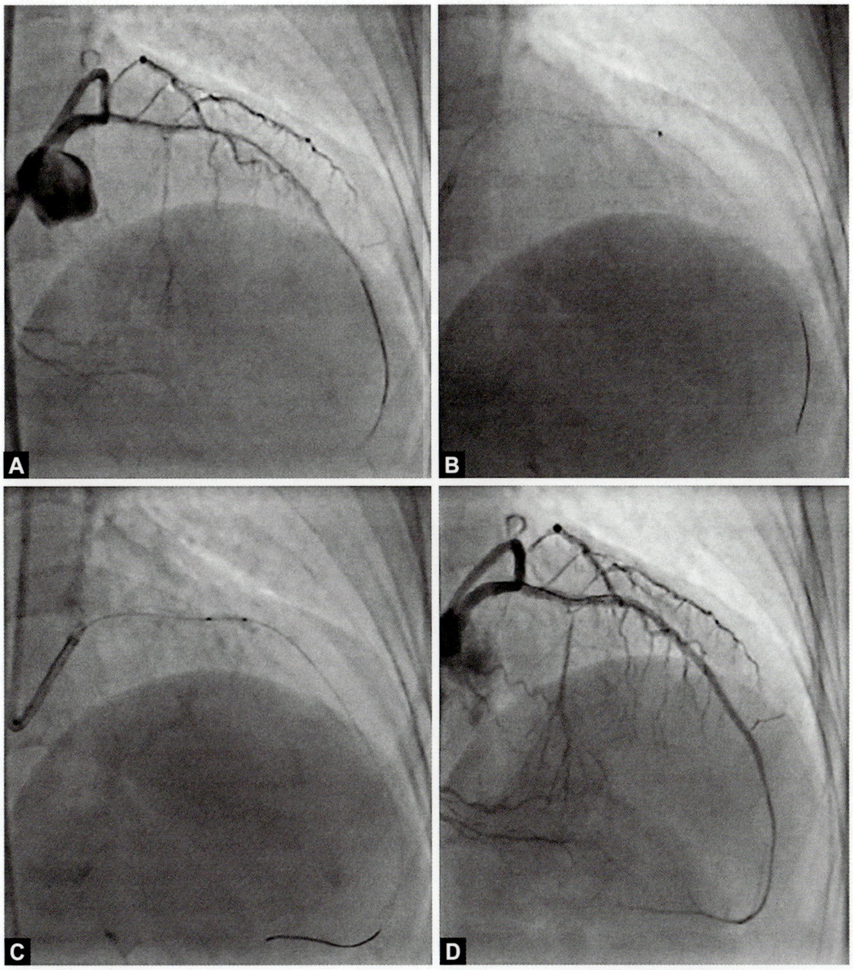

FIGS. 3A TO D: Undilatable lesion—excimer laser coronary angioplasty (ELCA)-OPN.

Undilatable Lesion: Underexpanded Stent

Very limited PCI tools are available to address underexpansion of a deployed stent. Stent underexpansion is a precursor for stent thrombosis. The other PCI tools like aggressive or high pressure/diameter balloon dilatation risks vessel damage and rotational atherectomy risks distal embolization and burr stalling. ELCA again comes out as the only technique to ablate resistant atheroma without tumultuous effect on the stent integrity. Though the laser excludes effect on the calcification itself, it modifies the plaque beyond the stent to accomplish complete stent expansion. The high power lasing in the absence of saline or magnifies safely the ablative effect in a contrast-milieu (contrast grenadoplasty). The ELLEMENT registry of 28 patients showed 96.4% procedural success with a low associated major adverse cardiovascular event (MACE) rate.[6]

Application

The application of contrast grenadoplasty awaits occurrence at Advanced Cardiac Institute, Pt J N M Medical College, Raipur, India.

Uncrossable Lesion: Chronic Total Occlusions

The first randomized trial comparing ELCA with balloon angioplasty [Amsterdam-Rotterdam (AMRO) trial] had one-third lesions as CTO and determined no significant advantage of excimer laser angioplasty over balloon angioplasty.[7] In a similar manner, the initial attempts prior to proper technical expertise with excimer laser for CTO PCI were not encouraging.[8] However, Shen in their four years experience with excimer LASER in 33 cases without the saline flush reported a success in 90% cases without serious complications.[9] In one of the largest series of ELCA for balloon failure lesions with a large proportion of CTO cases, ELCA enabled successful PCI in over 90%.[6] A study of 100 lesions in 80 subjects [LEONARDO study—early outcome of high energy Laser (Excimer) facilitated coronary angioplasty ON hARD and complex calcified and balloOn-resistant coronary lesions] reported 93.7% success rate with no complications. The most common indication (43.8%) for the use of ELCA among veterans was balloon uncrossable lesions and ELCA yielded 87.8% technical and 83.7% procedural success. Judit Karacsonyi reviewed 4,845 CTO lesions to observe that 15.5% of them were balloon uncrossable or balloon undilatable. The use of excimer laser in such cases had a greater technical (91.5% vs. 83.1%, $p = 0.010$) and procedural (88.9% vs. 81.6%, $p = 0.033$) success rates while a similar MACE incidence (3.92% vs. 3.51%, $p = 0.805$).[10]

The excimer laser is safest bail out device for uncrossable proximal cap after attaining distal wire passage as it possesses the antithrombotic and platelet-inactivation effects. The saline flush is not utilized to prevent extension of dissection and the improbable amount of saline reaching the laser-CTO interface.[2] Another caution is to avoid the use of high powered ELCA over polymer-jacketed wires that may sustain structural disintegrity in the process.[11]

Application

The patient was a bidi smoker male in mid-50s with diabetes and hypertension and old anterior and recent inferior wall myocardial infarction and recovered left hemiparesis. His diagnostic angiography revealed a diffuse critical triple vessel disease with CTO of the left anterior descending artery. He underwent lasing to the chronically occlusive left anterior descending artery and the diffusely diseased right coronary with 45 mJ/mm × 25 Hz. The stent implantation was successfully done to the three coronary arteries ***(Figs. 4A and B)****.*

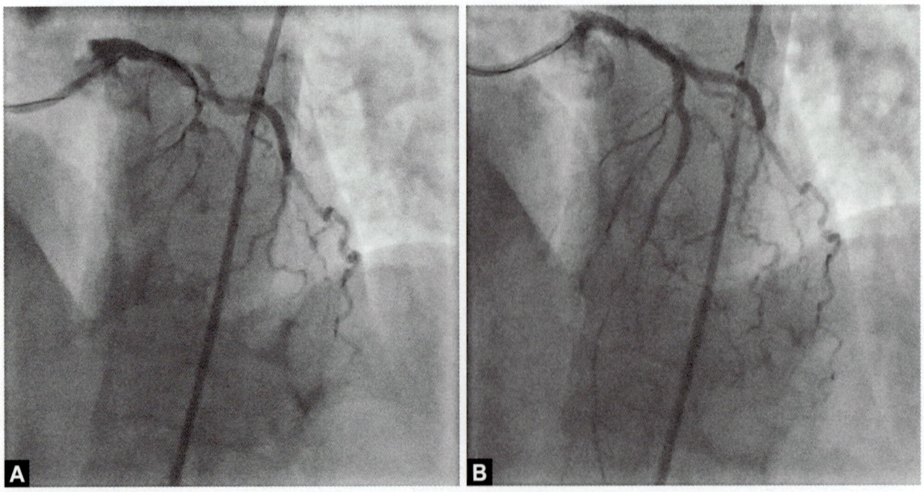

FIGS. 4A AND B: Uncrossable lesion—chronic total occlusions.

Uncrossable Lesion: RASER Percutaneous Coronary Intervention

The laser comes to rescue when even a very thin (0.09″) Rota guidewire would not track through a severe lesion. The complications after laser treatment were limited, gravest being vessel dissection, while perforations, spasm, and no reflow phenomenon were not observed. The other PCI devices utilized in similar pathology have a steep learning curve and a risk of grievous complications, such as no reflow/slow flow phenomenon, entrapment of rotablator burr, wire fracture, and coronary perforations.[12] RASER is the combination of ELCA and rotational atherectomy utilized in such unwieldy cases. The 0.9-mm X-80 catheter is exploited to provide the widest range of power and repetition rate to maximize the chances of procedural success even through a 6Fr radial access.[2]

Application

The application of RASER PCI awaits occurrence at Advanced Cardiac Institute, Pt J N M Medical College, Raipur, India.

Uncrossable Lesion: Takayasu Aortoarteritis

The ELCA use started with initial application for ablating peripheral artery lesions. The Peripheral Excimer Laser Angioplasty (PELA 2001) study randomized 251 superficial femoral artery occlusions to either laser-assisted angioplasty or balloon angioplasty alone. The ELCA group received significantly fewer stents (42% vs. 59%), though the outcomes were similar after 1 year. The Laser Angioplasty for Critical Ischemia (LACI 2006) gauzed effectiveness of laser angioplasty in 155 critically ischemic limbs to report a limb salvage in 92% patients after 6 months. The other similar studies LACI CIS, LACI Belgium, and LACI-RTO (refractory total occlusions) also delivered above 90% limb salvage rates. The latest CLiRpath Excimer Laser System to Enlarge Lumen Openings (CELLO 2009) evaluated Turbo Elite Laser Catheter System in 65 de novo lesions showing safety and successful revascularization 76.9% at 12 months. The more recent single-center studies are attesting possible application of excimer laser ablation in patients with diabetes with critical limb ischemia, in hemodialysis access intervention, Chen proposed that the "Lyse and Lase" technique of thrombolysis before laser ablation after a retrospective study of >450 critically ischemic limbs to minimizing distal embolization.[13]

Application

This young lady in her mid-40s was referred with anterior wall myocardial infarction and supposed cardiogenic shock as her peripheral arteries were not palpable. The attempted catheter coronary angiography failed through right radial and femoral routes, subsequent CT coronary angiography revealed middle aorta Takayasu aortoarteritis total occlusive calcified lesions that only permitted a coronary guidewire to track the 17 mm infrarenal calcified occlusion. The ELCA 1.4 mm was utilized at 45 mJ × 25 Hz and 60 mJ × 30 Hz to pave way for final 40 mm × 10 mm + 50 mm × 20 mm balloon in balloon angioplasty to equalize the pressure difference across the lesion. This is first in world use of excimer laser in a middle arch Takayasu aortoarteritis treatment ***(Figs. 5A to D)****.*

Long and Diffuse Atherosclerotic Lesions

In a study for safety and effectiveness of 100 complex coronary lesions laser had a procedural success rate of 92% and a clinical success rate of 91%.[14]

Application

A diabetic hypertensive, smoker male in mid 50s and with an old anterior and recent non ST elevation myocardial infarction. His diagnostic angiography revealed a diffuse calcified right coronary artery. He underwent lasing to diffusely diseased right coronary artery with 45 mJ/mm × 25 Hz. The stents were implanted successfully to the three coronary arteries ***(Figs. 6A to C)****.*

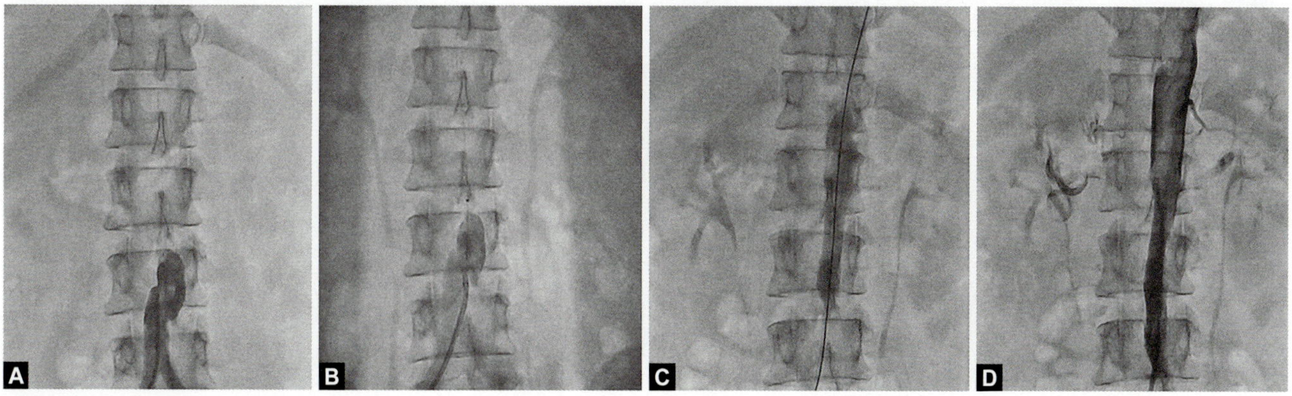

FIGS. 5A TO D: Uncrossable lesion—Takayasu aortoarteritis.

Moderately Calcified Lesions

Though the success with the laser has an inverse relation with the extent and degree of calcification (calcified 79% vs. noncalcified 96%; $p < 0.05$). The laser in almost all cases ablates at least the proximal calcified cap enough to permit further successful PCI. Bilodeau reported a procedural success rate of 93% with a clinical success rate of 86% excimer laser use in a subgroup with extremely complex lesions.[5]

Application

This smoker hypertensive and diabetic patient admitted with acute inferior and old anterior wall myocardial infarction underwent successful lasing and PCI to the mid-left anterior descending artery moderately calcified lesion barricading even small balloon passage ***(Figs. 7A to D)****. The right coronary artery calcified disease was in a nondiabetic hypertensive male patient in mid-70s with angina on exertion. The right coronary artery was lased with 45 mJ × 25 Hz and 50 mJ × 25 Hz power with guide extension catheter support to track 3.0 mm × 28 mm and 3.0 mm × 18 mm stents for successful deployment* ***(Figs. 7E and F)****.*

In-stent Restenosis (Due to Excessive Neointimal Proliferation)

Though the in-stent restenosis rate has reduced from 10 to 50% in the bare metal stent era with increasing utilization of drug eluting technology. ELCA, unlike other PCI devices, offers a safe and effective way to treat in-stent restenosis, as it leaves the stent unaltered. ELCA creates a greater IVUS cross-sectional area and luminal gain, with enhanced ablation of intimal hyperplasia as witnessed in a study of 107 in-stent restenosis lesions compared to balloon angioplasty alone. The optical coherence tomography (OCT) and optical frequency domain imaging also corroborated that the laser therapy ablates both the luminal and abluminal atherosclerotic material permitting further expansion of partly underexpanded stent.[2] In a comparison of the neointimal alteration with ELCA and scoring balloon predilution versus scoring balloon alone in in-stent restenosis, ELCA typically results in superior acute gain by neointima debulking but similar late angiographic and clinical outcome.[15] Radke showed that ELCA use in

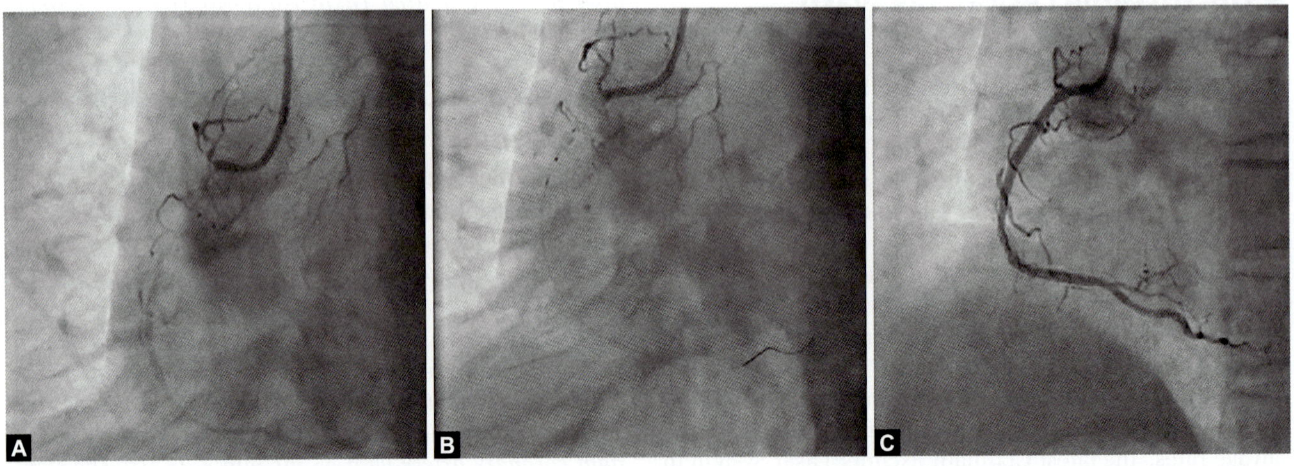

FIGS. 6A TO C: Long and diffuse atherosclerotic lesions.

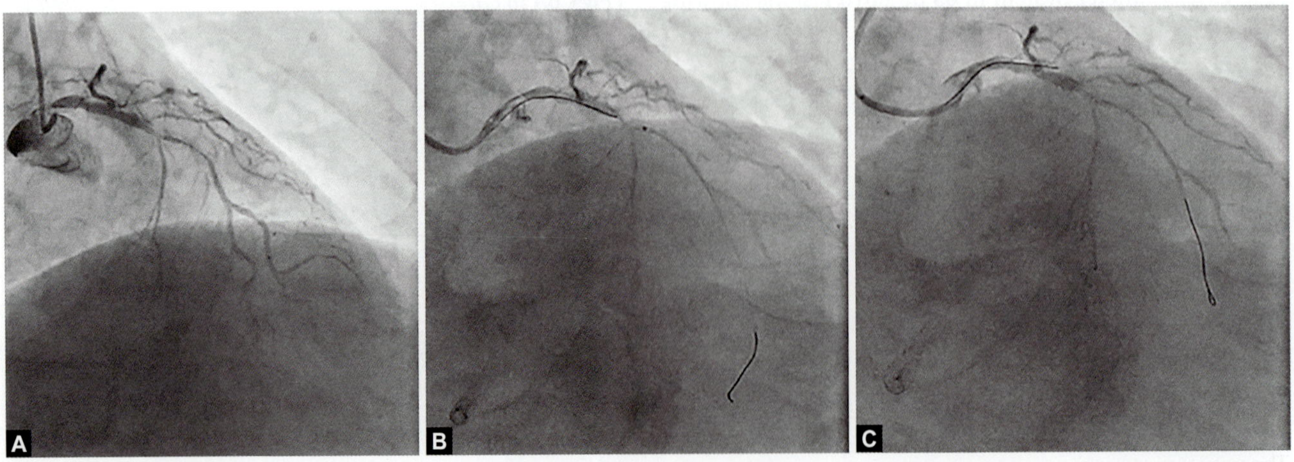

FIGS. 7A TO F: *Continued*

Continued

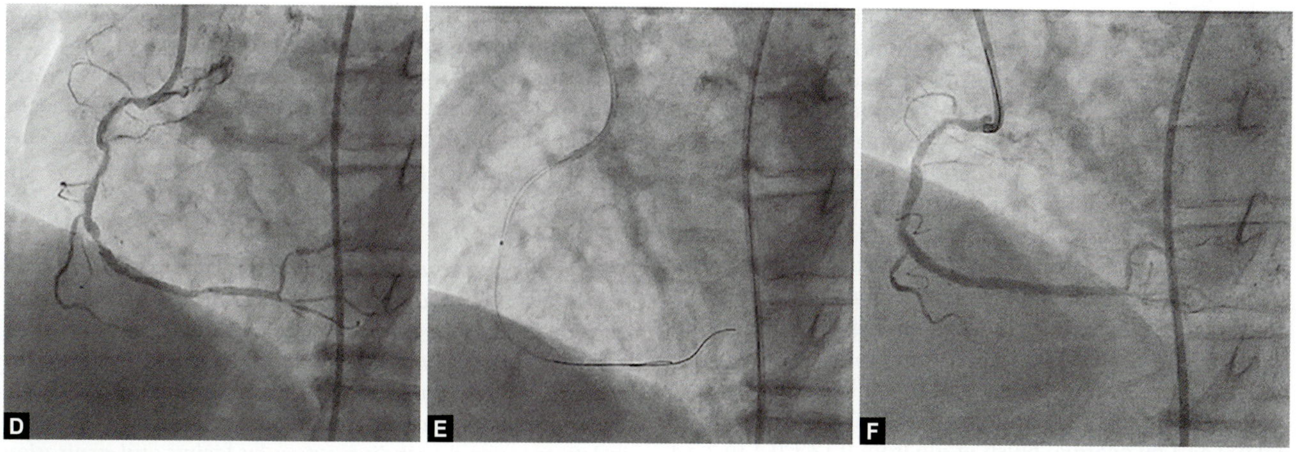

FIGS. 7A TO F: Moderately calcified lesions.

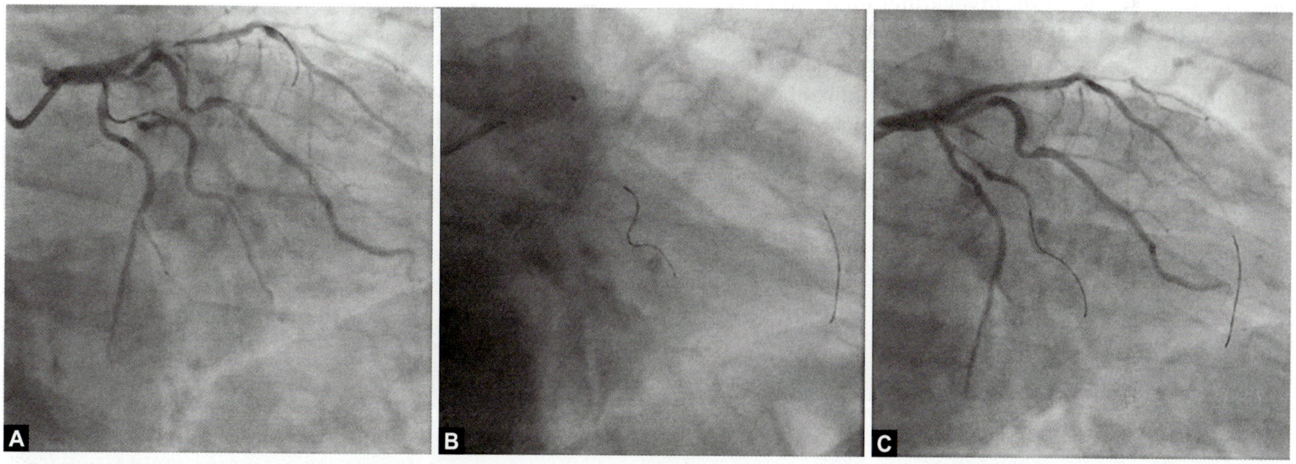

FIGS. 8A TO C: In-stent restenosis (due to excessive neointimal proliferation).

474 patients is associated with a higher probability of MACE (34.8%) in a meta-analysis of 3,012 in-stent restenosis patients; however, the drug eluting balloons were not used in this observation.[16]

Application

*This nondiabetic hypertensive patient had been implanted with a bare metal stent 21 years ago, now presented with angina on exertion CCS class III. He underwent IVUS determined lasing at 45 mJ × 25 Hz and 60 mJ × 25 Hz and a drug-eluting balloon expansion to the organic stent occlusion **(Figs. 8A to C)**.*

Acute Stent Thrombosis (Post Coronavirus Disease)

The use of ELCA increased from 2012 to 2019, with lesser use during the coronavirus disease-2019 (COVID-19) epidemic. The use is now trending up again.[10]

Application

*The COVID-negative alcohol user hypertensive patient initially presented after thrombolysis with streptokinase for anterior wall myocardial infarction, and underwent a successful rescue stent implantation to the ostial left anterior descending artery. He presented after 1 month again with COVID-19 and reinfarction in left anterior descending artery territory. The angiography revealed acute stent thrombosis that was then lased with 1.4 mm × 45 mJ × 25 Hz and balloon angioplasty for a successful treatment of the occlusion **(Figs. 9A to C)**.*

Primary Percutaneous Coronary Intervention with Large Thrombus Burden

Excimer laser coronary angioplasty among all ablative PCI devices is unique for effective thrombus removal with boosting fibrinolysis, platelet-inhibition, and concomitant plaque ablation. ELCA has excellent effectiveness in ablating the large onus of intracoronary thrombus to achieve an excellent immediate and long-term results.[2] The Cohort of Acute Revascularization of Myocardial infarction with Excimer Laser (CARMEL) multicenter registry is the largest study to have recruited 151 acute myocardial infarction (AMI) patients, majority having large thrombus burden. The use of ELCA increased thrombolysis in myocardial infarction (TIMI) flow grade from 1.2 to 2.8, shrunk angiographic stenosis from 83 to 52% and reduced major adverse coronary events (8.6%), especially in large angiographic thrombus burden. The laser AMI (LAMI) randomized study on 66 patients demonstrated safety and feasibility of ELCA, with an increase in the TIMI score from 0.2 ± 0.4 to 2.65 ± 0.5 ($p < 0.01$) and myocardial blush grade from 0.12 ± 0.4 to 2.5 ± 0.6 and excellent safety.[17] Shibata evaluated the impact of ELCA on myocardial salvage using nuclear scintigraphy in patients with ST-elevation myocardial infarction (STEMI) and described the advantages of ELCA in use of shorter stent lengths, fewer balloons, and increased direct stent implantation. The myocardial salvage index and the final TIMI-3 flow (67.1% vs. 45.7%, $p = 0.01$) were significantly better in the ELCA group. The Japanese ULTRAMAN registry demonstrated a better success rate and similar low complications for acute coronary syndrome (ACS) (175 patients) compared to the CAMEL study. Tomoyuki Arai studied 113 consecutive ACS patients to find a significant difference in peak creatine kinase-myocardial band and in-hospital major adverse cardiac events.[18]

Application

*This young man in late 20s with no known cardiac risks presented within 30 minutes of severe angina to be taken up immediately for primary PCI. The angiography revealed a thrombotic occlusion from ostial to distal left anterior descending artery without a stenotic lesion on IVUS. He underwent a very successful resolution of the entire thrombus in left anterior descending artery by lasing and aspiration **(Figs. 10A to D).***

Pacemaker Lead Extraction

The numbers of cardiac implantable electronic devices (CIEDs) are increasing and so are the CIED-related complications leading to the necessity of transvenous lead extraction

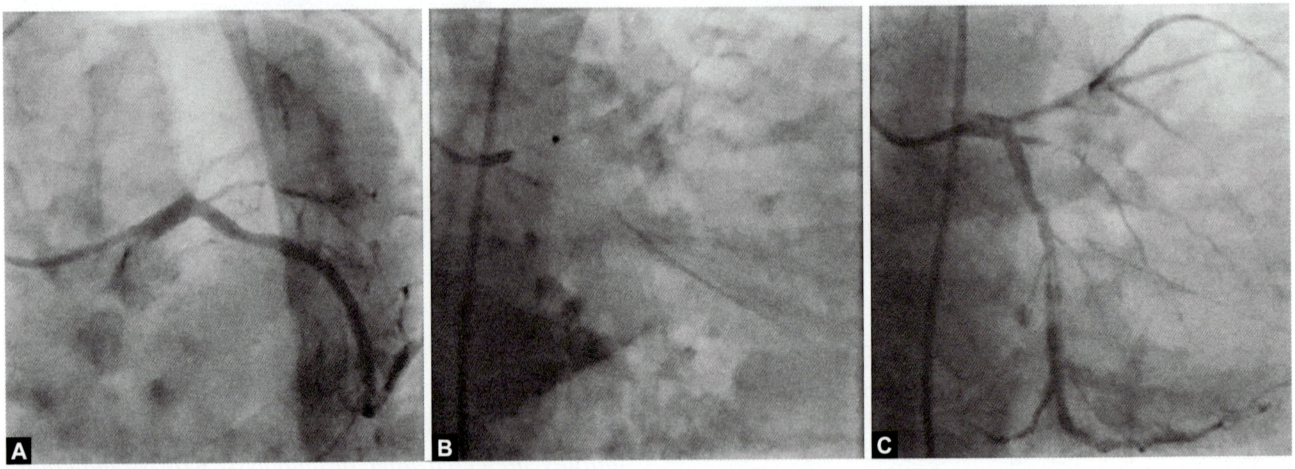

FIGS. 9A TO C: Acute stent thrombosis (post coronavirus disease).

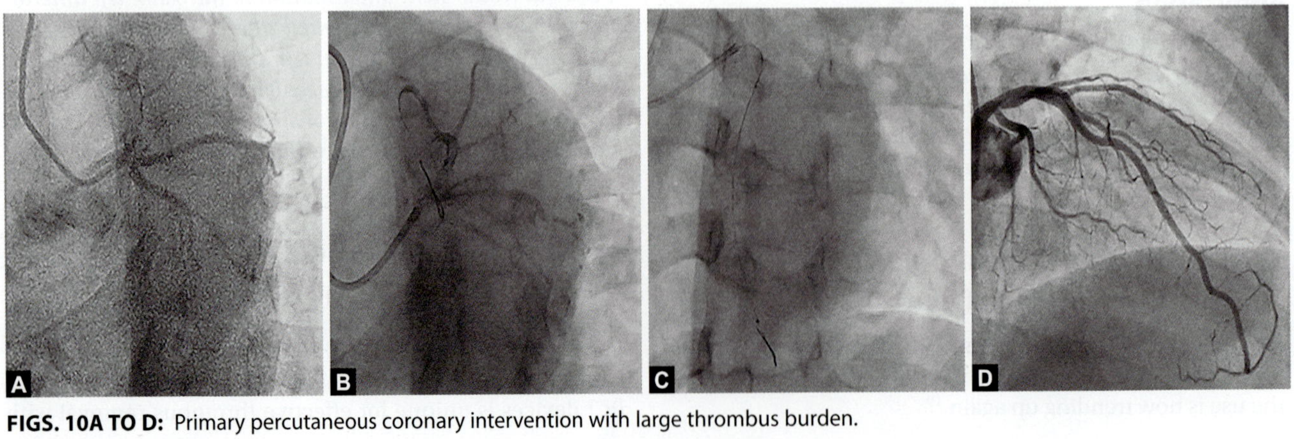

FIGS. 10A TO D: Primary percutaneous coronary intervention with large thrombus burden.

(TLE) to increase in proportion as well. Transvenous leads as a major risk factor for systemic infection bear an indication for a timely extraction. Lead-associated vascular pathology and longer lead dwell time in an ageing population impart a complexity and complication in lead extraction. The application of excimer laser powered extraction tools can be of help in these situations, and has shown good safety and efficacy.[19] In a single-center study of consecutive 1,725 lead extraction procedures in 775 patients, employing direct traction for 588 leads, and surgery for 22 leads. The remainder utilized a laser assisted removal for 190 leads, the femoral approach extraction in 717 leads, and rotating mechanical sheaths removal for 208 leads. The study concluded that major complications were associated with the laser sheath use than with the femoral approach or rotating mechanical sheaths (8.4, 0.5, and 1.2%, respectively, $p < 0.001$).[20] Misra extracted 575 leads from 372 patients to achieve an overall success rate of 97%. They utilized TightRail™ as the first tool used in 180 (31.3%) leads with success rate of 61.7%; laser sheaths were the first tool in 395 leads (68.7%) with success rate of 67.8%. However, the final extraction outcomes did not differ based on the modality employed used (adjusted odds ratio = 0.94; 95% confidence interval = 0.59–1.50).[21] Okada established that ELCA is equally safe in young and elderly patients for TLE for cardiac implantable electronic devices.[22]

Application

This patient with symptomatic complete heart block received a pacemaker in 2007 and subsequent two revisions (second one for infection at access site) at another center in 2019. The patient was referred by the plastic surgery department after four failed attempts to apply a graft at the exposed implant site. The patient underwent successful laser lead extraction and migration to a contralateral pacemaker implantation site. This represented the first in India outside license trial study laser lead extraction. However, 6 months later the contralateral site also showed signs of infection and the lead was extracted with laser catheter and a leadless pacemaker was implanted for the patient. This is the second in world reported case after a first Chinese implant of a leadless pacemaker in a laser lead extraction of an infected lead pacemaker case ***(Figs. 11A to F)****.*

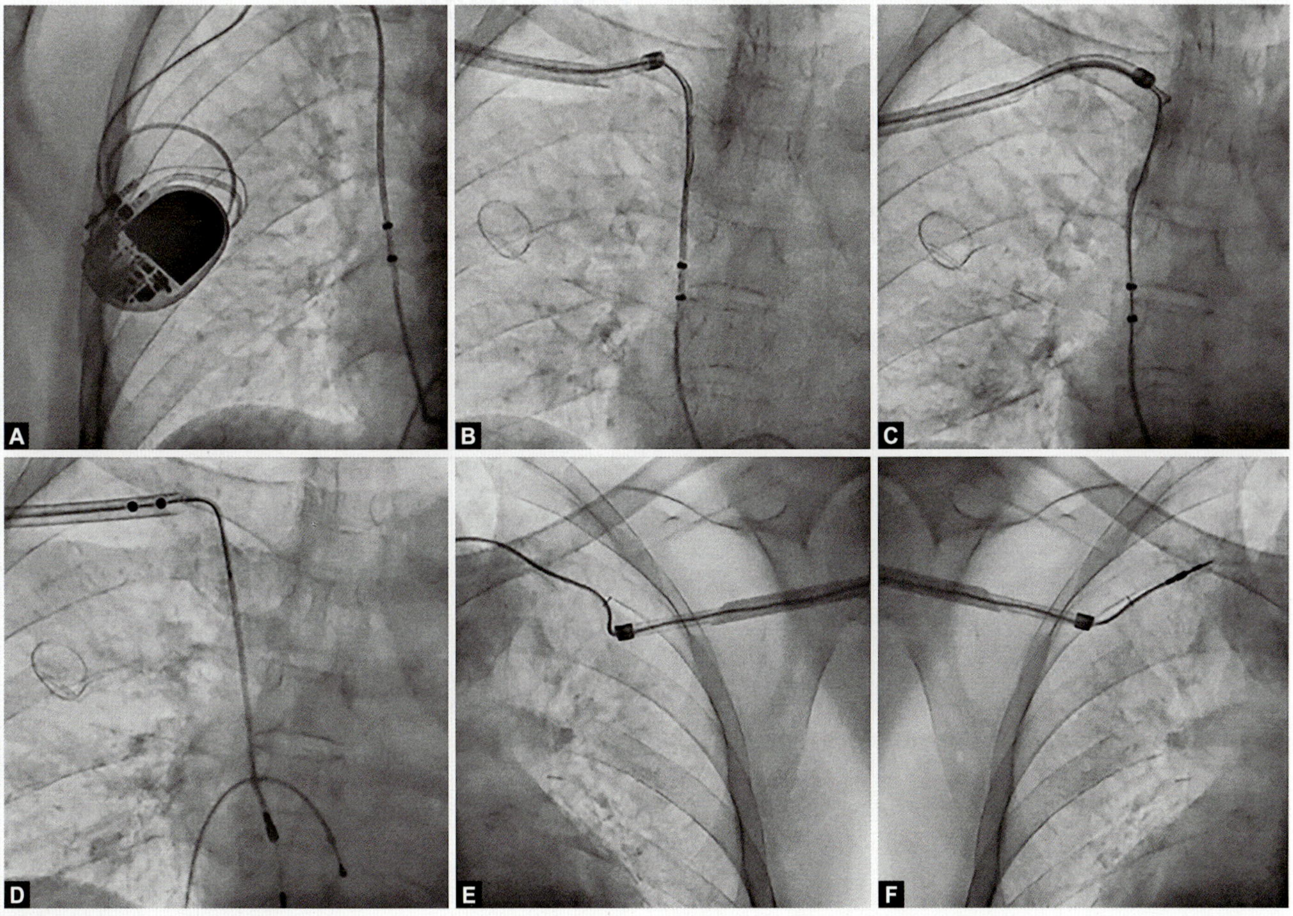

FIGS. 11A TO F: Pacemaker lead extraction.

Thrombus Annihilation/Restenosis in Saphenous Vein Graft

Litvack reported the first successful percutaneous excimer laser angioplasty of multiple restenosis of vein graft lesions.[23] Bittl showed in 495 patients with 545 lesions in SVGs treated with excimer laser angioplasty in the Percutaneous Excimer Laser Coronary Angioplasty registry embolization of thrombus or atheromatous material occurs in 2–17% of patients, and restenosis at the treated site appears in 50–80%.[24] The CORAL (COronary graft Results following Atherectomy with Laser) registry demonstrated smaller venous grafts and heavy thrombus load, nonsignificant rate of no reflow (5.1% vs. 3%, $p = .37$) and abrupt closure (3% vs. 1.7%, $p = 0.40$) compared to the distal protection in SAFER DPD study. SVGs occlusions frequently coexist with degenerative diffuse plaques and containing thrombus. The distal protection devices are bulky to allow distal delivery. Therefore ELCA comes out safer alternative for rescue in SVG interventions to preclude the need for routine DPD.[25]

Application

*This alcohol user, smoker, hypertensive, and diabetic male patient in early 70s had spontaneous resolution of an acute inferior wall myocardial infarction SVG to right PDA, diagonal and obtuse marginal artery grafts. The angiography revealed severe diffuse native triple vessels disease and patent left internal mammary artery to left anterior descending artery and SVG to obtuse marginal graft. However, the SVG to the right posterior descending artery (PDA) had thrombotic 90% stenosis and totally occluded SVG to diagonal artery graft. The SVG to right PDA thrombus was annihilated with laser at 45 mJ/mm × 25 Hz and subsequently stent of 3.0 × 36 mm was deployed successfully without the need for distal protection device **(Figs. 12A to D)**.*

Ostial or Bifurcation Lesions Requiring Ablative Plaque Modification

Though for coronary bifurcation lesions the best approach advocated is to stent the main vessel only. However, side branch mandates treatment, ELCA can safely debulk the side branch lesion to allow more foreseeable success with the main vessel-only approach.[2]

Application

*This tobacco chewer hypertensive male in late 40s presented with recent anterior wall myocardial infarction and a Medina (1, 1, 1) severe disease in left anterior descending artery and small diameter diagonal. The diagonal and the left anterior descending artery arteries underwent lasing with 0.9 mm × 45 mJ × 25 Hz followed by drug eluting balloon angioplasty to diagonal artery and stent implantation in left anterior descending artery **(Figs. 13A to D)**.*

CONCLUSION

The ELCA made a late entry into India and is on a way to become a first aid tool in cardiovascular interventions. The different applications of excimer laser in cardiovascular interventions can help draw interventional cardiologists to practice widely a safe yet high powered tool. The excimer laser like all other tools occupies more complimentary roles than competitive roles.

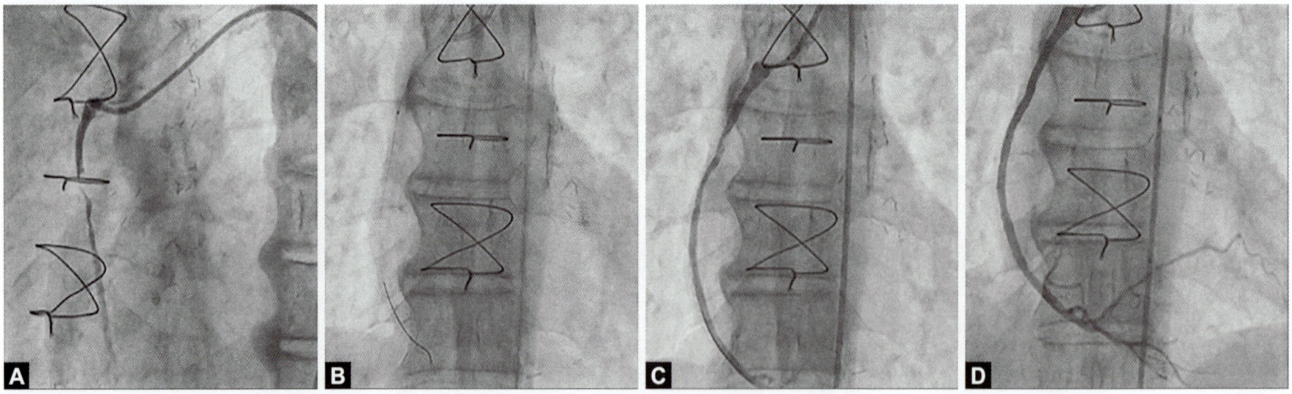

FIGS. 12A TO D: Thrombus annihilation/restenosis in saphenous vein graft (SVG).

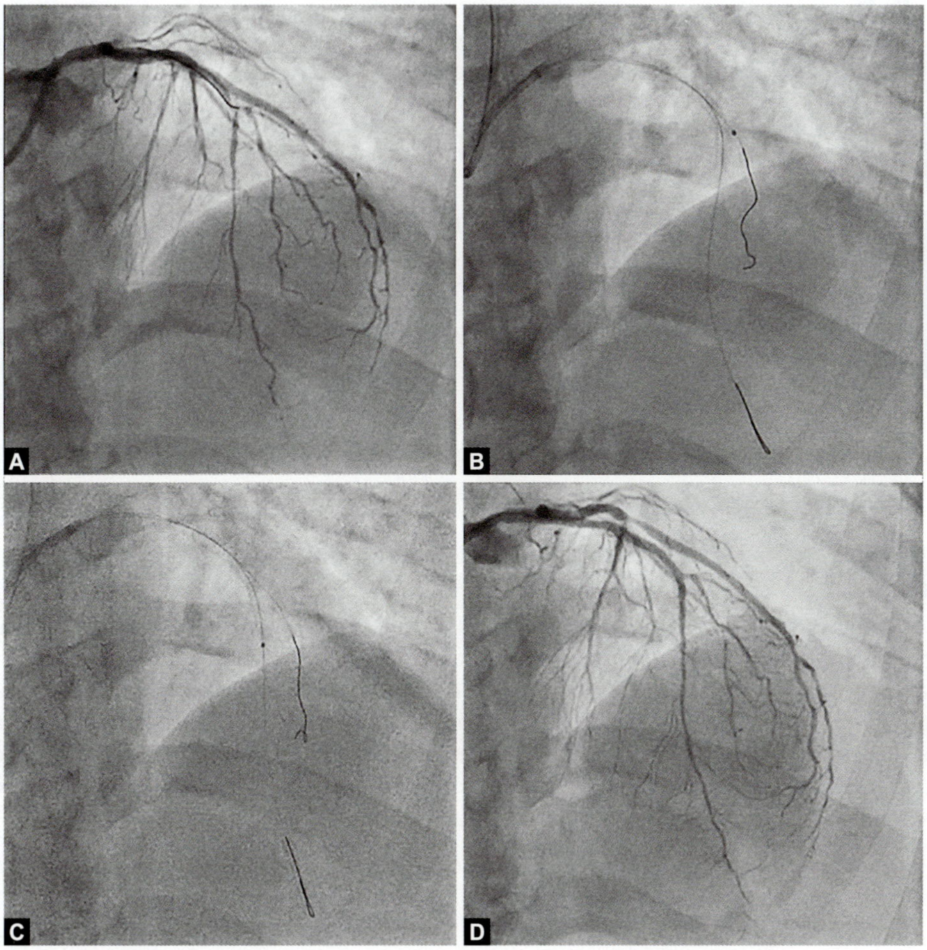

FIGS. 13A TO D: Ostial or bifurcation lesions requiring ablative plaque modification.

ONLINE REFERENCES

Please scan the QR code provided at the end of the table of contents for References of this chapter.

CHAPTER

152 Safety and Efficacy of Intravascular Lithotripsy in Coronary Interventions

Viveka Kumar, Purneshwar Kumar Pandey, Santosh Kumar Singh

ABSTRACT

The presence of coronary calcified lesions often challenges percutaneous coronary intervention, increases the risk of procedural complications resulting in suboptimal outcomes, and subsequently leads to future adverse cardiac events. The currently available calcium-modifying devices are based on debulking or tissue compression, with the aim of rupturing calcium and subsequently facilitating the deployment of optimal stent. However, the coronary intravascular lithotripsy (IVL) technique is based on the delivery of unfocused, circumferential, and pulsatile sonic pressure to the site of target lesions in order to fracture the vascular calcium safely from coronary and peripheral vessels. This chapter summarizes the available studies and evidences on the safety and efficacy of IVL in coronary interventions.

Keywords: Coronary calcification, coronary interventions, coronary lithotripsy, coronary plaque modification, intravascular lithotripsy system, lithotripsy.

INTRODUCTION

Coronary artery calcification (CAC) and its quantity have been known to exacerbate with age and presence of comorbidities and cardiovascular risk factors.[1,2] The prevalence of CAC is also known to be gender dependent, occurring in >90% of men and around 67% of women aged >70 years.[3] CAC often hinders around 20% of the percutaneous coronary intervention (PCI) procedures by impairment of device crossing and delamination of drug-eluting polymer, thereby altering the drug delivery and elution kinetics. It also leads to impairment of stent apposition and expansion. Stent underexpansion is associated with subsequent stent thrombosis and/or the need for target lesion revascularization. This cumulatively leads to lower procedural success rate, increased periprocedural adverse events, and unfavorable clinical outcomes compared with noncalcific plaques. Several studies have shown CAC as an independent predictor of PCI failure and for adverse events in later life.[4,5] The procedural success, its complexity, and time are influenced by the lesion calcification, its localization, either deep or superficial, thickness, and distribution (circumferential, focal, and longitudinal).[6]

Presently, numerous techniques are available and have been shown to treat calcified lesions including atherectomy devices, cutting/scoring balloons, high-pressure and super-high-pressure noncompliant balloons, both rotational and orbital, and excimer lasers.[7] However, these procedures are based on tissue debulking or tissue compression and are known to have increased rates of complications, such as distal embolization, dissections, and perforations. In addition, the success rate of these procedures decreased with the thick, eccentric, and deep calcifications and the induction of tissue injury sometimes led to hasten unrestrained neointimal growth and restenosis.[8] So far, high-pressure noncompliant balloons are known to be superior to specialty balloons and atherectomy devices based on improved clinical outcomes.[9,10]

Recently, a breakthrough novel strategy among interventional armamentarium, to fracture coronary calcium, has been developed which is based on the lithotripsy concept.

The novel technique is based on the established treatment procedures for ureterorenal calculi. The intravascular lithotripsy (IVL) system (Shockwave Medical, Santa Clara, California) is used to convert electrical energy into mechanical energy, i.e., pulsatile sonic pressure waves during low-pressure balloon inflation.[11]

The IVL technique is based on sonic waves instead of direct coronary tissue injury for calcium lesions modification. These sonic waves emitted from multiple lithotripsy emitters mounted on a catheter travel from the catheter to the surrounding vascular tissue to safely break calcium deposits present deep and superficial without tissue impairment and improving coronary vessel compliance. Moreover, the resulting calcium fragments after IVL therapy remained in situ, decreasing the risk of distal embolization. The prospective single-arm studies have demonstrated the safety and efficacy of IVL with reduced vascular tissue injury during the treatment of moderately calcified lesions to severe type in peripheral artery disease.[12-14] Also, the safety and feasibility of the shockwave lithoplasty system have been shown in the trials for the treatment of peripheral vascular stenosis.[15]

MECHANISM OF INTRAVASCULAR LITHOTRIPSY

Intravascular lithotripsy as a novel therapy is used for the treatment of vascular calcification. The mechanism of IVL is analogous to the well-established therapeutic strategy of using acoustic pressure waves to treat renal calculi.[16]

Extracorporeal shock wave lithotripsy (ESWL), since its introduction in the 1980s, uses pulsatile sonic pressure waves generated by the spark gap discharge between two electrodes within the transmitting medium. These emitted pulsatile pressure waves increase spherically. Further, the plasma vapor bubble forms by the energy discharged from the spark gap between the electrodes subsequently following the primary acoustic shockwave. Also, the rapid increase and breakdown of the vapor bubble, also known as a cavitation bubble, lead to secondary shockwaves resulting in calcium breakdown on encountering the differing acoustic resistances.

Although the electrohydraulic lithotripsy (EHL) spark gap technique was applicable to use in IVL, several amendments were made to make it safe and effective for intravascular interventions: (1) For the longitudinal therapy of calcium deposit vessel, multiple emitters are mounted on the shaft of the angioplasty catheter. (2) Tissue-safe positive- and negative-pressure pulses, delivered by IVL pressure waves, allow adequate coronary vessel compliance to fracture coronary calcium. This facilitates in mitigating vascular tissue injury due to tensile pressure. (3) To mitigate thermal injury, pressure wave emitters are surrounded within fluid-filled inflated balloons.

In contrast to ESWL, the IVL shockwaves are unfocused, which generates very low acoustic energy. Minimum energy is required to target vascular calcium because IVL shockwave initiates in the proximity of target tissue. The integrated semi-compliant balloon with emitters mounted on the shaft of catheter in IVL has various advantages. The heat produced during the formation of vapor bubble is dissipated by the fluid medium in the balloon and prevents direct contact of emitters and vascular vessel walls. Balloon deflation during every two cycles facilitates in dissipation of heat, and residual vapor bubbles allow perfusion of tissue hence averting ischemia. Integrated semi-compliant balloon during IVL therapy also provides mechanical support that reduces the risk of tissue deformation. The integrated semi-compliant balloon is thin and transparent which provides adequate pulse propagation from the emitter to the vascular vessel wall. Intriguingly, barotraumas are also averted due to an appropriate size of the IVL balloon catheter which inflates at subnominal pressure (4 atm) and generates circumferential rings to fracture calcium.

Coronary Intravascular Lithotripsy System

The IVL system comprises a portable IVL generator, connector cable, and IVL catheter **(Fig. 1)**. The IVL generator is user-friendly with two buttons (power on and other for delivering energy) and a rechargeable orthogonal "box" of size 28.0 cm × 15.2 cm × 29.2 cm and weighs around 6.8 kg. The color coding is given in the generator that represents the number of pulses that remained after each cycle.[17,18] The IVL generator generates pulses of electrical energy of 3,000 V. The discharge frequency is 1 Hz, and the number of pulses per cycle is fixed and relies on the type of catheter used in the IVL system. The IVL generator is connected to the IVL connector cable. The IVL connector cable has two magnetic poles, one connected to the generator and the other pole connected to the proximal part of the catheter. The size of the connector table is around 1.53 m in length that creates routes between generator and catheter and facilitates electrical energy transfer. The IVL catheters are angioplasty catheter and are of different sizes and internal designs. A series of EHL emitters are mounted on their shaft which transform electrical energy into sonic pressure waves. The sonic pressure pulses are unfocused, travel circumferentially, and generate 50 atm pressure in the spherical fields. These unfocused circumferential pulses selectively break the calcium and modify vessel compliance with minimum injury and preserving the integrity of vessel wall.

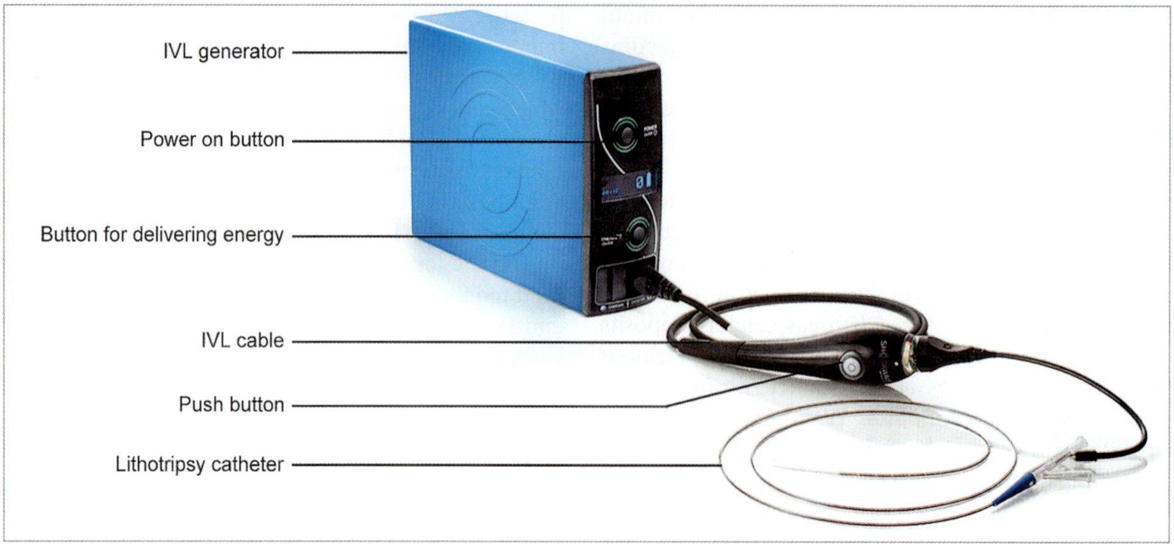

FIG. 1: Coronary intravascular lithotripsy system (IVL).

Source: Adapted from Shockwave Medical. [online] Available from https://shockwavemedical.com/technology/intravascular-lithotripsy-ivl/ [Last accessed September, 2023].

OVERVIEW OF THE CLINICAL STUDIES ON THE SAFETY AND EFFICACY OF INTRACORONARY INTRAVASCULAR LITHOTRIPSY

Various trials and studies have demonstrated the safety and efficacy of IVL in coronary interventions **(Table 1)**.

DISRUPT Coronary Artery Disease I Trial

A prospective multicenter, single-arm study was done by Brinton et al. to evaluate the feasibility of coronary IVL in 60 patients with heavily calcified atherosclerotic plaques.[19] The outcomes (clinical, device, and stent delivery success rate) were defined as residual stenosis <50% and delivery of device at target lesions. The clinical success rate, device success rate, and stunt delivery rate were found as high as 95, 98, and 100%, respectively. The major adverse cardiac events (MACE) were also assessed after 30 days and 6 months and defined by cardiac death, myocardial infarction (MI), and target vessel revascularization (TVR). Overall, the incidence of adverse cardiac events was found to be low as 5 and 8% after 30 days and 6 months, respectively. Optical coherence tomography (OCT) was used to decipher the mechanisms of calcium modifications.

DISRUPT Coronary Artery Disease II Trial

The other trial was conducted at 15 hospitals in nine countries involving 120 patients to investigate the safety and effectiveness of IVL.[20] The primary endpoint was MACE (cardiac death, MI, and TVR) in hospital, and OCT was done to evaluate the quantification of CAC's characteristics and calcium plaque. The incidence of MACE was found in 5.8 and 7.6% of patients in hospitals and after 30 days, respectively. The clinical success rate, device success rate, and stunt delivery rates were found as high as 94.2, 100, and 100%, respectively. The PCI OCT exposed 78.7% of calcium fracture.

DISRUPT Coronary Artery Disease III Trial

This trial was a prospective, multicentric international study intended to find out the regulatory approval of IVL for coronary interventions.[21] This trial was conducted by Hill et al. group including 431 patients from 47 sites in 4 countries with heavily calcified plaque. The primary safety and effectiveness endpoints were MACE at 30 days and procedural success, respectively. The safety and effectiveness were found to be 90.2 and 92.4%, respectively. An OCT study confirmed the multiplane and longitudinal calcium fractures post IVL in 67.4% of lesions.

DISRUPT Coronary Artery Disease IV Trial

This prospective study was conducted in Japanese population with the aim to evaluate the safety and effectiveness of IVL therapy of de novo stenoses in patients with severely calcified vessels.[22] The primary safety and efficacy endpoints were freedom from MACE at 30 days and procedural success (residual stenosis <50%), respectively. The safety and effectiveness were found to be 93.8 and 93.8%, respectively, in comparison to propensity-matched historical control group where freedom from MACE at 30 days was 91.2% and procedural success rate was 91.6%.

TABLE 1: Overview of studies with IVL in coronary interventions.[17]

Clinical trials	Number of patients	Calcification at baseline (%)	Primary endpoint	Outcome	Luminal gain post-IVL	Luminal gain poststent delivery	Residual stenosis	Calcium fracture evaluated using OCT (%)	References
Disrupt CAD I	60	100	MACE in 30 days and 6 months	5 and 8% MACE observed	–	1.7 mm	<50% in 100% lesions; <30% in 92% lesions	78	19
Disrupt CAD II	120	94.2	MACE in hospital and 30 days MACE	5.8 and 7.6% MACE observed	0.83 ± 0.47 mm		<50% in 100% lesions; <30% in 100% lesions	78.7	20
Disrupt CAD III	431	100	Safety by MACE in 30 days and effectiveness by procedural success	92.2% safety and 92.4% effectiveness of IVL was observed	–	1.7 mm	<50% in 100% lesions; <30% in 99.5% lesions	67.4	21
Disrupt CAD IV	64	100	Safety by MACE in 30 days and effectiveness by procedural success	93.8% safety and 93.8% effectiveness of IVL was observed	1.42 ± 0.42 mm	1.67 ± 0.37 mm	<50% in 98.4% lesions; <30% in 98.4% lesions	53.5	22
Pooled analysis of disrupt studies	628	97	Safety by MACE in 30 days and effectiveness by procedural success	92.7% safety and 92.4% effectiveness of IVL was observed	0.82 ± 0.48 mm	1.68 ± 0.47 mm	<50% in 93.2% lesions; <30% in 92.4% lesions	–	23
Registries	78	82.1	Safety by MACE in-hospital and strategy success (stent expansion with <20%)	100% safety and high procedural success observed (84.6, 77.3, and 64.7% for groups 1, 2, and 3, respectively)	0.89 ± 0.76 mm	1.87 ± 0.60 mm	–	–	24
Registries	45	97.8	Clinical success and angiographic success	90% clinical success and 94% angiographic success observed	1.90 ± 0.5 mm	2.80 ± 0.50 mm	–	–	25

(CAD: coronary artery disease; IVL: intravascular lithotripsy; MACE: major adverse cardiovascular events; OCT: optical coherence tomography)

Kereiakes et al. assessed the cumulative safety and efficacy of IVL.[23] A total of 628 patients with severe calcification from 12 countries participated in this study. The primary endpoints of safety and effectiveness were found in 92.7 and 92.4% of patients, respectively. Adverse events such as target lesion failure, stent thrombosis, and cardiac death were found to be 7.2, 0.8, and 0.5%, respectively, at 30 days. The rates of serious angiographic complications were found to be very low and consistent with IVL's mechanism of action. A follow-up for 1 year was also collected by Kereiakes and his group.[24] The rate of MACE was found to be low (13.8%). Similarly, the rate of cardiac death and stent thrombosis was found to be low at 1.1% each. The rate of repeat revascularization was also found to be low (4.3% for the target lesion and 6% for the target coronary vessel).

A prospective registry determined the success and safety of IVL.[25] 78 patients with severe coronary calcium plaque were enrolled at three different centers for this in the study. Patients were divided into three groups based on the therapy, namely group A: primary IVL therapy with calcium lesions ($n = 39$), group B: secondary IVL therapy for patients with failed dilation of lesion with noncompliant balloon ($n = 22$), and group C: tertiary IVL therapy for patients with stent underexpansion after previous stenting ($n = 17$). The primary endpoint was success (stent expansion with <20% in-stent residual stenosis) and safety outcomes (procedural complications and in-hospital MACE). The mean diameter of the post-IVL stenosis was found to be 45.1% ± 17.4% which was further reduced to 17.5% ± 15.2% post stenting. Likewise, the mean minimal lumen diameter increases post IVL and post stenting. The procedural success rates were found to be 84.6, 77.3, and 64.7% for group A, group B, and group C, respectively, without any in-hospital MACE.[25] Another research group also performed registry to determine the clinical and angiographic outcomes of IVL used for coronary interventions in patients with moderate-to-severe calcified lesions.[26] The primary outcome was in-hospital MACE and the secondary outcome was clinical success and angiographic success with stent expansion < 30% stent restenosis. A total of 45 patients with 50 calcified lesions were treated using IVL and divided into three groups based on their therapy, namely group 1: primary IVL therapy ($n = 23$), group 2: secondary IVL therapy ($n = 15$), and group 3: tertiary IVL therapy ($n = 12$). Overall, the clinical and angiographic success rates were high (90 and 94%, respectively).[26]

Sattar et al. meta-analyzed four studies comprising 282 patients with severely calcified coronary undergoing IVL therapy. The study demonstrated a significant improvement in the size of lumen to aid coronary stent deployment. The post-IVL mean lumen diameter was significantly high (2.70 mm), while before IVL diameter was 1.01 mm.[27] Another systematic review of cases was also performed by Sattar et al. including 24 patients from series and case reports.[28] The study showed 100% success rate in achieving stent implantations using IVL therapy without complications. Also, there was no significant difference observed among mortality rates of patients who underwent left circumflex coronary, IVL for left anterior descending (LAD), and left main coronary artery. It was observed that mortality rates were high among patients who had prior comorbid conditions and required less than three cycles of IVL.[28] Furthermore, a comprehensive literature-based study including eight single-arm observational studies was done by Mhanna et al. to elucidate the utility of adjunctive IVL.[29] A total of 980 patients were enrolled and had 97% severe calcifications. Clinical success and angiographic success were attained in 95.4 and 97% of patients, respectively. Overall, the IVL therapy significantly improves the lumen area and facilitates in reduction of calcium thickness.[29] Intriguingly, a study by Kaul et al. reported the comparison between IVL and traditional rotational atherectomy in severely calcified coronary plaque. The study demonstrated that IVL is much safer as it has reduced risk for atheromatous embolization along with better outcomes (post-IVL acute lumen gain, residual stenosis, and calcium fracturing). In contrast, the in-hospital MACE outcome was found to be better with rotational atherectomy than IVL.[30] Indian doctors also shared their experience on IVL in calcified coronary lesions.[31] IVL-assisted PCI was used to treat 25 patients and 30 coronary lesions in a tertiary care center. Overall, IVL was found to be a safe and effective method in fracturing the coronary calcium in order to deploy stent with minimal MACE.[31]

Khan et al. reported an elderly female patient aged 78 years with a history of surgical closure of atrial septal defect (ASD) 28 years ago who had undergone IVL for severely calcified plaque modifications.[3] Post-IVL and OCT images showed fracturing of calcium with good lumen gain for the deployment of stent. Further, patients followed up for 9 months and were found stable, implicating the safety of IVL for coronary interventions without complications.[3] We have our single-center experience of >50 IVL-assisted PCI with good result. One of the examples of IVL-assisted PCI at our center with good result is shown in **Figures 2A to D**.

CONCLUSION

The coronary IVL technique is a novel promising approach with a minimal risk of complications and the highest rate of success to treat moderate calcified coronary lesions to severe type. IVL can offer a substantial improvement in the coronary vessel lumen that aids in delivery of stunt and deployments in CAC. Plethora of studies and clinical data evaluated the safety and efficacy of IVL technique with respect to its effects on vessel healing response and cardiac conduction. In patients with either moderate or severe CAC who needed coronary revascularization, IVL was found to be the safely performed procedure with a high success rate and low risk of complications. However, evidences from long-term follow-up and randomized controlled trials (RCTs) are needed to review IVL efficacy, to advocate its superiority over presently available plaque-modifying strategies, and to its use in CAC patients routinely.

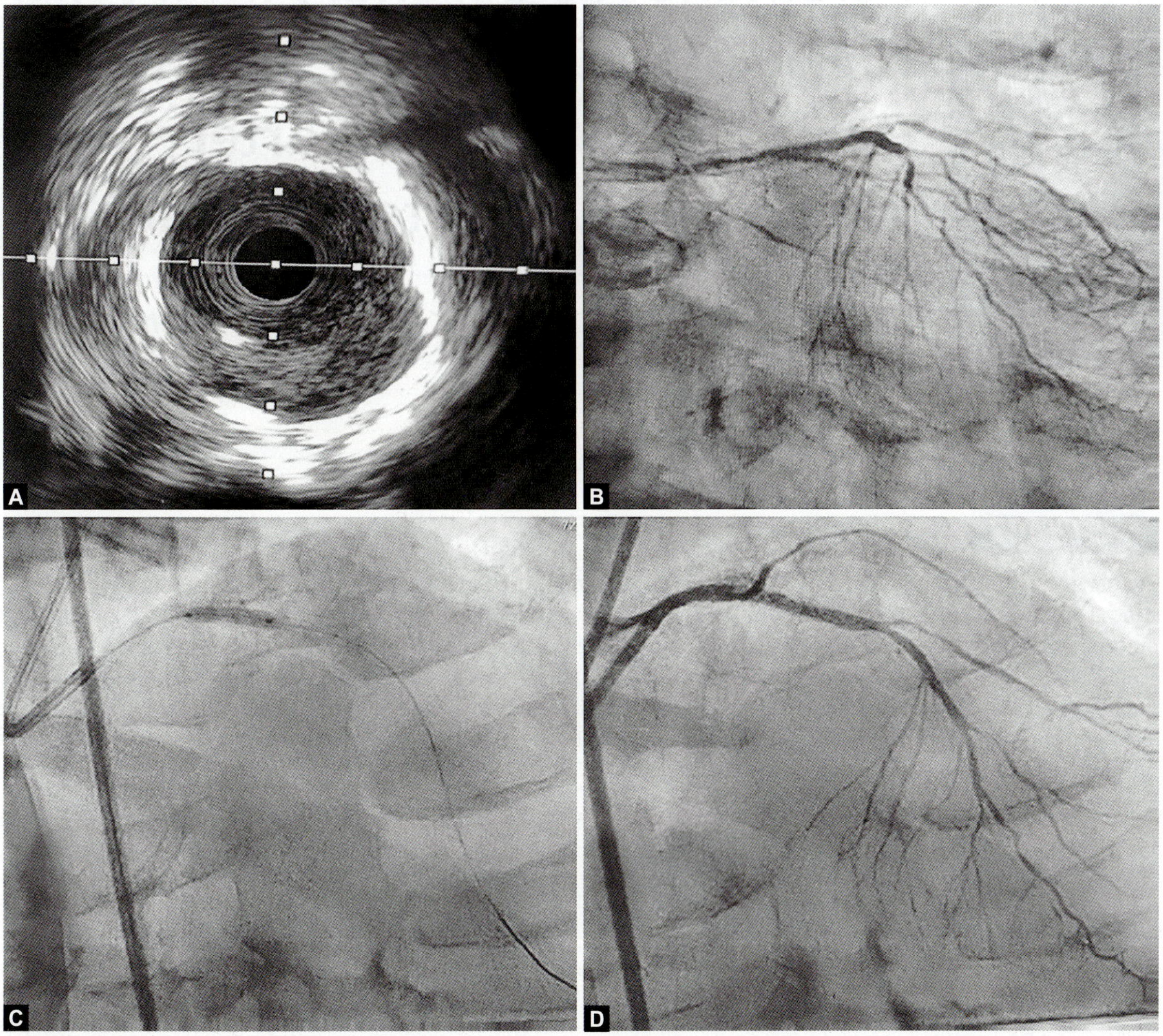

FIGS. 2A TO D: IVL-associated angioplasty. (A) IVUS image showing 360° severe calcification. (B) Coronary angiogram showing distal left main and LAD stenosis. (C) IVL therapy using 3.0 × 12 mm balloon. (D) Postangioplasty angiogram.

(IVL: intravascular lithotripsy; IVUS: intravascular ultrasound; LAD: left anterior descending)

ONLINE REFERENCES

Please scan the QR code provided at the end of the table of contents for References of this chapter.

CHAPTER

153

Percutaneous Coronary Intervention for Isolated Ostial Left Anterior Descending Coronary Artery Lesions: How Best to Approach?

Badrinarayana Tumula, Pradeep Kumar, Shabbir Ali Shaik

ABSTRACT

Percutaneous coronary intervention (PCI) of ostial left anterior descending (LAD) coronary artery lesion is challenging because of its location, area of myocardial supply, stent struts protrusion into LM (left main), and risk of side branch compromise. Different techniques for ostial LAD PCI include isolated ostial only stenting, crossover technique (floating technique). Use of imaging modalities increases the procedural success and final outcomes. In conclusion, intravascular imaging and crossover stenting followed by proximal optimization technique (POT) may be an optimal approach for the treatment of most ostial LAD lesions based on available data. Moreover, treatment strategies must be patient specific considering various clinical situations.

Keywords: Percutaneous coronary intervention, drug-eluting stents.

INTRODUCTION

An ostial lesion refers to part of coronary artery that lies within 3 mm of its origin.[1] Isolated ostial left anterior descending (LAD) coronary artery lesion is classified as distal left main (LM) bifurcation Medina 0, 1, 0.[2] Morphologically ostial lesions are mostly fibrotic or calcific in nature due to local flow disturbances and endothelial shear stress (ESS).[3] Ostial lesion of LAD is a complex coronary lesion requiring expertise in percutaneous coronary intervention (PCI) on LM and left circumflex arteries (LCX). Previously, coronary artery bypass graft (CABG) was a preferred choice of treatment because of high restenosis rates with PCI.[4] The meticulous positioning of stent in ostium of LAD without struts getting protruded into LM bifurcation and compromising LCX flow is quite challenging. Current advancement in stent technology, advent of newer generation drug-eluting stents, and availability of imaging modalities have made PCI safer and effective treatment strategy in isolated ostial LAD lesions.[5,6] There are very few studies comparing ostial stenting and crossover stenting.

OSTIAL LAD PCI TECHNIQUES

Intravascular Imaging

Incomplete lesion coverage is one of the main reasons for high restenosis rates in ostial stenting, others include technical difficulties. Rarely, ostial lesions are only confined to LAD and atherosclerotic plaques extend from LM to LAD in >90% of lesions as documented in intravascular ultrasound (IVUS) studies,[7-9] therefore, angiographically they are to be seen as LM lesions involving ostioproximal LAD. The best predictor of restenosis and stent thrombosis is post-PCI minimal stent area.[10-12] Intravascular imaging such as IVUS and optical coherence tomography (OCT) helps in planning appropriate plaque modification strategy, selecting appropriate stent size, length, and also useful in achieving optimal stent expansion.

Crossover Stenting or Floating Stent Struts

For ostial stenting, some of the stent struts should not be attached to the vessel wall. As the atherosclerotic plaque usually extends into the LM, crossover stenting technique is preferred. This has shown less target lesion revascularization (TLR) rates. The J-Cypher registry has shown that in terms of both safety and efficacy, 3-year outcomes of PCI using sirolimus eluting stents for ostial LAD lesions, crossover stenting across the LCX with a 1-stent approach is a better option. The 2-stent approach for bifurcation was associated with higher rate of TLR than the 1-stent approach.

Kissing Balloon or Nonkissing Balloon

In most of ostial LAD lesion PCI, the ostium of LCX is rarely affected. So, kissing balloon causes distortion of LM stent struts. In single stent crossover technique, routine kissing balloon is not recommended. Few studies have shown that kissing balloon did not improve incidence of death, MI, and TLR in bifurcation procedures.[13-15]

Proximal Optimization Technique in Crossover Stenting

European Bifurcation Club recommends ostial only stenting in lesions which are favorable without LM and LCX involvement and good bifurcation angle. In other situations, crossover stenting followed by proximal optimization technique (POT) and provisional kissing balloon should be preferred.[16] The POT is advised in crossover stenting technique to optimize proximal stent and improve long-term outcomes. In POT, a short balloon is inflated just proximal to carina, this prevents malapposition of the stent in the proximal vessel. In this technique as a single stent is used, the reference diameter of the stent should of proximal LAD. Many studies have shown that placing a stent from the distal LM to the ostium of the LAD (cross-over technique) has better results in terms of restenosis and TLR compared with ostial stenting.

Only Drug-coated Balloon Technique

It is an emerging angioplasty technique. It reduces neointimal hyperplasia without implanting protruding strut eliminating risk of late stent thrombosis. SPARTAN DCB study showed results with paclitaxel DCB had comparable long-term mortality rates with second-generation drug-eluting stents.[17]

CONCLUSION

In conclusion, crossover stenting followed by POT assisted by intravascular imaging may be an ideal approach for the treatment of most ostial LAD lesions based on available data. Imaging increases procedural success rates and decreases TLR. Moreover, treatment strategies must be patient specific considering anatomical lesion and various clinical situations.

ONLINE REFERENCES

Please scan the QR code provided at the end of the table of contents for References of this chapter.

CHAPTER

154 Approach to Coronary Aneurysm and Ectasia

Kesavamoorthy, Sabari Krishnan, Kousalya Gopalsamy

ABSTRACT

The coronary aneurysm is the abnormal focal dilatation of the epicardial coronary artery. Its diameter is 1.5 times greater than the distal reference lumen diameter. Its incidences vary in different studies. Since, the interventional era in cardiology has grown, the incidence of coronary aneurysms and ectasia has kept increasing. Its main causative factors are atherosclerosis, inflammatory, and noninflammatory, such as congenital and genetic factors. Even with these advancements in interventional cardiology, the management is still controversial. The prognosis remains nonpromising. This chapter deals with the overall approach to coronary aneurysms and ectasia.

Keywords: Coronary ectasia, coronary aneurysm, covered stent.

INTRODUCTION

Coronary artery aneurysm (CAA) is the abnormal focal dilatation of the epicardial coronary artery 1.5-fold greater than the regular adjacent segment. Coronary artery ectasia appears as diffuse arterial dilatation, where the length of dilatation exceeds 50% of its reference lumen diameter. Its incidence ranges from 0.3 to 0.5% in patients undergoing diagnostic coronary angiography **(Table 1)**.[1]

VESSEL WALL STRUCTURE BY INTRAVASCULAR ULTRASOUND (BOX 1)

- True aneurysm—all three-vessel wall integrity present
- Pseudoaneurysm—loss of vessel wall integrity
- Complex plaque with aneurysm appearance—stenosis with ruptured plaque or spontaneous or healed dissections
- Normal segment with aneurysmal appearance—normal segment adjacent to stenosis

TABLE 1: Definition and classification of coronary artery aneurysm (CAA).

Definition	Types and classification
Coronary aneurysm: Focal dilation at least 1.5 times the normal segment	*Morphology*: • Saccular aneurysm—transverse > longitudinal diameter • Fusiform aneurysm—transverse < longitudinal diameter

ANATOMICAL DISTRIBUTION

Coronary artery aneurysms are the most common in the proximal and mid part of the epicardial coronary arteries. The most frequent in the right coronary artery (RCA) is 68%, followed by the left anterior descending (LAD) artery at 60% and the left circumflex (LCX) first artery at 50%. It is rare in the left main, accounting for 0.1%.[2]

BOX 1 Coronary artery ectasia.

- *Type 1*: Diffuse ectasia of two or three vessels
- *Type 2*: Diffuse disease in one vessel and localized disease in another vessel
- *Type 3*: Diffuse ectasia in one vessel
- *Type 4*: Local or segmental ectasia

PATHOGENESIS AND ETIOLOGY

Coronary Artery Aneurysm and Coronary Artery Disease

The most common cause of CAAs is atherosclerosis, accounting for 50% of CAAs in adults. In the coronary artery surgery study (CASS) registry, the prevalence of CAA is 4.9%. Patients with aneurysms and concomitant coronary artery disease (CAD) were compared with coronary artery stenosis alone without an aneurysm; most were males, had a myocardial infarction in the past, and were associated with triple vessel disease. Histological examination of atherosclerosis CAAs revealed hyalinization and lipid deposition leading to weakness of intimal and medial layers of the vessel wall and destruction of the muscular elastic component. Such deficiency and decrease in the wall elasticity ultimately reduce the vessel tolerance to luminal pressure, predisposing to dilatation, and aneurysm formation.[3]

Genetic Association of Coronary Artery Aneurysms

Several genomic studies showed the association of variants on *chromosome 9p21.3* with CAD, and this locus was associated with an increased risk of intracranial aneurysm and abdominal aneurysm—the *9p21.3* linked to altered proliferative phenotypes that promote adverse vascular remodeling.[4]

Coronary Artery Aneurysm and Stent Implantation

Current literature shows that the incidence of CAA in stent implantation varies from 1.35 to 4%.[5] Several mechanisms have been proposed to elucidate the formation of stent-related CAAs, including stent implantation-induced coronary dissection and malapposition. Drug-eluting stent (DES) with various antiproliferative drugs has shown to be the risk of CAAs because of the mechanism of delayed neointimal healing and re-endothelization.[6] These drugs local hypersensitivity and cytotoxicity effects contribute to the weakness of all three arterial wall layers leading to aneurysmal in the epicardial arteries.

Vasculitis

Vasculitis is one of the important causes of CAAs. Among vasculitis, Kawasaki disease (KD) is the most common cause of CAAs in children and the second most common cause in adults. Acute coronary vasculitis in KD leads to dilatation and aneurysm formation. CAAs occur in around 10–15% of patients during the acute phase of the KD.[7] Takayasu arteritis (TA) is primary systemic vasculitis involving great arteries and branches. <10% have coronary involvement. There are three main types of lesions in TA—(1) stenosis or occlusion of the coronary ostia, (2) focal or diffuse coronary arteritis, and (3) coronary aneurysm.[8] Systemic lupus erythematosus, polyarteritis nodosa, and rheumatoid arthritis are other vasculitis diseases that can lead to CAA.[9]

Infections and Drug Use

Bacterial, fungal, syphilitic, mycobacterial, septic emboli, mycotic aneurysms, and human immunodeficiency virus (HIV) infections can cause CAA. Direct invasion of pathogens or immune complex deposition on the vessel wall can lead to mycotic lesions. Using drugs such as cocaine, amphetamine, and protease inhibitor can lead to CAA. Cocaine usage can cause vasoconstriction, leading to severe hypertensive crisis and direct endothelial damage, predisposing to CAA.[10]

CLINICAL PRESENTATION

Most CAAs are asymptomatic and few are symptomatic; symptoms are mainly due to underlying causes. Most clinical presentations of CAAs are similar to those of CAD. A frequent finding is the presence of thrombi in the aneurysm, and slow blood flow on the irregular surface of the aneurysm causes angina, dyspnea, myocardial infarction, and sudden death.[11] Rupture of CAAs is rare. Patients with a giant aneurysm can present in different ways, such as mediastinal mass or superior vena cava syndrome, often misdiagnosed as a tumor.[12,13]

DIAGNOSIS

Mostly diagnosed using imaging studies, the ideal methods should include evaluating the number, size, distribution, extension, presence, and absence of intra-aneurysmal thrombus. CAAs should be assessed for associated complications such as embolization, myocardial infarction, and rupture. Most CAAs are detected by diagnostic coronary angiography. Noninvasive imaging such as echocardiography, computed tomography (CT), and magnetic resonance imaging may also see them.[14]

CORONARY ANGIOGRAPHY

Coronary angiography provides information about the aneurysm's number, location, size, and shape. It details the severity of atherosclerosis, coronary stenosis, and collateral formation. Coronary angiography may not provide detail about the small aneurysms and mild ectasia. Major role in complex coronary aneurysm. As it is a lumenogram, it may not give information on the vessel wall or the actual aneurysm size. It also has limitations in detecting true and pseudoaneurysms.[15]

Computed Tomography Angiography

Multidetector computed tomography (MDCT) has been increasingly used for noninvasive coronary angiography.

MDCT has increased the incidental finding of CAA and ectasia. CT data were reconstructed to provide details about location, number, size, shape, morphology, concomitant coronary stenosis, and plaque composition. CT coronary angiography (CTCA) provides a rapid three-dimensional evaluation that helps understand the complex anatomy of cardiac structures, such as those seen in ectasia associated with coronary fistulas as well as the lumen composition and vessel wall can be assessed. Coronary angiography allows both diagnosis and treatment of CAAs; CTCA can be used to follow-up patients with treated or suspected CAAs.[16]

Intravascular Ultrasound

Intravascular ultrasound (IVUS) is the gold standard for providing critical anatomical information to address the diagnostic limitation of evaluating the coronary aneurysm during conventional coronary angiography.[17] It gives the transmural information of the coronary arterial wall and helps to differentiate the true and pseudoaneurysm. Pseudoaneurysms are characterized by the loss in the vessel wall integrity, prone to high risk of rupture, whereas poststent intervention aneurysms are true ones that follow the healed dissection.[18] IVUS on the angiographically regressed coronary aneurysm demonstrated the thickened intima-media complex and decreased vasoactive response to the vasodilators. IVUS, also used in treating CAAs, is essential in guiding the complete coverage of the aneurysm.[18]

Echocardiology

Transthoracic echocardiography and transesophageal echocardiography have high sensitivity and specificity in identifying the proximal aneurysm in left main coronary artery (LMCA) and RCA, making the ideal assessment for the diagnosing and following up the aneurysm in KD in children. It provides information about the location of the aneurysm and the presence or absence of thrombi.[19]

Coronary Magnetic Resonance Angiography

Coronary magnetic resonance angiography (MRA) is a valuable alternative for those for whom other noninvasive modalities are contraindicated. A series of KD patients demonstrated coronary MRA's ability to effectively diagnose all CAAs, occlusion, and stenosis found on coronary angiography.[20] Current literature supports the usage of coronary MRA in the proximal segments of the coronary artery; its resolution is reduced in the smaller distal segments, so additional studies are needed on coronary MRA to study the lesion in the distal segments.[21]

TREATMENT

The treatment option for CCAs is medical, percutaneous, and surgical approach. The disease's natural course and prognosis are related to many factors, based on symptoms, etiology, number, aneurysmal size, location, presence of thrombus, infection, atherosclerosis, and stenosis.

Medical Treatment

Coronary artery aneurysm is associated with higher mortality and adverse cardiac events. A study showed that 54% of major adverse cardiac events (MACE) rate at 4.5 years of follows-up. CAA following the coronary intervention, 27% MACE at 3 years. CAA treatment is individualized based on the patient's characteristics, presentation, characteristics of CAAs, and their association with the acute cardiac event. The main aim of management in CAA is to identify the etiology and prevent the progression of CAAs and their associated complication. Atherosclerosis is the main causative factor causing CAAs. Aggressive atherosclerotic management and risk factor control are essential in managing CAAs.

Statins are shown to inhibit the metalloproteinase secretion 1, 2, 3, and 9 from the vascular smooth cells and the macrophages, thereby preventing the progression of CAAs. Statins help control lipid levels, as atherosclerosis is a significant risk factor for CAAs.[22]

Angiotensin-converting-enzyme inhibitors (ACEI) help slow the progression of CAAs by inhibiting the transforming growth factor-beta (TGF-β).[23] Aspirin is prescribed for all patients, as the coexistence of atherosclerotic coronary obstruction has a higher risk of myocardial infarction. The role of dual antiplatelets is doubtful, and no data to support that warfarin and novel anticoagulant have been shown to improve the flow in the ectatic and aneurysmal segment. However, no data support this. Anticoagulants are recommended in patients with multivessel disease and recurrent events despite the dual antiplatelet. Vasodilators such as nitrates should be avoided as they increase myocardial ischemia.

In acute KD, intravenous (IV) immunoglobulin plays an essential role in the management; it results in regression of the aneurysm and lower MACE—limited evidence of anticoagulant and antithrombotic therapy in the prevention of thrombotic events in acute KD.

Percutaneous Intervention

Most of the data are from the patient who presented with acute coronary syndrome. An asymptomatic patient who is found incidentally requires no treatment unless it is DES-related aneurysm or a giant aneurysm that is more prone to rupture.

In symptomatic patients, the main aim of the treatment is to achieve thrombolysis in myocardial infarction grade 3 (TIMI 3) flow in ischemia-related arteries with CAAs. It is usually associated with a high thrombus burden that requires multiple runs of thrombus aspiration and intracoronary glycoprotein IIb/IIIa (GPIIb/IIIa) inhibitors. Despite all these efforts, slow flow and no flow are common.

The treatment modality differs with the shape and extent of the aneurysm:

- Saccular and focal aneurysms can be treated with a covered stent; however, short-term and long-term results are not promising.[24] We successfully treated a large poststenting aneurysm in the LCX with two overlapping covered stents **(Figs. 1A to E)**. Another patient with RCA is a diffusely ectatic vessel with distal stenosis and was successfully treated with a DES stent **(Figs. 2A and B)**.
- Saccular or fusiform aneurysms involving major side branches can be treated with a balloon, stent-assisted embolization, or surgical excision.

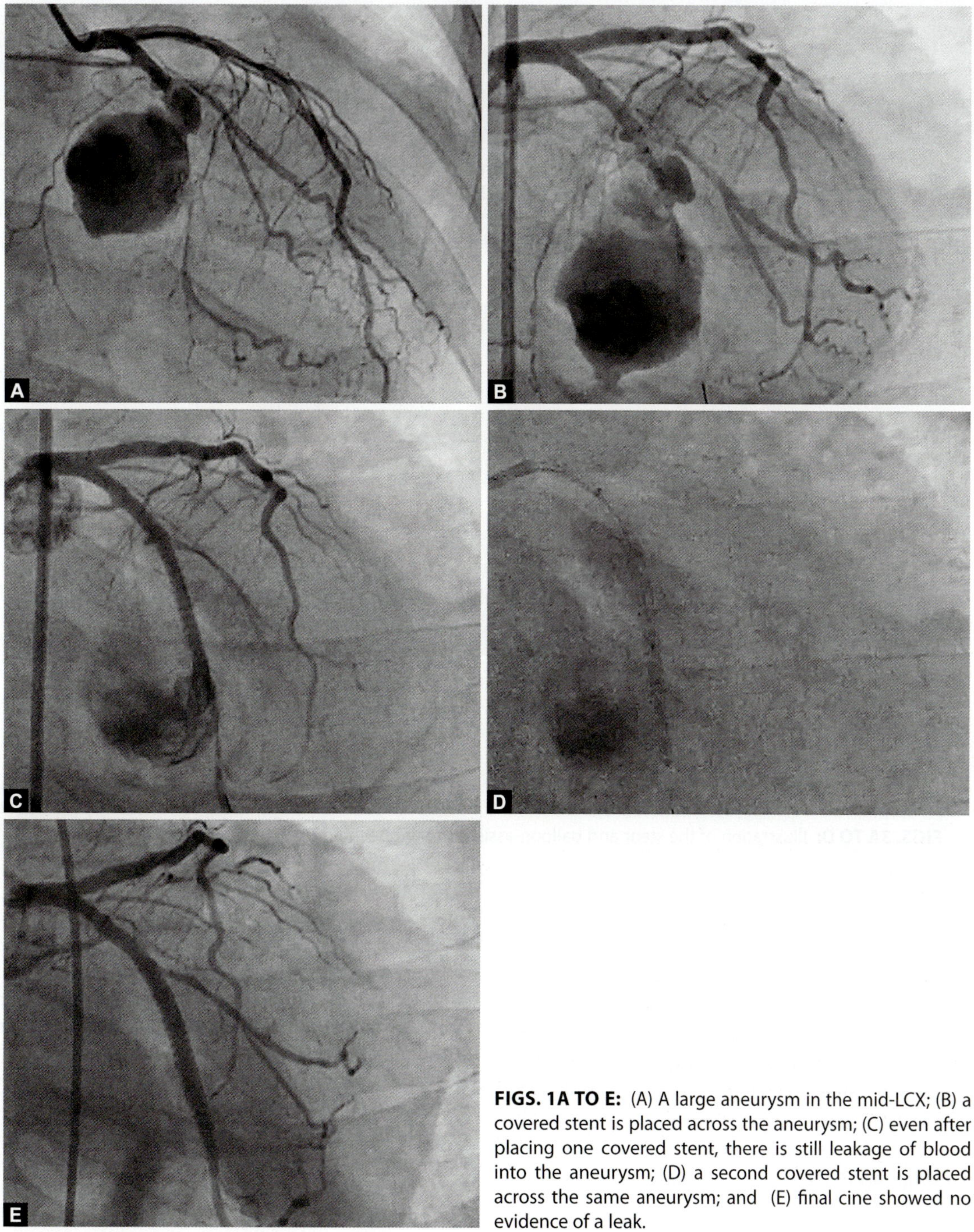

FIGS. 1A TO E: (A) A large aneurysm in the mid-LCX; (B) a covered stent is placed across the aneurysm; (C) even after placing one covered stent, there is still leakage of blood into the aneurysm; (D) a second covered stent is placed across the same aneurysm; and (E) final cine showed no evidence of a leak.

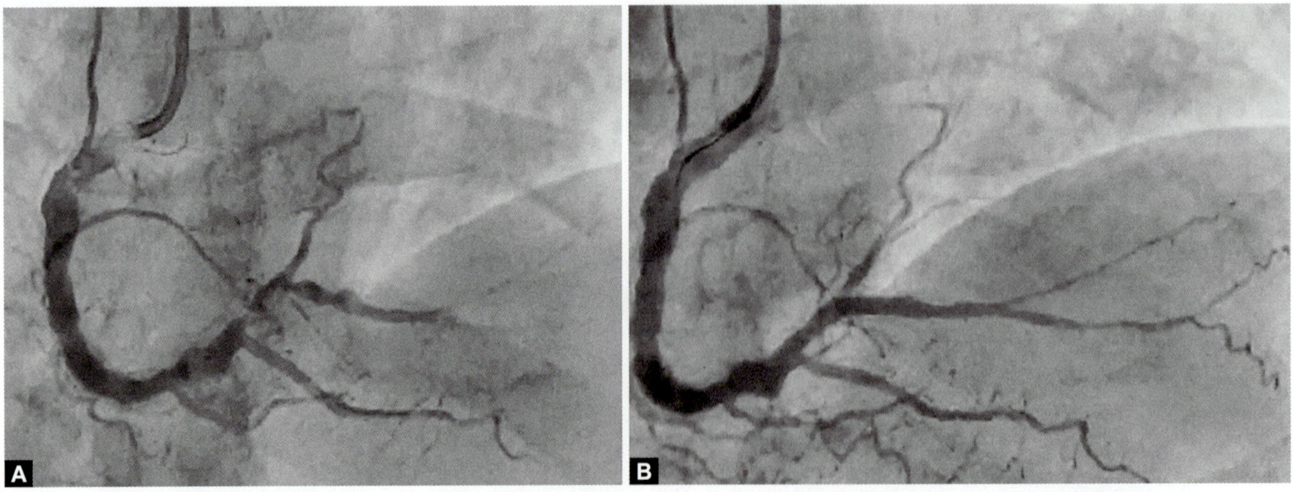

FIGS. 2A AND B: Diffuse ectasia in the right coronary artery associated with significant stenosis in the PLV branch, which was treated with DES.
(DES: drug-eluting stent; PLV: posterior left ventricular)

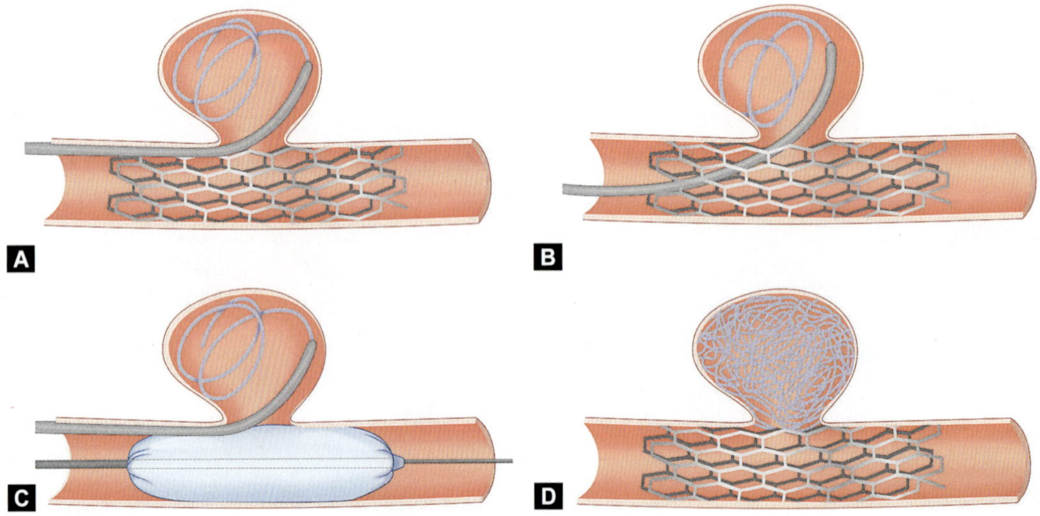

FIGS. 3A TO D: Illustration of the stent and balloon-assisted coiling technique.

- CAAs involving left main or multiple giant aneurysms (20 mm or more than four times of distal reference), surgical excision is the treatment of choice.
- Rapidly expanding saphenous vein graft (SVG) graft or those causing mechanical symptoms such as external compression of underlying structures, percutaneous closure with Amplatzer Occluders, or coil embolization with or without percutaneous coronary intervention (PCI) of the native vessel is a possible alternative to the surgery **(Figs. 3A to D)**.

Surgery

Surgery is the alternative treatment for patients who cannot be treated with percutaneous intervention and is usually done for a patient with an obstructive coronary lesion with a large saccular aneurysm with a high risk of rupture. Resection of the aneurysm, proximal and distal ligation, aneurysmal thrombectomy, and aneurysmectomy with or without bypass graft can be done to treat the aneurysm **(Flowchart 1)**.[25]

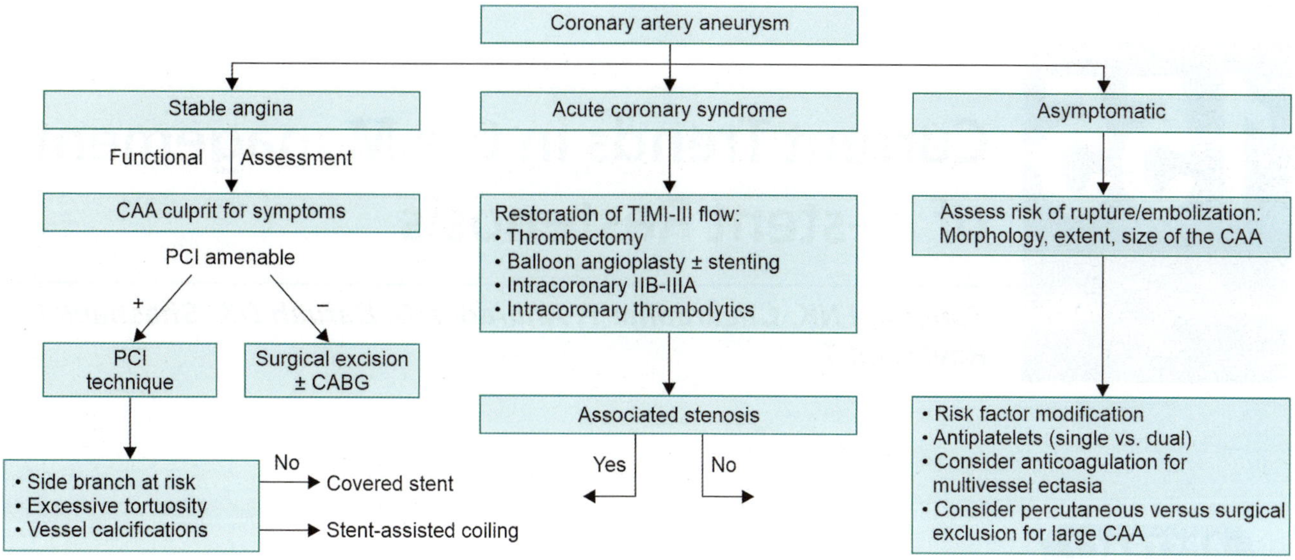

FLOWCHART 1: Suggested algorithm for managing patients with coronary ectasia and aneurysm.
(CAA: coronary artery aneurysm; CABG: coronary artery bypass grafting; PCI: percutaneous coronary intervention; TIMI: thrombolysis in myocardial infarction)

CONCLUSION

Coronary artery aneurysms are not uncommon and are usually associated with risk factors such as atherosclerosis and hypertension. Most of the aneurysm are asymptomatic. If a CAA presents with ACS, traditionally associated with a significant thrombus burden. During percutaneous intervention, slow-flow and no-flow are common. A focal coronary aneurysm can be stented with a covered stent; a large aneurysm with a side branch can be treated with a stent or balloon-assisted coil embolization. Symptomatic aneurysms that are not amenable to percutaneous intervention are dealt with surgically. Long-term prognosis of these treated patients is not promising.

ONLINE REFERENCES

Please scan the QR code provided at the end of the table of contents for References of this chapter.

CHAPTER

155

Current Trends in the Management of In-stent Restenosis

Panigrahi NK, Chakradhar P, Anuradha D, Baruah DK, Shashank C, Ravi Kant T

ABSTRACT

Target lesion revascularization after current generation of drug-eluting stent (DES) implantation continues to occur at a rate of 1–2% per year even up to a decade. In-stent restenosis (ISR) is the most common cause of stent failure. The clinical definition of ISR requires the presence of >50% diameter in-stent stenosis and one of the following: clinical symptoms of recurrent angina, objective signs of ischemia [electrocardiogram (ECG) changes], hemodynamic assessment with fractional flow reserve (FFR) < 0.80, intravascular ultrasound minimum cross-sectional area < 4 mm^2, or restenosis with ≥70% reduction in lumen diameter even in the absence of clinical symptoms or signs. Though the migration of smooth muscle cells begins as a process to re-endothelize the struts, neointimal hyperplasia toward the endoluminal sides of the stent creates the matrix for ISR and the underlying mechanical factors causing underexpansion of stent remain as nidus for recurrence. Intravascular imaging identifies the substrate and guides what interventional tools to be used and optimizes the post-percutaneous coronary intervention (PCI) results. Aggressive lesion preparation with cutting balloon/high-pressure balloon/intravascular lithotripsy balloon for calcified vessel wall and calcified neointima is mandatory before final therapy by drug-eluting balloon or DES. Laser or rotational atherectomy gives a niche in the recalcitrant, diffuse ISR. Intravascular brachy therapy offers limited solution with high chance of recurrence. Bypass surgery is the best option with left main ISR or ISR with associated multivessel disease.

Keywords: In-stent restenosis (ISR), target lesion revascularization, intravascular imaging (IVI), under-expanded stent, DES, drug-eluting ballon (DEB).

INTRODUCTION

Despite the widespread use of current third generation of drug-eluting stent (DES) platforms, in-stent restenosis (ISR) emerged as a specific subset of disease, the treatment of which is accounting for 5–10% of all percutaneous coronary intervention (PCI).[1] In the clinical trials involving contemporary DES, the criteria to measure clinical restenosis is defined as ischemia-driven target lesion revascularization (TLR) occurring at a rate of <3% at 1 year and 10% at 5 years.[2] However, angiographic assessment reveals higher rate of restenosis which remains a binary event defined as a stenosis of >50% of the stented segment.

Currently, optimization of PCI by intravascular imaging (IVI) is expected to impact long-term outcome of PCI. In recently completed RENNOVATE-complex PCI trial, the rate of clinically driven target vessel revascularization (TVR) at 2 years remained as 3.4% in IVI arm and 5.5% in angiographic arm.[3] Annually, a total of >7.5 lakhs stents are implanted in India (National Intervention Council of India, 2023 report). Globally, the penetration of IVI during PCI is around 13.9% and India is trialing currently at 5.5%.[4,5] Hence, the burden of ischemia-driven ISR is high and it is a challenging disease, subset to manage.

DEFINITION OF IN-STENT RESTENOSIS

Angiography: According to Academic Research Consortium (ARC) definition, angiographic restenosis is defined as luminal narrowing at least ≥50% of vessel diameter in stented segment or within 5 mm of its edge and with clinical or functional evidence of ischemia.

Intravascular imaging: ISR is defined as luminal cross-sectional area renarrowing of >75% of the reference vessel. In intravascular ultrasound (IVUS), minimum lumen area

(MLA) of <5 mm^2 is the cutoff value for stent underexpansion. In optical coherence tomography (OCT), at least 50% of the neointimal tissue volume at the site of MLA is significant neointimal hyperplasia (NIH).

Clinical re-stenosis: ISR associated with signs and symptoms of ischemia (ischemia driven). TLR is the measure of ISR in the clinical trial.

Silent restenosis: It is ISR without signs and symptoms of ischemia.

CLINICAL IMPACT OF IN-STENT RESTENOSIS

Although ISR is insidious in its progression and stable course, it does not seem to be innocuous. In the CathPCI registry, among 542,112 patients who underwent ISR-PCI, 25% presented with acute myocardial infarction.[1] Neoatherosclerosis (NA) and subsequent plaque rupture can coexist within the DES-ISR. Those who present as acute coronary syndrome (ACS) suffer higher major adverse cardiac events (MACE) and recurrent ISR.

MECHANISM OF IN-STENT RESTENOSIS

Mechanical and biological substrates ***(Fig. 1):*** The substrate associated with ISR could be biological and mechanical or both. The mechanical factors include stent undersizing and underexpansion, stent fracture, stent deformation and foreshortening, stent overlap, and geographic miss.[6] Mechanical issues remain as a trigger for recurrent ISR. Calcification of the vessel wall and calcific nodules in the neoatheroma mostly limit the subsequent expansion during second stent deployment.

Neointimal hyperplasia is the central biological mechanism of ISR, which comprises accumulation of smooth muscle cells and extracellular matrix in the neointima, covering the luminal side of the stent.[7,8] Unlike bare-metal stent (BMS)-ISR, DES-ISR is more focal and continues to occur beyond 6 months.

Neoatherosclerosis, a characteristic of DES-ISR, occurs beyond 1 year by accumulation of foam cells with or without necrotic lipid core. The calcification of neointima contributes for thrombotic stent occlusion, particularly 1 year after the stent implantation. In an IVI study involving DES-ISR, 40% of lesions in the IVUS show a minimum stent area (MSA) of <5 mm^2 and 66% had >50% NIH volume which indicate that both pathologies are commonly encountered even in second-generation DES-ISR.[9]

Stent failure: ISR is the most common cause. Late thrombosis can develop without ISR. Though ISR is the most common cause of stent failure, late and very late stent thrombosis could contribute for the stent occlusion. The incorporation of antiproliferative drugs into the stent platform with or without biodegradable polymers to prevent NIH resulting into delayed healing and incomplete stent strut coverage, predispose to late and very late stent thrombosis and is responsible for TLR occurring at a rate 1–2% per year beyond 1 year without reaching the plateau upto 10 years.[10] Addition of thrombotic complication into the NA makes ISR due to NIH and stent thrombosis inseparable.

Repeat revascularization (RR): TLR is the measure of ISR. RR in the clinical trials can be defined as TLR of stented segment or within 5 mm of its edge in the target vessel or as TVR of nonstented segment (5 mm beyond the stent edge) in the target vessel or non-TVR due to the progression of atherothrombotic disease in the nonstented vessel. TLR is the measure of clinical stent restenosis.

Recurrence of ISR: ISR begets ISR. Despite development in the treatment, the rate of recurrent ISR is high. In a follow-up

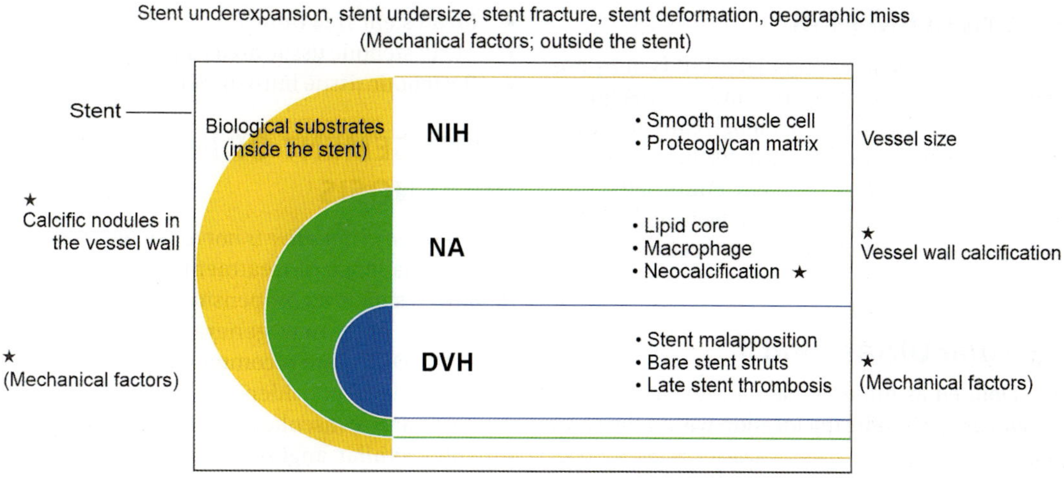

FIG. 1: Pathogenesis of stent failure.

(DVH: delayed vascular healing; NA: neoatherosclerosis; NIH: neointimal hyperplasia; Star: mechanical factors)

for 15 years including 48,000 patients, the recurrence of ISR after first, second, and third intervention was 8.3%, 17.1%, and 22.8%, respectively.[11] Mortality in the left main (LM)-ISR revascularization with repeat PCI is unacceptably high.

CLASSIFICATION OF IN-STENT RESTENOSIS

Angiographic: Prognostic Value of Angiographic Pattern for Subsequent Target Lesion Revascularization

Mehran et al. divided the angiographic pattern of ISR seen in the BMS into four groups as follows:[12]

- *Type I (focal ISR)*: Focal Lesions are ≤10 mm in length and are placed at—
  - *Type IA*: The unstented segment (articulation or gap)
  - *Type IB*: The body of the stent
  - *Type IC*: The proximal or distal margin
  - *Type ID*: A combination of these sites ("multifocal ISR")
- *Type II (diffuse ISR within stent)*: Lesions are >10 mm in length and are confined to the stented segment, without extending outside the margin(s).
- *Type III (diffuse proliferative within and beyond stent)*: Lesions are >10 mm in length and extend beyond the margin(s) of the stented segment.
- *Type IV (occlusive)*

The distribution of different patterns of angiographic ISR is as follows: Type I (65%), type 2 (25%), type 3 (6%), and type 4 (4%).[13] This classification bears a prognostic value for subsequent TLR, diffuse and occlusive ISR being forerunner of worst post-PCI results. The rates of TLR were 19%, 35%, 50%, and 83% in classes I (focal) to IV (occlusive), respectively.[14]

Histomorphometry: DES-ISR is Different than BMS-ISR

Unlike BMS-ISR, current generation of DES-ISR is morphologically more focal, looks more layered and heterogenous, shows lesser cellularity and more proteoglycans in histopathology[15,16] with less frequent peri-struts fibrin and inflammation, associated with complete stent endothelization within 3–6 months, and developing NA and neocalcifications over long run and ongoing late luminal loss occurring up to years.[15,17]

Intravascular Ultrasound[18]

- *Focal ISR*: Defined as lumen area < 4 mm^2 and length < 10 mm, subcategorized by the location within the stent as follows:
  - *Focal body type*: Confined to the body of stent
  - *Focal marginal type*: Extending to the margins of stent
- *Multifocal ISR*: Defined as the presence of multiple focal lesions, with subcategories as follows:
  - *Multifocal body type*: Confined to the body of the stent
  - *Multifocal marginal type*: Involving stent margins
- *Diffuse ISR*: Defined as MLA < 4 mm^2 and length > 10 mm, with subcategories as follows:
  - *Diffuse body type*: Confined to the stent body
  - *Diffuse marginal type*: Associated with stent involvement

Optical Coherence Tomography (Fig. 2)[19,20]

- *According to OCT appearance, ISR can be classified qualitatively into four groups as follows*:
  i. Homogeneous: Uniform high optical signal intensity without focal back scattering. Typical representation of areas of high distribution of smooth muscle cell
  ii. Heterogeneous: Mixed optical signal intensity and variegated back scattering; representative of proteoglycan-rich neointima or early neoatherosclerotic plaque
  iii. Attenuated: Superficial high signal intensity, high backscatter, indicative of lipid-rich core
  iv. Layered: Abluminal alternating high- and low-scattering layers most frequently seen in the peri-strut areas
- *According to the lumen shapes, ISR can be classified into two types*:
  i. Regular: Luminal border is sharp, smooth, and circular.
  ii. Irregular: Luminal border is irregular and marked by tissue protrusion from the wall.
- *According to visible intraluminal material*: Present or absent

Quantitative information:

- Mean lumen area (mm^2)
- Mean stent area (mm^2)
- Mean stenotic tissue area (mm^2)
- Restenotic tissue burden (%)

MANAGEMENT OF IN-STENT RESTENOSIS

The procedural objective is not to fail for the second time.

The challenge of treatment DES-ISR in comparison to de novo lesion is its propensity of subsequent recurrence.[21] Currently, both new generation DES and drug-coated balloons (DCBs) are recommended for the treatment of ISR as Class I (level of evidence A) by the European guidelines on coronary revascularization.[22] Either of this treatment provides similar angiographic net gain (acute gain—late luminal loss) and acceptable long-term clinical outcome. However, complex substrate DES ensures favorable clinical outcome and reduce the need for repeat intervention.[21,23]

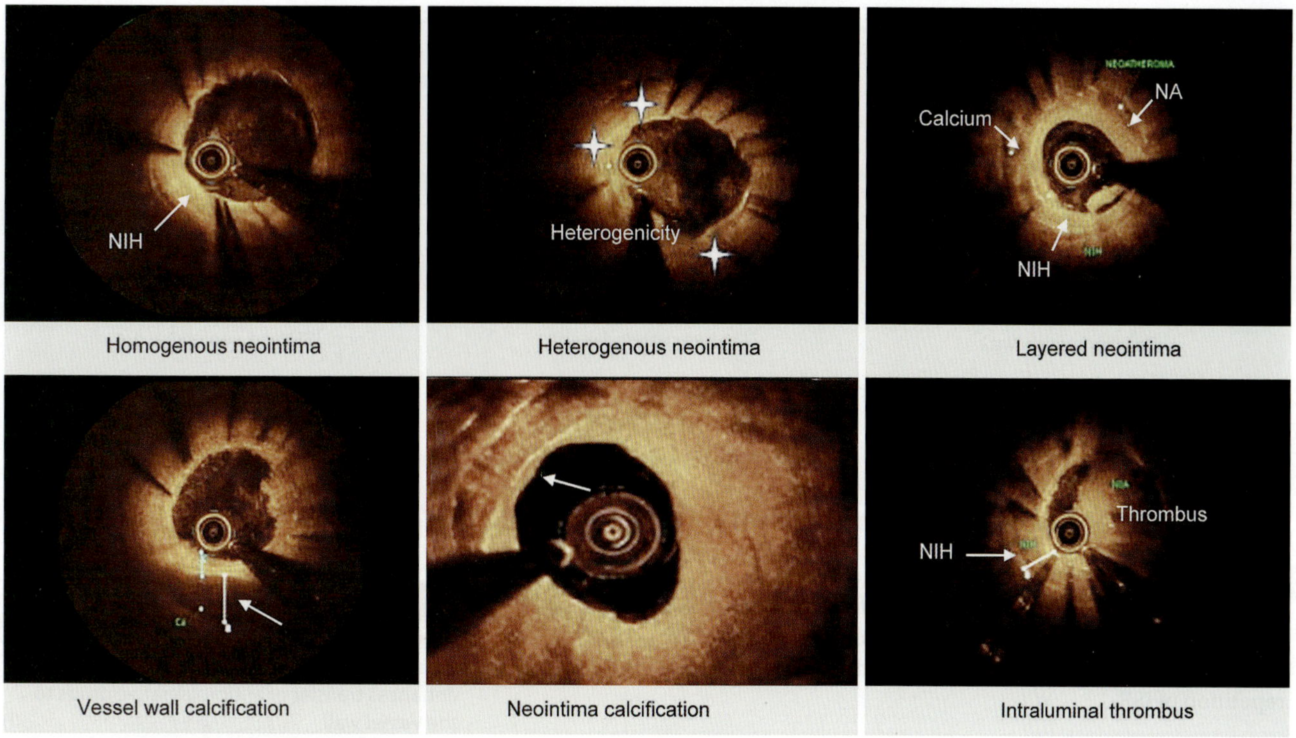

FIG. 2: Classification of OCT images in ISR.
(ISR: in-stent restenosis; NA: neoatherosclerosis; NIH: neointimal hyperplasia; OCT: optical coherence tomography)

Prediction Model for Recurrence of In-stent Restenosis: "The ISAR Score"

Recently, Coughlan et al. proposed a clinical score (the ISAR score) which comprises four variables and each having a score of 1 derived from 1,986 patients followed up retrospectively for a period of 7.4 years—(1) a nonfocal, <10 mm ISR pattern, (2) time interval to ISR <6 months, (3) ISR in the left circumflex coronary artery (LCx) particularly the ostium, and (4) ISR in a calcified vessel—were associated with repeat PCI for recurrent DES-ISR at 1 year [hazard ratio (HR) 0.60; confidence interval (CI) 0.57-0.63][24] However, a "diffuse" angiographic pattern, early presentation within 6 months, calcification of the vessel wall and resistant underexpansion (calcified nodules in the vessel wall), and neointima calcification which constitutes 4.9% of ISR lesions[23] are the strongest predictors of recurrences and markers of an aggressive vascular response.

Imaging

The objectives are: (1) to identify the substrate of ISR, (2) to aggressively address the mechanical issues, (3) guidance for selecting the devices, and (4) to optimize the postprocedure results.

Stent Boost (Figs. 3A to C)

Stent boost is a useful tool which can be performed readily in the catheterization laboratory to identify stent underexpansion, stent fracture, stent deformation, and geographic miss between the two stents. Stent fracture is delineated better with the stent boost imaging.

Intravascular Imaging

Intravascular ultrasound and OCT help in identifying the underlying multiple mechanism of ISR and provide guidance for which of the interventional tools is beneficial and assess the optimization of stenting after PCI. Despite the efficacy of IVI to improve the clinical outcome after PCI with ISR, current guideline recommendation is class II (level of evidence C).[22]

Does the morphologic pattern of OCT images guide the choice between drug-eluting balloon (DEB) or DES treatment? There was no difference in MACE and TLR after DEB or DES between the OCT finding with low inhomogeneity (homogenous means NIH). However, the difference exists favoring DES over DEB in treating lesion with high inhomogeneity (heterogenous means NA).[25]

Fractional Flow Reserve

As in the de novo lesion, a borderline ISR with 40–70% luminal diameter stenosis or if patient is oligosymptomatic, FFR value of >0.75 is safe to manage with medications.[26] However, there are no randomized data supporting an FFR-guided post-stent optimization after PCI for the ISR treatment strategy.

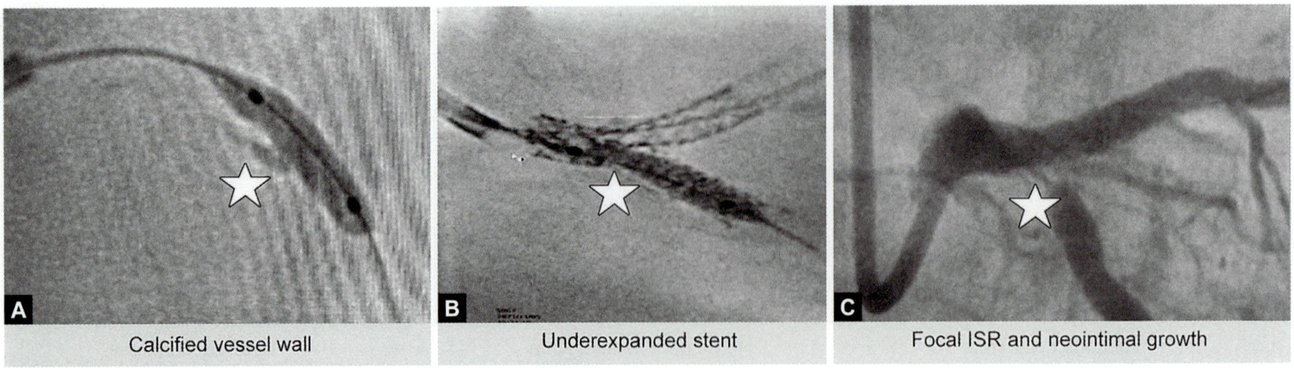

FIGS. 3A TO C: Utility of images enhancement and stent boost.
(ISR: in-stent restenosis)

Interventional Tools for the Lesion Preparation (Table 1)

Aggressive lesion preparation is the foundation of ISR treatment. Before delivering a definitive device such as DES or DEB, the mechanical cause must be addressed to prevent repetition of ISR.

High-pressure Balloon

Noncompliant (NC) high-pressure balloon (HPB) is to be used routinely for the aggressive predilatation of under-expanded or collapsed stent. It is seldom used primarily for the sole treatment of ISR. The problem faced during balloon dilatation is watermelon seeding phenomena due to slimy NIH.

Cutting/Scoring Balloon

In the cutting balloon (CB), the attached metallic blades incise the NIH in the target lesion. In the scoring balloon (SB), mounted spiral nitinol wire makes deep cut in the plaque-favoring tissue extrusion.[27] Creating the mechanical cleavage by this system provides the following advantages: (1) During preparation of the lesion, the deep cuts anchor the NC balloon and prevent watermelon seeding effect and allows subsequent aggressive HPB dilatation[28] and (2) allows lipophilic antiproliferative drug of DEB to penetrate deep into hyperplastic neointimal tissue and vessel wall.

Intravascular Lithotripsy Balloon

Intravascular lithotripsy (IVL) facilitates stent expansion of undilatable ISR by generating expanding shock waves at 50 atm pressure. Currently, data is limited and indicated as an off-label strategy. The safety and ease of handling this device makes it an attractive alternative. It is indicated in calcium-mediated unexpanded stent; the presence of calcified neo-atheroma in which high-pressure noncompliant balloon (HBP) and CB dilatation at higher pressure may predispose higher risk of vessel perforation and suboptimal results.[29]

TABLE 1: Mechanism of action of the interventional tools.

Interventional tools	Mechanism of action
CB/SB	• Cuts NIH tissue, facilitates tissue to extrude, and enhances transfer of antiproliferative drugs to the vessel wall • Modifies neointimal calcification
HPB	Dilates the underexpanded stent, disrupts NIH tissue, and modifies the calcium in the vessel wall and neointima
IVL	Expands undilatable stent, cracks the calcium underlying the unexpanded stent, and modifies neointimal calcium. Generates heat
LA	• Coagulates NIH tissue, generates heat, and facilitates recalcitrant stent • To expand and modify vessel wall and neointimal calcium
RA	• Ablates NIH tissue, modifies neointimal calcium, generates heat, and stent ablation • Facilitates stent to expand by HPB dilatation
DES	No additional stent layer, delivers antiproliferative drugs, and always to do CB dilatation and to address mechanical substrate before DEB
DEB	• Provides radial support and delivers antiproliferative drugs • Makes deep cuts in the NIH tissue

(CB: cutting balloon; DEB: drug-eluting balloon; DES: drug-eluting stent; HBP: high-pressure noncompliant balloon; IVL: intravascular lithotripsy; IVBT: intravascular brachy therapy; LA: laser atherectomy; NIH: neointimal hyperplasia; RA: rotational atherectomy; SB: scoring balloon)

Tracking the IVL balloon through calcified, undilatable ISR is the major hindrance. It requires to be negotiated after adequate predilatation and/or with the help of guide extension catheter.

Ablative Devices: Give a Niche in Diffuse, Recalcitrant In-stent Restenosis

Rotational atherectomy (RA) and excimer laser coronary atherectomy (ELCA) devices are used for the ablation of obstructive restenotic tissue. They play a decisive role in the preparation of a recalcitrant, particularly neoatherosclerotic calcified ISR lesion.[30]

Excimer laser coronary atherectomy device uses ultraviolet wavelength and generates both heat and shock wave to ablate tissue.[31] It is indicated in (1) recurrent ISR with severe vessel wall calcification (2) undilatable ISR because of severely underexpanded stent due to underlying severe vessel wall calcification,[32] and (3) diffuse ISR.

Excimer laser is used as an adjunct device to debulk the NIH tissue in diffuse ISR and facilitates further expansion of stent with open NC balloon dilatation. In a severely underexpanded stent, RA can do metallic stent ablation but may be associated with significant complication of burr entrapment and vessel perforation.[33] The benefit of routine ablation of tissue in diffuse ISR before DEB/DES is doubtful.[34] There are no randomized data for the use of RA in the treatment of DES-ISR.

DEFINITIVE TREATMENT: DEB OR DES—WHAT TO CHOOSE (FLOWCHART 1)

Drug-eluting Balloon

Drug-eluting balloon is coated with a matrix of lipophilic drugs (paclitaxel or sirolimus) and an excipient which facilitates rapid transfer and retention of antiproliferative drugs into the neohyperplastic tissue and the vessel wall.[35]

The advantages are as follows: (1) It is effective with less acute gain but also less late luminal loss (means equivalent net gain in comparison to re-DES); (2) does not require introduction of additional layer of metal stent; (3) Suitable in the smooth muscle-rich ISR (NIH) characterized in the OCT as homogenous neointimal proliferation;[22] and (4) can be managed with shortened course of DAPT in patient with high risk of bleeding.

It is indicated in the following scenario: (1) Focal ISR, (2) first ISR, (3) ISR of the side branch or ISR of the main vessel with a large side branch to prevent jailing, (4) ISR of the BMS), and (5) patients of ISR in whom bleeding risk with DAPT is high.

However, the success of DEB depends upon CB dilatation, and aggressive open NC balloon dilatation to achieve complete expansion of the stent without significant residual stenosis with adequate luminal area.[36] According to the consensus statement, DEB cannot be the sole armamentarium if angiographic result is suboptimal (residual stenosis of >30%, flow limiting dissection, and FFR < 0.80).[37]

Drug-eluting Stents

Based on randomized clinical trials and network meta-analysis,[38,39] the implantation of second DES achieves more angiographic success and is marginally more effective in reducing TLR in comparison to DEB.[40]

European guidelines recommend both repeat DES and DEB as first-line therapy for ISR (class I recommendation and level of evidence A for both).[22] However, the operator's decision to use either strategy depends upon the underlying

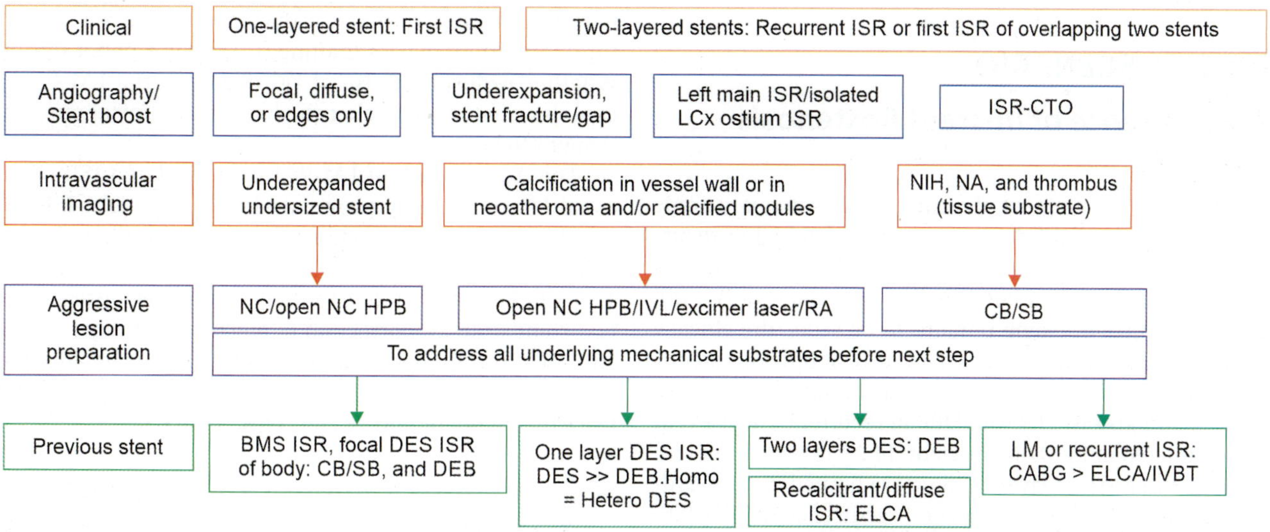

FLOWCHART 1: Treatment for ISR.

(BMS: bare-metal stent; CABG: coronary artery bypass grafting; CB: cutting balloon; CTO: chronic total occlusion; DEB: drug-eluting balloon; DES: drug-eluting stent; ELCA: excimer laser coronary atherectomy device; ISR: in-stent restenosis; IVBT: intravascular brachy therapy; IVL: intravascular lithotripsy; LCx: left circumflex artery; LM: left main; NA: neoatherosclerosis; NC HPB: noncompliant high-pressure dilatation; NIH: neointimal hyperplasia; RA: rotational atherectomy; SB: scoring balloon) substrates. While treating ISR, the focus should be on the restenotic segment and not on the entire length of the previous stent.

Repeat DES is the preferred option in the following circumstances: (1) Loss of mechanical integrity of stent such as fracture, gap between the stent, and stent collapse, (2) first DES-ISR, (3) diffuse DES-ISR, (4) ISR involving the stent edges, (5) suboptimal angiographic results (>50% residual stenosis) after repeated high-pressure NC balloon dilatation, (6) failed DEB strategy, (7) large dissection (longitudinal extension 2 mm or lateral extension > 60°), and (8) multiple layers (≥3) of stents.[37]

MEDICAL MANAGEMENT

Guideline-directed medical treatment including maximization of anti-ischemic drugs could be considered in the isolated side branch ISR in the non-LM anatomy, single vessel disease including ISR-chronic total occlusion (CTO) in the territory other than ostial left anterior descending (LAD), and ISR in the infarct-related artery without viable myocardium.

Antiplatelet Drugs to be Used after In-stent Restenosis-percutaneous Coronary Intervention

After PCI of ISR for stable coronary artery disease, dual antiplatelet therapy (DAPT) is continued for ≥3 months after DEB/CB, ≥1 year after re-DES or IVBT. In patient presenting with ACS, DAPT is to be continued for longer period, ≥6 months after DEB/CB and ≥1 year after re-DES.

In those presenting with ACS and receiving aspirin and clopidogrel, it is preferred to switch over to prasugrel daily or ticagrelor twice daily.

SPECIAL SCENARIO

Recurrence of In-stent Restenosis (Fig. 4)

The challenge of treatment of recurrent ISR is that it not only carries high rate of third recurrence but also higher recurrent TLR and MACE. The underexpanded stent remains as the trigger for recurrent ISR. Whether liberal use of IVL will alter the clinical outcome remains to be seen. The efficacy of DEB is better with one or two layering of previous stents. DEB in the treatment of three-layered scenario has the least favorable prognosis. TLR with DEB in recurrent ISR at 1 year is encountered in 14.5% in one stent, 14.9% in two stents, and 41.5% in three-stents layer.[41] There are limited data regarding what is to be done with second recurrence of DES-ISR. DES is found to be safe in more than two layers of stents[42] and offers a better option than balloon angioplasty in recurrence of ISR following DES.

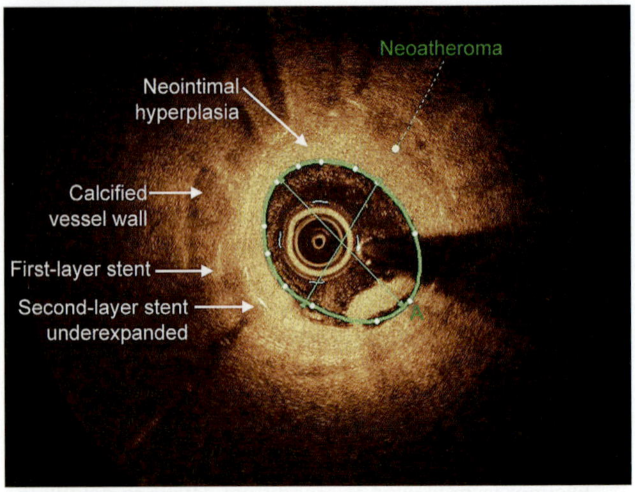

FIG. 4: Mechanism of recurrent in-stent restenosis (ISR)—multiple substrates coexist.

Intravascular brachy therapy (IVBT) has been recommended as Class IIb feasible option in American College of Cardiology/American Heart Association (ACC/AHA) guidelines in treatment of recurrent or two layers DES-ISR.[43] It can be utilized in conjunction with ISR debulking with RA and ELCA. However, the recurrence of TLR within 2 years following IVBT is very high (26.7%).[44,45]

Left Main In-stent Restenosis

Though repeat PCI can be done in majority of the case of LM-ISR,[46] mortality after TLR in LM stent failure is exceedingly high (30.2% in those with TLR compared to 17.3% without TLR). In the pooled analysis of ISAR MAIN and ISAR MAIN 2 study, the mortality in LM restenosis depends on patient-related factors more than procedural variables.[47] Coronary artery bypass grafting (CABG) is a better option. Whether widespread use of IVI during initial LM-PCI in complex anatomy will alter the long-term clinical outcome remains to be seen.

The Achilles hill of LM-PCI is the isolated ISR of the ostial LCx. Following provisional one stent, LCx-ISR can be addressed with correction of mechanical trigger by CB/HPB/IVL and final kissing with two DEB or converting into T-/TAP stenting or Culotte stenting. In the previously treated two-stent strategy, correction of mechanical trigger by CB/HPB/IVL and final kissing with two DEB can be adopted. However, mortality following TLR for failed LM stent is twice that of not requiring TLR **(Figs. 5A to C)**.

Saphenous Veinous Graft In-stent Restenosis

In DIVA trial, the prevalence of ISR in saphenous veinous graft (SVG) is 21%.[48] As the complication during PCI of

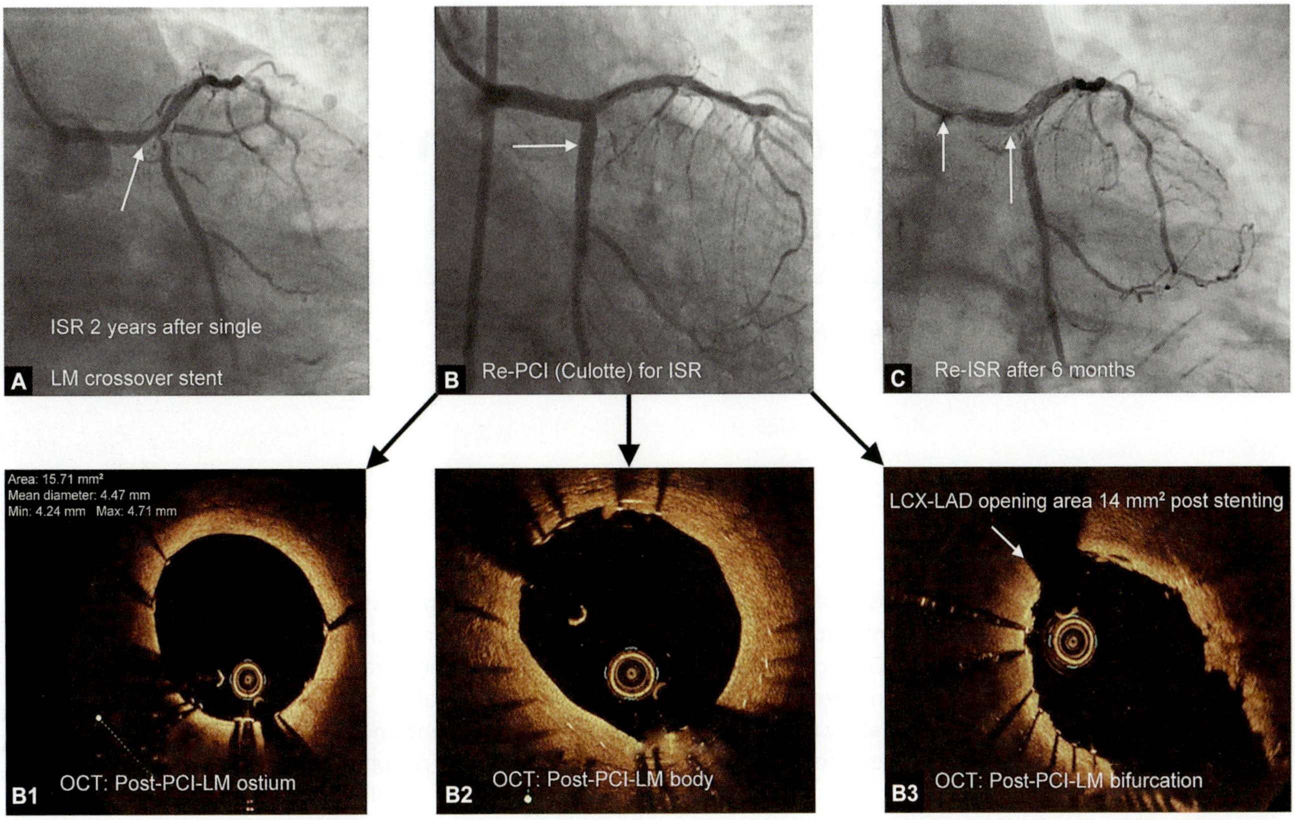

FIGS. 5A TO C: Recurrent ISR following left main TLR: (A) Isolated LCx ostial stenosis following provisional stenting to LM to LAD. (B) OCT-guided conversion to Culotte stenting with the second stent into LCx-LM during first occurrence; (B1) Post-PCI MSA of 15.5 mm^2 at the LM ostium; (B2) Post-PCI MSA of 14.78 mm^2 at the LM body; (B3) Post-PCI MSA of 14 mm^2 at the LM bifurcation. (C) Second recurrence of ISR at the ostium and bifurcation after 6 months.

(ISR: in-stent restenosis; LCx: left circumflex coronary artery; LM: left main; MSA: mean stent area; OCT: optical coherence tomography; PCI: percutaneous coronary intervention; TLR: target lesion revascularization)

SVG-ISR is remarkably high, the revascularization of the native vessel is preferred.[49]

Coronary Artery Bypass Grafting

There is no randomized trial comparing clinical outcome of CABG with PCI involving revascularization for ISR. In an observational study in whom CABG for ISR is advised 85% had multivessel disease. CABG is a reasonable option in selected patients with: (1) ISR of the body of the LM,[50] (2) recalcitrant symptomatic ISR in a major vessel, (3) ISR associated with multivessel disease,[51] or (4) ISR located in the ostial LAD.

CONCLUSION

Drug-eluting stent-ISR has emerged as a specific disease entity. The recurrence of second ISR following PCI is occurring in the tune of 1 in 5 with propensity for higher mortality in the LM-ISR. The underlying mechanism is multifactorial with mechanical issues remaining as the most important trigger for the recurrence. The definitive therapy such as DEB or DES cannot be effective without correction of mechanical causes. In case of recurrent ISR-associated LM or with multivessel disease, surgical revascularization remains the best option.

ONLINE REFERENCES

Please scan the QR code provided at the end of the table of contents for References of this chapter.

CHAPTER 156

Drug-coated Balloons: Current and Evolving Indications

Karunakar Rapolu, Siddharth Bajaj

ABSTRACT

Plain balloon angioplasty is still considered in some scenarios where stent implantation is not desirable (very small vessels, diffuse lesions, large resistant thrombus burden, side branches of bifurcations). This technique is associated with a relatively high restenosis risk. Drug-coated balloons (DCBs) have become an attractive tool for the "leave nothing behind" strategy. Studies have demonstrated that DCB are indeed effective and safe.

Emerging data suggest that DCBs allow for vasomotion, late lumen enlargement, and reduced stents-related adverse events. They have also gained major evidence supporting their clinical efficacy in peripheral arteries.

We describe the scenarios of clinical application, and available data from clinical trials in various indications.

Keywords: Bare metal stent (BMS), below the knee (BTK), dual antiplatelet therapy (DAPT), drug-coated balloons, drug-eluting stents (DESs), everolimus-eluting stents (EESs), in-stent restenosis (ISR), late lumen loss (LLL), major adverse cardiac event (MACE), percutaneous coronary intervention (PCI), percutaneous transluminal angioplasty (PTA), percutaneous transluminal coronary angioplasty (PTCA), superficial femoral artery (SFA), small-vessel disease (SVD), target lesion revascularization (TLR).

INTRODUCTION

The drug-eluting balloon (DEB) has demonstrated safety and efficacy for treatment of restenosed and de novo lesions in coronary artery disease in several clinical trials. Late lumen loss (LLL) at follow-up is consistently low (~0.2 mm), and no thrombotic event has been reported when using the DEB (SeQuent® Please) as a stand-alone therapy.

The concept behind drug-coated balloons (DCBs) was born in 2000. Despite a short contact time, the possibility to achieve a long-lasting biological effect was demonstrated with the experience with contrast media–taxane formulation. Initially in an animal study, balloon coating with only paclitaxel and a solvent had no effect in the porcine coronary stent model.[1] But coating with paclitaxel and iopromide (the X-ray contrast agent) as excipient showed a dose-dependent pronounced reduction of neointimal formation even after 4 weeks.[1]

For a long-time only drug used in DCBs was paclitaxel due to its high lipophilicity and favorable binding properties. However, the safety and effectiveness of sirolimus and its analogs on drug-eluting stents (DESs) encouraged the development of novel technologies.[2-4] Compared with those of paclitaxel-coated balloons, early small trials of sirolimus-coated balloons showed noninferior outcomes,[5,6] and hence some sirolimus-coated balloons are currently approved for clinical use in certain countries. Preclinical studies with zotarolimus-coated balloons demonstrated promising findings and recently, a biolimus-coated balloon was approved for clinical use.[7-9]

DRUG-COATED BALLOON ANGIOPLASTY

The rationale for use of DCB for angioplasty relies on the advantage of delivering an antiproliferative medication without implantation of a permanent metallic device.[1,10-12] Due to the absence of permanent metallic implants, the use of DCB has advantages over the midterm and long-term, including a mitigation of mechanisms that are stent-related leading to restenosis, thrombosis, and accelerated neoatherosclerosis. Also the antiproliferative effects of the drug delivered on the endothelial tissue reduces exaggerated neointimal hyperplasia after coronary artery disease treatment-related vessel wall injury.[1,10-16]

Small-vessel disease (SVD), in-stent restenosis (ISR), and bifurcation disease involving the side branch ostium are typical scenarios where the implantation of stents may not lead to sustained successful revascularization at a midterm or long-term follow-up.[17-19] and are associated with higher rates of restenosis and thrombosis after stenting than those with more common and less complex patterns of coronary artery disease.

Drug-coated balloons are rapid-exchange semicompliant balloon catheters with their surface coated with a formulation of an antiproliferative drug which is mainly paclitaxel and more recently sirolimus in combination with an excipient or carrier that regulates and facilitates the delivery.[1,12] Inhibition of cell division, ultimately leading to decreased neointima formation, is the primary mechanism of the antirestenotic effect of paclitaxel and sirolimus.[20]

Paclitaxel acts by irreversible binding to and stabilizing microtubules through a blockade of cell cycle progression during mitosis.[21] In contrast, sirolimus (rapamycin) forms a complex with an intracellular cytosolic protein (FKBP12) that binds to a 282-kDa serine/threonine protein kinase, reversibly inhibiting this protein, called mTOR (mammalian target of rapamycin) resulting in immunosuppression and inhibition of cell proliferation. Preclinical studies have demonstrated that DCB technology requires only 30–60 seconds of contact between the inflated balloon catheter and the vessel surface to allow an effective local intracellular drug transfer.[12,22,23] The short time of contact between vessel wall and device has proven to be enough to transfer an appropriate amount of drug inside the endothelial cells and available coatings preserve medication on DCB before delivery.[1,23,24]

Carriers that are clinically proven are iopromide, a low-osmolality contrast medium, and urea, an endogenous metabolite.[12,25] Later on, devices used other spacers, such as shellac, butyryl trihexyl citrate, acetyl tributyl citrate, resveratrol, and polyethylene glycol **(Figs. 1 to 4)**.[12,23,25]

Efficiency of DCB can be increased by the following:

- Adequate vessel preparation with predilation balloon 0.5–1.0 mm smaller than intended DEB
- Ensure 1:1 sizing between vessel and DEB [intravascular ultrasound (IVUS) in coronaries, extravascular ultrasound (EVUS) in peripherals].
- Transfer time from access sheath to DEB inflation must be short.
- For complete drug release, single prolonged inflation till manufacturer's recommended time (60 or 30 seconds)—if not tolerated, fractional release in quick intermittent inflations till recommended time is complete

Late Lumen Enlargement and Vasomotion

Balloon angioplasty alone can rarely achieve a result stent-like. A residual stenosis usually remains, which must not exceed 30% post lesion preparation.[26] Thereafter, late lumen enlargement described for paclitaxel-coated balloons[14,27] allows for angiographic results comparable with those of DES after a few months.[28] The most important mechanism for lumen improvement is the increase in the total vessel cross-sectional area.[14,29] Recent data also show that there may be a reduction of atherosclerotic plaque area in a portion of patients.[30]

Limus-coated Balloons

The comparisons between the first-generation paclitaxel-eluting and sirolimus-eluting stents have led to the doctrine that sirolimus and its analogs are the preferred drugs for local vascular therapy.[31] Owing to insufficient tissue uptake

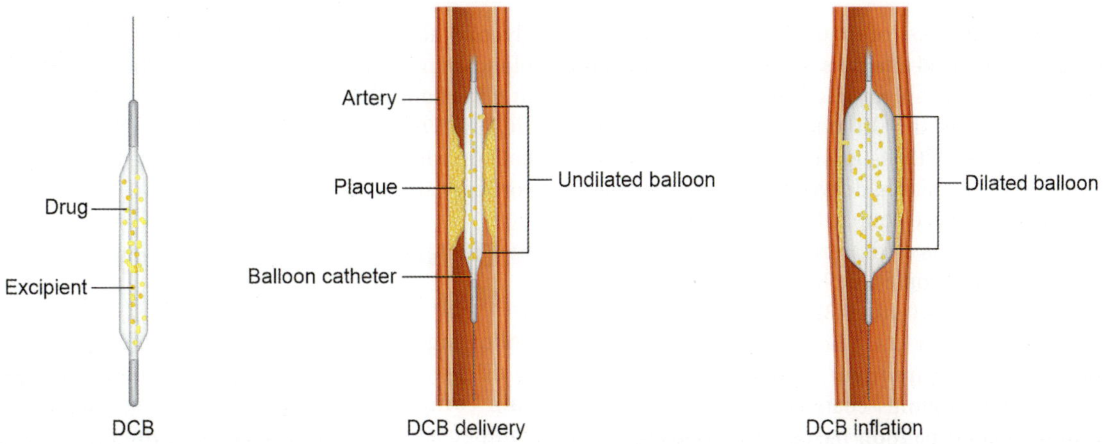

FIG. 1: Drug-coated balloon (DCB).

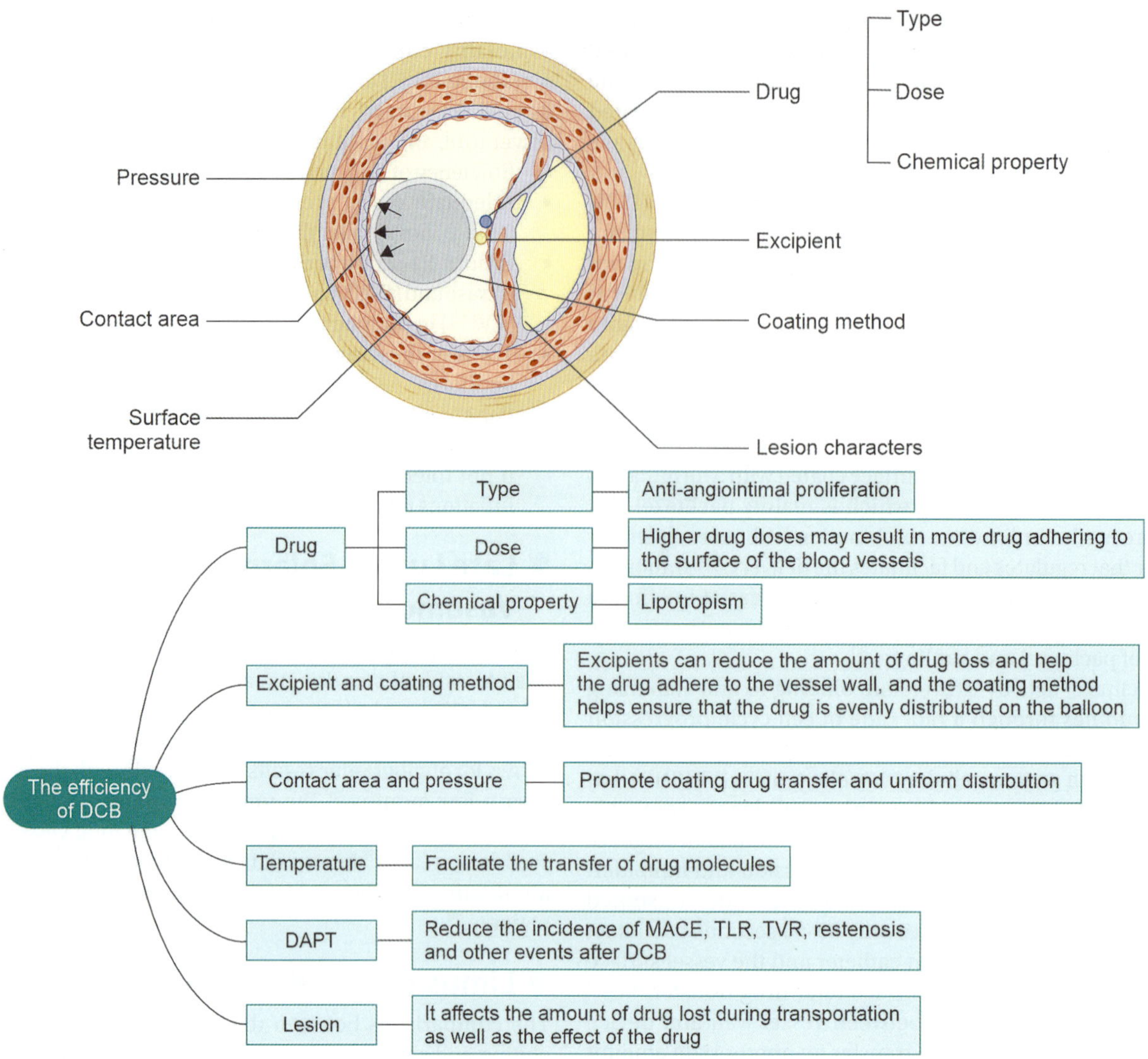

FIG. 2: Drug-coated balloon (DCB) structure and factors effecting efficiency of DCB.
(DAPT: dual antiplatelet therapy; MACE: major adverse cardiac event; TLR: target lesion revascularization; TVR: target vessel revascularization)

and shorter tissue retention of limus drugs compared with paclitaxel, early preclinical attempts to deliver sirolimus and its analogs with the technology used for paclitaxel-coated balloon were unsuccessful.[7,8] In modified crystal structure, a crystalline coating with 4-μg sirolimus/mm^2 balloon surface allowed for a high drug delivery and simultaneously, sufficient tissue persistence of up to 50% after 4 weeks.[2]

A trial of 70 patients with coronary de novo lesions showed that sirolimus-coated balloon was noninferior to paclitaxel-coated balloon (0.10 ± 0.32 mm vs 0.01 ± 0.33 mm) with regard to in-segment LLL. The in-segment late lumen enlargement was more frequent with paclitaxel-coated balloon compared to sirolimus-coated balloon.[6]

A sirolimus-coated balloon based on microreservoirs that consist of a biodegradable polymer poly(lactic-co-glycolic acid) and sirolimus coated with a phospholipid blend (amphipathic membrane) is being tested currently in a randomized clinical trial (RCT) (SELUTION DeNovo, NCT04859985) of 3,326 comparing this sirolimus-coated balloon with contemporary DES for the treatment of de novo coronary artery disease.

De Novo Coronary Artery Disease (Fig. 5)

Following the concept of DCB-alone strategy, treatment of de novo lesions accepts an inferior angiographic acute gain compared with that of stenting with a subsequent compensation of this advantage primarily by reduced LLL and sometimes, positive remodeling at follow-up.[10,29-34]

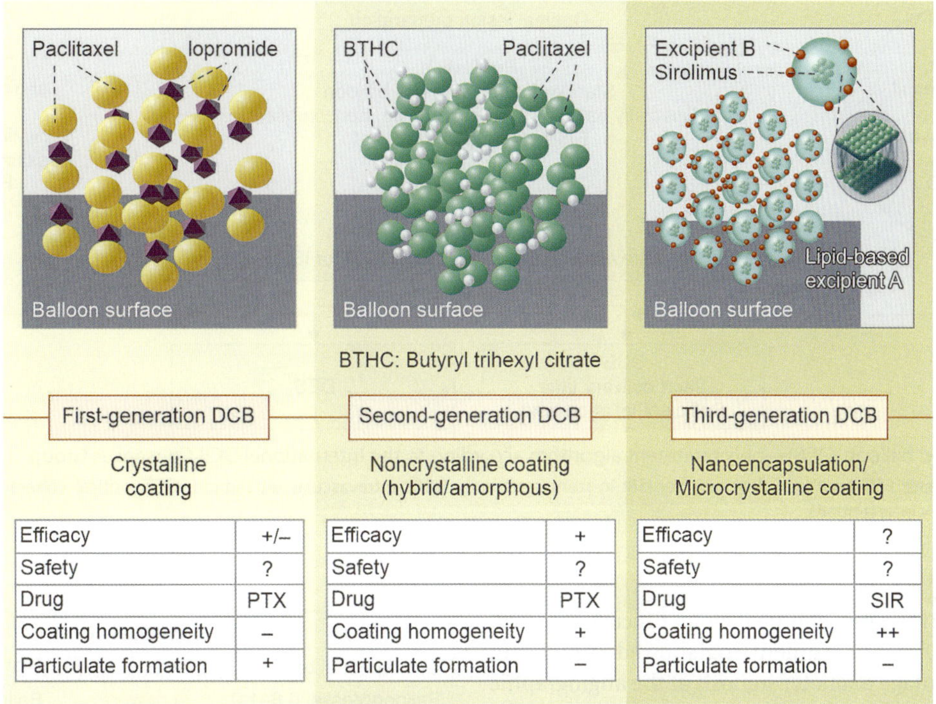

FIG. 3: Comparison between different generations of drug-coated balloon (DCB). The first and second generation of DCB employed paclitaxel (PTX) as the antiproliferative drug and the crystallinity of the coating played a role in the extent of particulate generation. The third generation is moving toward the use of sirolimus (SIR), which is less cytotoxic.

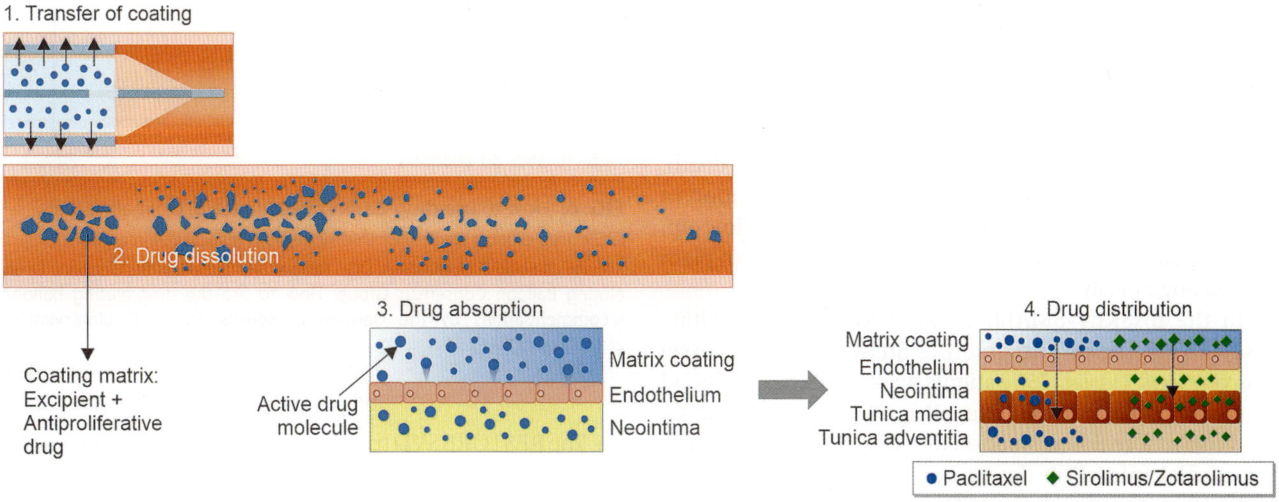

FIG. 4: The concept of drug release from drug-coated balloon (DCB); the transfer of balloon coating occurs by physical contact with the vessel wall, followed by eluting of drug from the coating and subsequent absorption into the tissue. Paclitaxel is expected to be predominantly transferred to the tunica adventitia while the limus-analogs, such as sirolimus, have been found to be equally distributed in the tunica media and adventitia layer.

Small Vessel

Due to reduced restenosis and target lesion thrombosis, DCB angioplasty for SVD is an attractive treatment option as it avoids the implantation of a permanent metallic layer. Several clinical studies on DCBs were conducted with the objective to address these hypotheses **(Table 1)**, and the definitions used to identify small vessels generally included coronary segments with reference diameter 2.75, <2.80, or 3.00 mm, depending on the study **(Fig. 6 and Table 1)**.[35-40]

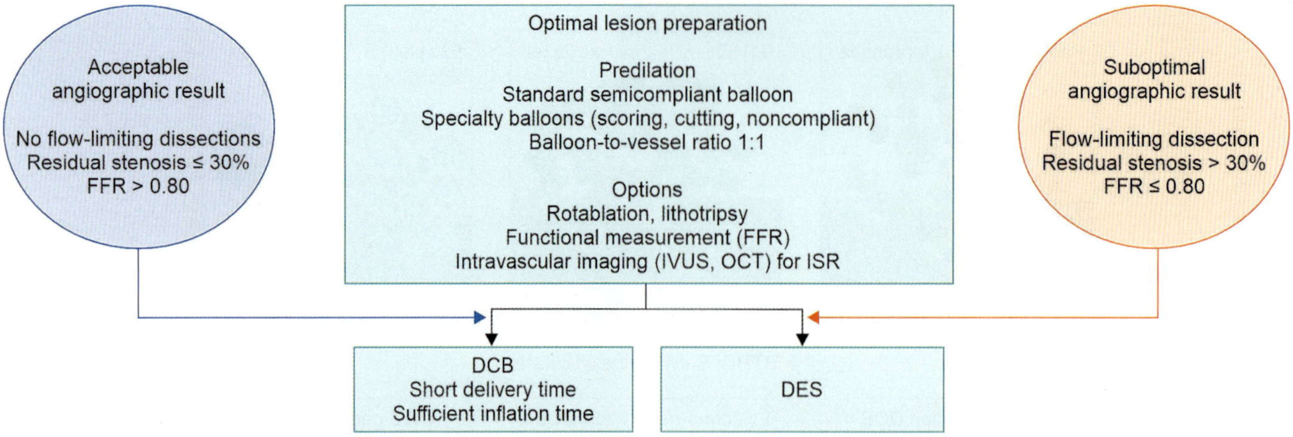

FIG. 5: Drug-coated balloon (DCB)—only treatment algorithm according to the International DCB Consensus Group.
(DES: drug-eluting stent; FFR: fractional flow reserve; ISR: in-stent restenosis; IVUS: intravascular ultrasound; OCT: optical coherence tomography; PCI: percutaneous coronary intervention)

The PICCOLETO (Drug Eluting Balloon Efficacy for Small Coronary Vessel Disease Treatment) trial showed a significant increase in percentage diameter stenosis at the angiographic follow-up with DCB.[36] Due to these unfavorable results, the trial was terminated.[36]

In the BELLO (Balloon Elution and Late Loss Optimization) trial, 182 patients with SVD randomly were assigned to DCB angioplasty or paclitaxel-eluting stent implantation. It demonstrated that at the 6-month angiographic follow-up, DCB results were not only noninferior but also superior to DES in the primary end point of LLL.[38] At 12 months no safety concerns related to DCB technology were observed, and the subsequent 24- and 36-month analyses showed significantly lower cumulative incidence of all-cause death, myocardial infarction, or target vessel revascularization in the DCB group.[41] In the 6-month angiographic follow-up, DCB angioplasty was associated with a lower LLL than plain balloon angioplasty.[16]

In the BASKET-SMALL 2 (Basel Kosten Effektivitäts Trial—DCBs versus Drug-eluting Stents in Small Vessel Interventions 2) trial, 758 patients were randomly assigned to DCB angioplasty or DES after adequate lesion preparation resulting in a residual stenosis of <30%, a thrombolysis in myocardial infarction flow grade 3. At 12 months, DCB angioplasty was noninferior to DES implantation in the per-protocol cohort.[42] The results of the intention-to-treat analysis were consistent.[37] The incidence of the individual end points of cardiac death , nonfatal myocardial infarction, and target vessel revascularization did not significantly differ between DCB angioplasty and DES implantation.[37] The results were consistent in subgroup analyses of diabetes mellitus,[43] acute coronary syndrome,[44] renal failure,[45] and high bleeding risk (HBR) with a concomitant trend toward lower bleeding risk[46] and significantly fewer vascular occlusions after DCB.[47]

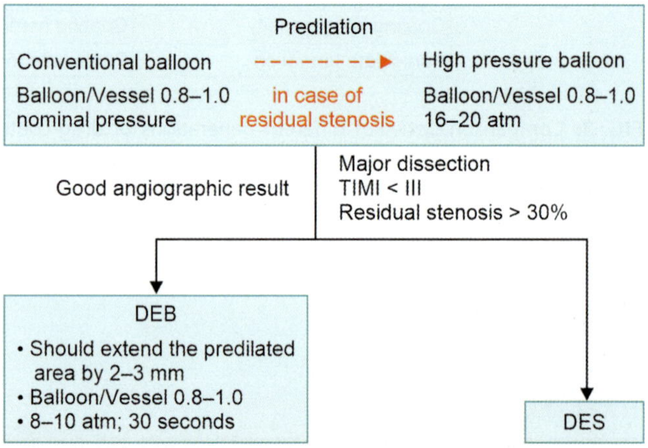

FIG. 6: How to use drug-eluting balloon (DEB) in small vessels.
(DES: drug-eluting stent; TIMI: thrombolysis in myocardial infarction)
Source: Kleber FX, Mathey DG, Rittger H, Scheller B; German Drug-eluting Balloon Consensus Group. How to use the drug-eluting balloon: recommendations by the German consensus group. EuroIntervention. 2011;7 Suppl K:K125-8.

The RESTORE SVD trial, including 230 patients presenting with de novo disease of small vessels randomized to paclitaxel-coated balloons or second-generation zotarolimus-eluting stents, showed at the 9-month angiographic follow-up that DCB angioplasty was noninferior to DES implantation regarding the primary end point of in-segment percentage diameter stenosis.[39] Results were unchanged at per-lesion and as-treated analyses.[39] However, the DCB group exhibited a smaller in-segment minimum lumen diameter and similar LLL than the DES group.[39] At 12 and 24 months, there were no differences between DCB and DES in cardiac death, target vessel myocardial infarction, or target lesion

TABLE 1: Main randomized clinical trials comparing drug-coated balloon (DCB) with drug-eluting stent (DES) for the treatment of small-vessel disease.

	PICCOLETO		BELLO		BASKET-SMALL 2		RESTORE SVD		PICCOLETO II	
Vessel size	≤2.75		<2.80		2.00–3.00		2.25–2.75		≤2.75	
Sample size	57		182		758		230		232	
DCB	Paclitaxel microcrystals on nanoporous surface		Urea–paclitaxel		Iopromide–paclitaxel		Shellac–paclitaxel		Dextran–paclitaxel	
DES	Paclitaxel-eluting durable-polymer stainless steel (97 μm)		Paclitaxel-eluting durable-polymer stainless steel (97 μm)		Paclitaxel-eluting durable-polymer platinum–chromium (81 μm) and zotarolimus-eluting durable-polymer cobalt–chromium (91 μm)		Zotarolimus-eluting durable-polymer cobalt–chromium (91 μm)		Everolimus-eluting durable-polymer cobalt–chromium (81 μm)	
Primary end point	In-lesion % diameter stenosis		In-lesion late lumen loss		Cardiac death, nonfatal myocardial infarction, or target vessel revascularization		In-segment % diameter stenosis		In-lesion late lumen loss	
Primary follow-up (months)	6		6		12		9		6	
Angiographic follow-up	Yes		Yes		No		Yes		Yes	
Maximum follow-up	9		36		36		24		12	
Design	Noninferiority		Noninferiority		Noninferiority		Noninferiority		Noninferiority	
Period	August 2007 to August 2008		Before July 2012		April 2012 to February 2017		August 2016 to June 2017		May 2015 to May 2018	
Region	Italy		Italy		Switzerland, Germany, and Austria		China		Italy and Spain	
Centers	1		15		14		12		5	
Registration*	EudraCT 2009-012268-15		NCT01086579		NCT01574534		NCT02946307		NCT03899818	
	DCB	DES	DCB	DES	DCB	DES	DCB	DES	DCB	DES
Patients/lesions[†]	28/28	29/29	90/81	92/82	382	376	116/100	114/93	118/105	114/104
In-segment % diameter stenosis	43.6 ± 27.4[‡]	24.3 ± 25.1[‡]	35.0 ± 16.0	33.3 ± 20.0	–	–	29.3 ± 20.2	23.9 ± 15.9	36.6 ± 21	32.2 ± 19
In-segment late lumen loss	NA	NA	0.05 ± 0.37	0.17 ± 0.45	–	–	0.25 ± 0.42	0.27 ± 0.36	0.01 ± 0.25[‡]	0.14 ± 0.38[‡]
In-segment binary restenosis	9(32.1)[‡]	3(10.3)[‡]	8(10.0)	12(14.6)	–	–	11(11.0)	8(8.6)	11(10.5)	10(9.6)

Continued

Continued

	PICCOLETO		BELLO		BASKET-SMALL 2		RESTORE SVD		PICCOLETO II	
Target lesion revascularization	9(32.1)	3(10.3)	6M: 4(4.4)	6M: 7(7.6)	NA	NA	12M: 5(4.4)	12: 3(2.6)	6(5.6)	6(5.6)
			36M: 6(6.7)	36M: 12(13.0)			24M 6(5.2)	36: 3(2.8)		
Target lesion thrombosis	0	0	6M: 0	6M: 0	12M: 2(1)	12M: 4(1)	12M: 0	12M: 0	0	2(1.9)
			36M: 0	36M: 0	36M: 2(1)	36M: 6(2)	24M: 0	36M: 0		
MACE§	10(35.7)	4(13.8)	6M: 9(10.0)	6M: 15(16.3)	12M: 28(8)	12M: 28(7)	12M: 11(9.6)	12M: 11(9.6)	6(5.6)	8(7.5)
			36M: 13(14.4)‡	36M: 28(30.4)‡	36M: 53(15)	36M: 53(15)	36M: 14 (12.2)	36M: 14(12.2)		
Dual antiplatelet therapy	• Stable angina: 1 month (3 months for bailout stenting) • Unstable angina: 12 months	12 months	1 month (3 month for bailout stenting)	12 months	• Stable angina: 1 month (3 months for bailout stenting with BMS and 6 months for bailout stenting with DES) • Acute coronary syndrome: 12 months	• Stable angina 6 months • Acute coronary syndrome 12 months	≥6 months	≥6 months	• Stable angina: 1 month • Acute coronary syndrome 12 months	• Stable angina: 6 months • Acute coronary syndrome 12 months
Main conclusions	DCB angioplasty showed a lower antirestenotic efficacy than DES implantation		DCB angioplasty was associated with improved angiographic and clinical results compared with DES implantations		DCB angioplasty was associated with similar clinical effectiveness and safety compared with DES implantation		DCB angioplasty was associated with noninferior angiographic effectiveness compared with DES implantation		DCB angioplasty is associated with a lower late lumen loss than DES implantation	

Note: Late lumen loss and percentage diameter stenosis are means and standard deviations. Binary restenosis and clinical outcomes are counts and rates.

*Registration in ClinicalTrials.gov except for the PICCOLETO trial that was registered with the European Union Drug Regulating Authorities Clinical Trials Database registry

†Patients analyzed at the clinical follow-up/lesions analyzed at the angiographic follow-up.

‡Significant differences.

§PICCOLETO: all-cause death, new ST-segment elevation myocardial infarction, or target lesion revascularization; BELLO: all-cause death, myocardial infarction, or target vessel revascularization; BASKET-SMALL 2: cardiac death, nonfatal myocardial infarction, or target vessel revascularization; RESTORE SVD: all-cause death, myocardial infarction, or repeat revascularization; PICCOLETO II: cardiac death, myocardial infarction, or target lesion revascularization.

(BMS: bare metal stent; EudraCT: European Union Drug Regulating Authorities Clinical Trials Database; MACE: major adverse cardiac events; NA: not available)

revascularization (TLR) and in each individual component of the composite end point.

Latest trial on the topic, namely the PICCOLETO II trial, showed that at a median angiographic follow-up of 189 days, a paclitaxel-coated balloon was noninferior and superior to a second-generation everolimus-eluting stent (EES) in the primary end point of in-lesion LLL.[35]

Bifurcation

Treatment of bifurcation lesions remains fraught with suboptimal results, particularly at the level of the side branch, which set the main rationale of studies investigating DCB in this setting **(Fig. 7)**.

The DEBIUT (Drug-Eluting Balloon in Bifurcations Trial) 117 patients were 1:1:1 randomly assigned to DCB angioplasty of both branches, followed by bare metal stent (BMS) implantation in the main vessel, and plain balloon angioplasty of the side branch, or paclitaxel-DES implantation in the main vessel and plain balloon angioplasty of the side branch.[48] Kissing balloon after provisional stenting was recommended regardless of the strategy assigned.[48] At the 6-month angiographic follow-up, the strategy based on DCB failed to show significant differences compared with the BMS-based strategy and resulted to be less effective than the DES-based strategy.[48]

In the BABILON (Paclitaxel-Coated Balloon in Bifurcated Lesions) trial, 108 patients were randomized to sequential predilation and DCB angioplasty of both branches, followed by provisional BMS implantation of main branch or sequential predilation of both branches, then by provisional EES implantation of the main branch.[49] The DCB plus BMS strategy was associated with a 9-month in-segment LLL noninferior to the DES-alone strategy.[49] Of note, the side-branch LLL was not significantly different between DCB and DES.

In a registry encompassing 127 patients, ~54% of all bifurcations could be treated by DCB-alone strategy with low event rates at 9 months and no thrombosis.[50]

In-stent Restenosis

In-stent restenosis is traditionally defined as a reduction in the luminal diameter of >50% within a previously stented segment or the 5-mm segments proximal and distal to the stent (stent edges). Despite substantial medical and technological advances, approximately 5–10% of contemporary percutaneous coronary interventions (PCIs) are performed for ISR **(Fig. 8)**.

Bare Metal Stent Restenosis

In PACCOCATH-ISR [Treatment of In-Stent Restenosis by Paclitaxel Coated Percutaneous Transluminal Coronary Angioplasty (PTCA) Balloons] trial, 52 patients with BMS-ISR were randomly assigned to angioplasty with either plain balloon or DCB. The primary angiographic end point of 6-month in-segment LLL was significantly lower in the DCB group.[51] The rates of 6-month binary restenosis and 12-month major adverse cardiac events (MACEs) were consistently lower in the DCB arm.[51]

PEPCAD II (Paclitaxel-Eluting PTCA-Balloon Catheter in Coronary Artery Disease II) trial showed that in 131 patients with BMS-ISR, DCB was associated with a significant

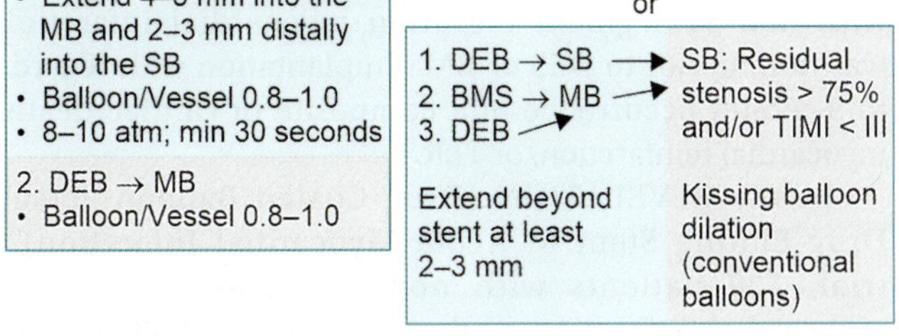

FIG. 7: How to use drug-eluting balloon (DEB) in bifurcation lesions.
(BMS: bare metal stents; MB: main branch; SB: side branch; TIMI: thrombolysis in myocardial infarction)
Source: Kleber FX, Mathey DG, Rittger H, Scheller B; German Drug-eluting Balloon Consensus Group. How to use the drug-eluting balloon: recommendations by the German consensus group. EuroIntervention. 2011;7 Suppl K:K125-8.

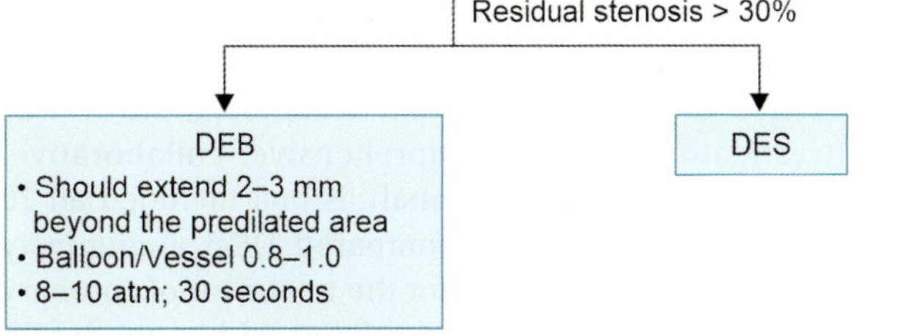

FIG. 8: How to use drug-eluting balloon (DEB) in in-stent restenosis (ISR).
(DES: drug-eluting stent; TIMI: thrombolysis in myocardial infarction)
Source: Kleber FX, Mathey DG, Rittger H, Scheller B; German Drug-eluting Balloon Consensus Group. How to use the drug-eluting balloon: recommendations by the German consensus group. EuroIntervention. 2011;7 Suppl K:K125-8.

reduction in the primary end point of 6-month LLL compared with first-generation paclitaxel-eluting stents.[52] No significant differences in the 6-month minimal lumen diameter and percentage diameter stenosis and the 12-month TLR were observed between DCBs and paclitaxel-eluting stents.[52] Of note, at the 3-year follow-up, there was no additional TLR.[53]

The TIS (Treatment of In-Stent Restenosis) trial provided consistent results by comparing paclitaxel-coated balloon versus second-generation EES in 136 patients with BMS-ISR. At 12-month angiography, patients treated by DCB showed a lower in-segment LLL and numerically lower binary restenosis.[54] At the 3-year follow-up, results were unchanged, and no safety concerns emerged in the DCB and DES groups with comparable rates of MACEs.[55]

Drug-eluting Stent Restenosis

The PEPCAD-DES (Treatment of DES-ISR With SeQuent Please Paclitaxel Eluting PTCA Catheter) trial comprising 110 patients confirmed that with respect to both LLL and TLR with any-type DES-ISR, DCB angioplasty is significantly more effective than plain balloon angioplasty, without late no catchup at the 3-year follow-up.[56,57]

The ISAR-DESIRE 3 (Randomised Trial of Paclitaxel-Eluting Balloon, Paclitaxel-Eluting Stent and Plain Balloon Angioplasty for Restenosis in "Limus"-Eluting Coronary Stents) trial assessed the comparison of plain balloon versus paclitaxel-coated balloon versus paclitaxel-eluting stent, in patients with limus-DES-ISR, concluding that DCB was noninferior to DES regarding in-segment percentage diameter stenosis, and both these devices were superior to plain balloon angioplasty,[42] but there was no significant difference was observed between the DCB and DES groups. At the 10-year follow-up, when compared with DCB numerical excess in cardiac death associated with DES was observed.[58]

In the RIBS IV (Restenosis Intra-stent of Drug-eluting Stents: Paclitaxel-eluting Balloon vs. Everolimus-eluting Stent IV) trial, when compared with EES, DCB was associated with inferior in-segment minimal lumen diameter and percentage diameter stenosis[59] due to increased incidence of TLR with DCB at 1 and 3 years' follow-up **(Table 2)**.

The DAEDALUS (Difference in Antirestenotic Effectiveness of Drug-eluting stent and DCB AngiopLasty for the occurrence of coronary in-Stent restenosis) study was an investigator-initiated comprehensive, collaborative, individual patient data meta-analysis that included all 10 available RCTs. This study compared DCB angioplasty with repeat stenting with DES for the treatment of coronary ISR.[60,61] Of note, DCB was associated with a moderate increase in the risk of TLR compared with DES at 3 years **(Fig. 9)**.[60]

Specific extensive patient-level analysis on ISR type supported very similar efficacy and safety of DCB and DES in the management of BMS-ISR.[61] Hence DCB may be the preferred treatment strategy for BMS-ISR, in light of these results. In contrast, repeat DES implantation was moderately more effective than DCB angioplasty in the treatment of DES-ISR.[61] This result, however, occurred at the cost of a numerical excess in the composite end point of all-cause death, target lesion thrombosis, or myocardial infarction with known limitations in the statistical power of subgroup analyses.[61] Differences in the individual susceptibility to antiproliferative drug-mediated suppression of neointimal growth and neoatherosclerosis may be partially responsible for the different efficacy of DCB between DES-ISR and BMS-ISR. A proportion of DES-ISR lesions may be due to the failure of the antiproliferative drug eluted post implantation, whereas BMS-ISR lesions may be still susceptible to the effects.

ACUTE CORONARY SYNDROME

In this setting, the rationale for a DCB-based strategy relies on the possible observation of nonsignificantly obstructive ulcerated lesions, which cause an acute coronary syndrome and often selecting stents with an inappropriate size owing to acute-phase dynamic vessel wall changes, mostly vasoconstriction and plaque remodeling.

The use of DCBs should be discouraged in significant thrombus burden due to the potential risk of abrupt vessel closure as there is absence of entrapment of thrombus by stenting. Owing to the limitations of drug delivery when thrombus is interposed between device and vessel wall, there may possibly be a lower antirestenotic effect of DCBs.

The DEB-AMI (Drug-Eluting Balloon in Acute ST-Segment Elevation Myocardial Infarction) was a three-arm trial which compared BMS implantation, DCB followed by BMS implantation, and DES implantation in 150 patients who presented with ST-segment elevation acute myocardial infarction.[62] In DEB-AMI trial, DCB followed by BMS implantation failed to show angiographic superiority to the DES and BMS-only groups.[62]

The PEPCAD NSTEMI (Bare Metal or Drug-Eluting Stent versus Drug Coated Balloon with Provisional Stenting in Non-ST-Elevation Myocardial Infarction) trial done in 210 patients showed that a DCB-only strategy presenting with non-ST-segment elevation myocardial infarction was noninferior to DES or BMS implantation with regards to 9-month occurrence of a composite of cardiac death, myocardial reinfarction, or TLR.[63]

In the REVELATION (Drug-Coated Balloon versus Drug-Eluting Stent in Acute Myocardial Infarction)[64] trial, 120 patients with non-ST-segment elevation myocardial infarction undergoing primary PCIs were randomly assigned DCB or DES with the objective of assessing the infarct-related lesion by a fractional flow reserve at 9 months.[64] No significant differences were observed in the fractional flow reserve at the follow-up, between DCB and DES.

TABLES 2: Main randomized clinical trials comparing drug-coated balloon (DCB) with drug-eluting stent (DES) for the treatment of in-stent restenosis (ISR).

	PEPCAD II		SAR-DESIRE 3*		PEPCAD China ISR		RIBS V		SEDUCE	
ISR type	BMS		DES		DES		BMS		BMS	
Sample size	131		268*		215†		189		50	
DCB	Iopromide–paclitaxel		Iopromide–paclitaxel		Iopromide–paclitaxel		Iopromide–paclitaxel		Iopromide–paclitaxel	
DES	Paclitaxel-eluting durable-polymer stainless steel (97 µm)		Paclitaxel-eluting durable-polymer stainless steel (97 µm)		Paclitaxel-eluting durable-polymer		Everolimus-eluting durable-polymer cobalt–chromium (81 µm)		Everolimus-eluting durable-polymer cobalt–chromium (81 µm)	
Primary end point	In-segment late lumen loss		In-segment % diameter stenosis		In-segment late lumen loss		In-segment minimum lumen diameter		% Uncovered struts‡	
Primary follow-up (months)	6		6–8		9		6–9		9	
Angiographic follow-up	Yes		Yes		Yes		Yes		Yes	
Maximum follow-up (months)	36		36		24		36		12	
Design	Nonequality		Noninferiority		Noninferiority		Nonequality		Nonequality	
Period	January 2006 to December 2006		August 2009 to October 2011		March 2011 to April 2012		January 2010 to January 2012		June 2009 to October 2011	
Region	Germany		Germany		China		Spain		Belgium	
Centers	10		4		17		25		2	
Registration§	NCT00393315		NCT00987324		NCT01622075		NCT01239953		NCT01065532	
	DCB	DES	DCB*	DES*	DCB	DES	DCB	DES	DCB	DES
Patients/lesions†	66/57	65/59	137/147	131/142	109/93	106/82	95/84	94/86	25/22	25/22
In-segment % diameter stenosis	29.4 ± 17.5	34.2 ± 24.3	38.0 ± 21.5	37.4 ± 21.8	29.0 ± 21.3	30.8 ± 25.3	24 ± 20‖	13 ± 17‖	31.8 ± 14.9	26.6 ± 14.6
In-segment late lumen loss	0.17 ± 10.42	0.38 ± 10.61	0.37 ± 0.59	0.34 ± 0.61	0.46 ± 0.51	0.55 ± 0.61	0.14 ± 0.5	0.04 ± 0.5	0.16 ± 0.49	0.08 ± 0.40
In-segment binary restenosis	4(7.0)	12(20.3)‖	39(26.5)	34(23.9)	18(18.6)	20(23.8)	8(9.5)	4(4.7)	2(9.1)	1(4.6)
Target lesion revascularization	12M: 4(6.3)	12M: 10(15.4)	12M: 30(22.1)	12M: 17(13.5)	12M: 17(15.6)	12M: 13(12.3)	12M: 6(6)	12M: 2(2)	1(4.2)	2(8.0)
	36M: 4(6.3)	36M: 10(15.4)	36M: 44(33.3)	36M: 29(24.2)	36M: 17(15.9)	36M: 14(13.7)	36M: 8(8)‖	36M: 2(2)‖		
Target lesion thrombosis	12M: 0	12M: 0	12M: 1(0.7)	12M: 1(0.8)	12M 1(0.9)	12M: 1(0.9)	12M: 1(1)	12M: 0	0	1(4.0)
	36M: 0	36M: 0	36M: 1(0.8)	36M: 2(1.6)	36M: 1(0.9)	36M: 3(2.9)	36M: 1(1)	36M: 0		

Continued

Continued

	PEPCAD II		SAR-DESIRE 3*		PEPCAD China ISR		RIBS V		SEDUCE	
MACE[¶]	12M: 6(9.1)	12M: 14(21.5)	12M: 32(23.5)	12M: 25(19.3)	12M: 26(23.9)	12M: 25(23.6)	12M: 11(12)	12M : 6(6)	NA	MA
	36M: 23(34.8)	36M: 27(41.5)	36M: 51(38.0)	36M: 48(37.7)	36M: 27(25.2)	36M: 31(30.4)	36M: 15(16)	36M: 10(11)		
Dual antiplatelet therapy (months)	6	12	>6	≥6	≥6	≥6	3	12	NA	MA
Main conclusion	DCB angioplasty reduced late lumen loss and binary restenosis compared with DES implantation		DCB was associated with noninferior effectiveness compared with DES implantation. At a long-term follow-up, DCB was associated with a trend toward an increased incidence of target lesion revascularization and a reduced mortality compared with DES		DCB angioplasty was associated with noninferior angiographic effectiveness compared with DES implantation. At a long-term follow-up, DCB was associated with a lower mortality than DES		DES was associated with superior angiographic effectiveness and superior long-term incidence of target lesion revascularization compared with DCB		DCB was associated with a lower percentage of uncovered struts at optical coherence tomography follow-up than DES implantation. However, in-stent percentage diameter stenosis at angiographic follow-up was higher after DCB angioplasty than that after DES implantation	
	RIBS IV		**TIS**		**DARE**		**RESTORE**		**BIOLUX-RCT**	
ISR type	DES		BMS		BMS: 120(45.8) DES:142(54.2)		DES		BMS: 86(35.7) DES: 155(64.3)	
Sample size	309		136		278		172		229	
DCB	Iopromide–paclitaxel (3 μg/mm²)		Iopromide–paclitaxel (3 μg/mm²)		Iopromide–paclitaxel (3 μg/mm²)		Iopromide–paclitaxel (3 μg/mm²)		Butyryl trihexyl citrate–paclitaxel (3 μg/mm²)	
DES	Everolimus-eluting durable-polymer cobalt–chromium (81 μm)		Everolimus-eluting durable-polymer cobalt–chromium (81 μm)		Everolimus-eluting durable-polymer cobalt–chromium (81 μm)		Everolimus-eluting durable-polymer cobalt–chromium (81 μm)		Sirolimus-eluting bioresorbable polymer cobalt–chromium (60–80 μm)	
Primary end point	In-segment late lumen loss		In-segment late lumen loss		In-segment minimum lumen diameter		In-segment late lumen loss		In-segment late lumen loss	
Primary follow-up (months)	6–9		12		6		9		6	
Angiographic	Yes		Yes		Yes		Yes		Yes	
Maximum follow-up (months)	36		36		12		12		18	
Design	Nonequality		Noninferiority		Noninferiority		Nonequality		Noninferiority	
Period	January 2010 to August 2013		January 2012 to August 2014		May 2010 to June 2015		April 2013 to October 2016		August 2012 to January 2015	

Continued

Continued

	RIBS IV		TIS		DARE		RESTORE		BIOCUX-RCT	
Region	Spain		Czech Republic		The Netherlands		South Korea		Germany and Latvia	
Centers	23		1		8		10		14	
Registration§	NCT01239940		NCT01735825		NTR2189		NCT01967199		NCT01651390	
	DCB	DES	DCB	DES	DCB	DES	DCB	DES	DCB	DES
Patients/Lesion†	154/139	155/133	68/74	68/74	137/105	141/115	86/38	86/36	157/128	72/59
In-segment % diameter stenosis	30 ± 22‖	23 ± 22‖	26.2 ± 18.0	30.9 ± 24.6	36.1 ± 15.5	33.8 ± 18.6	34 ± 21‖	26 ± 15‖	31.6 ± 12.8	32.0 ± 23.8
In-segment late lumen loss	0.30 ± 0.6‖	0.18 ± 0.6‖	0.09 ± 0.44	0.44 ± 0.73	0.17 ± 0.41	0.45 ± 0.47	0.15 ± 0.49	0.19 ± 0.41	−0.03 ± 0.38	0.13 ± 0.67
In-segment binary restenosis	27(19)	15(11)	6(8.7)	13(19.1)	19(18.1)	24(20.9)	8(19.5)	2(5.6)	NA	NA
Target lesion revascularization	12M: 20(13.0)‖	12M: 7(4.5)‖	12M: 5(7.4)	12M: 11(16.2)	12M: 11(8.1)	12M:7 (5.0)	12M: 5(5.8)	12M: 1(1.2)	12M: 18(12.5)	12M: 7(10.1)
	36M: 24(15.6)‖	36M: 11(7.1)‖	36M: 8(12.9)	36M: 14(22.2)					18M: 19(13.5)	18M: 8(11.6)
Target lesion thrombosis	12M: 3(1.9)	12M: 2(1.3)	12M: 1(1.5)	12M: 0	12M: 0	12M: 0	12M: 0	12M: 0	12M: 1(0.7)	12M: 2(2.9)
	36M: 4(2.6)	36M: 2(1.3)	36M: 2(2.9)	36M: 0					18M: 1(0.7)	36M: 2(2.9)
MACE¶	12M: 24(16.0)‖	12M: 10(7.0)‖	12M: 7(10.3)	12M: 13(19.1)	12M: 15(10.9)	12M: 13(9.2)	12M: 6(7.0)	12M: 4(4–7)	12M: 25(16.9)	12M: 10 (14.3)
	36M: 38(24.7)	36M: 24(15.5)‖	36M: 13(19.1)	36M: 20(29.4)					18M: 26(17.9)	18M: 13(18.6)
Dual antiplatelet therapy (months)	3	12	≥6	≥6	12	12	≥6	≥6	NA	NA
Main conclusion	DES was angiographically and clinically more effective than DCB angioplasty		DCB was associated with noninferior angiographic effectiveness compared with DES implantation		DCB angioplasty was associated with noninferior angiographic effectiveness compared with DES implantation		DES was associated with superior angiographic effectiveness compared with DCB		DCB was associated with noninferior angiographic effectiveness compared with DES implantation	

Note: Late lumen loss and percentage diameter stenosis are means and standard deviations. Binary restenosis and clinical outcomes are counts and rates.

*Only DCB and DES arms are reported. The ISAR-DESIRE 3 was a three-arm trial also including 134 patients randomly assigned to plain balloon angioplasty.

†Patients analyzed at the clinical follow-up/lesions analyzed at the angiographic follow-up.

‡As assessed by optical coherence tomography.

§Registration in ClinicalTrials.gov except for the DARE trial that was registered with the Netherland trials registry.

‖Significant differences.

¶RIBS IV: all-cause death, myocardial infarction, or target lesion revascularization; ISAR-DESIRE 3: all-cause death, myocardial infarction, or target lesion revascularization; PEPCAD China ISR: all-cause death, myocardial infarction, or any revascularization; RIBS V; all-cause death, myocardial infarction, or target vessel revascularization; SEDUCE; cardiac death, myocardial infarction, or target lesion revascularization, RIBS V: all-cause death, myocardial infarction, or target lesion revascularization; TIS: cardiovascular death, myocardial infarction, or target vessel revascularization; DARE: all-cause death, target vessel-related myocardial infarction, or target vessel revascularization; RESTORE; all-cause death, myocardial infarction, or target lesion revascularization; BIOLUX-RCT: cardiac death, myocardial infarction, or target lesion revascularization.

(BMS: bare metal stent; MACE: major adverse cardiac events; NA: not available)

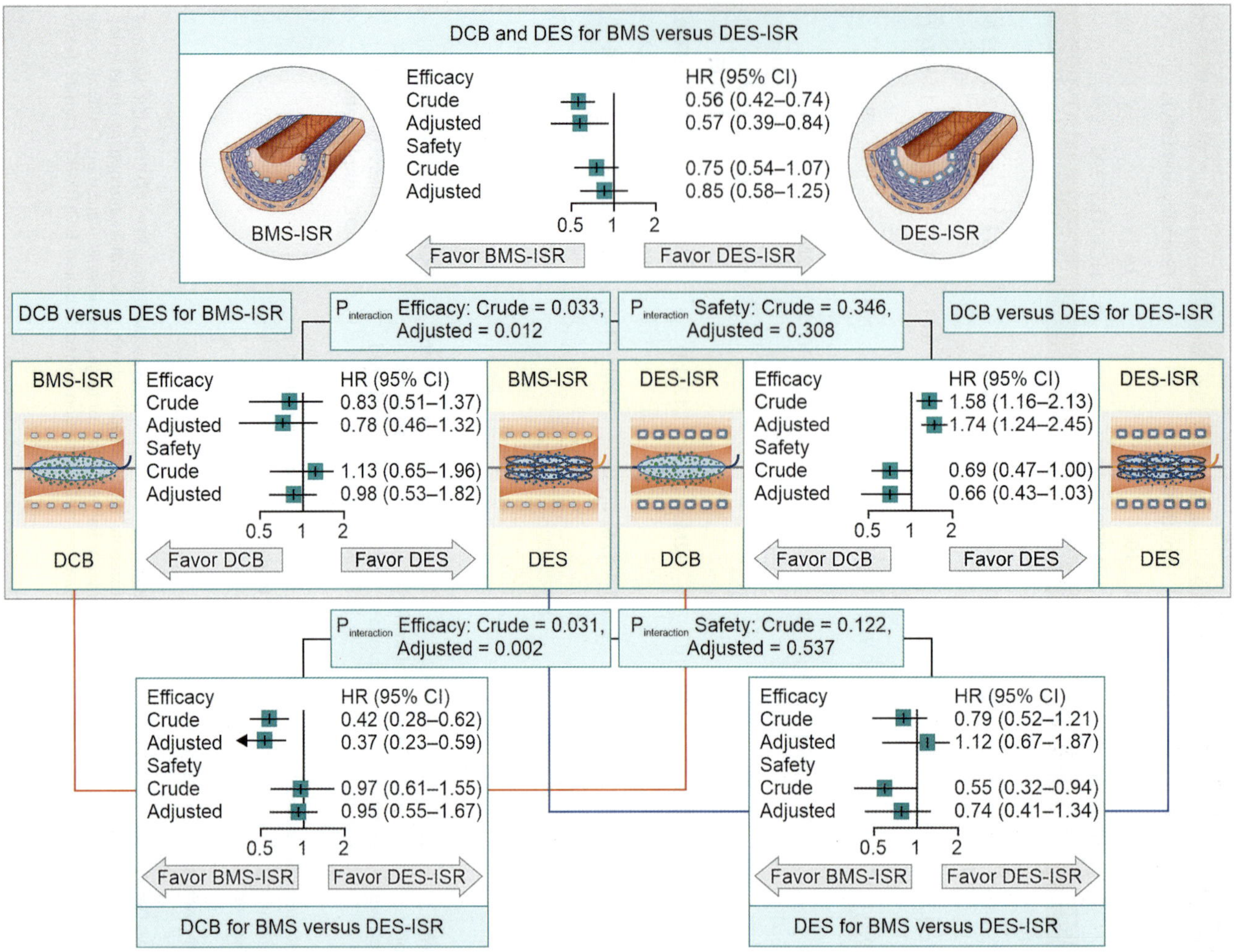

FIG. 9: Primary efficacy and safety endpoint risk of the DAEDALUS patient-level meta-analysis in clinical trials comparing drug-coated balloon (DCB) and drug-eluting stent (DES) in in-stent restenosis (ISR).

(BMS: bare metal stent; CI: confidence interval; DAEDALUS: Difference in Antirestenotic Effectiveness of Drug-eluting stent and DCB AngiopLasty for the occurrence of coronary in-Stent restenosis; HR: hazard ratio)

HIGH BLEEDING RISK

Several DES trials investigated HBR patients with 1 month of dual antiplatelet therapy (DAPT) in patients.[65-67] The DEBUT trial compared DCB treatment for de novo lesions with BMS implantation in an HBR population. Comparing well with the corresponding event rates for DES in LEADERS FREE,[65] SENIOR,[66] or ONYX ONE,[67] at 9 months, target lesion failure occurred in 14% in the BMS group. But by comparison, in DEBUT the primary end point in the DCB group occurred only in 4% of cases (one patient) after 1 year **(Fig. 10)**.[68]

PERIPHERAL ARTERIES

Superficial Femoral Artery

In the THUNDER trial, 154 patients were treated with conventional percutaneous transluminal angioplasty (PTA), Paccocath DCB, or a third arm with paclitaxel dissolved in the contrast medium. After 6 months, treatment with Paccocath DCB was associated with significant reductions in LLL compared to patients in the uncoated balloon group or patients treated with paclitaxel dissolved in the contrast medium.[69] Importantly, the rate of TLR remained significantly lower in the Paccocath group up to 5 years of follow-up.[63] The FemPac (Femoral Paclitaxel) trial confirmed the superiority of Paccocath DCB over PTA in the superficial femoral artery (SFA).[62]

The Orchid® DCB (Acotec Scientific, Beijing, China) is coated with 3 µg/mm² paclitaxel and magnesium stearate. In the AcoArt trial, relatively long lesions were treated (about 15 cm on average). LLL was 0.05 mm with coated balloons versus 1.15 mm with uncoated balloons ($p < 0.001$). At 1 year, the rates of TLR were 7.2% and 39.6%, respectively ($p < 0.001$).[68]

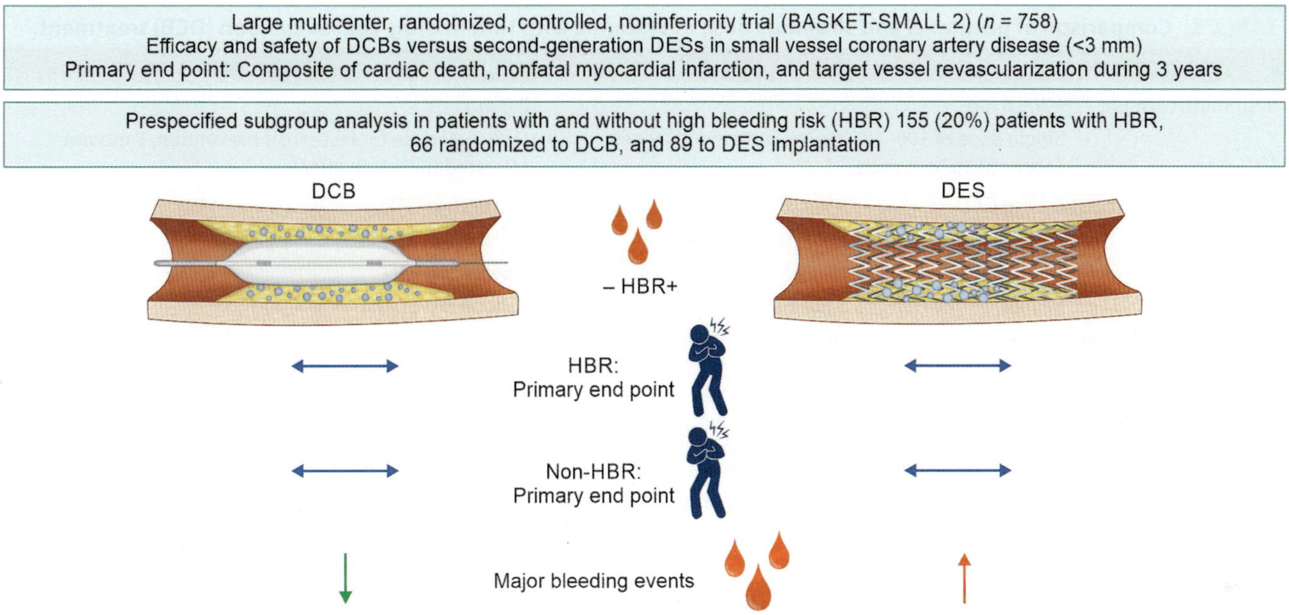

FIG. 10: Drug-coated balloon (DCB) versus drug-eluting stents (DESs) in small coronary artery disease with and without high bleeding risk. (BASKET-SMALL 2: Basel Kosten Effektivitats Trial-DCBs versus Drug-eluting Stents in Small Vessel Interventions 2)

The LEVANT I trial investigated a DCB coated with 2 μg/mm^2 paclitaxel using polysorbate and sorbitol as excipients (Moxy; Lutonix, Maple Grove, MN, USA). LLL at 6 months was significantly reduced (0.46 mm vs. 1.09 mm) by Moxy whereas TLR did not differ significantly between the two treatments (13% vs. 22%).[70]

In the LEVANT II pivotal trial including 476 patients, primary patency at 12 months was 65.2% for the DCB and 52.6% for control angioplasty. Freedom from clinically driven TLR was similar in both groups (38.0% vs. 37.5%).

Clinically established excipient-based paclitaxel coatings cause a dose-dependent suppression of neointimal formation with a maximal effect at about 3–4 μg/mm^2. A recent meta-analysis reported a significant reduction of restenosis [rate ratio (RR) 2.1; 95% confidence interval (CI) 1.2–3.4; $p < 0.001$] and TLR (RR 2.5; 95% CI 1.9–3.8; $p < 0.001$) by DCB with a regular dose of 3.0–3.5 μg/mm^2 compared to low-dose DCB with 2 μg/mm^2.[71]

Femoropopliteal Artery

Due to the high restenosis rates (20–40%) after stenting, endovascular therapy is challenging in femoropopliteal arteries. With respect to treatment effect for TLR due to the LEVANT I and II studies, there was a significant heterogeneity, suggesting a differential efficacy profile associated with the DCB platform used in these trials. The Lutonix DCB (Bard PV, Tempe, AZ, USA), which was considered to have a lower efficacy compared to other DCB, was the DCB investigated in the LEVANT studies.

In comparison to IN.PACT (Medtronic, Minneapolis MN, USA) and Stellarex DCB (Philips, Amsterdam, The Netherlands) after 28 days, the pharmacokinetic profile of Lutonix was found to have a lower paclitaxel tissue bioavailability.

For the treatment of symptomatic femoropopliteal lesions, the COMPARE multicenter RCT (NCT02701543) examined two DCBs and demonstrated that the Ranger DCB (Boston Scientific, Marlborough, MA, USA) was comparable with the IN.PACT DCB.

Below the Knee

Restenosis rates in infratibial artery disease range from 42% at 12 months for short lesions to 69% at 3 months for a lesion length of >18 cm. Initial nonrandomized series and one randomized study indicated favorable outcomes with the IN.PACT Amphirion DCB in this challenging scenario.[72,73]

However, the IN.PACT DEEP trial using the same device could not confirm these findings. Compared to PTA, no biological effect was seen in terms of LLL or TLR. Furthermore, there was a statistical trend in terms of major amputations at 1 year (8.8% vs. 3.6%; $p = 0.08$).[74] Several factors have been discussed as reasons for these findings, such as different protocols for wound care in higher Rutherford classes, device-specific issues such as drug loss on the way to the lesion, or simply (by chance) the best ever reported PTA outcomes in such a patient population.

A 2016 meta-analysis (five trials, 641 patients) reported that in below the knee (BTK) lesions DCB has superior angiographic performance and similar clinical efficacy when compared with balloon angioplasty or DES at 1-year follow-up. The analysis showed that treatment with DCB led to relatively lower LLL, without improvement in clinical

TABLE 3: Comparison of paclitaxel and sirolimus dose in systemic with that in drug-coated balloon (DCB) treatment.

	Paclitaxel	Sirolimus
Systemic treatment	~300.0 mg Single dose of 100–175 mg/m^2 intravenously per cancer treatment cycle	2.0 mg Daily oral dose for restenosis prevention, 5 mg not tolerated (67% side effects)
DCB treatment	0.4 mg CAD Balloon 3.0/20 mm @ 3 μg/mm^2 5.5 mg PAD Balloon 5.0/80 mm @ 3.5 μg/mm^2	0.2–0.6 mg CAD Balloon 3.0/20 mm @ 1–4 μg/mm^2 1.6–6.4 mg PAD Balloon 5.0/80 mm @ 1–4 μg/mm^2

(CAD: coronary artery disease; PAD: peripheral artery disease)

outcomes such as amputation and wound healing. The study concluded that a dedicated wound care management should be implemented for all patients with advanced-stage atherosclerotic BTK disease in order to evaluate the net clinical benefit of different revascularization strategies.

ANTIPROLIFERATIVE DRUG TOXICITY AND LONG-TERM MORTALITY (FLOWCHART 1)

Sirolimus and paclitaxel show a different dose-response relationship for apoptosis and parameters describing cytotoxicity and histopathologic changes. Increased apoptosis and histopathologic changes were observed only at high paclitaxel concentrations, which are found typically near the stent struts in the case of DES. Sirolimus is cytostatic but paclitaxel is cytotoxic.

For the treatment of femoropopliteal disease, paclitaxel concentrations are well below those at which cytotoxic effects are observed. Regardless of the concentration of paclitaxel on the balloon surface, ranging from 2 to 3 μg/mm^2, tissue levels of approximately 50–60 ng/mg occurred in the first hours after application, 5–20 ng/mg after 1 day, 2–10 ng/mg 1 week later, and decreasing further thereafter until disappearance after 30–45 days.

The dose of paclitaxel commonly used for cancer treatment is a single dose of 100–175 mg/m^2 intravenous per treatment cycle, with a typical systemic dose being ~300 mg.

A coronary balloon coated with paclitaxel 3.0 × 20 mm and concentration of 3 μg/mm^2 of paclitaxel on the surface is coated with approximately 0.4 mg of the antiproliferative drug, corresponding to a ratio of 750 between the systemic dose and the amount of drug needed for the local treatment of coronary artery disease. However, in peripheral artery disease, this ratio is 1:55 as the required paclitaxel-coated balloons are significantly longer than those needed for coronary artery disease.

Observation in analysis of 1,649 patients who were treated with paclitaxel-coated balloons for femoropopliteal artery disease revealed no significant difference in all-

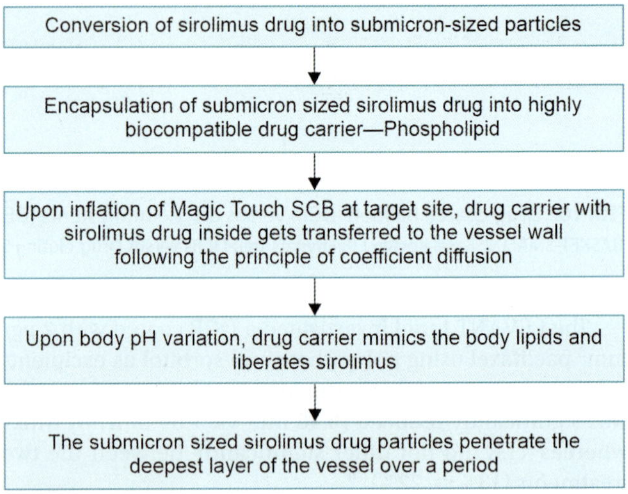

FLOWCHART 1: Magic Touch technology.

(SCB: sirolimus-coated balloon)

cause mortality across tertiles of nominal paclitaxel doses at crude and inverse probability of treatment weighting analyses.[75]

In the coronary artery disease setting, safety concerns associated with DCB angioplasty were not detected. In the pairwise comparisons of paclitaxel-coated balloon and paclitaxel-eluting stent groups in the 10-year outcomes analysis of the ISAR-DESIRE 3 trial, plain balloon group were not associated with an increased risk of death **(Table 3)**.

CONCLUSION

- Theoretical advantages of DCBs over DESs include broad surface contact, homogenous drug distribution, absence of stent footprint or polymer residue, and restoration of normal vessel anatomy and function.
- DCB delivery of paclitaxel combined with a hydrophilic spacer (excipient) results in clinically effective local tissue drug concentrations and sustained inhibition of neointimal growth.

- Among patients with coronary BMS or DES restenosis, DCBs show similar results to standard-of-care treatment (repeat stenting with a DES) and obviate the need for further stent implants.
- Among patients with de novo coronary artery disease, convincing data from randomized trials to support DCB therapy is lacking, and the use of DCBs for this indication requires further investigation.
- In peripheral artery disease, DCB therapy has proven superior to balloon angioplasty for treatment of de novo femoropopliteal and BTK disease.

ONLINE REFERENCES

Please scan the QR code provided at the end of the table of contents for References of this chapter.

CHAPTER 157

Zero-contrast/Ultra-low Contrast Percutaneous Coronary Intervention: Tips and Tricks

Prathap Kumar, Manu Rajendran, Blessvin Jino

ABSTRACT

Percutaneous coronary intervention (PCI) in chronic kidney disease (CKD) carries a high risk of contrast-induced acute kidney injury (CI-AKI). It is estimated that around 50% of deaths in advanced CKD are due to cardiovascular diseases. PCI is often denied in these patients due to the fear of precipitating CI-AKI. Zero or ultra-low contrast PCI is a newer technique to prevent CI-AKI in these patients. Though intravascular ultrasound (IVUS) and optical coherence tomography (OCT) can both be used for zero-contrast PCI, IVUS is frequently used. In this review, step-by-step details of zero-contrast PCI are described.

Keywords: Intravascular ultrasound, contrast induced acute kidney injury, zero-contrast percutaneous coronary intervention.

INTRODUCTION

Contrast-induced acute kidney injury (CI-AKI) is a serious complication of percutaneous coronary intervention (PCI), and it is often underdiagnosed. The Kidney Disease: Improving Global Outcomes (KDIGO) defines it as an increase in serum creatinine by ≥0.3 mg/dL within 48 hours of contrast administration or ≥50% increase within 7 days.[1] Recently, the term "contrast-associated AKI (CA-AKI)" is frequently used, since the postprocedural worsening of the renal function may also be caused by hypotension, drugs, and atheroembolism. Important risk factors for CI-AKI include cardiogenic shock, ST-elevation myocardial infarction (STEMI), acute heart failure, anemia, advanced age, preexisting renal dysfunction, low ejection fraction (EF), diabetes mellitus, and volume depletion. Though there is a descending trend in the incidence of acute kidney injury (AKI) among patients hospitalized with acute myocardial infarction,[2] the incidence of AKI among patients undergoing percutaneous coronary procedures has increased significantly.[3] Furthermore, the AKI-related incremental cost is estimated to be around $8,416 and $580 per inpatient procedure during index hospitalization and readmissions, respectively.[3] Additionally, CI-AKI is associated with increased mortality, with 36% and 12% chances of death during hospitalization and within 1 year of discharge, respectively.[4,5] There is a large variation in the volume of contrast used among operators. Data from the National Cardiovascular Data Registry Cath-PCI (NCDR Cath-PCI) registry showed that this variation was around 23% among operators,[6] and the CI-AKI risk had increased by 42% for every 75 mL of incremental contrast used. Hence, reducing the contrast usage during a procedure is an important way to reduce the risk of CI-AKI. The MOZART trial showed that the intravascular ultrasound (IVUS) guidance in PCI decreases the contrast volume (CV) requirement during PCI.[7] Moreover, recent studies have shown that ultra-low contrast [CV < estimated glomerular filtration rate (eGFR)] reduces the CI-AKI risk. Zero-contrast PCI is a novel method that requires extremely skilled PCI operators and meticulous analysis of intracoronary imaging for its successful clinical application, and it is a high-potential strategy to prevent CI-AKI and improve survival after PCI.

ZERO-CONTRAST PERCUTANEOUS CORONARY INTERVENTION

Though iodinated contrast media is considered essential to perform coronary procedures, these procedures may also be done without contrast media. Zero-contrast PCI is feasible with the use of intracoronary imaging. Though both IVUS and optical coherence tomography (OCT) may be used for zero-contrast PCI guidance, IVUS is commonly used. The first feasibility study on IVUS-guided zero-contrast PCI was done by Ali et al. among patients with advanced renal dysfunction, and none of these patients developed CI-AKI or major adverse cardiac events (MACE) on follow-up.[8] However, their study was done on a relatively fewer complex lesions, with a median synergy between PCI with taxus and cardiac surgery score of 12, and most of the patients received a single stent. Further studies with more complex lesions were done later, and most of these studies had high success rates and good short-term outcomes.[9,10] Apart from these, many case reports on highly complex lesions such as rotational atherectomy, left main bifurcation PCI, and chronic total occlusion (CTO) have been published, and all these suggest that even in complex lesion subsets, zero-contrast PCI is feasible.[11-13] Zero-contrast PCI under OCT guidance may also be done using dextran 40 or hydroxyethyl starch.[14,15]

Patient Selection and Preparation

We followed a simple approach for patient selection in our study[9] where patients with renal dysfunction were considered for zero-contrast PCI when they had met the following criteria:

- eGFR < 30 mL/min/1.73 m^2
- Serum creatinine > 1.5 mg/dL or eGFR 30–45 mL/min/1.73 m^2 and any of the following:
  - Age > 75 years
  - Left ventricular ejection fraction (LVEF) < 35%
  - Diabetes mellitus
  - Recent hypotension or shock

There are no universally accepted criteria for selecting patients for zero-contrast PCI, and it is the treating heart team's decision to choose the best possible method of revascularization. Although chronic kidney disease (CKD) patients who are not on maintenance dialysis are benefited the most, zero-contrast PCI is also useful in patients who are already on hemodialysis as it preserves the residual renal function. The BMC2 risk score is a reliable tool to predict CI-AKI in patients undergoing PCI. It can be calculated before PCI, and an online calculator is available. Predicted risk of <1%, 1–7%, and >7% are considered as low risk, intermediate risk, and high risk, respectively.[16] Patients with predicted risk > 7% may also be offered zero-contrast PCI. Even when zero-contrast PCI is planned, all patients require adequate hydration with isotonic saline before the procedure as per local institutional protocol. The POSEIDON trial showed that left ventricular end-diastolic pressure (LVEDP)-based intravenous fluid administration prevents CI-AKI effectively. All patients need to undergo routine baseline electrocardiogram (ECG) and echocardiographic examination before the procedure. This is important to compare and identify any new changes during the procedure.

CORONARY ANGIOGRAM

Although both radial and femoral accesses are feasible for zero-contrast PCI, femoral access allows preservation of the radial arteries for future dialysis. Moreover, larger-sized catheters can be used (>7 F) in the femoral approach, which give better support and larger lumen for multiple wires and IVUS runs. Many CKD patients have heavily calcified vessels, which often need rotational atherectomy for lesion preparation. Hence, femoral access is preferred by many operators. Though higher frames are preferred by some, we generally use 15 frames/s acquisition. For the left system, right anterior oblique (RAO) caudal and anteroposterior (AP)/RAO cranial projections are sufficient in most cases. For the right system, left anterior oblique (LAO) cranial is the preferred projection. A 5F catheter with smaller-sized syringes (5–10 mL) is preferred to minimize contrast use. Catheters without side holes should be used always. Biplane angiography reduces the contrast usage much. Similarly, diluted contrast can help in many cases, and higher acquisition rates may improve the image quality when diluted contrast is used. Unnecessary contrast puffing in between catheter engagement should be avoided.

Timing of the Procedure

An initial coronary angiogram should be performed with ultra-low CV (CV < eGFR), and subsequent PCI can be staged in stable patients. The duration between a coronary angiogram and subsequent zero-contrast PCI is variable and is dependent on the patient's clinical condition and the operator's preference. There is no uniform time interval followed in most of the studies, but many studies had an average time interval of 1 week.[8,10] Most of the low-osmolar contrast media have a half-life of 2 hours, and in patients with normal renal function, it takes 20 hours for the contrast to be eliminated. Hence, it is logical to give an interval of at least 24 hours, but this interval is not recommended by the American College of Radiology (ACR) committee on contrast media.[17] Furthermore, this interval may vary in patients with renal dysfunction. Hence, this approach cannot be universalized. Additionally, patients with acute coronary syndrome and ongoing angina may require urgent revascularization, and we have demonstrated in our study that immediate zero-contrast PCI following coronary angiography is feasible and is associated with a low incidence of CI-AKI.[9] Hence, a personalized decision should be taken regarding the time interval between the coronary angiogram and zero-contrast PCI.

Catheter Engagement and Wiring

Before inserting the guidewires into the guiding catheter, contrast in the guiding catheter should be removed by back bleeding or by aspiration. This step is needed in cases in which the guiding catheter is taken for coronary angiogram. Calcified vessels allow visualization of the arterial course and facilitate easier catheter engagement in many cases. Even in noncalcified vessels, catheter engagement poses little challenge for experienced operators. Once catheter engagement is done, it can be confirmed by inserting the guidewire into the coronary. Although ECG repolarization changes on saline injection into the coronaries have been described as a method of confirmation of catheter engagement, the earlier one is an easier method. It is essential to have previous coronary angiographic views as roadmap, as further steps such as guidewire crossing, lesion preparation, and stent deployment need the roadmap to identify the vessel course, lesion area, and landing zones. Hence, it is advisable to use the same fluoroscopic projections as coronary angiogram in all the steps.

Marker Wires and Metallic Silhouette

After catheter engagement and lesion crossing, the main operating wire may be parked as distal as possible. If possible, creating a loop in the distal tip of the guidewire is preferred, as the looped wire usually courses along the main vessel and is also atraumatic most of the time. Following this, additional guidewires (preferably hydrophilic) should be inserted into the major branches of the main vessel (marker wires), and this should be done in the same fluoroscopic projection as the angiogram. The left circumflex artery (LCX), major septal artery, and major diagonal artery are wired in cases where left anterior descending artery (LAD) stenting is planned. Similarly, for LCX stenting, at least one obtuse marginal (OM) branch and LAD are wired. The conus branch, right ventricular (RV) branch, right posterior descending branch (RPDA), and right posterolateral branch (RPLB) are the preferred side branches to be wired in cases where right coronary artery (RCA) stenting is planned. Importantly, in aorto-ostial stenting, one wire is placed in the aorta to mark the vessel ostium. The number of marker wires and the branches to be wired are selected according to the lesion and the discretion of the operator. Metallic silhouette is created to identify the proximal and distal landing zones easily and to position the stent correctly in the landing zones. Meticulous attention should be given while inserting multiple wires to prevent wire wrap, as these marker wires need to be in place till stent deployment.

INITIAL INTRAVASCULAR ULTRASOUND AND LESION PREPARATION

Once the metallic silhouette is created, initial IVUS run should be done. Sometimes, lesions are hard to be crossed by the IVUS probe, and predilatation may be needed. The operator experience is needed for predilatation before the IVUS run, as subintimal tracking of wire is possible in complex cases. Most experienced operators can identify this by tactile sensation. It is advisable to use smaller-sized balloons, such as 1.25–1.5 mm, to predilate before IVUS. Then the IVUS probe should be inserted as distal as possible, as angiographically normal areas may have significant disease on IVUS. Commercially available IVUS imaging systems have 100–150-mm pullback length, which is sufficient for most cases. During the initial IVUS run, it is essential to confirm the wire's position in the true lumen first. Then, minimal luminal area, proximal and distal reference vessel diameters, lesion length, and calcium arc and length are measured, along with the identification of proximal and distal landing zones. During IVUS pullback, whenever good landing zones are seen, "cine" store should be done, which can guide the stent placement. Lesion preparation is done as per the operator's discretion.

REPEAT INTRAVASCULAR ULTRASOUND AND STENT SIZING

Whenever possible, repeat IVUS run after initial lesion preparation is needed. This is to identify the dissection extent, if any, and to assess the adequacy of lesion preparation as well as to confirm the lesion length again, which guides in appropriate stent selection. Conventionally, stent size is selected according to the distal reference vessel diameter, and the length is selected according to the IVUS measured length. In tortuous vessels, it is important to keep in mind that 'IVUS-measured' length between proximal landing zone and distal landing zone may be different from the actual length because of wire bias. Additionally, when two stents are selected, stent overlap length should be considered, and in aorto-ostial stenting, stent protrusion into the aorta should be considered while selecting stent length. During IVUS analysis, the length between the distal landing zone and the distal-most marker wire and the length between the proximal landing zone and the proximal-most marker wire should be measured clearly. This helps in positioning the stent fluoroscopically. Additionally, some fluoroscopic markers such as the catheter tip, vessel calcium, rib margin, and diaphragm margin in a particular projection may aid in positioning the stent correctly. But stent positioning based on the marker wires is probably the best method. In cases in which two stents are required, repeat IVUS may be done after the first stent deployment, whenever possible. This is to select the second stent length more accurately, which is measured from the first stent edge to the proximal/distal landing zones. "Stent boost"/"clear stent" technologies can help us to position the second stent fluoroscopically.

POST-INTRAVASCULAR ULTRASOUND AND STENT OPTIMIZATION

After stenting, IVUS run is done to identify the adequacy of stent expansion, malapposition, edge dissection, minimal stent area (MSA), and ostial coverage in cases in which the vessel ostium is planned to be covered. Stent optimization is done as per the operator's discretion, and final IVUS run is done to confirm the optimization. Finally, MSA > 80% of the average reference lumen area, or MSA > 5.5 mm^2 in non-left main coronary artery (LMCA) and >8 mm^2 in LMCA without significant edge dissection or malapposition, without using contrast, is considered as a technically successful procedure. Final angiographic thrombolysis in myocardial infarction (TIMI) flow is a strong predictor of the long-term outcome after PCI and cannot be graded in IVUS. The long-term outcome of this zero-contrast PCI is still not known and needs further large studies.

COMPLICATION MANAGEMENT

Though complication management is common to all PCI procedures, meticulous attention is warranted during "zero-contrast PCI." Any new onset or worsening angina, hypotension, and fresh ECG changes should alert the operating team about the possible complications. Whenever hypotension occurs during the procedure, echocardiography should be done immediately to rule out vessel perforation. Check angiogram with minimal contrast may be used whenever complications are suspected. Even after the successful completion of the procedure, serial echocardiography is needed to identify distal wire perforation. As many CKD patients have complex coronary anatomy, aggressive preparation of the vessel and optimization of stent are needed, and complications should always be expected by the operating team. Final check coronary angiogram is advised by many operators, although it is not mandatory. Before commencing the procedure, there should be a "shared decision-making" between the heart team and the patient regarding this final check angiogram. This helps to avoid legal problems.

CASE EXAMPLE

A 48-year-old male presented with non-STEMI (NSTEMI). Echocardiogram showed left ventricular anterior wall hypokinesia with EF of 44%. The patient was a case of diabetes, hypertension, and CKD. His serum creatinine and eGFR were 2.4 mg/dL and 32 mL/min/1.73 m^2, respectively. The coronary angiogram showed total occlusion of the LAD **(Figs. 1A to H)**. He was planned for ad hoc zero-contrast PCI. The left system was engaged with a 7F JL guide catheter, and the LAD lesion and LCX were wired with Fielder FC guidewires. Then, the lesion was dilated with 1.25 × 10 mm balloon, and the diagonal was wired with another Fielder FC guidewire. Pre-IVUS run was done, and it showed proximal and mid-LAD vessel diameters of 4.5 and 3.5 mm, respectively **(Figs. 2A and B)**. Lesion length was 22 mm, and the proximal landing zone was 7.5 mm away from the LAD ostium and the distal landing zone was 9.5 mm away from the diagonal ostium. The lesion was stented with 3.5 × 26 mm drug-eluting stent (DES), and postdilatation was done with 4 × 12 mm non-compliant (NC) balloon. Poststenting IVUS run showed MSA of 7.8 mm^2 and a well-apposed and expanded stent.

CONCLUSION

Patients with CKD are at a high risk of cardiovascular events, and 50% of all deaths in stage 4 and 5 of CKD patients are due to cardiovascular mortality. However, the utilization of coronary angiogram and PCI is less among CKD patients, particularly those who are not on renal replacement therapy. Fear of precipitating CI-AKI is the predominant reason for this underutilization of the revascularization procedure. Advances in technology and intracoronary imaging help modern operators to perform PCI without contrast media. Operator experience in understanding the coronary anatomy, tactile feedback of guidewires, and intracoronary image interpretation are essential for the successful completion of this procedure. The widespread use of this technique has the potential to decrease mortality by reducing CI-AKI and to provide a better quality of life for patients with advanced CKD.

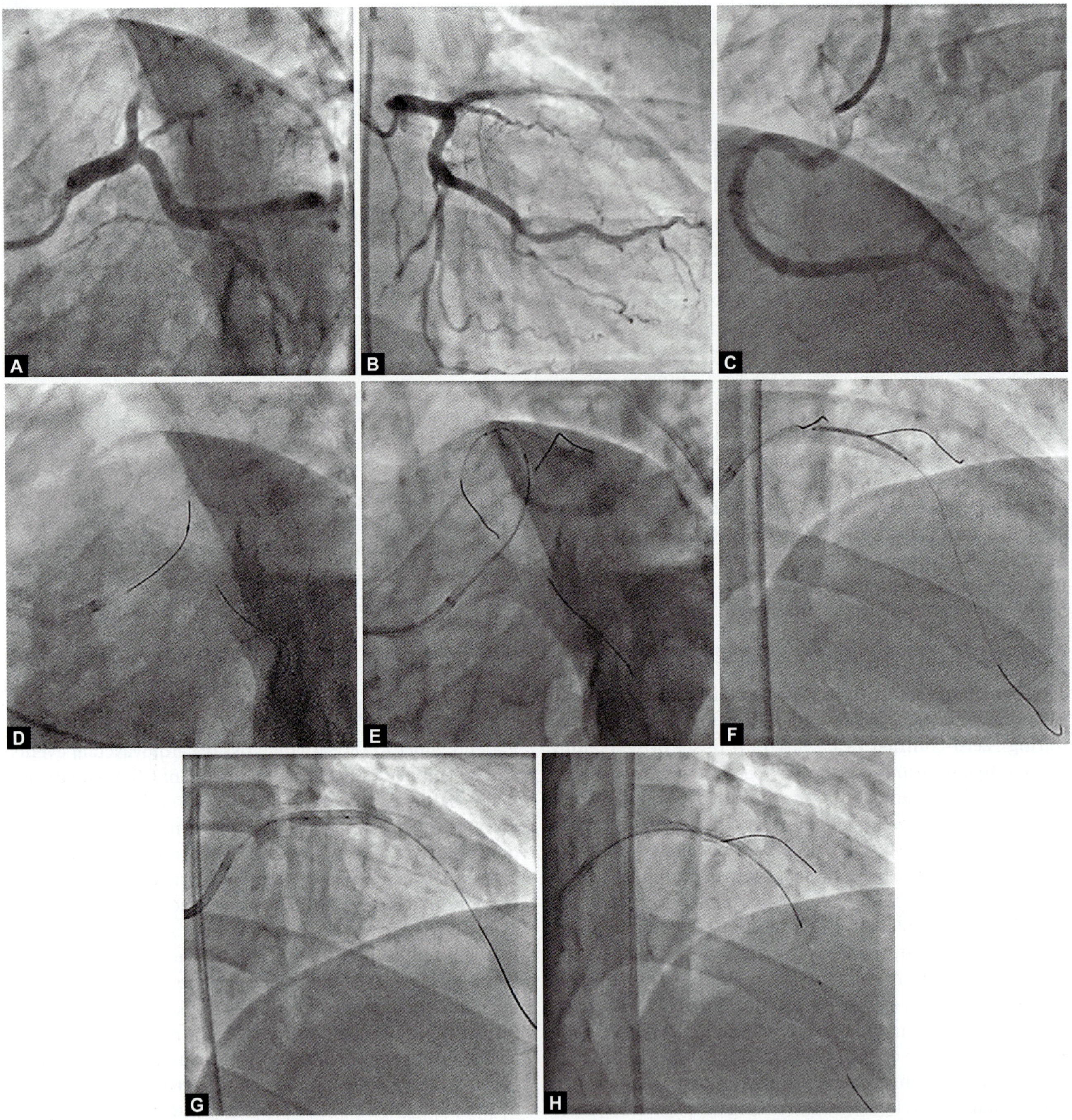

FIGS. 1A TO H: Angiographic images of zero-contrast percutaneous coronary intervention (PCI) to left anterior descending (LAD). Left anterior oblique (LAO) caudal and right anterior oblique (RAO) caudal views show proximal LAD total occlusion (A and B), and the LAO cranial view shows no significant lesion in the right coronary artery (RCA) (C). A 7F JL 4 guiding catheter was used to engage the left main coronary artery (LMCA). Fielder FC guidewire was used for crossing the LAD lesion, and another Fielder FC guidewire was parked in the left circumflex (LCX) as a marker wire to detect LAD ostium (D). Then, initial intravascular ultrasound (IVUS) run was done after predilatation with 1.25 × 10 mm balloon (E), and the stent was selected according to the IVUS measurements (IVUS images for stent selection are shown in Figs. 2A and B). A 3.5 × 26 mm drug-eluting stent (DES) was positioned across the LAD lesion as guided by the IVUS measurements, and the stent was deployed. Postdilatation was done with 4 × 12 mm balloon (F and G). Final IVUS run was done (H), which showed a well-expanded stent with minimal stent area (MSA) of 7.8 mm2 and no edge dissection or malapposition.

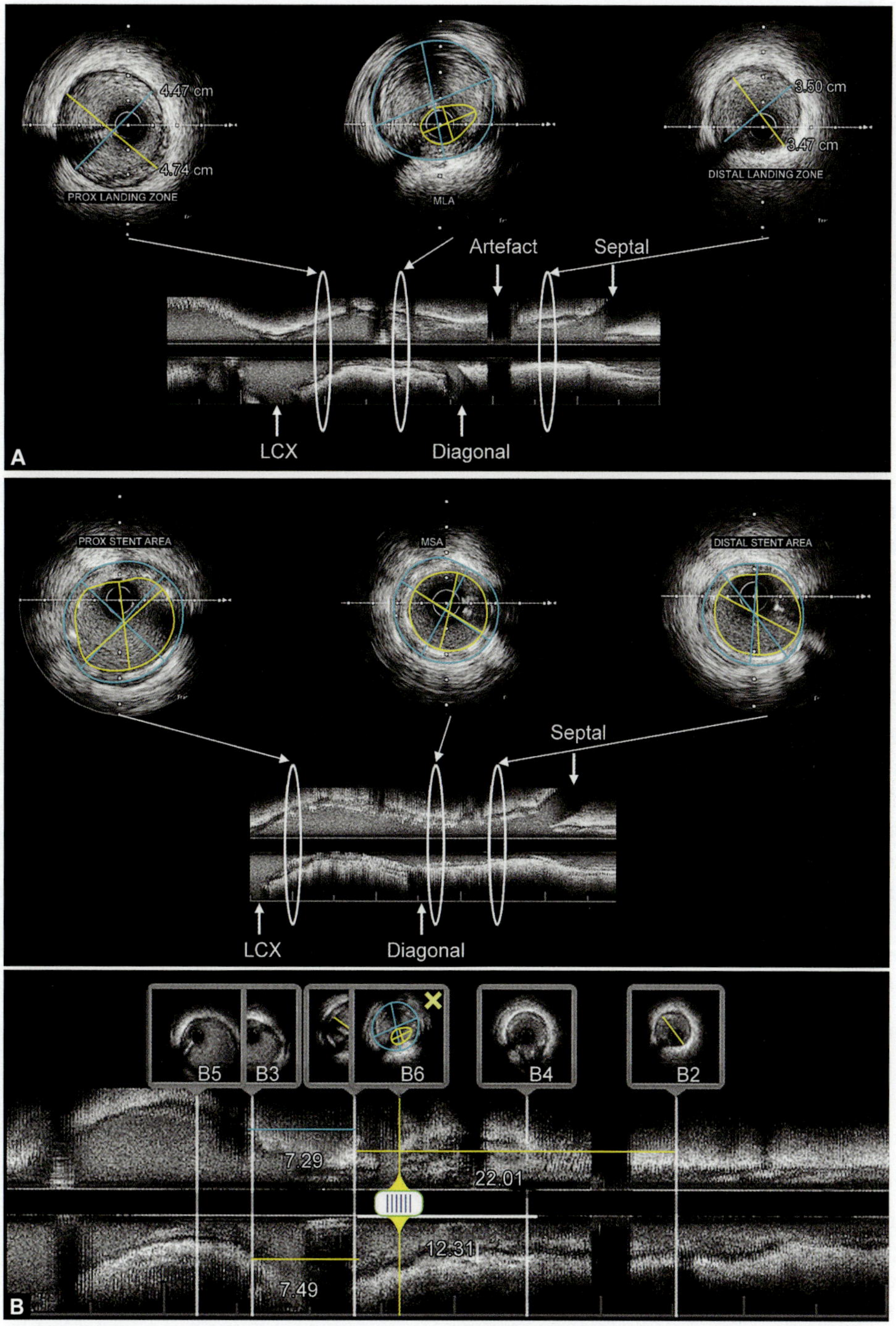

FIGS. 2A AND B: Pre- and post-intravascular ultrasound (IVUS) runs.
(LCX: left circumflex; MLA: minimal lumen area; MSA: minimal stent area)

ONLINE REFERENCES

Please scan the QR code provided at the end of the table of contents for References of this chapter.

CHAPTER

158 Percutaneous Coronary Intervention in Chronic Kidney Disease Patients

Panchanan Sahoo, Ritesh Acharya

ABSTRACT

Cardiovascular disease (CVD) is the major cause of morbidity and mortality in chronic kidney disease (CKD). CVD and CKD have been showing an increasing prevalence and drawing global attention in the last two decades. Patients with CKD are at an increased risk of developing CVD, and diagnosed CVD cases are at a higher risk of developing acute kidney injury (AKI) and progress to end-stage renal disease (ESRD) and renal replacement therapy (RRT). Although 30–40% of all patients undergoing percutaneous coronary intervention (PCI) have concomitant CKD, data on optimum treatment strategy in this population remain scarce as in most randomized controlled trials (RCTs) and research protocols, CKD and ESRD patients are excluded due to their higher ischemic bleeding risks, higher contrast-induced nephropathy (CIN), and short- and long-term worsened prognosis.

A large number of CKD patients are now undergoing coronary and peripheral angiography and catheter-based or surgical revascularization and treatment for heart valve diseases. In recent years, the utilization of advanced imaging procedures such as intravascular ultrasound (IVUS), fractional flow reserve (FFR), dynamic road maps, and physiology guidance has resulted in zero or ultralow contrast use, thereby preventing CIN.

The chapter aims to discuss of latest therapeutics and the best use of novel hard wires and treatment algorithms to prevent CIN and mortality in CKD patients.

Keywords: Cardiovascular disease, chronic kidney disease, contrast-induced nephropathy, acute kidney injury, coronary angiography, percutaneous coronary intervention.

CASE SCENARIO

At the outset, let me explain one case scenario: A 68-year-old male with multiple comorbidities such as hypothyroidism, diabetic, hypertensive, and chronic kidney disease (CKD) for 10 years presented to the emergency with lower limb swelling, shortness of breath, and atypical chest pain since 6 hours. His routine blood examination upon admission showed urea 96 mg/dL, creatinine 10.89 mg/dL, serum Na^+ 128, K^+ 6.4 mEq/L and troponin I 0.06 ng/mL. Hemodialysis was done on day 1, in view of atypical angina and rising titre troponin I to 1.35 and 6.9 ng/mL on day 2 and 3. Coronary angiography was done and found to have left main coronary artery (LMCA) 70% stenosis, left anterior descending artery ostium to mid-diffuse stenosis, left circumflex artery ostial 90%, and right coronary artery (RCA) mid-stenosis 90% **(Figs. 1 and 2)**. In view of the complexity of left-side lesions, RCA stenting was done with low osmolar contrast use **(Fig. 3)**. Percutaneous coronary intervention (PCI) has always been a challenge in CKD and end-stage renal disease (ESRD) in view of fear of contrast-induced nephropathy (CIN) and worsened prognosis.

INTRODUCTION

Cardiovascular disease (CVD) is the leading cause of morbidity and mortality among patients with CKD. The mortality rate for patients on hemodialysis is 20% per year, with approximately 50% attributable to a cardiovascular cause.[1] CVD prevalence and mortality increase with the progression of the severity of CKD based on the estimated glomerular filtration rate (eGFR) and the level of albuminuria.[2] Lower eGFR is associated with an increase in total CVD-related mortality and risk of acute coronary

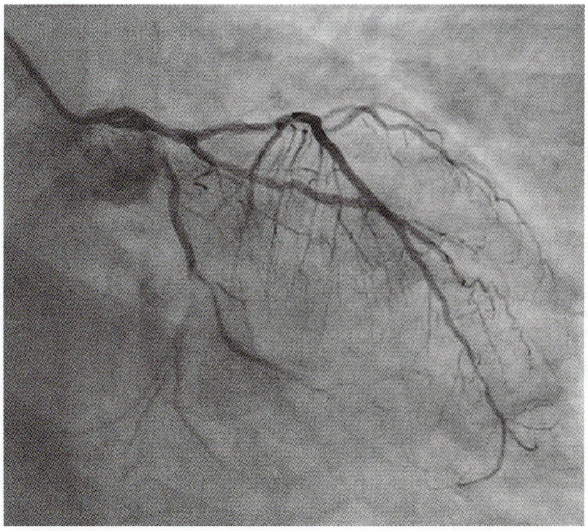

FIG. 1: Coronary angiogram (CAG) showing left main coronary artery (LMCA) 70% stenosis, left anterior descending (LAD) artery ostium to mid-diffuse stenosis, and left circumflex (LCX) ostial 90% stenosis in a chronic kidney disease (CKD) patient.

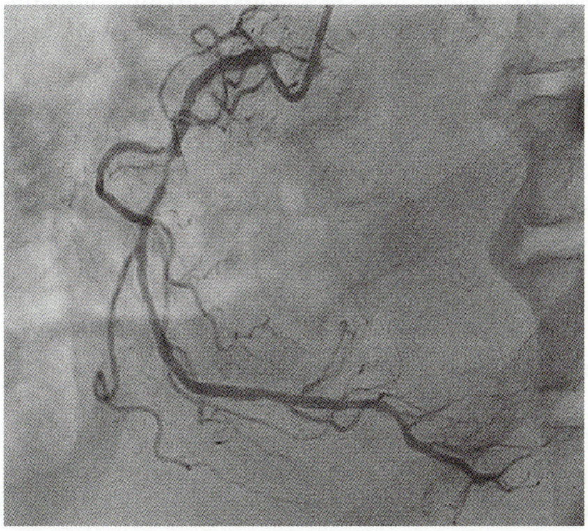

FIG. 2: Coronary angiogram (CAG) showing mid-right coronary artery 90% stenosis.

syndrome (ACS).[2] Even after adjustment for conventional risk factors, including diabetes and hypertension, the risk of mortality progressively increases with worsening CKD.[3]

With an increase in the global prevalence of CKD risk factors such as aging, obesity, diabetes, and hypertension, more CKD patients are now undergoing PCI.[2] Despite 30–40% of all patients undergoing PCI having concomitant CKD, data on optimal management strategies are scarce because most randomized controlled trials (RCTs) have usually excluded patients with severe CKD. Patients with CKD who present with ACS are less likely to receive guideline-directed medical therapy (GDMT) or invasive angiography, and the trend to avoid coronary interventions increases with increasing severity of CKD.[4]

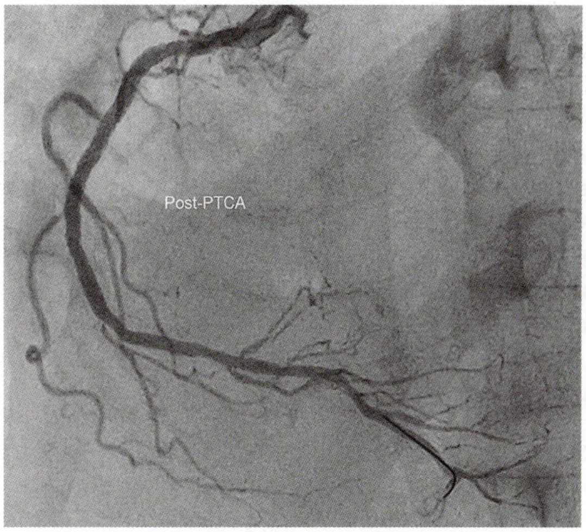

FIG. 3: Post percutaneous transluminal coronary angioplasty (PTCA) to right coronary artery (RCA) showing good result [thrombolysis in myocardial infarction (TIMI) 3 flow].

WHAT MAKES CORONARY ARTERY DISEASE IN CHRONIC KIDNEY DISEASE DIFFERENT?

An "oligosymptomatic" presentation is common; only 44% of patients with moderate-to-severe CKD or who are on dialysis, presenting with ACS, report typical pain. Coronary artery disease (CAD) in CKD usually presents in an atypical manner, more often with anginal equivalents such as shortness of breath or fatigue, which may be neglected.[3] Low functional capacity in severe CKD patients further limits the expression of angina.[3]

Acute coronary syndrome is a more common presentation in CKD in comparison to chronic coronary syndrome (CCS), but it is more likely to be a non-ST-segment elevation myocardial infarction (STEMI).[3] The potential reasons may be supply–demand mismatch, ischemic preconditioning, collateralization of blood vessels, and higher prevalence of left ventricular hypertrophy (LVH) altering the electrocardiographic findings.[3]

With worsening of glomerular filtration rate (GFR), the clinical manifestations of CAD become more prevalent, in parallel with the prevalence of large-vessel coronary disease, arteriosclerosis, microvascular disease, LVH, and myocardial fibrosis. Cardiovascular abnormalities in CKD are associated with traditional (diabetes and hypertension), nontraditional CKD-related CVD risk factors (anemia, inflammation, and oxidative stress), and dialysis-related factors (type and frequency of dialysis and dialysate composition).[3] Atherosclerosis in early CKD is driven by traditional risk factors, whereas nontraditional risk factors play a predominant role with progressive decline in GFR.[3] A higher prevalence of fibrocalcific and advanced atherosclerotic plaques with increased inflammation has been seen in autopsy studies of CKD versus non-CKD.[3]

Despite the high prevalence, the diagnosis of CAD in patients with CKD may be challenging, as both mild elevations in cardiac troponin and electrocardiogram (ECG) abnormalities are frequent.[5] Therefore, dynamic changes in ECG or cardiac troponin should be assessed to diagnose myocardial infarction (MI). High-sensitive troponin assays maintain high diagnostic and prognostic accuracy even in patients with renal dysfunction.[5]

WHOM TO INTERVENE?

Percutaneous coronary intervention improves survival in ACS and helps to control anginal symptoms in CCS; however, its net benefit among patients with CKD is less well established.[6] It is unclear whether medical therapy is as efficacious in patients with CKD due to underlying differences in the risk and benefit balance with underlying kidney disease.

Until sufficient evidence is garnered from well-conducted RCTs, patients with CKD should receive similar treatment to patients without CKD. A team-based approach, including cardiologists and nephrologists, with shared decision-making, would be advantageous, especially when considering revascularization for which decreased short-term risk must be balanced with long-term benefit.[1]

In the ISCHEMIA-CKD trial, among patients with CCS, advanced CKD, and moderate or severe ischemia, an initial invasive strategy when compared with an initial conservative strategy did not reduce the risk of death or nonfatal MI, suggesting that revascularization is beneficial only when the patient remains symptomatic despite medical therapy, clarifying conflicting data from previous studies.[7]

Current American College of Cardiology (ACC)/Society of Cardiovascular Angiography and Interventions (SCAI) guidelines, therefore, give a class III recommendation to routine coronary interventions in asymptomatic CCS patients with CKD.[4]

The TACTICS-TIMI 18 and FRISC II trials demonstrated that early invasive treatment reduced death and rates of MI in CKD patients with unstable CAD when compared with conservative medical management.[8,9] Long-term survival was significantly better in patients with CKD during the treatment of ACS by PCI, rather than conservative treatment.[10] Hence, early revascularization should never be delayed in patients with CKD presenting as ACS. ACC/SCAI recommendations have given STEMI and high-risk non-ST-segment elevation acute coronary syndrome (NSTEACS) in CKD a class I and IIa recommendation, respectively, for undergoing coronary angiography and revascularization.[4]

POSSIBLE COMPLICATIONS AND HOW TO ENSURE SAFETY?

The PCI benefit window for CKD patients is narrow. The issues in intervention for CAD in a CKD patient include:

- Development of CIN
- Suboptimal revascularization
- Effect of medications

Contrast-induced Nephropathy/Acute Kidney Injury

Contrast-induced nephropathy is defined as the impairment of renal function, with either a relative 25% increase or an absolute 0.5 mg/dL increase within 48–72 hours of intravenous (IV) contrast administration.[11]

Preexisting renal failure represents the most common predisposition to the development of CIN. The incidence of CIN increases significantly among patients with CKD, ranging between 12 and 50%.[12]

Patients with CKD have defective antioxidant systems, increased oxidative stress associated with inflammation, and endothelial dysfunction.[13] Contrast exerts direct renal toxicity mediated by free radicals and oxidative stress or indirect toxicity through medullary hypoxia by vasoconstriction.[6] CKD patients with post-PCI CIN have poorer short- and long-term outcomes regarding survival and renal function.[14] Currently, there is no specific treatment for contrast-induced acute kidney injury (CI-AKI) once the injury has occurred; therefore, it is critical to stratify the risk and implement all measures to prevent CI-AKI, especially in CKD.[14]

Risk Factors for Contrast-induced Nephropathy

Risk factors for CIN may be fixed, such as CKD, diabetes mellitus, female sex, age, and congestive heart failure (CHF), or modifiable, such as hypotension, contrast type and volume, anemia, nephrotoxic drugs, hypercholesterolemia, periprocedural dehydration/hypovolemia, and periprocedural hyperglycemia.[15]

Need for a Standard Protocol

When protocols were standardized and teams were coached to implement those protocols, AKI was reduced by 28% in patients with preexisting CKD. Various risk prediction tools such as the Mehran risk score, the ACC NCDR risk score, the ADVANCIS score, and the revised Mehran score have been proposed.[2] The Mehran model includes both clinical and periprocedural risk factors: CHF (5 points), hypotension (5 points), eGFR (4 points), age > 75 years (4 points), diabetes (3 points), anemia (3 points), and contrast volume (1 point for every 100 cc used).[15] No single scoring system was recommended over another, but the consistent use of a validated risk assessment tool helps in better awareness and identifying high-risk patients for stringent prevention strategies and closer follow-up.[2]

How to Minimize Contrast-induced Nephropathy?

Hydration

Periprocedural IV fluids remain the cornerstone treatment for the prevention of CI-AKI, especially in CKD. In euvolemic or hypovolemic patients, volume expansion with IV normal saline is recommended. Tailoring administration by giving more fluid to hypovolemic patients and less to those at risk of volume overload or pulmonary edema is the best approach and has been given a class IIa recommendation by the European Society of Cardiology (ESC) to prevent CIN.[2,5,16]

Volume expansion and AKI prevention are achieved by dilution of tubular contrast concentrations, increased urine flow rates and subsequent "clearing" of contrast from the kidneys, and potentially improved renal oxygen delivery.[2]

Current clinical practice guidelines and consensus statements recommend IV isotonic saline (1.0–1.5 mL/kg/h) started 3–12 hours before the procedure and continued for 12–24 hours after the exposure to contrast. In the case of a same-day procedure, faster hydration (3 mL/kg/h) can be used at least 1–3 hours before and 6 hours after the procedure.[15]

Intravenous hydration has been found to be more effective in reducing CIN than oral hydration, and hydration with 0.9% isotonic saline was found to be more effective in CIN reduction when compared to other solutions.[6]

To prevent CIN, pre- and posthydration with isotonic saline has been given a class IIa recommendation by ESC, especially if the expected contrast volume is >100 mL.[5,16]

Targeted hydration regimen [left ventricular end-diastolic pressure (LVEDP)],[16] noninvasive imaging assessments of volume status such as inferior vena cava dimensions,[2] and controlled hydration with forced diuresis and matched saline infusion using an automated system[16] (REMEDIAL II STUDY) represent valuable alternatives to standard hydration.

The Prevention of Contrast Renal Injury with Different Hydration Strategies (POSEIDON) trial showed that fluid administration guided by LVEDP reduced all-cause mortality, MI, or renal replacement therapy (RRT) significantly.[6]

Given the high rate of CIN among patients treated with saline hydration alone (15–20%), especially among patients with advanced CKD (grade ≥ 3b), it appears that saline hydration alone is not sufficient to prevent CIN.[17]

Sequential minimal contrast diagnostic angiography using ultra-low volume, followed by staged physiology- and intravascular ultrasound (IVUS)/optical coherence tomography (OCT)-guided zero-contrast PCI in patients with advanced CKD, facilitates better procedural planning and minimizes the contrast volume administration.[18]

Access

Nephroprotective effect of transradial approach (TRA) over transfemoral approach (TFA), including a lower incidence of major bleeding, embolization, hypotension and a lower use of contrast agents have made it the preferred route for interventions in CKD.[6] TRA was associated with a lower occurrence of acute kidney injury after coronary angiography or PCI, compared to TFA.[6] TFA may increase the risk of atheroemboli because of the proximity to renal arteries, thereby increasing the risk of AKI.[4] The 2021 ACC/American Heart Association Coronary Revascularization Guidelines state to "use radial artery access if feasible."[19] The AKI-MATRIX study failed to show a reduction in AKI with radial access when the KDIGO criteria were used as an outcome.[20] Further research is needed to identify which patients benefit from TRA with respect to AKI outcomes.

Contrast

The half-life of contrast medium is approximately 2 hours in patients with normal renal function and >30 hours in advanced CKD patients.[14]

The maximum acceptable contrast dose [5 mL × body weight (kg)/baseline serum creatinine (mg/dL)] should never be exceeded.[15] The ratio of contrast media volume (CMV) used to estimated creatinine clearance (CMV/CrC) is a valid and independent predictor of CI-AKI.[15] In CKD patients undergoing coronary interventions, minimal contrast use to prevent the occurrence of CI-AKI has been given a class I recommendation by ACC/SCAI/ESC.[4,5,16] A contrast volume to eGFR ratio of 3.7 as an upper dose limit is recommended, but practically, a ratio of <2 may be preferred.[2]

Technical advancements such as automated contrast injectors and smart manifold syringes reduce contrast volume delivery.[2]

The type of contrast is also very important. Low-osmolar contrast media (LOCM) and iso-osmolar contrast media (IOCM) are less nephrotoxic and are given a class I recommendation in CKD patients undergoing coronary interventions.[5,16]

Meta-analyses have shown a minor benefit of iso-osmolar media over low-osmolar agents in high-risk patients. Studies have shown that iso-osmolar dyes, by unknown mechanisms, prevent limb pain during peripheral angiography and potentially reduce composite renal and cardiovascular events.[2] Iodixanol (IOCM) and iopamidol (LOCM) appear to be contrast agents of choice to reduce the risk of CIN.[13]

Coronary Angiogram

- A total of 15 mL of contrast is usually sufficient for a reliable coronary angiogram (CAG) (2–3 mL of contrast to visualize the left coronary artery and 2 mL for the RCA).[6]
- Smaller catheters (5–6 Fr) without side holes ensure maximum opacification of the vessels with each contrast

injection.[21] Coronary calcium as a guide to locate the coronary artery ostia and as a landmark within the vessel to guide stent placement has also been suggested.
- Contrast medium should be removed from the catheter prior to every drug administration or catheter exchange.[6]
- T wave amplitude changes are seen in a significant number of patients when coronary artery was injected with 0.9% saline. By injecting 10–20 mL of 0.9% saline through the catheter, correct positioning of the catheter can be confirmed, with T wave changes, in addition to ST-segment depression or elevation.[6]
- Avoid low-magnification angiograms as these may be used as road map during PCI.[6]
- Using diluted contrast (1:1 or 1:2 ratio of saline to contrast) allows more contrast injection runs at the expense of luminal opacification.[6]
- Using higher frame rates may aid the operator to maximize visualization of the coronary anatomy with each injection.[6]
- The use of physiology or image guidance must be considered rather than additional angiographic views to determine whether the intervention is needed for a lesion.[6]

When clear angiographic images are available, PCI without contrast may be attempted. PCI should be planned at least after 1 week of CAG because CIN typically occurs during this period.[18] Systemic clearance of the contrast material via renal excretion, although markedly slower in severe CKD, is expected to be almost complete within this time period.[18] Although atheroemboli have been shown to contribute to nearly 10% of AKI post-PCI, the lack of worsening renal function following staged PCI strongly suggests that CIN is the major cause, and staged zero-contrast PCI would be a favorable approach in this extremely high-risk group.[18]

The use of imaging guidance, intracoronary pressure wires, coregistration of multimodality imaging, and road mapping could reduce contrast delivery to patients during PCI. The concept of "zero" or ultralow (total volume < 1 × eGFR) contrast volume PCI has been shown to be feasible in selected patients.[2]

Percutaneous Coronary Intervention

- It is preferable to use large guiding catheters (7 Fr or more) for stable support and to accommodate multiple guidewires, stents, and IVUS probes.[6]
- Diagnostic cine images displayed in real time may act as a road map for catheter engagement and intervention during PCI.[6]
- Tracing the course of the vessels on the reference angiography, multiple guidewires can act as a map to track major reference points during PCI (e.g., ostia, bifurcations, etc.).[6]
- Once the guidewire is placed correctly, IVUS/OCT may be used to accurately define plaque burden and reference vessel dimensions, allowing the selection of the optimal stent size.[6]
- Optimal stent expansion and possible dissections can be assessed by IVUS/OCT. Coregistration to merge angiography and intravascular probe position further increases PCI accuracy.[6]
- The physiological evaluation like FFR/instantaneous flow reserve (iFR) can be used to guide the procedure and confirm the effectiveness of the intervention.[6]
- Rotational atherectomy can be performed without contrast by taking wall calcification as guide.[6]
- Drug-eluting stent implantation showed better clinical outcomes than the bare-metal stent in reducing MI and mortality after PCI. No differences in the long-term clinical outcomes between the zotarolimus-eluting stent (ZES), everolimus-eluting stent (EES), and biolimus-eluting stent (BES) groups in acute MI in renal insufficiency patients undergoing PCI were found, except for nonfatal MI where ZES was found to be better.[22]
- For complications such as vessel perforation or distal embolization that cannot be ruled out by IVUS or functional tests, a small contrast injection may be used.[6]

A minimum assessment at 24 hours and ideally at 48–72 hours should be considered in patients with a high risk of AKI, especially inpatients.[2]

Biplane cineangiography may reduce contrast delivery or AKI risk though studies are sparse in CKD.[2]

Use of the DyeVert PLUS system (Osprey Medical) led to a 15.5% relative reduction in contrast volume; however, this did not translate into a reduction of CIN.[21]

As reactive oxygen species (ROS) play an important role in CI-AKI, the use of antioxidant agents has been evaluated over the years.
- High-dose statins before diagnostic catheterization reduce the occurrence of CI-AKI because of their pleiotropic effects, which reduce systemic inflammation, possibly by reducing the synthesis of endothelin-1 and inhibiting tissue-factor expression of macrophages.[4] In statin-naïve patients undergoing coronary angiography, pretreatment with high-intensity atorvastatin or rosuvastatin has been given a class IIa recommendation by ESC to reduce CIN.[5,16,23] Premedication with statins has been demonstrated to prevent CIN post-PCI independent of the hydration protocol.[24]
- Hemodialysis and hemofiltration have been proposed for CIN prevention in patients with CKD by removing contrast from circulation.[6] Hemodialysis has failed to show benefit in trials potentially due to the nephrotoxicity caused by a proinflammatory, procoagulative, hypotensive, and hypovolemic effect.[6] Hemofiltration can remove fluid and solutes with better volume control and hemodynamic stability.[6] Hemofiltration reduces CIN occurrence and 1-year mortality in patients with severe CKD, especially when hemofiltration is done before and after the procedure.[6] Currently, prophylactic

hemofiltration 6 hours before complex PCI has a class IIb recommendation, but hemodialysis has been given a class III recommendation by ESC to prevent CIN.[5,16]

Continuous hemofiltration takes a long time (≥18 hours) due to its low removal efficiency, which may be unrealistic in patients. The novel high-flow volume intermittent hemodiafiltration (HF-IHDF) can remove contrast medium from the blood six times faster than standard continuous hemodiafiltration (CHDF).[17] In addition, the levels of administered sodium bicarbonate are high with HF-IHDF, which may reduce oxidative stress within the kidney and also maintain fluid volume to avoid renal ischemia.[17] HF-IHDF has the potential to prevent CIN more effectively than other RRTs.[17] The CIN rates 2–3 days and 1 month after the interventional procedure were lower in patients treated with HF-IHDF than in the saline group, irrespective of the contrast volume/creatinine clearance ratio, suggesting that HF-IHDF may increase the tolerance to contrast agents.[17]

- N-acetylcysteine (NAC) is a potent scavenger of ROS and improves endothelium-dependent vasodilation. Although promising in animal models, NAC failed to prove a clinical benefit in the prevention of CI-AKI, even when used in IV preparations. Being inexpensive and safe at the doses used for CI-AKI prevention, it may be considered in intermediate–high-risk patients despite the inconclusive evidence.[15]
- Ascorbic acid and fenoldopam, although promising, could not provide encouraging results in trials.[15]
- Although a mild nephroprotective effect has been observed in a few clinical trials, the potential cardiovascular side effects and drug interactions currently limit the use of theophylline.[15]
- Recent studies have shown promising results with febuxostat, which reduced the incidence of CIN as well as postoperative serum uric acid levels, especially in CKD patients undergoing PCI.[25,26]

Dual Antiplatelets

Chronic kidney disease patients carry both a higher ischemic and bleeding risk.[6] Multiple studies have shown a high platelet reactivity in patients with CKD.[6] Dual antiplatelet (DAPT) duration should be individualized based on clinical characteristics and CKD.[6] In a post hoc analysis of the PRODIGY trial, CKD did not appear to affect ischemic events depending on DAPT duration, but a longer DAPT was associated with excessive bleeding in moderate and severe CKD.[27] But CKD has been included as a criterion in several risk scores for increased ischemic and bleeding risk. In a subanalysis of the PRECISE-DAPT population, shorter-term DAPT improved outcomes for patients with higher ischemic and bleeding risk, supporting the concept that bleeding risk prevention with shorter-term DAPT is preferred when both ischemic and bleeding risk are high.[28]

Recently published post hoc analysis of the HOST-REDUCE-POLYTECH-ACS trial showed that although the rates of both bleeding and ischemic events increased as renal function decreased, prasugrel dose de-escalation significantly reduced bleeding risk without a significant increase in ischemic events, regardless of the renal function.[29]

Patients with atrial fibrillation and CKD undergoing PCI are an increasingly large group, and properly tailored antithrombotic treatment is a must in view of high bleeding risk.[6]

Hemodynamic Support

The incidence of AKI ranges from 20 to 60% in STEMI with cardiogenic shock and is an independent predictor of RRT and mortality.[2] Baseline comorbidities, acute left ventricular dysfunction, and hypotension requiring vasopressor support increase the risk of AKI in these patients.[2] Intra-aortic balloon pump (IABP) may preserve renal function by improving forward cardiac output, renal perfusion, and coronary perfusion.[2] But the potential for vascular site bleeding, renal artery obstruction in cases of caudal migration of the IABP, and atheroembolism may worsen kidney function.[2] In high-risk PCIs, studies have been inconclusive regarding the risk of AKI when Impella catheters are used for support.[2] The impact of hemodynamic support devices on renal function, therefore, remains an ongoing area of investigation.

Anemia is associated with a higher incidence of CIN in patients with moderate renal dysfunction. Kidney is a highly oxygen-sensitive organ. In anemia, the decrease in oxygen transport of blood, reduced blood volume, and insufficient effective circulation would increase the consumption of oxygen and injury of oxidative stress in renal tubule cells.[30] Anemia also increases oxygen-free radical damage and the imbalance of vasoactive substances, which promote apoptosis and immune injury of kidney cells.[30] Therefore, correction of anemia in CKD patients undergoing coronary interventions must be ensured to prevent CIN.

Renal Guard System[6]

The Renal Guard system, an automated hydration system, along with increased diuresis, was associated with a statistically significant reduction in CIN and the need for RRT.

Cardiopulmonary Bypass Graft

It has been advised to delay cardiopulmonary bypass graft (CABG) in stable patients for 24 hours after CAG when suitable for better major adverse cardiovascular and cerebrovascular events (MACCE) outcomes.[4]

The in-hospital mortality rate was higher in CABG than PCI in CKD patients undergoing revascularization.[31] At the 1-year follow-up, CABG was associated with a lower survival rate than PCI, although at 5-year follow-up, the freedom from

MACCEs was also better in the patients of CABG compared with the patients of PCI.[31] PCI compared with CABG was associated with a significantly higher risk for all-cause death regardless of the stages of CKD without any significant interaction.[32] In CKD requiring LMCA intervention, CABG is associated with a lower risk of MACCE, MI, and repeat revascularization, but an increased risk of cerebrovascular accidents when compared to patients who received PCI therapy.[33] In the EXCEL trial, AKI occurred less frequently after PCI compared with CABG. There were no significant differences between PCI and CABG in terms of MACE events at 3 years in patients with and without CKD.[34]

Preferring CABG over PCI in patients with multivessel CAD whose surgical profile is acceptable and life expectancy is >1 year has been given a class IIa recommendation by ESC to minimize CIN.[5,16]

CONCLUSION

Although, in a patient with CKD, a standard protocol based approach helps in better outcomes of coronary interventions, individualized modifications depending upon the complex and versatile nature of patients with CKD presenting with CAD should be encouraged too. There is always a scope for research and advancement in this traditionally neglected patient population and the field would definitely continue to grow positively in future.

ONLINE REFERENCES

Please scan the QR code provided at the end of the table of contents for References of this chapter.

CHAPTER

159 Chronic Total Occlusion Retrograde Technique: Tips and Tricks

V Suryaprakasa Rao, PLN Kapardhi, Santosh Palled, Kiran Kumar G

ABSTRACT

Chronic total occlusion percutaneous coronary intervention (CTO PCI) poses a formidable challenge in the field of interventional cardiology, requiring advanced techniques to revascularize completely occluded coronary arteries. The *retrograde approach* has emerged as a crucial strategy to overcome these complex subset of CTO lesions when other methods in *hybrid algorithm* prove difficult or fail. This chapter highlights the essential tips and tricks of retrograde CTO PCI.

Keywords: Chronic total occlusion, controlled antegrade and retrograde tracking (CART), antegrade dissection and reentry (ADR), percutaneous coronary intervention, retrograde approach.

INTRODUCTION

Successful chronic total occlusion (CTO) recanalization, the last frontier in percutaneous coronary intervention (PCI), improves quality of life. There is significant reduction in angina, arrythmias burden, improved exercise tolerance and left ventricular ejection fraction especially in left anterior descending (LAD) territory.[1-3]

Crossing the wire in direction of blood flow is called antegrade approach and to that of opposite is called retrograde approach. The distal cap of CTO exposed to lower pressures and its tapered configuration with less fibrotic content, makes it often easier to cross.[4]

HISTORICAL PERSPECTIVE

The retrograde CTO approach originated in Japan, later extended to rest of world.[5] The first reported case of CTO (a balloon angioplasty of LAD) done in 1990 by Kahn and Hartzler via saphenous venous graft (SVG).[6] The success rate of CTO increased from ≈70 to 90% over last two decades;[7] however, this comes at a cost of increased complications. CTO's needs to be performed by experienced operators following a standard protocol and algorithms.

INDICATIONS OF THE RETROGRADE APPROACH

- *Primary (upfront) indication in following cases:*[8]
  - Proximal cap ambiguity
  - CTOs with bifurcation at distal cap, to ensure recanalization of both branches
  - Diffusely diseased or poorly visible distal vessel, where in distal reentry is challenging especially in case of subintimal wire entry
  - Aorto-ostial CTOs
  - Difficult to engage CTOs especially anomalous coronaries
- *Secondary indication*: Failed antegrade approach and retry

IDENTIFYING AND CROSSING THE COLLATERALS

Three types of collaterals can be used for CTOs, viz., bypass grafts, septal, and epicardial collaterals. Most commonly used are septal collaterals in nearly 50–60% cases as documented in various PCI CTO registries. saphenous vein graft (SVG) either occluded or patent acts as excellent conduit due to large size, lack of tortuosity, and no side branches.[9]

Based on diameter and collateral connection (CC), Werner classified CC into three categories, viz., CC-0 stands for no angiographically visible connection; CC-1 stands for a threadlike connection (<0.4 mm in diameter); and CC-2 stands for branch-like connection (>0.4 mm in diameter). CC-1 and CC-2 are prerequisite for successful wire crossing. With difficulty CC-0 can also be crossed with "trial and error" or "septal surfing" technique **(Fig. 1)**.[10]

Tip: Order of preference in selecting collaterals

Septal collaterals > SVGs > epicardial collaterals > arterial grafts [e.g., left internal mammary artery (LIMA)][11]

Trick: Ensure adequate vasodilatation followed by dual injection (donor artery first) with projection in right anterior oblique (RAO) cranial, anteroposterior (AP) caudal (do not pan); can excellently delineate septal collaterals and help to understand the entry and exit points.

Collaterals Crossing by Two Methods in CC-0

- Contrast injection (3 cc Luer lock syringe, aspirate blood before injecting) to establish connection (selective and super selective injection)
- "Trial and Error" or "Septal Surfing" technique—blindly crossing without contrast injection

Choice of Guidewire[12]

SUOH 03: This is a wire of choice in our practice for tortuous septal collaterals; It is atraumatic, with SLIP-COAT technology, spring coil, hydrophilic, 3 cm radiopaque segment, and preshaped with 1:1 torque.

Sion Blue (Asahi Intecc Co., Japan) is first choice for selecting the collaterals. A tip load of 0.7 g can be easily and smoothly advanced. Tip is coated with hydrophilic coating and rope coil technology. It facilitates advanced torque, guidewire retention, and flexible atraumatic tip.

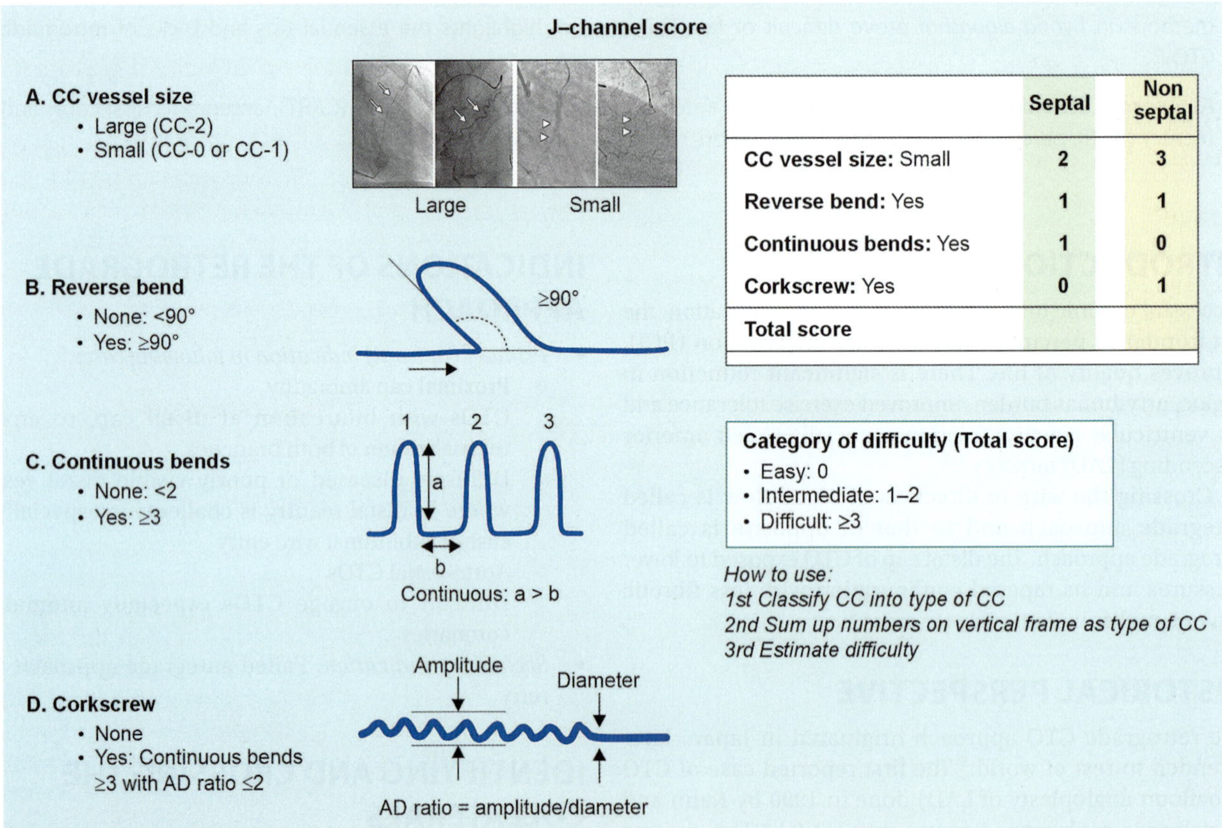

FIG. 1: J-channel scoring system for collateral connections (CC).
(AD: amplitude diameter ratio)

The *Sion Black* wire, is polymer jacketed, and has slip coating with rope coil structure of tip. This makes it better in sliding small channels in smoothly fashion.

Other wire which can be used for fine collaterals is *Fielder XTR* guidewire (Asahi Intecc Co.), which has polymer jacket coating with 0.010 inch tapered tip. This wire is also useful for *septal surfing* (a method used when collaterals are invisible CC-0 angiographically).

Tip: Wiring collaterals is done in a different manner as compared to CTO wiring. While tracking collaterals, wire should be rotated gently to straighten the collaterals while minimizing the forward/backward movements, supported by microcatheters.

- In case of any resistance which is felt during the wiring, always check anatomy in multiple angles (RAO cranial, RAO caudal or laterals), to look for bends and also ectopics. Avoid blind wiring. Injection should be done after checking back flow, for checking the connection at the exit point.

Choice of Microcatheter

Corsair

The Corsair is a first choice in septal collaterals; it includes a hybrid catheter with a polymer coating, tungsten braiding, SHINKA shaft technology with 150-mm length with tapered soft tip.

Caravel

The Caravel is Frontline microcatheter ideal for the navigation of tortuous vessels to facilitate wire exchange. It has hydrophilic coating, 0.019″ tip entry profile, ACTONE Technology braided shaft, and 150-mm working length.

Finecross MG (Terumo Corporation)

The Finecross MG microcatheter is designed with a hydrophilic coating and a tapered tip, facilitating smooth navigation through tortuous vessels. Its enhanced steerability allows for precise lesion crossing during retrograde PCI procedures, improving procedural success rates.

Corsair Pro 150 (Asahi Intecc Co., Ltd.)

The Corsair microcatheter features a unique flat-wire braid technology, 150 cm, providing excellent torque control and flexibility. Its slim profile allows compatibility with various guidewires, enabling deep-seated lesion penetration in complex retrograde PCI cases.

Corsair Pro XS

This is a well-balanced shaft stiffness and SHINKA-shaft, 1.3 Fr tip-entry profile, 150-cm length (85-cm hydrophilic coating), increased tip trackability via more flexible tip, and 10× torque and improved torque transmission.

Turnpike Spiral (Vascular Solutions Inc., now Part of Teleflex)

The Turnpike Spiral microcatheter incorporates a retractable, rotating, and kink-resistant tip, facilitating quick lesion access and minimizing vessel trauma during retrograde PCI procedures.

In difficult entry angulation of septals, a *Crusade* or *Sasuke (dual lumen)* microcatheters or *angulated microcatheters* (*super cross 90° or 120°*) can be used.

In case of difficulty in delivering the microcatheter to distal true lumen following things needs to considered in the order of preference:

- Extra backup for pushability
- Change of microcatheter
- Change of collateral channel

Approach: Bifemoral (7F, 8F), femororadial or biradial

Guide catheters:

- Left—extra back up (EBU)/Xtra back up (XBU); right—amplatz left (AL) (0.75/1/2) (side holes, to prevent conal artery ischemia)
- Retrograde guide catheter ideally be short (90 cm); long epicardial collateral; donor vessel being SVG or LIMA, large heart with high left ventricular diastolic pressure (LVDP)

Activated clotting time (ACT): Using unfractionated heparin, maintain ACT between 300 and 350 seconds. Check ACT every 30 minutes to avoid potential thrombotic complications in donor vessel.

CROSSING THE CHRONIC TOTAL OCCLUSION

Retrograde Wire Escalation

True-to-true (intraplaque crossing) used as a first approach in short-segment CTO (<20 mm), especially when distal tip is tapered; it is the final successful CTO strategy only in 5–10% CTOs.[13,14] Distal cap of CTO is less fibrous than proximal cap, hence easier to cross retrogradely.

Active wire control, is important principle to cross CTO, in this wire follows the true lumen though the lesion by using a guidewire with good trackability.[12] Crossing the CTO without entering subintimal space not only carries a long-term patency but also better safety.

Firstly, soft guidewire such as Fielder XT/XTR/XTA (polymer jacket wires) is attempted.

If polymer jacket wires cannot cross the CTO, wire is escalated to more penetrating wires (GAIA 2, GAIA 3 or ULTIMATEbros-3 (Asahi Intecc Co.)

ULTIMATEbros-3 has long hydrophilic coating except for its wire tip and its torque response is better than miracle 3 g wire.

If CTO is highly calcified then Conquest Pro 12/20, Pilot 200 (Abbott Co.), Hornet (Boston Scientific) can be used.

Recently, Gladius MG/Gladius EX are used to penetrate the distal cap and has an additional advantage of forming a knuckle for retrograde cross.

Retrograde Dissection and Reentry

Reverse controlled antegrade and retrograde tracking (CART) is most commonly used retrograde technique. The antegrade wire is introduced into CTO segment, and balloon dilatation is done on this wire, either in vessel or in subintimal space. Following this, the antegrade subintimal space is automatically connected with retrograde subintimal space, if retrograde wire has already created subintimal dissection.[12] Intravascular ultrasound (IVUS) in antegrade plays important role in determining the position of wires. If both wires obstructed in same plane (intimal or subintimal), then reverse CART technique becomes easy. If one wire is in intimal space and another wire in subintimal space, in this particular subset it is difficult to establish the connection, and one needs to use larger balloon antegradely to create a connection between these spaces **(Figs. 2 and 3)**.

In Knuckle wire technique, we advance retrograde wire with a knuckled tip into subintimal space.

Note: Polymer-jacketed wires like Fielder XT and other wires like Sion Black and Gladius MG are most commonly used for Knuckle technique.

In *directed* reverse CART small balloons are used to minimize vessel damage and in *extended* reverse CART reentry occurs more distally or proximally to occluded segment.

On comparison to reverse CART, in CART technique a balloon is inflated over retrograde wire followed by antegrade wire crossing.

Note: This technique is less frequently used nowadays.

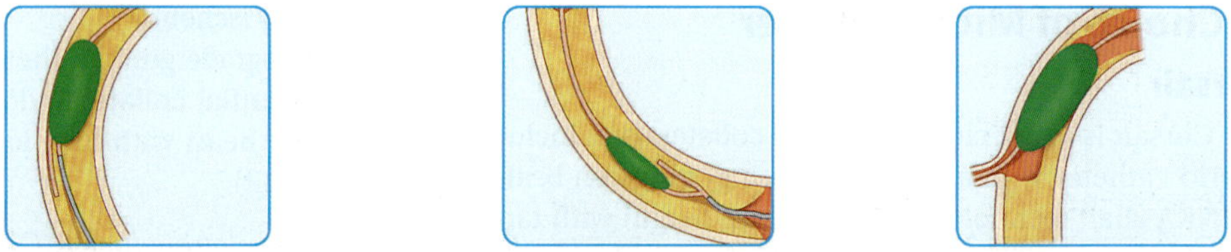

	Conventional	"Directed"	"Extended"
Extent of the intimal/ subintimal space	Within the CTO segment	Within the CTO segment	Beyond the CTO segment (Proximal or distal)
Prior CTO wiring	Antegrade or retrograde	Antegrade	Antegrade or retrograde
Knuckle wire technique (antegrade or retrograde)	Suitable	Unsuitable	Suitable
Antegrade balloon size	Large	Small	Large
Retrograde guidewire	Usually low to intermediate penetration force wire. However, high penetration force wire is required if the antegrade wire is in the subintima and the retrograde wire is in the intima	GAIA series of guidewires (Asahi Intecc)	Proximal extended reverse CART: Low to intermediate penetration force wire, distal extended reverse CART: high penetration force wire
IVUS guidance	Not routinely used, but should be considered if there is difficulty in achieving reverse CART	Not usually needed	Not routinely used, but should be considered if there is difficulty in achieving reverse CART
Suitable cases	CTOs which require bidirectional wiring and which are not suitable for "directed" reverse CART	CTOs with clear proximal cap and occlusion course without heavy calcification, and severe tortuosity	CTOs in which antegrade or retrograde cap penetration is not possible due to ambiguity or calcification
Unsuitable cases	None	CTOs with proximal cap and/or CTO course ambiguity, heavy calcification, and severe tortuosity, short occlusion length (<15 mm), poor retrograde wire control, use of knuckle wire	CTOs with a significant side branch close to the site where extended reverse CART to be performed

FIG. 2: Overview of the three subtypes of the reverse controlled antegrade and retrograde tracking (CART) technique. The essential elements of each technique are described in terms of extent of intimal/subintimal space, prior chronic total occlusion (CTO) wiring, use of knuckle wire technique, antegrade balloon size, necessity of intravascular ultrasound (IVUS) guidance, and suitable and unsuitable cases.[15]

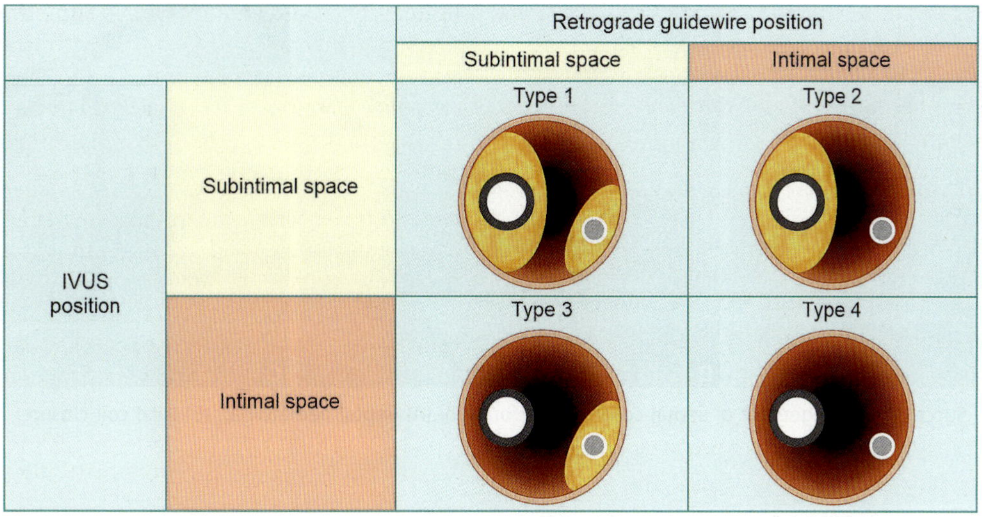

FIG. 3: Intravascular ultrasound (IVUS) position depicting the different planes of antegrade and retrograde wires.

Kissing Wire Technique[12]

If direct retrograde wiring is not possible or microcatheter is not reaching the lumen distal to the CTO, here one can use retrograde wire as a marker for antegrade wiring. In kissing wire technique (KWT) technique, retrograde wire remains intimal and acts as a landmark; whereas antegrade wire is advanced within CTO segment, and meets the retrograde wire at same point, checking in multiple views, and ensures the wire remains intimal.

EXTERNALIZATION OF WIRE AND DRUG-ELUTING STENT DEPLOYMENT

- Once the wire entered the antegrade guide catheter, balloon traps it (2.5 mm balloon for 7F) to facilitate tracking the microcatheter into antegrade catheter.

  Note: Using guide extension catheter in antegrade catheter for wire entry ensure that wire is not subintimal.
- Exchange this wire over microcatheter with most commonly used externalization wire RG3 (Asahi Intecc; 330 cm long, 0.010″)

  Note: The collaterals are always need to be protected by microcatheter while advancing or withdrawal of this wire.
- The externalized RG3 wire is followed on fluoroscopy along the common iliac region. The Y connector is unlocked and then detached from the guiding catheter hub. The retrograde wire is drawn carefully into copilot and then Y connector is reattached to guiding catheter hub. Flushing of the guide should be strictly avoided at this step and 20–30 cm of wire is externalized beyond the Y connector.
- Microcatheter slowly withdrawn into collaterals; now RG3 gives good support to work on the lesion and then stent deployment.
- Before advancing balloon/stenting from antegrade guide over RG3, make sure to disengage the retrograde guide catheter. A torquer should be placed on retrograde end of wire to prevent excessive pull of wire from antegrade side.
- In case of difficulty in microcatheter reaching the antegrade catheter, one can use rendezvous method.[16] In this method, antegrade or retrograde wire is carefully negotiated from one microcatheter to another.
- Under IVUS guidance, drug-eluting stent (DES) deployed over RG3; once procedure is done, a workhorse wire is placed in stented vessel. Carefully microcatheter is withdrawn into donor vessel, a check shoot to confirm any injury to collaterals, and place microcatheter back into septal, over which the RG3 wire is removed.

  Note: At this stage both antegrade and retrograde guide catheters are disengaged to prevent guide catheter induced dissection.

COMPLICATIONS

Donor Vessel Complications

The complications are mainly dissection and thrombosis; dissection is prevented by carefully disengaging catheter while withdrawing retrograde wire/microcatheter or during advancing balloon/stent antegradely. Ensuring adequate ACT of 300–350 seconds during procedure, and checking ACT every 30 minutes helps in preventing thrombosis.

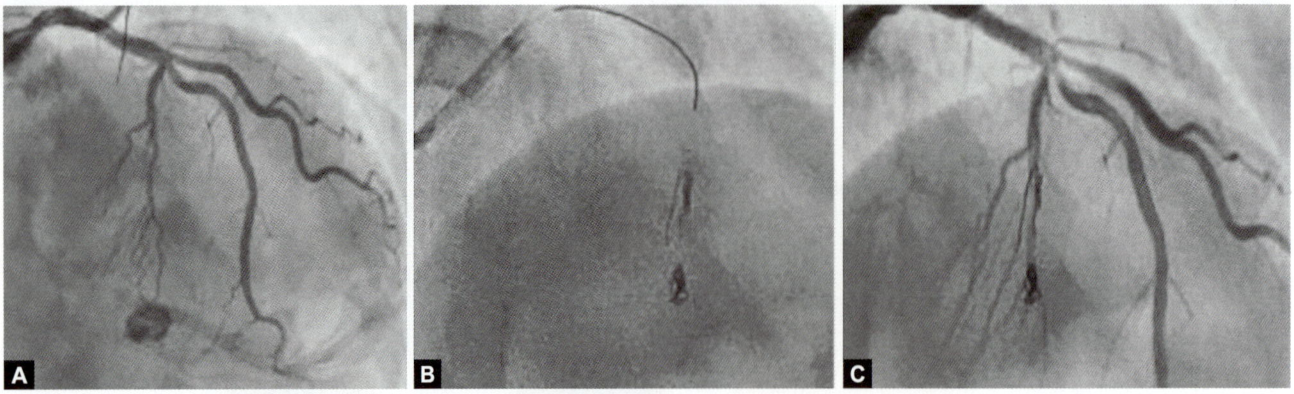

FIGS. 4A TO C: Successful management of septal collateral perforation; (A) Septal hematoma; (B) Hilal coil closure; (C) Sealed septal perforation.

Collaterals Damage

Large epicardial collaterals dissection and impaired flow can result in periprocedural myocardial infarction (MI). Perforation of epicardial collaterals often leads to cardiac tamponade needing pericardiocentesis. The perforation can be sealed by coils (Cook; Hilal 2 mm, 3 mm coils) or thrombin or subcutaneous fat, from both the ends. Never reverse anticoagulation with coronary hardware's inside.

Septal collaterals' perforation is often benign, small perforation needs serial echocardiographic monitoring. However, rapidly expanding septal hematomas can result in impeding ventricular filling[17] which needs prompt sealing using coils, fat or thrombin. The Hilal coils (Cook Medical) can be delivered through Finecross catheter.

Figures 4A to C demonstrate the successful management of rapidly expanding septal hematoma following septal collaterals perforation. Here, 2-mm coils (Cook, Hilal) placed over Finecross 130-cm microcatheter.

Large femoral access puncture should be done with micropuncture technique either fluoroscopy or ultrasonography guided. At the end of procedure access needs to be closed by vascular closure devices (ProGlide or Angio-Seal)

CONCLUSION

Recent advances in retrograde approach made CTO PCI more successful. One needs to be thorough in customary antegrade CTO approach before embarking upon retrograde approach. The limitations and complications associated with CTO PCI indeed call for adequate proctorship and training from an experienced CTO operator.

ONLINE REFERENCES

Please scan the QR code provided at the end of the table of contents for References of this chapter.

CHAPTER

160 Bioresorbable Scaffolds: Present Status

Brian Pinto, Surendra Poonia

ABSTRACT

Percutaneous coronary intervention, which is safe and effective, has become main treatment for coronary artery diseases and has been used widely in clinical practice. Fully bioresorbable scaffolds (BRSs) were designed to overcome the limitations of metallic drug-eluting stent (DES), which permanently cages the vessel wall, thereby preventing normal coronary vasomotion and precludes bypass grafting. A first-generation BRS has been demonstrated to be noninferior to a metallic DES for overall 1-year patient-oriented and device-oriented outcomes. Increased rates of scaffold thrombosis and target vessel-related myocardial infarction were noted that may be mitigated by improved patient and lesion selection criteria and procedural techniques. Large-scale, randomized, clinical trials are ongoing to determine the long-term relative efficacy and safety of BRSs compared with present metallic DES.

Keywords: Bioresorbable scaffolds, percutaneous coronary intervention, coronary artery diseases.

INTRODUCTION

The term "bioresorption" implies the complete elimination of a substance from the body through natural routes (such as kidney or lungs) by dissolution, assimilation, and excretion.[1] It is often confused with the term "bioabsorption." However, both the terms have distinct meanings. "Bioabsorption" in general, means conversion of a compound into another substance. It might not necessarily mean "degradation" or even "elimination from the body".[2] The word "scaffold" in English means a framework or support. In interventional cardiology, the term "vascular scaffold" is used for devices that provide "temporary" arterial support. However, scaffolds are distinct from stents. Stents are not temporary and continue to remain inside the vessels, once implanted.[2] The term "bioresorbable scaffold" (BRS) is used for devices that provide temporary arterial support when implanted and are completely eliminated from the body after a prespecified duration.

WHY BIORESORBABLE SCAFFOLD WAS INTRODUCED FOR TREATING IN CORONARY ARTERY DISEASE AND POTENTIAL ADVANTAGES OF BIORESORBABLE SCAFFOLD?

Simple angioplasty with balloon dilation, which was the first percutaneous treatment for obstructive coronary artery disease was associated with several challenges, such as vascular recoil and acute vessel closure due to occlusive coronary dissection.[3,4] Bare-metal stents (BMSs), which followed, also had significant rates of in-stent restenosis.[5] Moreover, the rate of neointimal hyperplasia inside the stent was even higher than that with plain balloon angioplasty, again requiring repeat procedures in several patients.[1] Further advancements led to the development of drug-eluting stents (DESs), which have further evolved with the use of more biocompatible or biodegradable polymers, thinner struts, and new antiproliferative drugs. Nevertheless, concerns about late and very late stent thrombosis (VLST) continue. It is presumed that this might be due to the continued presence of a permanent metallic foreign body in the coronary arteries.[2] Hence, the concept of a device that does the job, means provides short-term vessel support and inhibits early constrictive remodeling and then disappears, started the journey of BRS.

Bioresorbable scaffolds have obvious potential advantages over current metallic DES technology, as indicated below:

- A lower incidence of adverse events such as ST. With BRS, drug elution and scaffolding are temporary and provided by the device only until the vessel has healed. No foreign material, such as nonendothelialized struts and drug polymers, remains behind over the long term. Since these are potential triggers for ST, elimination of these materials reduces the rate of ST.[1]
- A stented vessel is subjected to rigid caging. However, with BRS the caging ceases to persist once the scaffold is bioresorbable. This can facilitate resumption of vessel vasomotion, adaptive shear stress, late luminal enlargement, and late expansive remodeling.[1]
- *Fewer bleeding complications*: It is assumed that once bioresorption of the temporary scaffold has been completed, long-term dual antiplatelet therapy (DAPT) might not be required. This is especially important in case of elderly patients who are at the highest risk of bleeding.[6]
- *A potential for providing better treatment options in the future*: Many patients have complex multivessel disease, for which multiple and long DES are often used. These patients are also likely to require repeat percutaneous or surgical revascularization in the future. The repeat procedures are potentially challenging because of the metallic cages formed by previously implanted DES. The absence of cages with the use of BRS is likely to ease the procedures for future revascularization.[5]
- The use of BRS also makes it feasible to use noninvasive imaging techniques such as computed tomography (CT) angiography or magnetic resonance imaging (MRI) for follow-up.[8] Even for BRSs that use metallic materials, CT or MRI can be performed once bioresorption has been completed. The currently used metallic stents can cause a blooming effect with these imaging modalities, making interpretation more difficult.
- The use of BRS alleviates concerns that some patients have about having an implant in their bodies for the rest of their lives.[2]

A comparison of advantages and disadvantages of metallic stents, DES, and BRS is shown in **Table 1**.

A general timeline of biovascular scaffold (BVS) resorption and its interactions with the vessel wall is shown in **Figure 1**.

HISTORY OF BIORESORBABLE SCAFFOLD

The efforts to create BRS started about 30 years ago. The first experimental studies used nonbiodegradable polyethylene terephthalate braided mesh stents in porcine animal models in 1992.[9] Later, in 1996, the Wiktor stent was implanted in porcine coronary arteries. This stent was coated with five different types of biodegradable polymers (polyglycolic acid/polylactic acid copolymer, poly caprolactone, polyorthoester, polyhydroxybutyrate/valerate copolymer and polyethylene oxide/polybutylene terephthalate). However, it led to marked inflammation inside the arteries leading to neointimal hyperplasia and/or thrombus formation.[10] Subsequently, Lincoff et al., compared the outcomes of a stent coated with high-molecular weight poly-L-lactic acid (PLLA) (321 kD) versus those with low-molecular weight PLLA (~ 80 kD) implanted in a porcine model. They found that the stent with high-molecular weight PLLA was well tolerated and effective, while that with low-molecular weight PLLA was associated with an intense inflammatory neointimal response. They also

TABLE 1: Potential advantage of bioresorbable scaffold.[2]

	Balloon angioplasty	Bare-metal stent	Drug-eluting metallic stent	Bioresorbable scaffold
Acute occlusion	–	+	+	+
Acute stent/scaffold thrombosis	Na	–	±	+
Subacute stent/scaffold thrombosis	Na	–	–	+
Acute recoil	–	+	+	+
Constrictive remodeling	–	+	+	+
Neointimal hyperplasia	–	–	+	+
Expansive remodeling	+	–	–	+
Late luminal enlargement	+	–	–	+
Late stent/scaffold thrombosis	Na	–	–	+

Note: "+" implies prevented or not restricted, while "–" implies not prevented, or restricted. Na = not applicable because of absence of stent.

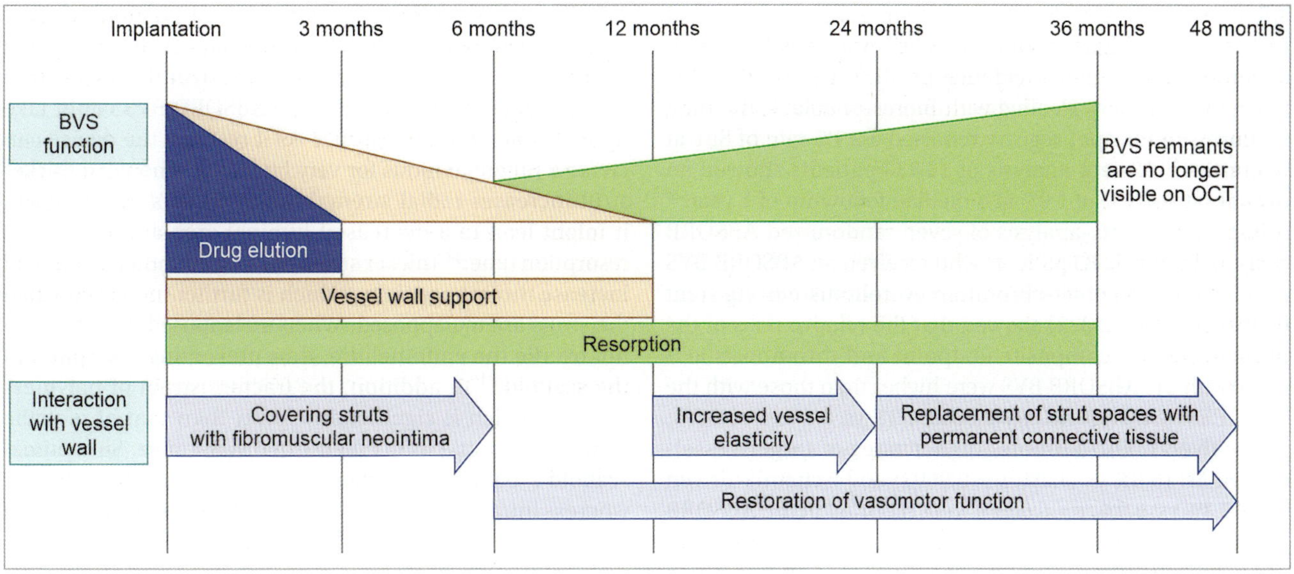

FIG. 1: A general timeline of bioresorbable vascular scaffolds (BVS) resorption and its interactions with vessel wall.[32]

proved the feasibility of drug-elution from PLLA, although no suppression of neointimal hyperplasia was reported.[11] Subsequently, in 1998, Yamakawa et al. reported that a fully biodegradable PLLA stent with a tyrosine kinase inhibitor effectively suppressed proliferative stimuli caused by balloon injury in a porcine model.[12]

In 2000, the Igaki-Tamai PLLA-based scaffold was the first BRS to be implanted in humans. Tamai et al. reported initial results from 15 patients in whom 25 scaffolds were successfully implanted. At 6 months, the restenosis rate and target lesion revascularization (TLR) rate per lesion were 10.5%; the rates per patient were 6.7%.[13] Long-term data with >10 years of follow-up of 50 patients implanted with 84 Igaki-Tamai biodegradable stents showed high cumulative TLR of 16% after 1 year, 18% after 5 years, and 28% after 10 years. Further development of this BRS was discontinued because it required a large 8-French guide catheter for delivery. Moreover, there was a potential for vessel wall injury from this heat-treated, self-expandable device.[14]

Nevertheless, researchers continued to refine the BRS technology leading to the development of the ABSORB BVS in 2009. The first-generation device (BVS 1.0) was tested in the ABSORB Cohort A in 30 patients. The 2-year cumulative incidence of major adverse cardiovascular events (MACE), including the composite of cardiac death, myocardial infarction (MI), and TLR was 3.4%, with no scaffold thrombosis (ScT). The in-stent late loss of 0.48 mm and the diameter stenosis of 27% did not differ from the findings at 6 months. Moreover, 34.5% of struts were not seen on optical coherence tomography (OCT), and the remaining visible struts were fully apposed. The study proved that BRS was noninferior to the best available DES during the resorption phase.[15,16] Further, the 5-year clinical follow-up also showed no ScT, only one case of non-Q-wave MI, and a MACE rate of 3.4%. This showed that the risk of occurrence of cardiac events was theoretically neutral once the scaffold had been fully resorbed after 3 years.[17,18] The second-generation BVS (BVS version 1.1) was tested in the ABSORB cohort B trial in 101 patients who had simple atherosclerotic lesions. At 6-month follow-up, 45 of the 101 patients included in the trial (cohort B1) showed a modest reduction in lumen area on intravascular ultrasound (IVUS) and OCT.[19] These favorable results persisted at the 12-month follow-up of the remaining 56 patients (cohort B2).[20] IVUS and OCT reports at baseline and at 12-month follow-up showed that the scaffold area remained unchanged. 5-year OCT follow-up of 53 patients in cohort B without TLR showed no visible struts. There was formation of a neointimal layer resembling a thick fibrous cap during the vascular healing process, which suggested that ABSORB BVS might facilitate the formation of stable endothelium.[21] Based on these favorable outcomes of observational trials and multiple randomized clinical trials, absorb BVS received the CE mark in 2011.[22] The device was also approved by the US Food and Drug Administration (FDA) in 2016.[23] However, these early studies of the ABSORB BVS only included patients with stable angina and largely excluded patients with complicated lesions.[24] Subsequently, the ABSORB II trial comparing ABSORB BVS versus XIENCE everolimus-eluting metallic stent showed a higher rate of composite endpoint due to target vessel MI, including periprocedural MI, in the ABSORB group. The patient-oriented composite endpoint, anginal status, and exercise testing were not statistically different between both devices at 3 years.[25] Similarly, the AIDA (Amsterdam Investigator-Initiated Absorb Strategy All-Comers Trial) that compared the ABSORB BVS with everolimus-eluting metallic stent in a real-world patient population, the rate of definite or probable device thrombosis in the scaffold group was about

3.5 times higher than that in the stent group over a period of 2 years. The higher incidence of ScT was associated with a significantly higher incidence of MI.[26] The GHOST-EU (Gauging Coronary Healing with Bioresorbable Scaffolding Platforms in Europe) registry reported a 2.1% rate of ScT at 6 months.[27] A meta-analysis of 16,830 patients showed an overall rate of ScT of 1.8% at a median follow-up of 1 year.[28] A large-scale meta-analysis of seven randomized ABSORB trials including 5,583 patients who received an ABSORB BVS (n = 3,261) or a cobalt-chromium everolimus-eluting stent (CoCr-EES) (n = 2,322) showed that the relative risks of the device-oriented composite endpoint and thrombosis at 2 years with the ABSORB BVS were higher than those with the CoCr-EES (9.4% vs. 7.4%, $p = 0.0059$, 2.3% vs. 0.7%, $p < 0.0001$, respectively). Furthermore, higher rates of target vessel-related MI (5.8% vs. 3.2%, p = 0.0003) and ischemia-driven TLR (5.3% vs. 3.9%, $p = 0.0090$) were reported in the ABSORB BVS groups, with similar levels of cardiac mortality in both groups.[29] Furthermore, in the ABSORB Japan trial, definite ScT occurred in 1.6% of the patients between the first and second year after implantation.[30] Cases of ScT have also been reported as late as 44 months after implantation.[31] These induced the manufacturer, Abbott Vascular, to discontinue the commercialization of ABSORB BVS.[32] Nevertheless, one recently reported trend from the later analyses of ABSORB III and ABSORB Japan trials is that period of excess risk ends with the time point of complete resorption of ABSORB BVS within ~3 years. Moreover, there seems to be no sign of a high rate of all patient- and device-oriented endpoints for the ABSORB BVS over the CoCr-EES between 3 and 5 years.

WHY THE FIRST BIORESORBABLE SCAFFOLD FAILED?

The most prominent feature of a BRS is bioresorption. Therefore, it is essential that materials used in the manufacture of BRS should have high biocompatibility and flexibility as well as mechanical properties to prevent scaffold fractures during implantation. It should also be able to allow some elastic shrinkage in later stages. Moreover, the process of degradation of BRS needs to match the time taken for the healing of coronary artery lesions. Hence, the BRS needs to provide effective support to the arterial wall for at least 6 months after implantation.[33]

The early BRSs were mainly composed of PLLA monopolymer. PLLA is a type of semicrystalline polymer that usually requires 2–3 years to be almost completely resorbed in vivo.[34] However, compared with traditional stent materials, such as steel or CoCr, PLLA has poorer mechanical properties such as stiffness and ductility. Its elasticity, which is important for providing radial strength is 66 times lesser than that of CoCr.[35] Inadequate ductility affects the crimping ability of BRS and limits its expansion range because the polymer can easily break during deployment.[36] Hence, to be able to provide support to the vessel equivalent to that by metallic stents, scaffolds prepared from PLLA have thicker struts to compensate for the reduced tensile and radial strength.[34] Absorb BVS had a 157 µm strut thickness. Due to the higher strut thickness, the ABSORB BVS could take up to 4 years to fully resorb.[37] As it resorbs, the device can create a potential nidus for very late ScT.[24] Though a thicker strut increases radial strength and prevents vessel recoil, it might lead to a decreased luminal area and prolonged resorption time.[38] Thicker struts prolong endothelization and increase thrombogenicity, which is further increased when the struts are malapposed. When malapposed, the struts do not overlie the endothelium, thus preventing resorption of the scaffold.[24] In addition, the fracture strain of polymers is 2–6%, which is significantly lower than that of metallic stents at 40%, and limits their expansion range. Suboptimal scaffold expansion and malapposition can lead to early ScT, whereas intraluminal scaffold dismantling might be the main mechanisms leading to late or very late ScT.[36]

FURTHER EVOLUTION OF BIORESORBABLE SCAFFOLD

Contemporary BRS devices are made of either a metallic alloy (magnesium or iron alloy) or L-isomer PLLA polymeric platform, covered with a polymer and an anti-proliferative drug. Recently, Zn alloy (Zn-3Ag) has also been suggested to be a promising material for BRS devices.[7] The new-generation BRSs use materials that are absorbable and have stronger mechanical properties. Use of such materials allows the manufacturers to provide thinner struts and smaller crossing profiles.[34] The latest generations of BRS (®MeRes100, Meril Life Science, Gujarat, India; ®Mirage, Manli Cardiology, Singapore; ®MAGNITUDE, Amaranth Medical, Mountain View, CA, USA; and ®Firesorb, MicroPort, Shanghai, China) have considerably lesser strut thickness through innovations in design.[40] Thinner struts facilitate easier delivery, reduce shear stress on the vessel wall, reduce blood flow turbulence, improve endothelization, and reduce thrombus formation. Thinner struts have also been shown to reduce restenosis and periprocedural MI rates. Through these innovations in stent and strut design, lower-profile scaffolds have been made possible without compromising on radial strength.[39]

Key design characteristics of current BRS technologies are shown in **Table 2**. As of now, six BRS devices have received the CE mark, namely, ABSORB (Abbott), Magmaris (Biotronik), Fantom (REVA Medical), DESolve (Elixir Medical), MeRes100 (Meril Life Sciences), and ART Pure (Arterial Remodeling Technologies). Outcomes of clinical trials with the new generation BRSs are shown in **Table 3**. As of now, 2-year outcomes are available for most of them, and some of them have shown promise with no cases of ScT and TLR at 2 years.

The 2018 European Society of Cardiology (ESC) guidelines on myocardial revascularization recommended that any BRS should not be used outside well-controlled clinical studies.[41]

TABLE 2: Key design characteristics of current bioresorbable scaffold technologies.[2]

SCAFFOLD	Manu-facturer	Strut material	Coating material	Eluted drug	Strut thickness (µm)	Crossing profile	Radio-pacity	Scaffold absorption (MONTHS)	Drug dose and release kinetics
Igaki-Tamai	Kyoto Medical	PLLA	None	None	170	N/A	Gold markers	24–36	NA
BVS 1.1 (Absorb GT1)	Abbott Vascular	PLLA	PDLLA (7 µm)	Everolimus	156	1.4 mm	Platinum markers	24–36	75% of drug eluted within 30 days Drug dose: 100 µg/cm²
DREAMS-2 (Magmaris)	Biotronik	93% Mg+ 7% rare earth elements	PLLA (1 µm)	Sirolimus	150	1.7 mm	Metallic markers	9	100% of drug eluted in 3-6 month Drug dose: 1.4 µg/mm²
Fantom	Reva Medical	Iodinated. Des-amino-tyrosine polycarbonate	Same as backbone (NA)	Sirolimus	125	1.3 mm	Intrinsic radio-pacity	36–48	60% of drug eluted within 30 days Drug dose: 197 mg/cm²
DESolve Nx (First gen)	Elixir	PLLA	BD polymer and drug matrix (<3µm)	Novolimus	150	1.5 mm	Metallic markers	12–24	>85% of drug eluted within 30 days Drug dose: 3 mg/mm
DESolve Cx (Second gen)					120	1.3 mm	Metallic markers	12–24	>85% of drug eluted within 30 days Drug dose: 5 mg/mm
MeRes 100	Meril Life Sciences	PLLA	PDLLA (3–4 µm)	Sirolimus	100	1.2 mm	Platinum markers	Up to 24	100% of drug eluted within 90 d Drug dose: 1.25 µg/mn²
ART Pure	ART	PDLLA	None	None	170	6-Fr compatible	None	18–24	NA
Mirage	Manli cardiology	PLLA	PLLA (NA)	Sirolimus	125 (<3 mm) 150 (>3.5 mm)	1.12–1.47 mm	Metallic markers	14	NA
Fortitude	Amaranth	Ultra-high-molecular-weight PLLA	PDLLA	Sirolimus	150	6-Fr compatible	None	10	Drug release profile: N/A
Firesorb	Shanghai Micro-Port Medical	PLLA	PDLLA (<5 µm)	Sirolimus	100–125	NA	Metallic markers	36	Drug dose: 4 µg/mm

Continued

Continued

SCAFFOLD	Manu-facturer	Strut material	Coating material	Eluted drug	Strut thickness (µm)	Crossing profile	Radio-pacity	Scaffold absorption (MONTHS)	Drug dose and release kinetics
Xinsorb	Shandong Huaan Bio-technology	PLA, PCL, PGA	PDLLA and PLLA	Sirolimus	160	NA	Platinum markers	24–36	70% of drug eluted within 30 days
			(NA)						Drug dose: 140 µg/mm^2
NeoVas	Lepu	PLLA	PDLA	Sirolimus	170	NA	Platinum markers	24	Drug dose: 15.3 µg/mm
			(NA)						
IBS	Life Tech	Nitrided iron	PLA	Sirolimus	70	5-Fr compatible	Gold	Effective support for 6 months and complete degradation in about 18 months	Drug dose: 5 µg/mm
IDEAL BioStent	Xenogenics	PLA	(NA)	Salicylate and sirolimus	200	NA	NA	9 months	Drug dose: 8.3 µg/mm
ArterioSorb	Arterius Ltd	PLLA	PDLA	Sirolimus	95	1.2 mm	Platinum	18–24 months	
HARTSORB	Hartlon	PLLA	None	None	90	1.3 mm	NA	Not available	NA
Bioheart	Bioheart	PLLA	PCL	Sirolimus	125	NA	NA	NA	NA
JMDT	JMDT	Magnesium	(NA)	Sirolimus	100	1.2 mm	NA	12 months	NA

[PCL: polycaprolactone; PDLLA: Poly(D,L-lactic acid); PGA: poly(glycolic) acid; PLA: poly lactic acid; PLLA: poly-L-lactic acid]

TABLE 3: Clinical trials of various bioresorbable scaffold.[39,49]

	No. of patients	Angiographic follow-up	LLL (months)	Clinical follow-up (months)	Scaffold thrombosis (%)	TLR (%)
MeRes 100	108	6	0.15 ± 0.23	24	0	0
Mirage	35	12	0.37 ± 0.14	12	3.4	7.2
Aptitude	60	9	0.33 ± 0.36	24	0	0
Magnitude	70	9	0.19 ± 0.16	9	0	0
Neovas	31	6	0.26 ± 0.32	24	0.4	3.2
Xinsorb	27	6	0.18 ± 0.21	30	3.3	3.3
Firesorb	45	6	0.15 ± 0.11	24	0	0
DESolve NX	122	6	0.20 ± 0.32	60	7.4	0
Fortitude	63	24	0.27 ± 0.37	24	4.9	1.8
Fantom	117	6	0.25 ± 0.40	24	4.2	0.8
Magmaris	1,075	12	0.52 ± 0.39	36	4.3	0.5

Some recently published systematic reviews and meta-analyses have shown poor outcomes of BRS versus DES. This might be possibly because most studies included in the meta-analyses used the ABSORB stent. In a 2022 systematic review and meta-analysis of 17 studies by Smith et al. comparing outcomes of BRS (n = 6,438) versus DES (n = 5,481), 91% of the BRS population studied received ABSORB. They found that ScT following BRS implantation was significant (3.47 times higher than that with DES at 2 years), started early (the first 30 days), and remained durable throughout the 5 years of follow-up (2.99 times greater risk than that with DES at 5 years). However, while there was an increased relative risk of ScT with BRS versus DES, the overall incidence of this complication was low (2.05% and 0.69% at latest follow-up, respectively), and its overall clinical relevance was limited, with equivocal all-cause mortality and revascularization rates observed across all time points. Moreover, the primary outcomes demonstrated a relative plateau in the total event rate in the BRS group after the dissolution period. There was a decrease in the relative risk between the 3-year and 5-year follow-ups.[42] In 2023, Sharifkazemi et al. investigated randomized clinical trials conducted over the last 10 years to compare the incidence rates of VLST with BRSs versus DESs. They included 11 studies; however, out of the 4,615 patients who received BRS, 3,085 (69%) received ABSORB. Thus, the outcomes of ABSORB had a significant influence on the results of the meta-analysis. The findings of this systematic review showed that the frequency of VLST was the same in the two groups in most of the investigated studies, and a significant difference was observed in this respect in only three RCTs. The results of the BIOFLOW V study ($n = 884$ received BRS, $n = 450$ received DES), which was included in this meta-analysis showed the superiority of BRS over DES, as no patient in the BRS group suffered ScT in the 1- to 3-year follow-up, while VLST was reported in 0.7% of the patients in the DES group. Meanwhile, the incidence of some clinical complications, including target vessel MI, ischemia-driven TLR, cardiac death or any MI, and composite of major adverse clinical event was reportedly higher in the 3-year follow-up of the DES group compared to that in the BRS group.[43]

It is important to remember that BRS has a lifespan of almost 3 years;[44] thus, the incidence of thrombosis will remain unchanged after the scaffolds are absorbed, and BRSs could perhaps prove superior with longer follow-ups.[43] The availability of later follow-up data from more recent and long-term follow-ups of the new generation BRSs is awaited.

OPTIMAL BRS DEPLOYMENT

Besides the drawbacks of the BRS design and material, the adverse outcomes in early clinical trials were attributed to two common procedure related factors, such as underexpansion and malapposition.[45] Several studies have reported that stent undersizing is a key factor for ST among patients receiving DES or BRS.[46-48] BRS struts are 150 μm thick, which is approximately 65–70% more thicker than DES and that makes it difficult to expand. In addition, in contrast to DES, BRS cannot be overexpanded. Therefore, more precise device sizing by intravascular imaging is essential. Other possible mechanisms of failure of BRS include (1) limited visibility of BRS preventing the operators from performing adequate postdilation; (2) BRS deployment in small vessels (reference vessel diameters of < 2.25 mm); and (3) strut fracture either due to disruption of the plastic scaffold, malapposition, or prolapse of struts into the lumen during the dissolving process.[49]

In order to deploy BRS optimally and to reduce complications, an algorithm was developed called *"five P's"*—(1) *p*roper sizing of the vessel by intravascular imaging; (2) *p*reparation of the lesion; (3) *p*aying attention to the expansion limits; (4) *p*ostdilation using an optimally sized noncompliant balloon; and (5) DAPT *p*ostprocedure.[49] In the ABSORB III trial, postdilation was performed in only 60% of patients after BRS deployment. In addition, intravascular imaging was performed in only 11% of patients to optimize BRS deployment. This further contributed significantly to the failure of the device apart from the PLLA-only material and strut thickness.[49]

1. *Proper sizing of the vessel by intravascular imaging*: Accurate assessment of the vessel size, plaque properties, and lesion characteristics is a crucial step before BRS implantation.[49] It is very important to select the appropriate scaffold size to match the coronary artery lesions. Implantation of an undersized and presumably malapposed scaffold might affect endothelial healing, as a result of which the scaffold is at risk for collapsing into the lumen and dragging the associated tissue, accelerates the formation of ScT.[34] Coronary angiography is associated with a tendency toward underestimation of the vessel size as compared with intravascular imaging.[50] Under coronary angiography, BRS has poor visibility, and the extent of stent degradation and vascular repair cannot be accurately judged, making it difficult to conduct the risk stratification of ScT and optimization of an antithrombotic treatment strategy.[34] Intravascular imaging is helpful in vessel sizing before implanting the BRS. Moreover, during the implantation process, intravascular imaging can help in obtaining the best vascular imaging results and detect immediate conditions such as the adherence of scaffolds, inadequate expansion, and edge dissection.[34] OCT as an intracoronary imaging modality allows for more accurate detection and quantification of BRS malapposition, underexpansion, tissue prolapse, and stent edge dissection. The four sides of the BRS struts can be seen on OCT.[49] A study demonstrated that OCT imaging guidance had a great influence in making decisions, with 16.4% of OCT pullbacks indicating the need for a different scaffold size. Subsequently, all patients underwent a postexpansion strategy under the guidance of aggressive systematic angiography; nevertheless, 31.8% of lesions still needed additional expansion when OCT was used after BVS deployment. OCT-guided postdilation led to a minimal scaffold area increase of 0.8 mm^2 (12.7%) and corrected the malapposition in nearly one-third of lesions.[51] Thus, OCT seems imperative for proper vessel sizing before BRS implantation and reliance on angiography might not be appropriate.
2. *Preparation of the lesion*: Before inserting the BRS, an appropriate size of noncompliant balloon should be used to predilate the vessel with a ≥1:1 balloon-to-reference vessel diameter ratio to obtain residual 20–40%

stenosis in two orthogonal views. This greatly reduces the risk of thrombosis. Additionally, the use of a cutting/scoring balloon facilitates BRS sizing and achieving optimal scaffold expansion in complex lesions prior to BRS implantation.[52] A meta-analysis of the data from the 5 ABSORB prospective studies demonstrated that aggressive predilation with a ≥1:1 balloon-to-artery ratio and optimal postdilation were independent predictors of freedom from ScT and TLF between 1 and 3 years [hazard ratio (HR) 0.44; $p = 0.03$, and HR 0.55; $p = 0.05$, respectively].[53]

3. *Paying attention to the expansion limits*: The time of balloon expansion should be extended to 30 seconds during stent deployment, which could fully expand BVS and allow obtaining a larger luminal diameter.[34]
4. *Postdilation*: A retrospective study showed that underexpansion (11.8%) was one of the common causes of ScT.[54] As per recent recommendations, a noncompliant balloon should be inflated up to 16–25 atm, with a nominal diameter up to 0.25–0.50 mm larger than that of the scaffold size. Postdilation should result in residual stenosis <10% in two orthogonal views and ensures that the entire scaffold opposes to the vessel wall.[34]
5. *Post-PCI DAPT*: After BRS implantation, the optimal duration of DAPT has yet to be determined.[49] According to current guidelines, the duration of DAPT after DES implantation in patients with stable ischemic heart diseases should be at least 6–12 months. For acute coronary syndrome patients, 12 months of DAPT is advised. Since scaffolds gradually degrade overtime, they avoid permanent implant residuals in blood vessels and theoretically shorten the time course of DAPT. There is no large-scale prospective randomized trial that support short duration of DAPT following BRS stenting will produce adverse effects.[34]

Follow-up of BRS after deployment by OCT may be required to determine the percentages of covered struts, the extent of neointimal coverage, and struts dismantling. OCT is a key imaging technique for the accurate assessment of scaffold absorption during follow-up.[49]

CONSIDERATIONS ON PATIENT AND LESION-SPECIFIC CHARACTERISTICS

Patient-related Characteristics

There are many patient-related factors involved in ST of DES have been reported. The clinical factors linked with ST vary in different time intervals. For early ST, MI and heart failure are major risk predictors.[55] Cardiogenic shock is especially predisposing condition because it adds insufficient coronary perfusion, liver dysfunction, and impaired drug absorption.[56] For late ST, renal failure and diabetes mellitus are predisposing factors, and history of malignancy is the strongest predictor of late ST [odds ratio (OR) 17.5; 95% confidence interval (CI) 4.7–65.3] because of a prothrombotic state and a high risk of DAPT-related bleeding.[7] As these predisposing factors affect the overall condition of the patient, confirmation of a similar association with ScT after BRS implantation can be expected.

Lesion-related Characteristics

ST is more common in complex lesion subsets after DES implantation. A study showed that lesion complexity was correlated significantly with early ST (adjusted OR 2.33; 95% CI 1.40–3.89).[57] Similarly, the challenge of lesion complexity remains with BRSs and may even be increased.

According to the recent clinical experience, implanting vessels with reference diameters of <2.25 mm and >3.75 mm is not recommended. Since BRSs tend to have thicker and wider scaffolds, ScT risk is increased after BRS implantation in small vessels (<2.25 mm).[53] Moreover, we should be cautious to avoid scaffold dislocation in regard to BRS implantation in large diameter vessels.

The BRS implantation in bifurcated lesions with already increased risk of ScT is challenging. A substudy from the GHOST-EU registry showed that ScT rate (2.5%) with BRSs was higher than that with contemporary DES in bifurcation lesions. It is suggested that the operator should make the decision on BRS size according to the proximal or distal reference diameter of the individual patient. BRS implantation in the main branch was performed before the proximal optimization technique. Side branch side opening, proximal optimization technique, and final proximal optimization technique are recommended when required.[58] Furthermore, due to the bulky design of BRSs, it is relatively difficult to put BRS into side branch through main branch-BRS struts. A conventional DES is usually the first choice if side branch stent is required.[59]

Calcified lesions commonly lead to underexpansion, an important contributory factor causing to ScT. Based on present clinical experience, calcification is not a contraindication for BRS implantation. Panoulas et al. have now proven that it is allowable to implant BRSs in adequately prepared calcified lesions and indicated that the cumulative 14-month rates of MACE were similar in noncalcified lesions (12.9% vs. 10.9%, $p = 0.546$).[60] However, BRS implantation is not recommended for heavily calcified lesions that are unlikely to be properly dilated.

Ostial lesions also represent a challenging subset due to concerns for acute recoil and restenosis in long term. The GHOST-EU registry demonstrated that treatment of coronary ostial lesions was an independent predictor of device-oriented composite endpoint [$p = 0.0025$; HR 2.65 (1.41–4.97)]. The risk of ScT at 12 months was significantly higher than that in nonostial lesions (4.9% vs. 2.0%, $p = 0.005$). Notably, the unsatisfactory incidence of ScT in ostial lesions might be due to a low rate of intravascular imaging guidance (32%) and postdilation (43%), which could lead to malapposition and under expansion of scaffolds.[61]

Presently, the clinical application of BRSs is commonly limited to simple lesions, and data among the high-risk population about the performance of BRS are mostly blocked. This leads to a lack of recommendations on approaches for complex lesions. Future clinical trials should have less exclusion criteria for evaluating the safety and effectiveness of BRSs and gaining more clinical experiences.

CURRENT LIMITATIONS

Few possible benefits of BRS are only seen in animal testing or small human cohorts, for example, the effect of restoring vasomotion. Most data are being derived from small, nonrandomized studies on patients with stable coronary artery disease. Hence, relatively few patients were treated and experience in complex lesions (e.g., bifurcation and ostial lesions, relatively long lesions, and small diameter vessels) or other clinical scenarios (e.g., acute coronary syndrome) are limited. In complex lesions, intravascular imaging should aid BRS implantation.

There is concern regarding strut thickness, which is greater than in conventional stents and may lead to vessel wall injury, platelet aggregation, nonlaminar flow, and poor deliverability. Thus, mechanical considerations seem more challenging when calcification or tortuosity is present. As it requires predilation and postdilation, prolonged balloon inflation time more induced myocardial ischemia might be associated with BRS implantation as compared to DES. Some BRS has low radial strength and poor deliverability in complex lesions; prolonged and more predilation is required, which can lead to higher risk of dissections that might require longer and/or multiple stents. Due to increased risk of scaffold fracture with overdilation, significant upsizing of BRS is not possible. Other limitations are availability of scaffold sizes, and need of special facilities for storage of some of BVS. In addition to this, the total cost and duration of PCI with a BRS are much higher than with a conventional DES.

At present, the optimal duration of DAPT with BRS implantation is not clearly recommended.

Multiple processes, including release of active drugs and polymer resorption, could adversely affect metal DES. This is illustrated by acquired malapposition, in the sense of defective healing, compared with the lack of stent strut apposition at the end of the procedure. Thus, defective healing and late adverse reactions may not be completely avoided with BRS.

Present BRS limitations will be possibly resolved in the near future. Although BRS's have more advantages than their disadvantages but still large randomized controlled trials are needed to support their use in complex lesions.

FUTURE

Recent data from the new-generation BRS shows the potential clinical benefits of contemporary BRS. Going ahead, the thinner struts of contemporary BRS devices and the use of routine intravascular imaging for optimal deployment might improve outcomes further. For optimal outcomes, thinner struts, newer design characteristics, appropriate patient selection, and standardized techniques of implantation guided by intravascular imaging seem to be the way forward. BRS is considered as a promising treatment option for ST-elevation myocardial infarction (STEMI) patients because these patients are often young and the ruptured plaques are usually soft with a small plaque burden. However, the results with the first-generation BRS in this population were not encouraging.[62-66] Results of the new-generation BVS in STEMI patients are awaited.

Other than coronary artery disease, the use BRS is also extending to peripheral arteries and gastrointestinal system. In the gastrointestinal system, the implantation of BRS can avoid repeated stent implantation and removal to drain obstructed biliary or pancreatic ducts in patients with obstructive biliary disease.[36] Other studies have reported promising outcomes with the use of BRS in peripheral arterial disease.[67-71]

CONCLUSION

In conclusion, the BRS technology holds promise. The long-term outcomes of future and currently ongoing trials with new-generation BRSs as well as ongoing device development focusing on new materials and thinner struts is likely to lead to its wider adoption in real-world practice.

ONLINE REFERENCES

Please scan the QR code provided at the end of the table of contents for References of this chapter.

CHAPTER

161

Multivessel Coronary Artery Disease with Left Ventricular Dysfunction: Management Strategies

Dev Pahlajani

ABSTRACT

Coronary artery disease is one of the most common lifestyle diseases in developed and developing countries. Despite the fact that an increasing number of acute myocardial infarction (AMI) patients are being treated by primary percutaneous coronary intervention (PCI) or fibrinolytic therapy, about 30% of patients have residual left ventricular dysfunction associated with significant obstructive coronary artery disease. About 60% of patients with left ventricular dysfunction have associated coronary artery disease. Several observational and randomized trials have been reported to compare the outcomes of treatment in this subset of patients. Three modalities of treatment have been the subject of such studies: (1) Medical treatment that essentially consists of guidelines-directed medical treatment (GDMT) with diuretics, renin–angiotensin receptor blockers, angiotensin receptor neprilysin inhibitors along with antiplatelets and statins and, whenever needed, cardiac resynchronization therapy with defibrillator (CRTD); (2) surgical treatment that consists of coronary artery bypass graft (CABG) with or without surgical ventricular reconstruction (SVR), with mitral valve replacement whenever indicated; and (3) PCI. Several of these studies have indicated that CABG is associated with a reduced risk of death, MI, or revascularization and rehospitalization when compared to PCI. The STITCH trial that compared CABG with GDMT failed to show advantage of CABG over medical treatment over 6-year follow-up. However, further 10-year follow-up has shown that CABG was associated with better outcomes as compared to medical treatment, particularly in younger patients. The recently published REVIVED-BCIS2 trial enrolled 700 patients and compared outcomes of all-cause death or hospitalization for heart failure with PCI and optimum medical therapy. At a median follow-up of 41 months, the incidence of PCI failed to show benefit over medical treatment. Therefore, the weight of evidence seems to be optimized for medical treatment, and in the event the patient continues to experience symptoms, CABG could offer a better quality of life.

Keywords: Heart failure, left ventricular dysfunction, coronary artery disease, coronary artery byass graft surgery, percutaneous coronary artery intervention.

INTRODUCTION

Coronary artery disease is the most common cause of left ventricular dysfunction (LVD). Despite advances in percutaneous coronary interventional (PCI) treatment and coronary artery bypass graft (CABG), a significant number of patients have residual scar and/or hibernating myocardium following episodes of acute coronary syndrome (ACS) or acute myocardial infarction (AMI). Any busy cardiovascular (CV) surgical or PCI team will encounter 25–30% of patients with multivessel coronary artery obstruction with reduced ejection fraction (EF) in their departments. The incidence of significant coronary artery disease and heart failure is being more commonly observed due to the improved survival following an episode of AMI or ACS. Subsequent to an attack of AMI, residual left ventricular ejection fraction (LVEF) of <50% is reported in about 75% of patients.[1] It is estimated that the prevalence of heart failure in the developed and developing world is 2–2.5% of the population, and in about 60% of them, ischemic heart disease happens to be the culprit. These patients have higher mortality than those with nonischemic LVD.

THERAPEUTIC OPTIONS

Since coronary artery obstruction is responsible for LVD in this subset of patients, it would seem logical that revascularization with CABG or PCI will improve left ventricular function and CV outcomes. With this assumption, several patients have been subjected to CABG or PCI. A question also arose whether it is important to perform viability studies with positron emission tomography (PET) scan, magnetic resonance imaging (MRI), or dobutamine stress echo and the choice of appropriate and reliable viability studies. The data from observational and randomized trials has been conflicting.

One must not forget the fact that several of these patients have complex coronary artery disease such as chronic total occlusion, diffuse and calcified vessels, and associated comorbidities such as diabetes, hypertension, and renal dysfunction. In such patients it may not be possible to achieve complete revascularization and high risk of stroke following CABG could be responsible for post procedural adverse outcomes.

There are several other factors that are responsible for suboptimal outcomes following revascularization. These patients have microvascular dysfunction, reduced coronary blood flow reserve, mitochondrial dysfunction, anaerobic metabolism, and increased diastolic blood pressure resulting in additional myocardial ischemia. Usual viability studies will fail to unmask such factors.

Left ventricular remodeling and loss of normal geometry are considered as some of the major risk factors for severe LVD, and unless surgical left ventricular reconstruction is performed at the time of CABG, results will be suboptimal. Scar tissue and/or changes in the refractoriness of the conduction system of the left ventricle could be responsible for life-threatening arrhythmias and sudden death.

EARLIER TRIALS

Most of the earlier trials comparing medical versus surgical treatment have been observational and retrospective and were conducted with the assumption that CABG will improve outcomes by as much as 50% over medical treatment in patients with LVD and coronary artery disease. However, it would be unfair to extrapolate their conclusions to contemporary medical treatment since drugs such as angiotensin receptor blockers, beta-blockers, and aggressive lipid-lowering did not form the part of medical treatment. Today, the thrust of the medical treatment for LVD and coronary artery disease has been on diuretics, beta-blockers, renin-angiotensin-aldosterone blockers, and angiotensin receptor neprilysin inhibitor (ARNI). Such guideline-directed medical treatment (GDMT) has certainly made a favorable impact on reducing mortality, decreasing hospitalizations, and improving symptoms. Automatic implantable cardioverter-defibrillator (AICD) or cardiac resynchronization therapy with a defibrillator could be added tools to nonsurgical treatment to improve outcomes.

Most of the earlier trials of medical versus surgical treatment or CABG versus PCI excluded patients with low EF. The COURAGE[2] trial excluded patients with severe LVD. In the very early stages, the CASS study conducted by the National Heart and Lung Institute that compared medical versus surgical treatment excluded patients with <35% EF. In a subgroup of 78 selected patients with three-vessel disease and LVEF of 35–50%, the 5-year mortality was 10% with CABG and 19% when assigned to medical treatment.[3] Even among one of the most studied contemporary trials - SYNTAX trial enrolled 2% of patients who had LVEF of <35%. FREEDOM trial enrolled only 32 patients who had EF of <40%. The ISCHEMIA trial was the only earlier trial that showed some benefit of invasive approach. This trial reported a reduced incidence of cardiac events in patients with ischemia on imaging tests and heart failure with EF of 35–40% **(Fig. 1)**.[5] Those with moderate ischemia without heart failure had no statistical difference in major cardiac events between invasive and conservative treatment.

Moreover, data that favored CABG over GDMT came from observational and retrospective studies.

COMPARING SURGICAL VERSUS PERCUTANEOUS CORONARY INTERVENTION

Most of the trials that compared CABG versus PCI enrolled very few patients with reduced EF. In the BARI trial,[6] there were only 22% of patients with low EF. However, this was in the era when the drug-eluting stents (DES) were not available. In these trials, data on the subset of patients with LVD and coronary artery revascularization versus medical treatment is lacking.

DATA FROM THE STITCH TRIAL

The STITCH trial was the first prospective randomized controlled trial to investigate whether CABG in patients with LVEF <35% will improve outcomes in the patients who were receiving GDMT.[7] Patients with Canadian Heart Association Functional class 3 or 4 angina and those with left main coronary artery stenosis were excluded from surgical revascularization. The trial enrolled 1,212 patients with EF of 35% or less and coronary artery disease from 99 sites in 22 countries. GDMT patients received renin-angiotensin-aldosterone inhibitors, beta-blockers, antiplatelet agents, and statins, with digoxin and diuretics when needed. 602 patients received medical therapy alone and 610 were randomized to medical therapy and CABG. The primary outcome was death from any cause, and secondary outcomes included rates of deaths from CV cases and death from any hospitalization from any cause. The trial, in its earlier follow-up of 56 months,

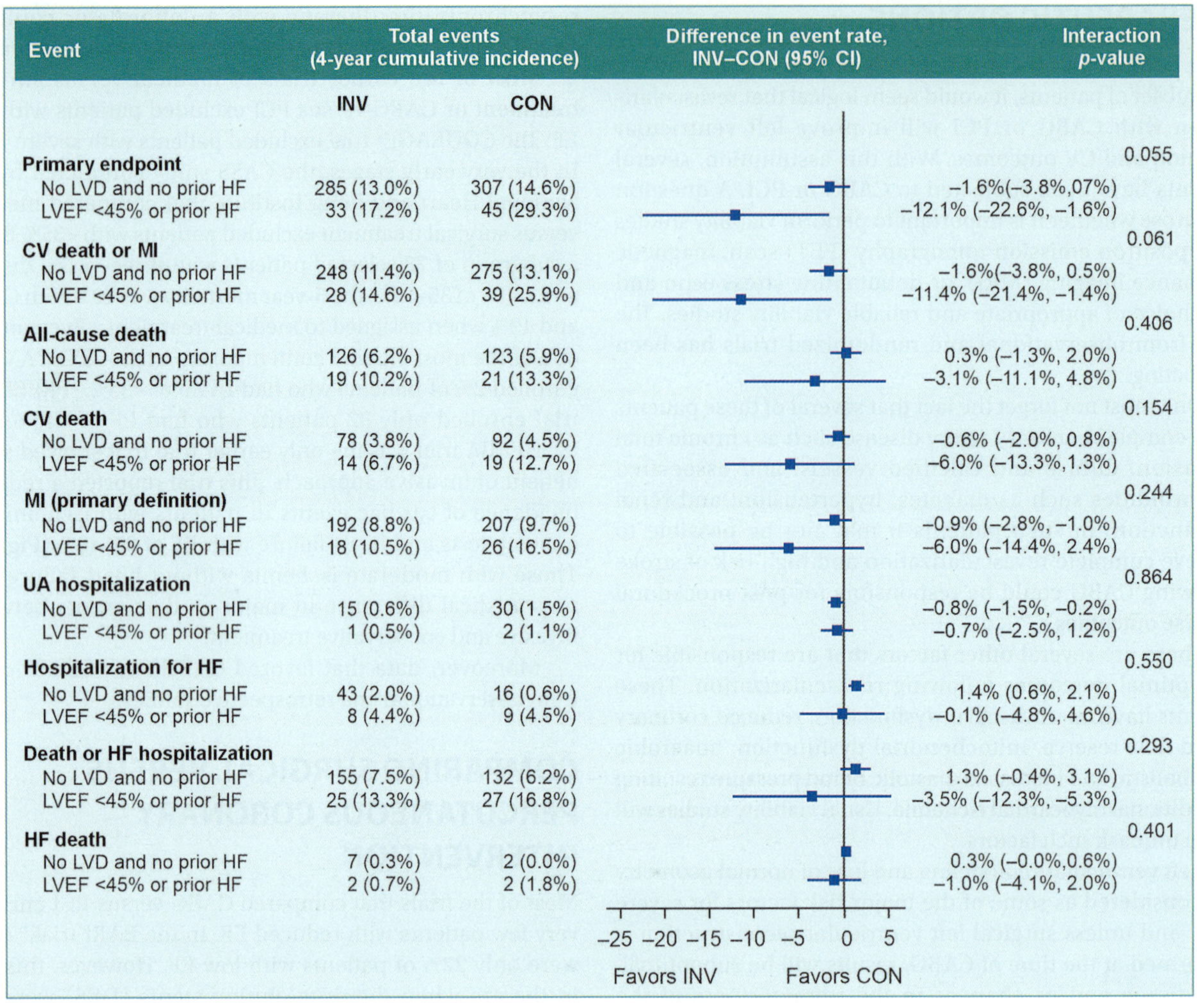

Event	Total events (4-year cumulative incidence) INV	CON	Difference in event rate, INV–CON (95% CI)	Interaction p-value
Primary endpoint				0.055
No LVD and no prior HF	285 (13.0%)	307 (14.6%)	−1.6%(−3.8%,07%)	
LVEF <45% or prior HF	33 (17.2%)	45 (29.3%)	−12.1% (−22.6%, −1.6%)	
CV death or MI				0.061
No LVD and no prior HF	248 (11.4%)	275 (13.1%)	−1.6%(−3.8%, 0.5%)	
LVEF <45% or prior HF	28 (14.6%)	39 (25.9%)	−11.4% (−21.4%, −1.4%)	
All-cause death				0.406
No LVD and no prior HF	126 (6.2%)	123 (5.9%)	0.3% (−1.3%, 2.0%)	
LVEF <45% or prior HF	19 (10.2%)	21 (13.3%)	−3.1% (−11.1%, 4.8%)	
CV death				0.154
No LVD and no prior HF	78 (3.8%)	92 (4.5%)	−0.6% (−2.0%, 0.8%)	
LVEF <45% or prior HF	14 (6.7%)	19 (12.7%)	−6.0% (−13.3%,1.3%)	
MI (primary definition)				0.244
No LVD and no prior HF	192 (8.8%)	207 (9.7%)	−0.9% (−2.8%, −1.0%)	
LVEF <45% or prior HF	18 (10.5%)	26 (16.5%)	−6.0% (−14.4%, 2.4%)	
UA hospitalization				0.864
No LVD and no prior HF	15 (0.6%)	30 (1.5%)	−0.8% (−1.5%, −0.2%)	
LVEF <45% or prior HF	1 (0.5%)	2 (1.1%)	−0.7% (−2.5%, 1.2%)	
Hospitalization for HF				0.550
No LVD and no prior HF	43 (2.0%)	16 (0.6%)	1.4% (0.6%, 2.1%)	
LVEF <45% or prior HF	8 (4.4%)	9 (4.5%)	−0.1% (−4.8%, 4.6%)	
Death or HF hospitalization				0.293
No LVD and no prior HF	155 (7.5%)	132 (6.2%)	1.3% (−0.4%, 3.1%)	
LVEF <45% or prior HF	25 (13.3%)	27 (16.8%)	−3.5% (−12.3%, −5.3%)	
HF death				0.401
No LVD and no prior HF	7 (0.3%)	2 (0.0%)	0.3% (−0.0%,0.6%)	
LVEF <45% or prior HF	2 (0.7%)	2 (1.8%)	−1.0% (−4.1%, 2.0%)	

FIG. 1: ISCHEMIA trial improved outcome with surgical treatment in reduced ejection fraction (EF).

(CON: conservative; CV: cardiovascular; HF: heart failure; INV: invasive; LVD: left ventricular dysfunction; LVEF: left ventricular ejection fraction; MI: myocardial infarction; UA: unstable angina)

Source: With permission from Lopes et al. (2020).[5]

found no significant difference between surgically treated patients and those treated with medical treatment. The primary outcome occurred in 41% of the medically treated group and 36% in the CABG group [hazard ratio (HR) with CABG 0.86% and $p = 0.12$] **(Figs. 2 and 3)**. However, patients assigned to CABG had lower rates of death from CV causes and death from any cause or hospitalization from CV causes as compared to medical treatment (HR with CABG 0.74% and p value = <0.001). When taking into account crossover as per protocol, there was an overall benefit of CABG when compared with medical treatment only. Further, CABG resulted in better quality of life and symptom relief. Subsequently, 10-year follow-up of patients in the STITCH trial demonstrated a reduction in all-cause mortality in patients with heart failure who received CABG and medical treatment versus GDMT only. The reduction in all-cause mortality in CABG was most pronounced in younger patients, whereas the beneficial effect on CV mortality was found to be consistent in all ages **(Figs. 4A to F)**.[8]

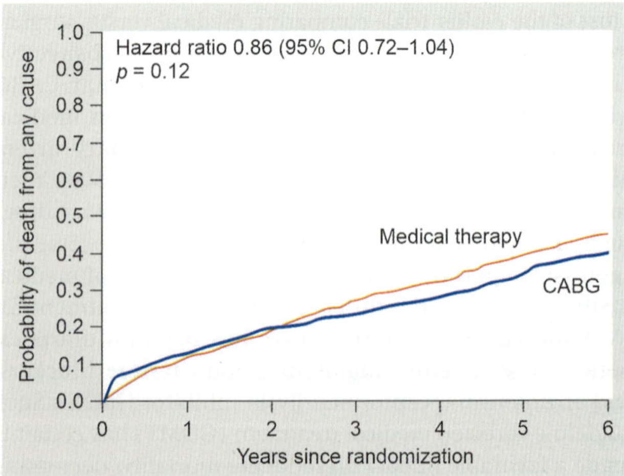

FIG. 2: STITCH trial. Kaplan–Meier curves for probability of death from any cause.

(CABG: coronary artery bypass graft; CI: confidence interval)

Source: With permission from Velazquez et al. (2011).[7]

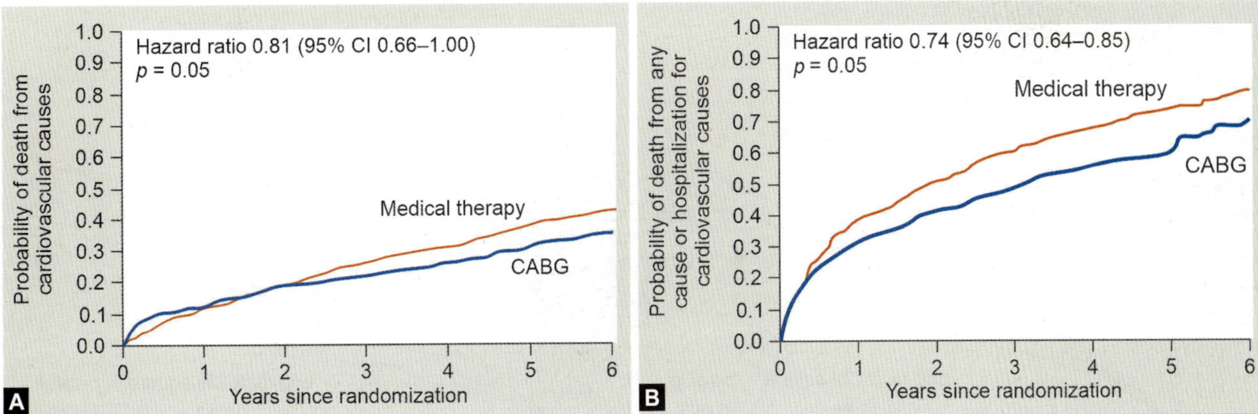

No. at risk (A)

Medical therapy	602	532	487	435	312	154	80
CABG	610	532	486	459	340	174	91

No. at risk (B)

Medical therapy	602	387	315	260	158	65	28
CABG	610	431	375	334	221	100	43

FIGS. 3A AND B: STITCH trial. Probability of death from cardiovascular cause and hospitalization.
(CABG: coronary artery bypass graft; CI: confidence interval)
Source: With permission from Velazquez et al. (2011).[7]

A meta-analysis of 21 studies by Wolff et al.[9] included 16,191 patients that compared the outcomes of patients with EF < 40% with coronary artery disease. Compared with medical treatment, there was a significant reduction in mortality with CABG [HR 0.73; 0.66, 95% confidence interval (CI) 0.62–0.85; $p < 0.001$] and PCI (HR 0.73; 95% CI 0.62–0.85; $p < 0.001$). CABG showed better survival as compared to PCI.

CORONARY ARTERY BYPASS GRAFT VERSUS PERCUTANEOUS CORONARY INTERVENTIONAL

While the results of CABG in patients with LVD and coronary artery disease have been equivocal, there have been studies to compare the role of PCI versus CABG. Cummings et al. from the United Kingdom[10] reported their data of 321 patients with multivessel coronary artery disease and LVEF of <30%.

This was a retrospective study wherein 214 underwent CABG (94 on-pump and 120 off-pump), and 107 had PCI with second-generation DES. Patients who underwent PCI had higher 10-year mortality compared to CABG. Patients operated by off-pump surgery had better outcomes than on-pump surgery (HR = 1.86 with p value <0.012 for on-pump CABG; HR = 2.32 with p value of 0.001 for off-pump CABG).

Bangalore et al.[11] compared CABG with PCI in patients with severe LVD. This, again, was not a randomized trial, and patients were selected from the New York state for PCI system and cardiac surgery reporting system registries. They identified 4,616 patients and studied the outcomes with everolimus-eluting stent in 1,351 patients and CABG in 3,265 patients. PCI was associated with a lower risk of stroke when compared to CABG. Death was similar in both groups. However, there was a higher risk of myocardial infarction (MI) and a higher risk of repeat revascularization in the PCI group **(Figs. 4A to F)**.

Sun et al.[12] retrospectively analyzed outcomes in 12,113 patients with LVEF < 35%. 2,397 underwent PCI, and 2,397 underwent CABG. The median follow-up was 5.2 years. Patients who underwent PCI had significantly higher mortality, death from CV disease and subsequent revascularization, and hospitalization for MI and heart failure as compared to matched surgically treated patients.

Similarly, Nagendra et al.,[13] from Alberta, Canada, analyzed outcomes of propensity-matched 2,925 patients, out of whom 1,326 underwent CABG and 1,599 received PCI. At 1, 5, 10, and 15 years, CABG had better survival and less repeat revascularization as compared to PCI.

Recently, Perera et al. published their data from the REVIVED-BCIS2 trial.[14] The aim was to ascertain whether multivessel PCI would improve event-free survival in LVD with coronary artery disease. This was a randomized trial that included 700 patients and randomized 347 to either PCI or 353 to optimum medical treatment. 39% were diabetics. The primary composite outcome was death from any cause or hospitalization for heart failure. Major secondary outcomes were LVEF at 6 and 12 months and quality of life scores. Over a median of 41 months, the primary outcome of all-cause mortality or hospitalization for heart failure occurred in 37.2% of the PCI group compared to 38.0% of optimal medical treatment ($p = 0.96$). All-cause mortality in the PCI group was 31.7% and 32.6% in the medical treatment group. There was no significant difference in LVEF at 1 year in both the groups **(Fig. 5)**.

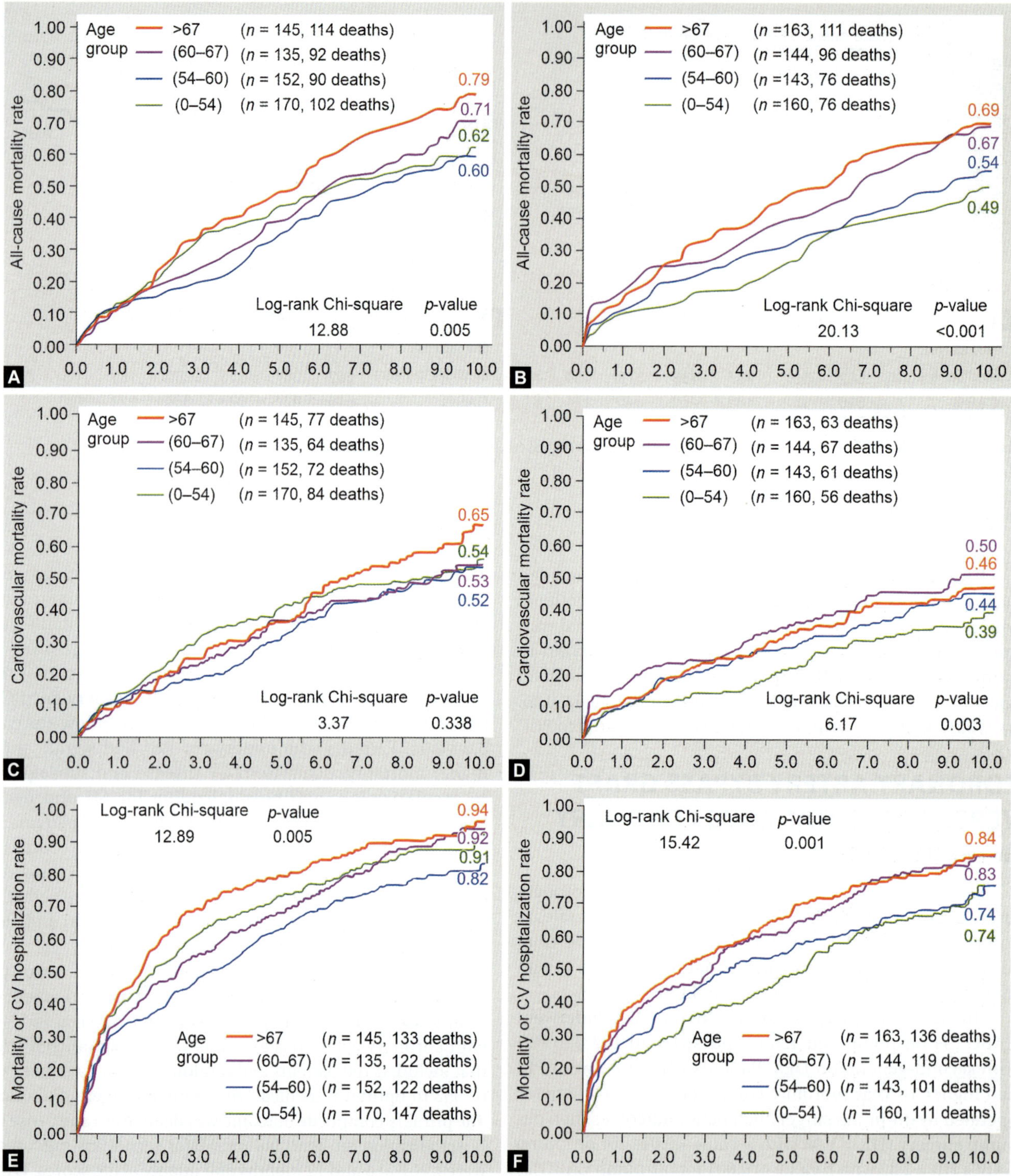

FIGS. 4A TO F: STITCH trial: 10-year follow-up for all cause—cardiovascular (CV) death as per age.

(CABG: coronary artery bypass graft; CI: confidence interval)

Source: With permission from Petrie et al. (2016).[8]

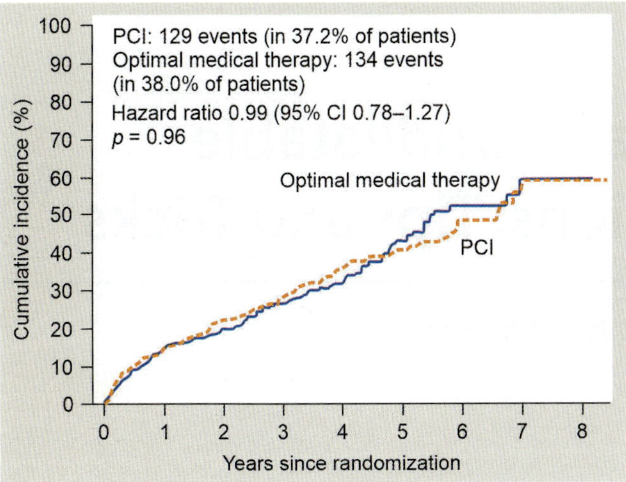

FIG. 5: REVIVED-BCIS2 trial.

(CI: confidence interval; PCI: percutaneous coronary intervention)

Source: With permission from Perera et al. (2022).[14]

ROLE OF VIABILITY

There has been a plethora of work done to assess whether viability studies by single-photon emission computed tomography (SPECT), PET or cardiac magnetic resonance imaging (CMRI), or a simpler inexpensive test like dobutamine stress echo could provide adequate information on the presence or absence of viable myocardium in the setting of reduced left ventricular function. Presence of viable muscle could be attributed to stunned or hibernating myocardium. Hibernating myocardium is defined as hypocontractile myocardium due to persistently low blood supply, while stunned myocardium is hypocontractile myocardium due to transient ischemia followed by reperfusion that usually exists for several hours or days. Enough information is available that ischemia-guided revascularization would provide greater benefit in reducing symptoms, death, and revascularization. One of the most valuable indicators of viability would be the presence of angina symptoms. However, other pathophysiological factors could be responsible for angina, namely microvascular disease, ventricular dilatations, left ventricular remodeling, and reduced cardiac output. Patients in the STITCH trial were enrolled regardless of viability. Initially, SPECT was required to be enrolled in the study. Subsequently, due to low recruitment, the protocol was revised to accept patients who also underwent low-dose dobutamine echo testing. Only 601 patients underwent viability testing. Viability testing failed to identify patients who would benefit from CABG. Myocardial viability was not associated with improved survival. This indicates that several other factors such as patient comorbidities, arrhythmias, and left ventricular remodeling are also very important factors for mortality in these patients.

The American College of Cardiology/American Heart Association 2013 guidelines for the management of heart failure indicate that, in the absence of angina, CABG may be considered for improving survival in patients with ischemic heart disease who have severe LVD, whether or not viable muscle is present (class IIB, level of evidence B).[15]

In light of the scientific data available, it seems that patients with coronary artery disease and LVD should be given a chance of CABG, may be along with surgical ventricular reconstruction (SVR) and mitral valve replacement.

The European Society of Cardiology, in its 2021 guidelines, has given class IIa with level of evidence B to CABG for patients suitable for surgery, especially those with diabetes and multivessel disease, and for those with persistent angina and coronary anatomy suitable for revascularization despite GDMT.[16]

Those with suitable anatomy and major left anterior descending (LAD) and left main obstruction may be subjected to revascularization after careful evaluation and involvement of the heart team.

The role of viability testing is limited.

Coronary artery bypass graft seems to be a preferred mode of revascularization compared to PCI.

As per the data available so far, PCI has not shown superiority over optimum medical therapy.

CONCLUSION

The data shows that surgical treatment with CABG, along with SVR and/or mitral valve replacement, has an edge over medical treatment. PCI has failed to show superiority over medical treatment. However, whenever the patient has symptoms with associated comorbidities and frailty, whether surgery may carry higher operative mortality, PCI will give a good option to give relief to the operated patient. Viability studies have failed to make a choice between GDMT and revascularization strategy. CABG, if performed at a younger age, is associated with better outcomes over 10-year follow-up as shown in the STITCH trial.

ONLINE REFERENCES

Please scan the QR code provided at the end of the table of contents for References of this chapter.

CHAPTER

162 Uncrossable and Undilatable Coronary Lesions: Tips and Tricks

Anil Sharma, Anushree D Kumbhalkar

ABSTRACT

The uncrossable coronary lesions are those lesions that cannot be crossed with a balloon after successful guidewire crossing. These lesions are challenging and are commonly encountered in tortuous and calcified arteries as well as chronic total occlusions. These procedures utilize longer procedural times, radiation dose, and contrast volumes with a lower likelihood of procedural success. Various step-by-step algorithmic strategies have been described to treat balloon uncrossable lesions, which usually starts with a simple cost-effective technique such as the use of a small, low-profile balloon followed by techniques that increase guide catheter support, for example, use of a buddy or extra supportive wire, guide extension catheter, or balloon anchor technique. The final approach includes various complex strategies of plaque modification, such as the use of microcatheters, wire cutting or puncture techniques, atherectomy, laser, and subintimal modification techniques. Sequential and simultaneous application of these techniques can result in the successful treatment of these challenging lesions. Furthermore, some of these lesions, even when crossed by balloon, may remain difficult to dilate and prepare for stenting.

In this chapter, we describe the tips and tricks for managing balloon uncrossable and/or undilatable coronary lesions utilizing various treatment modalities.

Keywords: Balloon uncrossable coronary lesions, undilatable coronary lesions, chronic total occlusion.

INTRODUCTION

The balloon uncrossable lesions are defined as lesions that cannot be crossed with a balloon after successful guidewire crossing and confirmation of the guidewire position in the true lumen. These lesions are challenging and are commonly encountered in day-to-day percutaneous coronary interventions (PCIs), particularly in tortuous and calcified arteries as well as chronic total occlusions (CTOs), particularly with higher Japanese chronic total occlusion (J-CTO) score.[1] In the PROGRESS-CTO registry, the prevalence of balloon uncrossable lesions following successful guidewire crossing was 9.0%, whereas the prevalence of balloon uncrossable or balloon undilatable lesions was 15.5%, and the prevalence of balloon undilatable lesions was 8.5%.[2]

These lesions require multiple treatment modalities and were associated with longer procedural times, radiation dose, and contrast volumes with a lower likelihood of procedural success. Several stepwise algorithms are available **(Flowchart 1)** for treating balloon uncrossable lesions and can be broadly categorized into (1) small balloon techniques, (2) techniques that increase guide catheter support, (3) various advanced plaque modification strategies, such as the use of microcatheters, atherectomy, laser, and (4) subintimal modification techniques.[3] Sequential and simultaneous application of these techniques can result in successful treatment of these challenging lesions.[4]

BALLOON UNCROSSABLE LESIONS

First-line Strategies: Balloon Selection

Small Balloon or Balloon Wedge (Nose Dive) Technique

Adequate lesion preparation requires an expanded noncompliant (NC) balloon sized 1:1 with the arterial

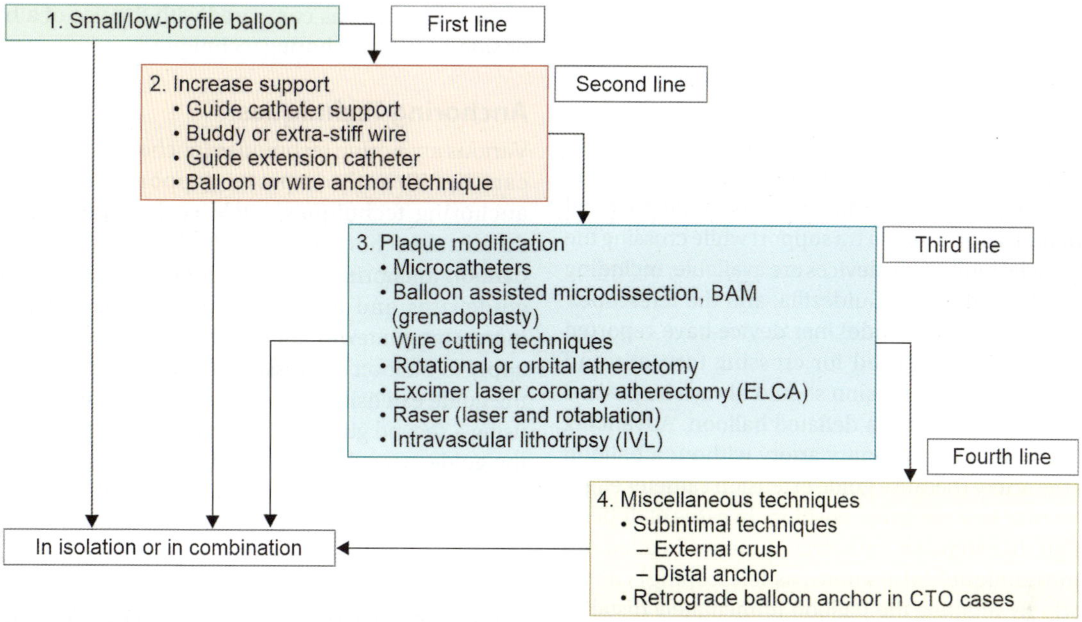

FLOWCHART 1: Stepwise algorithm for an approach to balloon uncrossable lesion.
(BAM: balloon-assisted microdissection; CTO: chronic total occlusion)

diameter. When an NC balloon fails to cross a lesion, the first step in most cases is to use a low-profile semi-compliant balloon with lubricious coatings. Examples include the 1.0 mm Sapphire Pro, 1.2 mm Mini-Trek, 0.85 mm Nano, Sprinter Legend, Across CTO, Apex Push, and chocolate balloons. Oscillating the balloon in a forward and backward motion is a technique based upon the physical principle that dynamic friction is less than static friction and may help with crossing resistant lesions.[1]

If the balloon stops advancing, it can be inflated while maintaining continuous forward pressure on the balloon with a little pull on the wire. We advise maintaining continuous forward pressure while deflating the balloon to facilitate balloon advancement. This may dilate the entry (modify proximal cap) into the lesion and allow crossing, sometimes with the same balloon (balloon-wedge technique). Alternatively, another new balloon can be used.[5] Slight balloon rotation may help sometimes, but care has to be taken to avoid balloon entrapment. Sometimes, reshaping of balloon tip or use of a new balloon from some other manufacturer may work. Be gentle in applying pressure because too much pressure may result in losing the guidewire, and ostial or distal dissection/perforation.

Sometimes, inflation with a larger diameter balloon just proximal to the lesion may disrupt the architecture of the proximal cap enough to allow subsequent passage of a small-profile balloon or microcatheter.[6] A new ultralow-profile balloon for resistant uncrossable lesions, particularly in CTO PCI, has been introduced, the blimp balloon. However, limited experience exists so far.[1]

Second-line Strategies: Increase Support

Guide Catheter Support

The use of a supportive guide catheter can be the difference between success and failure. Active and passive support can be increased by selecting different-shaped guides (for coaxial engagement) or those with larger diameters (7Fr or 8Fr).[1] Supportive guiding catheters [such as Amplatz left (AL) catheter for the right coronary artery (RCA) and extra-backup (EBU/XB) catheter for the left coronary artery] use the support of the contralateral wall of the aorta and help with coaxial alignment. Alternatively, coaxial guide engagement can be achieved by keeping a deflated balloon on a buddy wire such that half of its length remains inside the guiding catheter. Deep engagement of the guiding catheter into the artery provides active support. However, as the catheter size increases, there is potential for complications from dissection and pressure damping.[7] Refrain from injecting contrast in case of pressure damping. Femoral access may be better than radial access for using larger guiding catheters in complex procedures. Alternatively, a long sheath can be used to increase guide support. In case of ostial dissection, follow three fundamental steps: (1) Stop injecting dye, (2) do not lose the wire position, and (3) immediately do ostial stenting before dealing with a distal lesion.

Wire-based Support Techniques

An extra supportive wire, for example the Wiggle wire, can be used while dealing with balloon uncrossable lesions.[1]

The buddy wire technique requires negotiating a second wire through the lesion to enhance support, straighten tortuous bends, and reduce friction from wire bias.[1]

Guide Catheter Extensions

Guide catheter extensions allow deep engagement into the artery, traversing calcification and tortuosity in the proximal artery segment. This provides extra support while crossing the highly resistant lesions. Many devices are available, including the Heartrail II, GuideLiner, Guidezilla, and the telescope.[1] Two case series using the GuideLiner device have reported a 93% success rate when used for crossing tortuous and calcified lesions.[8] Guide extension should always be pushed into the coronary artery over a deflated balloon. Advancing guide extension into the coronary artery without a balloon can dissect the artery (because guide extension catheter edges are sharp) or may lose the guide position. In cases of difficult delivery of guide extension catheters, a method called the "inch-worm technique" (also known as telescoping) can be used. It works by inflating the balloon immediately distal to the guide extension catheter, and as the balloon is deflating, the guide extension catheter is advanced. The balloon is then further advanced, and the steps are repeated until the guide extension catheter is past the lesion. This is usually the most efficient way to advance the guide extension catheter. Another balloon anchoring technique (applicable in balloon undilatable and not in balloon uncrossable lesions) includes inflating the balloon distal to the lesion and advancing the GuideLiner while the balloon is still inflated. A guide extension catheter and an anchor balloon can also be used with two French discrepancies (i.e., 8Fr with 6Fr or less).[1] While injecting contrast through the guide extension, make sure that you have reduced the flow rate, contrast volume, and pressure settings on the power injector.

In a randomized trial, the use of a 5-in-6 (Fr) guide extension catheter was more effective and efficient in facilitating the success of transradial PCI for complex coronary lesions, as compared with the use of a buddy wire or side-branch anchoring technique.[9]

Anchoring Techniques

Various anchoring techniques (anchor wire/anchor balloon) can significantly improve support. There are various anchoring techniques, such as the side branch anchor, the distal anchor, and the coaxial anchor technique. Distal balloon anchoring requires crossing of the lesion with two guidewires and a balloon, and coaxial anchoring is for increasing guidewire support; hence, those techniques do not apply to balloon uncrossable lesions.[4] Coaxial anchoring of the guide extension catheter can sometimes be employed by using a second guide catheter to advance a balloon alongside the guide extension catheter; balloon inflation increases the support of the guide extension, further enhancing equipment delivery.[4] The side branch anchor technique **(Figs. 1A and B)** involves the advancement of a workhorse guidewire into a side branch (usually a conus or acute marginal branch for the RCA or a diagonal for the left anterior descending artery or obtuse marginal for circumflex artery), followed by a small balloon (usually 1.5–2.0 mm in diameter depending on side branch vessel size). The balloon is inflated, usually at 6–8 atm, anchoring the guide into the vessel and enhancing the advancement of balloons or microcatheters.[4] It may cause chest pain. Appropriate sizing of the anchor balloon is crucial to prevent side-branch dissection or perforation. An optimal anchor balloon needs to be large enough so that it does not slip.

A wire anchor can be used by inserting an extra supportive guidewire in a side branch, which will stabilize the guiding catheter and offer some support.[1]

Buddy wire stent anchor: If the proximal vessel needs stenting, a buddy wire can be inserted and a stent deployed over the first wire, effectively trapping the buddy wire, which then provides strong guide catheter support.[4] Tu et al. reported

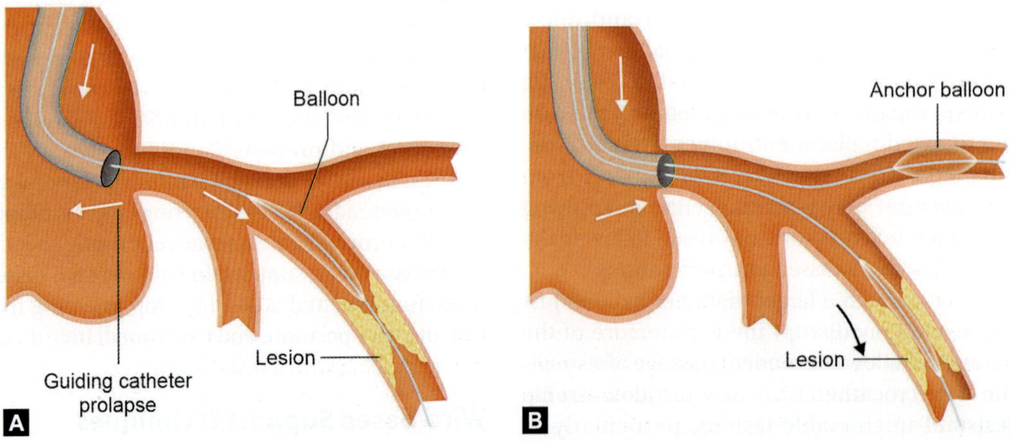

FIGS. 1A AND B: Illustration of the side branch anchor technique for treating a balloon uncrossable lesion. (A) Guiding catheter prolapse while the balloon is being negotiated across the lesion. (B) Facilitated balloon advancement across the lesion with the help of the side branch balloon anchor technique.

successful balloon and stent delivery in 86.7% of patients with the use of the "buddy-in-jail" technique.[10]

Deep wire crossing technique: A hydrophilic, polymer-jacketed guidewire crosses the lesion and advances into the ventricle/aorta through arterioluminal communications, providing strong support for the entire system and helping advance the balloon to the target segment.[4] Khelimskii et al.[11] reported the successful application of the deep wire crossing technique in 77.9% of patients with a 3.2% incidence of in-hospital major adverse cardiac events (MACE).

Third-line strategies: Plaque Modification

Microcatheters

Microcatheters are pushable devices that can create a small channel in the lesion, by virtue of their ability to transmit torque into and beyond resistant lesions. Coiled microcatheters should be spun quickly to reduce friction in the proximal artery and to build up torque while crossing resistant lesions.[1] Braided and coiled microcatheters are best suited for crossing challenging lesions as they can be rotated to minimize friction and facilitate advancement.[4]

Depending on the task at hand, a range of microcatheters with different design properties are available including Tornus, Corsair, Finecross, Turnpike, Turnpike LP, Turnpike Spiral, Turnpike Gold, and Mamba.[1] The Tornus catheter is a metal exchange penetration catheter comprising eight individual larger wires stranded together to form a spiral [0.12 mm in Tornus (2.1F) and 0.18 mm in Tornus 88Flex (2.6F)].[12] This results in a highly pushable device making it useful in calcified and difficult-to-penetrate lesions, while the thick wires, high tip stiffness, and screw pitch design of the Tornus 88Flex make it a more forceful, penetrating microcatheter. It should be advanced using counterclockwise rotation and withdrawn using clockwise rotation.[4] Its contribution to case completion by enhancing lesion crossing has been established in multiple small case series.[13] Fang et al.[14] reported successful crossing in 71.4% of patients with balloon uncrossable lesions with 87.5% final procedural success.

The hybrid microcatheters (e.g., Corsair and Caravel microcatheters) are useful for antegrade and retrograde CTO PCI.[15] The "Shinka" shaft of the Corsair microcatheter is made of two larger stainless steel wires wrapped around eight smaller wires, allowing pushability, flexibility, and transmission of force.[1]

The Turnpike family of microcatheters (Turnpike, Turnpike Spiral, Turnpike LP, Turnpike Gold) has a multi-layered shaft to enhance torque, flexibility, and tracking, while the hydrophilic coating over the distal 60 cm enhances lubricity.[16] The Turnpike Gold has a threaded metal tip enhancing penetrative capability by screwing through resistant lesions. The Turnpike Spiral has a soft nylon outer coil that provides rotational assistance for forward progression through lesions when rotated clockwise.[1] In contrast to the Tornus catheter, it is advanced by turning clockwise and withdrawn by turning counterclockwise.[4] We suggest avoiding rotation in only one direction or over-rotation to prevent microcatheter entrapment.

If the successful advancement of a microcatheter is achieved, a balloon can often subsequently cross the lesion. Alternatively, the guidewire could be exchanged for an extra supportive guidewire or an atherectomy guidewire for further lesion preparation.[4]

Grenadoplasty (Balloon-assisted Microdissection)

A small balloon (1.0–1.5 mm) is advanced as far as possible into the lesion and inflated at high pressure until it ruptures. The balloon rupture creates a contrast jet that creates microdissections and modifies the lesion such that another balloon can pass or make a subintimal entry possible, allowing reentry distal to the lesion.[1,4] This technique is easy and cost-effective with up to 50% success rate documented by Vo et al.[17] There is a small risk of dissection or perforation with this technique.[1] We recommend preparing the balloon well to prevent air embolism. Once the balloon ruptures, immediate suction should be applied with an inflating device.

Wire-based Techniques

Hu et al. have described the so-called *wire-cutting technique* in which a second wire is used to modify resistant lesions **(Fig. 2A)**.[18] In this technique, two guidewires are passed into the distal vessel, and a balloon is advanced to the site of the lesion abutting the uncrossable segment. The balloon is then inflated, jailing the second guidewire between the balloon and the lesion. This guidewire is then rapidly withdrawn producing a cutting effect on the lesion to facilitate balloon crossing.[1]

A modified version of this technique is the "seesaw balloon-wire cutting" technique **(Figs. 2B and C)**. In this technique, two balloons are advanced over the two guidewires (one balloon over each wire). One of the balloons is first advanced as distally as possible and inflated, pressing the other wire against the proximal cap. The balloon is deflated and withdrawn, and the other balloon is advanced distally and inflated, producing a similar cutting effect to modify the cap on the other side. This process is repeated multiple times until one of the balloons crosses the lesion.[4]

There are two other similar techniques for wire cutting, the *multi-wire plaque crushing* and the *crowbar effect technique*. In the *multi-wire plaque crushing technique*, one or two wires are inserted along the original wire and are then withdrawn in order to enlarge the lumen inside of the occlusion segment, facilitating balloon crossing.[4] In the *crowbar technique*, a soft guidewire (i.e., Fielder XT, XTA, Gaia first) is inserted through the balloon uncrossable lesion, followed by insertion of a second (i.e., Miracle 3, 6, Gaia

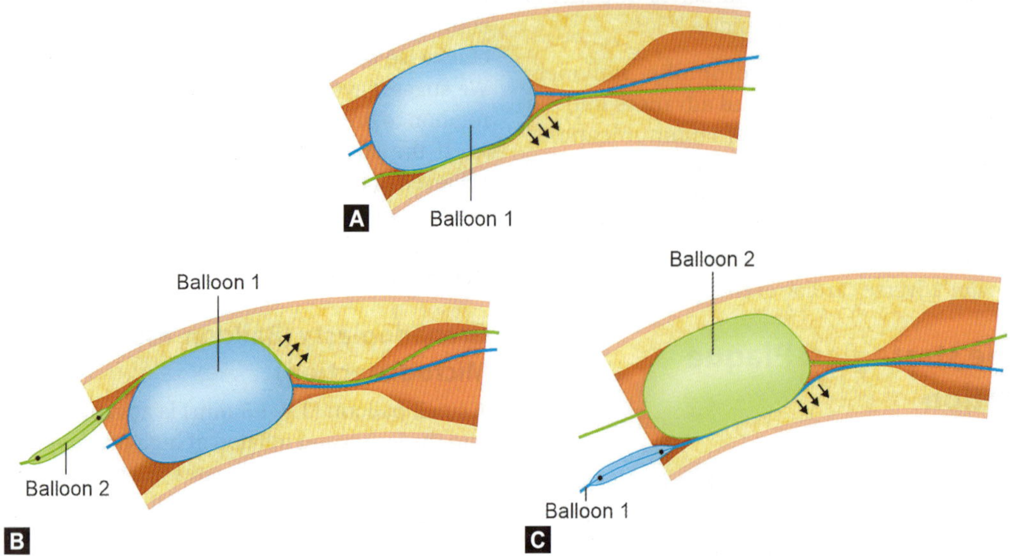

FIGS. 2A TO C: Illustrations of the (A) wire-cutting and (B and C) seesaw wire-cutting techniques.

second) and third stiffer (i.e., Miracle 12, Conquest Pro 12, Gaia second, Gaia third) guidewire along the trace of the first guidewire into the distal vessel true lumen. A small balloon (1.25–1.5 mm) is repeatedly inflated at high pressure (14–16 atm), which moves the balloon forward 2–3 mm with each inflation until it crosses the occlusion. The second and third guidewires are then withdrawn and a bigger balloon with a diameter of 2.0 mm or larger is inserted along the retained soft guidewire. The created channel is inflated further with the balloon, and stenting is performed.[4]

Atherectomy (Rotational or Orbital)

Rotational or orbital atherectomy can greatly facilitate lesion crossing with a balloon.[4] Thinning of the calcium with atherectomy that allows its fracture with dilatation is thought to be the mechanism of action.[1] However, these forms of atherectomy require wire exchange for a thinner (0.009″ for rotational and 0.012″ for orbital atherectomy) dedicated guidewire, which may not always be feasible through the balloon uncrossable lesion. If no other maneuver is successful in crossing the lesion, it is sometimes possible to "burry" a microcatheter as far as possible into the lesion, pull the wire, and attempt to rewire the lesion with a dedicated atherectomy guidewire. If rewiring is successful, atherectomy can be performed.[4] Introduction of novel atherectomy guidewires, such as the ViperWire Advance flex-tip with improved handling characteristics, can facilitate early atherectomy of balloon uncrossable lesions.[19] Atherectomy is challenging in tortuous vessels and should be avoided in case of large dissection or thrombotic lesions.

Rotational atherectomy helps to crack the calcium before complete debulking is attempted with a balloon. A floppy RotaWire is commonly used, which has a diameter of 0.009″ and ends in 0.014″. This wire is flimsy and noncoated with high chances of kinking. The extra-support RotaWire is used for ostial and tortuous lesions. If the RotaWire is unable to cross the lesion, try using a workhorse wire and advance a microcatheter deep into the lesion, and again attempt wiring with RotaWire. Burr sizes from 1.25 mm are commonly available. The ideal burr-to-artery ratio is kept between 0.4 and 0.6. The ideal distance to be maintained between the burr and wire tip is up to 30 mm and never <10 mm. The recommended speed of rotablation is between 140 and 160K rpm and that of the dynaglide is 70K rpm. It should be advanced with pecking movements for 10–15 seconds with a gap of 30–60 seconds between two rotablation cycles. This allows the flushing of debris distally either with flush or contrast and also brings down the local temperature. This process can be repeated 5–10 times as per the requirement. Temporary pacing is recommended while performing rotablation in RCA, dominant left circumflex (LCX) artery, and left coronary vessel with RCA CTO. Rotablation for distal lesions is riskier and should be performed with caution. The complications include dissection, especially when rotablation is attempted in tortuous vessels, burr entrapment, no reflow, and perforation. Burr entrapment can be managed by (1) increasing the speed of the Rotablator to 200K rpm with pushing and pulling of the catheter, (2) passing a buddy wire and dilatation with a small-sized balloon, (3) cutting the catheter and removing the Teflon sheath and advancing a guide extension catheter over the entrapped burr and removing the assembly en masse.

Excimer Laser Coronary Atherectomy

Excimer laser coronary atherectomy (ELCA) uses heat energy and a beam of monochromatic light to modify plaque by photochemical (fracture of molecular bonds), photothermal (tissue vaporization), and photokinetic (clearance of by-products) mechanisms. The predominant photoacoustic mechanism creates fractures in the calcium and facilitates lesion preparation.[1] It can be advanced over any 0.014″ coronary guidewire and is performed under continuous saline infusion.[4] The laser machine emits energy between 30 and 80 mJ/mm^2 and a repetition rate of 25–80 pulses/s through a multitude of catheters ranging from 0.9 to 2.0 mm in diameter. In highly resistant lesions, activation in the contrast medium potentiates the formation of larger bubbles to modify plaque but is associated with an increased risk of perforation.[20,21]

RASER angioplasty technique includes the combination of RA (rotational atherectomy) and ELCA (Excimer laser coronary atherectomy) to fully debulk the lesion. In this technique, ELCA creates a "pilot hole" that facilitates passage of RotaWire either independently or via microcatheter exchange to permit subsequent rotational atherectomy.[22]

Fourth-line Strategies: Dissection Re-entry

Subintimal External Crush Technique

In this technique, a wire is left in the true lumen to minimize the risk of vessel occlusion, and it can be used as a landmark for re-entry. A "scratch and go" technique is applied where a stiff wire is used to penetrate the subintimal space followed by a softer wire that can knuckle or track around the lesion.[1] Another option is the balloon-assisted subintimal entry technique in which a balloon sized 1:1 with the reference diameter of the vessel is inflated proximal to the lesion.[23] It creates dissections that act as an entry point to the subintimal space, through which wires and subsequently balloons can be passed around the lesion into the distal true lumen. Later on, access to the distal true lumen can be regained with a stiff wire or the Stingray re-entry balloon. This approach should be reserved as a last resort only by experienced operators.[1]

Subintimal Distal Anchor Technique

In this technique, a second guidewire is advanced subintimally distal to the CTO. A balloon is advanced over the subintimal guidewire distal to the CTO. The balloon is inflated distally, anchoring the true lumen guidewire, and enabling antegrade delivery of a balloon over the true lumen guidewire.[4]

BALLOON UNDILATABLE LESIONS

A balloon undilatable lesion is a lesion that cannot be expanded despite high-pressure multiple balloon inflations and shows "dog boning" with a central lesion on fluoroscopy.

Adequate lesion preparation before stent implantation is essential to achieve the best results. Stent deployment before adequate lesion preparation leads to stent under-expansion and suboptimal results. The achieved luminal diameter and minimal stent area are significant factors in determining the incidence of in-stent restenosis (ISR) and stent thrombosis. Hence, a stepwise approach **(Flowchart 2)** to lesion preparation and modification should be used, starting with the commonly available and least invasive strategy.[1]

Noncompliant Balloon

The NC balloons apply high pressures to resistant lesions without volume change, therefore focusing the pressure within the lesion rather than transmitting it to other parts of the artery. Their use is limited in eccentric calcific plaque due to guidewire bias, which directs transmission of force away

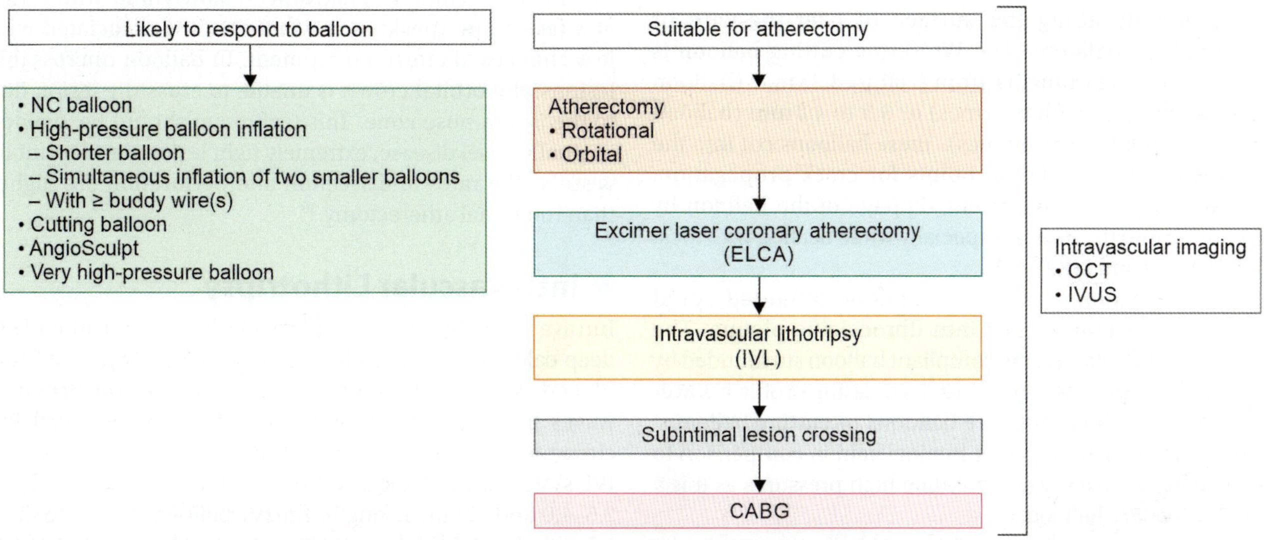

FLOWCHART 2: Stepwise algorithm for an approach to a de novo balloon undilatable lesion.
(CABG: coronary artery bypass graft; IVUS: intravascular ultrasound; NC: noncompliant; OCT: optical coherence tomography)

from the calcified segment. Many lesions may fail to dilate with these high-pressure NC balloons and require more aggressive strategies.[24] Prolonged (up to 60 seconds) inflation with high pressure can work too. Sometimes, inflating a 1:1 size balloon to high pressure (20 atm), then reducing (to 12 atm), and then inflating it again (20 atm) in an oscillating manner (inflate/deflate) can be a game changer. It is advised not to exceed 1:1 balloon size to prevent balloon/vessel perforation or air embolism. We recommend the use of a shorter NC balloon, which helps to focus the applied pressure at a desired point. On occasions, inflating two smaller sized balloons in the lesion simultaneously can produce a positive outcome.[1]

Ultrahigh-pressure Noncompliant Balloons

These balloons can deliver pressures of up to 40 atm with very little change in diameter. A notable example is the OPN NC balloon, which has a unique twin-layer construction allowing transmission of ultrahigh pressure with a low incidence of balloon rupture (factory-tested rated burst pressure is 42 atm). Their safety and efficacy have been established with a low incidence of complications such as perforation.[25] It has limited utility in crossing resistant lesions due to its bulky profile.[1] The size of the OPN balloon should be 0.25 mm smaller than the artery size to prevent perforation. It is available in 10, 15, 20 mm lengths and 1.5–4.0 mm diameters with 0.5-mm intervals.[25] OPN balloon rupture is linear and less risky than NC balloon rupture if it is less than 1:1 size. For the expansion of underexpanded stents, the OPN NC balloon is an effective modality.

Cutting/Scoring Balloons

The key characteristic of the cutting balloons is the presence of atherotomes (microsurgical blades) mounted longitudinally along the surface of over-the-wire or monorail NC balloons. The Wolverine cutting balloon is available in sizes ranging from 2.00 to 3.25 mm (balloon models with three atherotomes) or 3.5 to 4.0 mm (balloon models with four atherotomes). These balloons cut into the plaque, creating initiation points for crack propagation. The atherotomes also prevent slippage of the balloon by anchoring into the intima, especially while dealing with focal short lesions and ISR.[26]

Scoring balloons comprise balloon-mounted spiral scoring wires that anchor into fibrocalcific plaque. The AngioSculpt RX has a semi-compliant balloon surrounded by three nitinol spiral scoring wires. Its crossing profile is lower than OPN ultrahigh-pressure balloons or cutting balloons, and it helps to achieve larger luminal gain in comparison to NC balloons.[26] We suggest avoiding high pressures as it is a semi-compliant balloon.

These cutting balloons and scoring balloons can also be used to improve stent expansion after stent deployment and are a useful adjunct in treating ISR.[27]

Cutting and scoring balloon cut precisely (preferred during predilatation) unlike OPN NC balloon which causes uncontrolled dilatation (preferred in under-expanded stent). Cutting balloon is for plaque modification and not for expansion.

Excimer Laser Coronary Atherectomy

The excimer laser can be used to modify undilatable lesions through photothermal, photochemical, and photomechanical disruption of resistant plaque. After adequate plaque modification with laser, balloon dilatation with an NC balloon sized 1:1 with the lumen diameter should be used to ensure adequate expansion. Excimer laser with or without contrast is a safe and viable method to achieve adequate stent expansion in underexpanded stents.[28,29] High cost may be a limiting factor for the use of this technique.

Atherectomy (Rotational or Orbital)

Atherectomy is a fundamental technique to enhance lesion crossing as a debulking device.[1] It is less bulky than other modalities such as intravascular lithotripsy (IVL) and cutting balloon but is challenging in torturous vessels. Debulking and fracturing heavy superficial calcification enhance lesion crossing and expansion. Balloon dilatation with an NC balloon sized 1:1 with the artery is essential following atherectomy to ensure effective calcium modification, fracture, and lesion expansion before stent implantation.[1]

Orbital atherectomy can be performed in undilatable lesions, including ostial lesions. It causes forward and backward cutting in contrast to rotational atherectomy which only cuts in a forward direction. The crown size of 1.25 mm is available, which is rotated at either 80K rpm or 120K rpm. The catheter is to be advanced slowly and withdrawn slowly in contrast to rotational atherectomy in which the catheter is advanced slowly and withdrawn at a faster rate (pecking movement). It is associated with less chances of crown entrapment. In balloon uncrossable lesions, the orbital crown is unable to cross the lesion due to the 5-mm nose cone. This technique should be avoided in small-vessel disease, extremely tight lesions, and tortuous vessels. The rates of dissection and perforation are higher than rotational atherectomy.[30]

Intravascular Lithotripsy

Intravascular lithotripsy is particularly ideal for fracturing deep calcium. IVL uses electrohydraulic lithotripsy emitters placed within a balloon to create ultrasonic pressure waves that dissipate through the calcific plaque, causing circumferential fractures in multiple planes. The shockwave IVL system is available in various balloon sizes ranging from 2.5–4.0 and 12 mm in length. The IVL balloon should be sized 1:1 with the vessel reference diameter. The balloon catheter is connected to a generator that delivers 10 pulses of ultrasonic energy over 10 seconds, with a maximum of 8 cycles per balloon. IVL causes effective plaque modification, especially in cases with circumferential arc of calcium (>270°) as the ultrasonic waves reverberate to cause fractures in calcium. Further predilatation with an NC balloon may or may not be required. However, many operators use an NC balloon for optimal expansion and lesion preparation. In the DISRUPT CAD I trial, IVL-treated calcified lesions had multiple fracture lines in calcific plaque on optical coherence tomography (OCT) and reduced residual stenosis without any MACE.[31] IVL is easy to use, has a low crossing profile, and has very few complications.[1] High cost may be a limiting factor for the use of this technique.

Imaging

The role of intracoronary imaging such as OCT or intravascular ultrasound (IVUS) in the treatment of balloon undilatable lesions cannot be overemphasized. It can help to identify challenges with lesion expansion before treatment and also ensure that an optimal result has been achieved after treatment.

However, in the absence of imaging, adequate dilatation of every lesion must be confirmed by visualizing a dilated NC balloon in two perpendicular views. Never deploy a stent in an unyielded lesion.

MONITORING DURING PROCEDURE

Activated clotting time (ACT) should be checked every 20–30 minutes with a target ACT of 250–300 seconds as multiple devices increase the risk of thrombus formation. The patient should be monitored clinically, especially for any cardiac or neurological symptoms. Hemodynamic and electrocardiogram (ECG) monitoring should be strictly done during the procedure.

The possible complications expected during such PCI include loss of guide or guidewire position, ostial dissection, distal guidewire perforation, and balloon entrapment. Make sure that the guiding catheter tip and guidewire tip are in an appropriate position.

CONCLUSION

The balloon uncrossable lesions are commonly encountered during routine and CTO PCI and are a potential barrier to successful revascularization. In a contemporary registry, the prevalence of balloon uncrossable lesions following successful guidewire crossing was 9.0%, whereas the prevalence of balloon uncrossable or balloon undilatable lesions was 15.5%, and the prevalence of balloon undilatable lesions was 8.5%. Balloon uncrossable and/or balloon undilatable lesions have lower procedural success and higher complication rates compared to balloon crossable lesions. Guide catheter support and advanced plaque modification techniques for crossing resistant lesions increase the likelihood of successful lesion crossing. Once a balloon has crossed the lesion, the lesion must be adequately prepared and expanded before stent implantation.

The balloon undilatable coronary lesions are notorious and technically challenging. These lesions preclude optimal stent expansion, which can result in ISR and stent thrombosis. A meticulous approach by using appropriate techniques is the key to adequate lesion preparation and debulking to achieve the best results and clinical outcomes. It is important to understand that these techniques that either increase guide catheter support or modify plaque are interchangeable and can be used in any order (sequential or simultaneous) depending on availability and operator experience to achieve a successful PCI outcome.

ONLINE REFERENCES

Please scan the QR code provided at the end of the table of contents for References of this chapter.

CHAPTER 163

Appropriate Use of Imaging in PCI: IVUS and OCT

Debdatta Bhattacharyya, Saurabh Dhumale

ABSTRACT

Intravascular ultrasound (IVUS) and optical coherence tomography (OCT) have revolutionized cardiology and vascular medicine since their inception. IVUS, dating back to the 1970s, provided real-time cross-sectional images of coronary arteries, surpassing traditional angiography's limitations. OCT, emerging in the 1990s, utilized near-infrared light to create high-resolution cross-sectional images. Both technologies have played crucial roles in optimizing percutaneous coronary interventions (PCIs) and improving long-term outcomes, particularly in complex coronary interventions.

Several trials, such as ADAPT-DES and ULTIMATE, demonstrated that IVUS-guided PCI led to reduced adverse events. Similarly, the ILUMIEN series of trials have proved that OCT-guided PCI is beneficial in assessing plaque characteristics, optimizing stent deployment, and detecting complications such as dissection. However, the adoption of intravascular imaging remains limited, with data indicating underutilization, especially in regions such as India and the United States (US).

This chapter provides a comprehensive overview of IVUS and OCT, their principles, clinical applications, advantages, and limitations. It highlights the need for increased awareness and appropriate usage of intravascular imaging during PCI to enhance patient outcomes.

Keywords: Intravascular ultrasound, optical coherence tomography, intravascular imaging (IVI), complex percutaneous coronary intervention.

INTRODUCTION

Intravascular ultrasound (IVUS) and optical coherence tomography (OCT) are two advanced medical imaging technologies that have significantly transformed the field of cardiology and vascular medicine. After Andreas Grüntzig performed the first balloon angioplasty in 1977, there was a revolution in transcatheter/intravascular therapies for coronary artery disease. Balloon angioplasty was followed by advent of bare-metal stents, which made percutaneous transluminal coronary angioplasty (PTCA) a procedure with predictable acute outcomes. Next came the drug-eluting stents (DES) which drastically reduced the recurrence rates. Along with the remarkable developments in DES, a parallel revolution occurred in the field of intracoronary imaging, which improved our knowledge of composition of obstructive coronary lesions which aided in bed preparation prior to the PTCA as well as stent sizing and optimization after stent implantation.

HISTORY AND DEVELOPMENT OF INTRAVASCULAR IMAGING

Intravascular ultrasound was one of the earlier innovations, with its roots dating back to 1971, when Bom and colleagues developed one of the first catheter-based real-time imaging technique to be used in cardiac system, followed by Yock et al. in the 1980s at Stanford, when the team there introduced IVUS as a novel intravascular imaging (IVI) device. The initial concept involved the insertion of a catheter equipped with a miniaturized ultrasound transducer into the coronary arteries to obtain cross-sectional images of vessel walls. This was a substantial improvement over traditional angiography, which is essentially a luminogram and only provided two-dimensional (2D) images and lacked detailed information about plaque composition and vessel structure. Over the next few decades, IVUS technology underwent numerous improvements with the introduction of intracoronary transducers with higher frequencies and better image resolution. Additionally, the advent of motorized pullback systems enabled the acquisition of longitudinal images along the entire length of the vessel, enabling comprehensive assessment of lesions and stenosis.

Optical coherence tomography emerged later, in the early 1990s, as an optical analogue to IVUS. Although the two modalities have the same basic principles of emitting and receiving signals to create a visual image, OCT utilizes near-infrared light to create high-resolution, cross-sectional images of the coronary arteries. The development of OCT was initially motivated by the need for better resolution to accurately visualize the intricate microstructure of the arterial walls and identify vulnerable plaques. The earlier versions of OCT faced challenges, such as limited imaging depth and vulnerability to blood interference. However, ongoing research and technological advancements led to significant improvements in OCT's performance. The introduction of Fourier-domain OCT (FD-OCT) and swept-source OCT (SS-OCT) brought faster image acquisition and superior imaging quality, making it an invaluable tool in clinical cardiology.

The encouraging long-term success rates with DES emboldened interventionists to treat more complex lesions such as bifurcation stenosis, left main (LM) coronary stenosis, chronic total occlusions (CTOs), calcified lesions, and bifurcation stenosis. IVI has played a pivotal role in understanding how to plan and optimize stent implantation in these cases, thereby improving long-term outcomes.

Kang et al.[1] back in 2011 helped formulate predetermined IVUS targets for better long-term results. In their study of LM bifurcation angioplasty, a total of 403 patients treated with single- or two-stent strategies (crushing and T-stent) had immediate post-stenting IVUS and 9-month follow-up angiography. Post-stenting minimal stent area (MSA) was measured in each of the four segments—ostial left anterior descending (LAD), ostial left circumflex (LCX) polygon of confluence [(POC)—confluence zone of LAD and LCX], and proximal LM above the POC. Overall, 46 (11.4%) showed angiographic restenosis at 9 months: 3 of 67 (4.5%) nonbifurcation lesions were treated with a single stent, 14 of 222 (6.3%) bifurcation lesions were treated with single-stent crossover, and 29 of 114 (25.4%) of bifurcation lesions were treated with two stents. The MSA cut-offs that best-predicted in-stent restenosis (ISR) on a segmental basis were 5.0 mm^2 (ostial LCX ISR), 6.3 mm^2 (ostial LAD ISR), 7.2 mm^2 (ISR within the POC), and 8.2 mm^2 (ISR within the LM above the POC). Using these criteria, 133 (33.8%) had underexpansion of at least one segment. Angiographic ISR (at any location) was more frequent in lesions with underexpansion of at least one segment versus lesions with no underexpansion (24.1% vs. 5.4%, $p < 0.001$). 2-year major adverse coronary event-

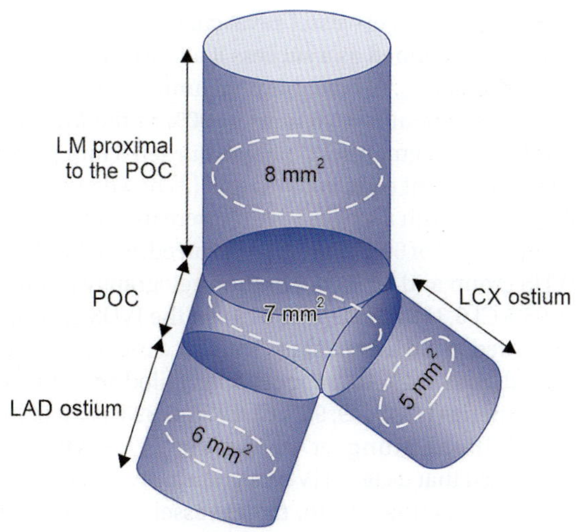

FIG. 1: The 5-6-7-8 criteria for left main bifurcation introduced by Kang et al.

(LAD: left anterior descending; LCX: left circumflex; LM: left main; POC: polygon of confluence)

free survival rate was significantly lower in patients with underexpansion of at least one segment versus lesions with no underexpansion (90 ± 3% vs. 98 ± 1%, log-rank $p < 0.001$), and post-stenting underexpansion was an independent predictor for major adverse cardiac events (MACE) [adjusted hazard ratio (HR) 5.56; 95% confidence interval (CI) 1.99–15.49; $p = 0.001$]. This resulted in the oft-quoted 5-6-7-8 formula **(Fig. 1)** for LM bifurcation stenting.

The ADAPT-DES trial[2] was a prospective, multicenter, nonrandomized all-comers study of 8,582 consecutive patients at 11 US and German sites designed to determine the frequency, timing, and correlates of adverse events after DES. At 2 years, IVUS guidance ($n = 3,361$; 39%) compared with angiography guidance ($n = 5,221$; 61%) was associated with reduced rates of (1) MACE [cardiac death, myocardial infarction (MI), or stent thrombosis; 4.9% vs. 7.5%; adjusted HR 0.72; 95% CI 0.59–0.89; $p = 0.003$], (2) definite/probable stent thrombosis (0.55% vs. 1.16%; adjusted HR 0.40; 95% CI 0.22–0.73; $p = 0.003$), and (3) MI (3.5% vs. 5.6%; adjusted HR 0.65; 95% CI 0.51–0.83; $p = 0.0006$). By landmark analysis, IVUS guidance compared with angiography guidance was also associated with significantly reduced rates of MACE, MI, stent thrombosis, and clinically driven target lesion revascularization between 1 and 2 years after DES implantation. The number needed to treat with IVUS guidance to prevent one major adverse cardiac event was reduced from 64 (42–137) at 1 year to 41 (29–69) at 2 years.

In the ULTIMATE[3] (Intravascular Ultrasound-Guided Drug-Eluting Stents Implantation in "All-Comers" Coronary Lesions) trial, a total of 1,448 all-comer patients who required DES implantation were randomly assigned (1:1 ratio) to either an IVUS guidance or angiography guidance group. The primary endpoint was target-vessel failure (TVF) at 12 months, including cardiac death, target-vessel MI, and clinically driven target-vessel revascularization (TVR). The procedure was defined as a success if all three IVUS-defined optimal criteria [i.e., (1) the minimal luminal area (MLA) in the stented segment is >5.0 mm^2 or 90% of the MLA at the distal reference segments; (2) plaque burden 5 mm proximal or distal to the stent edge is <50%; and (3) no edge dissection involves media with a length >3 mm] were met. At 12 months follow-up, a total of 60 TVFs (4.2%) occurred, with 21 (2.9%) in the IVUS group and 39 (5.4%) in the angiography group (HR 0.530; 95% CI 0.312–0.901; $p = 0.019$). In the IVUS group, TVF was recorded in 1.6% of patients with successful procedures, compared with 4.4% in patients who failed to achieve all optimal criteria (HR 0.349; 95% CI 0.135–0.898; $p = 0.029$).

In addition, Hong et al. in the IVUS-XPL[4] trial, demonstrated that usage of IVUS significantly reduced 1- and 5-year MACE (cardiac death, target vessel MI, or ischemic-driven target-lesion revascularization) in patients with long lesions implanted with second-generation DES, which proved the efficacy and safety of the usage of IVUS in complex percutaneous coronary intervention (PCI).

The first in-man OCT study was conducted in 2002. In the ILUMIEN II[5] study, OCT-guided stent implantation showed comparable stent expansions compared to those reported in the IVUS-guided group of the ADAPT-DES study. Thereafter, in the ILUMIEN III: OPTIMIZE[6] PCI-randomized study, the OCT-guided PCI, using an external elastic lamina-based protocol, was compared to operator-directed IVUS-guided or angiography-guided PCI. Target-lesion failure (TLF) and MACE at 12 months were adjudicated. There were no significant differences in the rates of TLF (2.0% OCT, 3.7% IVUS, and 1.4% angiography), MACE (9.8% OCT, 9.1% IVUS, and 7.9% angiography), or any of the individual components of these outcomes among the groups. No independent predictors of 12-month stent-related clinical events were identified from final OCT. In this underpowered study, OCT-guided PCI of noncomplex lesions did not show a statistical difference in clinical outcomes at 12 months compared with IVUS or angiography guidance. An appropriately powered trial, including only complex patients and lesions, was carried out subsequently (ILUMIEN IV).

The recently published ILUMIEN IV[7] trial was conducted at 80 sites in 18 countries. In this prospective, randomized, single-blind trial, they randomly assigned patients with medication-treated diabetes or complex coronary artery lesions to undergo OCT-guided PCI or angiography-guided PCI. A total of 2,487 patients underwent randomization: 1,233 patients were assigned to undergo OCT-guided PCI and 1,254 to undergo angiography-guided PCI. The minimum stent area after PCI was 5.72 ± 2.04 mm^2 in the OCT group and 5.36 ± 1.87 mm^2 in the angiography group (mean difference 0.36 mm^2; 95% CI 0.21–0.51; $p < 0.001$). TVF within 2 years occurred in 88 patients in the OCT group and in 99 patients in the angiography group (Kaplan–Meier estimates—7.4% and 8.2%, respectively; HR 0.90; 95% CI 0.67–1.19; $p = 0.45$). OCT-related adverse events occurred in one patient in the OCT group and in two patients in the angiography group. Stent thrombosis within 2 years occurred in six patients (0.5%) in the OCT group and in 17 patients (1.4%) in the angiography group.

Several trials conducted over decades have proven time and again that employing IVI (IVUS or OCT) during PCI helps in improving immediate and long-term outcomes. Despite this fact, while Japan has a very high IVI usage, recent data from the US by Truesdell et al.[8] suggested that overall IVI usage in PCIs was <20%. The National Informatics Centre (NIC) 2023 DATA suggests that IVUS was used in only 4.01%, while OCT was used in just 1.86% of PCIs performed in India in the year 2022. We here have tried to underline the benefits and highlight the appropriate usage of the two primary IVI modalities in hope to increase awareness and push for greater usage of IVI-assisted PCI for better outcomes.

SECTION 1: INTRAVASCULAR ULTRASOUND

Principles of Intravascular Ultrasound

Intravascular ultrasound is a catheter-based imaging technique that employs high-frequency sound waves from a piezoelectric crystal (10–40 MHz) to penetrate tissue and reflect off vascular structures to generate real-time cross-sectional images of coronary arteries. A specially designed catheter with a miniature ultrasound transducer at its tip is advanced through the coronary arteries, over a 0.014-inch coronary guidewire through a 5 French (F) or larger guide. The motorized pullback retracts the catheter at approximately 0.5 mm/s; manual pullback can be performed too. Tissue penetration is approximately 4–8 mm. The collected data is processed to create detailed images, offering valuable insights into the coronary artery anatomy and pathology. The axial resolution of IVUS images is currently 100–150 microns.

Clinical Applications of Intravascular Ultrasound

Assessment of coronary plaque composition: IVUS allows for accurate identification and classification of different plaque components, such as fibrous tissue, lipidic plaque, calcifications, and necrotic cores. The PROSPECT (Providing Regional Observations to Study Predictors of Events in the Coronary Tree) trial utilized IVUS to identify vulnerable plaques and found that plaques with large necrotic cores and thin fibrous caps were associated with future MACE.

Calcification: Although the conventional belief says that OCT is superior to IVUS in assessment of calcified arteries, it can still be employed to great use in optimizing results in calcified arteries. IVUS elegantly images coronary calcium and gives reliable information about:

- The arc of calcium **(Figs. 2A to C)**
- The length of calcium affecting the vessel
- Thickness of calcium in IVUS cannot always be measured due to acoustic shadowing from the calcific plaque;

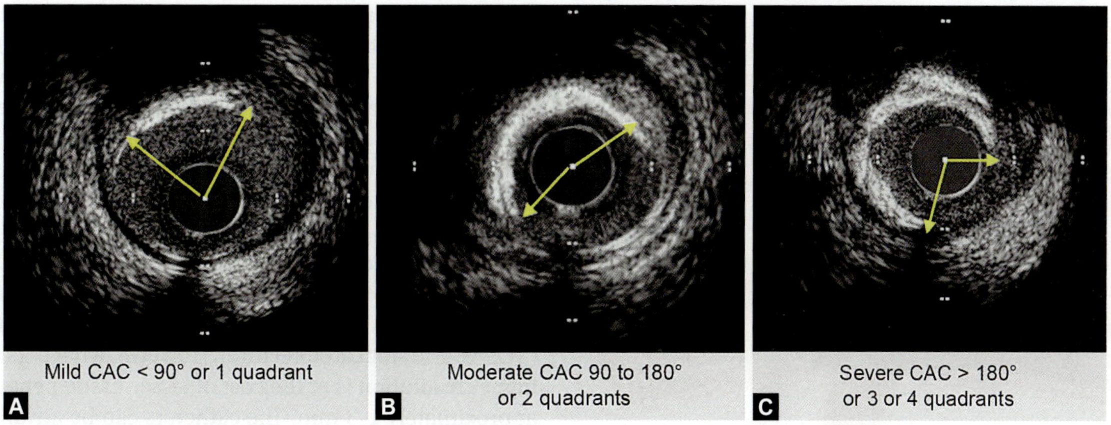

FIGS. 2A TO C: Arc of calcium calculated with the IVUS.
(CAC: coronary artery calcium; IVUS: intravascular ultrasound)
Courtesy: Boston Scientific.

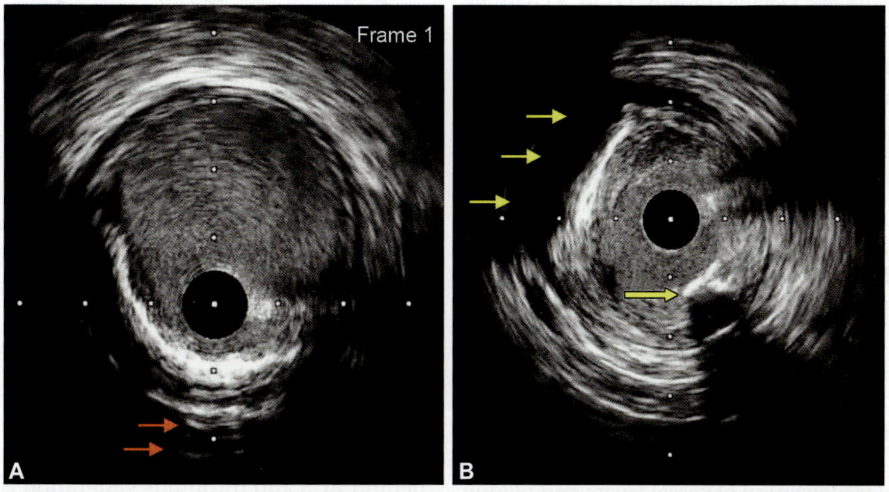

FIGS. 3A AND B: Thickness of the calcium based on presence and absence of reverberations on IVUS. (A) Likely thin calcium with presence of reverberations (arrows); (B) Likely thick plate of calcium (multiple arrows) and a calcific nodule (single large arrow).

however, based on presence or absence of reverberations, one can make assumptions if the calcific plaque is thin or thick **(Figs. 3A and B)**.

Guidance for PCI: IVUS is excellent in determining the vessel size (media to media), lumen area, and lesion length (if using motorized pullback or coregistration. IVUS-guided PCI has shown benefits in multiple trials, including the ADAPT-DES and the IVUS-XPL trials. IVUS also helps in evaluation of the etiology of acute complications (dissection, thrombus, intramural hematoma, and tissue protrusion) and guides in management of said complications.

Evaluation of bifurcation lesions: IVUS has proven beneficial in the evaluation of bifurcation lesions and guiding the selection of appropriate bifurcation stenting techniques. Especially during LM bifurcation PCI, it helps to ensure adequate MSA in the LM, carina, ostial LAD, and ostial LCX coronary arteries, while it also helps in assessment of patent side branch ostia during provisional stenting. IVUS in LM-PCI was found to have a mortality benefit in a study by Park et al. as early as 2004. The much discussed and seminal paper of Kang et al. established the 5-6-7-8 criteria for distal LM stenting. This criteria has been further refined by data analyzed from the EXCEL trial by Mintz et al.[9] who have suggested 7-8-9-10 instead of previous 5-6-7-8 criteria.

CTO PCI: IVUS is invaluable in all stages of CTO PCI for appropriate stent sizing despite heavy plaque burden, and especially in locating the ambiguous wire position (true lumen vs. subintimal). It also helps in IVUS-guided real-time proximal cap puncture with the IVUS catheter parked in the side branch looking at the proximal cap or with specialized

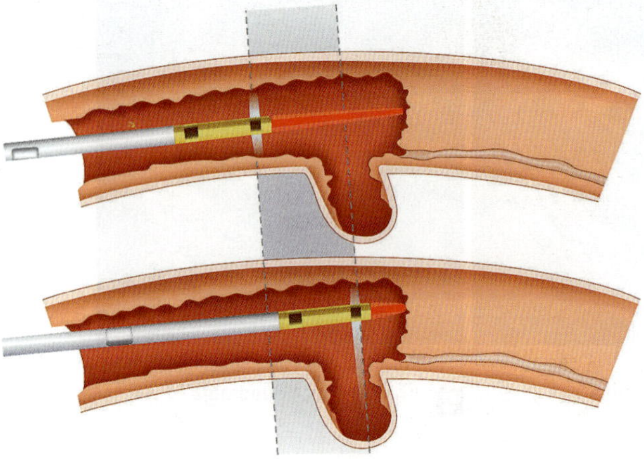

FIG. 4: The Eagle Eye Catheter (Phillips™).

catheters such as Eagle Eye Device (Phillips) **(Fig. 4)** with its shorter-tip design allowing for further advancement of the transducer in a highly stenosed or distal vessel, allowing the operator to image more distally.

Low-contrast PCI: Its useful in low-contrast/zero-contrast PCI to conserve contrast in patients with advanced renal insufficiency.

Advantages and Limitations of Intravascular Ultrasound

Advantages

- Real-time imaging during procedures
- Accurate assessment of vessel dimensions and plaque burden
- Greater depth of visualization of vessel layers and plaque components
- Facilitation of optimized stent deployment and improved clinical outcomes even in larger vessels >5 mm.
- No contrast used in the process, allowing multiple runs without the fear of contrast-induced nephropathy (CIN)
- Ostial LM assessment

Limitations

- Relatively lower resolution compared to OCT
- Limited penetration in heavily calcified plaques
- Requires expertise in image interpretation

SECTION 2: OPTICAL COHERENCE TOMOGRAPHY

Principles of Optical Coherence Tomography

Optical coherence tomography images are obtained using near-infrared light (~1,300 nm) emitted from a single fiber optic wire that reflects off vascular structures and returns to a detector. The interference patterns produced by the reflected light during the postprocessing create detailed images with micrometer level resolution. OCT has the highest resolution among all the contemporary available coronary imaging modalities (axial 10–20 µm and lateral 20–90 µm), which is ~10 times greater than that of IVUS (axial 100–150 µm and lateral 150–300 µm). The higher resolution of OCT enables more detailed evaluation than IVUS at the endoluminal level and for the superficial plaque [e.g., in detecting cavity formation of a plaque rupture, thin-cap fibroatheroma (TCFA), and stent architecture]. However, what is gained with higher resolution is at the cost of lesser tissue penetration of approximately 1–3 mm. The catheters can be advanced over a 0.014-inch coronary guidewire through at least a 5 F guide; although 6 F is preferable.[10]

Clinical Applications of Optical Coherence Tomography

Several clinical trials have highlighted the clinical utility of OCT in intravascular coronary imaging:

Assessment of plaque characteristics and vulnerability: TCFA is defined as a lipid plaque in which the minimum thickness of the fibrous cap is <65 µm and lipid occupies >90° in circumference. Other than thin cap, characteristics involving vulnerable plaque includes macrophage infiltration, neovascularization, large lipid core, and spotty calcifications. OCT is clearly superior to any other modality due to its higher resolution, in delineating all of these characteristics, and identifying a vulnerable plaque.

Acute coronary syndromes (ACSs): Several postmortem studies have established that the primary pathophysiology behind ACS and thrombus generation is a ruptured fibrous cap (RFC). Many modalities namely angioscopy, IVUS, near-infrared spectroscopy (NIRS), and near-infrared fluorescence may be used for imaging RFCs; however, OCT can most reliably identify culprit plaques with ruptured cap. While each modality is unique in its ability to visualize coronary lesions with different characteristics, OCT is particularly superior in delineating intraluminal mechanisms leading to ACS, like thrombus (red/white) and dissection flap in cases of spontaneous coronary artery dissection (SCAD) which are often missed on angiography **(Figs. 5A and B)**.

Calcified plaque: They are signal-poor regions with sharply delineated borders and limited shadowing. Light penetrates calcium; therefore, unlike IVUS, OCT can be used to quantify both the arc and thickness. Calcification thickness can be measured only when both the leading and trailing edges are visible. Calcium deposit length is measured on the longitudinal view. A calcium scoring system **(Table 1)** was introduced in 2019 by Fujino et al.[11] in which two points are given for a maximum angle > 180°, one point for maximum calcium thickness > 0.5 mm, and one point for calcium

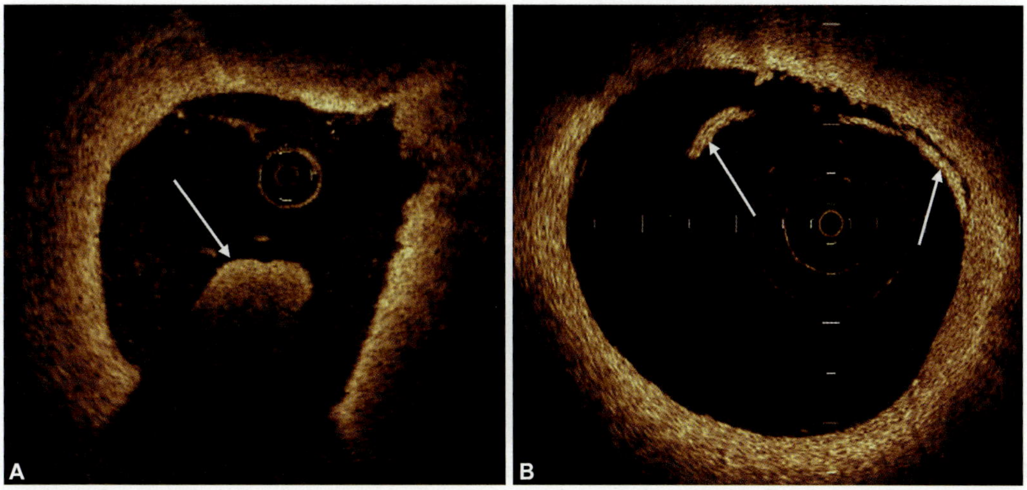

FIGS. 5A AND B: (A) Red thrombus, due to presence of red blood cells' components, causes a marked signal attenuation (arrow), while (B) white thrombus is platelet rich and exhibits a low-signal attenuation (arrows).
Courtesy: Abott Vascular Ltd.

TABLE 1: Optical coherence tomography (OCT)-based calcium volume index score proposed by Fujino et al.[11]

Maximum calcium angle (°)	≤ 90°	0 point
	>90° angle ≤ 180°	1 point
	>180°	2 points
Maximum calcium thickness (mm)	≤0.5 mm	0 point
	>0.5 mm	1 point
Calcium length (mm)	≤5.0 mm	0 point
	>5.0 mm	1 point
Total score	0–4 points	

deposit length > 5 mm. Lesions with a score of 4 points had poor stent expansion. OCT is superior to IVUS in identifying eruptive/noneruptive calcium nodules **(Figs. 6A and B)**.

Stent optimization: OCT is an excellent imaging modality for pre- and post-PCI assessment and stent optimization. It helps in appropriate stent sizing, detecting calcium, and other detractors of optimal stent expansion and their management prior to stenting, post-stenting stent underexpansion/ malapposition, tissue prolapse, and medial edge dissection. MLD-MAX is a unique algorithm **(Fig. 7)** designed to optimize the results of OCT-guided PCI. The rapidity with which OCT

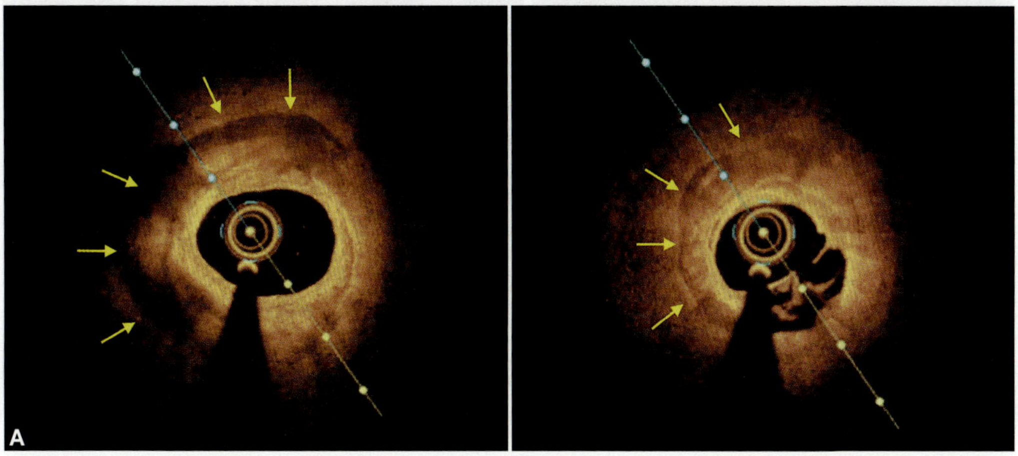

FIGS. 6A AND B: *Continued*

Continued

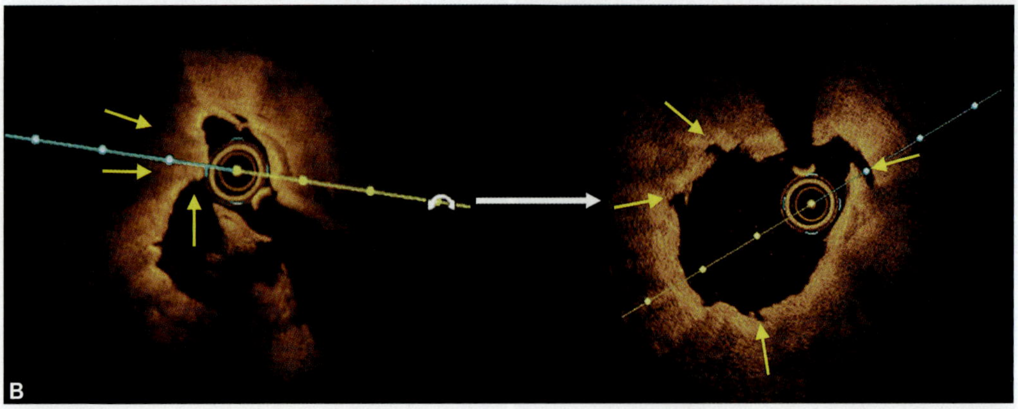

FIGS. 6A AND B: (A) An optical coherence tomography (OCT) cross-sectional image showing thick plate of calcium (arrows pointing). (B) The OCT image on the left shows calcific plaque with a nodule (arrows), while the one on the right shows cracks in the calcium (arrows) postmodification with intravascular lithotripsy.

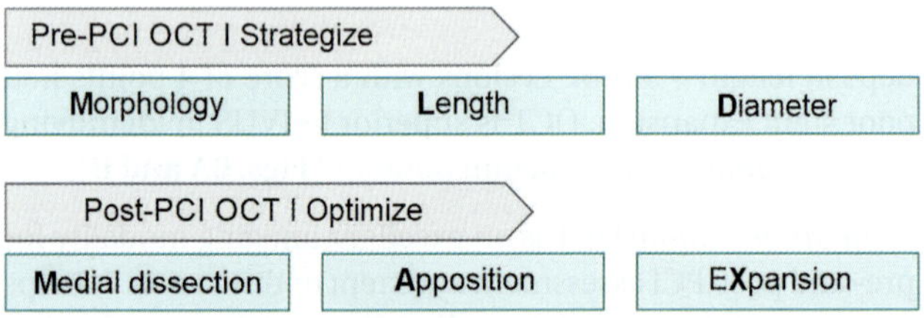

FIG. 7: The MLD-MAX algorithm.

(OCT: optical coherence tomography; PCI: percutaneous coronary intervention)

images are available post-stenting **(Fig. 8)**, complete with apposition and expansion indicators, makes it easier for the operator to analyze compared to the IVUS.

Bifurcation lesions: OCT provides useful guidance for the treatment of bifurcation lesions. It helps in excellent visualization of the side branch ostium, especially in 3D reconstruction **(Fig. 9)**. It also helps delineate the position of wire crossing through appropriate stent struts and identifying strut crowding in front of side branch ostium.

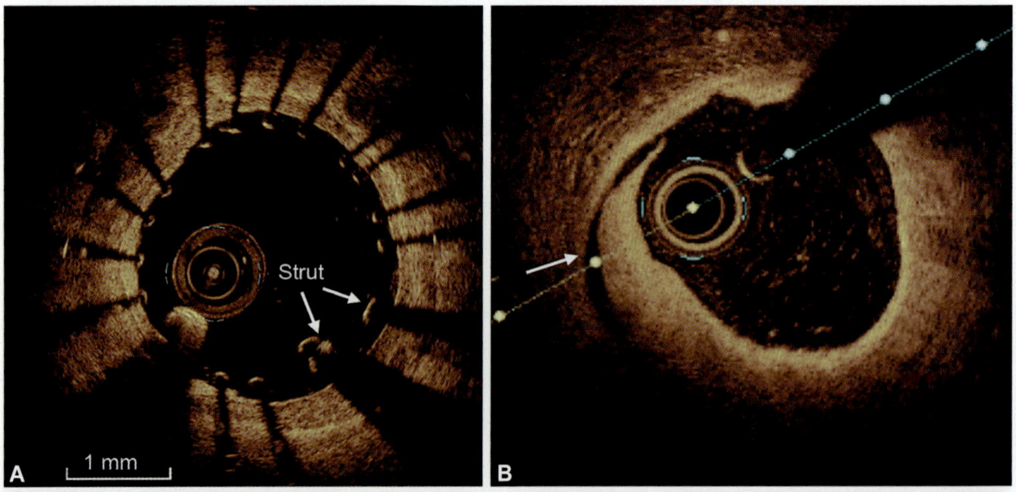

FIGS. 8A AND B: Optical coherence tomography (OCT) images showing (A) medial dissection and (B) stent malapposition.

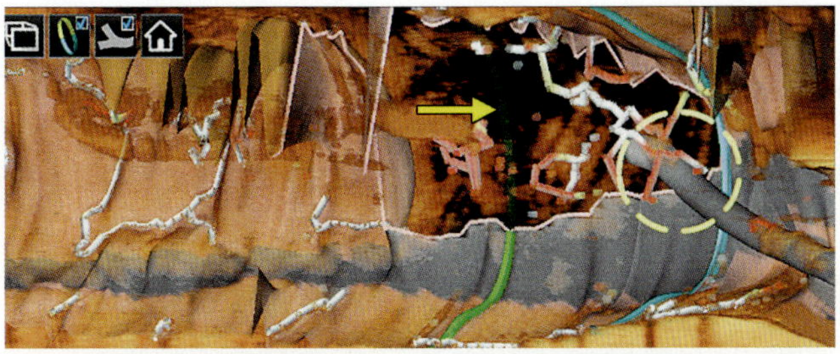

FIG. 9: A 3D reconstructed optical coherence tomography (OCT) image showing wire crossing into the side branch through crowded stent strut area (dotted circle), while the actual orifice free from struts depicted by thick arrow.

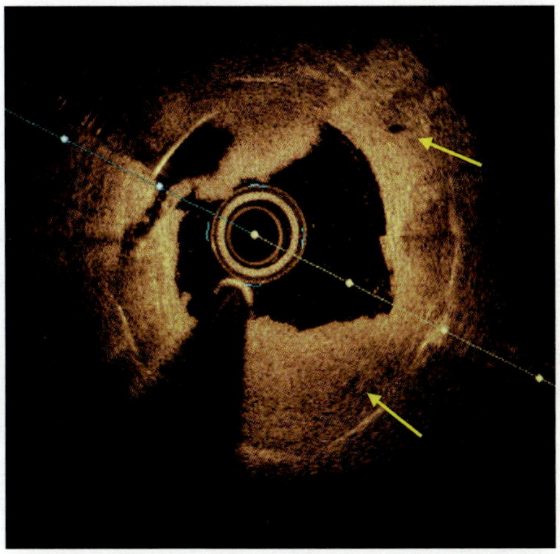

FIG. 10: Optical coherence tomography (OCT) cross-section from a case of in-stent restenosis showing thrombus and neoatherosclerosis.

ISR: OCT is superior to IVUS in delineating late stent changes and etiology of ISR. Not only it is excellent in visualizing the pathology of ISR, namely neointimal hyperplasia and neoatherosclerosis **(Fig. 10)**, but it also aids in delineating the etiology of ISR in the form of previous stent undersizing/malapposition. While approaching the reprocedure in such patients, it not only helps us in eliminating the previous etiology for ISR (undersizing/malapposition), but it also helps in visualizing calcific ISR and preemptive use of specialized devices during bed preparation.

Advantages and Limitations of OCT

Advantages

- Superior resolution (~10–20 μm)
- Detailed visualization of plaque composition and stent apposition
- Precise measurement of MLA and stent dimensions
- 3D reconstruction is superior technology and can be used for several causes.
- Superior identification of intraluminal structures (thrombus/flaps/calcific nodules)

Limitations

- Longer procedure time compared to IVUS
- Contrast-use limitation in patients with renal dysfunction
- LM (ostial or >5 mm vessel) is a bane for OCT
- Limited penetration in heavily calcified vessels

TABLE 2: Head-to-head comparison between IVUS and OCT in various situations.

Intravascular imaging systems: IVUS versus OCT		
Type of lesion	**IVUS**	**OCT**
Thrombus	✓	✓✓
Calcified	✓✓	✓
Stent opposition	✓	✓✓
Dissection	✓	✓✓
Neointimal hyperplasia	✓	✓✓
Thin-capped atheroma	×	✓✓
Ostial left main	✓✓	×
Vessel diameter > 5.0 mm	✓✓	✓

Note:
✓✓ Excellent lesion assessment
✓ Good lesion assessment
× Difficult lesion assessment
(IVUS: intravascular ultrasound; OCT: optical coherence tomography)

CONCLUSION

Intravascular coronary imaging with IVUS and OCT has significantly enhanced our understanding and management of coronary artery disease. IVUS provides real-time feedback, accurate measurements, and optimized stent deployment, while OCT offers superior resolution and detailed visualization of plaque morphology and stent apposition. Clinical trials have consistently demonstrated the benefits of both modalities in guiding interventions and improving patient outcomes. The selection between IVUS and OCT has to be nuanced and depends on the specific clinical scenario. As technology continues to advance, intravascular coronary imaging will remain pivotal in shaping the future of interventional cardiology, further improving patient care and outcomes **(Table 2)**.

ONLINE REFERENCES

Please scan the QR code provided at the end of the table of contents for References of this chapter.

CHAPTER 164

Coronary Lesion Assessment: Intravascular Ultrasound versus Optical Coherence Tomography

Sanjeeb Roy, Roopali Khanna, Arun Mohanty, Nishit Chandra

ABSTRACT

Intracoronary imaging goes beyond conventional angiography to overcome the well-established limitations of angiography. Intracoronary imaging by intravascular ultrasound (IVUS) and optical coherence tomography (OCT) is done either during diagnostic catheterization to assess the diseased vessel (native or graft or stent failure) or during the percutaneous coronary intervention (PCI) to provide valuable incremental decision-making information that can be used clinically for intervention strategy and optimization of stent implanted and minimize stent-related complications. Intracoronary imaging during PCI is now algorithmic protocol driven—assessing the lesion morphology, the length of lesion and vessel diameter in pre-intervention and in post-intervention assessing the stent expansion, apposition and stent-related complications like edge dissections. During the intervention in complex anatomy, often imaging is done to assess the adequacy of plaque modification technique adapted and escalate (if need be) or like in bifurcation lesions, ensure proper wire crossing to side branch (SB). Use of intravascular imaging has been supported by numerous studies, for complex lesion PCI in particular, and has shown to make an impact on outcome more so with IVUS (than OCT). The use of both modalities, with their advantages and disadvantages, in various clinical scenarios has been discussed in this brief discourse.

Keywords: Intravascular imaging, vulnerable plaque, bifurcation lesion, left main bifurcation, chronic total occlusions, acute coronary syndrome, bypass graft, primary PCI, calcified lesion and in-stent restenosis.

INTRODUCTION

Angiography is the cornerstone imaging modality for delineating coronary anatomy, diagnosing coronary artery disease (CAD), and guiding therapeutic interventions. Angiography is just a planar projection of contrast-filled lumen of otherwise a 3D coronary anatomy.[1] Various angles of planar projections are acquired and analyzed to overcome the foreshortening and overlapping, to virtually conceive 3D coronary anatomy. Therefore, it can at best be considered a lumenogram or shadowgraph, as it does not depict the vessel wall pathology and details of intraluminal defects in coronaries—native, stented, or grafted.

Intracoronary imaging goes beyond conventional angiography to overcome the well-established limitations of angiography. It elucidates the intraluminal and transmural anatomy of the native or stented coronary vessel or the coronary bypass grafts—profiling both in cross-section and longitudinal extent. Intravascular imaging (IVI) has undergone a sea change since its inception nearly three decades ago as a research tool, in terms of availability, ease of use, and the interpretation of information gathered. IVI helps to differentiate the normal and diseased vessels, provide information about the extent, nature, and severity of the disease, and serial monitoring of disease progression. In diseased vessel, it can identify plaque morphology, decide the coronary intervention strategy, selection and sizing of the stent, its optimization, and long-term follow-up. It impacts the clinical outcome—more so in complex procedures such as left main disease, chronic total occlusion (CTO), bifurcation diffuse disease, and heavily calcified lesions.

The two modalities of IVI that are available are intravascular ultrasound (IVUS) and optical coherence tomography (OCT). Near-infrared spectroscopy–IVUS (NIRS-IVUS) is a novel catheter-based IVI modality that provides a chemogram of the coronary artery wall, enabling the detection of lipid core and specific quantification of lipid accumulation measured as the lipid-core burden index (LCBI). An integrated OCT and IVUS in a single hybrid catheter system are under development. Micro-OCT is a recent technology that constructs 3D imaging of tissue with axial resolution <1 µm and lateral resolution <2 µm which will improve the identification of vulnerable plaque.

BASIC PRINCIPLES

Intravascular imaging is done either during diagnostic catheterization to assess the diseased vessel (native or graft or stent failure) or during the percutaneous coronary intervention (PCI) as a decision-making to intervention strategy and to optimize the stent result. The quality of the image in IVI is defined in terms of resolution and penetration.[2]

Intravascular ultrasound uses the principle of ultrasound imaging where transducer elements are mounted on the tip of a dedicated catheter, which emits ultrasound pulses, which are reflected from the tissue surface to produce gray-scale images. Current IVUS catheters have axial resolution of 80–100 µm, lateral resolution of 250 µm, and tissue penetration of 4–8 mm.[2] Frequency of ultrasound emitted is changed from 20 to 40 MHz and 60 MHz. High-definition IVUS (HD-IVUS) uses 60 MHz and has improved the resolution to around 30 µm.

Optical coherence tomography is based on optical interference of near-infrared light. OCT has a higher axial resolution of 10–15 µm, but poorer penetration (up to 1–2 mm).[2] Both modalities use short monorail catheters to emit waves directed at the vessel wall. The reflected beams to the monorail catheters are then analyzed and cross-sectional images are generated. Frequent flushing with contrast (or saline) is required to displace blood during OCT acquisition,[3] as blood strongly scatters light and attenuates the OCT signal. Superior resolution and obligatory flushing of the lumen make automatic measurements in OCT more accurate than IVUS which frequently need correction.

IMAGE INTERPRETATION

Intravascular Ultrasound

The basic principle of IVUS is that high-frequency sound waves are sent from a transducer and echo off-vessel walls are sent back to the system which are then system processed electronically to form the image. A structure's acoustic impedance (density) determines if ultrasound is reflected. Structures that reflect will appear in varying shades of "white" on the screen, e.g., calcium appears bright white because it reflects all ultrasound and produces acoustic shadows. Soft tissue will absorb the ultrasound and appear as a darker image on the screen. The IVUS terminology used for tissue characterization is enlisted in **Table 1**.

TABLE 1: Terminology for IVUS findings.

Echogenicity	Compared to the echogenicity of adventitia (hypoechoic and hyperechoic)
Shadowing	Complete reflection of sound waves from the surface (cannot see behind the structure)
Attenuation	Reduction in intensity of sound as it passes through the tissue due to absorption or scattering (intensity of signal varies)
Reverberation	Ghost images from repetitive reflections (>double images)

(IVUS: intravascular ultrasound)

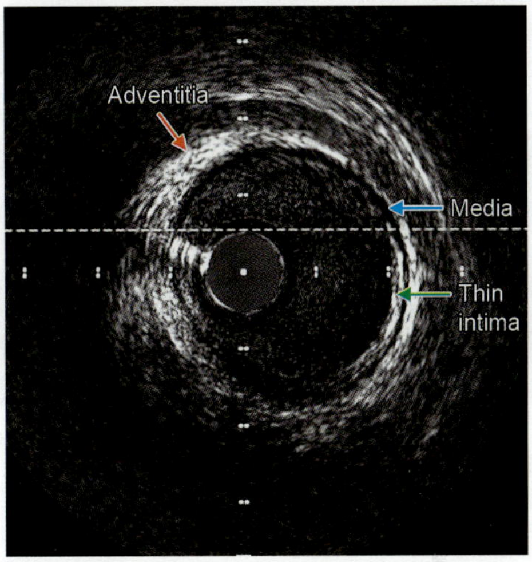

FIG. 1: IVUS: IVUS shows the three layers intima, media, and adventitia as labeled.
(IVUS: intravascular ultrasound)

The IVUS shows the three-layer structure of the artery—the echo-dense intima, the echo-lucent media, and the more echo-dense adventitia **(Fig. 1)**. Blood, fat, and smooth muscle reflect ultrasound poorly and appear dark in color. Coronary atheroma lies between the intima and media layers **(Fig. 1)**. Normal intimal thickness is <150–300 µm, intimal thickness is defined as >300–600 µm, and fibrous plaque intima is >600 µm. Different plaque morphology as assessed by IVUS is summarized in **Table 2** and **Figure 2**.

Optical Coherence Tomography

Optical coherence tomography is an IVI modality akin to IVUS. It utilizes light waves instead of sound waves for image acquisition and consequently provides a quantum leap in coaxial resolution. Light waves near the infrared range (1,300-nm wavelength) are projected around the imaged structure and the reflected backscattered light signals form the images for analysis. The OCT terminology used for tissue characterization is enlisted in **Table 3**.

TABLE 2: Plaque characteristics on IVUS: IVUS image interpretation terminology.

	Echogenicity	Attenuation	Reverberations	Shadowing
Fibrous plaque	Echo/Hyperechogenic	No	No	No
Lipidic plaque	Hypoechogenic	Yes	No	No
Necrotic plaque	Hypoechogenic	Yes	No	No
Calcified plaque	Hyperechogenic	No	Yes	Yes

(IVUS: intravascular ultrasound)

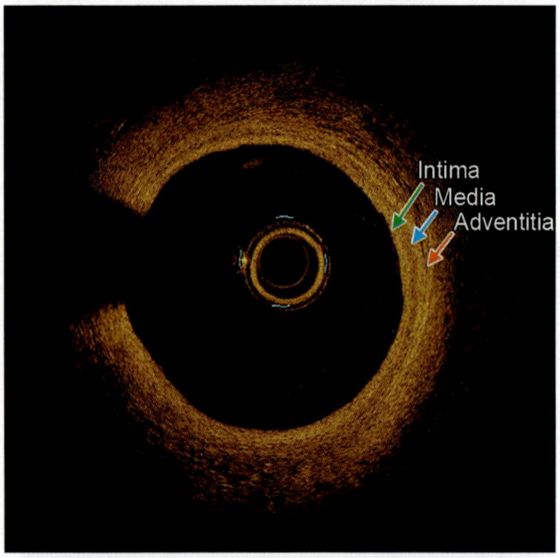

FIG. 2: OCT: OCT shows the three layers intima, media, and adventitia as labeled.

(OCT: optical coherence tomography)

TABLE 3: Terminology for OCT findings.

Backscatter	• Reflection of light waves from the tissue • *High backscatter*: Brighter pixel, also described as a "signal-rich" region • *Low backscatter*: Darker pixel, also described as a "signal-poor" region
Attenuation	• Reduction in the intensity of the light waves as they pass through tissue due to absorption or scattering • *High attenuation*: Light cannot penetrate very deep • *Low attenuation*: Light can pass through to allow visualization of deeper tissue
Borders	Borders can be sharp or diffuse

(OCT: optical coherence tomography)

The three-layered structure on OCT: The media appears to signal poor structure positioned between the thin backscattering intima layer and a heterogenous high backscattering adventitia layer. The dark band of media is surrounded by the internal elastic membrane and external elastic membrane **(Fig. 3)**. Different plaque morphology as assessed by OCT is summarized in **Table 4** and **Figure 2**.

There are certain limitations with both the modalities of imaging. Due to poor penetration depth of OCT (1.5–2 mm), it is difficult to visualize the whole vessel, arterial remodeling, and plaque burden measurement by OCT. In IVUS due to poor resolution, to detect plaque vulnerability is a challenge. Due to acoustic shadowing of calcium on IVUS, the calcium thickness cannot be assessed by IVUS which hinders to assess the severity of calcium.

CLINICAL UTILITY OF INTRAVASCULAR IMAGING

Intracoronary imaging by IVUS and OCT provides valuable incremental information that can be used clinically to optimize stent implantation and minimize stent-related problems **(Table 5)**. Preintervention imaging helps to identify the lesion characteristics and its severity and accordingly strategize the vessel preparation. Postintervention imaging helps to optimize the result and detect the complications of the procedure if any. PCI guidance with IVI is now an algorithm-step approach using either IVUS or OCT (summarized as mnemonic IVUS 1-2-3 Essentials and MLD MAX for OCT) **(Figs. 4 and 5)**. OCT-based measurements in early studies were found similar to phantom models while IVUS overestimated.[4] More contemporary studies show OCT and HD-IVUS measurements to be similar.[5,6]

Preprocedure Assessment

Preintervention imaging helps to identify the lesion characteristics and its severity and accordingly strategize the vessel preparation **(Figs. 6 and 7)**.

Lesion Severity

Lesion severity is assessed by minimum lumen area (MLA) and it fairly correlates with ischemia. For non-left main coronary artery (LMCA) lesions, IVUS MLA cut-off ranges from 2.1 to 4.1 mm^2 and OCT MLA cut-off ranges from 1.6 to 2.4 mm^2 as reported in various studies.[7-9] The vessel size is reported to be smaller in Asians than Western population. Meta-analyses suggest a cut-off of 2.8–2.9 mm^2 with IVUS and 2.0 mm^2 with OCT for Asian patients.[7-9] These have high

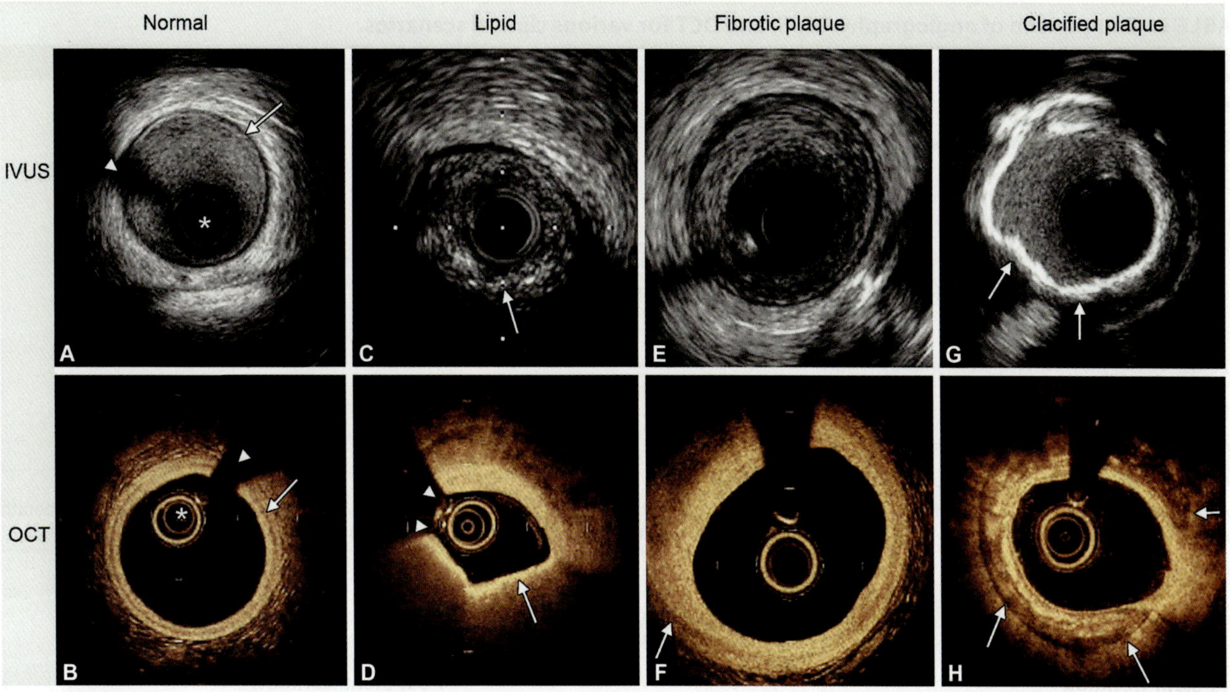

FIGS. 3A TO H: Lesion morphology appearance with intravascular imaging. Normal vessel on IVUS (A) and OCT (B). White arrow points to media and asterisk to lumen catheter. Arrowhead points to image catheter artefact. Lipid plaque on IVUS (C), and IVUS appears as attenuated (arrow) behind a signal-rich fibrous cap. (D) Media is less well visualized behind lipid in OCT (arrowhead). Fibrous plaque appears as intermediate echogenic (like adventitia) on IVUS (E) and homogenous with high back scatter and low attenuation on OCT (F) (arrow). Calcium bright on IVUS (G) (arrow) with acoustic shadowing and heterogenous on OCT with low back scatter and low attenuation and clear demarcation (H).

(IVUS: intravascular ultrasound; OCT: optical coherence tomography)

Source: Shlofmitz E, Ali ZA, Maehara A, Mintz GS, Shlofmitz R, Jeremias A. Intravascular Imaging-Guided Percutaneous Coronary Intervention. A Universal Approach for Optimization of Stent Implantation. Circ Cardiovasc Interv. 2020;13:e008686.

TABLE 4: Plaque characteristics on OCT: OCT image interpretation terminology.

	Backscatter	Attenuation	Edge	Texture
Fibrous plaque	Bright	Low	–	Homogenous
Lipidic plaque	Darker	High	Diffuse	Homogenous
Necrotic plaque	Darker	High	Diffuse	Heterogenous
Calcified plaque	Darker	Low	Sharp	Heterogenous

(OCT: optical coherence tomography)

negative predictive values but low positive predictive values. Deferral strategy based on IVI assessment has been found to be as good as FFR—as shown with the use of OCT in the FORZA study.[10] Positive remodeling or negative remodeling and the plaque burden can be better assessed using IVUS and limited in OCT **(Fig. 8)**.

Lesion Length

The lesion length is assessed on IVI by identifying healthy segments (landing zones) on either side. In diffusely diseased vessels, relatively healthy segments are identified with IVUS as plaque burden of <50% in IVUS and with OCT >180° of external elastic lamina (EEL) visible. The distance between the proximal and distal landing zones thus identified is the lesion length. Overall, <10% of the angiographically normal reference segment is disease free with <50% plaque burden.[11] Lipid-rich plaque [attenuated plaque on IVUS and thin-cap fibroatheroma (TCFA) on OCT], significant superficial calcium, or a muscle bridge is to be avoided when considering landing zones.[3]

Vessel Diameter

The vessel diameter is assessed by EEM–EEM diameter (when EEM visible) or lumen diameter (when EEM not visible), measured in two orthogonal planes and averaged as "reference vessel diameter". These measurements help in the choice of size of the stent and the diameter of the balloon for preparation (predilatation) and optimization

TABLE 5: Comparison of angiography, IVUS, and OCT for various clinical scenarios.

Indication	Angiography	IVUS	OCT
Assessment of left main coronary artery stenosis	+	+++	+
Assessment of non-left main coronary artery stenosis	++	++	+++
Localize the culprit lesion	+	++	+++
Identify a vulnerable plaque	–	++ (VH-IVUS)	+++
Determine the likelihood of distal embolization and periprocedural MI	–	+++ (VH-IVUS)	++
Size the vessel undergoing stent implantation	++	+++	+++
Optimize stent results	+	+++	+++
Evaluate stent thrombosis or restenosis	+	++	+++

(IVUS: intravascular ultrasound; OCT: optical coherence tomography)

Source: Parviz Y, Shlofmitz E, Fall KN, Konigstein M, Maehara A, Jeremias A, et al. Utility of intracoronary imaging in the catheterization laboratory: comprehensive evaluation with intravascular ultrasound and optical coherence tomography. Br Med Bull. 2018;125:79-90.

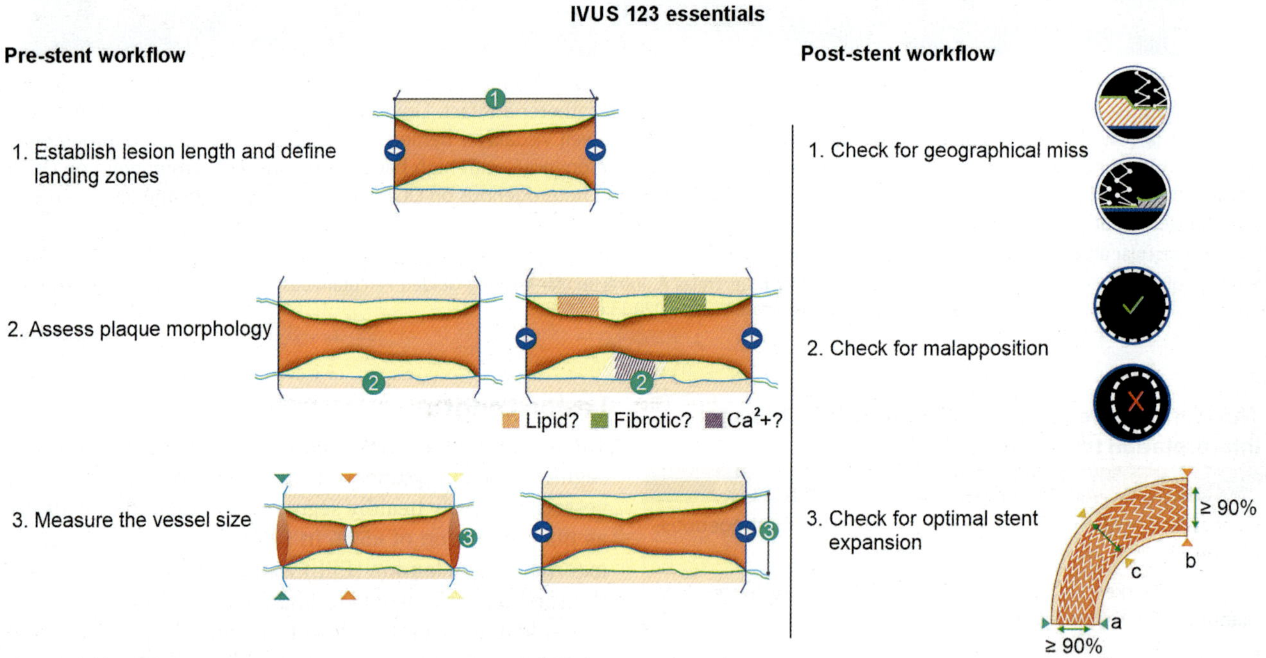

FIG. 4: Intravascular ultrasound (IVUS) algorithm (1-2-3 essential).

(postdilatation). The stent is sized according to distal reference (scaled down by 0.25 mm from EEM–EEM diameter or scaled up by 0.25 mm from lumen diameter). The balloon for optimization is according to distal and proximal reference vessel diameters (DOT—distal optimization technique and POT—proximal optimization technique).

Plaque Morphology

Plaque morphology is the next important step. IVI can differentiate the plaque as lipid, fibrotic, or calcified and the luminal contents **(Fig. 2)**. Lipid-rich plaque, IVUS-attenuated plaque (necrotic core with thin cap) or OCT TCFA, or plaque rupture has been associated with no- or slow-flow and periprocedural myocardial infarction. In setting of acute coronary syndrome (ACS), however, the positive predictive value is low and the negative predictive value is high. Presence of calcium hinders stent expansion and can be better visualized by imaging than by angiography.[12-14] Imaging helps to differentiate calcification as superficial or deep calcium, protruding nodular calcium or plate, eccentric

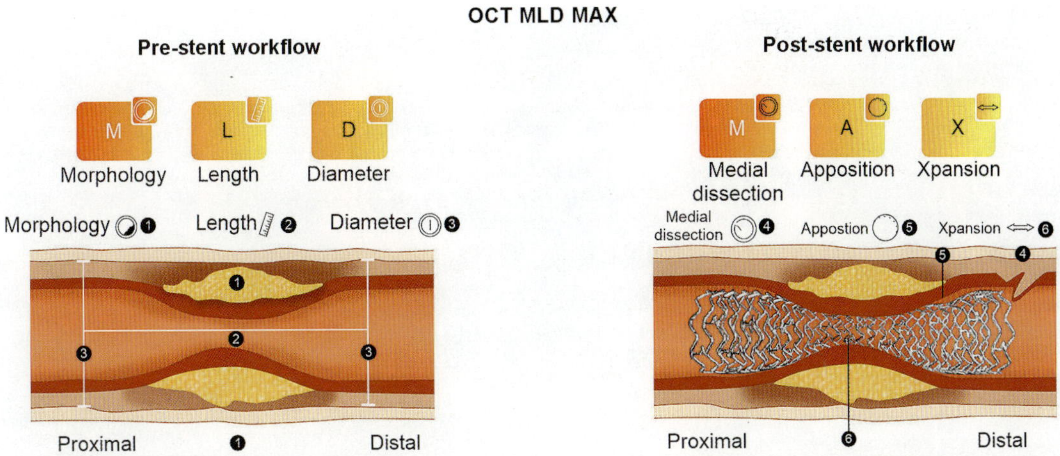

M Characterization of plaque and search for high calcium
L Select landing zone (based on healthy tissue/EEL visualization) and measure the length in between
D Measure the vessel diameter at landing zone and select balloon and stent size in accordance

M Address significant edge dissection >45° and >2 mm in length with medial extension
A Address gross malapposition (<0.5 mm axial distance and <2 mm long
X Confirm expansion (>90% of reference segment)

FIG. 5: OCT algorithm (MLD-MAX).
(EEL: external elastic lamina; OCT: optical coherence tomography)

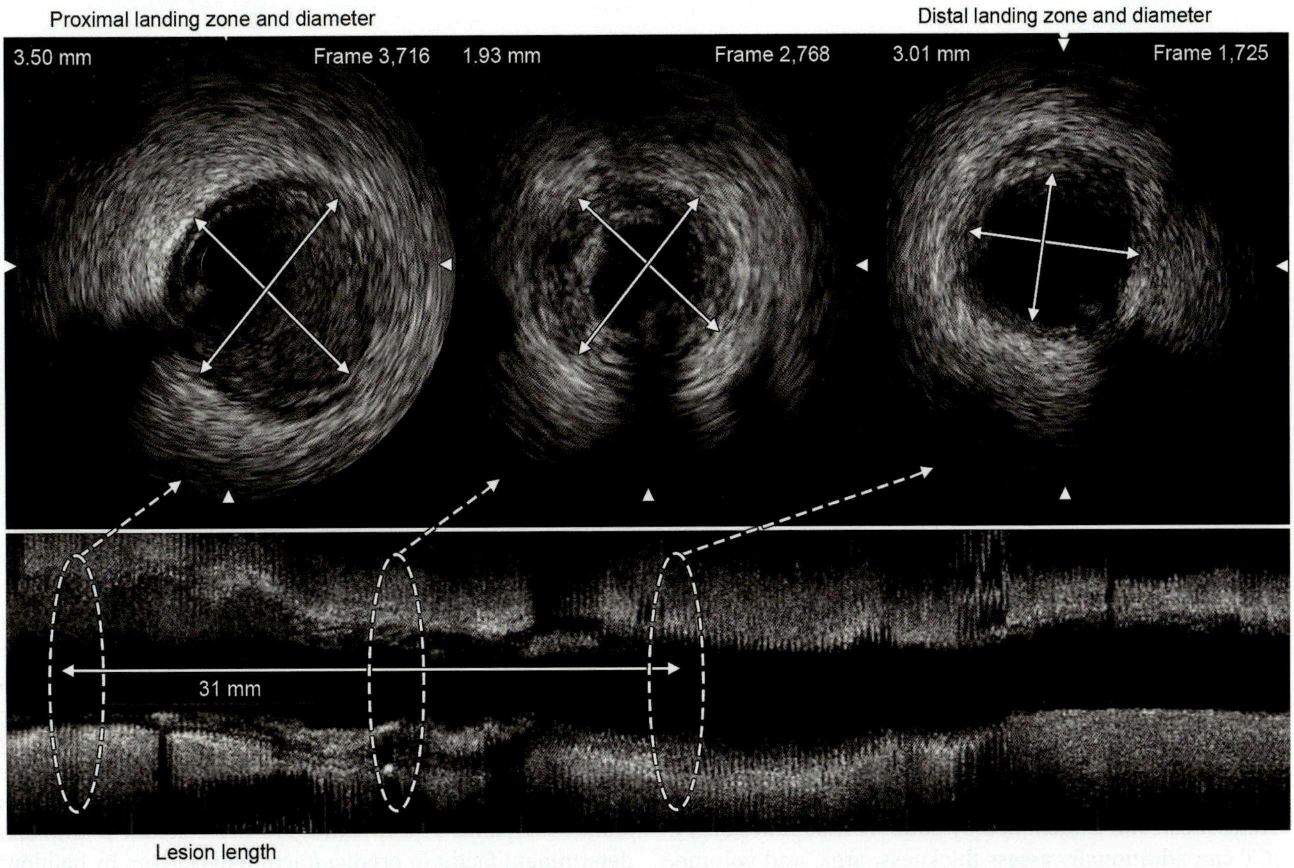

FIG. 6: Intravascular ultrasound assessment of landing zone, lesion length, vessel diameter, and lesion morphology at diseased segment.

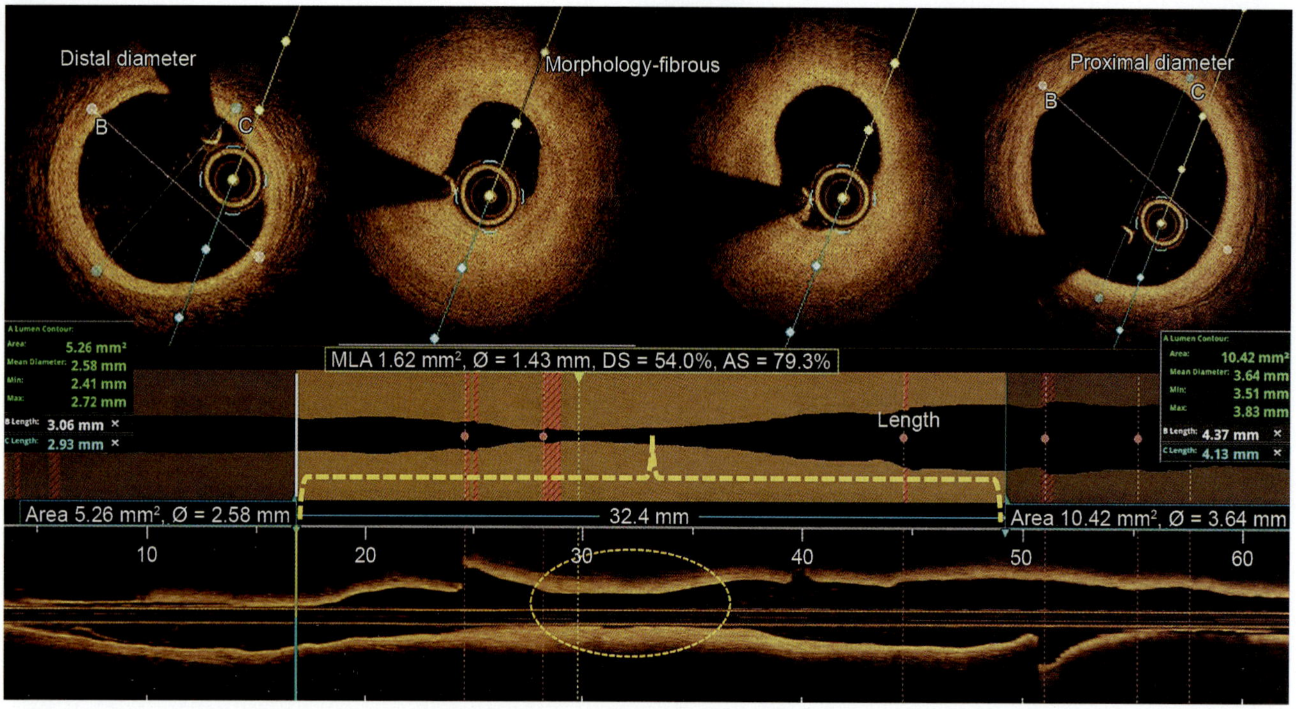

FIG. 7: OCT assessment of landing zone, lesion length, vessel diameter, and lesion morphology at diseased segment.
(DS: diameter stenosis; MLA: minimum lumen area; OCT: optical coherence tomography)

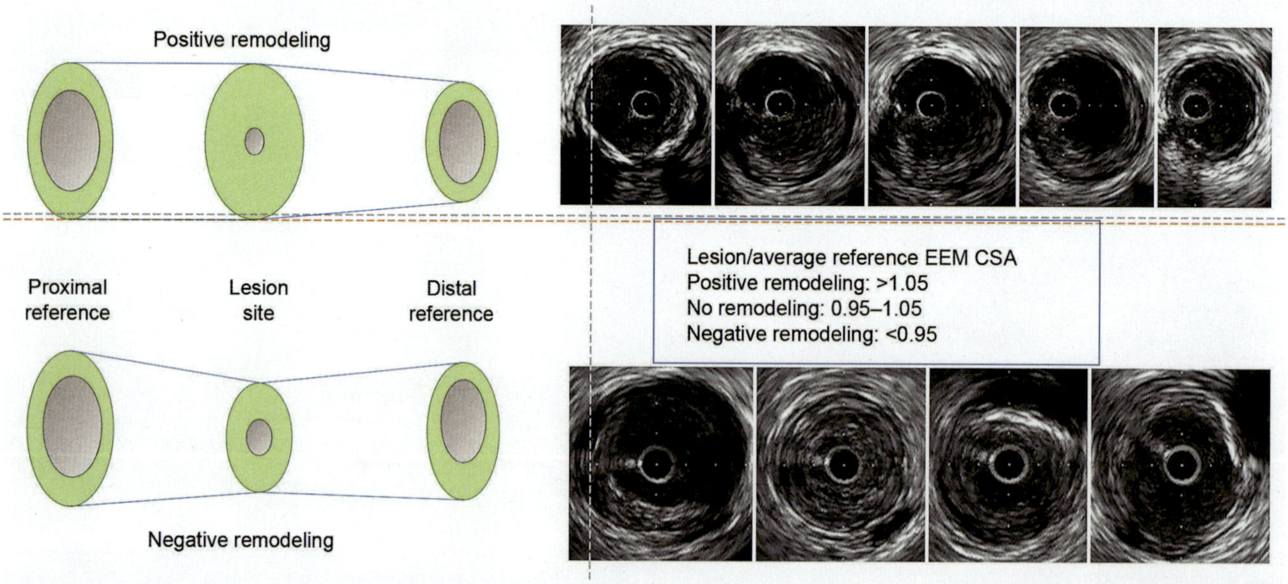

FIG. 8: Positive and negative remodeling.

or concentric, quadratic, hemispherical, or circumferential **(Fig. 9)**. The circumferential distribution and longitudinal extent of calcium is identified by both the modalities of IVI. OCT can additionally assess thickness, area, and volume, but will miss calcium behind lipid. The calcium distribution identified by imaging helps to select tools for the plaque modification. Identification of fractures on imaging after use of these tools ensures adequate preparation for the stent to expand. The thickness of the calcium is the key determinant factor to predict fracture of calcium by balloon and a thickness of 0.5 mm by OCT being the predictive threshold.[15,16] Calcium scoring has been developed for OCT

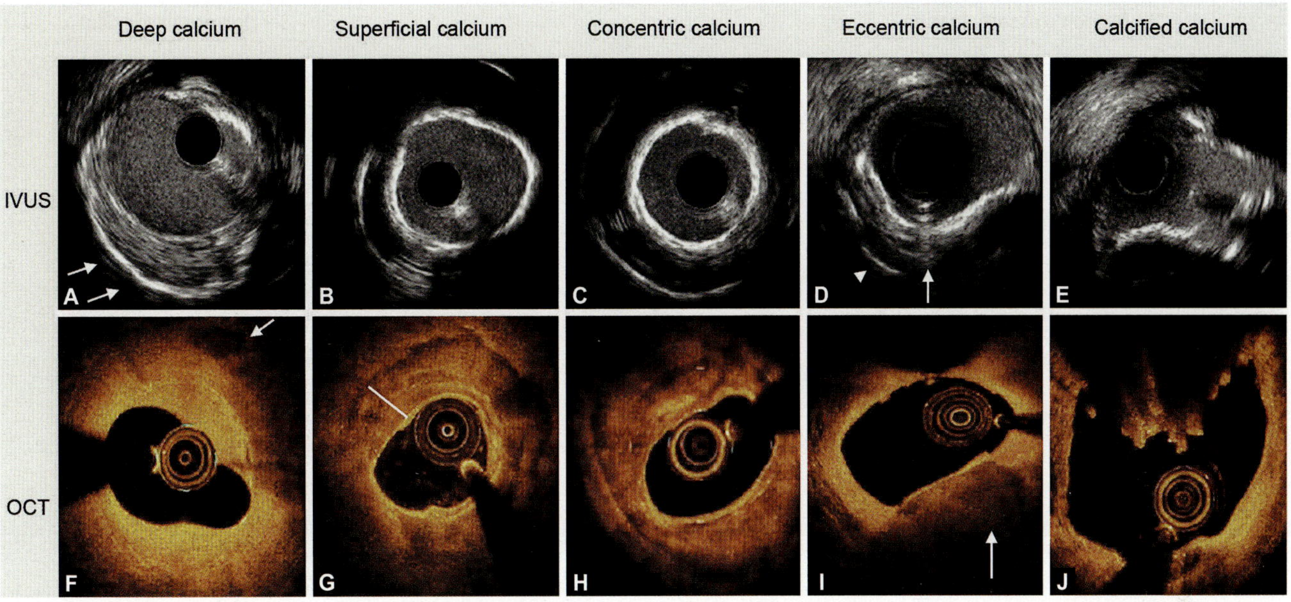

FIGS. 9A TO J: Coronary calcium. IVUS cross-section of: (A) deep calcium with arrows demonstrating the arc of calcium, (B) superficial calcium, (C) concentric calcium, (D) eccentric calcium with an arrow highlighting the arc of calcium with reverberations present (arrowhead), and (E) calcified nodule. OCT cross-section of (F) deep calcium with an arrow at the calcified plaque, (G) superficial calcium with calcium thickness easily assessed (line), (H) concentric calcium, (I) eccentric calcium with an arrow highlighting the calcium, and (J) calcified nodule.

(IVUS: intravascular ultrasound; OCT: optical coherence tomography)

Source: Shlofmitz E, Ali ZA, Maehara A, Mintz GS, Shlofmitz R, Jeremias A. Intravascular Imaging-Guided Percutaneous Coronary Intervention. A Universal Approach for Optimization of Stent Implantation. Circ Cardiovasc Interv. 2020;13:e008686.

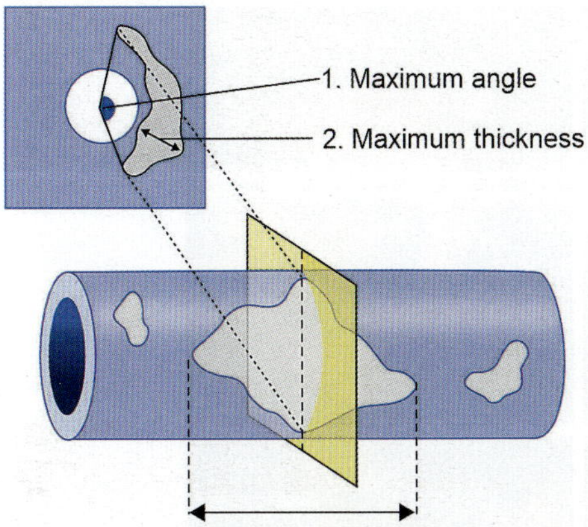

Severity	OCT criteria (0–4)		IVUS criteria (0–4)	
	Predictors of underexpansion			
	Calcium angle	≤ 00° = 0 ≤180° = 1 >180° = 2	Calcium angle	>360° = 1 >270° for ≥5 mm = 1
	Calcium length	≤5.0 mm = 0 >5.0 mm = 1	Calcium nodule	=1
	Calcium thickness	≤0.5 mm = 0 >0.5 mm = 1	Vessel diameter <3.5mm	=1
Mild to moderate	0–3		0–1	
Severe	4		≥2	

FIG. 10: Assessment of calcium distribution and severity. (A) Cross section view (B) Longitudinal view.

(IVUS: intravascular ultrasound; OCT: optical coherence tomography)

Source: Angsubakorn N, Kang N, Fearon C, Techorueangwiwat C, Swamy P, Brilakis ES, et al. Contemporary management of severely calcified coronary lesions. J Pers Med. 2022;12:1638.

(arc > 180°, thickness > 0.5 mm, length > 5 mm) and IVUS (arc > 270° or circumferential, presence of calcium nodule or vessel diameter of <3.5 mm) **(Fig. 10)**.[17,18] Calcium modification algorithms are in accordance **(Fig. 11)**. Adequacy of the plaque modification techniques can be assessed with imaging **(Fig. 12)**.

Postprocedure Assessment

Postprocedure imaging is performed after stent deployment and optimization to get desired angiographic result and to rule out various complications **(Figs. 13 to 15)**.

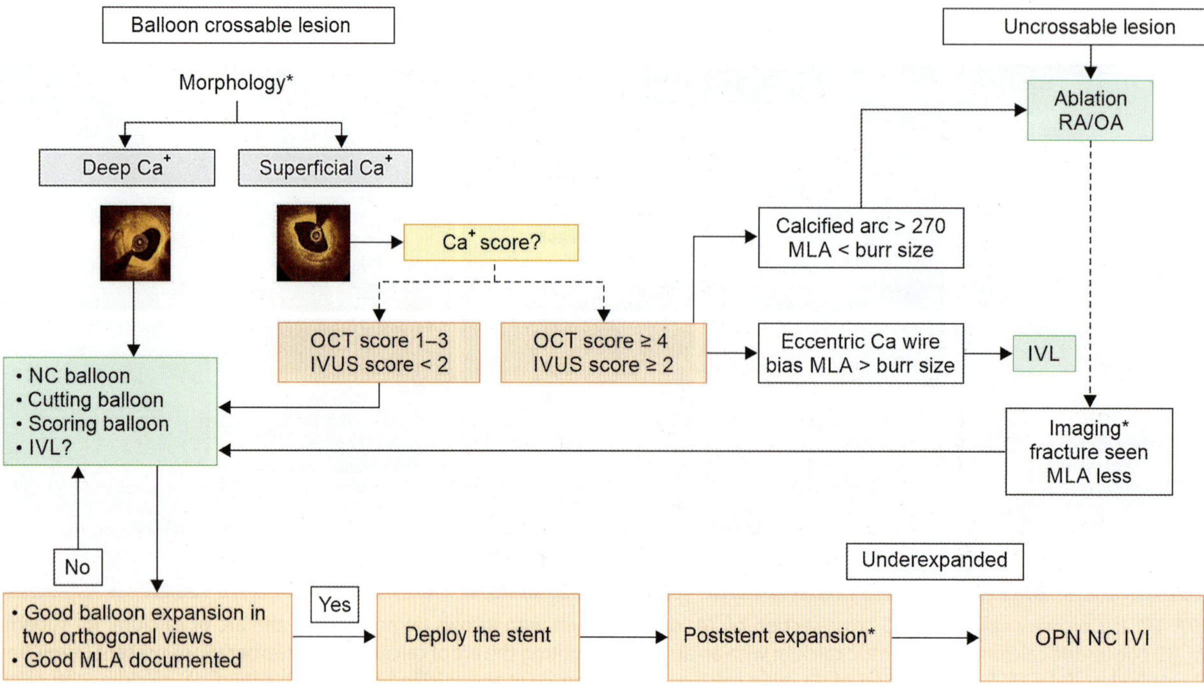

FIG. 11: Algorithm: Approach to calcified lesion.

[Ca+: calcium; RA: rotational atherectomy; OA: orbital atherectomy; IVL: intravascular lithotripsy; NC: noncompliant; MLA: minimal lumen area; OPN balloon (SIS MEdical)]

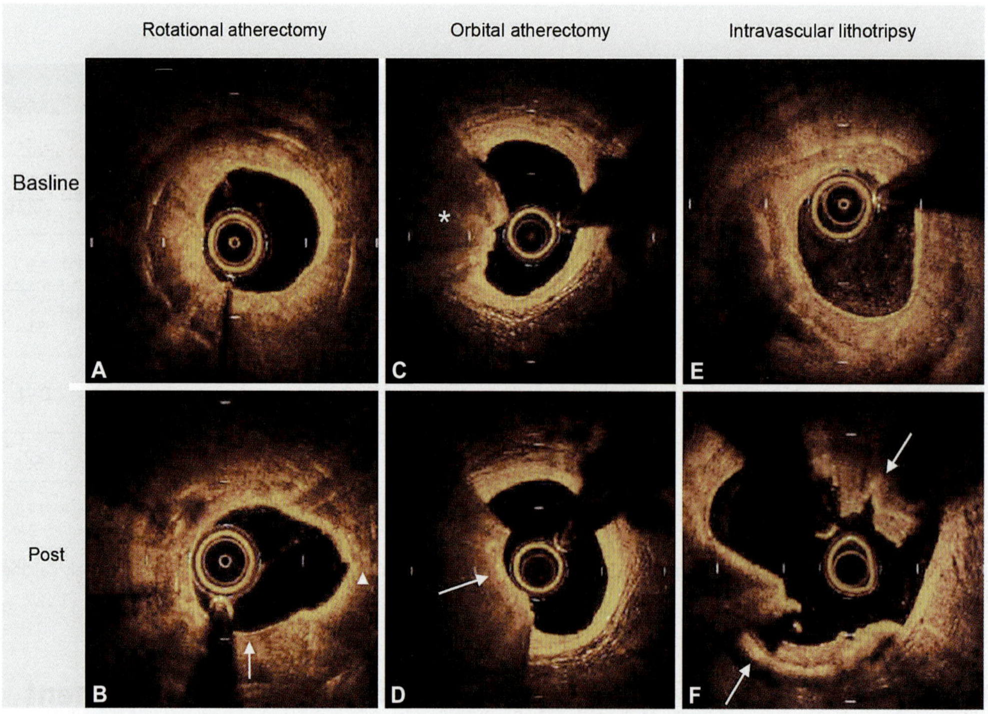

FIGS. 12A TO F: Impact of lesion preparation for circumferential calcium as assessed by optical coherence tomography (OCT). OCT cross-section: (A) circumferential calcium and (B) following treatment with rotational atherectomy (arrow). (C) Calcified nodule (asterisk), with eccentric plaque protruding into the lumen and (D) following ablation with orbital atherectomy demonstrating the characteristic smooth, concentric plaque modification. (E) Concentric, superficial calcification and (F) following treatment with intravascular lithotripsy, multiple calcium fractures are observed.

Source: Shlofmitz E, Ali ZA, Maehara A, Mintz GS, Shlofmitz R, Jeremias A. Intravascular imaging-guided percutaneous coronary intervention. A Universal Approach for Optimization of Stent Implantation. Circ Cardiovasc Interv. 2020;13:e008686.

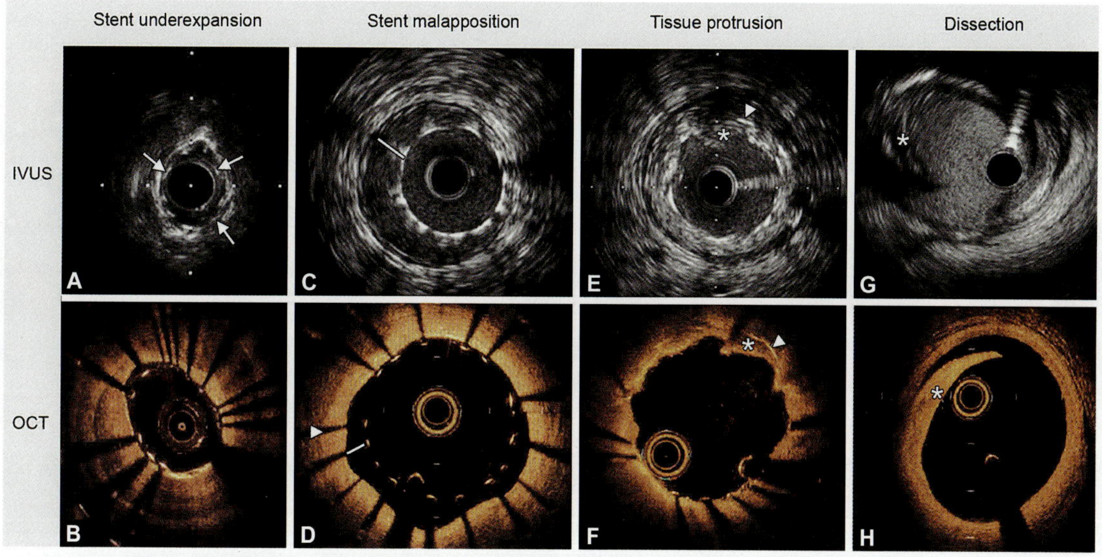

FIGS. 13A TO H: Post-stent assessment by intravascular imaging. IVUS cross-section with: (A) underexpanded stent strut in the setting of circumferential calcification, (C) stent malapposition with stent struts a significant distance (line) from the vessel wall, (E) tissue protrusion (asterisk) protruding into the lumen, beyond the stent struts that appear bright (arrowhead), (G) dissection flap (asterisk) extends into the lumen. OCT cross-section with: (B) underexpanded stent, (D) stent malapposition with stent struts a significant distance (line) from the vessel wall, (F) tissue protrusion (asterisk) protruding into the lumen, beyond the stent struts that appear bright (arrowhead). (H) Dissection flap (asterisk) extends into the lumen.

(IVUS: intravascular ultrasound; OCT: optical coherence tomography)

Source: Shlofmitz E, Ali ZA, Maehara A, Mintz GS, Shlofmitz R, Jeremias A. Intravascular imaging-guided percutaneous coronary intervention. A Universal Approach for Optimization of Stent Implantation. Circ Cardiovasc Interv. 2020;13:e008686.

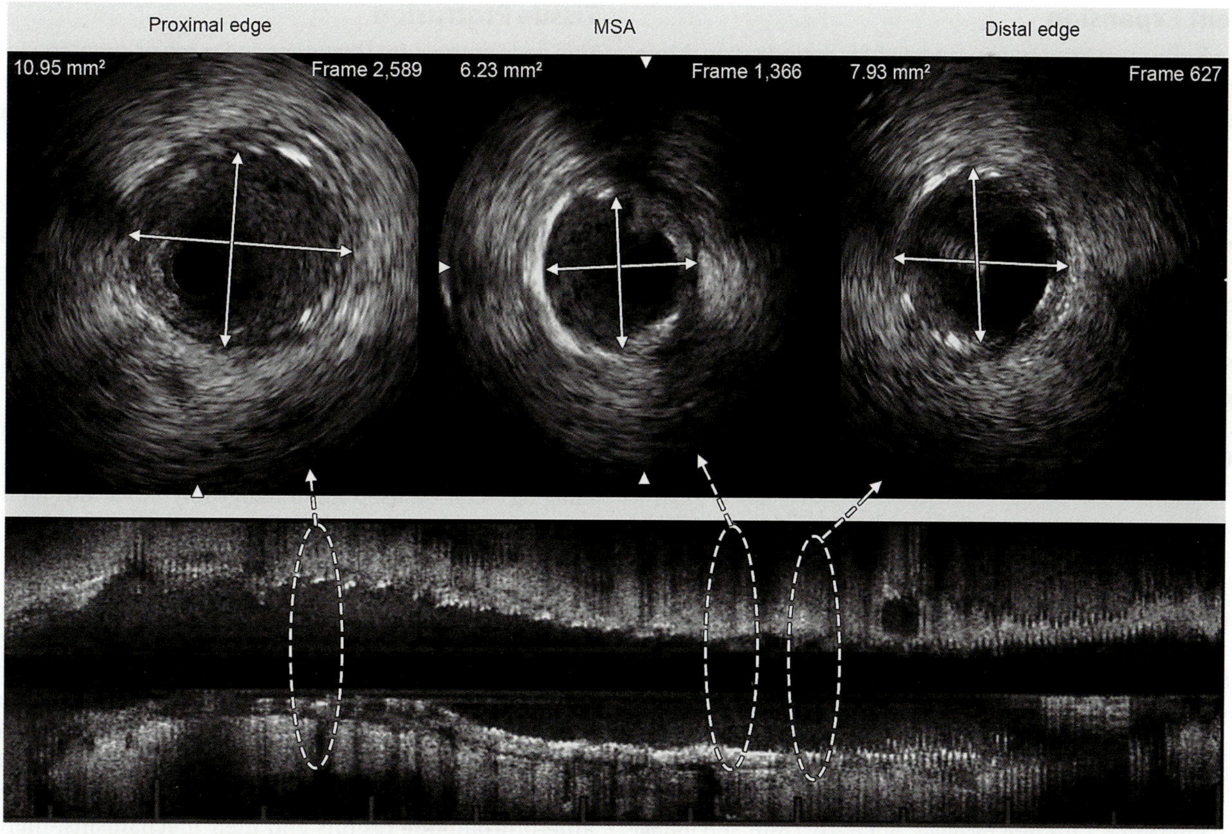

FIG. 14: IVUS-guided stent optimization. Well-expanded and apposed stent with no edge dissection or tissue protrusion in IVUS.

(IVUS: intravascular ultrasound; MSA: minimum stent area)

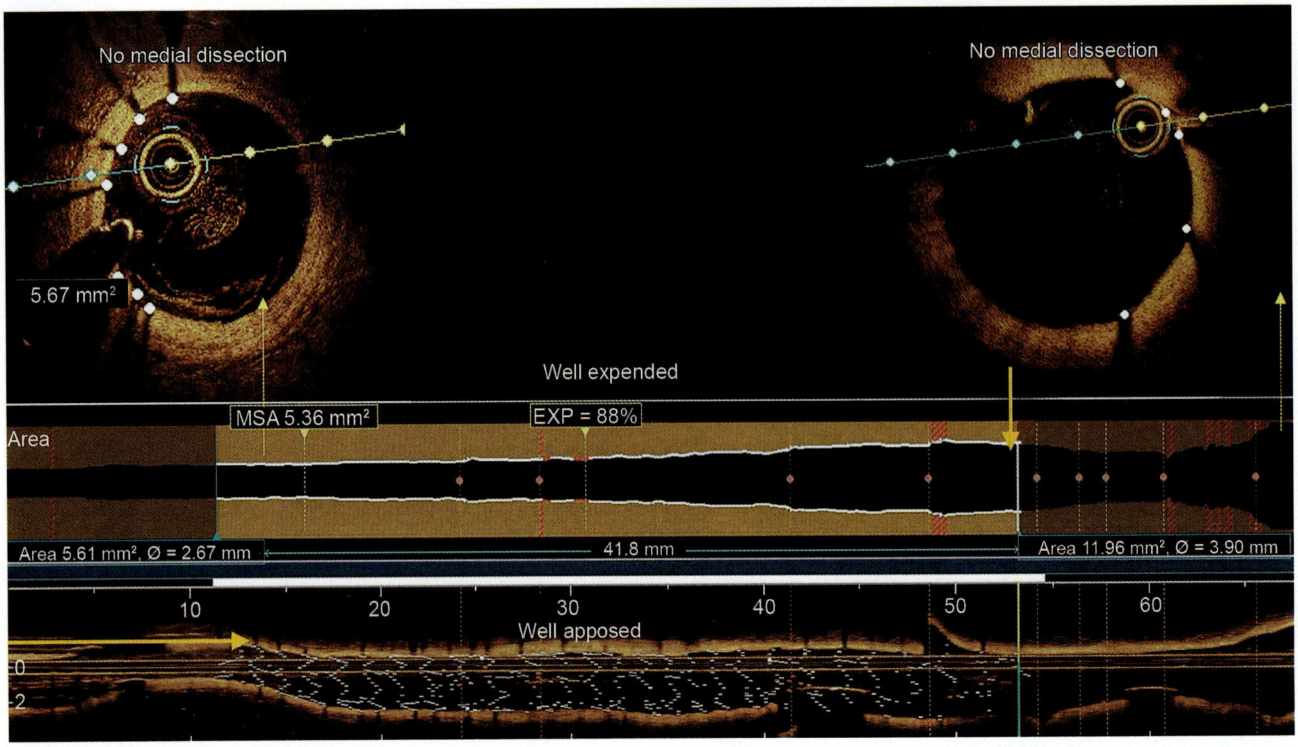

FIG. 15: OCT-guided stent optimization. Well expanded and apposed stent with no edge dissection or tissue protrusion on OCT. (MSA: minimum stent area; OCT: optical coherence tomography)

Stent Expansion

This is the most important parameter for optimization. More than 30 studies of IVI have shown that stent underexpansion is the consistent predictor for stent thrombosis or restenosis. For non-LMCA lesion, stent expansion of 5.5 mm^2 by IVUS or 4.5 mm^2 by OCT or minimum stent area (MSA) of >90% of distal reference area in non-LMCA lesion is considered optimal or if ideal MSA cannot be measured, an MSA of >40% of the lesion EEL area can be considered.[19-23] In long stenosis and stented segment, stent length is divided into two halves—proximal and distal, and the target optimization MSA is 90% of nearby reference proximal or distal reference segment areas.[20]

Geographical Miss

This is uncovered segment with >50% plaque burden, reduced lumen area, or significant lipid.[14] *Edge dissections* are more evident by IVI but mostly clinically silent. It is considered significant requiring additional stent when it extends to media or adventitia in depth, >2 mm in length or of >60° arc in lateral extension.[22] *Acute stent malapposition* is more frequently appreciated by OCT than IVUS. It has not been proven to be associated with any adverse events, except at proximal edge—more with bifurcation lesion—as wire recross could be abluminal and could cause serious stent deformation during attempts to cross with balloon. Acute malapposition > 0.3 mm resolves, but if > 0.3 mm and longer than 1 mm, then additional postdilatation considered.

Tissue Protrusion

This does not require treatment and resolves spontaneously. Tissue or thrombus prolapse especially in ACS if significantly compromises, the lumen will need additional treatment. The eccentricity or asymmetry of stent has not been proven to be of any clinical relevance.[14]

Final imaging run ensures proper optimization of stent deployment with stent area (MSA) of >90% of reference vessel area (>80% acceptable) and no major edge dissection or geographical miss **(Figs. 14 and 15)**.

USE OF INTRAVASCULAR IMAGING IN VARIOUS CLINICAL SETTINGS

Intravascular ultrasound and OCT—both modalities of imaging—can be used interchangeably in various clinical situations. Both are safe, effective, and efficient to use.

Acute Coronary Syndrome

Intravascular imaging in ACS helps to identify culprit lesions. OCT with its superior resolution and the need for flushing helps better visualization of plaque rupture, plaque erosion, thrombus (red and white), calcified lesion, and spontaneous coronary artery dissection (SCAD).[24] The imaging protocol in ACS helps in identifying atherothrombotic lesions and their mechanisms, thereby enabling tailored therapy **(Figs. 16 to 18)**.

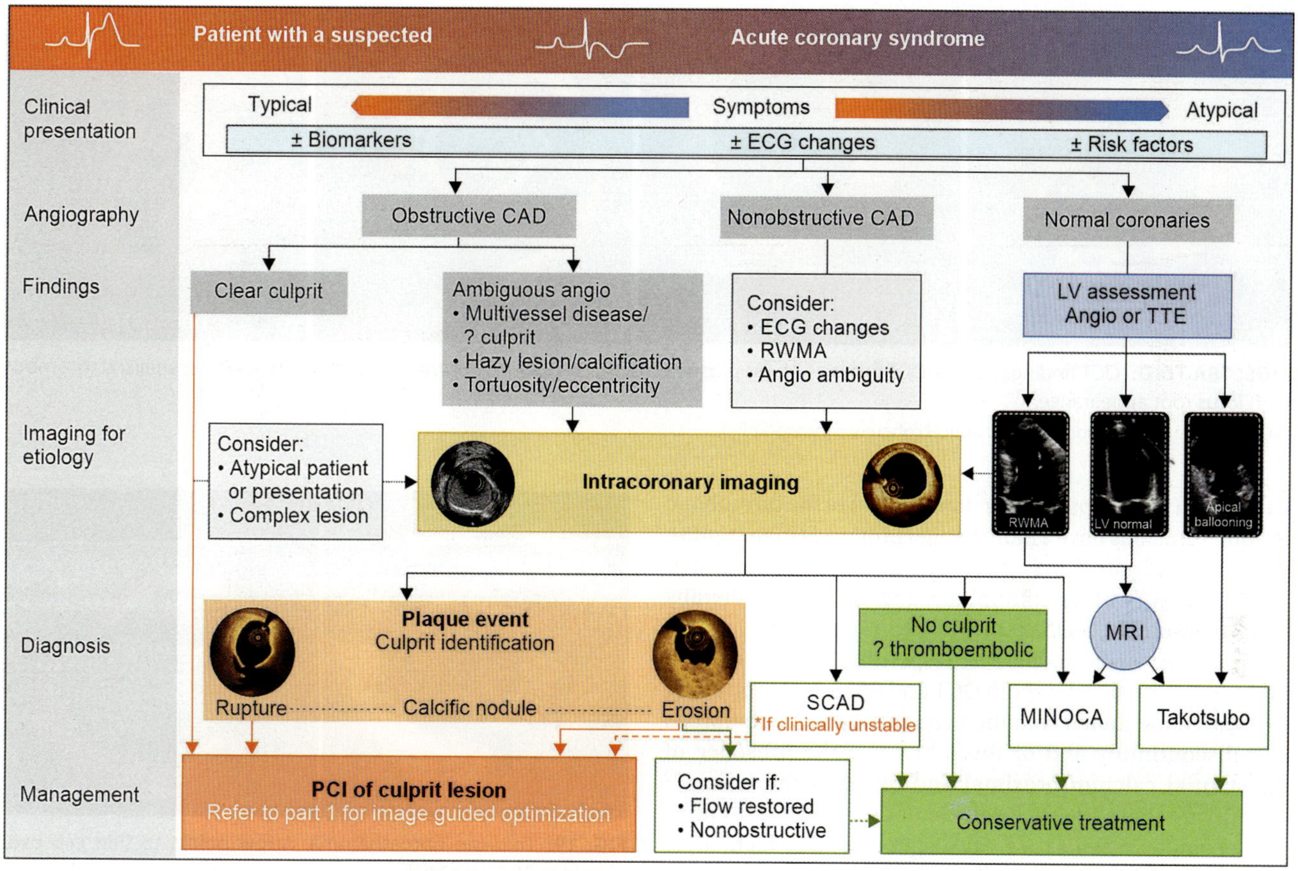

FIG. 16: Treatment algorithm based on intravascular imaging in ACS.

(ACS: acute coronary syndrome; CAD: coronary artery disease; ECG: electrocardiogram; LV: left ventricle; MINOCA: myocardial infarction with nonobstructive coronary artery; RWMA: regional wall motion abnormality; SCAD: spontaneous coronary artery dissection; TTE: transthoracic echocardiography)

Source: Johnson TW, Räber L, Di Mario C, Bourantas CV, Jia H, Mattesini A, et al. Clinical use of intracoronary imaging. Part 2: acute coronary syndromes, ambiguous coronary angiography findings, and guiding interventional decision making: an expert consensus document of the European Association of Percutaneous Cardiovascular Interventions. EuroIntervention. 2019;15:434-51.

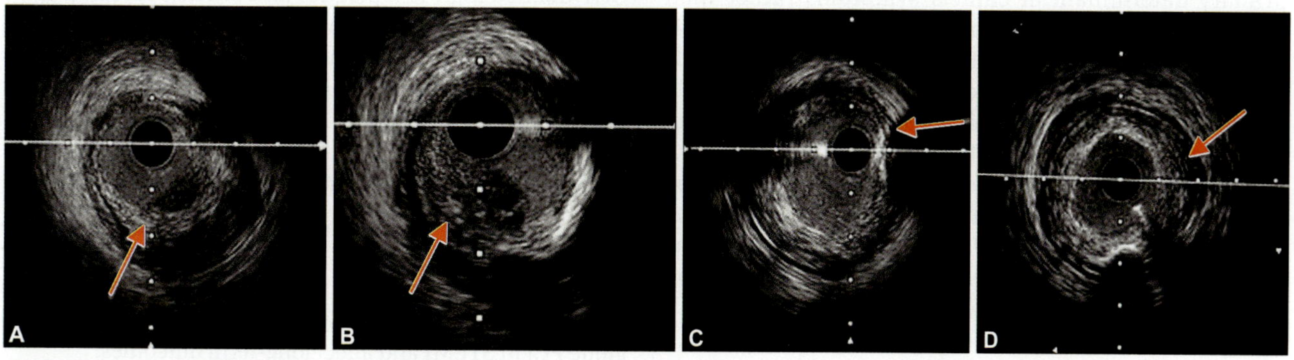

FIGS. 17A TO D: IVUS findings in ACS: (A) red thrombus, (B) mixed thrombus, (C) calcium nodule, and (D) intramural hematoma.

(ACS: acute coronary syndrome; IVUS: intravascular ultrasound)

Plaque rupture has discontinuity of fibrous cap overlying a lipid-rich core. The presence of thrombus overlying ruptured segments often precludes the identification of underlying lipid-rich core.[24] Hallmark features of plaque rupture of culprit lesion are the presence of thrombus, small lumen area, and greater plaque burden at culprit lesion. Ruptures could sometimes be multiple.[25]

In plaque erosion, there is denudation of endothelium, undetectable by IVI. It is diagnosed by exclusion, better with OCT. It is labeled as "definite erosion" in a nondisrupted plaque, mostly fibrous and with an overlying white thrombus. "Probable erosion" may lack thrombus but with an irregular luminal surface or there might be a thrombus with attenuation of plaque but no evidence of lipid/superficial

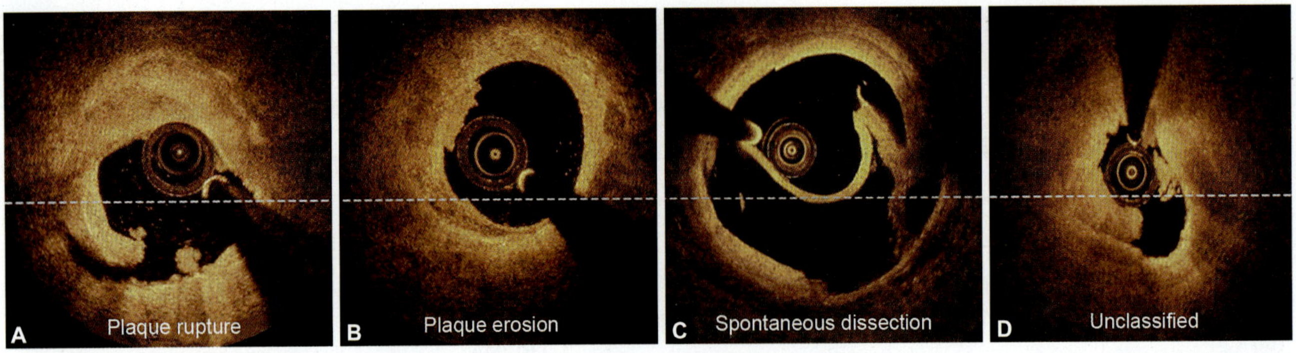

FIGS. 18A TO D: OCT findings in ACS. OCT findings of: (A) plaque erosion, (B) plaque rupture, (C) red thrombus, (D) recanalized thrombus with lotus root appearance.
(ACS: acute coronary syndrome; OCT: optical coherence tomography)

calcium on either upstream or downstream of the thrombotic lesion.[26] Erosions have a more benign prognosis than rupture and if luminal narrowing < 70% stenosis, these can be treated conservatively with antithrombotic and antiplatelet therapy with stenting (EROSION studies).[27-29]

Eruptive calcific nodules are responsible for 2–7% of ACS and can be visualized by both OCT and IVUS. It is protruding calcium in the lumen with the irregular surface with fibrous cap discontinuity and/or thrombus and the presence of substantial calcium proximal and distal to the lesion.[30] Identifying these eruptive calcific nodules is important as these complex lesions pose challenges and carry high target vessel revascularization rate.[31]

In ACS, imaging plays an important role in identifying nonatherosclerotic causes of ACS. IVUS and OCT help to identify the vasospastic segments.[32,33] Imaging helps to identify muscle bridges that could be angiographically silent. Restricted arterial relaxation in diastole is the primary determinant of clinical symptoms rather than systolic compression.[34] When SCAD is suspected, IVUS is the preferred modality as OCT needs flushing. Many SCAD patients when identified can be managed medically.[14]

Intravascular imaging with cardiac MRI is helpful in identifying the etiology of myocardial infarction with nonobstructed coronary arteries (MINOCAs). These could be myocarditis, takotsubo syndrome, and cardiomyopathy in the subacute phase.[35-38] NIRS-IVUS proves helpful in identifying culprit lesions in ST-segment elevation myocardial infarction (STEMI) and guides clinical therapy.[38,39]

Vulnerable Plaque

Vulnerable plaques are defined as plaques prone to rupture leading to arterial thrombosis in patients with ACS. The detection of vulnerable plaques OCT is superior to IVUS due to its better resolution **(Fig. 19)**. Vulnerable plaque is characterized by (1) thin fibrous cap (<65 μm) with underlying lipid-rich necrotic area, (2) activated macrophages near fibrous cap, (3) cholesterol crystals, and (4) neo angiogenesis.[40,41]

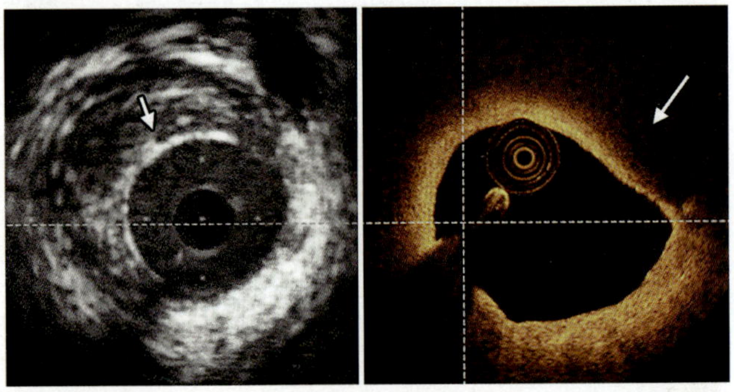

FIG. 19: Thin-cap fibroatheroma. Arrow points to thin cap over plaque in IVUS and OCT.
(IVUS: intravascular ultrasound; OCT: optical coherence tomography)

The CLIMA study is a prospective observational study and was conducted to explore the correlation between OCT-defined high-risk plaques and the risk of future acute coronary events. The presence of features of high-risk OCT plaques, including TCFA and macrophage infiltration, was found to be associated with a higher risk of major coronary events.[42]

Guidance of Primary PCI

The ability of IVI to determine the site of plaque rupture versus erosion, thrombus burden, and the longitudinal extent of underlying plaque, as well as to measure reference lumen and vessel diameters, underlies the potential utility to guide PCI in STEMI and affect long-term outcomes.

The HORIZON-AMI IVUS substudy showed smaller IVUS MSA that was an independent predictor of angiographic restenosis after primary PCI in patients with STEMI.[43] The randomized DOCTORS (Does Optical Coherence Tomography Optimize Results of Stenting) study showed that higher post-PCI FFR values were achieved with optical coherence tomographic guidance as compared to angiography guidance in 240 patients with non-STEMI (0.94 ± 0.04 vs. 0.92 ± 0.05; $p = 0.005$).[44]

Bifurcation Lesion

Imaging plays an important role in bifurcation PCI. The 3D reconstruction of OCT makes it more helpful in this complex anatomy. It allows reasonable profiling of SB ostia from the main branch (MB) pullback **(Figs. 20 to 22)**.[45-47]

The predictors of SB compromise can then be assessed. Narrow carina angle—"eyebrow" sign in IVUS or carina-tip angle <50° and carina tip-bifurcation point (CT-BP) distance <1.5 mm by OCT is important of all other predictors[38] **(Fig. 23)**. The stent should cover at least 6–8 mm proximal to the SB to accommodate the shortest POT balloon.[45-47]

During intervention, OCT helps to visualize the wire and rule out abluminal wiring. Prior to kissing balloon, it is important to visualize the strut crossed with the SB wire.

Poststenting imaging is helpful for optimization. Acute malapposition in bifurcation needs correction by adequate postdilatation, else rewiring SB carries risk of abluminal wiring.[46,47]

Left Main Assessment

For LMCA lesions, preintervention IVI is done to assess the severity and extent of the disease (lumen area, plaque burden,

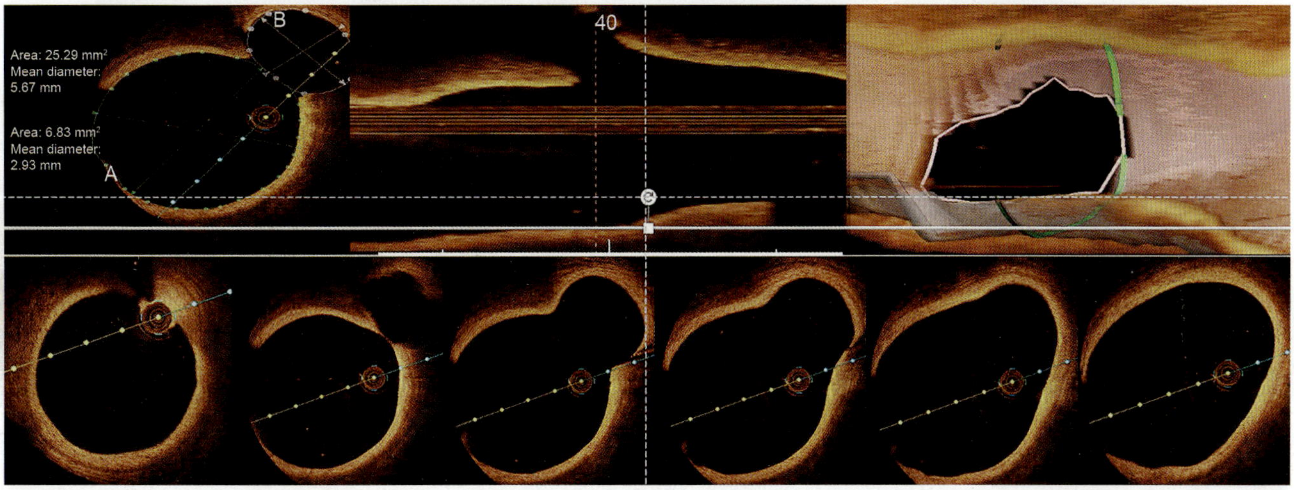

FIG. 20: Optical coherence tomography (OCT) imaging with 3D profiling of bifurcation lesion. OCT pullback in main branch (LAD) profiling the side branch (diagonal).

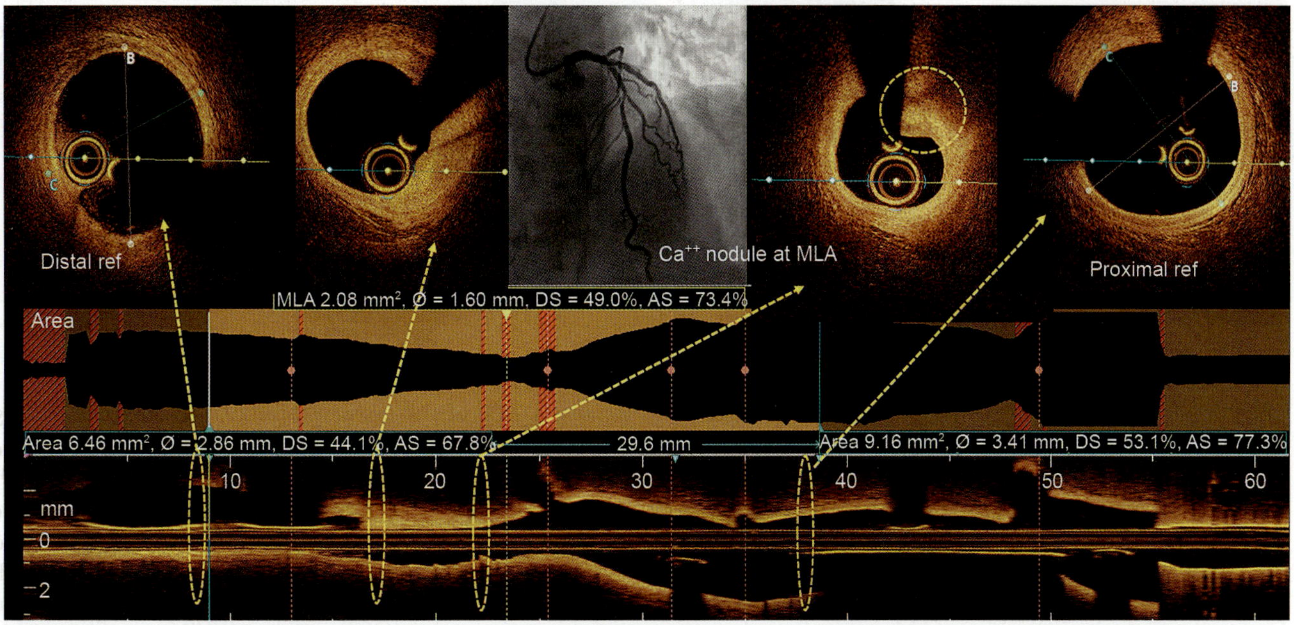

FIG. 21: OCT profiling of bifurcation lesion and presence of calcific nodule.

(AS: aortic stenosis; DS: diameter stenosis; MLA: minimal lumen area; OCT: optical coherence tomography)

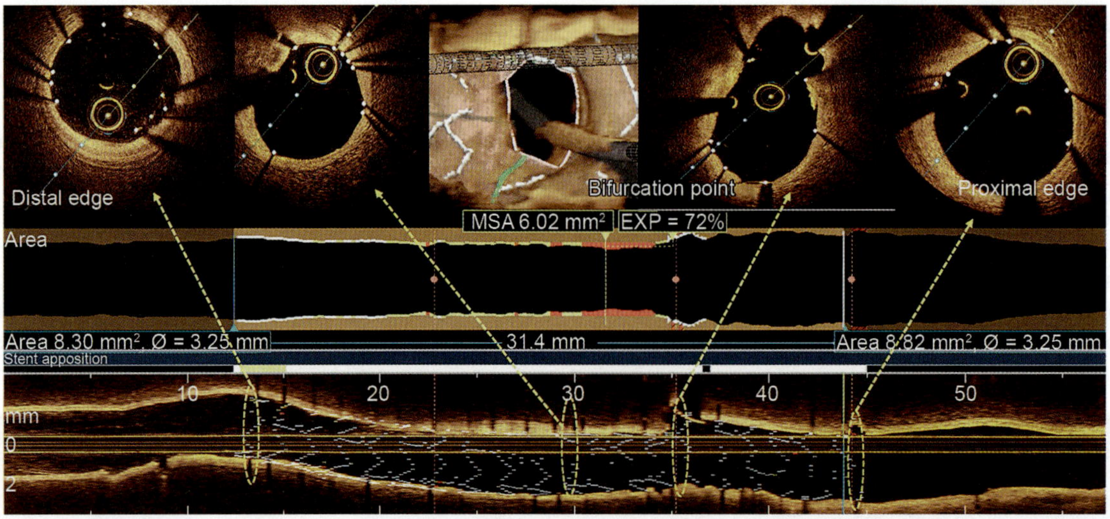

FIG. 22: Optical coherence tomography profiling of bifurcation lesion after stenting profiling the distribution of struts across the side branch ostia.

(MSA: minimum stent area)

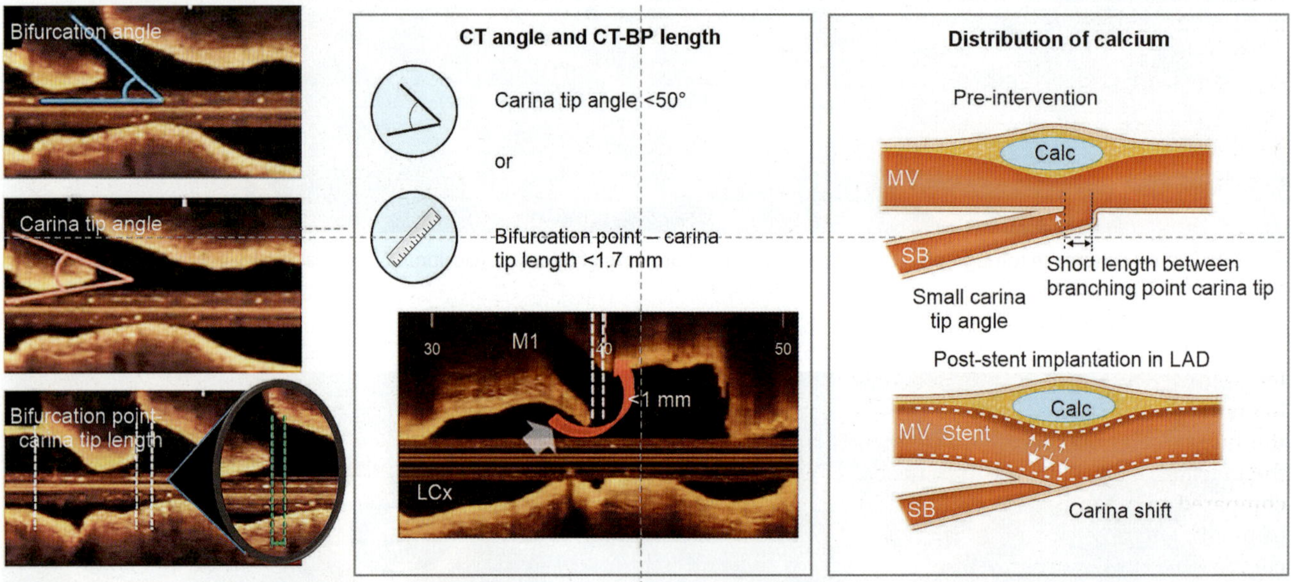

FIG. 23: Predictors of side branch occlusion on imaging—bifurcation angle, carina-tip (CT) angle, and bifurcation point-carina tip (CT-BP) length. Presence of calcium on contralateral of side branch ostia is predictor of carina shift.

(LAD: left anterior descending; LCx: left circumflex; MV: main vessel; SB: side branch)

and distribution) involving the Ostia, the stem, and at the bifurcation and direct imaging of the disease extension to left anterior descending (LAD) and left circumflex (LCx).[14,48-50] The strategy of LM PCI depends on LCx ostial involvement. Diffuse involvement of LM is difficult to pick up.[51] This IVI assessment helps to decide the intervention strategy—need for plaque modification, one-stent or two-stent strategy, stent and postdilatation balloon sizing, and optimization. Due to the disparity in the size of LM and its branches, the choice of stent-make and its size will depend on its expansion limits, radial strength, and SB access.

The cross-sectional area of nonatherosclerotic LM in Asians is 75% of the cross-sectional area of the Western population.[51] Suggested MLA cut-off values for lesion significance are smaller for Asians than the Western population. The LM MLA of <6.0 mm² correlated with ischemia in Western while MLA of >4.5–4.8 mm² is considered adequate in Asians.[14]

The IVUS scores over OCT for assessment of aortic–ostial junction, while OCT matches IVUS in profiling mid and distal LM. But, the OCT has an advantage in better profiling of the side-branch wire cross. Wire cross position is to be ascertained prior to kissing balloon to have optimal scaffolding of SB in single stent cross-over strategy and to get optimal MSA at the bifurcation in two-stent strategy.

Side branch assessment (LCx) after single stent cross-over strategy needs utmost caution. This is to avoid trapping of IVI catheter in jail struts during pullback. The final assessment of optimization of LM PCI result is crucial as in-stent restenosis (ISR) is associated with 30% of all causes and 23% of cardiac mortality.[52-54]

Chronic Total Occlusion

In CTO, imaging has important and multiple roles.[55] IVUS has an edge over OCT as it is not flow-dependent. In OCT, the need for blood clearance and contrast injection makes it not only difficult for use in CTO but could also worsen the intentional subintimal dissection, thereby making re-entry difficult.

During antegrade wire cross, IVUS helps in the assessment of the proximal cap when ambiguous, facilitates re-entry of wire when subintimal, and confirms distal true lumen position after wire cross. IVUS-guided penetration of the proximal cap is facilitated by the positioning of the catheter in the SB if present, else would need a front-looking catheter.

In retrograde approach, IVUS catheter on antegrade wire can facilitate retrograde wire entry to true lumen. IVUS assessment helps in profiling lesions and the need for plaque modification and vessel sizing. The CTO segments and distal vessels are often negatively remodeled.

Bypass Graft

Saphenous vein graft (SVG) amounts for the majority of coronary artery bypass graft (CABG) surgery conduits with higher rate of graft failure as compared to arterial grafts in long-term follow-up. The pathophysiology of SVG graft failure has not been well studied. Intracoronary imaging particularly the high-resolution OCT has vital role in understanding the mechanism of SVG failure. A freshly harvested SVG as compared to a native coronary artery has very thin layer of media and a thickened intima as compared to native coronary artery **(Fig. 24)**.

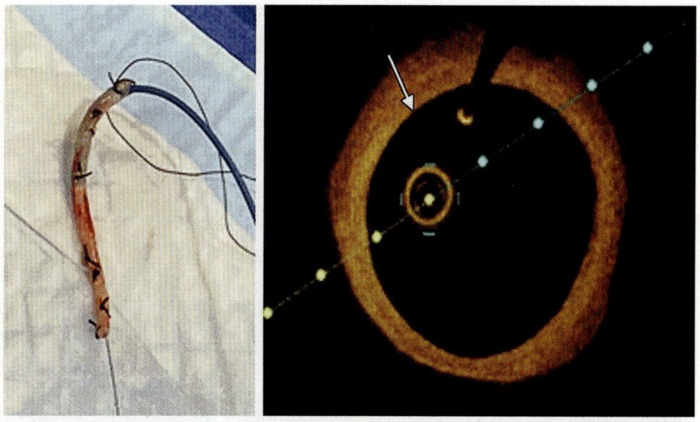

FIG. 24: Vein graft imaging (ex vivo). Freshly harvested graft with ex vivo imaging that shows thin media and intima (white arrow)
Courtesy: Dr Arun Mohanty unpublished series from SGR Hospital, New Delhi.

Adaptive remodeling occurs after grafting. The media becomes thicker with thick fibrocellular neo intima, a process known as arterialization of vein grafts **(Fig. 25)**. In asymptomatic CABG patients, OCT and IVUS performed after 3 years show areas of atherosclerotic degeneration with lipid pool and TCFA in 40% vein grafts (by OCT but not by IVUS). There were also adherent thrombi in 25% of the SVG studied.[56] This suggests that SVG degeneration starts as early as 3 years after CABG and continues further leading to graft degeneration in long-term follow-up.

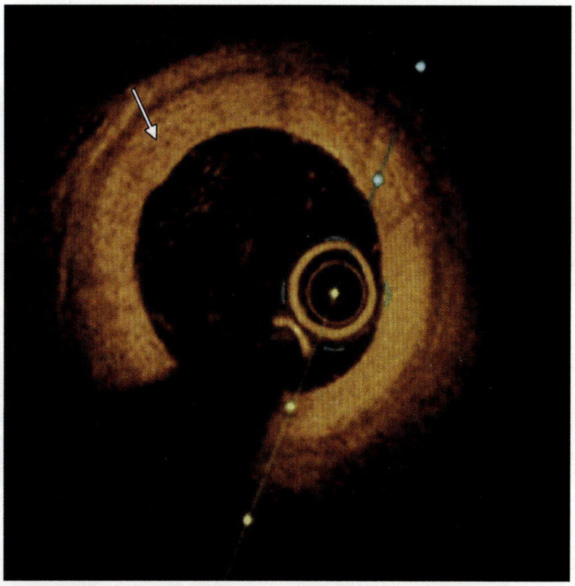

FIG. 25: Arterialized vein graft shows thick media and hypertrophied neointima (white arrow).

Marco T et al. in their IVUS study of 334 SVG grafts demonstrated calcification in 40% of degenerated SVG grafts.[57] Calcification was superficial in 40% and deep in 60% and calcification was predominantly located at SVG wall and not at the plaque. Another study involving IVUS and virtual histology involving 54 SVG grafts showed very rare incidence of dense calcification.[58] CABG patients presenting with acute coronary syndrome in 18 patients were studied at SGR Hospital, New Delhi. OCT imaging of these SVG grafts which were 7–14 years old, showed diffuse areas of degeneration with TCFA **(Fig. 26A)** and large areas of lipid pool and necrotic core and macrophages. There were areas of intimal loosening, plaque rupture **(Fig. 26B)**, and subintimal vacuolation, which were unique to SVG graft and usually not seen in native coronary lesions with ACS **(Fig. 26C)**. Red thrombi and white thrombi were seen in OCT imaging in our patients; however, calcification and fibrotic plaques were rarely seen.

Post PCI Follow-up

Stent Failure (Stent Thrombosis and Restenosis)

Intravascular imaging has helped to elucidate the events occurring within the stent. Stent thrombosis and restenosis

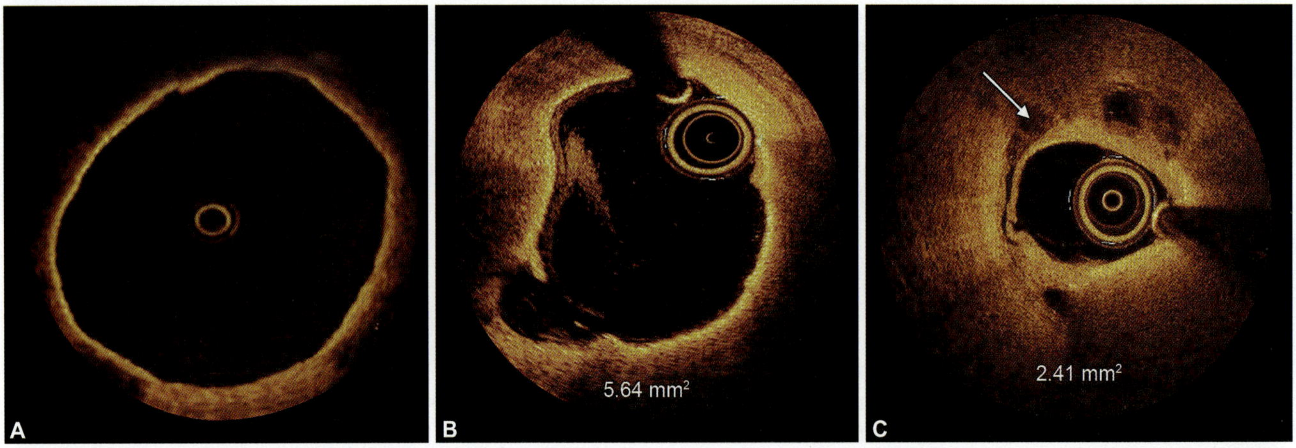

FIGS. 26A TO C: (A) Thin cap fibroatheroma, (B) ruptured plaque, and (C) degenerated vein graft with intimal loosening and vacuolation and large necrotic core.

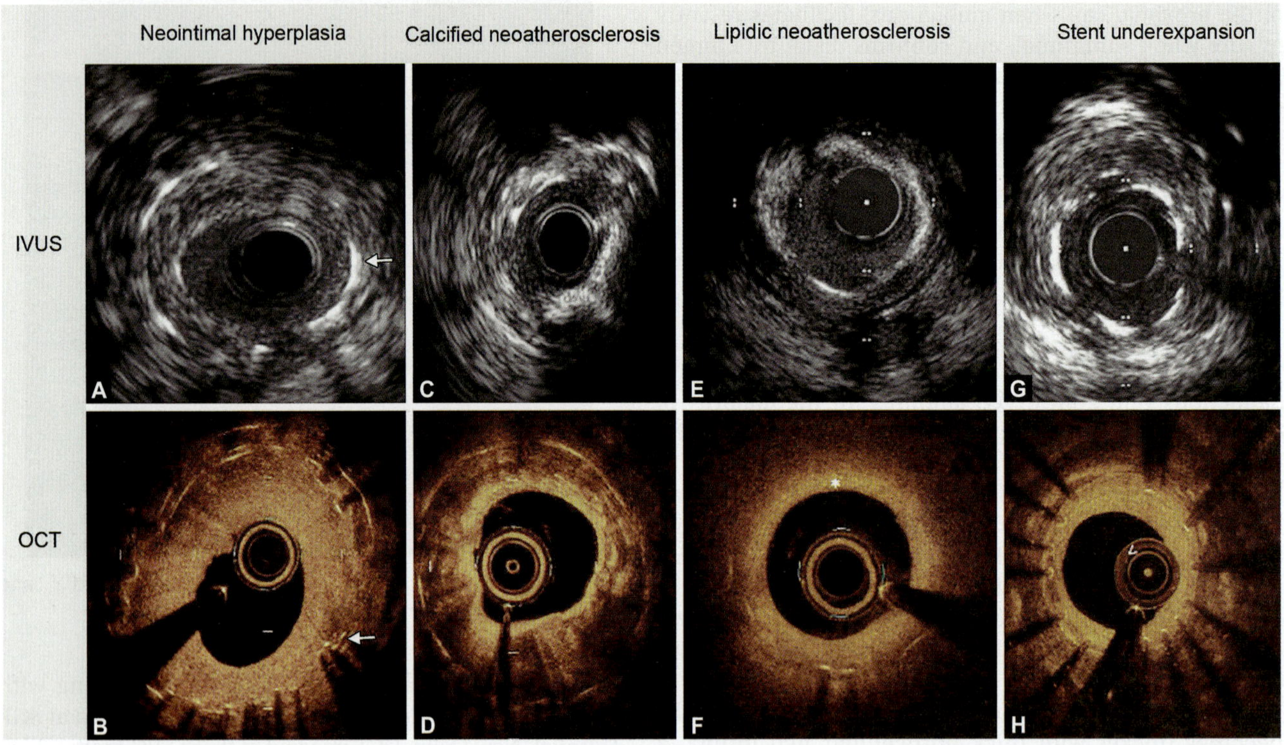

FIGS. 27A TO H: Intravascular imaging of stent restenosis. (A) Circumferential, neointimal tissue growth covering the stent struts (arrows) on IVUS. (B) OCT shows characteristic homogenous and bright appearance. (C) Calcified neoatherosclerosis appears bright on IVUS with shadowing beyond the calcium, obscuring visualization of stent struts. (D) OCT shows calcified neoatherosclerosis has a heterogenous appearance and has well-defined borders, with stent struts still visible. (E) Lipidic neoatherosclerosis appears as high attenuation both on IVUS. (F) OCT lipid atherosclerosis obscures visualization of stent struts but with an easily visualized fibrous cap (asterisk). (G) Stent underexpansion, on IVUS. (H) Stent underexpansion in OCT with blood is present within the OCT catheter (arrowhead).

Source: Shlofmitz E, Ali ZA, Maehara A, Mintz GS, Shlofmitz R, Jeremias A. Intravascular Imaging-Guided Percutaneous Coronary Intervention. A Universal Approach for Optimization of Stent Implantation. Circ Cardiovasc Interv. 2020;13:e008686.

have been attributed to multiple factors be it related to patient, device, or procedure (mechanical).[59] OCT is considered better than IVUS to ascertain the mechanism of in-stent thrombosis or restenosis, since IVUS has poorer resolution and cannot detect strut coverage, differentiate neointima from neoatherosclerosis, or identify thrombus accurately **(Fig. 27)**. Based on imaging and possible mechanisms, Waksman had classified ISR into several categories based on image-guided assessment of underlying cause **(Fig. 28)** and the management is algorithm driven **(Flowchart 1)**. In the prospective PESTO (Morphological Parameters Explaining Stent Thrombosis Assessed by OCT) registry of 120 patients

Type	Definition		Therapeutic guidance
I	Mechanical	Stent underexpansion (Type I A)	High pressure balloon, ELCA, or IVL. Underexpansion must be treated prior to further stent implantation
		Stent fracture (Type I B)	DES
II	Biologic	Neointimal hyperplasia (Type II A)	Balloon, DCB, DES, or VBT
		Neoatherosclerosis, noncalcified (Type II B)	DCB, or DES
		Neoatherosclerosis, calcified (Type II C)	Scoring balloon, ELCA, OA or RA prior to DES
III	Mixed pattern: Combined mechanical and biologic etiology		High-pressure NC balloon with DCB, DES, or VBT
IV	Chronic total occlusion		DCB or DES; VBT for multiple layers, CABG as needed
V	> 2 layers of stent		Balloon, DCB, VBT, or CABG

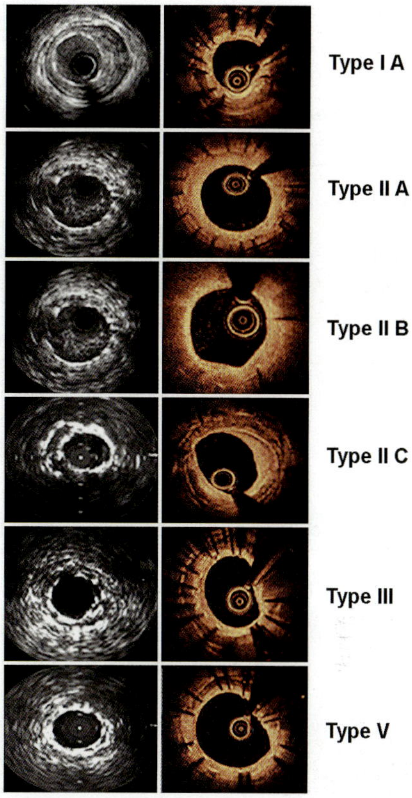

FIG. 28: Waksman classification of in-stent restenosis.

(CABG: coronary artery bypass graft; DCB: drug coated balloon; DES: drug-eluting stent; ELCA: excimer laser coronary atherectomy; IVUS: intravascular ultrasound; OA: orbital atherectomy; OCT: optical coherence tomography RA: rotational atherectomy; VBT: vascular brachytherapy)

Source: Shlofmitz E, Iantorno M, Waksman R. Restenosis of drug-eluting stents: a new classification system based on disease mechanism to guide treatment and state-of-the- art review. Circ Cardiovasc Interv. 2019;12:e007023.

with definite ST after metallic drug-eluting stent (DES) placement, strut malapposition (48%) and underexpansion (26%) were associated with acute ST and subacute ST, whereas malapposition (31%) and NA (28%) were associated with late ST and very late ST (>12 months).[60]

Composition of neoatherosclerosis can be better assessed by OCT (including calcification) and its lipid content by NIR-IVUS. IVI guidance in ISR helps to understand the underlying mechanism and to strategize. It is associated with improved outcome.[62-67]

Positive remodeling can lead to late stent malapposition, while negative remodeling contributes to restenosis. Uncovered stent struts, late acquired malapposition, and rupture of neoatherosclerotic lipid-rich plaque have been important causes of stent thrombosis.[61,62]

Impact of Intravascular Imaging on Outcome of PCI

There have been several randomized controlled trials (RCTs) (nearly 24 RCTs), registries (nearly 30), and 34 meta-analyses comparing IVI-guided PCI with angiography-guided PCI.[14] IVI has been shown to reduce adverse events, myocardial infarction, stent thrombosis, and mortality (both cardiac and all-cause). Clinical data with use of IVUS is more robust, while that of OCT emerging, but found at par with IVUS. Use of IVI yielded larger MSA with fewer complications but more number or use of longer stents.

The IVUS-XPL trial in 1,448 patients showed MACE (cardiac death, target lesion-related myocardial infarction, and ischemia-driven target lesion revascularization) reduction from 5.8 to 2.9%. At 5 years, reduction in events was maintained (10.7% vs. 6.6%).[68] In ULTIMATE trial, in 1,400 patients, target vessel failure (cardiac death, target vessel myocardial infarction, and clinically driven target vessel revascularization) reduced from 5.4 to 2.9%. At 3 years, the event rate was maintained (10.7% vs. 6.6%).[69,70] In these two studies, using IVUS guidance in PCI, 3-year mortality was reduced by 50% and mortality rate to 0.15% per year when optimal result achieved.[73]

In LM PCI, there are no large, randomized trial, but two RCTs, nearly 16 registries, and several meta-analyses have reported mortality advantage with use of IVUS guidance.[14] In EXCEL study and another Korean study, restenosis was correlated with stent expansion (MSA) in two different ethnic population with different cut offs.[71,72] In CTO PCI, use

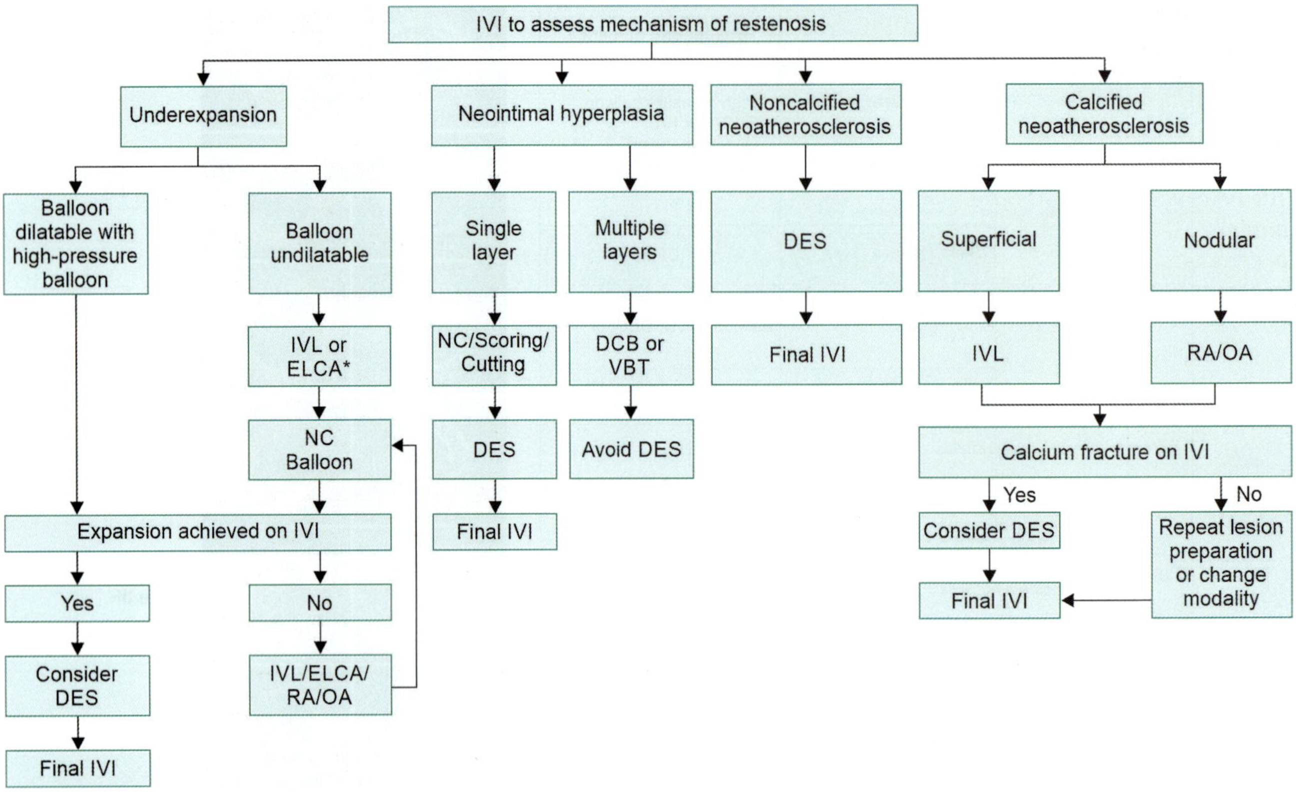

*If unsuccessful expansion with excimer laser coronary atherectomy (ELCA), contrast injection during ELCA can be used.

FLOWCHART 1: Algorithmic approach for treatment of in-stent restenosis (ISR) based on imaging-guided interpretation of underlying cause.

(DCB: drug-coated balloon; DES: drug-eluting stent; IVI: intravascular imaging; IVL: intravascular lithotripsy; NC: noncompliant; OA: orbital atherectomy; RA: rotational atherectomy; VBT: vascular brachytherapy)

Source: Shlofmitz E, Ali ZA, Maehara A, Mintz GS, Shlofmitz R, Jeremias A. Intravascular imaging-guided percutaneous coronary intervention. A Universal Approach for Optimization of Stent Implantation. Circ Cardiovasc Interv. 2020;13:e008686.

BOX 1 **EAPCI (2018) recommendations on the adjunctive use of intravascular imaging for diagnostic evaluation of coronary artery disease, guidance, and optimization of PCIs.**

Diagnosis assessment of coronary lesions:
- *Consensus opinion*:
  - Angiographically unclear/ambiguous findings (e.g., dissection, thrombus, and calcified nodule)
  - Assessment of left main stenosis
  - Complex bifurcation lesions
  - Suspected culprit lesion of acute coronary syndrome

PCI guidance and optimization:
- *RCT evidence*:
  - Long lesions
  - Chronic total occlusions
- *Consensus opinion*:
  - Patients with acute coronary syndrome
  - Left main coronary artery lesions
  - Two-stent bifurcation
  - Implantation of bioresorbable scaffolds
  - Patients with renal dysfunction (IVUS)

Continued

Continued

Identification of mechanism of stent failure:
- Restenosis
- Stent thrombosis

(EAPCI: European Association of Percutaneous Cardiovascular Intervention; IVUS: intravascular ultrasound; PCI: percutaneous coronary intervention; RCT: randomized controlled trial)

of IVUS guidance reduced composite of death/MI in CTO-PCI randomized trial.[73] Ongoing studies such as ILUMIEN IV: OPTIMAL PCI, IMPROVE, OCTIVUS, and GUIDE-DES will further elucidate and strengthen the role of imaging in various subsets.

GUIDELINE RECOMMENDATIONS

The European Association of Percutaneous Coronary Intervention (EAPCI) (2018) consensus document recommends IVI in selected scenarios **(Box 1)**.[74] In 2021, American College of Cardiology (ACC) coronary revascularization guideline gave class IIa recommendation use of IVUS for procedural guidance, particularly in cases of left main or complex coronary artery stenting, to reduce ischemic events.[75] It gave class IIa recommendation for OCT as a reasonable alternative to IVUS for procedural guidance, except in the ostial left main disease.

CONCLUSION

The IVUS and OCT both complement each other as imaging modalities. IVUS has a poor resolution but higher tissue penetration, whereas OCT has a good resolution but poorer penetration. With their inherent strength and limitations, the combined IVUS and OCT probes will be complementary and work synergistically to enable a comprehensive depiction of the coronary artery. Several RCTs, registries, and meta-analyses comparing IVI-guided PCI with angiography-guided PCI have shown that use of IVI reduces adverse events, myocardial infarction, stent thrombosis, and mortality (both cardiac and all-cause). Clinical data with use of IVUS is more robust, while that of OCT emerging [ILUMIEN IV and OCTIVUS data to be presented in European Society of Cardiology (ESC) congress 2023].

ONLINE REFERENCES

Please scan the QR code provided at the end of the table of contents for References of this chapter.

CHAPTER 165

Optical Coherence Tomography and Intravascular Ultrasound-guided Stenting: Sizing and Expansion Criteria

Image more-Optimize expansion-Improve outcomes

Gopala krishna Koduru, Raghuram Palaparti, Venkata RS Subrahmanya Sarma

ABSTRACT

Intracoronary imaging (ICI) has emerged as an important adjunct to percutaneous coronary intervention (PCI) to improve outcomes in the last two decades.[1] Avoidance of stent underexpansion (SU), significant plaque or lipid pool at stent edge, edge dissection, malapposition, and extensive tissue protrusion is the key to achieve a lasting result in image-guided PCI algorithm.[2] Stent sizing by conventional angiogram does not correlate well with imaging-based sizing. Minimal stent area (MSA) by intravascular ultrasound (IVUS) has been shown to be the strongest predictor of in-stent restenosis and stent thrombosis following stent optimization.[1] But, in real world practice, it is difficult to achieve predefined MSA by imaging in more than one-third of the patients. Hence, it is necessary to have an understanding of stent sizing and expansion criteria by ICI for every interventional cardiologist (IC).

Keywords: Intra coronary imaging, minimal stent area, percutaneous intervention, intravascular ultrasound, optical coherence tomography (OCT).

INTRODUCTION

Conventional coronary angiography (CA) has been the gold standard for diagnosis of coronary artery disease and guidance during percutaneous coronary intervention (PCI). Adjunctive use of intracoronary imaging (ICI) precisely characterizes plaque morphology, lesion length, and reference vessel diameter before PCI and optimizes the result after stent implantation. A recent network meta-analysis[3] of 28 randomized controlled trials (RCTs) **(Fig. 1)** has shown that the use of intravascular ultrasound (IVUS) or optical coherence tomography (OCT) compared with CA in PCI guidance provides a significant benefit by reducing major adverse cardiac event (MACE), cardiac death, and target vessel/lesion revascularization (TVR/TLR).

EVIDENCE FOR IMAGING-GUIDED PCI

Intravascular Ultrasound-guided PCI

Early trials with drug-eluting stents have demonstrated lower in-stent restenosis (ISR) and TLR rates with IVUS guidance.[4,5] Subsequently, RCTs comparing angiography-guided PCI with image guidance, such as ULTIMATE,[6,7] IVS-XPL,[7,8] RENOVATE-COMPLEX-PCI,[9] have demonstrated a significant reduction in MACE, death, TVR, and TLR during a follow-up of 2–5 years **(Fig. 2)**. IMPROVE (NCT04221815) is an ongoing study evaluating the clinical outcomes and cost-effectiveness of IVUS versus angiography-guided PCI in complex lesions in 2,500 to 3,000 patients with an expected follow-up of 4–5 years and the results are expected in late 2025.

Optical Coherence Tomography-guided PCI

The DOCTORS[12] and OCTACS[13] studies have shown improvement in surrogate endpoints such as postprocedural fractional flow reserve (FFR)[12] and strut coverage.[13] The ILUMIEN III trial[14] compared minimal stent area (MSA) by OCT, IVUS, and angiography. Minimum and mean stent expansions with OCT were noninferior to IVUS-guided PCI, but not superior to angiography alone. The ongoing OCTOBER trial (NCT03171311) is comparing angiography-guided PCI and optional use of IVUS with OCT-guided PCI in patients requiring complex bifurcation stent implantation and ILUMIEN IV (NCT03507777) is prospectively looking at

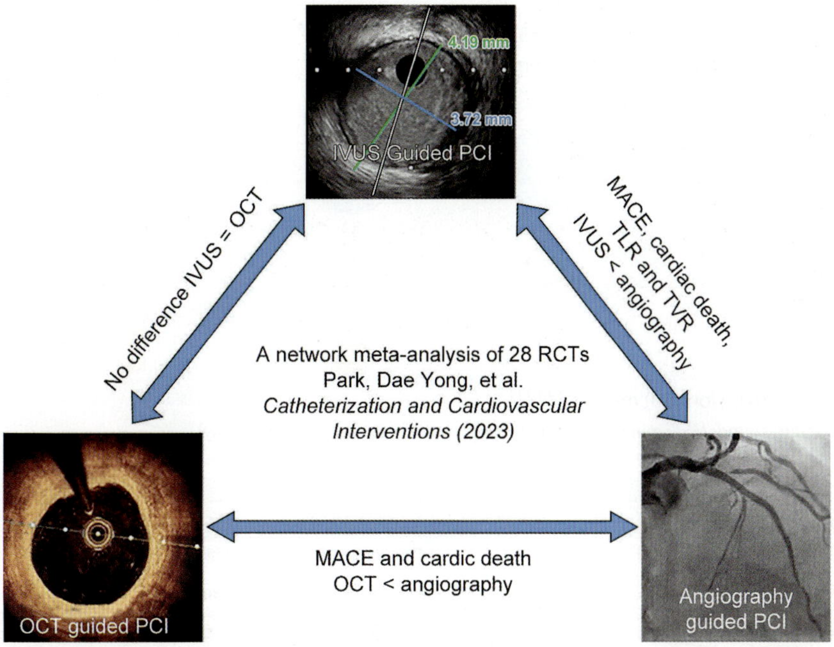

FIG. 1: Comparison of IVUS and OCT with conventional angiography (CA) PCI: A network meta-analysis of 28 RCTs.

(IVUS: intravascular ultrasound; MACE: major adverse cardiac event; OCT: optical coherence tomography; PCI: percutaneous coronary intervention; RCT: randomized controlled trial)

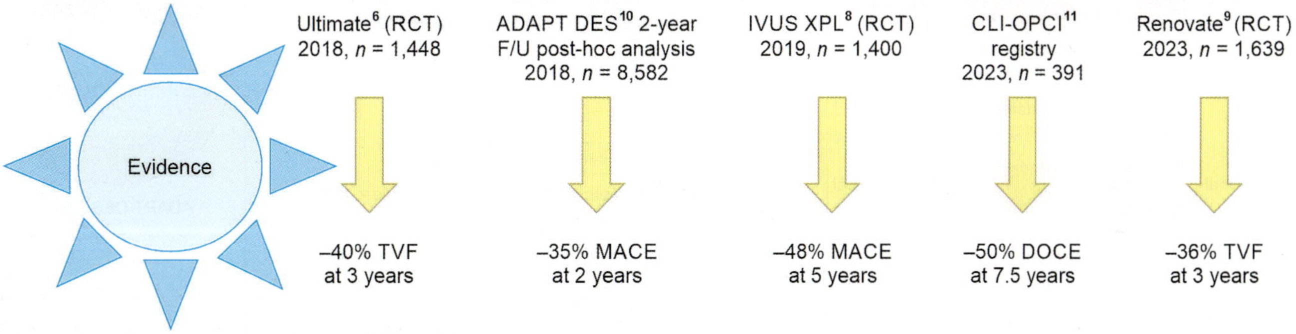

FIG. 2: Evidence in favor of image-guided PCI.[6,8-11]

(DOCE: device-oriented cardiovascular event; MACE: major adverse cardiac event; PCI: percutaneous coronary intervention; RCT: randomized controlled trial; TVF: target vessel failure)

the superiority of an OCT-guided strategy as compared to an angiography-guided stent implantation strategy in achieving larger post-PCI lumen dimensions and improving clinical outcomes in patients with high-risk clinical characteristics and/or with high-risk angiographic lesions. The results of these two studies are expected by the end of 2023.

Stent Expansion

Stent expansion has been described as the MSA, either as an absolute expansion or compared with the predefined reference lumen area (relative expansion). K Fujii et al.[1] showed that stent underexpansion (SU) and residual reference segment stenosis were associated with stent thrombosis after successful sirolimus-eluting stent implantation. Subsequently, Song HG et al.[4] showed an optimal cut-off value of post-stenting MSA of 5.5 mm^2 (IVUS or OCT) in preventing ISR across various DES platforms **(Fig. 3)**. ADAPT-DES IVUS substudy[10] has assessed various stent expansion indices and concluded that stent/vessel area at the MSA site >38.9% **(Figs. 4A to D)**, an index of relative stent expansion, was superior to absolute MSA and other expansion indices in predicting 2-year clinically driven TLR or definite stent thrombosis. CLI-OPCI[11] registry has revealed that an absolute MLA of 4.5 mm^2 is the best cut-off value for OCT to identify patients with device-oriented cardiovascular events (DOCE) and not relative stent expansion. According

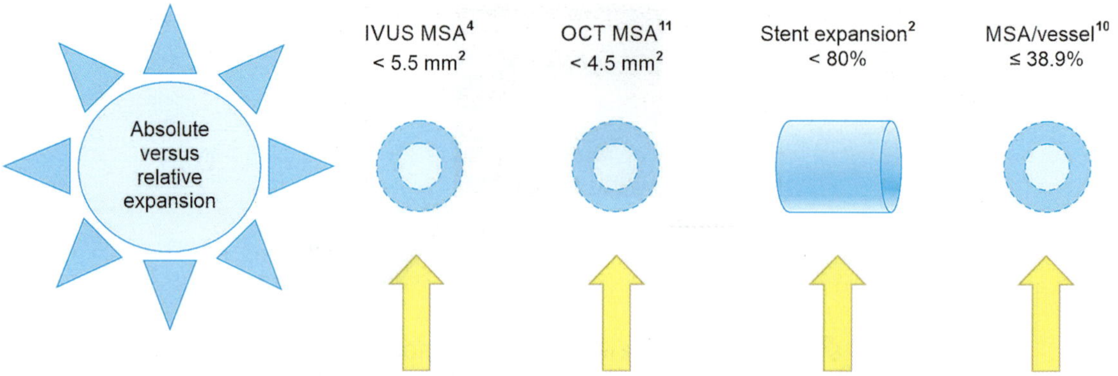

FIG. 3: Stent underexpansion (SU) metrics.[2,4,10,11]
(IVUS: intravascular ultrasound; MSA: minimal stent area; OCT: optical coherence tomography)

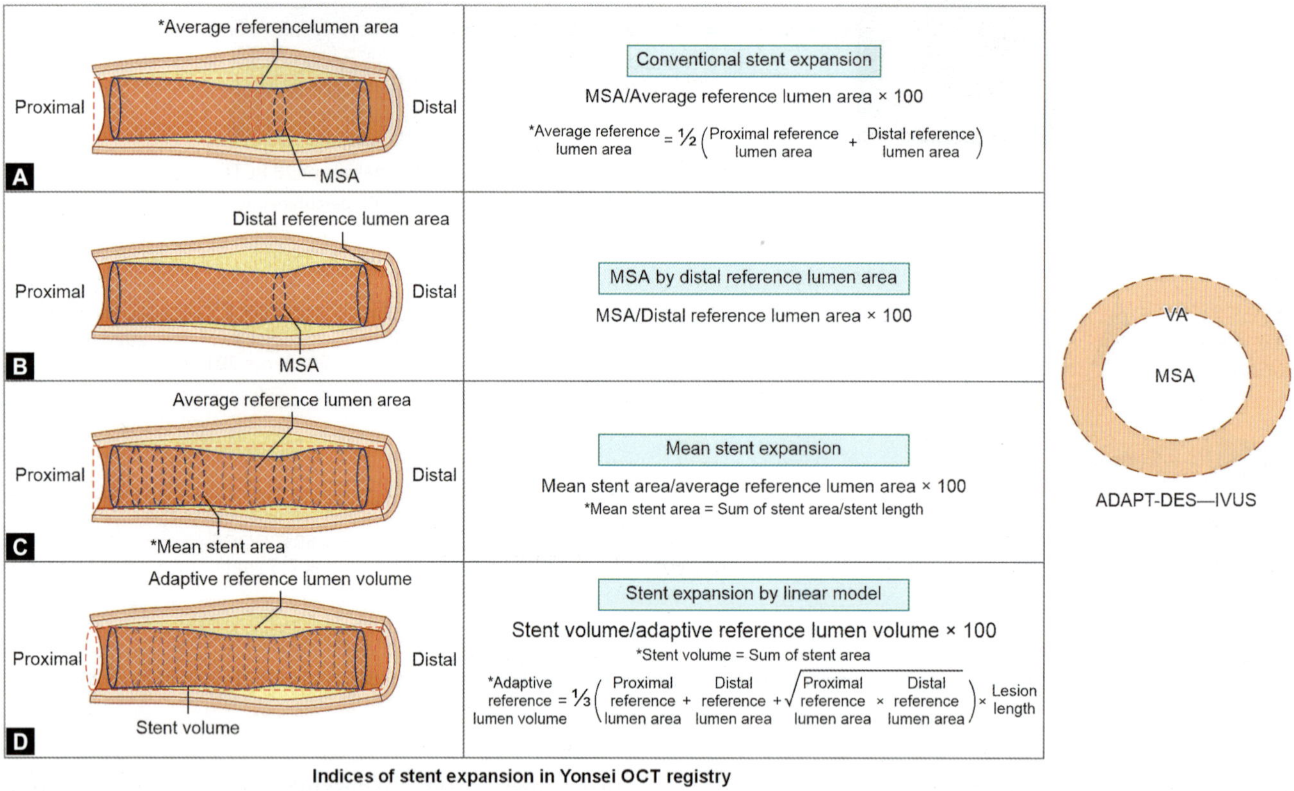

FIGS. 4A TO D: Relative stent expansion metrics.
(MSA: minimal stent area)
Source: With permission from Fujimura et al. (2021)[10] and Lee et al. (2023).[16]

to the European consensus document,[2] avoidance of SU is the most relevant target for PCI guidance. Greater absolute stent expansion has been associated with better long-term stent patency and MSA of <4.5 (OCT) or 5.4 mm^2 (IVUS) in non-left main (LM) lesions is an independent predictor of subsequent events. European expert group[2] believes that the cut-off >80% for the MSA (relative to average reference lumen area) appears to be a reasonable approach to adopt in clinical practice. A plethora of data supports the concept that the MSA is the most powerful predictor of long-term outcomes.

But RCTs, registries, expert opinions, and real-world practice continue to use relative stent expansion criteria for measuring stent expansion as the application of an MSA absolute cut-off value seems illogical **(Figs. 5A to C)** in the presence of small, large, and diffusely diseased vessels.

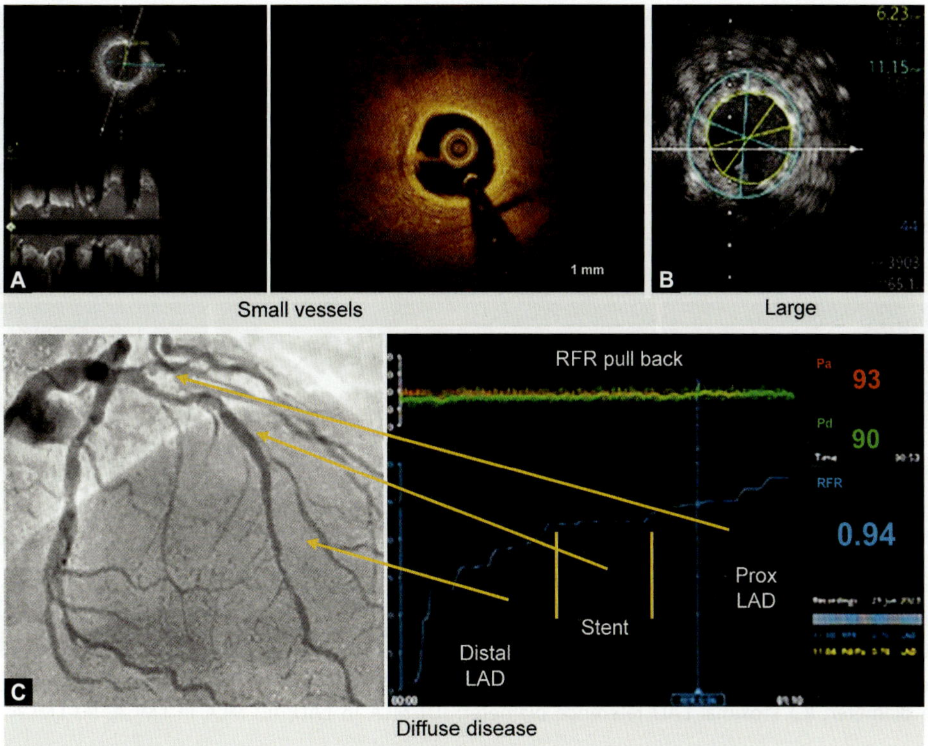

FIGS. 5A TO C: (A) MSA cutoff value is not achieved if the distal reference diameter <2.5 mm. (B) In large vessels, supplying large amount of myocardium MSA cutoff value is not sufficient. (C) In diffuse diseased small vessels, distal reference areas are not reliable. Postprocedural physiological studies help in making decisions.

(MSA: minimal stent area)

PROCEDURAL GUIDANCE OF IMAGING

Pre-PCI Assessment

The IVUS or OCT helps in assessing lesion morphology and length and reference vessel diameters in choosing plaque modification technique and the size of the stent to be deployed by applying the MLD algorithm **(Figs. 6A to G)**. Several imaging strategies have been proposed for the selection of stent diameter based on mean reference lumen, largest reference lumen, mean mid-wall reference, smallest reference external elastic lamina (EEL), or EEL-to-EEL distance. In the ILUMIEN III: OPTIMIZE PCI,[14] an EEL-based stent sizing was used while OPINION trial[15] used a lumen-based stent sizing.

Post-PCI Assessment

Post-procedure imaging is used to exclude SU and significant plaque burden or lipid pool at the stent edges, edge dissections, malapposition, and tissue prolapse using MAX algorithm **(Figs. 7 to 9)**. The IVUS criteria for optimization used in the ULTIMATE trial[6] include the following: (1) minimum lumen area (MLA) in the stented segment >5.0 mm^2 or 90% of the MLA at the distal reference segments; (2) <50% plaque burden within 5 mm proximal or distal to the stent edge; and (3) no edge dissection involving the media with a length >3 mm. The correlation of malapposition and tissue protrusion to subsequent events has not been well established.

THE BIGGER THE BETTER APPROACH: A WORD OF CAUTION

In Yonsei OCT registry,[15] stent expansion by linear model ≥65.0% was independently associated with DOCE. In CLI-OPCI registry,[11] stent overexpansion was significantly associated with an increased risk of edge dissection >200 μm and edge narrowing determining an increased risk of stent failure at follow-up. Earlier PCI studies have demonstrated that vessel wall injury by balloon overstretch or stenting during the procedure can promote intimal hyperplasia. Previous serial IVUS observational study[17] showed that an increase of total vascular area rather than lumen or plaque area was highly related to the magnitude of in-stent neointimal growth, suggesting that stretch or injury to the adventitia rather than intima affects neointimal hyperplasia. Therefore, there is a trade-off between a gain of a larger acute lumen area and the degree of vascular injury during PCI.

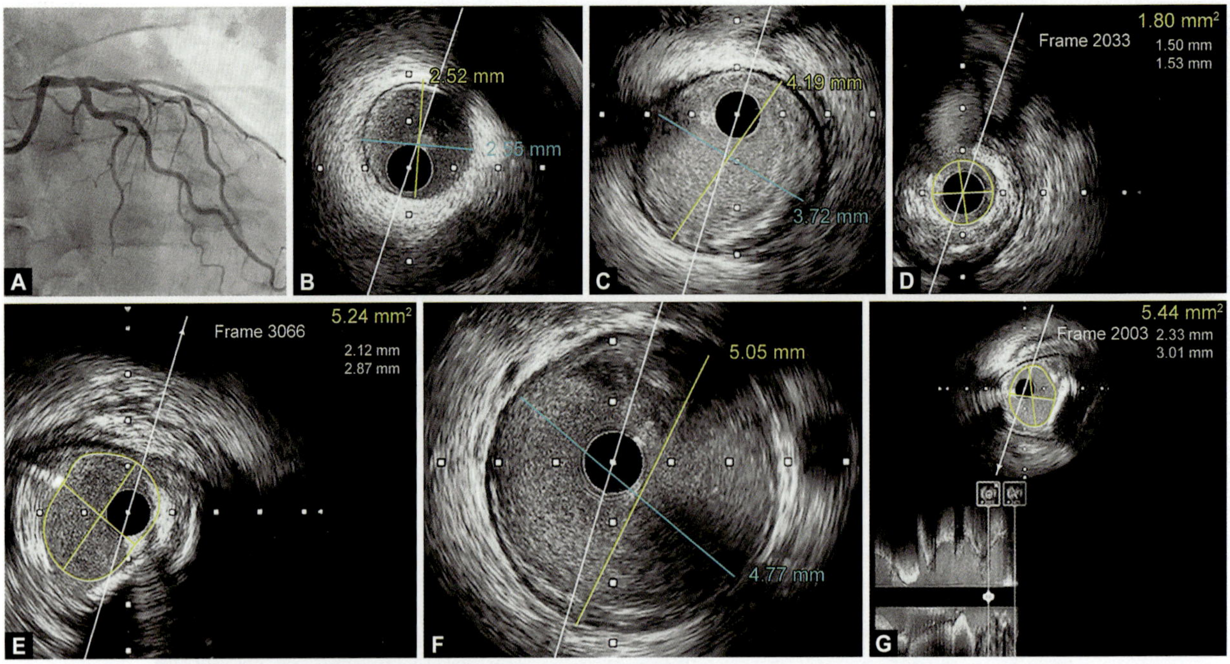

FIGS. 6A TO G: Pre-PCI IVUS assessment in a representative case showing: (A) Baseline coronary angiogram of the representative patient; (B) Distal reference diameter; (C) Proximal LAD reference diameter; (D) MLA in LAD; (E) MLA in LMCA; (F) LMCA reference diameter; (G) Ostial LCX.

(CAG: coronary angiography; IVUS: intravascular ultrasound; LAD: left anterior descending; LCX: left circumflex; LMCA: left main coronary artery; MLA: minimum lumen area; PCI: percutaneous coronary intervention)

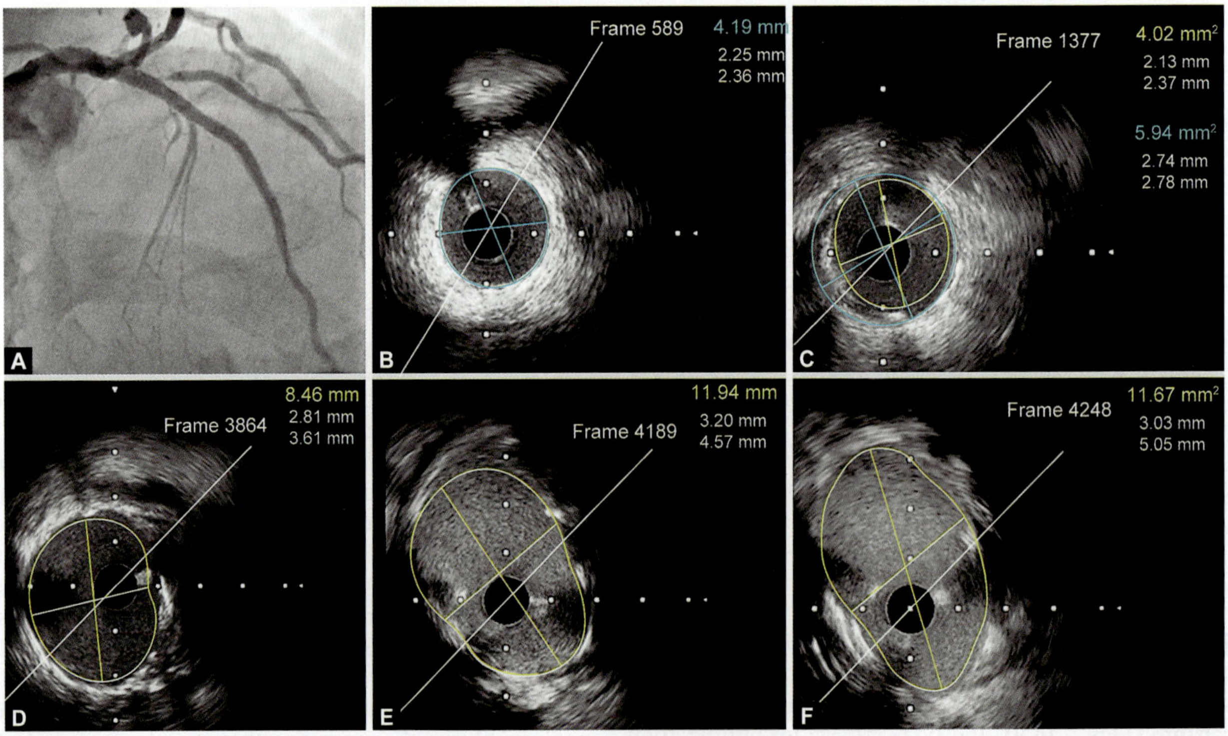

FIGS. 7A TO F: (A) Post-PCI IVUS assessment; (B) Distal reference area; (C) MSA in mid-LAD; (D) MSA in proximal LAD; (E) MSA at confluence; (F) MSA in LMCA.

Note: Relative expansion criteria were met but absolute MSA cutoff value was not achieved.

(CAG: coronary angiography; IVUS: intravascular ultrasound; LAD: left anterior descending; LMCA: left main coronary artery; MSA: minimal stent area; PCI: percutaneous coronary intervention)

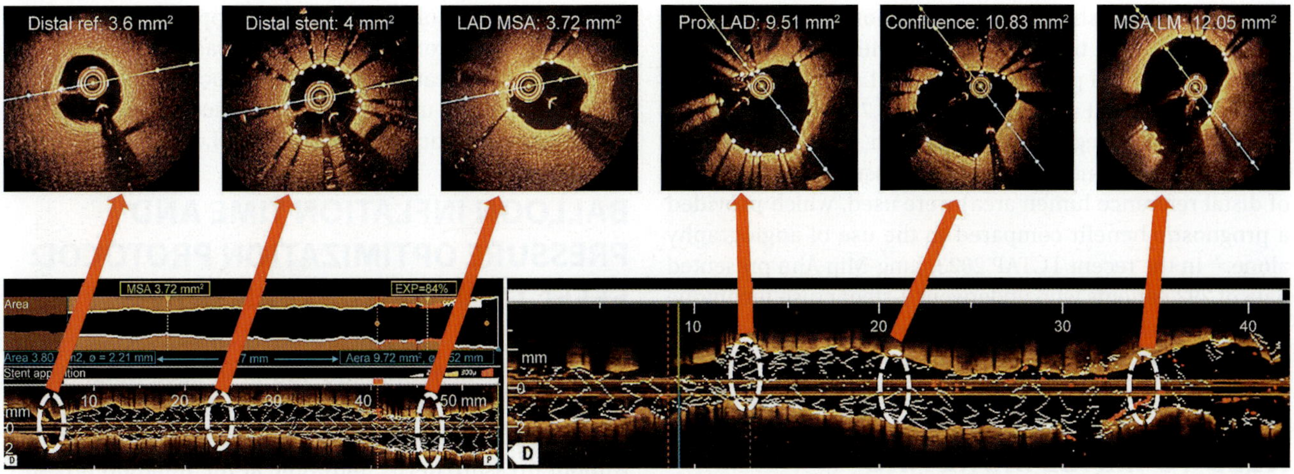

FIG. 8: Post-PCI OCT assessment of the same patient showing areas achieved in mid- and proximal LAD and LM.

Note: Relative expansion criteria were met but absolute MSA is 3.72 mm² falling short of cut-off value of 4.5 mm².

(LAD: left anterior descending; MSA: minimal stent area; OCT: optical coherence tomography; PCI: percutaneous coronary intervention)

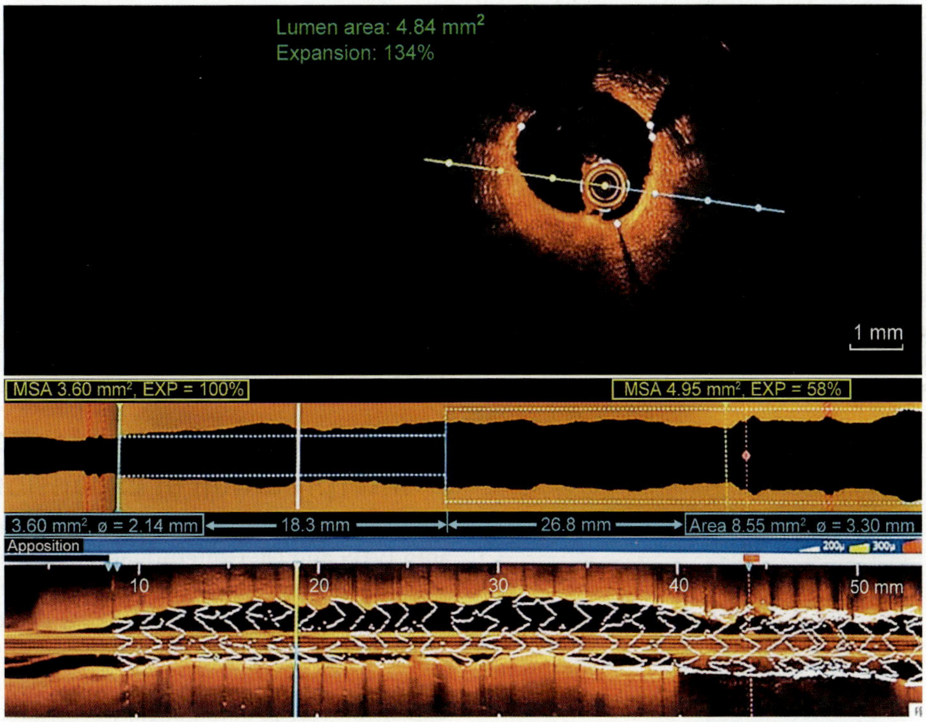

FIG. 9: Post-PCI OCT assessment after larger NC balloon dilatation achieving MSA of 4.72 mm².

(MSA: minimal stent area; NC: noncompliant; OCT: optical coherence tomography; PCI: percutaneous coronary intervention)

LEFT MAIN PCI STENT EXPANSION CRITERIA: HOW MUCH IS ENOUGH?

Both MSA and relative expansion criteria have been proposed to optimize left main (LM) PCI, especially with 2-stent strategies. Kang SJ et al.[18] studied IVUS in LM PCI in 403 patients treated with single or 2-stent strategies (crushing and T-stent) who had immediate post-stenting IVUS and 9-month follow-up angiography. The MSA cut-offs that best predicted ISR on a segmental basis were 5.0 mm² (ostial LCX ISR), 6.3 mm² [ostial left anterior descending (LAD) ISR], 7.2 mm² [ISR within the polygon of confluence (POC)], and 8.2 mm² (ISR within the LM above the POC). This led to the well-known 5-6-7-8 algorithm for LM PCI. This is no longer accepted by the key opinion leaders because of the smaller BSAs of Asian population compared to their western counterparts and short follow-up (9 months). In the IVUS substudy of EXCEL trial[19] by Fujino A, with 3-year follow-up, the MSA cut-offs of proximal LM, ostial LAD, and ostial LCX for predicting MACEs were 9.8, 7.3, and 5.7 mm^2, respectively. In the Spanish registry published in 2020, predefined relative stent expansion criteria (e.g., ostial LM MSA >90% of distal reference lumen area) were used, which provided a prognostic benefit compared to the use of angiography alone.[20] In the recent TCTAP 2023, Jung-Min Ahn presented data of 292 patients who underwent 2-stent crush technique at LM bifurcation and found that the optimal MSAs of left main coronary artery (LMCA), LAD, and LCX were 11.8, 8.3, and 5.7, respectively **(Fig. 10)**.

NEED TO IMAGE MORE AND IMAGINE LESS

The purpose of PCI with stenting is not only to alleviate symptoms and resolve myocardial ischemia with good angiographic result acutely but also to enhance patient prognosis in the long run by optimizing PCI beyond conventional angiography. In the evolution of interventional cardiology, after primary PCI, image-guided PCI is one modality that prevents MACE and saves lives (ULTIMATE,[6] IVUS XPL,[8] RENOVATE-COMPLEX-PCI,[9] ADAPT DES,[10] and CLI-OPCI[11]). Even though optimal expansion criteria (MSA >5.5 mm^2 or >80% reference MLA) achieved in only 60% of the randomized patients, they were able to reduce the MACE, death, and TVR rates close to 40% in those who underwent Image guided PCI. Image guided PCI is one among the few interventions in PCI to reduce the MACE rates close to 40%.[2] In RENOVATE-COMPLEX-PCI,[9] ICI-defined optimization occurred only in 45.4% of patients **(Fig. 11)**.

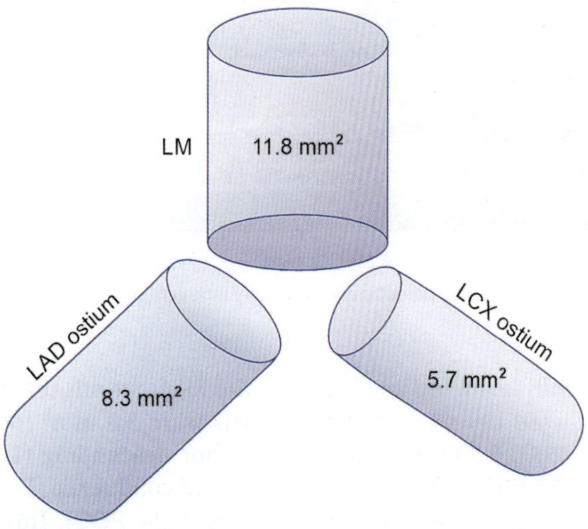

FIG. 10: Optimal cutoff points for MSA by IVUS in distal LM bifurcation lesions treated by 2 stent crush technique: Jung-Min Ahn et al.

(LAD: left anterior descending; LCX: left circumflex; LM: left main)

Post-PCI physiological assessment provides information about the functional results of revascularization and prognostic stratification after PCI.[21] Hence, there is a certain need for increased usage of ICI and intracoronary physiology in real-world practice for optimizing PCI.

BALLOON INFLATION TIME AND PRESSURE OPTIMIZATION PROTOCOL: EFFECT ON STENT EXPANSION

Earlier studies have shown that stent expansion can be optimized by high pressure and prolonged inflation.[22,23] The pressure optimization protocol (POP) describes the method of prolonged inflation with stability of 30 seconds without pressure decay allowable at the inflation pressure provided.[24] The POP has been demonstrated by imaging using OCT to fully expand stents compared to shorter inflation time (15–30 seconds) and to improve long-term outcomes, especially target vessel revascularization.[23,24]

OPERATOR EXPERIENCE: DOES IT MATTER?

A recent study by Choi KH et al.[25] in 6,005 patients who underwent PCI with drug-eluting stents for complex lesions demonstrated that PCI by experienced operators and the use of IVUS during complex PCI were independently associated with lower long-term risks of cardiac death or target vessel myocardial infarction (TVMI). The beneficial effects of IVUS were more prominent for less experienced operators.

WHAT IS NEW?

Artificial Intelligence for Rapid Interpretation of Expansion Metrics

Artificial intelligence (AI) algorithms are being incorporated into IVUS and OCT interpretation for stent sizing, plaque assessment, and measuring expansion metrics. The current OPTIS OCT system enables the easy detection of MSA and relative stent expansion by automated measurements after the stent deployment. The MSA and percentage of the stent expansion can be automatically calculated and highlighted after assigning markers for the site of interest that are close to the proximal and distal edges of the stent translating into a user-friendly tool during PCI. Ultreon™ software powered by AI from Abbott Vascular helps to guide physicians through PCI step-by-step for more accurate decision-making and an updated version Ultreon™ 2.0 has been launched recently.

Three-dimensional Stent

Three-dimensional (3D) stent feature from GE HealthCare is an innovative, intraprocedural 3D stent reconstruction leveraging on clinical micro-computerized tomography (CMCT) imaging. It does not require any imaging catheter

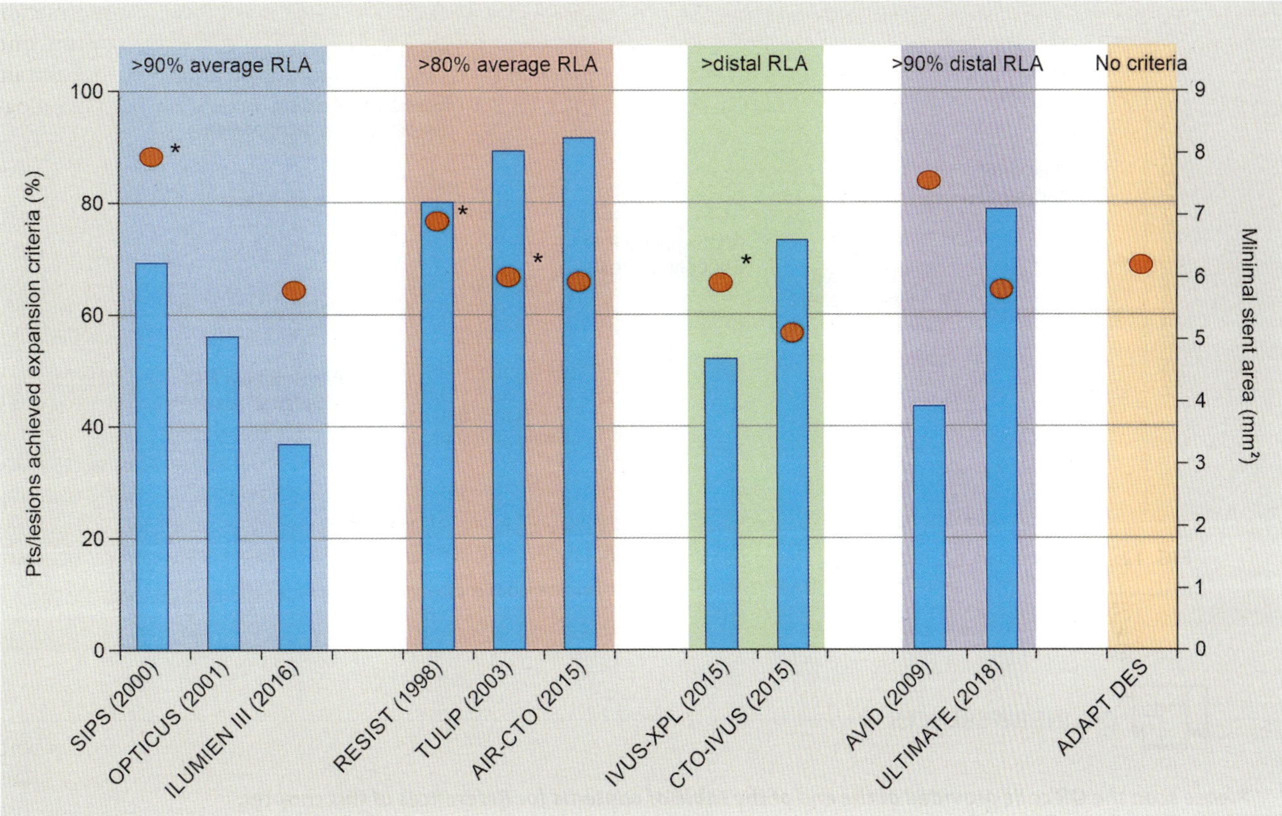

*Minimal lumen area.

FIG. 11: Even in RCTs, expansion criteria were met in <60% of patients. Red dots indicate % of patients achieving predefined MSA. Black bars indicate % of patients achieving predefined expansion criteria.

(MSA: minimal stent area; RCT: randomized controlled trial; RLA: reference lumen area)

and can give comparable results. However, it has limitations such as inability to assess stent apposition and dissections, high radiation, poor image resolution in high body mass index patients, and is yet to be validated in larger cohorts.

Intracoronary Imaging and Physiological Assessment Integration

The relationship between the OCT-guided PCI and FFR has been evaluated in a few studies. In the DOCTORS study,[12] OCT-guided stent optimization compared to angiography guidance led to significantly higher post-PCI FFR value. In the ongoing FUSION study (NCT04356027), the diagnostic performance of OCT pullback and corresponding virtual flow reserve (VFR) is being compared against a reference standard, FFR. A recent study assessed IVUS-based virtual FFR (IVUS-FFR) and found a good correlation with invasive FFR.[26]

CONCLUSION

- The RCT data with >12,000 patients has shown that image-guided PCI improves MACE and saves lives.
- Among the predefined criteria for image-guided PCI, adequate stent expansion correlates well with clinical outcomes.
- A plethora of data supports absolute MSA as the most powerful predictor of long-term outcomes.
- But RCTs, registries, and real-world practice continue to use relative stent expansion criteria for measuring stent expansion as the application of MSA has limitations.
- The question should not be whether to use IVUS or OCT but aiming for optimal PCI outcomes defined by validated imaging criteria **(Fig. 12)**.[27]
- The addition of post-PCI physiology in selected patients may contribute to favorable outcomes.

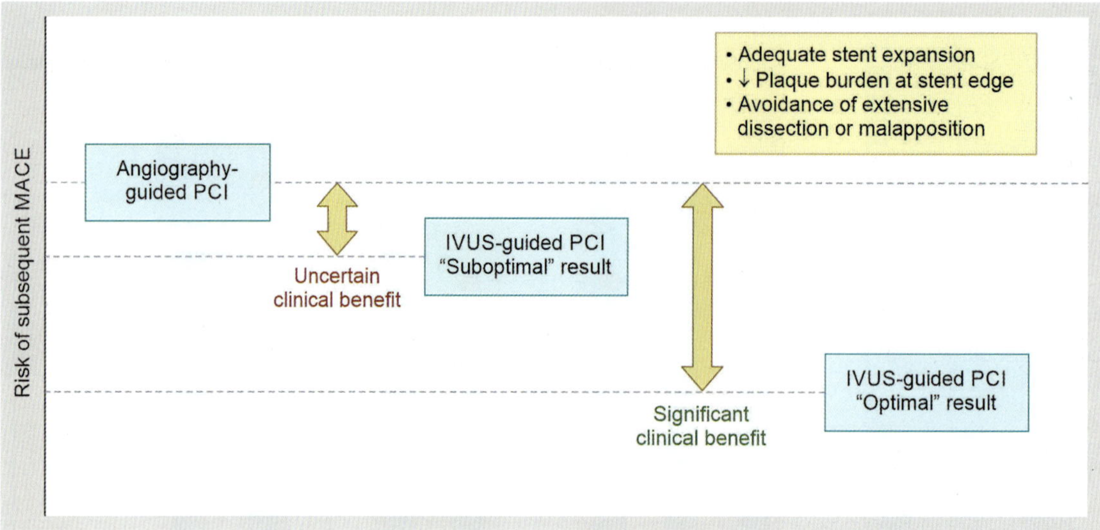

FIG. 12: Image guidance is not enough. The result is to be optimal.[27]

(IVUS: intravascular ultrasound; MACE: major adverse cardiac event; PCI: percutaneous coronary intervention)

ONLINE REFERENCES

Please scan the QR code provided at the end of the table of contents for References of this chapter.

CHAPTER

166 Intravascular Ultrasound in Contemporary Practice

Karthikeyan Balakrishnan, Sai Satish, Vijayakumar Subban

ABSTRACT

Coronary intravascular ultrasound (IVUS), with its ability to produce high-quality cross-sectional images of the coronary arteries, overcomes the limitations of coronary angiogram. It assists in assessment of plaque morphology, identification of vulnerable plaque, and evaluation of intermediate lesion in left main territory. It helps in rational decision-making regarding plaque modification, identification of appropriate landing zones, and stent size selection. Further, it also aids stent optimization. Current evidence supports the utility of IVUS in improving percutaneous coronary intervention (PCI) outcomes. IVUS plays a major role for procedure planning and stent optimization in complex PCI and understand the mechanism of stent failure.

Keywords: Intravascular imaging, PCI optimization, stent failure.

INTRODUCTION

Coronary angiography (CAG) remains the standard imaging modality for invasive assessment of coronary artery disease (CAD) and percutaneous coronary intervention (PCI). However, it is limited by its poor resolution, angle dependency, vessel overlap, foreshortening, and significant inter-and intra-observer variability. Further, CAG is a lumenogram and does not provide adequate information about the vessel wall and plaque characteristics.[1] Coronary intravascular ultrasound (IVUS), with its ability to produce high-quality cross-sectional images of the coronary arteries, allows tissue characterization and complement CAG in the qualitative and quantitative assessment of CAD. Further, it also aids in PCI by providing accurate vessel dimensions for device sizing and guiding stent optimization.

IMAGING PRINCIPLE AND SYSTEMS

Intravascular ultrasound works by the same principle as with any other ultrasound-based imaging modality. A miniature ultrasound transducer positioned at the tip of the imaging catheter emits high frequency ultrasound waves which get reflected from the tissue interfaces in the vessel wall. The imaging console processes these signals into two-dimensional cross-sectional images of the vessel analogous to histological cross-sections.

There are two basic IVUS systems in current use. The mechanical systems (Opticross^{TM} imaging catheter, Boston Scientific, Santa Clara, California; Revolution catheter, Volcano Corp, Rancho Cordova, California; View IT, Terumo Corp, Tokyo, Japan) consist of a single transducer element located at the tip of a flexible drive cable housed in a protective sheath and operated by an external motor drive unit. The transducer rotates at 1,800 rpm to produce cross-sectional images of the vessel wall. The imaging catheters operate at a central frequency of 40 MHz or 45 MHz and are 5F or 6F compatible. Recently, high definition (HD) mechanical systems (Opticross^{TM} HD imaging catheter) with central frequency of 60 MHz have been introduced for clinical use and provide resolution closer to that of Optical coherence tomography without compromising the depth penetration. In the solid-state system (Eagle Eye Catheter, Volcano Corp), there are no rotating components. There are 64 transducer elements mounted circumferentially around the tip of the catheter. The transducer elements are sequentially activated with different time delays to produce an ultrasound beam that sweeps around the vessel circumference. The catheter works at a central frequency of 20 MHz and is 5F compatible.[2,3]

Image Interpretation

Image interpretation by IVUS is based on the variations in the echo reflectivity of different vessel wall structures. Normal adult coronary arteries have a three-layered architecture on IVUS imaging—the echogenic intima, echolucent media, and echogenic adventitia (bright-dark-bright pattern). Plaque characterization by gray scale IVUS is based on the echogenicity of the plaque with reference to the echogenicity of the adventitia: (1) calcified plaque (hyperechoic to adventitia with acoustic shadowing and reverberations), (2) fibrous plaque (isoechoic to adventitia), (3) soft plaque (hypoechoic to adventitia), (4) mixed plaque (no single acoustic type constituting >80% of the plaque) (5) attenuated plaque (signal attenuation in the absence of superficial calcium) and (6) echolucent plaque (plaque with intraplaque echolucency) **(Figs. 1A to G)**. There are two interfaces in the IVUS images—blood/lumen interface and the plaque and media/adventitia interface—that are used for cross-sectional measurements. Length is estimated from the automatic pullback (pullback rate × duration of pullback). Images are described as if viewing the face of a clock, and there is no specific rotational orientation. The side branches and perivascular landmarks (pericardium, pericardial spaces, myocardium, and venous structures) are used to identify the axial position and rotational orientation within the vessel.[2,3]

CLINICAL APPLICATION OF INTRAVASCULAR ULTRASOUND

Assessment of Lesion Severity

Intravascular ultrasound minimal lumen area (MLA) has been compared to fractional flow reserve (FFR) in multiple studies for the assessment of lesion severity in non-left main coronary artery (LMCA) territory. The MLA cut-off value varied between 2.4 to 4 mm^2 in different studies, and the accuracy was only moderate limiting its application in routine practice.[4] The restriction of flow across stenosis depends on various parameters such as lesion eccentricity, amount of myocardium supplied, and length of the lesion, in addition to MLA, it is unlikely that a single parameter could accurately estimate the functional significance.[4]

ASSESSMENT OF PLAQUE VULNERABILITY

Vulnerable plaque is an atherosclerotic plaque which is prone to produce clinical events either from rapid progression or from thrombosis. It is characterized by large lipid content/necrotic core, thin fibrous cap, expansive remodeling, inflammation, spotty calcification, intraplaque hemorrhage, and neoangiogenesis. Identification of such plaques may guide the implementation of treatment strategies that reduce the future adverse outcomes.[5] The grayscale IVUS features of vulnerability are large eccentric plaque, positive remodeling,

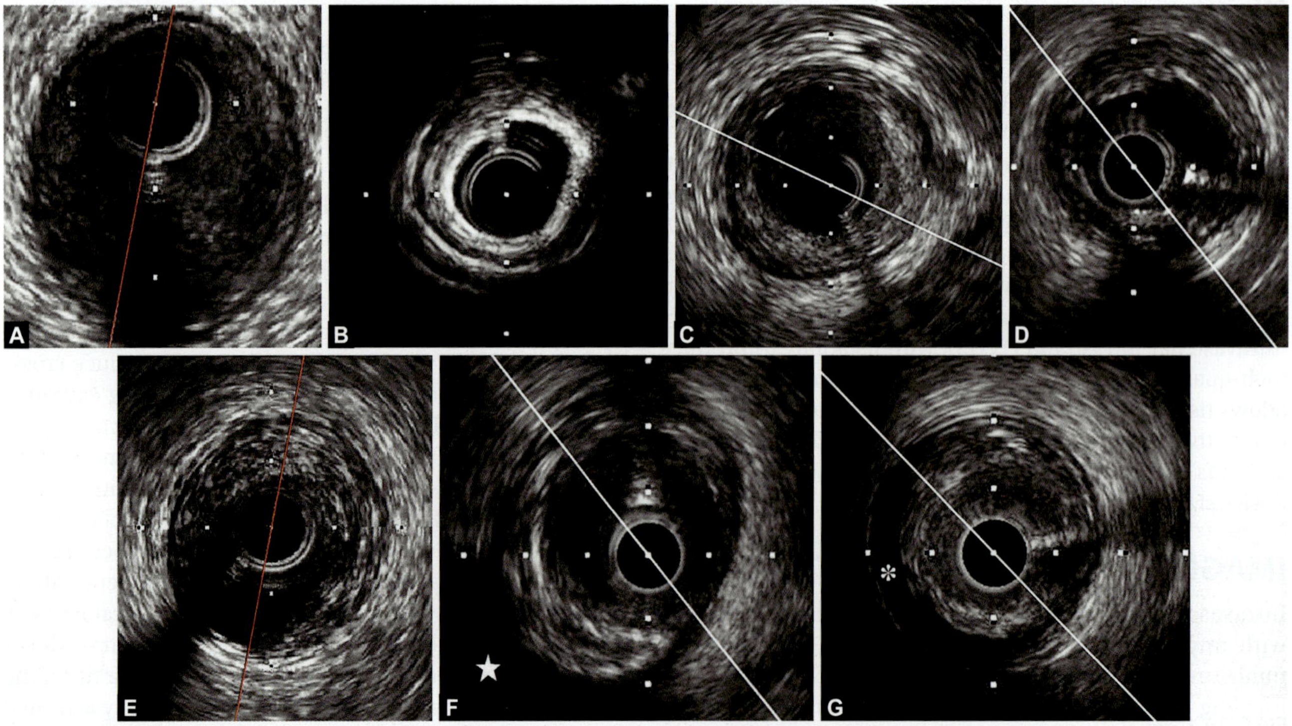

FIGS. 1A TO G: Intravascular ultrasound images of (A) three-layered appearance of coronary artery (bright-dark-bright); (B) Calcific plaque with acoustic shadowing and reverberations; (C) Fibrous plaque; (D) Soft plaque; (E) Mixed plaque with mixture of fibrous and soft elements; (F) Attenuated plaque (isoechoic plaque with shadowing, star); (G) Intraplaque echolucency (*).

attenuated plaque, spotty calcification, and intraplaque echolucency.[5] A recent histological study that validated these grayscale IVUS features, showed a high likelihood of necrotic core in plaques with signal attenuation in the absence of calcification (attenuated plaques), particularly in those with superficial attenuation and in plaques with areas of intraplaque echolucency **(Figs. 1F and G)**.[6]

Pre-percutaneous Coronary Intervention Assessment

The pre-stent assessment focuses on the following parameters.

- Plaque morphology
- Reference landing zones
- Stent sizing

Lesion characteristics influence intervention in two ways; firstly, with distal embolization and resultant no-reflow and secondly, by posing resistance to stent expansion. Various IVUS features such as, attenuated plaque, intraplaque echolucency, and positive remodeling have been linked with distal embolization during the intervention.

Lesion preparation depends on the plaque characteristics. Direct stenting may be preferred in the presence of soft plaque/attenuated plaque to reduce the incidence of distal embolization and no-reflow. Fibrous and fibrocalcific lesions require pretreatment with specialty scoring/cutting/high pressure balloon or rotational atherectomy. Further, IVUS also helps in verifying the adequacy of lesion preparation, particularly in calcified lesions. Imaging of the vessel proximal to the lesion detects any occult stenosis not identified by CAG. In addition, it also demonstrates any hindrance to device delivery such as calcified plaque.

The most important function of preprocedural imaging is appropriate device selection. Once the lesion assessment is completed, the vessel proximal and distal to the lesion is assessed and appropriate reference sites are identified. The reference sites are ones with no or minimal disease. In case of diffuse disease, a site with a plaque burden of <50% is selected as reference site. Then, the maximum, minimum, and average diameters of the external elastic lamina (EEL) and lumen are measured at the reference sites. The stent sizing is based on the smallest average reference diameter. The stent is downsized to the nearest 0.25 mm in case of EEL based approach and upsized to the nearest 0.25 mm in case of lumen-based approach. The distance between the reference segments provides the stent length **(Fig. 2)**.[7]

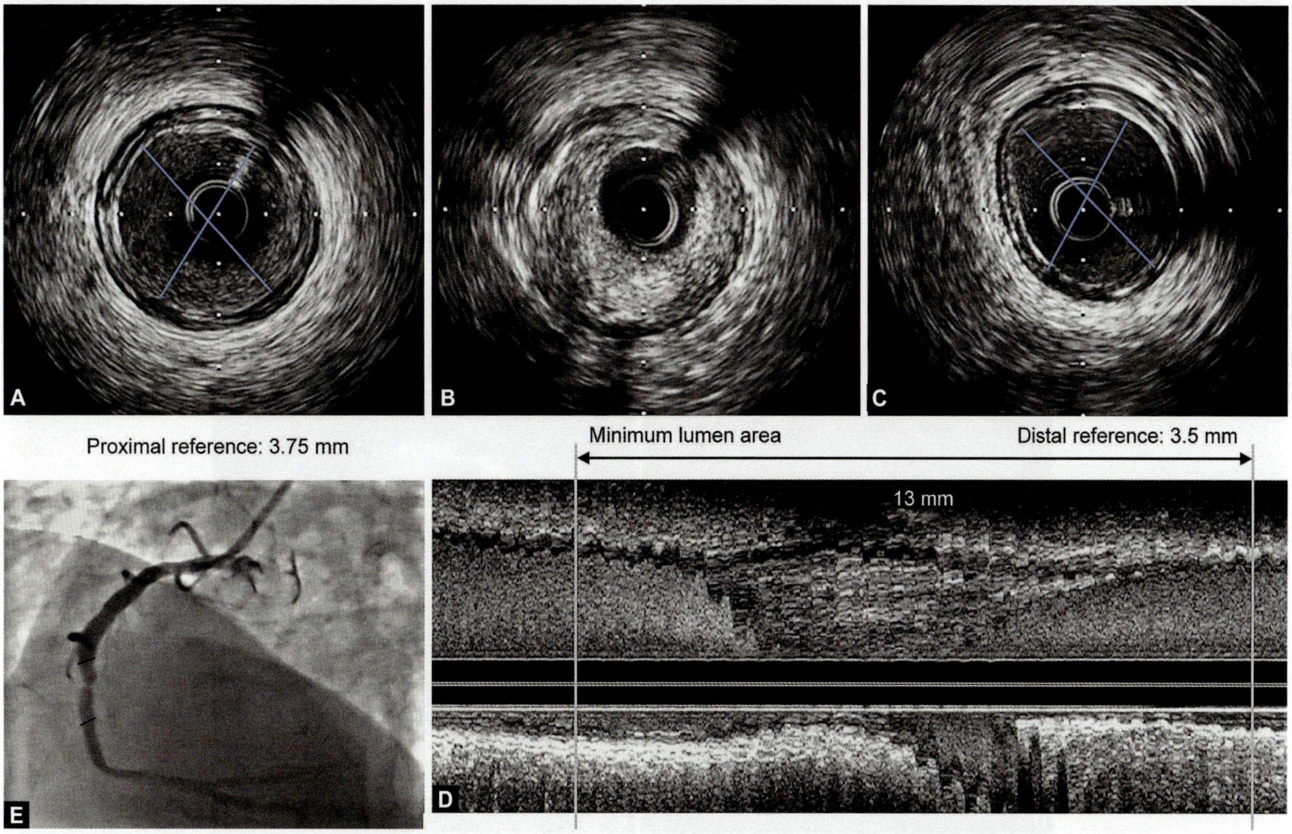

FIGS. 2A TO E: Intravascular ultrasound (IVUS) guided stent sizing. IVUS images showing the lesion (B), plaque free proximal (A) and distal (C) references and respective diameters. The length of the stent is based on the distance between the proximal and distal references (D). Here a 3.5 × 15 mm stent was selected based on the IVUS measurements. (E) Reference angiographic image.

Post-stent Assessment

Post-stent imaging is performed to verify the precision of stent implantation. It assesses stent expansion, apposition, stent edge abnormalities (geographic miss, edge dissection, and hematoma) and intrastent prolapse **(Figs. 3A to E)**.[3]

Stent Expansion

Stent expansion (SE) is the single most important predictor of both in-stent restenosis and stent thrombosis.[8,9] Quantification of SE is based on the minimum stent area (MSA) and is expressed as an absolute value or relative to the reference vessel lumen area or vessel area at the site of the MSA. The current consensus document recommends an absolute MSA >5.5 mm^2 or a relative stent expansion of 80% of the average reference lumen area for non-LMCA lesions.[7] A recent study showed MSA ≤38.9% of the vessel area at that site as a predictor of stent related outcomes.[10]

Malapposition

Malapposition is defined as the lack of contact between the stent strut and the luminal surface not overlying a side branch.[2] Acute malapposition results from one of the three reasons: (1) stent under-sizing, (2) stent under-deployment, or (3) underlying calcified plaque. IVUS identifies malapposition by the presence of blood speckles behind the stent struts.[2] The incidence of acute malapposition varied between 8 and 42% in different IVUS studies. With the available evidence so far, acute malapposition has not been associated with adverse events if the stent is well expanded.[11-15] In contrast to these prospective follow-up studies, malapposition is an important observation in patients presenting with stent thrombosis. The consensus statement recommends treatment of malappositions with incomplete apposition distance of >400 μ and a length >1 mm.[7]

Geographic Miss

Coronary atherosclerosis is a diffuse process and is mostly angiographically silent. In IVUS studies evaluating edge restenosis, the reference segment plaque burden that predicted edge restenosis varied from 47 to 57% between different stent types.[16] The current consensus recommends a landing zone with a plaque burden of <50% and absence of lipid rich plaque.

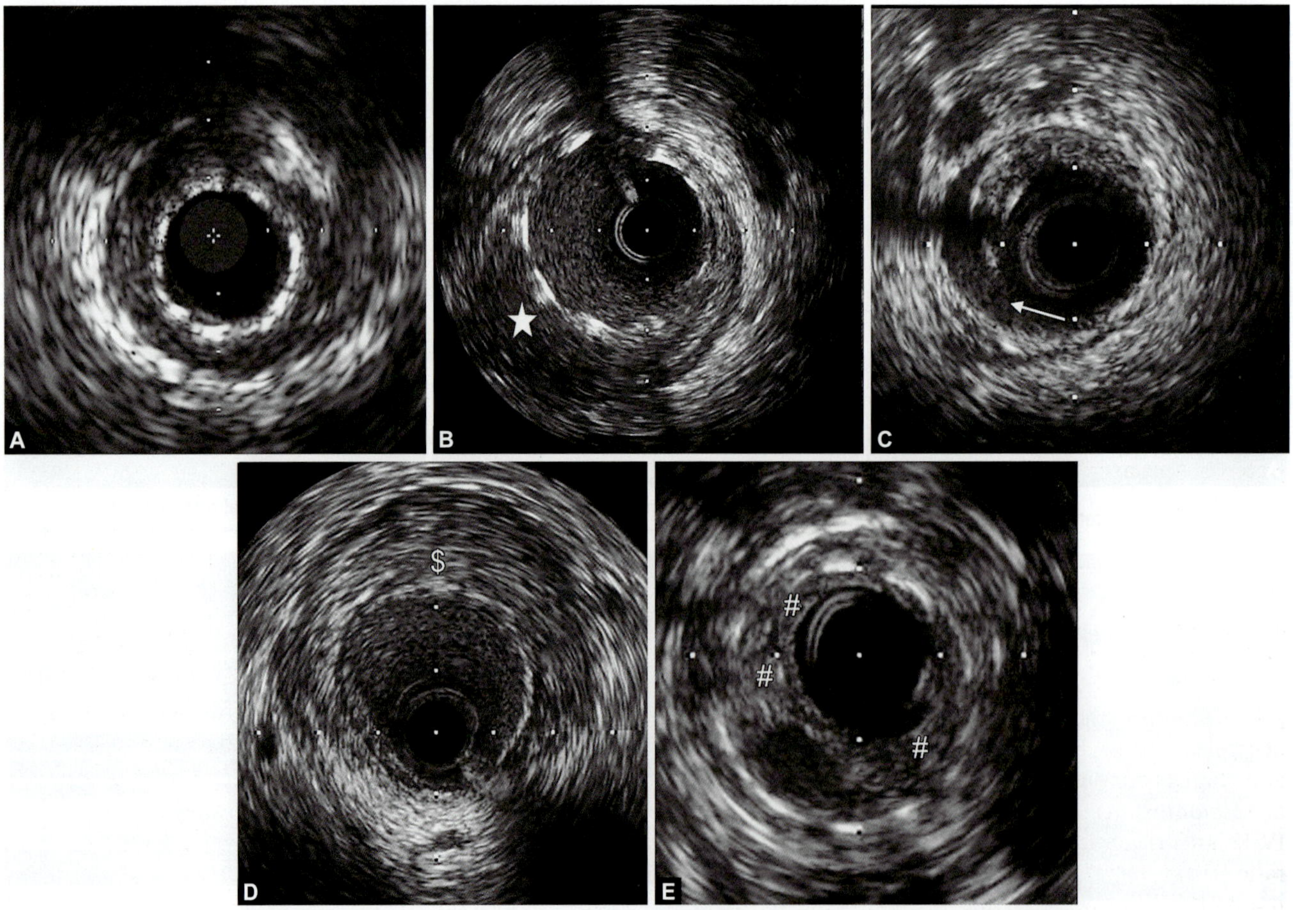

FIGS. 3A TO E: Examples of post-stenting abnormalities. (A) Underexpansion (3-mm stent with an area of 4.3 mm^2). (B) Malapposition (large gap between stent and vessel wall, star). (C) Edge dissection (disruption of intimal continuity, arrow). (D) Intramural hematoma (blood in the medial space, $). (E) Tissue prolapse (intra-stent material, #).

Dissections and Hematoma

Edge dissections commonly result from the landing stents in diseased reference segments, or implantation of oversized stents. IVUS with its high resolution detects a far greater number of edge dissections that are angiographically invisible. Most of the IVUS-detected edge dissections are minor (angiographically silent and no lumen compromise by IVUS) and can be left alone safely. The current consensus document recommends treating dissections meeting the following criteria—dissection with a large residual plaque burden, lateral extent of >60°, longitudinal extent of >2 mm, extension into the media, and location at the distal stent edge.[7]

Intramural hematoma (IMH) is an accumulation of blood within the medial space displacing the internal elastic lamina inward and EEL outward at the edges of the stent. In an IVUS study, it was associated with high incidence of non-Q wave myocardial infarction (MI), need for repeat revascularization, and sudden death.[17]

Tissue Prolapse

Prolapse of the thrombus or plaque material may occur following stent implantation in patients with acute coronary syndrome (ACS).[18] Minor tissue prolapse is a common finding with IVI and usually resolves without any consequences.[19] However, major tissue prolapse may be associated early stent thrombosis.[20]

CLINICAL EVIDENCE FOR INTRAVASCULAR ULTRASOUND-GUIDED CORONARY INTERVENTION

Intravascular ultrasound has played a tremendous role in understanding the mechanisms of balloon angioplasty, stent implantation, and stent failure. This understanding led to the modification of the stent optimization techniques with resultant improvement in patient outcomes. Although there were conflicting results in the earlier small, randomized studies, recent large, randomized trials comparing IVUS versus angiography-guided PCI in complex lesion subsets have shown improved outcomes with the use of IVUS. The ULTIMATE (Intravascular Ultrasound Guided Drug Eluting Stents Implantation in "All Comers" Coronary Lesions) study randomly assigned 1,448 all-comer patients to either an IVUS guidance or angiography guidance group (1:1 ratio). The primary endpoint of target vessel failure [TVF, a composite of cardiac death, target vessel myocardial infarction (TVMI), and clinically driven target vessel revascularization (TVR)] at 12 months, occurred in 21 (2.9%) and 39 (5.4%) in the IVUS and the angiography group respectively [hazard ratio (HR) 0.530; 95% confidence interval (CI) 0.312–0.901; p = 0.019].[21] The TVF continued to be better in the IVUS group at 3 years follow-up (6.6% vs. 10.7%, p = 0.01).[22] The IVUS-XPL (Impact of Intravascular Ultrasound Guidance on the Outcomes of Xience Prime Stents in Long Lesions) trial randomly designated 1,400 patients with long lesions between IVUS guidance and angiography guidance (1:1 ratio). The composite of major adverse cardiac events (MACE, cardiac death, TVMI, or ischemia-driven TLR) at 1 year, was significantly better in the IVUS-guided group (2.9% vs. 5.8%, p = 0.007).[23] At 5 years follow-up, MACE continued to be better with IVUS guidance (5.6% vs. 10.7%, p = 0.001).[24] In both the studies, when optimal IVUS criteria were met the event rate was as low as 1.5%.[21,22] In addition, multiple meta-analyses of randomized studies with DES showed lower incidence of overall MACE, death, TVMI, TLR, TVR, and stent thrombosis.[25-28] Further, in the recent ADAPT-DES study of 3,349 all-comer patient population, the IVUS guidance was associated with better outcomes in all patient subgroups with major benefit in patients with ACS and complex lesions.[29] In the pooled analysis of the above two randomized trials, IVUS guidance was associated with significant reduction in cardiac death (1% vs. 2.2%, HR 0.43; 95% CI 0.22–0.84; p = 0.011. In addition there was significant reduction in ischemia-driven target lesion revascularization in the IVUS group 3.8% vs. 6.5%, HR 0.57; 77% CI 0.40–0.82; p = 0.002).[30]

INTRAVASCULAR ULTRASOUND IN SPECIFIC LESION SUBSETS

Stent Failure

In-stent Restenosis

In-stent restenosis (ISR) remains the interventionist's major challenge even in the era of modern drug-eluting stents (DES) and results mainly from stent underexpansion and excessive neointimal growth.

Gross underexpansion of the stent may result in lumen compromise in the presence of normal neointimal growth. The immediate post-stenting MSA has repeatedly been shown to be an important predictor of ISR. With bare metal stents (BMS), a post-stenting MLA of <6.5 mm^2 identified ISR at follow-up.[20,31,32] In addition, the incidence of ISR decreased by 19% for every 1 mm^2 increase in the lumen area.[33] This led to the concept of "bigger is better" with BMS implantation. Though DES have suppressed neointimal hyperplasia significantly, MLA continues to be an important determinant of ISR. The IVUS MLA cut off which predicted DES restenosis at 9 months varied between 5 and 5.7 mm^2 among different DES.[31,32,34,35] In addition to MLA, the length of the stent >40 mm has also been associated with increased incidence of restenosis. Further, longer stents are also associated with higher incidence of underexpansion.[36]

Very Late Stent Thrombosis

Very late stent thrombosis (VLST) is a vexing problem with DES and continues to occur even with the second-generation stents, though at a lower rate. Pathological studies have demonstrated vessel wall inflammation, incomplete stent apposition, incomplete stent strut coverage, stent fracture and neoatherosclerosis in patients with VLST. IVUS has played a major role in understanding the pathophysiology of VLST in vivo.[37,38]

Late incomplete stent apposition (LISA) has been identified by IVUS in about three-fourths of the patients with VLST. LISA may be a persistent malapposition that existed at the time of stent implantation or develops later from either thrombus resolution or from vessel wall inflammation and positive remodeling. The cause-and-effect association between LISA and VLST is yet to be demonstrated conclusively. LISA, particularly the large ones or aneurysms, may be one of the several factors involved in the pathophysiology of VLST. It is postulated that vessel wall inflammation may be the initial event in the pathogenesis of VLST. ISA and resultant flow disturbance and poor stent strut coverage may culminate in thrombosis.[37,38]

Neoatherosclerosis

The development of atherosclerotic changes in the neointimal tissue is increasingly being recognized as an important cause of very late stent failure with both BMS and DES. Dysfunctional endothelium covering the neointimal tissue promoting alteration in the composition of the extracellular matrix and lipid accumulation has been proposed as the possible cause of neoatherosclerosis. This may result either in a progressive increase in the atherosclerotic tissue volume and in-stent restenosis or plaque rupture and stent thrombosis. Though these changes have initially been reported with pathological studies of very late stent failure, with the availability of IVUS tissue characterization algorithms, it is currently possible to diagnose neoatherosclerosis in vivo. It is characterized by lipid-laden intima, intimal rupture, and luminal thrombus. Though the exact management of neoatherosclerosis is largely unknown, aggressive antiatherosclerotic treatment as with native coronary atherosclerosis may be beneficial.[39]

Bifurcation Intervention

The various roles of IVUS during bifurcation PCI are identification of cause of side branch narrowing, selection of stenting strategy, predicting the chance of side branch compromise, and stent optimization.

Intravascular ultrasound helps in identifying the exact cause of angiographic side branch ostial narrowing before stenting. The most common mechanisms are (1) true atherosclerotic ostial disease, (2) atherosclerotic plaque in the main vessel without true involvement of the ostium, or (3) negative remodeling without much atherosclerotic plaque burden. The latter two are associated with lower incidence of side branch compromise following single stent crossover technique.[40] A preprocedure SB ostial MLA of <2.4 mm^2 and a plaque burden of >50% have been associated with postprocedure SB compromise and may benefit from elective two-stent strategy rather than a provisional strategy.[41] The IVUS predictors of side branch compromise following main vessel stenting are presence of a carina with a spiky morphology ("eyebrow" sign), absence of plaque at the carina, and eccentric plaque accumulation opposite to the carina.[42]

Left Main Intervention

The utility of IVUS during left main coronary artery (LMCA) intervention are: (1) intermediate lesion assessment, (2) clarifying angiographic ambiguity, (3) selection of stenting strategy, and (4) stent optimization.

Intermediate lesion assessment: In contrast to non-LMCA territory, with its little anatomical variability and relatively constant myocardial volume of supply, there is good correlation between IVUS and FFR in the LMCA segment.[4] Revascularization is recommended when the IVUS MLA is <4.5 mm^2 and deferred when it is >6 mm^2 and clinical judgment or some other form of assessment is recommended for an in-between MLA.[43]

Clarifying angiographic ambiguity: Angiographic haziness may result from thrombus, calcified nodule, or ruptured plaque. IVUS by characterizing them accurately helps in management decisions.

Selecting the stenting strategy: Stenting technique depends on the distribution plaque in different regions of LMCA. In ostial and shaft regions, IVUS helps in sizing the stent appropriately and identifies the landing zones with minimum plaque burden.[43] In case of distal LMCA disease, IVUS shows the extension of disease into the side branches. Severity and extent of disease at the ostium of LCX determines the stenting strategy. An LCX ostial plaque burden of 56% and area of <3.7 mm^2 identified postprocedure FFR of <0.80 in a study.[44] These lesions may need upfront two-stent strategy and others may be managed with single stent crossover technique.

Stent optimization: In a single center observational study of 403 patients treated with elective two-stent strategy, the optimal IVUS MLA cut off values that predicted restenosis were 5.0 mm^2, 6.3 mm^2, 7.2 mm^2, and 8.2 mm^2 at ostial left circumflex coronary artery, ostial left anterior descending coronary artery, polygon of confluence, and distal LMCA respectively.[45]

Chronic Total Occlusion Intervention

Intravascular imagine plays two important roles during CTO revascularization: (1) assists wire crossing when angiographic information alone is inadequate, (2) facilitates stent optimization as in any other PCI.

Angiographic imaging remains the cornerstone for wire handling during CTO PCI. However, this information is inadequate when the proximal occlusion site is blunt without a clear entry point or when the wire enters the subintimal space and results in collapsing of the distal true lumen. In the first situation, IVUS can be used to identify the optimal entry point when a suitable side branch is available. The IVUS catheter is introduced into the side branch and slowly pulled back proximally till the main branch is visible. Then the optimal entry site is identified (middle of the intimal plaque) and an angiographic image is obtained. The position of the IVUS catheter is marked on the angiogram and targeted for the wire entry. Once the wire enters the proximal cap, IVUS is again used to confirm the correct position of the wire. In the second situation, the subintimal space is enlarged with a small balloon and IVUS is introduced into the subintimal space to locate the site of wire entry from intimal plaque into the subintimal space and then a stronger second wire is directed into the intimal plaque and into the distal true lumen under IVUS guidance.[46-48]

During retrograde CTO PCI, the most common mode of recanalization is the reverse CART (controlled antegrade and retrograde subintimal tracking) technique. There are two important caveats for a successful reverse CART technique. First, both the antegrade and retrograde wires should be in the subintimal space or in the true lumen for effective wire crossing after balloon dilatation. The presence of antegrade wire in the true lumen and retrograde wire in the subintimal space results in a significant amount of intimal tissue between the wires and a larger balloon is required to break the tissue and connect the spaces. When the antegrade wire is in the subintimal space and the retrograde wire in the true lumen, the wire crossing is extremely difficult particularly in the presence of intervening calcified intimal tissue. Second, the balloon size should match the vessel size to effectively break the intervening tissue and connect the wires. When there is difficulty in wire crossing after antegrade balloon dilatation, IVUS helps in identifying the exact location of the antegrade and retrograde wires, the morphology of the intervening plaque and the true vessel size, so that the strategy may be appropriately altered to facilitate wire crossing into the proximal true lumen.[46-48]

Calcified Lesion Intervention

Coronary angiography is less sensitive to detect calcification. IVUS identifies calcification with a high degree of accuracy. It also clearly delineates the location, circumferential and longitudinal extent of calcification. This information is of potential importance during PCI to select the appropriate debulking strategy. The response to the balloon dilatation depends on the position of the calcium, whether superficial (close to the lumen) or deep (adventitial). Adventitial calcium may not pose much threat to the balloon dilatation or stent expansion.

Zhang et al. devised an IVUS-based calcium to predict stent expansion in calcified lesions. They used the following four characteristics: (1) Superficial calcium angle >270° longer than 5 mm, (2) 360° superficial calcium, (3) calcified nodule, and (4) vessel diameter <3.5 mm. Presence of each of these characteristics was given one point. A score of >2 predicted stent underexpansion and the need for atherectomy.[49]

CONCLUSION

Intravascular ultrasound supplements CAG in the evaluation of CAD. It provides valuable information on lesion severity, plaque vulnerability, lesion preparation, stent optimization, and understanding of stent failure. Data from randomized studies and registries have shown improved clinical outcomes with IVUS guidance for PCI compared to angiography guidance alone.

ONLINE REFERENCES

Please scan the QR code provided at the end of the table of contents for References of this chapter.

CHAPTER 167

Intravascular Ultrasound versus Fractional Flow Reserve in Guiding Percutaneous Coronary Intervention: A Comprehensive Comparison

Prasant Kumar Sahoo, Shyam Prasad Sahoo, Subasis Dash

ABSTRACT

In interventional cardiology, precise evaluation of coronary lesions is crucial for effective percutaneous coronary intervention (PCI) and improved patient outcomes. Intravascular ultrasound (IVUS) provides detailed anatomical information, aiding in stent sizing, deployment, and assessing stent expansion. Fractional flow reserve (FFR) measures the functional significance of lesions, guiding revascularization decisions based on their hemodynamic impact. The integration of IVUS and FFR offers a comprehensive approach to coronary lesion assessment, combining anatomical and functional information for optimal treatment decisions. The advantages of using IVUS and FFR in PCI include improved procedural success, reduced complications, and enhanced long-term outcomes. By combining both modalities, interventional cardiologists can confidently navigate through challenging clinical scenarios, such as left main coronary artery disease (CAD) and multivessel disease, ensuring targeted revascularization and minimizing adverse events. This chapter summarizes the significance of IVUS, FFR, and their integration in complex coronary cases, emphasizing the benefits of personalized treatment strategies based on individual patient characteristics.

Keywords: Percutaneous coronary intervention, intravascular ultrasound, optical coherence tomography, fractional flow reserve, coronary artery disease, interventional cardiology.

INTRODUCTION

Importance of Guiding Percutaneous Coronary Intervention with Imaging and Functional Assessments

Percutaneous coronary interventions (PCI) with imaging and functional assessments is crucial for effectively managing coronary artery disease (CAD) and achieving optimal outcomes. Intravascular imaging techniques such as intravascular ultrasound (IVUS) and optical coherence tomography (OCT) offer high-resolution views of the coronary arteries, aiding accurate lesion characterization and optimal stent deployment.[1,2] IVUS provides precise vessel measurements for improved stent placement, reducing adverse events and leading to better long-term results.[1] It has applications in understanding plaque burden and its composition and in determining the reference diameter for appropriate placement of the stent after PCI.[3] Integrating IVUS into PCI procedures has been associated with decreased late stent thrombosis and improved clinical outcomes in complex cases.[4,5]

The fractional flow reserve (FFR) is calculated by placing a pressure transducer across a lesion to induce maximal flow of blood pharmacologically. FFR in a normal coronary artery is 1.0. An FFR value of 0.80 or less indicates significant coronary stenosis with an accuracy of >90%.[6,7] Thus, FFR identifies hemodynamically significant lesions that benefit from stenting and plays a vital role in PCI decision-making.[8,9] FFR-guided PCI has demonstrated superior outcomes (reduced adverse events and reduced need for repeat revascularizations) compared to angiography-guided PCI.[10]

Combining IVUS with FFR can further enhance the procedural success rate and individualized treatment strategies. However, it is important to consider practicality and cost implications when integrating both IVUS and FFR.[11] Integrating both techniques requires two disposables and double instrumentations to obtain both IVUS and FFR, which is not practical in clinical routine use.[12] For particular complex situations such as bifurcation lesions and chronic total occlusions (CTO), combined modalities are often considered.[4,9]

INTRAVASCULAR ULTRASOUND: TECHNOLOGY AND APPLICATIONS

Intravascular ultrasound, a sophisticated imaging technology that uses high-frequency sound waves to provide high-resolution, real-time images of the vessel walls and the lumen, is extensively utilized in PCI procedures.[13] The procedure involves inserting a catheter with a miniature ultrasound transducer into the coronary arteries for a detailed assessment of plaque morphology, lesion length, and vessel dimensions. This facilitates precise lesion characterization and optimal stent sizing and placement.[1,13] IVUS provides valuable insights into stent apposition and expansion, enabling interventional cardiologists to ensure accurate stent deployment and reduce the risk of complications.[1]

Historical Perspective and Clinical Evidence for Intravascular Ultrasound-guided Percutaneous Coronary Intervention

Over the years, numerous clinical studies and trials have demonstrated the clinical utility of IVUS in guiding PCI procedures. A meta-analysis of such studies reported that IVUS-guided PCI was associated with a significant reduction in the risk of major adverse cardiac events (MACE), highlighting the value of IVUS in enhancing patient outcomes.[10]

Advantages of Intravascular Ultrasound in Guiding Percutaneous Coronary Intervention

Intravascular ultrasound can provide information on vessel morphology (size and subsequent layers) and plaque characteristics in real time and is not prone to technical errors.[3] IVUS is versatile and complements other imaging modalities, making it indispensable for optimizing treatment strategies for CAD. Additionally, IVUS assists in identifying vulnerable plaques and guiding appropriate therapeutic interventions to improve patient outcomes.[14] IVUS provides a tomographic image of the lumen and vessel wall; it can identify low-grade plaques prior to causing luminal narrowing, unlike the two-dimensional images seen on coronary angiography, which may not discern these lesions.

Limitations of Intravascular Ultrasound in Guiding Percutaneous Coronary Intervention

Intravascular ultrasound cannot provide information on coronary physiology. IVUS requires specialized training and expertise for accurate image interpretation during PCI procedures.[1] It is an invasive procedure that may be time-consuming and relatively expensive, limiting its widespread use in some healthcare settings.[1,11] Interventional cardiologists can still effectively utilize IVUS to enhance the precision and success of PCI procedures, benefiting patients with CAD.

FRACTIONAL FLOW RESERVE: PRINCIPLES AND APPLICATIONS

Fractional flow reserve is a tool in CAD management that assesses the functional significance based on blood flow measurements in stenotic coronary arteries. FFR-guided PCI allows for a targeted approach, optimizing revascularization strategies and minimizing unnecessary interventions. Clinical studies conducted after 2010[7,8,15-17] have consistently demonstrated the clinical utility of FFR in guiding PCI procedures, and FFR remains a cornerstone in interventional cardiology.

Fractional Flow Reserve-guided Percutaneous Coronary Intervention: Clinical Evidence and Outcomes

Fractional flow reserve-guided PCI has consistently demonstrated its effectiveness in improving patient outcomes. Studies, including FAME II and meta-analyses, have shown reduced adverse events and improved cost-effectiveness compared to angiography-guided PCI.[18,19]

Fractional Flow Reserve versus Noninvasive Functional Testing in Coronary Artery Disease Evaluation

Fractional flow reserve is superior to noninvasive stress testing in identifying coronary lesions that benefit from revascularization in patients with CAD. It directly assesses functional significance, providing precise information on ischemia and guiding optimal treatment decisions, leading to improved diagnostic accuracy and better outcomes.[7]

Advantages and Limitations of Fractional Flow Reserve in Guiding Percutaneous Coronary Intervention

Fractional flow reserve usage in guiding PCI provides objective, quantitative, and reproducible data and helps

TABLE 1: Advantages and limitations of intravascular ultrasound (IVUS) and fractional flow reserve (FFR) in percutaneous coronary intervention (PCI) guidance.

Criteria	IVUS[13,14]	FFR[16]
Lesion assessment	Detailed plaque morphology and vessel dimensions	Identification of hemodynamically significant lesions
Stent optimization	Precise stent sizing and deployment	Functional evaluation for appropriate stent placement
Lesion characterization	Assessment of plaque burden and remodeling	Functional impact on blood flow in coronary stenosis
Vulnerable plaque	Identification of vulnerable plaques	N/A (focuses on functional significance)
Complementing imaging	Complements other imaging modalities	N/A (a functional assessment, not imaging)

TABLE 2: Intravascular ultrasound (IVUS) versus fractional flow reserve (FFR): A comparative analysis based on inferences from observational studies and randomized trial.

Study	IVUS-guided PCI	FFR-guided PCI
Lesion assessment[17,20]	Anatomical information	Functional information
PCI decision-making[17,21]	Lesion characterization and stent deployment optimization	Identification of hemodynamically significant lesions
Clinical outcomes[20,22]	Improved procedural outcomes and reduced adverse events	Lower rates of major adverse cardiac events and revascularizations
Resource utilization[6,7]	It may increase procedure time and cost	Reduced need for unnecessary interventions
Long-term benefits[15,18]	Improved long-term outcomes	Better patient outcomes with reduced repeat revascularizations

(PCI: percutaneous coronary intervention)

identify hemodynamically significant lesions and optimize resource utilization.[6] FFR guides stent sizing and placement, reducing complications and improving patient outcomes.[6] However, limitations include the need for adenosine-induced hyperemia, which can be time-consuming and costly, and its inability to assess diffuse disease effects in certain patient subgroups.[6,7] **Table 1** shows the criteria for significance in IVUS and FFR in PCI guidance.

INTRAVASCULAR ULTRASOUND VERSUS FRACTIONAL FLOW RESERVE: COMPARATIVE ANALYSIS

Intravascular Ultrasound and Fractional Flow Reserve as Complementary Tools in Percutaneous Coronary Intervention

In the realm of PCI, IVUS and FFR serve as valuable complementary tools. **Table 2** provides an overview of the benefits and clinical outcomes associated with each approach from real-world studies.

Intravascular Ultrasound-guided versus Fractional Flow Reserve-guided Percutaneous Coronary Intervention: Head-to-Head Studies

Several head-to-head studies have compared the clinical outcomes of IVUS-guided and FFR-guided PCI. For instance, a study by Koo et al. demonstrated that IVUS-guided PCI improved procedural outcomes by providing more accurate lesion assessment and optimizing stent deployment.[1] Further, a systematic review on the impact of IVUS-guided PCI found that IVUS guidance for PCI was associated with significantly lower all-cause mortality, MACE, and reduced target vessel revascularization compared to angiography-guided PCI.[23] Similarly, the landmark FAME study compared FFR-guided PCI with angiography-guided PCI, showing that FFR guidance led to reduced MACE and revascularization rates.[24] In a study conducted by Sawant et al. to determine the reason for improved outcomes with FFR, post-PCI ischemia, a strong predictor of worse survival, and MACE was significantly reduced among patients who underwent FFR-guided PCI over angiography-guided PCI.[25] These studies highlight the significance of IVUS and FFR in improving PCI success and patient outcomes.[1]

Meta-analyses and Systematic Reviews on Intravascular Ultrasound and Fractional Flow Reserve in Percutaneous Coronary Intervention

Numerous meta-analyses and systematic reviews have shown the benefits of IVUS and FFR in PCI. Darmoch et al. demonstrated improved clinical outcomes with IVUS-guided PCI,[10] while De Bruyne et al. highlighted the superiority of FFR-guided PCI over medical therapy alone.[7] These findings emphasize the importance of using IVUS and FFR to optimize treatment strategies in PCI decision-making.

TABLE 3: Current guidelines and recommendations for the use of intravascular ultrasound (IVUS) and fractional flow reserve (FFR) in percutaneous coronary intervention (PCI).

Guideline/Recommendation	IVUS use in PCI	FFR use in PCI
ESC guidelines 2021[29]	Class IIa recommendation for IVUS guidance in complex PCI cases, including left main, bifurcation, and CTO lesions	Class I recommendation for FFR assessment in coronary stenoses of intermediate severity (FFR 0.80–0.85)
ACC/AHA guidelines 2020[30]	Class IIb recommendation for IVUS use in selected PCI procedures	Class I recommendation for FFR-guided assessment of hemodynamically significant coronary lesions
NICE guidelines 2021[31]	Recommends considering IVUS to optimize stent deployment in complex lesions	Suggests considering FFR in patients with stable angina and intermediate coronary stenosis
Japanese Circulation Society 2020[32]	Class IIb recommendation for IVUS use in complex and high-risk PCI	Class I recommendation for FFR use to guide treatment decisions in patients with intermediate coronary stenosis
EAPCI Expert Consensus 2019[33]	Supports IVUS use in PCI for optimization of stent implantation	Strongly recommends FFR use in coronary stenosis with intermediate severity (FFR 0.80–0.82)

(ACC/AHA: American College of Cardiology/American Heart Association; CTO: chronic total occlusion; EAPCI: European Association of Percutaneous Cardiovascular Interventions; ESC: European Society of Cardiology; NICE: National Institute for Health and Care Excellence)

Cost-effectiveness Considerations: Intravascular Ultrasound versus Fractional Flow Reserve

Cost-effectiveness is a crucial aspect when considering the adoption of IVUS and FFR in PCI practice. An Italian economic analysis has considered IVUS-guided PCI to be cost-effective, especially among those with high risk for cardiac events such as co-morbid diabetes, acute coronary syndrome, and renal insufficiency.[26] This, in countries with high incidences of diabetes and renal abnormalities, IVUS-guided PCI could be extremely effective in improving clinical outcomes. In a study, FFR-based management of CAD found that >40% of lesions identified significant by angiography were otherwise not. This led to changes in management strategies and led to a net cost benefit of $15,600.[27] These investigations have demonstrated the potential benefits of FFR and IVUS in reducing adverse events and optimizing resource utilization, thus improving patient outcomes, alongside their cost-effectiveness. These findings emphasize the long-term value of incorporating IVUS and FFR in guiding PCI procedures.

Current Guidelines and Recommendations for Intravascular Ultrasound and Fractional Flow Reserve Use in Percutaneous Coronary Intervention

Guidelines stress the significance of imaging and functional assessments in precise lesion evaluation and personalized treatment planning.[1,5] Expert consensus recommendations by Stone et al. advocate for appropriate IVUS utilization in PCI to enhance procedural outcomes.[14] Levine et al. (2019) guideline highlights FFR's clinical indications in CAD management, supporting its integration into PCI decision-making.[28] **Table 3** presents a summary of the current guidelines and recommendations for IVUS and FFR use in PCI.

INTEGRATING INTRAVASCULAR ULTRASOUND AND FRACTIONAL FLOW RESERVE IN COMPLEX PERCUTANEOUS CORONARY INTERVENTION CASES

Complex Lesion Assessment with Combined Intravascular Ultrasound and Fractional Flow Reserve

The integration of IVUS and FFR has shown significant value in the assessment of complex lesions during PCI procedures. By combining IVUS and FFR, interventional cardiologists can obtain a comprehensive understanding of lesion characteristics and hemodynamic significance.[1] This synergistic approach allows for more precise identification of functionally significant lesions, guiding appropriate treatment strategies in complex PCI cases.

Optimizing Stent Deployment and Post-percutaneous Coronary Intervention Assessment

The combination of IVUS and FFR optimizes stent deployment during PCI by guiding appropriate stent sizing and identifying hemodynamically significant lesions.[1,7] IVUS aids in assessing lesion morphology and confirming stent apposition, while FFR provides functional validation, ensuring hemodynamic improvement post-PCI.[1] This integrated approach enhances post-PCI assessment, leading to improved procedural success and patient outcomes.

Managing Bifurcation Lesions with Intravascular Ultrasound and Fractional Flow Reserve Guidance

Coronary bifurcations, which make up 15–20% of PCI, are one of the most puzzling lesions to treat in interventional cardiology in terms of improving procedural success and reducing cardiac events. Intracoronary imaging techniques such as IVUS and endovascular tools such as FFR can help achieve optimal results.[34] The integration of IVUS and FFR guidance proves valuable in managing bifurcation lesions during PCI. IVUS aids in visualizing the bifurcation anatomy and guiding stent strategy selection, while FFR helps identify the hemodynamically significant side branch for appropriate treatment decisions.[9] By using both IVUS and FFR in bifurcation PCI, interventional cardiologists can achieve optimal lesion assessment and stent strategy selection, reducing complications and enhancing procedural success.[9] This integrated approach ensures a comprehensive evaluation of the bifurcation lesion, leading to improved outcomes and minimized risks.

Fractional Flow Reserve and Intravascular Ultrasound in Coronary Artery Lesions beyond the Left Main

Fractional flow reserve and IVUS play vital roles in guiding PCI for coronary artery lesions beyond the left main coronary artery. FFR and IVUS are employed for improved clinical outcomes, especially in patients with multivessel CAD. IVUS-guided PCI was found to significantly improve clinical outcomes as compared to other treatments for multivessel disease.[35] Selective PCI conducted using FFR-guided for effective decision-making for the treatment of noninfarct-related artery lesions found superior outcomes in terms of the risk of death, myocardial infarction, or repeat revascularization.[36] The combination of both modalities provides a comprehensive evaluation of lesion severity and functional significance, enabling tailored treatment strategies and optimizing PCI outcomes. Integrating FFR and IVUS enhances decision-making in complex CAD cases, ensuring improved patient care and procedural success.[13,16]

CLINICAL DECISION-MAKING AND INDIVIDUALIZING PERCUTANEOUS CORONARY INTERVENTION STRATEGIES

Role of Intravascular Ultrasound and Fractional Flow Reserve in Patient Selection for Percutaneous Coronary Intervention

From preinterventional lesion evaluation, such as plaque morphology, lesion length, and reference vessel diameter, to postinterventional IVUS to assess the stent result, including minimal stent area and stent expansion, IVUS offers detailed guidance of PCI.[13] FFR offers functional insights, identifying hemodynamically significant lesions that may benefit from revascularization.[1,7] By combining IVUS and FFR data, interventional cardiologists can make well-informed decisions, tailoring treatment strategies for each patient based on their specific anatomical and functional characteristics.

Tailoring Treatment Based on Intravascular Ultrasound and Fractional Flow Reserve Findings

Treatment personalization based on IVUS and FFR findings is an essential aspect of PCI in patients with CAD. IVUS plays a crucial role in providing comprehensive anatomical insights, facilitating precise stent sizing, optimal deployment, and evaluation of stent expansion.[13] FFR offers functional insights by identifying hemodynamically significant lesions that may benefit from revascularization.[28] By integrating IVUS and FFR data, interventional cardiologists can customize PCI strategies according to individual anatomical and functional characteristics, resulting in improved procedural success and reduced risks.

Adapting to Challenging Clinical Scenarios with Integrated Data

The integration of IVUS and FFR data provides valuable support in adapting to challenging clinical scenarios during PCI.[19] IVUS offers detailed anatomical information, enabling precise lesion assessment, stent size selection, optimal deployment, and assessment of stent expansion.[13] Complementing this, FFR aids in identifying the functional impact of lesions, ensuring optimal treatment decisions.[7] In complex lesions, IVUS helps guide appropriate lesion preparation and stent selection, while FFR assists in identifying hemodynamically significant branches and choosing suitable stenting techniques.[9] Moreover, the integration of IVUS and FFR data has demonstrated benefits in cases of bifurcation lesions, providing valuable guidance in selecting the most suitable stenting approach.[9] By leveraging these combined insights, interventional cardiologists can confidently navigate challenging clinical scenarios, optimizing procedural outcomes and patient satisfaction.[7,9,13]

Optimal Technique Selection for Guiding Percutaneous Coronary Intervention: Considering Clinical Scenarios and Patient Factors

Optimal technique selection for guiding PCI involves careful consideration of various clinical scenarios and patient factors. One of the key determinants is the type and complexity of the coronary lesion. In cases of simple lesions with clear anatomy, standard angiography may be sufficient for decision-making. However, in complex lesions, additional intravascular imaging techniques such as IVUS and OCT can provide detailed anatomical information, aiding in lesion assessment, stent sizing, and deployment optimization.[1] Furthermore, functional assessment using FFR plays a crucial role in identifying hemodynamically significant lesions that may benefit from revascularization. The integration of IVUS and FFR data offers comprehensive insights into both the anatomical and functional aspects of coronary lesions, enabling interventional cardiologists to tailor treatment strategies accordingly.[1] Apart from lesion characteristics, patient factors also play a vital role in technique selection. Individual patients' comorbidities, age, overall health status, and willingness to comply with postprocedural care are essential considerations. Additionally, operator experience and expertise in using IVUS and FFR must be taken into account. Proper training and familiarity with the devices and interpretation of results are crucial for successful utilization and decision-making during PCI.[12] Furthermore, economic considerations and resource availability should be considered when selecting the optimal technique for PCI.

Complex Lesions and Anatomical Assessment

Complex lesions in coronary arteries pose unique challenges during PCI, and anatomical assessment plays a critical role in guiding the treatment strategy. Conventional angiography may not provide sufficient information to fully understand the intricacies of these lesions. Therefore, advanced intravascular imaging techniques such as IVUS and OCT are frequently employed to obtain detailed anatomical information.[13] IVUS allows for the visualization of vessel dimensions, plaque morphology, and the extent of disease, aiding in lesion assessment and determining the appropriate stent size and length. Additionally, FFR is used to assess the functional significance of these lesions **(Flowcharts 1A and B)**.[7]

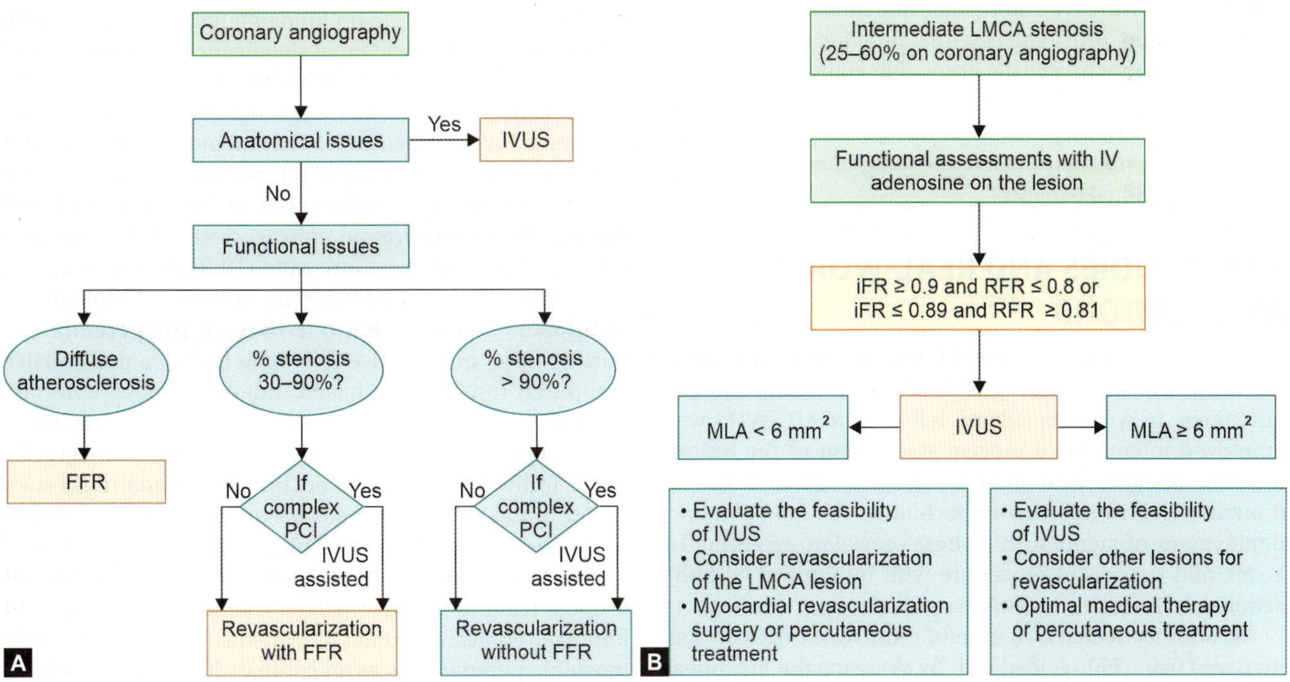

FLOWCHARTS 1A AND B: Depiction of intravascular ultrasound (IVUS) versus fractional flow reserve (FFR) in decision-making of percutaneous coronary intervention (PCI): (A) Simple PCI; (B) Complex PCI.

(iFR: instantaneous wave-free ratio; IV: intravenous; LMCA: left main coronary artery; MLA: minimal lumen area; RFR: resting full cycle ratio)

Functional Assessment of Hemodynamically Significant Lesions

Hemodynamically significant lesions in coronary arteries are those that impede blood flow to a degree that affects the myocardial perfusion, leading to ischemia and potentially causing symptoms such as angina or even myocardial infarction. Both IVUS and FFR play crucial roles in identifying and assessing the functional significance of these lesions.

Intravascular ultrasound provides detailed anatomical information, allowing visualization of plaque burden, vessel dimensions, and lesion characteristics.[13] While IVUS can accurately quantify the extent of atherosclerotic plaque, it alone does not provide direct functional information about the impact of the lesion on blood flow.

In contrast, FFR is a pressure-derived index that measures the functional significance of coronary stenosis by assessing the pressure drop across the lesion during maximum hyperemia.[7] FFR values < 0.80 are commonly used as a threshold to define hemodynamically significant lesions, indicating that the stenosis is causing a significant reduction in blood flow.

Resource Availability and Cost Considerations

Fractional flow reserve is favored over IVUS due to its cost-effectiveness in guiding PCI procedures. Studies have shown that FFR-guided PCI leads to substantial cost savings, approximately 1.5–2 times compared to angiography-guided PCI, with FFR-guided procedures costing around $2,000–3,000 less per patient.[7,11] The lower cost of FFR, which involves a pressure wire and adenosine infusion, makes it a valuable option, providing essential functional information while being more financially accessible compared to IVUS, which requires specialized catheters and imaging equipment. However, it is crucial to consider the specific clinical needs and available resources when choosing between FFR and IVUS for individual patients.

CASE STUDIES AND REAL-WORLD APPLICATIONS

Intravascular ultrasound and FFR have proven to be indispensable tools in guiding PCI and optimizing patient outcomes. In a case involving left main CAD, IVUS was employed to conduct a precise assessment of the lesion, offering insights into plaque morphology and vessel dimensions. This information facilitated the selection and deployment of stents with utmost precision, resulting in a safe and successful procedure with minimized complications and favorable long-term results.[4]

In another scenario, a case of multivessel disease was managed using FFR-guided PCI. By assessing the functional significance of individual lesions, FFR enabled interventional cardiologists to make informed decisions regarding revascularization, ensuring that only hemodynamically significant lesions were targeted. This approach optimized resource utilization and led to improved patient outcomes while maintaining cost-effectiveness.[7]

Moreover, in a complex CTO intervention, a combined approach involving both IVUS and FFR was employed. IVUS provided detailed visualization for lesion assessment and facilitated guidewire crossing, while FFR measurements guided decision-making during the intervention. The integration of IVUS and FFR data contributed to the successful revascularization of the challenging CTO lesion, resulting in improved procedural outcomes.[9] **Table 4** shows the comparison of real-world applications of IVUS and FFR in interventional cardiology.

INTEGRATING PHYSIOLOGICAL ASSESSMENT WITH IMAGING MODALITIES (BEYOND FRACTIONAL FLOW RESERVE)

The assessment of coronary artery lesions involves a range of physiological and nonhyperemic indices, as well as hyperemic indices, to guide treatment decisions effectively. Current coronary invasive evaluation methods are generally distinguished by FFR, OCT, and IVUS. Angiography, which is a commonly observed benchmark in the field of anatomic imaging, is becoming the sole exception.[44] Hyperemic indices such as FFR remain fundamental, providing crucial information on the functional significance of lesions during maximal hyperemia.[7] Additionally, contrast-based FFR (cFFR) allows for noninvasive functional evaluation without the need for adenosine. Instantaneous wave-free ratio (iFR) offers a nonhyperemic alternative, assessing lesion significance during a specific phase of the cardiac cycle.[45,46] Among the nonhyperemic indices, resting full cycle ratio (RFR) and diastolic pressure ratio (DFR) provide valuable assessments at rest, aiding in identifying physiologically significant stenoses without inducing hyperemia.[47,48] Furthermore, quantitative flow ratio (QFR), a noninvasive computed tomography-based index, evaluates coronary stenosis by computing flow patterns, allowing for a nonhyperemic assessment of lesion severity.[49] Integrating these indices with advanced imaging modalities, such as IVUS and OCT, enhances lesion characterization and facilitates optimal treatment planning.[17] This multimodal approach enables a comprehensive evaluation of coronary lesions, leading to personalized treatment strategies and improved clinical outcomes for patients. **Table 5** summarizes the nonhyperemic indices for coronary lesion assessment.

TABLE 4: Real-world applications of intravascular ultrasound (IVUS) and fractional flow reserve (FFR) in interventional cardiology.

Application	IVUS	FFR
Coronary assessment[37]	Provides detailed cross-sectional images of coronary arteries, aiding in the visual assessment of plaque burden, morphology, and stenosis severity	Measures the pressure drop across coronary artery stenosis, assessing the functional significance of the lesion
Guidance during PCI[38]	Assists in guiding stent size selection, stent placement, and optimizing stent expansion to improve procedural outcomes	Helps in identifying hemodynamically significant stenoses that would benefit from PCI, avoiding unnecessary interventions
Assessing plaque stability[39]	Enables the visualization of plaque characteristics (e.g., fibrous, calcified, or lipid-rich plaques), aiding in identifying high-risk plaques prone to rupture	Identifies functionally significant stenoses that may lead to myocardial ischemia and guide revascularization decisions
Post-PCI assessment[40]	Allows assessment of stent apposition, expansion, and complications (e.g., edge dissections, malposition) post-PCI	Evaluates the functional result of PCI, ensuring that the procedure successfully improves blood flow to the myocardium
Bifurcation lesions[41]	Helps in evaluating complex bifurcation lesions, optimizing stent placement, and assessing the side branch compromise	Assists in determining if the side branch of a bifurcation lesion is functionally significant and requires treatment
Atherosclerosis research[42]	Used in research to study disease progression, regression, and the effects of various treatment strategies on plaque morphology	Facilitates research on the physiological significance of coronary stenoses, guiding the development of evidence-based treatment strategies
Assessment in ACS[43]	Provides insights into plaque characteristics in ACS and helps guide immediate treatment decisions	Assists in identifying culprit lesions responsible for ACS by determining the functional significance of coronary stenoses

(ACS: acute coronary syndromes; PCI: percutaneous coronary intervention)

TABLE 5: Nonhyperemic indices for coronary lesion assessment.

Index	Definition	Clinical application
RFR[47]	Ratio of mean distal coronary pressure to mean aortic pressure during diastole, measured at rest	Assessing lesion significance without the need for hyperemia *(Cutoff value: 0.89)*
DFR[48,50]	Ratio of distal coronary pressure to aortic pressure during diastole, measured at rest	Nonhyperemic assessment for identifying physiologically significant stenosis *(Cutoff value: 0.89)*
iFR[45,46]	Ratio of distal coronary pressure to aortic pressure during a specific period of the cardiac cycle without inducing hyperemia	Assessing lesion significance without adenosine-induced hyperemia *(Cutoff value: 0.89)*
QFR[49]	Noninvasive computed tomography (CT)-based index that evaluates coronary stenosis by computing flow patterns	Nonhyperemic assessment to determine the functional severity of coronary lesions *(Cutoff value: 0.80)*

(DFR: diastolic pressure ratio; iFR: instantaneous wave-free ratio; QFR: quantitative flow ratio; RFR: resting full cycle ratio)

TABLE 6: Intravascular ultrasound (IVUS) versus fractional flow reserve (FFR): Practical numbers to remember.[51]

Left main	MLA > 6 mm^2
Nonleft main	MLA ≥ 4 mm^2
Safe to defer stenting	MLA < 4 mm^2 ≠ FFR < 0.8
In the absence of FFR	
Proximal LAD correlates with FFR <0.8	MLA < 3 mm^2
LAD after the second diagonal	MLA < 2.75 mm^2
Non-LAD vessels may predict FFR <0.8	MLA < 2.4 mm^2
Transplant coronary vasculopathy	Intima thickness > 0.5 mm

LAD: left anterior descending; MLA: minimum lumen area)

CASE REPORTS—EXAMPLES

Case reports of borderline lesion in left circumflex (LCx) and LMCA shaft lesion are shown in **Figures 1 and 2**, respectively.

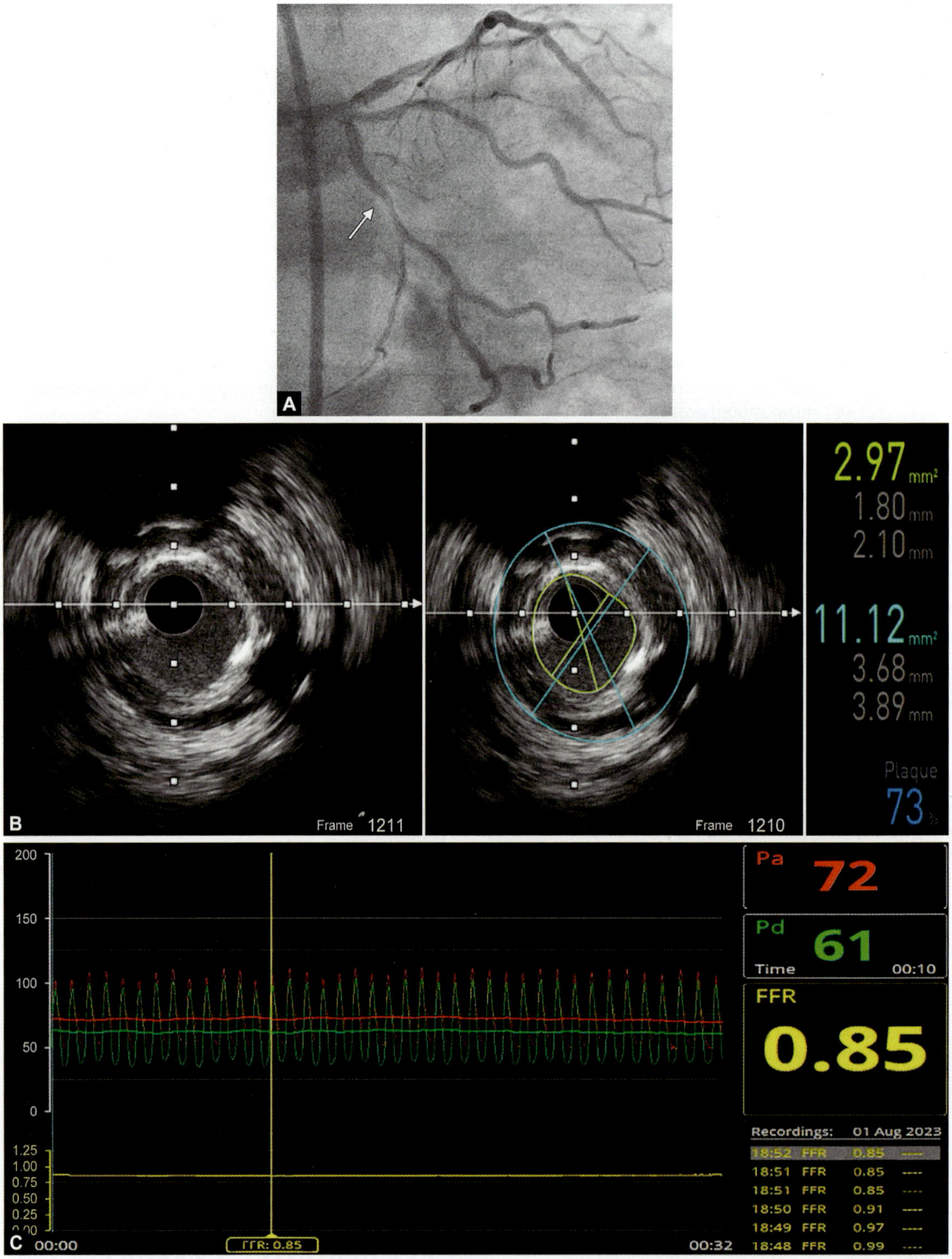

FIGS. 1A TO C: Case of PCI to LCx (IVUS vs. FFR): Borderline lesion in left circumflex (LCx). (A) Angiogram (approximately 70%); (B) Intravascular ultrasound (IVUS) images (plaque burden 73%); (C) fractional flow reserve (FFR) (nonsignificant). Final strategy: Medical management.

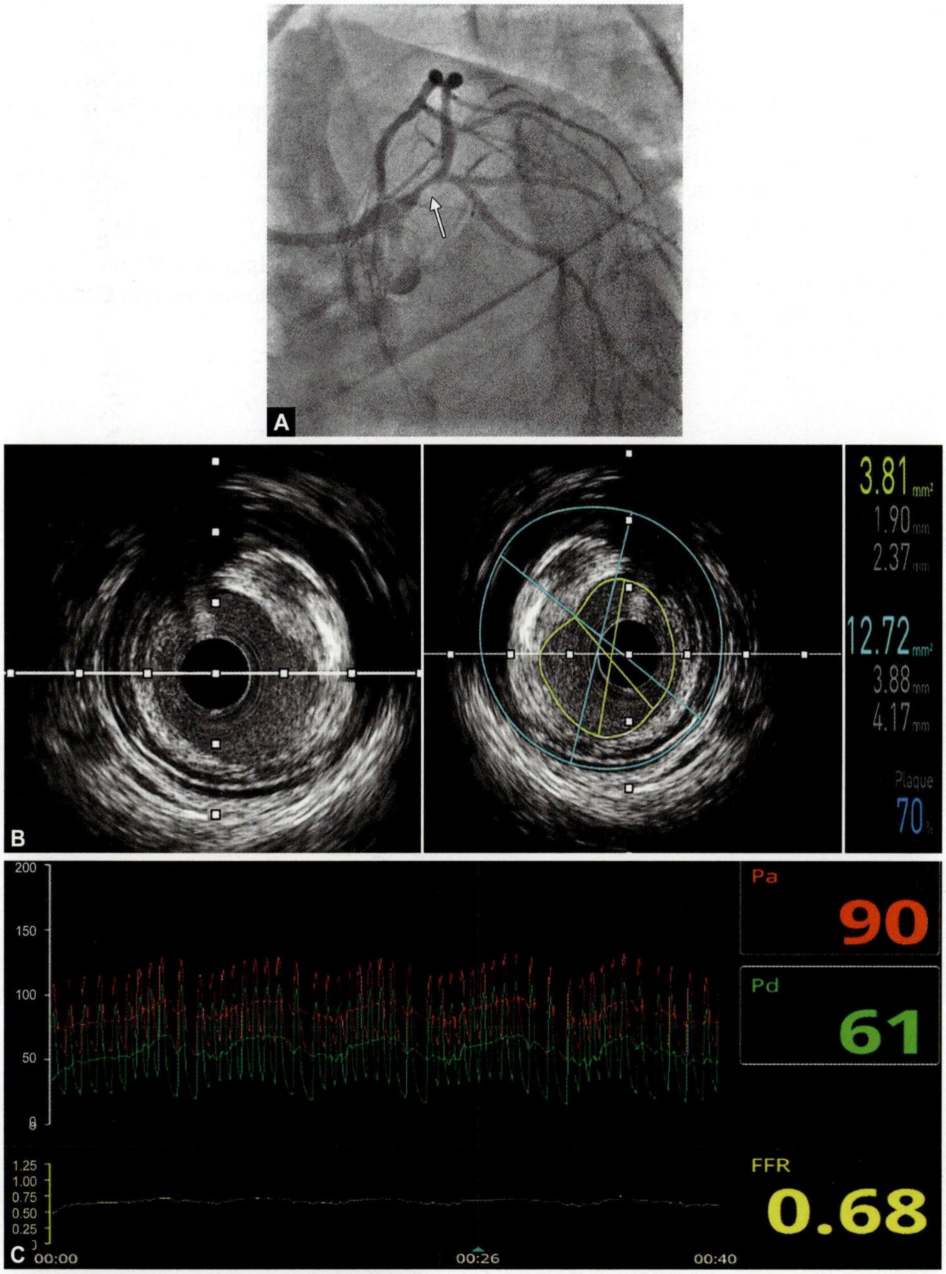

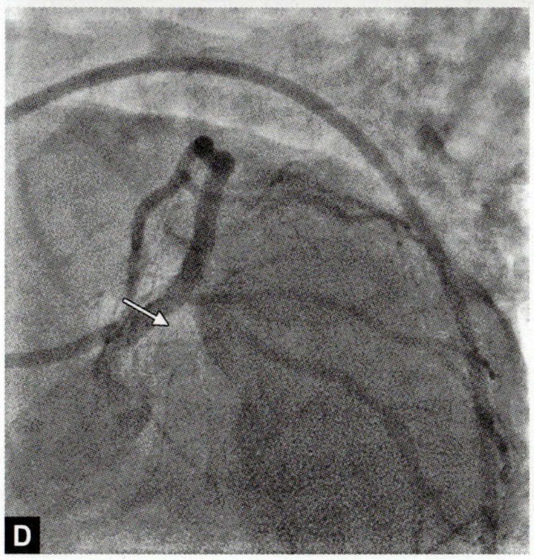

FIGS. 2A TO D: Case of PCI to LMCA (IVUS vs. FFR): Left main coronary artery (LMCA) shaft lesion. (A) Angiogram (approximately 70–80% lesion); (B) Intravascular ultrasound (IVUS) evaluation (significant plaque burden); (C) Fractional flow reserve (FFR) (significant values). Final strategy: LMCA stenting. (D) Poststenting results (single stent strategy).

CONCLUSION

The integration of IVUS and FFR has emerged as a powerful and transformative approach in the field of interventional cardiology. By combining high-resolution imaging with functional assessment, IVUS and FFR offer a comprehensive evaluation of CAD lesions, enabling precise lesion characterization, optimal stent sizing, and functional significance determination. This multimodal approach has been shown to enhance procedural success, improve patient outcomes, and reduce adverse events in PCI procedures. IVUS provides valuable anatomical insights, while FFR offers functional validation, guiding appropriate treatment decisions. The use of IVUS and FFR in complex cases, such as bifurcation lesions and CTO, further highlights their significance in managing challenging clinical scenarios. However, it is essential to consider practicality, resource availability, and operator expertise when implementing these technologies. Despite some challenges, the combined use of IVUS and FFR represents a promising paradigm in CAD management, ushering in an era of more personalized and effective care for patients undergoing PCI.

ONLINE REFERENCES

Please scan the QR code provided at the end of the table of contents for References of this chapter.

CHAPTER

168 Optical Coherence Tomography: What is New and What is the Future?

Mahesh Nalin Kumar, Ankush Gupta, Ashwin Mahesh, Abhinav Shrivastava

ABSTRACT

Intravascular imaging is becoming a crucial component of coronary intervention. In addition to the traditional longitudinal coronary artery angiography, intracoronary imaging employing intravascular ultrasound (IVUS) and optical coherence tomography (OCT) gives the interventionist simultaneous cross-sectional views of the coronary artery, provides a distinct advantage over IVUS in many imaging and procedural aspects due to its better resolution, accurate estimation of calcified lesion, and better stent failure evaluation and its three-dimensional (3D) reconstruction.

Keywords: Optical coherence tomography, intravascular imaging, stent optimization, stent failure, bifurcation, saline OCT.

INTRODUCTION

Optical coherence tomography (OCT) for stent optimization was upgraded to a class IIa recommendation in the most recent European Society of Cardiology (ESC)/European Association for Cardio-Thoracic Surgery (EACTS) guidelines, which is the same level of recommendation as intravascular ultrasound (IVUS).[1,2]

Both clinically and in significant studies conducted over a long period of time, OCT provides clear advantages over angiographic guidance **(Table 1)**. Studies have shown improved survival and reduced major adverse cardiovascular events (MACEs) in patients undergoing OCT-guided percutaneous coronary intervention (PCI) optimization compared with angiography only.[3,4] Following stent implantation and during PCI planning, OCT dramatically altered operator approach.[5-7] OCT-guided PCI optimization resulted in significantly higher post-PCI fractional flow reserve (FFR),[5,8] stent strut coverage,[9] and stent expansion.[6,10] OCT-guided PCI results in smaller minimum stent areas (MSAs) and stent expansions when compared to IVUS **(Table 2)**, despite having comparable rates of target vessel failure (TVF) and restenosis during a 12-month follow-up.[12] The stent sizing methodology changed due to this and moving from initial lumen sizes to reference external elastic lamina (EEL)-based sizes, resulting in MSA and stent expansion that are comparable to those of IVUS.[6,10,13] Phantom model tests revealed that IVUS underestimated the lumen area of the phantom model whereas OCT measured it on average to be equal to it.[14] Comparing OCT to IVUS, it was also discovered that OCT was more sensitive in stent edge dissection, inadequate stent apposition, intrastent tissue protrusion, and thrombus detection.[6,10,14]

PERCUTANEOUS CORONARY INTERVENTION OPTIMIZATION FOR OPTICAL COHERENCE TOMOGRAPHY

In addition to angiography, intracoronary OCT offers a better delineation of the artery wall and lumen and morphology of the plaque. To determine the appropriate stent size, lesion length and coronary diameter can be precisely determined using EEL. Stent apposition, stent expansion, substantial edge dissection, geographical miss, and plaque prolapse are all evaluated as part of post-PCI optimization **(Flowchart 1)**.

TABLE 1: The studies done for comparison between optical coherence tomography (OCT) and angiography for percutaneous coronary intervention (PCI) optimization.

Study/Journal/ Year/Design	Sample size	Primary end point	Result	Conclusion
CLI-OPCI EuroIntervention 2012 Retrospective, multicenter	• $n = 670$ • 335 in the OCT group • 335 in the angio group	1-year rate of cardiac death or MI	OCT group versus angio group: • Cardiac death (1.2% vs. 4.5%, $p = 0.010$) • Cardiac death or MI (6.6% vs. 13.0%, $p = 0.006$) • Composite of cardiac death, MI, or repeat revascularization (9.6% vs. 14.8%, $p = 0.044$) • Post-PCI OCT in the OCT group revealed adverse features requiring further interventions in 34.7% patients (one-third)	OCT-guided optimization can improve clinical outcomes of patients undergoing PCI
CLI-OPCI II (JACC Cardiovasc Imaging) 2015 Retrospective analysis, multicenter	1,002 lesions (832 patients)	• 1-year MACE [composite of all-cause mortality, MI, and target lesion revascularization (TLR)] • Association of suboptimal stent deployment as assessed by offline OCT with MACE at 1 year	Suboptimal stent deployment required the presence of at least one of the OCT findings: • *Edge dissection*: Presence of a linear rim of tissue with clear separation and a width >200 mm (<5 mm) to a stent edge • *Malapposition*: Stent-adjacent vessel lumen distance >200 mm • In-stent minimum lumen area (MLA) < 4.5 mm^2 • In-stent MLA <70% of the average reference lumen area • Intrastent plaque/thrombus protrusion >500 mm in thickness Suboptimal stent seen in 31.0% patients Independent predictors of MACE In-stent MLA < 4.5 mm^2 (p - 0.040), dissection >200 mm at the distal stent edge (p - 0.004), and reference lumen area <4.5 mm^2 at either distal ($p < 0.001$) or proximal ($p < 0.001$) stent edges	• Suboptimal stent deployment was associated with an increased risk of MACE • Presence of at least one significant criterion for suboptimal OCT stent deployment was confirmed as an independent predictor of MACE (HR 3.53, $p < 0.001$) • MACE group had significantly more findings of suboptimal stent deployment (59.2% vs. 26.9%; $p < 0.001$)
OCTACS study Circulation: Cardiovascular interventions 2015 RCT, single center	• 100 patients 1:1 • OCT-guided versus angio-guided Nobori biolimus-eluting DES implantation	Difference in percentage of uncovered struts in the OCT-guided versus the angio-guided group at 6-months	OCT-guided PCI resulted in a lower proportion of uncovered struts (4.3% vs. 9.0%, $p < 0.01$) and more number of completely covered stents (17.5% vs. 2.2%, $p = 0.02$)	OCT-guided optimization of DES improves strut coverage in comparison with angiographic guidance alone

Continued

Continued

Study/Journal/ Year/Design	Sample size	Primary end point	Result	Conclusion
ILUMIEN I European Heart Journal 2015 Prospective, nonrandomized, observational	418 patients (467 stenosis)	• Impact of OCT on physician decision-making • MACE at 30 days (cardiac death, MI, and TLR)	*Pre-PCI–OCT:* • Altered strategy in 55% of patients (57% stenosis) • Selecting different stent lengths (shorter in 25%, longer in 43%) *Post-PCI OCT:* • Unsatisfactory result in 25% of patients (27% stenosis) • 14.5% malapposition • 7.6% underexpansion • 2.7% edge dissection	• Decision-making was affected by OCT imaging prior to PCI in 55% and post-PCI in 25% patients • MACE events at 30 days were low: death 0.25%, MI 7.7%, repeat PCI 1.7%, and stent thrombosis 0.25%
DOCTORS Circulation 2016 RCT, multicenter	• $n = 240$ (NSTEMI–ACS) • 120 in the OCT group • 120 in the angio group	FFR post-PCI	• Significantly higher FFR in OCT group (0.94 ± 0.04 vs. 0.92 ± 0.05, $p = 0.005$) compared to angiographic-guided group • OCT led to altered procedural strategy in 55% patients *Post-PCI OCT revealed:* • Stent underexpansion 42% • Stent malapposition 32% • Incomplete lesion coverage in 20% • Edge dissection in 37.5% Led to the more frequent use of poststent dilation in the OCT-guided group versus the angiography-guided group (43% vs. 12.5%, $p < 0.0001$) with lower residual stenosis (7.0% vs. 8.7%, $p = 0.01$)	• OCT-guided PCI is associated with higher post-procedure FFR • There is no significant difference in the rate of procedural MI or complications
ILUMIEN III Lancet 2016 RCT, multicenter	• $n = 450$ • 158 (35%) in OCT • 146 (32%) in IVUS • 146 (32%) angiographic guidance • *Exclusion*: LM or ostial RCA, bypass graft stenosis, CTO, planned two-stent bifurcations, and ISR	• Post-PCI MSA as assessed by OCT Tested noninferiority of OCT guidance to IVUS guidance Superiority of OCT guidance to angiography guidance • Superiority of OCT guidance to IVUS guidance	• Final median MSA was 5.79 mm^2 with OCT and 5.49 mm^2 with angiography guidance. OCT guidance was not superior to angiography guidance ($p = 0.12$) • Minimum and mean stent expansion was significantly improved by OCT (87.6% and 105.8%) as compared with angiography (82.9%, $p = 0.02$ and 101.4%, $p = 0.001$ respectively) • Untreated major dissections at end of procedure and major malapposition were significantly less in OCT-guided group (28% and 11%) compared with angiography group (44%, $p = 0.006$ and 31%, $p < 0.0001$)	• OCT-guided stent placement was not superior to angiography-guided stent placement in terms of MSA • Minimum and mean stent expansions were significantly greater while untreated major dissections and major malapposition were significantly less in OCT than with angiography-guided PCI

Continued

Continued

Study/Journal/ Year/Design	Sample size	Primary end point	Result	Conclusion
LONDON PCI COHORT JACC: Cardiovascular interventions 2018 Registry (observational)	OCT in 1,149 (1.3%) patients, IVUS in 10,971 (12.6%) patients angiography alone in 75,046 patients	All-cause mortality at a median of 4.8 years	OCT-guided PCI was associated with significantly reduced mortality rates when compared with angiography alone (9.60% vs. 16.80%; $p < 0.0001$)	OCT-guided PCI was associated with improved MACE and long-term survival compared with angiography-guided PCI
iSIGHT Circulation: Cardiovascular interventions 2021 RCT	• $n = 156$ lesions • OCT [51 lesions (32.7%)] • IVUS [52 lesions (33.3%)] angiography [53 lesions (34.0%)]	Stent expansion (MSA ≥ 90% of the average reference lumen area)	Stent expansion with OCT guidance (98.01 ± 16.14%) was superior to angiography (90.53 ± 14.84%, $p = 0.041$)	Stent expansion with OCT guidance was superior to an optimized angiographic strategy

(ACS: acute coronary syndrome; CTO: chronic total occlusion; DES: drug-eluting stent; DOCTORS: Does Optical Coherence Tomography Optimize Results of Stenting; FFR: fractional flow reserve; HR: hazard ratio; ISR: in-stent restenosis; IVUS: intravascular ultrasound; LM: left main; MACE: major adverse cardiovascular event; MI: myocardial infarction; MSA: minimum stent area; NSTEMI: non-ST-segment elevation myocardial infarction; RCA: right coronary artery; RCT: randomized controlled trial)

TABLE 2: The studies done for comparison between optical coherence tomography (OCT) and intravascular ultrasound (IVUS) for percutaneous coronary intervention (IVUS) optimization.

Study/Journal/ Year/Design	Sample size	Primary endpoint	Stent sizing criteria in OCT guidance	Result	Conclusion
Habara et al.[11] Circulation: Cardiovascular interventions 2012 RCT, single center	• $n = 70$ • OCT group $n = 35$, IVUS group $n = 35$	Stent expansion analyzed by IVUS	Lumen diameter	• Focal and diffuse stent expansion were smaller (64.7% vs. 80.3%, 84.2% vs. 98.8%, $p < 0.05$, respectively) in OCT versus IVUS group • Minimum and mean stent area was smaller (6.1 vs. 7.1 mm^2 and 7.5 ± 2.5 vs. 8.7 ± 2.4 mm) under OCT versus IVUS	OCT guidance for stent implantation was associated with smaller stent expansion compared with conventional IVUS guidance
OPUS-CLASS JACC: Cardiovascular Imaging 2013 Prospective, multicenter	$n = 100$ Angiography performed in all Followed by OCT and IVUS in: • Pre-PCI—20 • Pre- and post-PCI—60 • Post-PCI follow-up—20	Comparison of lumen dimensions measurement with OCT versus IVUS versus angiography (QCA) in patient and in phantom model	Lumen diameter	• Mean minimum lumen diameter measured by QCA was significantly smaller than that measured by FD-OCT (1.81 vs. 1.91 mm; $p < 0.001$) • The minimum lumen area measured by IVUS was significantly greater than that by FD-OCT (3.68 mm^2 vs. 3.27 mm^2; $p < 0.001$) • In a phantom model, the mean lumen area according to OCT was equal to the actual lumen area of the phantom model; IVUS overestimated the lumen area	• OCT provided accurate measurements of coronary lumen with excellent intraobserver reproducibility • OCT is much more sensitive in detecting intrastent tissue protrusion, incomplete stent apposition, stent edge dissection, and intrastent thrombus compared with IVUS
ILUMIEN II JACC: Cardiovascular interventions 2015 Post-hoc analysis of two prospective studies	OCT-guided stenting in patients in the ILUMIEN I, $n = 354$ versus IVUS-guided stenting in the ADAPT-DES, $n = 586$	Post-PCI stent expansion (%) defined as the MSA divided by the mean reference lumen area	Lumen diameter	Degree of stent expansion was not significantly different between OCT and IVUS guidance 72.8% versus 70.6% respectively, p - 0.29	OCT and IVUS guidance resulted in a comparable degree of stent expansion

Continued

Continued

Study/Journal/ Year/Design	Sample size	Primary end point	Stent sizing criteria in OCT guidance	Result	Conclusion
OPINION European Heart Journal 2017 RCT, multicenter, noninferiority trial	• $n = 829$ • OCT-guided PCI, $n = 414$ • IVUS-guided PCI, $n = 415$	Target vessel failure (TVF) defined as a composite of cardiac death, MI, and ischemia-driven target vessel revascularization until 12 months after the PCI	Lumen diameter	• TVF occurred in 21 (5.2%) undergoing OCT-guided PCI and 19 (4.9%) undergoing IVUS-guided PCI (noninferiority = 0.042) • Rate of binary restenosis was comparable between OCT-guided PCI and IVUS-guided PCI (in-stent: 1.6% vs. 1.6%, $p = 1.00$; and in-segment: 6.2% vs. 6.0%, $p = 1.00$)	• OCT-guided PCI was noninferior to that of patients undergoing IVUS-guided PCI • Stent sizes were smaller in the OCT arm compared with the IVUS arm (2.92 vs. 2.99 mm; $p = 0.005$)
ILUMIEN III Lancet 2016 RCT, multicenter	• $n = 450$ • 158 (35%) in OCT • 146 (32%) in IVUS • 146 (32%) angiographic guidance	Post-PCI MSA as assessed by OCT	Proximal or distal normal segment EEL diameter (whichever is lesser) rounded down to the nearest 0.25 mm	• Final median MSA was 5.79 mm^2 with OCT and 5.89 mm^2 with IVUS guidance • OCT guidance was noninferior to IVUS guidance ($p = 0.001$), but not superior ($p = 0.42$) • Untreated dissections and major malapposition were significantly less frequent in OCT group compared with IVUS group	OCT-guided PCI using reference segment EEL-based stent optimization strategy was safe and resulted in similar MSA to that of IVUS-guided PCI
MISTIC-1 Circulation: Cardiovascular Interventions 2020 RCT, multicenter, noninferiority trial	• $n = 109$ • OCT—54 patients with 62 lesions • IVUS—55 patients with 64 lesions	In-segment MLA assessed using OCT at the 8-month follow-up	Lumen up-size for OCT guidance (10% or 0.25 mm larger than mean lumen diameter at reference sites)	• Postprocedural minimum stent area was 6.31 mm^2 and 6.72 ± 2.08 mm^2 in OCT and IVUS group, respectively ($p = 0.26$) • 8-month follow-up, in-segment MLA was 4.56 mm^2 and 4.13 mm^2 in OCT and IVUS group, respectively (noninferiority <0.001)	• OCT-guided PCI was not inferior to IVUS-guided PCI in terms of in-segment MLA at 8 months • Clinical outcomes at 3 years follow-up did not differ between the two groups
iSIGHT Circulation: Cardiovascular Interventions 2021 RCT	• $n = 156$ lesions • OCT [51 lesions (32.7%)] • IVUS [52 lesions (33.3%)] angiography [53 lesions (34.0%)]	Stent expansion (MSA ≥ 90% of the average reference lumen area)	• When EEL was visible in ≥180° of the vessel circumference, the reference was sized to the mean EEL diameter • Otherwise, the largest lumen diameter was used	Stent expansion with OCT guidance (98.01 ± 16.14%) was noninferior to IVUS (91.69 ± 15.75%, noninferiority <0.001)	Stent expansion with OCT guidance using a dedicated EEL-based sizing strategy was noninferior to that achieved with IVUS

(EEL: external elastic lamina; FD: frequency domain; MSA: minimum stent area; RCT: randomized controlled trial)

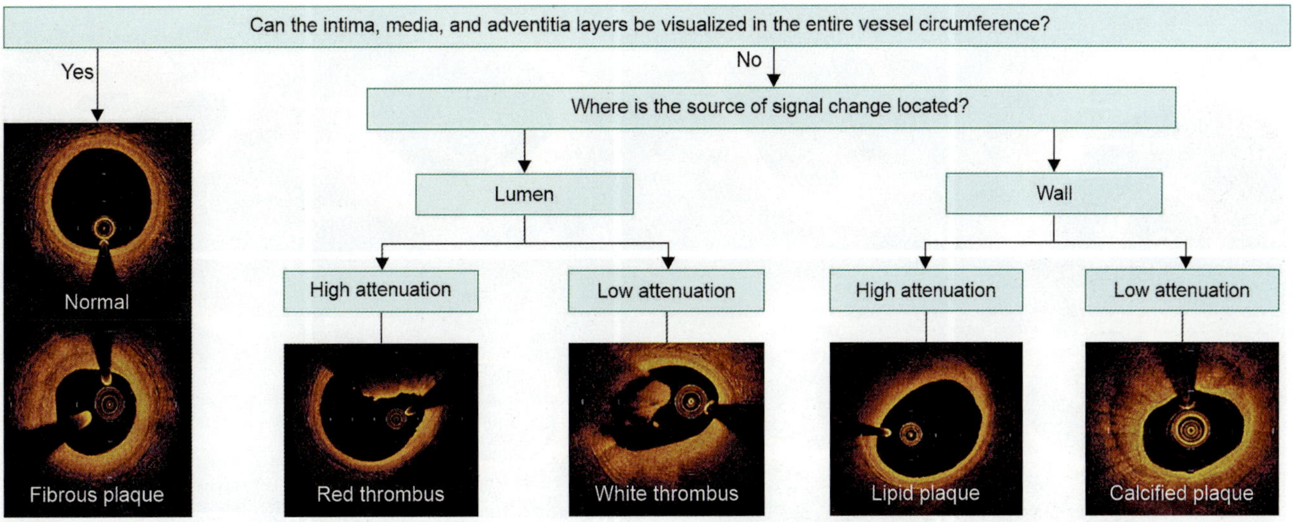

FLOWCHART 1: Algorithmic approach to optical coherence tomography image interpretation of common morphologies.[11]

PRE-PERCUTANEOUS CORONARY INTERVENTION EVALUATION (FIGS. 1A TO L)

Plaque Modification According to Morphology

- *Lipid-rich plaque (LRP)*: Fibroatheromas are lesions mostly made up of a necrotic lipid core with a fibrous top. The covering cap's risk of rupture depends on its thickness, and pathologic data have shown that thin-cap fibroatheroma (TCFA) with a thickness of <65 µm is particularly vulnerable to rupture. Significant stenoses caused mostly by LRPs and TCFAs **(Figs. 1B and G)** can be treated without predilatation by direct stenting.
- *Fibrotic plaque*: On OCT, fibrotic plaques feature a homogenous backscatter that is rich in signal because they are often rich in collagen or smooth muscle cells **(Fig. 1C)**. Fiber-rich plaques are mostly characterized as stable plaques, and the risk of rupture is inversely correlated with the degree of internal lipid accumulation.
- *Vulnerable plaques*: On OCT, the most vulnerable plaques can be identified by their substantial lipid cores (lipid in at least two quadrants of any picture), which are surrounded by a thin fibrous cap (<65 µm).[15] Multiple punctate signal-rich patches near the fibrous cap are a marker of TCFA-induced stenosis and a plaque's enhanced susceptibility to inflammation, i.e., macrophage infiltration **(Fig. 1L)**.[16-18] A high-risk vulnerable plaque was defined by the CLIMA study in 2019[19] as meeting four criteria: (1) a minimum lumen area (MLA) of 3.5 mm^2 or less; (2) a fibrous cap thickness of no >75 µm; (3) a lipid core with a lipid arc extension of >180°; and (4) the presence of macrophage clusters within the plaque. Even in intermediate lesions with a negative FFR have seen unfavorable outcomes in diabetic patients with TCFAs.[20]
- *Calcified lesion*: The most frequent cause of under-expanded stents (UESs), which leads to both acute and chronic stent failure, is calcified lesions that result in severe stenosis. For imaging of calcified lesions, OCT is clearly superior to IVUS. **Figures 1D to F** classify calcium deposition in a lesion into superficial, deep, and nodular calcium. The likelihood of stent underexpansion in calcified lesions has been established and verified using an OCT-based calcium score.[21] Maximum thickness >0.5 mm (1 point), contiguous length of calcium >5 mm (1 point), and maximum arc >50% or >180° (2 points) make up this "rule of 5s" score. When the score was below 3, the stent expanded as expected; however, when the score was higher than 4, calcium alteration during lesion creation was required **(Figs. 2A to E)**. The goal of modification should be calcium fracture, which is easily visible in OCT.[22]

Estimation of Lesion Length

The OCT pullback's L-mode view, which makes use of the pullback speed and frame rate for calculations, is used to determine the length. The proximal and distal stent landing zones are chosen as the normal-appearing segments within 5 mm of the stenotic lesion in the L-mode image. Segments exhibiting OCT markers of stable plaque-like thick fibrous cap atheroma and calcified plaque are chosen as landing zones in the case of diffusely diseased coronaries.

Estimating the Diameter

For stent sizing, EEL-based measurements at the distal landing zone should be used. The mean of two distinct diameter measurements obtained at least one quadrant

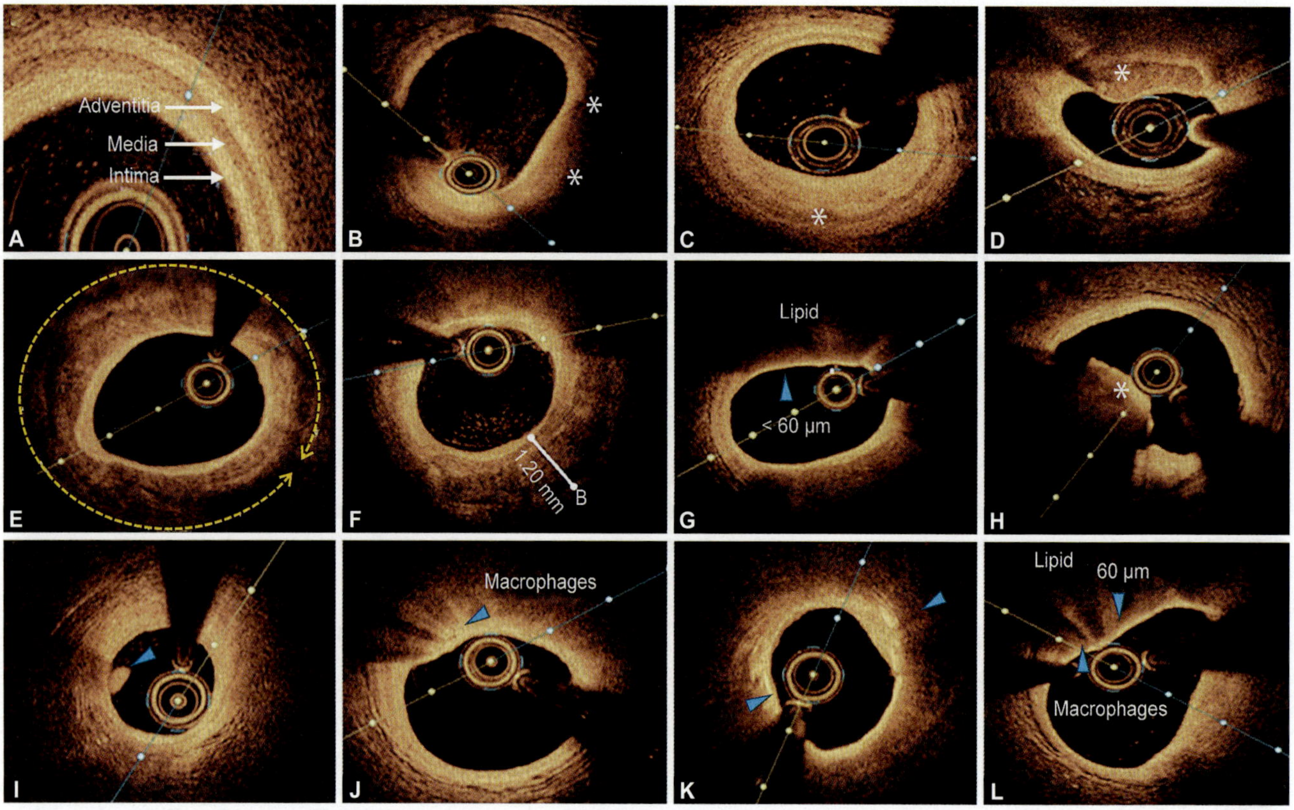

FIGS. 1A TO L: Representative optical coherence tomography (OCT) images with various plaque morphologies. (A) Normal coronary; (B) Lipid-rich plaque (LRP); (C) Fibrotic plaque; (D) Calcific nodule; (E) Near 360° arc of calcific plaque; (F) Deep calcium deposition; (G) Thin-cap fibroatheroma (TCFA); (H) Intraluminal red thrombus; (I) Intraluminal white thrombus; (J) Bright spots or bands at the boundary between the fibrous cap and lipid core suggestive of macrophages; (K) Bright signal-rich cholesterol crystals; and (L) Vulnerable plaque formed by a large lipid pool covered by TCFA with macrophage infiltration; areas of interest were highlighted by arrows and asterisks.

apart should be rounded down by 0.25 mm to the available stent size.[6] The mean lumen diameter is used for stent sizing and should be rounded up between 0.25 and 0.5 mm to calculate the stent size[12] if the EEL is not sufficiently visualized.

Functional Assessment

Another choice that cardiologists must make is whether to perform PCI on an intermediate lesion. OCT can be used to evaluate coronary lesions functionally, since it can characterize them precisely in a 3D image. There are very few direct comparisons between FFR and OCT for the functional assessment of an intermediate lesion, even though FFROCT (computational FFR using the OCT data) demonstrated good correlation and agreement with invasively recorded FFR ($r = 0.72$, p 0.001),[23] head-to-head comparisons between FFR and OCT for functional assessment of an intermediate lesion are very limited. The FORZA (Fractional Flow Reserve vs. Optical Coherence Tomography to Guide Revascularization of Intermediate Coronary Stenoses) trial[24] evaluated FFR and OCT guidance. If at least one of the following conditions was met, PCI was carried out in an intermediate lesion under OCT guidance: (1) area stenosis (AS) > 75%; (2) AS between 50 and 75% with MLA 2.5 mm^2; or (3) AS between 50 and 75% and plaque rupture. PCI was carried out in the FFR arm when the lesion was <0.80 on FFR. The study's 13-month follow-up revealed that OCT was safe but increased the need for PCI operations. After 13 months, it was connected to a decreased incidence of the combined outcome of MACE or severe angina, nevertheless. FFR led to more cautious patient management, which was related with lower costs, but it also had a greater incidence of revascularizations.

Optical Coherence Tomography and Stent Deployment

Optical coherence tomography angiography co-registration (ACR) capability helps in identifying stent edge landing zones and thus eliminating ambiguity in visually selecting "normal-appearing" reference segments on angiography. It offers a visual link between the real-time coronary angiography and the OCT pictures, which can be used for planning and executing the plan, respectively. Major edge

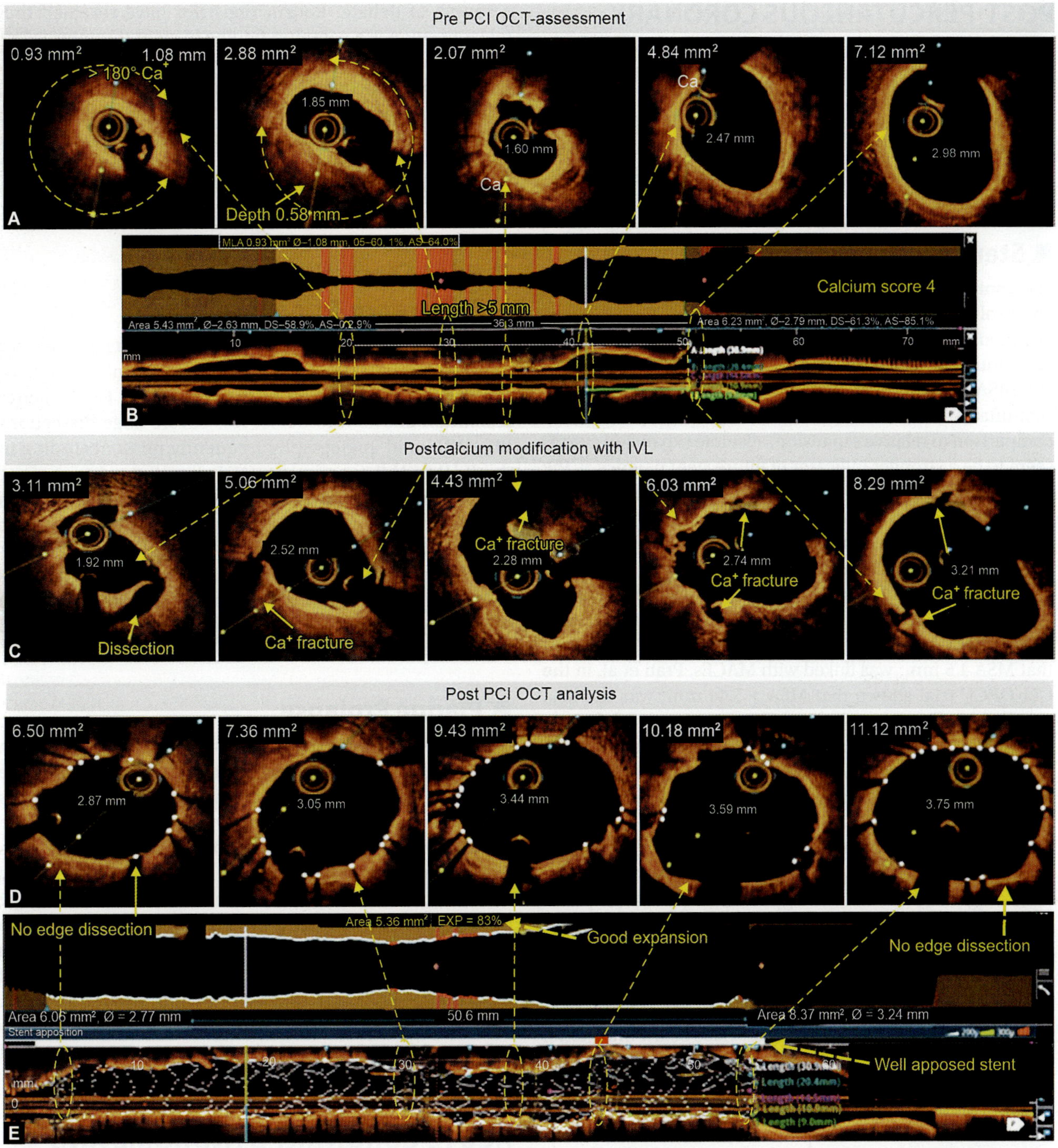

FIGS. 2A TO E: Optical coherence tomography (OCT)-guided management of calcified left anterior descending (LAD). (A and B) Pre-percutaneous coronary intervention (PCI) assessment showed a heavily calcified LAD with a calcium arc >180°, a calcium thickness of 0.58 mm, and a length of >5 mm resulting in a calcium score of 4. (C) Fractures in the calcium after modification with intravascular lithotripsy (IVL); (D and E) Post-PCI assessment showed 83% stent expansion, no edge dissection, and a well-apposed stent.

dissection and/or geographical miss were substantially less common in ACR-guided PCI than in OCT-guided PCI without ACR, according to Schneider et al.[25] study [(4.2% vs. 19.1%), $p = 0.03$]. According to Koyama et al.[26] there was a tendency for less major distal stent edge dissections when ACR was used (11.1% vs. 20.8%, $p = 0.07$).There was a tendency for less major distal stent edge dissections when ACR was used (11.1% vs. 20.8%, $p = 0.07$).

POST-PERCUTANEOUS CORONARY INTERVENTION OPTICAL COHERENCE TOMOGRAPHY

The estimation of stent expansion, stent apposition, substantial edge dissection, plaque prolapse, and geographic miss are all included in OCT-guided post-PCI stent optimization.

Stent Expansion

The minimal stent cross-sectional area is calculated as either an absolute value (absolute expansion) or as a percentage of a predetermined lumen area, such as the proximal, distal, maximum, or average lumen area (relative expansion). The MSA is frequently divided by the mean luminal cross-sectional area to determine relative stent expansion. In comparison to relative expansion, absolute expansion cutoffs seem to be a stronger indicator of future stent patency.[27] The best and most reliable parameter to predict both restenosis and stent thrombosis has been post-PCI MSA.[28] According to Soeda et al.[29] with an MSA cutoff value of 5.0 mm^2 for drug-eluting stent (DES), OCT-MSA was a reliable predictor of clinical outcomes and target lesion revascularization (TLR). Although the DOCTORS (Does Optical Coherence Tomography Optimize Results of Stenting) trial[8] determined that MSA 4.5 mm^2 was linked with MACEs, Prati et al. in the CLI-OPCI[3] trial shown that MSA > 5.44 mm^2 was the best cutoff to predict postprocedural FFR > 0.90 in non-left main (LM) arteries. On OCT, UES is identified when the MSA is <4.5 mm^2 and/or 80% of the mean lumen area **(Figs. 3A and B)**.[27] Greater absolute stent expansion has been linked to better long-term stent patency, better clinical outcomes, and a decreased chance of stent failure.[28,30-34] In addition to diagnosis, OCT also guides the management of UES by providing insights into etiology, such as poorly prepared calcified bed **(Figs. 3B to D)**.[34]

Stent Malapposition

Stent malapposition is defined by a lack of contact between at least one stent strut and the intimal surface below the arterial wall in a segment not above the side branch (SB) **(Figs. 3E and G)**. It may be either acute (found at the time of stenting) or late (found during a later follow-up). It is a frequent discovery during post-PCI optimization, detected in 15% of stents by IVUS imaging[35] and at a higher rate of 50% by OCT imaging,[36] possibly due to superior spatial resolution. In the generated stent image, OCT automatically identifies apposed **(Fig. 3F)** and malapposed stent struts and highlights them in white and red, respectively. In the apposition indicator in L mode, this can also be seen as a red bar **(Fig. 3E)**. Due to the lack of a definitive connection between acute malapposition and stent failure in some prospective studies.[37-39] The effect of acute stent malapposition on stent failure rates [i.e., in-stent restenosis (ISR) and stent thrombosis] has been a source of debate. Recent registries have revealed that malapposition is a common finding in stent thrombosis.[40,41] Small malapposition may therefore be less important. Because spontaneous neointimal integration is anticipated, acute malapposition of 400 mm with longitudinal extension of 1 mm should not be addressed, according to EAPCI (European Association of Percutaneous Cardiovascular Interventions) investigators, in the absence of prospective validation.[27]

Edge Dissection in Optical Coherence Tomography

When a stent is deployed in a coronary artery, it is possible for the vessel wall next to the struts to rupture unintentionally, leading to the dissection of the stent edge. OCT's better resolution allows it to detect less severe edge dissections that IVUS and angiography frequently miss. According to the ILUMIEN-3 experiment, OCT detected twice as many dissections as IVUS did. The incidence of edge dissection revealed by OCT ranged as high as 37.8% overall, and the majority (84%) were not visible on angiography.[42] Poor outcomes have been linked to major stent edge dissections **(Figs. 3H to J)**, which are characterized by their depth (disrupting at least the medial layer), lateral extension (>60°), and length (>2 mm).

Plaque Prolapse

In comparison to IVUS, OCT's superior axial resolution allows for crisper and more frequent visualization of tissue prolapse **(Fig. 3K)**. Plaque rupture, intracoronary thrombus development, and TCFA frequency all increase in proportion to the size of the prolapse. Plaque prolapse is associated with worse short-term prognoses after PCI and has been found to be a predictor of early stent thrombosis.[43,44] According to their intensity, the three types of plaque prolapse are smooth protrusion, disrupted fibrous tissue protrusion, and irregular protrusion. Irregular protrusion has a high risk of medial disruption and lipid core penetration. It has been demonstrated that irregular protrusions, predominantly influenced by TLR, are an independent predictor of clinical outcomes at 1 year.

ACUTE CORONARY SYNDROME AND OPTICAL COHERENCE TOMOGRAPHY

Optical coherence tomography can help overcome some of the difficulties seen during PCI in a patient with acute coronary syndrome (ACS). Approximately 4–10% of ST-segment elevation myocardial infarction (STEMI) patients, >30% of NSTEMI patients, and >10% of patients may have several culprit lesions on angiography present without a clear culprit lesion. Plaque rupture and erosion are the two most frequent causes of ACS, but calcified nodules, spontaneous

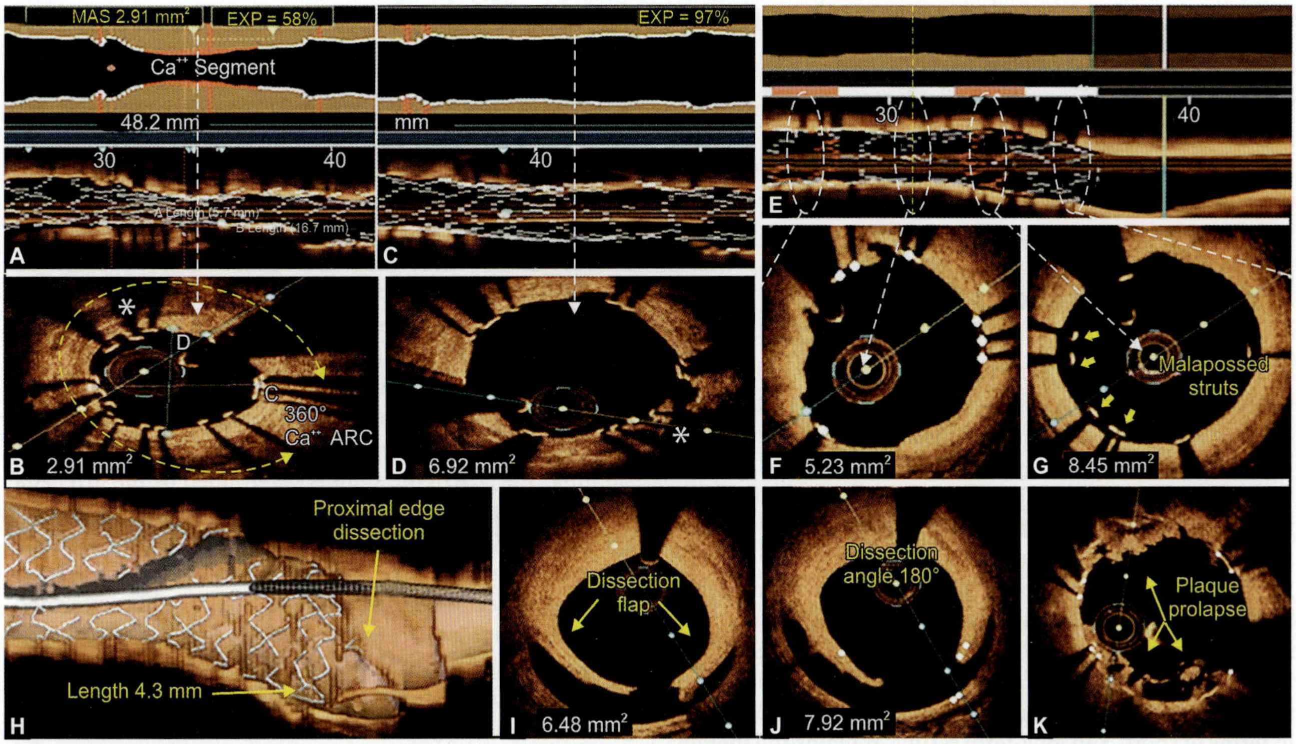

FIGS. 3A TO K: Post-percutaneous coronary intervention (PCI) assessment by optical coherence tomography (OCT). (A) Lumenogram and L mode showed under-expanded stent (UES) with minimum stent area (MSA) of 2.91 mm^2 and 58% stent expansion. (B) Cross-sectional image at MSA revealed 360° arc of calcium as a cause of UES. (C) Lumenogram and L mode showed 97% stent expansion after the treatment of UES with ultra-high-pressure balloon dilatation. (D) A cross-sectional image shows the fracture of the calcium arc resulting in the resolution of the UES. (E) A rendered stent view shows well-apposed stent struts (white) and malapposed stent struts (red) corresponding to the white and red bars in the apposition indicator. Apposition (F) and mal-apposition (G) of the stent struts can also be well-appreciated on respective cross-sectional images. (H to J) Major proximal stent edge dissection is seen with the dissection flap extending to media, dissection angle of 180° and 4.3 mm dissection length on three-dimensional (3D) reconstruction. OCT with its better axial resolution enables clearer and more frequent visualization of in-stent tissue prolapse (K).

dissection, and stent thrombosis are less frequent causes. OCT has a definite advantage over IVUS in detecting these pathogenic mechanisms of ACS because of its better resolution. It is easier to see the ruptured plaque with OCT because it has a discontinuity in the fibrous cap that covers a lipid-rich core. In contrast to erosion, which is more frequent in individuals with NSTEMI, or calcified nodules, which are only seen in NSTEMI, plaque rupture is the more frequent cause of ACS in STEMIs.

Plaque erosion on OCT is defined as the absence of fibrous cap disruption by Jia et al.[45] and is further divided into two categories: (1) definite OCT erosion, which is the presence of attached white thrombus overlying an intact and visible plaque, and (2) probable OCT erosion, which is either (i) luminal surface irregularity at the lesion site in the absence of thrombus or (ii), the attenuation of underlying plaque by thrombus. Patients with plaque erosion typically present with NSTEMI. Plaque erosion, on the other hand, appears to lead to a bigger residual lumen, the maintenance of vascular integrity, and a lower thrombus burden. Therefore, stent implantation can be avoided if plaque erosion is managed with vigorous antithrombotic therapy, minimizing both early and late problems related to stents. According to the erosion research,[46] in 7–10% of ACS patients, calcified lesions with fibrous cap disruption and no lipid core rupture are seen.

Spontaneous Dissection

A uncommon occurrence that can result in an ACS is spontaneous coronary artery dissection (SCAD). OCT is very helpful in making the diagnosis because it makes it simple to observe the multiple lumen morphology in the vessel wall that is typical of this disorder. However, there are dangers involved in conducting an OCT in SCAD. OCT can cause the dissection to spread and worsen the problem because it entails injecting contrast into the coronary stream. As a result, dye injection should be done with extreme caution and at modest flow rates. When an angiographic diagnosis is questionable, intravascular imaging can be helpful, according to a recent ESC/Acute Cardiac Care Association (ACCA) position paper on SCAD.[47]

OPTICAL COHERENCE TOMOGRAPHY FOR STENT FAILURE

The investigation of choice in the evaluation of stent failure is OCT. The main reasons for stent failure include scaffold thrombosis, ISR, and stent thrombosis. OCT pictures help in the selection of a suitable management approach by offering insights into the mechanism of stent failure.

In-stent Restenosis

The best method to study arterial healing following stenting is OCT. ISR is the most prevalent reason for stent failure. The etiology of an ISR, such as underexpansion, malapposition, or strut fracture, can be identified by OCT. Neointimal hyperplasia (NIH) or neo-atherosclerosis may also be used to describe ISR. NIH connected to bare-metal stent (BMS) is homogenous, compared to NIH connected to DES, which is more heterogeneous. As a cause of ISR, neo-atherosclerotic hyperplasia is characterized by lipid and/or calcium accumulation, a necrotic core, and even macrophage infiltration. In rare circumstances, it can be challenging to tell a DES-related ISR from TCFA lesions in native plaques. The implantation of DES proven to be superior than drug-eluting balloon (DEB) in terms of short- and long-term results, remains the therapy of choice for ISR.[48,49] The DES implantation's inclusion of a second metallic layer may also be unwelcome in some patients, by recent bioresorbable vascular scaffold (BVS). To maximize the acute luminal benefit without adding an additional permanent layer of metal, BVS offers a transient vascular scaffolding. For BVS implantation and to examine tissue coverage in a follow-up, OCT is preferred over IVUS. A 3-year follow-up intracoronary OCT examination showed that the scaffold was completely covered by tissue.[50] Another investigation employing BVS for ISR treatment and a 1-year follow-up revealed a nonsignificantly greater rate of device-related cardiovascular events compared to EES (10.1% vs. 5.2%, $p = 0.27$).[51] BVS indeed looks to be a viable option in the treatment of ISR. However, further studies have shown an increasing incidence of BVS-related thrombosis and myocardial infarction (MI) between 1 and 3 years.[52-54] The ABSORB III trial's 5-year follow-up revealed recently that the BVS period of elevated risk terminated at 3 years, which also happened to be the time of the scaffold's complete resorption.[55] ISR following BVS implantation, 3-year incidence gets comparable to that connected with DES implantation.[56]

Stent Thrombosis

Stent thrombosis is one of the most dangerous side effects of stent placement, as it can shorten life expectancy and cause MI. It has been demonstrated that OCT is practical in the presence of acute or subacute stent thrombosis. Underexpansion of the stented coronary segment and the presence of uncovered and malpositioned struts are the most frequent findings in these situations.

OPTICAL COHERENCE TOMOGRAPHY IN BIFURCATION LESIONS

Bifurcation lesions, which make up 15–20% of all PCI procedures and are frequently difficult, and provide special procedural and outcome problems. Plaque distribution is in relation to SB ostium, carina tip (CT) angle, and CT to bifurcation point (BP) length, which are the three crucial characteristics that must be recorded for provisional bifurcation angioplasty in addition to regular pre-PCI OCT assessment. In the provisional technique, it has been discovered that CT angle 50° and CT–BP length 1.7 mm are independent predictors of SB problems.[57] Due to carinal displacement, mostly calcified plaque opposite the SB ostia is a predictor of SB impairment after main branch (MB) stenting. The size of the stent is determined by the MB distal reference diameter, and the size of the proximal optimization technique (POT) balloon is determined by the MB proximal reference diameter. To evaluate stent extension, apposition, and edge dissection, post-PCI MB OCT pullback is performed. The bifurcation's 3D reconstruction clearly measures the stent struts over the SB ostium, determines if the carina is linked or not, and aids in the recrossing of the distal guidewire. Although it did not translate into better clinical outcomes, a few studies have showed that link-free carina with distal SB wiring resulted in the least amount of incorrect stent apposition or neocarina across the SB ostium after kissing balloon inflating (KBI).[58] Pre-PCI OCT examination is carried out in both the SB and MB for the upfront two-stent approach. Both stent sizes are determined by the distal reference diameter of SB and MB, while the POT balloon's size is determined by the proximal reference diameter of MB. In order to evaluate stent growth, apposition, edge dissection, and plaque protrusion, post-PCI OCT pullbacks of both MB and SB are collected. The SB ostium should be examined with the MB OCT pullback following the last KBI. Stent struts suspended over the SB ostium may act as a nidus for SB restenosis brought on by endothelization. Therefore, it must be guaranteed that the SB ostium is clear of any protruding stent struts.

Recently, it has been demonstrated that evaluating the SB ostium utilizing "cut plane analysis" through specialized "QAngioOCT" software dramatically reduces assessment error and yields measurements that are incredibly consistent and repeatable.

OPTICAL COHERENCE TOMOGRAPHY IN LEFT MAIN BIFURCATION LESIONS

Main branch and SB diameter disparities, tapering architecture, plaque eccentricity, and a higher likelihood of calcifications are among the distinctive characteristics of LM lesions that make accurate analysis using angiography challenging. Because of OCT's potential difficulties in imaging the LM body due to its larger size and the LM ostia due to poor blood clearance, guidelines prescribe IVUS for

LM angioplasty. OCT-guided mid and distal LM PCI has recently been the subject of numerous trials, with results equivalent to, if not better than, IVUS.[59,60] and demonstrated that 81% of OCT image frames in LM PCI were analyzable and that most of the nonanalyzable, artifact frames were in the proximal LM.

A significant amount of acute strut malapposition and stent underexpansion in bifurcation stenting were seen under OCT guidance, according to the ROCK-1[61] retrospective analysis. Late lumen loss in a 6-month follow-up tended to be lower in the OCT group (0.12 ± 0.41 vs. 0.26 ± 0.52 mm, $p = 0.10$), and was significantly reduced in the distal portion of the main vessel (0.03 ± 0.45 vs. 0.24 ± 0.53 mm, $p = 0.025$)). The LEMON study,[62] which examined the viability, safety, and effects of OCT-guided LM PCI, included 70 patients in its final analysis, of which 86% of the individuals met the primary endpoint of procedural success. 86% of the patients showed adequate stent expansion, 30% had considerable edge dissection, and 24% still had severe strut malapposition. OCT guidance changed the operators' strategy in one out of every four cases. The 1-year survival rate without significant clinical adverse effects was 98.6%. Because OCT can photograph most LM diameters encountered by the interventionist and has the advantage of post-PCI SB ostial optimization compared with IVUS, we advise using it for distal LM bifurcation angioplasty carried out either provisionally or with a two-stent technique upfront.

Recent research has shown that an aorto-ostial lesion, which has been a major obstacle to OCT, can now be seen using the soft polymer tip of the "Telescope" guide-extension catheter from Medtronic Cardiovascular in Santa Rosa, California, USA. This catheter's helical coil construction and relatively large gap allow infrared (IR) light to pass through the soft polymer. By inserting a guidewire into the aorta and lining up the guide catheter with the coronary ostia, it is also possible to scan the LM ostia.

CONTRAST SPARING OPTICAL COHERENCE TOMOGRAPHY

Novel contrast sparing strategies have been developed to enable the use of OCT in coronary revascularization in patients who have baseline renal impairment or are at a higher pre-procedural risk of developing contrast-induced nephropathy. The coronary blood field has been cleared using low-molecular-weight dextran (LMWD), and the same image quality and quantitative assessment have been accomplished.[63] However, its use is restricted by the availability and risk of anaphylactoid reactions. The use of OCT with LMWD has also been studied in patients with chronic kidney disease (CKD), in whom the use of LMWD did not adversely affect renal function and achieved similar short- and long-term clinical outcomes compared to IVUS-guided PCI. Heparinized saline is another medium that has been investigated as an alternative to contrast, and it has recently been shown to be practical and safe with good image quality.[64] One study saline OCT may be utilized as a contrast alternative for coronary OCT during PCI optimization; according to one study the coronary dimensions assessed using the technique were comparable to those obtained with contrast **(Fig. 4)**.[65,66] Further studies in this field are needed to provide firm evidence on the feasibility of saline as a flushing media. For solid proof that using saline as a flushing media is feasible, more research in this area is required.

FUTURE OF OPTICAL COHERENCE TOMOGRAPHY

Artificial Intelligence

For autonomous plaque characterization in OCT, a novel artificial intelligence (AI) framework has been created, and AI has largely emerged to favorably impact the way we work, especially in the field of imaging. Using Ultreon 1.0 software, the vessel diameter is determined and the amount of calcium in lesions is accurately assessed **(Fig. 5)**. The combination of OCT and FFR may also be utilized to characterize plaques. Additionally using a lumen profile, the virtual FFR produced by OCT is shown as a colored map, indicating simultaneously FFR for the entire vessel (blue arrows) and possible ischemia (yellow). Additionally, confirmation from the inside as well as the outside has been attained. Chu et al. found that AI-enabled OCT exhibited outstanding consistency in determining plaque burden when compared with human measures.[67]

Hybrid IVUS–OCT Catheter

As guiding tools, OCT and IVUS both have some drawbacks. The most complete intracoronary imaging guidance, nevertheless, could potentially be produced by merging the advantages of the two imaging methods into one. The initial prototypes had been in development since 2011, and Sheth et al.[68] first used a hybrid IVUS-OCT catheter in a clinical setting in 2018. The IVUS and OCT beams were aligned with one another, enabling immediate simultaneous image acquisition and review as well as inherent co-registration. While calcifications, stent struts, and very small dissections were clearer to see with OCT imaging, lipid-laden plaques, BPs, and deeper tissues were easier to see with IVUS. The system is not yet capable of supporting stand-alone OCT acquisition. The ability of the two techniques to work together synergistically to characterizes coronary atherosclerosis and produces high-quality co-registered images with clinically suitable standards in terms of the dimensions, speed, and resolution have been shown by this catheter powered by Novasight system technology (Conavi Medical, Inc Toronto, Canada) **(Fig. 6)**. Another hybrid IVUS–OCT catheter system with dual sensors in a sequential arrangement consisting of an IVUS transducer and an optical lens has been developed by TERUMO (Tokyo, Japan) by merging IVUS and optical

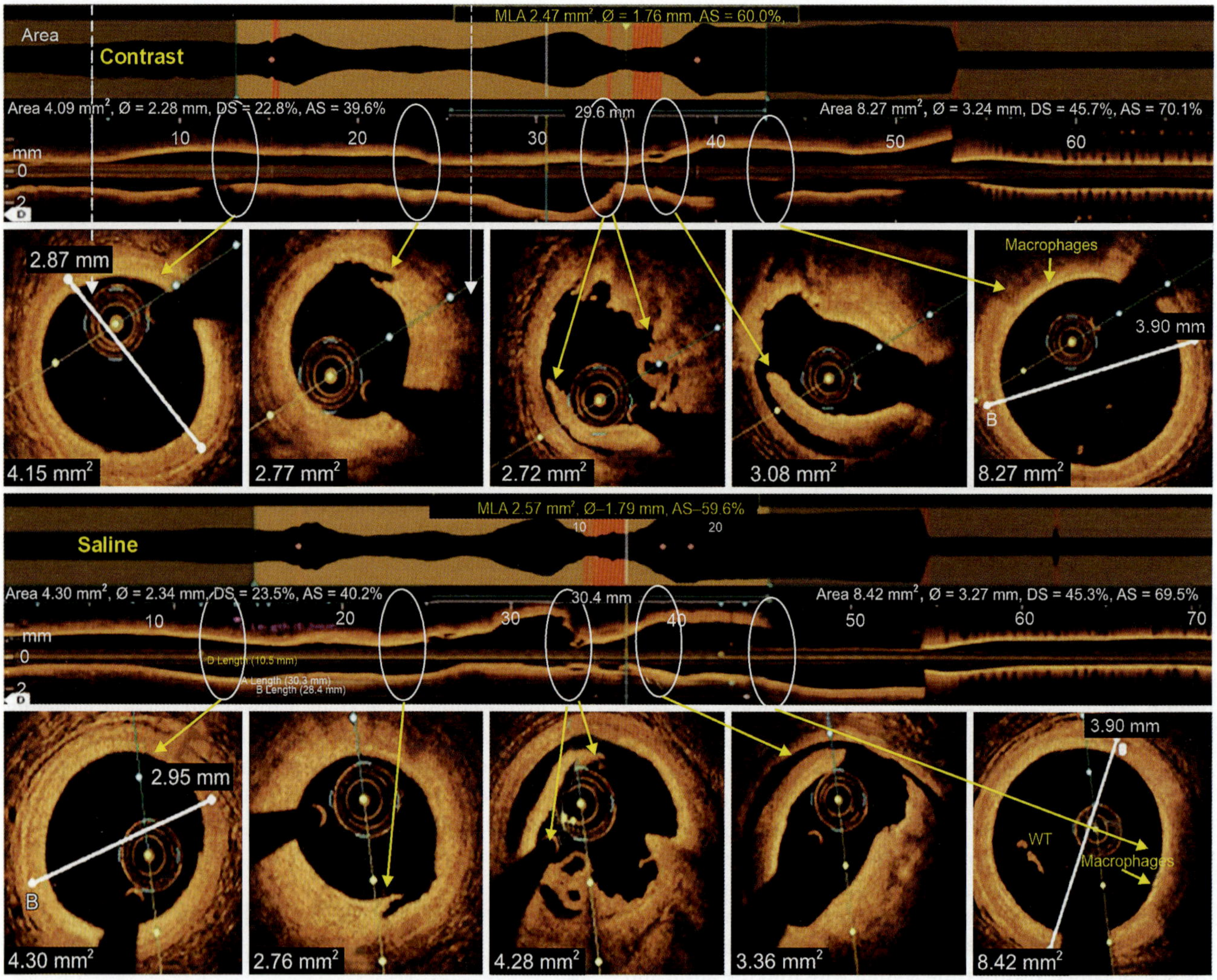

FIG. 4: Comparison between saline and contrast optical coherence tomography (OCT). The upper panel shows pre-percutaneous coronary intervention (PCI) run of right coronary artery (RCA) using contrast as a flushing media and in the lower panel the same vessel is imaged using saline as a flushing media for OCT and compared for image quality. All the lesion morphologies (including plaque rupture, dissections, recanalized thrombus, and macrophages) seen in contrast OCT are clearly seen with saline OCT (marked by yellow arrows at the same level).

frequency domain imaging (OFDI) probes. In this hybrid catheter, IVUS or OCT can be used separately according to the circumstances during the procedure

The first-in-human application study of the novel hybrid imaging system was done recently by Jia et al.[69] In addition to its good performance in image acquisition, the hybrid imaging catheter had a higher pullback speed, up to 40 mm/s, and a longer pullback length, up to 150 mm. It was concluded that the novel hybrid IVUS-OCT had achieved good clinical performance and reliability.

CONCLUSION

The use of intracoronary OCT has been proved to be undoubtedly superior to angiographic guidance, and even though the clinical outcomes are like those of IVUS guidance, OCT's detailed data and enhanced visualization of the lesion morphology promote better intraprocedural decision-making. When compared to IVUS, OCT is more successful at recognizing vulnerable plaques, quantifying calcified lesions, directing SB recrossing while bifurcation stenting, detecting intrastent tissue protrusion, detecting incomplete stent apposition, detecting stent edge dissections, and detecting intrastent thrombus. The ongoing large-scale ILUMIEN IV and OCTOBER trials are expected to provide additional evidence on the clinical and long-term advantages of OCT guidance. Saline-based OCT and the "telescope" catheter, though still in the early phases of development, provide ostial LM imaging, enabling OCT to overcome its traditional limitations. The use of this imaging technique in clinical practice should expand due to improved clinical outcomes and interventional knowledge.

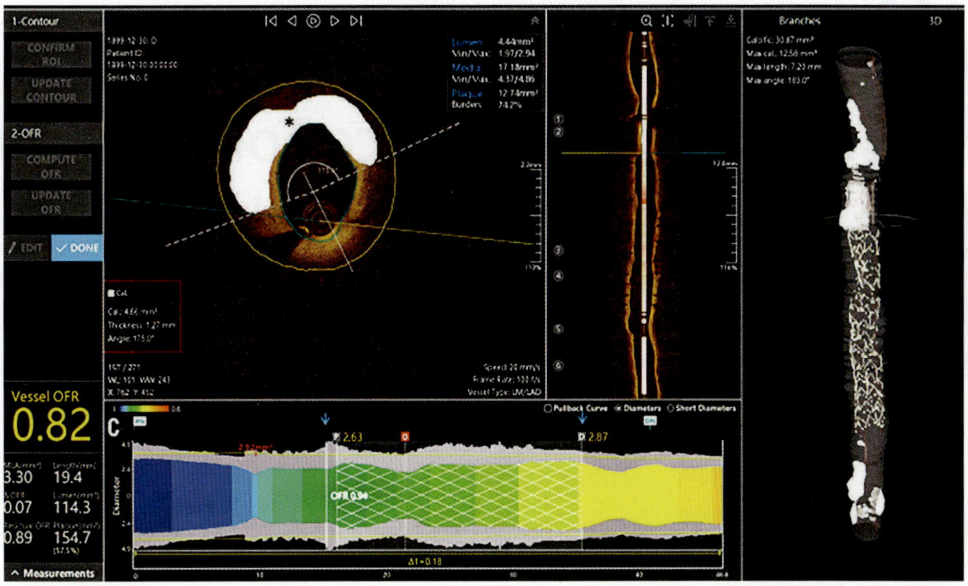

FIG. 5: Ultreon 1.0 software automatically detects the severity of calcium in lesions and measures the vessel diameter.

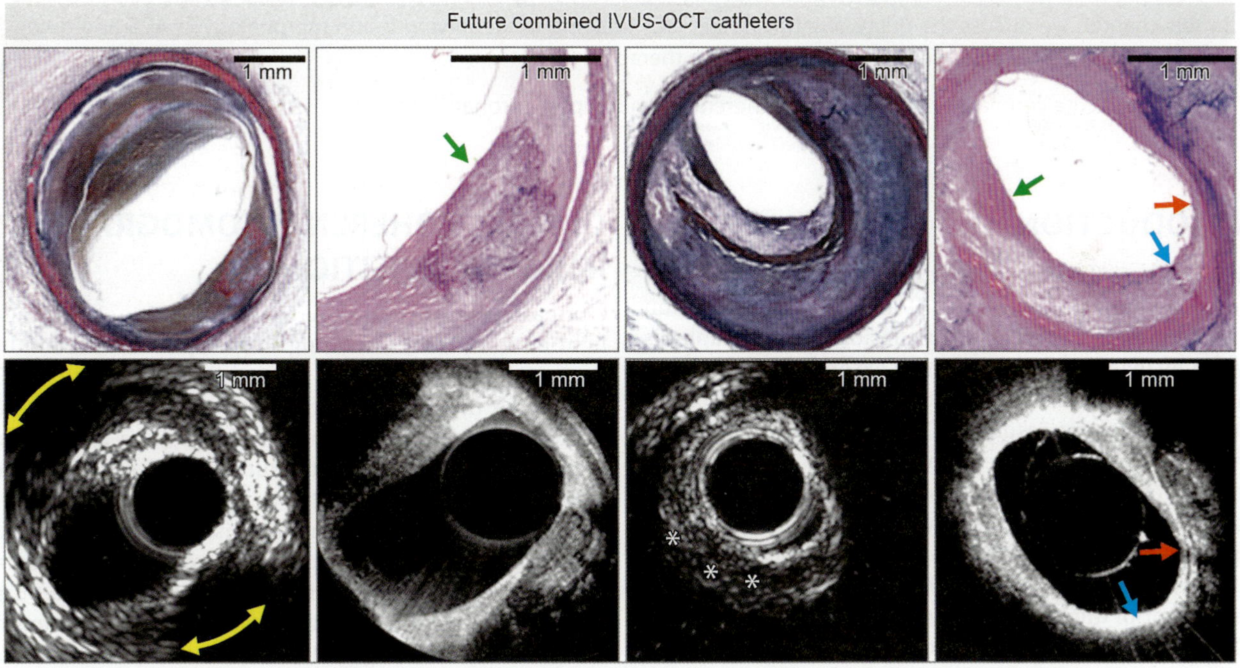

FIG. 6: Catheter powered by Novasight system technology (Conavi Medical, Inc Toronto, Canada) demonstrated the synergistic ability of the two modalities to characterize coronary atherosclerosis and produce high-quality co-registered images with clinically acceptable specifications with respect to the dimensions, speed, and resolution.

(IVUS: intravascular ultrasound; OCT: optical coherence tomography)

ONLINE REFERENCES

Please scan the QR code provided at the end of the table of contents for References of this chapter.

CHAPTER

169 Optical Coherence Tomography in Acute Coronary Syndrome

Rony Mathew, Musna PJ, Jo Joseph

ABSTRACT

The most common substrates for acute coronary syndromes (ACS) are plaque rupture, plaque erosion, and eruptive calcific nodule, while the less common etiologies are coronary artery dissection, coronary artery spasm, and coronary embolism. Optical coherence tomography (OCT) due to its innate ability for high-resolution intravascular imaging has the capability to identify these pathologies, enabling identification and tailoring therapy based on the culprit lesion. In this chapter, we discuss the utility of intravascular OCT imaging in identifying lesion morphology in ACS and guide percutaneous coronary intervention (PCI) for effective therapy.

Keywords: Acute coronary syndrome, optic coherence tomography, coronary imaging.

INTRODUCTION

Angiography is the most used imaging tool for patients with acute coronary syndrome (ACS) and stent implantation is recommended to treat culprit lesions. Angiography is limited by inaccurate assessment of lesion morphology and underlying mechanisms of ACS and suboptimal identification of poststent results.[1] "One-size-fits-all" approach may not be the best choice for patients with ACS caused by plaque erosion and nonatherosclerotic mechanisms, such as spontaneous coronary artery dissection (SCAD).[2,3] The very high resolution (10–15 mm) of intravascular optical coherence tomography (OCT) imaging allows accurate assessment of different underlying mechanisms of STEMI (ST-segment elevation myocardial infarction), potentially leading to tailored therapy. The high resolution of OCT enables identification of the details relevant to PCI strategy in ACS, such as plaque rupture, erosion, thrombotic debris, dissection, calcified nodules, calcium requiring lesion preparation, and thin cap fibroatheroma (TCFA).[4,5] We discuss how intravascular imaging may be used to optimize the outcomes of percutaneous coronary intervention (PCI) in ACS.

OPTICAL COHERENCE TOMOGRAPHIC IMAGE ACQUISITION

Optical coherence tomography utilizes near-infrared light emitted from a rotating single optical fiber and has an imaging lens within a monorail imaging sheath. By measuring the amplitude and delay of the backscattered light, OCT generates cross-sectional and three-dimensional images of the vessel microstructure. OCT gives greater axial resolution (10–20 μm), but lower penetration depth (1–2 mm). OCT imaging systems consist of an OCT imaging catheter, a drive motor operating control, and imaging software. The imaging catheter is attached to the purge syringe and flushed with the same material planned for coronary flushing and attached to the drive motor operating control. Intracoronary nitroglycerine is given before OCT imaging to eliminate spasm. To achieve blood clearance during catheter pullback, the guiding catheter at the coronary ostium should be properly engaged. Deep seating of the guide should be avoided as contrast injection may eject the guide, causing suboptimal image quality. In severely stenotic lesions, predilation should be performed to get blood clearance. The contrast flush rate of 4 mL/s for a total volume of 14–16 mL is needed for the left coronary artery and 3 mL/s for a total volume of 12–14 mL for the right coronary artery and the pressure limit of 300 psi if an automated injector is used. Contrast injection should stop immediately as the guide catheter is seen on the pullback image to minimize contrast use. Cine angiography should be performed during pullback to utilize contrast injection for angiography and OCT coregistration.[6]

LESION CHARACTERIZATION AND DECISION-MAKING

Normal vessel wall will be visualized by OCT as three-layered structure which represents intima, media, and adventitia **(Fig. 1)**. The internal elastic lamina is a signal-rich thick band that lies inside the dark band of the media and the external elastic lamina (EEL) lies in the outer border of the media.[7]

ATHEROSCLEROTIC CORONARY ARTERY DISEASE

A fibrous plaque will show a homogenous, high-signal region with low attenuation **(Fig. 2)**. A calcified plaque will have low-signal regions with low attenuation of light and may have sharp well-delineated borders **(Fig. 3)**, and a lipid-rich plaque will show low-signal regions with high attenuation of light signals (light does not penetrate through lipid) with diffuse borders covered with fibrous cap **(Fig. 4)**. OCT cannot be used to measure the depth or volume of lipid pools due to high attenuation behind. OCT-defined TCFA was a lipid-rich plaque with lipid arc within the plaque in more than two quadrants (>1,800) with a thin fibrous cap with thickness at the thinnest segment of <75 µm **(Fig. 5)**. Irregular intraluminal masses (>250 µm) with low attenuation are white thrombus and the red thrombus is high-attenuating which casts a shadow on the vessel wall and obscures the vessel wall behind.[8,9]

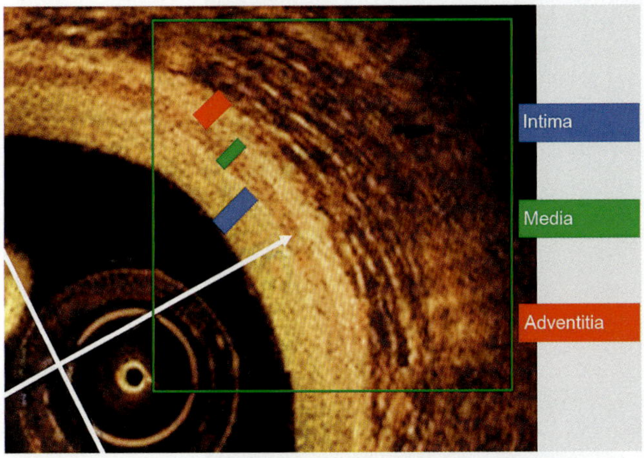

FIG. 1: Normal vessel wall structure.

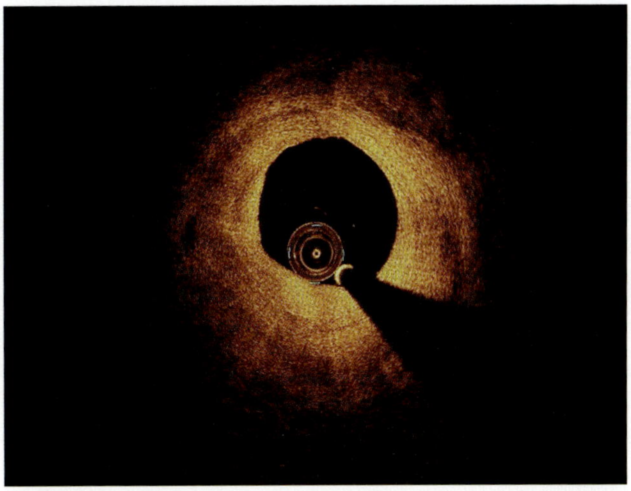

FIG. 2: Fibrous plaque.

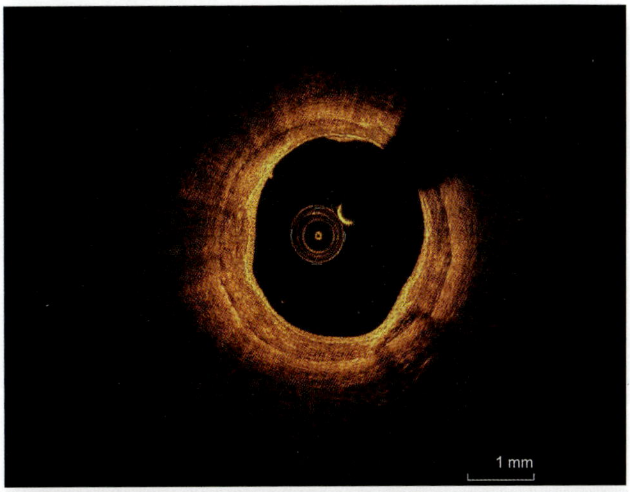

FIG. 3: Calcific plaque.

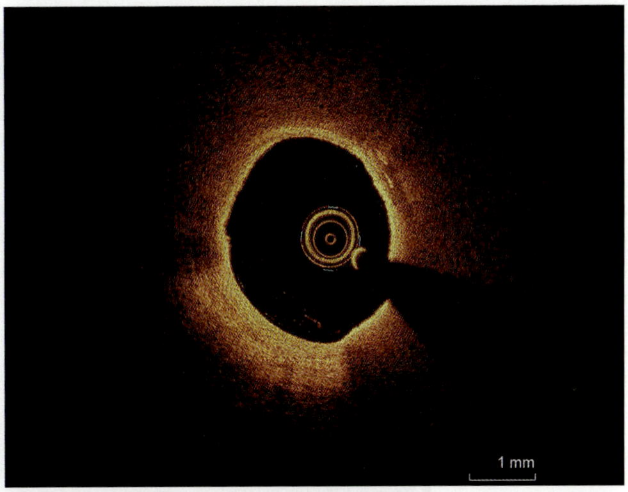

FIG. 4: Lipid plaque, with macrophages.

PLAQUE RUPTURE, PLAQUE EROSION, AND CALCIFIED NODULES: COMMON MECHANISM OF ACS

The most common underlying culprit lesion for ACS in patients with obstructive atherosclerotic coronary disease is a ruptured lipid-rich plaque, followed by plaque erosion and calcified nodule. Other uncommon mechanisms are tight stenosis, dissection, intramural hematoma, coronary spasm, and intimal fissures.[10,11]

Plaque Rupture

Optical coherence tomography-defined plaque rupture will have disrupted fibrous cap associated with a cavity and an underlying lipid plaque. Overhanging thrombus will be present in acute presentations **(Figs. 6 and 7)**. But with the early use of antithrombotic and antiplatelet drugs, the thrombus may dissolve before coronary catheterization or thrombi may be removed by aspiration. TCFAs rupture because of turbulent blood flow and inflammatory process activated by macrophages. The microcalcification generated by necrotic macrophages or smooth muscle cells makes plaques vulnerable to rupture under high radial strain.[12,13] The shoulder region of fibrous cap is the most vulnerable region at rest and the mid-fibrous cap during exercise. Rupture of the fibrous cap leads to exposure of highly thrombogenic necrotic core which leads to the formation of mainly the red thrombus.[14-16]

Plaque Erosion

Erosion by OCT is a diagnosis of exclusion in most of the cases. OCT erosion is defined by the absence of fibrous cap disruption and the presence of thrombus, usually white thrombus, or luminal surface irregularity in the absence

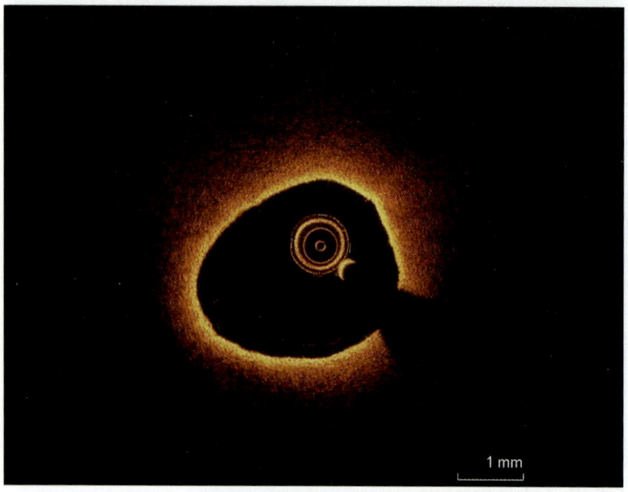

FIG. 5: Thin fibrous cap atheroma.

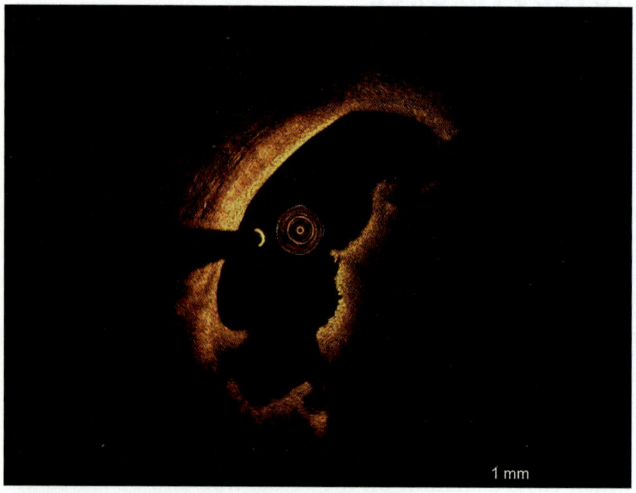

FIG. 6: Plaque rupture with red thrombus.

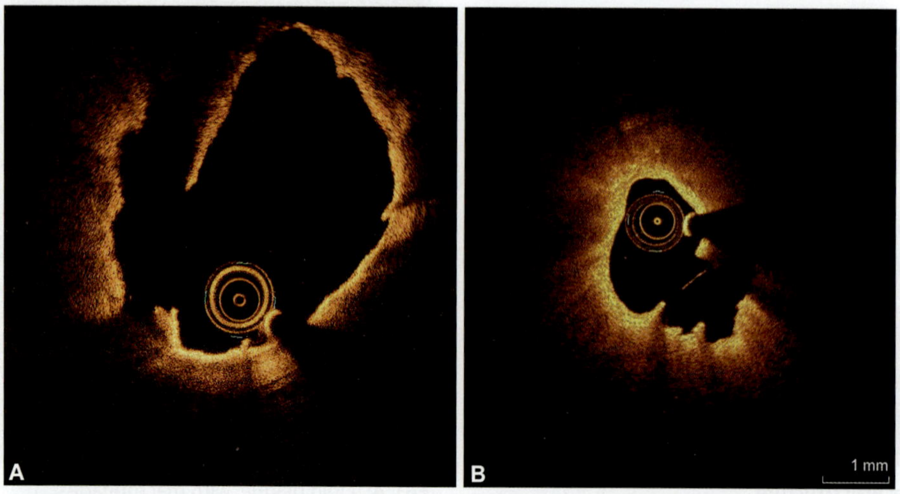

FIGS. 7A AND B: Ruptured plaques with empty cavity.

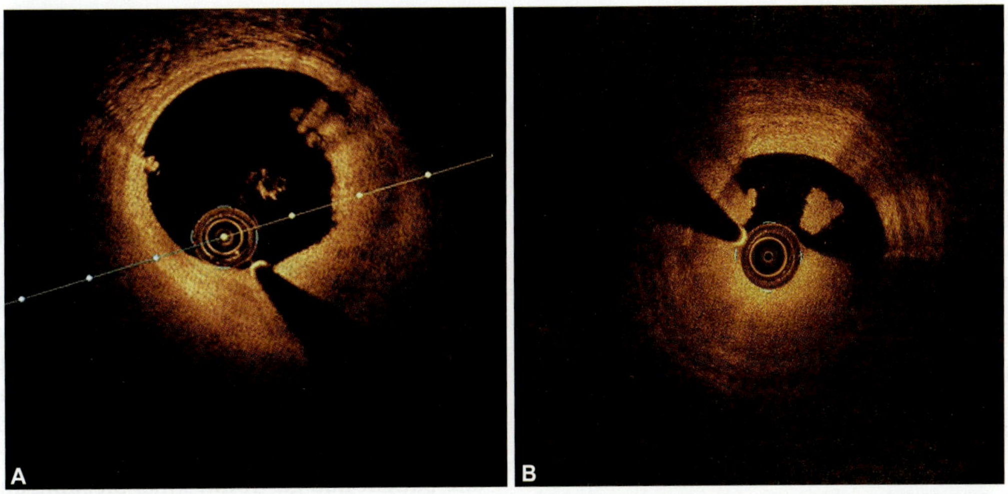

FIGS. 8A AND B: Plaque erosions with attached white thrombus; (A) without obstructive luminal narrowing; (B) with significant luminal narrowing.

of thrombus. In OCT erosion, there will be attenuation of underlying plaque by thrombus without superficial lipid or calcification immediately proximal or distal to the attached thrombus.[4] Definite OCT erosion was identified by the presence of attached thrombus overlying an intact visualized plaque. Probable OCT erosion was defined as either with luminal surface irregularity in the absence of thrombus or attenuation of underlying plaque by the thrombus without superficial lipid or calcifications proximal or distal to the thrombus.[9] On OCT, plaque erosion tends to have less diameter stenosis, thicker caps, smaller lipid arcs lower lipid content, and less calcification than ruptured plaque **(Figs. 8A and B)**. Plaque erosions are usually associated with negative remodeling of vessel wall.[17]Approximately two-thirds of plaque erosion cases presented as non-STEMI (NSTEMI).[18]

Calcified Nodule

Calcified nodules are the least common atherothrombotic cause of ACS.[9] At the site of culprit lesions, three different types of calcific plaques are described. Those are calcified protrusions **(Fig. 9)**, eruptive calcified nodules **(Fig. 10)**, and superficial calcific sheet with a prevalence of 25.5%, 7.1%, and 67.4% respectively. Eruptive calcified nodules are shown to be responsible for ACS.[19]

If the underlying plaque is calcium, with a disrupted fibrous cap and protruding nodular calcium, and if there is superficial calcium or sustentative calcium proximal and distal to the lesion, it is defined as OCT-calcified nodule.[9] Calcified protrusion is a calcific mass that is covered by a smooth fibrous surface. Eruptive calcified nodules are frequently located in the mid-right coronary artery where cyclic hinge movement leads to weakening and fracture of calcified plaque. Cyclic torsion could fragment sheets of calcium, resulting in small nodular calcium protrusions

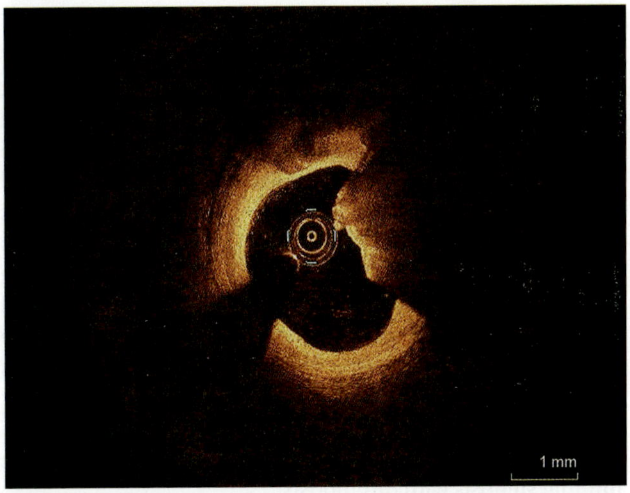

FIG. 9: Calcified protrusions.

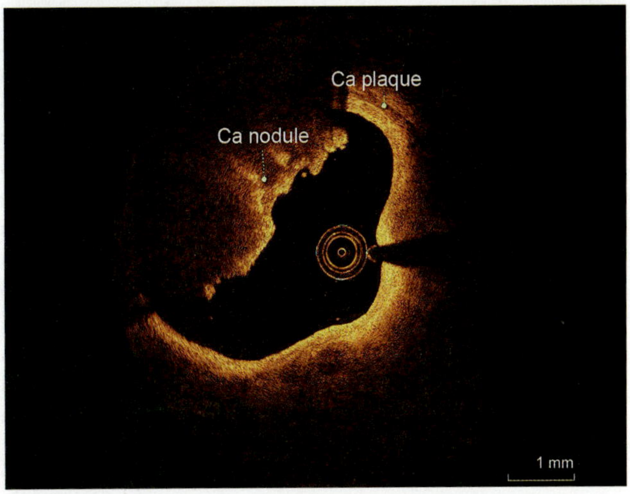

FIG. 10: Eruptive calcified nodule.

that are surrounded by fibrin. The calcium eventually erupts through the fibrin, disrupting the endothelium with the formation of overlying microthrombi.[19]

NONATHEROTHROMBOTIC LESSIONS

Spontaneous dissections and intramural hematoma are readily identified on OCT and are occasionally found in patients presenting with ACS.[5] OCT discovers the double-lumen morphology, with false and true lumen and the entry tear, and the circumferential and longitudinal extent of the disease.[20]

In patients presenting with vasospastic angina, OCT imaging will show bumping of the intima, which causes luminal irregularity. Erosion could be the secondary pathology at sites of vasospasm as erosion with thrombus was found in one quarter of spastic sites on imaging. In coronary embolism when OCT done after thrombectomy will not show any underlying atherosclerosis to precipitate an ACS.[20]

MANAGEMENT STRATEGIES

Current guidelines recommend stent implantation to treat culprit lesions in patients with STEMI. However, recent studies suggest that conservative medical therapy might be considered in cases caused by plaque erosion, SCAD, and coronary spasm. OCT which is key to the definitive diagnosis in these subsets of patients. The luminal stenosis is always not significant in lesions with intact fibrous cap. Considering the risks of in-stent thrombosis and restenosis and the need for prolonged dual antiplatelet therapy, a conservative nonstenting strategy was recommended in plaque erosions and in SCAD and can be considered in certain ruptures without dissection and/or hematoma. Such an approach may improve long-term outcome in patients who have lesser luminal stenosis with thrombosis.

Plaque erosion was found to have better long-term prognosis with PCI compared to plaque rupture in 18 months follow-up.[21] However, plaque erosion has been associated with poor vascular healing compared with plaque rupture at 6 months.[22] The TOTAL OCT study showed most lesions with intact fibrous cap in STEMI are severely stenotic and have significant residual stenosis after thrombectomy, irrespective of the presence of plaque rupture or intact fibrous cap. This study has shown that both intact fibrous cap and plaque rupture culprit lesions are advanced atherosclerotic lesions which may merit similar treatment strategies.[23] In an observational study of 31 patients with plaque erosion who had undergone thrombectomy, 40% of them were managed on dual antiplatelet therapy alone and rest of them ended in PCI. All of them were asymptomatic during follow-up period of 2 years, which suggested that deferred stenting is feasible in selected cases of plaque erosion.[24]

Erosion trial was the first landmark prospective study which proved the concept of deferred stenting in STEMI with plaque erosion. In this trial 25% of the STEMI cases were found to be due to plaque erosion. Plaque erosion with <70% luminal narrowing by OCT with TIMI 3 (thrombolysis in myocardial infarction 3) flow, stenting was deferred in the culprit vessel. At 1 month, follow-up OCT revealed greater than 50% reduction in thrombus volume and except two cases, all of them were asymptomatic during follow-up.[25] Tirofiban infusion was proved to have additional benefit on further analysis.[25,26] Out of 55 patients, 53 patients who underwent OCT at 1 year showed significant reduction in thrombus volume and complete thrombus resolution in half of patients, three patients underwent target vessel revascularization for angina.[26] 52 patients finished 4-year follow-up and all patients were free from death, myocardial infarction (MI), stroke, bypass surgery, or heart failure. Only one patient had gastrointestinal bleeding and 11 patients underwent target vessel revascularization. Patients in the nonrevascularized group had more reduction of thrombus at 1 month.[27] In conservatively managed patients with plaque erosion thrombus resolution with Tirofiban was also reported by Sugayama et al.[28] In the absence of plaque rupture with <70% narrowing of the culprit vessel, stenting was avoided in the OCT-guided prospective study by Souteyrand et al.[29] Patients were treated with two-step treatment strategy of primary PCI and delayed coronary angiograms and OCT after a mean period of 6 days. 23 patients were benefited from this approach, over a mean follow-up of 171 days and the mean luminal area was found to be increased and at 1 year only two patients underwent stenting for angina.[29]

Erosion III trial included patients with STEMI with nonobstructive culprit lesions with angiographic diameter stenosis of <70% and TIMI 3 flow after wiring or thrombectomy were randomized to either OCT or angiographic-guided treatment. A conservative nonstenting strategy was adopted in plaque erosions, certain ruptures without dissection or hematoma and SCAD. 116 of the 226 patients (51.3%) were treated with stent implantation. Compared to angiographic guidance group the rate of stent implantation in the OCT guidance group was 15% lower (43.8% vs. 58.8%; $p = 0.024$). In the OCT guidance group, 25 of 29 patients with culprit erosions and 30 of 74 culprit ruptures were treated medically. In the median follow-up of 369 days, five patients at 1 month had events, including one rehospitalization due to unstable angina and four cardiac deaths. The three of the four cardiac deaths were in the angiographic group. Recurrent MI and target lesion revascularizations were not observed in either group. This study demonstrated a crucial role for OCT in the decision-making process in STEMI.[30]

Assessment of lesion morphology on OCT can guide lesion preparation. Predilatation with an undersized balloon or a direct stenting approach may be appropriate in the presence of largely fibrous or lipid-rich plaques. In severely calcified lesions, noncompliant balloon dilation, use of a cutting or scoring balloon, atherectomy, or intravascular lithotripsy can be considered. In calcified lesions, an OCT-based scoring system has been validated to determine the lesions lead to stent underexpansion which can be easily recalled as the "rule of 5". 1 point for the maximum thickness of calcium >500 µm, 1 point for the length of calcium >5 mm, and 1 point for maximum arc >50% (>180° of the circumference) of the circumference of the vessel. A total score of ≥3 suggests that calcium modification with atherectomy or intravascular lithotripsy may be needed, whereas stent expansion in lesions with scores of ≤2 was generally acceptable.[31,32] When there is a maximum calcium arc >50% of the vessel circumference, lesions with calcium fracture have better stent expansion than those without calcium fracture.[33] All three calcific plaque types were associated with more periprocedural complications and suboptimal PCI results compared with noncalcified culprit plaques. The calcified nodules are challenging to treat and associated with smaller stent areas because of the eccentric rigidity of nodules which interferes with the symmetric stent expansion.[34] Eruptive nodules are associated with an increase in procedural complications, such as stent malapposition and stent edge dissection. Calcific sheets are associated with the smallest post-stent lumen area mainly due to inadequate lesion preparation during acute MI presentation.[35] Atherectomy may be needed to optimize outcomes in calcified lesions. Intravascular lithotripsy should be considered as atherectomy is contraindicated in thrombotic lesions in ACS.[36]

PRE-PERCUTANEOUS CORONARY INTERVENTION GUIDANCE

Length of the Stent

The most "normal" appearing segments within 5 mm are selected as proximal and distal reference frames where there is minimal atherosclerotic plaque, no TCFA or significant lipid, and where medial and adventitial layers are visible, and length of the stent is adjusted to available stent length.[6]

Diameter of the Stent

External elastic lamina-based measurements if EEL is visible in >180° or lumen-based measurements can be used if EEL visualization is insufficient. Stent size should be rounded down by 0.25 mm if EEL-based measurements are used; if lumen-based measurements are used it should be rounded up, between 0.25 and 0.5 mm, to determine the stent size.[6]

Angiographic Co-registration

It helps in precise stent positioning. The software will clearly show the selected distal and proximal landing zone on the co-registered angiography. In a randomized study, OCT-angiography co-registration resulted in a trend toward reducing major stent edge dissection compared to angiography guidance.[24] More recently, bifurcation and ostial OCT mapping (BOOM) has been described which helps in mapping of the side branch ostium to minimize protrusion of stent struts into the main branch and ensuring full coverage of the ostium of the side branch.[6]

POST-PERCUTANEOUS CORONARY INTERVENTION GUIDANCE

Post-PCI OCT run will be taken to assess the intramural hematoma and medial dissection, expansion, and malapposition.

Medial Dissection

ILUMIEN IV study classified major dissections as those with medial dissection and intramural hematoma ≥60° in arc from the center of the vessel and ≥3 mm in length from the edge of the stent.[6] In the CLI-OPCI registry, a linear tissue rim with width >200 µm was considered a major dissection. Distal edge dissection was associated with a 2.5-fold hazard of major adverse cardiac events (death, MI, target lesion revascularization), but not at the proximal edge.[36,37] In a detailed analysis the dissection depth at the distal edge, reference lumen area at the proximal edge, and overall dissection length were predictors of composite endpoint of cardiac death, target lesion MI, target vessel revascularization.[36-38]

Malapposition

Optical coherence tomography can identify malapposition which is absence of full contact between vessel wall and stent struts. Malapposition with incomplete stent apposition (ISA) distance of <400 µm and length of <1 mm requires no treatment and it heals by neointimal proliferation behind the stent struts. Malapposition associated with underexpansion and long malappositions >3 mm need correction. To correct malapposition lower pressure dilation will be done with semi-compliant balloon.[6]

Expansion

The current European consensus is that a minimal stent area (MSA) ≥80% of the mean reference lumen area and/or >4.5 mm^2 on OCT is considered acceptable. The proximal and distal reference segments (within 5 mm from the edges of the stent) are examined for inflow/outflow disease. If both the proximal and distal reference segments have a minimal lumen area (MLA) ≥ 4.5 mm^2, no further treatment is necessary. If there is untreated disease at the reference segment, defined as a focal MLA < 4.5 mm^2, it may need additional drug-eluting stent (DES) unless anatomy is not suitable (vessel tapering, diffuse disease, or no landing zone).[6,37,38]

OPTICAL COHERENCE TOMOGRAPHY: HIGH-RISK PLAQUE

Optical coherence tomography can identify vulnerable plaque characterized by TCFA, high lipid burden, macrophage infiltration, and cholesterol crystals **(Fig. 11)**. CLIMA trial included 1,003 patients of which the highly vulnerable features associated with hard events are MLA < 3.5 mm^2, lipid arc >180°, TCFA with a cap thickness of <75 μm, and macrophage infiltration.[39] Studies have shown that lipid plaques are associated with adverse cardiac events on follow-up compared to nonlipid plaques.[40] However, the prognostic impact of detecting vulnerable plaque remains unresolved **(Figs. 12A and B)**. The detection of vulnerable plaques in selected high-risk patients with prior ACS or diabetics may be of clinical significance. The OCT substudy of the COMPLETE (Complete vs. Culprit-Only Revascularization to Treat Multi-Vessel Disease After Early PCI for STEMI) trial showed that nearly 50% of patients had at least one obstructive nonculprit lesion containing TCFA. These obstructive lesions more commonly have vulnerable plaque morphology, including TCFA, high lipid burden, macrophages, and cholesterol crystals compared to nonobstructive lesions. Hence routine PCI of the obstructive nonculprit lesions in patients with STEMI and multivessel disease may be beneficial.[41] COMBINE OCT-FFR study conducted in diabetic patients with intermediate lesions and fractional flow reserve >0.80 showed that the presence of TCFA was associated with a 4.7-fold increase in the primary endpoint of cardiac death, MI, target lesion revascularization, or hospitalization for angina, which was driven mostly by higher rates of target lesion revascularization for MI and hospitalization for angina (4.1%).[42]

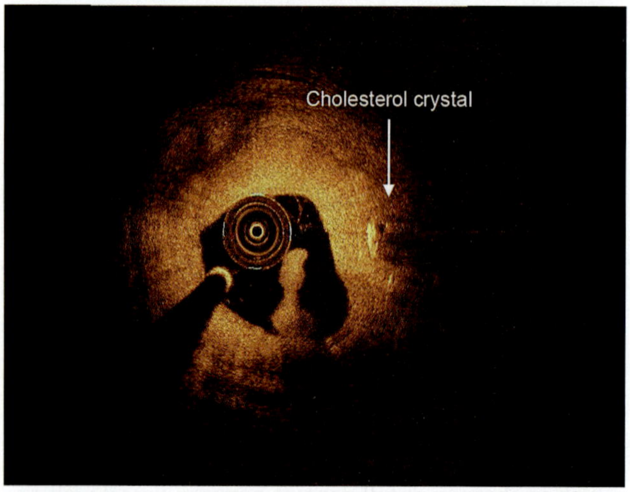

FIG. 11: Cholesterol crystals.

MYOCARDIAL INFARCTION WITH NONOBSTRUCTIVE CORONARY ARTERIES

Optical coherence tomography is an indispensable tool in the diagnostic work-up of MI with nonobstructive coronary arteries (MINOCA). The combination of OCT with cardiac magnetic resonance imaging (MRI) can help us to reach a definite diagnosis in the majority of MINOCA cases **(Flowchart 1)**. OCT could pick up an etiological lesion in around 50–80% of cases demonstrated by a few observational studies.[43-45] Blind three-vessel OCT is not practically

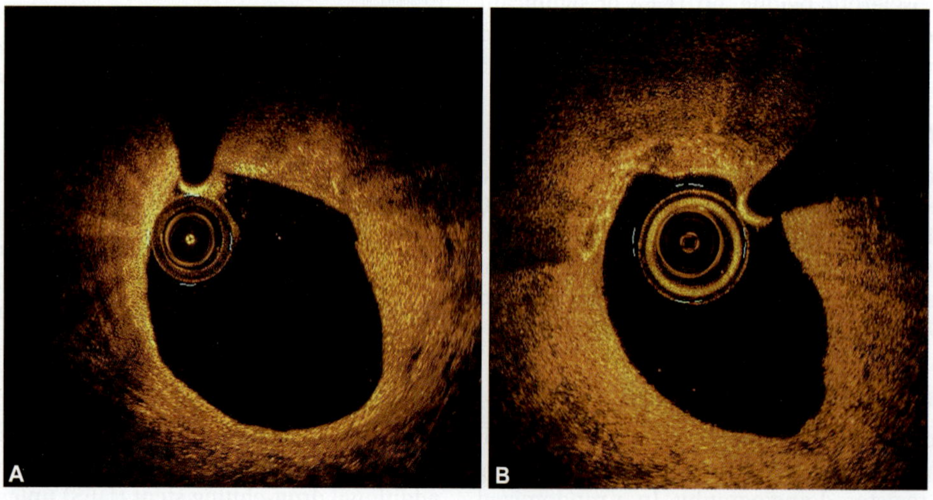

FIGS. 12A AND B: Macrophages.

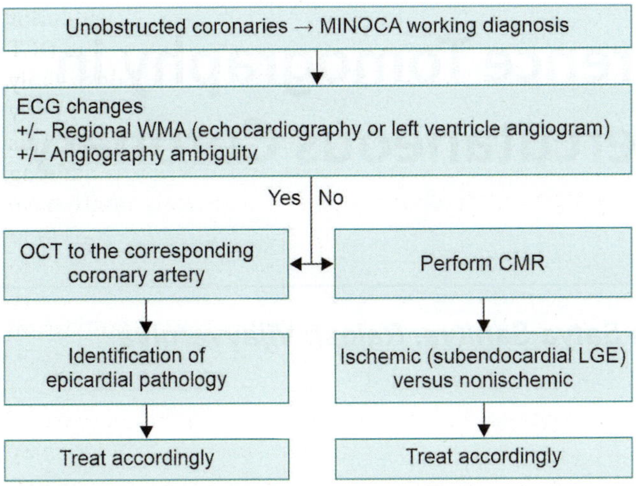

FLOWCHART 1: Clinical algorithm for the use of optical coherence tomography (OCT) in MINOCA (myocardial infarction with non-obstructive coronary arteries).

(CMR: cardiac magnetic resonance; ECG: electrocardiogram; LGE: late gadolinium enhancement; WMA: wall motion abnormality)

feasible and the diagnostic yield of such an approach is low. Plaque rupture and plaque erosions were the common diagnosis in MINOCA. Those patients with high-risk lesions had recurrent ACS events on follow-up and the events recurred at the segment where the high-risk lesions were identified and presented with obstructive coronary lesions. Nonatherosclerotic causes can be identified which will help in decisions regarding further management including antiplatelet therapy.[45]

CONCLUSION

Intravascular OCT imaging provides an abundance of data on coronary structures and pathologies, which will help in the diagnosis and management of ACS. Systematic efforts are ongoing to formulate the appropriate use and interpretation of OCT images, using practical algorithmic approaches. Robust evidence from the ongoing trials on the impact of OCT guidance could increase the adoption of this imaging modality in clinical practice.

ONLINE REFERENCES

Please scan the QR code provided at the end of the table of contents for References of this chapter.

CHAPTER

170 Optical Coherence Tomography in Bifurcation Percutaneous Coronary Intervention

Ankush Gupta, Mandava Satya Sahitya, Rajesh Vijayvergiya

ABSTRACT

Coronary bifurcation angioplasty constitutes a complex coronary intervention. It is associated with lower procedural success and higher complication rates. Contemporary evidence suggests better short- and long-term outcomes if bifurcation percutaneous coronary intervention (PCI) is done under image guidance as compared to angiography guidance. Guidelines recommend both intravascular ultrasound (IVUS) and optical coherence tomography (OCT) for PCI optimization in selected cases such as left main bifurcation disease. Higher resolution and three-dimensional (3D) reconstruction with OCT makes it a better imaging modality than IVUS for bifurcation angioplasty. 3D reconstruction of the side branch ostium after main branch stenting and proximal optimization technique (POT) is useful for guiding the optimum position of guidewire recross to improve long-term side branch outcome. The chapter describes the usefulness of OCT in bifurcation lesions including the left main disease.

Keywords: Intravascular ultrasound, main vessel (MV), optical coherence tomography, percutaneous coronary intervention, proximal optimization, side branch (SB).

INTRODUCTION

Coronary bifurcation lesion is a complex subset and constitutes 15–20% of percutaneous coronary intervention (PCI).[1,2] The procedural success rate is lower, and the complications are higher with PCI of bifurcation lesions. A coronary bifurcation lesion is defined as an atherosclerotic disease occurring adjacent or close to a major side branch (SB). The Medina classification is commonly used to define bifurcation anatomy. The key principle of bifurcation PCI is to keep it simple by using provisional stenting in which the main vessel (MV) is stented, and the SB is assessed and intervened if required. The criteria for SB intervention are angiographic stenosis of >70%, major dissection, TIMI flow < III grade, or fractional flow reserve (FFR) < 0.8. This is based upon evidence from randomized studies that did not show any benefit of two-stent strategies over single-stent strategies.[3] Provisional stenting has shown improved mortality, reduced major adverse cardiovascular events (MACE), lower incidence of stent thrombosis, and target lesion failure. An upfront two-stent strategy is used for important SB, its dimension of >2.5 mm and disease segment length of >10 mm, with true bifurcation lesions (Medina 1,1,1; 1,0,1; 0,1,1), narrow bifurcation angle (<70°), and predicted unfavorable recrossing after MV stenting. For the two-stent strategy, meta-analysis has shown that the double-kissing (DK) crush technique is superior to others when parameters such as MACE and target lesion revascularization (TLR) are considered, especially for left main (LM) bifurcation disease.

Contemporary guidelines advocate the use of intravascular imaging, i.e., intravascular ultrasound (IVUS) and optical coherence tomography (OCT) during PCI of selected cases like bifurcation lesions.[4] Both imaging modalities have shown to be superior to conventional angiography for the optimization of PCI. Higher resolution and three-dimensional (3D) reconstruction by OCT makes it superior to IVUS during bifurcation PCI. Studies have shown improved survival and reduced MACE in patients undergoing OCT-guided PCI optimization compared with angiography only.[5,6] Compared with IVUS, OCT-guided PCI initially resulted in smaller minimum stent area (MSA), stent expansions,[7] and stent diameters, albeit with similar rates of target vessel failure (TVF) and restenosis in a 12-month follow-up.[8] As part of the evolution of OCT, the stent sizing protocol evolved from initial lumen sizes to reference external elastic lamina (EEL)-based sizes resulting in MSA and stent expansion comparable to those of IVUS.[9-11] Phantom model trials showed that the mean lumen area measured by OCT was equal to the actual lumen area of the phantom model while IVUS overestimated it.[12] In a prospective observational study of IVUS versus angiography-guided bifurcation PCI, MACE and mortality benefits were more favorable with IVUS arm, extended up to 7 years of follow-up.[13] In this chapter, we will learn about the use of OCT in both LM and non-LM bifurcation PCI.

OPTICAL COHERENCE TOMOGRAPHY FOR NON-LEFT MAIN BIFURCATION PERCUTANEOUS CORONARY INTERVENTION

Pre-percutaneous Coronary Intervention Imaging

Angiography has inherent limitations to assess bifurcation anatomy due to overlapping and foreshortening. OCT clearly defines the bifurcation lesions, overcoming the misleading angiographic two-dimensional appearance. Pre-PCI pullback is taken from both main branch (MB) and SB for assessing the plaque morphology to choose a device for bed preparation and for measurement of vessel dimensions including lesion length. For provisional bifurcation angioplasty, in addition to routine pre-PCI OCT assessment, the three important parameters that need to be recorded are plaque distribution in relation to SB ostium, carina tip (CT) angle, and CT to bifurcation point (BP) length **(Figs. 1A to J)**. CT angle < 50° and CT-BP length < 1.7 mm have been found to be independent predictors of SB complications in the provisional strategy.[14] Predominantly, calcified plaque opposite to SB ostia is a predictor of SB compromise after MB stenting due to carinal shift. MB distal reference diameter guides the stent size while the proximal reference diameter guides the size of the proximal optimization technique (POT) balloon. For upfront two-stent strategy, pre-PCI OCT assessment is done in both SB and MB. The distal reference diameter of both SB and MB is used to decide the size of both stents and the proximal reference diameter of MB is used for sizing of the POT balloon, which is measured by EEL distance. In case EEL is not visible in at least 180° arc due to high plaque burden, lipidic plaque, or large vessel size, lumen-based stent sizing has to be done.[15-17] The stent length is at par with proximal and distal reference points. The MV stent should have a proximal extent of at least 6–8 mm from the bifurcation carina point so that proximal balloon optimization (POT) can be performed with the shortest available balloon. OCT can assess the SB by reconstructing a 3D image of the bifurcation from a MV pullback. In case of a conflicting wire shadow, the wire can be repositioned and repeat pullback must be taken. A new OCT-validated software "QAngioOCT" can reconstruct the cross-sections perpendicular to the SB central line and enable a more accurate assessment of SB ostia from MB pullbacks.[18]

OPTICAL COHERENCE TOMOGRAPHY DURING BIFURCATION PERCUTANEOUS CORONARY INTERVENTION

In provisional bifurcation angioplasty, after MB stenting and POT, wire recrossing of SB is required for kissing balloon inflation (KBI). 3D reconstruction at the bifurcation clearly quantifies the stent struts across SB ostium, identifies whether carina is link-free or not **(Figs. 1A to J)**, and helps in identifying the position of guidewire recrossing before KBI. A few studies have shown that link-free carina with distal SB wiring resulted in minimum inappropriate stent apposition or neocarina across the SB ostium after KBI although it did not translate into improved clinical outcomes[19] in provisional bifurcation angioplasty. In upfront two-stent strategy like DK crush technique, MB OCT pullback may be used to assess the appropriateness of SB stent crushing before the first proximal recross, thereby preventing the abluminal SB guidewire recross before the first KBI. OCT may again be used for guiding the distal SB recross before the second KBI, thereby reducing the length of neo-metallic carina that may translate into better long-term SB outcome. OCT guidance had a significantly lower number of malapposed stent struts compared to angiography guidance (7.5% vs. 15.8%; $p = 0.0009$).[20] Viceconte et al. found a lower rate of malapposition in the OCT arm in comparison to the angiography arm (7.1% vs. 17.5%; $p = 0.005$).[21]

OPTICAL COHERENCE TOMOGRAPHY AFTER BIFURCATION PERCUTANEOUS CORONARY INTERVENTION

After stenting of the bifurcation, OCT is useful in assessing the stent expansion, malapposition, tissue prolapse, geographical miss, and edge dissection. The bifurcation lesions have a fractal anatomy and the minimal stent area (MSA) should be assessed with respect to the proximal, distal, and SB reference lumen areas. Malapposition is more common at the proximal stent and edge dissection and tissue prolapse are more common at distal stent. It has been shown that OCT-guided final KBI resulted in better anatomical and functional results at the SB ostium.[22] Additional postdilatation is required if there is malapposition of >300 μm with a longitudinal length of >1 mm.

In provisional bifurcation strategy, the final MB pullback is taken for stent expansion proximal and distal to carina, for malapposition, edge dissection, plaque prolapse, and geographical miss. SB pullback is only recommended if KBI is done to document balloon dissections if present. For

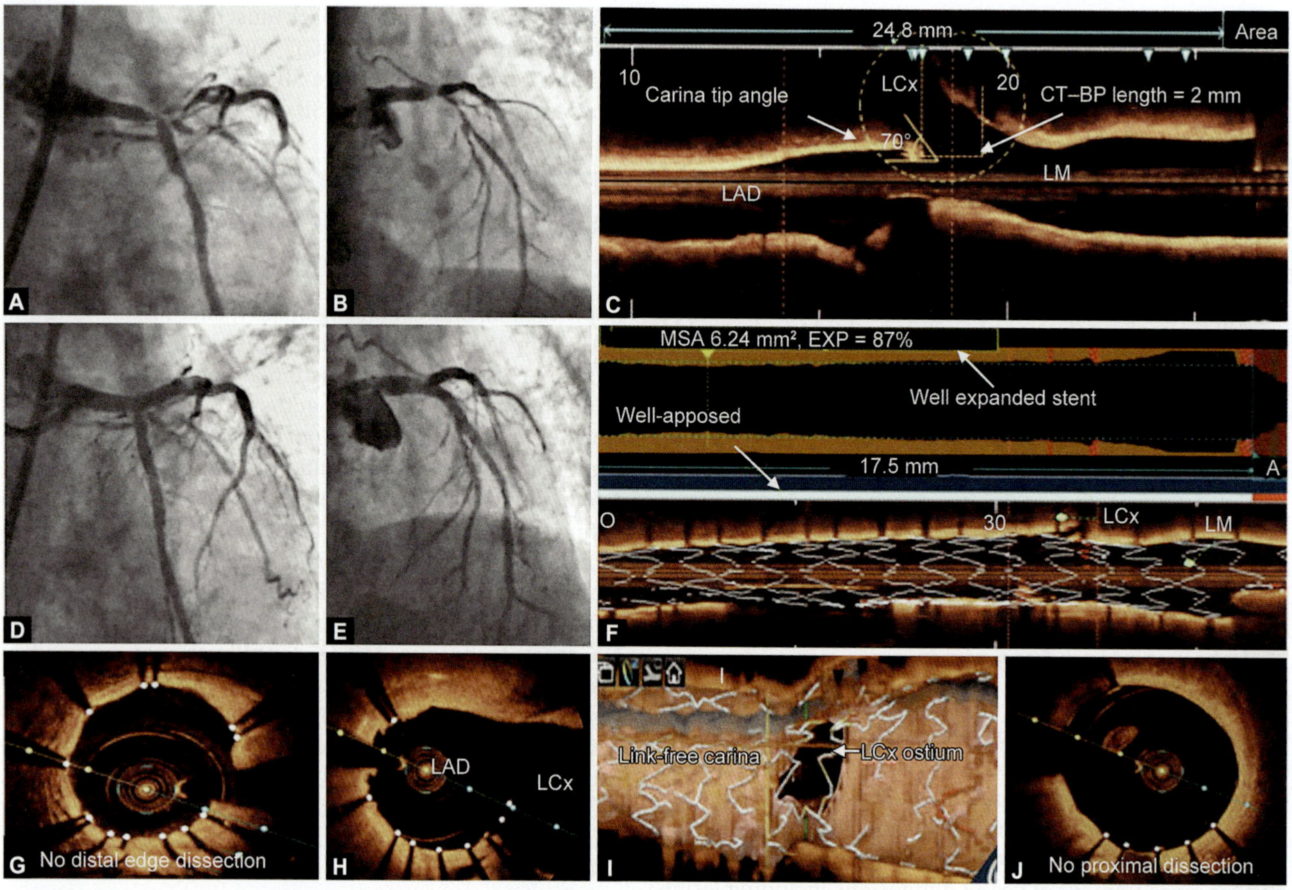

FIGS. 1A TO J: Optical coherence tomography (OCT) in bifurcation angioplasty. (A and B) Coronary angiography showed a significant left main (LM) bifurcation lesion (Medina 1,1,1). (C) Pre-percutaneous coronary intervention (PCI) OCT showed the carina tip (CT) angle of 70° and CT to bifurcation point (CT-BP length) of 2 mm suggestive of a bifurcation lesion suitable for provisional stenting without the risk of side branch (SB) compromise. (D) An OCT-guided LM-left anterior descending (LAD) crossover stenting was done followed by the proximal optimization technique (POT) with balloons of appropriate size. (E) Post-PCI angiography showed TIMI III flow in the left coronary system without left circumflex (LCx) compromise. Post-PCI OCT showed well-apposed stent with 87% expansion (F), without proximal or distal edge dissection (G and J), and minimal stent struts across LCx ostium (H). Three-dimensional (3D) reconstruction showed minimal inappropriate stent apposition across LCx ostium with link-free carina (I).

upfront two-stent strategy, both MB and SB OCT pullback are taken to assess segmental stent expansion, edge dissection, and apposition. MB OCT pullback after the final KBI is used to analyze the SB ostium. Hanging stent struts across the SB ostium can serve as a nidus for SB restenosis due to endothelization **(Figs. 2A to G)**. Hence, it should be ensured that SB ostium is free from hanging stent struts in the 3D reconstruction, with minimal neo-metallic carinal length in the L mode and the dumbbell sign or clear figure of 8 sign adjacent to the native carina in the B mode **(Figs. 3A to G)**.[23]

OPTICAL COHERENCE TOMOGRAPHY IN LEFT MAIN BIFURCATION PERCUTANEOUS CORONARY INTERVENTION

Left main lesions display specific features (diameter discrepancies between MB and SB, tapered anatomy, plaque eccentricity, and increased likelihood of calcifications) that are difficult to analyze correctly with angiography alone. Guidelines recommend IVUS for LM angioplasty, principally because of the theoretical limitations of OCT in imaging the LM body due to its bigger size and the LM ostia due to poor blood clearance. Recently, many trials have investigated OCT-guided mid and distal LM PCI with the results comparable, if not superior, to IVUS[24,25] and also demonstrated that 81% of OCT image frames in LM PCI were analyzable and that most of the nonanalyzable, artifact frames were in the proximal LM.[24]

The ROCK-1[26] retrospective study demonstrated that a substantial number of acute strut malapposition and stent underexpansion in bifurcation stenting were detected under OCT guidance. Compared with standard angiographic guidance alone, late lumen loss in a 6-month follow-up tended to be lower in the OCT group (0.12 ± 0.41 vs. 0.26 ± 0.52 mm, $p = 0.10$) and was significantly reduced in the distal portion of the MV (0.03 ± 0.45 vs. 0.24 ± 0.53 mm,

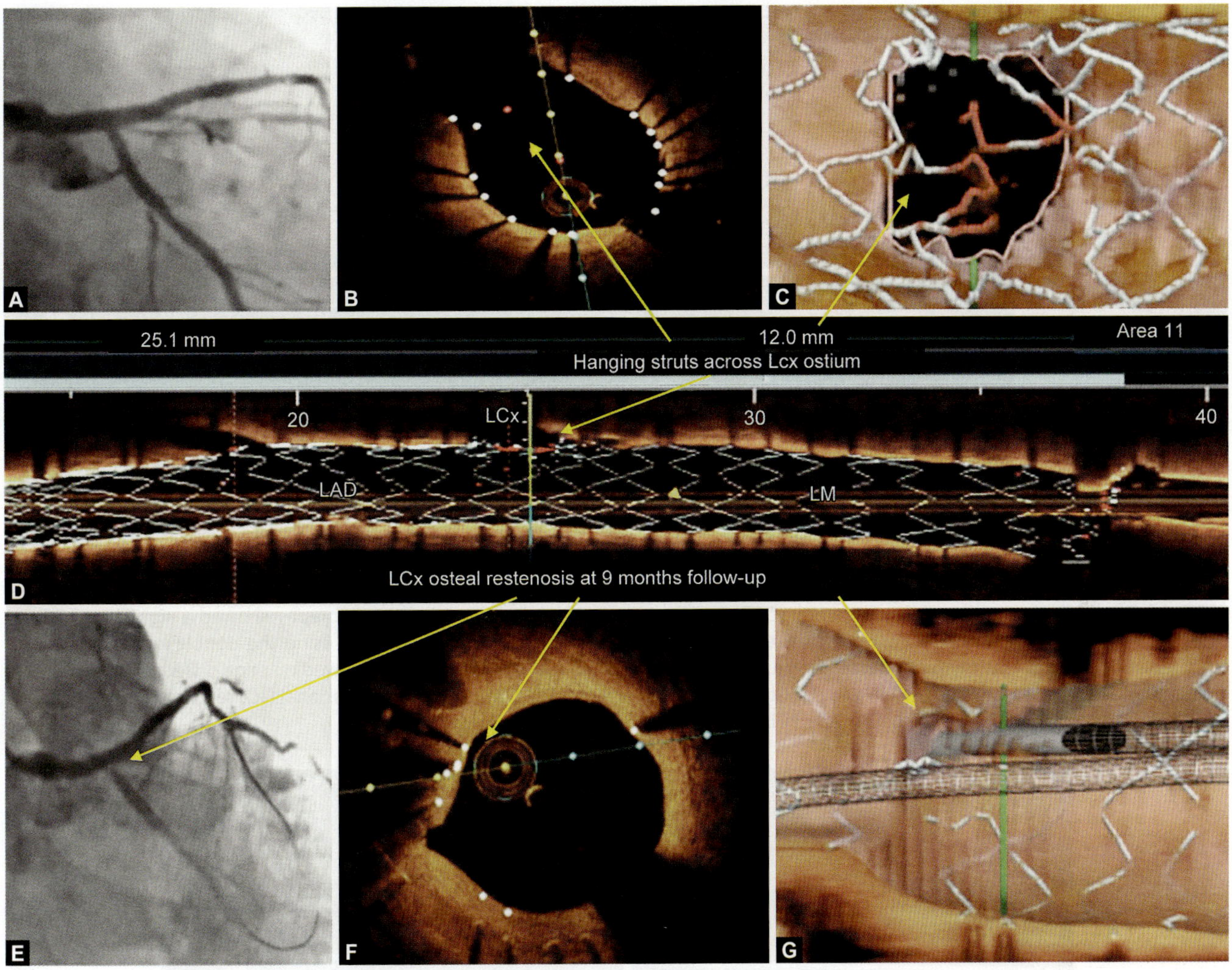

FIGS. 2A TO G: Optical coherence tomography (OCT) in bifurcation angioplasty. (A) The final angiogram picture after left main (LM) bifurcation angioplasty with two stents using the double kissing (DK) crush technique. The angiographic result for left circumflex (LCx) ostium was satisfactory, but OCT pullback of the main branch (MB) after final kissing balloon inflation (KBI) showed hanging stent struts (red) across LCx ostium on the cross-sectional view (B), on three-dimensional (3D) reconstruction (C), and on the rendered stent view (D). The same patient presented with crescendo angina after 9 months, and angiography showed LCx ostial in-stent restenosis (ISR) (E). OCT pullback of MB showed complete endothelization of hanging stent struts across LCx as a cause of ostial ISR (F and G).

(LAD: left anterior descending)

$p = 0.025$). In the 70 patients included in the final analysis of the LEMON study,[27] which aimed to analyze the feasibility, safety, and impact of OCT-guided LM PCI, the primary endpoint of procedural success was achieved in 86% of subjects. Adequate stent expansion was observed in 86%, significant edge dissection in 30%, and residual significant strut malapposition in 24% of the cases. OCT guidance modified operators' strategy in one out of four despite experienced operators and acceptable angiographic results. Additionally, 1-year survival free from major clinical adverse events was 98.6%. Therefore, we recommend OCT for distal LM bifurcation angioplasty performed either provisionally or with a two-stent strategy upfront as it can image most sizes of LM encountered by the interventionalist and has the distinct advantage of post-PCI SB ostial optimization compared with IVUS.

An aorto-ostial lesion, which has been a significant limitation of OCT, has recently been observed with the help of the soft polymer tip of the guide-extension catheter named "Telescope" (Medtronic Cardiovascular, Santa Rosa, CA, USA). This catheter has a helical coil constitution with a relatively wide gap that enables the penetration of infrared (IR) light through the soft polymer. It is certainly a step forward into the uncharted territory of OCT-guided ostial LM stenting. LM ostia can also be imaged by placing a guidewire in the aorta and aligning the guide catheter to the coronary ostia **(Figs. 4A to C)**.[23]

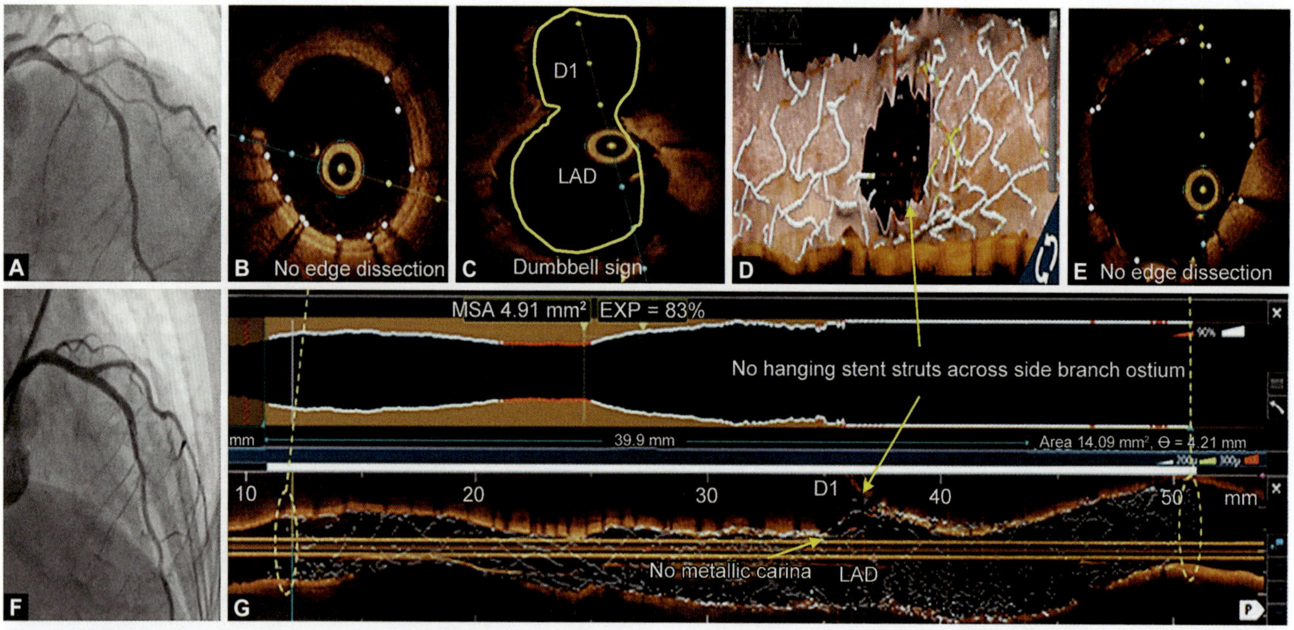

FIGS. 3A TO G: Optical coherence tomography (OCT) in bifurcation angioplasty. Coronary angiography showed a significant LAD/D1 stenosis (A) with Medina class (1,1,1). Patient underwent bifurcation angioplasty with two stents using the double kissing (DK) crush technique (F). OCT run of left anterior descending (LAD) after final kissing balloon inflation (KBI) showed no edge dissection (B and E) and clear figure of 8 or dumbbell sign (C). No hanging stent struts seen across D1 ostium on three-dimensional (3D) reconstruction (D) and on L mode (G). No neo-metallic carina seen at LAD/D1 bifurcation on the rendered stent view (G).

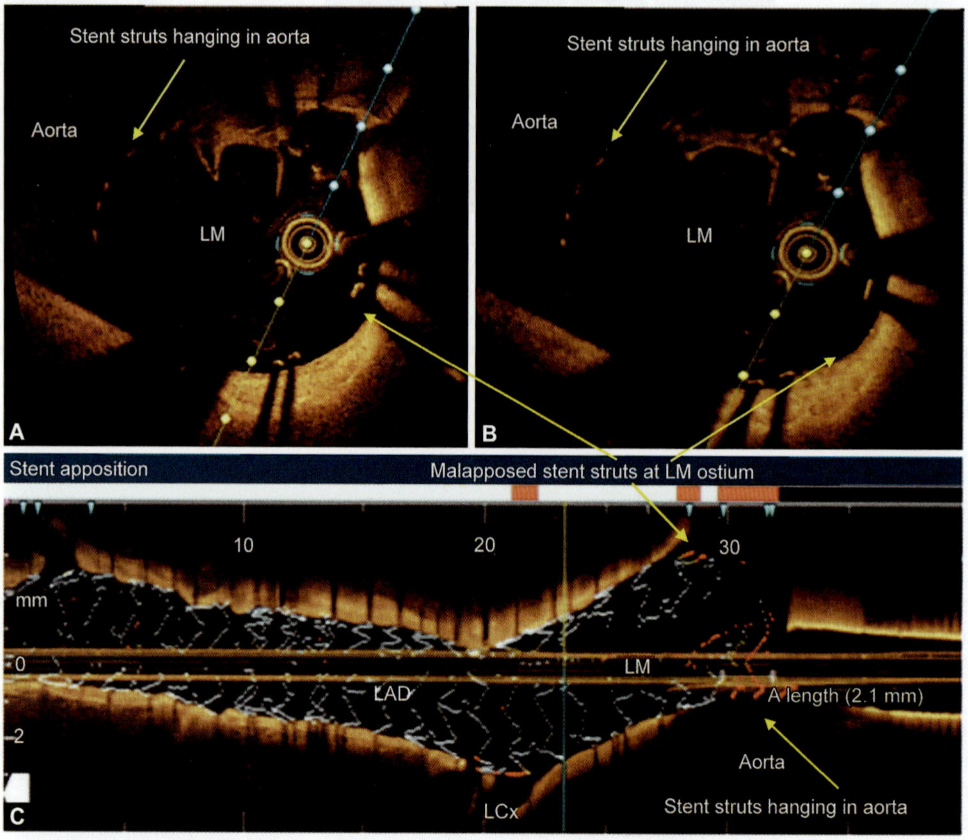

FIGS. 4A TO C: Left main ostial imaging with optical coherence tomography (OCT). OCT pullback from left anterior descending (LAD) to left main (LM) after provisional LM ostial to LAD crossover angioplasty with one wire in the aorta. Hanging stent struts in the aorta (suggestive of LM ostial coverage) can be clearly seen along with some malapposed struts in both the cross-sectional and rendered stent views.

(LCx: left circumflex)

TRIALS IN PROGRESS

There are multiple trials in progress evaluating the use of OCT in coronary bifurcation lesions. The OCTOBER and DOCTORS-Recross trials compare the OCT-guided bifurcation PCI with the standard angiography-guided PCI. The OPTIMUM trial assesses the 3D optical frequency domain imaging with angiography in bifurcation PCI.

CONCLUSION

Bifurcation PCI should be done under image guidance. High resolution and 3D reconstruction ability of OCT makes it superior to IVUS for bifurcation PCI. 3D OCT-guided optimization of SB ostium during two-stent strategy for complex LM bifurcation angioplasty is expected to improve the long-term SB outcomes.

ONLINE REFERENCES

Please scan the QR code provided at the end of the table of contents for References of this chapter.

CHAPTER

171

Optical Coherence Tomography in Stent Failure

Selvamani S, Thomas Xavier Paulsingh JS

ABSTRACT

The field of interventional cardiology started its career in 1977 by Andreas Gruentzig who did the first coronary balloon angioplasty. The arterial restenosis rate was high with plain balloon angioplasty due to elastic recoiling; bare metal stents (BMSs) were discovered to overcome this issue. But they were more prone for neointimal hyperplasia (NIH)-induced in-stent restenosis (ISR). This led to the discovery of drug-eluting stents (DESs). Even with the latest generation DES, the prevalence of stent failure due to restenosis and stent thrombosis (ST) is relatively unchanged.

Optical coherence tomography (OCT) is the best imaging technology to find out the mechanisms of stent failure to guide the further mode of treatment.

Keywords: Stent thrombosis, neointimal hyperplasia, minimum luminal area (MLA).

INTRODUCTION

Coronary stents played important role in the management of acute coronary syndrome (ACS) and chronic coronary syndrome with large ischemic burden. The latest generation drug-eluting stents (DESs) are having better long-term results compared to the older generation DES and bare metal stents (BMSs). Stent failure is the term used to describe the earlier and late complications associated with stenting. It includes in-stent restenosis (ISR) and stent thrombosis (ST). Both remain a challenge in interventional cardiology and both are associated with recurrence of symptoms and may need re-intervention with either re-percutaneous coronary intervention (PCI) or bypass graft. The prevalence of stent failure or target lesion revascularization is up to 20% in various registries.[1-4] Intravascular imaging has major role in the treatment of stent failure. The routine use of intravascular imaging has IIa/C indication in the European Society of Cardiology guidelines for detecting causes of stent failure.[5]

IN-STENT RESTENOSIS

The incidence of ISR is up to 10% with second-generation DES.[6,7] It is defined as a luminal narrowing with >50% diameter stenosis of a stented coronary segment or within 5 mm of a stent edge.[8] Intravascular imaging criteria for ISR is >70% reduction in luminal area **(Box 1)**.[9]

Factors Influencing In-stent Restenosis

Box 1 shows the factors influencing ISR.

Role of Optical Coherence Tomography

Intravascular imaging is essential to identify the pathogenesis of ISR which is essential to guide treatment strategy. As optical coherence tomography (OCT) has higher resolution compared with intravascular ultrasound (IVUS), it clearly identifies the pathogenesis of ISR.[10,11] Waksman classified ISR into five types based on the disease process in intravascular imaging **(Table 1)**.[12]

Stent Underexpansion (Type I A)

It is defined as stent expansion <80% minimum stent area (MSA) compared with average reference lumen area or MSA < 4.5 mm^2 by OCT.[13] Identifying the tissue composition can guide device selection. Soft tissue responds to high-pressure balloon dilatation. Calcified tissue may require rotablation, intravascular lithotripsy (IVL), or laser **(Fig. 1)**.[14]

BOX 1 Factors influencing in-stent restenosis.

- *Pharmacological:*
  - Drug resistance (dual antiplatelet therapy)
  - Hypersensitivity to drug
  - Hypersensitivity to polymer
- *Biological:*
  - Plasma proteolytic enzymes
  - Matrix metalloproteinases
- *Patient:*
  - Diabetes
  - Older age
  - Female
  - Genetic
- *Mechanical:*
  - Stent malapposition
  - Stent underexpansion
  - Edge trauma
  - Geographical miss
  - Stent fracture
- *Lesion:*
  - Type B/C
  - Long >20 mm
  - Small vessel <3 mm
  - Calcified
  - Bifurcation disease
  - Chronic total occlusion
  - Ostial or tortuous segment

Stent Fracture (Type I B)

Absence of metal scaffolding and limited drug delivery provide the substrate for neointima proliferation. Risk factors are tortuous vessels, right coronary artery, and longer stents. 3D reconstructed OCT images clearly identify stent fracture.[15,16]

Treatment: Percutaneous transluminal coronary angioplasty (PTCA) **(Figs. 2A and B)**.

Neointimal Hyperplasia (Type II A)

It is one of the most common causes of ISR of DES. Homogenous bright uniform layer is characterized of neointimal hyperplasia (NIH). Treatment often involves

TABLE 1: Waksman in-stent restenosis classification.

Type	Definition	
I	Mechanical	Underexpansion (Type I A)
		Stent fracture (Type I B)
II	Biologic	Intimal hyperplasia (Type II A)
		Neoatherosclerosis, noncalcified (Type II B)
		Neoatherosclerosis, calcified (Type II C)
III	Mixed pattern: Combined mechanical and biologic etiology	
IV	Chronic total occlusion	
V	More than two layers of stent	

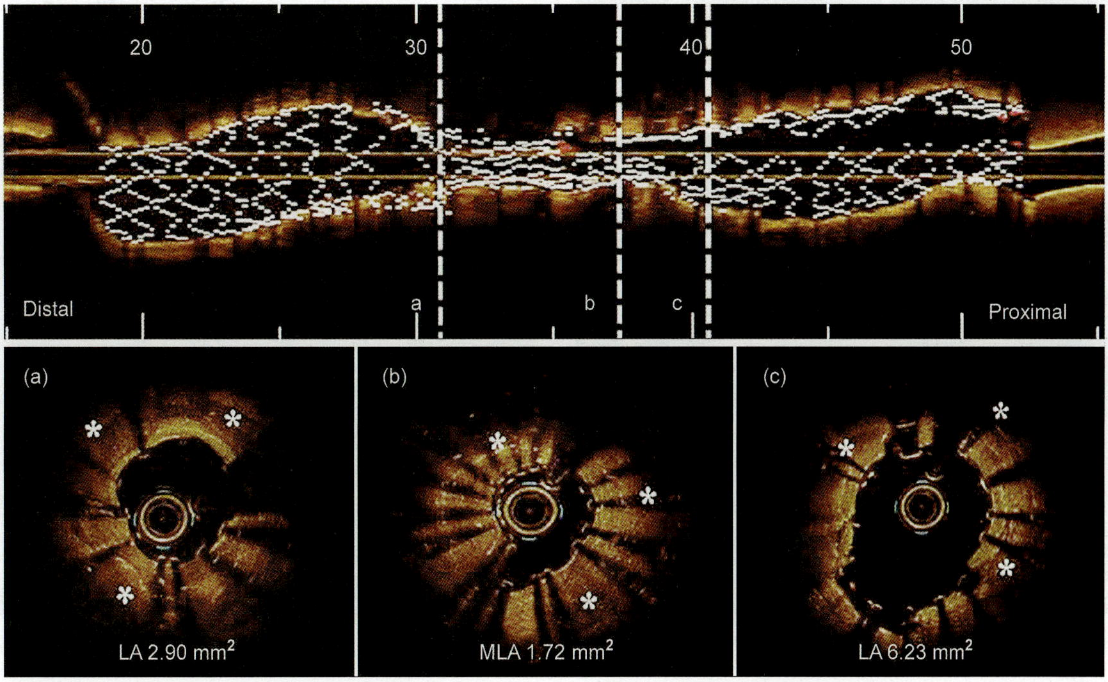

FIG. 1: Stent underexpansion.
(LA: lumen area; MLA: minimum lumen area)

balloon angioplasty with specialty balloons including cutting or scoring balloons to modify the neointimal tissue. Following modification, drug-eluting balloon (DEB) or DES should be used. Vascular brachytherapy (VBT) plays main role in the management of recurrent NIH **(Fig. 3)**.[17-20]

Neoatherosclerosis (Type II B and C)

Characteristic feature is heterogeneous pattern with lipid or thin cap fibroatheroma (TCFA). It may be noncalcified or calcified. Treatment is based on the underlying plaque morphology and it should be treated like de novo lesions. Calcified lesions may require special devices **(Fig. 4)**.

Mixed Pattern (Type III)

Combined mechanical and biologic patterns of restenosis are common in a single lesion.

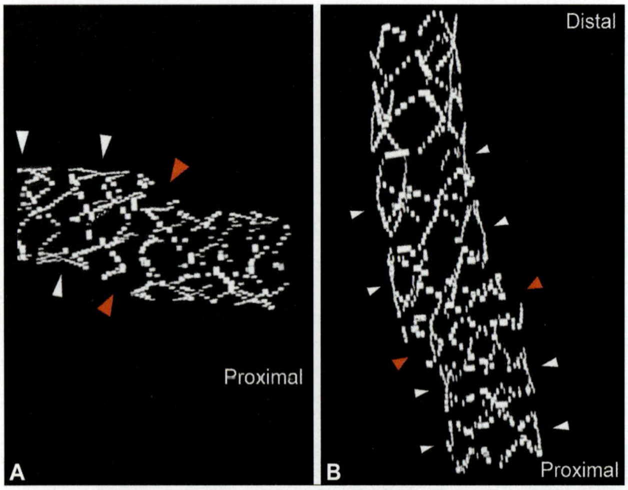

FIGS. 2A AND B: Stent fracture.

Treatment: High-pressure noncompliant (NC) balloon with DCB, DES, or vascular brachytherapy (VBT).

Chronic Total Occlusion (Type IV)

Following recanalization, they should be treated according to the underlying lesion morphology.

Preferred treatment: DCB or DES, VBT for multiple layers, coronary artery bypass graft (CABG) as needed.

Recurrent Restenosis (Type V)

Treatment of recurrent ISR is challenging because event rate is up to 20 % in 1-year follow-up. VBT should be considered in patients who had more than two layers of stent.

Edge Dissection or Increased Plaque at Stent Edge

Increased plaque (>54.5%) or lipid burden (>185°) at the edges of stent and the presence of edge dissections are predictors of ISR. ISR with residual plaque at the stent edge or major edge dissections with length >3 mm or circumferential extent >60° should be treated by another stent **(Flowchart 1)**.[21,22]

STENT THROMBOSIS

Stent thrombosis is a serious complication following coronary intervention. It usually presents like STEMI (ST-segment elevation myocardial infarction), non-STEMI (NSTEMI), or sudden cardiac death. Rarely, it will be asymptomatic due to collaterals **(Figs. 5 and 6 and Table 2)**.

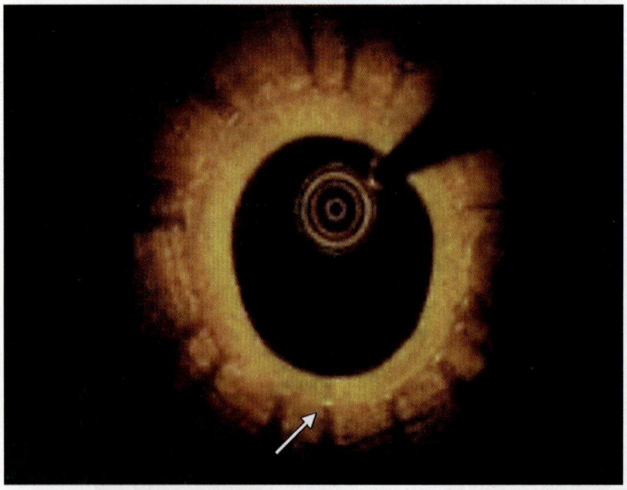

FIG. 3: Neointimal hyperplasia.

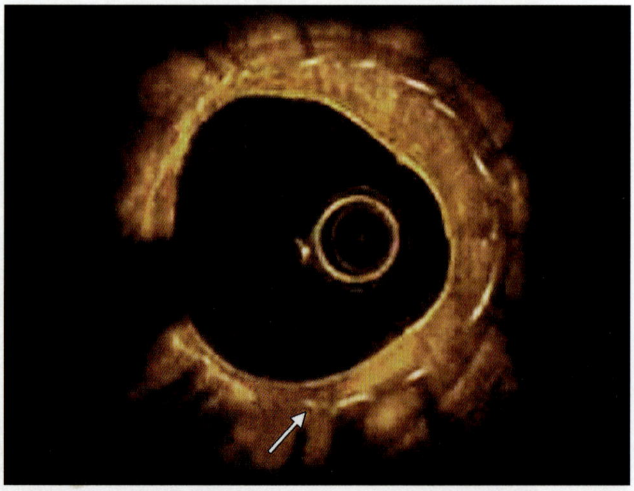

FIG. 4: Neoatherosclerosis.

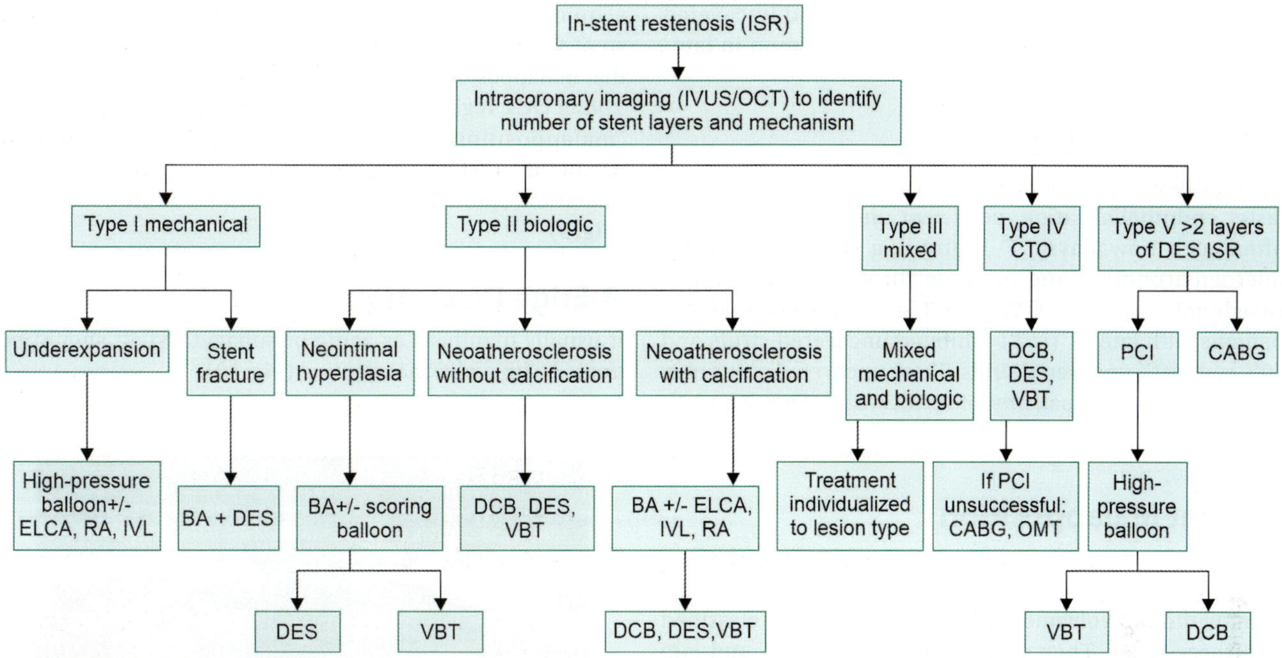

FLOWCHART 1: In-stent restenosis.

(BA: balloon angioplasty; CABG: coronary artery bypass graft; CTO: chronic total occlusion; DCB: drug-coated balloon; DES: drug-eluting stent; ELCA: excimer laser coronary atherectomy; IVL: intravascular lithotripsy; IVUS: intravascular ultrasound; OCT: optical coherence tomography; OMT: optimal medical therapy; PCI: percutaneous coronary intervention; RA: rotational atherectomy; VBT: vascular brachytherapy)

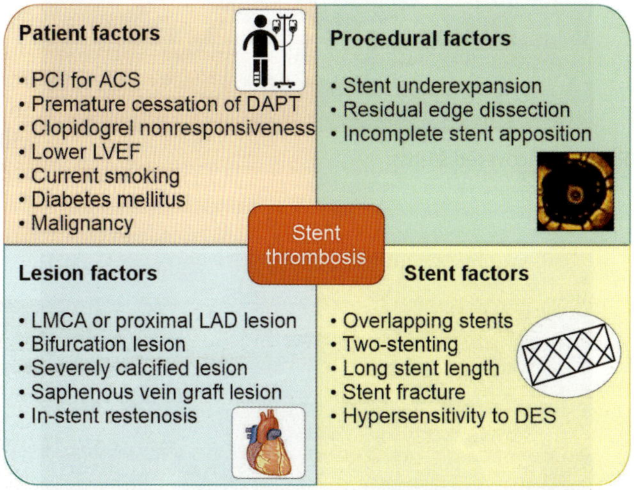

FIG. 5: Stent thrombosis.

(ACS: acute coronary syndrome; DAPT: dual antiplatelet therapy; LAD: left anterior descending; LMCA: left main coronary artery; LVEF: left ventricular ejection fraction; PCI: percutaneous coronary intervention)

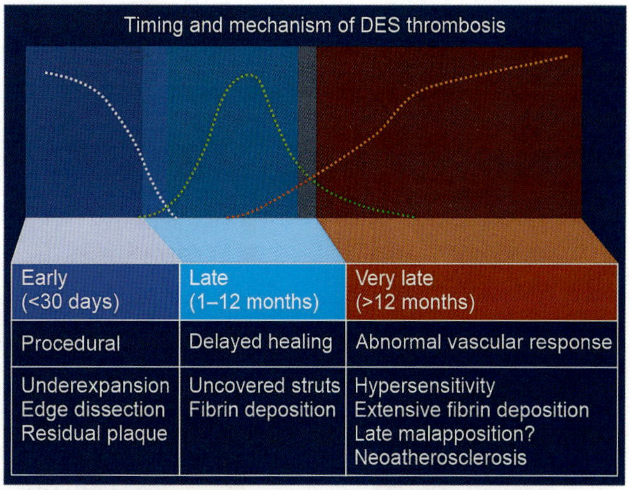

FIG. 6: Timing and mechanisms of stent thrombosis (ST).

(DES: drug-eluting stent)

TABLE 2: Classification of stent thrombosis (ST) in correlation with time frame.

Timing	Stent thrombosis	Time frame
Early	Acute ST	<24 hours
	Subacute ST	24 hours to 30 days
Late ST		31 days to 1 year
Very late ST		>1 year

Role of Optical Coherence Tomography in Stent Thrombosis

Intravascular OCT may provide insights into mechanistic processes leading to ST. *PRESGTIGE* registry collected the OCT findings in patients presented with ST. Uncovered and malapposed struts were frequently observed and the prevalence of both decreased with increasing time interval from the index stenting. Uncovered struts and underexpansion were most common in acute/subacute ST, and uncovered struts and neoatherosclerosis were most common in late/very late ST.[23]

Uncovered Stents

Though newer generation thin strut stents have enabled faster endothelialization, persistent uncovered stents are often seen nowadays.[24,25] Protruding struts affect local microenvironment and promote thrombus formation.[26] Guagliumi et al. in JACC 2012 OCT study revealed that 80% patients with late ST (LST) exhibited uncovered struts and 70% had >30% uncovered struts. These uncovered struts may persist in 20% of the patients for up to 2 years **(Figs. 7 and 8)**.

Treatment: Optimize dual antiplatelet therapy (DAPT).

Stent Malapposition

It is defined as separation of at least one strut from the intimal surface of the arterial wall with evidence of blood behind the strut, without involvement of side branches. It is classified into three types. They are early, late persistent, and late acquired. OCT clearly differentiated from well-expanded stent with positive remodeling. DETECT OCT trial found that malapposition distance >0.4 mm is a risk factor for ST.[27] *Yonsei* OCT registry showed that significant malapposition (malapposition volume ≥7 mm^3) is an independent predictor of ST.[28] Treatment should focus on aggressive dilatation. Another stent implantation should be avoided **(Fig. 9)**.[13]

Edge Dissection

It usually manifests as acute or subacute ST. It should be treated with additional stenting **(Fig. 10)**.[29]

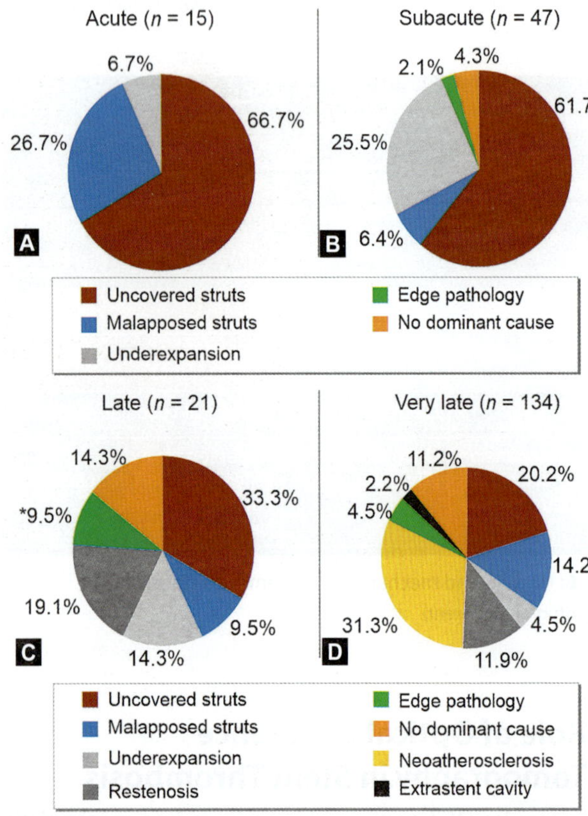

FIGS. 7A TO D: Findings of Prestige registry.[23]

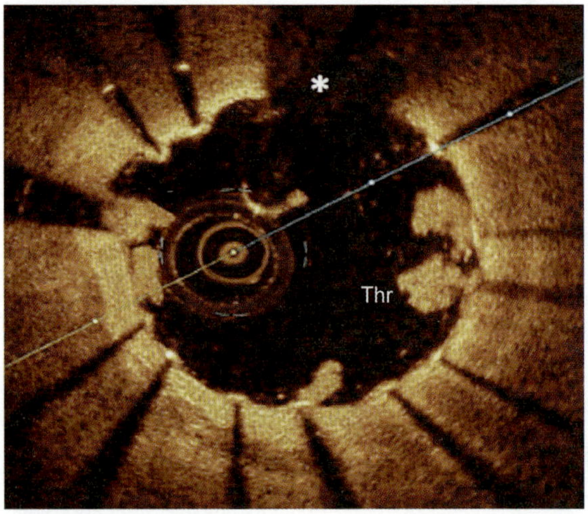

FIG. 8: Uncovered stents.

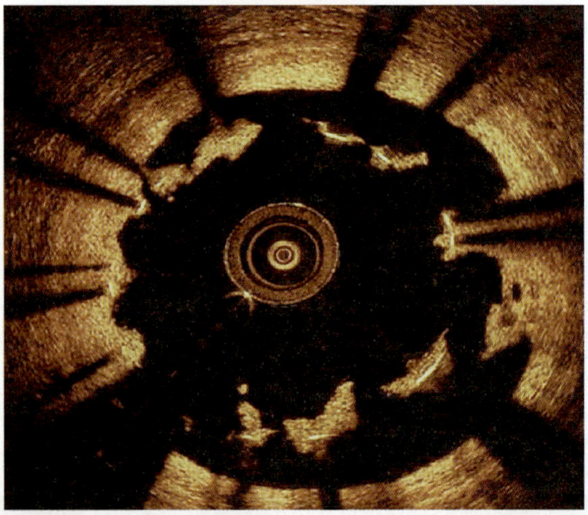

FIG. 9: Stent malapposition.

Underexpansion and Undersized Stent

Proper prestenting analysis is essential to prevent this complication. It can be treated with aggressive postdilatation.[30]

Neoatherosclerosis

It is one of the most common causes of late and very late ST.[31] OCT is superior to IVUS to diagnose neoatherosclerosis and superimposed thrombus.[32] Treatment is similar to de novo lesions **(Fig. 11)**.[33]

CONCLUSION

Stent failure secondary to ISR and ST remains a challenging clinical problem. Utilization of diagnostic tools such as intravascular imaging (OCT or IVUS) and intravascular imaging (OCT or IVUS) and fractional flow reserve (FFR), provides better insights compared with angiography alone, and permits more focused therapies to treat these lesions. There is no universal single line of treatment and patients may require special devices for long-term good result **(Flowchart 2 and 3)**.

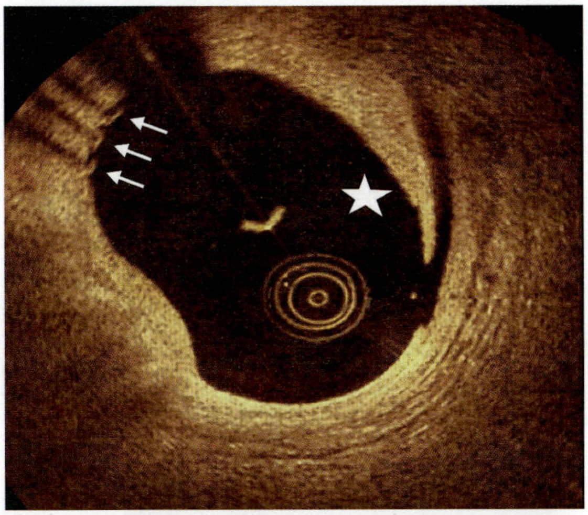

FIG. 10: Edge dissection.

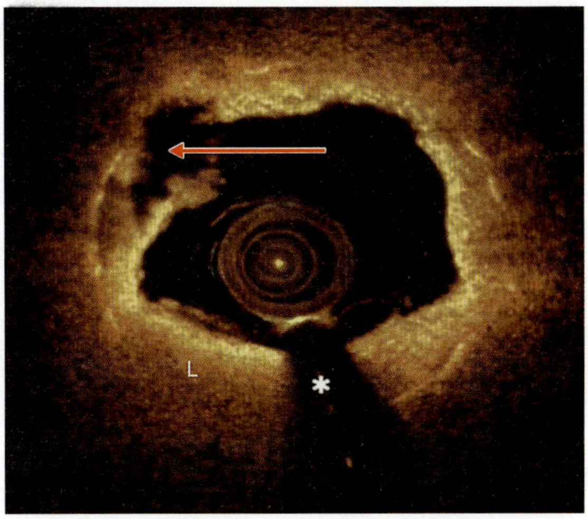

FIG. 11: New atherosclerosis with lipid rich plaque.

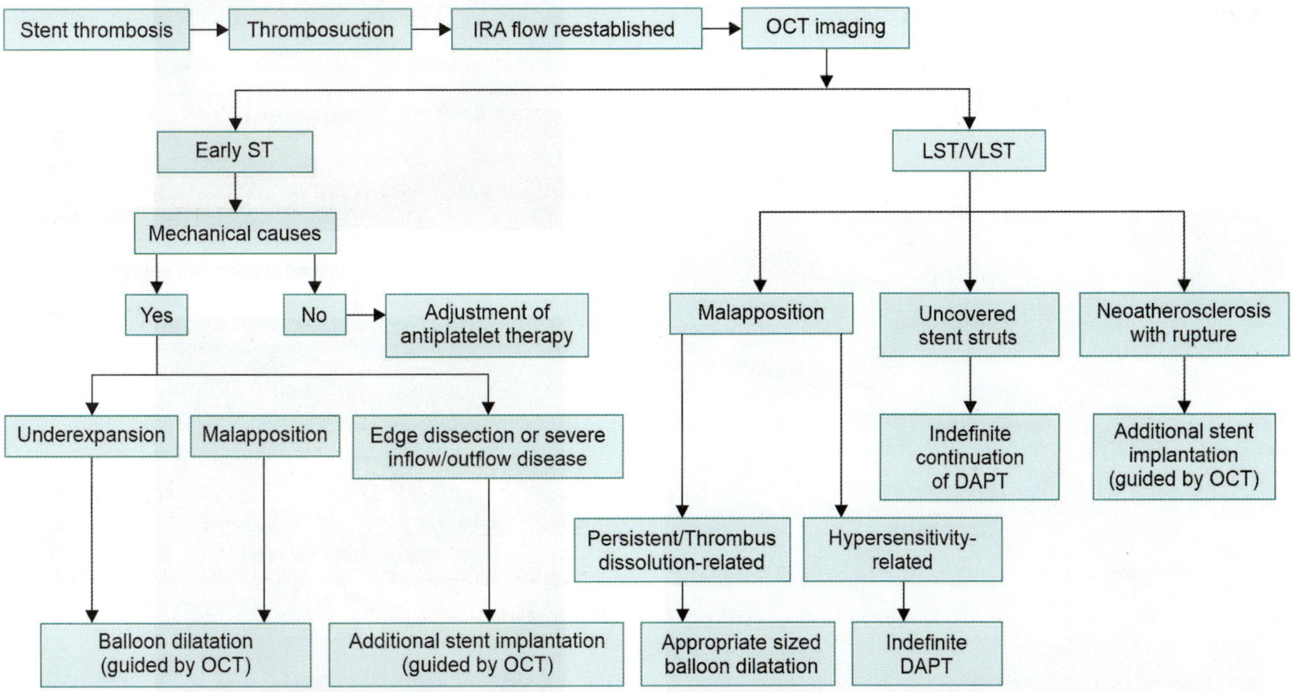

FLOWCHART 2: Algorithm for stent thrombosis (ST).[34]

(DAPT: dual antiplatelet therapy; IRA: infarct-related artery; LST: late stent thrombosis; OCT: optical coherence tomography; VLST: very late stent thrombosis)

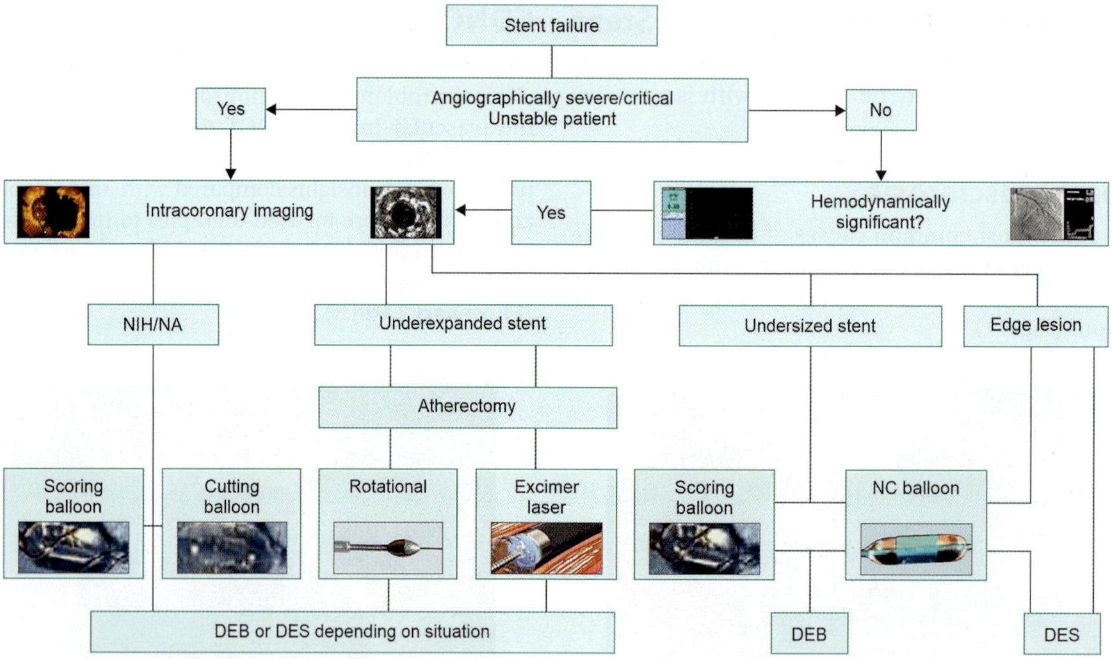

FLOWCHART 3: Algorithm for stent failure.[35]
(DEB: drug-eluting balloon; DES: drug-eluting stent; NA: neoatherosclerosis; NC: noncompliant; NIH: neointimal hyperplasia)

CASE 1 (FIGS. 12 TO 14)

A 63-year-old diabetic male S/P PTCA to left anterior descending (LAD) 3 years back presented with rest angina.

CASE 2 (FIGS. 15 AND 16)

A 65-year-old male, recent anterior wall myocardial infarction (AWMI), S/P PTCA to LAD 1 month back presented with ACS–NSTEMI.

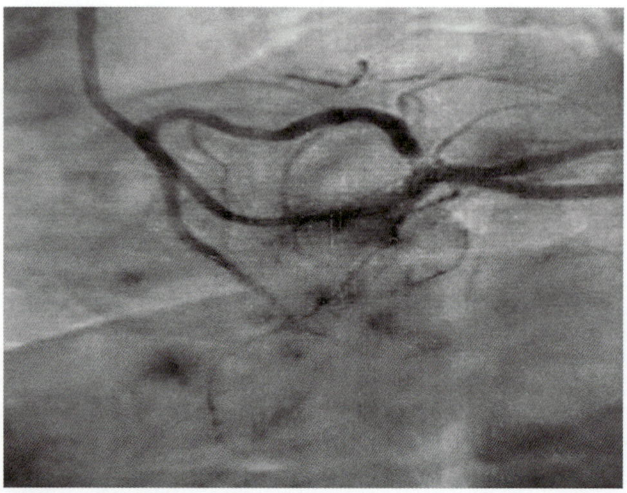

FIG. 12: Coronary angiography (CAG): In-stent restenosis (ISR) of left anterior descending (LAD) stent.

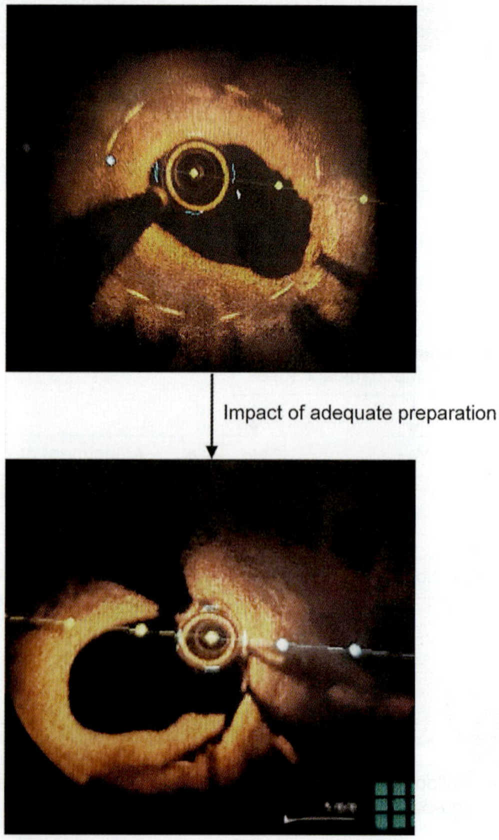

FIG. 13: Optical coherence tomography (OCT)—heterogeneous growth and impact of adequate preparation with cutting balloon.

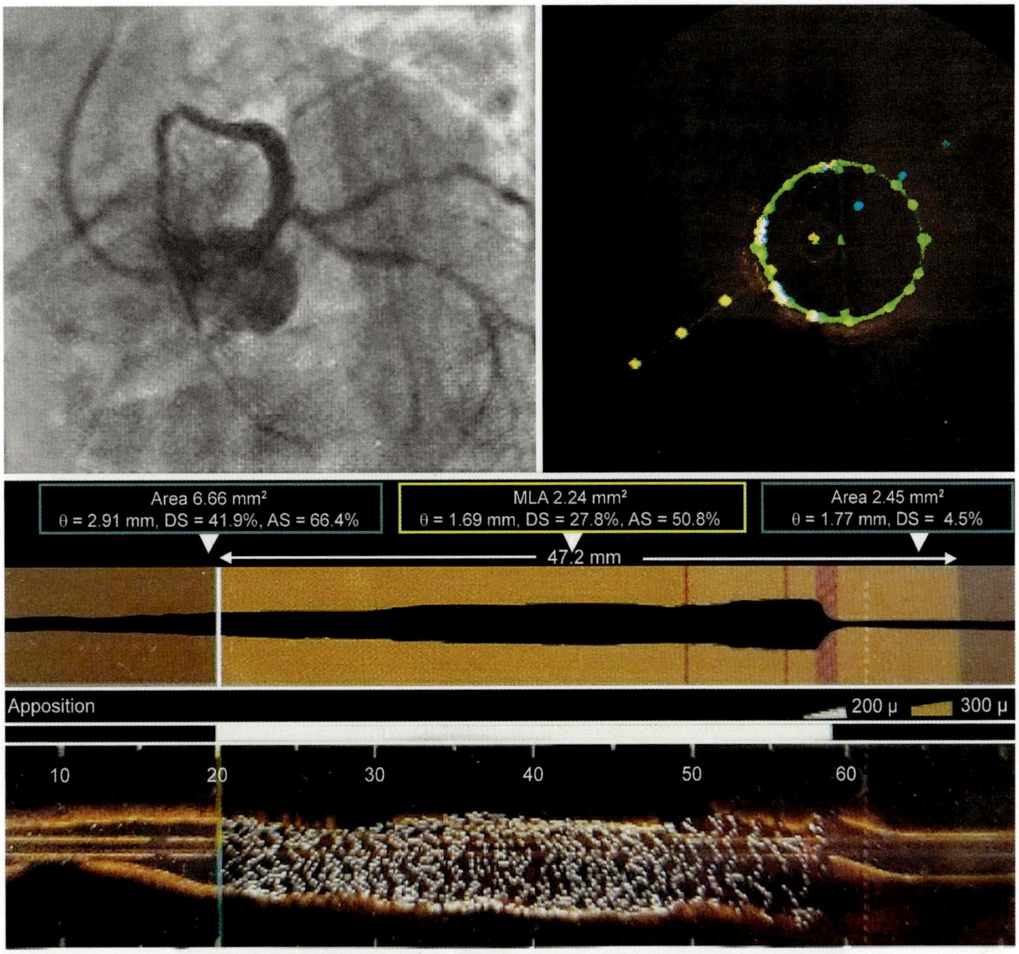

FIG. 14: Final result—left main coronary artery (LMCA) to left anterior descending (LAD) stenting.

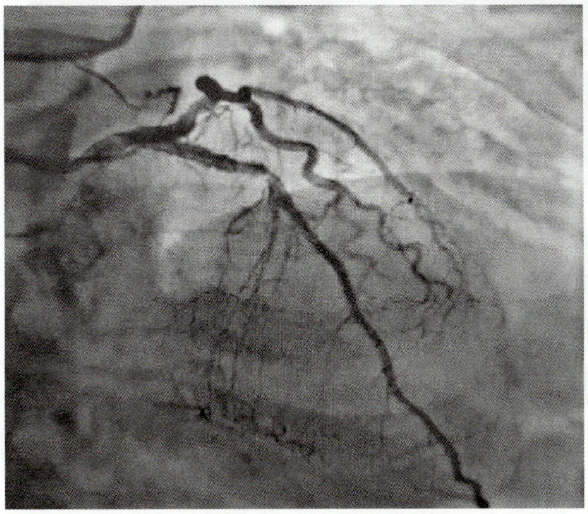

FIG. 15: Coronary angiography (CAG)—suspected thrombus in left anterior descending (LAD) stent.

CASE 3 (FIG. 17)

A 50-year-old male who developed acute ST following PTCA to left circumflex (LCX) 10 hours back has been referred here for image-guided further management.

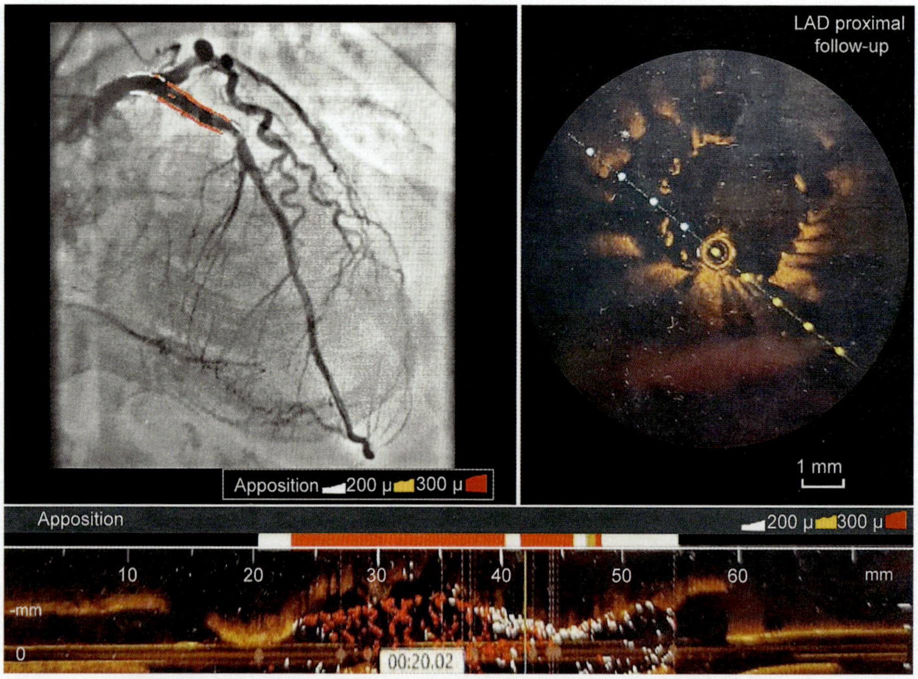

FIG. 16: Optical coherence tomography (OCT)—stent thrombosis due to polymer reaction.

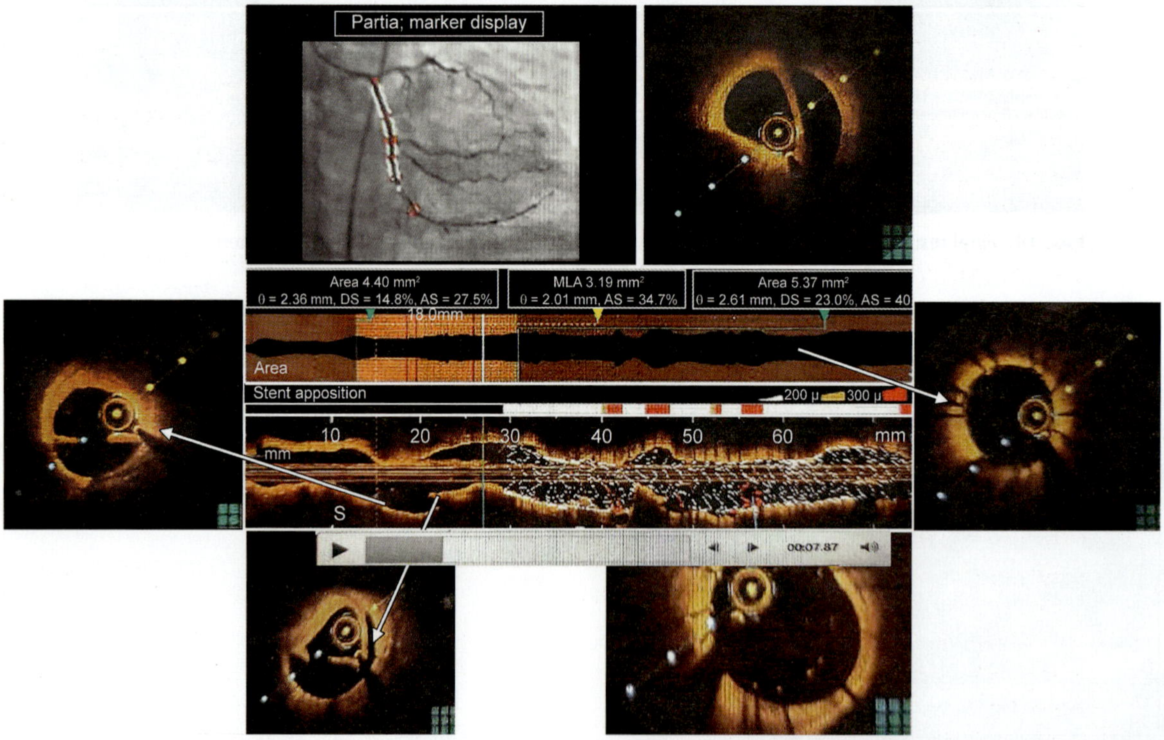

FIG. 17: Optical coherence tomography (OCT)—distal edge dissection, middle significant malapposition, and proximal underexpansion. A case of ST with multiple risk factors.

(ST: stent thrombosis)

ONLINE REFERENCES

Please scan the QR code provided at the end of the table of contents for References of this chapter.

SECTION 20

Structural Intervention

CHAPTER

172

Imaging in TAVR

Manoj Kumar Agarwala, Siddharth Bajaj

ABSTRACT

The most commonly acquired valve disease is aortic valve stenosis. Transcatheter aortic valve replacement (TAVR) offers treatment of severe aortic stenosis to those at high surgical risk. As there is no direct visualization of the valve, TAVR relies on meticulous preprocedure imaging to preplan implant selection and form a virtual roadmap of the truncal vasculature and the access pathway. Multidetector computed tomography (MDCT), a well-validated tool, is the gold standard in preprocedure planning for TAVR. For annular sizing, calcium burden, morphology of leaflet, and coronary assessment-gated sequencing is used, while for noncardiac structures, ungated imaging is sufficient.

Keywords: Multidetector computed tomography, aortic stenosis (AS), sinus of valsalva (SOV), sinotubular junction (STJ), transcatheter aortic valve implantation (TAVI), transcatheter aortic valve replacement, electrocardiogram (ECG).

INTRODUCTION

In his chapter, we discuss the important aspects of imaging for transcatheter aortic valve replacement (TAVR) in the native aortic valve.

AORTIC ANNULUS

The annulus mentioned in computed tomography (CT) TAVR measurements is not an anatomic annulus but a virtual annulus—a ring that is formed by the basal hinge points of the valve cusps,[1] measured with multiplanar reconstruction. The annulus is ovoid in most cases rather than circular[2] **(Figs. 1A and B)**.

Identification and positioning of the annular plane can be performed as follows **(Table 1)**:

- Manually utilizing standard multiplanar reformats
- Utilizing a software-based facilitating workflow along with manual identification of the basal hinge points, then placing marker points with subsequent positioning of the plane by the software

ANNULAR DYNAMISM AND PHASE SELECTION

Measurements of the annulus should be performed using electrocardiogram (ECG)-synchronized, ideally multiphasic dataset.

The anatomy of the aortic annulus should be reviewed throughout the cardiac cycle and importantly the phase that yields the largest dimensions with adequate image quality should be identified. There is decrease in ellipticity as well as stretch of the annular contour and hence resulting in larger dimensions in systole than diastole, in parts due to bulging of the aortomitral continuity toward the left atrium in systole and flattening in diastole. In septal hypertrophy, due to bulging of the basal septum into the annulus during systole, annular dimensions are smaller in systole than diastole.

Perimeter or Area

Having an appreciation of the anatomy of the aortic valve, its elliptical profile, and its potential to change geometrically

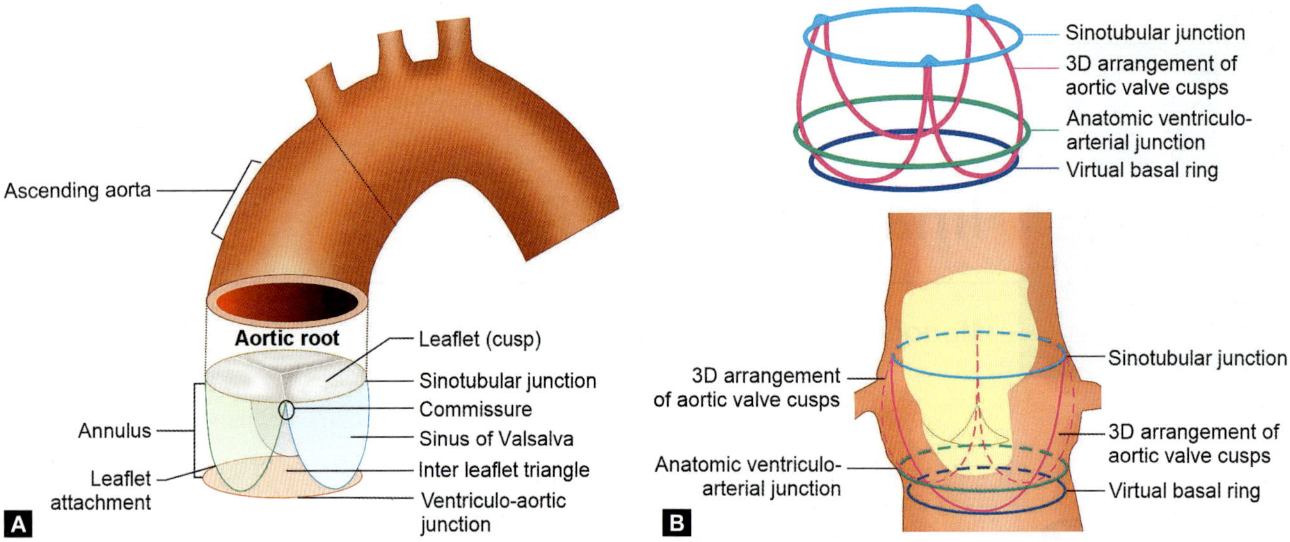

FIGS. 1A AND B: Aortic annulus (on the left) and aortic root (on the right) with all their components. The measured annulus in transcatheter aortic valve replacement (TAVR) sizing is the virtual ring formed by the basal hinge points of the valve cusps.

TABLE 1: To identify the annular plane.

Steps and descriptions	Multiplanar reformats
Step 1: Start out with multiplanar images in default axial, sagittal, and coronal orientation; center crosshairs onto the aortic valve	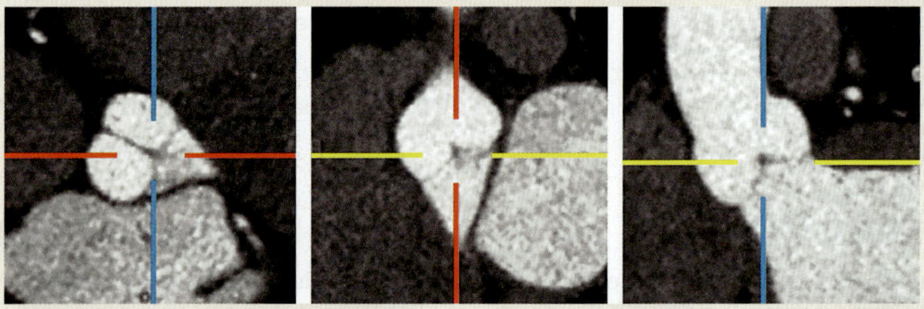
Step 2: Align the crosshairs in the sagittal and coronal views with the long axis of the aortic root; the resulting double oblique transverse view will depict the aortic valve en face	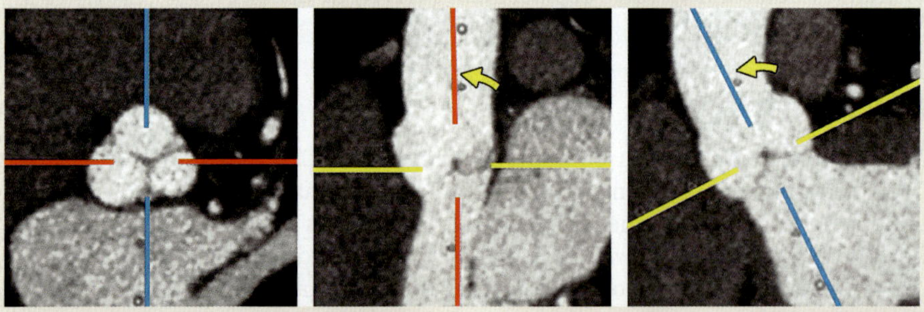
Step 3: Move the double-oblique transverse plane up and down to identify the lowest insertion point of the right coronary cusp which is usually located at about 1 o'clock. Position the center of the crosshairs exactly at the most basal insertion point of the right coronary cusp (white arrowhead)	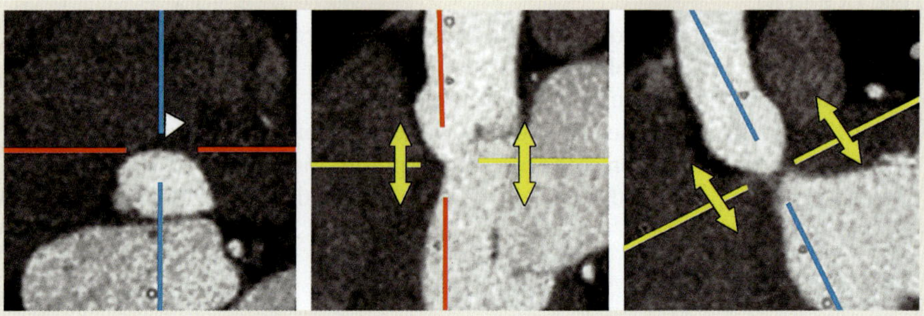

Continued

Continued

Steps and descriptions	Multiplanar reformats
Step 4: Rotate the crosshairs counterclockwise without moving up and down while maintaining its center position so that the formerly coronal view (here red crosshair) transects the lowest insertion point of the noncoronary cusp, which is located at approximately 8 o'clock (white arrowhead)	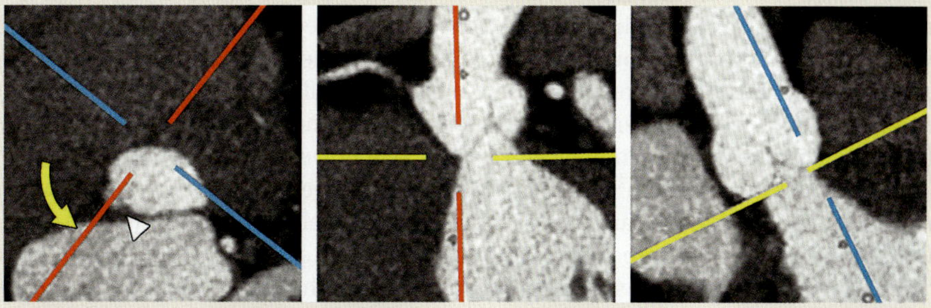
Step 5: The formerly coronal, now double-oblique view will show the lowest insertion point both of the right coronary cusp and the noncoronary cusp (white arrow heads). In this view, rotate the (here orange) crosshair, indicating the double-oblique transverse view to transect exactly through the most basal insertion point of the non-coronary cusps. Once this is achieved, the transverse double-oblique plane will contain two of the three lowest cusp insertion points	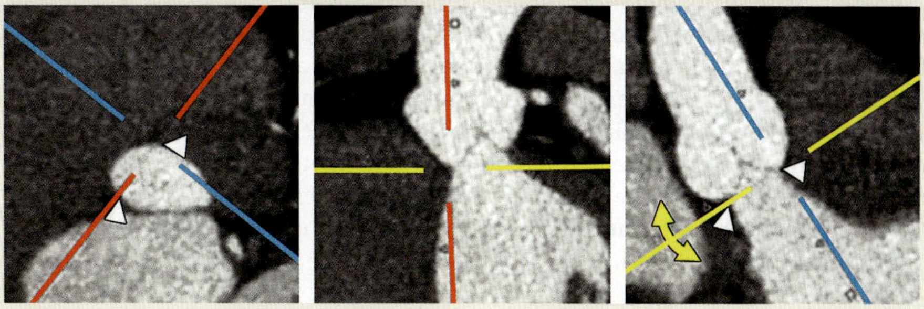
Step 6: In the formerly sagittal view, rotate (without moving it) the crosshair of the transverse double-oblique plane (here orange) until the lowest insertion point of the left coronary cusp just barely appears in the double-oblique transverse view (white arrowhead). Now, the formerly axial plane is exactly aligned with the lowest cusp insertion points of all three aortic cusps and represents both the orientation as well as the level of the annular plane	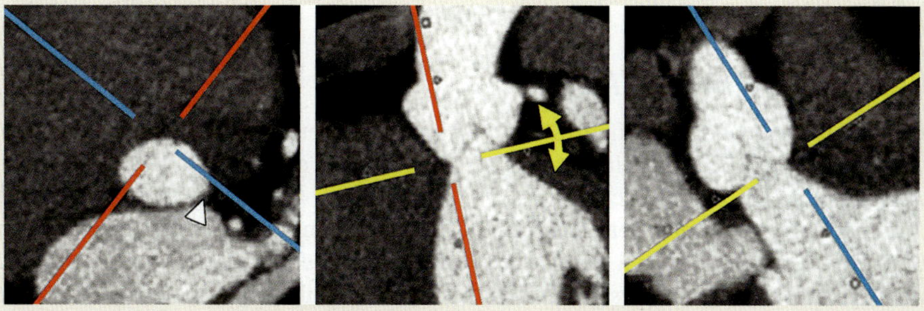
Step 7: Measurements of aortic annulus dimensions should be performed in the annular plane by means of a contouring tool	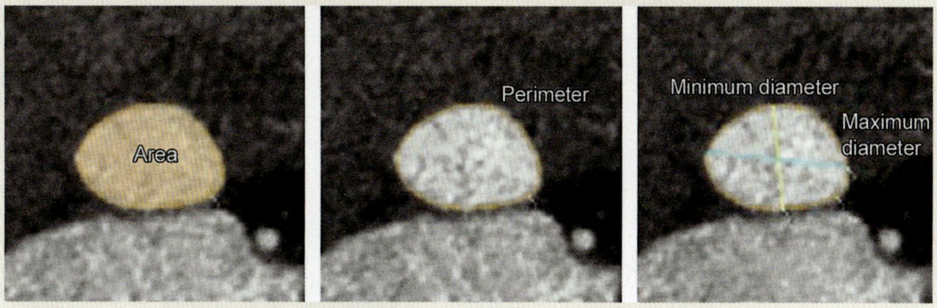

during the cardiac cycle, it is then interesting to consider the impact of these characteristics on annular sizing. Recent sizing charts for commercially available, implantable valves are based on three-dimensional (3D) area-derived measurements. There is, however, debate as to whether perimeter is actually the more appropriate measure. While good correlation has been demonstrated between area and perimeter measures with seemingly equal predictive power for paravalvular regurgitation[2,3] there are logical advantages in adopting the latter. As the annulus becomes progressively oval, area measurements are subject to potentially greater error as the area reduces in size disproportionately to the perimeter, leading to potential underestimation of the true annular dimensions, an important potential source of unintentional undersizing.[4] It is important to note that oversizing may impinge on the conduction system, increasing the risk of bundle branch block or complete heart block or less commonly disrupt the aortic root, rarely leading to rupture. With self-expandable devices relying on perimeter, balloon-expandable devices are largely sized on the basis of annular area **(Figs. 2A and B)**.

Valve Morphology

- Tricuspid or bicuspid
- Bicuspid aortic valves (BAVs) are associated with low TAVR success rates.

BICUSPID AORTIC VALVE

Commonly followed classification for BAV are Sievers classifications which essentially focus on the number of raphes (0, 1, or 2 for the respective types).

Depending on the number of commissures (2 vs. 3) and the presence or absence of a raphe, BAV can be classified into three broad morphologies: (1) tricommissural, clinically often referred to as "functional" or "acquired" BAV (it is not a part of Sievers classification); (2) bicommissural raphe-type (which is equivalent to Sievers type 1); and (3) bicommissural nonraphe-type (which is equivalent to Sievers type 0).[5] Ascending aortic dilation and aneurysms are more common in "bicommissural" BAV than "tricommissural" BAV. Within "bicommissural" BAV, the nonraphe type BAV exhibits smaller annuli with larger sinus diameters. For bicommissural raphe-type BAV, raphe characteristics including raphe length and raphe calcium are important.[5] In BAV, especially in Sievers type 0 BAV (only two hinge points to define the annular plane), defining the annulus may be a challenge. Annulus size is measured in similar fashion as for tricuspid valves **(Table 2 and Fig. 3)**.

By scrolling the CT images in the axial view, evaluation of the supra-annular space is done to identify different bicuspid configurations (tube, flared, and tapered) **(Fig. 4)**.

Valve Calcium

Similar to the protocol used in calculating the coronary artery calcium score by the Agatston method [unenhanced, ECG-synchronized CT angiography (CTA)], aortic valve calcification scores of ≥1,600 in women and ≥3,000 in men increase the likelihood of severe aortic stenosis. In annular calcification, irrespective of protruding distribution or crescent, the contour is drawn as if no calcium is present in a harmonic fashion.

Annular calcification (within the annular plane) and subannular calcification (the upper 4–5 mm of the LVOT with which device gets into contact) is described in a subjective, qualitative fashion and graded as none, mild, moderate, and severe based on the extent circumferentially, the thickness of the calcium that radially projects into the LVOT and the depth of calcium extension inferiorly into the LVOT.[6]

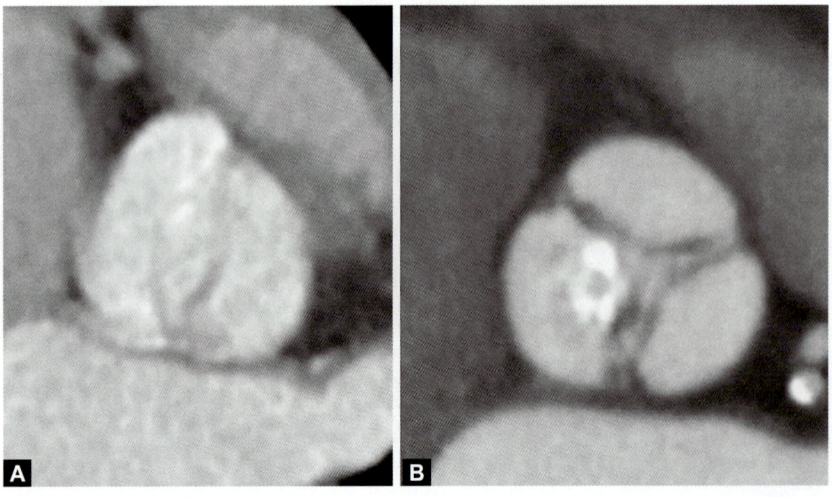

FIGS. 2A AND B: Valve morphology.

TABLE 2: Spectrum of morphology of bicuspid aorta.

Classifications	Characteristics	Double oblique transverse MPR	Volume-rendered en face-view systole	Volume-rendered en face-view diastole
Sievers type 0 bicommissural nonraphe type	• Two fairly symmetric cusps and two commissures • Each cusp has one most basal insertion point; thus, there is a total of two most basal insertion points	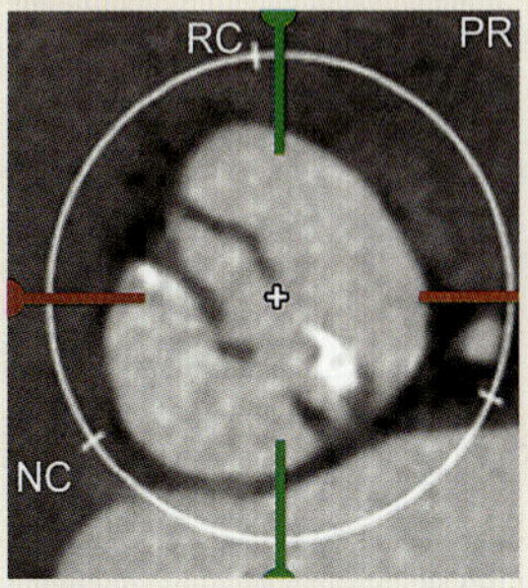	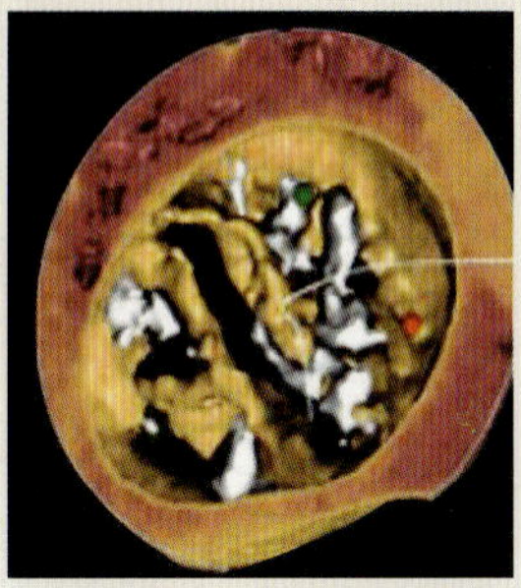	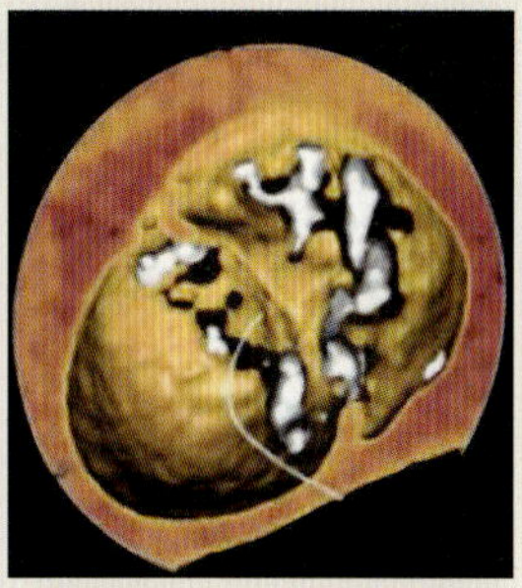
Sievers type 1/ bicommissural raphe type	• Two of three cusps are conjoined by a raphe • Asymmetric cusp sizes with the cusp opposing the raphe (i.e., cusp not participating in raphe formation) being larger than in a tricuspid aortic valve • Raphe does not extend to the level of the STJ which is the distinguishing characteristics to a nonopening commisure • Size of raphe and degree of calcification can vary • Upper row—noncalcified raphe; middle row–moderately calcified raphe; lower row—severely calcified raphe	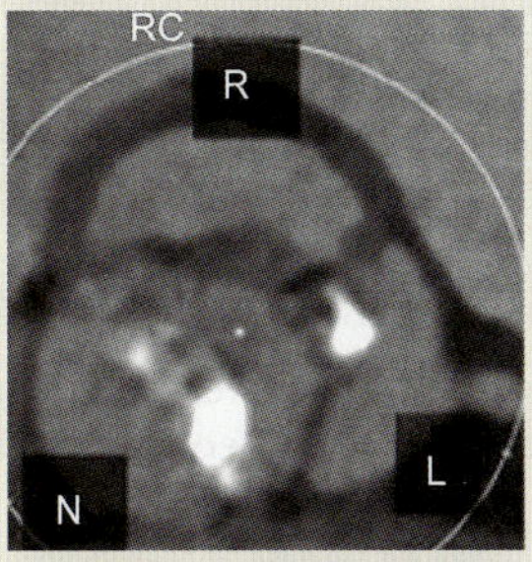 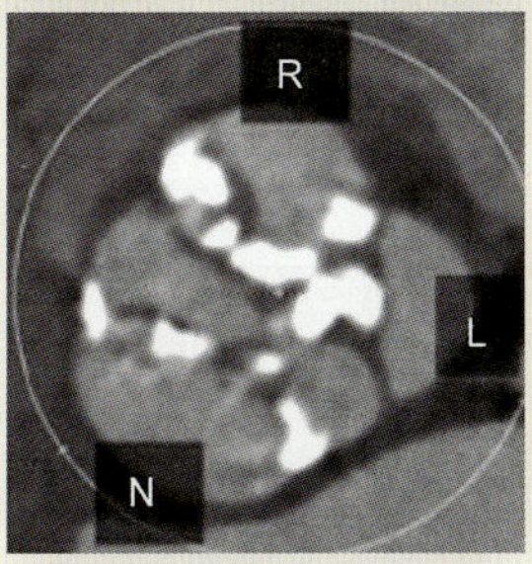 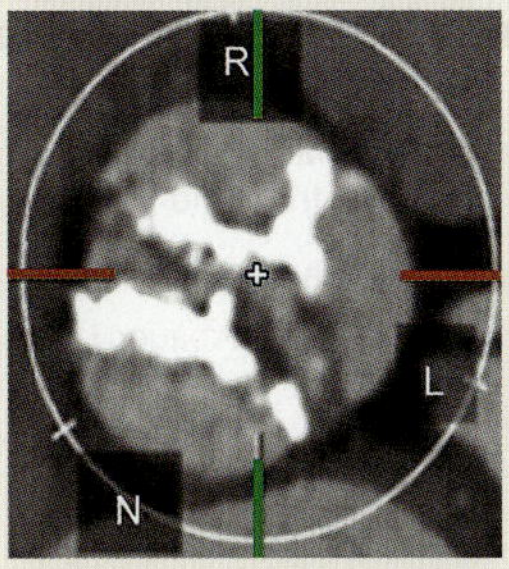	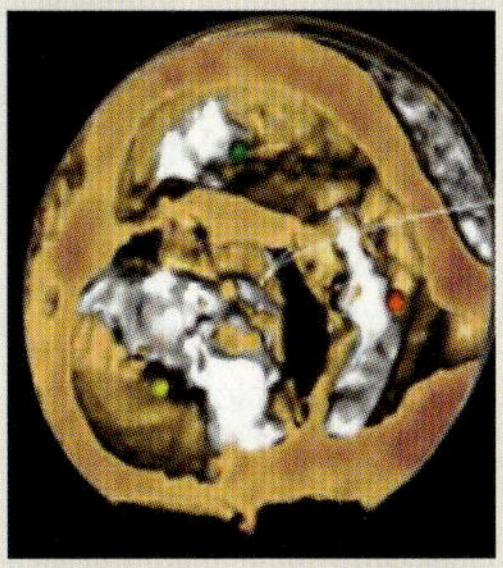 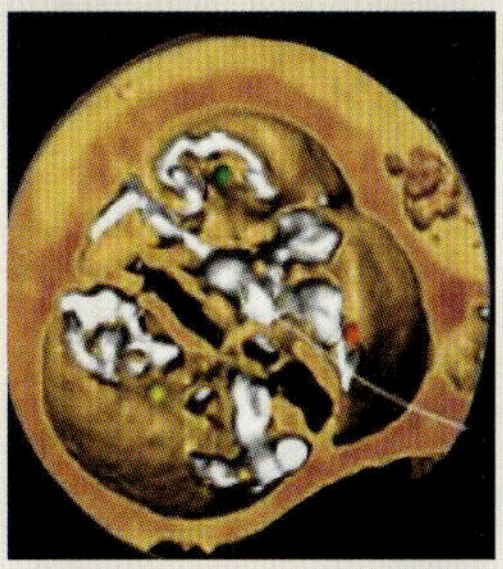 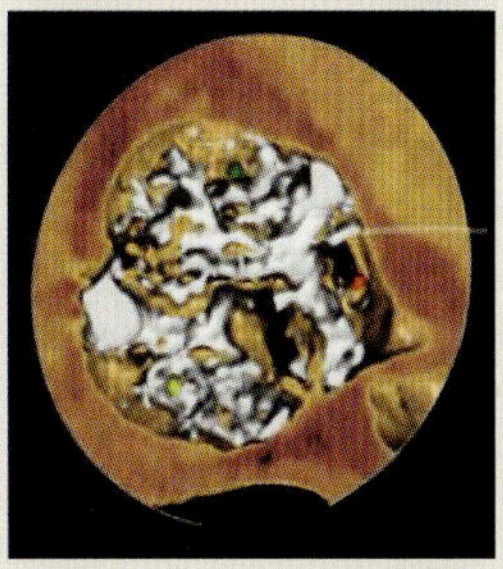	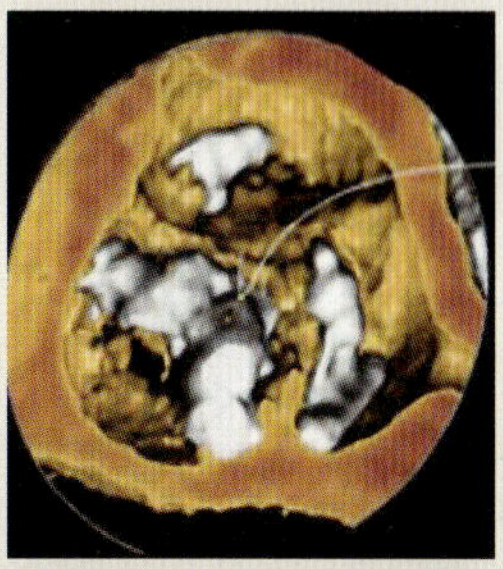 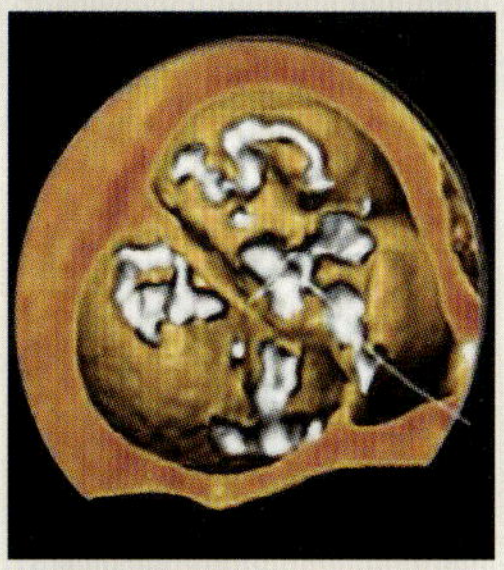 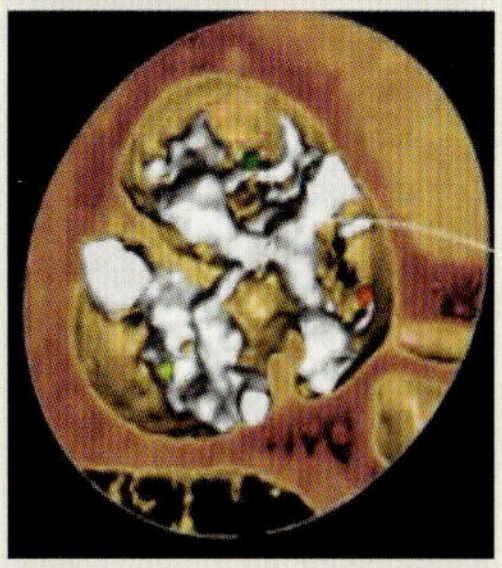
Acquired/ functional bicuspid valve (underlying tricuspid anatomy)	• Underlying tricuspid anatomy with symmetric sinus of Valsalva • Nonopening commissure due to degenerative changes (here RL commissure) • Nonopening commissure reaches STJ, which is the distinguishing factor compared to a raphe	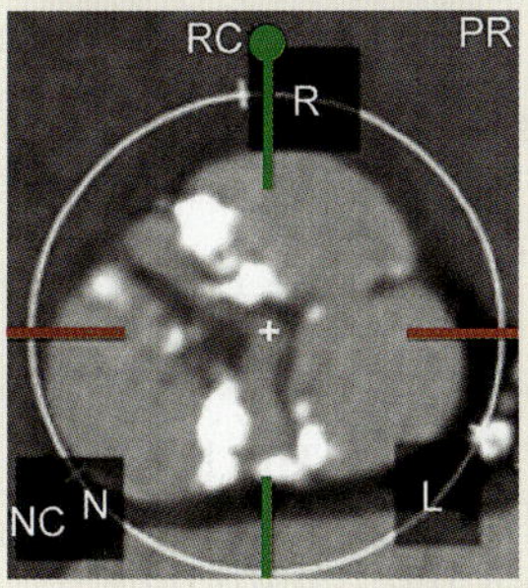	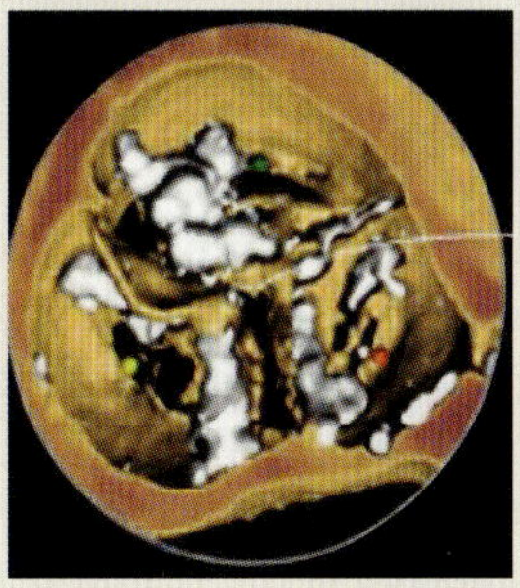	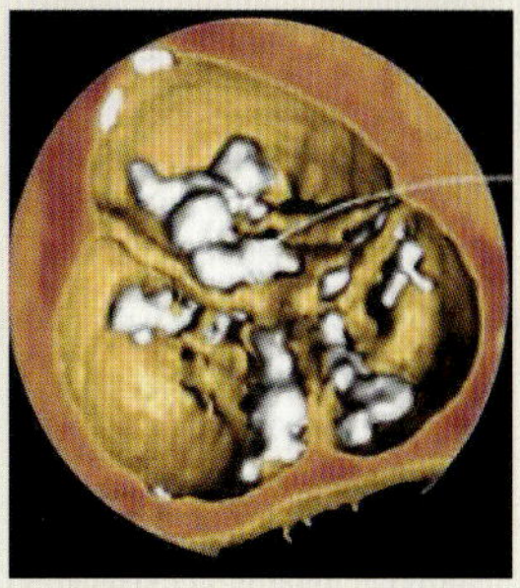

(MPR: multiplanar reformat; STJ: sinotubular junction)

Source: Blanke P, Weir-McCall JR, Achenbach S, Delgado V, Hausleiter J, Jilaihawi H, et al. Computed Tomography Imaging in the Context of Transcatheter Aortic Valve Implantation (TAVI)/Transcatheter Aortic Valve Replacement (TAVR): An Expert Consensus Document of the Society of Cardiovascular Computed Tomography. JACC Cardiovasc Imaging. 2019;12(1):1-24.

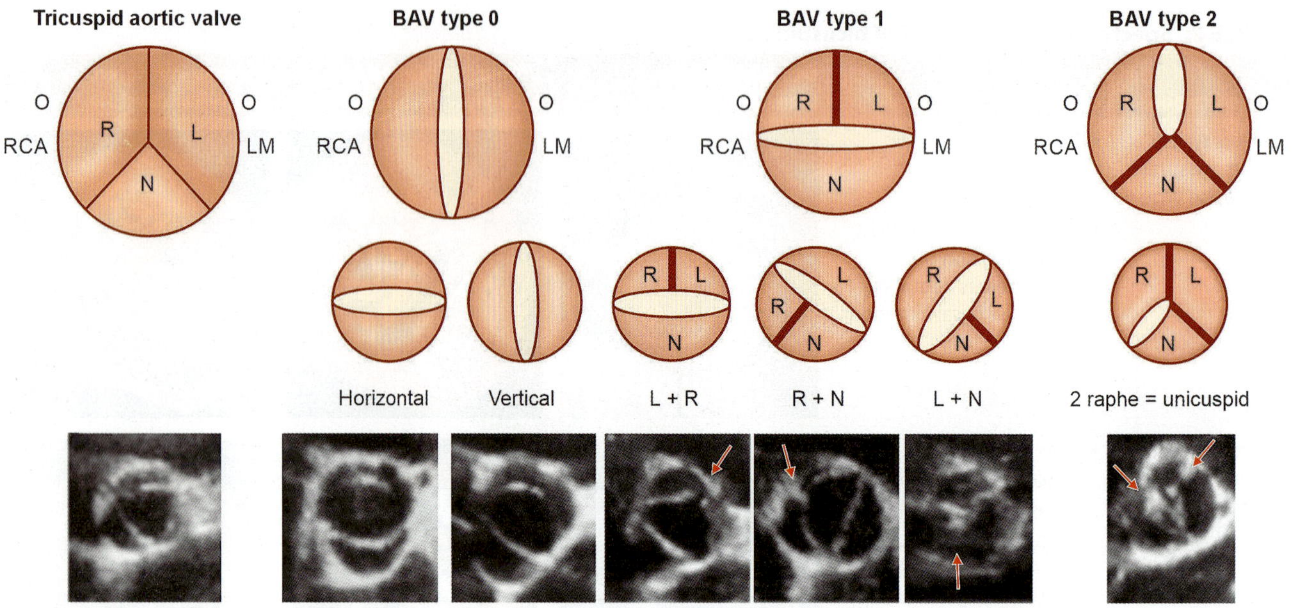

FIG. 3: Bicuspid aortic valve (BAV) morphology. Sievers classification and echocardiographic images are shown. Red bands and arrows represent the raphe or commissural fusion. The ostium of right coronary artery (RCA) is depicted on the left and the left main (LM) is on the right.

Source: Liu T, Xie M, Lv Q, Li Y, Fang L, Zhang L, et al. Bicuspid Aortic Valve: An Update in Morphology, Genetics, Biomarker, Complications, Imaging Diagnosis, and Treatment. Front Physiol. 2019;9:1921.

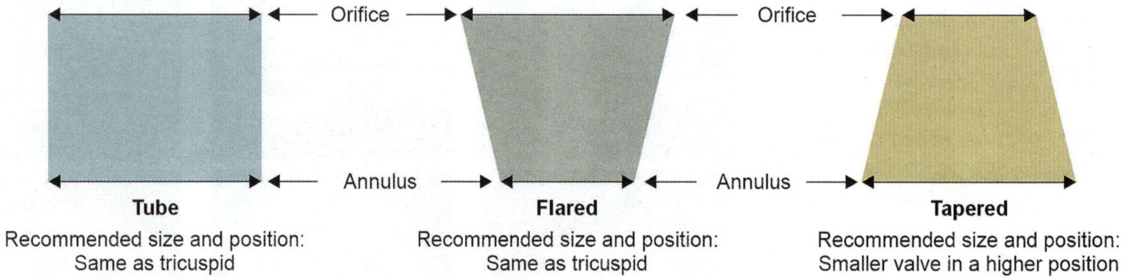

FIG. 4: Configurations during evaluation of supra-annular space.

Source: Blackman D, Gabbieri D, Del Blanco BG, Kempfert J, Laine M, Mascherbauer J, et al. Expert Consensus on Sizing and Positioning of SAPIEN 3/Ultra in Bicuspid Aortic Valves. Cardiol Ther. 2021;10(2):277-88.

Left Ventricular Outflow Tract

The landing zone of the device encompasses the aortic valve cusps, the annulus, and the LVOT.

The presence of severe calcification of the LVOT and aortic valve is demonstrated to be associated with increased risk of paravalvular regurgitation especially when calcium protrudes into the LVOT.[7-10] Within the LVOT, the location of calcification varies significantly across severe aortic stenosis patients. Most frequently affected is the region below the noncoronary cusp and the left coronary cusp, including the intervalvular fibrosa. The risk of annular rupture increases with large, protruding nodules of calcification, particularly with balloon-expandable valves. Severe calcification of the subannular device-landing zone increases the risk of complete heart block.[11,12]

Coronary Ostial Height and Sinus of Valsalva Diameter

The height of the coronary ostium should be measured perpendicularly from the annular plane to the lower edge of the ostium.[13]

There is an increased risk of coronary occlusion with low coronary ostial height (<12 mm) from the annulus and narrow sinus of Valsalva diameter **(Figs. 5 and 6)**.

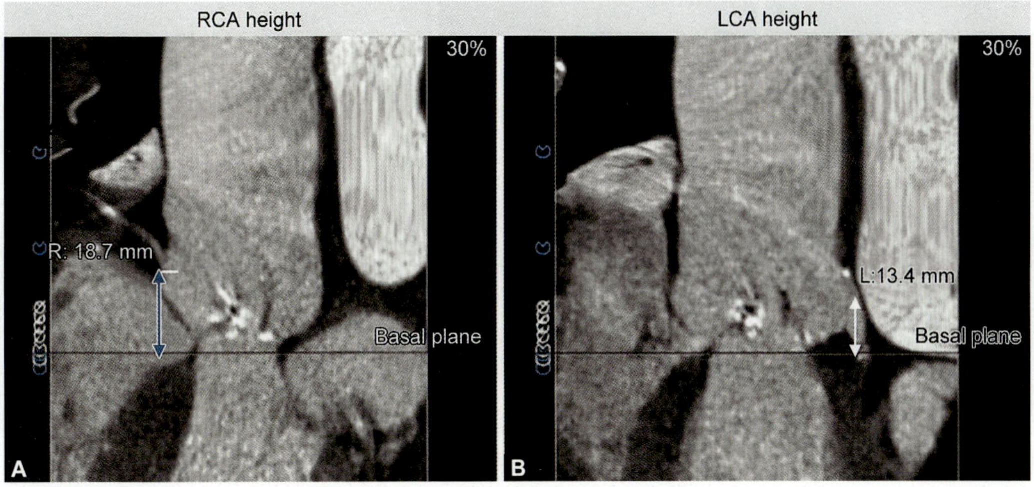

FIGS. 5A AND B: Coronary heights.
(LCA: left coronary artery; RCA: right coronary artery)

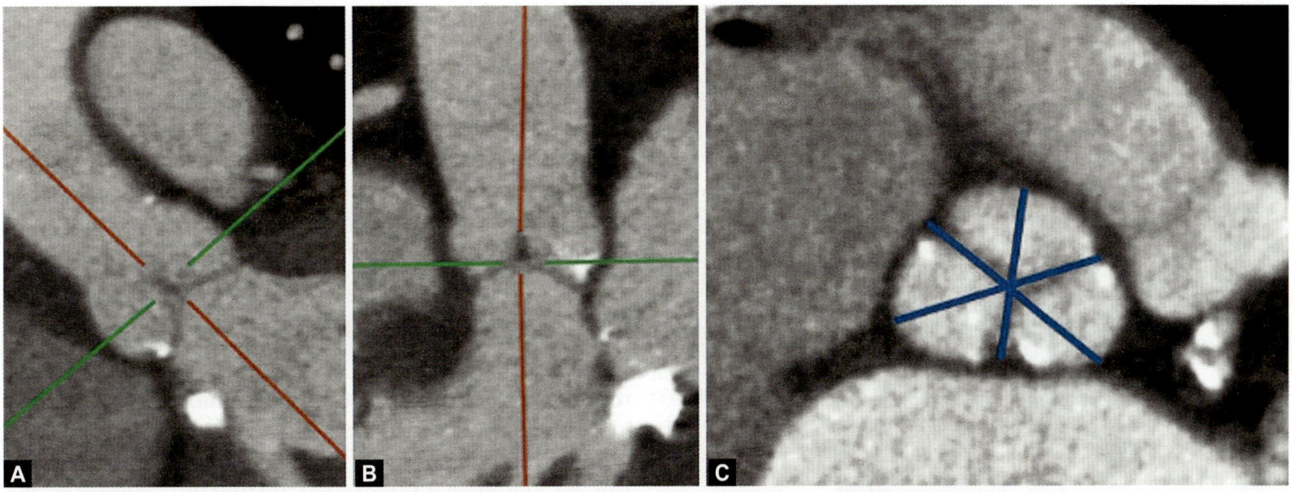

FIGS. 6A TO C: The plane where the sinus of Valsalva is measured (A and B). The measurements from cusp to commissure are shown in blue (C). Measurements are performed in triplicate and the average of the three measurements can be reported (if anatomy is symmetric). There is a greater likelihood of coronary occlusion with a sinus of Valsalva with a small diameter.

Source: Pontes ÍCM, Guimarães CPBF, Fonseca EKUN, Silva MMA, Sasdelli Neto R, Ishikawa WY. Computed tomography angiography in the planning of transcatheter aortic valve replacement: a step-by-step approach. Radiol Bras. 2022;55(6):373-9.

Diameter of the Sinotubular Junction

The sinotubular junction diameter should be measured in a transverse oblique plane **(Figs. 7A to C)**.

Height of the Sinotubular Junction

The sinotubular junction height should be measured from the annular plane to the lowest edge of the junction, perpendicular to the annular plane **(Fig. 8)**.[13]

Diameter of the Ascending Aorta

The ascending aorta diameter should be measured at the level of its greatest width or at the level of the main pulmonary artery[13] in its true axial plane **(Figs. 9A to C)**.

Optimal Projection Curve

Transcatheter aortic valve replacement is performed with fluoroscopy angulations, providing a coplanar view of the

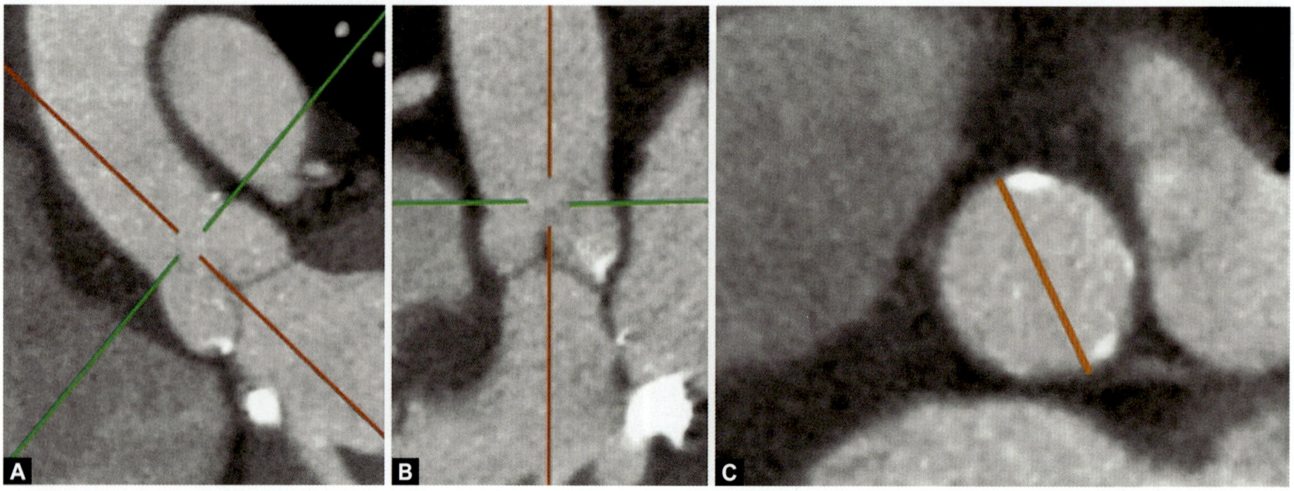

FIGS. 7A TO C: Plane of the sinotubular junction diameter (A and B). Orange is the sinotubular junction diameter (C).

Source: Pontes ÍCM, Guimarães CPBF, Fonseca EKUN, Silva MMA, Sasdelli Neto R, Ishikawa WY. Computed tomography angiography in the planning of transcatheter aortic valve replacement: a step-by-step approach. Radiol Bras. 2022;55(6):373-9.

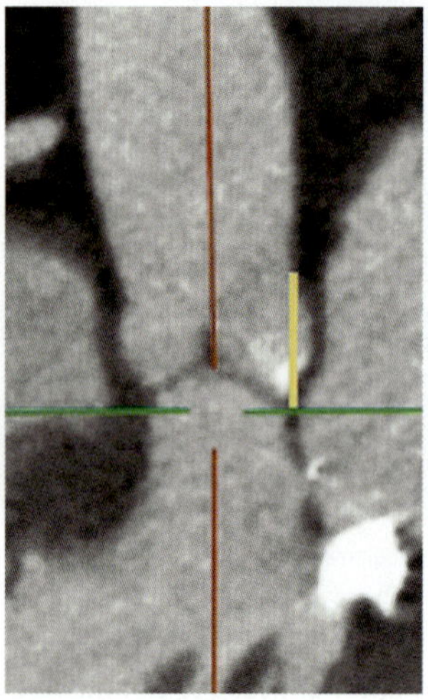

FIG. 8: Plane of the sinotubular junction height and the corresponding measurement shown in yellow.

Source: Pontes ÍCM, Guimarães CPBF, Fonseca EKUN, Silva MMA, Sasdelli Neto R, Ishikawa WY. Computed tomography angiography in the planning of transcatheter aortic valve replacement: a step-by-step approach. Radiol Bras. 2022;55(6):373-9.

aortic annulus without parallax. CT-derived angulations allow to optimize initial predeployment fluoroscopic angulation, thereby reducing the need for repeated root shots before deployment, thereby reducing procedure time, radiation exposure, and contrast usage.

Vascular Access Planning

The rate of vascular access complications during TAVR has been ranging between 6.3 and 30.7%.[14]

AORTA

The anatomy of the aortic arch including its branching should be described (especially when considering subclavian access), along with extent of the calcifications in the aorta, as well as aneurysm, tortuosity, any intraluminal obstruction, and thrombosis.[15]

Iliofemoral Vasculature

Iliofemoral vasculature is the most commonly used route. A virtual roadmap of the iliofemoral access allows identification of vessel size, tortuosity, calcification, and minimal lumen and helps to decide if transfemoral access can be achieved.[3] Significant tortuosity—increases the risk of trauma with the TAVR catheter system. Eccentric calcification—associated with easier access than circumferential calcification.

A scanner with a spatial resolution of 0.5–0.6 mm and at least 64 detectors and together with analysis on a workstation offering 3D manipulation[16] is recommended pre-TAVR.

Contraindications to transfemoral access—when the external sheath diameter exceeds the minimum artery diameter, peripheral artery disease, severe calcification, and significant vessel tortuosity **(Figs. 10 and 11)**.[17]

Cardiac Findings

The extent and degree of left ventricular hypertrophy or dilation, identification of left atrial appendage occlusion, and thrombus in the wall of the left ventricle must be reported and evaluated.[17]

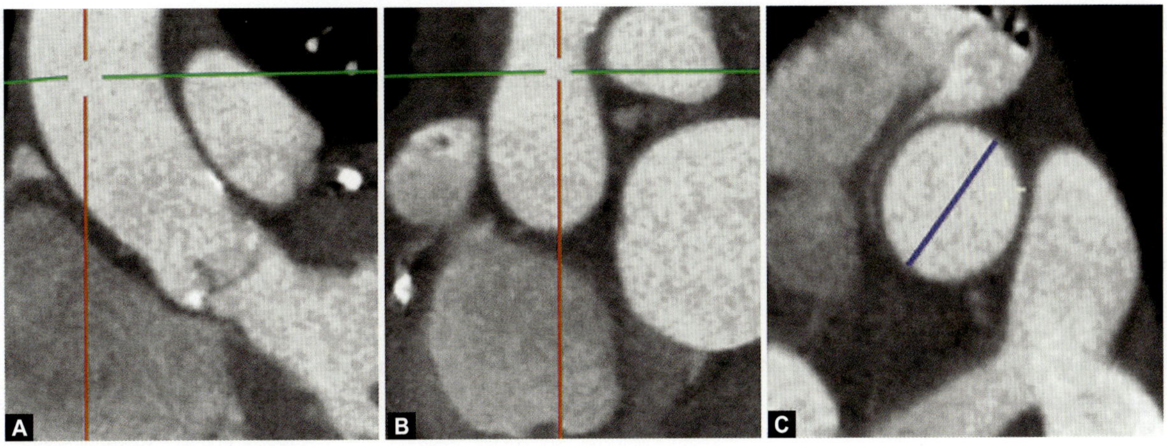

FIGS. 9A TO C: Plane of the ascending aorta and the corresponding measurement.

Source: Pontes ÍCM, Guimarães CPBF, Fonseca EKUN, Silva MMA, Sasdelli Neto R, Ishikawa WY. Computed tomography angiography in the planning of transcatheter aortic valve replacement: a step-by-step approach. Radiol Bras. 2022;55(6):373-9.

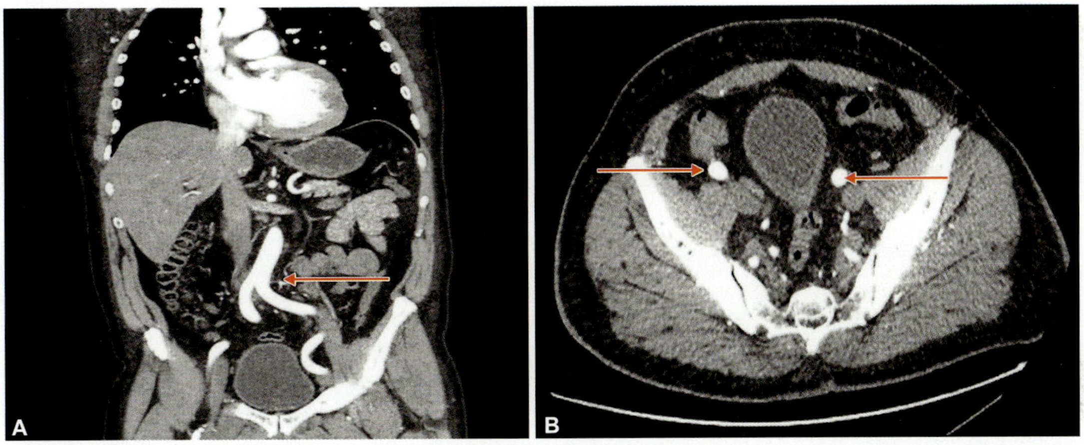

FIGS. 10A AND B: (A) Coronal image showing aortofemoral bifurcation and (B) the left and right femoral arteries in the axial image.

Source: Bleakley C, Monaghan MJ. The Pivotal Role of Imaging in TAVR Procedures. Curr Cardiol Rep. 2018;20(2):9.

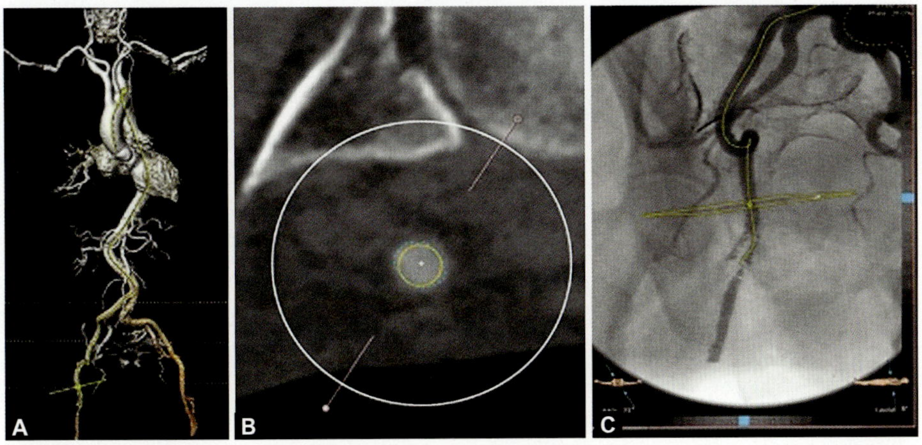

FIGS. 11A TO C: Three-dimensional (3D) reconstruction of the arterial system (A) and cross-section of the common right femoral artery at the optimal puncture site (B). The artery shows a good caliber (exceeding 6.5 mm as evident from the yellow circle) and no calcifications. Moderate tortuosity of the superficial iliac artery is evident at both 3D and angio reconstruction (C). In particular, the angio reconstruction allows for the fluoro-guided detection of the optimal access cite, based on its relationship with the femoral head.

Source: Pontes ÍCM, Guimarães CPBF, Fonseca EKUN, Silva MMA, Sasdelli Neto R, Ishikawa WY. Computed tomography angiography in the planning of transcatheter aortic valve replacement: a step-by-step approach. Radiol Bras. 2022;55(6):373-9.

CONCLUSION

Conventional sizing and positioning remain the most appropriate strategy when contemplating TAVI especially in challenging anatomies. Based on currently guidelines and evidence CT is the gold standard tool for pre-TAVR imaging assessment, and plays an important role in patient selection, improving outcomes and reducing the rates of paravalvular regurgitation . Imaging specialists who are responsible for CT interpretation should be made an integral part of the heart team.

ONLINE REFERENCES

Please scan the QR code provided at the end of the table of contents for References of this chapter.

CHAPTER

173 Large-bore Vascular Access and Closure

Shabbir Ali Shaik, BVA Ranga Reddy, Pratap Chandra Rath

ABSTRACT

Percutaneous transcatheter interventions such as endovascular repair of aortic aneurysm/type B (Stanford) aortic dissections, transcatheter aortic valve implantation has become alternative to conventional surgery and percutaneous mechanical circulatory support systems usage has been increased widely nowadays. These procedures require large-bore access into the femoral artery, and hence increase risk of vascular complications. Meticulous access site management is crucial for safe implementation of large-bore technologies and includes accurate puncture technique and reliable percutaneous closure devices. This chapter elucidates different techniques for obtaining femoral access and various strategies for percutaneous closure.

Keywords: Transcatheter aortic valve implantation (TAVI), endovascular aneurysm repair (EVAR), mechanical circulatory support (MCS), vascular access, vascular closure device (VCD).

INTRODUCTION

Cardiac catheterization has progressed to a wide range of diagnostic and interventional procedures in coronary, peripheral, endovascular, and structural heart disease interventions. Minimally invasive procedures such as endovascular aneurysm repair (EVAR), transcatheter aortic valve implantation (TAVI), and implantation of mechanical circulatory support (MCS) are gaining ground on traditional surgery.[1-3] These procedures require large-bore access, which is associated with increased risk of vascular complications. Despite the reduction in size of these devices **(Table 1)**, vascular and bleeding complications are still as high as 20% in TAVI and 12–22% in EVAR.[4-7] There was increased risk of morbidity and mortality.[8] Vascular complications are higher in females, obese individuals, renal failure, and those on anticoagulation use.[9-10]

TABLE 1: Risk of retroperitoneal hemorrhage with vascular closure device compared with manual compression.

Study	OR	95% CI
Farouque et al.	2.13	0.62–7.33
Ellis et al.	2.80	1.95–4.00
Farouque et al.	1.27	0.31–5.26

(CI: confidence interval; OR: odds ratio)

STRATEGIES FOR OBTAINING PERIPHERAL ACCESS

Good closure starts with good access. The ideal puncture site of common femoral artery is located between the lower border of the inferior epigastric artery (IEA) (marker for retroperitoneal space) and above the femoral bifurcation. Therefore, higher punctures are difficult to compress and increase risk of retroperitoneal bleeding.[11] Punctures below the femoral bifurcation are difficult in navigating the larger sheaths and cannot be closed with vascular closure devices (VCDs). There are different strategies for obtaining peripheral access for large-bore devices.

- *Anatomical landmarks*: First, identify the inguinal ligament between the anterior-superior iliac spine and symphysis pubis. Palpate the femoral pulse just below the inguinal ligament and puncture the common femoral artery through needle **(Fig. 1)**. It was highly operator dependent and usage was decreased and more preference was for radial artery.[12,13] It was shown in a small study by Pitta et al. that the actual puncture site is located outside the ideal location in nearly 13% cases, while anatomical landmarks are alone taken into consideration. Any vascular access obtained outside the desired location was associated with increased vascular complications.[14]

- *Ultrasound-guided access*: In this access, first the common femoral artery bifurcation should be seen in longitudinal view to know the exact site of bifurcation and extent of arterial wall calcifications. After that, the probe is turned counterclockwise to get a cross-sectional view above the bifurcation point. To differentiate artery from vein, color Doppler or compression test can be used. The anterior wall of common femoral artery is punctured at 45° angle and needle pathway and entry into vessel are seen in real time through ultrasound **(Figs. 2A and B)**. It precludes radiation and reduces the number of attempts and median time to access when compared with fluroscopy.[15,16]
- *Fluoroscopic-guided access*: This access shows spatial relationship between the common femoral artery and femoral head.[17] Under X-ray, a radiopaque instrument, such as a hemostat or puncture needle, is placed over the femoral head and puncture the femoral artery **(Figs. 3A and B)**. Alternatively, a wire or (e.g., pigtail) catheter can be placed from a contralateral access till level of the ipsilateral femoral head which serves as marker under fluoroscopy for puncture. One of the best method was to give a small contrast injection through the catheter from the opposite side, which is a bull's eye for the operator. Fluoroscopy-guided arterial puncture is an effective method with lower vascular complications and is superior than using anatomical landmarks.[18-20]
- *Surgical cut-down*: In this technique, common femoral artery puncture and closure are done under direct vision. Surgical cut-down is associated with a longer procedure time and duration of hospital stay and also increased chance of wound infection.[21-24]

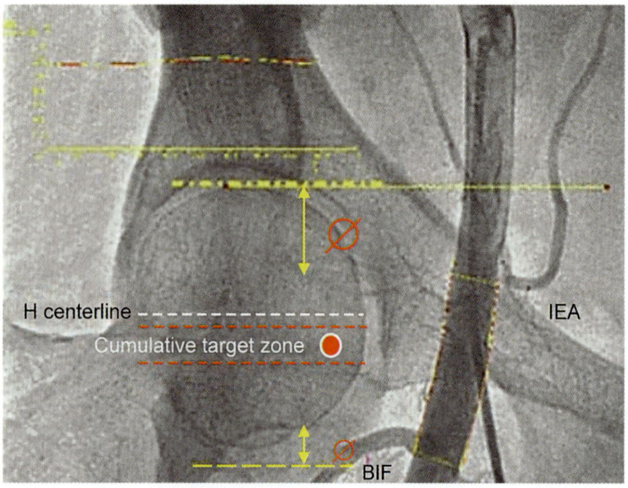

FIG. 1: Still-frame femoral artery angiogram, depicting the relationship of the FH and common femoral artery, demarcated by the inferior epigastric artery (above) and the BIF (below). The cumulative target zone identifies the location over the FH with the highest likelihood of common femoral artery access.

(BIF: femoral artery bifurcation; FH: femoral head; IEA: inferior epigastric artery).

Source: With permission form Turi (2005).[27]

Vascular Closure

- *Surgical closure*: Surgical closure is done after surgical cut-down for femoral access. Nowadays, most TAVI and EVAR procedures are performed in a total percutaneous manner except in few-selected patients with extreme obesity and those having femoral grafts or stents.[25]

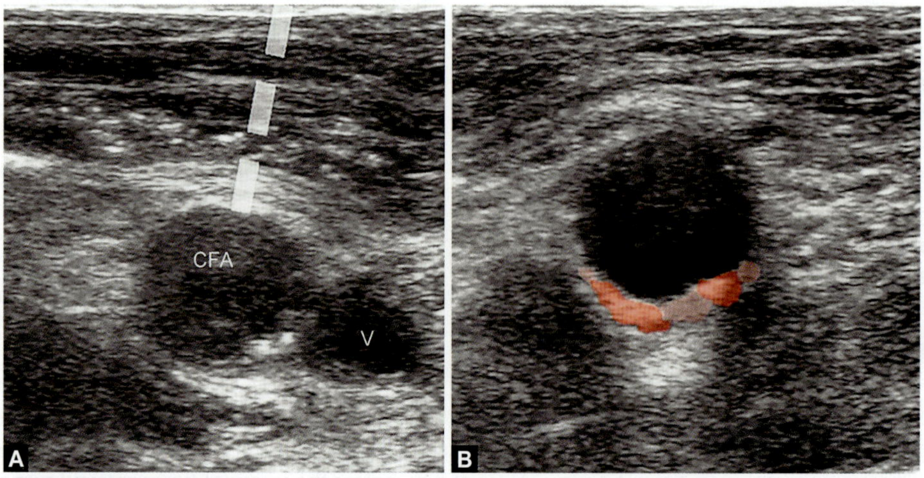

FIGS. 2A AND B: Ultrasound-guided access. (A) Common femoral artery and femoral vein (semicompressed). Dashed line—needle pathway. (B) Calcification of the posterior arterial wall marked in red.

(CFA: common femoral artery; V: femoral vein)

- *Suture-based closure devices*: The vast majority of large-bore vessel closure is performed by percutaneous suture-based techniques such as the Prostar® XL and multiple ProGlide® (Abbott Vascular) VCDs **(Fig. 4)**. Both devices are inserted using a preclosure technique.
    - *Prostar XL*: This device is inserted over the guidewire and its position in the artery is confirmed through the pulsatile flow from the main tube. The four prepared sutures inside the device are pulled out while maintaining the device in the same position

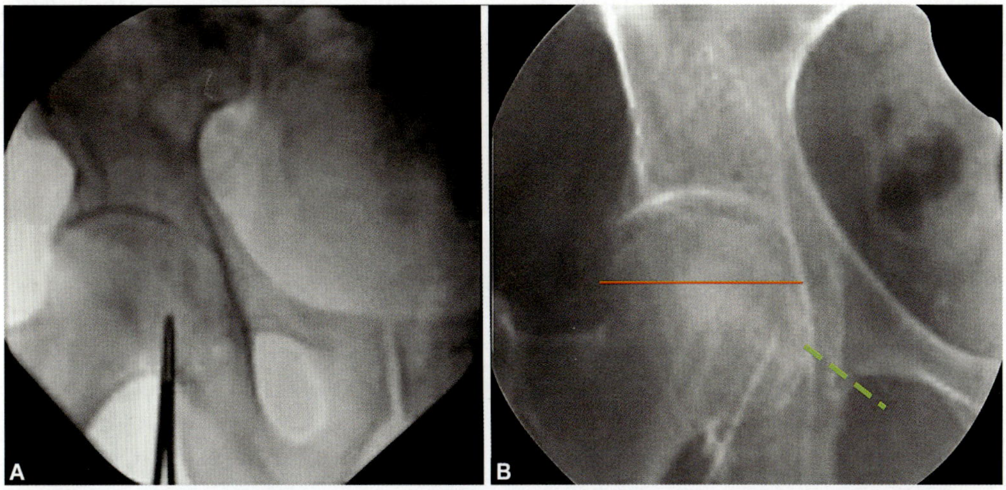

FIGS. 3A AND B: Still-frame fluoroscopic images in an anterior–posterior angulation just above the femoral head. (A) Hemostats are placed on the skin corresponding to the inferior-most border of the femoral head seen by fluoroscopy. (B) A needle is inserted at the tip of the hemostats and fluoroscopy is obtained just prior to arterial access to identify the anticipated point of arterial entry in relation to the femoral head.

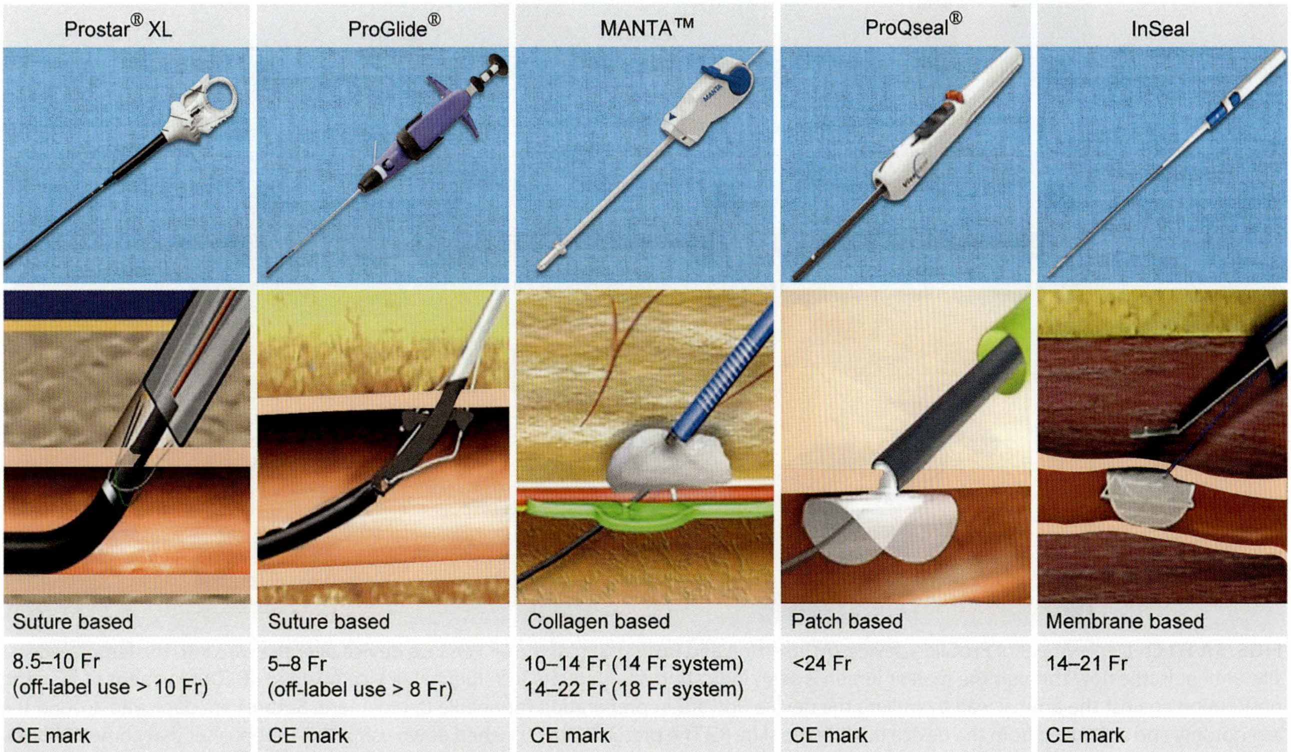

FIG. 4: Commercially available vascular closure devices.

Source: Abbott Vascular, Essential Medical, InSeal Medical, and Vivasure Medical.

so that the needles are pulled back, leaving behind the sutures in place. The arteriotomy site is closed by pulling the sutures and closing the knots **(Fig. 4)**.

- *ProGlide*: This device is inserted over the guidewire before inserting the sheath and deployed. Usually, there are two devices for large-bore arteriotomies and they are deployed at 10 O'clock and 2 O'clock position. After the procedure is completed, the sheath is removed and sutures are approximated with knot pusher and the vessel wall is closed **(Figs. 5A to C)**.[26]

Both suture-based techniques were performed with guidewire in place and hence, additional suture- or plug-based closure devices can be used if there is incomplete closure of large-bore vascular access.

The vascular complication rates are relatively lesser with usage of VCD when compared with surgical cut-down and shorter procedural time (91 min ± 32 vs. 153 min ± 112; $p < 0.05$).[28,29] In a study by Barbash et al., the major vascular complications were less with ProGlide when compared to Prostar XL (1.9% vs. 7.4%; $p < 0.001$) and less incidence of

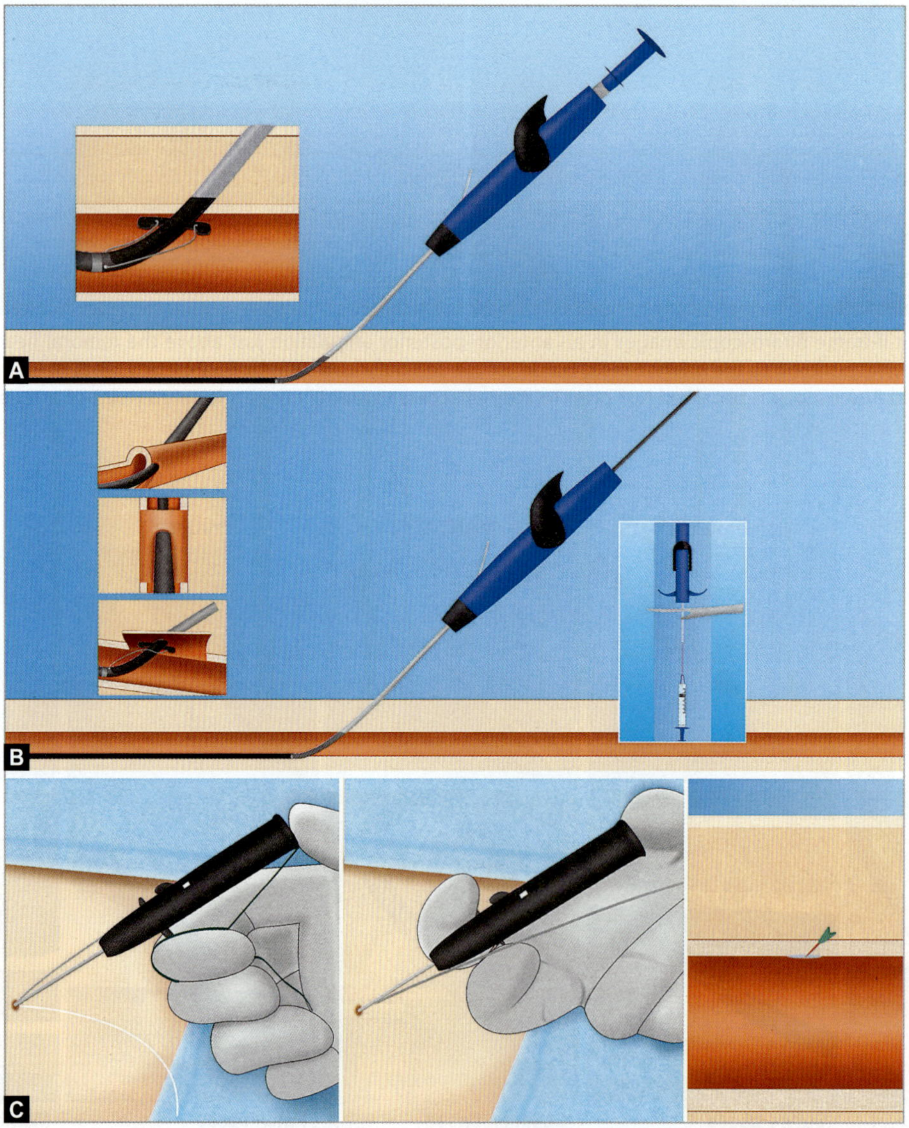

FIGS. 5A TO C: Deployment of ProGlide device. (A) Insertion and positioning of the 6F Perclose device over the wire into the femoral access site until pulsatile flow through the marker lumen is seen indicating an adequate intraluminal device position. (B) Deployment of foot and positioning against the arterial wall by pulling the device upward in preparation for needle deployment. Sutures are deployed around the arteriotomy and are pulled from the device outside the skin. (C) The pretied knot is pushed down using the knot pusher that comes with the device. Once hemostasis is achieved, the suture is cut using a knot cutter. The final suture lies securely around the arteriotomy to achieve hemostasis.

both major (3.2% vs. 16.7%; $p < 0.001$) and minor bleeding (8.9% vs. 13.6%; $p = 0.032$).[7] However, in an Italian study, ProGlide has showed more vascular complications than Prostar XL closure (24.0% vs. 11.4%; $p = 0.007$).[30] For proper execution of suture-based closure, VCDs require good learning curve. Suture-based VCDs can be safely used to close large-bore vascular access alternative to femoral access such as axillary and subclavian arteries.[31,32]

- *Collagen-based closure*:
    - *MANTA*: The MANTA™ VCD (Essential Medical) is a collagen-based VCD **(Fig. 4)**. It consists of a poly (lactic-co-glycolic) toggle within the artery that is attached to bovine collagen plug outside the vessel wall. The arteriotomy site is closed by sandwiching it between the toggle and the collagen. The operator holds the device handle and has to apply sufficient tension till the green marker is visible. The toggle and collagen plug takes 6 months to get absorbed.[33] The MANTA has a 14 Fr and 18 Fr version for arteriotomy closure between 10 and 14 Fr and 14 and 22 Fr, respectively. The MANTA has also been applied for completely percutaneous closure of axillary arteriotomies after TAVI.[34,35]
    - *Angio-Seal*: The Angio-Seal™ device (St Jude Medical, St Paul, MN) is the most common VCD used worldwide.[36] The procedural success rate is very high with short learning curve. The device consists of an intraluminal anchor and an extravascular collagen sponge—both are attached together with a bioresorbable suture. All components are bioresorbable and get resorbed completely by 3 months. Hemostasis is achieved by sandwiching the arteriotomy site between sandwich with the anchor and collagen sponge **(Figs. 6A to C)**. It has a delivery sheath and is available in 6 and 8 Fr sizes. The 8 Fr Angio-Seal device has more collagen in the sponge (28 g) than the 6 Fr device (18 g). In a small study where 1,004 patients underwent both diagnostic and interventional coronary procedures, vascular closure done with Angio-Seal device showed about 99% deployment success, with major vascular complications only in 0.4%.[37] One can close large-bore (>8 Fr) arteriotomies with more than one Angio-Seal using a "double wire" technique.
    - *EXOSEAL*: The EXOSEAL (Cordis) device consists of a plug applier and a bioabsorbable polyglycolic acid (PGA) plug. It is available in sizes 5, 6, and 7 F. It is inserted into the sheath and pulled along with sheath slowly to stop the bleeding from the marker lumen. Then the PGA plug was positioned outside the vessel wall, but underneath the vessel fascia. After pressing the deployment button, the plug extends and closes the branch canal **(Figs. 7A to D)**. EXOSEAL is the safest device with high success rate and lesser number of complications. In a small study of 168 patients, the device was successfully deployed in 166 patients (98.8%). Postprocedural complications were noted in 7.2% of patients with three pseudoaneurysms (1.8%) and nine hematomas (5.4%).[38]

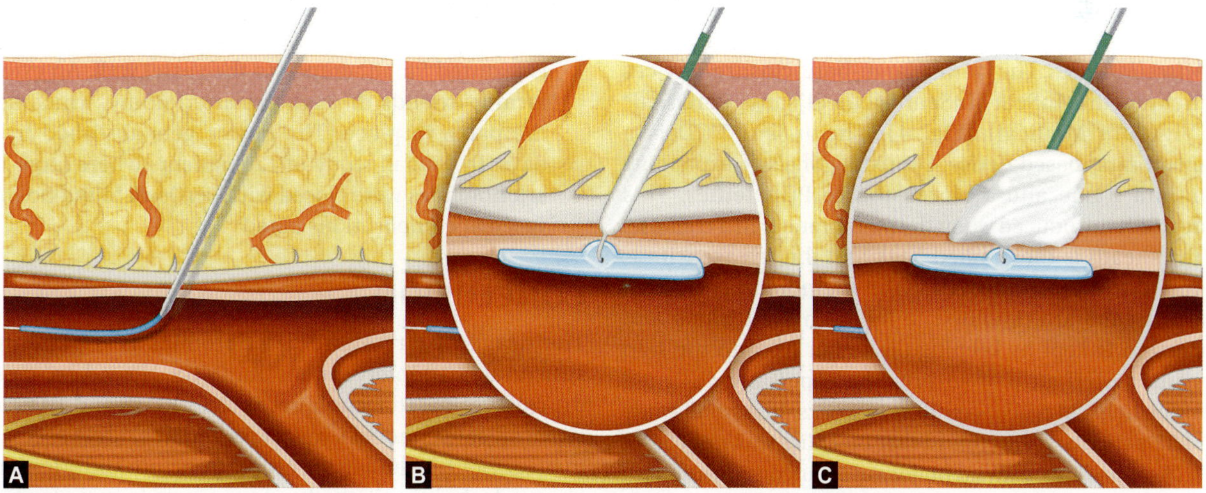

FIGS. 6A TO C: Deployment of Angio-Seal closure device. (A) The Angio-Seal sheath is placed within the vessel via the existing guidewire. It is advanced until blood flows out through the exit hole in the dilator as shown. It is then withdrawn until blood flow ceases and is advanced until the blood flow restarts. (B) Locator and guidewire are removed. The Angio-Seal is inserted fully into the sheath with two arrows on the sheath and device assembly meeting. The anchor will then be released beyond the sheath tip. The barrel of the device is retracted with a double "click," and the whole assembly is then withdrawn. The anchor will be fixed against the inside of the vessel by gentle traction. A tamper becomes visible on the suture as the sheath is removed. (C) Once fully visible, the tamper is advanced forward to tie a knot over the collagen plug, which becomes compressed against the puncture site. The suture is then cut above the tamper and the tamper is removed.

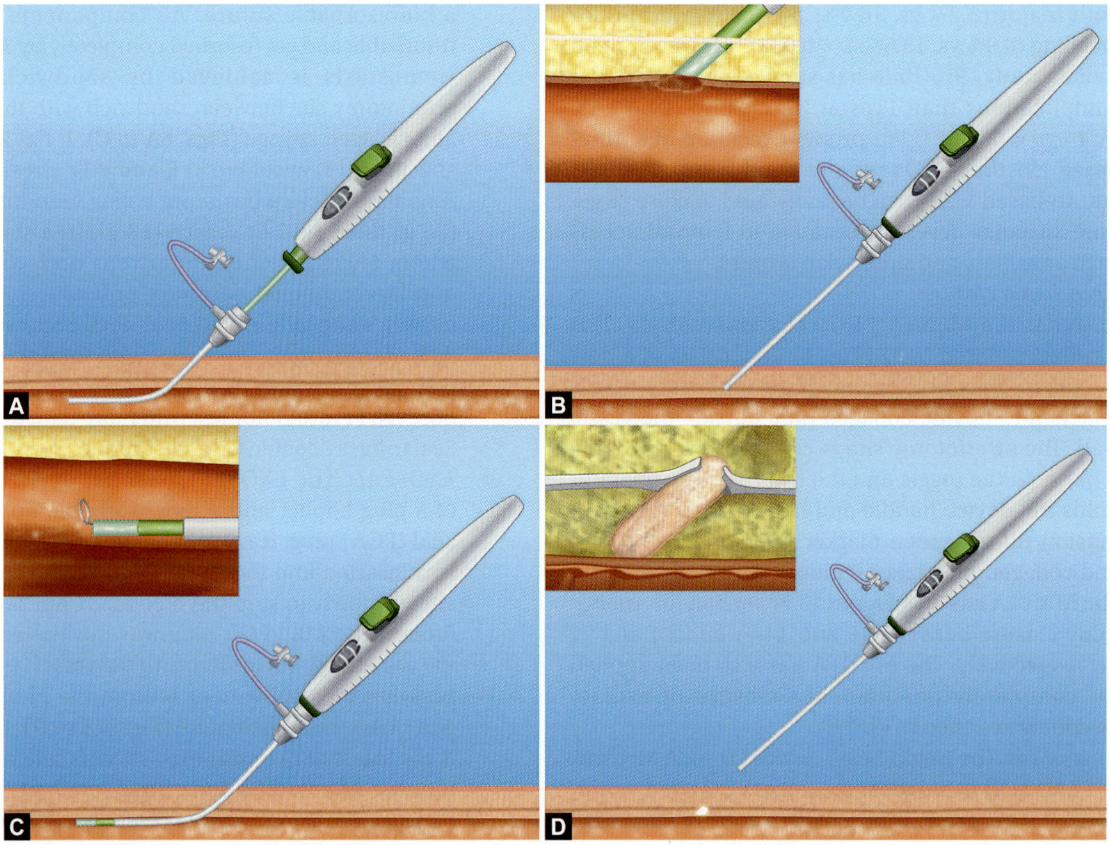

FIGS. 7A TO D: EXOSEAL device deployment. EXOSEAL deployment, using a dissolvable polyglycolic acid (PGA) plug, involves first inserting the device into the femoral sheath (A) and securing it to the sheath to allow for intraluminal deployment of an indicator wire (B). The sheath and device are pulled back until the indicator wire is at the arteriotomy (C), and the PGA sealant is then delivered to produce permanent hemostasis and the device is removed (D).

Courtesy: Cordis Corporation.

- *Miscellaneous*: The newer large-bore closure devices include the InSeal (InSeal Medical) and PerQseal® (Vivasure Medical) **(Fig. 4)**. The *InSeal VCD* is a membrane-based device, consisting of a self-expanding nitinol frame and a bioresorbable PGA tether. This device is introduced when the membrane is in a collapse. The sheath is then pulled back and the release wire is pulled to deploy the VCD. The membrane is pushed against the arteriotomy site by the nitinol frame and traction is kept by keeping the tether fixed to the skin using a Steri strip or suture. The especially designed frame helps in reaccess within 26 weeks. In a small study of 52 patients, it was found that bleeding was noticed in 7.7% of patients with no major vascular complications.[39] The *PerQseal VCD* consists of an intravascular patch which is supported by a scaffold. The surface of the patch is textured for adherence to the vessel wall. An external locator extends through the arteriotomy, which keeps the patch in place. The device gets absorbed by 180 days. In a small study of 120 patients where large-bore arteriotomies were closed with PerQseal found no major vascular complications noted.[40]

CONCLUSION

The usage of large-bore arteriotomies is expanding in structural heart interventions and MCS. Nowadays, most of the catheter-based techniques such as EVAR and TAVI have replaced conventional surgical procedures. Ideal access site management, including the proper puncture and arteriotomy closure technique, is the key for success in catheter-based therapies in clinical practice.

ONLINE REFERENCES

Please scan the QR code provided at the end of the table of contents for References of this chapter.

CHAPTER

174

Choice of Valves in Transcatheter Aortic Valve Implantation

Vijay Kumar, Vishal Rastogi, Ashok Seth

ABSTRACT

Transcatheter aortic valve implantation (TAVI) technology is rapidly evolving. The newer generation valves are addressing the main drawbacks and complications of the first and second generation transcatheter heart valves. There are numerous valves available in both balloon and self-expanding valve platforms with wider spectrum of sizes, better profile, easily deliverable, deployable, least paravalvular leak and pacemaker implantation rates and giving best hemodynamics and better durability. The decision about choice of valve in a particular patient is essential and governed by patient factors, design of the valve, ease of implantation, durability and the data supporting the various clinical outcomes. This chapter will elaborate the characteristics of the transcatheter heart valves entering into contemporary clinical practice and in pipe line of this ever-extending armamentarium and a discussion on how patient factors and device factors influence the choice of selection of a valve in a patient today especially in focus to life time management of severe aortic stenosis.

Keywords: Choice of valves, aortic stenosis (AS), transcatheter aortic valve implantation.

INTRODUCTION

In the last two decades, transcatheter aortic valve implantation (TAVI) has revolutionized the management of symptomatic severe aortic stenosis (AS) by becoming a standard of care across the entire spectrum of surgical risks. It has now expanded to young, low-risk patients with longer life expectancies, early asymptomatic severe AS patients, those with pure aortic regurgitation (AR), surgical tissue valves that have failed and for failed transcatheter heart valves (THVs). There has been a continuous evolution in device technology with several new generation of THVs to minimize procedural complications and improve patient outcomes. Choice of valves in a patient today is thus no more simple and straightforward.[1-10]

NEW-GENERATION TRANSCATHETER HEART VALVES, BIOPROSTHETIC, AND POLYMER-BASED LEAFLETS (TABLE 1 AND FIGS. 1 TO 12)

The armamentarium of transcatheter heart valves is ever expanding and we have today numerous valves and devices with better features than the older generation valves.[11-16] Two broad types of valves are Food and Drug Administration (FDA) approved for clinical use—(1) the balloon expanding valve (BEV) SAPIEN family (Edwards Lifesciences) and (2) the self-expanding valve (SEV) CoreValve family of valves (Medtronic) **(Fig. 1)**. The SAPIEN and SAPIEN XT are older generations of the SAPIEN family, whereas the current

TABLE 1: Current generation of transcatheter heart valves.

Current generation transcatheter heart valves	Type	Remarks
SAPIEN 3 (Edward Lifesciences)	BEV	Excellent sealing
SAPIEN 3 Ultra (Edward Lifesciences)	BEV	Excellent sealing
Myval Octacor (Meril Lifesciences)	BEV	Extralarge sizes
Myval (Meril Lifesciences)	BEV	Intermediate sizes available
Evolut R, Pro, and Pro+	SEV	Good sealing
Evolut FX (flex catheter designed)	SEV	Excellent flexibility and atraumatic nose cone
ACURATE neo 2 and (Boston Scientific)	SEV	Two-step deployment
Portico	SEV	Easy deployment
Navitor (Abbott) SEV	SEV	Intra-annular
Allegra (New Valve technology)	SEV	
Vienna valve (Relisys Medical Devices, India)	SEV	Fully premounted ready for deployment
LOTUS Edge (Boston Scientific)	Mechanically expandable	Needs more modifications

(BEV: balloon expanding valve; SEV: self-expanding valve)

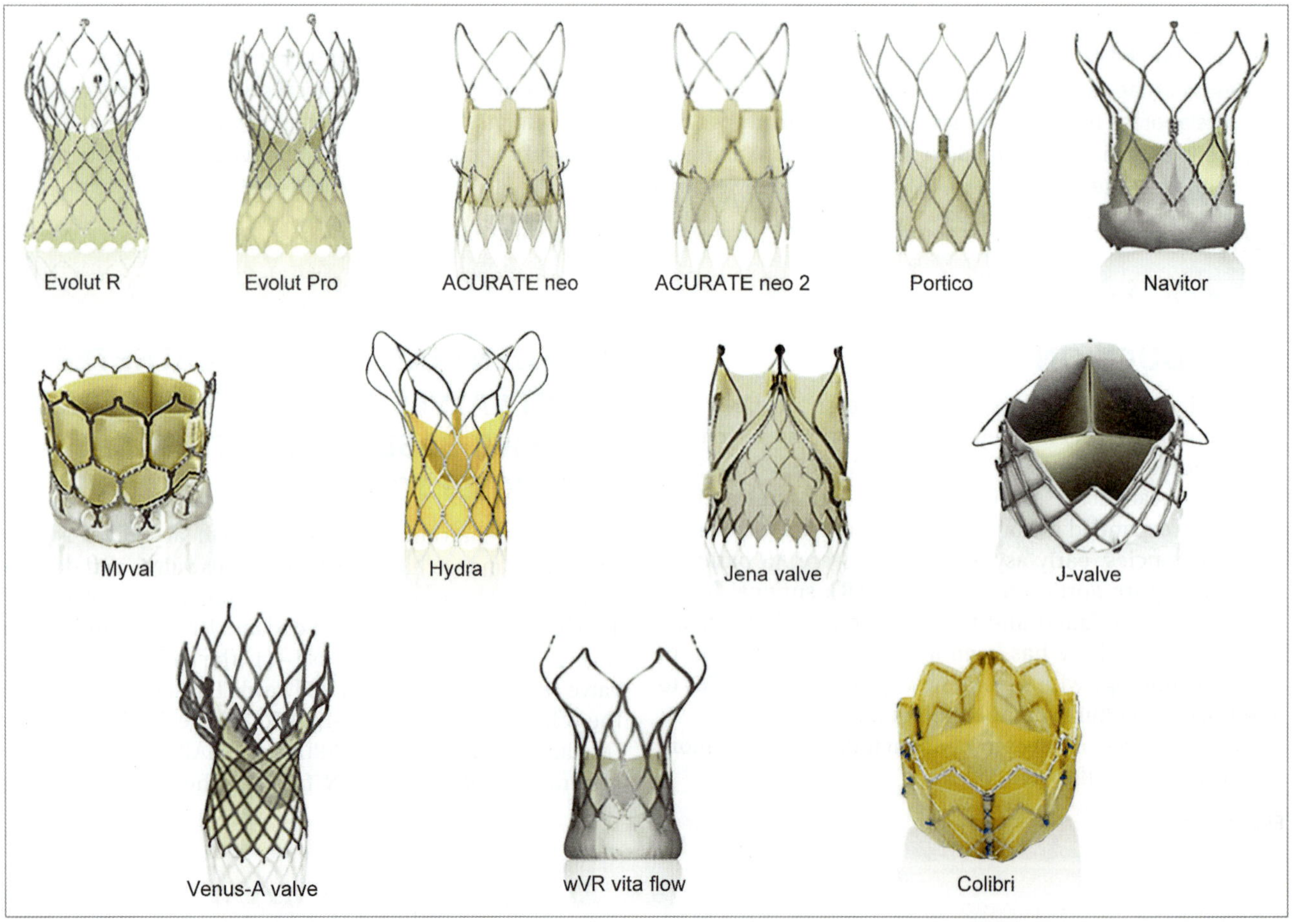

FIG. 1: New-generation transcatheter heart valves.

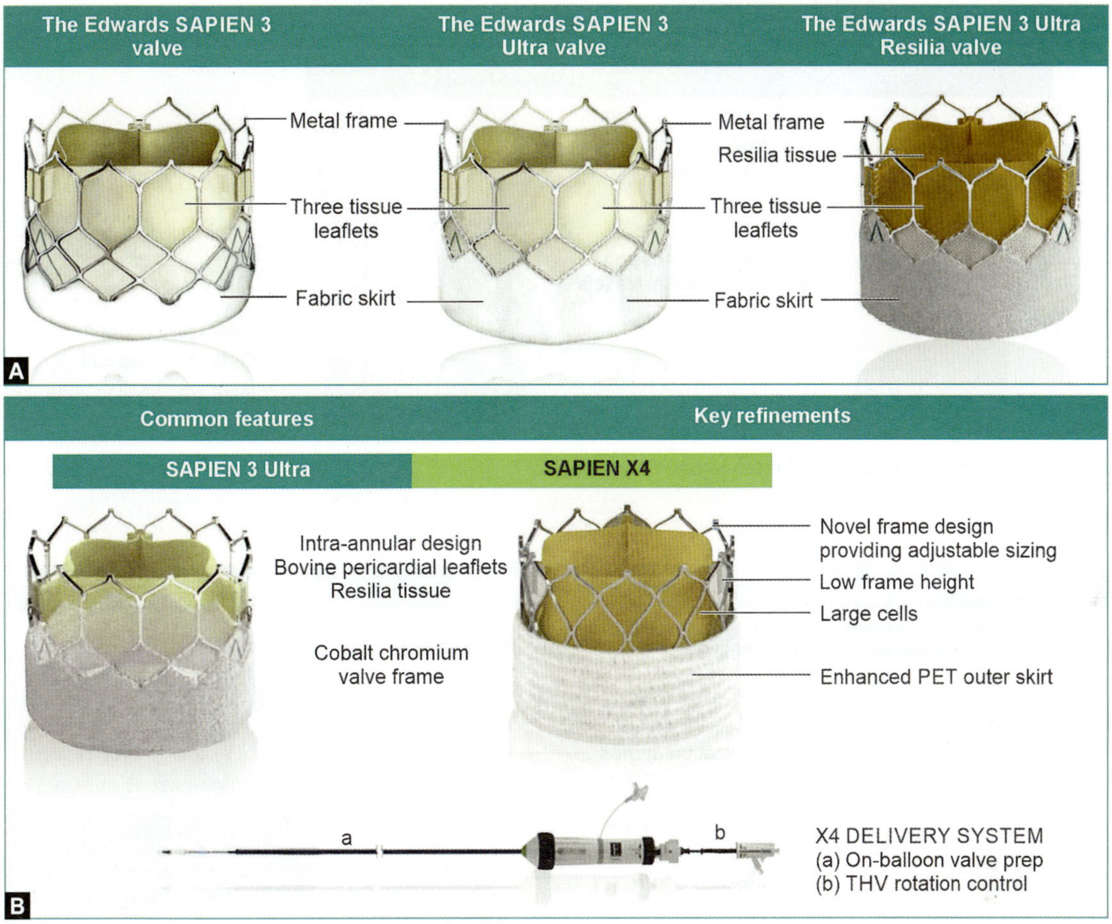

FIGS. 2A AND B: The latest Generation SAPIEN BEV platform SAPIEN 3 Ultra and ×4.

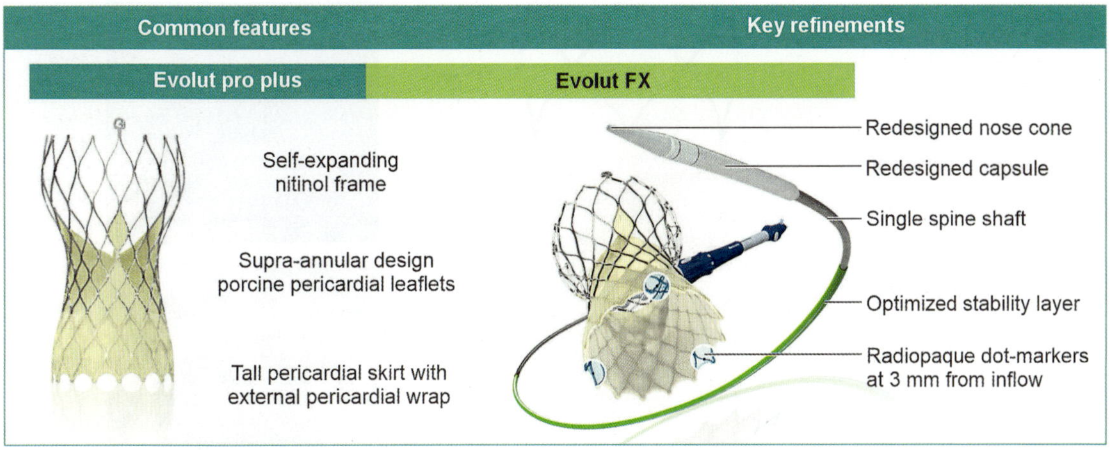

FIG. 3: Evolut Pro+ and FX—the new-generation Evolut platform.

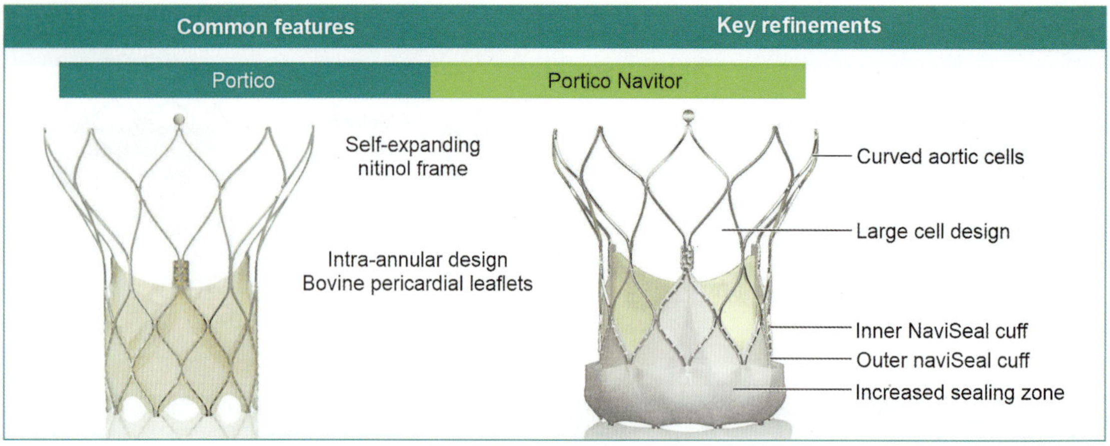

FIG. 4: Portico and Navitor—the intra-annular self-expanding valve (SEV).

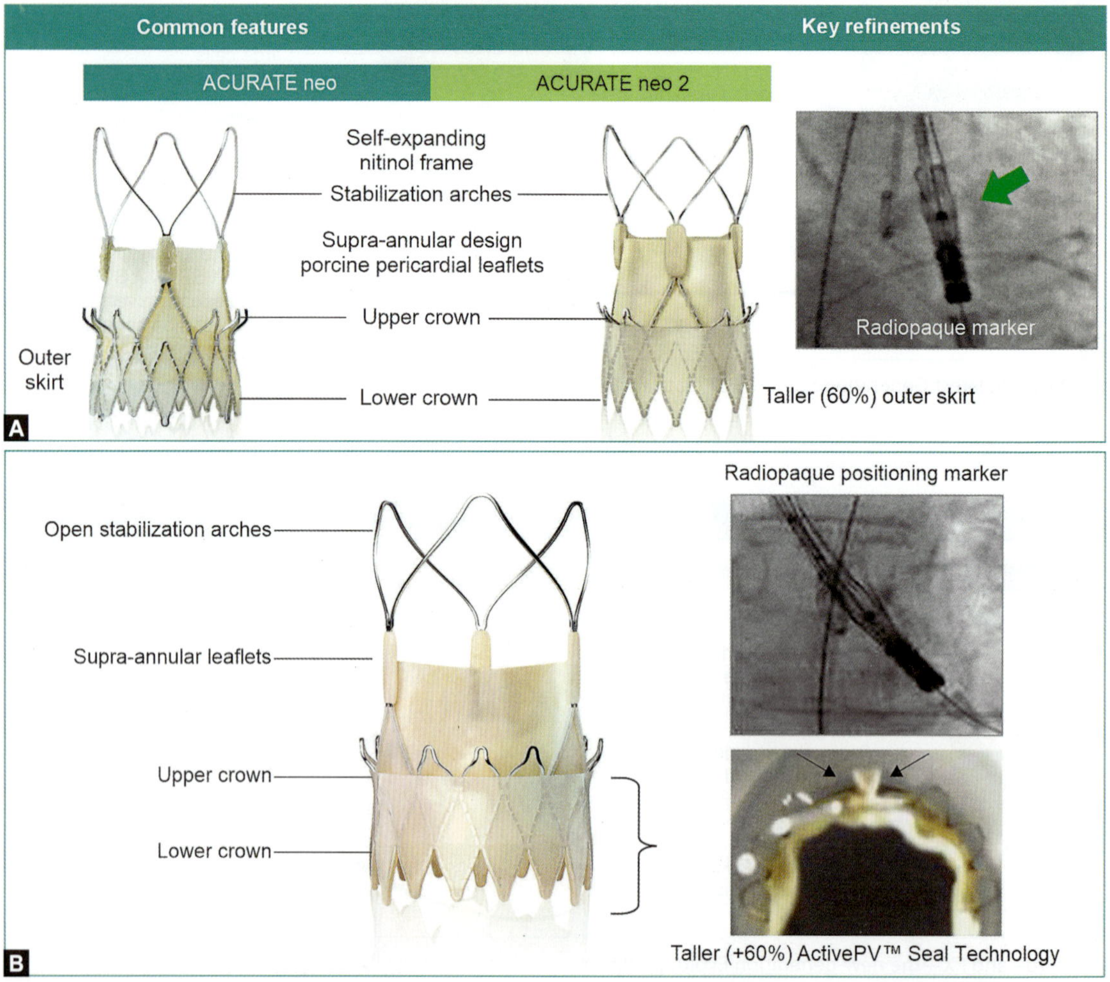

FIGS. 5A AND B: ACURATE neo and ACURATE neo 2: Refinements in ACURATE platform.

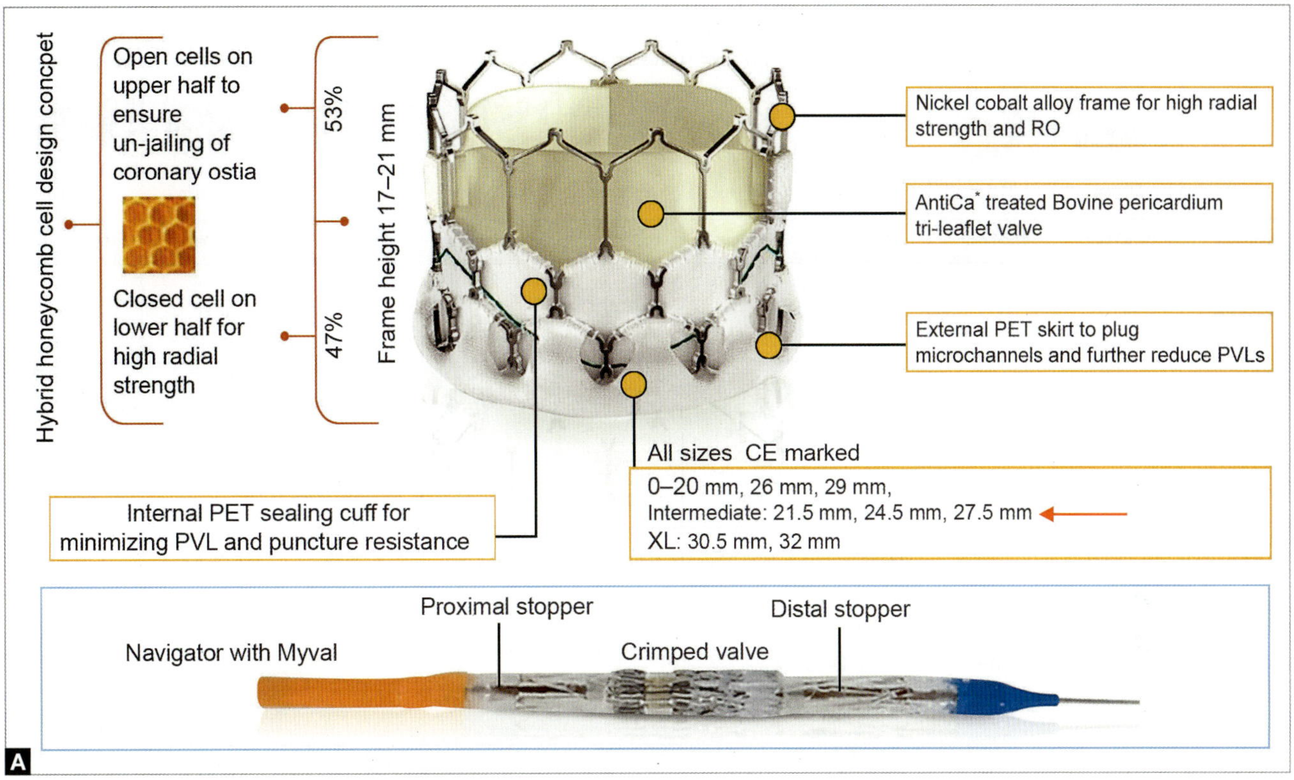

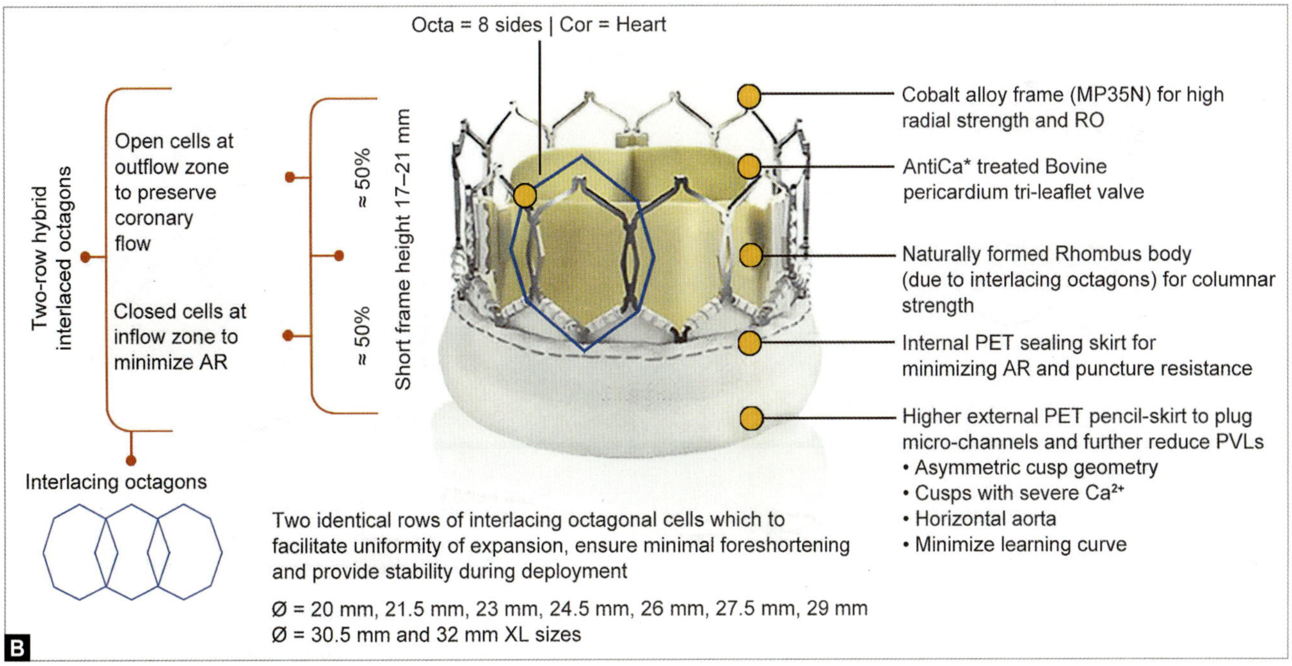

FIGS. 6A TO C: *Continued*

Continued

	Area 314 mm^2 17.35 mm 20 mm	Area 363 mm^2 18.35 mm 21.5 mm	Area 415 mm^2 17.85 mm 23 mm	Area 471 mm^2 18.75 mm 24.5 mm	Area 531 mm^2 18.85 mm 26 mm	Area 594 mm^2 19.25 mm 27.5 mm	Area 661 mm^2 20.35 mm 29 mm	Area 731 mm^2 20.90 mm 30.5 mm	Area 804 mm^2 21.14 mm 32 mm
Perimeter	62.83 mm	67.54 mm	72.26 mm	76.97 mm	81.68 mm	86.39 mm	91.11 mm	95.82 mm	100.53 mm
Python expandable introducer sheath	14 Fr	14 Fr	14 Fr	14 Fr	14 Fr	14 Fr	14 Fr	14 Fr	14 Fr
Native annulus area (CT derived)	270–330 mm^2	314–380 mm^2	360–440 mm^2	410–500 mm^2	460–560 mm^2	510–630 mm^2	570–700 mm^2	630–770 mm^2	700–840 mm^2
Area–derived diameter	18.5–20.5 mm	20.0–22.0 mm	21.4–23.7 mm	22.8–25.2 mm	24.2–26.7 mm	25.5–28.3 mm	26.9–29.9 mm	28.3–31.3 mm	29.9–32.7 mm
Native annulus size by TEE	16–19 mm	17.5–20.5 mm	18–22 mm	19.5–23.5 mm	21–25 mm	22.5–26.5 mm	24–28 mm	25.5–29.5 mm	27–31 mm

C

AntiCa*: Meril's proprietary anti-calcification treatment technology.

FIGS. 6A TO C: Myval and the new-generation Octacor.

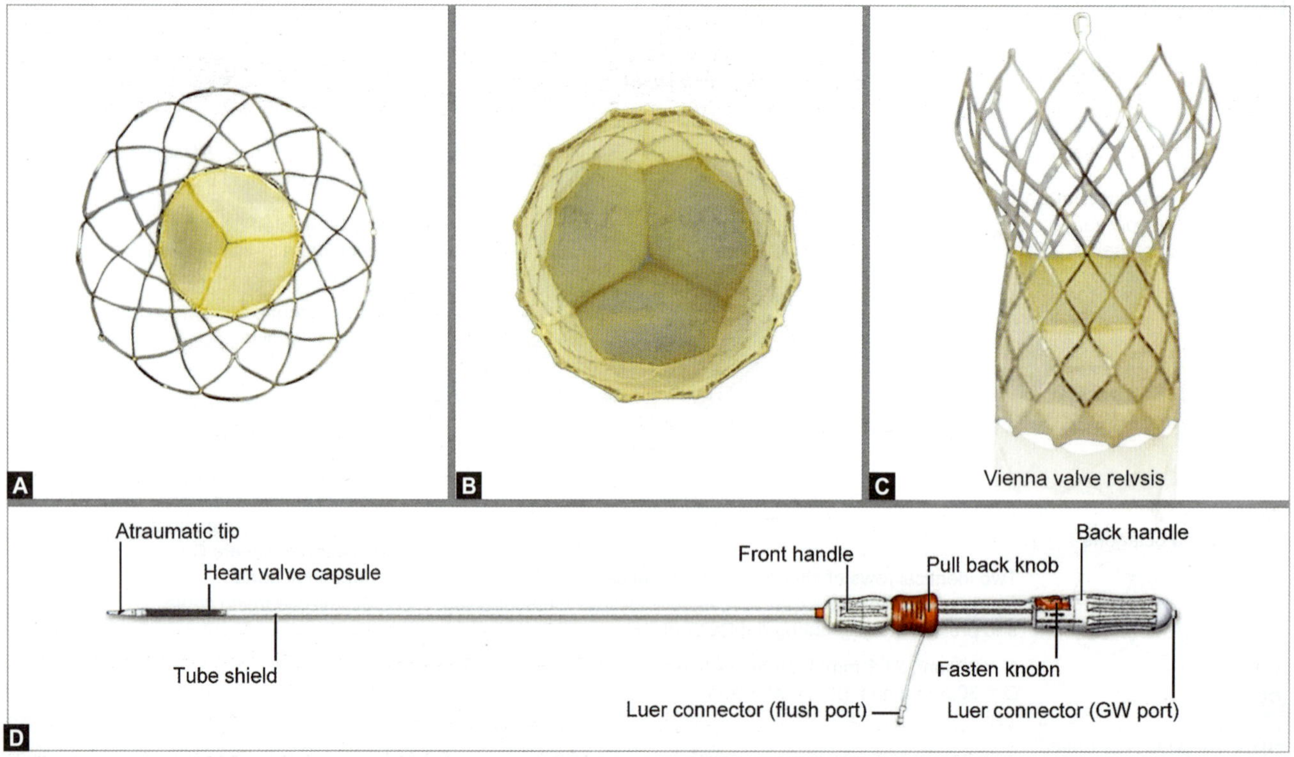

FIGS. 7A TO D: Vienna valve—dry premounted (A) outflow, (B) inflow, (C) side view, (D) catheter delivery system.

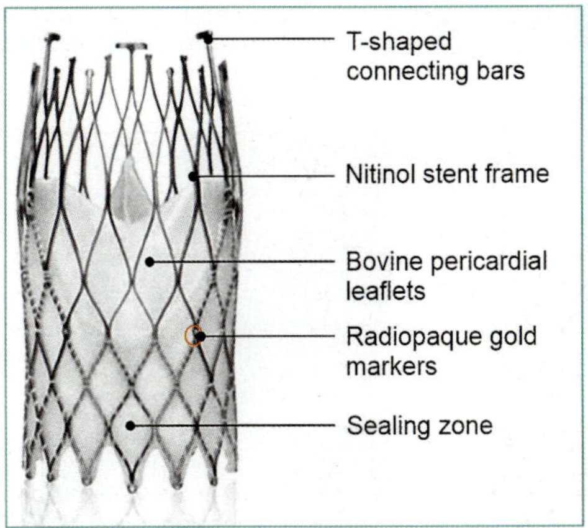

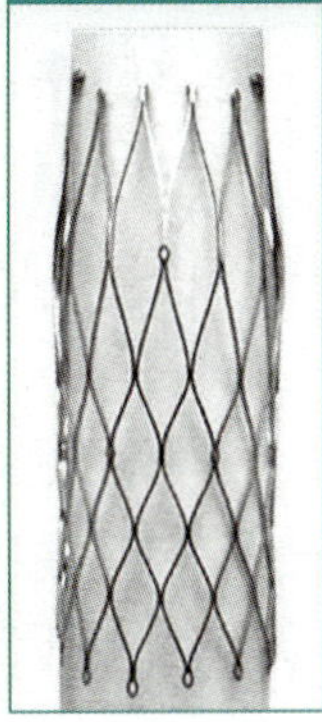

(mm)	NVT allegra 23 mm	NVT allegra 27 mm	NVT allegra 31 mm
Frame height	37.3	41.3	45.3
Frame inflow diameter	23.8	27.4	31.0
Frame outflow diameter	20.8	24.0	27.1
Annulus diameter	19–22 mm	22–25 mm	25–29 mm

FIG. 8: New valve technology Allegra SEV good for valve-in-valve.

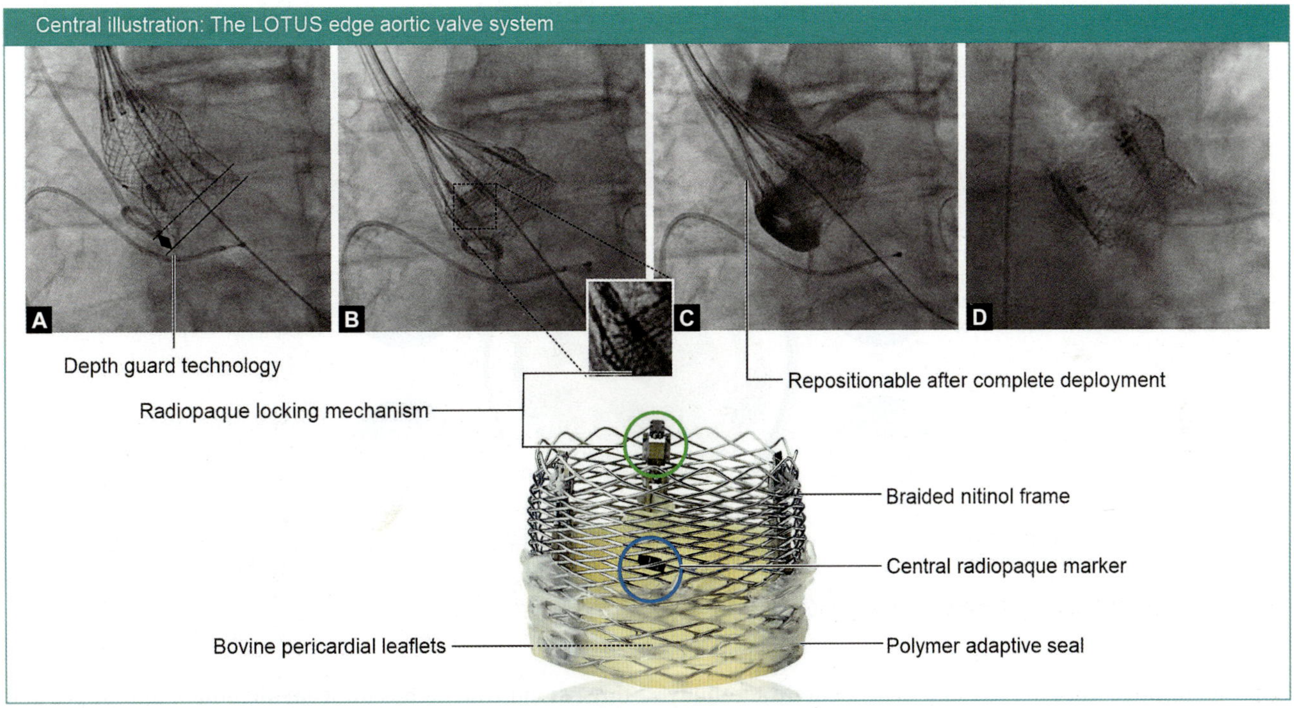

FIGS. 9A TO D: The LOTUS edge valve system from Boston Scientific.
Source: With permission from Armario X, et al. J Am Coll Cardiol Intv. 2021;14(2):172-81.

generation SAPIEN 3 and SAPIEN 3 Ultra (SAPIEN 3U) are the only two FDA approved BEVs. These are intra-annular designed valves and have bovine pericardium mounted on cobalt chromium frame **(Figs. 2A and B)**. The CoreValve, Evolut R, and Evolut Pro and Pro+ are supra-annular in design and consist of porcine pericardium sewn to self-expanding nitinol frame **(Fig. 3)**. The mechanically expandable LOTUS valve was recalled due to complexity of delivery system but newer iterations are now giving good results.

SAPIEN 3U, the fourth-generation SAPIEN platform has a 40% higher sealing skirt level above the valve inflow; *SAPIEN X4* with Resilia valve is the fifth-generation prosthesis with an outer skirt and leaflets treated with enhanced anticalcification technology to increase its longevity, dry storage, maintained thickness, and elasticity. It has delivery system with features to control THV rotation that enables commissural alignment for future coronary re access **(Figs. 2A and B)**. The ALLIANCE study is assessing the safety and efficacy.[13,14]

Evolut Fx (EFx) is the fourth-generation SEV from Medtronic with improvised features over fourth-generation *Evolut Pro and Pro+* **(Fig. 3)**. The EFx has single spine as

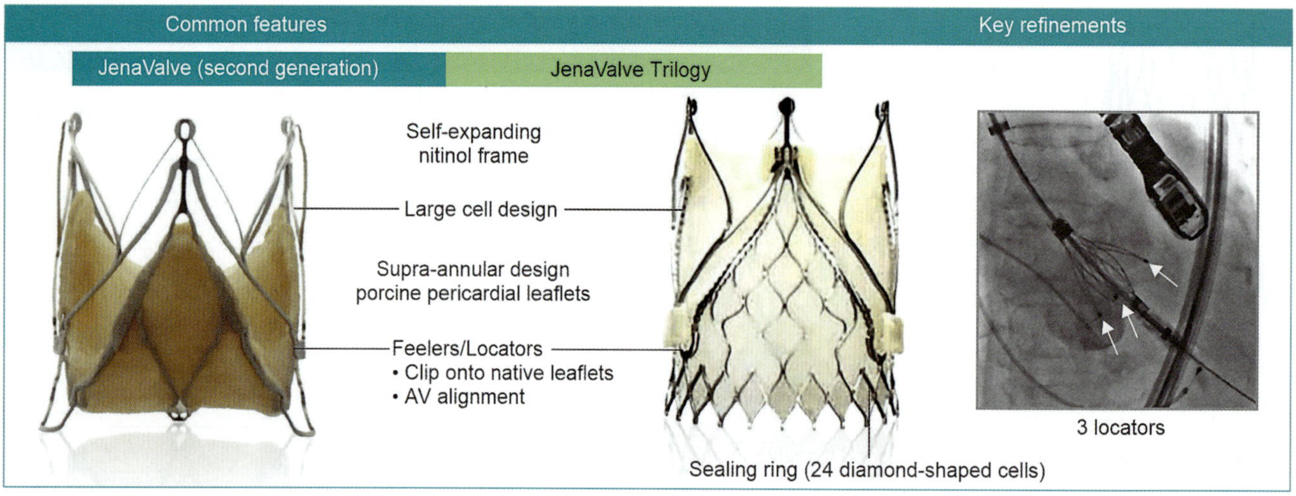

FIG. 10: Common features, key refinements of second generation JenaValve and JenaValve Trilogy.

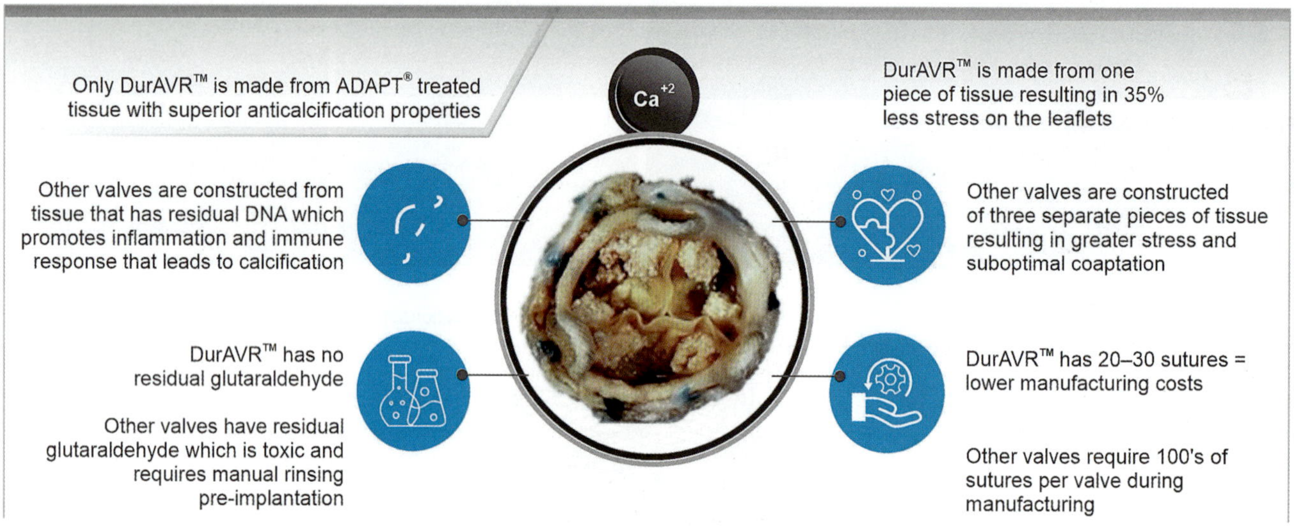

FIG. 11: The DurAVR system (Anteris Technologies).

opposed to two spines in Pro+ and helps better trackability and flexibility, an improved nose cone that makes it atraumatic, has three dot markers to identify three commissural locations and help symmetric deployment.

Portico Navitor, the third-generation Navitor[15] from Abbott structural heart has large cell design for coronary access and curved aortic cells to reduce injury, dedicated NaviSeal fabric cuffs which sync with cardiac cycle to fill the calcification-related gaps between THV and virtual basal ring and a landing zone without cut outs to reduce paravalvular leak (PVL) **(Fig. 4)**.

ACURATE neo 2 is an iteration of self-expanding supra-annular valve ACURATE neo (from Boston Scientific), has 60% taller sealing skirt extending to the upper crown reaching the waist of the stent, radiopaque positioning marker, and flexible catheter with less traumatic tip.[16] It has three stabilizing arches for axial alignment and upper and lower anchoring crowns for accurate positioning during a top to bottom deployment. The open upper frame provides unrestricted coronary access **(Figs. 5A and B)**.

Indigenous Valves from India

The first made in India valve was *Myval* (Meril life sciences, Vapi, Gujrat, India), is a BEV available in multiple sizes (20, 21.5, 23, 24.5, 26, 27.5, 29, 30.5, and 32 mm) for annulus range of (18.5–32.7 mm) (270–840 mm^2). It differs from SAPIEN 3 and ultra in terms of its frame that is made of nickel-cobalt and has a complete honeycomb design. It is available in 1.5-mm increments and thus precise size selection with minimized over- or undersizing is possible **(Figs. 6A to C)**.

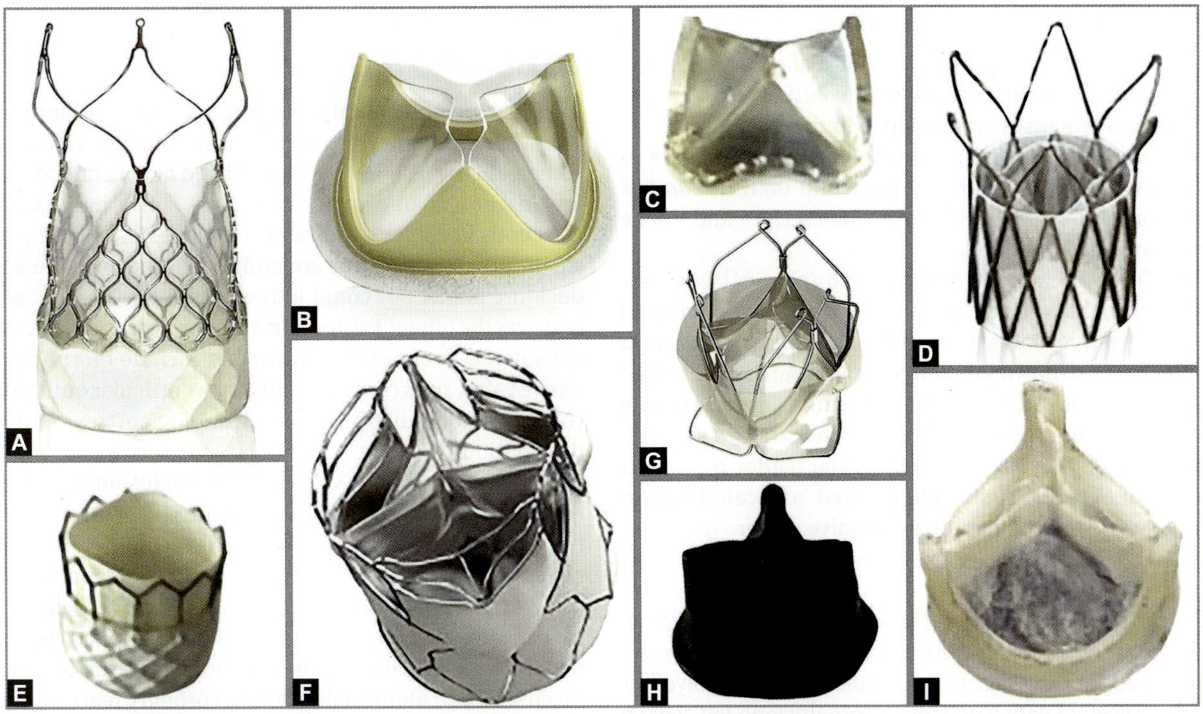

FIGS. 12A TO I: Selected polymeric heart prostheses—(A) Foldax TRIA TAVR; (B) Foldax TRIA SAVR A-M; (C) PoliValve; (D) Polynova TAVR; (E) Inflow TAVR; (F) SAT TAVR; (G) Triskele TAVR; (H) Hastalex; and (I) Innovia.

The *Myval Octacor* is a new generation of the Myval where the multirow cell design of TAVI scaffolds has been transformed to a two-row octagonal cell design concept from the previous generation Myval which had a three-row hybrid honeycomb hexagonal cell geometry **(Figs. 6A to C)**. Octacor has two rows of tessellating, geometrically identical octagons stacked one above the other forming the inflow and outflow zone. Each row is an interesting play of interlaced octagons, naturally incorporating a rhombus body at each intersection. It has least foreshortening compared to the previous generation Myval, minimal LVOT footprint and a sound platform for future valve in valve. XL sizing, unique to Octacor, includes 30.5- and 32-mm valves and is meant for those 10% real world scenarios of large annuli for whom there is no true XL valve available as of now. A 32-mm valve is good for 840-mm^2 area of annulus. It is directly crimped on the balloon of the delivery system maintaining the clock angle so that commissural alignment is achievable. This is the only BEV where commissural and coronary alignment features have been added and thus likely to be very useful in future coronary re-access. It is CE marked.[17-20]

The Myval platform has been successfully deployed in cases of pure AR by 10-20% oversizing them with good results and no valve embolization. The *Vienna valve*[21] from Relisys is another THV from Hyderabad India. It is a self-expanding nitinol frame, with bovine tissue, premounted features and ready to be used from the shelf directly. It is based on a dry valve technology and can be used as an off-shelf valve during emergency situations as well **(Figs. 7A to D)**.

The *ALLEGRA* (New Valve Technology Hechingen, Germany)[22] is again a trileaflet supra-annular SEV equipped with six gold markers on the frame that indicate the new valve plane and the delivery system provides an occlusion free implantation in three steps without fast pacing during implantation. This has potential to be used for valve in valve settings **(Fig. 8)**.

Mechanically expandable valves such as *LOTUS Edge* **(Figs. 9A to D)** from Boston Scientific Marlborough, MA USA has the so-called depth guard technology that facilitates early anchoring in order to limit the depth of implantation.[23] The mechanical principle of stent expansion and the outer adaptive seal ensures a surgery like result with regard to PVL and thus appears to be a good choice for bicuspid anatomy or severe calcification.

JenaValve **(Fig. 10)** which provides reliable annular anchoring system in the absence of AV calcification; it is supra-annular valve, mounted on self-expanding nitinol frame with large cell design, three integrated radiopaque locators called *feelers* meant for precise visualization while deployment and also serves in clipping the device to native leaflets thereby firmly anchoring the THV independent of calcification. It has a sealing ring of 24 diamond-shaped cells and THV securement with minimal protrusion into the LVOT. TAVI for pure AR is feasible by this dedicated valve and has good data to support.[24]

New Bioprosthetic Leaflets[24-30]

Resilia, Anteris DurAVR (single piece 3D leaflets), and *Foldax* have improved durability through prevention of structural deterioration processes involved in their manufacturing.

Resilia tissue showed good results through 5 years in COMMENCE trial[30] for surgical valve and then *Resilia* has been incorporated in the *SAPIEN 3U Resilia valve* and will be incorporated in *SX4* as well.

The DurAVR system (Anteris Technologies) is a new BEV platform, has a single piece of 3D tissue leaflet molded to mimic native valve **(Fig. 11)**. Computational fluid remodeling has shown greater coaptation area and height with a more uniform distribution of leaflet stress resulting in optimal laminar flow and lesser leaflet strain. *DNA and glutaraldehyde free acellular* pericardial leaflet treatment along with *ADAPT* tissue engineered anticalcification technology provides durability to the valve leaflet.

Foldax TRIA heart valve uses polymer-based leaflet that would last lifetime in a patient without deterioration and ensure physiological function **(Figs. 12A to I)**. A biomedical grade *Siloxane-based polyurethane-urea (TRIA life polymer)* is under study in vitro and in vivo. It is mounted on a polyether ether ketone stent with a polytetrafluoroethylene felt sewing ring. It is stored in a dry state and needs no preparation before implantation. *TRIA* LP heart valve has shown encouraging results at 3 years in human studies.

EVIDENCE OF SUPERIORITY OF ONE VALVE OVER THE OTHER

No evidence through any large-scale randomized head-to-head comparison is available to say that one valve is superior over the other. Head-to-head trials which have been done did not constitute challenging real-world cases but were designed with ideal TAVI patients. Results of regulatory approval trials cannot be encouraged because of the differences in patient population, their risk profile and the variety of device iterations. The CHOICE[31] (randomized comparison of THVs in high-risk patients) trial with severe AS showed no differences in the clinical outcomes of CoreValve versus SAPIEN XT at 5 years follow-up. Hemodynamics favored SEVs but valve deterioration was more with BEVs. Similarly, The SOLVE TAVI trial[32] (The Comparison of second-generation SEVs vs. the BEVs and general vs. local anesthesia in TAVI) found equivalent clinical outcomes with newer-generation S3 and self-expanding Evolut R devices at 30 days. A primary endpoint composed of all-cause mortality, stroke, significant PVL, and permanent pacemaker implantation (PPI) occurred in 25.9% BE group and 28.4% SE group. However, one-year stroke rate was significantly higher with the S3 group and moderate-to-severe PVL was more with the Evolut R group.

Large randomized long-term trials comparing head-to-head would be needed to establish the superiority of one valve over the other and till then no valve can be considered to be superior over the other.

CHOICE OF ONE VALVE OVER THE OTHER: HOW DO WE DECIDE?

Most patients are suitable for any valve but still in the real life, we decide one valve over the other taking into account some patient specific or device-related factors due to certain advantages of one over the other. These may result in variations in efficacy and safety outcomes in specific patient subgroups. These factors are numerous, not always make the deciding points but could influence the decision in favor of one over the other **(Tables 1 and 2)**. Certain factors are always considered in choosing a valve and include morphology of native valve, sizes of the annulus, left ventricular outflow tract (LVOT), sinotubular junction, ascending aorta, severity and distribution of calcium at annular and device landing zone, the aortic angulation (AA), coronary occlusion risk, and the evaluation of access vessel size, tortuosity, and calcification. An ideal valve theoretically should have low profile size, covers a wide range of annular sizes, be repositionable and retrievable, achieves optimal effective orifice area (EOA), single digit or zero residual gradient, has consistent neocommissural alignment, induces least residual PVL and no conduction abnormality, future coronary reaccess should be feasible with ease, and not the least it should be durable one. Lifetime management of AS with these valves will be an essential feature of evaluation and consideration whenever a decision of valve choice will be there for young and low-risk population. Till now, no such ideal valve exists and hence specific scenarios may favor one valve over the other from amongst the currently available valves and their newer iterations in the future.

CHANGING PRACTICES IN VALVE SELECTION FROM PAST TO THE PRESENT

Device selection in the beginning years of TAVI was largely based on the size of iliofemoral arteries (favoring the SEV in small-sized femoral and iliac) and the size of native annulus favoring (the BEV in large anatomies). In those early years, selection was mainly governed by the dimensions and specifications of the delivery sheath, the delivery catheter, and the anatomical limitations of the available valve sizes.

In subsequent years, full size matrix of THVs was available for both BEVs and SEVs. Choice of valve was then made on operators' familiarity with the device and on certain anatomical and clinical factors. Recognition of the complex aortic root anatomy sparked a shift in preprocedural imaging toward 3D ECG-gated multislice computed tomography (MSCT) scan which helped in reduction of complications with both the valves. With >20 years of TAVI now, experience and learning have increased, newer devices, dedicated valves, and delivery systems are available; newer deployment techniques, adoption of safety measures, and a possibility of customization by 3D printing exist in the pre-TAVR work

TABLE 2: Factors influencing transcatheter heart valve selection.

Factors decisive in choosing valve		First choice of valve	Not a preferred valve	Remarks about the choice of valve
Anatomical features				
	Small annulus	SEV	BEV	Supra-annular valves preferred for large effective orifice area and good hemodynamics
	Large annulus	BEV/SEV	–	Consider other factors to choose one
	Severe calcification	SEV	BEV	Over sizing in BEV dangerous
	Low coronary ostia height	BEV/SEV	Avoid valves with high skirt, small cells	Other factors of coronary occlusion to be kept in mind
	Horizontal aorta	BEV/SEV with flex catheters	SEV without flexing features	Stiff wires, buddy balloon or upfront snare techniques can help
	Bicuspid morphology	BEV/SEV	Never small valves	Valve sizing, raphe calcium, and leaflet length are important points
	Tricuspid morphology	SEV/BEV	–	Other factors decide
	Access vessel size			
	Small iliofemoral diameter	Valves having low profile delivery sheaths	Larger sheath valves	Low profile inline sheath, E sheaths
	Tortuous vessels	BEV	SEV	Stiff wires used to straighten
	Heavily calcified	SEV having low profile	BEV with large sheaths	Intravascular lithotripsy assisted or alternate access
Degenerated surgical valves		Supra-annular valve	BEV	Which valve has degenerated/fracturing required or not
Degenerated TAVI valves		Different from first THV		Data scarce, coronary occlusion, reaccess, and leaflet electrosurgical treatment
Comorbid conditions				
	Coronary artery burden and need for future visits	BEV	SEV	Coronary alignment and commissural alignment achievable or not
	Left ventricular dysfunction	BEV/SEV	SEV	All other factors to be seen
	RBBB	BEV	SEV	Better techniques and features of new-generation SEV also used
	Renal failure	BEV	SEV	Contrast lowest
Implantation ease	Operators ease and learning curve			
Alternate access	BEV can be only used for antegrade and transapical approach			
Rate of RV pacing	High rate of RV pacing needed for balloon expanding valves but caution in severe LV dysfunction patients			
Risk of pacemaker	Avoid SEV if high risk of PPI likely and choose supra-annular valve deployed by special techniques at a shallow depth			
Radiation risks	BEV	BEV	SEV/BEV with too many steps	Important for younger patients
Low risk and young	BEV/SEV		SEV new generation	EOA, hemodynamics, durability, PPI risk, stroke risk, and PVL
Low risk and elderly	SEV/BEV		–	Other factors
Life expectancy < 1 year	Not done			

(BEV: balloon expanding valve; SEV: self-expanding valve)

up. The principles of valve selection today have been further understood, more MSCT parameters and multiple factors are taken into account in order to achieve large EOAs, best hemodynamics, least patient prosthesis mismatch (PPM), least risk of PPI, no PVL, and have maximum durability. Keeping in mind the life expectancy of an individual, choice of valve is no more based on a simple considerations as in the past. According to the current practices, multifactorial determinants influence the decision of valve selection.

FACTORS INFLUENCING VALVE SELECTION (TABLE 2)[31-47]

Anatomical Factors

These include the morphology of aortic valve, dimensions of the annulus (AA), sinus of Valsalva (SOV), sinotubular junction (STJ), ascending aorta, and the LVOT. Annulus-based sizing of the valve is most reproducible and preferred option but needs to be correlated with morphological and other anatomical factors interplaying and influencing what size and type of valve one would be choosing for a patient. These factors constitute information about the distribution and severity of calcium in the device landing zone, coronary ostia heights, size of the native leaflets, and calcium chunks present in specific locations such as SOV, STJ, LVOT, around the coronary ostia, or the arch of aorta. Information about membranous septum length, septal bulge, hypertrophied ventricle, and aortopathy are other important inputs in valve selection so that procedural complications do not occur and the best results are achievable. TAVI in bicuspid morphology is totally a different ball game, as the same principles of valve selection and sizing do not apply which are meant for a tricuspid aortic valve. The ideal and perfect way of sizing in a bicuspid anatomy is still not definitive and valve selection principles not standardized, but with the current sizing algorithms and types of valves available, good outcomes similar to tricuspid valves have been seen in the large registries.

Annulus Size

Most devices are suitable for an annulus with average diameter of 16–30 mm. Larger dimensions can be catered by SAPIEN 3, 29 mm for 29.5-mm annulus, Evolut R 34 mm for 30-mm annulus and Myval Octacor up to 32-mm annulus. Use of S3 in >683-mm^2 area and Evolut R > 95-mm perimeter with a 34-mm Evolut R can be done but is considered off label use for the extralarge annulus. Both devices can be used for very large annulus as well up to 852 mm^2 by S3 and 100-mm perimeter annulus by 34-mm Evolut R. Most operators use overfilled S3 for very large annuli. 5 mL of extra can be added in S3 for very large annuli, but overexpansion of a smaller sized prosthesis will risk acute leaflet failure and reduced durability. Small annuli ≤23 mm or <400 mm^2 have high residual gradients and PPM with intra-annular devices and hence supra-annular THVs should be preferred. CHOICE trial had shown better EOA and gradients with SEV than BEVs at 5 years follow-up. Other patients in whom the supra-annular design may be favorable are those at increased risk of PPM, e.g., those going for valve in valve, TAVI for small surgical valves (21 mm or less), and obese patients with high body mass index (BMI) for their annuli. In borderline annuli, if SEV is chosen, higher degree of overexpansion can be done but if BEV is chosen, less oversizing should be done. Annulus rupture traditionally occurs more with BEVs but if postdilation is done with an oversized balloon the risk of rupture is more with SEVs.

- *Coronary burden and occlusion risk*: Coronary ostial occlusions more likely to occur if anatomical risk factors such as lower coronary ostial heights from annulus, shorter sinus heights, and a shallow effaced (SOV are present. Nonanatomical factors such as age, female sex, no previous bypass graft, implantation of s-exp valves, and valve-in-valve for failed surgical tissue valve could be potential risk for coronary occlusion. The coronary occlusion risk could be lowered by selecting a SEV with specific anchoring features as that of the upper crown of ACURATE neo 2 that keeps the native leaflets away or the THVs can be repositioned and retrieved before final release or the BEVs with large open cells and shorter frame heights are chosen.
- *Calcification*: Calcium is needed in the device landing zone but excess of it in the subannular plane and STJ affects the procedural outcomes and complications such as PVL and aortic annulus rupture are more likely to occur. Need for postdilation with both the s-exp and b-exp valves is seen to be there in some cases. Asymmetrical calcification, protruding chunks into LVOT, or annulus would need valves with advanced and extrasealing skirts to prevent significant residual PVL. New-generation valves of both types have circumferential sealing skirts to protect against PVL. Annulus rupture is likely to occur with oversized BEV in the presence of large protruding calcium and in this scenario SEV is advised to be selected. In a study patient with LVOT/annular rupture the BEV had ≥20% annular area oversizing more frequently. In extensive calcium anatomy, caution with both the valves is mandated.
- *Bicuspid morphology:* The unique anatomy of larger annuli dimensions, extensive and complex calcification patterns, asymmetric fish mouth orifice, and a dilated aortic root and ascending aorta combined with horizontal angulations in many make TAVI challenging. Bicuspid valve for TAVI is thus a relative contraindication for TAVI by the current guidelines despite favorable data coming up in recent years from registries-based analysis showing feasibility, safety, and good outcomes with present new generation of valves. Existing data are not consistent and do not allow us to make firm conclusions. Makkar et al.[42] found no significant data in mortality but increased 30-day rates of stroke with SAPIEN valves. Research in terms of differential device selection and long-term durability

are required because bicuspid anatomies are seen more in younger-aged patients who are being referred for TAVI.

- *Aortic angulation and horizontality*: It poses significant challenge to optimal delivery, positioning, and deployment of the TAVI valve. AA > 70° was excluded for early generation SEVs and BEV was preferred when there was increased AA >50°. Walksman[43] showed that AA > 48° did not influence with new-generation SE or BE valves. Despite the new-generation SEVs with flexing catheters the practice of using BEV for horizontal anatomy is preferred. CoreValve manufacturers recommend use only if <70° when using iliofemoral and left axillary route, <30° with right axillary approach and any angle with direct aortic approach. Flexibility capacity of the delivery system is the basic difference between the two valves. Active flexion and extension during valve delivery optimize the coaxial alignment of the BEV. Conversely, there is no control on flexion in the SEV. Noncoaxial approach can cause cross ability of valve challenges. Recent iterations of SEV delivery system have two shaft spines improving strength and 1:1 torque response. The long length of the stent frame of SEV results in symmetrical position and incomplete sealing of the paravalvular space. The shorter stent of BEV has nearly no intersection with the aorta. Sealing skirts in both have reduced PVL rates. Short stent frames and delivery systems with dual articulation and distal flexing features common to BEVs are preferred because they allow crossing of the arch, the valve, and easy positioning and deployment. Self-alignment after release of the stabilization arches makes ACURATE neo 2 a good SEV for horizontal configuration; EFx the latest generation of Medtronic CoreValve family has ability to flex and can be used in horizontal anatomy successfully.
- *Access route*: It is an important factor in deciding the THV. SAPIEN 3 and the ACURATE neo are only valves that can be implanted by transapical and transvascular route. Diameter of the sheath or the delivery system (in sheathless devices) is very important parameter that determines the choice of THV. Very small vessel < 5-mm femorals are suitable for Evolut R because of its lowest profile or the sheathless part of Portico can also be chosen. Sheaths size declared represent inner diameters and maximum outer diameters can be considerably more, especially upon insertion of delivery system and the valve. Rarely in tall individuals with very tortuous vessels, the delivery system may fall short in length. Abdominal aortic aneurysm does not preclude a transfemoral TAVI and tortuous arteries can be straightened with stiff wires.

Patient Factors Affecting Choice of Valves

- *Preexisting conduction disturbances*: Preexisting right bundle branch block (RBBB) conduction defect is an independent risk factor for need of PPI. Left bundle branch block (LBBB) and other conduction disturbances also increase the chance of PPI. Factors such as porcelain aorta, absence of prior valve surgery, septal hypertrophy, calcification of the left or noncoronary cusp, device landing zone, prosthesis implantation depth in LVOT, and larger or significantly oversized valve all can be associated with occurrence of advanced conduction block requiring PPI. The rate of PPI after TAVI varies as function of the type of valve. Early-generation SEV had 25–28% patients needing PPI and 5–7% for the BEV group. Drastic reduction of PPI after TAVI has not been seen with either valve despite new iterations. Overall, the PPI rate is variable, SEVs are associated with more PPI because of the radial force on the ventricular side and a deeper implant. Evolut Pro implantation depth can be planned according to the membranous septum length and shallower implantation targeted by using cuspal overlap technique reduces the risk of conduction disturbances and need of PPI. Similarly, ACURATE neo 2 and Navitor have shown lower PPI rates.
- *Burden of coronary artery disease (CAD) and future reaccess*:[46] 30% of patients going for TAVI have concomitant CAD. Outcomes are dependent upon the burden of CAD. Most adopt complete revascularization before TAVI but in elderlies, revascularization can be targeted and not total. Significant proportion of patients will need coronary angiography and PCI after TAVR at some point in their life. Technical complexity of coronary reaccess would occur if CoreValve family of SEV can occur because the taller stent is barrier to selective engagement of coronary ostia with regular diagnostic catheters. Height of Evolut Pro+ is 45 mm whereas height of S3 is 15.5–22.5 mm. The concave design of central part of avoids the contact of frame with the coronary ostia and the size of cells is accommodative of 10-French catheters but struts of the frame affects coaxial engagement. Height of the sealing skirt is 13–14 mm in Evolut whereas it is 11.6 mm for the inner sealing skirt and an outer skirt covers 8.1 mm of the lower third of the frame. For both valves, the relationship between final depth, skirt height and height of native coronary ostia plays role during reaccess of the coronaries. If anticipation of a future coronary intervention is there and access could be challenging with certain TAVI valves in situ, then choose valves such as SAPIEN 3, Myval Octacor, and ACURATE neo 2 which have large cells that allow unrestricted future coronary reaccess. Attention to improve neo commissural alignment with the native aortic valve commissures to facilitate coronary reaccess should be tried. Commissural alignment is critical when the proximal edge of the stent frame of the selected valve is higher than the coronary ostia. For both valves, commissural alignment has been described. Commissural alignment if not achieved then commissures will fall in front of the coronary ostia making

coaxial engagement almost impossible and coronary ostia can be engaged noncoaxially from diamonds on either side of the ostium. If risk is high for coronary occlusion due to risk factors but within the recommended measurement of the manufacturer then SEV is recommended because of its retrievability and repositionability. Coronary protection with wire, guides, and stents is done routinely where stenting could be required or a pre-emptive leaflet laceration by electrosurgery is conducted in valve-in-valve cases when native or prosthetic leaflets pose a risk to occlude the ostia of coronary arteries.

- *Patient prosthesis mismatch*: Supra-annular valves have lower residual gradients and least PPM. In clinical practice, special attention is to be kept because PPM would affect the long-term outcomes in a young low-risk patient.
- *Left ventricular systolic dysfunction*: THVs that would not require rapid pacing during deployment (e.g., SEV) should be chosen and those likely to end up having increased incidence of advanced conduction disturbances, significant PVL, and high residual gradients should not be selected in a patient or else, any of these happening to a patient would only deteriorate the clinical condition and affect outcomes in long term. If PPI is needed, a cardiac resynchronization therapy with defibrillator (CRTD) would be appropriate in the setting of severe LV dysfunction.
- *TAVI in renal failure patients:* BEVs need less or no contrast for deployment and should be preferred in the patients of CKD. The new-generation SEV, ACURATE neo 2 has stabilizing arches and crowns that reduce the need for high pacing and eliminate the acute renal insult by pacing. Longer pacing and repeated pacing with drop of blood pressure could cause acute kidney injury and could happen with either valves.

Rapid Pacing Tolerability Factor

Balloon expanding valves are deployed using rapid pacing but cannot be then tolerated by severe LV dysfunction patients or patients with huge ischemia burden. SEVs are deployed with very slow rapid or no pacing and could be the choice of THV in these patients.

Device Feasibility and Access Feasibility Factor

A BEV device can be used via an antegrade transeptal approach because the valve can be mounted and crimped with a reverse orientation on the balloon. A SEV cannot be loaded with a reversed orientation therefore a theoretical case when femoral access is not suitable there is no alternate access other than femoral vein, a BEV with antegrade transseptal approach may be best option.

- *Implanters experience with a device*: With increasing new devices available, the operator has to learn and adapt to new techniques and understand new mechanics. The ease of use and familiarity with a device are often an underestimated factor in procedural success and complications. Human error and technical failure increase with complexity of procedural steps and hence valve selection is also influenced by ease and familiarity of the prosthesis by the implanter and what he chooses for his patient.
- *Radiation dose* during TAVI procedure is not much. It is increased with complexity of the procedural steps requiring predilation, postdilation maneuvers to position, resheath recapture, etc., and would expose to greater radiation that could harm the young low-risk patients and hence becomes another matrix in deciding which valve for these young people going for TAVI procedure would appear safer against radiation hazards.
- *Valve durability factor*: It is going to be a major decisive factor in valve selection for the young low-risk patients who have long years of life ahead, but at the present there is no comparative long-term data on durability and hence differential selection based on this ground is not possible with the current generation of valves.

NEWER INPUTS FROM THE IMAGING MODALITIES FOR CHOICE OF VALVES IN TAVI

Miscellaneous new CT parameters that influence valve selection are membranous septal length, septal bulge, leaflet length and virtual THV to coronary ostia distance (VTC) for coronary occlusion risk in stented surgical valves and in valve in valve cases. These would favor then one valve over the other. Recently, patient-specific parametric modeling and 3D printing models have been created for pre-TAVI work-up, device sizing, bench top prediction of complications, planning for valve-in-valve and bicuspid aortic valves for better results and least chance of complications. It predicts how a THV will interact with a specific aortic anatomy even before the actual procedure is performed. Bench top predicted "best fit" valve showed statistically significant correlation with gold standard CT measurements.

LIFETIME MANAGEMENT FOR AORTIC STENOSIS—A NEW CONCEPT: AN IMPORTANT DETERMINANT IN VALVE SELECTION[47]

Landmark trials demonstrated noninferiority or even superiority of transfemoral TAVI and paved the way of TAVI to intermediate and low-risk patients. The low-risk patients who are young are likely to outlive their THVs and hence a greater emphasis is now on the planning a lifetime management best suited sequence in terms of surgery versus TAVI as the first procedure and then right prosthesis at the right time in the patients whole of life when the need for valve replacement arises. The choice of first procedure would pave the way for second and third procedures. It is thus very important to now decide what advice is ideal for a young patient of AS who needs valve replacement as the decision will predict the future challenges and or ease of managing his aortic valve disease. Factors such as feasibility of second and a third procedure of valve in valve when the first or second valves degenerate and need implantation of a new valve must be studied more extensively before making a final consensus. Coronary reaccess through struts and then the layers of frames will be a major challenge for future coronary intervention. The new-generation valves are targeting for techniques that will help and identify neo commissural alignment at time of deployment and make coronary reaccess easy keeping in mind the young and low-risk population. The increasing risk of coronary occlusion with leaflets of the older valve or the large bulky valves of some bicuspid cases needs complex electrosurgical techniques to rectify or prevent coronary occlusion. The learning curve for these techniques would be additional procedural steps for the operators. On the other hand, advancements in leaflet material and design of TAVI valves are being aimed to achieve an ideal valve that would last for patients' lifetime and in the eventuality of structural degeneration and failing TAVI valves there should not be a hindrance to implantation of the second or third valve if the need arises.

SELECTION OF TRANSCATHETER HEART VALVE: WHERE DO WE STAND TODAY?

Transcatheter heart valve selection was mainly dictated by the dimensions and specifications of the delivery sheath catheter and anatomical limitations in early days but in contemporary clinical practice operators are focusing on the prosthesis specifications such as frame height, design, radial force, anatomical characteristics, suitability for future coronary reaccess, use as second or third valve, and the leaflet characteristics for durability. Large multicenter registries and randomized controlled trial (RCT) have provided evidence necessary to ensure optimal use and patient outcomes after TAVI. The evidence for transfemoral TAVI shows that both BE and new-generation SE valves allow precise positioning and have good outcomes in a wide range of patients and anatomies with less need of pacemakers, lesser PVL, and good outcomes; however, device iterations today aim at improved hemodynamics, durability, and further reduction of stroke rates. There are so many valves available today and are approved or in way of approval that would make valve selection more difficult and confusing in the future. The newcomers have the same basic fundamental characteristics and are supported by a modest amount of scientific data. Majority of TAVI patients will probably be treated with one valve type, nevertheless a vast armamentarium is going to be useful for treatment of the complete spectrum of patients going for TAVI. Additionally, operator experience at the local expertise has to be also considered an important factor in ultimate success when selecting the valve type.

CONCLUSION

Choice of valve in TAVI is the key to success of the procedure. It should be governed by individualized approach that should take into consideration imaging-guided measurements, clinical profile of the patient, and the characteristics of the contemporary prosthesis available. Supporting data for TAVI in young low-risk patients and bicuspid anatomy are coming up with evidence of noninferior or superior outcomes and safety as that of surgical aortic valve replacement but more data needs to be available with regard to best hemodynamics and durability in order to make it standard of care for this population.

ONLINE REFERENCES

Please scan the QR code provided at the end of the table of contents for References of this chapter.

CHAPTER 175

Transcatheter Aortic Valve Replacement: Where Do We Stand in 2023?

Nagendra Boopathy Senguttuvan, Ravinder Singh Rao

ABSTRACT

Aortic stenosis (AS) affects 2–5% of the older adults after 70 years. Transcatheter aortic valve replacement (TAVR) is approved for the patients with severe AS, irrespective of their surgical risk. More and more younger patients will be treated by TAVR in the future. Various devices are available now. Cardiology community should work along with the surgeons to identify the right form of therapy for the patients. Lifetime management of the patients with severe AS starts from the first valve to be implanted; hence, significant thought process needs to considered before deciding which valve for which patient.

Keywords: Aortic stenosis, TAVR, SAVR, long-term outcomes.

INTRODUCTION

Aortic stenosis (AS) affects 2–5% of the older adults after 70 years. The prevalence of the same increases as age increases. The most common etiology is degenerative aortic valve disease across the world. Regarding the morphology, two-thirds < 70 years have bicuspid while 40% of >70 years have bicuspid valve morphology. Transcatheter aortic valve replacement (TAVR) is approved for the patients with severe AS irrespective of their surgical risk. In this chapter, we will discuss about the role of TAVR in 2023.

What is an ideal valve?

An ideal TAVR valve is yet to be identified. However, an ideal valve should have the features as described in **Box 1**.

When not to a TAVR in 2023?

"Primum non-nocere" or "first, do no harm" is the statement proposed by Hippocrates. In order to execute the same, we should know when not to consider TAVR in 2023.

In general, TAVR can be considered in patients with an estimated survival of >20 years. In addition, multiple factors such as the patient's anatomical factors, patient's personal preferences, and associated diseases along with the surgical risk of the patient's needs to be considered **(Fig. 1 and Table 1)**.

BOX 1 **Ideal transcatheter aortic valve replacement (TAVR) valve.**

- Minimal vascular access size
- Durable long term results
- Optimal effective orifice area
- Minimal paravalvular leak
- Suitable for wide range of annulus sizes
- Repositionable and retrievable
- Low risk of permanent pacemaker implant and/or new permanent conduction abnormalities
- Easy coronary reaccess
- Consistent commissural alignment
- Minimal need of contrast use
- Simple-to-use delivery system
- Suitable for use in patients with low ejection fraction (EF)
- Suitable for different aortic valve pathologies such as aortic regurgitation and bicuspid anatomy
- Should come with in-built system to prevent stroke

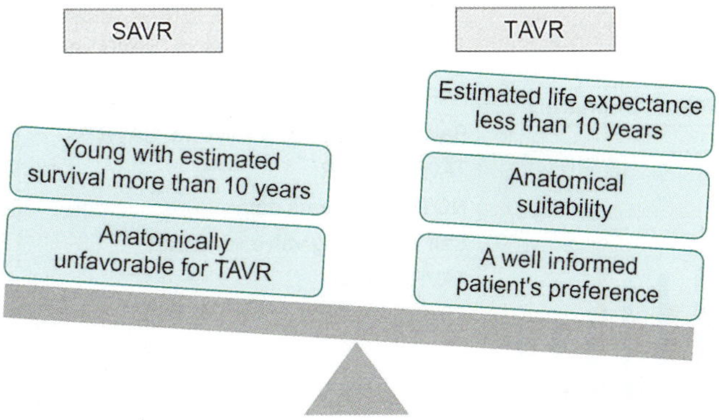

FIG. 1: Comparison of SAVR and TAVR.

(TAVR: transcatheter aortic valve replacement; SAVR: surgical aortic valve replacement)

LIFETIME MANAGEMENT OF TRANSCATHETER AORTIC VALVE REPLACEMENT

It is imperative to know when not to do rather than when to do. The utilization of TAVR in younger patients will create an epidemic of redo aortic valve replacement (AVR) which may be TAV in TAV (TAVR in TAVR) or surgical AVR in TAV after a decade. "With great power comes great responsibility"—Superman. We should not forget that EXPLANT TAVR registry have found a dangerously high-mortality rate of 25% at 1 month and 35% at 1 year; hence, such advanced therapies should be judiciously used for appropriate patients.

The most important factor that determines surgical aortic valve replacement (SAVR) or TAVR in an individual patient is the winner over the contest between expected longevity of an individual and durability of the valve. In 2023, age of the patient is the most important criteria for selecting a procedure of choice. It varies from 65 years in the USA to 75 years in the Europe, and 80 years in the Japan.[1] The expected longevity of the different race which varies from country to country, for example, in India the expected survival of an average male and female are 17.5 and 19.2 years respectively at the age of 60 years **(Fig. 2)**.[2]

The second most important factor that determines the selection of procedure is the durability of the TAVR valves as compared with the surgical valves. As of 2023, we have the longest follow-up of 8 years for the self-expanding

TABLE 1: Characteristics of TAVR and SAVR.

Characteristics	TAVR	SAVR	Unknown
Estimated survival of the patient > 10 years	+	+++	
Anatomical factors Severe LVOT calcification	+	+++	
Severe CAD (triple vessel/distal LM disease)	+	+++	
Bicuspid valve	+	+++	
Unicuspid valve	–	+++	
Porcelain aorta	+++	–	
Low coronary heights in low, intermediate or high-risk patients	–	+++	
Low coronary heights in prohibitively high-risk or high-risk patients	++ (basilica or chimney)	+	TAVR vs. SAVR
Highly unfavorable femoral anatomy in a low or intermediate-risk patient	+	+++	
Severe carotid disease		–	
Isolated aortic regurgitation		+++	
Significant multivalvular disease	+	+++	
Associated subvalvular LV outflow obstruction	+	+++	
Patient-related factors			
Frailty	+++	+	
Patients preference	+++	+	
Highly unfavorable femoral anatomy in a high-risk risk patient	++ (alternate access)	+	
Associated infective endocarditis	–	+++	
End stage or severe disease of any one organs (lung/liver/kidney)	+++	+	

(LVOT: left ventricular outflow tract; SVAR: surgical aortic valve replacement; TAVR: transcatheter aortic valve replacement)

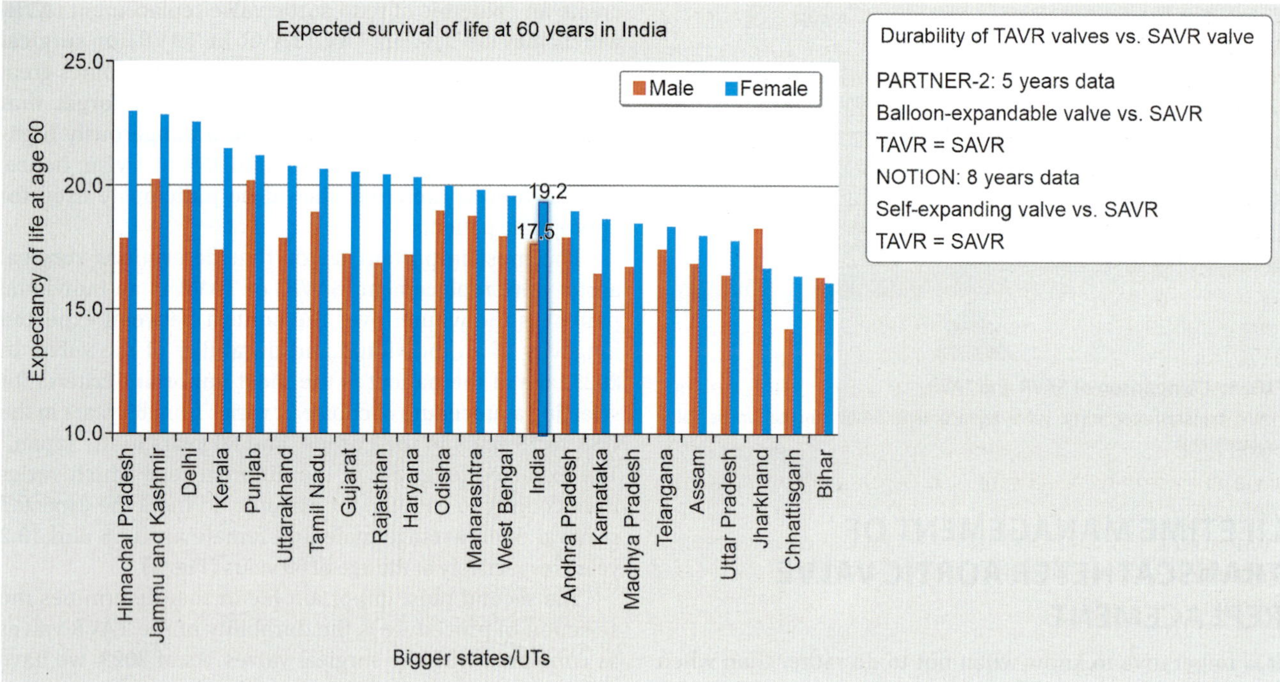

FIG. 2: Life-expectancy in TAVR and SAVR.
(transcatheter aortic valve replacement; SAVR: surgical aortic valve replacement)

valves (SEVs) from the NOTION study[3] and 5 years for the balloon-expandable valves (BEV) from the PARTNER-2 trial,[4] respectively. An expected mean survival of a surgical AVR from the Valve-in-Valve International Data (VIVID) registry was 9 years.[5] In general, age cut-off point for the Indian patient may be considered as 70 years from the author's perspective. Performing a TAVR inside a failed TAVR is much more difficult as compared with a TAVR inside a failed surgical valve due to various reasons such as coronary reaccess and acute closure of the coronary vessels.[6] Though randomized studies did not find a difference between BEV versus SEV, a recent meta-analysis found reduction in all-cause mortality with BEV as compared with SEV.[7] A shared-decision process involving a heart team that comprises of interventional cardiologist, imaging cardiologist, anesthesiologist and a cardiac surgeon is recommended in selecting the appropriate procedure taking into consideration the wishes and preferences of the patients.

"MINIMALISTIC" TRANSCATHETER AORTIC VALVE REPLACEMENT

Monitored anesthesia care (conscious sedation with a local anesthesia) is the norm of TAVR. Transfemoral access is the success of TAVR over SAVR. If a femoral arterial accesses is not available, then an extrathoracic access should be considered over intrathoracic access. Each center should have one alternate access which is comfortable for them. The data on alternate access for TAVR is not robust, however, percutaneous axillary, surgical carotid, or percutaneous transcaval are the commonly utilized access across the world. A percutaneous coronary intervention (PCI)-like TAVR procedures is considered in selected centers with which the author do not agree at present as the data for the same is not strong.

Aortic Valve Replacement in Asymptomatic Individual with Severe Aortic Stenosis

Asymptomatic patients with severe AS having low surgical risk with one of the following factors:

- With positive exercise stress test
- With elevated BNP (three times normal)
- With rapid disease progressions (increase in velocity of >0.5 m/s/year)
- Peak velocity of >5 m/s

Two recent randomized studies addressing the same question of early AVR in asymptomatic patients with severe AS and normal LV function needs emphasis here.[8,9] They randomized 145 patients to either early surgery versus the conservative management. The median time from randomization to AVR in the early surgery and conservative arms was 23 days and 700 days, respectively. With a median follow-up of 6.2 years and 6.1 years in the early surgery and conservative group, respectively, cardiovascular (CV) death was observed in 1% in the early surgery group and 15% in the conservative group. In the AVATAR (Aortic

Valve Replacement versus Conservative Treatment in Asymptomatic Severe Aortic Stenosis) trial, Banovic et al., randomized 157 patients with asymptomatic severe AS (exercise test negative) to early AVR (78 patients) versus conservative treatment (79 patients). The median time from randomization to SAVR in the early surgery group was 55 days, and 400 days in the conservative group. The study was stopped as advised by the data and safety monitoring board (DSMB). The primary outcome [the composite of all-cause mortality, myocardial infarction (MI), stroke, or unplanned hospitalization for the heart failure] was lower in the early AVR group as compared with the conservative group (15.2% vs. 34.7%, HR 0.46; 95% CI 0.23–0.90; $p = 0.020$). However, no difference in all-cause mortality was noted. Such a positive result of SAVR over medical therapy in patients with asymptomatic severe AS cannot be extrapolated to patients undergoing TAVR.[10] The EARLY TAVR (Evaluation of TAVR Compared to Surveillance for Patients With Asymptomatic Severe Aortic Stenosis) trial is being done, which may answer the above question.[11]

COMMISSURAL ALIGNMENT

Aligning the TAVR valve commissures with the native valve enable us to have good coronary reaccess in the future. It has also been shown that alignment of BEV with commissures provided some hemodynamic advantage to those who did not have. Commissural alignment in BEV is random until recent. However, OctoCor and Meril Life have produced intentional commissural alignment of BEV using a "clock method." Commissural alignment in SEVs use the saline port position. With Evolut series, the flush port should be at 3 o'clock while for ACURATE neo2 series the flush port should be in the 6 o'clock position. Commissural alignment with Navitor is still under the process. It is proposed that efforts should be made from the device industry and the scientific committee to make the process of commissural alignment more predictable, easily adaptable and reproducible.[12]

Coronary Reaccess

Aortic stenosis and coronary artery disease (CAD) are frequent occurrence in the same patient. Most of the trials involving high-risk and intermediate-risk groups of patients showed the presence of concomitant CAD in 63–75% of the patients.[13,14] In a small randomized study, it was shown that performing PCI before TAVR as compared with doing TAVR alone did not make a significant impact on death or rehospitalization for 1 year.[15] It has been shown in a recent study that outcomes of the patients who have CAD is worse than those without CAD.[16] In the same context, patient with more severe CAD have higher events as compared with those with less severe CAD. However, performing revascularization did not change the clinical outcomes in such patients.

Also, coronary access post-TAVR is a very challenging one leading to nonselective angiograms in many of the cases.[17] Recently, Faroux et al. found that PCI failure occurred significantly more commonly in patients with previous TAVR, predominantly due to failure to engage the coronary ostia.[18] Hence, a valve with a shorter frame such as BEVs and larger cells like ACURATE neo2 with reasonably predictable commissural alignment may be preferred in those patients who have severe CAD and are undergoing TAVR.

REDUCE CONDUCTION DISTURBANCE AND PACEMKAER

A recent meta-analysis concluded that the principle independent predictors for proton pump inhibitor (PPI) following TAVI are right bundle branch block (RBBB), SEV type, left bundle branch block (LBBB), age, and valve implantation depth.[19]

The incidence of permanent pacemaker implantation (PPI) requirement varies from valve to valve. It is higher with SEV. Point to remember is that having a new onset persistent LBBB [new-onset persistent (NOP)-LBBB] post-TAVR is not innocuous. Faroux et al. found that NOP-LBBB is associated with cardiac death and PPI within 1 year. Similarly, NOP-LBBB and PPI are associated with increased all-cause mortality and heart failure-related hospitalization in 1 year. Hence, we need to prevent the occurrence of conduction disturbance post-TAVR. For SEV, deploying the valve in cusp-overlap view [usually right anterior oblique (RAO) caudal] ensure high deployment of the valve.[20] Also, using a Minimizing Depth According to the Membranous Septum (MIDAS) strategy based on membranous septum length[21] has been proposed to reduce pacemaker occurrence. For BEV, deploying the valve in RAO caudal (cusp-overlap) has been shown to be associated with reduced occurrence of PPI.[22,23]

REDUCING STROKE

Mortality post-TAVR with stroke is very high. Outcome of TAVR has improved significantly over a period of time. In spite of such a positive effect, the incidence of stroke after TAVR is unchanged. It remains as 2% in most of the studies. Various devices are under study to prevent it. The most commonly used device is the Sentinel which protects one-half of the cerebral circulation (left vertebral is not protected). PROTECTED TAVR trial showed no overall benefit of Sentinel, however, it reduces disabling stroke.[24] The cost of the device remains a major concern in our country. However, the author believes it should be considered more frequently in valve in valve, severe calcified valve, young patients and bicuspid anatomy. **Figure 3** shows sentinel in a patient undergoing TAVR and the material obtained in the filter.

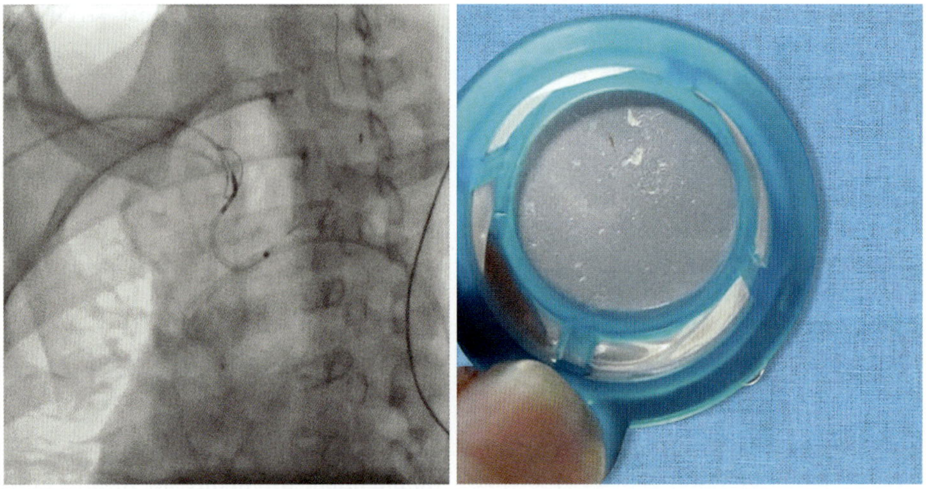

FIG. 3: Sentinel in a patient undergoing transcatheter aortic valve replacement (TAVR) and the material obtained in the filter.

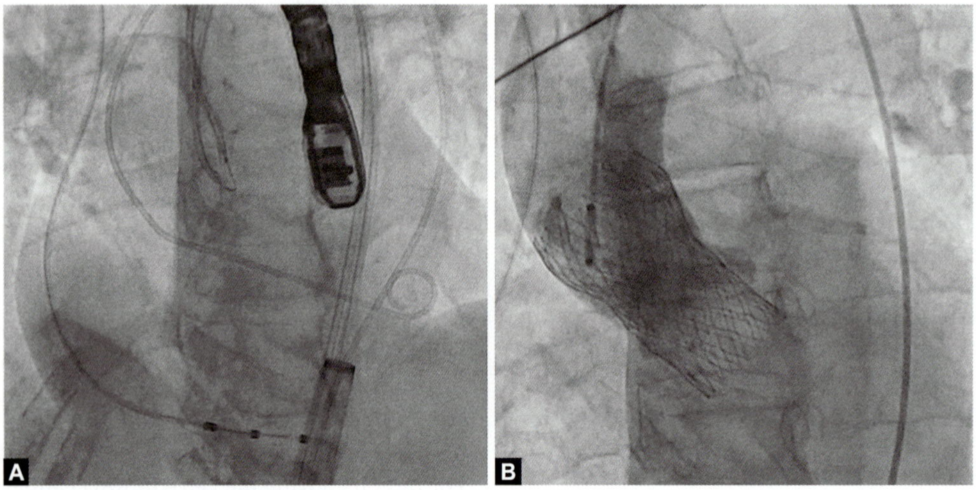

FIGS. 4A AND B: (A) Flying V Basilica and (B) Final aortogram.

ELECTROCAUTERY PROCEDURE FOR TRANSCATHETER AORTIC VALVE REPLACEMENT

The BASILICA (Bioprosthetic or Native Aortic Scallop Intentional Laceration to Prevent Iatrogenic Coronary Artery Obstruction) is considered to be the procedure of choice in patients who are high risk for acute coronary occlusion immediately post-TAVR. A piggyback catheter with a Astato 20 guidewire is electrocauterized to puncture the leaflet base and to cut the leaflet after snaring the wire in the left ventricular outflow tract (LVOT) **(Figs. 4A and B)**. A recent study has compared basilica with chimney stenting and found that the freedom from clinically relevant or complete coronary obstruction was same for both at 1 year.[25] However, chimney technique was associated with a higher risk of periprocedural complications.

Future

Dedicated devices for aortic regurgitation will become commonly available. The JenaValve and J Valve are the one currently available in Europe; however, they are not available in India. The Jena valve with its hooks to hold the valve acts like an anchor to hold the valve in situ and prevent any leaflet-related coronary occlusion.[26] Primary concern in doing valve in valve which can be TAV in SAV or TAV in TAV is the acute coronary occlusion. A dedicated device like shortcut device to cut the leaflet before deploying the new valve has been reported.[27]

CONCLUSION

Transcatheter aortic valve replacement is and will remain the treatment of the elderly patients with severe AS. It is imperative for the cardiology community to learn the nuances of the same. “Heart team approach” and “shared decision making” are the keys in selecting the treatment modality. First valve determines the feasibility of TAV in TAV in future. Hence, lifetime management of AS patients is an important entity to be considered.

ONLINE REFERENCES

Please scan the QR code provided at the end of the table of contents for References of this chapter.

CHAPTER 176

A Promising Odyssey: Transcatheter Aortic Valve Implantation's Advancements and Expectations for the Next 20 Years

Alain Cribier

ABSTRACT

The 20th anniversary of transcatheter aortic valve implantation (TAVI), a therapeutic innovation initiated by our group in 2002, was enthusiastically celebrated around the world last year. This technique consists of implanting a valve prosthesis within the native aortic valve of adults suffering from degenerative calcific aortic stenosis (AS) using usual cardiac catheterization techniques. AS is the most frequently acquired valvular disease in adults. For decades, many patients could not benefit from the only possible life-saving treatment, surgical aortic valve replacement (SAVR), because of old age or comorbidities. All these patients were doomed to early death. This has motivated our interest in the development of less-invasive interventional techniques, balloon aortic valvuloplasty in 1985, then TAVI, aimed at palliating the limitations of the first approach.

The development of TAVI was a fascinating 20-year odyssey, which, despite the worst initial criticisms, resulted in an extraordinary achievement. At present, more than two million patients have been treated with TAVI worldwide. This resulted from the combination of continuous technological advances and rigorous scientific evaluation, including several evidence-based trials comparing TAVI to SAVR in patients at decreasing surgical risk that demonstrated the noninferiority or superiority of TAVI on a patient's improvement and mortality at mid- and long-term. This led to a change in paradigm for the treatment of AS. The indication for TAVI, originally limited to "compassionate" use in high surgical risk patients, has been validated to include patients at intermediate risk and, finally, at low surgical risk as well. Since 2019, the number of TAVI procedures now exceeds the number of SAVR in numerous countries.

A continuous expansion of TAVI can be predicted in the next 20 years for many reasons, including aging population, increased number of qualified centers, advanced technologies, new indications, and a desirable reduction in the cost of TAVI. Remaining issues such as the long-term durability of TAVI valves and the management of structural valve dysfunction in the context of a younger population are under evaluation.

Keywords: Aortic valve stenosis, transcatheter aortic valve replacement, cardiac catheterization, outcomes.

INTRODUCTION

Transcatheter aortic valve implantation (TAVI) has experienced considerable global expansion in the world since 2002. The 20th anniversary of the first case performed by our team in 2002 was amply celebrated last year, with many moving celebrations highlighting the enormous interest aroused by this disruptive technique and the importance it has taken in medical practice. As in most countries, the rise of TAVI in India is actually very impressive, with a continual growth in the number of centers and operators. Over 20 years, TAVI has become a simpler, faster, and safer procedure as technology has advanced. Nevertheless, it remains essential for new operators to understand all aspects of this therapeutic modality, including indications, preclinical evaluation, techniques, and "tips and tricks" associated with different valve models, prevention and treatment of complications, and lifetime management; all these aspects will be discussed in the course of this 2023 CSI annual meet. TAVI is a magnificent technique that deserves to be learned and performed with great care, especially as it concerns increasingly younger patients with increased longevity, in whom complications considered minor and acceptable in the elderly may be impactful on the long term.

Before addressing the question of the place of TAVI now and in the future, it may be interesting to briefly recall here the key phases of TAVI development by our team, because this true odyssey can inspire all those who wish to innovate in medicine. Never getting discouraged despite difficulties and criticisms is the key message.

The only possible and live-saving treatment of degenerative aortic stenosis (AS) has long been surgical aortic valve replacement (SAVR) by mechanical valve and then increasingly by bioprosthetic valves, a heavy open-heart operation, of which many patients were deemed too old or too frail to undergo or incapable of surviving if they did. In the 2000s, only one-third of symptomatic patients were operated on in Europe.[1] This was particularly true in the 1980s since age per se, over 70 years, was a regular contraindication to open-heart surgery. Finding at this time for these patients a less-invasive alternative solution than SAVR became our priority.

FIRST STEPS OF TRANSCATHETER AORTIC VALVE IMPLANTATION DEVELOPMENT

We first developed in Rouen in 1985 the technique of balloon aortic valvuloplasty (BAV), a simple percutaneous procedure consisting of opening the calcified aortic valve with a balloon. The uneventful world premiere that resulted in an amazing clinical improvement was followed by a first series of inoperable patients, the publication of which in The Lancet[2] had a bomb effect in the medical community. BAV was rapidly adopted worldwide, but after tens of thousands of patients were treated, the enthusiasm declined due to unacceptable early valve restenosis. As there is always something good to keep from a failure, we are happy to see that BAV still exists, with specific validated indications, and it has known an impressive rebirth with the onset of TAVI since it is used daily all over the world, for valve predilation or post-dilation of transcatheter heart valves (THVs). BAV must be considered a preliminary and crucial step on the route to TAVI.

This failure that could have ended the story pushed us on the contrary to find a solution against restenosis, and this went through the concept of a percutaneous balloon-expandable stented-aortic valve, implantable by cardiac catheterization, under local anesthesia, a project announced since 1987. Despite the unfavorable opinion of all experts, the concept was validated by a landmark autopsy study in a fresh specimen of AS, conducted in Rouen in 1994. Without it, it is likely that TAVI would not exist today. Large-size (23 mm) Palmaz balloon-expandable stents could be fully expanded within all 12 calcified valves, and the optimal stent's dimensions (15–17 mm in length) avoiding any damage to the surrounding structures (mitral valve, coronary ostia, His bundle) were determined. Furthermore, the stents were strongly anchored within the calcified valves, thus decreasing the risk of secondary device embolization. Nevertheless, during 5 years, the search for industrial support was a total failure, the project appearing inconceivable and unrealistic to all experts ("the stupidest project ever presented..."), which would have discouraged many. In 1999, we finally created a startup company [Percutaneous Valve Technologies (PVT), NJ, USA] with two engineers and a renowned cardiologist, Martin Leon, who was clearly seduced by the project despite acknowledging its low chance of success. A biomedical partnership in Israel (ARAN R&D) allowed us to obtain prototypes of a THV, a 23-mm stainless steel stent containing a tricuspid valve made of polymer and later of equine pericardium. These prototypes, as well as the crimping device and the delivery systems, were constantly improved and extensively tested in the laboratory and on animal models. With my colleague Helene Eltchaninoff, a hundred implantations at various cardiac sites were performed in the sheep model to refine all technical aspects of THV implantation and to confirm the integrity of valvular structure and function at 5 months' follow-up, a crucial observation for a hypothetical approval for human use in the future.[3] However, succeeding TAVI in humans remained totally uncertain, and the decision of a first-in-human use was particularly difficult to take.

MOVING FROM DREAM TO REALITY

The first-in-man TAVI was a memorable event. It was performed in Rouen on April 16, 2002, as a last-resort option on a 57-year-old dying patient, in cardiogenic shock, with 12% left ventricular ejection fraction, with severe AS on a bicuspid valve, turned down for surgery due to multiple comorbidities. TAVI could only be attempted using a challenging trans-septal approach due to obstructed aortoiliac bypasses (the patient presented with subacute leg ischemia). The procedure was amazingly carried out without complication, followed by a real resuscitation on the table, followed by amazing clinical improvement. The publication of this case[4] was a resounding success in the medical community.

A first series of 38 cases could then be conducted in our center after 1 year of heavy discussion with the French High Health Authority whose experts (cardiac surgeons) imposed a drastic limitation of indication to inoperable dying patients with the use of the transseptal approach, as for the first case! With 85% procedural success, this challenging study confirmed the feasibility of TAVI and the reliability of implantation. Some patients' improvement was very impressive. One of these patients, an 83-year-old woman, was able to travel to Washington, DC, 1 year after implantation to express her feelings about TAVI at the 2004 Transcatheter Cardiovascular Therapeutics (TCT) meeting, to thousands of dazzled cardiologists. She did survive 6.5 years with no symptom and unchanged THV function.

The first-ever planned retrograde transfemoral (TF) approach was performed in a patient of this series having contraindication to the trans-septal approach. Despite the lack of any specific delivery system, the procedure was remarkably fast, easy, and uneventful, which gave us a good vision of how the procedure should be performed in the future. This patient had a 5-year uneventful follow-up before dying of noncardiac cause. Such clinical examples played an important role in the early acceptance of TAVI. The publication of our results[5,6] was decisive for the flight of TAVI abroad. In 2005, a total number of 100 cases had been performed in Europe and the USA.

In 2004, the acquisition of PVT by the company Edwards Lifesciences (Irvine, CA, USA) accelerated the evolution of TAVI with the creation of the Edward-SAPIEN valve and new delivery systems allowing its implantation by the retrograde TF approach,[7] and 1 year later by a less-invasive surgical transapical route,[8] an interesting alternative in case of an unusable femoral artery. With these two approaches, TAVI was covering the needs of almost all inoperable patients. In 2006, a competing valve appeared, the self-expandable CoreValve, later acquired by Medtronic (Minneapolis, MN, USA).[9] It is indisputable that the still ongoing competition between the two TAVI systems significantly accelerated the large expansion of the technique.

TRANSCATHETER AORTIC VALVE IMPLANTATION TAKES ITS FLIGHT IN THE WORLD: TECHNOLOGICAL ADVANCES AND EVIDENCE-BASED EVALUATION

At this point, no one could have predicted the extraordinary acceptance and expansion of TAVI over 20 years. This has resulted from constant technological advances with both valve TAVI systems and an outstanding scientific evaluation.

Technological and Procedural Advances

The step-by-step improvement of the valves and delivery systems, in particular the reduction of arterial introducers' caliber and the launch of multiple THV sizes, greatly facilitated and secured the TAVI procedures, enabling it to be realized today using the simpler and safer retrograde TF route in 95% of cases. A technique called "minimalist TF" (limited team in the room, local anesthesia, no periprocedural transesophageal echocardiography, limitation of arteriovenous lines, and short hospitalization with early discharge home) was initiated by our team in 2012[10] with the Edwards' second-generation valve (SAPIEN XT). Initially considered nonethical, it is now adopted worldwide. Other routes remain currently possible in case of an unusable femoral approach: Transapical, subclavian, transcarotid, transaortic, and even transcaval. This concerns a very limited percentage of cases.

With growing teams' experience, accurate anatomical evaluation by multislice computer tomography (MSCT), and the latest advanced TAVI systems **(Figs. 1 and 2)**, the success rate of TAVI now exceeds 95%, and severe complications have markedly decreased, in particular perivalvular leak (PVL), stroke, and conduction disorders requiring a permanent pacemaker. Today, a patient with symptomatic AS can be treated in 30–40 minutes, under local anesthesia, and return home within 2–3 days under simple antiplatelet therapy in the majority of cases, without a scar and without the need for rehabilitation. Follow-up is provided by consultation and ultrasound in the first month and every year. Thus, the difference with SAVR is major and explains the enthusiasm of patients for TAVI.

In 20 years, more than 20 medical companies stimulated by the success of TAVI have created other TAVI systems, of which very few have crossed the bar of human implantation. In Europe, till date, three other TAVI systems are marketed: Two self-expandable devices from Boston Scientific (Natick, MA, USA) and Abbott (Plymouth, MN, USA) and one promising balloon-expandable device from India (Meril Life, Vapi, India), which is the subject of an ongoing randomized trial versus the two historical models. Other THVs from Asia or South America are currently under clinical investigation.

Outstanding Scientific Evaluation

The amazing TAVI acceptance and expansion were also based on scientific rigor that fulfills the most stringent requirements of medicine. In 2007, obtaining the CE mark (European conformity) of the two TAVI systems was quickly followed by multiple national and international controlled registries on inoperable or high surgical risk patients,[11-15] resulting in the first expansion of TAVI in the world. Many national registries followed, including patients at high and then lower surgical risk, for instance, in France, the FRANCE, FRANCE 2,[16,17] and FRANCE-TAVI registries,[18] in which our group was much involved.

But the decisive steps were three rounds of randomized trials versus SAVR with both the Edwards and Medtronic valves, including thousands of patients and leading to the proof that a treatment, originally limited to "compassionate" or high surgical risk patients,[19-21] could be enlarged to patients at intermediate risk,[22,23] and finally, since 2019, to low surgical risk patients, 10 years younger, as well.[24,25] A wide superiority of TAVI was demonstrated with the Edwards device over medical treatment in inoperable patients, as well as noninferiority or superiority of TAVI regardless of the surgical risk over mortality, stroke, delay to functional improvement, and rehospitalization, at short- and mid-term with the two TAVI systems. Of note, in low-risk patients, more permanent pacemakers were required after implantation of self-expandable THV. These successive

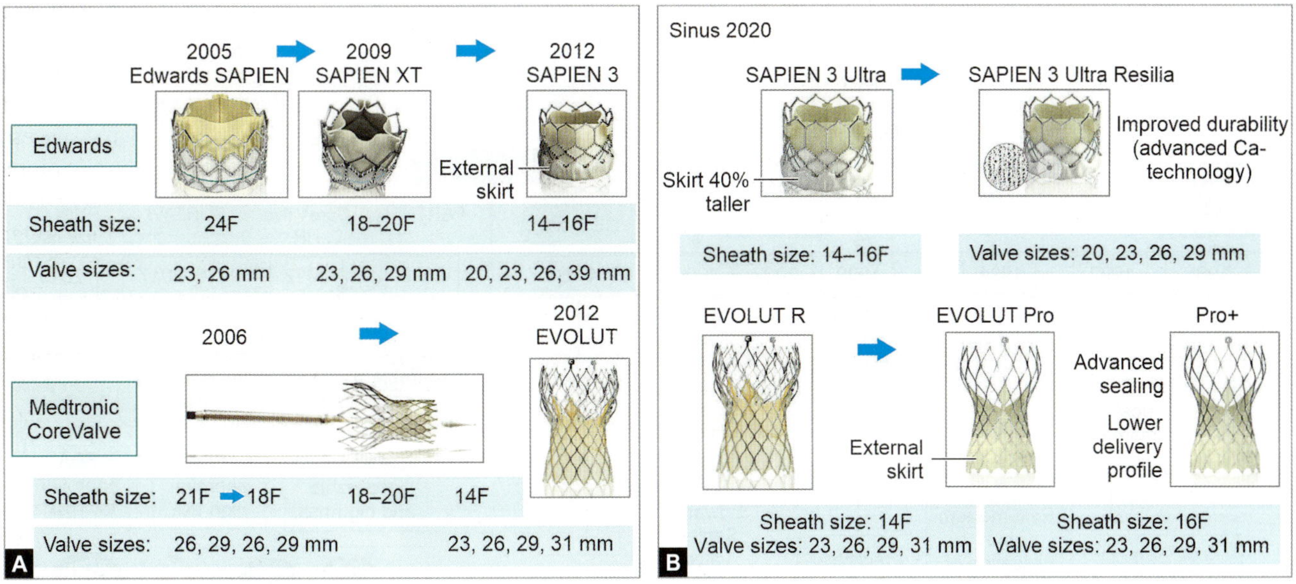

FIGS. 1A AND B: Advanced transcatheter heart valve (THV) technology over time, with the historical transcatheter aortic valve implantation (TAVI) systems from Edwards Lifesciences and Medtronic CoreValve.

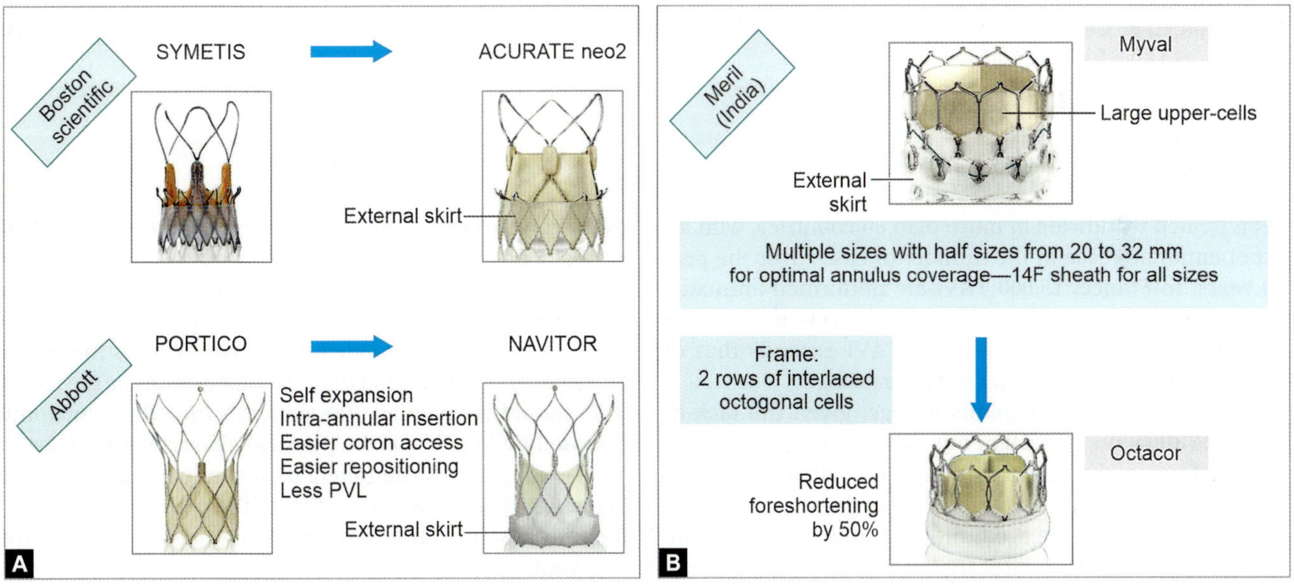

FIGS. 2A AND B: Advanced transcatheter heart valve (THV) technology over time since the late 2000 with the newer generations of transcatheter aortic valve implantation (TAVI) system from Boston Scientific, Abbott, and Meril Life.

indications were validated very soon after the reports by the scientific societies in the USA and Europe. A multidisciplinary discussion of each case (Heart Team) for the selection of patients appeared essential that deeply marked the medical culture.

The long road of TAVI development is summarized in **Figure 3**.

CURRENT PLACE OF TRANSCATHETER AORTIC VALVE IMPLANTATION AND LIFETIME MANAGEMENT

Transcatheter aortic valve implantation can today be considered as the reference treatment for patients with symptomatic AS. Currently, nearly two million patients have

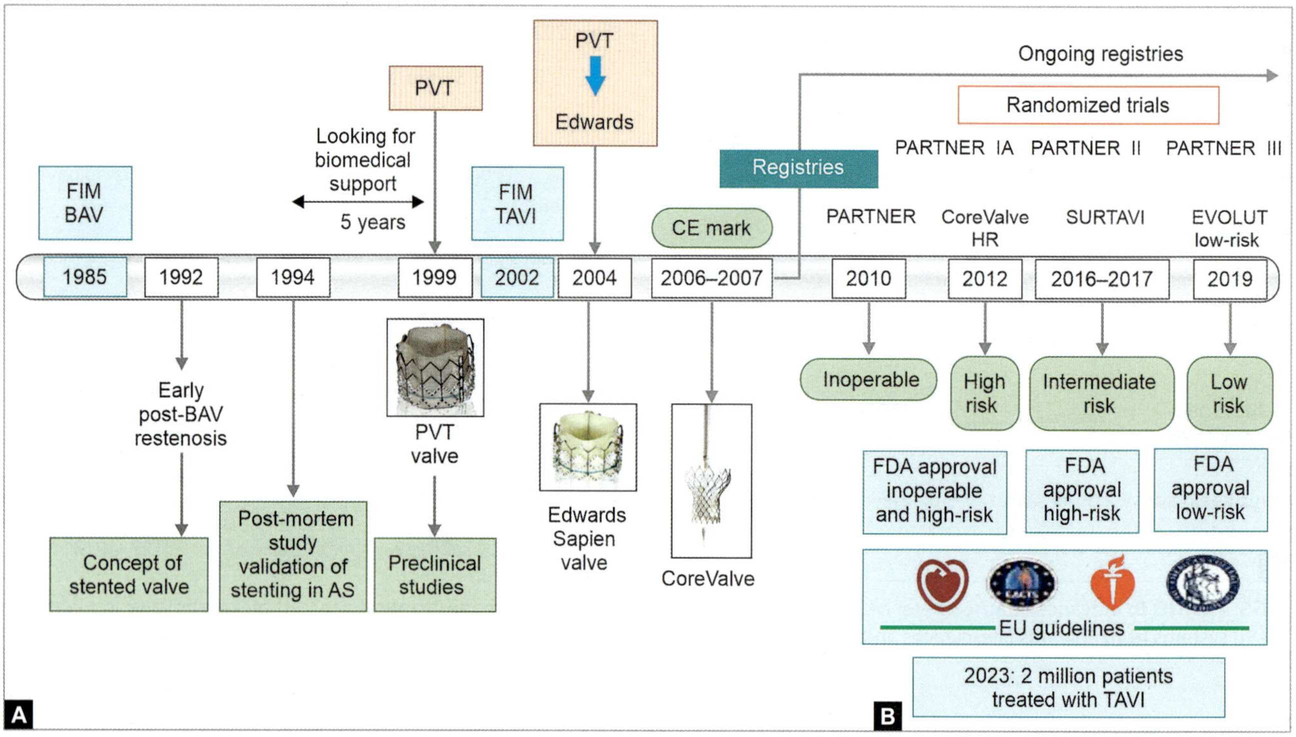

FIGS. 3A AND B: General overview of the long journey of TAVI development. The PARTNER trials are the randomized trials from Edwards Lifesciences. Other trials are from Medtronic CoreValve.

(AS: aortic stenosis; BAV: balloon aortic valvuloplasty; EU: European Union; FDA: Food and Drug Administration; FIM: first-in-man; PVT: Percutaneous Valve Technologies; TAVI: transcatheter aortic valve implantation)

been treated worldwide in more than 80 countries, with an exponential increase in the number of cases over the past 20 years. In France, 15,000 TAVI are performed annually, 20,000 in Germany, and 75,000 in the USA. In many European and US countries, the number of TAVI exceeds that of SAVR since 2019 and the gap keeps increasing.

Indication mainly depends on age, given the lack of accurate data on percutaneous valves' durability after 5 years. Despite the absence of alarm on still limited series of follow-up beyond 5 years,[26-28] the question remains posed and explains the age limit of 65 and 75 years in the low-risk population, as indicated in the US and European recommendations, respectively.

As with surgical bioprosthetic valves, structural valve dysfunction (SVD) may occur during follow-up. The rate of SVD has been shown to be low (below 2%) at 5 years in the first randomized trials and even lower after SAVR at 8 years (14% vs. 28%) in another randomized trial (NOTION trial) in all-comers treated with the Medtronic CoreValve.[29] SVD can be treated by redo-TAVI that has demonstrated to be feasible and effective or by secondary conversion to surgery. The choice of the first strategy has become crucial, especially in the youngest population, whose longer life span increases the probability of SVD. The issue of reaccessing the coronary arteries has become important, especially in younger patients with coronary artery disease (CAD) or having the risk of developing CAD in the future. THV with lower valve insertion might be privileged in first intention and tall-frame THVs avoided. Patient–prosthesis mismatch and THV underexpansion that potentially increase the risk of SVD should be avoided. The patient's individual anatomy assessed by MSCT and the physical characteristics of each THV platform must definitely be taken into consideration before TAVI since the protection of the coronaries is essential, more particularly in redo-TAVI. Furthermore, a third intervention (surgery or TAVI) may become necessary in the youngest patients, which deserves to be considered by the Heart Team and explained to the patient before deciding the first strategy. Thus, a tailored approach should be considered according to the patient's clinical status and anatomy. This is particularly true in bicuspid valves, observed in about 50% of young and low-risk patients. Even though the clinical outcome compared to tricuspid valves appears similar in carefully selected patients, the best strategy (surgery or TAVI) should be based on careful screening. Valve size selection, valve positioning, and expansion are more challenging in bicuspid valves, and the risk of coronary occlusion or PVL is higher, more particularly in the absence of valve raphe and severe calcification, often associated with aortic disease. Long-term outcomes remain uncertain in this population. Surgery, especially using the Ross procedure, may be considered the best option in challenging cases. Patient safety must always remain the priority.

HOW CAN WE SEE THE FUTURE OF TRANSCATHETER AORTIC VALVE IMPLANTATION?

The continued expansion of TAVI with an annual growth of 4–10% per year can easily be expected in the coming years for many reasons. The first one is the aging population. AS is typically a disease of the elderly with a prevalence increasing with age, of the order of 7% beyond 75 years, and the population older than 60 years will have doubled in 2050. This will justify the increasing number of operators and centers that are already in progress. The growing interest of cardiac surgeons themselves who wish to perform this procedure, the creation of an "interventional" surgical subspecialty, and the certification of some selected centers without cardiac surgery "on board" (a currently mandatory condition) would further promote the growth and expansion of TAVI, and this makes even more essential the continuation and multiplication of training programs by experienced operators.

Other indications of TAVI might appear in the future, such as TAVI in moderate AS and heart failure, moderate but symptomatic AS or asymptomatic severe AS. These indications are currently evaluated in several evidence-based studies with the two historical THV platforms. The results expected in the coming years might have unimaginable effects on TAVI expansion.

In parallel to the continuous refinement of the current THV platforms, the arrival of new generations of valves made of nonbiologic materials less prone to deterioration, currently in development, might also impact the future of TAVI.

It is to be noted that new technologies designed to improve the function of calcified aortic valves with non-invasive ultrasound therapy could find a place in the future for the treatment of AS patients as a bridge to SAVR or TAVI or in case of ineligibility for these therapeutic options.[30]

Finally, the cost of TAVI will remain a limiting factor, especially in countries with limited resources, but this might improve, as always, with increased demand and industrial competition.

CONCLUSION

The evolution of TAVI over the last 20 years is nothing less than a revolution in the practice of cardiology. 20 years after the first case, TAVI has become the treatment of choice for a majority of patients with degenerative AS, and the indications should explode in the future. The initial goal of treating inoperable patients has been far exceeded, resulting in a paradigm shift. Currently, surgery is reserved for patients for whom TAVI is not the ideal solution. TAVI has galvanized interest in structural heart disease that has led to promising percutaneous transcatheter treatments of the mitral and tricuspid valves, essential developments in cardiac imaging, and changes in the way specialists work together through the Heart Team. It was a long and bumpy road to get there, but the effort was worth it.

This shows how, leaving no room for luck, an idea, a concept, and a group of experienced individuals could meet a challenge and lead to a great therapeutic innovation to improve the lives of our patients.

ONLINE REFERENCES

Please scan the QR code provided at the end of the table of contents for References of this chapter.

CHAPTER 177

Evaluation and Management of Severe Aortic Stenosis with Multivalvular Disease and Coronary Artery Disease

Sreenivas Kumar A, Ramakrishna Janapati, Neusha Gopal

ABSTRACT

A significant proportion of aortic stenosis patients will have multivalvular disease and have concomitant coronary artery disease (CAD) as noted in approximately 50% of patients going for aortic valve replacement procedures. Age is a common risk factor for both CAD and valvular degeneration along with other common pathophysiologic factors. Management of these patients is guided by the individual physician discretion, patient comorbidities, patient preferences, and severity of valvular and vascular disease. We do come across such patients in our clinical practice and in this chapter, we will discuss the impact on clinical outcomes and various treatment strategies in this complex subset of patients.

Keywords: Coronary artery disease, aortic stenosis, valvular heart disease, transcatheter aortic valve implantation, PTCA, percutaneous coronary intervention.

INTRODUCTION

Aortic stenosis (AS) is the most common valvular disease in the western world, affecting 2% of the population between 65 and 75 years and 6% of those older than 75 years and is frequently associated with other valvular disease or mixed with some degree of aortic regurgitation (AR).[1] In developing countries such as India and other underdeveloped countries, rheumatic heart disease is still the most common cause of AS and mitral valve involvement invariably accompanies rheumatic AS. In the western world, isolated aortic valve disease primarily occurs due to a degenerative calcific disease of a native trileaflet valve or a congenitally bicuspid valve. In India, rheumatic AS is most common with a reported prevalence of 4.54 per 1,000 people.[2] From one study published from north India, the etiological distribution of all valvular heart diseases (VHDs) included rheumatic AS (83.1%), congenital AS (7.9%), and degenerative AS (6.6%).[3] It is difficult to measure the actual burden of AS in India due to lack of population-based epidemiological studies. With increasing life expectancy in Indian population, age-related degenerative valvular AS has now emerged as the most common cause of isolated AS in India.[4] With the advent of transcatheter valve replacement and its rapid expanded indications for low-risk population, the transcatheter aortic valve replacement (TAVR) is being offered to many elderly patients across the centers. Treating the multivalvular lesions with various combinations of transcatheter therapies is increasingly common in high-risk population apart from surgical therapy.[5]

Multivalvular disease (MVD) is defined as the combination of stenotic or regurgitant lesions of two or more cardiac valves and is increasingly prevalent in clinical practice, presenting in 10% of patients undergoing valvular surgery.[6] In MVD, rheumatic etiology is predominant in young people from Asian descent, while calcific or degenerative VHD is more common in older people.[4]

Prevalence of coronary artery disease (CAD) in VHD varies widely from 45 to 75%.[7] This prevalence is higher in degenerative VHD, especially in AS than in other groups; these two entities share common pathophysiologic risk factors such as aging, systemic hypertension, and degeneration, leading to frequent coexistence of both these conditions in the same patient.[8]

SYMPTOMS OF CORONARY ARTERY DISEASE IN AORTIC STENOSIS PATIENTS

Shortness of breath and exertional angina are the most common presenting symptoms in both these conditions, so the symptoms have limited utility in differentiating severity of both these conditions. Exercise stress testing is contraindicated in the presence of severe AS. In patients with left ventricular outflow tract (LVOT) obstruction and angina but without significant CAD on angiogram, it has been proposed that diminished coronary flow reserve (CFR) leads to an imbalance between myocardial oxygen supply and demand, resulting in ischemia or diffuse microvascular dysfunction. Coronary angiogram or computed tomography (CT) coronary angiogram is indicated in patients undergoing aortic valve replacement (AVR) with other coronary risk factors.[9]

CORONARY ARTERY DISEASE AND SURGICAL AORTIC VALVE REPLACEMENT

According to a large-scale Swedish registry, the prevalence of CAD varies from <10% in <50 years, 30% in 51–60 years, 41% in 61–70 years, and 51% in ≥71 years age group who underwent concomitant coronary artery bypass grafting (CABG) at the time of surgical AVR (SAVR).[10] In octogenarians undergoing SAVR, almost 60% patients had significant CAD requiring revascularization.[6,11] The presence of CAD is associated with impaired both short- and long-term outcomes among patients undergoing SAVR and even untreated CAD increases the mortality among patients undergoing isolated SAVR.[12] The risk of periprocedural events, such as bleeding, stroke, and postoperative atrial fibrillation, were significantly higher with CABG + AVR when compared to isolated SAVR and risk increases steeply in elderly patients above 80 years of age. Moreover, concomitant CABG was identified as an independent predictor of short- and long-term mortality among patients undergoing SAVR.[13] CABG is recommended (class I, level of evidence C) in patients with a primary indication for aortic valve surgery with a coronary stenosis ≥70% (≥50% in case of left main stenosis) as per both the American College of Cardiology/American heart association (ACC/AHA) and the European society of cardiology (ESC) guidelines for management of these patients.[9]

CORONARY ARTERY DISEASE AND TRANSCATHETER AORTIC VALVE REPLACEMENT

The prevalence of CAD is high with approximately 50% patients undergoing TAVR having CAD as seen in multiple studies.[14] As these population were elderly with other combined comorbid conditions beyond CAD, such as impaired left ventricular (LV) function, previous cardiac surgery, diabetes, pulmonary hypertension, and chronic kidney disease. The initial studies excluded CAD patients from TAVR studies as these studies included selective patients with high surgical risk for AVR. With TAVR being offered to low-risk patient population with more recent studies, the prevalence of CAD is also reduced significantly. The involvement of the left main and left anterior descending (LAD) artery in 11% and 50% of patients was reported in a recently published study on 4,000 TAVR recipients with CAD.[14] The presence of significant CAD adversely affects the long-term outcomes, even though there was no significant difference at 1-year follow-up of TAVR patients and previous studies reported controversial results based on the presence and severity of CAD and appropriate revascularization strategies.[15,16] However, significant CAD is an independent predictor of long-term mortality as TAVR is being offered to relatively low-risk population.[15,17] There was lack of uniformity on the definition of significant coronary artery stenosis and completeness of revascularization and lack of physiological assessment with the use of fractional flow reserve (FFR) or instantaneous wave-free ratio (IFR) in all the studies. The clinical management of AS patient with CAD needs heart team discussion with global evaluation of comorbid conditions.

Patients with severe AS presenting with acute coronary syndromes (ACSs) have a clear indication to undergo revascularization with percutaneous coronary intervention (PCI). In the presence of stable CAD, the randomized clinical trials failed to show clear beneficial effects with routine PCI pre-TAVR.[18,19] However, at this point in time, it is unclear whether complete revascularization of all angiographically significant coronary stenoses should be performed in patients undergoing transcatheter aortic valve implantation (TAVI). Indeed, a more selective strategy with PCI limited to significant stenosis of proximal segments of major epicardial vessels may be a valid alternative, allowing procedure time to be shortened, the use of contrast media to be optimized, and the risk of procedural complications to be reduced.

Timing of Percutaneous Coronary Intervention in Transcatheter Aortic Valve Replacement Patients

The optimal timing of PCI in TAVR patients is unclear, but majority of operators will perform PCI before TAVR. With this approach, patients will be subjected to repeated procedures, vascular access, and contrast media utilization and they need to be on dual antiplatelet therapy during TAVR procedure. One study comparing performing PCI < 30 days versus >30 days before TAVR did not show any significant difference with overall mortality at 2-year follow-up except increase in vascular complications and bleeding in <30 days group.[20] Another study by Singh et al. showed that patients had higher inhospital mortality with PCI and TAVR during same hospitalization.[21] Performing PCI of type A single-vessel disease and TAVI during the same session may be a practical solution and does not expose patients to risks associated with a second invasive procedure **(Figs. 1A to E)**. But if the CAD involves left main or multivessel disease, it is better to stage

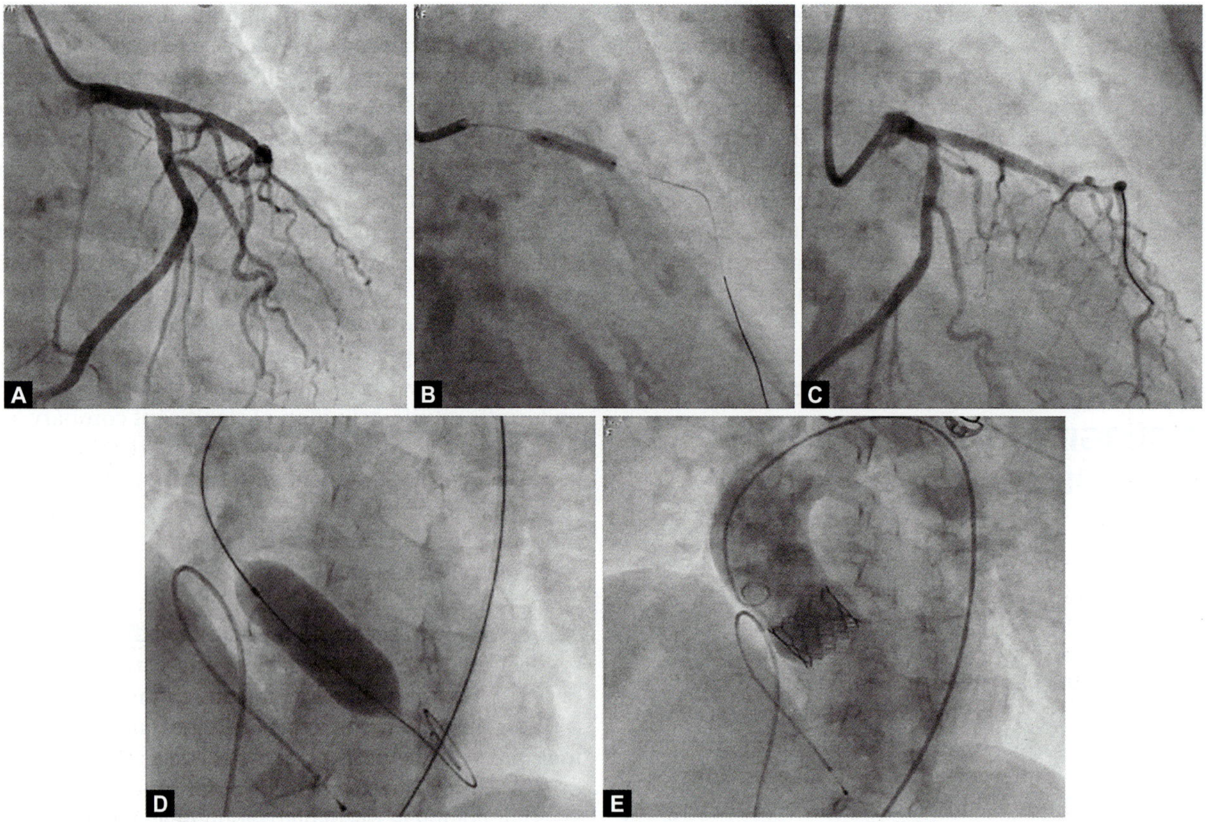

FIGS. 1A TO E: PCI and TAVR are being performed by the same procedure. (A) Proximal LAD type A lesion; (B) Balloon inflation, and (C) post-PTCA with DES; (D) Aortic valve predilatation with Z-MED balloon; (E) Balloon-expandable valve deployed with aortic root angiogram with pigtail catheter.

(DES: drug-eluting stent; LAD: left anterior descending; PCI: percutaneous coronary intervention; PTCA: percutaneous transluminal coronary angioplasty; TAVR: transcatheter aortic valve replacement)

the procedures depending upon the clinical presentation of the patient **(Figs. 2A to D)**. If patient presents with ACS or ST-segment elevation myocardial infarction (STEMI), the coronary revascularization should be done before TAVI, whereas if the patient presents with heart failure or symptoms of LV dysfunction, the TAVI should be done prior to revascularization, as this helps to improve LV function immediately post-TAVR and patient tolerates complex PCI procedure well without precipitation of LV failure (LVF) **(Figs. 3A to H)**.

On the other hand, a staged strategy—with PCI and TAVI performed in separate sessions—allows reduction of the procedure duration as well as contrast volume used during TAVI. At this point in time, PCI timing strategies are different among centers.

Taking into consideration the lack of evidence, it appears feasible to perform concomitant PCI and TAVI in patients with CAD, requiring revascularization if PCI complexity is expected to be low. Conversely, staged interventions may be a valuable option among patients with a greater extent of CAD for which a higher PCI complexity is foreseen **(Figs. 2A to D)**. Considering the complexity of decision-making in each patient, which vessel lesion to be treated and extent of treatment is left to the discretion of operator and heart team of that particular center **(Table 1)**.

CORONARY ARTERY DISEASE AFTER TRANSCATHETER AORTIC VALVE REPLACEMENT

The prevalence of CAD and acute coronary events in post-TAVR is limited to small studies and individual centers data. The predominant reasons for post-TAVR coronary events were related to atherothrombosis related to progression of preexisting CAD, previous stent failure, or coronary embolism from valve bioprosthesis. Other reasons for coronary occlusion will be impaired coronary flow dynamics due to TAVR valve and valve struts across the coronary ostia with low coronary heights from annulus. The presence of a TAVR valve could make the selective catheterization of coronary ostia difficult or even impossible during emergency PCI for patients presenting with acute coronary events. The selective engagement becomes more difficult with supra-annular,

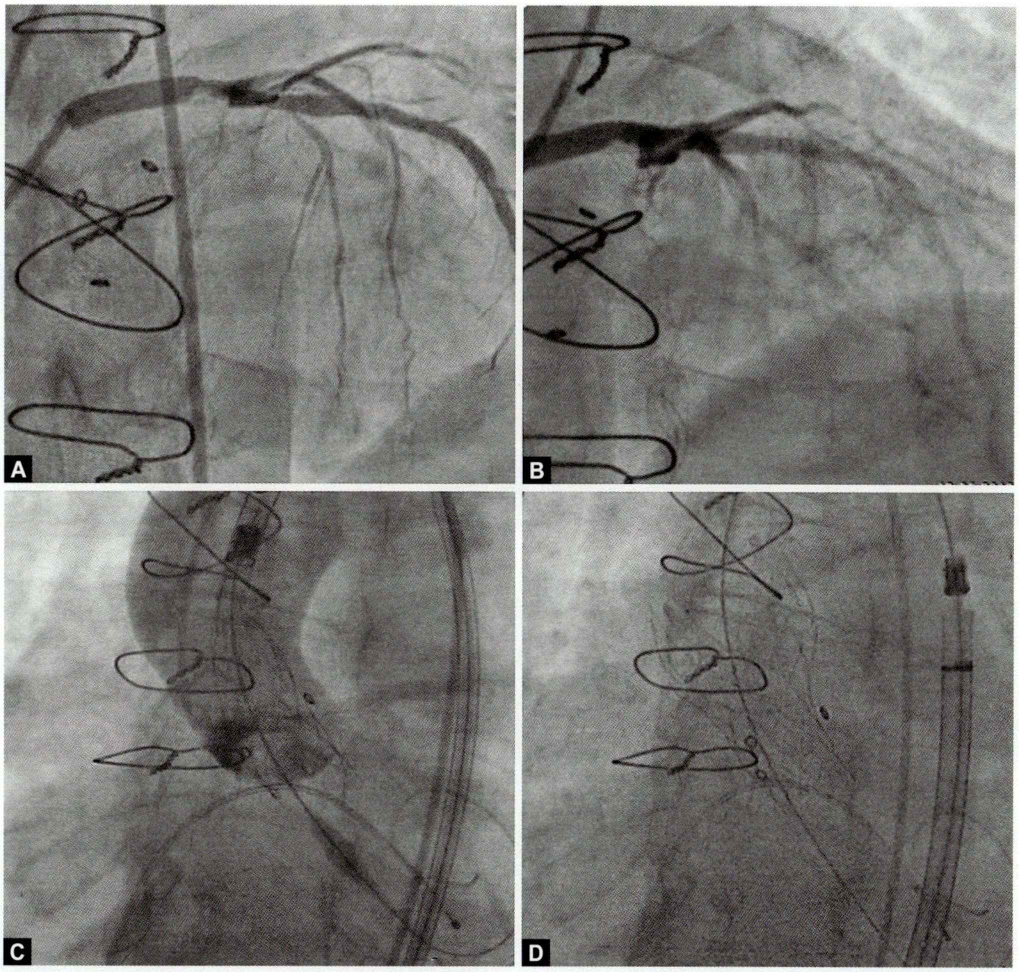

FIGS. 2A TO D: PTCA and stenting of distal LMCA lesion before TAVR in a post-CABG patient. (A) Distal LMCA eccentric stenosis; (B) After stenting of distal LMCA with DES; (C and D) Self-expanding valve being deployed across the degenerative aortic valve.

(CABG: coronary artery bypass grafting; DES: drug-eluting stent; LMCA: left main coronary artery; PTCA: percutaneous transluminal coronary angioplasty; TAVR: transcatheter aortic valve replacement)

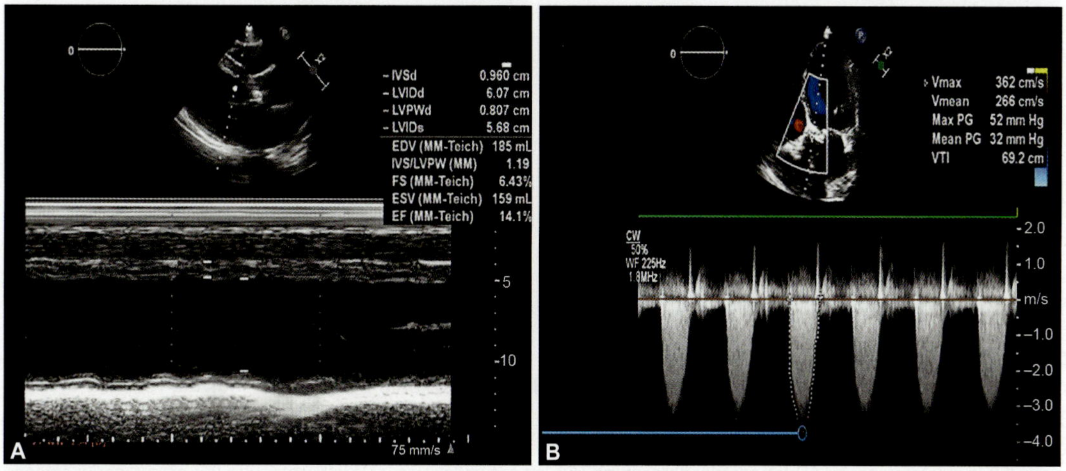

FIGS. 3A TO H: *Continued*

Continued

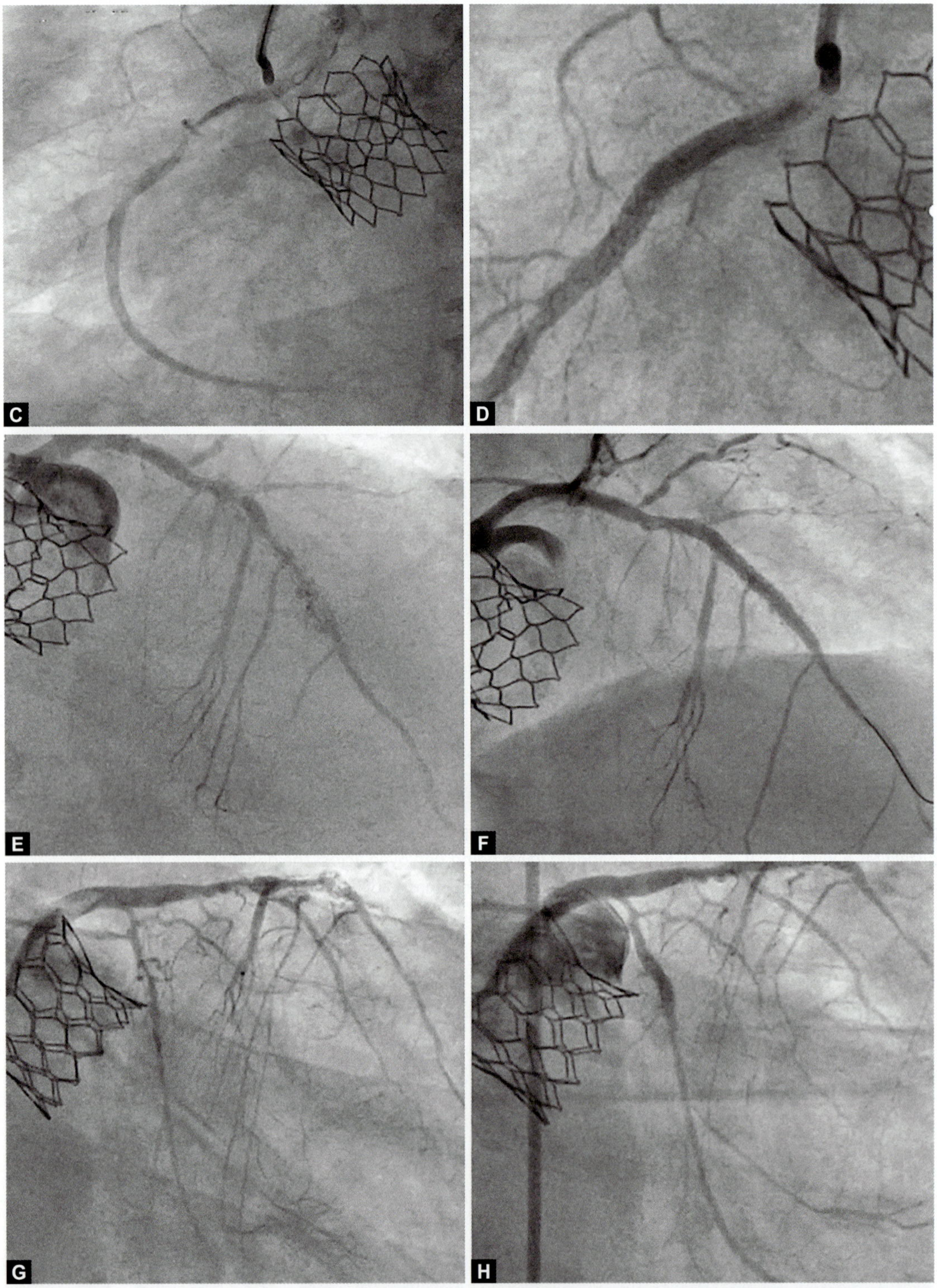

FIGS. 3A TO H: Post-TAVR (balloon-expandable valve) low-contrast multivessel PCI in a patient with ischemic severe LV dysfunction and low-flow–low-gradient, severe AS with chronic kidney disease. (A) Two-dimensional echo image showing reduced LV contractility with severe LV dysfunction; (B) Aortic valve gradients; (C and D) Proximal RCA lesion before and after angioplasty; (E and F) Mid-LAD ISR with long-segment disease before and after angioplasty; (G and H) LCx lesion before and after angioplasty.

(AS: aortic stenosis; ISR: in-stent restenosis; LAD: left anterior descending; LCx: left circumflex artery; LV: left ventricular; PCI: percutaneous coronary intervention; RCA: right coronary artery; TAVR: transcatheter aortic valve implantation)

TABLE 1: Timing of PCI with severe AS undergoing TAVR.

Timing of PCI	Advantages	Disadvantages	Clinical scenario
Simultaneous PCI and TAVI	• No need for additional vascular access • Shorter hospital stay • Less additional cost	• Higher contrast media load • Higher radiation dose and long duration procedure	• Simple coronary lesion • Normal kidney function
Pre-TAVI-staged PCI	• Possible lower risk of coronary events during TAVI procedure • Easy access for coronary • Prevent ischemia during rapid pacing during TAVI	• Risk of hemodynamic collapse during high-risk PCI procedures • Increased bleeding risk • Ostial stent struts can get crushed with TAVR valve frame	• Acute coronary syndromes • Ostial LMCA lesion and proximal coronary lesions • Complex coronary lesions • Type of valve, valve-in-valve procedures
Post-TAVI-staged PCI	• More reliable physiological assessment of borderline lesions • Better hemodynamics during PCI • Possible lower risk of bleeding related to lack of pre-TAVI dual antiplatelet therapy	• Difficult access to coronary ostia • Risk of ischemia during TAVI	Borderline coronary lesions

(AS: aortic stenosis; LMCA: left main coronary artery; PCI: percutaneous coronary intervention; TAVI: transcatheter aortic valve implantation; TAVR: transcatheter aortic valve replacement)

self-expanding valves and even more difficult with valve-in-valve TAVR. Various operators reported significantly higher radiation dosage, fluoroscopic times, and contrast medium use when compared with coronary angiography performed before TAVR.[22] With increasing number of TAVR being done in low- and intermediate-risk patients, these patients may present with future coronary events. The operators need to have understanding of the TAVR valve anatomy and challenges of coronary angiogram and PCI in this patient population **(Flowcharts 1 and 2)**.[22]

Some useful tips for selective engagement of coronaries in post-TAVR patients were shown in **Flowcharts 1 and 2** for self-expanding and balloon-expandable valves, respectively.

AORTIC STENOSIS AND MITRAL REGURGITATION

Mitral regurgitation (MR) frequently coexists with AS in patients undergoing AVR. According to different studies, MR is reported in 20–80% of patients with AS. In the PARTNER trial, about 20% of patients undergoing transcatheter or surgical AVR for severe AS presented with concomitant-moderate to severe MR. Presence of residual moderate to severe MR in patients undergoing surgical or TAVR is associated with higher mortality.[23]

Functional MR is present in around 60% of patients with AS and is likely to improve after AVR more significantly than degenerative MR. Thus, a careful evaluation of the MR mechanism is crucial for the decision of whether a simultaneous operation on the mitral valve is necessary considering that mixed mechanisms are frequent. Especially in older patients with heavy mitral valve calcification and wall motion abnormalities, the combined valvular lesions are frequent. The other condition that needs careful evaluation is ischemic MR which may be reversible with pre-TAVR revascularization of left circumflex artery (LCx) or right coronary artery (RCA) lesions. Physiologically, AS is associated with increased afterload, but when MR is present, the left ventricle is somewhat larger as volume overload is also present. The presence of MR may falsely underestimate the transvalvular aortic valvular gradient as MR reduces the stroke volume significantly and produces a low-flow–low-gradient AS. Severe MR also reduces the afterload along with reduced stroke volume; the assessment of AS severity needs to be carefully evaluated **(Figs. 4A to D)**.

Both these combined valvular lesions may precipitate atrial fibrillation subsequently with preload impairment due to loss of the "atrial kick," which is very poorly tolerated, leading to frequent symptoms of heart failure. Generally, symptoms do not always correlate with the AS severity and LV function with MR; concomitant MR is associated with poorer outcomes in AS patients undergoing AVR.[23,24]

AORTIC STENOSIS AND TRICUSPID REGURGITATION

Tricuspid regurgitation (TR) is common in patients with left-side valvular disease and more specifically in 40% of patients with severe degenerative AS.[24] Severe AS can lead to elevated LV end-diastolic pressures and increased left atrial pressures. Chronic high left atrial pressure leads to remodeling of the alveolar–capillary membrane and development of pulmonary hypertension. Pulmonary hypertension can lead to right ventricular (RV) pressure overload and right

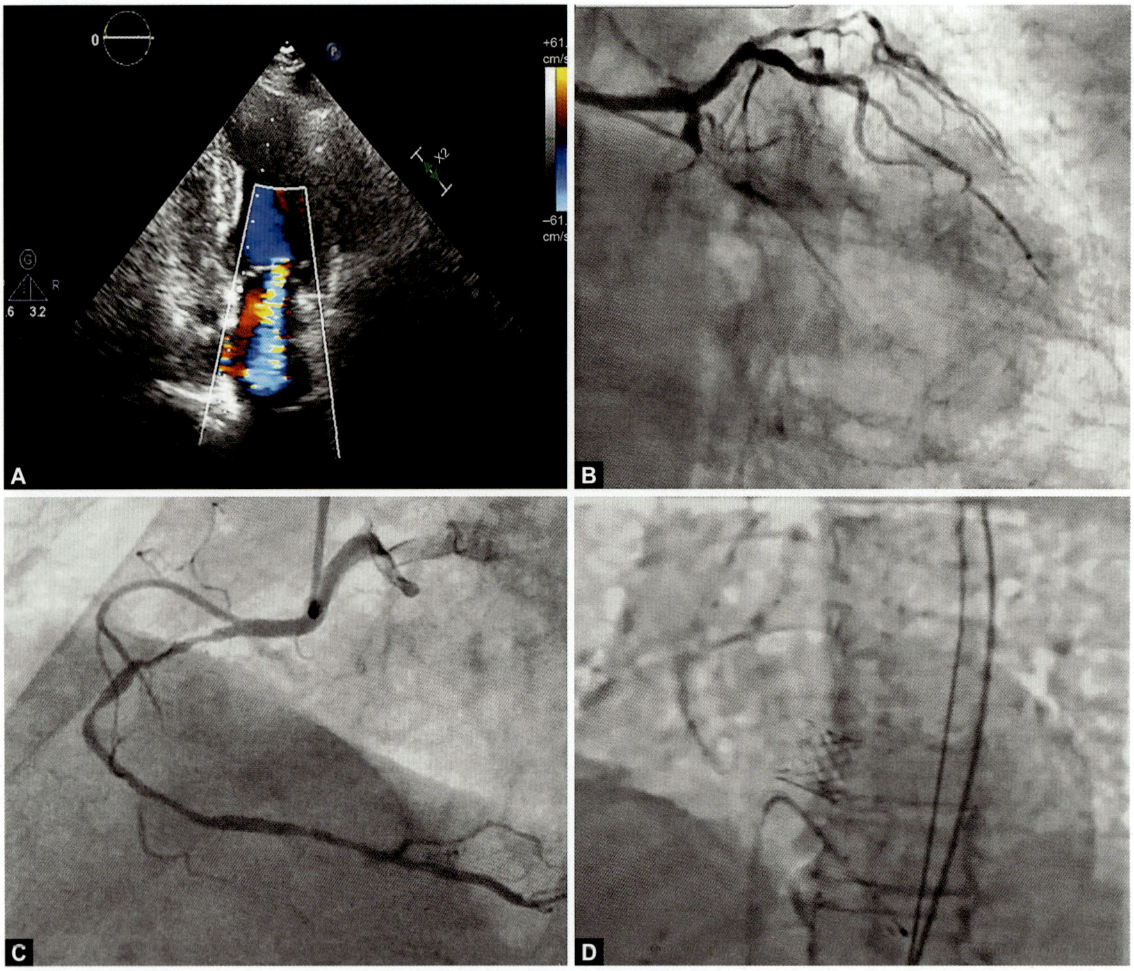

FIGS. 4A TO D: Severe MR with severe AS. Relieving ischemia and LVOT obstruction with PCI and TAVR leads to complete disappearance of MR in the same patient. (A) Echo image showing severe MR; (B and C) Significant narrowing of LCx and RCA lesion; and (D) Post-TAVR with balloon-expandable valve.

(AS: aortic stenosis; LCx: left circumflex artery; LVOT: left ventricular outflow tract; MR: mitral regurgitation; PCI: percutaneous coronary intervention; RCA: right coronary artery; TAVR: transcatheter aortic valve replacement)

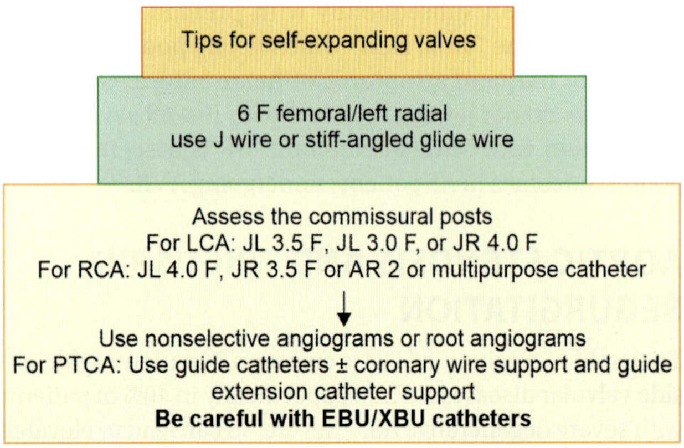

FLOWCHART 1: Tips and tricks for coronary access after self-expanding TAVR valves.

(AR: aortic regurgitation; EBU/XBU: extra-backup; JL: Judkin's left; JR: Judkin's right; LCA: left coronary artery; RCA: right coronary artery; PTCA: percutaneous transluminal coronary angioplasty; TAVR: transcatheter aortic valve replacement)

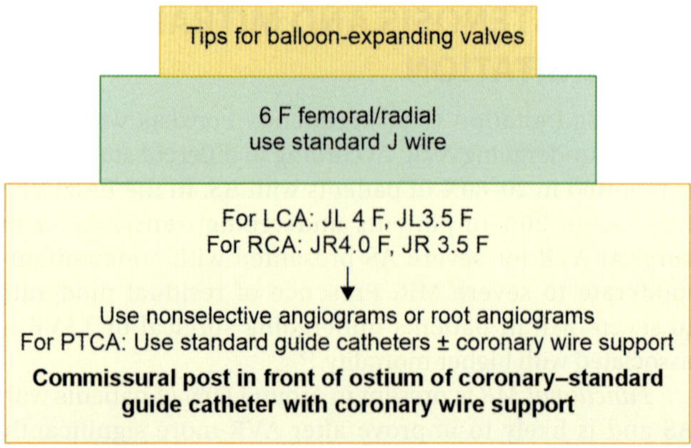

FLOWCHART 2: Tips and tricks for coronary access after balloon-expandable TAVR valves.

(JL: Judkin's left; JR: Judkin's right; LCA: left coronary artery; RCA: right coronary artery; PTCA: percutaneous transluminal coronary angioplasty) atrial (RA) dilation and TR. In advanced stages of right heart failure, it can create a low-flow–low-gradient AS.[24,25] Apart from this, involvement of tricuspid valve and at advanced stages even RV dysfunction is associated with adverse clinical outcomes in AS patients undergoing AVR. There is another classification proposed based on extent of extra-aortic valve involvement in AS patients undergoing as described in **Table 2.**[26]

AORTIC STENOSIS AND MITRAL STENOSIS

The association of mitral stenosis (MS) and AS is mostly due to rheumatic in origin or the combination of degenerative calcific disease-causing restricted mobility of the mitral valve leaflets and the aortic cusps, leading to degenerative MS and AS. In patients undergoing TAVI, concomitant MS is reported in 18–20% of patients mostly due to valvular degeneration and calcification.[27]

This combination of MS and AS in series is hemodynamically poorly tolerated and usually, patients become symptomatic at an early stage of the disease. Severe MS will severely impair LV preload and LV filling, leading to a reduction in cardiac output and a paradoxical low-flow condition, leading to underestimation of AS severity. Correction of severe MS without correcting severe AS can lead to sudden increase in LV filling pressures and pulmonary edema. The presence of residual MS with or without atrial fibrillation post-SAVR or TAVR is associated with poor long-term outcomes.[28]

AORTIC STENOSIS AND AORTIC REGURGITATION

The mixed aortic valve disease with a combination of AS and AR is seen in about 78% of patients with a primary diagnosis of predominant AS.[29] Conversely, 18% of patients with predominant AR have AS.[24] Combined lesions of AS and AR are frequently observed in cases of rheumatic heart disease and in bicuspid aortic valve disease. The degenerative aortic valve disease is a slowly progressive lesion with dominant stenosis with some degree of regurgitation. The management of this condition is frequently determined by the severity of the dominant lesion. Predominant regurgitation is associated with LV volume overload, where stenotic lesion causes pressure overload. Severe AR patients were excluded from pivotal TAVR clinical trials and reports on outcomes in the MVD population are limited. Based on previous studies and from meta-analyses, MR and TR have been associated with increased long-term mortality after TAVR, whereas preexisting AR does not increase mortality and may confer a survival benefit at 1 year among patients with MVD relative to patients with isolated AS.[30] With increasing operator experience, TAVR is being offered even for predominant AR lesions with some degree of aortic valve calcification.

TABLE 2: Stratification of AS based on extent of extra-aortic valve involvement.

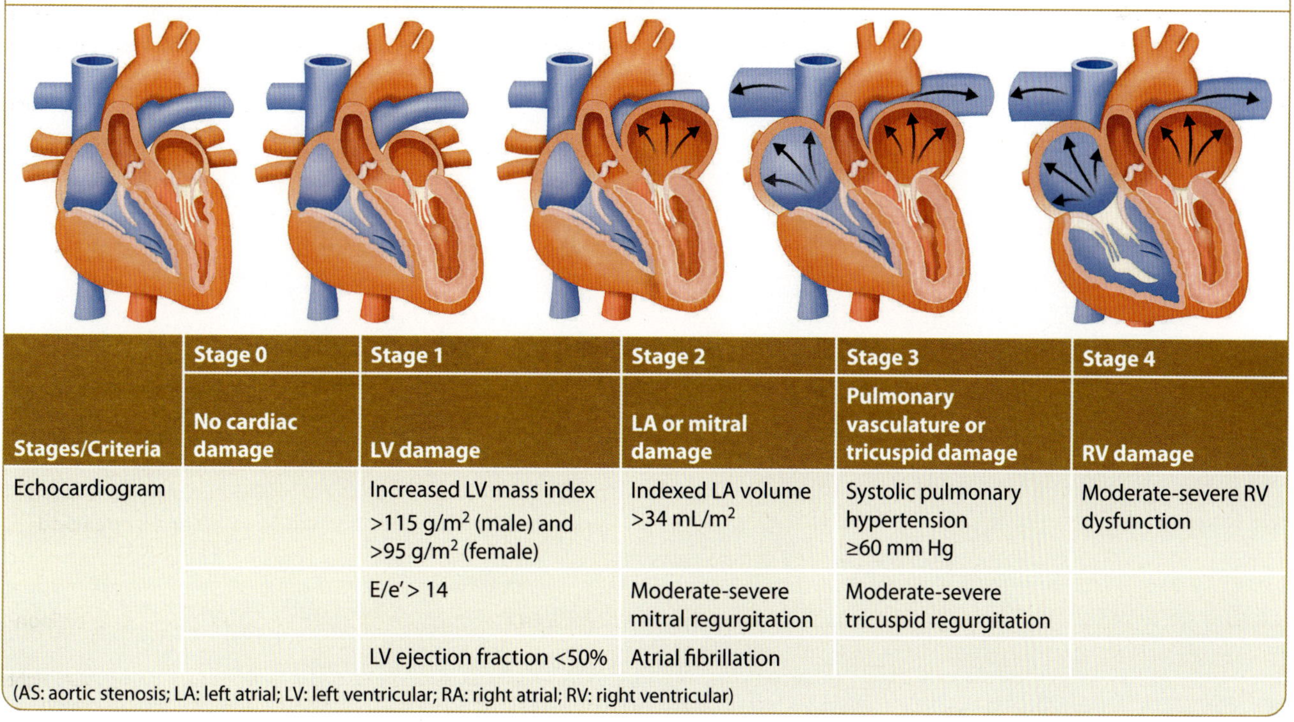

	Stage 0	Stage 1	Stage 2	Stage 3	Stage 4
Stages/Criteria	**No cardiac damage**	**LV damage**	**LA or mitral damage**	**Pulmonary vasculature or tricuspid damage**	**RV damage**
Echocardiogram		Increased LV mass index >115 g/m² (male) and >95 g/m² (female)	Indexed LA volume >34 mL/m²	Systolic pulmonary hypertension ≥60 mm Hg	Moderate-severe RV dysfunction
		E/e' > 14	Moderate-severe mitral regurgitation	Moderate-severe tricuspid regurgitation	
		LV ejection fraction <50%	Atrial fibrillation		

(AS: aortic stenosis; LA: left atrial; LV: left ventricular; RA: right atrial; RV: right ventricular)

CONCLUSION

Coronary artery disease incidence is quite common in severe AS patients undergoing TAVI. Significant CAD involving left main coronary artery (LMCA) or proximal LAD lesions needs PCI before TAVR. Patients with ischemic LVF/ACS need PCI before TAVR. Patients presenting as heart failure with severe LV dysfunction and CAD may benefit by initial TAVR followed by stabilization of LV and then staged PCI. In some patients with simple type A coronary artery lesions, performing simultaneous procedures during the same day could be beneficial in avoiding the risk of multiple procedures and saving some costs to the patient. Apart from this, AS is also associated with other valvular lesions which have significant impact on long-term outcomes of these patients. Individualized decision-making involving the entire heart team is important, keeping in view of clinical presentation of the patient and also based on combined valvular and vascular lesion severities and with equal importance being given to patient preferences.

ONLINE REFERENCES

Please scan the QR code provided at the end of the table of contents for References of this chapter.

CHAPTER

178 Transcatheter Heart Valve: Made in India

John Jose, Paul V George

ABSTRACT

Transcatheter aortic valve implantation (TAVI) is the treatment of choice for severe calcific aortic stenosis (AS) in elderly patients. Several devices are now available for TAVI, with each iteration of device technologies focused on making TAVI simpler, more effective, and safe procedure. In recent times, Indian manufactures have started developing transcatheter valve technologies with an aim to improve upon existing devices. Myval and Myval Octacor (Meril Lifesciences) are new-generation made-in-India balloon-expandable (BE) transcatheter heart valves, which are designed to simplify the procedure and facilitate precise valve deployment. Hydra valve [Vascular Innovations Company Limited, Nonthaburi, a subsidiary of Sahajanand Medical Technologies (SMT), India] is a novel self-expanding valve designed to have optimal hemodynamic performance, low pacemaker rate, and easy access to coronary arteries. This article focuses on technological aspects and clinical evidence for made-in-India transcatheter heart valves.

Keywords: Aortic stenosis, TAVI, Myval, Octacor, Hydra, balloon expandable, self expanding, transcatheter heart valve.

INTRODUCTION

Since the first human transcatheter aortic valve implantation (TAVI) two decades ago by Professor Alain Cribier,[1] transcatheter heart valve (THV) technologies have become increasingly popular and globally, it is estimated that over 200,000 TAVI procedures are performed annually. It is anticipated that TAVI procedures will continue to grow at 15% compound annual growth rate (CAGR) resulting in close to 500,000 TAVI procedures performed in the next 10 years globally. In India, TAVI procedures are being done since 2011, and currently over 2,400 procedures are being done annually involving 200 hospitals with close to 20 hospitals performing them regularly with sound clinical outcomes. With increasing awareness, lowering of procedural and device cost driven by indigenously manufactured devices, and an increase in reimbursement of the procedure, India is expected to perform > 10,000 TAVI procedures annually in the next 3–5 years. While TAVI is currently performed routinely for high surgical-risk symptomatic severe aortic stenosis (AS) patients who are 75 years of age and older, it is anticipated that in the upcoming years, it will also be routinely performed in the following cohort of patients:

- Very low surgical risk [Society of Thoracic Surgeons (STS) < 4%] population
- Low flow/low gradient AS
- Younger patient population
- Bicuspid aortic valve (BAV) anatomy
- Highly calcified aortic root complex
- Valve-in-valve (ViV) interventions
  - TAVI-in-surgical bioprosthesis
  - TAVI-in-THV
- Symptomatic moderate AS
- Asymptomatic severe AS
- Aortic regurgitation (AR)

Thus, in order to accommodate this potential large influx of TAVI cases, the learning curve and procedural time should reduce to accommodate procedural growth. Some of the features that contribute to predictive TAVI outcomes and reduce operator learning curve are:

- Precision placement, accuracy of deployment
- Availability of wide size matrix—conventional, intermediate, and extra-large sizes
- Direct crimping of THV on its delivery system for balloon-expandable (BE) valves

- Flexible delivery system which caters to variety of arch anatomies
- Low profile introducer sheath with ability to retrieve an undeployed THV
- Possibility to close the access site with fewer vascular closure devices
- High rate of device success, low postprocedure gradients, low rates of paravalvular leak (PVL), heart blocks, and permanent pacemaker implantation (PPI).

The "Make in India" drive and the aforementioned considerations have led Indian manufacturers to recently begin producing THVs for treating AS. In 2018, Meril Life Sciences launched their first indigenously designed and manufactured THV-Myval. In 2019, the HYDRA-THV (Vascular Innovations Company Limited, Nonthaburi—presently a subsidiary of SMT, India) received its Conformité Européenne (CE mark) as well as approval by the Indian regulatory body.

MYVAL SERIES

The generation-next BE THVs—Myval and Octacor (Meril Life Sciences Private Limited Vapi, India) were indigenously developed to address the existing and future unmet clinical needs in TAVI **(Figs. 1 and 2) (Table 1)**. The central driving principle of the Myval THV series (Generation-1 and -2) technology—includes the ability of THV to be positioned across the aortic root with precision and to be implanted with high degree of accuracy involving minimal foreshortening. Myval series also focused on a wider size matrix (THV diameters that include conventional, three intermediate, and two extra-large THV sizes) which allows the operators to have the bioprosthetic valve diameter matched with better approximation to the patients' native annulus without having to excessively over or under dilate as required by the previous and most current generation THVs. Another important mandate while designing Myval THV series was to allow the operator to directly mount the valve on its balloon delivery system in order to avoid any in situ maneuvering and thus minimize procedural steps and ensure procedural success with less effort. Complementing the TAVI effort, the low profile 14-French Python THV introducer sheath which is compliant to all the THV diameters (from 20 to 32 mm) allows full retrievability of the valve. The first-generation Myval THV technology was developed with this philosophy, which culminated in robust clinical data **(Table 2)**. So far, 76 articles including original research, review articles, case series/reports, abstracts, editorials, scientific letters, study protocol, and preclinical abstracts have been published across geographies demonstrating the wide clinical acceptance of the Myval THV technology. These academic publications establish the clinical evidence on Myval THV in diverse global populations and highlight the applicability of Myval THV in various off-label indications, as well.

Initially, the BE Myval THV was evaluated in the MyVal-1 study, which included intermediate and high-risk patients (n = 30) with severe symptomatic native AS. This first-in-human study of Myval THV showed acceptable clinical safety and efficacy, with no patients requiring new PPI up to 12-month follow-up.[2] Further on, numerous investigator-initiated and core laboratory-initiated studies were conducted to evaluate different TAVI outcome predictors—new PPI rates, conduction disturbance event

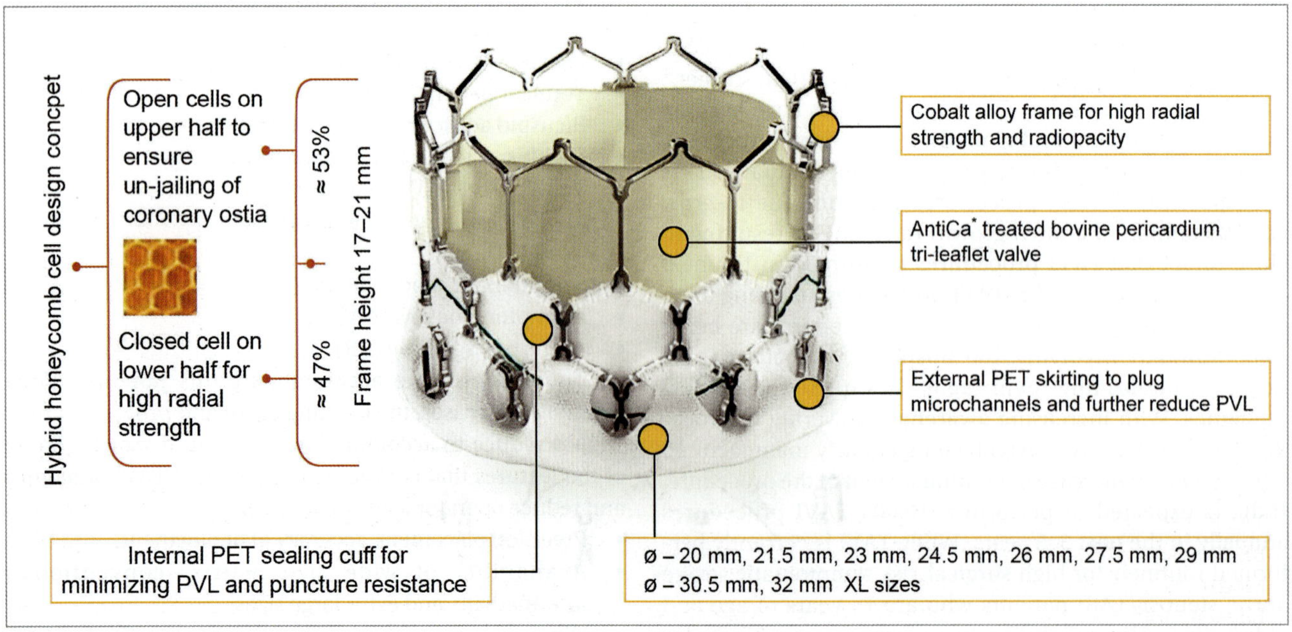

*Calcium

FIG. 1: Myval transcatheter heart valve.

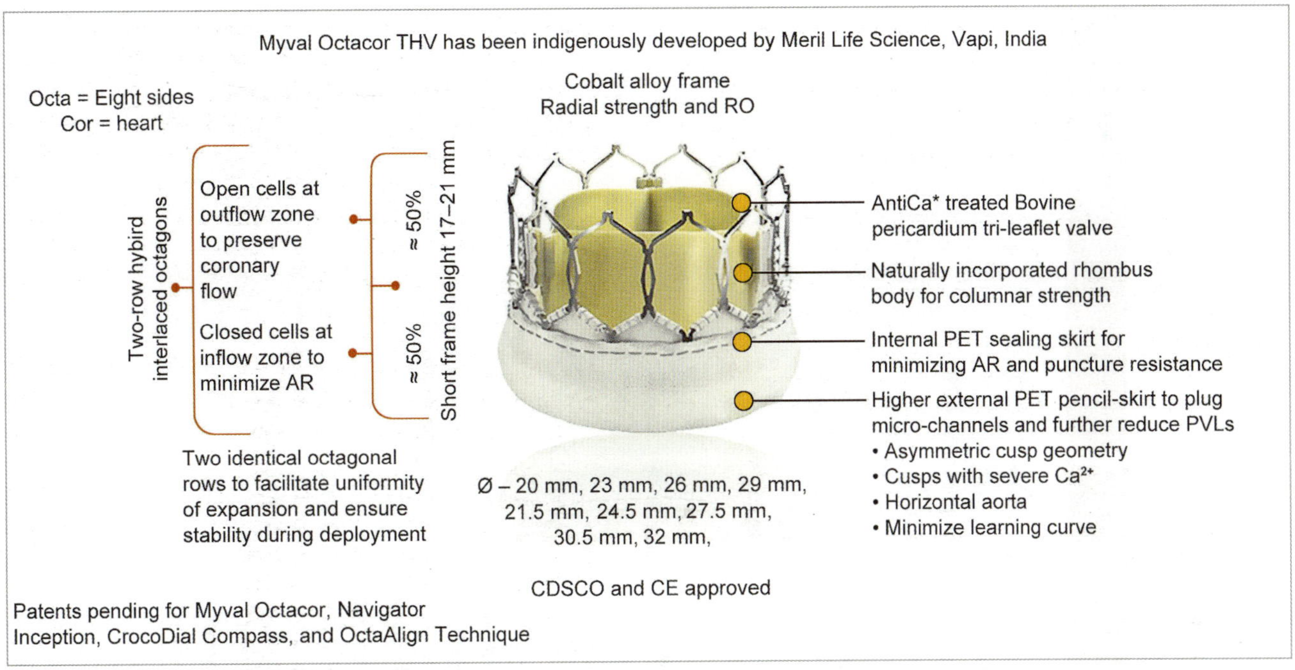

*AntiCa—Meril's proprietary tissue anticalcification technology.

FIG. 2: Myval Octacor transcatheter heart valve.

(AR: aortic regurgitation; PET: positron emission tomography; PVLs: paravalvular leaks)

TABLE 1: Unique features of Myval THV.

Myval THV—key unique features	Procedural benefits	Potential clinical implications
Unique, hybrid-honeycomb cell design (only three rows of hexagons)	Enhanced accuracy of placement due to "dark and light" bands and predictive deployment	Propensity to minimize both PVL and iatrogenic damage to conduction system
Large size matrix—conventional, intermediate, and extra large—XL	Better size approximation—avoids empirical over/under dilatation and reduced PPM	• Minimize potential aortic root damage • Optimal hemodynamics • Propensity to minimize both PVL and iatrogenic damage to conduction system
Direct crimping of THV on delivery balloon	• Eliminates need to maneuver the THV in situ • Minimal operator distraction and learning curve	Reduced procedural steps and associated inconvenience
Low profile, expandable 14 Fr introducer sheath for all THV diameters (20–32 mm)	• Low entry profile • Ease of closure • Full retrievability of undeployed Myval THV	• Minimal propensity for vascular injury • No need to deploy the THV at any undesired/unplanned heterotopic location

(PPM: permanent pacemaker; PVL: paravalvular leak; THV: transcatheter heart valve)

rates, coronary obstruction event rates, reduction of PVL), and have demonstrated favorable outcomes following TAVI utilizing the Myval THV. A single-operator, single-center retrospective study was conducted in patients (n = 105) with severe AS to assess the effect of minimalistic transfemoral TAVR under conscious sedation. Self-expandable (SE) and BE valves were implanted in 40% (Evolut R and CoreValve, Medtronic, Minneapolis) and 60% (Sapien 3, Edwards Lifesciences, California, US; and Myval) of the patients, respectively. The procedural success was achieved in 99%. Transfemoral TAVI under conscious sedation was regarded as safe and effective with low rate of all-cause mortality being 0.9%, stroke 1.9%, new PPI rate 5.7%, and 89.5% had no PVL at 30-day follow-up.[3] In another multicenter, retrospective study by Garcia-Gomez et al. Myval THV was proven to be safe and effective in patients (n = 100) with low predicted risk of intraoperative or the 30-day mortality.[2,4]

In a prospective, single-center study in The Netherlands, Halim et al.,[5] analyzed patients (n = 120) with severe symptomatic AS who received the Myval THV. At the 30-day follow-up, periprocedural stroke and the need for a PPI were observed in 3.3% of patients (in both cases) with improved

TABLE 2: Clinical summary of Myval transcatheter heart valve.

Study name	Study design	Patient population	Number of subjects	Major outcomes	Reference(s)
MyVal-1 study	First-in-human, prospective, multicenter, single-arm, and open-label study	Severe symptomatic AS	30	At 30-day follow-up: • *All-cause mortality*: 3.3% • *PPI and MI*: 0% • *Major vascular complications*: 6.7% At 12-month follow-up: • *All-cause mortality*: 13.3% • *PPI and MI*: 0% • *Major vascular complications*: 6.7% • *Device success*: 100.0% • *Procedural success*: 96.7%	Sharma et al. 2020[2]
Single-center experience of 105-minimalist transfemoral transcatheter aortic valve replacement and its outcome	Retrospective study	Severe AS	*105 (SE CoreValve and Evolut R)*: 40%, BE (Sapien 3: 31% and Myval: 29%)	At 30-day follow-up: • *Procedural success*: 99% • *All-cause mortality*: 0.9% • *Stroke*: 1.9% • *New PPI rate*: 5.7% • *Moderate to severe PVL*: 0.9% • *Valve thrombosis*: 0%	Rao et al. 2021[3]
Myval low-risk registry	Retrospective registry	Patients with calcified severe AS (low predicted operative mortality risk according to STS and EuroScore-II)	100	Postprocedural outcomes: • *Valve embolization, coronary artery occlusion, annulus rupture, or procedural death*: 0% • *Definitive PPI*: 8% At 30-day follow-up: • AVA (0.7 ± 0.2 vs. 2.1 ± 0.6 cm^2) and mean aortic valve gradient (43.4 ± 11.1 vs. 9.0 ± 3.7 mm Hg) improved significantly ($p < 0.001$) • *Moderate AR*: 4% • *Early safety*: 3% • *Clinical efficacy*: 1%	García-Gómez et al. 2022[4]

Continued

Continued

Study name	Study design	Patient population	Number of subjects	Major outcomes	Reference(s)
Short-term outcome after TAVR with a novel balloon-expandable valve	Prospective and single-center study	Native, severe symptomatic AS	120	Postprocedural outcomes: • *Successful implantation*: 98.3% • *Moderate or severe PVL*: 0% At 30-day follow-up: • *All-cause death*: 2.5% • *New PPI*: 3.3% • *All-stroke*: 3.3% • *Acute kidney injury*: 4.2% • *Moderate or severe PVL*: 0% At 6-month follow-up: • *All-cause death*: 5.8% • *Cardiac death*: 0.8% • *All-stroke*: 5.8%	Halim et al. 2022[5]
Balloon-expandable TAVR bioprostheses: Area or perimeter sizing? A prospective pilot study	Prospective and single-center pilot study	Symptomatic severe AS	60	At 30-day follow-up: • *Cardiac death, moderate to severe PVL, and major life-threatening bleeding*: 0% • *Aortic valve area*: 2.06 ± 0.4 cm^2 (baseline: 0.75 ± 0.2 cm^2) • *Aortic valve mean gradient*: 7.7 ± 3.5 mm Hg (baseline: 37.7 ± 12.4 mm Hg) • *New PPI*: 2% At 1-year follow-up: • *All-cause death*: 10% • *Cardiac death*: 3% • *New PPI*: 2%	Halim et al. 2022[6]
A propensity-matched study	Retrospective and single-center study	Severe AS	223 (Myval: 120, Evolut: 103)	At 30-day follow-up (Myval vs. Evolut): • *Cardiac death*: 1% vs. 2%, $p = 0.56$ • *All stroke*: 2% vs. 4%, $p = 0.41$ • *MI*: 1% vs. 3%, $p = 0.31$ • *New PPI*: 4% vs. 15%, $p = 0.01$ • *Moderate or severe PVL*: 1% vs. 4%, $p = 0.17$ At 1-year follow-up (Myval vs. Evolut): • *Cardiac death*: 2% vs. 4%, $p = 0.41$ • *All stroke*: 7% vs. 5%, $p = 0.76$	Halim et al. 2023[7]

Continued

Continued

Study name	Study design	Patient population	Number of subjects	Major outcomes	Reference(s)
Safety and performance parameters of the Myval transcatheter aortic valve bioprosthesis: The SAPPHIRE prospective registry	Single-arm and prospective registry	Severe AS	100	Postprocedural outcomes: • *Device success*: 100% • *Technical success*: 100% At 1-year follow-up: • *All-cause mortality*: 8% • *Cardiovascular mortality*: 5% • *New PPI*: 9% • *Stroke*: 3% At 2-year follow-up: • *All-cause mortality*: 12% • *Cardiovascular mortality*: 7% • *Stroke*: 3% • *Cerebrovascular events, renal failure, MI, and structural valve deterioration*: 0%	Testa et al. 2023[8]
Early outcomes of a next-generation balloon-expandable transcatheter heart valve—the Myval System: A single-center experience from Serbia	Prospective study	Symptomatic AS	13	Postprocedural outcomes: • *Procedural success*: 100% At 30-day follow-up: • *All-cause mortality*: 0% • *Early device success*: 100% • *Clinically significant AR or moderate/severe PVL*: 0% • *Stroke, bleeding, device-related vascular complications, or a new PPI*: 0%	Boljevic et al. 2023[9]
MATCH-BALL study	Prospective study	Symptomatic patients with severe AS	416 (Matched cohort: Myval = 103 and Sapien 3 = 103)	• *Postprocedural outcomes*: (Sapien 3 vs. Myval) • *Procedural success*: 94.2% vs. 93.2%, $p = 0.219$ At 30-day follow-up: • *Mortality*: 2.9% vs. 0.97%, $p = 0.625$ • *Clinical efficacy*: 12.6% vs. 4.9%, $p = 0.057$ • *Early safety*: 12.6% vs. 4.9%, $p = 0.096$ • *New PPI*: 15.5% vs. 5.8%, $p = 0.020$ • *Mean aortic gradient*: 12 mm Hg vs. 8 mm Hg • *Major bleeding*: 1% vs. 3.9% • *Major vascular complications*: 4.9% vs. 0% • *AKI*: 1% vs. 2.9%	Delgado-Arana et al. 2022[10]

Continued

Continued

Study name	Study design	Patient population	Number of subjects	Major outcomes	Reference(s)
The EVAL Registry	Retrospective and single-center study	Severe symptomatic AS	166 (Evolut R = 108, Myval = 58)	At 30-day follow-up (Myval vs. Evolut R): • *Device success*: 94.8% vs. 83.3% • *More than mild PVL*: 3.4% vs. 14.8%, $p = 0.03$ • *All-cause mortality*: 1.7% vs. 2.8% • *Bleeding*: 20.7% vs. 17.6% • *AKI*: 1.7% vs. 1.8% • *Nondisabling stroke*: 1.75% vs. 0.9% • *PPI*: 11% vs. 24.2% At 6-month follow-up: • *PVL*: 26% vs. 53.8% • *New PPI*: 11% vs. 27.5% • *All-cause mortality*: 5.2% vs. 12.3% • *More than mild PVL*: 7% vs. 19.8%, $p = 0.0396$	Barki et al. 2022[11]
Quantitative angiographic assessment of AR after TAVI: A comparative analysis	Retrospective core laboratory analysis	Patients underwent TAVI with BE valve	Myval ($n = 108$); Sapien 3 ($n = 397$); Sapien XT ($n = 239$)	• Mean angiographic quantitative AR: 6.3 ± 6.3% vs. 7.6 ± 7.1% vs. 8.8 ± 7.5% (Myval vs. Sapien 3 vs. Sapien XT) • *Percentages of moderate/severe angiographic quantitative AR*: 2.8% vs. 8.3% vs. 10.9% (Myval vs. Sapien 3 vs. Sapien XT)	Kawashima et al. 2021[12]
Post TAVI conduction disturbances: A retrospective core laboratory analysis	Core laboratory-based evaluation	Severe aortic stenosis who underwent TAVI	1,131 (Myval: 135, Sapien 3: 290, Evolut: 298, Accurate: 180, Portico: 125, and Allegra: 103)	• *New PPI*: Evolut—18.5%, Portico—29.5%, Allegra—22%, Acurate neo—9.1%, Sapien 3—13.4%, Myval—7.4% • Myval was associated with one of the lowest rates of conduction disturbances	Santos-Martinez et al. 2022[13]
Myval in bicuspid aortic valve stenosis	Retrospective study	Severe bicuspid AS	68	Postprocedural outcomes: • *None/trace AR*: 76.5%, mild AR: 20.5% and moderate AR: 3% • *Major vascular complications*: 1.5% • *Life-threatening bleeding*: 1.5% At 30-day follow-up: • *All-cause death*: 3% • *New PPI*: 8.5% • *All stroke*: 0% • *AKI (stage III–IV)*: 0% • *Mean transvalvular gradient*: 9.8 ± 4.5 mm Hg • *EOA*: 1.8 ± 0.4 cm^2	Elkoumy et al. 2022[14]

Continued

Continued

Study name	Study design	Patient population	Number of subjects	Major outcomes	Reference(s)
One-year outcomes after Myval implantation in patients with bicuspid aortic valve stenosis—a multicenter: Real-world experience	Retrospective study	Severe bicuspid AS	68	At 1-year follow-up: • *All-cause mortality*: 11.3% • *All-stroke*: 3.2% • *Major bleeding*: 1.6% • *PPI*: 8.3% • *Mean pressure gradient*: 10 mm Hg • *EOA*: 1.7 cm^2 • *Moderate AR*: 2% • *Valve thrombosis*: 1.6%	Elkoumy et al. 2023[15]
Transcatheter aortic valve implantation for severe bicuspid aortic stenosis—2 years follow-up experience from India	Retrospective study	Bicuspid AS	70 (30% BE Myval and Sapien; 70% SE CoreValve and Evolut R)	Postprocedural outcomes: • *Procedural success*: 98.2% • *PPI*: SE—16.32% and BE—4.7% 30-day follow-up: • *Procedural mortality*: 2.86% • *CHB needing PPI*: SE—16.32% and BE—4.7% • *Nondisabling stroke*: SE—8.16% and BE—14.29% At 2-year follow-up: • *Mild PVL*: 5% • *AKI*: 4.29% • *Valve degeneration and failure or infective endocarditis*: 0% • *THV thrombosis*: 1.43% • *Procedural mortality*: 2.86%	Kumar et al. 2022[16]
Comparison of latest-generation balloon and self-expandable transcatheter heart valves for the treatment of severe bicuspid aortic valve stenosis: Triton study	Retrospective and multicenter registry	Bicuspid aortic stenosis	360 (Myval = 122, Sapien 3 Ultra = 129 and Evolut Pro+ = 109)	Inhospital: • *Procedural and technical success*: 100% vs. 100% vs. 93.8% (Myval vs. S3U vs. EP+) At 30-day follow-up (Myval vs. S3U vs. EP+): • *Device success*: 100% vs. 87.5% vs. 81.3% • *All-cause mortality*: 0% vs. 2.5% vs. 3.8% • *Stroke*: 1.3% vs. 7.5% vs. 3.8% • *Bleeding*: 0% vs. 6.3% vs. 6.3% • *Early safety*: 85% vs. 70% vs. 67.5% • *New PPI*: 10% vs. 12.5% vs. 18.8% • *AKI*: 0% vs. 7.5% vs. 18.8%	Amat-Santos et al. 2023[17]

Continued

Continued

Study name	Study design	Patient population	Number of subjects	Major outcomes	Reference(s)
Transcatheter ViV/ViR implantation with Myval THV 1-year follow-up from a multicenter experience	Prospective, multicenter, and international registry	Patients with severe symptomatic aortic BHVs failure and mitral BHVs or annuloplasty ring failure undergoing transcatheter aortic ViV and mitral ViV or ViR implantation with BE Myval	97 [aortic ViV (n = 33), mitral ViV (n = 64)]	At 30-day follow-up: • *Technical success*: 98% • *All-cause death*: 1% • *Cardiovascular death*: 0% • *Stroke*: 1% • *New PPI*: 0% • *Major bleeding*: 1.1% • *Moderate to severe PVL*: 4.5%	Moscarella et al. 2023[18]
Valve-in-valve TMVR	Retrospective and multicenter registry	Mitral bioprosthesis degeneration underwent ViV TMVR with the BE Myval	11	At 30-day follow-up: • *Technical success*: 100% • Peak gradient: 7.2 ± 2.7 mm Hg • *Mean gradient*: 3.4 ± 1.7 mm Hg • *Procedural complications*: 0% At 6-month follow-up: • *LVOT obstruction, migration, PVL, and stroke*: 0%	Blasco-Turrión et al. 2022[19]
Early multicenter experience of a new balloon-expandable MyVal transcatheter heart valve in dysfunctional stenosed right ventricular outflow tract conduits	Retrospective and multicenter study	Patients who underwent TPVI with Myval THV for dysfunctional RVOT	7	• All patients experienced improved physical activity, with normal RV systolic function • *Pulmonary regurgitation, arrhythmias, infective endocarditis, and clotting or valve dysfunction*: 0% • *Pulmonary gradient*: 12.5 ± 5.8 mm Hg • *Valve related adverse events*: 0%	Sivaprakasam et al. 2021[20]
Feasibility of precise commissural and coronary alignment with Myval THV	Prospective study and *in silico* simulation based	Severe AS	10	• *Mean commissural misalignment*: 16.72 ± 8° • *Correct alignment*: Six cases • *Mild misalignment*: Four cases • *Moderate or severe misalignment*: 0 cases • The *in silico* model accurately predicted final in vivo position with correlation coefficient of 0.983 (95% CI 0.966–0.992), $p < 0.001$ • *Severe coronary overlap (CO)*: Three cases • *Mean transaortic gradient*: 6.1 ± 3.3 mm Hg • *Moderate-severe PVL*: None	Santos-Martínez et al. 2023[21]

Continued

Continued

Study name	Study design	Patient population	Number of subjects	Major outcomes	Reference(s)
The LANDMARK trial	Prospective, multicenter, multinational, randomized, open-label, and noninferiority trial	Symptomatic severe AS	768 [Myval THV series ($n = 384$), Sapien or Evolut THV series ($n = 384$)]	*Status*: As of 09th August 2023, 556 subjects are enrolled	• Kawashima et al. 2021[22] • ClinicalTrial.gov - NCT04275726[23]
The Compare-TAVI trial	Prospective and randomized study	Severe symptomatic AS	1,062 (Sapien: 531, Myval: 531)	*Status*: As of 31st July 2023, 895 subjects are enrolled	ClinicalTrial.gov - NCT04443023[24]
Myval intermediate-size study	Retrospective and core laboratory survey	Patients treated with TAVI using Myval	1,115	• Myval intermediate-size THVs were used in 468 (42.0%) patients • The availability of the intermediate-size THVs could mitigate the hazardous selection of grossly undersized or oversized valve, thereby reducing PVR, conduction disturbances, and life-threatening aortic annular rupture	Kawashima et al. 2021[25]
Angiographic quantification of aortic regurgitation following Myval Octacor implantation; independent core laboratory adjudication	Retrospective and core laboratory analysis	Severe symptomatic AS	103	• *The median absolute RF percentage*: 2% • *Moderate or higher AR*: 1.9% • *Mild AR*: 20.4% • *Minimal or no AR*: 77.7%	Elkoumy et al. 2023[15]

(AKI: acute kidney injury; AR: aortic regurgitation; AS: aortic stenosis; BE: balloon-expandable; BHVs: bioprosthetic heart valves; CHB: complete heart block; EOA: effective orifice area; MI: myocardial infarction; PVL: paravalvular leak; PVR: paravalvular regurgitation; PPI: permanent pacemaker implantation; RV: right ventricular; RVOT: right ventricular outflow tract; SE: systolic excursion; STS: Society of Thoracic Surgeons; TAVI: transcatheter aortic valve implantation; THV: transcatheter heart valve; ViV: valve-in-valve; ViR: valve-in-ring) valve function and the absence of moderate to severe PVL. At 6 months, the all-cause death and cardiac death rates were 5.8% and 0.8%, respectively. In another prospective single-center pilot study, at a 1-year follow-up (n = 60), only 2% of the patients needed PPI and 3% of the patients experienced stroke with no cases of cardiac death or moderate/severe PVL. Notably, in about one-third of the patients (33.3%), a larger valve size was implanted compared to the valve size calculated by area sizing, suggesting that perimeter sizing might offer advantages in certain cases.[6] Recently, these authors have conducted another comparative study to evaluate the safety and efficacy of SE Evolut (n = 103) and Myval THV (n = 120) in patients with tricuspid AS. There were no significant differences observed in cardiac death, stroke, or myocardial infarction between the two groups; the Myval group showed significantly lower rate of PPI (4% vs. 15%, p = 0.01) at the 30-day follow-up. Cardiac death, stroke rates, and moderate/severe PVL were comparable in both the groups at 1-year follow-up.[7]

In the SAPPHIRE prospective registry, TAVI was performed on consecutive patients (n = 100) with severe native AS at two Italian centers. The technical success was found to be 100% with no intrahospital mortality, and the clinical outcome was achieved without annular rupture, and without peri- and/or postprocedural coronary obstruction. At a 2-year follow-up, none/mild PVL was seen in the 95% of the patients, all-cause death rate was 12%, stable mean gradient and the structural integrity of the valve has not been deteriorated over the time showing a favorable safety and efficacy profile of Myval THV.[8] Recently, Darko et al., have reported their first-hand experience with Myval THV system in patients (n = 13) with symptomatic AS at a single-center in Serbia and demonstrated a favorable safety/efficacy profile of Myval THV in Serbian population.[9]

The positive attributes of Myval THV over contemporary THV systems are compared in the following trials:

- The MATCH-BALL trial—an investigator-initiated retrospective study, compared the early clinical (30-day) and matched hemodynamic outcomes of real-world consecutive patients (n = 416) with symptomatic AS treated with Sapien 3 (n = 286) or Myval THV (n = 130). Based on the blinded echocardiographic assessment, in terms of safety, decreased rate of PPI (15.5% vs. 5.8%), PVL, and residual gradient, the Myval THV was found to be preferable.[10] The EVAL registry was a comparative investigation on the Myval (n = 58) and Evolut (108) THVs in patients having severe AS with the Valve Academic Research Consortium 3 (VARC-3) device success as the primary composite endpoint. Inhospital outcomes and predischarge echocardiographic evaluation showed good abilities of Myval THV in preventing severe and moderate PVL (3.4% vs. 14.8%, p = 0.03) and obtaining a high VARC-3 device success (Myval vs. Evolut: 94.8% vs. 83.3%) as well as lower rate of PPI (11% vs. 24.2%, p = 0.05) compared to Evolut at a 30-day follow-up. At a 6-month follow-up, the moderate or severe PVL (6.9% vs. 19.8%, p = 0.0396) and PPI (11% vs. 27.5%, p = 0.02) was reported to be less in Myval group compared to Evolut THV.[11] Moreover, a retrospective study by Kawashima et al. focused on the quantitative angiographic data of AR following TAVI comparing three BE [Myval (n = 108); vs. Sapien 3 (n = 397) and Sapien XT (n = 239)] THVs. After the evaluation of 108 analyzable aortograms, when compared to the Sapien 3 (8.3%) and Sapien XT (10.9%) THVs, the incidence of moderate or severe post-TAVI AR was low in the Myval THV group (2.8%, p = 0.049).[12]
- Another study based on a core laboratory-based evaluation of ECGs from 9 European centers (n = 1,131 patients) compared the early conduction disturbances across Myval (n = 135) and contemporary THVs [Sapien 3 (n = 290); Evolut (n = 298); Acurate Neo (n = 180) (Boston Scientific, Marlborough, MA, USA); Allegra (n = 103) (NVT AG, Switzerland and Biosensors, Singapore); and Portico (n = 125) (Abbott Structural Heart, MN, USA)]. Compared to other THVs, the Myval THV system demonstrated reduced rates of early conduction disturbances. In case of Myval THV, there were similar procedural and inhospital outcomes occurred compared to its contemporary THVs. Similar rates of early new PPI were observed among Myval (7.4%), Sapien-3 (13.4%), and Acurate (9.1%), but Evolut, Portico, and Allegra presented significantly higher rates (18.5%, p = 0.003; 29.5% p < 0.001 and 22%, p = 0.001, respectively) of new PPI. The central analysis of the electrocardiograms revealed significant prolongation of the PR segment with Evolut, Portico, and Allegra THVs, whereas Evolut, Acurate, and Portico showed significant QRS widening compared to Myval.[13]

Myval THV system exhibited positive outcomes not only in tricuspid aortic anatomy but also in the circumstances of BAV. In the case of BAV, due to its complex anatomical features, dedicated trials and registries are carried out to validate the safety and efficacy of Myval THV in this patient population. In the study conducted by Elkoumy et al. Myval THV proved to be safe and effective in patients with severe bicuspid AS (n = 68).[14] This has been further linked to improved 30-day hemodynamic and 1-year clinical outcomes (n = 62).[14,15] BAV is comparatively prevalent among Indian patients experiencing AS. The use of TAVI in BAV cases in India has been explored by Kumar et al. The SE CoreValve, Evolut R, BE Sapien 3, and Myval THVs were used in this study. The procedural outcomes and imaging data (inhospital) were assessed in patients (n = 70) with BAV anatomy. After 2 years of follow-up, both SE and BE THVs were found to be effective in offering adequate hemodynamics, and reduced the PVL, PPI, and stroke rates.[16] To provide larger evidence volumes on BAV patients, the TRITON TAVI registry was undertaken at 12 global institutions by an independent investigators group. In this registry, patients (n = 360) with severe BAV stenosis who underwent TAVI were analyzed with the propensity-matched comparison on currently available latest iterations of BE and SE THVs. In total, the three arms comprised patients implanted with Myval THV ($n = 122$), Sapien 3 Ultra ($n = 129$), and Evolut Pro+ ($n = 109$). At the 30-day echocardiographic follow-up, the Myval group had satisfactory hemodynamic improvement with aortic valve area of 1.89 ± 0.37, and mean aortic valve pressure gradient of 9.9 ± 4.4 mm Hg. In terms of the safety outcomes, the primary endpoint assessment showed 100% device success in the Myval group, as compared to 87.5% ($p = 0.002$) and 81.3% ($p < 0.001$) in the Sapien 3 Ultra and Evolut Pro+ groups. Only 3.4% cases of moderate residual AR were observed in the Myval group in comparison to 24% in the Evolut Pro+ group and 0% in the Sapien 3 Ultra group. In this study, 0% PVL, 99.2% technical success, and 9.9% cases of new PPI were reported for BAV patients with AS compared to the Sapien 3 Ultra or the Evolut Pro+ THVs (10.9% and 18.3%, respectively).[17] The combined findings from the aforementioned studies/trials suggest that BE Myval THV may be an acceptable option for treating patients with severe BAV stenosis.

- Moscarella et al.[18] conducted a prospective, multicenter investigation on the safety and efficacy outcomes of Myval THV implantation in patients (total $n = 97$) with symptomatic AS ($n = 33$) and mitral ($n = 64$) bioprosthesis heart valves (BHVs)/ring dysfunction. Following ViV/valve-in-ring (ViR) implantation, procedural complications were found to be low (3%), which aligns with rates reported in other studies using different THVs. The patients experienced significant symptomatic improvement, with 90% of them achieving NYHA class I–II at follow-up. The 30-day follow-up revealed significant improvements in valve areas and reduced pressure gradients resulting in satisfactory outcomes, and the acceptable mortality rate (11%) was observed even in high-risk patient population involved in the study. In a registry-based study by Blasco-Turrión et al. ViV implantation was carried out using Myval THV in high surgical risk patients ($n = 11$) with mitral bioprosthesis deterioration. Procedural success was achieved in 100% of the patients with no major complications including stroke, device embolization, left ventricular outflow tract (LVOT) obstruction and new PVL were observed at the 6-month follow-up. There was no requirement for a second transcatheter mitral valve replacement (TMVR) implantation during index procedure in any of the patients, and no intraprocedural mortality or conversion to open heart surgery.[19]
- A multicenter study was conducted on seven patients suffering from right ventricular outflow tract (RVOT) conduits to assess the clinical performance of Myval THV in dysfunctional RVOT conduits. This was the first instance of using Myval THV in a pulmonary valve and the patients were followed up for a duration of 16 months. All patients experienced improved physical activity, with normal RV systolic function, no pulmonary regurgitation, no arrhythmias, and no instances of infective endocarditis, and clotting or valve dysfunction occurred. These median clinical follow-up outcomes for a small group of patients were found to be encouraging.[20] Furthermore, in order to explore the feasibility and preliminary outcomes of commissural alignment (CA) for the Myval THV, a prospective study was conducted in patients ($n = 10$) with tricuspid severe AS undergoing TAVI. CA was previously predicted by in silico biomodeling for all the enrolled patients and the software calculated rotation was applied during crimping. Degrees of coronary overlap and CA were used as the primary outcome indicators at one month. Mean commissural misalignment was found to be 16.7 ± 8°, mean transaortic gradient was 6.1 ± 3.3 mm Hg with no PVL. Thus, commissural misalignment and coronary overlap can be avoided, if patient specific CA based on computed tomography (CT) analysis is obtained.[21]
- In addition, two large-scale prospective, randomized studies are ongoing which would allow for the Myval THV series to be enrolled. The next-generation Myval Octacor THV, has been successfully selected for participation in the UK NHS Framework Agreement, is also being used in these large studies. The LANDMARK trial[22] (ClinicalTrials.gov NCT04275726, EudraCT number 2020-000,137-40) is a prospective, multinational, multicenter, randomized, open-label, and non-inferiority trial involving approximately 768 patients [Myval THV series ($n = 384$) and the contemporary Sapien or Evolut THV series ($n = 384$)] treated with TAVI through the transfemoral approach. The primary endpoint is the assessment of safety and efficacy through multiple predictors at the 30-day follow-up, including mortality, stroke, bleeding, acute kidney injury, vascular complications, valve regurgitation, and conduction disturbances requiring a new PPI. Additionally, the patients will be followed-up for up to 10 years after the TAVI procedure to gain insights into long-term outcomes and potential complications.[22,23] As of 4th August 2023, 552 subjects are enrolled in the LANDMARK trial.
- The Compare-TAVI trial[24] (ClinicalTrials.gov NCT04443023) is a prospective, randomized, investigator-initiated study that will be conducted in Denmark with the goal of enrolling 1,062 patients undergoing TAVI with different THVs (Cohort A: Sapien or the Accurate neo 2; Cohort B: Sapien or the Myval TAVI valve). The primary endpoint is a composite of MACE, which includes mortality, stroke, moderate/major PVL, and moderate/severe aortic device stenosis after 1 year of treatment. Additionally, the study will assess various other short- and long-term TAVI-related complications, major vascular access site and access-related complications, occurrence of valve thrombosis or severe stenosis, PVL, PPI, and other relevant parameters.

Registry-based follow-up will be conducted at 30-day, 1-year, 5 years, and 10 years. The next generation Myval Octacor THV is being used in this study as well. As of 4th August 2023, 895 subjects are enrolled in the Compare-TAVI study.

The expanded size matrix of Myval THV was designed with the intention of being appropriate for patients with annular areas between 270 and 840 mm^2 to avoid the requirement for over- or undersized THVs. To test this hypothesis, a large observational retrospective study was conducted by Kawashima et al.[25] globally in 27 countries with patients (n = 1,115) who underwent TAVI with Myval THV. The selection of appropriate size was based on multislice computed tomography (MSCT) data, annular dimension and degree of calcification. The results revealed that about 41% of the patients were implanted with appropriate intermediate-sized Myval THV, thus indicating operator's preference of using appropriate size than using over/undersized conventional THVs.

MYVAL OCTACOR TRANSCATHETER HEART VALVE

Myval Octacor THV is a trileaflet valve manufactured using bovine pericardium tissue that is decellularized using Meril's proprietary AntiCa treatment. Myval Octacor THV frame incorporates just two rows of tessellating, geometrically identical octagons stacked one above the other—forming the inflow and the outflow zone. Each row is an interesting play of interlaced octagons, naturally incorporating a rhombus body at each intersection **(Fig. 3)**.

Octacor has specifically retained the original characteristic features of its predecessor technology:

- Myval Octacor THV is the same genre as before—a BE THV
- Myval Octacor THV is also directly crimped on Navigator Inception THV balloon delivery system prior to its introduction within the 14 Fr Python introducer sheath
- The size matrix of Myval Octacor THV includes conventional (20, 23, 26, and 29 mm), intermediate (21.5, 24.5, and 27.5 mm) and extra-large (30.5 and 32 mm) diameters and is identical to the predecessor **(Table 3)**.
- All sizes of Myval Octacor THV ranging from 20 to 32 mm are compatible with 14F Python introducer sheath
- All diameters of an undeployed Myval Octacor THV may be fully retrieved from the 14 Fr Python introducer sheath in case there is a difficulty in crossing the annulus **(Fig. 4)**
- The Myval Octacor THV retains the similar short, expanded frame height as that of its predecessor technology
- Myval Octacor THV is manufactured from the same cobalt alloy (MP35N) like Myval THV for optimal radial strength and radiopacity

Myval Octacor THV has meaningful features which facilitate precise positioning and deployment. The two rows of cells design of Octacor as opposed to three rows of Myval THV reduces frame foreshortening during expansion and facilitate accuracy of deployment. Myval Octacor THV favorably foreshortens 25% less as compared to Generation-1 BE THV and 50% less as compared to Generation-1 self-expanding THV technologies. The external skirt in Myval Octacor THV is up to 50% of the frame height which minimizes propensity for PVLs. The Navigator Inception THV delivery system has a landing zone marker toward the ventricular end that facilitates precise positioning of Myval Octacor at the annulus **(Fig. 5)**. Thus, the newer-generation Myval Octacor THV, that has retained the salient features of Myval THV, aims to achieve precise positioning and deployment of the THV **(Figs. 6A to C)**.

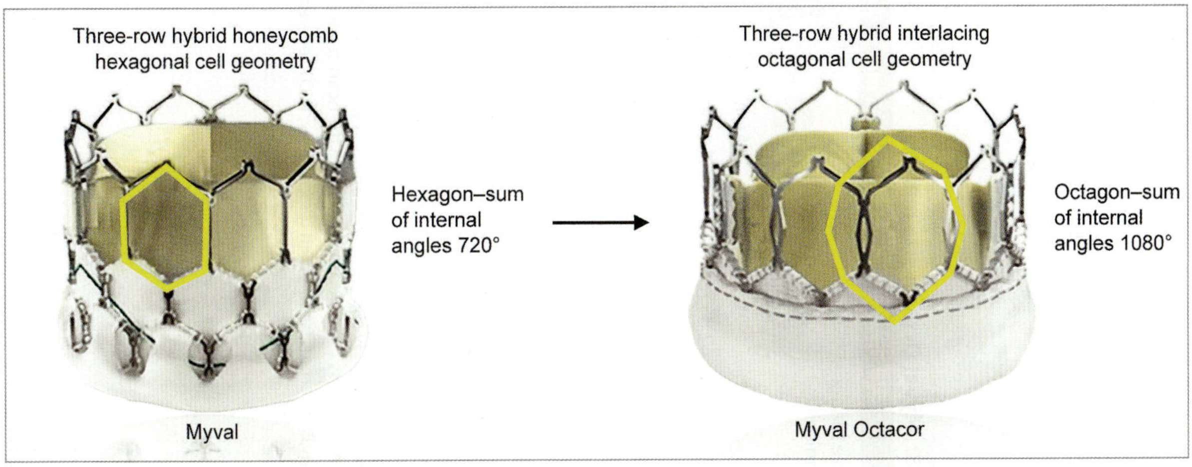

FIG. 3: Myval Octacor transcatheter heart valve cell design.

TABLE 3: Myval Octacor size matrix.

	Area 314 mm²	Area 363 mm²	Area 415 mm²	Area 471 mm²	Area 531 mm²	Area 594 mm²	Area 661 mm²	Area 731 mm²	Area 804 mm²
Myval Size Matrix and Technical Specs	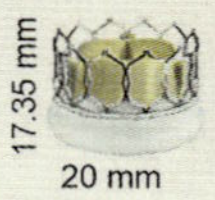	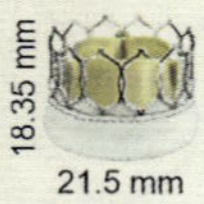	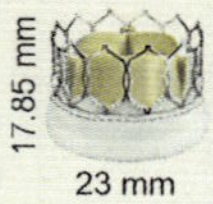	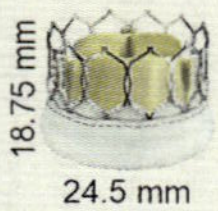	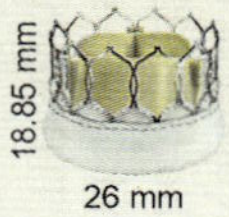	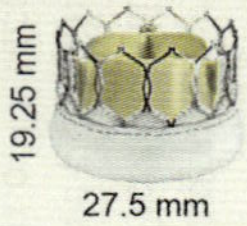	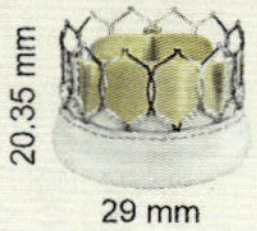	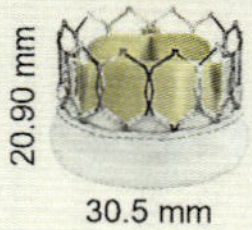	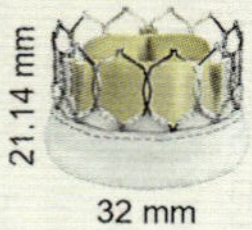
Perimeter	62.83 mm	67.54 mm	72.26 mm	76.97 mm	81.68 mm	86.39 mm	91.11 mm	95.82 mm	100.53 mm
Python expandable introducer sheath	14 Fr	14 Fr	14 Fr	14 Fr	14 Fr	14 Fr	14 Fr	14 Fr	14 Fr
Native annulus area (CT-derived)	270–330 mm²	314–380 mm²	360–440 mm²	410–500 mm²	460–560 mm²	510–630 mm²	570–700 mm²	630–770 mm²	700–840 mm²
Area-derived diameter	18.5–20.5 mm	20.0–22.0 mm	21.4–23.7 mm	22.8–25.2 mm	24.2–26.7 mm	25.5–28.3 mm	26.9–29.9 mm	28.3–31.3 mm	29.9–32.7 mm
Native annulus size by TEE	16–19 mm	17.5–20.5 mm	18–22 mm	19.5–23.5 mm	21–25 mm	22.5–26.5 mm	24–28 mm	25.5–29.5 mm	27–31 mm

Note: Sizing of Myval THV should be in correlation with cross-sectional CT images/measurement of AAo/STJ/SOV/annulus/LVOT/coronary ostia heights/valve anatomy (tricuspid/bicuspid)/Ca^{2+} score and dispersion across the root complex during the heart team meeting prior to procedure.

(AAo: ascending aorta; CT: computed tomography; LVOT: left ventricular outflow tract; SOV: sinus of Valsalva; STJ: sinotubular junction; TEE: transesophageal echocardiogram; THV: transcatheter heart valve)

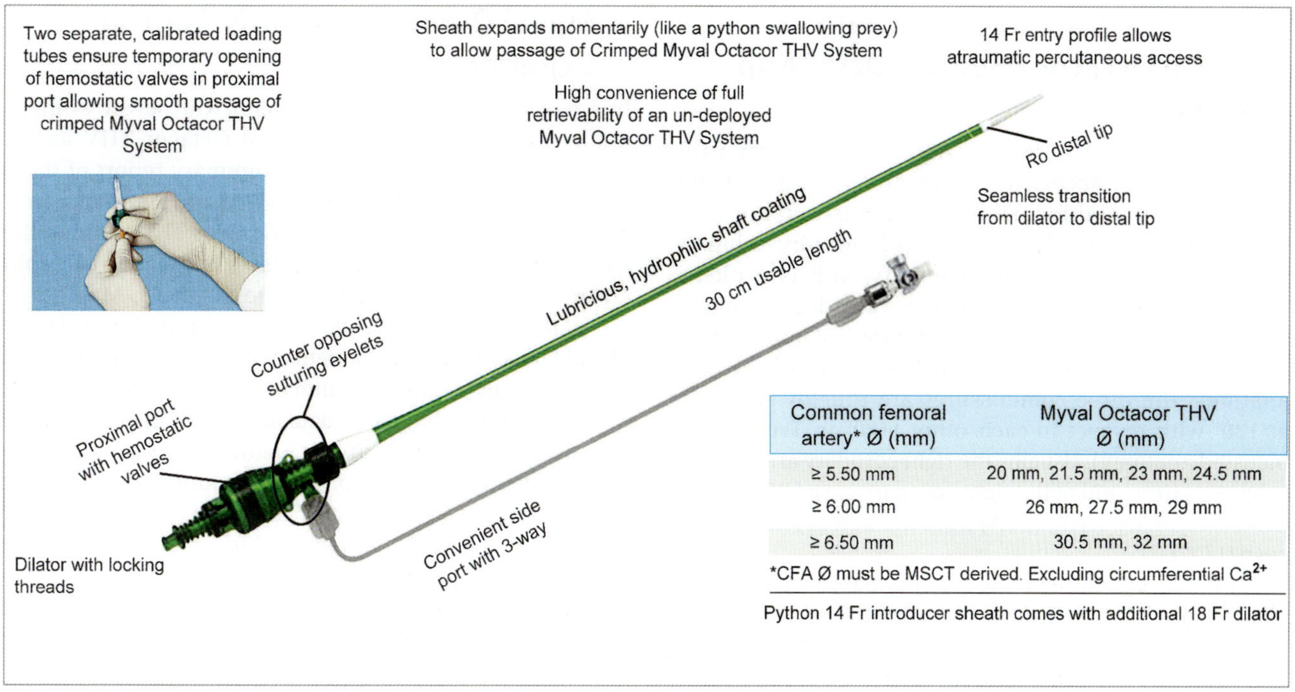

Common femoral artery* Ø (mm)	Myval Octacor THV Ø (mm)
≥ 5.50 mm	20 mm, 21.5 mm, 23 mm, 24.5 mm
≥ 6.00 mm	26 mm, 27.5 mm, 29 mm
≥ 6.50 mm	30.5 mm, 32 mm

*CFA Ø must be MSCT derived. Excluding circumferential Ca^{2+}

Python 14 Fr introducer sheath comes with additional 18 Fr dilator

FIG. 4: Python sheath.

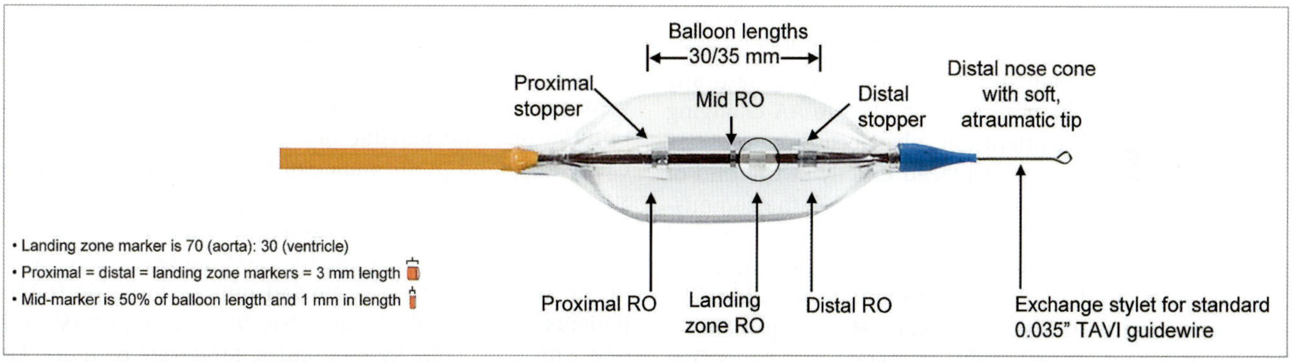

FIG. 5: Navigator delivery system of Octacor valve showing radiopaque (RO) markers.

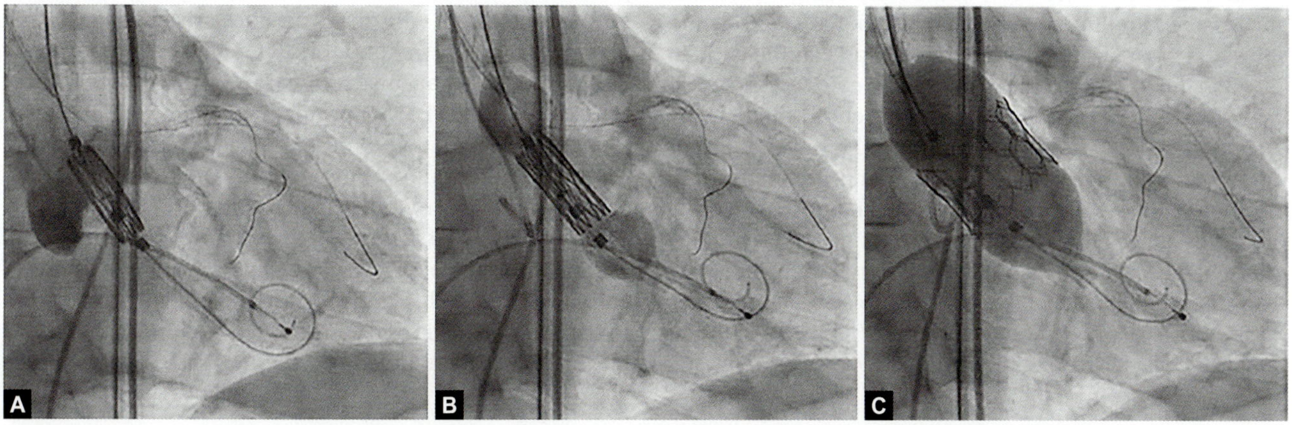

FIGS. 6A TO C: Fluoroscopy images showing precise deployment of Myval Octacor.

Commissural Alignment with Myval Octacor THV: The OctaAlign Technique

Commissural and coronary alignment impacts valve hemodynamics, access to the coronary ostia and flow following TAVI and redo-TAVI.[26] Commissural misalignment increases leaflet stress, and nonphysiological vorticity, increased thrombogenicity, and late plaque formation, potentially leading to early valve degeneration.[27] CA has the advantage of enabling future ViV interventions using the BASILICA method. In native tricuspid valve anatomy, the three commissures are roughly separated at 120° with respect to each other (180° in True Type-0 bicuspid anatomy). Usually, the right coronary artery (RCA) originates from mid of the right coronary cusp (RCC), while the left coronary artery (LCA) from the mid of left coronary cusp (LCC).

The novel OctaAlign approach is based on two established facts: (1) MSCT view is a horizontal mirror image of the anatomic/anteroposterior (AP) view; (2) a bioprosthetic THV with just one commissural postaligned at midpoint of RCC as per the MSCT view, will deploy anatomically toward the LCC-noncoronary cusp (NCC) commissure with minimal misalignment under fluoroscopic guidance. For device deployment, it is essential to note that aortic arch forms 180° turn between ascending aorta (AA) and descending thoracic aorta (DTA). The crimped Myval Octacor THV naturally rotates 180° during its passage from DTA to AA changing its orientation AP. We orient the valve according to MSCT view with commissural post placed exactly at the mid of RCC (origin of RCA). As the valve rotates 180°, the commissural post of the THV which was positioned at the mid of the RCC will be positioned at the NCC/LCC commissure with minimal misalignment. This technique is undertaken in conjunction with Myval Octacor THV components—Navigator Inception THV delivery system and CrocoDial Compass crimping tool. Using this technique, it is possible to predictably ensure the minimal misalignment between commissural posts of THV and commissures of native aortic valve. Preliminary experience using Myval Octacor, showed that the OctaAlign technique worked efficiently in 25 (83%) out of first 30 cases. CA in all 30 cases was assessed using the MSCT scan. The aligners present in the delivery system visually assist in maintaining the upward orientation and intuitively assists in preventing any inadvertent torquing of the system during insertion and further tracking the device across the aortic anatomy. Using the technique, crimped THV was prepared for loading within the 14 Fr Python introducer sheath (compatible to all diameters, i.e., 20–32 mm) keeping the navigator THV delivery catheter handle logo facing upward.[28]

Myval Octacor THV Early Clinical Experience

In a real-world scenario, 125 patients with severe symptomatic AS were treated with Myval Octacor THV across 18 centers in India. The internal summary report of these 125 patients (mean age: 69.95 ± 8.43 years) showed promising clinical outcomes of Myval Octacor THV. Among the study patients, 59% and 41% patients had native tricuspid aortic valve and BAV anatomies, respectively. Majority of the patients received 23 mm (24%) and 24.5 mm (19%) Myval Octacor THV; 10 patients received 29 and 30.5 mm and 10 patients required 20 mm of Myval Octacor THV. In a matched echocardiography data analysis of 21 patients, the effective orifice area at 30-day follow-up (1.81 ± 0.45 cm^2) improved more than twofolds as compared to that at preprocedure (0.65 ± 0.22 cm^2). The mean pressure gradient (51.75 ± 15.19 mm Hg at preprocedure vs. 10.76 ± 5.00 mm Hg at 30-day follow-up) and peak velocity (4.40 ± 0.83 m/s at preprocedure vs 2.11 ± 0.46 m/s at 30-day follow-up) also reduced markedly. These findings suggest satisfactory hemodynamic performance of the Myval Octacor THV through 30-day follow-up. No event of stroke was reported through the 30-day follow-up with the prosthetic aortic valve functioning normally. New significant conduction disturbances leading to new PPI were reported in nine patients and additionally five patients with preexisting conduction disturbances were implanted with new PPI. There were two reports of cardiac death in these 125 patients population. The satisfactory and clinically acceptable early safety and performance of Myval Octacor THV were successfully demonstrated. Videodensitometric assessment (an independent core laboratory analysis) of 103 analyzable aortograms of 125 patients who underwent TAVI with Myval Octacor THV was carried out. In total, 64 (62%) patients had tricuspid aortic valve, 38 (37%) with BAV, and one with unicuspid AV anatomies. Moderate or more AR incidence was 1.9% (observed in BAV group only), mild AR in 20.4%, and none or trace AR in 77.7%. The results are promising with Myval Octacor THV by limiting the rates of moderate or more AR.[28,29] As per these recent reports, the Myval Octacor THV shows the ability of its newer two-row design to control against residual PVL. The device's lower row composed of PET fabric and the external circumferential PET skirt are aimed at increasing the surface contact with the surrounding annular tissue, thus offering better resistance to less than moderate regurgitation levels.[30] Myval Octacor THV is also associated with a novel technique of OctaAlign for the operators that allow versatility in terms of coronary and CA that impacts valve hemodynamics, access to the coronary ostia and coronary flow following TAVI. This technique facilitates precise positioning and deployment.[31]

Conclusion

In a nutshell, both the first- and second-generation Myval THVs demonstrate the class effect of the BE valve genre. This is reflected amply in the early data that has been generated with Myval devices. With the OctaAlign technique, the valve aims for better precision and reduction in the incidences of new PPI. The OctaAlign technique is simple and easily applicable to current clinical practice without additional hardware or software or analysis.

HYDRA SELF-EXPANDING TRANSCATHETER AORTIC VALVE

The HYDRA THV [Vascular Innovations Company Limited, Nonthaburi, a subsidiary of Sahajanand Medical Technologies (SMT), India] is a novel bioprosthetic aortic valve consisting of a SE nitinol stent frame and three bovine pericardium leaflets placed supra-annularly that provide a large effective orifice area and low transvalvular pressure gradient **(Fig. 7)**. The stent frame includes a high sealing skirt at the inflow section to minimize PVLs. A nonflared inflow part aims to reduce interference with the conduction system and prevent new conduction abnormalities. The outflow part of the stent frame has three tentacles that serve as anchors to the delivery catheter and allow proper alignment and conformability to the shape of the aorta. The mid frame features large open cells (≥15 F) for easy access to the coronary arteries and high flexibility of the HYDRA delivery catheter. The stent frame also includes two sets of markers for precise guidance during valve implantation at the intended landing zone. The frame exerts varying radial force, with high force at the inflow section for secure anchoring, low force at the outflow section for better flexibility, and high hoop strength in the middle portion to accommodate various shapes and dimensions. The HYDRA THV is available in three sizes (22, 26, and 30 mm), covering a range of native aortic annulus diameters from 17 to 27 mm. The bovine pericardium leaflet tissue is treated with anticalcification technology. The HYDRA Aortic Valve Loading System securely crimps the THV into the capsule at the distal end of the delivery catheter (compatible with a 0.035″ guidewire), ensuring minimal damage to the valve leaflets. All three sizes of the HYDRA THV utilize the same delivery catheter with an outer diameter of 18 F, featuring a radiopaque nose cone at the distal end. The catheter shaft includes a stability layer to prevent movement of the valve toward the left ventricle during deployment. The HYDRA THV can be recaptured, retrieved, and repositioned during deployment until reaching 80% of its full deployment.

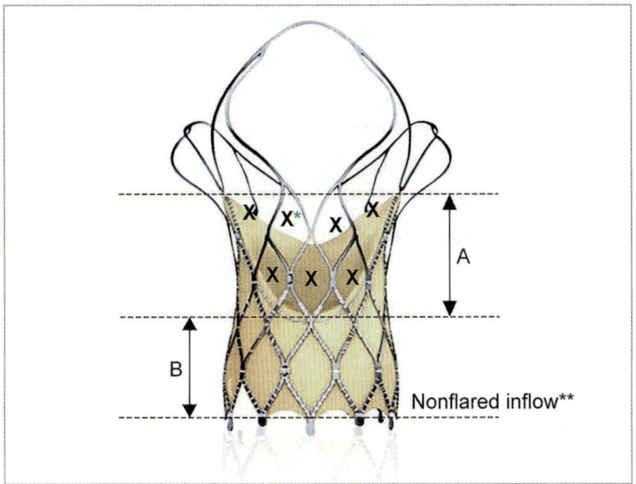

X*: Large cells facilitates easy access to the coronary arteries and flexibility of the delivery catheter.
A: Supra-annular position of leaflets provides large effective orifice area and low transvalvular gradient.
B: High sealing skirt mitigates paravalvular leak.
** Nonflared inflow part of stent frame reduces conduction abnormality.

FIG. 7: Hydra transcatheter heart valve.

The clinical safety and performance of the HYDRA THV has been established by three clinical studies. Preliminary evaluation of safety and performance of HYDRA THV was evaluated in first-in-man study.[32] Safety and performance of the HYDRA THV was further confirmed by GENESIS trial[33] and HYDRA CE study[34] which were conducted in patients with severe degenerative AS presenting a high predictable surgical mortality risk. The detailed descriptions baseline characteristics of patients enrolled in GENESIS trial and HYDRA CE study are enumerated **Table 4.**

The GENESIS trial was a prospective, multicenter, single-arm, and 6-month follow up study conducted in India. The objective of this study was to evaluate the safety and performance of the self-expanding HYDRA THV in the treatment of symptomatic severe AS in patients at high or extreme surgical risk. The primary safety endpoint was all-cause mortality at 30 days and the primary performance endpoint was device success defined as per VARC-II criteria. The GENESIS trial demonstrated a favorable and sustained 6-month safety and performance outcomes of the self-expanding HYDRA THV in patients with symptomatic severe AS who were at high or extreme surgical risk **(Table 5)**. Lower rates of paravalvular regurgitation and pacemaker suggest optimal anchoring and sealing without excessive radial pressure on the annulus or the outflow tract.

The HYDRA CE study was a premarket, prospective, multicenter, single-arm study conducted across 18 study centers in Europe and Asia-Pacific countries. The primary objective of this study was to evaluate the safety and performance of the self-expanding HYDRA THV in the treatment of symptomatic severe AS in patients at high or extreme surgical risk. The results of the HYDRA CE study demonstrated favorable and sustained 1-year efficacy providing large effective orifice area and low transvalvular gradient as well as high survival rates and low complication rates with regards to PVL, new permanent pacemaker, stroke, major vascular complications, and bleeding with the HYDRA THV in patients with symptomatic severe AS and high or extreme surgical risk **(Table 5)**.

TABLE 4: Baseline characteristics of patients enrolled in GENESIS trial and HYDRA CE study.

Characteristics	The GENESIS trial (*n* = 40)	The HYDRA CE study (*n* = 157)
Male	24 (60)	65 (41.4)
Coronary artery disease	19 (47.5)	65 (41.4)
Previous CABG/PCI	2 (5.0)/3 (7.5)	22 (14.0)/38 (24.2)
Peripheral artery disease	–	4 (2.5)
Permanent pacemaker	00	12 (7.6)
Diabetes mellitus	15 (37.5)	48 (30.6)
Hypertension	23 (57.5)	125 (79.6)
Pulmonary hypertension	3 (7.5)	19 (12.1)
Moderate or severe aortic regurgitation	–	17 (10.8)
STS score, %	–	4.7 ± 3.4
EuroSCORE II	–	5.1 ± 4.9
Mean aortic gradient, mm Hg	53.5 ± 18.1	49.5 ± 18.5
Aortic valve area, cm^2	-	0.7 ± 0.2

Note: Data expressed as mean ± standard deviation or as frequency (percentages).

(CABG: coronary artery bypass grafting; PCI: percutaneous coronary intervention; STS: Society of Thoracic Surgeons score)

The self-expanding HYDRA THV is useful for transcatheter treatment of severe AS. Initial results indicate a high hemodynamic performance and complication rates similar to those reported for second-generation transcatheter aortic bioprosthesis. However, long-term follow-up of GENESIS trial (up to 5 years) and ongoing GENESIS-II trial will provide clear understanding about its efficacy over an extended period.

CONCLUSION

Transcatheter heart valves that are globally competitive and efficient are now available and manufactured in India. The safety and effectiveness of made-in-India balloon expandable platform (Myval Generation-1 and 2) and self-expanding HYDRA THV have been proven in multicenter and worldwide clinical studies. With the widespread availability of these Indian made valves, the prospect is bright for affordable care for patients with severe AS who are eligible for TAVI in our country.

TABLE 5: 30 days and 1-year clinical outcomes of patients enrolled in GENESIS trial and HYDRA CE study.

Outcomes	The GENESIS trial	The HYDRA CE study
30-day clinical outcomes		
All-cause mortality	10.0	7.0
Cardiovascular mortality	7.5	5.7
All stroke	00	0.6
Major vascular complications	2.5	4.5
New permanent pacemaker implantation	7.5	11.7
Moderate or severe paravalvular leak	00	6.3
Mean aortic gradient, mm Hg	6.7 ± 2.8	8.1 ± 3.7
Effective orifice area, cm^2	2.3 ± 0.6	1.9 ± 0.6
6 months clinical outcomes		
All-cause mortality	17.5	NA
Cardiovascular mortality	7.5	
All stroke	00	
Major vascular complications	2.5	
New permanent pacemaker implantation	7.5	
Moderate or severe paravalvular leak	00	
Mean aortic gradient, mm Hg	7.6 ± 2.7	8.0 ± 3.6
Effective orifice area, cm^2	2.2 ± 0.7	1.8 ± 0.6
1-year clinical outcomes		
All-cause mortality	NA	14.6
Cardiovascular mortality		8.3
All stroke		0.6
Major vascular complications		4.5
New permanent pacemaker implantation		12.4
Moderate or severe paravalvular leak		6.9
Mean aortic gradient, mm Hg		8.8 ± 4.7
Effective orifice area, cm^2		1.7 ± 0.5

Note: Data expressed as mean ± standard deviation or as frequency (percentages).

ONLINE REFERENCES

Please scan the QR code provided at the end of the table of contents for References of this chapter.

CHAPTER

179 Transcatheter Aortic Valve Implantation in Bicuspid Aortic Valve Stenosis

Pratap Chandra Rath, Shabbir Ali Shaik, Pradeep Kumar

ABSTRACT

Bicuspid aortic valve (BAV) is the most common congenital valvular heart disease with an average prevalence of 0.5–2% in general population. The first in-human transcatheter aortic valve implantation (TAVI) by Cribier and colleagues in 2002 was actually performed in a patient with BAV. TAVI in BAV had been associated with anatomical complexity and procedural complications due to asymmetry of annulus to supra-annular structures, presence of raphe, excessive leaflet calcification, and aortopathy. Transcatheter heart valve (THV) sizing is based on considering both annulus and supra-annular dimensions. Earlier trials had excluded aortic stenosis (AS) with BAV, but recent trials have shown excellent results with TAVI in BAV group. There are no randomized trials comparing balloon-expandable versus self-expandable valves and no definitive recommendation has been formulated; however, various registries have shown that both the types are effective. Therefore, selection of THV is a patient-tailored approach, based on different THV features, geometries, and interactions with the surrounding anatomy. In this chapter, we have described the BAV diagnosis, classification, sizing, and selection of transcatheter valve, including technical challenges and procedural details.

Keywords: Transcatheter aortic valve implantation, bicuspid aortic valve, aortic stenosis, multidetector computed tomography (MDCT), virtual basal ring (VBR), virtual raphe ring (VRR), transcatheter heart valve, paravalvular leak (PVL).

INTRODUCTION

Bicuspid aortic valve (BAV) is the most common congenital valvular heart disease. It accounts for 0.5–2% in the general population and about 20% in octo- and nonagenarians who are referred for aortic valve surgery.[1] Transcatheter aortic valve implantation (TAVI) has become the gold standard procedure for elderly with severe aortic stenosis (AS) not only in inoperable, high-risk patients but also for intermediate-to-low-risk group. TAVI in man for the first time was introduced by Cribier and his colleagues in April 2002, which was performed in a patient with a BAV.[2] Initial randomized trials on TAVI have excluded AS with BAV, but present trials revealed good results and favorable outcomes even in BAV group.[3]

DIAGNOSIS OF BICUSPID AORTIC VALVE

It is difficult to diagnose BAV; however, one should consider both transthoracic echocardiography and multidetector computed tomography (MDCT) to confirm the diagnosis. Sievers and Schmidtke first classified BAV (surgical classification) into three categories based on the leaflet distribution and the number of raphe—type 0, type 1, and type 2.[4] Jilaihawi et al. classified based on MDCT into three patterns, namely (1) the bicommissural nonraphe type, (2) the bicommissural raphe type, and (3) the tricommissural or functional tricuspid.[5] Irrespective of the type of classification, there is no correlation with clinical outcomes following TAVI **(Figs. 1A and B)**.

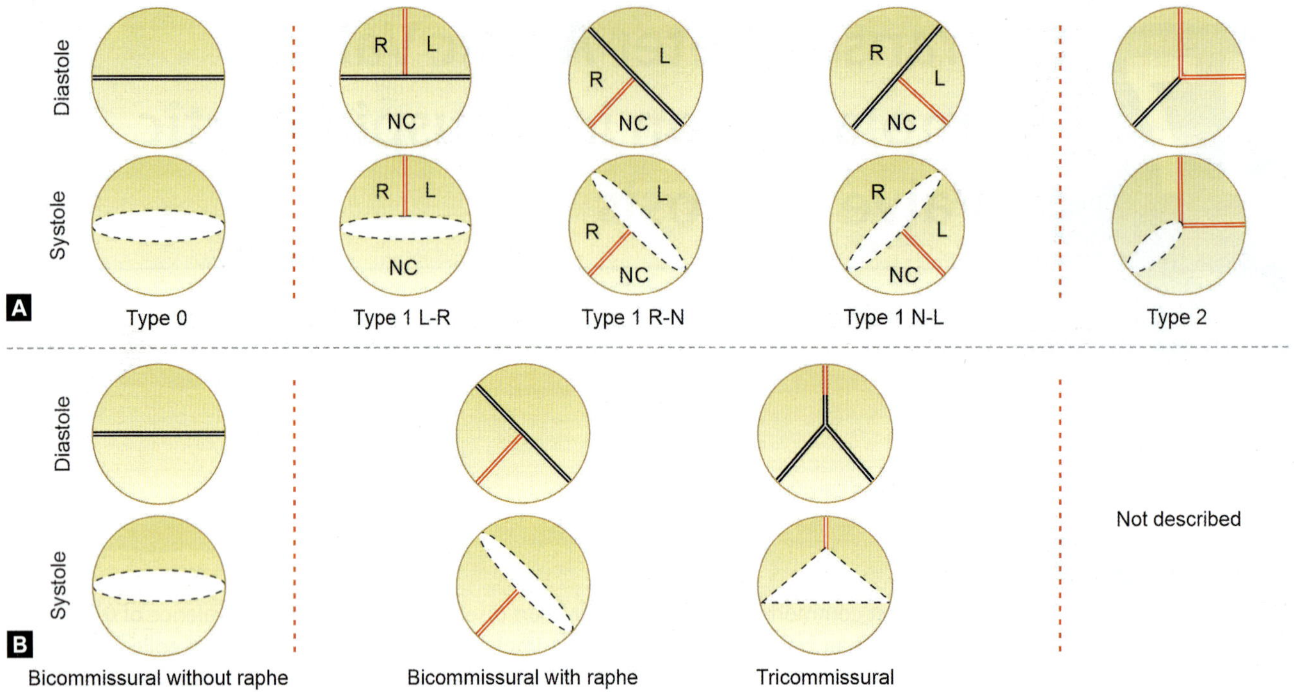

FIGS. 1A AND B: Classification of bicuspid aortic valve anatomy.
(L: left coronary cusp; N: noncoronary cusp; R: right coronary cusp)
Source: With permission from (A) Sievers and Schmidtke (2007)[4]; (B) Jilaihawi et al. (2016).[5]

CHALLENGES DURING TRANSCATHETER AORTIC VALVE IMPLANTATION IN BICUSPID AORTIC VALVE ANATOMY

Bicuspid Aortic Valve Anatomical Evaluation

In most of earlier randomized TAVI trials, bicuspid anatomy has been excluded in view of anatomical complexity and high procedural complications. Problems that commonly encounter during TAVI in BAV anatomy include:

- Larger annulus size compared with tricuspid valve[6,7]
- Aortic annulus is circular in shape but supra-annular structures are elliptical, giving rise to nontubular nature of atrioventricular (AV) complex (from the annulus to the leaflet tips) and so the narrowest diameter (point of highest resistance) is located above the annulus at commissural level.[8-11] Hence, sizing based on annulus causes transcatheter heart valve (THV) oversizing and leads to risk of underexpansion and complications such as annulus dissection/tear.[12,13]
- The leaflets of BAV are heavily calcified and more eccentric with asymmetrical distribution of calcium.[6]
- Presence of a calcified raphe which will prevent the adequate THV expansion.[6] Raphe present between noncoronary cusp (NCC) and left coronary cusp (LCC) nearer to His bundle causes conduction abnormalities.[14]
- Incidence of coronary anomalies are higher in BAV, like left dominance and separate origin of left main and circumflex artery. Location of coronary ostia near to the commissure along with thickened, lengthy, and calcific cusps predispose to coronary obstruction during TAVI.[15]
- Due to vertical annulus, aorta will become more horizontal, very challenging for the exact positioning of THV.[10]
- Lastly, aortopathy associated commonly with BAV cannot be managed by TAVI alone.

Transcatheter Heart Valve Sizing in Bicuspid Aortic Valve

Annular and Supra-annular Evaluation

Annulus also called as virtual basal ring (VBR) is the narrowest dimension of the aortic root, where the THV will anchor and seal in TAV.[16] However in BAV, the exact definition of VBR is difficult. In bicommissural raphe-type and in tricommissural type, the VBR is identified at the nadir of three cusps, whereas in BAV without raphe type where there are only two hinge points, demonstration of VBR is questionable. For THV sizing, we can derive annular diameters using

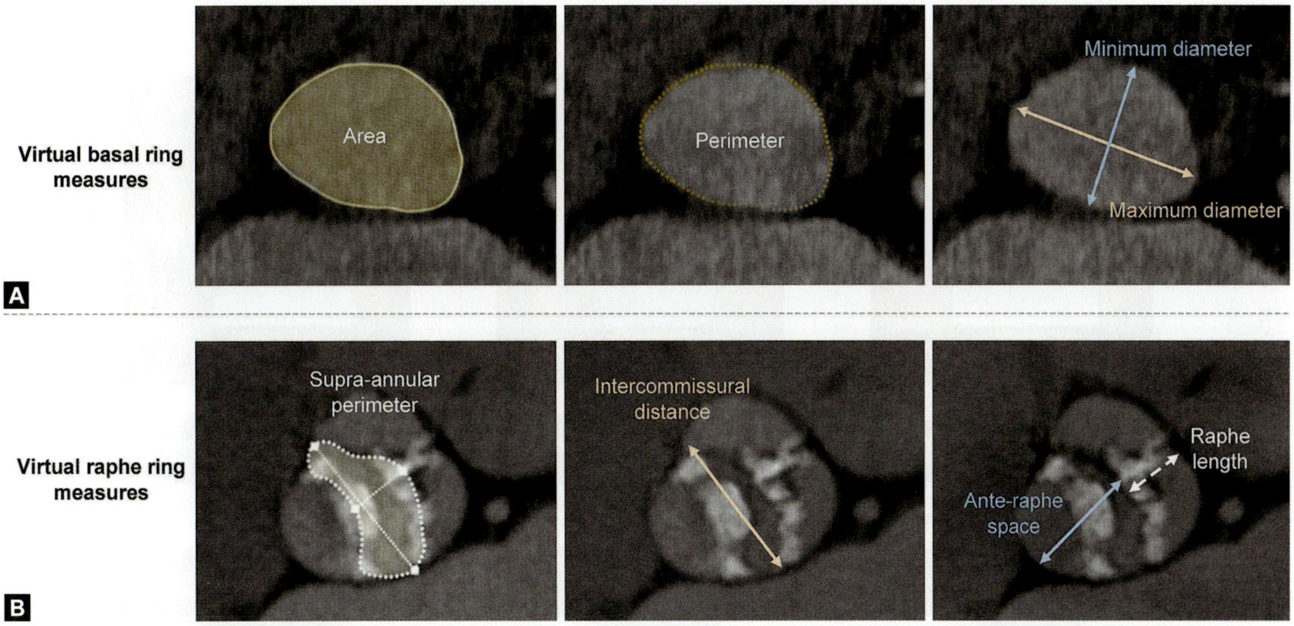

FIGS. 2A AND B: Sizing strategies in bicuspid aortic valve. (A) Standard computed tomography (CT)-based measurements at virtual basal ring and (B) Proposed CT-based measurements at virtual raphe ring.

MSCT[17] by calculating from area, perimeter, and mean diameter value (major and minor axis in eccentric annulus), shown in **Figure 2A**. Supra-annular sizing in BAV constitutes virtual raphe ring (VRR) evaluation because the narrowest dimension is at raphe plane rather than at annular plane.[13] Multiple parameters are used for supra-annular sizing, as shown in **Figure 2B**, which are as follows:

- *Supra-annular perimeter*: It is the perimeter-derived diameter calculated by taking the inner margin of leaflets during systole, excluding the calcified raphe and leaflet calcification.
- Intercommissural distance (corresponding to the major supra-annular diameter)
- Ante-raphe space (corresponding to the minor supra-annular diameter)
- *Raphe-specific measurements (length, degree, and distribution of calcification)*: Any raphe length > 50% of annulus diameter with calcium burden (>300 mm^3) limits the adequate expansion of THV.[16]

Based on VRR and VBR, three morphological aortic root patterns were described, namely **(Figs. 3A to C)**:[6,11,18]

1. *Codominant configuration*: VBR and VRR are equal in size **(Fig. 3A)**
2. *Annular or VBR-dominant configuration*: VBR is smaller in size than VRR **(Fig. 3B)**
3. *Raphe or VRR-dominant configuration*: VRR is smaller in size than VBR **(Fig. 3C)**

In codominant and VBR-dominant configurations, THV size is based on annulus. However, in VRR-dominant configuration with heavily calcific raphe, supra-annular sizing is recommended to overcome the problem of THV underexpansion.

Sizing of valve for MDCT-based (Jilaihawi et al.) classification:

- *Bicommissural nonraphe type*: In this type, both codominant and VBR-dominant patterns are equally found. Therefore, annular-based THV sizing is recommended.[11,18]
- *Bicommissural raphe-type*: Mostly codominant and VBR-dominant patterns are found; hence, annular-based sizing strategy is frequent, but in nearly 20% of cases, VRR-dominant pattern will be encountered, requiring supra-annular sizing strategy.[6,11,18]
- *Tricommissural BAV*: THV sizing depends on length, degree, and extent of calcification of the raphe; most of them are VRR-dominant and require supra-annular sizing strategy.[6,11,18]

Selection of Type of Transcatheter Heart Valve

There are no randomized trials comparing the balloon expandable versus self-expandable valves and no definitive recommendation has been formulated. Selection of valve should be a patient-centered approach, including THV design, multislice computed tomography (MSCT) data, and interactions with the surrounding structures.

- *Balloon-expandable valves*: The newer generation SAPIEN 3 valve has good external sealing skirt which reduces the risk of paravalvular leak (PVL) in challenging anatomies like BAV. The high radial strength of the valve provides adequate expansion in irregular geometries, but this is associated with increased risk of aortic injury. In the bicuspid arm of the low-risk transcatheter aortic

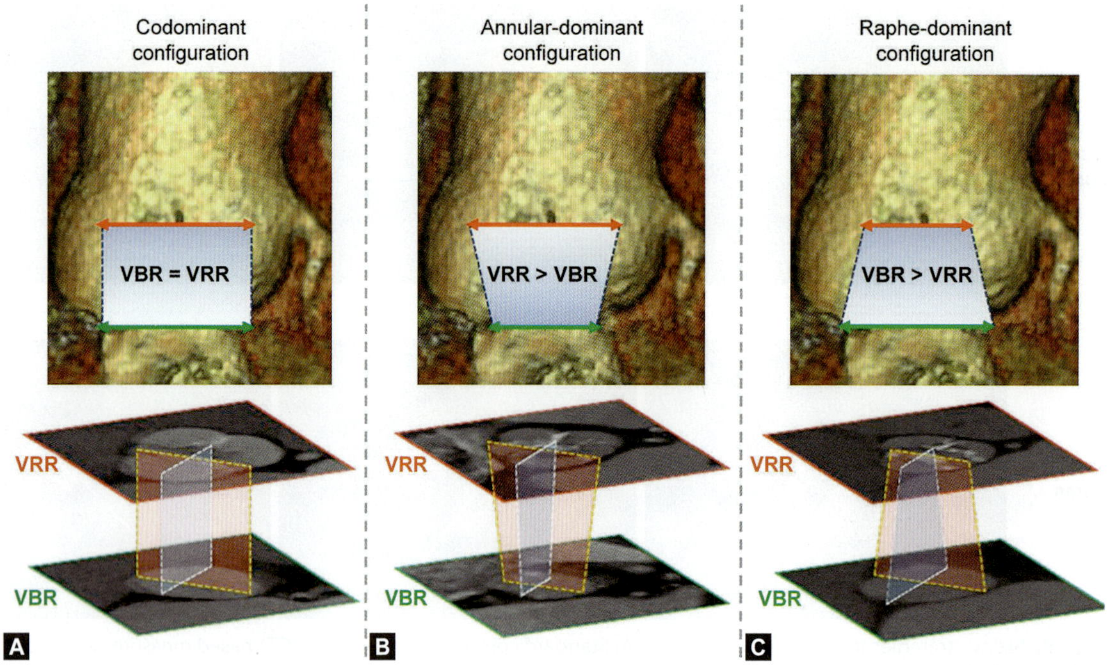

FIGS. 3A TO C: THV sizing in BAV. Different patterns of landing zone in BAV. (A) Codominant and (B) annular-dominant with standard annular-sizing strategy. (C) Raphe-dominant with advised supra-annular sizing strategy.
(BAV: bicuspid aortic valve; THV: transcatheter heart valve; VBR: virtual basal ring; VRR: virtual raphe ring)

valve replacement (TAVR) trial, where 74% of patients received the SAPIEN 3 THV, zero mortality, and no disabling strokes were reported in 30 days, with low rates of procedure-related complications, and excellent hemodynamic performance.[19]

- *Self-expandable valves*: The newer-generation self-expandable valves have good adaptability to the irregularly shaped landing zone, especially in BAV. The additional supra-annular design of the valve provides better hemodynamic performance despite under- or asymmetrical expansion at the inflow portion.[20] Lastly, the repositioning and recapturing nature of self-expandable valve helps in accurate positioning. In low-risk bicuspid study,[21] TAVR with the Evolut R/PRO THVs achieved favorable 30-day results, with low rates of death and stroke and high device success rate.[21]

In the BEAT (Balloon versus Self-Expandable Valve for the Treatment of Bicuspid Aortic Valve Stenosis) registry, the balloon-expandable valves (SAPIEN 3) had higher post-valve gradients and increased rates of annular rupture, while the self-expandable valves (Evolut R/PRO) had higher rates of moderate or severe PVL.[22] In a European registry, TAVI with accurate neo in BAV showed 30-day clinical endpoints were similar to that of TAV.[23]

Balloon Aortic Valvuloplasty

Balloon aortic predilatation is required in almost all BAV. It allows to (1) facilitate THV crossing and proper positioning, (2) test raphe's resistance, predicting THV expansion, (3) sizing of the THV. If the balloon indentation (waist sign) at the level above the annulus without contrast regurgitation guides, supra-annular sealing is required and it helps in THV sizing and implantation depth (VRR dominant) assessment,[24] and (4) predicting the risk of coronary occlusion and PVL with simultaneous aortogram during predilatation.

Transcatheter Heart Valve Implantation Technique

Two different landing zones were described for three morphological aortic root patterns as depicted in **Figure 4**.

- *Annular landing zone*: In codominant and VBR-dominant configurations **(Fig. 4A)**
- *Supra-annular landing zone*: In VRR-dominant configurations **(Fig. 4B)**. In this technique, valve implantation height should be targeted for good supra-annular sealing.[6,25] Caution with respect to device migration and coronary obstruction depending on aortic root anatomy.

Balloon Postdilatation

Balloon postdilatation should be restricted only when there is residual significant PVL or high post-valve gradients. The postdilatation balloon size should be the VBR or VRR, whichever has the smallest diameter to avoid balloon-related complications. The rate of postdilatation was significantly higher with the self-expandable Evolut R/PRO THVs compared with balloon-expandable SAPIEN 3 valve.[22]

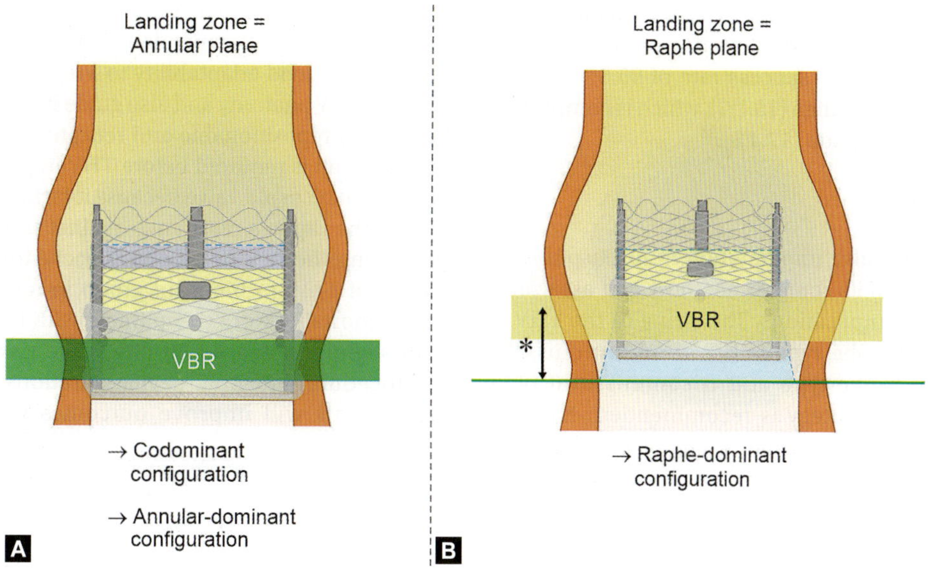

*CT-based VBR–VRR distance or "waist sign" location of balloon sizing.

FIGS. 4A AND B: THV positioning in bicuspid aortic valve. (A) Standard THV implantation at annular plane in case of codominant or annular-dominant shapes, (B) Optional higher THV implantation at supra-annular plane (raphe plane) in case of raphe-dominant shape.
(CT: computed tomography; THV: transcatheter heart valve; VBR: virtual basal ring; VRR: virtual raphe ring)

Cerebral Embolic Protection in Bicuspid Aortic Valve

Transcatheter aortic valve implantation in BAV is associated with an increased risk of stroke compared with tricuspid AS.[26] The possible contributing factors include higher calcium burden of valve, frequent balloon predilatation, and postdilatation.[22] Further studies are required to establish the actual role of cerebral embolic protection devices during TAVI in BAV subset.

Coronary Protection in Bicuspid Aortic Valve

The risk of coronary obstruction during TAVI in BAV is higher than tricuspid AS despite larger sinuses of Valsalva and higher coronary takeoff due to anatomical issues such as bulky leaflets and calcified raphe. Presence of calcific raphe between the NCC and right coronary cusp causes asymmetrical displacement of the THV and leaflets toward the left coronary artery ostium, leading to an increased risk of coronary obstruction, mostly when leaflets are long and bulky. Hence in all cases, balloon aortic valvuloplasty with simultaneous aortography will identify the patient at risk of coronary occlusion. In such cases, upfront coronary protection, after engaging the guide catheter it should pulled back into ascending aorta and with wire with device (balloon/stent) parked in the distal coronary bed.

Coronary Access

The use of low frame profile THV or alternatively the commissural alignment technique for supra-annular devices may increase the chance for selective coronary engagement.[27,28] Coronary reaccess is challenging specifically in valve-in-valve procedures. The BASILICA (Bioprosthetic Aortic Scallop Intentional Laceration to Prevent Iatrogenic Coronary Artery Obstruction) procedure to split the leaflets of native BAV (before TAVR) or THV (before TAVR-in-TAVR) might prevent the obstruction of coronary ostia and facilitate the coronary access (CA).[29]

TRANSCATHETER AORTIC VALVE IMPLANTATION OUTCOMES IN BICUSPID AORTIC VALVE

In 2017, Yoon et al. studied the outcomes of TAVI in BAV group with tricuspid AS and showed that 2-year mortality was similar (17.2% vs. 19.4%; $p = 0.280$) but with low procedural success and increased requirement of surgery (2% vs. 0.2%; $p = 0.006$) and more PVL in BAV group. There was no change in the pacemaker requirement.[30] In a study by Makkar et al., BAV treated with SAPIEN 3 valve compared the outcomes with tricuspid AS and showed that there was no difference in the 30-day (2.6% vs. 2.5%; $p = 0.82$) or 1-year mortality (12.9% vs. 14.1%; $p = 0.74$) but slightly higher risk of stroke (2.5% vs. 1.6%; $p = 0.02$) and pacemaker requirement (9.1% vs. 7.5%; $p = 0.03$) at 30 days. However at 1 year, the stroke rates were similar (3.4% vs. 3.1%; $p = 0.16$).[26] In a study by Forrest et al., BAV patients treated with Evolut-R/Pro found that there was no difference between the two groups in terms of 30-day or 1-year mortality (10.4% vs. 12.4%; $p = 0.63$), device success (96.5% vs. 96.4%; $p = 0.88$), surgical conversion (0.6% vs. 0.2%; $p = 0.29$), or pacemaker requirement (15.4% vs. 13.7%; $p = 0.30$) and stroke rates (3.9% vs. 4.4%; $p = 0.63$)[21] when compared with tricuspid AS. In low-risk bicuspid study, evaluating Evolut-R/Pro in BAV low-risk patients, 30-day results showed high device success rate of 95.3%, but the pacemaker requirement is high (15.1%), which is comparable to low-risk tricuspid AS group (17.4%).[31]

CONCLUSION

Transcatheter aortic valve implantation in biscuspid AS is challenging because of its complex anatomy and associated risk of procedural complications. The sizing of the THV in bicommissural nonraphe type is based on annulus, but in bicommissural raphe-type and tricommissural type, supra-annular sizing strategy is recommended. Balloon-expandable valves have high radial strength, which provide adequate expansion in BAV and external sealing skirt reduces the risk of PVL. Self-expandable valves with supra-annular design have good adaptability to irregularly shaped landing zones of BAV anatomy and also guide in accurate positioning because of repositionable and recapturable nature. Balloon predilatation is required before THV implantation in almost all cases of bicuspid valve because it facilitates THV crossing, testing the raphe's resistance against valve expansion and predicting the risk of coronary occlusion. The long-term results of TAVI in bicuspid group in terms of 30-day and 1-year mortality were comparable with tricuspid AS except with slightly increased 30-day strike risk. Advancements in procedural imaging, device iterations, and procedural refinements will improve outcomes with TAVI in BAV anatomy.

ONLINE REFERENCES

Please scan the QR code provided at the end of the table of contents for References of this chapter.

CHAPTER

180 Small Aortic Annuli and Horizontal Aorta

Praveen Chandra, Nagendra Singh Chouhan, Siddarth Varshney

ABSTRACT

Transcatheter aortic valve replacement (TAVR) is a recommended treatment for severe symptomatic native calcific stenosis in low to prohibitive surgical risk patients. As the number of TAVR being performed is increasing exponentially, interventional cardiologists are encountering complex anatomies which impair procedural success. Horizontal aorta (HA) and small aortic annulus (SAA) are two such frequently seen aortic anatomies. With meticulous preprocedural planning, TAVR outcomes are remarkable in these patients. We, in this chapter discuss in detail these two complex clinical scenarios.

Keywords: TAVR in complex anatomy, small aortic annuli, horizontal aorta.

INTRODUCTION

Transcatheter aortic valve replacement (TAVR) is a recommended treatment for severe symptomatic native calcific stenosis in low to prohibitive surgical risk patients. The heart team decides for each patient after assessment for surgical aortic valve replacement (SAVR) risk versus TAVR risk. TAVR risk is mainly dependent on patient's vascular anatomy, i.e., the aortic valve apparatus and the vascular access. There are certain aortic anatomic and valvular characteristics which may affect device success. Coronary occlusion and vascular complications are two most fearsome complications of TAVR in unsuitable anatomy. Other important determinants are heavy calcification, horizontal aorta (HA), and small aortic annulus (SAA) which are frequently encountered and make aortic valve replacement (AVR) technically more challenging. We will focus on SAA and HA in this chapter.

SMALL AORTIC ANNULUS

The presence of a SAA poses a major challenge in treatment of patients with severe calcific aortic stenosis (AS). This condition is frequently encountered in elderly women. The optimal approach for these patients remains controversial. Several surgical modifications such as aortic root enlargement (ARE), the development of stented prostheses implanted in a supra-annular position, stentless bioprosthetic, and more recently, sutureless bioprostheses. TAVR has emerged as a therapeutic alternative in patients with severe AS and is particularly beneficial in patients with SAA. It provides better valve hemodynamics and outcomes in SAA patients.[1]

Though there is no clear consensus regarding cutoff value which defines SAA but it is most frequently defined as an annulus that would not accommodate a prosthetic valve of size > 21 mm^2. Alternatively, it is also defined as an aortic annulus ≤ 23 mm, measured by echocardiography preoperatively or by direct sizing intraoperatively.[2] The more practical definition would be the annulus size disproportionately small to the patient's body surface area causing prosthesis–patient mismatch (PPM).

Clinical Implications of Small Aortic Annulus

- Females have more prevalence of SAA.
- SAA patients have higher surgical risk profile as determined by Society of Thoracic Surgeons (STS) and Logistic EuroScore (European System for Cardiac Operative Risk Evaluation).

- They have a lower body surface area.
- These patients have high prevalence of comorbidities such as obesity, diabetes mellitus, atrial fibrillation, and chronic kidney disease.
- Geographically, Asian populations have a smaller aortic annulus diameter than Europeans.
- SAA patients have more incidence of PPM.

Prosthesis–Patient Mismatch

Prosthesis-patient mismatch occurs when the effective orifice area (EOA) of a normally functioning prosthetic valve is small in relation to body size. Thus, prosthetic heart valve is unable to meet the patient's cardiac output requirements at rest and/or during exercise. In general, EOA of <0.85 cm^2/m^2 is considered to be the threshold for PPM, values between 0.65 and 0.85 cm^2/m^2 being categorized as moderate PPM and <0.65 cm^2/m^2 as severe PPM.

Small aortic annulus patients who undergo SAVR are more prone to receive smaller prostheses, and hence are at higher risk of developing PPM. Thus, there is less regression of left ventricular mass after AVR and this may also compromise the postoperative normalization of coronary flow reserve with a negative effect on left ventricular function. PPM is an independent predictor of long-term mortality, proportional to its severity and also has been linked to an increase in the incidences of structural valve deterioration (SVD). In patients with small annulus, a root enhancement surgery is recommended along with AVR.

Transcatheter Aortic Valve Replacement in Small Aortic Annulus

In patients with SAA and severe AS, increasing evidence exists that TAVR offers superior hemodynamic results than a SAVR alone. Clavel et al. compared balloon-expandable valves (BEVs) with surgical valves (stented and stentless) and showed that TAVR valves have lower transvalvular gradients, higher indexed EOA values, and reduced PPM rates, with the hemodynamic differences between valves particularly related to those patients with SAA.[3]

In a substudy of the PARTNER (Placement of Aortic Transcatheter Valve) I trial, patients with SAA had larger EOA with TAVR valve when compared with SAVR valves, this translated into a reduced rate of PPM.[4] The rate of moderate-to-severe aortic insufficiency was lower in patients with SAA undergoing TAVR, in comparison with those who have a larger annulus (9%).[1] The PARTNER I trial substudy showed no differences in mortality rates between TAVR and SAVR, based on aortic annulus size.[4] However, in patients with SAA, a higher incidence of major vascular complications and stroke was reported in the TAVR group compared to the SAVR group.

Small aortic annulus patients in general have higher periprocedural complications such as coronary obstruction and annular rupture therefore the meticulous planning and implementation of measures for the prevention of coronary obstruction, such as a careful evaluation of coronary ostium height, sinus diameter, and proper device selection, are of great importance in this subgroup of patients. Use of (SEVs) is preferred as they have better hemodynamics than a BEV and can be retrieved if coronary obstruction occurs after 80% deployment.

Rogers et al. showed that the SEV CoreValve system (CoreValve or Evolut R) was associated with lower peak velocity and have lower mean gradients in comparison to the Sapien valve. However, no statistically significant differences were noted in incidence of PPM between groups. The incidence of moderate-to-severe paraprosthetic aortic regurgitation was more frequent in patients who received the CoreValve system.[4] Data regarding hemodynamic performance of new generation valves is lacking. **Flowchart 1** shows proposed algorithm for management of patients with SAA.[2]

TAVI-SMALL2 registry[5] concluded that in SAA, implantation of supra-annular valve (SAV) and SEV was associated with a more favorable, forward, and hemodynamic profile than after intra-annular valve (IAV) and BEV implantation, respectively. SEV was found to be associated with more paravalvular leak as compared to BEV.

Okuno et al.[6] examined data from the Bern TAVR registry and the Swiss TAVR registry and concluded that using SEVs in patients with small annuli was associated with an improvement in hemodynamic parameters compared with BEVs, but this did not translate into better clinical outcomes with follow-up till 5 years.

Clinical case: A 56-year-old female presented to us with classical triad of angina, dyspnea, and syncope. She was found to have severe AS of type-0 bicuspid valve with annulus to left ventricular outflow tract (LVOT) calcium. Her perimeter-derived aortic annulus size was 22.8 mm **(Figs. 1A to D)**. After meticulous planning she underwent TAVR using 23-mm self-expandable SAV **(Figs. 2A and B)**. Her maximum and mean post-procedural gradient across aortic valve were 9 and 4 mm Hg, respectively with no valvular or paravalvular leak. She was discharged the very next day in satisfactory condition.

HORIZONTAL AORTA

Horizontal aorta is defined as increased aortic angulation (≥49°) or unfolding of the ascending aorta and aortic root. It is one of these anatomical challenges, particularly for the transfemoral approach for TAVR. HA makes TAVR technically more difficult by:

- Hampering valve crossing
- Impairing valve delivery
- Preventing coaxial alignment and optimal positioning of the valve within the aortic annulus **(Fig. 3)**
- Decreasing the overall control on important procedural steps

Extreme HA (>70°) is considered off-label for TAVR by transfemoral access as it was an exclusion in all TAVR trials.

Many previous reports have documented an association between increasing aortic root angulation and procedural failure using first-generation transcatheter heart valve (THV) devices. In addition, the risk of procedural failure in a HA seemed to be confined to the use of self-expanding valves as opposed to balloon-expandable ones. In cases of HA, coaxial alignment may not be perfectly achieved with a long stent frame with a nonsteerable delivery catheter in SEV as opposed to a short device with a steerable delivery system in BEV.

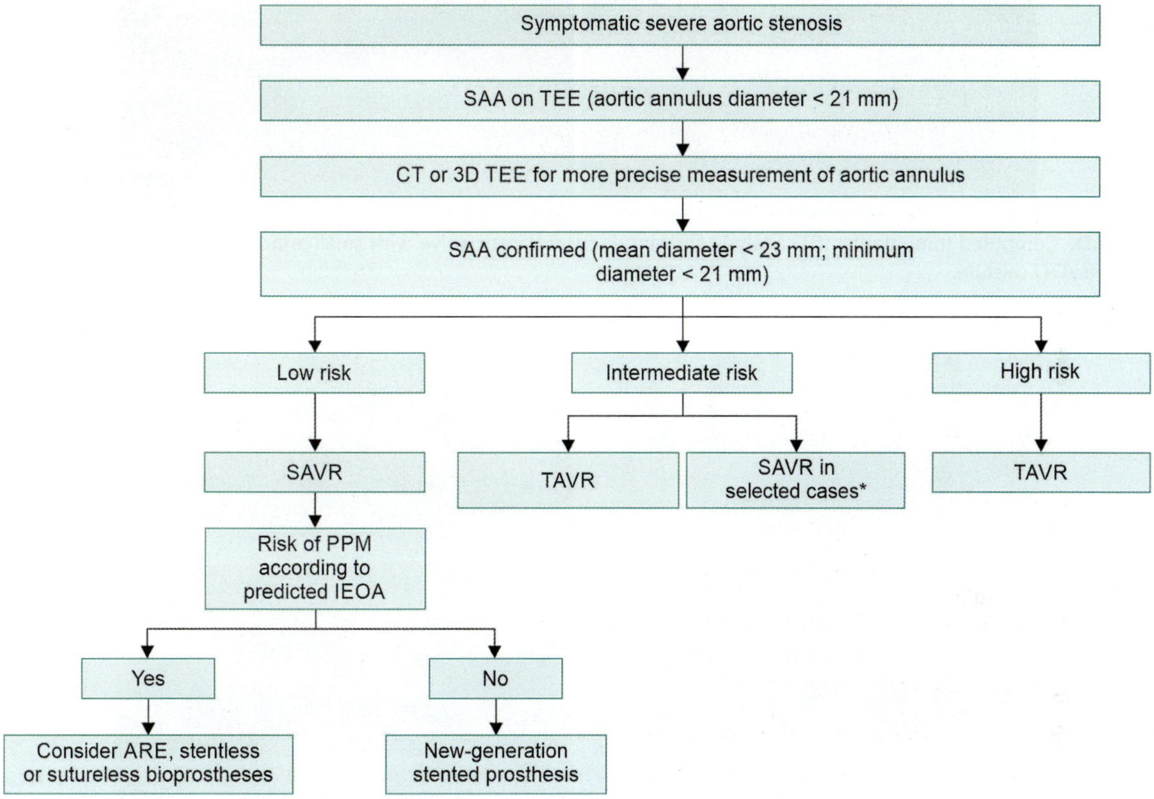

*Need for concomitant procedures, unfavorable anatomic characteristics for TAVR.

FLOWCHART 1: Proposed algorithm for management of patients with small aortic annulus (SAA).

(AA: aortic annulus; ARE: aortic root enlargement; BSA: body surface area; CT: computed tomography; iEOA: index effective orifice area; PPM: prosthesis–patient mismatch; SAVR: surgical aortic valve replacement; TAVR: transcatheter aortic valve replacement; TEE: transesophageal echocardiography; TTE: transthoracic echocardiography)

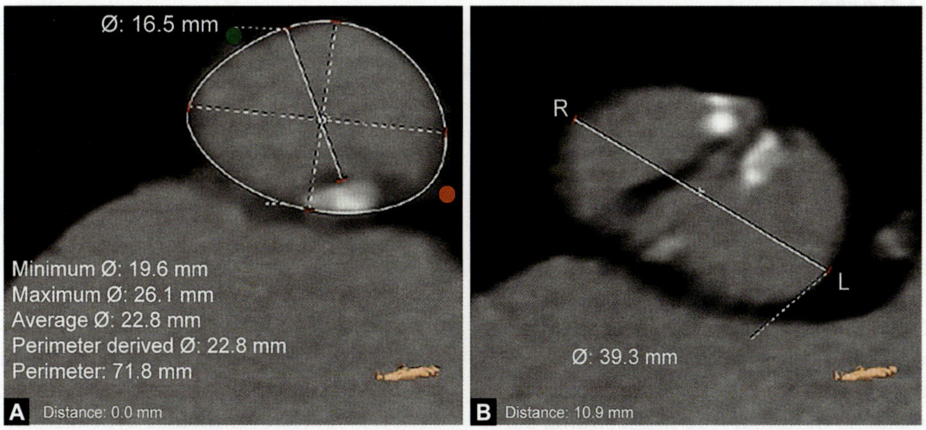

FIGS. 1A TO D: *Continued*

Continued

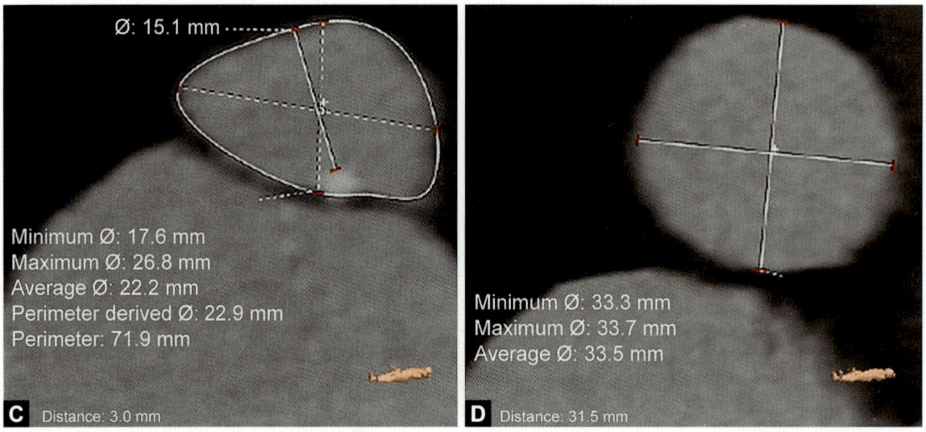

FIGS. 1A TO D: Computed tomography (CT) analysis showing bicuspid aortic valve with small annulus and annulus to left ventricular outflow tract (LVOT) calcium.

(SOV: sinus of Valsalva)

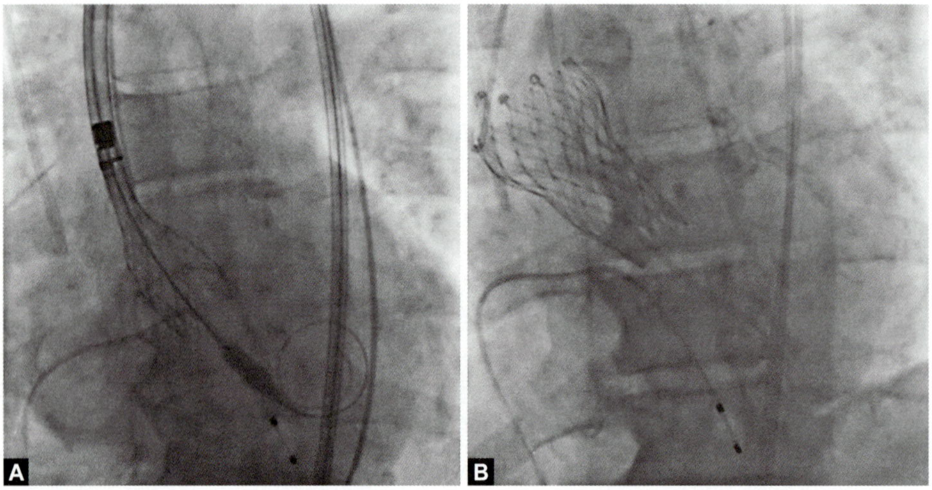

FIGS. 2A AND B: Transcatheter aortic valve replacement (TAVR) using self-expandable valve in a patient with bicuspid aortic valve and small annuli.

Strategies to Overcome Horizontal Aorta

- *Buddy balloon technique*:[7]
  - An additional stiff wire is advanced to the aortic root and a peripheral balloon is used as a shoehorn to allow sliding of valve over it.
  - This facilitates delivery of valve across the aorta.
- *Loop snare technique*:[8]
  - Prosthetic valve is parked in aorta.
  - A nitinol hydrophilic wire is advanced to ascending aorta using 4F internal mammary catheter via opposite femoral artery access (8F sheath) which is later removed.
  - A goose snare is advanced through the 8F sheath to snare the distal tip of nitinol wire in ascending aorta and a loop is made around TAVR valve **(Fig. 4)**.
  - The snared end of hydrophilic wire is externalized.
  - 8F Judkins right 4 (JR4) guiding catheter is advanced to ascending aorta over the both ends of externalized nitinol wire while clinching a loop around body of TAVR valve.
  - One operator advances the valve across native valve while another operator pulls the loop snare. This makes alignment and position more favorable.
  - After successful crossing of TAVR valve, JR4 and nitinol wire are removed and valve is deployed.

Clinical case: A 47-year-old, former smoker, diabetic male presented to us with New York Heart Association (NYHA) class 2 dyspnea. Upon evaluation, he was found to have severe AS in unicuspidal aortic valve, moderate aortic insufficiency, global left ventricular hypokinesia, and dilated aorta. His preprocedural computed tomography (CT) aortogram

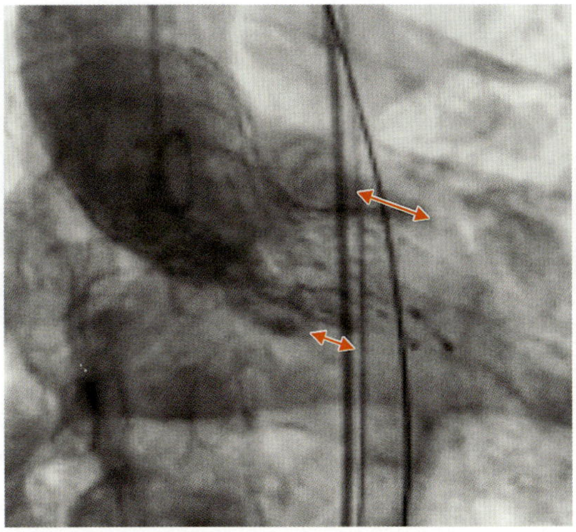

FIG 3: Oblique alignment of valve in a horizontal aorta: On one side the valve is 4 mm below annulus (small red arrow) while on other side it is around 8 mm deep (large red arrow).

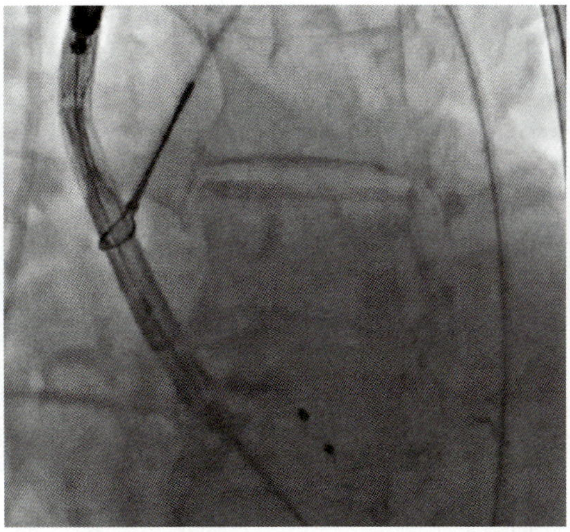

FIG. 4: Loop snare technique.

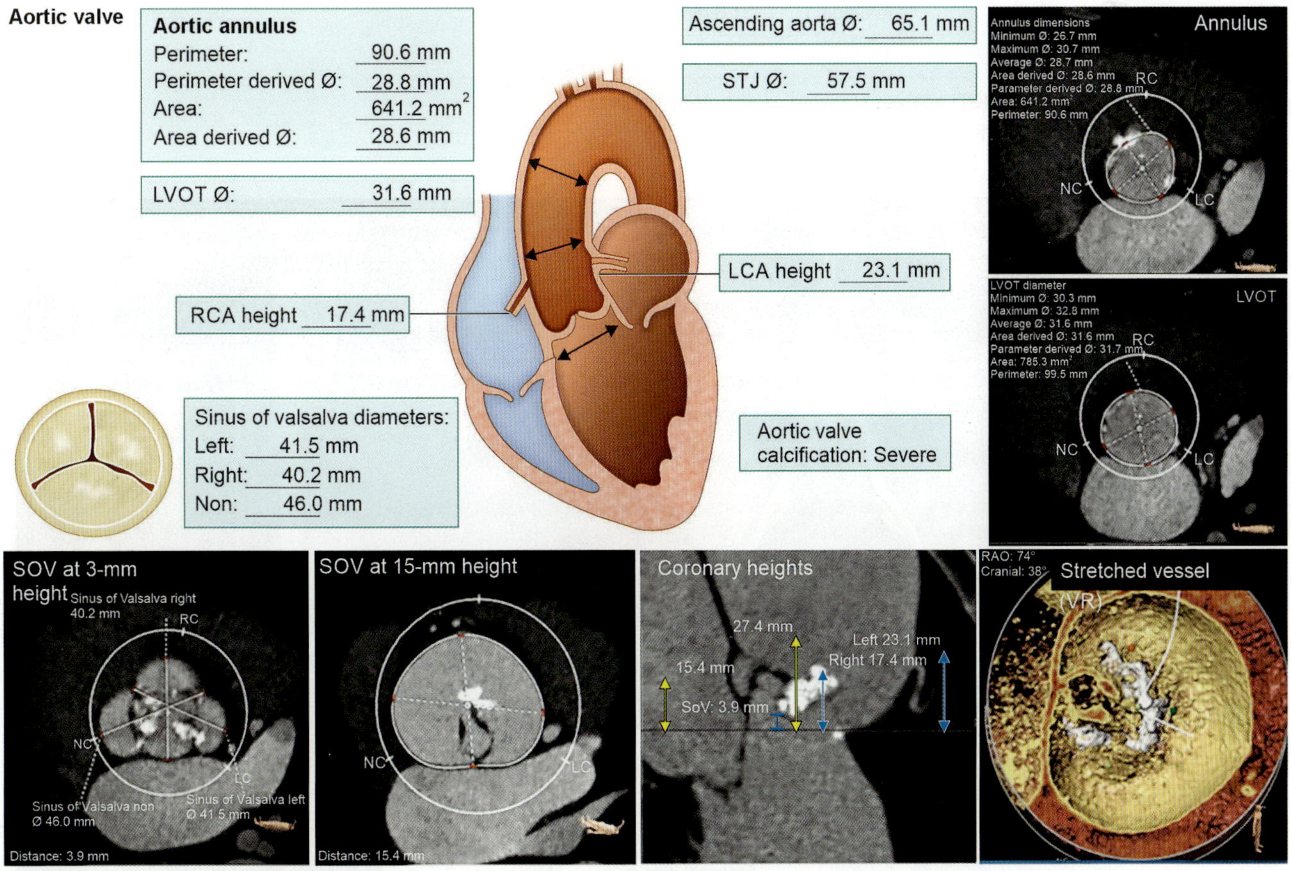

FIG. 5: Computerized tomography (CT) analysis showing aortic valve morphology.

(LCA: left coronary artery; LVOT: left ventricular outflow tract; RCA: right coronary artery; STJ: sinotubular junction; VR: volume rendering)

analyses are summarized in **Figures 5 to 7**. Patient had aortic angulation of 49°. After detailed analysis of his CT parameters, he was planned for balloon expandable 29-mm Octacor valve using "comalign" technique **(Figs. 8 and 9)**. Postprocedure his hemodynamics improved and we were able to get single-digit gradients across aortic valve **(Figs. 10A and B)**.

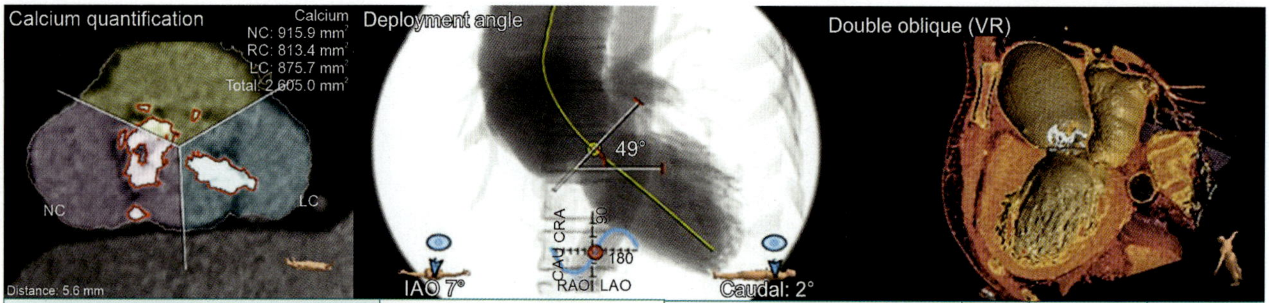

Ascending aorta Ø	Minimum: 62.6 mm Maximum: 67.5 mm Average: 65.1 mm
Sinotubular junction Ø	Minimum: 53.4 mm Maximum: 61.5 mm Average: 57.5 mm
Aortic annulus	Minimum Ø: 26.7 mm Maximum Ø: 30.7 mm Average Ø: 28.7 mm Eccentricity Ø: 0.13
LVOT Ø	Minimum: 30.3 mm Maximum: 32.8 mm Average: 31.6 mm
Sinus of valsalva height	3.9 mm

3D annular area mm²		641.2
3D area derived diameter mm		28.6
% annular area over/under	20 mm	–51.0%
	21.5 mm	–43.4%
	23 mm	–35.2%
	24.5 mm	–26.5%
	26 mm	–17.2%
Unicuspid aortic valve, 25-mm Mammoth, 29-mm Myval octacor →	27.5 mm	–7.4%
	29 mm	3.0%
	30.5 mm	13.9%
	32 mm	25.4%

FIG. 6: Computed tomography (CT) analysis showing morphology of aorta.
(LVOT: left ventricular outflow tract; VR: volume rendering)

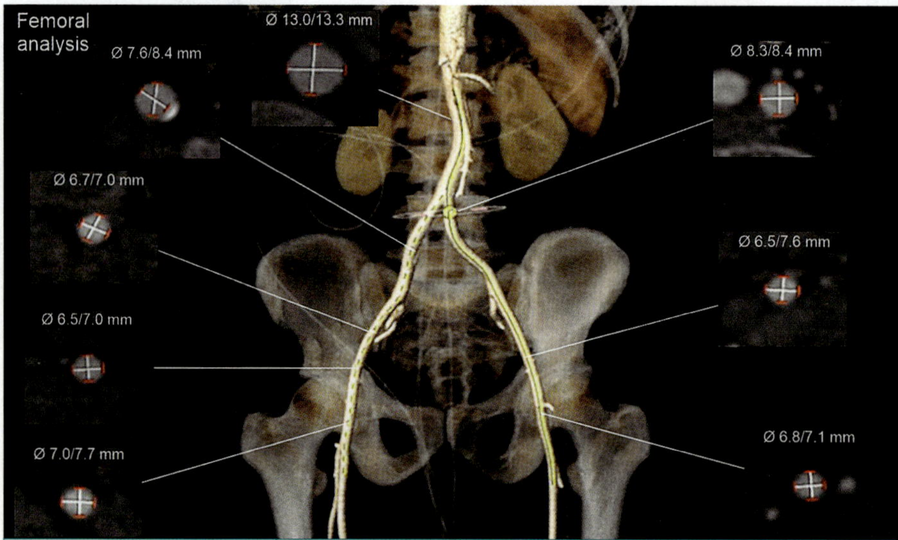

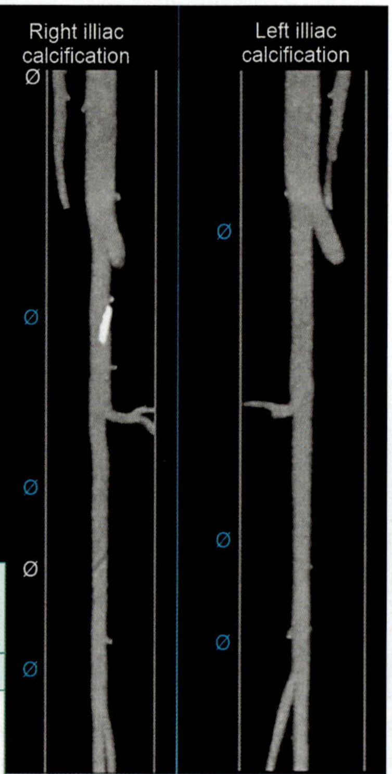

Right access dimensions	Minimum: 7.6 mm Maximum: 8.4 mm Average: 8.0 mm	Left access dimensions	Minimum: 8.3 mm Maximum: 8.4 mm Average: 8.4 mm
Common iliac calcification	Mild	Common iliac calcification	None
External iliac ø	Minimum: 6.7 mm Maximum: 7.0 mm Average: 6.8 mm	External iliac ø	Minimum: 6.5 mm Maximum: 7.6 mm Average: 7.0 mm
External iliac calcification	None	External iliac calcification	None
Femoral ø	Minimum: 7.0 mm Maximum: 7.7 mm Average: 7.3 mm	Femoral ø	Minimum: 6.8 mm Maximum: 7.1 mm Average: 7.0 mm

FIG. 7: Computed tomography (CT) analysis of peripheral vessels.

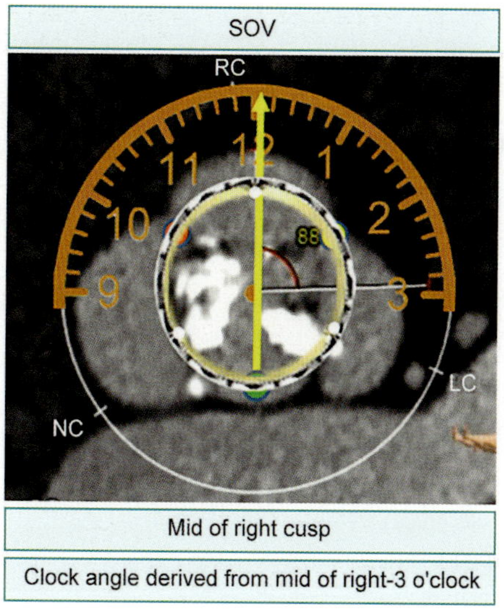

FIG. 8: Computed tomography (CT)-derived clock angle.
(LC: left coronary cusp; NC: noncoronary cusp; RC: right coronary cusp; SOV: sinus of Valsalva)

CONCLUSION

Transcatheter aortic valve replacement has revolutionized the treatment of aortic valve stenosis in patients with small annuli and HA. The unique design and features of these valves, including larger EOA, anchoring and sealing mechanisms, transcatheter approach, flexibility, and adaptability, make them well-suited for patients with these anatomical variations. TAVR offers a less invasive alternative with improved outcomes for high-risk patients who would not be suitable candidates for conventional surgical interventions. The evidence indicates that it provides excellent clinical outcomes, improved durability, enhanced valve function, and better hemodynamic performance compared to SAVR in patients with small annuli and HA.

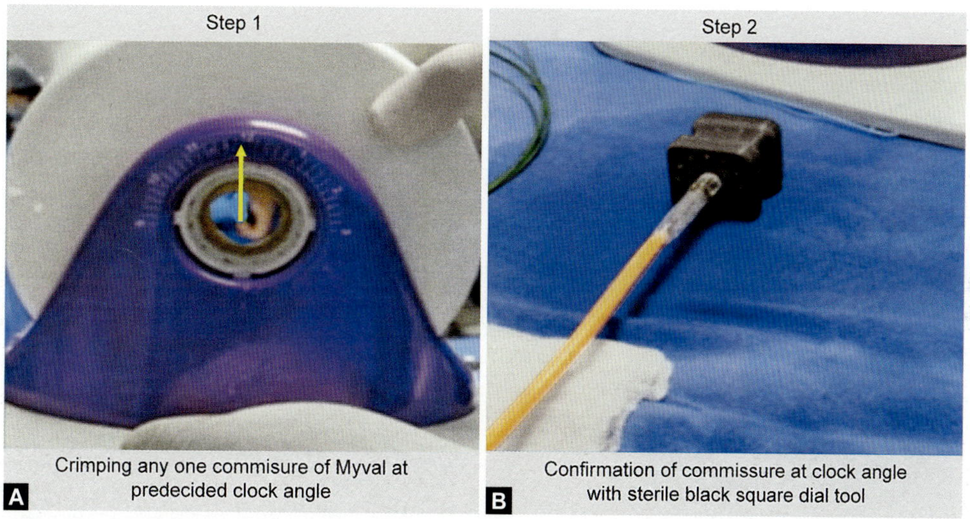

FIGS. 9A AND B: Steps of "comalign" technique.

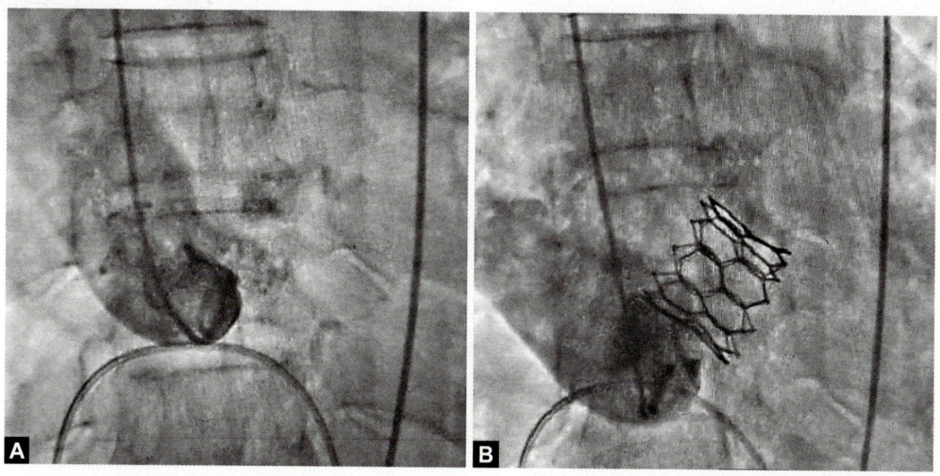

FIGS. 10A AND B: (A) Baseline aortogram; (B) aortogram after balloon-expandable valve (BEV) deployment.

ONLINE REFERENCES

Please scan the QR code provided at the end of the table of contents for References of this chapter.

CHAPTER

181 Protected Transcatheter Aortic Valve Replacement

Manik Chopra, Varun Bhatia

ABSTRACT

Stroke is the most feared, unpredictable, and underrecognized complication of transcatheter aortic valve replacement (TAVR), which has not decreased with the refinement of TAVR technology. It has a significant impact on quality of life and socioeconomic impact. Cerebral atheroembolism is mainly responsible for these strokes. Cerebral embolic protection devices (CEPDs) target to prevent or reduce this cerebral atheroembolism. SENTINEL CEPD is the only CEPD available in India. The PROTECTED TAVR trial showed that SENTINEL CEPD has an excellent safety record and appears to prevent disabling stroke. However, the evidence for constant reduction in periprocedural stroke is inadequate.

Keywords: TAVR, stroke, cerebral embolic protection devices, SENTINEL.

INTRODUCTION

Transcatheter aortic valve replacement (TAVR) via transfemoral access is a standard therapy for patients with severe aortic stenosis (AS) in elderly across the entire surgical risk spectrum.[1,2] Though the rate of complications related to TAVR are on a decreasing trend due to refinement of the technique, stroke rates remain the same at 2–4%.[3,4] However, the stroke rates are often underreported as neurological examination by neurologist and/or imaging were not part of majority of clinical studies and not routinely done in clinical practice. It is devastating and the most feared complication of TAVR also from patients' perspective. It increases mortality and morbidity substantially and has significant impact on socioeconomic aspects and quality of life. Cerebral embolic protection devices (CEPDs) were developed to mitigate TAVR-related stroke along with the burden of cerebral embolic debris and have been shown to be safe in various clinical settings. However, their true efficacy in stroke prevention during TAVR remains to be demonstrated.

CLINICAL MANIFESTATIONS OF STROKE RELATED TO TAVR

Major/clinically disabling strokes are clinically apparent. However, minor strokes, transient ischemic attacks and neurocognitive decline are subtle and are often undetected. Silent cerebral infarcts go undetected unless imaging is done.

ETIOLOGY AND TIMING OF STROKE DURING TAVR

Periprocedural or early strokes are mainly caused by athero- or thromboembolic events provoked by the disruption of atheromatous or calcific debris arising during several procedural steps. A prior history of stroke, arterial/valvular calcium burden, bicuspid aortic valves, aortic valve pre-/postdilatation and valve-in-valve procedures have been identified as risk factors for the same.[3,5] Late strokes may be related to calcified native valve disruption, incomplete endothelialization of the valve stent, suboptimal antiplatelet effect, new-onset atrial fibrillation, and patient's overall atherothrombotic burden. Reduced renal function, diabetes mellitus, and increasing age were found to be related to the incidence of late stroke.[6]

HISTOPATHOLOGY OF THE EMBOLIC DEBRIS

Cerebral embolic debris is generated in at least 99% of TAVI patients and includes pieces of calcium, valve and aortic tissue, myocardium, or other organic or foreign matter.[7] One in four patients have an average of 25 pieces of debris ≥0.5 mm headed to the brain. Debris of this size has the potential to occlude cerebral arteries [e.g., middle cerebral artery (MCA), anterior cerebral artery (ACA), posterior cerebral artery (PCA), and basilar artery (BA)].

CEREBRAL EMBOLIC PROTECTION DEVICES

According to mechanism of action, CEPDs can be classified into two groups: devices that capture (totally or partially) debris within the aorta before it reaches the brain and renal or peripheral arteries; or deflectors of debris from the aortic arch and its branches. The former may be positioned along the aortic arch and/or descending aorta or within the brachiocephalic trunk and/or common carotid arteries, while the latter are typically positioned along the roof of the aortic arch.

Devices can also be classified into partial capture devices (SENTINEL), full capture devices [Emblok (Innovative Cardiovascular Solutions)], Emboliner (Emboline), FLOWer (AorticLab)], primarily deflective devices with small capture capacity [TriGUARD 3 (Keystone Heart/Venus Medtech), ProtEmbo (Protembis), POINT-GUARD (Transverse Medical)], and deflection and capture devices [CAPTIS (Filterlex)].

Currently, only SENTINEL is available in India for clinical use.

SENTINEL

The SENTINEL Cerebral Protection System is a Certifications Experts (CE) and United States Food and Drug Administration (USFDA)-approved device which consists of two polyurethane filters with 140 mm diameter pores fixed in a flexible nitinol radiopaque frame, advanced from a 6 Fr sheath through the right radial or right brachial artery and deployed into the ostia of brachiocephalic trunk and left common carotid artery. It is designed to capture emboli passing into the cerebral circulation in two of the three branches of the aortic arch but not the left subclavian, leaving the left vertebral circulation unprotected.

The SENTINEL device has been studied in four randomized clinical trials (RCTs), MISTRAL-C (MRI Investigation in TAVI with Claret) trial, the CLEAN-TAVI (Claret Embolic Protection and TAVI) trial, SENTINEL trial, and the PROTECTED-TAVR (Stroke Protection with Sentinel during Transcatheter Aortic Valve Replacement) trial.

The US SENTINEL IDE study[7] was a larger multicenter study in which the authors reported debris in 99% of the filters. Despite a numerical reduction in all-cause stroke at 30 days, statistical significance was not met. Also, the median total new lesion volume in protected territories evaluated by diffusion-weighted MRI (DW-MRI) 2–7 days post-TAVR did not differ significantly between the control and the CEPD groups. The CEPD group demonstrated a reduction in stroke within 72 hours after TAVR [classified as procedural stroke by the Neurologic Academic Research Consortium (NeuroARC) definitions] when compared to the unprotected group (3.0% vs. 8.2%; $p = 0.053$).

The recently published PROTECTED TAVR trial[8] was the first randomized, open-label, multicenter, all-comer trial powered for clinical endpoints. It enrolled 3,000 patients undergoing transfemoral TAVR with all commercially available transcatheter heart valves, to receive TAVR plus the SENTINEL device (CEPD group: 1,501 patients) or TAVR with no CEPD (control group: 1,499 patients). The primary endpoint was all stroke (hemorrhagic, ischemic, or undetermined status—disabling or nondisabling) up to 72 hours post-TAVR procedure or hospital discharge using NeuroARC definitions. Successful device deployment was achieved in 94.4% of patients. SENTINEL use did not significantly reduce the incidence of stroke within 72 hours post-TAVR or before-hospital discharge compared to the control group. Disabling stroke (a secondary endpoint) was less frequent in the CEPD group (0.5%) compared to the control group (1.3%). The number needed to treat to prevent one disabling stroke was 125 patients. Although the device proved to be safe and a possible effect on disabling strokes (a secondary endpoint) was seen, clear clinical benefit is yet to be demonstrated.

ONGOING TRIALS

The BHF PROTECT-TAVI[9] (British Heart Foundation Randomized Trial of Routine Cerebral Embolic Protection in Transcatheter Aortic Valve Implantation) (n = 7,730) is an open label, outcome-adjudicated, multicenter, all-comer RCT in the United Kingdom (UK) that will randomize patients undergoing TAVR by any access route to CEPD (with the SENTINEL CEPD) or no CEPD, with no specific exclusion criteria. The primary outcome measure is stroke at 72 hours post-TAVR. Amongst a range of secondary outcome measures, a cost-effectiveness analysis at 12 months will be performed. Results are expected by July 2026.

CONCLUSION

Stroke following TAVR occurs at a constant rate despite advancement of TAVR technology; it is underrecognized and is the most feared complication with significant socioeconomic impact. It remains largely unpredictable with majority of periprocedural strokes due to cerebral embolization. Evidence of the same is present in majority of TAVR patients. SENTINEL CEPD has an excellent safety record and appears to prevent disabling stroke. However, the evidence for constant reduction in periprocedural stroke is inadequate. Ongoing and upcoming trials will address it further.

ONLINE REFERENCES

Please scan the QR code provided at the end of the table of contents for References of this chapter.

CHAPTER 182

BASILICA: Bioprosthetic or Native Aortic Scallop Intentional Laceration to Prevent Coronary Artery Obstruction

Ajoe John Kattoor, Vijay Iyer

ABSTRACT

Coronary artery obstruction remains a significant concern post transcatheter aortic valve replacement (TAVR), with potentially fatal implications. This chapter discusses the Bioprosthetic or Native Aortic Scallop Intentional Laceration to prevent Iatrogenic Coronary Artery obstruction (BASILICA) procedure, an innovative approach to mitigate these risks. We discuss patient selection, predictors of obstruction, detailed procedural description, and its limitations. Data from the BASILICA Investigational Device Exemption (IDE) trial and the multicenter International BASILICA registry demonstrate the efficacy of the procedure, with 94–95% successful leaflet traversal and laceration. There was a 10% stroke rate in the smaller BASILICA trial, but the larger BASILICA registry data revealed a 30-day stroke rate of 3%. Despite these promising results, the procedure does not eliminate the risk of coronary obstruction entirely as some of the factors that cause coronary obstruction are still out of the operator's control. Coronary obstruction was observed in 5% of patients from the BASILICA registry. The development of dedicated electrosurgical devices, as well as the introduction of newer devices such as the ShortCut (Pi-Cardia), which is currently under clinical trial, is expected to make the procedure more straightforward and safer.

Keywords: TAVR, BASILICA, aortic stenosis.

INTRODUCTION

Coronary artery obstruction has an incidence of around 0.7% in all transcatheter aortic valve replacement (TAVR) cases and 2.3% in valve-in-valve TAVR cases.[1,2] Coronary artery obstruction after TAVR has a high mortality up to 50%.[1,2] Coronary artery obstruction occurs due to the sequestration of the sinus of Valsalva at sinotubular junction (STJ), direct obstruction due to deficient sinus of Valsalva and displaced leaflet of native or bioprosthetic valve after TAVR, direct obstruction of the ostium of the coronaries from the displaced leaflet mass typically calcific nodule, embolization of thrombus or degenerative material or from TAVR skirt or commissural posts.[3] For patients at risk of coronary obstruction post TAVR, options include surgical valve replacement, palliative management, or interventional methods to prevent coronary artery obstruction. The interventional methods include traditional Chimney-Snorkel technique or the use of electrosurgical laceration of aortic scallop using BASILICA procedure. In this chapter, our goal is to present a discussion on the BASILICA procedure, aiming to provide clinicians with a clear understanding of its role, applicability, and outcomes in managing patients susceptible to coronary artery obstruction following TAVR.

Why is BASILICA needed?

The traditional approach to protect coronaries from obstruction post TAVR valve deployment involves prophylactically placing a guidewire and stent in the at-risk coronary. The stent is deployed in the coronary artery after pulling back and extended into the aorta, should coronary obstruction occur post TAVR valve placement.[4] However, the catheter and stent can become pinned between the TAVR valve and the aortic root, and they may often have to be deployed regardless of coronary obstruction to avoid being stripped of the balloon. Cyclic compression and abnormal flow mechanics around the snorkeled stent can lead to stent deformation and stent thrombosis, respectively. Additionally, accessing the coronaries can be extremely challenging through the snorkeled stent.[3] Orthotopic stent implantation through the cells of the TAVR valve has been reported and is thought to prevent stent deformation and reduce abnormal flow conditions which may occur with the traditional snorkel technique.[5] BASILICA procedure aims to address these shortcomings, provide a more durable result avoiding coronary obstruction, and, if needed, permitting orthotopic stent implantation.

SELECTION OF PATIENTS AND PREDICTION OF OBSTRUCTION

Accurate prediction of coronary obstruction is challenging, even with CT evaluation. A leaflet length less than the height of the coronary ostium from the annular plane suggests a lower likelihood of coronary obstruction. Long leaflets extending higher than the STJ can be obstructive when the STJ is narrow compared to the intended TAVR valve. Presence of calcific masses on the leaflet increases risk for obstruction and may even preclude performance of BASILICA procedure.[3] Data from Valve-in-Valve International Data (VIVID) registry revealed that coronary obstruction is more common in stented bioprosthesis with externally mounted leaflets and stentless bioprosthesis when compared to stented bioprosthesis with internally mounted valve leaflets (6.1% vs. 3.7% vs. 0.8%; $p < 0.001$). A shorter virtual valve-to-coronary (VTC) distance predicted increased risk for coronary obstruction (odds ratio 7.67; 95% confidence interval 3.14–18.7; $p < 0.001$) with an optimal cut off level of 4 mm.[2] Khan et al. recently developed and validated a multivariate prediction model for coronary obstruction after TAVR in native aortic stenosis. The study was performed on 60 patients with angiography-confirmed coronary obstruction and compared with 1,381 patients without obstruction. The authors concluded that the model best predicted coronary obstruction if cusp height > coronary height AND VTC ≤ 4 mm OR culprit leaflet calcium volume >600 mm^3.[6] Additionally, implantation characteristics such as depth of implantation, canting angle, TAVR device rotational alignment, and TAVR device flaring—many of which cannot be easily controlled during implantation—can affect risk for coronary obstruction, thus making accurate prediction difficult.[7]

Not all coronary obstructions post TAVR are amenable to the BASILICA procedure. Deficient sinus (direct obstruction by leaflet from obliteration of the sinus of Valsalva) and sequestered sinus (leaflet blocking the entire sinus of Valsalva, most commonly in valve-in-valve TAVR) are the only two types of coronary obstructions that may be amenable to BASILICA **(Fig. 1)**.[3]

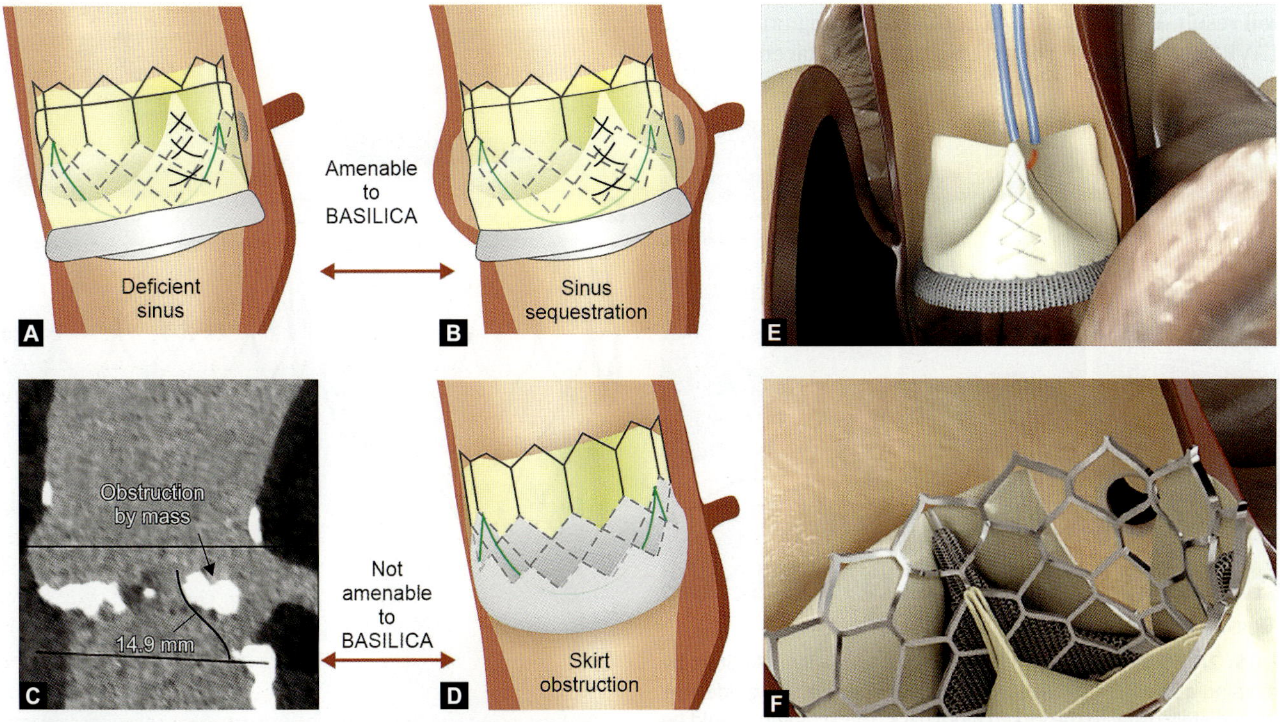

FIGS. 1A TO F: Mechanisms of transcatheter aortic valve replacement (TAVR)-induced coronary obstruction and mitigation by bioprosthetic or native aortic scallop intentional laceration to prevent iatrogenic coronary artery obstruction during TAVR (BASILICA). (A) Outward displacement of the aortic valve leaflets during TAVR can directly obstruct the coronary artery ostium if patient has a deficient sinus of Valsalva. (B) The displaced aortic valve leaflets indirectly cause obstruction of the coronary ostium by sequestering the sinus. (C) Direct obstruction of the coronary ostia by a bulky leaflet mass/calcium. (D) Fabric-covered frame or skirt obstructing coronary artery ostium in low coronary ostia. (E) In the BASILICA procedure, an electrified guidewire is used to lacerate the prior aortic valve leaflets. (F) After the BASILICA procedure, the TAVR implant can splay the lacerated leaflets, ensuring that blood can flow into the potentially threatened coronary ostium.
Source: With permission from Lederman et al. (2019).[3]

PRINCIPLE OF BASILICA PROCEDURE

The BASILICA procedure involves the intentional laceration of the native or bioprosthetic aortic leaflet using electrosurgery. This allows the leaflet to splay open after TAVR valve implantation, ensuring blood flow into the coronaries. This is achieved by concentrating an electrical charge on the leaflet tissue, causing it to vaporize. An electrical current path is created by connecting a guidewire and a dispersive electrode on the patient to an electrosurgery generator.[8] Charge concentration at the tissue to be lacerated is achieved by focally denuding the insulating polymer of a stiff coronary wire for a length of 2–3 mm and then kinking the guidewire in the form of a "V" so as to straddle the leaflet sides **(Figs. 2A to C)**. 5% dextrose solution which is a nonionic solution is injected through the catheter to flood the field of laceration so as to prevent char formation and thrombosis and also to avoid charge dispersion and thereby improving the efficiency of laceration.[3,8]

The lacerated leaflet should splay open once the TAVR valve is deployed, allowing blood from the aorta to fill the sinus of Valsalva and reach the coronaries. Adequate splaying may not occur if the laceration is too close to the leaflet tip or too far from the leaflet midline. In patients with a deficient sinus, the leaflet laceration must align exactly with the coronary ostium; otherwise, coronary obstruction will result. It is important to note that the alignment of the TAVR valve and skirt should also match the laceration. For example, the BASILICA procedure is likely to be futile if the TAVR commissural post overlies the area of laceration, as this could continue to cause coronary obstruction **(Figs. 3A to D)**.

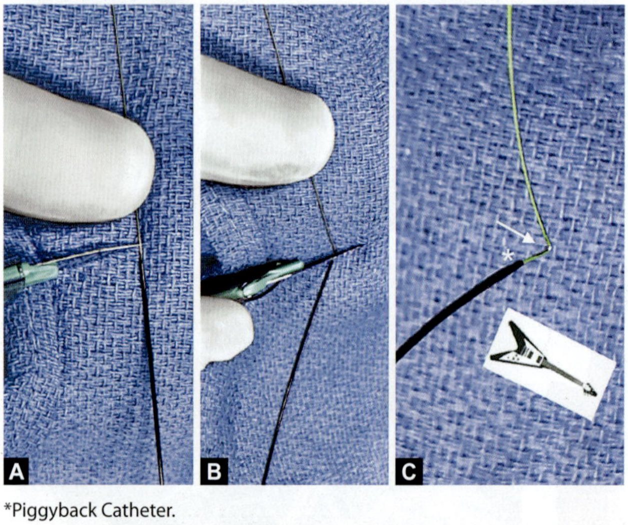

*Piggyback Catheter.

FIGS. 2A TO C: Creation of flying "V" for laceration. (A) Start by scraping a small section (around 2–3 millimeters) of the guidewire, immediately distal to the locked Piggyback. This scraping should be done noncircumferentially. (B) After scraping, use the back end of a scalpel to create a kink in the guidewire. (C) The noncircumferential inner-surface denudation (indicated by the arrow) near the Piggyback creates a V-shaped formation. This specific structure helps to facilitate the laceration of the aortic valve leaflets in the BASILICA procedure.

Source: With permission from Lederman et al. (2019).[3]

PROCEDURAL DESCRIPTION

The BASILICA procedure is typically performed under general anesthesia, using transesophageal echocardiography (TEE) and fluoroscopy for guidance. First, vascular access is established, including the placement of the TAVR sheath access. The GORE DrySEAL sheath is often utilized as the large-bore access sheath, as it can accommodate multiple catheters while maintaining hemostasis. The catheters used for laceration can be advanced through the same large-bore access sheath or through sheaths placed in different arterial accesses.

The stenosed aortic valve is first crossed, following which a 6-Fr guiding catheter (like a JR-4 or multipurpose) is placed in the left ventricle (LV). A gooseneck snare, typically around 2 cm in diameter, is introduced through the catheter and placed in the left ventricular outflow tract (LVOT). The guide

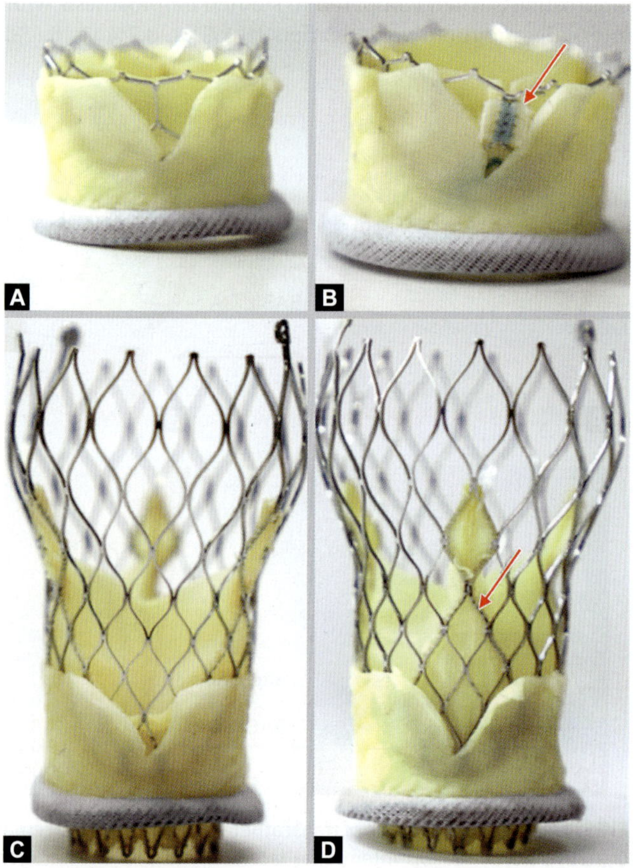

FIGS. 3A TO D: Transcatheter aortic valve replacement (TAVR) device commissures aligned with the laceration (B and D) likely to cause continued coronary obstruction (red arrow) when compared to commissural post away from the laceration (A and C).

Source: With permission from Lederman et al. (2019).[3]

catheter may be stabilized using a rigid guidewire anchor placed in the LV, however, should be removed immediately prior to laceration. Then, a second guide catheter, which aids in traversing the leaflet, is introduced.

The traversal guide catheter should contact the leaflet at the base and point toward the LVOT. An 8-Fr guide catheter is usually employed to enhance ease of manipulation. The newer elephant trunk or pachyderm-shaped guiding catheters (PAL1, PAL2, PAL3, Launcher for left and PJR4 for right coronary cusp) can significantly reduce the leaflet time-to-traversal during the BASILICA procedure.[9] Otherwise, coaxial catheter pairs or an oversized catheter such as AL2, AL3, AL4, for the left and MP for right can be selected.[10]

A stiff conductive guidewire (typically an Astato XS-20, 0.014 inch × 300 cm, Asahi-Intecc) is introduced into a PiggyBack wire converter (Teleflex), which provides insulation to the wire within the body. The system is then advanced to the tip of the traversal guide catheter. The external end of the Astato wire is clamped onto the electrosurgery pencil using hemostatic forceps after a 1 cm insulating coating of the wire is denuded with a scalpel. The traversal guiding catheter is then positioned in the mid base of the leaflet usually under fluoroscopy and TEE guidance and the Astato guidewire tip is then exposed. Fluoroscopic projection angles for BASILICA can be preselected from cardiac CT review.[7]

Radiofrequency energy is then applied for <1 second in pure cut mode (50 W) and the guidewire is advanced gently for 2–5 mm through the leaflet pointing to the LVOT. Calcification can prevent leaflet traversal in which case slight repositioning may be required. Once leaflet is traversed, it is further advanced without application of energy. The guidewire is then snared approximately 10–15 mm from its tip using the snare that was positioned in the LVOT. Once the snare grasp is confirmed, the Piggyback wire converter is withdrawn outside the body **(Figs. 4A to F)**. A flying "V" is created as described before **(Figs. 2A to C)**. The Piggyback wire converter is advanced close to the Flying "V" and locked in position. The flying "V" is then simultaneously advanced through the guide catheter and its hemostatic valve from one end and the snare is pulled out from the other guide catheter until the flying "V" straddles the leaflet sides for laceration.

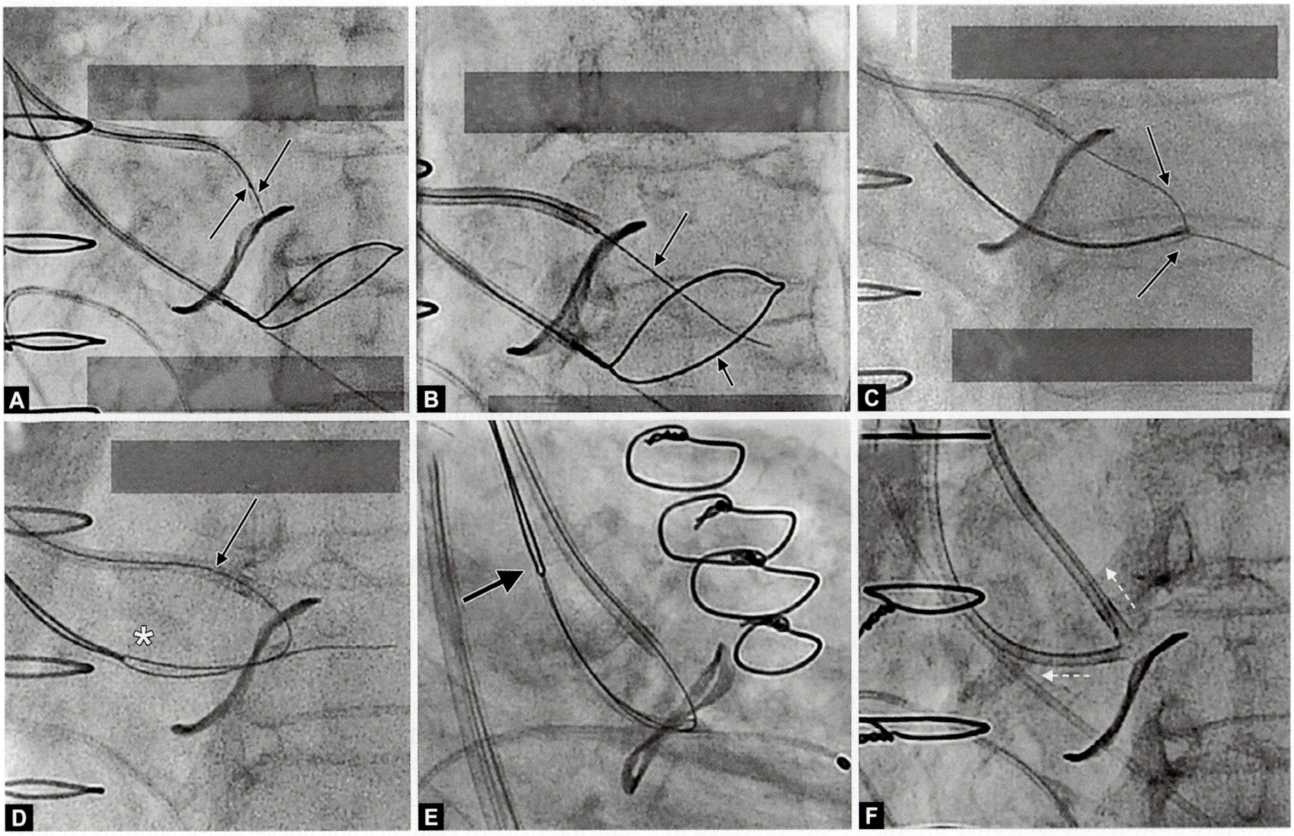

FIGS. 4A TO F: (A to C) Astato guidewire traversed through the leaflet and being snared in the left ventricular outflow tract (LVOT) using the prepositioned LVOT snare. (B) The Piggyback wire converter is pulled back. The stabilizing guidewire removed from the snare guide catheter. The flying "V" is then made outside the body. (C) The flying "V" is advanced from outside while simultaneously externalizing the Astato wire using the snare from the other guide catheter. (D) The flying "V" is positioned straddling the leaflet. (E) Flying tensioning the leaflet. (F) Laceration of leaflet with electrocautery.

Source: With permission from Komatsu et al. (2019).[10]

Once the flying "V" is apposed to the leaflet and guide catheters tips placed close to it, the relative position of the guide catheter with respect to the wire is locked using a compatible torquer or mosquito clamps placed close to the hemostatic valves of guide catheter. A pigtail catheter is also inserted through the TAVR access sheath into the LV so that rapid deployment of TAVR valve can be performed in the event of severe regurgitation or hemodynamic instability after laceration. Then, 5% dextrose solution is infused using two large syringes and simultaneously, the guidewire is electrified using 70-W energy in pure cutting mode and tensed. Care must be taken to avoid heavy traction force as it may cause mechanical avulsion rather than laceration. Once the leaflet is lacerated, the guiding catheters are removed one by one after releasing the lock and removal of Astato guidewire from the catheter. TAVR valve placement then proceeds in the usual fashion after placing a TAVR guidewire through the previously placed pigtail catheter in the LV.

If dual (left and right coronary leaflet) BASILICA is planned, the steps up to the advancement of the flying V to the leaflet are performed for each of the leaflets. The lacerations are then performed one by one. This is to avoid delays between the laceration of the leaflet and the valve deployment, as a long delay may risk hemodynamic deterioration.[3,10]

OUTCOMES DATA

The first study to evaluate the safety and feasibility of the BASILICA procedure was the BASILICA IDE (Investigational Device Exemption) trial.[11] The study included 30 patients with severe native or bioprosthetic aortic valve disease with high or extreme risk for surgery and high risk for coronary artery obstruction. The results were promising, with a 95% success rate for leaflet traversal and laceration and 100% freedom from coronary obstruction and reintervention at 30 days. There was one death and three strokes (10%) within this period.[11] At the 1-year mark, there were no additional strokes or myocardial infarctions, but there were two additional deaths, resulting in a total mortality rate of 10% for the first year.[12]

The multicenter International BASILICA registry built upon these findings. This registry included 214 patients from 25 centers in North America and Europe. The findings were consistent with those of the BASILICA IDE trial, with a 94% successful leaflet traversal and laceration and an 87% success rate for the BASILICA procedure without coronary obstruction, mortality, or reintervention. Partial or complete coronary obstruction even after BASILICA was observed in 5% of patients. At the 30-day mark, the mortality rate was 3% and the stroke rate was also 3%. The 1-year survival rate was 84%. Larger trials especially comparing the BASILICA with snorkel stenting technique are needed to definitely establish the safety and efficacy of BASILICA procedure.

PITFALLS

While the BASILICA procedure has been promising in many instances, it is important to recognize that it does have certain limitations and potential pitfalls. One notable limitation is that it does not completely eliminate the risk of coronary obstruction, as 5% of patients in the BASILICA registry still experienced this coronary obstruction after the procedure. In selected cases, it may be reasonable to consider coronary protection using guidewire and stent, in addition to BASILICA. Moreover, BASILICA may help to facilitate orthotopic stent placement rather than limiting options to a chimney-snorkel technique, potentially preserving future coronary access and possibly reducing the risk for stent thrombosis. However, this potential advantage also needs to be further studied and confirmed in clinical trials.[13] Another potential pitfall of the BASILICA procedure is related to the positioning of the stent post of the prior bioprosthetic valve or transcatheter valve. If these are situated directly in front of the coronary ostium, or if the coronary ostia is eccentrically located away from the midline of leaflet, BASILICA may not be able to prevent obstruction.[14] In addition, aligning the TAVR valve commissural post away from the site of laceration is essential to prevent continued coronary obstruction post-TAVR. However, several of the widely used current-generation valves lack markers for commissural alignment. Consequently, ensuring successful post TAVR outcomes can become dependent on factors outside the operator's control.

Interestingly, BASILICA may not reliably prevent coronary obstruction in certain TAVR-in-TAVR patients. In vitro studies suggest that with newer generation valves such as SAPIEN 3 and Evolut TAVR, the leaflets may not splay adequately with TAVR valve placement, even after laceration, thereby rendering laceration ineffective.[15] A newer technique, referred to as Balloon-assisted BASILICA, which involves dilating the leaflet traversal point with a 5-mm noncompliant balloon prior to laceration, has been proposed to improve leaflet splay in such instances.[16] There are also reports of leaflet prolapse/protrusion even after BASILICA causing coronary obstruction.[17]

RECENT ADVANCES

Dedicated electrosurgical devices are in development to facilitate leaflet laceration and traversal. A newer ShortCut (Pi-Cardia) device designed to split the bioprosthetic aortic valve leaflets is currently under clinical trial (ShortCut Study).[18] ShortCut device involves mechanical splitting of the leaflet using a splitting element and positioning arm. The positioning arm is positioned on the target leaflet under TEE and fluoroscopy guidance and engaged. The splitting element is then activated traversing the leaflet toward its base after which the device is pulled lacerating the leaflet from base to tip. As the field continues to advance, we anticipate that these dedicated devices will make the BASILICA procedure more straightforward and safer.

CONCLUSION

Coronary obstruction post TAVR carries a high mortality. CT can predict risk for coronary obstruction; however, it is not infallible, particularly due to variation in implantation characteristics. BASILICA procedure can help to prevent TAVR-related coronary obstruction; its limitations and potential pitfalls need to be carefully considered. More research is needed to optimize the procedure and develop additional strategies to ensure the best outcomes for patients. In future, dedicated devices may reduce the procedural expertise required for these types of procedures, potentially increasing their safety and efficacy.

ONLINE REFERENCES

Please scan the QR code provided at the end of the table of contents for References of this chapter.

CHAPTER

183 Commissural Alignment: Why and How?

Anantharaman Rajaram, Sai Satish, Vijayakumar Subban

ABSTRACT

Transcatheter aortic valve implantation (TAVI) is an established treatment for patients with severe symptomatic aortic stenosis (AS). As TAVI is increasingly being used in younger patients, most of these patients require lifetime management, in the form of redo valve replacement and treatment of associated coronary artery disease (CAD). These mandate optimal planning and execution of the first implant with best possible results. Commissural alignment (CA), a routine practice during surgical aortic valve replacement (SAVR), is gaining importance during TAVI to facilitate future coronary access and redo transcatheter aortic valve replacement (TAVR). This chapter aims to provide a brief overview of implications, definitions, computed tomography (CT) planning, CA with different technologies, and post TAVI assessment of CA.

Keywords: Transcatheter aortic valve replacement, commissural alignment, coronary alignment, coronary access.

INTRODUCTION

Transcatheter aortic valve implantation (TAVI) is an established treatment for patients with severe symptomatic aortic stenosis (AS). Even though it initially started as an alternative treatment for those with very high surgical risk, improvement in device technology, increasing operator experience, and voluminous data accumulated over the past two decades have expanded this technology to entire spectrum of patients with degenerative AS. As TAVI is increasingly being used in younger patients, most of these patients require lifetime management, in the form of redo valve replacement and treatment of associated coronary artery disease (CAD).[1,2] These mandate optimal planning and execution of the first implant with best possible results. Commissural alignment (CA), a routine practice during surgical aortic valve replacement (SAVR), is gaining importance during TAVI to facilitate future coronary access and redo transcatheter aortic valve replacement (TAVR).[3] This chapter aims to provide a brief overview of implications, definitions, computed tomography (CT) planning, CA with different technologies, and post TAVI assessment of CA.

WHY DO WE NEED TO ALIGN THE COMMISSURES?

The various possible implications of CA are (1) coronary access, (2) TAVR-in-TAVR, and (3) hemodynamic performance of the transcatheter heart valve (THV).

Coronary Access

Coronary artery disease and AS often coexist, approximately 50% of the patients undergoing TAVR have associated CAD.[4] About 10% of the patients present with acute coronary syndrome at 2 years post TAVI.[5] ST-segment elevation myocardial infarction (STEMI) in post TAVI patients has been associated with longer door-to-balloon times, higher primary percutaneous intervention failure rates, increased incidence of major adverse cardiovascular and cerebrovascular events, and mortality.[6]

Coronary access is less challenging following TAVI with balloon expandable THVs (BE-THVs) with shorter stent frames. However, it is a significant challenge in patients implanted with self-expandable THVs (SE-THV). In addition to taller stent frames, higher sealing skirts, supra-annular leaflet positioning, and higher implants, CA is a major predictor of failed coronary access. In nonselected patients with standard THV deployment CA was observed only in about 20% of the patients.[7]

The RE-ACCESS (Reobtain Coronary Ostia Cannulation Beyond Transcatheter Aortic Valve Stent) study systematically evaluated the feasibility of coronary access following THV implantation. Selective coronary cannulation was not successful in 7.7% of the population. The major predictors of failure were supra-annular THV design, higher implants, and higher THV to sinus of Valsalva ratio.[8]

The ALIGN-ACCESS (TAVR with Commissural Alignment Followed by Coronary Access) study evaluated the impact of CA on the feasibility of coronary access after TAVR in a population 206 patients implanted with either intra-annular BE-THV (SAPIEN 3, Edwards Lifesciences, Irvine, CA, USA) or supra-annular SE-THV (Evolut R/Pro, Medtronic, Minneapolis, MN, USA or ACURATE neo2, Boston Scientific, Marlborough, MA, USA). It showed that CA significantly improved with coronary access with supra-annular SE-THV.[9]

TAVI-in-TAVI

As progressively younger patients with longer life expectancy are being implanted with THV, many of them require redo valve replacement in their lifetime. TAVI-in-TAVI is a promising option for those with suitable anatomy.

During TAVI-in-TAVI, the degenerated leaflets of the first THV are sandwiched between the stent frames that convert the first THV into a covered cylinder, referred to as "neo-skirt". The height of the "neo-skirt" depends on the type of stent frame and the position of the leaflets. If the top of the neo-skirt is below the level of sinotubular junction (STJ) and native sinuses are wide, blood flows freely around the THV into the sinuses and coronaries remain perfused after implantation of the second THV. However, if the STJ is narrow and the neo-skirt is extending above the STJ, it causes sinus sequestration and severe impairment in coronary flow. Leaflet modification strategies, such as BASILICA (Bioprosthetic or native aortic scallop intentional leaflet laceration to prevent iatrogenic coronary obstruction) have been used effectively to prevent coronary obstruction during redo TAVR. However, for the leaflet modification to be effective there should be acceptable CA without overlap between commissural post and the coronary origin.[10]

Transcatheter Heart Valve Performance

Apart from its effect on coronary access and future TAVI-in-TAVI, commissural misalignment may adversely impact THV hemodynamics and durability. Commissural misalignment can create abnormal flow dynamics that in turn increases leaflet stress and blood stagnation inside the neo-sinuses. This blood stagnation may promote thrombus/plaque formation, and potentially premature valve degeneration.[3]

Bailey et al.,[11] in their experiments with computational models, simulated varying degrees of rotational alignment of THV and assessed the stress on the leaflets of the THV. When there was moderate-to-severe commissural misalignment, there was decrease in the distance between the prosthetic commissures. This in turn resulted in increased transvalvular shear stress. The protentional role of alterations in transvalvular flow conditions and accelerated THV degeneration is yet to be evaluated.

Subclinical leaflet thrombosis is commonly observed with both surgical and transcatheter prosthetic valves. Commissural misalignment may result in low flow conditions and blood stagnation inside the neo-sinuses. This in turn may promote leaflet thrombosis. In the LTR (Low-Risk TAVR) trial, commissural misalignment was associated with increased incidence of hypoattenuated leaflet thickening (HALT) compared to those with CA (40% vs. 28%).[12] The possible association of commissural malalignment with HALT and its impact on valve durability mandates further investigation.

The relationship between CA and hemodynamic performance of the THV was assessed in the RESOLVE registry. In this registry, although there was no difference in the baseline gradient between those with CA and commissural malalignment, there was a relative increase of >50% from the baseline gradient was observed in the group with commissural malalignment at 30-day follow-up.[13] In addition, commissural misalignment may result suboptimal leaflet closure and transvalvular aortic regurgitation. In a registry of 212 patients with both balloon and self-expandable valves, moderate-to-severe commissural misalignment was associated with increased incidence of central aortic regurgitation at discharge and at 3-month follow-up.[7]

TERMINOLOGIES AND DEFINITIONS: ALIGN TAVR CONSORTIUM

Recently, ALIGN TAVR consortium proposed standardized definitions for cusp symmetry, coronary ostial eccentricity, and CA **(Figs. 1A to C)**.[3]

Cusp symmetry is assessed on pre-TAVR CT. The annular plane is defined in the standard fashion and a parallel plane depicting all three commissures clearly is identified. Then the angle between the commissures of each cusp is measured and the largest cusp is identified. Based on the intercommissural angle of the largest cusp, the symmetry is classified into four categories: symmetric (120–125°), mildly asymmetric (125–130°), moderately asymmetric (130–135°), and severely asymmetric (>135°).

Coronary ostial eccentricity is defined based on the angular distance of the coronary ostium from the center of the respective cusp. The ostium is considered centered, mildly eccentric, moderately eccentric, and severely eccentric when

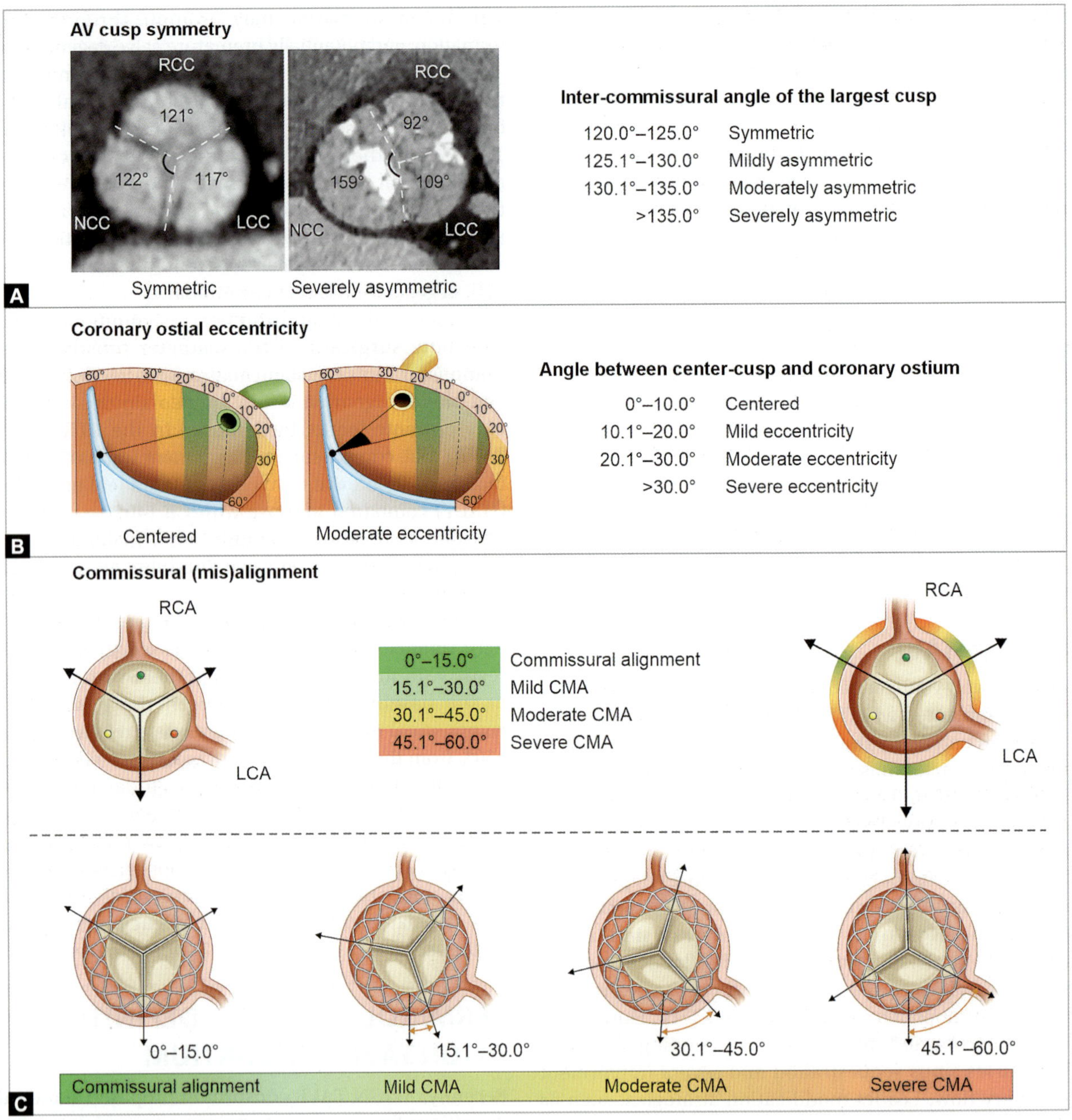

FIGS. 1A TO C: Proposed standardized definitions from the ALIGN-TAVR consortium. Proposed standardized definitions of (A) AV cusp symmetry; (B) coronary ostial eccentricity; and (C) commissural (mis)alignment to harmonize reporting in future literature and clinical trials in TAVR.

(AV: aortic valve; CMA: commissural alignment; LCA: left coronary artery; LCC: left coronary cusp; NCC: noncoronary cusp; RCA: right coronary artery; RCC: right coronary cusp; TAVR: transcatheter aortic valve replacement)

Source: With permission from Tang et al. (2022).[3]

the angle is between 0 and 10.0°, 10.1 and 20.0°, 20.1 and 30.0°, and >30.0°, respectively.[3]

Commissural alignment is assessed by measuring the pre- and postprocedure commissural positions in relation to the right coronary artery (RCA). In the preprocedure CT, RCA is rotated to 12 O'clock position in the cross-sectional image in the aortic centerline. A vertical line is then drawn through the RCA to the center of the aorta. The angle of each native commissure is measured clockwise from this vertical centerline at the level of aortic leaflet coaptation. Similarly, the angular locations of the neo-commissures are measured from the RCA in the postprocedure CT aortogram. The difference in the angular position of each native commissure and the neo-commissure is calculated. The average of the three values provides the degree of commissural misalignment. A THV is considered aligned if the average angle is 0–15°. A deviation of 15–30°, 30–45°, and 45–60° indicate mild, moderate, and severe misalignment, respectively.[7]

COMPUTED TOMOGRAPHY PLANNING FOR COMMISSURAL ALIGNMENT

A CT provides high-resolution volumetric images of the aortic root and has become the cornerstone of TAVI planning. It helps in planning CA in two ways: (1) it provides patient specific C-arm angles to facilitate CA and (2) CT-based simulations that predict rotational orientation of the device to enable CA.

Computed Tomography Predicted C-arm Angles for Commissural Alignment

A CT analysis helps in predicting C-arm angles that isolate one of the commissures that could be targeted during the procedure. When we move from left to right on the annulus "S" curve, it provides three important C-arm angles that help in CA: (1) right coronary cusp (RCC) and left coronary cusp (LCC) overlap view, usually in the right anterior oblique/caudal (RAO/CAU) projection, isolates RCC/noncoronary cusp (NCC) commissure on the right side of the fluoroscopic screen, (2) right and NCC overlap view, usually in the left anterior oblique/cranial (LAO/CRA) projection, isolates the RCC/NCC commissure on the left side of the screen, and (3) in between these two projections, the cusps are aligned side by side, the so-called three-cusp or coplanar view, where the LCC/NCC commissure is located in the middle and posterior, RCC/NCC commissure on the left side and RCC/LCC commissure on the right side. The current generation THVs are provided with fluoroscopic markers on the commissural posts and one of these markers can be aligned to the isolated commissure fluoroscopically to obtain CA. In case of eccentric coronary origin, coronary alignment instead of CA may be achieved by identifying fluoroscopic view that overlaps the coronary arteries. When one of the commissures is aligned to the right at this angle during deployment, this commissures lands in the midway between the coronaries.[14]

Computed Tomography-based Simulations to Predict Patient-specific Rotational Orientation

Redondo et al.,[15] described a CT simulation-based method to predict patient-specific rotational orientation of THV to achieve CA. In this technique, preprocedure TAVR CT data is used to create an aortic biomodel of the patient using Slicer. Aortic centerline from descending aorta to aortic root is calculated. The aortic biomodel mesh and centerline data are imported to computer-assisted design software. The method assumes that valve trajectory follows aortic centerline and THV rotations occur perpendicular to the centerline. The system estimates the relationship of the THV within the aortic root and location of the sinuses and coronary ostia. Then 3D model of the THV is positioned with one of the commissures at 12 O'clock position in the descending aorta. The virtual valve is then advanced into the aortic root following the central line and THV is implanted in the standard fashion. Optimal rotational orientation of the THV to achieve CA is then estimated by using controlled rotation of the THV model to align the commissural posts of the THV with native commissures. This method provides patient-specific rotational orientation of delivery catheter and reduces the need for rotation in the aortic root. The authors demonstrated enhanced CA with both self-expanding and balloon expanding THV using this technique.[16]

Crimping of the balloon expandable THV in a specific orientation based on the patient's aortic root anatomy has been described with MyVal THV. This method uses the mirror image relationship between cross-sectional CT image and fluoroscopic anteroposterior image. If one of the THV commissure is aligned to the middle of the RCC ex vivo based on the CT image, this commissure automatically deploys toward the LCC/NCC commissure in vivo. In this method, a circle is drawn around the cross-sectional image at the level of middle of the sinus of Valsalva. Horizontal and vertical center lines are drawn through the circle and the geometric center of the sinuses is located at the intersection of these lines. A line is drawn from this geometric center to the midpoint of the RCC. The angle between this line and the horizontal center line is the "angle of commissural alignment (AoCA)". A clock face is superimposed on this image to derive the clock angle. One of the commissures is crimped at this angle to derive CA **(Figs. 2A to D)**.[17]

COMMISSURAL ALIGNMENT WITH DIFFERENT TRANSCATHETER HEART VALVE PLATFORMS (FIGS. 3A TO L)

Balloon Expandable Valves

Balloon expandable THVs (SAPIEN 3 and MyVal, Meril Lifesciences, India) have three fluoroscopic commissural markers in the form of dual struts. Although easily identified after deployment, they are difficult to visualize once crimped on the delivery system. There is no specific recommendation on the crimping orientation of the SAPIEN THV as there was no improvement in the CA with different crimped orientations. The newer SAPIEN X4 valve design is expected

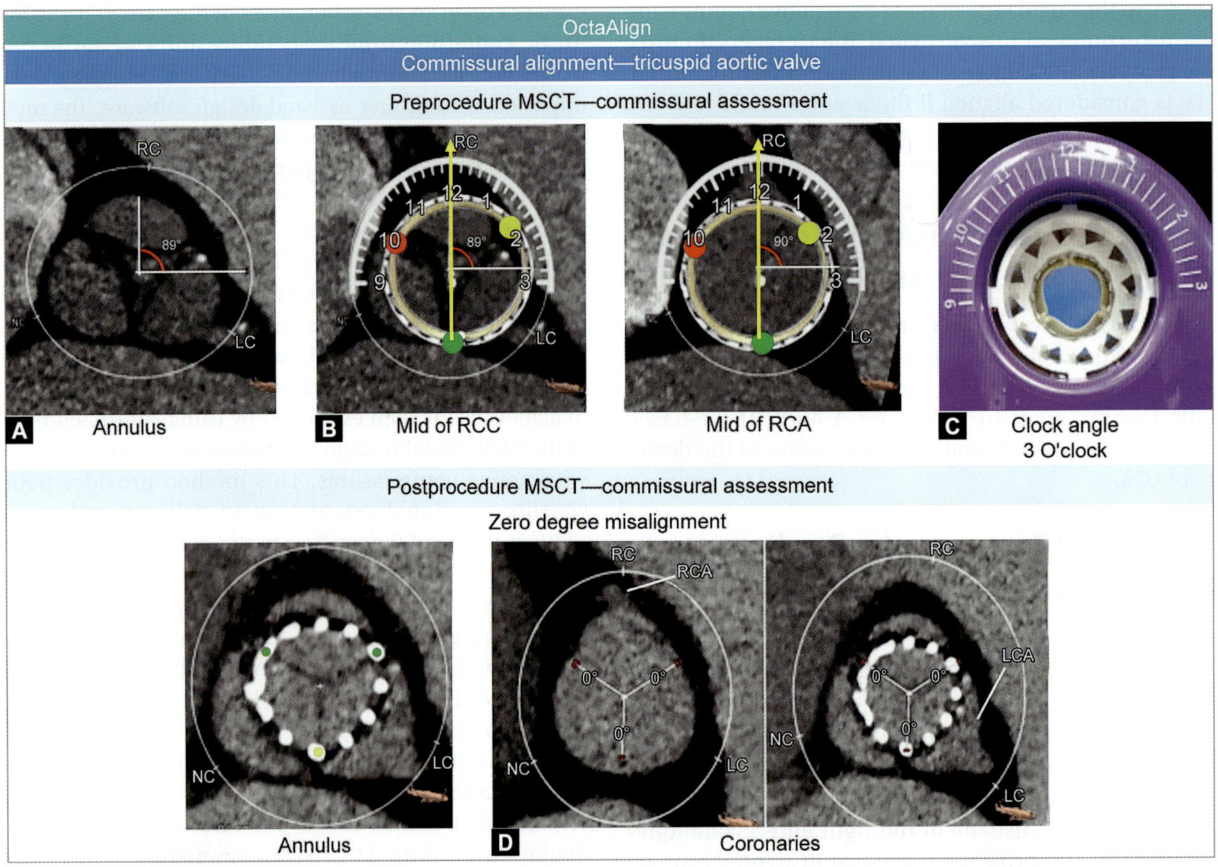

FIGS. 2A TO D: Commissural alignment with Octacor THV. (A) A circle is drawn around the cross-sectional image at the level of middle of the sinus of Valsalva. Horizontal and vertical center lines are drawn through the circle and the geometric center of the sinuses is located at the intersection of these lines. (B) A line is drawn from this geometric center to the midpoint of the RCC. The angle between this line and the horizontal center line is the "angle of commissural alignment". (C) A clock face is superimposed on this image to derive the clock angle. One of the commissures is crimped at this angle to derive CA. (D) Commissural alignment postprocedure.

(CA: commissural alignment; MSCT: multislice spiral computed tomography; RCA: right coronary artery; RCC: right coronary cusp; THV: transcatheter heart valve)

Courtesy: Meril Life Sciences.

to provide design features that improve CA.[3] The second generation of the Meril THV, the Octacor (Meril Lifesciences), provides four alignment markers on the delivery system to improve CA. The OCT ALIGN is currently investigating the CA with this valve using the crimping technique described earlier.[17]

Evolut Transcatheter Heart Valve

Evolut THV is a self-expanding supra-annular valve. It has a radio-opaque "C"-tab marking one of the commissures. When mounted on the delivery system, the "C"-tab is oriented 90° clockwise from the radiopaque hat marker. The delivery system is advanced with flush port rotated to 3 O'clock position and the hat marker is oriented along the outer curve of the aorta. For successful CA, the hat marker should be oriented center front and "C"-tab on the inner curve of the aorta in the cusp overlap view **(Fig. 3A)**.[3]

ACURATE Neo2–Transcatheter Heart Valve

The ACURATE neo2 THV is a self-expanding supra-annular valve. Its commissures can easily be identified by the presence of radiopaque commissural posts and free stent struts. In addition, the delivery system allows rotation after delivering the valve into position in the aortic root. CA with ACURATE neo2 follows a well-defined sequence of four steps: (1) the delivery system is inserted with the flush port pointing at 6 O'clock position; (2) the valve is delivered to the aortic root to position the radio-opaque marker at the top of the pigtail catheter; (3) configuration of the commissural posts is assessed in three-cusp co-planner view to determine the rotational direction: (i) 2:1 configuration—delivery catheter is rotated clockwise, (ii) 1:2 configuration—delivery catheter is rotated counterclockwise, and (iii) 1-1-1 configuration—no further rotation; and (4) C-arm is moved to RCC/LCC

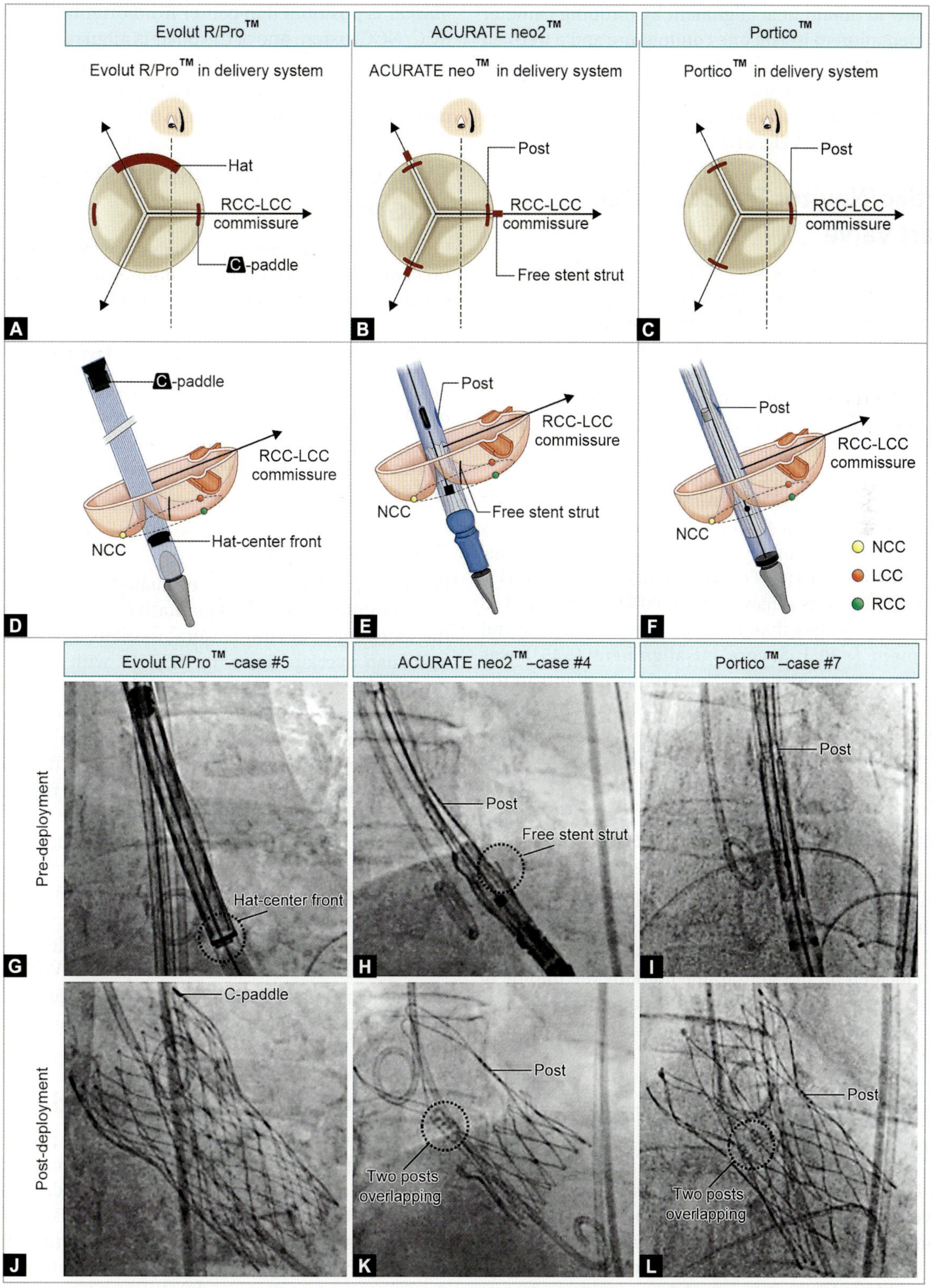

FIGS. 3A TO L: Neo-commissural alignment for self-expanding THVs: THV-specific orientations for implantation in RCC/LCC cusp overlap view. Illustration of how the radiopaque THV commissural markers should be oriented in a transversal plane (A to C) and from a fluoroscopic perspective using the RCC/LCC cusp overlap view (D to F) in order to obtain neo-commissural alignment— for the Evolut R/PRO (left column), ACURATE neo2 (middle column), and Portico valve (right column). (G to L) Fluoroscopic images from an RCC/LCC cusp overlap view illustrating the THV-specific implantation technique to obtain neo-commissural alignment.

(THV: transcatheter heart valve; LCC: left coronary cusp; NCC: noncoronary cusp; RCC: right coronary cusp)

Source: With permission from Bieliauskas et al. (2021).[14]

overlap view to obtain final alignment by torquing catheter to a 2-1 orientation to isolate one commissure and a free cell on the right side. The C-arm is rotated back to the co-planner view to confirm the 1-1-1 orientation and deployment. Once deployment is completed, the success of CA is assessed in the RCC/LCC overlap view **(Fig. 3B)**.[3]

Portico/Navitor Transcatheter Heart Valve

Navitor is self-expanding intra-annular THV. The stent frame is designed with three fluoroscopic markers positioned midway between the inflow and outflow portions of the THV. To attain CA, the flush port of the FlexNav delivery catheter is oriented at 12 O'clock position while being advanced through the aorta. Once the system is in position above the annulus, the location of the commissural posts is assessed in cusp overlap view and rotated as required to align one of the posts on the right side of the screen.[3]

The COMALIGN (COMmissural ALIGNment) study[14] prospectively evaluated CA by using the above delivery system orientation technique in a population of 60 patients, 20 each of Evoult, ACURATE neo2, and Portico SE THVs. Optimal CA (<15°) was achieved in 36 (60%) patients and 53 patients (88%) had less than or equal to mild commissural misalignment (≤30°). Severe misalignment (>45°) was observed in only two patients. None of the patients in the ACURATE neo2 group had more than or equal to moderate CMA. When optimal orientation was achieved before deployment, less than or equal to mild CMA could be achieved 98% of the patients **(Fig. 3C)**.

Hydra Transcatheter Heart Valve

Hydra THV (Sahajanand Medical Technologies, Wakhariawadi, India) is a self-expanding intra-annular THV. It has three tentacle-shaped arches with commissural posts in between. There are six fluoroscopic markers in two rows located on the stent frame marking the middle of each cusp. In contrast to other self-expanding THVs, the markers overlapped on the right of the screen (1:2 pattern) to achieve CA.[18]

COMMISSURAL ALIGNMENT IN BICUSPID AORTIC VALVE

Bicuspid aortic valve (BAV) anatomy is often associated with asymmetric cusp anatomy and hence there is a high likelihood of commissural misalignment. In type 1 BAV with RCC/LCC fusion, the delivery catheter orientation is like tricuspid anatomy with one of the commissural posts aligned on the right side in cusp overlap view and the hat marker is positioned in center front orientation. In case of RCC/NCC fusion, one of the posts is aligned on the left side and the hat marker is positioned in center back orientation. Coronary alignment rather than CA may be considered in patients with eccentric origin of the coronary arteries.[3]

EVALUATION OF COMMISSURAL ALIGNMENT

Commissural alignment is evaluated postprocedure by using pre- and post-TAVI CT imaging, fluoroscopy or coregistration of fluoroscopic images with pre-TAVI CT images.

Computed Tomography Imaging

Postprocedure CT is the standard modality for the assessment of CA. Fuchs et al.[7] have described a method that measures the pre- and postprocedure commissural positions in relation to the RCA as described earlier in the terminology and definition section.

Fluoroscopy

Fluoroscopy can be used to evaluate CA both qualitatively and semiquantitatively. Qualitative method depends on the assessment of commissural markers in the three-cusp and cusp overlap views. In BE-THV with three markers, one marker in the middle and two markers on either side in three-cusp view and two markers overlapped on the left and one marker isolated on the right side indicates CA. In case of correct position of the markers in the three-cusp view, and two markers overlapped on the right indicates severe commissural malalignment.[19] In case of SE-THVs, isolation of a commissural marker on the right side or C-tab on the right side in cusp overlap view indicates CA. In the semiquantitative method, pre- and post-TAVI images are obtained in the optimized three-cusp view.[3] The distance between the centerline and posterior middle commissural marker of the valve is measured in the post-TAVR fluoroscopy. Assuming circular THV deployment, the angular distance is derived by applying trigonometrical method using an arcsine function.[20]

Fluoroscopic–CT Coregistration

In fluoroscopic–CT coregistration method, pre- and post-TAVI images are acquired in the three-cusp coplanar view. Similar view is derived on pre-TAVI dataset using a dedicated 3-mensio valve software. A 2D THV frame is then superimposed on the axial section at the annular and aortic root level matching the commissural orientation seen on fluoroscopic view. The angular distance between the native and THV commissures is then measured.[21]

COMMISSURAL ALIGNMENT VERSUS CORONARY ALIGNMENT

Wang et al.[22] systematically evaluated the impact of cusp asymmetry and coronary eccentricity on coronary access in a population of 400 patients (200 tricuspid aortic valve and 200 BAV), using preprocedure cardiac CT. In their analysis, BAV was more often associated with cusp asymmetry compared to tricuspid aortic valve (52.5% vs. 2.5%, $p < 0.001$) and right coronary origin was more often eccentric than left coronary origin (28% vs. 6%, $p < 0.001$). They then simulated CA and coronary alignment fluoroscopic views and estimated the angular difference between them. The CA view and coronary overlap view differed by <20° in 95% of the patients [transcatheter aortic valve (TAV), 97% and BAV, 93%]. In a similar study, Redondo et al.[23] assessed the incidence of coronary overlap with simulated CA and coronary alignment in a population of 100 patients. RCA was more eccentric then LCA (18.50 vs. 6.50, $p < 0.001$) and the mean intercoronary angle was 140° ± 18.7°. Moderate-to-severe coronary overlap occurred in 32 patients despite optimal CA and larger coronary eccentricity (RCA >24.5° and LCA >19°) and extreme intercoronary angles (>147.5° or <103°) predicted coronary overlap. Coronary alignment virtually eliminated severe coronary overlap and reduced the incidence of moderate coronary overlap from 27 to 5% ($p < 0.001$). Although patient-specific coronary alignment appears to be a promising strategy, there are some limitations to this approach: (1) it often requires extreme RAO/CAU C-arm angulations compared to CA which are not always feasible during the procedure, (2) although it improves access to RCA, it may paradoxically make LCA access difficult, and (3) it may have adverse effects on THV function and durability compared to CA.[19] Further, the superiority of coronary alignment over CA on coronary access and TAVR in TAVR needs further evaluation.

CONCLUSION

Transcatheter aortic valve implantation is much more than successful implantation of the THV as younger patients with longer life expectancy are being treated. Although CA is feasible to a certain extent with current generation systems, there are many limitations. In the future, modifications in the device design and implantation techniques may help in improving CA.

ONLINE REFERENCES

Please scan the QR code provided at the end of the table of contents for References of this chapter.

CHAPTER 184

Cuspal Overlap Technique Transcatheter Aortic Valve Replacement: Why, How, and Where?

Sanjay Mehrotra

ABSTRACT

Transcatheter aortic valve replacement (TAVR) has rapidly evolved to become the standard of care for the treatment of severe aortic stenosis, which is now substantiated by its superiority over surgical aortic valve replacement (SAVR) in extreme-risk and intermediate-risk patients with severe aortic stenosis.

Keywords: Cuspal overlap, aortic stenosis, depth of implantation, pacemaker implantation, high deployment, transcatheter aortic valve.

INTRODUCTION

In extreme-risk patients who are not suitable for surgical treatment, TAVR reduced the rate of death from any cause or rehospitalization and cardiac symptoms (PARTNER trial).[1]

In high-risk patients with Society of Thoracic Surgery (STS) scores >8, with severe aortic stenosis, the outcomes were noninferior to the surgical aortic valve replacement although there was higher risk of stroke, paravalvular leak (PVL), and vascular complications.[2]

In the PARTNER II trial when TAVR was compared to SAVR in intermediate risk patients (STS score 4–8%), TAVR showed noninferiority and in the transfemoral group, TAVR was better when compared with respect to quality of life and mortality at 30 days and 1 year.[3]

Similar results were seen in SURTAVI trial, in self-expanding platform, where TAVR was noninferior to SAVR and using the transfemoral access cohort, TAVR resulted in a lower rate of death or disabling stroke than surgery [hazard ratio 0.79; 95% confidence interval (CI) 0.62–1.00; $p = 0.05$].[4]

Then came the low-risk patients where the STS score was <4%, TAVR resulted in shorter index hospitalization as compared to surgery in about 1,000 patients, when endpoint of composite of death, major stroke, and rehospitalization at 1 year was significantly lower in the TAVR group than in the surgery group (8.5% vs. 15.1%; –10.8 to –2.5; $p < 0.001$ for noninferiority).[5]

As we go to lower age group and younger patients (the mean age in PARTNER 3 trial was 70 years), the concerns which are raised are about the durability, life expectancy, risk of permanent pacemaker, PVL, coronary artery access in the future, and surgical risk of explantation.

Patients, who are undergoing this treatment for severe aortic stenosis, besides durability of the valve, the development of conduction abnormality has long-term implications due to not only issues related to permanent pacemaker implantation but also related to development of left bundle branch block, which results in dyssynchronous left ventricular contraction causing gradual deterioration of left ventricular functions.

This happens due to proximity of the conduction system to new deployed valve which may cause conduction disturbances ranging from complete atrioventricular (AV) conduction block to left bundle branch or prolongation of QRS interval.

With expanding use of TAVR in younger population with severe aortic stenosis, the need to optimize the treatment has become extremely important.

Multimodality approach for optimization includes reducing the need for permanent pacemaker and bundle branch block after deployment of the valve.

This started with shallow deployment technique especially for self-expanding valves (SEVs) but also for balloon-expanding valves to reduce the interaction of transcatheter heart valve (THV) with the conduction system. Later on, this got translated into concerns about future coronary access, especially when performing the procedure in younger patients with severe aortic stenosis, where on one end the concern is to avoid development of the conduction defect and a higher implant but it may result in difficult access to coronary, if required in the future.

The patients who do require permanent pacemaker which effects the ventricular functions, especially when right ventricular apex is used for the pacing.

Development of conduction abnormalities results in increase in duration of stay in the hospital and morbidity and mortality increases.

Why cuspal overlap technique?

Before we discuss why cusp overlap technique, we should understand the anatomy of the conduction system and strategies to minimize the damage to the conduction system.[6]

Aortic annulus, which is oval in shape and during the sizing, the measurement is done at the lowest hinge point where the leaflets arise from, in systole **(Figs. 1A and B)**.

Atrioventricular node which is located in the triangle of Koch and extends into the His bundle, which runs left of the central fibrous body and divides into the left bundle and right bundle.

The left bundle is very close to noncoronary cusp (NCC) and the right coronary cusp (RCC). Here, the strategies to reduce the interaction between devices, such as a catheter, dilation balloon, and the delivery sheath with the valve loaded, will reduce the chances of damage to the conduction system.

This interaction was not very well understood in the era of Medtronic Core valve and Sapien XT valve; hence, the pacemaker requirement was very high, which subsequently reduced with the usage of current generation of THV.

With the advent of retrievability of Evolute R and repositionability, the rate of permanent pacemaker implantation has reduced.

A recently published meta-analysis of 15 studies reported a pacemaker rate of 16.5% with Evolute SEV, 11.55%, and with ACURATE SEV it was 9.7%.[7]

Cusp overlap technique was suggested to reduce the risk of development of complete heart block or left bundle branch block, by reducing the interaction of the THV with the conduction system.[8]

Jilaihawi et al. described that the development of complete heart block or conduction abnormalities is dependent on the depth of the implant of the valve and length of the membranous septum. When the valve is deployed below the membranous septum, the risk of complete heart block is higher. The odds ratio of PPMI increased with difference between membranous septal length and implantation depth ($p < 0.001$).[9]

Core valve THV implantation depths were recommended to be 3–5 mm below the annular plane. The challenge lies in assessing the depths of implantation on aortography. If a Multislice CT is compared to aortography in estimating the depth, it fares better in correlating with the risk of need for pacemaker.[10]

What is double S curve?

The double S curve technique identifies a viewing angle which is at the intersection of the S-curve (the set of coplanar viewing angles) for the aortic annulus and self-expanding THV.

Multislice computed tomography (MSCT) can be used to define the direction of structures and produce an optimal projection curve which can be utilized to see a certain plane. This curve helps to eliminate the foreshortening of the valve catheter and the aortic annulus. This helps to predict an optimal projection curve prior to the procedure based on the CT scan but while doing the procedure, the optimal projection curve should be confirmed **(Fig. 2)**.

What is cuspal overlap technique?

It is a fluoroscopic method, which involves positioning the c-arm in such a way that it overlaps left coronary cusp (LCC) over the RCC, which helps in isolating the NCC.

The NCC is the most inferior cusp in the left ventricular outflow tract (LVOT) and this allows to position the valve in relation to this, which allows the operator to be highest location sufficient enough to avoid the injury to the conduction system and also have sufficient interaction of the frame with the annulus, without the risk of valve popping out. **Figure 3** attached explains the technique.

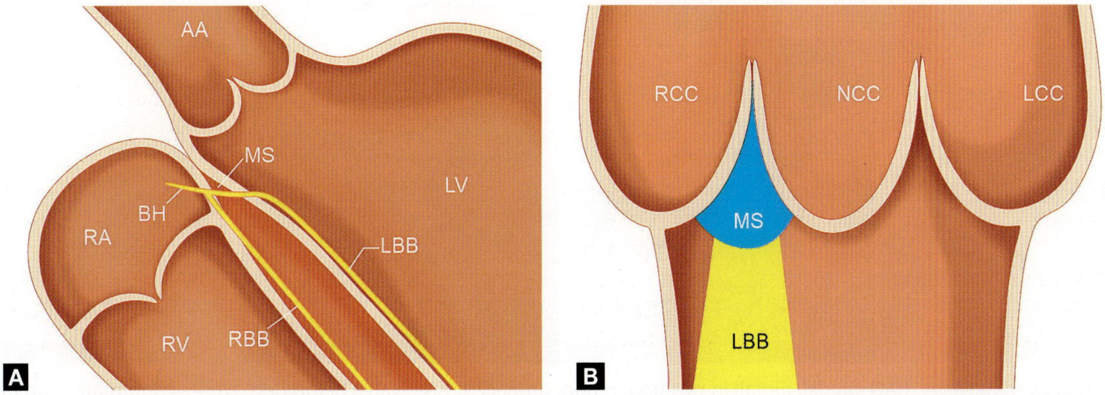

FIGS. 1A AND B: Conduction system in relation to membranous septum and the right coronary cusp (RCC) and noncoronary cusp (NCC).
(AA: ascending aorta; BH: bundle of His; MS: membranous septum; LBB: left bundle branch; LCC: left coronary cusp; LV: left ventricular; RA: right atrium; RBB: right bundle branch; RV: right ventricular)

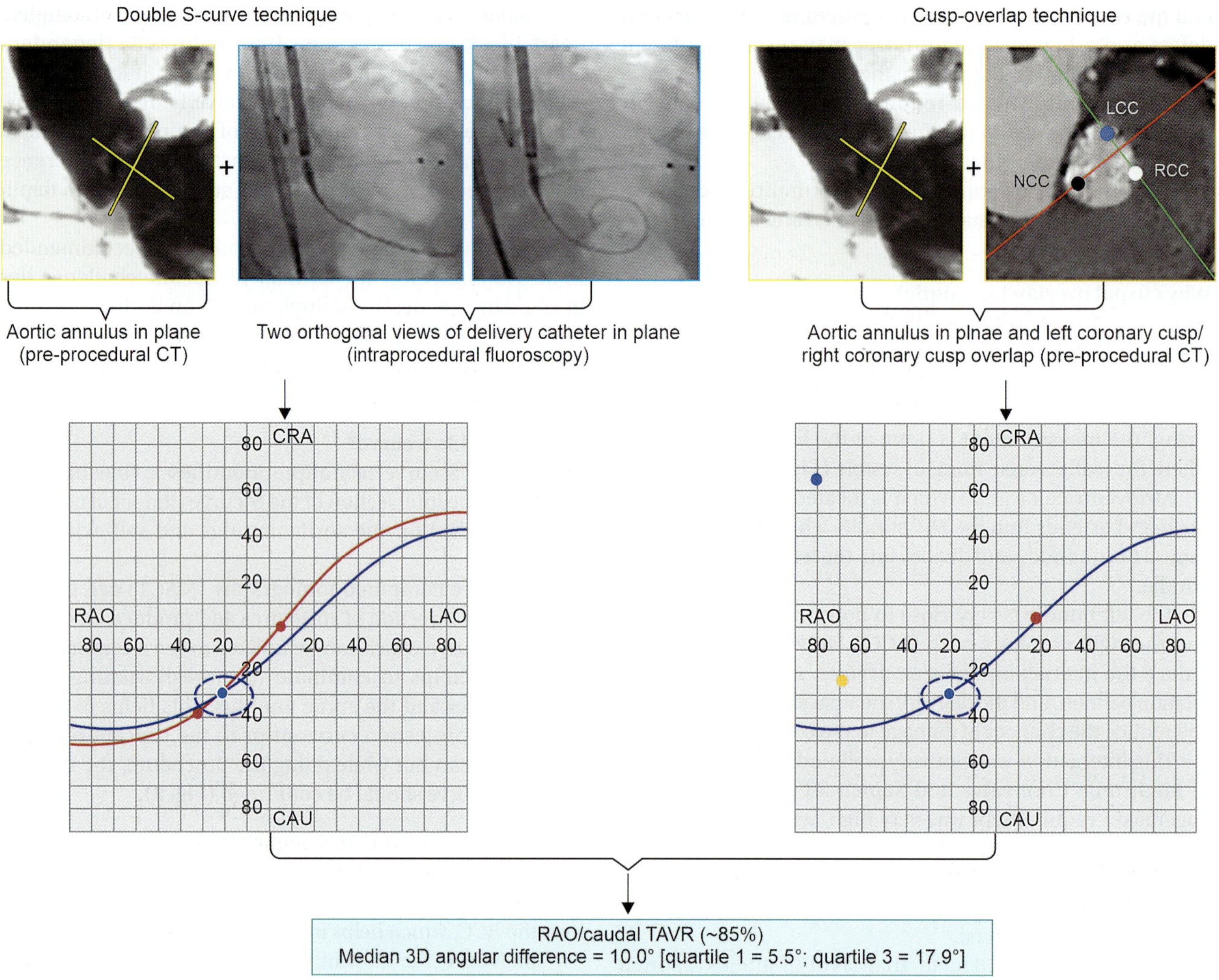

FIG. 2: Double S curve technique and RAO caudal view—derived on MSCT which need to be confirmed on fluoroscopy during the procedure. In 90% patients, MSCT-projected view corresponds with the fluoroscopy.

(MSCT: multislice computed tomography; RAO: right anterior oblique; TAVR: transcatheter aortic valve replacement)

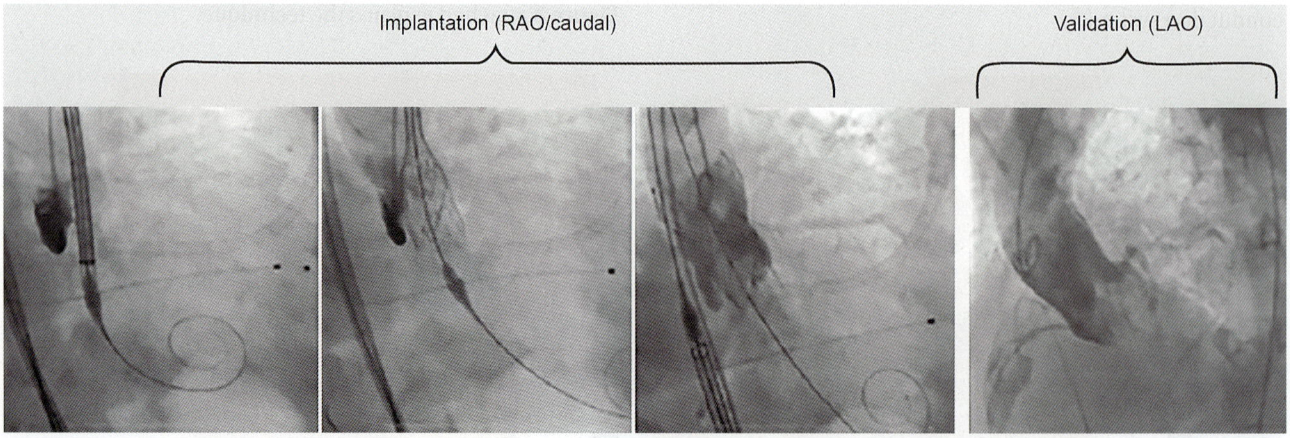

FIG. 3: Cuspal overlap view—RAO caudal, pigtail in position in noncoronary sinus—valve being deployed—confirmation on fluoroscopy LAO view to confirm the valve lower frame is below the left side annular plane.

(RAO: right anterior oblique; LAO: left anterior oblique)

There are some other important points which are required to be understood, while deploying especially Medtronic Evolute platform valve.

The stepwise methods to achieve best deployment without causing conduction defect and injury to the conduction system in causing left bundle branch block are as follows:

1. There should be efforts to avoid entering the left ventricle with the valve, so the efforts should be to do a top-down deployment which means the valve should be kept above the pigtail catheter which has been positioned in the noncoronary sinus and lower limit is assessed by the right cuspal overlap view.
2. The lower ring of the evolute valve has a ring which is usually aligned to a straight line in most cases in right cuspal overlap view.
3. Once the lower edge of the frame is deployed in cuspal overlap view, the lower frame alignment can be seen by going to left anterior oblique view to see that the lower frame is below the left cusp; here, it is important to see that the lower frame is below the annular plane.
4. The operator preferences are different for deploying the rest of the valve with or without rapid pacing to reduce the left ventricular pressure, till the position of retrievability.
5. The depth of the lower frame in the cuspal overlap view is about 3 mm which avoids the trauma to the conduction system.
6. Some operator use Lunderquist wire to increase the stability of the wire to achieve the stability of the THV while deploying.
7. The deployment may be even higher in patients with bicuspid aortic stenosis patients as the point of coaptation in such patients is even higher, although a predilatation of the aortic valve may be a better approach in such patients as need for a postdilatation, in case of significant PVL may carry some risks of valve dislodgement.

The above steps have led to better pacemaker rates and ease of procedure and have resulted in better outcomes with self-expanding Evolute valve.

Balloon expandable valves BEV have also utilized the right cuspal overlap view to achieve a state of valve deployment to reduce the interaction with the conduction system and have led to further reduction in pacemaker rates.

The valve angles generated by double S curve technique by MSCT and its utilization while using cuspal overlap technique were similar in 92% of patients in study reported by Ben-Shoshan et al.[11]

In vast majority of cases (>80%), this was in right anterior oblique (RAO) and caudal view, which provides maximum elongation of the LVOT and delivery catheter.

HIGH IMPLANTATION OF A BALLOON-EXPANDABLE VALVE

High implantation of a balloon-expandable valve has been traditionally done in coplanar view or the three cusps view. There may be added advantage of deploying the BEV also in RAO/CAUDAL projection to achieve a higher deployment which resulted in even further reduction of pacemaker rates.[12]

The authors reported significantly smaller implantation depths and lower rates of pacemaker (5.5% vs. 13.1%; $p < 0.001$) compared to conventional technique without any adverse outcomes of PVL or valve embolization.

BENEFITS AND ADVANTAGES OF CUSPAL OVERLAP TECHNIQUES IN TAVR

- *Preservation of cardiac conduction*: By avoiding interference with the AV node, the cuspal overlap technique may preserve the native cardiac conduction system more effectively.
- *Reduced mechanical stress*: Aligning the new valve with the native valve's cusps can reduce mechanical stresses on the implanted valve, potentially increasing its longevity.
- *Improved hemodynamic profile*: Proper alignment can optimize blood flow across the new valve, providing a more physiological flow profile.
- *Reduced PVL*: Properly aligning the new valve can minimize gaps between the native and new valves, reducing the risk of PVL.

While shallow deployment of THV is helpful in avoiding conduction disturbances and need for the pacemaker, there may be some limitations which one may encounter as touched upon earlier, for example, the risk of valve embolization may be the most serious one, although the evidence is <1%.

The operators using cusp overlap should be able to handle the complications which may arise as valve embolization, PVL, leaving a constrained valve.

Shallow implants may risk or future valve in valve options, especially if done in a younger patient who is low risk for otherwise surgical valve replacement, also there can be a potential risk of leaflet, obstructing the coronary arteries by creation of a neoskirt.

Access to coronary arteries in the future is a major concern when the indication TAVR has to be extended to the younger age and low-risk patients.

In the RE-ACCESS study of 300 patients, 7.7% patients had difficulty to cannulate the coronary arteries (left coronary artery in 4.7% and right coronary artery in 4.0% patients, while there was no difficulty prior to TAVR). The coronary access is even more difficult with evolute platform of THV when used as an implant depth of <6 mm.

The issue of commissural alignment is becoming more and more important, with valve technology both for BEV and SEV. The new device development is looking for improvement in these above-mentioned areas for the use of TAVR in low-risk younger patients.

Talking about this aspect is out of per view of this writing **(Fig. 4)**.

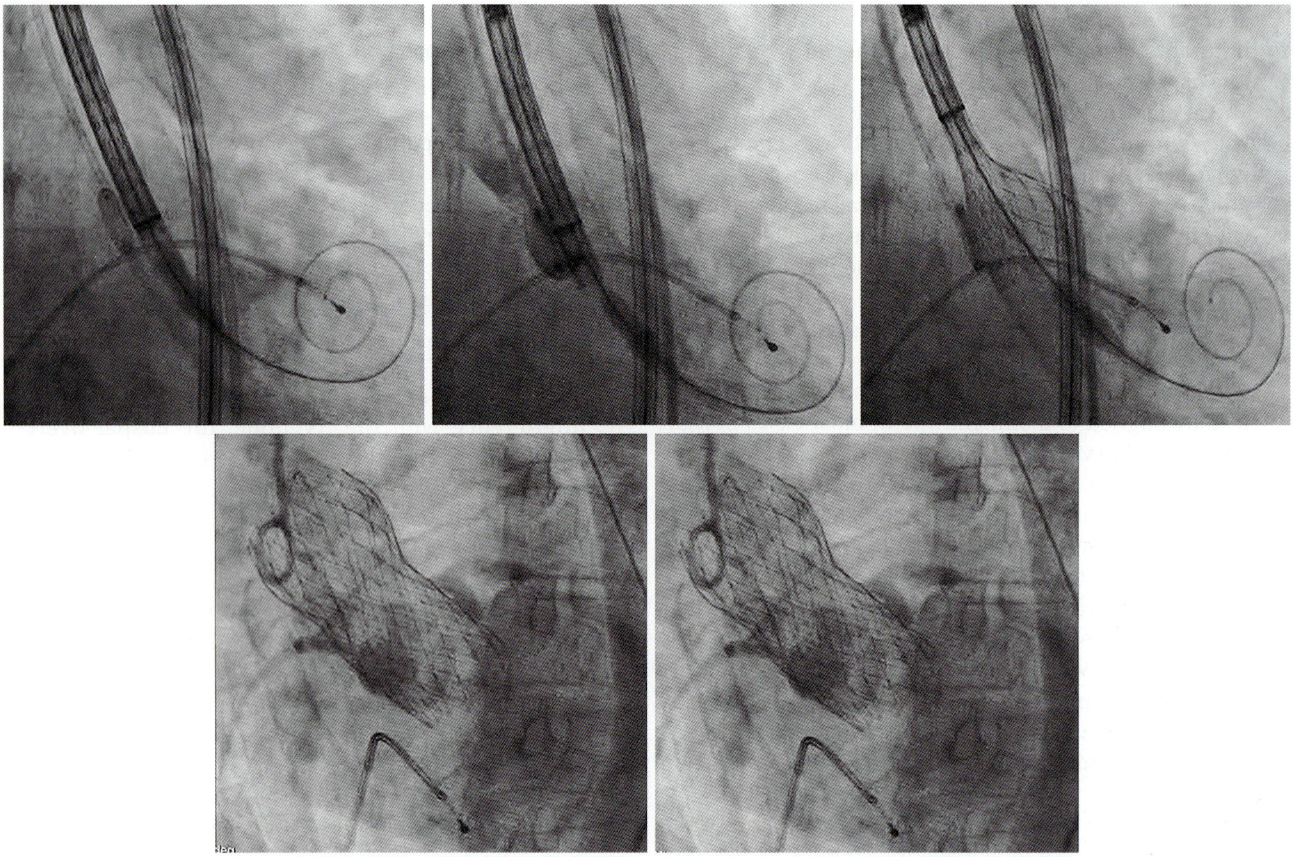

FIG. 4: Cuspal overlap view—RAO 9 CAUDAL 29—The valve is positioned at the lower level of pigtail in the cuspal overlap view and gradually released maintaining a depth of 3–4 mm and deployed after the frame alignment in LAO view to see that the left side of frame is below the left annular plane.

CONCLUSION

Imaging using multiple methods plays a very important role in deciding the size, positioning, and risk of PVL in choosing a THV.

Better hemodynamics and avoiding patient prosthesis mismatch, future coronary access, are increasingly recognized as significant aspect of sizing, designing, and structure of the valve.

Conduction abnormalities remain a major concern following TAVR as its incidence is higher, as compared to SAVR.

Need to avoid PPI and conduction abnormalities have led to understanding of shallow deployment combined with cuspal overlap technique.

This has reduced the injury to the conduction system and better outcomes in patients who are specially treated with SEVs.

Fluoroscopic cusp overlap technique added with MSCT double S-curve allows a view of LVOT and delivery catheter without foreshortening, which helps in shallow deployments and thus reduced rate of PPI. This was initially designed for SEV but its application in deploying even for BEV has resulted better results and lesser PPI requirement as an extended use.

ONLINE REFERENCES

Please scan the QR code provided at the end of the table of contents for References of this chapter.

CHAPTER

185 Conduction Abnormalities after Structural Heart Intervention

Ashraf SM, Thajfeer UM

ABSTRACT

Among structural heart interventions, transcatheter aortic valve replacement (TAVR) has maximum incidence of permanent conduction abnormalities. After TAVR procedure, conduction abnormality requiring permanent pacemaker implantation (PPI) is much higher than surgical aortic valve replacement (SAVR). Most of the conduction abnormalities occur during periprocedural period. The depth of transcatheter aortic valve implantation (TAVI) prosthesis implantation into the left ventricular outflow tract (LVOT) is the most important risk factor identified. Newer-generation TAVI valves proved to decrease periprocedural complications like paravalvular leak but not the PPI requirement.

Keywords: TAVR, LBBB, HAVB, PPI, SAVR.

INTRODUCTION

Among structural heart interventions, transcatheter intervention of aortic valve has maximum incidence of permanent conduction abnormalities. Transcatheter aortic valve replacement (TAVR) has been an alternative to surgical valve implantation in patients with high surgical risk patients. The most common permanent arrhythmic complications following TAVR are high-degree atrioventricular block (HAVB) and new-onset left bundle branch block (LBBB) requiring permanent pacemaker implantation (PPI). Surgical aortic valve replacement (SAVR) has lesser incidence of procedure related heart block than TAVR (3–6.9% vs. 17%).[1]

MECHANISM OF CONDUCTION INJURY AFTER TAVR

The His bundle penetrates membranous interventricular septum and emerges on the ventricular left side, directly within the aortic root and left ventricular outflow tract (LVOT), positioned superficially on the crest of the muscular septum. From this point, the left bundle fascicle originates which is directly related to the base of the interleaflet triangle which separates the right coronary leaflets of the aortic valve.[2] Conduction tissue injury can easily arise in TAVR once the prosthetic valve or calcific nodule on native aortic valve or LVOT exerts pressure on the related tissues. Postprocedure autopsy studies in TAVR patients showed local edema, hematoma, and infarction with compression of the His bundle causing conduction disorder.

Anatomical close relationship of conduction tissue with aortic valve complex, negative influence of aging on conduction tissue, and calcium deposition in both conduction tissue and aortic valve complex make vulnerable atmosphere in both TAVR and SAVR. In TAVR, most of patient subsets are older, have more pre-existing diseases such as renal dysfunction and impingement of valve material directly on conduction fibers in LVOT make even more vulnerable to heart block **(Fig. 1)**.

New development of LBBB is either temporary or permanent and can be either during or post procedure. Risk factors mainly procedure-related and patient-related factors. Deeper implantation of TAVR prosthesis leads to higher incidence of LBBB.[3]

Most well studied valves used in TAVR are Medtronic Evolute valve (self-expandable) and Edward Sapien valve (balloon-expandable). Compared to balloon-expandable prosthesis, self-expandable valves have higher incidence of LBBB since the radial force generated at membranous septum and ventricular side than annulus of aorta. We can also predict peri- and postprocedural LBBB by looking at QRS width, severe aortic valvular and LVOT calcification.[4]

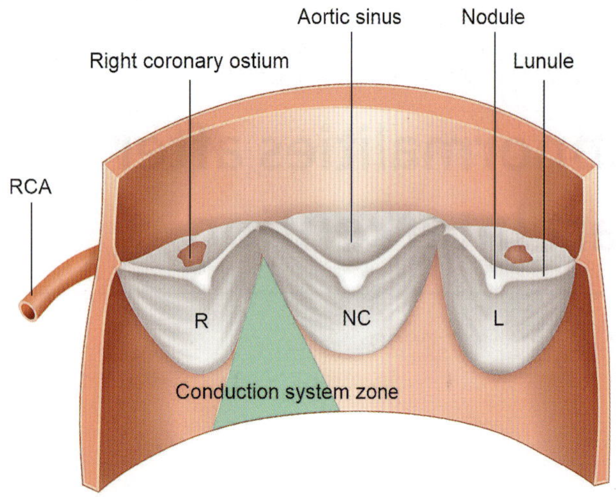

FIG. 1: Spatial relationship of conduction tissue with aortic valve.
(RCA: right coronary artery)

TABLE 1: Risk factors for conduction block after TAVR.

Anatomical	Patient related	Procedure related
Severe calcification of: • Aortic annulus and LVOT • Small LVOT diameter • Short membranous septum	• Female gender • Diabetes mellitus • Prolonged QRS	• Implantation depth • Use of self-expandable valve • Overexpansion of aortic annulus • Oversized valve • Balloon valvuloplasty

(LVOT: left ventricular outflow tract; TAVR: transcatheter aortic valve replacement)

Patient-related factors such as small aortic annulus, small LVOT diameter, and procedure-related factors like oversizing are also risk factors **(Table 1)**.

The HAVB develops during or after TAVR procedure with frequency around 2–7%.[5] Majority of HAVB occurs within 2–3 days and as many as half to three quarters of cases develop during procedure and majority require PPI. Very late development (after discharge) is very rare. Risk factors are similar to LBBB with additional risk factors such as pre-existing right bundle branch, PR prolongation, and fascicular block. Transient conduction disturbance during crossing with wires and exchanging catheters are often benign and not require PPI.

There is no increased cardiac mortality observed after post TAVR PPI during initial follow-up.

But heart failure and left ventricular dysfunction may develop due to long-term right ventricular pacing.[6]

OTHER STRUCTURAL INTERVENTIONS

Percutaneous perimembranous ventricular septal defect (VSD) device closure may lead to adverse heart events such as bundle branch block and atrioventricular block. Incidence is generally between 1 and 5% of procedures. Most likely mechanisms are mechanical compression of device at conduction tissue at defect margin and associated inflammatory edema of conduction tissue. 60% of cases are transient and often restored by inhibition of inflammation. Recurrent and late-onset conduction blocks are not reversible. Oversizing, device-related factors are major risk factors.

In patients undergoing transcatheter mitral valve repair (TMVR), MitraClip underlying conduction abnormalities can increase the risk of heart block because of close proximity with mitral valve (MV) apparatus especially posterior fascicle. But, incidence is very rare. Conduction abnormalities can appear in other valve and device implantations during procedures due to catheter movements, but often transient.

CONCLUSION

New-onset LBBB and HAVB are observed frequently following TAVR procedure despite improvement in device characteristics. Several anatomical, patient- and procedure-related factors may predict which patients are vulnerable to conduction block after TAVR. The best predictive risk factors are preexisting right bundle branch, deep implantation of device into LVOT, oversizing, and use of self-expandable valves.

ONLINE REFERENCES

Please scan the QR code provided at the end of the table of contents for References of this chapter.

CHAPTER

186 Coronary Interventions after Transcatheter Aortic Valve Implantation

Ashish Kumar, Himanshu Dabral, Rajneesh Kapoor

ABSTRACT

Transcatheter aortic valve implantation (TAVI) has emerged as a revolutionary intervention for severe aortic valve stenosis. However, concomitant coronary artery disease (CAD) poses unique challenges in the management of these patients. Currently, the indication for TAVI has expanded toward young patients who are at low surgical risk. Given the progressive nature of CAD, the necessity for coronary interventions will subsequently increase in TAVI patients in the future. This chapter explores the intricacies of coronary interventions after TAVI, emphasizing the importance of optimizing patient outcomes. We delve into the assessment of coronary anatomy, determination of the need for interventions, technical considerations, clinical outcomes, and future directions. By comprehensively examining these aspects, clinicians can make informed decisions and improve patient care. The optimal timing of percutaneous coronary intervention (PCI) remains unclear due to a lack of evidence. Depending on the valve type, position, and axial alignment of the implanted valve, coronary intervention after TAVI can be challenging. Hence, every cardiologist should be familiar with the different types of transcatheter heart valves and their characteristics and technical issues that can arise during invasive coronary procedures.

Keywords: Coronary angiography, PCI/PTCA, TAVI/TAVR, aortic stenosis.

INTRODUCTION

Transcatheter aortic valve implantation (TAVI) has transformed the treatment landscape for severe aortic stenosis (AS), offering a minimally invasive alternative to traditional surgical approaches. As TAVI procedures increase, clinicians encounter an evolving patient population with concomitant coronary artery disease (CAD). The optimal management of CAD in TAVI patients involves meticulous assessment of coronary anatomy, determination of the need for revascularization, and implementation of appropriate interventions. This chapter aims to provide a comprehensive overview of coronary interventions after TAVI, exploring technical considerations, clinical outcomes, and future directions for improving patient care.

ASSESSMENT OF CORONARY ANATOMY AND PHYSIOLOGY

Regarding diagnosis, both anatomical and hemodynamic assessments are the mainstay of CAD evaluation. Coronary angiography (CA) remains the standard anatomical test for CAD in TAVI patents. At the same time, computed tomography angiography is routinely used in preoperative planning and emerges as a necessary tool for the diagnosis of CAD before TAVI. Few data available on hemodynamic assessment of CAD in TAVI patients by fraction flow reserve (FFR) or instantaneous wave free ratio (iFR). The choice between ischemia-guided and anatomy-guided revascularization depends on patient-specific factors and lesion characteristics. Fractional flow reserve-computed tomography (FFR-CT) provides both anatomical and functional assessment of CAD and substantially improved diagnostic accuracy in a recent prospective comparison with invasive FFR in 42 patients (68 vessels) with severe AS. The CT data were interpretable in 92.3% of patients; sensitivity, specificity, positive predictive value (PPV) and negative predictive value (NPV) were 73.9%, 78.4%, 68.0%, and 82.9%, respectively. These data suggest that CTCA can be combined with FFR CT which may provide good results in terms of time, cost, and risk and may be an alternative first-line screening method in selected AS patient groups.[1]

OPTIMAL TIMING OF PERCUTANEOUS CORONARY INTERVENTION IN TAVI PATIENTS

Determining the optimal timing for percutaneous coronary intervention (PCI) in patients undergoing TAVI is a critical decision that requires careful evaluation. The timing of PCI should take into account factors such as the severity of CAD, clinical stability, and the risk-benefit ratio of revascularization. This section discusses the considerations for determining the optimal timing of PCI in TAVI patients.

Pre-TAVI PCI

In selected cases, a pre-TAVI PCI strategy may be employed to optimize coronary perfusion and reduce the burden of untreated CAD before the TAVI procedure.

Pre-TAVI PCI is typically considered for patients with severe CAD and significant myocardial ischemia who are suitable candidates for revascularization. The decision to perform pre-TAVI PCI should involve a multidisciplinary heart team discussion considering the complexity of the lesions, clinical stability, and procedural considerations.

Hybrid Approach

A hybrid approach, involving simultaneous TAVI and PCI procedures, can be considered in patients with significant CAD and symptomatic myocardial ischemia. This approach allows for immediate revascularization of significant coronary lesions during the TAVI procedure, minimizing the need for separate interventions, and potentially reducing the overall procedural risk. A collaborative effort between interventional cardiologists and structural heart specialists is essential to determine the feasibility and safety of the hybrid approach on a case-by-case basis.

Post-TAVI PCI

Post-TAVI PCI may be indicated when significant coronary lesions are identified during or after the TAVI procedure. The decision for post-TAVI PCI should be based on clinical judgment, considering factors such as residual angina, evidence of myocardial ischemia, or hemodynamically significant stenosis. The timing of post-TAVI PCI should be individualized, taking into account the complexity of the lesions, patient's clinical stability, and the need for additional antiplatelet therapy.

Serial Revascularization

In some cases, a staged approach to revascularization may be appropriate, particularly when the extent of CAD is extensive or complex. Serial revascularization involves performing PCI either before or after the TAVI procedure in a staged manner. This approach allows for a comprehensive evaluation of coronary anatomy and optimization of the revascularization strategy. The decision for staged revascularization should consider the patient's clinical status, hemodynamic stability, and the potential impact on procedural success and outcomes.

The optimal timing of PCI in TAVI patients requires a multidisciplinary approach and careful consideration of patient-specific factors. The decision should be based on the severity of CAD, clinical stability, procedural feasibility, and the risk-benefit ratio of revascularization. Individualized decision-making, considering the collaborative input of interventional cardiologists, cardiac surgeons, and other specialists, is crucial to achieve optimal outcomes in TAVI patients requiring PCI. In addition, the European guidelines for the management of valvular diseases state that the timing of intervention and the need for PCI should be individually discussed in patients planning to undergo TAVI as per the patient's medical condition and myocardium area at risk.[2] PCI before TAVI is a critical consideration, especially for stenosis >70% in major epicardial vessels and the left main coronary artery. When these stenoses are severe and pose a significant risk of myocardial ischemia, performing PCI prior to TAVI may be warranted. However, the decision to proceed with PCI should carefully weigh the potential benefits against the procedural risks, ensuring that the overall risk-benefit profile remains favorable. On the other hand, for stenosis located at mid or distal segments of the coronary vasculature or stenosis associated with small areas of ischemia, the urgency of PCI may be less pronounced. In such cases, it may be reasonable to defer PCI until after the TAVI procedure, provided that coronary access remains technically feasible after the valve implantation.[3]

REPORTED OUTCOMES OF CORONARY INTERVENTIONS IN PATIENTS WITH AORTIC STENOSIS

Goel et al.[4] showed that when PCI was performed in AS patients, there was no association of short-term mortality or procedural complications compared to compliant patients without AS. The research group includes 254 patients. Indications are acute coronary syndrome (ACS), congestive heart failure, or severe angina, and symptoms are thought to be caused by CAD, not AS. Patients with a left ventricular ejection fraction (LVEF) <30% and a Society of Thoracic Surgeons (STS) score >10 have a higher risk of death 30 days after PCI.

Gasparetto et al.[5] reported a prospective registry (PUREVALVE registry) of 191 consecutive patients with severe AS presenting for transcatheter aortic valve replacement (TAVR). PCI is indicated only for stenosis in the proximal or middle of the great arteries. PCI was performed after evaluation of symptoms, degree of myocardial risk, diagnosis-confirmed ischemia, and the technical feasibility of PCI. Chronic total occlusions and lesions in small vessels (reference diameters <2.5 mm) were not considered for PCI. Of the 191 patients who underwent TAVR, CAD was present in 113 (59.2%) and PCI was performed before TAVR in 39 (20.4%). Although this was a small observational study, the overall 30-day mortality did not differ significantly between patients with CAD post-PCI versus no CAD (5.7% vs. 2.9%). These results suggest that a selective, clinically focused PCI strategy prior to TAVR may be a reasonable strategy.

In a study conducted by Abdel-Wahab et al.,[6] they investigated two groups of patients who underwent different procedures. The first group consisted of 55 patients who underwent PCI with the CoreValve (Medtronic) prior to TAVR. The second group included 70 patients who underwent TAVR alone without prior PCI. The study findings revealed that there were no significant differences between the two groups regarding various clinical outcomes. Specifically, there were no significant differences in terms of 30-day mortality, incidence of myocardial infarction, major bleeding events, major vascular events, composite safety factors, or side effects at 6 months postprocedure. These results indicate that performing PCI with the CoreValve before TAVR did not confer additional risks or adverse events compared to TAVR performed alone. The study suggests that the approach of performing PCI prior to TAVR is feasible and safe in the selected patient population, without compromising clinical outcomes.

In another single study, Wendt et al.[7] compared 184 patients who received Surgical Aortic Valve Replacement (SAVR) plus coronary artery bypass grafting (CABG) with 59 patients who received TAVR plus PCI over 12 months. Despite the higher risk in the TAVR group, inhospital mortality rates were similar for TAVR plus PCI and SAVR plus CABG. Only LVEF predicted outcome.

According to Nai Fovino et al.,[8] in a group of 912 people, the frequency of CA was found to be 5.3% in a 2.1-year follow-up after TAVI. Of these, 35% of CAs were due to ACS and 54% of patients underwent PCI. Independent markers of CA were younger age, prior PCI, and prior CABG.

Vilalta et al.[9] reported a 10% ACS rate in a TAVI cohort (n = 774) during a median follow-up time of 25 months. The majority had a non-ST-segment elevation myocardial infarction (NSTEMI) (64.1%) and approximately 39% of those patients underwent PCI.

In a follow-up study from the SOURCE 3 registry[10] comprising 1,936 patients who were exclusively treated with the SAPIEN 3 transcatheter heart valve (THV), the rate of CA during a follow-up period of 3 years was 3.5% with a mean time from TAVI to CA of 441 days. Indications for CA were stable CAD (36.8%), NSTEMI (26.5%), and STEMI (11.8%); 69% of those patients underwent PCI **(Table 1)**.

TABLE 1: Overview of studies on coronary angiography (± PCI) after TAVI.

References	THV	Sample size	CA/PCI (%) performed	Indication for CA/PCI	Median time from TAVI in days	Success rate for PCI (%)
Perrin et al.[11]	• Evolut R: 9 • CoreValve: 7 • SAPIEN: 2 • Evolut Pro: 1	424	20 (4.7)/11 (55)	• ACS: 8 • CCS: 9 • Other: 3	464	11/11 (100)
Boukantar et al.[12]	CoreValve	550	16 (2.9)/7 (43.8)	• ACS: 7 • CCS: 3 • Others: 6	157	6/7 (85.7)
Nai Fovino et al.[8]	• SAPIEN XT: 21 • SAPIEN 3: 15 • CoreValve: 6 • Evolut Pro: 2 • JenaValve: 2 • Lotus: 2	912	48 (5.9)/26 (54)	• ACS: 17 • CCS: 8 • Others: 23	769	25/26 (95.2)
Blumenstein et al.[13]	• Edwards SAPIEN XT: 16 • CoreValve: 10 • Symetis ACURATE: 4 • Portico: 1	1,000	31 (3.1)/7 (22.6)	• ACS: 4 • CCS: N/A • Others: N/A	233	7/7 (100)

Continued

Continued

References	THV	Sample size	CA/PCI (%) performed	Indication for CA/PCI	Median time from TAVI in days	Success rate for PCI (%)
Vilalta et al.[9]	N/A	78	53 (67.9)/30 (56.6)	Only ACS patients included	300	N/A
Tarantini et al.[10]	Edwards SAPIEN 3 only	1,936	68 (3.5)/47 (69.1)	• ACS: 26 • CCS: 25 • Others: 17	441	46/47 (97.9)

(ACS: acute coronary syndrome; CA: coronary angiography; CCS: chronic coronary syndrome; PCI: percutaneous coronary intervention; TAVI: transcatheter aortic valve implantation; THV: transcatheter heart valve)

CORONARY ACCESS IN BALLOON-EXPANDABLE VALVES

Coronary access in patients with balloon-expandable valves is technically less challenging than with self-expanding valves, mainly due to the lower stent frame that in most cases does not protrude beyond the coronary ostium. However, there is a trend toward using high implantation depth, as studies over the last few years have shown that a lower device position increases the need for permanent pacemaker implantation.[14,15] In addition, the newer generations of balloon-expandable valves, e.g., the SAPIEN 3 and SAPIEN 3 Ultra, feature a taller stent frame than the precursor SAPIEN XT, thus increasing the probability of partially or totally covering the coronary ostia **(Fig. 1)**. On the other hand, the cells in the upper row have a 38% larger area than the SAPIEN XT, which makes it easier to engage the catheter through the struts and possibly compensates for the higher rate of supraostial positioning.[16] The new model SAPIEN 3 Ultra has a 40% higher skirt compared to SAPIEN 3 and is made of textured polyethylene terephthalate (PET) designed to support the healing process and improve sealing.

Faroux et al. analyzed angiographic and computed tomography data of 553 patients for the position of the THV relative to the coronary ostia who underwent successful implantation of SAPIEN XT and SAPIEN 3.[17,18] It was found that left main ostia was completely covered in 27% of cases, with a significantly higher proportion when the newer-generation SAPIEN 3 was implanted (43% vs. 12%). Nearly 10% of patients underwent CA [with or without percutaneous transluminal coronary angioplasty (PTCA)] after TAVI, and no difference was found in relation to valve position.

Another aspect to be taken into account in post-TAVI patients is a possible commissural misalignment in relation to the coronary ostia. In contrast to SAVR, where the valve commissures can be properly aligned with respect to native coronaries ostium, proper alignment is difficult in TAVI patients. Tang et al.[19] performed CT scans before and after TAVI to examine the anatomical relationship between the neocommissures and coronary ostia in 70 patients ($n = 53$ with SAPIEN, SAPIEN XT, or SAPIEN 3; $n = 17$ with Evolut R). They found that in >50% of patients, the neocommissures overlapped with the ostium of the left coronary artery (LCA) or the right coronary artery (RCA), or both. There is no difference in overlap between balloon-expandable and self-expandable THVs. However, the effect of this close anatomic relationship is currently unclear and the authors did not provide any information on interference with catheter coaptation.

The Myval device[20] (Meril Life Sciences, Gujarat, India) is a CE-marked, new-generation balloon-expandable THV. The valve consists of a three bovine pericardial tissue leaflets fixed to three vertical commissural posts (separated by 120°) on the metal frame. The nickel–cobalt stent frame has a hexagonal design cells that are arranged in such a fashion that large open cells occupy 53% of the frame toward the aortic end and small closed cells occupy 47% of the frame toward the ventricular end **(Fig. 2)**. The open cells in the upper half ensure optimal perfusion to the coronaries, whereas the closed cells in the lower half provide high radial strength. The valve frame, upon crimping under fluoroscopy gives rise to a unique pattern of alternating dark and light stripes. The second dark band from the ventricular end serves as the marker for precise positioning and deployment of the valve at desired location. The Myval THV is available in a range of sizes to accommodate different patient anatomies. The available sizes include normal (20.0, 23.0, 26.0, and 29.0 mm), medium (21.5, 24.5, and 27.5 mm), and extra-large (30.5 and 32.0 mm). Notably, the Myval's treatable range can further expand up to 32.7 mm with the extra-large size option. Despite its availability in multiple sizes, data on CA and/or PCI for this specific THV are limited. More research and clinical studies are needed to gather comprehensive data on the safety and efficacy of Myval in patients who require CA and/or PCI in conjunction with the THV procedure. Additional studies will help establish a better understanding of its performance in complex anatomies and guide clinical decision-making for the optimal treatment of patients.

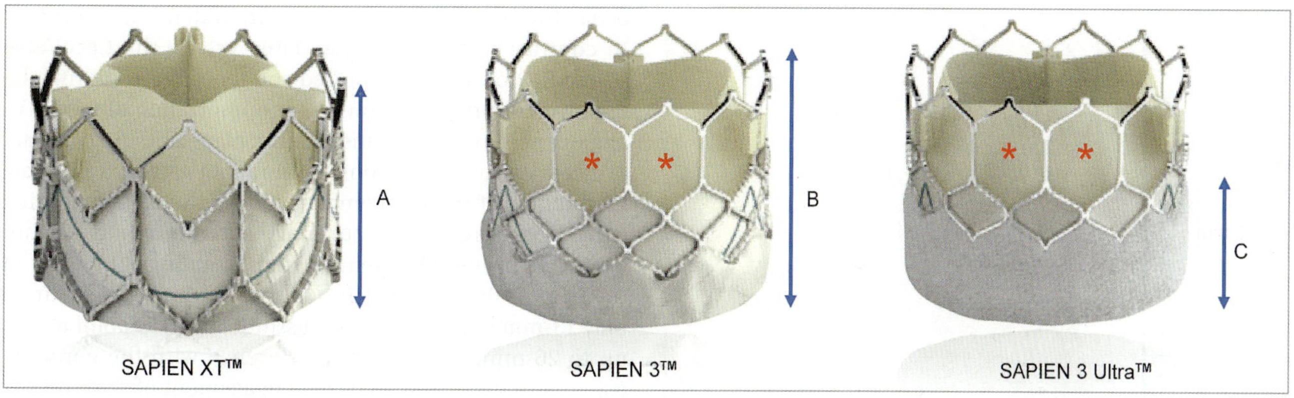

FIG. 1: Differences in frame height and cell dimensions between SAPIEN XT and SAPIEN 3/SAPIEN 3 Ultra. Compared with SAPIEN XT, the frame height (A and B) of SAPIEN 3 and SAPIEN 3 Ultra is taller, potentially leading to more interference with the coronary ostia, but the cells in the upper row are bigger thereby facilitating coronary access (red asterisk). The newer SAPIEN 3 Ultra retains the SAPIEN 3 stent frame design, but its outer skirt is 40% higher to provide a better sealing (C).

Courtesy: Edwards Lifesciences Corporation.

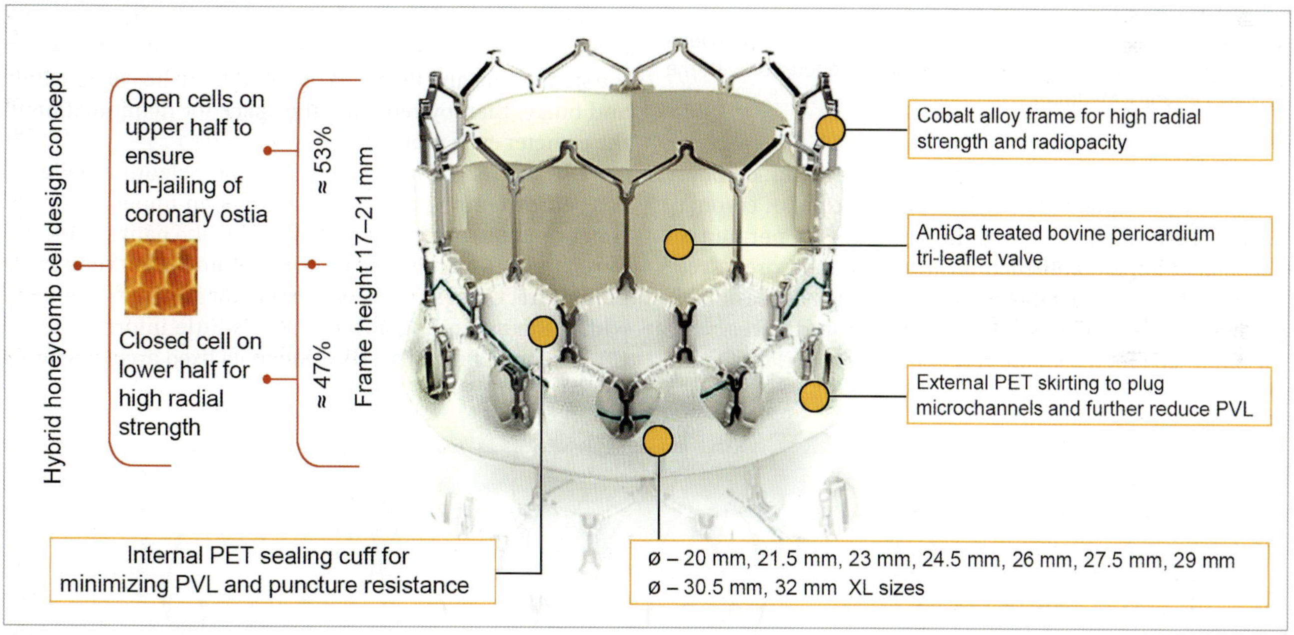

FIG. 2: Dimensions of MYVALVE.

(PET: polyethylene terephthalate; PVL: paravalvular leak)

Courtesy: Meril Life Sciences.

CORONARY ACCESS IN SELF-EXPANDING VALVES

In contrast to balloon-expandable valves, the proper engagement of the coronary ostia in patients with self-expanding valves is more challenging, and semiselective, or even unselective angiograms as well as unsuccessful PCIs are much more common than in cases with balloon-expandable valves.[12,13,21] There are several reasons why these THVs cause coronary access problems.

COREVALVE EVOLUT R/PRO

The Evolut R/Pro is a supra-annular valve with a shaft length of 45–46 mm that invariably extends over the coronary ostia. It has an inflow portion with high radial force that retains the valve in the annular plane, a concave waist that leaves enough space between the valve frame and the coronary ostia, and an outflow part situated in the aorta **(Fig. 3)**.[16]

Yudi et al.[16] recently published a report on the geometric interaction between the Evolut R/Pro and the coronary ostia.

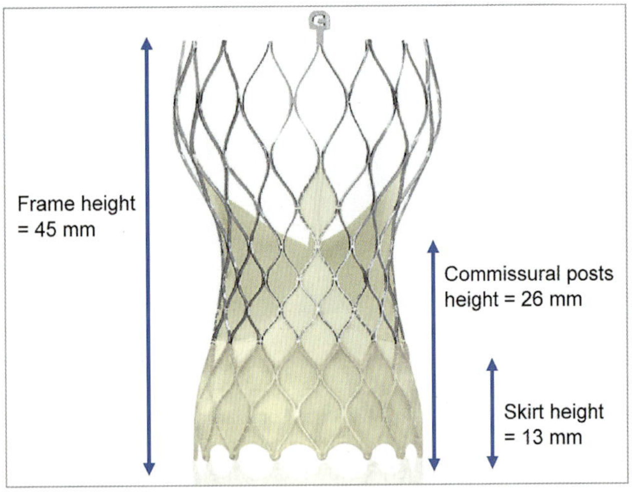

FIG. 3: The CoreValve Evolut Pro valve prosthesis consists of specific dimensions for the frame, skirt, and commissural post heights. The frame height measures 45 mm, and this design ensures that the CoreValve Evolut Pro surpasses the coronary ostia. The presence of a "waist" in the stent frame allows for adequate space between the coronary ostia and the valve, preventing interference with the coronary arteries (Medtronic).

The skirt height is 13 mm, which may interfere with coronary ostium when implanted at high depth or height of coronary ostia (<10 mm). Due to the higher rates of permanent pacemaker implantation demonstrated for the CoreValve,[22] the operators tend to implant the valve as high as reasonably possible to reduce the risk of conduction disturbances,[23] but this approach increases the risk of the skirt overlapping the ostia. The recommended implantation depth is 3–5 mm.[16] In contrast to balloon-expandable valves, the CoreValve Evolut R/Pro can be recaptured and repositioned during the deployment process, allowing for optimization of the THVs alignment in relation to the annular plane and the coronary orifices. As for the balloon-expandable valves, a possible interaction of the neocommissures of the self-expanding valve with the native coronary arteries could further aggravate proper engagement of the guiding catheter;[16] in the case of the Evolut R/Pro, although the sealing skirt is only 13-mm high, at the commissural insertion point it rises up to 26 mm, making an interference with the coronary ostia more likely and a coaxial engagement of the catheter more challenging. **Figures 4A to C** depicts three different scenarios for the relationship between the coronary ostium and the skirt and the stent frame struts of the Evolut R/Pro. Finally, the more shallow the sinus of Valsalva, the lesser the space that lies between the coronary ostia and the stent frame, making it more difficult to manipulate the catheter and properly engage the orifice. This is even more challenging when the native valve leaflets captured between the stent frame and the sinus of Valsalva are heavily calcified and bulky, thereby reducing the space for manipulation of the catheter even more.[16]

The ACURATE neo valve[24] (Boston Scientific) **(Fig. 5)** is a self-expanding valve consisting of an upper crown for supra-annular anchoring and capturing the native leaflets, a lower crown with minimal protrusion into the left ventricular outflow tract, and stabilization arches for axial self-alignment within the ascending aorta. There is little information on CA and/or PCI for this THV. Due to its fixed arch extending

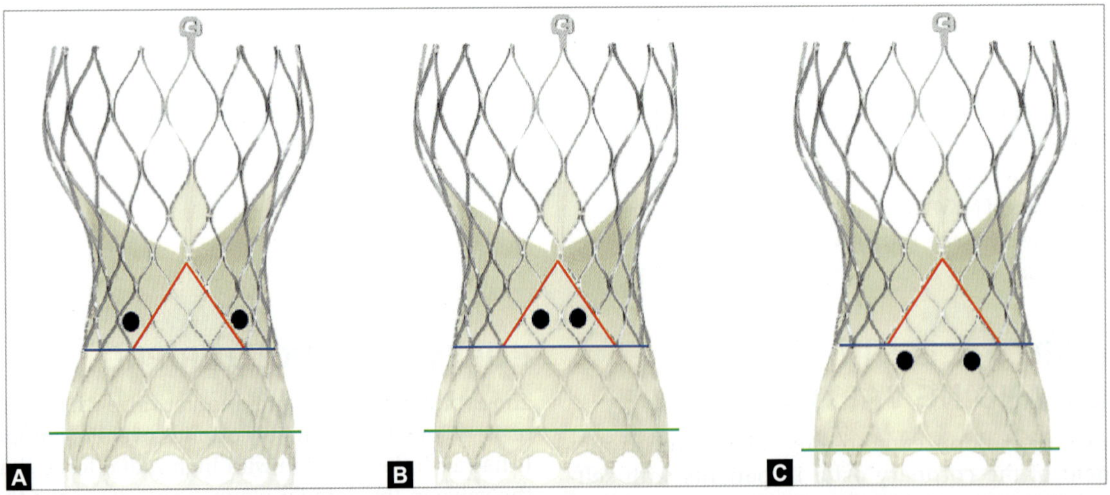

FIGS. 4A TO C: A schematic diagram illustrates various positions of the coronary ostium concerning the skirt and commissural posts in Evolut Pro. The diagram includes black dots representing two examples of coronary ostia positions. The annular plane is indicated by a green line, the upper limit of the sealing skirt by a blue line, and the skirt's course rising up with the commissural post by a red line. In scenario (A), the coronary orifices lie beyond the skirt and commissural posts, allowing for a likely coaxial intubation. In scenario (B), the coronary ostia are positioned in front of the commissural post, necessitating cannulation through an adjacent diamond. Scenario (C) displays an instance of low-lying coronary ostia and low implantation depth, with the sealing skirt facing the coronary ostia. For coronary engagement, cannulation should be performed from a diamond above.

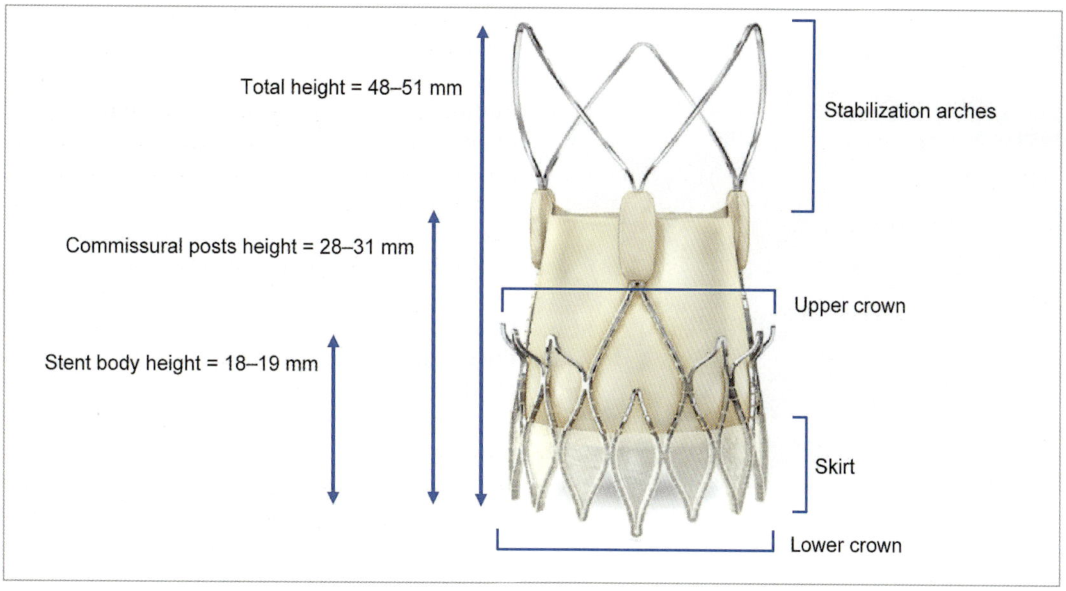

FIG. 5: The ACURATE neo valve prosthesis features specific dimensions for the total height, stent body height, and commissural post height. The upper crown of the stent body is designed to secure the native leaflets and anchor the device supra-annually. Additionally, the inclusion of stabilization arches aids in axial self-alignment within the ascending aorta (Boston Scientific).

into the ascending aorta the device will definitely protrude beyond the coronary ostium, thus impeding with the passage of the catheter.

In addition, the commissural post height (28–31 mm, depending on the valve size) is quite high and a commissural tab might randomly be positioned in front of the coronary ostia during implantation. Thus far, only one study has provided data on CA and PCI in patients with this valve; Blumenstein et al. reported on four patients with the precursor model of ACURATE valve.[13] Selective coronary access was possible in two patients; in the other two, semi-selective CA was done. One patient underwent PCI of the left anterior descending (LAD) artery, which was achieved by using an AL2 guiding catheter. However, intubation with that guiding catheter was initially semiselective and subsequent guidewire advancement led to proper engagement and successful PCI.[13]

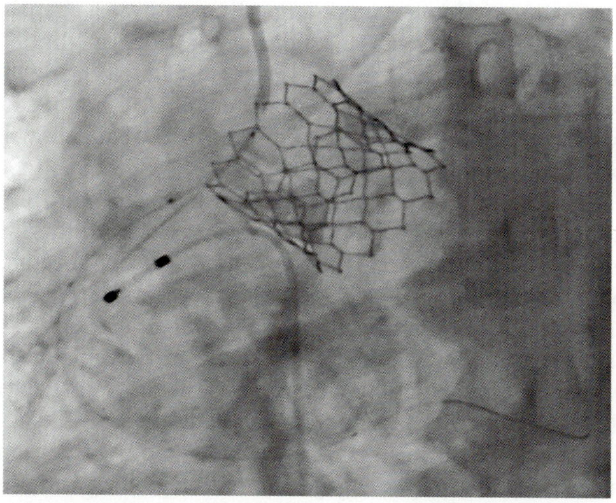

FIG. 6: Engagement of right coronary artery (RCA) in a patient with prior MYVALVE.

ENGAGEMENT OF GUIDING CATHETERS

Balloon-expandable Valves

Mostly the outflow part of the valve stent frame will be located below the coronary ostia; coronary cannulation with the guide catheters will be uncomplicated and may not differ from the situation with a native valve. If the stent frame protrudes beyond the coronary ostia, engagement of the guiding catheter must be performed through the stent cells near the coronary ostia, ideally in a coaxial orientation. If the coronary ostium is covered by the skirt or a commissural tab, catheter engagement should be done across the cell that is most adjacent to the coronary orifice. For guide catheter engagement of the LCA, a Judkins left (JL) 4 or JL 3.5 or an extra backup (EBU) catheter 3.5/3.75 can be used; for the RCA, usually a Judkins right 4 (JR4) is appropriate. **Figure 6** showing a patient with prior MYVALVE who had ACS having culprit lesion in RCA. Ostial engagement of RCA done with JR 3.5.

Self-expanding Valves

Since the stent frame of the self-expanding valves always extends beyond the coronary ostia, the guiding catheter is required to pass through the stent struts to successfully intubate the coronary arteries. If possible, the intubation of the coronary ostium should be performed coaxially through a stent cell at the level of the coronary orifice. Due to the

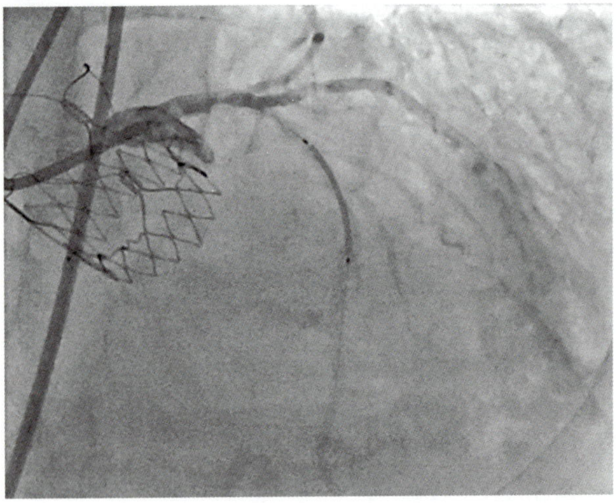

FIG. 7: Selective and supravalvular engagement of left coronary artery (LCA) in a patient with prior ACURATE neo 2 valve using extra backup (EBU) 3.0 catheter.

"waist" of the self-expanding valves, which measures 20–24 mm depending on the valve size, the space to manipulate the catheter is clearly smaller than the native aortic root dimensions. Hence, smaller guiding catheters for the LCA, like JL 3.5 or even JL 3.0 instead of JL 4.0, might be a better choice for successful engagement. **Figure 7** showing selective and supravalvular engagement of LCA in a patient with prior ACURATE neo 2 valve using EBU 3.0 catheter who presented with ACS.

For the RCA, a JR 4 guide catheter is mostly sufficient, although, when the sinus of Valsalva is wide and there is enough space between the stent frame and the coronary ostia, a longer-tipped guide catheter such as an Amplatzer right (AR) 2 or even a multipurpose catheter can be used. In certain cases when neocommissures or portions of the valve skirt extend in front of the ostia, engagement through a diamond cell near the ostium is recommended.

The use of EBU catheters for the LCA requires caution. In cases where proper engagement of the guiding catheter poses challenges, alternative techniques can be employed to facilitate access to the coronary ostium. One method involves advancing a coronary wire into the coronary artery, which acts as a guide to "rail" the EBU catheter into the ostium. Additionally, a small balloon can be positioned in the left main coronary artery to aid in guiding the catheter (balloon-assisted tracking). Careful inflation of the balloon in a more peripheral position in the coronary artery can also help "pull" the catheter into the ostium (anchoring balloon technique).[11]

In situations where difficulties persist, a bailout strategy involves cautiously advancing an extension catheter, such as GuideLiner or Guidezilla, into the coronary ostium to guide the guiding catheter into the correct position (mother-and-child technique).

In certain cases, the guide catheter might not be advancing into the coronary ostium, either due to interference of the stent frame or lack of coaxial alignment of the guide catheter to the ostium. Here, the guiding catheter extension can be used for the selective cannulation and the procedure can be performed solely through the guiding catheter extension device properly inserted into the coronary ostium.

CONCLUSION

Coronary interventions after TAVI play a crucial role in optimizing patient outcomes in the presence of concomitant CAD. By carefully assessing coronary anatomy, determining the need for revascularization, and addressing technical considerations, clinicians can navigate the complexities associated with these interventions. Ongoing advancements, future research, and multidisciplinary collaborations will further refine management strategies, enhancing the long-term prognosis for TAVI patients with concomitant CAD. TAVI is increasingly being performed in younger patients with a lower surgical risk due to widening indication and longer survival. As CAD is a progressive disease, the impact on TAVI patients will become more frequent in the future. Knowledge of the differences between THVs, their structure and function, and how they may interact with the coronary ostia is important to the operator. More research efforts are needed in order to define better and safe techniques for coronary interventions in TAVI patients.

ONLINE REFERENCES

Please scan the QR code provided at the end of the table of contents for References of this chapter.

CHAPTER 187

Antithrombotic Therapy in Patients with Transcatheter Aortic Valve Implantation

Anoop Agrawal

ABSTRACT

Transcatheter aortic valve implantation (TAVI) has largely replaced surgical aortic valve implantation in patients with severe aortic stenosis who are considered a high or intermediate risk for surgery and an excellent minimally invasive alternative for low surgical risk patients who are >65 years of age. As more patients adopt TAVI as the primary therapy, there is a palpable need to standardize antithrombotic therapy. Periprocedure antithrombotic therapy aims at reducing thromboembolic complications, which are often the major determinant of morbidity and mortality. For short-term and long-term time horizons, antithrombotic therapy is positioned to reduce leaflet thrombosis and prophylaxis against stroke in high-risk subsets. Preventing leaflet thrombosis may be of particular concern since it is often implicated in accelerated valve degeneration as well as higher cerebrovascular events. Conversely, TAVI patients often have a high bleeding risk, which needs to be factored in as well. This chapter delves into the nuances of antithrombotic therapy in TAVI patients by consolidating the available clinical data and societal guidelines.

Keywords: Transcatheter aortic valve implantation, transcatheter aortic valve replacement (TAVR), antithrombotic therapy, antiplatelet therapy, single antiplatelet therapy (SAPT), dual antiplatelet therapy (DAPT), leaflet thrombosis, bioprosthetic valve thrombosis (BVT), hypoattenuating leaflet thickening (HALT), reduced leaflet motion (RELM), hypoattenuating affecting motion (HAM).

INTRODUCTION

Since the first transcatheter aortic valve implantation (TAVI) for compassionate use in a human by Dr Alain Cribier in the year 2002, TAVI has evolved to become the preferred treatment option in patients with severe aortic stenosis who are at high or extreme surgical risk for surgical aortic valve replacement (SAVR) and an attractive alternative for those at a lower surgical risk spectrum.[1] Despite multiple iterative advancements in the transcatheter heart valve (THV) design, TAVI procedure, and standardization of patient care algorithms, much controversy exists regarding optimal antithrombotic strategy before, during, and after a TAVI procedure. The need for antithrombotic therapy in patients with an intravascular implant may seem obvious. However, it needs to be weighed against the bleeding risk since the TAVI patient subset is typically older and has one or more comorbidities rendering them a high bleeding risk. The incidence of late major bleeding can be as high as 11% at 1-year follow-up, the majority being gastrointestinal and associated with higher mortality.[2,3]

ROLE OF ANTITHROMBOTIC THERAPY BEFORE AND DURING TRANSCATHETER AORTIC VALVE IMPLANTATION PROCEDURE

Antiplatelet therapy and intravenous anticoagulants are routinely used during intravascular procedures such as angioplasty, and the same was traditionally extended to TAVI as well. The premise was to prevent catheter-induced thrombosis and related embolism. Although best practices in TAVI techniques led to a reduction in perioperative complications, the 30-day stroke rate saw only a marginal decline from 2.75 to 2.3% over the last decade.[4] An optimized antithrombotic regimen should aim to reduce the stroke rate further and minimize periprocedural bleeding and related morbidity and mortality.

The conventional practice of preloading with dual antiplatelet agents was challenged in BRAVO 3 substudy, which demonstrated that clopidogrel loading was associated with higher major vascular bleeding without any benefit in ischemic outcomes.[5] It is recommended that a single antiplatelet agent, typically a low-dose aspirin, should be started much before the anticipated TAVI procedure and continued during the perioperative period.[3]

In patients who are already on an oral anticoagulant (OAC) therapy pre-TAVI, a strategy to continue with the TAVI procedure without OAC interruption is not only safe, but also reduces periprocedural stroke as well as the need for blood transfusion.[6] If a patient takes a vitamin K antagonist (VKA), maintaining an international normalized ratio (INR) close to 2 is suggested. On the other hand, if a novel oral anticoagulant (NOAC) is continued, it is advisable to time the TAVI procedure at the anticipated trough level of the NOAC. Results from the randomized dataset of the POPular PAUSE TAVI (NCT04437303) trial looking at the safety of continued versus interrupted OAC are awaited. If OAC is continued perioperative, there is no role for concurrent antiplatelet therapy unless the patient has had a recent coronary angioplasty. In addition to OAC, the role of long-term aspirin is being evaluated in the AVATAR trial (NCT02735902), the results of which are not published yet.

The need to maintain intraprocedural activated clotting time (ACT) of >300 ms was relooked into, and the recent European Association of Percutaneous Cardiovascular Interventions (EAPCI) 2021 guidelines recommend maintaining an ACT of 250–300 ms.[3] Replacing heparin with bivalirudin did not reduce periprocedural bleeding events.[7] Hence, bivalirudin should be reserved for those with documented heparin allergy or heparin-induced thrombocytopenia. Routine use of protamine sulfate to reverse the heparin effect was associated with reduced bleeding complications without an increased risk of stroke or myocardial infarction.[8] One milligram of protamine neutralizes the anticoagulant effect of 100 units of heparin. Following the administration of heparin bolus, much of the heparin is metabolized over time during the procedure. Hence, by the end of the procedure, a lower dose of protamine is required to reverse the effect of the remaining heparin activity. Protamine can be dosed according to the final ACT or based on the time elapsed since the heparin bolus.[9] A simplified approach would be to calculate the amount of protamine required based purely on the total heparin administered and give half that dose at the end of the procedure.

ROLE OF ANTITHROMBOTIC THERAPY AFTER TRANSCATHETER AORTIC VALVE IMPLANTATION PROCEDURE

The rationale for continuing antithrombotic therapy post TAVI is based on the observation that thromboembolic events and bioprosthetic valve thrombosis (BVT) are known to occur post TAVI. Stroke or transient ischemic attack (TIA) risk, for example, seems to be elevated for up to 2 years following TAVI, after which the event rate stabilizes at around 2–3% annually, higher than age-matched peers likely due to comorbidities.[10,11] The local prothrombotic milieu that can be implicated for a higher thrombosis risk includes raw leaflet surface of the THV, de-endothelialized native leaflets exposing tissue factor, altered flow dynamics in and around neo-sinus leading to flow stasis, or deranged hemodynamic shear forces.[12-16] Continuing antithrombotic therapy for the duration it takes for the THV to endothelialize may partially help mitigate the thrombosis risk. For this hypothesis, earlier expert consensus recommended short-term OAC or dual antiplatelet therapy (DAPT). Clinical factors such as atrial fibrillation (AF), atherosclerotic cardiovascular disease, or poor left ventricular systolic function impose additional thrombotic risk, which must be dealt with as per the standard practice guidelines. Unfortunately, other than continuing OAC in AF, the role of antithrombotic therapy in preventing thromboembolism post TAVI is not well established.

Overview of Bioprosthetic Valve Thrombosis

Unlike thrombosis of mechanical prosthetic valves, BVT typically presents as focal or diffuse leaflet thickening, which may or may not impact leaflet motion. On a four-dimensional (4D) computed tomography (CT) scan, BVT can be seen as hypoattenuating leaflet thickening (HALT), which may be associated with a reduction in leaflet motion (RELM), in which case HALT is classified as hypoattenuation affecting motion (HAM) when >50% of leaflet motion is affected.[17] BVT can be categorized as clinical if associated with elevated transvalvular gradients or thromboembolism, or subclinical if diagnosed incidentally on imaging.

While BVT can be seen in 7–40% of all TAVI cases, only 3% or less are associated with altered valve hemodynamics or embolism. Risk factors for BVT include valve-in-valve TAVI, balloon expandable (intra-annular) THV, >20% oversizing of the THV, patient–prosthesis mismatch, and large sinuses of Valsalva. Additionally, male gender and obesity have also been found to increase the risk of leaflet thrombosis.[18] BVT can be seen as early as 3 days post THV implantation or may occur very late in the course, and at times resolves without any intervention.[18-20] The clinical impact of BVT has yet to be fully elucidated. Few observational studies correlated BVT with higher transvalvular gradients and early valve degeneration.[21-23] Conversely, substudies of landmark randomized trials and, most recently, 2-year follow-up data from the LRT study did not show such a signal.[24] A histological study suggested a time-dependent leaflet thickening in all explanted valves, likely resulting in early valve degeneration.[25] Concern for BVT associated with a higher incidence of thromboembolism was raised in a substudy of the PARTNER 3 trial, while data from Evolut Low Risk trial showed the contrary.[19,20] A subsequent meta-analysis of 3,621 patients demonstrated that BVT was associated with a 2.6-fold higher risk of cerebrovascular events.[18]

To summarize, the majority of BVT seen post TAVI are subclinical. The impact of BVT on both short-term and long-term valve function remains undetermined. Similarly, an association between BVT and cerebrovascular events needs to be better established. It is prudent to start OAC in clinical valve thrombosis, accounting for 0.6–2.8% of all TAVI cases. However, uncertainty exists in defining treatment goals for subclinical BVT cases and the net clinical implication of OAC therapy in this patient subset. Accumulated evidence does suggest that upfront OAC leads to reduced incidence of BVT, but its effect on clinical endpoints such as valve degeneration or reduction in thromboembolism remains to be seen.

Oral Anticoagulants in Post-transcatheter Aortic Valve Implantation Patients without an Existing Indication

Oral anticoagulant was found to reduce the incidence of BVT by >50% and may lead to a marginally lower decrease in the aortic valve area but similar short-term valve performance and clinical outcome without an increase in major bleeding complications.[18,26-28] In patients with BVT, the use of OAC is associated with the resolution of leaflet thrombosis in 94% of the cases, as opposed to spontaneous resolution in only 8% of the patients.[18] The patient cohort of the PARTNER 2 trial who continued VKA therapy had a lower stroke rate at 6 months without a corresponding increase in bleeding events.[27] The LRT 2.0 trial showed that warfarin, added to aspirin therapy, led to a lower incidence of composite clinical outcome, driven mainly by a lower incidence of HALT, RELM, and HAM without a decrease in hemodynamic gradient or higher bleeding complications.[28] Based on these observations, many early operators chose to prescribe OAC for 3–6 months post TAVI. Nevertheless, over time, it was learned that VKA use was associated with a higher risk of significant bleeding and possibly mortality, which must be weighed against its anticipated benefits.[21,23]

Observational data from RESOLVE and SAVORY registries showed similar efficacy of NOAC and VKA in reducing BVT, although the registries had patients with varied comorbidities, including AF.[22] The GALILEO trial tested the role of low-dose rivaroxaban (10 mg daily) combined with aspirin in patients post TAVI who lacked an established indication for OAC. The trial was stopped early due to a higher risk of death, thrombosis, and bleeding in the treatment arm.[29] Edoxaban use, compared to DAPT in the ADAPT-TAVI trial, was associated with a lower incidence of BVT but no difference in clinical outcomes.[30] REDOX-TAVI is an ongoing study evaluating the role of Edoxaban in this subset (NCT04171726).

Overall, data consistently shows that OAC reduces the incidence of subclinical BVT, but the clinical outcome remains unchanged. Added to the fact that OAC is associated with higher bleeding and mortality, a risk–reward ratio does not favor its use in all post-TAVI patients. Using OAC in a selective subgroup with a high thrombotic risk profile may be intuitive. However, such risk criteria are not well defined. The current guidelines have a weak recommendation or recommend against using OAC in patients who otherwise do not have a concurrent condition requiring long-term OAC. Antithrombotic strategies and key excerpts of recent guidelines are mentioned in **Box 1**.

Antiplatelet Agents in Post-transcatheter Aortic Valve Implantation Patients without an Existing Indication

Observations from randomized clinical trials as well as meta-analyses failed to show any benefit of DAPT over single antiplatelet therapy (SAPT) in reducing BVT or thromboembolic events such as stroke or myocardial infarction. SAPT may even reduce net adverse clinical events by reducing the risk of bleeding.[18,31-34] Consistently, a recent meta-analysis showed that SAPT reduced the risk of bleeding by more than half when compared to DAPT or OAC, without a corresponding increase in ischemic events.[35]

The older expert consensus recommendation of DAPT for 3–6 months post TAVI was primarily deductive in nature. The recent guidelines took cognizance of the available data, following which DAPT has been retroceded to a class 2b indication in the 2020 American College of Cardiology/American Heart Association (ACC/AHA) guidelines.[1] The 2021 European Society of Cardiology (ESC) guidelines too recommended SAPT as a class 1 recommendation,[36] modified from the older version when DAPT was the preferred option.[37]

The choice of a single antiplatelet agent remains unsettled. Low-dose aspirin had traditionally been the drug of choice for antiplatelet monotherapy, but recent insights from the OCEAN-TAVI registry pointed out that clopidogrel monotherapy may be superior to aspirin monotherapy, with or without an OAC, in reducing cardiovascular mortality.[38] Newer antiplatelet agents, namely ticagrelor or prasugrel, are associated with sustained suppression of high platelet reactivity, which in turn is associated with higher bleeding

BOX 1 Summary of antithrombotic therapy in patients with transcatheter aortic valve implantation.

Preoperative

- SAPT, preferably low-dose aspirin, to be started much before anticipated TAVI procedure[3]
- Clopidogrel loading before procedure likely of no benefit[5]
- If patient is already on long-term OAC, no need for therapy interruption[6]
  - In such cases, antiplatelet therapy does not need to be added unless recent ACS or PCI
- Newer antiplatelets agents likely of no benefit and may cause harm[39]

Intraoperative

- Maintain a target ACT between 250 and 300 ms[3]
- No benefit of bivalirudin over heparin; use only in true heparin allergy[7]
- Heparin reversal using time-adjusted or ACT-adjusted protamine dosing may be beneficial[8]

Postoperative and long-term

No baseline indication for antithrombotic therapy:

- SAPT, preferably low-dose aspirin lifelong[1,3,36]
- DAPT or VKA for the first 3 months if low bleeding risk (LOR 2b).[1] The ESC recommends against routine use of OAC (LOR 3)[36]
- Rivaroxaban 10 mg daily in combination with low-dose aspirin is contraindicated[1]

Baseline indications for OAC present:

- VKA may be preferred over NOAC for the first 3 months, particularly if new-onset AF (LOR 2a)[1]
- NOAC after 3 months of TAVI may be reasonable. This suggestion is an extension based on the original recommendation in the SAVR subset[1,36]
- No need for antiplatelet therapy unless recent ACS or PCI[3,36]

Baseline indications for antiplatelets present:

- Antiplatelet therapy should be chosen based on the underlying condition, as per relevant guidelines
- Abbreviated DAPT therapy may be preferred wherever feasible

Baseline indications for antiplatelets and OAC present:

- If perceived bleeding risk is higher than that of stent thrombosis:[3,36]
  - Aspirin to be stopped in ≤7 days
  - P2Y12 inhibitor (preferably clopidogrel) for 6 months (12 months in case of ACS) (a shorter therapy duration of clopidogrel for 1–3 months for CCS and 3–6 months for ACS may be chosen for highest bleeding risk subset)
- If perceived stent thrombosis risk is high: Triple therapy with aspirin, clopidogrel, and OAC should be <1 month[36]
- In patients receiving OAC, antiplatelet therapy should be discontinued beyond 12 months of therapy[36]

Miscellaneous

- If patients develop stroke after TAVI while being on antiplatelet agents, VKA therapy can be considered (LOR 2b)[1]
- Selective use of OAC in patients with confirmed HALT and restricted leaflet motion with elevated gradients should be considered (LOR 2a)[36]

(ACS: acute coronary syndrome; ACT: activated clotting time; AF: atrial fibrillation; CCS: chronic coronary syndrome; DAPT: dual antiplatelet therapy; ESC: European Society of Cardiology; HALT: hypoattenuating leaflet thickening; LOR: level of recommendation; NOAC: novel oral anticoagulant; OAC: oral anticoagulant therapy; PCI: percutaneous coronary intervention; SAPT: single antiplatelet therapy; SAVR: surgical aortic valve replacement; TAVI: transcatheter aortic valve implantation; VKA: vitamin K antagonist)

events.[39,40] Caution is advised against using these newer drugs in TAVI patients at high bleeding risk. Results from the REACTIC-TAVI trial proposing ticagrelor monotherapy post TAVI are awaited (NCT02817789).

Most recently, a registry analysis called into question the very need for any antithrombotic therapy following TAVI. The study showed that patients who did not receive antithrombotic therapy, compared to those who did, had a similar net adverse clinical event.[41] Findings from this study may support a clinical decision to defer antithrombotic therapy altogether in patients post TAVI who are deemed very high bleeding risk.

Oral Anticoagulants in Post-transcatheter Aortic Valve Implantation Patients with an Existing Indication

Atrial fibrillation remains the most common indication for long-term OAC therapy post TAVI. VKA or NOAC can be used for stroke prevention in patients with nonvalvular AF, whereas VKA is the preferred agent in valvular AF. Recent data supported the use of NOAC in patients with AF with a bioprosthetic surgical valve replacement or a repair.[42] While large observational and registry-based data[43-45] suggested that NOAC may be associated with a lower bleeding risk in patients with AF and TAVI, recent randomized trials failed to show such benefit.[29,30,46] Apixaban in patients post TAVI with an established indication for OAC led to reduced BVT but higher noncardiovascular mortality and no difference in a composite endpoint of ischemic and bleeding events.[46] Similarly, edoxaban was associated with higher bleeding compared to VKA with similar efficacy endpoints.[47]

When added to VKA or OAC, antiplatelet therapy adds bleeding risk without concomitant benefit in ischemic events.[48,49] The ESC guidelines recommend OAC alone unless the patient had a recent coronary intervention and do not give any preference to VKA or NOAC. The ACC/AHA guidelines recommend VKA in patients with new-onset AF within 3 months of the TAVI procedure.[1] In patients with a surgical bioprosthesis, NOAC is recommended over VKA after 3 months following surgical implantation of the valve.[1,36] Deducing a similar analogy, it may be prudent to continue VKA for a minimum of 3 months following TAVI, after which consideration to switch from VKA to NOAC can be given.

Antiplatelet Agents in Post-transcatheter Aortic Valve Implantation Patients with an Existing Indication

Patients who underwent a recent coronary intervention should continue antiplatelet therapy per the established guidelines. Limiting DAPT for 6 months in case of chronic coronary syndrome (CCS) and for 12 months in acute coronary syndrome (ACS) seems reasonable unless the perceived risk for stent thrombosis is very high. If additional therapy with an OAC is desired for a baseline indication as well, it is advisable to limit the duration of triple therapy to the shortest possible time.[3] Typically, aspirin is stopped in ≤7 days while clopidogrel and OAC are continued. It is recommended that OAC alone should be continued beyond 12 months. Refer to **Box 1** for further details.

CONCLUSION

Longevity of the THV and cerebrovascular events remain the Achilles heel of expanding TAVI use in the low-risk patient subset. By virtue of preventing thrombosis, antithrombotic therapy is poised to address both concerns. Unfortunately, the clinical results from the available data have been underwhelming. Propensity-matched data would suggest that midterm thromboembolic outcomes in TAVI patients may be attributed to baseline comorbidities. This also supports the hypothesis that TAVI-related thrombosis is multifactorial and antithrombotic therapy in itself is less likely to have a significant impact on clinical outcome. Added to the fact that TAVI patients are at higher risk for bleeding, the theme of "less is more" seems wise. A multipronged approach addressing a patient's clinical aspects in a longitudinal fashion using robust scientific vigor is the need of the hour. Above all, we should follow the dictum of primum non nocere.

ONLINE REFERENCES

Please scan the QR code provided at the end of the table of contents for References of this chapter.

CHAPTER 188

Complications of Transcatheter Aortic Valve Implantation and its Management

Sengottuvelu G, Senthilraj Thangasami

ABSTRACT

Since the first-in-man experience in 2002, transcatheter aortic valve replacement (TAVR) has revolutionized the treatment of severe symptomatic aortic stenosis. With progressive improvement in pertinent equipment and techniques, transcatheter aortic valve implantation (TAVI) has become a widely accepted procedure with the application of newer strategies such as routine use of conscious sedation, single arterial access approach, newer implantation techniques, use of novel technologies such as intravascular lithotripsy, and refinement of valve-bioprosthesis devices and has resulted in a dramatic reduction of complications. As the indication for TAVR is steadily moving toward lower-risk patients, an even stronger focus on the early diagnosis, adequate management, and prevention of these complications will be required for comparable results with surgical aortic valve replacement (SAVR). We hereby aim to summarize the most common complications associated with TAVR, their effective management, and their prevention.

Keywords: TAVI, complications, vascular access, preplanning TAVI.

INTRODUCTION

In the past few decades, transcatheter aortic valve replacement (TAVR) has been established as a standard therapy for patients with severe aortic stenosis (AS) across the entire spectrum of surgical risk patients. The advancement in device engineering and operator experience has made TAVR a safe procedure, resulting in a broader indication for patients undergoing valve replacement. However, perioperative complications still can occur with resultant significant mortality and morbidity. Knowledge of prevention and management of complications can have a significant impact on procedural success. In this chapter, we review the possible complications of the TAVR procedure **(Flowchart 1)** with a specific focus on strategies for their prevention and management.

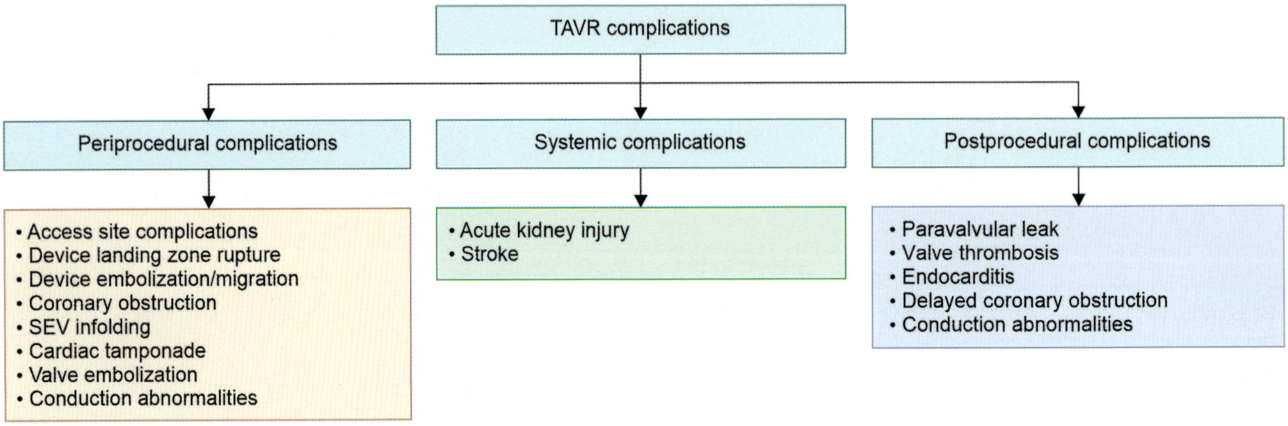

FLOWCHART 1: Schematic representation of transcatheter aortic valve replacement (TAVR) complications.

(SEV: self-expandable valve)

ACCESS SITE COMPLICATIONS

Establishing safe vascular access marks the first step in a successful TAVR procedure. The most common approach is the transfemoral approach, which has been shown to reduce morbidity and mortality in TAVR. In patients who are not suitable for transfemoral access, other approaches available include transaxillary/subclavian, transcarotid, transapical, and transcaval approaches.[1] As large-bore sheaths are used for vascular access, vascular complications are one of the major concerns in TAVR. According to the updated standard Valve Academic Research Consortium (VARC) definitions, vascular complication rates during TAVR range between 10 and 20%.[2] Vascular access complications **(Table 1)** can have a major influence on adverse outcomes after TAVR. Female gender, peripheral vascular disease with a decreased femoral diameter and/or circumferential calcification patterns, a sheath-to-femoral artery ratio of <1.05 or if the sheath diameter is more than the minimal femoral diameter, severe iliofemoral tortuosity with score > 21.2, operator experience, and planned surgical cut-down are considered independent predictors of vascular complications.[3]

Vessel dissection, vessel rupture, access site hematoma, and pseudoaneurysms are all possible complications encountered during or after TAVR **(Figs. 1 and 2)**. The incidence of dissection of the common femoral artery (CFA) or iliac arteries ranges between 1.6 and 21.4% for a complete percutaneous transfemoral approach and 2 and 7% for a surgical cut-down approach.[5] Dissections occur most likely in the external iliac artery during initial vascular access or while advancing the delivery system. They may not be observed until sheath withdrawal, and retrograde or contralateral antegrade angiography prior to completion of TAVR usually reveals these access site injuries. Fatal iliofemoral rupture is observed in 0.7% to up to 9.3% of TAVR procedures.[6] When a large-bore sheath is inserted in small, calcified vessels, it can lead to arterial avulsion and is often detected after sheath withdrawal, as the sheath usually seals the tear during the valve implantation. Access site hematomas are relatively common, with an incidence of 2.2–12.5%. Retroperitoneal hematoma or hemorrhage occurs with an overall incidence of up to 2.2%, and it can be due to aortic, iliac, inferior epigastric, or femoral injury and often presents with nonspecific symptoms of groin, flank, or back pain with or without hemodynamic changes. Pseudoaneurysm formation can occur in 2–6% of cases due to contained rupture with extravascular bleeding into a pseudo-capsule and present with a pulsatile mass in the groin. Access site infections range up to 6.3%. Closure device failure can occur in up to 4.4–8.7% of cases and can cause arterial dissection, rupture, and vascular constriction or

TABLE 1: Valve Academic Research Consortium-2 classification of vascular access site and access-related complications.[4]

Complication	Definition
Major vascular complications	• Any aortic dissection, aortic rupture, annulus rupture, left ventricle perforation, or new apical aneurysm/pseudoaneurysm • Access site or access-related vascular injury (dissection, stenosis, perforation, rupture, arteriovenous fistula, pseudoaneurysm, hematoma, irreversible nerve injury, compartment syndrome, percutaneous closure device failure) leading to death, life-threatening or major bleeding*, visceral ischemia, or neurological impairment • Distal embolization (noncerebral) from a vascular source requiring surgery or resulting in amputation or irreversible* end-organ damage • The use of unplanned endovascular or surgical intervention associated with death, major bleeding, visceral ischemia, or neurological impairment • Any new ipsilateral lower extremity ischemia documented by patient symptoms, physical exam, and/or decreased or absent blood flow on lower extremity angiogram • Surgery for access site-related nerve injury or permanent access site-related nerve injury
Minor vascular complications	• Access site or access-related vascular injury (dissection, stenosis, perforation, rupture, arteriovenous fistula, pseudoaneurysm, hematomas, percutaneous closure device failure leading to death, life-threatening or major bleeding visceral ischemia, or neurological impairment) • Distal embolization treated with embolectomy and/or thrombectomy and not resulting in amputation or irreversible end-organ damage • Any unplanned endovascular stenting or unplanned surgical intervention not meeting the criteria for a major vascular complication • Vascular repair or the need for vascular repair (via surgery, ultrasound-guided compression, transcatheter embolization, or stent graft)
Percutaneous closure device failure	Failure of a closure device to achieve hemostasis at the arteriotomy site leading to alternate treatment (other than manual compression or adjunctive endovascular ballooning)

*Refer to standard VARC Bleeding definition.[4]

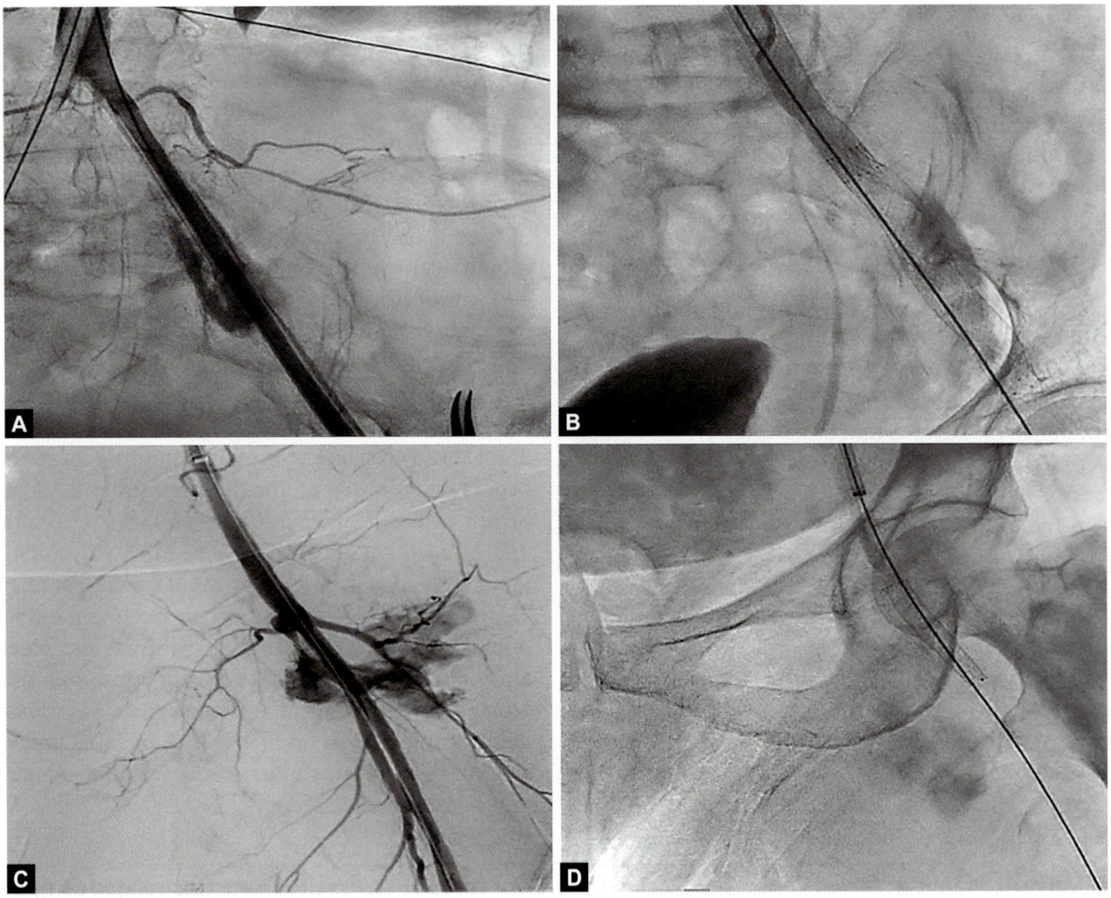

FIGS. 1A TO D: (A and B) Left common iliac artery rupture sealed by two covered stents. (C and D) Left deep femoral artery perforation sealed by covered stent.
Courtesy: Dr Sengottuvelu G, Apollo Hospitals, Chennai, India.

occlusion.[1] A desired approach to locate the optimal zone for arterial puncture is ultrasound-guided access. A linear ultrasound probe can help determine the height of the femoral bifurcation and exclude anterior wall calcification in the puncture zone. Compressibility of the femoral vein helps in differentiating from the artery. Real-time needle guidance can reduce the risk of a posterior wall or sidewall puncture. The fluoroscopic target zone for safe CFA puncture **(Figs. 3A to C)** can be done in anterior-posterior projection between the centerline of the femoral head and a caudal 14-mm margin avoiding both the femoral bifurcation and retroperitoneal vessels **(Figs. 3A to C)**. Additionally, a pigtail catheter positioned from contralateral access can act as a marker for safe puncture.[7] A low puncture distal to the femoral bifurcation should be avoided, as it bears a risk for pseudoaneurysm, arteriovenous fistula, dissection, rupture, or thrombus formation. A high puncture involving the external iliac artery or inferior epigastric artery will prevent achieving adequate hemostasis and can increase the risk of retroperitoneal bleeding by 18-fold. Primary vascular access should usually be performed using a micropuncture needle and a 4–5 F sheath to avoid large-bore needle trauma in case of an unsuccessful puncture. After confirmation of proper puncture, larger sheaths can be exchanged over a standard guidewire. Subclavian access is a frequent alternative site in patients with difficult femoral sites and is usually performed from the left side for better valve alignment. The transaxillary approach is commonly performed through a surgical cut-down, although a fully percutaneous method is feasible by puncturing the proximal one-third of the axillary artery.[8] The main advantage of the transcarotid approach is the short distance to the native aortic valve with anatomically facilitated coaxial alignment, but there is a risk of stroke, injury to nerve structures, and the respiratory tract in proximity. Transaortic access is performed through a right anterior minithoracotomy or a median hemisternotomy. Transcaval access is done via femoral venous access. At the level of the inferior vena cava, an arteriovenous fistula is created by using electrocautery over a coronary guidewire, and the transcatheter valve implantation is then carried out in a standard manner. The iatrogenic fistula can be closed with an Amplatzer PDA occluder or a covered stent. Vascular complications with the transcaval approach can range up to 20%.[1]

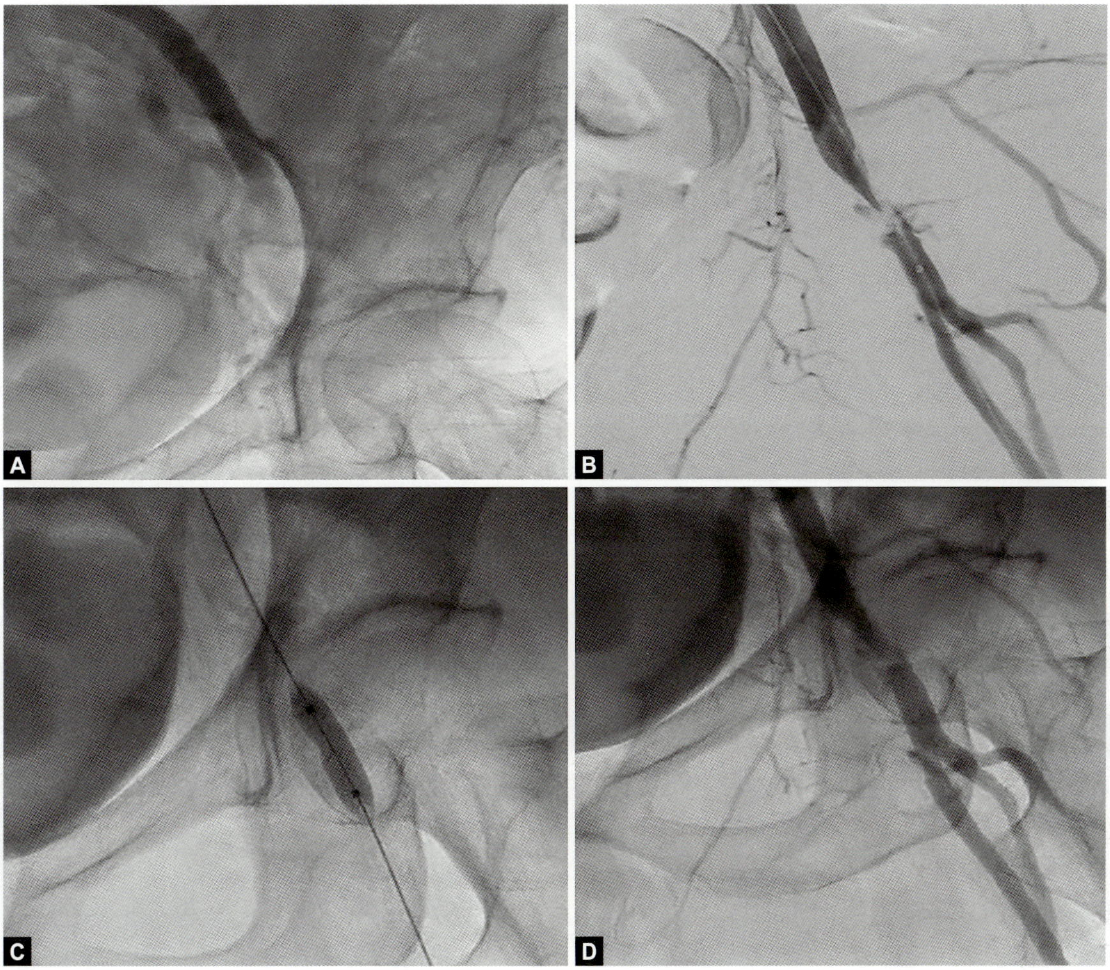

FIGS. 2A TO D: Left femoral artery occlusion after using two proglides, treated with prolonged balloon dilatation.
Courtesy: Dr Sengottuvelu G, Apollo Hospitals, Chennai, India.

Prevention and Management

Preprocedural assessment of the access arteries plays a key role in selecting the best strategy and in minimizing vascular complications. Contrast-enhanced multidetector computed tomography (MDCT) helps in deciding the safe access by assessing the tortuosity, skin-to-artery distance, iliofemoral vessel minimal lumen diameters > 5.5 mm, the position of the femoral bifurcation relative to the femoral head, calcification load, and the pattern of distribution. When feasible, transradial access can be considered for aortography and pigtail positioning. In comparison to the conventional bifemoral approach, using a transradial approach is associated with a significant reduction in vascular complications. In the presence of iliofemoral severe calcific stenosis, peripheral intravascular shockwave lithotripsy (IVL) can facilitate transfemoral access. Computed tomography (CT) evaluation of alternative access sites should be undertaken in case both iliofemoral arteries are not suitable for access. The routine practice of diagnostic crossover angiography to assess aortic or iliofemoral vascular complications after sheath removal aids in the prompt diagnosis of access site complications.[9] Arteriotomy closure devices, either suture-based or plug-based devices, should be used to close the access site securely.[8] These devices have been shown to shorten the time to hemostasis and time to ambulation. Vascular Doppler, CT aortogram, or angiography should be performed if there are clinical signs of ischemia, acute-onset leg or back pain, or hemodynamic deterioration. Asymptomatic small dissections with no flow limitation can be managed conservatively with close follow-up. If there is a compromised blood flow, angioplasty with prolonged balloon inflation may suffice for intima-media reapposition. However, extensive dissection requires uncovered or covered stent implantation or surgical exploration. Fatal iliofemoral rupture warrants immediate covered stent-graft implantation, interposition grafting, or a surgical patch repair. Bleeding from smaller tears can resolve in a couple of minutes with occlusion and anticoagulation reversal. Access site hematomas can appear either immediately after reversal or gradually over hours

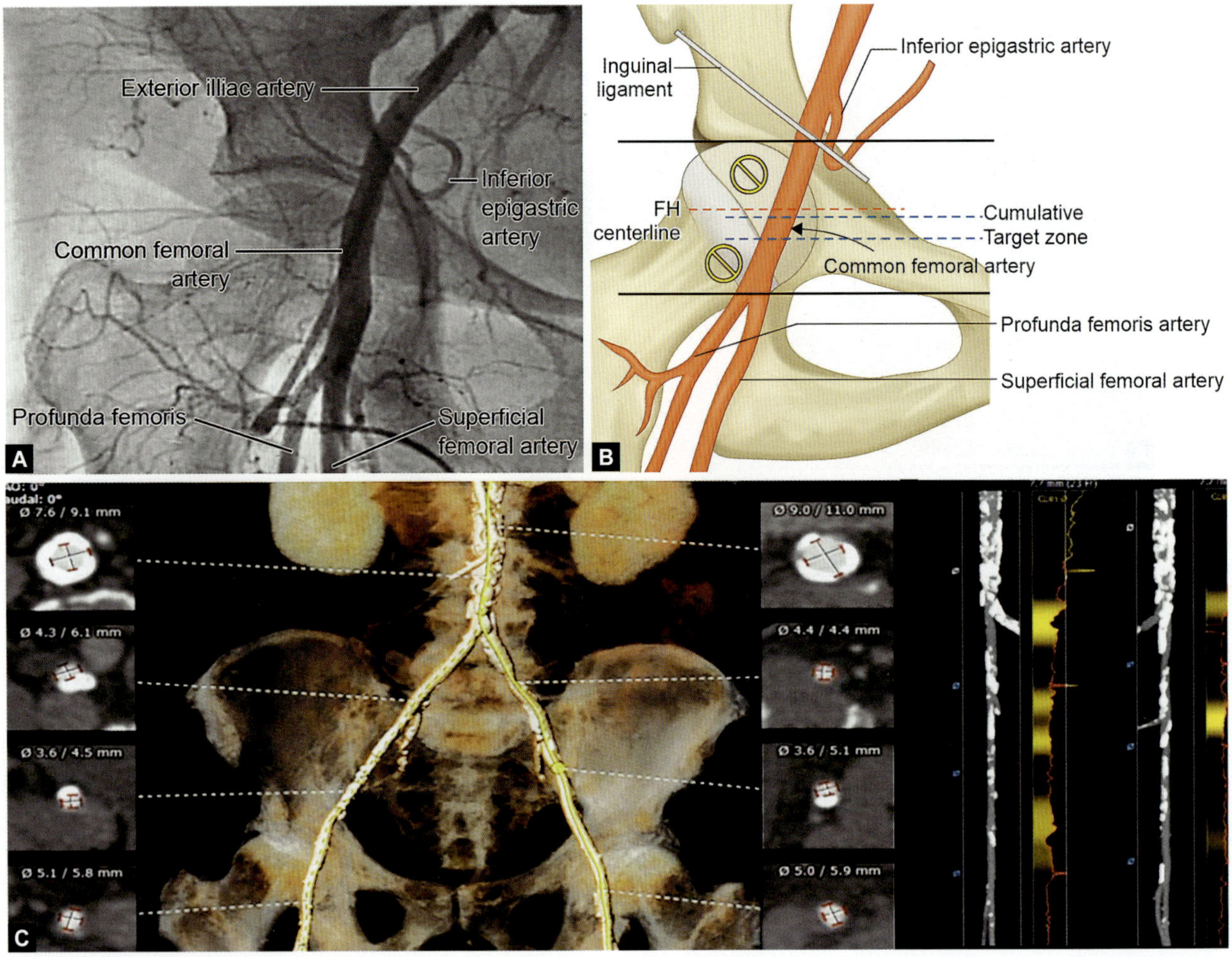

FIGS. 3A TO C: (A) Fluoroscopic and (B) schematic illustration of the ideal common femoral artery puncture site. (C) Heavily calcified femoral arteries precluding transfemoral transcatheter aortic valve replacement (TAVR).

Source: (A and B) With permission from Mach et al. (2021).[1]

to days after the procedure, despite manual compression and anticoagulation reversal. They are generally benign, with spontaneous resolution over weeks, but can lead to secondary infection, prolonged hospital stays, need for blood transfusion, and increased mortality. Hematomas can be managed conservatively in most cases. If oozing or active bleeding from the puncture site is apparent, manual compression and anticoagulation reversal should be performed immediately.[5] In case of a retroperitoneal hemorrhage, depending on the size and location of the bleeding, coil embolization for ruptured small vessels and covert stent-graft implantation or surgical repair in case of larger ruptures are indicated. Spontaneous thrombosis is common in patients with small pseudoaneurysms (3.0–3.5 cm), without the need for anticoagulation. Large pseudoaneurysms can cause progressive discomfort, septic embolism, local infection, and rupture. Ultrasound-guided thrombin injection is favored over ultrasound-guided compression in treating large pseudoaneurysms. A larger pseudoaneurysm is not amenable to thrombin injection and requires interventional or surgical occlusion. Access site superficial infections respond well to local or systemic therapy if treated early. Surgical debridement and vacuum-assisted therapy are the main therapeutic treatment options for deep wound infections. In case of closure device failure, manual compression alone is sufficient in most cases. If limb ischemia is suspected, vascular Doppler, CT angiography, or angiography may be needed to verify unrestricted blood flow. Stent deployment or balloon angioplasty may be indicated in case of severe vascular stenosis or bleeding.[1]

DEVICE LANDING ZONE RUPTURE

Device landing zone (DLZ) encompasses the aortic annulus, aortic sinus, aortic root, and left ventricular outflow tract (LVOT). Injuries to the DLZ **(Figs. 4A to D)** are one of the most feared TAVR complications because they can lead to immediate hemodynamic collapse with high mortality. The

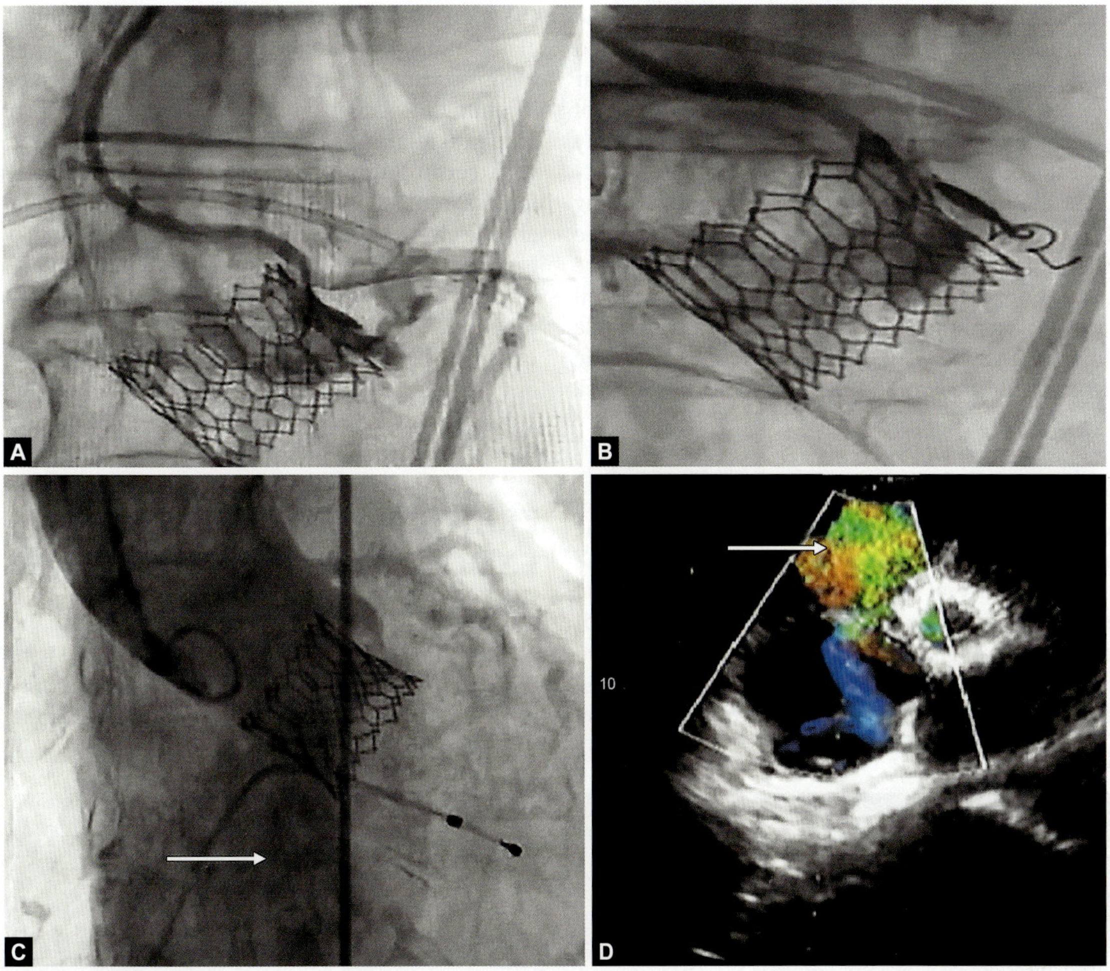

FIGS. 4A TO D: (A and B) Annular rupture caused by balloon-expandable valve treated with coil embolization. (C and D) Angiography and echocardiogram showing right coronary cusp rupture to right ventricle.

Courtesy: (A and B) Dr John Jose, Christian Medical College, Vellore. (C and D) Dr Sengottuvelu G, Apollo Hospitals, Chennai, India.

reported incidence of DLZ rupture is up to 0.5–1%. The most common anatomic site of rupture is the aortic annulus, followed by the sinus of Valsalva (16%), LVOT (10%), and sinotubular junction (6%). Self-expanding valves (SEVs) have a lesser chance of landing zone rupture in comparison to balloon-expandable valves (BEVs). Risk factors for rupture include heavy DLZ calcifications, shallow sinuses of Valsalva, small aortic annulus (<20 mm), bicuspid aortic valve, device over-sizing (>20%), annular eccentricity, long-term immunosuppressive therapy, and severe asymmetric subannular left ventricle (LV) hypertrophy along with LVOT calcification.[10] Annular rupture can occur with frank extravasation or be contained, as manifested by new periaortic hematoma. DLZ injury and rupture may occur during predilatation of the native aortic valve with a balloon, prosthetic valve deployment, or during post-dilatation of the valve for paravalvular leakage (PVL).[11]

Strategies to Prevent Device Landing Zone Rupture

The accurate annulus and landing zone sizing is a critical step during the preprocedure assessment. Each transcatheter heart valve (THV) is designed with specific annular dimensions. Annulus estimation by a 2D transthoracic echocardiogram can result in inaccurate measurements due to the asymmetric shape. Cardiac CT sizing and 3D transesophageal echocardiography (TEE) is the preferred technique and gives accurate, reproducible measurements for annular sizing. The maximum and minimum annulus areas should be assessed and measured, typically in a systolic phase. Cardiac magnetic resonance imaging (MRI) has an emerging role in annular sizing, especially in patients with renal dysfunction. In cases where multislice computed tomography (MSCT) measurements are not possible, aortography and balloon sizing can be performed to confirm the absence of lateral aortic regurgitation (AR) with fully inflated balloons of known sizes.[12] All THVs are sized by the annular area or perimeter. Additional measurements of the sinus of Valsalva diameter and height from the annular plane may be required in some cases. In high-risk anatomies, a self-expandable valve is preferred with exercising caution during pre- and post-dilatation. If a BEV is required, then a degree of underfilling should be considered. In patients with severe LVOT calcification, high implantation should be considered to decrease the radial force of the valve on the vulnerable LVOT. Valve oversizing (>20%) is a risk factor for aortic rupture and should be avoided in patients with high-risk features.[11]

Diagnosis and Management

The clinical manifestation can range from asymptomatic to immediate hemodynamic collapse, depending on the location and severity of the injury. Rupture should be suspected if there is a new-onset pericardial effusion, hemodynamic changes, aortic wall thickening or dissection, hematoma between the aorta and pulmonary artery, or a new intracardiac shunt such as a ventricular septal defect (VSD). TEE can identify annular rupture as well as associated paravalvular regurgitation. Angiography can also help identify ruptures. The treatment for rupture depends on the location, the sequelae of the injury, and the type of rupture. The immediate goal is to maintain hemodynamic stability, with cardiopulmonary bypass initiation, usually via the femoral route. For uncontained ruptures, surgical repair and aortic valve replacement are the preferred strategy.[13] In the case of supra-annular injury, aorta repair is needed, and in the case of subannular injury, LVOT repair with patching is required. For small lesions, such as a periaortic hematoma, conservative therapy may be considered, with reversal of anticoagulation and close surveillance. Percutaneous coil embolization or the use of vascular plugs is amenable in select cases and should be considered if feasible.[11]

TRANSCATHETER VALVE EMBOLIZATION/TRANSCATHETER VALVE MIGRATION

Transcatheter valve embolization (TVE) **(Figs. 5A to F)** is defined as the permanent loss of contact of the valve prosthesis with the annulus afterdeployment. The reported

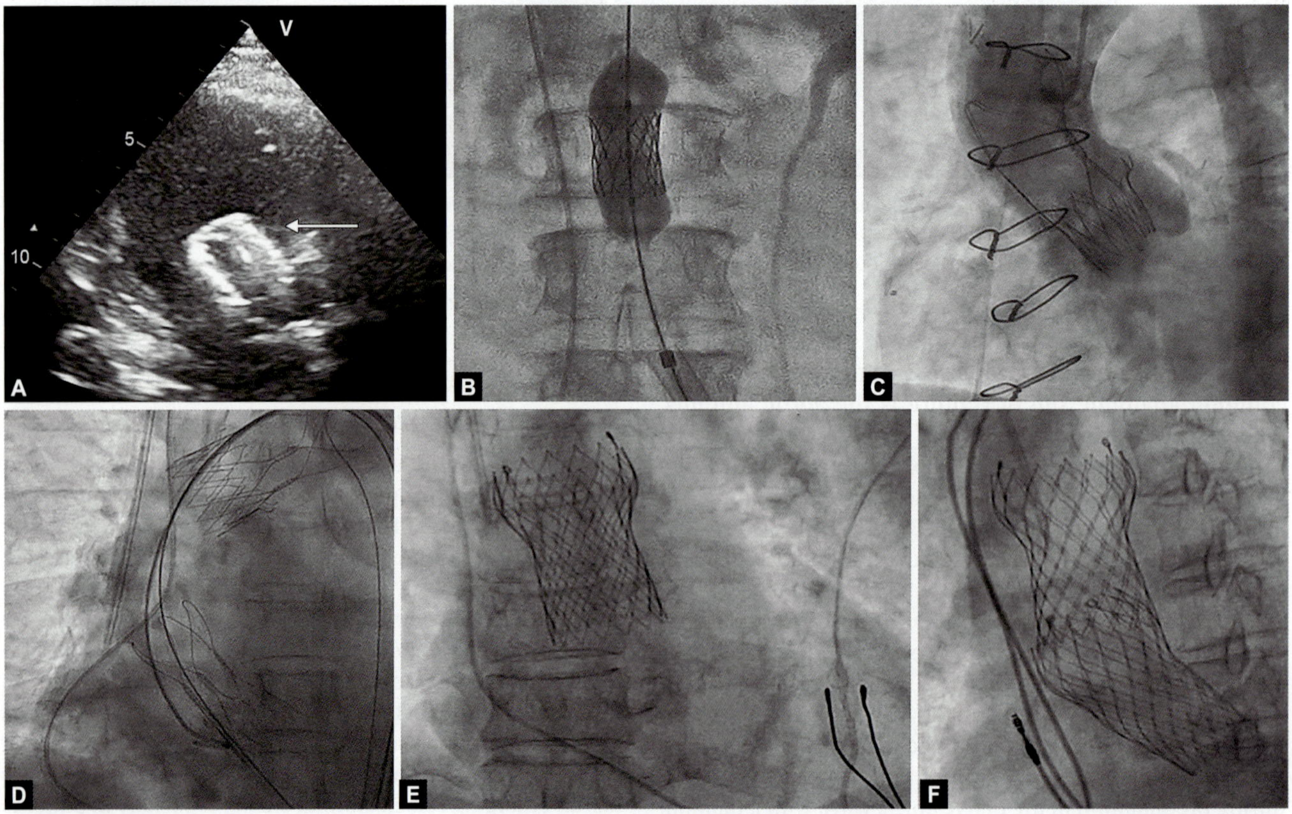

FIGS. 5A TO F: (A) Echo showing embolized valve in the left ventricle (LV). (B) Embolized balloon-expandable valve deployed in infrarenal abdominal aorta. (C) ACURATE neo 2 valve migration just above annulus. (C and D) ACURATE neo 2 valve pop-out managed with another ACURATE neo 2 valve. (E and F) Evolut R embolization in aorta side managed with another valve.

Courtesy: Dr Sengottuvelu G, Apollo Hospitals, Chennai, India.

incidence is up to 1% and is associated with a high risk of postprocedural morbidity, mortality, and the need for conversion to open heart surgery. TVE can occur in either the ventricular or the aortic direction and commonly occurs during the periprocedural period, although delayed migration (>24 hours post-procedure) has also been reported. The valve most commonly embolizes to the ascending aorta but can also embolize to the LV or descending aorta. The risk factors for embolization include significant aortic tortuosity, excessively small or large annuli, LVOT hypertrophy, complete absence of calcification, or the presence of heavy calcification and pure AR.[14]

Transcatheter heart valve migration (TVM) is the displacement of the valve from the deployed position with varying degrees. It can occur within minutes or even days after implantation. Malpositioning accounts for 50% of the cases of THV migration/embolization and is the most common cause. Other causes are improper valve manipulation and the delivery system, improper positioning of the wire, bicuspid valve, significant valve undersizing, and rapid pacing failure. Aortic embolization occurs as a result of the valve deployment in a high position and/or poor coaxial alignment of the device to the valve plane during implantation. Caudal migration toward the ventricle side usually occurs because of low implantation depth, eccentric and asymmetric calcification, and rarely because of the device undersizing.[15]

Prevention and Management

As most of the causes are technical, embolization/migration can be avoided with proper planning and precautionary measures. Ensuring a stable temporary pacemaker lead position and capture before valve crossing and deployment is essential to avoid loss of capture during valve deployment. Avoiding valve undersizing by proper MSCT assessment is essential. When encountering bicuspid aortic valve stenosis with heavy calcifications, THV with increased radial strength should be selected to avoid device underexpansion and subsequent risk of TVE/TVM. Following valve deployment, caution should be taken during retraction of the device's nose cone as well as the jailed pigtail catheter, which should be removed with the aid of a 0.035″ wire.[16]

The treatment strategy depends on the embolized location. If embolization is complicated by obstruction of coronaries, immediate proximal retraction of the device should be performed. If the valve has embolized to the LV, open surgery is required for removal; however, there are reports of balloon-assisted retrieval and a second attempt at reimplantation after identifying the cause. A BEV can typically be maneuvered with a balloon in place, while SEVs usually require snares. During the repositioning of an embolized BEV, the ventricular guidewire position should always be maintained within the valve to prevent valve inversion and potential flow obstruction. In prohibitive surgical risk patients, where surgery is not an option, dragging the embolized valve into a subannular position using a partially inflated balloon and deploying under rapid ventricular pacing can be an option. Maintaining coaxial wire positioning is of utmost importance during this maneuver.[11] A second valve can then be implanted, partially overlapping and anchoring the dislocated valve to prevent distal migration. The preferred location to deploy an embolized aortic valve on the aortic side is the descending aorta, distal to the left subclavian artery such that major aortic branches are avoided. However, in tortuous, heavily diseased or calcified aortas, the risk of aortic injury during repositioning maneuvers is high, and deploying the valve at a more proximal position can be considered and was found to not be associated with an elevated stroke risk. There are few reports of implanting a covered stent across the embolized valve, but this is not typically required as the second prosthesis in the aorta does not appear to cause any hemodynamic consequences. After the embolized valve is deployed in a stable position, a second THV implantation can be tried by traversing through the first valve and realigning with the annulus.[17]

CORONARY OBSTRUCTION

The coronary obstruction incidence is <1% for native valve TAVR and increases up to 3.5% for valve-in-valve (ViV TAVR). It presents acutely during the procedure with hypotension, ischemic electrocardiogram (ECG) changes in 50% of cases and ventricular arrhythmias in 25% of cases. Most of the cases usually involve the left coronary ostium. Acute coronary obstruction after TAVR is a potentially devasting complication **(Figs. 6A to C)**, with as much as 50% mortality. High-risk anatomical features for coronary obstruction include the presence of narrow shallow aortic sinuses (<30 mm) and low coronary ostia (<10 mm). For patients undergoing ViV TAVR, the surgically implanted valves with the highest risk of coronary obstruction include stented bioprostheses with externally mounted leaflets (e.g., St Jude Medical Trifecta, Sorin Mitroflow) and stentless bioprosthesis (e.g., Sorin Freedom, St Jude Medical Toronto SPV, Medtronic Freestyle). Stented bioprostheses with internally mounted leaflets (e.g., Edwards Lifesciences PERIMOUNT and Magna, Medtronic Hancock, St Jude Medical Epic and Mosaic) have the lowest risk of coronary obstruction.[18] The main factor implicated in coronary obstruction is the proximity of the coronary ostia to the final anticipated position of the displaced surgical valve leaflets after valve implantation. The mechanisms for coronary artery obstruction include displacement of a native/surgical valve leaflet toward the coronary ostium blocking the ostium, sinus of Valsalva sequestration by the displacement of native or surgical valve leaflets which can obstruct the entire sinus in an aortic root with a low and narrow sinotubular junction, mass obstruction of the coronary artery by a calcium deposit that is deflected during valve deployment, embolization of thrombus or degenerative

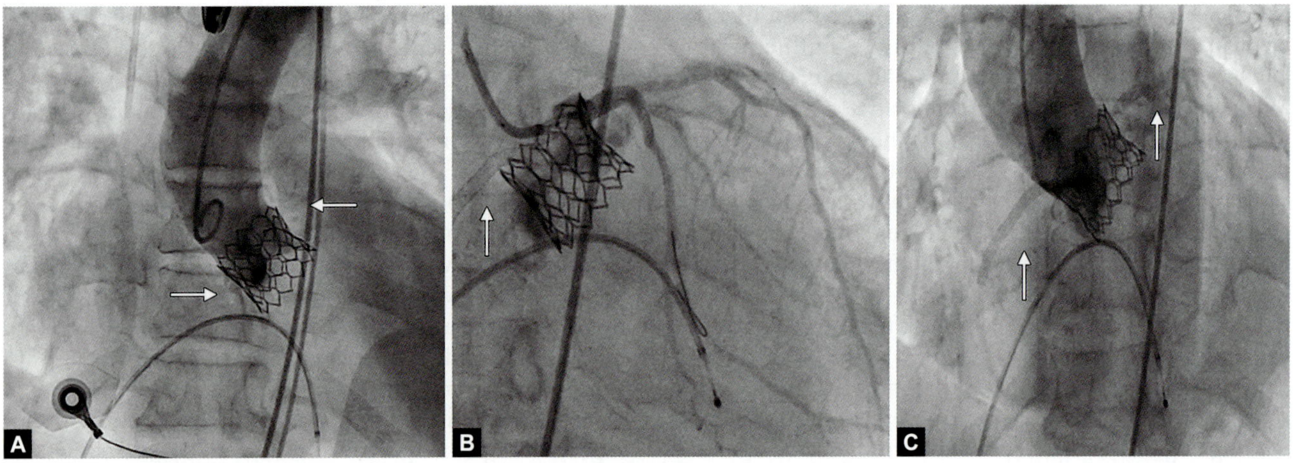

FIGS. 6A TO C: Both coronary occlusions in a patient after deploying balloon-expandable valve. Stenting of both the left coronary artery (LCA) and right coronary artery (RCA) restored flow.

Courtesy: Dr Sengottuvelu G, Apollo Hospitals, Chennai, India.

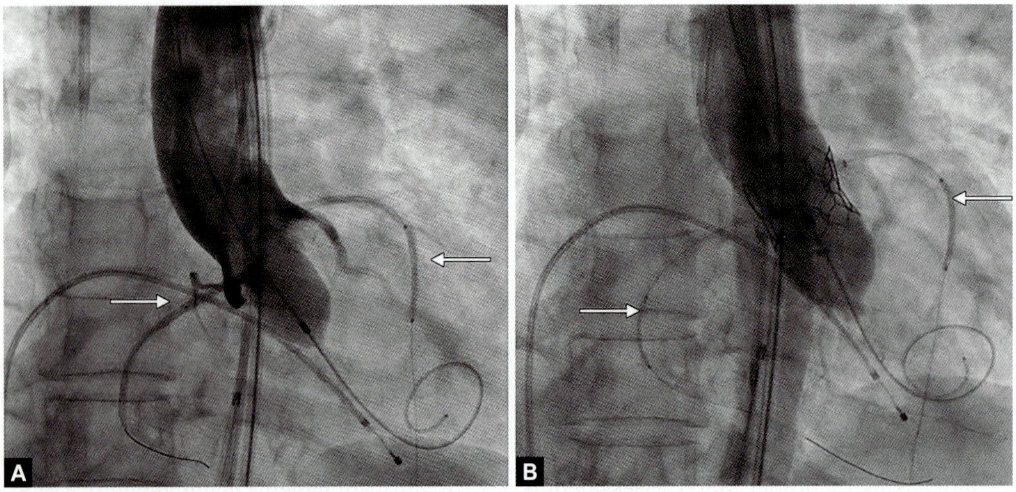

FIGS. 7A AND B: Bilateral coronary protection with stents in both the left anterior descending (LAD) artery and right coronary artery (RCA) of a patient with low coronary heights of both left coronary artery (LCA) and RCA during predilation and during valve deployment. Stents removed after confirming unobstructed flow in both vessels.

Courtesy: Dr Sengottuvelu G, Apollo Hospitals, Chennai, India.

material in the aortic root or on the TAVR device to cause coronary obstruction, valve skirt obstruction, where the valve prosthesis reaches high enough that the skirt covers the coronary ostium, aortic dissection with continuity of the rupture into the intima of one of the coronary ostia with resultant obstruction, and coronary air embolism.[19]

Prevention of Coronary Obstruction

Preprocedural cardiac MSCT is critical to identify the risk of coronary occlusion by measurement of the height of the coronary ostia in relation to the aortic annulus, the width of the sinotubular junction, and the width and height of the sinus of Valsalva. These measurements should be interpreted in the context of annular dimensions, overall aortic root dimensions, and anticipated THV valve size. For patients undergoing ViV TAVR implantation, the height of the coronary ostia in relation to the sewing ring, the virtual THV to coronary distance (VTC) measurement which is obtained by superimposing a virtual ring simulating the anticipated diameter of the fully expanded TAVR valve along the geometric center of the surgical valve, followed by a linear measurement from the ring to the coronary ostium, is required.[14] A VTC < 4 mm is associated with an increased risk of coronary obstruction. For patients at an increased risk of coronary obstruction, coronary protection with a standard 0.014-inch guidewire is advisable to help prevent and treat potential occlusion **(Figs. 7A and B)**. In some cases, a pre-emptive coronary balloon or stent with a high radial force can be mounted on a guidewire with a guide extension support and advanced in the left anterior descending artery and/or right coronary artery during valve deployment. If the coronaries get occluded, the stent can be pulled back and deployed in a "chimney" technique or "snorkel" technique to maintain coronary patency. Use of a fully or a partially recapturable THV (Evolut-R/PRO, Portico) or a THV with a favorable open-cell design (ACURATE neo, NAVITOR), achieving commissural alignment (Evolut and ACURATE neo), can minimize risk in select cases, although there are no prospective data. An alternative electrosurgical technique is the bioprosthetic aortic scallop intentional laceration to prevent iatrogenic coronary artery obstruction (BASILICA) technique to split either native or bioprosthetic aortic valve leaflets before THV implantation to maintain blood flow into the coronary sinus.[19] The procedure involves the intentional laceration of the leaflets using radiofrequency energy delivered to a guidewire suspended between two guiding catheters.[20]

Management

After coronary obstruction, severe cardiac depression can predispose the patient to cardiogenic shock and hemodynamic collapse. In cases of suspected coronary obstruction, a bolus angiogram of the aortic root may reveal which coronary vessel is involved. After that, selective intubation of the vessel, followed by balloon dilatation or stenting of the coronary ostium, should be considered. If the valve is implanted too high and coronary flow is obstructed by the valve skirt, the prostheses should be immediately retracted into the ascending aorta to relieve the obstruction. If the situation cannot be resolved percutaneously, then emergent open-heart bypass remains the bailout option.[21]

DELAYED CORONARY OBSTRUCTION

Delayed coronary artery obstruction **(Flowchart 2)** is a rare complication with a incidence of 0.2%. It is more likely to occur after "ViV" procedures and self-expandable valves. Most cases of delayed coronary obstruction occur within 7 days, but it can present after several months. Patients presenting within 7 days presented with either cardiac arrest or ST-segment elevation myocardial infarction (STEMI), and the proposed mechanism is the displacement of calcified native or surgical valve leaflet, while patients after 7 days mostly presented with stable or unstable angina with the proposed mechanism being the endothelization of bioprosthetic valve with some degree of coronary obstruction. Intravascular ultrasound (IVUS) may be helpful in doubtful cases.[22]

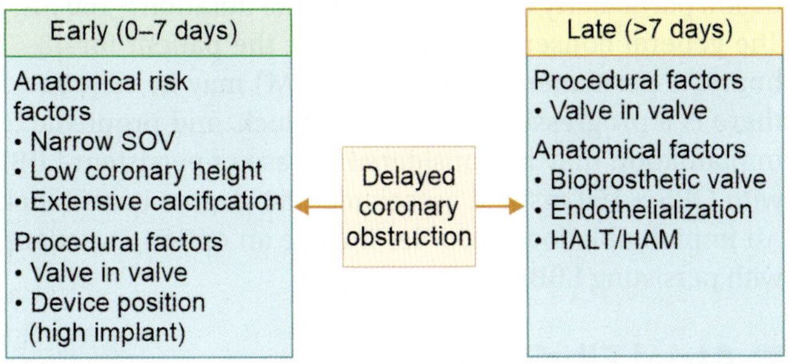

FLOWCHART 2: Etiology and risk factors for delayed coronary obstruction.

(HALT: hypo-attenuating leaflet thickening; HAM: hypo-attenuation affecting motion; SOV: sinus of Valsalva)

SELF-EXPANDABLE VALVE INFOLDING

Prosthetic valve infolding is a rare complication seen only with the use of SEVs. It is the wrinkling along the valve frame during deployment with secondary distortion and malfunctioning of the prosthesis leading to severe intravalvular and PVL with hemodynamic collapse. Infolding is also associated with the risk of periprocedural stroke. The mechanism for infolding is not clear but is likely related to the low radial force of the nitinol frame and is more relevant with larger valves because they have lower radial force. Risk factors for infolding include valve-related characteristics such as re-sheathing, larger valves (≥29 mm), and patient-related characteristics such as bicuspid valves, high ellipticity of the annulus, and heavy calcification.[23,24] Valve infolding should be suspected if there is a severe PVL and/or hemodynamic instability after SEV deployment. Signs of valve infolding can be seen on fluoroscopy, including a narrower-than-expected valve prosthesis and a vertical line along the valve frame. Careful attention to evaluate the valve frame with multiple fluoroscopic angles or the cusp-overlap view before release is mandatory, if infolding is suspected. Right anterior oblique (RAO) cranial view looking down the valve on the short axis can also confirm this diagnosis. On TEE, the infolded valve is easily recognized, particularly on the mid-esophageal short axis termed "Pac-Man sign."[25] If valve infolding is recognized before release, recapture, retrieve, and replacement with another THV is preferred. If infolding is noticed after valve deployment, immediate postdilatation is required to restore the valve function and avoid hemodynamic collapse. Typically, postdilatation can eliminate the infolding. If this is unsuccessful, retrieval and deployment of a new valve are required.[26]

PERICARDIAL EFFUSION/CARDIAC TAMPONADE

Cardiac tamponade can occur due to perforation of any of these structures: Right ventricle (RV), LV, ascending aorta, or aortic root. It can occur at any time during the procedure. Iatrogenic aortic dissection is quite common while manipulating devices in heavily tortuous, calcified, and diseased aortic anatomies. Ventricular perforation has been reported at around 1% in most of the series. Overall, RV perforation accounts for the majority of ventricular perforations and can occur due to the placement of the temporary pacing wire. Injury to the LV may result from perforation by the stiff guidewire or by the catheters used during valve passage. Aortic root rupture can occur while balloon valvuloplasty or after valve implantation, commonly in elderly women with fragile tissue where bulky calcifications can perforate the aortic root.[22]

Preventive Measures

Care should be taken during device and sheath manipulation in unfavorable anatomy and minimize wire and catheter exchanges. In a tortuous or horizontal aorta, an additional stiff wire advanced into the aortic root will enhance the support and deliverability of the THV. In cases of extremely hostile aortas, alternative access routes should be considered. Balloon-tipped pacing catheters, instead of screw-in leads or a direct LV pacing via the standard delivery wire, can also avoid pacing lead in the RV and minimize RV perforation. The use of a dedicated TAVR wire (e.g., Safari or Confida) is likely safer than self-shaped stiff support wires in avoiding LV perforation. Carefully monitor wire position during manipulations and balloon inflation.[13]

Diagnosis and Management

All patients should undergo echocardiography to rule out pericardial effusion at the end of the implantation procedure. Small effusions < 10 mm without hemodynamic impairment can be monitored with an echocardiogram at close intervals. Patients with rapidly increasing effusions and effusions with hemodynamic impairment should undergo pericardiocentesis. Full reversal of the anticoagulation state by protamine should be considered on a case-by-case basis as it can risk thrombus formation. RV perforations are almost always managed conservatively or with pericardiocentesis and rarely require surgical repair. However, in the case of a posterior effusion, these may be difficult to access from a percutaneous approach, and an emergent surgical sternotomy should be considered in such cases. For LV perforations, management depends on the clinical status, type, extent of injury, and operative candidacy. In free LV perforations, rapid hemodynamic instability can occur needing immediate intervention with cardiopulmonary bypass, sternotomy, and open repair. If there is a small LV perforation, percutaneous drainage still may be possible. In cases of LV pseudoaneurysm, percutaneous plug placement can be considered.[27]

CONDUCTION ABNORMALITIES

The incidence of rhythm abnormalities is highly variable, ranging from 5.7 to 45.2%.[28] Patients with severe AS can have baseline myocardial or conduction disease due to the calcium deposits predisposing them to cardiac dysrhythmias post TAVR. Moreover, there is a close anatomical relationship between the aortic valve **(Fig. 8)**, the aortic annulus, and the conduction system. The bundle of His is located just below the aortic leaflets, just below the level of the membranous septum. This becomes more superficial at the crest of the interventricular septum, giving rise to the left bundle. The left bundle is more superficial at the basal attachment of the right and noncoronary commissures, which makes it more vulnerable to mechanical interaction during TAVR and can cause trauma and potential damage leading to tissue injuries such as hematoma, edema, necrosis, or compression.[29] The common dysrhythmias post TAVR include left bundle branch block (LBBB) **(Flowchart 3)**, high-grade atrioventricular (AV) block, and atrial fibrillation.[22]

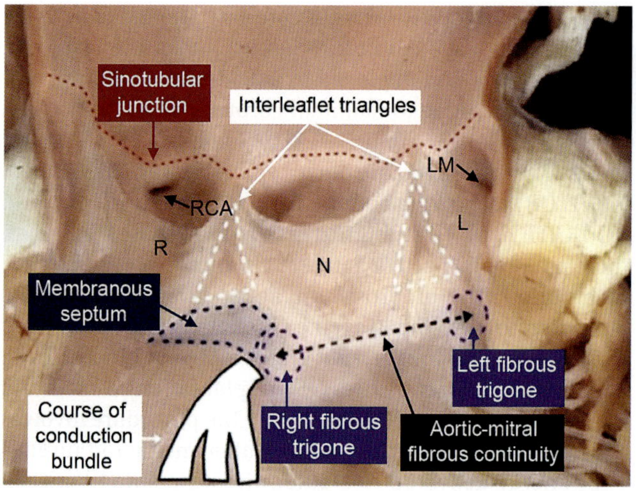

FIG. 8: Relationship between the aortic valve structures and annulus with the conduction system.
(LM: left main; RCA: right coronary artery)
Source: With permission from Chen et al. (2020).[30]

Left Bundle Branch Block

Developing a new-onset LBBB is more frequent after TAVR than SAVR. It usually occurs within 24 hours and resolves within a month, but it persists in 55% of the cases. New-onset LBBB causes ventricular dyssynchrony that can negatively impact left ventricular function and also predisposes to ventricular arrhythmias and sudden cardiac death, particularly if preprocedural QRS duration > 160 ms.[31] The general consensus is to monitor the patient for 48–72 hours. A permanent pacemaker (PPM) may be required if there is a progression to AV nodal block, and prophylactic implantation may be considered in case of persistent LBBB with QRS > 160 ms and associated first-degree heart block. An implantable loop recorder may be an option in patients with persisting LBBB.[32]

Atrial Fibrillation

Aortic stenosis results in pressure overload and related stretch of the left-sided chambers predisposing these patients to the risk of atrial fibrillation. Preexisting atrial

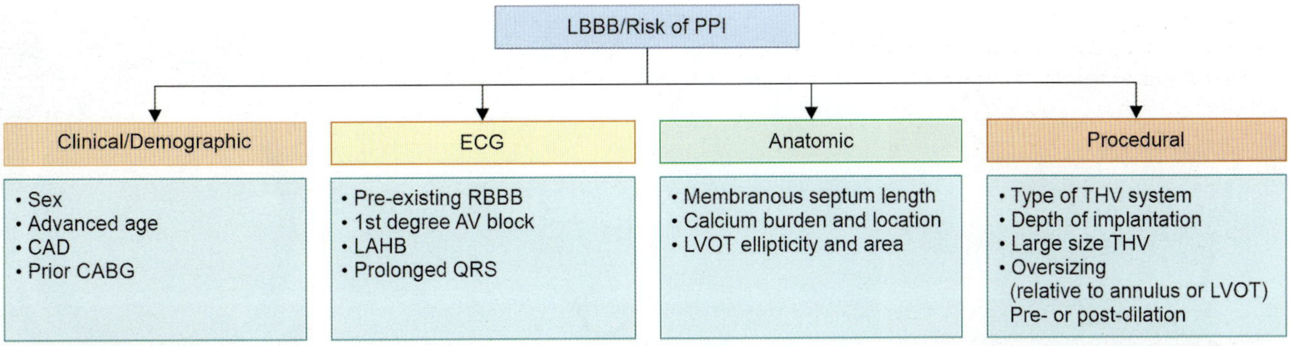

FLOWCHART 3: Predictors of permanent pacemaker implantation (PPI) and new-onset left bundle branch block (LBBB) after transcatheter aortic valve replacement.

(AV: atrioventricular; CABG: coronary artery bypass grafting; CAD: coronary artery disease; ECG: electrocardiogram; LAHB: left anterior hemiblock; LVOT: left ventricular outflow tract; RBBB: right bundle branch block; THV: transcatheter heart valve)

fibrillation is common in these patients. A meta-analysis of over 30,000 patients reported new-onset atrial fibrillation with an incidence of 11%, 14%, 14%, and 25% during in-hospital, 30-day, 1-year, and 2-year follow-ups, respectively.[22]

High-grade Atrioventricular Block

High-grade AV block is the most common reason for PPM placement and usually occurs immediately after the TAVR procedure. The STS TVT Registry reported that 60–96% of high-grade AV blocks occur within 24 hours. AV blocks may develop after 48 hours of procedure in 2–7% of the cases. Right bundle branch block (RBBB) may be associated with delayed-onset heart block with a median onset at 6 days post procedure. In patients with normal sinus rhythm and no new conduction disturbances on immediate postprocedure ECG, the risk of developing delayed AV block is <1%.[11]

Strategies to Avoid Pacemaker Implantation

Right bundle branch block is one of the most consistent and strong predictors of PPI. Increased calcium burden and distribution in the DLZ, as well as deeper implantation, are associated with the risk of postprocedural PPI. Thus, a right ventricular temporary pacing wire should be preferred in patients at high risk of periprocedural conduction disturbances instead of using LV wire pacing. Prophylactic PPM can also be considered in patients with preexisting high-grade conduction abnormalities. During the procedure, rapid atrial pacing can also be performed to risk-stratify patients. Those developing atrial-pacing-induced Wenckebach AV block are at a high risk for PPI. The choice of valve prosthesis can impact the rates of PPI. Lower PPI rates were seen with the use of BEV compared to SEV. Latest generation valves, such as the ACURATE neo, have low radial strength and are associated with a low PPI rate. The cusp overlap technique involves overlapping the left and right coronary cusps to isolate the noncoronary cusp and helps in achieving higher implantation, which can reduce PPM implantation rates. Preprocedural CT can measure the membranous septum length, and achieving an implantation depth less than the length of the membranous septum can reduce PPI rates.[33,34]

STROKE

Cerebrovascular events are serious complications, affecting patient survival with potentially devastating neurological sequelae. TAVR-related stroke risk is lower than that found for SAVR and is reported to occur in about 2% of TAVR procedures.[35] A periprocedural stroke occurs during the first 48 hours and accounts for about half of TAVR-related strokes. These events can occur due to thrombi, bleeding, embolic debris liberated from the native aortic valve, and hemodynamic instability. Occult atrial fibrillation or subclinical valve thrombosis associated with emboli and ischemic stroke accounts for the other 50% of cerebrovascular accidents. Studies suggest that the highest rate of embolism during TAVR is during valve positioning and deployment, followed by during balloon aortic valvuloplasty. In addition to clinically apparent strokes, studies suggest that up to 84% of patients have new silent ischemic lesions post TAVR. These studies have shown that patients develop multiple cerebral lesions spread across both cerebral hemispheres, consistent with embolic showering events, and can be diagnosed using diffusion-weighted MRI.[14]

Prevention and Management

Optimal anticoagulation throughout the procedure is of utmost importance to minimize thrombus formation. Unfractionated heparin remains the routine anticoagulant during TAVR, with a parenteral bolus followed by additional doses to achieve an activated clotting time of 250–300 seconds. Multiple cerebral embolic protection devices (CEPD) are in use during TAVR to reduce embolic strokes **(Figs. 9A to C)**. These devices positioned across the origins of the supra-aortic vessels can capture or deflect embolic debris away from the cerebral blood flow and can effectively

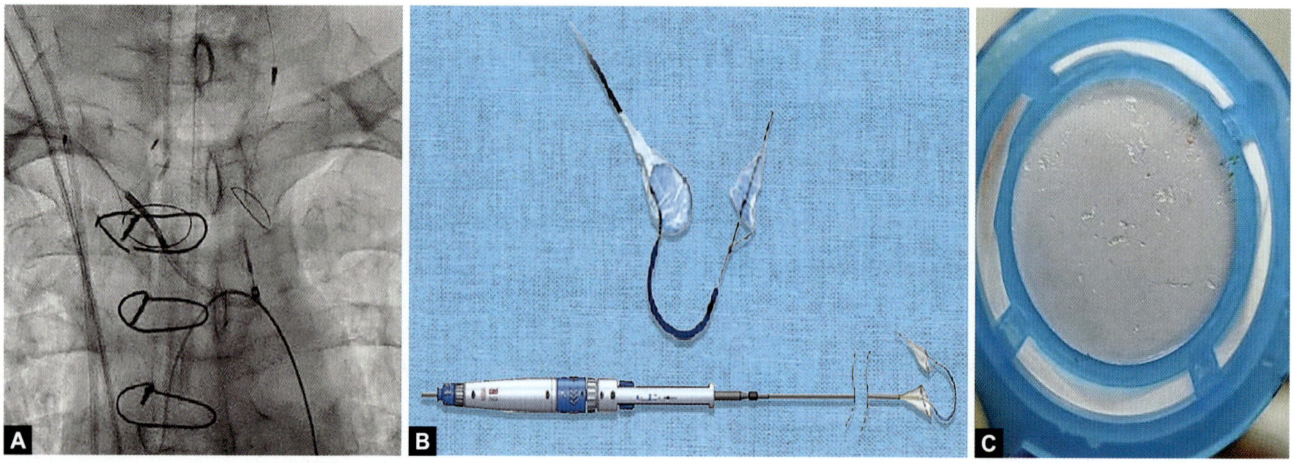

FIGS. 9A TO C: (A) Protection with Sentinel device in a patient with bovine aortic arch; (B) Sentinel device; (C) Collected debris.
Courtesy: Dr Sengottuvelu G, Apollo Hospitals, India.

reduce the burden of ischemic strokes during TAVR.[36] The Sentinel Cerebral Protection System consists of two interconnected filters that are deployed with one filter in the brachiocephalic trunk and the other in the left common carotid artery through the right radial artery before TAVR. These filters trap emboli flowing through these arteries during TAVR and are removed after the procedure. As most of the TAVR procedures are done under general anesthesia or conscious sedation, the diagnosis of periprocedural stroke is often delayed. When a stroke is suspected, immediate assessment by a dedicated stroke team and prompt access to CT of the brain, CT cerebral angiography, and MRI brain are essential.[37]

ACUTE KIDNEY INJURY

The overall incidence of acute kidney injury (AKI) in patients undergoing TAVR ranges between 10 and 40%, with stage 3 AKI comprising 1%. Multiple patient and procedural-related factors are implicated in the development of post-TAVR AKI. Baseline renal dysfunction is the strongest independent risk factor for the long-term mortality and development of post-TAVR AKI.[38] Other risk factors include the presence of other comorbid illnesses such as diabetes, anemia, chronic obstructive pulmonary disease (COPD), severe inflammatory response syndrome, and peripheral vascular disease. Procedural factors include hemodynamic instability during rapid pacing, direct apical or aortic access, significant bleeding, embolism of atherosclerotic or calcific microfragments during catheter manipulation, increased use of contrast, conversion to general anesthesia or open-heart surgery, and the need for blood cell transfusions.[39]

Prevention

Prior identification of patients at high risk for AKI and following appropriate prevention strategies can reduce the risk of AKI. The ratio of contrast volume to glomerular filtration rate (GFR) > 3.2 and the threshold value of contrast volume × serum creatinine to body weight of 2.7 are cutoffs to identify patients at risk for the development of AKI. For these high-risk patients, adequate prehydration and the use of the RenalGuard system are important.[40] Contrast-sparing strategies, including the use of alternative imaging modalities, such as MRI or three-dimensional TEE, for preprocedural planning and intraprocedural guidance in patients with baseline renal dysfunction, should be considered. Low-contrast volume CT protocols with ECG gating can provide an adequate assessment of aortic, peripheral vessels, and coronary arteries, obviating the need for invasive angiography. Alternatively, echocardiography, gadolinium-free cardiac MRI, color Doppler of peripheral vessels, and fusion angiography can be used with procedural adaptions to perform a zero-contrast procedure.[14] Using a self-expandable valve allows less precise sizing than a balloon-expandable THV and can be beneficial in renal dysfunction patients. Using multiple 0.035 guidewires as markers in the annulus and annular calcification as markers can guide valve positioning and deployment without contrast, and the final result and access site can be assessed by imaging rather than contrast injections **(Figs. 10A and B)**.

PARAVALVULAR LEAK

Blood flowing through a channel between the implanted valve and the cardiac tissue as a result of a lack of appropriate sealing is referred to as PVL **(Figs. 11A to G)**. PVL has been observed to occur more frequently after TAVR than SAVR.[41] A patient with PVL can present with new or worsening heart failure or hemolysis. Studies show the incidence of mild PVL in 7.8–40.8%, moderate PVL in 8.2–11.8%, and severe PVL in 3.5–12.2%. A recent meta-analysis of 38 studies comprising about 25,000 patients showed that even mild PVL can increase the risk of all-cause mortality, rehospitalization, and cardiovascular mortality following

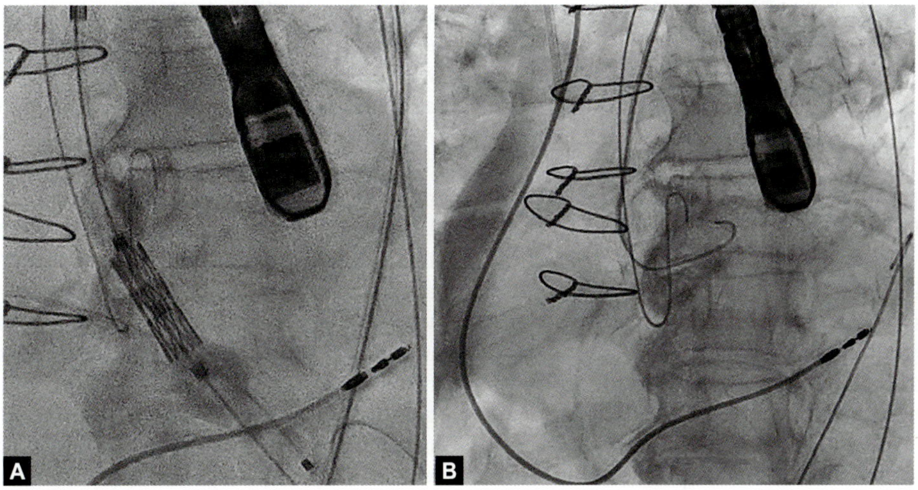

FIGS. 10A AND B: (A) Guidewire positioned in the noncoronary cusp in coplanar view acts as a marker during valve implantation. (B) Two guidewires to mark the left coronary cusp (LCC) and noncoronary cusp (NCC) aligning the annular plane.
Courtesy: Dr Sengottuvelu G, Apollo Hospitals, India.

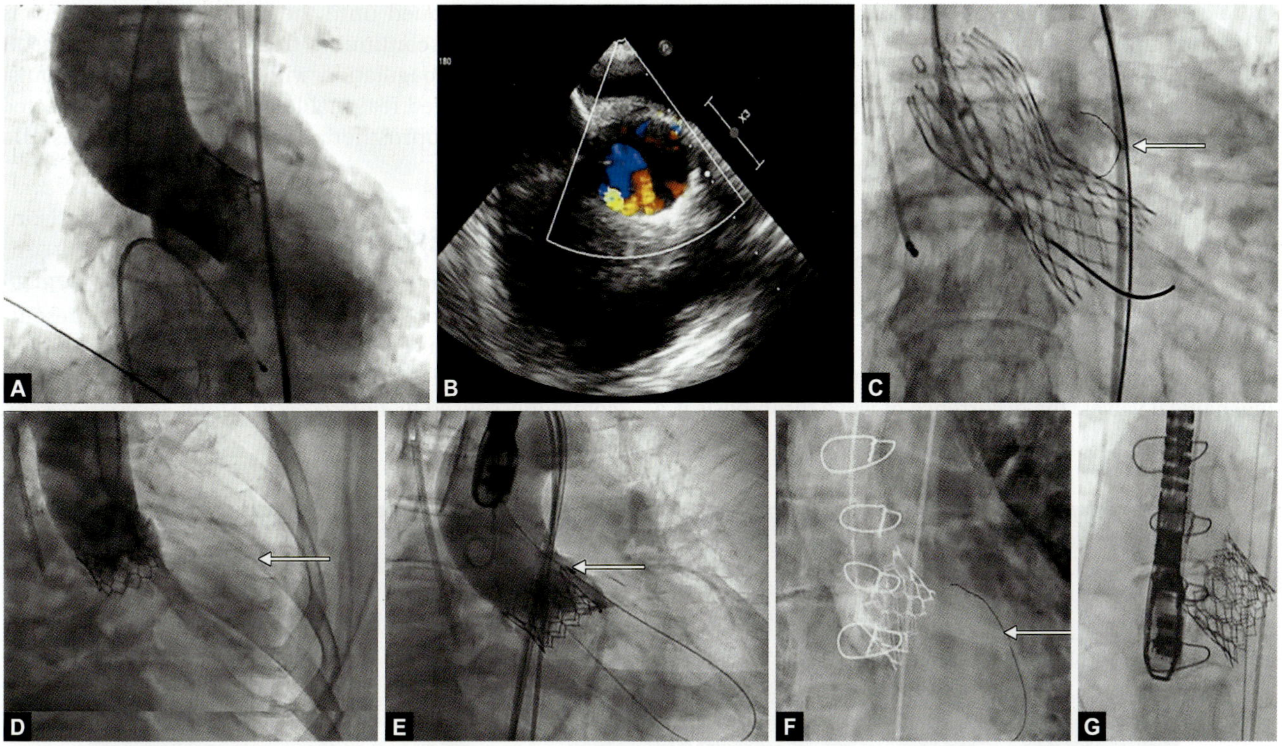

FIGS. 11A TO G: (A) Aortogram showing paravalvular leak (PVL). (B) Multiple PVL jet around the valve. (C) Mispositioning deep into left ventricular outflow tract (LVOT) causing PVL. (D and E) PVL closed by vascular plug. (F and G) PVL treated with transcatheter aortic valve (TAV) in TAV.

TAVI. Residual moderate-to-severe PVL is a strong independent predictor for mortality. High-risk features for PVL include undersizing of THV and heavy annular and/or leaflet calcification, which may lead to valve underexpansion or malpositioning. Therefore, particularly for younger patients undergoing TAVR, the aim should be to achieve minimal to no residual leak.[22]

Prevention, Diagnosis, and Treatment

Accurate preprocedural CT analysis can identify high-risk individuals, and appropriate device selection plays a key role in minimizing PVL. Use of newer generation valves such as Sapien 3 Ultra (Edwards Lifesciences), Evolut Plus (Medtronic), and ACURATE neo 2 (Boston Scientific) valves with an additional sealing skirt and the NAVITOR (Abbott) valve with a dynamic sealing skirt can minimize PVL in high-risk anatomy.

Currently, the gold standard for the evaluation of PVL is echocardiography and color Doppler evaluation. However, conventional aortography, quantitative video densitometry, and hemodynamic indices such as AR index (ARI) calculated as LVEDP—diastolic blood pressure/systolic blood pressure may be useful. ARI can indicate severity with ARI < 25 being associated with higher mortality. Hemodynamic indices may be limited by heart rate variations, atrial fibrillation, and altered hemodynamic conditions due to sedation and/or anesthesia. Balloon postdilatation is the mainstay of treatment with balloon sizing based on preprocedural CT measurements of the annulus. The use of repeated aggressive balloon dilatation to correct PVL must be balanced against the risk of subsequent aortic injury, annular rupture, or stroke, especially in patients with heavy or nodular calcification. The degree of preprocedure AR can be a useful guide to deciding on aggressive postdilatation post-TAVR. Patients with a mixed aortic valve disease have more compliant ventricles and can tolerate postprocedural AR better than those with smaller, stiffer ventricles, as with isolated AS without regurgitation. If despite balloon dilatation, PVL is severe along with significant hemodynamic compromise, then a second THV can be implanted as a TAVR-in-TAVR procedure, with a BEV being preferred. Snares can be used if there is an inadequate depth of implantation. In more stable cases, or if diagnosed later postprocedurally, elective closure with vascular plugs can be considered.[42]

VALVE THROMBOSIS

Although bioprosthetic valves are less thrombogenic than mechanical valves, the occurrence of valve thrombosis is a serious issue. Clinical valve thrombosis is defined as prosthetic valve dysfunction with a typical thrombus on the valve with an elevated transvalvular gradient ≥ 20 mm Hg and often with symptoms of heart failure or left-sided thromboembolic events. The incidence is estimated to be between 0.6 and 2.8%. Echocardiography or MDCT demonstrates a mobile mass or thrombus on the prosthetic valve. Subclinical leaflet thrombosis, also called hypoattenuating leaflet thickening (HALT), is described as a hypoattenuating lesion on the aortic side of the leaflets as seen on MDCT. If the valve leaflet motion is affected, it is called hypoattenuation affecting motion (HAM).[43] Predictors of bioprosthetic valve thrombosis include (1) >50% increase in mean transvalvular gradient, (2) increased leaflet thickness, (3) abnormal leaflet mobility, (4) presence of atrial fibrillation, (5) small valve size and (6) underexpansion, (7) aggressive postdilatation, (8) geometric deformation of THV, and (9) the underlying thrombophilia.[44] Patients with clinical valve thrombosis are treated with direct oral anticoagulants for 1-6 months with high success rates. For the most optimal outcome, treatment should be continued until the transvalvular gradient is reduced, and discontinuing treatment prior may result in relapse. Anticoagulation with a vitamin K antagonist (VKA) is considered reasonable in patients with suspected or confirmed bioprosthetic valve thrombosis (class IIa indication).[45]

INFECTIVE ENDOCARDITIS

Endocarditis post-TAVR infective endocarditis (TAVR-IE) is a rare but serious complication that typically presents several months after the procedure **(Fig. 12)**. The incidence of TAVR-IE is low, approximately 2%. It is most commonly caused by *Enterococcus*, *Staphylococcus aureus*,

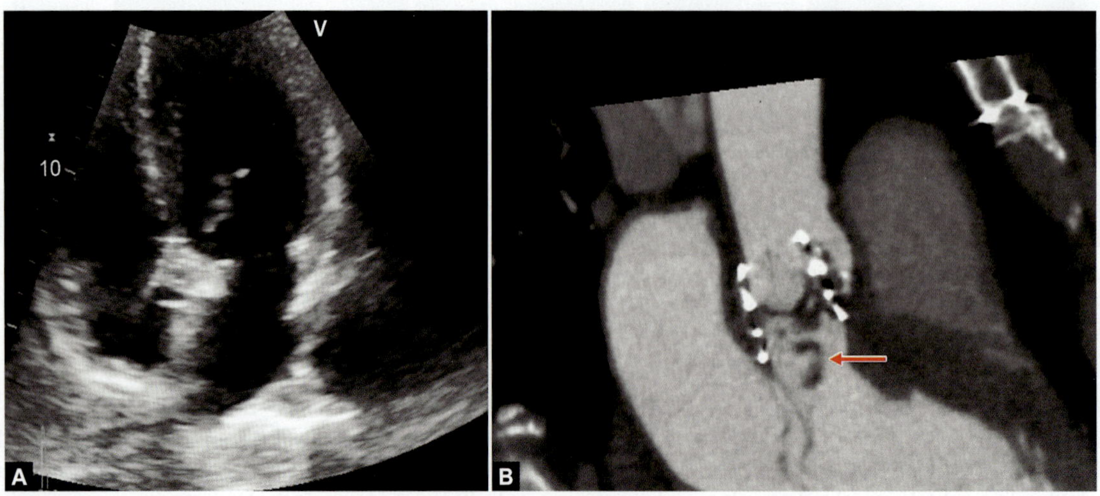

FIGS. 12A AND B: Infective endocarditis of transcatheter aortic valve replacement (TAVR) valve with freely mobile vegetation in echo and computed tomography (CT).

Courtesy: Dr Sengottuvelu G, Apollo Hospitals, Chennai, India.

and coagulase-negative *Staphylococcus* and is associated with high mortality with rates of in-hospital mortality of 36% and a 2-year mortality rate of 66.7%.[46] Modified Duke criteria have lower diagnostic accuracy in these cases because of the high incidence of negative blood cultures and difficult transthoracic echo. Therefore, multiple imaging techniques such as CT or positron emission tomography (PET) scans can have a role in this population. Risk factors for IE after TAVR include patient factors such as younger age, male, higher body mass index, diabetes, COPD, chronic kidney disease (CKD), prior history of IE, pulmonary hypertension, coagulopathy, liver disease, atrial fibrillation, peripheral vascular disease, blood transfusion during hospitalization, critical preoperative state, and anemia. Procedural factors include residual AR, low TAVR placement, bleeding complication, implantation of more than one valve, and ViV procedure.[47] Antibiotic therapy guidelines are the same as those recommended for prosthetic valve endocarditis. Conservative treatment with antibiotics is the most advocated strategy. The role of surgery and the timing of surgery are still under debate.[48]

Prevention

The ESC guidelines (2015) propose that antimicrobial prophylaxis should be initiated before TAVR and discontinued 48 hours afterward. Periprocedural antibiotic prophylaxis with cephalosporin monotherapy is the most commonly used regimen. A recent review of recommendations proposed switching from cephalosporin to amoxicillin/clavulanic acid, given its great efficacy against enterococci, or adding teicoplanin or vancomycin in addition to cephalosporins to cover methicillin-resistant staphylococci.[49]

CONCLUSION

With rapid advances in device technology and refinements in techniques, procedural morbidities and complications during or immediately after TAVR have reduced drastically. However, if complications occur, they remain major factors affecting the success of the procedure and carry a significant morbidity and mortality risk. Meticulous preprocedural planning, appropriate patient selection and evaluation, and determining procedural difficulties before the procedure may help reduce the complications.

ONLINE REFERENCES

Please scan the QR code provided at the end of the table of contents for References of this chapter.

CHAPTER

189 Durability of Transcatheter Aortic Valves

Amit Kumar Chaurasia, Yogesh Om Sharma, Nitin Kumar Parashar

ABSTRACT

Transcatheter aortic valve replacement (TAVR) is a percutaneous minimally invasive procedure, an alternative to surgical aortic valve replacement (SAVR), for the treatment of severe aortic stenosis in indicated patients. The safety of TAVR procedure has been documented in multiple trials but little is known about the long-term durability of these valves. The indications for TAVR are expanding to a larger number of patients including younger and lower-risk patients. So, it becomes imperative to study degeneration rates and long-term durability of transcatheter aortic valves. TAVR valves have bioprosthetic leaflets which are prone to degeneration. The prosthetic valvular dysfunction has been categorized as structural valve deterioration (SVD) and non-SVD. This article reviews the potential mechanisms, definitions, and rates of transcatheter aortic valvular dysfunction compared with SAVR.

Keywords: TAVR, SVD, durability.

INTRODUCTION

The first transcatheter aortic valve replacement (TAVR) was done by Alain Cribier in the year 2002.[1] In a short span of two decades, transcatheter aortic valve implantation (TAVI) has become the standard-of-care for patients with severe aortic stenosis.[2-7] There is no doubt that TAVR should be the standard of care for patients with prohibitive-risk, high-risk, and intermediate-risk patients. This has been well endorsed by various guidelines as well. European Society of Cardiology (ESC) gives class I indication for TAVR for all patients above 75 years of age who require aortic valve replacement, whereas the American College of Cardiology (ACC) and American Heart Association (AHA) give class I indication for anyone above 80 years of age.[8,9] Though the age group 65–80 years gets a class I indication as per AHA/ACC guidelines, it also says that patients should be given the choice of TAVR as well as surgical aortic valve replacement (SAVR). What is clear is that any patient who is <65 years of age and suitable for SAVR should always undergo SAVR. With encouraging results from low-risk trials, one should not feel that TAVR can replace SAVR. One should understand that low-risk trials were done in a certain population, which holds for only the population included in the trial.[5,6] Severe aortic stenosis with the bicuspid aortic valve, age <65 years, significant coronary artery disease, unfavorable anatomy like too small annuli or with excessive calcification in left ventricular outflow tract (LVOT), those suitable for mechanical valve, or any other associated procedures were excluded from the trial. In other words, a huge population with severe aortic stenosis has been excluded from the trials. The debate about who is the ideal candidate for low-risk TAVR will keep continuing and one should not forget that at the center of this debate is the patient; for him, the durability of the valve is what matters the most.

CHALLENGES WITH SURGICAL AORTIC VALVE DURABILITY

Any new therapy is always compared with an established one and in the case of TAVR, the established therapy is SAVR. So, we need to understand the durability of SAVR valves. Most SAVR bioprosthetic valve mentions the durability of 15–25 years but the truth is far from reality.[10-13] Most of the SAVR durability trials have freedom from redo surgery as their clinical endpoint. Patients who are at high risk for redo SAVR may not be offered SAVR at all and many of these patients may die without being included in the outcome study. This may be one of the reasons why many trials that have looked into 15 or 20 years of durability data have so low number needed to be treated at the end. There are other surgical bioprosthetic valves like the Trifecta which have shown degeneration at even 1 year.[14] In simple words, bioprosthetic valve dysfunction (BVD) defines the durability of the valves. BVD can either be structural valve deterioration (SVD) which is due to the defect in the prosthetic material such as leaflet tear, stent fracture, or leaflet calcification and non-SVD, which is due to some secondary process such as patient prosthesis mismatch (PPM), paravalvular leak (PVL), pannus in growth, valve thrombosis, or endocarditis. Before 2017, there was no standard definition for SVD and different trials had different definitions; so, there was no uniformity in reported trial data. Most TAVR operators aspire to have a single-digit postprocedure gradient, whereas the usual mean gradient post-SAVR is 15–20 mm Hg. This creates a bias in comparing TAVR with SAVR durability.

STANDARDIZED DEFINITIONS

In 2017, a consensus statement from the European Association of Percutaneous Cardiovascular Interventions (EAPCI), the ESC, and the European Association for Cardiothoracic Surgery (EACTS) was published which divided valve durability by valve dysfunction and valve failure.[15] BVD was classified into four categories. Category I consisted of patients with SVD defined as moderate when the mean aortic valve gradient was >20 mm Hg or at 3 months follow-up if the mean gradient increased by 10 mm Hg or if the patient had moderate intravalvular aortic regurgitation; and severe, if the mean gradient was >40 mm Hg or at 3 months, follow-up if the gradient increased by 20 mm Hg or if the patient had severe intravalvular aortic regurgitation. Category II consisted of patients with non-SVD defined as patients with PPM: moderate ([indexed effective orifice area (iEOA) ≤ 0.85 cm^2/m^2 after 3 months postprocedure] and severe (iEOA ≤ 0.65 cm^2/m^2 after 3 months postprocedure). Category 3 consisted of patients with bioprosthetic valve thrombosis leading to valve dysfunction and category 4 consisted of patients with BVD secondary to infective endocarditis. Bioprosthetic valve failure was defined as valve-related death or severe hemodynamic deterioration of the valve leading to reintervention of the valve.

A white paper on the Standardized Definition of SVD for Surgical and Transcatheter Bioprosthetic Aortic Valves was published in 2018.[16] Today, the most widely accepted definition is by Valve Academic Research Consortium (VARC), which published the last update in 2021. The VARC-3 criteria were published in 2021 and provide the most recent insight into SVD.[17] VARC-3 criteria require both permanent morphologic change in the valve and hemodynamic change in the valve. So essentially, VARC-3 criteria combine both structural as well as non-SVD. VARC classifies SVD into four stages. Stage 1 has only morphological changes without any hemodynamic consequences. Stage 2 has hemodynamic changes when echocardiography is done at 1–3 months. Either there should be an increase in mean gradient by 10 mm Hg which should increase the overall mean gradient by >20 mm Hg with an associated decrease in effective orifice area (EOA) ≥0.3 cm^2 or ≥25% or a decrease in Doppler velocity index (DVI) by 0.1 or by 20%. If there is an increase in intravalvular regurgitation by one grade overall leading to intravalvular regurgitation more than moderate is also regarded as stage 2. Stage 3 is when there is an increase in mean gradient by 20 mm Hg leading to an overall mean gradient of >30 mm Hg with an associated decrease in EOA by 0.3 cm^2 or >25% from the previous echocardiogram and or decrease in DVI by 0.1 or 20%. It also says an increase in aortic regurgitation grade by 2 or severe aortic regurgitation will be regarded as Stage 3 **(Table 1)**.

COMPARISON OF BALLOON-EXPANDABLE VALVES TO SURGICAL VALVES

Due to variability in the definition of SVD in the early days and different trials utilizing different definitions, the true incidence of SVD would always be questionable. One would be surprised to see that PARTNER 1B trial showed no SVD at 5 years.[7] Patient survival in very high-risk cases was also low. However, we should keep in mind that the patients recruited were octogenarians, had multiple comorbid conditions, and hence they would have died due to the natural cause than due to the valve conditions themselves. As for the PARTNER 1A trial, at 5 years, the echocardiographic parameters such as EOA and mean transvalvular aortic gradient were similar.[2] The outcome was also similar despite moderate-to-severe PVL. This does not mean that a PVL does not have adverse effects on the outcome. These patients had many comorbidities and many have died as a result of natural processes. PARTNER 2 trial randomized about 2,032 patients to either TAVR (1,011 patients) or SAVR (1,021 patients).[18] The mean STS score ranged between 5 and 8% in both groups. There was no difference in the groups as far as the primary outcome of death or disabling stroke was concerned. However, one should note that this was the only trial in which the primary outcome was marginally better in the SAVR group than in the TAVR group, although this was not statistically significant. Rehospitalization and reintervention were more in TAVR than SAVR group. Though reintervention was very few in the TAVR group, the main causes were progressive stenosis or increased regurgitation which indirectly indicates SVD. However, we should be cautious in deriving this association as this was not the aim of this study. A proper subset analysis should be done in this regard with a longer duration of follow-up. PARTNER 3 data will throw light on the actual durability of the self-expandable valve in low-risk patient.[5]

TABLE 1: Consensus statements.

ESC and EAPCI (2017)	VARC-3
Category 1: SVD— • Moderate SVD: ○ Mean AVG ≥ 20 mm Hg ○ 3 months FU mean AVG increased by 10 mm Hg ○ Moderate intravalvular AR • Severe SVD: ○ Mean AVG ≥ 40 mm Hg ○ 3 months FU mean AVG increased by 20 mm Hg ○ Severe intravalvular AR *Category 2*: Non-SVD— • Patient with PPM: ○ Moderate iEOA ≤ 0.85 cm^2/m^2 post 3 months of procedure ○ Severe iEOA ≤ 0.65 cm^2/m^2 post 3 months of procedure *Category 3*: Valve thrombosis leading to valve dysfunction *Category 4*: IE leading to valve dysfunction	*Stage 1*: • Morphological changes • No hemodynamic changes *Stage 2*: • Morphological changes • Hemodynamic changes: ○ Mean AVG increased by 10 mm Hg ○ Overall AVG if increased >20 mm Hg • ≥0.3 cm^2 or >25% EOA decrease • DVI decreased by 0.1 or 20% • Intravalvular AR increases by one grade or more than moderate AR *Stage 3*: • Morphologic changes • Hemodynamic changes: ○ Mean AVG increases by 20 mm Hg ○ Overall AVG increased by 30 mm Hg ○ ≥0.3 cm^2 or >25% EOA decreases from the previous ECHO ○ DVI decreases by 0.1 or 20% ○ AR increases by 2 grades or more than severe AR

(AR: aortic regurgitation; DVI: Doppler velocity index; EOA: effective orifice area; ESC: European Society of Cardiology; EAPCI: European Association of Percutaneous Cardiovascular Intervention; iEOA: indexed effective orifice area; PPM: patient prosthesis mismatch; SVD: structural valvular deterioration; VARC: Valve Academic Research Consortium)

COMPARISON OF SELF-EXPANDABLE TAVR VALVE TO SURGICAL AORTIC VALVE

The NOTION trial is the only trial that has looked into the durability of the TAVR valve beyond years. This was a low-risk trial as the STS score for mortality was 3 ± 1.7 years; however, the mean age of the patient was 79.1 ± 4.8 years.[19] Again, since the mean age was high, the same cannot be extrapolated to younger patients. Also, many of these patients would die of natural causes in the due course of time and hence longer durability of the valve cannot be ascertained. However, this was a randomized trial between TAVR and SAVR and would provide a good comparison between the two. At 5 years, EOA was larger for TAVR than SAVR (1.7 vs. 1.2 cm^2, $p < 0.001$) and transvalvular aortic gradient was lower with TAVR in comparison to SAVR (8.2 vs. 13.7 mm Hg; $p < 0.001$). However, moderate-to-severe PVL was more in TAVR than SAVR (8.2% vs. 0%, $p < 0.001$). At 8 years, the TAVR group has significantly lower SVD (13.9% vs. 28.3%, $p = 0.0017$); however, the BVF was similar (8.7% vs. 10.5%, $p = 0.61$) in both TAVR and SAVR groups.[20] There was no incidence of clinical valve thrombosis and the incidence of endocarditis was similar in both the groups. Many would argue that the power of study would not be adequate for the outcome analysis done. What we need to note is that despite the use of CoreValve in this study, TAVR has fared better than SAVR in that particular age group of patients and since the older generation valve was used in this study, it should not be a surprise that the TAVR group had a higher rate of moderate-to-severe PVL. As mentioned earlier, it would not be possible to know the exact durability of the TAVR valve in this study, as the mean age of the patients was almost 80 years and these patients would die of natural processes and also they would not exert themselves so much to tell about the real stress-related degeneration of the TAVR valve in the human body. Analysis was done by pooling data from CoreValve US High-Risk Pivotal and SURTAVI intermediate-risk patients and presented at the CRT conference, which showed significantly lower BVD in TAVR with self-expandable valve than SAVR at 5 years [7.8% vs. 14.2%; hazard ratio (HR) $p < 0.001$]. The SVD (2.2% vs. 4.4%; HR 0.46; $p < 0.004$) and 30-day PPM (3.7% vs. 11.8%; HR 0.29; $p < 0.001$) both were lower in the TAVR group in comparison to SAVR, although 88% of the valve used was older generation CoreValve and only 12% was Evolut R in the TAVR group. A standardized definition of valve durability was used in this analysis. Long-term follow-up data from Evolut's low-risk TAVR study will help us in understanding the long-term durability of these patients.

Registries such as FRANCE 2, Finnish, and OBSERVANT have also looked into the durability of TAVR and SAVR.[21-24] They may provide real-life data regarding durability; however, we should keep in mind that these were patients from prohibitive-risk or high-risk areas and trying to extrapolate that data may not be a good idea. The FRANCE 2 registry tried to compare the durability data between self-expandable and balloon-expandable valves. But it should be kept in mind that in real-life cases, interventionists tend to choose a self-expandable platform for heavily calcified valves and hence this platform may have more PVL. It would be interesting to see despite these limitations if the self-expandable platform can perform as well as balloon expandable.

COMPARISON OF SELF-EXPANDABLE WITH BALLOON-EXPANDABLE TAVR VALVE

With two distinctive types of TAVR platforms, it should not be a surprise if there arises a debate as to which platform is better and with the standardization of definitions of SVD and BVF, the comparison between the two platforms also makes sense. The CHOICE trial which consisted of 241 patients compared self-expandable (Medtronic CoreValve) with balloon-expandable (Edwards Sapien XT).[25,26] Although at 30 days, the incidence of a permanent pacemaker, more than mild PVL and need for implantation of more than one valve was more self-expandable; however, at 5 years, there was no significant difference in mortality, CV death, stroke rate, or rate of rehospitalization. It was surprising to note that BVF was also similar in both groups. Please note that this was a trial with the older generation in both groups. CoreValve was used as a self-expandable valve which was a nonretrievable system. The Solve TAVI trial compared Sapien 3 and Evolut R platform. There was lower all-cause mortality and stroke rate with self-expandable than balloon expandable. There was significantly lower moderate-to-severe PVL with self-expandable; and a very important change; the rate of pacemaker had come down for self-expandable platform. The reason for this could be standardization of the technique and more operators excepting the cuspal-overlap technique which eventually lead to higher implantation of the valves and lesser requirement of permanent pacemaker. In 300 patients, Deutsch et al., at 7.14 years median follow-up, showed significantly lower SVD with SE than BE (11.8% vs. 22.6%, $p = 0.01$).[27] Barbanti et al. at 8 years showed higher SVD with CoreValve than with Sapien XT. Eltchaninoff et al. found the incidence of SVD and BVF to be 3.2% and 0.6% at 8 years.[28] In one of the earliest studies (between 2007 and 2011) with CoreValve that had 88% echocardiographic follow-up, no case of SVD was noted; however, 3.3% of patients had to redo TAVR due to severe PVL.[29] Again, one should note due to lack of standard definition there was this variability. The UK TAVI registry with a median follow-up of 5.8 years showed moderate and severe SVD of 8.7% and 0.4% respectively and there was no significant difference between SE or BE valves.[30]

WHAT THE FUTURE HOLDS?

Transcatheter aortic valve implantation is an evolving field. Over the years, newer generation valves have been developed and the results with these newer generation valves have been better than the previous generation valves. On average new generation, valves have been introduced every 4–5 years. By the time, we start getting long-term data about these valves, it is time to test the durability of the newer generation valve. Nevertheless, trials have shown that the new generation Sapien 3 valve had lesser SVD in comparison to the older generation Sapien XT. Looking at SAVR durability data, we can expect the average life of the TAVR valves to be around 10–15 years. As guidelines now endorse low-risk TAVR in the selected group of patients, the durability of these valves will become of utmost importance. In pursuit of lifetime management of aortic valve disease, there has been a search for material that would make ideal valve tissue. The following would make the ideal tissue material for the valve— (1) biocompatible, (2) have low thrombogenicity, (3) have optimal hemodynamic performance, (4) low cost to produce, (5) finally have TAVR applicability. The first-generation polymer valves were made up of—(1) polysiloxanes, (2) polytetrafluoroethylene, (3) polyurethanes.[31] The first-generation polymer valve did not last for long. The main causes of failure of these polymers were—(1) pressure overload causing mechanical degeneration of the valve, (2) degradation of the polymer under physiological conditions, (3) high thrombogenicity, (4) rapid calcification, and (5) early pannus formation on the valve. The following polymers are the most promising polymers that can be used for valve development. These polymers have superior mechanical properties and biocompatibility in comparison to first-generation polymers—(1) Polyhedral oligomeric silsesquioxane poly(carbonate-urea) urethane (POSS-PCU); (2) Nanocomposite graphene–PCU polymer (FGO-PCU, Hastalex); (3) Siloxane poly(urethane–urea) (SiPUU, LifePolymer); (4) Poly(styrene-b-isobutylene-b-styrene) (SIBS) and poly(styrene-b-4-vinylbenzocyclobutene-b-isobutylene-b-styrene-b-4-vinylbenzocyclobutene) (xSIBS); (5) Nanocomposite polyvinyl alcohol (PVA) and bacterial cellulose (PVA-BC); (6) Linear-low-density polyethene (LLDPE) and hyaluronan-enhanced linear-low-density polyethene (HA-LLDPE).[32] These polymers have been used in both TAVR as well has SAVR valves. Some of the polymeric TAVR valves that have been developed and undergoing in vivo as well as in vitro studies have been summarized in the **Table 2**.

TABLE 2: Polymer-based TAVR valves under developmental stage.

Device name	Leaflet material	Features	Development stage
Foldax Tria (Foldax Inc)	SiPUU [LifePolymer (LP)]	No need for lifetime anticoagulation; NiTinol frame, 19F OD delivery system which may be decreased to 12F	Preclinical testing—completed pilot study in sheep model. Larger preclinical study may begin in 2022 which may eventually lead to a first-in-human study
Inflow (I4HV Inc)	Copolymers of PU-PUS	Polymeric valve with cobalt-chrome alloy frame; 15–16 F OD	Animal trial in sheep model completed. Large GLP animal trial planned followed by a first-in-human study
SAT (Strait Access Technologies Inc)	Triblock polyurethane combining siloxane and carbonate segments (Carbosil)	Intercommissural anchoring arms with nickel–cobalt–chromium frame, AR patients can be treated	In vitro testing
Triskele (UCL Cardiovascular Engineering Laboratory)	Urethane (POSS-PCU) polymer	Fully retrievable NiTinol frame system	Animal trial completed. First-in-human study in Q1 2023

(AR: aortic regurgitation)

CONCLUSION

The indications of TAVR have been progressively expanded to include all spectrum of surgical risk patients based on the safety documented in various clinical trials in comparison with surgery. While short-term and medium-term results following TAVR demonstrate favorable outcomes, long-term durability still remains unclear. Long-term durability is particularly important for younger patients as they will outlive the prosthetic valve and require repeat intervention. The release of standardized definitions of SVD allows data comparison from different places with the aim of obtaining better insight into real-world data. Although short-term and medium-term follow-up results are favorable, it is imperative to collect long-term data on these valves before the wider adaptation of TAVR in guidelines.

ONLINE REFERENCES

Please scan the QR code provided at the end of the table of contents for References of this chapter.

CHAPTER

190 Valve-in-valve Transcatheter Aortic Valve Replacement

Vigyan Vijay Bang

ABSTRACT

Valve-in-valve transcatheter aortic valve replacement (ViV TAVR) has become an alternative to reoperative surgery in patients with structural valve degeneration. This procedure can be associated with unique technical challenges. Procedure planning is the cornerstone of success. It involves reviewing the index presentation and identifying the type and size of bioprosthesis implanted, knowing the unique characteristics of the prosthesis, and understanding the mechanism of valve failure, reviewing serial echocardiograms to identify the evolution of valve performance, and, finally, anticipating unique complication associated with ViV TAVR, such as coronary obstruction/sinus sequestration and patient–prosthesis mismatch. This procedure is in its nascent stage, and more work is required to understand its long-term clinical implications, particularly in patients at lower risk for reoperative surgical aortic valve replacement.

Keywords: Valve-in-valve TAVR, THV-in-THV, bioprosthetic valve fracture.

INTRODUCTION

Valve-in-valve transcatheter aortic valve replacement (ViV TAVR) has become an alternative to reoperative surgery in patients with structural valve degeneration (SVD). Bioprosthetic valves now represent majority of surgical aortic valve replacement (SAVR) in younger patients, who can expect a valve reintervention within their lifetime.[1] ViV TAVR can be associated with unique technical challenges. Here, we review some of the key considerations of this procedure.

CHARACTERISTICS OF SURGICAL VALVES AND STRUCTURAL VALVE DEGENERATION

Understanding the characteristics of the implanted surgical prosthesis is key. This includes valve manufacturer and size, fracturability or expansibility, leaflet mounting—external versus internal, and the true internal diameter of the prosthesis.

Historically, bioprosthetic valve failure of surgically implanted valves has been defined as the rate of reoperation. This has been criticized since SVD may go unnoticed in the absence of well-defined echocardiographic parameters to identify severity. Additionally, patients may not be suitable candidates for a reoperation or elect not to undergo another surgery despite SVD. Therefore, and in the era of transcatheter valve interventions, a standardized definition of SVD has been proposed.[2] This includes both morphologic and hemodynamic characteristics of failing bioprostheses **(Table 1)**.

This may help in the uniform assessment of SVD in surgical and transcatheter bioprosthetic valves. Ultimately, accurate data comparing the durability of SAVR and TAVR will come from long-term follow-up of randomized trials comparing patients at low surgical risk.[3,4]

Safety of Redo Surgical Aortic Valve Replacement and Valve-in-valve Transcatheter Aortic Valve Replacement

Mortality of ViV TAVR has been captured in the Valve-In-Valve International Data (VIVID) and Transcatheter Valve Therapies (TVT) registries.[5,6] 30-day mortality was 4.6% in the VIVID registry and 2.1% in the TVT registry. Small surgical valves and aortic stenosis as the cause for SVD (rather than

TABLE 1: Structural valve degeneration (SVD) definition.

SVD stage	SVD definition
Stage 0	No significant change from immediate postimplantation
Stage 1	Morphologic leaflet abnormality (such as leaflet thickening, calcification, or new leaflet motion disorder) without significant hemodynamic changes
Stage 2S	*Moderate stenosis*: >10 mm Hg increase from baseline with decrease in EOA and DVI
Stage 2R	Moderate valvular regurgitation (paravalvular regurgitation should not be considered as SVD)
Stage 2RS	Moderate stenosis and regurgitation
Stage 3	Severe stenosis and/or severe regurgitation

Notes: This SVD definition excludes infective endocarditis, valve thrombosis, isolated patient–prosthesis mismatch without deterioration in valve function, isolated paravalvular regurgitation, and frame distortion without abnormal leaflet function. These conditions may account for stage 1 SVD because these bioprostheses could be prone to early SVD.

(EOA: effective orifice area; DVI: Doppler velocity index)

regurgitation) were associated with higher mortality in the VIVID registry.[5] On the other hand, the mortality for patients included in the Society of Thoracic Surgeons (STS) database after redo SAVR was 4.7%.[7] However, these comparisons are limited by the bias of patients with higher surgical risk and comorbidities undergoing ViV TAVR.

CORONARY OBSTRUCTION

Coronary obstruction during TAVR can be catastrophic with an ~50% mortality rate. It occurs more often in ViV TAVR for failed surgical bioprosthesis (2.35%) than native valve TAVR (<1%).[8] The incidence of left coronary obstruction is most common (72%), followed by both coronary arteries (20%). Isolated right coronary artery obstruction is the least common (8%). In terms of timing, coronary obstruction occurs most commonly during the TAVR (64%) but can occur within the first 24 hours after TAVR (22%) or later (14%). Obstruction can be partial or complete and is typically associated with persistent hypotension. Coronary obstruction after ViV TAVR is eight times more likely to occur in stentless valves or those with externally mounted leaflets, compared with ViV TAVR for valve with internally mounted leaflets [odds ratio (OR) 7.67].[8]

Computed tomography (CT) angiogram is the cornerstone of TAVR planning and is helpful in identifying the risk of coronary obstruction by measuring the virtual transcatheter valve to coronary ostia (VTC) distance. It is measured by placing a virtual cylinder of the diameter of the planned TAVR in the center of the degenerated bioprosthetic valve frame. The distance between the virtual valve and the coronary ostia is defined as the VTC. A VTC of <4 mm is highly predictive of coronary obstruction (area under curve 0.943, $p < 0.0001$).[8] Another important mechanism of coronary obstruction in ViV TAVR includes sinus sequestration where the leaflets of the degenerated bioprosthesis reach the sinotubular junction (STJ). In such anatomy, if the diameter of the STJ approximates the TAVR, there is a risk of sealing the STJ, precluding coronary filling. Features that mitigate this risk include internally mounted leaflets on the degenerated prosthesis and patent coronary bypass grafts.

Salvage percutaneous coronary intervention after TAVR is technically difficult and was unsuccessful in 18% of cases in a large series.[9] Despite successful revascularization, the mortality was 22%. Emergency coronary artery bypass grafting (CABG) carried a mortality of 50%, and unsuccessful revascularization was fatal in 100% of cases.

Identification of a high risk of coronary obstruction should prompt a reconsideration of redo SAVR or adoption of alternative strategies for coronary protection. These include "chimney" stenting and Bioprosthetic or native Aortic Scallop Intentional Laceration to prevent Iatrogenic Coronary Artery obstruction (BASILICA). The former technique involves deploying a prepositioned stent at the ostium of the obstructed coronary artery, extending into the sinus/aortic root, behind the TAVR frame, with the ability to retract the undeployed stent if there is no compromise of coronary artery flow. Stenting was required in 20% of the cases when this strategy was employed, with 100% procedural success, even though the long-term patency of this strategy remains unclear.[10] BASILICA offers an alternative strategy where the leaflets that threaten to obstruct coronary flow are lacerated by transcatheter electrocautery, preserving access and blood flow to the coronary artery. The BASILICA IDE trial demonstrated 86.9% procedural success.[11]

Bioprosthetic Valve Fracture

Valve-in-valve transcatheter aortic valve replacement performed in small surgical prostheses, typically <21 mm, are associated with high transvalvular gradients.[5] Consideration must be given to redo SAVR with annular enlargement techniques to facilitate placement of a larger prosthesis. Bioprosthetic valve fracture (BVF) is an alternative to reoperative surgery. It is performed using a high-pressure noncompliant balloon, usually with a coronary indeflator connected to the balloon using a three-way stopcock to deliver additional high pressure to a fully inflated balloon. Notably, the Abbott Trifecta and Medtronic Hancock II valves are not fracturable.[12]

This has been shown to be a safe and effective technique with no adverse complications and improved valve performance. The mean gradient decreased from 20.5 to 6.7 mm Hg ($p < 0.001$) with an increased effective orifice area from 1 to 1.8 cm^2 ($p < 0.001$).[13] BVF may be performed before or after ViV TAVR. There may be a theoretical advantage to BVF after ViV TAVR in expansion of the newly implanted prosthesis, lower risk of debris embolization, and prevention of hemodynamic collapse from aortic leaflet avulsion and subsequent aortic regurgitation. Alternatively, BVF prior to ViV TAVR may prevent subclinical leaflet injury of the newly implanted prosthesis. There have been case reports of BVF leading to annular rupture and should be used with caution in patients with heavy annular and left ventricular outflow tract (LVOT) calcification.[14]

TAVR-in-TAVR

While TAVR-in-TAVR is a relatively uncommon procedure currently, with the indication of TAVR expanded to low-risk patients, the volume is expected to increase over time. It may be required acutely due to valve embolization during index valve deployment. Alternatively, ViV TAVR might be required to treat failed transcatheter heart valves (THV), in the setting of either SVD or non-SVD (such as significant paravalvular regurgitation). The outcomes to treat failed THV are available in small case series but appear to be feasible.[15]

Typically, the valve size is similar to the index THV, with the exception of an inappropriately sized index THV. Therefore, assessing the original computed tomography angiography (CTA) can offer valuable insight into the mechanism of valve failure. If the size of the index THV is unknown, it may be estimated on multidetector computed tomography (MDCT) using the true internal diameter of the prosthesis at the level on the annulus. Positioning of the THV in THV is typically done by aligning outflow to outflow but should be chosen on a case-by-case basis. For example, we chose to implant deeper in a patient with THV failure due to non-SVD etiology of significant paravalvular regurgitation caused by incomplete seal due to severe raphae and annular calcification, successfully sealing the paravalvular leakage (PVL) (see **Figs. 1A to D**). A balloon-expandable THV is theoretically advantageous in such a setting, due to higher radial force. Conceptually, the assessment of risk for coronary obstruction is similar to ViV TAVR, as above.

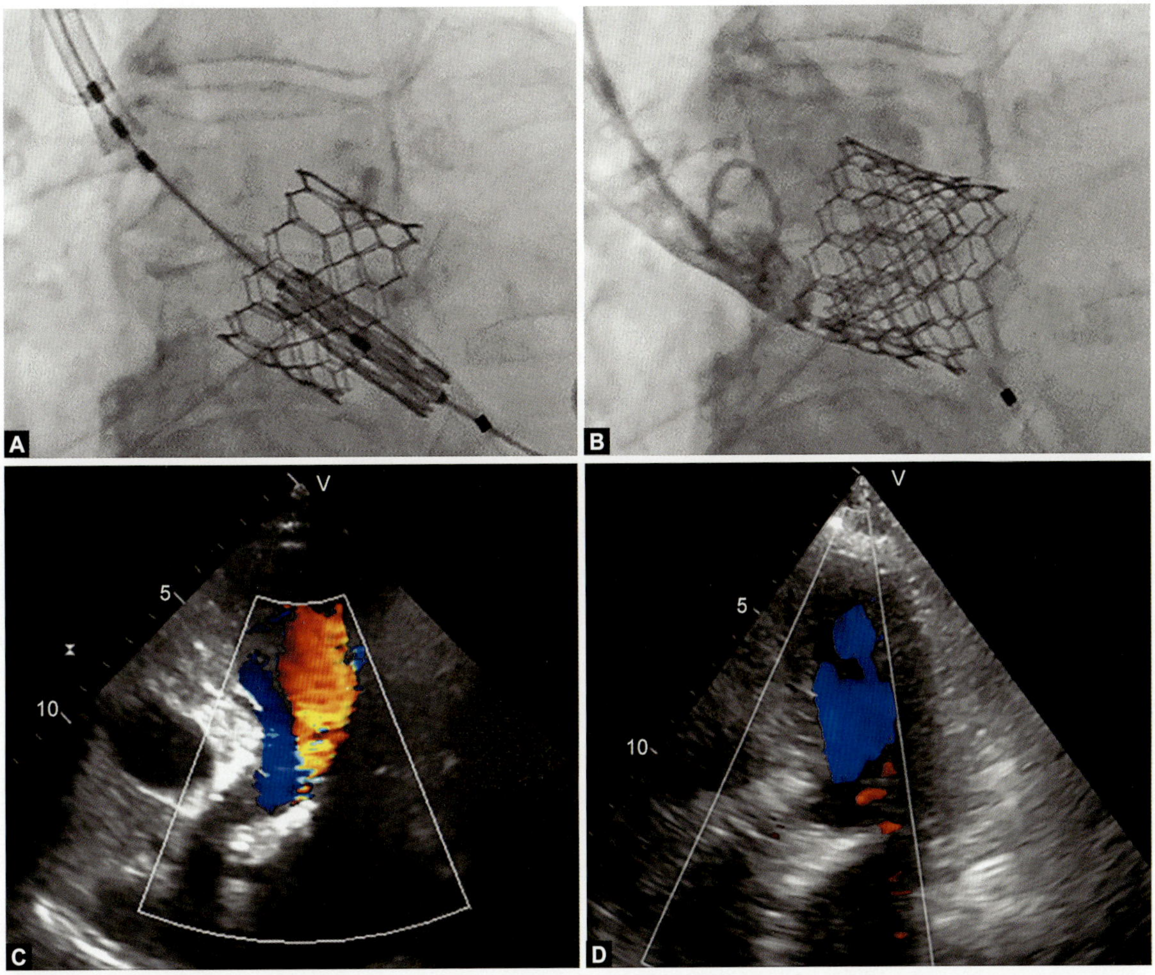

FIGS. 1A TO D: Cineangiography and echocardiogram assessment of TAVR in TAVR to address symptomatic severe paravalvular regurgitation after index TAVR. (A) TAVR in TAVR to treat severe PVL. Top of valve frame aligned below the outflow of the index prosthesis to address mechanism of non-SVD valve failure. (B) Complete resolution of PVL after TAVR in TAVR. (C) Severe PVL after index TAVR. (D) Trivial PVL after TAVR in TAVR.

(PVL: paravalvular leakage; SVD: structural valve degeneration; TAVR: transcatheter aortic valve replacement)

CONCLUSION

Valve-in-valve transcatheter aortic valve replacement is an excellent treatment strategy for failed bioprosthetic surgical valves. In the absence of randomized data, ViV TAVR should be weighed against reoperative SAVR as an alternative, particularly in lower risk patients. Adjunctive strategies to optimize outcomes include procedures such as BASILICA to prevent coronary obstruction and BVF to optimize valve hemodynamics, and a patient–prosthesis mismatch should be carefully considered.

ONLINE REFERENCES

Please scan the QR code provided at the end of the table of contents for References of this chapter.

CHAPTER

191

Transcatheter Aortic Valve Replacement for Pure Aortic Regurgitation

Kayan Siodia, Srinivas Kudva, Haresh G Mehta

ABSTRACT

Transcatheter aortic valve implantation (TAVI) is increasingly becoming the standard therapy for severe aortic stenosis. Over the years, the indication has expanded from extreme/high risk to intermediate- and low-risk group population as well.

As a standard and safety guideline, currently only calcified severe aortic stenosis or combination of stenosis and regurgitation/insufficiency can undergo a TAVI; however, there have been a few off-label TAVI use reported in pure isolated aortic regurgitation (AR) in patients who are at high risk for surgery.

In this chapter, we highlight some of the considerations for performing TAVI in pure AR anatomy including tips and tricks that have been used to safely deploy the valve giving optimum clinical results. This also highlights the risk to be aware of during execution of the case.

Keywords: Severe aortic stenosis, aortic regurgitation, aortic insufficiency, native aortic pure aortic regurgitation.

INTRODUCTION

Over the past decade, percutaneous treatment of calcified severe aortic stenosis has been widely accepted [transcatheter aortic valve implantation (TAVI)]. The various improvements in the valve technology have encouraged skilled operators to widen the indication. In some such attempts, there have been few patients treated with TAVI for pure aortic regurgitation (AR) anatomy as an off-label use.

The anatomy of patients with pure AR is different than that of calcified aortic stenosis. Therefore, the operators come across unique challenges in using TAVI for these patients.

With careful consideration, planning, and execution, there is now some understanding on how a TAVI valve can be safely deployed with the currently available nondedicated devices for pure AR anatomy. This chapter focuses on planning and execution tips and tricks learnt from real-life experiences using TAVI in pure AR anatomy.

PREVALENCE

The prevalence of AR in native aortic valve increases with age. In the United States, it is reported to be between 4.9 and 10%. AR is common among males as compared to females. The Framingham Heart Study, a prospective epidemiological study, evaluated the prevalence and severity of AR and other valvular diseases by color Doppler examinations in 1,696 men and 1,893 women. The study revealed that the prevalence of AR (ranging in severity from trace to ≥ moderate regurgitation) is 13.0% in men and 8.5% in women. Worldwide, the most common cause of AR is rheumatic heart disease, particularly in Asia, Middle East, and North Africa.[1]

CAUSES

Aortic regurgitation can be due to malfunction in the coaptation of the leaflets or a dysfunction of the supporting structures such as the aortic root or the annulus or both.

The two major types of diseases due to which AR occurs are described here.

Valve Disease

- *Infective endocarditis* changes the anatomy of leaflets, which leads to prolapse due to loss of commissural support.

- *Bicuspid aortic valve (BAV)* is a congenital defect which can cause AR due to underdeveloped cusps.
- *Rheumatic disease* can lead to fibrous infiltration of the cusps that can prevent proper opening and closure of the leaflets.
- *Pre-existing bioprosthetic valves* with structural deterioration can lead to AR.

Aortic Root Complex Disease

Dilation of the annular root complex many a time leads to separation of the leaflets that results in AR. This etiology could be age related, retrograde dissection, or severe chronic systemic hypertenstion.[2-4]

CHANGES IN PHYSIOLOGY DUE TO AR

Patients with AR can be asymptomatic for years. However, there is progressive left ventricular (LV) dilation and dysfunction.

Progression of the disease is related to the severity of regurgitation, the etiology of aortic valve disease, the presence of symptoms, and the size and function of the LV.

There is an overload of the left ventricle due to the AR. An increase in LV end-diastolic volume causes dilation and eccentric hypertrophy of the LV. This allows ejection of a larger stroke volume. The function of the LV could be compensated by LV dilation and hypertrophy. Over time, wall thickening fails to keep pace with the hemodynamic load resulting in a decline in systolic function and ejection fraction.

In advanced stages, symptoms of heart failure develop.

Increase in the LV mass leads to an increased need for oxygen by the myocardium. Further, there is reduction in the coronary perfusion pressures causing myocardial ischemia and chest pain due to exertion.

The annual mortality in patients with symptomatic severe AR can be as high as 25%.[5]

STAGES OF AR

The 2020 American College of Cardiology (ACC)/American Heart Association (AHA) Guideline for the management of patients with valvular heart disease has categorized the AR in various stages, to be precise in four stages.

Ranging from patients at risk of AR (Stage A) or with progressive mild-to-moderate AR (Stage B) to severe asymptomatic (Stage C) and symptomatic (Stage D) AR. Each of these stages is defined by valve anatomy, valve hemodynamics, severity of LV dilation, and LV systolic function, as well as by patient symptoms.[6]

OUTCOME OF UNTREATED AR

Early stages of AR may not show any symptoms. As it progresses, it affects the hemodynamics and functioning of the heart muscle. In absence of any treatment, heart failure, ischemic cardiomyopathy, arrhythmia, and even sudden death can ensue.

Surgery has shown to benefit these patients with symptoms. Therefore, it is well justified to have valve replacement (surgically or transcatheter) to prevent complications.[7]

TREATING TEAM

A heart team including an experienced cardiac surgeon, a structural interventional cardiologist, and the other supporting staff should be a mandate when planning for treatment of pure AR cases especially using transcatheter options.

CHOICE OF TREATMENT

Surgical aortic valve repair or replacement (SAVR) is the conventional treatment. However, the Euro Heart Survey showed that valve intervention was "underutilized" in approximately 8% of patients because of an elevated risk of perioperative mortality due to advanced age or multiple comorbidities. This rate was even higher in patients with lower left ventricular ejection fraction (LVEF).

As per guideline and good clinical practice, if patients with isolated severe AR who have indications for SAVR and are candidates for surgery, TAVI is a contraindication due to the technical challenges imposed by the absence of anchoring aortic valve calcification. The 2020 ACC/AHA Valvular Heart Disease Guidelines strongly advise against use of TAVI in patients with isolated severe AR.[8]

CONCERNS USING TAVI FOR PURE AR

Transcatheter aortic valve implantation is not encouraged in pure AR because of challenges that could compromise procedural success.[9,10] The absence of calcification of the aortic annulus and the frequent coexistence of aortic root dilation poses significant difficulties for positioning and anchoring of transcatheter heart valves (THVs), and absence of an anchoring factor (calcium) leads to increased risk of no or inadequate sealing causing significant amount of paravalvular leak (PVL) and/or embolization.

As a practice when planning a TAVI in pure AR patient, one should look to oversize THVs a minimum of 20% to enable valve sealing. With this amount of oversizing, the risk of annular rupture and need for a pacemaker also increase. The AR increases the chances of THV embolization. Pure AR patients have advanced cardiac problems such as LV dysfunction and impaired hemodynamics, adding an incremental risk of procedural complications.

LITERATURE FOR TAVI IN PURE AR

There is no randomized clinical trial that has compared TAVI with SAVR for the treatment of pure AR or compared specific THVs. The data available today are mostly case reports, single center experiences, or meta-analysis.

With this data, the literature supports feasibility of TAVI in patients with pure AR with the currently available devices; however, it comes with several technical challenges and risk of complications to be managed.

Haddad et al. reported a systematic review and meta-analysis to summarize the available evidence on the use of TAVI in patients with pure AR and compared outcomes between first- and second-generation valves. The main outcome of interest was all-cause mortality at 30 days. A total of 638 patients across 12 studies were included. Mean age ranged from 68 to 84. Society of Thoracic Surgeons score ranged from 5.4 to 13.1% and Logistic EuroSCORE ranged from 18.2 to 33%. The incidence rate of all-cause mortality at 30 days was found to be 11% [95% confidence interval (CI) 7–16%; I^2 = 20.86%]. All-cause mortality at 30 days for first generation valves had an incidence rate of 15% (95% CI 10–20%; I^2 = 10%) compared to 7% (95% CI 3–13%; I^2 = 37%) in second generation valves with subgroup interaction analysis p = 0.059. Device success incidence rate in second-generation valves was 92% (95% CI 83–99%; I^2 = 67%) versus 68% (95% CI 59–77%; I^2 = 53%) in first-generation valves with p = 0.001. TAVI appears to be a feasible treatment choice for pure AR patients at high risk for surgical valve replacement. Second-generation valves show promising results in terms of short-term outcomes.[11]

One of the largest series to date, reported by Yoon et al., included patients treated with first- and second-generation THV and with new-generation devices [Evolut R (Medtronic) and SAPIEN 3 (Edwards Lifesciences)]. This study showed that the use of new-generation devices was associated with improved procedural outcomes. The difference was mainly driven by lower rates of need for a second implant and significant residual AR.[12]

Similar conclusions were yielded by a meta-analysis published in 2018 by Rawasia et al. The group receiving a new-generation device had lower 30-day mortality [9.1% (6.8–11.7%) vs. 15.3% (10.3–21.1%)] and higher device success rate [92.8% (86.6–97.2%) vs. 75.2% (63.6–85.2%)] compared to the group receiving old-generation devices. Although the outcomes for patients undergoing TAVI for severe AR remain worse when compared with those undergoing TAVI for on-label indications, the difference continues to narrow.[13]

In a recent international, multicenter, observational study that enrolled all consecutive patients with symptomatic severe noncalcified AR undergoing TAVR with the Myval device (Made in India Balloon Expandable Valve), a total of 113 patient were recruited. The annular area was beyond the recommended range for extra-large sizes in 2.6% of cases, and additional volume was added in 92% (median 4 cc, up to 9 cc). The extra-large sizes were used in 95 patients (84.1%), and the mean oversizing was 17.9 ± 11.0%. The technical success rate was 94.7%; the rate of residual ≥ moderate AR was 8.9%, and the pacemaker rate was 22.2%. There were no cases of annular rupture, cardiac tamponade, or aortic dissection, but in 4 patients (3.5%), valve embolization occurred **(Fig. 1)**. 30-day and 1-year mortalities were 5.3% and 9.7%, respectively **(Figs. 2 and 3)**. Technical success

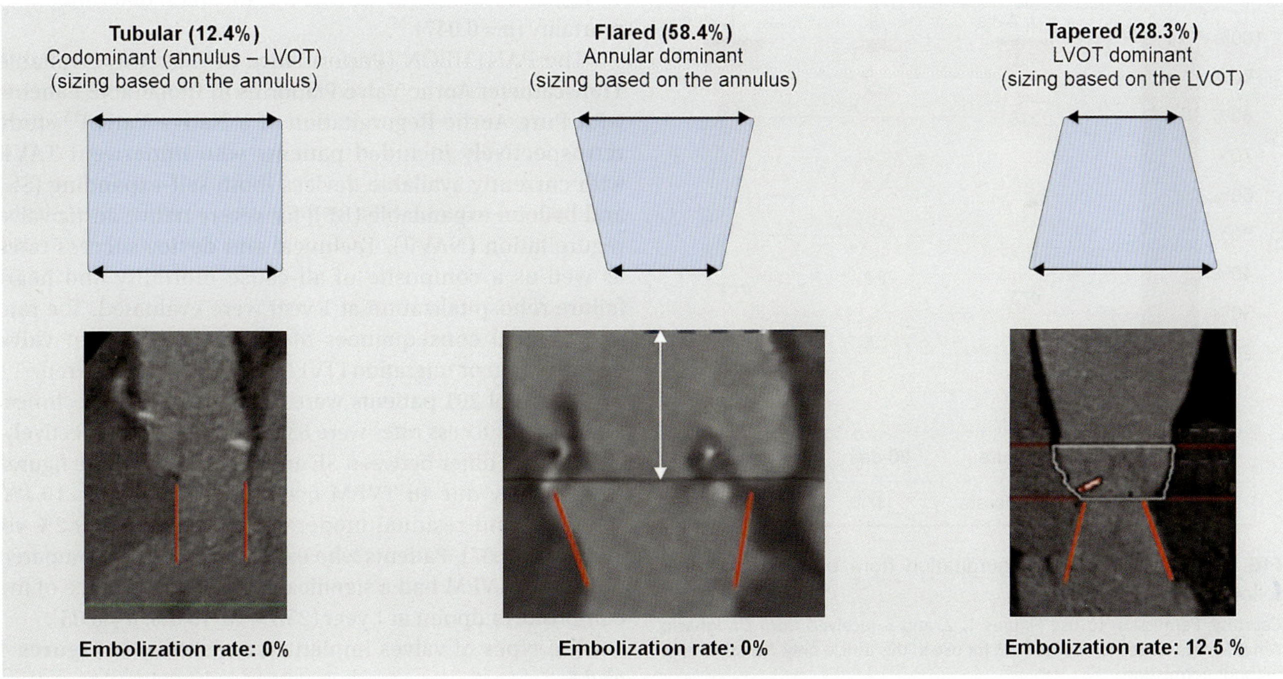

FIG. 1: Rate of device embolization according to the morphology of left ventricular outflow tract (LVOT).

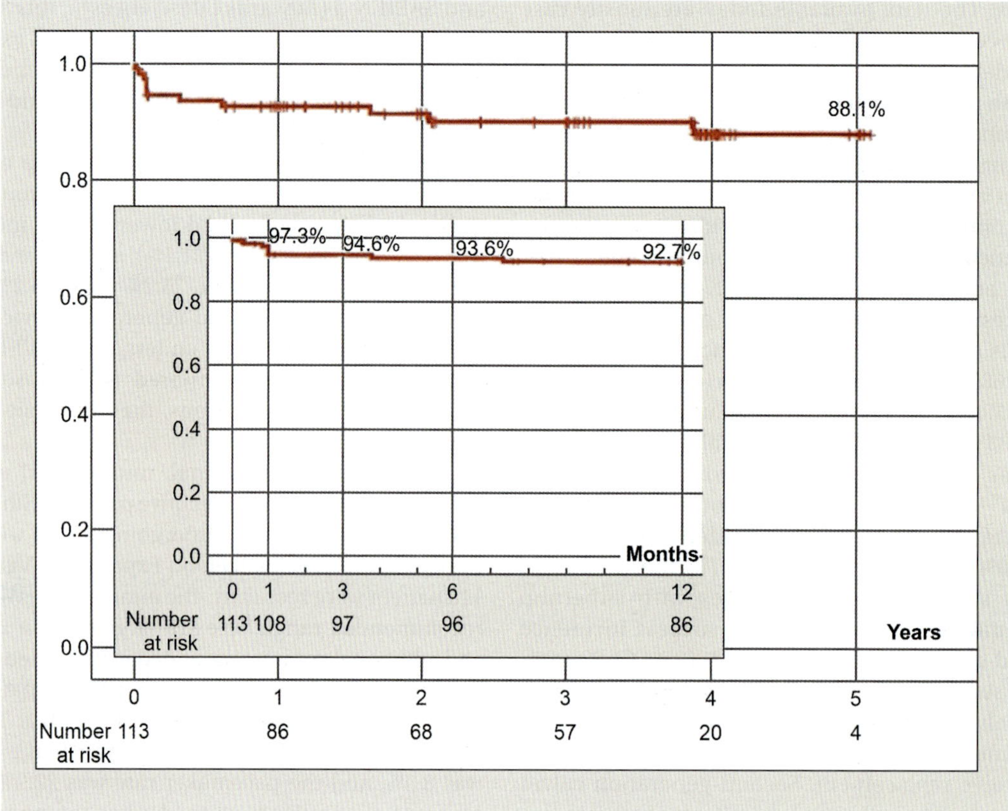

FIG. 2: All-cause mortality through 5 years follow-up.

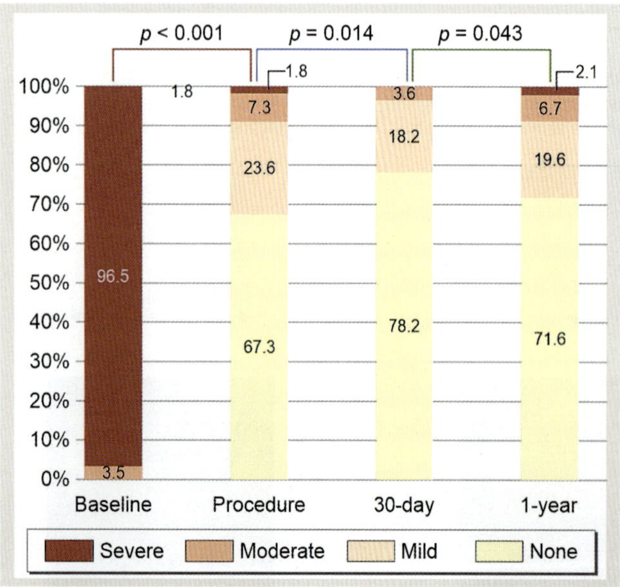

FIG. 3: Degree of aortic regurgitation from baseline to 1-year follow-up.

Courtesy: Permission to use Figures 1, 2, and 3 received from Dr. Ignacio Amat Santos on September 6, 2023 for use in this article only. No other uses without permission.

was associated with better survival (97.1% *vs.* 72.7%; $p = 0.012$), and valve embolization was the main determinant of mortality ($p = 0.047$).[14]

The PANTHEON (Performance of Currently Available Transcatheter Aortic Valve Platforms in Inoperable Patients with Pure Aortic Regurgitation of a Native Valve)[13] study retrospectively included patients who underwent TAVR with currently available devices [both self-expanding (SE) and balloon expandable (BE)] for severe native aortic valve regurgitation (NAVR). Technical and device success rates as well as a composite of all-cause mortality and heart failure rehospitalization at 1 year were evaluated. The rate and clinical consequences of acute transcatheter valve embolization or migration (TVEM) were also considered.

A total of 201 patients were included. Overall technical and device success rates were 83.6% and 76.1%, respectively, and did not differ between SE and BE devices. These figures were mostly due to TVEM occurrence (14.6% vs. 16.1%; $p = 0.47$) and residual moderate or greater AR (9.2% vs. 10.1%; $p = 0.87$). Patients who experienced TVEM compared to without TVEM had a significantly higher incidence of the composite endpoint at 1 year (25.7% vs. 15.8%; $p = 0.05$).

The types of valves implanted are shown in **Figures 4 and 5**.

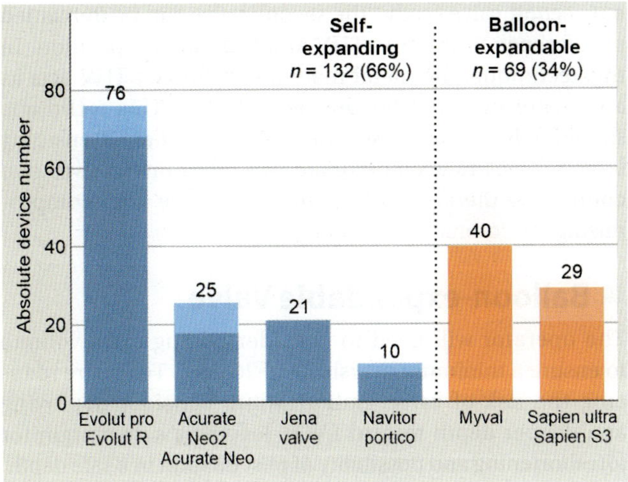

FIG. 4: The histogram shows the transcatheter heart valves used in The PANTHEON study.

WHICH DEVICE IS PREFERRED?

Initial experiences resulted in poor outcomes with TAVI in pure AR with higher rates of device embolization, higher mortality, higher rates of 2nd valve implantation, and higher unacceptable amount of PVL.

Early experience with first-generation self-expanding valves which were favored initially because it was thought to facilitate safe anchoring by oversizing without increased risk for annular disruption had disappointing results.

The use of second-generation balloon-expandable and self-expanding TAVI systems demonstrated improved outcomes in patients; however, higher than acceptable procedural complications and mortality rates were observed.[15,16]

JenaValve (Jena Valve Technology) and J-Valve (JC Medical) are two investigational devices undergoing feasibility studies in the US.

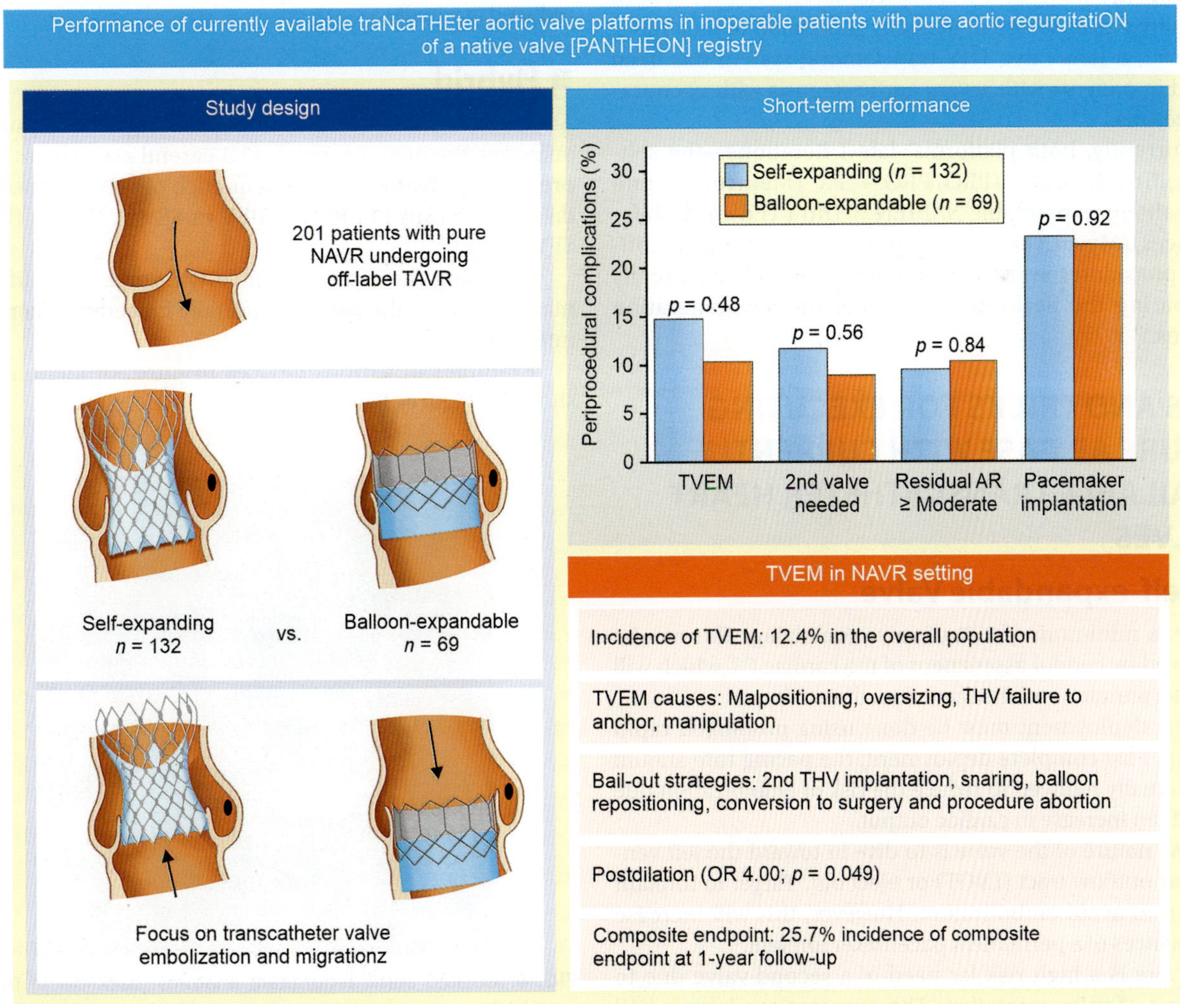

FIG. 5: Comparison between the performance and short-term results of self-expanding (SE) and balloon-expandable (BE) THVs appeared to be similar. Transcatheter valve embolization and migration (TVEM) remained the most frequent complication and had a significant impact on outcomes in both the short-term and during the 1-year follow-up period.

(AR: aortic regurgitation; NAVR: native aortic valve regurgitation; TAVR: transcatheter aortic valve replacement; THV: transcatheter heart valve)

Courtesy: Permission to use Figure 4 and 5 received from Dr. Luca Testa on September 6, 2023 for use in this article only. No other uses without permission.

The JenaValve THV is made up of self-expanding nitinol stent with a porcine pericardial valve. There is a presence of "locators" attached to the valve frame that clip onto the leaflets upon deployment, facilitating anchoring without relying on annular calcification or the need for oversizing. The other positive features of this TAVI system are: (1) the supra-annular location of the actual valve, theoretically improving hemodynamics; and (2) the presence of large cells at its aortic end and the possibility of anatomically correct alignment with native sinuses, facilitating coronary access. A potentially negative feature is the lack of a dedicated sealing skirt, which might increase the risk for significant post-procedure PVL.

The initial experience in Europe using the JenaValve THV for pure severe AR was encouraging, with the valve being successfully implanted via a transapical approach in >96% of patients. However, a high mortality of 20% was observed in patients at 1-year follow-up.

With the need of a transapical access, higher risk of mortality was observed in the early generation of JenaValve; however, a JenaValve THV transfemoral system has been tested in patients with severe aortic stenosis with encouraging results.[17,18]

Currently, both platforms' latest iterations—the self-expanding Evolut R/PRO/PRO +/FX (Medtronic) and the balloon-expandable SAPIEN 3/Ultra (Edwards Lifesciences)/Myval (Meril Lifesciences)—are used for off-label procedures in pure AR. There is no evidence currently comparing the performance of specific new-generation devices.[19-21]

TIPS AND TRICKS FOR EXECUTING A PURE AR CASE WITH CURRENTLY AVAILABLE TRANSCATHETER HEART VALVES

Self-expandable Valve

Target a minimum of 25% of valve oversizing. This can be achieved by careful assessment of the cardiac CT which will give the annulus and the aortic root dimensions.

The deployment must be done using prolonged rapid pacing. Post complete deployment, the pacing rate should be gradually reduced to reduce the risk of embolization due to sudden increase in cardiac output.

The nature of the valve is to dive in toward the left ventricular outflow tract (LVOT) or eject out. Target to implant deeper to avoid embolization. However, this will increase the chances of a permanent pacemaker implant.

There is a high risk for need of a second valve due to chances of valve migration. The operator can have a bail out second valve ready. The second valve can be implanted in reference to the first THV at a little higher position. In this technique, the metal material of the first THV acts as an anchoring agent for the second THV. This technique should only be used post careful assessment of CT ensuring large sinuses to accommodate two tall frames valves and confirming there is no formation of a tube graft compromising the coronary perfusion.

Balloon-expandable Valve

The operator will need to consider adding extra volume to ensure a minimum oversizing of 20–25%. To ensure reducing the risk of valve embolization, consider deploying at a deeper depth toward LVOT leaving a safe margin for foreshortening and possibility of post dilation in a safe depth. The above-mentioned use of two valves can be employed in balloon-expandable valves (BEVs) also.

Post complete deployment, the pacing rate must be reduced gradually.

Hybrid

As the rate of second valve implant is higher in a pure AR anatomy, the operator must do a careful assessment of CT pre case to ensure the best sequence of valve [self-expandable valve (SEV) in BEV or BEV in SEV or BEV in BEV or SEV in SEV].

Choosing the right sequence will impact the lifelong management of the patient especially if needing a coronary intervention.

Examples of various devices in pure AR anatomy are shown in **Figures 6 to 13**.

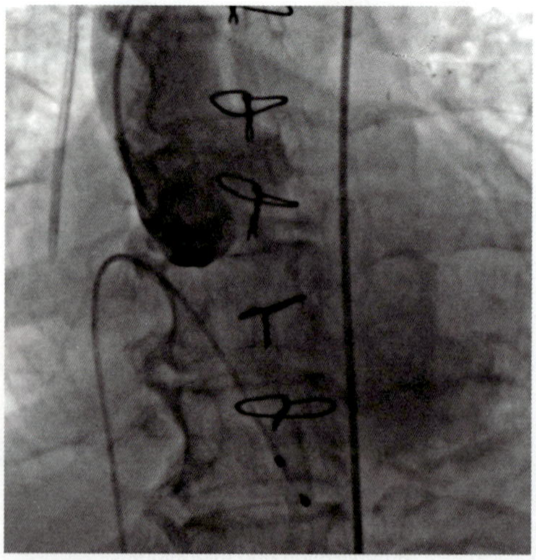

FIG. 6: Isolated aortic regurgitant anatomy (backflow in the left ventricle).

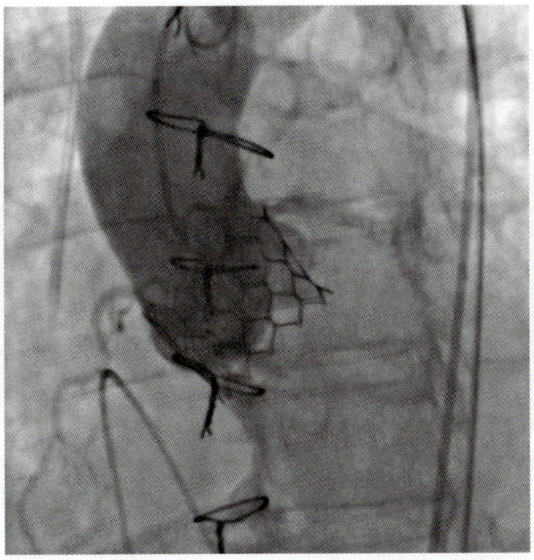

FIG. 7: Balloon expandable valve post implant.

MANAGING PURE AR IN THE COMING TIMES

Pure AR anatomy remains to be a challenging anatomy to be treated and needs different strategies and expertise for optimum clinical outcomes.

There is a need for developing dedicated valve and delivery system, which can ensure a safe and predictable outcome for patient undergoing a transcatheter-based treatment modality.

In August 2023, J-Valve transfemoral (TF) system by Genesis MedTech **(Fig. 14)** has been granted breakthrough device designation by the US Food and Drug Administration (FDA). The grant is for treatment of pure AR and AR-dominant mixed aortic valve disease. Currently, any patient's eligibility for this device must be evaluated and confirmed by a heart team approach and must be confirmed to be a high

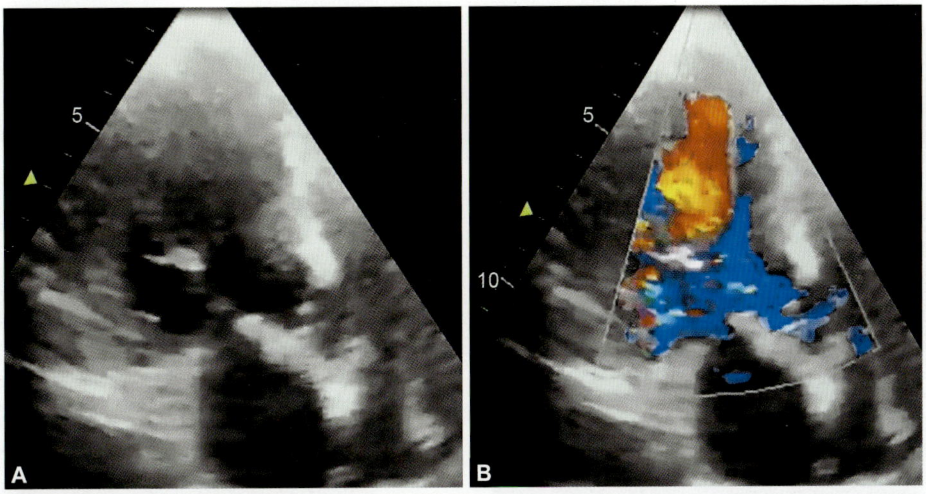

FIGS. 8A AND B: Echocardiogram of a pure aortic regurgitation anatomy.

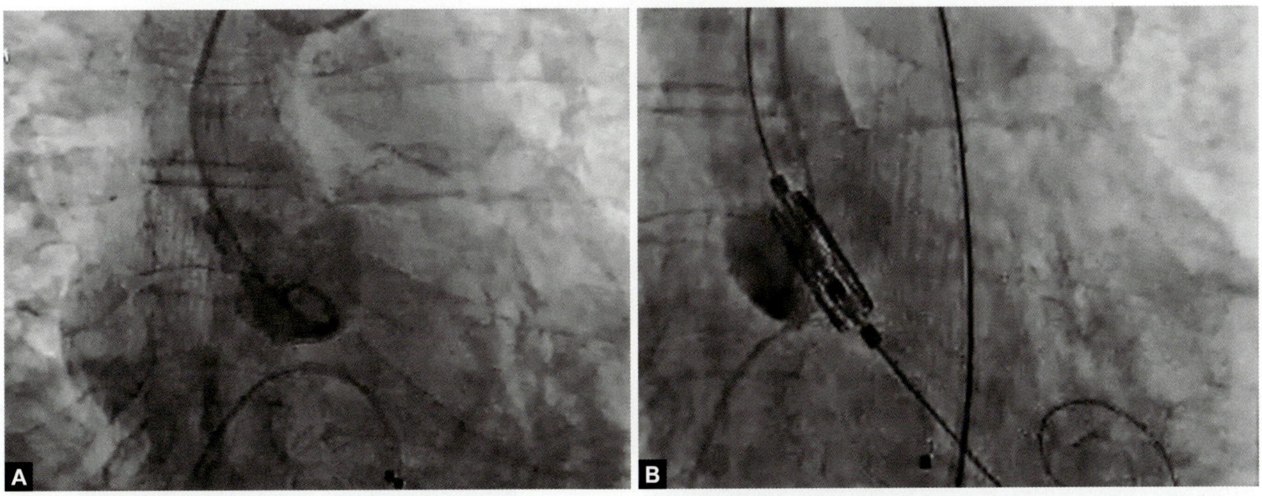

FIGS. 9A TO D: *Continued*

Continued

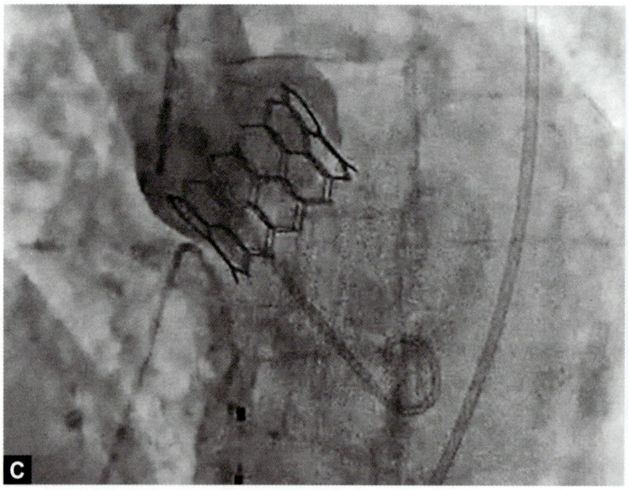

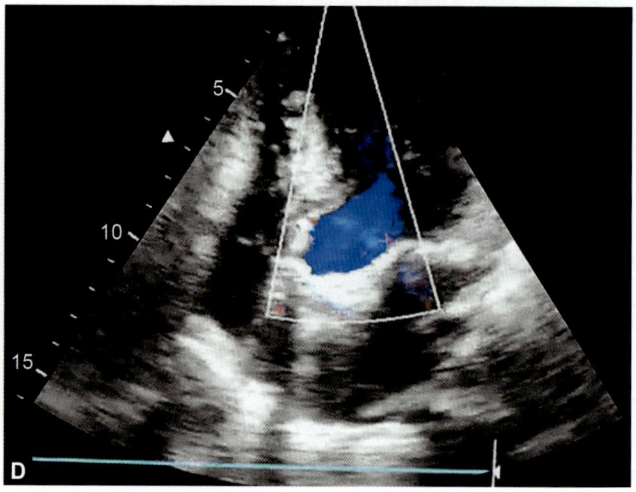

FIGS. 9A TO D: Transcatheter aortic valve implantation of balloon-expandable valve with post echocardiogram image.

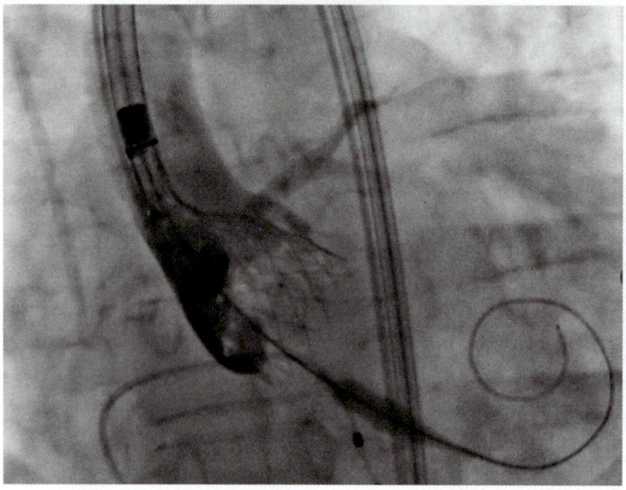

FIG. 10: Self-expandable valve in a pure aortic regurgitation anatomy at point of no capture.

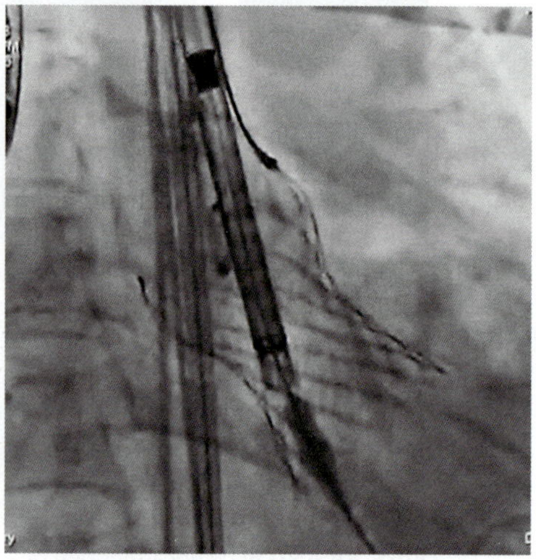

FIG. 12: Self-expandable in self-expandable valve.

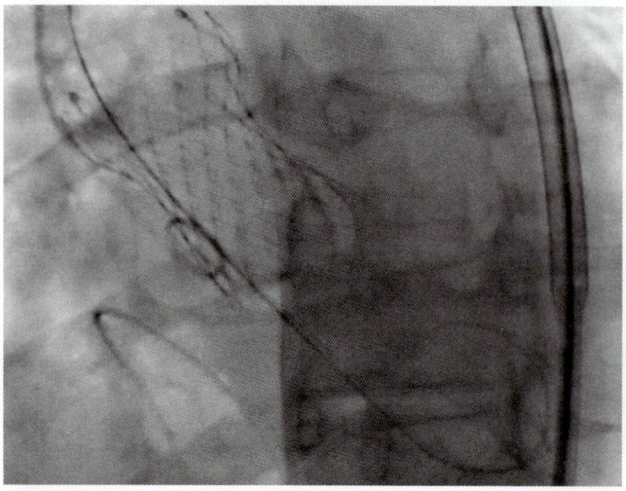

FIG. 11: Post full deployment (deeper than usually recommended by IFU).

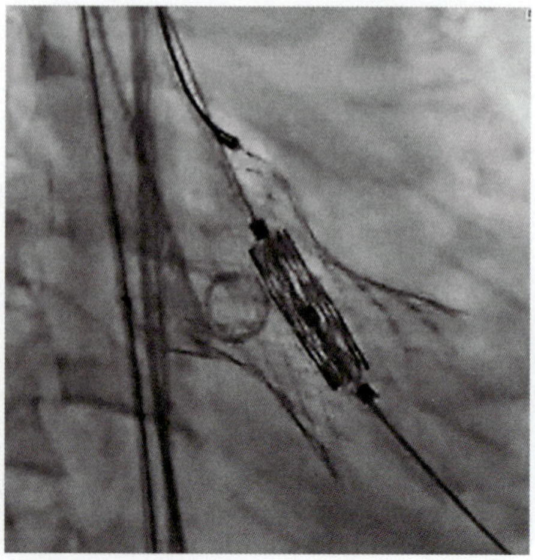

FIG. 13: Balloon-expandable in self-expandable valve.

Courtesy: Data received from Dr. Praveen Chandra at Medanta The Medicity Gurgaon on August 14, 2023. For personal use only. No other uses without permission.

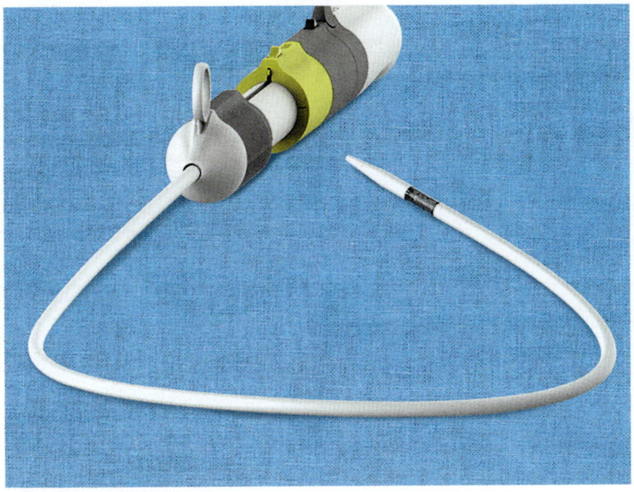

FIG. 14: J-valve transfemoral (TF) system.

Source: Downloaded from Cardiovascular News. (2023). Transfemoral TAVI device gains US FDA breakthrough status for aortic regurgitation. [online] Available from https://cardiovascularnews.com/transfemoral-tavi-device-aortic-regurgitation-us-fda-breakthrough/. [Last accessed September, 2023] for personal use only. Not other uses without permission.

risk for SAVR. The system utilizes an anchor mechanism and a stent frame that expands to attach the device to a failing valve. The system includes two components including the bioprosthesis and the delivery device. The bioprosthesis is made up of bovine pericardium leaflets, a nitinol stent frame covered with polyester fabric and a nitinol anchor ring. The delivery device is used to position the bioprosthesis in the native aortic valve.[22,23]

With wide use of this device, further evolving devices developed for managing pure AR may make treatment of this challenging anatomy more feasible in the coming times.

CONCLUSION

Transcatheter aortic valve implantation is a very well-accepted treatment modality for calcified severe aortic stenosis and in combination with mild-to-severe AR. However, in pure AR, it is still an off-label use. With the currently available valves, there have been cases performed with optimal results. However, it must be attempted only by skilled operators with good amount of experience in handling devices and managing complications like embolization.

The new devices show good promise in having a more predictable and safe deployment of a transcatheter valve. However, long-term study results are awaited before it can be approved in various countries and widely accepted as a treatment of choice.

ONLINE REFERENCES

Please scan the QR code provided at the end of the table of contents for References of this chapter.

CHAPTER 192

A Tale of Two Leaflets: The Evolution of MitraClip Transcatheter Edge-to-edge Repair

Saro Avedikian, Saibal Kar

ABSTRACT

Mitral regurgitation (MR) represents a significant challenge which has been traditionally addressed through surgical MR repair. However, the last two decades have witnessed an evolution in the treatment approach with the introduction and refinement of the MitraClip system for transcatheter edge-to-edge repair (TEER). The EVEREST II trial highlighted the potential of percutaneous repair using the first-generation MitraClip, even though conventional surgery initially exhibited higher effectiveness. The subsequent COAPT trial confirmed the superiority of the second generation MitraClip to medical treatment alone for the treatment of secondary MR. The third-generation MitraClip, included two different sizes of clips in addition to changes in the delivery system. The one year results of the EXPAND registry utilizing the third generation devices showed a significant improvement of regurgitation grades in comparison to the previous studies. The fourth-generation MitraClip has expanded its anatomical reach and offers enhanced procedural efficacy. Current clinical guidelines have established TEER for treatment of patients with secondary MR, optimized on medical treatment as well as for patients with chronic primary MR who face prohibitive surgical risk. The encouraging contemporary results of TEER, has lead the pathway to the ongoing REPAIR MR trial, which is prospective multicenter randomized study, comparing TEER versus conventional surgical repair for intermediate surgical risk patients with primary MR. Collectively, the advancements in MitraClip technology combined with heightened operator expertise suggest a transformative shift in MR treatment strategy, with forthcoming trials set to clarify patient selection for TEER versus surgical solutions.

Keywords: Mitral regurgitation, MitraClip TEER, EVEREST II trial.

INTRODUCTION

The mitral valve (MV), nestled between the left atrium and the left ventricle of the heart, is an intricate structure with dynamic function. The architecture of the MV encompasses two leaflets, anterior and posterior, which open like doors during diastole to allow blood flow from the left atrium to the left ventricle and form a tight seal during systole to prevent backflow as the left ventricle contracts to deliver blood to the systemic circulation. The base of the MV leaflets is the annulus, a fibrous D-shaped ring which provides structural integrity with its dynamic shape, changing throughout the cardiac cycle. The leaflets are attached to the anterolateral and the posteromedial papillary muscles housed in the left ventricle by thin, fibrous tendrils called the chordae tendineae. Each cord is meticulously designed and positioned to distribute even tension and maintain the competency of the valve. This complex system is designed to ensure efficient unidirectional blood flow during the cardiac cycle. However, given its delicate architecture as well as its structural dependence on left ventricular integrity, the MV has a propensity for disease and malfunction.

HISTORICAL PROGRESSIONS

Mitral valve regurgitation is generally classified as primary/degenerative or secondary/functional. Primary/degenerative mitral regurgitation (PMR) results from an intrinsic leaflet abnormality, whereas secondary/functional mitral regurgitation (SMR) results from the inability of structurally normal leaflets to coapt completely due to the distortion of the supporting architecture in the left ventricle as a result of ischemic or dilated cardiomyopathy.

Historically, surgical MV repair was the standard of care for treatment of severe or moderate-to-severe mitral regurgitation (MR).[1] In the early 1990s, Alfieri et al. demonstrated the effectiveness and durability of a central double-orifice stitch by approximation of the mitral leaflets **(Fig. 1)**. Influenced by the principle of the Alfieri stitch, first-generation endovascular devices began to emerge that demonstrated the safety and efficacy of endovascular double-orifice edge-to-edge MV repair in porcine models.[2,3]

A decade later, Feldman et al. led the initial human clinical experience in the EVEREST phase I feasibility study (Endovascular Valve Edge-to-Edge Repair Study) and demonstrated that percutaneous edge-to-edge MV repair using the first-generation MitraClip system can be performed safely to reduce the degree of MR and that the reduction can be sustained at 6 and 12 months **(Fig. 2)**.[4] The inclusion criteria of these patients included a minimum of three of six criteria for moderate-to-severe (3+) or severe (4+) MR, a flail segment width < 1.5 cm, and a regurgitant jet origin from within the central two-thirds of the line of leaflet coaptation. This phase I study of only 27 patients was not associated with any procedural complications and moderate efficacy at 6 months. These findings set the stage for risk-benefit comparison of percutaneous MV repair with conventional surgical repair in the EVEREST phase II trial.[4]

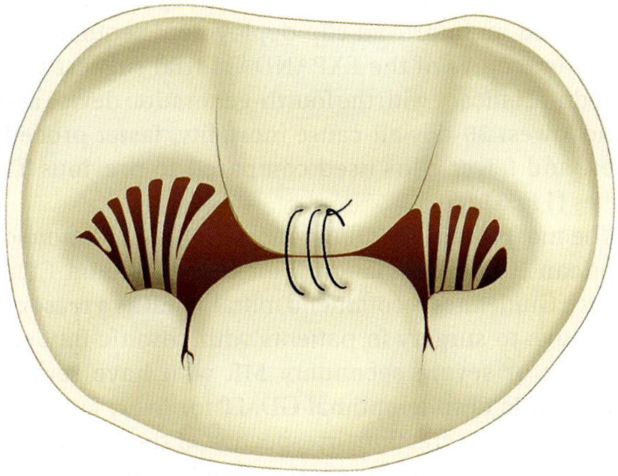

FIG. 1: Alfieri technique involves suturing together anterior and posterior leaflets at a single point midway between the circumferences of the leaflets.

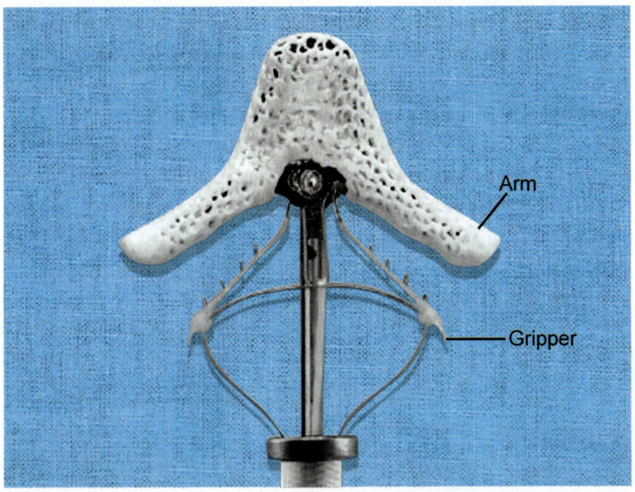

FIG. 2: The first-generation MitraClip device used in EVEREST I and II trials.

In the EVEREST II, percutaneous repair with transcatheter edge-to-edge repair (TEER) was compared to conventional surgery for PMR and SMR in patients who were classified as low risk for surgery. Patients with moderate-severe (grade +3) or severe (grade +4) MR were randomly assigned in a 2:1 ratio to undergo either percutaneous repair with the first-generation MitraClip or conventional surgery for MV repair or replacement. The primary effectiveness outcome was a composite of freedom from death, from surgery for MV dysfunction, and from moderate-to-severe (3+) or severe (4+) MR at 12 months. The study found that percutaneous repair was less effective than conventional surgery at reducing MR and the primary effectiveness outcome at 12 months favored conventional surgery. However, patients who underwent percutaneous repair had improved safety outcomes at 30 days and beyond 12 months, the need for surgery or the rates of moderate-to-severe MR were similar for both groups.

Although there were no prespecified formal subgroup analyses, exploratory intention-to-treat subgroup analyses suggested that in three subgroups, patients ≥ 70 years of age, those with SMR, and for those with left ventricular ejection fraction (LVEF) < 60%, surgery was not superior to percutaneous repair with regard to efficacy. This paved the revolution in the technology of TEER of MR and robust studies specifically in patients with SMR were underway.

The second-generation NT clip (Abbott) was used in the landmark COAPT (Cardiovascular Outcomes Assessment of the MitraClip in Patients with Heart Failure and Secondary Mitral Regurgitation) trial.[5] Patients with heart failure with reduced ejection fraction (mean LVEF 31%) resulting in moderate-to-severe (3+) or severe (4+) SMR on optimal guideline-directed medical therapy (GDMT) were randomized to treatment with percutaneous TEER with MitraClip plus medical therapy or to medical therapy alone. Exclusion criteria included vertical coaptation length < 2 mm in valves with leaflet tethering, evidence of calcification in the grasping area of the A2 or P2 scallops, presence of a significant cleft of the A2 or P2 scallops, and lack of both primary and secondary chordal support.[5] The study illustrated that the device group had a 32.1% absolute reduction in heart failure hospitalization at 24 months compared to medical therapy alone. The TEER group was also associated with a 16% absolute reduction in all-cause death, and the prespecified safety criteria were met at 12 months **(Fig. 3)**. The superiority of MitraClip over medical therapy alone in patients with SMR

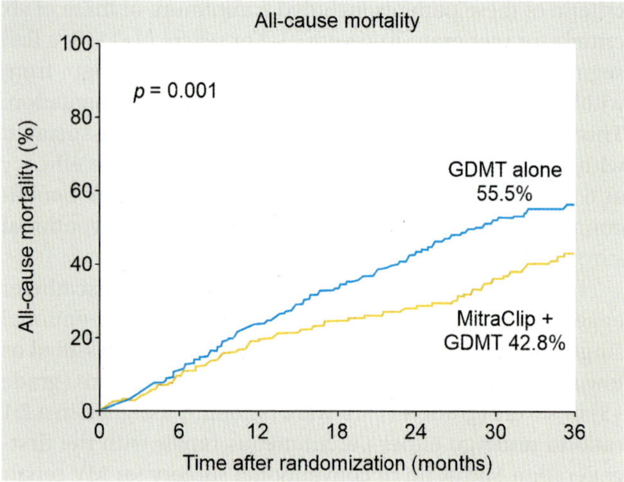

FIG. 3: All-cause mortality from the COAPT trial (MitraClip, Abbott). (GDMT: guideline-directed medical therapy)

was reconfirmed with the COAPT-5 (Five-Year Follow-up after Transcatheter Repair of Secondary Mitral Regurgitation) study which remonstrated risk reduction for heart failure hospitalization as well as for death from any cause across all patient subgroups.[6]

The technological advancement of TEER continued to trailblaze with the third-generation MitraClip system (G3) including NTR (9 mm arm length) and XTR (12 mm arm length), which allowed operators to address a wider range of MV anatomies and improved the ease of use with the modified delivery catheter, allowing for increased precision and predictability during steering. Although the efficacy of TEER was demonstrated in treatment of SMR in COAPT and COAPT-5, the gold standard for PMR remained conventional surgery.[5,6] In 2023, Kar et al. challenged this notion with the report of the 1-year outcomes from the EXPAND (Contemporary Outcomes Following Transcatheter Edge-to-Edge Repair) study.[7] Of the 1,041 enrolled patients, half had PMR or mixed etiology, which more closely represented real-world selection criteria. The investigators demonstrated a significant leap in MR reduction and improvement of patient-reported outcomes; 96% of patients experienced MR reduction ≤2+ upon clip implantation, and only 1.9% of patients required surgical MV replacement in the first 12 months.[7] Not only did the study demonstrate the efficacy and safety of the G3 MitraClip system in the acute procedural setting, the reduction in MR was sustained with 84.5% of patients with PMR and 93% of patients with SMR maintaining MR severity of 1+ at 12-month follow-up **(Figs. 4A to F)**. Furthermore, all-cause mortality and heart failure hospitalizations at 12-months were 14.9% in the PMR group and 18.9% in the SMR group, which were significantly lower than the rates in previous studies.[7] Overall, the study suggested that technological advancements of the device as well as increasing operator experience and proficiency contributed to significantly improved clinical and quality of life outcomes across a broad range of MV anatomies in both PMR and SMR compared to results with earlier-generation MitraClip systems.

The TEER revolution continues with the fourth-generation (G4) MitraClip **(Fig. 5)**. The MitraClip G4 system further expands its scope for MV anatomies with two additional 50% wider clip sizes (NTW and XTW). The MitraClip G4 system also utilizes an independent grasping feature and an improved clip deployment sequence.[8] The 30-day outcomes of the EXPAND G4 trial suggest further procedural efficacy with the fourth-generation device as well as the lowest 30-day all-cause mortality, faster procedure times, and fewer clips used compared to previous TEER studies **(Fig.6)**.[8]

The most recent (2020) American College of Cardiology/American Heart Association Joint Committee on Clinical Practice Guidelines recommend mitral TEER as a reasonable alternative to surgery in patients with chronic moderate-to-severe or severe secondary MR who have remained symptomatic despite optimal GDMT for heart failure with reduced ejection fraction, irrespective of the surgical risk.[9] On the hand, the guidelines recommend the use of TEER for patients with chronic primary MR who are at prohibitive risk for surgery. In reality, most of the cases of surgical repair are offered to patients who are at low risk for surgery. As a result, there are large proportions of patients who are not offered surgical treatment because of age and other comorbidities. This unmet need, along with the excellent contemporary results of the fourth-generation TEER device have paved the path for a new prospective randomized clinical trial, the REPAIR MR (Percutaneous MitraClip Device or Surgical Mitral Valve Repair in Patients with Primary Mitral Regurgitation who are Candidates for Surgery), which will compare the clinical outcomes of MitraClip TEER to conventional surgical repair for PMR patients with moderate surgical risk in a broad population of patients.

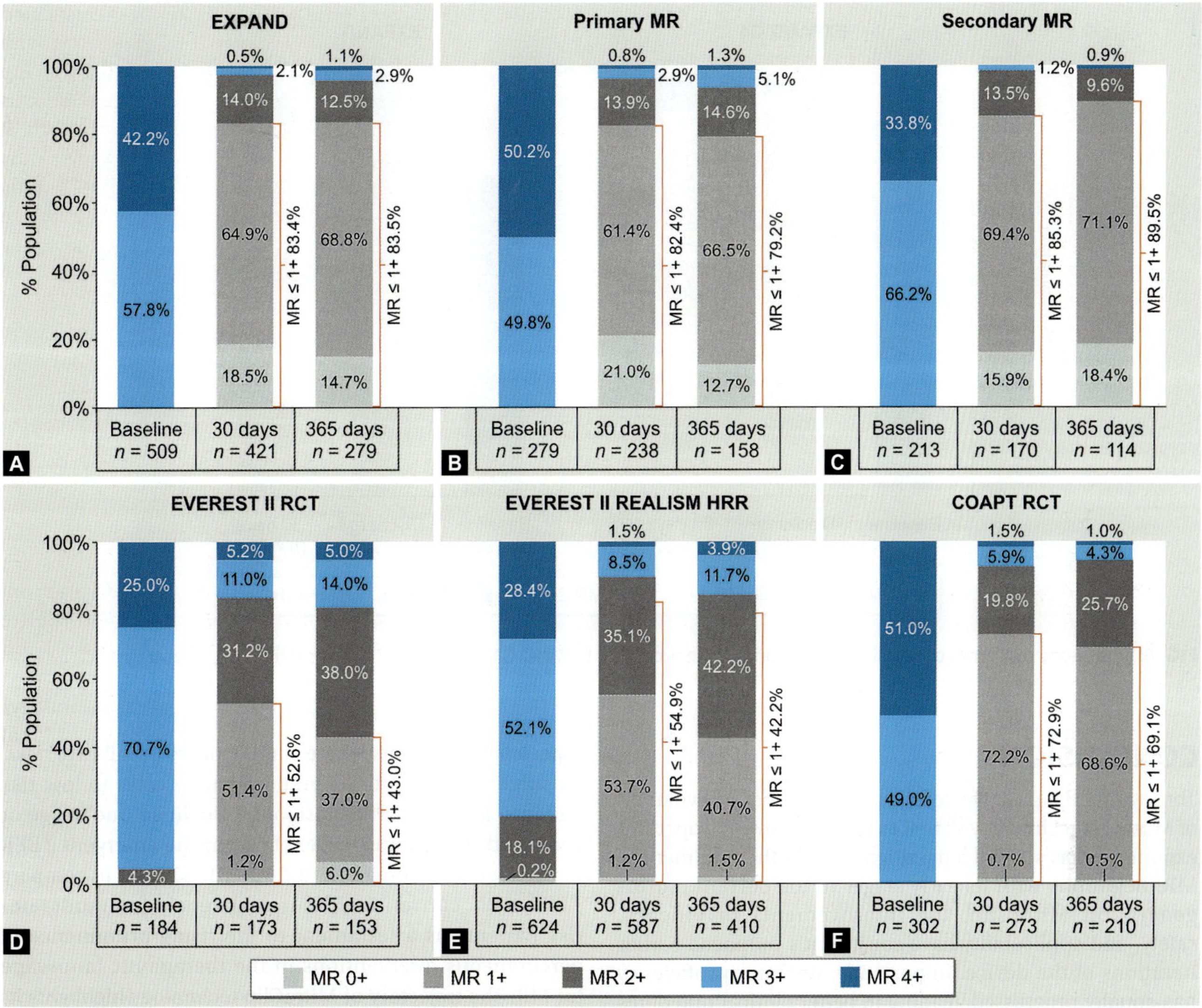

FIGS. 4A TO F: Echo core lab (ECL) adjudicated MR severity assessments across baseline, 30-day, and 1-year follow-up for EXPAND all subjects (A), primary MR subjects (B), and secondary MR subjects (C). The overall reduction in MR in EXPAND, which is higher than that reported in historical trials: EVEREST II RCT (D), EVEREST II REALISM HHR (E), and COAPT RCT (F).

(HHR: hypertrophic heart rate; MR: mitral regurgitation; RCT: randomized clinical trial)

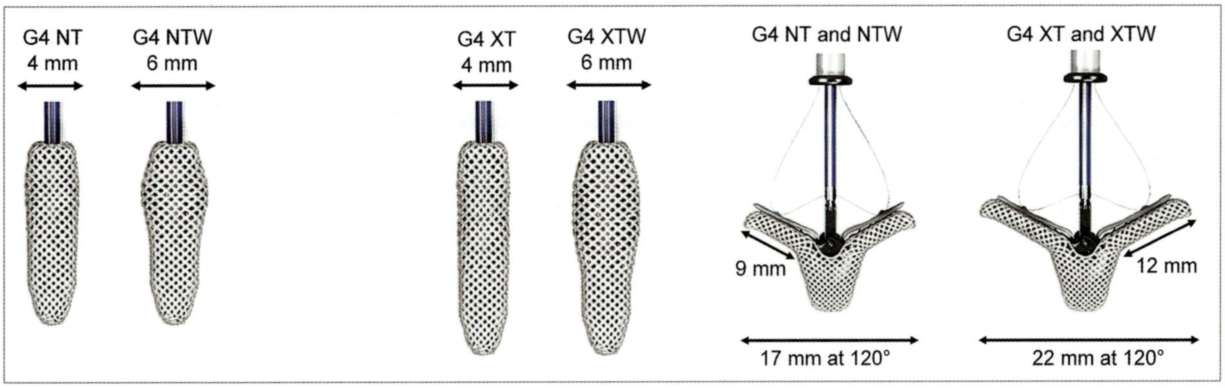

FIG. 5: The fourth-generation (G4) MitraClip, showing the four sizes (MitraClip, Abbott).

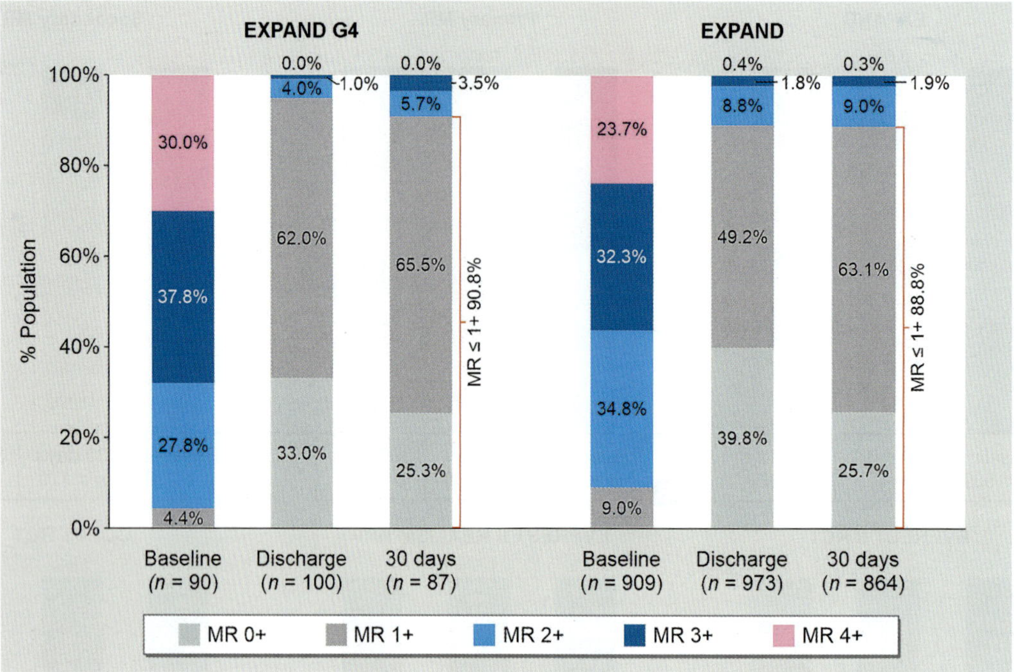

FIG. 6: Thirty-day outcomes of mitral regurgitation (MR) reduction in EXPAND G4 versus EXPAND trials (MitraClip, Abbott).

CONCLUSION

Throughout the past two decades, the tremendous evolution of MitraClip technology as well as the vast growth of operator experience has steered a paradigm shift in the treatment of MR. Beginning with its early stages to the current fourth-generation MitraClip, the improvements in efficacy, safety, and applicability have consistently outpaced earlier iterations of the device. Importantly, operator proficiency has equally progressed, leading to better clinical outcomes across a spectrum of MR anatomies, encompassing both primary and secondary types. These advancements have been acknowledged and endorsed by notable clinical guidelines, pointing to TEER as a viable alternative, especially for patients where surgery poses prohibitive risks. As surgical interventions predominantly cater to low-risk patients, a significant cohort, often sidelined due to age or comorbidities, stands to benefit from the emergent TEER technology. The imminent REPAIR MR trial, set to compare TEER with conventional surgical repair for moderate-risk patients, is a testament to the rising prominence of percutaneous interventions in the therapeutic landscape for MR. The trajectory of MitraClip technology highlights its potential in redefining the gold standard for MR treatment; the stage is now set for new, large, randomized trials to delineate the MR patients who would gain additional benefit from TEER as opposed to surgery.

ONLINE REFERENCES

Please scan the QR code provided at the end of the table of contents for References of this chapter.

CHAPTER 193

Transcatheter Mitral Valve Implantation: Technique, Present Status, and Future Directions

Nandhakumar Vasu, Ajit S Mullasari

ABSTRACT

Degenerated mitral bioprosthetic valve patients requiring repeat surgical valve replacement can be treated with a transcatheter mitral valve-in-valve procedure with good mid-term outcomes using balloon-expandable valves, which were originally designed for transcatheter aortic valve implantation. The same technique is used in the mitral valve-in-ring and valve-in-mitral annular calcium anatomy but with suboptimal mid-term outcomes. Transcatheter mitral valve replacement in native mitral valve pathology is under investigation with at least nine upcoming transcatheter mitral valves. We describe the computed tomography planning, transcatheter mitral valve-in-valve procedure, expected complications, and its management in this chapter.

Keywords: Transcatheter mitral valve implantation, mitral valve-in-valve, transseptal access, neo-left ventricular outflow tract obstruction, commissural alignment, complications.

INTRODUCTION

The paradigm shift in managing valvular heart disease from surgical methods to transcatheter therapy happened in 2002 after Alain Cribier described the first-in-human percutaneous transcatheter implantation of aortic valve prosthesis.[1] Though the techniques were born at the aortic position, evolution rapidly brought these techniques to the mitral valve. Mitral valve pathologies vary widely. Various transcatheter repair techniques are available for mitral regurgitation and mitral stenosis, including the time-tested percutaneous transvenous mitral commissurotomy. Transcatheter mitral valve implantation (TMVI) is being performed in four scenarios: (1) Native mitral valve without annular calcium, (2) valve-in-mitral annular calcification (ViMAC), (3) valve-in-ring (ViR), and (4) valve-in-valve (ViV). This chapter elaborates on transcatheter mitral ViV. The techniques that are mentioned in this chapter are those followed at our center.

COMPUTED TOMOGRAPHY ASSESSMENT OF MITRAL VALVE ANATOMY

Electrocardiography (ECG)-gated, contrast-enhanced cardiac computed tomography (CT) is used to find the ideal landing zone for the transcatheter mitral valve prosthesis; size the valve; check the possibility of neo-left ventricular outflow tract (LVOT) obstruction and possibility of paravalvular, inter-ring valvular or intervalvular leak, or identification of the ideal septal puncture site; plan for prophylactic electrosurgical technique to prevent neo-LVOT obstruction or bailout procedures if neo-LVOT obstruction develops; and assess the feasibility of bioprosthetic valve fracture if patient-prosthesis mismatch (PPM) is a concern. Approximately 50–70 mL of iodinated contrast, depending on the body surface area, is required to get good images. Heart rate in sinus rhythm should be <70 beats per minute

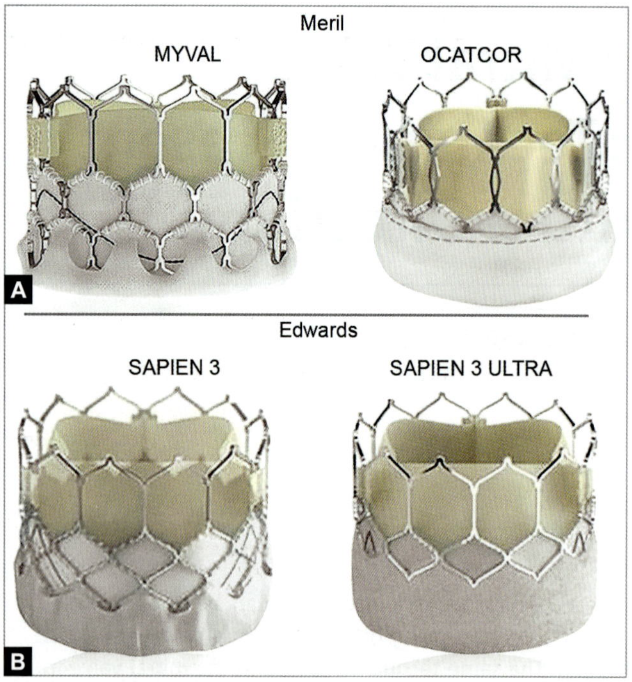

FIGS. 1A AND B: (A) MERIL MYVAL and OCTACOR valves and (B) EDWARDS SAPIEN3 and SAPIEN3 ULTRA valves. Note the additional external sealing skirt in OCTACOR and SAPIEN3 ULTRA valves to reduce paravalvular leak.

(bpm) to get the optimal images. But given the clinical scenario, sometimes it may be difficult to bring down the heart rate to <70 bpm, where reasonable images can be obtained with 71–90 bpm also. In atrial fibrillation or frequent atrial and ventricular ectopics, the R–R interval varies; hence, ECG gating may not be accurate. The reconstructed images are available in 5% intervals from 0 to 100% of the cardiac cycle. Mitral valve sizing is usually done at 75% of the cardiac cycle in diastole, and neo-LVOT measurements are done at 35% of the cardiac cycle in systole. The CT images are assessed on a dedicated structural heart segmentation software, 3mensio, Pie Medical.[2]

Mitral Valve-in-Valve

In a degenerated bioprosthetic valve, identification of the sewing ring and/or stent posts is the first step to measuring the landing zone area. Since only balloon-expandable circular valves from two manufacturers (MYVAL™ and OCTACOR™ from MERIL and SAPIEN3™ and SAPIEN3 ULTRA™ from EDWARDS) are currently available **(Figs. 1A and B)** for transcatheter mitral VIV procedure, annulus area measurement is the key to size the valve. Dedicated mobile applications are available to know the true inner diameter (ID) of the previous surgical or transcatheter valves and suggest ideal sizes for EDWARDS valves. Nevertheless, measuring the ID and area at the landing zone is prudent, since the old valve's tissue ingrowth and calcified degenerated material may further reduce the ID, which is known as

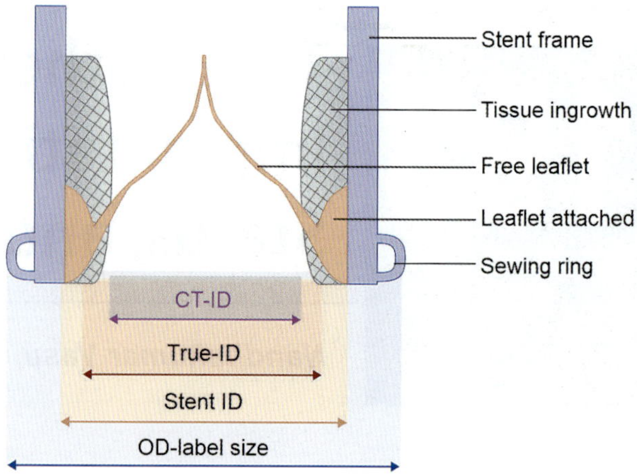

FIG. 2: Sizing nomenclatures of various measurements in the surgical bioprosthetic valve.
(CT: computed tomography; ID: inner diameter; OD: outer diameter)

CT-ID **(Fig. 2)**. Moreover, the MERIL manufacturer comes with the option of intermediate sizes 21.5, 24.5, and 27.5 mm and extra-large sizes 30.5 and 32 mm in addition to the conventional sizes 20, 23, 26, and 29 mm. But in the dedicated applications today, it is only for the EDWARDS valve that recommended sizes are available. These intermediate sizes of MERIL valves may play a crucial role in anatomies with neo-LVOT < 200 mm^2 to prevent LVOT obstruction, though no shreds of evidence are available at present.

While measuring the annulus of a mitral bioprosthetic valve, blooming artifact should be kept in our mind. The contrast of the CT image has to be adjusted to remove the blooming artifact. **Figures 3A and B** show the 27-mm Perimount valve with a blooming artifact with its exaggerated outer area derived diameter (ADD) of 31 mm and undermeasured inner ADD of 22.8 mm. After eliminating the blooming artifact, **Figures 3C and D** show the real inner and outer ADD as 24.8 and 28.5, respectively. The mitral ViV mobile application shows the true ID of the 27-mm Perimount valve as 25 mm. After completion of tracing the mitral annulus in a degenerated mitral bioprosthesis, three automated measurements appear, namely anterior-posterior (AP) diameter, trigone to trigone (TT) diameter, and commissure to commissure (CC) diameter **(Fig. 3E)**. In a circular bioprosthetic valve sewing ring, all three measurements are the same. We recommend 5–20% oversizing by area for the ViV mitral procedure whereas aggressive oversizing beyond 20% by area should be cautiously done only in rare scenarios such as expected PPM, by the experienced operator, where the operator plans bioprosthetic valve fracture after cautiously ruling out the possibility of annular rupture.

The aorto-mitral angle is the angle between the perpendicular line drawn from the aortic annulus and mitral annulus, whereas the angle between the virtual aortic and mitral annular planes is known as the inverse angle **(Fig. 3F)**.

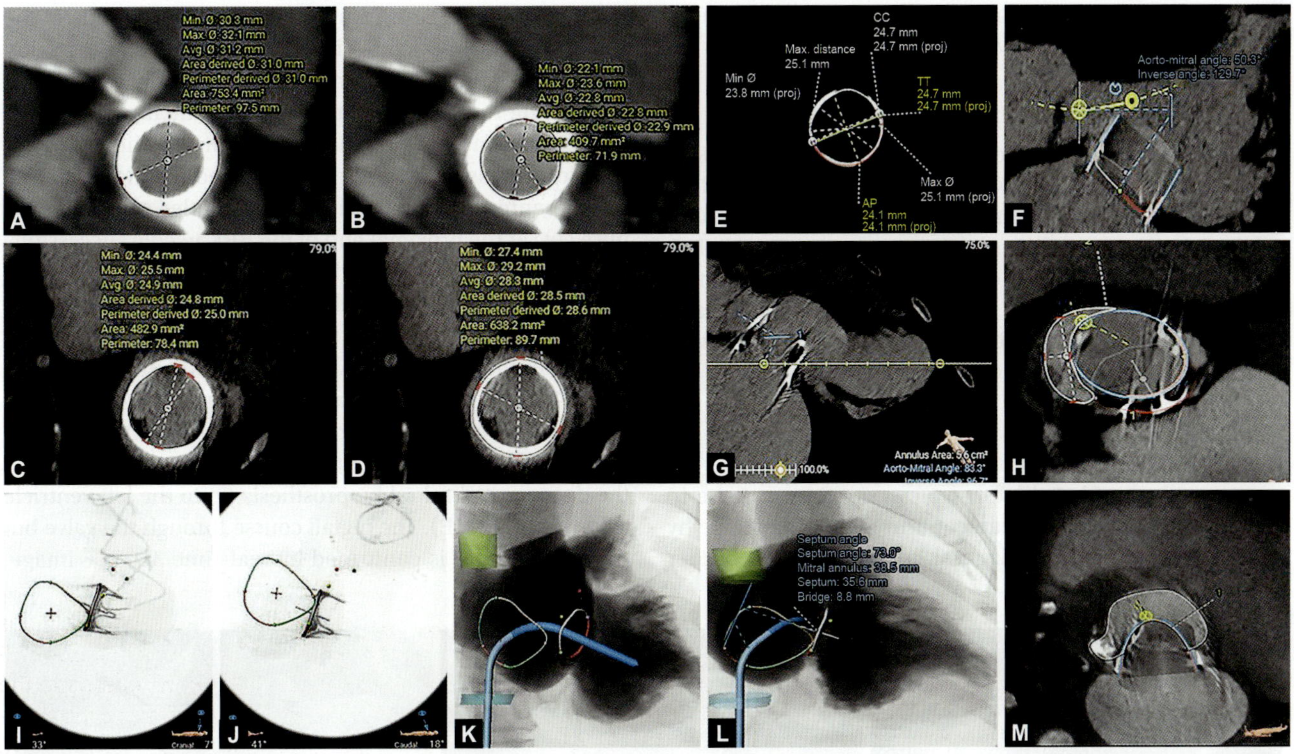

FIGS. 3A TO M: Computed tomography assessment for the mitral valve-in-valve procedure. (A and B) Blooming artifact exaggerated the measurement of outer and inner diameters. (C and D) The correct measurement of outer and inner diameter after eliminating the blooming artifact. (E) Automated measurements of commissure to commissure (CC), trigone to trigone (TT), and anterior–posterior (AP) diameters. All are equal for a circular bioprosthetic surgical valve. (F) Aorto-mitral angle and inverse angle. (G) Acute aorto-mitral angle predicts neo-left ventricular outflow tract (LVOT) obstruction. (H) Critical neo-LVOT area of 190 mm^2. (I) Coplanar view where all the three commissural posts are in a single line with equidistance. (J) Cusp overlap or two commissure post view. (K) Catheter course from inferior vena cava through the inferoposterior part of the interatrial septum into the mitral valve. (L) Acute septum-mitral angle predicts difficult tracking of the delivery system. (M) Ideal neo-LVOT area of >250 mm^2.

If the inverse angle is closer to 90°, the chances of neo-LVOT obstruction are maximum, which means the trajectory of the mitral valve and the LVOT is perpendicular **(Fig. 3G)**. If the inverse angle is 180° theoretically, the chance of neo-LVOT obstruction is nil, which means both trajectories are parallel, but this is never the case in reality. The probability of neo-LVOT obstruction proportionately increases as the angle comes down from 180° to 90° and reaches the maximum at 90°.[3] This can be predicted by calculating the neo-LVOT area in end systole and if the area is <200 mm^2 (**Fig. 3H** shows the neo-LVOT area of 190 mm^2), preventive or bailout strategies need to be planned to prevent LVOT obstruction.[4,5] The good size neo-LVOT area of 420 mm^2 is given in **Figure 3M** for comparison. The coplanar view, where all three commissural posts are seen in one line with equidistance or the bicommissural view, can be identified with the CT images **(Figs. 3I and J)**. Another important angle is the septal-mitral angle. This angle is formed between the inferior vena cava (IVC)—septal puncture line and the mitral annulus—septal puncture line **(Fig. 3L)**. The valve delivery catheter course can be drawn, and the ideal septal puncture can be chosen **(Fig. 3K)**. This angle predicts the difficulty of tracking the valve delivery system. If the angle becomes <90°, the difficulty of tracking the delivery system is much higher.

TECHNIQUE

Vascular Access

The procedure is done under general anesthesia since transesophageal echocardiogram (TEE) guidance is needed at several steps, and rapid pacing is necessary during valve deployment to make the heart standstill for a period of 10–20 seconds usually. The vascular access site for valve delivery is usually taken at the right common femoral vein (CFV). If right CFV access is not available due to deep vein thrombosis or vein stenosis, then left CFV is taken. Ultrasonogram-guided puncture over the right CFV, at least 1 cm above the saphenofemoral junction, is chosen. After the puncture, a single Proglide™ (Abbott) is deployed to secure the vein. A 9F short sheath is inserted to secure venous access. On the opposite side, a 6F short sheath is inserted at the common femoral artery. The right internal jugular vein or left femoral vein 6F access is taken to position the temporary pacemaker at the right ventricular apex as rapid ventricular pacing is needed during valve deployment.

Transseptal Access

Interatrial septal (IAS) puncture is taken using 8F SWARTZ SL-1 sheath with BRK, BRK2, or BRK1 needle, depending on the left atrial size and the distance between the IVC-right atrial junction and the septal puncture site. The 3D TEE probe is positioned at mid-esophageal 90° with mild retroflexion to show the bicaval view **(Fig. 4B)** and the X-plane cursor was placed across the junction of the upper two-thirds and lower one-third of the septum. This will give the anteroposterior projection of the septum with the aortic valve anteriorly **(Fig. 4A)**. The ideal puncture site is the inferior and posterior part of the IAS, and by tenting the septum with the SL-1 dilator, we can confirm our site in TEE. Fluoroscopically, we can confirm the puncture site by drawing an imaginary horizontal line at the lower border of the valve sewing ring and vertically at the midline of the spine. The ideal puncture site falls right off the intersection on the horizontal line (green rectangle; **Fig. 4C**). After confirming the right puncture site, advancing the needle generally punctures the IAS. Though a radiofrequency ablation transseptal needle is suggested for the thick IAS, at our center, the application of a unipolar cautery (40 W pure cut) at the proximal end of the BRK needle successfully punctured the thick IAS where the needle alone failed to puncture. A 0.025-inch coiled spring wire is placed in the left atrium (LA), and an 8.5F Agilis™ (Abbott) deflectable sheath is placed in the LA over the coiled spring wire **(Fig. 4D)**. In the coplanar view, the Agilis catheter is deflected toward the center of the mitral annulus, and a 6F pigtail with a 0.035-inch J tip Teflon wire is passed across the degenerated mitral bioprosthesis up to the left ventricle (LV) apex **(Fig. 4E)**. The pigtail course through the valve but not paravalvular is confirmed by real-time 3D-TEE image.

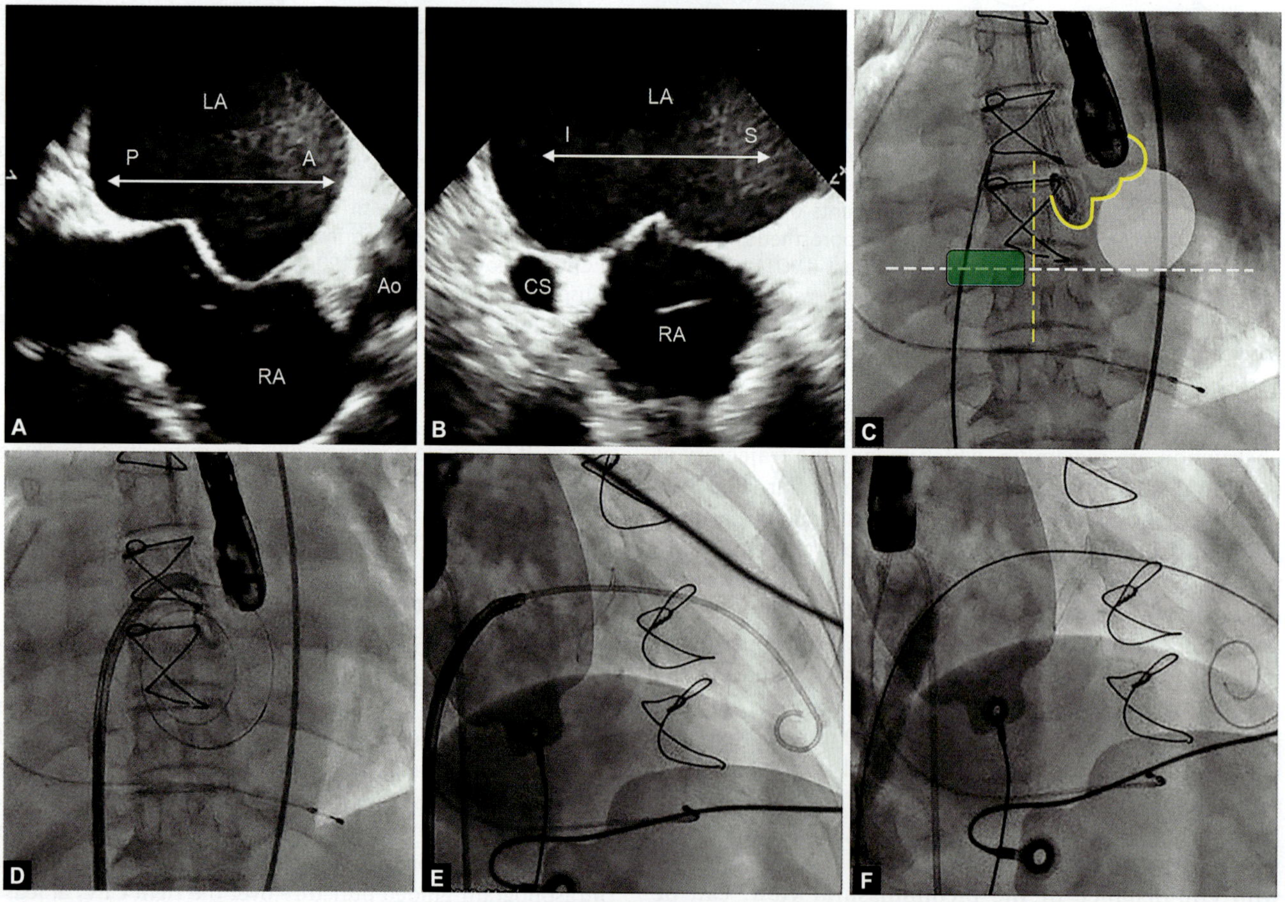

FIGS. 4A TO F: Procedural steps of transseptal access. (A) Transesophageal echocardiogram with mid-esophageal 45° view shows the tenting of the septum away from the anterior aorta (Ao). (B) Transesophageal echocardiogram with mid-esophageal 90° bicaval view shows inferior septal tenting closer to coronary sinus (CS). (C) Posteroanterior fluoroscopy shows the ideal puncture site for mitral valve-in-valve (ViV) procedure as the green rectangle. White circle denotes Epic mitral valve and yellow denotes aortic cusps. (D) Agilis™ deflectable sheath is railed over a 0.025-inch coiled spring wire. (E) A 6F pigtail from the Agilis sheath in the left atrium (LA) crosses the mitral valve and is kept at the left ventricle (LV) apex. (F) A 14-mm Z-MED II balloon dilates the interatrial septum.

(RA: right atrium)

A safari-2™ extra small curve (2.9 × 3.2 cm) wire (Boston Scientific) is placed in the LV apex through the pigtail catheter. The 9F sheath is removed, and over the safari-2™ wire, a 14F MERIL Python™ sheath or EDWARDS 14F or 16F e-sheath™ is inserted, the tip of which is generally positioned just below the IVC–right atrium (RA) junction. A 14 mm diameter with 4 cm length noncompliant balloon is used to dilate the IAS in order to facilitate the tracking of the valve delivery system **(Fig. 4F)**.

Preparing the Transcatheter Valve with the Delivery System

The crimping of the valve in vitro is done in a reverse position compared to retrograde transfemoral transcatheter aortic valve implantation (TAVI). The sealing skirt of the valve is positioned proximally for percutaneous transvenous transseptal TMVI during crimping. For transapical retrograde TMVI, the sealing skirt of the valve is positioned distally while crimping.

During transseptal mitral TMVI, the in vivo positioning of the crimped valve over the balloon by the pusher of the commander delivery system in EDWARDS valves can be done in the IVC by slightly withdrawing the e-sheath; otherwise, in vitro direct crimping of the valve over the balloon is also suggested. For MERIL valves, direct crimping of the valve as usual is followed.

Aligning Commissures

Like in TAVI, the commissural alignments are important in TMVI. The need for commissural alignment in TAVI is for coronary perfusion, whereas it is important in TMVI to prevent neo-LVOT obstruction, specifically in ViR or ViMAC where the neo-LVOT area is critically narrow. The idea is that commissural posts should not fall on the LVOT. To achieve this, we follow the below-mentioned protocol at our center. While crimping the valve, one of the commissures is crimped at the 12 o'clock position in both manufacturers' valves. During the insertion of the valve delivery system through the sheath, the delivery system turned 180° upside down (MERIL or EDWARDS logo facing down) to facilitate the flex system toward the left side of the patient. Hence, one of the commissures is facing the 6 o'clock position. The "roll" of the MERIL Navigator™ or EDWARDS Commander™ delivery system finally positions one of the commissures at the mitral annulus posteriorly. Since the LVOT is anterior at 12 o'clock, and the three commissures are separated at 120° apart, none of the commissures falls on the LVOT.

Valve Tracking and Deployment

While crossing the IVC–RA junction, the flex system of the delivery system (Navigator or Commander) is actuated. Based on the septal-mitral angle, some degrees of counterclockwise rotation of the delivery system are required to track the valve. If the septal-mitral angle is acute, <90°, the tracking of the valve may be difficult. As we try to push the valve across the mitral bioprosthesis, the valve may buckle upward due to noncoaxial pushing force **(Fig. 5A)**. Once the operator notices the upward buckling, the operator should stop further push because of two reasons. Either inadvertent buckling of safari-2 wire into the LA from LV or a sudden jump of the valve into the LV cavity can happen. The former needs the removal of the valve with the delivery system and repeating the procedure from introducing the Agilis™ sheath and valve cross with pigtail. The latter may lead to LV perforation. If the septal-mitral angle is acute and delivery system tracking fails despite counterclockwise rotation, POULEZ (Preparation of U-stitch to correct Lateral deflection for Endovascular mitral replacement in short landing Zone) technique or LV rail through percutaneous LV apical access helps in successful tracking of the transcatheter valve across the mitral annulus.[2,6]

The positioning of the transcatheter valves is guided by the proximal edge of the central marker of the balloon to be aligned with the sewing ring **(Fig. 5B)** if it is visible without stent posts (e.g., Biocor, Epic) or the distal edge of the transcatheter valve stent frame to be aligned with the edges of the older valve commissural posts in coplanar view if older valve commissural posts alone are visible (e.g., Mosaic valve). If both are visible, we advise choosing the sewing ring alignment, as the foreshortening happens at the atrial side alone during deployment. The final target is 80:20 (LV:LA) positioning with a flare at the LV side. In a critical neo-LVOT, 70:30 positioning is accepted. The valve is deployed during rapid ventricular pacing at 180–200 bpm by making the heart standstill. The tension in the delivery system is removed and checked with test rapid pacing for 3–5 seconds. The valve is deployed in a slow fashion over 15–20 seconds by two operators in synchrony with each other. First, the dumbbell of the balloon is inflated by the second operator, and the stability of the valve position is confirmed. If the valve moves, the first operator makes adjustments by holding the wire in the right hand and the delivery system in the left hand. Since the valve at the beginning of the deployment is always at the anterolateral commissure **(Fig. 5B)**, while inflating the balloon the posteromedial commissural positioning needs to be carefully watched and a final gentle push by the first operator is needed to seat the valve coaxially **(Fig. 5C)**. Rapid pacing is stopped only after deflating the balloon and pulling back it into the LA. The expansion of the valve stent frame in the coplanar view and in the en-face view is confirmed **(Figs. 5D and E)**. The functioning of the transcatheter valve, intervalvular or paravalvular leak is checked in the TEE image. The gradient across the new mitral valve, effective orifice area index, and LVOT gradient are measured. A small hemodynamically insignificant residual IAS defect with a left-to-right shunt measuring 5–8 mm is usually seen at the end of the procedure **(Fig. 5F)**. Usually, it spontaneously closes in 3 months' time. **Figures 5G and H** show the 3D-TEE image of the 26 mm MERIL MYVAL

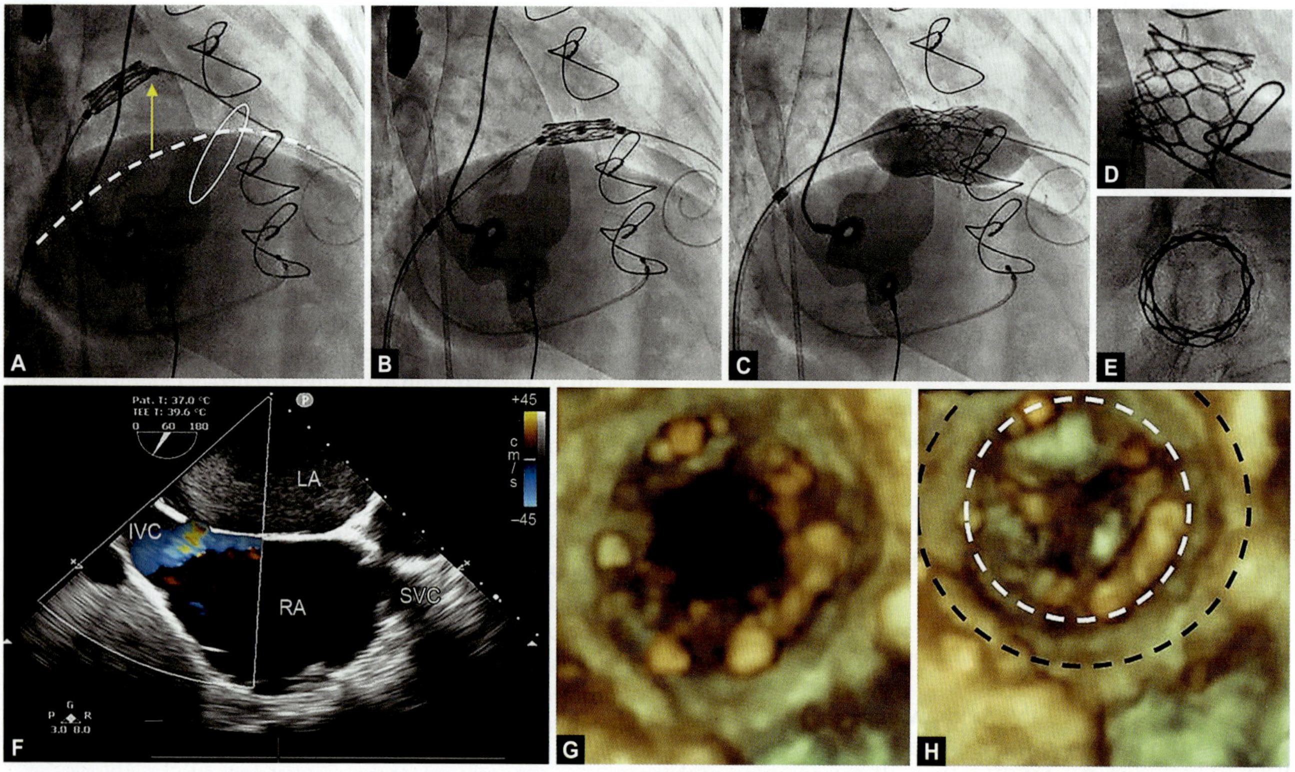

FIGS. 5A TO H: Procedural steps of MERIL MYVAL deployment. (A) Upward buckling of the navigator delivery system due to acute septal-mitral angle. White oval—Epic mitral valve. Yellow dotted lines represent the correct course of the wire and delivery system. (B) 26 mm MERIL MYVAL positioned by keeping the proximal edge of the middle balloon marker on the anterolateral commissure of the sewing ring. (C) Deployment of the 26 mm MERIL MYVAL in an 80:20 fashion. (D and E) 26 mm MERIL MYVAL seen in coplanar and en-face views. (F) Residual left-to-right shunt across the 5-mm atrial septal defect at the end of the procedure. (G) 3D transesophageal echocardiogram at end-diastole shows the complete opening of all three leaflets. (H) 3D transesophageal echocardiogram at end-systole shows normal coaptation of all three leaflets. The 12 o'clock (LVOT) is free of commissure.

(IVC: inferior vena cava; LA: left atrium; LVOT: left ventricular outflow tract; RA: right atrium; SVC: superior vena cava)

in diastole with a complete opening of all three leaflets and normal closure of all the leaflets in systole, respectively. **Figure 5H** shows the mitral valve in systole at 12 o'clock free of commissural post against the LVOT. The black circle marks the sewing ring outer border of the 27 mm Epic bioprosthetic valve and the white circle marks the transcatheter valve stent frame.

Access Closure

The large-bore venous access is closed with a single Proglide. If Proglide is not used at the beginning of the procedure or gets cut during closure, a figure-of-eight stitch is applied to close the access. The 6F arterial access is closed by manual compression. The temporary pacing catheter is removed at the end of the procedure.

Management of Complications

Ventricular Embolization

Deep implantation or movement of the valve while deploying, either due to the tension in the delivery system or due to loss of rapid ventricular pacing, leads to embolization of the valve into the LV. Maintaining the LV wire in position is of paramount importance during this nightmare as the embolized valve is still over the LV wire. Inflating the balloon inside the valve and gently pulling inside the previous valve stent posts can be done. It is impossible to replace it in the landing zone. Once the embolized valve is anchored in the stent post, a new transcatheter valve can be deployed at the right landing zone, anchoring the trapped embolized valve inside the older valve stent posts. If the case is mitral ViR or ViMAC, bioptome forceps can be used to hold the embolized valve just below the mitral annulus while deploying the new transcatheter valve to trap the embolized one.[7] LVOT obstruction is possible in critical neo-LVOT area patients.

Atrial Embolization

Inadvertent LA embolization of the valve is common in ViR or ViMAC procedures. If it happens, the LV wire is carefully withdrawn into the LA by maintaining the embolized valve rail over the wire. The wire can be changed over a pigtail catheter into an Amplatzer superstiff™ wire, and the wire tip is placed in the left upper pulmonary vein. A new valve is deployed through a new transseptal access at the mitral annulus. Following this, the embolized valve can be anchored to the IAS with an Amplatzer atrial septal occlude device.[2]

LVOT Obstruction

If the LVOT gradient after TMVI is >30 mm Hg peak to peak by catheter hemodynamic measurement at the end of the procedure, it is considered as severe LVOT obstruction. Usually, this is a complication of ViR or ViMAC. Alcohol septal ablation can be used as a bailout with 1 mL of ethanol into the first large septal perforator branch of the left anterior descending coronary artery. The immediate stunning and delayed remodeling of the septum give a generally decent reduction of the LVOT gradient. Atrioventricular nodal blocks are a possibility, and the patient may require a permanent pacemaker. More than 1 mL of ethanol injection may lead to ventricular septal rupture. Radiofrequency ablation of the septum at LVOT is another bailout option. If the native anterior mitral leaflet is the reason for the LVOT obstruction, rescue tip to base LAMPOON (Laceration of the Anterior Mitral leaflet to Prevent LVOT ObstructioN) can be used as the bailout.[2,8] The kissing balloon technique can be used to maintain the mitral annulus to LV apex trajectory while deploying the balloon-expandable valve to prevent LVOT obstruction.[9] Various LAMPOON techniques, namely antegrade LAMPOON, balloon-assisted LAMPOON, tip-to-base LAMPOON, and retrograde lampoon techniques, are used to lacerate the anterior mitral leaflet to prevent LVOT obstruction. Sometimes, alcohol septal ablation is also used as a pre-emptive measure to prevent this complication.[10]

Intervalvular and Paravalvular Leak

A leak between the transcatheter mitral valve and the sewing ring of degenerated mitral bioprosthesis is known as intervalvular leak. It is due to calcified bioprosthesis, which prevents proper sealing of the skirt of the transcatheter valve onto the sewing ring. Trivial or 1+ leak settles down on its own after reversing the heparin. 2+ or more leaks can be managed with a postdilatation by adding 1 or 2 cc volume extra in the same delivery catheter balloon. A paravalvular leak in a mitral ViV is defined as a leak between the native mitral annulus and the older bioprosthetic valve's sewing ring, which can be identified during CT evaluation. The paravalvular leak is much more common during ViR or ViMAC procedures. This can be addressed after completing the TMVI procedure using dedicated Amplatzer Vascular Plug™ devices.[11]

FOLLOW-UP CARE

Extubation is usually done after 1 hour of the procedure, and 24-hour intensive care unit monitoring is sufficient. However, prolonged monitoring for 2–3 days is mandatory in patients with severe pulmonary hypertension, right ventricular dysfunction, suspected intravascular hemolysis due to LVOT obstruction or paravalvular leak, and prolonged procedure > 2 hours.

Patients are usually discharged on the fifth postprocedure day with the advice of 1 month, 3 months, 6 months, and 1 year followed by a once-in-a-year follow-up. Anticoagulation with vitamin K antagonists is recommended unless there is a contraindication in patients with atrial fibrillation, whereas direct oral anticoagulants are recommended for those in sinus rhythm.

SHORT-TERM AND MID-TERM OUTCOMES

The largest ViV and ViR patient data with 4-year outcomes is available from the VIVID registry.[12] A total of 1,079 patients who underwent mitral ViV (n = 857) and ViR (n = 222) from 90 centers across the old were enrolled in this registry. The most frequently used valve was SAPIEN3, and the most frequent access site was transapical (61.6%), with transseptal access use only 36.9%. Technical success was achieved in 93.5% of ViV and 82% of ViR. The device failure rate with the criteria of postprocedure mean gradient ≥ 5 mm Hg was present in 61.4%, and with the revised criteria of ≥10 mm Hg, the device failure rate decreased to 8.9%. Major stroke and LVOT obstruction were seen in 1.2% and 2.6% of the patients, respectively. The rate of anticoagulation was 71.9%. Severe PPM was seen in 24.5% of the patients. More than or equal to moderate mitral regurgitation post procedure was seen in 5.9%.[12]

At 30 days, the mortality was 6.5% in ViV and 8.6% in ViR group. 1-year and 4-year survival for ViV was 86.2% and 62.5%, and for ViR, it was 76.8% and 49.7%, respectively.

A multivariate analysis showed independent correlates of mortality to be highest with chronic kidney disease and chronic lung disease [hazard ratio (HR) 1.9 for each], NYHA class IV and ViR (HR 1.5 for each), and pulmonary artery systolic pressure, age (HR 1 for each).[12]

CONCLUSION

Currently used MERIL and EDWARDS balloon-expandable valves were originally designed for TAVI procedures with tri-leaflet valves. Off-label we are currently using these circular devices for TMVI procedures. This may be suitable for the ViV procedure as the landing zone is circular. However, these valves are not ideal for ViR and ViMAC. There are many dedicated devices for native mitral valve pathology with and without mitral annular calcium that are currently under clinical trials. Three transfemoral TMVI systems, namely SAPIEN M3 dock and valve system (Edwards Lifesciences, Irvine, California), the EVOQUE system (Edwards Lifesciences) with a self-expanding nitinol frame, and three bovine pericardial leaflets, the Cephea TMVR system (Abbott, Menlo Park, California), are of importance. There are at least six transapical or transapical-transfemoral TMVR systems that are under investigation, namely Tendyne system (Abbott, Menlo Park, California), TIARA system (Neovasc Inc, Richmond, Canada), Intrepid system (Medtronic, Minneapolis, Minnesota), Highlife system (Highlife SAS, Irvine, California), Cardiovalve (Cardiovalve, Or Yehuda, Israel), and AltaValve system (4C Medical Technologies, Minneapolis, Minnesota).[13]

ONLINE REFERENCES

Please scan the QR code provided at the end of the table of contents for References of this chapter.

CHAPTER

194

Transcatheter Mitral Valve Replacement

Abdul S Talpur, Mustafa Sajjad Cheema, Yasar Satar, Shirley Adivi, Ramesh Daggubati

ABSTRACT

In the field of symptomatic mitral valve regurgitation management, transcatheter mitral valve replacement (TMVR) technology is rapidly gaining prominence as a primary therapeutic approach, particularly for patients who are deemed unsuitable for surgery or present with a high degree of surgical risk. This chapter offers a detailed look at TMVR, an important treatment option for mitral valve disease. It traces the history and development of TMVR and compares its results with traditional surgery. The chapter also discusses the possible risks of TMVR. It pays particular attention to the use of TMVR in high-risk patients and those with complex cases while discussing new technologies and ongoing research on TMVR.

Keywords: TMVR, mitral stenosis, mitral regurgitation, mitral annular calcification.

INTRODUCTION

Mitral regurgitation (MR), the third most prevalent form of valvular heart disease, afflicts approximately 24.2 million individuals globally.[1] Given its predominance among older adults, MR accounted for an estimated 0.88 million disability-adjusted life years (DALYs) and 34,000 fatalities in 2019.[2,3] The prevalence of MR is either balanced between genders or slightly higher in males. Notably, the incidence of mitral valve prolapse (MVP), a significant contributor to MR, is markedly higher in white patients compared to their black counterparts.[1] MR, whether primary or degenerative, is predominantly a consequence of myxomatous degeneration and MVP.[1] MVP, as the most common cardiac mitral valvular pathology worldwide, affects 2–3% of the global population.[1] In developing nations, rheumatic heart disease (RHD) remains a significant concern and is the leading cause of mitral valvular pathology necessitating hospital admissions.[1]

Historically, surgical repair has been the preferred approach over replacement in primary MR due to superior outcomes.[4] However, the best approach to secondary MR remains to be debated. With a decreasing incidence in mitral stenosis due to RHD and significant improvements in outcomes after open heart surgery, mitral valve disease—specifically primary MR—is now treated primarily with open surgery.[4] However, in countries such as the USA, where the population continues to age and the prevalence of comorbidities correspondingly rises, a substantial number of patients are either not recommended for, or are precluded from, surgical intervention.[4-6]

The emergence of transcatheter mitral valve replacement (TMVR) therapies has introduced viable and safe alternatives to traditional medical and surgical treatments.[4] This is particularly beneficial for those patients who are deemed unsuitable candidates for conventional mitral valve surgery.[4] The earliest transcatheter mitral valve repair (TMVr) technology to be developed was the MitraClip, implanted in a human for the first time in 2003.[7] Since then, it has grown its market share steadily and to date over 25,000 patients have been treated with this method worldwide.[4] Other devices that have completed the various steps of development up to CE mark approval include NeoChord, Valtech Cardioband, and the Mitralign device.[4]

Transcatheter mitral edge-to-edge repair has emerged as the most successful and widely adopted TMVr therapy to date, with significant device iterations and enhancements observed in 2020.[4] In addition to mitral edge-to-edge repair, there is an increasing body of evidence supporting therapeutic strategies that target the mitral annulus (MA) and mitral valve chordae.[4] However, the number of TMVRs using a dedicated mitral prosthesis in a native mitral valve has remained relatively limited so far.[4] Conversely, other valves, including the Neovasc Tiara, Medtronic Intrepid, and Boston Scientific MValve devices, have entered various stages of clinical trials.[4] These devices are vying with Tendyne to secure the first commercial approval for TMVR in Europe, followed by the US.[4]

MITRAL VALVE ANATOMY, PATHOPHYSIOLOGY AND CLASSIFICATION

The MA, a dynamic structure, undergoes changes throughout the cardiac cycle.[8] It is characterized by parallel collagen fibers and a saddle-like shape, with the anterior portion forming the most atrial part of this saddle.[8] The posterior MA, less anchored, allows for more movement during myocardial contraction and relaxation.[8] The mitral valve leaflets, designed to withstand billions of cycles of opening and closing, work in unison to occlude medial and lateral gaps.[8] The optimal ratio of MA to mitral leaflet area, crucial for preventing significant MR, falls between 1.5 and 2.0.[8] The chordae tendineae, fibrous cords extending from the papillary muscle (PM) tips, insert into the ventricular aspects of the leaflets.[8] Lastly, the PMs, originating from the apical one-third of the LV wall, control the distance between the MA and the PM tips, ensuring the proper functioning of the mitral valve.[8]

Mitral regurgitation is a complex condition that can arise from various failures within the mitral valve apparatus and the left ventricle (LV).[9] It is typically classified as either primary (degenerative or organic) or secondary (functional).[9]

Primary MR is predominantly due to abnormalities in the mitral valve leaflets.[9] It is associated with conditions such as myxomatous degeneration, leaflet flail, MVP, rheumatic valve disease, and connective tissue disorders, which directly affect the structural integrity of the leaflets.[9] Secondary MR, on the other hand, is typically a consequence of diseases affecting the left atrium and LV, sparing the mitral valve leaflets.[9] However, various components of the mitral valve apparatus can be compromised.[9] Left ventricular cardiomyopathies, either ischemic or nonischemic, can lead to tethering of the mitral valve leaflets due to regional wall motion abnormalities or LV remodeling.[9] Annular dilatation can occur as a result of left atrial or LV dilatation, and dysfunctional mitral valve closure can be related to reduced LV contractility or dyssynchrony.[9] Although the leaflets are generally unaffected in secondary MR, compensatory changes such as leaflet thickening and increased leaflet area can occur, leading to a mixed disease that exhibits characteristics of both primary and secondary MR.[9]

Mitral regurgitation can also be classified according to the Carpentier's classification based on leaflet mobility. Type I MR is characterized by normal leaflet mobility, but inadequate coaptation due to annular dilation or leaflet perforation.[8] This type is often associated with conditions such as chronic atrial fibrillation, endocarditis, iatrogenic trauma, or congenital disease.[8]

In the context of type I MR, despite normal leaflet mobility, significant MR can occur due to annular dilation.[8] This is predominantly observed in elderly patients with atrial fibrillation.[8] However, the precise mechanisms and potential therapeutic interventions for this type of MR remain elusive and necessitate further investigation.[8] Existing research indicates that mitral annular dimension is the sole independent echocardiographic predictor of MR in these cases.[8] Type II MR is characterized by excessive leaflet mobility due to prolapse or ruptured chordae, commonly seen in conditions such as MVP and fibroelastic deficiency (FED).[8] The two phenotypes of type II MR, FED and myxomatous disease (MD), exhibit distinct physiological differences.[8] FED is localized and involves ruptured chords with leaflet redundancy, while MD is characterized by generalized redundancy and thickening of both leaflets.[8]

The dynamics of type II MR annular are a subject of ongoing debate.[8] While some studies suggest normal annular dynamics, others have observed abnormal early-systolic annular dynamics in patients with type II MR.[8] These patients exhibit reduced anteroposterior contraction combined with simultaneous enlargement of intercommissural diameter, resulting in diminished annular area contraction.[8] Type III MR is associated with restricted leaflet mobility, leading to leaflet coaptation at the ventricular level. This can occur in both diastolic and systolic phases (type IIIa) or only in systole (type IIIb).[8] Type IIIb functional MR occurs despite structurally normal mitral leaflets and is a consequence of LV dysfunction.[8] It is unequivocally associated with LV remodeling and enlargement.[8]

TRANSCATHETER MITRAL VALVE REPLACEMENT RATIONALE AND INDICATIONS

Data extracted from the Society of Thoracic Surgeons Adult Cardiac Surgery Database reveals that in 2016, around 18,000 isolated mitral surgeries were executed in the United States, a 24% rise compared to the figures from 2011.[10] The division of surgical approaches was skewed toward mitral valve repair, employed in two-thirds of patients, while the remaining one-third were subjected to surgical mitral valve replacement, predominantly with bioprostheses.[10] These statistics are of particular importance given the average age of patients receiving a bioprosthesis is 66 years, and the median time to mitral valve degeneration is approximately 15 years.[10,11] Consequently, an estimated 2,000 patients per year would require reintervention due to bioprosthesis degeneration, and this could present a high risk of death owing to advanced age and the reoperation itself.[10,11]

The gold standard care for primary MR patients eligible for intervention is surgical mitral valve repair.[12,13] This method involves the restoration of physiological leaflet motion (when the disease primarily affects the leaflets) through several technical procedures such as leaflet resection, chordal transposition, annuloplasty repair, and the implantation of artificial chordae.[9] Although these techniques may be challenging, at expert mitral valve surgical centers with a high volume of cases, over 95% of primary MR cases can be successfully repaired.[9]

Patients who are symptomatic, considered at high surgical risk, and have suitable anatomy might be eligible for TMVr.[11] The strategy for those patients with primary MR at low surgical risk would ideally involve mitral valve repair , followed by surgical mitral valve replacement when repair is unfeasible.[9] All patients with MR, stenosis, or mixed mitral valve disease could potentially be candidates for TMVR.[11] European guidelines suggest TMVR as viable alternatives to surgery for patients facing an increased surgical risk.[11] However, no explicit recommendations for TMVR are present in the most recent update of American guidelines.[11]

In the case of secondary MR, the optimal surgical approach is less defined.[9] While surgical mitral valve repair is favored in treating primary MR, the secondary form presents a more varied national approach towards surgical methods, either repair or replacement.[9]

The Cardiothoracic Surgical Trials Network (CTSN) conducted a large randomized trial to address this issue, with 251 patients randomized to either mitral valve repair or chordal-sparing replacement.[14] Upon the completion of 1 year postoperation, the mortality rates exhibited no significant deviation between the two groups.[14] However, the incidence of recurring moderate or severe MR was observably diminished within the group that had undergone valve replacement.[14] Conversely, when considering a composite endpoint that amalgamates major adverse cardiac or cerebrovascular events, quality of life indicators, and functional status, the statistical disparity between the two groups remained inconspicuous.[14] Given these results, both mitral valve repair and mitral valve replacement seem reasonable surgical options for patients with secondary MR who carry an acceptable surgical risk.[14]

Transcatheter Valve Therapy registry data show that between 2013 and 2017 in the United States, 803 patients with failing bioprostheses or rings underwent TMVR.[15] Considering the high-risk profile of patients with secondary MR, combined with a lack of evidence for surgery's impact on hard outcomes, a less invasive transcatheter approach for treating severe secondary MR may be advantageous.[16]

Mitral annular calcification (MAC) is a condition that transpires due to the accumulation of calcium deposits along the MA, a physiological process that bears notable similarity with the pathophysiological mechanisms observed in atherosclerosis.[17] Despite the pervasive nature of MAC within the general populace, especially amongst the demographic groups of women and older individuals, establishing an accurate prevalence has proven elusive.[11] This uncertainty arises from the lack of standardized definitions for the condition, the constraints associated with the echocardiographic assessment of calcifications, and the nonuniform implementation of computed tomography (CT) examinations.[11] Despite the challenges and risk of perioperative complications associated with mitral surgery for patients with MAC, TMVR using transcatheter aortic valve replacement (TAVR) has been proposed for these patients, albeit its application is currently restricted to a limited number of candidates.[11]

PRELIMINARY COMPREHENSIVE EVALUATION FOR TRANSCATHETER MITRAL VALVE REPLACEMENT

Prior to implementing TMVR, a thorough examination is mandatory to exclude severe coexisting conditions or anatomical findings that may either contraindicate or render the intervention futile.[11] Alongside establishing the patient's suitability for the procedure, this preoperative evaluation facilitates intervention strategy planning, deciding on the most appropriate operative route, and determining the size of the transcatheter aortic valve (TAV).[11]

Essential clinical assessments include transthoracic and two-and-three-dimensional transesophageal echocardiograms and contrast CT.[18,19] These investigations enable confirmation of the mitral valve disease severity, characterization of the mitral valve, especially the leaflets and subvalvular apparatus, and the exclusion of active endocarditis, prosthesis or ring disinsertion, paravalvular leaks, or valve thrombosis.[11] Additionally, contrast CT provides valuable insights into mitral valve morphology, facilitates the determination of MA dimensions, and enables a precise evaluation of the risk of left ventricular outflow tract (LVOT) obstruction.[11]

There are key specific anatomical features to consider before TMVR:

Mitral valve complex morphology: A comprehensive assessment of the radiopacity and position of bioprostheses and surgical rings, the completeness and flexibility of surgical rings, the anterior leaflet morphology, and the severity and extension of calcifications in patients with MAC is vital. These features significantly influence TMVR results and help determine the procedural strategy and intervention risk.[11]

Mitral annulus, bioprosthesis, or ring dimensions: For precise sizing of the transcatheter heart valve and confirming TMVR eligibility using aortic valves, an accurate evaluation of the MA dimensions is crucial.[11] Especially in patients with degenerated bioprostheses, the "true internal diameter" is generally smaller by at least 1 mm than the manufacturer-provided internal diameter, and the discrepancies vary according to the prosthesis type.[11]

Risk assessment of LVOT obstruction: A comprehensive evaluation of the dimensions of the neo-LVOT postsimulation of a right-sized THV on CT images in systole best predicts the risk of LVOT obstruction following TMVR.[11]

Other anatomic features: Morphology of the interatrial septum and the dimensions of the left atrium must be meticulously evaluated as they significantly influence procedural planning.[11]

Patient Selection

Eligibility for TMVR depends on clinical and anatomic factors along with bioprostheses/rings specific characteristics. To derive benefits from TMVR, patients' symptoms should be attributed to mitral valve disease.[11] However, patients with active endocarditis, prosthesis/ring disinsertion, paravalvular leaks, or valve thrombosis as the primary causes of mitral valve dysfunction are ineligible for TMVR. Moreover, patients with advanced heart disease may not benefit from TMVR.[11]

Anatomically, patients with an excessively large MA as per currently available sizes of aortic valves and TMVR candidates with insufficient extension of calcifications might not be suitable due to a high risk of valve embolization.[11] Similarly, patients at high risk for LVOT obstruction might be denied intervention.[11]

Lastly, specific prosthesis and ring factors influence the patient's eligibility. Patients with small surgical prostheses or rings or those with prosthesis-patient mismatch after surgery might not benefit from TMVR.[11] Conversely, most patients with bioprosthesis failure are real candidates for TMVR, the primary limitation being the bioprosthesis size.[11]

TRANSCATHETER MITRAL VALVE REPLACEMENT TECHNIQUES AND THEIR EFFICACY (TABLE 1)

Transcatheter mitral valve replacement techniques include the following:

- Transcatheter mitral annuloplasty
    - Indirect mitral annuloplasty
        - Carillon mitral contour system
        - ARTO system
    - Direct mitral annuloplasty
        - Cardioband mitral system
        - Millipede transcatheter mitral annuloplasty system
- Transcatheter edge-to-edge mitral valve repair
    - MitraClip G4 system
    - PASCAL transcatheter valve repair system
- Transcatheter mitral valve chordal repair
    - NeoChord
    - HARPOON mitral valve repair system (MVRS)

TRANSCATHETER MITRAL ANNULOPLASTY

Surgical and transcatheter mitral annuloplasty aim to reduce the circumference of the MA and improve the coaptation of the mitral leaflets.[20] Transcatheter approaches can be categorized as indirect or direct, based on their relation to the MA.[20]

Indirect transcatheter mitral annuloplasty methods utilize the coronary sinus (CS) as a reference point to the MA.[20] Two examples are the Carillon Mitral Contour System (Cardiac Dimensions, Washington, DC, USA) and the ARTO system (MVRx, California, USA), both of which received CE mark approval and were studied in the Mitral Valve Repair Clinical (MAVERIC) CE Mark trial.[20] Direct transcatheter mitral annuloplasty provides an alternative to the CS approach, though it involves a more complex procedural technique.[20] Two systems that closely resemble surgical mitral annuloplasty are the Cardioband mitral system (Edwards Lifesciences, California, USA) and the Millipede mitral annuloplasty system (Boston Scientific, Massachusetts, USA). Both systems use a transseptal approach with a steerable guide catheter.[20]

Carillon Mitral Contour System

The Carillon mitral contour system obtained CE approval in 2011 for use in patients with functional MR who remain symptomatic despite guideline-directed medical therapy (GDMT) and have significant MR caused by annulus dilatation.[20] The Carillon system consists of three components—the sizing catheter, the delivery system, and the Carillon implant.[20] The sizing catheter estimates the dimensions of the CS and great cardiac vein (GCV) to select

TABLE 1: Transcatheter mitral valve replacement (TMVR) techniques.

TMVR techniques	TMVR techniques subcategories and examples	References
Transcatheter mitral annuloplasty	• Indirect mitral annuloplasty ○ Carillon mitral contour system ○ ARTO system • Direct mitral annuloplasty ○ Cardioband mitral System ○ Millipede transcatheter mitral annuloplasty system	[20]
Transcatheter edge-to-edge mitral valve repair	• MitraClip G4 system • PASCAL transcatheter valve repair system	[20]
Transcatheter mitral valve chordal repair	• NeoChord • HARPOON mitral valve repair system	[20]

an appropriate-sized implant.[20] Percutaneous delivery of the implant and its engagement with the locking mechanism are facilitated by the delivery system. The Carillon XE2 implant comprises a distal anchor (in the GCV), a proximal anchor (in the CS), a ribbon connector, and proximal and distal crimp tubes.[20]

The implant is deployed, tensioned, and secured in the coronary vein, leading to immediate reduction of MR, which can be adjusted during the catheterization procedure in the cardiac catheterization lab.[20] The procedure is performed via jugular venous access and is typically conducted without general anesthesia.[20] Limitations of the Carillon system include the distance between the CS and the MA, which may limit its therapeutic effectiveness, and the risk of compression on the left circumflex coronary artery by the distal anchor.[20] However, the device can be repositioned or retrieved if needed.[20] The Carillon system is not recommended for patients with a cardiac resynchronization therapy (CRT) device or pacing lead in the CS.[20]

Results from the REDUCE FMR trial demonstrated that the Carillon device significantly reduced MR volumes and LV volumes in symptomatic patients with functional MR despite GDMT.[21] A total of 5-year follow-up data indicated sustained functional improvement and favorable survival rates after treatment with the Carillon system.[21]

ARTO System

The ARTO system is a transcatheter indirect mitral annuloplasty device designed to improve mitral leaflet coaptation and reduce functional MR. It accomplishes this by connecting anchors placed in the GCV and the atrial septum with a "bridge suture".[20] Using fluoroscopy, the ARTO system is delivered through venous access to the right atrium.[20] The procedure involves two steps: (1) cannulation of the CS from the right jugular vein and deployment of a T-bar implant in the lateral wall via the GCV, and (2) deployment of an atrial septal implant through a transseptal puncture.[20] The "bridge suture" between these two anchors facilitates inward displacement and subsequent reduction of the mitral annular anteroposterior diameter.[20]

The bridge length can be adjusted to achieve optimal MR reduction.[20] It is feasible to perform a MitraClip treatment after ARTO, even in the presence of the bridge.[20] The ARTO system's safety and efficacy were demonstrated in the MAVERIC CE Mark trial, which enrolled 45 patients with functional MR.[20] Results showed a decrease in MR severity and significant improvement in functional status, quality of life, and exercise capacity up to 1 year postprocedure.[20] Larger randomized controlled trials are needed to further study the safety and efficacy of the ARTO system.[20]

Cardioband Mitral System

The Cardioband mitral system is a transcatheter, transseptal adjustable direct mitral annuloplasty device designed to reduce the mitral annular circumference, and improve leaflet coaptation.[20] The Cardioband implant is a polyester sleeve with radiopaque markers, covering the delivery system that deploys screw anchors.[20] Proper positioning of the first anchor is essential, and multiplanar transesophageal echocardiography (TEE) and 3D-TEE views are utilized to verify its correct placement.[20] The first anchor is placed lateral and anterior in the MA, and coronary angiography confirms the absence of damage to the left circumflex coronary artery.[20] Anchors are then placed along the posterior side of the MA until the medial side is reached.[20] A contraction wire following the sleeve's path is connected to an adjusting spool, cinching the Cardioband device and reducing the mitral annular diameter. The implant is available in different sizes.[20]

The Cardioband mitral system gained CE mark approval for treating functional MR in 2016.[20] In a single-arm, multicenter prospective study, 60 consecutive patients with moderate or severe functional MR were treated with the Cardioband system.[20] Although technical challenges were observed, the system demonstrated reasonable performance and safety. Further larger randomized controlled trials are needed to assess the safety and efficacy of the Cardioband mitral system comprehensively.[20]

Millipede Transcatheter Mitral Annuloplasty System

The Millipede system is an innovative transcatheter, transseptal direct mitral annuloplasty device currently in development and investigation.[20] This system has demonstrated proof-of-concept in more than 20 human clinical procedures and is currently enrolling patients for a global feasibility study.[22-24]

The design of the Millipede device consists of a complete semi-rigid ring, conceptually following the full-ring surgical predicates commonly used as a stand-alone mitral valve repair for patients with functional MR.[20] The core of the device features a nitinol zig-zag stent frame, which is circumferentially fixed to the MA by eight helical anchors, ensuring secure positioning.[20]

The unique feature of the Millipede technology lies in its eight slider components located at the top of the frame.[20] These slider components can be individually cinched to achieve tailored downsizing of the MA.[20] This adjustability allows for precise customization, leading to optimal mitral valve repair.[20] The delivery catheter used for the Millipede system is designed for transvenous transseptal delivery, involving a 27 Fr profile.[20] This delivery approach enables the system to be introduced through the veins and across the septum, reaching the mitral valve without the need for open-heart surgery.[20] An additional advancement in the Millipede system is the integration of an intracardiac echocardiography catheter through the central lumen of the delivery catheter.[20] This feature provides unobstructed near-field imaging of the MA, crucial for real-time control and precision during device anchoring.[20]

Transcatheter Mitral Valve Chordal Repair Systems

NeoChord Artificial Chordae Delivery System

The NeoChord system is designed to treat severe degenerative MR due to prolapse or flail of posterior, anterior, or both mitral valve leaflets.[20] The best candidates for NeoChord treatment are patients with a central posterior leaflet (P2) prolapse or flail, and the procedure is ideally performed at an early stage of mitral valve pathology before annular dilatation occurs.[25,26] The NeoChord procedure is performed under general anesthesia with intraprocedural TEE guidance.[20] After a standard left lateral mini thoracotomy, the apical access site is confirmed through real-time 2D-TEE imaging.[20] The device is navigated to the mitral valve, and the leaflet edge is grasped, creating a loop of suture and a girth hitch knot through the mitral leaflet.[20] Typically, 3–4 neo-chordae are implanted, and their length can be adjusted to achieve maximal MR reduction under normal LV filling conditions.[20] The neo-chordae are then tied to the left ventricular epicardial pledget.[20]

Clinical studies, including the Transapical Artificial Chordae Tendineae trial, have demonstrated the immediate safety and efficacy of the NeoChord system, leading to CE approval.[20] Ongoing trials, such as the RECHORD trial, aim to provide more long-term outcome data.[20]

HARPOON Mitral Valve Repair System

The HARPOON MVRS is intended to reduce the degree of MR in patients with severe degenerative MR caused by posterior mitral leaflet prolapse.[20] It achieves this by delivering and anchoring ePTFE chords to the prolapsed mitral valve leaflet in a beating heart.[20] The HARPOON procedure is performed under general anesthesia using a left lateral thoracotomy incision.[20] Once TEE confirms the correct position of the delivery system and end effector on the targeted site of the mitral leaflet, the plunger is released to deploy a double-helical knot through the free edge of the leaflet.[20] The procedure is repeated until the desired number of ePTFE chords have been implanted. The ePTFE chords are passed through a stiff Teflon pledget and simultaneously tensioned to achieve the desired leaflet coaptation.[20]

The HARPOON system has shown satisfying immediate safety and efficacy in clinical trials, leading to CE approval.[20] The ongoing RESTORE IDE pivotal trial aims to evaluate the safety and effectiveness of the HARPOON MVRS in patients with severe degenerative MR.[20]

TRANSCATHETER MITRAL VALVE REPLACEMENT DEVICES UNDER DEVELOPMENT AND THEIR EFFICACY (TABLE 2)

There are several TMVR devices under clinical evaluation or development:

- CardiAQ/EVOQUE, under development, and clinical evaluation by Edwards Lifesciences Inc.
- Tiara, currently being developed and clinically evaluated by Neovasc Inc.
- FORTIS, a device under development, and clinical assessment by Edwards Lifesciences Inc.
- Tendyne, under the development and clinical trial process by Abbott Inc.
- Intrepid, currently under development and clinical evaluation by Medtronic Inc.
- Caisson, under development and clinical evaluation by LivaNova.
- HighLife Bioprosthesis and Subannular Implant, devices currently in development and clinical evaluation by HighLife SAS.
- SAPIEN M3, under development and clinical trial by Edwards Lifesciences Inc.
- Cardiovalve, presently under development and clinical assessment by Cardiovalve.
- NaviGate, a device under development, and clinical evaluation by NaviGate Cardiac Structures Inc.

TABLE 2: Transcatheter mitral valve replacement (TMVR) devices.

Name	Description	References
CardiAQ/EVOQUE	Under development and clinical evaluation by Edwards Lifesciences Inc	[9, 27]
Tiara	Currently being developed and clinically evaluated by Neovasc Inc	[9, 27]
FORTIS	Device under development and clinical assessment by Edwards Lifesciences Inc	[9, 27]
Tendyne	Under the development and clinical trial process by Abbott Inc	[9, 27]
Intrepid	Currently under development and clinical evaluation by Medtronic Inc	[9, 27]
Caisson	Under development and clinical evaluation by LivaNova	[9, 27]
HighLife Bioprosthesis and Subannular Implant	HighLife Bioprosthesis and Subannular Implant, devices currently in development and clinical evaluation by HighLife SAS	[9, 27]
Cardiovalve	Presently under development and clinical assessment by Cardiovalve	[9, 27]
NaviGate	A device under development and clinical evaluation by NaviGate Cardiac Structures Inc	[9, 27]

Transcatheter mitral valve replacement technologies are instrumental in the quest to provide less invasive solutions to patients with severe MR.[9] The Tendyne MV system, created by Abbott Structural (Santa Clara, CA, USA), employs a trileaflet porcine pericardial valve encased on a nitinol frame.[9] This self-expanding valve is installed via a transapical approach and can be both repositioned and retrieved after implantation.[9,27] Its nitinol stent, bearing a D-shape, complements the native mitral valve's anatomy, and its inclusion of an atrial sealing cuff aids in minimizing paravalvular leak.[9] Early studies on the Tendyne MV system reported promising outcomes, resulting in its CE Mark approval in January 2020.[28,29] Currently, the SUMMIT trial is being conducted to evaluate the Tendyne system's efficacy compared to the MitraClip, with a portion of the trial involving the Tendyne system's application in severe MAC.[9]

Neovasc Inc, based in Richmond, Canada, has developed the Tiara transcatheter mitral valve.[9,27]

Similar to the Tendyne system, it uses a self-expanding trileaflet bovine pericardial valve, which is placed on a nitinol frame.[9] A unique feature of the Tiara is its large atrial skirt, which not only helps position the device but also curbs paravalvular leak.[9,27] It was first implanted in 2014, and its early feasibility trial is ongoing.[30]

The Intrepid valve system, created by Medtronic Inc (Redwood City, CA, USA), is another self-expanding trileaflet bovine pericardial valve mounted on a nitinol frame, installed via the transapical approach.[9,27] Its unique design featuring a large atrial portion ensures optimal seating of the device and adequate sealing to the native annulus.[9] Following successful early trials, the APOLLO trial was conceived to explore the Intrepid system's efficacy in patients with severe MR.[9,27] The trial design has recently been revised to include the MitraClip in the control arm and to incorporate a transseptal new valve design platform.[9]

Among the transfemoral/transseptal devices, the CardiAQ valve was initially designed for both transapical and transfemoral/transseptal access.[27,31] While the initial version of the CardiAQ valve met with mixed results, the insights gleaned from its deployment have informed the design of the EVOQUE valve, the successor of the CardiAQ valve.[9] The EVOQUE system boasts a trileaflet bovine pericardial valve on a nitinol frame, featuring an intra-annular skirt to minimize paravalvular leak and is available in two sizes.[9]

The Caisson TMVR system, developed by LivaNova (Maple Grove, MN, USA), encompasses a self-expanding trileaflet porcine valve on a nitinol frame.[9,27] Its D-shaped anchor design conforms to the mitral valve annulus, ensuring a secure fit.[8] However, this device has recently been discontinued.[9,27]

The Sapien M3 system by Edwards Lifesciences (Irvine, CA, USA) combines a modified Sapien 3 TAVR valve and a coiling nitinol docking system.[9,27] This balloon-expandable bovine pericardial valve is placed on a cobalt-chromium stent frame and delivered via the transfemoral, transseptal approach.[9,27] Initial trials of this device have reported highly successful implantations and significant reductions in MR without notable adverse events.[32]

In hindsight, the evolution of TMVR technologies presents significant strides in the management of severe MR. However, it is important to note that these technologies are continually being refined and that new entrants, such as the HighLife valve, Cardiovalve, Cephea Valve, AltaValve, NSCI NaviGate valve, and the MValve, are being developed.[9,27] Although their efficacy is yet to be ascertained, their development contributes to the breadth and depth of TMVR options available, improving the prognosis and quality of life of patients with severe MR.[9,27]

CHALLENGES AND RISKS IN TRANSCATHETER MITRAL VALVE REPLACEMENT (FIG. 1)

Transcatheter mitral valve replacement, though a promising procedure, presents several challenges and

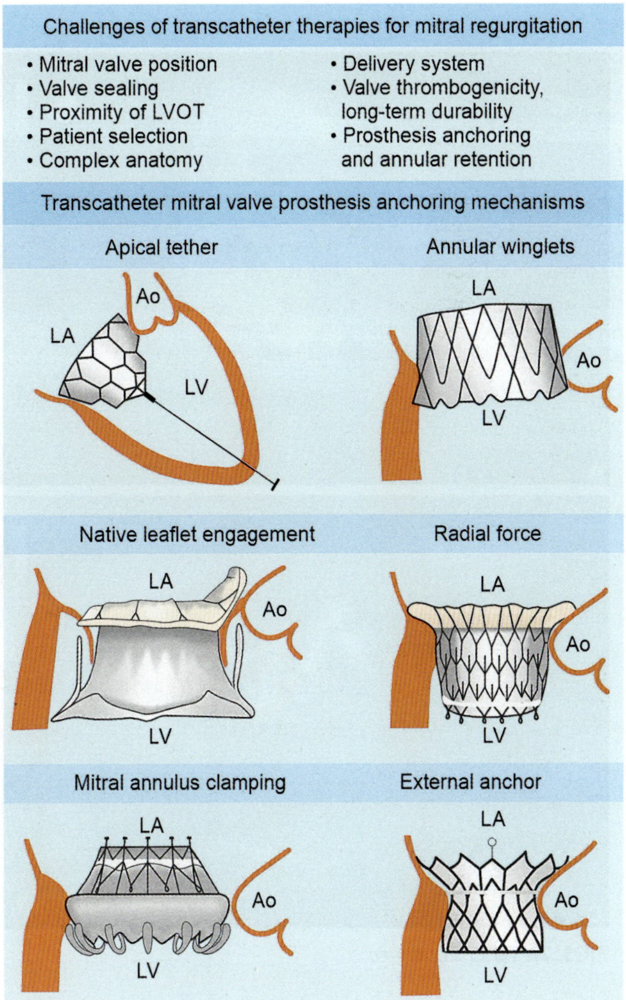

FIG. 1: Challenges and types of TMVR.

Source: Regueiro A, Granada JF, Dagenais F, Rodés-Cabau J. Transcatheter mitral valve replacement: insights from early clinical experience and future challenges. J Am Cardiol. 2017;69(17):2175-92.

risks. There are various potential impediments to consider, from the risk of a futile intervention to the possibility of periprocedural complications, and even the longevity of the prosthesis.[9,11]

The futility of intervention is an imminent risk, particularly in frail patients with severe comorbidities and advanced heart disease, as well as those afflicted with concurrent valve diseases such as MAC and aortic stenosis.[11] A noteworthy fact is that patients with severe MAC, despite an acceptable 30-day mortality risk, have an alarming half of them dying within a year, with MAC being a considerable independent predictor of mortality.[11,33]

The possibility of complications during the procedure also poses significant concern.[11] Obstruction of the LVOT, defined by an intraventricular gradient increase of at least 10 mm Hg, is one such complication.[9,11] This obstruction can occur due to the displacement of the anterior leaflet or protrusion of the transcatheter heart valve into the LVOT, with a concerning correlation with a death risk exceeding 50%.[11] The risk is particularly elevated in patients undergoing valve-in-ring or valve-in-MAC procedures.[11]

Anchoring and migration of the prosthesis in the mitral position is another potential challenge due to significant forces.[9,11] In addition, the consequences of suboptimal outcomes such as prosthesis-patient mismatch due to an internal diameter of the prosthesis/ring <22 mm or oversizing >20%, and paravalvular leaks must be considered.[11]

Furthermore, the risk of valve thrombosis, especially within the first 3 months postimplantation, is significant and tends to reduce following valve endothelialization.[11] Mitral bioprostheses and TAVR devices present higher risks compared to their surgical counterparts.[34,35] Even though valve thrombosis incidence appears low, it potentially contributes to the degenerative process of the valve.[11] Despite the myriad challenges and risks, TMVR continues to hold promise for patients who are unsuitable for conventional surgery, and ongoing research and development may help mitigate these risks **(Fig. 2)**.[11]

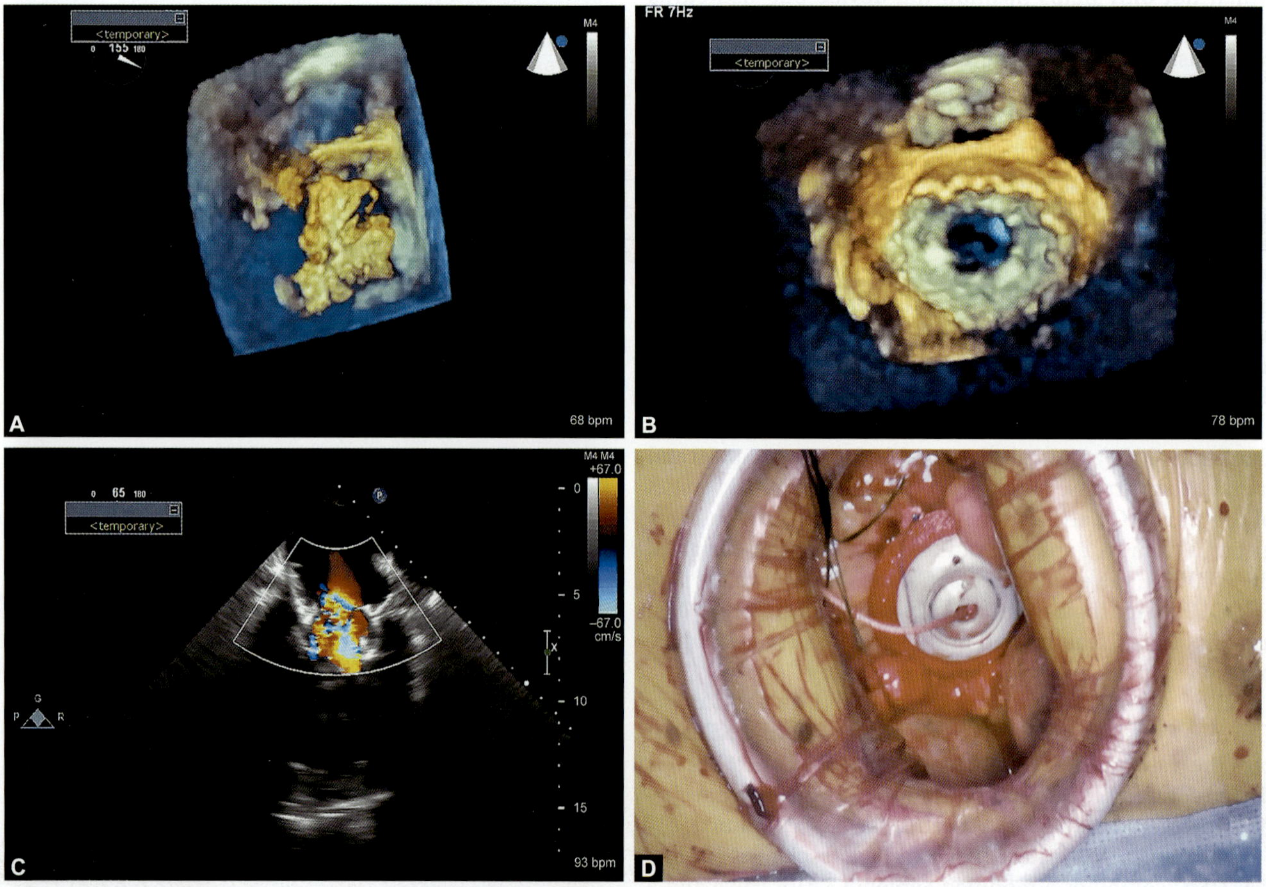

FIGS. 2A TO E: *Continued.*

Continued

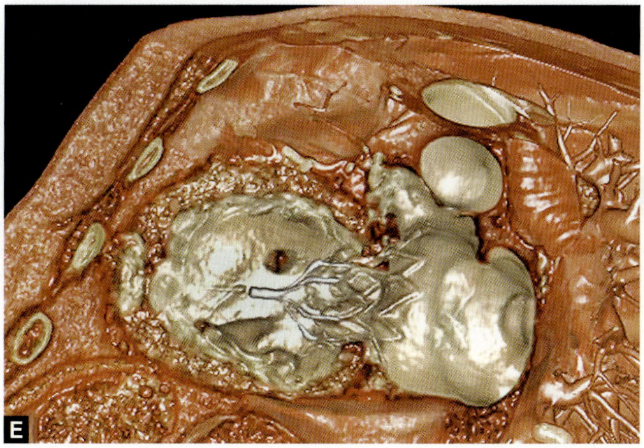

FIGS. 2A TO E: Illustrations of a Tendyne transcatheter mitral valve replacement in a patient with severe mitral regurgitation.

CONCLUSION

Transcatheter mitral valve replacement has emerged as a promising and transformative approach for managing symptomatic mitral valve regurgitation, providing viable alternatives to traditional surgical interventions for high-risk patients. TMVR technology, exemplified by various devices, has expanded treatment options and offered hope for complex mitral valve diseases. While surgical repair yields good outcomes, TMVR addresses the unmet need for patients with prohibitive surgical risks. Ongoing research and development in the field have the potential to revolutionize mitral valve disease management by improving patients' quality of life and extending therapeutic options for this challenging condition.

ONLINE REFERENCES

Please scan the QR code provided at the end of the table of contents for References of this chapter.

CHAPTER

195 Transcatheter Therapy for Tricuspid Valve Regurgitation

Rajendra Kumar Jain, B Srinivas, Shirisha Reddy Kommareddy

ABSTRACT

Tricuspid regurgitation (TR) causes progressive right heart failure and carries poor long-term outcomes. Therapy is often limited to diuretics and surgery during concomitant left-sided surgery. Isolated TR surgeries are rare and carry high mortality.[1] In view of recent advances in transcatheter procedures for other valve lesions like aortic stenosis (AS) and mitral regurgitation (MR), a renewed interest in TR and its therapies has evolved. Transcatheter therapies have been shown to reduce TR severity and improve quality of life. We reviewed the anatomy, etiology, classification, and available transcatheter therapies for TR.

Keywords: Tricuspid regurgitation, transcatheter tricuspid valve repair, transcatheter tricuspid valve replacement.

INTRODUCTION

Tricuspid regurgitation (TR) is a common finding in echocardiography (echo) in the adult population.[2] TR is caused by pathology involving tricuspid valve (TV) (primary) and functional (secondary). TR severity can be classified as mild, moderate, and severe according to the American Society of Echocardiography. TR of more than moderate severity is associated with significant mortality and morbidity. Progressive TR leads to right ventricular (RV) dysfunction, heart failure, and death. TR can itself be a predictor of adverse events independent of left heart disease, left ventricular ejection fraction (LVEF), pulmonary hypertension (PH), and RV dysfunction.[3]

Therapy for TR involved medical therapy like diuretics, guideline-directed medical therapy (GDMT) to improve LVEF and rhythm control for atrial fibrillation (AF) or surgery during concomitant left-sided valve surgery. Isolated TR surgery carried a high mortality risk as it was often considered at a very late stage in disease course. In recent times, transcatheter therapies for TR are evolving and can reduce TR severity and improve quality of life.

Tricuspid valve is often called the forgotten valve. Recent advances in imaging, understanding TR mechanism, and improved outcomes with TR therapies have led to renewed interest in transcatheter therapies for TR.

ANATOMY OF TRICUSPID VALVE

Tricuspid valve complex consists of leaflets, tricuspid annulus (TA), chordae tendineae, papillary muscles, and right atrial (RA) and ventricular myocardium. The TV usually has three leaflets, septal, anterior, and posterior as shown in **Figure 1A**. The anterior leaflet extends from anteroseptal commissure to anterolateral papillary muscle. The septal leaflet is inserted into the fibrous portion of the TA. Posterior leaflet is inserted into lower RV myocardium and its expansion is limited by diaphragm and hence TA dilation occurs predominantly in anterolateral direction.[4] The number of leaflets is variable. One study showed that three leaflets were seen in only 54% of the patients and four leaflets were seen in 39% of the patients, two leaflet configuration in 4.5% of the patients and five leaflets in 2.4% of the patients.[5] Wider coaptation distance, smaller leaflet grasp area, and complex subvalvular anatomy with multiple jets may be some of the problems encountered during intervention with additional leaflets.

Tricuspid annulus is an elliptical structure and its posteroseptal portion is more apical than anteroseptal one. The papillary muscles that support the leaflets are multiple and variably subdivided. Each papillary muscle connects to the homolateral leaflet by chordae tendineae. This is unlike left ventricular (LV) papillary muscles wherein each supplies

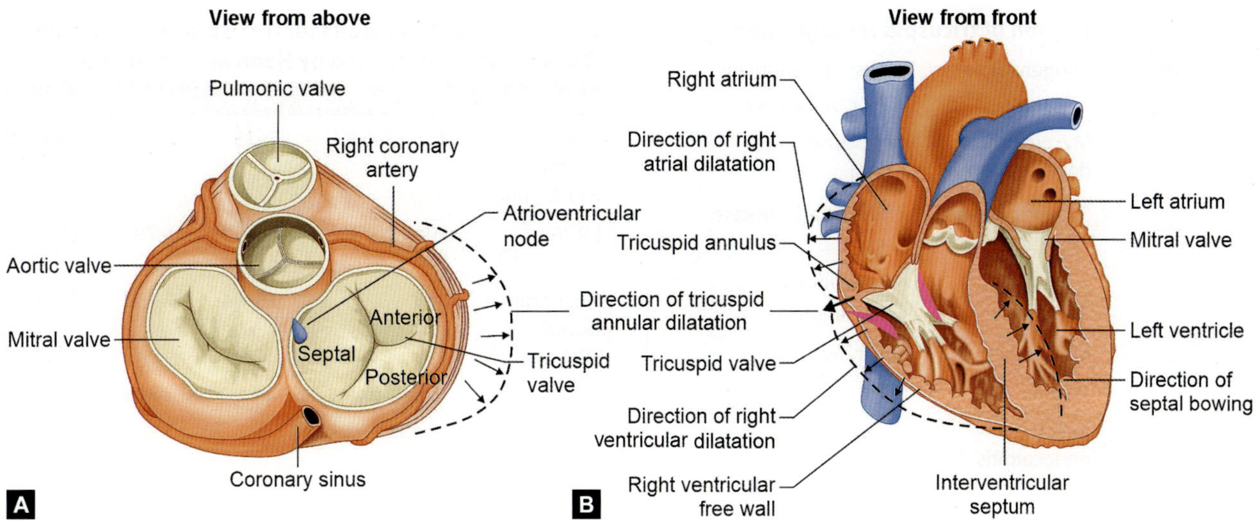

FIGS. 1A AND B: Anatomy of tricuspid valve and surrounding structures.
Source: With permission form Dahou et al. (2019).[6]

both leaflets. This leads to easy expansion of TA leading to functional tricuspid regurgitation (FTR).

Important structures like the right coronary artery (RCA), and atrioventricular (AV) node lie close to TV and can be damaged during the procedures as given in **Figure 1B**.

ETIOLOGY AND CLASSIFICATION OF TRICUSPID VALVE REGURGITATION

Tricuspid regurgitation has been classified traditionally as primary and secondary. Primary TR occurs due to intrinsic valve abnormality and FTR or secondary TR due to RA or ventricular abnormality. Primary TR is caused by rheumatic disease, infective endocarditis, and connective tissue diseases like Marfan syndrome, Ebstein's anomaly, carcinoid, radiation, and rheumatoid arthritis.

Secondary TR develops due to structural alterations in RA and RV myocardium leading to annular dilation and leaflet tethering. Left heart diseases like mitral regurgitation (MR), mitral stenosis (MS), aortic stenosis (AS), PH, atriogenic TR (AF causing TR or isolated atrial enlargement) and RV dysfunction due to RV infarction and arrhythmogenic right ventricular dysplasia (ARVD) are some of the causes of secondary TR.

A recent classification scheme identifies different morphologic entities of atrial and ventricular secondary TR and a new category called cardiac implantable electronic device (CIED)-related TR as shown in **Table 1**.

Tricuspid regurgitation is seen in heart failure with reduced ejection fraction (HFrEF) patients. One study showed prevalence of moderate-to-severe TR in these patients of about 23%. Female gender, age, and AF were associated with TR in this group. The presence of TR was associated with increased mortality. In patients with heart failure with preserved ejection fraction (HFpEF) TR of moderate-to-severe degree was seen in 11–51% and was associated with increased adverse events.

Cardiac implantable electronic device-induced TR has an incidence of 38% after lead placement. It is one of the most common causes of acquired TR and has a mortality of 10–20%.

PATHOPHYSIOLOGY OF SECONDARY OR FUNCTIONAL TRICUSPID REGURGITATION

Functional tricuspid regurgitation is caused due to alterations in RA and ventricular myocardium leading to TA dilation and/or leaflet tethering. Most common causes of FTR are LV dysfunction or left heart disease leading to left atrial dilation, increased pulmonary wedge pressure, and RV afterload.[4]

Coaptation is the contact surface between leaflets during systole. Greater the coaptation, lesser the TR. In severe cases of TR due to dilation of annulus or severe tethering of leaflets, no coaptation occurs. Normal coaptation occurs at TA level or just below it toward the apex. Coaptation height is the distance between plane of TA and leaflet coaptation point. The area between leaflets and the annular plane is called the tethering area.

Most common cause of FTR is PH. PH causes RV dysfunction, papillary muscle displacement, and leaflet tethering. RV eccentricity index > 2 [indicates an increase of anteroposterior (AP) diameter] predicts the severity of TR.[8] With increase in TR, RV dilates and the systolic function worsens thereby increasing RV diastolic pressure and interventricular septum shifts to left ventricle. Thus, TR begets TR.

TABLE 1: Classification of tricuspid regurgitation.

Primary TR (10–15%)	Congenital	• Ebstein's anomaly • AV canal defects
	Myxomatous degeneration	• Prolapse • Flail
	Systemic disease	• Rheumatic disease • SLE • Sarcoidosis • Radiation
	Malignancy	Carcinoid
	Trauma	Chest wall
	Infective endocarditis	
	Iatrogenic	RV biopsy
	Drugs	• Fenfluramine • Methysergide
Secondary/ Functional TR (80%)	Atrial secondary TR	• Chronic AF • Heart failure with preserved ejection fraction
	Ventricular secondary TR	• LV systolic dysfunction • Aortic and mitral valve disease • Primary PAH • RV dysfunction—myocardial diseases, ischemic heart disease, ARVD
CIED-induced TR (5%)		

(AF: atrial fibrillation; ARVD: arrhythmogenic right ventricular dysplasia; AV: atrioventricular; CIED: cardiac implantable electronic device; LV: left ventricular; PAH: pulmonary arterial hypertension; RV: right ventricular; SLE: systemic lupus erythematosus; TR: tricuspid regurgitation)
Source: With permission form Hahn et al. (2022).[7]

Idiopathic FTR is related to RA abnormality, TA, and basal RV dilation. AF leads to structural and electrical left atrial and RA remodeling leading to idiopathic FTR. Schlotter and colleagues defined atrial secondary TR as TV tenting height of 10 mm or lesser, mid-ventricular RV diameter of 38 mm or lesser, and LVEF > 50%.[9]

Tricuspid regurgitation is influenced by preload conditions. Small changes in RV preload caused by inspiration may lead to doubling effective regurgitant orifice area (EROA) and regurgitant volume.

Clinical Presentation of Tricuspid Regurgitation

Symptoms of TR are often nonspecific and present late in the disease course. Symptoms of TR due to AF include fatigue, exercise intolerance, and venous congestion.

TABLE 2: Updated cutoffs for tricuspid regurgitation (TR) severity as proposed by Hahn and Zamorano.[11]

Parameters	Mild	Moderate	Severe	Massive	Torrential
Biplane vena contracta width (mm)	<3	3–6.9	7–13	14–20	≥21
EROA by PISA (mm^2)	<20	20–39	40–59	60–79	≥80
Quantitative Doppler EROA (mm^2)			75–94	95–114	≥115

(EROA: effective regurgitant orifice area; PISA: proximal isovelocity surface area)

Long-standing TR with RV remodeling may present with right heart failure signs like ascites, loss of appetite, and hepatic dysfunction. Cardiohepatic syndrome (CHS) is seen in patients with TR and elevated RA pressure and can be acute/ischemic known as type 1 and chronic/congestive known as type 2. CHS is often associated with cardiorenal syndrome. TV interventions have not shown to reduce hepatic or renal dysfunction and hence risk stratification of patients before intervention is required.[10]

Multimodality Imaging

Echocardiography is an important tool for estimating severity, etiology, and grading of TR. New grading of TR extends the severity to "massive" and "torrential "as shown in **Table 2**. TR can be assessed by qualitative, semiquantitative, and quantitative measures. Qualitative methods include color Doppler jet area and continuous wave (CW) signal density and morphology. Semiquantitative methods include vena contracta width, proximal isovelocity surface area (PISA) radius, and hepatic vein flow as shown in **Figures 2A to E**. Quantitative measures are EROA and regurgitant volume. 2D echo also helps assess RV function, left-sided structures, and superior vena cava (SVC) and inferior vena cava (IVC) evaluation. 3D echo which is available recently helps in better evaluation of morphology of leaflets and surrounding structures and helps in choosing best therapy.

The presence of RV dysfunction with TR is considered high risk for transcatheter tricuspid valve intervention (TTVI) and may lead to RV and PA uncoupling. RV function can be assessed by tricuspid annular plane systolic excursion (TAPSE), fractional area change (FAC), RV myocardial performance index, lateral annulus peak systolic velocity (RV S′) and RV dP/dt. 3D right ventricular ejection fraction (RVEF) and RV strain are also used to assess RV function.

Presence of PH is common in patients with TR and is associated with an adverse outcome following intervention. Pulmonary artery systolic pressure (PASP) evaluation is important. Right heart catheterization is rarely done in cases to evaluate patients with TR. It is done in severe PH cases to

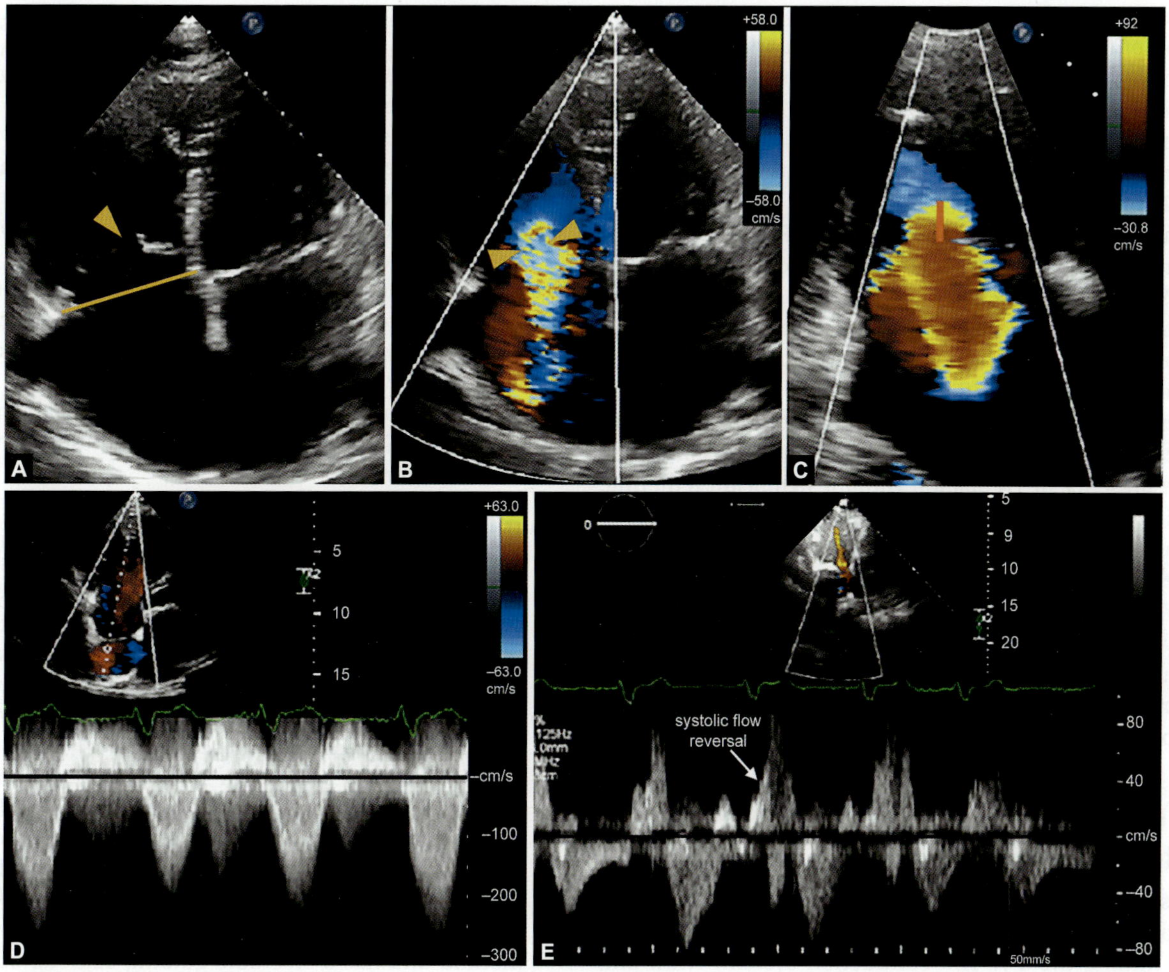

FIGS. 2A TO E: The echocardiographic assessment of severe tricuspid regurgitation (TR). (A) The right heart chambers are both dilated, with apical tethering of the tricuspid leaflets and central coaptation gap (arrowhead), vena contracta width (B), and proximal isovelocity surface area (PISA) radius (C) are indicative of severe TR. (D) The continuous wave Doppler demonstrates a dense, triangular waveform, and there is evidence of systolic flow reversal in the hepatic veins (E).

Source: With permission from Yucel et al. (2020).[12]

plan TR therapies. RCA angiography can be done to look for any injury post procedure.

Transesophageal echocardiogram (TEE) is used to assess TV leaflets, subvalvular apparatus, left-sided structures, and surrounding structures.

Intracardiac imaging [intracardiac echocardiography (ICE)] catheter is introduced via femoral vein and navigated into heart for obtaining 2D and 3D images. Provides additional benefit during procedures.

Computed tomography (CT) is useful in patients undergoing direct suture or tricuspid ring annuloplasty and for transcatheter tricuspid valve replacement (TTVR). It helps in evaluating TA size and location, surrounding structures like RCA, and also identifies fluoroscopy planes. SVC and IVC and their surrounding structures can be studied which is important in procedures like caval valve implantation (CAVI).

Cardiac magnetic resonance (CMR) aids in accurate assessment of RV function, volume, fibrosis, and tissue characterization. Leaflet length, thickening, prolapse, etc., can also be studied. Arrhythmias may cause difficulty in image acquisition and the presence of pacemaker may produce artifacts.

MANAGEMENT OF TRICUSPID REGURGITATION

Surgical Therapy for Tricuspid Regurgitation

The treatment of choice for severe TR is surgical repair. According to the American College of Cardiology (ACC) guidelines, surgical repair is indicated in the following conditions:[13]

- In patients with severe TR at the time of left-sided valve surgery
- In symptomatic patients with primary severe TR

- In symptomatic patients with FTR poorly responsive to optimal medical therapy, in which annular dilation coexist, in absence of severe PH or left-sided disease
- In patients with progressive TR at the time of left-sided valve surgery if they have suffered from right heart failure or in case of coexistent annular dilations ≥40 mm or ≥21 mm/m^2
- In symptomatic patients with severe TR, who underwent prior left-sided valve surgery, in absence of severe PH or RV systolic dysfunction
- In asymptomatic patients with severe primary TR and progressive RV dilation or systolic dysfunction

Surgical repair at the time of left-sided surgery is associated with RV reverse remodeling and improvement of clinical status. Annuloplasty with prosthetic ring is preferred in the presence of TA dilation without significant tethering. Predictors of TR relapse include TA dilation, RV dilation/dysfunction, LV dysfunction, PH, permanent AF, and the presence of pacing lead. Annuloplasty with direct suture (De Vega or Kay—bicuspidalization of the TV) is preferred in unfavorable morphology.

Surgical TV replacement if indicated is done by a bioprosthetic valve due to its lower thromboembolic complication risk.

Transcatheter Therapies for Tricuspid Regurgitation

Transcatheter therapies are challenging due to the complex anatomy, angle between SVC/IVC and the TA, and structures surrounding the TV. The conduction system, RCA, and coronary sinus are at risk during the procedure. At present, transcatheter interventions are broadly divided into two groups as shown in **Figure 3**.

1. Transcatheter tricuspid valve repair (TTVr) systems—coaptation device, annuloplasty systems
2. TTVR systems—heterotopic or orthotopic valves

Transcatheter tricuspid valve repair systems include coaptation devices that increase native leaflet coaptation or fill the orifice area and annuloplasty devices. Annuloplasty devices are modeled after surgical repair procedures which are used to reduce annulus size. Three broad categories of annuloplasty are direct ring annuloplasty, indirect ring annuloplasty, and direct suture annuloplasty. TTVR includes replacing the valve.

Currently available devices and their mechanisms are summarized in **Table 3**. Images of some of these devices are depicted in **Figure 4**.

Coaptation Devices

- *MitraClip system*: It is the most common TTVr system used due to familiarity of use in MR patients.[4] It is a cobalt chromium polyester-covered system with two arms to grasp two leaflets. It uses a 24-Fr delivery system and can be delivered through transfemoral or trans-jugular access. Newer MitraClip G4 is available now and allows for independent leaflet capture.

  Predictors of success of MitraClip on TR include primary TR with valve prolapse or secondary TR with normal leaflets, central/anterolateral jet, coaptation depth < 10 mm, coaptation gap < 7.2 mm, leaflet length > 10 mm, and absence of global RV dysfunction.[16-18]
- *TriClip*: It is similar to MitraClip using leaflet grasp method and has a steerable guiding catheter suitable for the right heart.

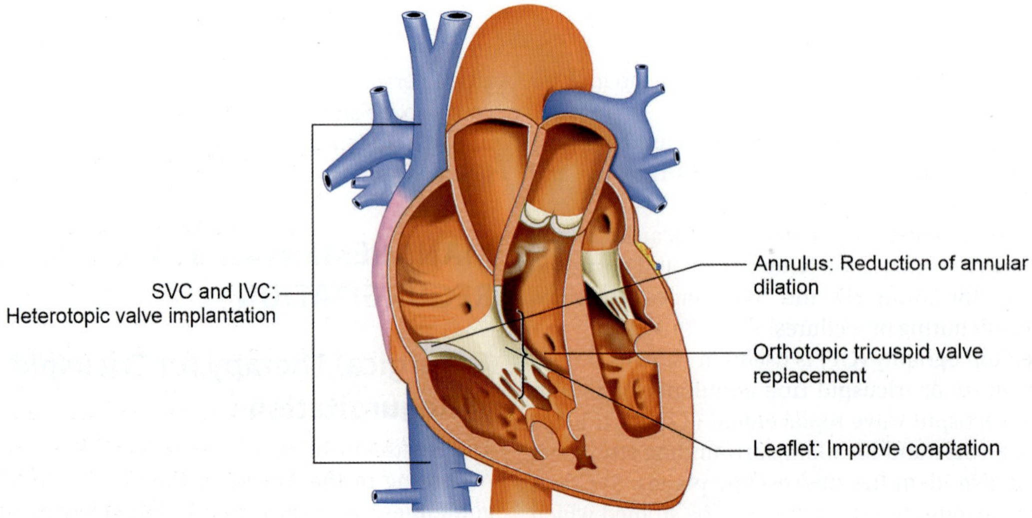

FIG. 3: Targets of tricuspid valve intervention.
(IVC: inferior vena cava; SVC: superior vena cava)

TABLE 3: Current available transcatheter tricuspid regurgitation (TR) therapies and related trials.[4,14]

Mechanism		Device	Study/Trial
Coaptation devices	Edge-to-edge repair	MitraClip	
		TriClip	TRILUMINATE
		PASCAL	CLASP TR
		Mistral	
	Spacer devices	FORMA	SPACER
Annuloplasty devices	Direct ring	Cardioband	TRI-REPAIR, TriBAND
		IRIS Millipede Ring	
	Indirect ring	TRAIPTA (transatrial intrapericardial tricuspid annuloplasty)	
	Direct suture	Trialign	SCOUT
		TriCinch	PREVENT
		PASTA (pledge-assisted suture tricuspid valve annuloplasty)	
Tricuspid valve replacement (TVR) devices	Orthotopic valves	NaviGate	
		TriSOL	
		LUX-Valve	
		TriCares	
		EVO-QUE	TRISCEND
		Intrepid	
	Heterotropic valves	Sapien	
		TricValve	TRICUS
		Tricento	

TRILUMINATE[19] trial is a prospective, single-center study for evaluating the TriClip TTVr system. Symptomatic patients with moderate or higher TR, no indication for left-sided or pulmonary valve correction, and high surgical risk were included. This system showed durable repair in 87% patients with sustained reduction in TR of >1 grade and 74% of them having moderate or lower TR at 1 year.[20] Torrential TR at baseline is a predictor of failure of TriClip system. It worked well in reducing semiquantitative echo parameters of TR like EROA (0.65 vs. 0.32), regurgitant volume (52 vs. 27 mL/beat) between baseline and 1 year follow-up. Quality of life was assessed by Kansas City Cardiomyopathy Questionnaire which showed an increase of 20 points from baseline and improvement in New York Heart Association (NYHA) class and 6-minute walk test was also noted.

- *PASCAL device*: It is a 10-mm central nitinol woven spacer that acts as a filler in regurgitant orifice. It has contoured broad paddles for leaflet grasping. It uses a 22-Fr delivery system.

  The CLASP TR trial done on 34 patients showed procedural success in 85%, and 70% patients had at least 2 TR grade reduction at 30 days. Improvement was noted in echo parameters, specifically the PISA, EROA, and vena contracta width.[21]
- *FORMA spacer device*: FORMA spacer device is a foam-filled polymer balloon that provides surface for native leaflets to coapt.[22] It is delivered from the left subclavian vein through a rail anchored at the septal portion of the RV apex.[23] The rail is also anchored to the subclavian vein. This was studied in 29 patients. 27 were implanted, two devices were explanted, one due to migration, and the other due to infection.[24] 31% of major adverse events (MAE) occurred at 30-day follow-up. Improvement in TR and echo (EROA, vena contracta width) parameters is shown.

Emerging coaptation devices:
- *Mistral device*: The spiral-shaped Mistral device improves leaflet coaptation by grasping the subvalvular apparatus. The device is advanced transfemorally using a 8.5-Fr delivery system into RV. The spiral is anchored and tightened around the chordae tendineae of two adjacent leaflets. Results showed reduction in 1 TR grade, no MAE and improvement in echo parameters, and functional status at 30 days.
- *Cerclage-TR block*: Its concept is based on mitral loop annuloplasty device which has shown reduction in MR.
- *CroíValve*: It assists coaptation in dilated TA. It uses a coaptation valve as well as a prosthetic valve that works in conjunction with native valve. It has an anchor system in SVC that locks the position of coaptation valve using a stent in SVC.

Annuloplasty Devices

Direct Ring Annuloplasty

- *Cardioband*: This device **(Figs. 5 and 6)** improves TR via annular size reduction. It consists of a polyester sleeve with radiopaque markers. 12–17 stainless steel anchors are implanted through the sleeve along the annulus. The implant is cinched to reduce the size of annulus. It was previously used for patients with functional MR.

  TRI-REPAIR trial was conducted on 30 patients over a period of 6 months. Device was successfully implanted in all the patients. Complications included three deaths (one device-related due to RV obstruction), cardiac tamponade, pacemaker requirement, ventricular tachycardia (VT), stroke, renal failure, and bleeding. The TriBAND trial also showed favorable outcomes at discharge and at 30 days.

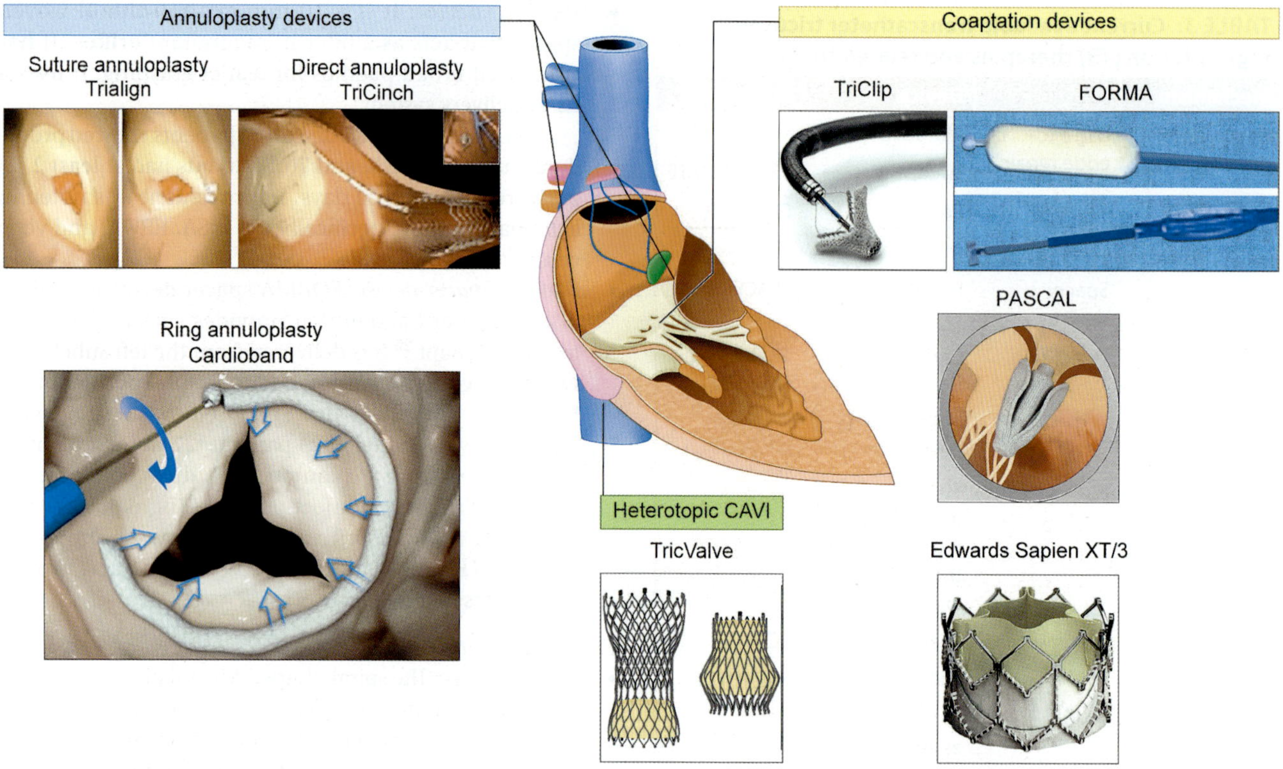

FIG. 4: Various types of devices for tricuspid regurgitation (TR) reduction.
(CAVI: caval valve implantation)
Source: With permission from Besler et al. (2018).[15]

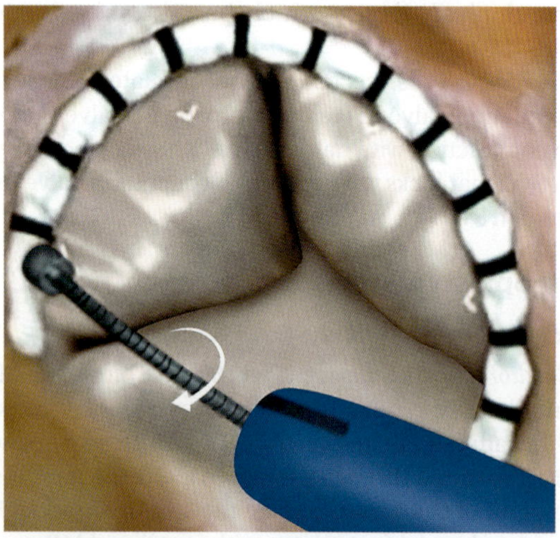

FIG. 5: Cardioband device.
Source: With permission from Arnold et al. (2021).[25]

- *IRIS Millipede ring*: The IRIS Millipede ring is a complete semirigid annuloplasty ring made of nitinol. It has eight anchors that fix the device to the TA. It has integrated ICE. This device is currently under development.[27]

Indirect Annuloplasty

TRAIPTA (transatrial intrapericardial tricuspid annuloplasty): It is a circumferential implant and exerts a compressive force to reduce the TA size[4,28] as shown in **Figure 7**. The pericardium is accessed by puncturing the RA appendage, and nitinol loop of the device is opened inside the pericardium to encircle the heart. The RA appendage defect is closed by a closure device.

Direct Suture Annuloplasty

- *Trialign system*: It mimics the modified Kay surgical technique that is obliteration of the posterior leaflet making a TV into a bicuspid valve. Pledgets are fixed at the posteroseptal and AP commissure and cinched resulting in plication of posterior leaflets. RCA angiography is performed to check for complications. The SCOUT trial[30] enrolled 15 patients. One patient required RCA stenting, and three pledget detachments occurred in remaining patients. Reduction of TR is noted and increase in LV stroke volume was observed.
- *TriCinch system*: The TriCinch system consists of two components—stainless steel screw that is placed in the anterior–posterior portion of the TA and self-expandable nitinol stent. This device is placed via transfemoral

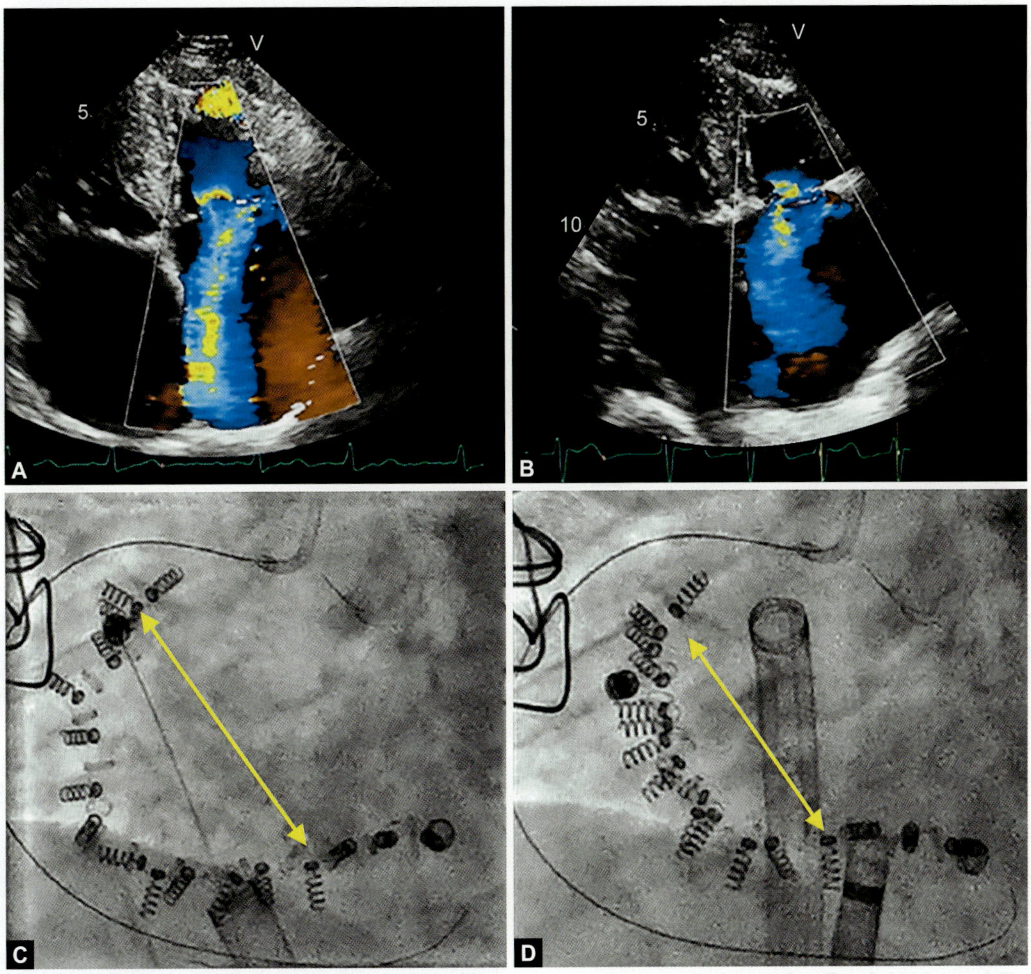

FIGS. 6A TO D: Apical four-chamber view showing severe tricuspid regurgitation at baseline. (A) Reduced to mild immediately after implantation; (B) left anterior oblique projection demonstrating the direct annuloplasty implanted before (C) and after (D) contraction with resulting decrease in the annular size (shown in yellow arrows).

Source: With permission from Simard et al. (2021).[26]

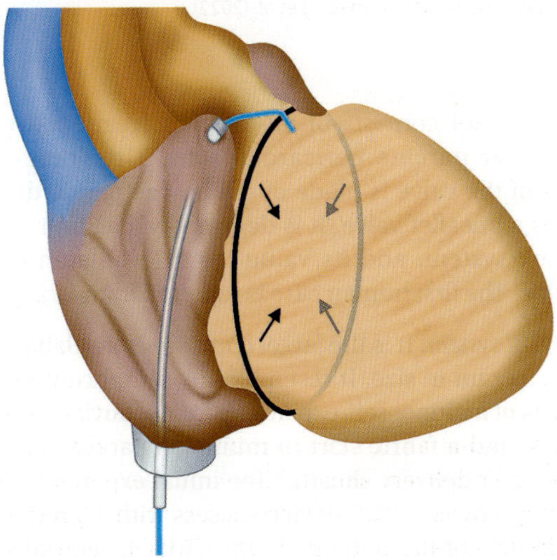

FIG. 7: Transatrial intrapericardial tricuspid annuloplasty (TRAIPTA).

Source: With permission from Asmarats et al. (2018).[29]

route. RCA angiography is needed to rule out RCA damage. The PREVENT[31] study was done in 24 patients and successfully implanted in 18 patients. 1 TR grade reduction is observed in 94%. Complications like hemopericardium (2), RCA damage (1), late annular detachment (5) were noted.

- *Minimally invasive annuloplasty-tricuspid (MIA-T)*: MIA-T consists of ultralow-mass polymeric, biocompatible PolyCor anchors that are tensed by thermoplastic myolast polymer. It is designed to obliterate the posterior leaflet.
- *Pledge-assisted suture tricuspid valve annuloplasty (PASTA)*: PASTA is similar to the Hetzer double orifice suture technique. This was first implanted in an 84-year-old man, with torrential TR and RV dysfunction. The patient was discharged with recurrence of severe TR.[32]
- *DaVingi TR system*: This system offers a two-stage procedure to reduce the tricuspid annular size. In the

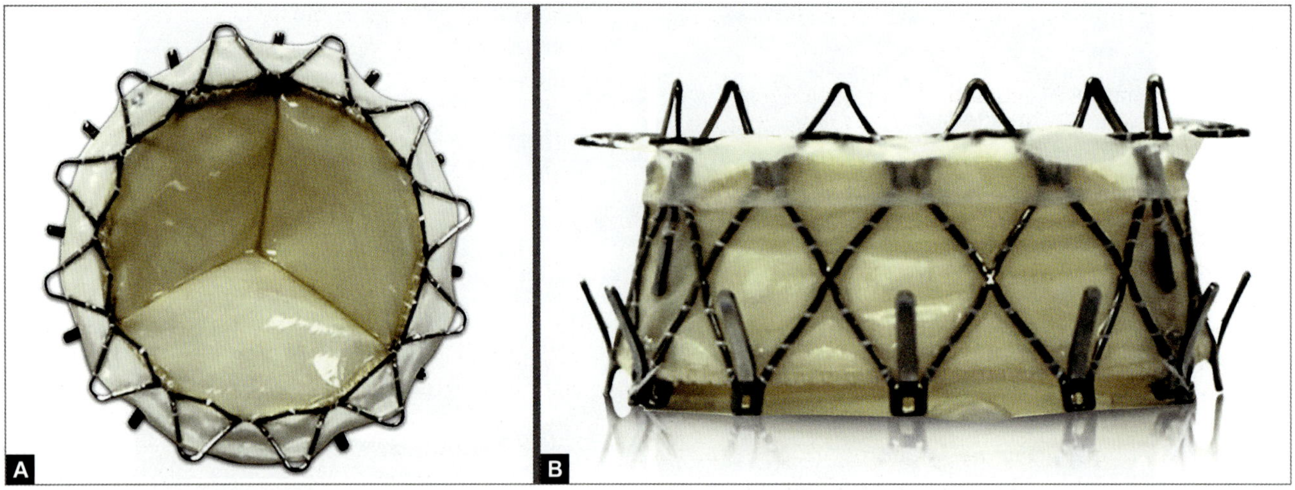

FIGS. 8A AND B: NaviGate inflow and lateral views.
Source: With permission from Asmarats et al. (2018).[29]

first part, a flexible ring is placed in the annulus featuring a balloon and by firing all the anchors simultaneously, and the adjustment chord is fixed at internal jugular vein (IJV). The chronic healing secures the implant to the tissue. In the second part, cinching of the annulus is performed using a 16-Fr adjustment tool.

Transcatheter Tricuspid Valve Replacement

There are two types of TTVR: orthotropic and heterotropic. Orthotropic involves placing a prosthetic valve in TA, and heterotropic is placing prosthetic valve in SVC or IVC.

Orthotropic Tricuspid Valve Replacement

- NaviGate
- TriSol valve
- LUX-Valve
- TRiCares Valve
- EVOQUE TV
- The Intrepid

Navigate: It is a self-expanding tricuspid bioprosthesis as shown in **Figures 8A and B**. It is an atrioventricular valved stent with trileaflet design. It is conical in shape and reduces transvalvular gradient and minimizes right ventricular outflow tract (RVOT) obstruction. It requires a 42-Fr delivery catheter via transtubular access. Transatrial approach can also be done through minimally invasive thoracotomy.

LUX valve: It is a self-expanding bovine valve that is a radial force-independent TTVR device as depicted in **Figure 9**. It consists of four components—trileaflet prosthetic valve, self-expandable nitinol stent, interventricular septal anchor, and two graspers for leaflet fixation. Valve is delivered via mini thoracotomy using a transatrial approach. This device was implanted in 12 patients with good procedural success and 90% had a mild TR and significant symptomatic improvement.

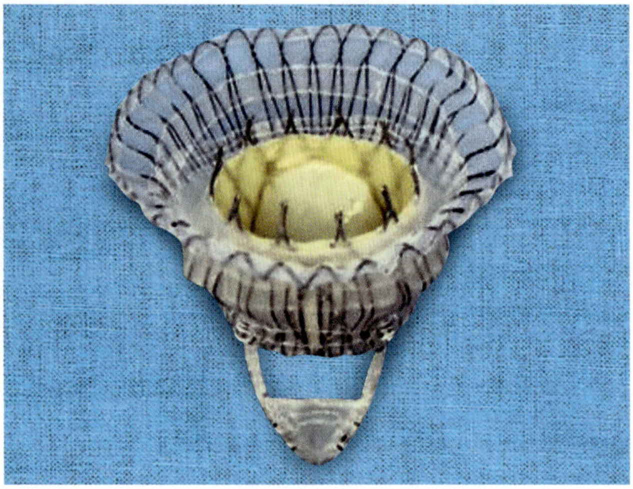

FIG. 9: Atrial view of LUX-Valve.
Source: With permission from Ning et al. (2022).[33]

TriSol: TriSol consists of an atrial polyester skirt and a ventricular porcine pericardial skirt. The dome-shaped leaflet of the valve is made of the bovine pericardium and creates a bileaflet valve. It is delivered via a 30-Fr steerable delivery system, and its value is retrievable and repositionable. The first human case is reported from Israel.

EVOQUE system: It is the largest prosthesis available in trials and is 52 mm in size. It resembles its mitral counterpart. It consists of a nitinol self-expanding frame, bovine pericardial leaflets, and a fabric skirt to minimize paravalvular leaks. It has 28-Fr delivery sheath.[4] The initial experience with 25 patients showed a 92% device success with TR reduction to <1% in 92% of the patients.[34] The TRISCEND trial showed 3.2% all-cause mortality at 6 months in 132 patients. 100% of the patients are with mild or less TR post procedure.

Improvement in quality of life and NYHA class was also noted.

Intrepid: The Intrepid is composed of a nitinol frame with trileaflet bovine pericardium. It uses a 35-Fr sheath. It is first presented as a compassionate use in three patients.

Heterotropic Valves

In this strategy, the valve is deployed in the SVC or IVC to limit the effects of severe TR on surrounding organs but sparing the right atrium. CAVI uses both self-expandable and balloon-expandable devices. The backflow into the SVC is low compared to the IVC due to the hydrostatic pressure. Hence, CAVI with balloon-expandable valves is performed only into the IVC. CAVI suitability includes the presence of pulsatile caval backflow and adequate venae cavae measurements (<30 mm for balloon-expandable and <42 mm for self-expandable valves).

Some of the heterotopic valves are:

- Sapien valve
- TricValve
- TriCentro

- *Sapien valve*: It is used for severe AS patients and is a balloon-expandable valve. It has been implanted either in SVC or both in SVC and IVC after deploying a stent in venae cavae for anchoring. This was an off-label use. TRICAVAL study compared CAVI versus GDMT in patients with severe TR, high surgical risk, and NYHA class > 2. Patients with severe LV dysfunction and CKD and IVC landing zone diameter exceeding 31 mm were excluded. Prosthesis was successfully installed in all the patients. The trial was stopped prematurely due to high failure rates.
- *TricValve*: As depicted in **Figure 10,** the TricValve device consists of two pericardial tissue, self-expandable valves on nitinol stent frame, one for SVC and another for IVC. The IVC valve has an upper segment protruding into the right atrium and the biological valve located above the diaphragm to prevent backflow into hepatic veins. For the SVC valve, the stent frame has a funnel shape with upper and lower segments tapered to facilitate fixation at cavoatrial inflow. The proximal stent segment is mounted with a trileaflet woven pericardial valve.
- *TriCentro*: The TriCentro CAVI device consists of a bicavally anchored nitinol stent deployed top-down from SVC into IVC. A lateral bicuspid porcine pericardial valve allows implant into the right atrium. The device needs to be custom-made for each patient.

Device selection: Assessment of anatomic and physiological factors helps us in choosing the right device. An algorithm for the same is described in **Flowchart 1**.

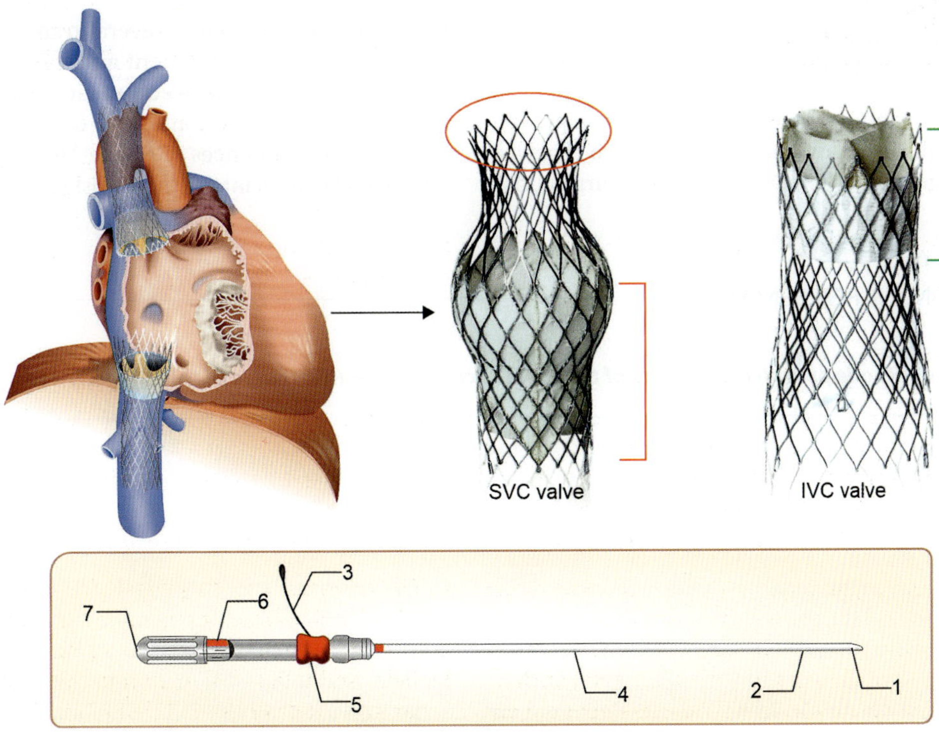

FIG. 10: Components of TricValve and its delivery system.

(IVC: inferior vena cava; SVC: superior vena cava)

Source: With permission from Wong et al. (2022).[35]

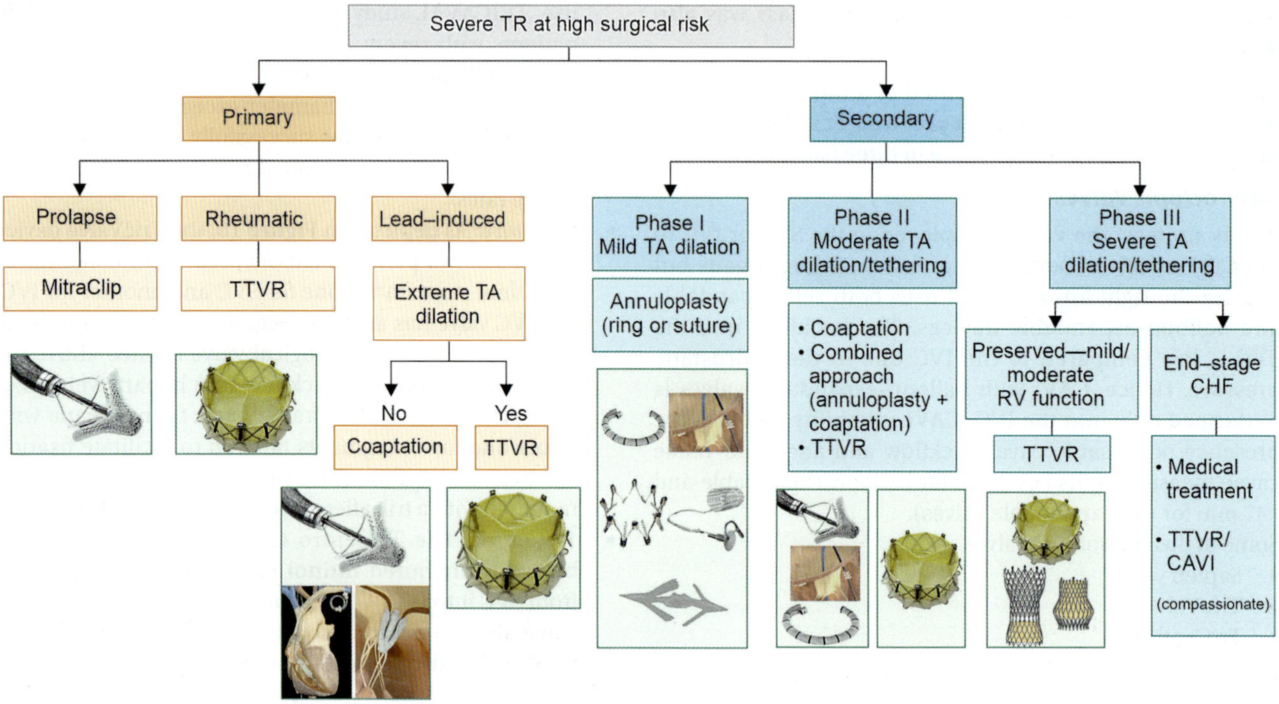

FLOWCHART 1: Algorithm for choosing the right device for patients with severe tricuspid regurgitation (TR).
(CAVI: caval valve implantation; CHF: congestive heart failure; RV: right ventricular; TA: tricuspid annulus; TTVR: transcatheter tricuspid valve replacement)
Source: With permission from Asmarats et al. (2018).[29]

CONCLUSION

Severe tricuspid regurgitation is a common problem with considerable morbidity. In recent years, improvement in understanding the complex anatomy, pathophysiology, and availability of multi-modality imaging have led to renewed interest in management of TR. Due to the high surgical risk of most of these patients, several transcatheter therapies are under active development and have shown to reduce severity of TR and improved functional status and quality of life. TTVR should be considered early in the course of the disease as consequences of severe TR like liver and kidney disease make these interventions risky.

ONLINE REFERENCES

Please scan the QR code provided at the end of the table of contents for References of this chapter.

CHAPTER

196 Percutaneous Pulmonary Valve Implantation

K Sivakumar

ABSTRACT

In the last three decades, significant progress made in imaging, surgical techniques, and intensive care management has permitted adult survival of most congenital heart diseases. As the repaired outflow tracts often progressively develop stenosis or regurgitation, these patients need competent pulmonary valves to sustain the right ventricular function. Redo surgeries carry significant morbidity as well as shorter longevity of hemodynamic improvement. This opened the role of percutaneous pulmonary valve implantation in most of these patients. This chapter discusses the current role of this therapy and the different valves available for use in India.

Keywords: Right ventricular dysfunction, pulmonary regurgitation, venus P valve, Melody valve, Myval heart valve, Sapien S3 heart valve.

INTRODUCTION

Survival to adulthood has improved in most cyanotic congenital heart diseases due to progress made in diagnostic imaging, surgical techniques, refined anesthesia, and intensive care, as well as meticulous surveillance of operated patients. Cyanotic malformations associated with varying forms of pulmonary outflow obstructions often permit survival beyond neonatal period and are amenable to various types of palliative and corrective surgical interventions.

TETRALOGY OF FALLOT: THE PROTOTYPE

Tetralogy of Fallot—the classical prototype of such a malformation is the most common cyanotic heart diseases beyond infancy. Surgical correction relieves the hypoxia, thereby allowing survival to adolescence, though varying degrees of pulmonary stenosis and regurgitation cause deleterious effects in the long term.[1] Chronic right ventricular (RV) pressure and volume overload lead to ventricular dysfunction as well as life-threatening arrhythmias.

NATURAL HISTORY OF RIGHT VENTRICULAR DYSFUNCTION

When patients with tetralogy of Fallot are operated with transannular patch, incidence of significant pulmonary regurgitation identified in the immediate postoperative echocardiography at the time of discharge from hospital is 48% and this increases to 85% when the patients are evaluated 2 years later. This indicates that the progress of pulmonary regurgitation is almost universal in every patient with a transannular patch.[2] However, if patients are operated with a valved homograft, dysfunction of the conduit manifesting as significant pulmonary stenosis and/or regurgitation is identified in half of the patients at a time frame of 10 years after the surgical correction. When they are reoperated for a conduit change, the degeneration of the conduit is accelerated and significant dysfunction is identified within 5 years.

DOES RIGHT VENTRICULAR DYSFUNCTION LEAD TO DEATH?

Pulmonary regurgitation with dilated right ventricle leads to heart failure, arrhythmia, and sudden cardiac death. RV dysfunction is often asymptomatic in the first few years, with symptoms occurring only in 6% of the patients at the end of 20 years of surgery. But almost 30% of patients become symptomatic when the patients are followed after 40 years.[3] Once they become symptomatic, death occurs within a short period and symptoms are a clear indication for surgery. Symptoms such as fatigue, edema, and arrhythmia indicate failure of compensatory mechanisms and are clear evidences of irreversible dysfunction.

OTHER CYANOTIC HEART DISEASES

Few other less common cyanotic anomalies such as truncus arteriosus, dextro-transposition (d-transposition) of great arteries with ventricular septal defect and pulmonary stenosis, and double outlet right ventricle with pulmonary stenosis; some forms of corrected transpositions are managed in early life with placement of a homograft or xenograft conduit from right ventricle to pulmonary artery to relieve the obstructed outflow. These conduits degenerate and dysfunction over time to cause a similar sequel on the right ventricle.

BICUSPID AORTIC VALVE AND ROSS SURGERY

Among acyanotic congenital heart diseases, the most common among them is a bicuspid aortic valve. Young patients presenting with aortic valve dysfunction with aortic annulus that do not permit a prosthetic valve insertion are treated with Ross procedure that involves placement of a similar conduit. All these patients often require a replacement of the pulmonary valve in their second-to-fourth decade.

WHY TRANSCATHETER THERAPY INSTEAD OF SURGERY?

Repeat surgeries for surgical pulmonary valve replacement through redo sternotomies carry additional surgical risks due to bleeding, repeated RV incisions, effect of cardiopulmonary bypass, and myocardial ischemia.[4] Percutaneous pulmonary valve implantation was the first transcatheter valve therapy introduced to clinical practice 25 years ago.[5] The last two decades saw significant progress in different designs of transcatheter pulmonary valves, preprocedural assessment with three-dimensional imaging tools, recognition of the common adverse events and overcoming them, as well as postintervention surveillance.

AIMS AND OBJECTIVES OF THIS REVIEW

Indications for transcatheter pulmonary valve implantation in patients with pulmonary stenosis and pulmonary regurgitation have different clinical basis. Different types of valves available for clinical use will be discussed. The procedural steps, key information obtained from the different imaging tools, techniques of implantation of different valves, and assessment of the outcomes are discussed.

INDICATIONS IN PATIENTS WITH PREDOMINANT STENOSIS

Any symptomatic severe pulmonary stenosis with gradient exceeding 50 mm Hg and RV systolic pressures exceeding two-thirds systemic pressures are clear indications for intervention. In asymptomatic patients, RV dysfunction defined as ejection fraction <47%, systemic venous congestion, ventricular arrhythmias, and secondary tricuspid regurgitation are additional indications for intervention. In younger patients, the relief of pulmonary stenosis may be achieved by balloon or stent angioplasty; however, this leads to free pulmonary regurgitation that will ultimately need a competent pulmonary valve.

INDICATIONS IN PATIENTS WITH PULMONARY REGURGITATION

While symptomatic pulmonary regurgitation is universally accepted as an indication for pulmonary valve implantation, asymptomatic patients benefit by arrest of progressive RV dilatation. Beyond a threshold, if the right ventricle dilates, delayed valve implantation may not offer a significant advantage.[6] Certain indices used in patient selection include indexed RV end-diastolic and end-systolic volumes of 160 mL and 80 mL, respectively. Dilated right ventricle with twice the volume of the left ventricle, right ventricle ejection fraction <45%, and progressive new onset of tricuspid regurgitation.[7] Progressive widening of the QRS complexes in electrocardiogram and ventricular arrhythmias are additional indications for implantation of pulmonary valves.

ROLE OF HEART TEAMS

Even though the cardiac anatomy of a patient is suited for both surgical and percutaneous valve implantations, certain clinical guidelines should direct the most optimal approach. They include ability of the procedure to achieve the best hemodynamics, a sufficiently large valve that allows higher cardiac output during exercise, avoiding interactions with neighboring structures such as coronaries or aortic root, sternal compression, relief of all distal stenosis, and closure of residual septal defects. History of previous endocarditis should also influence the decision-making.

ROLE OF ADULT CONGENITAL HEART DISEASE SPECIALIST

While adult cardiologists or pediatric cardiologists currently handle most structural interventions, the physician performing these interventions should be aware of the nominal size of conduits and tissue valves, as well as the common forms of coronary anomalies in each clinical situation. Associations of aortic root dilatation and aortic valve regurgitation, identification of pulmonary artery kinks and stenosis, and recognition of residual ventricular or atrial septal defects that may not show any color Doppler flows due to elevation in right heart pressures are better identified by adult congenital heart disease (ACHD) specialists and they should be part of each heart team.

TYPES OF VALVES

There are two forms of percutaneous pulmonary valves. Balloon-expandable valves are ideally suited for narrowed conduits or narrowed native outflow tracts. They often need prestenting to relieve the stenosis, followed by implantation of pulmonary valves within these stents that act as landing zones. Such valves include Melody (Medtronic Inc, Minneapolis, MN), Sapien S3 (Edwards Lifesciences LLC, Irvine, CA), and Myval (Meril Lifesciences, Vapi, India). Self-expanding valves are typically recommended in native-dilated outflow tracts. These valves are often larger in profile and cannot be implanted in stented outflow tracts. Examples of these valves include Venus-P (Venus MedTech, Shanghai, PRC), Medzenith PT (Medzenith, Beijing, PRC), Pulsta (Taewoongmedical, South Korea), Inovare (Braile Biomedica, Brazil), and Harmony (Medtronic Inc, Minneapolis, MN).

Venus P-valve

This self-expandable nitinol framework with a trileaflet porcine pericardial valve is available in straight and flared designs.[8] The latter design that is commonly used is available in diameters of 18–36 mm in 2 mm increments. The flared design of the valve has five open cells in distal flare that connect all the sharp edges to the outer wire frame. The valve is rinsed to remove the glutaraldehyde preservative and crimped in ice-cold saline to reduce the nitinol memory, using a proprietary compression device and loaded on the 22 or 24F delivery system **(Figs. 1A and B)**.

Myval Transcatheter Valve

Myval transcatheter valve is structured on a nickel–cobalt alloy frame with a unique honeycomb design comprising of hexagonal elements.[9] The valve consists of decellularized bovine pericardial tissue crafted into a trileaflet valve on the metal frame that has a skirt of polyethylene terephthalate to retard deposition of calcium and minimize paravalvular regurgitation. The valve is crimped on a unique hi-flex, over-the-wire navigator balloon using a mechanical crimping tool Val-de-Crimp™, prior to insertion into the systemic circulation. The broad size matrix of Myval THV (20, 21.5, 23, 24.5, 26, 27.5, 29, 30.5, and 32 mm) facilitates the optimal sizing of the transcatheter heart valve (THV). A 14F Python™ introducer sheath suitable for all the sizes of Myval THV ensures uneventful retrieval of undeployed THV in adverse conditions. While the same valve used in aortic position is utilized for pulmonary position too, the differences in pulmonary deployment from aortic deployment include mounting and crimping the valve in reverse position to allow antegrade pulmonary blood flow and anteflexion at

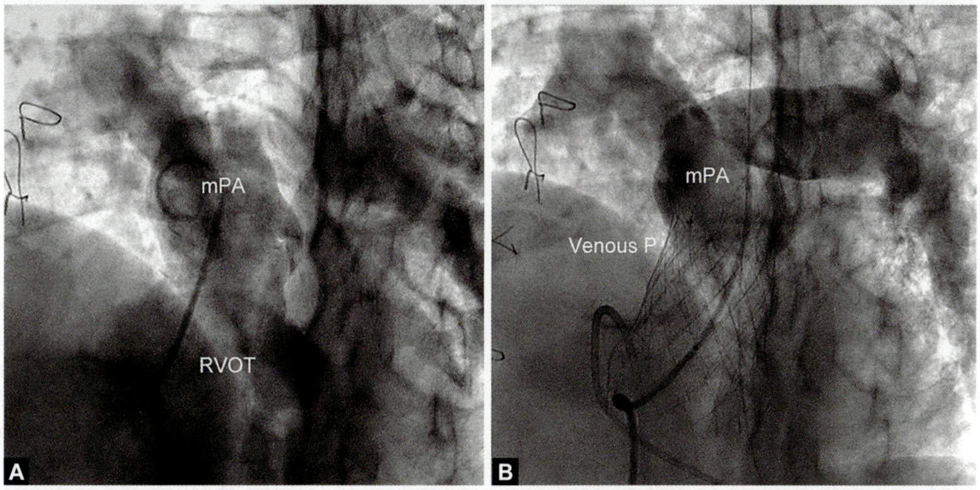

FIGS. 1A AND B: Venus P-valve. Free pulmonary regurgitation after transannular repair of Fallot tetralogy (A) results in dilated main pulmonary artery (mPA) and right ventricular outflow tract (RVOT). Venus P-valve implantation (B) resulted in correction of pulmonary regurgitation.

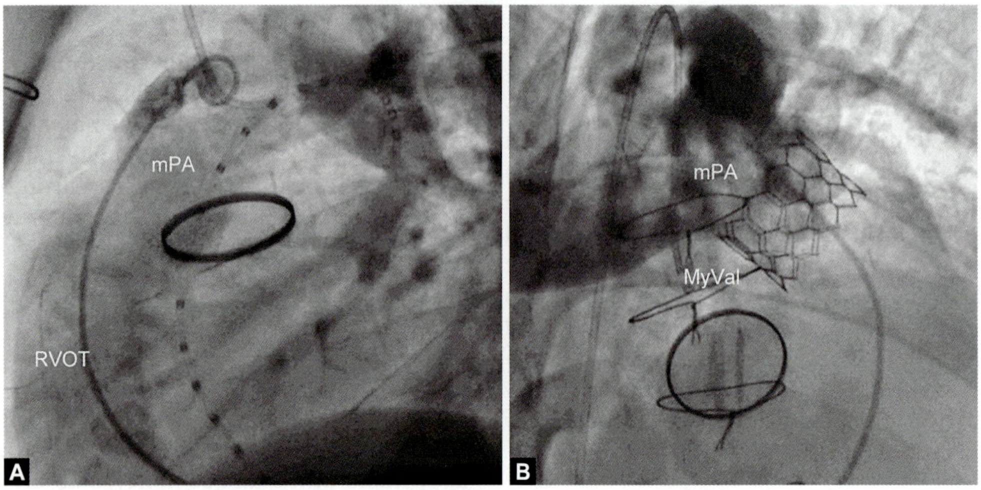

FIGS. 2A AND B: Myval valve. Free pulmonary regurgitation after transannular repair of Fallot tetralogy (A) results in dilated main pulmonary artery (mPA) and right ventricular outflow tract (RVOT). Myval valve implantation (B) resulted in correction of pulmonary regurgitation.

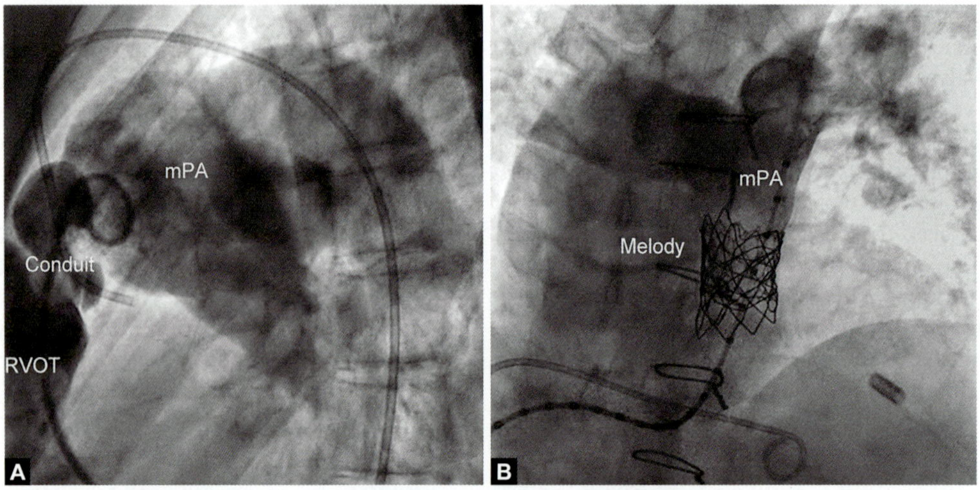

FIGS. 3A AND B: Melody valve. Severe stenosis of the conduit (A) placed from right ventricular outflow tract (RVOT) and main pulmonary artery (mPA) is corrected by Melody valve implantation (B).

the tricuspid valve contrary to retroflexion at the aortic arch **(Figs. 2A and B)**.

Melody Valve

The Melody valve consists of a valve-containing bovine jugular vein, sewn inside a balloon-expandable 8-zig Cheatham platinum-iridium stent.[10] The valve is delivered via a 22 Fr system and can be expanded up to a diameter of 22 mm. The Ensemble delivery system consists of a balloon-in-balloon in diameters of 18–22 mm. This valve is relatively simpler to mount and very flexible to use in tortuous conduits. Introduced in 2000, this valve has the longest clinical experience among all the transcatheter valves **(Figs. 3A and B)**.

Sapien Valve

Sapien valve is made of three bovine pericardial leaflets sewn inside a 14 mm-long stainless-steel stent.[11] The ventricular two-thirds of the stent is covered with a fabric-sealing cuff designed to reduce the potential for paravalvular leaks. The valve is currently available in diameters of 23, 26, and 29 mm. It is mounted on a 3 cm-long, high-pressure balloon and is delivered via a 24–26 Fr sheath. The valve was initially designed for aortic valve replacement via an antegrade or retrograde approach. To facilitate delivery of the valve in a retrograde fashion through the tortuous aortic arch, a specially designed Retroflex catheter is used. The Retroflex catheter is also helpful for negotiating the venous system and the right-sided heart chambers **(Figs. 4A and B)**.

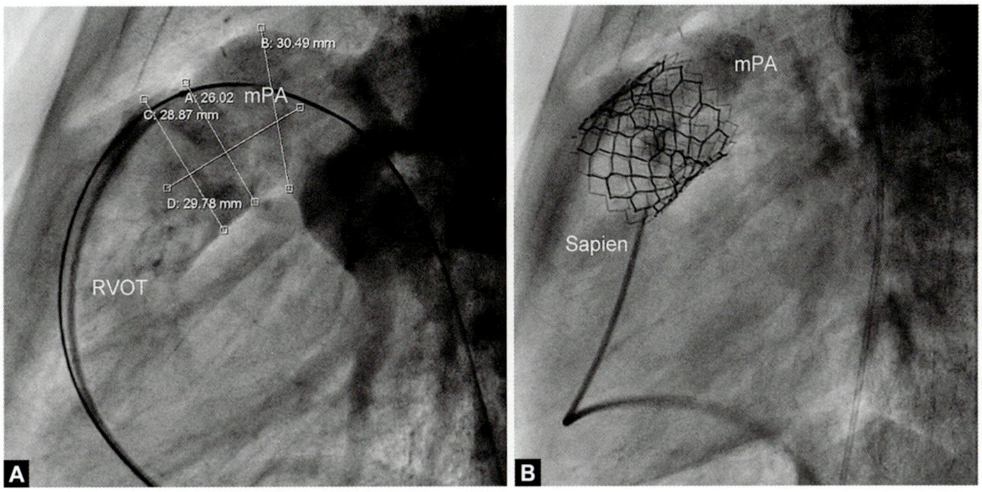

FIGS. 4A AND B: Sapien valve. Free pulmonary regurgitation after transannular repair of Fallot tetralogy (A) results in dilated main pulmonary artery (mPA) and right ventricular outflow tract (RVOT). Sapien S3 implantation (B) resulted in correction of pulmonary regurgitation.

Harmony Valve

This is a porcine pericardial tissue valve sewn onto a self-expanding nitinol frame covered in a polyester knit fabric.[12] It has an asymmetrical hourglass shape with a slightly wider inflow than outflow end. The valve is treated to mitigate leaflet calcification and sterilized using 0.2% glutaraldehyde. The Harmony thermophotovoltaic (TPV) device is commercially available with a 22- or 25-mm valve diameter. The TPV25 is shorter in length than the TPV22 and has a wider diameter at the inflow and outflow ends. A single 25F delivery system with a coil-loading catheter is used for all valve sizes.

PROCEDURAL DETAILS

The procedure is often performed on general anesthesia, biplane fluoroscopy from femoral vein access, or rarely jugular vein access. Prior three-dimensional imaging with computed tomography often typically guides initial angiograms in orthogonal projections. Baseline pressures are recorded in right heart chambers to exclude branch pulmonary artery stenosis. Oximetry excludes atrial or ventricular residual septal defects. Balloon interrogation to study coronary compression is dependent on the compliance and calcifications in the conduit. Conduit preparation and creation of landing zones involve deploying covered stents within the narrowed segments.

CORONARY AND AORTIC ROOT TESTING

Since conduits may be very closely related to left or right coronary artery, stenting of these conduits might compromise the coronary flows. Anomalous coronary arteries such as left anterior descending coronary arising from right coronary artery as well as anomalously implanted coronaries after Ross procedure may be at additional risks. While selective coronary angiogram is more definite in identifying an interaction between the interrogating balloon and the coronary flows, aortic root angiogram will additionally identify aortic root distortion and creation of aortic insufficiency.

PROCEDURAL PROBLEMS FROM PERCUTANEOUS PULMONARY VALVE IMPLANTATION

Percutaneous pulmonary valve implantation is consistently reported to have a very low periprocedural complication rate of 3–6%.[13] Coronary artery compression is the most catastrophic complication. 5–6% of patients have anomalous coronary anatomy that makes them more amenable for coronary compression with a prestenting of the conduit. Homograft rupture may occur in calcified conduits with high-pressure balloon dilatation. Covered stents are recommended in this situation. Stent migration is a problem in borderline dilated outflow tracts. Tricuspid valve damage is also reported during passage of delivery system.[14]

EARLY AND LATE PROCEDURAL RESULTS

Following valve implantation, improvement in RV outflow gradient and pulmonary regurgitation is almost always noted. Improvement of RV volumes and RV function as well as improvement in left ventricular ejection fraction is accompanied by improvement in New York Heart Association (NYHA) functional class and exercise performance.[15] Late problems are related to stent compression, stent fracture, endocarditis.[16] Valve leaflet thrombosis may be prevented by long-term antiplatelets or anticoagulation.[17]

CONCLUSION

Different transcatheter valve designs have improved the applicability of percutaneous pulmonary valve implantation in most patients with repaired RV outflow tract. Even though indications for this expensive therapy are very clear and proven in symptomatic patients, asymptomatic patients are often considered for this therapy using different imaging and hemodynamic criteria. Establishing procedural safety is mandatory when such asymptomatic patients are included. Patients with challenging anatomy and physiology are now amenable for percutaneous pulmonary valves as more and more valve designs are emerging for clinical use.

ONLINE REFERENCES

Please scan the QR code provided at the end of the table of contents for References of this chapter.

CHAPTER

197 Left Atrial Appendage Occlusion: Current Indications and Technical Challenges

Bharat Vijay Purohit, Meeraji Rao

ABSTRACT

Atrial fibrillation (AF) is most common arrhythmia especially in an elderly associated with significant risk of causing ischemic stroke. The mainstay of treatment to prevent stroke is oral anticoagulant (OAC) [especially direct oral anticoagulants (DOACs)]. Despite the usefulness, a significant number of patients either do not take the drugs or are ineligible for drug therapy or have recurrences of stroke despite adequate therapy. Left atrial appendage (LAA) occlusion (LAAO) is a novel therapy to prevent stroke especially in nonvalvular atrial fibrillation (NVAF). It is slowly establishing itself as alternate to drugs in select subset of patients. Various devices are available to occlude LAA with subtle differences in their mechanism of occlusion, method of implantation, and post-procedure antithrombotic regimen. The key to development of therapy is to assess appendage properly by transesophageal echocardiography (TEE)/computed tomography (CT) or intracardiac echocardiography (ICE) for suitability of device therapy and minimize procedural/postprocedural complications and selecting optimal size to occlude the appendage effectively. A lot of research is ongoing to address various aspects of device therapy.

Keywords: Atrial fibrillation, LA appendage occlusion, device therapy.

INTRODUCTION

Atrial fibrillation (AF) is one of the most common arrhythmias affecting almost 2–4% of the population with increasing incidence as age advances.[1] Above the age of 55 years, it is estimated to affect one in five individuals or one in three if associated with at least one of these risk factors such as smoking, alcohol consumption, body mass index, blood pressure, diabetes, and history of heart failure or myocardial infarction.[2]

Most dreaded complication of AF is development of stroke due to thrombus formation in left atrium (LA) or left atrial appendage (LAA). In a patient with nonvalvular atrial fibrillation (NVAF) (i.e., AF in conditions other than in those with moderate or severe mitral stenosis or post valve replacement) 89% of times the thrombus forms in LAA.[3]

ANATOMY OF LEFT ATRIAL APPENDAGE

Left atrial appendage is not a fixed structure. It is a finger-like projection from LA with considerable variations in its size, shape, and relationship to surrounding structures. LAA is situated at the anterior and the lateral walls of the LA, with its tip directed anterosuperiorly. It overlies important structures like left border of the right ventricular outflow tract or the pulmonary trunk and left main coronary artery or left circumflex (LCX) artery and the left lateral ridge separates the orifices of the left pulmonary veins from the LAA orifice.[4] LAA is divided into three parts: orifice (it is quite variable ranging from elliptical, round, triangular, water drop, foot, or irregular), neck region which is smooth, and then body which is 10–12 mm away from ostium and is trabeculated and lobulated. In most cases there are two lobes (54%), followed by three lobes (23%), one lobe (20%), and four lobes (3%).[5]

Based on computed tomography (CT) and magnetic resonance imaging (MRI) images, LAA has been divided into four major categories; these are *chicken wing* (48%), *cactus* (30%), *windsock* (19%), and *cauliflower* (3%).[6] Among these, cauliflower variety has highest probability of developing stroke and chicken wing variety has least probability for developing stroke.[6]

Stroke prevention is a major goal of therapy in a patient with AF. It is done by either converting it to sinus rhythm or by drugs [oral anticoagulant (OAC)] or by closure of LAA (either surgically or by device).

DEVICES FOR LEFT ATRIAL APPENDAGE CLOSURE

Devices available for LAA closure (LAAC) are based on the principle that 90% of thrombus forms in appendage and hence its closure will obviate the need for anticoagulant and patient can be managed with antiplatelets. The devices for LAAC are basically of three types:[7]

1. *Plug*: These have a lobe or umbrella which closes the neck of the LAA [WATCHMAN™ (Boston Scientific, Marlborough, MA, USA), WaveCrest® (Biosense Webster, Diamond Bar, CA, USA)].
2. *Pacifier principle*: This device has a lobe or umbrella and an additional disc to seal the ostium of the LAA [Amplatzer™ Cardiac Plug (ACP), Amulet™ (both Abbott Vascular, Santa Clara, CA, USA) Ultraseal (Cardia, Inc, Eagan, MN, USA), LAmbre™ (Lifetech, Shenzhen, China)].
3. *Ligation*: LARIAT® (SentreHEART, Inc, Redwood City, CA, USA) e Sierra Ligation System [epicardial ligation device (Aegis Medical Innovations Inc, Vancouver, BC, Canada)]. Here, LAA is closed by use of snare to ligate the body of the LAA using an endocardial and epicardial approach.

Recently, a new device CLAAS (Conformal LAA Seal) device has been developed to overcome the limitation of conventional devices. It has a foam cup, with a *nitinol* endoskeleton with an expanded polytetrafluoroethylene cover. It comes in just two sizes for all LAA, regular for LAA ostium ≤25 mm and large for LAA ostium ≤32 mm. This obviates the need for very accurate sizings and simplifies the implant procedure and does not need very precise coaxial deployment (as needed in other devices), thereby reducing peridevice leaks. The device is attached by a tether mechanism (instead of rod mechanism) obviating the need for screwing mechanism thereby reducing device-related thrombus (DRT) formation and obviates the need for OAC post procedure.[8]

At present in India the available devices are Watchmen/FLX, Amulet/ACP, and LAmbre device. **Figures 1A to E** depict some of these devices. The Watchman/Watchman FLX and Amplatzer Amulet are Food and Drug Administration (FDA)-approved. Choice of device depends predominantly on operator preferences. Majority of LAA can be closed by any of the devices. There are no large randomized trials comparing various devices. In the AMULET IDE trial which compared Amulet with Watchman, Amulet device was found to be noninferior to Watchman device in terms of primary safety (composite of procedure-related complications, all-cause death, or major bleeding at 12 months) or primary efficacy endpoint [ischemic stroke or systemic embolism (ISSE) at 18 months].[9] The Amulet arm had slightly higher procedure-related complications mainly

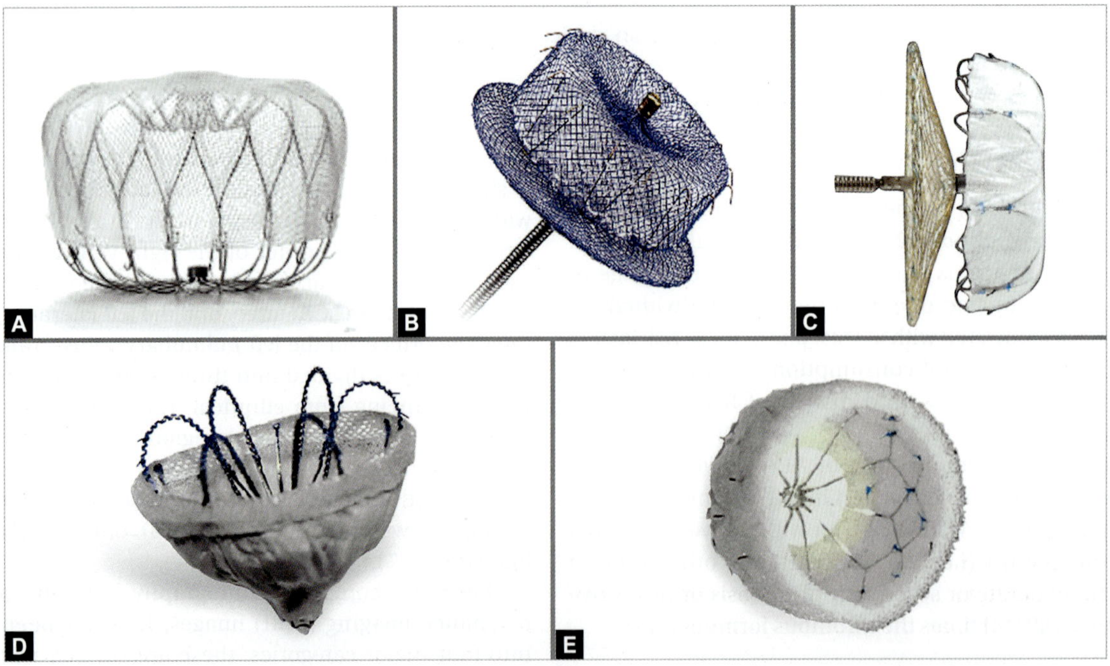

FIGS. 1A TO E: Devices for left atrial appendage occlusion (LAAO). (A) Watchman FLX; (B) Amulet; (C) LAmbre; (D) Wavecrest; (E) Conformal LAA Seal.

Source: Saw J, Holmes DR, Cavalcante JL, Freeman JV, Goldsweig AM, Kavinsky CJ, et al. SCAI/HRS Expert Consensus Statement on Transcatheter Left Atrial Appendage Closure. J Am Coll Cardiol Intv. 2023;16(11):1384-400.

related to higher device embolization and tamponade (4.5% vs. 2.5%). This happened in the initial learning phase of operator.[8] In the trial LAA occlusion (LAAO) was higher in Amulet arm compared to Watchman (98.9% vs. 96.8%; $p < 0.001$ for noninferiority and $p = 0.003$) for superiority. The SWISS APERO trial also compared Amulet with Watchman/FLX and found that by 45 days there was no difference in clinical outcome between the two, however, Amulet had higher procedure-related complication (9.0% vs. 2.7%; $p = 0.047$) driven mainly by higher bleeding complication in Amulet arm (7.2% vs. 1.8%) but peridevice leaks were higher in Watchman arm (27.5% vs. 13.5%; $p = 0.020$), however, none was >5 mm.[10] In another retrospective study comparing Watchman, ACP/Amulet, and LAmbre device at mean follow-up duration 28.3 ± 24.4 months found no difference between the three devices in terms of safety (bleeding risk or procedural complication) and efficacy (ischemic stroke prevention) with similar success rate in terms of implantation of device.[11] Wavecrest 2 trial comparing Wavecrest device with watchman device is ongoing.

EVIDENCE FOR LEFT ATRIAL APPENDAGE OCCLUSION

The concept of LAAO came in the year 1949 when Madden did resection of LAA in patient with rheumatic valvular disease and AF.[12] A meta-analysis of five trials of surgical exclusion of LAA had mixed result mainly due to incomplete exclusion of LAA.[13] In the most recent LAAOS III (Left Atrial Appendage Occlusion Study III) trial patients with AF who were undergoing cardiac surgery on cardiopulmonary bypass were randomized to undergo LAAO or no occlusion in 1:1 fashion.[13] Over a mean follow-up period of 3.8 years, the primary outcome (first occurrence of ischemic stroke) occurred more in nonocclusion group then occlusion group (7.0% vs. 4.8%; $p = 0.001$).[14]

In current scenario, still mainstay of stroke prevention in AF is by use of anticoagulation [warfarin or direct oral anticoagulant (DOAC), e.g., apixaban, rivaroxaban, dabigatran, endoxaban]. Based on current evidence DOACs are found superior to warfarin in stroke prevention and accordingly have been given class 1 indication for stroke prevention in all the guidelines in patient with NVAF.[15] Despite superior safety and efficacy of DOAC over warfarin still a lot of patients do not receive DOAC or receive it at inappropriate dose due to fear of higher bleeding risk, compliance issue (related to long-term use), need for dose adjustment in patient with renal/liver disease, advanced age, and higher cost. In a recent meta-analysis of 23 studies involving 162,474 AF patients almost 24% patient received off-label dose (under or overdose of DOAC).[15] In Asian countries, almost 32% patient were prescribed underdose.[16] This brings in the necessity of an alternate therapy in such patients where OACs are contraindicated or not used or have doubtful efficacy.

Left atrial appendage occlusion is a safe and effective alternative to use of OAC. Since first publication of use of LAAO in 2002 by Sievert et al. a lot of data has emerged establishing the safety and efficacy of the therapy.[17] Early trials with Watchman device, the PROTECT AF (WATCHMAN Left Atrial Appendage System for Embolic Protection in Patients With Atrial Fibrillation) and PREVAIL (Evaluation of the WATCHMAN LAA Closure Device in Patients With Atrial Fibrillation Versus Long Term Warfarin Therapy) trials, compared the device with warfarin. The 5-year data showed similar rate of all-stroke or systemic embolism (SE) between groups [hazard ratio (HR) 0.96; 95% confidence interval (CI) 0.60–1.54; $p = 0.87$].[18] However, incidence of hemorrhagic stroke was significantly lower in device arm (HR 0.20; 95% CI 0.07–0.56; $p = 0.0022$).[17] These data were further supported by result of EWOLUTION registry (from Europe) which analyzed real-world data on use of Watchman device. Over 2-year follow-up device arm conferred a 80% relative risk reduction (RRR) for the combined endpoint of ischemic stroke/transient ischemic attack (TIA)/SE compared to historical group.[18] Similarly, looking at bleeding risk the device group conferred a 46% RRR compared to historical group.[19] In this registry a subgroup analysis was done to assess long-term safety efficacy of device by analyzing patients who were switched to single antiplatelet or no therapy after 6 months of device implantation.[19] Of total 1,005 patients receiving Watchman, it was seen 766 patients were switched to either single-antiplatelet therapy (SAPT; $n = 639$) or no therapy ($n = 127$). Over follow-up these patients had ischemic stroke rate of 1.4 strokes/100 patient-years ($n = 14$ strokes) at 2 years. The expected historical rate for this cohort was 7 strokes/100 patient-years (conferring a 80% RRR). Similarly, the bleeding rate was 1.3 bleeds/100 patient-years ($n = 14$ major nonprocedural bleeds) at 2 years with an expected bleeding rate in historical cohort of 4.9 bleeds/100 patient-years (conferring a 73% RRR).[20] There are no large randomized trials comparing device with DOAC. In one study clinical outcomes among AF patients having LAAO after enrollment in the Amulet Observational Study ($n = 1,078$) versus propensity score-matched AF patients treated by DOACs were compared.[20] The annualized event rate was significantly lower for the LAAO cohort (14.5; 95% CI 12.8–16.5) than for the DOAC cohort (25.7; 95% CI 22.1–30.0) the risk of ischemic stroke was similar between both but risk of bleeding was significantly lower in LAAO group.[21] The only study comparing directly LAAO with DOAC was PRAGUE 17 (Left Atrial Appendage Closure vs. Novel Anticoagulation Agents in Atrial Fibrillation) trial.[22] In this study the primary outcome, i.e., composite of safety and efficacy of both strategies: (1) stroke (ischemic or hemorrhagic) or TIA; (2) SE; (3) clinically significant bleeding; (4) cardiovascular death; or (5) a significant periprocedural or device-related complications, was similar in both LAAO (10.99% per 100 patient-years) and DOAC group [13.42% per 100 patient-years; subdistribution hazard ratio (sHR) 0.84; 95% CI

0.53–1.31; $p = 0.44$].[22] The annualized all stroke/TIA rates were 2.60% with LAAC and 2.57% with DOACs (sHR 1.00; 95% CI 0.40–2.51) and the annualized bleeding [of International Society on Thrombosis and Hemostasis (ISTH) major/nonmajor clinically relevant bleeding (NMCRB)] risk was also similar in both group 5.50% with LAAC compared with 7.42% with DOAC (sHR 0.81; 95% CI 0.44–1.52) annualized cardiovascular mortality was also similar in both groups 3.18% with LAAC compared to 4.28% with DOACs (sHR 0.75; 95% CI 0.34–1.62) suggesting that LAAC was non-inferior to DOAC ($p = 0.004$).[22] Another subset of AF patient where LAAO can be considered is AF patient who cannot take OAC and those on hemodialysis where anticoagulant benefit is uncertain.

In the small ASAP trial, a four-center, nonrandomized study of Watchman LAAO implantation in 150 warfarin-ineligible patients with nonvalvular AF treated with postimplantation only aspirin and clopidogrel for 6 months and aspirin thereafter. After a median follow-up of 55.4 months (range 1.2–75.6 months), the annualized ISSE rate was 1.8% (95% CI 0.9–3.3%). This rate was 75% lower than the annual 7.3% rate expected for this cohort if they were receiving aspirin alone.[23] In a meta-analysis of 29 observational studies including 7,951 individuals with contraindication of OAC use of LAAO was associated with 74% RRR in stroke reduction.[24] In an Italian multicenter study on *dialysis* patients treated with LAAC at 2-year follow-up, no event was observed in patients who underwent the procedure compared to an incidence of 4% in oral anticoagulant therapy (OAT) patients and 8% in patients not taking OAT. Long-term hemorrhagic events are significantly less frequent in LAAO patients compared to group taking OAT, and the No-therapy cohort (10.6%, 19.5%, and 16.7% at 2 years, respectively).[25]

Despite the promise of therapy lack of large randomized studies have prevented the endorsement of therapy by all major guidelines. Most of the data have come from smaller studies or observational studies. Some of the issues still needing answer are being addressed by ongoing trials such as CHAMPION AF (comparing Watchman/FLX with DOAC in NVAF eligible for DOAC), OCCLUSION AF (comparing Amulet/Watchman with DOAC in NVAF eligible for DOAC), ASAP-TOO study (assessing Watchman device in patients with nonvalvular AF who are deemed ineligible for OAC), trial which is stopped prematurely, CLOSURE AF (assessing role of LAAO in high bleeding risk or contraindication to OAC), COMPARE LAAO (comparing LAAO with antiplatelet/or no therapy in NVAF with contraindication to OAC) STROKECLOSE [assessing role of LAAO in NVAF with intracranial hemorrhage (ICH) within 12 months], CLEARANCE (role of LAAO in NVAF with history of ICH), and WATCH-TAVR [comparing LAAO with medical therapy in patient NVAF patient undergoing transcatheter aortic valve replacement (TAVR)].[26]

PROCEDURAL CONSIDERATION

Transesophageal Echo

Imaging modality of choice is transesophageal 2D and/or 3D echo which is beneficial to assess other valvular pathology (especially mitral stenosis), obtaining LAA dimension (orifice, landing zone, depth, assessment of lobe, and any anatomical variability), and in thrombus/spontaneous echo contrast assessment.

For sizing, measurements taken in multiple planes and highest dimension are chosen as size. Usually, dimensions are measured in four different midesophageal views: (1) four-chamber view (0°–20°), (2) 45°–60° view at the level of the aortic valve, (3) in an apical two-chamber view at approximately 90°, and (4) long-axis view (120°–135°).

Figures 2A and B depict transesophageal echocardiography (TEE) and CT images in assessing orifice, landing zone, and depth of LAA for assessing suitability for LAAO, and choosing right size device.

Computed Tomography

At least a 64-slice CT with electrocardiogram (ECG) gating is needed for analyzing LAA. Unlike TEE, CT is noninvasive and does not need sedation. CT is comparable or may be better to TEE for providing detailed information on variable size and shape of the LAA and its surrounding structures, and for accurate device sizing, and for the evaluation of extracardiac structures. To identify thrombus, a delayed phase imaging is needed. TEE is considered superior to CT in assessing presence or absence of thrombus.

Patient should be properly hydrated to get adequate left atrial mean pressure. In order to get adequate images preferably give 500 mL saline before CT.

Computed tomography is good in identifying characteristic features which makes epicardial LAA difficult like pericarditis and pericardial adhesions from previous surgery or radiation, pericardial thickening, calcifications, effusions, pectus excavatum, a posteriorly rotated heart, and an LAA positioned behind the pulmonary trunk or adjacent to a coronary bypass graft.

For orifice measurement, cardiac phase at which the LAA ostium is the largest is chosen (ventricular end systolic phase, i.e., 30–40% R-R interval). It is measured in long-axis view as distance between LCX artery and the *coumadin* ridge. Landing zone varies depending on device used. For Watchman device landing zone is distance between LCX and another point 10–20 mm inside coumadin ridge. For ACP/Amulet device the landing zone is 10 mm and 12–15 mm inside of the LAA orifice, respectively, perpendicular to the walls of the LAA.

Generally, CT images are 0.7–5.2 mm larger than TEE, and 2–4 mm larger than fluoroscopy measurements. In the event of variation in TEE and CT measurements, the larger of the two measurements is used.

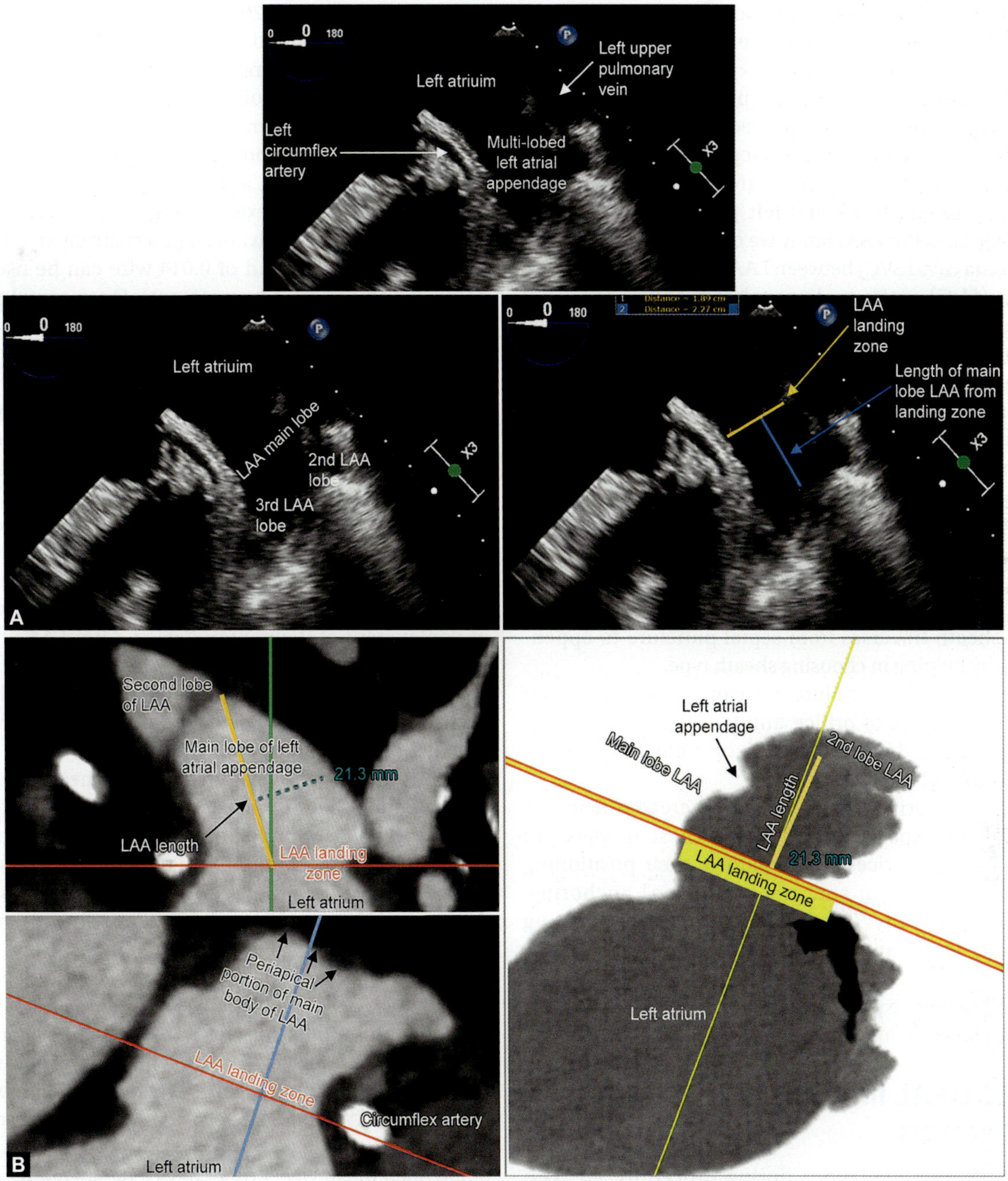

FIGS. 2A AND B: Transesophageal echocardiogram (TEE) and computed tomography angiography (CTA) images of the left atrial appendage (LAA) landing zone and definition of optimal LAA length measurements. (A) TEE images demonstrate the multilobed LAA that emanates from a larger body of the main lobe of the LAA. The landing zone is depicted by an yellow line measured at the level of the circumflex artery. The length of the main lobe of the LAA is depicted by the blue line measured from the centroid of the LAA landing zone (yellow line) to the center of the periapical region of the main body of the LAA. Care is taken to avoid measuring lengths to accessory LAA lobes as this may not accurately mimic the ability of current generation LAA occlusion (LAAO) devices to fully expand within very narrow portions of the distal lobes of the LAA. (B) CTA images demonstrate the multilobed LAA that emanates from a larger body of the main lobe of the LAA. The landing zone is depicted by a red line measured from the centroid of the LAA landing zone (demarcated by solid yellow line), to the center of the periapical region of the main body of the LAA. Care is taken to avoid measuring lengths to accessory LAA lobes as this may not accurately mimic the ability of current generation LAAO devices to fully expand within very narrow portions of the distal lobes of the LAA.

Source: Saw J, Holmes DR, Cavalcante JL, Freeman JV, Goldsweig AM, Kavinsky CJ, et al. SCAI/HRS Expert Consensus Statement on Transcatheter Left Atrial Appendage Closure J Am Coll Cardiol Intv. 2023;16(11):1384-400.

Computed tomography images identify any anatomical variation in LA (e.g., presence of left atrial diverticula or accessory appendage). They also identify surrounding structures clearly, and thereby predict any potential complication during or after procedure. Most important are identifying relation of left superior pulmonary vein (LSPV) and LAA, LCX artery and great cardiac vein are inferior to LAA, pulmonary trunk and left pulmonary artery are posteroinferior to the LAA; rarely we can see a persistent left superior vena cava (SVC) between LAA and LSPV, saphenous vein graft (SVG) grafts to diagonal and obtuse marginal (OM) are also close to LAA, and left phrenic nerve is located posterolateral to LAA close to tip or neck of LAA. If planning epicardial closure then relation of left internal mammary and inferior epigastric artery is also important to avoid injury.

Interatrial septum assessment is also very important. Good septal puncture is essential for success of LAAO. Ideal puncture site is posteroinferior margin. CT/TEE can give us idea about presence of atrial septal defect/patent foramen ovale (PFO), septal aneurysm, or any previous septal occluder or surgical patch which can make septal puncture challenging. It can give a virtual imaging of septal puncture and how sheath traverses from septal puncture to appendage thereby helping in choosing sheath type.

Similar to TAVR procedure, CT can also give coplanar view for assessment of orifice and landing zone thereby choosing proper device size and optimal fluoroscopy views for device placement.

Recently 3D printed models can be created from CT images by using specialized software. These models can help test various devices with regard to their positioning (depth of implantation and any angulation) anchoring, sealing, and stability. These models help in selecting appropriate device and its size, shorten procedure time, reduce contrast use, and reduce radiation dose. These have been found to reduce postprocedural complications such as peridevice leaks and incomplete closures.

PROCEDURAL IMAGING AND DEVICE DEPLOYMENT

Principle imaging modalities during procedure are TEE and fluoroscopy. Recently intracardiac echocardiography (ICE) is also used. Advantage of ICE is it avoids general anesthesia, no need for additional operator, and more precise images of LA/LAA and septum.

Under fluoroscopy and echo guidance femoral vein/femoral artery is accessed and pigtail is kept in aortic sinus to help in septal puncture. Then septal puncture catheter [Mullins sheath or transseptal puncture sheath from Abbott (SL-1) sheath] with Brockenbrough (BRK) needle advanced to left subclavian vein and pulled down with clockwise rotation. Under fluoroscopy and TEE guidance posteroinferior margin of septum is identified and puncture needle is advanced. TEE imaging (~45°) short-axis view at base is used for anteroposterior (AP) direction, and a bicaval view (90°–120°) with long-axis view used for identifying craniocaudal directions. Nowadays instead of manual advancement to puncture the septum we use cautery. Proximal end of puncture needle is touched with 15–20 W of radiofrequency (RF) catheter for 1 second. The septal puncture is positioned at the posteroinferior margin, stylet is then advanced, and cautery is connected to it; this punctures the septum exactly at the place; over this needle and septal catheter is advanced (alternatively stylet provided with needle or back end of 0.014 wire can be used for RF delivery and needle advancement). Once septal puncture done 5,000 unit heparin is given intravenously. Then pigtail is introduced to LA and advanced to LSPV or inside the appendage. Then angiogram is taken of LAA in RAO 30° cranial 20° and RAO 30° caudal 20° view. AP cranial view corresponds to TEE 0°, TEE 90° corresponds to RAO 30°, the RAO 30° cranial 20° view corresponds to TEE images at 45° and RAO 30° caudal 20° view corresponds to TEE 135° images. The RAO cranial view gives better idea of orifice of LAA and landing zone and is used in deploying the Amplatzer Amulet device or LAmbre device whereas RAO caudal view gives better image of body and lobes and helps in deployment of Watchman device. After LAA angiogram for Amplatzer Amulet or LAmbre device pigtail is kept in LSPV and then stiff wire (Amplatz extra stiff wire) is used to exchange pigtail to device delivery sheath. For watchman deployment pigtail is inserted deep into body of LAA and sheath is advanced over it to keep the sheath deep inside the appendage. For Amplatzer Amulet device after insertion of device sheath is pulled back to LA and by clockwise or counterclockwise rotation is aligned to LAA axis and then device is advanced by creating a bulb and pushing the device slightly out of sheath and then sheath along with bulb is advanced inside LAA till landing zone and then the distal disk is pushed for deployment. Distal disk should be kept in such a way that it is just inside the LCX, i.e., two-third inside and one-third outside LCX margin (for LAmbre the umbrella is deployed just beyond LCX. Then sheath is pulled back by holding the device and proximal disk is released. For Watchman device, the device is pushed to tip of sheath and then keeping the device still the sheath is pulled out to open the device. Proper device deployment is checked by various tests such as PASS/CLOSE or COST depending on device. For Watchman device typical strawberry form suggest proper sizing and then PASS criteria is used: Position (device just protruding into the LA), Anchoring (tug test), Size adequate (strawberry shape, at least 10% compression), and Sealing (<5 mm peridevice leak). For Amplatzer Amulet, CLOSE criteria is used: Circumflex two-third of device distal to LCX, Lobe should be compressed properly (10–20% compression) giving it a tire shape, Orientation of device should be aligned to axis of appendage, Separation between device lobe and disk should be proper, Elliptical—the outer disk should be concave or elliptical. For LAmbre, we use COST criteria: Circumflex artery, device umbrella should be beyond LCX artery, Open umbrella—

umbrella is fully open (nadir of claws is at same level as the radiopaque marker connecting umbrella and cover), Sealing is optimal (leak <3-5 mm), Tug test to test device stability.

Once these criteria are met the device is released. And sheath removed and femoral vein is closed by figure-of-eight suture or using *perclose* device.

POST PROCEDURE

Anticoagulant/Antiplatelet Regimen Post Procedure

For Watchman/Watchman FLX anticoagulant (DOAC/ warfarin) and aspirin (75–325 mg) are given for 6 weeks after procedure and a follow-up TEE at 45 days if shows minimal residual peridevice flow and no DRT then warfarin is stopped and dual antiplatelet with aspirin 81–150 mg + clopidogrel 75 mg daily given for 6 months and then single antiplatelet with aspirin 81–150 mg is continued. Trials are ongoing to assess if 6 months of antiplatelet is enough or need to continue beyond 6 months also.

For Amulet/LAmbre device dual antiplatelet with aspirin 75–325 mg + clopidogrel 75 mg daily is given for 1–6 months followed by single antiplatelet aspirin 81–150 mg daily is continued.

Any DRT should be treated with anticoagulation. And *repeat* imaging at 45- to 90-day intervals is performed to assess for resolution of thrombus so that anticoagulation can be stopped and antiplatelets continued.

Post Procedure Imaging

Immediately post procedure we look for delayed pericardial tamponade or device embolization.

Follow-up imaging is recommended at 6–24 weeks and again after 12 months. We do a TEE or CT to assess peridevice leak or DRT formation. For assessing significant peridevice leak (>5 mm) both CT and TEE are equally sensitive. However, CT is more accurate in DRT assessment. Once DRT is seen anticoagulation regimen is intensified as mentioned above. As per studies 2–4% of cases have DRT. Presence of DRT confers a higher risk of stroke. There are various factors for development of DRT which could be patient-related [e.g., poor left ventricular ejection fraction (LVEF), irregular antithrombotic treatment, smoking, spontaneous echo contrast, and history of thromboembolism] and implant-related (e.g., deep implantation, improper size, peridevice leak, or LAA patency). Any peridevice leak is seen in 15–30% of cases of ACP or Watchman cases; however, significant leak (>5 mm) is seen in 1–2% cases. Most of the time peridevice leak is due to *off-axis* deployment of device or improper size of device. Significant leak can be sealed by coils.

INDICATION FOR LEFT ATRIAL APPENDAGE CLOSURE

As per both European and American guidelines, it is a class IIb indication for use in patients ineligible for OAC.[27,28]

As per European Heart Rhythm Association (EHRA)/ European Association of Percutaneous Cardiovascular Interventions (EAPCI) consensus document subset of patients where LAAO can be suggested are:[7]

- Patients with NVAF eligible for OAC should be given OAC (preferably DOAC). However, in these subsets if there is a patient who despite explaining the advantage of OAC is unwilling for any form of anticoagulant should be offered LAAO instead of no anticoagulant.
- In those having contraindication for anticoagulant (e.g., ICH/intraspinal hemorrhage, either due to diffuse amyloid angiopathy or untreatable vascular malformation) severe gastrointestinal (e.g., diffuse angiodysplasia) pulmonary or urogenital source of bleeding that cannot be corrected or those with severe side effects under vitamin K antagonists and/or contraindication for NOAC.
- Those with higher major bleeding risk on long-term anticoagulation (e.g., those on hemodialysis, post-OAC intracranial or major bleed).
- In those noncompliant to OAC (here every effort should be made to improve compliance to OAC and if it fails LAAO can be offered after detailed discussion of risk and benefit and efficacy), caution is exercised and LAAO should not be offered as a simple, safe, and equally effective alternate to OAC in these subsets.
- In select cases with high recurrent stroke despite on OAC with malignant LAA morphology instead of intensifying antithrombotic regimen LAAO can be offered.

CONCLUSION

Left atrial appendage occlusion is a promising therapy for stroke prevention in AF who are ineligible for OAC. Proper procedural planning using TEE/CT or ICE helps in selecting appropriate device and can identify as well as prevent complications. Operator experience is very important to avoid periprocedural complications and improve success. Results of various ongoing studies will clarify a lot of unsolved issues which can help in wider acceptance of therapy.

ONLINE REFERENCES

Please scan the QR code provided at the end of the table of contents for References of this chapter.

SECTION 21

Endovascular and Peripheral

CHAPTER 198

Endovascular Treatment of Abdominal Aortic Aneurysm with Hostile Neck Anatomy

Manoj Kumar Agarwala, Mohammed Abdul Azeez Asad

ABSTRACT

Endovascular aneurysm repair (EVAR) of abdominal aortic aneurysms (AAAs) has emerged as potentially the first choice of management of these lesions with widespread acceptability among physicians as well as patients alike, due to its minimally invasive nature with lesser rates of perioperative morbidity and mortality. However, as many as one-fourth of patients with AAA, present with a challenging anatomy ranging from short and angulated neck to different shapes and characteristics. This hostile neck anatomy (HNA) has its own technical difficulties and can be overcome with meticulous planning and adaptation of special modified strategies. In order to prevent future endoleaks and other complications that can lead to failure of the endovascular graft and potentially aneurysmal enlargement, rupture, and death, these special techniques utilized may be hybrid (using mini or total laparotomy or laparoscopy) or totally percutaneous, depending on the patient anatomy as well as expertise and equipment available.

Keywords: Abdominal aortic aneurysm, endovascular aneurysm repair, hostile neck.

INTRODUCTION

Abdominal aortic aneurysm (AAA) is most commonly defined as a maximum abdominal aortic diameter ≥3.0 cm, which typically is >2 standard deviations over the mean diameter among men. A smaller diameter threshold may be considered in women and some Asian populations. In other definitions, it has been defined as maximum diameter of abdominal aorta that is ≥50% greater than that of suprarenal diameter.[1] The estimated prevalence of AAA is about 1.7% in men over 65 years of age. This goes up to 3.3% in men between ages of 65 and 74 years.[2,3]

Endovascular aneurysm repair (EVAR) has emerged as potentially the first choice of management of these lesions. It has gained widespread acceptability among physicians as well as patients alike, being minimally invasive with lesser rates of perioperative morbidity and mortality.[4] However, endovascular repair becomes technically difficult and challenging in certain anatomical subsets. The most important segment that decides feasibility of EVAR is the neck of the aneurysm, which is the aortic segment between the lowest renal artery and the aneurysmal sac. This is the portion that works as the landing zone during EVAR.

The characteristics of the aneurysmal neck like its length, breadth, shape, and its angle with the main aneurysmal sac are important determinants of a successful implantation of a stent graft.[5] A difficult or hostile neck can predispose the patient to future complications ranging from type 1 endoleak and loss of endograft fixation or seal to device migration, sac enlargement, and, eventually, aneurysm rupture and death.[6] Other factors seen to have worse outcomes are suprarenal angulation and presence of calcification, or thrombus in the neck lumen.[7]

Also, to be noted is the fact that maximum neck diameters and minimum neck lengths vary according to different manufacturers as per their instructions for use (IFU) for the various stent graft models. The newer grafts like Endurant or Ovation model can be accommodated in neck lengths between 10 and 15 mm. The suprarenal as well as infrarenal angulation is also different as per IFU for these models. For example, Anaconda endovascular graft from Vascutek can be accommodated with neck angulations up to 90°, unlike most other grafts which are best suited for angles up to 60°.

WHAT IS HOSTILE NECK?

Different definitions have been used to identify difficult or hostile neck. The most commonly used criteria for hostile neck anatomy (HNA) for AAAs were reported by Stather et al. in a 2013 review and meta-analysis of patient outcomes undergoing EVAR in patients who have HNA compared with those with favorable neck anatomy. Patients whose anatomy met one or more criteria of neck length <15 mm, neck diameter >28 mm, and angulation >60° had increased 30-day mortality following EVAR as well as 30-day migration rate and decreased technical success rates when all three criteria were met.[8]

However, the presence of short and angulated aneurysmal neck also happens to be a major risk factor for perioperative mortality after open surgical correction of AAAs as well as renal impairment in the long-term. Hence, there have been many modifications to traditional EVAR to improve the outcomes in such patients with a short aneurysmal neck.[6]

Types of Hostile Neck Anatomy

- *Short neck*: The distance between the lowest renal artery and the aneurysm sac proper is <15 mm.
- *Conical neck*: Also referred to as reverse tapered, this is the most frequently encountered hostile neck.[5]
- *Angulated neck*: Aortic neck angulation is defined as the angle between the axes of the proximal infrarenal aorta and the longitudinal axis of the aneurysm. It is classified as: mildly angulated <40°, moderately angulated <60°, and severely angulated as >60°.[9]
- *Reverse conical neck*: Also referred to as tapered neck, this has a broader proximal segment and narrows down near the actual sac.
- *Barrel-shaped neck*: There is an additional bulge involving the renal arteries.
- *Dumbbell or double barrel-shaped neck*: This has a double bulge involving the renal arteries along with a constriction before the aneurysmal sac **(Figs. 1A to F)**.

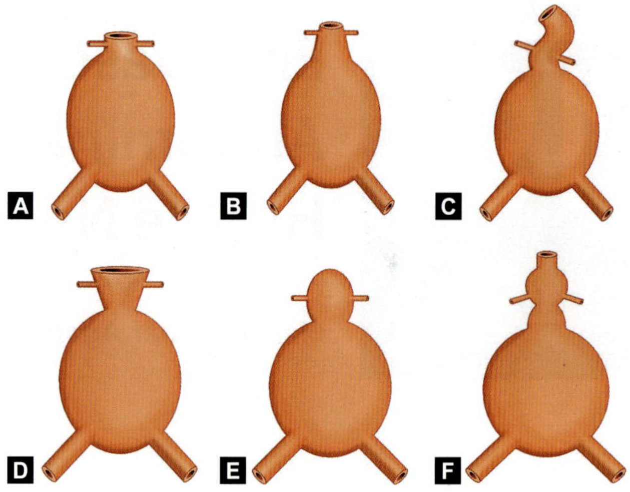

FIGS. 1A TO F: Different shapes of hostile necks. (A) Short neck; (B) Conical/reverse tapered; (C) Angulated; (D) Tapered or reverse conical; (E) Barrel-shaped; (F) dumbbell or double barrel-shaped.[5]

OVERCOMING THE HOSTILE NECK

The presence of HNA can be overcome using modified strategies for EVAR. Some of these use hybrid approach with either open or laparoscopic modification. Others depend on total endovascular techniques.

Hybrid Techniques

- *Renal debranching using extra-anatomic bypass*: The endograft is percutaneously placed more proximally, covering both the renal arteries. Extra-anatomic bypass is provided by a laparotomy with a hepatorenal bypass for the right renal artery and splenorenal bypass for the left renal artery.[10] This revascularization procedure is typically staged before the endovascular procedure to avoid renal ischemia. Iliorenal grafts can also be done in a similar fashion if the anatomy is suitable.[6]
- *VORTEC (Viabahn Open Revascularization Technique)*: This hybrid procedure again utilizes a laparotomy. The debranching is achieved with the help of covered stents or stent grafts, which are placed using Seldinger technique into the target branch artery. The proximal portion of the graft that remains outside the branch artery is directly sutured to the proximal portion of the native artery as seen in **Figures 2A to I**.[11] Utilizing the stent graft preserves the target vessels, which may be difficult to dissect surgically and maybe covered in scar tissue.[6]
- *Proximal aortic neck banding*: This hybrid procedure utilizes a mini-laparotomy or laparoscopic techniques. A part of the infrarenal aorta, including a small proximal portion of the aneurysmal sac is reinforced using a strip of Dacron felt. Within this banded proximal aortic neck, endograft is placed and its proximal end is anchored, thus preserving the target branches.[6,12]

Endovascular Techniques

- *Chimney or snorkel technique*: This total endovascular technique is simpler than dedicated, but more expensive than, custom-made fenestrated and branched devices. This has become a well-established strategy in patients with hostile neck, particularly in emergency situations as it can be made readily "off the shelf".[5,12] In this technique, a covered stent is positioned across the target renal or visceral artery, with its distal end in the target branch and its proximal part within the proximal aortic segment,

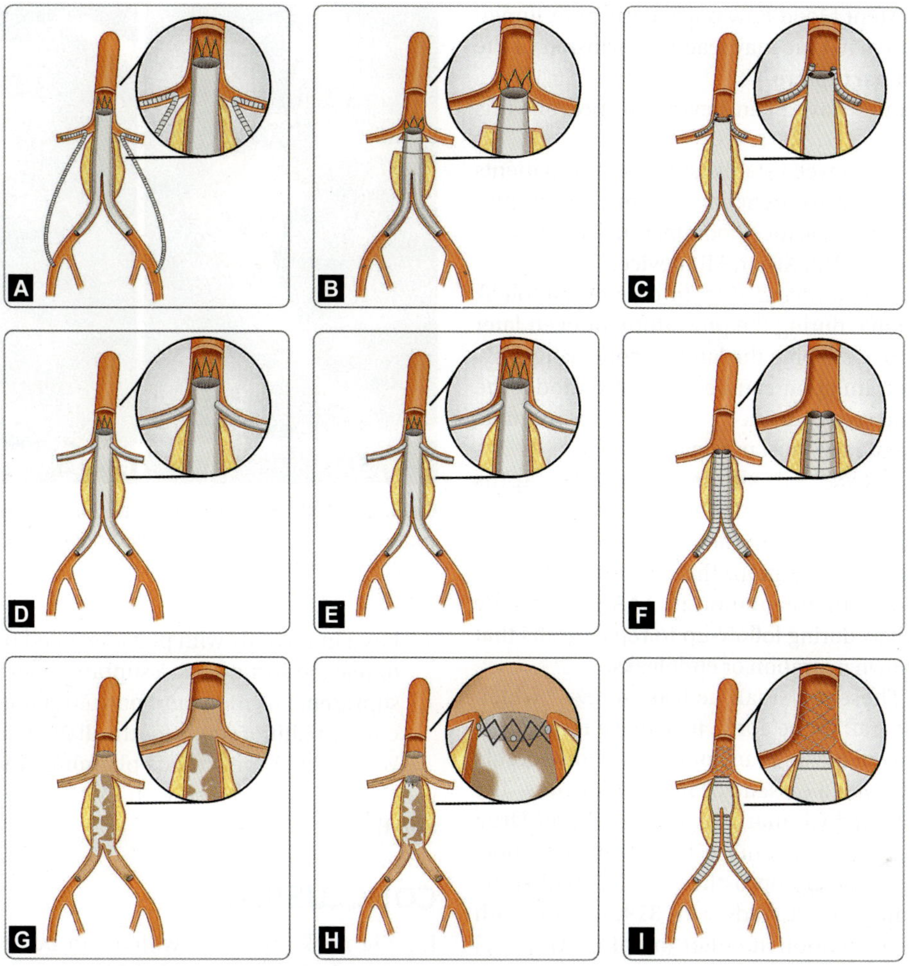

FIGS. 2A TO I: Abdominal aortic aneurysm (AAA) repair techniques for hostile proximal neck. (A) Viabahn Open Revascularization Technique (VORTEC); (B) Neck banding; (C) Chimney; (D) Fenestrated; (E) Branched; (F) Nellix; (G) Multilayer; (H) Endostapling; (I) Ovation.[6]

parallel to the aorta. EVAR is then performed positioning the proximal end of the main body of the endograft alongside the branch stent. This branch stent creates a dual channel flow, perfusing the target organ whilst acting as a "chimney" or "snorkel".[13,14]

- *Fenestrated or branched grafts*: Fenestrated EVAR or FEVAR has become the gold standard in patients with short-necked or juxtarenal aneurysms.[15] These are custom-made stent grafts with complete or partial holes or prefabricated branches for the visceral arteries within the main device. Once the main body of the endograft is deployed, these are accessed percutaneously. A covered stent, which is balloon-expandable, is positioned across the fenestration and flared against the internal aspect of the stent graft to provide a complete seal of the branch vessel.[6]
- *Dedicated devices*: These special dedicated devices treat complex AAAs using a totally different model.

The NELLIX System (Endologix, Irvine, CA) consists of two balloon-expandable endoframes. These are surrounded by polymer-filled endobags. The endobags fill up and obliterate the aneurysm sac, thereby maintaining endograft position. It is intended for use in both favorable and hostile anatomy, including short neck length <10 mm and severely angulated neck >60°.[16]

Multilayer system: The Cardiatis (Isnes, Belgium) is a 3D multilayer braided stent that is constructed in multiple interlocking layers; this arrangement apparently decreases the transgraft flow by up to 90%, reducing sac pressure and risk of rupture, but also maintains flow in branches.[17]

ENDOLEAK: PREVENTION AND TREATMENT

One of the most frequently encountered complications of EVAR is type 1a endoleak, with an overall incidence reported to be about 5.4%, increasing to 9.2% in AAA with hostile neck as reported in the ANCHOR (Aneurysm Treatment Using the Heli-FX Aortic Securement System Global Registry) study.[9,18] Type 1a endoleak is a leaking channel between the aortic wall and the graft fabric near the proximal attachment site of the graft. This persistent blood flow outside the graft lumen but within the aneurysmal sac may lead to expansion of the aneurysm and eventual rupture.[9]

Several techniques have been devised to prevent this complication.

- Fenestrated EVAR, is well established option in patients with short-necked or juxtarenal aneurysms.[15] Examples are Zenith (Cook Medical Inc, Bloomington, IN), Jotec, or Anaconda (Terumo, Ann Arbor, MI) devices.
- *Low-pressure balloon remodeling*: In case an endoleak is detected on table during the procedure, or even later during follow-up, reshaping the landing zone using low-pressure balloon inflation can be done to remodel the landing zone and create an effective seal. This is a simple and effective method in most patients.[5]
- *Endostapling systems*, initially introduced by Aptus Endosystems, have helical staples that mimic hand sutures to enhance sealing at the proximal attachment site as well as prevent migration. This can be done during the initial endograft implantation in AAA with hostile anatomy as well as during follow-up to repair grafts that have already shown migration or endoleaks.
- *EndoAnchors*: These are small helical "screws" which secure the endograft to the aorta, to achieve transmural fixation. The system includes an applicator and steerable sheath (16/18 F) with a cassette of 10 EndoAnchors. The system has obtained CE marking and Food and Drug Administration approval and is indicated for Cook, Gore, and Medtronic endoprostheses. ANCHOR study was a multicenter cohort study with 319 patients with EndoAnchor implantation at either initial EVAR (76%) or during follow-up for neck complications (24%). Implantation of EndoAnchors was technically successful in 98% of patients. Freedom from type 1a endoleak at 1 year was seen in 95% of patients in the primary group and 77% in the revision group. There were no surgical conversions, aneurysm-related deaths, or aneurysm ruptures during follow-up.[7,19,20]
- *Ovation*: The Ovation Abdominal Stent Graft System (TriVascular Inc Santa Rosa, CA) is a dedicated device that has a main body with polymer-filled rings on its top used to seal the aortic neck, a suprarenal stent with anchors for suprarenal fixation, and polytetrafluoroethylene (PTFE)-covered nitinol stents for the iliac vessels.[6]

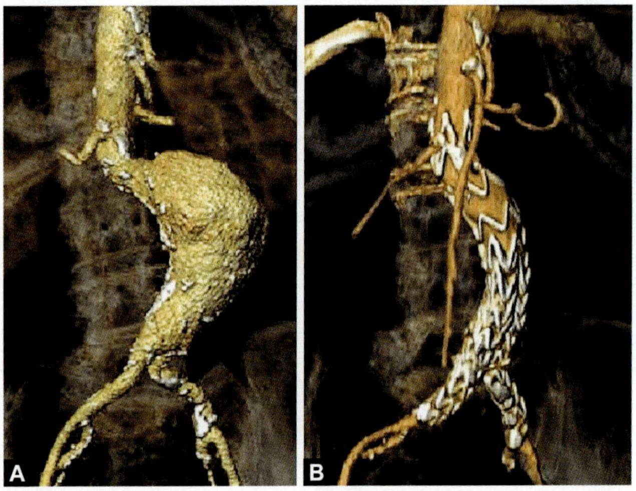

FIGS. 3A AND B: Example of abdominal aortic aneurysm with short as well as severely angulated neck treated with endovascular repair with stent graft.

With proper meticulous planning, AAAs with seemingly very HNA can be treated with EVAR as shown in **Figures 3A and B**.

CONCLUSION

Hostile neck anatomy, which can be seen in as many as one-fourth of patients with AAA, present unique difficulties and challenges to repair using standard EVAR techniques. Special techniques and strategies have been developed to overcome these challenges. One area of major focus in their management should be prevention and treatment of endoleaks, particularly type 1a endoleaks. With proper planning and execution, successful EVAR can be performed in these challenging subsets of patients in order to improve patient outcomes.

ONLINE REFERENCES

Please scan the QR code provided at the end of the table of contents for References of this chapter.

CHAPTER

199 Renal Artery Stenosis: When and How to Stent?

NN Khanna, Swati Singh, Sushant Mishra

ABSTRACT

Renal artery stenosis is one of the common causes of secondary hypertension and can lead to refractory and resistant hypertension while on maximally tolerated medical therapy, progressive decline in renal function, and cardiac destabilization syndromes such as flash pulmonary edema. Even though randomized trials so far have failed to show any benefit of revascularization over optimal medical therapy, these trials are now being questioned as there are several unaddressed biases in inclusion criteria of these studies and they have failed to include the subset of patient who would have derived maximum benefit from revascularization. The authors address two basic questions pertaining to renal artery revascularization, namely when and how to stent renal arteries. The authors also review the existing guidelines and various techniques to optimize patient selection, avoid complications, and provide a durable outcome.

Keywords: Renal artery stenting, renal artery stenosis, renovascular hypertension.

INTRODUCTION

Renal artery stenosis (RAS) is a spectrum of disease that involves, but is not limited to, renal vasculature. Renovascular hypertension is one of its multiple manifestations; other major ones being progressive decline of renal function, flash pulmonary edema, cerebrovascular accident (CVA), recurrent congestive heart failure, and aortic and acute coronary syndromes. Early observational studies showed promising results of renal artery revascularization, which led to initial extensive efforts by surgeons/interventionists to identify the candidates for revascularization; however, randomized trials comparing percutaneous renal artery stenting versus guideline-directed medical therapy (GDMT) showed no difference in the final outcome, which later resulted in relative "inertia" in renal artery intervention.[1-4] However, lately after the significant flaws in design of these trials are being apparent, there is recent reemergence in interest in this intervention.[5,6] In this chapter, we will attempt to simplify this controversial topic and try to address two basic questions pertaining to renal artery stenting, namely "when" and "how" to revascularize renal arteries.

DEFINITIONS

Renovascular hypertension: It represents one manifestation of a spectrum of clinical syndromes associated with renovascular disease.[7] Two most common causes of same being atherosclerotic renovascular disease (ARVD) and fibromuscular dysplasia (FMD). It is defined as a type of secondary hypertension resulting from occlusion in renal arteries.

Ischemic nephropathy: It can be understood as end stage, likely irreversible, manifestation of renovascular hypertension, resulting in loss of renal mass, extensive fibrosis, and loss of glomerular filtration rate (GFR). It is important to understand the difference between the abovementioned two definitions in order to answer our first question, i.e., "when" to revascularize renal arteries, as latter is the situation where revascularization would offer no benefit and in the former we need to selectively choose the subset which would benefit the most from revascularization.

EPIDEMIOLOGY

The prevalence of renovascular hypertension, as a cause of secondary hypertension, ranges from 0.1 to 5% in various studies.[8-10] There is a correlation between increasing severity of hypertension and prevalence of ARVD. It is noted in up to one-fourth (14–24%) of patients with resistant hypertension undergoing coronary angiography for suspected coronary atherosclerosis.[11-13] The prevalence of atherosclerotic RAS (ARAS) is somewhat higher (30–40%) in patients with peripheral arterial disease and abdominal aortic aneurysm.[14,15] ARAS is found to be more common in people with atherosclerosis in any other vascular bed.[16]

Overall, RAS is predominantly due to atherosclerosis (>90%) in adult population, whereas FMD is more common in young females.[17] FMD is a congenital condition, with female preponderance, mostly nonatherosclerotic, noninflammatory, with fibroplasia in multiple arteries, commonly carotid, femoral, and renal.[18] FMD commonly involves mid-to-distal portions of renal arteries and is described angiographically as "string of pearls" because of its beaded appearance. FMD can be flow limiting, frequently leading to hypertension, and can be multifocal (commonly) or focal; the latter shows promising results with balloon (only) angioplasty. One-third of multifocal FMD also responds well to intervention.[19]

Other rarer causes of renovascular hypertension include, but are not limited to, renal artery dissection (spontaneous/iatrogenic), renal artery jailing by stent grafts during aortic interventions, renal artery aneurysm, dissection, extravascular compression, mid-aortic coarctation, allograft inflow obstruction, and anatomic variants.

DIAGNOSIS

Noninvasive

1. *Renal artery Doppler*: It is initial investigation of choice. It is commonly offered to all young patients who present with hypertension as a part of workup for etiology.

Diagnostic Criteria

- Peak systolic velocity (PSV) of >200 cm/s (95% sensitivity and 90% specificity for >50% stenosis)
- A ratio of renal artery PSV to the PSV of the aorta of >3.5 (92% sensitivity for >60% diameter stenosis)[20,21]

Disadvantages: Ultrasound examination is operator dependent and bowel gas or bulky body habitus may obscure imaging.

2. *Computed tomography angiography (CTA) and magnetic resonance angiography (MRA)*: CT and MR imaging can be advised when ultrasonography (USG) is unable to confirm the presence/severity of RAS. The sensitivity of CTA is 90–100% and specificity 97% for stenosis > 50%. The sensitivity of MRA is 92–97%, with specificity of 73–93%.[21]

Disadvantages: Higher cost, lesser availability of these tests, and detrimental effect of contrast agents used on overall renal function.

3. *Split renal function*: It is a form of nuclear study using 99mTc diethylenetriaminepentaacetic acid which assesses the impact of hemodynamically significant unilateral RAS on overall renal function.

Invasive Stenosis Assessment

Angiographic ARAS > 70% diameter stenosis is severe or significant and diameter stenosis of 50–70% is considered moderate stenosis. For the latter subset, confirmation of the hemodynamic severity of the RAS is recommended prior to stenting.[20] A resting or hyperemic translesional systolic gradient of 20 mm Hg, a resting or hyperemic mean translesional gradient of 10 mm Hg, or a renal fractional flow reserve (RFFR) 0.8 will confirm hemodynamically significant ARAS.

Disadvantages: Bleeding risk, radiation exposure, and contrast-induced nephropathy (CIN).

Now addressing the first basic question of this chapter, i.e., when to revascularize/stent a RAS. Based on the recommendations by the American Heart Association (AHA)/American College of Cardiology (ACC) **(Table 1)**, subset of patients who would benefit the most from revascularization and those who would not has been identified and summarized as given in **Boxes 1 and 2**.

PATIENT POPULATION/CHARACTERISTICS THAT WARRANT REVASCULARIZATION

- *Congestive heart failure*: The classical "flash pulmonary edema" due to noncardiac cause is often described in setting of ARAS and is a strong indication for revascularization. There are several case series to support revascularization in such patients.[22,23] As high as 75% of all such patients showed no further episodes after revascularization.[23,24] Recurrent congestive heart failure and pulmonary edema are considered indications of stenting on the basis of expert opinion and observational studies.[24]
- *Refractory hypertension*: It is defined as either hypertension not controlled by three or more different classes of drugs including a diuretic or that controlled by four or more classes of antihypertensives. Secondary hypertension is more common in this subset. 14–23% of such cases can be attributed to ARAS.[11,12] Although controlled trials failed to show any benefit of renal artery

TABLE 1: Current American Heart Association/American College of Cardiology guidelines for renal artery stenting.

Clinical scenario	Recommendations
Cardiac destabilization syndrome (flash pulmonary edema and acute coronary syndrome) with either severe RAS or moderate RAS with translesional gradient ≥ 10 mm Hg	Class I, level of evidence: B Class IIa, Level of evidence: B (unstable angina)
Class IV CKD patient with bilateral moderate RAS with resting translesional gradient ≥ 10 mm Hg with pole-to-pole length of kidney 7 cm	Class IIa, level of evidence: B
CKD stage IV patients with bilateral severe RAS or severe unilateral RAS in solitary kidney	Class IIb, level of evidence: B
Resistant hypertension with bilateral RAS or solitary severe RAS	Class IIa, level of evidence: B
Recurrent CHF with unilateral moderate RAS with translesional gradient ≥ 10 mm Hg	Class I, level of evidence: B
Resistant hypertension with unilateral severe RAS	Class IIa, level of evidence: B
Asymptomatic patient with unilateral or bilateral or solitary kidney with hemodynamically significant RAS	Class IIb, level of evidence: C

(CHF: congestive heart failure; CKD: chronic kidney disease; RAS: renal artery stenosis)

BOX 1 Patients likely to benefit.

Hemodynamically significant RAS with:
- Sudden flash pulmonary edema
- Recurrent CHF
- Refractory ACS
- Refractory hypertension who fail GDMT
- Progressive renal disease (AKI/CKD) due to bilateral or unilateral ARAS
- Fibromuscular dysplasia with hypertension (balloon angioplasty only)
- Bilateral renal artery stenosis with progressive loss of renal functional mass
- Single native kidney renal artery stenosis
- Renal allograft—transplant renal artery stenosis
- Aortic disease with renovascular protection as a part of endovascular repair
- Pediatric mid-aortic syndromes
- Radiation-induced renovascular disease with clinical syndromes

(ACS: acute coronary syndrome; AKI: acute kidney injury; ARAS: atherosclerotic renal artery stenosis; CHF: congestive heart failure; CKD: chronic kidney disease; GDMT: guideline-directed medical therapy)

BOX 2 Patients not likely to benefit.

- Asymptomatic patients
- Causality of symptoms not established (RAS is an innocent bystander)
- Hypertensives who are not on maximally tolerated medical therapy
- CKD with small kidneys (pole-to-pole size < 7 mm)
- Hemodialysis > 3 months

(CKD: chronic kidney disease; RAS: renal artery stenosis)

stenting in such cases, the trials had their own inherent flaws in their design. Older retrospective studies did favor revascularization in such cases.[25]

- *Progressive decline in kidney function*: Out of all patients requiring initiation of hemodialysis, 11–22% can be attributed to bilateral ARAS[26] and a subset of such patients have shown favorable recovery of renal function after undergoing revascularization.[26,27] When measured kidney volume is more than that expected on the basis of GFR, kidney may be in the state of "hibernation" which can be understood as a state similar to hibernating myocardium in coronary artery diseases and revascularization in such cases is often fruitful.
- *FMD*: FMD-related hypertension should be suspected especially in young females (<50 years) with early-onset, accelerated hypertension. Prevalence of FMD in such population is as high as 7.5%.[28] Whenever FMD-related hypertension is suspected, most such cases require invasive hemodynamic assessment to determine the need for revascularization. Balloon angioplasty without stenting is treatment of choice in such cases.[29] Such treatment is more effective in unifocal (vs. multifocal) disease. Even though no randomized controlled trial (RCT) is available to support this form of treatment, observational studies have shown promising results in terms of cure of/improvement in control of hypertension.[30]

Characteristics Suggesting Clinical Benefit from Revascularization

- *Nonproteinuric hypertension with unilateral RAS*: Significant proteinuria indicates irreversible renal injury. Post-hoc analysis of the CORAL (Cardiovascular Outcomes for Renal Atherosclerotic Lesions) trial supports the hypothesis that revascularization offered better outcome in the presence of less proteinuria (measured as urine albumin to creatinine ratio).[31]
- *New-onset hypertension*: Shorter duration of hypertension is more likely to be cured by revascularization. A duration of hypertension <1 year was associated with a nearly

twofold higher rate of cure or improvement compared with failure or death.[32]

- *Renin activation*: Although controversial, early studies showed significant reduction in blood pressure (BP) when plasma/ipsilateral renal vein renin activity study revealed a "lateralization," i.e., stenotic-contralateral ratio 1.55–1.80.[33,34]

ANALYSIS OF EXISTING EVIDENCE

As discussed earlier, several prospective randomized trials, particularly those limited to ARVD, have not shown any significant benefit after successful revascularization. So, an updated systematic review published by the Agency for Health Care Research and Quality stated that the "strength of evidence" for selecting modalities for therapy is low.[6] However, unfortunately, all these trials have considerable limitations.[35-37]

Observational/Nonrandomized Trials

- *The ASPIRE-2 (Evaluation of the Safety and Effectiveness of Renal Artery Stenting After Unsuccessful Balloon Angioplasty)*: A balloon-expandable stent was used if angioplasty failed to achieve <50% stenosis in patients with aorto-ostial ARAS, causing hypertension. Systolic BP decreased from 168 ± 25 mm Hg to 149 ± 25 mm Hg and diastolic BP decreased from 82 ± 13 mm Hg to 77 ± 12 mm Hg at 24 months ($p < 0.001$).[38]
- *The HERCULES (Herculink Elite Renal Stent to Treat Renal Artery Stenosis) trial*: It showed a significant reduction in SBP in patients with significant ARAS and uncontrolled hypertension who underwent renal artery stenting.[39]

Randomized Controlled Trials

There are four major RCTs related to revascularization in RAS:

1. *The DRASTIC (Dutch Renal Artery Stenosis) study*: It assigned 106 patients with ARVD with normal or mildly impaired renal function to revascularization via balloon angioplasty or medical therapy alone. The study revealed no difference in the primary outcome of SBP control at 12 months. However, 44% of the patients from the medical therapy group crossed over to the intervention group.[40]

- *The STAR (Stent Placement for Atherosclerotic Stenosis of Renal Artery)*:[1] 140 patients with normal or impaired renal function and stable hypertension were assigned into medical therapy versus intervention which included balloon angioplasty with stenting. Patients were recruited on the basis of only 50% stenosis. After 2 years of follow-up, the trial failed to show any difference between intervention and medical therapy alone in the primary outcome. However, there were many limitations of this trial worth mentioning. One-third of patients in the medical therapy group and 44% in the stent group had arterial occlusion to a small kidney or shrunken kidney, although renal size < 8 cm was an exclusion. Half the patients were on fewer than three medications for hypertension.
- *The ASTRAL (Angioplasty and Stenting for Renal Artery Lesions)*:[2] It included 806 patients. 60% of the patients had stenosis of >70%. The trial showed no difference in the outcomes of renal function decline, renal events, cardiovascular events, or death. The trial failed to answer the question of intervention in severe ARVD. 40% of the patients in this trial did not meet the entry criteria for severe RAS on angiography.
- *The CORAL trial*:[3] It included 931 patients to compare revascularization versus optimized therapy with blockade of the renin-angiotensin-aldosterone system for RAS with high BP, chronic kidney disease (CKD), or both. The trials showed no differences in individual primary outcomes, major cardiovascular events, kidney events (progressive CKD, the provision of renal replacement therapy, or death attributable to kidney disease), or a composite outcome. The subjects of this trial had a mean RAS by computer-assisted angiography of 67% with <50% having severe disease. Because the patients with hemodynamic lesion severity of moderate (50–70% diameter stenosis) lesions was not hemodynamically confirmed, it is very likely that many patients with nonobstructive ARAS were enrolled in the trial.[3] Hypertension was not required, and entry SBP was 150 mm Hg on two antihypertensive agents with >25% already at goal. The trial did not confer a significant benefit with respect to prevention of clinical events. Later, a post-hoc analysis of the CORAL data after 5 years of follow-up did show that individuals with minimal proteinuria experienced improved event-free survival from the composite end point cardiovascular death, progressive renal insufficiency, and overall survival at 5 years.[41]

In summary **(Table 2)**, these trials indicate that most patients with RAS would not benefit from revascularization when compared head-to-head with medical therapy alone. However, these studies had many unaddressed biases. Most of these trials excluded the patients with clinical conditions and also did not clarify criteria for hemodynamically severe renal artery occlusive disease who may benefit the most from revascularization. This bias in election may have prevented the enrollment of the most eligible patients who would have benefitted from revascularization, e.g., those with "flash" pulmonary edema or refractory hypertension or those with very severe stenosis and uncontrolled BP. **Table 3** summarizes major limitations of these trials.

Having addressed the question of appropriate patient selection, we now move to our second question, i.e., how to revascularize renal arteries. We will be discussing the procedural details as well as potential complications and ways to minimize them.

TABLE 2: Comparison of various trials of renal artery intervention.

Trials	STAR	ASTRAL	CORAL
Year	2009	2009	2014
Number of patients	140	806	947
Inclusion criteria	• eGFR < 80 • Ostial ARAS > 50% (CTA, MRA, and DSA) • Controlled BP < 140/90 mm Hg	• Atherosclerotic renal artery disease in >1 renal artery amenable to revascularization • Clinician unsure if revascularization would provide clear benefit	• Severe RAS (angiographically >60% but <100%) • Hypertension with systolic BP ≥ 155 mm Hg on ≥2 agents or CKD with eGFR < 60 mL/min/1.73 m^2
Exclusion criteria	• Renal size < 8 cm • Renal artery < 4 mm • eGFR < 15 • T2DM with proteinuria > 3 g/day • Malignant hypertension	• Disease needing surgical revascularization • High likelihood of requiring revascularization in next 6 months • Nonatheromatous disease • Prior renal artery revascularization	• FMD • CKD not due to ischemic nephropathy • Serum creatinine > 4 • Kidney size < 7 cm • Lesions that could not be treated with one stent
Intervention	PTRA with stenting with GDMT versus GDMT alone	PTRA with or without stenting with GDMT versus GDMT alone	PTRA with stenting with GDMT versus GDMT alone
Primary endpoint	Worsening renal function (>20% decrease in eGFR)	Slope of the reciprocal of creatinine over 5 years	• Time to major renal or cardiovascular event (CVA, MI, CHF hospitalization, or progressive renal dysfunction) • Need for dialysis
Result	• No significant difference in GDMT only versus intervention group • Procedure-related complications reported in intervention group	• No significant difference in GDMT only versus intervention group for BP reduction, renal events, major cardiovascular events, or death • Serious complications reported in intervention group	No significant difference in GDMT only versus intervention group for primary endpoint or all-cause mortality
Shortcomings	• Small cohort • Exclusion of high-risk RAS patients • Patients had controlled BP • Majority of participants had <50% stenosis	• Lack of equipoise in recruitment • Higher than reported complication rate • Inadequate use of antihypertensive agents in intervention group • Diagnosis of RAS made with noninvasive tests • Patients with insignificant lesions included	• Antihypertensive therapy not optimized • Inclusion of patients with mild stenosis • Only moderate correlation between angiography and hemodynamically significant stenosis

(ARAS: atherosclerotic renal artery stenosis; BP: blood pressure; CHF: congestive heart failure; CKD: chronic kidney disease; CTA: computed tomography angiography; CVA: cerebrovascular accident; DSA: digital subtraction angiography; eGFR: estimated glomerular filtration rate; FMD: fibromuscular dysplasia; GDMT: guideline-directed medical therapy; MI: myocardial infarction; MRA: magnetic resonance angiography; PTRA: percutaneous transluminal renal angioplasty; RAS: renal artery stenosis; T2DM: type 2 diabetes mellitus)

TABLE 3: Limitations of trials comparing medical therapy alone to renal artery intervention.

	DRASTIC	STAR	ASTRAL	CORAL
Inclusion of patients without hemodynamically significant severe RAS	+	+	+	+
Inclusion of patients without hypertension or without proper antihypertensive medicine optimization	+	+	–	+
Inclusion of patients without progressive renal insufficiency	–	+	+	–
Recruitment bias	–	–	+	+

Vascular Access

Depending on operator's comfort, either of radial, femoral, or brachial access can be used. However, there is a strong consideration for radial access to prevent vascular access site complications[42] and it is especially useful in heavily diseased abdominal aorta and downwardly originating renal arteries. While taking radial route, it is to be kept in mind that either radial can be taken, but while left radial has shorter distance to renal arteries especially in tortuous aorta thus important in taller patients, right radial access is more comfortable and exposes to lesser radiation to operator.[43] In radial access, routine 100 cm-long guides and 135 cm-long balloons may prove short in tall patients or tortuous aorta, so occasionally 110 or 125 cm guide catheters and 150 cm balloons may be required.[43]

Renal Angiography

Renal angiography must be performed in appropriately indicated patients only, to avoid unnecessary intervention and procedural complications. Most of patients for renal angiography have already diagnosed significant renal stenosis on noninvasive investigations or have nondiagnostic noninvasive test results. Previous noninvasive tests must be carefully reviewed for helpful information such as presence of atherosclerosis, FMD, accessory renal arteries, location and angulation of renal arteries, aortic aneurysm, aortic calcification or thrombus, and iliac artery disease. Radial and femoral access both can be used for renal artery angiography and stenting. Radial route may be preferred to avoid access site complications. Adequate prehydration is important to prevent CIN. Always attempt to reduce use of iodinated contrast. Limited abdominal nonselective arteriography can be done with contrast or CO_2. Digital subtraction angiography (DSA) is also recommended for same. Selective renal angiography can be done via using aortic and renal artery calcification as landmarks to reduce contrast use.

Translesional Gradient

Translesional pressure gradient should be used to assess angiographically moderate stenosis. Resting translesional pressure gradient of ≥10 mm Hg and hyperemic gradient of ≥20 mm Hg with Pd/Pa of <0.8 defines significant stenosis. Here, papaverine (30 mg renal intra-arterial bolus) or dopamine (50 mcg/kg renal intra-arterial bolus) can be used as vasodilators and not adenosine as adenosine is a renal vasoconstrictor.[44-46]

Intravascular Ultrasound-guided Sizing

Intravascular ultrasound (IVUS) can be used for precise stent sizing as undersizing may lead to restenosis and oversizing may lead to complications. IVUS also helps in optimizing stent apposition, documenting complete ostial coverage, any dissections, and reducing contrast use. However, it is not routinely recommended as it has not shown to improved renal outcomes.[46]

PREVENTING ATHEROEMBOLISM

One of the major consideration in renal stenting is to prevent renal atheroembolism as it has been associated with significant increase in morbidity and decrease in 5-year survival (54% vs. 85%; $p < 0.011$).[47] To prevent atheroembolism and thus preventing ischemic damage to kidney, "no touch technique"[48] or catheter-in-catheter or telescoping technique[49] is recommended. **Figures 1A to E** demonstrate these techniques.

In no touch technique, a 0.035 guidewire is introduced in guide catheter past its tip to avoid scraping of aortic wall. Once renal artery is selectively engaged and 0.014 angioplasty guidewire is introduced in renal artery and has crossed the lesion, 0.035 guidewire is removed and renal angioplasty is completed.

In telescoping, a 4 or 5 F diagnostic catheter is placed inside a guide catheter 2 F larger and once guidewire crosses the lesion, guide advanced to engage coronary and diagnostic catheter is removed.

Embolic protection devices (EPDs) have also been used to prevent renal atheroembolism. A small RCT with 100 patients compared renal outcomes with renal stenting alone, stenting with EPD, stenting with glycoprotein IIb/IIIa, and stenting with EPD and glycoprotein IIb/IIIa both. It showed that only the group with renal stenting with both EPD and glycoprotein IIb/IIIa has shown improved renal outcomes ($p < 0.01$).[40] As of now, there is insufficient evidence to recommend use of glycoprotein IIb/IIIa and EPD in renal artery stenting.

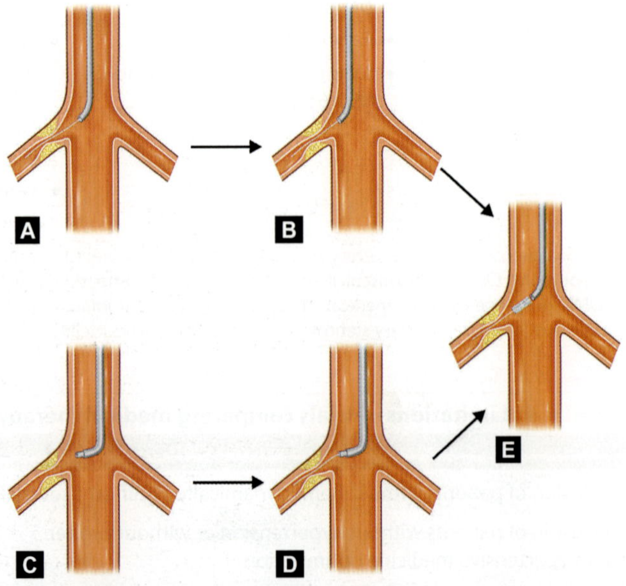

FIGS. 1A TO E: (A and B) No touch technique; (C and D) Telescoping technique; and (E) Stent placement.

They may be used in selected patients with worsening renal function as an aid to prevent ischemic damage to kidney.

RENAL ANGIOPLASTY PROCEDURE

Various CT studies have shown that right renal artery is best visualized in straight anteroposterior (AP), while left renal artery is best seen in 20–40° left anterior oblique (LAO) projection as it arises obliquely from aortic axis.[50] So, initial angiography is done in 15° LAO view.[51] In ostial disease, it is important to accurately identify true ostium in multiple-angulated views **(Figs. 2A and B)**. Sheath size of 6 or 7 F can be taken depending on selected stent size and type (covered or uncovered). Patients are routinely anticoagulated with heparin. Multipurpose catheter from left radial give optimal alignment to engage renal arteries. Also multipurpose angiographic (MPA) or Judkins Right 4 (JR4) guide catheter can be used from radial site. If femoral access is chosen, IMA catheter, renal standard curve or renal double curve (RDC), or hockey stick catheters can be used.[52] A 0.014 wire is used to cross the lesion and tip is kept in first or second order renal artery branches during all steps of procedure, else it may advance and cause cortical perforation or retroperitoneal hematoma. If EPD is being used, it can be positioned at this time. Appropriate stent sizing is crucial to prevent procedural complications and restenosis. IVUS provides excellent guide for sizing. Also, preprocedural CTA or MRA can also be used to choose appropriate stent sizing. Balloon should be undersized, its length should be limited to only slightly longer than the lesion and dilatation should not be performed beyond 1 cm distal to lesion to avoid distal dissections. Balloon inflation should be done for 20–30 seconds. Stent should be chosen 1:1 to reference vessel and avoid choosing poststenotic dilatation as reference diameter. Aim is to avoid under- and oversizing with reducing angiographic RAS to ≤30% and abolishing intralesional gradient. Stent should cover lesion completely and slightly extend (1–3 mm) in abdominal aorta. Excessive pain while deploying stent indicate overstretching adventitia and may mark impending rupture, so instantly deflate balloon if severe pain occurs. Stent balloon can be used to flare renal artery ostium in aorta. In **Figures 3 and 4**, we can see bilateral RAS with bilateral renal artery stenting.

COMPLICATIONS

Complication rate is ≤2% and mainly comprise femoral vascular site complications. Other complications are renal atheroembolism and azotemia, arterial or aortic dissection, renal artery subcapsular hematoma due to reperfusion injury, and occasionally renal artery rupture has been reported.

POSTPROCEDURAL CARE

All patients undergoing renal intervention should receive antiplatelet therapy for at least several months. Clopidogrel is most commonly used in these patients and is the standard of care. Some people also prefer to give dual antiplatelet therapy for 1 month and then switching to single antiplatelet treatment. Antihypertensive medications need optimization in follow-up.

RESTENOSIS

Renal artery stents have excellent long-term patency rates. In long-term, large diameter vessels with good luminal gain have lower rates of restenosis as compared to smaller vessels and stents. In a patient series of renal artery stenting, 1-year follow-up angiography showed 36% restenosis rate for <4.5 mm vessel, 16% for 4.5–6 mm vessel, and 6.5% restenosis rate in vessels >6 mm diameter.[53] Bare-metal stents (BMSs) have 79–85% primary patency and >92–98% secondary patency rates over 5-year follow-up.[54]

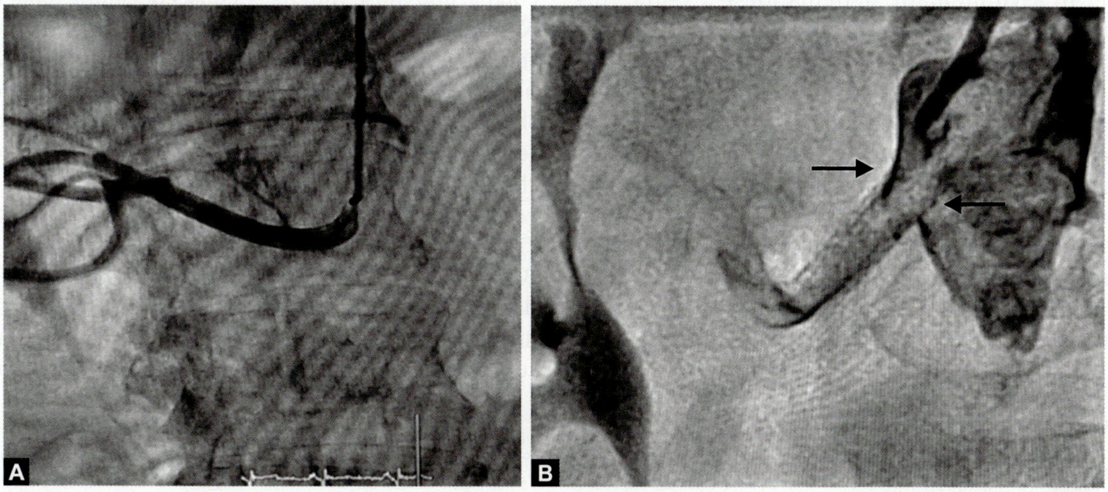

FIGS. 2A AND B: (A) Renal artery ostium is not well defined in anteroposterior (AP) view as it appears arising posteriorly and at an acute angle pointing downward. (B) For exact ostial placement of stent, left anterior oblique (LAO) view is helpful as it clearly defines the ostium.

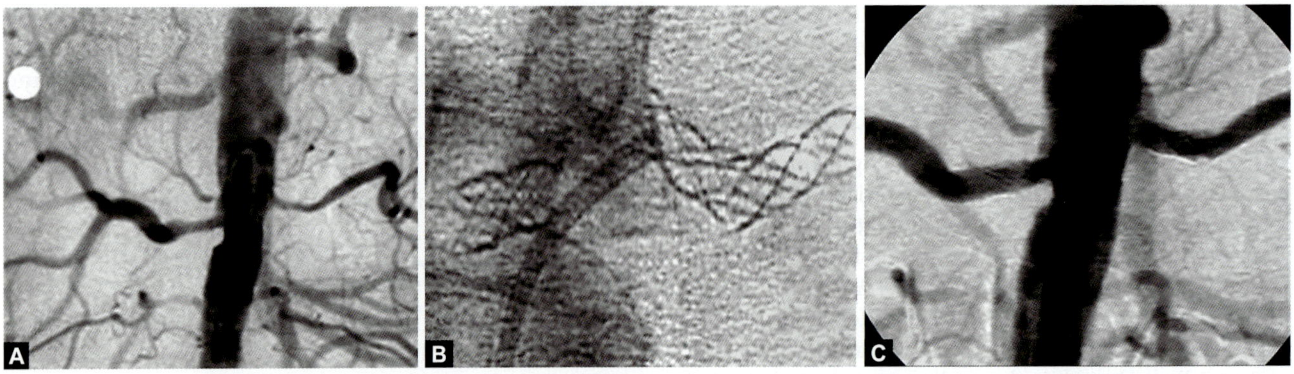

FIGS. 3A TO C: (A) Bilateral renal artery stenosis; (B) Perfectly expanded stents; (C) Successfully placed bilateral renal stent.

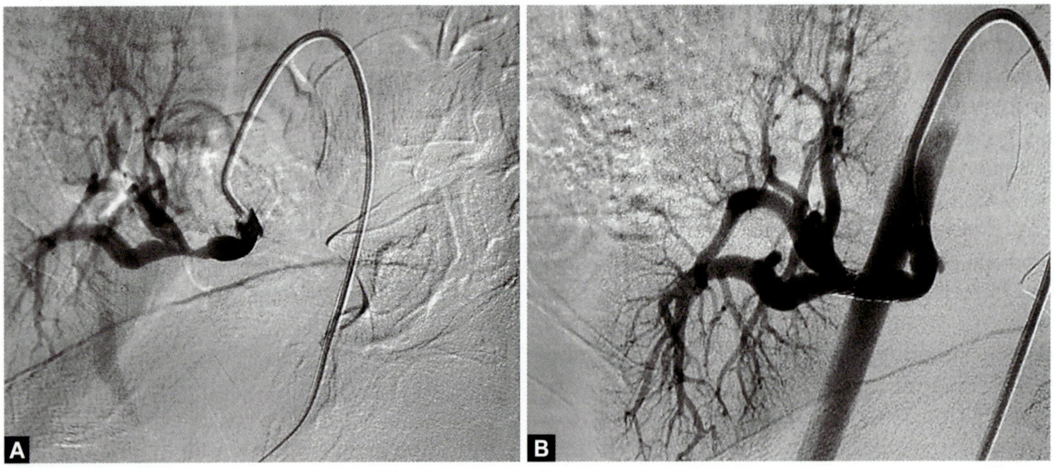

FIGS. 4A AND B: (A) Anastomotic site stenosis in postrenal transplant renal artery and (B) Postrenal artery stenting in transplanted kidney renal artery stenosis.

FOLLOW-UP

There are no unified guidelines for follow-up after renal artery stenting. In most recent appropriate use (AU) guidelines, renal artery duplex USG is advised after 1–2 weeks of stenting, then after 3–6 months, and annually thereafter in asymptomatic patients for 3–5 years. Any recurrence of hypertension or worsening of renal function necessitates duplex USG to look for stent restenosis.[55,56] If stenosis is suspected on duplex USG, clinical evaluation for recurrence of symptoms should be done. As next step, CTA is preferred over MRA to look for in-stent restenosis (ISR) as it avoids metal artifact.[57,58] If all imaging is inconclusive and there is recurrence of symptoms, repeat angiography with hemodynamic evaluation is warranted. Repeat stenting of ISR is preferred over balloon angioplasty given 58% lower recurrent restenosis rates with stent.[59]

CONCLUSION

Renal artery stenting should be offered to most symptomatic patients with hemodynamically significant moderate-to-severe RAS, causing resistant hypertension on maximally tolerated medical therapy, those with flash pulmonary edema, and those with recent onset declining renal function. Noninvasive assessment via renal artery Doppler ultrasound should be the initial diagnostic test and CTA or MRA should be reserved for ambiguous cases. Invasive assessment should be offered for severe cases who are candidates for revascularization. Hemodynamic pressure assessment should be done for indeterminate (50–70%) cases. Stenting with appropriately sized BMS is the procedure of choice. Treating RAS for indications mentioned here results in better BP control and better clinical outcome. Although RCTs till date fail to confirm this hypothesis, these trials had their own limitations. More studies are needed which include patient subsets which derive maximum benefit from this intervention.

ONLINE REFERENCES

Please scan the QR code provided at the end of the table of contents for References of this chapter.

CHAPTER

200

Carotid Artery Stenting in Asymptomatic Carotid Stenosis

Ashish Jai Kishan, Atul Mathur

ABSTRACT

Unlike symptomatic carotid artery stenosis, making a clinical decision to treat asymptomatic carotid stenosis is a challenge. Based on analogous findings of efficacy and safety in various randomized control trials while comparing carotid endarterectomy (CEA) with carotid artery stenting (CAS), the latter is now recommended as an alternative to CEA. Also in many countries, now CAS is more frequently performed for asymptomatic carotid artery stenosis compared to CEA. On the other hand, recent reports have shown that CAS is not superior with respect to best medical treatment (BMT) in asymptomatic carotid stenosis. Because of this confusion, the role of CAS needs to be reevaluated in patients with asymptomatic carotid. Several clinical factors need to be assessed while considering the appropriate mode of treatment of asymptomatic carotid stenosis including stenosis degree, stroke risk by medical treatment, patient life expectancy, and high risk for CEA or CAS. The aim of this article is to review pragmatically the information available and help reach to a clinical decision on CAS in asymptomatic carotid stenosis.

Keywords: Carotid endarterectomy, carotid artery stenting.

INTRODUCTION

The journey, which began with coronary artery intervention, has now over several decades progressed to incorporate therapies for peripheral vascular diseases. However, with regards to the asymptomatic carotid artery stenosis, there has been a challenge.[1-3] The controversy is not only with regards whether to revascularize these asymptomatic patients but also pertaining to the revascularization procedure that needs to be performed.[4,5]

Patients are considered as asymptomatic carotid artery stenosis if they lack a recent history (<6 months) of ipsilateral ischemic stroke or transient ischemic attack.[1] 10–15% of all the ischemic strokes are due to asymptomatic carotid artery stenosis (lesion > 50%).[6] Thus, asymptomatic carotid artery stenosis does represent a great prospect for prestroke intermediation. The important question now is which intervention is preferred. The gold standard for treatment of carotid artery stenosis has been carotid endarterectomy (CEA),[7] however, with recent advances with regards to carotid artery stenting (CAS) and dual antiplatelet therapy, the optimal management of carotid artery stenosis in general and especially asymptomatic carotid artery stenosis has been questioned. As per American Heart Association (AHA) 2014 guidelines, patients with >70% internal carotid artery stenosis, CEA is recommended if they are deemed to have low risk for myocardial infraction, perioperative stoke, or death.[8] The Heart and Stroke Foundation of Canada, The UK National Institute for Health and Clinical Excellence as well as the US Society for Vascular Surgery all do recommend CEA for such patients who are asymptomatic and requiring revascularization.[9-11] Between these two treatment options, various randomized control trials have shown equivalence, there still exist certain subgroups that have had significant different outcomes.[12]

CAROTID ARTERY STENTING

The proposal for carotid angioplasty came from 1977 to 1979 after experiments on animal models proved to be successful.[13,14] In 1980, the first carotid angioplasty was performed to treat atherosclerotic stenosis. The endovascular approach, however, was beset with issues of acute elastic recoil, restenosis, and dissections. This impediment was taken care of by carotid stent placement which was performed for the first time in 1989 to treat the intimal flap following carotid angioplasty.[15] The procedure of CAS has since then increased exponentially due to its minimally invasive nature in comparison to CEA. One of major safety challenges faced initially during the early days of carotid stenting was propagation of the emboli from the stenotic segment, distally. This technical issue was dealt with the use of distal occlusive balloon inflation. The balloon was placed distally to the stenotic lesion and aspiration was done after angioplasty, thereby preventing the distal embolization of atheromatous materials to the cerebral circulation.[16,17] Embolic protection device has since then evolved and now use of various types of protection devices has been widely accepted during carotid stenting.

CAROTID ENDARTERECTOMY

Nearly 30 years prior to carotid angioplasty, the origin of CEA was seen in the year 1954, and since then it has been a mainstay of treatment for carotid artery stenosis.[18] In 1991, the North American Symptomatic Carotid Endarterectomy Trial (NASCET) which was a randomized control trial, proved the efficacy of CEA. The trial had randomized the eligible patient with 70–99% carotid artery stenosis and recent history of transient ischemic stroke or nondisabling stroke into groups of best medical management with or without CEA. Those who underwent surgery had significantly lower rates of stokes and lower rates of major or fatal strokes on ipsilateral side of surgery.[7]

With the documented success in the symptomatic carotid stenosis patients, investigators tested the hypothesis of beneficial role of CEA in patients with asymptomatic carotid artery stenosis. Asymptomatic Carotid Atherosclerosis Study (ACAS), in 1995 was a randomized control trial which provided the answer. It had enrolled asymptomatic carotid patients with stenosis ≥ 60% and randomized to best medical management with or without CEA.[19] At the end of follow-up period, surgical arm patients had lower rates of ipsilateral stroke or death in comparison to only medically treated arm. Asymptomatic Carotid Surgery Trial (ACST) was another randomized control trial which also reaffirmed the benefit of CEA in asymptomatic carotid artery stenosis patients. It too had enrolled patients with carotid stenosis ≥60% and at the end of follow-up of 5 years, showed lower rates of strokes compared to those in medical arm.[20]

Carotid Artery Stenting versus Carotid Endarterectomy

There are five large, randomized control clinical landmark trials that have compared CAS with CEA. These are Asymptomatic Carotid Trial (ACT), ACST-2, Stent-Protected Angioplasty versus Carotid Endarterectomy-2 (SPACE-2), Stenting and Angioplasty with Protection in Patients at High Risk for Endarterectomy (SAPPHIRE), and Carotid Revascularization Endarterectomy versus Stenting Trial (CREST) **(Table 1)**.[21-25] Patients enrolled in ACT, ACST-2, and SPACE-2 trials exclusively included patients with asymptomatic carotid stenosis, whereas SAPPHIRE and CREST trials had included patients with asymptomatic as well as symptomatic carotid artery stenosis. Various primary and secondary outcomes of clinical trials have been described in **Table 2**.

TABLE 1: Carotid revascularization—clinical trials.

Carotid stenosis—type	CEA vs. BMT	CAS vs. BMT	CAS vs. CET
Asymptomatic	• VACS (1993) • ACAS (1995) • ACST (2004) • SPACE-2 (2022) • CREST-2 (ongoing) • ACTRIS (ongoing)	• SPACE-2 (2022) • CREST-2 (ongoing)	• ACT (2016) • ACT-2 (2021) • SPACE-2 (2022)
Symptomatic	• NASCET (1991) • ECST (1998)		• EVA-3S (2006) • SPACE (2006) • ICSS (2010) • CAVATS (2010)
Mixed	ECST-2	ECST-2	• SAPPHIRE (2004 and 2008) • CREST (2010)

(ACT: Asymptomatic Carotid Trial; ACAS: Asymptomatic Carotid Atherosclerosis Study; ACST: Asymptomatic Carotid Surgery Trial; ACTRIS: Asymptomatic Severe Atherosclerotic Carotid Artery Stenosis at Higher than Average Risk of Ipsilateral Stroke; BMT: best medical treatment; CAS: carotid artery stenting; CAVATAS: Carotid and Vertebral Artery Transluminal Angioplasty Study; CEA: carotid endarterectomy; CREST: Carotid Revascularization Endarterectomy versus Stenting Trial; ECST: European Carotid Surgery Trial; EVA-3S: Endarterectomy versus Stenting in patients with Symptomatic Severe carotid Stenosis; ICSS: International Carotid Stenting Study; NASCET: North American Symptomatic Carotid Endarterectomy Trial; SAPPHIRE: Stenting and Angioplasty with Protection in Patients at High Risk for Endarterectomy; SPACE: Stent-Protected Angioplasty versus Carotid Endarterectomy; VACS: Veterans Affairs Carotid Study)

Between CAS and CEA, periprocedural outcomes (myocardial infraction, stroke, or death within 30 days of postprocedure) did not differ significantly in SAPPHIRE, CREST, ACT, and ACST-2 trials. The event rates post-CAS in asymptomatic carotid stenosis were <4% which were slightly lower when compared to those that partially included symptomatic carotid stenosis (5%). Amongst CAS and CEA, there were no significant difference in most other periprocedural events (stroke or death). In CREST, however, periprocedural stroke or death were significantly more frequent. These trials principally also evaluated long-term composite outcomes of periprocedural stroke, postprocedural ipsilateral—stroke, myocardial infraction, or death up to 4 years after carotid interventional therapy. CAS was found to be noninferior to CEA for the composite outcomes in first year in both SAPPHIRE trial ($p = 0.004$ for

TABLE 2: CAS versus CEA clinical trials primary and secondary outcomes.

Characteristic	SAPPHIRE	CREST	ACT	ACT-2	SPACE-2
Year of publication	2004*; 2008†	2010	2016	2021	2022
Number of patients included	334*; 260†	2,502	1,453	3,625	513
Asymptomatic cases	70.1%	47.2%	100%	100%	100%
Number of patients with CAS	167*; 143†	1,262	1,089	1,811	197
Stenosis cutoff for trial inclusion‡	≥80%§	≥60% or ≥70%‖	≥70%¶	≥60%§	≥50%§,**
Periprocedural (or procedural) outcome†					
Stroke, myocardial infarction, or death	4.8% ↔ 9.8% ($p = 0.09$)	5.2% ↔ 4.5% ($p = 0.38$)	3.3% ↔ 2.6% ($p = 0.60$)	3.9% ↔ 3.2% ($p = 0.26$)	2.5% ↔ 2.5% ($p = 0.96$)§§
Stroke or death		4.4% ↔ 2.3% ($p < 0.01$)‡‡	2.9% ↔ 1.7% ($p = 0.33$)		
Disabling stroke or death				0.9% ↔ 1.0% ($p = 0.77$)	0.5% ↔ 0.5% ($p = 0.98$)
Stroke		4.1% ↔ 2.3% ($p = 0.01$)	2.8% ↔ 1.4% ($p = 0.23$)	3.6% ↔ 2.4% ($p = 0.06$)	
Death		0.7% ↔ 0.3% ($p = 0.18$)	0.1% ↔ 0.3% ($p = 0.43$)		
Long-term outcome					
Follow-up period	1 year* and 3 years†	4 years	1 year* and 5 years‖	5 years	5 years
All events					
Composite outcomes					
• Periprocedural stroke, myocardial infarction, or death or postprocedural ipsilateral stroke	12.2% ↔ 20.1%; $p < 0.01$ for noninferiority of CAS*,¶¶ 24.6% ↔ 26.9% ($p = 0.71$)†	7.2% ↔ 6.8% ($p = 0.51$)¶¶	3.8% ↔ 3.4%; $p = 0.01$ for noninferiority of CAS*,¶¶		
• Periprocedural stroke or death or postprocedural ipsilateral stroke		6.4% ↔ 4.7% ($p = 0.03$)			4.4% ↔ 2.5% ($p = 0.37$)¶¶,***
• Periprocedural stroke or postprocedural ipsilateral stroke		6.2% ↔ 4.7% ($p = 0.04$)			
Individual outcomes					
• Any stroke		10.2% ↔ 7.9% ($p = 0.03$)	6.9% ↔ 5.3% ($p = 0.44$)‖		9.2% ↔ 5.3% ($p = 0.19$)
• Ipsilateral stroke					4.4% ↔ 2.0% ($p = 0.23$)
• Death		11.3% ↔ 12.6% ($p = 0.45$)	12.9% ↔ 10.6% ($p = 0.21$)‖		9.3% ↔ 7.6% ($p = 0.62$)

Continued

Continued

Characteristic	SAPPHIRE	CREST	ACT	ACT-2	SPACE-2
Postprocedural events					
Stroke				5.2% ↔ 4.5% ($p = 0.33$)¶¶	
Ipsilateral stroke		2.0% ↔ 2.5% ($p = 0.85$)	2.2% ↔ 2.7% ($p = 0.51$)‖		
Fatal or disabling stroke				2.4% ↔ 2.5% ($p = 0.91$)	

Event frequencies represented by "% in CAS ↔ % in CEA group (*p*-value)"
*1-year outcome.
†3-year outcome.
‡For asymptomatic stenosis.
§On duplex ultrasonography.
‖≥60% on angiography or ≥70% on ultrasonography.
¶On ultrasonography or angiography.
**≥50% according to North American Symptomatic Carotid Endarterectomy Trial (NASCET) criteria and ≥70% according to European Carotid Surgery Trial (ECST) criteria.
††Outcomes within 30 days after treatment procedure.
‡‡Values did not correspond with summation of separate values of stroke and death.
§§Only stroke occurred periprocedurally, so incidences of stroke or death and stroke were same with the incidence of stroke, myocardial infarction, or death.
‖‖5-year outcome.
¶¶Primary or main outcome.
***Specifically, any ischemic or hemorrhagic stroke or death from any cause within 30 days, or any ipsilateral ischemic stroke within 5 years of follow-up, contrary to other trials that did not specify the type of stroke.
(CT: Asymptomatic Carotid Trial; ACST: Asymptomatic Carotid Surgery Trial; SPACE, Stent-Protected Angioplasty versus Carotid Endarterectomy; CAS: carotid artery stenting; CEA: carotid endarterectomy; CREST: Carotid Revascularization Endarterectomy *vs.* Stenting Trial; SAPPHIRE: Stenting and Angioplasty with Protection in Patients at High Risk for Endarterectomy)

noninferiority) and ACT trial ($p = 0.01$ for noninferiority). During follow-up of 3 years in SAPPHIRE and 4 years in CREST trial, the cumulative incidences of composite outcome were not significantly different between CAS and CEA groups ($p = 0.71$ and 0.51, respectively). With respect to stroke related long-term outcomes, CREST trial showed unfavorable results after CAS; significantly more frequent any stroke ($p = 0.03$) and periprocedural and postprocedural ipsilateral stroke ($p = 0.04$).

The 1-year outcome of various trials including ACT, SAPPHIRE, CREST, ACST-2, and SPACE-2 was done in a recent meta-analysis which showed significant difference in periprocedural stroke, myocardial infarction, or death when CAS was compared with CEA. Similarly, the long-term stroke, myocardial infarction, or death was not different significantly in both these groups. However, CAS group had a higher risk of any stroke during the perioperative period versus CEA ($p = 0.004$).[26]

Carotid Artery Stenting versus Best Medical Treatment

To date, SPACE-2 is the only randomized control trial which has compared CAS with BMT in asymptomatic carotid artery stenosis. Originally, it was designed to allocate patients into three groups of (1) CEA plus BMT, (2) CAS plus BMT, and (3) BMT alone randomly. However, due to slow recruitment, the study protocol was amended to randomize the patients to either CEA versus BMT (SPACE-2a) or CAS versus BMT (SPACE-2b).[27] The patients enrolled were asymptomatic within last 180 days for the study. The uniqueness of the study was that there were specified treatment targets for BMT which included physical activity ≥30 minutes at least three times a week, blood pressure ≤130/85 or 130/80 mm Hg, limited alcohol consumption (e.g., <30 g/day for males), smoking cessation, improved lipid profiles (e.g., low density lipoprotein <130 or 100 mg/dL according to comorbidities), glycated hemoglobin (HbA1c) <7%, and body mass index <25 kg/m^2. Of total 513 patients enrolled in the study, there were no significant difference in the primary outcomes (periprocedural any stroke/death or postprocedural ipsilateral ischemic stroke within 5 years) between CAS and BMT ($p = 0.52$).

Analysis

In asymptomatic carotid artery stenosis patients, CAS as a modality of revascularization is comparable to CEA. This can be based on the results of 1-year outcome data of SAPPHIRE and ACT trial. Also, findings of the recent meta-analysis showed comparable peri procedural as well as long-term outcomes of CAS and CEA.[26] However, with respect to data of CREST trial, one must interpret its data cautiously as it had shown unfavorable results in CAS group. Since it had included >50% symptomatic carotid artery stenosis study population, those adverse outcomes might not be applicable to asymptomatic carotid artery stenosis.

Based on the conclusion of SPACE-2 trial, neither CAS nor CEA was found to be superior to intensive medical treatment in asymptomatic carotid artery stenosis, with no difference in periprocedural and long-term outcomes. Historically, the annual stroke-related event rates in 1980s had been 4%, which by 2000s was merely <2%, irrespective of stenosis degree. This can probably be explained by advancement of medical strategies in primary prevention of stroke. The SPACE-2 trial was also remarkable as it was the first to set specifically designed BMT, where all the patients had received detailed lifestyle coaching including smoking cessation, weight loss, and regular physical activities along with medications. A cautious approach should be taken while interpreting the results of SPACE-2 as adherence to the BMT as needed in not possible in the real clinical practice. Even target blood pressure as well as the weight reduction were accomplished only in 25% study group. Also, 36% of the study population had nonhigh-grade level of carotid stenosis [as per European Carotid Surgery Trial (ECST) and NASCET criteria]; such mild nature of disease might exaggerate the effect of BMT. Finally, the SPACE-2 trial had to be terminated early as fewer number of patients were enrolled than planned.

Another trial conducted was ECST-2, in which patient with carotid artery stenosis ≥50% and low-to-intermediate risk of stroke were enrolled. They were randomized into two groups, one in BMT and the other with BMT along with carotid revascularization mainly by CEA. The recent interim results are suggestive of no significant difference in outcomes. The composite rate of periprocedural death, stroke, or MI at the end of 2 years in combined BMT and carotid revascularization was 10.0% whereas in 10.3% in BMT alone group. Moreover, these finding were regardless of the whether patients were asymptomatic or symptomatic.

Decisive Factors for CAS in Asymptomatic Carotid Artery Stenosis

Clinical factors to be considered for CAS in asymptomatic carotid artery stenosis are (1) degree of stenosis, (2) stroke risk by medical treatment, (3) patient's life expectancy, and (4) high risk for CEA or CAS.

Degree of Stenosis

One of the most important criteria deemed as the necessity of vascularization in the treatment of asymptomatic carotid artery stenosis is the stenosis degree. Various randomized control trials have set the cutoff of the stenosis as ≥50–80%.[21-23,25] Since SPACE-2 trial did not show a clear advantage of CAS in asymptomatic carotid artery stenosis with ≥50% stenosis, the relevant stenosis degree can now be considered in a range of ≥60–80%.[6,11,28-38] Presently, all the guidelines have recommended CAS for asymptomatic carotid artery stenosis ≥60–80%. Guidelines that have clearly indicated stenosis degree eligible to CAS are Society of Vascular Surgery (SVS, 2021), German Austrian Society (2020), European Society for Vascular Surgeon (ESVS, 2017), and American Stroke Association/AHA (ASA/AHA, 2011; 2014). On the other hand, guidelines which recommended CAS just as an alternative to CEA without specifying stenosis degree for CAS were European Stroke Organization (ESO, 2011), European Stroke of Cardiology (ESC, 2011), and ESVS (2009).

Various diagnostic modalities are available for assessment of degree of stenosis including duplex ultrasonography (DUS), computed tomography angiography (CTA), magnetic resonance angiography (MRA), or catheter angiography. CAS was indicated as ≥60% carotid stenosis determined by catheter angiography in the AHA/ASA guidelines. Similarly, in asymptomatic carotid stenosis, CAS was recommended for ≥70% by DUS or ≥80% by CTA or MRA if DUS revealed stenosis ≥50–69%.

The most preferable and widely used modality to assess stenosis degree is DUS.[37] However, catheter angiography is recommended in ASA/AHA (2011; 2014) guidelines and it was also utilized in the CREST and ACT trials. Similarly based on ESC (2011) guideline and ESVS (2017) guideline, CTA or MRA can be used equally with DUS. In conditions where results are equivocal or inaccurate stenosis on DUS, CTA or MRA can be added based on AHA/ASA (2011; 2014) guidelines, German/Austrian (2020) guideline, and SVS (2021) guideline. When there is asymptomatic carotid stenosis ≥60%, use of all modalities is possible to evaluate degree of stenosis. For stenosis ≥70%, DUS is mostly preferable modality.

Throughout the historical trials, the degree of stenosis degree for CAS has not been consistent, however, the most recent guidelines primarily recommend CEA at the cutoff of ≥60% or ≥70% for asymptomatic carotid stenosis.[6,35,37,38] In American guidelines, the cutoff of ≥70% was adopted, whereas European guidelines had preferably adopted ≥60%. Exceptionally, ≥60% stenosis by catheter angiography has been considered as eligible criteria for CAS in AHA/ASA (2014) guideline.

Stroke Risk by Medical Treatment

The primary goal of revascularization treatment of carotid stenosis is to prevent the development of future stroke. In comparison to symptomatic carotid stenosis, the risk of occurrence of future stroke by medical treatment should be more thoroughly assessed in asymptomatic carotid artery stenosis. Variety of clinical and imaging features are associated with the risk of future stroke in asymptomatic carotid stenosis including—(1) plaque characteristics including morphology, size, and vulnerability, (2) stenosis progression, and (3) microembolization. If the stenosis progresses by 10%, the risk of future stroke doubles.[39-41] On imaging, various features which are associated with vulnerable plaque are noted, which includes intraplaque hemorrhage, plaque ulceration, plaque neovascularity, thin/ruptured fibrous cap, and presence of a lipid-rich necrotic core.[42] The risk of future stroke increases by more than two to three times when there is echolucent plaque or intraplaque hemorrhage.[43-45] Also documented is the risk more than three times when there is silent infarction or contralateral transient cerebral ischemic attack or stroke.[46,47] European guidelines have especially recommended to consider risk of future stroke in the decision-making process of revascularization treatment.[6,38] Revascularization treatment should be actively considered if asymptomatic carotid stenosis patient has at least one of the above features which can increase the risk of future stroke.[6,48]

Life Expectancy of Patient

Although, this feature is most overlooked one, patient's life expectancy is a major consideration in the decision of revascularization therapy in asymptomatic carotid stenosis. Specific criteria of patient's life expectancy for inclusion have been used in major clinical trials had a specific criterion, including—minimum of 1 year in SAPPHIRE, 3 years in ACT, and 5 years in SPACE-2 and CREST trial.[21,23-25] Guidelines now commonly recommend revascularization on a patient with life expectancy ≥3 or 5 years.

High Risk for CEA or CAS

As CAS is considered an alternative to patients who are deemed ineligible for CEA, high-risk features for CEA should be examined. Nonvascular features for high-risk CEA are the high cervical lesions and complicated surgical fields. Commonly, above C2 level carotid lesions are interpreted to be unsuitable to CEA. With exposure of carotid artery at a higher level, there is an increased risk of cranial nerve injury especially vagus nerve. Past history of neck surgery or irradiation can result in fibrotic or scarred changes of surrounding connective tissues, causing surgical dissection more tough during CEA. CEA is more challenging when there is spinal immobility by previous cervical fusion, arthritis, or kyphosis; even obese patient with short neck possesses a significant hurdle. Patients with contralateral laryngeal nerve palsy or vocal cord injury are regarded to be ineligible for CEA as the procedure has an apparent risk of cranial nerve injury.

In presence of contralateral carotid occlusion, the data on CEA is a bit conflicting. Several studies have shown that post-CEA, there is significantly increased in perioperative stroke risk with contralateral carotid occlusion.[49] However, this increase was very modest. Furthermore, in another randomized study it was seen post-CEA stroke-free survival being comparable between patients with and those without contralateral carotid occlusion.[50] There is also a higher risk of stroke after CEA in presence of a tandem lesion, this might be due to increased chance of hemodynamic compromise during general anesthesia and CEA.

With respect to CAS, it is the tortuosity of aortic arch, common carotid artery, and internal carotid artery, which is not only associated with technical failure, but also there is an increased risk of stroke and death.[51,52] In tortuous course of internal carotid artery, especially, it is difficult to negotiate a distal embolic protection device at an appropriate location. In CAS, the periprocedural risk is directly associated with atherosclerotic burden. With increase in catheter manipulation in aortic arch as well as in target arteries that carries a high atherosclerotic burden, there is increased chances of embolic stroke.[52] The periprocedural outcomes in CAS are also affected by the lesion morphology. The passage of the endovascular devices gets disturbed in presence of heavily calcific and long complex lesion.[51,52] There is high risk of stent fracture or deformation in heavily calcified lesions.[53] Similarly with long and complex stenosis there is an increased risk of embolic stroke during endovascular manipulation.[51]

With age perspective, usually patients who are >80 years old, have a higher risk of stroke in CAS than in CEA.[25,54] The risk of stroke was higher in patients aged >70 years after CAS in CREST trial.[25] Correspondingly, higher risk of stroke is also noted in older age for the candidates who underwent CEA. Benefits of CEA were only observed in patients <75 years, and not in ≥75 years (p for interaction by age = 0.04) in ACST-1 trial.[55] This, however, could be explained due to more comorbidities afflicting the older patients which would increase the risk of stroke post-CEA.[37] These comorbidities include severe cardiac and pulmonary diseases and renal failure; and they are expected to increase the risk of stroke postrevascularization in both CEA and CAS. However, there is little evidence to support the association of the comorbidities. In view of relatively lower risk of cardiac or pulmonary events, CAS is preferred over CEA in presence of severe cardiac or pulmonary comorbidities. Since chronic renal insufficiency could also affect the risk of stroke post both the modes of revascularization, in such predicament, medical treatment can be preferred.[56]

In asymptomatic carotid stenosis, the current position of CAS is somewhat limited. In all the recent guidelines, revascularization method preferred for asymptomatic carotid stenosis is CEA. It is only where CEA is deemed as high risk or not suitable, CAS recommended. Unlike the distinct association between CEA and CAS, the role of CAS in comparison to medical therapy alone, has not yet been settled. In AHA/ASA (2014) guideline, it only states that there is lack of evidence regarding the effectiveness of

CAS versus with medical treatment alone.[35] In ESO (2021) guideline, which is based on short-term interim results of SPACE-2 trial, it recommends against CAS as a routine alternative to medical therapy alone.[38] However, considering the limitations of the SPACE-2 trial, it is not appropriate yet to reduce the role of CAS in asymptomatic carotid stenosis, rather further studies should be conducted to confirm it.

CONCLUSION

In asymptomatic carotid stenosis, it can be acknowledged, CAS is comparable to CEA regarding outcomes including efficacy and safety. On the other hand, role of CAS compared to BMT in asymptomatic carotid stenosis should be reevaluated as per SPACE-2 trial. However, considering some limitations of SPACE-2 trial, it is too early to assert that CAS is no longer beneficial under the intense and systematic medical treatment. Alternatively, the need of the hour is to reevaluate the clinical as well as imaging features which are associated with high risk of future strokes in asymptomatic carotid stenosis. Hence, while deciding to perform CAS in asymptomatic carotid stenosis, a more thorough approach should be taken to assess the high-risk features.

ONLINE REFERENCES

Please scan the QR code provided at the end of the table of contents for References of this chapter.

CHAPTER

201 Interventional Therapies in Acute Pulmonary Embolism

BC Srinivas, Shanmugam K, Arun Kumar

ABSTRACT

Pulmonary embolism is the leading cause of preventable death in hospitalized patients. Even though huge advances in prevention and treatment have come in the last two decades, still the mortality is significant. Intravenous thrombolysis has greatly improved mortality and morbidity in the last two decades with probably lesser incidence of chronic thromboembolic pulmonary hypertension (CTEPH). Newer interventional therapies such as catheter-directed lysis and mechanical thrombectomy offer a new hope for these groups of patients with possibly lesser risks. Surgery is traditionally done for patients with contraindications to lysis with its attendant risks. Mechanical thrombectomy offers a new first-line therapy for these patients with contraindications to lysis.

Keywords: Pulmonary embolism, thrombolysis, catheter-directed lysis, ultrasound-assisted catheter-directed lysis, Inari FlowTriever, indigo aspiration, penumbra, lightning aspiration, mechanical thrombectomy, rheolytic thrombectomy.

INTRODUCTION

Pulmonary embolism (PE) remains the most common cause of preventable deaths in hospitalized patients and is the third most common cause of cardiovascular deaths after myocardial infarction and stroke.[1] Despite progress in treatment, mortality still remains high.[2] First line of treatment for massive PE remains thrombolysis based on small randomized controlled trial (RCT) or surgery where lysis is contraindicated. Interventional therapies are upcoming and could pave a way in future for treatment of PE, possibly with lesser risks and better outcomes. In this chapter, let us review the established interventional devices and the emerging ones.

PATHOPHYSIOLOGY

Obstruction to the pulmonary arteries raises pulmonary artery pressure (PAP) proximal to the obstruction and reduced pulmonary flow distal to the obstruction with vasoconstriction due to metabolites and pulmonary infarction in a minority. Sudden increase in right-sided cardiac afterload results in acute right heart failure, hypoxemia, and decreased cardiac output, leading to cardiogenic shock.

RISK STRATIFICATION

Pulmonary embolism can have a myriad variety of presentation, ranging from dyspnea and syncope to profound shock. Geneva and Wells rule and its simplified versions are the most frequently used prediction scores. D-dimer testing is advocated in low clinical probability setting due to high negative predictive value, whereas computed tomography (CT) pulmonary angiogram is advocated in high clinical probability to rule in PE.

Once PE is confirmed, risk stratification for mortality is done. The European Society of Cardiology (ESC) guidelines 2019 are commonly followed as given in **Table 1**.[3]

TREATMENT

The treatment of PE is based on risk stratification. In high risk, thrombolysis or emergency surgery is recommended in case of contraindications to lysis as the first line of treatment.

TABLE 1: Risk stratification of PE—the ESC guidelines 2019.

Early mortality risk	Indicators of risk			
	Hemodynamic instability	Clinical parameters of PE severity and/or comorbidity: PESI class III–V or sPESI ≥ 1	RV dysfunction on TTE or CTPA	Elevated cardiac troponin levels
High	+	+	+	+
Intermediate–high	–	+	+	+
Intermediate–low	–	+	One or none positive	
Low	–	–	–	– (optional)

(CTPA: computed tomography pulmonary angiogram; ESC: European Society of Cardiology; PE: pulmonary embolism; PESI: pulmonary embolism severity index; RV: right ventricular; sPESI: simplified PESI; TTE: transthoracic echocardiography)

Thrombolysis

Treatment can be given up to 14 days of symptom onset, though the maximum benefit is seen within 2 days.[4] Recombinant tissue plasminogen activator (rtPA), streptokinase, urokinase, tenecteplase, and reteplase—all have been tried in PE, though head-to-head trials for superiority of one regimen over the other is lacking. The Food and Drug Administration (FDA)-approved regimens are recommended for high-risk PE. Thrombolysis even though leads to fast improvement in majority of patients, a minority of patients continue to have persistent right ventricular (RV) dysfunction and no clinical improvement in up to 8% of patients.[5] These patients were traditionally treated with surgery rather than repeat thrombolysis; newer interventional therapies can be of benefit in these groups of patients. Thrombolysis is also limited due to its feared side effect of major bleeding in particular intracranial bleeding which can occur in up to 1.7% of patients. Benefit in mortality is seen only in high-risk group with hemodynamic instability.[6]

Surgical Embolectomy

Surgical pulmonary embolectomy is generally reserved for patients with contraindications or failed lysis.[7] Some potential indications are those with impending cardiopulmonary arrest in surgical centers and RV clot in transit.[8] Even though inhospital mortality is high given their high initial risk, low incidence of chronic thromboembolic pulmonary hypertension (CTEPH) on follow-up and low risk of pulmonary hemorrhage make this procedure an established option in higher centers.[9]

Interventional Therapies

To address the growing unmet need of patients and to prevent complications associated with treatment, new interventional treatments are upcoming. These can be broadly divided into two classes—facilitation of thrombolysis with lesser doses and manual aspiration of thrombus. All of these procedures are primarily intended to reduce the thrombus burden rather than complete removal, improve RV hemodynamics, and possibly prevent CTEPH in the long term.

Facilitation of Thrombolysis

One method to decrease dose of lytic drugs will be to deliver them directly into the vessels involved and thrombus itself. Besides having a huge thrombus burden, longer infusions of lytic drugs may result in better efficacy and possibly reduce complications as in prosthetic heart valve thrombosis.

Catheter-directed Lysis

Simpler method of facilitating lysis is delivering the drugs directly on the thrombus through perfusion catheters with multiple side holes. Commercially available catheters include Unifuse, Cragg-McNamara, and Fountain infusion system. Multipurpose or Judkins right catheter is used in some centers due to cost benefits with multiple side holes made manually. The SUNSET sPE (Standard vs. Ultrasound-Assisted Catheter Thrombolysis for Submassive Pulmonary Embolism) trial showed catheter-directed lysis to be as equivalent to ultrasound catheter guided with similar reductions in pulmonary pressure, RV size reduction, and comparable lytic doses.[10]

Ultrasound-assisted Catheter-directed Thrombolysis

In this technique, both lytic drug and ultrasound waves are directed into thrombus by way of a single catheter with a microsonic core wire. Ultrasound in vitro studies have shown that it facilitates lytic drug entry and reversible disaggregation of fibrin fibers which are not crosslinked.[11] EkoSonic endovascular system is commercially available and efficacy has been proven in multiple trials. The ULTIMA trial which enrolled patients with submassive PE showed decrease in pulmonary artery systolic pressure, RV/left ventricular (LV) ratio, and Miller score which measures pulmonary clot burden compared to standard anticoagulation alone.[12] Multiple single-arm trials also consistently showed efficacy and safety of this system with probably lesser bleeding.[13,14] Slow lysis with this system may preclude its use in massive PE and impending circulatory arrest.[15]

Mechanical Removal of Thrombus

Mechanical removal of thrombus can be done by large- or small-bore catheters. Principle is not for complete removal, rather to improve hemodynamics. Advantage will be minimal bleeding risk with disadvantages being of vascular access complications and mechanical injuries to cardiac structures and pulmonary vasculature.

Pigtail Thrombectomy

Simple method of fragmentation of thrombus is to take a standard pigtail and fragment the thrombus by rotation or smaller peripheral balloons to restore flow to branches. Efficacy of these simple methods are limited to case reports and case series and thrombus removal is actually not done, rather fragmentation is done with distal embolization being a concern. These procedures can be done in addition to local thrombolysis.

Rheolytic Thrombectomy

AngioJet catheter is used that uses high speed saline jets for fragmentation of thrombus by creating vacuum. The same catheter can also be used for local thrombolysis.[16] Side effects include hematuria, thrombocytopenia, anemia, acute kidney injury, and bradyarrhythmias.[17] These safety concerns have limited its use currently.

Inari FlowTriever Device

In this, the actual extraction of thrombus is done. Catheters are available in 16, 20, and 24 French (24 F) sizes. Direct manual aspiration is done usually through a FlowTriever which has three self-expanding nitinol mesh disks to retrieve the thrombus into the suction catheter as shown in **Figure 1**. Large catheter size limits its use in distal vessels and efficacy is proven in single-arm studies. Future RCT is needed to establish its role as an alternative to thrombolysis.

The FLARE study was a single-arm prospective company-sponsored trial in which 106 intermediate-risk PE patients were enrolled and average RV/LV reduction of 0.38 was noted. No device-related complication was noted, but four procedure-related complications were observed, including one case of reperfusion pulmonary hemorrhage requiring lobectomy.[18] Single-center retrospective study analyzed 46 patients with 100% technical success and two major adverse events with hemoptysis and blood loss requiring transfusion.[19] Recently published FLASH registry, enrolling up to 1,000 patients, which analyzed 800 patients in the United States (US) cohort, significant reductions in RV/LV ratio (0.25 at 48 hours), reduction in mean PAP (23%) and dyspnea were observed (66–15%). Major adverse events were observed in 1.8% of patients including 11 major bleeds and three intraprocedural adverse events with one tricuspid valve injury.[20]

Indigo Aspiration System

Indigo aspiration system (Penumbra) with associated tubing and separator has got FDA clearance for pulmonary embolectomy as shown in **Figures 2A and B**. Initial trials done with 8 F system have shown promising results in single-arm trials. The EXTRACT-PE trial done in submassive PE on 119 patients showed significant reduction in mean RV/LV ratio from 1.47–1.04. There was 1.7% rate of major adverse events including one device-related death due to

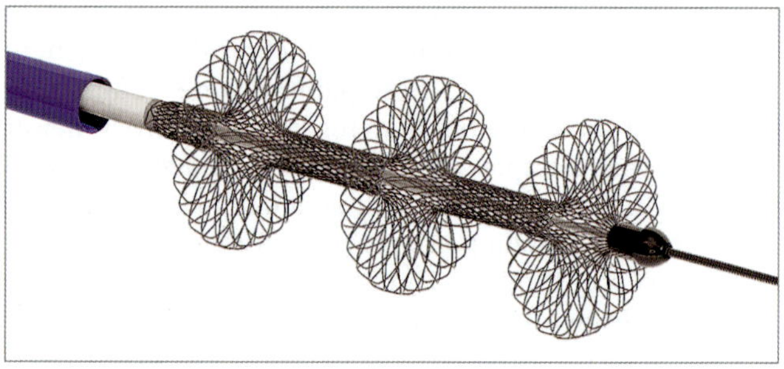

FIG. 1: Inari FlowTriever catheter.

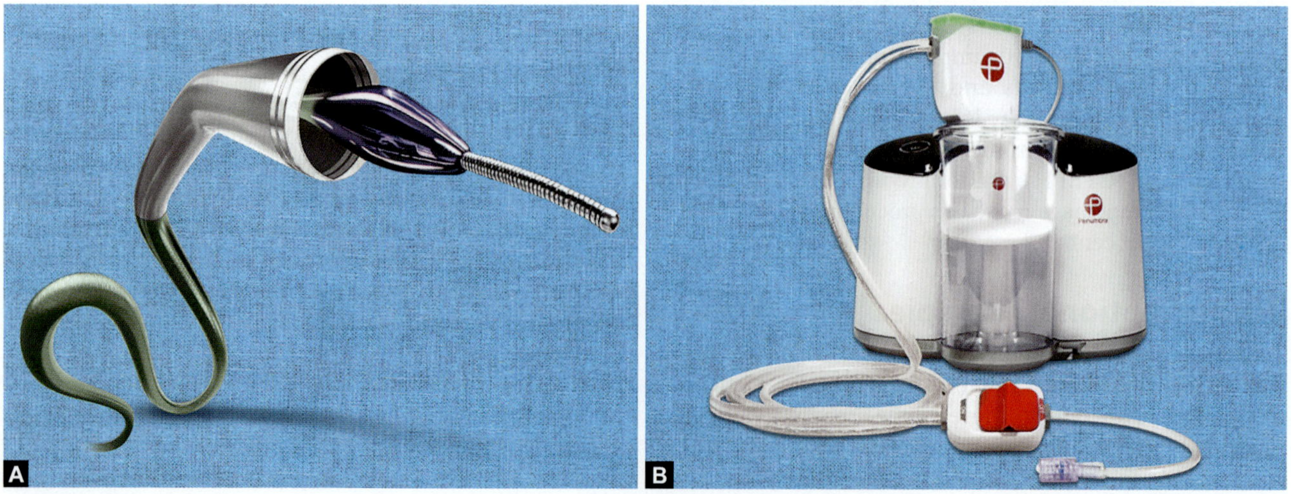

FIGS. 2A AND B: Indigo aspiration system. (A) Lightning 12 aspiration catheter and separator 12; (B) Penumbra ENGINE and lightning aspiration tubing.

sustained ventricular tachycardia (VT) after hemoptysis periprocedure.[21] Many small center trials have shown efficacy of this system in intermediate–high-risk PE.

Newer device with 12 F system is in early trials currently.[22]

CONCLUSION

Newer interventional therapies, predominantly mechanical thrombectomy, offers a new hope for patients with contraindications to lysis. Larger RCTs are needed to establish its efficacy in intermediate high-risk pulmonary thromboembolism (PTE) as an alternative to catheter-directed or systemic lysis. These devices may in the future lead to decreased incidence of chronic thromboembolic PE. Whether adding both mechanical plus low-dose catheter-directed lysis to achieve dual benefits in both large and small pulmonary arteries needs to be evaluated in future trials.

ONLINE REFERENCES

Please scan the QR code provided at the end of the table of contents for References of this chapter.

CHAPTER

202 Interventional Approach to Central Vein Occlusions

CM Nagesh, Vijaykumar JR, Babu Reddy, BC Srinivas

ABSTRACT

The chronic kidney disease is a major health problem with significant morbidity and mortality. The creation and maintenance of the hemodialysis access are crucial for renal replacement therapy, but <50% of these accesses remain patent for 3 years. Central venous obstruction (stenosis or occlusion; CVO) is a common and significant cause of access failure in hemodialysis-dependent chronic kidney disease patients. The incidence of CVO is reported in up to 40% patients and has increased over the past decade mainly due to long-term use of the central venous catheters. CVO causes venous hypertension with or without debilitating symptoms. The surgical reconstruction has high patency rates of 80–90% at 1 year, but it is associated with significantly high rate of perioperative mortality and morbidity due to the intrathoracic location of deep veins. Endovascular intervention being less invasive, safer with good success rate has evolved as the first-line treatment. The role of the primary stenting and the type of stent in every patient is still controversial.

Keywords: Central venous obstruction, endovascular therapy, balloon angioplasty, Central vein occlusion, chronic kidney disease, hemodialysis, venous intervention.

INTRODUCTION

Central venous obstruction (stenosis or occlusion; CVO) is common condition associated with chronic kidney disease (CKD) leading to significant morbidity and mortality. Approximately, 1.8 million patients worldwide are receiving renal replacement therapy and the number is increasing at a rate of 7% every year.[1] Maintenance of the hemodialysis access is crucial for renal replacement therapy, because of <50% patency rate at 3 years.[2] CVO is a most common cause of access failure in hemodialysis-dependent CKD patients. Long-term use of central venous catheters has increased the incidence of CVO in up to 40% patients in the past decade.[3,4] CVO causes venous hypertension resulting in asymptomatic to debilitating symptoms such as respiratory distress. The surgical reconstruction is associated with high perioperative morbidity and mortality due to intrathoracic location of deep veins, but have 1-year high patency rates of 80–90%.[4] Endovascular intervention being less invasive, safer with good success rate has evolved as the first-line treatment. The role of the primary stenting and the type of stent in every patient are still controversial. Crossing the occluded vessel remains the most challenging step and traditional blunt and sharp recanalization techniques are used to cross the occluded vessels. It requires lot of expertise in the field of venous intervention for the successful recanalization. Newer advanced techniques such as radiofrequency guidewires help in 18% of cases where traditional methods fail.[5] This review mainly focuses on thoracic central veins occlusions.

BACKGROUND

Central venous obstruction is defined as significant narrowing of the venous lumen leading to impedance of blood flow. The thoracic central veins include the superior vena cava, both brachiocephalic veins, thoracic segments of internal jugular vein, and suprahepatic inferior vena cava (IVC). There is strong association of CVO with previous placement of central venous catheters.[6] The incidence of CVO is significantly higher in patients with a history of subclavian catheterization (42–50%) as compared to internal jugular vein use.[6,7] The factors responsible for CVO include the number and duration of central vein catheters, left-sided catheterization, and the number of catheter-related infections.[7] Main mechanisms of CVO are:

- External compression by musculoskeletal and vascular structures
- Venous wall thickening owing to organized thrombus, fibrosis, or endovenous interventions
- Intraluminal obstruction

CLINICAL FEATURES

Clinical spectrum varies from being asymptomatic identified incidentally on radiography to severe disability. It should be suspected in patients presenting with ipsilateral limb swelling in existing dialysis catheter. Many of them become symptomatic after the fistula creation because of the increased flow, worsens the venous hypertension and the patients develop the signs and symptoms of venous obstruction including incapacitating arm edema, ulceration, tissue loss, varicosity, and pain. The symptoms depend on the site of stenosis or obstruction. subclavian vein occlusions most commonly present with edema of the corresponding extremity and breast. Innominate vein stenosis or occlusion affects blood flow from the same side of the face as well as the upper extremity and breast. Patients with bilateral innominate vein obstruction presents such as superior vena caval syndrome with upper limb edema, facial puffiness, and neck engorgement. Some patients with severe edema are so symptomatic that they are unable to lie down and used to sleep in sitting posture. In extreme cases, patient can have cellulitis, gangrene, and ultimately amputation of the limb adding to severe disability.

DIAGNOSIS

The diagnosis of CVO requires both clinical and imaging findings. History of previous central venous catheter placement, with ipsilateral arm, breast, face, or neck swelling gives clue to the diagnosis. Many patients will have evidence of arteriovenous (AV) access dysfunction, with decreased access flows. Numerous dilated collaterals in the neck or chest and arm edema, on the side of the cardiovascular disease (CVD) on examination.

Duplex ultrasound is the initial modality used for diagnosing CVO. Absence of normal respiratory variation in the diameter of central veins and polyphasic atrial waves is diagnostic. Disadvantage of duplex ultrasound is that it is difficult to visualize the central veins with high body mass index or significant chest musculature. Digital subtraction central venography is the gold standard for the diagnosis of CVD, and is more sensitive than duplex ultrasound. Computed tomography (CT) venogram and magnetic resonance (MR) venogram also help in diagnosis, knowing lesion anatomy and procedural planning.

ENDOVASCULAR INTERVENTION

Endovascular intervention was first reported by Glanz et al. in 1984.[8] Percutaneous transluminal angioplasty (PTA) with or without stent implantation is currently the first line to treat the CVO because it is less invasive, safe and maintains the patency of vascular access, and relieves the symptoms. The PTA has demonstrated a variable technical success rate ranging from 70 to 90%.[8] The procedure failure is mainly related to inability to cross the long segments of total occlusion. Short-segment obstruction and focal restenosis can be managed with plain balloon angioplasty alone. Recoiling of the vessel is more commonly seen after the balloon angioplasty and the restenosis rate is also high with plain balloon angioplasty. Primary stent implantation has got the advantage of reducing the number of repeat interventions required for maintaining the patency. Both bare metal stents and recently covered stents are used. The primary patency rates at 3 months, 6 months, and 12 months in various studies were ranged between 65 and 95%, 54 and 90%, and 33 and 70%, respectively as shown in **Table 1**. The assisted patency rate varies between 85 and 100%. Following successful intervention, the limb edema resolved over 1 week in majority of the patients and facilitated the use of fistula for dialysis.

The recurrence of CVO following intervention usually occurs either due to intimal hyperplasia causing in-stent restenosis or progression of remote lesion. Stent fracture, foreshortening, and stent migration are the rare causes of restenosis.[9,10] Choosing the appropriate diameter of the stent and precise placement of the stent are important to prevent foreshortening and migration. The collapsing and expansion of the central veins during respiration may also facilitate both the stent shortening and stent migration.[9] Adequate predilatation, proper lesion assessment, and advising the patient to refrain from taking deep breaths at the time of stent deployment are very essential in preventing the stent migration and displacement.

Surgical options for CVD are associated with significant morbidity in patients with CVD and are a second-line treatment alternative in patient's refractory to percutaneous endovascular treatment options.

Our Experience

We have done endovascular intervention in 315 cases of central vein occlusions from January 2011 to May 2023. Technical success was achieved in about 94% of the patients during the index procedure. In 6% of cases, we failed to cross the lesion despite sharp recanalization techniques. Balloon angioplasty alone achieved satisfactory result in 66.5% of patients. In 33.5% patients, due to suboptimal result or long-segment total occlusion, we have used self-expanding stents. Primary patency rate in our experience is 85%, 70%, and 61% at 3 months, 6 months, and 1 year, respectively. Assisted

TABLE 1: Comparison of stent patency rates in various studies.

Study	Total patients	Repeat procedures	Technical success	3-month stent patency rates		6-month stent patency rates		1-year stent patency rates	
				Primary	Assisted	Primary	Assisted	Primary	Assisted
Haage et al. (1999)	50	73 with 19 additional stents	NA	92%	NA	84%	97%	56%	97%
Vogel et al. (2004)	15	NA	NA	81%	NA	74%	NA	67%	NA
Aytekin et al. (2004)	14	22 repeats in 9 pts	100%	85.7%	88.8%	50%	55.5%	14.3%	33.3%
Christiduo et al. (2006)	22	17 stents in 13	95.4%	88.3%	95.4%	65.3%	79%	45.6%	74%
Bakken et al. (2007)	26	17 stents in 10 of 13 repeat procedure patients	96%	65%	72%	54%	55%	45%	46%
Ozyer et al. (2009)	43	80 repeat procedures	NA	85%	98%	68%	91%	33%	67%
Kim YC et al. (2009)	15	14 patients	NA	NA	NA	NA	NA	46.7%	60%
Shi Ya-xue (2013)	11	NA	83.3%	NA	NA	90%	NA	77%	83.3%
Our experience	315	105	94%	85%	100%	70%	94%	61%	86%

patency rate are 100%, 95%, and 86% at 3 months, 6 months, and 1 year, respectively. Limb edema resolved rapidly over next 2–5 days in majority of patients. Some of them needed intensive dialysis to remove the fluid shifted from third space to intravascular compartment over the next 1–2 weeks.

PROCEDURAL STEPS IN THE PERCUTANEOUS INTERVENTION OF CENTRAL VENOUS OCCLUSIONS

Several key points that can help during the procedure and improve the success and patency rates are as follows:

- Lesion anatomy using appropriate imaging techniques such as CT venography, MR venography, or conventional venogram helps in planning the procedure such as the venous access, the size, and number of stents required.
- Vascular access is important as the coaxial approach using the antegrade puncture of brachial, cephalic, axillary vein, subclavian vein, and external or internal jugular vein can facilitate the lesion crossing, which is the most important step for successful intervention **(Figs. 1A to F)**. The antegrade puncture can be performed successfully by the using fluoroscopic guidance during levophase of brachial artery angiogram and by feeling the engorged veins with bruit. The knowledge and the use of both the antegrade and retrograde approach can increase the success rate.
- There are two ways of crossing the lesion—(1) blunt and (2) sharp recanalization methods. For simple lesions, Terumo hydrophilic wire along with angled catheter with slow drilling can be used to cross lesions which is called blunt recanalization.
- In case of resistant tough lesion either the hard end of the guidewire, TIPS needle or occasionally Brockenbrough septal puncture needle can be used **(Figs. 2A to D)**. This method is called sharp recanalization. Recently, power wire devices and radiofrequency ablation using electrified wires can be used to cross tough lesions.
- Always create a venovenous loop as the lesions are usually hard with extensive fibrosis. The loop will provide adequate support to push the balloon and the stent across the lesions.
- The lesions should be adequately predilated.
- We recommend that primary stent deployment should be done in all cases because the stent will prevent the recoil by providing effective mechanical support. The various studies including our study have shown better follow-up patency rates when stents are used. Also, if the restenosis occurs, the stent can act as roadmap for the intervention.
- The choice of stent is also important. The central veins in these patients are tortuous and have larger diameter making the self-expandable stents more suitable for these patients. The stent shortening and movement should be carefully seen and the missed lesion should be covered by the additional stent if required.
- Bilateral innominate vein occlusion treated with simultaneous kissing balloon angioplasty using self-expanding stents **(Figs. 2A to D)**.
- Immediate resolution of limb swelling, facial puffiness can be noted before discharge and on follow-up **(Figs. 3A to D)**.
- Complications such as venous perforation or rupture **(Figs. 2A to D)** do occur during predilatation and can be managed with prolonged balloon dilatation with or

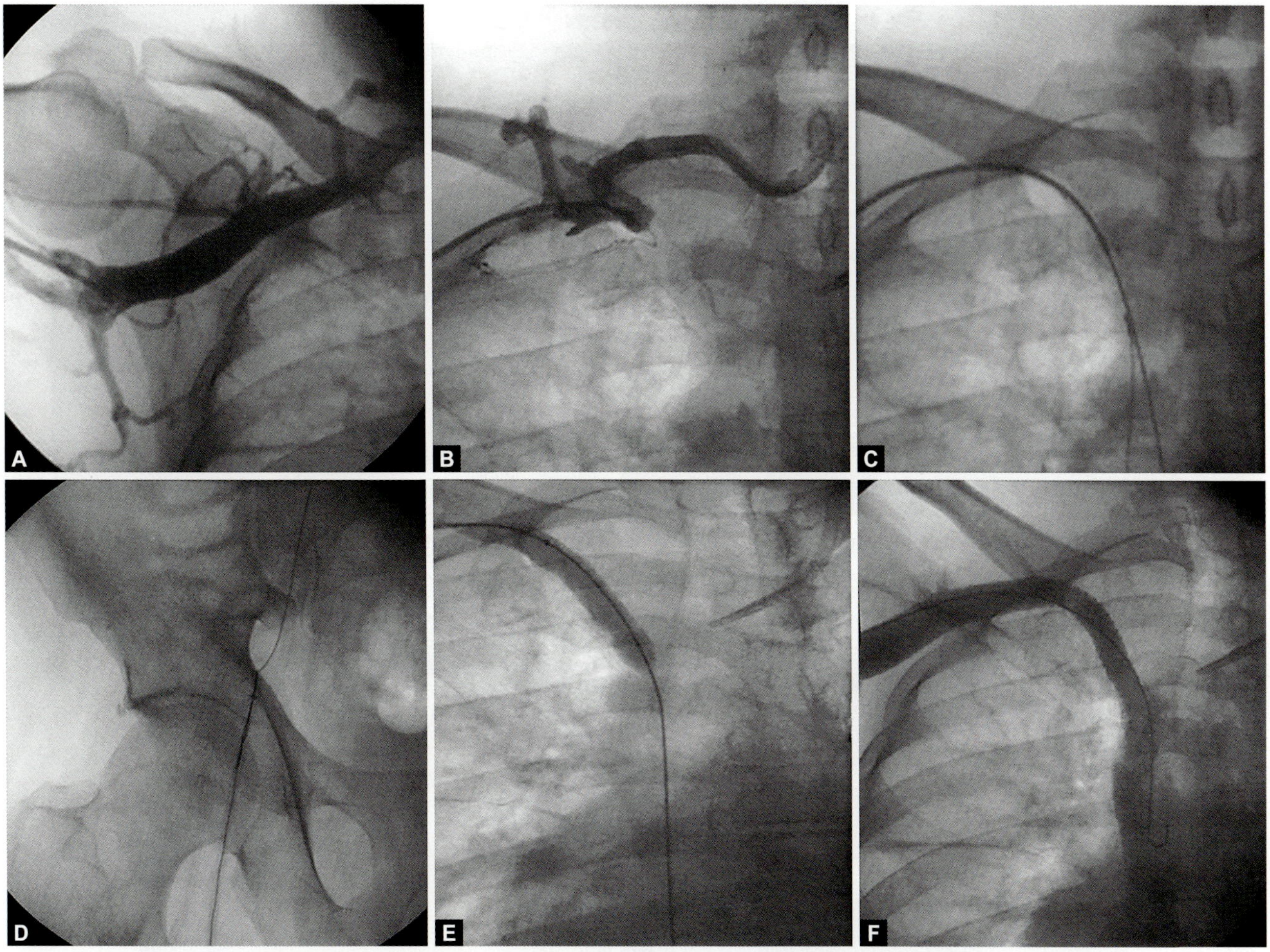

FIGS. 1A TO F: Brachial artery injection in levophase showed subclavian vein total occlusion—(A) accessing the Axillary vein by antegrade puncture technique. (B) Attempt to cross the lesion with multipurpose catheter and straight Terumo Assembly, the lesion is hard. (C) Finally, we crossed the lesion with same assembly. (D) Wire was snared from the right femoral vein, thereby creating the venovenous loop. (E) Lesion was predilated with 8 × 40 mm peripheral balloon. (F) Final result after deployment of 10 × 60 mm self-expanding nitinol stent and poststenting dilatation.

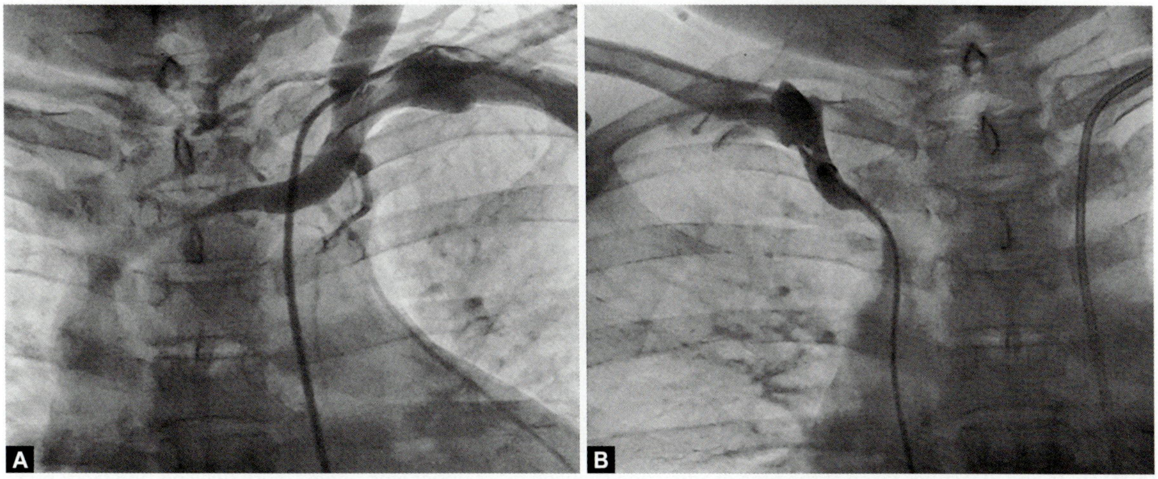

FIGS. 2A TO D: *Continued*

Continued

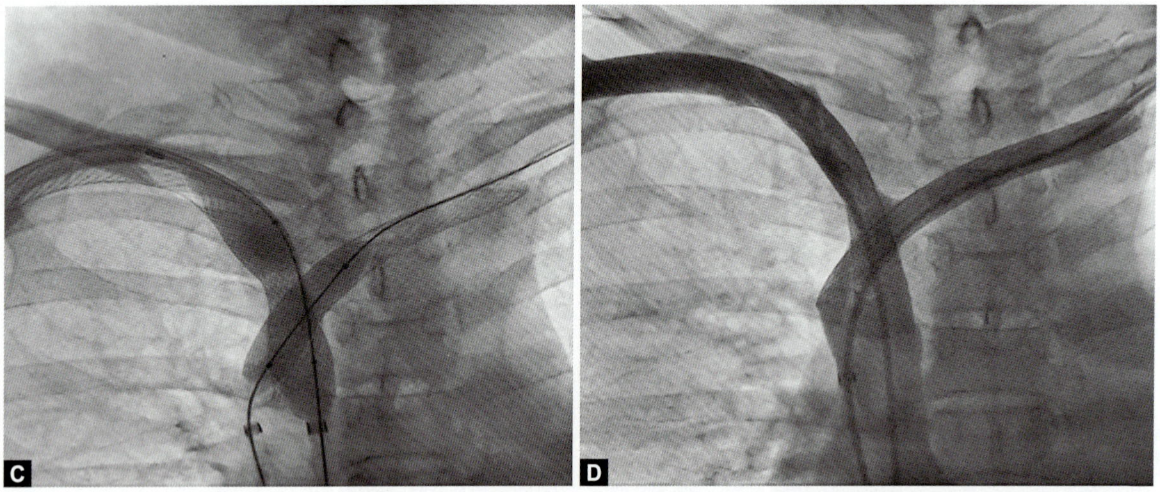

FIGS. 2A TO D: Simultaneous kissing balloon angioplasty done pre- and poststenting in bilateral innominate vein occlusions.

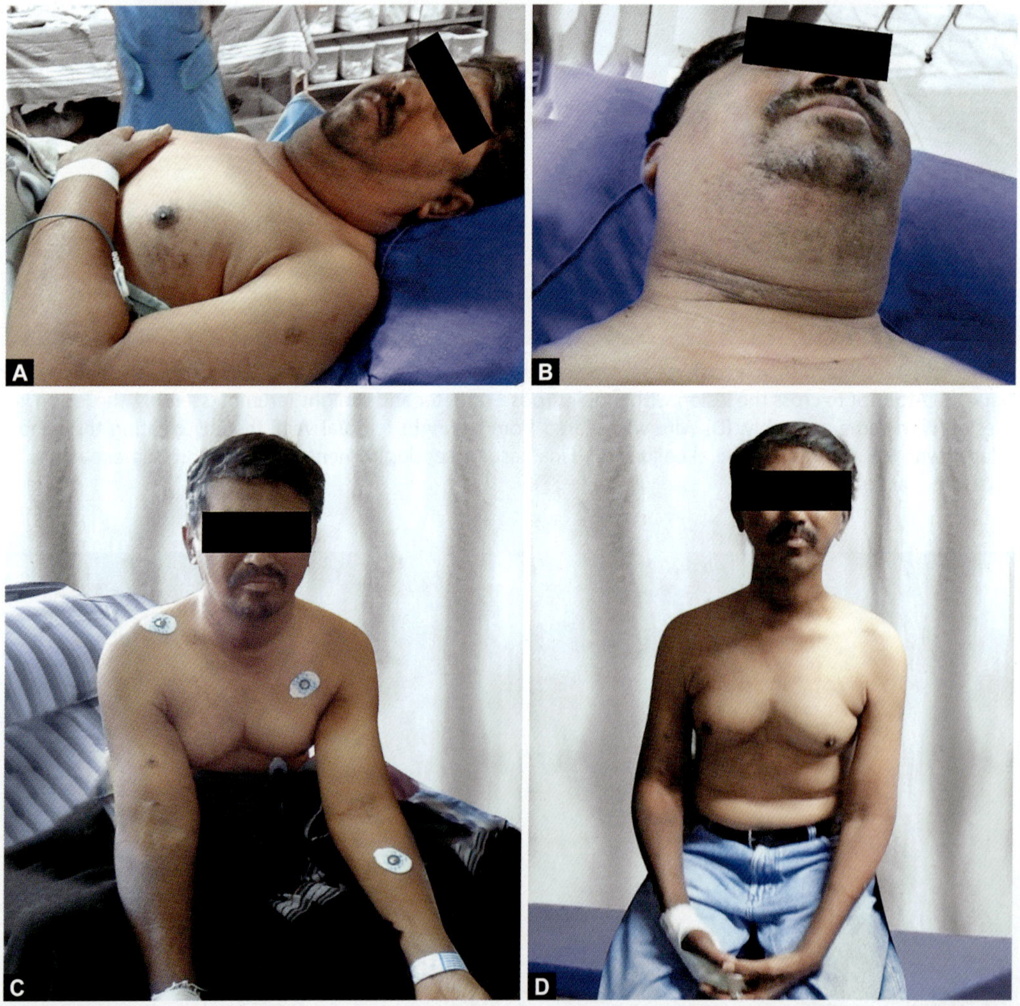

FIGS. 3A TO D: (A and B) Pictures taken at the time of admission showing gross upper limb edema, neck swelling, and facial puffiness, (C) at discharge, (D) 1-month follow-up.

without stenting, urgent pericardiocentesis, and autologous blood transfusion as in our case **(Figs. 4A to M)**.

- The importance of the patience, perseverance, and knowing different approaches cannot be underestimated in these cases.

The covered stents and the drug-eluting stents are under evaluation and may be helpful for reducing the restenosis rates in this subset of patients.

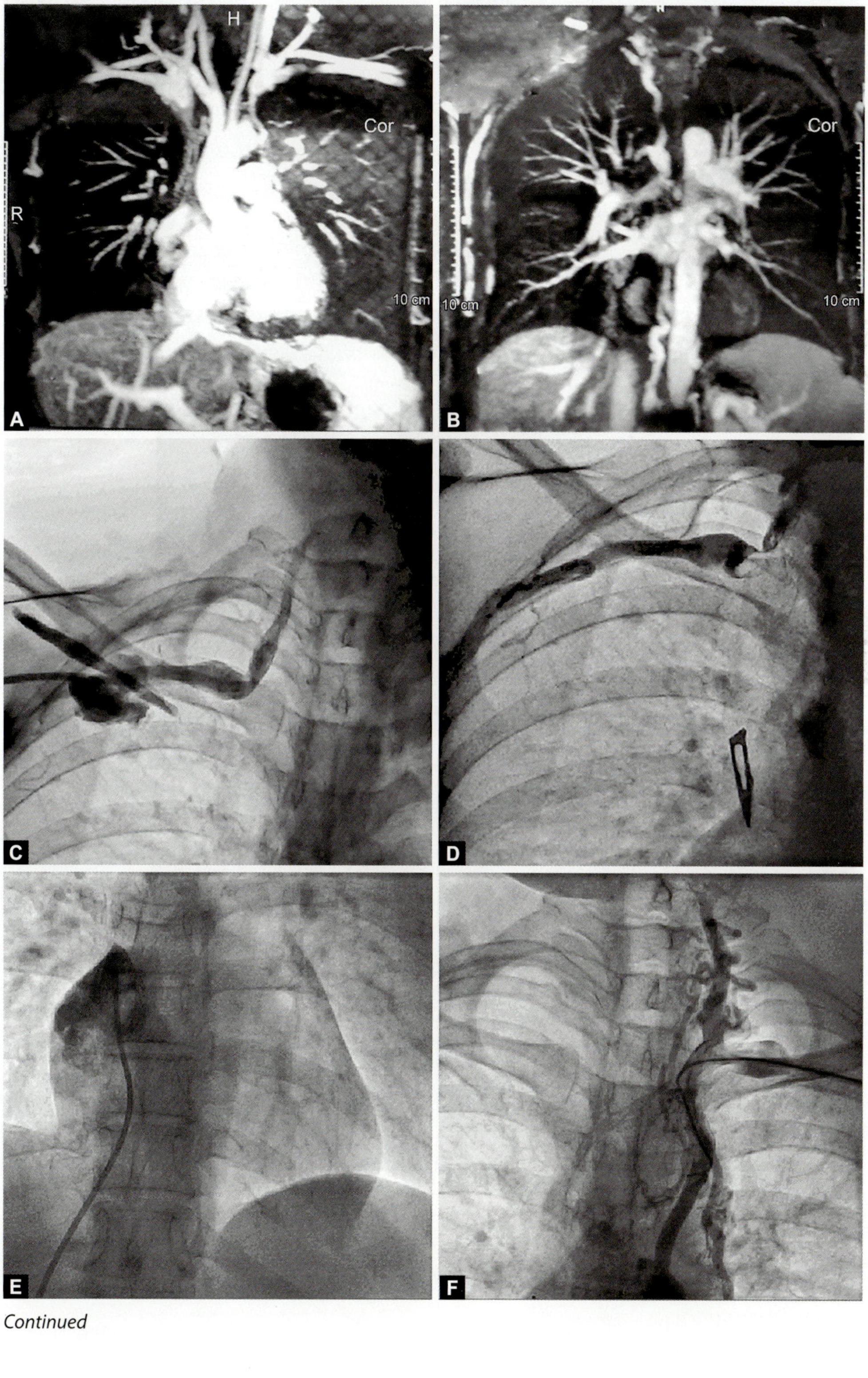

FIGS. 4A TO M: *Continued*

Continued

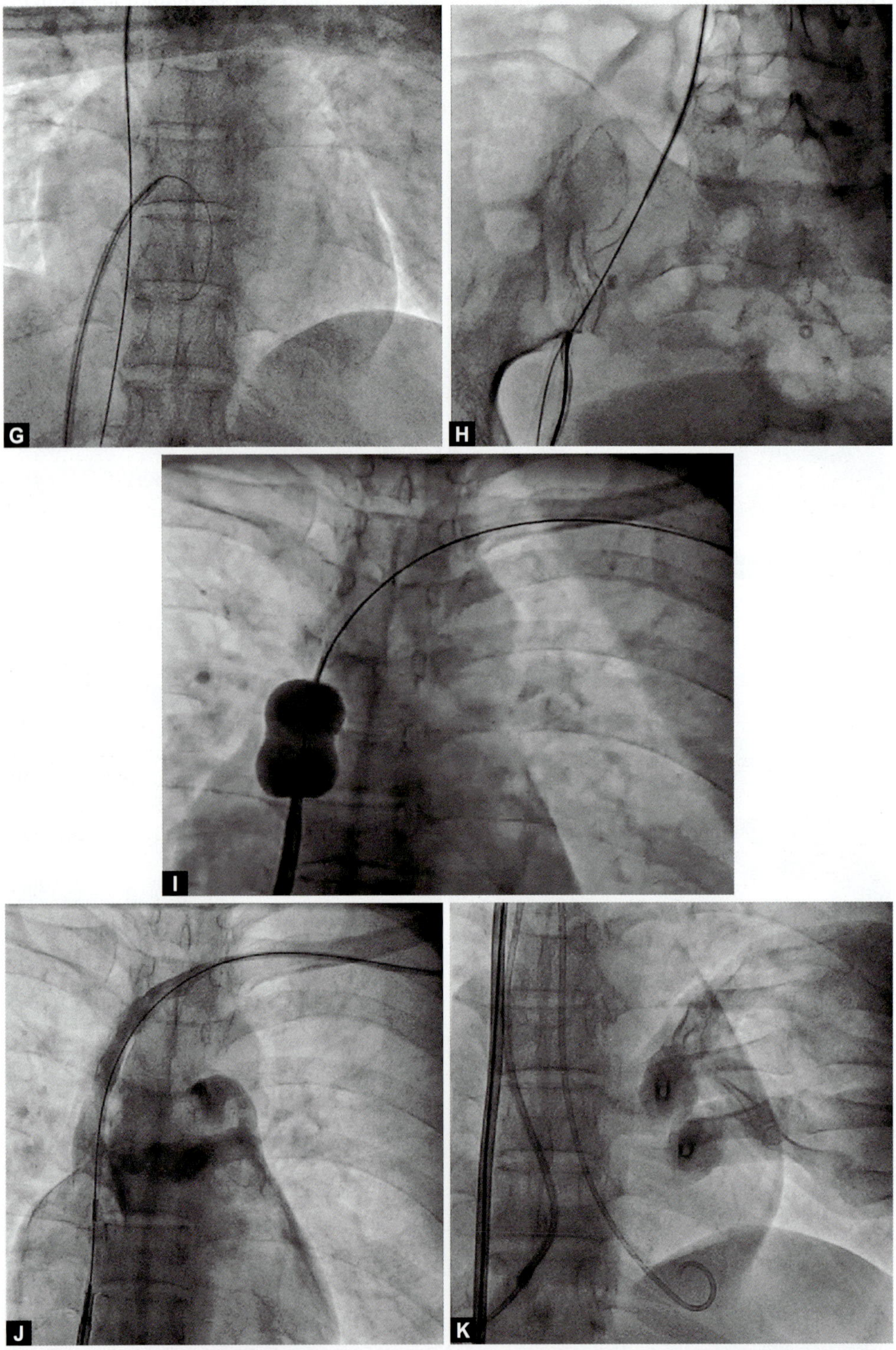

FIGS. 4A TO M: *Continued*

Continued

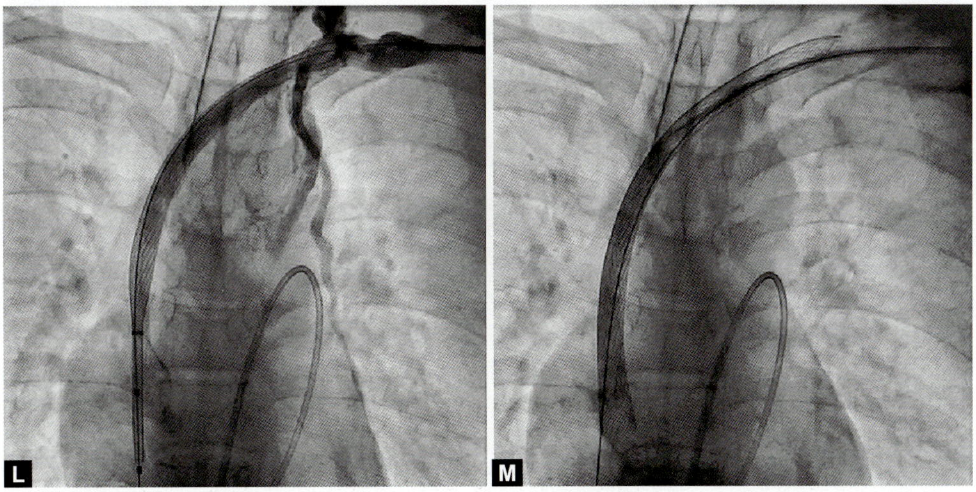

FIGS. 4A TO M: (A and B) CT venogram showing SVC occlusion with significant collaterals. (C and D) Contrast injection by subclavian venous and right internal jugular vein showed occlusion of SVC. (E) Contrast injection by multipurpose catheter at right atrium with SVC obstruction showed proximal extent of obstruction. (F) Trying to cross via left subclavian venous approach. (G and H) Terumo wire crossed by loop method from left subclavian vein and snared through right femoral vein using goose neck snare. (I) Predilatation using 22-mm accura balloon. (J) SVC rupture leading to large pericardial effusion. (K) Pigtail in situ, with simultaneous aspiration and autotransfusion done. (L and M) 8 × 60 mm wall stent deployed and perforation sealed.

ENDOVASCULAR MANAGEMENT OF IVC AND HEPATIC VENOUS OBSTRUCTION

Inferior vena cava obstruction results from thrombosis secondary to hypercoagulable disorders, extrinsic compression by tumors, infective phlebitis, inflammation, trauma, surgery or in many number of cases, and idiopathic. Budd–Chiari syndrome is a heterogeneous group of disorders resulting in obstruction of hepatic venous outflow from the level of hepatic venules, main hepatic veins (HVs) to suprahepatic IVC till IVC-right atrial (RA) junction.[11,12] Okuda in 2001 emphasized that the classic hepatic venous outflow obstruction (HVOO) also called hepatic vein thrombosis (HVT) and membranous obstruction of vena cava (MVOC) are epidemiologically, pathologically, and clinically different and should be treated as two different clinical entities.

Membrane such as obstruction found angiographically is found to consist of organized old thrombus arranged in layers of different ages. The clinical onset is mild and causes liver damage by congestion. A distinct pattern of subcutaneous venous collaterals typically develops together with retroperitoneal collaterals through the ascending lumbar and the iliolumbar veins into the hemiazygos and azygos veins (Fig.). In longstanding cases, it results in swelling of extremities, pain, venous ulceration, ascites, impaired liver, and renal functions. The course of the disease can be confused with other causes of cirrhosis and portal hypertension.

DIAGNOSIS

Established by high clinical suspicion and physical findings. CT angiography helps in understanding the lesion characteristics including the thrombus at the lesion site.

Treatment of IVC obstruction includes:

- Surgical (direct visualization of obstruction and removal or venous bypass grafts)
- Interventional (balloon dilatation ± stenting)

The decision of stenting the IVC is often individualized. However, it is particularly useful in the following cases:

- Long segment of obstruction or multiple segments of obstruction
- Restenosis after balloon angioplasty
- Enlarged caudate lobe of liver or extrinsic tumor compression on IVC (e.g., hepatoma).

In cases with associated HV obstruction (all three HVs), angioplasty and stent implantation of the HV lesion are performed in the same setting or sometimes staged 1–2 weeks later. HV occlusion is approached mostly from the right jugular vein. Once the lesion is crossed with guidewire, balloon angioplasty is performed with 6–8 mm × 30 mm balloon. These lesions are primarily stented using either balloon expandable stents or self-expandable stents **(Figs. 5A to D)**. If the lesion cannot be crossed from the IVC end, ultrasound-guided percutaneous puncture of HVs is performed to enter into the HVs. This approach facilitates crossing the HV occlusion, as the lesion becomes nearer and coaxial. Once, the lesion is crossed, guidewire is

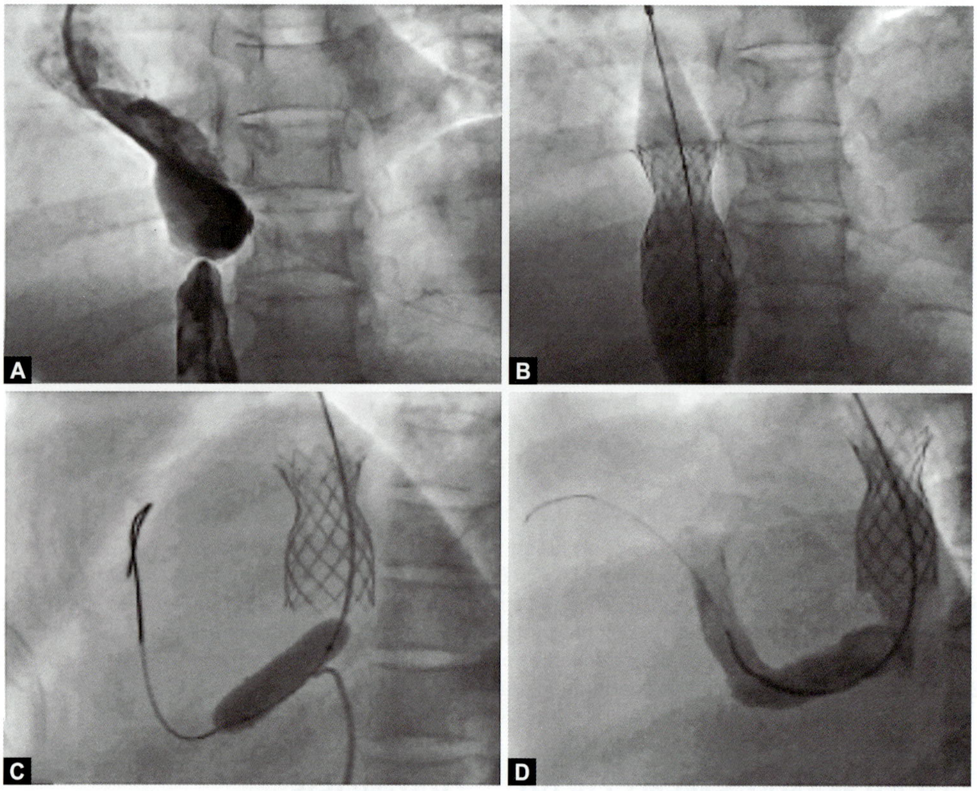

FIGS. 5A TO D: Intervention in a case of combined inferior vena cava (IVC) and hepatic vein (HV) obstruction. (A and B) Initially IVC is intervened and balloon dilatation and stenting done from femoral vein approach. (C) Next HV is approached through IJV and intervened and stented. (D) Final result reveal patent IVC and hepatic vein.

snared from the jugular or femoral venous approach and balloon angioplasty and stent implantation is performed. Subsequently, the track through the hepatic parenchyma is closed with coil or gel foam to prevent bleeding.

CONCLUSION

Central venous occlusion is an important cause of dialysis failure in CKD patients on maintenance hemodialysis. Repetitive/prolonged central vein catheterization predisposes to CVO. Balloon angioplasty with or without stent implantation has shown good procedural outcomes, however, high restenosis rate in intermediate and long-term which necessitates repetitive reinterventions. Endovascular management is technically challenging and demanding including sharp recanalization techniques in up to one-third of cases. Maintaining central vein access facilitates long-term dialysis. Long-term outcomes are determined by associated comorbidities.

Balloon angioplasty and stent implantation are safe and effective in relieving IVC and HV obstruction with minimal morbidity whenever anatomy is suitable.

ONLINE REFERENCES

Please scan the QR code provided at the end of the table of contents for References of this chapter.

CHAPTER

203

Takayasu Arteritis: An Overview

Syed Imamuddin

ABSTRACT

Takayasu arteritis is a condition characterized by granulomatous inflammation affecting large blood vessels, primarily the aorta, its proximal branches, and the pulmonary arteries. This inflammatory process can lead to various vascular abnormalities, including stenosis, occlusion, dilation, or the formation of aneurysms.[1] Uncontrolled progression of Takayasu arteritis could result in crippling morbidities such as stroke, blindness, refractory hypertension, heart failure, and death.

Keywords: Heart, inflammation, Takayasu arteritis, vasculitis.

INTRODUCTION

The history of Takayasu arteritis dates back to the early 20th century when it was first described by Dr Mikito Takayasu, a Japanese ophthalmologist. In 1908, Dr Takayasu reported a case of a young female patient with unusual retinal findings and absent radial pulses as "a case of peculiar changes in the central retinal vessels".[2] He recognized the systemic nature of the disease, involving large arteries beyond the ophthalmic vessels. He published his observations in the Japanese medical literature, coining the term "aortitis syndrome" to describe the condition.

In 1948, Shimizu and Sano coined this pathological condition "pulseless disease." Since then, the disease has been recognized to involve not only the aortic arch and its primary branches but also various other arteries throughout the body. Lesions associated with Takayasu arteritis have been detected in vessels such as the abdominal aorta and renal arteries, highlighting the systemic nature of the disease. In the following years, more cases of this rare disease were reported in Japan and other parts of the world. In the 1950s, the name "Takayasu arteritis" was established to honor Dr Takayasu's pioneering work in recognizing and characterizing the condition.[3]

INCIDENCE AND PREVALENCE

Even though the disease is widespread throughout the world, Takayasu arteritis is known to exhibit significant variations in its prevalence across different populations. Higher prevalence rates have been observed in the Asian population, with Japan reporting the highest known prevalence of approximately 40 cases per million. In contrast, the United States has reported the lowest known frequency, with an estimated prevalence of 0.9 cases per million.[4] Based on a recent systematic review, the prevalence of Takayasu arteritis has been reported to range from 3.2 to 40.0 cases per million worldwide. Similarly, the annual incidence has been estimated to be between 0.4 and 2.6 cases per million.[5] It is more frequently observed in women, presenting up to 90% of cases in adults; however, a series on childhood Takayasu arteritis have shown variable female/male ratios: 6.9:1 in Mexico, 4.3:1 in Korea, 3.2:1 in the USA, 2.8:1 in Turkey, 1.9:1 in India, 1.7:1 in South Africa, and 1.2:1 in Israel. Mortality rates in children with Takayasu arteritis have been reported up to 35%.[6]

WHY IS TAKAYASU ARTERITIS LABELED AS PULSELESS DISEASE?

In Takayasu arteritis, the affected blood vessels experience ongoing and continuous inflammation, resulting in the development of narrow areas (stenotic lesions) and the formation of aneurysms. Consequently, the affected tissue receives inadequate blood flow, leading to reduced perfusion. Due to this characteristic, Takayasu arteritis has been labeled as the "pulseless disease."

During the initial acute phase, which is alternatively referred to as the prepulseless or active inflammatory stage, there is a noticeable thickening of the aortic wall. This thickening can occur with or without changes in the arterial lumen, indicating the presence of inflammation. In the subsequent phase of the disease, referred to as the chronic pulseless phase or sclerotic phase, the ongoing inflammatory process becomes more apparent. This is characterized by the development of granulomas, which are composed of macrophages, epithelioid cells, and giant cells. In the final stage, known as the pulseless end-stage sclerotic phase, notable changes occur in the arterial lumen. This phase is characterized by stenosis observed in 90–100% of patients, along with occurrences of occlusion or thrombosis, atypical coarctation, dilation, and/or aneurysms.[7]

DIAGNOSTIC CRITERIA

Takayasu arteritis is often suspected based on certain clinical manifestations, including hypertension, vascular bruits, asymmetrical blood pressure between limbs, or uneven arterial pulses in the extremities. Patients may also experience accompanying symptoms such as fever, malaise, or musculoskeletal issues. Laboratory tests during active disease phases may reveal elevated acute-phase proteins, although sometimes results may appear normal.

The definitive diagnosis of Takayasu arteritis relies on visualizing lesions in the aorta or its major branches. Therefore, a comprehensive evaluation of the entire aorta and its primary branches, including cranial vessels (regardless of the presence of neurological symptoms), should be performed. Moreover, other causes of aortic and large-vessel involvement ought to be excluded. The differential diagnoses of Takayasu arteritis include congenital disorders (such as aortic coarctation, Marfan syndrome, and fibromuscular dysplasia), other primary vasculitides, and secondary vasculitides (both infectious and autoimmune).[8,9]

In 1988, Ishikawa proposed the initial diagnostic criteria for Takayasu arteritis, which included an obligatory criterion of age <40 years at the time of diagnosis or onset of characteristic symptoms/signs.[10] In 1995, modifications **(Table 1)** to the Ishikawa diagnostic criteria were put forward, which removed the age criterion, thus increased the sensitivity and specificity to 92.5% and 95%, respectively.[11]

TABLE 1: Modified Ishikawa criteria for diagnosis of Takayasu arteritis.[11]

Brief description	
Major criteria:	
Left midsubclavian artery lesion	Most severe obstruction between points 1 cm proximal and 3 cm distal to the left vertebral artery ostium
Right midsubclavian artery lesion	Most severe obstruction between the right vertebral artery ostium and a point 3 cm distal to it
Characteristic signs and symptoms of at least 1-month duration	Limb claudication, pulselessness or pulse differences in limbs, unobtainable BP or systolic BP difference 10 mm Hg in limb, fever, neck pain, transient amaurosis, blurred vision, syncope, dyspnea, or palpitations
Minor criteria:	
High ESR	Unexplained ESR >20 mm/h at diagnosis or evidence in patient's history
Carotid artery tenderness	Unilateral or bilateral common carotid artery tenderness
Hypertension	Persistent BP >140/90 mm Hg brachial/>160/90 popliteal
Aortic regurgitation or annuloaortic ectasia	By auscultation, Doppler/2-dimensional echocardiography, or angiography
Pulmonary artery lesion	Lobar or segmental arterial occlusion on angiography or perfusion scintigraphy, or presence of stenosis aneurysm, luminal irregularity on angiography
Left mid common carotid lesion	Most severe obstruction in the 5-cm length from a point 2 cm distal to its ostium
Brachiocephalic trunk lesion	Most severe obstruction in the distal third
Descending thoracic aorta lesion	Narrowing, dilation or aneurysm, luminal irregularity: tortuosity alone is unacceptable
Abdominal aorta lesion	Narrowing, dilation or aneurysm, and luminal irregularity
Coronary artery lesion	Documented before the age of 30 years, absence of risk factors such as hyperlipidemia or diabetes mellitus

Note: The presence of two major or one major and two minor or four minor criteria suggests a high probability of Takayasu arteritis.

(BP: blood pressure; ESR: erythrocyte sedimentation rate)

CLINICAL FEATURES

Takayasu arteritis presents with a wide spectrum of manifestations, varying from asymptomatic cases, where the condition is incidentally discovered due to impalpable pulses or bruits, to severe neurological impairments. The disease progression is often described as a two-stage process. The initial "prepulseless" phase is characterized by nonspecific inflammatory features, which may include systemic symptoms. This is followed by a chronic phase where vascular insufficiency develops, sometimes accompanied by intermittent disease flares.[12] The disease typically manifests during the second or third decade of life, and it is not uncommon to be a significant delay in diagnosis from the onset of initial symptoms. This delay can range from months to even years before the condition is properly recognized and diagnosed.

Nonspecific features of Takayasu arteritis include fever, night sweats, malaise, weight loss, arthralgia, myalgia, and mild anemia.[12] With the progress of inflammation and development of stenoses, more characteristic features become apparent, influenced by the development of collateral circulation.[9]

Characteristic features of Takayasu arteritis:[9]

- Diminished or absent pulses associated with limb claudication and blood pressure discrepancies
- Vascular bruits, often multiple, and particularly affecting the carotids, subclavian, and abdominal vessels
- Hypertension, generally reflecting renal artery stenosis
- Takayasu retinopathy
- Aortic regurgitation resulting from dilatation of the ascending aorta, separation of the valve leaflets, and valve thickening
- Congestive cardiac failure associated with hypertension, aortic regurgitation, and dilated cardiomyopathy
- Neurological features secondary to hypertension and/or ischemia, including postural dizziness, seizures, and amaurosis
- Other symptoms include dyspnea, headaches, carotidynia, myocardial ischemia, chest wall pain, and erythema nodosum.

However, clinical features may vary depending on stage of the disease and involvement of particular vascular regions. **Table 2** outlines clinical manifestations of Takayasu arteritis according to vascular region involved.

TABLE 2: Clinical manifestations of Takayasu arteritis according to vascular region involved.

Symptoms and signs	
General:	
Constitutional symptoms	Fatigue, low-grade fever, night sweats, and weight loss >2 kg
Other symptoms of active disease	Myalgia, arthralgia, arthritis, and abdominal pain
Vascular involvement	Weak or missing pulses, vascular bruit, and vascular tenderness
Specific:	
Carotid arteries	Dizziness, amaurosis fugax, vision loss, transient ischemic attacks, and stroke
Subclavian arteries	Arm claudication, inter-arm blood pressure difference > 10 mm Hg. Proximal subclavian obstruction can cause subclavian steal
Vertebral arteries	Stenosis/occlusion can cause vertigo or contribute to cerebral ischemic symptoms when multiple arch branches are obstructed
Ascending and arch of aorta	Aortic regurgitation due to aortic dilation, aneurysm, and rarely aorta stenosis
Descending aorta	Systemic hypertension, dyspnea, and heart failure due to aorta stenosis and aneurysm
Abdominal aorta	Systemic hypertension, lower limb claudication, and aneurysm
Renal arteries	Systemic hypertension and renal failure
Mesenteric arteries	Postprandial abdominal pain, weight loss, sitophobia, gastrointestinal hemorrhage
Iliac and femoral arteries	Lower limb claudication or fatigue
Coronary arteries	Angina, heart failure, and myocardial infarction
Pulmonary arteries	Dyspnea, cough, chest pain, and pulmonary hypertension

PATHOPHYSIOLOGY

Takayasu arteritis is characterized by the presence of advanced lesions that exhibit panarteritis with intimal proliferation. The inflammatory process gives rise to a variety of vascular lesions, which can be stenotic, occlusive, or aneurysmal in nature. It is important to note that aneurysmal lesions may also feature areas of arterial narrowing. These vascular changes contribute to several significant complications associated with Takayasu arteritis. Hypertension is a common complication, primarily resulting from renal artery stenosis, or less frequently, stenosis of the suprarenal aorta. Aortic valve involvement can lead to aortic insufficiency, while pulmonary hypertension and the development of aortic or arterial aneurysms are also observed. Congestive heart failure is frequently encountered in Takayasu arteritis, whereas dilated cardiomyopathy, myocarditis, and pericarditis have been reported but are less prevalent.[13]

In the chronic phase of Takayasu arteritis, macroscopic examination reveals thickening of the aorta due to fibrosis affecting all three layers of the vessel. The narrowing of the lumen occurs in a patchy pattern, often affecting multiple areas. In cases where the disease progresses rapidly, insufficient fibrosis may lead to the formation of aneurysms. The intima of the affected vessels may display a ridged appearance resembling "tree bark," a characteristic feature shared by several types of aortitis.[14]

Microscopically, Takayasu arteritis exhibits distinct histopathological features that can be categorized into two phases: (1) the acute florid inflammatory phase and (2) the healed fibrotic phase. During the acute phase, vasa vasorum, characterized by inflammation in the adventitia, can be observed. The media of the affected vessels shows infiltration of lymphocytes and occasional giant cells, accompanied by neovascularization. The intima thickens due to the accumulation of mucopolysaccharides, smooth muscle cells, and fibroblasts. In the chronic phase, fibrosis occurs, leading to the destruction of elastic tissue. It is important to note that similar histopathological findings can be observed in giant cell arteritis, making it challenging to differentiate between these two vasculitis conditions based solely on biopsy results. However, the clinical manifestations experienced by the patient often provide crucial information for the accurate diagnosis of Takayasu arteritis.[15]

CLASSIFICATION

The first clinical classification of Takayasu arteritis based on vessel involvement was proposed in 1978 by Ishikawa which was based on 96 patients aged <30 years.[16] Later in 1990, a new classification criterion was developed and published by the American College of Rheumatology (ACR) to simplify the clinical diagnosis. Six criteria were selected for the traditional classification: onset at age <40 years, claudication of an extremity, decreased brachial artery pulse, >10 mm Hg difference in systolic blood pressure between arms, a bruit over the subclavian arteries or the aorta, and arteriographic evidence of narrowing or occlusion of the entire aorta, its primary branches, or large arteries in the proximal upper or lower extremities.[17]

In 2007, the Pediatric Rheumatology European Society proposed consensus criteria for classifying various subtypes of vasculitis in children, including Takayasu arteritis. These criteria were later supported by the European League Against Rheumatism (EULAR).[18,19] According to these criteria, the diagnosis of childhood Takayasu arteritis requires the presence of angiographic abnormalities along with at least one of the following indicators: reduced peripheral artery pulses or claudication of extremities, a blood pressure difference exceeding 10 mm Hg, the presence of bruits over the aorta or its major branches, or hypertension **(Fig. 1)**.

Recently, the ACR/EULAR has endorsed a classification criteria for Takayasu arteritis in 2022 **(Table 3)**. This classification has been validated for use in research.[21]

PECULIARITIES OF TAKAYASU ARTERITIS IN INDIAN SUBSET

Although more prevalent in young women (with a male-to-female ratio of 1:8) and typically manifesting between the ages of 25 and 30, Takayasu's arteritis is recognized as a significant contributor to renovascular hypertension in India.[22] In Japan, the condition tends to affect the aortic arch more frequently, while Indian and Korean patients commonly exhibit greater involvement of the abdominal aorta.[23]

The new angiographic classification of Takayasu's arteritis, established during the Takayasu conference in 1994, reveals that Japanese patients primarily experience involvement of the aortic arch and its branches, categorized as type I and IIa. However, determining the most prevalent type in India has been a subject of controversy. Some authors suggest it is type IV, while others argue in favor of type V.[24,25] Nonetheless, a recent retrospective study has provided clarity by demonstrating that type V is indeed the

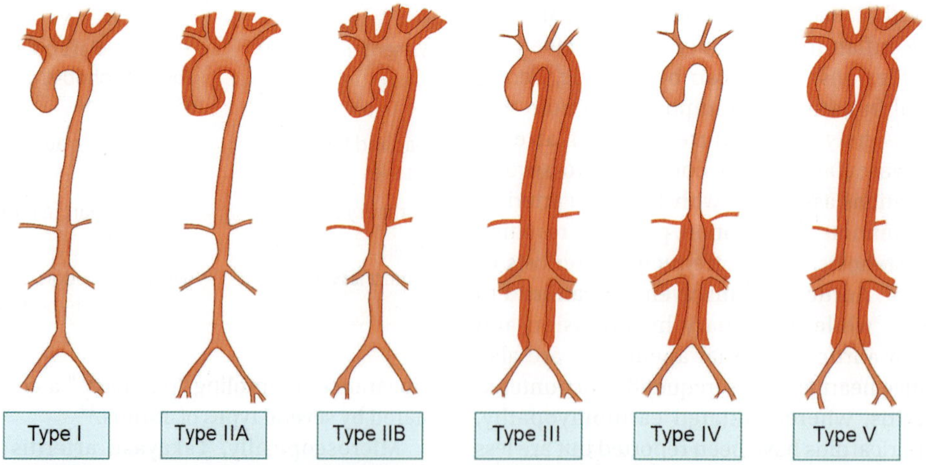

Type I	Branches from the aortic arch
Type IIA	Ascending aorta, aortic arch and its branches
Type IIB	Ascending aorta, aortic arch and its branches, thoracic descending aorta
Type III	Thoracic descending, aorta, abdominal aorta, and/or renal arteries
Type IV	Abdominal aorta and/or renal arteries
Type V	Combined features of types IIb and IV

FIG. 1: Classification of Takayasu arteritis and distribution of the cases for each type.[20]

TABLE 3: The 2022 American College of Rheumatology/EULAR classification criteria for Takayasu arteritis.[21]

Considerations when applying these criteria:	
• These classification criteria should be applied to classify the patient as having Takayasu arteritis when a diagnosis of medium-vessel or large-vessel vasculitis has been made	
• Alternate diagnoses mimicking vasculitis should be excluded prior to applying the criteria	
Absolute requirements:	
• Age ≤ 60 years at time of diagnosis	
• Evidence of vasculitis on imaging[1]	
Additional clinical criteria:	
• Female sex	+1
• Angina or ischemic cardiac pain	+2
• Arm or leg claudication	+2
• Vascular bruit[2]	+2
• Reduced pulse in upper extremity[3]	+2
• Carotid artery abnormality[4]	+2
• Systolic blood pressure difference in arms ≥ 20 mm Hg	+1
Additional imaging criteria:	
• Number of affected arterial territories (select one):[5]	
○ One arterial territory	+1
○ Two arterial territories	+2
○ Three or more arterial territories	+3
• Symmetric involvement of paired arteries[6]	+1
• Abdominal aorta involvement with renal or mesenteric involvement[7]	+3
Sum the scores for 10 items, if present. A score of ≥ 5 points is needed for the classification of Takayasu arteritis	

1.	Evidence of vasculitis in the aorta or branch arteries must be confirmed by vascular imaging (e.g., computed tomographic/catheter-based/magnetic resonance angiography, ultrasound, and positron emission tomography)	5.	Number of arterial territories with luminal damage (e.g., stenosis, occlusion, or aneurysm) detected by angiography or ultrasonography from the following nine territories: thoracic aorta, abdominal aorta, mesenteric, left or right carotid, left or right subclavian, left or right renal arteries
2.	Bruit detected by auscultation of a large artery, including the aorta, carotid, subclavian, axillary, brachial, renal, or iliofemoral arteries	6.	Bilateral luminal damage (stenosis, occlusion, or aneurysm) detected by angiography or ultrasonography in any of the following paired vascular territories: carotid, subclavian, or renal arteries
3.	Reduction or absence of pulse by physical examination of the axillary, brachial, or radial arteries	7.	Luminal damage (stenosis, occlusion, and aneurysm) detected by angiography or ultrasonography involving the abdominal aorta and either the renal or mesenteric arteries.
4.	Reduction or absence of pulse of the carotid artery or tenderness of the carotid artery		

(EULAR: European League Against Rheumatism)

most common classification observed in India.[26] In South-East Asia and Africa, the prevailing type is type III, which is often referred to as "middle aortic syndrome".

There is a causal association between Takayasu's arteritis and tuberculosis (TB). One key factor of interest is a 65-kDa heat shock protein (HSP), which is an immunogenic component of *Mycobacterium tuberculosis*. It has been observed that the expression of HSP is significantly increased in aortic tissue, potentially due to molecular mimicry. This suggests that antibodies produced in response to bacterial HSP exposure in the human host might cross-react with the human homologue of HSP-65, which is present on the surface of stressed endothelial cells. This interaction with endothelial HSP could trigger an immune response that plays a role in the development of Takayasu arteritis lesions.[27,28] Moreover, a notable and robust positive reaction to tuberculin, along with the results of multiple tests assessing cell-mediated immunity (CMI), provides further evidence of exaggerated T-cell responses in individuals with Takayasu's arteritis.[29]

EVOLUTION OF MARKERS IN TAKAYASU ARTERITIS

The absence of specific laboratory tests or validated biomarkers for Takayasu arteritis poses a challenge in clinical practice and research settings. It is noteworthy that around one-third of patients do not exhibit elevated inflammatory markers upon initial evaluation. Monitoring disease progression often relies on nonimaging tests such as erythrocyte sedimentation rate (ESR) and C-reactive protein (CRP), which are considered essential acute phase reactants.[6]

Studies report that patients with active disease had higher ESR and CRP levels as compared with patients with stable/inactive disease (ESR: 5–115 mm/h vs. 1–43 mm/h and CRP: 0.1–99.1 mg/dL vs. 0.06–7.77 mg/dL for active vs. stable disease, respectively).[30-33] Patients with active disease often exhibit higher levels of circulating interleukin-6 (IL-6)[32,34,35] and IL-18[34] compared to individuals with stable, inactive disease or those who are in a healthy state.[36]

Researchers have explored serum autoantibodies such as antiendothelial cell antibody (AECA), circulating endothelial cells, and serum proteins such as vascular endothelial growth factor, matrix metalloproteinase-9, IL-6, and IL-18 as potential biomarkers for assessing disease activity in Takayasu arteritis. However, the findings thus far have been inconclusive. Some studies have suggested a correlation between serum levels of pentraxin 3 (PTX-3) and active disease in Takayasu arteritis.[37,38] The PTX-3 levels are raised in patients with Takayasu arteritis than in controls,[39] but within patients with Takayasu arteritis, differences according to disease activity were observed to be inconsistent.[39,40]

INVESTIGATIONS

Accurate diagnosis and ongoing monitoring of Takayasu arteritis necessitate imaging techniques to visualize the affected blood vessels. Various modalities such as conventional angiography, contrast-enhanced magnetic resonance angiography (MRA), and computed tomography angiography (CTA) are utilized, each with its own set of advantages and limitations **(Table 4)**.[6]

The nuclear magnetic resonance (NMR) has emerged as an alternative method to CT, especially angio-NMR, being equally sensitive to angiography in detecting lesions

TABLE 4: Imaging modalities in the evaluation of Takayasu arteritis patients.[6]

Modality	Advantages	Disadvantages
Digital subtraction angiography	• Excellent morphological definition (lumen) • Allows vision of distal vessels	• Invasive • Radiation • Low sensitivity for assessment of disease activity • Does not provide information about vessel wall
Magnetic resonance angiography	• Good morphological definition (lumen) • Fairly good measurements of arterial wall thickness • Allows vision of arterial wall edema • Provides information on gadolinium uptake in vessel wall • Good sensitivity for assessment of inflammation • No radiation	• Does not allow vision of small vessels • It may overestimate stenosis • Expensive
Computed tomography angiography	• Good morphological definition (lumen) • Fairly good measurement of arterial wall thickness • Good imaging of arterial lumen	• Radiation • Low sensitivity for assessment of disease activity • Does not allow vision of small vessels
Doppler ultrasound	• Very good measurement of arterial wall thickness • Provides fair definition of anatomical details • Inexpensive • Fair sensitivity for assessment of disease activity • No radiation • Noninvasive	• Operator-dependent • Poor definition of descending aorta • No direct measure of inflammation
[^{18}F]Fluorodeoxyglucose position emission tomography	Good sensitivity for early assessment of inflammation	• Very poor definition of anatomic details • Radiation • Expensive • It may underestimate activity

of large vessels. However, its sensitivity reduces in case of smaller branch involvement and may overestimate the degree of stenosis in renal and subclavian arteries.[41] Recently, fluorodeoxyglucose positron emission tomography (FDG-PET) has come up as a promising technique in the early diagnosis and assessment of response to treatment in Takayasu arteritis as well as in other large-vessel vasculitis, as it is more sensitive method than conventional clinical methods in terms of evaluating ongoing vascular inflammation.[42]

MEDICAL MANAGEMENT

Systemic glucocorticoids (GCs) are the primary therapeutic approach to induce remission in patients with Takayasu arteritis. The commonly prescribed initial dosage of prednisone is 0.5–1 mg/kg/day. According to the 2018 recommendations from the EULAR, most patients should receive an initial dose of 40–60 mg/day. Thus far, there is no evidence indicating that a higher starting dose improves treatment outcomes.[43] The 2021 guidelines from the ACR also recommend a high initial dose of GC due to the potential for organ damage and life-threatening events associated with Takayasu arteritis onset. However, the ACR guidelines allow for lower doses to be considered in patients with newly active, nonsevere diseases, such as those experiencing constitutional symptoms without limb ischemia.[44]

The 2018 EULAR recommendations advised selecting a conventional synthetic disease-modifying antirheumatic drug (csDMARD) as the initial treatment option for patients, with options including methotrexate, azathioprine, mycophenolate mofetil, or leflunomide. If a patient experiences intolerance to the first choice csDMARD, switching to another csDMARD is considered a viable alternative. Moreover, major progress has been made in development of targeted biological disease-modifying antirheumatic drugs (bDMARDs). Tumor necrosis factor-α (TNF-α) and IL-6 seem to be very promising therapeutic targets.[45] **Figure 2** summarizes selections to assess disease activity and therapeutic strategies in Takayasu arteritis.

According to the 2018 EULAR guidelines,[43] the pharmacologic treatment approach for Takayasu arteritis involves a two-phase strategy. In phase I, a combination of glucocorticoids and conventional synthetic disease-modifying antirheumatic drugs (DMARDs) is recommended. If a relapse occurs, phase II involves the addition of a biologic DMARD to the treatment regimen **(Fig. 3)**.

INTERVENTIONS

During the chronic phases of Takayasu arteritis, a key aspect of treatment involves restoring blood flow to the affected organs through either surgical procedures or endovascular interventions such as balloon angioplasty, stent placement, or stent graft replacement. It is generally recommended that both surgical and endovascular approaches are attempted only after the inflammation in the vessel wall has been effectively suppressed.[46]

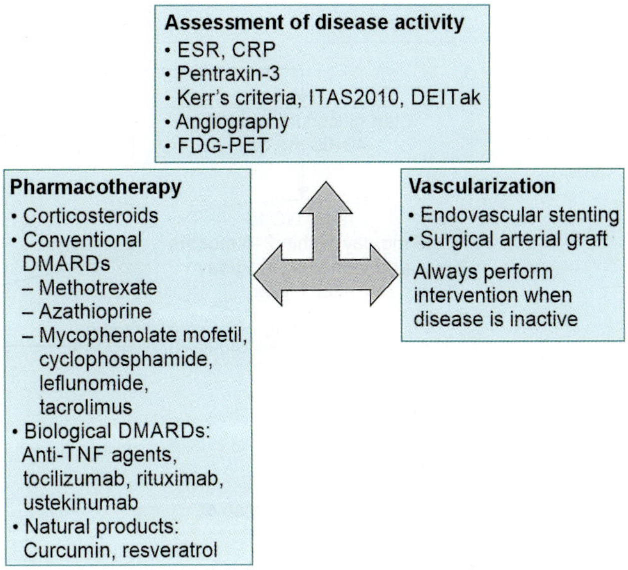

FIG. 2: Opportunities to assess disease activity and therapeutic strategies in Takayasu arteritis.

(CRP: C-reactive protein; ESR: erythrocyte sedimentation rate; DMARD: disease-modifying antirheumatic drug; FDG-PET: fluorodeoxyglucose positron emission tomography)

According to the guidelines provided by EULAR, ACR, ESC (European Society of Cardiology), and ESVS (European Society for Vascular Surgery), it is advisable to carry out elective endovascular interventions or reconstructive surgery when the patient is in a stable remission state.[43,44,47,48] Performing surgical procedures on patients with active disease poses a higher risk of complications and increases the likelihood of needing further revisions due to relapse or progression of symptomatic disease.[49,50]

The choice of vascular interventions for patients with Takayasu arteritis depends on various factors such as the location of the vascular damage, disease activity, timing, and other considerations. The decision-making process should involve collaboration between vascular surgeons and rheumatologists.[45] In recent years, percutaneous endoluminal angioplasty has gained popularity as a method of choice for Takayasu arteritis patients due to advancements in endovascular treatment. This approach is particularly suitable for treating stenotic lesions in areas like the supra-aortic, iliac, and renal arteries.[51,52] Conversely, for inflammatory thoracic aortic aneurysms, the standard first-line treatment still involves open surgery with resection and replacement of the affected aorta. However, there have been promising outcomes reported for thoracic endovascular aortic repair (TEVAR), suggesting that it may become a less

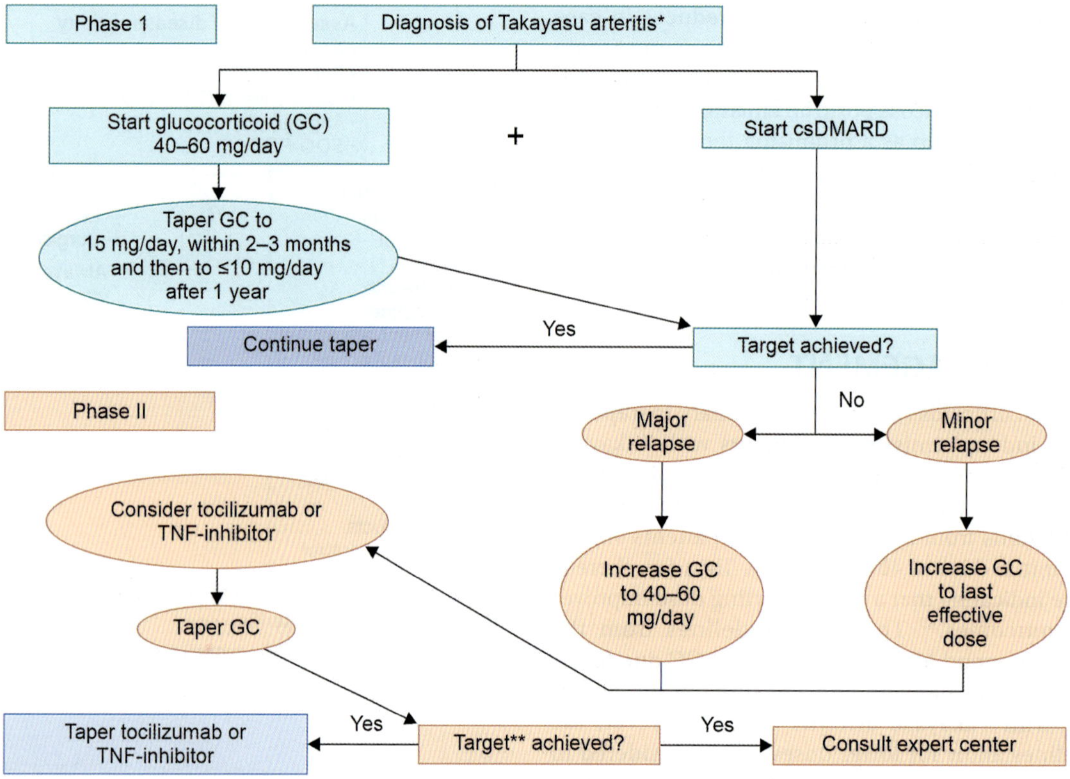

*The clinical diagnosis of Takayasu arteritis should be confirmed by imaging.
**The treatment target is sustained remission plus the ability to taper GCs to the specified target without relapse.

FIG. 3: The 2018 EULAR algorithm for pharmacologic treatment of Takayasu arteritis.
(csDMARD: conventional synthetic disease-modifying antirheumatic drug; EULAR: European League Against Rheumatism; GCs: glucocorticoids; TNF: tumor necrosis factor)

invasive alternative for selected patients in the future.[53] Interventional strategies in specific lesions and arteries are described in **Table 5**.[11]

PROGNOSIS

Literature states variable survival rates for the patients with Takayasu arteritis. At 15 years, the prognosis was found to be significantly worse when major complications were present and the disease showed a progressive course, with an estimated survival rate of only 43%.[54] However, some studies have reported the 10-year survival rate as 81.4%, and the 20-year rate as 73.5%.[55,56] In the study conducted by Comarmond et al., they found that the 5-year and 10-year complication-free survival rates in Takayasu arteritis were reported as 70% and 54%, respectively.[54] Several factors have contributed to the prognosis of patients with Takayasu arteritis in recent years (**Fig. 4**).[11] Risk factors for vascular complications included a progressive clinical course (<1 year from symptom onset to diagnosis), involvement of the thoracic aorta, and the presence of retinopathy. Furthermore, the prognosis was found to be worse in patients with pulmonary artery involvement who also had pulmonary hypertension, compared to those without pulmonary hypertension.[57]

FUTURE

There is a need to address the deficiencies in managing Takayasu arteritis, which could be the subject of future research. Two significant gaps are the absence of well-defined, universally accepted criteria for diagnosing Takayasu arteritis and determining disease activity. Additionally, there is a need for reliable biomarkers to differentiate various forms of large-vessel vasculitis, evaluate disease activity, and predict treatment response. Another area that requires attention is the development of safe imaging techniques with high accuracy in detecting vascular inflammation. By gaining a better understanding of the underlying mechanisms of Takayasu arteritis, new opportunities for effective drug development may emerge. Enhancing the management of advanced vascular disease necessitates a greater level of clarity, potentially through the implementation of randomized trials to address unresolved matters. An optimal approach could involve the establishment of a global registry to comprehensively

TABLE 5: Interventional strategies in specific lesions and arteries.[11]

	Strategy	Comment
Aortic/Mitral regurgitation	Valve replacement surgery	Hospital mortality 4.8% with aortic valve replacement, late dilatation of ascending aorta 11.1%
Coronary artery occlusion/stenosis	Coronary artery bypass surgery if refractory to medical treatment	PCI is associated with 39% restenosis compared with 9% with bypass surgery
Carotid artery occlusion/stenosis	Balloon angioplasty ± adjunctive stenting, or bypass surgery	High incidence of brain hyperperfusion after carotid artery bypass surgery
Subclavian artery occlusion/stenosis	Balloon angioplasty ± adjunctive stenting in short lesions (<8 cm); conservative Rx in long lesions	High restenosis rates in long lesions distal anastomosis to small arteries may impact bypass surgery results
Descending thoracic stenosis	Endovascular therapy/bypass surgery	Long endografts enable safe high-pressure lesion dilatation
Visceral aorta occlusion or stenosis	Endovascular therapy/bypass surgery	Access to aortic side branches is possible via braided self-expanding stent struts
Infrarenal aorta and iliac occlusions/stenosis	Endovascular therapy/aorto-bi-iliac or -femoral bypass surgery	Covered stents are preferred in occlusions to avoid rupture and bare stents for stenosis
Mesenteric/renal aorto-ostial occlusion/stenosis	Balloon angioplasty ± adjunctive stenting or elective covered stent	Bypass surgery/renal autotransplant if endovascular therapy is not feasible
Pulmonary artery occlusion/stenosis	Balloon angioplasty ± adjunctive stenting; staged revascularization	Angioplasty improves survival in patients with pulmonary hypertension
Aortic aneurysms	Open surgery/Bentall procedure/endovascular therapy	• Hospital mortality 7.4% with Bentall procedure • 93% 5-year survival in a recent hybrid series of thoracic aortic aneurysms

(PCI: percutaneous coronary intervention; Rx: treatment)

Sources:

1. Matsuura K, Ogino H, Kobayashi J, Ishibashi-Ueda H, Matsuda H, Minatoya K, et al. Surgical treatment of aortic regurgitation due to Takayasu arteritis: long-term morbidity and mortality. Circulation. 2005;112:3707-12.
2. Huang Z, Zhang H, Wang M, Yang W, Qiao S, Hu F. Revascularization versus medical therapy in Takayasu's arteritis patients with coronary artery involvement. Rheumatol Ther. 2021;8:119-33.
3. Luo XY, Wu QH, Zhang FX. Open and endovascular management of severe cerebral ischemia in Takayasu's arteritis. Ann Vasc Surg. 2017;42:101-110.
4. Porter A, Mason JC. Intervention in Takayasu aortitis: when, where, and how? Hearts. 2020;1:62-74.
5. Joseph G, George PV, Pati PK, Chandy ST. Feasibility of angioplasty and stenting for abdominal aortic lesions adjacent to previously stented visceral artery lesions in patients with Takayasu arteritis. Cardiovasc Intervent Radiol. 2007;30:293-6.
6. Zhou YP, Wei YP, Yang YJ, Xu XQ, Wu T, Liu C, et al. Percutaneous pulmonary angioplasty for patients with Takayasu arteritis and pulmonary hypertension. J Am Coll Cardiol. 2022;79:1477-88.
7. With permission from Oishi et al. (2022).[53]

document the heterogeneity observed in Takayasu arteritis across different regions of the world.[11]

TRIALS

Several ongoing clinical trials are currently focused on Takayasu arteritis, a rare form of large-vessel vasculitis. These trials aim to address various aspects of Takayasu arteritis management, including improving diagnostic criteria, determining optimal treatment strategies, and assessing the effectiveness of new therapeutic interventions. Some trials are investigating the use of biologic agents, such as TNF inhibitors and IL-6 inhibitors, to control disease activity and reduce inflammation in Takayasu arteritis patients. Other trials are exploring the potential of different imaging techniques, such as PET scans, to accurately diagnose and monitor disease progression. Additionally, there are ongoing efforts to establish international registries to gather comprehensive data on Takayasu arteritis patients, enabling a better understanding of the disease's heterogeneity and aiding in the development of personalized treatment approaches. These ongoing trials hold promise for advancing our knowledge and improving the management of Takayasu arteritis in the future. **Table 6** outlines new targeted therapies in Takayasu arteritis with recent trial evidence.[45]

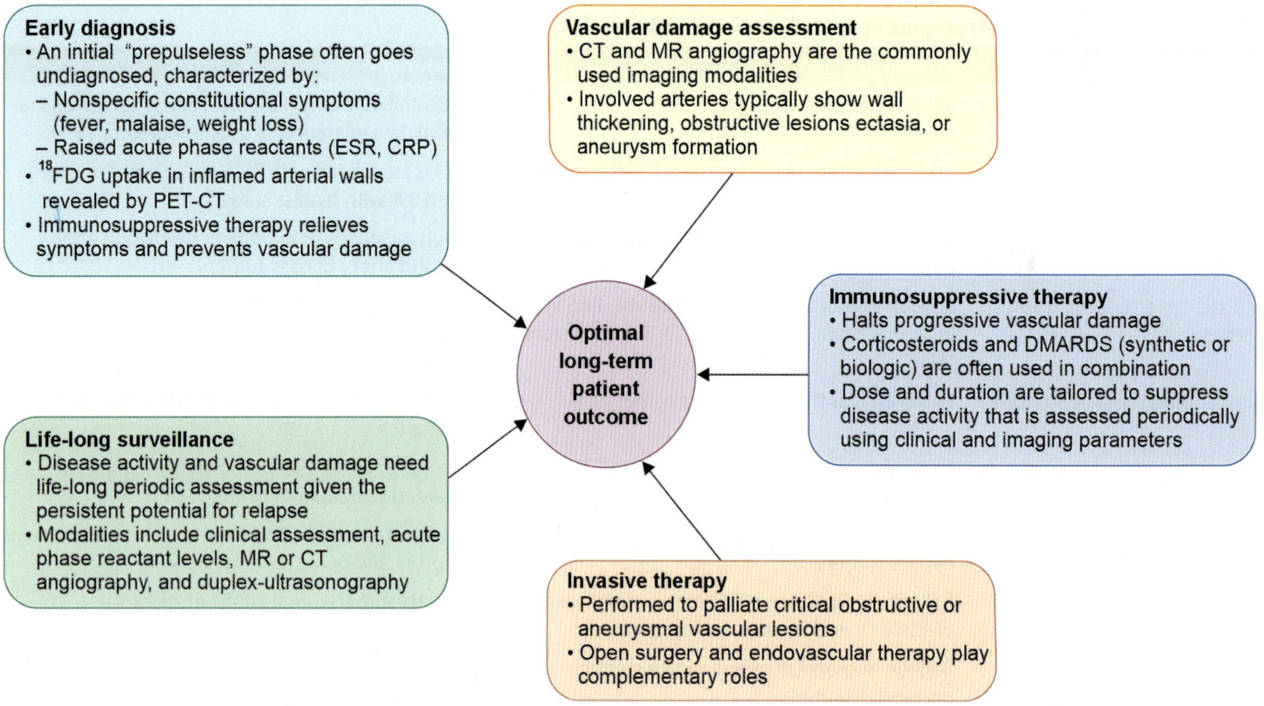

FIG. 4: Components of patient care in Takayasu arteritis.[11]

TABLE 6: New targeted therapies and evidence in Takayasu arteritis.[45]

Drug	Pathogenetic basis	Evidence in Takayasu arteritis	Recommendations and clinical use
TNF-α inhibitors (infliximab, etanercept, adalimumab, golimumab, certolizumab pegol)	*Inhibitors of TNF-α (bDMARDs):* • TNF-α has a major role in the development of Takayasu arteritis granulomatous inflammation • In active Takayasu arteritis higher serum levels of TNF-α and higher mRNA expression and intracellular production by T cells	• Cohort studies and open-label prospective study, showing positive results in Takayasu arteritis patients (clinical improvement, GC-sparing effect, higher sustained remission rate compared to cDMARDs) • No RCTs • Meta-analysis with 19 observational studies, showing >80% of treated patients attaining at least partial clinical response • Good safety profile in cohort studies	• *2018 EULAR recommendations:* TNF-α inhibitors as second-line treatment in Takayasu arteritis patients resistant to csDMARD • *2021 ACR guidelines*: TNF-α inhibitors as first-line treatment, such as methotrexate and azathioprine
Tocilizumab	*Anti-IL-6r (bDMARD):* • IL-6 is a proinflammatory cytokine • Higher IL-6 levels in Takayasu arteritis patients compared to HC and in Takayasu arteritis patients with active disease compared to patients with low-disease activity	• Cohort studies, showing positive results in Takayasu arteritis patients (clinical improvement, GC sparing effect, higher sustained remission rate compared to cDMARDs) • Meta-analysis with 22 observational studies, showing more than 87% of treated patients attaining at least partial clinical response • *One RCT (Takayasu arteritis T study)*: Relapse-free survival tended to be improved in treated patients, but no statistical significance. Longer-term open-label extension showed GC-sparing effect, lower radiological disease progression, better PROs • Good safety profile in cohort studies and RCT	• *2018 EULAR recommendations:* Tocilizumab as second-line treatment in Takayasu arteritis patients resistant to csDMARD • *2021 ACR guidelines*: Tocilizumab as second-line treatment in patients with inadequate response to other immunosuppressive therapies

Continued

Continued

Drug	Pathogenetic basis	Evidence in Takayasu arteritis	Recommendations and clinical use
JAK-inhibitors (tofacitinib, upadacitinib)	*Inhibitors of JAK-STAT signaling pathway (tsDMARDs):* • Block signaling of cytokine implicated in Takayasu arteritis pathogenesis (type 1 and 2 interferons, IL-6, IL-12, IL-17, and IL-23) • Suppress tissue-resident memory T cells and reduce inflammatory-related vascular damage	*Tofacitinib*: • Case reports and one prospective observational study, showing positive results in Takayasu arteritis patients (clinical improvement, lower radiological disease progression, superior to methotrexate) • Good safety profile • One ongoing RCT (NCT04299971) *Upadacitinib:* • One ongoing RCT (NCT04161898) • No data on other JAK-inhibitors	• Only case reports • Not included in 2018 EULAR recommendations or 2021 ACR guidelines
Rituximab	*Anti-CD20 (bDMARD):* • In Takayasu arteritis patients B-cells infiltrates in the inflamed arteries adventitia and high levels of activated B-cell subsets in the peripheral blood • Rituximab blocks B cell differentiation and B-T cell stimulation	• Isolated case reports on rituximab in Takayasu arteritis with contradictory results • No RCTs, no meta-analysis, no ongoing trial	• Very limited evidence with contradictory results • Only case reports • Not included in 2018 EULAR recommendations or 2021 ACR guidelines
Abatacept	*Soluble fusion protein CTLA4-Ig (bDMARD):* • In Takayasu arteritis patients B-cells infiltrates in the inflamed arteries adventitia and high levels of activated B-cell subsets in the peripheral blood • Abatacept blocks B-T cell costimulation	• *One RCT with 34 Takayasu arteritis patients:* Abatacept not associated with a longer median duration of remission compared to placebo	• *2021 ACR guidelines*: Abatacept is not recommended in Takayasu arteritis
Ustekinumab	*Anti-p40, IL-12, and IL-23 inhibitor (bDMARD):* • Th17 and Th1 pathways contribute to Takayasu arteritis pathogenesis • Ustekinumab target p40, a common subunit of IL-12 and IL-23 (main cytokines involved in Th17 and Th1 pathways)	• A small prospective observational study (improvement in clinical symptoms but no changes in intramural enhancement on MRA) • One ongoing RCT (NCT04882072)	• Very limited evidence • Not included in 2018 EULAR recommendations or 2021 ACR guidelines

(ACR: American College of Rheumatology; bDMARD: biological disease-modifying antirheumatic drug; EULAR: European League Against Rheumatism; GC: glucocorticoid; IL: interleukin; JAK-STAT: Janus kinase/signal transducers and activators of transcription; MRA: magnetic resonance angiography; RCT: randomized controlled trial; TNF: tumor necrosis factor)

CONCLUSION

In conclusion, the overview of Takayasu arteritis presented in this chapter has provided a comprehensive understanding of this rare and enigmatic disease. Takayasu arteritis, often referred to as "pulseless disease," poses significant challenges in diagnosis, treatment, and management due to its complex and variable clinical manifestations. This chapter has highlighted the key aspects of the disease, including its incidence, pathophysiology, clinical presentation, diagnostic criteria, and treatment options.

Various studies on Takayasu arteritis are ongoing, and there is much more to be learned about this complex disease. By doing so, we can ultimately improve the quality of life for individuals living with Takayasu arteritis and work toward a future where this condition is better understood and managed.

ONLINE REFERENCES

Please scan the QR code provided at the end of the table of contents for References of this chapter.

SECTION 22

Mechanical Circulatory Support

CHAPTER

204 Cardiogenic Shock: Risk Stratification and Management

Swasthi S Kumar, Harikrishnan S

ABSTRACT

Cardiogenic shock is a state of reduced cardiac output. Trials have defined cardiogenic shock as systolic blood pressure of <90 mm Hg despite fluid resuscitation resulting in tissue hypoperfusion. In-hospital mortality with the best available management is reported to be as high as 50%. Inotropes and vasopressors form the main pillars of the treatment strategy. We have summarized the available evidence and guidelines regarding the risk stratification and management of cardiogenic shock.

Keywords: Cardiogenic shock, vasopressors, inotropes, shock, mechanical circulatory support.

INTRODUCTION

Cardiogenic shock (CS) is a state of reduced cardiac output resulting in tissue hypoperfusion. If not appropriately managed, it can lead to a downhill trajectory, with the patient developing multiorgan dysfunction syndrome. Left ventricular (LV) dysfunction secondary to acute myocardial infarction (AMI) is the most common cause. In-hospital mortality with the best available management is as high as 50%. However, studies show a trend toward reduction in CS-related in-hospital mortality.[1]

The definition of CS requires persistent hypotension with evidence of hypoperfusion **(Table 1)**. Trials like the SHOCK and IABP shock trials are frequently quoted while defining CS. Hypotension has been variably defined as systolic blood pressure (SBP) <90 mm Hg lasting for 30 minutes or more or SBP <90 mm Hg despite adequate fluid therapy or requirement of inotrope support to maintain the same. Hypoperfusion has been defined in various trials as reduced urine output <30 mL/h, rising creatinine, altered mental status, cold and clammy extremities, lactate >2 mmol/L and metabolic acidosis. SHOCK trial has defined CS hemodynamically as a cardiac index (CI) <2.2 L/min/m^2 and pulmonary capillary wedge pressure (PCWP) >15 mm Hg.[2] Other hemodynamic parameters such as cardiac power output (CPO), cardiac power index (obtained by dividing CPO by body surface area), and pulmonary artery pulsatility index (PAPi) have also been used in the diagnosis of CS.[3] CPO, which indicates the pumping capability of the heart and the resistance of the conducting vessels, is calculated by multiplying cardiac output (L/min) with mean arterial pressure divided by 451. PAPi, the ratio of pulmonary artery pulse pressure to right atrial pressure (PASP-PADP/RAP), is a hemodynamic parameter indicating right ventricular function.

RISK STRATIFICATION OF CARDIOGENIC SHOCK

Due to the high mortality associated with it, risk stratification and prognostication are crucial in patients with CS. It must be communicated to the family whether the patient is expected to improve with inotropic support, will require mechanical support devices, or is unlikely to benefit from any management strategy. The requirement of multiple inotropes, mechanical support devices, and multiorgan dysfunction, particularly renal dysfunction, portends a poor prognosis. Lower hemoglobin and albumin levels, higher glucose, troponin, NT-ProBNP levels, and inflammatory markers have also been shown to foreshadow a worse prognosis. Several scoring systems incorporating such variables have been developed to help with risk stratification

TABLE 1: Definition of cardiogenic shock as used in the SHOCK trial[2], IABP-SHOCK II trial,[4] and ESC guidelines.[5]

Definition of cardiogenic shock	
SHOCK trial	*Clinical criteria*: • SBP <90 mm Hg for ≥30 min OR requirement of inotropic support to maintain SBP ≥90 mm Hg • Hypoperfusion: Urine output <30 mL/h, or cool extremities *Hemodynamic criteria*: • CI of ≤2.2 L/min/m^2 • PCWP ≥15 mm Hg
IABP-SHOCK II trial	*Clinical criteria*: • SBP <90 mm Hg for ≥30 min OR catecholamines to maintain SBP >90 mm Hg • Pulmonary congestion • Hypoperfusion: Altered mental status, cold/clammy skin and extremities, urine output <30 mL/h, or lactate >2.0 mmol/L
ESC guidelines	• SBP <90 mm Hg with adequate volume • Hypoperfusion *Clinical*: Cold extremities, oliguria, mental confusion, dizziness, narrow pulse pressure *Laboratory*: Metabolic acidosis, elevated serum lactate or creatinine

(CI: cardiac index; PCWP: pulmonary capillary wedge pressure; SBP: systolic blood pressure)

TABLE 2: IABP-SHOCK II score for risk stratification of cardiogenic shock associated with acute myocardial infarction.

IABP-SHOCK II score	
Variable	**Points**
Age >73 years	1
History of stroke	2
Glucose >191 mg/dL	1
Creatinine >1.5 mg/dL	1
Arterial lactate >5 mmol/L	2
TIMI flow grade <3 after PCI	2
Total	9

Low risk: 0–2; intermediate risk: 3–4; high risk: 5–9 points

TABLE 3: CardShock risk score.

CardShock risk score	
Variable	**Points**
Age >75 years	1
Confusion at presentation	1
Previous MI or CABG	1
ACS etiology	1
LVEF <40%	1
Blood lactate	
<2 mmol/L	0
2–4 mmol/L	1
>4 mmol/L	2
eGFR	
>60 mL/min/1.73 m^2	0
30–60 mL/min/1.73 m^2	1
<30 mL/min/1.7 3 m^2	2

Low risk: 0–3 (mortality risk ≤10%); intermediate risk: 4–5 (mortality risk 30–40%); high risk: 7–9 points (mortality risk >70%)

in CS. The IABP-SHOCK II score, CardShock score, and SCAI (Society for Cardiovascular Imaging and Interventions) staging system are the most discussed in the literature.

The IABP-SHOCK II score was derived from the IABP Shock II trial by multivariate regression analysis, in which six variables were independent predictors of 30-day mortality. Post-percutaneous coronary intervention (PCI) thrombolysis in myocardial infarction (TIMI) flow is one of the components, and this score is specifically for AMI associated CS. It has been validated in the IABP-SHOCK II registry, and further external validation was done in the CardShock trial. The 30-day mortality in patients in the low-risk, intermediate-risk and high-risk categories are 23.8%, 49.2%, and 76.6%, respectively **(Table 2)**.

The CardShock study enrolled patients with CS due to both acute coronary syndrome (ACS) and non-ACS-related causes. CS associated with myocardial infarction (MI) was found to be independently associated with increased mortality compared to other etiologies. ACS-related CS, age, history of prior MI or coronary artery bypass graft surgery (CABG), LV systolic dysfunction and elevated blood lactate levels were independent predictors of mortality, and the CardShock risk score was put forward, including these variables to predict short-term (in-hospital) mortality. All the variables are easily obtained by clinical assessment, and the score can be calculated in the early period after the presentation of shock, facilitating early risk stratification **(Table 3)**.[6]

The Society for Cardiovascular Imaging and Interventions has described the five stages of CS based on clinical signs and symptoms, biochemical markers, and hemodynamic parameters **(Fig. 1)**.[7]

- *Stage A*: "At risk" of developing CS. For example, Patients with AMI. They have no hypotension or hypoperfusion and have normal blood lactate levels and normal hemodynamic parameters (cardiac index ≥2.5 L/min/m^2, CVP ≤10 mm Hg, PCWP ≤15 mm Hg, PA saturation >65%).

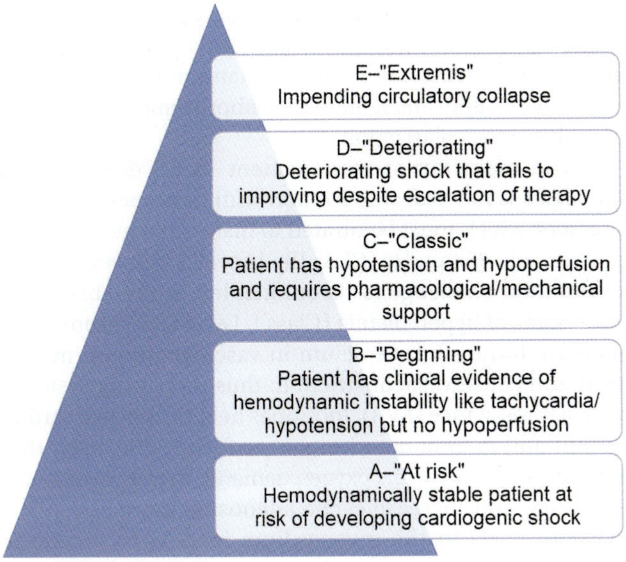

FIG. 1: SCAI stages of cardiogenic shock.[7]
(SCAI: Society for Cardiovascular Imaging and Interventions)

TABLE 4: Scoring systems to predict survival from cardiogenic shock after VA-ECMO.

SAVE score		ENCOURAGE score
• Etiology of cardiogenic shock (myocarditis, refractory VT/VF, congenital heart diseases) • Age • Body weight • Pre-ECMO organ failure • Duration of intubation prior to ECMO (hours)	• Peak inspiratory pressure ≤20 cmH_2O • Pre-ECMO cardiac arrest • Diastolic blood pressure before ECMO ≥40 mm Hg • Pulse pressure before ECMO ≤20 mm Hg • HCO_3 before ECMO ≤15 mmol/L	• Age ≥60 years • Female gender • Body mass index >25 kg/m^2 • Glasgow coma score <6 • Creatinine >150 µmol/L • Lactate (<2, 2–8, or >8 mmol/L) • Prothrombin activity <50%

- *Stage B*: "Beginning CS"—the patient has hemodynamic instability in the form of hypotension and tachycardia without any evidence of hypoperfusion (normal blood lactate levels).
- *Stage C*: "Classic CS"—the patient has hypotension with associated hypoperfusion (lactate ≥2 mmol/L, cold and clammy extremities, reduced urine output, deranged renal and hepatic functions) and requires one pharmacological or mechanical intervention beyond fluid resuscitation. Hemodynamic parameters are deranged (cardiac index <2.2 L/min/m^2, PCWP >15 mm Hg).
- *Stage D*: "Deteriorating CS"—patient fails to respond to initial interventions and requires escalating doses of pharmacological agents. The patient has multiorgan dysfunction at this stage.
- *Stage E*: "Extremis"—impending circulatory collapse. The patient has profound hypotension despite maximal hemodynamic support. The patient develops multiple arrhythmias such as ventricular tachycardia/fibrillation requiring defibrillation. Blood lactate levels are over 8 mmol/L, and the patient has a severe metabolic acidosis.

The Inova group suggested an algorithm for diagnosis and management of CS which includes activation of Shock team upon the diagnosis of CS based on clinical evidence; early patient transfer to a cardiac catheterization laboratory or intensive care unit; echo and right heart catheterization for acute decompensated heart failure related CS and right heart catheterization along with coronary angiography and revascularization in ACS related CS; establishing hemodynamic criteria for CS based on cardiac index, PCWP, PAPi, and CPO; and early institution of mechanical circulatory support (MCS). Lower values of CPO and cardiac power index and PAPi are important predictors of adverse cardiac outcomes. The Inova group developed a scoring system for predicting short-term mortality in CS, including hemodynamic parameters. This scoring system, however, makes cardiac catheterization mandatory and remains to be validated in further studies.[3] Several other scoring systems are also available, such as the CLIP score, a biomarker-based risk score (cystatin C, lactate, interleukin-6, N-terminal pro-BNP) for AMI-related CS[8] and CS score (CSS).[9]

Two scoring systems for the early identification of patients who might benefit from extracorporeal membrane oxygenation (ECMO) are the SAVE (survival after veno-arterial ECMO) and ENCOURAGE score **(Table 4)**. The SAVE score was developed based on data extracted from the ELSO registry (Extracorporeal Life Support Organization). It included parameters such as age, weight, etiology of CS, pre-ECMO organ failures, and duration of mechanical ventilation before ECMO. SAVE score gives importance to the etiology of CS (e.g., myocarditis +3 points, congenital heart disease -3 points). The total score varies from –35 to +17 and divides patients into five risk classes.[10] ENCOURAGE score was developed to predict mortality in AMI-associated CS who received VA-ECMO and included seven readily available variables (age, gender, BMI, Glasgow coma score, creatinine, lactate, and prothrombin activity).[11]

MANAGEMENT OF CARDIOGENIC SHOCK

Patients diagnosed with CS require urgent transfer to a tertiary care center with a cardiac catheterization laboratory and intensive care unit. A quick analysis of the presenting symptoms and clinical signs, along with basic investigations such as ECG, ECHO and cardiac biomarkers, help identify the etiology in most cases such as AMI, arrhythmias, myocarditis, end-stage cardiomyopathy or pulmonary embolism. Critically ill patients must be intubated and mechanically ventilated, and acid-base parameters must be optimized.

Cardiogenic shock secondary to AMI behaves differently in the acute setting than other etiologies and needs immediate coronary angiography within 2 hours of hospital admission (Class Ic).[5] Patients with AMI with CS, when randomized to medical stabilization or early revascularization with PCI or CABG in the SHOCK trial, the early revascularization group had significantly lower 6-month mortality. However, the 30-day mortality did not differ between the two groups.[2] More than half the patients presenting with CS have triple vessel disease, and mortality varies based on the culprit lesion, being as high as 80% in left main lesions to close to 40% in culprit lesions involving LAD, LCX, or RCA.[12] The age-old concept of revascularizing both culprit and nonculprit lesions has taken a turn following the CULPRIT SHOCK trial.[13] Patients with CS complicating AMI when randomized to culprit vessel PCI (with staged revascularization of nonculprit vessels) or multiple vessel PCI of both culprit and nonculprit vessels, the primary composite outcome of 30-day mortality and renal failure requiring hemodialysis was significantly lower in culprit vessel group. These findings have been challenged by the results of the KAMIR-NIH registry, which has shown lower all-cause mortality, re-MIs, and repeat revascularizations in the multivessel PCI group.[14] One practical way of making a decision is to reassess the clinical status after culprit vessel revascularization, and if there is no improvement, proceed to complete revascularization.

The mainstay of management in CS due to other etiologies is medical stabilization with inotropes and vasopressors, which must be titrated to maintain a mean arterial pressure of >65 mm Hg (Class IIb, Level C).[5] However, a trial of the fluid challenge is recommended in the absence of overt signs of hypervolemia (Class I, Level C).[5] Vasopressors increase intracellular calcium in vascular smooth muscle cells and cause vasoconstriction, thus increasing systemic vascular resistance (SVR). Inotropes help to improve cardiac output and maintain end-organ perfusion. However, they increase the myocardial oxygen demand, thereby worsening ischemia; and increase cyclic adenosine monophosphate (cAMP) levels in the myocardium leading to increased intracellular calcium levels, which may predispose to arrhythmias. So, they must be titrated for the shortest possible duration in the lowest possible doses to maintain end-organ perfusion. The available pharmacological agents, their recommended dosed and adverse events have been summarized in **Table 5**.

TABLE 5: The available pharmacological vasopressors and inotropes for managing cardiogenic shock and their recommended doses and adverse events.

Drug	Receptor				Dose	Adverse effects
Catecholamines	α1	β1	β2	DA		
• Noradrenaline	+++++	+++	++	–	0.05–0.4 μg/kg/min	Hypertension, peripheral ischemia, arrhythmias (less when compared to epinephrine, dopamine)
• Adrenaline	+++++	++++	+++	–	0.01–0.5 μg/kg/min	Arrhythmias, hypertension, cardiac ischemia, splanchnic vasoconstriction, lactic acidosis
• Dopamine	+++	++++	++	+++++	• Low dose (2–5 μg/kg/min)- vasodilation via DA receptor • Intermediate dose (5–10 μg/kg/min)–promotes noradrenaline release and increases cardiac output via β1 • High dose (10–20 μg/kg/min)–vasoconstriction via α1 receptors	Arrhythmias, hypertension
• Dobutamine	+	+++++	+++	–	0.5–20 μg/kg/min	Hypotension, tachycardia, ventricular arrhythmias, cardiac ischemia, eosinophilic myocarditis
Milrinone	PDE3 inhibitor				50 μg/kg bolus f/b 0.375 –0.75 μg/kg/min	Ventricular arrhythmias, hypotension, torsades de pointes
Enoximone	PDE3 inhibitor				0.5 mg/kg bolus f/b 2–10 μg/kg/min	Hypotension, bradycardia, transient atrial fibrillation
Levosimendan	Calcium sensitizer				6–24 μg/kg bolus followed by a 6-h intravenous infusion at 0.1–0.4 μg/kg/min	Hypotension, tachycardia

- *Catecholamines*: The endogenous catecholamines therapeutically used in CS are norepinephrine, epinephrine, dopamine, and dobutamine.
    - Norepinephrine, through its predominant action via the α1 receptor, is a potent vasoconstrictor and is the first-line vasopressor agent used in CS. It increases blood pressure without much effect on cardiac output. It also has minimal chronotropic impact compared to other catecholamines and is less prone to cause arrhythmias. Being a potent peripheral vasoconstrictor, ischemic necrosis of digital extremities is a rare but severe complication seen more with norepinephrine than with other agents **(Fig. 2)**.
    - Adrenaline has predominant β1 action at lower doses, thus increasing cardiac output. At higher doses, it increases SVR by its dominant α1 action. The skeletal muscle glycolysis caused by adrenaline and the reduced hepatic lactic uptake due to splanchnic vasoconstriction predisposes to lactic acidosis in patients treated with adrenaline infusions.[16] Hence, arterial blood gas lactate levels may be a poor indicator of changes in hemodynamic status in patients treated with adrenaline infusions. Epinephrine is equal to norepinephrine in improving cardiac index, however, at the cost of rising heart rate and lactic acidosis.[17] Compared to other drug regimens in CS, epinephrine has also been shown to have up to three times higher risk of mortality.[18] Hence, it is now considered a second-line agent in CS.
    - Dopamine at low doses binds to presynaptic D2 and postsynaptic D1 receptors in the coronary, renal, and mesenteric vasculature and causes vasodilation. It attaches to β1 in higher doses and promotes noradrenaline release, causing vasoconstriction. Further increases in doses cause α1 mediated vasoconstriction. SOAP II trial, which randomized patients with shock to receive either norepinephrine or dopamine, showed more significant 28-day mortality in the subset of patients with CS. Dopamine was also associated with a greater risk of arrhythmias.[19] This was further substantiated in a meta-analysis that showed that nor-epinephrine was superior in terms of mortality risk and arrhythmias.[20]
    - Dobutamine, via its intense action on β1 receptors, increases cardiac output and is the inotrope of choice in CS. At lower doses <5 μg/kg/min, it causes peripheral vasodilatation through its action on β2 receptors and may cause a fall in BP. At doses >5 μg/kg/min, its predominant activity is on the α1 receptor and causes vasoconstriction. The combination of norepinephrine and dobutamine is safer regarding the risk of arrhythmias, lactic acidosis, and gastric mucosal perfusion than epinephrine.[21]
    - Phenylephrine is an α1 agonist; currently, no data supports its use in CS.

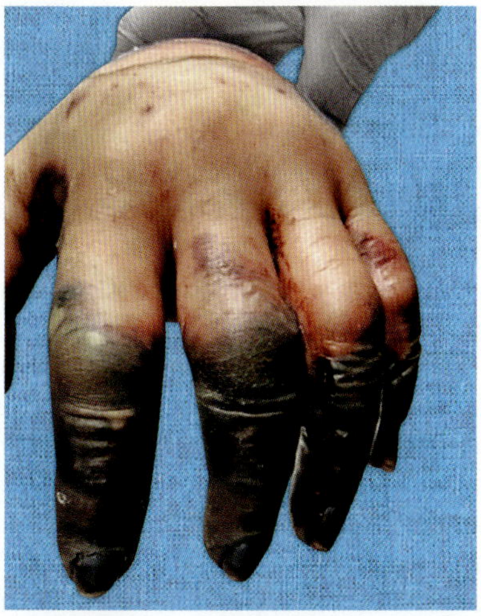

FIG. 2: Digital ischemia in a patient treated with norepinephrine and vasopressin infusion.

Source: With permission from Jesani et al. (2021).[15]

- *Vasopressin*: Vasopressin causes vasoconstriction via V1 receptors. Compared to epinephrine and norepinephrine, vasopressin does not cause constriction of the pulmonary vascular bed. It is postulated to be helpful in right ventricular failure, but this needs to be further studied. In patients with refractory CS following AMI, vasopressin helped increase the mean arterial pressure without any added adverse events.[22] The maintenance dose of vasopressin ranges from 0.01 to 0.04 units/min.

    In patients with chronic heart failure, adrenergic receptors are desensitized, making them unresponsive to catecholamines in CS. Most patients with ventricular dysfunction are on long-term beta blockers, which again restrict the activity of these agents. The newer agents such as milrinone and levosimendan, which act via pathways independent of catecholaminergic receptors, come into play in such scenarios.
- Levosimendan is an inodilator. It acts as a calcium sensitizer that increases the sensitivity of troponin C to intracellular calcium in the myocardium. It also works on ATP-dependent potassium channels, leading to the relaxation of vascular smooth muscle and hence causing coronary and peripheral vasodilation. Levosimendan does not increase intracellular calcium levels. Thus it neither increases myocardial oxygen consumption nor possesses proarrhythmic effects. Hemodynamic effects can last up to 7–9 days, so infusions of >24 hours are not necessary.[23] Renal dose modification is recommended for levosimendan. Levosimendan may be considered a rescue therapy in patients with CS who fail to respond to dobutamine and may help wean such patients off catecholamines.

- Milrinone and enoximone are phosphodiesterase-3 (PDE3) inhibitors. They increase cAMP levels, thus increasing calcium influx into myocytes and, thereby, cardiac contractility. They also inhibit vascular phosphodiesterase and act as a potent vasodilator. In the DOREMI trial, milrinone was not found to be superior to dobutamine in terms of mortality, MIs, cardiac arrest, stroke or renal replacement therapy.[24] A head-to-head comparison of enoximone and levosimendan in patients with refractory CS favored levosimendan in terms of survival at 30 days.[25]
- *Newer agents*: NOS inhibitors

Systemic inflammation and nitric oxide-induced vasodilation have been postulated as a mechanism for persistent CS, and the role of nitric oxide synthase (NOS) inhibitors has been an emerging interest. However, the TRIUMPH trial, which studied tilarginine acetate, an NOS inhibitor, in CS secondary to AMI, failed to show any benefit.[26]

MECHANICAL SUPPORT DEVICES IN CARDIOGENIC SHOCK

In refractory CS not responding to medical management, the short-term use of mechanical support devices has been given a Class IIb Level C recommendation.[5] MCS offers cardiovascular support without the added risk of arrhythmias and worsening myocardial ischemia, as seen with inotropes and vasopressors.

The intra-aortic balloon pump (IABP), developed by Dr Adrian Kantrowitz and his team in 1967, is the most commonly used one. If inserted via the femoral access, the radio-opaque marker tip of the IABP balloon should lie 1–2 cm below the left subclavian artery (which corresponds to the second to third intercostal space in chest X-ray), and the lower end of the balloon should be above the renal arteries. IABP works on the principle of counterpulsation. The balloon inflates at the beginning of diastole, corresponding to the dicrotic notch in arterial pressure tracings or the middle of the T wave in ECG, causing "diastolic augmentation" and improving coronary perfusion. The balloon deflates at the onset of systole, corresponding to the peak of the R wave in ECG or before the upstroke in arterial pressure tracing, causing "systolic unloading", improving the forward flow. It was initially given a Class I recommendation in the ESC and AHA guidelines.[27,28] IABP SHOCK II trial, which randomized patients with CS complicating AMI who received early revascularization by CABG or PCI into the IABP group or medical stabilization, showed no difference in 30-day all-cause mortality or mortality on 6-year follow-up.[4] There was no difference in reinfarctions, repeat revascularizations or quality of life. In the newer ESC guidelines, the routine use of IABP has been downgraded to a Class III Level B recommendation.[5] The use of IABP is contraindicated in the presence of significant aortic regurgitation or aortic dissection. Complications include limb ischemia due to mechanical obstruction of the left subclavian artery by the IABP balloon or thrombosis, aortic dissection during insertion of the guide wire and balloon rupture and helium embolization. IABP use requires regular monitoring of left upper limb pulse and saturation for early detection of proximal migration of balloon and monitoring of renal functions and urine output to detect distal migration. Once a mean arterial pressure of 65 mm Hg and cardiac index >2 L/min/m^2 is achieved, the patient may be weaned off IABP by either reducing the ratio of augmented to non-augmented beats every 1–6 hours (1:1 → 1:2 → 1:3) or by decreasing the balloon filling volume by 10 mL every 1–6 hours till 20 mL. If a ratio of 1:3 is tolerated for more than 6 hours, the device may be removed.

Impella is a continuous flow device with an axial pump. The inner cannula is placed 3.5 cm below the aortic valve, and the outer cannula is just above the aortic valve; it carries oxygenated blood from the LV to the ascending aorta and provides a circulation "in series" to the normal circulation. The various Impella devices available are Impella 2.5, Impella CP, and Impella 5 for the unloading of LV, which provide a maximum flow of 2.5 L/min, 3–4 L/min, and 5 L/min, respectively and Impella RP for the support of RV with a maximum flow of 4 L/min. The IMPRESS trial compared patients with CS complicating AMI treated with Impella with patients on IABP from the IABP SHOCK II trial. There was no difference in 30-day mortality between the two groups. However, complications such as bleeding and peripheral vascular complications were more common in the Impella group.[29] ISAR-SHOCK also compared Impella 2.5 L to IABP in patients with CS complicating AMI; Impella showed superior hemodynamics regarding an increase in cardiac index 30 minutes after implantation.[30] Thirty-day mortality was comparable in both groups. This was a small study conducted on 26 patients, and Impella 2.5 is a small LVSD with a pump flow of only 2.5 L/min; hence it is hard to draw meaningful conclusions. Patients with left main or complex triple vessel disease with severe LV dysfunction undergoing high-risk PCI in the PROTECT trial, when randomized to IABP or Impella, the Impella group showed a more remarkable improvement in CPO and a trend toward lesser major adverse cardiac events at 90 days. However, these patients were not in CS.[31] The Danish cardiogenic shock trial (DanShock trial) compares Impella and conventional therapy in AMI and is currently underway.

Tandem heart is a continuous flow device with a centrifugal pump which unloads the LA into the abdominal aorta or iliac arteries, thus providing a "parallel circulation". It is a partial support device (2–4 L/min). Theme registry studied patients with CS supported with Tandem heart within 48 hours of diagnosis; there was a significant improvement in cardiac index and lactate clearance in these patients, and the survival at 6 months was >60%.[32] Smaller randomized trials that compared Tandem heart with IABP have shown superior hemodynamics with the former at the cost of more complications like bleeding, without any difference in 30-day survival.[33,34]

Centrimag is an extracorporeal full support (with flow rate up to 9.9 L/min) continuous flow device with a centrifugal pump and a magnetically levitated impeller. It can be used as an RV, LV or biventricular support device. It can also be used along with an oxygenator for ECMO. A retrospective analysis of Centrimag in critical CS secondary to myocarditis, ischemic cardiomyopathy, dilated cardiomyopathy and other causes excluding post-cardiac surgery showed a 55% survival to discharge and 46% 5-year survival.[35] Small studies have shown a benefit of a combined Centrimag and ECMO strategy termed Ec-VAD in CS.[36,37]

Venoarterial ECMO or ECLS (extracorporeal life support) helps deliver venous blood from the right atria or femoral vein to an oxygenator and returns the oxygenated blood with the help of a centrifugal pump back into the aorta or femoral artery. Most of the data on ECMO in CS comes from small retrospective studies. A meta-analysis of over 12,000 patients managed with VA-ECMO showed in-hospital mortality as high as 60%.[38] ELCS-SHOCK, EURO-SHOCK, and ANCHOR were three large RCTs planned to study the role of VA-ECMO in CS. EURO-SHOCK studied the use of ECMO in patients with CS persisting 30 minutes after primary PCI of the culprit vessel. There was no difference in 30-day all-cause mortality, and vascular and bleeding complications were more common in the ECMO group. Recruitment in the trial was affected by the COVID-19 pandemic, and the trial was prematurely terminated.[39] ANCHOR and ELCS-SHOCK trials are currently underway.

The current guidelines recommend initiating MCS only in CS not responding to pharmacological therapy. The National Cardiogenic Shock Initiative studied the role of early initiation of MCS in CS. Patients admitted with acute MI-related CS were managed with early insertion of MCS (mean door-to-support time was 85 minutes). The survival to explant was 72%.[40] ECMO-CS trial studied the early initiation of ECMO versus conservative strategy with downstream initiation of ECMO in case of worsening hemodynamic status. The 30-day incidence of all-cause mortality, resuscitated cardiac arrest or use of other MCS was not statistically different between the two groups.[41] Whether early MCS confers, any real benefit remains to be further studied.

CONCLUSION

Cardiogenic shock is a medical emergency warranting early recognition, risk stratification, and initiation of treatment. Scores such as IABP shock II in MI-related CS and CardShock score help identify patients with a high mortality risk. SAVE and ENCOURAGE scores identify patients who will benefit from ECMO. After a quick fluid challenge in patients without overt hypovolemia, patients must be started on vasopressors and inotropes. The combination of noradrenaline and dobutamine is the recommended first-line therapy; adrenaline and dopamine are second-line agents in CS due to the higher risk of arrhythmias and mortality demonstrated in trials. Vasopressin has been postulated to be helpful, particularly in right heart failure, but it needs further study. In patients with chronic heart failure with desensitization of catecholaminergic receptors and who are on long-term beta-blocker therapy, newer agents such as levosimendan and milrinone act independently of the catecholaminergic pathway are attractive options. The routine use of MCS devices is not recommended. The short-term use of mechanical support devices may be considered in refractory CS not responding to medical management. Even with the best available management, mortality risk remains high in CS.

ONLINE REFERENCES

Please scan the QR code provided at the end of the table of contents for References of this chapter.

CHAPTER

205

Mechanical Circulatory Support during PCI of Cardiogenic Shock and High-risk PCI

Sridhar Kasturi

ABSTRACT

Application of mechanical circulatory support (MCS) is gaining momentum in the recent times to maintain adequate systemic and myocardial perfusion while performing percutaneous coronary intervention (PCI) of patients with cardiogenic shock (CS) and protected PCI. Before commencing MCS, patients must be evaluated with appropriate steps to determine prognosis based on clinal, hemodynamic criteria and relevant diagnostic tests to proceed with emergency or high-risk revascularization strategies with necessary inotropic and MCS support. Early staging and detection of phenotype of CS with respect to the congestion profile may be associated with improved clinical outcomes. It is often useful for patients with de novo or refractory CS by providing short-term hemodynamic support, as a bridge to decision, a bridge to recovery, or a bridge to a more durable platform [left ventricular assist device (LVAD) or transplantation]. Sometimes, combination of various MCS platforms is also being used to take the synergistic benefits of different devices such as ECPella/BiPella/venoarterial extracorporeal membrane oxygenation (VA-ECMO) and intra-aortic balloon pump (IABP). Escalation and de-escalation of MCS should be considered in appropriately selected patients based on clinical, hemodynamic, and other diagnostic parameters during MCS support for the extension of support as long as it is necessary with careful consideration of the risks versus benefits.

Keywords: MCS, ECMO, IABP, impella, cardiogenic shock.

INTRODUCTION

Cardiogenic shock (CS) manifests as tissue hypoperfusion with hypoxia caused due to a primary cardiac dysfunction which is seen in about 5–10% of patients presenting with acute myocardial infarction (AMI), more often in ST-elevation myocardial infarction (STEMI) patients. Although many advances took place in the management, still the incidence of CS in the past few years have remained unchanged. Even though early revascularization remains the main management option with proven reduced mortality in the long term, a delay in the decision-making and treatment may lead to further progression of clinical and hemodynamic deterioration, which may lead to about 50% inhospital mortality even with advanced tertiary care services despite the best interventional and surgical strategies. The recent evidence supports the implementation of a shock protocol and early escalation of mechanical circulatory support (MCS) support prior to percutaneous coronary intervention (PCI) in CS of STEMI is associated with increased survival rate to hospital discharge (74%), and patients who underwent right heart catheterization with proper hemodynamic evaluation showed lowest inhospital death rate compared to those without.[1]

Mechanical circulatory support improves hemodynamic status of patients of CS and protected PCI, hence allows the operator to do complete revascularization of high-risk, complex PCI. MCS increases the systemic perfusion, coronary perfusion, decreases left ventricle (LV) filling pressures, LV wall stress, and myocardial oxygen consumption. During the management of patients with CS, it should be initiated as early as possible, preferably prior to starting PCI procedure, and the appropriate escalation and de-escalation strategies are useful to provide the maximum benefits with minimal complications.

DEFINITION

Cardiogenic shock diagnostic criteria includes systolic blood pressure (SBP) < 90 mm Hg for ≥30 minutes (or support in order to maintain blood pressure), a cardiac index (CI) ≤ 2.2 L/min/m², pulmonary capillary wedge pressure (PCWP) ≥ 15 mm Hg, and markers of end-organ hypoperfusion (urine output < 30 mL/h, altered mental status, cool extremities, lactate > 2.0 mmol/L).[2] Heart failure guidelines include clinical criteria along with hemodynamic criteria in the definition of CS: SBP < 90 mm Hg despite appropriate fluid resuscitation with clinical and laboratory evidence of end-organ damage.

ROLE OF INOTROPIC SUPPORT

Almost all patients of CS require early initiation of inotropic support which can augment cardiac output (CO) and increase blood pressure to more or less normal ranges but increase myocardial oxygen consumption. Inotropic therapy increases LV afterload and worsens microvascular congestion, and therefore reduces CO and deterioration of the hemodynamic and metabolic status of CS **(Figs. 1A and B)**; it must be aimed at achieving the adequate tissue perfusion without significantly increasing cardiac work; and it should be used for the shortest duration and with the lowest possible doses and number of inotropic drugs.

PREPROCEDURAL EVALUATION

Before the initiation of MCS, assess the ability of MCS to provide hemodynamic or circulatory support in terms of only LV or right ventricular (RV) support versus biventricular support and effect on cardiac power output (CPO) and pulmonary artery pulsatility index (PAPi), coronary perfusion, myocardial protection ability of MCS to offload the ventricle while providing support, ease of use in terms of insertion and operation, contraindications or limitations, and potential complications with reasonable alternative plans of backup strategies.

Prior to the commencement of the MCS, it is also essential to rule out absolute contraindications which include irreversible cardiac failure with a lack of an exit strategy (i.e., heart transplantation or durable MCS) and concomitant irreversible, noncardiac, multi-organ failure or other terminal illnesses. Patients with relative contraindications should be carefully evaluated for risk versus benefit of MCS with alternative backup plan if any complications would develop.

Evaluation of Clinical, Biochemical, and Hemodynamic Parameters for Assessing Severity and Guiding Management (Table 1)[3]

Physical: Tachycardia, extensive rales, hypotension with low systolic and mean BP, elevated jugular venous pressure

TABLE 1: Hemodynamic parameters assisting device selection.

RV failure	LV failure
CVP ≥ 15 mm Hg	SBP <90 mm Hg or MAP < 60 or >30 mm Hg drop and inotropes/vasopressors
PAPi ≤ 1.85	• CI < 2.2 L/min/m² • CPO < 0.6 W
RA/PCWP ratio ≥ 0.8	LVEDP > 15 mm Hg
Deteriorating shock (SCAI C and D stages)-Failure to respond to initial therapy with clinical signs of hypoperfusion.	

(CI: cardiac index; CPO: cardiac power output; CVP: central venous pressure; LV: left ventricular; LVEDP: LV end-diastolic pressure; MAP: mean arterial pressure; PAPi: pulmonary artery pulsatility index; PCWP: pulmonary capillary wedge pressure; RA: right atrial; RV: right ventricular; SBP: systolic blood pressure; SCAI: Society for Cardiovascular Angiography and Interventions)

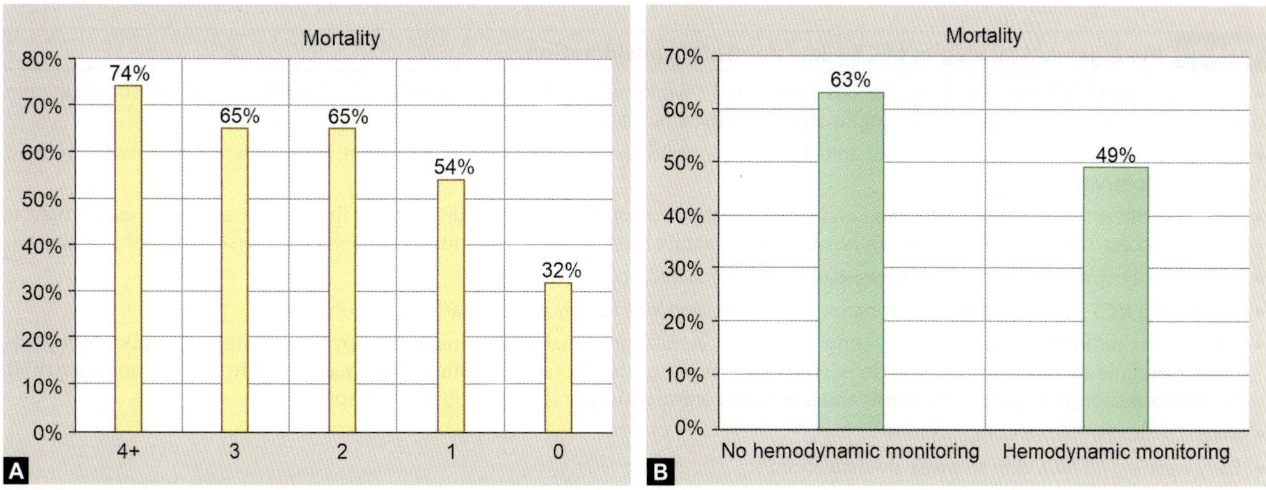

FIGS. 1A AND B: Invasive hemodynamics and decreased inotropes associated with survival in acute myocardial infarction/cardiogenic shock (AMI/CGS).

(JVP), increased capillary refill time, oliguria, alteration in mental status, mottled, and cold and clammy extremities.

Investigations: Increased serum creatinine (S. cr), low-estimated glomerular filtration rate (e-GFR), increased lactate and decreased lactate clearance, low serum bicarbonate, increased base deficit, and increased venous arterial carbon dioxide gap [P(v-a) CO_2].

Hemodynamic: CI, pulmonary artery compliance, CPO, left ventricular end-diastolic pressure (LVEDP), mean arterial pressure (MAP), PAPi, and low central venous oxygen saturation ($ScvO_2$)/mixed venous oxygen saturation (SvO_2).

Ventilatory: Partial pressure of end-tidal carbon dioxide partial pressure ($PETCO_2$).

Mechanical circulatory support should be aimed at improving CO and reducing LVEDP **(Fig. 2)** to relieve ischemia and to provide adequate tissue perfusion and oxygenation to avert hemodynamic and metabolic consequences of shock which lead to multi-organ dysfunction. CS associated **(Box 1)** with multi-organ dysfunction is associated with very high mortality compared to without (31% vs. 48%).[4]

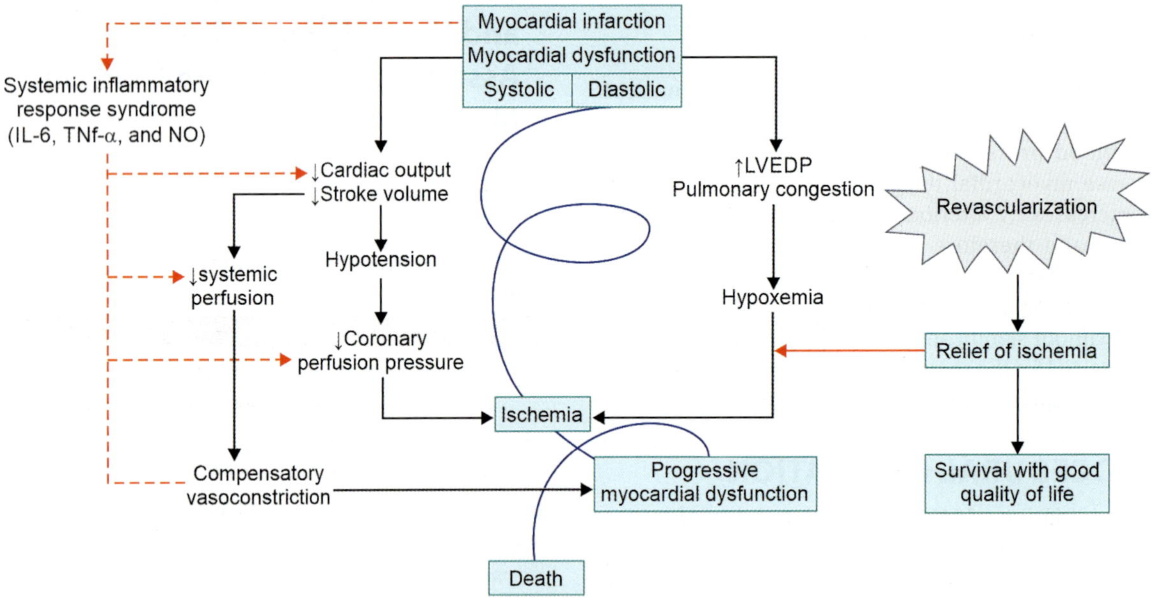

FIG. 2: Classic shock paradigm.

(IL-6: interleukin 6; LVEDP: left ventricular end-diastolic pressure; NO: nitric oxide; TNF-α: tumor necrosis factor alpha)

Source: Adapted from van Diepen S, Katz JN, Albert NM, Henry TD, Jacobs AK, Kapur NK, et al.; American Heart Association Council on Clinical Cardiology; Council on Cardiovascular and Stroke Nursing; Council on Quality of Care and Outcomes Research; and Mission: Lifeline. Contemporary Management of Cardiogenic Shock: A Scientific Statement From the American Heart Association. Circulation. 2017;136(16):e232-68.

BOX 1 Management strategies of CS—key points for consideration.

- *Early recognition ACS with CS*: Assess various causes and severity of CS, clinical examination, ECG, lactate, urine output, creatinine, echocardiography, and invasive angiography with hemodynamic data
- *Assessment of staging and severity of shock*: Initial stabilization with oxygenation, ventilator support, fluid challenge of no overt overload, and inotropes/vasopressors
- *Early catheterization laboratory activation and initial of early and optimal MCS*: Multidisciplinary shock team approach, assessment of vascular access, CPO < 0.6 W, CI < 2.2 L/min/m^2, elevated lactate levels > 4, rule out anoxic brain injury/irreversible end-organ failure
- Plan for early optimal culprit vessel PCI result/repair of mechanical complications
- Monitoring MCS using invasive hemodynamic parameters and look for any need of early escalation of MCS
- *Initiate optimal intensive care support*: Lung protective ventilation, renal replacement therapy if indicated, thromboprophylaxis, norepinephrine and other vasopressors as per the requirement, gastric protection, optimal glycemic control, frequent monitoring of Hb for any correction, and look for any sepsis and adequate control with appropriate antibiotic therapy
- Minimize device-related complications
- Early weaning off MCS with stepwise de-escalation
- Discuss and plan for an alternative strategy for patients with multiple failed weaning attempts of MCS

(ACS: acute coronary syndrome; CI: cardiac index; CPO: cardiac power output; CS: cardiogenic shock; ECG: electrocardiogram; Hb: hemoglobin; MCS: mechanical circulatory support; PCI: percutaneous coronary intervention)

CLASSIFICATION OF CARDIOGENIC SHOCK

Patients with CS must be evaluated with appropriate steps to determine prognosis and staging of shock based on clinical, hemodynamic criteria and relevant diagnostic tests to proceed with emergency revascularization strategies with necessary inotropic and MCS support **(Table 2)**.

ASSESSMENT OF PHENOTYPE OF CARDIOGENIC SHOCK

Identification of the CS phenotype with respect to the congestion profile may be associated with improved short-term outcomes.[6] It can be classified based on the ventricle affected: (1) LV dominant, (2) RV dominant, or (3) biventricular failure.

Cardiogenic shock with LV-dominant type: It is characterized by high PCWP (>18 mm Hg) with normal or reduced central venous pressure (CVP) (14 mm Hg) with normal or reduced pulmonary artery pressure and PCWP (14 mm Hg), normal or elevated PCWP (>18 mm Hg) and hypotension, along with reduced LV function. At least 40% of patients diagnosed with LV-dominant CS, in fact, have biventricular failure.

Right ventricular-dominant type of CS is characterized by a relatively normal PCWP in the setting of an elevated right atrial (RA) pressure (>15 mm Hg) and an elevated ratio of RA pressure to PCWP (>0.63 or 0.86 mm Hg), which should trigger further evaluation for RV failure. The cutoff for an abnormal RA/PCWP has been described as >0.86 in AMI, but the RA/PCWP ratio exists on a spectrum with higher levels predictive at higher sensitivity and specificity of RV failure. RV function can be quantified by measuring RV stroke work, RV stroke work index, and CVP/PCWP ratio. A CVP/PCWP ratio > 0.86 signifies impaired RV function, provided CVP is elevated above normal. In addition, the PAPi [pulmonary arterial systolic pressure–pulmonary arterial diastolic pressure (PASP–PADP)/CVP]

TABLE 2: SCAI expert consensus statement on the classification of cardiogenic shock.[5]

SCAI shock stages	Physical team	Biochemical markers	Hemodynamics
A	• Normal JVP • Lung sounds clear • Strong distal pulses • Normal mentation	• Normal renal function • Normal lactic acid	• Normotensive (SBP > 100 or normal for point) *If hemodynamics done*: • Cardiac index > 2.5 L/min/m² • CVP < 10 • PA sat > 65%
B	• Elevated JVP • Rales in lung fields • Strong distal pulses • Normal mentation	• Normal lactate • Minimal renal function impairment • Elevated BNP	SBP < 90 or MAP < 60 or >30 mm Hg drop *If hemodynamics done*: • Cardiac index > 2.2 L/min/m² • PA sat > 65%
C	• Ashen, mottled, dusky • Volume overload • Extensive rales • Killip class III or IV • BiPAP or mechanical ventilation • Acute alteration in mental status	• Lactate > 2 • Creatinine doubling or >50% drop in GFR • Increases LFTs • Elevated BNP • Urine output < 30 mL/h	• Drugs/device used to maintain BP above stage B values • Cardiac index < 2.2 L/min/m², PCWP > 15 mm Hg, RAP/PCWP > 0.8, PAPi < 1.85, and cardiac power output < 0.6 W
D	Any of stage C	• Any of stage C *and* • Deteriorating	• Any of stage C and • Requiring multiple pressors or addition of mechanical circulatory support devices to maintain perfusion
E	• Near pulselessness • Cardiac collapses • Mechanical ventilation • Defibrillator used	• Lactate > 5 • pH < 7.2	• No SBP without resuscitation • PEA or refractory VT/VF • Hypotension despite maximal support

(BiPAP: bilevel positive airway pressure; BNP: brain natriuretic peptide; BP: blood pressure; CVP: central venous pressure; GFR: glomerular filtration rate; JVP: jugular venous pressure; LFTs: liver function tests; MAP: mean arterial pressure; PA sat: pulmonary artery saturation; PAPi: pulmonary artery pulsatility index; PCWP: pulmonary capillary wedge pressure; PEA: pulseless electrical activity; RAP: right atrial pressure; SBP: systolic blood pressure; SCAI: Society for Cardiovascular Angiography and Interventions; VT/VF: ventricular tachycardia/ventricular fibrillation)

BOX 2 Evaluation and prognostication of CS-proposed criteria of SCAI.

- *Shock severity*:
  - Staging of SCAI shock
  - Hemodynamic assessment
  - Assessment of metabolic derangements
  - Assess vasopressor toxicity
- *Risk modifiers*:
  - Nonmodifiable risk factors, e.g., age and comorbidities
  - Cardiac arrest with coma
  - Presence/reversibility of organ failure
  - Systemic inflammatory response
  - Frailty/risk of complications
- *Phenotype and etiology*:
  - Acute versus acute-on-chronic
  - Clinical etiology of CS
  - RV versus LV versus BIV systolic dysfunction
  - Cardiac versus cardiopulmonary failure
  - Congestion profile
  - Biochemical phenotype

(BIV: biventricular; CS: cardiogenic shock; LV: left ventricular; RV: right ventricular; SCAI: Society for Cardiovascular Angiography and Interventions)

has been found to be more specific for evaluation of the degree of RV dysfunction. The predictive value regarding inhospital mortality of RV dysfunction has been examined in AMI-CS and acute decompensated heart failure; the retrospective study by Jain et al. found higher RAP, RA/PCWP, and lower PAPi and RV stroke work index values in nonsurvivors than those in survivors.[7] At present, there is no hemodynamic gold standard for defining RV failure because the aforementioned hemodynamic values can be influenced by volume resuscitation, passive congestion, or concurrent valvular disease (i.e., tricuspid stenosis, tricuspid regurgitation, pulmonic stenosis, and pulmonic regurgitation). Therefore, the diagnosis of RV or biventricular failure require consideration of both invasive hemodynamic assessment of RV failure and noninvasive cardiac imaging (i.e., echocardiography) **(Box 2)**. In clinical practice, it is essential to consider the RA/PCWP along with other hemodynamic, clinical, biochemical, and imaging parameters on a spectrum of severity to take appropriate escalation and de-escalation steps.

SELECTION OF TYPE OF MECHANICAL CIRCULATORY SUPPORT DEVICE FOR CARDIOGENIC SHOCK

Principles of shock management aim at ensuring adequate systemic perfusion with minimal complications with clear exit plan up to recovery or alternative heart replacement therapies **(Tables 3 and 4)**.

Mechanical circulatory support is often useful for patients with de novo or refractory CS by providing short-term hemodynamic support, as a bridge to decision, a bridge to recovery, or a bridge to a more durable platform [left ventricular assist device (LVAD) or transplantation]. Sometimes, combination of various MCS platforms is also being used to take the synergistic benefits of different devices such as ECPella—combination of venoarterial extracorporeal membrane oxygenation (VA-ECMO) with an Impella for LV decompression, VA-ECMO with an intra-aortic balloon pump (IABP), BiPella—left-sided support with an Impella 2.5/CP/5.5 and right-sided support with an Impella RP, and right-sided TandemHeart with an LV Impella. If pulmonary support is needed, an oxygenator can be added to an extracorporeal RV assist device (TandemHeart or surgical RV assist device) or a TandemHeart LVAD, and alternatively VA-ECMO can also be considered.

MECHANICAL CIRCULATORY SUPPORT FOR HIGH-RISK PERCUTANEOUS CORONARY INTERVENTION

Mechanical circulatory support **(Fig. 3)** may be considered in patients who are surgically unsuitable or at high risk due to associated comorbidities, complex coronary disease of left main (LM), microvascular disease (MVD), and severely calcified lesions requiring plaque modification devices, severe LV dysfunction—ejection fraction (EF) < 25%, SBP 100 mm Hg, and LVEDP > 25 mm Hg.

Complex High-risk Indicated PCI (CHIP) score is based on baseline patient characteristics and procedural variables, which is used to predict risk and major adverse cardiac and cerebrovascular events (MACCE) rate of patients undergoing CHIP-PCI which include[8] seven patient-related factors, such as (1) age > 80 years, (2) female, (3) previous myocardial infarction, (4) previous stroke, (5) peripheral vascular disease (PVD), (6) EF < 30%, and (7) chronic kidney disease (CKD), and six procedural factors, such as (1) rotational atherectomy (ROTA), (2) left main coronary artery (LMCA), (3) MVD, (4) dual arterial access, (5) LV MCS, (6) total lesion length > 60 mm. As per the analysis in >3 lakh patients who underwent PCI in the United Kingdom (UK), there was an exponential increase in MACCE rate and other adverse events with the increase in CHIP score.

Mechanical circulatory support during high-risk PCIs should be based on LV dysfunction and complexity of coronary anatomy and disease. It offloads LV by maintaining balance between myocardial oxygen demand and supply, and thereby maintains CO, end-organ perfusion, relieves tissue hypoxia, and allows recovery of ischemic but viable myocardium. IABP support may be considered for patients with EF 30–40%, low syntax score < 32/Society of Thoracic Surgeons (STS) < 5 and without any plan for extensive revascularization. Impella acts as a more effective MCS device when EF < 30%, syntax score >32/STS > 5, and extensive

TABLE 3: CS—evaluate for hemodynamic criteria before choosing the MCS device.

	CVP (mm Hg)	PCWP (mm Hg)	CVP/PCWP	PAPi	RV failure
RV dominant shock	>14	<18	>0.86	<1.5	• Short or intermediate term ○ Impella RP ○ TandemHeart ○ ECMO ○ Protek Duo • Post cardiac surgery ○ Impella RP ○ TandemHeart ○ CentriMag/RotaFlow
LV dominant shock	<14	>18	<0.86	>1.5	• Short term ○ Impella ○ TandemHeart ○ ECMO ○ Protek Duo • Intermediate term ○ Impella 5.0 ○ TandemHeart • Postcardiac surgery ○ CentriMag/RotaFlow
Biventricular shock	>14	Variable	>0.86	<1.5	• Short or intermediate term ○ Peripheral ECMO • Intermediate term ○ Impella CP/RP ○ LV assist device/Protek Duo ○ TandemHeart • Postcardiac surgery ○ Central ECMO ○ CentriMag/RotaFlow

(CS: cardiogenic shock; CVP: central venous pressure; ECMO: extracorporeal membrane oxygenation; MCS: mechanical circulatory support; PAPi: pulmonary artery pulsatility index; PCWP: pulmonary capillary wedge pressure; RV: right ventricular)

TABLE 4: Comparison of different mechanical support devices.

MCS device	IABP	IMPELLA	TandemHeart	VA-ECMO
CO (L/min)	0.5–1.0	2.5/3.0–4.0/5.0	4.0–5.0	4.0–10.0
Mechanism of action	Balloon inflation–deflation (aortic)	Axial flow continuous pump (LV-to-Ao)	Centrifugal flow continuous pump (LA-to-Ao)	Centrifugal flow continuous pump (RA-to-Ao)
Flow rate	NA	2.5–5.5 L/min	Maximum 4.0 L/min	Maximum 7.0 L/min
Access site	Femoral artery/ axillary artery	Femoral artery/axillary artery	Femoral artery/Femoral vein	Femoral artery/Femoral vein
Cannula size	7–8 Fr arterial	13–21 Fr arterial	• 12–19 Fr arterial • 21 Fr venous	• 14–19 Fr arterial • 17–21 Fr venous
LV preload	–	↓↓	↓↓	↓↓
LVEDP	↓	↓↓	↓↓	↔
Afterload	↓	↓	↑	↑↑↑
PCWP	↓	↓↓	↓↓	↔

Continued

Continued

MCS device	IABP	IMPELLA	TandemHeart	VA-ECMO
Coronary perfusion	↑	?	?	?
Myocardium O_2 demand	↓	↓	↓↔	↔
TPR	↓	↓	↑	↑↑
Hemodynamic support	+	++	+++	+++
Contraindications:				
Vascular	Severe PAD	Severe PAD	Severe PAD	Severe PAD
Valve	Moderate-severe AR	• Mechanical aortic valve • Moderate-severe AR, AS with AVA < 0.6 cm^2	Severe AR	Moderate-severe AR
Structural	Significant aortic disease, i.e., aortic aneurysm/dissection	LV thrombus	LA thrombus and VSD	Unrepaired aortic dissection
Complications:				
Bleeding	Low	Moderate	Very high	High to very high risk
Vascular	Low	Moderate–High	High	Very high
Hemolysis	No	Yes	Yes	Yes
Device related	Balloon rupture	Device migration/malfunction	Device migration	Device malfunction
Rare	Aortic dissection/ rupture, and thrombocytopenia	Aortic valve injury	Cardiac tamponade	Thrombocytopenia and neurological injury
Advantages	• Simple cannulation • ≤8 Fr arterial access	• Simple cannulation • Direct LV unloading • Antegrade (physiologic flow)	• Direct LA loading • Indirect LV unloading	• Simple cannulation • Biventricular support • Oxygenation support
Disadvantages	• Low cost • Minimum of cardiac function and competent aortic valve required • Modest ventricular unloading	• Expensive • Hemolysis • Frequent monitoring of device position with bedside echocardiography	• Requires transseptal access • Retrograde (nonphysiologic) blood flow	• Labor intensive • Complex patient management • Immobilized patient • Dual vessel access • Nonpulsatile flow • Cerebral hypoxia • Limb ischemia

(Ao: aortic; AR: aortic regurgitation; AS: aortic stenosis; AVA: aortic valve stenosis; IABP: intra-aortic balloon pressure; LA: left atrial; LV: left ventricular; LVEDP: LV end-diastolic pressure; MCS: mechanical circulatory support; NA: not applicable; PAD: peripheral artery disease; PCWP: pulmonary capillary wedge pressure; RA: right atrial; TPR: total peripheral resistance; VA-ECMO: venoarterial extracorporeal membrane oxygenation; VSD: ventricular septal defect)

revascularization is to be performed, whereas ECMO is more useful for patients with cardiac arrest and severe hypoxia.

SALIENT FEATURES OF DIFFERENT MECHANICAL CIRCULATORY SUPPORT DEVICES

Intra-aortic balloon pump: It increases diastolic blood pressure (DBP), reduces mean arterial BP, decreases afterload, decreases myocardial oxygen consumption, increases coronary artery perfusion, and moderately enhances CO. Presence of some level of LV function and electrical stability is essential to make it more effective, as increase in CO is dependent on the work of the heart itself.[9] IABP requires adequate LV function for its efficacy, and it will become less ineffective as the LV function deteriorates. It consists of a flexible catheter with one lumen that allows for either distal aspiration/flushing or pressure monitoring, and available in sizes between 25 and 50 cc. Additionally, it has a mobile console that contains the system for helium transfer, and computer control of the inflation and deflation cycle.

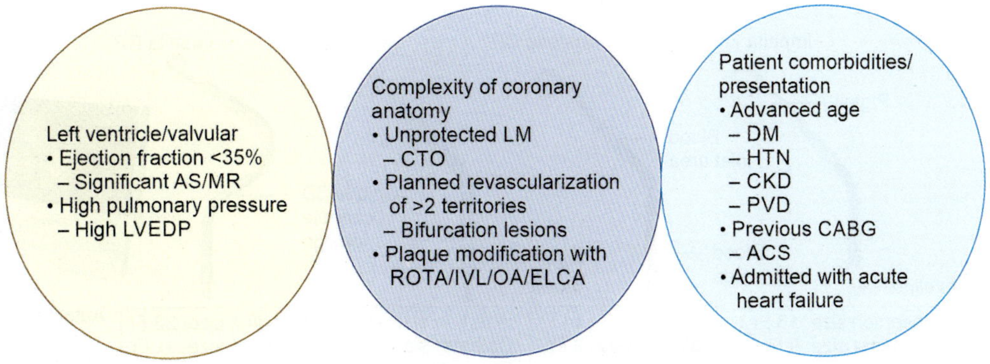

FIG. 3: High-risk PCI characteristics.

(ACS: acute coronary syndrome; AS: aortic stenosis; CABG: coronary artery bypass grafting; CKD: chronic kidney disease; CTO: chronic total occlusion; DM: diabetes mellitus; ELCA: excimer laser coronary atherectomy; HTN: hypertension; IVL: intravascular lithotripsy; LM: left main; LVEDP: left ventricular end-diastolic pressure; MR: mitral regurgitation; OA: orbital atherectomy; PVD: peripheral vascular disease; ROTA: rotational atherectomy)

TABLE 5: Selected randomized trials of circulatory device therapy and indications.

Trials	Study devices	Indications	Primary outcomes
IABP SHOCK II	IABP	Cardiogenic shock	No difference in 30-day mortality or secondary endpoints
CRISP	IABP	Acute anterior myocardial infarction	Trend toward higher infarct size and vascular complications with IABP
PROTECT II	Impella 2.5 versus IABP	High-risk PCI	No difference in 30-day MAE; halted for futility and DSMB concerns for safety trends
BCIS	IABP	High-risk PCI	No difference in inhospital MACCE; improved 5-year survival
IMPRESS	Impella CP versus IABP	Cardiogenic shock	No difference in 30-day mortality or secondary endpoints

(DSMB: Data and Safety Monitoring Board; IABP: intra-aortic balloon pressure; MACCE: major adverse cardiac and cerebrovascular events; MAE: major adverse events; PCI: percutaneous coronary intervention)

IABP requires only a small arteriotomy of 7.5 Fr, increases CO by 0.5–1 L/min, is simple to use, less expensive, and widely available. Although it has been in the clinical practice with a backup of vast real-world experience in CS, refractory angina, and high-risk PCI due to hemodynamic effects; however, no clinical outcome improvement in many studies and guidelines downgraded recommendations or even discouraged its usage. Failure of IABP **(Table 5)** in the clinical trials should not be treated as against use of IABP therapy itself, especially in hospitals with unavailability of other advanced MCS systems, especially when operating high-risk subset patients and expedite steps for early revascularization of culprit vessel to improve survival rate.[10] While performing revascularization of CS, patients preferable to use limited and adequate hydration as per the LVEDP are advisable to reduce mortality and morbidity associated with contrast-induced nephropathy (CIN). It should be avoided in patients with PVD, aortic aneurysm, and aortic regurgitations (ARs) **(Table 5)**.

Impella: It is a percutaneously axial flow pump **(Fig. 4)**, used for short-term MCS (<1–6 days) of patients undergoing protected PCI, and ongoing CS as a result of isolated left ventricular failure that is not responding to conventional treatment measures with or without an IABP.[11] It is the most effective MCS when procedural time of PCI is prolonged with large area of myocardium at ischemic risk. It sucks blood from the LV through inflow part, thereby unloads LV, reduces LVEDP, LV end-diastolic volume (LVEDV), and LV wall stress, and reduces oxygen demand and pumps blood into ascending aorta, hence increases mean systolic pressure, increases myocardial oxygen supply, CO, and end-organ perfusion.

The USpella registry, a retrospective study of 154 patients of AMI-CS, highlighted that early initiation of Impella 2.5 prior to PCI improved survival rates and also complete revascularization compared with those who received it post-PCI.[12] The IMPRESS trial of 24 patients of severe CS with acute STEMI managed with primary PCI, compared effectiveness of Impella versus IABP in reducing mortality in STEMI found no difference in 30-day and 6-month mortality between the two groups.[13] The ISAR-SHOCK (Efficacy Study of LV Assist Device to Treat Patients with Cardiogenic Shock) trial of 25 patients with AMI-CS were randomized to receive either Impella 2.5 (n = 12) or IABP (n = 13), Impella 2.5 was

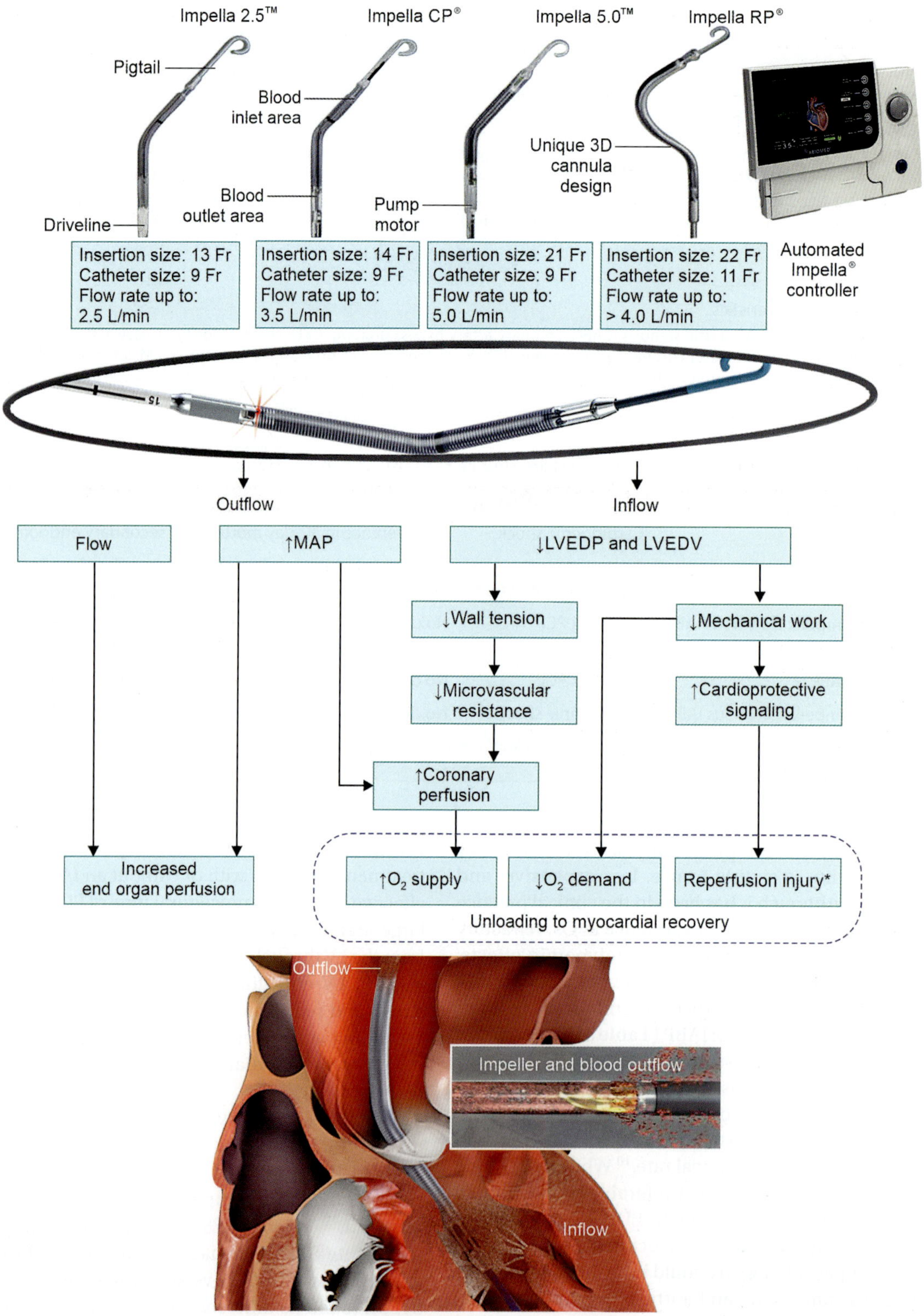

FIG. 4: Impella.

(3D: three dimensional; MAP: mean arterial pressure; LVEDP: left ventricular end-diastolic pressure; LVEDV: left ventricular end-diastolic volume) associated with greater increase in CI, although there was no difference in 30-day mortality between the two groups. However, the small sample sizes of these earlier studies preclude any definitive conclusions regarding the use of either of these devices in AMI-CS.[14]

The PROTECT II trial, one of the largest randomized controlled trials (RCTs) in patients with high-risk PCI, randomized 452 patients to receive the Impella 2.5 ($n = 226$) or IABP ($n = 226$) during high-risk PCI. Although the trial was not completed due to futility, the primary endpoint of a 30-day composite outcome of adverse events was not significantly different between the two groups.[15] As per the PROTECT II trial, the procedural benefits of hemodynamically protected PCI with Impella are fewer hypotensive events, higher CPO, and facilitation of more extensive atherectomy. The clinical benefit of Impella-protected PCI was a reduction of major adverse events postdischarge accompanied with an improvement in ventricular function and heart failure symptoms, and these postdischarge clinical benefits were more pronounced in patients who underwent more complete revascularization with Impella support.

The PROTECT III[16] study, conducted as a part of postmarketing surveillance of the Impella 2.5/Impella CP for high-risk PCI, showed that there was a lower composite endpoint of MACCE with both the Impella 2.5 and Impella CP, compared with such events observed among the PROTECT II trial participants who received the Impella. The ongoing PROTECT IV is currently enrolling patients who will be randomized[17] to undergo high-risk PCI with or without the Impella 2.5. Based on the overall evidence provided, the Food and Drug Administration (FDA) approved Impella 2.5 system for patients undergoing high-risk PCI with significant LV dysfunction to allow a longer and more thorough procedure by preventing episodes of hemodynamic instability.

HeartMate percutaneous heart pump: It is delivered percutaneously into the femoral artery via an integrated 14 Fr sheath. The pump expands to 24 Fr once it is placed across the aortic valve and pumps the blood from LV to the aorta.

Extracorporeal membrane oxygenation ***(Fig. 5A)***: It provides biventricular and pulmonary support and carries some of the disadvantageous-like dual-vessel access with large-sized cannulas, nonpulsatile flow, distension of the LV limiting its recovery and pulmonary hemorrhage, aortic thrombus, cerebral hypoxia, and limb ischemia. It augments CO by 0.4.5 L/min, can be used for several weeks, and does not require sinus rhythm for effective function. Unlike the Impella or the TandemHeart, there is no need for transseptal puncture or crossing of the aortic valve.

There are two varieties of ECMO systems available: (1) veno-venous (VV) ECMO and (2) VA-ECMO.

The device configuration includes three components: (1) Membrane oxygenator and heat exchanger, (2) centrifugal or roller pump, and (3) drainage or perfusion cannula, and cannulation can be done centrally or peripherally. Central cannulation includes a drainage cannula in the right atrium and a perfusion cannula in the ascending aorta. Peripheral cannulation includes a drainage cannula in the jugular or femoral vein, and a perfusion cannula in the femoral, axillary, subclavian or sometimes in the carotid artery. The blood is drawn from the venous system at the right atrium or inferior vena cava and returned to the arterial system through a central or peripheral cannulation site after gas exchange. As a result, there is an increase in afterload and stroke work without any significant reduction of LV wall stress. Therefore, venting is often required to decompress the LV and prevent dilation, which can be managed with some additional strategies such as atrial septostomy, surgical LV vent, IABP, or percutaneous LVAD. Other complications include upper body hypoxemia, bleeding, infection, and limb ischemia. Harlequin syndrome, which is reported in 8.8% of cases, is observed in patients with preserved LV EF when the mixing point of oxygenated blood from ECMO and deoxygenated blood from native LV is below the level of origin of the left carotid artery. This clinical syndrome is also referred to as differential hypoxia and North–South syndrome.[18]

Although no RCTs have evaluated ECMO, observational data from large registries such as the Extracorporeal Life Support Organization showed a survival-to-hospital-discharge rate of 40.2% among 756 patients who received ECMO for AMI-CS.[18] In another study using data from the same registry, the survival-to-hospital-discharge rate was 29% among 2,885 adults who received ECMO for extracorporeal cardiopulmonary resuscitation (CPR).[19]

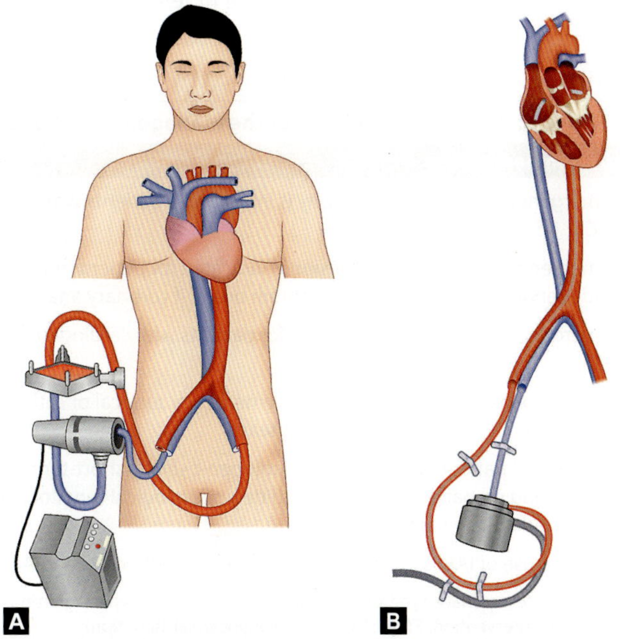

FIGS. 5A AND B: (A) Extracorporeal membrane oxygenation (ECMO) and (B) TandemHeart.

Venoarterial-ECMO is also useful to provide support for patients of CS refractory to conventional medical therapy, and ECMO-CPR is inclusion of ECMO with CPR for patients who do not attain sustained return of spontaneous circulation after cardiac arrest. Conventional CPR is associated with survival of 15–17% for in-hospital cardiac arrest and 8–10% for out-of-hospital cardiac arrest, whereas ECMO-CPR rapidly establishes circulation and improve the outcome. VA-ECMO provides advantage of maintaining oxygenation as well as perfusion pressure unlike Impella and IABP, particularly if there is a very high risk of cardiac arrest-asystole/ventricular tachycardia (VT) and ventricular fibrillation (VF).

TandemHeart: It **(Fig. 5B)** is a centrifugal continuous flow pump [left atrium-to-aortic (LA-to-AO)] which requires transseptal puncture through femoral vein and femoral artery sites that provides direct LA unloading and indirect LV volume unloading and additional pulmonary support by retrograde (nonphysiological) blood flow. It drains with 21 Fr cannula from LA and returns oxygenated blood through 12–19 Fr arterial cannula and generates about 4.0–5.0 L/min of CO. MCS with truncus arteriosus associated with complications such as cardiac perforation, tamponade, air embolism, and residual atrial septal defect (ASD) related to septal puncture and contraindicated in patients who have ventricular septal defect (VSD), significant AR, and LA thrombus.

COMPLICATIONS RELATED TO ACCESS SITE PUNCTURE

Major complications of MCS are due to access related to bleeding, hence meticulous puncture of femoral site using femoral head bony landmarks/intravascular ultrasound (IVUS)/microneedle puncture is essential; avoid puncture site at calcified and diseased segments and if possible, assess iliofemoral anatomy with computed tomography (CT) angiography evaluation prior to procedure **(Table 6)**, especially for elderly patients with PVD. Maintain adequate limb flow during MCS, especially with ECMO/Impella to avoid limb ischemia by various measures such as placing antegrade superficial femoral artery (SFA) sheath and contralateral limb perfusion (external femoral–SFA).

HOW AND WHEN TO ESCALATE MECHANICAL CIRCULATORY SUPPORT

It should be considered in appropriately selected patients with evidence of clinical hypoperfusion or hemodynamic deterioration de novo, while on inotropes, or during initial MCS support. Possible indicators of ongoing severe CS may include (1) persistently low CI (< 2.2 L/min/m^2); (2) CPO < 0.6 W; (3) hypotension (SBP < 90 mm Hg or MAP < 65 mm Hg); (4) inadequate lactate clearance and lactate > 2 mmol/L; (5) evidence of RV failure, including a ratio of RA to PCWP > 0.86 or PAPi ≤ 0.9; (6) profound hypoxemia; or (7) recurrent VT or VF. Early recognition of appropriate patients who can be considered for escalation to MCS may lead to improved survival. MCS in appropriately selected candidates should be initiated as soon as possible with sufficient support to fully reverse the potential hemometabolic consequences of shock. If there is a delay in the early initiation of MCS, it would cause worsening of end-organ perfusion and further metabolic derangements which may make ineffective attempts of future-escalating MCS strategies.

TABLE 6: Recommendations for the management of patients with cardiogenic shock.

Recommendations	Class	Level
Emergency coronary angiography is indicated in patients with acute heart failure or cardiogenic shock complicating ACS	I	B
Emergency PCI of the culprit lesion is indicated for patients with cardiogenic shock due to STEMI or NSTE-ACS, independent of time delay of symptom onset, if coronary anatomy is amenable to PCI	I	B
Emergency CABG is recommended for patients with cardiogenic shock if the coronary anatomy is not amenable to PCI	I	B
In cases of hemodynamic instability, emergency surgical or catheter-based repair of mechanical complications of ACS is indicated, as decided by the heart team	I	C
In selected patients with ACS and cardiogenic shock, short-term mechanical circulatory support may be considered, depending on patient age, comorbidities, neurological function, and the prospects for long-term survival and predicted quality of life	IIb	C
Routine use of IABPs in patients with cardiogenic shock due to ACS is not recommended	III	B

(ACS: acute coronary syndrome; CABG: coronary artery bypass grafting; IABPs: intra-aortic balloon pump; NSTE: non-ST-elevation; PCI: percutaneous coronary intervention; STEMI: ST-elevation myocardial infarction)

HOW AND WHEN TO DE-ESCALATE MECHANICAL CIRCULATORY SUPPORT

Percutaneous coronary intervention with MCS is associated with high rate of complications; it requires constant hourly and day-to-day monitoring which includes physical, diagnostic, and hemodynamic criteria for assessing any worsening or improvement of clinical situation to take appropriate steps regarding escalation or de-escalation strategies. Higher number of complications are anticipated when it is extended for long duration; therefore, carefully assess to minimize the duration of MCS, balancing the risk versus benefit to stabilize patients with lower morbidity and mortality. De-escalation of MCS should be planned as per the device-specific stepwise decrease protocol with careful monitoring of any deterioration at the time of weaning of the MCS to assess any need to extend further or re-escalation of the device or additional MCS support. MCS patients of multiple failed attempts at weaning should be encouraged for durable MCS/cardiac transplantation or palliation management. Evaluate daily for de-escalation of MCS based on clinical, hemodynamic, and other appropriate criteria and it should be considered whenever evidence of full or partial recovery myocardial dysfunction, requiring only minimal intravenous (IV) inotropic support, improved contractility on echocardiography, and improvement in end-organ hypoperfusion is present. Sometimes, MCS-related complications such as vascular injury and bleeding may compel for early withdrawal of MCS. IABP should be weaned at inflation timing of 1:2 or 1:3 or with 10–25% volume decrease and lowest level before removing IABP should be at 1:3 or 75% reduction in volume. Impella CP/5.5/RP requires weaning to the lowest level of P2 before removing with stepwise reduction of 2,000–3,000 revolution per minute (RPM) per step.

Venoarterial-ECMO should be weaned off with increment of 0.5–1.0 L/min at 2–3 hours interval and lowest level before decannulation to be maintained at 2 L/min as a standard protocol and 30 minutes intervals for rapid de-escalation protocol. If unable to wean off/from MCS, patients can be considered for an LVAD/transplant management or palliative care.

We are showcasing two case-based examples of PCI with MCS support about its usefulness in our day-to-day clinical practice and its role in improving the outcome of very high-risk interventional procedures as mentioned further.

CASE 1: PRIMARY PCI WITH ECMO SUPPORT–STEMI WITH CARDIOGENIC SHOCK

Clinical History

A 32-year-old female presented with one episode of chest pain, shortness of breath (SOB), and sweating early morning on the day of admission. Patient was accompanying her father-in-law to get him admitted into the hospital who had been suffering from chronic obstructive pulmonary disease (COPD). She suddenly collapsed outside the causality while waiting for admission of her father-in-law. Patient had sudden onset of seizure and cardiovascular (CV) collapse and decreased responsiveness, intubated and resuscitated in emergency room [CPR was carried out for 30 minutes as per advanced cardiovascular life support (ACLS) and direct current (DC) shock delivered five shocks for recurrent VT/VF episodes]. ECG—anterior wall myocardial infarction with wide QRS complexes **(Fig. 6A)**. 2D echo—akinetic apical interventricular septum (IVS), and apical anterior wall, hypokinesia of mid IVS, anterolateral wall regional wall motion abnormalities (RWMA) with well-preserved thickness of infarcted segments, severe LV dysfunction, EF 30%. Investigations: C-reactive protein (CRP) 66 mg/L, hemoglobin (Hb) 11.5 g/dL, blood urea 17 mg/dL, S. Cr 0.7 mg/dL, eGFR 102 mL/min, troponin-I >24 ng/mL, random blood sugar (RBS) 310 mg/dL, N-terminal prohormone of brain natriuretic peptide (NT-proBNP) 3,962 pg/mL, D-dimer 1,653 ng/mL. ECMO support **(Figs. 6B to D and Table 7)** was carried out using right femoral vein and left femoral artery sites, angiography was done through radiofrequency ablation (RFA), which showed LMCA normal, left anterior descending (LAD)—total thrombotic occlusion of proximal LAD, left circumflex artery (LCX)—normal, right coronary artery (RCA)—proximal-to-mid 30% stenosis. Posterior descending artery (PDA) and Posterior Left Ventricular branch-(PLVB)—normal **(Figs. 7A and B)**.

Procedure

Radiofrequency ablation route, using 7 Fr extra-backup (EBU) 3.5 guiding catheter, angiogram revealed LAD proximal total thrombotic occlusion. LAD lesion was crossed with 0.014" × 190 cm BMW wire. Predilatation done with 2.5 × 15 mm Tazuna balloon to establish antegrade flow and to relieve ongoing myocardial ischemia. Optical coherence tomography (OCT) was done to assess the cause of AMI in young female, which showed long-segment fibrolipid plaque, extending from proximal to distal LAD with plaque rupture (PR) associated with red thrombus in the mid-LAD segment **(Fig. 8)**.

Proximal LAD stenting was done with 3.0 × 26 mm Resolute Onyx stent. Post-OCT showed long-segment fibrolipid plaque with PR distal to the stent. Mid-LAD stenting was done with 2.75 × 38 mm Resolute Onyx stent. Postdilatation was done with 3.0 × 12 mm NC Trek Balloon. Post-OCT showed more than 50% plaque burden in the distal landing zone, fibrotic plaque distal to stent. Hence, distal LAD stenting was done with 2.5 × 15 mm Resolute Onyx stent. Postprocedure angiographic view showed well-implanted stents with thrombolysis in myocardial infarction III (TIMI-III) flow without any dissection. Final Post-OCT run showed well-apposed and expanded stent without any dissection **(Fig. 9)**.

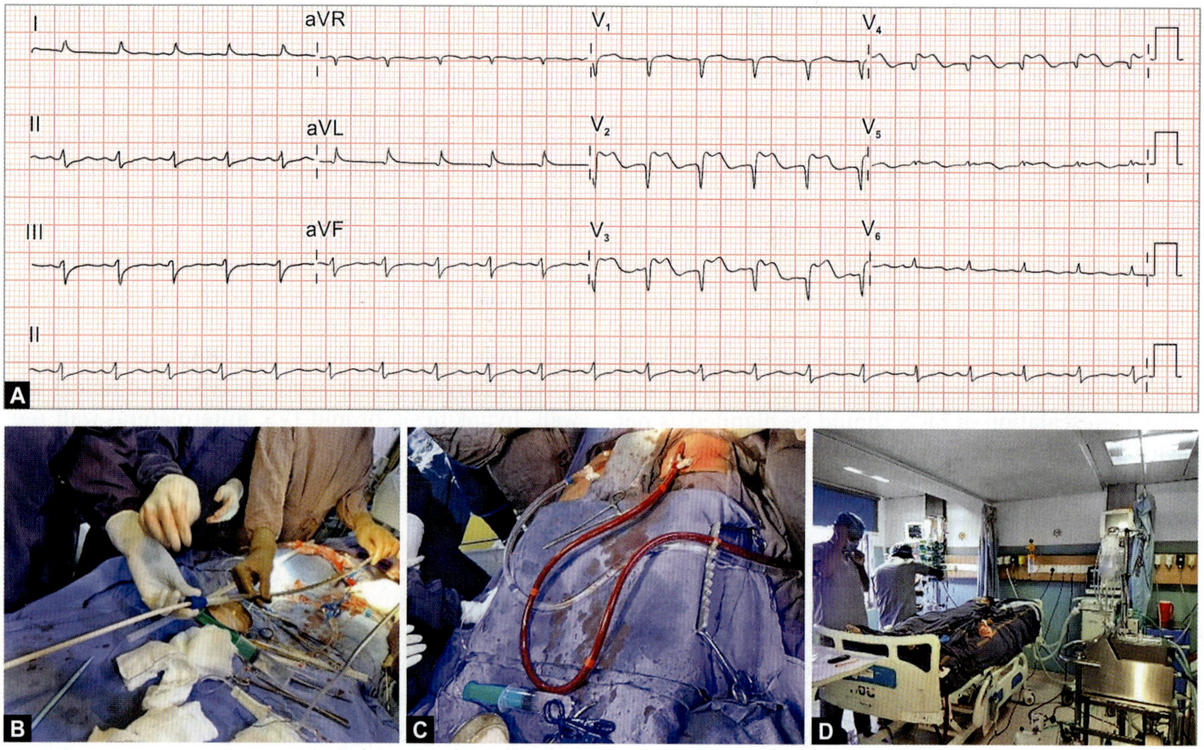

FIGS. 6A TO D: (A) Electrocardiogram (ECG) and (B to D) extracorporeal membrane oxygenation (ECMO).

TABLE 7: Indications for percutaneous biventricular assist devices in CS.

Devices	Indications
VA ECMO: Based on the evidence from registry data, case reports	May be used in case of: • Combined LV and RV failure • Combined LV and ventilation/oxygenation failure • Combined ventilation/oxygenation and RV failure • Refractory cardiac arrest
Impella: Based on the evidence from registry data, case reports	VA ECMO and LV unloading
BiPella: Based on the evidence from registry data, case reports	May be used in RV and LV failure without pulmonary failure

(CS: cardiogenic shock; LV: left ventricular; RV: right ventricular; VA-ECMO: venoarterial extracorporeal membrane oxygenation)

The patient developed repeated episodes of VT during the first 48 hours which were treated with IV-Cordarone and $MgSO_4$ infusions and DC shocks. Repeat check angiography was performed on the second day due to re-elevation of ST-segment in anterior leads to rule out any stent thrombosis which revealed patent stents, no ST with good antegrade flow. The patient was weaned off from inotropic and ECMO support 4 days later due to hemodynamic and clinical improvement.

The patient developed right upper limb venous thrombosis, and thereby produced right upper arm venous edema, treated with IV-heparin and nonvitamin K antagonist oral anticoagulants (NOACs). The patient developed right leg massive hematoma due to oozing from perivenous sheath of ECMO resulting in elevated bilirubin, significant fall of Hb (5.5 g%) requiring multiple blood transfusions. MCS was weaned off gradually from 3 to 2 liters before removing ECMO support on the fourthpost-PCI day with repair of arterial and venous insertion sites at the groins. The patient was discharged on the 12th postprocedure day in a stable status with relief of right upper limb edema and complete relief of CV symptoms. Follow-up visits of first, second, and third year showed excellent exercise capacity, no recurrence of symptoms, good LV function, EF 50%, and without any significant RWMA.

CASE 2

A 74-year-old male, presented with ACS-NSTEMI, with history of sudden onset of class IV SOB due to heart failure with reduced EF (HFrEF) [rapid antigen test (RAT) positive and reverse transcription-polymerase chain reaction (RT-PCR) negative]. ECG—anterolateral ST depressions, 2D echo—RWMA of anterolateral wall and moderate LV dysfunction with EF 36%. Investigation: Hb serial testing

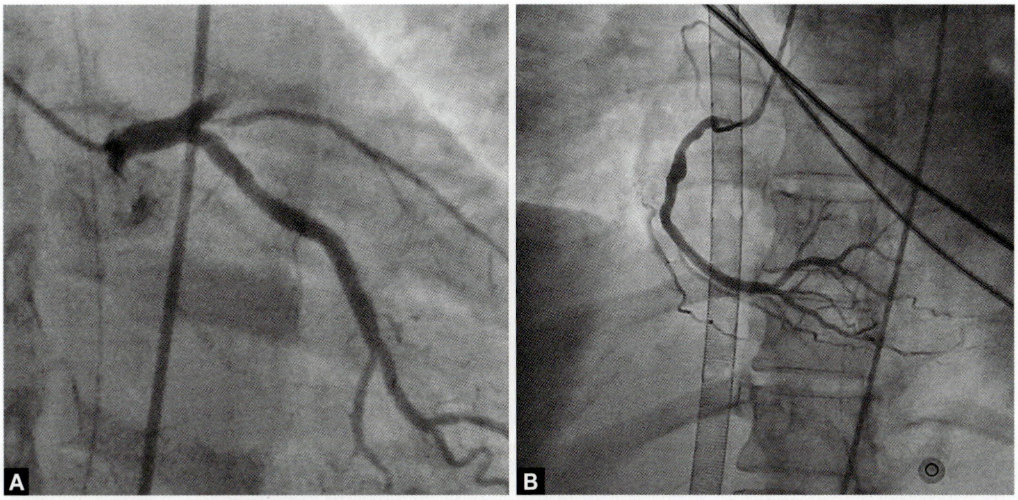

FIGS. 7A AND B: Coronary angiogram.

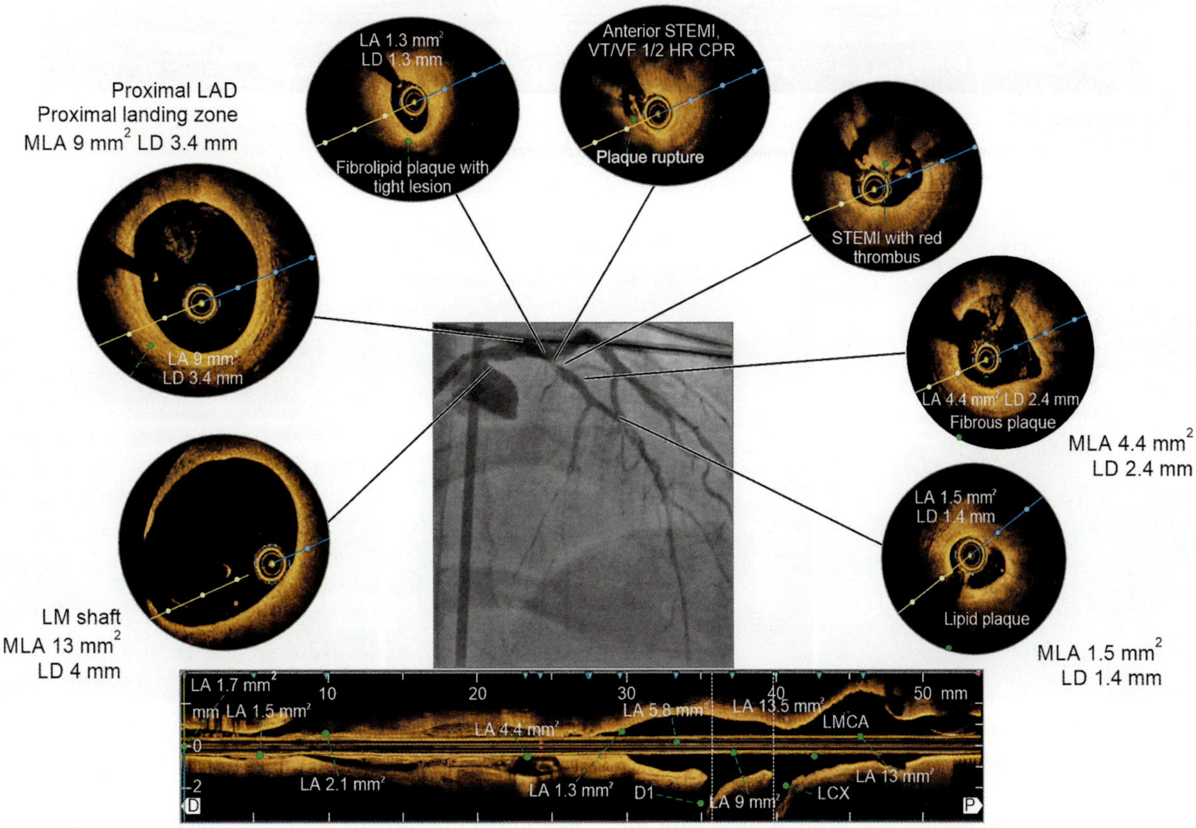

FIG. 8: Presstenting OCT assessment.

(LA: left artery; LAD: left anterior descending; LCX: left circumflex artery; LD: lumen diameter; LM: left main; LMCA: left main coronary artery; MLA: minimal lumen area; OCT: optical coherence tomography)

showed elevated values of S. Cr 1.2 → 1.32 → 1.13 mg/dL, NT-proBNP 11,847 → 7,747 pg/mL, troponin 1,617 → 7,638 → 11,096 ng/mL, and CRP 41 → 36 → 27 mg/L.

Coronary angiogram (CAG): LAD—D1 bifurcation eccentric critical (90%) stenosis with TIMI grade I flow, RCA—proximal 90% lesion and distal 70–80% lesion, procedure planned was LM bifurcation PCI + stent to LAD—D1 and RCA with Impella support, CABG was differed due to recent history of coronavirus disease 2019 (COVID-19) infection and congestive cardiac failure (CCF) **(Figs. 10A to C)**.

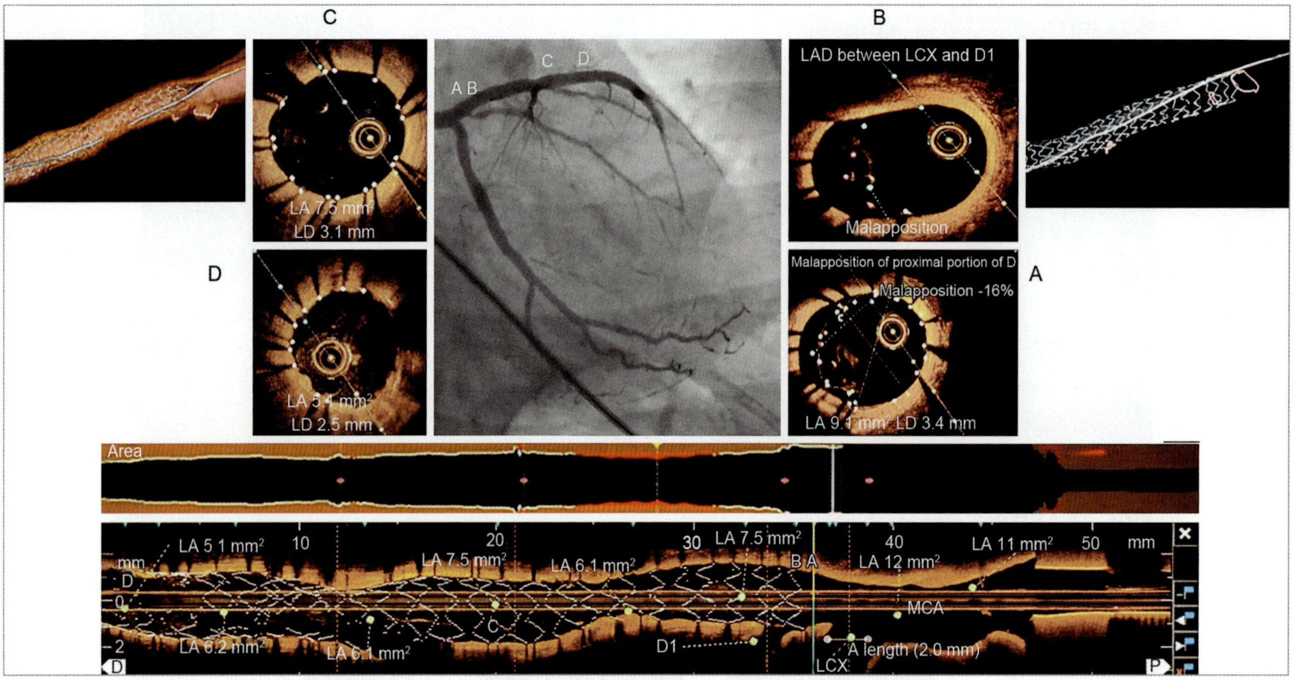

FIG. 9: Poststenting OCT.

(LA: left artery; LD: lumen diameter; LMCA: left main coronary artery; OCT: optical coherence tomography)

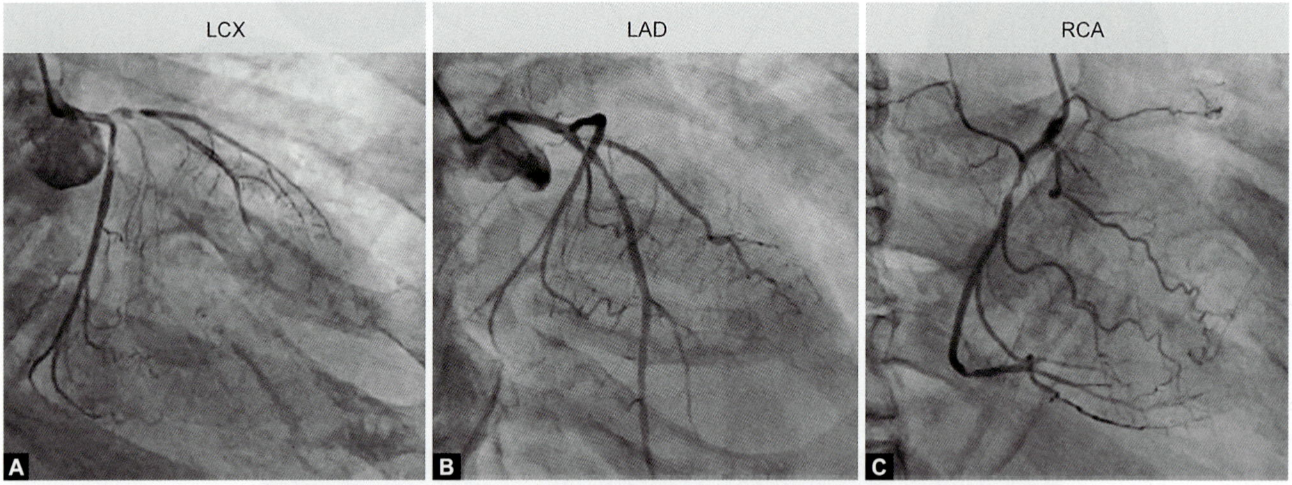

FIGS. 10A TO C: Coronary angiogram.

(LAD: left anterior descending; LCX: left circumflex artery; RCA: right coronary artery)

Right femoral artery access was used, 6 Fr sheath for percutaneous transluminal coronary angioplasty (PTCA). Right femoral vein: 7 Fr sheath, left femoral artery: 7 Fr sheath, exchanged with 13 Fr sheath for the insertion of Impella device through left femoral artery. Pigtail catheter with exchange length 0.035- inch wire was placed in the LV. The regular 0.035- inch wire was exchanged with 0.018- inch wire which was shaped distally with semicircular curve before inserting into the LV. The Impella device was introduced over the 0.018- inch wire which was placed across aortic valve with inlet portion in the LV and outlet portion in the aortic root under fluoroscopy guidance. The device was connected externally to the controller after checking all necessary precautions. CO of around 2.5 liters was maintained after starting device with a MAP about 80–85 mm Hg **(Tables 8 and 9)**.

Right coronary artery was engaged with Judkins right (JR) 3.5, 6 Fr guiding catheter through RFA route. RCA lesion was crossed with 0.014" BMW wire, predilated with 2.0 × 10 mm Ryurei balloon. Then, mid-RCA stenting was done with 2.75 × 28 mm Xience Xpedition Stent at 12 atms. Postdilatation was done with 3.0 × 10 mm NC Balloon at 12 atms. Post-stent

TABLE 8: Indication for pVAD in HR-AMI without CS.

Device and evidence	Indication
IABP CRISP-AMI and PAMI-II	It is not suggested
Impella Pre-clinical studies and pilot trial	Impella CP usage is feasible as a preventive unloading strategy; currently, there is no data showing an advantage for this approach
VA-ECMO No data available	Should not be used, increasing afterload in the setting of acute coronary ischemia might be useful

(AMI: acute myocardial infarction; CRISP-AMI: Counterpulsation to Reduce Infarct Size Pre-PCI-AMI; CS: cardiogenic shock; HR-AMI: Heart Rate-AMI; PAMI-II: Primary Angioplasty in Myocardial Infarction; pVAD: percutaneous ventricular assist device; VA-ECMO: venoarterial extracorporeal membrane oxygenation)

TABLE 9: Selected nonrandomized studies of MCS in AMI cardiogenic shock.

Investigators Trials	Study device, methods	Indications	Primary outcomes
Schrage et al.	IABP, Impella; propensity match	Cardiogenic shock	No difference in 30-day mortality; significantly higher bleeding and vascular complications with Impella; no difference in survival pre- versus post-PCI implantation
Amin et al.	IABP, Impella; risk adjusted	Cardiogenic shock	Significantly higher risk-adjusted inhospital death, bleeding, and stroke with Impella versus IABP
Dhruva et al.	IABP, Impella; risk adjusted	Cardiogenic shock and AMI	Significantly higher risk-adjusted inhospital death and bleeding with Impella versus IABP both pre- versus post-PCI implantation

(AMI: acute myocardial infarction; IABP: intra-aortic balloon pump; MCS: mechanical circulatory support; PCI: percutaneous coronary interventions)

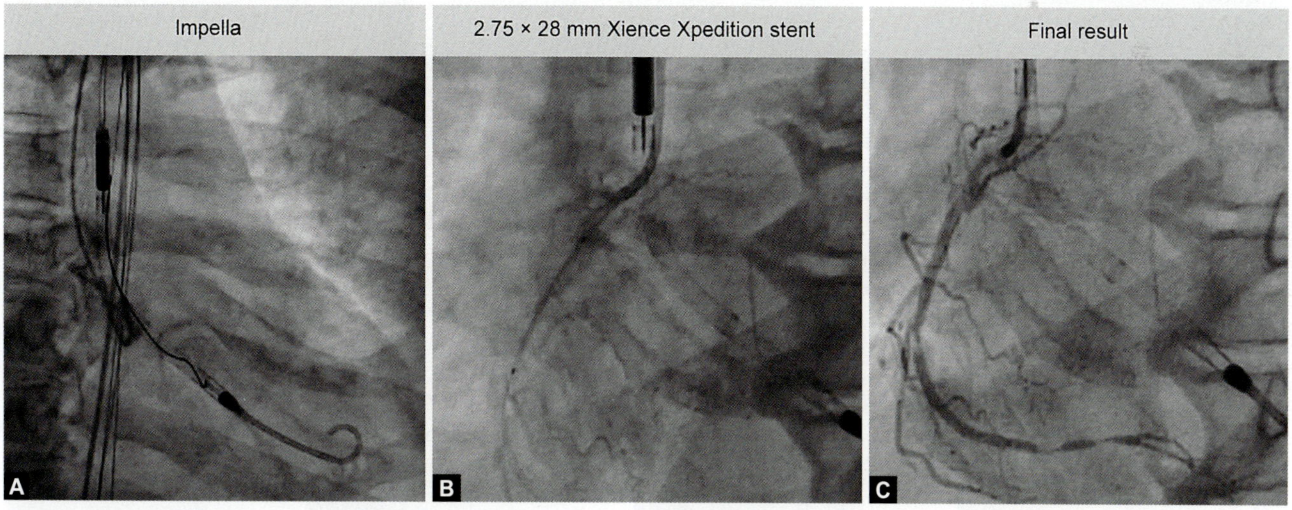

FIGS. 11A TO C: Right coronary artery (RCA) stenting with Impella supported.

angiography showed distal diffuse narrowing with haziness at the distal edge of stent, which could be due to spasm or intramural hematoma (IMH) with distal extension. The patient was treated with intra coronary (IC) nitroglycerin (NTG) and Nikoran injections and repeat angiogram showed markedly improved vessel size and distal flow with small area of haziness distal to the stent. Then, planned for recheck angiogram of RCA after PCI of LM to LAD provisional stenting to verify spasm versus distal dissection and any need for distal RCA stenting **(Figs. 11A to C)**.

Left main coronary artery was engaged with EBU 3.5–6 Fr guiding catheter. Initially, we faced a lot of difficulties to enter LAD with guide wires. Finally, a BMW wire was placed in D1 with the help of SuperCross micro catheter support and GW was entering into the D1 but could not enter LAD bifurcation lesion due to eccentric and critical lesion. Then, Crusade dual lumen catheter was exchanged with SuperCross microcatheter and it was placed into the LAD/D1 bifurcation site and the second BMW wire passed through crusade and its tip was redirected successfully to cross the lesion and finally, it was placed in the distal LAD. Runthrough wire was placed in the LCX to protect LCX while performing LM to LAD provisional stenting. LAD was predilated with 2.0 × 10 mm Ryurei Balloon at 12 atms and 2.5 × 12 mm NC Balloon at 12–14 atms. Predilatation of diagonal was done with 2.0 × 10 mm Ryurei Balloon at 08–10 atms. Then LMCA to proximal LAD stenting done with 3.0 × 38 mm Xience Xpedition Stent deployed at 12 atms. Postdilatation of LAD-stented segment was done with 3.0 × 12 mm NC Balloon at 14–16 atms. The proximal optimization technique (POT) of LMCA was done with 4.5 × 10 mm NC Balloon at 08–10 atms. Poststenting IVUS study of LAD to LM showed well-deployed stent with good expansion and apposition without any medial edge dissection. Final angiographic views showed excellent end result without any complications **(Figs. 12A to C)**.

After PCI of LM, an attempt was made to reengage RCA for checking angiogram. But the patient suddenly developed ST elevations in inferior leads with severe hypotension and SBP of 40 mm Hg on Impella. Angiography of RCA showed total occlusion of RCA, crossed with guide wire, and dilated with 2.0 × 10 mm Balloon at 10 atms, then 2.75 × 23 mm Xience Xpedition Stent was deployed distal to the mid-RCA to cover IMH with dissection. Finally, an entire stented segment was postdilated with 3.0 × 10 mm NC Balloon at 10 atms. One more additional stent 2.25 × 18 mm Xience Xpedition was deployed by overlapping the second stent extending into the PDA. The final angiographic views showed excellent end result without any dissection or residual stenosis and TIMI III flow **(Figs. 13A to D)**.

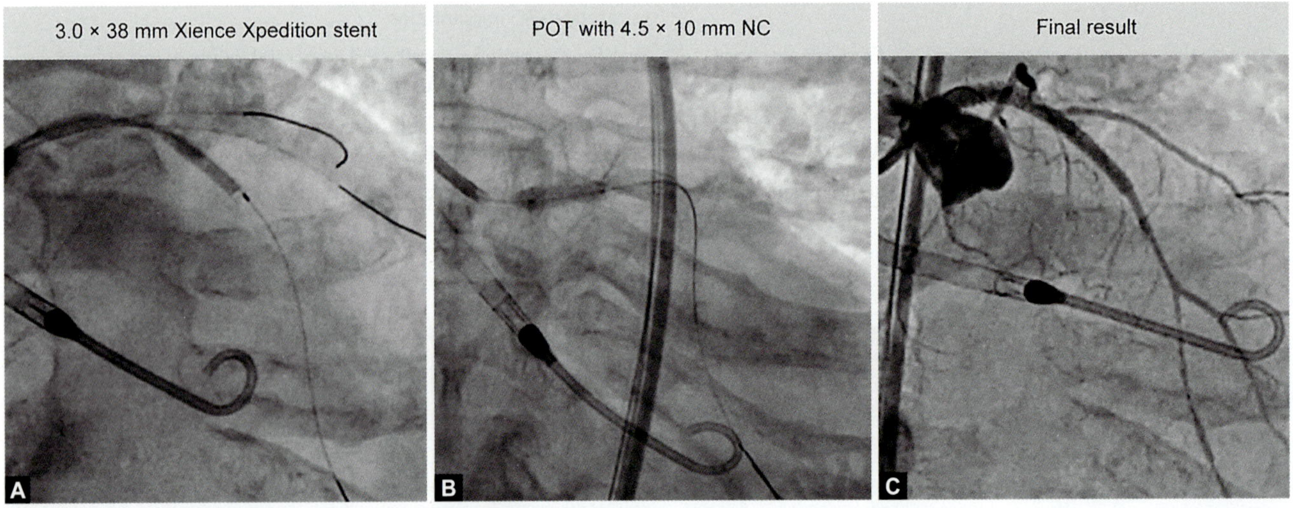

FIGS. 12A TO C: LAD stenting with Impella supported.
(LAD: left anterior descending; POT: proximal optimization technique)

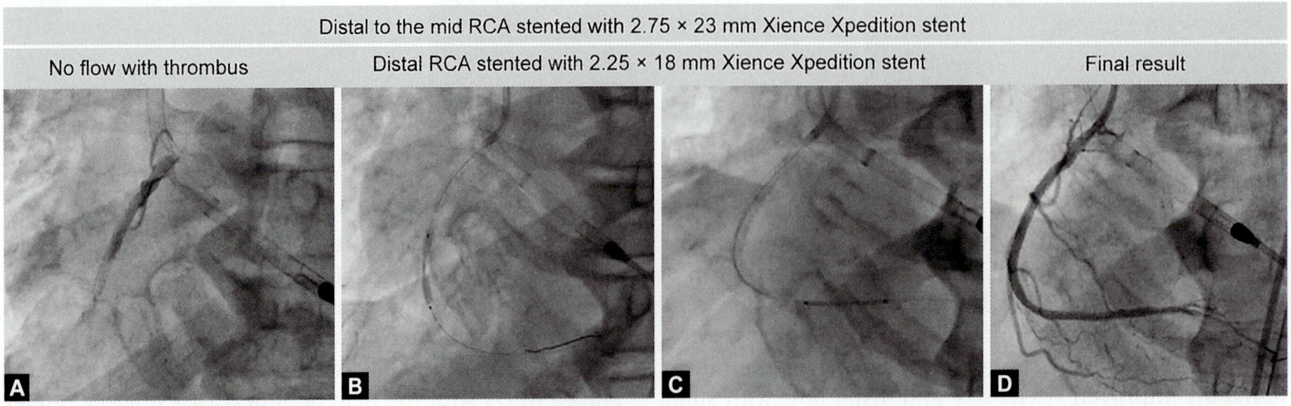

FIGS. 13A TO D: Additional stenting of right coronary artery (RCA).

CONCLUSION

Hemodynamic support is crucial to maintain adequate systemic and myocardial perfusion while performing PCI of patients with CS and protected-PCI. Impella is the most effective MCS is recommended when procedural time is longer with high myocardial ischemic burden to allow complete revascularization or high-risk interventions. In contrast to Impella and IABP, ECMO provides advantage of maintaining oxygenation as well as perfusion pressure, particularly if there is very high risk of cardiac arrest due to ventricular arrhythmias or asystole. Although augmentation of CO and hemodynamic support with IABP is only 0.5 liter, still it is more often and widely used in many centers across the world because of its cost and availability.

ONLINE REFERENCES

Please scan the QR code provided at the end of the table of contents for References of this chapter.

CHAPTER

206 Hemodynamics of Cardiogenic Shock

Anil Dhall, Mahendra Chouhan, Jasneet Singh

ABSTRACT

Monitoring in cardiogenic shock (CS) involves clinical, noninvasive, and invasive modalities, including clinical parameters, echocardiography, arterial catheterization, central venous pressure, and advanced hemodynamic monitoring for appropriate diagnosis, timely intervention, circulatory support, escalation, and de-escalation.

First-line monitoring is crucial for evaluating indicators of reduced blood flow and assessing symptoms. Continuous monitoring of physiological indicators is essential in cases of cardiovascular surgery, intervention, and critical care. Echocardiography can identify etiologies such as left or right systolic dysfunction, severe valvular disease, or left ventricular (LV) outflow tract obstruction. Advanced hemodynamic monitoring, such as pulmonary artery catheterization (PAC), is recommended for patients nonresponsive to initial therapies or those with right ventricular (RV) dysfunction.

Pulmonary artery catheterization is the mainstay of invasive hemodynamic monitoring, accurately determining filling pressures, diagnosing CS, and identifying normotensive CS in patients with clinical hypoperfusion and systolic blood pressure (SBP) > 90 mm Hg.

Keywords: Hemodynamic monitoring, cardiogenic shock, pulmonary artery catheterization, mechanical circulatory support, monitoring in CS, management of CS.

INTRODUCTION

Hemodynamic monitoring in cardiogenic shock (CS) is cornerstone in its management. Though CS can have diverse etiologies but classically, there are two major subsets of CS, i.e., ST-elevation myocardial infarction/acute coronary syndrome (STEMI/ACS) shock and decompensated heart failure (HF) shock. The widespread use of mechanical circulatory support (MCS) is changing CS management and outcomes. Effective hemodynamic monitoring with a pulmonary artery catheterization (PAC) can guide clinical decision-making for optimizing therapies for CS patients. In individual cases, PAC was helpful to decide the diagnosis, prognosis and also, guide the treatment by escalation and de-escalation of supportive or primary therapies. However, with the advent of echocardiography, many hemodynamic variables could be assessed noninvasively. Along with development of echocardiography, rampant use of PAC without standardized protocols with its inability to constructively use its hemodynamic data led to its failure to alter outcomes in clinical trials. The ESCAPE trial highlighted the same. The invasive and noninvasive data needed to be used in complimentary fashion and it may be noted that ESCAPE trial did not recruit patients with CS. However, this had a demoralizing effect on routine PAC use in CS. This has been advent of better supportive therapies such as complex high-risk indicated percutaneous coronary intervention (CHIP PCI), Impella, venoarterial extracorporeal membrane oxygenation (VA-ECMO), Tandem heart, and others. They require frequent careful adjustments, monitoring, escalation, and de-escalation, and PAC use has staged a comeback and now, serial studies are actually proving its benefits.

CARDIOGENIC SHOCK

Cardiogenic shock is defined by a cardiac index (CI) of <1.8 L/min/m^2 without support, and <2.0–2.2 L/min/m^2 with support. Additionally, it is characterized by a systolic blood pressure (SBP) below 90 mm Hg and indications of systemic hypoperfusion, such as elevated lactic acid levels, in the absence of hypovolemia. The condition being referred to is characterized by a persistent decrease in BP and inadequate blood flow throughout the body, which can be attributed to impaired functioning of either the left ventricle, right ventricle, or both ventricles. CS may arise due to various dysfunctions, including myocardial, valvular, electrical, pulmonary arterial, or pericardial abnormalities, either individually or in combination. The initiation of CS elicits a cascade of compensatory mechanisms that lead to alterations in various physiological parameters, including heart rate, pulmonary and systemic vascular resistance (SVR), tissue microcirculation, renal function, volume status, and myocardial contractility. These adjustments aim to restore adequate tissue perfusion.[1]

Patients with CS can use pharmacotherapies such as inotropes and vasopressors, as well as MCS devices to improve hemodynamics and contractility. Optimizing hemodynamic profile in pharmacologic and mechanical therapies presents challenges for clinicians. Therapeutic approach for CS patients varies significantly among institutions and clinicians, affecting indications, timing, and choice of MCS devices. MCS devices have evolved as novel treatments to restore systemic perfusion for cardiac recovery in the short term or as durable support devices for refractory HF. Right heart catheterization hemodynamic parameters help choose an MCS device and escalate mechanical support.

MONITORING IN CARDIOGENIC SHOCK

Clinical, noninvasive, and invasive modalities are used to determine the hemodynamic status of the patient. They are used in a systematic manner as described in **Flowchart 1**. Clinical parameters are based on assessment of volume status, BP, congestion, and organ perfusion or organ system dysfunction. The clinical assessment alone can have several limitations.

Goals of Monitoring

- Characterization of the type of cardiac dysfunction and the degree of its severity
- Very early detection of associated vasoplegia
- Detection and monitoring of organ dysfunction and tissue oxygenation
- Guidance of the introduction and optimization of inotropes and vasopressors as well as the timing of mechanical support

First-line Monitoring

Initial assessment and subsequent clinical tests are essential for the evaluation of indicators of reduced blood flow, such as mottling. Symptoms such as cold and hot extremities, disorientation, and mental confusion are observed and can estimate the volume status as discussed in **Table 1**.

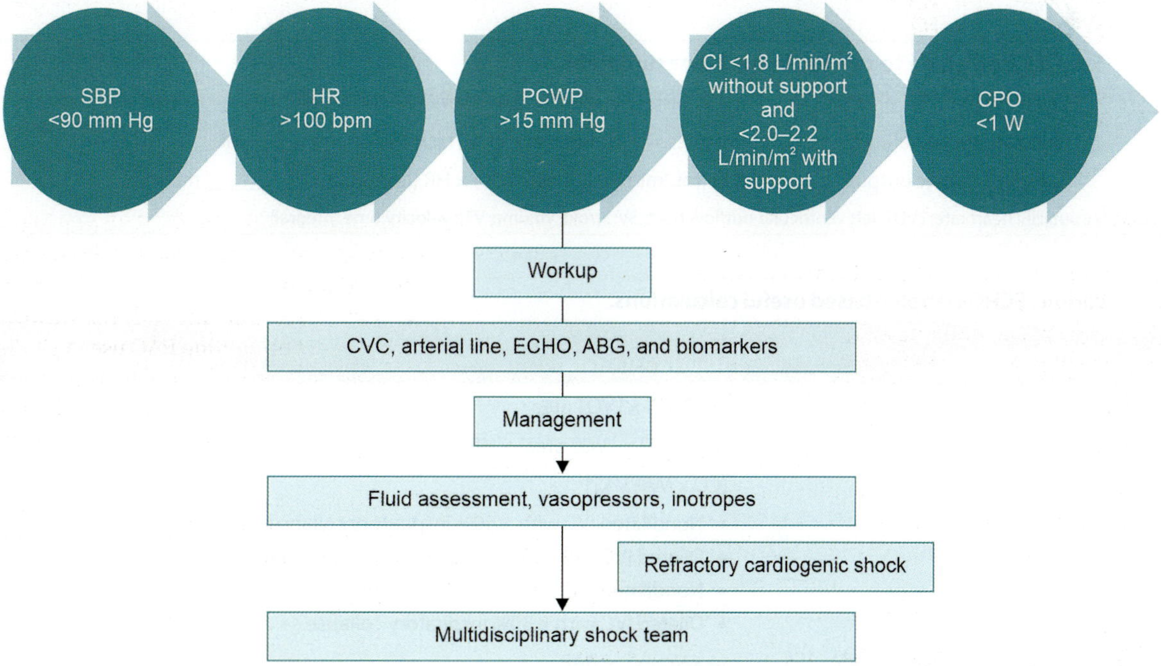

FLOWCHART 1: Diagnosis and management of cardiogenic shock.

(ABG: arterial blood gas; CPO: cardiac power output; CVC: central venous catheter; ECHO: echocardiogram; HR: heart rate; PCWP: pulmonary capillary wedge pressure; SBP: systolic blood pressure)

Furthermore, it is imperative to promptly implement the continuous monitoring of essential physiological indicators, such as pulse oximetry, BP, respiratory rate, and heart rhythm, at the patient's bedside in cases of cardiovascular surgery. In addition, it is essential to monitor urine output and conduct frequent electrocardiograms. Nevertheless, clinical examinations may be unable to estimate cardiac output, which is an essential parameter in the management of CS patients.[2] The ability to determine cardiac output, a crucial parameter in the care of patients with CS, is currently lacking. Diastolic arterial pressure, mean arterial pressure (MAP), pulse pressure variation, and systolic arterial pressure must be monitored. Elevated jugular venous pressure (JVP) with clear lung fields could point to severe acute right ventricular (RV) dysfunction.

TABLE 1: 2 × 2 matrix for evaluation of cardiogenic shock.

Peripheral circulation	Volume status: Wet	Volume status: Dry
Cold	Classic cardiogenic shock (↓CI; ↑SVRI; ↑PCWP)	Euvolemic cardiogenic shock (↓CI; ↑SVRI; ↔PCWP)
Warm	Vasodilatory cardiogenic shock or Mixed shock (↓CI; ↓/↔SVRI; ↑PCWP)	Vasodilatory shock (not cardiogenic shock) (↑CI; ↓/SVRI; ↓/PCWP)

(CI: cardiac index; SVRI: systemic vascular resistance index; PCWP: pulmonary capillary wedge pressure)

Echocardiography

Echocardiography can identify the etiology, such as left or right systolic dysfunction [secondary to acute myocardial infarction (AMI), myocarditis, acute or chronic HF, or rhythm or conduction disturbances], severe valvular disease (endocarditis, aortic dissection, or chordae or papillary muscle rupture), or LV outflow tract obstruction. For patients who do not react to early medication, routine cardiac output assessment is recommended. Echocardiography is favored over more intrusive modalities to identify CS and choose appropriate treatment, consider clinical and hemodynamic parameters. Invasive hemodynamic data can determent in the management, but PACs have increased in-hospital mortality risk, therefore, noninvasive echocardiography data can optimize treatment without complications, offering advantages such as wide availability, low cost, and noninvasiveness. **Tables 2 and 3** describe the steps and calculations involved in cardiac output measurements.

Echocardiography measures right and left filling pressures, fluid responsiveness, and pulmonary artery (PA) pressure (**Fig. 1** highlights few of these such as LV ejection fraction, stroke volume, cardiac output, etc.). While most CS patients have increased LV end-diastolic pressure (LVEDP), hypovolemia may also be present in some situations. The assessment of right (inferior vena cava diameter, respiratory

TABLE 2: Step by step guide to cardiac output measurement.

Step 1	Calculate the LVOT area	LVOT area = π × (LVOT diameter/2) 2 LVOT area = _________ cm^2
Step 2	Calculate stroke volume	SV (mL) = LVOT area (cm^2) × VTI (cm) SV = _________ mL
Step 3	Calculate cardiac output	CO (mL/min) = SV (mL/cycle) × HR (bpm) CO = _________ mL/min

(CO: cardiac output; HR: heart rate; LVOT: left ventricular outflow tract; SV: stroke volume; VTI: velocity time integral)

TABLE 3: Various ECHO Doppler-based useful calculations.

Echocardiography parameters	How to calculate	Normal values
Stroke volume (SV)	LVOT VTI × LVOT area	50–100 mL
Cardiac output (CO)	(LVOT VTI × LVOT area) × HR	5–6 L/ min
CPO	(CO x MAP)/451	1 w
RAP	• Nondilated IVC with > 50% inspiratory collapse → 3–5 mm Hg • Dilated IVC with > 50% inspiratory collapse → 8–10 mm Hg • Nondilated IVC with < 50% inspiratory collapse → 8–10 mm Hg • Dilated IVC with < 50% inspiratory collapse → 13–15 mm Hg	3–5
Pulmonary artery systolic pressure (PAPS)	(4 × $Vmax^2$) + RAP	<35
LV filling pressure [medial early mitral valve inflow velocity to early diastolic annular velocity ratio (E/e' ratio)]	E/e'	<14

(CPO: cardiac power output; CO: cardiac output; HR: heart rate; IVC: inferior vena cava; LVOT: left ventricular outflow tract; MAP: mean arterial pressure; RAP: right atrial pressure; VTI: velocity time integral)

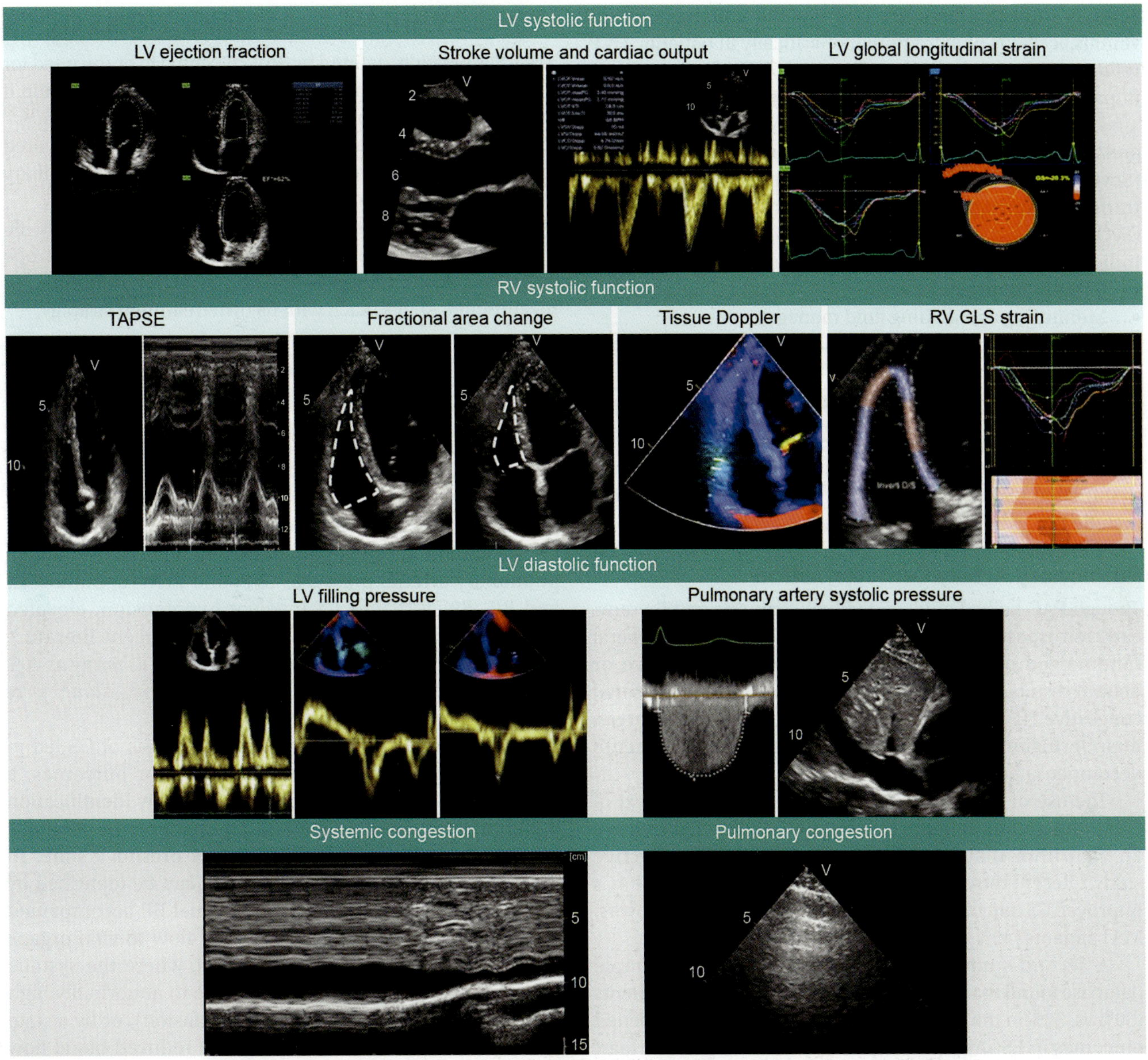

FIG. 1: Some measurements in echocardiography.
(LV: left ventricular; RV: right ventricular; TAPSE: tricuspid annular plane systolic excursion)

changes, and hepatic vein) and left (mitral E/A and E/é) congestive symptoms is crucial for personalizing treatment and assessing diuretic need.[3,4] Additionally, repeated echocardiography can identify mechanical problems in AMI, including LV or RV free wall rupture, interventricular communication, mitral chordae or papillary muscle rupture, or mechanical cardiac support difficulties.

Arterial Catheterization

While the utilization of cuff arm pressure in a noninvasive manner is generally effective in evaluating MAP, it is important to note that instances of severe hypotension and hypothermia can impact the consistency between noninvasive and invasive MAP measurements. A study conducted by Burstein et al. demonstrated that a MAP below 65 mm Hg, as measured using a combination of invasive and noninvasive methods, within the initial 24 hours of care for patients with CS, was correlated with an increased death risk.[5]

Central Venous Pressure

The central venous pressure (CVP) reflects the pressure in the central veins, usually measured in the thoracic cavity, when they enter the right atrium. CVP fluctuates with respiration, so the time of measurement can be important. Normally, CVP should be measured in the end-expiratory state. CVP actually indicates pressure and not the volume. Central venous access is often required for critically ill patients. CVP reflects RV preload and function, high CVP always reflects impaired cardiac function (or hypervolemia or tamponade), affected by intrathoracic pressures (mechanical ventilation), and allows measurement of central venous oxygen saturation ($ScvO_2$) that provides information on adequacy of oxygen transport [surrogate of mixed venous oxygen saturation (SvO_2)].

Indications for CVP measurements include:

- Diagnostic measurements
- Monitoring and guiding fluid management
- Monitoring and guiding pharmacological interventions

Advanced Hemodynamic Monitoring

Advanced hemodynamic monitoring is recommended for patients nonresponsive to initial therapies or those with RV dysfunction.[2] Some of the widely used advanced monitoring include PAC.

Pulmonary Artery Catheterization

Though PAC helped guide individual diagnosis and therapy, early retrospective registries showed no PAC benefit. Several randomized controlled trials followed with negative or neutral results. The PAC did not help acute decompensated congestive HF patients either. CS patients have multiorgan hypoperfusion or elevated lactate levels, unlike acute decompensated congestive HF.

The use of PAC has not been studied in the context of CS, evaluated in patients receiving MCS, or used to drive an algorithm that improves outcomes in a prospective study.[6] Recent retrospective registry studies found that PACs improved CS outcomes in Impella pump (Abiomed, Danvers, MA) patients (49% vs. 63%).[7,8]

A second study using the National Inpatient Sample database found that PAC use improved survival in CS patients (30% vs. 38% in the most recent year analyzed) but worsened outcomes in ESCAPE (Evaluation Study of Congestive Heart Failure and Pulmonary Artery Catheterization Effectiveness)–acute decompensated congestive HF patients.[9] Based on such findings, PACs are being added to CS treatment algorithms being evaluated at US centers.[10,11] Current society guidelines and scientific statements recommend limited PAC use in cardiovascular disease and CS (with or without MCS) patients due to limited evidence.

Factors influencing utility of PAC in CS:

- Importance of accurate pressure signal acquisition and interpretation
- *Characterizing different phenotypes of CS*: LV-dominant, RV-dominant, or biventricular shock
- Understanding hemodynamics for selection and management of MCS devices using PAC derived data to drive a treatment algorithm.

HEMODYNAMIC CLASSIFICATIONS OF CS

The CS is typically defined by SBP < 90 mm Hg or the need for inotropic, vasopressor, or mechanical support to maintain it above 90 mm Hg, along with end-organ hypoperfusion.[12,13] It requires an abnormally low CI and normal or elevated intracardiac filling pressures [CVP and pulmonary capillary wedge pressure (PCWP)].

Medically refractory CS doesn't resolve within 30–60 minutes of volume optimization and recommended inotrope or pressor doses. CS can be LV-dominant, RV-dominant, or biventricular shock, each with its own treatment strategy.

Hemodynamic Profiles in Cardiogenic Shock

As described in **Table 4**, *LV-dominant CS* has high PCWP and normal or reduced CVP in reduced LV function. *RV-dominant CS* has elevated CVP, normal to low PA pressure, PCWP, and preserved LV function. RV-dominant CS is a variant affecting patient with PA hypertension, high pulmonary arterial pressure, CVP, and PCWPs, but low CI and BP. *Biventricular CS* involves hypotension, elevated CVP, PCWP, and reduced LV function. Recent literature suggests that *biventricular shock is present in as many as 40% of patients who, based on clinical assessments alone, were suspected of having LV-dominant CS.*[14]

Lack of robust criteria for early diagnosis of CS led to delays in initiation of treatment and poor outcomes, a concept of preshock was introduced for early identification if patients requiring escalation. The patients in preshock may exhibit symptoms indicative of a preshock state. In the suitable clinical context, preshock can be identified by the presence of either a relatively normal BP accompanied by early indications of reduced blood flow to vital organs (such as the accumulation of lactate), where the systolic BP is maintained above 90 mm Hg due to abnormally high SVR (known as normotensive hypoperfusion), or by a state of relative low BP without any signs of reduced blood flow

TABLE 4: Hemodynamic profiles in cardiogenic shock.

	RV-dominant shock	Biventricular shock	LV-dominant shock
CVP (mm Hg)	>14	>14	>14
PCWP (mm Hg)	<18	Variable	>18
CVP/PCWP	>0.86	>0.86	<0.86
PAPi	<1.5	<1.5	>1.5

(CVP: central venous pressure; LV: left ventricle; PAPi: pulmonary artery pulsatility index; PCWP: pulmonary capillary wedge pressure; RV: right ventricle)

to vital organs (referred to as hypotensive normoperfusion). Further investigation may be necessary to determine the ability to accurately identify patients with hypotension and normoperfusion. This is due to the limited availability of clinical and biochemical criteria and tools for establishing normoperfusion.

In the classic paradigm of CS, the depression of cardiac output after AMI causes intense systemic vasoconstriction and an initial elevation of SVR. This was not observed in the SHOCK trial, even in patients without sepsis. All patient groups had similar mean heart rates and CIs, but the median SVR was significantly lower in patients with systemic inflammatory response syndrome (SIRS) despite a high rate of vasopressor drug use inappropriate vasodilation caused by SIRS has also been reported in CS, resulting in confused hemodynamic parameters with low CI and SVR.[15]

SCAI Classification

The Society for Cardiovascular Angiography and Interventions (SCAI) classification of CS **(Table 5)** aims to provide a simple schema for clear communication and clinical trials to differentiate patients. 2019 SCAI Clinical Expert Consensus Statement on Classification of CS was developed based on physical examination in conjunction with biochemical and invasive hemodynamic data. Signs and symptoms of systemic and pulmonary congestion and hypoperfusion are considered to classify the worsening SCAI stages of CS. Although physical examination plays a pivotal role in the initial identification and classification of CS, has been shown to have low accuracy, and is less adequate to identify the cause of shock and for risk stratification than invasive parameters. The classification system should be simple, intuitive, and suitable for rapid assessment, as shock patients often deteriorate abruptly. The new schema should be applied at the bedside upon patient presentation and allows reassessment as the patient progresses.

Biomarkers assess myocardial dysfunction severity and response to hypoperfusion, supporting cardiac diagnosis and prognosis, with frequency varying depending on clinical scenario. Electrolytes, renal function, and liver function markers indicate hypoperfusion. A creatinine of >1.33 had a significantly higher mortality in the IABP-SHOCK II (Intra-aortic Balloon Pump in Cardiogenic Shock II) trial, serum lactate is an early marker of mitochondrial dysfunction, associated with adverse outcomes in CS treatment.

Arterial blood gas tests assess patient's clinical status. Severe acidosis impairs myocardial contractility and vasopressor response. A base deficit abnormality predicts shock occurrence and severity. Serum bicarbonate

TABLE 5: 2019 SCAI classification of cardiogenic shock.

Stage of shock	Biochemical markers	Hemodynamics	Description
A Stage A "At risk"	Normal renal function and lactate	• Normotensive CI ≥ 2.5 L/min/m² • CVP < 10 mm Hg • PA sat ≥ 65%	Patients currently not in CS, but are at risk of developing CS. These include those with STEMI, NSTEMI, and acute or acute-on-chronic CHF
B Stage B "Beginning" cardiogenic Shock	Normal renal function and lactate; elevated BNP	• SBP < 90 or MAP < 60 or > 30 mm Hg drop from baseline • Pulse ≥ 100 bpm • CI ≥ 22.2 L/min/m² • PA sat ≥ 65%	Clinical evidence of hypotension or tachycardia without hypoperfusion
C Stage C "Classic" cardiogenic shock	*Lactate ≥ 2 mmol/L:* Serum creatinine doubling or >50% drop in GFR; elevated LFTs and BNP	• SBP < 90; MAP < 60 or >30 mm Hg drop from these targets • CI <2.2 L/min/m² • PCWP > 15 mm Hg • RAP/PCWP ≥ 20.8 • PAPi <1.85 • CPO ≤50.6 W/m²	Clinical evidence of hypoperfusion requiring baseline and medications/MCS beyond volume resuscitation to restore perfusion
D Stage D "Deteriorating or doom"	Stage C and deteriorating	Stage C + requiring multiple pressors or MCS devices to maintain perfusion	Like stage C, but getting worse and failed to respond to initial interventions
E Stage E "Extremis"	pH ≤ 7.2 Lactate > 5 mmol/L	Hypotensive despite maximal support	Cardiac arrest (PEA or refractory VT/F) with ongoing CPR or ECLS placement

(BNP: brain natriuretic peptide; BP: blood pressure; bpm: beats per minute; CHF: congestive heart failure; CI: cardiac index; CPO: cardiac power output; CPR: cardiopulmonary resuscitation; CS: cardiogenic shock; CVP: central venous pressure; ECLS: extracorporeal life support; GFR: glomerular filtration rate; LFT: liver function test; MAP: mean arterial pressure; MCS: mechanical circulatory support; NSTEMI: non-ST elevation myocardial infarction; PA: pulmonary artery; PAPi: pulmonary artery pulsatility index; PCWP: pulmonary capillary wedge pressure; PEA: pulseless electrical activity; RAP: right atrial pressure; sat: saturation; SBP: systolic blood pressure; STEMI: ST elevation myocardial infarction; VF: ventricular fibrillation; VT: ventricular tachycardia) assessment in CS patients may predict prognosis and is an important marker to follow during shock resuscitation to assess therapy response. Study finds serum bicarbonate drops before lactate rises.

HEMODYNAMIC MONITORING USING PULMONARY ARTERY CATHETERIZATION

Pulmonary artery catheterization is the mainstay of invasive hemodynamic monitoring. Although their value in the past has been questioned due to potential complications, more recent studies have shown that they may improve prognosis. PA catheters can accurately determine filling pressures, diagnose CS versus other shocks, and identify normotensive CS in patients with clinical hypoperfusion and SBP > 90 mm Hg. PA catheter hemodynamics can also assess RV involvement in myocardial infarction (MI), distinguish classic cardiogenic from mixed shock, help choose or titrate vasopressor or inotropic drugs, select patients who may benefit from MCS, and guide weaning. The saturation of PA blood, CI, and cardiac power output (CPO) can also help determine prognosis.

Direct Parameters

While the act of performing right heart catheterization alone does not appear to provide any mortality advantage, the hemodynamic measurements derived from this procedure, including CVP, pulmonary artery systolic pressure (PASP), pulmonary artery diastolic pressure (PADP), PA occlusion pressure or PCWP, and cardiac output/CI, have demonstrated associations with mortality outcomes. The parameters can be utilized for the computation of pulmonary vascular resistance and the quantification of right ventricle functionality.

Derived Parameters

Cardiac Power Output

Tan et al.[16] has shown that the resting CPO for a hemodynamically stable average sized adult is approximately 1 W. However, during stress or exercise, cardiac power reserve can be recruited to increase the heart's pumping ability up to 6 W. In patients with chronic HF, this recruitable reserve is significantly diminished and is strongly correlated with outcome.

Cardiac power is a novel hemodynamic measure. By incorporating both flow and pressure domains, it represents the cardiac pumping ability. Cardiac power is the strongest hemodynamic correlate of outcome for patients in CS. Increasing age and female gender are independently associated with lower cardiac power **(Fig. 2)**.

$$\text{Cardiac power index} = \frac{\text{MAP} \times \text{CI}}{451}$$

(Cutoff; 0.32 w/m²)

Cardiac Power Index $= \frac{\text{MAP} <55}{451}$

TABLE: Cardiac Power Index (Cutoff: 0.32 W/m²)

MAP ≤55

CI ≤1.7

	Mean Arterial Pressure						
Fick CI	85	80	75	70	65	60	55
2.6	0.49	0.46	0.43	0.40	0.37	0.35	0.32
2.4	0.45	0.43	0.40	0.37	0.35	0.32	0.29
2.2	0.41	0.39	0.37	0.34	0.32	0.29	0.27
2.0	0.38	0.35	0.33	0.31	0.29	0.27	0.24
1.8	0.34	0.32	0.30	0.28	0.26	0.24	0.22
1.6	0.30	0.28	0.27	0.25	0.23	0.21	0.20

FIG. 2: Cardiac power index.

Cardiac power output and cardiac power index (CPI) are two significant derived parameters that have demonstrated a robust correlation with the risk of in-hospital mortality in CS.[17] The concepts of CPO and CPI are utilized to measure and assess the amount of external mechanical work performed by the left ventricle. A CPO value below 0.6 W, calculated as the difference between MAP and right atrial pressure multiplied by cardiac output, is indicative of poorer prognoses in patients with AMI complicated by CS, even when receiving treatment in accordance with established guidelines.

Similarly, to how the indices function as substitutes for LV function, indices such as RV stroke work, RV stroke work index, and the ratio of CVP to PCWP serve to quantify RV function. An elevated CVP/PCWP ratio > 0.86 indicates impaired RV function, if the CVP is also above the normal range. In a similar vein, RV CPO and RV CPI can be quantified, albeit to a lesser extent, and akin to LV parameters.

The utilization of PA catheters holds significant importance in differentiating CS from other etiologies of shock, identifying normotensive CS in patients experiencing clinical hypoperfusion and systolic BP above 90 mm Hg, and precisely assessing filling pressures. PA catheter hemodynamics play a crucial role in evaluating RV participation in MI, differentiating between classic CS and a mixed shock presentation, aiding in the selection or adjustment of vasopressor or inotropic medications, identifying patients who may derive benefits from MCS, and providing guidance for the gradual withdrawal of pharmacological or mechanical support. The assessment of PA blood saturation, along with CI and CPO, is instrumental in determining the prognosis.

The evaluation of systemic blood flow can be accomplished through the utilization of thermodilution or Fick methods, both of which assess cardiac output. CI, which is calculated by dividing cardiac output by body surface area, is a valuable metric for normalizing cardiac output. Additionally, SvO_2 serves as an indicator of systemic blood flow. The parameters discussed may not provide a direct indication of perfusion at the end-organ or tissue level due Postcardiac to the presence of concurrent microvascular dysfunction that occurs during the later stages of CS.

Right Ventricular Function Assessment

The SHOCK trial registry data suggests that cardiac power is the strongest hemodynamic parameter to correlate of mortality in cardiogenic shock.

The indices of RV function encompass RV stroke work, RV stroke work index, and the ratio of CVP to PCWP. In typical circumstances, CVP is notably lower than PCWP. A CVP/PCWP ratio > 0.86 indicates potential impairment of RV function. However, this ratio is more accurate in identifying RV dysfunction when CVP is elevated beyond the normal range. In recent times, the utilization of the pulmonary artery pulsatility index [PAPi = (PAS – PAD)/CVP] has demonstrated its utility in providing a more precise assessment of RV dysfunction. A PAPi value of <0.9 is indicative of a notable decline in RV function. When combined with other observations, this finding may imply the necessity for additional RV support.[16]

Right ventricular failure remains a major cause of morbidity and mortality. Percutaneous RV support devices play an important role in the management of RV failure with the ability to rapidly stabilize patients with CS involving the RV. The role of RV-AMCS devices will be as a bridge to therapy or recovery while advancements in coronary intervention, pulmonary hypertension, cardiac surgery, transplantation medicine, and ventricular assist device (VAD) technology offer options for patients who survive CS. As RV devices become more commonly used, their role in the management of RV failure will be less dependent on operator skill and more dependent on improved algorithms for the early detection of RV failure, device selection, patient monitoring, and weaning protocols for both isolated RV failure and biventricular failure.[18] PAC measurements help differentiate CS subtypes and tailor therapies based on shock subtypes, aiming to resolve hemodynamic profile and prevent sequelae.

MECHANICAL CIRCULATORY SUPPORT DEVICES

Mechanical circulatory support devices have evolved as novel treatments to restore systemic perfusion for cardiac recovery in the short term or as durable support devices for refractory HF. CS has a growing number and variety of MCS devices to improve efficacy or replace pharmacotherapy to avoid side effects to improve efficacy or replace pharmacotherapy to avoid side effects. Data indicates that higher inotrope and vasopressor usage negatively impacts CS outcomes, with survival rates for patients requiring 0–4 drugs at 68%, 46%, 35%, and 26%, respectively. Severe CS treatment is futile especially when multiple drugs are needed. Flowchart for selection of temporary MCS in management of CS shown in **Flowchart 2**.

Right heart catheterization with a PAC is the cornerstone of a standard clinical hemodynamic evaluation of patients undergoing MCS. However, widespread routine use of PAC has declined over the past decade and there is no consensus on systematic use of PAC data.

Various devices utilized in the medical field for cardiovascular support include aortic counter pulsation pumps, transvalvular percutaneous left ventricular assist devices (pLVADs), percutaneous left atrial decompression devices, and ECMO devices. It is worth mentioning that although various types of MCS have similar impacts on BP and cardiac output, they can have distinct effects on the heart and lungs. This is particularly evident when considering PCWP, which is associated with LVEDP, and myocardial oxygen demand (MVO_2).

The lack of effectiveness of the IABP, coupled with the difficulties encountered during the implantation of percutaneous left atrial decompression devices, has led to the predominant utilization of pLVADs and ECMO as the most commonly employed MCS devices in cases of CS. IABP works by diastolic augmentation but manages to increase cardiac output to a maximum of 0.5.

The utilization of ECMO in the context of severe LV dysfunction has the potential to elevate LVEDP and PCWP due to the rise in afterload pressure. Consequently, this may

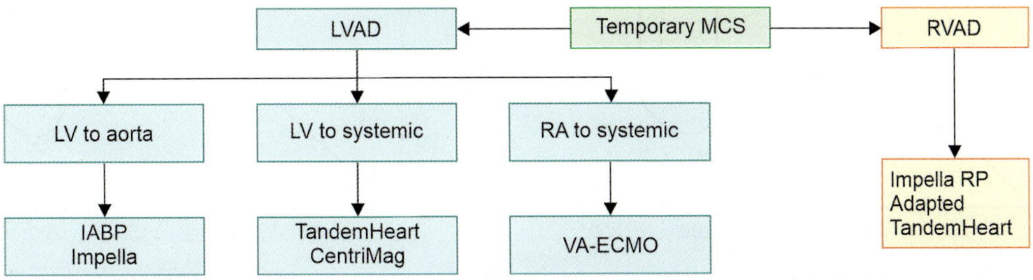

FLOWCHART 2: Use of temporary MCS in CS.

(IABP: intra-aortic balloon pump; LVAD: left ventricular assist device; MCS: mechanical circulatory support; RVAD: right ventricular assist device; VA-ECMO: venoarterial extracorporeal membrane oxygenation)

lead to the development or exacerbation of pulmonary edema in certain instances. Elevated LV afterload has the potential to induce the closure of the aortic valve, thereby increasing the likelihood of thrombus formation in either the aortic root or the ventricle. ECMO is good for the organs but bad for the heart and can create harlequin or North-South syndrome.

On the other hand, pLVADs can directly alleviate the workload on the left ventricle, resulting in a simultaneous decrease in PCWP and LVEDP. ECMO circumvents the left ventricle (and right ventricle) and augments the overall pressure-volume area, which exhibits a positive correlation with elevated MVO_2. Consequently, the addition of a pLVAD is frequently employed in conjunction with ECMO in order to mitigate the adverse effects on LV and pulmonary function. MCS devices can be categorized according to their mechanism of action, the specific anatomical locations from which blood is extracted from the body, the site where the blood is reintroduced, and whether they facilitate the exchange of oxygen and carbon dioxide gases. Sometimes combinations may be needed such as ECPella, BiPella, and Impella + IABP depending on hemodynamic parameters.

The pressure-volume analysis **(Figs. 3 and 4)** is the most explicit method for depicting the hemodynamics of MCS. While the direct application of this format in clinical practice is limited, valuable insights can be obtained from the observation that fundamental parameters derived from PAC are directly associated with characteristics of the pressure-volume loop. By utilizing these parameters in conjunction with basic measurements of LV and RV size, it becomes possible to analyze the principal attributes of LV and RV pressure-volume loops. The association of these measurements with "single beat" estimations of ventricular end-systolic and end-diastolic pressure-volume relationships offers valuable insights into the mechanics and hemodynamics of CS.

The utilization of PACs is crucial in the management of patients receiving MCS, as the hemodynamic effects and individual patient responses can vary significantly across different forms of MCS.

Cardiovascular pressure measurements, such as CVP and PCWP, in patients with cardiovascular disease can exhibit rapid fluctuations because of various factors, including underlying medical conditions, medication dosages, and the response to MCS. The reliability of clinical assessment is questionable, whereas PACs offer precise measurements. Laboratory and bedside evaluations, including measurements of urine output, serum creatinine level, and lactic acid level, are essential for determining the severity and predicting the outcome of CS. However, it is important to note that these assessments may not immediately reflect hemodynamic changes, as the timing of their response can vary depending on the degree of hemodynamic impairment, autoregulation of organ vasculature, and the presence of pre-existing chronic organ dysfunction. Like other laboratory tests, no test is used in isolation. The sequential increase in lactate levels, along with the presence of additional clinical indicators of reduced blood flow to vital organs, can serve as a valuable indicator for determining the necessity of transferring a patient to a specialized facility that can provide advanced medical interventions for individuals with CS.

Hemodynamic-based MCS Selection

Identifying the shock subtype and considering device impact on parameters such as cardiac output, PCWP, CVP, and MAP helps practitioners choose the best device or combination for a patient. Real-time hemodynamic data from the PAC, trends, and metabolic signals provide a powerful combination for appropriate MCS selection and timely management of CS. MCS selection is often influenced by clinical factors like body size, vascular access, physician preference, institutional

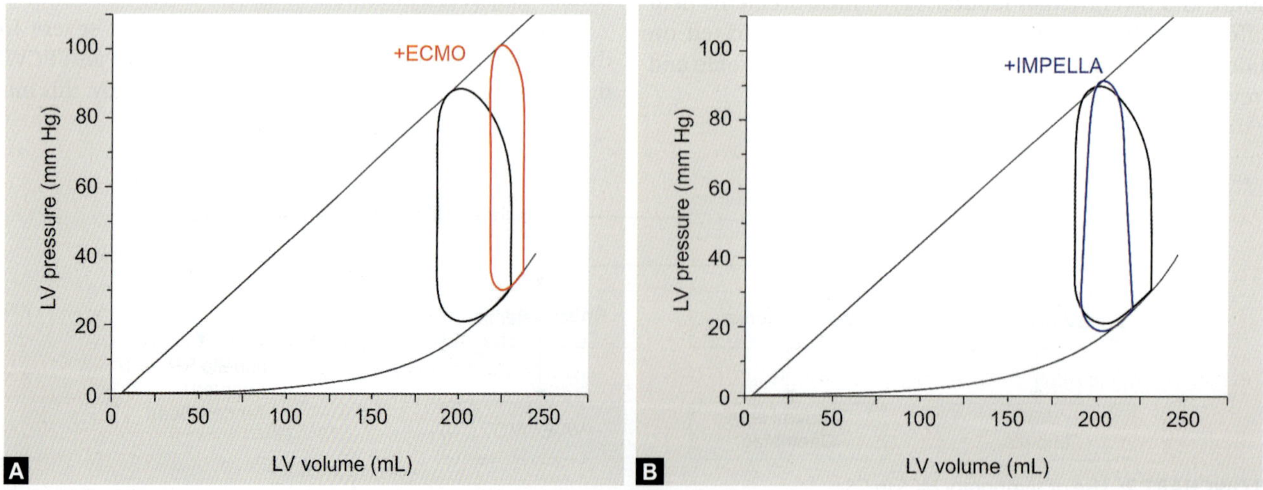

FIGS. 3A AND B: Pressure volume loops to analyze ECMO and Impella.
(ECMO: extracorporeal membrane oxygenation; LV: left ventricular)

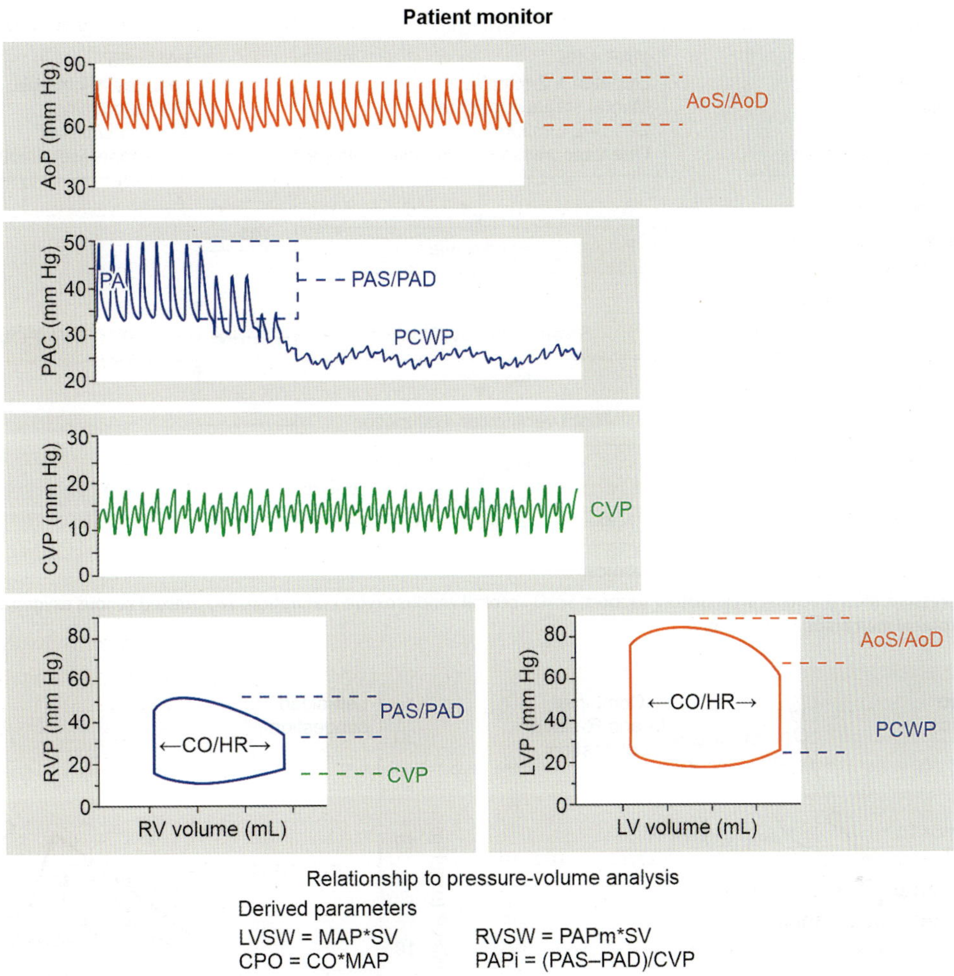

FIG. 4: Relation of pressure–volume analysis to hemodynamic parameters. In addition to standard arterial blood pressure and heart rate (HR) monitoring, basic parameters obtained from the pulmonary artery catheterization (PAC) include pulmonary artery systolic (PAS) pressure, pulmonary artery diastolic (PAD) pressure, pulmonary capillary wedge pressure (PCWP), and central venous pressure (CVP). Cardiac output (CO) is obtained by thermodilution or Fick principle; CO/HR yields stroke volume. The parameters link directly to key features of right and left ventricular pressure-volume loops. This can be combined with basic information of right- and left-ventricular size, providing even more specificity to the loop. Other parameters can be obtained as detailed in supplemental AoD indicates aortic diastolic pressure.

(AoD: aortic diastolic pressure; AoS: aortic systolic pressure; CPO: cardiac power output; EDV: end-diastolic volume; LVP: left ventricular pressure; LVSW: left ventricle stroke work; MAP: mean arterial pressure; PAPi: pulmonary artery pulsatility index; PAPm: mean pulmonary artery pressure; RVP: right ventricular pressure; RVSW: right ventricle stroke work; SV: stroke volume)

resources, support goals, metabolic and respiratory status, concurrent infection, and device adverse event profile, in addition to anticipated hemodynamic effects as discussed in **Flowchart 3**.

HEMODYNAMIC-BASED PATIENT MANAGEMENT DURING MCS

The use of MCS is dependent on the hemodynamics derived from PAC. Cardiac output and CI are utilized to evaluate the sufficiency of blood flow from both artificial devices and the patient's own heart, taking into consideration the individual's body size. SvO_2 offers supplementary assessment of flow adequacy in relation to the physiological condition. The measurement of serum lactate offers additional information; however, the time it takes for lactate to be cleared from the body and the delay in obtaining laboratory results make the measurement of SvO_2 more advantageous in terms of guiding therapeutic interventions.

The measurement of PCWP holds significance in assessing both the extent of pulmonary venous congestion and LVEDP. The monitoring of PCWP during MCS serves as a valuable tool in assessing LV decongestion and unloading. However, it is important to note that PCWP measurements may be influenced by various factors, such as pulmonary venous disease, atrial abnormalities, and mitral valve stenosis. As a result, pulmonary arterial pressure (PAD) is often utilized as a substitute for PCWP in clinical practice.

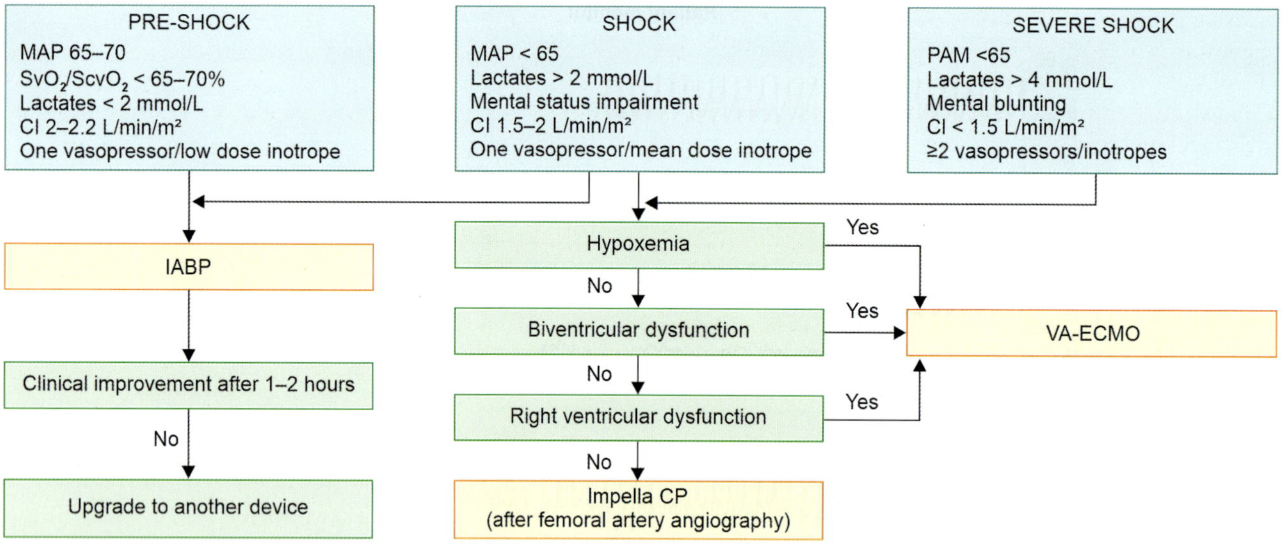

FLOWCHART 3: MCS selection based on hemodynamics.

(MAP: mean arterial pressure; MCS: mechanical circulatory support; $ScvO_2$: central venous oxygen saturation; SvO_2: mixed venous oxygen saturation; VA-ECMO: venoarterial extracorporeal membrane oxygenation)

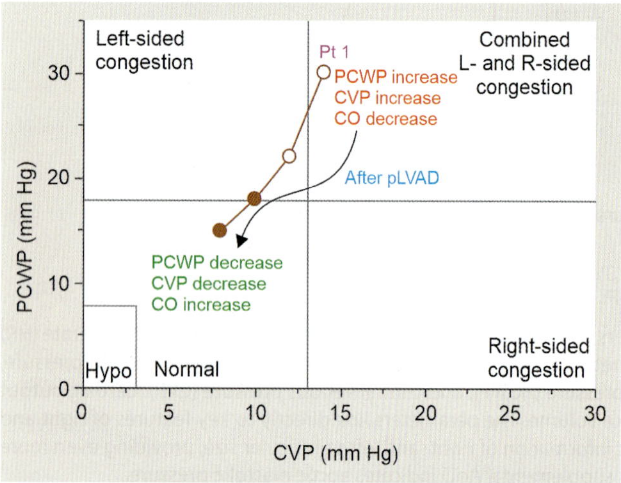

FIG. 5A: Case of patient 1 presenting with hypotension and decreased cardiac index despite inotropic support. Use of PACs allows for customization of therapy.

(CVP: central venous pressure; CO: cardiac output; PAC: pulmonary artery catheterization; PCWP: pulmonary capillary wedge pressure)

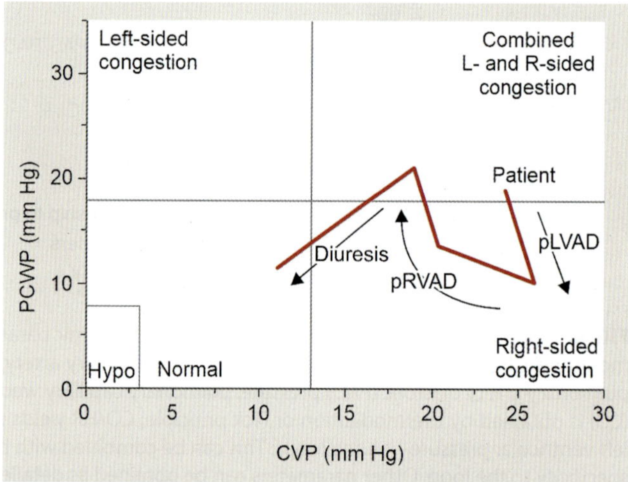

FIG. 5B: Case of patient 2 presenting with hypotension and decreased cardiac index despite inotropic support. Use of PACs allows for customization of therapy.

(CVP: central venous pressure; CO: cardiac output; PAC: pulmonary artery catheterization; PCWP: pulmonary capillary wedge pressure; pLVAD: percutaneous left ventricular assist device; pRVAD: percutaneous right ventricular assist device)

There may be discrepancies between PADP and PCWP, particularly in patients with pulmonary hypertension or mitral insufficiency, or when PAC measurements are not obtained from pulmonary functional zone III. It is recommended to measure the PCWP concurrently with the insertion of PAC to accurately determine the disparity between the PADP and the PCWP. This disparity can serve as a reference point for subsequent measurements of PAD pressure.

The primary objective of MCS approaches is to enhance cardiac output. However, it is important to note that the effects of these approaches on the hemodynamic profile can exhibit substantial variability, both across different devices and among individual patients.

Patient Examples

Patient 1 **(Fig. 5A)** exemplifies a prototypical case of a patient presenting with primary left HF. Initially, the PCWP exhibits a significant increase, the CVP is elevated, and the cardiac output experiences a decrease. The introduction and subsequent escalation of pLVAD support have been observed to result in a decrease in PCWP and an increase in cardiac output. The reduction in PCWP leads to a decrease in RV afterload, subsequently causing a secondary decrease in CVP.

Patient 2 **(Fig. 5B)** exhibits a prevailing condition of congestion on the right side, accompanied by a slight increase in PCWP. The measured PA pressure is 30/20 mm Hg, with a calculated PAPi of approximately 0.5. These findings suggest the presence of notable RV dysfunction. However, due to the patient's decreased CI and elevated PCWP (which is above the upper limit of normal), the logical initial intervention would be the implantation of a pLVAD. Nevertheless, upon the implementation and subsequent escalation of pLVAD power, there was a significant decline in PCWP, accompanied by a further elevation in CVP. This observation suggests that the RV is unable to adequately match the flow generated by the pLVAD. Upon the initiation of peripheral venoarterial cannulation [percutaneous RV assist device (pRVAD)], there is an observed increase in PCWP. This increase in PCWP subsequently leads to an augmentation in LV filling, resulting in an overall increase in CI. Despite being reduced, CVP still remains significantly elevated. When diuresis is increased, both PCWP and CVP decrease to levels that are within the normal range. While multiple therapeutic approaches exist for each of the three patients, the PAC data was utilized to assess the hemodynamic efficacy of the chosen treatments and identified the necessity to address their volume status.

ESCALATION OF MCS

Escalation refers to the process of transitioning from one MCS to another that has a greater flow capacity. This transition may also involve the addition or removal of a secondary device, which is necessitated by insufficient support provided by the initial MCS. When contemplating the escalation of therapy, it is imperative to acknowledge that as the duration of critical illness extends, there is an increased probability of advancing toward multiorgan failure. This is based on the type of failure as described in **Figure 6**.

The PAC offers real-time and continuous data to assess the effectiveness of pharmacologic and mechanical support strategies. Additionally, it presents clinically significant trends that, when appropriately analyzed, may indicate the need for an escalation of medical intervention. If the PAC data indicates that the level of support offered by the initially selected form of MCS is insufficient, it may be necessary to quickly increase the intensity of therapy. The potential increase in assistance for unintentional hemodynamic impacts should be taken into account.

It can be questioned whether such rapid and decisive clinical decision making can be made without a PAC in place.

This phenomenon is exemplified in the PCWP tracings in **Figure 7**, It can be questioned whether such rapid and decisive clinical decision making can be made without a PAC in place. which depict a case study of a patient who exhibited CS

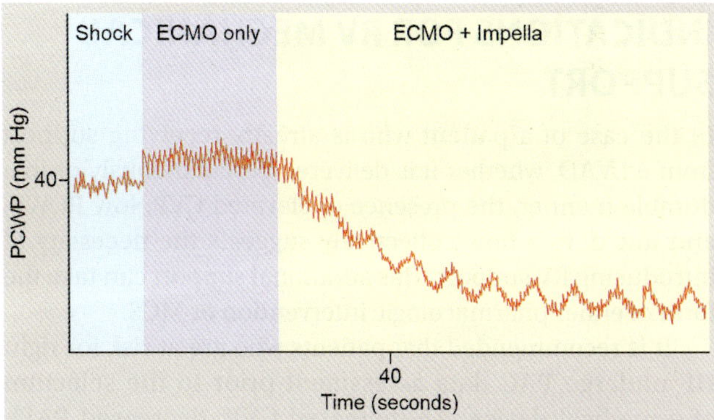

FIG. 7: Changes in pulmonary capillary wedge pressure (PCWP) with extracorporeal membrane oxygenation (ECMO) and Impella. PCWP at the time of presentation in cardiogenic shock, which increases after initiation of ECMO and rapidly decreases with the initiation of Impella support.

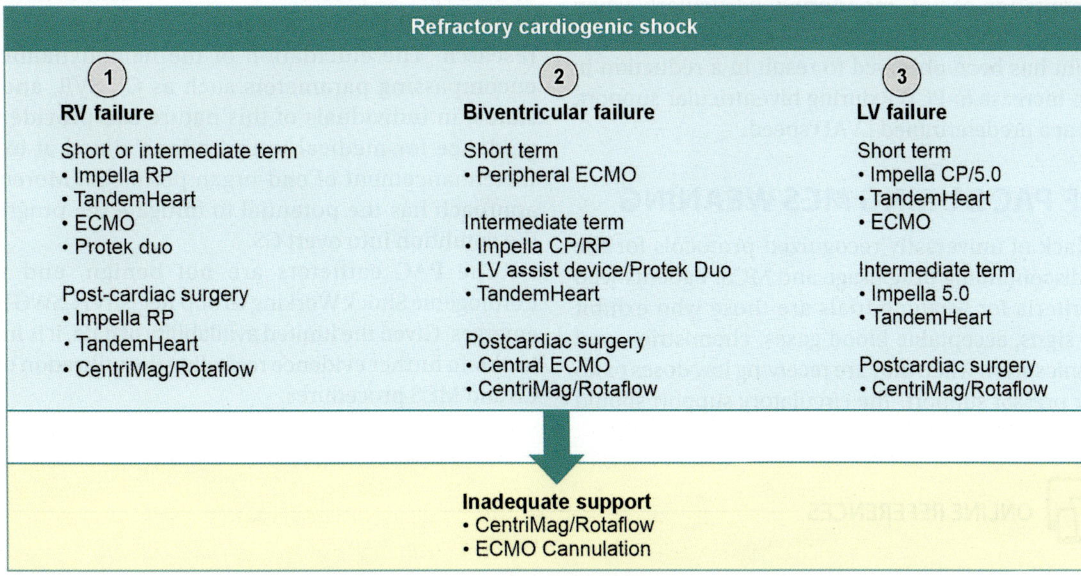

FIG. 6: MCS selection in refractory CS.

(CS: cardiogenic shock; ECMO: extracorporeal membrane oxygenation; LV: left ventricular; MCS: mechanical circulatory support)

accompanied by increased PCWP and subsequently received ECMO therapy. The PCWP exhibited a further increase, thereby indicating the necessity for LV decompression. The initiation of percutaneous VAD (pVAD) support resulted in a swift reduction in PCWP, leading to decompression of both the LV and the lungs.

In a broader sense, this case demonstrates the effectiveness of utilizing the PAC in achieving several important outcomes:

- Prompt detection of elevated PCWP upon admission
- Prompt identification of worsening hemodynamic condition following the initiation of the initial MCS in the form of ECMO
- The ability to determine the appropriate intervention, which in this instance involved escalating the level of support and incorporating Impella
- Confirmation of the swift resolution of the issue

INDICATIONS FOR RV MECHANICAL SUPPORT

In the case of a patient who is already receiving support from a LVAD, whether it is delivered percutaneously or in a durable manner, the presence of elevated CVP, low PCWP, and low device flow collectively suggests the necessity of introducing RV support. This additional support can take the form of either pharmacologic intervention or MCS.

It is recommended that patients who are at risk for right HF undergo PAC data assessment prior to the selection of a medical device. An increased CVP, decreased PAPi, and diminished PCWP collectively suggest the necessity for prompt RV assist device (RVAD) assistance. In certain instances, RVAD support alone may be warranted, without the need for LVAD support.

The optimization of RVAD output is enhanced through the implementation of PAC monitoring, particularly when it is combined with LVAD support. The augmentation of RVAD output has been observed to result in a reduction in CVP and an increase in PCWP during biventricular support, specifically at a predetermined LVAD speed.

ROLE OF PAC DURING MCS WEANING

There is a lack of universally recognized protocols for the process of discontinuing drug usage and MCS. Patients who meet the criteria for weaning trials are those who exhibit stable vital signs, acceptable blood gases, chemistries, and hemodynamics, even when they are receiving low doses or no inotropic or pressor support. The circulatory support should be gradually decreased while closely monitoring vital signs and hemodynamics, with particular attention to PCWP, CVP, and cardiac output. It is important to ensure appropriate BP, heart rate, and cardiac output throughout each stage of the process. The maintenance of hemodynamic stability, as determined by parameters derived from PAC, along with the clinical evaluation of peripheral perfusion, is deemed sufficient. As the reduction of support continues, it is done so gradually until the flow levels recommended specifically for the device reach a minimum threshold, at which point the device is removed.[19]

CONCLUSION

The facilitation of MCS and device escalation optimization is achieved through the utilization of hemodynamic parameters derived from PAC, which enable the identification of volume status, cardiac biventricular function, CPI, etc. This identification allows for the appropriate administration of appropriate therapy.

The utilization of percutaneous assist devices, or PAC, presents the opportunity to effectively diagnose, guide, optimize, and gradually discontinue therapies in the context of CS, regardless of the presence or absence of MCS.

The measurement of CVP and PCWP, either separately or in conjunction with other parameters such as the CVP/PCWP ratio, PAPi, RV stroke work, and RV stroke work index, offers crucial insights into volume status and the extent of RV dysfunction. This information can help determine the necessity for fluid administration, diuretic therapy, renal replacement therapy, or the initiation of RV mechanical support.

The investigation and consideration of the utilization of percutaneous assist devices in individuals with persistent normotensive-hypoperfusion preshock, characterized by systolic BP above 90 mm Hg without the administration of inotropes or pressors, but with evident deterioration in end-organ function, is warranted and merits additional research. The elucidation of the hemodynamic profile, encompassing parameters such as CI, SVR, and volume status, in individuals of this nature can provide valuable guidance for medical interventions aimed at expediting the enhancement of end-organ perfusion. Moreover, this approach has the potential to mitigate the progression of the condition into overt CS.

The PAC catheters are not benign, and we avail Cardiogenic Shock Working Group Registry (CSWG) data as it emerges. Given the limited availability of data, it is imperative to obtain further evidence regarding the utilization of PACs in CS and MCS procedures.

ONLINE REFERENCES

Please scan the QR code provided at the end of the table of contents for References of this chapter.

CHAPTER

207

Temporary and Durable Ventricular Assist Devices: Current Status

Aditi Singhvi, Bagirath Raghuraman

ABSTRACT

End-stage heart failure (HF) and cardiogenic shock (CS) have a high mortality. Durable left ventricular assist devices (LVADs) are a viable option for improving quantity and quality of life in those with end-stage HF. With the advent of the HeartMate 3 (HM3) device, incidence of adverse events (AEs) has reduced significantly. There have also been advances in patient selection, surgical techniques, and long-term management. All of these have contributed to improved outcomes in LVAD recipients. An array of temporary mechanical circulatory support (TMCS) devices is available, and these can improve the condition of patients with CS, if instituted in a timely manner. They can also be used to bridge patients to recovery, durable LVAD, or heart transplantation (HT). There has been a shift in using TMCS for critical patients and reserving LVADs for less acutely ill advanced HF patients. Efforts are underway to refine patient selection, optimize management of patients with LVAD and TMCS, and enhance device technology.

Keywords: Durable left ventricular assist device, temporary mechanical circulatory support, end-stage heart failure, cardiogenic shock, bridge to transplant.

INTRODUCTION

Heart failure (HF) affects 8–10 million individuals in India, of whom 1–5% will progress to end-stage disease.[1] Treatment options for these individuals include heart transplantation (HT) or durable left ventricular assist devices (LVADs).

Advancements in LVADs have made these devices an increasingly viable and life-saving option for patients with end-stage HF who are not suitable candidates for HT or are at a high risk of waitlist mortality. LVADs can be employed either as a bridge to transplantation (BTT) or as a long-term solution [destination therapy (DT)].

Temporary mechanical circulatory support (TMCS) devices are used to provide short-term support while determining if a patient can recover or requires durable LVAD or HT. Early use of TMCS can lead to better outcomes.[2] The aim of this chapter is to highlight recent trends in the field of LVAD and TMCS, patient outcomes, and explore future directions.

DURABLE LEFT VENTRICULAR ASSIST DEVICES

Evolution

The first-generation pulsatile LVADs were volume-displacement pumps. They were bulky, noisy, and had frequent mechanical failures. Continuous-flow (CF) LVADs with smaller profile and improved durability were subsequently developed. Examples include, HeartMate II (HMII) and HM3 (Abbott Laboratories), HeartWare Ventricular Assist Device (HVAD) (Medtronic), and EvaHeart (EvaHeart). Total artificial hearts have also been developed, like SynCardia (SynCardia Systems), which is a pneumatically driven pulsatile system.

Engineering and Pump Technology

Contemporary LVADs are CF pumps with an inflow cannula implanted in the left ventricular (LV) apex, a rotor propels blood, and an outflow graft returns blood to the ascending aorta. Modern LVADs are contact-free, using magnetic and/or hydrodynamic systems instead of mechanical bearings and an impeller. This reduces the risk of thrombosis and improves hemocompatibility.

Of the contemporary LVADs, HMII is an axial-flow pump, and the HM3 and Evaheart are centrifugal-flow pumps. The HMII is larger and requires implantation in a preperitoneal pocket, while the centrifugal-flow pumps are compact and implanted in the pericardial space. Hydrodynamic performance of the two differs as well. There is less change in flow with axial-flow pumps and a larger change with centrifugal-flow pumps for a given change in pressure gradient across the pump. Pressure gradient is determined by the systemic blood pressure (BP), therefore strict BP management is imperative for normal functioning of centrifugal-flow pumps.

Left Ventricular Assist Device Recipient Epidemiology and Outcomes

The number of LVADs implanted annually worldwide has been steadily increasing, to about 5,000 per year, with the greatest increase in North America.[3]

The International Registry for Mechanically Assisted Circulatory Support (IMACS) database now includes 25,000 patients with global representation, and one-third of recipients are non-white.[3] Contemporary LVAD recipients have more comorbidities, more social issues hindering direct transplant candidacy, and are sicker at the time of implant, with more than half in cardiogenic shock (CS).[3,4] This suggests increasing referral for LVAD therapy, possibly more late referrals and/or increasing expertise leading to willingness to take on sicker cases.

Recently in USA, >70% of LVAD implants have been DT. However, in non-North American-based registries, less than half are DT implants.[3,5] Even if patients are listed for transplant, the rate of HT is low (28% at 1 year).[3] Additionally, some patients implanted as DT may achieve sufficient improvements to become transplant eligible, whereas others implanted as BTT may develop contraindications to HT. Therefore, distinguishing between DT and BTT indications is less relevant in the contemporary era. Most implants nowadays are HM3. HVAD has been withdrawn from the market due to a higher incidence of strokes and pump thrombosis (PT).[6]

Long-term outcomes for patients on LVAD support is improving, despite increasing preimplant disease severity. Recent Interagency Registry for Mechanically Assisted Circulatory Support (INTERMACS) data reports overall survival for patients on CF-LVAD at 1, 2, and 5 years of 82, 73, and 47%, respectively.[4,7] 5-year survival in BTT patients was 52%, and 44% in DT.[4] More contemporary HM3 data show an even better survival of 80% at 2 years, which is comparable to HT and about 60% at 5 years, with similar outcomes in DT and BTT recipients.[8-11]

Patient Selection

The first step in assessing candidacy for durable LVAD is evaluating the patient's risk of morbidity and mortality from HF with continued medical management. Chronic HF patients with recurrent HF hospitalizations, high diuretic requirement, hemodynamic instability, progressive end-organ dysfunction, inotrope dependence, frequent ventricular arrhythmias, despite maximally tolerated goal-directed medical therapy (GDMT) or inability to tolerate GDMT should be evaluated for LVAD. Cardiopulmonary exercise testing and risk scores such as the Seattle Heart Failure Model and Heart Failure Survival Score can help prognosticate ambulatory patients.[12-14]

In patients with noninotrope-dependent, ambulatory systolic HF, INTERMACS 4 patients are likely to experience improved survival and quality of life with LVAD compared to medical therapy, but not INTERMACS 5–7.[15] However, these data are with HMII. These findings may change further in favor of LVAD with HM3, which has less adverse events (AEs).

Recent cancer is not a contraindication for LVAD implantation, unlike for HT. Psychosocial evaluation is also crucial.

Perioperative Mortality Assessment

The operative period carries the highest risk for patients undergoing LVAD implants. Predicting this risk is challenging; age, comorbidities, preoperative right ventricular (RV) dysfunction, renal dysfunction, liver dysfunction, and frailty are risk factors for mortality after LVAD. The preoperative INTERMACS profile appears to be one of the most important prognostic factors, with INTERMACS profile 1 and 2 having higher mortality.[16] The Model for End-Stage Liver Disease (MELD) and the MELD-XI [excluding international normalized ratio (INR)] also have prognostic value.[17] The HMII Risk Score (age, albumin, creatinine, INR, and center volume) has been developed to stratify risk post-HMII.[18]

Long-term Survival Assessment

Few studies have examined long-term survival predictors post-LVAD. The risk of hemocompatibility-related events in a particular patient is also difficult to predict. Operative survival is obligatory for long-term survival, so the abovementioned factors remain relevant. Of the HMII Risk Score, center volume is the only variable independently associated with long-term survival.[18] HM3 Survival Risk Score [age, prior cardiac surgery, sodium, blood urea nitrogen, LV end-diastolic dimension, right atrial (RA) to pulmonary capillary wedge pressure (PCWP) ratio] has been devised to estimate 1- and 2-year survival post-HM3.[19]

Right Ventricular Function Assessment and Management

Right ventricular failure (RVF) prediction is challenging and requires comprehensive assessment, including:[20-22]

- Signs of right-sided volume overload
- Assessment of nutritional status, and renal and hepatic function
- Echocardiographic parameters of qualitative and quantitative RV function, RV to LV diameter ratio, and tricuspid regurgitation (TR) severity
- Hemodynamic parameters:
    - RA pressure ≥ 18 mm Hg
    - RA pressure to PCWP ratio > 0.63
    - Pulmonary artery pulsatility index < 0.9
    - Right ventricular stroke work index < 0.25

Multiple risk scores have been developed, all with modest predictive value.[23] The EUROMACS-RHF (European Registry for Patients with Mechanical Circulatory Support-Right-sided Heart Failure) Risk Score (INTERMACS class, inotrope use, severe RV dysfunction by echocardiogram, RA to PCWP ratio, and hemoglobin) outperforms others.[24]

Right ventricular function optimization prior to LVAD implant is the key. Diuretics, ultrafiltration, and inotrope support may decrease RVF risk. Preoperative use of intra-aortic balloon pump (IABP) can stabilize patients with RVF and improve post-LVAD outcomes.[25] Elective RV assist device (RVAD) implantation can be considered in high-risk patients.[26]

Left Ventricular Assist Device Implantation

Hemodynamic stabilization pre-LVAD is essential as patients in CS prior to implant have worse outcomes. TMCS should be considered for stabilization. Nutrition, coagulopathy, infection, and renal and liver function should also be addressed prior to surgery.

Minimally invasive surgical techniques have been used for LVAD implantation with positive outcomes.[27] Other considerations during implantation include, anesthesia management, addressing significant TR and aortic regurgitation (AR), weaning from cardiopulmonary bypass, and transesophageal echocardiogram-guided LVAD speed adjustment. Diligent postoperative management is key to support RV function, end-organ recovery, and identify complications.

Long-term Management

A structured and specialized ambulatory management plan is essential for favorable outcomes post-LVAD. There are several unique aspects to managing LVAD recipients like altered physiology due to CF, assessment for normal LVAD function, and complications.

International Society for Heart and Lung Transplantation (ISHLT) guidelines recommend a mean arterial pressure (MAP) goal of ≤80 mm Hg for patients with CF-LVAD.[28] HF medications are the preferred agents for hypertension; and they may even improve survival.[29] Data on the mortality benefit of implantable cardioverter-defibrillators (ICDs) in CF-LVAD patients is inconsistent.[30] In patients without an existing ICD at the time of implant, most centers will implant one only if there is a history of ventricular arrhythmias. Continuing cardiac resynchronization therapy (CRT) after LVAD implantation does not have a well-defined role.[31]

Antithrombotic Therapy

Left ventricular assist device patients require anticoagulant and antiplatelet treatment to prevent PT and stroke. Aspirin 81–100 mg is recommended for HeartMate devices. The goal INR is 2.0–3.0, but adjustments may be made based on the patient's history.[28] Direct oral anticoagulants should be avoided due to increased thromboembolic events.[32] Low-molecular-weight heparin may be used cautiously for bridging subtherapeutic INR, but it carries risks of bleeding and thromboembolism.[33] Given the significantly reduced PT risk with HM3, lower intensity anticoagulation (INR target 1.5–1.9) has been studied and short-term safety was demonstrated.[34]

Complications

Adverse events remain prevalent, with the most common being infection (40% at 1-year post-LVAD), major bleeding [33% at 1-year post-LVAD; half is gastrointestinal (GI)] and stroke (13% at 1-year post-LVAD).[4] AE rates are highest in the 90-days postimplant, and then decline significantly, except device-specific infections, which have a constant incidence. Leading causes of death post-LVAD are multiorgan failure (16%), neurologic dysfunction (16%), and HF (13%).

Hemocompatibility-related Adverse Events

These include PT, stroke, and spontaneous nonsurgical bleeding and are thought to be a result of CF, shear stress, and antithrombotic therapy. PT rates with HVAD and HMII were 8–10% at 1 year, but only 1.4% with HM3 in the MOMENTUM trial.[35] Optimal implant technique, early postoperative initiation of anticoagulation with heparin bridging, speed optimization, and maintaining MAP ≤ 90 mm Hg have been shown to reduce thrombosis.[36] Monitoring serum lactate dehydrogenase levels for hemolysis is recommended. PT should be suspected if there is evidence of hemolysis and/or suboptimal pump performance.

Neurological Complications

These include hemorrhagic and ischemic strokes, majority of which are cardioembolic. Traditional risk factors such as atrial fibrillation, prior stroke, and diabetes, and LVAD-related complications can increase the risk of stroke, like inflow or outflow blockages, inadequate anticoagulation, reduction of anticoagulation due to GI bleed, and LVAD infection.[37-39] Strict BP management is essential to reduce the risk of hemorrhagic stroke.[40] Notably, beyond 6 months, HM3 recipients had a 77% lower stroke risk than HMII recipients supporting the pump's improved hemocompatibility.[41]

Bleeding

Bleeding is caused by the use of antithrombotic therapy, LVAD-mediated acquired von Willebrand factor deficiency, CF, and aberrations in angiogenesis.[42,43] About one-third of GI bleeds are related to arteriovenous malformations. Endoscopy can be diagnostic and therapeutic.[44] Despite intervention, recurrence occurs in about 25% of patients. Pharmacologic therapies to prevent GI bleed, such as angiotensin-converting enzyme inhibitors, octreotide, thalidomide, danazol, and digoxin, have had mixed results.[45]

Left Ventricular Assist Device Infection

The driveline remains the Achilles heel of LVAD therapy, and is the cause of most LVAD-specific infections. 1-year mortality with LVAD infections is fivefold higher.[46] LVAD infections also increase risk of PT, bleeding, stroke, hospitalization, and failure to achieve transplantation.[47] Trauma to the exit site, younger age, overweight, and exposed driveline velour increase the risk of infection.[48] Therefore, meticulous exit site and driveline care and driveline immobilization are crucial. Positron emission tomography imaging with F-18 labeled fluoro-2-deoxyglucose can help evaluate the presence and extent of infection.[49] Pump exchange may be required in case of persistent bacteremia though recurrence even following exchange is high, especially with candidemia and if coexisting ICD/CRT is not removed. HT should be pursued with increased urgency, if feasible. Importantly, post-transplant survival is not negatively affected by the presence of LVAD infection.[50]

Right Ventricular Failure

Right ventricular failure may occur early postoperatively or late. Incidence of acute or early RV failure post-LVAD implant is 10–40% and leads to higher perioperative and 1-year mortality.[51,52] Causes include changes in RV geometry, loss of septal contribution to RV contraction, and increased RV preload due to augmented cardiac output (CO) post-LVAD, and operative insults such as vasoplegia, right coronary artery ischemia, blood loss, volume resuscitation, hypoxia, and acidosis. Timely use of temporary RVADs is essential. Percutaneous RVADs have also been used successfully.[53] Diuresis, inotropes, and pulmonary vasodilators are helpful.[54] Late or chronic RVF is a distinct entity, and associated with high morbidity and mortality. Management is challenging, consists of mainly diuresis, and has consideration for HT. It is unclear whether chronic pulmonary vasodilator use improves symptoms, reduces PT, reduces late RVF, or facilitates eventual HT listing.[55,56]

Left Ventricular Failure

Causes of LV failure post-LVAD, include hypertension, LVAD dysfunction (due to PT or technical fault), AR, and inadequate LV unloading.

Significant AR post-LVAD implant increases morbidity and mortality.[57] AR develops because of reduced aortic valve opening with subsequent commissural fusion and high proximal aortic afterload causing increased transvalvular pressure gradients. Surgical correction of preexisting significant AR at time of implantation is recommended.[58] Adjustment of LVAD speed to allow for intermittent aortic valve opening may be preventive. In patients who develop refractory AR, surgical or transcatheter aortic valve replacement should be considered.[59]

If volume overload is due to inadequate LV unloading, increasing the LVAD speed may help. Hemodynamic optimization with ramp testing has been shown to decrease hospitalizations.[60]

Myocardial Recovery and Explantation

Hemodynamic unloading on LVAD support can enhance reverse myocardial remodeling, and improve LV function. Incidence of contractility improvement is high, but real-world LVAD explantation rate is 1–2%.[61] A recent study demonstrated that optimized unloading with GDMT increased LVAD explantation in a preselected patient population. Mortality in those who were weaned from LVAD was similar to those who underwent HT.[62] The INTERMACS Cardiac Recovery Score (I-CARS) can be used to predict probability of myocardial recovery.[63]

Shared Decision-making

When contemplating LVAD implantation, the potential for improved survival and quality of life must be weighed against risks of AEs and burdens placed on patients and caregivers.[64] Clinician education and decision aids for patients and caregivers considering LVAD can facilitate shared decision-making.[65] Assessment and provision of adequate psychosocial support for LVAD patients and caregivers is essential.[66]

Left Ventricular Assist Device Use in India

The first modern LVAD was implanted in 2012. Given the relatively shorter wait time for HT and high cost, most durable LVAD implants in India have been used for patients who are ineligible for HT due to factors like age, or foreign nationals. There is no national registry for LVADs. Single-center reports show that the early outcomes with LVAD are inferior to HT, with 1-year survival at 72%, and 5-year survival of 50%.[67] Long-term management is challenging. Patients tend to return to their community and most centers do not have experience with LVAD therapy. Patients tend to monitor

BP themselves and INR with point-of-care devices, which are unreliable. Driveline infections are common because of the weather. Strokes are an important cause of morbidity, and management is difficult because of the limited availability of interventional neurology facilities. PT is usually managed with thrombolytics, as pump exchange is not feasible financially.

Left Ventricular Assist Device as Bridge to Transplant

High cost is essentially prohibitive for durable LVAD followed by HT in India. The current donor heart allocation system in India stratifies patients based on illness severity. Those managed with nondischargeable TMCS devices like extracorporeal membrane oxygenation (ECMO) are given preference over stable patients with durable LVADs. Therefore, LVAD recipients will tend to undergo HT only in case of a device-related complication, rather than when ambulatory and stable. LVAD patients also experience more vasoplegia and bleeding with HT surgery. Nonetheless, durable LVAD may offer a safer strategy for long-term survival in patients who are deteriorating on TMCS or are not receiving HT offers even after prolonged duration of TMCS support. Additionally, total survival may be better with a period on LVAD followed by HT as survival after HT is relatively unchanged due to complications such as cardiac allograft vasculopathy and renal failure.

Future Directions

Current focus in LVAD technology is on generating pulsatility, miniaturization, total implantability,[68] remote monitoring, optimizing antithrombotic regimen, and reducing AEs. Efforts to get insurance coverage for LVAD therapy in India are ongoing.

TEMPORARY MECHANICAL CIRCULATORY SUPPORT

Despite recent advances, mortality in CS is high, 40–50%, in CS complicating acute myocardial infarction (AMI) and 50% in chronic HF with CS.[69,70] CS is caused by low CO and coronary and systemic hypoperfusion; leads to a vicious spiral of worsening myocardial dysfunction, neurohormonal activation, and increased myocardial oxygen demand; and eventually causes end-organ failure, systemic inflammatory response, circulatory collapse, and death if left untreated. Prevention of multiorgan dysfunction syndrome (MODS) is critical to improving outcomes in CS. Mortality is higher with more inotropes, as they worsen myocardial oxygen demand, worsen peripheral perfusion, are proarrhythmic, and generally ineffective in increasing CO substantially.[2] TMCS devices improve peripheral perfusion without increasing myocardial oxygen demand. Early use of TMCS can avoid progression to MODS, which is superior to medical management and associated with improved survival.[2,71-73]

In USA, approximately 2,000 TMCS device implants are performed annually.[74] Usage in India is low, despite availability and supportive evidence. A single center in India has reported their use of 24 TMCS devices over a period of 5 years to bridge patients to HT resulting in improved outcomes.[70]

Indications

Initial management of CS generally involves addressing the underlying etiology, like performing percutaneous coronary intervention (PCI) in case of AMI, and using vasopressors and inotropes. TMCS is indicated for CS (from any etiology, like AMI, mechanical complications of AMI, postcardiotomy, acute on chronic HF, restrictive cardiomyopathy, myocarditis, HT graft failure or rejection, valvular disease, cardiac tamponade, drug overdose) unresponsive to medical therapy. However, the decision regarding when to upgrade to TMCS can be challenging.

In AMI-CS, decision-making based on cardiac power output (CPO) <0.6 [(MAP × CO)/450] and lactate >4 mmol/L has been shown to improve survival.[71] An algorithmic approach with serial evaluation and institution of TMCS accordingly is advised. This has demonstrated improved survival in AMI-CS.[71,75,76] Invasive hemodynamic monitoring-guided TMCS initiation and management has also been shown to reduce mortality.[77-79] Of note, chronic HF-CS patients tend to have higher filling pressures, lower mixed venous oxygen, less pH derangement, and normal lactate, as they have compensated to a chronic low CO state, compared to AMI-CS.[80] Therefore, multiple variables, including hemodynamics, measures of systemic perfusion, and end-organ function should be utilized in decision-making about TMCS. The Society of Cardiovascular Angiography and Interventions (SCAI) classification of CS can be used to facilitate prompt recognition of phenotypic severity, and institute treatment in a timely manner to improve outcomes.[81] The use of TMCS device provides time to determine whether the patient can improve and recover from the initial insult, or whether they will require durable support like an LVAD or HT.

Temporary mechanical circulatory support can also be used for refractory myocardial ischemia, for support during high-risk PCI, in patients with low ejection fraction (EF) awaiting cardiac surgery or intervention for valvular disease, refractory ventricular arrhythmias, during ventricular tachycardia ablation, and as a bridge to HT.

Steps for Temporary Mechanical Circulatory Support Selection

A multidisciplinary team-based approach is critical in determining timing of intervention and appropriate patient and device selection. Considerations include:

- Likelihood of recovery and expected duration of support
- Expected degree of circulatory support

- Need for RV, LV, or biventricular support
- Oxygenation status
- Vascular access
- Availability of TMCS devices at one's institution, experience of the team and available resources
- Cost-effectiveness

Temporary Mechanical Circulatory Support Options

Percutaneous TMCS devices include IABP, Impella devices, TandemHeart, and peripheral venoarterial extracorporeal membrane oxygenation (VA ECMO). Right-sided support options include Impella RP, Tandem RVAD, and ProtekDuo. Surgical options are CentriMag and central VA ECMO. The key characteristics and differences are highlighted in **Table 1** and complications in **Table 2**.

Contraindications

Absolute contraindications include:

- Nonrecoverable neurologic injury
- Malignancy or noncardiac disease with life expectancy <1 year
- Nonrecoverable CS patients who are not candidates for durable LVAD or HT

Relative contraindications are:

- Advanced age
- Significant peripheral vascular disease
- Significant ongoing bleeding
- Inability to receive anticoagulation
- Sepsis

Intra-aortic Balloon Pump

Intra-aortic balloon pump is the most commonly used TMCS device. It consists of a balloon that inflates during diastole and deflates just prior to systole. The counterpulsation reduces LV afterload and improves coronary perfusion. There is only a modest increase in CO. The largest randomized trial of IABP in AMI-CS as well as a meta-analysis failed to demonstrate survival benefit.[82-84] Therefore, guidelines recommend against the routine use of IABP in AMI-CS.[85,86] However, chronic HF patients with severely reduced CO, mitral regurgitation (MR) and elevated systemic vascular resistance experience significant hemodynamic improvement.[87] Therefore, there is increasing use of IABP in stabilizing chronic HF patients and bridging to HT or LVAD.[88] Percutaneous axillary approach for IABP placement has been shown to be a feasible strategy for bridging to HT and permits ambulation.[89] IABP is quick and easy to deploy, has a low complication rate, is widely available, and there is widespread familiarity with it; therefore, it will continue to be used in clinical practice, at least as a first step to stabilizing patients in CS, awaiting coronary artery bypass surgery, refractory ventricular arrhythmias, etc., and particularly to bridge patients to HT.

Impella® Devices

The Impella devices (Abiomed) are micro-axial CF pumps that are placed across the aortic valve into the LV. The motor rotating at high speeds pulls blood out of the LV and ejects it into the aorta. This directly unloads the LV, reduces wall stress and myocardial oxygen demand, improves coronary perfusion and augments CO. Impella can facilitate myocardial recovery and improve end-organ perfusion. Impella devices include (1) Impella 2.5 (flow 2–2.5 L/min, 12 Fr system), (2) Impella cardiac power (CP) (flow 3.5–4 L/min, 14 Fr system), (3) Impella 5.0 (flow 5 L/min, 21 Fr system), (4) Impella 5.5 for left-sided support and, (5) Impella RP for right-sided support [pulls blood out of inferior vena cava (IVC)/RA and ejects into the pulmonary artery (PA)] (flow 4L/min, 22 Fr system). The pump is connected to a console which displays relevant data and allows adjustment of power level. The left-sided devices are inserted through the femoral artery (FA). The Impella 5.0 can be inserted via the axillary artery too. Impella RP is inserted via the femoral vein. Routine echocardiographic evaluation is needed to confirm position, as malposition or migration can lead to hemolysis and/or ineffective unloading. Advantages of Impella are peripheral insertion, LV unloading, up to 21 days of support, and ability to ambulate patients with axillary cannulation. Disadvantages are immobilization with femoral cannulation, expense, catheter migration, need for frequent repositioning, risk of hemolysis, mitral valve impingement, and PT. The device is contraindicated in the presence of LV thrombus, severe AR, mechanical aortic valve, ventricular septal defect, and LV free wall rupture. The device is preload-dependent so hypovolemia and small LV cavity size, like in restrictive cardiomyopathy, can lead to suction.

Clinical trials with Impella 2.5[2] or registry data[84] have not demonstrated any mortality benefit, but it has been shown to be beneficial for high-risk PCI.[90] Of note, the more robust devices, Impella CP and 5.0, have not been evaluated in randomized trials. A meta-analysis demonstrated an overall survival to discharge of 74% with Impella 5.0 in the setting of CS related to various etiologies, with the highest rates of recovery in patients with postcardiotomy shock and AMI-CS and survival to definitive therapy of 74% in those with chronic HF with CS.[91] Impella 5.0 has been successfully used for bridging patients with CS to HT or durable LVAD.[92] The Impella RP is effective for RVF following cardiac surgery, and post-LVAD.[93] There are reports of biventricular Impella being used successfully.[94]

TandemHeart®

TandemHeart is an extracorporeal, centrifugal, CF pump, with an inflow cannula inserted via the femoral vein, and placed in the left atrium (LA) via transseptal puncture

TABLE 1: Temporary mechanical circulatory device options and their key characteristics and differences.

	Left ventricular support						Right ventricular support			Biventricular support
	IABP	Impella 2.5	Impella CP	Impella 5.0	TandemHeart	CentriMag	ProtekDuo	Impella RP	CentriMag	VA ECMO
Pump mechanism	Pneumatic	Axial flow	Axial flow	Axial flow	Centrifugal flow	Centrifugal flow	Centrifugal flow	Axial flow	Centrifugal flow	Centrifugal flow
Pump location	Extra-corporeal	Intra-corporeal	Intra-corporeal	Intra-corporeal	Paracorporeal	Paracorporeal	Paracorporeal	Intracorporeal	Paracorporeal	Paracorporeal
Cannula size	8 Fr	13 Fr	14 Fr	22 Fr	• Inflow 21 Fr • Outflow 15–19 Fr	Variable	21 Fr	23 Fr	Variable	• Venous 18–21 Fr • Arterial 15–22 Fr
Placement	Per-cutaneous	Per-cutaneous	Per-cutaneous	Per-cutaneous	Percutaneous	Percutaneous or sternotomy	Percutaneous	Percutaneous	Percutaneous or sternotomy	Peripheral or central
Inflow	N/A	LV	LV	LV	LA	LA or LV	RA	IVC/RA	RA	IVC/RA
Outflow	N/A	Aorta	Aorta	Aorta	Aorta	Aorta	PA	PA	PA	Femoral or axillary artery/aorta
Effect on LV afterload	Decrease	Decrease	Decrease	Decrease	Increase	Increase	None	None	None	Increase
Effect on PCWP	Slightly reduced	Reduced	Reduced	Reduced	Reduced	Reduced	None	None	None	Increased
Maximum flow (L/min)	1	~2	~3–3.5	~4–4.5	4	>5	~5	~4	>5	>5
Time to initiation	Very low	Medium	Medium	High	High	High	Moderate	Moderate	High	Low to medium
Ability to cannu-late at bedside?	Yes	No	No	No	No	No	By experie-nced providers	No	No	Yes, if peripheral; No, if central
Ability to be mobile?	No, if femo-ral; Yes, if axillary	No	No	Yes	No	Yes	Yes	No	Yes	Yes, if central; No, if peripheral
Intensity of anticoagulation	Low	Low	Low	Low	High	Moderate	High	Low	Moderate	High
Duration of support	Hours to days	Hours to days	Days	Days to weeks	Days to weeks	Days to weeks	Days to weeks	Days	Days to weeks	Days to weeks
Hemolysis	Rare	Moderate	Moderate	Low	Low	Low-to-moderate	Low	Low-to-moderate	Low	Low-to-moderate
Bleeding risk	Low	Low	Low	Moderate	Moderate	Moderate-high	Moderate	Low	Moderate-to-high	High
Risk of limb ischemia	Low	Low	Moderate	Low	Low	Low	None	None	None	High, if peripheral
Cost	Low	High	High	High	High	Medium	Medium	High	Medium	Medium

(CP: cardiac power; IABP: intra-aortic balloon pump; IVC: inferior vena cava; LA: left atrial; LV: left ventricular; N/A: not available; PA: pulmonary artery; PCWP: pulmonary capillary wedge pressure; RA: right atrial; VA ECMO: venoarterial extracorporeal membrane oxygenation)

TABLE 2: Complications with temporary mechanical circulatory support devices.

IABP	Impella	TandemHeart	CentriMag	VA ECMO
• Limb ischemia • Bleeding • Infection • Hematoma • Vascular injury • Thrombocytopenia • Aortic dissection • Bowel ischemia • Thromboembolism • Stroke	• Bleeding • Hematoma • Tamponade • Infection • Stroke • Hemolysis and pigment-induced nephropathy • Aortic valve injury • Mitral valve injury • Limb ischemia • Thrombocytopenia • Vascular injury • Aortic dissection • Pseudoaneurysm	• Perforation of the posterior wall, aortic root, or the coronary sinus • Tamponade • Vascular injury • Thrombocytopenia • Bleeding • Infection • Arrhythmias • Air embolism	• Bleeding • Mediastinal bleeding requiring re-exploration • Tamponade • Infection • Hemolysis • Thrombocytopenia • Stroke	• Lower limb ischemia, including requiring amputation • Upper extremity, head and neck hypoxia • LV distension and pulmonary edema • LV thrombosis • Bleeding • Compartment syndrome • Vascular injury—dissection, pseudoaneurysm, arteriovenous fistula • Stroke • Infection • Neurological complications • Thrombosis of circuit • Arterial and venous thrombosis

(IABP: intra-aortic balloon pump; LV: left ventricular; VA ECMO: venoarterial extracorporeal membrane oxygenation)

and outflow cannula in the FA. It aspirates blood from the LA and returns it to the FA, and can provide up to 5L/min flow. It bypasses the LV, so can be used in case of LV thrombus, ventricular septal rupture, or mechanical aortic valve. Regular monitoring is needed to ensure the catheter tip does not migrate from the LA into the RA, which can be catastrophic. Small studies have demonstrated greater hemodynamic improvement with TandemHeart compared to IABP in AMI-CS; however, without any mortality benefit.[95] It is recommended for CS unresponsive to Impella and acute mechanical complications of MI such as acute MR and ventricular septal rupture.[96]

CentriMag® and Rotaflow®

The CentriMag (Abbott Laboratories) and Rotaflow (Maquet Cardiopulmonary AG) are extracorporeal, magnetically levitated, centrifugal, CF pumps that can provide up to 10 L/min flow. Both require surgical cutdown. The pumps can be used for LV support with LA or LV to aortic cannulation, for RV support with RA to PA cannulation or for biventricular support. The device directly unloads the ventricle reducing myocardial oxygen demand. The device is preload and afterload sensitive. Echocardiography is helpful in speed optimization. Available data is mostly observational. A meta-analysis showed a 62–83% survival on support depending on the indication.[97] Reports of patients bridged to LVAD or HT or recovery on CentriMag, demonstrate 59–74% survival to discharge, and 68% 1-year survival.[98,99] CentriMag is being increasingly used for postcardiotomy CS or as an upgrade if there is worsening despite percutaneous devices.

ProtekDuo®

The TandemLife ProtekDuo is a dual-lumen cannula with the inflow in the RA and outflow in the PA. Blood is pulled out from the RA and delivered to the PA. An oxygenator can also be added. It has been successfully used for severe RVF post-LVAD surgery,[100] and in the setting of AMI, acute myocarditis, severe pulmonary hypertension, and HT with severe graft dysfunction.

Venoarterial Extracorporeal Membrane Oxygenation

Extracorporeal membrane oxygenation is a method of providing circulatory and/or respiratory support. It aims to restore the ratio of oxygen delivery to consumption. It is an extracorporeal setup consisting of a CF, centrifugal or servo-modified roller pump, membrane oxygenator and heat exchanger with drainage cannulae. Cannulation can be:

- *Central*: Generally in patients who cannot be weaned off from cardiopulmonary bypass; it requires a sternotomy or thoracotomy, and inflow cannula is placed in the RA and outflow in the ascending aorta.
- *Peripheral*: Inflow is placed in a peripheral vein, like the jugular or femoral and outflow in one of the large peripheral arteries, like the femoral, axillary, or subclavian artery.

Deoxygenated blood is removed from the venous system, passed through an oxygenator, and returned to the arterial system, providing complete cardiopulmonary support. CardioHelp (Maquet Getinge Group, New Jersey) is a new, compact system, convenient for transport, allows rapid priming, and has the ability to monitor various parameters.

In ECMO, blood is returned to the aorta increasing LV afterload, which increases myocardial oxygen demand. If LV contractility is poor, LV filling pressures can increase leading to pulmonary edema, and stagnation causing clotting. To reduce these risks, LV decompression is often needed, either via inotropes, or mechanically with IABP, Impella (ECPELLA), atrial septostomy, or surgical LV vent. Another potential risk, if lung function is poor, and mixing of the blood ejected by the LV and extracorporeal flow is in the descending aorta, is that the right arm, brain, and coronaries will be perfused with deoxygenated blood ejected by the native LV. This is called Harlequin or north-south syndrome. Therefore, blood gases should be checked from the right arm. This can be addressed by the addition of another cannula from the perfusion cannula (containing oxygenated blood) to the venous side, referred to as venoarteriovenous ECMO. Limb ischemia is common with femoral cannulation, therefore an antegrade perfusion catheter should always be used. Adequate anticoagulation is essential, as there is a high chance of clot formation within the circuit, particularly the oxygenator. If a simple, closed circuit without connectors and coated circuit tubing with improved biocompatibility are used, clotting risk is reduced.

The decision regarding when to place patients on ECMO therapy is challenging. Guidelines endorse the use of VA ECMO for CS refractory to initial therapy, CS with respiratory failure, and for cardiac arrest.[77] Risk scores can be used to predict mortality of patients with ECMO therapy.[101] In a small, randomized trial, immediate implementation of VA ECMO in patients with rapidly deteriorating or severe CS did not improve clinical outcomes compared with an early conservative strategy with upgrade to VA ECMO in case of deterioration.[102] Maintaining patients on ECMO requires an expert, multidisciplinary team, monitoring of hemodynamics, cardiac and respiratory status, coagulation parameters, hemolysis markers, and neurological status. Within a few days of ECMO support, it should be apparent whether the patient has stabilized or is deteriorating because of irreversible multiorgan failure, in which case palliative measures should be pursued. After stabilization, the possibility of recovery versus requirement of permanent support with LVAD or HT should be determined. Weaning should be attempted systematically using echocardiography and hemodynamics, once end-organ function has recovered, patient is euvolemic and on minimal inotropes.[103] Levosimendan can increase chance of success of weaning from VA ECMO.[104]

There are no large, randomized trials with ECMO. However, ECMO use is increasing, and registry date shows an overall survival to discharge of 42%.[105] Centers have even reported a 30-day survival of 80%.[106] ECMO is increasingly being used as a bridge to LVAD or HT with a survival rate of about 70%.[107] The ECLS-SHOCK trial (Extracorporeal Life Support in Cardiogenic Shock; ClinicalTrials.gov identifier: NCT03637205) will evaluate the efficacy of VA ECMO in addition to revascularization in patients with AMI-CS.

Future Directions

Temporary mechanical circulatory support development is focusing on smaller devices, lower AE profile, ability to deploy rapidly and easily at the bedside. There needs to be a change in outlook of management of CS, with earlier upgrade to TMCS to avoid irreversible organ failure and use of hemodynamic profiling to guide decision-making. The Cardiogenic Shock Working Group and European Mechanical Circulatory Support Summit are academic consortiums studying management of CS and optimization of TMCS use. Randomized clinical trials are needed to determine the safety and effectiveness of TMCS.

CONCLUSION

The burden of advanced HF is increasing. Durable LVADs offer a viable option for patients with end-stage HF. In the contemporary era, outcomes with LVADs are approaching those with HT, though AEs remain prevalent. TMCS devices can improve outcomes in more acutely ill patients and provide support till recovery, if feasible or bridge patients to durable LVAD or HT. A systematic, data-driven, and multidisciplinary team-based approach is essential to guide decision-making regarding TMCS and enhance outcomes. Opportunities for improvement in the field of LVAD and TMCS are device technology, better patient selection, and optimizing medical and surgical management.

ONLINE REFERENCES

Please scan the QR code provided at the end of the table of contents for References of this chapter.

CHAPTER

208

Extracorporeal Membrane Oxygenation in Cardiogenic Shock

Dilip Kumar, Dipanjan Chatterjee, Debopriyo Mondal, Rana Rathor Roy, Ashesh Halder, Sourav Das

ABSTRACT

Venoarterial extracorporeal membrane oxygenation (VA-ECMO) is a form of temporary mechanical circulatory support. It provides both respiratory and hemodynamic support. Also known as extracorporeal life support, ECMO is capable of providing efficient cardiopulmonary support and it can buy time for other treatments to promote recovery in patients with cardiogenic shock, even cardiac arrest refractory to conventional therapies. It can act as a bridge to a more durable mechanical solution in the setting of acute or acute on chronic cardiopulmonary failure. In this chapter, we will provide a brief overview of VA-ECMO, the associated physiological considerations of peripheral VA-ECMO, and its complications. We will also provide process for weaning from VA-ECMO.

Keywords: Cardiogenic shock, MCS, VA-ECMO, cardiopulmonary support.

INTRODUCTION

Cardiogenic shock is commonly defined as a state of low cardiac output that is inadequate to support the systemic perfusion requirements. Organ hypoperfusion is a central feature of cardiogenic shock. Cardiogenic shock is an acute emergency, which is classically managed by medical support with inotropes or vasopressors and frequently requires invasive ventilation. However, both catecholamines and ventilation are associated with a worse prognosis and many patients deteriorate despite all efforts. Mechanical circulatory support (MCS) is increasingly considered to allow for recovery or to bridge until making a decision or definite treatment. Various MCS devices have been manufactured with the main motto to provide various levels of hemodynamic support for reduction of devastating morbidity and mortality in patients with cardiogenic shock. The main mechanism of action is to reduce myocardial wall stress and oxygen consumption vis-à-vis increasing end-organ perfusion. Extracorporeal membrane oxygenation (ECMO) is most commonly used among all MCS devices.

CARDIOGENIC SHOCK

In patients with acute myocardial infarction, cardiogenic shock is the main cause of early mortality. Acutely decompensated chronic heart failure, decompensated valvular heart disease, myocarditis, takotsubo syndrome, acute pulmonary embolism, acute allograft failure, incessant arrhythmia, peripartum cardiomyopathy, etc., comprise the conditions which can lead to cardiogenic shock.[1]

VENOARTERIAL-ECMO

Venoarterial ECMO (VA-ECMO) is a form of temporary MCS and simultaneous extracorporeal gas exchange. It is used as a salvage intervention in patients with cardiogenic shock. Even cardiac arrest refractory to standard therapies, ECMO can provide hemodynamic support and can buy time for other treatments to promote recovery. ECMO can work as a bridge to a more durable mechanical solution in the setting of acute or acute on chronic cardiopulmonary failure.

The VA-ECMO system contains (1) an inflow/drainage cannula transporting blood from a central vein [usually inferior vena cava/right atrium (IVC/RA)] to the pump, (2) a centrifugal pump to keep hemolysis to a minimum, (3) a membrane oxygenator able to fully undertake oxygenation and decarboxylation of the blood, (4) a blood warmer, and (5) an outflow/return cannula leading to a central artery. VA-ECMO can be established via peripheral or central access. Central VA-ECMO is primarily implemented in the operating room and provides short-term support, often in postcardiotomy patients unable to wean from cardiopulmonary bypass (via RA and aorta or subclavian artery). Additionally, severe peripheral vascular disease can be an indication for central cannulation.[2] Peripheral VA-ECMO is initiated percutaneously or by surgical cut down outside of the operating room for patients with refractory cardiogenic shock and cardiac arrest via femoral vein—IVC (drainage) and for return usually via femoral arterial access or arterial return to a graft placed on the subclavian artery. The major advantage of peripheral access is the avoidance of invasive thoracic surgical intervention. The standard approach for percutaneous VA-ECMO is femoral artery and vein cannulation, and in adults, the tip of an 18–28 Fr cannula is used to drain deoxygenated venous blood, which is positioned in the mid RA. The oxygenated and decarboxylated blood is returned back to the systemic circulation via a 15–19 Fr arterial cannula with its tip typically positioned in the iliac artery after passing through the "membrane lung." Selection of cannulas with appropriate diameters is crucial not only to reduce the risk of vascular injury but also to avoid significant negative inflow (preferably <50 mm Hg) and high outflow pressure (<300 mm Hg) and to achieve adequate flow. A 7 or 8 Fr distal reperfusion cannula is routinely inserted into the superficial femoral artery with tip directed toward the foot to mitigate the risk of distal limb ischemia.[3] The sidearm of the distal perfusion sheath is connected with short tubing using a male-to-male connector to the vent port of the arterial cannula. VA-ECMO can thus provide biventricular support as well as gaseous exchange, which are big advantages over other MCS devices. Even in the presence of low cardiac function, organ perfusion can be maintained by providing large volume oxygenated blood flow. In contrast with intra-aortic balloon pump (IABP) and some percutaneous ventricular assist devices (pVADs), the native right ventricular function is not as critical to the provision of systemic perfusion due to the lessened reliance on transpulmonary flow with VA-ECMO.[3] The goal is to maintain systemic oxygen delivery at least three times the oxygen consumption (the DO_2:VO_2 ratio is >3).[4] During VA-ECMO therapy, continuous parenteral anticoagulation is mandatory to avoid thrombotic complications, but it can result in bleeding complications **(Figs. 1 and 2)**.

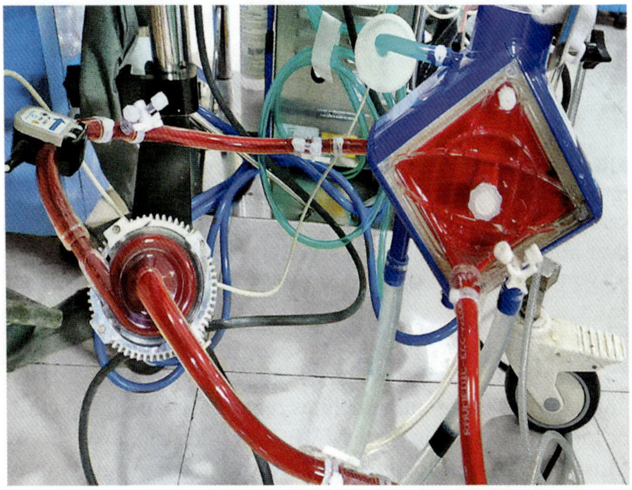

FIG. 2: Oxygenator circuit venoarterial extracorporeal membrane oxygenation (VA-ECMO).

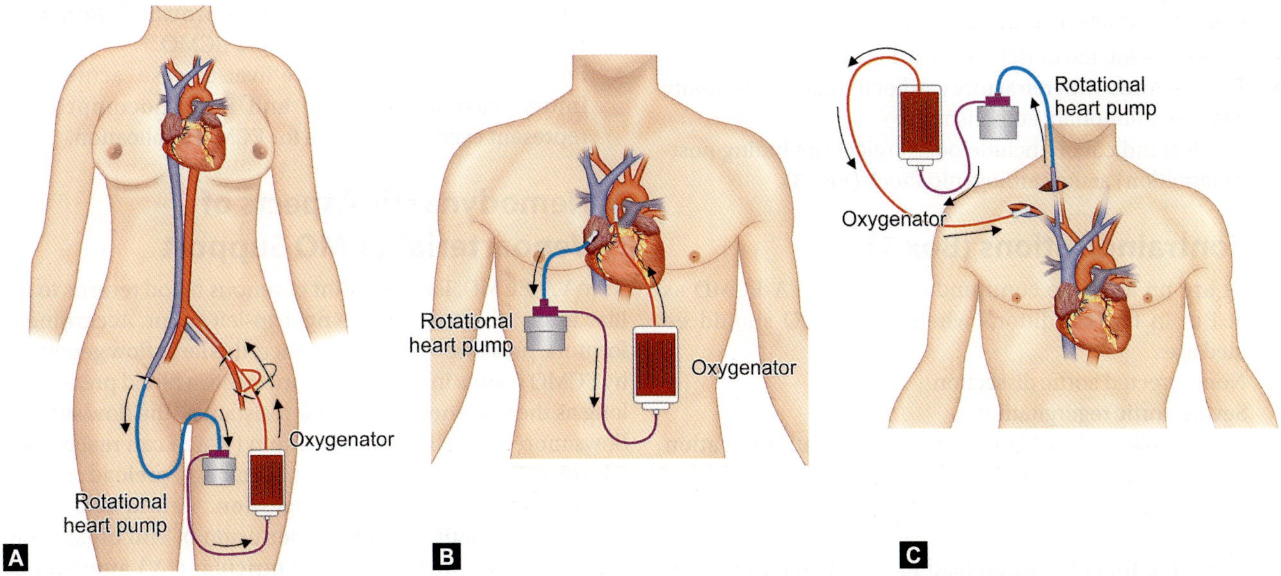

FIGS. 1A TO C: Central and peripheral venoarterial extracorporeal membrane oxygenation (VA-ECMO) cannulation strategies. (A) Peripheral VA-ECMO (femoro-femoral configuration); (B) Central VA-ECMO; (C) Peripheral VA-ECMO.[5]

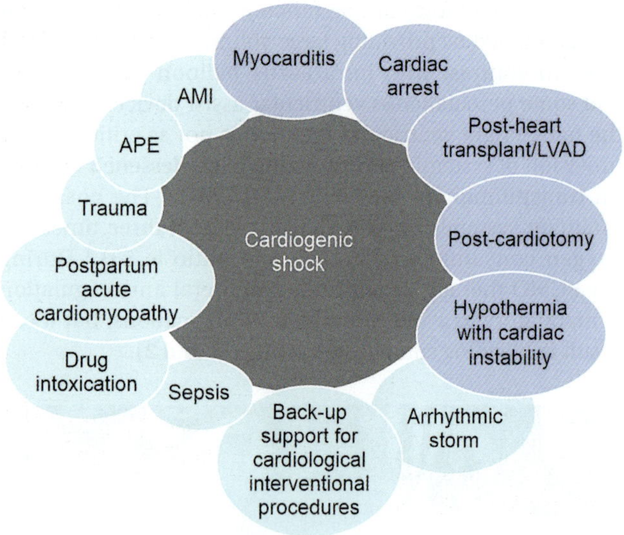

FIG. 3: Common (dark blue) and emerging situations (light blue) for venoarterial extracorporeal life support in the context of cardiogenic shock.[4,6]

(AMI: acute myocardial infarction; APE: acute pulmonary embolism; LVAD: left ventricular assist device; Sepsis: sepsis-associated cardiomyopathy)

Patient Selection

There are no clear cut guidelines regarding patient selection or indications for the use of VA-ECMO in cardiogenic shock. Most patients in Society for Cardiovascular Angiography and Interventions (SCAI) classification stage D and E can be treated with VA-ECMO. Common medical conditions for ECMO are as follows:

- Acute myocardial infarction
- Fulminant myocarditis
- Intoxication with cardiotoxic drugs
- End-stage dilated or ischemic cardiomyopathy
- Hypothermia with refractory cardiocirculatory instability
- Massive pulmonary embolism

Surgical indication include postsurgical (including post-transplantation) acute cardiogenic shock **(Fig. 3)**.

Contraindications (Box 1)

There are no absolute contraindications for VA-ECMO as such. But in few conditions where VA-ECMO should be avoided are:

- Noncorrected aortic dissection
- Severe aortic regurgitation
- Uncontrolled bleeding constituting a contraindication for parenteral anticoagulation
- Cases where acute or chronic conditions make the recovery unlikely
- When the therapy cannot lead to a next step in patient care (bridge to recovery, permanent MCS, or transplant)

BOX 1 Contraindications.[4]

- Cardiac recovery unlikely and no indication for heart transplant or durable left ventricular (LV) assist device
- Poor life expectancy (end-stage peripheral-organ diseases, malignant tumor, massive pulmonary embolisms in cancer patients, chemotherapy-induced chronic cardiomyopathy, etc.)
- Severe aortic valve regurgitation
- Severe vascular disease with extensive aortic and peripheral vessel involvement (calcification, stenosis, and closure), including axillary arteries
- Acute type A or B aortic dissection with extensive aortic branches (ascending, supra-aortic, and femoral) involvement (preoperatively)
- Severe neurologic impairment (i.e., prolonged anoxic brain damage, extensive trauma, and bleeding)
- Severe immunologic disease with marked blood and coagulation disorders
- Liver cirrhosis (Child–Pugh class B and C)

Recommendations[4]

- VA-ECMO should be considered for cardiogenic shock within 6 hours of its occurrence, refractory to conventional pharmacological and fluid therapy, and in patients with reversible cardiocirculatory collapse or those eligible for alternative cardiocirculatory assistance, for example, VADs or transplantation.
- Etiologies compromising appropriate ECMO function (aortic insufficiency) should be considered to represent potential contraindications.
- Age, per se, should not be used as an absolute contraindication.
- Prognostic score may be used to provide information regarding decision-making before ECMO.
- Poor life expectancy, severe liver disease, acute brain injury, vascular disease, and immunocompromise represent exclusion criteria for ECMO application.

Hemodynamic Aspects of Venoarterial-ECMO Support

As in VA-ECMO, large amount of venous blood returns to the iliac artery, there is massive right-to-left shunt. According to formula, pressure = flow × resistance, this large flow generated by ECMO results in a significant increase in blood pressure as long as there is enough vascular resistance. The flow support flows more typically run ≈3–4 L/min (which can reach up to 7 L/min). Because of huge venous drainage, preload reduces which leads to venous decongestion. Reinfusion to the systemic circulation increases perfusion of end organs, but subsequently it increases left ventricular (LV) afterload by retrograde flow support.

Complications of VA-ECMO Therapy

Bleeding/Clotting

Maintaining hemostatic balance in VA-ECMO is very challenging. As large foreign surface has to be kept for long time so anticoagulation is necessary to prevent thrombus formation. Unfractionated heparin (UFH) is used (alternatively, low molecular weight heparins or direct thrombin inhibitors—bivalirudin/argatroban can be used). With UFH, the aim is to keep an activated partial thromboplastin time of 1.5–2 times above the upper limit. Thrombus formation can occur in the circuit or in the vascular system (left ventricle, proximal aorta due to stasis of blood), leading to systemic thromboembolic infarct or stroke.

Because of the presence of ECMO, circuit bleeding risk already increased due to large synthetic surface, endothelial injury, and shear stress in the extracorporeal circuit, causing consumption of clotting factors. On top of this, use of anticoagulation increases bleeding risk. Also, usually necessary administration of transfusion of blood components leads to immunological responses, which intensifies bleeding risk. Bleeding sites are most often seen in cannula insertion sites, but other sites are also documented. In large registries, bleeding complications are found in up to 44% of VA-ECMO patients, with approximately 2% suffering intracranial hemorrhage.

Hemolysis

Hemolysis is due to increased shear stress in the ECMO circuit. In most cases, hemolysis is low level, especially since the widespread use of centrifugal pumps.

But in presence of the following risk factors, severe hemolysis can occur, reported in up to 5% of patients:

- Insufficient flow in the outflow cannula, leading to a rise in the negative pump head pressure
- Development of pump head thrombosis

Hemolysis leads to the release of free hemoglobin (Hb) in plasma, which is toxic and leads to acute renal failure. Peak plasma free Hb > 500 mg/L is an independent predictor of worse outcome and needs to be addressed urgently.

Limb Ischemia

Limb ischemia is a well-known complication with peripheral VA-ECMO cannulation and can occur in about 3.6% of patients. As a solution to it, positioning of an additional antegrade sheath should be performed to allow distal limb perfusion. Flow measurement to be done to ensure adequate tissue perfusion, which is around 100 mL/min. Initial ultrasound-guided cannulation provides further reduction in access-related complications. Regular monitoring of the cannulated lower limb and comparing to the noncannulated limb clinically (color, temperature, diameter at calf, movement of feet, and tone of calf muscles), measuring flow in popliteal artery by ultrasound can guide in diagnosing limb ischemia. Comparing near-infrared spectroscopy (NIRS) over calf muscles can give very early indication of limb ischemia. Tissue saturation by NIRS should be above 50%, preferably 60%, and there should be <20% difference between the two extremities **(Fig. 4)**.

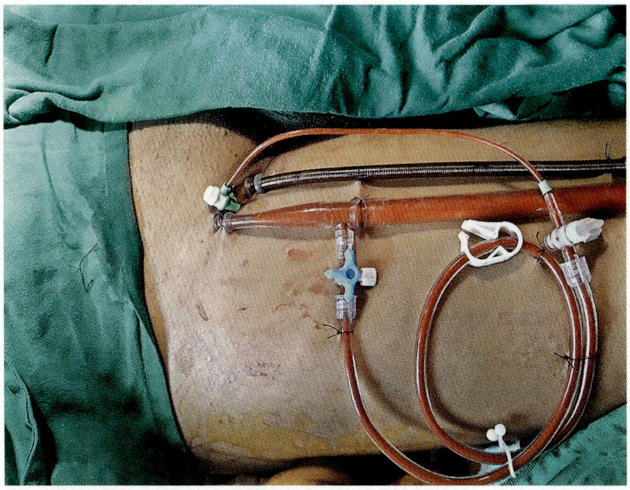

FIG. 4: Distal limb perfusion.

Inadequate Left Ventricular Unloading—Left Ventricular Distention

Our main aim after heart failure is myocardial recovery. For myocardial recovery, stroke work and myocardial oxygen consumption has to be reduced. VA-ECMO reduces preload and increases afterload due to retrograde aortic flow which in turn, causes an increase in left ventricular end-diastolic pressure (LVEDP) and LV volume. This results in increased LV filling pressures, wall stress, and severe pulmonary congestion. Increase in LVEDP causes decrease in coronary perfusion pressure which leads to decreased myocardial perfusion. In patients with extremely low systolic LV function and in all patients with ongoing arrest, VA-ECMO support results in a functionally closed aortic valve without relevant transaortic blood flow. This potentially results in severe LV distension and pulmonary congestion, stasis of blood in the LV, and proximal aorta (risk of clot formation in these sites) in the presence of sufficient systemic circulation. This problem aggravates with higher VA-ECMO flows. Hence, ECMO flow should be such that it allows adequate tissue perfusion as well as allows LV ejection with every beat **(Figs. 5 to 7)**.

Thus, LV unloading, prevention of LV distension, reduction of myocardial wall stress, and enhancement of coronary perfusion are important goals during MCS for bridge-to-recovery. Unloading (= "venting") can be achieved by different methods.

Table 1 shows options, procedures available to pursue, or favoring LV unloading during venoarterial extracorporeal life support.

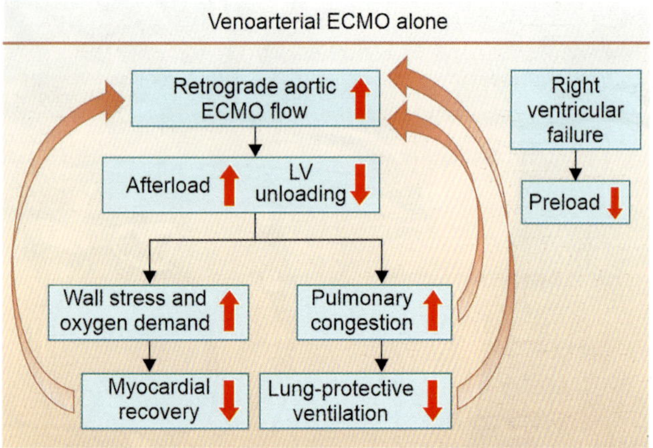

FIG. 5: The vicious circle in patients undergoing venoarterial extracorporeal membrane oxygenation (ECMO) therapy in cardiogenic shock resulting from the development of severe pulmonary edema and acute lung injury due to an increase in afterload and insufficient left ventricular (LV) unloading resulting from retrograde aortic flow.[6]

North–South (Harlequin) Syndrome

In VA-ECMO, there is formation of a watershed zone due to antegrade LV flow and retrograde ECMO flow, which occurs usually between the aortic root and the diaphragm **(Fig. 8)**. But watershed depends upon native LV output.

North–South syndrome or differential hypoxia is a complication unique to peripheral VA-ECMO. It can develop when native LV partially regains its function but lungs do not. Then, deoxygenated blood travels through the pulmonary circulation and into the LV, which is then ejected into the ascending aorta. So, a mixing area is formed by the deoxygenated antegrade blood from native LV and oxygenated blood from pump. The location of this mixing area depends upon the native LV function and pump flow. So, areas perfused by deoxygenated blood remain in risk of ischemia including myocardium and brain. That is why arterial oxygen saturation is to be taken from right radial artery to early detection of mismatch. Cerebral oximetry (NIRS) can be used to detect cerebral oxygenation and perfusion. If the differential cyanosis cannot be resolved by increasing the circuit flow, an additional cannula may be placed into the right internal jugular vein to achieve a hybrid configuration [venoarterial-venous ECMO (VAV-ECMO)]. In this case, oxygenated blood will be directed toward the RA by incorporating a "Y" connector into the arterial limb of the ECMO circuit. The oxygen-rich blood will cross the pulmonary circulation, thereby improving saturation in the proximal branches of the aorta **(Figs. 8 and 9, Table 2, and Boxes 2 and 3)**.[3]

Weaning from VA-ECMO

Weaning is a tricky job in VA-ECMO. Consider the following:

- Patients have experienced sufficient cardiac recovery

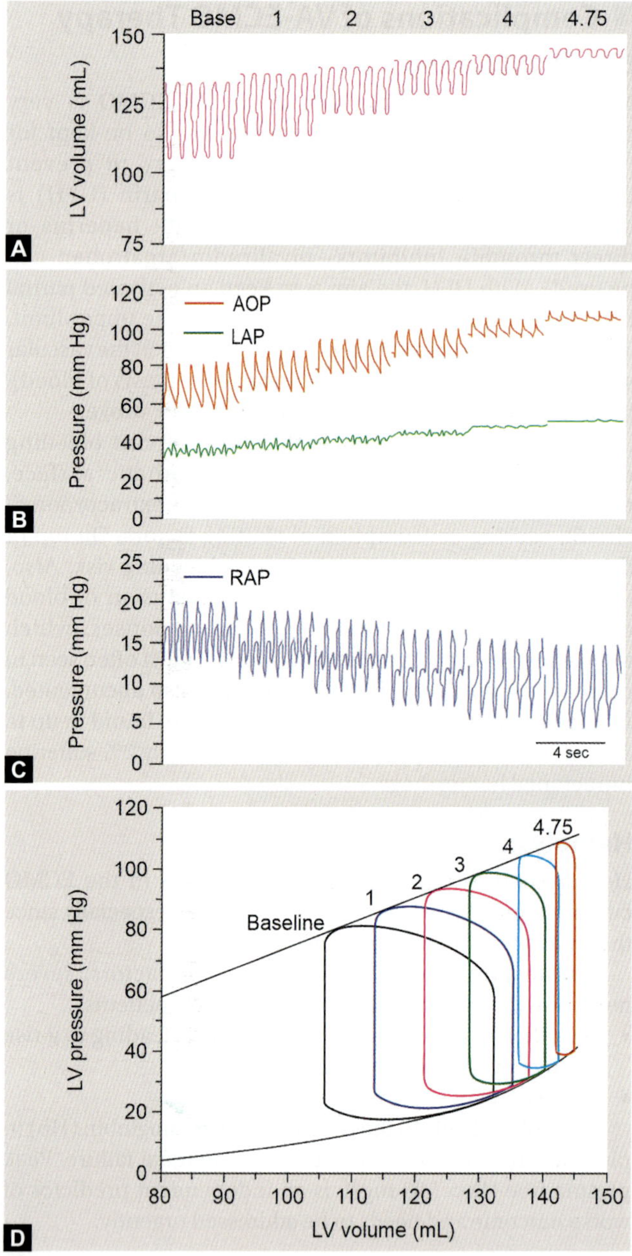

FIGS. 6A TO D: Hemodynamic changes that occur during acute cardiogenic shock and peripheral VA-ECMO at increasing flow rates (1, 2, 3, 4, 4.75 L/min) with an unvented LV: (A) LV volume and pressure increases; (B) AOP and LAP increase; (C) RAP decreases; (D) Pressure–volume loops generated during acute cardiogenic shock and VA-ECMO at increasing flow rates. With increasing ECMO flow rates there is an increase in aortic pressure and afterload (slope of the arterial elastance and end-systolic pressure). There is a concomitant decrease in stroke volume (represented by the width of the pressure–volume loop) and an increase in LV volume (LV distention) and LAP. As stroke volume approaches zero, this would clinically correspond to the aortic valve remaining closed throughout the cardiac cycle.

(AOP: aortic pressure; LAP: left atrial pressure; LV: left ventricle; RAP: right atrial pressure; VA-ECMO: venoarterial extracorporeal membrane oxygenation)

Method	Factor	Grade of severity		
Arterial line	Arterial pulsatility	Mild weakness	Moderate weakness	Almost pulseless
Central venous line	$ScvO_2$	75–55%	55–45%	<45%
	CVP	8–12 mm Hg	12–16 mm Hg	>20 mm Hg
Echocardiogram	AV	Opening every 2 beats/min	Opening every 3–4 beats/min	Closure
	LV distension	Mild	Moderate	Severe
	LA distension	Mild	Moderate	Severe
	"Smoke-like" effect	Mild	Moderate	Severe
	IVC dilatation[1]	1.5 to 2.5 cm	>2.5 cm	>2.5 cm
	IVC collapse[2]	<50%	<50%	No change
Swan-Ganz catheter	PCWP	13–18 mm Hg	18–25 mm Hg	>25 mm Hg
Chest X-ray	Congestion[3]	Alveolar edema	Interstitial edema	Redistribution
		Less-invasive LV unloading Maneuvers To be applied	IABP + less-invasive LV unloading Maneuvers To be applied	Invasive catheter-based LV-unloading Maneuvers To be applied

FIG. 7: Criteria to be used for the assessment of LV unloading need.[7]

(AV: aortic valve; CVP: central venous pressure; IABP: intra-aortic balloon pump; IVC: inferior vena cava; LA: left atrial; LV: left ventricular; PCWP: postcapillary wedge pressure; $ScvO_2$: central venous oxygen saturation)

TABLE 1: LV unloading strategies during VA-ECMO support.

Strategies	Advantages	Disadvantages
Inotropes	Simple to implement	Limited LV unloading; increases myocardial oxygen consumption
Vasodilators	Simple to implement	Limited LV unloading; blood pressure may not be sufficient
IABP	Bedside implementation possible; increased coronary blood flow	Unreliable degree of unloading
Balloon atrial septostomy	Bedside implementation possible	Indirect LV unloading; possible need for ASD closure after decannulation
LA→aortic cannula connected to venous port of ECMO circuit	More controlled LA decompression than septostomy	Indirect LV unloading; possible need for ASD closure after decannulation
Surgical LV vent	Direct LV venting; provides reliable LV unloading	Requires surgical placement and removal; impacts apex of the heart; blood stasis in proximal aorta still possible
Percutaneous LV vent	Bedside implementation possible; direct LV unloading; provides reliable LV unloading	Limited LV unloading compared with surgical LV vent; blood stasis in proximal aorta still possible
Percutaneous ventricular support	Impella FDA approved for this indication; direct LV unloading; antegrade flow support; aortic root washing; offers the possibility for ECMO to be weaned with continued circulatory support	North–South syndrome still possible
Off-pump central VA-ECMO	Direct LV unloading; total antegrade flow support; allows for ambulation; minimizes risk of vascular injury	Requires surgical placement and removal; impacts apex of the heart

(ASD: atrial septal defect; FDA: Food and Drug Administration; IABP: intra-aortic balloon pump; LA: left atrial; LV: left ventricular; VA-ECMO: venoarterial extracorporeal membrane oxygenation)

- The need for minimal vasoactive, inotropic support to maintain an adequate pulse pressure (PP) > 10 mm Hg, mean arterial pressure (MAP) of >65 mm Hg

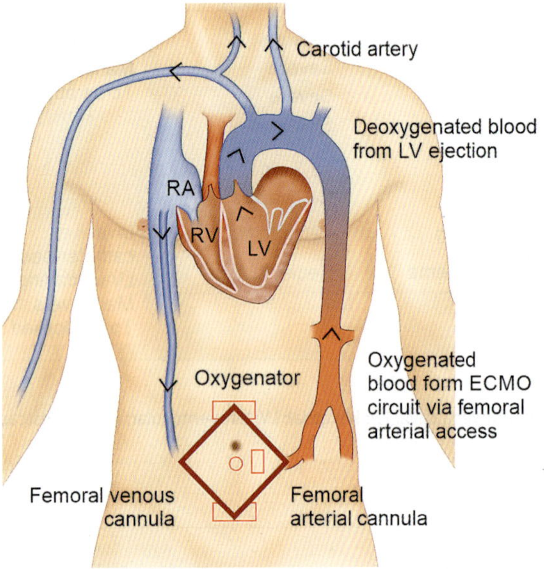

FIG. 8: Differential hypoxia.
(ECMO: extracorporeal membrane oxygenation; LV: left ventricular; RA: right atrial; RV: right ventricular)

- An acceptable mixed venous/central saturation at 1–1.5 L/min of VA-ECMO flow
- A higher arterial systolic and PP
- Aortic velocity time integral (VTI) (≥10 cm), left ventricular ejection fraction (LVEF) (<20–25%), lateral mitral annulus peak systolic velocity (TDSa, ≥6 cm/s).[9]

Before starting the weaning process, detailed assessment of myocardial recovery and end-organ function is to be done. Invasive hemodynamic monitoring and echocardiography is needed before starting weaning. Different algorithms are there but none of them is superior. Systematic approach to be followed with clinical judgment. A stepwise reduction in ECMO flow by 0.5 L/min to a final flow rate of ~1–1.5 L/min with monitoring of the following parameters:

- Close control of MAP
- PP
- Oxygenation
- Lactate levels
- Need for inotropes and vasopressors and close echocardiographic monitoring of myocardial function

In a simple rule, with an ECMO flow <1.5 L/min, mixed venous saturation is to be kept above 65% and arterial saturation above 90%. After achievement of lowest ECMO flow, 12-hour stable hemodynamics is required. After that, final decannulation to be done by surgical exposure and direct closure. In case of insufficient myocardial recovery, ECMO can work as a bridge directly to long-term mechanical solutions or heart transplantation.

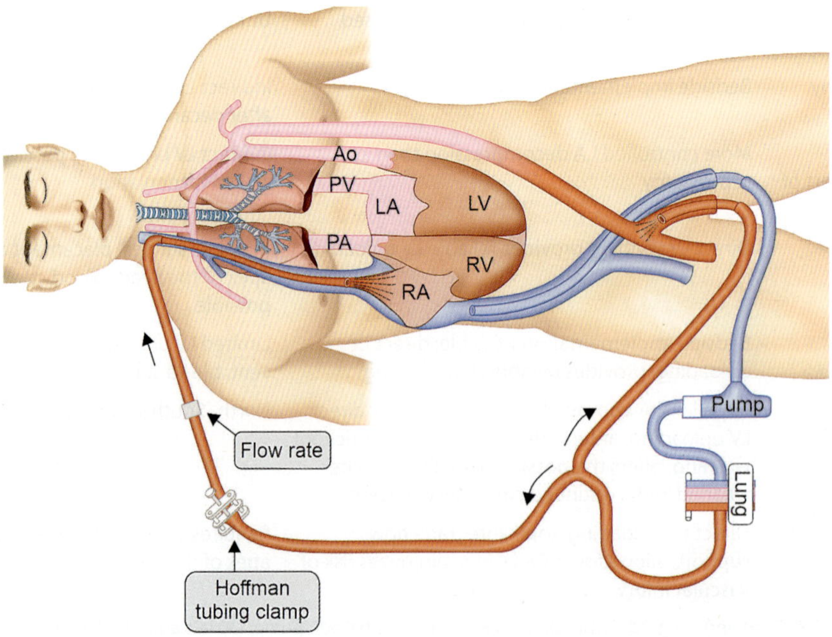

FIG. 9: Venoarterial-venous ECMO (VAV-ECMO).[8]
(Ao: aorta; LA: left atrial; LV: left ventricular; PA: pulmonary artery; PV: pulmonary vein; RA: right atrial; RV: right ventricular)

TABLE 2: Major complications of VA-ECMO and suggested management.[4]

Complications	Management
Malpositioning of cannula	Routine use of ultrasound/fluoroscopy for cannulation procedure
Ischemia of cannulated leg	• Prophylactic use of small antegrade perfusion cannula • NIRS monitoring of calf muscle before, during, and after VA-ECMO oximetry, pulse Doppler of cannulated leg
Deep vein thrombosis of femoral/caval vein	• Adequate anticoagulation during and after VA-ECMO • Ultrasound control of vessels after decannulation
Overloading of LV	• Reduce MAP to lowest acceptable value • Use small dose of inotropes and avoid vasopressors if possible • Use PAC and end-tidal CO_2 for monitoring of pulmonary perfusion • Regular echocardiography • Venting of LV when indicated (see proper table)
Differential oxygenation	• Monitoring of BGA and saturation on right arm • NIRS monitoring of the brain and lower limbs • Optimize ventilation • VAV cannulation only if necessary
Lower body hyperoxemia/hypocapnia	• BGA post-membrane after every change in ECMO settings • Adjust gas flow and blender settings to achieve normocapnia and slight hyperoxemia (150 mm Hg) after the oxygenator
Device clotting	• Adequate anticoagulation • Regular maintenance by control of aPTT or ACT, D-dimers, transmembrane pressure and gas transfer capacity—if relevant, and timely system replacement
Hemorrhage	• Adequate anticoagulation (reduced or stop heparin administration in case of excessive bleeding or life-threatening hemorrhage) • Regular control of aPTT or ACT, platelets, and fibrinogen • NIRS monitoring of brain • Avoid every unnecessary invasive procedure

(ACT: activated clotting time; aPTT: activated partial thromboplastin time; BGA: blood gas analysis; ECMO: extracorporeal membrane oxygenation; LV: left ventricle; MAP: mean arterial pressure; PAC: pulmonary artery catheter; NIRS: near-infrared spectroscopy; VAV: venoarterial-venous)

BOX 2 Clinical monitoring during venoarterial extracorporeal membrane oxygenation (VA-ECMO).[4]

Invasive arterial blood pressure monitoring/right radial artery:
- Pulse pressure—measure of native contractility versus ECMO blood flow
- Oxygen saturation—measure of oxygenation in proximal aortic arch/detection of differential oxygenation

Pulse oximetry/right hand: Oxygen saturation—measure of oxygenation in proximal aortic arch/detection of differential oxygenation

Pulmonary artery catheter:
- Detect elevated left-sided filling pressure
- Support indication for adjunct left ventricular (LV) unloading
- Continuous cardiac output monitoring as indication of residual pulmonary artery flow (alternatively, residual pulmonary artery flow can be monitored by measuring end-tidal CO_2)

Echocardiography:
- Early cardiac diagnostics and identification of contraindications to VA-ECMO
- Visualization of proper vascular access and guidance cannulation
- Optimal tailoring of ECMO support
- Serial assessment of hemodynamic and cardiac conditions
- Cardiac assessment during weaning trial

Electrocardiography: Consider continuous, multilead electrocardiographic monitoring

Near-infrared spectroscopy (NIRS): Monitoring of limb (single and bilateral comparison) and brain perfusion

BOX 3 Clinical management during venoarterial-ECMO.[4]

Mechanical ventilation:
- Apply lung-protective ventilation strategy with tidal volume 6–8 mL/kg ideal body weight
- Avoid pulmonary edema (LV distension monitoring and prevention, pulse pressure >10 mm Hg and aortic valve opening assessment, higher PEEP, vasodilators, ECMO flow adjustment, moderate inotropes, diuretics, or venting strategies as indicated and according to local expertise and resources)
- Promote mobilization
- Consider extubation

General critical care management:
- Protocolize anticoagulation therapy and monitoring
- Consider multimodal neuromonitoring/neuroimaging
- Close monitoring and aggressive treatment of lower limb ischemia, including embolectomy, vessel repair, revascularization, and fasciotomy
- Consider altered pharmacokinetics/drug dosing
- Strive for a neutral/negative fluid balance
- Connect CRRT device to ECMO circuit, if required

(CRRT: continuous renal replacement therapy; ECMO: extracorporeal membrane oxygenation; LV: left ventricular; PEEP: positive end-expiratory pressure)

CONCLUSION

We can utilize peripheral VA-ECMO as a short-term support for managing patients with cardiac arrest, severe biventricular failure, and cardiogenic shock irrespective of etiology. It can be initiated safely in the cardiac catheterization laboratory by experienced interventional cardiologists with very short door to support time, even during ongoing cardiopulmonary resuscitation (CPR). It may also be instituted in the field (mobile ECMO programs), at bedside in the intensive care unit (ICU), or in the operating room. Full VA-ECMO support not only allows time to perform diagnostic and therapeutic interventions while maintaining appropriate hemodynamics and gas exchange, but also provides time for potential organ recovery.

ONLINE REFERENCES

Please scan the QR code provided at the end of the table of contents for References of this chapter.

CHAPTER 209

Cardiac Transplantation: Indications, Eligibility, and Current Outcomes

Alla Gopala Krishna Gokhale, Siddharth Chinta, Mrinalini Alla

ABSTRACT

Cardiac transplantation is a proven treatment for advanced heart failure. Even though advanced heart failure is a major problem in India, many patients do not get this benefit. Apart from low organ donation rates, one of the main reasons is the lack of clarity to the referral doctors about the role of heart transplantation in the plethora of treatment options available. This chapter aims at giving some clarity on indications for heart transplantation and when to refer patients with advanced heart failure for heart transplantation and its current outcomes.

Keywords: Heart transplant, indications, when to refer, long term results.

INTRODUCTION

Heart failure affects about 1% of the population in India.[1] Of these, ≈5% of patients are expected to end in stage D heart failure [advanced heart failure (AHF)].[2] With an expected population of nearly 1.4 billion, this means the burden of AHF in India is nearly 0.7 million.[3] Of these, nearly 50,000 people need heart transplantation.[4] During the period of 2016–2018, the average heart transplantation rate in India was 0.2 per million population compared to the global average of 1.09.[5] Till April 2021, 1,113 heart transplants were done in India.[6] Even though heart transplantation is accepted as the gold standard treatment for AHF with a 1-year survival of ≈90% and a median survival of ≈13 years,[7] the main factors that contribute to the low rate of heart transplantation include low organ donation rate, affordability, and very low referral to the heart transplantation centers.

Orthotopic heart transplantation by bicaval technique is used in most of the patients after excision of the native recipient heart. It is preferred over the orthotopic biatrial method because of the lesser incidence of atrial arrhythmias and the need for permanent pacemakers. Another technique practiced rarely in special situations is heterotopic heart transplantation where the donor heart is piggybacked onto the native heart to assist it.

INDICATIONS FOR HEART TRANSPLANTATION

- The most common indication is when a patient remains in AHF (stage D) in spite of being on recommended/maximum tolerated doses of drugs proven to reduce mortality and improve the New York Heart Association (NYHA) class and other proven interventions like resynchronization therapy. Surgeries that can reverse heart failure, such as coronary artery bypass surgery, valve surgeries, and correction of congenital defects, were ineffective or not indicated. Without advanced therapies such as heart transplantation or ventricular assist device, they are at a very high risk of death (up to 75% in 1 year).[8] When a treating physician has any doubt about the timing of referral to the transplant centers, the following can help them in taking the decision:
    - I NEED HELP:[9] Presence of the following indicates AHF.
        - I: Inotropic requirements
        - N: New York Heart Association (NYHA) functional class III/IV in spite of guideline-directed therapy
        - E: End-organ dysfunction like renal/hepatic dysfunction due to heart failure or treatment

  - E: Ejection fraction (EF) < 25%
  - D: Defibrillation needed repeatedly
  - H: Hospitalizations frequently (at least one heart failure rehospitalization in the last 12 months)
  - E: Edema persisting in spite of increasing diuretic dosages
  - L: Low blood pressure
  - P: Prognostic medications cannot be uptitrated anymore
- Measuring peak volume of oxygen consumption VO_2 max thresholds in cardiopulmonary stress testing can also help. The numbers favoring listing for heart transplantation are as follows:[10]
  - VO_2 max ≤12 mL/kg/min on beta-blocker
  - VO_2 max ≤14 mL/kg/min if not on beta-blocker
  - VO_2 max <50% of predicted VO_2 in younger patients and women
  - If VO_2 max is between 12 and 14 mL/kg/min, heart failure prognostic scores such as Seattle Heart Failure Model (SHFM) and Heart Failure Survival Score (HFSS) can help to some extent.[11]
- Significant angina or its equivalent in patients with coronary artery disease, including transplant cardiac allograft vasculopathy, not amenable to medical treatment and where percutaneous or surgical revascularization is not possible
- Less common indications are patients with recurrent ventricular arrhythmias not amenable to medical therapy or to interventions, such as ablation and defibrillator implantation, or ablative surgery, and patients with cardiogenic shock after cardiac surgery or myocardial infarction who are dependent on continuous intravenous ionotropic support and circulatory support devices to keep adequate tissue perfusion.

For optimal results to the patients and their families and for better resource utilization, referral should be in the golden window period wherein the patient has AHF and yet is not so advanced that irreversible end-organ damage has happened.[12]

CONTRAINDICATIONS FOR HEART TRANSPLANTATION[10]

With increasing experience, many contraindications have become relative over time and only few remain absolute contraindications.

Absolute Contraindications

- Expected life span of <2 years in spite of heart transplantation
- Severe irreversible pulmonary artery hypertension (unless combined heart and lung transplantation is planned)
- Advanced cerebrovascular disease

Relative Contraindications

- Age >70 years
- Severe obesity [body mass index (BMI) > 35 kg/m^2] or frailty
- Diabetes mellitus with significant end-organ damage
- Severe renal, hepatic, or pulmonary dysfunction unless a combined transplant is planned
- Recent cancers
- Active infection
- Pulmonary embolism in the last 6–8 weeks
- History of drug abuse in the last 6 months
- Inadequate social support
- Psychological abnormalities interfering with the ability to follow advice
- Severe peripheral vascular disease

ASSESSMENT OF POTENTIAL RECIPIENT

For optimal results, it is very important to evaluate the potential recipient for exclusion of any reversible causes and to ensure that the patient needs and is fit for transplantation. Apart from routine presurgical tests, the two most important tests needed are diagnostic right heart catheterization (RHC) and detection of any antibodies [panel reactive antibodies (PRA)] in the recipient that can result in rejection.

- *RHC*: This is to be done to assess pulmonary artery pressures, cardiac output, transpulmonary gradient (TPG), and pulmonary vascular resistance (PVR). If the pulmonary artery systolic pressures are >50 mm Hg, PVR is >3 wood units, and/or TPG is >15 mm Hg, then postoperatively there are higher chances for right heart failure, increasing the perioperative mortality and morbidity. In that situation, a vasodilator challenge should be done for reversibility with drugs such as sodium nitroprusside, inhaled nitric oxide, milrinone, prostacyclin inhalation, or prostaglandin E1 (PGE1) infusions before listing the patient for heart transplantation.[10,11] This should be repeated every 3–6 months to ensure that readings are within operative range.
- *PRA*: This gives an indication of the presence of preformed circulating antibodies to human leukocyte antigens (HLA class I and II). PRA > 10% is considered positive. Their presence increases the risk of intra- and postoperative rejection and coronary artery vasculopathy in the long term. If these antibodies are high, interventions such as plasmapheresis, intravenous immunoglobulins, and treatment with rituximab may be needed for desensitization. Prospective cross-matching or virtual cross-matching is needed in these patients.

POST-TRANSPLANTATION COURSE AND OUTCOMES

- Careful monitoring in the postoperative course and immunosuppression are critical for good long-term outcomes. With increasing experience and present immunosuppressive therapy, median survival after heart transplantation is getting better. As per International Society for Heart and Lung Transplantation (ISHLT) 2017 registry,[13] 1-year survival is nearly 85% and median survival exceeds 12 years, and for those who survive at the end of 1 year, median survival is around 13–14 years with excellent quality of life for most. The predominant causes of mortality in these patients are graft failure in the first 1 month infections in the first year and chronic allograft vasculopathy (CAV) and renal failure in the long term. Apart from monitoring the clinical condition regularly, they also need monitoring for rejection and immunosuppressive drug optimal doses.

Monitoring for graft rejection: Routine periodic endomyocardial biopsy remains the gold standard for monitoring rejection in the first few years. The frequency of biopsies is coming down in many places due to its invasiveness and potential complications, and noninvasive modalities are being looked into. Some of the potential new modalities are as follows:

- Gene expression profiling for cell-mediated rejection: It is useful in excluding cell-mediated rejection. It has a negative predictive value of 99.6% for moderate-to-severe cellular rejection, but its positive predictive value remains low and its utility in antibody-mediated rejection is unclear.[14] AlloMap (CareDx) is an approved gene expression test for low-risk patients for acute cellular rejection.
- Donor-derived cell-free deoxyribonucleic acid (DNA): One of the studies has shown that detection of ≥0.25% donor-derived cell-free DNA has a very high negative predictive value of 99.2% for acute cellular and antibody-mediated rejections.[15] However, its positive predictive value still remains low.
- Cardiac magnetic resonance (CMR): The study by Anthony et al. suggests that this can be a safer and accurate alternative to endomyocardial biopsy.[16] CMR allows for the assessment of structure, function, and characterization of myocardial tissue.

However, more studies are needed before routine adoption of these alternative monitoring methods in place of endomyocardial biopsy.

- *Immunosuppression*: Lifelong immunosuppression in the right doses is the key for preventing rejection and improving long-term survival. In fact, it is only after the discovery of cyclosporine A that heart transplantation results got better. There are two categories of immunosuppression used—induction and maintenance immunosuppression. Induction therapy is not used by most centers on a regular basis. It is used to decrease acute perioperative immune response to the graft in specific situations. Antithymocyte globulin or basiliximab is used for induction. Using them can help in delaying the start of calcineurin inhibitors. Maintenance immunosuppression is with a triple-drug regimen—combination of calcineurin inhibitor (cyclosporin or tacrolimus—tacrolimus is used more widely these days), antimetabolites (azathioprine or mycophenolate—mycophenolate is preferred by most centers), and steroids. Steroids are usually weaned off in a few months, leaving only calcineurin inhibitor and antimetabolite lifelong. In those with coronary artery vasculopathy or who develop nephrotoxicity after transplant related to tacrolimus, tacrolimus may need to be replaced with mammalian target of rapamycin (mTOR) inhibitors such as everolimus or sirolimus.
- *Early postoperative complications*: Apart from postoperative bleeding, pericardial effusion, arrhythmias, etc., some important complications are as follows:
  - Primary graft dysfunction: It is the most common cause of mortality in the first month after the surgery. Mortality in 30 days is 30% and is seen in 7.4% of patients.[17] Risk factors include older recipient age, older donor age, donor–recipient size mismatch, prolonged ischemic time, female donor, etc.
  - Acute right ventricular failure is seen in 2–3% of patients but has a very high mortality. Etiology is often multifactorial including high pulmonary artery pressures in the recipient, volume overload, suboptimal myocardial protection, small-sized heart for the recipient, etc.

    Their management starts from the preoperative period like optimization of control of heart failure in the recipient, making sure that pulmonary hypertension is not irreversible, protecting the donor heart with good myocardial protection, and keeping the ischemic time to the minimum. Early identification of the problem and aggressive treatment with inotropes and, if needed, with temporary ventricular support are the keys to saving these patients.
  - Cardiac rejection: Two types of rejections can happen in the early postoperative period after heart transplantation.
    - Hyperacute rejection: It happens immediately after the removal of the aortic cross-clamp due to the presence of preformed antibodies to the donor heart. These days, it is extremely rare as the recipient is checked for any antibodies in the preoperative evaluation and cross-matching is done often before surgery.
    - Acute rejection: Cell-mediated acute rejection is more common than antibody-mediated rejection (20–40% vs. 10–20%). Diagnosis is confirmed by endomyocardial biopsy and by the presence of inflammatory infiltrate

or by immunohistochemical staining. Cell-mediated rejection is generally treated with steroids. Antibody-mediated rejection often needs addition of drugs such as rituximab, bortezomib, plasmapheresis, and/or intravenous immunoglobulins.

- *Late complications*:
  - *CAV*: This is a very common complication with an incidence of nearly 8% in the first year, 30% at 3 years, and >50% at 10 years.[18] This is accelerated atherosclerosis affecting smaller arteries and often not amenable to angioplasty or bypass surgery. Patients present with atypical symptoms such as heart failure, arrhythmias, or sudden death. The International Society of Heart and Lung Transplantation recommends intravascular ultrasound with coronary angiogram as a regular screening test for early detection. Alternative modalities sometimes used for diagnosis are computed tomographic angiography and dobutamine echocardiography. Treatment options include optimizing immunosuppression, considering the use of everolimus, increasing doses of statins, angioplasty or bypass surgery in select patients, and rarely retransplantation.
  - Infections: Due to immunosuppression, infections remain a major concern leading to 30% mortality in the first year and 10–13% per year after that.[19] In the first few months, it is bacterial septicemia and pulmonary infections. Most pneumonias are caused by opportunistic organisms such as cytomegalovirus, *Aspergillus* species, and pneumocystis. Typically, preventive vaccination for pneumococcal pneumonia, influenza, and hepatitis B is done before transplantation. Preventive vaccination with live vaccines is not recommended to these patients after transplant as they are on immunosuppressants.
  - Chronic kidney disease due to calcineurin inhibitor is seen in nearly 50% in 5 years post transplant follow-up.
  - The incidence of malignancies is nearly 28%. Specifically, skin cancers and lymphoma are a risk after heart transplantation due to immunosuppression.

RECENT ADVANCES HAPPENING

Two developments are worth mentioning in the area of increasing the donor pool for transplantation:

1. *Ex vivo perfusion systems*: Cold storage is the standard technique used for preservation and transportation of the donor heart. But it has limited ischemia time, usually 4 hours or less to have good results. Ex vivo perfusion systems like Organ Care System (OCS) perfuse the coronaries and keep the heart beating and warm, permitting transport of the organ in a more physiological condition, allowing (1) extension of the time between harvesting and implantation of heart safely allowing transporting of organ over longer distances with lesser concern about ischemic times and harvesting of hearts in donation after circulatory death (DCD) and (2) assessment and possible improvement of function in marginal hearts.[20] Both of these are likely to result in increasing the number of donor hearts.
2. *Opt-out method of organ donation*: In most countries including India, the present system of organ donation is opt-in where organs are harvested from a suitable donor only if the attendants of the donor agree to donate. In some countries such as Spain, and a recent addition to these is the United Kingdom, they have opt-out method. In this, all suitable donors are considered for organ harvesting unless the attendants of the donor refuse. This has increased the number of available organs by nearly 25–30% in these countries.

CONCLUSION

For many patients with end-stage AHF, heart transplantation remains the gold standard. Median survival of the recipients is steadily increasing proper selection of patients, and their postoperative management is very critical for the success. Apart from alternative developments like mechanical assist devices, developments like newer immunosuppressive drugs, ex vivo perfusion systems, DCD, and opt-out method of donations, better critical care facilities are likely to increase the availability of this life-saving procedure to the needy. It is very important that physicians treating these heart failure patients refer them in the golden window period to advanced centers with heart transplantation facilities.

ONLINE REFERENCES

Please scan the QR code provided at the end of the table of contents for References of this chapter.

CHAPTER

210 Heart Transplant: Pre- and Postmanagement

R Ravi Kumar, Sarumathi Thangavel

ABSTRACT

Cardiac transplant is one of the treatment options for selective few patients with advanced heart failure. As the field of thoracic transplantation is rapidly evolving in India, it is imperative that cardiologists and cardiothoracic surgeons become familiar with the pretransplant evaluation process and perioperative and post-transplant management of cardiac transplant recipients. The purpose of the article is to discuss a brief overview of cardiac transplantation in India.

Keywords: Cardiac transplant, immunosuppression management, advanced heart failure therapy.

INTRODUCTION

Advanced heart failure is associated with significant morbidity and mortality. Approximately 5% of the patients with heart failure proceed to have an advanced heart failure. Heart transplantation is the gold standard treatment of choice for those selective few patients with progressive heart failure refractory to optimized medical and device therapy. The purpose of this review is to familiarize cardiologists and cardiothoracic surgeons involved with cardiac transplantation with the decision-making process in assessing for candidacy for advanced therapies such as heart transplant and left ventricular assist device (LVAD), listing patients for cardiac transplantation, optimizing patients prior to cardiac transplantation, and to provide guidance and insight on the posttransplant management of patients receiving a cardiac transplant.

The need for effective heart transplants in a large country like India is incontestable with experts estimating that there might be a burden of at least 2.5 million end-stage heart failure patients in India, with estimated prevalence of 2–3/1,000 population.[1] Inclusion and listing criteria for heart transplantation have evolved over the last few decades and have been influenced by expansion of the donor heart pool, utilization of marginal donor, donation after circulatory death (DCD), improvements in immunosuppression, better logistics available for transport of donor organ and better perioperative management of adverse factors affecting outcome. The modern guidelines on this subject are provided by the International Society for Heart and Lung Transplantation (ISHLT) which was first published in 2010 with the most recent update in 2022.[2]

BRIEF HISTORY OF CARDIAC TRANSPLANTATION IN INDIA[3-5]

Routine heart transplantation using modern methods after the brain death law was introduced in 1993. Heart transplantation was performed by Dr Venugopal, Dr KM Cherian, and others in the 1990, but there were far and few transplants in between due to the absence of an efficient national procurement registry and donor allocation system. The path-breaking initiative came about in 2008 with the establishment of the transplant authority of Tamil Nadu (TRANSTAN) which has allowed 575 heart transplants in the state between 2008 and 2023. This initiated the process of organ sharing registries in Kerala, Karnataka, Maharashtra, Gujarat, Andhra Pradesh, and the NOTTO in New Delhi. The long-term Indian experience and registry data from the Indian Society for Heart and Lung Transplantation has been recently published.

Pretransplant Evaluation

Indications

In the current era, the most common indication for cardiac transplantation in India and around the world is dilated cardiomyopathy. With the advances in the management of coronary artery disease (CAD) with percutaneous coronary intervention and medical therapy, the numbers of patients requiring heart transplant for ischemic cardiomyopathy has decreased over the last decade, but this has in turn led to an increase in cardiac transplant in patients with restrictive cardiomyopathy (has recently gained more recognition), hypertrophic cardiomyopathy, arrhythmogenic right ventricular dysplasia (ARVD), congenital heart disease and patient's requiring retransplantation. Patients with refractory angina or arrhythmias are also eligible for the heart transplant if symptoms are persistent despite percutaneous coronary intervention/ablation/medical therapies leading to poor quality of life. Concomitant liver transplantation might be required for patients with a failing Fontan with chronic hepatic congestion leading to cardiac cirrhosis.

Identifying Patients with Advanced Heart Failure

Clinicians should utilize the acronym "I NEED HELP" to identify patients with advanced symptoms[6] as enumerated in **Table 1**. The clinical cues that helps physicians identify patients with advanced heart failure are those with inability to tolerate guideline-directed medical therapy for heart failure secondary to hypotension or renal dysfunction, those who have persistent fluid overload despite escalating doses of diuretics, those who present with recurrent defibrillator shocks, those with persistent New York Heart Association (NYHA) class IV symptoms, those with worsening liver and renal dysfunction, those with recurrent hospitalizations or emergency room visits for heart failure exacerbations and those requiring continuous inotropes such as dobutamine or milrinone.

The echocardiographic parameters that help identify such patients are marked left ventricular cavity dilatation of over 7–8 cm, significant secondary mitral regurgitation from mitral annulus dilation, restrictive mitral inflow pattern, concomitant right ventricular failure, and pulmonary hypertension. Other parameters that help in terms of obtaining more objective data in addition to echocardiogram are elevated filling pressures on right heart catheterization, low cardiac index (<2.2 L/min/m^2), peak oxygen consumption (VO_2) < 14 mL/kg/min and (<12 mL/kg/min for those on β-blockers) on cardiopulmonary exercise testing performed by a bicycle ergometer. Once these patients are identified, they must be referred to a cardiac transplantation center for further evaluation. A sample for the suggested workflow that should be followed in the cardiac transplantation center (or advanced heart failure center as called in the United States) issued by the American Heart Association is depicted in **Flowchart 1**.

TABLE 1: The "I NEED HELP" acronym for markers of advanced HF.

I	Inotropes	Previous or ongoing use of inotropic support
N	NYHA class/natriuretic peptides	Persistent NYHA class III or IV symptoms
E	End-organ dysfunction	Worsening renal or liver function
E	Ejection fraction	Very low ejection fraction <20%
D	Defibrillator shocks	Recurrent defibrillator shocks for ventricular tachyarrhythmia
H	Hospitalizations	More than 1 hospitalization in 12 months
E	Edema/escalating diuretics	Persistent fluid overload and/or increasing diuretic requirements
L	Low blood pressure	SBP consistently <90 mm Hg
P	Prognostic medication	Inability to tolerate ACEI/ARB/ARNI or β-blocker

(ACEI: angiotensin-converting enzyme inhibitor; ARB: angiotensin receptor blocker; ARNI: angiotensin receptor–neprilysin inhibitor; HF: heart failure; NYHA: New York Heart Association; SBP: systolic blood pressure)

Benefits of Early Referral and the Golden Window for Referral

There certainly is a golden window of referral for patients **(Fig. 1)**.[7] These are the patients who have low cardiac index based on their right heart catheterization but do not have hypotension or end-organ dysfunction secondary to their cardiac dysfunction. These patients benefit the most since they have higher probability of achieving guideline-directed medical therapy, they have access to hemodynamic monitoring and to specialized diagnostic techniques such as cardiac magnetic resonance imaging, pyrophosphate (PYP) scan, and positron emission tomography (PET) scan for cardiac sarcoidosis to help identify their etiology of heart failure. They will also have access to additional therapeutic options such as cardiac resynchronization therapy, transcatheter edge-to-edge repair of mitral valve, pulmonary artery hemodynamic monitoring, etc. These patients will also have their comorbidities well managed which might otherwise limit their functional improvement after cardiac transplantation.

Disadvantages of a Late Referral

Patients who are not referred in a timely fashion, often present with cardiac cachexia and progressive multiorgan dysfunction which makes them ineligible for cardiac transplantation. These patients often require temporary mechanical support with a very high risk of progressive deterioration resulting in pump failure and death.

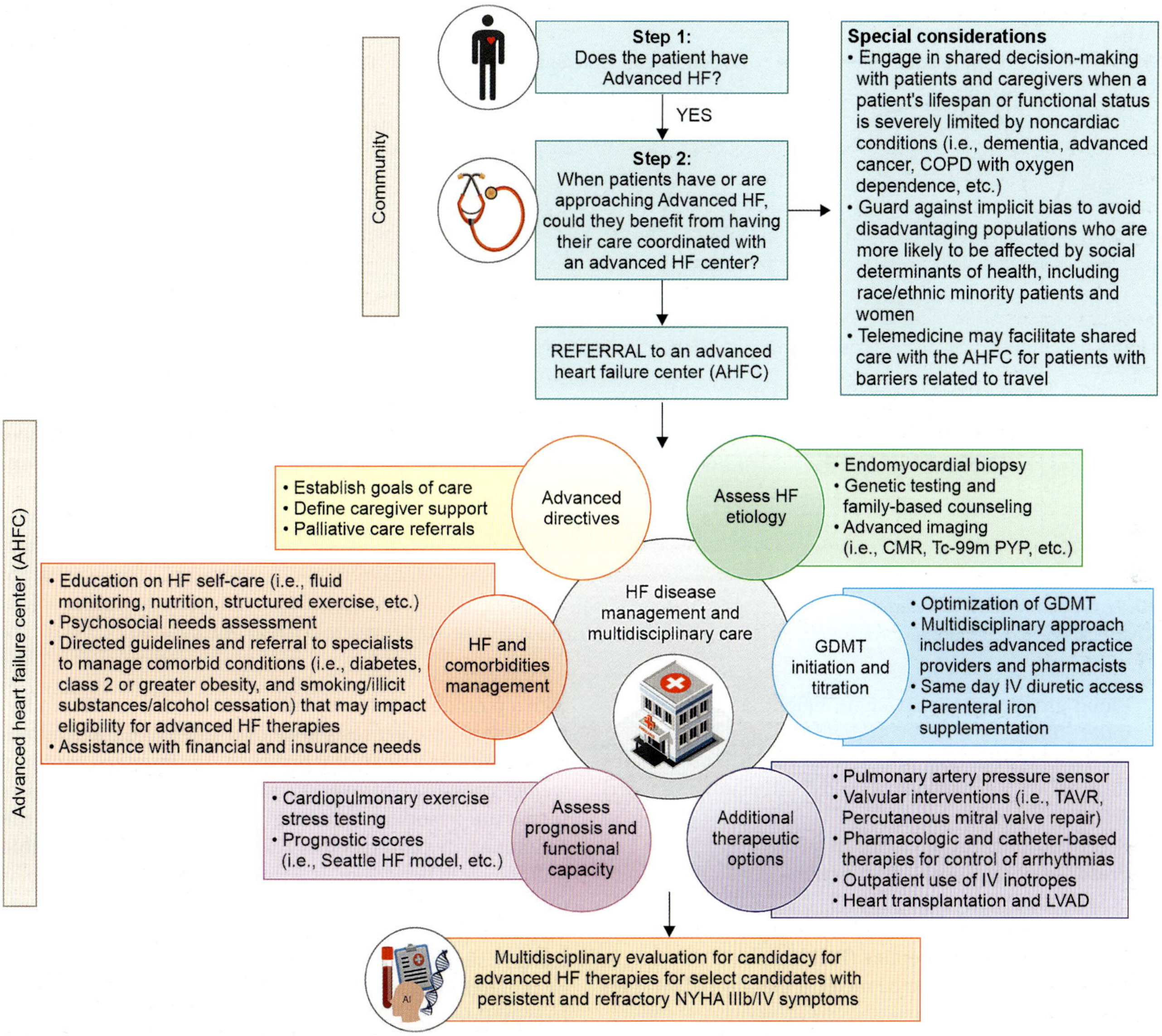

FLOWCHART 1: Algorithm for advance heart failure center.

(COPD: chronic obstructive pulmonary disease; CMR: cardiac magnetic resonance; HF: heart failure; GDMT: guideline-directed medical therapy; IV: intravenous; LVAD: left ventricular assist device; NYHA: New York Heart Association; TAVR: transcatheter aortic valve replacement; Tc-99m PYP: technetium-99m pyrophosphate)

Evaluation of Heart Transplant Candidacy

The goal of evaluation is threefold. (1) To ensure that there are no alternative medical/surgical therapies available for treating heart failure other than cardiac transplant, (2) to ensure that the patient does not have any end-organ dysfunction secondary to cardiac or noncardiac etiology which will in turn affect the overall outcome posttransplantation, and (3) to ensure that there are no other nonmedical limitations such as medical nonadherence, substance abuse disorder or lack of social support which will prevent the patient from having a good outcome after cardiac transplantation. Decisions are usually taken by a multidisciplinary team comprising of a heart failure cardiologist, cardiac surgeon, medical subspecialists and transplant coordinators. The discussion is usually focused on the management of patient's comorbidities such as hepatic and renal dysfunction, pulmonary hypertension, diabetes mellitus, obesity, history of malignancy, hematological disorders, and infectious diseases. Usually a multidisciplinary approach is needed where a specialist along with the advanced heart failure team will help comanage the patient before and after cardiac transplantation if their condition is reversible.

Pretransplant basic assessment in clinic includes:

- Diagnosis—ischemic or nonischemic, infiltrative, restrictive, ARVD, hypertrophic obstructive cardiomyopathy (HOCM), refractory angina, and congenital heart disease

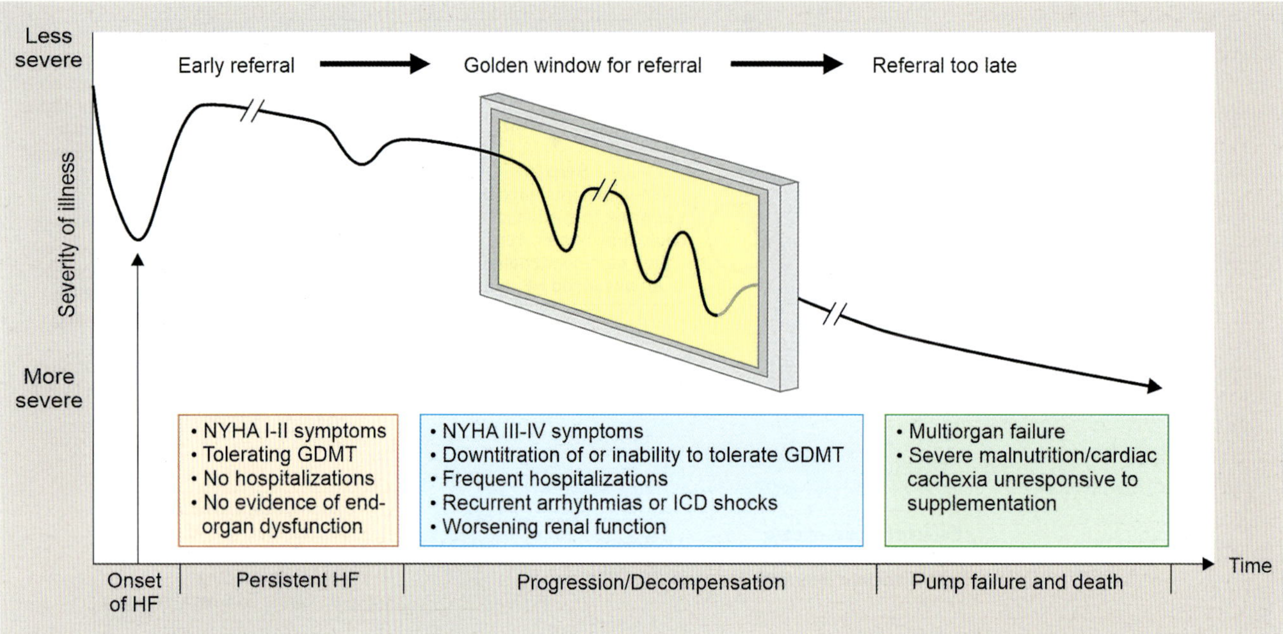

FIG. 1: Golden window for referral.
(GDMT: guideline-directed medical therapy; HF: heart failure; ICD: implantable cardioverter-defibrillator; NYHA: New York Heart Association)

- Blood group, age, sex, weight, height, and body mass index (BMI)
- NYHA classification and INTERMACS (Interagency Registry for Mechanically Assisted Circulatory Support) grading
- Recent hospitalizations for heart failure
- Presence of end-organ dysfunction—renal, hepatic, or pulmonary
- Peak VO_2—performed with a bicycle ergometer
- Pro-brain natriuretic peptide (BNP) levels
- Current guideline-directed medical therapy (GDMT) for heart failure
- Echocardiographic parameters needed—left ventricular ejection fraction (LVEF), left ventricle end diastolic dimension (LVEDD), mitral regurgitation (MR) grading, right ventricular (RV) function, tricuspid regurgitation (TR) grading, pulmonary artery systolic pressure (PASP) using TR gradient and inferior vena cava (IVC) diameter and collapsibility, and pericardial effusion
- Chest X-ray and electrocardiogram
- Right heart catheterization
- Panel reactive antibody screening by Luminex to measure antibodies against human leukocyte antigen (HLA) (class I and class II)
- HLA typing
- Viral markers

Right Heart Catheterization

A right heart catheterization is mandatory prior to listing the patient for cardiac transplantation. Pulmonary hypertension with a pulmonary artery systolic pressure of over 50 mm Hg, pulmonary vascular resistance over three and transpulmonary gradient (mean PA pressure—pulmonary capillary wedge pressure) of over 12 should trigger cardiologists to pursue vasodilator testing to determine whether the pulmonary hypertension is reversible or not. Irreversible pulmonary hypertension is a risk factor for right ventricular dysfunction of the cardiac allograft in the immediate postoperative period. Vasodilator testing can be performed by using IV sildenafil, IV milrinone, or IV nitroprusside infusion or inhaled nitric oxide. If the pulmonary hypertension is irreversible even after a vasodilator challenge then the patient should be considered for a combined heart-lung transplantation.

Contraindications for Cardiac Transplantation

Absolute Contraindications for Cardiac Transplantation

- Major systemic illness with a life expectancy of <2 years despite heart transplantation
- Active substance (tobacco, drug, or alcohol) abuse
- Multisystem disease with severe extracardiac organ dysfunction
- Severe symptomatic cerebrovascular disease
- Irreversible pulmonary hypertension with pulmonary vascular resistance of >3–6 Wood units
- Major psychiatric illness or active substance abuse that cannot be managed sufficiently to allow posttransplant care and safety

Relative Contraindications

- Age >70 years (carefully selected patients who are >70 years may be considered)
- Infection
- Acute pulmonary thromboembolism within 6–8 weeks
- Morbid obesity (BMI > 35 kg/m^2)
- Tobacco use within 6 months
- Recent past (within 6 months) substance (drug or alcohol) abuse
- Irreversible hepatic dysfunction with bilirubin of >2.5 mg/dL and/or transaminases >2 × normal, or cirrhosis on biopsy
- Irreversible renal dysfunction with estimated glomerular filtration rate (eGFR) <30 mL/min/1.73 m^2. Kidney transplantation can be considered in such patients
- Other conditions that increase the risk of perioperative complications or limit tolerance of immunosuppression or rehabilitation (e.g., peripheral vascular disease that would limit rehabilitation and is not amenable to revascularization, active peptic ulcer disease, cholelithiasis, diverticulosis, and advanced hepatic disease)
- Neoplasm (requires individualized assessment of severity, treatment options, and prognosis)
- Insulin-requiring diabetes mellitus with end-organ damage (other than nonproliferative retinopathy) or persistent poor glycemic control glycated hemoglobin (HbA1c) >7.5% despite optimal efforts
- Inadequate social support or cognitive behavioral disability that would prevent compliant care
- Human immunodeficiency virus (HIV)

For those patients with relative contraindications, a permanent left ventricular assist device can be considered to stabilize the patient while waiting for the patient to be optimized for cardiac transplantation such as severe pulmonary hypertension, obesity or recent remission from malignancy.

Management of Patients during Waiting Period Prior to Cardiac Transplantation

Once the patient is registered for transplantation, he/she should follow-up every week or every other week with regular laboratory testing (electrolytes and liver and renal function every 2 weeks) to help optimize patient's volume status, nutrition and other comorbidities which in turns leads to good outcome after cardiac transplantation.

- *Sensitized patients*: Patients with panel reactive antibody (PRA) >40% will need to undergo desensitization with Rituximab prior to transplantation to avoid acute rejection. Elevated PRA is usually secondary to multiple blood transfusions, pregnancy, prior organ transplant, presence of homograft, and presence of durable or temporary LVAD. The PRAs associated with durable LVADs decline rapidly in the postoperative period following transplant upon explant of the LVAD.

Matching of Donors versus Recipients

As per the standard international criteria following matching procedures are obligatory between recipient and donor.

- *Immunological match*: The immune response to a solid transplanted organ critically depends on the level of allele match in the major histocompatibility antigens present in the short arm of chromosome 6. These HLA sites are further classified into HLA class 1 (A, B, and C) and HLA class 2 (DQ, DR, and DB). For a variety of reasons, full house of HLA match is not necessary for heart transplant unlike kidney transplant. HLA antigens play an important part in late rejection and tests like single antigen bead anti-HLA antibodies measured by immunofluorescence are routinely used to rule out antibody-mediated rejection. Human leukocyte antigen typing of the donor is not routinely performed but a complement-dependent cytotoxic assay [complement-dependent cytotoxicity (CDC) assay] is performed between the donor serum and the recipient lymphocytes.
- *Blood group match*: The rules of blood group match the same as blood transfusion except the fact that rhesus positive and negative factors are not important for heart matching. So, an O group recipient can accept only an O group donor, while AB group recipient can accept any blood group donor. A and B groups can accept their own group or O donors. AB donors can donate only to AB recipients.
- *Weight matching*: As per ISHLT guidelines, 15–20% oversizing of donors is permissible (in practice this depends on surgeon's skills and may get stretched to 30% for pediatric recipients and young adult donors). Under sizing of up to 10% is permissible. In cases where the recipient pulmonary vascular resistance is high (in the 3–5 Wood unit range), an oversized donor is required which helps the donor right ventricle overcome the higher pulmonary compliance without overt RV failure.

Preservation and Transport of Donor Organ

The present standard of care for preservation and transport of the donor organ involves, cross clamp and introduction of crystalloid long-duration cardioplegia using solutions such as histidine-tryptophan ketoglutarate (HTK) and Custodiol solution. Then the donor heart is transported in ice cold saline at temperatures of 1–4°C. This cold ischemic nonbeating heart survives anaerobic energy generation but at low levels of metabolism. Since there is loss of tissue adenosine 5′-triphosphate (ATP) levels along with cold injury during transportation, the maximum tolerated cold ischemic time is 4 hours, from the time of cross-clamp in the donor body to removal of cross clamp in the recipient.

Organ Care Systems and Normothermic Donor Organ Transport[8,9]

TransMedics Inc. has now introduced a normothermic, beating heart, ex vivo organ care system for donor heart transport, which can extend the ex vivo warm ischemic time up to 8–9 hours after explanting the organ by providing warm blood perfusion to the beating heart.

Post-transplant Management

Immunosuppression Protocols

Steroid Dosing

The standard US immunosuppression protocols involve 1,000 mg IV Solu-Medrol at the time of first anastomosis, followed by 125 mg IV every 8 hours × three doses, followed by 1 mg/kg dosing oral prednisone daily with reduction by 10 mg every week. Considering higher infection risks with these high steroid doses and higher chance of gastrointestinal (GI) bleeding, most of the Indian protocols now use much lower long-term dose of prednisolone, 5–10 mg/day up to the first 6 months after heart transplant. These lower doses seem to be extremely safe with very low incidence of rejection comparable to western figures, 88% survival in 1 year and seem to have lowered the risks of infection and GI bleeding.

Immunosuppression Protocols—Induction Therapy[10-14]

One practical problem faced early on by the transplant teams was the higher increasing creatinine in the early postoperative period after heart transplant. This is due to a variety of factors like higher preoperative creatinine, cardiopulmonary bypass, catabolism, surgical inflammatory syndrome (SIRS), etc. Under such a situation, initiation of postoperative calcineurin inhibitor (CNI) drugs like tacrolimus was a big challenge since CNI agents themselves are nephrotoxic. To circumvent this problem, the modified protocol of "induction therapy" was introduced. The common induction agent used in the US protocols was antithymocyte globulin (ATG), needed to be given daily for 7–10 days, thus increasing the complexity and cost of treatment. The bolus injectable "induction" drug basiliximab (Simulect) 10–20 mg given in two doses; one just before going on bypass and next after 4 days was found to be effective, simple to use and safe as an induction agent in the Indian context. After 20 mg IV Simulect, there is a luxury of starting tacrolimus anytime in the first week with reduced risk of renal failure and low rates of acute rejection. Hence, the typical combination immunosuppression regimen in India would be 1–2 mg bid of tacrolimus, 720 mg bid of mycophenolate, and 5 mg of prednisone in the first 6 months. Such low-dose immunosuppression protocols are now increasingly adopted in Europe. Such low-dose steroid protocols also seem to have obviated the need for antifungal prophylaxis. In case of persistent higher creatinine a month after heart transplantation, selected patients will benefit from substitution of sirolimus instead of nephrotoxic CNIs such as tacrolimus and cyclosporine.

Immediate Postoperative Management in the Intensive Care Unit

- Patient is managed as in any postcardiac surgery with broad-spectrum antibiotic coverage, ventilator management, and chest tube drainage.
- Patient is also monitored with hemodynamic monitoring of pulmonary artery pressures and right atrial pressures along with cardiac output. This helps in early recognition of primary or secondary graft dysfunction.
- Patient is kept on intravenous isoprenaline infusion for first 3–4 days to keep the heart rate above 100 BPM. Other inotropes such as adrenaline, milrinone, and dopamine are given as necessary to maintain systemic pressures. Inhaled nitric oxide is often used for higher pulmonary pressures with a NO delivery system. A cheaper alternative for inhaled nitric oxide would be oral sildenafil in the perioperative period to reduce pulmonary artery pressures and prevent right ventricular dysfunction.
- Patient is closely monitored with daily bedside echocardiography to assess graft function.
- Close monitoring of serum urea, creatinine, white blood cell (WBC) count and platelet count are done and immunosuppression drugs are tailored accordingly.
- Close monitoring of infection by routinely checking blood and urine cultures and biomarkers like procalcitonin.
- Monitoring and treatment of blood loss and coagulation problems.
- Once the patient is extubated and off inotropes, then early initiation of physiotherapy to fasten recovery is recommended.
- An endomyocardial biopsy is usually performed around day 7–10 for surveillance of rejection.

Early Perioperative Complications

- *Acute graft failure*: It happens in the immediate postoperative period and it can happen for any number of reasons such as poor donor quality, donor recipient size mismatch, procurement techniques, ischemia reperfusion injury, hyper acute rejection, RV dysfunction secondary to pulmonary hypertension, severe vasoplegia (in patients with long standing LVAD) refractory to vasopressor support. In such cases temporary mechanical support will be required and often patients with acute graft failure come out of the operating room on peripheral or central venoarterial extracorporeal membrane oxygenation (VA-ECMO).
- *Primary graft dysfunction*: Primary graft dysfunction (PGD) is a diagnosis of exclusion and can be made only after surgical complications, hyperacute rejection, bleeding, size-mismatch, and other causes causing acute graft failure are ruled out. Primary graft dysfunction can

TABLE 2: Criteria for grading PGD.

Ventricle	Severity	Criteria
PGD—left ventricle	*Mild*: One of the mentioned criteria must be met	LVEF ≤ 40% by echocardiography, or hemodynamics with RAP > 15 mm Hg, PCWP > 20 mm Hg, CI < 2.0 L/min^2 (>1 hour) requiring low dose inotropes
	Moderate: Must meet one criterion from (1) and another criterion from (2)	1. LVEF ≤ 40%, or hemodynamic compromise with RAP > 15 mm Hg, PCWP > 20 mm Hg, CI < 2.0 L/min^2, MAP < 70 mm Hg (>1 hour) 2. High dose of inotropes, inotrope score >10* or newly placed IABP (regardless of inotropes)
	Severe	Dependence on left or biventricular mechanical support including ECMO, LVAD, BiVAD, or percutaneous LVAD. Excludes requirement for IABP
PGD—right ventricle	Diagnosis requires either both (1) and (2), or (3) alone	1. Hemodynamics with RAP > 15 mm Hg, PCWP < 15 mm Hg, CI <2.0 mL/min^1 2. TPG < 15 mm Hg and/or pulmonary artery systolic pressure < 50 mm Hg 3. Need for RVAD

*Inotrope score = dopamine (×1) + dobutamine (×1) + amrinone (×1) + milrinone (×15) + epinephrine (×100) + norepinephrine (×100) with each drug dosed in µg/kg/min.

(BiVAD: biventricular assist device; CI: cardiac index; ECMO: extracorporeal membrane oxygenation; IABP: intra-aortic balloon pump; LVAO: left ventricular assist device; LVEF: left ventricular ejection fraction; MAP: mean arterial pressure; PCWP: pulmonary capillary wedge pressure; PGD: primary graft dysfunction; RAP: right atrial pressure; RVAD: right ventricular assist device; TPG: transpulmonary pressure gradient)

be isolated involving only the right ventricle or it can involve both the right and left ventricle. Report from a consensus conference on primary graft dysfunction after cardiac transplantation[15] provides us with criteria for grading PGD as shown in **Table 2**.

Hematological Trend and Other Parameters in the Immediate Postoperative Period

- *WBC count*: We get a slightly higher WBC count around 15,000–18,000 in the postoperative period because of administration of high dose steroids which slowly falls to lower range of normal—about 5,000. Any abnormal daily fall or fall below 3,000 requires urgent action which includes but not limited to evaluating the patient for sepsis and reducing the immunosuppression.
- *Platelet count*: Levels are usually in the range of 50,000–80,000 immediately after surgery. In some patients, platelet counts drops to a nadir of 40,000 slowly over 3 days and then improves. Transfusion is generally not needed until and unless the platelet count drops to 20,000 or if there is any active evidence of bleeding.
- *Body temperature*: Mild temperature rise till 99°F is quite common. Some patients may have initial hypothermia. Any temperature above 100°F requires further evaluation.
- *Liver function*: Higher bilirubin generally directs up to 12 mg/dL is common in the first 4-5 days. Mild rise in serum glutamate pyruvate transaminase (SGPT) or gamma-glutamyl transferase (GGT) is also common. In patients with preoperative ECMO status, high bilirubin levels are very common. No action is generally necessary unless the levels down trend down around 7–10 days.
- *Renal function*: Renal dysfunction is common in the post-operative period and it is prudent to not introduce CNI in the immediate postoperative period if basiliximab is used for induction therapy. The ideal time to start CNI is when creatinine levels have normalized or trending down. This is usually around 3-4 days post-transplant.

Infection Prophylaxis in Transplant Recipients

In standard Indian protocols, the anticytomegalovirus (anti-CMV) agent valacyclovir 450 mg daily is given for the first 3 months and trimethoprim-sulfamethoxazole three times a week is given for 6–12 months. Antifungal prophylaxis is not routinely used in India as we use low dose steroids even in the immediate postoperative period.

Common Infections Detected in Indian Patients Following Heart Transplant

In one series of 80 patients from Chennai, five patients had significant CMV infection from a period of 4 weeks to 1 year after transplant. One patient died of mucormycosis. Three patients had overwhelming sepsis in the intensive care unit in the first few days after transplant. Two patients had pneumonia 3–5 months after transplant. One had a severe form of lymph node and gastrointestinal (GI) tuberculosis; two had mild candida infection involving the GI tract. Remaining patients were infection free after they were strictly counseled to follow an infection avoidance lifestyle and periodic monitoring for life-threatening infections like CMV.

Endomyocardial Biopsies for Surveillance of Rejection[16,17]

Endomyocardial (EM) biopsies are the current gold standard for rejection surveillance and they are routinely advocated every week for the first 3–4 weeks and then every month for 3 months and then every other month in the first year following heart transplant in the United States. Since cost of EM biopsies is prohibitively high in the India and recalling patients from far-flung areas is difficult, it is prudent to limit the EM biopsies to two in the first year. The first biopsy is usually performed around day 7–10 prior to discharge and another at the end of 1 year. This policy does not impact survival or rejection rates. In our series of 164 cases, clinical and biopsy proven rejection rates have remained very low (only eight clinical or biopsy-proven rejections in 164 in a 3-year period).[16] Extra care was taken during the EM biopsy to make the procedure low risk by adopting all precautions like using a 6F Mullins sheath to introduce the 5F bioptome and using echocardiography guidance to place the sheath oriented toward the septum. In the 130 EM biopsy procedures done, there were no cases of pericardial tamponade and only two cases of increased or new tricuspid regurgitation were identified. The EM biopsy samples are sent for both cell-mediated rejection (CMR) analysis and antibody-mediated rejection (AMR) analysis.

Noninvasive Allograft Rejection Monitoring[18-21]

Noninvasive markers for rejection surveillance now available are as follows:

- Single antigen bead assay anti-HLA class 1 or 2 antibody measurement using Luminex is useful in diagnosis of antibody-mediated rejection.
- Donor-derived cell-free deoxyribonucleic acid (DNA), one-point blood test for early diagnosis of rejection and has emerged as a potentially valuable biomarker. It is currently available in the United States with limited availability in India being done by few laboratories such as Trunome and Lal Path India.
- Cylex (ImmuKnow) test measures the activity of CD4+ levels. Levels of <130 units suggest over immunosuppression and >450 suggest under immunosuppression. This is based on the Eurofins Viracor Assay.
- *AlloMap* gene expression profile analysis 15/19 gene panel for rejection surveillance is currently only available in the United States. The combination of AlloMap and AlloSure has a greater area under the curve (AUC).

CONCLUSION

In a large but developing country like India with a total population of 1,407 million, an area of 3.2 million km^2, and limited resources, the logistics of creating a nationwide cadaveric organ procurement and sharing network is extremely challenging and daunting by any criteria. If you add the fact that health is a state subject under the Indian constitution, many states, although they have ratified the National Organ Transplant Act (amended) of 2014, are yet to form an efficient organ procurement and transplantation network. These include large states like West Bengal, Uttar Pradesh, Madhya Pradesh, and Bihar. Hence, given the fact that total heart transplants in the country, going by the availability of cadaveric organs, will be in the range of only maximum 150–200/year for the next 1–2 years, there is bound to be a huge gap between the availability of donor hearts and demand from dying patients with heart failure.

ACKNOWLEDGMENT

We thank Dr KR Balakrishnan Chairman of Division of Heart and Lung Transplant MGM Hospital Chennai and his Team for Academic advice and sharing the team data.

ONLINE REFERENCES

Please scan the QR code provided at the end of the table of contents for References of this chapter.

23 Electrophysiology

CHAPTER

211

ABC of Electrophysiology Study

VS Ramchandra

ABSTRACT

The goal of this chapter is to demystify the electrophysiology (EP) study. By understanding a few basics and following a quick set of pacing protocols, the diagnosis is glaringly evident in a few minutes. However, as the second component that usually follows suit, namely ablation, has a lot of variables such as the power delivered and catheter stability; a confident diagnosis helps us to persist with the ablation and obtain success.

Keywords: EPS, electrophysiology, ablation, pacing.

INTRODUCTION

Electrophysiology study (EPS) is the basis for all electrical interventions of the heart. Almost six decades into its first performance, the technique essentially remains the same, with improvements in signal quality, electronic review of recordings, specialized catheters that can locate the origin of a single ectopic beat, and electroanatomical mapping techniques—all making the study so much easier and fun.

Electrophysiology study is commonly and wrongly regarded as a very esoteric procedure in cardiology that needs a lot of patience and intelligence to interpret. The technology is quite empirical and same as the electrocardiogram (ECG). The ECG measures the voltage difference between two electrodes (bipoles). The voltage difference is created by the wavefront of electrical de-/repolarization that propagates through the heart muscle. As the distance between these bipoles is large (e.g., in lead 1, between the right and left arm), the ECG measures the sum total of the electrical activity in that direction at a particular point of time. Imagine these bipoles placed very closely on an EP catheter that can be inserted into different chambers of the heart. Because they are closely spaced, it measures only the local electric activity between the bipoles. By putting multiple poles on each catheter and multiple catheters in different chambers of the heart, and timing the electric signals from these large number of bipoles, a map of the electrical activation of the heart can be obtained. Impulses can also be delivered from these bipoles just like through a temporary pacemaker catheter.

The EP adventure starts with four catheters. Those with four poles each (two dipoles—proximal and distal) are called quadripolars. There is a catheter placed, touching the right atrial wall that shows an impulse corresponding to the P wave on the surface ECG and another in the right ventricle that shows a signal corresponding to the surface QRS. The His quadripolar is placed across the right atrioventricular (AV) groove and shows an atrial signal (termed A), followed by a sharp His spike (sharp as the conduction through His is fast), and followed by a large V potential. The time from start of the His spike to surface QRS (the start of the surface QRS shows the earliest ventricular depolarization, whereas the His catheter shows a signal when the depolarization wave front reaches the catheter tip, sometime later) is the His ventricular (HV) interval. A common indication for EPS is left bundle branch block (LBBB) or bifascicular block with syncope. Here the surface ECG tells us that two of the three fascicles are diseased. An HV > 100 ms indicates that the third fascicle is also conducting slowly and may totally block, producing a complete heart block (CHB). Therefore, the EPS tell us that a pacemaker is needed in this patient. This way we know that "intervals" are very important.[1] The fourth catheter is a decapolar placed in the coronary sinus (CS) that runs in the left AV groove. It shows both A and V potentials at multiple areas (wherever the bipole is situated) across the left AV groove. In a person with a left lateral concealed pathway, a signal from the ventricular catheter will show earliest A signal at the distal CS bipole. Therefore, the second important information we get from EPS is the "path of conduction" of electrical impulse. The impulse always takes the fastest and shortest path.

The third information is the "voltage or amplitude" of the signal that denotes the amount of tissue in contact with the bipole recording the signal. A voltage of <0.5 mV indicates scar. Low amplitude, fractionated, wide and late potentials indicate slow flow across diseased tissue. Mid-diastolic potentials are potentials between two impulses during tachycardia and indicate the same. Ablating these diseased areas is a mainstay of ventricular tachycardia (VT) and atrial fibrillation (AF), "complex fractionated atrial electrogram" (CAFÉ) ablation.

The fourth property that is measured in EPS is the "effective refractory period" (ERP). For example, to determine the refractory period of the AV node (AVN), a drive train of around eight impulses at a cycle length of 400 ms is delivered through the A catheter followed by a premature impulse, simulating an atrial ectopic at 300 ms after the eighth beat. If there is an A to His [atrial His (AH)] jump at 250 ms, it indicates that the refractory period of the fast pathway was reached and the impulse had to move through the slower conducting slow input pathway of the AVN. At 230 ms A1 A2 interval, the impulse in the atrium may not be followed by His or the V signal, indicating that the refractory period of the AVN has been attained. This shows that this patient has dual AV inputs that may predispose to AVN reentrant tachycardia (AVNRT). The refractory period is the time taken for the tissue to be excitable again after it was depolarized once. This is the time taken for the cell membrane to regain its original polarity. Therefore, the longer the action potential duration, the longer the refractory period. The drive train is used to stabilize the conduction properties before the premature impulse is put in. The refractory period of most tissues decreases with tachycardia to facilitate conduction. Therefore, it is mandatory to mention the drive train cycle length (therefore the term effective) when talking about ERP. The ERP of a tissue is noted when it cannot be captured (no local propagation of the depolarizing impulse). For example, at a drive train of 400 ms from the atrial catheter, if there is no atrial capture when a premature impulse is introduced at 200 ms, it means that at a drive train cycle length of 400 ms, the tissue at that area is refractory at 200 ms. Moving the catheter to an adjacent diseased area may show a refractory period of 300 ms. When adjacent areas have different refractory periods, a premature impulse reaching the area with a longer refractory period may be blocked and takes a different route to reach an area that is excitable and can conduct the impulse. Usually, areas with shorter refractory periods have longer conduction times. So by the time the impulse exits this area with shorter refractory period, the adjacent area's longer refractory period is over and the impulse can turn back, producing a re-entry circuit. This could be macro-reentry such as an AVNRT or a smaller one around a scar in the ventricle or a microreentry of a focal atrial tachycardia. This difference in refractory period of adjacent tissues is referred to as "dispersion of refractory period" which is a very important cause of AF. This change in refractory period may also happen with acute ischemia such as in the first few hours after myocardial infarction (MI) and is the main cause of sudden cardiac death (SCD).

Electroanatomical mapping systems create an electromagnetic or other three-dimensional (3D) fields through three or more sources around the patient's chest. Moving the catheter in this field while touching the walls of the heart chambers produces a 3D image of these chambers. Software combining this spatial location with timing and voltage of impulses at those points give a 3D voltage/scar map and the flow of the reentrant circuit around the scar. In a focal tachycardia such as an atrial tachycardia or a right ventricular outflow tract (RVOT) VT, there is a point source from which impulses move around like ripples from a stone thrown in a pond.

Talking about reentrant tachycardias, because the depolarizing wavefront (head) moves in circles, it leaves a tail of refractoriness. A premature impulse introduced in the "gap" between the head and tail will reset the tachycardia to a shorter cycle length. This is called entrainment. If the morphology of the tachycardia on the 12-lead ECG is the same during entrainment, it means that the same cycle is being followed. A postpacing interval that is the same as the tachycardia cycle length (TCL) means that the point is in the tachycardia circuit. Ablation at this point can terminate the tachycardia. Entrainment is a key maneuver used in location of reentrant tachycardias.[2]

The basic EP study usually is done in these steps:

1. The AH and HV intervals are noted.
2. A straight decremental pacing (pacing from the atrial catheter at cycle lengths decrementing by 10 ms, for example, 400-390-380...) is done till the atrium stops capturing. As the A-H interval prolongs (the HV interval cannot prolong as it does not have Wenckebach properties of the AVN), the AV interval surpasses the pacing cycle length. This is called crossover and indicates slow pathway conduction at the AVN. Later on at shorter cycle lengths, Wenckebach phenomenon happens in the AVN. If there is pre-excitation over a pathway that conducts faster than the AVN especially at faster rates, pre-excitation on the surface ECG increases and as AH prolongs without prolongation of AV, the His starts getting enveloped by the QRS on the His catheter. Therefore, atrial decremental pacing can (1) induce tachycardia, (2) show slow pathway conduction of AVN, and (3) unmask pre-excitation.

3. A extras to detect AVN ERP—here after a drive train to stabilize refractory periods, premature impulses are given in a decremental manner. For example, eight cycles at 400 ms (A1), an extra at 300 ms (A2). The AH and HV are noted. Next eight cycles at 400 ms are followed by an A extra at 290 ms. The AH prolongs but the HV does not. If at A1–A2 of 250 ms there is a jump of AH interval by 20 ms, it indicates that the ERP of the fast pathway of the AVN was attained and the conduction jumped to the slow pathway with a shorter ERP. This AH jump indicates dual AVN pathways. Many times, an AVNRT is initiated after the conduction moves to the slow pathway. Later at 220 ms, the extra may block at the AVN totally, which means that the ERP of the AVN at a drive train cycle length of 400 ms is 230 ms.

   If there is pre-excitation, there is increasing surface ECG pre-excitation with shorter A1–A2. When the pathway ERP is reached, the impulse goes down only through the AVN, the surface ECG of A2 narrows and an orthodromic AV re-entry tachycardia (AVRT) may be initiated as the impulse going down the AVN can go up into the atria via the pathway that had not conducted anterogradely. If the AVN ERP is longer than the anterograde pathway ERP, an antidromic (pre-excited) AVRT may be initiated.

   If the Infra-Hisian conduction system is diseased, the impulse conducted through the AVN may block after a His tracing is obtained. This is an Infra-Hisian block and is an indication for permanent pacemaker implantation (PPI).
4. V straight decremental pacing—here from say 400-390-380 ms...,V pacing is decremented till ventriculoatrial (VA) conduction blocks or V fails to capture. Normally there is concentric Retrograde VA conduction across the AVN because this is the only legitimate connection between the ventricles and the atria. Concentric means the A signal on the His catheter is earlier than any other A signal. The VA interval increases with faster V pacing due to Wenckebach properties of AVN. If there is a pathway that conducts retrogradely with a short and fixed VA conduction time, the VA conduction becomes eccentric, i.e., the right or left atrial signals are earlier than the His A signal if there is a right-sided or a left-sided pathway, respectively.
5. V extras (after a drive train to stabilize ERP)—here the VA interval may jump to slow retrograde VA conduction across the AVN, with a VA interval jump. Retrograde pathway conduction may become evident with eccentric conduction at shorter V_1–V_2 intervals.

   A VT study is done to reproducibly induce a VT with extras. As the V_1–V_2 or V_2–V_3 intervals are shortened, there is an R on T phenomenon with the extras falling in the relative refractory period of the previous beat. This facilitates slower conduction and induction of VT. A reproducibly inducible VT in a post-MI patient with moderate left ventricular (LV) dysfunction with nonsustained ventricular tachycardia (NSVT) on Holter or ECG, is a MADIT II indication for automatic implantable cardioverter defibrillator (AICD).

   Long-shorts, i.e., V_2–V_3 that is shorter than V_3–V_4, is used by some electrophysiologists to induce bundle branch re-entry VT.
6. Burst A pacing at shorter cycle lengths of 170–220 ms is used to induce atrial flutter or fibrillation.
7. Sinus node recovery time (SNRT) is the time the sinus node takes to recover and put out an impulse after it is suppressed with faster A pacing for a minute or two. If the sinus node takes a long pause to recover after overdrive suppression, it indicates sick sinus syndrome (SSS).

We will discuss a few maneuvers used after a paroxysmal supraventricular tachycardia (PSVT) is induced to differentiate between them.

- *Putting premature V during tachycardia*: Once the AVN and the His–Purkinje system have conducted a beat anterogradely, it is refractory for some time to conduction, and therefore will not allow the premature V to conduct to the atrium. However, a retrogradely conducting pathway will allow the premature beat to conduct to the atrium, which is recorded by the A catheter. However, an extremely premature V beat can conduct retrogradely through the His. Therefore it is important to time the premature V after the anterograde His signal on the His catheter, to prove that there is a concealed retrograde pathway.
- Entrainment from the V catheter is done by pacing continuously for a few beats at a cycle length shorter than the TCL. The A–A interval recorded on the A catheter is the same cycle length as V pacing (and the P wave morphology/activation is same as the original tachycardia, although this is difficult to see). Once V pacing is stopped, the original TCL is reinstated. The difference between VA during tachycardia versus during entrainment from the V is called VA differential. V and A that are simultaneous (VA < 50 ms) and a VA differential during entrainment > 100 ms indicates AVNRT. This is because during AVNRT, the A and V are activated simultaneously, but during V pacing, the signal has to travel through the V to get into the gap of the re-entry. However in AVRT which is a macroreentry through the A-AVN-V pathway, the V-pacing catheter is close to the circuit and the VA differential is less. A V-A-A-V response after terminating V pacing indicates atrial tachycardia. This is because if there are no two pathways between V and A (either a slow/fast VA in AVNRT or a concealed pathway in AVRT), when the V-paced beat moves through the AVN, it blocks the next atrial tachycardia signal, giving a V-A-A-V. VA dissociation when V is paced with continuation of tachycardia after pacing also indicates atrial tachycardia. The VAAV response is an extremely important maneuver to distinguish atrial tachycardias from atypical AVNRT.[3]

- If the VA interval of the tachycardia is >50 ms (or long RP tachycardias which means surface VA > AV), it may mean atrial tachycardia, concealed pathway AVRT, or atypical AVNRT with the retrograde conduction through slow pathway. It usually makes matters easy to put a CS decapolar and quickly map the right AV groove during tachycardia or V pacing to exclude a pathway. Although this may be an innocent bystander pathway, noninducibility of tachycardia after ablating the pathway indicated causality.
- *Atrial flutter versus atrial tachycardia*: In atrial flutter, the cycle length is usually <250 ms. There is no isoelectric line on the surface ECG and moving a catheter in relation to a fixed catheter can map the majority of the cycle length to either atrium. Electroanatomical mapping also shows the macroreentry. In atrial tachycardia, the cycle length varies by >10% of TCL and mapping shows a point source.
- Ventricular tachycardia is easy to diagnose as the QRS is usually broad and the retrograde His is absent or masked. There might be VA dissociation during tachycardia with V faster than A, making the diagnosis easy. In Mahaim and other pre-excitations, A pacing/extras produce pre-excited beats.

DIAGNOSIS AND ABLATION

- *AVNRT*: Here, there is simultaneous activation of V and A during tachycardia (VA < 50 ms) and His-A-V signals on the His catheter. Premature ventricular contractions (PVCs) with antegrade His on His catheter cannot pre-excite the A as the His is refractory to the PVC. Entrainment from V during tachycardia produces wide VA differential and VAV. Ablation is largely anatomical, at the apex of Koch's triangle although Jackman/Haissaguerre potentials or fragmented potentials may be useful. Having a larger V than A on the ablation catheter prevents AV block. Successful ablation always produces junctionals—the VA conduction is used as surrogate marker of intact AV conduction. Postablation endpoints include noninducibility, lack of crossover, slow conduction absent, and increase in AVN ERP.
- *Atypical AVNRT*: This is a long RP tachycardia. The same maneuvers as typical AVNRT are used.
- *Concealed pathway AVRT*: VA is >50 ms. Eccentric VA conduction is evident either on the CS decapolar or during mapping the right AV groove. A late PVC introduced during tachycardia after antegrade His can preexcite the A through the pathway. Para-Hisian pacing may be used for concealed septal pathways where VA conduction is not eccentric. Normally, pacing high output from the distal His captures the His right bundle, seen as a narrow antegrade QRS and stimulus atrial (SA) is short. Decreasing the output fails to capture the conduction system and the QRS broadens and SA increases. However, if there is a septal pathway, the SA remains the same both times as the impulse can conduct back to the atrium though the fast-conducting pathway whether or not the conduction system is captured. Endpoints after ablation include noninducibility, no eccentric VA conduction, or VA block. Some use adenosine, during VA conduction—this drug blocks the AVN but not the pathway—so persisting VA conduction indicates intact pathway.
- *Atrial tachycardia*: Discrete P waves with isoelectric segment between Ps is seen. There is V-A-A-V response on entrainment from the V. Tachycardia induction also does not start with a large AH jump. A focal source is identified when we map for the earliest point. Endpoint after ablation is noninducibility.
- *Atrial flutter*: Here there is continuous macroreentry and no isoelectric line. Mapping in relation to a reference catheter in the atrium shows that most of TCL can be mapped to a single atrium. After locating the isthmus (by entrainment or electroanatomical mapping), an ablation line with a cool tip catheter terminates the tachycardia. Differential pacing from both sides of the ablation line confirms bidirectional block. In most cases, a right-sided flutter involves the cavotricuspid isthmus; therefore, one may proceed directly with a cavotricuspid line ablation. In the left atrium, it may either be a roof or mitral annular flutter, in which cases either a roof line or a line from the left inferior pulmonary vein through the CS can terminate the tachycardia. Postsurgical rhythms are much more complicated and need painstaking mapping.
- *Atrial fibrillation*: This is again an anatomical ablation using wide area circumferential ablation (WACA) around the pulmonary veins. Endpoints are noninducibility and exit block from the pulmonary vein or no pulmonary vein potentials on a lasso catheter placed inside the pulmonary vein during sinus rhythm or A pacing.
- *Idiopathic VT*: Usually, these are RVOT or LV fascicular VTs. Diagnosis is made from the surface ECG. RVOT VT or PVCs are mapped to the earliest signal. Sometimes a 12/12 pacemapping congruence with the tachycardia ECG helps. A deep negative wave on a unipolar signal also denotes that the catheter is right on the spot of origin of tachycardia, as all signals are moving away and spreading from this spot. In LV fascicular VTs, a semianatomical approach with the catheter placed on the septum inferiorly and distally, tachycardia is induced and early signals or fascicular potentials are targeted.
- *Ischemic VT*: These are VTs secondary to scar and not really ischemic in nature. A voltage map is created with an electroanatomical system. Most tachycardias originate from the low voltage, fragmented, slow conduction areas around the scar. A totally "substrate-based ablation" can be done without inducing tachycardia in unstable

patients, by connecting scars with ablation lines and targeting fractionated and late potentials on the fringes of the scar. An attempt at tachycardia induction can be made at this point and if a stable VT is induced, this can be mapped to locate exit points or isthmuses or mid-diastolic potentials.

CONCLUSION

This chapter explains how an EPS is done and how with just two maneuvers (VPCs during tachycardia and entrainment from V) the vast majority of arrhythmias can be diagnosed and ablated.

ONLINE REFERENCES

Please scan the QR code provided at the end of the table of contents for References of this chapter.

CHAPTER 212

Basic and Advanced Electrophysiologic Mapping Techniques in Arrhythmias

Ajay Naik, Aarya Naik

ABSTRACT

Electrophysiological mapping techniques have evolved from electrode-based conventional mapping with fluoroscopic guidance to sophisticated three-dimensional electroanatomic mapping systems with near-zero fluoroscopic radiation exposure.

In the initial era, arrhythmias most likely to be amenable to cure with catheter ablation were those that had a focal origin or involved a narrow, anatomically defined isthmus. With the advent of sophisticated systems, even complex arrhythmias such as atrial fibrillation and scar-related ventricular arrhythmias can be managed effectively. Arrhythmias in complex anatomies including congenital heart disease and cardiomyopathies are also treated nowadays with excellent outcomes.

With continual advancements in electrophysiologic mapping and catheter ablation techniques, arrhythmia management has become a predictable, consistent, and effective science.

Keywords: Arrhythmia, electrophysiologic mapping, electroanatomic mapping, ablation.

INTRODUCTION

Cardiac arrhythmia management has evolved rapidly and immensely over the past few decades. Antiarrhythmic drug (AAD) therapy used to be the mainstay of arrhythmia management in the past. The therapeutic effect of AADs is not consistently predictable and efficacy is limited. Some drugs are associated with bothersome and even fatal side effects (e.g., ventricular proarrhythmia).[1]

Nonpharmacologic interventions for arrhythmia began with electrophysiologic (EP) mapping and surgical techniques in the 1970s. In the early ablation era, catheter ablation (CA) was performed primarily with high-energy direct current (DC) shocks. After 1989, radiofrequency catheter ablation (RFCA) emerged as an elegant solution for arrhythmia management.

Catheter ablation can be defined as the use of an electrode catheter to destroy (or deactivate) small areas of myocardial tissue or conduction system, or both, that are critical to the initiation or maintenance of cardiac arrhythmias.

CONVENTIONAL ELECTROPHYSIOLOGIC MAPPING AND ABLATION

Electrophysiology studies (EPS) and CA procedures are performed in a catheterization laboratory equipped with a specialized electrophysiology (EP) mapping system.

Among the earliest EP mapping systems was the Mingograf (Siemens–Elema AB), an analog-based system with an inkjet printer **(Fig. 1)**.

Digital revolution resulted in the computerization of EP mapping and recording systems, making them more efficient and user-friendly. Four major companies have dominated the conventional EP mapping ecosystem (sometimes called "2D mapping," in common parlance) **(Fig. 2)**, these are as follows:

1. Prucka (GE Healthcare)
2. Bard (Boston Scientific)
3. EP Tracer (Cardiotek)
4. Workmate Claris (Abbott)

Electrophysiologic Study and Catheter Ablation Procedure

The procedure can be performed on either an inpatient or outpatient basis. Patients may receive conscious sedation before and during the procedure.

Two or more multipolar electrode catheters are inserted percutaneously under local anesthesia into a femoral, subclavian, or internal jugular vein and positioned in the heart under fluoroscopic guidance **(Figs. 3A and B)**. Transeptal puncture is performed when necessary to access the left side of the heart. Arterial access may be needed for hemodynamic monitoring or retrograde transaortic route for catheter access to the left ventricle.

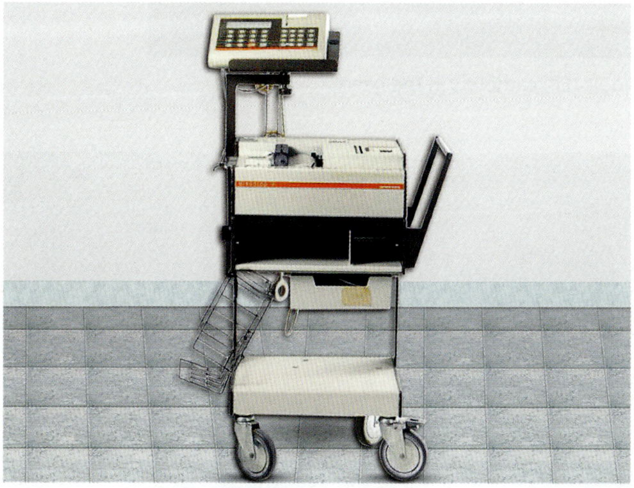

FIG. 1: Mingograf.

Each electrode catheter has four or more electrodes. Typically, the most distal electrode pair is used for electrical stimulation (pacing) and the delivery of critically timed extra stimuli, while the proximal electrodes are used to record electrograms (EGMs) from localized regions within the heart.

A diagnostic EPS is performed to define the arrhythmia mechanism, and subsequently, an ablation catheter is positioned at the arrhythmogenic substrate. Typically, diagnostic EPS is followed by ablation concurrently in the same procedure session.

Catheter ablation is performed primarily using radiofrequency energy (RFE). Up to 50 W of RFE is delivered for 30–60 seconds as a continuous, unmodulated, and sinusoidal waveform with a frequency of approximately 500,000 cycles/s, between the 4 mm tip of a deflectable ablation catheter and a ground plate positioned on the patient's back or thighs. Destruction or deactivation of tissue critical for arrhythmogenesis (such as an accessory pathway or an ectopic focus) and its subsequent replacement with scar eliminates arrhythmia.

Owing to its high success rate and low risks, RFCA has become the first-line treatment for many arrhythmias.[2]

Biophysics of Radiofrequency Ablation

The majority of CA systems in use today monitor the temperature of the ablation electrode and automatically adjust power output to achieve a targeted electrode

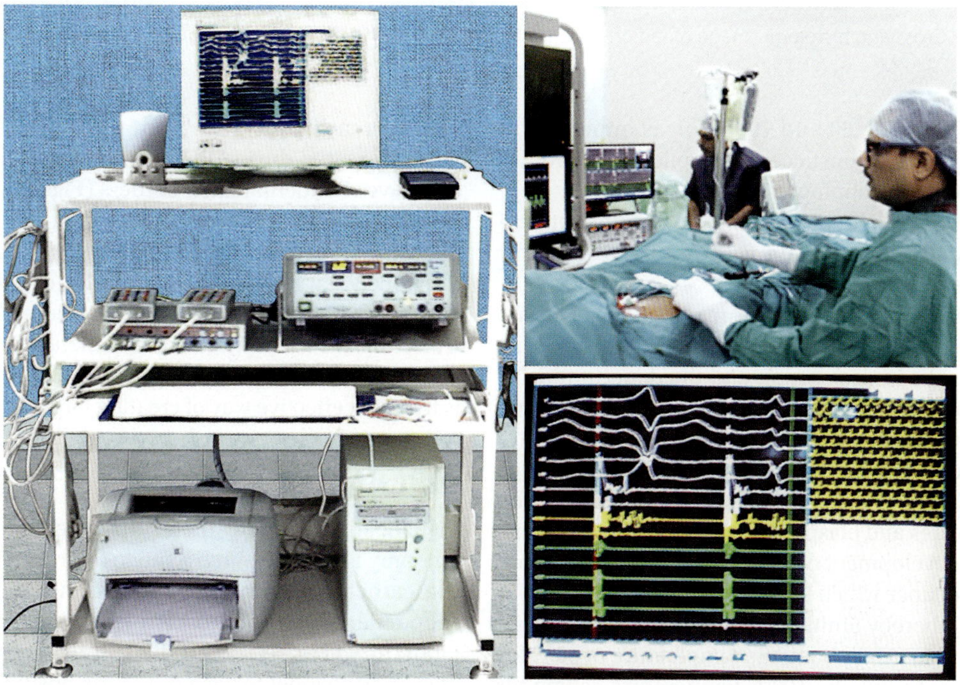

FIG. 2: Conventional electrophysiologic mapping system.

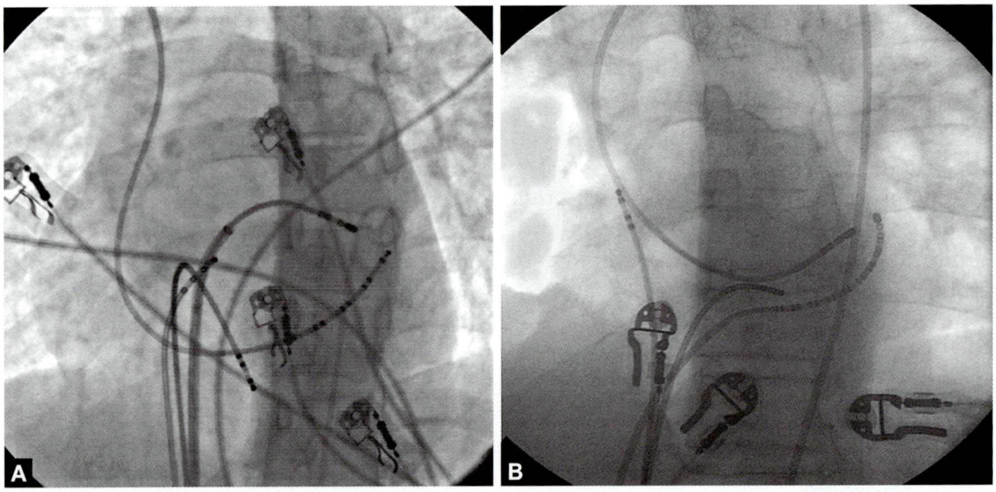

FIGS. 3A AND B: Fluoroscopic image of electrophysiologic (EP) catheters in the heart.

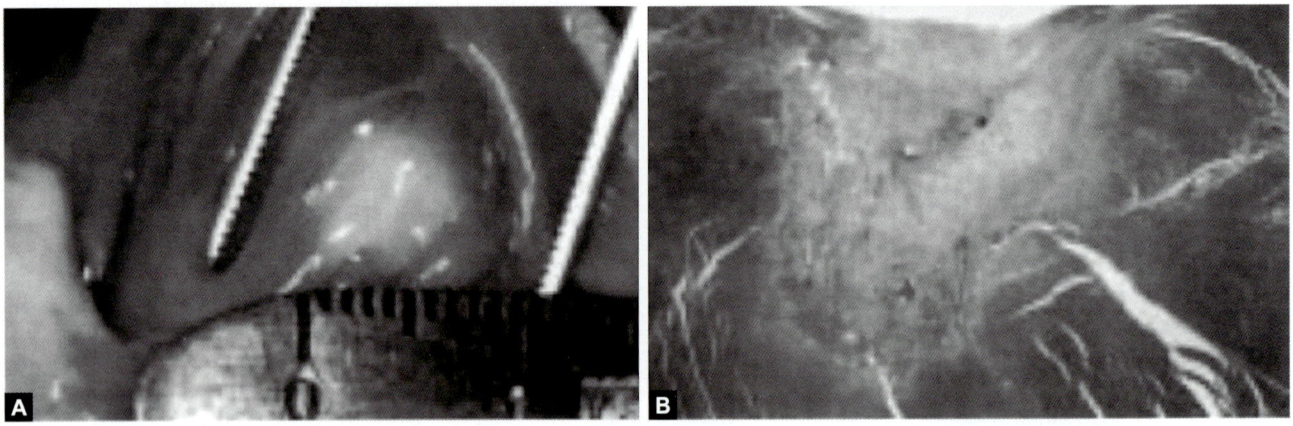

FIGS. 4A AND B: Gross and histologic image of radiofrequency lesion.[1]

temperature of between 60 and 70°C. This is important in determining whether an unsuccessful application of RFE is because of inaccurate mapping or inadequate heating.

In the event of inadequate heating, additional applications of energy at the same site with improved catheter stability may result in success.

Thermal injury is the principal mechanism of tissue destruction during RFCA procedures. Elevation of tissue temperature results in desiccation and the denaturation of proteins, and also in the coagulation of tissue and blood. Irreversible tissue injury occurs at temperatures above 50°C.

When the temperature at the electrode-tissue interface exceeds 100°C, the tissue immediately adjacent to the electrode desiccates and plasma proteins denature to form a coagulum. The development of a coagulum results in a rapid increase in impedance which leads to a dramatic decrease in current density, thereby limiting further lesion growth. As a result of the need to achieve a tissue temperature of 50°C for irreversible tissue injury, the 100°C temperature ceiling for tissue heating, and the rapid decrease in tissue temperature with increasing distance from the ablation electrode, the lesions created during RFCA procedures are small (5 mm) and have well-demarcated borders **(Figs. 4A and B)**.[1]

Methods for improved cooling of the electrode have been developed to allow the delivery of higher RF power. Previously, larger (8 mm) electrodes or dumbbell-shaped electrodes were used to increase surface area for RF delivery. Currently, the use of irrigated RF catheters, in which the distal electrode is actively cooled by saline (or half-saline) infusion is the most effective way of creating larger lesions.

BIPLANE FLUOROSCOPY

Visualization of the catheter tip in relation to the cardiac anatomy is crucial. Since a single fluoroscopic view displays the catheter in only one projection against the cardiac silhouette, biplane fluoroscopy is a useful addition to the EP laboratory **(Fig. 5)**. When the two fluoroscopic planes are placed orthogonal to each other, the position of the catheter in three-dimensional (3D) space can be inferred. There needs

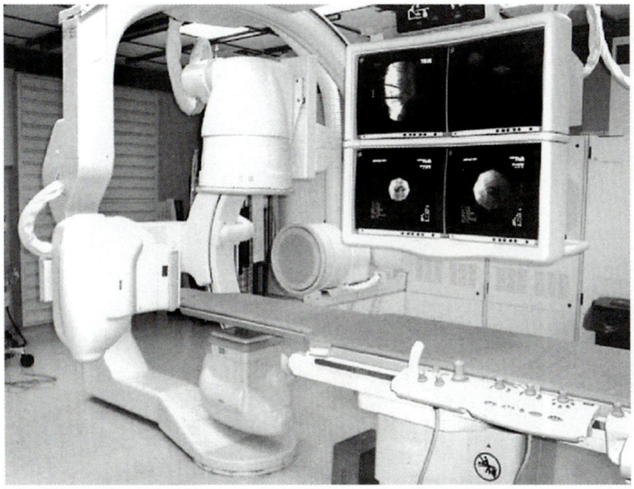

FIG. 5: Biplane fluoroscopy.

to be awareness about the inherent higher risk of exposure to radiation dose for both the operator and the patient.

NONFLUOROSCOPIC MAPPING TECHNIQUES

The improved understanding of the pathophysiological mechanisms of arrhythmias' induction and perpetuation has boosted catheter-based ablation of complex arrhythmias, such as atrial fibrillation (AF) and ventricular arrhythmias (VAs). Identification and modification of the complex arrhythmogenic substrates have resulted in prolonged procedure times and increased exposure to ionizing radiation for both operators and patients.

Electroanatomical mapping (EAM) was first introduced into clinical practice in 1997, thereafter, remarkable progress has been made in catheter infrastructure, signal recording and processing, catheter guidance and visualization, and simultaneous real-time depiction and processing of different types of critical information during an ablation procedure.

Nonfluoroscopic tracking of catheter tip position and orientation in 3D space using either magnetic fields or impedance technology has represented a major advancement. Contemporary 3D-EAMS have significantly reduced the need for fluoroscopic visualization of catheters, to the extent of achieving "zero-fluoroscopy" procedures. They have also created a precise and trustworthy "virtual environment" capable of guiding complex mapping and ablation procedures.

Furthermore, 3D EAM capability is enhanced by integrating data from other imaging modalities, such as computed tomography (CT) and cardiac magnetic resonance (CMR).

For most complex cases, contact-based EAM is the preferred technique. Noncontact mapping and/or multipolar catheters are required for high-density mapping of arrhythmias, especially those that are nonsustained or even infrequent ectopic beats.

Noninvasive mapping of arrhythmias is being attempted by high-density body surface electrocardiogram (ECG) maps projected onto reconstructed images of cardiac chambers created by CT and CMR.

CONTACT-BASED ELECTROANATOMIC MAPPING

The two most widely used contact-based EAM systems (EAMSs) worldwide are CARTO® (Biosense Webster Inc, Diamond Bar, CA, USA) and EnSite Precision™ Cardiac Mapping System (Abbott, Illinois, USA). Rhythmia HDx™ (Rhythmia Medical, Boston Scientific Inc, Marlborough, MA, USA) has also been recently introduced.

The EAMS depicts the EP catheters in a 3D geometric shell of the cardiac chamber created by nonfluoroscopic mapping. The spatiotemporal depiction of the catheters remains in memory and can be used to move the catheters to precise locations.

Electroanatomical mapping systems imply that the electrical signals at the points of contact of the mapping catheter are linked to anatomical points on the cardiac chamber. With rapid advancements in this field, it is possible to rapidly create a multipoint model by wide sweeps of multipolar or mapping catheters. (CARTO3® Fast Map Module and EnSite™ AutoMap module and TurboMap feature).

CARTO (Figs. 6A and B)

The CARTO system is based on three active weak magnetic fields (5×10^{-6} to 5×10^{-5} Tesla), produced by a three-coil location pad placed underneath the patient's thorax. Proprietary catheters have a magnetic minisensor at the tip that continually measures the strength of the magnetic field and calculates the catheter's exact position in the 3D space.

Current versions of CARTO are capable of concurrently displaying multiple catheters by a sophisticated current-based catheter location technology. Six electrode patches positioned at the patient's back and chest monitor the current emitted at a unique frequency by various catheter electrodes. The catheters are visualized in a 3D virtual area "matrix," which can be created only by a magnetic sensor-equipped proprietary catheter.

Ensite Precision (Figs. 7A and B)

EnSite technology uses six skin electrodes to create a high-frequency electric field (8.0 kHz) in three mutually orthogonal planes on the patient's thorax, a coordinate system in the three X/Y/Z axes.

Nonproprietary conventional EP catheters can be localized on the basis of an impedance gradient-calculation

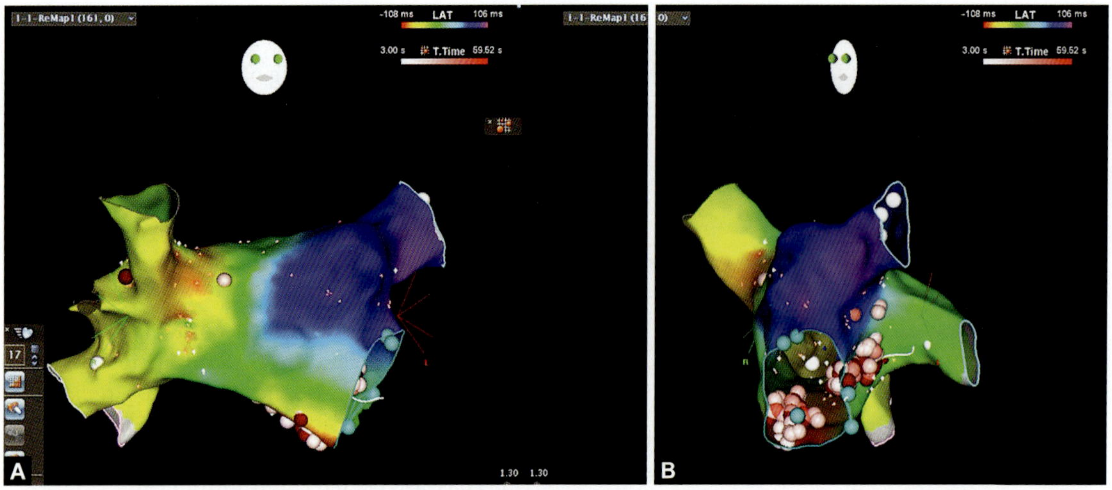

FIGS. 6A AND B: CARTO mapping during atrial flutter ablation.

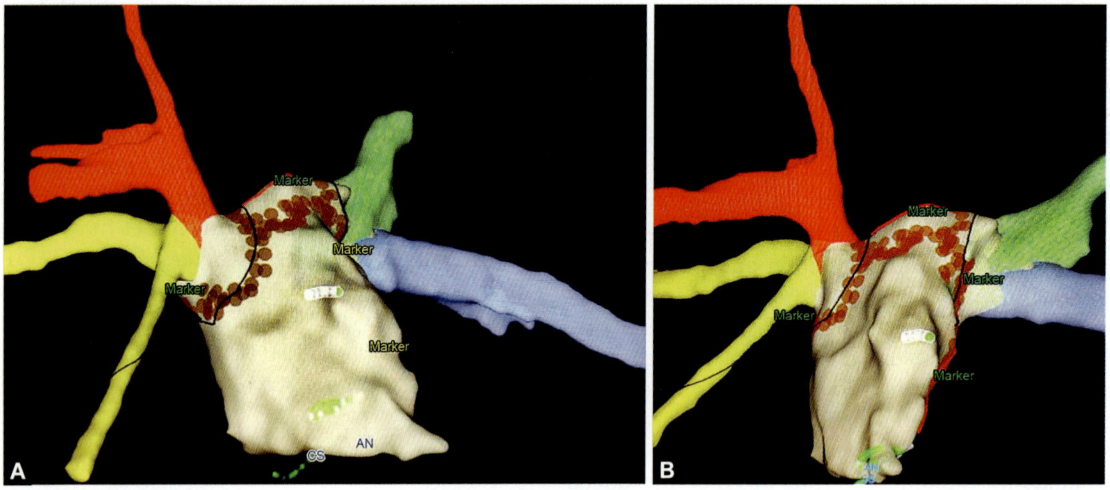

FIGS. 7A AND B: EnSite mapping during atrial fibrillation ablation.

system in relation to a reference electrode placed on the patient's body. The major advantage of the Ensite system is that it is an open system within which multiple catheters from different manufacturers can be displayed. It is not limited by proprietary catheter hardware.

Rhythmia (Figs. 8A and B)

Rhythmia HDx^{TM} Mapping system is a recently introduced technology that can simultaneously record large numbers of EGMs with a very high spatial resolution. It utilizes a mini basket bidirectional deflectable catheter (64-electrode IntellaMap Orion® High Resolution Mapping Catheter, Boston Scientific Inc) incorporating an electrode array in eight splines.

Each of the eight splines has eight small, low-impedance electrodes (64 electrodes in total). Electrode localization is done by a magnetic sensor in the distal region of the catheter along with impedance sensing on the 64 basket electrodes. Auto mode mapping enables rapid automatic annotation of activation times.

NONCONTACT MAPPING

In contact-based EAMS, manual point-by-point mapping is required to build a proper activation map of an ongoing tachycardia or extrasystoles. However, if the arrhythmia is not sustained or not hemodynamically tolerated, point-by-point mapping may be insufficient or even not feasible. A major advantage of noncontact mapping is that it can create a full map even from a single tachycardia beat.

EnSite Array® (St Jude Medical, Inc, St Paul, MN, US)[3] basket-catheter is the most common noncontact mapping system **(Fig. 9)**. A 3D EnSite reconstruction is created with a moving mapping catheter to project the shell. The multipolar noncontact catheter uses 64 unipolar electrodes, which record virtual unipolar far-field EGMs using a mathematical

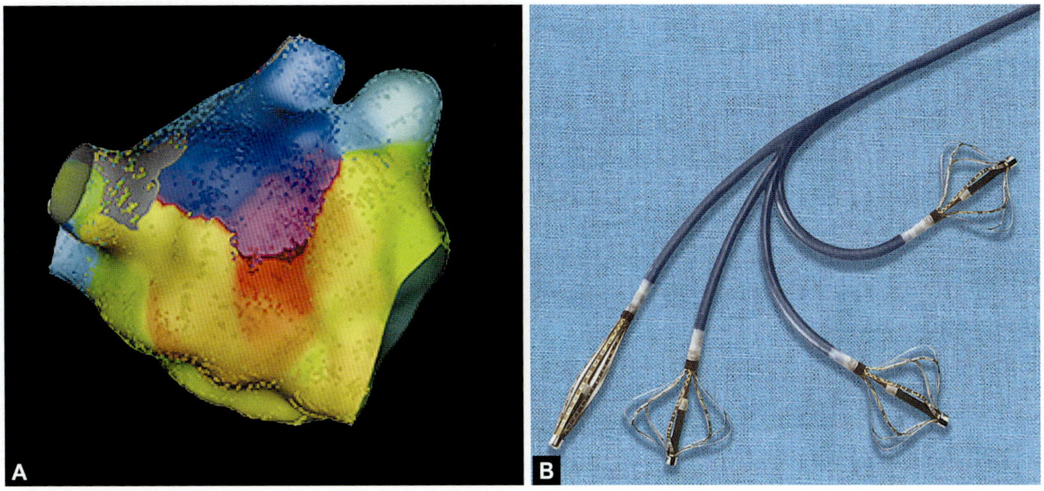

FIGS. 8A AND B: Rhythmia and Intellamap Orion® catheter.

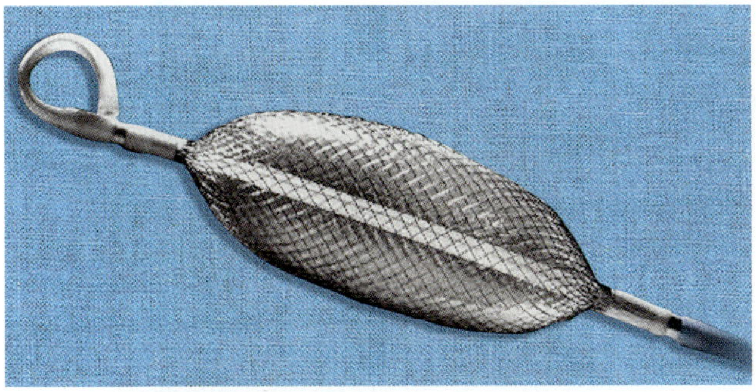

FIG. 9: EnSite Array® noncontact mapping catheter.

inverse solution of the Laplace's law and then project them (n = 3,360) on the 3D shell.

Virtual unipolar EGMs obtained at the earliest site of activation have a QS or rS morphology. Ectopic beats can be mapped by confirming early intrinsic deflection compared with adjacent site activation. The quality of recorded signals worsens with distances exceeding 40 mm from the center of the array. The basket catheter generally remains stable in the right atrium and right ventricle. The basket is less stable in the left ventricle.

MULTIELECTRODE MAPPING

The use of multielectrode catheters enable rapid high-density activation and substrate mapping through simultaneous multiple-point acquisition. Multielectrode contact-based catheters PentaRay® (Biosense Webster, Inc, Diamond Bar, CA, USA) and Advisor HD Grid® catheter (St Jude Medical, St Paul, MN, US) have been very useful in AF and VT ablation **(Figs. 10 and 11)**.

NONINVASIVE MAPPING

Noninvasive cardiac mapping provides information on the topography of arrhythmogenic foci preprocedurally, in order to reduce time-consuming mapping times. Body surface unipolar recordings are projected onto 3D reconstructed images of the heart derived from CT or CMR scans. Using complex mathematical equations, the torso potentials are related to the epicardial surface of the heart.

Body surface potential maps (BSPMs) have been used for approximating the site of origin of cardiac ectopic activity and propagation properties of ectopic beats **(Flowchart 1)**.

RIPPLE MAPPING

Established EAMS necessitates manual-based annotation and/or correction of acquired map points because automated annotation is prone to errors. On the other hand, manual point-by-point annotation can be fairly subjective. It can also lead to severe signal misjudgment and prolong the procedure times.

Ripple mapping is a software-based program to present the EGM location, timing, and amplitude on the 3D shell of the cardiac chamber of interest created by CARTO mapping **(Fig. 12)**. The EGMs are displayed in a unique manner as bars of varying colors and dimensions depending on voltages and activation times. The changing bar sizes and colors create a "wave-like" movement of the propagation, helping the recognition of activation pathways.

IMAGE INTEGRATION

Defining myocardial scar and better substrate definition is an important component of VT ablation procedures. In complex anatomies and myocardial substrates, the accuracy of scar mapping in both endocardial and epicardial regions is further improved by image integration of contrast-enhanced CT images with EAMS-generated shells **(Fig. 13)**. In patients with cardiac implantable electronic devices (CIEDs) undergoing VT ablation, late gadolinium enhancement (LGE) identification by CMR can further facilitate scar identification and mapping.

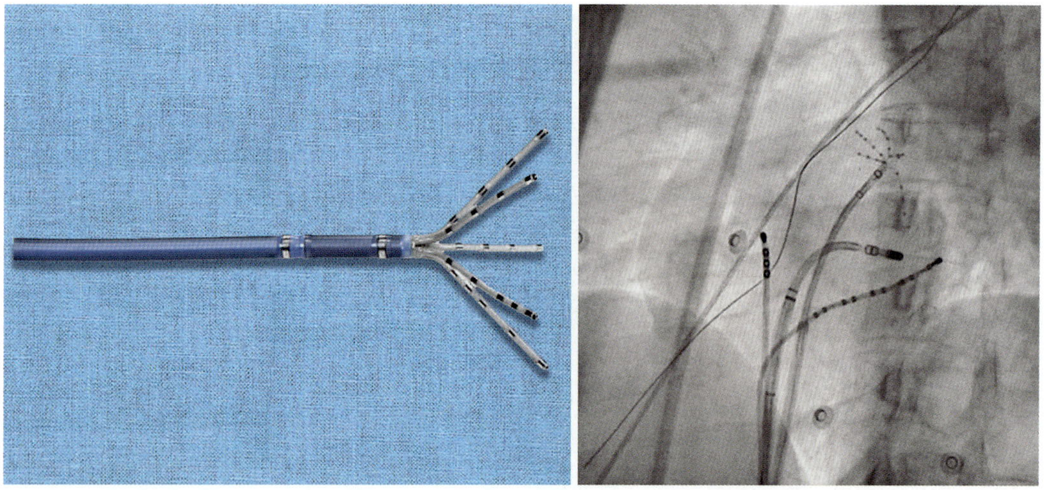

FIG. 10: PentaRay® catheter in the left atrium during intra-atrial reentrant tachycardia ablation.

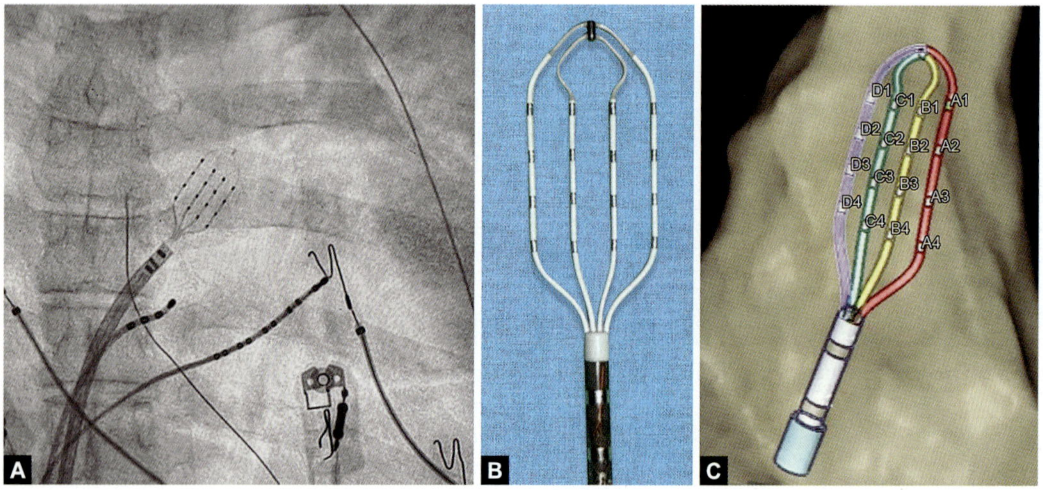

FIGS. 11A TO C: Advisor™ HD Grid catheter during atrial fibrillation ablation.

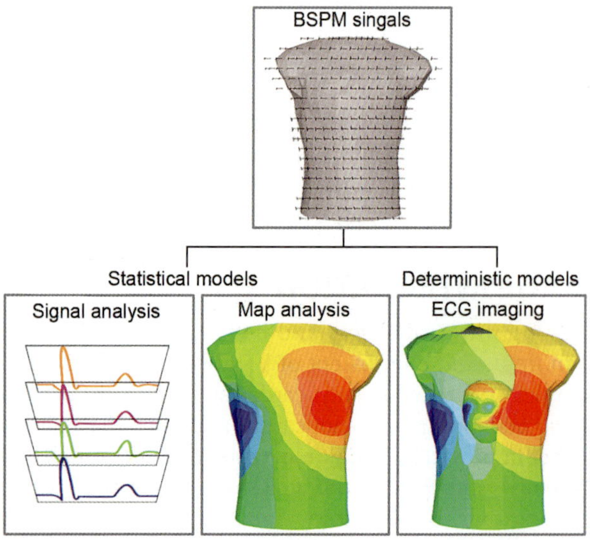

FLOWCHART 1: Body surface potential map.
(ECG: electrocardiogram; BSPM: body surface potential mapping)

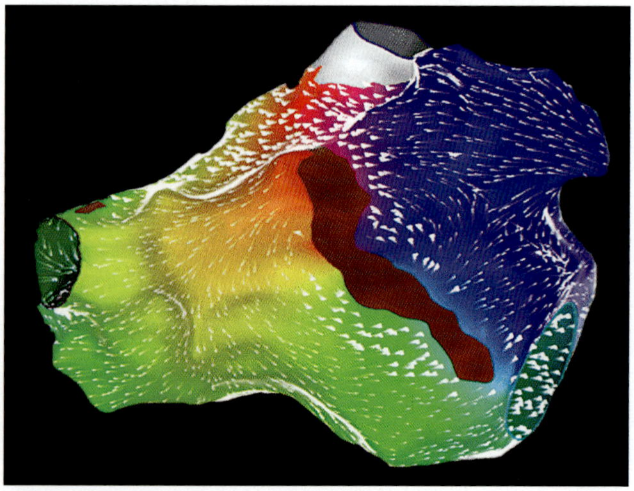

FIG. 12: Ripple mapping with CARTO.

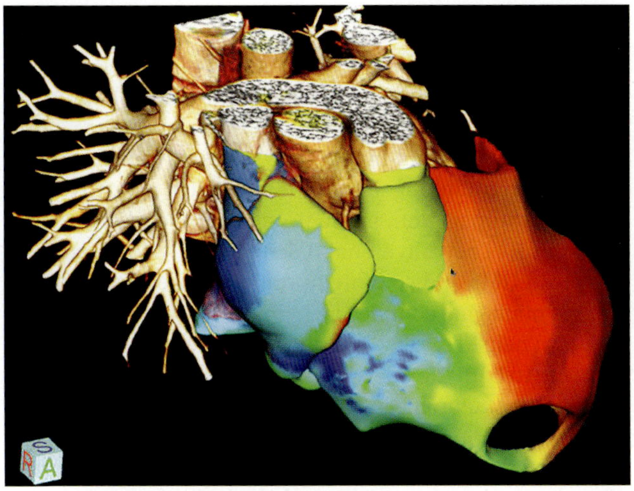

FIG. 13: CARTO–CT image integration.

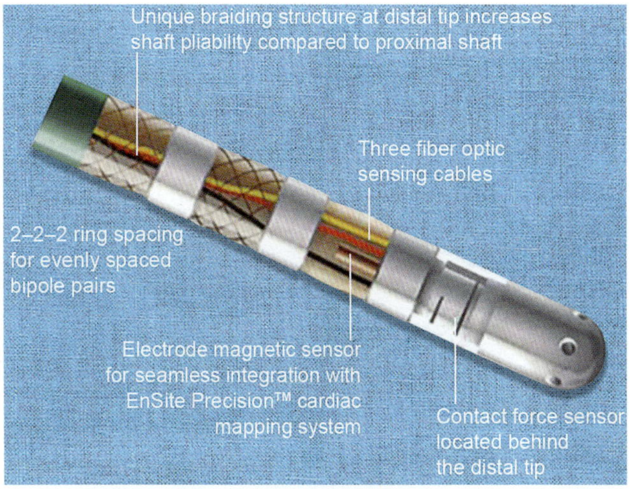

FIG. 14: TactiCath® contact force catheter.

Courtesy: TactiCath (Endosense, Geneva, Swizerland)

CONTACT FORCE

The distance and the orientation of the mapping catheter bipolar to the underlying tissue play a significant role in the qualitative and quantitative characteristics of the acquired signal, which in turn, influence the results of voltage-based substrate mapping. Adequate contact between the catheter and tissue is considered a determinant to credible characterization of the underlying arrhythmogenic substrate.

Also, lesion formation during ablation is evaluated through the fulfillment of certain criteria, including EGM amplitude reduction, initial impedance and impedance drop during ablation, and electrode temperature, the proper contact between tissue and the catheter can be guaranteed only through its direct measurement. Contact force (CF) is used to evaluate the contact between the tissue and the catheter tip. Adequate CF is crucial for RF lesion size, a CF of between 5 and 20 g is generally used as a guide for delivering an effective and safe lesion.

High power settings (45 W) and high pressures (>40 g) are likely to result in charring and crater formation at ablation sites. A CF > 100 g during ablation is associated with complications like perforation.

Three available technologies are able to directly measure CF during ablation procedures, these are:

1. *TactiCath® catheter* (Endosense, Geneva, Switzerland) **(Fig. 14)** incorporates a force sensor between the second and third electrode, consisting of a deformable body and three optical fibers to measure microdeformations. This correlates with the force applied to the catheter tip. Infrared laser light is emitted through the proximal end of the three optical fibers. CF applied to the tip changes the wavelength of this laser.
2. *ThermoCool SmartTouch®* ablation catheter (Biosense Webster Inc, Diamond Bar, CA, US) **(Fig. 15)** tip electrode is mounted on a precision spring that permits a small amount of electrode deflection. A transmitter coil that is coupled to the tip electrode emits a location reference signal. Location sensor coils placed at the proximal end of the spring detect micromovement of the transmitter coil at the tip electrode on the spring. The 3D-based system senses the location information of the sensor and calculates the associated force.
3. *IntelliSense®* (Hansen Medical Inc, Mount View, CA, US) **(Fig. 16)**, is used in conjunction with a dedicated robot system for CA.

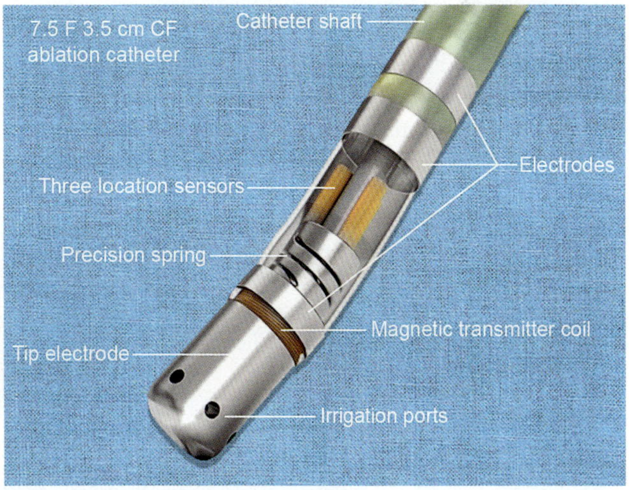

FIG. 15: SmartTouch® contract force catheter.

Courtesy: ThermoCool SmartTouch ablation catheter (Biosense, Webster Inc, Diamond Bar, CA, USA).

INTRACARDIAC ECHOCARDIOGRAPHY/ ULTRASOUND

Intracardiac echocardiography (ICE) may allow better imaging of the anatomic substrate relative to the ablation catheter **(Fig. 17)**. This is useful in procedures requiring arrhythmia mechanisms closely associated with intracardiac structures, such as papillary muscle or moderator band VT. It is also useful to reduce fluoroscopy and improve monitoring in procedures such as AF ablation.

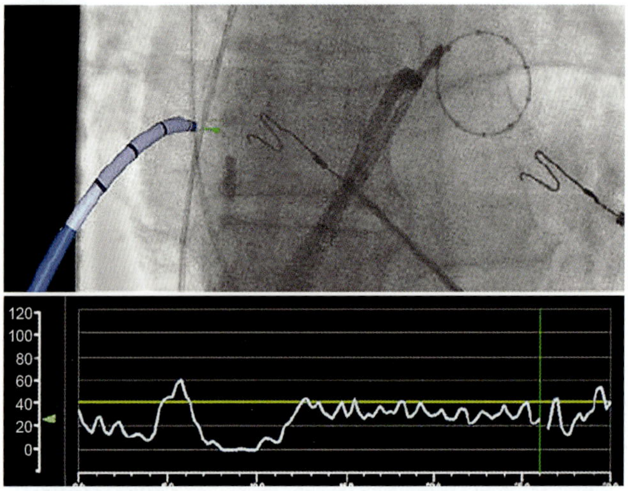

FIG. 16: IntelliSense catheter use during robotic mapping.

CONCLUSION

Arrhythmia management has become a refined science owing to significant innovations entering and shaping the clinical practice.

Electroanatomical mapping systems have been instrumental in enhancing our understanding of arrhythmia initiation, propagation, pathophysiological, and anatomical correlation. They have enabled real-time visualization of complex EGMs and spatiotemporal data, a critical requirement of managing complex arrhythmogenic substrates. They have also helped markedly reduce the fluoroscopic radiation exposure to both the operators and the patient.

Accurate mapping and demarcation of areas of scar, low-voltage, and border zone areas further enhances the ability to effectively modify or eliminate arrhythmogenic substrate. CF technology and multielectrode high-resolution mapping with rapid automatic point annotation have immensely improved mapping and ablation capabilities and safety.

Electrophysiologic mapping and concurrent therapeutic ablation interventions have remarkably benefited patients suffering from highly symptomatic complex supraventricular and VAs. Ongoing advancements in this field promise to improve patient outcomes even more in the near future.

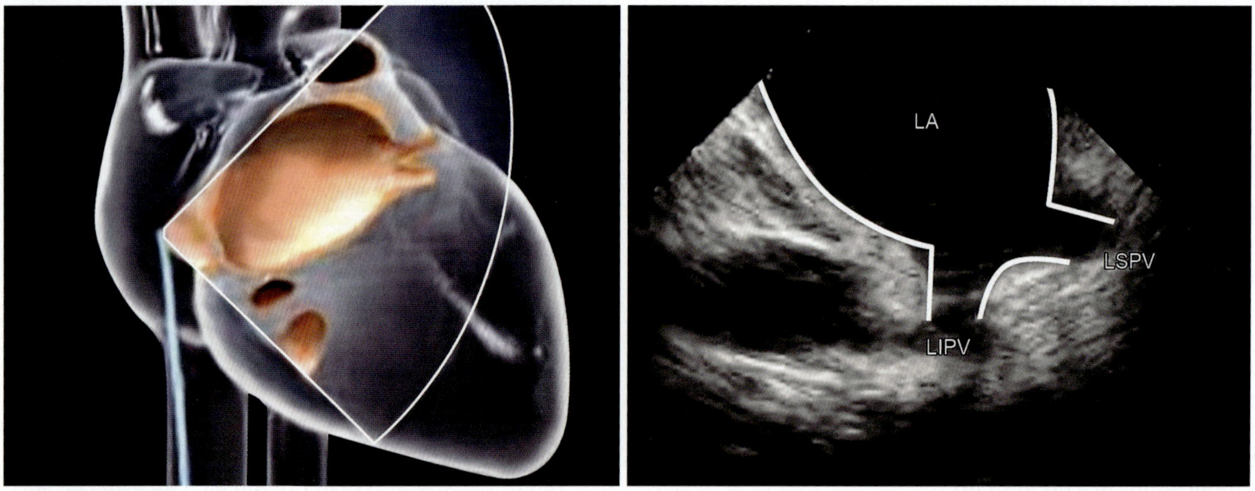

FIG. 17: Intracardiac echocardiography/ultrasound.

(LA: left atrium; LIPV: left inferior pulmonary vein; LSPV: left superior pulmonary vein)

ONLINE REFERENCES

Please scan the QR code provided at the end of the table of contents for References of this chapter.

CHAPTER

213 Catheter Ablation of Ventricular Arrhythmias in Ischemic and Nonischemic Cardiomyopathies

P Vijay Shekar, C Narasimhan

ABSTRACT

Catheter ablation for ventricular tachycardia (VT) in patients with structural heart disease (SHD) is an established and effective treatment strategy. Identification of the arrhythmogenic substrate (scar-related reentrant circuit) and targeting the critical components of the circuit (isthmus) forms the basis of catheter ablation. Mapping and ablation strategy primarily depends on patient's clinical profile and VT characteristics. Use of 3D electroanatomical mapping (EAM) tools, multielectrode catheters and contact force sensing catheters have resulted in shorter duration, better procedural outcomes, and improved safety of these procedures.

Keywords: Ventricular tachycardia, catheter ablation, scar-related reentry circuit, activation mapping; pace mapping, entrainment mapping, substrate mapping.

INTRODUCTION

Ventricular arrhythmias (VAs) in patients with structural heart disease (SHD) are associated with increased mortality and sudden cardiac arrest (SCA).[1] Radiofrequency ablation (RFA) is an effective and definitive therapy to control the arrhythmia in these patients. Over the past three decades, significant progress has led to better understanding of the pathophysiology of arrhythmias. Advancements in preprocedural imaging, especially cardiac magnetic resonance (CMR) imaging, improvement in mapping, and ablation strategies have improved the safety and efficacy of these procedures.[2-5]

HISTORY OF VENTRICULAR TACHYCARDIA ABLATION

Historically, VT ablation involved surgical resection of left ventricular (LV) aneurysm or endocardial encircling ventriculotomy to eliminate VT. Later, Josephson developed the technique of map-guided subendocardial resection. The procedure was based on the identifying "specific targets" during mapping—diastolic or presystolic electrical activation recorded during VT on the endocardium between the densely scarred myocardial tissue and more normal muscle (border zones). In 1983, the first endocardial ablation of VT using direct current (DC) energy electrical shock delivered via a standard quadripolar endocardial catheter positioned in the area of interest was described by Hartzler and colleagues. In the subsequent years, radiofrequency (RF) energy replaced DC energy for ablation of all arrhythmias by late 1980s. Since then, advanced mapping techniques and ablation tools have resulted in improved clinical outcomes.[6-9]

VENTRICULAR TACHYCARDIA IN STRUCTURAL HEART DISEASE

Patients with SHD can be broadly divided into two groups: (1) Ischemic cardiomyopathy (ICM) and (2) Nonischemic cardiomyopathy (NICM).

Ischemic Cardiomyopathy

Among patients presenting with VT due to SHD, ICM contributes to a vast majority, accounting for about three-fourths of all cases.[10] Patients with acute ischemia usually present with polymorphic VT (PMVT) and ventricular fibrillation (VF). Occasionally, acute ischemia can also lead to monomorphic VT (MMVT) due to reversible and transient slow conduction in the ischemic cells.

On the other hand, post-myocardial infarction (MI) patients typically present with MMVT due to presence of scar. Following a MI, infarcts may lead to arrhythmias through different mechanisms. Scar related reentrant VT accounts for >80% of MMVTs. Reentry involving the bundle branches or fascicles is encountered in up to 19% of patients, whereas focal VT mechanisms occur less frequently.

Surviving bundles of myocardium in a myocardial scar result in zig-zag slow conduction leading to reentrant VT.[11]

Nonischemic Cardiomyopathy

Patients with NICM represent a heterogeneous subset with varying etiologies, including idiopathic dilated NICM, valvular heart disease, hypertensive, hypertrophic, toxic, genetic, inflammatory, tachycardia-induced, peripartum, and infiltrative cardiomyopathy.

Among patients with NICM, VTs are more often pleomorphic and polymorphic; hemodynamically unstable; and are more difficult to induce compared with post MI VTs. The substrate is less well defined for ablation compared to ICM due to heterogeneous patchy scar, intramural location, and more involvement of the epicardium. Intramural location offers challenges in identifying the optimal ablation target site based on conventional mapping techniques.

UNDERSTANDING THE SUBSTRATE FOR ABLATION

Scar-related reentry is the most common mechanism of VT in both ICM and NICM patients. The myocardial scar is a heterogeneous structure, involving densely scarred tissue and tissues that contain surviving islands of myocardial cells **(Fig. 1)**. Slow conduction in these surviving myocardial channels (isthmus) allows part of the channel to recover from activation allowing the impulse to reenter the newly recovered tissue setting up a reentry circuit. These critical channels (isthmus) sustaining reentry can be deep within the scar or between the scar border and another anatomical barrier like a valve annulus and are the usual targets for ablation. Mapping involves identification of the critical channels.[10-14]

Multiple anatomical and functional models have been suggested for reentrant VT circuit. VT circuits are complex structures, which may have multiple entrances, exits, and dead ends of activation. It also comprises of other surviving myocardial tissues that include the outer loop, inner loop and bystander tracts **(Fig. 2)**.

INDICATIONS FOR CATHETER ABLATION[5]

According to the 2019 expert consensus document endorsed by the Heart Rhythm Society (HRS) and the European Heart Rhythm Association (EHRA), the following are recommendations for catheter ablation for VT.

Ischemic Cardiomyopathy Patients

- In patients with ischemic heart disease (IHD) who experience recurrent MMVT despite chronic amiodarone therapy, catheter ablation is recommended in preference to escalating antiarrhythmic drug (AAD) therapy. (Class I)
- In patients with IHD and recurrent symptomatic MMVT despite AAD therapy or when AAD therapy is contraindicated or not tolerated, catheter ablation is recommended to reduce recurrent VT. (Class I)
- In patients with IHD and VT storm refractory to AAD therapy, catheter ablation is recommended. (Class I)
- In patients with IHD and an implantable cardioverter defibrillator (ICD) who experience a first episode of MMVT, catheter ablation may be considered to reduce the risk of recurrent VT or ICD therapies. (Class II b)

Nonischemic Cardiomyopathy Patients

- In patients with NICM and recurrent sustained MMVT for whom antiarrhythmic medications are ineffective, contraindicated, or not tolerated, catheter ablation is useful for reducing recurrent VT and ICD shocks. (Class I)

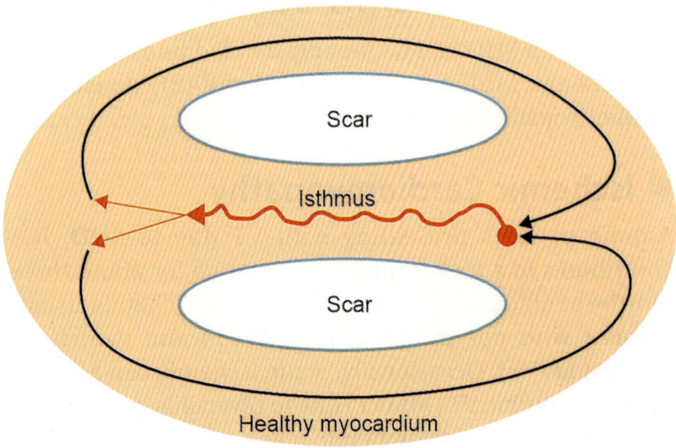

FIG. 1: Schematic representation of scar-related entrant circuit.

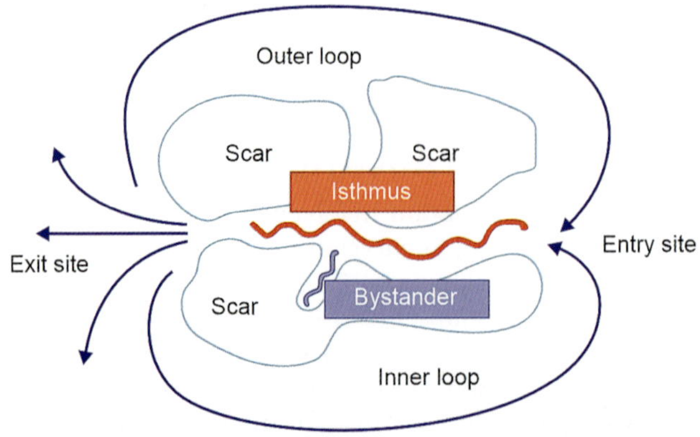

FIG. 2: Scar-related reentry ventricular tachycardia (VT) circuit and its components. The slow conducting "isthmus" should be the target of mapping and ablation.

- In patients with NICM and electrical storm refractory to AAD therapy, catheter ablation is useful for reducing recurrent VT and ICD shocks. (Class I)
- In patients with NICM, epicardial catheter ablation of VT can be useful after failure of endocardial ablation or as the initial ablation approach when there is a suspicion of an epicardial substrate or circuit. (Class II a)
- In patients with hypertrophic cardiomyopathy (HCM) and recurrent MMVT in whom AAD therapy is ineffective or not tolerated, catheter ablation can be useful. (Class I)
- In patients with cardiac sarcoidosis and recurrent VT despite medical therapy, catheter ablation can be useful to reduce the risk of VT recurrence and ICD shocks. (Class II a)
- In patients with NICM related to lamin A/C (LMNA) mutations and recurrent VT, catheter ablation may be considered as a palliative strategy for short-term arrhythmia control. (Class II b)

PREPROCEDURAL RISK ASSESSMENT

These patients have concomitant advanced heart failure and multiple comorbidities making them vulnerable for complications. A thorough preprocedural risk evaluation helps to minimize the risks associated with the procedure and improve outcomes. The *PAAINESD score* > 15–17 identifies patients with SHD and VT at particularly high risk of adverse periprocedural and postprocedural outcomes **(Table 1)**.[15]

ROLE OF 12-LEAD ELECTROCARDIOGRAM

Electrocardiogram (ECG) during VT allows for localization of the "exit site" of VTs with a predictive accuracy of >70% to guide initial mapping efforts. Several algorithms have been devised to predict the exit site in post-MI VT. These algorithms indicate the exit site of the circuit, but not the critical isthmus which should be the target for ablation. 12-lead ECG **(Fig. 3)** can also suggest the presence of epicardial substrate and thus guide mapping strategies **(Box 1)**.[16,17]

Electrocardiogram during sinus rhythm is helpful to evaluate the presence of underlying substrate and also helps to localize the scar and origin of the VAs. In patients with underlying SHD, parameters such as QRS duration, fragmentation, and the presence of conduction abnormalities provide prognostic information, including risk of sudden cardiac death.

Electrocardiographic imaging (ECGI) is a noninvasive mapping strategy that combines a computed tomography scan of the chest and with a continuous 256-lead ECG recorded by a multielectrode vest to accurately predict the exit site of ventricular tachycardia.

TABLE 1: The PAAINESD score, developed to predict the risk of periprocedural hemodynamic decompensation.

Variable	Points
Pulmonary disease (COPD)	5
Age > 60 years	3
General anesthesia	4
Ischemic cardiomyopathy	6
NYHA Class III/IV	6
EF < 25%	3
VT storm	5
Diabetes mellitus	3

(COPD: chronic obstructive pulmonary disease; EF: ejection fraction; NYHA: New York Heart Association; VT: ventricular tachycardia)

PERIPROCEDURAL IMAGING

Preprocedural transthoracic echocardiography (TTE) should be done to assess LV function, presence and localization of scar, and intracardiac thrombi. Presence of cardiac thrombi precludes catheter ablation and hence should be looked for.

Preprocedure CMR is an important imaging tool for patients undergoing VT ablation and late gadolinium enhancement (LGE)-CMR helps to localize the scar. By demonstrating location and extent of delayed enhancement, CMR helps in periprocedural planning including the need for epicardial access. Delayed gadolinium enhancement and gray border zones have good correlation with conducting channels and can identify critical isthmus sites in >70% of cases. Use of CMR for targeting the arrhythmogenic substrate has resulted in reduced VT recurrence and reduced mortality. CMR in addition to identifying the substrate will also be beneficial for to determine the etiology of NICM **(Figs. 4A to C)**.[18,19]

Computed tomography can be used as an alternative when MRI is not available. Though CT has higher spatial resolution than CMR, it has poor scar delineation owing to lower contrast to noise ratio. Cardiac anatomy and substrate characterization identified by CMR and CT imaging can be integrated into the EAM systems for guidance during the ablation procedure.

PROCEDURAL CONSIDERATIONS

Ultrasound guided vascular access (femoral vein access) is important to reduce vascular complications and should be routinely used.[20]

Depending on the patient profile, VT ablation can be usually performed either under general anesthesia (GA) or under monitored anesthesia care (MAC). Advantages of MAC with sedation are avoiding anesthetics that can potentially depress myocardial contractility and decrease the inducibility of VT. But however, for patients undergoing prolonged, complex procedures who have unstable rhythms or poor cardiopulmonary reserve, GA is preferred.[21]

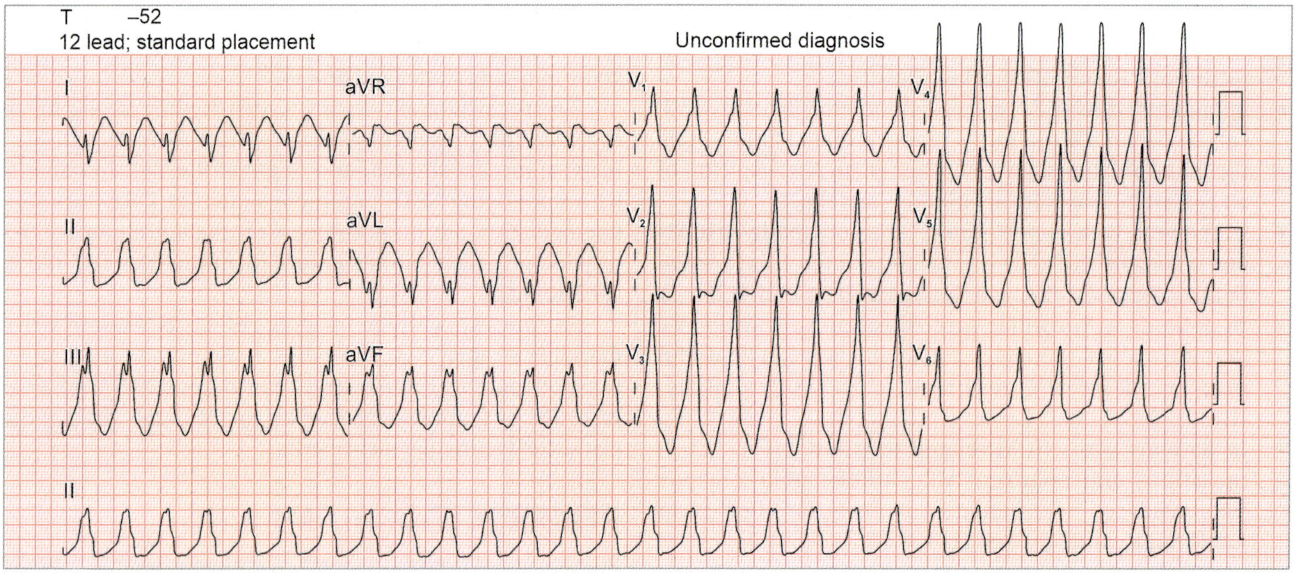

FIG. 3: 12-lead electrocardiogram (ECG) demonstrating monomorphic ventricular tachycardia (VT) with features of epicardial exit—presence of pseudo delta wave in V_1–V_6 measuring 70 ms, presence of q wave in I and absence of q waves in inferior leads.

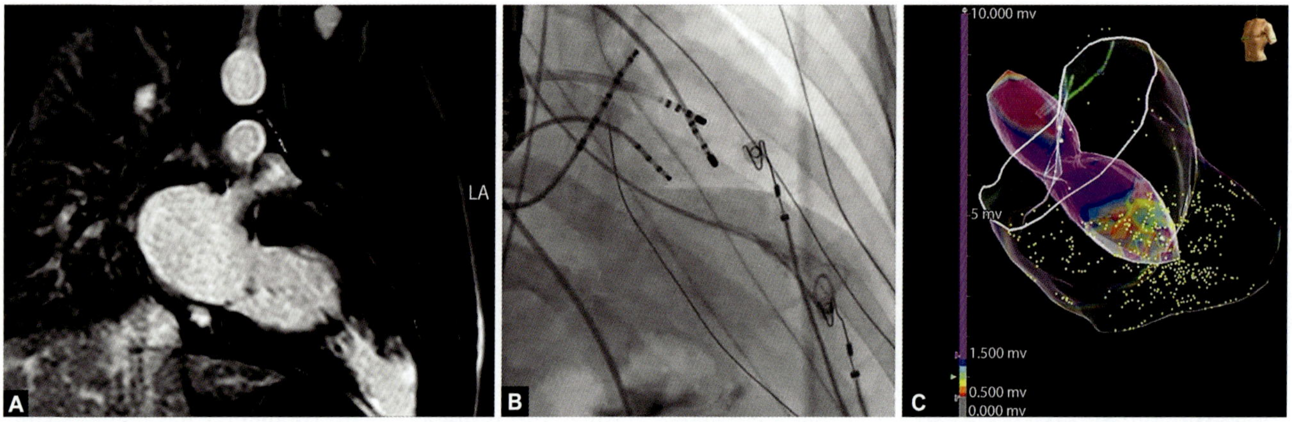

FIGS. 4A TO C: Preprocedural cardiac MRI (CMR) demonstrating mid-cavitary obstruction and left ventricular (LV) aneurysm in a hypertrophic cardiomyopathy (HCM) patient. LV angiogram using pigtail catheter and endocardial shell created using 3D electroanatomical mapping (EAM) correlates with CMR findings.

BOX 1 Electrocardiogram (ECG) criteria to suggest epicardial exit of the ventricular tachycardia (VT).

- Intrinsicoid deflection time ≥85 ms
- Shortest RS complex ≥121 ms
- Maximum deflection index ≥0.55
- Q waves in lead I and no q waves in inferior leads
- Pseudo delta wave ≥34 ms

In high-risk patients, especially in patients with unstable rhythms and hemodynamic compromise, mechanical circulatory support (MCS) can be used periprocedurally to aid VT ablation. Though Intra-aortic balloon pumps (IABPs), Impella, extracorporeal membrane oxygenation (ECMO), and other support devices have been used in VT ablation. Choice of MCS is a tailored decision and depends on the patient profile, availability, and expertise.[22]

Use of intracardiac echocardiography (ICE) during the procedure is beneficial to identify and target intracavitary structures like the papillary muscles for ablation. Catheter position and stability can be assessed with ICE and complications like pericardial effusion can be diagnosed early. Use of ICE limits radiation exposure.[23]

MAPPING TECHNIQUES (FLOWCHART 1)

Activation Mapping

Activation mapping is performed during VT and hence is suitable for hemodynamically stable arrhythmias. It involves recording of local electrograms from multiple sites during VT. In case of scar-related reentry, there is continuous excitation of the circuit throughout the tachycardia cycle length (TCL). In "exit sites", electrograms can be fractionated and immediately precede the onset of the QRS complex. Ablation at exit sites can terminate the tachycardia; however, it can also result in a change of the tachycardia exit resulting in a different configuration. Ablation of the diastolic pathway, "isthmus", is therefore a more desirable target, given it can eliminate the critical component required for reentry. Electrograms at isthmus sites are characterized by presence of very low-voltage amplitude (<0.5 mV), multiple fractionated potentials that occurs earlier during the diastole **(Fig. 5)**.[24,25]

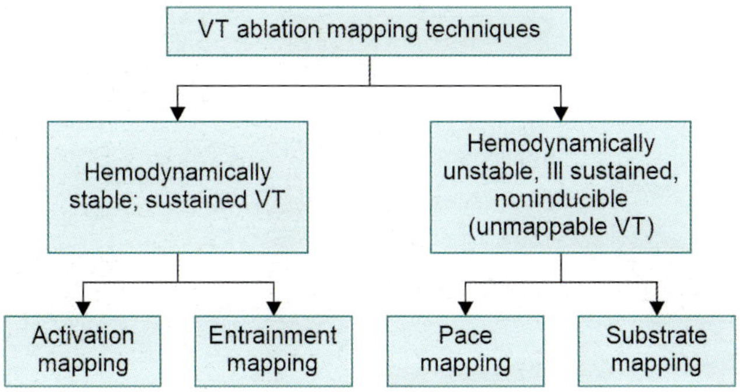

FLOWCHART 1: Mapping techniques.
(VT: ventricular tachycardia)

Activation mapping can be performed only in sustained and hemodynamically stable VTs. In patients with less tolerated VTs, limited activation mapping can be performed in conjunction with substrate, entrainment, and/or pace mapping **(Figs. 6A and B)**.

Entrainment Mapping

Entrainment is a pacing maneuver that helps establish reentry as the mechanism of the underlying tachycardia and can be used as an effective mapping tool to identify different components of the reentry circuit. Entrainment is performed by pacing from different sites (that are either within or outside the reentry circuit) at a rate slightly faster that the VT cycle length. During the entrainment maneuver, parameters such as QRS morphology, specific intervals, and morphology of electrograms are analyzed to identify critical components of the reentry circuit **(Fig. 7)**.[26,27] Entrainment mapping can be performed only during stable and sustained VTs.

Pace Mapping

Pace mapping is performed when the targeted arrhythmia is difficult to induce or is hemodynamically unstable. It is a technique used to locate the origin of VT by pacing the myocardium at different sites to reproduce the clinical 12-lead morphology. The paced 12-lead ECG morphology is compared with the clinical VT and the optimal site should exactly match the tachycardia QRS, including individual notches as well as major deflections **(Figs. 8A and B)**. Automated algorithms which express the match percentage are also available. Though pace mapping is commonly more

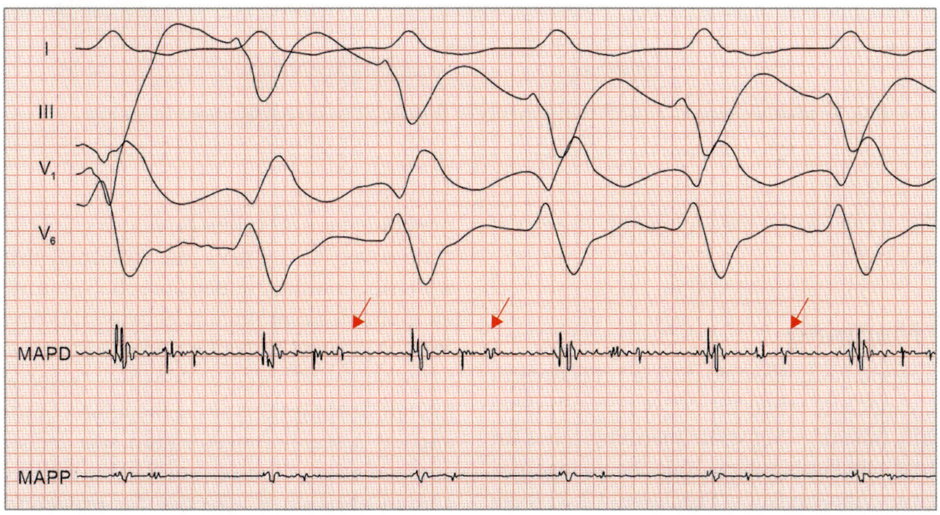

FIG. 5: Activation mapping during ventricular tachycardia (VT) demonstrating diastolic potentials (red arrows).

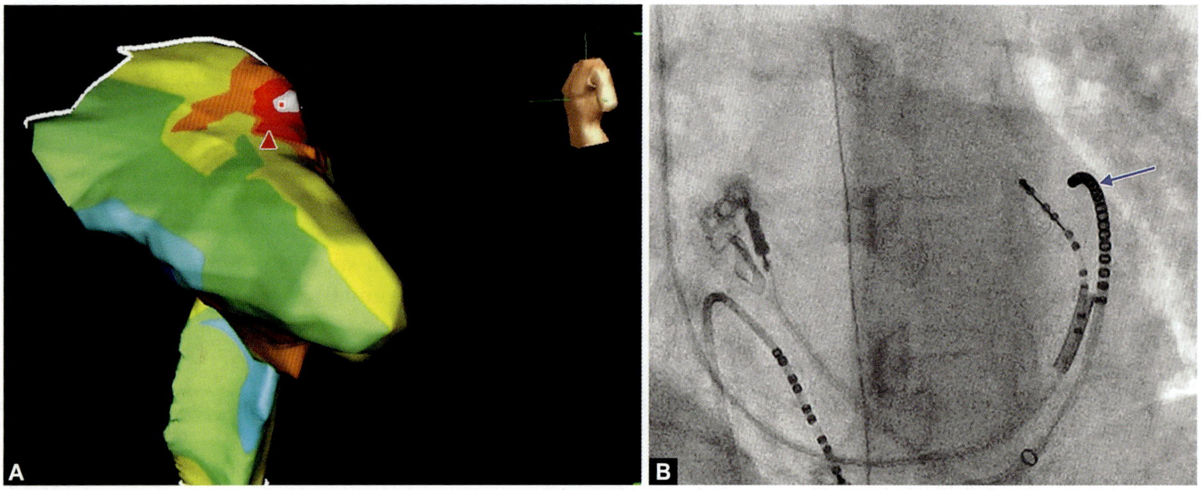

FIGS. 6A AND B: Activation mapping using 3D electroanatomical mapping (EAM) (EnSite Precision) and multipolar catheter in the epicardium (blue arrow) close to the mitral annulus demonstrating a focal site of ventricular tachycardia (VT) origin (epicardial) (white region indicated by red arrow).

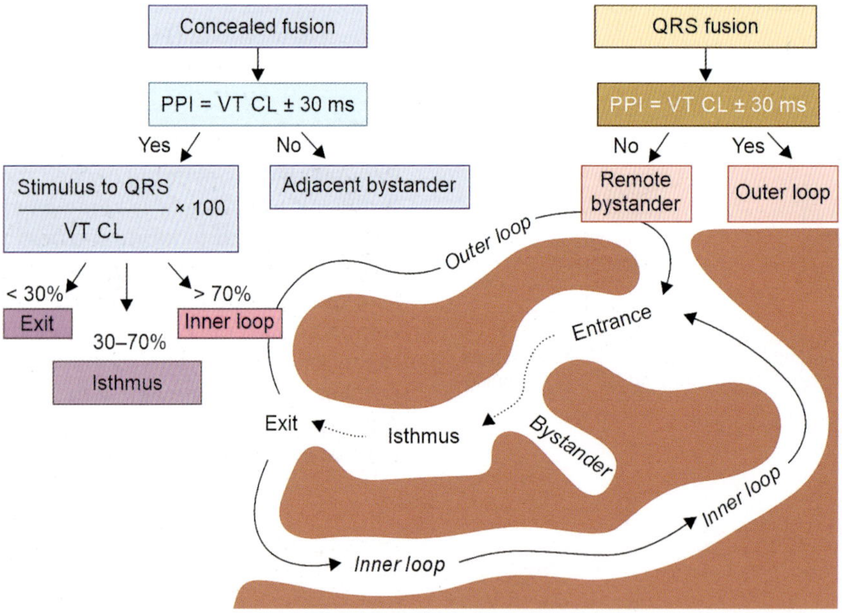

FIG. 7: Identification of critical components of the circuit using entrainment mapping.

helpful for focal VTs, it can also be used to identify the exit of the VT in reentrant VTs.[28,29]

Substrate Mapping

Substrate-guided mapping is performed during sinus rhythm or paced rhythm, especially when the VT is noninducible or hemodynamically unstable. Substrate mapping relies on identification of areas with low bipolar or unipolar voltage and abnormal electrogram characteristics **(Figs. 9A to C)**. Voltage mapping identifies arrhythmogenic substrate by using predefined cut off values for dense scar (<0.5 mV) and border zone areas (0.5–1.5 mV). The abnormal electrogram features, which include fragmented potentials, late potentials (LPs), and local abnormal ventricular activity (LAVA), represent areas of slow or delayed activation that constitute surrogate markers for potential VT circuits. Substrate-based ablation strategies include linear lesions along the infarct border, ablation of LPs and LAVA, scar homogenization, scar dechanneling, and scar/core isolation. Multiple studies have shown that substrate-guided ablation is effective for prevention of arrhythmia recurrences in scar-related unmappable VT.[30,31]

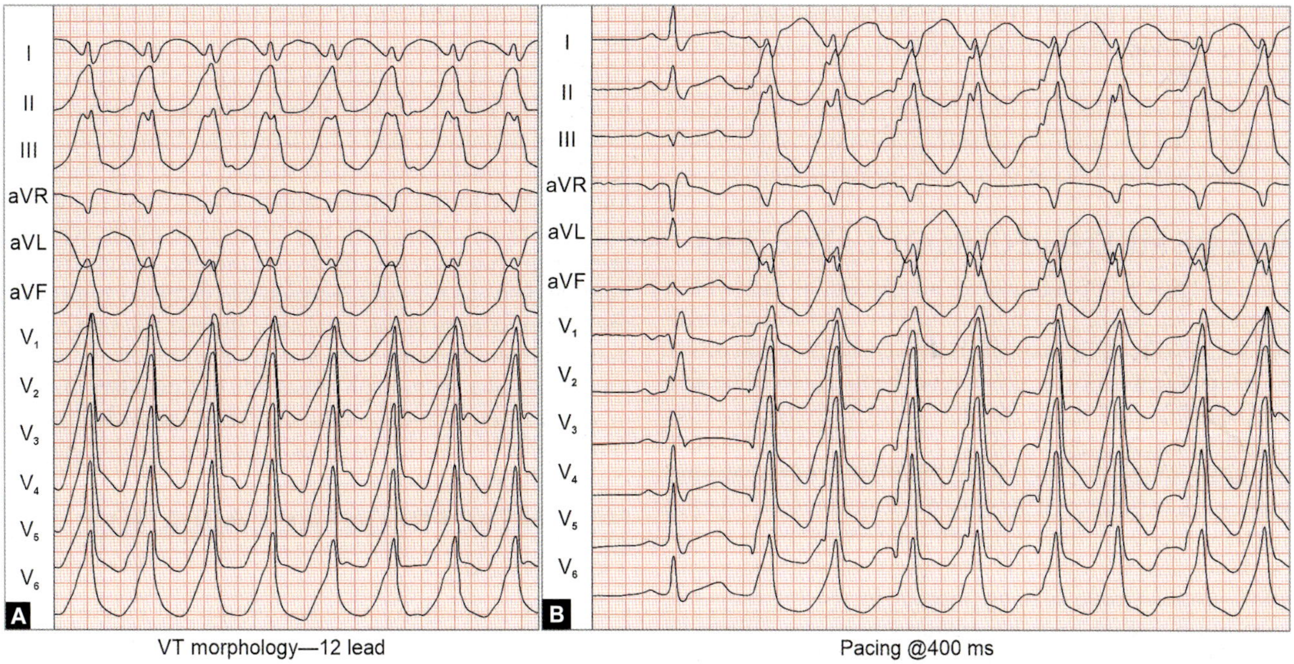

FIGS. 8A AND B: Pace mapping demonstrating comparison of ventricular tachycardia (VT) and paced morphology demonstrating a 11/12 match.

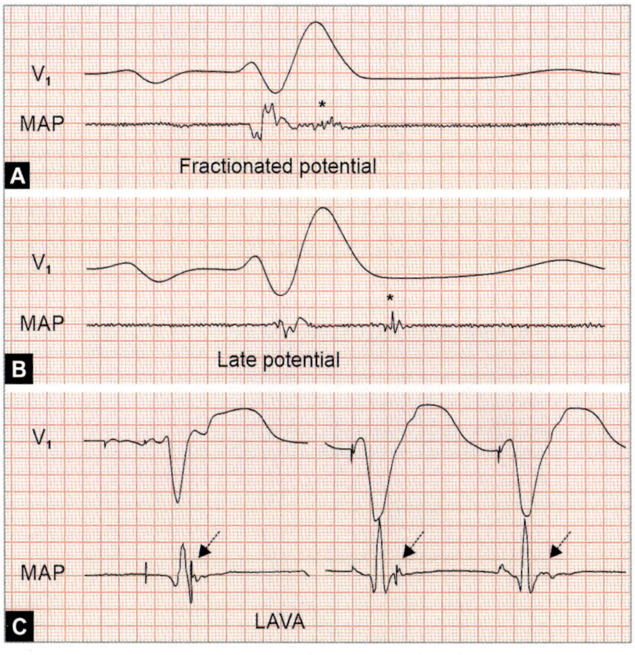

FIGS. 9A TO C: Surrogate markers of arrhythmogenic substrate during substrate mapping. (A) Fractionated potential; (B) Late potential (LP); (C) Local abnormal ventricular activity (LAVA).

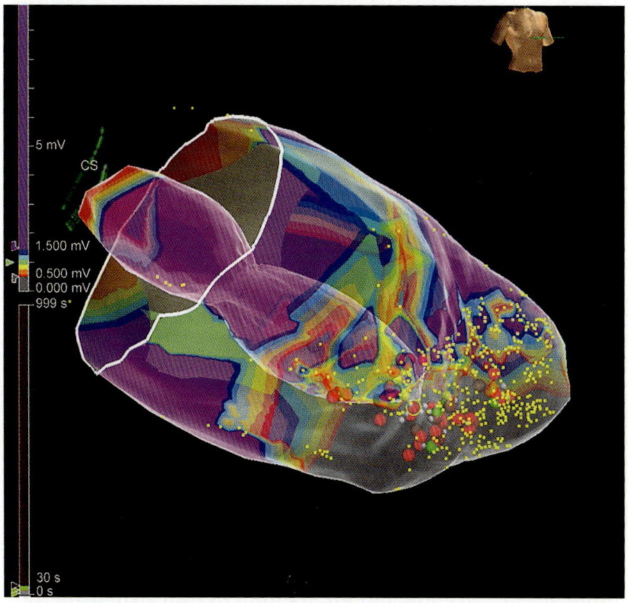

FIG. 10: Substrate mapping using 3D electroanatomical mapping (EAM) (EnSite Precision) demonstrating dense scar in the left ventricular (LV) apical region (gray areas) in a patient with mid-cavitary hypertrophic cardiomyopathy (HCM) and ventricular tachycardia (VT)—combined endocardial and epicardial approach. Red and green dots indicate sites of ablation. Yellow dots indicate mapping points. Purple regions indicate normal voltage areas and red/yellow/green areas represent border zones.

USE OF 3D ELECTROANATOMICAL MAPPING SYSTEMS

Electroanatomical mapping systems utilize information derived from catheter-mounted electrodes to reconstruct an 3D image of the targeted cardiac chamber **(Fig. 10)**. The current EAM systems use (1) impedance-based measurements and algorithms to recognize diagnostic and ablation catheters and (2) magnetic field-based localization of mapping and ablation catheters. EAM systems commonly used in India are the CARTO mapping system (Biosense

Webster, Diamond Bar, CA) and the EnSite Precision system (Abbott Laboratories, Abbott Park, IL, St Jude Medical, St Paul, MN).[32-34]

Regardless of the EAM technology, it offers advantages of decreased fluoroscopic time (radiation exposure), more precise mapping, and use of versatile mapping strategies.

USE OF MULTIELECTRODE CATHETERS

Conventional mapping involves acquisition of data with a point by point (PbP) method using a catheter with a single bipole. However, PbP mapping is time consuming and prone to errors due to catheter orientation, contact, electrode size and spacing, and other factors. Multielectrode mapping catheters are capable of acquiring data from multiple sites simultaneously for each beat. Multielectrode mapping catheters have improved the procedural outcomes by offering higher mapping density, resolution, and speed.

Multielectrode catheters often use small electrodes with short interelectrode spacing, thereby increasing mapping resolution, which can be advantageous for substrate mapping. These catheters can also be useful for activation mapping during VT, given they allow rapid acquisition of multiple sites at high spatial resolution that can facilitate identification of a reentry isthmus or VT focus. Currently, several multielectrode catheters are available. The Pentaray catheter (Biosense Webster, Diamond Bar, CA) is a flower-shaped catheter with five splines, each with four electrodes (a total of 20 electrodes). The Advisor HD Grid catheter (Abbott Laboratories, Abbott Park, IL) is a novel 4-by-4 unipolar electrode array with 1-mm (diameter) electrodes, equidistantly spaced 3 mm apart from each other.[35-37]

ABLATION TOOLS AND TECHNIQUES

Unipolar RFA remains the mainstay of ablation technology. Successful ablation to a large extent depends on the delivery of durable lesions at the site of interest. Use of irrigated tip catheters helps to improve power delivery and create deeper and larger lesions. Tissue heating at the electrode-tissue interface through continuous irrigation of saline helps to deliver higher power. Ablation lesion size increases with the duration of current application and although short duration applications are sufficient for ablation in thin structures, 60–90 seconds or longer applications are usually employed for VT.[38]

Lesion size is critically dependent on the contact of the ablating electrode with the tissue. Catheters with contact force sensors provide real-time information about the degree of contact (which is usually expressed in grams). RF applications with a mean contact force >10 g are more likely to result in electrical inexcitability in scar areas. Contact force sensor catheters in addition to ensuring durable lesions, also improves the safety of the procedure by preventing excess catheter contact and related complications. Contact force sensing has become an integral part of RF catheter ablation.

When the substrate is intramural (deep within the myocardium), lesions created by conventional ablation techniques may fail to reach the desired depth and hence fail to eliminate the VT. In such cases, alternate strategies such as use of hypotonic saline for irrigation, bipolar ablation, and needle ablation have been studied in clinical trials and found to be effective. Bipolar ablation is performed by with a second catheter that is closely opposed to tissue, with the target substrate between the two catheters. This technique helps to deliver RF lesions between two catheters improving the current density in this local area. Bipolar ablation can be delivered between catheters that are positioned across the interventricular septum, on either side of a papillary muscle, or with catheters in the endocardial and epicardial spaces **(Fig. 11)**.[38,39]

NONRADIOFREQUENCY ABLATION TECHNIQUES

Catheter cryoablation has been infrequently employed for treating VA. Cryo catheters become adherent to the tissue during lesion formation, which improves catheter stability and contact. Cryoablation has been found useful in the treatment of VT arising from highly mobile papillary muscles, which can be difficult to ablate using RF ablation catheters.[40]

Transvenous ethanol ablation involves creating controlled infarctions by injecting ethanol into the venous tributaries of the coronary sinus.[41,42]

Stereotactic radiotherapy involves use of stereotactic motion-gated external beam radiation for ablation. The therapy has been explored in animal models and its feasibility has been demonstrated in humans.[43]

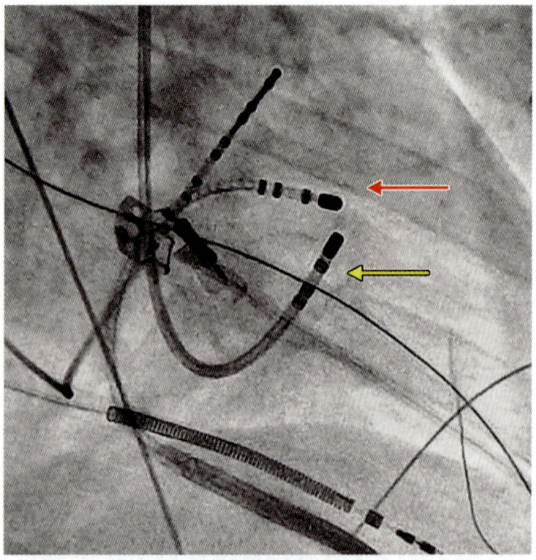

FIG. 11: Bipolar ablation (combined endoepicardial ablation) of ventricular tachycardia (VT) in a patient with nonischemic cardiomyopathy (NICM). Yellow arrow indicates ablation catheter in the left ventricular (LV) endocardium beneath the aortic valve. Red arrow indicates ablation catheter through subxiphoid approach in pericardial space.

COMPLICATIONS ASSOCIATED WITH CATHETER ABLATION

Complications, including vascular access bleeding, tamponade, and volume overload, are reported in 4–11% of patients. Other serious but infrequent complications include cardiac tamponade requiring surgery, phrenic nerve injury, and coronary artery injury. Percutaneous epicardial access is associated with risk of collateral injury during access to epicardium. Injury to liver, RV hematoma, tamponade, pericarditis, and coronary arterial injuries have been reported. Thromboembolic complications including pulmonary embolism are rare, can be prevented by meticulous attention to intra- and postprocedure anticoagulation, but can occur.[44-47]

Inhospital mortality is as high as 3% and has been reported due to refractory VT, refractory heart failure, and cardiac tamponade. Ablation that results in left bundle branch block (LBBB) or atrioventricular (AV) block can lead to hemodynamic deterioration due to cardiac dyssynchrony that can warrant implantation of pacemakers or cardiac resynchronization therapy (CRT).

OUTCOMES OF VENTRICULAR TACHYCARDIA ABLATION

The outcomes of VT ablation depend on the underlying substrate, the stage of the disease, and patient comorbidities.

The VANISH trial in ICM patients compared the strategies of escalating AAD therapy according to a predefined protocol versus catheter ablation in 259 patients and followed them for a mean duration of 27.9 ± 17.1 months. The composite primary endpoint of death, VT storm, or appropriate ICD shock was lower in the ablation arm. In the multicenter THERMOCOOL VT ablation trial, the number of VT episodes in the 6 months before and after ablation was reduced from a median of 11.5 to 0 episodes. However, data to support catheter ablation as a stand-alone therapy in patients with VT due to IHD is lacking, thus warranting an ICD implantation for secondary prevention.[5,44]

Catheter ablation of VT appears to be safe and effective in NICM, achieving long-term arrhythmia control in 50–70%, with a survival rate of 70%. However, NICM comprises of heterogeneous disorders and hence the outcomes and prognosis may vary accordingly. Ablation abolishes at least one inducible VT in 60–74% of patients and all inducible VTs in 43–72% of patients with dilated cardiomyopathy. During median follow-ups ranging from 15 to 48 months, approximately 31% of patients experience recurrence of at least one VT. Approximately half of those with recurrent VT experience fewer VT episodes after the ablation procedure. Recurrence of VT after ablation is more frequent among NICM compared to ICM.[45,46] In patients with VT circuits inaccessible to catheter ablation, hybrid surgical options can be considered.

SPECIFIC NONISCHEMIC CARDIOMYOPATHY SUBSTRATES

Cardiac Sarcoidosis

The mechanisms of VT in patients with cardiac sarcoidosis include abnormal automaticity and triggered activity during the inflammatory phase and predominantly scar-related reentry in the chronic phase. 18-fluorodeoxyglucose positron emission tomography-computed tomography (^{18}FDG PET-CT) is helpful in identifying the active inflammatory phase. When PET scanning identifies active inflammation during the acute phase, treatment with immunosuppressive agents and anti-arrhythmics is preferred over ablation. The ablation approach to scar-related reentrant VT in cardiac sarcoidosis is similar to that employed in other scar-related VTs.[48,49]

Arrhythmogenic Right Ventricular Cardiomyopathy

In patients with arrhythmogenic right ventricular cardiomyopathy (ARVC), scar location is heterogeneous based on the chamber (predominantly RV but can also involve the LV), the number of foci, and depth (epicardial and/or endocardial). A combined endocardial and epicardial substrate catheter ablation has improved acute success and lowered recurrence rates compared with endocardial-only catheter ablation and hence a combined endo-epi approach might be a reasonable first-line choice. Isolated epicardial involvement with a completely normal endocardial bipolar map has been observed in 26–40% of patients. Due to progressive nature of the disease, repeat procedures may be warranted.[50]

Hypertrophic Cardiomyopathy

Catheter ablation in HCM patients can be challenging due to the thickness of the myocardium, and epicardial access has been required in the majority of patients. VTs arising from apical aneurysms can be ablated from the endocardium. Overall, the results of ablation are encouraging, acutely eliminating VT in 80% of patients, with more than two-thirds of patients free of VT in the long-term follow-up. If catheter ablation is ineffective, other methods, including venous alcohol injection and surgical resection and ablation, may be considered.[47]

CONCLUSION

Catheter ablation is a safe and effective strategy for VT in patients with ICM and NICM. Optimal timing and mapping strategy needs more data. Patients with ICM seem to have better outcomes with ablation compared to NICM patients, which constitute a heterogeneous group. Scar-related reentry is the common mechanism of VT and understanding the substrate guides the mapping strategy. Preprocedural imaging, especially CMR with scar characterization, has a positive influence on VT ablation outcomes and hence is strongly recommended. Mapping strategy depends on the VT characteristics—sustained versus ill sustained, hemodynamically stable versus unstable, and inducible VT versus noninducible VT. Use of EAM, multipolar catheters, high resolution and high density mapping tools, and irrigated tip and contact force sensor ablation tools have significantly improved procedural outcomes of VT ablation.

Non-RF ablation techniques are employed when conventional ablation techniques fail to eliminate the VT.

ONLINE REFERENCES

Please scan the QR code provided at the end of the table of contents for References of this chapter.

CHAPTER

214 Conduction System Pacing: Where are We Today?

Shunmuga Sundaram Ponnusamy

ABSTRACT

With increasing number of pacemaker implants, soon it was realized that long-term right ventricular (RV) pacing has been associated with deleterious effects on left ventricle. Search for an ideal pacing site which would provide electrical and mechanical synchrony as close as to the normal ventricular activation resulted in direct capture of conduction system fibers. Both his bundle pacing (HBP) and left bundle branch pacing (LBBP) provide superior electrical resynchronization and prevent RV pacing-induced cardiomyopathy. Though HBP has been shown to be associated with frequent lead dislodgments and rise in pacing threshold, LBBP overcomes its limitations. LBBP could be considered as an excellent alternative for cardiac resynchronization therapy (CRT) as it provides better correction of distal conduction system disease in patients with wide QRS and LV dysfunction. Though LBBP has been shown to produce excellent electrical and mechanical resynchronization, the long-term safety data is lacking. Improvement in the sheath and lead design will help in making the procedure technically easy and improve the acute procedural success rate. Addressing the unmet needs in the future will help in establishing LBBP as a standard pacing strategy.

Keywords: Left bundle branch pacing, heart failure, cardiac resynchronization therapy, template beat, septal perforation.

INTRODUCTION

With the aging population, the indication for permanent pacing will continue to grow as it still remains the effective therapy for symptomatic bradyarrhythmia patients. For decades, right ventricular (RV) has been the standard site for deploying the pacing lead. It is a safe, time-tested, technically simple, and well-tolerated procedure complemented by plenty of clinical data. Ventricular-based single chamber pacing system with fixed rates was used initially which competed with intrinsic rhythm putting the patient at risk of ventricular fibrillation. Subsequently in early 1980s, dual-chamber demand mode pacemakers with long-lived lithium iodide batteries were introduced which were able to sense and pace in both atrium and ventricle allowing physiological rates and atrioventricular (AV) synchrony.

QUEST FOR PHYSIOLOGICAL PACING

With increasing number of implants, soon it was realized that long-term RV pacing has been associated with deleterious effects on left ventricle (LV). The prevalence of pacing-induced cardiomyopathy (PIC) varies between 5.9 and 39% based on the definitions used.[1] PIC is defined as a decline in LV ejection fraction (LVEF) of <50%, absolute decline of ≥10%, and/or new-onset heart failure (HF) symptoms or atrial fibrillation (AF) after pacing.[2] RV pacing produces left bundle branch block (LBBB) on the surface electrocardiography (ECG) resulting in pre-excitation of the interventricular septum and nonphysiological activation of the LV. Altered electrical activation results in myofibrillar disarray, increased fibrosis, perfusion defect, and dysfunction. Both interventricular and intraventricular dyssynchronies have been considered as an important etiological factor for PIC. Nonapical pacing sites have been studied extensively to overcome the limitations of RV apical pacing. However, pacing either the septum or outflow tract failed to show superiority over conventional apical pacing in terms of reduction in pacing-related complications.[3] Efforts were made to reduce the ventricular pacing by algorithms without much difference in clinical outcomes. Search for an ideal pacing site which would provide electrical and mechanical synchrony as close as to the normal ventricular activation resulted in direct capture of conduction system fibers.

HIS BUNDLE PACING

Though temporary His bundle pacing (HBP) has been attempted to correct wide QRS in patients with conduction system disease, clinical feasibility was first demonstrated by Deshmukh et al.[4] in the landmark study of patients with AF with HF. HBP was successful in 12 out of 14 patients using standard pacing leads by reshaping the stylet, which resulted in improvement in LVEF from 20 to 31% along with reduction in LV end-diastolic diameter (LVEDD). With the availability of specialized sheaths and pacing leads, support from several multicenter trials, and social media platform (#dontdisthehis), HBP gathered significant momentum and considered no longer a difficult procedure. HBP is performed with continuous recording of intracardiac electrograms and 12-lead ECG. His signals are recorded from pacing lead tip either in the electrophysiology system or in pacing system analyzer (PSA). The pacing lead along with the sheath is placed in the distal HB to obtain a small atrial electrogram, sharp His signal, and ventricular electrogram with a normal His electrogram to ventricular electrogram interval (35–55 ms). It is essential to ensure that the lead is positioned distal to site of the block before deploying it by four to five rapid rotations. Rebound of the lead after rapid rotations will confirm the penetration of membranous septum. Current of injury (COI) in the His signals from the lead tip electrogram predicts adequate penetration, lead stability, and stable capture threshold during follow-up. Unipolar capture threshold of <1.5 V at 1 ms pulse width and a sensed R-wave amplitude of >1.5–2 mV without atrial oversensing are considered as acceptable parameters. In patients with AV block, Vijayaraman et al.[5] showed 84% success rate for HBP with higher correction rate for AV nodal block (93%) as compared to those with infranodal block (76%). Similarly in patients eligible for cardiac resynchronization therapy (CRT), Sharma et al.[6] reported 90% procedural success with significant improvement LVEF and clinical symptoms. In patients with LBBB and LV dysfunction, Huang et al.[7] showed 76% success rate with >85% echocardiographic super-response rate. However, HBP has been shown to be associated with high capture threshold, lead dislodgment, atrial oversensing, ventricular undersensing, and premature battery depletion. An increase in pacing threshold by >1 V was observed in 12% of patients during 5-year follow-up.[8] Lead revisions may be required in 5–7% of patients.[9]

LEFT BUNDLE BRANCH PACING

With the pursuit to overcome the limitations of HBP, Huang et al.[10] suggested distal conduction system capture by deep sepal placement of the lead to directly pace the left bundle branch fibers. Left bundle branch pacing (LBBP) is defined as capture of proximal left bundle or one of its fascicles along with septal myocardium at a low capture threshold.[11] Left bundle branch area pacing (LBBAP) is defined as the capture left subendocardial area with or without simultaneous conduction system capture and includes LBBP, left fascicular pacing, and LV septal pacing (LVSP).[12] Anatomically, LBBP provides wide area of target as the fibers fan out as an extensive network on the LV subendocardium as compared to narrow band of HB. It is essential to confirm LBB capture and to differentiate it from LVSP to obtain better electrical and mechanical synchronization. LBB capture can be confirmed by paced QRS morphology of RBB delay pattern (qR/rSR in lead-V_1) along with one of the following criteria:[13]

- Demonstration of LBB potential
- Output-dependent change in QRS morphology—nonselective to selective or nonselective to septal transition at near threshold output
- Abrupt shortening of R-wave peak time (RWPT), as measured in lead V_5/V_6 (from the pacing artefact to the peak of R-wave) along with short and constant value at high- and low-pacing output.
- *Physiology-based ECG criteria*: Paced RWPT equals the native RWPT and paced RWPT equals the LBB potential to V_6
- V_6–V_1 interpeak interval >44 ms
- Programmed deep septal stimulation to demonstrate change in QRS morphology, duration, and axis

IMPLANTATION TECHNIQUE

The procedure is performed with continuous monitoring of intracardiac electrograms and 12-lead ECG. A preprocedural echocardiography will help in assessing the thickness of interventricular septum, scar, and dilatation of cardiac chambers. The tools required for implantation include sheath and pacing lead. Both fixed curve and deflectable sheaths are available for deploying the lead in the left bundle branch area. The most commonly used pacing lead is the lumenless 4.1-F sized SelectSecure™ lead (Medtronic Inc, Minneapolis) though conventional stylet-driven leads are also evaluated in various studies.

The distal extent of the His bundle is delineated by the temporary quadripolar catheter placed through femoral venous access or by the pacing lead. The delivery sheath along with the pacing lead is placed 1–1.5 cm apical to the His bundle along an imaginary line connecting the distal His signals to the RV apex **(Figs. 1A to C)**. The target area for deep septal deployment is identified by pace mapping from the right side of the septum to obtain a "W" pattern in lead-V_1, discordant QRS complexes in lead aVL and aVR. A tall R-wave in lead-II predicts proximal left bundle capture while a deep S-wave predicts posterior fascicular capture. It is essential to get a perpendicular sheath-septal orientation by

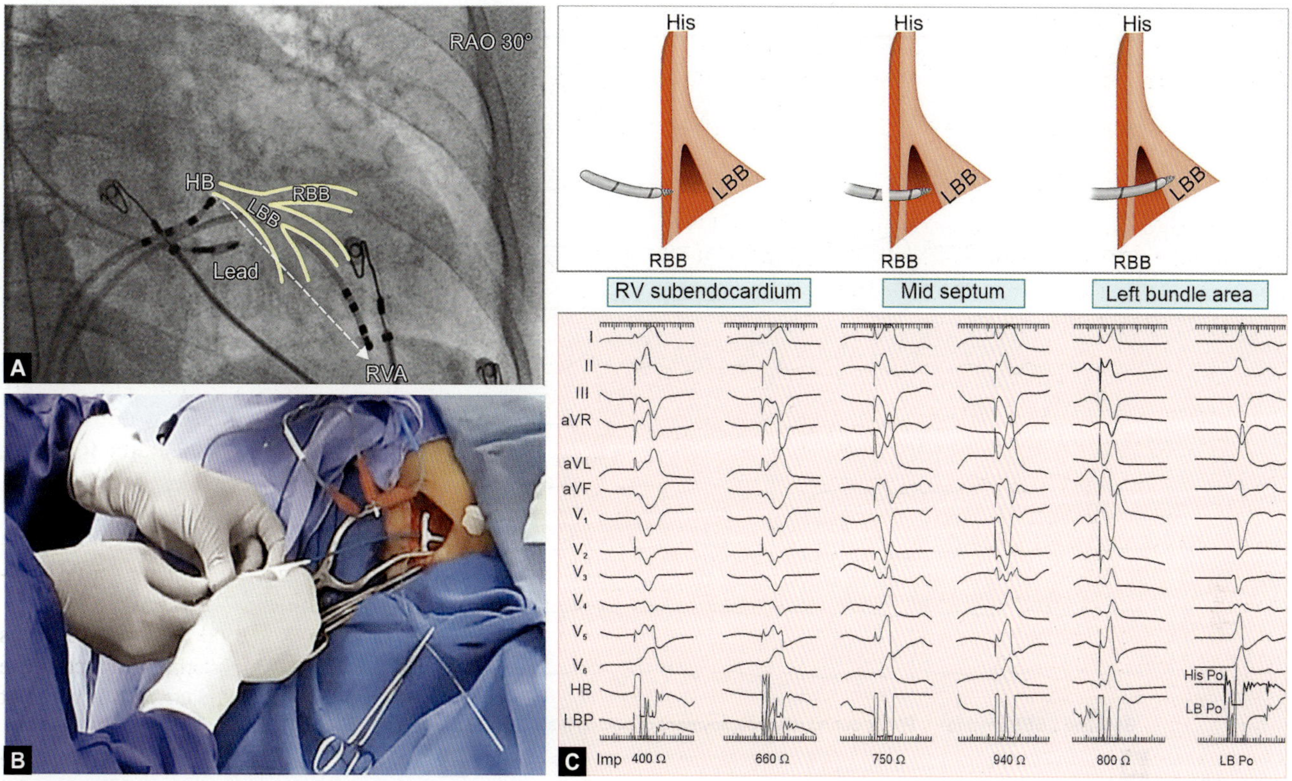

FIGS. 1A TO C: LBBP implantation technique. (A) Right anterior oblique (RAO) fluoroscopic view showing the target site for the placing the lead. (B) Rapid rotations to be given closer to the hub of the sheath with both the hands. (C) Changes in QRS morphology, duration, and unipolar impedance during the lead implantation. Note the notch in the nadir of V_1 gradually ascends up to form R-wave along with reduction in QRS duration.

(HB: His bundle; LBB: left bundle branch; LBBP: left bundle branch pacing; RBB: right bundle branch; RVA: right ventricle apex)

Source: With permission from Ponnusamy SS, Vijayaraman P. How to implant His bundle and left bundle pacing leads: Tips and Pearls. Cardiac Failure Review. 2021;7:e13.

gentle counter-clockwise torque of the sheath for successful lead deployment. After identifying the optimal target site, the lead deployment can be done by any one of the two techniques—(1) conventional method (gradual deployment with close monitoring of unipolar pacing impedance and paced QRS morphology), and (2) premature ventricular complex (PVC)-guided method (rapid deployment with monitoring of the PVC morphology.[14,15]

In conventional method, the lead is deployed gradually with monitoring of unipolar impedance (gradual rise before it drops by 100–150 Ohms as the pacing lead reaches LV subendocardium) and paced QRS morphology (gradual change in QRS morphology as the notch on the nadir of V_1 ascends up to form R-wave). In PVC-guided approach,[14,15] rapid rotations are given to deploy the lead in left anterior oblique (LAO) fluoroscopic view. PVCs are commonly generated during rapid lead movement. The morphology of PVCs changes from QS to qR/rSR in lead-V_1 as the lead traverses from right to left side of the septum **(Figs. 2A and B)**. Template beat is defined as PVC with right bundle branch delay (RBBD) pattern and QRS duration of <130 ms.[15] Rapid rotations should be stopped after observing the template beat as further rotation will result in perforation of the septum. A sharp high-frequency LBB potential preceding the local ventricular electrogram by 15–35 ms is seen in all patients with baseline non-LBBB morphology. Nonselective to selective capture transition is observed at near-threshold pacing output value **(Figs. 2A and B)**. Selective LB capture is characterized by change in QRS morphology (rSR in lead-V_1, increase in amplitude and duration of S-wave in lead-V_6, and rounded terminal-R wave in lead-aVR) and a distinct interval between pacing artefact and local ventricular electrogram. Nonselective LB capture is characterized by pseudo-delta wave on the surface ECG and pacing artefact immediately followed by local ventricular electrogram. R-wave peak time as measured in lead-V_6 from pacing artefact to peak of R-wave should be short and constant at high and low pacing output. After confirming LBB capture, the sheath is removed after providing adequate slack for the lead. Anodal capture threshold is measured by gradually reducing the pacing output in bipolar configuration.

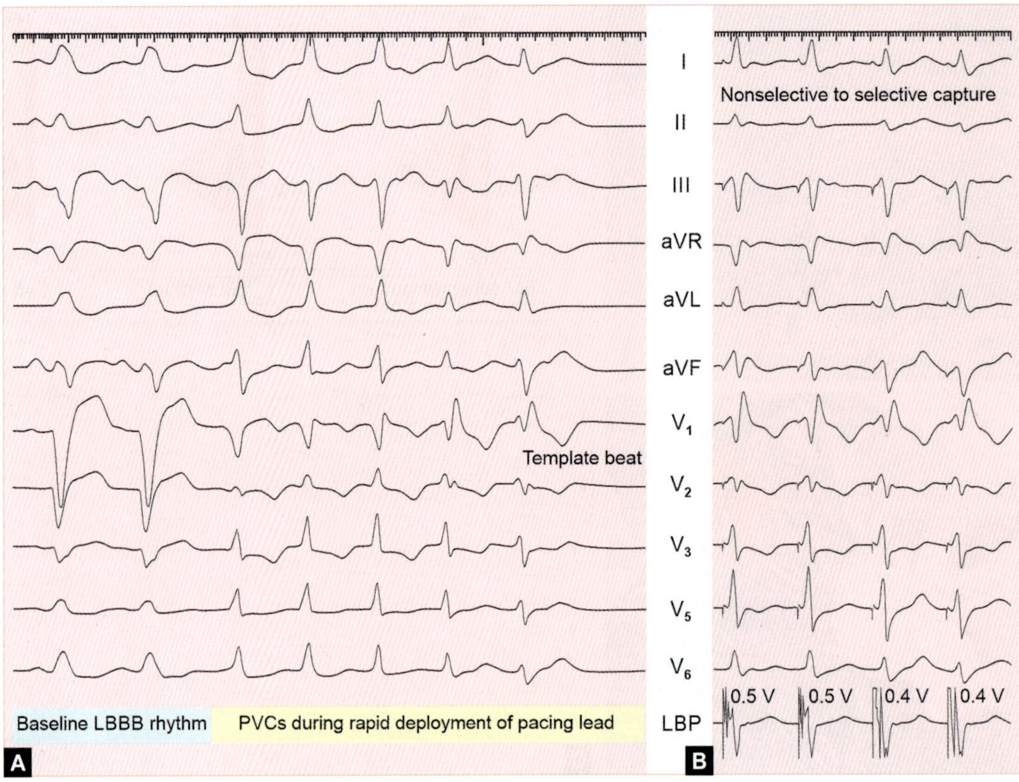

FIGS. 2A AND B: (A) Premature ventricular complexes during rapid lead deployment. Note the gradual change in the morphology of the PVCs from QS to rSR as the lead traverses from right to left side of the septum. (B) Output-dependent change in QRS morphology—nonselective to selective capture transition at near threshold pacing output.

(LBBB: left bundle branch block; PVC: premature ventricular complex)

Source: Modified with permission from Ponnusamy SS, Vijayaraman P. My preferred approach to left bundle branch pacing: Lumenless leads. Heart Rhythm O2. 2023;4(2):147-53.

SEPTAL PERFORATION

The incidence of septal perforation varies between 0.3 and 14.1%.[16] Unfiltered unipolar electrogram (0.5–500 Hz) from the lead tip is used to identify septal perforation during implantation. A significant drop in COI and presence of either type-I (QS) or type-II (RS) pattern in the unipolar electrogram will indicate septal perforation during implantation **(Figs. 3A and B)**. Complete perforation will show type-I pattern with complete loss of capture while partial perforation of helix into the LV cavity will show type-II pattern with intact capture of septal myocardium in majority of the patients. Unipolar pacing impedance of <450 Ohm has 100% sensitivity and 96.4% specificity for diagnosing septal perforation. It is essential to monitor unipolar parameters as bipolar might still show COI when the lead tip has already perforated. Lead has to be removed from the perforated site and repositioned at a different site. Accidental repositioning of the lead at the same site can be diagnosed by fluoroscopic landmark, absent template beats during deployment, similar paced QRS morphology, and hypertransmission of rotations to the lead tip inside the septum. Prompt identification of septal perforation and immediate repositioning of the lead at a different site will help in avoiding long-term complications.

LEFT BUNDLE BRANCH PACING IN SCARRED VENTRICLE

There is growing evidence to suggest that quantification of scar by cardiac magnetic resonance (CMR) imaging with late gadolinium enhancement (LGE) will guide in deployment of coronary sinus lead, assessing the scar burden, and long-term prognosis of patients with cardiomyopathy. Deployment of the coronary sinus lead in the scar will result in wide bizarre paced QRS morphology along with increased risk of ventricular arrhythmias. The response to CRT will be suboptimal in these subgroups of patients. Septal scar is considered as one of the limiting factors for successful LBBP **(Figs. 4A to D)**. In a retrospective observational study, Ponnusamy et al.[17] showed the efficacy of CMR in predicting procedural success in patients with scarred LV. The procedural success was low (64%) in cardiomyopathy patients with scar as demonstrated by LGE-CMR. A transmural scar in the LBBP zone defined as inferior aspect

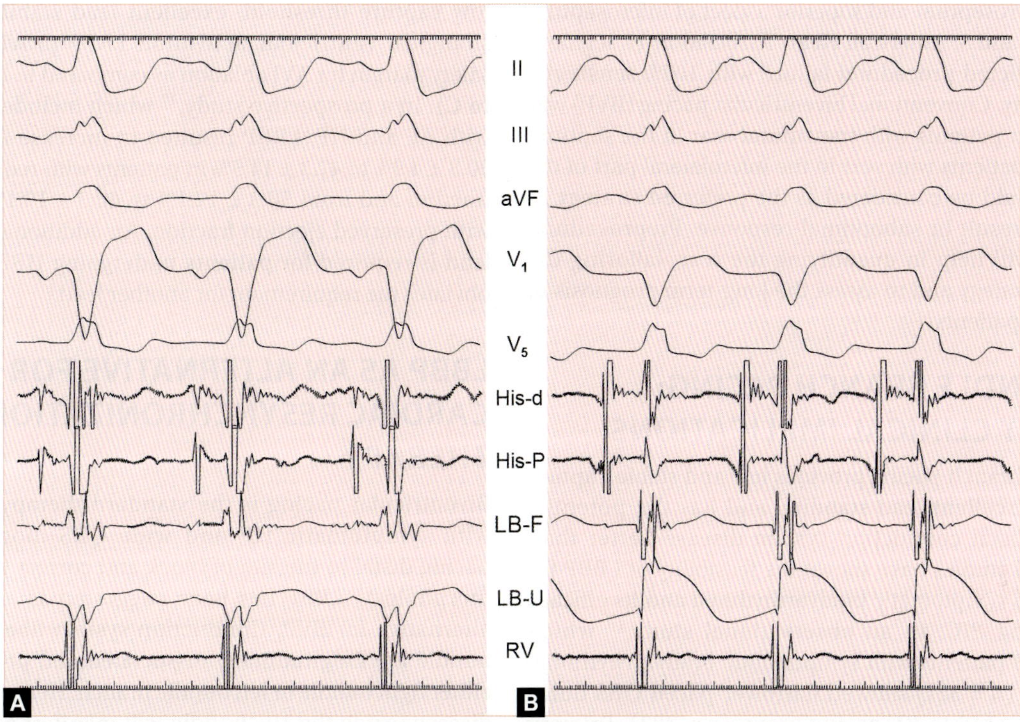

FIGS. 3A AND B: (A) Septal perforation during LBBP. Unfiltered unipolar electrogram (LB-U) showing QS pattern (type-a) along with absent current of injury (COI). (B) Lead repositioned at a different site showing significant COI.

(LB-F: filtered unipolar electrogram; LBBP: left bundle branch pacing; His-d and His-P: His bundle signals distal and proximal)

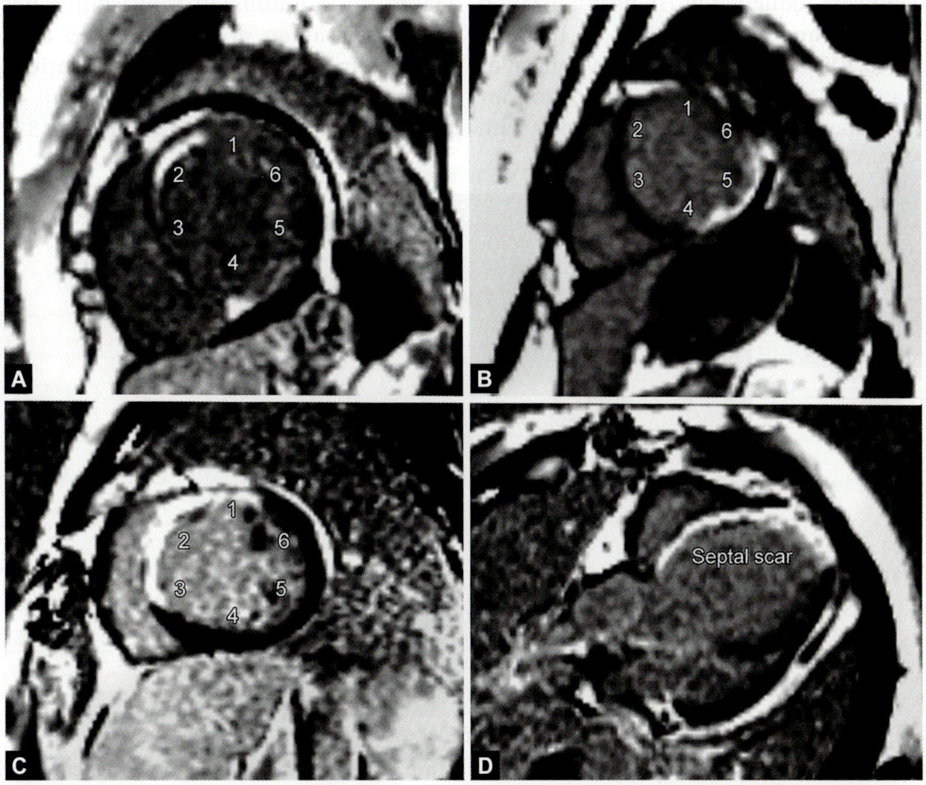

FIGS. 4A TO D: LBBP in scarred ventricle. (A and B) CMR showing LGE in superior aspect of segment 2 (A) and segments 4, 5, and 6 (B). Both these cases had a successful procedure as LBBP zone was free of scar. (C and D) CMR showing transmural scar in the interventricular septum resulting in procedural failure.

(CMR: cardiac magnetic resonance; LBBP: left bundle branch pacing; LGE: late gadolinium enhancement) of basal anteroseptum and superior aspect of inferoseptum (segments 2 and 3; American Heart Association 17 segment model) predicted procedural failure with 100% sensitivity and specificity. Conventional biventricular pacing (BVP) was performed in patients with transmural scar in the septum. Similarly in patients with scar in the inferolateral part of the LV, LBBP could be considered as the preferred strategy as BVP would result in suboptimal response. Preprocedural LGE-CMR will help in quantifying the scar, tailoring the treatment strategy and to assess the long-term prognosis of CRT eligible patients.

LEFT BUNDLE BRANCH PACING: CURRENT CLINICAL IMPLICATIONS

Left bundle branch pacing provides low and stable capture threshold, excellent lead stability, and has the potential to correct distal conduction system disease better than HBP. Several studies have shown the feasibility of LBBP for patients with symptomatic bradyarrhythmia and its efficacy in preventing PIC. In an observational study,[18] which included 703 patients with symptomatic bradyarrhythmia, LBBP group (n = 321) showed narrower-paced QRS duration as compared to RV pacing group (n = 382). Primary composite endpoint of all-cause mortality, HF hospitalization, or upgrade to BVP was significantly higher in RV pacing group (23.3%) as compared to LBBP (10%). LBBP was associated with significant reduction in HF hospitalization (37% vs. 10.5%; $p = 0.004$) and mortality (7.8% vs. 15%; $p = 0.03$) as compared to RV pacing group. Atrioventricular junction (AVJ) ablation is another evolving indication for LBBP in patients with permanent AF and HF. Along with low capture threshold, excellent lead stability and physiological ventricular activation LBBP provide adequate safety margin for AVJ ablation as compared to HBP **(Figs. 5A to C)**. In a prospective study,[19] which included 99 patients with AF and HF, LBBP resulted in increase in LVEF from 30.3 ± 4.9% to 47.3 ± 14.5% in patients with reduced ejection fraction and from 56.3 ± 12.1% to 62.3 ± 19.1% in patients with preserved ejection fraction. An additional back-up RV lead is required for patients undergoing HBP while LBBP obviates the requirement for another lead.

LBBP AS AN ALTERNATIVE FOR CARDIAC RESYNCHRONIZATION THERAPY

Biventricular pacing is the standard therapy for patients with symptomatic HF and wide QRS morphology. By pacing distal to the site of block and correct the wide QRS morphology, LBBP has been suggested as an acceptable alternative for BVP. Conduction system fibers inside His bundle are longitudinally dissociated and predestined for either right bundle or left bundle branch. Hence, a segmental disease inside the His bundle will manifest as either right bundle branch block (RBBB) or LBBB. Dyssynchronous activation of the ventricle due to LBBB can be corrected by direct capture of LBB fibers distal to site of the block. A large nonrandomized multicenter observational study by Vijayaraman et al.[20] reported 85% success rate for LBBP among 325 CRT eligible patients. LBBP resulted in improvement in LVEF from 33 to 44% ($p < 0.01$) and reducing in QRS duration from 152 ± 32 ms to 137 ± 22 ms

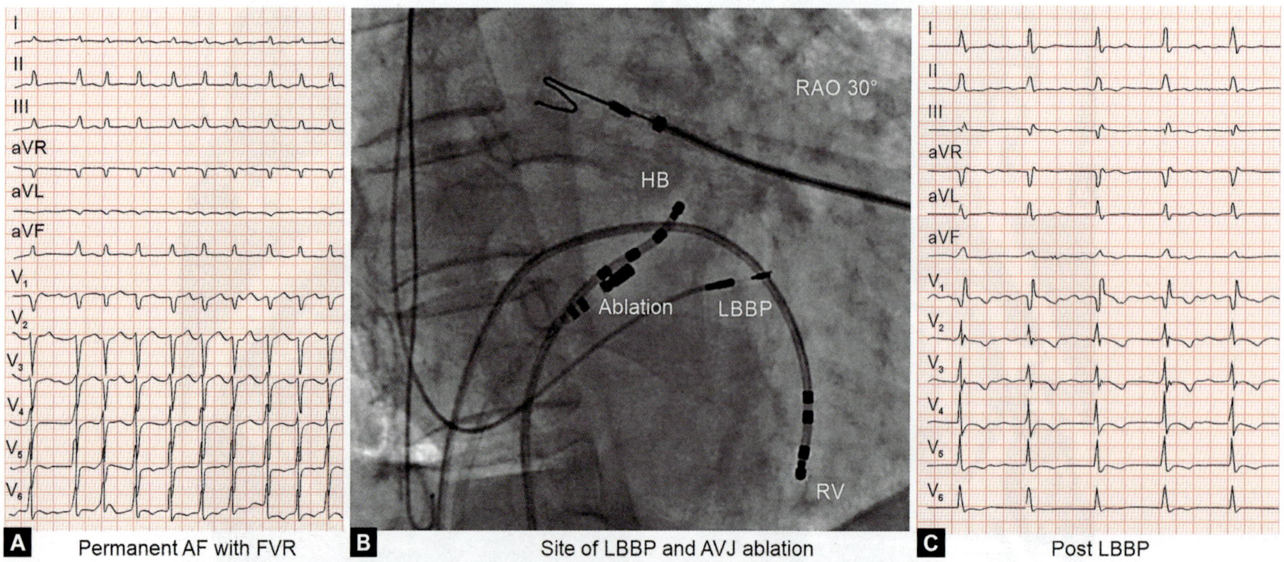

FIGS. 5A TO C: AVJ ablation with LBBP. Baseline ECG showing refractory fast ventricular rate with permanent atrial fibrillation (A). AVJ ablation was done after placing the LBBP lead (B). Note the safety margin provided by LBBP as the pacing lead is away from the site of ablation. Post AVJ ablation, ECG showing narrow paced QRS complex with right bundle branch delay pattern (C).

(AF: atrial fibrillation; AVJ: atrioventricular junction; ECG: electrocardiogram; HB: His bundle; LBBP: left bundle branch pacing; RAO: right anterior oblique; RV: right ventricular)

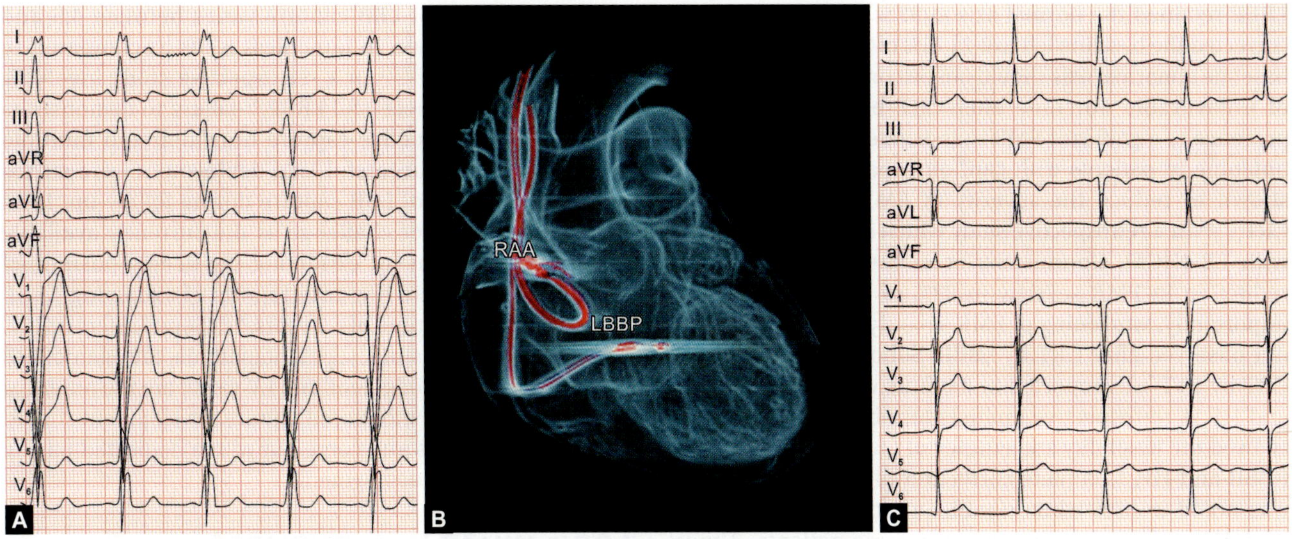

FIGS. 6A TO C: Left bundle branch pacing (LBBP) optimized dual chamber pacemaker (LOT-DDD). Baseline ECG (A) showing left bundle branch block. Pacing lead was deployed in the proximal interventricular 1.5 cm below the noncoronary cusp (B) resulted in complete correction of wide QRS (C). Note the right bundle branch delay pattern was corrected by optimizing the atrioventricular delay to achieve native AV nodal fusion.

(AV: atrioventricular; RAA: right atrial appendage)

($p < 0.01$). Another nonrandomized multicenter study[21] included 1,778 patients with class I or II indications for CRT at 15 international centers for comparing the clinical outcomes after LBBP and BVP. LBBP resulted in greater change in LVEF as compared to BVP (13 ± 12% vs. 10 ± 12%; $p < 0.001$). The primary outcome of composite endpoint of time to death or HF hospitalization was significantly reduced with LBBP as compared to BVP [20.8% vs. 28%; hazard ratio (HR) 1.495; 95% confidence interval (CI) 1.2–1.8; $p < 0.001$].

The feasibility of LBBP optimized dual chamber pacemaker (LOT-DDD) in LBBB-associated nonischemic cardiomyopathy (LB-NICM) was evaluated by Ponnusamy et al.[22] in MADURAI LBBP study **(Figs. 6A to C)**. Patients were categorized into low (<10%) or high (>10%) scar burden based on LGE quantification by CMR imaging. LOT-DDD resulted in complete correction of LBBB in 96% of study population with <10% scar burden (101/105 patients). Primary composite endpoint of death, HF hospitalization, or ventricular arrhythmias were observed in 3.8% in low scar burden as compared to 33.3% in patients with high scar burden ($p < 0.0001$). Normalization of LV function (LVEF ≥ 50%) was observed in 80% of patients with low scar burden as compared to 33.3% in high scar burden at the end of 1-year follow-up.

In a randomized trial designed[23] for showing noninferiority, 70 CRT eligible patients were randomized 1:1 to BVP or conduction system pacing. Both groups of patients showed similar reduction in LV end-systolic volume, left ventricular activation time, and rates of mortality or HF hospitalization. In another randomized trial comparing LBBP versus BVP by Wang et al.,[24] 40 patients with LBBB and NICM were included. Crossovers were observed in 10% of LBBP group as compared to 20% of BVP group. LBBP resulted in greater reductions in LV end-systolic volumes, NT-proBNP levels, and improvement in LVEF at 6 months follow-up.

LBBP FOR SUBOPTIMAL BVP RESPONDERS

A substantial proportion of patients undergoing BVP (30–50%) are considered as nonresponders to CRT therapy. Presence of significant functional mitral regurgitation (FMR), poor coronary sinus anatomy, abnormal baseline QRS axis, and non-LBBB morphology are some of the predictors of poor response to therapy. The lead may not be deployed in the optimal site inside the coronary sinus due to tortuous venous anatomy, small caliber, venous stenosis, or due to phrenic nerve stimulation in 5–7% of patients. Surgical placement of epicardial LV lead is suggested in these patients, which is associated with significant morbidity. In a multicenter study, Vijayaraman et al.[25] showed the feasibility and efficacy of LBBP in BVP failure patients. LBBP was successful in 200 out of 212 attempted patients (94% acute procedural success) and resulted in reduction in QRS duration from 170 ± 28 ms to 139 ± 25 ms ($p < 0.001$) along with improvement in LVEF from 29 ± 10% to 40 ± 12% ($p < 0.001$). Baseline abnormal axis in patients with cardiomyopathy is considered as a marker of poor prognosis and response to CRT. In a retrospective study by Ponnusamy et al.,[26] 64 consecutive patients with LB-NICM were included. Left axis deviation was noted in 37% of patients.

LBBP retained the normal axis in 93% of the patients and corrected the baseline left axis in 75% of the patients. Hence, baseline abnormal axis should not be considered as a marker of unfavorable outcome after CRT by LBBP. Similarly, presence of significant FMR is associated with unfavorable outcome in patients with cardiomyopathy. BVP has been shown to reduce the severity of FMR by 30–40% after CRT.[27,28] In a retrospective study which involved 79 patients with LB-NICM, Ponnusamy et al.[29] showed significant reduction in FMR severity in 82% of the patients. More importantly, worsening of FMR severity from baseline was not observed after CRT by LBBP. Suboptimal response to CRT by BVP was reported in patients with baseline RBBB and HF. A retrospective multicenter observational study[30] showed the feasibility and efficacy of LBBP for patients with RBBB and HF. Complete correction of RBBB morphology was noted in 33% while significant attenuation of RBBB morphology was noted in the remaining patients. Almost 61% of the patients showed ≥5% increase in LVEF from the baseline. Though LBBP is expected to produce RBB delay pattern, the mechanism of RBBB correction could be due to nonselective capture of septal myocardium along with LBB fibers and anodal capture. Future large-scale multicentric randomized trials comparing LBBP versus BVP will help in establishing LBBP as a first-line approach for CRT. Left versus left clinical trial (NCT05650658) is a multicenter randomized trial designed to compare CSP versus BVP among 2,136 CRT eligible patients and expected to start enrolling patients in the later part of this year.

LEFT BUNDLE BRANCH PACING: UNMET NEEDS

Though LBBP has been shown to produce excellent electrical and mechanical resynchronization, the long-term safety data is lacking. The effect of myocardial contractions on the lead insulation and helix tip is unknown. There are few reported cases of helix fracture.[31] There is no effective anchoring mechanism for the lead inside the septum. Periodic assessment in the device clinic at 3–6-month interval is warranted to assess the capture of LBB due to micro- or macrodislodgement during follow-up. The incidence of loss of LBB capture varies between 4.6 and 12%and less common in lumenless leads as compared to stylet-driven leads.[32,33] In a retrospective study involving 323 patients with successful LBBP,[32] failure to demonstrate nonselective to selective capture transition and multiple attempts (≥3) for successful lead deployment were strong predictors for loss of LBB capture during follow-up. Lead extraction is another challenge as the currently available tools are not meant for extracting the deeply positioned LBBP lead. There are few case reports of extracting LBBP leads with dwelling time of < 3 years.[34,35] Septal artery injury, coronary cameral fistula, septal hematoma, iatrogenic RBB injury, and lead dislodgment into LV cavity are the potential complications to be monitored. Future development should address these issues and come out with a dedicated pacing lead for deep septal deployment.

LBBP: WHAT IS IN FUTURE?

Improvement in the sheath and lead design will help in making the procedure technically easy and improve the acute procedural success rate. Leadless LBBP is an exciting technology, which combines two latest innovations in pacing. The efficacy of leadless CRT by WiSE-CRT has been reported in several observational studies.[36] All these patients received electrode in the LV lateral wall. Elliott et al.[37] showed the feasibility of LV septal endocardial pacing targeting the LBB area. The WiSE-CRT electrode has 3.6-mm tines which may be sufficient to penetrate the LV subendocardium to capture the LBB fibers. Biological pacemakers, the most physiological form of pacing, could be generated by reprogramming the somatic cells or pluripotent to generate spontaneous action potentials.[38] Biological pacing effectively avoids many of the complications of electronic pacemakers.

CONCLUSION

Conduction system pacing has gained significant momentum in the recent years. LBBP overcomes many of the limitations of HBP with better learning curve. Recent studies suggest LBBP as an acceptable alternative for providing CRT. Addressing the unmet needs in the future will help in establishing LBBP as a standard pacing strategy.

ONLINE REFERENCES

Please scan the QR code provided at the end of the table of contents for References of this chapter.

CHAPTER

215

Pacing-induced Cardiomyopathy

Anand M, John Roshan Jacob

ABSTRACT

Chronic right ventricular pacing (RVP) can lead to dyssynchronous activation of the left ventricle which over time can lead to ventricular dysfunction. Pacing-induced cardiomyopathy (PICM) is defined as either left ventricular ejection fraction (LVEF) <50% or an absolute decline in LVEF >10% with or without new-onset heart failure or atrial fibrillation in the presence of significant RVP burden and in the absence of an alternative cause. The risk factors for PICM include male sex, history of myocardial infarction, chronic kidney disease, atrial fibrillation, lower baseline LVEF, wider native QRS duration, higher RVP percentage, and wider paced QRS duration. The paced QRS duration being the only modifiable risk factor striving to achieve the narrowest QRS while placing the ventricular lead is crucial. Conduction system pacing (CSP) and algorithms to minimize RVP will help avert PICM. Cardiac resynchronization therapy (CRT) in those with ventricular dysfunction who need pacing helps prevent PICM. Besides CRT CSP is showing promise as a new modality to treat PICM.

Keywords: RV pacing, dyssynchrony, cardiomyopathy.

INTRODUCTION

Permanent pacemaker implantation is the standard treatment for symptomatic bradyarrhythmia. Conventionally endocardial right ventricular pacing (RVP) lead was placed in the RV apex in view of the simplicity of the procedure and lead stability concerns. However, chronic RVP can lead to dyssynchronous activation of the left ventricle which in the long term can lead to adverse left ventricular remodeling and dysfunction leading to pacing-induced cardiomyopathy (PICM).

DEFINITION OF PACING-INDUCED CARDIOMYOPATHY

Various studies have used different definitions to identify PICM. As a result, the prevalence reported in different studies varies from 10 to 20%. Some of the studies have used absolute left ventricular ejection fraction (LVEF) cut off <50% or 40% and a decline in LVEF by ≥10% or ≥5% with or without symptoms of heart failure in the presence of significant RVP burden.[1] In the meta-analysis by Somma et al., the most common definition used for the diagnosis of PICM was LVEF <50% or absolute decline in LVEF by ≥10%.[1] Kaye et al. compared the three different definitions of PICM to determine its prevalence: (a) LVEF ≤40%, if baseline LVEF was ≥50%, or absolute reduction in LVEF ≥5% if baseline was <50%; (b) LVEF ≤40%, if baseline LVEF was ≥50%, or absolute reduction in LVEF ≥10% if baseline was <50%; and (c) absolute reduction in LVEF ≥10%, regardless of baseline. The prevalence of PICM was highest by the third definition and it was 39% while it was 9.3% and 5.3% by the first and second definitions, respectively.[2] Of the 46 patients with PICM by the third definition, 31 patients had LVEF >50% even though there was an absolute reduction in LVEF by ≥10%. This study highlights the fact that decrement in LVEF to <50% or <40% may represent only the tip of the iceberg. Hence, using the absolute LVEF cut-off for defining PICM may underestimate the true incidence of PICM by failing to identify patients who had a clinically significant reduction in LVEF from baseline, but the absolute LVEF remained >50%.[3]

Although primarily a decrement in LVEF has been used to diagnose PICM, clinical features such as heart failure hospitalization (HFH) and the development of new-onset atrial fibrillation should be considered in diagnosing this clinical entity. In the MOST trial, >40% RVP burden was associated with a 2.5-fold increased incidence of heart failure. The rate of atrial fibrillation (AF) occurrence was also increased with RVP burden in this trial.[4] Hence, *the most acceptable definition of PICM is either LVEF <50% or absolute decline in LVEF ≥10% with or without new-onset heart failure or atrial fibrillation in the presence of significant RVP burden and in the absence of an alternative cause.*[5]

RISK FACTORS FOR PACING-INDUCED CARDIOMYOPATHY

In the meta-analysis by Somma et al., the risk factors for PICM were male sex, history of myocardial infarction, chronic kidney disease, atrial fibrillation, baseline LVEF, native QRS duration, RVP percentage, and paced QRS duration **(Fig. 1)**.[1] In a retrospective study by Perla et al. in patients who underwent pacemaker implantation, LVEF <55% at baseline, RVP percentage >33% and paced QRS duration >160 ms were associated with increased risk of PICM.[6] In this study, patients with two or more risk factors had higher risk of PICM (OR 11.62; 95% CI 4.62–29.21; p-value < 0.001) than those with one risk factor (OR 3.89; 95% CI 1.62–9.34; p-value 0.002). Among these risk factors for PICM, paced QRS duration is the only modifiable risk factor. Placing the lead to obtain the narrowest possible paced QRS duration would help reduce the incidence of PICM.[6]

RIGHT VENTRICULAR PACING BURDEN ON PACING-INDUCED CARDIOMYOPATHY

In the MOST trial, >40% RVP burden was associated with a 2.5-fold increased incidence of heart failure.[4] In the Dual Chamber and VVI Implantable Defibrillator (DAVID) trial, among candidates for defibrillator implantation, percent RVP as a continuous variable was correlated with death and HFH. As a dichotomous variable, DDDR RVP >40% was associated with an increased incidence of death or HFH when compared to DDDR RVP ≤40% (p = 0.025).[7] In the Multicenter Automatic Defibrillator Implantation Trial (MADIT) II study, patients with RVP burden >50% had a significantly higher risk of new or worsened heart failure [hazard ratio (HR) 1.93; p = 0.002] and ventricular tachycardia (VT)/ventricular fibrillation (VF) requiring implantable cardioverter defibrillator (ICD) therapy (HR 1.50; p = 0.02).[8] Kiehl et al. in 2016 showed that RVP percentage both as a continuous (HR 1.011 per 1% RVP; 95% CI 1.002–1.02; p = 0.021) and as a categorical (<20% or ≥20% RVP) (HR 6.76; 95% CI 2.08–22.0; p = 0.002) variable was independently associated with PICM.[9] All these studies reinforce the fact that the higher the RVP burden higher the risk for the development of PICM and ideally there is no absolute cut-off value.

Most of these studies on PICM had RV apical pacing. RV apical pacing is associated with wider-paced QRS and a higher degree of dyssynchrony when compared to RV septal pacing as septal pacing would lead to relatively earlier activation of the conduction system and be closer to physiological LV activation. Clinical studies on RV apical pacing versus non-apical RVP have shown equivocal results.[10,11] However, it is still best to avoid RV apical pacing for the abovementioned reason.

PATHOGENESIS OF PACING-INDUCED CARDIOMYOPATHY

High pacing burden is the major risk factor for the development of PICM. However, not all patients with high pacing burden develop PICM. It is not clear why some of these patients on long-term RVP do not develop ventricular dysfunction or symptoms of heart failure.

Left ventricular dyssynchrony is the main culprit behind the development of PICM. As the pacing lead does not activate the conduction system early, there is slow myocyte-to-myocyte propagation resulting in heterogeneity in myocardial activation across the ventricular septum, similar to left bundle branch block (LBBB). The latest activation site is the basal, inferior left ventricle.[12,13] This asynchronous activation and contraction will result in a redistribution of myocardial work and strain with less effective contraction.[12,14] These effects result in abnormal myocardial metabolism and altered regional perfusion, increased fibrosis and myofibrillar disarray, functional mitral regurgitation, reduced cardiac output, and increased filling pressures **(Fig. 1)**.[15-17] Adverse remodeling of the ventricles is regarded as a chronic process which generally takes months to years to manifest as cardiomyopathy. However, in a few patients there is a small but significant decrease in the LVEF which can be detected within a few hours of initiating RVP.[18] These acute effects are consistent with clinical studies wherein patients develop heart failure symptoms within a few weeks or months of high pacing burden.[19]

Merchant et al. described PICM as a dyssynchrony associated cardiomyopathy (DAC). They lumped it along with LBBB-cardiomyopathy and premature ventricular

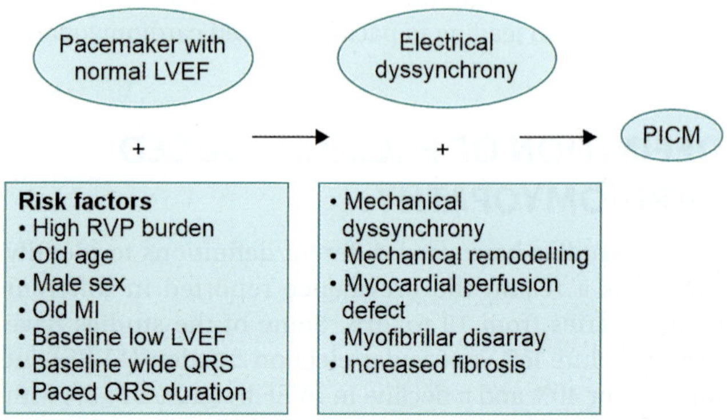

FIG. 1: Pathogenesis of PICM.

(LVEF: left ventricular ejection fraction; MI: myocardial infarction; PICM: pacing-induced cardiomyopathy; RVP: right ventricular pacing)

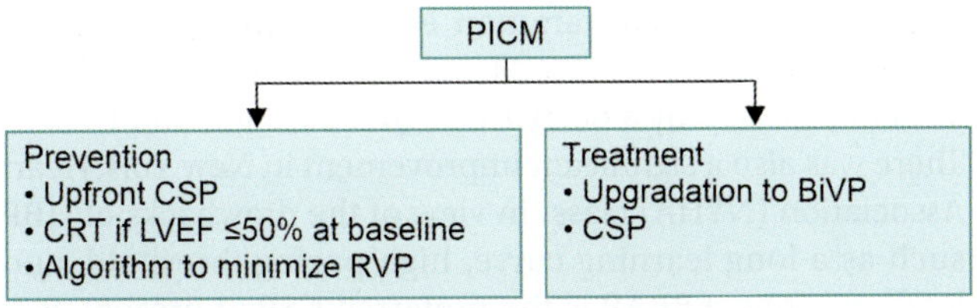

FLOWCHART 1: Prevention and treatment of PICM.

(BiVP: biventricular pacing; CRT: cardiac resynchronization therapy; CSP: conduction system pacing; LVEF: left ventricular ejection fraction; PICM: pacing-induced cardiomyopathy; RVP: right ventricular pacing)

TABLE 1: Preferred pacing strategy according to LVEF at the time of implantation.

LVEF	CSP	CRT
EF >50%	Preferred	No
EF 36–50%	Alternative	Preferred
LVEF ≤35%	Alternative	Preferred

(CRT: cardiac resynchronization therapy; CSP: conduction system pacing; EF: ejection fraction; LVEF: left ventricular ejection fraction)

contraction (PVC) induced cardiomyopathy.[3] All these three disease entities share some common features. They are:

- *Ventricular dyssynchrony*: In all three entities, intra-ventricular and interventricular dyssynchrony is the primary pathophysiological insult that can lead to left ventricular dysfunction.
- *Dose response relationship*: Several studies have shown that a higher pacing burden (generally >20%) and wider paced QRS duration is associated with the risk of PICM.[1,4,6-8] For LBBB-cardiomyopathy, the width of QRS is associated with more dyssynchrony and thereby increased risk of cardiomyopathy and its response to cardiac resynchronization therapy (CRT).[13] For PVC-induced cardiomyopathy, the burden of PVCs and the width of PVC-QRS reflect the dose of dyssynchrony and increase the likelihood of cardiomyopathy.[20,21]
- *Cardiomyopathy is reversible if dyssynchrony is eliminated*: For PICM, it can be accomplished through either reduction in RVP or upgrading to CRT with biventricular pacing (BiVP) or conduction system pacing (CSP) **(Flowchart 1)**.[22,23] For LBBB cardiomyopathy, LV function can be improved with either CRT or CSP.[13,24] For PVC-induced cardiomyopathy, LV function improves once the PVC burden is reduced either by antiarrhythmic medications or catheter ablation.[21,25,26]

PREVENTION OF PACING-INDUCED CARDIOMYOPATHY

At the Time of Pacemaker Implantation (Table 1)

- *Pacing with baseline LVEF >50%*: With the development of CSP, the paced QRS morphology is narrower and can correct LBBB or right bundle branch block (RBBB) aberrancy present at baseline. His bundle pacing (HBP) has its own limitations in the form of high pacing threshold, unstable sensing, premature battery depletion, and longer learning curve. On the other hand, left bundle branch area pacing (LBBAP) has a shorter learning curve. LBBAP has stable sensing and threshold, longer battery life and the need for lead revision is less.[5]

  In patients with anticipated high pacing burden and associated risk factors for PICM with normal LVEF, CSP should be attempted.[27] Abdelrahman et al. compared the clinical outcomes of HBP with RVP.[28] The study showed that the primary combined endpoint of death, HFH, or upgrade to BiVP was significantly reduced in the HBP group [83 of 332 patients (25%)] compared to RVP [137 of 433 patients (32%); HR 0.71; 95% CI 0.534–0.944; p = 0.02]. This difference was observed primarily in patients with ventricular pacing >20%. The incidence of HFH was also significantly reduced in HBP (12.4% vs. 17.6%; HR 0.63; 95% CI 0.430–0.931; p = 0.02). Similar results were reported by Sharma et al. for LBBAP.[29] The primary composite outcome of all-cause mortality, HFH, or upgrade to BiVP was significantly lower with LBBAP (10.0%) compared to RVP (23.3%) (HR 0.46; 95% power; CI 0.306–0.695; p < 0.001). Among patients with ventricular pacing burden >20%, LBBAP was associated with a significant reduction in the primary outcome compared to RVP. LBBAP was also associated with a significant reduction in mortality and HFH.

  His bundle pacing has been shown to improve diastolic function in patients with diastolic heart failure with RVP. Herweg et al. showed significant improvement in diastolic filling time, septal E′, and reduction in Tei Index after HBP in four out of five patients with RVP-induced diastolic heart failure.[30]

  The Biventricular Pacing for Atrioventricular Block to Prevent Cardiac Desynchronization Study (BioPACE trial) failed to demonstrate the superiority of BiVP over conventional RVP in patients with normal baseline LVEF.[31] There is limited evidence on upfront BiVP for baseline normal LVEF and currently, there is no recommendation for the same.
- *Pacing with baseline LVEF >35 to <50%*: In patients with anticipated high pacing burden with LVEF >35 to <50%, either CRT with BiVP or CSP should be done upfront.[27] In the BLOCK HF trial, Curtis et al. showed that upfront CRT when compared to standard RVP in patients with LVEF <50% with high degree AV block was associated with a significantly reduced composite endpoint of time to death from any cause, emergency visit for heart failure or increase in LV end-systolic volume index >15%.[32] Both HBP and LBBAP have been utilized as alternative or rescue options for CRT and the results have been non-inferior to CRT.[33-35]
- *Pacing indication with baseline LVEF <35%*: In patients with pacing indication and the LVEF <35%, CRT with

BiVP is the recommendation.[27] CSP with HBP or LBBAP can be used as a rescue strategy when the LV lead cannot be implanted, has a high threshold, or is non-responder to CRT.[33,35]

On Follow-up

Switching on algorithms to minimize RVP: As a high RVP burden is associated with an increased risk of PICM, algorithms have been developed to reduce RVP and promote native AV conduction in whom only intermittent pacing is required as in sinus node dysfunction and intermittent CHB. The negative impact of these algorithms is that they can allow excessively prolonged PR intervals which can lead to an increase in LA pressure, diastolic mitral regurgitation, impairment of LV function and potentially be proarrhythmic.[5] However, there is no robust evidence to support algorithms that minimize RVP, in having net clinical benefit in reducing HFH, new-onset AF incidence, and all-cause mortality. In a meta-analysis of seven randomized controlled trials (RCTs) to assess whether ventricular pacing reduction modalities (VPRM) influence hard clinical outcomes when compared to standard dual chamber pacing mode, there was no statistical difference in the hard clinical outcomes such as the prevalence of persistent/permanent AF, all-cause hospitalization and all-cause mortality between the two groups even though RVP percentage was significantly lower in the VPRM group.[36] Hence, on an individual basis VPRM may be switched on to prevent high pacing burden **(Flowchart 1)**.

TREATMENT OF PACING-INDUCED CARDIOMYOPATHY

As RVP-induced electrical and mechanical dyssynchrony is the major factor behind the development of PICM, resynchronizing the left ventricle by BiVP is the treatment of choice. BiVP has been shown to reverse LV dilatation, LV dysfunction, and reduce mitral regurgitation.[22,23,32] In a retrospective study of CRT procedures by Khurshid et al., 69 patients with PICM underwent upgradation to CRT.[37] LVEF improved from 29.3 to 45% over a median of 7 months. Most improvement in LVEF occurred in the first 3 months, although improvement continued over the remainder of the first year. In a meta-analysis based on three studies by Somma et al. the overall response rate to CRT was around 84–86%.[1]

Conduction system pacing, either HBP or LBBAP, also resynchronizes the left ventricle by activating the His-Purkinje system. Vijayaraman et al. showed that HBP is feasible in patients with PICM and induced reverse modeling as demonstrated by a decrease in QRS duration and LVEF.[38] There was also a significant improvement in New York Heart Association (NYHA) class. In view of the drawbacks of HBP such as a long learning curve, high pacing threshold, and lead revisions, LBBAP is the preferred CSP at present as it overcomes these limitations. Rademakers et al. showed that LBBAP is feasible for treating PICM.[39] 20 patients with PICM underwent LBBAP and there was a significant reduction in QRS duration, an increase in LVEF and NYHA class at 6 months. LBBAP as compared with HBP by pacing beyond the site of conduction system disease has a higher chance of correcting LBBB with low and stable pacing parameters along with better lead stability and learning curve. However long-term safety data on LBBAP is not yet available and there are reports of delayed septal perforation with loss of left bundle capture and distal conductor fracture which are unique to LBBAP.[40,41] Hence, CSP should be used as an alternative strategy for PICM in cases where LV lead cannot be implanted, has a high threshold, or is non-responder to CRT.

Hence, upgradation to CRT (or CSP in selected cases) is the treatment of choice for PICM. However, upgradation to CRT is associated with increased procedural complications, lead revisions, cardiovascular implantable electronic devices (CIEDs) infection, and mortality as compared to de novo procedures.[42,43] Hence, every attempt must be made at the time of pacemaker implantation to prevent pacing-induced cardiomyopathy as discussed in the previous section.

CONCLUSION

Pacing-induced cardiomyopathy is characterized by a decline in LVEF from the baseline with new-onset heart failure symptoms in the presence of a high RVP burden and the absence of an alternate cause. Male sex, old myocardial infarction (MI), chronic kidney disease, preimplant QRS duration, baseline LV function, paced QRS duration, and RVP burden are some of the important risk factors for the development of PICM. Treatment of choice once PICM develops is CRT with BiVP with CSP with LBBAP being an emerging alternative. CSP has been shown to prevent the development of PICM consistently in various studies.

Further work is needed in establishing why some individuals are at higher risk of developing PICM and devising preventive strategies for these individuals. More evidence is currently required before recommending CSP as the treatment of choice for PICM.

ONLINE REFERENCES

Please scan the QR code provided at the end of the table of contents for References of this chapter.

CHAPTER 216

Left Ventricular Dyssynchrony Assessment and Cardiac Resynchronization Therapy Optimization

Siddhartha Mani

ABSTRACT

Assessment of left ventricular mechanical dyssynchrony (LVMD) received great interest with the appearance of cardiac resynchronization therapy (CRT), although guidelines still keep QRS duration as the main selection criterion. Echocardiography with advanced imaging tools, e.g., color tissue Doppler, strain imaging, and speckle tracking can objectively assess the timing and sequence of different left ventricular (LV) segment contraction and thus locate the exact site of delayed activation and dyssynchrony. On the other hand, several formulas and algorithms have been developed for atrioventricular (AV) and ventriculoventricular (VV) delay optimization during CRT implantation based on echocardiography (e.g., Ritter's method and iterative method), intracardiac electrocardiogram, impedance cardiography (IC), acoustic cardiography, etc. The aim is to minimize the dyssynchrony and yield highest cardiac output as measured by LV dP/dt of mitral regurgitation (MR) jet or aortic velocity time integral (VTI). Finally, although it is evident that AV and VV optimization using the methods available can improve the acute hemodynamic response of CRT, long-term clinical improvement is much less convincing and we need more data for that.

Keywords: LV dyssynchrony, echocardiography assessment, CRT, AV delay optimization, VV delay optimization.

INTRODUCTION

Cardiac resynchronization therapy (CRT) has become an important treatment for the management of heart failure (HF) patients with left ventricular (LV) systolic dysfunction and a ventricular conduction delay. An optimal response to CRT is not guaranteed as approximately 30% of patients do not appear to experience significant clinical improvement. So clearly, there is enough scope to improve the effectiveness of this therapy. Improvements in patient selection and device optimization are two available strategies. Echocardiography seems to be a reliable tool for correctly evaluating LV mechanical dyssynchrony and identifying candidates for CRT and thus reducing the number of clinical nonresponders. Device optimization postimplantation includes individualized programming of the atrioventricular (AV) and ventriculoventricular (VV) delay to maximize the hemodynamic and, hopefully, clinical response to CRT. There are multiple strategies for AV and VV optimization without a clear "gold standard" for comparison. Guidelines for CRT also do not provide recommendations for optimization of these parameters, reflecting a lack of consensus on this issue. Despite these limitations, AV and VV optimization may prove useful in select patients with CRT, and a working understanding of the methods and controversies involved is important for all cardiologists who manage these patients.

LEFT VENTRICULAR ENDOCARDIAL ACTIVATION

Left ventricular endocardial activation begins at 0–15 ms after the onset of the QRS and the entire activation completes within 40 ms. The duration of LV endocardial activation ranges from 28 to 50 ms. Left bundle branch (LBB) activation precedes right bundle branch (RBB) activation by 10–20 ms. The inferior border of the middle septum is the earliest area of LV endocardial activation. The superior-basal aspect of the free wall is a second endocardial breakthrough site in the area of the insertion of the anterior papillary muscle. Activation then spreads radially from these breakthrough sites so that the apex is activated relatively late. The base at

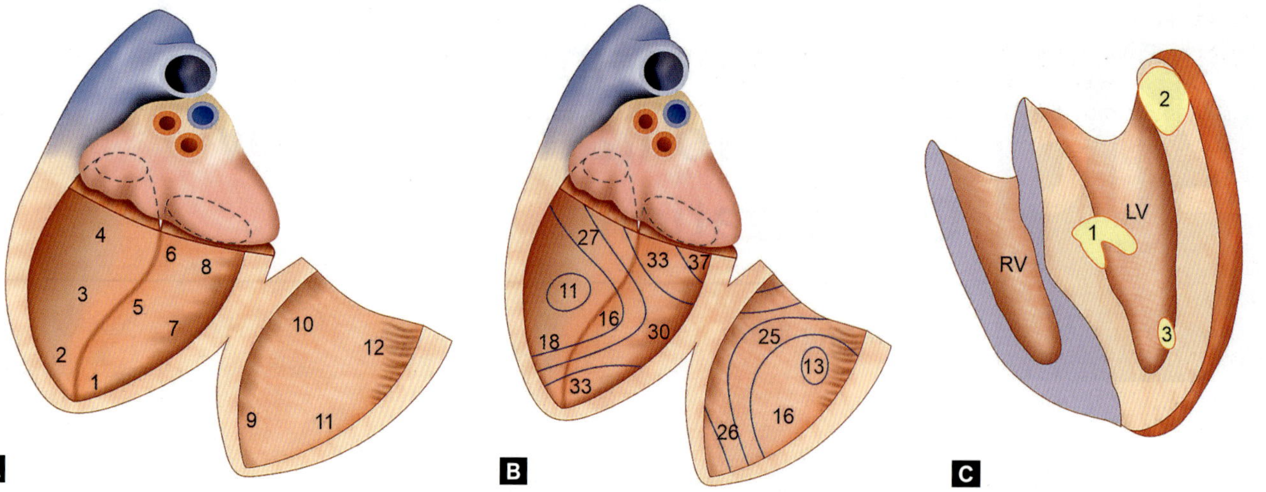

FIGS. 1A TO C: (A) Schema of mapping sites in the left ventricle: Site 1 is the apex; sites 2, 3, and 4 are on the septum; sites 5 and 7 are on the inferior wall; sites 6 and 8 are on the posterior base; sites 9 and 10 are on the lateral wall; and sites 11 and 12 are on the anterior wall. (B) Sinus rhythm isotonic map for entire group. Numbers represent mean values for local activation times for the entire group. (C) Endocardial breakthrough sites 1, 2, and 3 represents inferior border of middle septum and superior-basal aspect of the free wall and insertion of anterior papillary muscle.

(LV: left ventricle; RV: right ventricle)

the inferioposterior wall is consistently the last area to be activated. Activation of the septum is mainly left to right but does proceed in both directions. The more thinly walled right ventricle has an earlier epicardial breakthrough than the thicker LV wall. The last area of right ventricle to be activated is the pulmonary conus and postbasal region **(Figs. 1A to C)**.

LEFT VENTRICULAR CONTRACTION

Left ventricular contraction typically begins after the entire QRS is completed. It is a synchronous regional mechanical contraction with minimal difference in timings. LV systolic contraction is typically composed of three morphological events—thickening, translation, and torsion.

Thickening constitutes movement of endocardium toward the center of left ventricle. Proximal inferior-posterior and lateral wall contract relatively late. Absolute and percentage thickening is maximum at base than apex. Translation represents movement of center of left ventricle posterolaterally during systole. Due to torsion, left ventricle rotates clockwise as a whole in early systole. Then the base of the heart continues to rotate clockwise and apex starts to rotate anticlockwise. LV rotation measured by cardiac magnetic resonance (CMR) progressively decreases from apex to base. Torsion of the endocardium is greater than that of the epicardium by approximately twofold. Less torsion occurs in posterior and posteroseptal regions than in anterior and anterolateral regions.

WHAT HAPPENS IN LEFT BUNDLE BRANCH BLOCK?

The right side of the septum is activated first. Septal activation proceeds from right side (anterior) to left side (posterior). There is late activation of the posterior and lateral LV walls. The early septal contraction occurs before normal ejection when LV pressure is low and does not contribute to ejection. This process generates heterogeneous stress and strain in the left ventricle, with one wall exerting forces on the contralateral wall and resulting in stretching and thinning.

LEFT VENTRICULAR DYSSYNCHRONY

Left ventricular dyssynchrony can be intraventricular or interventricular. Not all patients with a wide QRS complex exhibit have evidence of mechanical dyssynchrony. Up to 30–50% of patients with a narrow QRS complex may have mechanical dyssynchrony measured by echocardiography.

Intraventricular Dyssynchrony (Echo Assessment)

Often dyssynchrony can be assessed visually as an early septal in-and-out motion described as septal flash or bounce.

Select either the parasternal long-axis or short-axis views. Position the M-mode cursor at the midventricular level (papillary muscle level). Set sweep speed to 50–100 mm/s. Identify the time delay from peak inward septal motion to peak inward posterior wall. Cutoff value of ≥130 ms is considered as a marker of LV dyssynchrony with a sensitivity of 100% and specificity of 63%. It predicts ≥15% decrease in LV end-systolic volume index and improvements in clinical outcome with CRT.[1]

Longer delays in septal to posterior wall motion delay were associated with greater reverse remodeling. Measurement of the septal-to-posterior wall motion delay by M-mode may be difficult in many patients because of complex septal motion–wall motion abnormalities involving the septum or posterior wall. CONTAK-Cd trial[2] and PROSPECT[3] study also identified a high degree of variability in analysis. Therefore, M-mode is not advocated to be used in isolation to quantify dyssynchrony but may be considered as supplemental to other approaches, such as tissue Doppler (TD).

Color TD M-mode is a useful adjunct to M-mode determination of LV dyssynchrony. Color-coded changes in direction help in identifying the transition from inward to outward motion in the septum and posterior wall **(Fig. 2)**.

Color Tissue Doppler

The largest body of literature to quantify dyssynchrony is represented by the assessment of longitudinal LV shortening

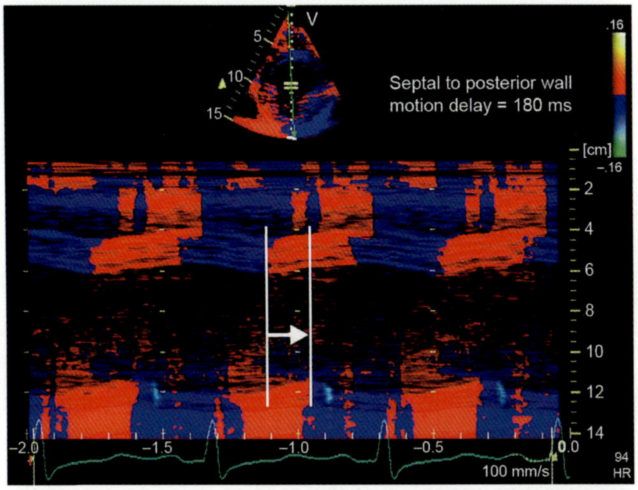

FIG. 2: Septal to posterior wall motion delay in Color TD-M mode.

velocities using TD from the apical windows. Position the left ventricle cavity in the center of the sector and align as vertically as possible. Set the depth to include the level of the mitral annulus. Patients are instructed to hold their breath transiently at end expiration, while a 3- to 5-beat digital capture is performed. Record three standard imaging planes: apical 4-chamber view, apical 2-chamber view, and apical long-axis view. Determine the LV ejection interval. This is usually done using pulsed Doppler from an apical 5-chamber or apical long-axis view, where the LV outflow tract is seen and velocity is recorded. The timing of beginning ejection to end ejection is then superimposed as the ejection interval on the subsequent time-velocity curve analysis. Size and place regions of interest in the basal and mid-region of opposing LV walls (four regions per view) to determine time-velocity plots. Manually adjust the regions of interest within the LV wall to identify the site where the peak velocity during ejection is most reproducible. Determine time from onset of the QRS complex to the peak systolic velocity for each region—four segments per view for each of the three views for a total of 12 segments. An alternative is to determine the difference in the time to peak S wave from opposing walls, as described in the opposing wall delay method **(Fig. 3)**.

Mechanical Dyssynchrony Index (Yu Index)

The 12-site standard deviation (SD) of the time-to-peak systolic velocity in the ejection phase with a cutoff value of ≥33 ms signifies mechanical dyssynchrony. To predict LV reverse remodeling (defined as a 15% reduction in LV end-systolic volume) in patients with a QRS duration > 150 ms, this cutoff value has a sensitivity of 100% and specificity of 78%.

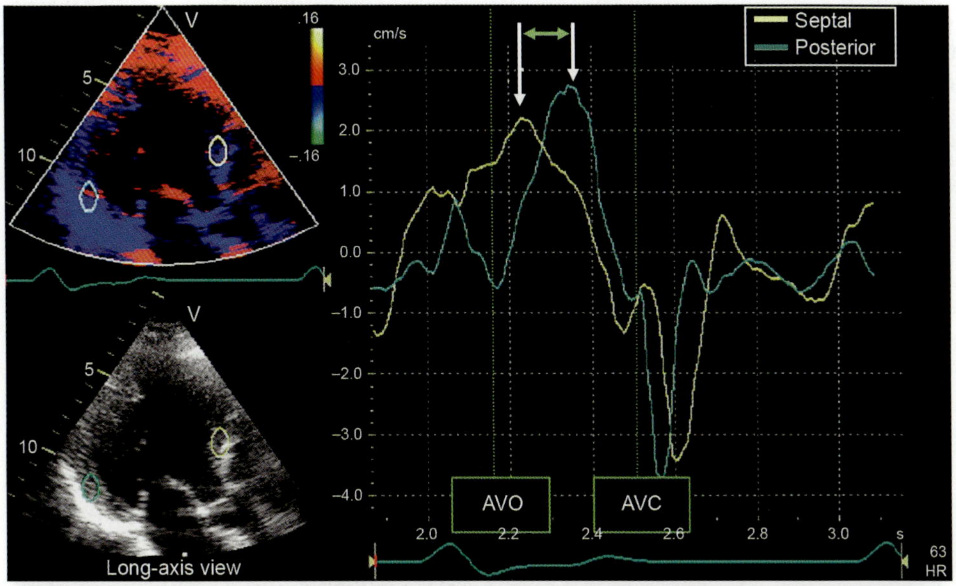

FIG. 3: Opposing wall delay method-difference in the time to peak S wave from opposing walls. (AVC: aortic valve closing; AVO: aortic valve opening)

An opposing wall peak systolic delay ≥ 65 ms is the cutoff for prediction of both clinical response to CRT and reverse remodeling. Analysis of TD data in atrial fibrillation is especially complex and problematic, and no data are currently available to support dyssynchrony analysis in this scenario.

Strain Rate Imaging and Speckle Tracking

Strain rate imaging and speckle tracking can differentiate active myocardial contraction from passive translational movement and have been utilized to identify dyssynchrony. However, TD longitudinal strain can be technically challenging because strain is calculated along scan lines, is Doppler angle dependent, and is difficult in patients with spherical LV geometry, often encountered in severe HF. Currently, TD strain rate is restricted by a poor signal-to-noise ratio. Radial thickening is a major vector of LV contraction, and short-axis dynamics are important markers of dyssynchrony. So, radial strain rate can be used to assess dyssynchrony. Speckle-tracking program is applied to routine gray-scale echocardiographic image. It determines longitudinal/radial strain from multiple points averaged to standard segments. It is not limited by Doppler angle of incidence **(Fig. 4)**.

Interventricular Dyssynchrony (Echo Assessment)

Interventricular dyssynchrony is not as useful in the prediction of response to CRT as LV intraventricular dyssynchrony. It is principally assessed as the interventricular mechanical delay (IVMD), i.e., the time difference between right ventricular (RV) and LV ejection, determined by the onset of pulsed Doppler flow velocities in the LV and RV outflow tracts, respectively. IVMD has been identified as a predictor of worsening symptom status and cardiac mortality in patients with HF and has been shown to be of prognostic value in patients with CRT (usually 40–50 ms).

CARDIAC RESYNCHRONIZATION THERAPY OPTIMIZATION

Criteria for optimal response to CRT are as follows:

- Reduction of LV end-systolic volume (LVESV) > 15%
- Percent change LV dP/d_{tmax} ≥ 25%
- 1–2 mL/kg/min improvement in peak VO_2
- One-step improvement in New York Heart Association (NYHA) class
- 10-point improvement in quality-of-life measures
- Improvement in 6-minute walking distance by 50–70 m
- Clinical responders
- Baseline QRSd > 155 ms
- Baseline LV dP/d_{tmax} of <700 mm Hg/s
- Improvement in echocardiographic indicators of LV dyssynchrony

Around 18–30% of patients fail to respond clinically to CRT; the causes being as follows:

- Suboptimal LV lead positions
- Inappropriate programming
- Lead dislodgement
- Myocardial scar
- Myocardial dysfunction

Lead Placement

Optimal LV lead placement is crucial for a favorable CRT response. In the absence of scarring, the optimal LV lead position is generally lateral or posterolateral. Apical pacing and pacing in a densely scarred region should be avoided. Multidetector computed tomography (CT) can be used for preoperative mapping of the cardiac veins to assess the availability of suitable veins in potential target segments prior to CRT implantation.[4] The CRT outcome can also be predicted by analyzing the three-dimensional (3D) coronary sinus lead-tip trajectory and optimizing its placement based on advanced imaging methods.[5] The introduction of a LV quadripolar lead provides multiple ways to pace the ventricle,

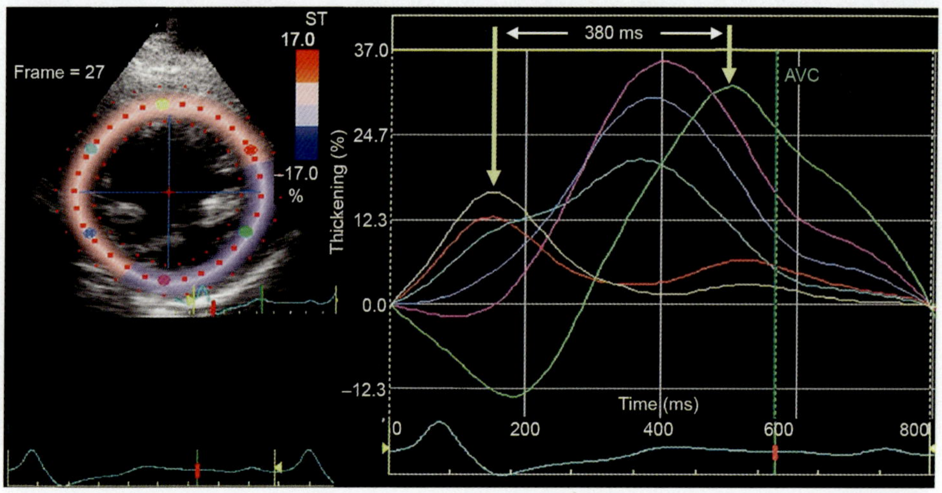

FIG. 4: Speckle tracking at multiple points to determine the radial strain.

and thus more options to avoid negative workload of the LV segments and achieve CRT optimization.[6]

Device optimization postimplantation includes individualized programming of the AV and VV delay to maximize the hemodynamic and, hopefully, clinical response to CRT. Considering additional variables such as the AV delay offset for atrial-sensed (AS) versus atrial-paced (AP) CRT and rate-adaptive AV delay modulation, the complexity of CRT programming is obvious. There are multiple strategies for AV and VV optimization without a clear "gold standard" for comparison, which make interpretation of available data challenging. Guidelines for CRT also do not provide recommendations for optimization of these parameters, reflecting a lack of consensus on this issue.[7] Despite these limitations, AV and VV optimization may prove useful in select patients with CRT, and a working understanding of the methods and controversies involved is important for all physicians who manage these patients.

ATRIOVENTRICULAR OPTIMIZATION

The importance of AV synchrony is intuitive, as preservation of both passive and active LV filling contribute to stroke volume and cardiac output. Interestingly, AV optimization may be more useful to resynchronize the left ventricle electrically than to optimize filling. Early studies in patients with complete heart block and dual-chamber pacemakers confirmed variation in stroke volume with changes in programmed AV delay.[7] In CRT, in which the majority of patients have preserved intrinsic AV nodal conduction but prolonged inter- and intraventricular conduction, AV delay programming has also been correlated with changes in LV systolic function, as measured invasively by dP/dt.[8] Furthermore, all of the major trials of CRT in HF patients, with the exception of the CONTAK-CD trial,[2] performed some method of AV delay optimization.

A pattern consistent with stage I diastolic filling (E wave lower than A wave) has not been shown to be improved on by AV alterations after CRT; hence, AV optimization is not required in these patients.

Atrioventricular optimization is recommended if:

- A wave is not identified.
- E and A waves are merged.
- A wave is truncated by mitral closure.
- If stage II (pseudonormal) or stage III (restrictive), diastolic dysfunction is present.
- Patients in atrial fibrillation or with frequent ventricular ectopy or tachycardia would not be appropriate candidates for AV optimization.

A relatively short AV delay may result in truncation of the A wave, representing atrial systole, while a prolonged AV delay can also result in shortening of total diastolic filling time.[8] One of the earliest and more commonly cited methods of AV delay optimization using mitral inflow is the Ritter method. Originally validated in patients with dual chamber pacemakers, this method involves measuring the interval from the QRS onset or pacing spike to the end of the A wave at relatively long and short AV delays, and the difference between these two is subtracted from the "long" AV delay to arrive at the optimal AV delay **(Figs. 5A and B)**.

This formula is intended to result in optimal diastolic filling time without truncation of the A wave. AV delays derived using this method have been shown to correlate with

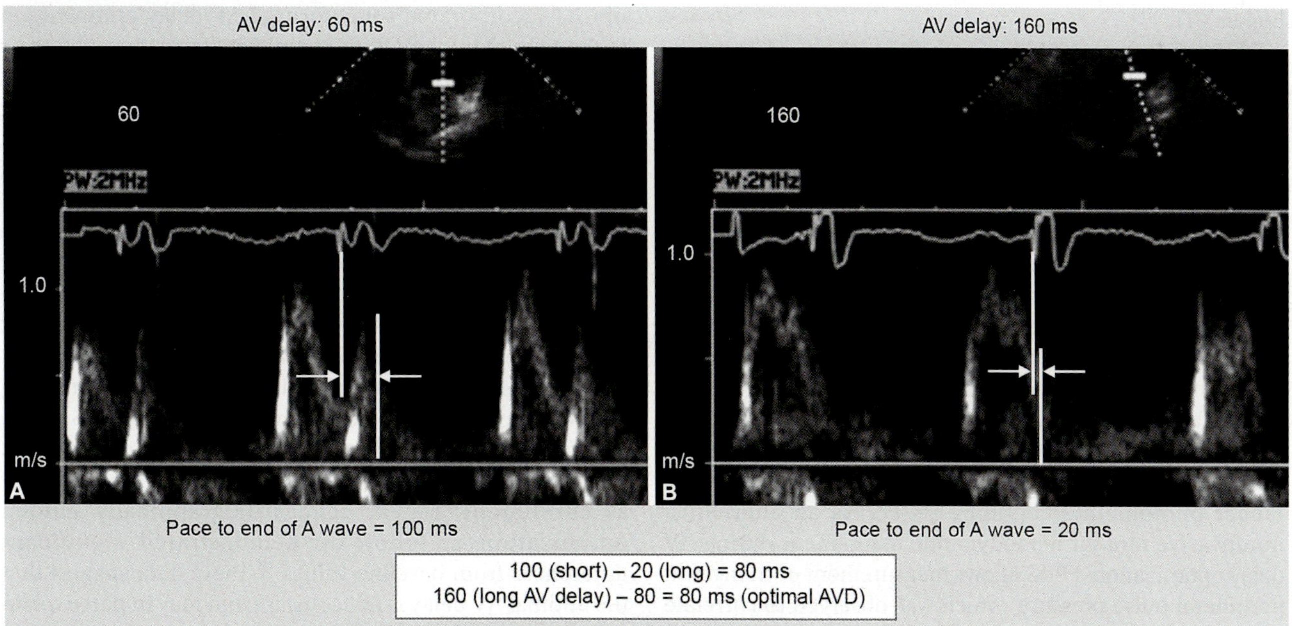

FIGS. 5A AND B: Ritter's method-optimization of AV delay.
(AV: atrioventricular; AVD: AV delay)

improvements in stroke volume [derived from impedance cardiography (IC)]. This was method of AV optimization used in the InSync III trial.[9]

Other strategies utilizing the mitral inflow pattern include a "fast and simple" approach and the iterative method.

The "fast and simple" method requires the presence of mitral regurgitation (MR) on the spectral Doppler pattern. The AV delay is set 5–10 ms below the longest AV delay, ensuring biventricular (BiV) capture. The time interval from the end of the A wave to the onset of high velocity MR (i.e., LV contraction) is subtracted from the long AV delay to arrive at the optimal AV delay. The optimal AV delay derived with this method has been shown to result in higher invasively measured cardiac output.[10]

The iterative method is the most common echocardiographic optimization technique and was used in the CARE-HF[11] and the SMART-AV[12] trials and involves programming a relatively long AV interval with gradual shortening in 20 ms steps. When truncation of the A wave is observed on the mitral inflow Doppler, the AV interval is gradually prolonged in 10 ms steps until the delay with maximal E and A wave separation is obtained. The reproducibility and consistency of measurement of this technique has been challenged despite its relative ease of use compared with other techniques.

Optimizing LV systolic performance by Doppler-derived measures of LV systolic function, e.g., LV dP/dt from the mitral regurgitant jet or aortic pulsed-wave Doppler velocity time integral (VTI) have also been applied to AV delay optimization.

In two small, nonrandomized comparisons of AV delay optimization by the aortic VTI method versus Ritter's method of mitral inflow, optimization by VTI was shown to result in a higher VTI.[13,14]

Mitral inflow VTI is another method of Doppler optimization of the AV delay.

Other Methods of Atrioventricular Optimization

All the earlier methods for AV delay optimization rely on echocardiography. While this has been the "gold standard", it requires significant training, skill, time, and healthcare resources. As a result, several alternative noninvasive tools have been developed for AV delay optimization. In general, these include noninvasive measures of hemodynamic optimization and device-based intracardiac electrogram (IEGM) algorithms. IC, for example, uses changes in transthoracic impedance to estimate stroke volume. Finger photoplethysmography (FPPG) is an alternative noninvasive tool for hemodynamic assessment during AV delay optimization. FPPG allows measurement of changes in peripheral pulse pressure, which was observed to correlate reasonably well with simultaneously measured central aortic pressure. The Finometer® (Finapres Medical Systems, Amsterdam, Holland) is a device that provides continuous, noninvasive measurement of arterial pressure through a finger cuff photoelectric plethysomgraph.[15]

Peak endocardial acceleration (PEA) is a device-based algorithm that has also been evaluated for AV delay optimization. The algorithm makes use of an accelerometer incorporated into a pacing lead behind the pacing electrode. The CLEAR trial randomized 238 patients with CRT to PEA-optimized AV/VV intervals or to "usual" optimization methods. At 1-year follow-up, response to CRT was significantly higher in the group optimized by PEA (76% vs. 62%), although this benefit was largely restricted to improvements in subjective endpoints.[16]

Finally, acoustic cardiography is another relatively new technique for AV optimization. This technology integrates the surface electrocardiogram and heart sound data to measure the intensity of S3, the electromechanical activation time (EMAT, representing the time from the QRS onset to S1), and LV systolic time (LVST, the time interval from S1 to S2). An AV delay tailored to optimize these parameters in CRT patients was comparable to the mitral inflow method.[17]

Intracardiac electrogram-based AV delay algorithms are clearly desirable given the potential for incorporation into device software for rapid optimization and potentially continuous modification. Such technology could reduce costs, time, and the possibility of user error introduced with more complex methods, such as echocardiography.

Areas of Uncertainty in Atrioventricular Optimization

It is evident that many issues regarding AV delay optimization remain unresolved. While the majority of the landmark trials of CRT incorporated some form of AV delay optimization at the time of implantation, definitive data supporting their superiority over an empiric, fixed AV delay are lacking. Most available data involve hemodynamic studies demonstrating an acute improvement with optimization. More relevant, however, are long-term, randomized, controlled studies of these interventions on clinical outcomes. With the exception of SMART-AV, comparative studies have been too small to draw meaningful conclusions. Indeed, SMART-AV suggests that empiric programming of a fixed AV delay results in similar clinical outcomes to an optimized AV delay, at least with the methods used in the trial.

Other areas of uncertainty in AV delay programming include the stability of the optimal AV delay, AP/AS offset, and rate-adaptive AV delay. In three independent studies of AV delay optimization using mitral inflow Doppler at enrollment, repeat echocardiographically guided optimization at follow-up demonstrated significant differences from baseline values.[18] These data suggest that the optimal AV delay is not constant and may in part explain the lack of long-term clinical benefit of optimization over an empiric AV delay in SMART-AV.

Given the increasing prevalence of both intrinsic and iatrogenic sinus node dysfunction in HF populations, atrial pacing is often clinically necessary and, at times, desirable. The optimal AV delay offset with AP has been shown to be patient specific and differ significantly from nominal device settings.

VENTRICULOVENTRICULAR OPTIMIZATION

From the foregoing discussion, it is clear that AV delay programming to ensure ventricular pre-excitation with optimal LV diastolic filling and systolic function is complex, and the optimal method that translates into improved patient outcomes is uncertain. These issues are even more apparent in studies of VV optimization. Several noninvasive approaches to VV optimization have been proposed, each with its own limitations. More recently, Abraham et al.[19] reported the results of a randomized study in 238 patients of simultaneous versus optimized sequential BiV pacing. The VV interval was adjusted to minimize the septal to posterior wall motion delay. At 6-month follow-up, significantly more patients had improved based on a clinical composite score with optimized sequential pacing (75%) than with simultaneous BiV pacing (65%). However, there were no significant differences in the 6-minute walk distances, quality of life, or HF event rates.

Dyssynchrony-guided Ventriculoventricular Optimization

As with AV optimization, VV optimization has most often been performed with echocardiography. VV optimization using echocardiographically derived markers of dyssynchrony is significantly limited by the time and expertise required. For example, in the PROSPECT trial to evaluate the predictive value of echocardiographic markers of dyssynchrony for response to CRT, there was significant variability in TD imaging (TDI) quality despite extensive training of study sites. More telling was a survey of AV/VV optimization practices at centers that involved the FREEDOM trial of the St Jude QuickOpt™ algorithm. The reported use of TDI was only 13.6% among centers.[20] Thus, the applicability of dyssynchrony optimization in a "real-world" clinical setting is questionable.

Aortic Velocity Time Integral Method

A simplified echocardiographic approach involves optimization of the VV interval using aortic VTI, similar to AV delay optimization. In this method, the aortic VTI is measured at varying intervals of RV and LV pre-excitation and that producing the highest VTI is used as the optimal VV delay. The InSync III trial compared the aortic VTI method of VV optimization in 422 patients using the MIRACLE study population as the control group. They demonstrated significant improvements in stroke volume and 6-minute walk distance with optimized VV pacing above simultaneous pacing alone, but there was no significant difference in improvement in NYHA class or quality of life. Subsequent studies have also failed to demonstrate an improvement in 6-month clinical outcomes with aortic VTI-optimized VV intervals over simultaneous BiV pacing.[21,22]

Other Methods of Ventriculoventricular Optimization

Despite limited data demonstrating improved outcomes with echocardiography-guided VV optimization, several other approaches have been developed. These include real-time intracardiac echocardiography during CRT implantation,[23] electroanatomic mapping,[24] radionuclide angiography,[25] the Finometer®,[26] PEA, and optimization using the surface QRS.[27,28] Several device-based IEGM algorithms for VV optimization have also been developed and evaluated.

The St Jude QuickOpt™ algorithm (St Jude Medical, Inc, St Paul, Minnesota, USA) calculates the optimal AV delay and VV offset based on IEGMs measured from the right atrial (RA), RV, and LV leads. The AV delay is determined from the duration of the sensed atrial electrogram—if >100 ms, 30 ms is added to calculate the optimal AV delay and if <100 ms, 60 ms is added. For the paced AV delay offset, 50 ms is added to the sensed AV delay. The VV offset determination is more complex. The time interval between sensed local activation between the RV and LV leads is first measured (Δ). The difference in conduction delay to the RV lead during LV pacing and LV lead during RV pacing is then calculated (ε). The estimated optimal VV offset is then given by the formula $VV = 0.5\ (\Delta + \varepsilon)$, with positive values indicating LV preactivation and negative values indicating RV preactivation. This algorithm was initially evaluated in 11 patients and found to correlate well with the optimal VV delay obtained using the aortic VTI method.[29] However, subsequent validation studies have shown conflicting results, with some demonstrating a good correlation with echocardiographically optimized VV delays and others suggesting inferior performance of the algorithm.[30] More importantly, there are no prospective data on the effect of this algorithm on long-term clinical outcomes.

Other IEGM-based algorithm utilized in Boston Scientific and Medtronic (Medtronic, Inc, Minneapolis, Minnesota, USA) devices has been evaluated as well. However, the studies do not prove either optimization strategy superior to empiric AV/VV delay programming.

Areas of Uncertainty in Ventriculoventricular Optimization

It is evident that while VV optimization using the methods available can improve the acute hemodynamic response of CRT, long-term clinical improvement above that derived from simultaneous BiV pacing has not been definitively proven. There are several possible explanations for this discrepancy in results. First, the methods used for VV optimization may be suboptimal to achieve adequate inter- and intraventricular resynchronization. As previously discussed, the technical difficulty of Doppler optimization methods introduces the possibility of operator error. IEGM-based algorithms do not account for LV lead location, which can influence the degree of pre-excitation required for maximum resynchronization. An additional methodological concern involves the sequence of AV and VV optimization. In almost all studies of VV optimization, AV delay optimization was performed, first followed by VV optimization. The utility of this strategy has been questioned by a study that determined the optimal AV/VV settings by testing 45 different combinations of AV and VV intervals. The optimal settings identified with this method were significantly different from a strategy of optimizing the AV or VV interval first. Secondly, the magnitude of hemodynamic improvement with optimized VV pacing may be too small to be clinically meaningful. Third, it has been repeatedly shown that the optimal VV delay, like the AV delay, varies over time and with exertion.[31] Programming a fixed, though optimized, VV interval at the time of implantation would then be similar to empiric programming at long-term follow-up.

CONCLUSION

Finally, it may be that VV optimization has been applied to the wrong population of patients. The majority of CRT recipients appear to benefit from BiV or LV pacing, particularly in the presence of a left bundle branch block (LBBB). Whereas VV optimization may not improve response rates in an unselected population of CRT patients, focused application in patients with a suboptimal response or non-LBBB morphologies could potentially be beneficial. This question was addressed in a study of 65 patients identified as "nonresponders" who were randomized to simultaneous BiV pacing or VV optimization. Response rates were 18.9% higher at 9-month follow-up in the optimized group, although this difference was not statistically significant and 50% of patients in the control group became responders.

ONLINE REFERENCES

Please scan the QR code provided at the end of the table of contents for References of this chapter.

CHAPTER

217 Sinus Node Disorder: Diagnosis and Management

Vijay Garg, Himanshu Jain, Shivangi Tiwari, Siddhant Gupta

ABSTRACT

Sinoatrial (SA) node is the natural pacemaker of heart, located in superior right atrium. The sinus node dysfunction (SND) is closely associated with risk factors such as atrial fibrillation and aging. The syndrome is commonly associated with disease in elderly individuals given the role of degenerative fibrosis and age-dependent alterations in its pathogenesis, presenting generally with lightheadedness, palpitations, presyncope, and syncope. Most common cause of SND is replacement of sinus node tissue by fibrous tissue; other causes include use of medications such as calcium channel blockers or β-blockers. Diagnosis of such patients is made on basis of surface ECG or 24-hour Holter monitoring. Treatment of sinus node disorders includes removal of extrinsic cause; however, the management is mostly medical, later stages may warrant the need of pacemaker placement.

Keywords: Pacemaker, atrial fibrillation, 24-hour Holter monitoring, sinus node dysfunction.

INTRODUCTION

The sinoatrial node (SAN) is a spindle-shaped structure composed of a fibrous tissue matrix with closely packed cells. It is 10–20 mm long and 2–3 mm wide and tends to narrow caudally toward the inferior vena cava (IVC). It lies <1 mm from the epicardial surface, laterally in the right atrial sulcus terminalis at the junction of the superior vena cava (SVC) and right atrium **(Fig. 1)**.[1]

Bachmann's bundle is a prominent interatrial muscle bridge that extends across the roof of the atria anterosuperior to the fossa ovalis. Conduction over Bachmann's bundle leads to early endocardial activation in the anterior left atrium in order to help facilitate interatrial synchrony. Normal conduction velocities within the sinus node are slow 2–5 cm/s, it increases the likelihood of intranodal conduction block.[1]

The term "sinus node dysfunction (SND)" was discovered in 1967 and initially, it represents the delayed functioning of the SAN in patients with electrocardioversion. Recently, SND is described as a group of disorders where the efferent functions of the SAN are malformed due to alterations in it and its associated tissues, thereby resulting in chronic arrhythmia with an inappropriate supply of blood to the heart, brain, and other parts of the body.[2,3]

In addition, supraventricular tachycardia occurs in around 50% of patients with SND syndrome and is a particular indicator of its occurrence.

In DANPACE trial study, report stated that the incidence, epidemiological, and prognostic significance of syncope in 1,415 patients with SND in a follow-up of 5 years show a higher mortality rate. The epidemiological studies reported that the age of occurrence of SND is between 20 and 90 with an increasing trend with age. The SND was reported more prevalent among older individuals with a 5-year survival rate between 62 and 65% and embolism incidence reported was 16%.[4] The incidence of SND has been showing increasing trends in United States since 2012, with an estimate of 75,000 individuals having SND every year. Around 1 in every 500 individuals above 65 years of age and suffering from a cardiovascular disorder was an SND patient. It was also projected that by the end of the year 2060, there will be more than 2 lakh new cases of SND in the United States every year.[5]

Till now, pacemaker implantation has been recognized as an efficient treatment strategy for SND, with >50% of pacemaker transplantation surgeries have occurred worldwide.[6] Nevertheless, there are still various patients for whom a pacemaker is suitable and also there are no reports available on mortality rate reduction among patients after

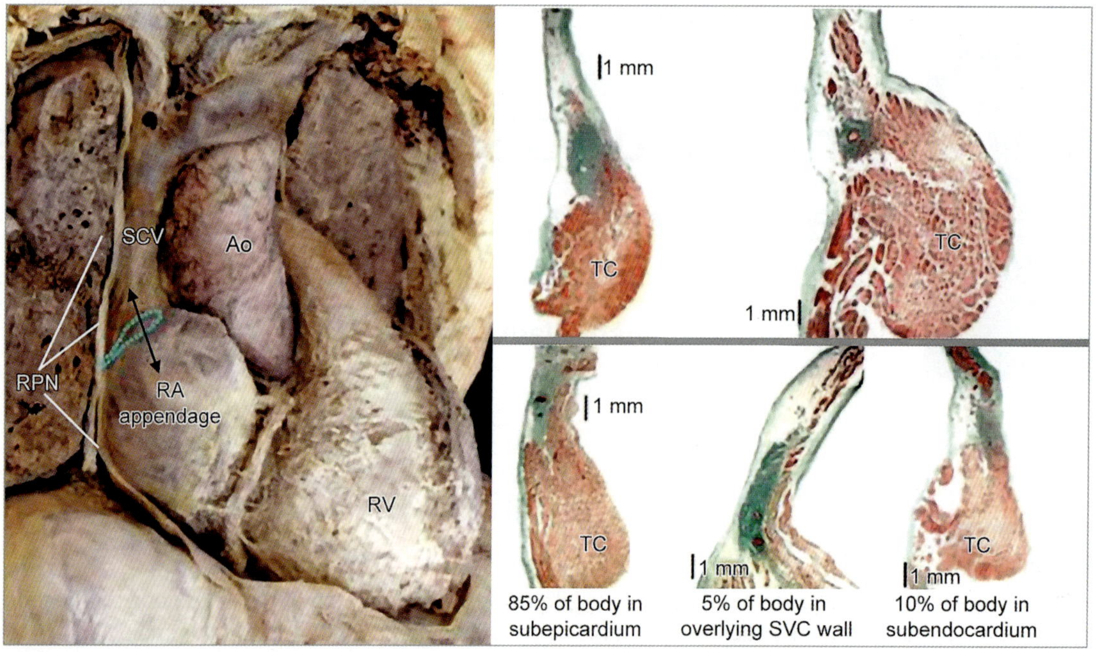

FIG. 1: Sinoatrial node.

pacemaker implantation.[7] In recent years, in order to oppress the drawbacks of conventional pacemaker implantation, more focused and well-detailed research is required on biological pacemakers which is becoming a research hotspot nowadays.[8]

FUNCTIONING OF SINOATRIAL NODE

Wit and Cranefield defined automatic activity as activity that arose in the absence of an external cause (i.e., activity that did not have to be triggered by a stimulated action potential). The prototypical example of automaticity is the spontaneous beating of the SA node. The sinoatrial (SA) node normally displays the highest intrinsic rate. All other pacemakers are referred to as subsidiary or latent pacemakers because they take over the function of initiating excitation of the heart only when the SA node is unable to generate impulses or when these impulses fail to propagate.[9]

The ionic mechanism(s) underlying SAN cell automaticity include(s) HCN channels in the surface membrane or intracellular Ca^{2+} oscillations affecting Ca^{2+}-sensitive ion channels and ion transporters in the cell surface membrane as the main regulators of the heart rate. Excess electrical coupling depresses SAN automaticity because the SAN membrane potential is damped by the surrounding atrial myocardium to a more negative potential than the normal maximal diastolic potential, thereby inhibiting spontaneous diastolic depolarization.[10]

Blood Supply

The artery supplying the SAN branches from the right (55–60% of the time) or the left (40–45%) circumflex coronary artery and approaches the node from a clockwise or counterclockwise direction around the junction of the SVC and right atrium **(Fig. 2)**.[11]

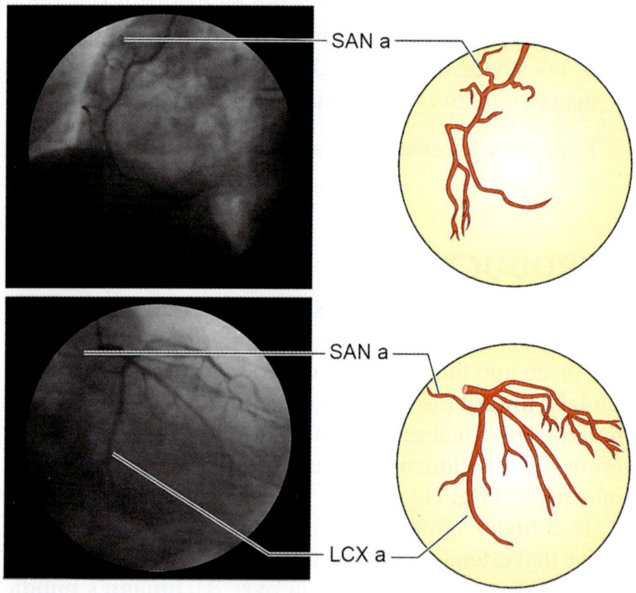

FIG. 2: Angiographic view of sinoatrial node (SAN) node blood supply. (LCX: left circumflex)

Source: Adapted from Ramanathan L, Shetty P, Nayak SR, Krishnamurthy A, Chettiar GK, Chockalingam A. Origin of the sinoatrial and atrioventricular nodal arteries in South Indians: an angiographic study. Arq Bras Cardiol. 2009;92:342-8.

SINUS NODE DISORDER

Figures 3 and 4 represent etiology of sinus node disorder.

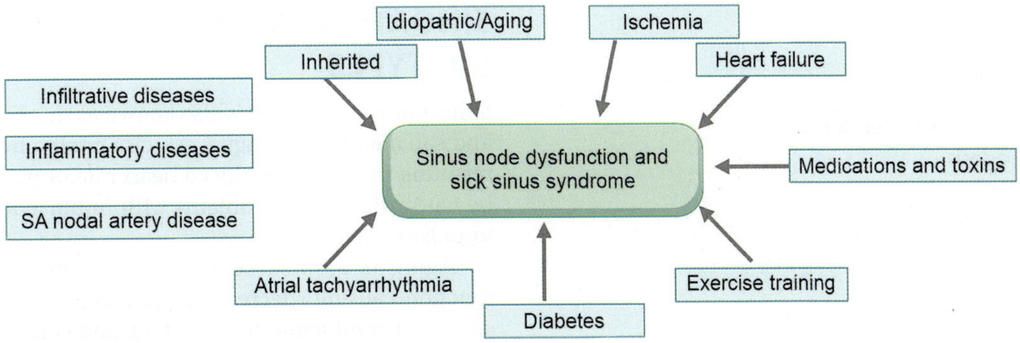

FIG. 3: Sinus node disorder.

Note: Examples of the types of ion channel remodeling seen in each case are shown. Further to our discussion, sinus node dysfunction is also seen in heart failure and diabetes. Atrial tachyarrhythmias include atrial fibrillation and atrial flutter.

(SA: sinoatrial)

Courtesy: Reproduced with permission from Wiley Periodicals, Inc.

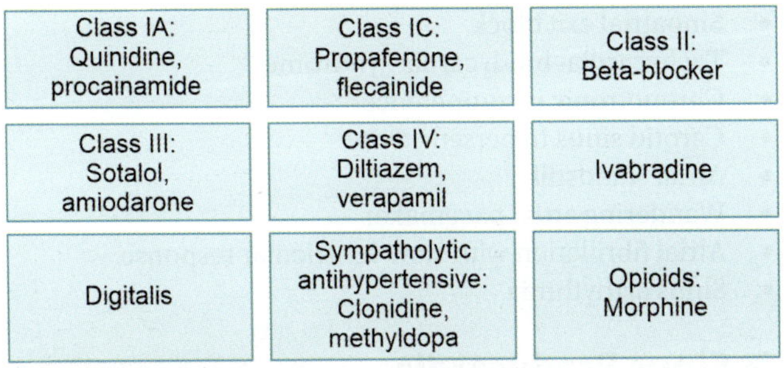

FIG. 4: Causes of extrinsic sinus node dysfunction: Drugs.

CONDITIONS ASSOCIATED WITH BRADYCARDIA

Conditions associated with bradycardia are given in **Box 1.** [12,13]

EPIDEMIOLOGY

It is estimated that the incidence of SND in the United States is approximately 1 in 600 cardiac patients aged >65 years. As it is related with advanced age, SND is more prevalent in countries where citizens have a longer life expectancy.[14]

Symptomatic patients are generally older, in seventh or eighth decade of life, with frequent comorbidities.

Risk factors associated with SND include higher body and mass index ratio, height, high blood pressure, right artery branch block, and extended QRS interval. The atrioventricular conduction disturbance can happen in patients with SND with respect to degenerative processes underlying both situations. The yearly prevalence of high-grade atrioventricular block following a pacemaker implant for SND is nearly 1.8%. The risk is higher among patients with pieces of evidence of conduction disturbances and with a prevalence of up to 35% within 5 years of pacemaker transplantation.

BOX 1 Conditions associated with bradycardia.[12,13]

Intrinsic:
- Cardiomyopathy (ischemic or nonischemic)
- Congenital heart disease
- Degenerative fibrosis infection/inflammation
- Chagas disease
- Diphtheria
- Infectious endocarditis
- Lyme disease
- Myocarditis
- Sarcoidosis
- Toxoplasmosis
- Infiltrative disorders
- Amyloidosis
- Hemochromatosis
- Lymphoma
- Ischemia/infarction
- Rheumatological conditions
- Rheumatoid arthritis
- Scleroderma
- Systemic lupus erythematosus
- Surgical or procedural trauma
- Cardiac procedures such as ablation or cardiac catheterization
- Congenital heart disease surgery
- Septal myomectomy for hypertrophic obstructive cardiomyopathy

Extrinsic:
- Autonomic perturbation
- Carotid sinus hypersensitivity
- Neurally mediated syncope/presyncope
- Physical conditioning
- Situational syncope
- Cough
- Defecation
- Glottic stimulation
- Medical procedures

Continued

Continued

- Micturition
- Vomiting
- Sleep (with or without sleep apnea)
- Metabolic acidosis
- Hyperkalemia
- Hypokalemia
- Hypothermia
- Hypothyroidism
- Hypoxia

PATHOPHYSIOLOGY

Sinus node dysfunction is described as a heterogenous clinical manifestation that describes the dysfunctioning of the sinus node and surrounding atrial myocardial entities to develop a heartbeat that meets the physiological requirements of a normal human being. Typical thresholds of SND include a sinus frequency of <50 beats per minute. However, examining such criteria alone is not sufficient for diagnosing SND.[15]

Nevertheless, the most distinct perception of chronotropic ineffectiveness better represents the inability of the heart to pump effectively with augmented activity or requirement.

The most prevalent cause of SND is gradual fibrosis of the sinus node and atrial fibrillation (AF), which finally obstructs impulse generation and transmission. The connective tissue encloses and shields the special pacemaker cardiomyocytes of the SAN; the increase in heart collagen portion with age is connected with decreased heart rate and sinus conduction times.[16] The histopathological findings further assist the connection between fibrillation and SND. Besides structural remodeling from fibrillation, age-associated molecular remodeling also subsidizes the pathophysiological characteristics of SND by alterations in the expression of ionic channels and clock genes in the sinus node.[17]

In addition, SND is linked with the disorders causing atrial myocardial malformations.

CLINICAL PRESENTATION OF SINOATRIAL NODAL DYSFUNCTION

It ranges from mild fatigue to frank syncope. Severity of clinical manifestations correlates with the heart rate or the pause duration. Patients with SND may manifest symptoms attributable to sinus bradycardia, sinus arrest, or SA exit block.

- Syncope
- Dyspnea on exertion due to chronotropic incompetence (CI)
- Lightheadedness and chronic fatigue
- Decreased exercise capacity and recurrent falls

Correlation between symptoms and bradycardia is considered to be the "gold standard" of diagnosis.

SINOATRIAL NODAL DYSFUNCTION SUBTYPES

Sinus node dysfunction is also known as sick sinus syndrome and can manifest as fatigue, exercise intolerance, or syncope resulting from either reduced heart rate or pauses. SND can be categorized into problems with impulse formation and impulse conduction.

Aging is associated with alterations in sinus node function, causing a decrease in the intrinsic HR, an increase in sinoatrial conduction time (SACT), and conduction slowing and voltage loss around the region of crista terminalis, and increases SACT. In the presence of clinically detectable SND, there is caudal shift of the leading pacemaker site within the SA node pacemaker complex:

- Sinus bradycardia
- Sinus pause, sinus arrest
- Sinoatrial exit block
- Tachycardia–bradycardia syndrome
- Chronotropic incompetence
- Carotid sinus hypersensitivity
- Atrial standstill
- Wandering atrial pacemaker
- Atrial fibrillation with slow ventricular response
- Sinus arrhythmia

Sinus Bradycardia

Sinus bradycardia is defined as a sinus rate <60 bpm. In most instances, sinus bradycardia is a benign arrhythmia **(Figs. 5A and B)**. In healthy young adults and trained athletes, resting sinus bradycardia may be a normal phenomenon caused by increased vagal tone. Sinus bradycardia is common during sleep in elderly individuals. Correlation of symptoms with sinus bradycardia is critical in the evaluation. Sinus bradycardia occurs in 10–15% of patients with acute myocardial infarction (MI), more prevalent when patients are seen in the early hours of infarction. Bradycardia that follows resuscitation from cardiac arrest is associated with a poor prognosis.[18]

Management

Treatment of sinus bradycardia is not usually necessary unless cardiac output is inadequate or arrhythmias result from the slow rate. Atropine (0.5 mg intravenously as an initial dose, repeated if necessary) is generally effective acutely; lower doses, particularly given subcutaneously or intramuscularly, can exert an initial parasympathomimetic effect, possibly by a central action. For recurrent symptomatic episodes, temporary or permanent pacing may be needed.[18]

Sinus Pause, Sinus Arrest

Sinus pause or arrest means failure of sinus node discharge with lack of atrial activation of sinus origin. It is a disorder of impulse formation resulting in absence of P waves

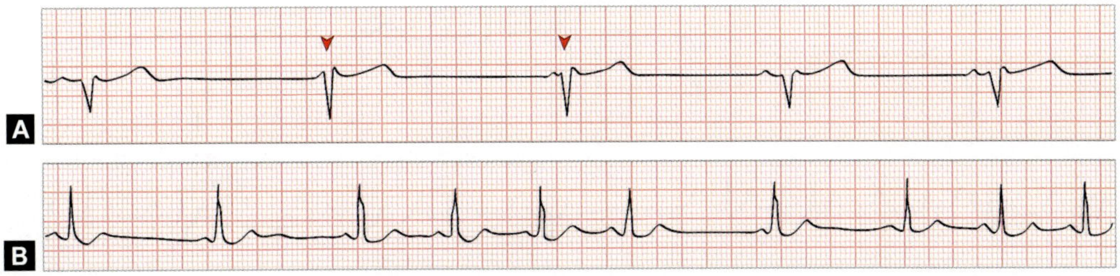

FIGS. 5A AND B: (A) Sinus bradycardia at a rate of 40–48 beats/min. The second and third QRS complexes (arrowheads) represent junctional escape beats. Note the P waves at the onset of QRS complex. (B) Nonrespiratory sinus arrhythmia occurring as a consequence of digitalis toxicity. Monitor leads were used.

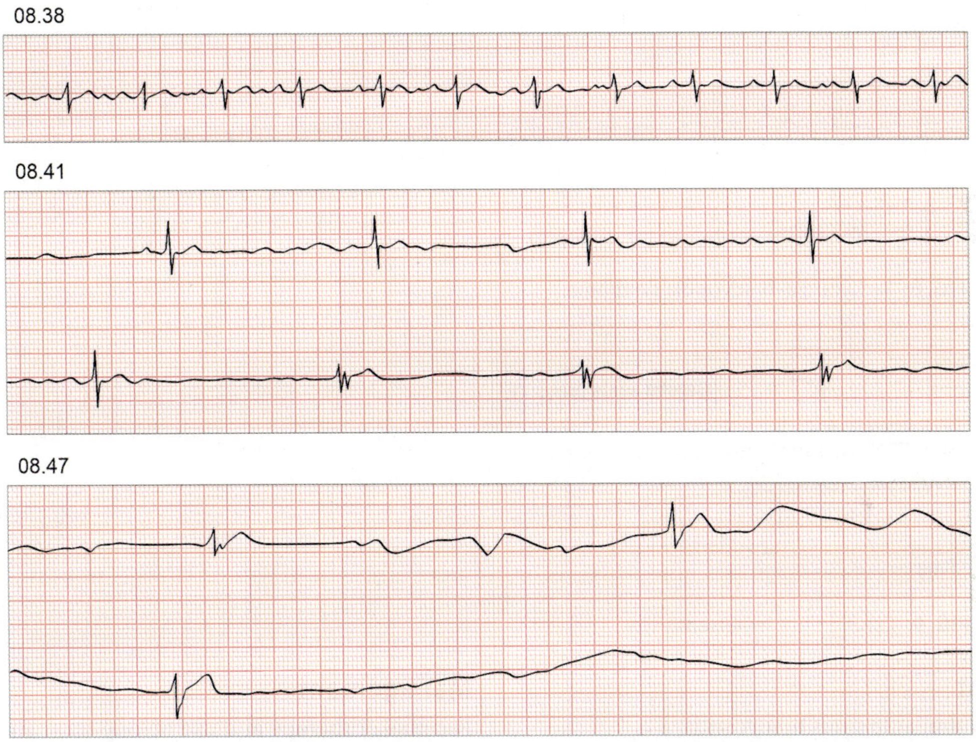

FIG. 6: Sinus arrest. The patient had a long-term electrocardiographic recorder connected when he died suddenly of cardiac standstill. The rhythms demonstrate progressive sinus bradycardia and sinus arrest at 8:41 AM. The rhythm then becomes a ventricular escape rhythm, which progressively slows and finally ceases at 8:47 AM. The paired electrocardiographic strips are continuous recordings.

and periods of ventricular asystole if lower pacemakers (junctional or ventricular) do not initiate escape beats. The resulting pause in sinus activity should not be in multiples of preceding sinus cycle length (P-P interval), which would indicate that SA exit block is present **(Fig. 6)**.[19]

Management

Chronic pacing (permanent) is indicated only in symptomatic patients or those with sinus pause exceeding 3 seconds.

Sinoatrial Exit Block

In SA exit block, the impulse is formed in the sinus node but fails to conduct to the atria. This particular arrhythmia is recognized on ECG by pauses resulting from the absence of normal P waves and the duration of the pause, measuring an exact multiple of the preceding P-P interval. In first-degree SA block, there is significant prolongation of the time for the sinus impulse to exit into the atria (SA conduction time). This cannot be identified clinically or electrocardiographically. Second-degree SA block can be type I (Wenckebach) or type II. Type I is defined as progressive prolongation of SA conduction, manifested on surface ECG as progressive shortening of P-P interval, before the pause created by loss of a P wave. While in type II SA exit block, the P-P intervals remain constant before the pause **(Figs. 7A and B)**. Third-degree or complete SA block will manifest as absence of P waves, with long pauses resulting in lower pacemaker escape rhythm; it is quite impossible to diagnose with certainty without invasive sinus node recordings.[20]

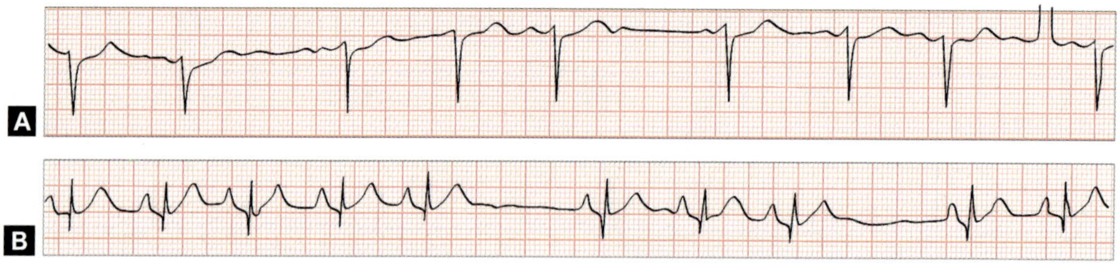

FIGS. 7A AND B: Sinus nodal exit block. (A) Type I sinoatrial (SA) nodal exit block has the following features. The P-P interval shortens from the first to the second cycle in each grouping, followed by a pause. The duration of the pause is less than twice the shortest cycle length, and the cycle after the pause exceeds the cycle before pause. The PR interval is normal and constant. Lead V_1 is shown. (B) The P-P interval varies slightly because of sinus arrhythmia. The two pauses in sinus nodal activity equal twice the basic P-P interval and are consistent with type II 2:1 SA nodal exit block. The PR interval is normal and constant. Lead III recording is shown.

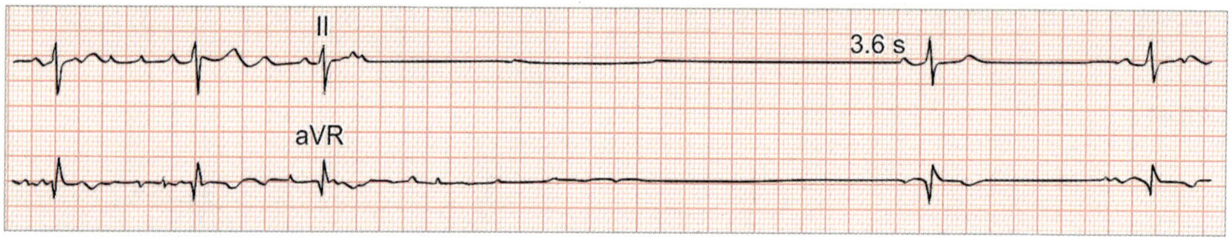

FIG. 8: Tachycardia–bradycardia syndrome.

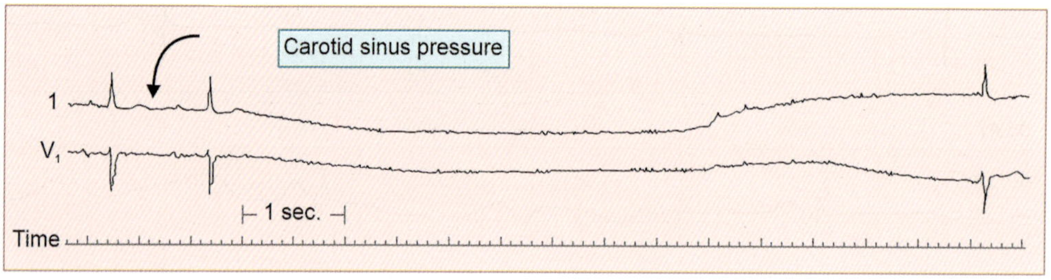

FIG. 9: Carotid sinus hypersensitivity.

Management

Management is similar to sinus bradycardia.

Tachycardia–Bradycardia Syndrome

Sinus bradycardia intertwingled with periods of atrial tachyarrhythmias is a common manifestation of SND. The atrial tachyarrhythmias usually range from paroxysmal atrial tachycardia to atrial flutter and AF. These patients most often experience prolonged sinus arrest and asystole upon termination of the atrial tachyarrhythmias, resulting from suppression of sinus node and secondary pacemakers. Long sinus pauses which occur after electrical cardioversion of AF and chronic AF with a slow ventricular response in the absence of AV nodal-blocking drugs are some other manifestations of SND **(Fig. 8)**. These patients may demonstrate very slow ventricular rates at rest or during sleep and occasionally have long pauses. They may also conduct rapidly and develop symptoms caused by tachycardia during exercise. Occasionally, they may develop complete AV block with junctional or ventricular escape rhythms.[21]

Management

Pacemaker therapy and use of long-term anticoagulation to prevent strokes.

Chronotropic Incompetence

Inability of the sinus node to achieve at least 85%, 80%, or less commonly 70% of the age-predicted maximal heart rate (APMHR, 220—age) obtained during an incremental dynamic exercise test. CI has also been determined from change in HR from rest to peak exercise during an exercise test, commonly referred to as the HR reserve. While the resting heart rates may be normal, these patients may have either the inability to increase their heart rate during exercise or have unpredictable fluctuations in heart rate during activity. Few patients may initially experience a normal increase in heart rate with exercise, which then plateaus or decreases inappropriately.[22]

Carotid Sinus Hypersensitivity

An abnormal response following carotid sinus massage (pause longer than 3 seconds) can indicate SND **(Fig. 9)**, but this response can also occur in asymptomatic older individuals.[23]

Atrial Standstill

Atrial standstill is a rare clinical syndrome in which there is no spontaneous atrial activity and the atria cannot be electrically stimulated. The surface ECG usually reveals junctional bradycardia without atrial activity **(Fig. 10)**. The atria are generally fibrotic and without any functional myocardium. Lack of mechanical atrial contraction poses a high risk for thromboembolism in these patients.[24]

Wandering Atrial Pacemaker

This is characterized by multiple P waves of varying morphology with a relatively normal or slow rate **(Fig. 11)**, caused by shifting of dominant pacemaker focus between sinus node and latent pacemakers in other atrial and AV junctional sites. The shift in pacemaker focus occurs gradually, over the course of several beats, so that only one pacemaker at a time controls the rhythm. Apart from change in wave morphology, the shift in pacemaker focus is usually associated with different PR interval (depending on its proximity to the AVN) and R-R intervals. By definition, wandering atrial

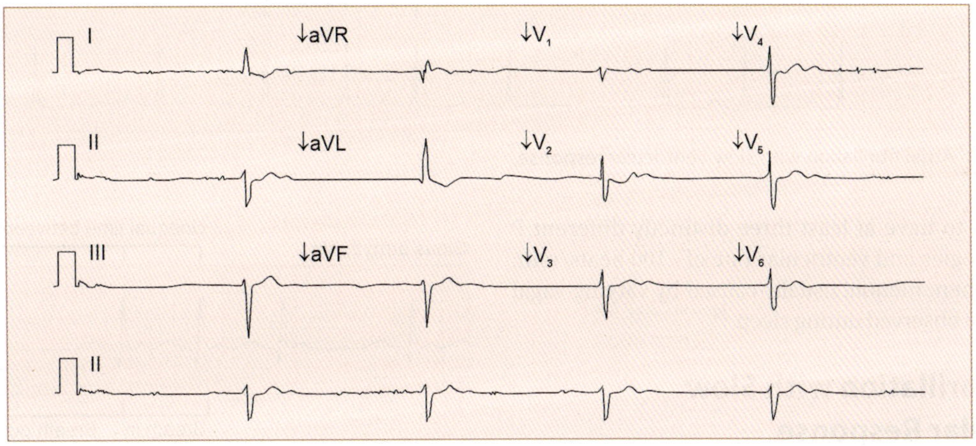

FIG. 10: Atrial standstill.

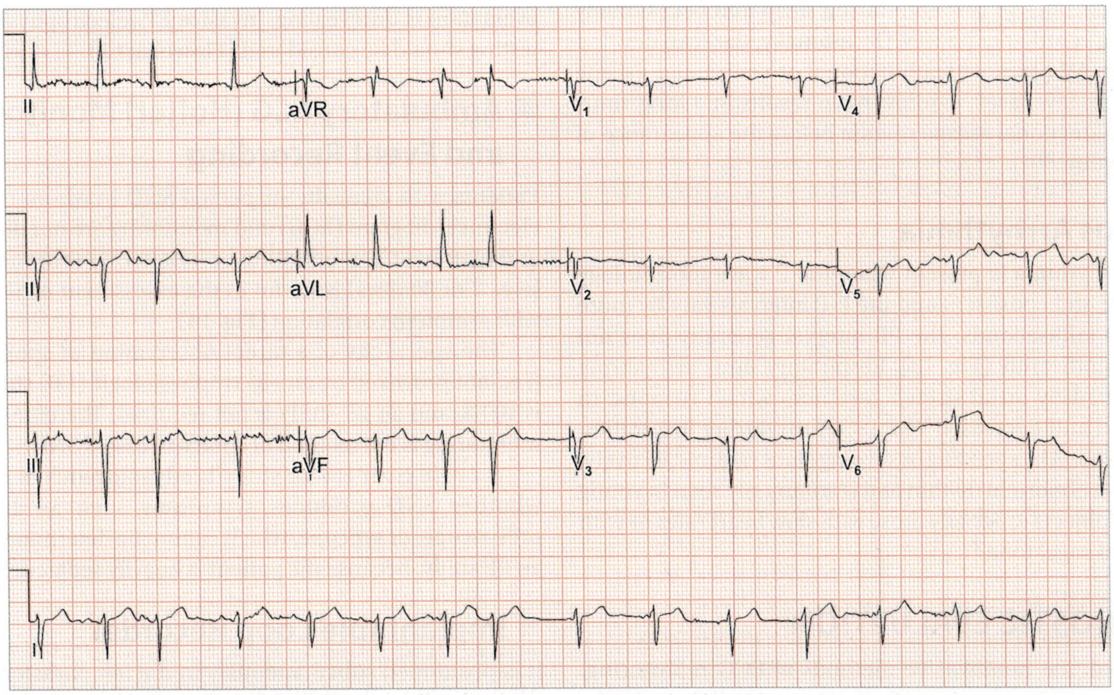

FIG. 11: Wandering atrial pacemaker.

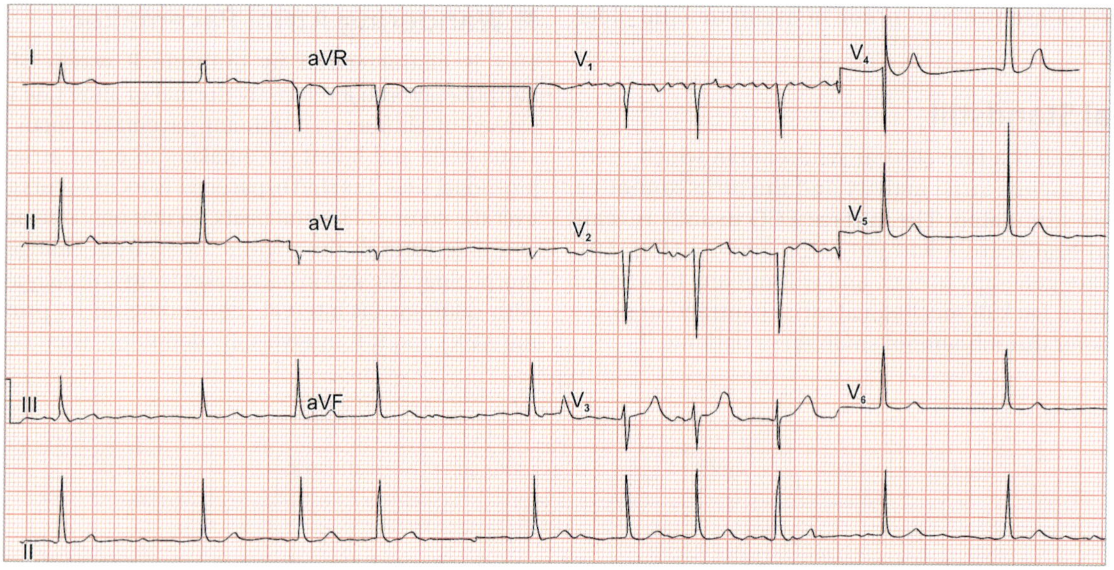

FIG. 12: Atrial fibrillation with slow ventricular response.

pacemaker has to have at least three distinctly different P waves morphologies and ventricular rate of <100 beats/min. It is a normal phenomenon, usually caused by varying vagal tone, and can be observed during sleep.[25]

Atrial Fibrillation with Slow Ventricular Response

Persistent AF with a slow ventricular response in the absence of AVN blocking drugs is often present in patients with SND **(Fig. 12)**. These patients can demonstrate very slow ventricular rates at rest and during sleep and occasionally have long ventricular pauses. Occasionally, they can develop complete AV block with a junctional or ventricular escape rhythm. In few cases, cardioversion results in a long sinus pause or junctional escape rhythm before the appearance of sinus rhythm.[26]

Sinus Arrhythmia

Sinus arrhythmia is present when the P wave morphology is normal and consistent and the P-P intervals vary by more than 120 milliseconds. The PR interval generally does not vary insignificantly **(Fig. 13)**. Respiratory sinus arrhythmia is mediated by atrial stretch receptors which respond to increased and decreased venous return during inspiration and expiration by speeding or slowing sinus rate, respectively. It is not an abnormal rhythm and is commonly seen in young healthy subjects especially those with slow heart rates or with enhanced vagal tone.[27]

DIAGNOSTIC EVALUATION

In general, the noninvasive methods of ECG monitoring, exercise testing, and autonomic testing are used first.

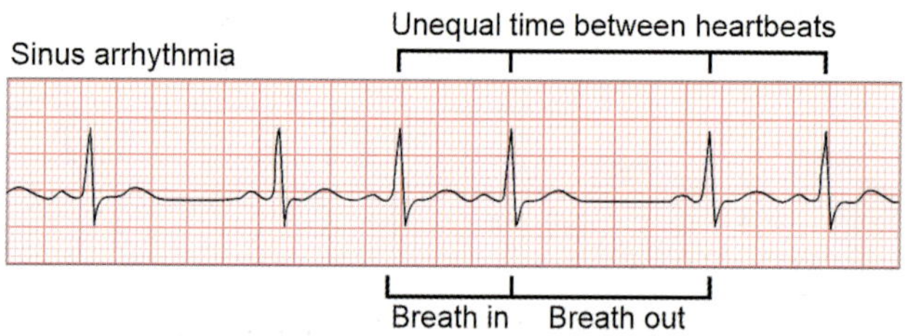

FIG. 13: Sinus arrhythmia.

However, if symptoms are infrequent and noninvasive evaluation is unrevealing, invasive EP (electrophysiological) testing should be considered **(Flowchart 1)**.

Ambulatory ECG (Holter) Monitoring and Event Recording

Patients with clinically suspected SND in whom the initial electrocardiogram (ECG) and monitoring are not diagnostic, ambulatory ECG monitoring or long-term event monitoring (e.g., 7 or 30 days) is useful in the assessment of SND along with symptom correlation **(Fig. 14)**.

The specificity of a direct observation of spontaneous [i.e., not provoked by an electrophysiologic (EP) study] SND is 100%, and an EP study is not required. Therefore, cardiac monitoring is the method of choice to assess SND.

A 24–48-hour Holter study is advantageous of revealing whether SND produces symptoms such as dizziness, presyncope, or syncope, which cannot be determined during an EP study, because the patient is heavily sedated.[28]

Implantable Loop Recorder

It is positioned subcutaneously in the left parasternal area at the level of the 4th–5th intercostal space under local

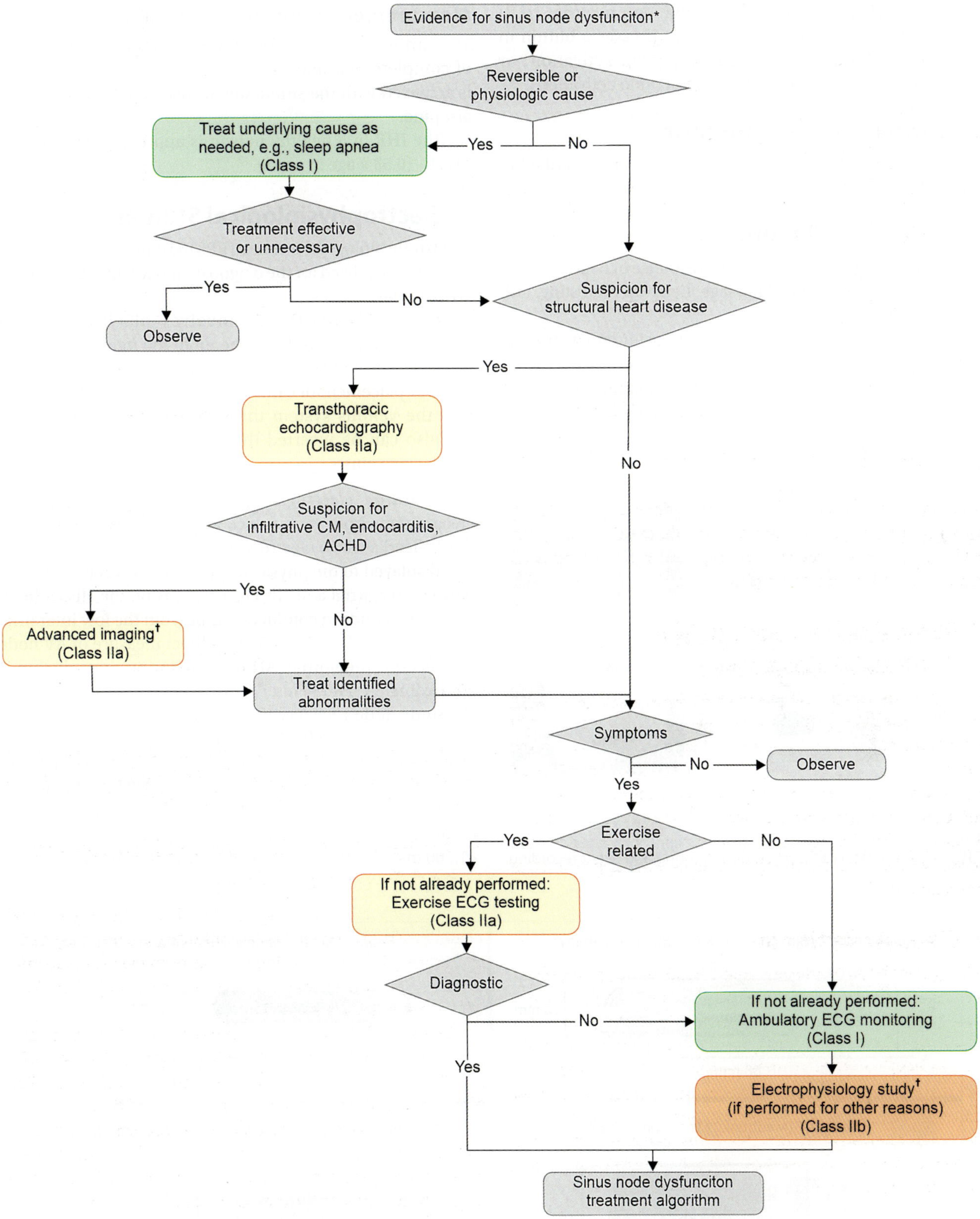

*Sinus pauses, sinus bradycardia, junctional rhythm, ectopic atrial rhythm (all with heart rate < 50 bpm) while awake.

†The electrophysiology test should not be done primarily for sinus node dysfunction.

FLOWCHART 1: Initial evaluation of suspected or documented sinus node dysfunction algorithm.

anesthesia **(Fig. 15)**. The implantable loop recorder (ILR) stores rhythm strips when the patient presses a button in response to symptom occurrence (patient activation) or when the heart rate meets a preset limit (auto activation).[29]

Cardiac Rhythm Monitor

Different types of cardiac rhythm monitors are described in **Table 1**.

Autonomic Testing

It can be assessed by observing the response of heart rate and rhythm with carotid sinus massage, head-up tilt testing, and Valsalva maneuver.

Pharmacological evaluation done by using either atropine (1 or 2 mg) or isoproterenol (2–3 μg/min) may be useful, as both agents normally increase the sinus rate. Abnormal response is an increase in the sinus rate of <25% above the baseline, or to a sinus rate <90 beats/min.[28]

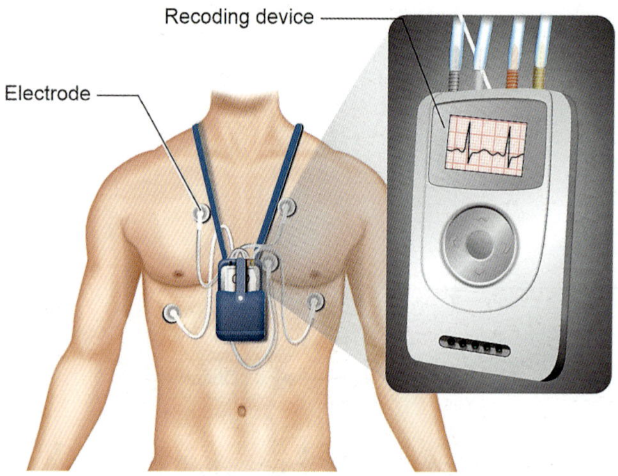

FIG. 14: Ambulatory ECG (Holter) monitoring and event recording.

Measurement of Intrinsic Heart Rate

The intrinsic heart rate (IHR) is the heart rate in the presence of complete pharmacologic denervation of the SN, which is achieved with the simultaneous use of beta-blockers and atropine.

The IHR in a healthy person is approximately equal to 117.2 – (0.53 × age in years).[30]

Electrophysiological Studies

Electrophysiological studies (EPS) are minimally invasive procedures utilized for the diagnosis and treatment of cardiac arrhythmias.

The TECHNIQUE-EPS involves placing catheters equipped with electrodes at the tip in the right atrium, right ventricle, coronary sinus, and the His region. Fluoroscopy is used for placement of catheters, which are typically inserted into the venous system through femoral venous access but also can be inserted through the internal jugular or subclavian veins.

Intracardiac electrograms: During EPS, intracardiac electrograms from various locations in the heart, along with the 12-lead surface electrocardiogram (ECG), are recorded and displayed to the physician. The AH interval is measured between the atrial and His electrograms on the His catheter and corresponds to conduction time from the low interatrial septum to the His, which is an indirect measure of AV node conduction. The normal AH interval during sinus rhythm is approximately 55–130 ms.[29]

Sinus node recovery time (SNRT) and corrected sinus node recovery time (CSNRT) are the most common means of assessing sinus node function. The SNRT is measured after pacing the atrium at different rates up to 300 bpm for at least 30 seconds. The interval between the last atrial paced beat to the first sinus beat is the SNRT. The normal SNRT value is <1,500 ms. The normal value for CSNRT is <525 ms.

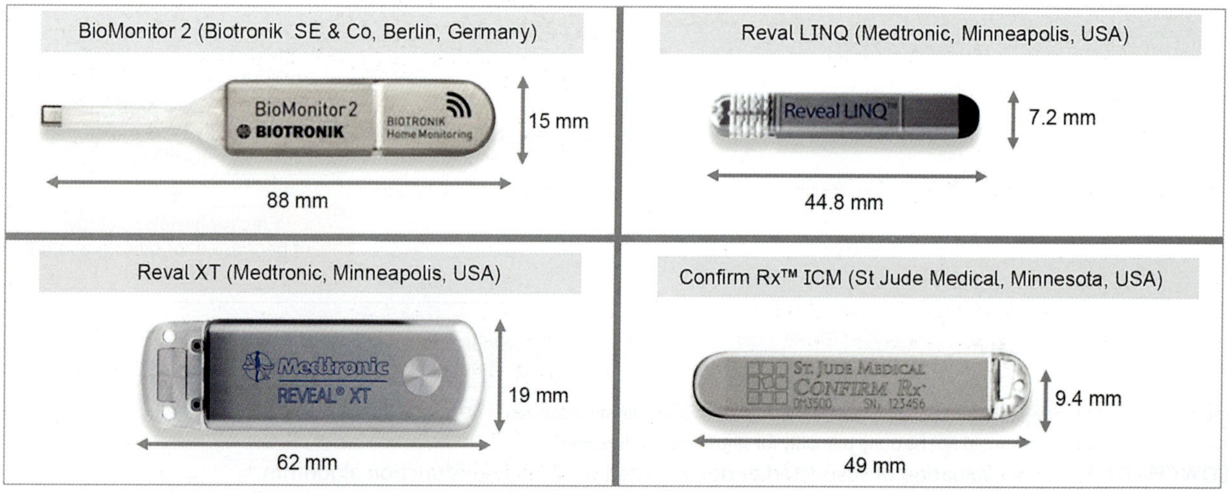

FIG. 15: Implantable loop recorder.

TABLE 1: Device description and patient selection based on types of monitor.[22]

Types of monitor	Device description	Patient selection
Nonphysician prescribed smartphone-based systems	Commercially available smartphone-based systems	Patient access to the technology
Holter monitor	Continuous recording for 24–72 hours; up to 2 weeks with newer models	Symptoms frequent enough to be detected within a short period (24–72 hours) of monitoring
Patient-activated, transtelephonic monitor (event monitor)	A recording device that transmits patient-activated data (live or stored) via an analog telephone line to a central remote monitoring station (e.g., physician office)	Frequent, spontaneous symptoms likely to recur within 2–6 weeks
External loop recorder (patient or auto-triggered)*	• A device that continuously records and stores rhythm data over weeks to months • Patient activated, or auto-triggered	Frequent, spontaneous symptoms potentially related to bradycardia or conduction disorder
External patch recorders	• Patch device that continuously records and stores rhythm data, with patient-trigger capability to allow for symptom-rhythm correlation • No leads or wires, and adhesive to chest wall/sternum	Can be considered as an alternative to external loop recorder
Mobile cardiac outpatient telemetry	Device that records and transmits data (up to 30 days) from preprogrammed arrhythmias or patient activation to a communication hub at the patient's home	Spontaneous symptoms, potentially related to bradycardia or conduction disorder, that are too brief, too subtle, or too infrequent to be readily documented with patient activated monitors
Implantable cardiac monitor	• Subcutaneously implanted device, with a battery life of 2–3 years • Triggered by the patient (or often family member witness) to store the event	Recurrent, infrequent, unexplained symptoms, potentially related to bradycardia

* Higher yield in patients who are able to record a diary to correlate with possible arrhythmia.

The sinoatrial conduction time (SACT), the time required for impulse propagation from sinus node to atrium, can be measured during EPS and represents another method to ascertain sinus node function. SACT is measured by direct (recording sinus node electrograms) and indirect (pacing maneuvers) methods.

ADDITIONAL INVESTIGATIONS

- *Laboratory studies*: Thyroid function testing and serum electrolyte testing (Na^+, K^+, and Ca^+)
- *Echocardiography*: This documents the presence of underlying valvular and ischemic heart disease, diagnosis of amyloid
- *Transesophageal atrial pacing*: Perform safely to determine SNRT in children
- Exercise stress testing **(Fig. 16)**

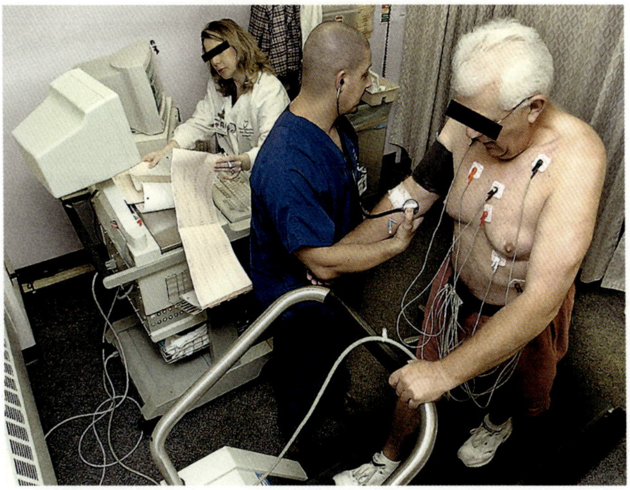

FIG. 16: Exercise stress testing.

MANAGEMENT

Acute Management (Flowchart 2 and Table 2)[31,32]

Drugs for bradycardia attributable to SND ***(Tables 3 and 4).***[33,34]

Patients with symptoms of SND secondary to relapse should be treated primarily with medical therapy to eliminate or reduce negative symptoms:

- Although pacing is the mainstay of treatment for symptomatic SND, temporary or reversible causes of SND must first be identified and treated.
- Before permanent treatment, discontinuation of an illicit drug, correction of electrolyte abnormalities, and treatment of an exogenous cause of SND (e.g., obstructive sleep apnea, hypothyroidism, and hypoxemia) should be considered.
- As a principle of SND, vagal hyperactivity is often suspected because of its transient nature and increased

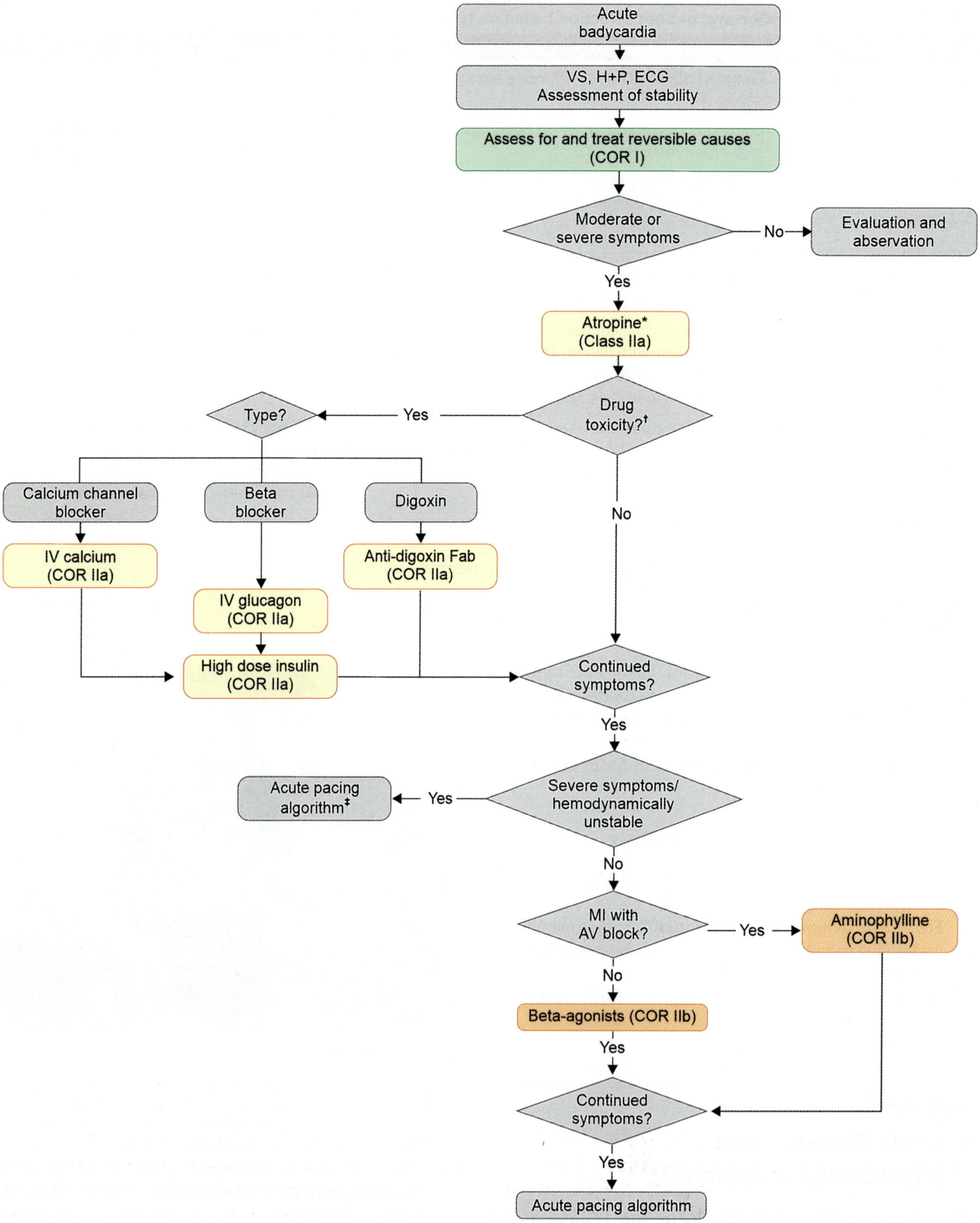

*Atropine should not be given in patients after heart transplant.

†In patients with drug toxicity and severe symptoms, preparation for pacing should proceed simultaneously with pharmacologic treatment of drug toxicity.

FLOWCHART 2: Acute management algorithm.[31]

(AV: atrioventricular; ECG: electrocardiography; MI: myocardial infarction)

TABLE 2: Acute medical therapy.[32]

Medication	Dosage	Comments
Symptomatic sinus bradycardia or atrioventricular block		
Atropine	0.5–1 mg IV (may be repeated every 3–5 minutes to a maximum dose of 3 mg)	
Dopamine	5–20 μg/kg/min IV, starting at 5 μg/kg/min and increasing by 5 μg/kg/min every 2 minutes	Dosages of >20 μg/kg/min may result in vasoconstriction or arrhythmias
Isoproterenol	20–60 μg IV bolus followed doses of 10–20 μg, or infusion of 1–20 μg/min based on heart rate response	Monitor for potential development of ischemic chest pain
Epinephrine	2–10 μg/min IV or 0.1–0.5 μg/kg/min IV titrated to desired effects	
Second- or third-degree atrioventricular block associated with acute inferior MI		
Aminophylline	250-mg IV bolus	
Calcium channel blocker overdose		
10% calcium chloride	1–2 g IV every 10–20 min or an infusion of 0.2–0.4 mL/kg/h	
10% calcium gluconate	3–6 g IV every 10–20 min or an infusion at 0.6–1.2 mL/kg/h	
Beta-blocker or calcium-channel blocker overdose		
Glucagon	3–10 mg IV with infusion of 3–5 mg/h	
High-dose insulin therapy	IV bolus of 1 unit/kg followed by an infusion of 0.5 units/kg/h	Follow glucose and potassium levels
Digoxin overdose		
Digoxin antibody fragment	Dosage is dependent on amount ingested or known digoxin concentration	• One vial binds approximately 0.5 mg of digoxin • Administer over at least 30 minutes • May be repeated
Post heart transplant		
Aminophylline	6 mg/kg in 100–200 mL of IV fluid over 20–30 minutes	
Theophylline	300 mg IV, followed by oral dose of 5–10 mg/kg/day titrated to effect	• Therapeutic serum levels range from 10–20 μg/mL • Usual posttransplant dosages average 450 mg ± 100 mg/day
Spinal cord injury		
Aminophylline	6 mg/kg in 100–200 mL of IV fluid over 20–30 minutes	
Theophylline	Oral dose of 5–10 mg/kg/day titrated to effect	Effective dosages often result in serum levels below the usual effective range of 10–20 μg/mL

(IV: intravenous)

TABLE 3: Recommendations for therapy of beta-blocker- and calcium channel blocker-mediated bradycardia.[33]

COR	LOE	Recommendations
IIa	C-LD	In patients with bradycardia associated with symptoms or hemodynamic compromise because of calcium channel blocker overdose, intravenous calcium is reasonable to increase heart rate and improve symptoms

(COR: class of recommendation; LOE: level of evidence)

TABLE 4: Recommendations for theophylline/aminophylline for bradycardia attributable to SND.[34]

COR	LOE	Recommendations
IIa	C-LD	In post heart transplant patients, aminophylline or theophylline is reasonable to increase heart rate if clinically indicated

(COR: class of recommendation; LOE: level of evidence; SND: sinus node dysfunction) vagal tone, as well as symptoms associated with certain medical conditions.

- SND from the vagus may respond to atropine but should be treated if the patient is symptomatic.
- Medical treatment (atropine and isoproterenol) can only be used as an emergency measure until it is done.
- In hemodynamically significant bradycardia, temporary percutaneous or transvenous pacing is indicated to provide immediate stabilization before permanent pacemaker (PPM) implantation.

Chronic Management (Flowchart 3)

*General principles of chronic therapy/management of bradycardia attributable to SND **(Table 5)**.*

In symptomatic patients with tachycardia-bradycardia syndrome, pacing may be required to prevent symptomatic bradycardia and allow the use of drug therapy for control of the tachycardia.[35]

Such patients are at increased risk for thromboembolism, and the issue of long-term anticoagulation for stroke prevention should be addressed.

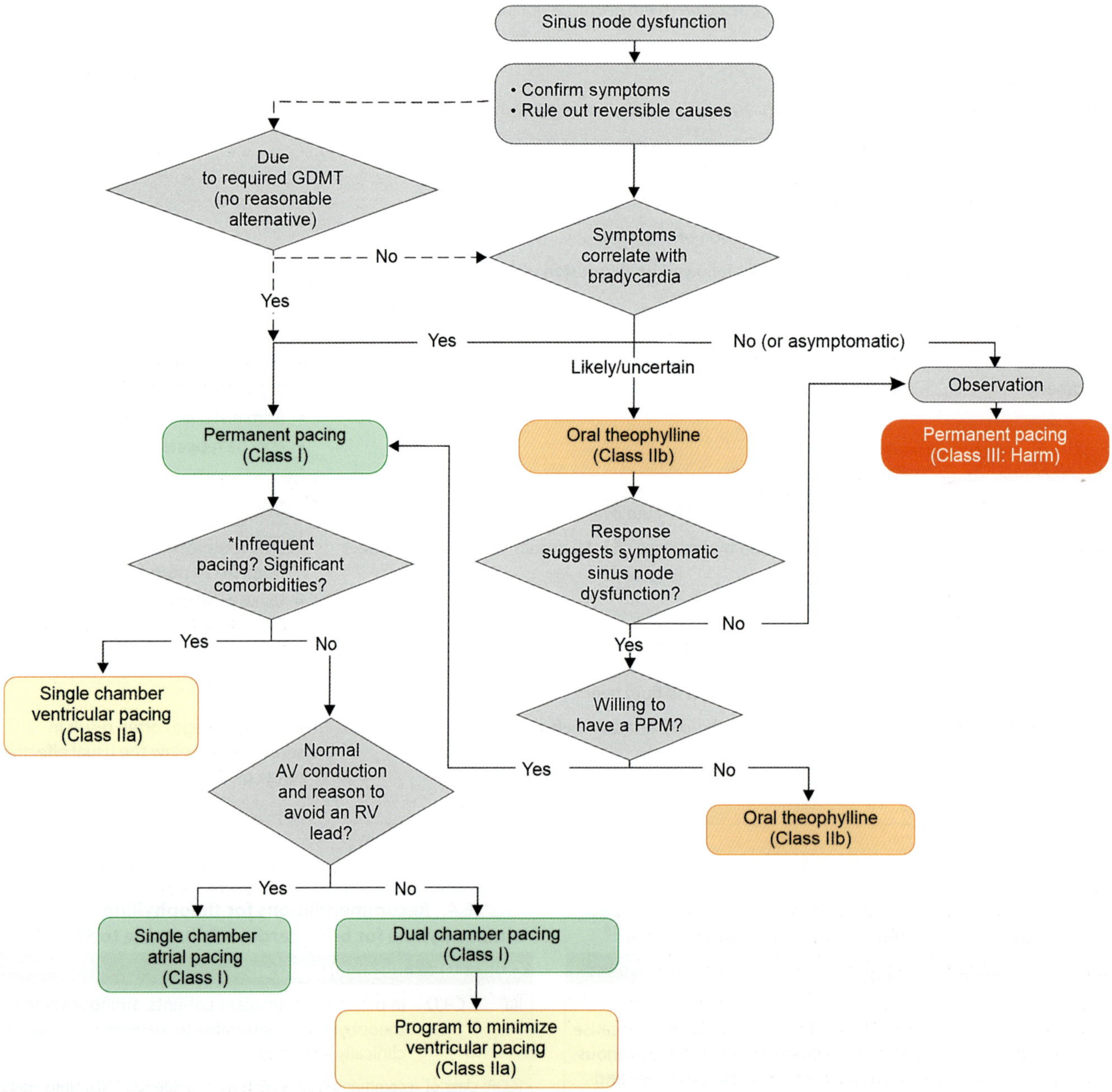

*Symptomatic patients with very infrequent need for pacing for rate support or patients with significant comorbidities.

FLOWCHART 3: Algorithm for chronic management.[29]

Note: Dashed lines indicate possible optional strategies based on the specific clinical situation.

(GDMT: guideline-directed medical therapy; PPM: permanent pacemaker; RV: right ventricular)

TABLE 5: Recommendations for general principles of chronic therapy/management of bradycardia attributable to SND.

COR	LOE	Recommendations
III: Harm	C-LD1	In asymptomatic individuals with sinus bradycardia or sinus pauses that are secondary to physiologically elevated parasympathetic tone, permanent pacing should not be performed

(COR: class of recommendation; LOE: level of evidence; SND: sinus node dysfunction)

TABLE 6: Recommendations for temporary pacing for bradycardia attributable to SND.

COR	LOE	Recommendations
IIa	C-LD	In patients with persistent hemodynamically unstable SND refractory to medical therapy, temporary transvenous pacing is reasonable to increase heart rate and improve symptoms until a permanent pacemaker is placed or the bradycardia resolve

(COR: class of recommendation; LOE: level of evidence; SND: sinus node dysfunction)

Importantly, in patients with symptomatic paroxysmal AF accompanied by prolonged sinus pauses on AF termination, catheter ablation of AF may be preferred to pacemaker implantation, as it can potentially eliminate the arrhythmia and the need for permanent pacing.

*Temporary pacing for bradycardia attributable to SND **(Table 6 and Box 2)**.*

Temporary pacing is used to acutely treat bradycardia causing hemodynamically significant instability, such as prolonged and symptomatic pauses, life-threatening ventricular arrhythmias mediated by bradycardia, or severe symptomatic bradycardia pertaining to a reversible cause with a goal to avoid PPM implantation.[36]

Temporary pacing can be implemented transcutaneously via a transesophageal approach or by insertion of a transvenous pacing electrode or pulmonary-arterial pacing catheter.

In patients with persistent hemodynamically unstable SND refractory to medical therapy, temporary transvenous pacing is reasonable to increase heart rate and improve symptoms until a PPM is placed or the bradycardia resolves. In patients with SND with severe symptoms or hemodynamic compromise, temporary transcutaneous pacing may be considered to increase heart rate and improve symptoms until a temporary transvenous or PPM is placed or the bradycardia resolves.

BOX 2 HRS/ACCF recommendations for pacemaker device and mode selection for SND.[30]

Class I:

- DDD or AAI is recommended over VVI in patient with SND and intact and intact AV conduction
- DDD is recommended over AAI in patient with SND

Class IIa:

- Rate adaptive pacing can be useful in patients with significant symptomatic chronotropic incompetence, and its need should be reevaluated during follow-up
- In patient with SND and intact AV conduction, programming dual-chamber pacemaker to minimize ventricular pacing can be useful for prevention od AF

Class IIb:

- AAI pacing may be considered in selected patients with normal AV and ventricular conduction
- Single-chamber VVI pacing may be considered in instances where frequent pacing is not expected or the patient has significant comorbidities that are likely to influence survival and clinical outcomes

CLASS III:

- DDD or AAI should not be used in patients in permanent or long-standing persistent AF where efforts to restore or maintain sinus rhythm are not planned

(AAI: single-chamber atrial pacing; ACCF: American College of Cardiology Foundation; AF: atrial fibrillation; AV: atrioventricular; DDD: dual-chamber pacing; HRS: Heart Rhythm Society; SND: sinus node dysfunction; VVI: single-chamber ventricular pacing)

TABLE 7: Recommendations for permanent pacing techniques and methods for chronic therapy/ management of bradycardia attributable to SND.[37]

COR	LOE	Recommendations
I	B-R	In symptomatic patients with SND, atrial-based pacing is recommended over single-chamber ventricular pacing
I	B-R	In symptomatic patients with SND and intact atrioventricular conduction without evidence of conduction abnormalities, dual-chamber or single-chamber atrial pacing is recommended

(COR: class of recommendation; LOE: level of evidence; SND: sinus node dysfunction)

*Permanent pacing for chronic therapy/management of bradycardia attributable to SND **(Table 7)**.*[37]

COMPLICATIONS OF SINOATRIAL NODAL DYSFUNCTION

- Sudden cardiac death
- Syncope
- Thromboembolic events, including stroke
- Congestive heart failure (CHF)
- Atrial tachyarrhythmias

PROGNOSIS

The prognosis of patients with SND is dependent on the underlying associated condition. There is low incidence of sudden cardiac death in patients with SND. Pacemaker therapy does not affect survival in patients with SND.

Patients with tachycardia-bradycardia syndrome have a worse prognosis as compared to patients with isolated SND. The overall prognosis depends on their underlying ventricular dysfunction.

FUTURE PROSPECTS OF RESEARCH AND DEVELOPMENT IN SINUS NODE DYSFUNCTION

The application of pacemaker implantation had improved the quality of life for many heart patients with SND, but it still faces issues with postinfections, postcardiac injuries, wire loss, and restrained electronic life. The biological pacemaker-built sinus node pacemaking cells perform normally in the heart specifically through regulating a single gene, multiple genes, and signaling pathways. Current evidences have reported that genes and signaling processes included in biological pacemaking include T-box gene 3, TBX 18, insulin growth factors, homeobox 2, Wnt-signaling pathway, and HCN-signaling pathway. Currently, there are various reports on Tbx family involving Tbx1, 3, 5, and 18. Insulin-like growth factors were one of the important markers involved in differentiating cardiac histocytes in the cardiac region, which promotes cardiac progression and differentiation.

The Wnt-signaling pathway is differentiated into classical and nonclassical Wnt-signaling pathway, with the former playing an important role in regulating the development of SAN. However, most of the research has been conducted on basic experiments, and efficiency of targeted differentiation of pacemaker cells through regulating genes and signaling pathways was generally limited. Moreover, there is an issue of causing inflammatory reactions and cytotoxicities in organisms, and more research is required in the near future to overcome such issues and to deliver scientific foundation for studying biological pacing in humans and its gradual clinical applications.

CONCLUSION

- Sinus node dysfunction is most often related to age-dependent progressive fibrosis of the sinus nodal leading to abnormalities of sinus.
- Both sleep disorders of breathing and nocturnal bradycardias are relatively common, and treatment of sleep apnea reduces the frequency of these arrhythmias along with cardiovascular benefits.
- The presence of left bundle branch block on electrocardiogram markedly increases the chances of underlying structural heart disease and of diagnosing left ventricular systolic dysfunction. Echocardiography is usually the most appropriate initial screening test.
- In patients having acquired second-degree Mobitz type II atrioventricular block, high-grade atrioventricular block, or third-degree atrioventricular block not caused by reversible or physiologic causes, permanent pacing is recommended regardless of symptoms.
- In patients with a left ventricular ejection fraction between 36 and 50% and atrioventricular block, who have an indication for permanent pacing, techniques which provide more physiologic ventricular activation (e.g., cardiac resynchronization therapy and His bundle pacing) are preferred over right ventricular pacing to prevent heart failure.
- In patients with bradycardia having indications for pacemaker implantation, shared decision-making and patient-centered care are followed.
- Identifying patient populations benefitted the most from emerging pacing technologies (e.g., His bundle pacing, transcatheter leadless pacing systems) will require further investigation as these modalities are incorporated into clinical practice.

ONLINE REFERENCES

Please scan the QR code provided at the end of the table of contents for References of this chapter.

INDEX

Page numbers followed by *b* refer to box, *f* refer to figure, *fc* refer to flowchart, and *t* refer to table.

A

D

E

F

G

H

I

J

K

L

M

P

Q

R

S

T

U

V